LeMone & Burke's
Medical-Surgical Nursing
Clinical Reasoning in Patient Care

Seventh Edition

Gerene Bauldoff, RN, PhD, FAAN
Professor of Clinical Nursing
The Ohio State University
College of Nursing
Columbus, Ohio

Paula Gubrud, RN, MS, EdD, FAAN
Associate Professor
School of Nursing
Oregon Health & Science University
Portland, Oregon

Margaret-Ann Carno, RN, MBA, MJ, PhD, CPNP, D,ABSM, FAAN
Professor of Clinical Nursing and Pediatrics
Co-Director Baccalaureate Programs
School of Nursing
University of Rochester
Rochester, New York

Pearson

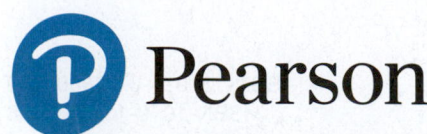

Director of Portfolio Management: Katrin Beacom
Executive Portfolio Manager: Pamela Fuller
Development Editor: Laura S. Horowitz, York Content Development
Portfolio Management Assistant: Erin Sullivan
Vice President, Content Production and Digital Studio: Paul DeLuca
Managing Producer, Health Science: Melissa Bashe
Content Producer: Michael Giacobbe
Creative Digital Lead: Mary Siener
Managing Producer, Digital Studio, Health Science: Amy Peltier
Digital Studio Producer, REVEL and e-text 2.0: Ellen Viganola
Digital Content Team Lead: Brian Prybella
Digital Content Project Lead: William Johnson
Vice President, Product Marketing: David Gesell
Executive Field Marketing Manager: Christopher Barry
Field Marketing Manager: Brittany Hammond
Full-Service Project Management and Composition: Pearson CSC
Project Manager: Emily Tamburri
Inventory Manager: Vatche Demirdjian
Interior Design: Studio Montage
Cover Design: Studio Montage
Printer/Binder: LSC Communications, Inc.
Cover Printer: LSC Communications, Inc.
Cover: Marco Govel/Shutterstock

Credits and acknowledgments borrowed from other sources and reproduced, with permission, in this textbook appear in the Credits section at the end of the book.

Notice: Care has been taken to confirm the accuracy of information presented in this book. The authors, editors, and the publisher, however, cannot accept any responsibility for errors or omissions or for consequences from application of the information in this book and make no warranty, express or implied, with respect to its contents.

The authors and publisher have exerted every effort to ensure that drug selections and dosages set forth in this text are in accord with current recommendations and practice at time of publication. However, in view of ongoing research, changes in government regulations, and the constant flow of information relating to drug therapy and drug reactions, the reader is urged to check the package inserts of all drugs for any change in indications of dosage and for added warnings and precautions. This is particularly important when the recommended agent is a new and/or infrequently employed drug.

Library of Congress Cataloging-in-Publication Data

Names: Bauldoff, Gerene, author. | Gubrud-Howe, Paula Marie, author. | Carno, Margaret-Ann, author. | Preceded by (work): LeMone, Priscilla. Medical-surgical nursing.
Title: LeMone & Burke's medical-surgical nursing : clinical reasoning in patient care / Gerene Bauldoff, Paula Gubrud, Margaret-Ann Carno.
Other titles: LeMone and Burke's medical-surgical nursing | Medical-surgical nursing
Description: Seventh edition. | Hoboken NJ : Pearson Education, [2020] | Preceded by: Medical-surgical nursing : critical reasoning in patient care / Priscilla LeMone, Karen Burke, Gerene Bauldoff, Paula Gubrud. Sixth edition. [2015]. | Includes bibliographical references and index.
Identifiers: LCCN 2018056118| ISBN 9780134868189 | ISBN 0134868188
Subjects: | MESH: Nursing Process | Nursing Care | Medical-Surgical Nursing--methods | Patient Care Planning
Classification: LCC RT41 | NLM WY 100.1 | DDC 617/.0231--dc23
LC record available at https://lccn.loc.gov/2018056118

Pearson

ISBN-13: 978-0-134868189
ISBN-10: 0-13-4868188

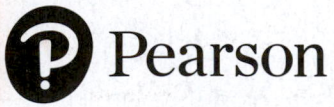

About the Authors

Gerene Bauldoff, RN, PhD, FAAN

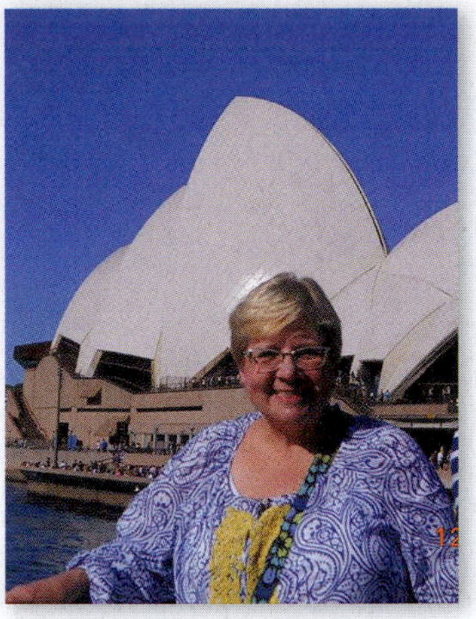

Gerene Bauldoff is a Professor of Clinical Nursing at The Ohio State University College of Nursing in Columbus, Ohio. She has been a nurse educator for 19 years, teaching medical-surgical nursing, clinical and research methods and measurement, and evidence-based practice courses at the baccalaureate, master's, and doctoral levels. Prior to her nursing educator role, her clinical background included home health nurse, lung transplant coordinator, and pulmonary rehabilitation coordinator. Dr. Bauldoff has a diploma from the Western Pennsylvania Hospital School of Nursing in Pittsburgh, Pennsylvania, and a BSN from LaRoche College in Pittsburgh. Her graduate education is from the University of Pittsburgh, with a MSN in medical-surgical nursing (cardiopulmonary clinical nurse specialist) and PhD in nursing in 2001, training under Leslie Hoffman, PhD, RN, FAAN.

Dr. Bauldoff is an active member of multiple professional organizations including the American Academy of Nursing (AAN), Sigma Theta Tau International Honor Society of Nursing, the American Association of Cardiovascular and Pulmonary Rehabilitation (AACVPR), the American Thoracic Society Nursing Assembly, and the American College of Chest Physicians (ACCP). She is a recognized expert in medical-surgical nursing, focusing on the care of the patient with chronic pulmonary disease, serving on committees focusing on international standards for and patient-centered outcomes in pulmonary rehabilitation. She has been honored with fellowships in AAN and ACCP and is a master fellow in AACVPR. Dr. Bauldoff has conducted several international presentations related to evidence-based practice and clinical outcomes.

Dr. Bauldoff considers nursing as the greatest profession, using scientific evidence to provide the highest quality of care while maintaining the personal relationship with patients and their families. Her experiences provide her with insights and lessons that she shares with her students.

Dr. Bauldoff resides in central Ohio. She enjoys international travel, walking, bicycling, golfing, and spending time with her family and friends.

I dedicate this book to the memory of my parents, to my sisters, and to my friends, especially Vicki von Sadovszky, Linda Daley, Patty Orndoff, and Eileen Collins—you are my touchstones to the world and are my greatest sounding boards. You help me keep my feet on the ground and my face turned toward new opportunities. You mean the world to me!

Paula Gubrud, RN, MS, EdD, FAAN

Paula Gubrud is Senior Associate Dean for Academic Affairs and an Associate Professor at Oregon Health and Science University (OHSU) School of Nursing. She has more than 25 years of experience as a nurse educator involving multiple levels of programs from LPN to doctoral education. Dr. Gubrud is a founding leader and co-director of the Oregon Consortium for Nursing Education, an award-winning consortium that includes the five campuses of OHSU and nine community colleges. She also has more than 20 years of experience in medical-surgical nursing, critical care, home health, and hospice. Dr. Gubrud earned a baccalaureate degree in nursing from Walla Walla University (1980), an MS in community-based nursing from OHSU (1993), and an EdD in postsecondary education from Portland State University (2008). She is a frequent invited speaker at national and international nursing education conferences and consults with other states and countries on the development of competency-based curriculum and nursing education consortiums designed to promote academic progression in nursing education. Her research activity is focused on clinical education redesign and the integration of simulation into nursing curriculum.

Dr. Gubrud is passionate about nursing and the opportunities it provides members of the profession. She values the sacred relationship nurses experience with patients as they promote health, treat illness, and provide comfort and palliative care. She believes the nation's health depends on highly qualified nurses who are dedicated to lifelong learning in pursuit of evidence-based, patient-centered care.

Dr. Gubrud lives in the Pacific Northwest and enjoys reading, camping, hiking, and fishing. She catches really big salmon year round!

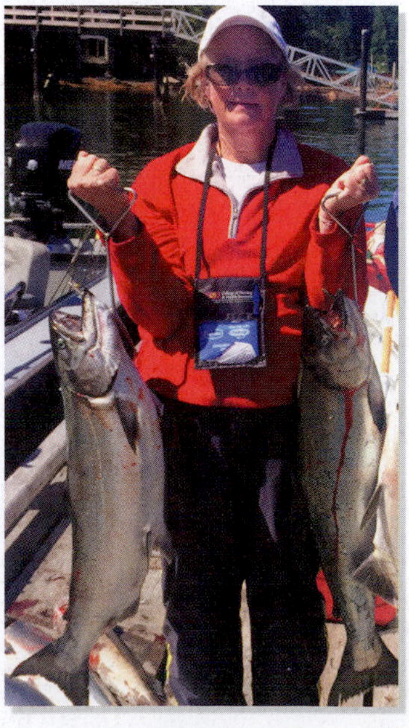

I dedicate this book to my husband Leland Howe and my children Elizabeth Gubrud-Howe, Gabriel Howe, and Caleb Howe for encouraging me to pursue my professional passions and goals. I also dedicate this book to my father, Allan Gubrud, who instilled insatiable curiosity, a love of learning, and a passion to teach.

Margaret-Ann Carno, PhD, MBA, MJ, RN, CPNP, D,ABSM, ATSF, FAAN

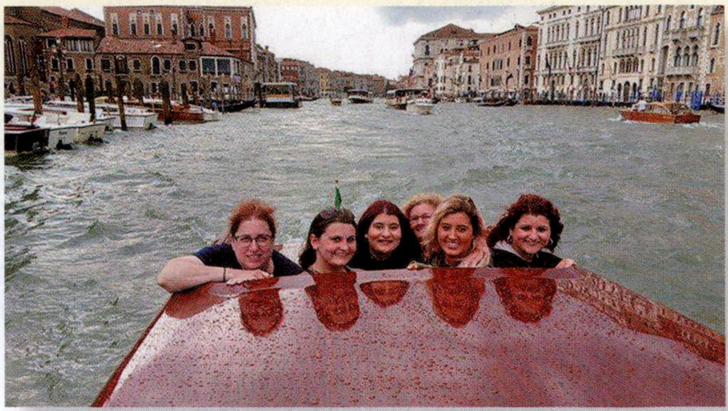

Margaret-Ann Carno is Professor of Clinical Nursing and Pediatrics as well as Co-Director of Baccalaureate Programs at the University of Rochester, School of Nursing. Dr. Carno has over 20 years of teaching across baccalaureate, master's, and doctoral levels of nursing education in medical-surgical nursing, pediatrics, ethics, health law, sleep across the lifespan, and research. Seeing students be successful gives Dr. Carno the greatest joy.

Dr. Carno earned her baccalaureate in nursing at Syracuse University and then went on to complete an MBA in Operations Management and an MS in Nursing (Pediatric Critical Care) also from Syracuse University. She received her PhD from the University of Pittsburgh under the guidance of Leslie Hoffman, PhD, RN, FAAN. Dr. Carno also holds a Masters in Jurisprudence in Health Law from University of Loyola–Chicago and a post Masters certification as a Pediatric Nurse Practitioner from the University of Rochester, School of Nursing. She is a Fellow of the American Academy of Nursing and of the American Thoracic Society. Dr Carno is a Diplomate of the American Board of Sleep Medicine.

When she is not teaching or working on other duties, Dr. Carno enjoys traveling the world with her beloved cousins as shown in the accompanying photo, where Dr. Carno is on the left.

I dedicate this book to my father Joseph, who while was in my life only a short time instilled the idea I could be anything I wanted and to never stop learning. Also to my mom, Libera, who has been my champion and support throughout my life.

Thank You

We wish to thank the editorial team. First and foremost, our intrepid publisher, Pamela Fuller, has provided fearless leadership and a forward-thinking strategy. This book would not exist without the expert editorial and organizational skills of Laura Horowitz, our development editor who brought this project to fruition with passion and graceful patience. The editorial assistance of Erin Sullivan who helped us keep all the balls in the air. We appreciate the work of Studio Montage on the cover and interior design. They brought the new structure to life! We also wish to thank our contributors and reviewers who shared their expert knowledge.

Gerene Bauldoff
Paula Gubrud
Margaret-Ann Carno

Contributors

Mei R. Fu, PhD, RN, FAAN
Associate Professor with Tenure
NYU Rory Meyers College of Nursing
New York University
New York, New York
(Chapter 14)

Maurade Gormley, MSN, CPNP, BSN
NYU Rory Meyers College of Nursing
New York University
New York, New York
(Chapter 14)

Lynne M. Hutchinson, DNP, FNP-BC
Assistant Professor of Nursing
University of South Carolina Beaufort
Bluffton, South Carolina
(Chapter 5)

Laura Mood, PhD, MSN, BSN, RN
Assistant Professor, School of Nursing,
University of Portland
Perioperative Nurse, Oregon Health & Science University
Portland, Oregon
(Chapters 2 and 4)

Pam Phillips, PhD, RN
Assistant Professor
University of South Carolina Beaufort
Hilton Head Island, South Carolina
(Chapter 6)

Kimberly Regis, RN, DNP, PNP-BC
Nationwide Children's Hospital
Ambulatory Specialty Clinics
Columbus, Ohio
(Chapter 8)

Matthew Sorenson, PhD, APN, ANP-C, FAAN
Director, School of Nursing
Associate Professor, Nursing
College of Science and Health
DePaul University
Chicago, Illinois
(Chapter 9)

Betsy Swinny, RN, MSN, APRN, FNP-C, CCRN
Associate Director
Baptist Health System, School of Nursing
San Antonio, Texas
(Chapters 18, 19, and 20)

Jill Volkerding, DNP, RN, CNL, CNE
Assistant Professor of Clinical Practice
College of Nursing
The Ohio State University
Columbus, Ohio
(Chapters 43 and 44)

Janice Wilcox, DNP, RN
Nurse Educator/Clinical Instructor
James Nursing Staff Development
College of Nursing
The Ohio State University
Columbus, Ohio
(Chapters 12 and 13)

Anita M. Zehala, MS, RN, ONC, APRN-CNS, CNE
Clinical Instructor of Practice
College of Nursing
The Ohio State University
Columbus, Ohio
(Chapters 39 and 40)

Reviewers

Wanda G. Barlow, MSN, RN, FNP-BC
Nursing Instructor
Winston Salem University
Winston Salem, North Carolina

Heidi L. Benavides, MSN, RN
Clinical Assistant Professor
University of Texas Health Science Center San Antonio
San Antonio, Texas

Angie Brindowski, MSN, BSN, RN
Department Chair
Clinical Assistant Professor
Carroll University
Waukesha, Wisconsin

Deborah Ellis, RN, MSN, FNP
Associate Professor of Nursing
Missouri Western State University
St. Joseph, Missouri

Shaana Escobar, DNP, RN
Assistant Professor
Department of Nursing
Arkansas Tech University
Russellville, Arkansas

Judith Faust, MSN, RN, CNE
Associate Professor
Ivy Tech Community College
Lafayette, Indiana

Jacqueline Guhde, MSN, RN, CNS
Senior Instructor
The University of Akron
Akron, Ohio

Anne Harner, EdD, MSN, RN
Assistant Professor
School of Nursing
Florida Gulf Coast University
Fort Myers, Florida

Shawna Harvey, MSN, RN
Dean of Nursing
Fortis College, Westerville
Newark, Ohio

Catherine Howell, RN, MSN
Professor, Nursing Education
San Diego City College
San Diego, California

Jamie L. Houchins, PhD, MSN, RN
Dean, School of Nursing
Ivy Tech Community College
Sellersburg, Indiana

Noreen C. Kostelecky, MSN, RN
Peoria, Illinois

Lee Ann Leech, DEd, MSN, RN, CRNI
Nursing Instructor
Edinboro University
Edinboro, Pennsylvania

Lynda S. Logan, MSN, RN
Assistant Professor, School of Nursing
Ivy Tech Community College
Lafayette, Indiana

Heidi Loucks, MS, RN, CNE
Nurse Educator
Casper College
Casper, Wyoming

Naomi Lungstrom, MN, ARNP, FNP
Clinical Assistant Professor
Washington State University
Spokane, Washington

Andrea R. Mann, MSN, RN, CNE
Third Level Chair and Instructor
Aria Health School of Nursing
Trevose, Pennsylvania

Greta I. Marek, DNP, RN, CNE
Assistant Professor
College of Nursing
East Tennessee State University
Johnson City, Tennessee

Mary Elizabeth McKenna-Dailey, FNP-BC
Professor, Nurse Education
North Shore Community College
Danvers, Massachusetts

Nancy Peifer Neil, RN, BSN, MSN, PhD
Palm Beach State College
Lake Worth, Florida

Sonia Rudolph, RN, MSN, APRN, FNP-BC
Nursing Division Chair
Jefferson Community & Technical College
Louisville, Kentucky

Donna Russo, RN, MSN, CCRN, CNE
Nursing Instructor
ARIA Health School of Nursing
Trevose, Pennsylvania

Laree J. Schoolmeesters, PhD, RN, CNL
Associate Professor
Presbyterian School of Nursing
Queens University of Charlotte
Charlotte, North Carolina

Marnie Lynn Sperling, DMD, MSN, RN
Clinical Assistant Professor
Henry P. Becton School of Nursing and Allied Health
Fairleigh Dickinson University
Florham Park, New Jersey

Marianne Swihart, MEd, MSN, BSN, AS
Associate Professor
Pasco Hernando Community College
New Port Richey, Florida

Preface

Why We Wrote This Book

Dr. LeMone-Koeplin developed the original vision for *Medical-Surgical Nursing: Clinical Reasoning in Patient Care* based on the belief that nursing is a holistic, evidence-based, person-centered profession. Nursing care, therefore, is provided for the whole person, not just for a malfunction of one or more body systems. We chose the cover and unit opener images to reflect this emphasis on the whole person.

The revisions and updates reflected in the seventh edition of *Medical-Surgical Nursing: Clinical Reasoning in Patient Care* further reflect our belief that nurses should possess the necessary knowledge, skills, and attitudes to continuously improve the quality and safety of care in healthcare systems. We believe that nurses need to be able to use evidence-based practice, apply clinical reasoning skills, and understand nursing care standards to safely perform complex skills and tasks. In Unit 1, *Dimensions of Medical-Surgical Nursing*, Chapter 2, Health and Illness in Adults, includes a section on critical care with a table to easily find critical care–related topics like shock and sepsis, burns, cardiac and pulmonary disorders, as well as disorders of the liver/pancreas, acute kidney injury, and spinal cord injury. Unit 2, *Alterations in Patterns of Health*, has been revised to include a new, comprehensive chapter on caring for the patient with alterations in sleep (Chapter 3) to emphasize the impact that inadequate sleep has on the patient in a multitude of ways.

In this textbook, discussions of the human responses to illness and disease are structured within the framework of clinical reasoning and the nursing process. Nursing care is presented within the context of nursing problems or diagnoses, emphasizing the importance of developing individualized evidence-based plans of care. The quality and safety implications for nursing care are addressed. Throughout the text, nursing care planning is based on a philosophy that individuals, their families, and communities are active participants in health and illness as well as consumers of healthcare services.

Regardless of the type of healthcare service or setting, medical-surgical nurses must use knowledge and skills to provide competent and safe patient care. The ability to effectively prioritize activities and patient care needs is critical. Nursing care is structured by the activities planned and carried out through clinical reasoning and multiple thinking strategies when applying the nursing process. Care of the medical-surgical patient is based on established professional ethics and standards and is focused on promoting or returning the patient to a state of functional health or providing palliative care at the end of life. Transitions of care are addressed for selected topics related to nursing based on prevention, acute, chronic, and end-of-life foci.

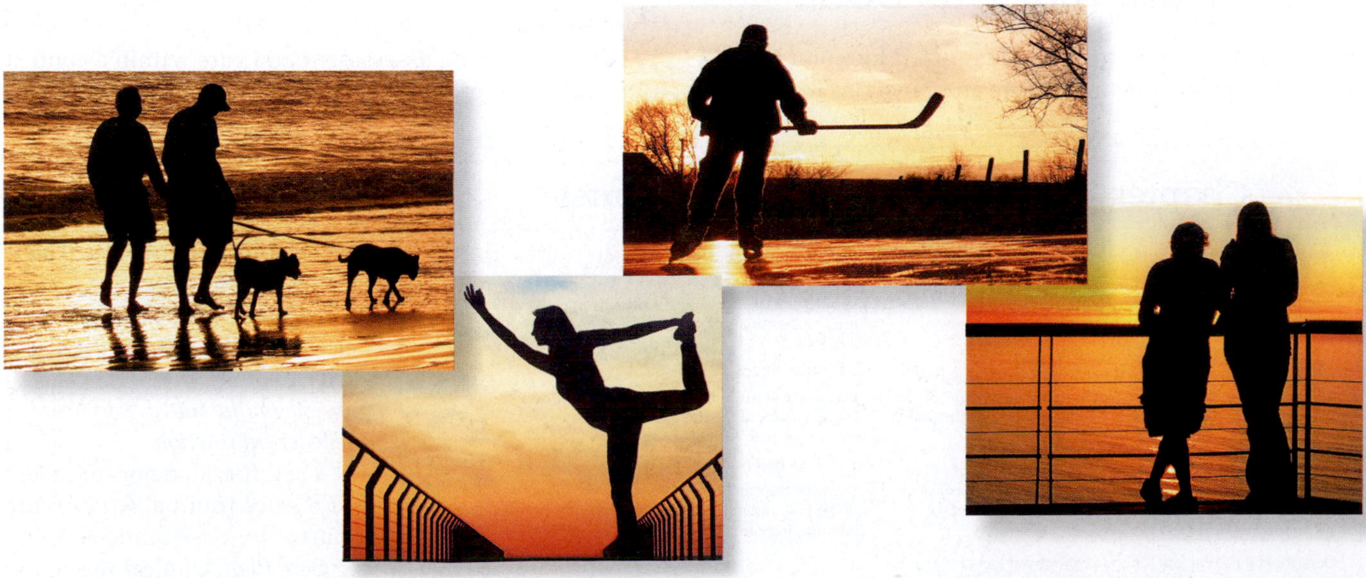

Throughout the text, we make every effort to communicate that both nurses and patients may be male or female and that patients require holistic, individualized care regardless of their age, gender, or racial, cultural, or socioeconomic background. Where indicated, we addressed issues related to special populations including older adults, the LGBTQI population, veterans, and adult survivors of pediatric conditions and congenital disorders. Our goal is to help students acquire the knowledge, resources, and competencies that ensure a solid base for clinical reasoning and that are applied to provide safe, individualized, and competent nursing care. We use understandable language and a consistent format, focusing on the most commonly encountered conditions. We have developed multiple learning strategies to facilitate success—audio, illustrations, teaching tips, and video and animation media.

Starting with the first edition, we have held fast to our vision that this textbook:

- Maintains a strong focus on nursing care as the essential element in learning and doing nursing, regardless of the gender, age, race, culture, or socioeconomic background of the patient or the setting for care.
- Provides a balance of pathophysiology, pharmacology, and interprofessional care to support interdependent and independent nursing interventions.
- Emphasizes the nurse's role as a caregiver, educator, advocate, leader and manager, and as an essential member of the interprofessional healthcare team.
- Uses functional health patterns and the nursing process as the structure for providing nursing care in today's world by prioritizing nursing interventions specific to altered responses to illness.
- Fosters clinical reasoning and decision making as the basis for safe, knowledgeable, individualized clinical practice.

Organization of This Book

The 50 chapters in this text are organized into units based on alterations in human structure and function. To increase student learning, each chapter in the book includes key terms, learning outcomes and clinical competencies, chapter highlights, test yourself NCLEX-type questions, and references with supporting evidence. Each chapter is grouped into sections, and each section has a learning outcome.

Each unit with a focus on altered health opens with an assessment chapter. This chapter draws on the student's prerequisite knowledge and serves to reinforce basic principles of anatomy and physiology as applied to assessment in both health and illness. Following the assessment chapter, nursing care chapters provide information about major illnesses and traumatic injuries. Each nursing care chapter follows a consistent format, including the following key components:

Pathophysiology and Risk Factors

The discussion of each *major* illness or injury begins with incidence and prevalence, risk factors, and an overview of pathophysiology, followed by manifestations (signs and symptoms) and complications. Selected *Focus on Cultural Diversity* boxes demonstrate how race, age, and gender affect differences in incidence, prevalence, and mortality.

Manifestations and Complications

To further describe *major* illnesses, manifestations including signs and symptoms, antecedents, and subsequent clinical symptoms commonly seen are described for each condition. Common complications are also described to provide important information to allow anticipation of potential problems.

Interprofessional Care

Interprofessional care considers diagnosis and treatment by the healthcare team. The section includes information, as appropriate, about specific tests necessary for diagnosis, medications, surgery and other treatments, fluid management, dietary management, and complementary and alternative therapies. Specific information with related nursing care is highlighted in *Medication Administration* boxes and boxes focused on the nursing care of patients having a specific treatment or surgery.

Nursing Care

We discuss nursing assessment and care within a context of priorities of care, diagnoses, outcomes, and interventions, with rationales provided for each intervention. Boxes throughout each illness discussion section present information essential to patient care. These features include *Nursing Care of the Patient*, *Genetic Considerations*, *Focus on Cultural Diversity*, *Safety Alerts*, *Multisystem Effects*, *Pathophysiology Illustrated*, and *Moving Evidence into Action*.

Last, for 80 major disorders or types of trauma, we provide a narrative *Case Study & Nursing Care Plan*. Clinical reasoning

Chapter Outline and Learning Outcomes

questions specific to the care plan are provided in a section called *Clinical Reasoning in Patient Care* (with suggestions for decision-making provided in Appendix B under *Evaluate Your Response to Clinical Reasoning in Patient Care*). The nursing care section ends with information about continuity of care with essential patient and caregiver education, and suggestions for referrals and additional patient resources.

Transitions of Care

New to the seventh edition, this section addresses critical issues for patients and families along the care continuum. For identified disorders, we describe care needs related to prevention, acute and chronic disease, and end-of-life considerations to support planning for and implementing comprehensive care transition.

End-of-Chapter Sections

Each chapter ends with *Chapter Highlights*, a bulleted list of key points for each section/learning outcome; *Test Yourself NCLEX-RN Review*, 10 NCLEX-style review questions that reinforce comprehension of the chapter content (the correct answers with rationales are found in Appendix B); *References* to support all evidence presented in the chapter; and *Additional Resources* for students who need or want additional study.

What's New in the Seventh Edition

We are delighted to welcome Margaret-Ann Carno as a coauthor of this book. Information about Dr. Carno is included in About the Authors on page x. New features of the seventh edition include:

- A consistent chapter structure with numbered sections, a matching learning outcome for each, and a new design that emphasizes the structure, making it easier for students to navigate the book.
- Chapter 3, *Nursing Care of the Patient with Alterations of Sleep*, which describes commonly seen sleep disorders. The greatest strength of the chapter is that it demonstrates the linkage between sleep and health and the bidirectional nature of sleep and health.
- Recognizing the overwhelming number and variety of medications nurses must safely administer, the most commonly prescribed drugs are printed in **blue type** in the *Medication Administration* features.
- *Transitions of Care* replaces the section previously titled Continuity of Care. This section focuses on the nurse's responsibility for preparing the patient and caregivers for transitions of care from one healthcare setting to another or to the home.

Chapter Features

Assessment Addressing the first step in the nursing process, the assessment feature provides a review of the objective and subjective data needed to provide a clear clinical picture of the condition. Techniques and normal findings are compared to abnormal findings. Selected assessments include detailed guidelines for psychomotor skills used to assess the organ system.

Integumentary Assessments

Technique and Normal Findings (*in italics*)	Abnormal Findings
Inspect skin color and note any odors coming from the skin. *Skin color should be even, appropriate to the age and race of the patient, without foul odors.*	■ A strong odor of perspiration may indicate poor hygiene and a need for patient teaching. A foul odor may indicate a disorder of the sweat glands. ■ Pallor and/or cyanosis are seen with exposure to cold and with decreased perfusion and oxygenation. In cyanotic dark-skinned patients, skin loses glow and appears dull. Cyanosis may be more visible in the mucous membranes and nail beds of these patients. ■ In dark-skinned patients, jaundice may be most apparent in the sclerae of the eyes. ■ Redness, swelling, and pain are seen with various rashes, inflammations, infections, and burns. First-degree (superficial) burns cause areas of painful erythema and swelling. Red, painful blisters appear in second-degree (partial-thickness) burns, whereas white or blackened areas are common in third-degree (full-thickness) burns. ■ Vitiligo, an abnormal loss of melanin in patches, typically occurs over the face, hands, or groin. Vitiligo is thought to be an autoimmune disorder.
Inspect the skin for lesions and alterations, including calluses, scars, tattoos, and piercings. Include inspection of skin creases and folds. *Skin should be intact without lesions.*	■ Primary, secondary, and vascular lesions are described and shown in Tables 15.4 through 15.6. ■ Pearly edged nodules with a central ulcer are seen in basal cell carcinoma. ■ Scaly, red, fast-growing papules are seen in squamous cell carcinoma. ■ Dark, asymmetric, multicolored patches (sometimes moles) with irregular edges appear in malignant melanoma. ■ Circular lesions are usually present in ringworm and in tinea versicolor. ■ Grouped vesicles may be seen in contact dermatitis. ■ Linear lesions appear in poison ivy and herpes zoster. ■ **Urticaria** (hives) appears as patches of pale, itchy wheals in an erythematous area. ■ In psoriasis, scaly red patches appear on the scalp, knees, back, and genitals. ■ In herpes zoster, vesicles appear along sensory nerve paths, turn into pustules, and then crust over. ■ Bruises (**ecchymosis**) are raised bluish or yellowish vascular lesions. Multiple bruises in various stages of healing suggest trauma or abuse.
Palpate skin temperature. *Skin should be warm.*	■ Skin is warm and red in inflammation and is generally warm with elevated body temperature. ■ Decreased blood flow decreases the skin temperature; this may be generalized, as in shock, or localized, as in arteriosclerosis.

Diagnostic Tests
of the Endocrine System

PITUITARY TESTS		
NAME OF TEST	PURPOSE AND DESCRIPTION	RELATED NURSING INTERVENTIONS
Growth hormone (GH), human growth hormone (hGH)	In this blood test, GH levels (affected by food, stress, and activity) are measured to identify GH deficiency (dwarfism) or GH excess (gigantism, acromegaly). Normal value: Men: <5 ng/mL Women: <10 ng/mL	Tell patient not to eat or drink 8–10 h prior to having blood drawn. Have patient rest for 30–60 min before blood is drawn.

Diagnostic Tests This feature identifies commonly used diagnostic tests for specific disorders. The tests are identified while the values of characteristics related to the specific disorder are emphasized, making a clear connection between the significance of the test and the disorder.

Genetic Considerations
Examples of Inherited Endocrine System Disorders

- Type 1 and type 2 diabetes mellitus are classified as multifactorial inheritance disorders because both genetic and environmental factors are necessary for onset of these disorders.
- Hashimoto disease (chronic thyroiditis) is believed to have a genetic component.
- Multiple endocrine neoplasia is a group of rare diseases caused by genetic defects leading to hyperplasia and hyperfunction of two or more components of the endocrine system (especially the parathyroid, pancreas, and pituitary glands).
- Fragile X syndrome is a genetic condition that causes developmental problems including learning disabilities and mental retardation. Males are usually more severely affected than females.

Genetic Considerations With the expanding knowledge of genetic impact on disease, the Genetics Considerations feature provides examples of system-specific disorders. This feature is found in both the assessment chapters as well as the detailed disorder chapters.

Focus on Cultural Diversity
Estimates of Prevalence of Diabetes Mellitus

- 15.1% of American Indians and Alaska Natives have DM. The rate varies; only 6% of Alaska natives have DM, whereas 22.2% of Native Americans in southern Arizona have DM.
- 12.7% of non-Hispanic Blacks ages 18 years or older have DM.
- 12.1% of Hispanic/Latino Americans ages 18 years or older have DM. Rates of diabetes are lower among Cuban Americans (9%) and Central and South Americans (8.5%) and higher for Mexican Americans (13.8%) and Puerto Rican Americans (12%).
- 8% of Asian Americans ages 18 years or older have DM.
- 7.4% of non-Hispanic Whites ages 18 years or older have DM (CDC, 2017b).

Focus on Cultural Diversity This feature provides essential guidelines for nurses to help them provide culturally sensitive care.

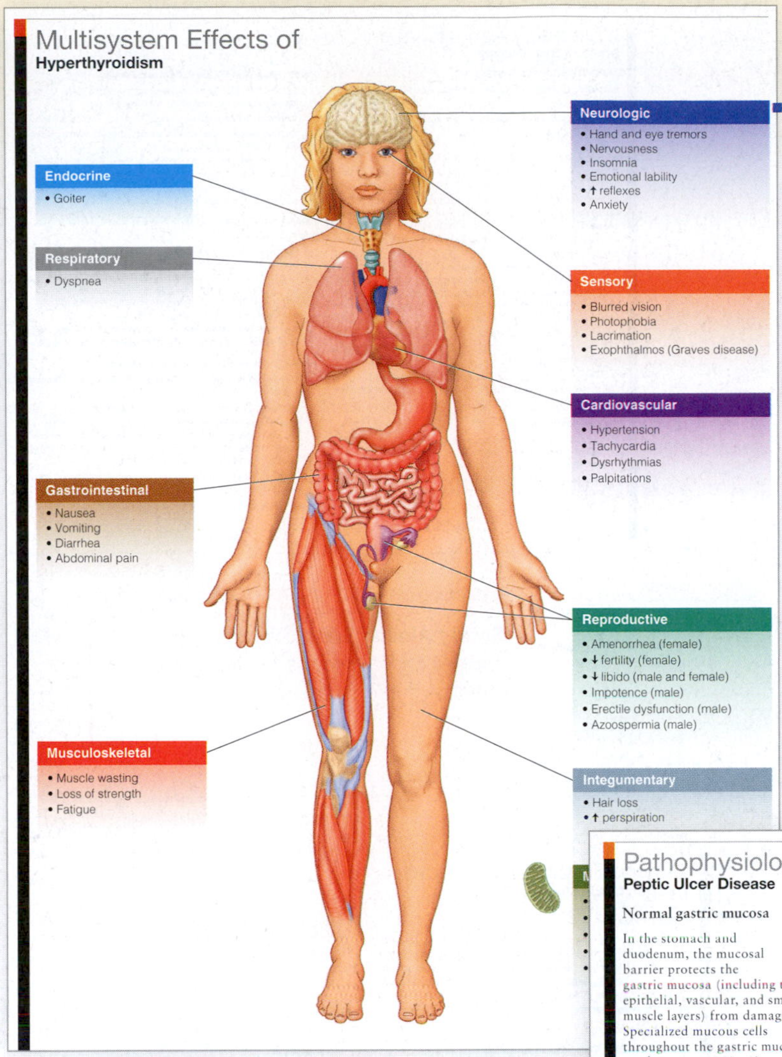
Multisystem Effects of
Hyperthyroidism
Endocrine
• Goiter
Respiratory
• Dyspnea
Gastrointestinal
• Nausea
• Vomiting
• Diarrhea
• Abdominal pain
Musculoskeletal
• Muscle wasting
• Loss of strength
• Fatigue
Neurologic
• Hand and eye tremors
• Nervousness
• Insomnia
• Emotional lability
• ↑ reflexes
• Anxiety
Sensory
• Blurred vision
• Photophobia
• Lacrimation
• Exophthalmos (Graves disease)
Cardiovascular
• Hypertension
• Tachycardia
• Dysrhythmias
• Palpitations
Reproductive
• Amenorrhea (female)
• ↓ fertility (female)
• ↓ libido (male and female)
• Impotence (male)
• Erectile dysfunction (male)
• Azoospermia (male)
Integumentary
• Hair loss
• ↑ perspiration

Multisystem Effects These new and updated illustrated features focus on a specific disorder describing manifestations and effects on body systems.

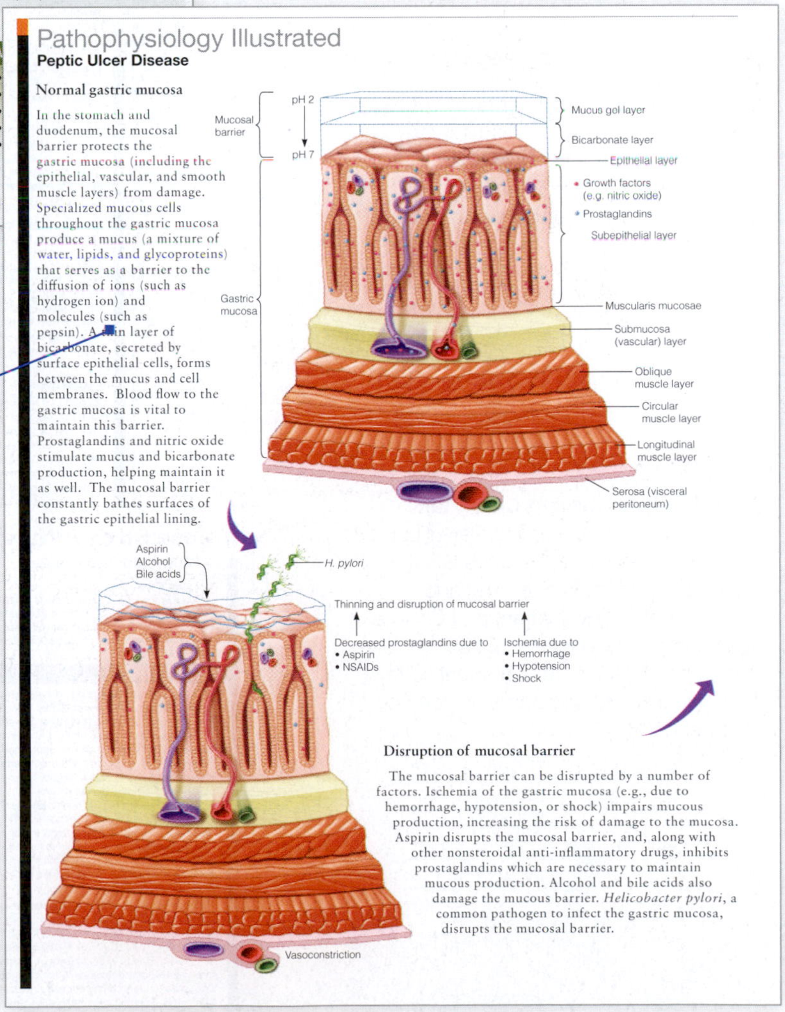
Pathophysiology Illustrated
Peptic Ulcer Disease
Normal gastric mucosa
In the stomach and duodenum, the mucosal barrier protects the gastric mucosa (including the epithelial, vascular, and smooth muscle layers) from damage. Specialized mucous cells throughout the gastric mucosa produce a mucus (a mixture of water, lipids, and glycoproteins) that serves as a barrier to the diffusion of ions (such as hydrogen ion) and molecules (such as pepsin). A thin layer of bicarbonate, secreted by surface epithelial cells, forms between the mucus and cell membranes. Blood flow to the gastric mucosa is vital to maintain this barrier. Prostaglandins and nitric oxide stimulate mucus and bicarbonate production, helping maintain it as well. The mucosal barrier constantly bathes surfaces of the gastric epithelial lining.
Mucosal barrier
pH 2
pH 7
Gastric mucosa
Mucus gel layer
Bicarbonate layer
Epithelial layer
• Growth factors (e.g. nitric oxide)
• Prostaglandins
Subepithelial layer
Muscularis mucosae
Submucosa (vascular) layer
Oblique muscle layer
Circular muscle layer
Longitudinal muscle layer
Serosa (visceral peritoneum)
Aspirin
Alcohol
Bile acids
H. pylori
Thinning and disruption of mucosal barrier
Decreased prostaglandins due to
• Aspirin
• NSAIDs
Ischemia due to
• Hemorrhage
• Hypotension
• Shock
Vasoconstriction
Disruption of mucosal barrier
The mucosal barrier can be disrupted by a number of factors. Ischemia of the gastric mucosa (e.g., due to hemorrhage, hypotension, or shock) impairs mucous production, increasing the risk of damage to the mucosa. Aspirin disrupts the mucosal barrier, and, along with other nonsteroidal anti-inflammatory drugs, inhibits prostaglandins which are necessary to maintain mucous production. Alcohol and bile acids also damage the mucous barrier. Helicobacter pylori, a common pathogen to infect the gastric mucosa, disrupts the mucosal barrier.

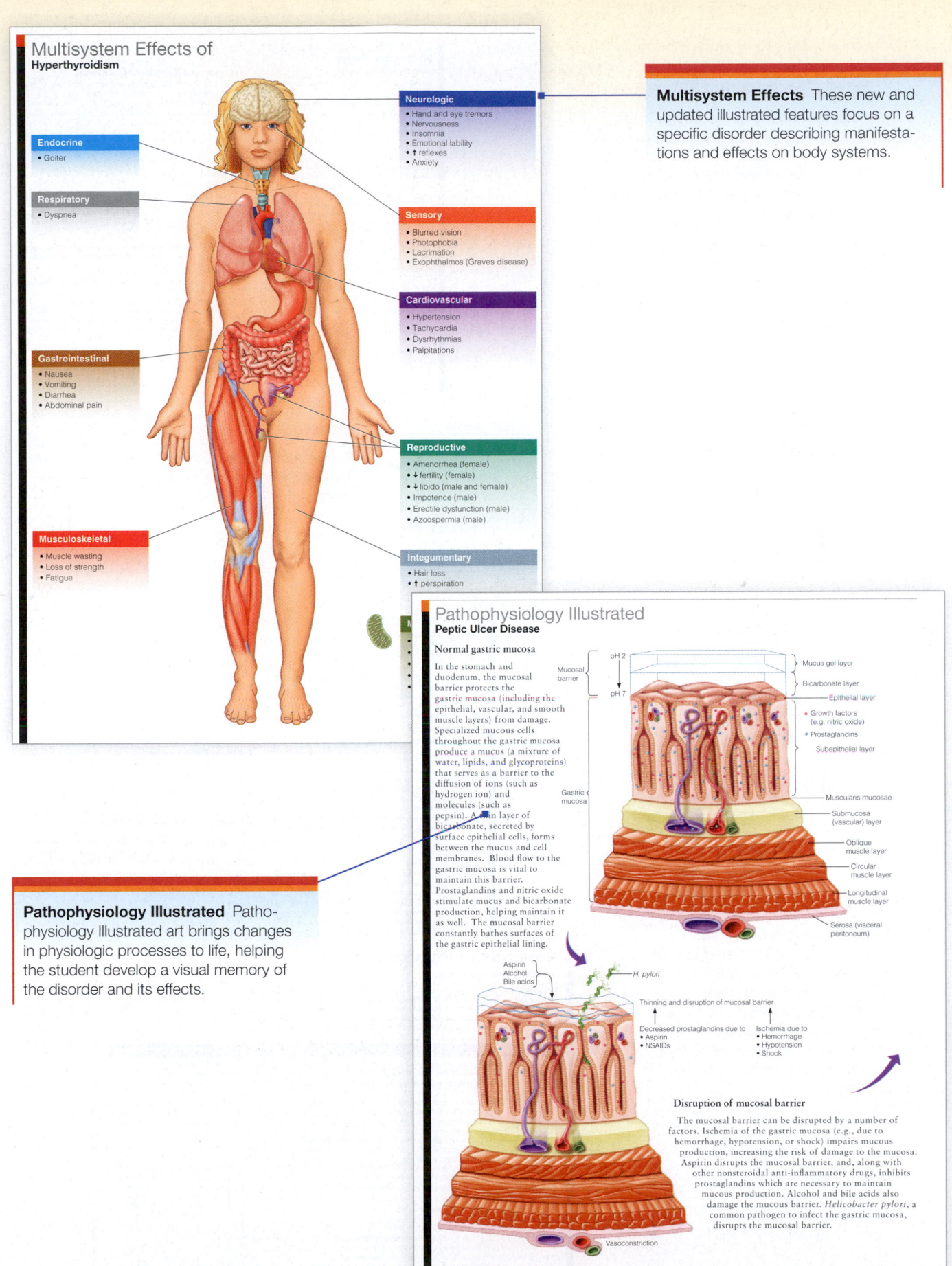

Pathophysiology Illustrated Pathophysiology Illustrated art brings changes in physiologic processes to life, helping the student develop a visual memory of the disorder and its effects.

Medication Administration Drugs appropriate for the chapter disorders are featured, as well as the related nursing responsibilities and patient/family teaching. The top 200 prescribed drugs are shown in blue type.

Medication Administration 22.A

Drugs to Treat Obesity

APPETITE SUPPRESSANTS

phentermine (Adipex-P, Fastin, Ionamin, Obestin-30, Oby-Trim, others)

phentermine and topiramate extended release (Qsymia)

lorcaserin (Belviq)

Phentermine acts directly on the appetite-control center in the CNS to suppress the appetite and reduce hunger. Topiramate increases feelings of fullness and increases calorie burning.

Liraglutide (Saxenda, Victoza) is a glucagon-like peptide 1 (GLP-1) that causes increased insulin release and decreased glucagon release. Liraglutide is approved for the treatment of Type 2 diabetes but it also delays gastric emptying so has an independent weight loss effect.

Bupropion and naltrexone (Contrave) is a combination medication—a dopamine and norepinephrine reuptake inhibitor and opioid receptor antagonist. The combination decreases the motivation/reinforcement that food provides (dopamine effect) and the pleasure/palatability of eating (opioid effect).

Lorcaserin (Belviq) activates the serotonin 5-HT 2c receptor in the brain, which causes a person to feel full after eating smaller amounts of food.

These drugs may be used to treat obesity in patients with a BMI > 30 and patients with a BMI > 27 who have risk factors such as diabetes or hypertension.

Nursing Responsibilities

- Assess for contraindications, such as pregnancy or lactation, use of other appetite suppressants, impaired liver or kidney function, history of CHD, or alcohol abuse.
- Regularly monitor blood pressure and heart rate during treatment. Increases may indicate need to reduce dose or discontinue treatment.

Health Education for the Patient and Family

- Take as directed; do not exceed recommended dose. Do not take if you may be pregnant or are nursing.
- Take your last dose no later than 4:00 p.m. to avoid insomnia.
- You may experience difficulty sleeping, nervousness, or palpitations while taking this drug.
- Increase your fluid intake to reduce possible side effects of dry mouth and constipation.
- This drug does not replace diet and exercise for weight loss; continue to follow your prescribed regimen.

LIPASE INHIBITOR

orlistat (Alli, Xenical)

Orlistat inhibits lipases necessary for the breakdown and absorption of fat, thus decreasing the absorption of dietary fat. Its action is primarily local, within the GI tract, with few systemic effects.

Nursing Responsibilities

- Administer with meals or up to 1 hour following a meal.
- Provide a fat-soluble vitamin supplement (A, D, E, and K) daily. Separate administration time from orlistat by at least 2 hours.

Health Education for the Patient and Family

- Take as directed; do not increase dose. You may skip a dose if you do not consume a meal.
- Use in conjunction with a low-calorie, low-fat diet.
- Common gastrointestinal side effects include oily or fatty stools, flatulence, oily discharge, or frequent stools with difficulty controlling defecation. These side effects may diminish with time or increase if a meal high in fat is consumed.
- Notify your healthcare provider if you become pregnant while taking this medication.

Note: Drugs identified in *blue* are among the 200 most commonly prescribed medications in the U.S.

Source: Data from Adams, Holland, & Urban, 2017.

SAFETY ALERT: Sublingual nitroglycerin tablets and nitroglycerin spray are the only medications appropriate to treat an acute anginal attack. ■

Safety Alerts Safety Alerts bring forward critical information for safe and effective nursing practice.

Moving Evidence into Action These boxes focus on evidence into specific topics and how the external evidence, internal evidence, and patient priorities and values are incorporated into high-quality care.

Moving Evidence into Action

Decision Making in Heart Failure

Clinical Issue

Heart failure is a major disease process impacting function throughout the world. As HF is a chronic illness, ongoing decisions must be made related to treatments, pharmacologic options, and other, more invasive therapeutic options like surgery. How patients make decisions is an important concept for nurses to understand.

External Evidence

Hamel, Gaugler, Porta, and Hadidi (2018) conducted a systematic review of the literature to examine complex decision making to clarify key decision points and identify commonalities. Their review included 12 studies. Themes identified included "processing the decision," "timing and prognostication," and "considering the future." Some of the subthemes focused on when and how information was received, making the treatment decision, the role of the "future" in their decisions, and the influence of life and death decisions. Common themes were timing of discussions, the delivery of information, and considerations of the future.

Internal Evidence

As part of the evaluation of internal evidence, one must consider the patient's "real-time" response to the clinical decisions that must be made, the proposed treatment plan, and identification of stakeholders that influence the patient decision-making process. One question to ask: Are there patients with heart failure who are confronted with significant decisions regarding treatment planning within the population of your care environment? Does the clinical environment support the information related to patient decision making? How does providing more support for HF patients decision making in your environment impact costs?

Patient Considerations

When considering use of a new practice (like additional supportive decision making for patients with HF), the nurse must consider the specific patient population where it will be used. Will patients and their families be amenable to additional information related to their decision making?

Putting the Pieces Together

In the ideal world, the patient is a partner with the healthcare team, especially when making decisions related to the therapeutic plan when faced with a chronic illness like heart failure. Knowing the common themes that make up patient decision making can allow the healthcare team to support effective decision making by the patient and his or her family. To effectively implement a plan, it is important to evaluate the external evidence and consider the internal implications and patient/family issues. With the use of decision-making themes, more effective patient decisions can be supported. This will lead to increased patient participation in his or her therapeutic plan and patient satisfaction.

Reference

Hamel, A. V., Gaugler, J. E., Porta, C. M., & Hadidi, N. N. (2018). Complex decision-making in heart failure: A systematic review and thematic analysis. *Journal of Cardiovascular Nursing, 33*(3), 225–231.

Case Study & Nursing Care Plan Each Case Study & Nursing Care Plan includes Assessment, Diagnoses, Expected Outcomes, Planning and Implementation, Evaluation, and Clinical Reasoning in Patient Care. Cues for students to evaluate their responses to the Clinical Reasoning items are located in Appendix B.

Case Study & Nursing Care Plan

A Patient with Hypertension

Margaret Spezia is a married, 49-year-old woman with eight children whose ages range from 3 to 18 years. For the past 2 months, Mrs. Spezia has had frequent morning headaches and occasional dizziness and blurred vision. At her annual physical examination 1 month ago, her blood pressure was 168/104 and 156/94 mmHg. She was instructed to reduce her fat and cholesterol intake, to avoid using salt at the table, and to start walking for 30 to 45 minutes daily. Mrs. Spezia returns to the clinic for a follow-up.

ASSESSMENT

While escorting Mrs. Spezia to the exam room and obtaining her weight, blood pressure, and history, Lisa Christos, RN, notices that Mrs. Spezia seems restless and upset. Ms. Christos says, "You look upset about something. Is everything OK?" Mrs. Spezia responds, "Well, my head is throbbing, and I'm sort of dizzy. I think I'm just overdoing it and not getting enough rest. You know, raising eight children is a lot of work and expense. I just started working part time so we wouldn't get behind in our bills. I thought the extra money might relieve some of my stress, but I'm not so sure that's really happening. I'm not getting any better and I'm worried that I'll lose my job or become disabled and that my husband won't be able to manage the children by himself. I really need to go home, but first, I want to get rid of this awful headache. Would you please get me a couple of aspirin or something?"

Mrs. Spezia's history shows a steady weight gain during the past 18 years. She has no known family history of hypertension. Physical findings include height 160 cm (63 in.); weight 102 kg (225 lb); T 37.2°C (99°F); P 100 bpm and regular; R 16/min; BP 180/115 (lying), 170/110 (sitting), 165/105 mmHg (standing); average 10-point difference in readings between right and left arm (lower on left). Skin cool and dry, capillary refill 4 seconds right hand, 3 seconds left hand. Mrs. Spezia's total serum cholesterol is 245 mg/dL (normal < 200 mg/dL). All other blood and urine studies are within normal limits. Based on analysis of the

DIAGNOSES

- Fatigue due to effects of hypertension and stresses of daily life
- Obesity related to excessive food intake
- Inability to maintain a healthy lifestyle
- Insufficient understanding of effects of prescribed treatment

EXPECTED OUTCOMES

- Patient will reduce blood pressure readings to < 150 systolic and 90 diastolic by return visit next week.
- Patient will incorporate low-sodium and low-fat foods into her diet from a provided list.
- Patient will develop a plan for regular exercise.
- Patient will verbalize understanding of the effects of prescribed drug, dietary restrictions, exercise, and follow-up visits to help control hypertension.

Visuals

The visuals in **LeMone & Burke's Medical-Surgical Nursing** have been updated for currency, accuracy, realism, and style. Visual learners in particular will be delighted to see the detailed illustrations, vivid photos, and numerous tables.

Table 15.2 Skin Color Assessment Variations in People with Light and Dark Skin

Disorder and Cause	Change in Light Skin	Change in Dark Skin
Pallor: *A decrease or absence in skin color as the result of a decrease in tissue perfusion; a decrease in shape, size, or amount of RBCs; or an absence of melanin (local or generalized).*		
Anemia (decreased or abnormal size and shape of RBCs)	Generalized paleness	Brown skin is dull and has a yellow cast; black skin is dull and has an ashen gray cast
Hemorrhage (decreased amount of circulating RBCs)	Generalized paleness	Brown skin is dull and has a yellow cast; black skin is dull and has an ashen gray cast
Shock (decreased amount of circulating RBCs or decreased perfusion)	Generalized paleness	Brown skin is dull and has a yellow cast; black skin is dull and has an ashen gray cast
Arterial insufficiency (trauma, acute arterial occlusion, or arteriosclerosis)	Local paleness	Dull, ashen gray
Vitiligo (patchy loss of melanocytes)	Patches of white spots, most often found over the skin of the face, hands, or groin	Patches of white spots, most often found over the skin of the face, hands, or groin
Albinism (total absence of melanin)	White/pink	Tan, cream, or white
Cyanosis: *A bluish discoloration of the skin and mucous membranes resulting from a local or generalized excess of deoxygenated hemoglobin or a structural defect in the hemoglobin molecule.*		
Acute and chronic disorders of the structure and function of the heart and lungs (arterial insufficiency; exposure to cold, hypothermia)	Dusky blue; color may be generalized or local, depending on cause	Skin may appear darker, but will be dull; cyanosis is more readily assessed in the nail beds, oral mucous membranes, and conjunctivae
Erythema: *Redness of the skin or mucous membranes that is the result of dilation and congestion of superficial capillaries.*		
Hyperemia (inflammation, increased body temperature, hot environmental temperature, embarrassment, alcohol ingestion)	Red or bright pink	Difficult to assess; skin may have a dark red cast
Carbon monoxide poisoning (carbon monoxide displaces oxygen on the hemoglobin molecule, causing hypoxia, carboxyhemoglobinemia)	Cherry red in face and upper torso	Cherry red lips, oral mucous membranes, and nail beds
Venous stasis (inability of veins to return blood to heart; may result from edema, varicose veins, or pressure)	Dusky red	Difficult to assess
Jaundice: *Yellowish discoloration of the skin, mucous membranes, and sclerae of the eyes, caused by increased amounts of bilirubin or other pigments in the blood.*		
Increased serum bilirubin to > 2–3 mg/100 mL (liver disease, pancreatic disease, gallbladder disease, hemolysis such as following blood transfusion, severe burns or infections)	Yellowing of skin follows yellowing of sclerae and mucous membranes; may also be assessed in the fingernails and palms of the hands	Yellowing is best assessed at the junction of the hard palate and the soft palate or on the palms of the hands; sclerae may be yellow near the limbus (do not confuse with normal yellow eye pigmentation)
Uremia (retained urochrome pigments in the blood)	Orange-green or gray cast to skin	Difficult to assess; may appear as yellowish-green color in the sclera of the eye

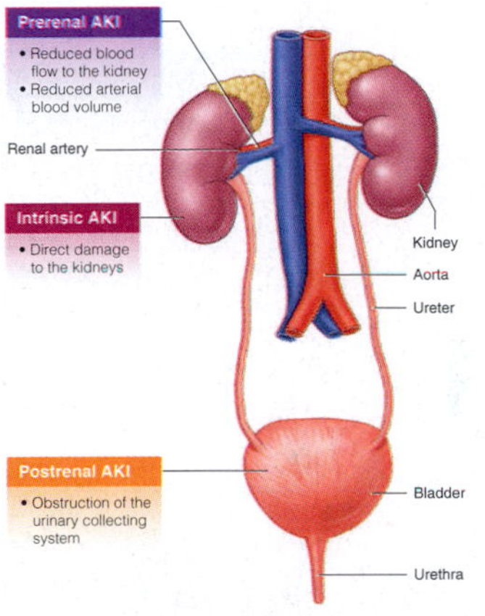

Prerenal AKI
• Reduced blood flow to the kidney
• Reduced arterial blood volume
Renal artery
Intrinsic AKI
• Direct damage to the kidneys
Kidney
Aorta
Ureter
Postrenal AKI
• Obstruction of the urinary collecting system
Bladder
Urethra

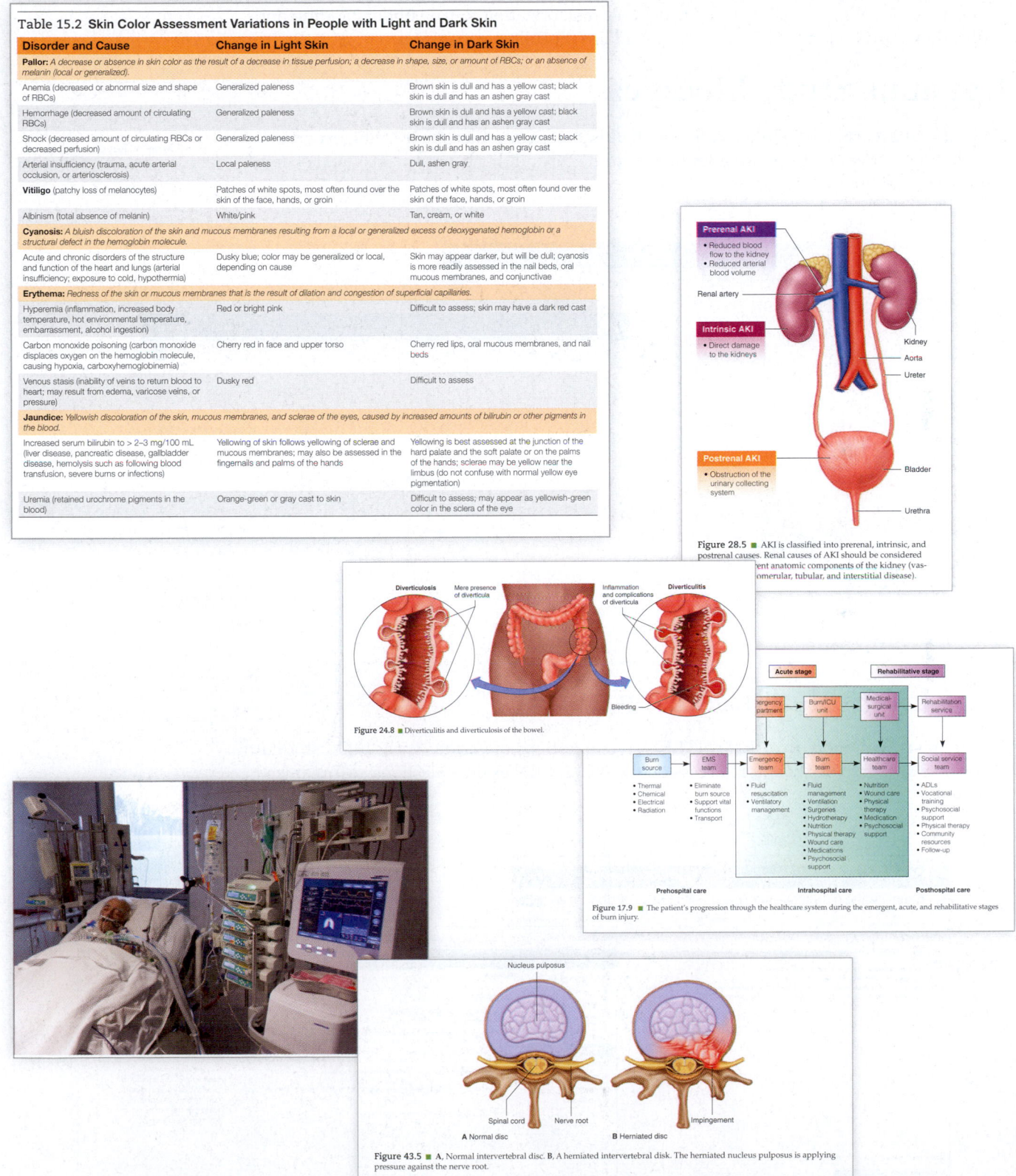

Figure 28.5 ■ AKI is classified into prerenal, intrinsic, and postrenal causes. Renal causes of AKI should be considered …ent anatomic components of the kidney (vas- …omerular, tubular, and interstitial disease).

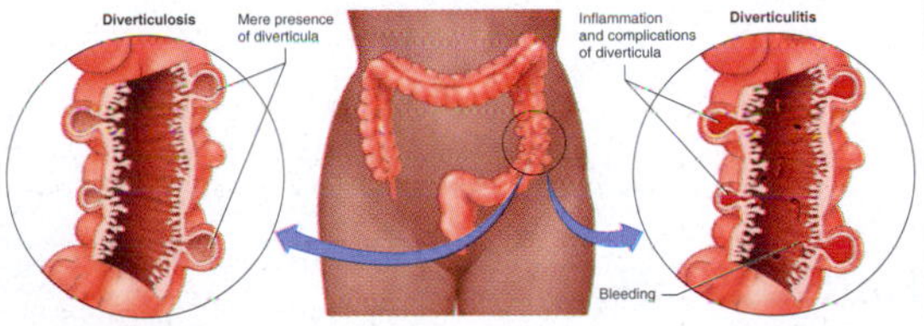

Diverticulosis
Mere presence of diverticula
Inflammation and complications of diverticula
Diverticulitis
Bleeding

Figure 24.8 ■ Diverticulitis and diverticulosis of the bowel.

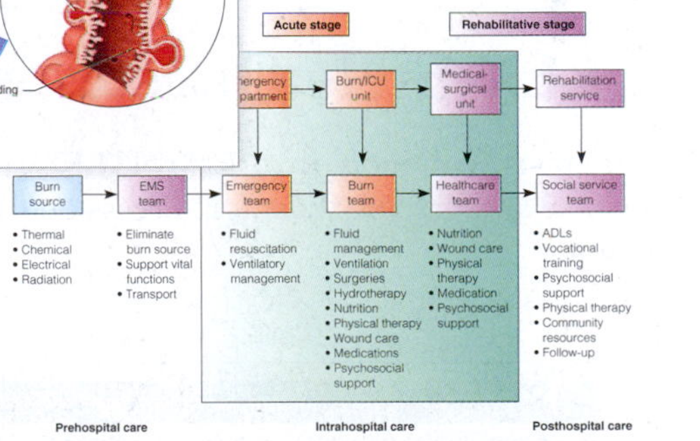

Acute stage
Rehabilitative stage
Burn/ICU unit
Medical-surgical unit
Rehabilitation service
Burn source
EMS team
Emergency team
Burn team
Healthcare team
Social service team
• Thermal
• Chemical
• Electrical
• Radiation
• Eliminate burn source
• Support vital functions
• Transport
• Fluid resuscitation
• Ventilatory management
• Fluid management
• Ventilation
• Surgeries
• Hydrotherapy
• Nutrition
• Physical therapy
• Wound care
• Medications
• Psychosocial support
• Nutrition
• Wound care
• Physical therapy
• Medication
• Psychosocial support
• ADLs
• Vocational training
• Psychosocial support
• Physical therapy
• Community resources
• Follow-up
Prehospital care
Intrahospital care
Posthospital care

Figure 17.9 ■ The patient's progression through the healthcare system during the emergent, acute, and rehabilitative stages of burn injury.

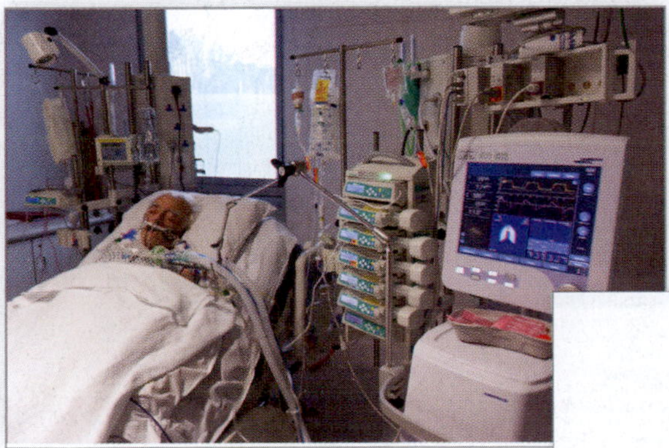

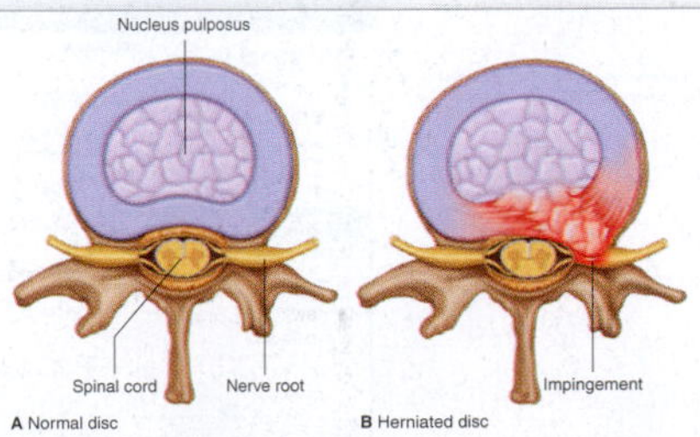

Nucleus pulposus
Spinal cord
Nerve root
Impingement
A Normal disc
B Herniated disc

Figure 43.5 ■ A, Normal intervertebral disc. B, A herniated intervertebral disk. The herniated nucleus pulposus is applying pressure against the nerve root.

MyLab Nursing

MyLab Nursing is an online learning and practice environment that works with the text to help students master key concepts, prepare for the NCLEX-RN exam, and develop clinical reasoning skills. Through a new mobile experience, students can study *LeMone & Burke's Medical-Surgical Nursing* anytime, anywhere. New adaptive technology with remediation personalizes learning, moving students beyond memorization to true understanding and application of the content. MyLab Nursing contains the following features:

Dynamic Study Modules

New adaptive learning modules with remediation that personalize the learning experience by allowing students to increase both their confidence and their performance while being assessed in real time.

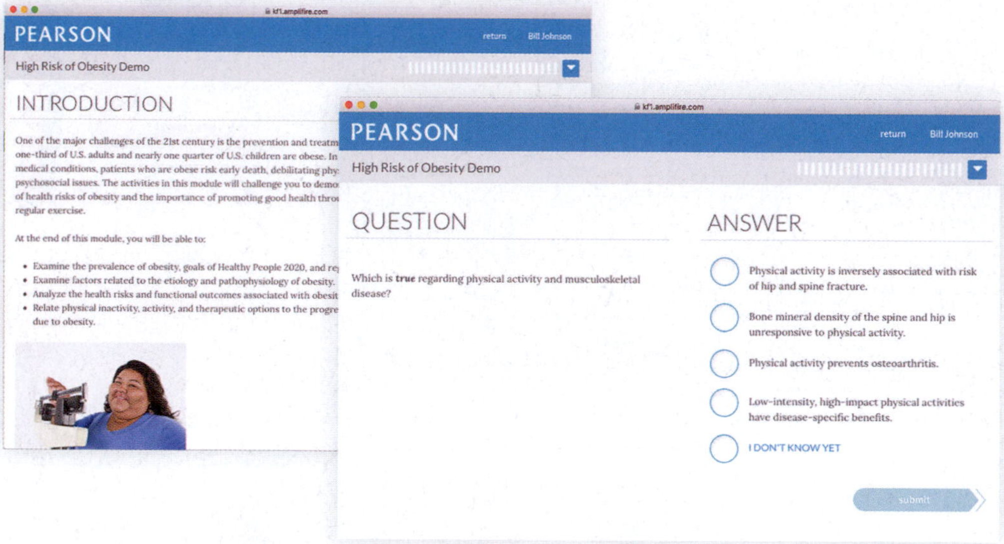

PEARSON
return
Bill Johnson
High Risk of Obesity Demo
INTRODUCTION
PEARSON
return
Bill Johnson
High Risk of Obesity Demo
QUESTION
ANSWER
Which is true regarding physical activity and musculoskeletal disease?
Physical activity is inversely associated with risk of hip and spine fracture.
Bone mineral density of the spine and hip is unresponsive to physical activity.
Physical activity prevents osteoarthritis.
Low-intensity, high-impact physical activities have disease-specific benefits.
I DON'T KNOW YET

NCLEX-Style Questions

Practice tests with more than 1000 NCLEX-style questions of various types build student confidence and prepare them for success on the NCLEX-RN exam. Questions are organized by chapter.

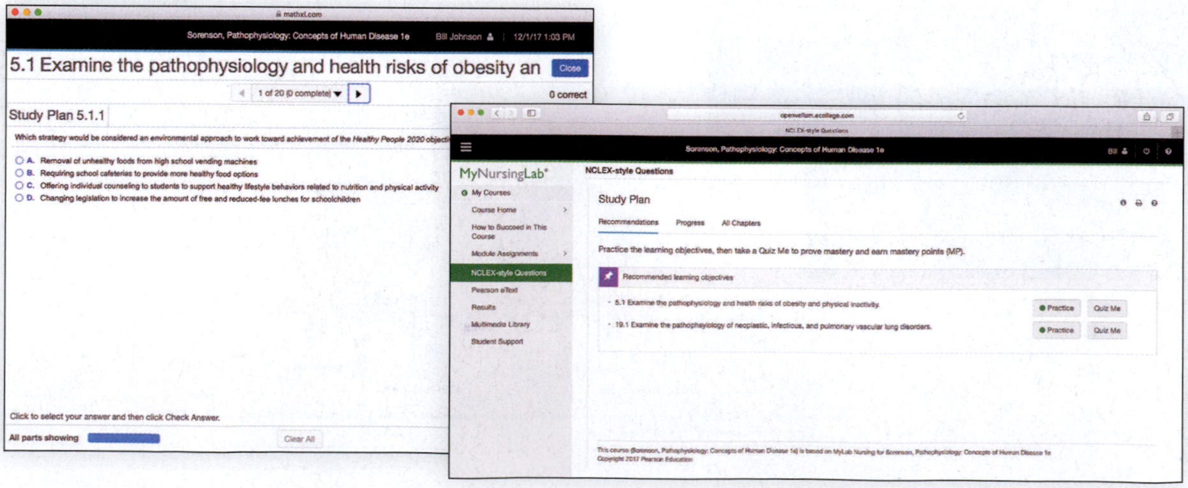

5.1 Examine the pathophysiology and health risks of obesity an
Close
Study Plan 5.1.1
0 correct
MyNursingLab
NCLEX-style Questions
Study Plan

Decision Making Cases

Clinical case studies that provide opportunities for students to practice analyzing information and making important decisions at key moments in patient care scenarios. These 15 unfolding case studies are designed to help prepare students for clinical practice.

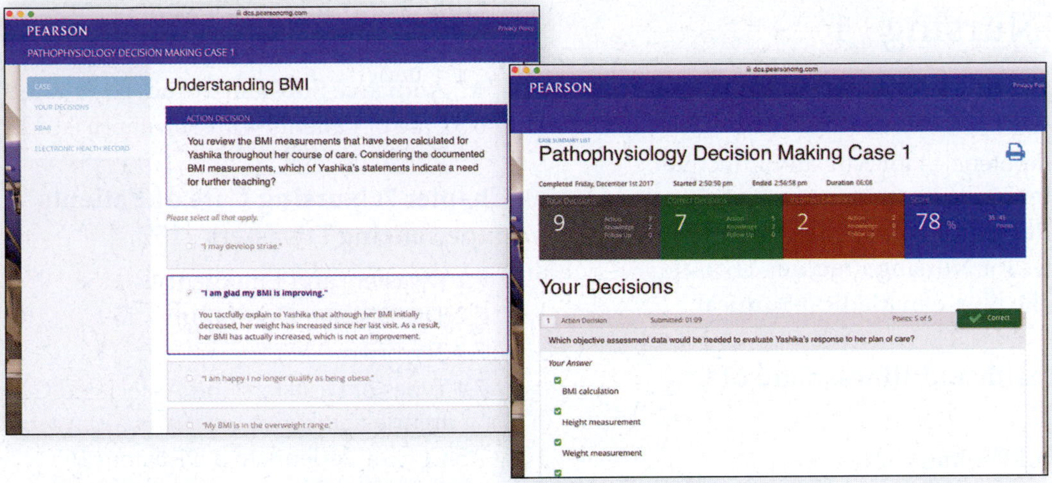
PEARSON
PATHOPHYSIOLOGY DECISION MAKING CASE 1
Understanding BMI
You review the BMI measurements that have been calculated for Yashika throughout her course of care. Considering the documented BMI measurements, which of Yashika's statements indicate a need for further teaching?
"I am glad my BMI is improving."
PEARSON
Pathophysiology Decision Making Case 1
9
7
2
78 %
Your Decisions
Which objective assessment data would be needed to evaluate Yashika's response to her plan of care?
BMI calculation
Height measurement
Weight measurement

Pearson eText

The eText enhances student learning both in and outside the classroom. Students can take notes, highlight, and bookmark important content, or engage with interactive and rich media to achieve greater conceptual understanding of the text content. Interactive features include audio clips, pop-up definitions, figures, questions and answers, the nursing process, hotspots, and video animations. Some examples of video animations include:

- **Congenital Heart Defect Animations** illustrate the many congenital heart defects that may occur in newborns and provide students the opportunity to see, hear, and understand how congenital heart defects impair the correct functioning of the heart and how they may be corrected.

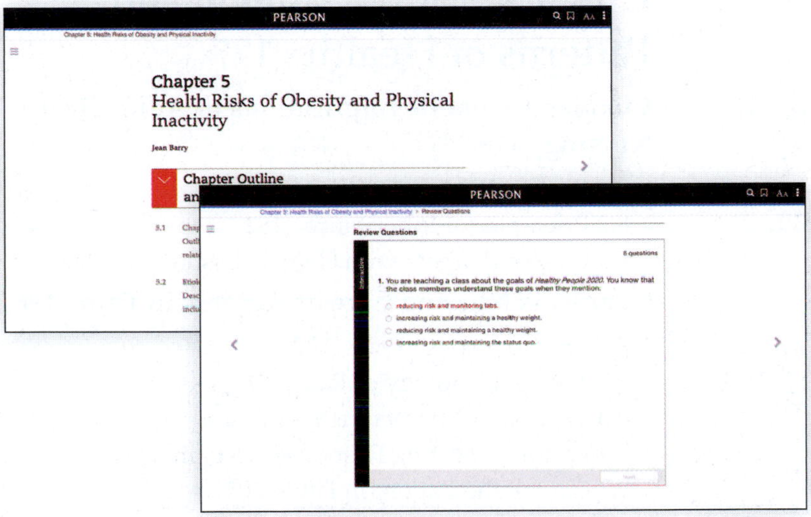
PEARSON
Chapter 5
Health Risks of Obesity and Physical Inactivity
Jean Barry
Chapter Outline
PEARSON
Review Questions

Instructor Resources

Instructor Resource Manual
Lecture Note PowerPoints
Test Bank

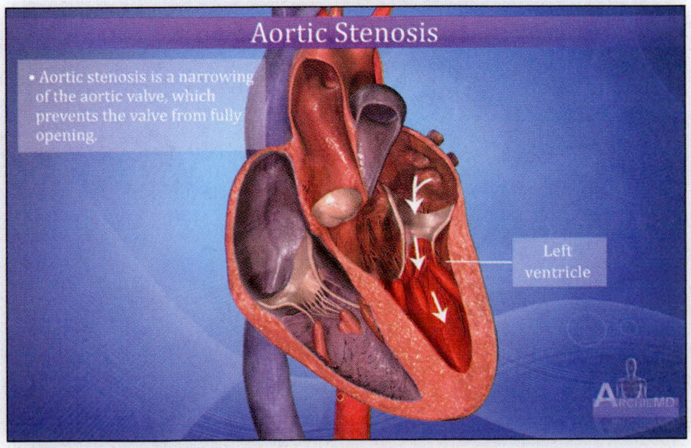
Aortic Stenosis
• Aortic stenosis is a narrowing of the aortic valve, which prevents the valve from fully opening.
Left ventricle

Contents

Unit

1

Dimensions of Medical-Surgical Nursing

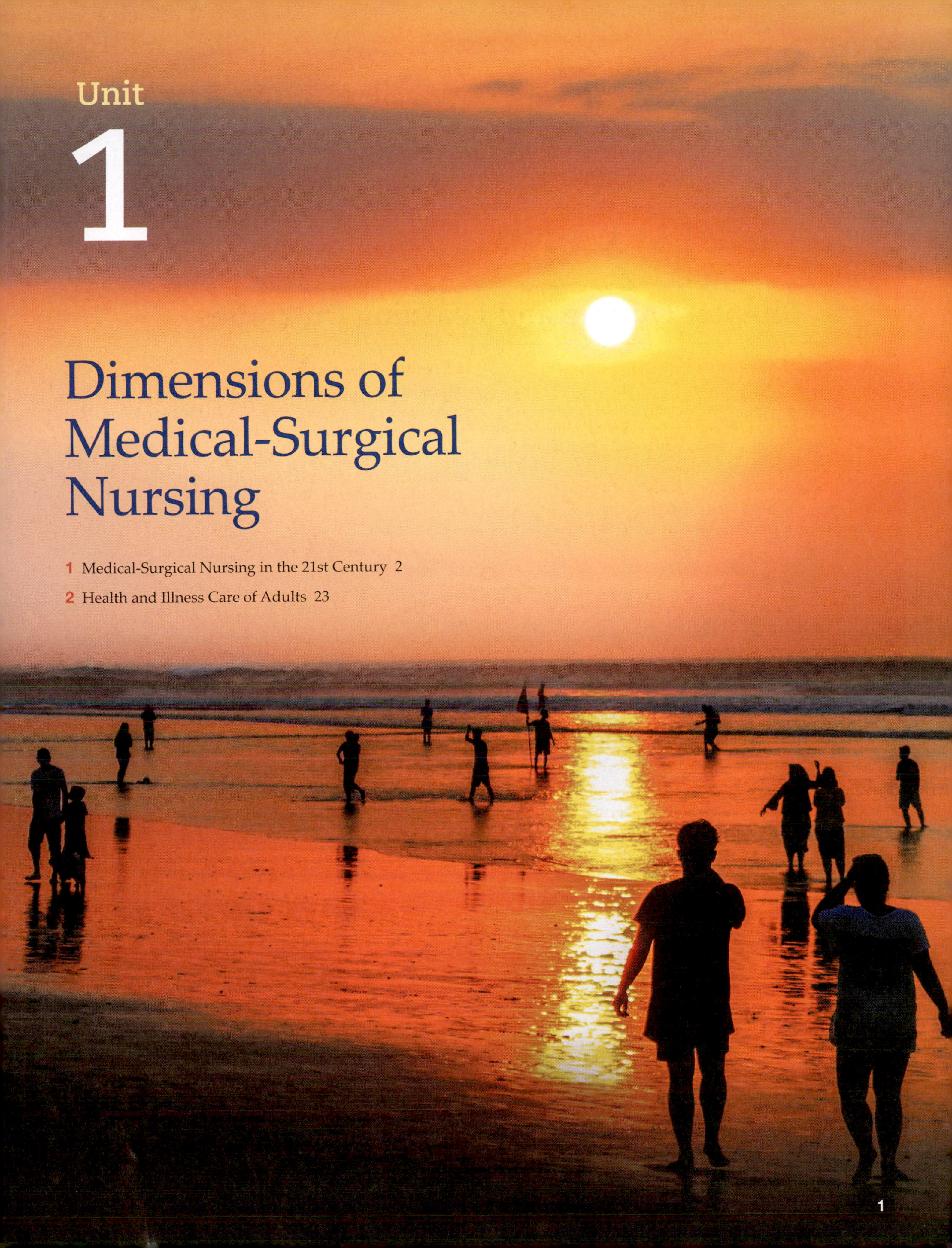

Chapter 1

Medical-Surgical Nursing in the 21st Century

Chapter Outline and Learning Outcomes

1.1 Core Competencies for Safe and Effective Healthcare 4

Describe the core competencies for healthcare professionals: Patient-centered care, interprofessional teams, evidence-based practice, quality improvement, safety, and health information technology.

1.2 Clinical Reasoning in the Nursing Process 4

Apply the attitudes, mental habits, and skills necessary for clinical reasoning when using the nursing process in patient care.

1.3 Guidelines for Nursing Practice 11

Explain the importance of nursing and interprofessional codes of ethics, standards of practice, and legal and ethical issues as guidelines for clinical nursing practice.

1.4 Roles of the Nurse in Medical-Surgical Practice 14

Explain the activities and characteristics of the nurse as caregiver, educator, advocate, leader and manager, and researcher.

CLINICAL COMPETENCIES

- Demonstrate clinical reasoning and apply critical thinking skills when using the nursing process to provide knowledgeable, safe, and patient-centered care.
- Use health systems technology to provide evidence-based, patient-centered care in all healthcare delivery settings.
- Provide clinical care that integrates the medical-surgical nursing roles of caregiver, educator, advocate, leader/manager, and researcher.
- Contribute nursing knowledge and expertise as a member of the interprofessional team to provide safe, quality, and affordable patient-centered care.

KEY TERMS

accountable care organization (ACA), 16
applicability, 18
appraisal, 18
care bundle, 9
clinical reasoning, 4
code of ethics, 11
core competencies, 4
delegation, 16
dilemma, 13
ethics, 11
evidence-based practice (EBP), 8
health literacy, 14
Health information technology (HIT), 17
interprofessional care, 9
medical-surgical nursing, 3
nursing process, 6
patient, 3
patient-centered medical home (PCMH), 16
Patient Protection and Affordable Care Act (ACA), 2
professional boundaries, 13
reliability, 18
standard, 12
Triple Aim, 4
validity, 18

As a new era of healthcare emerges in the 21st century, nursing must embrace the knowledge, skills, and values that define the profession while simultaneously developing roles and ideals based on emerging science, changes in the health concerns of populations, and emerging healthcare delivery models. The **Patient Protection and Affordable Care Act (ACA)**, enacted in 2010, created new expectations and responsibilities for nurses in all healthcare settings. The ACA was designed to provide access to healthcare services for more Americans and create new models of care. Despite controversy and multiple attempts to repeal, the ACA remains as the law governing health in the near future (National Council of State Boards of Nursing, 2018). The three main goals of the ACA were to improve access of healthcare for patients, elevate the quality of care, and reduce healthcare expenditures (Collins & Saylor, 2018). The original intent of the ACA continues to influence healthcare policy and reimbursement, and it is changing provider practice and the environment. The nursing profession is well positioned to respond to demands of a transitioning healthcare system that emphasize health promotion/disease prevention, management of chronic disease, complex acute care, and care coordination during transitions between care settings. As the acuity of hospitalized patients and the prevalence of chronic illness continue to increase, nurses must possess a vast array of knowledge; cognitive, communicative, and technical skills; and well-developed ethical comportment (National Council State Boards of Nursing 2018) (**Figure 1.1** ■).

Nursing, as defined by the American Nurses Association (ANA; 2015), "is the protection, promotion, and optimization of health and abilities, prevention of illness and injury, alleviation of suffering through the diagnosis and treatment of human response, and advocacy in the care of individuals, families, communities, and populations." **Medical-surgical nursing** is the health promotion, healthcare, and illness care of adults based on knowledge derived from the arts and sciences and shaped by knowledge (the science) of nursing. The adult **patient**—the person with whom and for whom nursing care is designed and implemented—ranges in age from the late teens to the early 100s. Medical-surgical nursing focuses on the adult patient's response to actual or potential alterations in health. Medical-surgical nurses must be knowledgeable about all body systems, the disorders that affect them, and the interrelatedness of body systems and health problems. Medical-surgical nurses need to be strong communicators who are able to effectively interact with other members of the healthcare team, patients, and their families (**Figure 1.2** ■). Medical-surgical nurses coordinate patient care during transitions between care settings and provide health education and coaching to promote healing and optimal function. Delegation to and management and supervision of nursing assistive personnel is an ever-increasing component of effective medical-surgical nursing care. Medical-surgical nurses need to be able to apply evidence-based practice, clinical reasoning skills, and nursing care standards to safely perform complex nursing care skills and tasks. Medical-surgical nurses provide individualized quality care while using

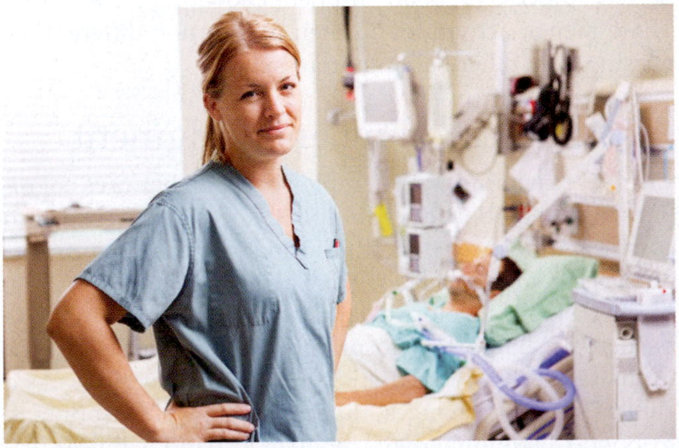

Figure 1.1 ■ Critical care nursing in an intensive care unit requires care of high-acuity patients.

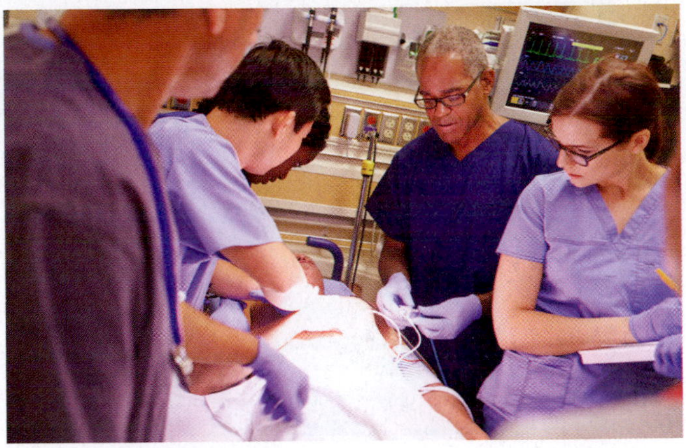

Figure 1.2 ■ In emergency departments, nurses function as members of a tight-knit, well-coordinated team to save the lives of patients.

resources responsibly with a goal of achieving optimal patient outcomes.

The wide range of ages and the variety of healthcare needs specific to individual patients make medical-surgical nursing an ever-changing and challenging area of nursing practice. The medical-surgical nurse must recognize that individual patients are part of families and live in communities. In some instances, nursing care is directed toward the family (for example, supporting the family of a dying individual) or even the community (for example, immunizing people to prevent an outbreak of hepatitis A).

In this textbook discussions of the human responses are structured within the framework of clinical reasoning and the nursing process. Nursing care is presented within the context of nursing problems or diagnoses, emphasizing the importance of developing individualized, evidence-based plans of care. The quality and safety implications for nursing care are addressed. Throughout the text, nursing care planning is based on a philosophy that individuals, their families, and communities are active participants in health and illness as well as consumers of healthcare services.

Nursing care is structured by the activities planned and carried out through clinical reasoning. Nurses use multiple thinking strategies when applying clinical reasoning to the nursing process. Care of the medical-surgical patient is based on ethics and standards established by nursing organizations and is focused on promoting or returning the patient to a state of functional health or providing palliative care at the end of life (**Figure 1.3** ■). No matter the type of healthcare service or setting, medical-surgical nurses must use their knowledge and skills to provide competent and safe patient care. The ability to effectively prioritize activities and patient care needs is critical. This chapter provides a broad overview of the clinical practice of medical-surgical nursing, including core competencies, a framework and guidelines for care delivery, and the roles of the nurse in medical-surgical care.

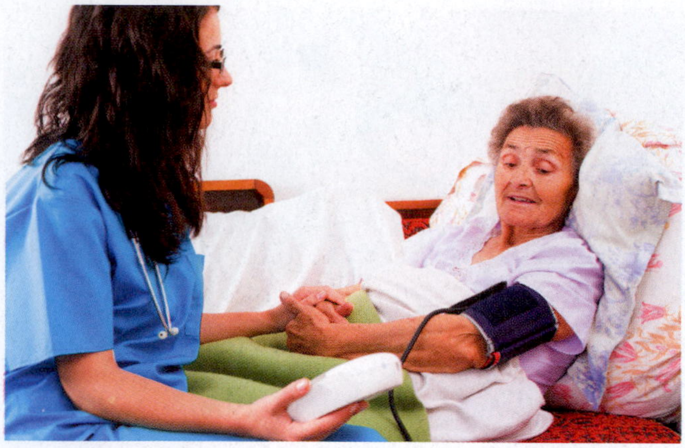

Figure 1.3 ■ This nurse on a palliative care team visits a patient in her home.

1.1 Core Competencies for Safe and Effective Healthcare

The healthcare system in the United States faces numerous challenges, including an increasingly older patient population, an increase in the prevalence of chronic illness, changing consumer desires and expectations, rapidly expanding information and technologies, and a focus on improving quality and safety of care (**Figure 1.4** ■). After examining a number of studies about these challenges, the Institute of Medicine (IOM; 2001) found that, although misuse of services and injuries resulting from errors are becoming more common, safety and quality problems exist largely because of problems within the system and not through the fault of highly dedicated healthcare professionals. The Institute of Health Improvement (IHI) launched the **Triple Aim** initiative in 2007 (Berwick, Nolan, & Whittington, 2008). The IHI posits that focusing on three critical objectives simultaneously will result in better models for providing healthcare. The three objectives are:

1. Improve the patient care experience (including quality and satisfaction).
2. Improve the health of populations.
3. Reduce the per capita costs of healthcare.

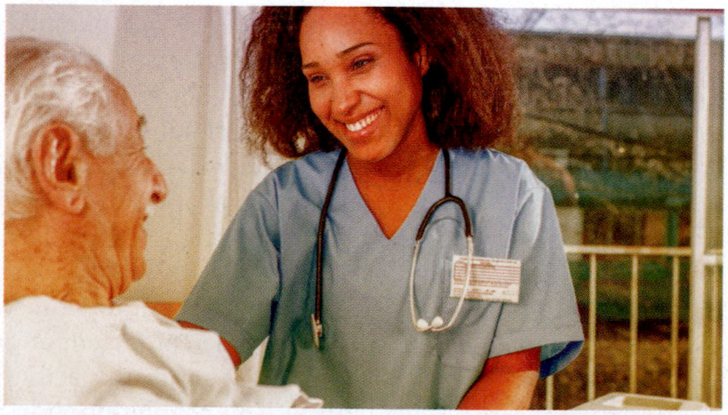

Figure 1.4 ■ In the United States, the population is growing older. In 2010, the U.S. population over age 65 was about 40 million. By 2030, the projected population of older adults will be over 70 million.

In 2003 the National Academy of Sciences proposed a set of five **core competencies** that all healthcare professionals should possess, regardless of their discipline, to meet the needs of the 21st-century health system. In 2011 major health professions organizations united to form the Interprofessional Education Collaborative (IPEC). It further refined the IOM core competencies and developed strategies for achieving them (Interprofessional Education Collaborative Expert Panel, 2011). The competencies are based on using communication, knowledge, technical skills, clinical reasoning, critical thinking, and values in clinical practice. The Quality and Safety Education for Nurses (QSEN) initiative (Cronenwett et al., 2007) focused on developing specific IOM competencies for nursing, with a major goal of providing nurses with the necessary knowledge, skills, and attitudes to continuously improve the quality and safety of care in healthcare systems (Stalter & Mota, 2018). The six QSEN competencies—patient-centered care, teamwork and collaboration, evidence-based practice (EBP), quality improvement, safety, and informatics—provide recommended competencies defining the knowledge, skills, and attitudes that all nurses should demonstrate for safe practice (Stalter & Mota, 2018). The definitions for each QSEN competency are provided in **Table 1.1**.

1.2 Clinical Reasoning in The Nursing Process

As nurses care for patients, they use clinical reasoning and judgment and multiple ways of thinking including critical thinking, analytical reasoning, creative thinking, and the nursing process (Benner, Sutphen, Leonard, & Day, 2010). These mental activities and their application differentiate nursing from other helping professions.

Clinical Reasoning and Judgment

Clinical reasoning is a "complex process that uses cognition, metacognition, and discipline-specific knowledge to gather and analyze patient information, evaluate its significance, and weigh alternative actions" (Simmons, 2010, p. 1151). Well-developed clinical reasoning abilities are particularly important to promote quality and safe care in the face of ill-defined and ambiguous situations. As a clinical situation changes, nurses use clinical reasoning to respond to the immediate problem at hand. Clinical reasoning involves complex and multiple cognitive processes, which integrates the unique context of a clinical situation

Table 1.1 Definition of QSEN Competencies

Competency	Definition
Patient-centered care	■ The nurse will recognize the patient as the source of control in the nurse-patient relationship and will provide compassionate and coordinated care based on respect for the patient's preferences, values, culture, and needs.
Teamwork and collaboration	■ The nurse will function within nursing teams and interprofessional teams with open communication and mutual respect, sharing decision making to achieve quality patient care.
Evidence-based practice (EBP)	■ The nurse will integrate current best evidence with clinical expertise to deliver optimal healthcare that is based on patient and family preferences.
Quality improvement (QI)	■ The nurse will use data to monitor the outcomes of care and continuously design and test changes to improve the quality and safety of healthcare systems.
Safety	■ The nurse will minimize risk of harm to patients, providers, and the interprofessional team through individual performance and by optimizing system effectiveness.
Informatics	■ The nurse will use information and technology to improve communication, manage knowledge, mitigate errors, and support decision making to achieve quality patient care.

Sources: Cronenwett et al., 2007; QSEN Institute, retrieved from http://qsen.org/competencies/pre-licensure-ksas.

Table 1.2 Foundational Knowledge Used in Clinical Reasoning

Foundational Sources of Knowledge	Definition
Knowing the profession	Knowledge of standards of practice, scope of practice, competencies, skills, and roles of nurses Application of the professions' values and ethics
Knowing self	Knowledge of one's own strengths, limitations, skills, experience, assumptions, preconceptions, learning, and other needs
Knowing the case	Knowledge of pathophysiology, patterns that exist in typical cases, evidence-based practices relevant to appropriate patient population, predicted trajectory, and predictable patient responses
Knowing the patient	Knowledge of a patient's baseline data, patterns that exist in laboratory or other data, and patterns in physiologic responses to pathology and treatment
Knowing the person	Knowledge of a patient's past experience in relation to health and illness, supports and resources, treatment preferences, and knowledge of the patient in the context of family and community

Source: Gillespie, M., & Patterson, B. (2009). Helping novice nurses make effective clinical decisions: The situated clinical decision-making framework. Nursing Education Perspectives, 30(3), 164–170. https://journals.lww.com/neponline/Abstract/2009/05000/Helping_Novice_Nurses_Make_Effective_Clinical.7.aspx

and addresses individual concerns of the patient and family (Benner et al., 2010). Clinical judgment is the outcome of the clinical reasoning process and is defined as " . . . an interpretation or conclusion about a patient's needs, concerns or health problems and/or the decision to take action (or not), and to use or modify standard approaches, or to improvise new ones as deemed appropriate by the patient's response" (Tanner, 2006, p. 204). Information and knowledge used in clinical reasoning and judgments are derived from knowing the patient as an individual; grasping baseline data; understanding the case; knowing one's self by assessing one's own assumptions, preconceptions, and biases (e.g., critical thinking skills); and knowing the professional standards of practices (Gillespie & Patterson, 2009). **Table 1.2** defines these foundational sources of knowledge that nurses use in the clinical reasoning process.

The experienced nurse uses numerous sources of knowledge and multiple reasoning strategies simultaneously when addressing a clinical or patient care problem. Student and novice nurses typically rely on fewer patient cues, limited sources of knowledge, and one or two reasoning processes to understand a particular patient problem and to decipher potential solutions (Simmons, 2010). As the nurse gains experience, research indicates nurses use heuristics (informal thinking strategies or cognitive shortcuts) to interpret complex clinical situations. Additionally, expert nurses rely heavily on reflecting-on-action as an aspect of clinical judgment as they create a repertoire of skillful judgment developed through the process of reflecting on paradigm cases (Boyer, Tardif, & Lefebvre, 2016; Tanner, 2006). Clinical reasoning is an iterative process using various sources of knowledge, multiple reasoning processes, and metacognition.

As you practice clinical reasoning, you will use:

- Knowledge gained through classroom studies, textbooks, and current resources and by interacting with experienced nurses.
- Experience gained by working with patients experiencing similar problems or disorders. Taking time to reflect on each patient encounter will help you develop clinical reasoning and judgment skills.
- An understanding of the patient as an individual, who presents with both current and previous illness experiences. Knowing your patient will help you notice what is salient to each individual patient and understand the situation holistically.

- Personal values and beliefs, including recognition of prejudices that may influence thinking (e.g., believing that all homeless people are dirty or that older adults cannot learn to care for themselves). Your personal values influence what you notice as salient issues for individual patients. Being aware of your biases will help you analyze situations objectively.
- An ability to identify possible options, evaluate the alternatives, and reach a conclusion.

It takes practice to make clinical reasoning an integral component of a nurse's ability to address complex and ill-defined situations. The beginning nurse uses a deliberate process of assessing, considering possible alternative causes and action options, and choosing the most appropriate of the alternatives considered. With knowledge and experience, the nurse recognizes expected patterns of response, deviations from the expected, and the probable meaning of the deviation. Clinical reasoning gradually becomes more internalized; the nurse begins thinking like a nurse. Thinking critically and creatively involves more than just cognitive (knowledge) skills. It is strongly influenced by one's attitudes and mental habits. To engage in sound clinical reasoning, you must be aware of your attitudes and how they affect your thinking (refer to **Table 1.2**). Case studies and questions designed to prompt critical reflection are included throughout this book to provide practice in clinical reasoning.

The Nursing Process

The **nursing process** is application of the scientific clinical reasoning nurses use as they provide care to patients (National Council of State Boards of Nursing [NCSBN], 2014). As nurses gain increasing autonomy in their practice, the nursing process helps them identify their independent practice domain. The nursing process provides a common reference system and a common terminology to serve as a base for improving clinical practice through research. In addition, the nursing process can serve as a framework for the evaluation of quality care.

The nursing process can be used in any setting. The purpose of care may be to promote wellness, maintain or restore health, or provide comfort and facilitate coping with disability or death. Regardless of the purpose of care, the planned process of nursing allows for the inclusion of specific, individualized, and holistic activities.

The nursing process also benefits the patient receiving care and the agency or institution providing that care. The patient receives planned, individualized interventions; participates in all steps of the process; and is assured continuity of care through the written care plan. The nursing process benefits the healthcare institution through better resource utilization, increased patient satisfaction, and improved documentation of care.

The five phases of the nursing process are assessment, diagnosis, planning, implementation, and evaluation. These phases are interrelated and interdependent. They are often used cyclically, with the patient central to all phases, as illustrated in **Figure 1.5** ■. Many state nursing practice acts and the national licensing examination are structured on a nursing model of care based on the nursing process (NCSBN, 2014).

This text assumes that the student already has a basic understanding of the nursing process and is now ready to expand and apply that knowledge to adult patients with medical-surgical health problems. The following discussion is intended to serve only as a review; for more information, consult books specifically focused on the use of the nursing process, and read the case studies in the nursing care chapters throughout this textbook.

Assessment

Assessment is a critical element in each phase of the nursing process. It begins with the patient's first encounter with the healthcare system and continues as long as the patient requires care. During assessment, data (pieces of information) about the patient's health status are collected, validated, organized, clustered into patterns, and communicated either verbally or in written form. Assessment serves as the basis for identifying nursing problems and/or deriving accurate nursing diagnoses, for planning and implementing both initial and ongoing individualized care, and for evaluating care.

The nurse collects holistic assessment data, considering all dimensions of the patient. The data collected are both objective and subjective. Information that the nurse perceives by the senses is *objective data*; it is seen, heard, touched, or smelled and can be verified by another person (e.g., blood pressure, temperature, pulse, or the presence of infected drainage). Information that is perceived only by the person experiencing it (e.g., pain, dizziness, anxiety) is *subjective data*.

Nurses conduct both initial and ongoing assessments. The initial assessment, conducted through a nursing history and physical assessment, is obtained to provide a comprehensive picture of the patient's health status. The initial assessment is sometimes referred to as the baseline assessment and is necessary to provide comprehensive data about the individual's health responses, identify specific factors that contribute to these responses, and facilitate mutually established goals and outcomes of care.

Focused assessments are ongoing and continuous, occurring whenever the nurse interacts with the patient. In a focused assessment, data are gathered about an identified or potential problem and then used to evaluate nursing actions and make decisions about whether to continue or change interventions to meet outcomes. Assessments provide structure for documenting nursing care. Focused assessments enable the nurse to identify responses to a disease process or treatment modality not present during the initial assessment and to identify new problems and concerns. Focused assessments are linked to clinical reasoning as the nurse attends to collecting and analyzing data related to the patient's immediate and salient health concerns.

To make accurate and holistic assessments, nurses must have and use a wide variety of knowledge and skills.

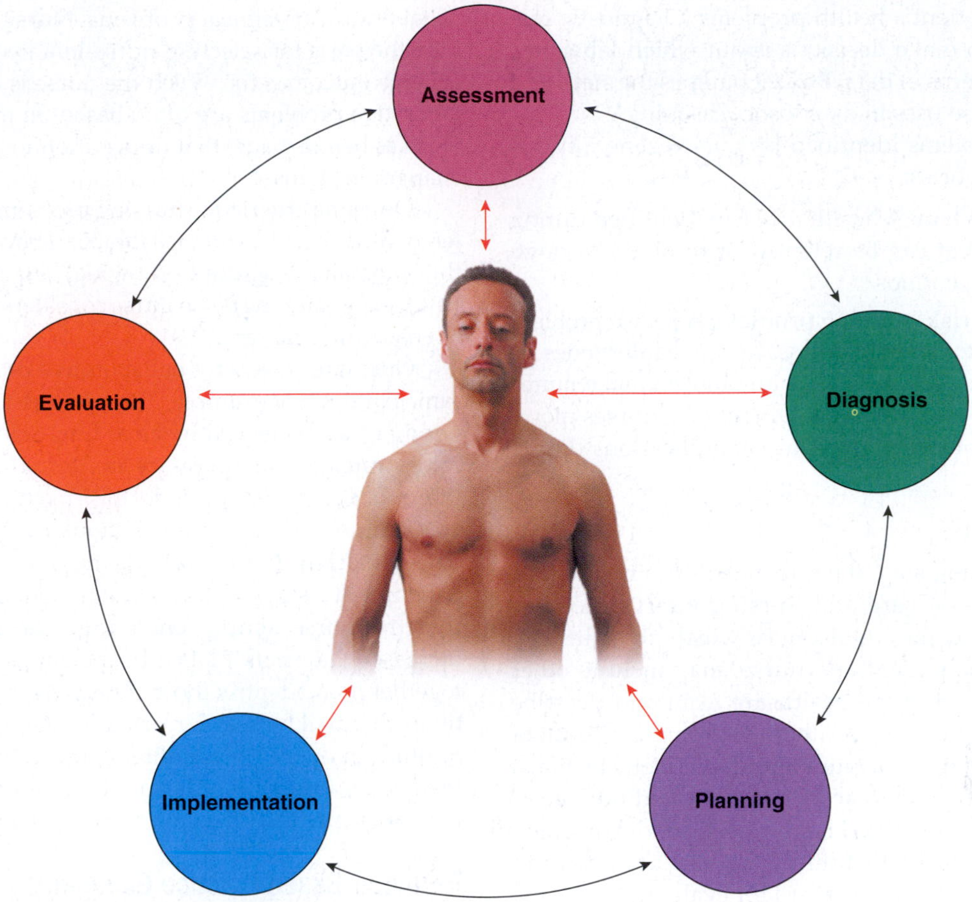
Assessment
Evaluation
Diagnosis
Implementation
Planning

Figure 1.5 ■ Steps of the nursing process. Notice that the steps are interrelated and interdependent. For example, evaluation of the patient might reveal the need for further assessment, additional nursing diagnoses, and/or a revision of the plan of care.

The ability to assess the physical status of the patient is essential, as is the ability to communicate effectively. Nurses must know and understand pathophysiology and pharmacology and be able to identify abnormal laboratory and diagnostic test data. Finally, nurses need a solid foundation of nursing knowledge and skill to interpret assessment data and to use that interpretation as the basis for individualized care.

Nurses use a number of clinical reasoning skills when assessing. An attitude of inquiry is used during data gathering. The nurse must distinguish relevant data from those that are irrelevant, as well as important data from unimportant data. In addition, the nurse identifies missing data and seeks additional information to fill in gaps (Wilkinson & Barcus, 2017).

Diagnosis

The term *diagnosis* (the act of identifying a disease, illness, or problem) is used in both medicine and nursing. The nursing process uses the term *diagnosis* for the step where a patient's problems are described. Many agencies use the term *nursing problem* to describe the problem identified in the assessment phase of the nursing process. Some agencies label this phase of the nursing process *nursing diagnosis* and use terminology approved by the International Nursing Knowledge Association (2018). With the increasing emphasis on interprofessional and patient-centered care, the practice of identifying health concerns by using brief problem statements is increasing because this approach provides a unified language that is recognized by multiple health disciplines and more understandable to patients than nursing diagnosis nomenclature. We use problem statements in this text to identify common nursing concerns related to health problems.

The nurse analyzes assessment data to support appropriate nursing problem statements and diagnoses. During analysis, the nurse organizes or categorizes data so that it can be used to identify actual or potential health problems. Data can be organized within a variety of frameworks. Methods commonly used are basic human needs (Maslow, 1970), body systems, human response patterns, and functional health patterns (Gordon, 1994). Gordon's (1994) functional health patterns are used in many healthcare systems to help nurses organize data and care. Identifying health concerns or needs and delineating a problem statement or making a diagnosis is a complex process that always involves uncertainty. Therefore, the nurse uses diagnostic reasoning to choose a problem statement that best defines the individual patient's health problems. Diagnostic reasoning is used to make decisions about which label best describes the patterns of data. **Box 1.1** outlines the steps and processes the nurse uses in diagnostic reasoning.

Nursing problems identified by nurses generally fall within three categories:

1. **Nursing problem:** A health problem identified during assessment that can be relieved or resolved through nursing interventions
2. **Potential (or risk) nursing problem:** A health problem that is likely to develop unless the nurse intervenes
3. **Collaborative problems:** A health problem that requires both medical and nursing interventions; nurses monitor for and intervene to reduce complications (Boyer et al., 2015).

Planning

During the planning step, the nurse identifies the desired patient outcomes of care and nursing interventions to achieve those outcomes. Outcomes, which are mutually established by the patient and nurse, may include other disciplines involved in the healthcare team and describe the expected patient responses that will occur as a result of the nursing interventions. Nursing interventions (actions) are specifically planned to achieve the desired outcomes. Both outcomes and nursing interventions are documented in a written plan of care that directs nursing activities and documentation and provides a tool for evaluation.

Nurses plan interventions for problems that require nursing management (stated as nursing diagnoses) and for collaborative or clinical problems. Nursing diagnoses provide the basis for selecting nurse-initiated interventions to achieve outcomes for which the nurse is accountable. Collaborative problems are often based on medical diagnoses (such as hemorrhage) that nurses monitor to detect onset or changes in status.

Outcome criteria for nursing problems are patient centered, time specific, and measurable. They are classified into three domains: Cognitive (knowing), affective (feeling), and psychomotor (doing). The nurse considers all three domains to ensure holistic care.

Outcome criteria for collaborative problems follow the same pattern. For example, "Respiratory complications will not occur as evidenced by clear lung sounds, pulse, respiratory rate, and temperature in normal range for patient throughout recovery period."

Planned nursing interventions must be specific and individualized. If, for example, the nurse identifies that a patient is at risk for a fluid volume deficit, it is not enough that the nurse simply encourage the patient to drink increased amounts of fluid. The nurse and the patient together must identify those liquids the patient prefers, the times that will be best for drinking them, and the amount of fluid (in ounces or milliliters); this information is documented as a nursing order on the written care plan. Only then does care truly become a part of the plan of care.

Evidence-Based Practice Guidelines

Evidence-based practice (EBP) is defined as the practice of nursing in which the nurse makes clinical decisions on

BOX 1.1
Overview of Diagnostic Reasoning

INTERPRET THE DATA

Level I—Recognize significant cues

1. *Organize data*, differentiating patient's subjective and objective assessment data.
2. *Compare patient's individual data to expected presentation* to identify significant cues.

Level II—Cluster cues and identify data gaps

3. *Cluster significant cues*; look for patterns and connections between clusters.
4. *Identify data gaps, unexpected and ambiguous findings.*

Level III—Draw conclusions about the present health status

5. *Consider explanations for each cue cluster. Identify the hypothesis best explains it.* (*Note:* You can sometimes identify both the problem and etiology in this step.)
6. *Identify problem or desired health outcome* (wellness goal, actual, potential, and possible nursing problem; collaborative problems; and medical problems).
7. *Identify patient and family strengths and challenges.*

Level IV—Determine etiologies and categorize problems

8. *Examine the possible etiologies of the problems.*
9. *Determine if there is a connection between etiologies for each identified problem.*
10. *Categorize problems according to illustrate connections.*

VERIFY THE PROBLEM/DIAGNOSES

11. *Verify the identified problems, strengths, and challenges* with the patient, family, other professionals, and references.

LABEL THE PROBLEM

12. *Choose a problem label.* The appropriate label will be contextual according to the setting and norms of the practice setting. Many use standard problem statements specific to the agency; others use NANDA diagnoses. Develop formal statements describing health status, nursing and wellness problem/diagnoses, and collaborative problems. Use format according to the agency policy.
13. *Prioritize the problems.*

RECORD THE DATA

14. *Record the problem statements* on the appropriate documents: patient care plan, electronic health record or other agency document.

Source: Wilkinson, Judith M., Nursing Process and Critical Thinking, 5th ed., © 2012b. Printed and Electronically reproduced by permission of Pearson Education, Inc., Upper Saddle River, New Jersey.

the basis of the best available current research evidence; his or her own clinical expertise, including internal evidence of patient findings; and the needs and preferences of the patient (Melnyk, Gallagher-Ford, & Fineout-Overholt, 2017). EBP uses careful and diligent decision making, taking into consideration each individual clinical situation.

Whenever possible, planned nursing interventions are based on evidence, that is, nursing research and nursing practice guidelines. The integration of electronic health records includes access to evidence-based nursing practice guidelines at the point of care (Kroning, 2018). Guidelines are collections of practical information used to help guide decisions related to specific circumstances (Caple & Karakashlan, 2017).

Nurses use guidelines to help identify appropriate interventions for a given nursing care problem or diagnosis. Evidence-based nursing care guidelines also show the strength of the evidence used, allowing nurses to evaluate the appropriateness of a given guideline for the individual circumstance. See **Box 1.2** for a brief history of EBP.

Overview of EBP

EBP has described as a problem-solving approach for clinical practice that includes three foundational legs:

1. **External evidence**—where nurses search, appraise, and synthesize the relevant research findings related to their clinical question. External evidence comes from well-designed research studies.
2. **Clinical expertise and internal evidence**—which includes nurses' own clinical expertise incorporating their patient assessments and evaluations as well as internal evidence, which is derived from quality improvement and outcomes evaluations.
3. **Patient preferences and values**—where nurses incorporate the individualization to their specific patient that is a benchmark for quality nursing care. It is the patient experience and circumstances that influence a nurse's choice of nursing intervention (Melnyk et al., 2017).

Evidence-based nursing guidelines are available through specialty nursing organizations, healthcare systems, on the Web, and in published resources and should be used in the care planning process.

Care Bundles

A **care bundle** is defined by the IHI (Institute for Healthcare Improvement, 2018) as a "small set of evidence-based interventions for a defined patient segment/population and care setting that, when implemented together, will result in significantly better outcomes than when implemented individually" (p. 2). Care bundles are **interprofessional care** standards that pull together a short list of interventions and treatments that are already recommended and are generally accepted in national guidelines. Examples of care bundles include the IHI Ventilator Bundle and the IHI Central Line Bundle (Salmond, Echevaria, & Allread, 2017). Care bundles were initially developed to address complex patients in critical care units but are now used in multiple settings (Clancy, 2017). The effectiveness of a bundle is based on the body of evidence behind it and the consistency in which the bundle is implemented (IHI, 2016). The IHI developed guidelines that the intraprofessional team should use when designing care bundles. **Box 1.3** outlines the IHI guidelines.

Implementation

The implementation step is the action or doing phase of the nursing process, during which the nurse carries

BOX 1.2
History and Factors That Promote EBP in Nursing

Nursing practice based on evidence extends back to Florence Nightingale, whose systematic assessment and evaluation of the environment and the impact on outcomes (mortality, etc.) are widely described. EBP is a problem-solving approach to clinical practice questions.

Evidence-based medicine (EBM) has been around for more than a century, but came into the modern medical lexicon in the early 1990s, arising out of Great Britain. Dr. Sackett and colleagues defined the attributes and exceptions to EBM in 1996, cautioning that EBM is not "cookbook medicine," where clinical care is based on general evidence without consideration of the practitioner's expertise or the patient's specific situation and values. Another important early innovator in EBP was Dr. Archie Cochrane, a British medical researcher who promoted the systematic evaluation of evidence to support the highest quality clinical decisions. Dr. Cochrane noted that with the limited resources available to the practitioner, an efficient and effective method was needed to evaluate evidence. The Cochrane Collaboration, named for Dr. Cochrane, is a worldwide network of clinical experts (more than 28,000 persons) who develop, publish, and update reviews of research literature related to specified topics. The Cochrane Collaboration databases are recognized for their high quality related to healthcare effectiveness.

EBP implementation has increased, with a stronger focus on quality of care by policymakers and healthcare reimbursement organizations like the Centers for Medicare and Medicaid Services. The Institute of Medicine (IOM), a part of the National Academy of Science, focuses on developing and recommending policies related to the health of the U.S. population. In 2007, the IOM set the goal that by 2020, 90% of all healthcare decisions will be based on evidence (IOM, 2007; Melnyk et al., 2017). Supporting the movement toward EBP, the ANA has included evidence-based practice and research as the ninth standard in the ANA's *Nursing Scope and Standards of Practice* (2016).

The use of EBP in nursing is imperative because it can help to (1) promote the best patient outcomes, (2) reduce costs, (3) reduce care variations due to geographic location, and (4) encourage healthcare worker retention.

Moving Evidence into Action

Impact of Integrated Electronic Health Records on Quality of Nursing Care and EBP

Clinical Issue

The adaptation of electronic health records (EHR) is becoming a standard for care across health settings and by all healthcare professionals. With successful adaptation, the use of EHR improves quality, safety, and efficiency, leading to improved health outcomes. EHR also provides decision support for national high-priority conditions such as sepsis and provides a means for communicating information needed for the care coordination process. Personal EHR can be accessed by patients, thereby promoting more engagement in care and providing access to self-management tools. EHR is becoming an integral part of patient care and is here to stay. However, incorporating EHR into nursing practice has been challenging. Nurses cite a multitude of perceptions related to using EHR indicating the process required to use a computer takes time away from patient care and depersonalizes the medical record, as the system can prohibit documentation of the patients' unique assessment information and response to nursing interventions (Kroning, 2018). Three in every four U.S. hospitals have an EHR system in place (Kroning, 2018).

External Evidence

A retrospective analysis was conducted in a large hospital with 10 medical surgical units and two critical care units to determine the effectiveness of incorporating electronic, evidence-based practice tools into the bedside nurse's workflow. The study explored the impact of adopting an integrated EHR system on the quality of nursing care, cost, and nurse turnover. A retrospective study examined quality nursing care outcomes (patient falls, select hospital-acquired infections, hospital-acquired pressure ulcer rate, ventilator-associated pneumonia) before and after the implementation of EHR (Walker-Czyz, 2016). The results of the study indicated incorporating EBP tools through EHR promotes decision making at the point of care and improves quality of care. However, cost indicators were negatively impacted during implementation. Nurse turnover increased and did not return to baseline (Walker-Czyz, 2016).

Internal Evidence

Duffy (2015) describes the pros and cons of using EHR and recommends a planned change strategy when implementing the conversion of paper documentation to an EHR. Strategies to facilitate the adaptation of EHR include increasing staffing during training and designing a systematic training program. Monitoring user satisfaction during implementation of EHR can facilitate effective adaptation (Jones & Stockman, 2018). Nurses should be involved in planning the implementation of EHR and participate in developing policies and procedures related to system security, patient privacy, and implications related to nursing workflow.

Patient Considerations

When considering the adaptation of EHR, the focus for implementation should be ensuring the process improves patient care outcomes and ensuring nursing care is not compromised during the transition.

Putting the Pieces Together

The design and implementation of EHR is essential in today's healthcare system. To effectively implement a plan, the external evidence demonstrating projected positive outcomes should be examined and a planned change strategy should be implemented. Patient care outcomes and nurses' satisfaction should be monitored and adjustments made in the EHR to ensure nurse workflow is improved, not hindered.

References

Duffy, M. (2015). Nurses and the migration to electronic health records. *American Journal of Nursing, 115*(12), 61–66.

Jones, N. T., & Stockman, C. (2018). Facilitating adaptation of an electronic documentation system. *Computers, Informatics Nursing, 36*(5), 225–231.

Kroning, M. (2018). 59 clicks in the EHR. *Nursing Management, 49*(5), 10–14.

Walker-Czyz, A. (2016). The impact of an integrated electronic health record adoption on nursing care quality. *Journal of Nursing Administration, 46*(7/8), 366–372.

out planned interventions. In some instances, the nurse assigns and supervises nursing assistive personnel in carrying out planned interventions. Ongoing assessment of the patient before, during, and after the intervention is an essential component of implementation in either case. Although the plan may be appropriate, many variables can modify or negate any planned intervention, making a change in the plan necessary. For example, the nurse would not be able to force fluids if the patient were nauseated or vomiting.

When implementing the planned interventions, the nurse follows several important principles:

- Set daily priorities, based on initial assessments and on the patient's condition as reported during the change of shift report and/or documented in the patient's chart. Ensure that critical assessments (such as status of invasive lines, fluids infusing, or changes in health status during the preceding shift) take first priority.
- Be aware of the interrelated nature of nursing interventions. For example, while giving a bath the nurse can also assess physical and psychologic status, use therapeutic communication, teach the patient, do range-of-motion exercises, and provide skin care.
- Determine the most appropriate interventions for each patient, based on health status and illness treatment. Examples of appropriate interventions include:
    a. Directly perform the activity for the patient.
    b. Assist the patient to perform the activity.
    c. Supervise the patient/family while they are performing the activity.
    d. Assign and supervise nursing assistive personnel to perform the activity.
    e. Teach the patient/family about healthcare.
    f. Monitor the patient at risk for potential complications or problems.

BOX 1.3
IHI Bundle Design Guidelines

- ***The bundle has three to five interventions (elements), with strong clinician agreements.*** The bundles integrate a short list of already recommended guidelines that are accepted nationally or through consensus by local clinicians.
- ***Each bundle is relatively independent.*** The bundle is developed so that if one of the interventions of care is not implemented it will not affect whether other bundle elements are implemented.
- ***The bundle is used with a defined patient population in one location.*** Evidence indicates a bundle is most successful if applied to a particular patient population in a defined location. For example, there are two bundles for patients experiencing sepsis. One bundle applies to managing patients in the emergency department and another for managing patients with sepsis in the critical care environment.
- ***The interprofessional team develops the bundle.*** Communication and teamwork are essential to successful implementation of a bundle.
- ***Bundle elements should be descriptive rather than prescriptive, to allow for local customization and appropriate clinical judgment.*** For instance, the interventions that address prophylactic treatment for deep venous thrombosis in the Ventilator Bundle do not specify the type of prophylaxis.
- ***Compliance with bundles is measured using all-or-nothing measurement, with a goal of 95% or greater.*** If any of the interventions are not documented, implementation of the bundle is considered incomplete and no partial credit is given.

- Use available resources to provide interventions that are realistic for the situation and practical in terms of equipment available, financial status of the patient, and resources available (including staff, agency, family, and community resources).

Documenting interventions is the final component of implementation, and it is a legal requirement. Care can be documented in many different ways. Narrative source-oriented and problem-oriented charting methods are used, as are focused charting, charting by exception, and computer-assisted documentation.

Evaluation

The *evaluation* step allows the nurse to determine whether the plan was effective, as well as determine whether to continue the plan, revise the plan, or terminate the plan. The outcome criteria that were established during the planning step provide the basis for evaluation. Evaluation takes place continuously throughout patient care, as illustrated earlier in Figure 1.5.

To evaluate a plan, the nurse collects data from the patient and the patient's chart. The nurse then compares the status of the patient with the written outcomes. If the outcomes have been accomplished, the nurse may either continue or terminate the plan. If the outcomes have not been accomplished, the nurse must modify the nursing problem/diagnoses, outcomes, or plan.

With experience, the nurse does not consciously stop and consider each step of the nursing process. Rather, using the process as a framework, care is based on the patient's specific, individualized needs. For example, when caring for a patient who is hemorrhaging, the nurse uses all five steps simultaneously to meet critical, life-threatening needs. In contrast, when considering long-term needs for a patient with a chronic illness or disability, the nurse makes in-depth assessments, mutually determines goals with the patient, and documents a written plan of care that is developed and revised as necessary by all nurses providing care. As a nurse becomes an expert practitioner, the nursing process becomes so much a part of the nurse that he or she may not even consciously consider it while providing care; the practice is the process (Benner, 1984).

1.3 Guidelines for Nursing Practice

Nursing practice is structured by codes of ethics and standards that guide nursing practice and protect the public. Individual nursing practice is held to these standards in a court of law. The guidelines are especially important because nurses encounter legal and ethical problems almost daily.

Codes for Nurses

An established **code of ethics** is one criterion that defines a profession. **Ethics** are principles of conduct. Ethical behavior is concerned with moral duty, values, obligations, and the distinction between right and wrong. Codes of ethics for nurses provide a frame of reference for "professionally valued and ideal nursing behaviors that are congruent with the principles expressed in the Code for Nurses" (Ketefian, 1987, p. 13).

The large number of ethical issues facing nurses in clinical practice makes the established codes for nurses critical to moral and ethical decision making. The codes also help to define the roles of nurses. The codes of ethics presented here were developed by and for members of the International Council of Nurses (ICN) and the American Nurses Association (ANA).

The ICN Code

The *ICN Code of Ethics for Nurses* (2012) helps guide nurses in setting priorities, making judgments, and taking action when they face ethical dilemmas in clinical practice. The ICN code specifies what nurses are accountable for in terms of people, practice, society, coworkers, and the profession. The philosophical basis for the ICN code establishes nurses are responsible for promoting health, preventing illness, and alleviating suffering.

The ANA Code

The ANA *Code of Ethics for Nurses* (2015) states principles of ethical concern, guiding the behavior of nurses and also defining nursing for the general public (**Box 1.4**). The ANA *Code of Ethics for Nurses* is a dynamic document that undergoes periodic updating; the most recent update was done using a consensus process. The professional registered nurse is responsible for ensuring that the ANA Code of Ethics is applied in daily practice and guides ethical behavior and comportment.

Standards of Nursing Practice

A **standard** is a statement or criterion that can be used by a profession and by the general public to measure the quality of practice. Established standards of nursing practice make each individual nurse accountable for practice. This means that each nurse providing care has the responsibility or obligation to account for his or her own behaviors within that role. Professional nursing organizations develop and implement standards of practice to identify clearly the nurse's responsibilities to society.

BOX 1.4
The American Nurses Association Code of Ethics for Nurses

1. The nurse practices with compassion and respect for the inherent dignity, worth, and uniqueness of every person.
2. The nurse's primary commitment is to the patient, whether an individual, family, group, community, or population.
3. The nurse promotes, advocates for, and protects the rights, health, and safety of the patient.
4. The nurse has authority, accountability, and responsibility for nursing practice; makes decisions; and takes action consistent with the obligation to promote health and to provide optimal care.
5. The nurse owes the same duties to self as others, including the responsibility to promote health and safety, preserve wholeness of character and integrity, maintain competence, and continue personal and professional growth.
6. The nurse, through individual and collective effort, established, maintains, and improves the ethical environment of the work setting and conditions of employment that are conducive to safe quality health care.
7. The nurse, in all roles and settings, advances the profession through research and scholarly inquiry, professional standards development, and the generation of both nursing and health policy.
8. The nurse collaborates with other health professionals and the public to protect human rights, promote health diplomacy, and reduce health disparities.
9. The profession of nursing, collectively through its professional organizations, must articulate nursing values, maintain integrity of the profession, and integrate principles of social justice into nursing and health policy.

Sources: Data from American Nurses Association, 2015; Lachman, Swanson, & Winland-Brown, 2015; Winland-Brown, Lachman, & Swanson, 2015.

The ANA Standards of Practice (2016) are outlined in **Box 1.5**. These standards allow objective evaluation of nursing licensure and certification, institutional accreditation, quality assurance, and public policy. The Standards of Professional Performance are listed in **Box 1.6**.

Health Information Privacy Rules

Although the right to privacy of health and other personal information is an accepted ethical principle of nurses and other healthcare providers, federal rules also govern what can be shared and with whom. The Health Insurance Portability and Accountability Act and the Standards for Privacy of Individually Identifiable Health Information, commonly referred to together as HIPAA, are designed to protect individuals' health information while allowing such information to be shared as needed for effective care. The rules apply to those who transmit health information electronically—including nurses and others employed in hospitals, clinics, and other settings.

While often misinterpreted, HIPAA rules allow disclosure of health information for treatment purposes, even without the patient's explicit consent. Although the patient's privacy is to be protected, safety protections such as posting the patient's name outside his or her room are allowed to help ensure that care is provided to the correct patient. Unless the patient specifically objects, health information can also be shared with family members who are involved in the patient's care. Other state or federal laws may override the patient's right to privacy of health information, for example, laws that require nurses and other healthcare providers to report evidence of child, older adult, or spousal abuse.

SAFETY ALERT: Posting information on social media about a patient may be viewed as a breach of privacy. You may NOT post pictures, patient names, or even small details that can be connected to a specific patient. Posting information about coworkers can also be

BOX 1.5
Standards of Practice

- ***Assessment:*** The nurse gathers data salient to the patient's health status.
- ***Problem Identification/Diagnosis:*** The nurse analyzes the assessment data to identify the nursing problems/diagnosis.
- ***Outcomes:*** The nurse develops patient-centered outcomes to address identified nursing problems/diagnosis.
- ***Planning:*** The nurse in collaboration with the patient, develops evidence-based interventions designed to achieve expected outcomes.
- ***Implementation:*** The nurse executes all phases of the plan, promotes health, coordinates care with other healthcare providers, facilitates a safe care environment and evaluates progress toward meeting expected outcomes revising the plan a needed.

Source: Based on *Nursing: Scope and Standards of Practice* © 2016 by American Nurses Association.

BOX 1.6
Standards of Professional Performance

- ***Ethics:*** The nurse uses ethical principles to guide all aspects of nursing practice.
- ***Intentional/Life Long Learner:*** The nurse engages in continuous learning to assure current knowledge and skills are used in practice.
- ***Professional Practice:*** The nurses uses professional practice standards, guidelines, regulatory rules and laws to execute and evaluate their own practice as a leader and is a contributor to the maintaining and improving standards of the profession.
- ***Evidence-Based Practice and Research:*** The nurse participates in efforts to improve the quality of nursing practice.
- ***Quality Nursing Practice:*** The nurse applies current evidence and research to plan and provide nursing care.
- ***Communication:*** The nurse uses appropriate communication skills with patients and other healthcare providers.
- ***Collaboration:*** The nurse collaborates with patients, families, healthcare providers and community members when planning, implementing and evaluating nursing care.
- ***Teamwork and Leadership:*** The nurse demonstrates effective teamwork behaviors and provides leadership in patient care situations.
- ***Stewardship:*** The nurses uses appropriate resources to provide nursing care assuring practice is safe, effective, avoids unnecessary waste and is fiscally responsible.
- ***Environment:*** The nurse advocates for care environments that are safe and healthy using renewable resources whenever possible.

Source: Based on *Nursing: Scope and Standards of Practice* © 2016 by American Nurses Association.

damaging. Keep current of agency policy, state laws, and your nurse practice act, as violation of regulations related to patient information or even organizational information can be grounds for discipline or dismissal (Mayan, 2018). ■

Professional Boundaries

Nurses are expected to act in the best interests of the patient. They must avoid use of their position for personal gain and not become involved in the patient's personal relationships. **Professional boundaries** are the borders between the vulnerability of the patient and the power of the nurse. The nurse as care provider and keeper of private information about the patient places the nurse in a position of power. It is vital that nurses recognize this relationship and establish boundaries to safely and effectively meet the patient's needs. Confusion between the needs of the nurse and those of the patient can result in boundary violations (NCSBN, 2014). It is the nurse's responsibility to establish and maintain professional boundaries, providing an appropriate level of involvement for effective care.

Legal and Ethical Issues in Nursing

A **dilemma** is a choice between two unpleasant, ethically troubling alternatives. Nurses who provide medical-surgical nursing care face dilemmas almost daily. Many commonly experienced dilemmas involve confidentiality, patient rights, and issues of dying and death. The nurse must use ethical and legal guidelines to make decisions about moral actions when providing care in these and in many other situations.

Nurses respect the right to confidentiality of patient information found in the patient's record or secured during interviews. However, an individual's right to privacy and confidentiality creates a dilemma when it conflicts with the nurse's right to information that may affect personal safety. The law in most states mandates that HIV test results can be given to another person only with the patient's written consent. Many healthcare providers believe that this law violates their own right to personal safety.

The right to refuse treatment (including surgery, medication, medical therapy, and nourishment) also raises nursing dilemmas (**Figure 1.6** ■). The situation, the alternatives, and the potential harm from refusal must be carefully explained. The nurse is faced with the dilemma of respecting the patient's autonomy or following the ethical principle of beneficence, doing what is best for the patient.

Issues surrounding dying and death have become increasingly pressing as advances in technology extend the lives of people with chronic, debilitating illness and major trauma. These changes have altered concepts of living and dying, resulting in ethical conflicts regarding quality of life and death with dignity versus technologic methods of preserving life in any form.

Even if the patient is competent and requests that no heroic measures be used to maintain life, many questions arise in nursing care. What constitutes a heroic measure?

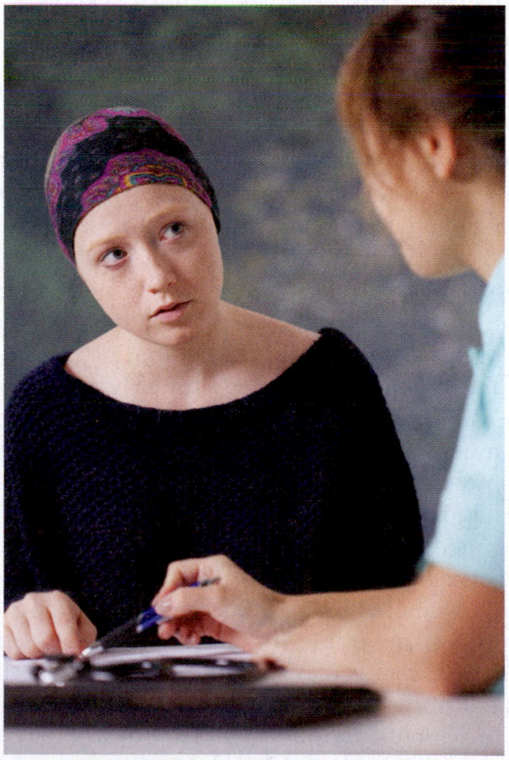

Figure 1.6 ■ One important nursing task is educating patients about upcoming procedures and obtaining their informed consent to proceed.

Should nursing interventions to provide comfort include administering narcotics at a level known to depress respirations? These and other questions are being debated not only within the healthcare system but also in the courts.

1.4 Roles of The Nurse in Medical-Surgical Practice

Healthcare today is embedded in a vast and complex system. It reflects changes in society, changes in the populations requiring nursing care, changes in reimbursement, and an emphasis on quality and safety and a philosophical shift toward health promotion rather than illness care. The roles of the medical-surgical nurse have broadened and expanded in response to these changes. Medical-surgical nurses are increasingly expected to be caregivers, educators, advocates, leaders and managers, and researchers. The nurse assumes these various roles to promote and maintain health, to prevent illness, and to facilitate coping with disability or death for the adult patient (an individual requiring healthcare services) in any setting.

The Nurse as Caregiver

Nurses have always been caregivers. However, the activities carried out within the caregiver role have changed tremendously in the 21st century. From 1900 to the 1960s, the nurse was regarded primarily as the person who gave personal care and carried out physicians' orders. This dependent role has changed as a result of the increased education of nurses, research in and the development of nursing knowledge, and the recognition that nurses are autonomous and informed professionals.

The caregiver role for the nurse today is both independent and collaborative. Nurses independently make assessments and plan and implement patient care based on nursing knowledge and skills. Nurses also collaborate with other members of the healthcare team to implement and evaluate care (**Figure 1.7** ■).

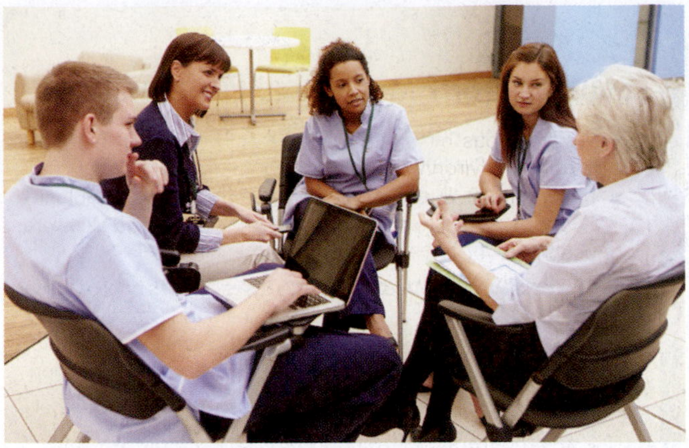

Figure 1.7 ■ Nurses are part of the interprofessional healthcare team that discusses the individualized plan of care and outcomes.

As a caregiver, the nurse practices both the science and the art of nursing. In medical-surgical nursing, the science requires a deep understanding of normal physiology and the pathophysiology underlying disease processes commonly affecting adults. Just as the pediatric nurse must understand the physical and psychosocial development of children, the medical-surgical nurse must understand the physical, psychosocial, economic, and developmental differences among adults spanning from the late teens to older adults who are living into their 80s, 90s, and even 100. Using clinical reasoning in the nursing process as the framework for care, the nurse provides interventions to meet not only the physical needs but also the psychosocial, cultural, spiritual, and environmental needs of patients and families. See **Box 1.7** for a discussion of culturally competent nursing care. Considering all aspects of the patient ensures a holistic approach to nursing. Holistic nursing care is based on a philosophical view that interacting wholes are greater than the sum of their parts. A holistic approach also emphasizes the uniqueness of the individual.

In providing comprehensive, individualized care, the nurse uses a variety of reasoning skills to analyze and synthesize knowledge from the arts, the sciences, and nursing research and theory. The science (knowledge base) of nursing is translated into the art of nursing through caring. Caring is the means by which the nurse is connected with and concerned for the patient (Benner & Wrubel, 1989). Thus, the nurse as caregiver is knowledgeable, skilled, empathic, and caring.

The Nurse as Educator

The nurse's role as educator is increasingly important for several reasons. Healthcare providers and consumers as well as local, state, and federal governments are placing greater emphasis on health promotion and illness prevention, hospital stays are shorter, and the number of individuals who are chronically ill in our society is increasing. Early discharge of patients from the hospital setting or rehabilitation facility to home care means that family caregivers must learn how to perform complex skills. All of these factors make the educator role essential to maintaining the health and well-being of patients.

Health literacy has become an increasing concern as patients take a more active role in their healthcare. Health literacy is the degree to which individuals have the capacity to obtain, process, and understand basic health information and services needed to make appropriate health decisions (U.S. Department of Health and Human Services, 2010). Medical-surgical nurses are instrumental in assessing the health literacy of patients and fulfilling the role of educator to ensure that patients have and can apply the health information required for achieving optimum health and healing. The framework for the role of educator is the teaching–learning process. Within this framework, the nurse assesses learning needs, plans and implements teaching methods to meet those needs and the patient's health literacy, and evaluates the effectiveness of

BOX 1.7
Culturally Competent Nursing

The primary focus of nursing care is the patient, as the patient relates to the environment and experiences events or situations related to health or illness. These experiences are given shape and personal meaning by culture—the socially inherited characteristics of a human group. These characteristics include the beliefs, practices, habits, likes, dislikes, customs, and rituals people learn from their families and pass on to their children. Cultural background is an essential component of an individual's ethnic identity. An individual's ethnic identity includes belonging to a social group within a culture and a social system and sharing a common religion, language, ancestry, and physical characteristics.

The healthcare system encompasses patients who are culturally diverse. This diversity includes differences in country of origin, health beliefs, sexual orientation, race, socioeconomic level, and age. Despite increasing diversity, nursing has been slow to address the need for culturally competent care. Many different factors account for this inattention, including ethnocentrism (people's belief that their own cultural group's beliefs and values are the only acceptable ones) and prejudice. The healthcare system is itself a culture, composed primarily of White middle-class people, and it often serves as a barrier to culturally competent care.

In 2015 a task force with membership representing several healthcare organizations developed guidelines for the provision of care regardless of geographic site. The 10 guidelines can be applied in the areas of clinical practice, nursing education, and research (Sullivan, 2015). The 10 guidelines address:

1. Knowledge of cultures
2. Education and gain in culturally competent care
3. Critical reflection
4. Cross cultural communication
5. Culturally competent practice
6. Cultural competence in healthcare organizations and systems
7. Patient advocacy and empowerment
8. Multicultural workforce
9. Cross cultural leadership
10. Evidence-based practice and research.

The American Academy of Nursing recommends the integration of these guidelines into nursing curricula, public health policy, and healthcare practice settings (Sullivan, 2015).

People of every culture have the right to have their cultural values known, respected, and addressed appropriately in nursing and other healthcare services (Leininger, 1991). To provide nursing care that is culturally competent, nurses must develop sensitivity to personal fundamental values about health and illness; must accept the existence of differing values; and must be respectful of, interested in, and understanding of other cultures without being judgmental.

the teaching. To be an effective educator, the nurse must have effective interpersonal skills and be familiar with adult learning principles (**Figure 1.8** ■).

A major component of the educator role today is discharge planning. Discharge planning, which begins on admission to a healthcare setting, is a systematic method of preparing the patient and family for exit from the healthcare agency and for maintaining continuity of care after the patient leaves the setting. Discharge planning also involves making referrals, identifying community and personal resources, and arranging for necessary equipment and supplies for home care. Changes in payment systems suggest that hospitals may not be reimbursed for readmission within 30 days of discharge. All of these changes in healthcare delivery are increasing the importance of providing comprehensive discharge planning and teaching.

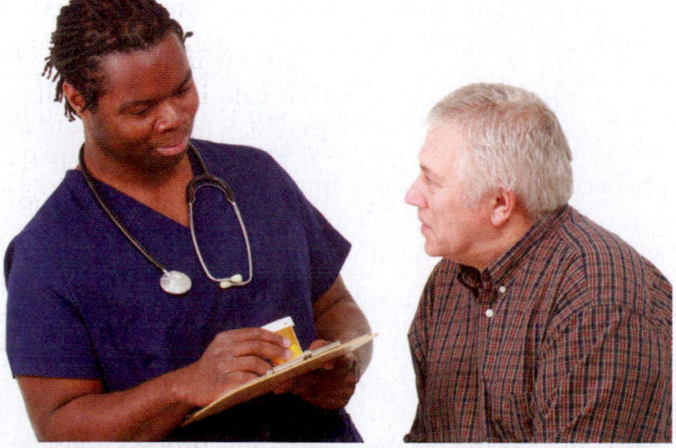

Figure 1.8 ■ The nurse's role as educator is an essential component of care. As part of the discharge planning process, the nurse is responsible for teaching for self-care at home.

The Nurse as Advocate

In its code of ethics, the ANA (2015) identifies the professional role of the nurse as an advocate and describes the responsibility to protect the rights of patients. The patient entering the healthcare system may be unprepared to make independent decisions. However, today's healthcare consumer is better educated about options for care and may have very definite opinions. The nurse as patient advocate actively promotes the patient's rights to autonomy and free choice. The goals of the nurse as advocate are to:

- Assess the need for advocacy.
- Communicate with other healthcare team members.
- Provide patient and family teaching.
- Assist and support patient decision making.
- Serve as a change agent in the healthcare system.
- Participate in health policy formulation.

The nurse must practice advocacy by believing that patients have the right to choose treatment options based on information about the results of accepting or rejecting the treatment, without coercion. The nurse must also accept and respect the decision of the patient, even though it may differ from the decision the nurse would make. Gerber (2018) outlines four stages of advocacy that can be used to guide the nurse when advocating for a patient.

1. The first stage involves assessing the patient's needs. The nurse should establish a therapeutic relationship and communicate with the patient to determine the patient's values and identify who they want involved in decision making.
2. The second stage involves identifying the patient's specific goals and empowering the patient's decision-making process.
3. The third stage involves implementing the patient's plan, which may involve facilitating communication with other members of the healthcare team to ensure the patient's choices are honored.
4. The fourth stage involves evaluating the outcome of the advocacy actions focusing on whether the patient's expected outcomes were realized.

The Nurse as Leader and Manager

All nurses are leaders and managers. They practice leadership and they manage time, people, resources, and the environment in which they provide care. Nurses carry out these roles by directing, delegating, supervising, and coordinating nursing activities. Nurses must be knowledgeable of how and when to delegate, as well as the legal requirements of delegation. Nurses also evaluate the quality of care provided.

Models of Care Delivery

Nurses are leaders and managers of patient care within a variety of models of care delivery. Examples are primary nursing, team nursing, and transitional care coordination. The nursing shortage made the combination of primary and team nursing more economically feasible.

Primary Nursing

Primary nursing allows the nurse to provide individualized direct care to a small number of patients during their entire inpatient stay. This model was developed to reduce the fragmentation of care experienced by patients and to facilitate family-centered continuity of care. In primary nursing, the nurse provides and coordinates care; communicates with patients, families, and other healthcare providers; and carries out discharge planning.

Team Nursing

Team nursing is practiced by teams of variously educated healthcare providers. For example, a team may consist of a registered nurse, a licensed practical nurse, and two unlicensed assistive personnel (UAPs). The registered nurse is the team leader. The team leader is responsible for making assignments and has overall responsibility for patient care by team members. All team members work together, each performing the activities for which he or she is best prepared.

Care Coordination

Care coordination focuses on management of a caseload (group) or panel of patients and the members of the healthcare team caring for those patients. The purpose of care coordination is to achieve the IHI's Triple Aim: To improve the patient care experience, to maximize positive outcomes, and to contain costs. The role of case manager is a similar position and is usually a clinical specialist. The emerging role of care coordination also involves managing a caseload or panel of patients that consists of patients with similar healthcare needs. As case manager or care coordinator, the nurse emphasizes continuity of care during transitions between healthcare settings. Coordinating care involves knowing the patient's nuanced responses to health problems and ensuring that critical information and care planning is continuous between settings, with an eye toward ensuring that the healthcare team works together to promote optimum outcomes (Izumi et al., 2018). Patients are at risk for experiencing complications and adverse events during transitions between settings or when care is transferred from one provider to another. Medications are sometimes administered or taken incorrectly when the patient is discharged to home. Critical signs and symptoms are overlooked and not reported. These disruptions in treatment plans lead to patient suffering, adverse effects on health, and increased healthcare costs (Izumi et al., 2018). The care coordinator may be part of the healthcare team within a **patient-centered medical home (PCMH)** or **accountable care organization (ACA)**. The PCMH/ACA healthcare team is led by the patient's primary care provider and includes a care coordinator who is often an RN. The physician or nurse who is the patient's primary care provider is responsible for leading the development of the plan of care with the patient and the family. The nurse performing the role of care coordinator collaborates with the patient and the rest of the healthcare team to implement and monitor the plan. The care coordinator makes appropriate referrals to other healthcare providers and manages the quality of care provided, including accuracy, timeliness, and cost. The care coordinator is also in contact with patients after discharge, ensuring continuity of care and health maintenance. The expansion of the Affordable Care Act is expanding the role of care coordination, especially in the management of patients with chronic disease and during transitions of care.

Delegation

Delegation is carried out when the nurse assigns appropriate and effective work activities to other members of the healthcare team. When the nurse delegates nursing care activities to another person, that person is authorized to act in the place of the nurse, while the nurse retains the accountability for the activities performed. Delegation skills are becoming increasingly important in healthcare as agencies restructure and implement cost containment measures. More categories of healthcare workers with minimal nursing education and experience are being hired to assist the registered nurse as *nurse extenders*, or *UAPs*. The Affordable Care Act includes provisions for an increase in the use of UAPs. Guidelines for delegation include:

- Consider the training, experience, and competence of each member of the healthcare team, the complexity of the task to be assigned, and the amount of time available to supervise the tasks.

- Determine the level of nursing judgment and evaluation required for the task.
- Consider the patient's condition and the potential harm and difficulty of performing the task.
- Know the state's nurse practice act and any practice limitations that may exist.
- Delegate only tasks that are within the scope of practice or authorized duties for each category of worker.
- Assign the right job to the right person. Tasks that are routine and standard are the best to assign to others.
- Know when it is appropriate to retain direct responsibility for care activities. The nurse should perform tasks that are complex or require a high level of nursing judgment.
- Give clear and complete directions for assignments. Ask questions to be sure directions have been understood.
- Give the team member the authority to complete the task while remaining accountable for the outcomes of care.
- Monitor the care provided and give constructive evaluation, if necessary.

Quality and Safety

As a major sector within the healthcare workforce, nurses have a significant responsibility for ensuring the quality and safety of care patients receive. This responsibility goes beyond ensuring that individual patients receive safe and effective patient-centered nursing care to recognizing healthcare system issues that impact quality of care. The current focus of safety initiatives is on minimizing the risk of harm to patients and providers by improving the performance and effectiveness of both individuals and healthcare systems (Lachman et al., 2015; Winland-Brown et al., 2015). All nurses must be prepared to understand, take seriously, and participate in quality and safety improvement strategies.

As a leader and manager, the nurse encourages the use of strategies such as standardized practices, checklists, and technology to improve safety and quality. When an error or near miss occurs, the nurse's focus is on reporting the incident to promote analysis of the factors and systems leading up to it, not on blaming the individuals involved.

In the role of leader and manager, the nurse is responsible for the quality of patient care through a process of quality improvement.

Quality improvement uses data to monitor the outcomes of care and the processes used to deliver that care. Changes to improve the quality and safety of healthcare systems are continuously designed and tested through quality improvement strategies and initiatives (Kiper, 2018; Oster & Deakins, 2018).

Quality improvement methods are used to evaluate patient care. Nurses commonly evaluate actual care against an established set of standards of care. Nurses and other healthcare providers make this evaluation by reviewing documentation, by conducting patient surveys and nurse interviews, and/or by direct observation of a nurse while patient care is being provided. The data are then used to identify differences between actual practice and established standards and to develop a plan of action to resolve the differences. The actions are then assessed through internal peer review or by an external medical review organization, called a utilization and quality control peer review organization (PRO), to determine whether they were effective in improving practice. **Health information technology (HIT)** is facilitating this process as systems include the patient electronic medical records and access to databases that provide standards of care and evidence-based practice guidelines.

The Nurse as Researcher

Nurses have always identified problems in patient care. Early nurse researchers showed the link between effective preoperative patient education and shorter postoperative hospital stays with fewer complications. Today, nurse researchers are studying a broad variety of questions and issues. To develop the science of nursing, nursing knowledge must be established through clinical research and then published so that the findings can be used by all nurses to provide evidence-based patient care.

With the integration of EBP into all aspects of care, the influence of nursing research is becoming apparent in the day-to-day practice of medical-surgical nursing. One approach is to develop the clinical question in a format that will support searching for answers in the literature. The PICOT question format has been well described by Melnyk and colleagues (2017). **PICOT** is an acronym for terms to be included in the clinical question. These include:

Patient population

Intervention or issue of interest

Comparison intervention or group

Outcome

Time frame.

PICOT questions can be framed to ask different types of questions about intervention, diagnosis, prognosis, etiology, or meaning.

Nursing Research as External Evidence

Well-conducted research studies make up the basis of external evidence. Many different approaches, designs, and methodologies are available that provide differing levels of reliable information. With generation of the PICOT question, the next step is to determine the level of evidence that best answers the question. Evidence is ranked hierarchically, with the strongest evidence at the peak of the pyramid, with lower levels for study designs with more risk for bias. The hierarchy includes seven levels:

Level I: Systematic reviews or meta-analyses of randomized controlled trials

Level II: Randomized controlled trials

Level III: Controlled trials without randomization

Level IV: Case control and cohort studies

Level V: Systematic reviews of descriptive and qualitative studies

Level VI: Single descriptive or qualitative studies

Level VII: Opinion of authorities and/or reports of expert committees.

Levels I and V are considered preappraised literature because these contain review and analysis of multiple studies. Levels II, III, IV, and VI are individual studies. Level VII is not actually data-based research, but evidence that is based on expert opinion. See **Figure 1.9** ■ for the evidence hierarchy pyramid.

Appraisal of the external evidence requires a discerning review of the strengths and weaknesses of the literature of interest. According to Melnyk et al. (2017), the focus of the process is to determine if the evidence being appraised is appropriate to use in clinical decision making. The validity and reliability of the evidence should be considered.

Validity is determined by evaluating the soundness of the scientific methods and the internal and external validity. *External validity* refers to how the results can be applied to others beyond the sample studies (generalization). External validity can be controlled by replication of the study. This is the underlying concept to the strength of meta-analyses and systematic reviews. Use of a control group also supports external validity.

Internal validity refers to the extent that you can be assured that the independent variable (intervention) actually influenced the dependent variable (outcome). To evaluate for internal validity, one must focus on how the study was conducted (Did it follow rigorous procedures?) and sampling. Problems with study procedures are called *bias*. Bias can be controlled through activities like blinding that prevent the investigator and/or the participants from knowing whether the experimental intervention or the non-intervention is assigned to a specific participant. A single-blind study is one in which the researchers collecting the data do not know group assignment; a double-blind study is one in which neither the researchers nor the participants know group assignment.

Reliability deals with the quantitative results. How large of an effect did the intervention have on the outcomes? How precise was the effect estimate? The type of data and the selected statistical tests are evaluated to determine reliability.

Reliability and validity can also refer to the quality of the instruments used in the research. Instrument validity is defined as the degree to which an instrument measures what it is supposed to measure. Instrument reliability refers to the consistency with which an instrument measures the topic of interest.

Applicability focuses on the extrapolation of research findings to your specific patient situation. Although the statistical analysis information may not be used to answer applicability, this is extremely important because it provides the support for using the evidence to individualize your patient care.

Relationship between Research Process and Nursing Process

The nursing process and the research process have many similarities. Both use a systematic approach, set goals, collect data used as evidence, analyze the data, and then evaluate the results of the process. See **Table 1.3** for a comparison of the nursing process and research process.

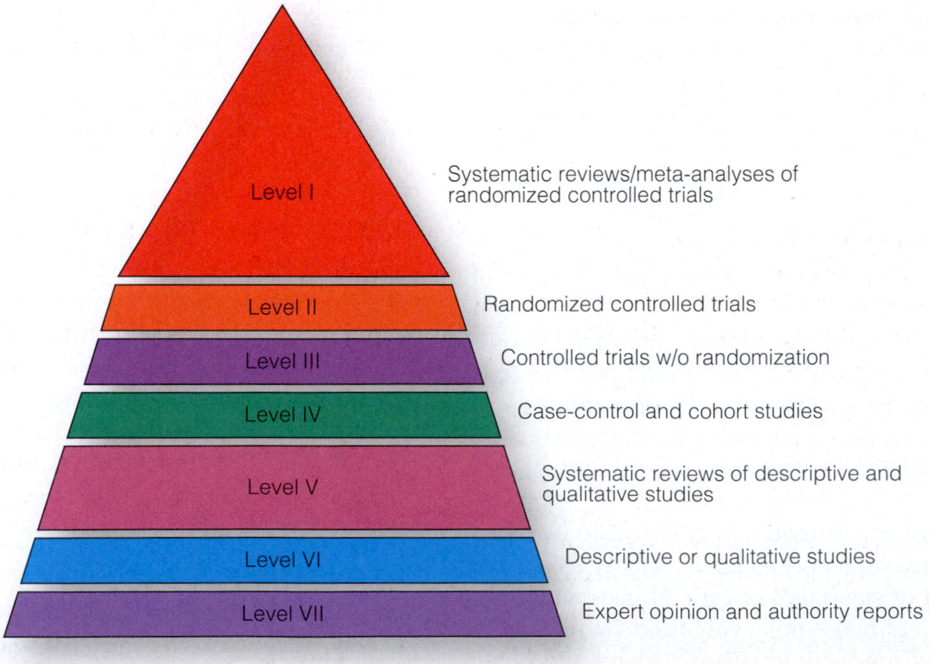
Level I
Systematic reviews/meta-analyses of randomized controlled trials
Level II
Randomized controlled trials
Level III
Controlled trials w/o randomization
Level IV
Case-control and cohort studies
Level V
Systematic reviews of descriptive and qualitative studies
Level VI
Descriptive or qualitative studies
Level VII
Expert opinion and authority reports

Figure 1.9 ■ Hierarchy of evidence.

Table 1.3 Comparison of the Nursing and Research Processes

Nursing Process	Research Process
Assessment ■ Data collection ■ Data interpretation	Problem/purpose identification ■ Identify research question ■ Knowledge of nursing ■ Clinical experiences
Nursing diagnosis	■ Conduct literature review ■ Choose a theory (if appropriate)
Planning ■ Setting goals ■ Planning interventions	Choose appropriate methods
Implementation	Collect information (data)
Evaluation	Conduct analysis (analyze results) Report findings

Use of Technology in EBP: Locating the Evidence

Effective literature searching is a necessary foundation to locating appropriate external evidence. With computerization of databases, searching no longer requires hours in the library culling through stacks of journals. Selection of an appropriate database is central to efficient literature searching. The terms from the PICOT question may be used as keywords. Additionally, databases often have the ability to use controlled vocabulary terms (medical subject heading [MeSH] terms). These terms are structured to retrieve the more specific terms that fall under a general term. MeSH terms are common in the large databases.

Examples of large databases include PubMed from the National Library of Medicine; Cumulative Index of Nursing and Allied Health Literature (CINAHL), and the Cochrane Collaboration. Subscriptions may be needed to access some benefits of the databases. Academic libraries as well as many medical and hospital libraries maintain such subscriptions. Additionally, public libraries may have access. Working with the librarian is the best source of specific information about available databases and other evidence resources. Some databases are specific to medical specialties. Additionally, the National Guideline Clearinghouse provides an open access database of clinical guidelines.

To be relevant, nursing research must have a goal to improve the care that nurses provide for patients. This means that all nurses must consider the researcher role to be integral to nursing practice. Summaries of relevant nursing research are included in almost all the nursing care chapters of this textbook. After the summary and discussion of each study, a clinical reasoning section specifically related to the findings of the study encourages the student to apply the findings to the clinical setting.

CHAPTER HIGHLIGHTS

1.1 Core Competencies for Safe and Effective Healthcare

Describe the core competencies for healthcare professionals: Patient-centered care, interprofessional teams, evidence-based practice, quality improvement, safety, and health information technology.

- The Patient Protection and Affordable Care Act will create new models of care and new roles for nurses that emphasize clinical reasoning, interprofessional teams, and knowledge-based technology.
- Recommended core competencies for all healthcare professionals include providing patient-centered care, working in interprofessional teams, using evidence-based practice, applying quality improvement, promoting safe healthcare systems, and using informatics.

1.2 Clinical Reasoning in the Nursing Process

Apply the attitudes, mental habits, and skills necessary for clinical reasoning when using the nursing process in patient care.

- The nursing process is the cyclical series of activities grounded in clinical reasoning and is used by nurses to provide patient care to promote wellness, maintain health, restore health, or facilitate coping with disability or death. The five interrelated phases of the nursing process are assessment, diagnosis, planning, implementation, and evaluation.

1.3 Guidelines for Nursing Practice

Explain the importance of nursing and interprofessional codes of ethics, standards of practice, and legal and ethical issues as guidelines for clinical nursing practice.

- The clinical practice of nursing is guided by codes for nurses and standards of practice.
- The human responses that nurses must consider when planning and implementing care result from changes in the structure and/or function of all body systems, as well as the effects of those changes on the psychosocial, cultural, spiritual, economic, and personal life of the patient.

1.4 Roles of the Nurse in Medical-Surgical Nursing

Explain the activities and characteristics of the nurse as caregiver, educator, advocate, leader and manager, and researcher.

- Nurses function as caregivers, educators, advocates, leaders and managers, and researchers to promote and maintain health, prevent illness, improve healthcare delivery and systems, and facilitate coping with disability or death for the adult patient.

TEST YOURSELF NCLEX-RN® REVIEW

1. The nurse is reviewing the Quality and Safety Education (QSEN) competencies for nurses. Which competency fosters open communication, mutual respect, and shared decision making to achieve quality patient care?
   A. Patient-centered care
   B. Quality improvement
   C. Evidence-based practice
   D. Teamwork and collaboration
2. When planning care for a patient, the nurse uses clinical reasoning based on which foundational knowledge? (Select all that apply.)
   A. Knowing the profession
   B. Knowing self
   C. Knowing financial restraints
   D. Knowing the patient
   E. Knowing the person
3. The nurse is identifying outcomes while planning a patient's care. What will the nurse do when selecting appropriate outcomes?
   A. Emphasize outcomes identified by the physician.
   B. Focus on outcomes requested by family members.
   C. Determine outcomes that are mutually agreeable with the patient.
   D. Select outcomes based on organizational policies and standards.
4. The nurse is using the nursing process when providing care to assigned patients. Place in order the steps in which the nurse will use this process.
   A. Planning
   B. Diagnosis
   C. Evaluation
   D. Assessment
   E. Implementation
5. The nurse focuses on the science of nursing before providing care to a newly admitted patient. On what is the nurse focusing?
   A. Holistic care
   B. Knowledge base
   C. Practice component
   D. Clinical competency
6. The nurse is determining appropriate information to include in a patient's discharge instructions. In what role is the nurse functioning at this time?
   A. Educator
   B. Advocate
   C. Caregiver
   D. Researcher
7. The nurse is advocating for a patient. What is the nurse doing?
   A. Performing range-of-motion exercises
   B. Analyzing the effectiveness of exercise
   C. Assisting and supporting patient decision making
   D. Delegating responsibilities for patient care to others
8. The nurse assigns patient care activities to other members of the team. In which role is the nurse functioning?
   A. Caregiver
   B. Advocate
   C. Researcher
   D. Leader/manager
9. The nurse manager is teaching staff about the use of newly adopted care bundles. Which information will the manager include? (Select all that apply.)
   A. Care bundles are specific to certain groups of patients in one location.
   B. Care bundles are a list of 10 or more interventions.
   C. These care bundles have been written by nursing administration.
   D. Compliance with bundles will be scored.
   E. The interventions in care bundles must be strictly followed.
10. The nurse delegates vital sign assessment to unlicensed assistive personnel (UAP). Who is accountable for the assessment findings?
    A. UAP
    B. Nurse
    C. Patient
    D. Physician

See Test Yourself answers in Appendix B.

REFERENCES

American Nurses Association (ANA). (2015). *Code of ethics for nurses with interpretive statements.* Silver Spring, MD: Author.

American Nurses Association (ANA). (2016). *Nursing: Scope and standards of practice* (3rd ed.). Silver Spring, MD: Author.

Benner, P. (1984). From novice to expert: Excellence and power in clinical nursing practice. *The American Journal of Nursing, 84*(12), 1480.

Benner, P., Sutphen, M., Leonard, B., & Day, L. (2010). *Educating nurses: A call for radical transformation.* San Francisco, CA: Jossey-Bass.

Benner, P., & Wrubel, J. (1989). *The primacy of caring: Stress and coping in health and illness.* Menlo Park, CA: Addison-Wesley.

Berwick, D. M., Nolan, T. W., & Whittington, J. (2008). The Triple Aim: Care, health, and cost. *Health Affairs, 27*(3), 759–769.

Boyer, L., Tardif, J., & Lefebvre, H. (2015). From a medical problem to a health experience: How nursing students think in clinical situations. *Journal of Nursing Education, 54*(11), 625–632.

Caple, C., & Karakashlan, A. (2017). *Care plans: Preparing.* Glendale, CA: Cinahl Information Systems.

Clancy, H. C. (2017). Care bundles: Easing the transition to long-term care. *Nursing Management, 48*(7), 14–16.

Collins, B. L., & Saylor, J. (2018). The Affordable Care Act: Where are we now? *Nursing, 46*(5), 43–47.

Cronenwett, L., Sherwood, G., Barnsteiner, J., Disch, J., Johnson, J., Mitchell, P., & Warren, J. (2007). Quality and safety education for nurses. *Nursing Outlook, 55*(3), 122–131.

Duffy, M. (2015). Nurses and the migration to electronic health records. *American Journal of Nursing, 115*(12), 61–66.

Gerber, L. (2018). Understanding the nurse's role as patient advocate. *Nursing, 48*(4), 55–58.

Gillespie, M., & Patterson, B. (2009). Helping novice nurses make effective clinical decisions: The situated clinical decision-making framework. *Nursing Education Perspectives, 30*(3), 164–170.

Gordon, M. (1994). *Nursing diagnosis: Process and application* (3rd ed.). St. Louis, MO: Mosby.

Institute for Healthcare Improvement (IHI). (2018). What is a bundle? Retrieved from http://www.ihi.org/resources/Pages/ImprovementStories/WhatIsaBundle.aspx.

Institute of Medicine (IOM). (2001). *Crossing the quality chasm: A new health system for the 21st century* (Committee on Quality of Health Care in America report). Washington, DC: National Academy Press.

International Council of Nurses. (2012). *The ICN code of ethics for nurses.* Geneva: Imprimerie Fornara.

Interprofessional Education Collaborative Expert Panel. (2011). *Core competencies for interprofessional collaborative practice: Report of an expert panel.* Washington, DC: Interprofessional Education Collaborative.

Izumi, S., Barfield, P. A., Basin, B., Mood, L., Neunzert, C., Tadesse, R., . . . Tanner. (2018). Care coordination: Identifying and connecting the most important care for patients. *Research in Nursing and Health, 41*(1), 49–56.

Jones, N. T., & Stockman, C. (2018). Facilitating adaptation of an electronic documentation system. *Computers, Informatics Nursing, 36*(5), 225–231.

Ketefian, S. (1987). A case study of theory development: Moral behavior in nursing. *Advances in Nursing Science, 9*(2), 10–19.

Kiper, V. (2018). Translating leadership into safe nursing practice. *Nursing Made Incredibly Easy, 16*(3), 48–51.

Kroning, M. (2018). 59 clicks in the EHR. *Nursing Management, 49*(5), 10–14.

Lachman, V. D., Swanson, E. O., & Winland-Brown, J. (2015). The new code of ethics for nurses with interpretive statements (2105): Practical application, part 2. *MedSurg Nursing, 24*(5), 363–368.

Leininger, M. (1991). Transcultural care principles, human rights, and ethical considerations. *Journal of Transcultural Nursing, 3*(1), 21–23.

Maslow, A. H. (1970). *Motivation and personality* (2nd ed.). New York, NY: Harper & Row.

Mayan, J. (2018). The social media conundrum. *Nursing Management,* 49(1), 8–9.

Melnyk B. M., Gallagher-Ford., L., & Fineout-Overholt, E. (2017). *Implementing evidence-based practice competencies in healthcare: A practical guide for improving quality, safety and outcomes.* Indianapolis, IN: Sigma Theta Tau International.

NANDA International. (2018). T. H. Herdman & S. Kamitsuru, Eds. *NANDA International, Inc. Nursing diagnoses: Definitions and classification. 2018–2020* (11th ed.). New York, NY: Thieme.

National Academy of Sciences. (2003). Executive summary. *Health professions education: A bridge to quality.* Retrieved from http://www.nap.edu.

National Council of State Boards of Nursing. (2014). *Professional boundaries: A nurse's guide to the importance of appropriate professional boundaries.* Chicago, IL: Author. Retrieved from https://www.ncsbn.org/Professional-Boundaries_Complete.pdf.

National Council of State Boards of Nursing. (2018). The nursing regulatory environment in 2018: Issues and challenges. *9*(1), 54–65.

Oster, C. A., & Deakins, S. (2018). Practical application of high-reliability principles in healthcare to optimize quality and safety outcomes. *Journal of Nursing Administration, 48*(1), 50–55.

Salmond, S. W., Echevaria, M., & Allread, (2017). Care bundles: Increasing consistency of care. *Orthopaedic Nursing, 36ci*(1), 45–48.

Simmons, B. (2010). Clinical reasoning: Concept analysis. *Journal of Advanced Nursing, 66*(5), 1151–1157.

Stalter, A. M., & Mota, A. (2018). Using systems thinking to envision quality and safety in healthcare. *Nursing Management, 49*(2), 32–38.

Sullivan, C. G. (2015). Implementing culturally competent care. *Nursing Outlook, 63,* 227–229.

Tanner, C. A. (2006). Thinking like a nurse: A research-based model of clinical judgment in nursing. *Journal of Nursing Education, 45*(6), 204–211.

U.S. Department of Health and Human Services, Office of Disease and Health Promotion. (2010). *National action plan to improve health literacy.* Washington, DC: Author.

Walker-Czyz, A. (2016). The impact of an integrated electronic health record adoption on nursing care quality. *Journal of Nursing Administration, 46*(7/78), 366–372.

Wilkinson, J.M., & Barcus, L., (2017). *Pearson Nursing Diagnosis Handbook* (11th ed.). Hoboken, NJ: Pearson Education.

Winland-Brown, J., Lachman, V. D., & Swanson, E. O. (2015). The new code of ethics for nurses with interpretive statements (2015): Practical application, part 1. *MedSurg Nursing, 24*(4), 268–271.

Chapter 2

Health and Illness Care of Adults

Chapter Outline and Learning Outcomes

2.1 Health and Wellness 24

Define health and the health–illness continuum, and discuss factors affecting the health of individuals, families, communities, and special populations.

2.2 Health Promotion and Maintenance 34

Compare and contrast health risks, assessment, and health promotion for the young adult, middle adult, and older adult.

2.3 Disease, Illness, and Injury 35

Differentiate between disease, illness, and injury, and describe illness behaviors and needs of the patient with acute, critical, and chronic illness.

2.4 Types of Nursing Care 40

Describe essential elements and goals of coordinated primary care models; the services, settings, and essential components of community-based care and home healthcare; and nursing interventions to deliver safe, effective, and competent care to patients in their homes.

CLINICAL COMPETENCIES

- Use knowledge of individual and family variables to promote, restore, and maintain health when planning and implementing patient-centered care for adults.
- Engage patients, family members, and other health team members in active partnerships to promote and maintain health and safety of the adult.
- Use high-quality electronic sources to plan and promote health for the adult.
- Base individualized plans to promote and maintain health status on patient values, current evidence, and standards of practice.
- Provide safe and effective individualized patient care in community-based settings and the home.
- Use quality measures to evaluate and improve community-based and home care for adults.

KEY TERMS

acute illness, 36
adverse childhood experience (ACE), 37
chronic illness, 37
community-based care, 41
critical illness, 36
disease, 35
exacerbation, 38
family, 25
health, 24
health–illness continuum, 24
holistic healthcare, 24
home healthcare, 42
hospice care, 45
illness, 36
late effects, 33
manifestations, 36
palliative care, 45
patient-centered medical home (PCMH), 41
primary care, 40
rehabilitation, 42
remission, 38
respite care, 45
social determinants of health, 24
transgender, 32
transitional care, 41
wellness, 24

Nurses promote and protect health as well as treat patient responses to disease and illness. The ever-increasing cost of illness care has resulted in initiatives to promote and maintain health in which nurses can and do play integral roles.

In the healthcare system of the 21st century, hospitals are primarily acute care providers with services focused on high-technology care for severely ill or injured people or for people having major surgery. Even those patients rarely remain in the hospital for long. They are transitioned as rapidly as possible to less acute care settings within the hospital and then to community-based and home care. In 2012, The Joint Commission released a white paper titled *Transitions of Care: The Need for a More Effective Approach to Continuing*

Patient Care. The white paper outlines the need to change from episodic care events to a model that focuses on coordinated care between settings. Healthcare is transforming and the roles and opportunity for nurses and the profession are changing at a rapid pace (National Council State Board of Nursing [NCSBN], 2018; Salmond & Echevarria, 2017).

2.1 Health and Wellness

In 1948, the World Health Organization (WHO) defined **health** as "a state of complete physical, mental, and social well-being, and not merely the absence of disease or infirmity." This definition, which WHO (1974) maintains to date, is multidimensional, addressing the importance of the physical, mental, emotional, and social components of health. Health is not just a state of being, but the resources (e.g., physical, personal, social) used by each person in dealing with the challenges of living.

The **health–illness continuum**, a conceptual model developed by Dunn (1959), represents health as a dynamic process, with high-level **wellness** at one extreme of the continuum and death at the opposite extreme (**Figure 2.1** ■). Individuals place themselves at different locations on the continuum at specific points in time. As commonly illustrated, the health–illness continuum fails to account for the complexity and interrelatedness of health and illness. Health does exist in individuals affected by disease, and people with no evidence of disease can have poor health. Pender, Murdaugh, and Parsons (2015) present a model with multiple parallel lines representing levels of health throughout the lifespan. Illnesses (acute or chronic) are shown as events occurring along the lines. An individual who has achieved optimum health may develop an acute or chronic illness. Illness, in turn, can either inhibit or promote the individual's desire and actions to achieve optimal wellness.

Factors Affecting Health

A variety of factors influence wellness, including self-concept, environment, culture, and spiritual values. These factors often interact to promote health or to become risk factors for alterations in health. The **social determinants of health** as defined by the World Health Organization are the conditions in which people are "born, grow, work, live, and age, and the wider set of forces and systems shaping the conditions of daily life" (WHO, 2018) There has been increased attention to these conditions that are thought to be the foundation of individuals' and communities' health. The social determinants of health are critical to understanding health inequity (Persoud, 2018).

Healthy People 2020 is a U.S. government initiative administered through the U.S. Office of Disease Prevention and Health Promotion that identifies health-related goals every 10 years. Healthy People 2020 (U.S. Department of Health and Human Services [HHS], 2018) identifies level of education as the leading predictor of health outcomes and have developed goals and subgoals that aim to promote education as means to improve individual and community health. **Holistic healthcare** considers all aspects of an individual (physical, psychosocial, cultural, spiritual, and intellectual) as essential components of individualized care.

Genetic Makeup

Each person's genetic makeup influences health status throughout life. Genetic makeup affects personality, temperament, body structure, intellectual potential, and susceptibility to alterations in health. Examples of chronic illnesses that are known to be associated with genetic makeup include sickle cell disease, hemophilia, diabetes mellitus, and cancer. Ongoing discoveries in genetics, which are changing the delivery of healthcare as treatment for disease, are designed to target specific genetic markers. See Chapter 8 for further discussion of the influence of genomics in healthcare and nursing.

Cognitive Abilities and Education

Although cognitive abilities are determined prior to adulthood, cognitive development affects whether people view themselves as healthy or ill; cognitive levels may also affect health practices. Injuries to and illnesses affecting the brain may alter cognitive abilities. Educational level affects the ability to understand and follow guidelines for health. Health literacy can be linked to cognitive abilities and level of education. Low health literacy can create challenges for patients in navigating the healthcare

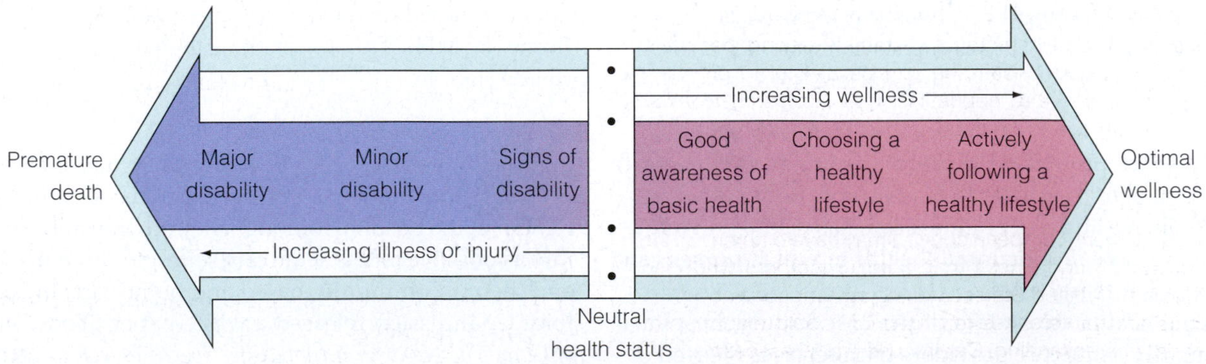
Increasing wellness
Premature death
Major disability
Minor disability
Signs of disability
Good awareness of basic health
Choosing a healthy lifestyle
Actively following a healthy lifestyle
Optimal wellness
Increasing illness or injury
Neutral health status

Figure 2.1 ■ An illness–wellness continuum.

system and self-managing chronic illness (Ingram & Kautz, 2018).

Ethnicity and Culture

Certain diseases have a higher rate of incidence in some cultural and ethnic groups than in others. For example, in the United States hypertension is more common in African Americans, diabetes mellitus and chronic liver disease are among the leading causes of illness in Native Americans, and eye disorders are more prevalent in Chinese Americans. The ethnic and cultural background of an individual also influences health values and behaviors, lifestyle, and illness behaviors. Every culture defines health and illness in a way that is unique. In addition, each culture may have health beliefs and illness treatment practices that influence a patient's choices.

Lifestyle and Environment

The components of an individual's lifestyle that affect health status include patterns of eating, use of chemical substances (alcohol, nicotine, caffeine, legal and illegal drugs), exercise and rest patterns, and coping methods. Examples include the relationship of obesity to hypertension, cigarette smoking to chronic obstructive pulmonary disease, and a sedentary lifestyle to heart disease and certain cancers. The link of sleep to overall health has been identified as a consideration that is especially relevant to nursing care planning. See Chapter 3 for more information about sleep. The environment has a major influence on health. Occupational exposure to toxic substances (such as asbestos and coal dust) increases the risk of pulmonary disorders. Air, water, and food pollution increase the risk of respiratory disorders, infectious diseases, and cancer. Environmental temperature variations can result in hypothermia or hyperthermia, especially in the older adult.

Socioeconomic Background

Both lifestyle and environmental influences are affected by income level. The culture of poverty, which crosses all racial and ethnic boundaries, negatively influences health status. Poverty and homelessness are social determinants of health that adversely affect health outcomes for individuals and communities (Olshansky, 2017). Needed medical care is often delayed or lacking, particularly among uninsured adults. As a result, illness may be more severe, the risk for complications greater, and hospital stays longer (National Center for Health Statistics [NCHS], 2017). Living at or below the poverty level may result in crowded living conditions, increasing the risk of contracting communicable diseases. Other problems include lack of infant and child care, inadequate nutrition, use of addictive substances, and violence.

Geographic Area

The geographic area in which one lives influences health status, health risks, and access to healthcare. Vector-borne diseases such as Rocky Mountain spotted fever (RMSF) and Lyme disease are more prevalent in certain regions of the United States (RMSF in south-central and southern states, Lyme disease in the eastern states). More healthcare providers, including specialists, are available in urban settings than in rural areas.

Family

Family structure and function affect the health status of individuals within the family unit. Although some people have no family ties, most have one or more significant individuals in their lives. A **family** is a social unit of two or more people who are emotionally involved with each other and who depend on one another for emotional, physical, and psychosocial support.

Although every family is unique and influenced by cultural values and beliefs, all families have certain structural and functional features in common. The family as a unit is responsible for the following (Pender et al., 2015):

- Developing self-care and dependent-care competencies of its members
- Fostering resilience of family members to include shared values and shared goals

Focus on Cultural Diversity

Genetic Differences Among Cultures

As genetic science and our understanding of disease and pathology have advanced, there is increasing recognition of differences and similarities among people across the globe. Certain diseases and conditions are more likely to develop in some groups than in others; for example, sickle cell disease occurs more frequently in people whose ancestors are from Central Africa, the Near East, the Mediterranean region, and parts of India; Caucasian American women of small stature and of Scandinavian heritage have a higher risk of developing osteoporosis. Biologic variations may also affect the way the body metabolizes drugs, leading to an effect that is either less than or greater than anticipated.

Biologic differences among people of various cultural groups may affect both food preferences and food tolerance. Mexican Americans, African Americans, Native Americans, and Asian Americans may be lactose intolerant; that is, they do not produce enough lactase to tolerate large amounts of dairy products. If too much milk is consumed, undigested lactose in the intestine causes manifestations such as cramping, flatulence, abdominal bloating, and diarrhea.

Although known biologic variables among people of different races and cultures can be helpful in providing individualized health education, it is important to avoid stereotyping based on racial and cultural differences. For example, a recent emigrant from Ethiopia has a significantly different cultural background than a person of color who was raised in the United States. Likewise, a recent emigrant from a northern European country may have different beliefs about health and illness than family members who were raised in the United States. Making assumptions about risk factors and preferences for treatment could lead to inappropriate care planning. Careful and tactful assessment will help the nurse understand how best to support patients.

- Providing social and physical resources to the family group
- Promoting healthy individuals while maintaining family cohesion.

Age, Gender, and Development

Age and gender are factors in health and illness. Cardiovascular disorders are uncommon in young adults, but the incidence increases after the age of 40. Myocardial infarctions are more common in men than in women until women are postmenopausal. Some diseases occur only in one gender or the other (e.g., prostate cancer in men, cervical cancer in women). The older adult often has increased incidence of chronic illness and increased potential for serious illness or death from infectious illnesses such as influenza and pneumonia.

The adult years are commonly divided into three stages: The young adult (age 18 to 40), the middle adult (age 40 to 65), and the older adult (over age 65). Although developmental markers are not as clearly delineated in the adult as in the infant or child, changes in physical status, psychosocial development, and major health risks do occur with aging.

The Young Adult

From age 18 to 25, the healthy young adult is at the peak of physical development. All body systems are functioning at maximum efficiency. Then, during the 30s, some normal physiologic changes begin to occur (**Figure 2.2** ■). **Table 2.1** summarizes physical characteristics typical of the young adult. Major health risks for the young adult include accidents, sexually transmitted infections, substance abuse, and physical or psychosocial stressors. These risk factors may be interrelated (see the Moving Evidence into Action feature).

Injuries

Unintentional injuries are the leading cause of injury and death in people between age 15 and 44 (NCHS, 2017). Most

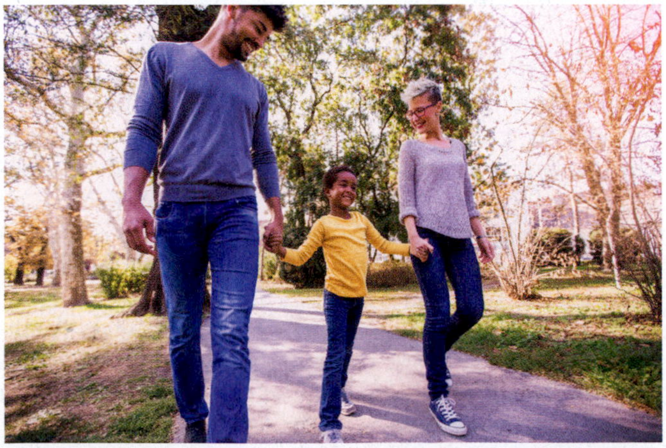

Figure 2.2 ■ Young adults are generally in good health although some normal physiologic changes begin to occur during the 30s.

Table 2.1 Physical Characteristics of the Young Adult Years

Assessment	Status
Skin	Smooth, even temperature; some wrinkles may appear
Hair	Slightly oily, shiny; graying may begin Balding may begin
Vision	Snellen 20/20
Musculoskeletal	Strong, coordinated
Cardiovascular	Maximum cardiac output Rate: 60–90 bpm Mean BP: 120/80 mmHg
Respiratory	Rate: 12.20/min Full vital capacity

injuries and fatalities occur as the result of motor vehicle crashes, but injuries and death also result from assaults (homicide), drowning, fire, guns, occupational accidents, and exposure to environmental hazards. Accidental injury or death is often associated with the use of alcohol or other chemical substances or with psychologic stress. Suicide is the third leading cause of death in those 15 to 24 years old, but drops to the fourth leading cause in those age 25 to 44. In both groups, the suicide rate is significantly higher in males than in females (NCHS, 2017).

Sexually Transmitted Infections

Sexually transmitted infections include genital herpes, chlamydia, gonorrhea, syphilis, and HIV/AIDS. The young adult who is sexually active with a variety of partners and who does not use barrier protection is at greatest risk for development of these diseases.

Substance Abuse

Substance abuse is a major cause for concern in the young adult population. Although alcohol abuse occurs at all ages, binge drinking (consuming four or more drinks in about 2 hours, leading to a blood alcohol concentration of 0.08%) is more common among young adults (Centers for Disease Control and Prevention [CDC], 2018a). Alcohol contributes to motor vehicle crashes and physical violence, and it is damaging to the developing fetus in pregnant women. It can also cause liver disease, contributing to chronic liver disease and cirrhosis, the sixth leading cause of death among young adults age 25 to 44 years (NCHS, 2017).

Other commonly abused substances include nicotine; marijuana; stimulants such as amphetamine, methamphetamine, and cocaine; and opioid pain relievers (National Institute on Drug Abuse, 2018). The misuse of and addiction to opioids including prescription pain relievers, heroin, and synthetic opioids such as fentanyl is a serious national crisis that affects individual and public health as well as social and economic welfare (National Institute on Drug

Abuse, 2018). See Chapter 6 for a more in-depth discussion of addiction and related nursing care.

Smoking increases the risk of respiratory and cardiovascular diseases. Marijuana can affect memory and learning for days to weeks after its use. Methamphetamine, a highly addictive substance, can lead to structural and functional changes in the areas of the brain associated with emotion and memory. Cocaine can cause death from cardiovascular effects (increased heart rate and ventricular dysrhythmias) and can lead to addiction and health problems in the baby born to an addicted mother. Opioid pain relievers cause drowsiness and impair coordination and can cause fatal overdose.

Physical and Psychosocial Stressors

Malignancies are among the top five leading causes of death in the young adult. For this reason, emphasizing the importance of attending to changes in their bodies is critical. Behavioral patterns established in young adulthood also impact the risk for many chronic diseases more commonly diagnosed in middle or late adulthood, including obesity, coronary heart disease, diabetes, chronic lung disease, and chronic liver disease. Health promotion for young adults must include teaching about healthy behaviors and eating habits associated with reduced risk for developing cancers and chronic diseases. See Chapter 21 for more on health promotion for nutrition.

The young adult is subject to physical stressors such as work-related risks (e.g., electrical hazards, mechanical injuries, exposure to hazardous materials), exposure to the sun, participation in high-risk activities (e.g., contact sports, driving too fast), ingestion of chemical substances (e.g., caffeine, alcohol, nicotine), and pregnancy.

Many different and individualized psychosocial stressors may affect the young adult. Choices about education, occupation, relationships, independence, and lifestyle affect both current and future health. The young adult without adequate education or job skills may face unemployment, poverty, homelessness, and limited access to healthcare. Young adults are more likely to be uninsured than are people in other age groups; as a result, they are more likely to delay or avoid needed medical care due to cost (NCHS, 2017).

The Middle Adult

The physical status and function of the middle adult, age 40 to 65, is similar to that of the young adult. However, many changes take place between age 40 and 65. **Table 2.2** lists the physical changes that normally occur in the middle years. The middle adult is at risk for alterations in health from obesity, cardiovascular disease, cancer, substance abuse, and physical and psychosocial stressors. These factors are often interrelated.

Obesity

Weight gain is common in middle adulthood, usually the result of continuing to consume the same number of calories while decreasing physical activity (**Figure 2.3** ■). Obesity affects all of the major organ systems of the body, increasing the risk of atherosclerosis, hypertension, elevated cholesterol and triglyceride levels, and diabetes. Obesity is also associated with cancer, osteoarthritis, fatty liver disease, and gallbladder disease.

Table 2.2 Physical Changes in the Middle Adult Years

Assessment	Changes
Skin	■ Decreased turgor, moisture, and subcutaneous fat result in wrinkles. ■ Fat is deposited in the abdominal and hip areas.
Hair	■ Loss of melanin in hair shaft causes graying. ■ Hairline recedes in males.
Sensory	■ Visual acuity for near vision decreases (presbyopia) during the 40s. ■ Auditory acuity for high-frequency sounds decreases (presbycusis); more common in men. ■ Sense of taste diminishes.
Musculoskeletal	■ Skeletal muscle mass decreases by about age 60. ■ Thinning of intervertebral disks results in loss of height (about 2.5 cm [1 in.]). ■ Postmenopausal women may develop low bone density or osteoporosis.
Cardiovascular	■ Blood vessels lose elasticity. ■ Systolic blood pressure may increase.
Respiratory	■ Loss of vital capacity (about 1 L from age 20 to 60) occurs.
Gastrointestinal	■ Large intestine gradually loses muscle tone; constipation may result. ■ Gastric secretions are decreased.
Genitourinary	■ Hormonal changes occur: Menopause, women (↓ estrogen) Andropause, men (↓ testosterone).
Endocrine	■ Gradual decrease in glucose tolerance occurs.

Cardiovascular Disease

Cardiovascular disease (CVD) ranks second only to cancer as the leading cause of death for middle-age adults

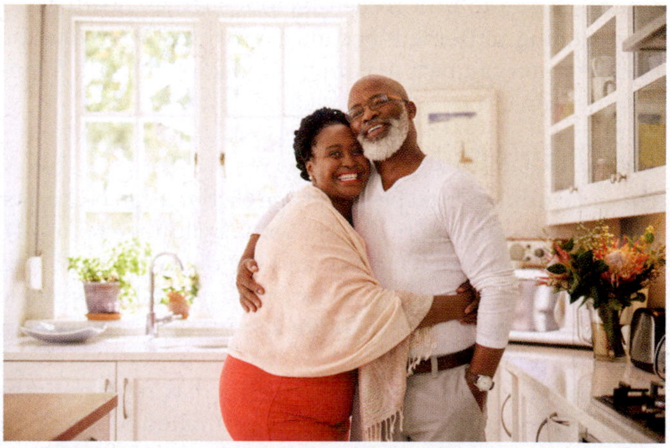

Figure 2.3 ■ Middle adults (age 40–65) are prone to weight gain due to decreased physical activity.

(NCHS, 2017). Diabetes, hypertension, and obesity, prevalent chronic diseases among this age group, are major risk factors for CVD, as are male gender, family history, physical inactivity, cigarette smoking, and elevated blood cholesterol levels. Stroke, kidney disease, hypertension, and peripheral vascular disease are other potential consequences of CVD.

Cancer

Cancer is the leading cause of death in adults between age 45 and 64 in the United States (American Cancer Society [ACS], 2018). Cancers of the breast, colon, lung, and reproductive system are common in the middle years. Prolonged exposure to environmental carcinogens and use of alcohol and nicotine are significant cancer risk factors for the middle adult.

Substance Abuse

Although the middle adult may abuse a variety of substances, the most commonly abused are alcohol, nicotine, and prescription drugs. Excess alcohol use in the middle adult contributes to an increased risk of liver cancer, cirrhosis, pancreatitis, hyperlipidemia, and anemia. Alcohol abuse also increases the risk of accidental injury or death and disrupts careers and relationships. Cigarette smoking increases the risk of cancers of the upper respiratory tract and lung, upper gastrointestinal tract, pancreas, bladder, and kidney. It is a major risk factor for chronic obstructive pulmonary disease and cardiovascular disease.

Physical and Psychosocial Stressors

The middle adult years are ones of change and transition, frequently resulting in stress. Both men and women must adapt to changes in physical appearance and function. Children may leave home or choose to remain at home longer than they are welcome. Parents are aging, with illness probable and death inevitable. The middle adult thus becomes part of what has been called the "sandwich generation," caught between the need to care for both children and aging parents. Career changes may occur by choice or due to unforeseen factors such as health, and approaching retirement becomes a reality. Divorce in the middle years can be a major emotional, social, and financial stressor.

The Older Adult

The older adult period begins at age 65, but it can be further divided into three periods: The young-old (age 65 to 74), the middle-old (age 75 to 84), and the old-old (age 85 and over). With increasing age, a number of normal physiologic changes occur, as listed in **Table 2.3**. See also Multisystem Effects of Aging.

The older adult population is increasing more rapidly than any other age group. An estimated 66.8 million older adults age 60 and over resided in the United States in 2015, comprising 21% of the population. There will be 79.7 million older adults by the year 2040, more than twice the number in 2000. In 2015, the average life expectancy in the United States was 78.8 years. Life expectancy for females is 4.8 years higher than for males (Administration on Aging [AOA], 2015; Kochanek, Murphy, Xu, & Tejada-Vera, 2016).

The increasing numbers of older adults have important implications for nursing. Patients in all healthcare settings will be older, with nursing care and teaching needs that differ from those of young and middle adults (**Figure 2.4** ■). Gerontologic nursing (care of the older adult) is a nursing specialty area; it is also an integral component of medical-surgical nursing.

The older adult is at risk for alterations in health from a variety of causes. The majority of older adults have one or more chronic health problems; many have multiple illnesses. The most frequently occurring conditions in the older adult are arthritis, heart disease, cancer, diabetes, and hypertension (AOA, 2015). The leading causes of death are heart disease, cancer, and chronic lower respiratory diseases. Like the middle adult, the older adult is at risk for alterations in health from obesity and a sedentary lifestyle. Other risk factors specific to this age group include accidental injuries, pharmacologic effects, and physical and psychosocial stress.

Injuries

Injuries in the older adult can lead to hospitalization, self-care deficits, loss of independence, and even death. The risk of injury is increased by normal physiologic changes that accompany aging, pathophysiologic alterations in health (e.g., cardiac irregularities, decreased sensation related to diabetes mellitus), environmental hazards, and lack of support systems. The three major causes of injury in the older adult are falls, fires, and motor vehicle crashes. Of these, falls with resultant hip fractures are the most significant in terms of long-term disability and death.

Pharmacologic Effects

A number of risk factors predispose the older adult to toxic drug effects. Age-related changes in tissue and organ structure and function alter the absorption of both oral and parenteral medications. Poor nutrition and decreased liver function may alter drug metabolism. The aging kidney may not excrete drugs at the normal rate. Self-administration of both prescribed and over-the-counter (OTC) medications presents risks for error resulting from confusion, forgetfulness, or misreading the directions. The older adult may require drugs for several chronic diseases, increasing the risk for adverse drug interactions. In addition, the older adult living on a fixed income may have to make a choice between buying medications or food, resulting in undermedication and ineffective treatment of an illness.

Physical and Psychosocial Stressors

The older adult is exposed to the same environmental hazards as the young and middle adult, but the effects of an

Table 2.3 Physical Changes in the Older Adult Years

Assessment	Changes
Skin	■ Decreased turgor and sebaceous gland activity result in dry, wrinkled skin. Melanocytes cluster, causing "age spots" or "liver spots."
Hair and nails	■ Scalp, axillary, and pubic hair thins; nose and ear hair thickens. ■ Women may develop facial hair. ■ Nails grow more slowly; may become thick and brittle.
Sensory	■ Visual field narrows, and depth perception is distorted. Cataracts may develop. ■ Pupils are smaller, reducing night vision. ■ Lenses yellow and become opaque, resulting in distortion of green, blue, and violet tones and increased sensitivity to glare. ■ Production of tears decreases. ■ Sense of smell decreases. ■ Age-related hearing loss progresses, involving middle- and low-frequency sounds. ■ Threshold for pain and touch increases. ■ Proprioception (sense of physical position) may be altered, increasing risk for falls.
Musculoskeletal	■ Loss of overall mass, strength, and movement of muscles occurs; tremors may occur. ■ Loss of bone structure and deterioration of joint cartilage results in kyphosis, increased risk of fractures, and restricted range of motion.
Cardiovascular	■ Systolic blood pressure rises. ■ Cardiac output decreases. ■ Peripheral resistance increases, and capillary walls thicken.
Respiratory	■ Continued loss of vital capacity occurs as the lungs become less elastic and more rigid. ■ Anteroposterior chest diameter and residual volume increase. ■ Although blood carbon dioxide levels remain relatively constant, blood oxygen levels decrease by 10 to 15%.
Gastrointestinal	■ Decreased saliva production affects dentition, and loss of taste buds decreases ability to taste salt and sweet. ■ Gag reflex is decreased, stomach motility reduced, and gastric emptying is delayed. ■ Both large and small intestines have some atrophy, with decreased peristalsis. ■ The liver decreases in weight and storage capacity; gallstones increase; pancreatic enzymes decrease.
Genitourinary	■ Kidneys lose mass, and the glomerular filtration rate is reduced (by nearly 50% from young adulthood to old age). ■ Bladder capacity decreases, and the micturition reflex is delayed. Urinary retention is more common. ■ Women may have stress incontinence; men may have an enlarged prostate gland. ■ Reproductive changes in men occur: a. Testosterone decreases. b. Sperm count decreases. c. Testes become smaller. d. Length of time to achieve an erection increases; erection is less full. ■ Reproductive changes in women occur: a. Estrogen levels decrease. b. Breast tissue decreases. c. Vagina, uterus, ovaries, and urethra atrophy. d. Vaginal lubrication decreases. e. Vaginal secretions become alkaline.
Endocrine	■ Pituitary gland loses weight and vascularity. ■ Thyroid gland becomes more fibrous, and plasma T_3 levels decrease. ■ Pancreas releases insulin more slowly; increased blood glucose levels are common. ■ Adrenal glands produce less cortisol.

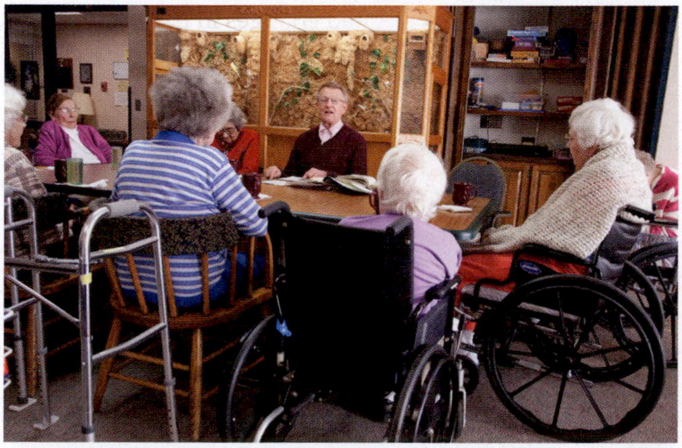

Figure 2.4 ■ The older adult population is increasing rapidly. This group of older women (in the middle-old and old-old periods) who live in a nursing home are listening to an author read from his book.

accumulation of years of exposure may now appear. For example, exposure to the sun in earlier years may be manifested by skin cancer, and the long-term effects of exposure to noise pollution can result in impaired hearing. The older adult is at increased risk for respiratory disorders as a result of years of smoking, occupational toxins, or environmental pollutants. Living conditions and economic constraints may prevent the older adult from having necessary heating and cooling, contributing to thermal-related illnesses and even death. Elder abuse and neglect further increase the risk of injury or illness.

Psychosocial stressors for the older adult include the illness or death of a spouse, decreased or limited income, retirement, isolation from friends and family because of lack of transportation or distance, return to the home of a child, or relocation to a long-term healthcare facility. A further stressor may be role loss or reversal—for example, when the wife becomes the caretaker of her chronically ill

Multisystem Effects of Aging

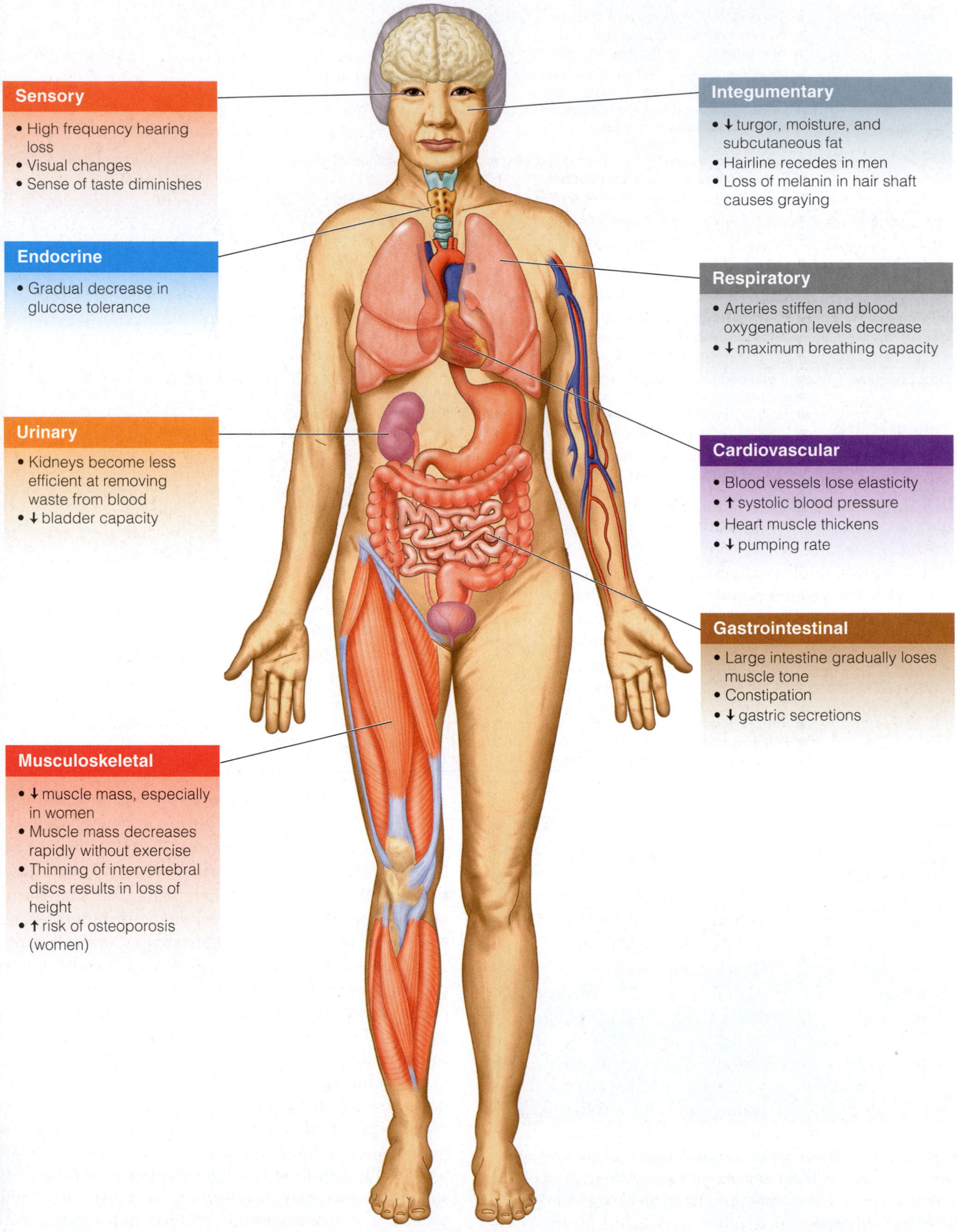

Sensory
• High frequency hearing loss
• Visual changes
• Sense of taste diminishes
Endocrine
• Gradual decrease in glucose tolerance
Urinary
• Kidneys become less efficient at removing waste from blood
• ↓ bladder capacity
Musculoskeletal
• ↓ muscle mass, especially in women
• Muscle mass decreases rapidly without exercise
• Thinning of intervertebral discs results in loss of height
• ↑ risk of osteoporosis (women)
Integumentary
• ↓ turgor, moisture, and subcutaneous fat
• Hairline recedes in men
• Loss of melanin in hair shaft causes graying
Respiratory
• Arteries stiffen and blood oxygenation levels decrease
• ↓ maximum breathing capacity
Cardiovascular
• Blood vessels lose elasticity
• ↑ systolic blood pressure
• Heart muscle thickens
• ↓ pumping rate
Gastrointestinal
• Large intestine gradually loses muscle tone
• Constipation
• ↓ gastric secretions

husband. Depression is a common problem among older adults; depressive symptoms increase with age, affecting 15% of people age 85 and older and suicide rates increase as well, especially in men (Federal Interagency Forum on Aging-Related Statistics, 2016).

Considerations for Special Populations

Military Service Members and Veterans

There are approximately 21 million veterans and 3 million active-duty and reserve members of the U.S. military. Less than half of this population use services provided by the Veterans Affairs (VA) health system (Woodall, 2017). This means that most are using civilian healthcare facilities, and that most nurses will at some time or another provide care for a member of this population. Thus, it is important for nurses to have some understanding of military culture, demographics, service-associated healthcare issues, and the implications of such in providing care to this unique population.

Demographics

Presently, there are 1.4 million persons in active-duty military positions in the United States. The Army is the largest branch of military service, followed by the Air Force, Navy, Marine Corps, and Coast Guard, respectively. Of the present-day active force, women now make up almost 15% of its total members, while persons of minority status comprise about 40%. The veteran population today includes persons who served in one or more U.S. conflicts, including World War II (1939–1945), the Korean War (1950–1953), Vietnam War (1964–1975), Desert Shield/Desert Storm (1990–1991), and the Global War on Terror, including Operation Enduring Freedom (OEF) and Operation Iraqi Freedom (OIF) (2001–present). The largest population of living veterans includes those who served in Desert Shield/Desert Storm (the Gulf War), followed by those who served during the Vietnam era. This is important information as those actively serving during these conflicts were potentially exposed to various health-related hazards as a result of their service (Smith & Harris, 2017).

Military Culture

U.S. active-duty military members and veterans are a unique population, multifaceted in their areas of service and experiences. However, all embrace similar views on what it means to be a part of military life. Military culture manifests in covert displays of service-related values, customs, traditions, philosophical principles, and/or behavioral standards (e.g., stoicism). Attributes common in this population include self-discipline, teamwork, loyalty, selfless duty to one's country, order, and procedure, as well as rank and obedience to authority. These attributes are markers of one who embraces military service as a component of his or her identity. Thus, it is critical that the nurse acknowledges the service of this population; offers compassion for those who have experienced, or are experiencing, service-related hardships; and extends respectful care to those seeking it in the healthcare setting.

Service-Related Healthcare Issues

Veterans experience or are at risk for a multitude of health concerns, including combat injuries, mental health issues, illness related to occupational exposure, and the development of chronic conditions.

World War II Veterans. From 1939 until 1945, World War II was fought on three fronts: Land, sea, and air. World War II veterans experience combat-related injuries and illness related to artillery blast injuries and combat fatigue, now termed *posttraumatic stress disorder (PTSD)*. Patients who served in World War II tend to be independent and may be reluctant to report symptoms or ask for help. Nurses need to assess these patients frequently, observe them closely, and support their independence while balancing the importance of safety (Smith & Harris, 2017).

Korean Conflict Veterans. These veterans fought from 1950 until 1953. The Korean conflict is sometimes referred to the Forgotten War. Frostbite was a common injury, resulting in limb loss. Other injuries and illnesses were related to small arms and artillery blasts, hearing loss, and PTSD. Veterans who fought in Korea perceive the conflict to be a full war, although it was not classified as a war. Respecting their service and, like World War II veterans, careful and frequent assessment while supporting autonomy is important (Smith & Harris, 2017).

Vietnam Veterans. Vietnam veterans fought from 1964 until 1973, resulting in over 58,000 deaths. These soldiers endured guerilla warfare, extreme heat, and exposure to Agent Orange, which was a toxic chemical used widely through the Vietnam war. This war was unpopular and soldiers did not receive the admiration and respect soldiers from other wars had experienced. Major injuries and illnesses experienced by Vietnam veterans include wounds from small arms, grenades, and artillery blasts. Significant numbers from this veteran population are also subject to PTSD, tobacco and substance abuse disorders, and hepatitis C. Vietnam veterans are from the Baby Boomer generation and have a strong need to feel valued. They may be more verbal about their needs (Smith & Harris, 2017).

Recent Veterans. Veterans of more recent wars have fought in the conflicts that began in 1990 and continue today. Soldiers fighting Middle East wars have experienced extreme environmental conditions, suffering through extreme heat, sandstorms, urban combat, and an elusive enemy. Many have been injured by improvised explosive devices, resulting in long-term injury related to burns, traumatic brain injury, and amputations. There is also increased prevalence of suicide and domestic violence in this veteran population. Most veterans fighting in the Middle Eastern conflicts come from Generation X and Generation Y. Veterans from these generations like flexibility and are more likely to question authority. The nurse should establish rapport, assess for suicidal ideation, and be prepared to establish boundaries (Smith & Harris, 2017).

Mental health or behavior adjustment issues as well as substance abuse disorders are common in the veteran population. More than 40% of veterans who obtain healthcare are known to have at least one mental or behavioral health disorder. PTSD is experienced by veterans four times more often than for persons who have no military history. PTSD generally occurs after witnessing or experiencing a traumatic event. It can be associated with traumatic brain injury, military sexual trauma, sleep problems, substance use, pain, and other psychiatric disorders.

Veterans who survived traumatic bodily injury or amputation may experience, in addition to mental health challenges, body image issues, sensory/functional deficits, and years of rehabilitative care, not to mention the social stigma and structural barriers associated with the acquisition of physical impairment and/or claiming a disabled identity. All of these service-specific stressors and physical and/or psychological traumas experienced by veterans during their tour(s) of duty make reintegration to civilian life extremely challenging, further compromising their health and access to treatment. In fact, veterans comprise almost 12% of the homeless adult population (Kip et al., 2016). Disability, unemployment (due to lack of skills transferrable to civilian work), mental and physical health issues, and substance abuse are primary factors that make it difficult for veterans to experience any sense of stability postdeployment. This situation has a direct impact on their health-seeking behaviors, access to healthcare, rehabilitation, healing treatments, and other care needed to restore and/or improve their health.

Many veterans were previously exposed to hazardous chemicals (Agent Orange, contaminated water), radiation (nuclear weapons, x-rays), air pollutants (burn pit smoke, dust), occupational hazards (asbestos, lead), warfare agents (chemical and biological weapons), excessive noise, and vibration from working with machinery (U.S. Department of Veterans Affairs, 2017). In addition, some veterans were given vaccinations for protection against hazardous exposures (e.g., anthrax vaccine), despite the lack of available evidence of long-term health consequences. As such, some vaccinations given to this population remain under investigation today as medically unexplainable health problems continue to arise and be reported by the veterans who received them.

Any of these hazardous exposures (including vaccination serums) may have immediate and/or long-term consequences for the health of the veteran who was exposed. Certain cancers, medically unexplained illnesses (Gulf War syndrome), infectious diseases, thyroid disease, ischemic heart disease, amyotrophic lateral sclerosis (ALS), type 2 diabetes, Parkinson disease, peripheral neuropathy, liver dysfunction, and other health problems are presumed associated with specific exposures during military service.

Nursing Implications

It is important for nurses caring for veterans to complete a military-specific, service-related health history to ascertain information on current physical, emotional, psychological, socio-cultural, and spiritual health issues. In addition, nurses need to assess patients who are veterans for historical hazardous exposures (type and duration) and consider their impact on the veteran's current health situation, surgical/treatment course, and/or future health status.

Gender and Sexual Minorities

More than 10 million people in the United States identify as being lesbian, gay, bisexual, transgender, queer, or intersex (LGBTQI), and this number is growing and becoming more visible based on prior years' population data, positive changes in societal attitudes, and the enactment of more inclusive state and federal laws (Woodall, 2017). However, individuals who are LGBTQI continue to experience health disparities due to historical and ongoing stigmatization, and this shapes how they perceive and interact with others, including healthcare professionals. In fact, many report reluctance to reveal their sexual orientation or gender identity to healthcare providers. Thus, it is important that healthcare professionals create a safe, affirming environment in which LGBTQI patients feel comfortable volunteering information.

Transgender is an umbrella term that covers a range of identities that transgress social gender norms. This group includes persons whose gender identity differs from their anatomical sex or whose gender expression varies significantly from what is traditionally associated with that sex. Importantly, transgender persons may vary from or reject traditional cultural conceptualizations of gender in terms of the male–female dichotomy, or "binary." As well, this population is varied in sexual expression and sexual orientation.

Nursing Implications

Nursing care specific to the LGBTQI population focuses on establishing a welcoming environment that facilitates nurse–patient trust building. Providing culturally competent, patient-centered care to members of the LGBTQI community is really no different than providing care to any other individuals. Moreover, the nurse working with *any* patient should use gender-neutral language and avoid unintentional assumptions of heterosexuality. During initial nurse–patient introductions, the nurse should ask the patient what name and pronoun the patient wants the healthcare team to use in speaking to or about the patient. Nurses should also avoid making assumptions about the gender, sexual orientation, and role/status of the patient's support persons or visitors. When completing a physical assessment, it is essential to structure it based on the patient's organs that are present, rather than by perceived or assumed gender. If gathering a health history, the nurse should ask about specific sexual activities in a nonjudgmental manner and assess risk behaviors. Transgender persons have higher rates of depression and anxiety compared to others. Therefore, the nurse should assess for such, implement the appropriate screening mechanisms, and ensure the patient receives necessary treatment if applicable and desired by the patient. Also, nurses need to keep in mind that signs and symptoms of depression and anxiety may be heightened for transgender persons who do not have adequate social support or who are unable to express their gender identity.

Hormone therapy is common within the transgender population, although evidence is lacking on the long-term effects of hormone therapy in this group. What is known is that testosterone can damage the liver, especially if taken in high doses or by mouth. Estrogen can increase blood pressure, blood glucose (sugar), and blood clotting. Antiandrogens, such as spironolactone, can lower blood pressure, disturb electrolytes, and dehydrate the body. It is important that the nurse has knowledge of whether or not the patient is on a hormone regimen.

In summary, culturally competent care necessitates that healthcare professionals conduct a critical self-assessment of their personal knowledge, attitudes, assumptions, and unconscious biases relevant to patients of different backgrounds than their own. The results of this self-assessment will assist the healthcare professional in identifying gaps in knowledge and opportunities for further exploration/education about the unique attributes and healthcare needs of various populations. Lifelong learning is a professional expectation of nurses. Thus, intentionally educating oneself about that which is unknown or foreign from one's own experience serves to enhance understanding and promote competence in providing patient-centered care to persons from a diverse array of communities/populations

Adults with Sequelae from Congenital/Childhood Conditions

During the last decades, dramatic progress has been made in the survival rates for children suffering from illnesses such as congenital heart defects, childhood cancers, and cystic fibrosis. Currently 1.4 million adults live with a congenital heart defect in the United States (Gilboa et al., 2016). More than 80% of children treated for pediatric malignancy survive into adulthood. In the past, children diagnosed with cystic fibrosis were not expected to survive past early adolescence. Now over 50% of people with cystic fibrosis are over 18 years old (Cystic Fibrosis Foundation, 2018). Surviving serious childhood illness has an impact on adult health.

Adults Surviving Childhood Cancers

The term **late effects** is used to describe health problems that occur months or years after the treatment for cancer has ended. Anywhere from 60% to more than 90% of survivors of childhood cancer go on to develop one or more chronic health conditions and 20 to 80% experience severe or life-threatening complications during adulthood (National Cancer Institute, 2018). There are three important factors that contribute to the increased risk of late effects:

1. Tumor-related factors
   - Type of cancer
   - Where the tumor was in the body
   - How the tumor affects the way tissue and organs function
2. Treatment-related factors
   - Type of surgery
   - Chemotherapy type, dose, and schedule
   - Type of radiation therapy
   - Stem cell transplant
   - Use of two or more treatments at a time
   - Blood product transfusion
   - Chronic graft-versus-host disease
3. Patient-related factors
   - Patient's sex
   - Other noncancer health problems
   - The age and developmental state of the patient when diagnosed and treated
   - Length of time since diagnosis and treatment
   - Changes in hormone levels
   - Inherent tissue sensitivities and capacity for normal tissue repair
   - Function of organs not affected by cancer treatment
   - Socioeconomic status
   - Health habits.

Adults with Congenital Heart Defects

Most patients with congestive heart defects (CHD) require lifelong cardiac care. Recent data indicate that more than 40% of adults with CHD report a gap of at least of 3 years (Gilboa et al., 2016). Adults with CHD need to be monitored for the development of complications such as arrhythmias and pulmonary hypertension and should receive follow-up in a regional center for adults with CHD at least once or twice annually (Gilboa et al., 2016).

Nursing Implications

The primary focus of long-term follow-up for patients who have survived serious childhood illness is to facilitate access to routine and comprehensive health screening to identify worsening comorbid chronic conditions or new complications. Typically, survivors need multidisciplinary long-term follow-up programs. The nurse should contribute to the development of a care plan that identifies personalized health screening recommendations and provides information about health promotion and lifestyle that modify risks. Identifying possible complications of serious childhood illness should be a focus when the survivor is hospitalized. Careful assessment and monitoring should be included in the care plan. Supporting the individual and family throughout acute episodic illness as adults should address the possible psychosocial influence of previous hospitalization and encounters with the healthcare system as a child.

Ensuring the patient has a comprehensive discharge plan and facilitating the transition from one setting to another includes implications of the childhood illness that should be considered in ongoing and comprehensive care.

2.2 Health Promotion and Maintenance

The U.S. Department of Health and Human Services has published national public health objectives each decade since 1980. *Healthy People 2020* (HHS, 2018) provides a foundation for disease prevention and wellness activities across public and private sectors, as well as a model for measuring achievement of identified goals and objectives. Broad goals for the current decade are described in **Box 2.1**.

The nurse promotes health by teaching the activities that maintain wellness:

- *Screening:* Reviewing the health screenings a patient should be accessing and facilitating referrals as appropriate
- *Immunization:* Reviewing immunization records and assisting the patient with access to immunizations as scheduled
- *Health teaching:* The nurse is critical to health promotion as an educator. Patient teaching is a crucial nursing action in every healthcare setting and in the majority of nurse–patient encounters.

Health teaching includes providing information about the characteristics and consequences of diseases when risk factors have been identified and by supplying specific information about decreasing risk factors (Pender et al., 2015). Teaching the side effects of treatments and medications, identifying complications, and providing reputable resources the patient can use and learn about to support healthy lifestyles and disease prevention (e.g., American Heart Association, American Cancer Society) are important health promotion interventions. Health teaching and coaching is an essential component of the nursing role for patients with chronic conditions.

The nurse also promotes health by following healthy practices and serving as a role model. Setting activity goals, self-monitoring, and prescribing exercise are examples of behavioral strategies.

Health promotion for individuals is directed at increasing well-being and maximizing potential (Pender et al., 2015). Health promotion goes beyond disease prevention (e.g., maintaining immunization status) and includes health screening, promoting healthy lifestyle, and managing chronic illness. Teaching health-promoting behaviors is an essential component of medical-surgical nursing.

Healthy behaviors that are known to promote health and wellness include:

- Eat a balanced diet, following two overarching concepts: (1) Maintain calorie balance over time to achieve and sustain a healthy weight; and (2) focus on consuming nutrient-dense foods and beverages. The U.S. Department of Agriculture provides a general guideline of what to eat each day in their MyPlate program (see Chapter 21).
- Exercise moderately and regularly, engaging in at least 30 minutes of continuous activity (such as walking) 5 or more days per week.
- Sleep 7 to 8 hours each day.
- Eliminate smoking and use of other tobacco products such as smokeless tobacco. Limit alcohol intake.

BOX 2.1
Healthy People 2020: Overarching Goals

With a vision of "a society in which all people live long, healthy lives" and the overall mission of improving the nation's health, *Healthy People 2020* has four major goals. These goals address factors that contribute to the health status of individuals or populations and include social and physical determinants of health.

OVERARCHING GOALS

- Attain high-quality, longer lives free of preventable disease, disability, injury, and premature death.
- Achieve health equity, eliminate disparities, and improve the health of all groups.
- Create social and physical environments that promote good health for all.
- Promote quality of life, healthy development, and healthy behaviors across all life stages.

Health Indicators

Health indicators address determinants of health and provide a means of assessing the nation's health. These are organized under 12 areas:

- Access to health services (people with health insurance, people with a usual primary care provider)
- Clinical preventive services (e.g., cancer screening, hypertension management)
- Environmental quality (air quality, exposure to secondhand smoke)
- Injury and violence
- Maternal, infant, and child health (infant deaths, preterm deaths)
- Mental health (suicides, major depressive episodes in adolescents)
- Nutrition, physical activity, and obesity (e.g., obesity in adults and children, vegetable intake)
- Oral health
- Reproductive and sexual health
- Social determinants (high school graduation rates)
- Substance abuse (e.g., binge drinking, alcohol or illicit drug use in adolescents)
- Tobacco use.

Source: HHS, 2018.

- Keep sun exposure to a minimum; use sunscreen liberally when out of doors.
- Practice safe sex (monogamy, use of barrier protection).
- Have regular dental examinations and cleanings.
- Maintain recommended immunizations (current recommendations can be accessed at *http://www.cdc.gov/vaccines/schedules/hcp/adult.html*.

Follow the guidelines for recommended health promotion activities in **Table 2.4**.

2.3 Disease, Illness, and Injury

Disease and *illness* are terms that are often used interchangeably, but in fact they have different meanings.

Disease

Disease (literally meaning "without ease") is defined as any alteration in a body system or organ structure or function.

Table 2.4 Recommended Health Promotion Activities for Adults

Age Group	Activity
Young adults	■ Routine physical examination (every 1–3 years for females; every 5 years for males) ■ Immunizations as recommended, such as tetanus-diphtheria boosters every 10 years, meningococcal vaccine if not given in early adolescence, annual influenza vaccines (CDC, 2018d), hepatitis B vaccine, and HPV vaccine (CDC, 2017c) ■ Alcohol and drug screening. ■ Regular dental assessments (every 6 months) ■ Risk-based assessment of vision at age 18 (AAP, 2015) ■ Professional breast examination every 1–3 years for women ■ Screening women for cervical dysplasia starting at 21 years old (AAP, 2015). Pap test pattern: Age 21–29 every 3 years, age 30–65 every 3 years or Pap and HPV test every 5 years (ACS, 2018) ■ Testicular examination every year for men ■ Screening for cardiovascular disease (e.g., cholesterol test every 5 years if results are normal; blood pressure to detect hypertension; baseline electrocardiogram at age 35 if indicated) ■ Diabetes mellitus screen every 3 years, if in high-risk group (National Diabetes Education Initiative [NDEI], 2016) ■ Smoking: History and counseling, if needed ■ Education about career efforts and personal balance, stress management, sexuality, safety promotion, and accident prevention
Middle adults	■ Physical examination (every 3–5 years until age 40, then annually) ■ Immunizations as recommended, such as a tetanus booster every 10 years and annual influenza vaccines (CDC, 2018d) ■ Regular dental assessments (e.g., every 6 months) ■ Tonometry for signs of glaucoma and other eye diseases every 2–3 years or annually, if indicated ■ Breast examination for women annually by primary care provider. For age 40–44, choice of getting mammogram; for age 45–54, annual mammogram; starting at age 55, mammogram annually or every 2 years (ACS, 2018) ■ Screen women for cervical dysplasia with a Pap test every 3 years until age 65 or Pap and HPV test every 5 years (ACS, 2018) ■ Testicular examination for men annually by primary care provider. PSA testing might start at age 50 or age 45 for African Americans with positive history (ACS, 2018) ■ Screenings for cardiovascular disease (e.g., blood pressure measurement; electrocardiogram and cholesterol test as directed by the primary care provider) ■ Diabetes mellitus screen every 3 years, if in high-risk group (NDEI, 2016) ■ Starting at age 45, screenings for colorectal cancer: Stool-based test or flexible sigmoidoscopy every 5 years or colonoscopy every 10 years (ACS, 2018) ■ Smoking: History and counseling, if needed. Starting at age 55, low-dose CT chest scan annually if 30 pack-year smoking history, current smoker, or quit within the last 15 years (ACS, 2018) ■ Education about adequate sleep, weight control, medication compliance, and accident prevention
Older adults	■ Regular dental assessments (e.g., every 6 months) ■ Tonometry for signs of glaucoma and other eye diseases every 2–3 years or annually, if indicated ■ Total cholesterol and high-density lipoprotein measurement every 3–5 years until age 75 ■ Aspirin, 81 mg daily, if in high-risk group ■ Diabetes mellitus screen every 3 years, if in high-risk group (NDEI, 2016) ■ Smoking: History and counseling, if needed. Until age 74, low-dose CT chest scan annually if 30 pack-year smoking history, current smoker, or quit within the last 15 years (ACS, 2018) ■ Breast examination for women annually by primary care provider; mammogram annually or every 2 years (ACS, 2018) ■ Pap smear (women) only if previous abnormal smears, serious cervical pre-cancer, or hysterectomy for malignancy (ACS, 2018) ■ Annual digital rectal exam ■ Testicular examination for men annually by primary care provider. PSA testing by choice, with repeat frequency depending on PSA level (ACS, 2018) ■ Annual guaiac-based fecal occult blood test (gFOBT) or fecal immunochemical test (FIT) or stool DNA test (sDNA) every 3 years (ACS, 2018) ■ Screenings for colorectal cancer: After age 75, discuss with provider; after age 85, colorectal screening is no longer needed (ACS, 2018) ■ Visual acuity and hearing screen annually ■ Depression screen and family violence screen periodically ■ Height and weight measurements annually ■ Sexually transmitted infection testing, if in high-risk group; screening for HIV and hepatitis C if indicated ■ Annual flu vaccine; high-dose vaccine if over age 65 or in high-risk group (CDC, 2018d) ■ Two pneumococcal vaccines, PCV13 and PPSV23, at 65 (CDC, 2017a) ■ Two doses of shingles vaccine for adults age 50 or older ■ Tetanus booster every 10 years ■ Education about restful sleep, adequate nutrition, maximization of strengths, medication compliance, and accident prevention

Diseases are characterized by identifiable signs and symptoms and usually a recognized pathophysiologic process and etiology, although the cause of many diseases is still unknown. Diseases are generally categorized as either congenital (present at birth) or acquired (caused by events that occur after birth) (Sorenson, Quinn, & Klein, 2019). We now recognize that many diseases involve the interaction of a genetic predisposition and environmental factors. Recognized causes of disease include:

- Genetic variations
- Environmental factors such as exposure to viruses, chemicals, or drugs that affect the developing fetus
- Infectious agents
- Tissue injury due to lack of oxygen, temperature extremes, radiation, or toxins (e.g., alcohol, drugs, cigarette smoke)
- Poor nutrition (obesity, malnutrition)
- Inadequate or disordered immune responses
- Neoplasia.

Diseases may be classified as acute or chronic, communicable, congenital, degenerative, functional, malignant, idiopathic, or iatrogenic. These classifications are defined in **Table 2.5**. In all types of disease, alterations in structure or function cause signs and symptoms (**manifestations**) that prompt an individual to seek treatment from a physician or traditional healer. Both subjective symptoms and objective signs are commonly present. Subjective symptoms may include such manifestations as nausea, general malaise, fatigue, chest pain, shortness of breath, or abdominal pain. Bleeding, vomiting, diarrhea, limited movement, swelling, and changes in elimination are all examples of objective signs. Pain (a subjective symptom) is often the primary reason that prompts an individual to seek healthcare.

Illness

Illness is the response an individual has to a disease. This response is highly individualized because the individual responds not only to his or her own perceptions of the disease but also to the perceptions of others. Illness integrates pathophysiologic alterations; the psychologic effects of those alterations; the effects on roles, relationships, and values; and cultural and spiritual beliefs. An individual may have a disease and not categorize him- or herself as ill or may validate feelings of illness through the comments of others ("You don't look as though you feel well today").

Acute Illness

An **acute illness** occurs rapidly, lasts for a relatively short time, and is self-limiting. The condition responds to self-treatment or to medical-surgical intervention. Patients with uncomplicated acute illnesses usually have full recovery and return to normal preillness functioning.

Critical illness is a subcategory of acute care. Critically ill patients typically require life-sustaining treatments and intense monitoring of vital signs and other complex physiological data involving specialized equipment. The American Association of Critical-Care Nurses (Harden & Kaplow, 2017) describes critically ill patients as individuals who are at high risk for actual or potential life-threatening health problems. The more critically ill the patient is, the more likely he or she to be highly vulnerable, unstable, complex, and in need of intensive and vigilant nursing care. Several common critical diseases and injuries are addressed in chapters related to the major systems involved (**Table 2.6**).

Illness behaviors are highly individualized and are influenced by age, gender, family values, socioeconomic status, culture, educational level, and mental status. The commonly recognized sequence of illness behaviors follows.

1. ***Experiencing symptoms.*** In the first stage of an acute illness, an individual experiences one or more manifestations such as pain, fever, bleeding, or swelling that prompt awareness of a change in normal health. If the manifestations are mild or are familiar (such as symptoms of the common cold or influenza), the individual usually uses a traditional remedy for self-treatment such as rest or OTC medications. If the symptoms are relieved, no further action is taken; however, if the symptoms are severe or become worse, the individual moves to the next stage.

Table 2.5 Disease Classifications and Definitions

Classification	Definition
Acute	A disease that has a rapid onset, lasts a relatively short time, and is self-limiting
Chronic	A disease that requires continuing management over a long period—years or even decades
Communicable	A disease that can spread from one person to another
Congenital	A disease or disorder that exists at or before birth
Degenerative	A disease that results from deterioration or impairment of organs or tissues
Functional	A disease that affects function or performance but does not have evidence of organic changes
Malignant	A disease that tends to become worse and cause death
Idiopathic	A disease that has an unknown cause
Iatrogenic	A disease that is caused by medical therapy

Table 2.6 Critical Illness Coverage

Critical Illness	Covered In
Acute heart failure	Chapter 31, Section 31.1, Heart Failure
Cancer	Chapter 14 for overall cancer care; specific cancers are covered in relevant chapters
End-stage renal disease	Chapter 28, Section 28.2, Kidney Failure; subsection The Patient with Chronic Kidney Disease
Major organ transplantation ▪ Heart transplantation ▪ Kidney transplantation	Chapter 31, Section 31.1, Heart Failure; subsection Cardiac Transplantation Chapter 28, Section 28.2, Kidney Failure, subsection Kidney Transplantation
Respiratory failure	Chapter 37, Section 37.4, Respiratory Failure
Severe burns	Chapter 17, Section 17.5, Major Burns
Shock	Chapter 11, Section 11.3, Shock, and Section 11.4, The Patient Experiencing Shock
Traumatic brain injury	Chapter 42, Section 42.6, Traumatic Brain Injury

2. ***Assuming the sick role.*** In the second stage of illness behavior, the individual assumes the sick role, accepting the symptoms as indicative of an illness. A focus on alterations in function resulting from the illness is characteristic of this stage. If the illness is resolved, the individual resumes normal activities; however, if manifestations remain or increase in severity, the individual moves to the next stage by seeking medical care.
3. ***Seeking medical care.*** In our society, a physician or other healthcare provider usually provides validation of illness. People who believe themselves to be ill (and who are encouraged by others to contact a healthcare provider) make the medical contact for diagnosis, prognosis, and treatment of the illness. If the medical diagnosis is of an illness, the individual moves to the next stage.
4. ***Assuming a dependent role.*** The stage of assuming a dependent role begins when an individual accepts the diagnosis and planned treatment of the illness. The responses of the individual to care depend on many different variables: The severity of the illness, the degree of anxiety or fear about the outcome, the loss of roles, the support systems available, individualized reactions to stress, and previous experiences with illness care. The cause and severity of the illness and the individual's resources affect whether the individual moves to the next stage, recovery and rehabilitation, or to chronic illness or even death.
5. ***Achieving recovery and rehabilitation.*** The final stage of an acute illness is recovery and rehabilitation. The individual gives up the dependent role and resumes normal roles and responsibilities.

Chronic Illness

Chronic illness is a term that encompasses many different long-term pathologic and psychologic alterations in health. It is the leading health problem in the world today, accounting for 70% of all deaths in the United States (CDC, 2017b). Nearly half of all adults in the United States have at least one chronic disease; many of those have multiple chronic diseases. As a result, chronic disease management and treatment account for more than 85% of healthcare spending (CDC, 2017b). The incidence and prevalence of chronic illness are increasing, and that trend is predicted to continue. Heart disease, cancer, and stroke cause more than 50% of all deaths annually. Current trends contributing to an increased incidence of chronic illnesses include an aging population, diseases of lifestyle and behavior (e.g., obesity, smoking), and environmental factors. The staggering physical, psychosocial, and economic costs of chronic illness have made its prevention and effective management a focus of the Affordable Care Act of 2010.

Chronic illness is defined as a condition that requires continuing management over a long period—years or even decades. Chronic diseases include communicable diseases such as tuberculosis and HIV infection and noncommunicable diseases such as cancer, heart disease, diabetes, and chronic lung disease; long-term mental health disorders such as schizophrenia; and physical, sensory, or structural impairments (e.g., arthritis, visual impairment). Four common behavioral risk factors account for most chronic disease: Lack of physical activity, poor nutrition, tobacco use, and excessive alcohol consumption (CDC, 2018a, 2018c).

Additionally, recent research has identified a link between **adverse childhood experience (ACE)** and chronic illness. The ACE study found a relationship between an accumulation of risky lifestyle behaviors and the development of chronic disease, disability, and early death (see **Figure 2.5** ■). The ACE screening questionnaire is used to calculate an ACE score and assesses childhood exposure to psychological, physical, and sexual abuse; household dysfunction; substance abuse; and mental illness. Witnessing domestic violence and or criminal behavior in the household as a child contributes to the ACE test score (CDC, 2016; Zarnello, 2018).

The intensity of a chronic illness and its related manifestations range from mild to severe. More than one body system is often affected. With effective management, many chronic diseases can remain stable for extended periods of time. Often, however, patients experience progressive symptoms and periodic acute crises. Some chronic diseases are characterized by periods of remission and exacerbation. During periods of **remission**, the individual does not experience symptoms, even though the disease is still clinically present. During periods of **exacerbation**, the symptoms reappear.

Each person with a chronic illness has a unique set of responses and needs. The response of the individual to the illness is influenced by factors such as the disease itself; the life state at which it develops; the effect of disease-related limitations on physical, psychologic, and social functioning; and emotional responses to the illness. These factors are highly complex and interrelated, resulting in individualized illness behaviors and needs. Although the experience of each person with a chronic illness is unique, people with chronic illness face common challenges, including:

- Recognizing and appropriately responding to symptoms
- Using medications effectively (**Figure 2.6** ■)
- Learning to manage an ongoing treatment plan
- Modifying lifestyle to adapt to and minimize the impact of the disease
- Developing effective strategies for coping with the psychosocial effects of chronic illness
- Maintaining a feeling of being in control
- Interacting effectively with the healthcare system on an ongoing basis.

Many people with chronic illness successfully manage health-related needs, whereas others do not. Research indicates that adaptation is influenced by variables such as anger, depression, denial, self-concept, locus of control, hardiness, and disability. Nurses play an increasingly important role in promoting independent functioning, reducing healthcare costs, and improving well-being and quality of life for patients with chronic illnesses.

Illness Prevention

In addition to health promotion goals and activities as outlined in *Healthy People 2020*, actions taken by the individual patient and healthcare provider to prevent illness and limit its progression are important. Three levels of illness prevention have been defined: Primary, secondary, and tertiary prevention.

1. ***Primary prevention*** focuses on activities and specific actions to prevent disease by eliminating risk factors for disease to the extent possible. Primary prevention often occurs within communities outside the healthcare system. In some cases, primary prevention measures are legislated, such as clean air and water standards and the use of seat belts in automobiles. Following are examples of primary prevention activities:
   - Eating nutritious foods and balancing calorie intake with energy expenditure
   - Reducing exposure to industrial hazards such as noise and dust
   - Practicing safer sex
   - Obtaining immunizations
   - Eliminating the use of alcohol and cigarettes
   - Avoiding cell phone use and texting while driving.
2. ***Secondary prevention***, which usually occurs within the healthcare system, involves activities that emphasize early diagnosis and treatment of disease to effect an early cure or prevent disease progression (Sorenson

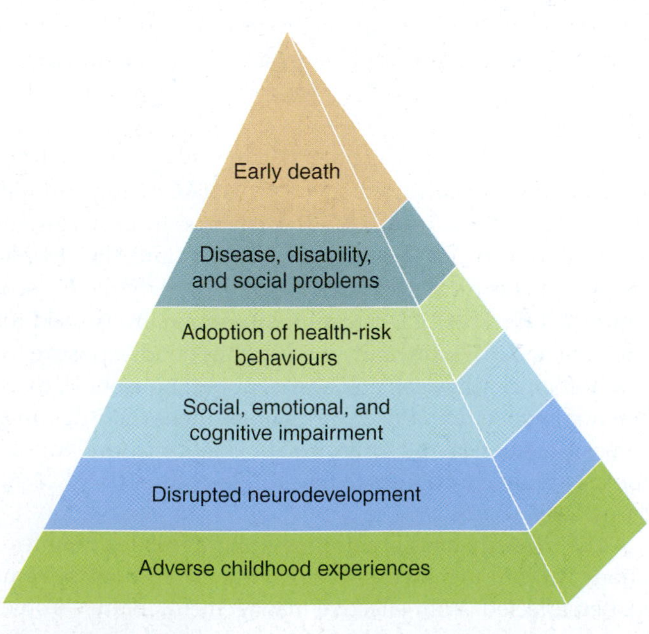
Death
Early death
Disease, disability, and social problems
Adoption of health-risk behaviours
Social, emotional, and cognitive impairment
Disrupted neurodevelopment
Adverse childhood experiences
Conception

Figure 2.5 ■ Adverse childhood experience (ACE) has been linked to chronic illness, disability, and early death.

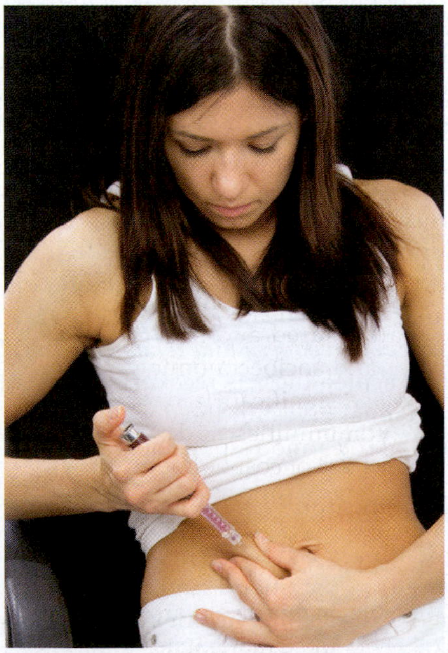

Figure 2.6 ■ Patients with a chronic illness such as diabetes must learn to manage their disorder, including using medications.

et al., 2019). Following are examples of secondary prevention activities:

- Screening for common diseases such as hypertension, diabetes mellitus, malignancies, and glaucoma
- Obtaining regular physical examinations
- Performing self-examination for breast and/or testicular cancer
- Obtaining specific treatment for illness (e.g., treatment of streptococcal infections of the throat helps prevent secondary disorders involving the heart and/or kidneys).

3. ***Tertiary prevention*** focuses on preventing further health decline and reducing complications associated with disease. The goal is to return and maintain the affected individual at his or her highest possible level of function. For acute illness, tertiary prevention activities primarily revolve around rehabilitation, such as:
   - Specific rehabilitation programs for cardiovascular problems, head injuries, and strokes
   - Work training programs following illness or injury
   - Educating the public to employ rehabilitated people to the fullest possible extent.
4. Tertiary prevention activities for the individual with chronic illness focus on effective disease management to promote high-level functioning and prevent acute crises. Recognition of spiraling costs has led to an increased focus on and initiatives to promote coordinated interprofessional primary care for patients with multiple chronic conditions and complex care needs. Nurses play a significant role in several evidence-based models for chronic care, as outlined in the following section of this chapter.

Injury and Violence

Injury and violence affect everyone and the medical-surgical nurse will provide care for patients and families experiencing health-related problems created by these unexpected and unintended events (**Figure 2.7** ■). In the first half of life, more Americans die from violence and injury than any other cause (CDC, 2018b). Approximately 214,000 people die from injury every year. Millions of people are injured and survive, facing life-long mental, physical, and socioeconomic challenges. Injury and violence have a significant economic impact on individuals, families, communities, and country. The CDC (2018b) estimated the total of cost of injury and violence in the United States was $671 billion in 2013. The CDC is focused on research and prevention strategies that address the following problems:

- Motor vehicle crashes are a leading cause of death and injury in the United States
- Opioid overdoses have quadrupled since 1999, with more than 15,000 people dying from prescription opioid overdoses in 2015

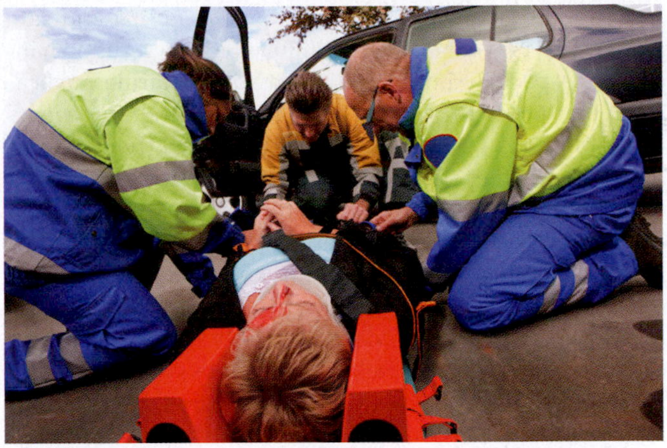

Figure 2.7 ■ Motor vehicle crashes are the leading cause of death and injury in the United States.

- 2.8 million older adults are treated in emergency departments for fall injuries
- On average, 20 people per minute are victims of physical violence by an intimate partner in the United States
- Nearly 1 in 5 women (18.3%) and 1 in 71 men (1.4%) have been raped in their lifetime.

Nurses and other healthcare professionals are at increased risk for occupational injury and workplace violence. The Occupational Safety and Health Administration (OSHA) (U.S. Department of Labor, n.d.) has identified healthcare workers as one of the most likely groups to experience some type of security-related incident. Most of the focus has been on violence-related experiences in acute care hospitals. However, OSHA has identified other settings in which workplace violence protocols should be implemented, including:

- Residential treatment settings such as nursing homes
- Nonresidential treatment/service settings such as small neighborhood clinics and mental health centers
- Community care settings such as residential facilities and group homes
- Fieldwork settings such as homes where healthcare nurses and other members of the team make visits.

Injury Prevention

Injury prevention involves patient teaching regarding safe practices in many areas; a common example is motor vehicle operation. Teaching patients the importance of wearing seat belts, obeying traffic laws, and avoiding driving while under the influence of alcohol and other substances are topics to be addressed. Reminders to avoid driving when sleep deprived and the correlation between fatigue and automobile crashes can be included when discussing injury prevention. Use of safety gear such as wearing a helmet when riding a bike or participating in high-speed sports such as downhill skiing should be emphasized.

Nurses should comply with agency policy and safe practices to prevent on-the-job injury. Safe medication handling is especially important when administering medications that are highly toxic, such as chemotherapy agents (Callahan, et al., 2016). Adherence to safe handling of needles and other sharps prevents harm to the nurse using such equipment and other personnel who can be exposed to equipment that has not been disposed of properly. Safe patient handling will prevent musculoskeletal injuries that can lead to chronic pain. The nursing leadership goals related to safety include adopting highly standardized processes such as safety checks, transparent communication including use of the SBAR format (situation, background, assessment, and recommendation, which is described in Chapter 4) when handing off care (Stewart & Hand, 2017), and interprofessional collaboration. A large multisite study demonstrated a strong positive correlation between nurses' perceptions of workforce safety and patient outcomes (Press Ganey, 2016).

2.4 Types of Nursing Care

Transformative changes are occurring in healthcare. Factors driving healthcare transformation include fragmented care between settings, access problems, unsustainable costs, and disparities in health outcomes among the population (Salmond & Echevarria, 2017). Greater coordination of care across providers and across settings will reduce hospitalizations due to poor management of chronic illness, and improve support and outcomes for patients managing complex self-care regimens. Because of the nursing role, respect for the profession, and their education and practice emphasizing holistic care, nurses are positioned to lead and perform as a full member of the healthcare team. As we shift from episodic, provider-based care to team-based, patient-centered care, new roles and practice settings for nurses will emerge (Salmond & Echevarria, 2017).

Payment systems for prevention, care coordination, and care management will solidify the roles that involve nursing interventions: New roles include focus of care on health promotion, disease prevention, and chronic disease management, with an emphasis of providing and coordinating care during acute care episodes and at the end of life. These foci of care will be delivered across settings with an aim toward seamless transition so patients receive a continuum of preventive and curative services according to their unique needs over time (WHO, 2008). Discussion of health problems throughout this text are organized according to these four roles of nursing care:

- *Health promotion and disease prevention* strategies address nursing action and role in preventing the health malady being discussed (e.g., dietary guidelines to prevent disease).
- *Acute care* nursing interventions focus on vigilant assessment for early recognition of complications and/or deteriorating condition, administering treatments to restore health and preparing patients for the next care setting once the disease/illness condition is stabilized.
- *Chronic care* is typically focused on care coordination and support of the patient and caregiver's self-care. Managing symptoms, preventing complications, and delaying disease progression through ongoing assessment, health teaching, and coaching are primary nursing care activities.
- *End-of-life care* focuses on symptom management that includes continuous nursing assessments and adjusting medications to achieve optimum pain control and comfort. Supporting the patient and caregivers and securing needed resources are important nursing actions throughout this phase of illness.

Emphasis on the nurse as a member of the interprofessional healthcare team applies across the focus of care and all healthcare settings.

In the healthcare system of the 21st century, hospitals are primarily acute care providers, but acute care is also provided in skilled nursing facilities, specialized clinics and in homes. Acute care services use high-technology care for ill or injured people or for people having surgery. Healthcare has become a managed care, community-based system, in which most healthcare services are provided outside the hospital. The Affordable Care Act of 2010 places increasing emphasis on effective patient management to prevent hospital admission or readmission following discharge. Discussion of selected current models and alternate settings of care follows. It is important to note that these models and settings are not mutually exclusive; for example, primary care is often delivered in community-based settings, and disease management often occurs within programs associated with acute medical centers.

Primary Care

Primary care is comprehensive first-contact health and illness care across the lifespan. Preventive care services as well as care for acute and chronic diseases are encompassed within the primary care model (Bauer & Bodenheimer, 2017). The American Academy of Ambulatory Care Nursing (2017) has developed core competencies to guide nursing practice in primary care settings.

Primary care settings are increasingly diverse. While traditionally delivered by physician-led teams within a physician's office or clinic, primary care increasingly occurs in retail walk-in clinics, hospital-affiliated practices, workplace settings, and in nonphysician provider practices (Bauer & Bodenheimer, 2017). Primary care is emphasizing health screening for underserved populations such as military veterans (Mohler & Sankey-Deemer, 2017) and also includes specialized care such as palliative care (Gorman, 2016). The nursing role is expanding in primary care, as a shortage of physician primary care providers increases. The nursing role in primary care is evolving to integrated nursing actions related to chronic care management and population health focus (Bauer & Bodenheimer, 2017).

The **patient-centered medical home (PCMH)**, also called a *healthcare home*, is a primary care model that focuses on all levels of illness prevention. The PCMH, led by a primary care provider (e.g., physician, nurse practitioner), is designed to provide accessible, comprehensive, and coordinated patient and family care within the community (Salmond & Echevarria, 2017; Spahr, Coddington, Edwards, & McComb, 2018). For people with chronic illnesses, the goal of the PCMH is to provide comprehensive care with a focus on preventing acute disease crises. In addition to the primary care provider, the PCMH interprofessional team often includes care coordinators or case managers, a role often filled by nurses, as well as social workers and rehabilitation therapists. Basic facets of the PCMH include an ongoing patient–primary care team relationship, responsibility for total patient care, improving access to care and reducing health disparities, increasing preventive services, and improving chronic disease management (Salmond & Echevarria, 2017; Spahr et al., 2018).

Care and Disease Management

In the care management model for chronically ill patients and their families, a nurse or social worker helps assess problems, communicate with healthcare providers, and navigate the healthcare system (Salmond & Echevarria, 2017). Under the care management model, patients report improved satisfaction and quality of care; quality of life and survival are also improved.

Improved patient outcomes are also demonstrated with the disease management model. This model focuses on providing education and instruction about the disease (e.g., heart failure, diabetes mellitus, chronic obstructive pulmonary disease), its management, self-monitoring, and interactions with healthcare providers.

Transitional Care

Transitional care focuses on interventions to facilitate transitions from one healthcare setting to another or to home (Elliott & DeAngelis, 2017). Transitional care interventions to prepare the patient and caregiver for transitions are typically led by a nurse or advanced practice nurse. Interventions include development of an evidence-based plan of care, ongoing support, and an emphasis on early identification of and response to risks and symptoms to avoid adverse events. The goal of transitional care is to improve the care and outcomes of chronically ill patients by streamlining plans of care, improving the ability of patients and caregivers to manage care needs, and interrupting patterns of frequent acute health crises (Elliot & DeAngelis, 2017; Salmond & Echevarria, 2017; Spahr et al., 2018).

Community-Based Care

Community-based care is a primary care model that centers on individual and family healthcare needs. In contrast to community health nursing, which focuses on the health of the community, the nurse in community-based care settings provides direct services to individuals to manage acute or chronic health problems and to promote self-care. The care is provided in the local community, is culturally competent, and is family centered. The philosophy of community-based nursing directs nursing care for patients wherever they are, including where they live, work, play, worship, and go to school (**Figure 2.8** ■).

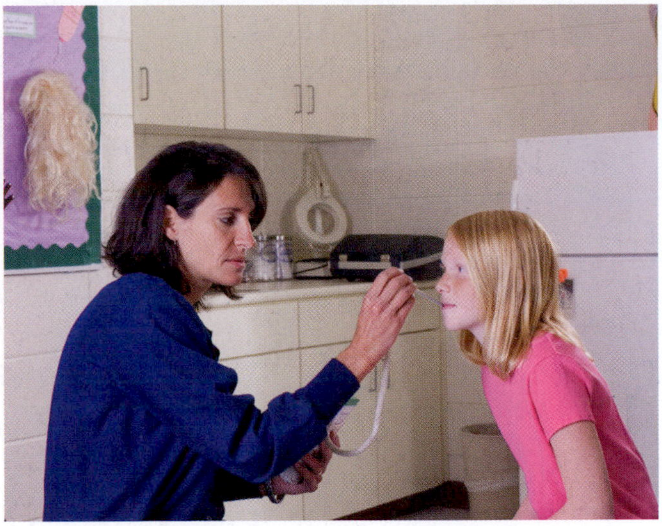

Figure 2.8 ■ According to the National Association of School Nurses (2017), there are over 90,000 full-time equivalent school nurses in the United States delivering care to students in grades K–12 in public and private schools.

Nurses provide community-based care in settings ranging from leading support groups in a hospital (for individuals and family members diagnosed with such illnesses as cancer or diabetes) to managing a freestanding clinic to providing care in the patient's home. Other community-based care settings include county health departments, religious parishes, schools, homeless shelters, mental health centers, ambulatory surgical centers, alcohol/drug rehabilitation facilities, manufacturing or other businesses, and jails/prisons.

Skilled Care and Extended Care

Skilled care in extended or long-term care facilities is often provided at multiple levels within the community. For example, skilled care is typically provided in a nursing home setting (**Figure 2.9** ■). Skilled care is reimbursed by Medicare and is used as a transition from the hospital or home. Skilled care requires a nursing care plan completed and evaluated by a registered nurse and often includes rehabilitation services such as physical and occupational therapy. Increasingly, intermediate or skilled care is provided for patients as an alternative to hospitalization (step-up care) or for rehabilitation as the patient transitions from acute care to home (step-down care).

Many extended care settings provide an aging-in-place model that allows older adults to remain on the same campus as independence diminishes and increasing levels of care are required.

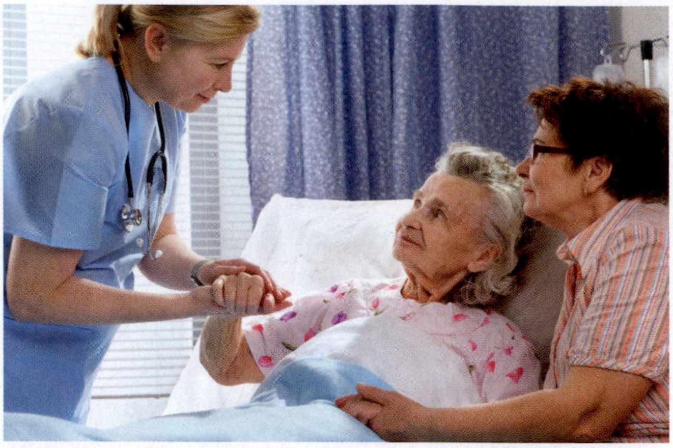

Figure 2.9 ■ Residents of nursing homes often require skilled care, which is reimbursed by Medicare.

Patient-centered primary care, often provided by a geriatric advanced practice nurse (nurse practitioner or clinical nurse specialist), within extended care has been shown to improve the quality of care and reduce emergency department visits and hospital admissions of residents. In this model, the nurse regularly assesses residents, trains caregivers to recognize and respond to changes, treats residents within the extended care setting, and communicates with families (Salmond & Echevarria, 2017).

Rehabilitation

Rehabilitation is the process of learning to live to one's maximum potential with a chronic impairment and its resultant functional disability. Rehabilitation nursing is based on a philosophy that each person has a unique set of strengths and abilities that can enable that person to live with dignity, self-worth, and independence. Nursing care to promote rehabilitation primarily focuses on patients with chronic illnesses or impairments. Rehabilitation most often begins in the acute phase of an illness or injury. Settings in which rehabilitation services are delivered include the patient's home, skilled care facilities, and specialty programs within medical centers or in the community.

Rehabilitation promotes reintegration into the patient's family and community through a team approach. Many different aspects of the patient's life are included in the plan of care: Physical function, mental health, interpersonal relationships, social interactions, family support, and vocational status. Assessment includes functional health level and self-care abilities, educational needs, psychosocial needs, and the home environment. It is critical to determine the priorities of needs from the patient and family perspective before establishing any plan of care.

Interventions are planned and implemented to prevent complications, assist in achieving a realistic level of independence, educate the patient and family about home care, and make referrals to community agencies (for nursing care, special equipment or supplies, support groups, counseling, therapy, vocational guidance, and assistance with daily living activities).

Home Healthcare

Home care is not simply illness care at home, nor is it the act of setting up a hospital room in someone's house. **Home healthcare** is the delivery of services to restore or maintain the health of individuals and families in the home (Guido, 2014). Home healthcare includes a variety of services, including skilled nursing, physical and occupational therapy, pharmacy services, and durable medical equipment such as ventilators and enteral feeding pumps. Home nursing care services include acute and chronic illness care and palliative care that reduces hospital admissions or readmissions (**Figure 2.10** ■).

Home healthcare services must be necessary and medically indicated and ordered by a qualified healthcare provider (e.g., physician, nurse practitioner) in order to qualify for reimbursement by private insurance, Medicare, or Medicaid. A physician, nurse, social worker, discharge planner, or family may make the referral for home care. Home healthcare agencies are public or private organizations that provide skilled nursing and other therapeutic services in the patient's home. These agencies primarily differ in the way their programs are organized and administered (e.g., private not-for-profit agencies, proprietary agencies, institution-based agencies). All home care agencies are similar in that they must meet uniform standards for licensing, certification, and accreditation.

Medicare is home healthcare's largest single reimbursement source, although other sources exist (Medicaid, other public funding, private insurance, and public donations). Medicare does not reimburse visits made to support general health maintenance, health promotion, or patients' emotional or socioeconomic needs. The patient must meet specific criteria to secure Medicare reimbursement:

- The physician must decide that the patient needs care at home and make a plan for home care.
- The patient must need at least one of the following: Intermittent (not full-time) skilled nursing care,

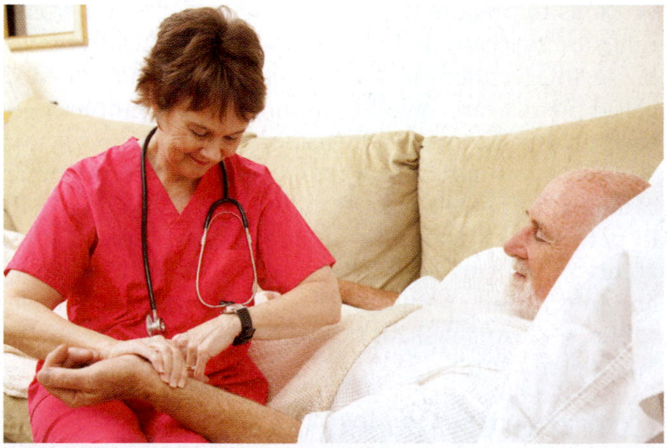

Figure 2.10 ■ Home healthcare nurses provide care for patients with acute and chronic conditions, and they provide palliative and hospice care for patients near or at the end of life.

physical therapy, speech-language pathology services, or occupational therapy.

- The patient must be homebound. This means leaving the home is a major effort. When leaving the home, it must be infrequent, for a short time, to get medical care, or to attend religious services.
- The home care agency must be Medicare approved.

Medicare will reimburse only when the skilled provider performs at least one of the following tasks:

- Teaching about a new or acute situation
- Assessing an acute process or a change in the patient's condition
- Performing a skilled procedure or a hands-on service requiring the professional skill, knowledge, ability, and judgment of a licensed nurse.

Home care encompasses both healthcare and social services provided in the home. Among patients who benefit from home care services are those who:

- Cannot live independently at home because of age, illness, or disability
- Have chronic, debilitating illnesses such as congestive heart failure, heart disease, kidney disease, respiratory diseases, diabetes mellitus, or muscle-nerve disorders
- Are terminally ill and want to die with comfort and dignity at home
- Do not need in-patient hospital or nursing home care but require additional assistance
- Need short-term help at home for postoperative care.

When a referral for home healthcare is made, an initial assessment visit by a registered nurse must occur within 48 hours. A comprehensive assessment, including review of all medications and their effects, must be completed within 5 days after the start of care (Guido, 2014). Licensed nurses provide nursing care based on physician orders. These nurses conduct initial and ongoing assessments, develop and implement plans of care, supervise other care providers, coordinate patient care with the physician, advocate for the patient and family, and teach family members and friends how to care for the patient when professional services are no longer necessary.

Nursing practice in the home is a unique experience that differs in many ways from nursing practice in a hospital setting. The individual receiving care and the family are the patients in home care. Nurses are invited into homes, meaning they are guests and cannot assume entry as they do in formal clinical settings. The environment belongs to the patient, who retains control. Every nursing action must communicate respect for these boundaries. To negotiate both repeated entry and a share of power in the patient's domain, the nurse must establish trust and rapport quickly. To do so, the nurse must communicate an understanding that she is a guest in the patient's home—offering suggestions in a way that acknowledges the patient's right to say no, sensing and honoring "where people are in their situation," maintaining a respectful distance, letting go of ethnocentric views ("My way is the best way"), and noticing and honoring family customs ("I see that no one wears shoes in your house; I'll take mine off, too."). Nurses should negotiate their schedules around the family's needs; nursing should enhance family coping, not complicate it.

Above all, the nurse should validate patients' illness experiences, remembering that everyone needs someone who is willing to listen and say, "I hear what you are saying, and I think I have a sense of how you feel." The nurse speaks slowly and directly to the patient, within the patient's range of vision (the patient may need to lip-read) and refrains from shouting at patients who have a hearing impairment.

On the first nursing visit, the nurse stresses the essential information and repeats it on subsequent visits to avoid overwhelming the patient with too much information. The nurse can suggest that patients have someone else present "to help listen." When making suggestions, the nurse offers patients the pluses and minuses of each alternative. Informed decisions are difficult to make if people are too overwhelmed to think of their options. The nurse must also allow time for families to process new information. See **Table 2.7** for additional suggestions when teaching and caring for the patient in the home.

It is important to avoid overwhelming families with numerous healthcare providers in the home. Most people dislike having strangers in their home, no matter how helpful they may seem to be. The nurse can help families manage moments of crisis by staying as close as possible. If abuse is suspected, the nurse must notify authorities and/or remove patients from potentially dangerous situations.

Safety

Performing a safety assessment in the home is a nursing responsibility and a legal requirement. Nurses cannot close their eyes to an unsafe environment. Upon entering the home and on a continuing basis, the nurse must alert the family to unsafe and hazardous conditions, suggest remedies, and document in the clinical record the family's response to the nurse's suggestions. See **Box 2.2** for a sample home safety assessment list. In addition, nurses must remain alert to the following:

- How patients ambulate and handle stairs
- How patients manage care when alone
- A supply of expired medications
- Inappropriate clothing or shoes
- Cooking habits that may precipitate a fire
- An inadequate food supply
- Poorly functioning utilities
- Signs of abusive behavior.

Although nurses cannot change the family's living space and lifestyle, they can register their concern and react appropriately if the risk for injury is significant or if abuse

Table 2.7 Interventions in Home Health Nursing

Intervention	Description
Set goals and boundaries	■ Explore the patients' and families' expectations of home care. ■ Explain the primary goal (to achieve self-care). ■ Define nurse and patient roles within this framework and discuss limitations (e.g., "No, a home care nurse is not the same as a private duty nurse"). ■ Stress mutual accountability, choice, and negotiation as part of the process.
Assess the home environment	■ Survey the environment and members of the household, noting hygiene and dress; verbal and nonverbal communication; significant relationships and visiting patterns; appearance of the house, yard, sidewalk, and neighborhood. ■ Assess the effect of illness on the family. ■ Ask questions and listen carefully to stories and offhand remarks.
Set priorities	■ Develop an initial plan to address issues of safety and those of greatest concern to the patient and family. ■ Mutually establish short-term and long-term goals, remembering that those priorities that primarily belong to the nurse may not be met. ■ Be prepared to modify the plan according to conditions within the home and family.
Promote learning	■ Actively promote learning by identifying what is most important to the patient. ■ Prioritize material on a need-to-know (e.g., information to ensure safety), want-to-know, ought-to-know basis, assessing and responding to learner readiness. ■ Timing is important; people who are not ready to listen cannot learn. ■ Allow sufficient time, teaching while providing care when possible. ■ Ask patients how and when they learn best, and use appropriate methods and materials when possible. ■ Capitalize on patients' frustrations and desires to regain control of self-care. ■ Empower learners by talking them through tasks, encouraging them to ask questions, and urging them to write thoughts and questions to discuss during the next visit or doctor's appointment.
Limit distractions	■ To the extent possible, limit distractions such as children, animals, noise, clutter, and mannerisms that are controlling, manipulative, or aggressive. ■ Elicit the patient's help by asking, for example, "May I please turn off your television while we visit?" or "I would like to schedule my next visit for a time when the children are in school. Is that all right with you?" ■ Do not debate the priority of the visit over the distraction (such as a favorite television show), which may risk losing the patient's trust and rapport. ■ Attend to environmental and behavioral distractions that can yield useful information; for example, a dirty house could indicate a lack of interest in housekeeping, outright neglect and abuse, depression, or increased disability. ■ Be truthful about allergies, fear of a patient's pet, or difficulty hearing in a particular room. ■ If all efforts at limiting distractions fail, leave the home and return on another day: "I can see this is not going to work for us today. I will need to leave." ■ Seek out a colleague to discuss personal distractions, such as fear of harm, reaction to the patient's lifestyle, preoccupation with role, or a feeling of being overwhelmed by the situation in the home.
Make do	■ Be resourceful and cost conscious with equipment, supplies, and services in the home. ■ When necessary to make do or improvise, do so in a low-key manner to avoid causing the family additional anxiety. ■ Make every effort to convey the message that the situation is under control; react as necessary after leaving the home.

or neglect is suspected. Ignoring an unsafe environment is considered nursing negligence.

The disposal of toxic medications and sharp objects (such as needles used for injections) is a safety issue in the home, especially if young children are present. The nurse must address this with the patient, demonstrate safe disposal, and provide the necessary equipment for safe disposal. Documentation should address what information the nurse has covered, the family's response to the teaching, and assessment of the family's ongoing practice of safety precautions.

Nurses must focus on personal safety and survival as well as their patients' safety and survival. When traveling in the community, the nurse takes such precautions as keeping car doors locked, having a cellular phone, keeping supplies out of sight, and staying inside the car in potentially dangerous situations. Colleagues, families, and community members can offer useful guidelines for maintaining safety and self-protection.

Infection Control

Infection control in the home centers on protecting patients, caregivers, and the community from the spread of disease. Within the home, nurses may encounter patients with infectious or communicable diseases, patients who are immunocompromised, and/or patients with multiple access devices, drainage tubes, or draining wounds. The home presents a challenging environment in which to practice infection control for several reasons: Families have habitual patterns of behavior; caregivers often lack any formal education on the subject; the setting itself may not be conducive; and facilities for even the most basic of aseptic practices (hand hygiene) may be lacking.

Health teaching is the single most important nursing intervention in controlling infection. Patients and caregivers need to know the importance of effective hand hygiene, the use of gloves, the disposal of wastes and soiled dressings, the handling of linens, and the practice of standard precautions. Unfortunately, teaching about infection control does not always bring about a change in behavior. Changing a family's values and behavior frequently demands a great deal of ingenuity from the nurse.

Teaching and supporting the caregiver is a significant aspect of home health nursing care. Caregiver burden is not easily hidden in the home. In the United States, an estimated 43.5 million people are taking care of relatives and friends

BOX 2.2
Home Safety Assessment Checklist

When preparing patients for discharge to home, the nurse focuses on safety first. Even when home care is planned, a day or two may elapse before services begin and patients must be able to manage until then. Information and supplies to get the patient through the first few days at home must be provided prior to discharge. Additionally, patients should have contact information for the nurse and physician, and complete written information about their medications and manifestations they should report. Finally, all patients should be able to perform necessary procedures safely and obtain necessary supplies in the community.

GENERAL HOUSEHOLD SAFETY

1. Do stairwells and halls have good lighting?
2. Do staircases have handrails on both sides?
3. Are rugs securely tacked down?
4. Is the telephone readily accessible? Are the numbers easy to read?
5. Are electrical cords in good condition and out of the way?
6. Is furniture sturdy?
7. Is the temperature of the home comfortable?
8. Are protective screens in front of fireplaces or heating devices?
9. Are smoke detectors and carbon monoxide detectors present and working?

BATHROOM

1. Are grab bars present in the tub and/or shower? Around the toilet?
2. Are toilet seats high enough?
3. Are nonskid materials (rugs, mats) on the floor, tub/shower?
4. Are medications stored safely? Out of the reach of children?
5. Is the water temperature safe?
6. Are electrical outlets and appliances a safe distance from the tub?

KITCHEN

1. Are floors slippery? Are nonskid rugs used?
2. Is the stove in good working order?
3. Is the refrigerator in good working order? Clean?
4. Are electrical outlets overloaded with appliance cords?
5. Are sharp objects kept in a special container or safe area?
6. Is food storage adequate? Clean?
7. Are cleaning materials stored safely?

who have disabilities (Family Caregiver Alliance, 2018). Many of these caregivers are themselves older adults. Caregiving has only recently been acknowledged as a complex activity, requiring adjustment in family living patterns, relationships, and finances. Early hospital discharge of family members with chronic conditions places enormous emotional, physical, and financial burdens on family caregivers. For some families, the crisis of caregiving is short lived, but for others it lasts for years. As a result, caregivers are at great risk for both physical and emotional illness. Because the success of home care depends heavily on the supports in place, addressing the needs of the support network is imperative.

Palliative and Hospice Care

Palliative care focuses on symptom management with intent of improving quality of life for patients with chronic illness. The patient receiving palliative care may seek lifesaving treatment in the event their condition becomes unstable. Patients receiving hospice services agree not to receive CPR and other lifesaving measures. See Chapter 5 for more information about hospice and palliative care.

Hospice care is a model of care delivered in many settings, from homes to skilled care and extended care settings, adult foster care homes, and specialized facilities such as hospice homes. Hospice care is designed to provide medical, nursing, social, psychologic, and spiritual care for terminally ill patients and their families. Hospice care relies on a philosophy of relieving pain and suffering and allowing the patient to die with dignity in a comfortable environment. Licensed nurses, medical social workers, physicians, occupational and physical therapists, and volunteers provide care. As the population ages, medical-surgical nurses will provide more palliative care in all settings.

Respite care provides short-term or intermittent home care, often using volunteers. These services exist primarily to give the family member or friend who is the primary caregiver some time away from care. Respite care does much to relieve the burden of full-time caregiving.

CHAPTER HIGHLIGHTS

2.1 Health and Wellness

Define health and the health–illness continuum, and discuss factors affecting the health of individuals, families, communities, and special populations.

- Health is a dynamic state influenced by multiple internal, external, physical, social, and mental factors.
- These factors include those that cannot be changed (e.g., genetic makeup, gender, age, ethnicity, and culture) as well as modifiable factors (e.g., lifestyle and environment).
- The health–illness continuum represents health as a dynamic process, with high-level wellness at one extreme of the continuum and death at the opposite extreme.

- The adult years are commonly divided into three stages: The young adult (age 18 to 40), the middle adult (age 40 to 65), and the older adult (over age 65).
- Young adults are at risk for alterations in health from injuries, sexually transmitted infections, substance abuse, and physical and psychologic stressors. Cancers are a leading cause of death, and behaviors established in young adulthood affect risk for developing common chronic diseases in the future.
- Middle adults are at risk for alterations in health from obesity, cardiovascular disease, cancer, substance abuse, and the stresses of change and transition.
- Older adults are at risk for alterations in health from chronic illnesses, injuries, drug toxicities, and changes in income and marital status.
- Community factors known as social determinants of health include social support systems, access to healthcare services, the environment, and economic resources.
- Populations that may require extra care include veterans, members of the LGBTQI community, and adult survivors of congenital/childhood conditions.

2.2 Health Promotion and Maintenance

Compare and contrast health risks, assessment, and health promotion for the young adult, middle adult, and older adult.

- *Healthy People 2020* provides a foundation for disease prevention and wellness activities across public and private sectors, as well as a model for measuring achievement of identified goals and objectives.
- Nurses play a major role in promoting the health of individuals, families, and communities. Health promotion focuses screening, immunizations, and health teaching.

2.3 Disease, Illness, and Injury

Differentiate between disease, illness, and injury, and describe illness behaviors and needs of the patient with acute, critical, and chronic illness.

- Disease, defined as any alteration in a body system or organ structure or function, are characterized by identifiable signs and symptoms and by specific recognized pathophysiologic processes and etiologies.
- Illness is the response an individual has to a disease; this response is highly individualized because the individual responds not only to his or her own perceptions of the disease but also to the perceptions of others. Illnesses can be acute or chronic.
- Injury and violence affect everyone and the medical-surgical nurse will provide care for patients and families experiencing health-related problems created by these unexpected and unintended events.
- The primary health risks for the individual and family vary, depending on age and developmental stage, among other factors. Behaviors to promote individual health, however, remain very consistent throughout the lifespan.

2.4 Types of Nursing Care

Describe essential elements and goals of coordinated primary care models; the services, settings, and essential components of community-based care and home healthcare; and nursing interventions to deliver safe, effective, and competent care to patients in their homes.

- Most health and illness care occurs outside the acute hospital environment, in community-based and primary care settings. Home healthcare is increasingly important as hospital stays become shorter or are avoided altogether.
- Primary care is comprehensive first-contact health and illness care across the lifespan. Preventive care services as well as care for acute and chronic diseases are encompassed within the primary care model.
- Transitional care focuses on interventions to facilitate transitions from one healthcare setting to another or to home. The steps of transitional care include health promotion, acute care, chronic care, and end-of-life care.
- Community-based care focuses on individual and family healthcare delivered in the local community.
- Skilled care, which is reimbursed by Medicare, is typically provided in extended care or long-term care facilities such as nursing homes. Rehabilitation nursing is based on a philosophy that each person has a unique set of strengths and abilities that can enable that person to live with dignity, self-worth, and independence.
- Ensuring safety and patient and family education are major responsibilities of the home healthcare nurse. In this setting, the patient and family are primary members of the team and are instrumental in establishing priorities of care.

TEST YOURSELF NCLEX-RN® REVIEW

1. During an assessment the nurse asks a patient to rate her current health status on a continuum from being well to being ill. Which health factor is the nurse assessing in this patient?
   A. Culture
   B. Genetic makeup
   C. Cognitive abilities
   D. Lifestyle and environment
2. The nurse is concerned that an older patient is at risk for a health problem because of psychosocial stressors. What did the nurse most likely assess in this patient?
   A. Caring for ailing spouse
   B. Recent fall resulting in a hip fracture
   C. Thirty-year history of smoking cigarettes
   D. Use of over-the-counter pain medication
3. The nurse is preparing an educational session that focuses on health promotion activities for the middle-aged adult. What is the purpose of this teaching?
   A. Diagnose diseases.
   B. Emphasize activities that maintain wellness.
   C. Explain success of medical treatments for illnesses.
   D. Focus on adhering to prescribed medication regimens.
4. The nurse is planning care to prevent the onset of illness for a patient with a chronic disease. Which secondary prevention activities would be appropriate for this patient? (Select all that apply.)
   A. Receiving recommended immunizations
   B. Scheduling regular physical examinations
   C. Eliminating the use of alcohol and cigarettes
   D. Obtaining specific treatment for illnesses
   E. Screening for common diseases
5. After seeing a healthcare provider for upper respiratory illness symptoms, a patient is being admitted to the hospital for care. The nurse will plan care for this patient experiencing which illness behavior?
   A. Seeking medical care
   B. Assuming the sick role
   C. Experiencing symptoms
   D. Assuming a dependent role
6. The nurse is participating in a conference to identify interventions for an older patient. The patient started hemodialysis while hospitalized and will be continuing hemodialysis once discharged. What is the ultimate goal for this planning session?
   A. Navigate through the healthcare system.
   B. Deliver services to maintain the patient's health in the home.
   C. Improve the patient and family's ability to manage care needs.
   D. Manage acute or chronic health problems and promote self-care.
7. A hospital committee is tasked with designing a patient-centered medical home to be implemented for newly discharged patients with chronic diseases. Which concept should the committee chair emphasize when reviewing the purpose of this primary care approach for these patients?
   A. Reduce health disparities.
   B. Prevent acute disease crises.
   C. Increase preventive services.
   D. Improve the patient–primary care relationship.
8. The nurse is determining if a patient with Medicare coverage is a candidate for home care. On which purpose should the nurse focus to determine if Medicare will cover this patient's home care services?
   A. Patient is recently widowed and is having difficulty spending time alone in the home.
   B. Patient is newly diagnosed with diabetes and is learning how to self-administer insulin.
   C. Patient has difficulty with bathing and needs assistance with clothing and home chores.
   D. Patient requests nursing visits to occur during meals to provide socialization while eating.
9. During a home visit the nurse sees that an older patient has a supply of expired antibiotics. What will the nurse do after making this discovery? (Select all that apply.)
   A. Recommend disposal of the medications.
   B. Explain how to safely dispose of these medications.
   C. Remind the patient to take medications that are not expired.
   D. Move the expired medications to the back of the medication area.
   E. Collect all expired medications and take them to be destroyed.
10. The nurse is making a home visit to a patient recovering from bacterial pneumonia. Which intervention is the most important to control infection in the home environment?
    A. Teaching the patient to conduct hand hygiene after expectorating into tissues
    B. Isolating the patient from family members while still taking prescribed antibiotics
    C. Separating the patient's bath towels and clothing from the rest of the family's items
    D. Reminding home caregivers to wash the patient's eating utensils in hot, soapy water

See Test Yourself answers in Appendix B.

REFERENCES

Administration on Aging. (2015). A profile of older Americans: 2015. Retrieved from https://www.acl.gov/sites/default/files/Aging%20and%20Disability%20in%20America/2015-Profile.pdf.

American Academy of Ambulatory Care Nursing. (2017). *Position paper: The role of the registered nurse in ambulatory care.* Retrieved from https://www.aaacn.org/sites/default/files/documents/RNRolePositionPaper.pdf.

American Academy of Pediatrics (AAP). (2015.) *AAP releases summary of updated preventive healthcare screening and assessment schedule for children's checkups.* Retrieved from https://www.aap.org/en-us/about-the-aap/aap-press-room/pages/AAP-Releases-Summary-of-Updated-Preventive-Health-Care-Screening-and-Assessment-Schedule-for-Children's-Checkups.aspx.

American Cancer Society (ACS). (2018). *American Cancer Society guidelines for the early detection of cancer.* Retrieved from www.cancer.org/healthy/findcancerearly/cancerscreeningguidelines/american-cancer-society-guidelines-for-the-early-detection-of-cancer.

Bauer L., & Bodenheimer, T. (2017). Expanded roles of registered nurses in primary care delivery of the future. *Nursing Outlook, 65,* 624–632.

Callahan, A., Ames, N. J., Manning M. L., Touchton-Leonard, K., Yang, L., & Wallen, G. R. (2016). Factors influencing nurses' use of hazardous drug safe-handling precautions. *Oncology Nursing Forum, 43*(3), 342–349.

Caregiver Action Network. (2016). *Caregiver statistics: Demographics.* Retrieved from https://www.caregiver.org/caregiver-statistics-demographics.

Centers for Disease Control and Prevention. (2016). *Adverse Childhood Experiences.* https://www.cdc.gov/violenceprevention/acestudy/.

Centers for Disease Control and Prevention. (2017a). *Adults: Protect yourself with pneumococcal vaccines.* Retrieved from www.cdc.gov/features/adult-pneumococcal/.

Centers for Disease Control and Prevention (CDC). (2017b). *Chronic diseases and health promotion.* Retrieved from www.cdc.gov/chronicdisease/overview.

Centers for Disease Control and Prevention. (2017c). *HPV vaccination information for young women.* Retrieved from www.cdc.gov/std/hpv/stdfact-hpv-vaccine-young-women.htm.

Centers for Disease Control and Prevention. (2018a). *Fact Sheets: Binge drinking.* Retrieved from www.cdc.gov/features/adult-pneumococcal/

Centers for Disease Control and Prevention (CDC). (2018b). *Key injury and violence data.* Retrieved from https://www.cdc.gov/injury/wisqars/overview/key_data.html.

Centers for Disease Control and Prevention. (2018c). *Physical activity.* Retrieved from www.cdc.gov/physicalactivity/.

Centers for Disease Control and Prevention. (2018d). *Recommended adult immunization schedule—United States 2014.* Retrieved from https://www.cdc.gov/vaccines/schedules/hcp/adult.html.

Cystic Fibrosis Foundation. (2018). *About cystic fibrosis.* Retrieved from https://www.cff.org/What-is-CF/About-Cystic-Fibrosis/?gclid=Cj0KCQjwgMnYBRDRARIsANC2dflqLh0Pi5G6AlL_DvESARr4gN5URqYx22JCvn4kld-LtJTuyxV0ZxogaAtYAEALw_wcB.

Dunn, H. L. (1959). High-level wellness for man and society. *American Journal of Public Health, 49*(6), 786 – 792.

Elliott, B., & DeAngelis, M. (2017). Improving patient transitions from hospital to home: Practical advice from nurses. *Nursing, 47*(11), 58–62.

Family Caregiver Alliance. (2018). *Fact sheet: Selected caregiver statistics.* Retrieved from www.caregiver.org/about.

Federal Interagency Forum on Aging-Related Statistics. (2016). *Aging stats.* Retrieved from https://agingstats.gov.

Gorman, R. D. (2016). Integrating palliative care into primary care. *Nursing Clinics of North America, 51*(3), 367–379.

Gilboa, S. M., Owen, J. D., Kucik, J. E., Oster, M. E., Riehle-Colarusso, T., Nembhard, W. N., . . . Marelli, A. J. (2016). Congenital heart defects in the United States: Estimating the magnitude of the affected population in 2010. *Circulation, 134,* 101–109.

Guido, G. (2014). *Legal and ethical issues in nursing* (6th ed.). Upper Saddle River, NJ: Pearson.

Harden, S. R., & Kaplow, R. (2017). *Synergy for clinical excellence: The AACN synergy model for patient care* (2nd ed.). Burlington MA: Jones & Bartlett.

Ingram, R., & Kautz, D. D. (2018). Creating "win-win" outcomes for patients with low health literacy: A nursing case study. *Medsurg Nursing, 27*(2), 132–134.

The Joint Commission. (2012). *Hot topics in healthcare. The transitions of care: The need for a more effective approach to continuing patient care.* Retrieved from https://www.jointcommission.org/assets/1/18/Hot_Topics_Transitions_of_Care.pdf.

Kip, K., D'Aoust, R. F., Hernandez, D. F., Girling, S. A., Cuttino, B., Long, M. K., . . . Rosenzweig, L. (2016). Evaluation of brief treatment of psychological trauma among veterans residing in a homeless shelter by use of accelerated resolution therapy. *Nursing Outlook, 64,* 411–423.

Kochanek, K. D., Murphy, S. L., Xu, J., & Tejada-Vera, B. (2016). Deaths: Final date for 2014. *National Vital Statistic Reports, 65* (4), 1–5.

Mohler, K. M., & Sankey-Deemer, C. (2017). Primary care providers and screening for military service and PTSD. *American Journal of Nursing, 117*(11), 22–28.

National Association of School Nurses (NASN). (2017). *2016 school nurse workforce study results.*

Retrieved from https://schoolnursenet.nasn.org/blogs/nasn-profile/2017/05/10/school-nurse-workforce-study-results

National Cancer Institute. (2018). *Late effects of treatment for childhood cancer (PDQ®)-Health Professional Version*. Retrieved from https://www.cancer.gov/types/childhood-cancers/late-effects-hp-pdq.

National Center for Health Statistics (NCHS). (2017). *NCHS fact sheets*. Hyattsville, MD: U.S. Department of Health and Human Services, Centers for Disease Control and Prevention. Retrieved from https://www.cdc.gov/nchs/about/fact_sheets.htm.

National Council State Board of Nursing (NCSBN). (2018). The NCSBN 2018 environmental scan. *Journal of Nursing Regulation, 8*(4), S3–20.

National Diabetes Education Initiative. (2016). *Diabetes management guidelines*. Retrieved from www.ndei.org/ADA-2013-Guidelines-Criteria-Diabetes-Diagnosis.aspx.html

National Institute on Drug Abuse. (2018). Retrieved from https://www.drugabuse.gov.

Olshansky, E. F. (2017). Social determinants of health: The role of nursing. *American Journal of Nursing, 117*(12), 11.

Pender, N., Murdaugh, C., & Parsons, M., (2015). *Health promotion in nursing practice* (7th ed.). Upper Saddle River, NJ: Pearson.

Persoud, S. (2018). Addressing social determinants of health through advocacy. *Nursing Administration Quarterly, 42*(2), 123–128.

Press Ganey. (2016). The role of workplace safety and surveillance capacity in driving nurse and patient outcomes. 2016 Nursing Special Report. Retrieved from http://www.pressganey.com/about/news/2016-nursing-special-report.

Salmond, S. W., & Echevarria, M. (2017). Healthcare transformation and changing roles for nursing. *Orthopaedic Nursing, 36*(1), 12–25.

Smith, C. J., & Harris, H. (2017). Caring for our veterans: A shared responsibility. *Nursing, 47*(11), 46–47.

Sorenson, M., Quinn, L., & Klein D. (2019). *Pathophysiology: Concepts of human disease*. Hoboken, NJ: Pearson Education.

Spahr, J., Coddington, J., Edwards, N., & McComb, S. (2018). Implementing comprehensive primary care referral tracking in a patient-centered medical home. *Journal of Nursing Care Quality, 33*(3), 255–262.

Stewart, K. R., & Hand, K. (2017). SBAR, communication, and patient safety: An integrated literature review. *Medsurg Nursing, 26*(5), 297–305.

U.S. Department of Health and Human Services. (2018). *Healthy People 2020*. Washington, DC: Author.

U.S. Department of Labor, Occupational Safety and Health Administration. (n.d.). *Guidelines for preventing workplace violence for healthcare and social service workers*. Retrieved from https://www.osha.gov/Publications/osha3148.pdf.

U.S. Department of Veterans Affairs. (2017). Public health: Vibration. Retrieved from https://www.publichealth.va.gov/exposures/vibration/index.asp.

Woodall, W. (2017). Care of LGBTQ patients. *Medsurg Nursing, 26*(2), 137–147.

World Health Organization. (1974). *Constitution of the World Health Organization: Chronicle of the World Health Organization*. Geneva: Author.

World Health Organization. (2008). *Integrated health services--What and why?* (Technical Brief No. 1). Retrieved from www.who.int/healthsystems/service_delivery_techbrief1.pdf.

World Health Organization (WHO). (2018). Social determinants of health. Retrieved from http://www.who.int/social_determinants/en/.

Zarnello, L., (2018). The case of adverse childhood experiences. *Nursing, 48*(4), 50–54.

ADDITIONAL RESOURCES

Administration on Aging: A Profile of Older Americans: 2015

www.acl.gov/sites/default/files/Aging%20and%20Disability%20in%20America/2015-Profile.pdf.

American Cancer Society: Guidelines for the Early Detection of Cancer

www.cancer.org/healthy/find-cancer-early/cancer-screening-guidelines/american-cancer-society-guidelines-for-the-early-detection-of-cancer.html

Centers for Disease Control and Prevention: Healthy Living

www.cdc.gov/healthyliving/index.html

Centers for Disease Control and Prevention: Chronic Disease Prevention and Health Promotion

www.cdc.gov/chronicdisease/index.htm

Elliott, B., & DeAngelis, M. (2017). Improving patient transitions from hospital to home: Practical advice from nurses. *Nursing, 47*(11), 58–62.

www.ncbi.nlm.nih.gov/pubmed/29069063

Healthy People 2020

www.healthypeople.gov/2020/topics-objectives

Healthy People 2030

www.healthypeople.gov/2020/About-Healthy-People/Development-Healthy-People-2030

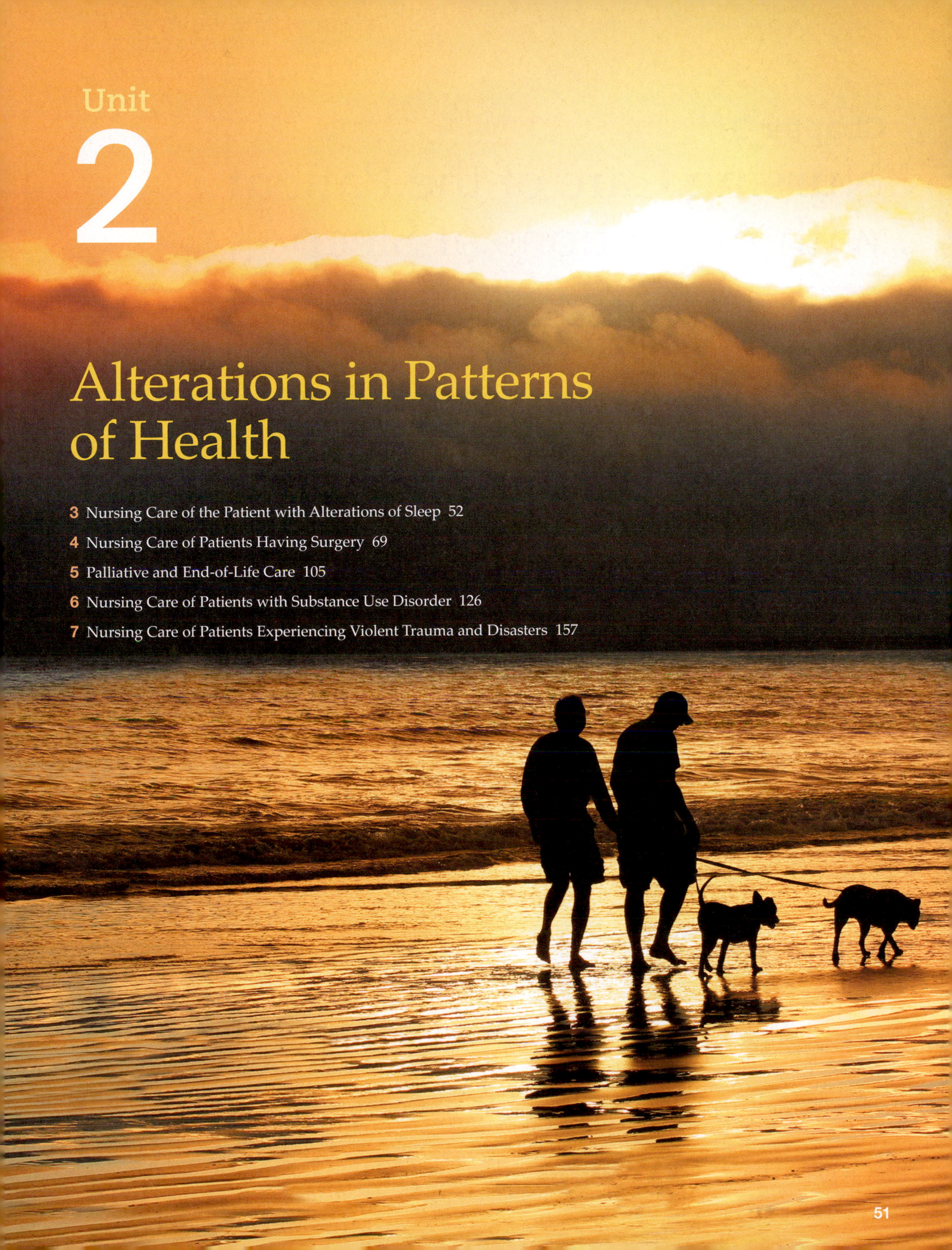

Unit

2

Alterations in Patterns of Health

Chapter 3

Nursing Care of the Patient with Alterations of Sleep

Chapter Outline and Learning Outcomes

3.1 Overview of Sleep and Rest 53

Describe the physiology of sleep, normal sleep patterns, and factors affecting sleep.

3.2 Health Promotion 56

Summarize topics that nurses teach to promote healthy sleep across the lifespan.

3.3 Assessing the Patient with Altered Sleep 57

Outline the components of the assessment of sleep including topics for the health assessment interview, techniques for physical assessment, and the diagnostic tests used in the assessment.

3.4 Assessment of Selected Populations 59

Differentiate considerations for assessing the sleep of older adults, veterans, and individuals in the LGBTQI population.

3.5 Sleep Deprivation 59

Describe the pathophysiology and manifestations of sleep deprivation, and outline the interprofessional care and nursing care of patients with this disorder.

3.6 Insomnia 59

Describe the pathophysiology and manifestations of insomnia, and outline the interprofessional care and nursing care of patients with this disorder.

3.7 Sleep-Disordered Breathing 62

Describe the pathophysiology and manifestations of sleep-disordered breathing, and outline the interprofessional care and nursing care of patients with this disorder.

3.8 Restless Legs Syndrome 64

Describe the pathophysiology and manifestations of restless legs syndrome, and outline the interprofessional care and nursing care of patients with this disorder.

CLINICAL COMPETENCIES

- Assess patients with sleep disturbances, using data to select and prioritize appropriate nursing diagnoses and identify desired outcomes of care.
- Identify the effects of sleep disorders on the functional health status of assigned patients.
- Use research and an evidence-based plan to provide individualized care for patients with sleep disorders.
- Collaborate with the interprofessional care team in planning and providing care for patients with sleep disorders.
- Safely and knowledgably administer medications and prescribed treatments for patients with sleep disorders.

KEY TERMS

actigraphy, 58
central sleep apnea (CSA), 63
insomnia, 59
obstructive sleep apnea (OSA), 62
rest, 52
restless legs syndrome, 64
sleep, 52
sleep hygiene, 56

Sleep is a fundamental process of all species, and in humans, sleep is one of the most important processes for survival. **Sleep** is a reversible disengagement from the environment that has some common characteristics: Most humans sleep with their eyes closed, in a recumbent position, with regular breathing. While observing a sleeping person, sleep can seem peaceful and restful, yet complex processes are going on in the body that are necessary for survival (Carskadon & Dement, 2017). **Rest** is a period of diminished activity, without disengagement from the environment, for mental and physical rejuvenation.

3.1 Overview of Sleep and Rest

Purpose and Use of Rest

Rest is the process of allowing the body time to recover and conserve energy. Rest is different than sleep, as during sleep hormones are released and short-term memories/learning are moved to long-term memories/learning. Also, during sleep, especially during REM sleep, glucose metabolism in the brain can be as high as in wakefulness (Maquet et al., 1990). In rest however, there is a conservation of energy and a relaxation of the brain where glucose is not being used as much as in strenuous thinking. When we talk about rest, we are talking about periods during the day where the patient is allowed some quiet time. It is known that prolonged bedrest can be harmful, especially for older patients (Tanner et al., 2015).

Physiology of Sleep

The physiology of sleep is complex, involving multiple body systems, including the immune, metabolic, and sympathetic and parasympathetic nervous systems. All body systems must work in concert for restful and restorative sleep to occur, and the reverse is also true: Restful sleep is needed for adequate body functions. For example, if the sympathetic nervous system (flight-or-fight response) does not down-regulate, then restorative sleep will not occur. This is because if the sympathetic nervous system is activated, the parasympathetic nervous system (energy conservation, reparative system) is not. During sleep it is the parasympathetic nervous system that is more active for the repair and maintenance of the human body.

It is known that changes in sleep patterns that decrease the quality and quantity of sleep affect many physiologic functions, including:

- Satiety, with overeating leading to obesity and cell insensitivity to insulin (Van Cauter & Tasali, 2017)
- Mood, including irritability and depression (Klumoers et al., 2015)
- Immune system function, including a decreased ability to fight off infection (Opp & Krueger, 2017)
- Cognitive functioning, such as decreased retention of new material (Peigneux, Fogel, & Smith, 2017).

Changes in sleep patterns can be caused by disease processes (such as pain syndromes and neurologic disorders) and medications that cross the blood–brain barrier, including those that are not usually thought to affect sleep. These medications include atenolol, procainamide, chlorothiazide, sertraline, and levothyroxine (Adams, Holland, & Urban, 2017). The reverse is also true: If sleep patterns are altered negatively, then treatment for disease processes such as depression, neurologic disorders, and chronic pain may not achieve the intended goals of treatment. It is important for nurses to assess for difficulties and potent sleep disorders because the interaction of sleep and other physiological processes is linked. This chapter focuses on common sleep disorders and the bidirectional nature of sleep and physiologic processes.

There are a number of models for the reasons why humans sleep (Achermann & Borbély, 2017). The most important one for nurses to know is the *two-process model*, which proposes an interaction between a homeostatic process (the buildup and release of sleepiness) and the circadian process of the body's natural cycle (the timing of sleep and the buildup of the need to sleep). This model is straightforward in the sense that during daytime the body builds up a need to sleep that is "released" during sleep. The circadian process times the sleep portion during the nighttime and the buildup of the pressure to sleep during the day (Achermann & Borbély, 2017). This is important for nurses to understand because patients who are not active during the daytime due to illness or disability may not have the buildup of pressure to sleep. This lack of buildup may make it difficult for the patient to have consolidated, quality sleep during the nighttime. Also if external cues for the circadian rhythm are disturbed (for example, in a hospital where lights are not turned off at night), then the patient may fall asleep at different hours.

Another consideration for understanding sleep is the relationship between sleep and the immune system. Both interleukin 1 (IL-1) and tumor necrosis factor (TNF) are involved with the regulation of sleep and also with the regulation of the immune response (Opp & Krueger, 2017). Changes in both of these cytokines have downstream effects on a number of other cytokines, which individually or in tandem will affect sleep. While the published studies are only correlative, there is research that suggests that recovery is aided by sleep (Opp & Krueger, 2017). This is another reason why it is important for nurses to understand sleep.

Normal Sleep Patterns

Most humans (except those who work "shiftwork") sleep when it is dark and are awake when it is light. Light is the most important regulator of sleep and circadian rhythms. Light is perceived by the retina and is transmitted through the retinohypothalamic tract to the suprachiasmatic nucleus (SCN) in the hypothalamus. The SCN projects into the pineal gland to either secrete or stop secreting melatonin, which is a hormone connected to sleep. **Figure 3.1** ■ demonstrates the physiological activities of the retinohypothalamic tract. When it becomes dimmer out, the pineal gland secretes melatonin, which in turn signals the body it is time to sleep. Light can affect the secretion of melatonin. This includes light from TVs, computers, cell phones, and tablets, which is a main reason for difficulty in falling asleep for a large portion of the population. This is also why it is hard for some people who work the night shift to sleep during the daytime even with eye masks.

The normal amount of sleep is about 8 hours of consolidated sleep per 24-hour day during the night time. This can vary based on the person. Sleep and the body's natural circadian rhythm work together. For example, sleep is easiest as the body temperature is decreasing. From a circadian rhythm perspective, decrease in body temperature occurs in the evening. This interaction between sleep and circadian

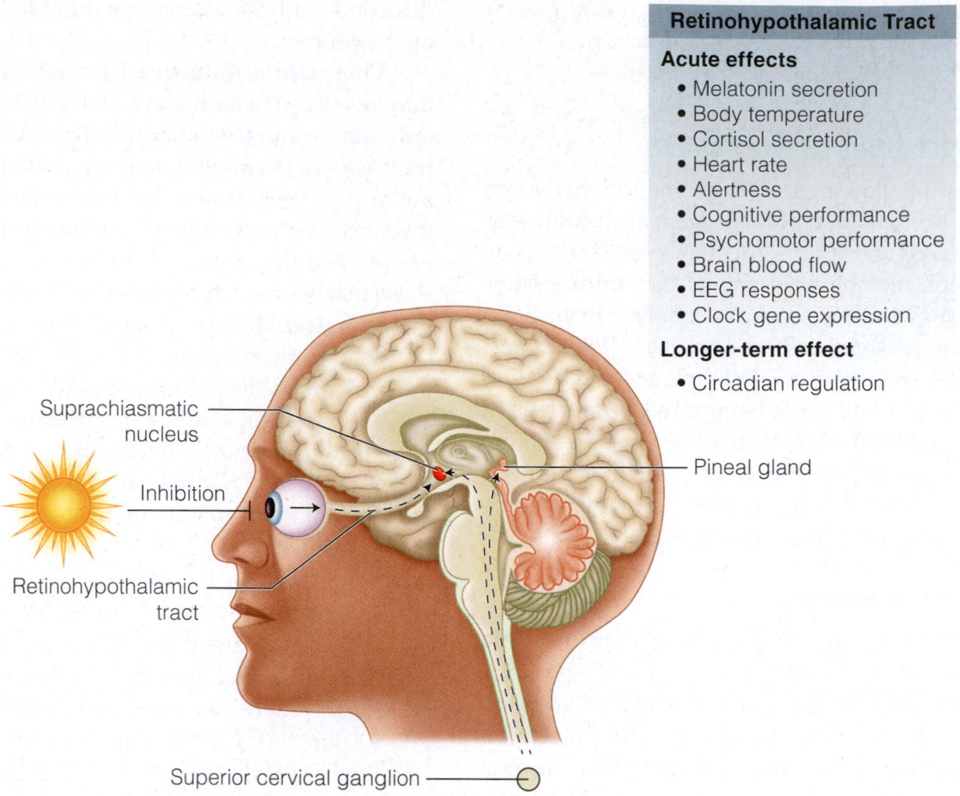

Retinohypothalamic Tract
Acute effects
• Melatonin secretion
• Body temperature
• Cortisol secretion
• Heart rate
• Alertness
• Cognitive performance
• Psychomotor performance
• Brain blood flow
• EEG responses
• Clock gene expression
Longer-term effect
• Circadian regulation
Suprachiasmatic nucleus
Inhibition
Retinohypothalamic tract
Pineal gland
Superior cervical ganglion

Figure 3.1 ■ The effect of light on the retinohypothalamic tract.

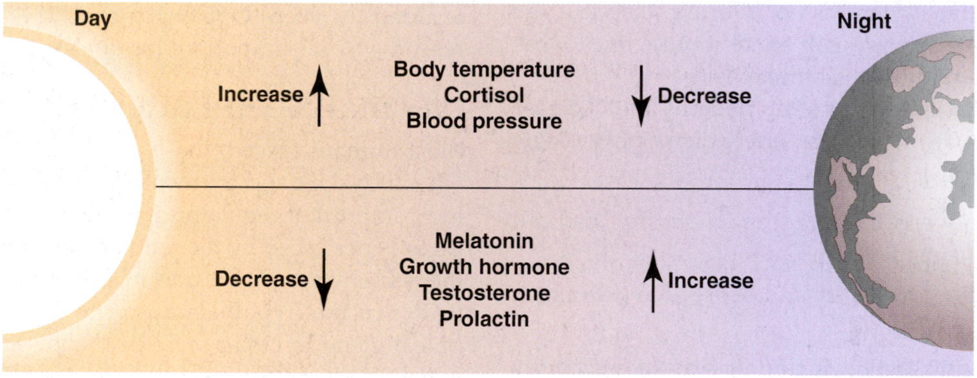

Day
Night
Increase
Body temperature
Cortisol
Blood pressure
Decrease
Decrease
Melatonin
Growth hormone
Testosterone
Prolactin
Increase

Figure 3.2 ■ Many physiologic functions follow a circadian pattern throughout the day and night.

rhythm is demonstrated in **Figure 3.2** ■. Also the relationship between the circadian rhythm and what is occurring in the body in relation to sleep and alertness is demonstrated in **Figure 3.3** ■. Current research is beginning to demonstrate the genetic basis for the amounts of sleep humans obtain along with the 24-hour rhythm of the human body (Vitaterna, Turek, & Jiang, 2017). The *CLOCK* and *PER* genes are thought to work in the tissue of the SCN, as destruction of the SCN eliminates a circadian rhythm in mammals and transplant of SCN tissue restores the circadian rhythm. While the genetic basis for most sleep disorders is not known, work continues in this area.

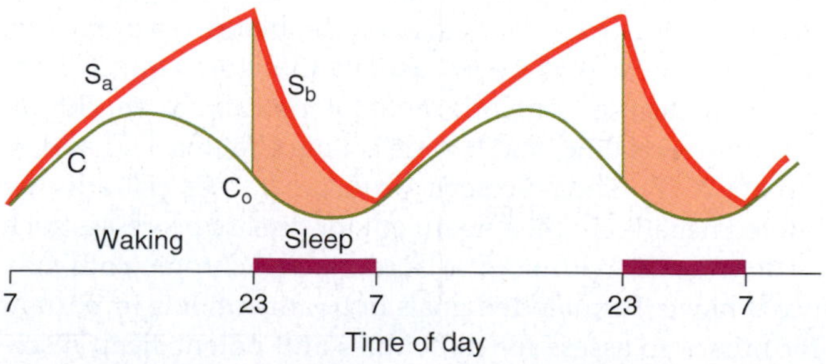

Sa
Sb
C
Co
Waking
Sleep
7
23
7
23
7
Time of day

Figure 3.3 ■ The two-process model for sleep. S, sleep pressure; C, circadian rhythm.

Sleep is divided into two main types, nonrapid eye movement (NREM) and rapid eye movement (REM). NREM sleep is further divided into three stages:

N1: Light sleep

N2: Slightly deeper sleep

N3: Deep or slow-wave sleep.

A person "cycles" through all stages of sleep every 90 to 120 minutes starting with NREM sleep (Carskadon & Dement, 2017). As the night progresses, less time is spent in N3 and more time is spent in REM sleep (**Figure 3.4** ■). N3 sleep is connected with growth hormone secretion. REM sleep is where memory consolidation occurs along with dreaming. There are specific electroencephalogram characteristics for each stage of sleep. Finally, during REM sleep, the body experiences muscle atonia. This prevents the sleeping individual from "acting out" his or her dreams. If this muscle atonia is lost, then a specific sleep disorder is present and can be indicative of a developing neurologic disorder such as Parkinson disease. There is no muscle atonia in the NREM stages of sleep. Patients with disrupted sleep may experience parasomnias, which are partial arousals from sleep where the person's brain is partially asleep and partially awake. Parasomnias include sleep walking, sleep talking, and night terrors.

SAFETY ALERT: For patients in the hospital setting, assessment for parasomnias is important as safety can become an issue. ■

Factors Affecting Sleep

Many factors can affect sleep. Some are intrinsic to the individual, some are behaviors of the individual, and some are medically related (such as different disease processes or medications). Intrinsic factors include the patient's baseline emotional state.

Extrinsic factors include noise, light, hunger, room temperature, and so on. Light, as described above, can affect sleep. Something as simple as a street light outside or the light in a hospital hallway can disrupt sleep. Sound is another important disruptor of sleep. In a typical hospital, noise is slightly decreased at night but is still above some patients' threshold for sleep. Finally, in the hospital, typical nursing actions during the evening and night (such as taking routine vital signs) will disrupt sleep.

Different disease processes (not necessarily sleep disorders) can affect sleep. Congestive heart failure is known to cause changes in breathing during the night, decreasing the quality and quantity of sleep. Anxiety can also affect sleep. If a person is anxious at bedtime and keeps thinking about distressing thoughts (called *rumination*), falling asleep will be delayed. As described later in the chapter, a number of medications usually not thought of as sleep interrupters can in fact disrupt sleep.

Bidirectional Nature of Sleep and Physiological Processes

Sleep has a bidirectional relationship with physiologic processes in the body. Sleep disorders such as obstructive sleep apnea can affect the cardiovascular, neurologic, respiratory, and emotional functions of the human body. This bidirectional interaction can be seen in many interactions and body systems. Common interactions are covered here.

Cardiovascular Disorders and Sleep

Inadequate sleep due to a sleep disorder such as obstructive sleep apnea, insomnia, or personal restrictions of sleep is correlated with hypertension, coronary artery disease, subclinical atherosclerotic disease, and cerebrovascular disease (St-Onge et al., 2016). The mechanisms by which inadequate sleep cause these issues are multifaceted. There is a disruption in the autonomic nervous system with a lack of parasympathetic relaxation and a continued high level of sympathetic activity. There can be changes in cytokine production and other pro-inflammatory changes. Sleep deficits from any reason also adversely affect glucose homeostasis and insulin sensitivity, leading to increased weight gain. This in turn leads to obesity and type 2 diabetes, which compound the cardiovascular risk.

Patients with congestive heart failure or other cardiovascular conditions can have issues with sleep. There can be metabolic changes within the sleep–wake system in relation to the cardiovascular disease, such as changes in catecholamine levels. Sleep deprivation can occur with cardiovascular diseases due to pain or difficulty breathing. Untreated or

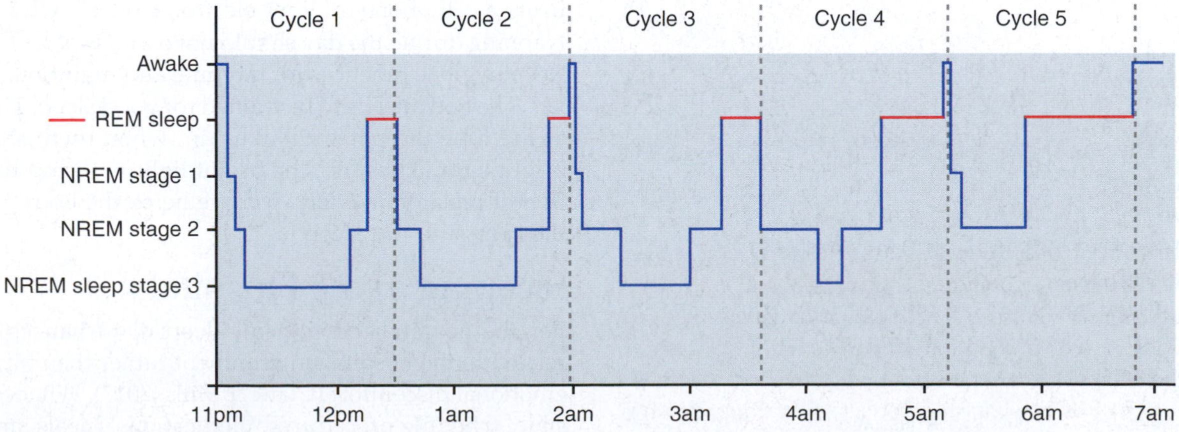
Cycle 1
Cycle 2
Cycle 3
Cycle 4
Cycle 5
Awake
REM sleep
NREM stage 1
NREM stage 2
NREM sleep stage 3
11pm
12pm
1am
2am
3am
4am
5am
6am
7am

Figure 3.4 ■ Typical pattern of sleep stages across the night.

poorly treated obstructive sleep apnea can lead to strokes, and strokes can lead to issues with sleeping (insomnia or excessive sleepiness) along with inducing OSA, depending on where the stroke occurred in the brain. This in turn can negatively affect the recovery of the person who has had a stroke.

Neurologic Disorders, Pain, and Sleep

Sleep disturbances can be a harbinger of degenerative neurologic disorders. REM behavior disorder has been linked with the development of Parkinson disease or related disorders (Silber, St. Louis, & Boeve, 2017). Sleep can also be affected by seizure disorders (i.e., sleep deprivation can induce seizures) and nighttime seizures can induce sleep deprivation. Any medication that crosses the blood–brain barrier can affect sleep. Some SSRIs will decrease the amount of REM sleep while others will increase the amount. Medications can also induce insomnia and exacerbate the underlying medical issue (Adams et al., 2017). Pain at nighttime has also been demonstrated to affect sleep quantity and quality. Common opioid analgesics used for pain control can have deleterious effects on sleep. Good sleep hygiene is important for all patients with medical conditions and/or taking medications that negatively affect sleep. **Table 3.1** lists selected medications that affect sleep.

Table 3.1 Selected Medications and Their Effect on Sleep

Class of Medication and Examples	Sleep Disruption
Cardiovascular Disorders	
Lipophilic beta blockers pindolol propranolol metrolprolol	■ Increase number of awakenings and total time awake at night ■ Potential to provoke nightmares
Antiarrhythmics procainamide quinidine disopyramide	■ Insomnia ■ Daytime sleepiness
Neurologic Disorders	
Selective serotonin reuptake inhibitors (SSRIs) fluoxetine escitalopram	■ Insomnia
Sedating tricyclic antidepressants amitriptyline	■ Daytime sleepiness
Activating tricyclic antidepressants imipramine	■ Insomnia
Anticholinergics tiotopium oxybutynin scopolamine	■ Daytime sleepiness
Levodopa or dopamine agonists	■ Daytime sleepiness
Respiratory Disorders	
Bronchodilators (both long and short acting) albuterol formoterol	■ Difficulty falling asleep ■ Insomnia
Corticosteroids	■ Insomnia

Sources: Data from Adams et al., 2017; Winchchniak, Wierzbicka, Walecka, & Jernajczk, 2017.

Respiratory Disorders and Sleep

Any respiratory disorder has the potential to affect sleep. Chronic coughing or wheezing during the night will either awaken the patient fully or cause an arousal or sleep stage change. Medications given to prevent wheezing or coughing at nighttime can also disrupt sleep. Bronchodilators used for both asthma and chronic obstructive pulmonary disease can delay sleep onset. Adults with chronic respiratory diseases state that difficulty falling asleep, staying asleep, and daytime sleepiness are related to their underlying disease process (Marin & Carrizo, 2017).

3.2 Health Promotion

Sleep is one of the fundamental processes of the human body. Promoting quality and appropriate quantity of sleep is an important role for nurses. As stated previously, when sleep is disrupted, most of the body systems are affected. Promoting quality and appropriate quantity of sleep involves patient education on the effects of sleep, how to obtain "good" sleep, and finally reviewing all medications and health issues to develop a plan of care to promote sleep and minimize issues with poor sleep.

The Importance of Rest

Rest can be promoted by helping the patient understand disease processes and how the body recovers. The hospitalized patient may need periods of no interruptions during the day to relax and allow the body to heal. It is a balancing act, though, because if the patient naps frequently during the daytime, then nighttime sleep can be adversely affected.

Sleep Hygiene

Sleep hygiene is a series of practices and habits that help an individual achieve quality sleep. Good sleep hygiene includes going to bed at the same time, awakening at the same time, exercising daily, being exposed to bright light in the morning, having proper nutrition, not eating immediately before bedtime, avoiding alcohol before bedtime, avoiding caffeine after mid-afternoon, avoiding use of electronic devices 1 to 2 hours before bedtime, and using the bedroom only for sleeping and other personal activities. Watching TV in bed is *not* good sleep hygiene and neither is using a cell phone or other electronic device while in bed. Napping during the day should not occur. **Box 3.1** lists good sleep hygiene practices for daytime and nighttime.

The body needs to be trained for good sleep. This starts at the time the patient wakes up, when there should be bright light exposure. The bright light will stop the secretion of melatonin. Daily exercise helps the body build up the "pressure" for sleep.

Sleeping in the Hospital

For the hospitalized patient, sleep disturbances may be related to the hospital environment rather than physical or emotional discomfort (Clark & Mills, 2017). Whenever possible, schedule procedures, medications, meals, and other activities around the patient's normal sleep schedule. Nurses

BOX 3.1
Good Sleep Hygiene

DAYTIME ACTIONS

Have a consistent wakeup time.

Get exposed to bright light upon awakening.

Exercise daily.

Do not nap during the day.

Limit caffeine in the afternoon.

Do not eat a heavy meal 1-2 hours before bedtime.

NIGHTTIME ACTIONS

Refrain from using electronics at least 1 hour before bedtime.

Have a consistent bedtime.

Have a consistent bedtime routine.

Keep the bedroom cool, dark, and quiet.

Do not keep or use TV or other electronics in the bedroom.

Use the bed only for sleep and sex.

should assess the patient's individual circadian rhythm because patients who normally go to sleep late may develop sleep disturbances if forced to attempt sleep before their normal bedtime. In contrast, patients who are early risers may prefer to have physical therapy first thing in the morning.

Once a sleep schedule is identified, bedtime rituals may include assisting the patient with hygiene activities such as toileting and a hand and face wash, offering a warm beverage or massage, and retrieving fresh pillows or extra blankets. Reduce environmental distractions such as noise and external light sources, as outlined in **Box 3.2**. If good sleep hygiene still does not produce a restful night of sleep, it may be appropriate to request an order for a sedative/hypnotic to help the patient sleep.

One aspect to also inquire about is "who" is usually in the patient's bedroom. Patients in the hospital may have problems falling asleep if they feel the lack of their usual sleep companion (human or animal). While not much can be done in the hospital setting concerning this, the information is still important to know as this could be a reason why the patient is not sleeping.

BOX 3.2
Minimizing Environmental Stimuli in the Hospital Setting

NOISE

- Place patients in single-bed rooms when possible instead of multiple-bed rooms. If a patient must be in a semiprivate or larger room, close the curtains between clients.
- Keep the patient's door closed to reduce hallway noise.
- Reduce excess noise at specified quiet hours (e.g., turn off televisions, lower the ringtone of telephones, reduce the volume or discontinue use of the paging system).
- Minimize noise from staff interactions and minimize use of the public address system.
- Perform only essential activities in the patient's room during sleeping hours.

LIGHT

- Adjust window coverings to block outside lights at night and to allow natural light during the day.
- At night, use a nightlight or turn on bathroom lights instead of overhead lighting.
- When entering a patient's darkened room, use a flashlight instead of turning on the room lights.

SURROUNDINGS

- Pleasant surroundings and color schemes can produce a calming environment, producing comfort and improved outcomes.
- Decrease use of bold, abstract picture hangings, as this can enhance agitation and inability to sleep.

3.3 Assessing the Patient with Altered Sleep

Health Assessment Interview

The interview for the patient with altered sleep needs to be comprehensive, as any major body system can have an impact on sleep. An example of this is uncontrolled asthma. Nighttime wheezing can prevent a patient from sleeping, yet using medications such as albuterol can excite the cardiac and nervous systems and prevent falling asleep. Besides the standard interview, the patient should be asked specific questions concerning sleep/wake habits and patterns, including:

- What time do you go to bed?
- What do you do the 2 hours before bedtime?
- What time do you wake up?
- Do you wake up to an alarm clock or spontaneously?
- Do your habits vary on weekdays versus weekends?
- Do you smoke, drink alcohol, or use substances before going to bed or at other times during the day?
- Do you take any prescription or over-the-counter (OTC) medications in general or specifically for sleep?
- Do you snore? Sleep walk? Sleep talk?
- How do you feel when you wake up?
- Do you ever fall asleep during the day? While driving?

Having the patient keep a sleep diary for a couple of days provides good information (see **Figure 3.5** ■).

Physical Examination

The majority of information for sleep disorders is found during the interview phase of an assessment as opposed to the physical examination. The nurse should pay attention to the oropharynx for "crowding" (small air space at the back of the throat) and neck size if obstructive sleep apnea is suspected. Weight and BMI should be calculated. Diagnostic tests ordered for patients with sleep alterations are listed in the Diagnostic Tests feature.

Sleep Diary	Name:						
	Week of:						
Morning Questions	Mon.	Tues.	Wed.	Thurs.	Fri.	Sat.	Sun.
What time did you go to bed last night?							
What time did you fall asleep?							
How many times did you wake up last night?							
How long were you awake during the night?							
Was your sleep good, fair, or poor?							
Did you wake up before your alarm?							
How many times did you hit the snooze button?							
How do you feel this morning?							
Evening Questions	Mon.	Tues.	Wed.	Thurs.	Fri.	Sat.	Sun.
Did you drink any caffeine today?							
How much?							
Did you exercise today?							
How many minutes?							
How many times did you nap today?							
Did you drink any alcohol today?							
How much?							

Figure 3.5 ■ Example of a sleep diary.

Diagnostic Tests

NAME OF TEST	PURPOSE AND DESCRIPTION	RELATED NURSING INTERVENTIONS
Polysomnography	A multichannel overnight study to assess sleep quality, type, and respiratory issues along with neurological issues	Education concerning the procedure; postexam education based on findings
Home sleep test	Limited study conducted at home to diagnosis OSA	Set-up and postexam education based on findings

Measurement of Sleep

Sleep is measured in a number of ways, and some are more accurate and objective than others. The usual questions asked of patients rely on the patient's recall and perception, so the responses may not be accurate. Asking a patient to keep a sleep diary will provide more accurate information if the patient truly fills out the form every day.

There are a number of questionnaires that assess for sleepiness and some sleep disorders, such as the Epworth Sleepiness Scale, which is readily available online, and the STOP-BANG questionnaire of obstructive sleep apnea in adults (University of Toronto, 2012). One way to measure sleep–wake over time is through the use of **actigraphy**, in which a small accelerometer is worn on the nondominant wrist to measure movement. Through computer algorithms, the output provides long-term data (usually for 2 to 3 weeks) of sleep–wake cycles. If the actigraphy is coupled with standardized sleep diaries, the combined data are more compelling. There are a number of personal devices, such as watches, that consumers wear that claim to measure sleep and even which sleep stage a person is in, but at the time of publication of this textbook most, if not all, have not been validated and should not be solely relied on for sleep issues. They are useful, though, in that information from these devices may bring patients in to seek treatment for sleep disorders.

Finally, for certain sleep disorders (such as obstructive sleep apnea), overnight polysomnography is used. This can be through a limited home sleep test where the patient wears some equipment at home or a full in-sleep lab. This is discussed more in Section 3.7. Assessments used to examine sleep are outlined in **Table 3.2**.

Table 3.2 Selected Sleep Assessments

Assessment	Description and Abnormal Findings
Examination of oropharynx	■ Examined with light and tonged depressor ■ Normal finding is a large, open area in the back of the throat ■ Abnormal finding is crowded small space in the back of the throat
Epworth Sleepiness Scale	■ This scale measures sleepiness during the day ■ A score of 0–10 is a normal level of daytime sleepiness ■ A score above 10 indicates excessive daytime sleepiness
STOP-BANG Questionnaire	■ This questionnaire helps determine the risk of obstructive sleep apnea ■ A score of less than 3 indicates a low risk for OSA ■ A score of 3–4 indicates intermediate risk of OSA ■ A score of 5–8 indicates a high risk of OSA
Actigraphy	■ A watchlike device that measures rest–activity levels continuously for up to 4 weeks ■ Demonstrates disrupted sleep
Sleep diary	■ A paper or digital form completed daily by the patient ■ Examines sleep across a typical week

3.4 Assessment of Selected Populations

When assessing sleep in older adults, the process is the same but the nurse must realize there are multiple factors that influence sleep. As humans age, there is a tendency for earlier bedtimes and then resultant earlier arise time, though the underlying physiological reasons for this are still to be elucidated. Lack of activity during the daytime due to illness or disability may not have the buildup of pressure to sleep (as described in Section 3.1). Older adults can have a number of sleep complaints. Some of these complaints can be from comorbid conditions such as pain syndromes or respiratory issues such as chronic obstructive pulmonary disease. Men with benign prostrate hyperplasia may need to frequently urinate at night. Women in menopause have a risk for OSA that is the same as men, due to changes in progesterone and fat redistribution (Baker, Joffe, & Lee, 2017). Finally, sleep difficulties in older adults can have profound implications such as social isolation, increased risk of fall, and in severe cases, delirium.

Changes in sleep patterns in veterans will depend on any injury or disease caused by being in service. For example, if the veteran suffers from posttraumatic stress disorder, then nightmares or insomnia may be present. If the veteran suffered an injury, then chronic pain could prevent quality sleep.

Patients in the LGBTQI community are more likely to suffer from stress, depression, and bullying, putting them at risk for poor sleep (quality and quantity) along with insomnia. Nurses should assess the patient for any sleep issues, mental health issues, and bullying. Providing them with resources to help with the issues is important. Mental health counselors or nurses with specialization in mental health issues should be recommended. Nurses should provide tips and techniques for good sleep and relaxation to help this vulnerable population of patients.

3.5 Sleep Deprivation

The Patient with a Sleep Deficit

Pathophysiology and Manifestations

As noted previously, sleep deficit can have profound effect on physiologic, emotional, and cognitive functioning. There is an increase in heart rate, decrease in concentration, slowing of reflexes, and irritability. The basis for most of these outward changes is changes in cytokine levels along with other neuroendocrine proteins. The cytokines that regulate sleep are also involved with the immune system. This is one of the reasons why when a person becomes sleep deprived, they have an increased risk of infection. Sleep deprivation changes the leptin/ghrelin and other regulators of satiety, making overeating and obesity an issue. Sleep deprivation increases insulin resistance along with A1C levels and impairs fasting glucose levels (St-Onge et al., 2016). It also causes an increase in proinflammatory markers and proinflammatory cytokines (St-Ogne et al., 2016).

Interprofessional and Nursing Care

Interprofessional care for all patients with sleep difficulties may involve psychotherapists, respiratory therapists, physicians, sleep technologists, and nurses. Each will have a different role. For example, with insomnia (described in the next section) cognitive-behavioral therapy is important. This type of therapy is provided by psychotherapists or nurse practitioners with special training in the therapy. If a patient suffers from sleep apnea, then a respiratory therapist may assist in the fitting and management of positive airway pressure treatment. Adherence to treatment is a major concern for almost all of the sleep disorders. To assist the patient in treatment adherence, a multidisciplinary team is almost always used. Nurses play a particularly important role. The nurse will provide follow-up on treatment adherence, offer support, and problem-solve with the patient on issues of treatment adherence. The nurse can help the patient overcome almost any difficulty with treatment and provide a holistic view of the patient's treatment.

3.6 Insomnia

Insomnia is the inability to fall asleep, stay asleep, or feel rested upon awakening. During the day, the patient with insomnia will feel tired or fatigued; have difficulties learning, paying attention, or concentrating; and may be irritable and prone to accidents (Sateia, 2014).

The Patient with Insomnia

The factors that perpetuate insomnia after the initial stressor include poor sleep habits, intrinsic arousals, and changes in cognition (Buysse & Harvey, 2017). Daytime consequences of insomnia include fatigue, mood changes, and performance issues at work. The daytime consequences can have a bidirectional relationship with emotional, cognitive, and physiologic arousals, which in turn have a bidirectional relationship with worry about sleep, rumination about not being able to sleep, and the consequences of not sleeping. Insomnia can become a perpetuating cycle that is difficult to break.

Insomnia has been shown to be a risk factor for the development of depression, anxiety, and headaches. Insomnia has also been shown to be associated with the development of fibromyalgia, rheumatoid arthritis, osteoporosis, and asthma (Slivertsen et al., 2014). While exact mechanisms are not known, it is postulated that neuroendocrine and immune system changes that are seen with sleep deprivation could be a reason. There is a strong relationship between insomnia and future development of depression (Buysee & Harvey, 2017). There is also some evidence that links shortened sleep with performance impairments and increase in mortality risk (Buysse & Harvey, 2017).

Pathophysiology and Manifestations

There are a number of models to describe the pathophysiology of insomnia. One model states that all individuals have predisposing factors for insomnia, then a precipitating factor will occur, such as a job change or other life stress, which will move the person over a threshold, and insomnia will occur. Depending on how the person reacts to the insomnia, it will either resolve or it will become chronic (**Figure 3.6** ■). Once the insomnia starts, it can become self-reinforcing, which will keep the insomnia going.

Interprofessional Care

Diagnosis

Diagnosis of insomnia is based on patient report as described above. The patient will report trouble falling asleep, staying asleep, or poor quality of sleep. There is no bloodwork or imaging tests for insomnia. Sometimes, actigraphy will be used to assess the patient's sleep patterns over a length of time. The results of the actigraphy are not used to confirm the diagnosis of insomnia but to elucidate further the degree of difficulty sleeping.

Medications

There are numerous medications for insomnia, both prescribed and over the counter. The key issue with medication use in insomnia is once the medication is stopped the insomnia will still be present. Medication for the treatment of insomnia should be used only short term while other proven therapies, such as cognitive-behavioral therapy, are implemented to help resolve the underlying issues of insomnia. Unfortunately, it is easier for some prescribers to keep patients on medications for insomnia as opposed to using other treatment modalities. A number of the medications used have significant side effects (tricyclics, trazadone, benzodiazepines, other sedating antidepressives). Even the medications with FDA approval for insomnia have serious reported side effects (see **Medication Administration 3.A**). Also most of these medications have the potential for significant daytime effects (sleepiness, poor coordination, poor judgment). Most OTC sleep aids contain diphenhydramine (Benadryl). Both prescribed and OTC agents for sleep can cause psychologic and physiologic dependency. Patient may be reluctant to stop using the medication due to the fear of not being able to sleep. This fear then becomes self-perpetuating if the person is unable to fall asleep. This is why assessment of any medication or supplements used for sleep is needed and why a plan should be developed to help the patient learn how to fall asleep independently. Melatonin, an OTC medication, is used by many patients, although its effectiveness may be inconsistent.. Melatonin is best used for inability to fall asleep and must be given approximately 30 minutes before bedtime. More than 5 mg of melatonin is not effective (National Center for Complementary and Integrative Health [NCCIH], 2017). The FDA considers melatonin a supplement, and it does not regulate supplements, so the doses and purity of them are not guaranteed. Finally, some patients use herbal remedies for sleep. The most common is valerian. There is limited information on the efficacy of this herbal supplement (NCCIH, 2016).

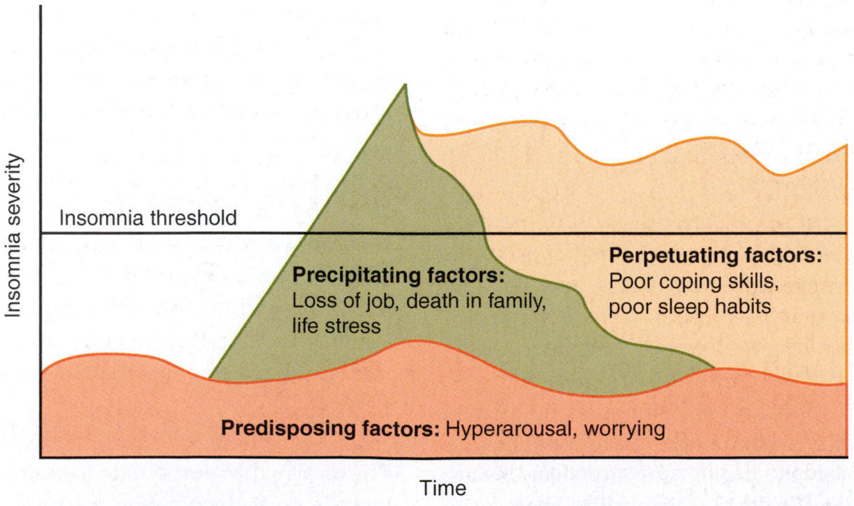
Insomnia severity
Insomnia threshold
Precipitating factors:
Loss of job, death in family, life stress
Perpetuating factors:
Poor coping skills, poor sleep habits
Predisposing factors: Hyperarousal, worrying
Time

Figure 3.6 ■ Predisposing, precipitating, and perpetuating model of insomnia.

Medication Administration 3.A

Sleep Agents

EXAMPLES

zaleplon (Sonata)

zolpidem (Ambien)

Sleep medications are used for short-term treatment of insomnia.

Nursing Responsibilities

- Monitor for changes in behavior.
- Monitor for tolerance, abuse, and dependence.
- Provide safe environment and monitor ambulation after drug ingestion.
- Monitor respiratory status in the presence of pre-existing pulmonary function compromise.
- Patient education is important on side effects and risks (see below).

Health Education for the Patient and Family

- Advise patients to get into bed immediately after taking medication.
- Can cause daytime drowsiness.
- Can cause amnesia, confusion, sleep walking, and hallucinations.
- Can cause suicide ideation.
- Do not take with alcohol and let provider know of any over-the-counter or supplements that are taken.
- Sleep walking and sleep driving have occurred, especially when used with other central nervous system depressants.

Note: Drugs identified in blue are among the 200 most commonly prescribed medications in the United States.

SOURCES: Data from Adams et al., 2017; Shields, Fox, & Liebrecht, 2018; prescribing information for zolpidem, *www.accessdata.fda.gov/drugsatfda_docs/label/2016/019908s037lbl.pdf*.

Nursing Care

Nurses must carefully ask why a patient is on a medication and also ask about any over-the-counter medications being used. Some patients will not think that what they take for sleep is a medication, so the nurse must question carefully. Nurses must be alert to the issue of dependency on medications for sleeping.

Sometimes a simple question from the nurse elucidates there is a sleep disorder. Every patient, whether in the hospital or in a clinic setting, should be assessed for sleep patterns. Teaching about good sleep hygiene should be conducted for every patient, no matter the age or presenting issue.

Moving Evidence into Action

Sleep in the Hospitalized Patient

Clinical Issue

Sleep in hospitalized patients is known to be disrupted. This can be due to comorbid sleep disorders, other medical disorders, or the hospital environment and medical/nursing treatments.

External Evidence

A number of studies have demonstrated disrupted sleep in hospitalized patients. The disruptions can be due to pain, light, noise, medication, and crowding of rooms (Clark & Mills, 2017). Clark and Mills (2017) developed a "sleep menu" for medical/surgical patients. The menu includes potential options to improve sleep with a follow-up section on what interventions worked and what interventions did not. Some of the interventions include eye shades, sound machines, fans, and aromatherapy. The results of the study demonstrated no significant differences due to small sample size and limited time frame; however, there were some important points made. Patients were satisfied that nurses were asking about sleep and that they were given options for improving their sleep. The majority of patients selected the following interventions: Closing the door to their room, dimming the lights, using a warmed blanket, and drinking a calming tea (Clark & Mills, 2017).

Internal Evidence

Each hospital floor needs to determine what is feasible based on severity of patients. However, simple interventions such as dimming the lights, decreasing noise, and providing eye shades can enhance sleep. Ear plugs are also an easy intervention to provide to patients. Implementing a questionnaire as described in the Clark and Mills article is also an easy implementation. The survey would need to be tailored to what is feasible in each specific hospital or unit. Also all staff need to be educated about the importance of sleep.

Considerations

Some patients may have a sleep disorder before coming in to the hospital. Also in hospital rooms where there are two patients, balancing the needs of both patients can be tricky. If one patient requires darkness and another needs a little light, offering eye shades to one may help.

Putting the Pieces Together

Using the information from patients on their normal sleep patterns along with offering different techniques for promoting sleep in the hospital may allow patients to achieve quality sleep while hospitalized.

Reference

Clark, A., & Mills, M. (2017). Can a sleep menu enhance the quality of sleep for a hospitalized patient? *Medsurg Nursing, 26*(4), 253–257.

3.7 Sleep-Disordered Breathing

The Patient with Obstructed Sleep Apnea

Pathophysiology

Obstructive sleep apnea (OSA) is a disorder of breathing during the night. OSA is caused by the airway either partially or completely collapsing during the nighttime. Respiratory effort continues but airflow is blocked. Eventually there is a change in blood chemistry, which signals the brain to "arouse" (not necessarily come to a complete awakening) enough for stimulation of the nerves controlling the function of the upper airway to cause the muscles to become more tight, which opens the airway, allowing airflow. This process causes the individual to snore, snort, or gasp repeatedly (hundreds of times) over the night, which in turn decreases restful sleep. Along with the repeated brain arousals, there is sympathetic nervous stimulation, including desaturations and changes in heart rate (first decrease then increase) and blood pressure (increase) due to the changes in the balance between the parasympathetic and sympathetic nervous systems. In adults during these periods of obstructive breaths, dysrhythmias, up to and including asystole, can be seen.

Risk Factors

Risk factors for OSA include obesity, large neck size, and male gender (until menopause for women, then incidence and risk factors are the same). Other risk factors are small oropharynx, small midface, and micrognathia.

Manifestations and Complications

The manifestations of OSA can be divided into nighttime and daytime symptoms. Nighttime symptoms include snoring, snorting, and gasping. Daytime symptoms include headache upon arising, daytime sleepiness, irritability, and inability to concentrate.

The complications of untreated or poorly treated OSA are numerous, ranging from poor daytime function (e.g., sleepiness, cognitive function) to hypertension, cardiovascular disease, and stroke due to the cyclical nature of the closing of the airway, which the brain tries to keep open by "arousing the body" and stimulating the sympathetic nervous system (Somers & Javaheri, 2017).

Interprofessional Care

Diagnosis

Diagnosis is based on either an overnight polysomnography or a limited home sleep study. There are specific criteria for scoring and interpreting the studies, which then leads to the diagnosis of OSA.

Nutrition

If the patient is overweight, the best treatment for OSA is weight loss. The patient does not need to be at ideal weight, but even a small percentage of weight loss can be effective. While this is the best treatment for OSA, it is also the hardest to accomplish and maintain. Nurses have a key role in weight reduction, helping patients to set goals and make appropriate food and activity choices while monitoring progress and offering encouragement.

Treatment for OSA

There are a number of different treatments for OSA: Weight loss, positional devices, oral devices, positive airway pressure, surgery, and a recently approved neurostimulator for select patients. For very mild sleep apnea, positional devices can be used so the patient maintains a side sleeping position, which helps prevent the patient from rolling on his or her back, allowing the airway to more easily obstruct. Oral devices, which look like mouth guards, help bring forward the jaw and tongue, which increases the diameter of the posterior oropharynx. *Continuous positive airway pressure (CPAP)* is a device that supplies a constant airflow through a patient interface. The amount of air pressure holds the airway open during the nighttime. Nurses play a vital role in assisting with adherence to the prescribed positive airway pressure. Troubleshooting, support, and active problem solving are all areas in which nursing plays a key role. **Figure 3.7** ■ demonstrates how continuous positive airway pressure works.

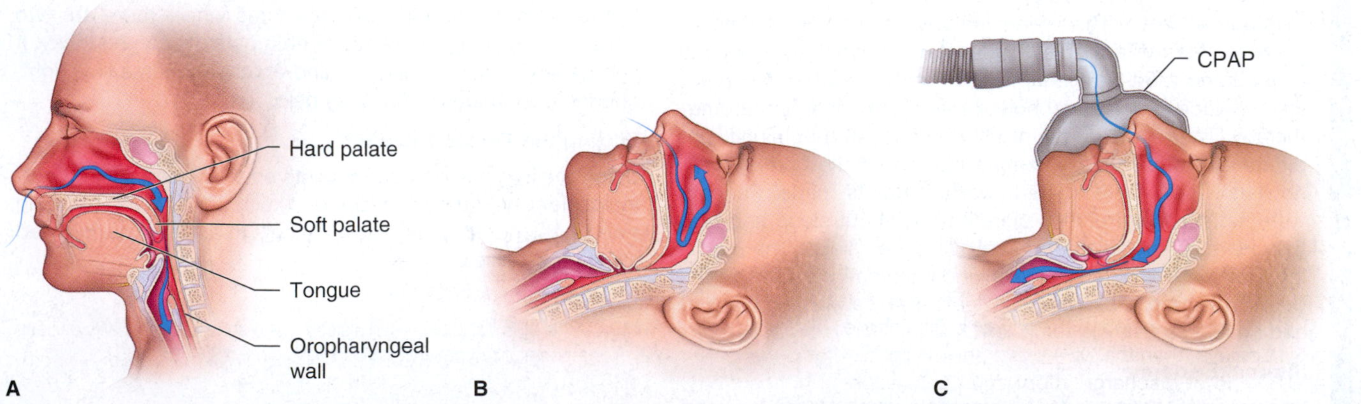
Hard palate
Soft palate
Tongue
Oropharyngeal wall
A
B
CPAP
C

Figure 3.7 ■ Nasal CPAP keeps the airway open during sleep. **A**, In awake individual, muscle tone maintains open airway against negative pressure during inspiration. **B**, When asleep, the tongue, soft palate, and oropharyngeal walls collapse, closing off the airway. **C**, Positive pressure, supplied by CPAP, acts as a splint to keep the airway open, regardless of the sleeper's position.

There are surgical procedures for the treatment of OSA, but success rates are low. The surgery is in three parts including a uvulopalatopharyngoplasty, followed by genioglossus advancement or hyoid myotomy and suspension, and then finally maxillomandibular advancement. The FDA has recently approved a hypoglossal nerve stimulator for selected patients, which stimulates the hypoglossal nerve to maintain upper airway patency during sleep. This is used for moderate to severe OSA in adults. Nurses are involved in the education of care after surgery, troubleshoot surgical complications, and monitor for other complications if there are comorbid conditions (which are likely to be present).

Nursing Care

Nurses play a vital role in assisting adherence to the prescribed positive airway pressure. Troubleshooting, support, and active problem solving are all areas in which nursing plays a key role. Education of the patients, support, and follow-up are very important.

Assessment

Assessment of a patient with OSA for nurses is asking about adherence to the treatment regimen and troubleshooting any issues. Some issues such as dry nose, excoriations on the face, and air swallowing are simple for the nurse to troubleshoot. The most important intervention a nurse can do is support the patient who is undergoing positive airway pressure and educate them on the importance of continued treatment to avoid the consequences of untreated OSA.

Priorities of Care

The main priority of care for nurses in most of the treatments for OSA is supporting the patient with adherence to treatment. Patients on PAP need support guidance and assistance with troubleshooting. With weight loss (which should be for every patient with OSA), support, encouragement, and education are nursing's priorities.

The Patient with Central Sleep Apnea

Pathophysiology

Central sleep apnea (CSA) is a consolidation of a couple of different types of apnea, including central sleep apnea with Cheyne-Stokes breathing (common with congestive heart failure); central apnea due to a medical disorder without Cheyne-Stokes breathing (due to failure of ventilatory control centers to initiate ventilator effort); and central sleep apnea due to a medication or substance abuse (Sateia, 2014).

Risk Factors

There are multiple risk factors for CSA. Medications, neurological diseases, heart failure, and obesity can all lead to some form of CSA. Some of these risk factors are nonmodifiable (muscular degenerative diseases) while some can be prevented (congestive heart failure).

Moving Evidence into Action

Preventing Complications of Surgery in Patients with OSA

Clinical Issue

Patients with OSA, whether diagnosed or not, have increased risk of complications during and after all surgical procedures. Screening for OSA is important before surgery

External Evidence

A multidisciplinary approach to screening for OSA was implemented in a perioperative setting (Lemus, McMullin, & Bailnowski, 2017). For the study, all patients who were undergoing orthopedic surgery were asked if they had OSA. If they reported an OSA history, the patients were asked to bring their positive airway pressure machine and interface along with a copy of the orders for the setting of the machine at the time of the scheduled surgery for use during hospitalization. By having the patient's own device and interface there would not need to be a period of acclimation to the interface or machine. The OSA protocol was then initiated, which included handoff information about the patient, OSA documentation in the EHR, modified pain management, and modified monitoring and discharge criteria. Patients who had not been diagnosed with OSA were screened with the STOP-BANG questionnaire. If the results of the questionnaire were positive, then the OSA protocol was initiated as described above, and at discharge information and teaching concerning OSA was given. Findings were a decrease of 12.4% in complications in patients with OSA or a positive STOP-BANG screen from the preintervention state (Lemus et al., 2017).

Internal Evidence

Screening for OSA is simple and can be added to most EHRs. This issue concerns what to do with the information. Follow-up is important as many patients do not feel OSA is an important disease to treat, and treatment has a high nonadherence rate. Strong support for teaching and follow-up is important for any setting where there is screening for OSA.

Patient Considerations

As stated above, adherence to positive airway pressure treatment is a challenge. Surgery is not always successful and weight loss is difficult. Those patients who are most likely to follow treatment recommendations are those who feel better early in treatment. Nurses need to support patients in a number of ways for success in OSA treatment.

Putting the Pieces Together

Nurses should be attuned to the risks of OSA in all their patients. Undiagnosed OSA can have significant short-term and long-term sequela in patients.

Reference

Lemus, L. P., McMullin, B., & Bailnowski, H. (2017). Don't ignore my snore: Reducing perioperative complications of obstructive sleep apnea. *Journal of PeriAnesthesia Nursing, 33*(3), 338–345.

Manifestations and Complications

The manifestations of central sleep apnea depend on the underlying cause. All patients with CSA will experience tiredness and sleepiness during the day. Symptoms during sleep will include pauses in breathing without any effort or waxing/waning respirations (e.g., Cheyne-Stokes breathing). Complications of all types of CSA include hypoxemia, hypercapnea, and worsening of underlying disease processes.

Interprofessional Care

Diagnosis

An overnight polysomnography is needed to diagnosis CSA. There are specific diagnostic criteria for each one of the subtypes of CSA.

Treatment

Treatment involves different types of positive airway pressure at night, sometimes supplemental oxygen, and in extreme cases noninvasive ventilation. There are no medications for treating CSA. If the CSA disorder is due to medications (primarily use of opioids and derivatives) then weaning from the medications (if possible) and/or switching medications can help decrease the number of central events during the night.

3.8 Restless Legs Syndrome

The Patient with Restless Legs Syndrome

Pathophysiology

Restless legs syndrome (RLS) is a common sleep disorder affecting 5 to 10% of adults. The pathophysiology of RLS relates to dopamine levels in the brain. The dopamine is needed for effective neuromuscular action and response. In the brain, one of the limiting factors for producing dopamine is iron. Patients with low iron stores are more likely to have RLS than those who do not.

Risk Factors

There are a few risk factors for RLS. One is a family history of RLS. The genetics have not been completely elucidated, but there is a familial relationship for RLS. Also any neuromuscular disease, including Parkinson disease, places a person at a higher risk for RLS. Finally, any disease process or health state that decreases iron stores places a person at higher risk for RLS, including chronic anemia, pregnancy, renal failure, and dialysis.

Manifestations and Complications

The manifestations of RLS are primarily a "creepy-crawly" or a "pins-and-needles" feeling in the legs, in the evening, which is relieved by movement. These abnormal feelings prevent the person from falling asleep as they must keep moving the legs (and sometimes arms) to relieve the feelings. The main complication from RLS is sleep disruption. Depending on the medication used to treat the symptoms of RLS, there can be a worsening of symptoms (called *augmentation*) over time. Also most medications used to treat RLS will have side effects and their potential complications.

Interprofessional Care

Diagnosis

Diagnosis is strictly based on patient report and a diagnosis of exclusion. The symptoms must be in the evening, relieved by movement, and not due to another disease process.

Medications

Medication treatment for RLS is done in a stepwise approach. Treatment first starts with gabapentin or like medications. If this class of medication does not work, then dopamine agonists are prescribed. The next step is dopamine precursors. Sometimes, benzodiazepines or opiates are used. Finally, iron supplementation is prescribed for patients with low iron stores.

The patient needs to be monitored for augmentation, which is increasing severity of symptoms after a length of time of being on a specific medication or with an increase in medication dosage as a way to control symptoms.

Nutrition

Increasing the iron content in the diet may help, as may iron supplements. If iron supplements are used, they should be taken with orange juice or other citrus juice to promote absorption. Milk and other drinks with calcium will bind with the iron and prevent absorption.

Integrative Therapies

There is little data that supports integrative therapies as a treatment for RLS. A healthy diet, daily exercise, decreasing stress, and good sleep hygiene are all needed in the treatment of RLS.

CHAPTER HIGHLIGHTS

3.1 Overview of Sleep

Describe the physiology of sleep, normal sleep patterns, and factors affecting sleep.

- Sleep is a reversible disengagement from the environment that has some common characteristics: Most humans sleep with their eyes closed, in a recumbent position, with regular breathing.
- One of the known purposes of sleep is to restore homeostasis along with mental and physical rejuvenation.
- Rest is a period of diminished activity, without disengagement from the environment, for mental and physical rejuvenation but does not necessarily restore homeostasis.
- The physiology of sleep is complex, involving multiple body systems, including the immune, metabolic, and sympathetic and parasympathetic nervous systems.

- Most humans sleep when it is dark and are awake when it is light. Light is the most important regulator of sleep and circadian rhythms.
- The normal amount of sleep is about 8 hours of consolidated sleep per 24-hour day during the nighttime. This can vary based on the person.
- Sleep is divided into two main types, nonrapid eye movement (NREM) and rapid eye movement (REM).
- NREM sleep is divided into three stages: N1, light sleep; N2, slightly deeper sleep; N3, deep or slow-wave sleep.
- Sleep has a bidirectional relationship with psychologic and physiologic processes in the body.
- Sleep disturbances can be a harbinger of degenerative neurologic disorders.

3.2 Health Promotion

Summarize topics that nurses teach to promote healthy sleep across the lifespan.

- Sleep is one of the fundamental processes of the human body. Promoting quality and appropriate quantity of sleep is an important role for nurses.
- Sleep hygiene is a series of practices and habits that help an individual achieve quality sleep. Good sleep hygiene includes going to bed at the same time, awakening at the same time, exercising daily, being exposed to bright light in the morning, having proper nutrition, not eating immediately before bedtime, avoiding alcohol before bedtime, avoiding caffeine after midafternoon, avoiding use of electronic devices 1 to 2 hours before bedtime, and using the bedroom only for sleeping and other personal activities.
- For the hospitalized patient, sleep disturbances may be related to the hospital environment rather than physical or emotional discomfort.

3.3 Assessing the Patient with Altered Sleep

Outline the components of the assessment of sleep including topics for the health assessment interview, techniques for physical assessment, and the diagnostic tests used in the assessment.

- The interview for the patient with altered sleep needs to be comprehensive, as any major body system can have an impact on sleep.
- The majority of information for sleep disorders is found during the interview phase of an assessment as opposed to the physical examination.
- Sleep is measured in a number of ways, and some are more accurate and objective than others. Questionnaires, sleep diaries, and polysomnography are all used to measure sleep.

3.4 Assessment of Selected Populations

Differentiate considerations for assessing the sleep of older adults, veterans, and individuals in the LGBTQI population.

- As humans age, there is a tendency for earlier bedtimes and then resultant earlier arise times, though the underlying physiological reasons for this are still to be elucidated. Lack of activity during the daytime due to illness or disability may not have the buildup of pressure to sleep.
- Veterans who suffer from PTSD may have nightmares or insomnia. Veterans that suffered an injury may have chronic pain that prevents quality sleep.
- Patients in the LGBTQI community are more likely to suffer stress, depression, and bullying, putting them at risk for poor sleep (quality and quantity) along with insomnia.

3.5 Sleep Deprivation

Describe the pathophysiology and manifestations of sleep deprivation, and outline the interprofessional care and nursing care of patients with this disorder.

- Sleep deficit can have a profound effect on physiologic, emotional, and cognitive functioning. There is an increase in heart rate, decrease in concentration, slowing of reflexes, and irritability.
- Interprofessional care for all patients with sleep difficulties may involve psychotherapists, respiratory therapists, physicians, sleep technologists, and nurses.

3.6 Insomnia

Describe the pathophysiology and manifestations of insomnia, and outline the interprofessional care and nursing care of patients with this disorder.

- Insomnia is the inability to fall asleep, stay asleep, or feel rested upon awakening. During the day, the patient with insomnia will feel tired or fatigued; have difficulties learning, paying attention, or concentrating; and may be irritable and prone to accidents.
- Insomnia has been shown to be a risk factor for the development of depression, anxiety, and headaches. Insomnia has also been shown to be associated with the development of fibromyalgia, rheumatoid arthritis, osteoporosis, and asthma.
- There are numerous medications for insomnia, both prescribed and over the counter. The key issue with medication use in insomnia is once the medication is stopped the insomnia will still be present.

3.7 Sleep-Disordered Breathing

Describe the pathophysiology and manifestations of sleep-disordered breathing, and outline the interprofessional care and nursing care of patients with this disorder.

- Obstructive sleep apnea (OSA) is a disorder of breathing during the night. OSA is caused by the airway either partially or completely collapsing during the nighttime. Respiratory effort continues but airflow is blocked. Complications of untreated or poorly treated OSA are numerous, ranging from poor daytime function to hypertension, cardiovascular disease, and stroke.
- Central sleep apnea (CSA) is a consolidation of a few types of apnea. The manifestations of CSA depend on the underlying cause.
- Treatment of sleep-disordered breathing involves different types of positive airway pressure at night, sometimes supplemental oxygen, and in extreme cases noninvasive ventilation.

3.8 Restless Legs Syndrome

Describe the pathophysiology and manifestations of restless legs syndrome, and outline the interprofessional care and nursing care of patients with this disorder.

- Restless leg syndrome (RLS) is a common sleep disorder effecting 5 to 10% of adults. The pathophysiology of RLS relates to dopamine levels in the brain.
- The manifestations of RLS are primarily a "creepy-crawly" or a "pins-and-needles" feeling in the legs, in the evening, which is relieved by movement.

TEST YOURSELF NCLEX-RN® REVIEW

1. A patient reports that he sleeps very little, preferring to "rest" several times each day. What does the nurse consider prior to replying to this remark?
   A. Rest and sleep have the same physiologic effects.
   B. Lack of sleep can interfere with learning.
   C. People disengage from their environment while resting.
   D. This type of resting should be done in a recumbent position with eyes closed.
2. A patient reports difficulty sleeping. Which suggestions will the nurse provide? (Select all that apply.)
   A. Drink a glass of wine right before going to bed.
   B. Exercise every day
   C. Avoid being exposed to bright light in the morning.
   D. Put electronic devices away 1 to 2 hours before bedtime.
   E. Watch TV in bed until sleepiness occurs.
3. A patient says that the fitness monitor he wears each night indicates that he does not sleep well. How does the nurse respond to this statement?
   A. "As long as these devices are worn on the dominant arm they are accurate."
   B. "Check to see if the devices counts your heart rate accurately to determine if it records other information correctly."
   C. "Tell me about how you feel you are sleeping."
   D. "These devices are not very accurate for recording how well you sleep."
4. A nurse has taken a job working the night shift in an assisted living facility for older adults. The nurse will expect which sleep patterns from the residents?
   A. They will sleep longer and better than younger persons.
   B. Men of this age will snore, but snoring is unusual in older adult women.
   C. As a group, older adults tend to go to bed earlier than younger persons.
   D. As a group, older adults tend to sleep later in the morning than younger persons.
5. A patient who is a war veteran has post-traumatic stress disorder (PTSD). As a result, the patient has frequent periods of awakening throughout the night and other nights of sleeplessness. The nurse will monitor this patient for which physiologic effects? (Select all that apply.)
   A. Bradycardia
   B. Slowing of reflexes
   C. Increased number of infections
   D. Decreased blood glucose
   E. Weight gain
6. A patient reports the development of insomnia following a stressful job change. Which information will the nurse provide?
   A. As long as the insomnia is only occasional, there is no need to worry.
   B. Some people are genetically inclined to be poor sleepers.
   C. Once insomnia develops it can becoming self-reinforcing.
   D. Chronic insomnia is very rare.
7. A patient reports having difficulty falling asleep and staying asleep that has been occurring for the last three months. The nurse reviews the medical record for which information to help validate the diagnosis of insomnia?
   A. The patient's report of sleeplessness
   B. Results of actigraphy
   C. Serotonin level
   D. Brain wave measurements

8. A patient was found to have obstructive sleep apnea (OSA), but does not wish to use a continuous positive airway pressure (CPAP) device. The nurse will suggest which alternative measures to decrease OSA? (Select all that apply.)
   A. Weight loss if the patient is obese
   B. Use of a device to prevent back-sleeping
   C. Use of an oral device to push the tongue back
   D. Maintaining a daily exercise routine
   E. Taking melatonin 30 minutes before bedtime
9. A patient reports being awakened at night by a "creepy-crawly" feeling in the legs that is only relieved by frequent positions changes. Which intervention will the nurse suggest?
   A. Sleep with only a light blanket over the legs.
   B. Drink a glass of milk with each meal.
   C. Sleep in a cool room.
   D. Increase dietary iron intake.
10. A patient will begin taking zolpidem for treatment of insomnia. The nurse determines that teaching about this medication is understood when the patient makes which statement?
   A. If this medication is effective, I can take it as long as necessary.
   B. If I drink a glass of wine with dinner, I must wait at least two hours before taking this medication.
   C. Sleep walking may occur while taking this medication.
   D. I should take this medication an hour before I plan to go to bed.

REFERENCES

Achermann, P., & Borbély, A. A. (2017). Sleep homeostasis and models of sleep regulation. In M. Kryger, T. Roth, & W. C. Dement (Eds.), *Principles and practice of sleep medicine* (6th ed.). pp. 377-387. Philadelphia, PA: Elsevier.

Adams, M. P., Holland, L.N., & Urban, C. (2017). *Pharmacology for nursing: A pathophysiologic approach* (5th ed.). Hoboken, NJ: Pearson Education.

Baker, F. C., Joffe, H., & Lee, K. A. (2017). Sleep and menopause. In M. Kryger, T. Roth, & W. C. Dement (Eds.), *Principles and practice of sleep medicine* (6th ed.). pp. 1553-1563. Philadelphia, PA: Elsevier.

Buysse, D. J., & Harvey, A. G. (2017). Insomnia: Recent developments and future directions. In M. Kryger, T. Roth, & W. C. Dement (Eds.), *Principles and practice of sleep medicine* (6th ed.). pp. 757-760. Philadelphia, PA: Elsevier.

Carskadon, M. A., & Dement, W. C. (2017). Normal human sleep: An overview. In M. Kryger, T. Roth, & W. C. Dement (Eds.), *Principles and practice of sleep medicine* (6th ed.). pp. 15-24. Philadelphia, PA: Elsevier.

Clark, A., & Mills, M. (2017). Can a sleep menu enhance the quality of sleep for a hospitalized patient? *Medsurg Nursing, 26*(4), 253–257.

Klumoer, U. M. H., Vellman, D. L., van Tol, M. J., Kloet R. W., Boellaard, R., Lammertsma, A. A., & Hoogendijk, W. J. G. (2015). Neurophysiological effects on sleep deprivation in healthy adults, a pilot study. *PLOS One, 10*(1), e011690.

Lemus, L. P., McMullin, B., & Bailnowski, H. (2017). Don't ignore my snore: Reducing perioperative complications of obstructive sleep apnea. *Journal of PeriAnesthesia Nursing, 33*(3), 338–345.

Marin, J. M., & Carrizo, S. J. (2017). Overlap syndromes of sleep and breathing disorders. In M. Kryger, T. Roth, & W. C. Dement (Eds.), *Principles and practice of sleep medicine* (6th ed.). pp. 1179-1188. Philadelphia, PA: Elsevier.

Maquet, P., Dive, D., Salmon, E., Sadzot, B., Franco, G., Poirrier, R., . . . Framck, G. (1990). Cerebral glucose utilization during sleep-wake cycle in man determined by positron emission tomography and [^{18}F]2-fluoro-2-deoxy-D-glucose method. *Brain Research, 513*(1), 139–143.

National Center for Complementary and Integrative Health. (2017). *Melatonin: In depth.* Retrieved from https://nccih.nih.gov/health/melatonin.

National Center for Complementary and Integrative Health. (2016). *Valerian.* Retrieved from https://nccih.nih.gov/health/valerian.

Opp, M. R., & Krueger, J. M. (2017). Sleep and host defense. In M. Kryger, T. Roth, & W. C. Dement (Eds.), *Principles and practice of sleep medicine* (6th ed.). pp 193-201. Philadelphia, PA: Elsevier.

Peigneux, P., Fogel, S., & Smith, C. (2017). Memory processing in relation to sleep. In M. Kryger, T. Roth, & W. C. Dement (Eds.), *Principles and practice of sleep medicine* (6th ed.). pp 229-238. Philadelphia, PA: Elsevier.

Sateia, M. (2014). *International classification of sleep disorders* (3rd ed.). Darien, IL: American Academy of Sleep Medicine.

Shields, K. M., Fox, K. L., & Liebrecht, C. (2018). *Pearson nurse's drug guide.* New York, NY: Pearson.

Silber, M. H., St. Louis, E. K., & Boeve, B. F. (2017). Rapid eye movement parasomnias M. Kryger, T. Roth, & W. C. Dement (Eds.), *Principles and practice of sleep medicine* (6th ed.). pp. 993-1001. Philadelphia, PA: Elsevier.

Slivertsen, B., Lallukka, T., Salo, P., Pallesen, S., Hysing, M., Krokstad, S., & Overland, S. (2014). Insomnia as a risk factor for ill health: Results from the large population-based prospective HUNT study in Norway. *Journal of Sleep Research, 23*, 124–132.

Somers, V. K., & Javaheri, S. (2017). Cardiovascular effects of sleep-related breathing disorders. In M. Kryger, T. Roth, & W. C. Dement (Eds.), *Principles and practice of sleep medicine* (6th ed.). pp. 1243-1252. Philadelphia, PA: Elsevier.

St-Onge, M. P., Grandner, M. A., Brown, D., Conroy, M. B., Jean-Louis, G., Coons, M., & Bhatt, D. L.(2016). Sleep duration and quality: Impact on lifestyle behaviors and cardiometabolic health. A scientific statement from the American Heart Association. *Circulation, 134*, e367–386.

Tanner, R. E., Brunker, L. B., Agergaard, J., Barrows, K. M., Briggs, R. A., Kwon, O. S., . . . Drummond, M. J. (2015) Age-related differences in lean mass, protein synthesis and skeletal muscle markers of proteolysis after bed-rest and exercise rehabilitation. *Journal of Physiology, 593*(18), 4259–4273.

University of Toronto. (2012). *The official STOP-BANG tool website.* Retrieved from www.stopbang.ca/index.php.

Van Cauter, E., & Tasali, E. (2017). Endocrine physiology in relation to sleep and sleep disturbances In M. Kryger, T. Roth, & W. C. Dement (Eds.), *Principles and practice of sleep medicine* (6th ed.). pp. 202-219. Philadelphia, PA: Elsevier.

Vitaterna, M. A., Turek F. W., & Jiang, P. (2017). Genetics and genomics of circadian clocks. In M. Kryger, T. Roth, & W. C. Dement (Eds.), *Principles and practice of sleep medicine* (6th ed.). pp. 272-280. Philadelphia, PA: Elsevier.

Winchniak, A., Wierzbicka, A., Walecka, M., & Jernajczk, W. (2017). Effects of antidepressants on sleep. *Current Psychiatry Reports, 19*(9), 63.

ADDITIONAL RESOURCES

American Academy of Sleep Medicine (AASM)
www.aasmnet.org

American Sleep Apnea Association
www.sleepapnea.org

National Sleep Foundation
www.sleepfoundation.org

Chapter 4

Nursing Care of Patients Having Surgery

Chapter Outline and Learning Outcomes

CLINICAL COMPETENCIES

- Assess the physiologic and psychosocial health status of patients scheduled for surgery to determine their ability to tolerate surgery and identify risks for complications.
- Develop an understanding of patient-centered perioperative care, integrating respect for individual patient preferences, values, and specific needs.
- Function effectively within an interprofessional team using written and structured verbal communication techniques to minimize risks associated with transitions in care of the perioperative patient.
- Observe and/or participate as appropriate in nursing responsibilities and evidence-based interventions that promote patient safety and quality care in the perioperative environment.
- Use the nursing process to provide safe and effective nursing care for patients in the preoperative, intraoperative, and postoperative phases of surgery.

KEY TERMS

anesthesia, 70
circulating nurse, 84
conscious sedation, 72
deep venous thrombosis (DVT), 97
dehiscence, 96
evisceration, 96
general anesthesia, 70
hemorrhage, 96
inflammatory phase, 94
intraoperative phase, 70
malignant hyperthermia, 72
perioperative nursing, 70
postanesthesia care unit (PACU), 90
postoperative phase, 70
preoperative phase, 70
proliferative phase, 95
pulmonary embolism (PE), 97
regional anesthesia, 71
remodeling phase, 96
scrub person, 84
shock, 97
surgery, 70
surgical site infection (SSI), 78

Perioperative nursing, care provided immediately before, during, and after surgery, is a specialized area of practice that requires knowledge and understanding of the following:

- Surgical anatomy
- Anticipated physiologic disruptions related to surgery and their potential consequences
- Potential injuries to the patient and strategies to prevent them
- Risk factors and potential complications of surgery
- Evidence-based nursing care to promote optimal patient outcomes
- Effects of surgery on the emotional, psychosocial, and spiritual status of the patient and family.

Perioperative nursing incorporates the three phases of the surgical experience: Preoperative, intraoperative, and postoperative. The **preoperative phase** begins when the decision for surgery is made and ends when the patient is transferred to the operating room. The **intraoperative phase** begins with the patient's entry into the operating room and ends with admittance to the postanesthesia care unit (PACU) or other recovery setting. The **postoperative phase** begins with the patient's admittance to the PACU or other recovery setting and ends with the patient's complete recovery from the surgical intervention.

4.1 Overview of Surgery

Surgery is an invasive procedure performed to diagnose and treat disease, repair injury, restore function, or aesthetically alter bodily features. It can be medically necessary or elective. Although surgery is a medical treatment, the perioperative nurse works in collaboration with the interprofessional team to identify and meet the patient's needs (**Figure 4.1** ■). The nurse has the primary responsibility and accountability for nursing care of patients undergoing surgery. Multidisciplinary teamwork and autonomous nursing care prevent surgical complications and promote optimal patient outcomes.

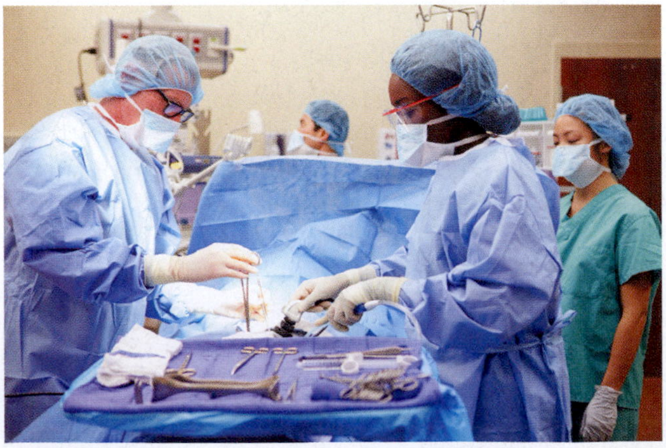

Figure 4.1 ■ Surgical team in the operating room.

Surgical Methods and Classifications

Many procedures may be performed using either an open technique or a minimally invasive approach based on the health status, condition, and purpose of the surgical intervention. Open invasive surgical procedures were traditionally the gold standard for successful outcomes. An open approach is generally used to see and ensure protection of vital structures surrounding a target organ. However, miniaturization and technology have reduced the numbers of open procedures done today. Now, minimally invasive techniques are preferred, if safe for the patient. These types of procedures are carried out through small incisions with the aid of cameras, scopes, and specialized instruments for incising and suturing.

Robot-assisted surgery is also a method of minimally invasive surgery used today. Robotic technology offers three-dimensional views of the target organ, whereas laparoscopic technology offers only two-dimensional views. With the robotic systems, instruments are easier for the surgeon to manipulate. However, robotic, computer-aided surgical systems are not independent systems: The primary surgeon operates the robotic controls and another surgeon at the patient's side exchanges sterile instruments, retracts patient tissues, and manipulates nonrobotic sterile instruments used to assist the procedure.

Minimally invasive surgery, whether performed robotically or laparoscopically, has advantages for patients. There is less operative trauma, leading to improved postoperative comfort and decreased pain. Although these procedures may take longer than similar open surgeries, they result in shorter hospital stays and fewer complications such as adhesions (bands of scar tissue).

Surgical procedures can be classified according to purpose, risk, technique, and urgency. See **Table 4.1** for detailed information on surgical classifications and examples of each.

Anesthesia for Surgery

Anesthesia is used to produce sedation, analgesia (freedom from pain), reflex loss, and muscle relaxation during a surgical procedure. An anesthesiologist (physician) or certified registered nurse anesthetist (CRNA) completes a preoperative anesthesia evaluation of the patient and administers anesthetics before and/or during the intraoperative phase of surgery. There are several kinds of anesthesia used in surgeries/procedures, but presently there is no known best prescriptive combination of anesthesia methods and medications for any given surgical procedure due to the vast variety of individual responses that occurs with anesthesia.

General Anesthesia

General anesthesia produces central nervous system depression that manifest as a state of unconsciousness, muscle relaxation, analgesia, and amnesia. It is most commonly administered by a combination of intravenous drugs and inhalation agents. With loss of consciousness, the patient does not perceive pain, the skeletal muscles relax, and

Table 4.1 **Classification of Surgical Procedures**

Classification	Function	Examples
Purpose		
Diagnostic	Determine or confirm a diagnosis	Breast biopsy, bronchoscopy, diagnostic laparoscopic procedure
Ablative	Remove diseased tissue, organ, or extremity	Appendectomy, amputation, radio-frequency ablation of tumor cells
Constructive	Build tissue/organs that are absent (congenital anomalies)	Repair of cleft palate
Reconstructive	Rebuild tissue/organ that has been damaged	Skin graft after a burn, total joint replacement
Palliative	Alleviate symptoms of a disease (not curative)	Bowel resection in patient with terminal cancer
Transplantation	Replace organs/tissue to restore function	Heart, lung, liver, kidney transplant
Risk		
Minor	Minimal physical assault with minimal risk	Removal of skin lesions, dilation and curettage (D&C), cataract extraction
Major	Extensive physical assault and/or serious risk	Transplantation, total joint replacement, thoracotomy, colostomy, nephrectomy
Technique		
Minimally invasive surgery (MIS)	Minimize incision and tissue disruption	Laparoscopic cholecystectomy, laparoscopic-assisted vaginal hysterectomy
Laser surgery	Minimize tissue damage	Laser iridotomy, laser polypectomy
Urgency		
Emergency	Performed immediately	Obstetric emergencies, bowel obstruction, ruptured aneurysm, life-threatening trauma
Urgent	Necessary to be performed within 1–2 days	Heart bypass surgery, amputation resulting from gangrene, closed fractures
Elective	Not urgent or emergent; scheduled for a predetermined date	Cosmetic surgery, cataract surgery, tubal ligation

reflexes diminish. Advantages to general anesthesia include rapid excretion of the anesthetic agent and prompt reversal of its effects when desired. Additionally, general anesthesia can be used with all age groups and any type of surgical procedure.

Disadvantages of general anesthesia include risks associated with circulatory, respiratory, hepatic, and renal side effects. Patients with serious respiratory or circulatory diseases, such as emphysema or congestive heart failure, are at greater risk for complications. Patients with renal or hepatic disease cannot metabolize and eliminate anesthetics safely. Inhalation agents can trigger malignant hyperthermia, so they are not used in patients who have experienced a prior malignant hyperthermia event or have excessive risk factors (see **Box 4.1**).

The phases of general anesthesia are divided into three distinct categories: Induction, maintenance, and emergence.

1. ***Induction:*** During the induction phase, the patient receives the anesthetic agent intravenously or by inhalation. Airway patency is achieved and maintained with endotracheal tube (ETT) intubation, the laryngeal mask airway (LMA), or esophageal-tracheal Combitube (see **Figure 4.2** ■). Various types of stylets with or without light guidance may be used as adjuncts to endotracheal intubation. In particular, lighted stylets and/or wands are useful when direct vision of the glottis and/or vocal cords is difficult or near impossible during induction procedures.
2. ***Maintenance:*** The next phase of general anesthesia is maintenance. During this period, the ETT or LMA is secured with tape, and the anesthesiologist maintains the proper depth of anesthesia while constantly monitoring physiologic parameters such as heart rate, blood pressure, respiratory rate, temperature, and oxygen and carbon dioxide levels while the surgery is underway.
3. ***Emergence:*** The final phase of general anesthesia is the patient's emergence from this altered physiologic state. As the anesthetic agents are withdrawn or the effects reversed pharmacologically, the patient begins to awaken. The ETT or LMA is removed once the patient is able to reestablish voluntary breathing. It is critical to ensure airway patency during this period because extubation (removal of the synthetic airway) may cause bronchospasm or laryngospasm.

Common side effects that may occur with general anesthesia include nausea and vomiting, a hangover effect, confusion, and amnesia. Adjunct medications including corticosteroids, antiemetics, and anxiolytics may be administered preoperatively and intraoperatively to reduce or prevent these side effects.

Regional Anesthesia

Regional anesthesia results in analgesia, reflex loss, and muscle relaxation in an area of the body but does not cause the patient to lose consciousness. It is the instillation of medication around the nerves to block transmission of

BOX 4.1
Malignant Hyperthermia

Malignant hyperthermia is a rare multifactorial genetic disorder that can be triggered by inhalational anesthetic gases and succinylcholine, a depolarizing neuromuscular blocker. The initial manifestations are an unexplained rise in end-tidal carbon dioxide that does not respond to ventilation and sustained skeletal muscle contraction (Riazi & Brandom, 2015). The temperature rises rapidly to as high as 43°C (109.4°F) as a result of sustained hypermetabolism. Cardiac dysrhythmias develop and oxygen and ATP are rapidly consumed. Lactate and carbon dioxide, by-products of metabolism, are produced in excess (Sorenson, Quinn, & Klein, 2019). If unchecked the condition will progress to hyperkalemia, myoglobinuria, disseminated intravascular coagulation, congestive heart failure, bowel ischemia, and compartment syndrome in the limbs.

Malignant hyperthermia can develop during or after surgery. If the early symptoms of malignant hyperthermia (e.g., increased carbon dioxide levels, tachycardia and tachypnea, muscle stiffness or rigidity, escalating temperature) are identified, suspected triggering agents are immediately discontinued. Oxygen is immediately administered with a nonrebreather mask. The patient should not be unattended, good IV access should be maintained. If signs and symptoms of malignant hyperthermia manifest postsurgery, the anesthesia provider should be summoned immediately. Dantrolene, a muscle relaxant, is administered and measures to decrease core body temperature should be started at once and continued until core temperature is 36.0°C (96.8°F). A urinary catheter should be placed to monitor urine output and blood should be drawn for testing. Blood gases should be drawn to measure pH; sodium bicarbonate is given to correct metabolic acidosis. Insulin may be ordered to decrease serum potassium. This patient may be transferred to the ICU for continued monitoring and doses of Dantrolene every 4.6 hours.

nerve impulses in a particular area. The patient is awake and conscious during the surgical procedure but does not perceive pain. Regional anesthesia may be used along or as an adjunct in combination with other types of anesthetics. Regional anesthesia may be classified in several ways:

- *Local nerve infiltration* is achieved by injecting lidocaine, bupivacaine, or tetracaine around a local nerve to suppress sensation over a limited area of the body. This technique may be used when a skin or muscle biopsy is obtained or when a small wound is sutured.
- *Nerve blocks* are accomplished by injecting an anesthetic agent at the nerve trunk to produce a lack of sensation over a specific larger area, such as an extremity.
- *Epidural blocks* are local anesthetic agents injected into the epidural space, outside the dura mater of the spinal cord. This type of intraspinal anesthesia provides safe and effective pain relief for patients of all ages with less risk of adverse effects than general anesthesia. It is indicated for surgeries of the arms and shoulders, thorax, abdomen, pelvis, and lower extremities. The epidural catheter is often left in place for pain relief in the postoperative period; it can also be used for chronic pain management.
- *Spinal anesthesia* is administered similarly to epidural except the anesthetic medication is infused in a single injection. Spinal anesthesia is effective for approximately 90 minutes. Surgeries of the lower abdomen, perineum, and lower extremities are likely to use this type of regional anesthesia. Leakage of cerebrospinal fluid (CSF) into the epidural space can cause reduced CSF pressure and postoperative headaches. Treatment may include hydration, caffeine, analgesics, or administration of an epidural blood patch. Hypotension is common with epidural and spinal anesthesia. Blood pressure should be monitored and, if critical hypotension occurs, the anesthesia provider should be alerted and expected to increase intravenous fluids and administer vasoactive medications.

Conscious/Moderate Sedation

An increasing number of surgical and diagnostic procedures are being performed using **conscious sedation**, also

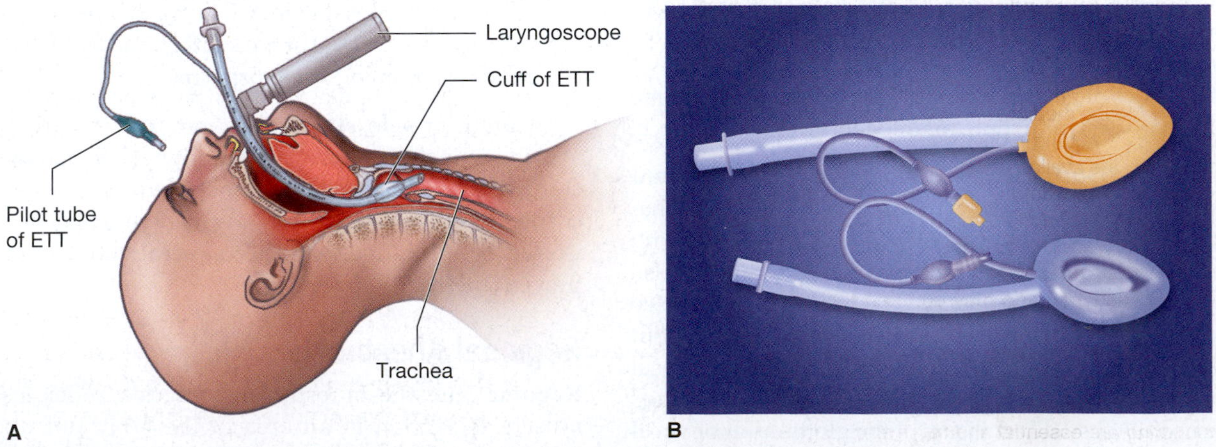
Laryngoscope
Cuff of ETT
Pilot tube of ETT
Trachea
A
B

Figure 4.2 ■ Airway management devices. **A**, Endotracheal tube (ETT). **B**, Laryngeal mask airway (LMA).

called *moderate sedation/analgesia*. This type of anesthesia provides analgesia, amnesia, and moderate sedation. The patient under conscious sedation has an altered level of consciousness but is still able to maintain a patent airway and respond to verbal and environmental stimuli (Stone, 2017). The pharmacologic effects are produced by administering a combination of intravenous medications with opioids (such as morphine sulfate or fentanyl [Sublimaze]) or sedatives (such as diazepam [Valium] and midazolam [Versed]). Propofol (Diprivan) is an anesthetic agent commonly used for conscious sedation. Physician supervision is always required and a registered nurse must be prepared to initiate rescue interventions if sedation becomes too deep or loss of protective reflexes occurs. See **Box 4.2** for implications related to the administration of midazolam and propofol. Institutions base their policies defining the qualifications of those who care for patients undergoing conscious sedation on professional standards, regulatory guidelines/mandates, and state law.

Assessment prior to conscious/moderate sedation includes evaluating the appropriateness of this type of sedation for the patient based on physical status. Patients with compromised circulation or airway, a history of sleep apnea or snoring, a history of problems with anesthesia or analgesia, or who use medications that would potentially interact with conscious/moderate analgesia medications may require the anesthesiologist to manage sedation procedures. Patients need to be appropriately fasting, and baseline vital signs must be taken prior to giving the sedative. The patient must sign a consent form, and a patent IV line must be in place. Equipment to rescue the patient should be available if sedation becomes too deep. Oxygen saturation, pulse, breathing, and level of consciousness must be monitored throughout the procedure. Common adverse effects include venous thrombosis, phlebitis, local irritation,

BOX 4.2
Safely Administering Midazolam and Propofol

Midazolam hydrochloride (Versed) is most commonly administered intravenously as a preoperative sedative or used in conjunction with opioids for sedative effects during conscious sedation. Preoperative doses range from 0.5 to 2 mg based on age, weight, and any comorbidities of the patient. Dosages used during conscious sedation are titrated in 0.5- to 1-mg increments based on the length and depth of sedation needed as well as the patient's response to the medication. Patients receiving midazolam should be in a care setting where continuous respiratory and cardiac monitoring are available.

Propofol (Diprivan) has a rapid onset (40 to 60 seconds) and short duration of action, making it one of the most commonly administered anesthetic agents in the United States. It is used for induction and maintenance of anesthesia and conscious/moderate sedation and may be used to sedate patients undergoing mechanical ventilation or other procedures. Intravenous doses used during conscious/moderate sedation range from 5 to 80 mcg/kg/min. Profound respiratory depression and hypotension can occur with Propofol; continuous respiratory and cardiac monitoring are essential and respiratory support must be immediately available.

confusion, drowsiness, hypotension, and apnea. Reversal agents (naloxone hydrochloride [Narcan] and flumazenil [Romazicon]) are used as needed to enhance the safety of conscious sedation.

Monitored Anesthesia Care

Monitored anesthesia care (MAC) is a physician service distinct from conscious/moderate sedation. It allows for the safe administration of a maximal depth of sedation in excess of that provided during conscious/moderate sedation. The ability to adjust the sedation level from full consciousness to general anesthesia during the course of a procedure provides maximal flexibility in matching sedation level to patient needs and procedural requirements. In situations where the procedure is more invasive or when the patient is especially fragile, optimizing sedation level is necessary to achieve ideal procedural conditions. The administration of sedatives, hypnotics, analgesics, and anesthetic drugs commonly used for the induction and maintenance of general anesthesia may, but not always, be a part of MAC.

Monitored anesthesia care may be indicated in situations where minimal sedation is the procedural standard. However, it is provided because small doses of medications used for sedation may precipitate adverse physiologic responses in certain patients, necessitating acute clinical intervention and/or resuscitation. In some cases, MAC is also indicated when a "deep" level of sedation is anticipated based on the patient's condition and/or procedural requirement. In these situations, there is always a possibility the patient may require a shift to general anesthesia. Due to the strong likelihood that "deep" sedation may, with or without intention, transition to general anesthesia, the skills of an anesthesia provider are necessary to manage the effects of general anesthesia on the patient as well as to return the patient quickly to a state of "deep" or lesser sedation. Like all anesthesia services, MAC includes a multitude of postprocedural responsibilities beyond the expectations of practitioners providing conscious/moderate sedation.

Settings for Surgery

Surgical patients may be inpatients or outpatients. The complexity of the surgery and recovery and the expected level of care needed on completion of the surgery are the major differences. Both inpatient and outpatient (or *ambulatory* or *same-day*) surgeries are performed in the operating rooms in many hospitals. Outpatient surgery is also performed in freestanding surgical facilities and in medical clinics. The number of outpatient surgeries has grown rapidly in the past decade as part of the effort to contain the high costs of surgery. Diagnostic procedures, minimally invasive and laparoscopic procedures, and biopsies are commonly performed as outpatient surgeries. Moreover, increasingly complex surgeries on patients with complicated medical problems are now frequently performed on an outpatient basis. This increase in the number of outpatient procedures and the acuity level of patients has presented a challenge to the nurse, the patient, and the family. The role of the nurse to assess, monitor, and/or educate the patient and his or her family pre-, intra-, and postoperatively is critical in preventing complications and poor outcomes.

Outpatient surgery offers several potential advantages:

- Decreased cost to the patient, hospital, and insuring agency
- Reduced risk of healthcare-associated infection
- Less interruption in the patient's and family's routine
- Possible reduction in time lost from work and/or other responsibilities
- Less physiologic stress on the patient and family.

In some ambulatory surgery centers, perioperative nurses (or OR nurses) may be cross-trained to provide care within all phases of the patient's surgical experience; however, in the hospital setting these nurses most often serve as circulating or scrub nurses within the intraoperative phase. As such, perianesthesia nurses perform in roles in the pre- and/or postoperative phases of surgery in most hospital settings. These nurses care for patients and their family members/significant others as they transition within the perianesthesia/periprocedural continuum of care. This continuum includes preanesthesia, postanesthesia phase I, postanesthesia phase II, and extended care. This chapter provides an overview of perioperative and perianesthesia nursing roles in promoting optimal surgical outcomes. For more in-depth information about the nursing standards and recommended practices relevant to each of these specialty nursing roles, visit their respective professional organizations. For operating room nurses, visit the Association for periOperative Nurses website (*www.aorn.org*); for perianesthesia nurses, visit the American Society of Perianesthesia Nurses website (*www.aspan.org*).

The care of the patient in the inpatient setting is similar but the underlying health condition of the patient, the complexity of the surgery, and the situation creates the need for skilled and continuous nursing care. Consequently, the nursing care team includes more members and care is provided across departments. Patients may be transferred to the perioperative setting from the emergency department, the intensive care unit, a procedural unit (e.g., labor and delivery), or any ward within the hospital. In nonemergent situations, the transferring nurse will begin the preoperative assessment and checklist before sending the patient to the surgical department. The inpatient nurse will then ensure informed consent and site marking for the procedure, educate the patient about the process, and perform required hygiene measures. After surgery, patients are transferred to the PACU and then assigned a unit and bed if staying overnight.

Patients undergoing urgent or elective surgery who have underlying complex health conditions will be managed in the inpatient setting, as the comorbidity of multiple diseases creates increased risk for complications. The nursing role focuses on continuous assessment to ensure complications are identified early and addressed immediately. Because the surgical experience occurs across departments when the patient is cared for in the in-patient setting, ensuring handoff communication, care coordination is consistent, and medication reconciliation is a critical nursing function.

Perioperative Patient Safety

Within perioperative settings, patient safety initiatives are generally driven by U.S. heathcare regulatory requirements and/or mandates. These are established standards to which all parties must adhere. When it comes to healthcare, the U.S. government often allows such regulatory requirements to be satisfied by a healthcare organization's adherence to standards established by professional associations or public and private agencies governed primarily by professionals. The Joint Commission is one of these; it is a not-for-profit organization and a primary driver of patient safety initiatives in various settings including hospitals, home care, ambulatory surgery centers, long-term care facilities, laboratories, and more. The organization provides accreditation and/or certification for healthcare facilities and programs that demonstrate a commitment to meeting patient safety via the implementation of specific performance standards. Accreditation and/or certification issued by The Joint Commission is recognized nationwide as an indicator of organizational or programmatic quality.

In 2002, The Joint Commission established the National Patient Safety Goals (NPSGs) program to help accredited organizations address specific areas of concern in regard to patient safety. Since that time, The Joint Commission has disseminated annually a list of NPSGs for organizations/programs to use as a guide in ensuring the safety and quality of their practices. For details on the development of NPSGs and the NPSGs designated for the current year, see *www.jointcommission.org/standards_information/npsgs.aspx*.

The Universal Protocol is another standard developed by the The Joint Commission. This standard is specifically intended to prevent wrong patient, wrong procedure, or wrong site surgeries and to promote the safety of patients having a surgery or other types of invasive procedures by improving team-based communication. Elements of the Universal Protocol include the implementation of a preprocedural verification process; surgical site marking; and a standardized time-out procedure that occurs immediately prior to surgery/procedure start time. For additional information, including the corresponding expectations relevant to each of these elements of the Universal Protocol, see *www.jointcommission.org/assets/1/18/UP_Poster1.PDF*.

Essentially, safety in the perioperative environment is the responsibility of all personnel involved in the patient's care. All members of the patient's care team have a part to play in preventing errors during the perioperative process. Following the Universal Protocol and speaking up for the benefit of patient and healthcare worker safety is critical in the surgical environment (Stone, 2017).

4.2 Patient Risks: Preoperative Considerations

Risks are inherent in all phases of surgery. For example, transporting the patient to and from the operating room (OR) requires assessment of the needs of the patient for supplemental oxygen, intravenous therapy, cardiac monitoring, and safety issues pertaining to the means of transport. Chemicals, electrical equipment, and environmental hazards in the surgical area have the potential to harm patients and must be monitored and maintained carefully. Nutritional status, skin integrity, and mobility status may play a role in the positioning of the patient for surgery and maintenance of skin integrity during the perioperative period. **Table 4.2** outlines patient-specific risk factors that have implications for perioperative nursing care.

Medication Interactions

Over-the-counter medicines and herbal preparations as well as prescription medications may interact with drugs

Table 4.2 Surgical Risk Factors and Corresponding Nursing Implications

Factor	Associated Risk	Nursing Implications
Advanced age	Age-related changes affect physiologic, cognitive, and psychosocial responses to the stress of surgery; decrease tolerance of general anesthesia and postoperative medications; and delay wound healing.	■ Selected nursing interventions are summarized in Table 4.6 later in the chapter. ■ Need to understand and develop an individualized plan of care addressing multiple comorbidities.
Malnutrition	Reserves may not be sufficient to allow the body to respond satisfactorily to the physical assault of surgery; organ failure and shock may result. Increased metabolic demands may result in poor wound healing and infection.	■ Promote weight gain by providing a well-balanced diet high in calories, protein, and vitamin C. ■ Administer parenteral nutrition, nutritional supplements, and enteral feedings as prescribed. ■ Daily weights and calorie counts may also be ordered.
Obesity	The patient with obesity is at increased risk for delayed wound healing, wound dehiscence, infection, pneumonia, atelectasis, thrombophlebitis, dysrhythmias, impaired skin integrity, and heart failure.	■ Promote weight reduction if time permits. ■ Monitor closely for wound, pulmonary, and cardiovascular complications. ■ Encourage coughing, turning, and breathing exercises and early ambulation.
Low socioeconomic status	Because of limited access to healthcare, pathology may be more advanced at diagnosis. Risk is greater for emotional stress, poor nutrition, lack of exercise, and poor social support systems.	■ Assess for undiagnosed chronic conditions and nutritional status. Involve social services for help with resources. ■ Low educational or reading level may require adaptation of discharge instructions or education.
Chronic Conditions		
Alcoholism/substance use	The patient may be malnourished and experience delirium tremens (acute withdrawal symptoms). More general anesthesia may be required. Altered coagulation, hemorrhage, and delayed wound healing can result from liver damage and poor nutritional status.	■ Monitor closely for signs of delirium tremens, responses to anesthesia and analgesia, bleeding, and wound complications. ■ Encourage well-balanced diet. Administer supplemental nutrients as ordered. ■ Administer antagonist medications such as naloxone or flumazenil with caution.
Arthritis	Inflammation or degenerative changes in joints limit mobility and comfort. Ask about timing of last dose of NSAID or ASA.	■ Position and pad arthritic joints, including the spine. ■ Handle joints gently to avoid strain on ligaments and tendons. ■ Monitor for bleeding.
Cardiovascular disorders	Cardiovascular disease increases the risk of heart failure, hemorrhage and shock, hypotension, venous thrombosis, pulmonary embolism, stroke (especially in the older patient), and fluid volume overload.	■ Diligently monitor vital signs, reporting changes such as tachycardia, dysrhythmias, tachypnea, or dyspnea. ■ Closely monitor fluid intake and output to prevent circulatory overload. ■ Assess skin color, oxygen saturation, and lung sounds. Report hypoxia, chest pain, lung congestion, or peripheral edema. Administer oxygen as ordered. ■ Promote early postoperative ambulation to reduce the risk of venous thrombosis and pulmonary embolism. ■ Determine that prescribed beta-blockers are given preoperatively.
Diabetes mellitus	Diabetes increases the risk for fluctuating blood glucose levels, which can lead to life-threatening hypoglycemia or ketoacidosis. Diabetes also increases the risk for cardiovascular disease, delayed wound healing, and wound infection.	■ Monitor blood glucose levels every 4 hours or as ordered; report levels of 180 mg/dL or higher or outside prescribed limits. ■ Administer insulin as prescribed. ■ Monitor for manifestations of hypoglycemia and hyperglycemia. ■ Encourage intake of food at the designated meal and snack times.
Immune suppression	Suppressed immunity impairs ability to resist infection and promote tissue repair. Advanced age, immune deficiency diseases, malnutrition, chronic disease, cancer treatment, and alcohol abuse compromise immunity.	■ Prevent hypothermia, maintain sterile fields, consistently prevent infection. ■ Nourishment and normoglycemia promote wound healing.
Nicotine use	Cigarette smokers are at increased risk for respiratory complications such as pneumonia, atelectasis, and bronchitis because of increased mucous secretions and a decreased ability to expel them.	■ Support efforts to quit smoking. ■ Monitor closely for respiratory difficulties. Encourage breathing, coughing, turning, and early ambulation. ■ Promote fluid intake to 2500–3000 mL (unless contraindicated) to help liquefy respiratory secretions. ■ A nicotine patch may reduce withdrawal symptoms during the postoperative period.

(continued)

Table 4.2 Surgical Risk Factors and Corresponding Nursing Implications (*countined*)

Factor	Associated Risk	Nursing Implications
Renal and liver disorders	Renal or liver dysfunction may affect the ability to tolerate general anesthesia, cause fluid/electrolyte and acid–base imbalances, decrease the metabolism and excretion of drugs, increase the risk for hemorrhage, and delay wound healing.	■ Monitor intake and output; fluid, electrolyte, and acid–base balance; and responses to medication. ■ Note that patients may require lower doses of medications due to renal or liver disease.
Respiratory disorders	Patients with pulmonary disease are at higher risk for developing respiratory complications such as atelectasis and pneumonia. Respiratory depression from general anesthesia and acid–base imbalance may also occur.	■ Closely monitor respirations, pulse, oxygen saturation, and breath sounds. ■ Also assess for hypoxia, dyspnea, lung congestion, and chest pain. ■ Encourage coughing, turning, and breathing exercises and early postoperative ambulation.
Medical Therapies		
Medications	Anesthesia interaction with some medications can cause respiratory depression, hypotension, and circulatory collapse. Other medications can produce side effects that increase surgical risk.	■ Inform the anesthesiologist of all prescribed and over-the-counter medications, as well as any herbal preparations.
Anticoagulants/platelet inhibitors	May cause intraoperative and postoperative hemorrhage.	■ Monitor for bleeding. ■ Assess prothrombin time (PT), partial thromboplastin time (PTT), and international normalized ratio (INR) values.
Antidepressants (particularly monoamine oxidase inhibitors)	Increase the hypotensive effects of anesthesia.	■ Closely monitor blood pressure.
Antihypertensives	Increase the hypotensive effects of anesthesia.	■ Closely monitor blood pressure.
Antibiotics (particularly the "mycin" group)	May cause apnea and respiratory paralysis.	■ Monitor respirations.
Diuretics	May lead to fluid and electrolyte imbalances, producing altered cardiovascular response and respiratory depression.	■ Monitor intake and output and electrolytes. ■ Assess cardiovascular and respiratory status.
Herbal supplements	Some may prolong the effects of anesthesia. Others may increase the risks of bleeding or raise blood pressure.	■ Inquire about the use of herbs or other dietary supplements. These should be discontinued at least 2 weeks before surgery.
Immunosuppressants	Steroids, drugs to treat cancer and autoimmune disorders, and transplant rejection drugs suppress the immune system and increase the risk of infection and hypothermia	■ Monitor CBC with differential for leukopenia. ■ Document current dosage of medications and time of last dose. ■ Administer prescribed steroids in the perioperative period to prevent adrenal crisis. ■ Prevent hypothermia and maintain asepsis. ■ Monitor wound healing.
Treatments	Radiation therapy	■ Tissue integrity may be compromised in targeted fields.
In the Operating Room		
Fluid/electrolyte imbalance	Depending on the type and extent of fluid and electrolyte imbalance, cardiac dysrhythmias or heart failure may occur. Liver and renal failure may also result.	■ Administer intravenous fluids as ordered. ■ Monitor intake and output. ■ Monitor patient for evidence of electrolyte imbalance.
Hypothermia/hyperthermia	Hypothermia or hyperthermia increase the risk for infection, cardiac morbidity, myocardial ischemia, surgical bleeding, skin damage, and patient discomfort.	■ Monitor core temperatures and prevent chilling or overheating. ■ Remove wet drapes and test the temperature of fluids used.
Surgical site infections	Sterile field contamination, opening body organs containing pathogens (e.g., the bowel) increases risk for infection.	■ Administer antibiotics prior to incision as ordered. ■ Carefully maintain sterile fields. ■ Monitor and sustain core body temperature between 36° and 38°C (96.8° and 100.4°F).
Venous stasis	Lower limbs, especially when tourniquets are applied, are susceptible to blood clotting. Patients with cancer have higher risks of blood clots.	■ Promote venous circulation with intermittent pneumatic compression devices as ordered. ■ Monitor circulation in arms and legs during surgery.

given during surgery, augmenting hemodynamic effects such as hypertension or hypotension. Some categories of medications require special consideration, including drugs that alter blood clotting, cardiovascular drugs, bronchodilators, drugs that affect neurologic or endocrine function, glaucoma drugs, and immune suppressants. Thus, at every transition point in the perioperative care continuum it is vital that the nurse gathers a complete history of medications, including herbal preparations, that the patient has been taking regularly.

Anticoagulant medications, including aspirin and nonsteroidal anti-inflammatory drugs (NSAIDS), should be discontinued prior to surgery to prevent excessive blood loss during surgery. A patient's surgery may be canceled if laboratory tests of bleeding time, prothrombin time (PT), partial thromboplastin time (PTT), and international normalized ratio (INR) are elevated. Guidelines for discontinuing use of anticoagulants vary according to the particular medication; it is generally recommended that aspirin or products containing aspirin, NSAIDs, and medications that alter platelet function and clotting be discontinued 5 days or longer before surgery. Similarly, herbs or nutritional supplements that impair clotting should be discontinued 2 weeks prior to surgery. The most common herbs and supplements that may inhibit coagulation are vitamin E, garlic, ginkgo, ginseng, fish oil, and chamomile. Many plants contain coumarins, so they have the potential to interact with warfarin and inhibit coagulation. Others inhibit platelet aggregation or prevent the conversion of fibrinogen to fibrin. Patients taking warfarin for the risk of blood clots due to atrial fibrillation will be counseled about the appropriate time to withdraw warfarin. If surgery is urgent due to trauma or sudden onset of morbidity, the impact of anticoagulants needs to be evaluated with PT, PTT, and INR before the operation and so that appropriate support for clotting is at the ready.

Herbal medicines or dietary supplements may also produce levels of chemicals that interact with conventional medications, exacerbating or impairing the intended effect. Anesthesia drugs often decrease hepatic blood flow and interfere with the metabolism and elimination of medications. This increases the risk of adverse drug–herbal supplement interactions during surgery. Cardiovascular instability, impaired glucose control, increased metabolism of perioperative medication, and unpredictable response to anesthesia are categories of adverse reactions of perioperative herbal use.

Transfer of Care

Poor communication during transitions from one care setting or team member to another can lead to confusion about the patient's condition and appropriate care. It may also contribute to duplicative tests, inconsistent patient monitoring, medical errors, and/or surgical delay. Such communication failures create serious patient safety, quality of care, and health outcome concerns. The transfer of essential information and the responsibility for care of the patient during transitions in care is vital for the safety of the patient and optimization of positive surgical/procedural outcomes. Within the healthcare setting, this critical transfer point is operationalized as a handoff (or handover). A handoff report during a transition in care provides essential, up-to-date, specific patient information and offers nurses the opportunity to ask and respond to questions. Effective communication is reflected by timely, accurate, complete, and clear information that is understood by the healthcare professional who is accepting responsibility for the patient's care. Healthcare personnel, including nurses, should use structured communication strategies and techniques such as SBAR (situation, background, assessment, and recommendations) to help ensure clarity in information transfer processes and reduce the risk for error in patient care (see **Figure 4.3** ■).

SBAR Report

Report given by:	Time :________________
Report received by:	Phone:________________

S	**Situation:** Patient name Age Location Code status Current vital signs and O_2 saturation Patient's current status
B	**Background:** Admitting date and diagnosis Allergies Diagnostic tests pending Patient's physical/mental status Oxygen in use or not
A	**Assessment:** Lungs, heart, neurologic status IV sites/fluids/rates Diet and intake/output Active precautions Isolation precautions Special care—tubes, wounds
R	**Recommendations:** Suggestions for diagnostic tests Treatments Transfer to critical care Come to see patient

Figure 4.3 ■ Information included in an SBAR handoff report.

Thromboembolism

Persons having surgery are at risk for thromboembolism. The duration of the procedure and the patient position during the procedure contribute to this risk for all patients. Yet certain patients may be at higher risk than others, depending on their medical history (e.g., venous injury, prolonged bedrest, or paralysis). Each patient's risk for developing deep vein thrombosis (DVT) needs to be assessed preoperatively and appropriate prophylaxis initiated when indicated. Prophylactic courses are generally dependent on the patient's health history, present status, and planned procedure. DVT can lead to pulmonary embolism (PE) and to significant patient morbidity, mortality, and increased healthcare costs. Patients at high risk for DVT may be prescribed low-dose unfractionated heparin, low-molecular-weight heparin, factor Xa, or warfarin, as well as the use of intermittent sequential compression devices (ISCDs) and graduated compression stockings during the perioperative period (**Figure 4.4** ■). Always, the risk of bleeding, perhaps complicated by anticoagulant therapies, must be balanced against the risk of postoperative DVT and thromboembolism.

Hypothermia

Hypothermia is a risk in the perioperative period as well. Research shows that normothermia (core body temperature in the range of 36.0° to 37.5°C [96.8° to 99.5°F]) in the patient reduces the risk for infection, cardiac morbidity, myocardial ischemia, surgical bleeding, and patient discomfort. Risk factors for the development of perioperative hypothermia include (1) older age (60 years or older); (2) low body weight/poor nutritional status; (3) preexisting

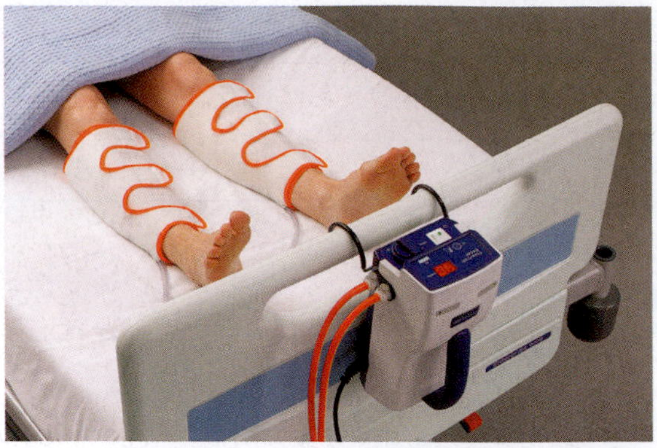

Figure 4.4 ■ Intermittent sequential compression devices (ISCDs).

diagnosis contributing to impaired thermoregulation (e.g., diabetes, hypothyroidism); (4) general anesthesia, especially if combined with regional anesthesia; (5) the nature, extent, and duration of surgery; (6) use of nonwarmed intraoperative fluids; and (7) the ambient temperature of the actual operating room. Methods to minimize the risk of intraoperative hypothermia include preoperative patient warming, limiting the amount of skin exposed, warming intravenous fluids, and continuous monitoring of the patient's temperature. Heating of fluids or the use of heating units with thermal blankets necessitates consistency in assessment of the patient's temperature and skin integrity throughout the perioperative period. The evidence to date is inconclusive regarding a preferred method for temperature monitoring. It is best practice to determine the method based on the clinical situation and to use the same method consistently throughout the perioperative period when clinically feasible.

Surgical Site Infection

Despite the carefully cleaned surgery environment and use of sterile equipment and specific surgical attire, a significant percentage of patients develop **surgical site infections (SSIs)**. Patients suffer increased morbidity and mortality and healthcare costs increase dramatically as a result of surgical site infections (SSIs). See **Box 4.3** for the Centers for Disease Control and Prevention (CDC) recommendations for prevention of SSI.

Positioning Injury/Pressure Injuries

Depending on the nature, extent, and duration of surgery, all patients are at risk for potential injury and/or the development of pressure injuries. The most common predictors of perioperative pressure injuries include being of an advanced age, having a diagnosis of diabetes or vascular disease, and undergoing a vascular procedure. Prevention of positioning injury requires anticipation of the positioning equipment necessary based on the patient's identified needs, the planned operative procedure, postoperative course, application of the principles of body mechanics and ergonomics, ongoing assessment throughout the perioperative period, and coordination with the entire perioperative team. Intraoperative planning related to patient positioning should focus on patient comfort and safety, surgical site access, and making possible the assessments of circulatory, respiratory, integumentary, musculoskeletal, and neurological structures.

Box 4.3
SSI Prevention

1. Patients should shower or bathe (full body) with soap (antimicrobial or nonantimicrobial) or an antiseptic agent on at least the night before surgery.
2. The appropriate parenteral prophylactic antimicrobial agents should be applied before skin incision in all cesarean section procedures.
3. Antimicrobial prophylaxis should be administered only when indicated and timed such that a bactericidal concentration of the agents is established in the serum and tissues when the incision is made.
4. Skin prep in the operating room (OR) should be done with an alcohol-based agent unless contraindicated.
5. For clean and clean-contaminated procedures, additional prophylactic antimicrobial agent doses should not be administered after the surgical incision is closed in the OR, even when a drain is being used.
6. Topical antimicrobial agents should not be applied to the surgical incision.
7. During surgery, glycemic control should be implemented using blood glucose target levels less than 200 mg/dL.
8. Normothermia should be maintained in all patients.
9. For patients with normal pulmonary function undergoing general anesthesia with ET intubation, increased fraction of inspired oxygen should be administered during surgery and immediately after extubation in postop.
10. Blood transfusions should not be withheld from surgical patients as a means to prevent SSIs.

Source: Data from CDC, 2017.

Cardiac Events

Myocardial infarction is a risk following major surgery. The circulatory system is stressed during surgery, increasing the risk for cardiac ischemia. Beta-blocker medications inhibit sympathetic nervous system stimulation of the myocardium and reduce oxygen demand, thereby reducing the risk for infarction. Any patient who is taking beta-blocker medication regularly needs to take the usual dose prior to any type of surgery. Interpreting and responding to identified risk factors requires nursing judgment. It is important to bring information to the attention of the surgeons and anesthesiologists prior to surgery so necessary modifications can be made for the patient.

4.3 Perianesthesia: Preoperative Nursing Care

Most patients undergoing elective surgery will have a preoperative/preadmission assessment to determine their fitness for surgery prior to the day of the procedure. This assessment is usually conducted by a perianesthesia nurse (or preadmission nurse) and an anesthesia provider in the preanesthesia phase of care.

Preanesthesia Phase

This phase includes two subphases: Preadmission and day of surgery/procedure. In the preadmission phase, the nurse focuses on physical, psychological, sociocultural, and spiritual preparation of the patient for the surgical experience. Interview and assessment techniques are used to identify potential and/or actual problems. To optimize patient outcomes, the nurse provides patient education and other essential interventions as needed.

Preadmission Testing

The role of the nurse in this phase is to complete a health history, physical examination, and psychosocial assessment; facilitate diagnostic testing and/or review results; and identify patient preferences (e.g., name, culture, language, learning style, advanced directive). As well, the nurse assesses the discharge plan and the patient's resources/ability to perform self-care postprocedure.

Preoperative teaching also occurs during this phase. Patient teaching is an essential nursing responsibility in the preanesthesia phase. Patient education and emotional support have a positive effect on the patient's physical and psychologic well-being and on family members, both before and after surgery. Although the time available for teaching patients undergoing ambulatory or outpatient surgery is limited, the responsibility of the patient and family for postoperative care and monitoring increases its importance. Because outpatient surgical stays are brief, it is valuable for nurses to be sensitive, perceptive, and able to listen to and identify the patient as an individual within a unique family.

Patient teaching should begin as soon as the patient learns of the upcoming surgery and may be done in the physician's office or at the time of preadmission testing. Although education continues in all stages of the perioperative process, most teaching is done before surgery because day of surgery anxiety, pain, and the effects of anesthesia can affect the patient's ability to learn.

The amount of information desired varies from patient to patient. Therefore, the nurse assesses the patient's need for and readiness to accept information. The teaching is in part directed by the particular surgical procedure being performed and by the type of anesthesia. The information in **Box 4.4** is relevant to most patients undergoing major surgery.

Box 4.4
Preoperative Patient Teaching

BREATHING AND COUGHING EXERCISES

Diaphragmatic (abdominal) breathing and coughing exercises help prevent pulmonary complications such as atelectasis and pneumonia. Risk factors for pulmonary complications include general anesthesia, abdominal or thoracic surgery, history of smoking, chronic lung disease, obesity, and advanced age. Diaphragmatic breathing promotes lung expansion and ventilation and enhances blood oxygenation, while coughing helps loosen, mobilize, and remove pulmonary secretions. Splinting an abdominal incision decreases the physical and psychologic discomfort associated with coughing. The nurse:

1. Assists the patient, as needed, to a sitting position.
2. Asks the patient to place the hands lightly on the abdomen.
3. Instructs to inhale deeply through the nose, so the chest and abdomen expand.
4. Instructs the patient to hold the breath for a count of five.
5. Instructs the patient to exhale completely through pursed (puckered) lips, so the chest and abdomen deflate.
6. Asks the patient to repeat for five deep breaths, and then to inhale deeply, holding the breath briefly, then coughing once or twice while contracting abdominal muscles.
7. Instruct the patient for whom coughing is painful to splint the incision with interlocked hands or a pillow.
8. Instructs or reminds the patient to repeat the exercises every 1 to 2 hours while awake, taking short rest periods between coughs, if necessary.

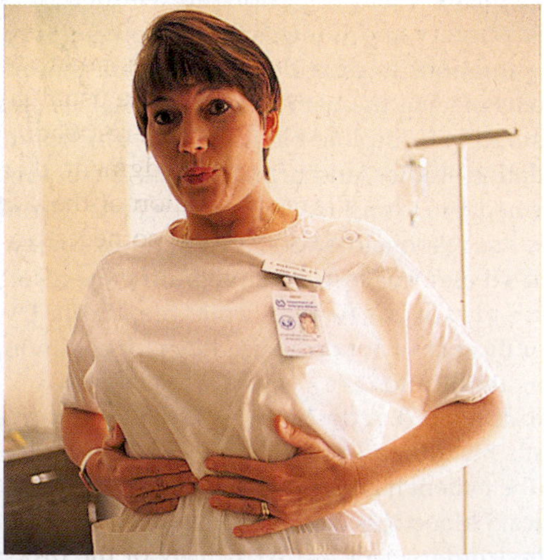

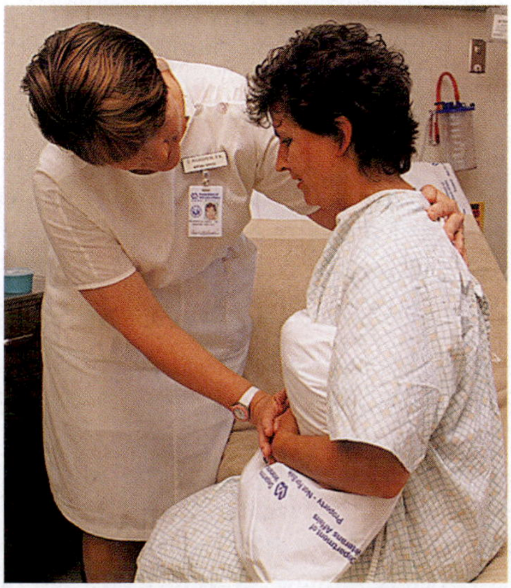

(continued)

SAFETY ALERT: Coughing may be contraindicated after some surgeries (such as neurosurgery). The nurse needs to pay close attention to orders and protocols for postoperative care as they relate to specific surgeries. ■

LEG, ANKLE, AND FOOT EXERCISES

Leg exercises are taught to the patient who is at risk for developing DVTs, or the formation of blood clots in a vein. Risk factors for DVT include decreased mobility; a history of circulatory disorders; and cardiovascular, pelvic, or lower extremity surgeries.

As the leg muscles contract and relax, blood is pumped back to the heart, promoting cardiac output and reducing venous stasis. These exercises also maintain muscle tone and range of motion, which facilitate early ambulation.

The nurse teaches the patient to perform the following exercises while lying in bed:

1. *Muscle pumping exercise:* Contract and relax calf and thigh muscles at least 10 times consecutively.
2. *Leg exercises:*
   a. Bend the knee and raise it toward the chest.

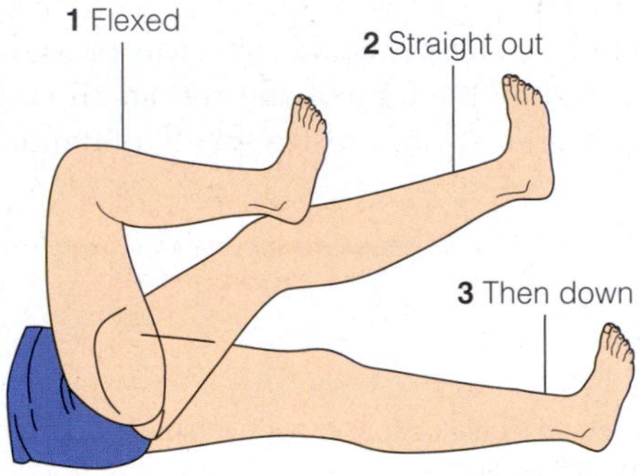
1 Flexed
2 Straight out
3 Then down

   b. Straighten leg and hold for a few seconds before lowering the leg back to the bed.
   c. Repeat exercise five times consecutively prior to alternating to the other foot.
3. *Ankle and foot exercises:*
   a. Rotate both ankles by making complete circles, first to the right and then to the left.
   b. Repeat five times and then relax.
   c. With feet together, point toes toward the head and then to the foot of the bed.
   d. Repeat this pumping action 10 times, and then relax.

Encourage the patient to perform leg, ankle, and foot exercises every 1 to 2 hours while awake, depending on the patient's needs and ambulatory status, the physician's preference, and institutional protocol.

TURNING IN BED

The patient may need to be taught to minimize discomfort when turning in bed. The patient may need to be advised that use of prescribed analgesics and splinting the incision with a hand and a small pillow or blanket will ease discomfort when turning. The nurse should encourage the patient to turn at least every 2 hours while awake. Specific patient instructions may include:

1. Instruct to grasp the side rail toward the direction to be turned, to rest the opposite foot on the mattress, and to bend the knee.
2. Instruct to roll over in one smooth motion by pulling on the side rail while pushing off with the bent knee.
3. Pillows may need to be positioned behind the patient's back to help maintain a sidelying position. The older patient may also need padding over pressure points between the knees and ankles to decrease the chance of decubitus ulcer formation from pressure.

In addition to teaching the patient and family about measures that will decrease the risk of complications, the nurse provides other preoperative information to prepare the patient and family for surgery. This information should include, but is not limited to:

- Diagnostic tests—reasons and preparations
- Arrival time if surgery is scheduled the day of admission
- Preparations for surgery, including fasting prior to surgery, skin preparation, indwelling catheter or bladder elimination, start of intravenous infusion, preoperative medication, handling of valuables (rings, watch, money)
- Instructions regarding current medications and any preoperative medications to be taken before admission
- Informed consent
- Expected timetable for surgery and the recovery room
- Location of the surgical waiting area and method to inform personal companions of progress throughout surgery
- Anticipated postoperative routine and devices or equipment (drains, tubes, equipment for IV infusions, oxygen or humidifying mask, dressings, splints, casts)
- Plans for postoperative pain control
- Appropriate clothing to wear after discharge from outpatient surgery.

It is also the nurse's role to ensure the patient understands where and when to arrive on the day of surgery and what actions are appropriate (or not) prior to surgery. Upon this preoperative preparation of the patient, the nurse is responsible for establishing, documenting, and communicating the plan of care to the perioperative team.

Diagnostic tests are performed within a week prior to elective surgery and immediately before surgery in emergency situations to provide baseline data that may reveal problems placing the patient at additional risk during and after surgery. Complete blood counts, electrolyte studies, coagulation studies, and urinalysis are the most commonly performed preadmission laboratory tests. Perianesthesia nurses are responsible for verifying and reviewing their patient's diagnostic tests and integrating the results into the patient's plan of care (where applicable). **Table 4.3** discusses the significance of abnormal findings for common tests and nursing implications.

Additional diagnostic tests may be performed as the patient's history and physical findings indicate. For example, if the patient has a low hemoglobin and hematocrit, and significant blood loss during surgery is anticipated, the surgeon may order a type and crossmatch of the patient's blood

Table 4.3 Common Laboratory Tests for Surgery

Test	Significance of Increased Values	Significance of Decreased Values	Nursing Implications
Hemoglobin (Hgb) and hematocrit (Hct)	Dehydration, excessive plasma loss, polycythemia	Fluid overload, excessive blood loss, anemia	■ Monitor oxygenation and vital signs. ■ Assess for bleeding.
Glucose and hemoglobin A1C (Hgb A1C)	Impaired glucose metabolism, stress, or infection	Inadequate glucose intake in relation to insulin	■ If decreased, monitor for manifestations of hypoglycemia. ■ Notify surgeon of glucose < 70 mg/dL or > 180 mg/dL.
White blood cell (WBC) count	Infectious/inflammatory processes, leukemia	Immune deficiencies	■ Monitor for manifestations of inflammation. ■ Monitor drainage, temperature, and pulse. ■ Use strict standard precautions.
Platelet count	Malignancies, polycythemia vera	Clotting deficiency disorders, chemotherapy	■ If decreased, assess for bleeding at incision sites and drainage tubes and assess for hematomas.
Carbon dioxide (CO_2)	Emphysema, chronic bronchitis, asthma, pneumonia, respiratory acidosis, vomiting, nasogastric suctioning	Metabolic acidosis, hyperventilation	■ Monitor respiratory status and ABGs.
Prothrombin time (Pro-Time, PT, INR) and partial thromboplastin time (PTT)	Defect in mechanism for blood clotting, anticoagulant therapy (aspirin, heparin, warfarin), potential effect of other drugs affecting clotting time	Hypercoagulability of the blood may lead to thrombus formation in the veins	■ If clotting time is elevated, monitor PT/PTT values. ■ Assess for bleeding at incision site and drainage tubes and for hematomas. ■ If clotting time is decreased, monitor for thrombus formation (pulmonary emboli, venous thrombosis), and evaluate PT and PTT values.
Urinalysis	Varied	Varied	■ Used to detect abnormal substances (e.g., protein, glucose, red blood cells, or bacteria) in the urine. ■ Notify surgeon if abnormalities are detected.
Serum creatinine, BUN	Renal dysfunction	Malnutrition, musculoskeletal wasting	■ Monitor urinary output. ■ Monitor wound healing.
Electrolytes			
Potassium (K^+)	Kidney dysfunction, dehydration, suctioning	Diuretic therapy, vomiting, NG suctioning	■ Monitor K^+ level, cardiac and neurologic function, and perioperative diuretic therapy.
Sodium (Na^+)	Kidney dysfunction, dehydration, saline-containing intravenous fluids	Diuretic therapy, vomiting, NG suctioning, fluid volume excess	■ Monitor Na^+ level and I&O. ■ Assess for peripheral edema and effects of perioperative diuretic therapy.
Chloride (Cl^-)	Kidney dysfunction, dehydration, alkalosis	Diuretic therapy, vomiting, NG suctioning	■ Monitor Cl^- level and I&O. ■ Assess for peripheral edema and perioperative diuretic therapy.

Note: ABGs, arterial blood gases; BUN, blood urea nitrogen; I&O, input and output; NG, nasogastric; PT, prothrombin time; PTT, partial thromboplastin time.

in anticipation of a possible transfusion. Another scenario may involve a patient who is susceptible to renal insufficiency, which increases risk for fluid volume overload in the perioperative period and for accumulation of metabolic by-products and medications dependent on renal clearance. When this risk is known, renal function testing may be performed preoperatively. It is evaluated on the basis of glomerular filtration rate (GFR), which is estimated by using serum creatinine (reported as the eGFR) or by measuring urinary creatinine. Creatinine is a stable product of muscle mass; it is filtered by the kidneys or secreted by the kidney tubules. In kidney failure, serum creatinine rises and the GFR is low. The best indicator of GFR is the creatinine clearance, a comparison of both serum and urinary creatinine levels.

In addition to laboratory tests, patients with risk factors related to heart and lung function typically have a chest x-ray. This radiologic procedure provides baseline information about the size, shape, and condition of the heart and lungs. Pulmonary complications such as lung disease or pneumonia may require that surgery be postponed to allow further evaluation or treatment. If findings are abnormal and the surgery cannot be postponed, information from the chest x-ray study can be used to determine the safest form of anesthesia. An electrocardiogram (ECG) is ordered routinely for patients undergoing general anesthesia when they are over 40 years of age or have cardiovascular disease. The ECG provides data for evaluation of either new or preexisting cardiac conditions. As well, pulmonary function studies are often performed to determine the extent of respiratory dysfunction in patients with congestive heart failure. The data gleaned from these tests informs the anesthetist before and during surgery in choosing the type of anesthetic to be used and guides the surgeon and nursing staff in the recovery phases. The patient's surgery may be canceled or postponed if any life-threatening conditions are discovered via preoperative testing.

Day of Surgery/Procedure

On the day of surgery/procedure, the perianesthesia nurse focuses on preoperatively validating existing information, including, but not limited to, verification of patient identification and the expected procedure, management of relevant preoperative status (e.g., allergies, mobility or sensory limitations, vital signs, lab results, IV therapy, medication administration, last food eaten, last void), and review and/or completion of the preadmission assessment, including, but not limited to, normothermia, skin integrity, pain/comfort, safety needs, spiritual needs, skin preparation, and availability of transport home at discharge.

During assessment processes on the day of surgery, the nurse identifies the patient's individual needs and the factors that may increase risks associated with surgery. The type of surgical procedure determines the assessment and interventions planned by the nurse. However, a complete history and assessment, including a review of medications, are also necessary for a risk assessment to determine the patient's overall health status. Table 4.2 lists common risk factors for the patient undergoing surgery and the related nursing interventions and implications. For example, when a patient is admitted for a right total knee arthroplasty, it should be of concern to the nurse if this patient has type 2 diabetes that requires insulin, smokes 1.5 packs of cigarettes per day, has numbness in the right foot, and is taking medication for hypertension. This information should be incorporated into a care plan, using appropriate nursing diagnoses and interventions to meet the patient's needs and assist the patient toward full postoperative recovery.

Importantly, the patient's response to planned surgery varies greatly. When planning and implementing nursing care, consider individual psychologic and physical differences, the type of surgery, and the circumstances surrounding the need for surgery. Having an operation is a significant and stressful event. Regardless of the nature of the surgery (whether major or minor), the patient and family will be anxious. The degree of anxiety they will feel is not necessarily proportional to the magnitude of the surgical procedure. For example, a patient scheduled to have a biopsy to rule out cancer, which is considered minor surgery, may be more anxious than a patient undergoing gallbladder removal, which is considered major surgery.

The nurse's ability to listen actively to both verbal and nonverbal messages is imperative to establishing a trusting relationship with the patient and family. Therapeutic communication can help the patient and family identify fears and concerns. The nurse can then plan nursing interventions and supportive care to reduce the patient's anxiety level and assist the patient to cope successfully with the stressors encountered during the perioperative period.

In most institutions, a surgical checklist serves as an outline for finalizing preparation of the patient for surgery. This checklist includes items that require attention by both the preoperative and intraoperative nurse prior to the patient's transfer to the operating room. The surgical checklist will look different in every facility, but its purpose is the same: To ensure the safety and effectiveness of the surgical process so that the best possible patient outcomes can be achieved and undue errors minimized.

Patient and Procedure Identification

One item generally listed on the surgical checklist is identification of the patient and procedure. The patient must be actively involved in identification procedures, and if the patient is not able to participate or if the patient's reliability is questioned, the family or designated caregiver is responsible for identifying the patient prior to the surgical procedure. The nurse identifies each patient using a minimum of two patient identifiers (e.g., name, birthdate, medical record number) as indicated per their facility's policy.

Informed Consent

Ensuring the completion of informed consent is another line item on most surgical checklists. The surgeon who performs a procedure is responsible for obtaining the patient's consent for care. The surgeon should discuss the procedure with the patient and family in language they can understand. Informed consent is disclosure to the patient of risks associated with the intended procedure or operation and is usually obtained by means of a legal document required for all invasive procedures or therapeutic measures, including surgery. The language of the document varies according to the statutory and common laws of each state. Informed consent includes the following information:

- Need for the procedure in relation to the diagnoses
- Description, purpose, and intended outcome of the proposed procedure
- Possible benefits and potential risks
- Likelihood of a successful outcome
- Alternative treatments or procedures available
- Anticipated risks should the procedure not be performed
- Physician's advice as to what is needed
- Right to refuse treatment or withdraw consent.

Ideally, the nurse should be present when the preceding information is provided. Later, the nurse can discuss the information with the patient and family, if necessary. If the patient has questions or concerns that were not discussed or made clear, or if the nurse questions the patient's understanding, the surgeon is responsible for supplying further information. If these situations arise, the nurse should contact the surgeon before the patient signs a consent form for the operation or special procedures.

Medication Administration

The patient having surgery receives medications before surgery to achieve specific therapeutic outcomes. A combination of preoperative drugs may be ordered to induce sedation; decrease anxiety; induce amnesia; increase comfort; reduce gastric acidity and volume; promote gastric emptying; decrease nausea and vomiting; and dry oral and respiratory secretions for purposes of reducing the risk of aspiration.

The surgical patient is generally given preoperative antibiotics within 1 hour of surgical site incision time as well. Any delay in administration should be reported promptly to the operating room team. Preoperative antibiotic prophylaxis is effective in the prevention of postoperative complications in many surgeries. This mirrors the goal of administering preoperative antibiotics, which is to guard against or prevent the patient from acquiring an SSI. **Table 4.4** outlines commonly prescribed preoperative medications including antibiotics.

Most surgical patients are required to refrain from eating meals or drinking milk for 6 hours before surgery and drinking clear liquids for 2 hours before surgery. This is stated as NPO, which stands for "nil per os," which is Latin for "nothing by mouth." It is important to note that these are general guidelines. Current evidence is mixed regarding best practices specific to preoperative fasting. Nurses need to know their organizations' policies. Preoperative fasting requirements in healthy patients undergoing elective procedures may contribute to withdrawal effects for those with caffeine addictions (e.g., headaches and irritability). Dehydration, hypovolemia, and hypoglycemia are other recognized side effects. Thirst, worry, and hunger are reported by patients to be related to fasting as well. Medications may be needed to facilitate patient comfort in these situations. In addition, throughout the preoperative fasting period, decisions about which of the patient's routine medications to administer require careful analysis. Importantly, there are certain medications that when stopped abruptly can have a negative effect on the patient (e.g., steroids, antiseizure medications, and tranquilizers). To reduce the patient's risk of an adverse surgical event and/or complication, the best guideline is to confer with the surgeon and anesthetist about specific medications and whether or not they should be given or discontinued prior to surgery.

Insulin is generally withheld when the patient is NPO, but depending on the anticipated length of the surgery, the dosage may be adjusted for the previous evening as well as

Table 4.4 Examples of Commonly Used Preoperative Medications

Generic Name	Trade Name	Action by Category	Nursing Implications
Antibiotics			
cefazolin	Ancef	Prevents SSIs in orthopedic and general surgeries and is associated with lower risk of mortality in older adult patients.	■ Patients with beta-lactam allergies receive vancomycin or clindamycin.
Benzodiazepines			
diazepam lorazepam midazolam	Valium Ativan Versed	Decreases anxiety and produces sedation to some extent. Induces amnesia. May induce substantial amnesia.	■ Monitor for respiratory depression, hypotension, drowsiness, and lack of coordination.
Opioid Analgesics			
fentanyl hydrocodone morphine oxycodone tramadol	Sublimaze Vicodin Morphine Roxicodone Ultram	Decreases anxiety, provides analgesia. Allows reduced anesthetic dose.	■ Monitor for respiratory depression and safety if ambulating. See Chapter 9 for nursing implications of specific opioid analgesics.
Antacids			
sodium citrate	Bicitra	Increases the pH and reduces volume of gastric fluid; used in patients with GERD. and/or trauma.	■ No significant factors in this setting.
H_2Receptor Antagonists			
cimetidine famotidine nizatidine ranitidine	Tagamet Pepcid Axid Zantac	Reduces gastric acid volume and concentration.	■ Monitor for confusion and dizziness in older adults.
Gastric Acid (Proton) Pump Inhibitors			
lansoprazole omeprazole pantoprazole	Prevacid Prilosec Protonix	Suppresses gastric acid secretion.	■ Monitor for dizziness and headache, rash, or thirst.
Antiemetics			
metoclopramide ondansetron	Reglan Zofran	Enhances gastric emptying. Affects the vomiting center in the brain.	■ Monitor for sedation and extrapyramidal symptoms (involuntary movement, muscle tone changes, and abnormal posture).
Anticholinergics			
atropine sulfate glycopyrrolate scopolamine	Atropine sulfate Robinul Scopolamine	Reduces oral and respiratory secretions to decrease risk of aspiration; decreases vomiting and laryngospasm.	■ Monitor for confusion, restlessness, and tachycardia. ■ Prepare patient to expect a dry mouth.

Note: Drugs identified in blue are among the 200 most commonly prescribed medications in the United States.

the morning of surgery. Under anesthesia, the manifestations of hypoglycemia (insulin reaction) are absent, so withholding insulin the morning of surgery when the patient is NPO is advisable. Blood glucose is monitored intermittently during surgery with the goal of maintaining normal blood sugar level (refer to Table 4.3). Patients who ordinarily manage their diabetes mellitus with oral medications may be placed on sliding-scale insulin to manage blood glucose during the perioperative experience. Evidence-based practice supports subcutaneous basal insulin administration for patients with hyperglycemia to maintain blood glucose levels below 180 mg/dL throughout the perioperative period. This practice is associated with better healing, fewer infections, and shorter hospital stays (Copanitsanou, Dafogianni, & Iraklianou, 2016).

Complimentary Care Interventions

Various complementary therapies may be implemented by nurses or other professionals across the perioperative continuum to decrease patient anxiety and/or promote comfort. There is evidence suggesting that there are positive benefits for surgical patients who receive complementary therapies including music, massage therapy, acupuncture or acupressure, aromatherapy, hypnosis therapy, Reiki therapy, guided imagery, relaxation audios, and/or essential oils. The perianesthesia and/or perioperative nurse should assess the patient's acceptance of and willingness to use available complementary interventions and obtain the patient's written consent as needed per facility policy. Persons providing such complementary therapies should have the education, competency, and appropriate certification or license to do so. This person may or may not be a perianesthesia or perioperative nurse, depending on the surgical facility or state regulation.

4.4 Surgery: Intraoperative Nursing Care

Care of the patient upon entry to the operating room consists of a flurry of critical activities that are accomplished in a coordinated and synchronous fashion by all members of the intraoperative team. This phase of care can be overwhelming for the patient, so it is important that members of the team inform the patient of their roles, actions, purpose, and what to expect during this time prior to the induction of anesthesia. The OR nurse facilitates these communications when necessary.

Members of the Intraoperative Team

The intraoperative (or surgical) team generally includes a surgeon, surgical assistant(s), anesthesiologist or CRNA, circulating registered nurse (RN), and a scrub nurse, certified surgical technologist (CST), surgical technologist, or operating room technician (ORT). Each member provides specialized skills and is essential to successful patient outcomes.

The surgeon is the physician performing the procedure. As head of the surgical team, the surgeon is responsible for all medical actions and judgments. Surgical assistants work closely with the surgeon in performing the operation. The number of assistants varies according to the complexity of the procedure. The assistant may be another physician, a certified first assistant, a physician assistant, or other trained person. Registered nurses may become certified to function as a first assistant (RNFA) through academic preparation and clinical training (Association of periOperative Registered Nurses [AORN], 2013). The assistant performs such duties as exposing the operative site, retracting nearby tissue, sponging and/or suctioning the wound, ligating bleeding vessels, and suturing or helping suture the surgical wound.

The anesthesiologist or CRNA administers anesthesia and assumes responsibility for the patient's general well-being during surgery. The anesthesiologist or CRNA evaluates the patient preoperatively, administers the anesthesia and other required medications, transfuses blood or other blood products, infuses intravenous fluids, continuously monitors the patient's physiologic status, alerts the surgeon to developing problems and treats them as they arise, and supervises the patient's immediate postoperative recovery.

The **circulating nurse** is a registered nurse who coordinates and manages a wide range of activities before, during, and after the surgical procedure. The circulating nurse coordinates the care of surgical patients, oversees the physical aspects of the operating room and required equipment, assists with transferring and positioning the patient, prepares the surgical site, ensures that no break in aseptic technique occurs, administers medications, handles surgical specimens, and counts all sponges, sharps, and instruments. This RN assists all other team members, including the surgeon, scrub person, and anesthesiologist or CRNA. It is also the responsibility of the circulating nurse to document intraoperative nursing activities, including, but not limited to, patient position, surgical pause or time-out, skin preparation, medications, placement of incisions, drains, catheters, implants, and other medical devices, as well as the start and end time of the procedure. Care planning based on physiologic and psychosocial assessments of the patient and evaluation of patient outcomes are other primary functions of the circulating nurse. Finally, the circulating nurse is at all times an advocate for the safety and well-being of the patient.

A **scrub person**, (an RN, ORT, or CST) generally handles sutures, instruments, and other equipment immediately adjacent to the sterile field (**Figure 4.5** ■). This role requires technical skills, manual dexterity, anticipatory thinking, and in-depth knowledge of the anatomic and mechanical aspects of a particular surgery.

In some settings, perioperative nurses as well as ORTs and CSTs may specialize within the already specialized field of surgical patient care. Many facilities have developed specialty surgical teams in response to the increasingly complex demands of technical surgeries. For example, a designated cardiac surgical team may be responsible for all open heart surgery cases and ordinarily not be involved with other procedures. The use of specialty surgical teams

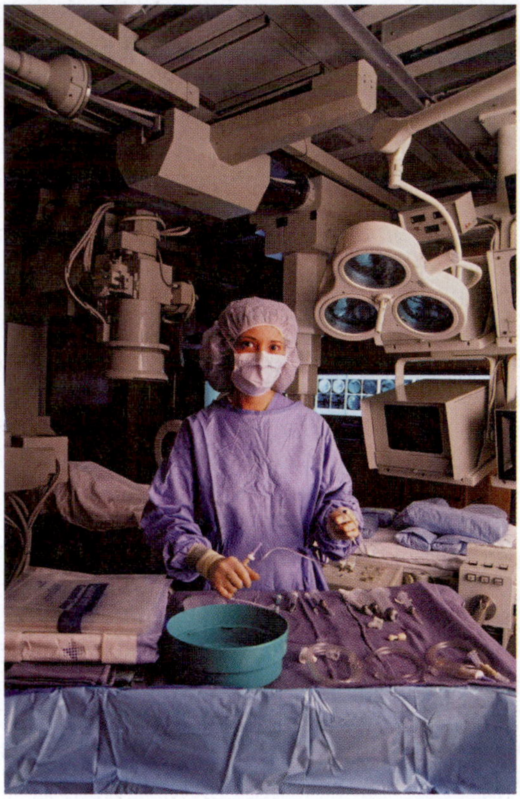

Figure 4.5 ■ A scrub nurse in the operating room.

allows RNs, ORTs, and CSTs to become highly skilled in a particular range of procedures.

Aseptic Practices

It is essential that environmental conditions promote the best possible surgical outcomes for patients. *Asepsis* is defined as not septic, or the absence of disease-causing organisms. Aseptic practice means to take all necessary steps to reduce the risk of bacterial, fungal, or viral contamination that may cause infection or septic disease. Moreover, *medical asepsis* is the absence of disease-causing microorganisms and is often referred to as a *clean state*, or more than sanitary. *Surgical asepsis*, however, is the absence of all microorganisms, and is otherwise known as *sterile*. Medical and surgical aseptic techniques are performed in the perioperative setting. The level of aseptic practice employed is indicated by the type of procedure the patient is having and its categorization.

Attire in the Surgical Environment

Strict dress codes in the surgical department promote asepsis, facilitate infection control, reduce cross-contamination between the surgery department and other patient care areas or departments, and promote the health and safety of patients and personnel. All personnel in the surgical department wear specific surgical attire to minimize bacterial shedding and reduce wound contamination. Surgical attire may include freshly laundered, nonsterile apparel designated for the surgical setting that includes a two-piece pantsuit, scrub dress, cover jacket, head covering, dedicated shoes, masks, and protective eyewear.

Expectations related to appropriate attire are dependent upon the *zone* in which personnel work. Importantly, the surgical department is divided into three zones: R*estricted*, *semirestricted*, and *unrestricted*. Restricted zones include the actual ORs where surgeries are performed by the intraoperative team. Semirestricted zones in the surgical setting include hallways, work areas, and sterile processing and storage rooms. In restricted and semirestricted areas, personnel wear surgical attire of a disposable type provided by the facility and/or a scrub suit laundered by a healthcare-accredited laundry facility. In these areas, personnel should also don a surgical cap that covers the head, hair, and ears. Facial hair, excluding eyebrows, is also covered as well with a facility-provided mustache/beard cover. In addition to this attire, in restricted zones, clean surgical masks are worn while in sterile surgical procedures and also in many clean procedures for personal protection (**Figure 4.6** ■). Perioperative staff who work in restricted zones should either wear shoe covers or shoes dedicated only for their intraoperative role. Unrestricted zones include all areas surrounding the semirestricted and restricted areas of the surgical setting (e.g., family waiting area, pre-/postoperative areas, staff lounges, locker

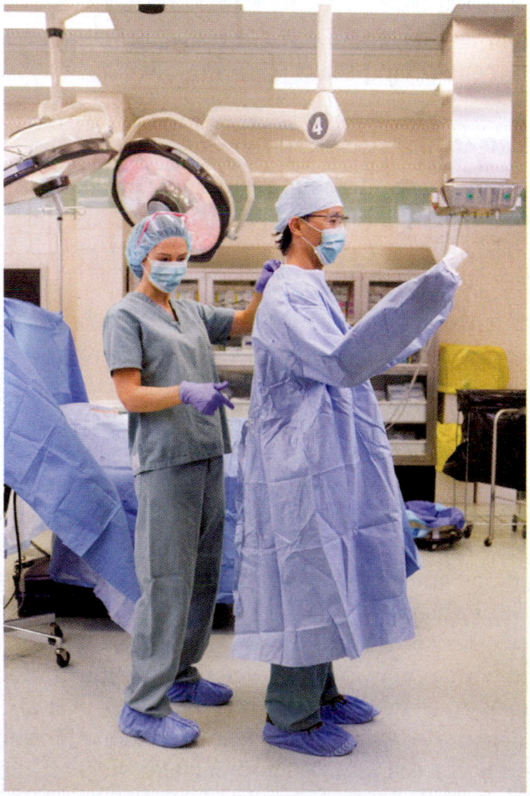

Figure 4.6 ■ Surgical attire. Scrub attire includes scrub suit, shoe covers, and cap or hood to cover hair, as shown on the left. Personnel in restricted zones also wear a mask, and those at the operating table wear a sterile gown and gloves over their scrub attire.

rooms). Scrub attire is not required in these areas. Thus, individuals in hospital uniforms and/or street clothes are permitted in the unrestricted zone.

Hand Hygiene

Hand hygiene is essential in preventing transmission of microorganisms from the hands of perioperative personnel to patients and/or the surgical environment. To reduce the patient's risk of developing a healthcare-acquired infection, a standardized hand hygiene protocol should be performed by perioperative personnel (1) before and after patient contact; (2) before carrying out a clean or sterile task; (3) after risk for blood or body fluid exposure; (4) after contact with patient's surroundings; (5) when hands are visibly soiled; (6) before and after eating; and (7) after using the restroom. An alcohol-based hand rub is also appropriate in certain situations where hands are not visibly soiled or dirty. Importantly, the use of gloves does not replace the need for hand hygiene as there is always a risk for glove failure.

Surgical Scrub

The surgical scrub is performed to render hands and arms as clean as possible in preparation for a procedure. All personnel who participate directly in the operative procedure must perform a surgical scrub with a sponge or brush and an antimicrobial agent or FDA-approved alcohol-based antiseptic surgical hand rub. Skin cannot be rendered sterile, but it is considered "surgically clean" following the scrub. The purpose of the surgical scrub is to:

- Remove dirt, skin oils, and transient microorganisms from nails, hands, and forearms.
- Increase patient safety by reducing the number of resident microorganisms on surgical personnel.
- Leave an antimicrobial residue on the skin to inhibit growth of microbes for several hours.

Sterile Technique

A sterile field is prepared by the scrub person for patients who are having a surgical or other invasive procedure. Perioperative personnel involved in such procedures perform a standardized surgical hand scrub and don a mask, eye protection, sterile gown, and gloves prior to setting up sterile supplies. Once sterile supplies are set up on a designated field (e.g., a table covered by a sterile drape), personnel use methods that maintain the sterility and integrity of additional items opened, dispensed, and/or transferred to the field. Sterile fields should never be left unattended. Perioperative personnel must constantly monitor sterile fields for contamination by visitors, vectors (e.g., insects), and/or any break in sterile technique. When a break in sterile technique occurs, personnel acknowledge the situation and then implement corrective action immediately, unless in doing so the patient may suffer undue harm.

Sterilization and Disinfection

Intraoperative nurses maintain knowledge of sterilization and disinfection procedures. In most surgical settings, there are typically sterile processing personnel who handle used/dirty instrumentation, disinfect instruments/devices, and reprocess or sterilize them for subsequent surgical cases. However, in some facilities, nurses may be responsible for disinfection procedures and the sterilization of surgical instruments/devices or the oversight of such. Intraoperative nurses, at minimum, are familiar with device category/classifications (e.g., critical, semicritical, and noncritical types), the level of disinfection required for each type, and the chemicals, processes, and conditions most effective for achieving disinfection and/or sterilization. Intraoperative nurses also understand how to determine if a specific surgical tool, instrument tray, or device has been cleaned and/or if it has met the conditions of sterilization. This knowledge is critical in the provision of perioperative nursing care as it potentiates appropriate aseptic practices and reduces the patient's risk for acquiring a SSI.

Patient and Worker Safety in the Operating Room

Intraoperative nurses maintain specialized knowledge about the surgical environment of care and evidence-based practices for mitigating risk of injury to self, team members, and patients. They are vigilant in the identification of potential safety issues, correcting them, and/or reporting them per organizational policy. Intraoperative nurses ensure a safe environment of care for both workers and patients by implementing nursing interventions that promote safe lifting and moving practices; the safe use of medical devices and personal protective equipment (PPE); appropriate identification of and response to clinical and alert alarms; the safe use of blanket- and solution-warming cabinets; fire prevention, suppression, and risk assessment; the safe use and handling of medical and anesthetic gases; proper handling and storage of all potentially hazardous chemicals; the identification of necessary latex precautions and appropriate response to latex-related reactions; and the proper disposal of hazardous and medical waste.

Other areas of potential risk of injury for both patients and intraoperative team members include medication administration, radiation exposure, counting of surgical items, sharps handling, specimen management, surgical smoke plume, and transmissible infections. Intraoperative nursing practice requires specific knowledge on risk reduction in all of these areas, a working understanding of specialty standards and practice recommendations produced by professional nursing organizations (e.g., Association of peri-Operative Nurses, American Society of Perianesthesia Nurses), and related facility policies and procedures.

Patient Care

All patients who enter the operating suite are at risk for unintended injury due to the complexities and hazards inherent in the surgical environment. Thus, it is the nurse's primary goal to reduce such risk and ensure the patient remains free from injury, taking into account the patient's health history and postoperative goals. This section describes, in brief, the activities of the intraoperative (or OR) nurse that are performed to reduce unintended patient injury and promote optimal surgical outcomes.

For cases involving general anesthesia, routine intraoperative nursing care provided upon entry of the patient to the OR and prior to induction usually includes (1) identifying the patient; (2) assisting the patient with transferring from a stretcher to the operating room table (if applicable for the case), and maintaining the patient's modesty in the process; (3) providing warm blankets to the patient and/or applying a forced-air warming blanket/device to promote normothermia; (4) ensuring the patient is comfortable and secured to the bed via a safety belt; (5) assisting the anesthetist with the application of patient monitors (e.g., ECG leads, BP cuff, pulse oximeter); and (6) applying ISCDs to the patient's lower extremities to reduce the risk of DVT, unless contraindicated.

Once the patient has been sufficiently oxygenated in preparation for the induction phase of anesthesia, the circulating nurse focuses all attention on the patient. At this point, the nurse remains ready to assist the anesthetist as needed throughout the induction phase and until the ETT (or other ventilation device) is fully functioning and secured in place. The transition from preinduction activities to the induction phase of anesthesia is one of the most critical points of the surgical process for the patient. After anesthetic medications have been given, the patient may appear oblivious to the surroundings; however, patients are particularly vulnerable to noise stress during induction and emergence from anesthesia. *Intraoperative awareness* is the patient's subconscious awareness of what is being said and done during surgery. Although most patients do not consciously remember what happened or what was said, psychologic trauma can result if conversations are unprofessional. Measures to reduce noise during the intraoperative phase include minimizing the number of people present, reducing voice volume, and minimizing conversations among surgical team members or use of the telephone. Importantly, all intraoperative team members are responsible for promoting a calming environment during induction of anesthesia that conveys to the patient (who is essentially transferring all control to the surgical team) that the team recognizes their collective protective responsibility to the patient and will take good care in performing their roles.

After the patient is unconscious and during the maintenance phase of anesthesia, the circulating nurse works with the intraoperative team to accomplish (1) positioning the patient as needed for access to the operative site; (2) hair removal by clippers or depilatory product (if required); (3) antimicrobial skin preparation; (4) application of a dispersive pad (if electrosurgery is planned); and (5) insertion of a urinary catheter (depending on the procedure and/or its expected duration). At this point, the nurse also ensures that baseline sharps, sponges, instruments, and other countable items have been documented, all local medications are available, and that the scrub person has everything needed for the surgical case.

When all activities have been completed to prepare the patient for the operation, the surgeon and assistants complete the necessary surgical scrub. The scrub person gowns and gloves the surgeon and assistants using sterile technique. The circulating nurse assists the team as needed in this process. Thereafter, the patient is draped, the circulating nurse makes all needed connections of sterile cords or tubing handed off the field to their respective end-unit (e.g., medical device/equipment), and then the surgical pause (or time-out) is conducted preincision. All members of the patient's intraoperative team participate in this activity. After any and all concerns raised during the time-out have been addressed, the surgeon makes the incision. Once the procedure is underway, the circulating nurse assists other members of the intraoperative team as needed throughout the case (e.g., troubleshooting of electrical equipment, dispensing of instruments/supplies to the sterile field, specimen collection/handling/documentation, updating surgical counts, providing surgical updates to the patient's family members, and otherwise coordinating patient care), vigilantly monitoring the patient's physiologic status and the sterile field and team members within it for potential breaks in asepsis and documenting all surgical activities performed.

At the end of the surgical procedure, the circulating nurse and scrub person concurrently ensures, via their facility's surgical count policy, that all counts are correct. If counts are incorrect upon closing of the surgical site, the intraoperative team implements appropriate procedures to resolve the discrepancy, and the circulating nurse documents the actions taken and the results of such.

When the surgical drapes are removed from the patient and the wound is cleaned and/or dressed, the circulating nurse remains ready to assist the anesthetist with emergence or extubation processes (as needed). It is important that the nurse is attentive during the patient's emergence from anesthesia as there are many possible complications that can arise (e.g., laryngospasms or bronchospasms leading to hypoxia, reduced airway reflexes, or physiological compromise in other systems).

After the patient is extubated, breathing independently, and maintaining adequate oxygenation with or without supplemental oxygen, the circulating nurse readies the patient for transfer to a stretcher or inpatient bed (if applicable) and assists in the actual process. Before the patient is transferred to PACU, ICU, or other recovery unit, the circulating nurse gives the requisite patient report to the receiving nurse per organizational policy. Once the patient leaves the operating suite, the circulating nurse completes any necessary follow-up activities (e.g., specimen transport, documentation, or other communication) to close out the case prior to preparing for the next. The scrub person deconstructs the sterile field, appropriately disposes of sharps and other items that cannot be decontaminated and reprocessed, and transports all dirty instrumentation to the decontamination area within the perioperative setting.

Every perioperative facility will have its own policies, norms, and/or routines regarding surgical process, Universal Protocol, and communication requirements specific to patient transitions in care across perioperative settings and beyond. Thus, it is important for all nurses who work within the perioperative setting to be aware of such and comply with facility policies and procedures, assuming they meet professional nursing standards and practice recommendations. If current policies/procedures do not meet or exceed professional nursing standards, it is the role of the perioperative nurse to voice concern and advocate/participate in institutional policy change.

Positioning

Proper surgical positioning is imperative to prevent injury to the patient. Pressure, rubbing, and/or shearing forces can cause injury to the tissue over bony prominences. Improper positioning can also lead to sensory and motor dysfunction, resulting in nerve damage and overstretched tendons and ligaments, causing muscle or joint injury. As well, pressure on peripheral blood vessels can decrease venous return to the heart and negatively affect the patient's blood pressure. If the patient is not properly positioned to promote lung expansion, oxygen desaturation can occur also. See **Table 4.5** for information about the most common surgical positions and their possible complications.

Surgical Counts

Surgical counts are done in the OR to prevent accidental retained foreign objects (items left in the surgical cavity) such as instruments, needles, or sponges. To prevent patient injury from the possible retention of foreign objects, the AORN (2017) recommends the following:

- A consistent multidisciplinary approach to preventing retained objects should be used and enforced during all surgical and invasive procedures.
- Radiopaque surgical soft goods (e.g., sponges, towels, textiles), sharps, and instruments should be counted for all procedures.
- Standardized measures for investigation and reconciliation of count discrepancies should be taken during the closing count and before the end of surgery. When a discrepancy in the count(s) is identified, the surgical team should carry out steps to locate the missing item.
- Perioperative staff members may consider the use of adjunct technologies to supplement manual count procedures and to ensure no unintended item remains.
- Measures taken for the prevention of retained objects should be documented in the patient's medical record.
- Policies and procedures for the prevention of retained objects, including device fragments, should be developed, reviewed periodically, revised as necessary, and readily available in the practice setting.

Table 4.5 **Common Surgical Positions**

Client Position	Steps to Be Taken to Safely Position Client
Supine The circulating nurse places the client on his or her back and ensures that the accompanying steps are completed. 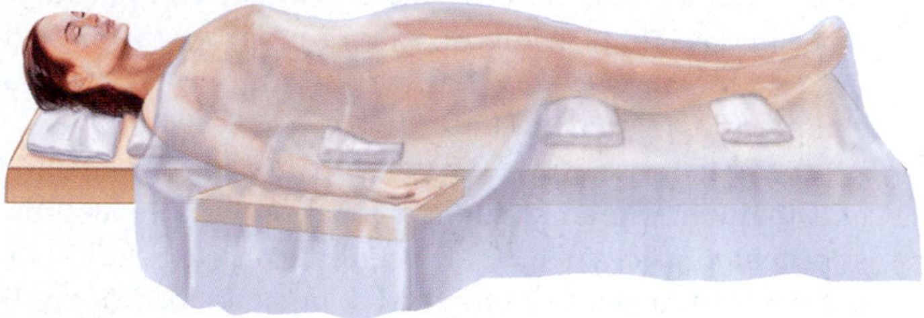	1. Arms are gently secured on padded arm boards at less than a 90-degree angle with palms up. 2. Alternatively, and only if necessary, tucked arms may be secured at the client's side with palms of hands facing in toward the thighs, elbows and hands protected and padded, and hands and wrists anatomically aligned. 3. Pillows are placed under the client's knees. 4. Bony prominences (e.g., heels) are elevated from the surface of the bed using pillows and a padded foot board for leg positioning. 5. A wedge is placed under a pregnant client's right hip/flanks to displace the uterus to the left.
Semi-Fowler (sitting) The circulating nurse places the client in the sitting position and ensures that the accompanying steps are completed. 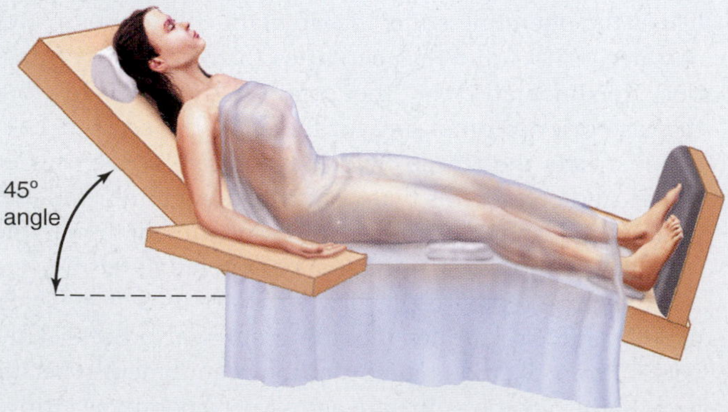45° angle	1. Arms are gently secured on padded arm boards at less than a 90-degree angle with palms up. 2. Pressure points are protected by properly positioning and padding the buttocks/sacrum and other bony prominences. 3. Bony prominences (e.g., heels) are elevated from the surface of the bed using pillows and a padded foot board for leg positioning. 4. The foot of the bed is lowered slightly to allow the knees to flex. 5. The client's feet are supported on a padded foot board to prevent plantar flexion and stretching of the tibial nerve. 6. The back of the operating room bed is raised to become the back rest, supporting the shoulders and torso with safety restraints.

Client Position	Steps to Be Taken to Safely Position Client
Prone and Jackknife The circulating nurse places the client on his or her stomach and ensures that the accompanying steps are completed. 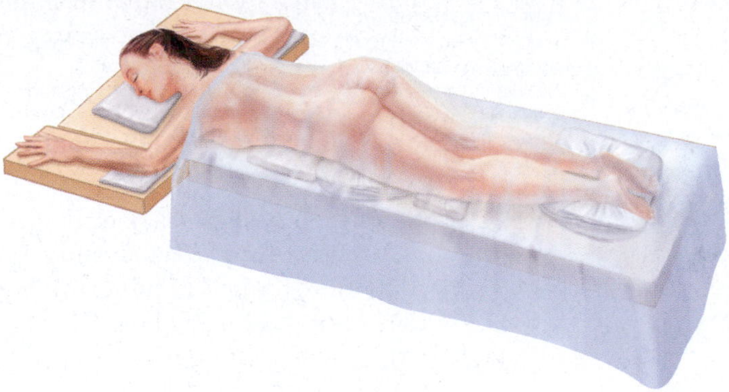 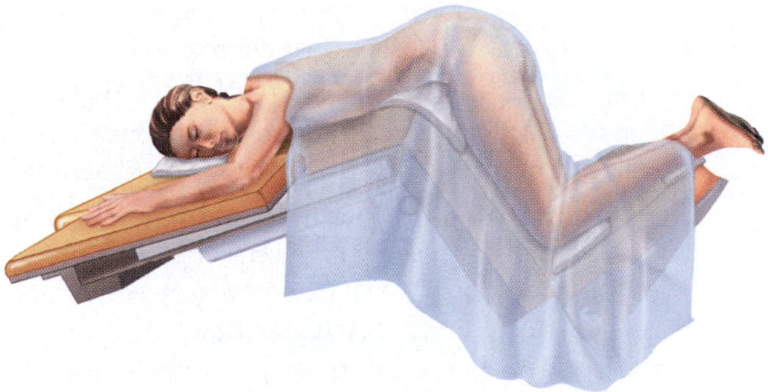	1. The cervical neck is maintained in alignment. 2. Toes are elevated from the surface of bed. 3. Eyes are protected to prevent ocular injury (e.g., pressure, corneal abrasion). 4. Female breasts and male genitalia are not compressed.
Lateral The circulating nurse places the client on his or her side (left or right) and ensures that the accompanying steps are completed. 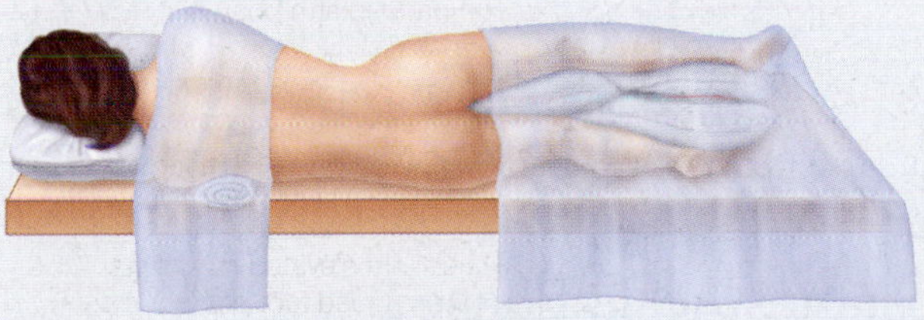	1. The correct surgical side is initialed before the client is transferred to the operating room. The initials must be visible after positioning, prepping, and draping. 2. The client is positioned on the nonoperative side. 3. Pressure points are padded on the dependent side (e.g., ear, acromion process, iliac crest, greater trochanter, lateral knee, malleolus). 4. Correct spinal alignment is maintained when the client is turned and stabilized in position. 5. Axillary rolls or other devices are needed to safely position arms and prevent brachial plexus injury.
Trendelenburg or Reverse Trendelenburg The circulating nurse places the client on his or her back with padded shoulder braces in place and ensures that the accompanying steps are completed. This position displaces the intestines into the upper abdomen. 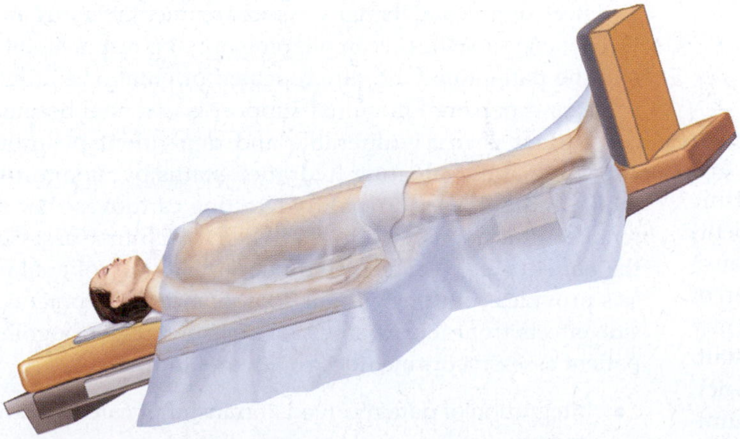	1. Time in the head-down position is monitored to identify physiological shifts. 2. The client is prevented from sliding and sheering injuries. 3. Injury to the client's shoulders is prevented. 4. The feet are supported on a padded foot board to prevent plantar flexion and stretching of the tibial nerve. 5. Injury to the client's brachial plexus is prevented. 6. Injury to the client's feet is prevented.

Client Position	Steps to Be Taken to Safely Position Client
Lithotomy This is a gynecological position. The circulating nurse places the client on her back with both legs elevated in stirrups and ensures that the accompanying steps are completed. 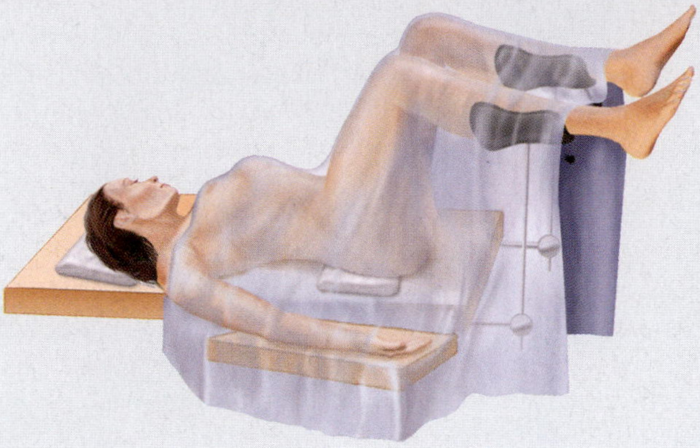	1. Ankles and heels are padded. 2. Stretching of the perineal nerve is prevented by ensuring that the hip and knee joints are not overextended. 3. Arms are padded on arm boards at less than a 90-degree angle with palms up. 4. The client's legs are removed from stirrups slowly and brought together simultaneously to prevent lumbosacral strain. 5. The client's legs are raised and lowered slowly and simultaneously to maintain hemodynamic status.
For All Procedures: Before draping the client, the circulating nurse must complete the accompanying steps for all surgical positions.	1. Pressure is evenly distributed over bony prominences. 2. The client's body alignment is always assessed to prevent musculoskeletal compromise. 3. Placement of safety straps is assessed. 4. Tissue perfusion is assessed. 5. The client's skin integrity is assessed, and the nurse ensures that there is no pooling of solutions or wet surfaces. 6. The client's circulatory, neurological, and respiratory systems are not compromised.
For each surgical procedure, the circulating nurse must evaluate the client postoperatively for injuries, covering all of the accompanying steps.	1. Skin injuries (e.g., reddened, bruised, tears) 2. Musculoskeletal and nerve injuries (e.g., aberrations in circulation, movement, and sensation) 3. Pressure ulcer development (e.g., identifies the stages of pressure ulcer development) 4. Eye injuries.

Source: PEARSON EDUCATION, . ., NURSING: A CONCEPT-BASED APPROACH TO LEARNING, VOLUME II, 3rd Ed., ©2019. Reprinted and Electronically reproduced by permission of Pearson Education, Inc., New York, NY.

While not all surgeries have equal risk for retained surgical items, those that do must include a careful count procedure with appropriate action if the count is incorrect. Stopping a closing procedure to recount and search for missing items increases anesthesia and wound exposure, but retained items contributes to serious infections and other potential liabilities.

4.5 Perianesthesia: Postoperative Nursing Care

Perianesthesia nurses apply the nursing process in their practice while preserving human dignity, autonomy, and confidentiality; protecting patient rights; and supporting the well-being of each patient. They provide care to patients in the immediate postanesthesia period (Phase I) and transition them to Phase II level of care, the inpatient setting, or to the intensive care setting for continued care. Each facility will have its own policies for perianesthesia nursing staffing requirements, assessments and their required frequency, patient discharge criteria, and documentation/communication. Nurses working in perianesthesia care settings are able to demonstrate phase-specific competencies and are familiar with their organization's policies and procedures that impact their practice.

Postanesthesia Phase I

Upon patient admission to the **postanesthesia care unit (PACU)**, the nurse immediately assesses the patient's airway and breathing and monitors vital signs and the surgical site to determine the response to the surgical procedure and to detect significant changes. Assessing mental status and level of consciousness is an ongoing nursing responsibility, and the patient may require repeated orientation to time, place, and person. Emotional support is essential because the patient is in a vulnerable and dependent position. Assessing and evaluating hydration status by monitoring intake and output is crucial to detecting cardiovascular or renal complications. In addition, the PACU nurse assesses the patient's pain level. Careful administration of analgesics provides comfort without compounding the potential side effects from the anesthesia. Other initial and ongoing patient assessments include, but are not limited to:

- Integration of data received at transfer of care from the operating suite
- Vital signs

- Comfort level
- Neurological function including level of consciousness and pupillary response
- Sensory and motor function
- Position of patient
- Skin integrity
- Patient safety needs
- Neurovascular (e.g., peripheral pulses, sensation in extremities)
- Condition of dressings and visible incisions
- Type, patency, and securement of drainage tubes, catheters, and receptacles
- Intravenous assessment.

Postsurgical Pain Management

Pain is expected after surgery. It is neither realistic nor practical to eliminate postoperative pain completely. Nevertheless, the patient should receive substantial relief from and control of this discomfort and experience minimal episodes of ineffective pain relief. Controlling postoperative pain not only promotes comfort but also facilitates coughing, turning, deep-breathing exercises, earlier ambulation, and decreased length of hospitalization, resulting in fewer postoperative complications and therefore reducing healthcare costs. Despite the apparent benefits and methods of effective pain control and improved understanding of pain physiology, pain control remains a challenge for many postoperative patients. Managing acute postoperative pain is an important nursing role before, during, and after surgery. Successful pain management involves the cooperative efforts of the patient, physician, and nurse. The patient's input and participation in assessing pain and pain relief are essential to developing a successful pain control regimen, including effective dosing and scheduling of postoperative analgesics. For example, the patient can rate pain using a standard pain scale. Perianesthesia nurses who work in recovery settings are competent in acute postoperative pain management, including assessing patients' pain level and administering pain medications.

At the end of a surgical procedure or immediately postoperatively, Ketorolac tromethamine (Toradol) is most commonly administered to assist with pain management. It is an NSAID that should be used with caution in patients over 65 years of age, those under 50 kg (110 lb), and those with reduced or potentially reduced renal function. The usual adult dose is 30 mg given intravenously every 6 hours for a period of 24 to 48 hours. This medication is given in conjunction with an opioid analgesic as well. Contraindications include hypersensitivity to aspirin or other NSAIDs, active GI bleeding, or peptic ulcer disease and pregnancy.

NSAIDs are used to treat mild to moderate postoperative pain. This category of drugs should be given soon after surgery (orally, parenterally, or rectally) along with opioids unless contraindicated. Although NSAIDs may not be sufficient to control pain, they allow lower doses of opioid analgesics and therefore fewer side effects. NSAIDs can be given safely to older patients, but they should be observed closely for side effects, particularly gastric and renal toxicity.

Opioid analgesics, such as morphine, are considered the foundation for managing moderate to severe postoperative pain. Opioid dosage requirements vary greatly from one patient to another, so the dosage must be individually tailored. In the immediate postoperative period, older adult patients benefit from the same protocol for morphine titration as do younger patients. Intravenous morphine may be initiated at a slightly reduced dose and then titrated to the same protocol as for younger patients. Morphine-related adverse effects such as nausea and vomiting, respiratory depression, constipation, urinary retention, pruritus, and allergy or sedation are similar among varying age groups. Patient-controlled epidural anesthesia (PCEA) may be more effective for older adult patients and is associated with earlier improved mental status and bowel activity.

Postanesthesia Phase II

During this phase of care, the perianesthesia nurse focuses on preparing the patient/family/significant other for care in the home or transition to an extended-care setting via appropriate patient assessment, planning, implementation, and evaluation for discharge. The nurse performs the same assessments as in Phase I, but has additional responsibilities of reviewing surgery discharge instructions with the patient and/or family/accompanying responsible adult as appropriate and facilitating follow-up to extended care, if indicated. For outpatient surgery, discharge criteria to home care includes:

- Patient is able to tolerate fluids or food without nausea and/or vomiting.
- Vital signs are stable and/or within approximately 10% of preoperative status.
- Patient is able to stand and begin to walk without dizziness or nausea.
- Pain is controlled or alleviated with oral medication that will be used after discharge.
- Patient is able to urinate.
- Patient is oriented or is at preoperative mental status.
- Patient and/or significant other demonstrates understanding of postoperative instructions.

Because the postoperative phase does not end until recovery is complete, the nurse's role as educator is vital as the patient nears discharge. As the patient prepares to recuperate at home, the nurse provides information and support as needed for self-care. Written guidelines, directions, and information should accompany all aspects of teaching. Opportunities for patient and family teaching are often brief, necessitating an organized, coordinated effort. The most common teaching needs include:

- ***Wound care:*** Demonstrate and explain the procedure, then encourage the patient and family to participate in the care. As time allows, have the patient or caregiver do a return demonstration of the procedure. Ideally, teaching is carried out over several days, evaluated, and reinforced.

- *Signs and symptoms of a wound infection:* The patient should be able to determine what is normal and what should be reported to the physician.
- *How and when to take one's temperature:* The patient and family should have an oral thermometer and know to report a temperature over 101°F. Older adults' baseline temperature is frequently below 98.6°F, so establishing a baseline temperature and instructing the patient to report an abnormal temperature is an important consideration.
- *Limitations or restrictions*: Describe any precautions related to activities of daily living such as driving and bathing.
- *Control of pain:* If analgesics are prescribed, teach the patient about the dosage, frequency, purpose, common side effects, and other side effects to report to the physician. Reinforce effective analgesic use and provide information on managing side effects such as gastric upset or constipation.

When the patient is discharged to a transitional, rehabilitation, or skilled-care facility for additional recovery before returning home, the nurse conveys information both verbally and in writing to the receiving facility. This report includes the following information:

- Patient name and identifying data; the surgery or procedure done, including any modifiers (e.g., right hip arthroplasty)
- Wound management, current medications and their purpose, prescribed activity and any limitations (e.g., limited weight bearing or restricted joint flexion)
- Current status, including vital signs and temperature; respiratory and circulatory status; pain level and management; fluid balance and nutrition; skin status; current activity level and degree of independence; pertinent cultural, emotional, psychosocial, or spiritual care needs; specific patient requests, needs, or values
- Specific rehabilitation orders and conditions for discharge from rehabilitation or skilled care (Amato-Vealey et al., 2008).

The nurse provides an opportunity to address any questions or concerns when handing off the patient to facility staff.

Extended Care

The nurse's role in this phase focuses on providing care when extended observation/intervention after discharge from Phase I or II is required. Components of nursing assessment and management in this setting are similar to those in Phase II, but also include a focus on nourishment, elimination patterns, and coordination of further care (if needed) and/or safe transport from the institution. Importantly, wound healing after surgery depends on adequate nutritional intake. Thus, it is important that oral fluids and feeding are resumed as soon as possible, based on the type of surgery performed, the patient's mental status, resumption of peristalsis (either audible bowel sounds or passage of flatus), and the patient's ability to tolerate liquids without nausea and vomiting.

For patients receiving extended care upon discharge from Phase II, postoperative analgesics should be administered at regular intervals around the clock (ATC) to maintain a therapeutic blood level. Administering analgesics as needed (PRN) lowers this therapeutic level; delays in medication administration further increase pain intensity. Therefore, PRN administration of analgesics is not recommended in the first 36 to 48 hours postoperatively. Patient-controlled analgesia (PCA) and patient-controlled epidural analgesia (PCEA) are often used for postsurgical pain patient control. The medication is administered using an intravenous infusion pump that is programmed to allow the patient to activate the administration of pain medication by pushing a button. Patients using PCA or PCEA following surgery need to be taught the importance of using the allowed dosages regularly to prevent increasing pain levels.

Only later in the postoperative recovery period should opioid analgesics (oral or parenteral) be given as needed. In this way, pain relief can be maintained, while the potential for drug side effects is decreased. Older adult patients often require fewer opioids than younger patients in the later postoperative period. When moving from parenteral analgesia to oral analgesics, it is essential for the nurse to remember that oral and parenteral doses may differ significantly. The oral dose of an opioid such as morphine, codeine, or hydromorphone may be two to five times higher than the parenteral dose to achieve equivalent pain relief.

Contrary to the belief of many healthcare providers (including nurses), physical dependence and tolerance to opioid analgesics rarely develops with short-term postoperative use. Instructing the patient on how to monitor pain and providing clear instructions for administering medication is important. Limiting prescriptions to the number of pills limits the risk of unnecessary prolonged use of medication and creates opportunity for a check-in if the patient needs to refill the prescription, as pain can be a warning side of complications. However, it is important to recognize that opioid analgesics, when used to treat acute pain, rarely lead to psychologic dependence and addiction. According to the WHO (2009) pain ladder, acute pain is appropriately treated with opioids, tapering to nonprescription analgesics as healing progresses (**Figure 4.7** ■).

Nutrition and Fluid Management

Fluids are commonly administered intravenously preoperatively and until the patient is fully awake after surgery and bowel sounds are present. Balanced electrolyte solutions are often used to prevent electrolyte imbalance related to presurgical fasting. Potassium chloride may be added to the intravenous solution if nasogastric suction is in place or fasting will be prolonged. Although intravenous fluids maintain hydration and electrolyte balance, they do not

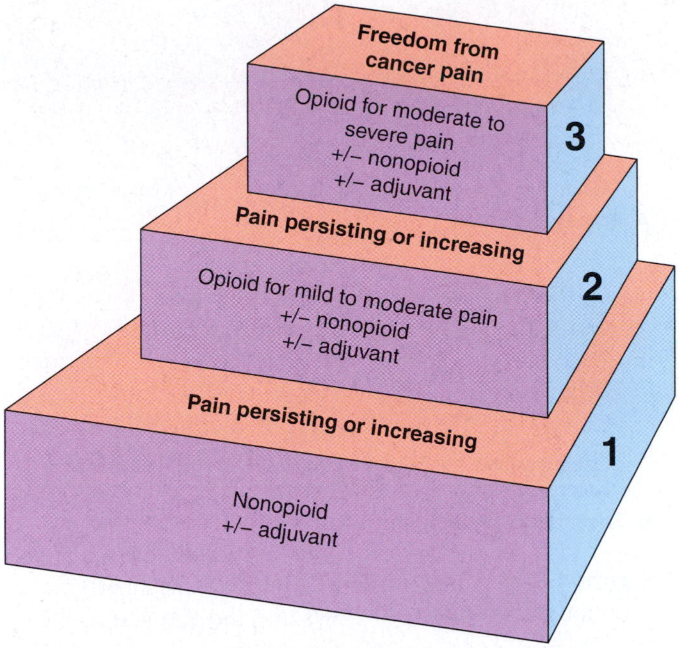
Freedom from cancer pain
Opioid for moderate to severe pain +/– nonopioid +/– adjuvant
3
Pain persisting or increasing
Opioid for mild to moderate pain +/– nonopioid +/– adjuvant
2
Pain persisting or increasing
1
Nonopioid +/– adjuvant

Figure 4.7 ■ WHO pain ladder.

provide nutrition. See Chapter 10 for more information about intravenous fluids and fluid balance.

Surgery is a physiologic insult that results in a hypercatabolic state with accelerated protein loss. Thus, patients are at risk following surgery for protein-calorie malnutrition (PCM) in the postoperative patient when fasting is prolonged for 12 or more hours. PCM slows wound healing and impairs immune defenses, increasing the risk for postoperative complications. Reestablishing food intake early in the postoperative period also supports gastrointestinal function. Enteral intake prompts blood flow and perfusion of the GI mucosa, maintaining its absorptive barrier and immunologic functions. With prolonged fasting, blood flow is diverted from the GI tract to organs such as the heart and brain during physiologic stress, which can lead to tissue ischemia and atrophy in the gut.

Unless balanced nutrition through gastrointestinal intake can be reestablished within 3 to 4 days, parenteral nutrition is critical for homeostasis and wound healing. Glucose solutions of up to 10% concentration can be administered peripherally (peripheral parenteral nutrition). Peripheral parenteral nutrition is used for short-term nutritional support (less than 7 days). These solutions, which contain glucose, amino acids, and electrolytes, are approximately isotonic to prevent damage to the veins. Despite this, phlebitis is a common complication of peripheral parenteral nutrition. When the need for parenteral nutritional support is prolonged, central vein access must be established. The large diameter and blood flow in central veins allows administration of high-calorie solutions with protein, carbohydrates, lipids, vitamins, and minerals (total parenteral nutrition). This is important for patients who have extended recovery periods without eating after surgery. Risks associated with parenteral nutrition include fluid and electrolyte imbalances, hyperglycemia, infection, and sepsis.

Transfer and Continued Care of Stable Postoperative Patients

When awake and after being stabilized, the patient may be transferred to a specific inpatient unit within the hospital. The PACU/perianesthesia nurse communicates information about the patient's condition and postoperative orders to the receiving inpatient unit RN prior to the patient's arrival. This report includes patient identifiers, the procedure performed, medications, blood and intravenous fluids administered, current vital signs, pain level, cardiorespiratory and neurologic status, and other pertinent information such as chronic diseases, cultural considerations, and other appropriate and necessary information. Provision of this data prepares the inpatient unit RN for additional problems or needed equipment.

Immediate and continuing assessment is essential to detect and/or prevent complications. In documenting assessment findings, the inpatient unit RN completes a flow record of the individual patient's situation. Baseline data are obtained and compared with preoperative data. Upon transfer, the receiving unit nurse performs a postoperative head-to-toe assessment that includes, but is not limited to:

- General appearance
- Vital signs
- Level of consciousness
- Emotional status
- Respiratory rate
- Skin color and temperature
- Discomfort/pain
- Nausea and/or vomiting
- Type of intravenous fluids and flow rate
- Dressing site
- Drainage on the dressing and/or bed linens
- Urinary output (catheter or ability to urinate)
- Ability to move all extremities.

Hospital policy or physician's orders dictate the frequency of follow-up assessments. After major surgery, the inpatient unit RN generally assesses the patient every 15 minutes during the first hour and, if the patient is stable, every 30 minutes for the next 2 hours, and then every hour during the subsequent 4 hours. Assessments are then carried out every 4 hours, subject to change according to the patient's condition and protocol for the particular surgical procedure. It is critically important to inform the surgeon immediately if the assessment reveals any signs of impending shock or other life-threatening changes.

After carrying out the initial assessment and ensuring the patient's safety by lowering the bed and placing the call light within reach, the inpatient unit RN notes the physician's postoperative orders. These orders guide the nurse in the care of the postoperative patient. For example, the orders specify activity level, diet, medications for pain and nausea, antibiotics, continuation of preoperative medications, frequency of vital sign assessments, administration of intravenous fluids, and laboratory tests such as hemoglobin and potassium level. In most institutions, orders written prior to surgery must be reordered following surgery because the patient's condition is presumed to have changed.

4.6 Patient Risks: Postsurgical Considerations

Nursing care before, during, and after surgery is aimed at preventing complications and/or minimizing their effects. Wound healing, and common postoperative wounds, cardiovascular and respiratory complications, and problems associated with elimination are discussed next.

Wound Healing

Normally surgical wounds heal by *primary* or *secondary intention* (**Figure 4.8** ■). Tissue healing by cell regeneration or primary intention occurs when the wound is uncomplicated and clean and has sustained little tissue loss. The edges of the incision are well approximated (have come together well) with sutures, staples, or surgical glue. This type of surgical incision heals quickly, and very little scarring is expected.

Healing by secondary intention occurs when the wound is large, gaping, and irregular. Tissue loss prevents wound edges from approximating; therefore, connective scar tissue (granulation tissue) fills in the wound to restore its structural integrity. This type of wound takes longer to heal, is more prone to infection, and develops more scar tissue. Tertiary intention occurs when the surgical wound becomes infected, often requiring debridement of necrotic tissue. Granulation tissue fills in the gaping wound and closure is prolonged, leaving a wide scar.

Wound healing occurs in three phases: The inflammatory phase, the proliferative phase, and the remodeling phase (**Figure 4.9** ■). Healing time varies according to factors such as age, nutritional status, general health, and the type and location of the wound.

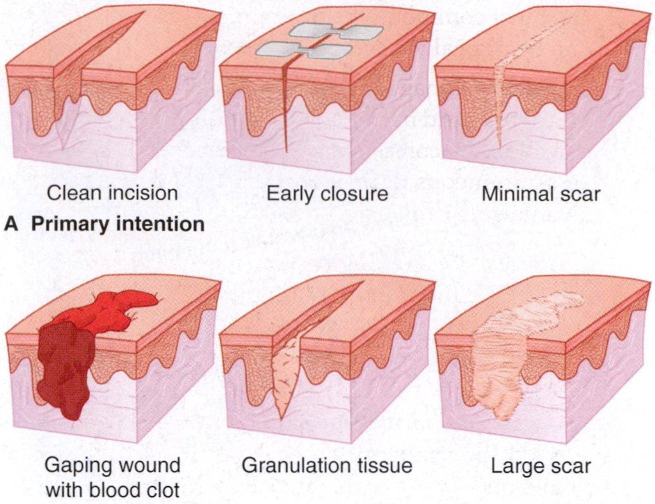
Clean incision
Early closure
Minimal scar
A Primary intention
Gaping wound with blood clot
Granulation tissue
Large scar
B Secondary intention

Figure 4.8 ■ Wound healing by intention. **A**, Primary intention. **B**, Secondary intention.

Inflammatory Phase

The **inflammatory phase** begins with the surgical incision. Physiologic mechanisms to maintain hemostasis and promote blood clotting are activated. Blood vessels initially constrict, then dilate and become more permeable to bring plasma and blood cells to the site. Phagocytic WBCs remove invading organisms and debris from the area. These cells also release growth factors to stimulate tissue repair.

Wound drainage (exudate) results from the inflammatory process during initial wound healing. The drainage is composed of escaped fluid and cells from the rich blood supply that surrounds the wound tissue. Wound drainage is described as serous, sanguineous, or purulent:

- Serous drainage contains mostly the clear serous portion of the blood. The drainage appears clear or slightly yellow and is thin in consistency.
- Sanguineous drainage contains both serum and red blood cells and has a thick, reddish appearance. This is

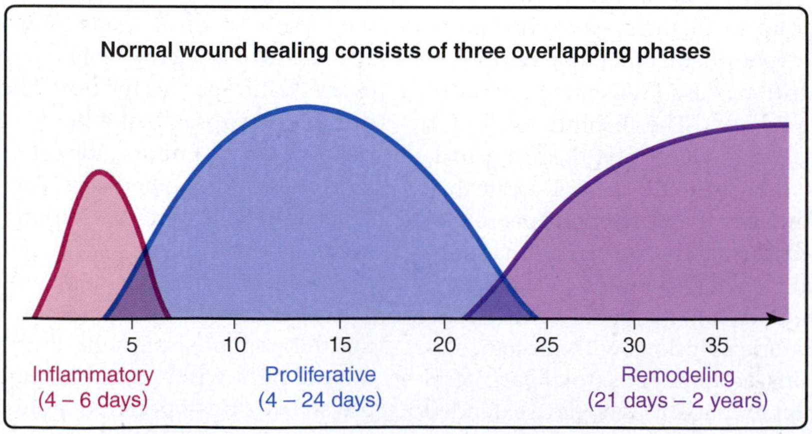
Normal wound healing consists of three overlapping phases
5
10
15
20
25
30
35
Inflammatory (4 – 6 days)
Proliferative (4 – 24 days)
Remodeling (21 days – 2 years)

Figure 4.9 ■ Timeline for inflammatory, proliferative, and remodeling stages of wound healing.

the most common type of drainage from an uncomplicated surgical wound.

- Purulent drainage is composed of white blood cells, tissue debris, and bacteria. Purulent drainage results from infection. Its consistency is greater than that of serous or sanguineous drainage, and the color and odor vary by infecting organism.

Wound drainage devices are used to decrease pressure in the wound area by removing excess fluid, which promotes healing and decreases complications (see **Figure 4.10** ■). Penrose drains (Figure 4.10C) promote healing from the inside to the outside and decrease the chance of abscess formation. Wound care focuses on cleaning around the drain with a prescribed solution, such as sterile normal saline, and replacing the dressing as necessary to keep the surrounding skin dry and encourage further drainage. An absorbent dressing is placed over the drain and gauze (not shown).

Wound suction devices promote drainage of fluid from the incision site, decreasing pressure on healing tissues and reducing abscess formation. Shown are the Jackson-Pratt and Hemovac wound suction devices (see Figure 4.10 A, B).

The frequency with which the device is emptied depends on the time elapsed since surgery, type of surgery, amount of drainage, and agency policy. For example, immediately after surgery the nurse may empty the device every 15 to 60 minutes. As drainage decreases, the device is emptied every 2 to 4 hours (per policy). Care is taken to maintain asepsis when emptying suction devices, avoiding contamination of the drain or the drain plug. Amount, color, consistency, and odor of drainage are documented. Usually, the drain is removed on the second to fourth day after surgery. Removal causes minor patient discomfort. After removal, the drain site is cleaned and a sterile dressing is applied.

Proliferative Phase

The **proliferative phase** begins within 2 to 3 days after surgery. Fibroblasts (connective tissue cells that synthesize collagen, growth factors, and other wound healing elements) and vascular endothelial cells proliferate to form granulation tissue (Sorenson et al., 2019). This tissue is initially fragile and bleeds easily. Epithelial cells proliferate at the wound edges to form a new surface.

Sutures or staples are removed during this phase of wound healing. Wound strength is only about 10% of normal

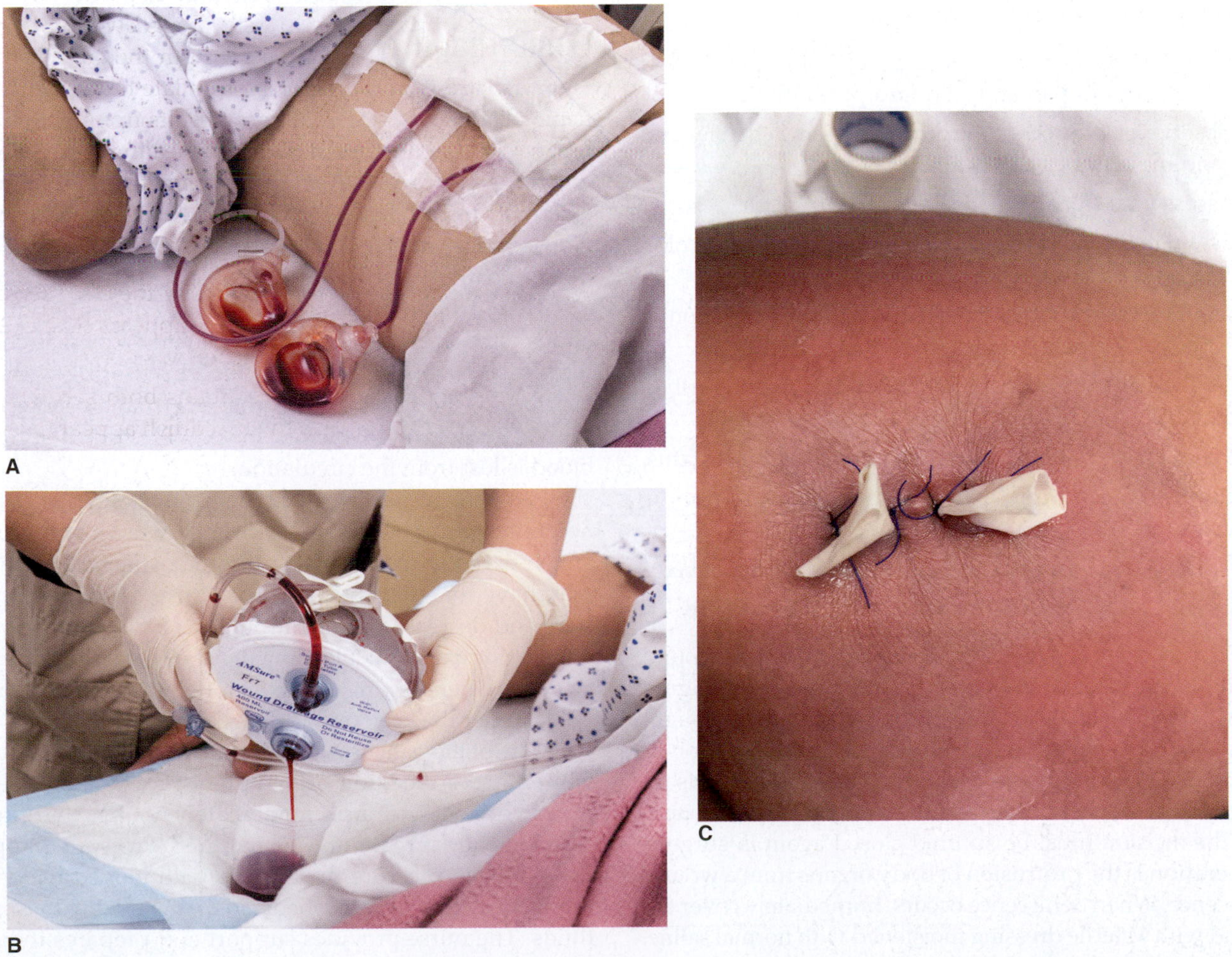
A
B
C

Figure 4.10 ■ Wound drainage devices. **A**, Jackson-Pratt drain. **B**, Hemovac drainage system. **C**, Penrose drain.

tissue strength at the time of their removal, but increases significantly during the next 4 weeks (Scott-Thomas et al., 2017). Sutures or staples may be removed over a period of several days, with initial removal of every third suture/staple, then half of the remaining sutures/staples, and finally all remaining. Wound closure strips (e.g., Steri-Strips) or surgical adhesives may be used to maintain approximation of wound edges that are not fully healed.

Remodeling Phase

During the **remodeling phase**, scar tissue is remodeled by a process of collagen synthesis and breakdown to increase its strength. This phase begins about 3 weeks after surgery and can continue for 6 or more months.

Nursing Care of Surgical Wounds

Nursing care of the postoperative patient with a surgical wound focuses on preventing and monitoring for wound complications. The nurse assumes a leading role in supporting the wound healing process, providing emotional support to the patient, and teaching wound care to the patient.

Common assessment findings of an infected wound include pain; purulent, odorous discharge and redness; warmth; tenderness; and edema around the edges of the incision. Additionally, the patient may have a fever, chills, and increased respiratory and pulse rates. Nursing care includes the following measures:

- Maintain medical asepsis (e.g., by using good hand hygiene technique) and standard precautions.
- Observe aseptic technique during dressing changes and handling of tubes and drains.
- Assess vital signs, especially temperature.
- Evaluate the characteristics of wound discharge (color, odor, and amount).
- Assess the condition of the incision (approximation of the edges, sutures, staples, or drains).
- Clean, irrigate, and pack the wound in the prescribed manner.
- Maintain the patient's hydration and nutritional status.
- Culture the wound prior to beginning antibiotic therapy.
- Administer antibiotics and antipyretics as prescribed.
- Provide supportive measures to patient and family.

Serious complications may result from delayed wound healing or may occur immediately following surgery (**Figure 4.11** ■). They also may occur after forceful straining (coughing, sneezing, or vomiting). **Dehiscence** is a separation in the layers of the incisional wound. Treatment depends on the extent of wound disruption. If the dehiscence is extensive, the incision must be sutured closed again in surgery. **Evisceration** is the protrusion of body organs from a wound dehiscence. When dehiscence occurs, immediately cover the wound with a sterile dressing moistened with normal saline. Emergency surgery is performed to repair these conditions.

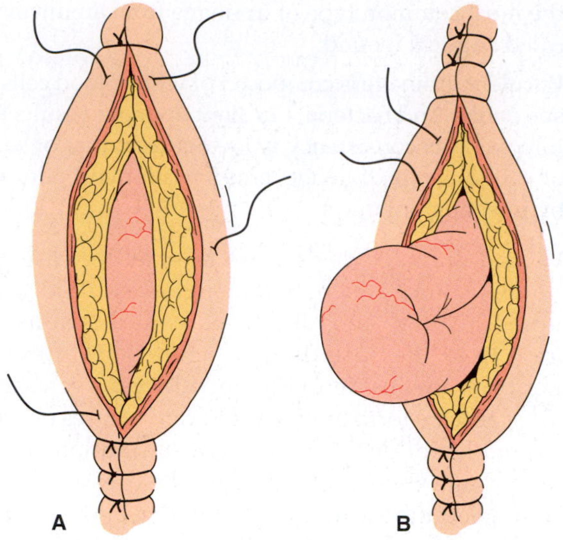
A
B

Figure 4.11 ■ Wound complications. **A**, Dehiscence is a disruption in the incision resulting in a separation of the layers of the wound. **B**, Evisceration is a protrusion of a body organ through a surgical incision.

Cardiac Events

Common postoperative cardiovascular complications include hemorrhage, shock, DVT, and PE.

Hemorrhage

Hemorrhage is an excessive loss of blood. A concealed hemorrhage occurs internally from a blood vessel that is no longer sutured or cauterized or from a drainage tube that has eroded a blood vessel. An obvious hemorrhage occurs externally from a dislodged or ill-formed clot at the wound. Hemorrhage may also result from clotting abnormalities due to a pathologic condition or adverse medication effects.

Hemorrhage from a venous source oozes out quickly and is dark red, whereas an arterial hemorrhage is characterized by bright red spurts of blood pulsating with each heartbeat. Whether the hemorrhage is from a venous or an arterial source, hypovolemic shock will occur if sufficient blood is lost from the circulation.

Assessment findings with hemorrhage depend on the amount and rate of blood loss. Restlessness and anxiety are observed in the early stage of hemorrhage. The patient may have manifestations such as tachycardia; cool, pale skin; and decreased urine output. The blood pressure may remain normal. Frank bleeding may be obvious or may only be noted when turning or repositioning the patient if blood pools under the back or buttocks.

Care of the patient who is hemorrhaging centers around stopping the bleeding and replenishing the circulating blood volume. The nurse immediately notifies the surgeon as emergency surgery may be required. Pressure is applied using a snug pressure dressing or with gloved hands. An intravenous line is established and maintained with isotonic fluids. The nurse provides support and prepares them for the possibility of emergency surgery.

Shock

Shock is a life-threatening postoperative complication. It results from an insufficient blood flow to vital organs, an inability to use oxygen and nutrients, or the inability to rid tissues of waste material. The most common type of shock in the postoperative patient is *hypovolemic shock*, which results from a decrease in circulating fluid volume due to blood or plasma loss or, less commonly, severe prolonged vomiting or diarrhea. Manifestations of hypovolemic shock include an altered level of consciousness, confusion, and restlessness; tachycardia and tachypnea, weak, thready pulses, and possible hypotension; decreased urine output; and cool, clammy, pale, or cyanotic skin. Chapter 11 provides a detailed discussion of nursing care of the patient with various types of shock.

Deep Venous Thrombosis

Deep venous thrombosis (DVT) is the formation of a thrombus (blood clot) in association with inflammation in deep veins. It is a complication that most often occurs in the lower extremities of the postoperative patient resulting from a combination of several factors, including vessel trauma during surgery and sluggish blood flow during and after surgery. Risk factors for postoperative DVT include:

- Orthopedic surgery to lower extremities; urologic, gynecologic, or obstetric surgeries; or neurosurgery
- Age over 40 years
- Pregnancy, varicose veins, hormone replacement therapy, or use of birth control pills
- History of previous DVT or pulmonary emboli
- Prolonged immobility
- Cigarette smoking
- Infection or sepsis
- Malignancy.

Prevention of venous stasis is an important nursing responsibility; it reduces adverse patient outcomes and decreases healthcare costs. Early ambulation is the key to preventing venous stasis. Anticoagulant medications such as low-molecular-weight heparin are used in high-risk populations. Effective prevention includes the use of mechanical prophylactic devices such as ISCDs on the foot, entire leg, or calf only is documented as effective prevention.

Common assessment findings specific to DVT reveal pain or cramping in the involved calf or thigh. Redness and edema may also occur along with a slightly elevated temperature. The patient may have a positive Homans sign (pain in the calf on dorsiflexion of the affected foot), although this is an unreliable sign of DVT.

Nursing care of the patient with DVT includes assessing the affected extremity, administering and monitoring the effects of prescribed anticoagulants, maintaining activity restrictions as ordered, and teaching and supporting the patient and family. See Chapter 32 for more information about caring for the patient with DVT.

Pulmonary Embolism

A **pulmonary embolism (PE)** is a dislodged blood clot or other substance that lodges in a pulmonary artery. DVT is the major risk factor for PE. Early detection of this potentially life-threatening complication depends on the nurse's astute, continuing assessment of the postoperative patient.

Common assessment findings of the patient experiencing a PE include mild to moderate or severe dyspnea, chest pain, diaphoresis, anxiety, restlessness, rapid respirations and pulse, dysrhythmias, cough, and cyanosis. The severity of the symptoms is determined by the degree of pulmonary vascular blockage. Sudden death can occur if a major pulmonary artery becomes completely blocked.

Stabilizing respiratory and cardiovascular functioning while preventing the formation of additional emboli is of utmost importance in the care of the patient with a pulmonary embolism. Nursing care includes prompt notification of the physician and frequent assessment of cardiac, respiratory, and neurologic status. Oxygen saturation is monitored, and supplemental oxygen may be administered. Intravenous access is maintained; anticoagulants and analgesics may be prescribed. The nurse also focuses on supporting the patient and family during this crisis. Chapter 37 provides more information about care of the patient experiencing pulmonary embolism.

Respiratory Events

Common postoperative respiratory complications include pneumonia and atelectasis. Pneumonia is inflammation of lung tissue. Inflammation is caused either by a microbial infection or by a foreign substance in the lung, which leads to inflammation. Numerous factors may be involved in the development of pneumonia, including aspiration of gastric contents, retained pulmonary secretions, impaired cough reflex, and decreased mobility.

Common assessment findings of the postoperative patient with pneumonia include:

- Chills and fever
- Tachycardia, tachypnea
- Cough, which may be productive
- Dyspnea
- Chest pain
- Crackles and wheezes.

Treating the pulmonary infection, supporting the patient's respiratory efforts, promoting lung expansion, and preventing the organisms' spread are the goals in the care of the patient with pneumonia. The nurse frequently assesses vital signs, oxygen saturation, and the patient's ability to tolerate activity. Interventions may include elevating the head of the bed and administering oxygen to support lung ventilation and gas exchange and administering medications per physician orders. The nurse may also encourage mobility as tolerated and the use of an incentive spirometer at least every 1 to 2 hours. Adequate hydration will help the patient to liquefy respiratory secretions as well. The nurse teaches to the patient proper disposal of tissues, to cover the mouth when coughing, and good hand hygiene technique. Care of the patient with pneumonia is discussed in Chapter 36.

Atelectasis is an incomplete expansion or collapse of lung tissue resulting in inadequate ventilation and retention of pulmonary secretions. Common assessment findings include dyspnea, diminished breath sounds over the affected area, anxiety, restlessness, crackles, and cyanosis.

Promoting lung expansion and systemic oxygenation of tissues is a goal in the care of the patient with atelectasis. Nursing care is similar to that provided for the patient with pneumonia as outlined above.

Elimination Issues

Common postoperative complications associated with elimination include urinary retention and altered bowel elimination. Urinary retention may occur postoperatively as a result of the recumbent position, effects of anesthesia and narcotics, inactivity, altered fluid balance, nervous tension, or surgical manipulation in the pelvic area.

The nurse assesses for bladder distention if the patient has not voided within 7 to 8 hours after surgery or if the patient is urinating small amounts frequently. A portable ultrasound scanner may be used to determine the amount of urine in the bladder. This noninvasive procedure provides information to prevent unnecessary catheterization and decreases the potential for urinary tract infections and urethral trauma from repeated catheterizations. The nurse promotes fluid intake as allowed, monitoring intake and output. Promoting normal urinary elimination requires the following nursing actions:

1. Provide privacy.
2. Assist the patient to use the bedside commode or walk to the bathroom.
3. Assist male patients to stand to void.
4. Pour a measured amount of warm water over the perineal area. (If urination occurs, subtract the amount of water from the total amount for an accurate output measurement.)

Bowel elimination is frequently altered after abdominal or pelvic surgery and sometimes after other surgeries. Return to normal gastrointestinal function may be delayed by general anesthesia, narcotic analgesia, decreased mobility, or altered fluid and food intake during the perioperative period.

Nursing care focuses on assessing for and promoting the return of normal bowel function. To assess for the return of peristalsis, the nurse asks the patient about the passage of flatus, auscultate bowel sounds every 4 hours while awake, assess the abdomen for distention, and monitor for defecation. A distended abdomen with absent bowel sounds may indicate paralytic ileus (impaired propulsion of intestinal contents). Measures to promote bowel function include encouraging ambulation, promoting fluid intake of 2500 to 3000 mL (unless contraindicated), and providing for privacy during elimination. The patient receiving opioid analgesics may require a stool softener or mild laxative to prevent constipation, a side effect of these drugs. If no bowel movement has occurred within 3 to 4 days after surgery, a suppository or an enema may be ordered.

4.7 Surgical Considerations for Special Populations

Nurses are expected to be culturally competent. As well, they have a duty to practice " . . . with compassion and respect for the inherent dignity, worth, and unique attributes of every person" (American Nurses Association, 2015). This means no matter the patient's social or economic status, personal attributes, life situation, and/or nature of health problem, the nurse is professionally obliged to treat every individual in a manner that serves to promote, protect, and restore health. This section calls attention to two specific populations and best practices in meeting their perioperative care needs.

Older Adults

With an ever-increasing population of adults of advanced age, the nurse must be aware of normal age-related changes experienced by older adults and modify nursing care accordingly in an effort to provide safe, supportive care. Certain physiologic, cognitive, and psychosocial changes associated with the aging process place older adults at increased risk for surgical complications.

Specifically, cardiovascular and tissue changes that result from aging place the older adult at increased risk for surgical complications, especially when long, complicated surgeries are planned (e.g., thoracic or abdominal open surgeries). The older adult is more prone to hypotension, hypothermia, and hypoxemia resulting from anesthesia and the cool temperature in the operating room.

Positioning may cause complications in the older adult as well. Intraoperative positioning of arthritic joints can cause postoperative joint pain unrelated to the operative site. The longer the surgery is, the greater the chance of decubitus ulcer formation. The older patient is at increased risk for developing decubitus ulcers because of decreased subcutaneous fat tissue and reduced peripheral circulation.

Immune function declines with aging too, increasing the risk for surgical infections in the older adult. The classic signs of infection, fever, redness, pain, and swelling may be diminished in the older adult patient; instead, manifestations such as confusion, lethargy, and anorexia

Table 4.6 **Nursing Interventions for Older Adults Undergoing Surgery**

System	Age-Related Changes	Nursing Interventions
Body composition	Decreased lean muscle mass and strength, increased body fat; decreased thirst	Assist to change positions frequently. Monitor I&O, assess for dehydration and fluid imbalance.
Nutrition-immune status	Decreased appetite, taste, and saliva production increase risk for malnutrition; immune function declines with aging	Assess for inflammation and wound healing; monitor temperature and laboratory values for evidence of infection, malnutrition; minimize duration of fasting.
Integument	Loss of subcutaneous fat, thinning of dermis and epidermis, decreased moisture and elasticity	Position carefully to prevent pressure ulcers. Avoid shearing forces, which can tear skin. Examine mucous membranes, laboratory studies, and urine output to evaluate hydration status.
Sensory-perceptual	Age-related vision and hearing impairment	Encourage patient to wear glasses and hearing aids whenever possible; speak clearly, not loud; minimize noise in environment; provide adequate room light; remain within patient's field of vision when speaking.
Respiratory	Decreased vital capacity and increased residual volume; increased ventilation/perfusion mismatch; diminished cough reflex	Assess baseline parameters and monitor respiratory status and lung sounds. Teach and encourage coughing and diaphragmatic breathing exercises. Encourage ambulation.
Cardiovascular	Decreased cardiac reserve; increased risk for postural hypotension	Monitor vital signs, pulse strength, skin color and temperature, and urine output. Assess for cardiac dysrhythmias and edema. Encourage ambulation and leg exercises to prevent DVT.
Gastrointestinal	Gum disease, loss of teeth, and dry mouth affect appetite and food intake; slowed GI motility contributes to early satiety and constipation	Provide mouth care; avoid alcohol-based products that dry mucous membranes. Encourage adequate fluid intake and small, frequent meals, soft diet. Monitor bowel function.
Genitourinary	Decreased kidney function; decreased bladder capacity; potential prostate enlargement in men	Monitor I&O, serum electrolyte, BUN, and creatinine levels. Assess for drug side effects. Assist to normal voiding position as needed.
Musculoskeletal	Decreased bone density; loss of muscle mass; increased joint stiffness	Carefully position on OR table. Move carefully and gently. Prevent pressure sores. Encourage and assist with postoperative ambulation.
Cognitive-psychologic	Cognition remains stable, but information processing slows; more difficulty with word retrieval, naming	Provide ample time for teaching and learning; encourage repetition; provide supplemental written materials and instructions.

may develop. The focus of care needs to be strongly on prevention.

Finally, the older adult often has some degree of hearing and/or visual impairment. These impairments coupled with a strange environment can make the operating room a frightening, disorienting place. By effectively communicating with the patient, the nurse can provide support and reassurance to minimize these factors. To decrease confusion and assist in communication, hearing aids and glasses should be used when appropriate and possible.

Advanced age alone is not a contraindication for surgery. Factors that contribute to successful surgical outcomes for older adults include stabilizing nutrition and hydration, controlling concurrent chronic conditions with appropriate medication reconciliation, and providing information for realistic expectations about the surgery and the recovery. **Table 4.6** shows a summary of age-related changes with selected nursing interventions.

Transgender Adults

Some transgender individuals undergo medical and/or surgical interventions to alter their sexual anatomy and physiology, and still others do not request these interventions. Transgender persons who undergo gender-affirming surgery (e.g., breast augmentation, mastectomy, genital reconfiguration, tracheal shaving, facial masculinization or feminization surgery) may have a medical diagnosis of gender dysphoria, meaning discomfort with one's sex assigned at birth.

Hormone therapy is common within the transgender population, though evidence is lacking on the long-term effects of hormone therapy in this group. What is known is that testosterone can damage the liver, especially if taken in high doses or by mouth. Estrogen can increase blood pressure, blood glucose (sugar), and blood clotting. Antiandrogens, such as spironolactone, can lower blood pressure, disturb electrolytes, and dehydrate the body. These risks associated with hormone therapy have obvious implications for transgender surgical patients, and especially for those having lengthy procedures (e.g., genital reconfiguration/reconstruction). Moreover, to minimize intraoperative and postoperative risks related to the combination of hormone use and the experience of surgery, it is important that the nurse has knowledge of whether or not the patient is on a hormone regimen.

Case Study & Nursing Care Plan

A Patient Having Surgery

Martha Overbeck is a 74-year-old widow who lives alone in a senior citizens' housing complex. She is active there, as well as in the Lutheran church. She has been in good health but has become progressively less active as a result of arthritic pain and stiffness. Mrs. Overbeck has degenerative joint changes that have particularly affected her right hip. On the recommendation of her physician and following a discussion with her friends, Mrs. Overbeck has been admitted to the hospital for an elective right total hip replacement. Her surgery has been scheduled for 8:00 a.m. the following day.

Mrs. Eva Jackson, a close friend and neighbor, accompanies Mrs. Overbeck to the hospital. Mrs. Overbeck explains that her friend will help in her home and assist her with the wound care and prescribed exercises.

ASSESSMENT

Gloria Nobis, RN, is assigned to Mrs. Overbeck's care on return to her room. Ms. Nobis performs a complete head-to-toe assessment and determines that Mrs. Overbeck is drowsy but oriented. Her skin is pale and slightly cool. Mrs. Overbeck states she is cold and requests additional covers. Ms. Nobis places a warmed cotton blanket next to Mrs. Overbeck's body, adds another blanket to her covers, and adjusts the room's thermostat to increase the room temperature. Mrs. Overbeck states that she is in no pain and would like to sleep. She has even, unlabored respirations and stable vital signs as compared to preoperative readings.

Mrs. Overbeck is NPO. An intravenous solution of dextrose and water is infusing at 100 mL/h per infusion pump. No redness or edema is noted at the infusion site. Ms. Nobis notes that the antibiotic ciprofloxacin hydrochloride (Cipro) is to be administered by mouth when the patient is able to tolerate fluids. Mrs. Overbeck has a large gauze dressing over her right upper lateral thigh and hip with no indications of drainage from the wound. Tubing protrudes from the distal end of the dressing and is attached to a passive suctioning device (Hemovac). Ms. Nobis empties 50 mL of dark red drainage from the suctioning device and records the amount and characteristics on a flow record. Mrs. Overbeck has a Foley catheter in place with 250 mL of clear, light amber urine in the dependent gravity drainage bag.

Mrs. Overbeck's feet are slightly cool and pale with rapid capillary refill time bilaterally. Dorsalis pedis and posterior tibial pulses are strong and equal bilaterally. Ms. Nobis notes slight pitting edema in the right foot and ankle as compared with the left extremity. She also notes sensation and ability to move both feet and toes, without numbness or tingling (paresthesias).

Ms. Nobis records these findings on the electronic medical record. After ensuring that Mrs. Overbeck is safely positioned and can reach her call light, Ms. Nobis gives Mrs. Overbeck's friend, Mrs. Jackson, a progress report.

DIAGNOSES

Ms. Nobis identifies the following postoperative priorities of care for Mrs. Overbeck:

- Potential infection of the surgical wound on the right hip
- Risk for injury of right hip prosthesis secondary to total hip replacement
- Pain related to right hip incision and positioning of arthritic joints during surgery
- Risk of sequelae related to immobility.

EXPECTED OUTCOMES

The expected outcomes established in the plan of care specify that Mrs. Overbeck will:

- Regain skin integrity of the right hip incision without experiencing signs or symptoms of infection.
- Verbalize signs and symptoms of infection to be reported to her physician.
- Describe measures to be taken to prevent dislocation of right hip prosthesis.
- Report control of pain at incision and in arthritic joints.
- Remain afebrile.
- Remain free of complications related to immobility.

PLANNING AND IMPLEMENTATION

Ms. Nobis develops a care plan that includes the following interventions to assist Mrs. Overbeck during her postoperative recovery:

- Use aseptic technique while changing dressing.
- Monitor temperature and pulse every 4 hours to assess for elevation.
- Assist to change positions frequently (q2h) and cough and deep-breathe. Assist with early ambulation.
- Assess wound every 8 hours for purulent drainage and odor. Assess edges of wound for approximation, edema, redness, or inflammation in excess of expected inflammatory response.
- Teach Mrs. Overbeck and Mrs. Jackson the signs and symptoms of infection and when to report findings to the physician.
- Review and discuss with Mrs. Overbeck the written materials on total hip replacement.
- Convey empathetic understanding of Mrs. Overbeck's incisional and arthritic joint pain.
- Medicate Mrs. Overbeck every 4 hours (or as ordered) to maintain a therapeutic analgesic blood level.

EVALUATION

Throughout hospitalization, Ms. Nobis works with Mrs. Overbeck and Mrs. Jackson to ensure that Mrs. Overbeck can care for herself after discharge from the hospital. Five days after her surgery, Mrs. Overbeck is discharged with a well-approximated incision with no indications of an infection. Prior to discharge, Ms. Nobis is confident that with Mrs. Jackson's help Mrs. Overbeck can properly assess the incision. She can cite the signs and symptoms of an infection, take her own oral temperature, and describe preventive measures to decrease the chances of dislocating her prosthetic hip. Because of her reduced mobility the past 5 days, Mrs. Overbeck says she can tell the arthritis in her "old bones" is "acting up." She reports less pain in her right hip than before the surgery. Mrs. Overbeck tells Ms. Nobis she will be back the following winter to have her left hip replaced.

CLINICAL REASONING IN PATIENT CARE

1. Describe risk factors for Mrs. Overbeck's safety. What changes in her home environment would you suggest to promote safety until she recovers more fully?
2. Why is Mrs. Overbeck placed on the antibiotic Cipro even though she has no indications of an infection? What teaching would you do?
3. Mrs. Overbeck's clotting time is slightly elevated as a result of an ordered anticoagulant. Why would this medication be ordered? Consider the patient's age and the area of surgery.
4. Mrs. Overbeck is 30 pounds above her ideal weight and has osteoarthritis. Develop a care plan related to intake in excess of metabolic requirements.

See Evaluating Your Response in Appendix B.

CHAPTER HIGHLIGHTS

4.1 Overview of Surgery

Compare various methods of and settings for surgical procedures, types of anesthesia, and perioperative patient safety.

- Surgery is a major physiologic and psychologic stressor that carries significant risks. Nurses have a critical role in identifying individual patient risks throughout the perioperative period. Nurses protect the safety of, maintain the physiologic and psychologic integrity of, advocate for, and promote recovery of the patient undergoing surgery.
- Surgeries take place in inpatient and outpatient settings, often with the use of minimally invasive procedures that expedite discharge, facilitate healing, and increase patient satisfaction.
- Surgery is an invasive procedure requiring that legal guidelines be followed to protect the patient and healthcare providers. The intraoperative team includes surgeons, anesthetists, nurses, and technicians; all are responsible for the safety of the patient and the progression of the surgery.

4.2 Patient Risks: Preoperative Considerations

Differentiate patient risks that can be mitigated in the preoperative stage.

- Systematic, structured, and effective communication among all members of the interprofessional team is essential for safe and effective perioperative care. Care transitions (preadmission to day of surgery care; day of surgery preoperative care to intraoperative care; intraoperative care to postanesthesia Phase I recovery; postanesthesia Phase I recovery to postoperative Phase II recovery; and postoperative Phase II recovery to home or extended care) present significant opportunities for errors, emphasizing the importance of effective communication.
- The focus on safety during surgery continues to increase, with attention directed to preventing wrong site and wrong patient surgeries (using the Universal Protocol), surgical site infections, DVT and PE, and adverse cardiac events. A team approach to safety works best; each member of the team must feel accountable for the results of the surgery and entitled and safe in sharing observations and concerns as the procedure progresses.
- Patient teaching prior to and following surgery empowers patients to achieve successful recovery, discharge, and rehabilitation. Most of the care patients receive as they heal from surgery is either provided by self or a caregiver outside the healthcare environment. Patients and their families need to know how to appropriately assess healing progress and access help if needed and when to report suspected complications.
- Assessing, coordinating, and implementing preoperative preparation, evaluating and ensuring the patient's readiness for surgery, and teaching are key preoperative nursing roles.

4.3 Perianesthesia: Preoperative Nursing Care

Describe the preanesthesia phase, preadmission testing, and procedures for the day of surgery.

- Operating room and perianesthesia care nursing are professional specialties that require unique orientation and education. These professionals make careful assessments of the risks each patient faces and make plans to ensure safe, successful surgical outcomes.

- Special attention is focused on early recognition of potential patient risks related to surgical experience and implementing nursing interventions to minimize risk and promote safety.

4.4 Surgery: Intraoperative Nursing Care

Outline aseptic practices, safety, and patient care during surgery.

- During the intraoperative phase, the nurse's focus is on identifying patient risks, taking into account each individual's health status and history, and implementing a nursing care plan intended to promote and maintain patient safety.
- Patient advocacy is a critical nursing role during this phase as well. When the patient is under anesthesia and/or unable to speak, it is up to the intraoperative nurse and team members to ensure the patient's needs and/or surgical expectations are met.

4.5 Perianesthesia: Postoperative Nursing Care

Describe postoperative nursing care including postanesthesia care, extended care, and transfers.

- During the postoperative phase, nurses are instrumental in promoting the patient's comfort and initial recovery, identifying and preventing potential complications, and teaching the patient and family or caregivers about continuing care needs.
- Pain management is offered prior to, during, and after surgery, with methods designed to stimulate best therapeutic response. Although acute pain may be associated with surgery, many patients also experience chronic pain that affects their response to pain management therapies.

4.6 Patient Risks: Postsurgical Considerations

Summarize postsurgical risks to patients including wound healing, cardiac events, respiratory events, and elimination issues.

- Wound healing occurs in three stages: Inflammatory, proliferative, and remodeling.
- Common postoperative cardiovascular complications include hemorrhage, shock, DVT, and PE.
- Hemorrhage, an excessive loss of blood, can be internal or obvious.
- Shock, which is a life-threatening postoperative complication, results from an insufficient blood flow to vital organs, an inability to use oxygen and nutrients, or the inability to rid tissues of waste material.
- Deep venous thrombosis (DVT) is the formation of a thrombus (blood clot) in association with inflammation in deep veins.
- A pulmonary embolism (PE) is a dislodged blood clot or other substance that lodges in a pulmonary artery.

4.7 Surgical Considerations for Special Populations

Differentiate considerations for perioperative care of older adults and transgender adults.

- Unique characteristics of older adult patients increases the need for individualized care. Assessment of physical, emotional, and spiritual status can be more difficult when patients have hearing or visual impairments or when individuals speak and understand a foreign language. Surgery can be frightening to patients and their families and they need reassurance and interventions to relieve anxiety, decrease pain, and promote healing.
- Some transgender individuals undergo medical and/or surgical interventions to alter their sexual anatomy and physiology, while others do not request these interventions. Hormone therapy has risk factors that impact surgery.

TEST YOURSELF NCLEX-RN® REVIEW

1. Which action should the nurse perform when implementing informed consent?
   A. Define the risks and benefits of the surgery.
   B. Witness the patient's signature on the consent form.
   C. Explain the right to refuse treatment or withdraw consent.
   D. Advise the patient and family about what is needed for the diagnosis.

2. The nurse is caring for a patient recovering from surgery provided through an outpatient surgical center. On what teaching should the nurse focus to assist this patient with her recovery?
   A. Nutritional needs
   B. Pain medication doses
   C. Identifying complications
   D. Fluid and hydration status

3. When providing patient-centered care to a patient recovering from surgery, why should the nurse provide nonsteroidal anti-inflammatory drugs?
   A. To increase amnesia
   B. To stimulate appetite
   C. To potentiate analgesia
   D. To improve renal function
4. When reviewing the medical record for a patient scheduled for surgery, the nurse notes abnormal laboratory values. Which value is the priority for the nurse to report to the healthcare provider?
   A. Increased chloride
   B. Decreased glucose
   C. Increased creatinine
   D. Decreased hemoglobin
5. The nurse is concerned that a patient who has undergone knee surgery is developing a vascular problem distal from the operative site. What did the nurse most likely assess in this patient? (Select all that apply.)
   A. Bounding pedal pulse
   B. Poor muscle tone in the foot
   C. Skin that is cool to the touch
   D. Redness or swelling in the calf
   E. Cramping in the lower leg
6. The nurse notes that a patient did not receive ordered medications prior to having surgery. What should the nurse do about the patient's medications?
   A. Resume them now.
   B. Decrease doses by half for 36 hours.
   C. Check for new orders before providing.
   D. Withhold until fully recovered from anesthesia.
7. The nurse is preparing a patient with type 1 diabetes mellitus for surgery and withholds the morning insulin dose. How will the nurse explain this action to the patient?
   A. "There is no risk that you will develop high blood glucose during surgery."
   B. "It will be better if your blood glucose is low during anesthesia.'
   C. "You received an extra dose of insulin last night."
   D. "Signs of low blood glucose are harder to recognize during surgery."
8. The nurse is reviewing the pain management orders for a patient who is recovering as expected from surgery done 1 week ago. What should the nurse anticipate regarding pain medications for the patient?
   A. Progress from NSAIDs to opioids
   B. Progress from oral to parenteral routes
   C. Given as needed rather than on a schedule
   D. Induce a strong sedative effect to decrease the risk of nausea
9. The nurse is preparing an older patient for a surgical procedure that is planned to take 8 hours. Which postoperative risk is this patient more prone to experiencing? (Select all that apply.)
   A. Memory loss due to blood loss
   B. Hearing loss due to extended anesthesia
   C. Hypothermia due to cool environment
   D. Pressure sores and joint pain from operative positioning
   E. Surgical site infection
10. A patient has just been admitted to the PACU. Why should the nurse provide interventions to reduce hypothermia in this patient? (Select all that apply.)
    A. To decrease cardiac ischemia
    B. To reduce the risk for wound infection
    C. To increase patient comfort and analgesia
    D. To reduce surgical bleeding
    E. To increase respiratory drive

See Test Yourself answers in Appendix B.

REFERENCES

Amato-Vealey, E.J., Barba, M.P., & Vealey, R.J. (2008). Hand-off communication: A requisite for perioperative patient safety. *AORN Journal, 88*(5), 763–770.

American Nurses Association. (2015). *Code of ethics for nurses with interpretive statements.* Silver Spring, MD: Author.

Association of periOperative Registered Nurses (AORN). (2013). *Registered nurse first assistant.* Retrieved from www.aorn.org/Advocacy/Issues_and_Initiatives/Legislative_Priorities/Registered_Nurse_First_Assistant.aspx.

Association of periOperative Registered Nurses (AORN). (2017). *Perioperative standards and recommended practices.* Denver, CO: Author.

Centers for Disease Control and Prevention (CDC). (2017). Centers for Disease Control and Prevention guideline for prevention of surgical site infection, 2017. *JAMA Surgery, 152*(8), 784–791. Retrieved from https://jamanetwork.com/journals/jamasurgery/fullarticle/2623725.

Copanitsanou, P., Dafogianni, C., & Iraklianou, S. (2016). Perioperative management of adult patients with diabetes mellitus. *International Journal of Caring Sciences, 9*(3), 1167–1176.

Pearson Education. (2018). *Nursing: A concepts-based approach to learning* (3rd ed.). Hoboken, NJ: Author.

Riazi, S., & Brandom, B.W. (2015). Malignant hyperthermia – An update for perioperative nurses. *ORNAC Journal, 33*(4), 16–26.

Scott-Thomas, J., Hayes, C., Ling, J., Fox, A., Boutflower, R., & Grahm, Y. (2017). A practical guide to systematic wound assessment to meet the 2017–2019 CQUIN target. *Journal of Community Nursing, 31*(5), 30–34.

Sorenson, M., Quinn, L., & Klein, D. (2019). *Pathophysiology: Concepts of human disease.* Hoboken, NJ: Pearson Education.

Stone, C. (2017). Procedural sedation and analgesia. In C. Stone & R. L. Humphries (Eds.), *Current diagnosis and treatment: Emergency medicine* (8th ed.). New York, NY: McGraw-Hill;. http://accessmedicine.mhmedical.com.liboff.ohsu.edu/content.aspx?bookid=2172&sectionid=165058258. Accessed May 12, 2018.

World Health Organization. (2009). *WHO's pain ladder.* Geneva: Author.

ADDITIONAL RESOURCES

Association for periOperative Nurses
www.aorn.org

American Society of Perianesthesia Nurses
www.aspan.org

National Patient Safety Goals
www.jointcommission.org/standards_information/npsgs.aspx

Universal Protocol
www.jointcommission.org/assets/1/18/UP_Poster1.PDF

Chapter 5

Palliative and End-of-Life Care

Chapter Outline and Learning Outcomes

CLINICAL COMPETENCIES

- Recognize physiologic changes in the dying patient.
- Use assessments, patient values, and evidence-based practice guidelines to provide nursing interventions that enhance quality of life and promote a comfortable and dignified death for patients and their families.
- Use principles of palliative care to manage pain and other symptoms associated with life-threatening illness and end-of-life needs.
- Communicate effectively with and function within the interprofessional team to plan and provide individualized care for patients and families experiencing loss, grief, and death.
- Integrate individual and cultural values and variations, as well as expressed needs and preferences, into the plan of care for patients and families experiencing loss, grief, and death.
- Identify self-care strategies to use when caring for patients and families experiencing loss, grief, and death.

KEY TERMS

advance directive, 114
aid in dying, 114
assisted suicide, 114
bereavement, 113
death, 106
death anxiety, 120
delirium, 116
do-not-resuscitate order (DNR), 114
durable power of attorney, 114
end of life, 112
euthanasia, 114
grief, 106
grieving, 106
healthcare surrogate, 114
hospice, 113
living will, 114
loss, 105
mourning, 106
palliative care, 111
physician orders for life-sustaining treatment (POLST), 114

Loss may be defined as an actual or potential situation in which a valued object, person, body part, or emotion that was formerly present is lost or changed and can no longer be seen, felt, heard, known, or experienced. A loss may be temporary or permanent, complete or partial, objectively verifiable or perceived, physical or symbolic. Only the individual who experiences the loss can determine the meaning of the loss (**Figure 5.1** ■). Although the order of importance varies with the individual, people most commonly fear the following losses:

- Death
- Health
- Body part
- Social status
- Lifestyle
- Marital relationship
- Reproductive function
- Sexual function.

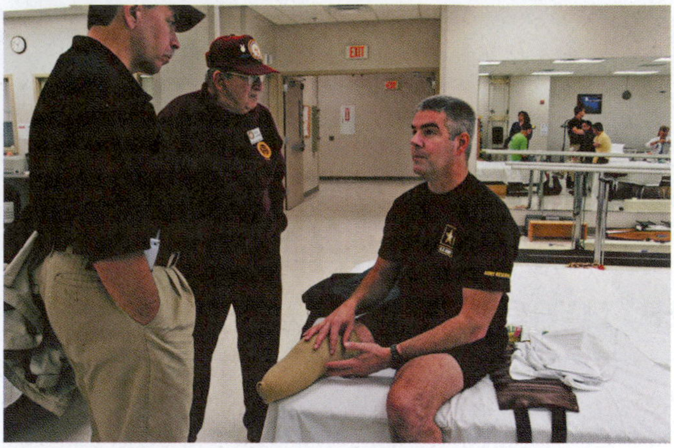

Figure 5.1 ■ Loss of a body part or a functional ability is one of the hazards of serving in combat. Only the individual who experiences the loss can determine the meaning of the loss.

Loss always results in change. The stress associated with the loss may be the precipitating factor leading to physiologic or psychologic change in the individual or family. The effective or ineffective resolution of feelings surrounding the loss determines the individual's ability to deal with the resulting changes. There are many different types of loss, with responses to the loss individualized within each person. This chapter considers loss from both a general and from a specific focus. There is, within the chapter, a greater emphasis on loss from death, as this is often a difficult situation because nurses care for the person who is dying and for the people who are left to experience the loss (**Figure 5.2** ■). Some of the terms used throughout the chapter are introduced in the following paragraphs.

Grief is the emotional response to loss and its accompanying changes. Grief as a response to loss is an inevitable dimension of the human experience. The loss of a job, a role (e.g., the loss of the role of spouse, as occurs in divorce), a goal, body integrity, a loved one, or the impending loss of one's own life or a loved one's life may trigger grief. Although death is the ultimate loss, losses that occur in any phase of the life cycle may produce grief responses as intensely painful as those observed in the death experience.

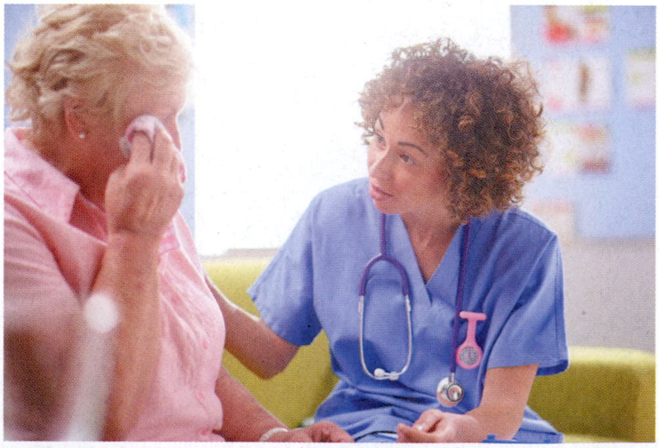

Figure 5.2 ■ A nurse comforts the wife of a dying man as she sits by his bed in the hospital.

Grieving may be thought of as the internal process the individual uses to work through the response to loss. **Mourning** describes the actions or expressions of the bereaved, including the symbols, clothing, and ceremonies that make up the outward manifestations of grief. Both grieving and mourning are healthy responses to loss because they ultimately lead the individual to invest energy in new relationships and to develop positive self-regard.

Death is defined in many ways. One commonly used definition of death is an irreversible cessation of circulatory and respiratory functions or irreversible cessation of all functions of the entire brain, including the brainstem. With the current life-support systems available, the most often used criterion for determining death is whole-brain death (permanent irreversible cessation of the functioning of all areas of the brain). The criteria for whole-brain death are listed in Chapter 11, Nursing Care of Patients Experiencing Trauma and Shock.

Although death is an inevitable part of life, it is often an immensely difficult loss for the person who is dying and for his or her loved ones. Death may be accidental (for example, from trauma); purposeful (from suicide); occur suddenly or at the end of a long and painful struggle with a chronic or terminal illness such as congestive heart failure, cancer, or chronic obstructive pulmonary disease; or be the natural end of the aging process.

5.1 Loss and Grief

Medical-surgical nurses often care for patients exhibiting responses typical of various stages of the grieving process. Highly individual in quality and duration, the grief process may range from discomforting to debilitating, and it may last a day or a lifetime, depending on what the loss means to the person experiencing it.

Theories of Loss, Grief, and Dying

Although each person experiences loss in a different manner, knowledge of some of the major theories of loss, grief, and dying can give the nurse a framework for holistic care of the patient and family anticipating or experiencing a loss.

Freud: Psychoanalytic Theory

Sigmund Freud (1917, 1957) wrote about grief and mourning as reactions to loss. Freud described the process of mourning as one in which the individual gradually withdraws attachment from the lost object or person. He observed that with normal grieving, this withdrawal of attachment is followed by a readiness to make new attachments. In comparing melancholia (prolonged gloominess, depression) with the normal emotions of grief and its expression in mourning, Freud observed that the "work of mourning" is a nonpathologic condition that reaches a state of completion after a period of inner labor.

Bowlby: Attachment Theory

John Bowlby (1973, 1980) believed that the grieving process initiated by a loss or separation from a loved object or person successfully ends when the grieving person experiences feelings of emancipation from the lost object or person. He divided the grieving process into three phases and identified behaviors characteristic of each phase:

- *Protest.* The protest phase is marked by a lack of acceptance of the loss. All energy is directed toward protesting the loss. The person experiences feelings of anger toward self and others, and feelings of ambivalence toward the lost object or person. Crying and angry behaviors characterize this phase.
- *Despair.* The person's behavior becomes disorganized. Despair mounts as efforts to deny the loss compete with acceptance of permanent loss. Crying and sadness, coupled with a desire for the lost object or person to return, result in disorganized thoughts as the patient recognizes the reality of the loss.
- *Detachment.* As the person realizes the permanence of the loss and gradually relinquishes attachment to the lost object, a reinvestment of energy occurs. Both the positive and negative aspects of the relationship are remembered. Expressions of hopefulness and readiness to move forward are characteristic of this phase.

Bowlby's theory was used as a base for a "continuing bonds" theory, developed by Field, Gao, and Paderna (2005). This theory poses the belief that mourners of loved ones lost by death continue to have memories of the deceased, feel their presence, and save meaningful belongings. These actions bring comfort to the bereaved and allow a new relationship to form with those lost by death. As a result, the mourners resolve their grief and accept the loss.

Engel: Acute Grief, Restitution, and Long-Term Grief

George Engel (1964) related the grief process to other methods of coping with stress: After the individual perceives and evaluates the loss (the stressful event), the individual adapts to it. Engel's recognition of the effect of cognitive factors on the grieving process was an important contribution to the understanding of grieving. The acute stage is initiated by shock and disbelief and may be manifested by denial, which in turn may help the individual to cope with the overwhelming pain. As the shock and disbelief begin to fade, the loss becomes a reality, and pain, anguish, anger, guilt, and blame surface. Culturally patterned behaviors, such as maintaining a stoic pose in public or weeping openly, characterize this phase. During restitution friends and family gather to support the grieving person through rituals dictated by their culture. The mourner continues to feel a painful void and is preoccupied with thoughts of the loss. The mourner may join a support group or seek other social support for coping with the loss. This stage lasts about 1 year, after which the mourner begins to come to terms with the loss and interests in people and activities are renewed.

Lindemann: Categories of Symptoms

Erich Lindemann (1944) interviewed people who had lost a loved one during the course of medical treatment, disaster victims, and relatives of members of the armed forces who had died. Lindemann's research led him to describe normal grief, anticipatory grieving, and morbid grief reactions. He placed symptoms characteristic of normal grief into categories of somatic (physical symptoms without an organic cause) distress, preoccupation with the image of the deceased, feelings of guilt, hostile reactions, and loss of patterns of conduct.

Anticipatory grieving was defined as a cluster of predictable responses to an anticipated loss. These responses include the range of feelings experienced by the individual or family preoccupied with an anticipated loss. The term *morbid grief reaction* described delayed and dysfunctional reactions to loss; a variety of debilitating health problems were seen in people who displayed excessive or delayed responses to loss.

Caplan: Stress and Loss

Gerald Caplan's (1990) theory of stress and its relationship to loss is useful in understanding the grief process. He expanded the focus of the grief process to include not only bereavement but also other episodes of stress that people experience, such as may result from surgery or childbirth. Caplan described three factors that influence the person's ability to deal with a loss. He believed these factors might cause distress for a year or more following the loss:

- The psychic pain of the broken bond and the agony of coming to terms with the loss
- Living without the assets and guidance of the lost person or resource
- The reduced cognitive and problem-solving effectiveness associated with the distressing emotional arousal.

Caplan described the process of building new attachments to replace those that have been lost as involving two elements: A feeling of hope and the assumption of regular activity as a form of participating in ordinary living.

Kübler-Ross: Stages of Coping with Loss

Elisabeth Kübler-Ross's (1969, 1978) research on death and dying provided a framework for gaining insight about the stages of coping with an impending or actual loss. According to Kübler-Ross, not all people dealing with a loss go through these stages, and those who do may not experience the stages in the sequence described. In identifying the stages of death and dying, Kübler-Ross stressed the danger of prematurely labeling a stage and emphasized that her goal was to describe her observations of how people come to terms with situations of loss.

Some or all of the following reactions may occur during the grieving process and may reappear as the person experiences the loss:

- *Denial.* A person may react with shock and disbelief after receiving word of an actual or potential loss. After receiving a terminal diagnosis, notification of a death, or other serious loss, people may make such statements as "This can't be happening to me" or "This can't be true."
- *Anger.* In the anger stage, the person resists the loss. The anger is often directed toward family and healthcare providers.
- *Bargaining.* The bargaining stage serves as an attempt to postpone the reality of the loss. The person makes a secret bargain with their god, expressing a willingness to do anything to postpone the loss or change the prognosis.
- *Depression.* The person enters a stage of depression as the full impact of the actual or perceived loss is realized. The person prepares for the impending loss by working through the struggle of separation. While grieving over "what cannot be," the person may either talk freely about the loss or withdraw from others.
- *Acceptance.* The person begins to come to terms with the loss and resumes activities with hopefulness for the future. Some dying people reach a stage of acceptance in which they may appear to be almost devoid of emotion. The struggle is past, and the emotional pain is gone.

Factors Affecting Responses to Loss

A variety of factors affect an individual's responses to loss. These include age, social support, families, culture and spiritual practices, and rituals of mourning.

Age

The understanding of and reaction to loss is influenced by the age of the person experiencing the loss. In general, as people experience life transitions, their ability to understand and accept the losses associated with the transitions increases. From the age of 3 years, the development of the concept of death as a loss proceeds rapidly. **Table 5.1** outlines the development of the concept of death throughout the lifespan.

Social Support

Grieving is painful and lonely. An individual's social support system is significant because of its potentially positive influence on the successful resolution of grief. Some losses may lead to social isolation, placing affected people at high risk for dysfunctional grief reactions. For example, partners of people who die with AIDS often report feeling excluded by the deceased person's family and by healthcare providers. Characteristic factors that can interfere with successful grieving include:

- Perceived inability to share the loss
- Lack of social recognition of the loss

Table 5.1 Development of the Concept of Death

Age	Beliefs/Attitudes About Death
3 years	■ Fears separation. ■ Lacks comprehension of permanent separation.
4–5 years	■ Believes death is like sleeping and is reversible. ■ Expresses curiosity about what happens to the body.
6–10 years	■ Understands finality of death. ■ Views own death as avoidable. ■ Associates death with violence. ■ Believes wishes can be responsible for death.
11–12 years	■ Reflects views of death expressed by parents. ■ Expresses interest in afterlife as an understanding of mortality develops. ■ Recognizes death as irreversible and inevitable.
13–21 years	■ Usually has a religious and philosophic view of death but seldom thinks about it. ■ Views own death as distant or a challenge, acting out defiance through reckless behavior. ■ Previously held developmental awareness of death may still be present.
22–45 years	■ Does not think about death unless confronted with it. ■ Emotionally distances self from death. ■ Attitude toward death influenced by religious and cultural beliefs.
46–65 years	■ Experiences the death of parents or friends. ■ Accepts own mortality. ■ Experiences waves of death anxiety. ■ Puts life in order to prepare for death and decrease anxiety.
66 years and older	■ Fears lingering, incapacitating illness. ■ Views death as inevitable but from a philosophical viewpoint, that is, as freedom from pain and illness or as a spiritual reunion with deceased friends and loved ones.

- Ambivalent relationships prior to the loss
- Traumatic circumstances of the loss.

A change in residence, a divorce, or even the death of a pet can cause an individual to feel extremely isolated, yet the person experiencing these types of loss does not ordinarily receive the same social support offered to the person mourning the death of a loved one. A woman having an abortion or giving up a child for adoption seldom receives the same social support as the mother of a child who died at birth. It is therefore especially important for nurses not to place a value on any patient's loss when assessing the need for support.

The painful nature of grief can cause the patient to withdraw from a previously established social support system, thereby increasing the feelings of loneliness caused by the loss. A recently widowed woman, for example, may refuse invitations involving married couples with whom she had socialized while her husband was alive, even though her needs for social interaction remain similar to those established before the loss.

Family

A well-functioning family usually rallies after the initial shock and disbelief and provides support for each other during all phases of the grieving process. After a loss, the functional family is able to shift roles, levels of responsibility, and ways of communicating.

The patient and family members are considered the unit of care when providing end-of-life care in any setting. Care that addresses the needs of both patient and family is complex. The family may have negative as well as positive effects on the patient. For example, the dying patient may request that someone the family perceives as an outsider be near, and the family may respond with anger to the perceived intrusion. Similarly, certain family members may express hurt feelings or anger if the patient is unresponsive to other family members. Well-meaning family members may also try to shield the patient from the pain of grieving. It is rare for the family and the patient to experience anger, denial, and acceptance in unison. While one member is in denial, another may be angry because "not enough is being done."

Culture and Spiritual Practices

The influence of culture and ethnic identity on communication, family values, and beliefs about and practices related to illness and death are important considerations when providing nursing care. There are countless ethnocultural and religious differences in the way people observe dying, death, and mourning. For example, differences in the way death is expressed in the United States include "passed away," "died peacefully," "departed this life," "went home to be with God," and "passed from this life." Objects such as masks, statues, and candles may be expressions of death and death rituals. Examples of religious traditions in mourning and end-of-life rituals include:

- ***Buddhism:*** Because Buddhist funeral customs vary by region or schools, nurses should consult with the patient or family and encourage communication with the patient's spiritual advisor. Nurses and other healthcare staff can support the Buddhist patient by reducing environmental stimuli, as death should take place in a peaceful atmosphere. Buddhists may wish to have a teacher or spiritual advisor with them during and in the period immediately following death. Because of this, they may ask for the body not to be touched or removed for several hours following death (The Buddhist Society, 2018).
- ***Catholicism:*** The patient or the family may request a priest to give Last Rites, special prayers offered for those who are dying. Autopsy and organ donation are at the discretion of the patient and family.
- ***Hinduism:*** According to Hindu belief, death is part of the process of spiritual evolution and leads to the next life or existence. Family members may be reluctant to disclose the severity of an illness or impending death, for fear that their loved one will lose hope. Following death, the body is prepared for cremation by performing ritual cleansing and dressing the deceased in new clothes.
- ***Islam:*** Families may refuse autopsy unless for the purpose of forensic or medical science. Organ donation and transplantation are acceptable. Use of advance directives is appropriate. If the patient is in serious condition, communicate bad news gradually with the help of a family elder or spokesperson. After death, the body is washed only by Muslims of the same gender.
- ***Judaism:*** Life-extending measures and euthanasia may be forbidden depending on the type of Judaism practiced. Autopsy is generally prohibited unless it is legally required (forensic) or it can save the life of another through organ donation. The body is ritually washed and burial occurs as soon as possible. There is a 7-day mourning period.
- ***Protestantism:*** Prolonging of life may have restrictions. Organ donation, autopsy, burial, and cremation are individual decisions.

The extent to which individuals and families follow religious traditions related to mourning and end-of-life issues varies greatly. Careful and tactful assessment will help the nurse understand how best to support patients who are dying and their families.

Spiritual Beliefs

Patients who are dying often ask questions of themselves and others as to what their life has meant, why this illness has affected them, and what will happen to them when they die. They may feel abandoned by God or worry that their behavior caused the illness resulting in death. These questions and concerns lead to spiritual distress, which if unresolved may lead to hopelessness, anxiety, and depression.

When spiritual distress is resolved, the patient can die more peacefully.

The principles, values, personal philosophy, and meaning of life by which the patient has pursued goals and self-actualization may be called into question when the patient responds to an actual or perceived loss. Because of a fear of intruding on the personal spiritual beliefs and practices of the patient, the nurse often feels uncertain about implementing interventions that would be helpful to the patient responding to a loss. The following questions using the mnemonic device **FICA©** may be used to assess a patient's spiritual or religious practices (George Washington Institute for Spirituality and Health, 2018):

Faith: What is your faith or belief? Do you consider yourself a spiritual or a religious person? Does religious faith or spirituality play an important part in your life? What do you believe gives your life meaning?

Influence: How does your religious faith or spirituality influence your thoughts about health? How does it affect the way that you take care of yourself?

Community: Do you consider yourself part of a spiritual or religious community or congregation? How is that community or congregation a source of support for you?

Address: Do you have any special religious or spiritual issues or concerns that you would like me to address with you? Is there someone else you would like to speak to about these matters?

It is often difficult for patients with an incurable illness to maintain hope and a sense that their lives have had meaning. To meet spiritual needs, nurses can help patients accept the uncertainty that comes with their illness and future death and respect the spiritual beliefs and practices of patients and their families. Patients who are religious need opportunities for prayer, devotions, and religious rituals. Other resources for spirituality include meditation, guided imagery, music, and art. Privacy and space for these activities should be provided without question.

Rituals of Mourning

Through participation in religious ceremonies such as baptism, confirmation, and bat or bar mitzvah, people joyously celebrate progression to a new stage of life and loss of a former way of being. The funeral ceremony serves many of the same purposes in meeting the needs of the bereaved as people gather to share loss. Through the ceremony, people symbolically express triumph over death and deny the fear of death. Culture is the primary factor that dictates the rituals of mourning (**Figure 5.3** ■). See the accompanying Focus on Cultural Diversity feature, which provides examples of values and rituals for death in selected groups of people.

Nurses' Response to Patients' Loss

Nurses care for patients and families at various stages of the grief process and may feel that crisis situations are not the time for self-reflection. However, because the nurse's conscious or unconscious reactions to the patient's responses to the loss will influence the outcome of any intervention, nurses need to take time to analyze their own feelings and values related to loss and the expression of grief. The nurse can promote self-awareness by reflecting on the following questions:

- What are my personal feelings about how grief should be expressed?
- Am I making judgments about the meaning of this loss to the patient?
- Are unresolved losses in my own life preventing me from relating therapeutically to the patient?

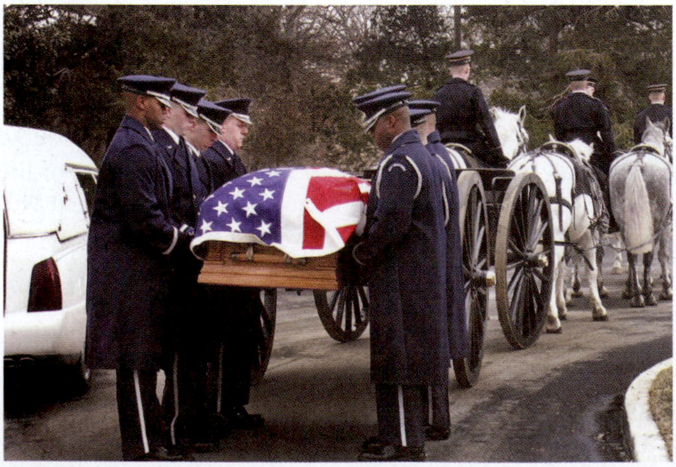

A

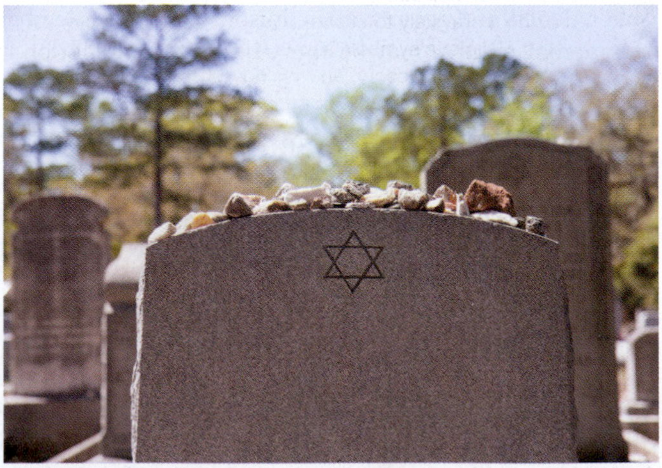

B

Figure 5.3 ■ Funeral, burial, and mourning customs vary widely. Examples shown here include: **A**, A military funeral with full honors at Arlington Cemetery, and **B**, a Jewish gravestone with memory stones left by mourners.

Focus on Cultural Diversity

Cultural and Ethnic Aspects of Terminal Illness Care

The extent to which individuals and families follow traditional cultural beliefs related to end-of-life care and mourning varies greatly. Careful and tactful assessment will help the nurse understand how best to support patients who are dying and their families. Examples of cultural/ethnic beliefs and practices include:

- ***Native American:*** Beliefs, practices, and rituals related to dying vary by tribe and depend on individual and familial circumstances. For example, traditional Navajos may refuse to touch the body both out of respect and out of a traditional fear of contamination. Family and close friends may be reluctant to discuss death and dying out of respect for the patient, but still may seek hospital care for a loved one with terminal illness (Giger, 2017).
- ***African American:*** Assess patient and family need to talk with an elder, minister, or other faith leader. Some patients and families may lean on faith leaders and family more than on healthcare professionals for care of those who are terminally ill (Giger, 2017).
- ***Chinese American:*** Ensure the head of the family is present when terminal illness is discussed. The patient may not want to discuss approaching death. Reluctance to speak about death may or may not be associated with a traditional Chinese taboo that views speaking of death as likely to bring bad luck to the family (Giger, 2017). Dying at home is likely to be viewed as more desirable than dying in a facility, as hospitals and other institutional settings are viewed as isolative (Spector, 2017).
- ***Iranian:*** Information about a terminal illness should be presented by a trusted member of the healthcare team to the family and never to the patient when he or she is alone. Decisions about life-saving measures are often made by the family. When death occurs, notify the family immediately. If the patient is Muslim, a Muslim family member of the same sex may need to bathe the body soon after death (Purnell, 2014).
- ***Mexican American:*** Many Mexican Americans have strong family ties. Religion (often Roman Catholicism) and faith play an important role in the life of many Mexican American families. Therefore, spiritual care may be a necessary component when caring for patients who are terminally ill. Because of their strong sense of family, Mexican Americans may be more likely to choose to be cared for and to die at home. Religious symbols and practices, such as iconography, saying the Rosary, and reciting specific prayers may be important (Giger, 2017; Spector, 2017).
- ***Vietnamese:*** No single religion is practiced by the Vietnamese people. Families may struggle with the decision to terminate life-saving measures already in place, as doing so may be considered taking a role in the patient's death. Provide factual information to the family and support during the decision-making process (Purnell, 2014). Patients often prefer to die at home. Spiritual/religious rites are often conducted in the room.

5.2 Palliative Care

Palliative care is an area of care that has evolved out of the hospice experience, but exists outside of hospice programs, is not restricted to the end of life, and is used earlier in the disease experience (**Figure 5.4** ■). The World Health Organization (WHO) defines palliative care as an approach to patient care that improves the quality of life of patients and their families who are facing problems associated with life-threatening illness. This is done through the prevention and relief of suffering by means of early identification, assessment, and treatment of pain and other physical, psychosocial, and spiritual problems (WHO, 2018). The American Nurses Association (ANA; 2016) supports the vision of the WHO with the position that nurses are obligated to provide comprehensive, compassionate, end-of-life care to their patients and families. Nurses and other healthcare providers have a responsibility to establish decision-making processes that reflect physiologic realities, patient preferences, and the recognition of what, clinically, may or may not be accomplished. Establishing goals of care for *this* patient at *this* time may provide a framework for discussion about what care should be provided. This process often involves collaboration with experts in decision making, such as ethics committees or palliative care teams. Palliative care can be used in all types of healthcare settings and is focused on the relief of physical, mental, and spiritual distress for individuals who have an incurable illness. The goal of palliative care is to prevent and relieve suffering by early assessment and treatment of pain and other physical, psychosocial, and spiritual needs to improve the patient's quality of life.

It has evolved into a specialized medical field and aims to relieve symptoms such as pain, nausea, respiratory distress, anxiety, agitation, delirium, and stress. The palliative care team provides symptom management related to serious chronic illness such as cancer, chronic obstructive pulmonary disease, congestive heart failure, kidney failure, Alzheimer disease, and dementia.

Although palliative care may be provided by a single person, it usually involves the combined efforts of an interprofessional team, including physicians, nurses, social workers, chaplains, home health aides, and volunteers. Care is provided at any stage of serious illness and the plan of care is continuous, following the patient between settings. Palliative care is the focus of end-of-life care. The expected outcomes of care are directed by interventions to manage current manifestations of the illness and to prevent new manifestations from occurring.

The Patient in Palliative Care

The patient receiving palliative care can receive this care in a variety of settings. These may include hospitals, skilled nursing centers, or at home. There are new and emerging outpatient practices specializing in palliative care. Some larger institutions have palliative care centers to promote the comprehensive nature of palliative care.

Interprofessional Care

Imperative to providing comprehensive palliative care to a patient is the concept of interdisciplinary collaboration. This is an approach to patient care that is based on communication and cooperation among the various disciplines on a health care team. Each discipline has a unique role on the healthcare team, providing a specific skill set, which

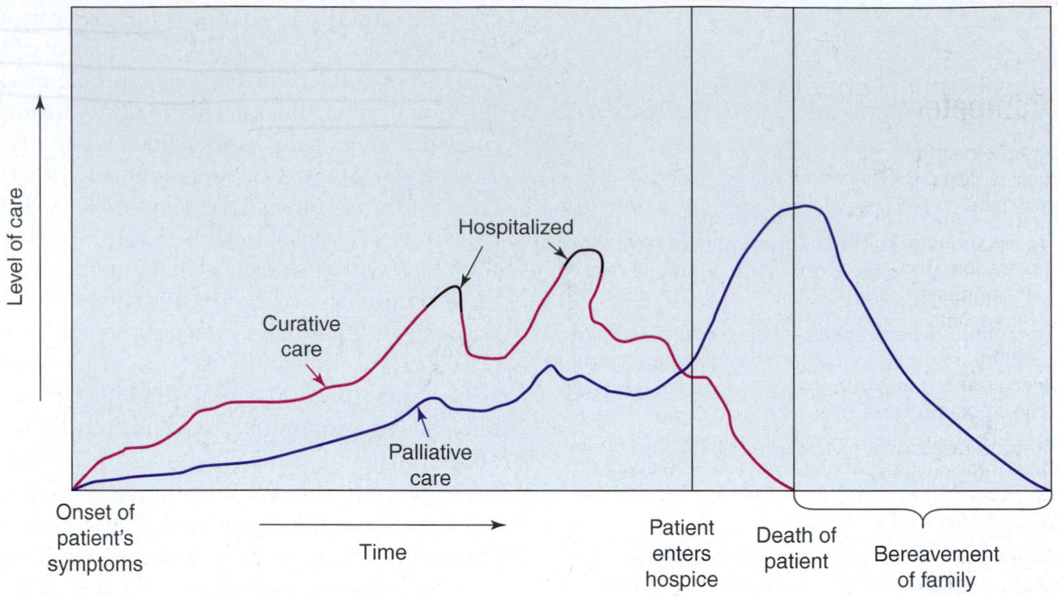
Level of care
Hospitalized
Curative care
Palliative care
Onset of patient's symptoms
Time
Patient enters hospice
Death of patient
Bereavement of family

Figure 5.4 ■ Integrated model of palliative care. Palliative care for individuals with a chronic life-threatening illness should begin with the onset of symptoms and take place concurrently with curative care. The levels of curative and palliative care vary over time depending on the patient's needs. When curative care is no longer effective or its burden on the patient outweighs its benefit, the focus shifts to mainly palliative care. The palliative care team continues to support the patient's family through the bereavement period after the death of their loved one.

contributes to a comprehensive, integrated plan of care. This is in contrast to what is the common practice of multidisciplinary care, which has multiple specialties providing care to the same patient, with multiple plans of care, which are often in contrast to each other and confusing to the patient (Dudley, Wallhagen, Ritchie, & Rehm, 2016).

Nursing Care

The professional nurse's role in providing palliative care for a patient is to support and enact the comprehensive, interdisciplinary plan of care. This care can come in the form of meeting physical, spiritual, or psychosocial needs of the patients. All steps of the nursing process, from assessment through intervention, will be used in the palliative care setting.

Assessment

Nurses are often the direct care providers to patients in a palliative care setting. Assessment is an important role for the nurse. Assessment can include the physical needs of the patient such as performing vital signs, skin assessment, and collecting data on the various body systems. In addition, the nurse will assess a patient's functional status, social support, cultural needs, spiritual strengths, and practices as well as psychological well-being. Documentation and communication of these findings to the other members of the health care team is an essential nursing function (National Consensus Project for Quality Palliative Care, 2013).

Priorities of Care

The priority of care for a patient in a palliative care setting should reflect goals set by the patient and family. These goals and priorities will change over time as the disease process evolves. The priorities of care are based on regular comprehensive evaluation of the patient (Agency for Healthcare Research and Quality [AHRQ], 2013).

Diagnoses, Outcomes, and Interventions

With the patient in palliative care, nursing care focuses on the concepts of pain control, prevention and management of complications from the primary disease process, maintaining quality of life, and assisting the patient and family in planning for end-of-life care (Carpenita, 2014).

Transitions of Care

Palliative care provides management of disease symptoms, family and patient psychosocial support, and the facilitation of a patient-centered, comprehensive plan of care. These patients face complex medical decisions. One of the most critical decisions is when to transition from palliative care to hospice or end-of-life care. At some point in the patient's care, there will be a critical change in condition, which will necessitate the decision to move from palliative care to hospice care. The nurse plays an important role in transitions of care, providing the communication and documentation necessary for patient understanding and palliative care team involvement (AHRQ, 2016).

5.3 End-of-Life Care

The term *end of life* refers to the final weeks of life when death is imminent. End-of-life nursing care that ensures a peaceful death was mandated by the International Council of Nurses in 1997 and further supported by the American Association of Colleges of Nursing (AACN) in 1999. **Box 5.1** outlines the competencies necessary for nurses to provide high-quality end-of-life care as defined by the AACN (2017).

BOX 5.1
Nursing Competencies for End-of-Life Care

1. Promote the need for palliative care for seriously ill patients and their families, from the time of diagnosis, as essential to quality care and an integral component of nursing care.
2. Identify the dynamic changes in population demographics, healthcare economics, service delivery, caregiving demands, and financial impact of serious illness on the patient and family that necessitate improved professional preparation for palliative care.
3. Recognize one's own ethical, cultural, and spiritual values and beliefs about serious illness and death.
4. Demonstrate respect for cultural, spiritual, and other forms of diversity for patients and their families in the provision of palliative care services.
5. Educate and communicate effectively and compassionately with the patient, family, health care team members, and the public about palliative care issues.
6. Collaborate with members of the interprofessional team to improve palliative care for patients with serious illness, to enhance the experience and outcomes from palliative care for patients and their families, and to ensure coordinated and efficient palliative care for the benefit of communities.
7. Elicit and demonstrate respect for the patient and family values, preferences, goals of care, and shared decision making during serious illness and at end of life.
8. Apply ethical principles in the care of patients with serious illness and their families.
9. Know, apply, and effectively communicate current state and federal legal guidelines relevant to the care of patients with serious illness and their families.
10. Perform a comprehensive assessment of pain and symptoms common in serious illness, using valid, standardized assessment tools and strong interviewing and clinical examination skills.
11. Analyze and communicate with the interprofessional team in planning and intervening in pain and symptom management, using evidence-based pharmacologic and nonpharmacologic approaches.
12. Assess, plan, and treat patients' physical, psychological, social, and spiritual needs to improve quality of life for patients with serious illness and their families.
13. Evaluate patient and family outcomes from palliative care within the context of patient goals of care, national quality standards, and value.
14. Provide competent, compassionate, and culturally sensitive care for patients and their families at the time of diagnosis of a serious illness through the end of life.
15. Implement self-care strategies to support coping with suffering, loss, moral distress, and compassion fatigue.
16. Assist the patient, family, informal caregivers, and professional colleagues to cope with and build resilience for dealing with suffering, grief, loss, and bereavement associated with serious illness.
17. Recognize the need to seek consultation (i.e., from advanced practice nursing specialists, specialty palliative care teams, ethics consultants, etc.) for complex patient and family needs.

Source: AACN, 2017, pp. 2–3.

Nurses care for the dying patient in critical care units, emergency departments, hospital units, long-term care facilities, and the home. Regardless of the setting, the patient's wishes about death should be respected. The Dying Person's Bill of Rights states that each person has "the right to be cared for by caring, sensitive, knowledgeable people who will attempt to understand my needs and will be able to gain some satisfaction in helping me face my death" (Barbus, 1975).

Settings and services for end-of-life care range from the critical care unit in a hospital to the patient's own home. Two methods of providing end-of-life care—hospice and palliative care—are described in this section.

Hospice

Hospice is a philosophy of care rather than a program of care. It is comprehensive and coordinated care for patients with limited life expectancy that reaffirms the right of every patient and family to fully participate in the final stages of life. Provided by hospice agency nurses and other members of a healthcare team (including social workers, clergy, home health aides, and volunteers), it is based on a philosophy of death with comfort and dignity, encompassing biomedical, psychosocial, and spiritual aspects of the dying experience. Although most hospice care is provided in the home, it may also be provided in hospitals, long-term care facilities, or other community-based settings.

There are more than 4000 hospice agencies in the United States, with services and care reimbursed by private insurance or a Medicare hospice benefit (Centers for Disease Control and Prevention, 2016). Services are reimbursed by Medicare for an initial 90-day period, followed by a subsequent 90-day period, and an unlimited number of 60-day periods as long as the patient continues to meet eligibility requirements (U.S. Centers for Medicare and Medicaid Services [CMS], 2018). The average length of service is 71 days, with 98% of the hospice care being provided was at the routine home care level (Hospice Association of America, 2018). Hospice services usually begin when the patient has 6 months or less to live and ends with the family 1 year after the death of the patient. This continuation of care for the family is called *bereavement care* (**bereavement** is the time of mourning experienced after a loss).

To be eligible for hospice benefits from Medicare or Medicaid, the patient must have a serious, progressive illness with a limited life expectancy. In most cases, a family (or other) caregiver must be continuously in the home with the patient. The patient must have Medicare, waive traditional Medicare benefits for the terminal illness, have physician certification of a terminal illness with a life expectancy of 6 months or less, and care must be provided by a Medicare-certified hospice agency or program. Hospice care under Medicare includes home care, inpatient care when needed, and a variety of services not otherwise covered by Medicare (CMS, 2018). The focus is on care, not cure.

Legal and Ethical Issues

Issues such as those involved in advance directives and living wills, euthanasia, and quality of life are especially important to nurses in upholding the specific care requests of their patients.

Advance Directives

Advance directives are legal documents, such as Five Wishes (*https://www.agingwithdignity.org/*), that allow an individual to plan for healthcare and/or financial affairs in the event of incapacity. They include living wills, healthcare surrogates, durable powers of attorney, and physician orders:

- **Living will**: A document that provides written directions about life-prolonging procedures to provide instructions when an individual can no longer communicate in a life-threatening situation.
- **Healthcare surrogate**: An individual selected to make medical decisions when an individual is no longer able to make them for him- or herself.
- **Durable power of attorney**: A document that can delegate the authority to make health, financial, and/or legal decisions on an individual's behalf. It must be in writing and must state that the designated person is authorized to make healthcare decisions.
- **Physician orders for life-sustaining treatment (POLST)**: A form for patients with serious, progressive, chronic illnesses that translates their wishes regarding life-sustaining treatment into actionable medical orders.

A living will is a legal document that formally expresses an individual's wishes regarding life-sustaining treatment in the event of terminal illness or permanent unconsciousness. It is not a type of durable power of attorney and usually does not designate a substitute decision maker. It is the responsibility of the nurse as an advocate to request and record the patient's preference for care and include it in the plan of care. The nurse's documentation helps communicate these preferences to the other members of the healthcare team.

Facilities that receive Medicare and Medicaid funds are required to provide all patients with written information and counseling about advance directives and the institution's policies governing them. The specific terms of this requirement are found in the Patient Self-Determination Act (PSDA). A copy of the signed advance directive must be kept in the patient's medical record, but patients do not have to sign it in order to be treated. Nurses are the healthcare providers in close contact with patients, so they often support patients and families with unresolved feelings about the moral, ethical, and legal aspects of their actions. Although advance directives do not ease the pain of seeing patients die, they do help facilitate patient-centered care by providing guidance so nurses can implement patient preferences for end-of-life care.

Do-Not-Resuscitate Orders

A **do-not-resuscitate order (DNR)**, or no-code, is written by the physician for the patient who has a terminal illness or is near death. This order is based on the wishes of the patient and family that no cardiopulmonary resuscitation be performed for respiratory or cardiac arrest. A "comfort measures only" order indicates that no further life-sustaining interventions are necessary and that the goal of care is a comfortable, dignified death. Agency protocols should be established defining comfort care for consistency in nursing care. Confusing or conflicting DNR orders create dilemmas because nurses are involved in resuscitation and either begin CPR or ensure that unwanted attempts do not occur. The American Nurses Association (ANA; 2012) recommends that the DNR order should be directed by what the informed patient wants or wanted. The ANA further recommends that guidelines and policies be developed to help resolve conflicts between patients and their families, between patients and healthcare professionals, and among healthcare professionals.

Euthanasia, Assisted Suicide, and Aid in Dying

Euthanasia (from the Greek for "painless," "easy," "gentle," or "good death") is the practice of intentionally ending a life to relieve pain and suffering. Many arguments are made for and against euthanasia, and nurses have often found themselves at the center of the debate. The ANA position statement titled *Euthanasia, Assisted Suicide, and Aid in Dying* (2013) opposes nurse participation in euthanasia and emphasizes the obligation of the nurse to provide compassionate end-of-life care aimed at promoting comfort, alleviating suffering, providing adequate pain control, and at times forgoing the provision of life-sustaining treatment. Additionally, nurses have pushed for the development of appropriate guidelines and procedures for DNR orders. When no such orders exist, the nurse faces a dilemma. Certainly, there are situations in which the nurse's role is clear. For example, it is considered malpractice to participate in slow codes (in which the nurse does not hurry to alert the emergency team when a terminally ill patient who does not have a DNR order stops breathing).

In **assisted suicide**, the means to end the patient's life is provided to the patient with knowledge of the patient's intention. In assisted suicide someone makes the means of death accessible but does not act as the direct agent of death. **Aid in dying** is an end-of-life care option in which mentally competent, terminally ill adults can ask their physician to provide a prescription for medication that the patient can self-administer to end life peacefully (ANA, 2013). Nurses should be aware of state laws governing this practice and be familiar with the laws and professional position statements regarding this practice in the state in which they are licensed. Because care settings offer many complex and technologic interventions, it is not likely that the ethical aspects of euthanasia, assisted suicide, and aid in dying will soon be resolved. However, advance directives do give patients a much more active role in decisions about their own care.

Physiologic Changes in the Dying Patient

Death is a highly individualized process and may occur rapidly or slowly. Physiologic changes are a part of the dying process. Although each person responds differently, certain manifestations are common in the dying process, regardless of the trauma or disease process that is causing death. These include:

- Difficulty talking or swallowing
- Nausea, flatus, abdominal distention
- Urinary and/or bowel incontinence, constipation
- Decreased sensation, taste, and smell
- Weak, slow, and/or irregular pulse
- Decreasing blood pressure
- Decreased, irregular, or Cheyne-Stokes respirations
- Changes in level of consciousness
- Restlessness, agitation
- Coolness, mottling, and cyanosis of the extremities.

The discussion that follows includes treatments and related nursing care.

Pain

Pain is a common problem for patients at the end of life, and what people often say they fear the most. Pain, a subjective experience, is influenced by the patient's emotions, previous experiences with pain, and family and culture (Sorenson, Quinn, & Klein, 2019). Unfortunately, pain is sometimes undertreated at the end of life because patients, families, physicians, and nurses fear that the high doses of opioids necessary to control pain will cause addiction or other harm. However, nearly all pain at the end of life can be managed without causing addiction or hastening death through respiratory depression. There is no maximum allowable dose for full agonist opioids such as morphine sulfate; the dose should be increased to whatever is necessary to relieve pain. It is of utmost importance to keep the patient comfortable by providing general comfort measures (**Box 5.2**) and by administering ordered medications for pain, neuropathic pain (which is rarely relieved by opioids), seizures, and/or anxiety. The pathophysiology, treatment, and nursing care of patients experiencing pain are fully described in Chapter 9, Nursing Care of Patients in Pain.

Dyspnea

Respiratory changes, including dyspnea, are normal as death nears. Dyspnea is a subjective experience, and the patient often reports having a feeling of suffocation, shortness of breath, or tightness in the chest. Up to 50% of dying patients have severe dyspnea, especially those with lung tumors (primary or metastatic), restrictive lung disease, or pleural effusion (Sorenson et al., 2019). Regardless of the terminal illness or fatal injury, the final cause of death is a lack of oxygen to the brain.

Morphine is the medication of choice for palliative treatment of dyspnea. It may be necessary to gently instruct the family that the patient is dying and will stop breathing as a result of the disease, not the morphine.

As death nears, respirations often become fast or slow, shallow, and labored. The patient may have apnea or Cheyne-Stokes respirations (regular periods of deep, rapid breathing followed by no breaths for 5 to 30 seconds). Fluid may accumulate in the lungs, causing crackles, especially in patients who are well hydrated and in those who are having difficulty swallowing or coughing. These sounds are not painful for the patient, but they may be treated with oxygen, opioids (to improve respirations and decrease anxiety), and medications to decrease secretions (atropine, scopolamine, hyoscyamine, or glycopyrrolate). Note that oxygen and suctioning are only temporary measures and (especially with suctioning) may even be traumatic for the patient. Nursing care to improve respirations include keeping the head of the bed elevated. Keeping the room cool and providing a breeze from a fan often makes the patient more comfortable.

> **BOX 5.2**
> **Providing Comfort for the Patient Nearing Death**
>
> - Maintain clean skin and bed linens.
> - Use a draw sheet to turn the patient as often as possible so the patient is comfortable.
> - Position the patient to promote comfort and protect bony areas with padding. Reposition the patient and raise the head of the bed if fluids accumulate in the upper airways and back of the throat.
> - Use bed pads or insert a Foley catheter (if ordered) for urinary incontinence.
> - Use gentle massage to improve circulation and shift edema.
> - Provide small, frequent sips of fluids, ice chips, or Popsicles.
> - Provide oral care, using a soft, moist brush.
> - Clean secretions from the eyes and nose.
> - Administer ordered pain medications as needed to maintain comfort.
> - Administer oxygen as prescribed to relieve dyspnea.

Anorexia, Nausea, and Dehydration

Although anorexia and a decrease in food and fluid intake are normal in the dying patient, the family often views this as giving up (Sorenson et al., 2019). Anorexia may be a protective mechanism; the breakdown of body fats results in ketosis, which leads to a sense of well-being and helps decrease pain. Parenteral or enteral feedings do not improve manifestations or prolong life and may actually cause discomfort. As weakness and difficulty swallowing progress, the gag reflex is decreased and patients are at increased risk for aspiration if oral foods are given.

Nausea, with or without vomiting, is a common problem in dying patients. Nausea and vomiting may be caused by reduced gastric emptying, constipation (a side effect of morphine), bowel obstruction, uremia, or hypercalcemia. If the patient is conscious and complains of nausea, antiemetics such as prochlorperazine (Compazine) or ondansetron (Zofran) should be administered (Adams, Holland, & Urban, 2017).

Dehydration is less of a problem than overhydration. Forcing fluids or initiating intravenous fluids for hydration may in turn increase fluid in the lungs, peripheral edema, ascites, and vomiting. Dehydration in the patient nearing death primarily causes discomfort from dry mouth and thirst. The patient should be given small sips of water or an atomizer can be used to spray the inside of the mouth. Oral care should be given at least every 2 hours and more often if the patient is breathing through his or her mouth.

Altered Levels of Consciousness

Neurologic dysfunction results from any or all of the following: Decreased cerebral perfusion, hypoxemia, metabolic acidosis, sepsis, an accumulation of toxins from liver and renal failure, the effects of medications, and disease-related factors. These changes may result in decreased level of consciousness, restlessness, or delirium (Sorenson et al., 2019). Patients with terminal **delirium** may be confused, restless, or agitated. Moaning, groaning, and grimacing often accompany the agitation and may be misinterpreted as pain. Level of consciousness often decreases to the point where the patient cannot be aroused. Terminal or agitated delirium can result from a variety of causes including pain, bladder distention and stool impaction, or unfinished business with family members. Although decreased consciousness and agitation are both normal states at the end of life, they are very distressing to the patient's family.

Several tools can be used to assess the underlying cause of delirium. These include the Mini-Mental State Examination, Confusion Assessment Method, Memorial Delirium Assessment Scale, and the Bedside Confusion Scale. Careful assessment will aid in identifying the underlying cause of terminal delirium, which will help determine patient-centered nursing actions (Sorenson et al., 2019).

Medications for treating terminal delirium include low doses of neuroleptics, tranquilizers, or antianxiety medications. A patient near death often has altered cerebral function, so the nurse must stand near the bedside and speak clearly. Hearing is thought to be the last sense a dying patient loses; the nurse should never whisper or engage in conversation with the family as if the patient were not there. Nursing care for the comatose patient is outlined in **Box 5.3**.

Hypotension

As death nears, the cardiac output decreases, as does intravascular blood volume. As a result, blood pressure gradually decreases and the pulse is often rapid and irregular. The extremities are cooler, and cyanosis is present in nail beds, skin, and lips. The skin on the legs and in dependent areas may become mottled in color. Renal perfusion decreases and the kidneys cease to function. Urinary output is scanty.

BOX 5.3
Nursing Care for the Patient in a Coma

- Instill artificial tears if the patient does not blink.
- Keep lights at a low level.
- Keep skin clean and dry.
- Cover the patient with a light blanket.
- Use adult incontinence pads or pants for incontinence.
- Turn every 2 hours and maintain joints in positions of comfort.

Psychosocial Support

As the patient's condition deteriorates, the nurse's knowledge of the patient and family guides the care provided. It may be necessary to provide opportunities for patients to express personal preferences about where they want to die and about funeral and burial arrangements. If the family feels that this is morbid, the nurse explains that it helps patients to keep a sense of control as they approach death.

The patient needs the opportunity to say good-bye to others. The nurse encourages and supports the patient and family as they terminate relationships as a necessary part of the grief process. The nurse acknowledges that termination is painful and, if the patient or family desires, stays with them during this time. Family members are often afraid to be present at the moment of death, yet dying alone is the greatest fear expressed by patients.

Death

The manifestations listed here are seen after death occurs, and they are the basis for pronouncing death. They appear gradually and not in any special order. To confirm death, a physician or other healthcare provider is legally required to pronounce death. The time of death, with any related data, is documented in the patient's chart. Manifestations of death include:

- Absence of respirations, pulse, and heartbeat
- Fixed and dilated pupils; eyes may stay open
- Release of stool and urine
- Waxen color (pallor) as blood settles to dependent areas
- Body temperature drops
- Lack of reflexes
- Flat encephalogram.

The nurse may fear being present at the moment of the patient's death. In fact, Kübler-Ross (1969) noted that the nurse's fear of death frequently interferes with the ability to provide support for the dying patient and family. Thoughts such as "Please, God, don't let him die on my shift" are common, and they express the nurse's emotional turmoil in dealing with the task. Nurses who have worked through their own feelings about death and dying are more at ease in assisting the dying patient toward a peaceful death.

After the death, the family is encouraged to acknowledge the pain of loss. The nurse's presence and support as the bereaved express their sorrow, anger, or guilt can help them resolve their grief. It is important for the bereaved not to suppress the pain of grieving with drugs. By accepting variations in the expression of grief, the nurse supports the family's grief reactions.

Resolution of grief begins with acceptance of the loss. The nurse can encourage this acceptance by maintaining open, honest dialogue and by providing the family with the opportunity to view, touch, hold, and kiss the person's body. As family members realize the finality of the death, they are often comforted by the presence of the nurse who cared for the patient during the final days.

Postmortem Care

The nurse documents the time of death (required for the death certificate and all official records), notifies the physician, and assists the family (if needed) in choice of a funeral home. If the patient dies at home, death must be pronounced before the body is removed. In some states and in some situations, nurses can pronounce death; for specifics, consult state practice acts, laws, and agency policy. All jewelry is removed and given to the family unless the request is made that it be left on. The body is kept in place until the family is ready and gives permission for it to be moved. If an autopsy is required or requested, the body must be left undisturbed (e.g., do not remove any tubes) for transportation to the medical examiner.

Documentation of the death is completed by sending a completed death certificate to the funeral home (for a death in the home) or by completing the required paperwork and sending the body to the morgue or funeral home (for a death in the hospital or long-term care setting).

Self-Care for the Nurse

Caring for dying patients and their families can be very stressful for the nurse. The nurse who has developed a close relationship with a patient who has died may experience strong feelings of grief. Crying with families, at one time considered unprofessional, is now recognized as an expression of empathy and caring. Sharing grief with the family after the death of a loved one helps both the nurse and family to cope with their feelings about the loss. Taking time to grieve after the death of a patient provides a release that can help prevent "blunting" of feelings, a problem often experienced by nurses who care for patients who are terminally ill. Debriefing with peers, communicating feelings, and identifying strategies that promote personal emotional health should become part of the nurse's self-care practices (**Figure 5.5** ■).

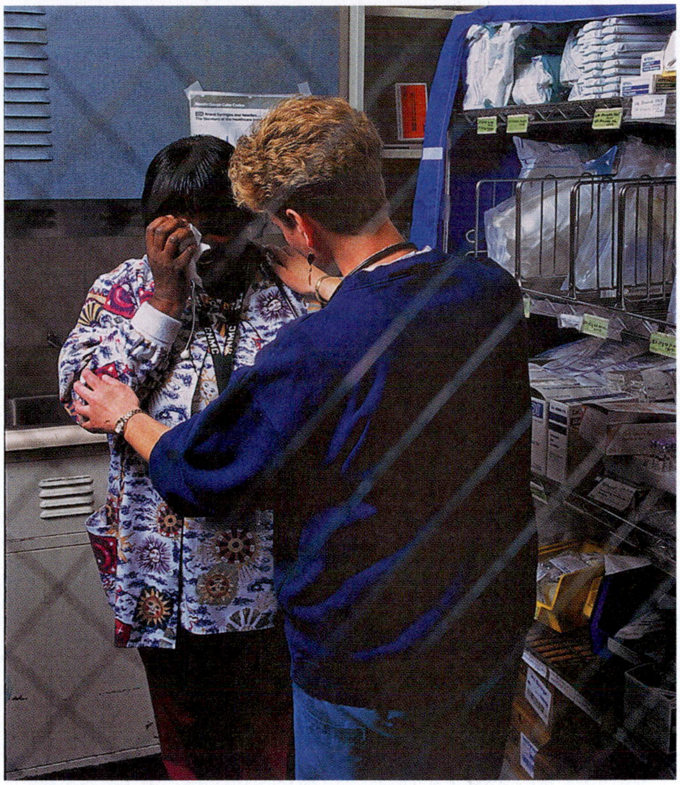

Figure 5.5 ■ Nurses need to express their own grief in a supportive environment. Sharing with colleagues the sadness and grief or futility of resuscitation efforts often helps nurses provide supportive care to the next family who needs it.

Nurses working with critically or terminally ill patients should be aware that witnessing a patient's death and the family's grief may reactivate feelings about some unresolved grief in their own lives. In these cases, nurses may need to reflect on their responses to their own losses. Also, nurses who work with dying patients need support from peers and other professionals to work through the often overwhelming feelings that result from dealing with death, grief, and loss.

The Patient Experiencing Grief

Grief is an important consideration when working with patients near the end of life and their families. Nurses need to understand the grieving process to help patients and their families work through the grieving process.

Interprofessional Care

Interventions for loss and grief may be planned and implemented by any or all members of the healthcare team. Nurses and social workers provide interventions to help patients or families adapt to a loss. They also make referrals to mental health professionals (grief counselors, social services), support groups, chaplains, and legal or financial assistance agencies.

Grieving patients frequently enter the healthcare system with significant somatic symptoms. In some cases, the symptoms of grief and loss are overlooked until the patient reaches a crisis state requiring psychiatric medical intervention. Collaborative care by the physician and the nurse early in the normal grieving process can help the patient achieve an early and effective resolution of grief and avoid physical or psychiatric health problems.

Nursing Care

Nurses practicing in all types of settings care for patients who are in various stages of the grieving process. Grief is highly individual. The grief process may range from uncomfortable to debilitating, and it may last for a day or a lifetime, depending on what the loss means to the person experiencing it. A case study and care plan for a patient who is grieving is included at the end of this section.

In planning and implementing nursing care for the patient experiencing a loss, the nurse considers the individual responses, which may vary greatly. In an era of short acute care stays for patients, nurses may feel that an elaborate grief assessment is impossible or, at the least, impractical. But research and clinical experience suggest that patients who delay the grieving process after a loss are prone to have health problems that may last a lifetime.

Assessment

Knowledge of the expected physical reactions to loss provides the nurse with a basis for identifying reactions requiring further assessment. To assess the extent of physical distress, the nurse observes for changes in sensory processes and asks questions about the patient's sleeping and eating patterns, activities of daily living, general health status, and pain.

Physical Assessment. People who experience a loss may experience one or more predictable somatic (physical) symptoms. Gastrointestinal manifestations such as indigestion, nausea or vomiting, anorexia, weight gain or loss, constipation, or diarrhea occur frequently. The shock and disbelief that accompany a loss may cause shortness of breath, a choking sensation, hyperventilation, or weakness. Some people also report insomnia, preoccupation with sleep, fatigue, and decreased or increased activity level.

Crying and sadness are observed during normal grief states. Crying may make the individual feel exhausted and interfere with carrying out activities of daily living. However, an individual who is unable to cry may have difficulty completing the mourning process. If the person does not express feelings of grief, somatic symptoms may increase.

Reactions to loss are not always obvious. For example, in patients who experience an illness following a serious loss, assessment may reveal somatic complaints related to the grief state as well as the illness. When an individual who has been healthy begins to develop patterns of increased illness, the nurse should be aware that this may signal dysfunctional grieving. This is especially common in the loss and grieving associated with a change in body image. In addition to making a physical assessment, assess the patient's perception of the alteration in body image. The loss of a body part, weight gain or loss, and scars from surgery or trauma can be difficult for a patient to accept. Some patients may grieve hair loss that accompanies chemotherapy used in cancer treatment.

It is imperative for the dying patient's concerns about pain to be assessed, especially if the patient has cancer or another painful illness. Knowledge of pain theories and pain assessment can help the nurse assess the need for pain medication (see Chapter 9). During the last stages of dying, the patient usually becomes very weak and sensations and reflexes decrease; these changes call for careful assessment of the patient's physical needs.

Spiritual Assessment. Because spiritual beliefs and practices greatly influence people's reaction to loss, it is important to explore them with the patient when assessing a loss. The spiritually healthy patient has inner resources that help work through the grief process. Faith, prayer, trust in God or a superior being, perception of a purpose in life, or belief in immortality are examples of the inner resources that may sustain the patient during an actual or perceived loss. Patients who had not considered themselves religious before the actual or perceived loss often turn to religion to seek comfort or to cope with feelings of despair, helplessness, hopelessness, or guilt.

Assessing the dying patient's spiritual life and its significance to the patient and family helps identify spiritual support systems. Some nurses are uncomfortable with assessing a patient's spiritual needs; the following questions may be helpful:

- What are the spiritual aspects of the patient's philosophy about life? Death?
- Are the values and beliefs about life and death congruent with those of people who are important to the patient?
- Which spiritual resources and rituals have significance for the patient?

Belief systems that are incompatible with those of family members can be an additional source of stress for patients dealing with a loss. The anger and resentment often observed among families faced with decisions concerning dying members may be avoided if the nurse assesses the potential effect of differing beliefs.

Patients coping with a loss often perceive that it is a punishment from their god for their wrongdoing or for their failure to remain faithful to their religious practices. Therefore, it is important to assess the level of guilt the patient or family expresses. Assessing the patient's comments regarding feelings of responsibility for the loss helps determine whether these feelings are an expected phase of grieving or indicate dysfunctional grieving.

Psychosocial Assessment. When working through the grief process, patients can be overwhelmed by the fears associated with the loss and the changes it will produce. The patient responding to an actual or perceived loss commonly expresses anxiety (fear of the unknown). An extreme level of anxiety can threaten the patient's well-being. Assessment includes helping patients openly acknowledge their fears. Some patients may fear the feelings they experience while proceeding through the grief process more than the loss itself. The most common fear expressed by patients facing a loss is that of losing self-control.

Talking with dying patients is often difficult. The following suggestions may be helpful:

- When patients initiate conversations about dying, you may feel unprepared for their questions. They can take you by surprise and may lead you to believe that the patient expects a crystal ball response. Remember that the purpose of all such discussions is to keep the lines of communication open with the patient. The idea is to make the subject of dying discussible and to communicate to the patient that it does not make you afraid to do so. An open-ended statement such as "Tell me what concerns you the most" provides a means of encouraging communication.
- Some patients may be too fearful to ask physicians such questions. They often approach staff who they perceive as less intimidating or more approachable. The question often comes in the middle of the night, when there are no distractions, when anxiety or pain may keep the patient awake, and when the patient may feel most alone with psychospiritual distress. In any case, the nurse may be the person present when questions about dying arise.
- Because of the surprising nature of such questions, you may feel tempted to escape ("I've got to go take that patient's vital signs right now") or pass the buck ("That sounds like a question for your doctor"). Be vigilant about such impulsive behavior and realize that it only serves your own need to reduce your anxiety, but does nothing to assist the patient with his or her anxiety. It is well within the scope of your professional practice as a competent nurse to provide counseling and death education, especially when the patient asks you for it or indicates an unmet need for such information and support. *When in doubt, ask a question in response, such as "Tell me how you feel about that" or "What have you been told already?"* This will accomplish several things. First, it will help you to regain your composure. The second point of asking a question is that it will give you more information about what is on the patient's mind so that your intervention can be as specific and responsive to that patient as possible.
- Do not provide false reassurance. It is important to remember that avoiding discussions about death robs the patient of precious time to accomplish goals that produce hope. Dying people hope for many things even when they cannot hope for a cure, such as hope for freedom from pain, to be surrounded by loved ones, and for the rest of their allotted time to be spent in meaningful pursuits.

Awareness of the altered sensorium observed during the stage of shock and disbelief provides parameters for assessment. The nurse may note in the patient feelings of numbness, unreality, and emotional distance, intense preoccupation with the lost person or object, helplessness, loneliness, and disorganization. As awareness of the loss begins to develop, preoccupation with the lost person or object may increase, and self-accusation and ambivalence toward the lost person or object may follow.

Priorities of Care

- Nursing interventions designed to achieve the optimum level of comfort are the priority in providing quality end-of-life care.
- Managing dyspnea is often a priority of care for terminal patients. A variety of interventions including oxygen, positioning, and administration of opiates and sedatives is common.
- Restlessness and delirium are common for actively dying patients and require aggressive intervention. Determining the cause of terminal delirium so the appropriate intervention can be identified is a nursing care priority.
- Providing time for the patient and family to be together is essential during end-of-life care.
- Providing emotional and spiritual support for patients and families experiencing grief and loss is important. A holistic approach that addresses physical, psychosocial, and spiritual needs of the patient and family is essential.

Diagnoses, Outcomes, and Interventions

A variety of nursing problems and/or diagnoses may be appropriate for the patient experiencing loss and grief, as well as for the patient who is nearing death. Nurses practicing medical-surgical nursing will often provide interventions to alleviate pain and symptoms associated with the end of life and interventions for grieving, chronic sorrow, and death anxiety.

Manage Pain and Other Symptoms. The focus of palliative care is to promote comfort by alleviating pain and other symptoms experienced because of terminal illness. Pain is the most common symptom, requiring aggressive management and monitoring. In addition to providing adequate pain control, nursing actions involve treating other symptoms such as nausea, dyspnea, and delirium.

Expected Outcome: Pain and other symptoms associated with end of life will be minimized as demonstrated by the patient's verbal description of comfort level or absence of nonverbal expressions and gestures commonly associated with discomfort.

The nurse will:

- Systematically assess pain and other symptoms related to serious and terminal illness. *Continuous assessment will facilitate early treatment of pain and other symptoms.*
- Advocate for adequate pain control for the patient including around-the-clock, scheduled, or continuous infusion of opioids. *Around-the-clock dosing provides optimal pain control and does not lead to addiction.*
- Avoid unnecessary procedures, tests, and activities for dying patients. Stop or modify vital signs for dying

patients. Stop or reduce tube feedings; turn off monitors and alarms. *Avoiding tests and procedures creates a calm environment and facilitates a peaceful death.*

- Provide time for the patient and family to be together. *Ensuring that the patient and family have the needed time to say good-bye will facilitate effective grieving.*
- Turn and reposition the patient only for comfort. Modify bathing routine or stop per family request. *Limiting interventions that do not promote comfort facilitates a peaceful death.*
- Provide frequent oral care. *Dry oral mucous membranes are a common source of discomfort for dying patients.*
- Explain mottling and cyanosis as part of the dying process to family members. *Family members may think the patient is cold. Explaining what a normal physiologic response is will reassure them that their loved one is being well cared for.*
- Provide temperature comfort measures such as a cool washcloth, warm blanket, or ice packs as appropriate. *Family can provide these simple measures and participating in care may be comforting.*
- Administer supplemental oxygen, provide optimal positioning to promote oxygenation (e.g., semi-Fowler), and consider use of oral suctioning as appropriate. *Dyspnea is common at end of life and treating these symptoms will promote a peaceful death.*
- Consider obtaining medication orders to treat dyspnea such as morphine, glycopyrrolate, scopolamine patch, Atropine 1% ophthalmic solution, and antianxiety agents. *These medications will reduce secretions.*
- Treat delirium and restlessness aggressively. Maintain a calm environment, minimize bright lights, talk softly to the patient, and use touch and presence. *Creating a calm environment will reduce the patient and family's anxiety.*

Support the Grieving Patient and Family. Grieving is a combination of intellectual and emotional responses and behaviors by which people adjust their self-concept in the face of an actual or potential loss. Grieving may be a response to one's own future death; to loss of body parts or functions; to loss of a significant person, animal, or possession; or to loss of a social role. Nursing interventions are designed to assist with grief resolution.

Expected Outcome: Patient/family will demonstrate successful adaptation to loss using effective and positive coping mechanisms.

The nurse will:

- Assess for factors causing or contributing to the grief. Ask about support systems, how many losses have occurred, relationship with the lost person, significance of the body part, and previous experiences with loss and grief. *Grief and mourning occur when an individual experiences any type of loss.*
- Use open-ended questions to encourage the person to share concerns and the possible effect on the family. *Grief resolution cannot occur until the patient acknowledges the loss.*
- Promote a trusting nurse–patient relationship: Allow enough time for communications; speak clearly, simply, and concisely; listen; be honest in responses to questions; do not give unrealistic hope; offer support; and demonstrate respect for the person's age, culture, religion, race, and values. *An effective nurse–patient relationship begins with acceptance of the patient's feelings, attitudes, and values related to the loss. If the patient is ready to talk, listening and being present are the most appropriate interventions.*
- Ask about strengths and weaknesses in coping with the other losses. *Current responses are influenced by past experiences with loss, illness, and death. Socioeconomic and cultural backgrounds, as well as cultural and spiritual beliefs and values, affect an individual's ability to adapt to loss.*
- Teach the patient and family the stages of grief. *This helps them to be aware of their emotions in each stage and reassures them that their reactions are normal.*
- Provide time for decision making. *In periods of stress, people may need extra time to make informed decisions.*
- Provide information about appropriate resources, including support from family, friends, support groups, community resources, and legal/financial aids. *Support from others decreases feelings of loneliness and isolation and facilitates grief work.*

Relieve Death Anxiety. **Death anxiety** is worry or fear related to death or dying. It may be present in patients who have an acute life-threatening illness, who have a terminal illness, who have experienced the death of a family member or friend, or who have experienced multiple deaths in the same family.

Expected Outcome: Patient or family will express fears related to death or dying and identify effective coping strategies that will minimize the adverse effects of uncontrolled anxiety.

The nurse will:

- Explore the patient's knowledge of the situation. For example, ask, "What has your doctor told you about your condition?" *This provides information about the patient's knowledge base about the condition and about his or her ability to make informed decisions.*
- Ask the patient to identify specific fears about death. *This provides data about any unrealistic expectations or misperceptions.*
- Determine the patient's perceptions of strengths and weakness in coping with death. *Identifying past strengths can help the patient cope with loss, illness, and death.*
- Ask the patient to identify needed help. *This determines whether available resources are adequate.*
- Encourage independence and control in decisions about treatment and care. *This promotes self-esteem, decreases feelings of powerlessness, and allows the patient to retain dignity in dying.*
- Facilitate access to culturally appropriate spiritual rituals and practices. *This provides spiritual comfort.*

- Explain advance directives and assist with them if necessary. *Advance directives help ensure that the patient's wishes for end-of-life care are carried out.*
- Encourage life review and reminiscence. *Life review is self-affirming.*
- Encourage activities such as listening to music, aromatherapy, massage, or relaxation exercises. *These activities decrease anxiety.*
- Suggest keeping a journal or leaving a written legacy. *A written document provides continuing support to others after death.*

Provide Patient Education. In addition to teaching patients and families to carry out the physical skills that are necessary to the patient's care, nurses also provide information on identifying signs of deterioration and additional sources of support.

Expected Outcome: Patient and family will understand the grieving process.

The nurse will:

- Encourage both children and adults to discuss expected or impending loss and to express feelings.
- Teach problem-solving skills. Define what the possible changes and problems are related to the predicted loss, develop potential strategies for dealing with problems, list pros and cons of each strategy, and decide which strategies might be most useful to try first to solve potential problems associated with loss.
- Teach individuals and families how to support a person who is dealing with an impending loss.
- Explain what to expect with a loss: Sadness, fear, rejection, anger, guilt, loneliness.
- Teach signs of grief resolution:

  a. No longer living in the past, becoming future oriented
  b. Breaking ties with the lost object or person (acute stage often shows signs of resolving in 6 to 12 months)
  c. The possibility of having painful waves of grief years after the loss, especially on the anniversary of the loss and in response to triggers such as pictures, events, songs, or memories.

Case Study & Nursing Care Plan

Loss and Grief

Pearl Rogers is a 79-year-old woman who is admitted to the Methodist Home Nursing Center. Mrs. Rogers lived with her husband of 58 years until his death 9 months ago. She had one son who died in an auto crash 2 years ago, and she has one daughter who lives nearby. After her husband's death, Mrs. Rogers lived with her daughter until her admission to the nursing center. Mrs. Rogers has become increasingly agitated and helpless, complaining constantly of pain. Her daughter states that Mrs. Rogers is chronically constipated, has difficulty sleeping, and has stopped engaging in all social activities, including weekly church services. She cries frequently. Extensive medical testing prior to her admission to the nursing center revealed Mrs. Rogers has arthritis but no other pathologic disorder.

ASSESSMENT	DIAGNOSES	EXPECTED OUTCOMES
On admission to the nursing center, Mrs. Rogers says, "I'm a sick woman, and no one will listen to me! I can't walk, I'm so weak. My head hurts, and I'm always sick to my stomach. I haven't had a bowel movement in a week, and I never sleep more than 3 hours a night." Physical assessment findings include swollen knees and ankles, with limited mobility of the lower extremities.	■ Grieving due to stress of husband's death ■ Insomnia related to grieving ■ Constipation related to inactivity	■ Engage in normal grief work: Work through grief process, discuss reality of losses, use nondestructive coping mechanisms, and discuss positive and negative aspects of the loss. ■ Experience adequate and restful sleep: Fall asleep 20 to 30 minutes after retiring and awaken feeling rested after 7 to 8 hours of sleep. ■ Have a bowel movement with soft, formed stools at least every other day.

PLANNING AND IMPLEMENTATION

- Promote trust: Show empathy and caring, demonstrate respect for Mrs. Rogers's culture and values, offer support and reassurance, be honest, and engage in active listening.
- Assist in labeling Mrs. Rogers's feelings: Anger, fear, loneliness, guilt, isolation.
- Explore previous losses and the ways in which the patient has coped.
- Encourage review of Mrs. Rogers's relationship with her dead husband.
- Reinforce expressions of behaviors associated with normal grieving.
- Encourage participation in usual spiritual practices.
- Encourage participation in a grief group that meets at the facility.
- Consult with the physical and recreational therapist to help the nursing staff provide afternoon activities.
- Provide measures that assist in bowel evacuation: Encourage exercise as tolerated, including walks and rocking in a rocking chair. Offer foods that stimulate bowel movements. Offer privacy: Close the door, ensuring that the emergency call bell is within reach, and do not interrupt.
- Administer a mild laxative and/or stool softener, if necessary, but discontinue as soon as possible.

(continued)

EVALUATION

After 4 weeks at the nursing center, Mrs. Rogers states, "I don't feel any better, but I know I have to accept my situation." Although Mrs. Rogers states that she doesn't feel better, she is walking the length of the hall, sleeping better, and having regular bowel movements. Mrs. Rogers is also less withdrawn and has openly discussed her feelings related to her husband's death, including her anger at the loss of her son and her husband less than 2 years apart. She has attended the grief group once and has attended chapel services on Sunday for the past 2 weeks. Her daughter visits her each Saturday and takes her in a wheelchair to the shopping mall.

CLINICAL REASONING IN PATIENT CARE

1. What common physical manifestations of grief did Mrs. Rogers experience?
2. How might Mrs. Rogers's daughter be more involved in developing and implementing her mother's plan of care?
3. Suppose Mrs. Rogers says that she does not want any help, that she just wants to be left alone to die. How would you respond?

See Evaluating Your Response in Appendix B.

CHAPTER HIGHLIGHTS

5.1 Loss and Grief

Differentiate theories of loss and grief and outline any factors affecting responses to loss.

- Caring for patients and families experiencing loss, grief, and death emphasizes integration of holistic nursing interventions focused on providing individualized patient-centered care.
- Providing direct patient care and coordinating, leading, and participating as a member of the interprofessional team is an essential role for the registered nurse when caring for this population.
- Grief is the emotional response to a loss, experienced by an individual as grieving. Bereavement, a form of depression accompanied by anxiety, is a common response to loss of a loved one by death. Death, although inevitable, is an immensely difficult loss.
- There are many different theories of how people respond to loss, grief, and death. These theories are useful when providing nursing care to patients and families.
- An individual's response to loss is influenced by age, social support, family members, cultural and spiritual beliefs, and rituals of mourning. Nurses need to assess the way in which they respond to loss to better care for patients.

5.2 Palliative Care

Explain the concept of palliative care and the nurse's role in care of the patient and family.

- Palliative care is an area of care that has evolved out of the hospice experience, but exists outside of hospice programs, is not restricted to the end of life, and is used earlier in the disease experience.
- Palliative care usually involves the combined efforts of an interprofessional team, including physicians, nurses, social workers, chaplains, home health aides, and volunteers.
- The expected outcomes of palliative care are directed by interventions to manage current manifestations of the illness and to prevent new manifestations from occurring.

5.3 End-of-Life Care

Outline the legal, ethical, and physiologic issues encountered when caring for the dying patient.

- Legal and ethical issues involved in end-of-life care include advance directives (living wills, healthcare surrogates, durable powers of attorney, physician orders for life-sustaining treatment), do-not-resuscitate orders, euthanasia, assisted suicide, and aid in dying.
- Hospice is a philosophy of care rather than a program of care. It is comprehensive and coordinated care for patients with limited life expectancy that reaffirms the right of every patient and family to fully participate in the final stages of life.
- To provide knowledgeable and compassionate care at the end of life, nurses must recognize physiologic changes as the patient nears death, support the patient and family, provide postmortem care, and resolve their own grief.
- Nursing care of patients experiencing an actual or potential loss includes accurate physical, spiritual, and psychosocial assessment. It also includes provision of interventions to alleviate pain and symptoms associated with the end of life and interventions for the human responses of grieving, chronic sorrow, and death anxiety.

TEST YOURSELF NCLEX-RN® REVIEW

1. The nurse is planning care for a patient whose spouse recently passed away. Which statement should the nurse keep in mind when planning care for this patient who has experienced a loss? (Select all that apply.)
   A. Loss always results in change.
   B. Grief and mourning are determined by one's cultural values.
   C. Successfully coping with loss is primarily dependent on the strength of an individual's social support system.
   D. The feelings associated with loss can only be determined by the person who experiences it.
   E. Grief may be mild.
2. A patient newly diagnosed with a terminal illness states, "I hate this cancer." According to Kübler-Ross, what stage of loss is being verbalized?
   A. Anger
   B. Denial
   C. Bargaining
   D. Depression
3. A 12-year-old has lost both parents in an automobile accident. Which statements, made by the child, does the nurse evaluate as age-appropriate grieving? (Select all that apply.)
   A. "I wish my parents would wake up."
   B. "I know we all die sometime."
   C. "I will always be careful so I will not die."
   D. "I think my parents went to heaven."
   E. "I did this when I told my dad I wished he would die."
4. A terminally ill patient has died and the nurse is waiting for the family to arrive before moving the patient. What is the primary factor that dictates this family's ritual of mourning?
   A. Age
   B. Culture
   C. Gender
   D. Social support
5. A patient says, "I don't want anything heroic done if I die. Just let me go." Which document should the patient complete that expresses wishes for life-sustaining treatment in the event of terminal illness or permanent unconsciousness?
   A. Living will
   B. No-code order
   C. Healthcare surrogate
   D. Durable power of attorney
6. A patient has been referred to hospice and asks what it means. What should the nurse respond to the patient about this type of care?
   A. It is a special place of care.
   B. It is a lifelong type of care.
   C. It is a model of care rather than a place of care.
   D. It is designed for patients with serious chronic illness.
7. A patient nearing death requests that no medication be given that would cause a loss of consciousness, including pain medication. What should the nurse do to provide the best end-of-life care for this patient?
   A. Give the medication; comfort is the highest priority.
   B. Give half the ordered dose to provide compassionate care.
   C. Discuss this with family members and follow their wishes.
   D. Respect the patient's wishes and withhold pain medications.
8. The nurse is caring for a patient who is dying. Which intervention supports the last sense typically lost in dying?
   A. The nurse uses essential oils to mask unpleasant smells in the room.
   B. The nurse encourages family to continue to touch the patient.
   C. The nurse dims the lights in the room.
   D. The nurse encourages the family to speak with the patient.
9. A patient with a terminal illness is demonstrating signs of imminent death. What should the nurse keep in mind about the treatment of pain at the end of life?
   A. Refrain from administering opioids to the dying patient.
   B. There is no maximum allowable dose for opioids during end-of-life care.
   C. As a patient nears death, no pain is perceived and no medications are necessary.
   D. It is important to withhold pain medications if the patient has respiratory changes.
10. A patient, recently widowed, tells the nurse, "I just can't even get out of bed in the mornings anymore." What response by the nurse would be most helpful in resolving the patient's grief?
    A. "I don't know why you feel that way."
    B. "This must be a difficult time for you."
    C. "Why do you think you feel this way?"
    D. "After you get up, you will feel better."

See Test Yourself answers in Appendix B.

REFERENCES

Adams, M. P., Holland, L. N., & Urban, C. (2017). *Pharmacology for nursing: A pathophysiologic approach* (5th ed.). Hoboken, NJ: Pearson Education.

Agency for Healthcare Research and Quality (AHRQ). (2013). *Guideline summary. Palliative care for adults* [NGC: 010131]. Rockville MD: Author. Retrieved from https://www.guideline.gov/summaries/summary/47629/palliative-care-for-adults.

Agency for Healthcare Research and Quality [AHRQ]. (2016). *Chartbook on care coordination. Transitions of care.* Retrieved from https://www.ahrq.gov/research/findings/nhqrdr/chartbooks/carecoordination/measure1.html.

American Association of Colleges of Nursing (AACN). (2017). *CARE: Competencies and recommendations for educating undergraduate nursing students. Preparing nurses to care for the seriously ill and their families.* Washington, DC: Author. Retrieved from www.aacnnursing.org/Portals/42/ELNEC/PDF/New-Palliative-Care-Competencies.pdf.

American Nurses Association. (2012). *Position statement: Nursing care and* do not resuscitate (DNR) and allow natural death (AND) decisions. Retrieved from https://www.nursingworld.org/~4af078/globalassets/docs/ana/ethics/endoflife-positionstatement.pdf.

American Nurses Association (ANA). (2013). *Position statements: Euthanasia, assisted suicide, and aid in dying.* Retrieved from www.nursingworld.org/MainMenuCategories/Policy-Advocacy/Positions-andResolutions/ANAPositionStatements.

American Nurses Association (ANA). (2016). *Position statement: Nurses' roles and responsibilities in providing care and support at the end of life.* Retrieved from https://www.nursingworld.org/~4ad4a8/globalassets/docs/ana/nursing-care-and-do-not-resuscitate-dnr-and-allow-natural-death-decisions.pdf.

Barbus, A. (1975). *Dying person's bill of rights.* Created at The Terminally Ill Patient and the Helping Person Workshop. Lansing, MI: South Western Michigan Inservice Education Council.

Bowlby, J. (1973). *Attachment and loss, separation, anxiety, and anger* (Vol. 2). New York, NY: Basic Books.

Bowlby, J. (1980). *Attachment and loss, loss, sadness, and depression* (Vol. 3). New York, NY: Basic Books.

Buddhist Society. (2018). *Buddhist funerals.* Retrieved from https://www.thebuddhistsociety.org/page/buddhist-funerals.

Caplan, G. (1990). Loss, stress, and mental health. *Community Mental Health Journal, 26*(1), 27–48.

Carpenita, L. J. (2014). *Nursing care plans. Transitional patient and family centered care* (6th ed.). New York, NY: Wolters Kluwer Health.

Centers for Disease Control and Prevention (CDC), National Center for Health Statistics. (2016). *Hospice care.* Retrieved from https://www.cdc.gov/nchs/fastats/hospice-care.htm.

Dudley, N., Wallhagen, M., Ritchie, C., & Rehm, R. (2016). Facilitators of and barriers to interdisciplinary communication and collaboration in palliative care and primary care. *Journal of Pain and Symptom Management, 51*(2), 442–443.

Engel, G. (1964). Grief and grieving. *American Journal of Nursing, 64*, 93.

Field, N., Gao, B., & Paderna, L. (2005). Continued bonds in bereavement: An attachment theory based perspective. *Death Studies, 29*(4), 277–299.

Freud, S. (1957). Mourning and melancholia. In J. Strachey & A. Tyson (Eds.), *The complete psychological works of Sigmund Freud* (Vol. 14). London: Hogarth Press. (Original work published 1917.)

George Washington Institute for Spirituality & Health. (n.d.). *FICA© spiritual history tool.* Retrieved from https://smhs.gwu.edu/gwish/clinical/fica/spiritual-history-tool.

Giger, J. N. (2017). *Transcultural nursing: Assessment and intervention* (7th ed.). St. Louis, MO: Elsevier.

Hospice Association of America. (2018). *Facts and figures: Hospice care in America.* Retrieved from https://www.nhpco.org/sites/default/files/public/Statistics_Research/2017_Facts_Figures.pdf.

Kübler-Ross, E. (1969). *On death and dying*. New York, NY: Macmillan.

Kübler-Ross, E. (1978). *To live until we say goodbye*. Englewood Cliffs, NJ: Prentice Hall.

Kübler-Ross, E. (1997). *On death and dying: What the dying have to teach doctors, nurses, clergy, and their own families.* New York, NY: Simon & Schuster.

Lindemann, E. (1944). Symptomatology and management of acute grief. *Amercan Journal of Psychiatry, 201*, 141–148.

National Consensus Project for Quality Palliative Care. (2013). *Clinical practice guidelines for quality palliative care* (3rd ed.). Pittsburgh, PA: Author.

Purnell, L. D. (2014). *Guide to culturally competent care* (3rd ed.). Philadelphia, PA: F. A. Davis.

Sorenson, M., Quinn, L., & Klein, D. (2019). *Pathophysiology: Concepts of human disease.* Hoboken, NJ: Pearson Education.

Spector, R. E. (2017). *Cultural diversity in health and illness* (9th ed.). Hoboken, NJ: Pearson Education.

U.S. Centers for Medicare and Medicaid Services. (2018). *How hospice works.* Retrieved from https://www.medicare.gov/what-medicare-covers/part-a/how-hospice-works.html.

World Health Organization. (2018). *WHO definition of palliative care.* Retrieved from http://www.who.int/cancer/palliative/definition/en/.

ADDITIONAL RESOURCES

Aging with Dignity
www.agingwithdignity.org

End-of-Life Nursing Education Consortium
www.aacnnursing.org/ELNEC

National Coalition for Hospice and Palliative Care
www.nationalcoalitionhpc.org

National Hospice and Palliative Care Organization
www.nhpco.org/learn-about-end-life-care

Chapter 6

Nursing Care of Patients with Problems of Substance Abuse

Chapter Outline and Learning Outcomes

Outline the pathophysiology, manifestations, and complications of substance abuse; the risk factors for substance abuse; and characteristics of individuals who abuse substances including nurses.

Differentiate the effects of selected addictive substances on physiologic, cognitive, psychologic, and social well-being.

Describe the interprofessional care, nursing care, and transitions of care for patients who abuse substances.

CLINICAL COMPETENCIES

- Assess and monitor the health status of patients with substance abuse or dependence.
- Monitor for signs of withdrawal and life-threatening conditions.
- Provide skilled nursing care during the detoxification period, respecting expressed needs, values, and preferences.
- Collaborate and coordinate with the patient and other members of the interprofessional team when caring for patients with substance abuse problems.
- Educate patients about stress management, coping skills, nutrition, relapse prevention, and healthy lifestyle choices.
- Using assessed data and current standards of practice, plan and implement individualized nursing care for patients experiencing problems with substance abuse.
- Evaluate patient responses to care, revising the plan of care as needed to promote, maintain, or restore functional health status to patients with substance abuse problems.
- Apply technology and information management tools to support safe processes of care for patients with substance abuse disorders.

KEY TERMS

alcohol, 132
amphetamine, 135
caffeine, 131
cannabis sativa, 134
central nervous system depressants, 135
cocaine, 135
co-occurring disorders, 127
delirium tremens (DT), 133
detoxification, 138
hallucinogens, 137
inhalants, 137
Korsakoff psychosis, 132
nicotine, 133
opiates, 136
psychostimulants, 135
substance abuse, 127
substance dependence, 127
substance use disorder (SUD), 127
tolerance, 127
Wernicke encephalopathy, 132
withdrawal, 127
withdrawal symptoms, 127

6.1 Overview of Substance Abuse Problems

Substance abuse refers to the use of any chemical in a fashion inconsistent with medical or culturally defined social norms despite physical, psychologic, or social adverse effects. Anxiety and depressive disorders frequently occur with substance abuse. More than 90% of people who commit suicide have a depressive or substance abuse disorder (National Alliance on Mental Illness, 2017). In 2016, 28.6 million people aged 12 or older used an illicit drug in the past 30 days, which corresponds to about 1 in 10 Americans overall (10.6%), but the number ranges as high as 1 in 4 for young adults aged 18 to 25 (Center for Behavioral Health Statistics and Quality [CBHSQ], 2017). Moreover, in 2016, 136.7 million Americans aged 12 or older reported current use of alcohol, including 65.3 million who reported binge alcohol use in the past month and 16.3 million who reported heavy alcohol use in the past month (CBHSQ, 2017).

The fifth edition of the *Diagnostic and Statistical Manual of Mental Disorders* (DSM-5; American Psychiatric Association [APA], 2013) includes classification criteria for distinguishing between substance abuse and substance dependence. **Substance dependence** refers to a severe condition occurring when the use of the chemical substance is no longer under an individual's control for at least 3 months. Continued use of the substance usually persists despite adverse effects on the person's physical condition, psychologic health, and interpersonal relationships. The DSM-5 criteria deal with the behavioral aspects and the maladaptive patterns of substance use, emphasizing the physical symptoms of tolerance and withdrawal. **Tolerance** is a cumulative state in which a particular dose of the chemical elicits a smaller response than before. With increased tolerance, the individual needs higher and higher doses to obtain the desired effect. When an individual is physically addicted to the drug and stops taking it, **withdrawal symptoms** can occur within hours. **Withdrawal** is an uncomfortable state lasting several days, manifested by tremors, diaphoresis, anxiety, high blood pressure, tachycardia, and possibly convulsions. **Substance use disorder (SUD)** is the term that encompasses abuse of addictive drugs and alcohol. SUD also includes gambling, which is a process (or behavioral) addiction (**Figure 6.1** ■). Drugs, alcohol, and process addictions all produce such an intense activation of the reward system that daily activities are neglected (APA, 2013).

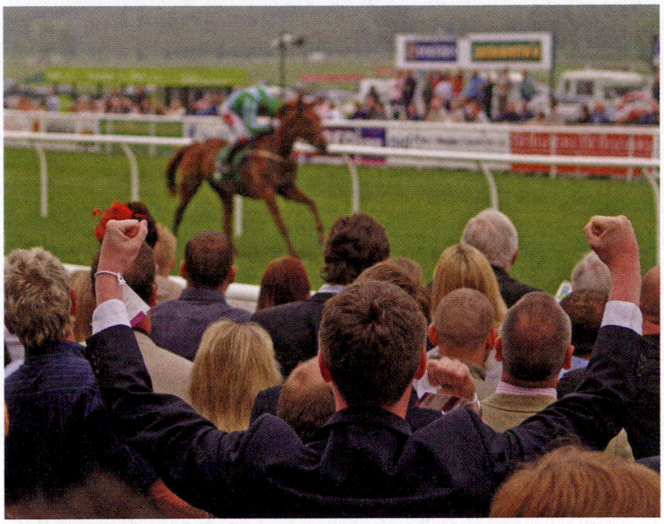

Figure 6.1 ■ Gambling disorder, one of the process disorders, produces behavioral symptoms comparable to those seen in substance use disorders.

Pathophysiology, Manifestations, and Complications

The human tendency to seek pleasure and avoid stress and pain is partially responsible for substance abuse. Evidence implicates the endogenous opioid system and other neurotransmitters in the development and maintenance of addictive behaviors. A person's experiences when using a drug or other substance reflects the function of the particular neurotransmitter it disrupts. Each individual neuron manufactures one or more neurotransmitters: Dopamine, glutamate, serotonin, acetylcholine, and others (National Institute on Drug Abuse [NIDA], 2014a, 2017a). Each neurotransmitter is associated with particular effects depending on its distribution among the brain's various functional areas. Dopamine, for example, is highly concentrated in regions that regulate motivation and feelings of reward and is a strong motivator for drug use. A neurotransmitter's impact also depends on whether it stimulates or dampens activity of its target neurons. Dopamine has been identified as the primary neurotransmitter responsible for sustaining the addictive quality of drugs and for increasing drug-seeking behavior (NIDA, 2017a). In alcohol abuse, the neurotransmitters of interest are dopamine, serotonin, GABA, and glutamate (Banerjee, 2014). In summary, the reinforcing properties of substances can create a pleasurable experience and reduce the intensity and perception of unpleasant experiences.

Manifestations of substance abuse include failure to meet major role obligations (e.g., work, education, family), engaging in hazardous activities while impaired, and a pattern of legal or interpersonal relationship problems (APA, 2013). Individuals with substance dependence use the drug in larger dosages and for longer than it is intended to be used and demonstrate tolerance to the drug and withdrawal symptoms when the drug is withheld or unavailable. These individuals often withdraw from family and friends, focusing instead on obtaining, taking, and recovering from the drug (APA, 2013).

People with mental health disorders are more likely than people without mental health disorders to experience an alcohol or substance use disorder (CBHSQ, 2015). **Co-occurring disorders** (previously called *dual diagnosis* or *dual disorders*) refer to the coexistence of substance abuse or dependence and a psychiatric disorder in one individual. One disorder can be an indication of another, such as the relationship between alcoholism and depression.

Alcohol dependence and major depression commonly occur together, each posing a significant risk for the development of the other. A depressed person may use self-medication in the form of alcohol to treat the depression, or the person with alcoholism may become depressed. Commonly co-occurring mental disorders in adults are alcohol abuse or alcohol dependence with depression, psychosis, and anxiety (Anker, Kushner, Thuras, Menk, & Unruh, 2016). In the United States, among adults aged 18 or older in 2014 with any mental illness in the past year, the percentage of adults who also had a co-occurring substance use disorder (SUD) was highest among those aged 18 to 25 (29.3%), followed by those aged 26 to 49 (20.8%), then by those aged 50 or older (10.3%) (CBHSQ, 2015). Globally, mental illness and SUDs cause disability and premature mortality and significantly challenge healthcare delivery systems; the global burden of mental and substance use disorders increased by 37.6% between 1990 and 2010 due to population growth and aging in developed and developing regions (Whiteford et al., 2013). **Table 6.1** lists terminology associated with substance abuse.

Risk Factors

Various risk factors help explain why one person becomes addicted while another does not. Genetic, biologic, psychologic, and sociocultural factors shed light on how an individual may abuse or become dependent on a substance:

- ***Genetic factors*** include an apparent hereditary factor, especially with alcohol use and dependence. Single-nucleotide polymorphism (SNP) analysis has shown that a dominant minor allele (DNA sequence) on the *DRD3* gene increases alcoholism susceptibility, a dominant minor allele on the *NTRK2* gene delays the alcoholism onset age, and minor alleles on other genes advance or shorten the alcoholism onset age (Yang et al., 2017). According to the American Society of Addiction Medicine (ASAM; 2017), there are multiple neurotransmitters and genes that influence the responses to alcohol, the manifestations of alcohol dependence, and the risk for developing the disease. While allele and gene mapping has produced interesting findings, it has not developed into an overarching explanation

Table 6.1 Terminology Associated with Substance Abuse

Term	Definition
Abstinence	Voluntarily going without drugs or alcohol.
Addiction	Disease process characterized by the continued use of a specific chemical substance despite physical, psychologic, or social harm (used interchangeably with substance dependence).
Codependence	Cluster of maladaptive behaviors exhibited by the significant others of an individual who abuses substances that serves to enable and protect the abuse at the expense of living a full and satisfying life.
Co-occurring disorders	Concurrent diagnosis of a substance use disorder and a psychiatric disorder. One disorder can precede and cause the other, such as the relationship between alcoholism and depression.
Cross-tolerance	Tolerance to one drug confers tolerance to another.
Delirium tremens	Medical emergency usually occurring 3 to 5 days following alcohol withdrawal and lasting 2 to 3 days. Characterized by paranoia, disorientation, delusions, visual hallucinations, elevated vital signs, vomiting, diarrhea, and diaphoresis.
Detoxification	Process through which an addicted individual withdraws from alcohol or other substance.
Dual diagnosis	Coexistence of substance abuse/dependence and a psychiatric disorder in one individual (used interchangeably with dual disorder and co-occurring disorders).
Kindling	Brain sensitization to events such as stress, trauma, or the effects of substance use.
Korsakoff psychosis	Secondary dementia caused by thiamine (B_1) deficiency that may be associated with chronic alcoholism; characterized by progressive cognitive deterioration, confabulation, peripheral neuropathy, and myopathy.
Physical dependence	State in which withdrawal syndrome will occur if substance use is discontinued.
Polysubstance abuse	Simultaneous use of many substances.
Psychologic dependence	Intensive subjective need for a particular psychoactive drug.
Substance abuse	Continued use of a chemical substance in a fashion inconsistent with medical or social norms, for at least 1 month, despite related problems.
Substance dependence	Severe condition occurring when the use of the chemical substance is no longer under control for at least 3 months; continued use persists despite adverse effects (used interchangeably with addiction).
Substance use disorder (SUD)	Disorder occurring when the recurrent use of alcohol and/or drugs causes clinically and functionally significant impairment, such as health problems, disability, and failure to meet major responsibilities at work, school, or home. According to DSM-5, the diagnosis of SUD is based on evidence of impaired control, social impairment, risky use, and pharmacological criteria.
Tolerance	State in which a particular dose elicits a smaller response than it formerly did. With increased tolerance the individual needs higher and higher doses to obtain the desired response.
Wernicke encephalopathy	Caused by thiamine (B_1) deficiency, characterized by nystagmus, ptosis, ataxia, confusion, coma, and possible death; the disorder is a medical emergency. Common in chronic alcoholism.
Withdrawal syndrome	Constellation of signs and symptoms that occurs in physically dependent individuals when they discontinue drug use.

of alcohol and substance use. Geneticists are now conducting longitudinal research to understand how genetic risk unfolds across development, especially vulnerabilities that may occur during transitions from early adolescence through young adulthood (Dick et al., 2014). Some of this research involves *epigenetics*, the study of changes in organisms caused by modification of gene expression rather than alteration of the genetic code (Deans & Maggert, 2015). See the Genetic Considerations box.

- ***Biologic factors*** were first identified by Jellinek (1946) in his disease model of alcoholism. He hypothesized that addiction to alcohol may have a biochemical basis and identified specific phases of the disease. Expanding on Jellinek's early work, researchers have implicated low levels of dopamine and serotonin in the development of alcohol dependence. Dopamine and dopamine receptor sites are intricately involved in the complex workings between the nervous system and abusive substances. Any drug's ability to have an impact on the biochemical mechanisms of the brain must be able to do so at a receptor site or at a number of receptor sites (**Figure 6.2** ■). Most abused substances either mimic or block the brain's most important neurotransmitters at their respective receptor sites. For example, heroin and other opiates mimic natural opiate-like neurotransmitters such as endorphin, enkephalin, and dynorphin. In contrast, cocaine and other stimulants block the reuptake of dopamine, serotonin, and norepinephrine (NIDA, 2014a).
- ***Psychologic factors*** attempt to explain substance abuse through a combination of psychoanalytic, behavioral, and family-system theories. Psychoanalytic theorists view substance abuse as a fixation at the oral stage of development, while behavioral theorists see addiction as a learned, maladaptive behavior. Family-system theory focuses on the pattern of family relationships throughout several generations. No addictive personality type has been identified; however, several common factors seem to exist among people with alcoholism and substance abuse problems. Many people with substance abuse problems have experienced sexual or physical abuse in their childhood or other trauma and as a result have low self-esteem and difficulty expressing emotions (Substance Abuse and Mental Health Services Administration [SAMHSA], 2014b). A link also exists between substance abuse and psychiatric disorders such as depression, anxiety, and antisocial and dependent personalities. The habit of using a substance becomes a form of self-medication to cope with day-to-day problems, and over time it develops into an addiction. Also, alcoholism can be environmentally influenced, as occurs on college campuses where harmful and underage drinking remain significant problems and lead to negative consequences such as binge drinking, alcohol poisoning, poor academic outcomes, impaired driving, unsafe sex, fights, sexual assaults, suicide attempts, unintentional injuries, overdoses, and death among college students (National Institute on Alcohol Abuse and Alcoholism [NIAAA], 2015b).
- ***Sociocultural factors*** often influence individuals' decisions as to when, what, and how they use substances. Ethnic differences in the way alcohol is metabolized may explain why some individuals choose not to drink. When alcohol is first metabolized, it is converted into a by-product known as acetaldehyde,

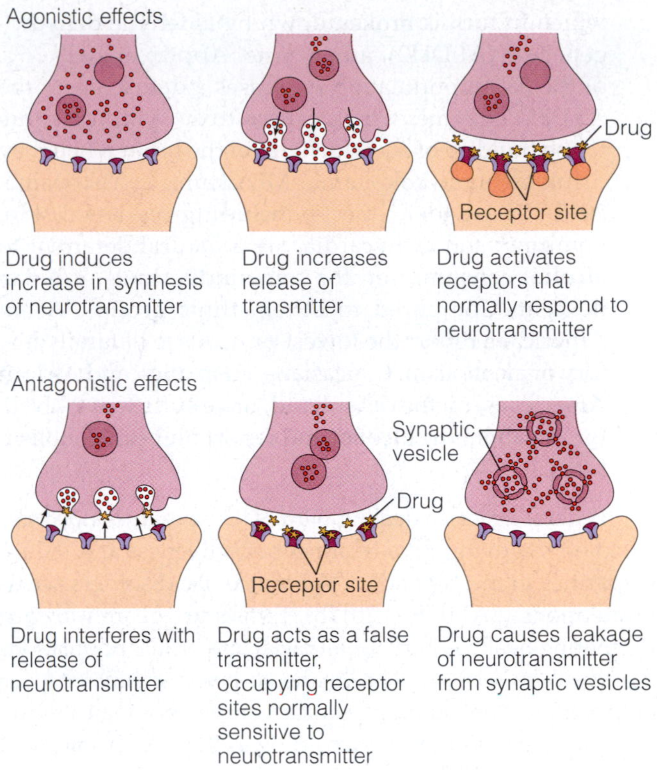

Agonistic effects
Drug
Receptor site
Drug induces increase in synthesis of neurotransmitter
Drug increases release of transmitter
Drug activates receptors that normally respond to neurotransmitter
Antagonistic effects
Synaptic vesicle
Drug
Receptor site
Drug interferes with release of neurotransmitter
Drug acts as a false transmitter, occupying receptor sites normally sensitive to neurotransmitter
Drug causes leakage of neurotransmitter from synaptic vesicles

Figure 6.2 ■ Action of abusive substances at brain receptor sites.

Genetic Considerations

Family Risk Factors for Alcoholism

Children of alcoholics (COAs) are about four times more likely to develop alcohol problems than children of nonalcoholics (National Association for Children of Alcoholics [NACOA], 2015). According to ASAM (2017), the single strongest predictor for risk for developing alcohol dependence is a male with a positive (particularly multigenerational) family history of male alcoholism. However, alcoholism is not solely determined by genetics; more than half of all COAs are not alcoholics. Research shows that many factors influence the risk of developing alcoholism. Some factors lower the risk, whereas others increase the risk. Researchers think an individual is at increased risk if the following situations are present:

- An alcoholic parent is depressed or has other psychological problems
- Both parents abuse alcohol and other drugs
- The parents' alcohol abuse is severe
- Conflicts lead to aggression and violence in the family (NACOA, 2015).

which in turn is broken down by aldehyde dehydrogenase 2 (ALDH2), an enzyme. Approximately 36% of the Asian population possesses a deficiency of the ALDH2 enzyme, which causes toxic symptoms due to the buildup of acetaldehyde in the brain when they drink alcohol (Yokoyama, Mizukami, & Yokoyama, 2015). These toxic effects, including reddened skin, vomiting, and tachycardia, are a natural deterrent to alcohol consumption for some individuals of Asian descent. Compared to other ethnic groups, Asian Americans report the lowest prevalence of family history of alcoholism. Caucasians, Hispanics, and African Americans, on the other hand, have sufficient ALDH2 for metabolizing alcohol and report higher alcoholism rates.

Federal agencies dealing with SUD have developed targeted efforts to improve treatment effectiveness and reduce disparities in mental and/or substance use disorders across populations (SAMHSA, 2017b). Efforts are geared toward promoting health equity for all racial and ethnic populations vulnerable to behavioral health disparities. A significant focus of this effort is encouraging clinical competence in healthcare providers such as nurses. According to the U.S. Department of Health and Human Services (HHS), cultural competence "refers to the ability to honor and respect the beliefs, languages, interpersonal styles, and behaviors of individuals and families receiving services, as well as staff members who are providing such services. Cultural competence is a dynamic, ongoing developmental process that requires a long-term commitment and is achieved over time" (SAMHSA, 2014c).

Many factors place an individual at risk for substance use, abuse, and dependence. No single cause can explain why one individual develops a pattern of drug use and another person does not. Thorough assessment of these factors is necessary to understand the whole person and plan appropriate interventions.

Characteristics of Individuals Who Abuse Substances

As mentioned, no addictive personality type exists; however, many individuals with substance abuse problems have several characteristics in common. Addictive behavior associated with alcoholism and other substances is characterized by compulsive preoccupation with obtaining the substance, loss of control over consumption, and development of tolerance and dependence as well as impaired social and occupational functioning (APA, 2013). People who abuse substances tend to indulge in impulsive, risk-taking behaviors and often have a low tolerance for frustration and pain. Often they rebel against social norms and engage in various antisocial and risky behaviors such as stealing, promiscuity, driving while intoxicated, and violence against others. There is also a tendency toward anxiety, anger, and low self-esteem in people with substance abuse problems. Many people have a desire for social acceptance and initiate drug use to fit in with a peer group. Others may suffer from social anxiety and use drugs or alcohol to feel less inhibited while interacting with others.

Impaired Nurses

By the nature of their roles, dentists, pharmacists, physicians, and nurses are in frequent contact with drugs and are at high risk for substance abuse problems. Healthcare professionals have a higher risk for opiate abuse than other professionals due to the accessibility of opiates in their line of work. Nurses experience many pressures in the workplace and often have easy access to drugs (American Nurses Association [ANA], 2017). This may result in greater vulnerability for substance abuse and dependence and can lead to impaired professional practice.

Nurses must act responsibly when coworkers display signs of substance use. If colleagues are showing signs of a substance abuse problem, information about impaired nurse programs is available through most state boards of nursing to help individual nurses. Nurses convicted of working or driving under the influence of alcohol, illegal substances, or nonmedical use of prescription drugs are subject to disciplinary action by their state board of nursing. Currently, 37 states offer some form of a substance abuse treatment program to direct nurses to treatment, monitor their reentry to work, and continue their license (ANA, 2017). However, a disciplinary hearing can be held and may result in censure, probation, or suspension of a professional license. The loss of professional licensure is the most severe form of disciplinary action and may prevent an individual from ever practicing nursing again. Warning signs of impaired nurses in the workplace are listed in **Table 6.2**.

Table 6.2 Warning Signs of Impaired Nurses in the Workplace

At-Risk Situations	Observable Warning Signs
Easy access to prescription drugs	▪ Inaccurate narcotic counts or frequent missing drugs ▪ Patients complain of ineffective pain control, deny receiving pain meds ▪ Excessive "wasting" of drugs ▪ Volunteering to give medications to patients ▪ Frequent trips to the bathroom
Role strain	▪ Frequent tardiness or absenteeism, especially before and after scheduled days off ▪ Haphazard, shoddy documentation ▪ Patient care judgment errors ▪ Unorganized, erratic behavior; unkempt appearance
Depression	▪ Irritability; unable to focus or concentrate ▪ Abrupt mood swings ▪ Isolating self; taking long breaks ▪ Apathetic, depressed, lethargic ▪ Unexplained absences from assigned unit
Signs of alcohol or drug use	▪ Smell of alcohol on breath ▪ Excessive use of perfumes, mouthwash, or mints ▪ Slurred speech, flushed face, reddened eyes, unsteady gait ▪ Wearing long sleeves in hot weather to cover up arms
Signs of withdrawal	▪ Tremors ▪ Restlessness ▪ Sweating ▪ Watery eyes ▪ Runny nose ▪ Stomachaches

6.2 Addictive Substances and Their Effects

Currently, in addition to collecting data on nicotine and alcohol, the federal government obtains information on 10 categories of drugs: Marijuana (including hashish), cocaine (including crack), heroin, hallucinogens, inhalants, methamphetamine, and the misuse of prescription-type pain relievers, tranquilizers, stimulants, and sedatives (CBHSQ, 2017). Following is a list that describes SUD usage taken from the *2016 National Survey on Drug Use and Health (NSDUH)* on trends in the behavioral health of people aged 12 years old or older in the civilian, noninstitutionalized population of the United States (CBHSQ, 2017).

- Alcohol is the most abused substance in the United States. There were 136.7 million current alcohol drinkers in 2016, including 65.3 million who were binge alcohol users and 16.3 million who were heavy alcohol users.
- An estimated 63.4 million people were current users of a tobacco product, including 51.3 million cigarette smokers. Across all age groups, tobacco use and cigarette use were lower in 2016 than in most years during the past decade.
- Some 28.6 million people used an illicit drug in the past 30 days, which corresponded to about 1 in 10 Americans, which was higher than usage in every year during the past decade. The increase was driven primarily by marijuana use and the nonmedical use of prescription pain relievers, such as opioids.
- Some 24 million people reported current marijuana use during the past 30 days. The percentage of people aged 12 or older who were current marijuana users in 2016 was higher than the percentages during the past decade.
- Some 6.2 million individuals (2.3%) misused prescription drugs. Prescription pain relievers were the most commonly misused drug, with 3.3 million people who misused prescription pain relievers.
- An estimated 2.0 million people (0.7%) were current nonmedical users of tranquilizers, which was a similar percentage to past years.
- About 1.9 million people aged 12 or older (0.7%) were current users of cocaine, including about 432,000 (0.2%) current users of crack. These numbers have been stable or slightly lower over the past decade.
- An estimated 1.7 million people (0.6% of the population) were current nonmedical users of stimulants.
- Several drugs are grouped under the category of hallucinogens, including LSD, PCP, peyote, mescaline, psilocybin mushrooms, "Ecstasy" (MDMA or "Molly"), ketamine, DMT/AMT/"Foxy," and Salvia divinorum. In 2016, an estimated 1.4 million people (0.5%) were current users of hallucinogens. Usage has been relatively stable, with recent increases as new substances have started to be used.
- In 2016, approximately 667,000 people (0.7%) aged 12 or older were current users of methamphetamine. Of note, most methamphetamine that is now used in the United States is produced and distributed illicitly rather than through the pharmaceutical industry.
- Inhalants include a variety of substances, such as nitrous oxide, amyl nitrite, cleaning fluids, gasoline, spray paint, computer keyboard cleaner, other aerosol sprays, felt-tip pens, and glue used to get high. In 2016, approximately 600,000 people (0.2%) were current users of inhalants.
- An estimated 497,000 people (0.2%) were current misusers of sedatives in 2016.
- About 475,000 people aged 12 or older were current heroin users in 2016, about 0.2% of the population. Despite the dangers associated with heroin, its use has increased in recent years, primarily due to decreased availability of prescribed opioids, which has caused addicted individuals to turn to heroin.

Since 2016, when this data was collected, the opioid epidemic occurred; at its peak, more than 90 Americans died each day after overdosing on opioids (NIDA, 2018). The misuse of and addiction to opioids—including prescription pain relievers, heroin, and synthetic opioids such as fentanyl—has been a serious national crisis that has affected public health as well as social and economic welfare. The Centers for Disease Control and Prevention (CDC) estimated that the total economic burden of prescription opioid misuse alone in the United States has been $78.5 billion annually, including the costs of healthcare, lost productivity, addiction treatment, and criminal justice involvement (Florence, Zhou, Luo, & Xu, 2016).

In the late 1990s, pharmaceutical companies reassured the medical community that patients would not become addicted to prescription opioid pain relievers, and healthcare providers began to prescribe them at greater rates (NIDA, 2018). This led to widespread diversion and misuse of these medications before it became clear that opioid medications were highly addictive. Opioid overdose rates began to increase. In 2015, more than 33,000 Americans died as a result of an opioid overdose, including prescription opioids, heroin, and illicitly manufactured fentanyl, a powerful synthetic opioid (NIDA, 2018). In 2016, approximately 11.8 million people (4.4%) aged 12 or older misused opioids in the past year (CBHSQ, 2017). Of concern has been the appeal of opioids to a younger population. About 891,000 adolescents aged 12 to 17 misused opioids (3.6%) during 2016; about 2.5 million young adults aged 18 to 25 (7.3% of all young adults) misused opioids in 2016 (CBHSQ, 2017).

Caffeine

Although it is not an illicit substance, **caffeine** is a stimulant that increases the heart rate and acts as a diuretic. Some 85% of the U.S. population consumes at least one caffeinated beverage per day, with caffeine intake highest among adults aged 50–64 years (Mitchell, Knight, Hockenberry, Teplansky, & Hartman, 2014). Older age groups primarily consume coffee, while carbonated soft drinks and tea provide a greater percentage of caffeine in younger adults. Although commonly consumed daily in soft drinks, coffee, tea, chocolate, and some pain relievers, an excessive amount of caffeine can cause negative physiologic effects, especially cardiac-related risks. Approximately 300 mg/day is safe for most people, but over 600 mg is considered excessive and not recommended (Potter & Moller, 2018). Individuals with a history of cardiac disease are advised to cut down or eliminate caffeine intake altogether. Caffeine, if consumed in large quantities, can also cause higher total cholesterol levels and insomnia (Schaefer & McDermott, 2016).

A caffeine-addicted person who abruptly withdraws from caffeine often experiences headaches and irritability. A rising number of adolescents are developing caffeine dependence by consuming sizable quantities of soft drinks and coffee. Also of concern with adolescents are energy drinks containing high concentrations of caffeine, which can cause adverse effects such as anxiety/nervousness, hyperactive behavior, disrupted sleep, seizures, nonventricular and ventricular dysrhythmias, and tachypnea (Seifert et al., 2013). Energy drink use has also been associated with alcohol and other substance misuse (Patrick & Maggs, 2014).

Alcohol

Alcohol is the most commonly used and abused legal substance in the United States. Alcohol and other CNS depressants act on neurotransmitters in the brain such as gamma-aminobutyric acid (GABA) (Potter & Moller, 2018). GABA is the most prevalent inhibitory neurotransmitter in the brain and has a major role in decreasing neuronal excitability. Alcohol creates an additive effect with GABA, further inhibiting arousal and depressing the autonomic nervous system. This may explain why cross-tolerance effects occur when alcohol and other CNS depressants are used in combination. When taken together, alcohol and other CNS depressants such as benzodiazepines and barbiturates can lead to respiratory depression and death (Potter & Moller, 2018).

Alcohol is the most abused substance in the United States, with slightly more than half (50.7%) of people aged 12 or older consuming alcohol. There were 136.7 million current alcohol drinkers in 2016, including 65.3 million who were binge alcohol users and 16.3 million who were heavy alcohol users (CBHSQ, 2017). Binge alcohol use is defined as drinking five or more drinks on the same occasion on at least 1 day in the past 30 days. Binge drinking for males is defined as drinking five or more drinks on the same occasion on at least 1 day in the past 30 days; binge alcohol use for females has been defined as drinking four or more drinks on the same occasion on at least 1 day in the past 30 days (CBHSQ, 2017). Heavy alcohol use is defined as binge drinking on 5 or more days in the past 30 days for males and females. Nearly half of current alcohol users reported binge alcohol use (47.8%), and one in eight current alcohol users reported heavy alcohol use (CBHSQ, 2017). There is considerable overlap among the various categories.

Although the legal drinking age in all 50 states is 21, many underage people use alcohol. By age 15, about 33% of teens have had at least one drink; by age 18, about 60% of teens have had at least one drink (NIAAA, 2017). People ages 12 through 20 drink 11% of all alcohol consumed in the United States. Although youth drink less often than adults do, when they do drink, they drink more, consuming more than 90% of their alcohol by binge drinking (NIAAA, 2017). In 2016, about 7.3 million people aged 12 to 20 reported drinking alcohol in the past month, including 4.5 million who reported binge alcohol use and 1.1 million who reported heavy alcohol use. Thus, about three-fifths of underage current drinkers (62.5%) were binge alcohol users, and about one in seven were heavy alcohol users (14.7%) (CBHSQ, 2017). Alcohol can be considered an entry point to other substance use, sometimes leading to initiation of tobacco or marijuana use (Barry et al., 2016). Nearly 140,000 alcohol-related emergency department (ED) visits were made during 2010 by patients under the age of 21 (SAMHSA, 2012). Almost one-third (31%) of those alcohol-related ED visits for minors involved other substances as well.

Alcohol is absorbed in the mouth, stomach, and digestive tract. The liver metabolizes approximately 95% of the ingested alcohol and the rest is excreted via the skin, kidney, and lungs (Wall, Luczak, & Hiller-Sturmhöfel, 2016). Generally, an individual can break down approximately 1 ounce of whiskey every 90 minutes. Factors such as body mass, food intake, and liver function can affect the rate of alcohol absorption.

When used in moderation, alcohol can have positive physiologic effects by increasing levels of desirable cholesterol (HDL) and lowering levels of bad cholesterol (LDL). Alcohol in moderation also decreases platelet aggregation, thereby decreasing coronary artery disease and protecting against stroke (Potter & Moller, 2018). However, when consumed in excess, alcohol can severely diminish one's ability to function and can ultimately lead to life-threatening conditions. Chronic use of alcohol can cause debilitating neurologic and psychiatric disorders. Damage to the liver occurs with chronic alcohol abuse and can progress from fatty liver to other liver diseases such as hepatitis or cirrhosis (NIAAA, 2015a). Chronic alcoholism is the major cause of fatal cirrhosis. Alcohol causes damaging effects to many other systems; its potential effects include myocardial disease, erosive gastritis, acute and chronic pancreatitis, sexual dysfunction, and an increased risk of breast cancer (NIDA, 2014b).

Malnutrition is another serious complication of chronic alcoholism, especially thiamine (B_1) deficiency, which can result in neurologic impairments. Thiamine depletion is thought to cause the Wernicke-Korsakoff syndrome observed in people with chronic alcoholism (Potter & Moller, 2018). Severe cognitive impairment is a principal feature of **Wernicke encephalopathy** and **Korsakoff psychosis**. Although these are sometimes considered to be two distinctive disorders, they are actually different phases of the same disease, commonly called *Wernicke-Korsakoff syndrome*. Wernicke encephalopathy indicates the acute, life-threatening stage of the illness, and Korsakoff psychosis indicates the chronic, later stage (NIDA, 2014b).

Although alcohol is a CNS depressant, it actually disrupts sleep, thus altering the sleep cycle, decreasing the quality of sleep, intensifying obstructive sleep apnea, and reducing total sleeping time. Heavy drinkers have a higher mortality rate and many fatalities occur from alcohol-related accidents (NIDA, 2014a). Blood alcohol levels (BALs) are highly predictive of CNS effects. Euphoria, reduced inhibitions, impaired judgment, and increased confidence are seen at 0.05%; the legal level of intoxication in many states is 0.08%. Toxic levels in excess of 0.5% can cause coma, respiratory depression, peripheral collapse, and death (NIAAA, 2015c; Potter & Moller, 2018). Of note, the National Academies of Science, Engineering, and Medicine (2018) recently issued a report recommending that state laws criminalizing alcohol-impaired driving lower the blood alcohol concentration (BAC) from 0.08 to 0.05%.

Chronic consumption of alcohol produces tolerance and creates cross-tolerance to general anesthetics, barbiturates, benzodiazepines, and other CNS depressants. If alcohol is withdrawn abruptly, the brain becomes overly excited because receptors previously inhibited are no longer inhibited. This hyperexcitability manifests clinically as anxiety, tachycardia, hypertension, diaphoresis, nausea and vomiting, tremors, sleeplessness, and irritability (SAMHSA, 2015a). Severe manifestations of alcohol withdrawal include seizures, convulsions, and **delirium tremens (DTs)**. Episodes of delirium tremens have a mortality rate of 1 to 5% (Schuckit, 2014).

Nicotine

Nicotine is found in tobacco and enters the system via the lungs (cigarettes and cigars) and oral mucous membranes (chewing tobacco as well as smoking). In low doses, nicotine stimulates nicotinic receptors in the brain to release norepinephrine and epinephrine, causing vasoconstriction. As a result, the heart rate accelerates and the force of ventricular contractions increases. Gastrointestinal (GI) effects include an increase in gastric acid secretion, increased tone and motility of GI smooth muscle, and promotion of vomiting. Nicotine acts on the central nervous system (CNS) as a stimulant, binding to acetylcholine receptors in the brain and causing the release of dopamine and norepinephrine (Mishra et al., 2015). This dopamine release reinforces the addictive craving for nicotine, increasing the difficulty of quitting smoking (Potter & Moller, 2018). Smoking cessation can pose a problem for hospitalized patients and individuals in the community (see the Moving Evidence into Action box).

Moving Evidence into Action

Smoking Cessation in Patients in Acute Care Settings and the Community

Clinical Issue

Despite the well-publicized deleterious health effects posed by cigarette smoking and the legally restricted access to cigarettes to minors, smoking remains a persistent problem. Smoking has been banned in stores, malls, hospitals, office buildings, college campuses, and restaurants.

External Evidence

A systematic review and meta-analysis provided evidence that brief interventions for smoking cessation have potential benefits (Aveyard, Begh, Parsons, & West, 2012). Nicotine replacement therapy (NRT) also increases quit rates with or without additional counseling. NRT aims to reduce withdrawal symptoms from tobacco products by replacing nicotine in the blood. All forms of NRT—available as chewing gum, skin patches, nose spray, inhalers, and tablets—increase the likelihood that an individual will succeed in quitting smoking (Chauhan, Dev, Desai, & Andhale, 2016). Medications such as varenicline (Chantix), nicotine receptor partial agonists, have been shown to be effective in reducing smoking (Cahill, Lindson-Hawley, Thomas, Fanshawe, & Lancaster, 2016). Moreover, research has shown that combining NRT with varenicline is more effective than the medication alone at achieving tobacco abstinence (Koegelenberg et al., 2014). Buproprion (Zyban) has also been used successfully to reduce cravings in smoking cessation (Cahill et al., 2016).

Internal Evidence

Most hospitals have a no-smoking policy. The nurse must know the organizational policy and be prepared to institute the standard of care for patients who smoke cigarettes. Familiarity with institutional standard of care for nicotine replacement therapy is especially important.

Patient Considerations

Patients will have varying physiologic and psychologic responses to lack of access to smoke while hospitalized. The nurse must enforce the no-smoking policy and approach the patient with nonjudgmental and empathetic communication to support the patient's difficulties with nicotine withdrawal. The nurse should advocate for nicotine replacement therapy for the patient if needed.

Putting the Pieces Together

Admission to the hospital provides an excellent opportunity for nurses to assist patients to quit smoking. Patients in hospitals may find it easier to quit in an environment where smoking is restricted or prohibited. In addition, individuals may be more open to cessation efforts when faced with the risks associated with surgery. Healthcare professionals, especially nurses, can be very instrumental in smoking-cessation efforts. Advising hospitalized smokers to quit and referring them to online and community resources to aid smoking cessation is an easy, cost-effective method to reduce tobacco dependence (Potter & Moller, 2018).

Effective nursing strategies include asking patients about their tobacco use, counseling those who want to quit, reinforcing cessation efforts, and early follow-up with those who quit smoking (CDC, 2016). This evidence points to the important role nurses possess to encourage their patients to quit smoking and the need for nurses to incorporate smoking-cessation interventions as part of their standard practice.

(continued)

In summary, the primary impetus for smoking cessation regardless of care setting comes from healthcare providers, such as physicians and nurses. According to the CDC (2017a), many smokers want to quit. Getting started often takes support and motivation from healthcare providers, who are willing to introduce the topic and provide information about NRT and other adjunct therapies to support smoking cessation. The CDC and partner organizations, such as the American Academy of Family Physicians (AAFP), American Association of Nurse Practitioners (AANP), American Academy of Pediatrics (AAP), and others, offer handouts and toolkits that can be used to educate and motivate patients.

References

Aveyard, P., Begh, R., Parsons, R., & West, P. (2012). Brief opportunistic smoking cessation interventions: A systematic review and meta-analysis to compare advice to quit and offer of assistance. *Addiction*, *107*(6), 1066–1073.

Cahill, K., Lindson-Hawley, N., Thomas, K. H., Fanshawe, T. R., & Lancaster, T. (2016). Nicotine receptor partial agonists for smoking cessation. *Cochrane Database of Systematic Reviews*, Issue 5, 1–151. doi: 10.1002/14651858.CD006103.pub7

Centers for Disease Control and Prevention. (2016). *Current cigarette smoking among adults in the United States.* Retrieved from https://www.cdc.gov/tobacco/data_statistics/fact_sheets/adult_data/cig_smoking/index.htm.

Centers for Disease Control and Prevention. (2017a). *Health care professionals: Help your patients quit smoking.* Retrieved from https://www.cdc.gov/tobacco/campaign/tips/partners/health/hcp/index.html.

Chauhan, P., Dev, A., Desai, S., & Andhale, V. (2016). Nicotine replacement therapy for smoking cessation. *Pharmaceutical and Biological Evaluations*, *3*(3), 305–312.

Koegelenberg, C. F., Noor, F., Bateman, E. D., van Zyl-Smit, R. N., Bruning, A., O'Brien, J. A., . . . Irusen, E. M. (2014). Efficacy of varenicline combined with nicotine replacement therapy vs varenicline alone for smoking cessation: A randomized clinical trial. *Journal of the American Medical Association*, *312*(2), 155–161.

Potter, M. L., & Moller, M. D. (Eds.). (2018). *Psychiatric-mental health nursing: From suffering to hope* (2nd ed.). Hoboken, NJ: Pearson Education.

Initially, nicotine increases respiration, mental alertness, and cognitive ability, but eventually depresses these responses (Potter & Moller, 2018). Moderate doses of nicotine can cause tremors. Tolerance can develop to nausea and dizziness, but not to the cardiovascular effects. High doses of nicotine, found in some insecticides, can cause acute poisoning, resulting in convulsions and death (National Institutes of Health, 2015).

Nicotine dependence results from chronic use with withdrawal seen as craving, nervousness, restlessness, irritability, impatience, increased hostility, insomnia, impaired concentration, increased appetite, and weight gain (Potter & Moller, 2018). Gradual reduction in nicotine use and use of nicotine replacement therapy (NRT) may help users quit using tobacco.

Chronic health problems from smoking have been well established in the form of cancer, heart disease, emphysema, hypertension, and death (Potter & Moller, 2018). Smoking is now the number-one cause of preventable death and disease among women. An estimated 15.1% of women (about 15 out of 100) in the United States are current smokers (Centers for Disease Control and Prevention [CDC], 2016). Far more women are dying of lung cancer than of breast cancer (CDC, 2017b). Women are also confronted with unique health concerns from smoking during pregnancy. Smoking during pregnancy leads to increased risks for infants such as low birth weight, stillbirth, preterm delivery, perinatal mortality, and sudden infant death syndrome (SAMHSA, 2015a). Secondhand effects from smoking have been demonstrated, especially to fetuses during pregnancy. Smoking also increases the risk for infertility. Postmenopausal women who smoke have lower bone density and higher risk for hip fracture than women who have never smoked (SAMHSA, 2015a).

Of increasing health concern is the electronic cigarette (eCig or e-cigarette), a battery-powered appliance that simulates cigarette smoking but administers nicotine through a vapor that resembles smoke (SAMHSA, 2014a). Individuals using an e-cigarette are "vaping"—not smoking, as with tobacco cigarettes. The device uses a liquid solution of nicotine and flavorings that are inhaled when the e-cigarette is used (**Figure 6.3** ■). Concerns emerged because the solutions used in vaping were unregulated until 2016 (Food and Drug Administration, 2017). E-cigarette use more than doubled among U.S. middle and high school students when e-cigarettes were introduced, increasing from 4.7% in 2011 to 10% in 2012 (SAMHSA, 2014a). A consensus report from the National Academies of Science, Engineering, and Medicine (2018) stated that "the evidence reviewed by the committee suggests that e-cigarettes are not without biological effects in humans."

Cannabis

Cannabis sativa is the source of marijuana. According to 2016 National Survey on Drug Use and Health (NSDUH) data, marijuana is the most commonly used drug with an estimated 24.0 million Americans aged 12 or older in 2016 currently using marijuana, or 8.9% of the population aged

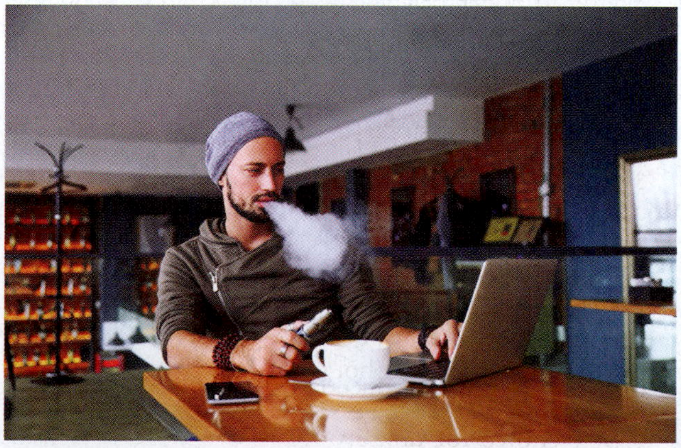

Figure 6.3 ■ While e-cigarettes are less harmful than combustible cigarettes, vaping does carry risks. Among them are the likeliness of transition to traditional smoking and an increased risk for myocardial infarction.

12 or older (CBHSQ, 2017). This percentage has steadily increased from 2002, reflecting legalization and decriminalization in some states. The greatest psychoactive substances are in the flowering tops of the cannabis plant. Marijuana (also known as *grass*, *weed*, *pot*, *dope*, *joint*, and *reefer*) and hashish are the most common derivatives (NIDA, 2015b). The psychoactive component of marijuana is an oily chemical known as delta-9-tetrahydrocannabinol (THC). THC activates specific cannabinoid receptors in the brain. Evidence suggests that marijuana may act like opioids and cocaine in producing a pleasurable sensation, probably by causing release of endogenous opioids and then dopamine (NIDA, 2015b).

The physiologic effects of cannabis are dose related and can cause an increase in heart rate and bronchodilation in short-term use. Chronic long-term use can lead to airway constriction, bronchitis, sinusitis, asthma, and increased risk for respiratory cancer (Potter & Moller, 2018). The reproductive system is also affected by marijuana; it causes decreased spermatogenesis and testosterone levels in males and suppresses follicle-stimulating, luteinizing, and prolactin hormones in females, impairing breast-feeding for new mothers. Birth defects may also be associated with cannabis use. Marijuana crosses the placental barrier and is spread to fetal tissues. When a pregnant woman smokes marijuana, she increases the risk of abnormalities in the fetus such as CNS disturbances, low birth weight, decreased length, smaller head circumference, and fetal death (NIDA, 2015b).

Subjective effects of marijuana include euphoria, sedation, and hallucinations. Chronic use of marijuana can result in amotivational behaviors such as apathy, dullness, poor grooming, reduced interest in achievement, and disinterest. At extremely high doses, tolerance and physical dependence result (Potter & Moller, 2018).

CNS Depressants

Central nervous system depressants, including barbiturates, benzodiazepines, paraldehyde, meprobamate, and chloral hydrate, are also subject to abuse. Cross-dependence exists among all CNS depressants and cross-tolerance can develop to alcohol and general anesthetics (Brust, 2014). Chronic users of barbiturates require progressively higher doses to achieve subjective effects as tolerance develops, but at greater risk of respiratory depression. The depressant effects related to barbiturates are dose dependent and range from mild sedation to sleep to coma to death. With larger doses over time and a combination of alcohol and barbiturates, the risk of death increases greatly. The risk of accidental overdose and death resulting from barbiturates has resulted in decreased prescription use, yet barbiturates are still clinically useful for seizure disorders and alcohol withdrawal (Brust, 2014).

Benzodiazepines have replaced barbiturates as the drugs of choice for anxiety-related disorders. Benzodiazepines alone are thought to be safer than barbiturates because of their more favorable efficacy and safety profile (Bhatia, Bhatia, & Kolli, 2017). However, CNS depressants when taken together (e.g., alcohol and benzodiazepines) can result in death related to respiratory depression (Potter & Moller, 2018).

Psychostimulants

Psychostimulants such as cocaine and amphetamines have a high potential for abuse (NIDA, 2017c). Euphoria is the main subjective effect associated with cocaine and amphetamines, leading to addiction. **Cocaine** powder has been snorted (inhaled through the nostrils) for thousands of years, but other methods of ingestion are also popular and potentially more dangerous. Freebased cocaine (also called *crack*) is heat stable and usually cooked in a baking soda solution and smoked (NIDA, 2016). Cocaine hydrochloride (HCl) is diluted or cut before sale, and the pure form (*rocks*) can be administered intranasally (snorted) or injected intravenously. *Skin popping*, or subcutaneous injection of cocaine, may lead to the formation of abscesses under the skin (NIDA, 2016).

Mild overdose of cocaine produces agitation, dizziness, tremor, and blurred vision. Major overdose produces anxiety, hyperpyrexia, convulsions, ventricular dysrhythmias, severe hypertension, and possible hemorrhagic stroke, angina, or myocardial infarction (MI) (Potter & Moller, 2018). The use of cocaine during pregnancy is especially problematic because the drug crosses the placenta and enters the fetal bloodstream. Spontaneous abortion, premature delivery, retardation of intrauterine growth, congenital abnormalities, and fetal addiction can result. Long-term intranasal use of cocaine can cause atrophy of the nasal mucosa, necrosis and perforation of the nasal septum, and lung damage (Potter & Moller, 2018).

With an estimated 2.6% of the U.S. population aged 13 years or older, or 6.6 million people who inject drugs (PWID) over their lifetimes, injection drug users (IDUs) in the United States are associated with increased rates of transmission of bloodborne viruses, including human immunodeficiency virus (HIV) and hepatitis C virus (Lansky et al., 2014). Infection can be traced to sharing of syringes and other injection equipment, such as cookers, cotton, or water (Broz et al., 2014). IDUs also exhibit significantly higher rates of other risky health behaviors, such as unprotected vaginal intercourse and unprotected anal sex (Broz et al., 2014). In summary, IDUs report higher rates of unsafe injection- and sex-related behaviors that non-injectors, resulting in more HIV and hepatitis B and C infections, as well as other skin and soft-tissue injuries (Broz et al., 2014).

Amphetamine use causes arousal and an elevation of mood with a sense of increased strength, mental capacity, and self-confidence, as well as a decreased need for food and sleep. These stimulant drugs, however, pose a severe health risk to society due to devastating physical and neurologic consequences, including amphetamine-induced mental disorders (Potter & Moller, 2018).

Methamphetamine, which is illegally manufactured, distributed, and abused, is a powerful stimulant drug commonly referred to as *speed*, *crystal*, *crank*, *go*, and *ice*. The manufacture of methamphetamine is a relatively simple process and can be carried out by individuals without special knowledge or expertise in chemistry (NIDA, 2017c). In 2016, approximately 667,000 people aged 12 or older were current users of methamphetamine, an estimated 0.2% of the population aged 12 or older (CBHSQ, 2017). In 2015, methamphetamine use was separated from surveillance of misuse of prescription stimulants, so meaningful data for trending is not currently available (CBHSQ, 2017). Methamphetamine is often taken in combination with other drugs such as cocaine and marijuana and, like heroin and cocaine, can be inhaled, injected, ingested, or smoked.

The highest percentage rates of methamphetamine use were found in the Midwest and West. Methamphetamine use has been linked with HIV and other bloodborne infections, likely due to injecting the drug, and high rates of STIs among both men and women (Maxwell, 2014). In one study, females reported significantly more benefits from methamphetamine use related to doing more housework, caring for the children, weight loss, relief from depression, and increased confidence, while enhanced sexual pleasure was the most significant benefit cited by males (Maxwell, 2014). The most common risks of methamphetamine use cited were in the areas of damage to the brain; mental health problems, such as anxiety, depression, and paranoia; social relationships; and problems with other aspects of their lives that resulted from drug use, including problems with social services, legal issues, and employment (Maxwell, 2014).

Methamphetamine users experience numerous physical symptoms including weight loss, tachycardia, tachypnea, hyperthermia, insomnia, and muscular tremors. The behavioral and psychiatric symptoms reported most often include violent behavior, repetitive activity, memory loss, paranoia, delusions of reference, auditory hallucinations, and confusion or fright (Potter & Moller, 2018). A psychotic state with hallucinations and paranoia is common with long-term use, requiring treatment similar to other psychotic disorders. The cardiovascular effects of amphetamines are comparable to those of cocaine, including vasoconstriction, tachycardia, hypertension, angina, and dysrhythmias. Tolerance to mood elevation, appetite suppression, and cardiovascular effects develops with amphetamines; however, dependence is more psychologic than physical (NIDA, 2017c).

Withdrawal from amphetamines produces dysphoria and craving with fatigue, prolonged sleep, excessive eating, and depression. The most effective treatments for methamphetamine addiction are currently behavioral therapies, such as cognitive-behavioral and contingency-management interventions (NIDA, 2017c). Although a large number of people cope with amphetamine and polysubstance dependence worldwide, limited evidence exists for effective pharmacologic treatment. One recent study found that among frequent methamphetamine users, oral naltrexone was associated with reductions in meth-using days (Saraiya, Campbell, & Hu, 2017); however, this is not yet standard treatment.

Opiates

Opiates such as morphine, codeine, hydrocodone, and oxycodone are narcotic analgesics. Examples of some common brand names include Vicodin, Percocet, and OxyContin. Narcotic analgesics are a type of pain reliever derived from natural or synthetic opiates. Many individuals were originally exposed to opiates in the context of prescription pain management; however, others use opiates under social or illicit circumstances. Opioid misuse (taking a legal prescription medication for a purpose other than the reason it was prescribed) has spread into the more rural areas of the South and Midwest, with overdose deaths occurring primarily among White, non-Hispanic men and women (Rudd, 2016). Misuse and use disorders were most commonly reported in adults who were uninsured, were unemployed, had low income, or had behavioral health problems (Han et al., 2017). However, opiates are used and abused by people of all socioeconomic statuses.

The problem of abuse of and addiction to prescribed narcotics is a major issue for the United States. In 2016, there were 11.8 million past-year opioid misusers aged 12 or older in the United States, the vast majority of whom misused prescription pain relievers (CBHSQ, 2017). This represented 4.4% of the population aged 12 or older. About 891,000 adolescents aged 12 to 17 misused opioids in the past year. About 2.5 million young adults aged 18 to 25 misused opioids in the past year, which corresponded to about 7.3% of young adults. An estimated 8.4 million adults aged 26 or older misused opioids in the past year, which represented 4.0% of this age group (CBHSQ, 2017).

The prevalence of prescription opiate abuse seems to reflect, in part, changes in medication prescribing practices, changes in drug formulations, and fairly easy access via the internet or from family and friends. More than half of persons abusing pain relievers reported that they did not have a prescription for the drug and the source of the drug was from a friend or relative for free (Han et al., 2017). More than 60% reported that they misused opioids to relieve physical pain (Han et al., 2017).

The most frequent opiates included methadone, oxycodone and its extended-release forms, and combination forms (e.g., hydrocodone with acetaminophen). In 2016, the CDC issued new guidelines for prescribing opioid medications for chronic pain to guide primary care providers to ensure safe and effective treatment for patients (Dowell, Haegerich, & Chou, 2016). Despite government interventions to curtail prescriptions of opioids, drug overdose deaths primarily due to opioids in 2016 exceeded 59,000, the largest annual jump ever recorded in the United States (Katz, 2017).

When denied prescription opioids, abusers have turned to an influx of illicitly manufactured fentanyl and similar drugs. The most deadly of the fentanyl analogues is carfentanil, a large animal tranquilizer 5,000 times stronger than heroin. Strength and quality of illicit opioids is uneven. For example, on the day that carfentanil hit the streets of Akron, Ohio, 17 people overdosed and one person died in a span of 9 hours; over the next 6 months there, 140 overdose deaths occurred of people testing positive for carfentanil (Katz, 2017). Drug overdoses from prescription opioids and illicit drugs are now the leading cause of death among Americans under age 50 (Katz, 2017).

Heroin, despite the dangers associated with it, has increased in use in recent years (CBHSQ, 2017). A highly addictive opioid that is illegal and has no accepted medical use in the United States, heroin has been abused for many centuries. It is usually administered intravenously. It induces a rush or *kick* that lasts less than a minute, followed by a sense of euphoria lasting several hours. Tolerance develops to the euphoria, respiratory depression, and nausea but not to constipation and miosis (excessive constriction of the pupil of the eye).

Physical dependence occurs with long-term use of opiates. Initial withdrawal symptoms such as drug craving, lacrimation, rhinorrhea, yawning, and diaphoresis usually take 10 days to run their course. The second phase of opiate withdrawal lasts for months, with insomnia, irritability, fatigue, and potential problems of GI hyperactivity and premature ejaculation (Potter & Moller, 2018). Methadone is a synthetic opiate used to treat chronic pain and addiction to other opiates. Methadone often enables patients to function productively while managing recovery and is a viable support for withdrawal (SAMHSA, 2015a).

Hallucinogens

Hallucinogens are also called *psychedelics* and include LSD (D-lysergic acid diethylamide), PCP (phencyclidine), peyote, mescaline, psilocybin mushrooms, "Ecstasy" (3,4-methylenedioxymethamphetamine; also known as *MDMA* or *Molly*), ketamine, DMT/AMT/Foxy (dimethyltryptamine) and *Salvia divinorum* (CBHSQ, 2017). Psychedelics bring on the same types of thoughts, perceptions, and feelings that occur in dreams. They are commonly divided into two broad categories: Classic hallucinogens (such as LSD) and dissociative drugs (such as PCP). When under the influence of either type of drug, people often report rapid, intense emotional swings and seeing images, hearing sounds, and feeling sensations that seem real but are not (NIDA, 2015a).

PCP (also called *angel dust*, *peace pill*, *ozone*, *rocket fuel*, *love boat*, *hog*, *embalming fluid*, or *superweed*) was developed in the 1950s as an anesthetic similar to ketamine, an often-abused medication used primarily during anesthesia. However, due to severe adverse effects its development for human use was discontinued. PCP is known for inducing violent behavior and negative physical reactions such as seizures, coma, and death. The most common route of administration is smoking tobacco, marijuana, or herbal cigarettes laced with PCP powder or the liquid form of PCP (NIDA, 2015a).

MDMA, commonly known as *Ecstasy* or *X*, was popular in the 1980s as a recreational drug associated with dance clubs and has reappeared in recent years as a date rape drug. In 2014, more than 17 million persons aged 12 or older reported using MDMA at least once in their lifetime (CBHSQ, 2015). MDMA is predominantly used by males between the ages of 18 and 25; most use typically begins at 21 years of age (NIDA, 2017d). Parties where other drugs such as marijuana or alcohol are present may lead to easier access or availability of Ecstasy, thereby increasing the chances for first-time Ecstasy use.

LSD, also known as *acid*, *blotter*, *doses*, *hits*, *microdots*, *sugar cubes*, *trips*, *tabs*, or *window panes*, was first used to simulate psychosis. It affects serotonin receptors at multiple sites in the brain and spinal cord. LSD, a clear or white, odorless, water-soluble material, is usually taken orally but can be injected or smoked in tobacco or marijuana cigarettes laced with LSD (NIDA, 2015a). An individual's response to a trip (the experience of being high on LSD) cannot be predicted and psychologic effects and flashbacks are common. Serotonin imbalance is thought to affect impulse control (Preller et al., 2017). LSD does adversely affect impulse control, with users reporting subjective well-being, happiness, closeness to others, openness, and trust (Schmid et al., 2015). Other hallucinogens are similar to LSD but with different potency and course of action. Because physical dependence to hallucinogens does not appear to occur, withdrawal symptoms are not present (Potter & Moller, 2018).

Inhalants

Inhalants, also known as *bold* (nitrites), *laughing gas* (nitrous oxide), *climax*, *locker room*, *poppers* (amyl nitrite and butyl nitrite), *rush* (nitrites), *snappers* (amyl nitrite), and *whippets* (fluorinated hydrocarbons), are categorized as solvents, aerosols, gases, or nitrites (NIDA, 2017b). Inhalants are often products easily bought and found in the home or workplace—such as spray paints, markers, glues, and cleaning fluid—-that have psychoactive properties when inhaled. Abusers may sniff or snort fumes from a container or dispenser (such as a glue bottle or a marking pen); spray aerosols (such as computer cleaning dusters) directly into the nose or mouth; *huff* from a chemical-soaked rag in the mouth; sniff or inhale fumes from chemicals sprayed or put inside a plastic or paper bag (*bagging*); or inhale from balloons filled with nitrous oxide, often called *laughing gas* (NIDA, 2017b).

Nitrous oxide (laughing gas) and ether are the most abused anesthetics. Amyl nitrite, butyl nitrite, and isobutyl nitrite are volatile nitrites used especially during sex to stimulate muscle relaxation and venous dilation, prolong erections, and increase libido (Zhang et al., 2016). Amyl nitrite is manufactured for medical use, but butyl and isobutyl nitrites are sold for recreational use. Long-term effects of inhalant use may include liver and kidney damage, hearing loss, bone marrow damage, loss of coordination and limb spasms from nerve damage, delayed behavioral development and brain damage from restricted oxygen flow to the brain (NIDA, 2017b).

Of particular concern is the use of a wide assortment of organic solvents that are available to and inhaled by young children. Organic solvents are often ingested by bagging, huffing, or sniffing. Common organic solvents are toluene, gasoline, lighter fluid, paint thinner, nail polish remover, benzene, acetone, chloroform, and model airplane glue. The effects from inhaling organic solvents produce a high and prolonged use can lead to increased risk for abusing other substances. Sniffing can cause the heart to stop within minutes, known as sudden sniffing death (NIDA, 2017b). The use of inhalants with a paper or plastic bag or in a closed area may cause death from suffocation.

6.3 Care of Patients with Substance Abuse Problems

Interprofessional Care

Effective treatment of substance abuse and dependence results from the efforts of an interprofessional team specializing in the treatment of psychiatric and substance abuse disorders. The interprofessional team often includes the nurse, physicians such as psychiatrists and addictionologists, psychologists, case managers, social workers, recreational therapists, and dietitians, among others. Substance dependency treatment occurs in two major phases: Acute and rehabilitation. Therapies may include detoxification, aversion therapy to maintain abstinence, group and/or individual psychotherapy, psychotropic medications, medication-assisted treatment (MAT), cognitive-behavioral strategies, family counseling, and self-help groups. Patients with substance abuse can be treated in either inpatient or outpatient settings.

Emergency Care

A substance overdose is a life-threatening condition that requires emergency treatment. The care of a patient who has overdosed on any substance is a serious medical emergency. A recent focus of harm reduction has been providing naloxone (Narcan), an opioid antagonist that can be used by police and emergency medical technicians (EMTs) in the field as well as by laypersons to reverse the effects of opioid overdose and reduce deaths. These opioid reversal devices are discussed in more detail later in this chapter; they are available for purchase over the counter and many have been distributed free of charge by advocacy groups (SAMHSA, 2015b). Respiratory depression may require mechanical ventilation. If overdose is not reversed in the field, the patient may become severely sedated and difficult to arouse (Potter & Moller, 2018). Every effort must be made to keep the patient awake; however, stupor and coma may often result. A seizure is another serious complication that requires emergency treatment. If the overdose was intentional, the patient must be constantly monitored for further signs of suicidal ideation. Never leave an actively suicidal patient alone.

SAFETY ALERT: There is an emerging practice of training healthcare providers to administer naloxone (Narcan) in community-based settings. Off-duty healthcare providers can carry doses of naloxone that can be administered if a drug-overdose situation is encountered outside of the healthcare setting. ■

Diagnostic Tests

Diagnostic tests can provide valuable information about the patient's physical condition and help determine the course for treatment.

The body fluids most often tested for drug content are blood and urine, although saliva, perspiration, and hair can be tested. The simplest method of detecting blood alcohol content is to use a Breathalyzer. Urine drug screens (UDSs) and/or blood alcohol levels (BALs) are the main biologic measures for assessment purposes (Potter & Moller, 2018).

Urine drug screening is noninvasive and the preferred method for detecting substances in the body. The length of time that drugs can be found in blood and urine varies according to dosage and metabolic properties of the drug. All traces of the drug may disappear within 24 hours or may still be detectable 30 days later. The psychoactive substance found in marijuana, THC, is stored in fatty tissues (especially the brain and reproductive system) and can be detected in the body for up to 6 weeks (Potter & Moller, 2018).

Knowledge of an individual's BAL is helpful to determine level of intoxication, level of tolerance, and whether the person accurately reported recent drinking. At 0.10% (after five to six drinks in 1 to 2 hours), voluntary motor action becomes clumsy and reaction time is impaired. The degree of impairment varies with gender, weight, and food ingestion. Small women who drink alcohol on an empty stomach will experience intoxication more rapidly than large males who have eaten a full meal. At 0.20% (after 10 to 12 drinks in 2 to 4 hours), function of the motor area in the brain is depressed, causing staggering and ataxia (Potter & Moller, 2018). A level above 0.10% without associated behavioral symptoms indicates the presence of tolerance. A BAL greater than 0.08% is considered legal intoxication in most states. High tolerance is a sign of physical dependence. Assessing for withdrawal symptoms is important when the BAL is high.

Treatment for Withdrawal

The patient who is intoxicated on entry into the hospital or treatment center requires **detoxification**, or removal of the substance from the body. The withdrawal syndrome also begins acutely, necessitating support by the interprofessional team.

Withdrawal symptoms from opiates and stimulants can be very unpleasant but are generally not life-threatening. The patient experiencing an acute phase of cocaine withdrawal may become suicidal.

Alcohol and CNS depressants such as benzodiazepines and barbiturates share a similar withdrawal syndrome. Manifestations of withdrawal syndrome include tremor, agitation, and anxiety, along with excessive autonomic nervous system activity: Tachycardia, a rapid respiratory rate, hyperthermia, and insomnia (Potter & Moller, 2018). Early signs of withdrawal appear within a few hours following cessation of the drug, peak after 24 to 48 hours, and then rapidly improve. Patients who have used higher quantities of alcohol, those who have abused additional drugs, and those with chronic diseases may experience a withdrawal seizure or *delirium tremens (DTs)* (Schuckit, 2014). Delirium tremens is a medical emergency that usually occurs 2 to 5 days following alcohol withdrawal and persists 2 to 3 days. Patients with DTs experience disorientation, paranoid delusions, visual hallucinations, and marked withdrawal symptoms.

In managing alcohol withdrawal, the goal is to minimize adverse outcomes, such as injury, seizures, delirium, and mortality. The patient is assessed for gastrointestinal bleeding, liver failure, cardiac dysrhythmias, glucose, and fluid and electrolyte imbalances (SAMHSA, 2015a).

Nutrition is assessed, and multiple B vitamins are administered orally. Thiamine (vitamin B_1) supplements are continued for a week or longer to prevent Wernicke's encephalopathy (SAMHSA, 2015a). Signs of overdose and withdrawal from major substances are summarized in **Table 6.3** along with recommended treatments.

Table 6.3 Signs and Treatment of Overdose and Withdrawal

Drug	Overdose		Withdrawal	
	Manifestations	Treatment	Manifestations	Treatment
CNS Depressants Alcohol Barbiturates Benzodiazepines	Cardiovascular or respiratory depression or arrest (mostly with barbiturates) Coma Shock Convulsions Death	Frequent VS and cardiorespiratory assessment ***If awake:*** Keep awake Induce vomiting Activated charcoal to absorb drug ***Coma:*** Clear airway, intubate IV fluids Gastric lavage Seizure precautions Possible hemo- or peritoneal dialysis	Nausea and vomiting Tachycardia Diaphoresis Anxiety or agitation Tremors Marked insomnia Grand mal seizures Delirium (after 5–15 years of heavy use)	Carefully titrated detoxification with indicated medication (if applicable) or gradual reduction of dose (benzodiazepines)
Stimulants Cocaine-crack Amphetamines	Respiratory distress Ataxia Hyperpyrexia Convulsions Coma Stroke Myocardial infarction (MI) Death	Medication management for 1. Hyperpyrexia 2. Convulsions 3. Respiratory distress 4. Hypertension 5. Dysrhythmias	Fatigue Depression Suicidal thoughts Agitation Apathy Anxiety Sleep disorders Disorientation Lethargy Craving	Antidepressants (if indicated) Medications for symptom relief
Opiates Heroin Morphine Methadone	Pupillary constriction Bradycardia Respiratory depression/arrest Coma Shock Convulsions Death	Narcotic antagonist (naloxone [Narcan]) quickly reverses CNS depression	Yawning, insomnia Irritability Rhinorrhea Panic Diaphoresis Cramps Nausea and vomiting Muscle aches Chills and fever Lacrimation Diarrhea	Methadone tapering Clonidine-naltrexone detoxification Buprenorphine substitution
Hallucinogens Lysergic acid diethylamide (LSD)	Panic episode Psychosis Brain damage	Low stimuli with minimal light, sound, activity Have one person "talk down patient," reassure Speak slowly and clearly Diazepam for anxiety	No pattern of withdrawal	
Phencyclidine piperidine (PCP)	Agitation Possible hypertensive crisis Respiratory arrest Hyperthermia Seizures Encephalopathy and coma	Gastric lavage Acidify urine to help excrete drug Minimal stimulus Do *not* attempt to talk down, speak slowly in low voice Diazepam or haloperidol (Haldol)		
Inhalants Volatile solvents such as butane, paint thinner, airplane glue, or nail polish remover	***Intoxication:*** Excitation Drowsiness Disinhibition Staggering Light-headedness Agitation ***Adverse effects:*** Damage to nervous system Death	Support affected systems	No pattern of withdrawal	
Nitrates	Enhance sexual pleasure	Neurologic symptoms may respond to vitamin B_{12} and folate		
Anesthetics such as nitrous oxide	Giggling, laughter Euphoria	Chronic users may experience polyneuropathy and myelopathy		

Medications

Close monitoring is essential to ensure protection of the patient. Critical care monitoring may be indicated to manage alcohol withdrawal delirium, particularly when very high doses of benzodiazepines are needed or when there are significant concurrent medical conditions. In addition to thiamine and multivitamins, benzodiazepines are used to manage symptoms associated with alcohol withdrawal and prevent serious adverse effects, such as seizures and aggressive behavior. The dosing needed to control agitation and insomnia can vary sharply among patients and can be unusually high (Schuckit, 2014). Antipsychotic medications such as haloperidol (Haldol) may be used for severe agitation or hallucinations, although they can prolong the QT interval and increase the likelihood of seizures (Schuckit, 2014). Alternative depressive-type drugs may also be used for uncomplicated withdrawal, including phenobarbital, clomethiazole, midazolam, carbamazepine, and oxcarbazepine (Schuckit, 2014). Common drugs used in the treatment of substance abuse and withdrawal are presented in **Table 6.4**.

SAFETY ALERT: Medications given to help manage craving symptoms post-withdrawal from alcohol are usually not started until the patient has completed detoxification or until the BAL is below a set norm (usually below 0.10%). The BAL may be repeated several times,

Table 6.4 Drugs Used in the Treatment of Substance Withdrawal/Abuse

Drug	Dose	Purpose
Benzodiazepines		
chlordiazepoxide (Librium) diazepam (Valium) lorazepam (Ativan) oxazepam (Serax)	50–100 mg 4–40 mg 2–6 mg 30–120 mg	Diminishes anxiety and has anticonvulsant qualities to provide safe withdrawal. May be ordered q4h or prn to manage adverse effects from withdrawal; then dose is tapered to zero.
Vitamins		
folic acid multivitamins thiamine (Vitamin B_1)	1 mg/day 1 tab/cap daily 100 mg/day*	Corrects vitamin deficiency caused by heavy long-term alcohol abuse. Prevents Wernicke's encephalopathy.
Anticonvulsants		
magnesium sulfate phenobarbital	1 g q6h 30–320 mg	Reduces postwithdrawal seizures. For seizure control and sedation.
Abstinence Medications		
acamprosate (Campral) buprenorphine/naloxone (Suboxone) disulfiram (Antabuse) methadone naltrexone (ReVia)	333–666 mg/tid 4/1–24/6 mg/day 125–500 mg/day 20–120 mg/day 50–150 mg/day	Diminishes cravings for alcohol. Blocks craving for opioids. Prevents breakdown of alcohol. Blocks craving for heroin. Diminishes cravings for alcohol and opioids.
Antidepressants		
fluoxetine (Prozac) sertraline (Zoloft)	20–80 mg/day 50–200 mg/day	Enhances and stabilizes mood and diminishes anxiety.
Antihypertensive		
clonidine	0.1–1.2 mg/day	Extensive off-label usage for treating withdrawal symptoms of heroin, methadone, and other opiates; relieves anxiety, agitation, elevated blood pressure, tachycardia, and tremor
Nicotine Replacement and Adjunct Therapy		
buproprion (Zyban)	150 mg PO daily, titrating up to 150 mg BID for 7–12 weeks	Selectively inhibits neuronal reuptake of dopamine Do not use in clients with eating disorders or seizure disorders; can cause seizures. *Has been associated with increased risk of suicidal behaviors in children adolescents, and young adults.*
NRT (gum, lozenges, inhalers, spray, transdermal patches)	Varies; patient should follow directions; often doses are reduced as patient proceeds through program	Ganglionic cholinergic receptor antagonists that have stimulant and depressant effects on peripheral and central nervous systems Contraindicated for patients with recent myocardial infarctions, life-threatening arrhythmias, temporomandibular joint disease, severe angina, and women with childbearing potential (should use contraception while using) Transient redness, itching, or burning is common with transdermal patches; caution patient to remove patch before placing a new one.
varenicline (Chantix)	0.5 mg/day PO, titrating up to 1 mg BID for 12 weeks; regimen may be repeated once	Partial agonist at nicotinic acetylcholine receptors, the sites responsible for the dopamine effects of nicotine *Can cause suicidal ideation.* Should not be used with chronic depression, renal impairment (adjust dosing), in older adults, or during pregnancy.

Note: Medications identified in blue are among the 200 most frequently prescribed drugs in the United States.

*Doses can go much higher when treatment is initiated, as high as 1000 mg/day for 3 days.

Sources: Data from Kampman & Jarvis, 2015; SAMHSA, 2015a, 2015b; Wilson, Shannon, & Shields, 2017.

several hours apart, to determine the body's metabolism of alcohol and when it is safe to give the patient medication to minimize the withdrawal symptoms. These medications include the opioid antagonist naltrexone (Revia, oral; Vivitrol, IV); disulfiram (Antabuse), which causes an aversive reaction if alcohol is consumed; and acamprosate (Campral). ■

Reducing fragmentation between different parts of the fragmented mental health system is a key priority for improving mental health outcomes. One of the largest problems is the disconnection of mental healthcare from the rest of the system (Das, Naylor, & Majeed, 2016). While mental health problems are very common in the community, the majority of adults with mental health problems are supported largely or exclusively by primary care providers (Hunter, Goodie, Oordt, & Dobmeyer, 2017). Mental health problems often coexist with physical health comorbidities, and many long-term conditions are also linked to anxiety, depression, or other mental health problems. In addition to diagnosable mental health problems coupled with complex physical comorbidities, the patients often also have challenging social circumstances, such as unemployment, poor housing, and substance abuse disorders (Das et al., 2016).

One of the answers is co-location (into the same or nearby office) for primary care providers, behavioral health providers, psychologists, and other support staff, such as social workers and case managers (Miller, Petterson, Burke, Phillips, & Green, 2014). Children and adolescents are a particularly underserved population, and integration of medical-behavioral primary care is essential to improve youth behavioral health outcomes (Asarnow, Rozenman, Wiblin, & Zeltzer, 2015). Many medical organizations have incorporated behavioral health services into the Patient-Centered Medical Home (PCMH), an evolving approach to providing comprehensive primary care for patients who need mental health care, substance abuse care, and health behavior change, as well as attention to family and other psychosocial factors (Baird et al., 2014). In this model, every patient in the PCMH has a personal physician who knows the patient's situation and biography and who is committed to the well-being of each patient, accepting responsibility for appropriate care (Baird et al., 2014).

Uniting behavioral health patients into a PCMH to integrate care has been difficult because nearly one in five U.S. residents lives in a rural area (SAMHSA, 2016c). Individuals living in rural locations experience mental and substance use disorders at rates that are similar to (and sometimes higher than) those of their urban counterparts. One answer to providing care to isolated individuals has been telehealth, using internet and communications technologies, such as videoconferencing, chat, and text messaging, to provide health information and treatments in real time. Telehealth also includes exchanging information and delivering services asynchronously, such as through secure email, webinars, or "store-and-forward" practices and by videotaping a client encounter and forwarding the video to a professional who is offsite, for analysis at a later time (SAMHSA, 2016c). As access to telehealth increases, the potential for improved treatment and treatment outcomes for behavioral health issues and substance abuse increases for rural patients.

Nursing Care

Assessment

A comprehensive approach to the assessment of substance use is essential to ensure adequate and appropriate intervention. Use therapeutic communication techniques to establish trust prior to the assessment process (Potter & Moller, 2018). Questions should be asked in a nonthreatening, matter-of-fact manner, phrased so as not to imply wrongdoing. For instance, a nonthreatening question such as "How much alcohol do you drink?" is preferable to the judgmental question "You don't drink too much alcohol, do you?" Open-ended questions that elicit more than a simple yes or no answer help to determine the direction of future counseling (Potter & Moller, 2018). Examples of open-ended questions include:

- "On average, how many days per week do you drink alcohol or use drugs?"
- "On a typical day when you use drugs or alcohol, how many hits or drinks do you have?"
- "What is the greatest number of drinks you have had at any one time during the past month?"
- "What drug(s) did you take before coming to the hospital or clinic?"
- "How long have you been using the substances?"
- "How often and how much do you usually use?"
- "What kinds of problems has substance use caused for you, your family, friends, finances, and health?"

A brief overview of the patient's current mental status is also significant. Again, questions should be open-ended, matter of fact, and not judgmental (Potter & Moller, 2018).

- "Is there a history of abuse (physical or sexual) or violence in your family?"
- "Have you ever tried to commit suicide?"
- "Are you currently having suicidal or homicidal ideation?"

Three important areas to assess are a history of the patient's past substance use, medical and psychiatric history, and the presence of psychosocial concerns.

Substance Use History. A thorough history of the patient's substance use is important to ascertain the possibility of tolerance, physical dependence, or withdrawal syndrome. The questions above are helpful in eliciting a pattern of substance use behavior (Potter & Moller, 2018) as well as detect polysubstance abuse.

Substance abuse in older adults is likely to increase over subsequent decades as baby boomers reach retirement age. People of any age can have substance abuse problems, but the consequences in older adults can be more critical (Kuerbis, Sacco, Blazer, & Moore, 2014). Falls and accidents can rob older adults of their independence, and substance abuse increases the risk of falls by affecting alertness, judgment, coordination, and reaction time. In addition, older adults (especially older women) are just as likely as younger people to use prescription or OTC medicines, especially opiates, which can be harmful when mixed with alcohol and/

or illicit drugs (West, Severtson, Green, & Dart, 2015). Alcohol and drug abuse can also make certain medical problems hard to diagnose, for example, by dulling a pain sensation that might warn of a heart attack.

Substance abuse and dependence is less likely to be recognized and can be difficult to detect in older adults because many of the symptoms of abuse (e.g., insomnia, depression, loss of memory, anxiety, musculoskeletal pain) may be confused with conditions commonly seen in older patients (West et al., 2015). Healthcare professionals frequently attribute these symptoms to the aging process and fail to address the misuse and abuse of substances. Often, the symptoms of substance abuse are treated rather than confronting the abuse itself. Alcohol negatively interacts with the natural aging process to increase risks for injuries, hypertension, cardiac dysrhythmias, cancers, gastrointestinal problems, cognitive deficits, bone loss, and emotional challenges such as depression in older adults (Potter & Moller, 2018). Because depression and alcohol abuse often accompany the grief and losses that occur for many older adults, nurses should routinely screen older adults for both substance abuse and mental disorders (Potter & Moller, 2018).

Medical and Psychiatric History. The patient's medical history is an important area for assessment and should include the existence of any concomitant physical or mental condition (e.g., HIV, hepatitis, cirrhosis, esophageal varices, pancreatitis, gastritis, Wernicke-Korsakoff syndrome, depression, schizophrenia, anxiety, or personality disorder) (SAMHSA, 2015a). Ask about prescribed and OTC medications as well as any allergies or sensitivity to drugs. A brief overview of the patient's current mental status is also significant (Potter & Moller, 2018).

Psychosocial Issues. Information about the patient's level of stress and other psychosocial concerns can help in the assessment of substance use problems. Some questions to ask patients might include:

- "Has substance use affected your ability to hold a job?"
- "Has substance use affected relationships with your spouse, family, friends, or coworkers?"
- "How do you usually cope with stress?"
- "Do you have a support system that helps in times of need?"
- "How do you spend your leisure time?"

Screening Tools. Several screening tools may help the nurse determine the degree of severity of substance abuse or dependence. These screening tools provide a nonjudgmental, brief, and easy method to ascertain patterns of substance abuse behaviors:

- *The Michigan Alcohol Screening Test (MAST) Brief Version* (Pokorny, Miller, & Kaplan, 1972) is a 10-question, dichotomous, self-administered questionnaire that takes 10 to 15 minutes to complete. An answer of yes to three or more questions indicates a potentially dangerous pattern of alcohol abuse.
- *The* **CAGE** *questionnaire* (Ewing, 1984) is more useful than the MAST when the patient may not recognize he or she has an alcohol problem or is uncomfortable acknowledging it. This questionnaire is designed to be a self-report of drinking behavior or may be administered by a professional. One affirmative response indicates the need for further discussion and follow-up. Two or more yes answers signify a problem with alcohol that may require treatment.

  Have you ever felt you should **C**ut down on your drinking?
  Have people **A**nnoyed you by criticizing your drinking?
  Have you ever felt bad or **G**uilty about your drinking?
  Have you ever had a drink first thing in the morning (an "**E**ye-opener") to steady your nerves or to get rid of a hangover?

- *The Brief Drug Abuse Screening Test (B-DAST)* (Skinner, 1982) is a yes/no self-administered questionnaire that is useful in identifying people who are possibly addicted to drugs other than alcohol. A positive response to one or more questions suggests significant drug abuse problems and warrants further evaluation. Because self-report tools are not always answered truthfully, all patients who screen positive for drug addiction should be evaluated according to other diagnostic criteria.

Physical Assessment. Focused physical assessment of the patient with substance abuse includes level of consciousness; orientation to time, place, and person; and mental status. Observe the patient's apparent general health (height and weight, balance, gait, skin color and condition, hair and nails), nutritional status, and for evidence of recent or past trauma. Obtain vital signs, including orthostatic vital signs, and blood glucose. Assess skin turgor and for presence of edema (Potter & Moller, 2018).

Withdrawal Assessment Tools. Nurses working in medical-surgical units, psychiatric units, and special substance abuse units routinely care for patients experiencing acute alcohol or opiate withdrawal. Several assessment tools are available to determine the severity of withdrawal symptoms and indicate the need for pharmacologic treatment to manage withdrawal symptoms. A symptom-triggered approach to the administration of benzodiazepines during alcohol withdrawal results in less total medication use and requires a shorter duration of treatment (Potter & Moller, 2018). Examples of withdrawal assessment tools include:

- *The Clinical Institute Withdrawal Assessment of Alcohol—Revised (CIWA-Ar)* (Sullivan et al., 1989) (**Figure 6.4** ■) is used widely in clinical and research settings for initial assessment and ongoing monitoring of alcohol withdrawal signs and symptoms (Keys, 2011). The CIWA-Ar scale is a validated 10-item assessment tool that can be used to monitor and medicate patients going through alcohol withdrawal. The CIWA-Ar assesses for several alcohol withdrawal symptoms (e.g., high blood pressure, rapid pulse and respirations, tremors, insomnia, irritability, sweating, and convulsions) and results in a score that is used to direct the administration of benzodiazepines or other drugs to relieve associated symptoms

Clinical Institute Withdrawal Assessment of Alcohol Scale, Revised (CIWA-Ar)

Patient:____________________ **Date:** ________________ **Time:** ____________ (24 hour clock, midnight = 00:00)

Pulse or heart rate, taken for one minute:____________________ **Blood pressure:**______

NAUSEA AND VOMITING -- Ask "Do you feel sick to your stomach? Have you vomited?" Observation.
0 no nausea and no vomiting
1 mild nausea with no vomiting
2
3
4 intermittent nausea with dry heaves
5
6
7 constant nausea, frequent dry heaves and vomiting

TREMOR -- Arms extended and fingers spread apart. Observation.
0 no tremor
1 not visible, but can be felt fingertip to fingertip
2
3
4 moderate, with patient's arms extended
5
6
7 severe, even with arms not extended

PAROXYSMAL SWEATS -- Observation.
0 no sweat visible
1 barely perceptible sweating, palms moist
2
3
4 beads of sweat obvious on forehead
5
6
7 drenching sweats

ANXIETY -- Ask "Do you feel nervous?" Observation.
0 no anxiety, at ease
1 mild anxious
2
3
4 moderately anxious, or guarded, so anxiety is inferred
5
6
7 equivalent to acute panic states as seen in severe delirium or acute schizophrenic reactions

AGITATION -- Observation.
0 normal activity
1 somewhat more than normal activity
2
3
4 moderately fidgety and restless
5
6
7 paces back and forth during most of the interview, or constantly thrashes about

TACTILE DISTURBANCES -- Ask "Have you any itching, pins and needles sensations, any burning, any numbness, or do you feel bugs crawling on or under your skin?" Observation.
0 none
1 very mild itching, pins and needles, burning or numbness
2 mild itching, pins and needles, burning or numbness
3 moderate itching, pins and needles, burning or numbness
4 moderately severe hallucinations
5 severe hallucinations
6 extremely severe hallucinations
7 continuous hallucinations

AUDITORY DISTURBANCES -- Ask "Are you more aware of sounds around you? Are they harsh? Do they frighten you? Are you hearing anything that is disturbing to you? Are you hearing things you know are not there?" Observation.
0 not present
1 very mild harshness or ability to frighten
2 mild harshness or ability to frighten
3 moderate harshness or ability to frighten
4 moderately severe hallucinations
5 severe hallucinations
6 extremely severe hallucinations
7 continuous hallucinations

VISUAL DISTURBANCES -- Ask "Does the light appear to be too bright? Is its color different? Does it hurt your eyes? Are you seeing anything that is disturbing to you? Are you seeing things you know are not there?" Observation.
0 not present
1 very mild sensitivity
2 mild sensitivity
3 moderate sensitivity
4 moderately severe hallucinations
5 severe hallucinations
6 extremely severe hallucinations
7 continuous hallucinations

HEADACHE, FULLNESS IN HEAD -- Ask "Does your head feel different? Does it feel like there is a band around your head?" Do not rate for dizziness or lightheadedness. Otherwise, rate severity.
0 not present
1 very mild
2 mild
3 moderate
4 moderately severe
5 severe
6 very severe
7 extremely severe

ORIENTATION AND CLOUDING OF SENSORIUM -- Ask "What day is this? Where are you? Who am I?"
0 oriented and can do serial additions
1 cannot do serial additions or is uncertain about date
2 disoriented for date by no more than 2 calendar days
3 disoriented for date by more than 2 calendar days
4 disoriented for place/or person

Total **CIWA-Ar** Score ______
Rater's Initials ______
Maximum Possible Score 67

*The **CIWA-Ar** is not* copyrighted and may be reproduced freely. This assessment for monitoring withdrawal symptoms requires approximately 5 minutes to administer. The maximum score is 67 (see instrument). Patients scoring less than 10 do not usually need additional medication for withdrawal.

Source: From Sullivan, J. T., Sykora, K., Schneiderman, J., Naranjo, C. A., and Sellers, E. M. Assessment of alcohol withdrawal: The revised Clinical Institute Withdrawal Assessment for Alcohol scale (**CIWA-Ar**). *British Journal of Addiction 84*:1353–1357, 1989.

Figure 6.4 ■ Assessment tool for alcohol withdrawal.

of withdrawal and prevent seizures. A score of 8 points or fewer corresponds to mild withdrawal symptoms. Scores of 9 to 15 points indicate moderate withdrawal, while a score of 16 or greater denotes severe withdrawal and an increased risk of delirium tremens and seizures.

- *The Clinical Opiate Withdrawal Scale (COWS)* (Wesson & Ling, 2003) rates 11 common signs or symptoms of opiate withdrawal. The summed total score of the 11 items can be used to assess the intensity of opiate withdrawal and determine the extent of a patient's physical dependence on opioids. A score of less than 12 on the COWS indicates mild or no opiate withdrawal symptoms, whereas a score of 13 or more indicates moderate to severe withdrawal symptoms.

Diagnoses, Interventions, and Outcomes

The primary nursing diagnoses, outcomes, and interventions for patients with substance abuse problems are listed in this section. Implications for nursing care in acute and home care settings are combined in this discussion (Potter & Moller, 2018). See the Case Study & Nursing Care Plan on page 146 for the patient experiencing withdrawal from alcohol.

Priorities of Care

Monitoring safety is the key component of care, as is protecting the patient from risk for injury (Potter & Moller, 2018). Helping patients cope with the results of their substance use—both physical and mental—is critical.

Reduce Risk for Injury. Patients who use or abuse substances are at increased risk for injury.

Expected Outcome: Patient will be free of injury as evidenced by steady gait and absence of subsequent falls (Potter & Moller, 2018).

The nurse will:

- Assess patient's level of consciousness and orientation to determine specific risks to safety. *Knowledge of the patient's level of cognitive functioning is essential to the development of an appropriate plan of care.*
- Obtain a drug history as well as urine and blood samples for laboratory analysis of substance content. *Subjective history is often not accurate and knowledge regarding substance use is important for accurate assessment.*
- Place patient in a quiet, private room to decrease excessive stimuli, but do not leave patient alone if excessive hyperactivity or suicidal ideation is present. *Excessive stimuli increase patient's agitation.*
- Frequently orient patient to reality and the environment, ensuring that potentially harmful objects are stored outside the patient's access. *Patient may harm self or others if disoriented and confused.*
- Monitor vital signs every 15 minutes until stable and assess for signs of intoxication or withdrawal. *The most reliable information about withdrawal symptoms is vital sign measurements; they provide information about the need for medication during detoxification.*

Promote Coping Strategies. Patients who use substances may have high levels of stress and often have maladaptive coping mechanisms.

Expected Outcomes: Patient will express true feelings associated with using substances and identify healthy adaptive methods of coping with stressful situations (Potter & Moller, 2018).

The nurse will:

- Establish trusting relationship. Be genuine, honest, and respectful of the patient. Keep all promises and convey an attitude of acceptance of the patient. *Trust is essential to the nurse–patient relationship. The development of a nonjudgmental, therapeutic nurse–patient relationship is essential to gain the patient's trust.*
- Encourage patient participation in therapeutic group activities such as cognitive-behavior therapy groups, support groups, or Alcoholics Anonymous meetings with other people who are experiencing or have experienced similar problems. *Peer feedback is often more accepted than feedback from authority figures.*
- Set limits on manipulative behavior and maintain consistency in responses. *Patient is unable to set own limits and must begin to accept responsibility without being manipulative.*
- Encourage patient to verbalize feelings, fears, or anxieties. Use attentive listening and validate patient's feelings with observations or statements that acknowledge feelings. *Verbalization of feelings helps patient to develop insight into behaviors and long-standing problems.*
- Encourage the patient to focus on strengths and accomplishments rather than weaknesses and failures. *Minimize attention to negative ruminations.*
- Encourage participation in therapeutic group activities. Offer recognition and positive feedback for actual achievements. *Success and recognition increase self-esteem.*

Promote Adequate Nutrition. Patients who abuse substances are often malnourished and require interprofessional care and education to maintain adequate nutrition.

Expected Outcomes: Patient will gain 0.45 kg (1 lb) per week without evidence of increased fluid retention. Serum albumin levels will return to normal range (Potter & Moller, 2018).

The nurse will:

- Administer vitamins and dietary supplements as ordered by physician. *Vitamin B_1 is necessary to prevent neurocognitive complications from chronic alcoholism such as Wernicke's syndrome.*
- Monitor labwork (e.g., total albumin, complete blood count, urinalysis, electrolytes, and liver enzymes) and report significant changes to physician. *Objective laboratory tests provide necessary information to determine the extent of malnourishment.*
- Collaborate with the dietitian to determine number of calories needed to provide adequate nutrition and realistic weight gain. Document intake, output, and calorie count. Weigh daily if condition warrants. *Weight loss or gain is important assessment information so that an appropriate plan of care can be developed.*
- Teach the importance of adequate nutrition by explaining a diet containing necessary nutrients and relating

the physical effects of malnutrition on body systems. *Patient may have inadequate knowledge of proper nutritional habits.*

Provide Patient Education. Educating patients about the negative effects, both physical and psychological, of their substance abuse is a priority for nurses.

Expected Outcome: Patient will verbalize the negative effects of substance abuse and agree to seek professional help to quit abusing substances (Potter & Moller, 2018).

The nurse will:

- Assess the patient's level of knowledge and readiness to learn the effects of drugs and alcohol on the body. *Baseline assessment is required to develop appropriate teaching material.*
- Develop a teaching plan that includes measurable objectives. Include significant others, if possible. *Lifestyle changes often affect all family members.*
- Begin with simple concepts and progress to more complex issues. Use interactive teaching strategies and written materials appropriate to the patient's educational level. Include information on physiologic effects of substances, the propensity for physical and psychologic dependence, and the risks to a fetus if the patient is pregnant. *Active participation and handouts enhance retention of important concepts.*
- Teach assertiveness techniques and effective communication techniques such as the use of "I feel" rather than "You make me feel" statements. *Previous patterns of communication may have been aggressive and accusatory, causing barriers to interpersonal relationships.*

Promote Orientation to Reality. Assess the patient's level of disorientation to determine specific risks to safety.

Expected Outcome: Patient will be alert and oriented to time, place, and person and free of hallucinations or delusions (Potter & Moller, 2018).

The nurse will:

- Observe for withdrawal symptoms, monitor vital signs, provide adequate nutrition and hydration, place on seizure precautions. *These actions provide supportive physical care during detoxification.*
- Assess level of orientation frequently; orient and reassure the patient of safety in presence of hallucinations, delusions, or illusions. *Patient may be frightened.*
- Explain all interventions before approaching the patient, avoid loud noises and talk softly to the patient, decrease external stimuli by dimming lights. *Excessive stimuli increase agitation.*
- Administer prn medications according to detoxification schedule. *Benzodiazepines, administered in the dosing suggested by withdrawal protocols, help to minimize the discomfort of withdrawal symptoms and prevent seizures in alcohol withdrawal.*
- Use simple, step-by-step instructions and face-to-face interaction when communicating with the patient. *Patient may be confused or disoriented.*
- Express reasonable doubt if the patient relays suspicious or paranoid beliefs. Reinforce accurate perception of people or situations. *Communicate that you do not share that false belief as reality.*
- Convey acceptance that the patient believes a situation (hallucination) to be true, but that the nurse does not see or hear what is not there. *Arguing with the patient or denying the belief serves no useful purpose because delusions are not eliminated.*
- Talk to the patient about real events and real people. Respond to feelings and reassure the patient that he or she is safe from harm. *Discussions that focus on the delusions may aggravate the condition. Verbalization of feelings in a nonthreatening environment may help the patient develop insight.*

Delegating Nursing Care Activities

As appropriate and allowed by the designated duties and responsibilities of unlicensed assistive personnel, nursing care activities such as monitoring vital signs, assessing for symptoms of withdrawal, obtaining daily weights, assisting with ADLs, and providing for safety monitoring and reorientation of the patient with acute withdrawal symptoms may be delegated (Potter & Moller, 2018).

Transitions of Care

Nurses may interact with patients experiencing substance abuse or substance dependence in a variety of settings in the hospital including emergency departments, medical/surgical units, and intensive care units (Potter & Moller, 2018). Urgent and ambulatory care centers and pain clinics are other settings in which patients with substance abuse disorders will frequently appear for minor health problems associated with chronic disorders related to substance abuse or dependence. Nursing care of the patient with substance abuse or dependence is challenging and requires a nonjudgmental atmosphere promoting trust and respect (Potter & Moller, 2018).

Health promotion efforts are aimed at preventing drug use among children and adolescents and reducing the risks among adults. Adolescence is the most common phase for the first experience with drugs (Potter & Moller, 2018); therefore, teenagers are a vulnerable population, often succumbing to peer pressure. Healthy lifestyles, parental support, stress management, good nutrition, and information about ways to steer clear of peer pressure are important topics for the nurse to provide in school programs.

Nurses should provide adults with information on healthy coping mechanisms, relaxation, and stress reduction techniques to decrease the risks of substance abuse (Potter & Moller, 2018). Nurses have a responsibility to educate their patients about the physiologic effects of substances on the body as well as ways to manage stress and anxiety. Nurses must encourage and support periods of abstinence while assisting patients to make major changes in lifestyles, habits, relationships, and coping methods (Potter & Moller, 2018).

Patients admitted to acute care settings with an acute illness or exacerbation of a chronic disease may have coexisting substance abuse or dependence. Patients with substance

Case Study & Nursing Care Plan

A Patient Withdrawing from Alcohol

George Russell, age 58, fell at home and broke his arm. His wife took him to the ED and an open reduction and internal fixation (ORIF) of his right wrist was performed under general anesthesia in the operating room. Rather than being discharged home, he was admitted to the postoperative unit for observation following surgery because he required large amounts of anesthesia during the procedure.

Mr. Russell has a ruddy complexion and looks older than his stated age. He discloses that he was laid off from his factory job 2 years ago and has been working odd jobs until last week when he was hired by a local assembly plant. His father was a recovering alcoholic and his 30-year-old son has been treated for alcohol abuse in the past. Mr. Russell states that he knows alcoholism runs in the family, but he feels that he has his drinking under control. However, he cannot remember the events that led up to his fall and how he might have broken his arm.

ASSESSMENT

During the nursing assessment, Mr. Russell is hesitant to provide information and refuses to make eye contact. Prior to surgery, a BAL was drawn because the ED nurse detected alcohol on his breath. His BAL was 0.40%, which is five times the legal limit for intoxication in many states. His vital signs are within the upper limits of normal, but he is confused and disoriented with slurred speech and a slight tremor of the hands. He is 6 feet tall and weighs 140 pounds. His total albumin is 2.9 mg and he has elevated liver enzymes. His wife states that he rarely eats the meals she prepares because he is usually drinking and has no appetite for food.

DIAGNOSES

- Poor coping skills
- Potential for injury
- Poor nutrition related to drinking and poor appetite

EXPECTED OUTCOMES

- Patient will express his true feelings associated with using alcohol as a method of coping with stressful situations.
- Patient will identify three adaptive coping mechanisms he can use as alternatives to alcohol in response to stress.
- Patient will verbalize the negative effects of alcohol and agree to seek professional help with his drinking.
- Patient will be free of injury as evidenced by steady gait and absence of subsequent falls.
- Patient will gain 0.45 kg (1 lb) per week without evidence of increased fluid retention. Serum albumin levels will return to normal range.

PLANNING AND IMPLEMENTATION

- Immediately consult with a physician regarding implementation of a detoxification protocol with scheduled medications to prevent seizures and delirium tremens (DTs), and observe and treat signs of withdrawal syndrome.
- Establish trusting relationship with patient and spend time with him discussing his feelings, fears, and anxieties.
- Explain the effects of alcohol abuse on the body and emphasize that prognosis is closely associated with abstinence.
- Teach a relaxation technique that the patient feels is useful.
- Provide community resource information about self-help groups and, if patient is receptive, a list of meeting times and phone numbers.
- Consult with a dietitian to determine number of calories needed to provide adequate nutrition and realistic weight gain. Document intake, output, and calorie count.
- Consult with physician to begin Vitamin B_1 (thiamine) and dietary supplements.
- Prior to discharge, arrange consultation with a health care provider who specializes in addictions so that patient can receive medication-assisted treatment (MAT) and be prescribed anticraving medications to facilitate recovery.

EVALUATION

Mr. Russell was successfully detoxed and discharged from the postoperative unit without complications. He contacted the employee assistance program (EAP) at his new place of employment. He was on medical leave while his arm completely healed and now attends Alcoholics Anonymous meetings 5 days a week. He reports that he enjoys taking long walks with his wife in the warm weather and that his appetite has returned. He has gained 10 pounds in the past 6 weeks and feels physically better than he has in many years.

CLINICAL REASONING IN PATIENT CARE

1. What factors could be contributing to Mr. Russell's unhealthy use of alcohol as a coping mechanism?
2. What safety issues should be addressed with Mr. Russell?
3. What teaching should be done to reduce Mr. Russell's future risk of alcohol-related diseases?
4. Explain why it would be important to include questions about Mr. Russell's medication history and his use of other medications during the initial nursing assessment.
5. Mr. Russell asks you to explain the risks of taking disulfiram (Antabuse). What should you tell him?
6. Develop a care plan for Mr. Russell to address the nursing problem of impaired nutrition. Why is this necessary?

See Evaluating Your Response in Appendix B.

abuse or dependence have impaired senses and risk-taking behaviors that lead to injuries from falls and accidents requiring medical attention. Nurses will frequently encounter these patients in hospital EDs as well as medical and surgical units. Key safety considerations for hospitalized patients with substance abuse problems include (Potter & Moller, 2018):

- Closely monitor patients admitted for a drug overdose for signs of suicidal ideation.
- Never leave an actively suicidal patient alone.
- During acute alcohol withdrawal (first 72 hours), assess for withdrawal symptoms and administer benzodiazepines as ordered.
- Monitor unconscious patients closely for possibility of aspiration. Never place an intoxicated, unconscious patient in a supine position.
- Seizure precautions are indicated for patients experiencing acute withdrawal symptoms.
- Follow detoxification and withdrawal protocols to prevent signs of delirium tremens from occurring after withdrawal from alcohol.
- Monitor patients for signs of hallucinations, delusions, or altered sensory perceptions that may lead to injuries.
- Assess for fall and choking risk. Provide one-to-one assistance as needed.
- Maintain fluid and electrolyte balance.

Nurses may also encounter patients in alcohol and drug abuse (ADA) treatment programs where patients are hospitalized for detoxification and in-patient therapy. These patients may be voluntarily admitted but many are court-ordered to undergo treatment after charges of driving under the influence (DUI) or driving while intoxicated (DWI) (Potter & Moller, 2018). Occupational nurses and community health nurses will also interact with patients who have substance abuse problems in employee assistance programs and community health departments. There has been an increase in home- and community-based detoxification programs because of cost advantages (Potter & Moller, 2018).

Rehabilitation from problems of substance abuse begins when detoxification is complete and the patient is abstinent. The recovery phase of treatment continues indefinitely.

Medications used to treat alcoholism are disulfiram (Antabuse), naltrexone (ReVia, Depade), and acamprosate (Campral) (Wilson et al., 2017). Disulfiram is a form of aversion therapy that prevents the breakdown of alcohol, causing physical illness (intense vomiting) if taken while drinking alcohol. It should never be given to a patient without their knowledge (Potter & Moller, 2018). All forms of alcohol, including mouth rinses and OTC cough and cold preparations, must be avoided.

Naltrexone (Vivitrol), a long-acting IM injectable opioid antagonist, is used along with counseling and social support to help people who have stopped drinking large amounts of alcohol or who have stopped abusing opiate medications or street drugs to avoid abusing these substances again (Wilson et al., 2017). Naltrexone (ReVia) is also available for oral administration. Naltrexone can help reduce the craving for alcohol by blocking the pathways to the brain that trigger a feeling of pleasure when alcohol and narcotics are used. Patients should discontinue all opiates 7 to 10 days before starting on naltrexone. Because naltrexone blocks opiate receptors, patients should avoid taking any narcotics, such as codeine, morphine, or heroin, while on naltrexone (Potter & Moller, 2018). It is recommended that patients wear a medical alert bracelet stating they are on naltrexone, in case of emergency medical treatment. While on disulfiram or naltrexone, psychosocial treatments such as Alcoholics Anonymous meetings, individual counseling, or group therapy are important because the desire to take a break from treatment can overcome the patient's motivation to continue taking the medication. Injectable naltrexone, which is administered by a HCP once every 4 weeks, has been shown to improve compliance with the recovery plan (Potter & Moller, 2018).

Acamprosate is another medication prescribed for patients who want to abstain from alcohol. The chemical structure of acamprosate is similar to GABA and glutamate neurotransmitters. Acamprosate is thought to block glutamate receptors while simultaneously activating GABA receptors in the brain, thus stabilizing the chemical imbalance that is disrupted by alcoholism (Wilson et al., 2017). Acamprosate is fairly effective in reducing cravings of alcohol-dependent patients when used in combination with psychosocial and other supportive interventions (Potter & Moller, 2018).

Buprenorphine (Buprenex, Subutex) is used solely for the treatment of opioid dependence. Buprenorphine has been used in detoxification treatment since the early 1980s. Suboxone (buprenorphine/naloxone) binds tightly to mu-opioid receptors and is not easily displaced by opioid antagonists, causing a longer duration of action (Wilson et al., 2017). This may explain the lack of significant withdrawal symptoms upon cessation of the drug and may also contribute to its effectiveness in opioid detoxification (Potter & Moller, 2018). However, buprenorphine treatment has some limitations. Limited numbers of physicians and other HCPs are certified to treat opioid dependence with Suboxone, which can make this type of treatment difficult to access. Access has been improved by recent legislation that extended prescribing and administering privileges to advanced practice nurses (APRNs) and physician assistants (PAs) in office-based settings (SAMHSA, 2017c). Because of buprenorphine's opioid effects, it can be misused, particularly by people who do not have an opioid dependency (SAMHSA, 2016a). It is also more expensive than traditional treatment with older medications such as clonidine (Wilson et al., 2017). In addition, patients complain about the expense of treatment, access issues, and the need to travel to access services. Suboxone is available in sublingual, film, and transmucosal products (Wilson et al., 2017).

Methadone is a medication used in medication-assisted treatment (MAT) to help people reduce or quit their use of heroin or other opiates. When taken as prescribed, it is safe and effective (SAMHSA, 2016b). Methadone works by changing how the brain and nervous system respond to pain; it lessens the painful symptoms of opiate withdrawal and blocks the euphoric effects of opiate drugs such as heroin, morphine, and codeine, as well as semi-synthetic opioids like oxycodone and hydrocodone (SAMHSA, 2016b). Methadone is offered in pill, liquid, and wafer forms. Methadone can be addictive, so it must be used exactly as prescribed; also it can cause overdose and interacts with many medications (Wilson et al., 2017). As with all medications used in medication-assisted treatment (MAT), methadone is to be prescribed as part of a comprehensive treatment plan that includes counseling and participation in social support programs (SAMHSA, 2016b).

Finally, a recent focus of harm reduction has been providing naloxone (Narcan), an opioid antagonist, in kit form to laypersons to reverse the effects of opioid overdose and reduce deaths. These opioid reversal devices have been found to be safe and cost-effective (Wheeler, Jones, Gilbert, & Davidson, 2015), and there have been many reports of overdose reversals since these kits have become available for purchase over the counter. Therefore, public health officials recommend providing naloxone kits to any laypersons who might witness an opioid overdose, to patients in substance use treatment programs, to persons leaving prison and jail, and as a component of responsible opioid prescribing (Wheeler et al., 2015).

The community provides many options for treating substance abuse, including a mixture of individual, group, and family therapy. Medical detoxification can occur in hospitals, psychiatric units, special substance abuse units, methadone clinics, or outpatient settings. Less restrictive environments include residential rehabilitation programs, halfway houses, and partial hospitalization programs (Potter & Moller, 2018). These programs provide structured environments for individuals recovering from substance abuse problems while maintaining a viable presence in the community. In addition, because of its privacy and low cost, home detox has become a more viable option (Muncie, Yasinian, & Oge, 2013). Patients can obtain vocational counseling, become involved in self-help groups such as Alcoholics Anonymous or Narcotics Anonymous, and receive drug and health education.

Teaching the patient and family includes:

- The negative effects of substance abuse, including physical and psychologic complications of substance abuse
- The signs of relapse and the importance of after-care programs and self-help groups to prevent relapse
- Information about specific medications that help to reduce the craving for alcohol and opiates (naltrexone [ReVia; Vivitrol] and acamprosate [Campral]) and maintain abstinence (disulfiram [Antabuse]), including their potential side effects, possible drug interactions, and any special precautions to be taken (e.g., avoiding OTC medications such as cough syrup that may have alcohol content)
- Ways to manage stress including techniques such as progressive muscle relaxation, abdominal breathing techniques, imagery, meditation, and effective coping skills.

In addition, suggest the following resources:

- Alcoholics Anonymous, Narcotics Anonymous, and other self-help groups
- Employee assistance programs
- Individual, group, and/or family counseling
- Community rehabilitation programs
- National Alliance on Mental Illness.

Patients are at highest risk for relapse within the first few months after stopping the abused substance. An acronym that can assist the patient in recognizing behaviors that lead to relapse is **HALT**:

Hungry

Angry

Lonely

Tired.

Nurses should emphasize the importance of a balanced diet, adequate sleep, healthy recreation activities, and a caring support system to prevent relapse.

In end-of-life care, nurses are often dealing primarily with older adults. Substance use among older adults is a public health concern that could increase in the future, especially as the baby boom generation ages. There are some areas of concern for this population: On an average day, 6 million older adults used alcohol and 132,000 older adults used marijuana (SAMHSA, 2017a). Alcohol can interact dangerously with medications taken by older adults, including over-the-counter drugs, herbal remedies, and prescriptions. Alcohol can also exacerbate common medical conditions in older adults, including stroke, high blood pressure, diabetes, osteoporosis, memory loss, and mood disorders (SAMHSA, 2017a).

Combining several medications or pairing medications with alcohol may affect older adults more strongly than younger adults and may necessitate visits to the ED. According to federal data, many ED visits by adults aged 65 or older involved illicit drug use, alcohol used in combination with other substances (visits for alcohol alone were not included for adults), or nonmedical use of pharmaceuticals (e.g., prescription medications, over-the-counter remedies, dietary supplements) (CBHSQ, 2017; SAMHSA, 2017a). Although this was not the chief cause of drug-related ED visits for this age group, use of illicit drugs, use of drugs combined with alcohol, and nonmedical use of pharmaceuticals typically result in an average 300 ED visits each day (SAMHSA, 2017a).

In the context of the opioid epidemic, where close monitoring of opioid prescription and use is being implemented, palliative care and hospice health care providers are concerned that patients with genuine pain issues may have trouble obtaining the medication they need. Also, as cancer treatment extends life, patients of all ages with advanced cancer will have pain requiring opioid therapy at some stage during their illness (Pinkerton & Hardy, 2017). The majority of patients will receive adequate pain relief from opioids with no short- or longer-term adverse outcomes; however, a small group of patients will develop substance misuse issues that will influence HCP management and prescribing practices (Pinkerton & Hardy, 2017).

Given the current climate, the potential ethical issues of limiting effective analgesia on the basis of addiction risk or history must be acknowledged. HCPs must be aware of the risk factors for opioid misuse, and before patients enter palliative care, they must screen for addiction issues prior to starting opioid therapy (Pinkerton & Hardy, 2017). HCPs must also be able to manage and monitor those identified as having an opioid misuse problem because the risks of medication diversion are well known. However, in the context of terminal or malignant pain, restricting of opiates in patients with addiction is considered neither achievable nor desirable (Dunlop, 2018).

In addition to increased screening for at-risk patients and issuing fewer prescriptions for opioids, HCPs are increasingly referring patients to pain management clinics for nonpharmacological treatments and to providers of complementary and integrative treatments (National Center for Complementary and Integrative Health, 2017). In summary, as more patients of all ages enter palliative care for management of chronic health issues, further research is needed to develop screening and management of addiction in patients with cancer-related and other chronic pain issues (Dunlop, 2018).

Care of Special Populations

Older Adults

Substance abuse among older adults is a rapidly growing health problem in the U.S. (Chhatre, Cook, Mallik, & Jayadevappa, 2017). The aging baby boomer population has had more exposure to tobacco, alcohol and drug from a younger age than previous generations. Exposure to the use of illicit drugs at a younger age is a risk factor for substance abuse in later life. Consequently, the use of illicit drugs among older adults does appears to be increasing (Chhatre, et al). Financial stress, mobility problems, social isolation, caregiver role strain are some of the many social factors that contribute to the development of substance abuse in older adults (Blow & Barry, 2014)

Due to stigma attached to substance abuse, this health problem can be undetected and undertreated in the older adult population. Consequently, accurate estimates of prevalence are unknown. Additionally, healthcare professionals may confuse the symptoms of substance abuse disorders with comorbidities and co-occurring conditions such as anxiety and depression and age-related physiological changes. As comorbidities increase with age, the presence of substance abuse can lead to worsening of consequences related to other health problems and have adverse impact outcomes of care.

Nurses are in a unique position to screen and intervene on behalf of older adult patients for problems with substance abuse. The nurse should conduct initial screening for substance abuse when assessing the older adult patient in both inpatient and community-based settings. If initial screening suggests there is a problem the patient should be referred for more extensive assessments that measure substance use severity, problems, and consequences associated with use of illicit substances (Blow & Barry, 2014). The nurse should approach the patient in nonjudgmental manner, be alert for factors that may be contributing to substance abuse, and use a holistic approach to developing interventions. The nurse should communicate findings of concern and facilitate referrals for substance abuse treatment that are sensitive to the unique needs of older adults.

Military Service Members and Veterans

The U.S. Department of Defense (DoD) and U.S. Department of Veterans Affairs (VA) report there are approximately 2.1 million current military service members and 21 million living veterans in the United States (Haibach, et al., 2017). When entering the service, military members typically are healthier than the general U.S. population. However, over time, long-term health status is worse when compared to the U.S. population especially in the areas of physical activity, nutrition, and tobacco and alcohol use (Hailbach, et al., 2017). Recent studies report some women in the military are engaging in a high rate of hazardous drinking in response to the prevalence of post-traumatic stress disorder (PTSD) related to *Operations Enduring Freedom and Iraqi Freedom* (Haun, et al., 2016). Veterans also have a high rate of nonmedical use of prescriptions, opioid misuse and abuse, and heroin addiction (Banerjee, et al., 2016). The etiology of the high prevalence of addiction in the veteran population involves multiple complex variables including underrecognition and undertreatment of chronic pain related to military-service injuries (Banerjee et al., 2016).

Nursing care of the veteran should include screening for signs of PTSD, pain, and illicit use of addictive substances. The nurse should approach the veteran in a caring and nonjudgmental manner and use therapeutic communication to obtain military history and in-depth psychosocial data. The VA/DoD has developed clinical practice guidelines for veterans with substance use disorders and the nurse can be a source for assisting veteran patients to access this care. The nurse should be familiar with local veteran-centric resources and the referral process used to help veterans access the VA healthcare system. Veteran patients are eligible for VA health benefits at no or very minimal cost, and high quality care for substance abuse is readily available once the patients are in the VA health system.

Gender and Sexual Minorities

Sexual and gender minority populations have long been assumed to be at greater risk for substance abuse than their heterosexual peers (Talley, et al., 2016). The landmark Institute of Medicine (IOM) report titled *The Health of Lesbian, Gay, Bisexual, and Transgender People: Building a Foundation for Better Understanding* published in 2011. The report uncovered that early research used to validate assumptions regarding substance abuse in gender minority populations should be questioned due to limitations of methodology, sample size, poor measures and lack of appropriate comparison groups. The IOM report also called for increased National Institutes of Health (NIH) funding dedicated to studying health concerns and health outcomes of this population. Many studies are currently in progress (Talley, et al., 2016). The increasing rate of substance abuse has become a major public health concern regardless of a person's sexuality (Taliaferro, et al., 2014)

Social stigma and discrimination due to homophobic practices by healthcare professionals requires the nurse to establish therapeutic relationships with patients from sexual and gender minority populations. Establishing trust using a nonjudgmental and caring person-centered approach is essential as the nurse conducts holistic assessment. Initial substance abuse screening for this population should be included in assessment in both inpatient and community settings. Nurses have an obligation to monitor current research findings and use emerging evidence-based practice standards that address the unique healthcare needs and interventions for LGBTQ persons.

CHAPTER HIGHLIGHTS

6.1 Overview of Substance Abuse Problems

Outline the pathophysiology, manifestations, and complications of substance abuse; the risk factors for substance abuse; and characteristics of individuals who abuse substances, including nurses.

- Substance abuse is the use of any chemical despite adverse effects on the individual's physical, psychologic, interpersonal, or social health.
- Substance dependence occurs when control over the chemical substance is lost and the individual must use increasing amounts to produce the desired effect (tolerance) and must use the substance to avoid or relieve uncomfortable symptoms (withdrawal).
- Combinations of genetic, biologic, psychologic, and sociocultural factors contribute to substance abuse or dependence. Addictive behavior has been linked to biochemical changes in dopamine and serotonin brain levels as well as to heredity, ethnicity, and peer pressure.
- Adolescents are particularly influenced by society and peers to use substances, predominantly tobacco, alcohol, and illicit drugs. A positive cultural identity and family environment act as protective deterrents for substance use.
- People with substance abuse problems have common characteristics including risk-taking behavior, low tolerance for frustration or pain, compulsive preoccupation with the substance, anxiety, anger, and low self-esteem. Stress management, anger control, social support, and counseling are helpful strategies to avoid substance abuse and dependence.

6.2 Addictive Substances and Their Effects

Differentiate the effects of selected addictive substances on physiologic, cognitive, psychologic, and social well-being.

- Alcohol is the most commonly used and abused legal substance in America; however, polysubstance abuse is frequent in many individuals. Marijuana is the most commonly used illicit drug. Substances such as cocaine and methamphetamine are often used in conjunction with alcohol. Abuse of prescription antianxiety agents and narcotic analgesics such as opioids is a significant problem.
- Although not an illicit substance, caffeine is a stimulant that increases the heart rate and acts as a diuretic. Some 85% of the U.S. population consumes at least one caffeinated beverage per day, with caffeine intake highest among adults ages 50 to 64 years.
- Alcohol is the most commonly used and abused legal substance in the United States. There were 136.7 million current alcohol drinkers in 2016, including 65.3 million who were binge alcohol users and 16.3 million who were heavy alcohol users.
- Binge drinking for males is defined as drinking five or more drinks on the same occasion on at least 1 day in the past 30 days, while binge alcohol use for females has been defined as drinking four or more drinks on the same occasion on at least 1 day in the past 30 days.
- Overuse of alcohol causes damaging effects to the liver and many other systems; its potential effects include myocardial disease, erosive gastritis, acute and chronic pancreatitis, sexual dysfunction, and an increased risk of breast cancer.
- Nicotine acts on the central nervous system (CNS) as a stimulant, binding to acetylcholine receptors in the brain and causing the release of dopamine and norepinephrine. Chronic health problems from smoking include cancer, heart disease, emphysema, hypertension, and death.
- Nicotine replacement therapy (NRT) and related medication may help users quit using tobacco.
- Marijuana is the most commonly used drug, with an estimated 24.0 million Americans aged 12 or older in 2016 currently using marijuana. The psychoactive component of marijuana is a chemical known as delta-9-tetrahydrocannabinol (THC), which activates specific cannabinoid receptors in the brain.
- Central nervous system depressants, including barbiturates, benzodiazepines, paraldehyde, meprobamate, and chloral hydrate, are also subject to abuse. Cross-dependence exists among all CNS depressants and cross-tolerance can develop to alcohol and general anesthetics.
- Depressant effects related to barbiturates are dose dependent and range from mild sedation to sleep to coma to death.
- Psychostimulants such as cocaine and amphetamines have a high potential for abuse. Euphoria is the main subjective effect associated with cocaine and amphetamines, leading to addiction. Cocaine overdose

produces anxiety, hyperpyrexia, convulsions, ventricular dysrhythmias, severe hypertension, and possible hemorrhagic stroke, angina, or myocardial infarction.

- Methamphetamine is often taken in combination with other drugs such as cocaine and marijuana and, like heroin and cocaine, can be inhaled, injected, ingested, or smoked. Methamphetamine users experience numerous physical symptoms including weight loss, tachycardia, tachypnea, hyperthermia, insomnia, and muscular tremors.
- Opiates such as morphine, meperidine, codeine, hydrocodone, and oxycodone are narcotic analgesics. Some individuals used opiates for prescription pain management; however, many others use opiates under social or illicit circumstances. In 2016, there were 11.8 million past-year opioid misusers aged 12 or older in the United States, the vast majority of whom misused prescription pain relievers.
- Hallucinogens are also called psychedelics and include a number of substances such as LSD, PCP, peyote, mescaline, psilocybin mushrooms, "Ecstasy," ketamine, and salvia. When under the influence of either type of drug, people often report rapid, intense emotional swings and seeing images, hearing sounds, and feeling sensations that seem real but are not.
- Inhalants are categorized into three types: Anesthetics; volatile nitrites; and organic solvents, solvents, aerosols, gases, or nitrites. Long-term effects of inhalant use may include liver and kidney damage, hearing loss, bone marrow damage, loss of coordination and limb spasms from nerve damage, delayed behavioral development, and brain damage from restricted oxygen flow to the brain.

6.3 Care of Patients with Substance Abuse Problems

Describe the interprofessional care, nursing care, and transitions of care for patients who abuse substances.

- Effective treatment of substance abuse and dependence results from the efforts of an interprofessional team specializing in the treatment of psychiatric and substance abuse disorders. Substance dependency treatment occurs in two major phases: Acute and rehabilitation.
- The interprofessional team often includes the nurse, physicians such as psychiatrists and addictionologists, psychologists, case managers, social workers, recreational therapists, and dietitians, among others.
- Nurses will interact with patients experiencing substance abuse or substance dependence in a variety of settings in the hospital including emergency departments, medical/surgical units, and intensive care units.
- Urgent and ambulatory care centers and pain clinics are other settings in which patients with substance abuse disorders will frequently appear for other health problems.
- Nursing care of patients experiencing substance abuse problems includes health promotion efforts to prevent substance abuse; comprehensive physical, spiritual, and psychosocial assessment; and interventions for the human responses of ineffective coping and denial, imbalanced nutrition, readiness for enhanced knowledge, acute confusion, and risk for injury or violence.
- Severe alcohol withdrawal or delirium tremens is a medical emergency that usually occurs 2 to 5 days following cessation of alcohol consumption. A symptom-triggered approach to the administration of benzodiazepines during alcohol withdrawal results in less total medication use and requires a shorter duration of treatment than other treatments.
- Nurses and other healthcare professionals are susceptible to substance abuse due to pressures in the workplace and easy access to drugs. Nurses need to assess their response to stress and seek early treatment for depressive symptoms to avoid practicing while impaired.
- Substance abuse among older adults is a growing health problem that can be confused with comorbidities and co-occurring conditions. There is a high prevalence of substance abuse among service members and veterans. LGBTQ patients may have experienced social stigma and discrimination within the healthcare systems. Nurses should approach all patients in a caring and nonjudgmental manner, use therapeutic communication to conduct a holistic assessment, communicate findings of concern to the healthcare team, and facilitate referrals for treatment.

TEST YOURSELF NCLEX-RN® REVIEW

1. The nurse is reviewing the laboratory values for a patient who is intoxicated. Which alcohol level is considered the minimum for an individual to be legally considered intoxicated?
   A. 0.05%
   B. 0.08%
   C. 0.50%
   D. 1.00%
2. Which question is the most appropriate for the nurse to use when interviewing a patient who is suspected of having alcohol abuse problems?
   A. "Have you been drinking lately?"
   B. "You don't drink much alcohol, do you?"
   C. "Typically, how many days per week do you drink alcoholic beverages?"
   D. "Has your drinking caused a lot of problems between you and your spouse?"

3. The nurse is caring for a patient with chronic alcoholism. Why should the nurse prepare to administer thiamine (vitamin B_1) for this patient?
   A. To prevent acute pancreatitis
   B. To prevent cirrhosis of the liver
   C. To prevent hepatic encephalopathy
   D. To prevent Wernicke's encephalopathy
4. The nurse is planning care for a patient who is demonstrating signs of substance withdrawal. Which substances present the highest medical danger during withdrawal?
   A. Opiates and marijuana
   B. Alcohol and CNS depressants
   C. Amphetamines and hallucinogens
   D. CNS stimulants and amphetamines
5. A patient with a history of alcohol abuse has been prescribed disulfiram (Antabuse). What should the nurse teach the patient about the purpose of this medication? (Select all that apply.)
   A. It decreases the discomfort of withdrawal symptoms.
   B. It decreases the pleasant, reinforcing effects of alcohol.
   C. It blocks the signs and symptoms of alcohol withdrawal.
   D. It prevents the breakdown of alcohol to inhibit impulsive drinking.
   E. It causes an aversive reaction if alcohol is consumed.
6. The nurse manager is concerned that a staff nurse has a substance abuse problem. What behaviors might lead the manager to this concern? (Select all that apply.)
   A. The nurse consistently has to work overtime to complete documentation.
   B. The nurse's personal hygiene has become poor.
   C. One of the nurse's patients reports that routine pain medications are not being given.
   D. The nurse made a medication error on a patient who was admitted at shift change.
   E. There have been two patient complaints about the amount of perfume the nurse wears.
7. The nurse is completing an education session on smoking cessation with a group of patients in a prenatal clinic. Which participant statement indicates that additional teaching is required?
   A. Lung cancer is second only to breast cancer as a cause of death in women.
   B. Women who smoke have an increased risk for stroke and heart disease.
   C. Women who smoke during pregnancy have a higher risk for infertility.
   D. Smoking is the leading known cause of preventable death and disease among women.
8. The nurse is teaching a patient with a history of substance abuse about the medication naltrexone (ReVia). Which patient statement indicates that teaching has been effective?
   A. "I should stop taking all pain medications before starting on naltrexone."
   B. "I should wear a medical alert bracelet that states I'm taking naltrexone."
   C. "I should read labels of OTC cold medicines to make sure they don't have alcohol."
   D. "I should go to my Narcotics Anonymous meetings for 1 month, then I can stop going."
9. The nurse and patient are establishing goals of care for a substance abuse problem. Which would be a realistic goal for this patient?
   A. The patient will be able to use alcohol or drugs in moderation.
   B. The patient will focus on negative aspects of past behaviors and interpersonal relationships.
   C. The patient will identify ways to deal with stressful situations instead of resorting to substance use.
   D. The patient will refrain from using substances until craving for the substance has been eliminated.
10. The nurse planning care for a patient with substance abuse will likely plan interventions for which patient problem?
    A. The patient is at risk of rapid cognitive decline due to the toxic effects of abused substances.
    B. The patient may become overhydrated from increased fluid intake.
    C. The patient's coping mechanisms are impaired due to the effects of substance abuse.
    D. The patient is at risk for weight gain due to overeating during withdrawal.

See Test Yourself answers in Appendix B.

REFERENCES

American Nurses Association. (2017). *What to do if you suspect a nurse is a substance abuser.* Retrieved from https://www.americannursetoday.com/the-impaired-nurse-would-you-know-what-to-do-if-you-suspected-substance-abuse/.

American Psychiatric Association. (2013). *Diagnostic and statistical manual of mental disorders* (5th ed.). Arlington, VA: American Psychiatric Association.

American Society of Addiction Medicine. (2017). *State of the art in genetics of addiction: A joint statement.* Retrieved from https://www.asam.org/advocacy/find-a-policy-statement/view-policy-statement/public-policy-statements/2011/12/15/state-of-the-art-in-genetics-of-addiction-a-joint-statement.

Anker, J. J., Kushner, M. G., Thuras, P., Menk, J., & Unruh, A. S. (2016). Drinking to cope with negative emotions moderates alcohol use disorder treatment response in patients with co-occurring anxiety disorder. *Drug and Alcohol Dependence, 159*(Suppl. C), 93–100.

Asarnow, J., Rozenman, M., Wiblin, J., & Zeltzer, L. (2015). Integrated medical-behavioral care compared with usual primary care for child and adolescent behavioral health: A meta-analysis. *JAMA Pediatrics, 169*(10), 929–937.

Aveyard, P., Begh, R., Parsons, R., & West, P. (2012). Brief opportunistic smoking cessation interventions: A systematic review and meta-analysis to compare advice to quit and offer of assistance. *Addiction, 107*(6), 1066–1073.

Baird, M., Blount, A., Brungardt, S., Dickinson, P., Dietrich, A., Epperly, T., . . . Korsen, N. (2014). Joint principles: Integrating behavioral health care into the patient-centered medical home. *Annals of Family Medicine, 12*(2), 183–185.

Banerjee, N. (2014). Neurotransmitters in alcoholism: A review of neurobiological and genetic studies. *Indian Journal of Human Genetics, 20*(1), 20–31.

Banerjee, G., Edelman, J., Barry, D. T., . . . Marshall, B. (2016). Non-medical use of prescription opioids is associate with heroin initiation among US veterans: a prospective cohort study. *Addiction, 111,* 2021-2031.

Barry, A. E., King, J., Sears, C., Harville, C., Bondoc, I., & Joseph, K. (2016). Prioritizing alcohol prevention: Establishing alcohol as the gateway drug and linking age of first drink with illicit drug use. *Journal of School Health, 86*(1), 31–38.

Bhatia, S. C., Bhatia, S. K., & Kolli, V. (2017). Sedative, hypnotic or anxiolytic-related disorders. In S. C. Bhatia (Ed.), *Substance and Nonsubstance Related Addiction Disorder: Diagnosis and Treatment* (pp. 175–187). Sharjah, United Arab Emirates: Bentham Science Publishers.

Blow, F. C. &. Barry K. L. (2014). Substance misuse and abuse in older adults: What do we need to know to help? *Generations: Journal of the American Society of Aging, 38* (3), 53-67.

Broz, D., Wejnert, C., Pham, H. T., DiNenno, E., Heffelfinger, J. D., Cribbin, M., . . . Taussig, J. (2014). HIV infection and risk, prevention, and testing behaviors among injecting drug users—National HIV Behavioral Surveillance System, 20 US cities, 2009. *MMWR Surveillance Summaries, 63*(1), 1–56.

Brust, J. C. (2014). Neurologic complications of illicit drug abuse. *CONTINUUM: Lifelong Learning in Neurology, 20*(3, Neurology of Systemic Disease), 642–656.

Cahill, K., Lindson-Hawley, N., Thomas, K. H., Fanshawe, T. R., & Lancaster, T. (2016). Nicotine receptor partial agonists for smoking cessation. *Cochrane Database of Systematic Reviews,* Issue 5, 1–151. doi: 10.1002/14651858.CD006103.pub7

Center for Behavioral Health Statistics and Quality. (2015). *Behavioral health trends in the United States: Results from the 2014 National Survey on Drug Use and Health* (HHS Publication No. SMA 15-4927). Rockville, MD: Substance Abuse and Mental Health Services Administration.

Center for Behavioral Health Statistics and Quality. (2017). *Key substance use and mental health indicators in the United States: Results from the 2016 National Survey on Drug Use and Health* (HHS Publication No. SMA 17-5044, NSDUH Series H-52). Rockville, MD: Substance Abuse and Mental Health Services Administration. Retrieved from https://www.samhsa.gov/data/.

Centers for Disease Control and Prevention. (2016). *Current cigarette smoking among adults in the United States.* Retrieved from https://www.cdc.gov/tobacco/data_statistics/fact_sheets/adult_data/cig_smoking/index.htm.

Centers for Disease Control and Prevention. (2017a). *Health care professionals: Help your patients quit smoking.* Retrieved from https://www.cdc.gov/tobacco/campaign/tips/partners/health/hcp/index.html.

Centers for Disease Control and Prevention. (2017b). *Leading causes of death in females, 2014 (current listing).* Retrieved from https://www.cdc.gov/women/lcod/2014/race-ethnicity/index.htm.

Chauhan, P., Dev, A., Desai, S., & Andhale, V. (2016). Nicotine replacement therapy for smoking cessation. *Pharmaceutical and Biological Evaluations, 3*(3), 305–312.

Chhatre, S., Cook, R., Mallik, E., & Jayadevappa, R. (2017). Trends in substance use admissions among older adults. *BMC Health Services Research, 17,* 584.

Das, P., Naylor, C., & Majeed, A. (2016). Bringing together physical and mental health within primary care: A new frontier for integrated care. *Journal of the Royal Society of Medicine, 109*(10), 364–366.

Deans, C., & Maggert, K. A. (2015). What do you mean, "epigenetic"? *Genetics, 199*(4), 887–896.

Dick, D. M., Cho, S. B., Latendresse, S. J., Aliev, F., Nurnberger, J. I., Edenberg, H. J., . . . Kuperman, S. (2014). Genetic influences on alcohol use across stages of development: GABRA2 and longitudinal trajectories of drunkenness from adolescence to young adulthood. *Addiction Biology, 19*(6), 1055–1064.

Dowell, D., Haegerich, T. M., & Chou, R. (2016). *CDC Guideline for Prescribing Opioids for Chronic Pain — United States, 2016.* (MMWR No. RR-1). Atlanta, GA: Centers for Disease Control.

Dunlop, A. S. (2018). Increasing awareness of addiction in palliative care: Applying best practice in an area of limited management guidance. *Internal Medicine Journal, 48*(1), 103–104.

Ewing, J. A. (1984). Detecting alcoholism: The CAGE questionnaire. *Journal of the American Medical Association, 252*(14), 1905–1907.

Florence, C. S., Zhou, C., Luo, F., & Xu, L. (2016). The economic burden of prescription opioid overdose, abuse, and dependence in the United States, 2013. *Medical Care, 54*(10), 901–906.

Food and Drug Administration. (2017). *FDA's new regulations for e-cigarettes, cigars, and all other tobacco products.* Retrieved from https://www.fda.gov/TobaccoProducts/Labeling/RulesRegulationsGuidance/ucm394909.htm.

Haibach, J.P., Haibach, M.A., Hall, K. S., & Goldstein, M. G. (2017). Military and veteran health behavior research and practice: challenges and opportunities. *Journal of Behavioral Medicine, 40,* 175-193.

Han, B., Compton, W. M., Blanco, C., Crane, E., Lee, J., & Jones, C. M. (2017). Prescription opioid use, misuse, and use disorders in U.S. adults: 2015 National Survey on Drug Use and Health. *Annals of Internal Medicine, 167*(5), 293–301.

Haun, J. N., Duffy, A., Lind. J. D., Kisala, P., & Luther, S. L. (2016). Qualitative inquiry explores health-related quality of life of female veterans with post-traumatic stress disorder. *Military Medicine, 181,* e1470-e1475.

Hunter, C. L., Goodie, J. L., Oordt, M. S., & Dobmeyer, A. C. (2017). *Integrated behavioral health in primary care: Step-by-step guidance for assessment and intervention* (2nd ed.). Washington, DC: American Psychological Association.

Institute of Medicine (IOM). The health of lesbian, gay, bisexual and transgender people: Building a foundation for better understanding. Washington DC: The National Academies Press, 2011.

Jellinek, E. (1946). *Phases in the drinking history of alcoholics.* New Haven, CT: Hillhouse Press.

Kampman, K., & Jarvis, M. (2015). American Society of Addiction Medicine (ASAM) National Practice Guideline for the use of medications in the treatment of addiction involving opioid use. *Journal of Addiction Medicine, 9*(5), 358–367.

Katz, J. (2017, June 5). Drug deaths in America are rising faster than ever. *New York Times.* Retrieved from https://www.nytimes.com/interactive/2017/06/05/upshot/opioid-epidemic-drug-overdose-deaths-are-rising-faster-than-ever.html.

Keys, V. A. (2011). Alcohol withdrawal during hospitalization. *American Journal of Nursing, 111*(1), 40–44.

Koegelenberg, C. F., Noor, F., Bateman, E. D., van Zyl-Smit, R. N., Bruning, A., O'Brien, J. A., . . . Irusen, E. M. (2014). Efficacy of varenicline combined with nicotine replacement therapy vs varenicline alone for smoking cessation: A randomized clinical trial. *Journal of the American Medical Association, 312*(2), 155–161.

Kuerbis, A., Sacco, P., Blazer, D. G., & Moore, A. A. (2014). Substance abuse among older adults. *Clinics in Geriatric Medicine, 30*(3), 629–654.

Lansky, A., Finlayson, T., Johnson, C., Holtzman, D., Wejnert, C., Mitsch, A., . . . Crepaz, N. (2014). Estimating the number of persons who inject drugs in the United States by meta-analysis to calculate national rates of HIV and hepatitis C virus ifections. *PLoS ONE, 9*(5), e97596.

Maxwell, J. C. (2014). A new survey of methamphetamine users in treatment: Who they are, why they like "meth," and why they need additional services. *Substance Use and Misuse, 49*(6), 639–644.

Miller, B. F., Petterson, S., Burke, B. T., Phillips, R. L., & Green, L. A. (2014). Proximity of providers: Colocating behavioral health and primary care and the prospects for an integrated workforce. *American Psychologist, 69*(4), 443–451.

Mishra, A., Chaturvedi, P., Datta, S., Sinukumar, S., Joshi, P., & Garg, A. (2015). Harmful effects of nicotine. *Indian Journal of Medical and Paediatric Oncology: Official Journal of Indian Society of Medical and Paediatric Oncology, 36*(1), 24–31.

Mitchell, D. C., Knight, C. A., Hockenberry, J., Teplansky, R., & Hartman, T. J. (2014). Beverage caffeine intakes in the U.S. *Food and Chemical Toxicology, 63*(Suppl. C), 136–142.

Muncie, H. L., Yasinian, Y., & Oge, L. (2013). Outpatient management of alcohol withdrawal syndrome. *American Family Physician, 88*(9), 590–595.

National Academies of Science, Engineering, and Medicine. (2018). *Public health consequences of e-cigarettes. Consensus study report: Highlights.* Retrieved from https://www.nap.edu/resource/24952/012318ecigaretteHighlights.pdf.

National Alliance on Mental Illness. (2017). *Risk of suicide.* Retrieved from https://www.nami.org/Learn-More/Mental-Health-Conditions/Related-Conditions/Suicide.

National Association for Children of Alcoholics. (2015). *Children of alcoholics: Important facts.* Retrieved from www.nacoa.net/impfacts.htm.

National Center for Complementary and Integrative Health. (2017). *Chronic pain: In depth.* Retrieved from https://nccih.nih.gov/health/pain/chronic.htm.

National Institute on Alcohol Abuse and Alcoholism. (2015a). *Beyond hangovers* (NIH Publication No. 15-7604). Rockville, MD: Author.

National Institute on Alcohol Abuse and Alcoholism. (2015b). *Planning alcohol interventions using NIAAA's College AIM (Alcohol Intervention Matrix)* (NIH Publication No. 15-AA-8017). Bethesda, MD: Author.

National Institute on Alcohol Abuse and Alcoholism. (2015c). *Rethinking drinking: Alcohol and your health.* (NIH Publication No. 15-3770). Bethesda, MD: Author.

National Institute on Alcohol Abuse and Alcoholism. (2017). *Underage drinking.* Retrieved from https://pubs.niaaa.nih.gov/publications/underagedrinking/Underage_Fact.pdf.

National Institute on Drug Abuse. (2014a). *Drugs, brains, and behavior: The science of addiction* (NIH Pub No. 14-5605). Rockville, MD: National Institutes of Health.

National Institute on Drug Abuse. (2014b). *Principles of adolescent substance use disorder treatment: A research-based guide* (NIH Publication Number 14-7953). Rockville, MD: National Institutes of Health.

National Institute on Drug Abuse. (2015a). *Hallucinogens and dissociative drugs: Including LSD, psilocybin, peyote, DMT, ayahuasca, PCP, ketamine, dextromethorphan, and salvia* (NIH Publication No. 15-4209). Rockville, MD: National Institutes for Health.

National Institute on Drug Abuse. (2015b). *Marijuana: Facts parents need to know* (NIH Publication No. 14-4036). Rockville, MD: National Institutes of Health.

National Institute on Drug Abuse. (2016). *What is cocaine?* Retrieved from https://www.drugabuse.gov/publications/drugfacts/cocaine.

National Institute on Drug Abuse. (2017a). *Impacts of drugs on neurotransmission.* Retrieved from https://www.drugabuse.gov/news-events/nida-notes/2017/03/impacts-drugs-neurotransmission.

National Institute on Drug Abuse. (2017b). *What are inhalants?* Retrieved from https://www.drugabuse.gov/publications/drugfacts/inhalants.

National Institute on Drug Abuse. (2017c). *What is methamphetamine?* Retrieved from https://www.drugabuse.gov/publications/drugfacts/methamphetamine.

National Institute on Drug Abuse. (2017d). *What is the scope of MDMA use in the United States?* Retrieved from https://www.drugabuse.gov/publications/research-reports/mdma-ecstasy-abuse/what-is-the-scope-of-mdma-use-in-the-united-states.

National Institute on Drug Abuse. (2018). *Opioid overdose crisis.* Retrieved from https://www.drugabuse.gov/drugs-abuse/opioids/opioid-overdose-crisis.

National Institutes of Health. (2015). *How smoking affects your health.* Retrieved from http://nihseniorhealth.gov/quittingsmoking/howsmokingaffectsyourhealth/01.html.

Patrick, M. E., & Maggs, J. L. (2014). Energy drinks and alcohol: Links to alcohol behaviors and consequences across 56 days. *Journal of Adolescent Health, 54*(4), 454–459.

Pinkerton, R., & Hardy, J. R. (2017). Opioid addiction and misuse in adult and adolescent patients with cancer. *Internal Medicine Journal, 47*(6), 632–636.

Pokorny, A. D., Miller, B. A., & Kaplan, H. B. (1972). The brief MAST: A shortened version of the Michigan Alcohol Screening Test. *American Journal of Psychiatry, 129*, 342–345.

Potter, M. L., & Moller, M. D. (Eds.). (2018). *Psychiatric-mental health nursing: From suffering to hope* (2nd ed.). Upper Saddle River, NJ: Pearson Education.

Preller, K. H., Herdener, M., Pokorny, T., Planzer, A., Kraehenmann, R., Stämpfli, P., . . . Vollenweider, F. X. (2017). The fabric of meaning and subjective effects in LSD-induced states depend on serotonin 2A receptor activation. *Current Biology, 27*(3), 451–457.

Rudd, R. A. (2016). Increases in drug and opioid-involved overdose deaths—United States, 2010–2015. *Morbidity and Mortality Weekly Report, 65*, 1445–1452.

Saraiya, T., Campbell, A., & Hu, M.-C. (2017). Predictors of internet-delivered drug treatment outcomes and acceptability among women. *Drug & Alcohol Dependence, 171*, e183–e184.

Schaefer, A., & McDermott, A. (2106). Coffee and cholesterol: Is there a link? *Healthline.* Retrieved from https://www.healthline.com/health/high-cholesterol/coffee-link

Schmid, Y., Enzler, F., Gasser, P., Grouzmann, E., Preller, K. H., Vollenweider, F. X., . . . Liechti, M. E. (2015). Acute effects of lysergic acid diethylamide in healthy subjects. *Biological Psychiatry, 78*(8), 544–553.

Schuckit, M. A. (2014). Recognition and management of withdrawal delirium (delirium tremens). *New England Journal of Medicine, 371*(22), 2109–2113.

Seifert, S. M., Seifert, S. A., Schaechter, J. L., Bronstein, A. C., Benson, B. E., Hershorin, E. R., . . . Lipshultz, S. E. (2013). An analysis of energy-drink toxicity in the National Poison Data System. *Clinical Toxicology, 51*(7), 566–574.

Skinner, H. A. (1982). *Drug Abuse Screening Test (DAST).* Langford Lance, UK: Elsevier Science.

Substance Abuse and Mental Health Services Administration (SAMHSA). (2012, July 2). Highlights of the 2010 drug abuse warning network (DAWN) findings on drug-related emergency department visits. *DAWN Report.* Rockville, MD: Author.

Substance Abuse and Mental Health Services Administration. (2014a). *E-cigarettes pose risks.* Retrieved from https://www.samhsa.gov/samhsaNewsLetter/Volume_22_Number_3/e_cigarettes/.

Substance Abuse and Mental Health Services Administration. (2014b). *Trauma-informed care in behavioral health services* (HHS Publication No. [SMA] 13-4801). Rockville, MD: Author.

Substance Abuse and Mental Health Services Administration. (2014c). *Treatment improvement protocol: Improving cultural competence* (SMA 14-4849). Rockville, MD: Author.

Substance Abuse and Mental Health Services Administration. (2015a). *Detoxification and substance abuse treatment: A treatment improvement protocol* (HHS Publication No. [SMA] 15-4131). Rockville, MD: Author.

Substance Abuse and Mental Health Services Administration. (2015b). *Medication for the treatment of alcohol use disorder: A brief guide* (HHS Publication No. [SMA] 15-4907). Rockville, MD: National Institutes of Health, National Institute on Alcohol Abuse and Alcoholism.

Substance Abuse and Mental Health Services Administration. (2016a). *Buprenorphine.* Retrieved from https://www.samhsa.gov/medication-assisted-treatment/treatment/buprenorphine.

Substance Abuse and Mental Health Services Administration. (2016b). *Methadone.* Retrieved from https://www.samhsa.gov/medication-assisted-treatment/treatment/methadone

Substance Abuse and Mental Health Services Administration. (2016c). *Rural behavioral health: Telehealth challenges and opportunities [In brief].* Rockville, MD: SAMHSA. Retrieved from https://store.samhsa.gov/shin/content/SMA16-4989/SMA16-4989.pdf.

Substance Abuse and Mental Health Services Administration. (2017a). *A day in the life of older adults: Substance use facts.* Retrieved from https://www.samhsa.gov/data/sites/default/files/report_2792/ShortReport-272.html.

Substance Abuse and Mental Health Services Administration. (2017b). *About the Office of Behavioral Health Equity (OBHE).* Retrieved from https://www.samhsa.gov/behavioral-health-equity/about#KEYS.

Substance Abuse and Mental Health Services Administration. (2017c). *Qualify for nurse Practitioners (NPs) and physician assistants (PAs) waiver.* Retrieved from https://www.samhsa.gov/medication-assisted-treatment/qualify-nps-pas-waivers.

Taliaferro, J. D., Lutz, B., Moore, A. K., & Scipien, K. (2014). Increasing cultural awareness and sensitivity: Effective substance treatment in the adult lesbian population. *Journal of Human Behavior in the Social Environment, 24,* 582-588.

Talley, A. M., Gilbert, P. A., Mitchell, J., Goldbach, J. Marshall, B.D.L., & Kaysen, D. (2016). Addressing the gaps on risk and resilience factors for alcohol use outcomes in sexual and gender minority populations. *Drug and Alcohol Review, 35,* 484-493.

Wall, T. L., Luczak, S. E., & Hiller-Sturmhöfel, S. (2016). Biology, genetics, and environment: Underlying factors influencing alcohol metabolism. *Alcohol Research: Current Reviews, 38*(1), 59.

Wesson, D. R., & Ling, W. (2003). The clinical opiate withdrawal scale (COWS). *Journal of Psychoactive Drugs, 35*(2), 253–259.

West, N. A., Severtson, S. G., Green, J. L., & Dart, R. C. (2015). Trends in abuse and misuse of prescription opioids among older adults. *Drug and Alcohol Dependence, 149,* 117–121.

Wheeler, E., Jones, T. S., Gilbert, M. K., & Davidson, P. J. (2015). Opioid overdose prevention programs providing naloxone to laypersons — United States, 2014. *Morbidity and Mortality Weekly Report, 64*(23), 631–635.

Whiteford, H. A., Degenhardt, L., Rehm, J., Baxter, A. J., Ferrari, A. J., Erskine, H. E., . . . Vos, T. (2013). Global burden of disease attributable to mental and substance use disorders: Gindings from the Global Burden of Disease Study 2010. *The Lancet, 382*(9904), 1575–1586.

Wilson, B. A., Shannon, M. T., & Shields, K. M. (2017). *Pearson nurse's drug guide 2017.* Upper Saddle River, NJ: Pearson Education.

Yang, H.-C., Chen, I.-C., Tsay, Y.-C., Li, Z.-R., Chen, C.-h., Hwu, H.-G., & Chen, C.-H. (2017). Using an event-history with risk-free model to study the genetics of alcoholism. *Scientific Reports, 7*(1975), 4–12.

Yokoyama, A., Mizukami, T., & Yokoyama, T. (2015). Genetic polymorphisms of alcohol dehydrogense-1B and aldehyde dehydrogenase-2, alcohol flushing, mean corpuscular volume, and aerodigestive tract neoplasia in Japanese drinkers. In V. Vasiliou, S. Zakhari, H. K. Seitz, & J. B. Hoek (Eds.), *Biological basis of alcohol-induced cancer* (pp. 265–279). Cham, Switzerland: Springer.

Zhang, H., Teng, T., Lu, H., Zhao, Y., Liu, H., Yin, L., . . . Vermund, S. H. (2016). Poppers use and risky sexual behaviors among men who have sex with men in Beijing, China. *Drug and Alcohol Dependence, 160*(Suppl. C), 42–48.

ADDITIONAL RESOURCES

American Society of Addiction Medicine
https://www.asam.org

National Institute on Alcohol Abuse and Alcoholism
https://www.niaaa.nih.gov

National Institute on Drug Abuse
https://www.drugabuse.gov

Substance Abuse and Mental Health Services Administration
https://www.samhsa.gov

Chapter 7

Nursing Care of Patients Experiencing Disasters

Chapter Outline and Learning Outcomes

Explain the difference between an emergency and a disaster.

Outline the five phases of the disaster continuum and discuss the nurse's role in each.

Describe the types of injuries and manifestations associated with biologic, chemical, or radiologic terrorism.

Differentiate the common injuries associated with various types of disasters.

Describe the interprofessional care and nursing care of patients in a disaster.

CLINICAL COMPETENCIES

- Activate a personal and family disaster plan to allow for your participation in disaster response.
- Apply accepted triage tools and systems adopted by local emergency medical services and hospitals to establish care based on disaster situation and available resources.
- Adapt evidence-based standards of nursing practice, based on resources available, to implement nursing care for patients with injuries suffered as a result of a disaster.
- Provide safe and knowledgeable nursing care to treat disaster-related injuries.
- Evaluate and revise plan of care to restore functional health status to patients who have sustained injuries due to a disaster.
- Maintain personal safety and the safety of others at the scene of a disaster.
- Provide education to promote participation in core preparedness activities.

KEY TERMS

bioterrorism, 161
cold zone, 167
conventional weapons, 161
disasters, 158
emergency, 158
evaluation phase, 161
hot zone, 167
human-generated disasters, 158
mass casualty events (MCEs), 158
mitigation, 160
natural disasters, 158
nonconventional terrorist weapons, 161
personal protective equipment (PPE), 167
preparedness, 159
radiation sickness, 165
recovery, 161
response, 160
reverse triage, 167
surge capacity, 160
terrorism, 161
triage, 167
warm zone, 167

Disasters occur nearly every day somewhere in the world with significant health consequences for individuals, families, healthcare systems, and communities. As the largest healthcare workforce, nurses are expected to know how to provide care for victims of disasters whether they work in acute care settings, ambulatory sites, long-term care facilities, or at home in their communities. There is no way to know where or when disasters may strike. Because of this, nurses must be prepared to develop a personal plan to protect their own family so they are available to assist patients, families, friends, healthcare workers, first responders, and communities in their recovery from disastrous events. The frequency of disasters is increasing.

There are a number of basic competencies that nurses should be cognizant of related to disaster preparedness. The World Health Organization (WHO) and International Council of Nurses (ICN) published the *ICN Framework of Disaster Nursing Competencies* (2009), which were validated in 2016 (Hutton, Veenema, & Gebbie, 2016) (**Box 7.1**). This framework defines competencies pertinent to all registered nurses and addresses nursing actions required in each phase of disaster management. Awareness of critical competencies prepares nurses to participate in disaster prevention/mitigation and preparedness, respond effectively to mass casualty events, and contribute nursing care during the recovery/rehabilitation phase. Nurses are expected to have sufficient knowledge to recognize the potential for a disaster event to occur; when such an event has occurred; and what they can do to protect themselves, family members, and community members from harm or from potential exacerbation of conditions. Nurses need to be aware of their role in disaster planning, response, mitigation, and recovery. Equally important, nurses must be aware of professional limitations and be able to respond to mass casualty events appropriately within the scope of nursing practice.

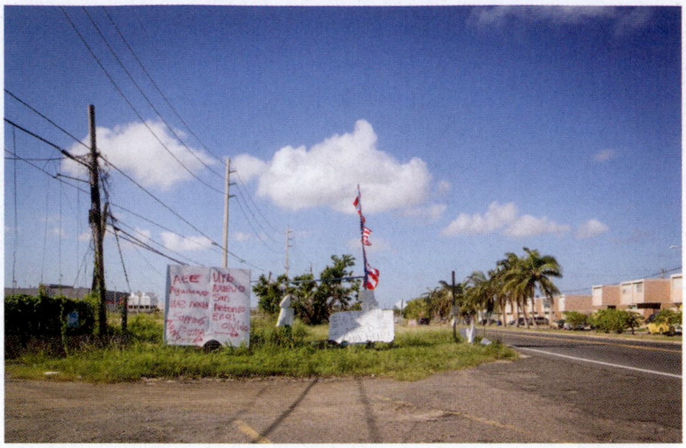

Figure 7.1 ■ Hurricane Maria inundated Puerto Rico on September 20, 2017, just 2 weeks after Hurricane Irma did the same. A total of 64 people died during the storm, but over 4600 people died from September 20 through the end of December 2017 due to effects of the storm. Reported issues include delayed medical care or no medical care at all, an inability to access medications for chronic conditions, and lack of electricity to run respiratory equipment (Kishore et al., 2018). This photo was taken on October 19, a month after the hurricane, showing people pleading for help.

7.1 Disasters and Emergencies

Veenema and Woolsey (2013) define a **disaster** as " . . . any destructive event that disrupts the normal functioning of a community" (p. 3). Disasters may be natural or human generated. **Natural disasters** are caused by acts of nature or emerging diseases. They may be unexpected or predictable through advanced meteorologic technologies. For example, in 2017 Hurricane Irma caused catastrophic damage in the Caribbean before hitting Florida, and an even worse storm, Hurricane Maria, hit Puerto Rico, the Dominican Republic, and the Virgin Islands, killing thousands of people (**Figure 7.1** ■). Puerto Rico lost its entire electric grid and months after the storm is still suffering from island-wide outages every few weeks (Holmes, 2018).

Human-generated disasters are designated into three broad categories: Complex emergencies, technologic disasters, and disasters that are not caused by natural hazards but occur in human settlements. Human-generated disasters are either accidental or intentional. Examples of human-generated disasters include mass shootings; war; chemical, biologic, radiologic, and nuclear terrorism; transportation accidents; group violence; food or water contamination; deforestation; and building collapse. Using bacteria or a toxin to contaminate large amounts of vegetables at a grocery store is an example of a deliberate or intentional human-generated disaster. A campfire that has been left unattended such that the embers are carried by high winds to the dry trees and brush nearby, creating a massive forest fire, is an example of a human-generated accidental disaster (**Figure 7.2** ■).

An **emergency** is distinguished from a disaster in that an emergency encompasses an unforeseen combination of circumstances calling for immediate action for a range of victims from one to many. For example, a motor vehicle crash may call for emergency assistance for a small number of individuals whose injuries are minor to very severe or fatal. Emergencies are generally accommodated within the emergency management system. Complex emergencies such as a multivehicle crash may be labeled as a multiple casualty event that does not exceed the capacity of local resources to provide needed medical care.

In contrast, disasters seldom involve a single victim. Instead, disasters are complex emergencies that significantly overwhelm available hospitals, emergency medical services, facilities, and resources. Disasters are typically labeled as **mass casualty events (MCEs)** because the event occurs quickly and suddenly and overwhelms local resources with many seriously ill or injured victims needing care. An example of a mass casualty event is that of an entire community affected by the release of a hazardous material, such as a chemical, as a result of a train derailment.

BOX 7.1
Disaster Nursing Competencies

1. Risk reduction, disease prevention, and health promotion
2. Policy development and planning
3. Ethical practice, legal practice, and accountability
4. Communication and information sharing
5. Education and preparedness
6. Care of communities
7. Care of individuals and families
8. Psychologic care
9. Care of vulnerable populations
10. Long-term care needs.

Source: WHO & ICN, 2009.

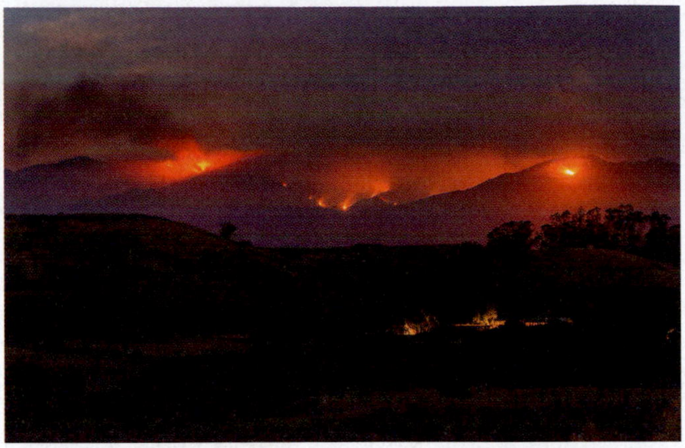

Figure 7.2 ■ Nationwide, over 80% of wildfires are started by humans. In California in 2017, over 1.3 million acres were burned in wildfires, more than 10,000 structures were damaged or destroyed, and 43 people were killed. The Whittier fire pictured here was accidentally started by teenager driving a vehicle through tall grass at a camp (Ferreira, 2018).

In summary, the key difference between an emergency and a disaster is that an emergency can be handled by the usual emergency management systems already in place, whereas a disaster overwhelms general emergency systems and requires additional resources.

7.2 The Disaster Continuum

The cycle of activity related to disaster is referred to as the *disaster continuum* (Veenema & Woolsey, 2013). This cycle occurs preimpact (before), impact (during), and postimpact (after) a disaster. The five basic phases of disaster management are preparedness, mitigation, response, recovery, and evaluation (Veenema, 2018) (**Figure 7.3** ■). Actions taken during each phase, in combination with the nature and scope of the preparedness, influence the extent of illness, injury, and death that occurs. It is important to understand that these phases do not necessarily happen in sequence; they may overlap or occur simultaneously.

Preparedness

Preparedness refers to proactive planning and preparation while the threat of a disaster is still in the future, and efforts are aimed at developing a disaster response prior to occurrence. Preparedness means having a comprehensive disaster plan in place that coordinates efforts among many people, agencies, and levels of government. The plan is based on familiarity with possible disaster agents based on previous experiences, as well as experiences of others from various regions and countries. It is imperative that all individuals and agencies who may be involved in the disaster response be involved in the planning. In this way, information is shared and representatives from each agency explain and offer their respective resources and expertise and note deficiencies in the plan. Planning committees will exist on all levels—federal, regional, state, local, and individual agencies.

In the United States, disaster preparedness has been a priority issue for government and military agencies. These efforts have been expanded to public and private healthcare sectors. Healthcare professionals are among the essential personnel in addressing disaster preparations and in dealing with the consequences of a disaster. Nurses comprise the largest group of healthcare professionals and will play key roles in disaster relief whether they work in hospitals, residential facilities, ambulatory care, schools, or at home in their communities. The general public looks to nurses for information and trusts that what nurses advise is true and accurate. Nurses have a responsibility to be educated and to assimilate the new skills and demands necessary to assist patients, families, and communities in preparing for and responding to disastrous situations effectively. National Incident Management System (NIMS) courses are offered free of charge through the Federal Emergency Management

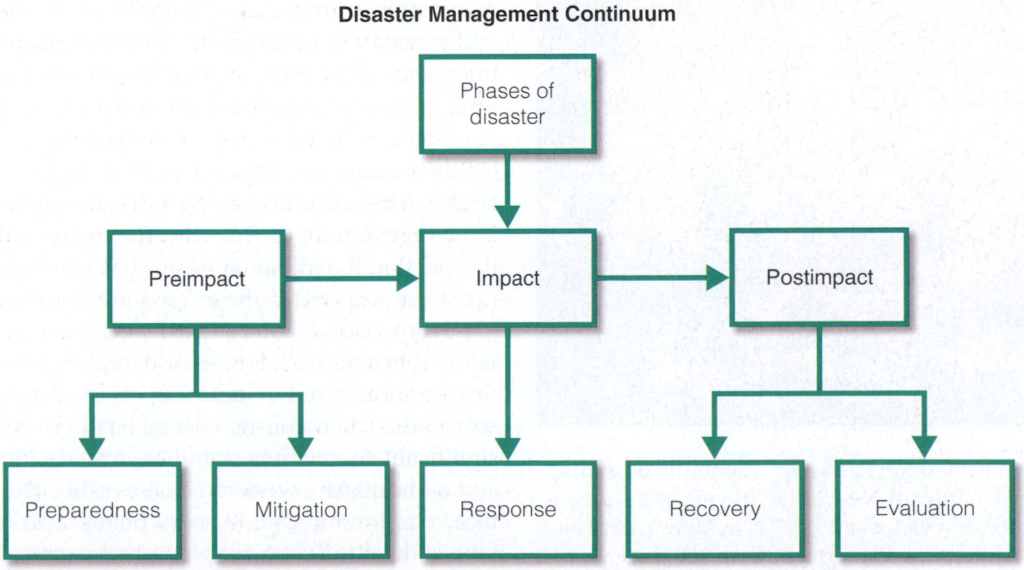
Disaster Management Continuum
Phases of disaster
Preimpact
Impact
Postimpact
Preparedness
Mitigation
Response
Recovery
Evaluation

Figure 7.3 ■ Disaster management is a process that includes preparedness, mitigation, response, recovery, and evaluation.

Agency (FEMA) and provide needed education to prepare nurses for providing care in disasters.

Numerous disaster agencies are involved in disaster planning, response, and mitigation depending on the severity of the disaster and the resultant necessary response. The U.S. National Response Framework (NRF) is a national effort designed to integrate resources of the local, state, and federal governments and includes voluntary relief agencies, the private sector, and international resources if needed to provide assistance to communities following natural or human-made disasters (Department of Homeland Security, 2016). The Department of Homeland Security (DHS) and FEMA coordinate the NRF to provide assistance when local and state resources are not sufficient to provide needed disaster response. The NRF and NIMS work together to facilitate the nation's incident management capacity and improve efficiency. NRF and NIMS ensure that jurisdictions and disciplines work together to respond to disasters by following standardized practices.

Local disaster response plans include action plans for various types of disaster situations, designation of the overall incident commander, and identification of community resources. The local emergency management agency is also represented in the state management planning efforts.

Hospitals and other healthcare agencies develop their own disaster plans. However, it is very important for each agency to understand its role within the larger community disaster plan. When disasters occur, competing healthcare systems must put the competition aside and work collaboratively in the response effort to ensure favorable outcomes following a disaster.

Nurses participate in disaster planning by having a nurse representative on the planning committee at least at the agency level. Disaster preparedness involves identifying potential vulnerabilities and anticipating the probability for a disaster to occur. For example, some geographic locations are prone to tornadoes so buildings are equipped with tornado shelters and citizens participate in tornado drills.

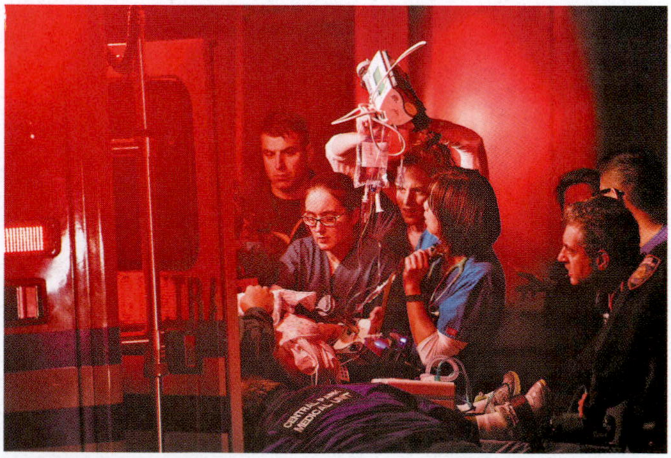

Figure 7.4 ■ Medical workers assist a patient into an ambulance during an evacuation of New York University's Langone Medical Center, Monday, October 29, 2012, in New York. The New York City hospital moved out more than 200 patients, including 20 infants from the NICU, after its backup generator failed when the power was knocked out by Hurricane Sandy.

Hospital disaster planners must prepare for the possibility that a disaster may involve the hospital. The hospital's response may include the evacuation of patients as well as relocating and operating from an independent facility (**Figure 7.4** ■). **Surge capacity** is the healthcare system's ability to rapidly expand beyond normal services to meet the increased demand for qualified personnel, medical care, and public health in the event of a large-scale disaster. Hospitals must be constantly aware of the number of beds available, which patients may be discharged, staffing, equipment, other resources, and their overall ability to manage casualties quickly.

Mitigation

The **mitigation** phase includes measures to reduce the harmful effects of a disaster and occurs when there is knowledge about an impending disaster that has not yet occurred. Activities during this stage include warning, pre-impact mobilization, and evacuation, if appropriate.

Response

The **response** phase happens after a disaster has occurred. It involves the immediate response to the effects of the disaster. National agencies have state and local offices that respond to disasters. However, the most immediate response is from the local groups and organizations. The community relies on local assistance or aid because outside sources of aid have not yet arrived. The local disaster response organizations include fire departments, police departments, public health departments, public works, emergency services, and the local branch of the American Red Cross. The community is rapidly assessed for damage, and the types and extent of injuries suffered as well as the immediate needs of the community determined.

Assistance from outside of the affected area arrives later, and search and rescue operations commence as well as first aid, emergency medical assistance, establishment or restoration of communication and transportation, assessment of infectious diseases and mental health problems, and evacuation of residents, if necessary. Individual states may request aid from neighboring states or the federal government if the disaster exceeds local and state resources.

Nurses should follow the disaster plan of their agencies, communities, and the local emergency management agency. This includes having a disaster plan for the nurse's immediate family. In this way, the nurse will feel secure in the fact that the immediate family is situated safely and the nurse can respond to the staging area to await instructions.

Nurses use a multitude of nursing knowledge and skills to assist in a disaster. Nurses use their expertise in infectious disease control and in assessing physical as well as psychosocial needs. In a disaster, mental health issues are extremely significant for victims, families, friends, first responders, and all healthcare workers. Nurses will ensure that patients receive follow-up care for both physical wounds and mental health concerns. Advanced practice nurses may take on significantly greater responsibilities, especially if they are competent and prepared in emergency and trauma care.

Protocols and standards of care are in place to guide the practice of all nurses. Nurses need to determine the boundaries of their practice in times of emergencies when mass numbers of victims must be treated without the luxury of an on-site physician.

Recovery

In the **recovery** and reconstruction phase, restoration and reconstitution take place. This stage involves rebuilding and returning to some semblance of normalcy. During this phase, restoration, reconstitution, and mitigation take place. Restoration includes rebuilding, replacing lost or damaged property, returning to school and work, and continuing life without those who were killed in the disaster. Reconstitution occurs when the life of the community returns to a new normal.

Evaluation

The final stage of recovery is the **evaluation phase** (Veenema, 2018). The evaluation phase involves determining what worked and what did not work and what anticipated and unanticipated issues and challenges emerged. Evaluation is also an activity in the preparation and planning aspects of the nondisaster stage. This illustrates the cyclical nature of planning and disaster response; the work is never complete. Future-oriented activities take place to prevent subsequent disasters or to minimize their effects. Some of these activities may include increased security and surveillance measures. Nurses may suggest ideas for responding to the victims of disasters more effectively and efficiently. For example, nurses may communicate the need for carts stocked with specific items that will assist them in treating patients faster. They may suggest a more efficient method of tracking patients as they enter the healthcare system and move from area to area based on the patients' acuity and condition.

7.3 Terrorism

Terrorism is defined by the U.S. Department of Defense (2018) as the "unlawful use of violence or the threat of violence, often motivated by religious, political, or other ideological beliefs, to instill fear and coerce governments or societies in pursuit of goals that are usually political." One of the goals of terrorism is to cause psychologic effects that reach a much wider audience than the immediate victims or object of an attack. High-profile acts draw attention to the terrorists and their cause. It is thought that terrorists seek to obtain leverage, influence, and power through the publicity generated by their violence (Wahedi, 2016).

The weapons terrorists use are often described as conventional and nonconventional. **Conventional weapons** include bombs and guns. Car/truck and package bombs have become powerful weapons in attacks such as the Boston Marathon bombing on April 15, 2013 (**Figure 7.5 ■**). Terrorists use explosive devices such as letters, parcels, pipes, pressure cookers, barometric and fertilizer truck bombs, as well as incendiary bombs such as Molotov cocktails. Other types of conventional terrorist weapons include handguns, rifles, semiautomatic weapons, hand grenades, rocket-propelled devices, and even surface-to-air, shoulder-fired missiles that can bring down helicopters, fighter aircraft, and civilian airliners.

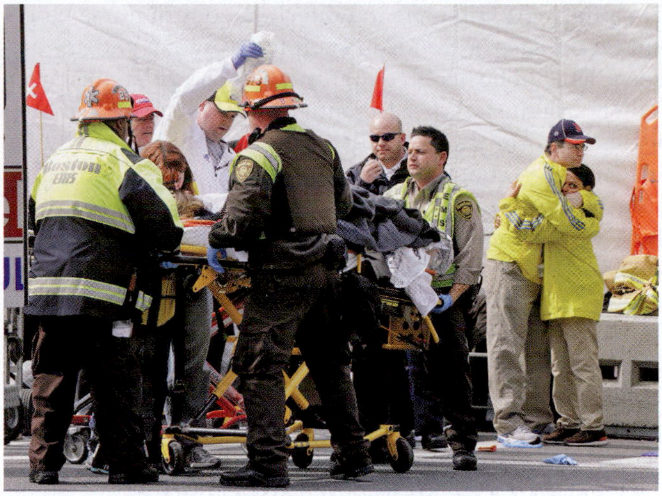

Figure 7.5 ■ EMS personnel and volunteer nurses helped care for hundreds of victims of the Boston Marathon bombings on April 15, 2013.

Nonconventional terrorist weapons include those in the chemical, biologic, and nuclear categories. Chemical terrorism attacks may manifest as the release of a toxin into highly populated areas, bodies of water, and unventilated areas. Another type of chemical terrorism is a specific attack on a particular product, especially a food product. This is accomplished by introducing a toxic chemical substance directly into the product.

Bioterrorism

Bioterrorism involves the use of etiologic agents (disease) with deliberate intent to cause illness or death in a population, food, and/or livestock. Bioterrorism includes the use of organisms such as bacteria, viruses, and rickettsia and the use of products of organisms—toxins. The main purpose of biologic weapon use is mass devastation. Unfortunately, it is not uncommon for the results of a biologic attack not to be known for several hours or days after the attack because aerosolized biologic particles are odorless, colorless, and tasteless. Unless the terrorists announce the biologic attack, its occurrence may remain unknown until patients begin to present at emergency departments or physicians' offices a few days or weeks after the release of the agent. Detection is difficult because of the numerous different healthcare facilities available for patient treatment. Surveillance is essential to detect such an event. The goal of the surveillance system is to determine the status of the public's health and detect any sudden change in that status. Fortunately, biologic weapons are not as common, accessible, or available as chemical weapons.

Healthcare providers must be alert to the recognition, reporting, and treatment of high-priority biologic agents. A disaster preparedness plan should be established in every healthcare facility to outline the protocol and procedures to be taken in response to a suspected bioterrorism attack.

Hospital staff will alert the infection control nurse when subtle changes or trends in symptoms among patients are seen. The public health department is also given this data. When an unusual disease pattern presents itself, laboratories perform tests on cultures that would normally be discarded as contaminants. Laboratory personnel report unusual clusters of laboratory results. Special laboratories have been established to perform a battery of tests on suspicious specimens of rarely seen bacteria, toxins, viruses, or increased numbers of a particular strain or specimen. The Centers for Disease Control and Prevention (CDC; 2018c) has created detailed planning and response toolkits about bioterrorism agents and diseases for healthcare providers.

Nuclear/Radiologic Terrorism

The nuclear category of nonconventional terrorist weapons encompasses the use of a nuclear device to cause mass murder and devastation. This category of terrorism includes the use, or threat of the use, of fissionable radioactive materials in an attack. A purposeful explosion at a nuclear power plant is an example of this type of terrorism. Using conventional weapons against one of the many nuclear reactors in the world could cause an explosion that would result in extensive and possibly irreversible environmental damage. Damage to the reactors could cause radioactive matter to be released into the atmosphere, potentially endangering large population centers.

The radiologic dispersion bomb is probably the most accessible nuclear device to be used by terrorists. Another name for this device is *dirty bomb* because it consists of a conventional explosive combined with radioactive waste by-products from nuclear reactors. The dirty bomb discharges deadly radioactive particles into the environment. It is cheaper to make than a nuclear bomb and radioactive waste material is relatively easy to obtain. Radioactive waste is found throughout the world and is typically not as well guarded as nuclear weapons. The CDC has created detailed planning and response toolkits about radiological terrorism (CDC, 2018d).

7.4 Types of Disasters and Associated Common Injuries

This section describes a variety of disasters and the injuries that are common to each specific disaster. **Table 7.1** outlines types of disasters with related injuries and nursing implications.

Hurricanes and Tornadoes

A *hurricane* is a type of tropical cyclone. It is a low-pressure system that generally forms in the tropics. Hurricanes can wreak havoc on coastlines as well as several hundred miles inland. Hurricanes and tropical storms can also spawn tornadoes, create storm surges along the coast, and cause extensive damage from heavy rainfall. Floods are deadly and destructive. Excessive rain can trigger landslides or

Table 7.1 Types of Disasters and Common Injuries

Type of Disaster	Common Injuries	Nursing Implications
Natural Disasters		
Hurricane-related injuries	Drowning; cleanup injuries; aggravation of chronic illnesses; stress-related symptoms; upper respiratory infections; gastrointestinal illnesses; animal, snake, and insect bites; obstetric complications; contaminated water supplies and insect-breeding grounds; heat-related illnesses; lack of sanitation and safe housing	■ Asphyxia; wounds; bone, joint, and muscle injuries; infections; skin irritations; waterborne and insect-borne diseases; dehydration; starvation or malnutrition; diseases may occur. ■ Evaluate for hidden injuries and responses, in addition to those that are apparent.
Tornado-related injuries	Flying debris; injuries similar to hurricane-related injuries	■ Injuries and fatalities can occur from direct impact from the storm or afterward when people walk in the debris and enter damaged buildings.
Thunderstorm-related injuries	Resistance of body tissues to electrical current *Least resistance:* Nerves, blood, mucous membranes, muscle *Intermediate resistance:* Dry skin *Most resistance:* Tendon, fat, bone	■ Potential for tissue destruction with longer duration of contact with high-voltage current; if energy current is dissipated at the skin surface, significant surface burns result, especially in calloused areas.
Earthquake-related injuries	High incidence of mortality and morbidity; explosions	■ May result in stress-related symptoms; wounds; bone, joint, and muscle injuries; cleanup injuries; gastrointestinal and respiratory problems; aggravation of chronic illnesses; obstetric complications; burns.
Tsunami-related injuries	"Tsunami lung," a severe infection caused by aspirating muddy, bacteria-laden water	■ Requires aggressive respiratory and ventilator management, blood transfusions, antibiotics, and other medical support.
Snowstorm-related injuries	Overexertion and exhaustion	■ Myocardial infarction can occur.
Disaster-related eye injuries	Specks of dust or debris; cuts, punctures, or stuck objects; blows to the eye	■ Administer eyewash or flushing versus rubbing; stabilize eye with rigid shield. ■ Apply cold compress, no pressure; patient should visit healthcare professional to rule out serious injury or internal eye damage.

Type of Disaster	Common Injuries	Nursing Implications
Traumatic Injuries		
Blast injuries	Auditory	■ Tympanic membrane rupture, ossicular disruption, and cochlear damage occur; damage from foreign body can occur.
	Eye, orbit, face	■ Perforated globe, air embolisms, fractures are common; damage from foreign body can occur.
	Respiratory	■ May result in blast lung, hemothorax, pneumothorax, pulmonary contusion and hemorrhage, atrioventricular fistulas (source of air embolism), airway epithelial damage, aspiration pneumonitis, sepsis.
	Digestive	■ May result in bowel perforation, hemorrhage, ruptured liver or spleen, sepsis, mesenteric ischemia from air embolism.
	Circulatory	■ Cardiac contusion, myocardial infarction from air embolism, shock, vasovagal hypotension, peripheral vascular injury, and air embolism–induced injury can occur.
	Central nervous system injury	■ Concussion, closed and open brain injury, stroke, spinal cord injury, air embolism–induced injury can occur.
	Renal injury	■ May result in renal contusion, laceration, acute kidney injury due to rhabdomyolysis, hypotension, and hypovolemia.
	Extremity injury	■ Traumatic amputation, fractures, crush injuries, compartment syndrome, burns, cuts, lacerations, acute arterial occlusion, air embolism–induced injury can occur.
Blunt trauma	Head and torso blunt trauma, penetrating trauma	■ Fractured limbs, spinal injury, pulmonary and cardiac contusions can occur.
Pressure trauma	Lungs	■ Tearing of the alveoli causes swelling, fluid accumulation, possible pulmonary emboli, eventual hypoxia.
	Ear injury: Ear pain, hearing loss	■ Keep auditory canal clean.
	Bowel injury	■ Make the patient comfortable.
Biologic, Radiologic, and Chemical Injuries		
Radiologic dispersion bomb (dirty bomb) blast	Radiation sickness	■ Get rid of contaminated clothes, shower, and evacuate the area within a day of a small or medium blast. Those close to the blast could suffer radiation sickness and require hospital care.
Nuclear detonation	Thermal burns	■ May involve only the epidermis and upper layers of dermis with short duration of heat exposure.
Bright light flash of nuclear detonation	Eye burn injuries	■ May blind the patient momentarily, effects will disappear with time, can impair a patient's ability to perform self-care and other ADLs.
Radiation exposure injury	Bone marrow and blood cell damage	■ A reduction in the blood's oxygen-carrying capacity results in nausea, fatigue, and a general feeling of malaise. Reduced platelet production causes clotting disorders and possibly hemorrhage. When the body's white blood cells are destroyed, it is important to reduce the patient's exposure to infection. Infection at the time of reduced WBC production can be severe and even fatal.
	Bowel	■ Cells that reproduce the bowel lining are damaged, resulting in nausea and vomiting, loss of appetite, diarrhea, fluid loss, and malaise in the acute stage; later, dehydration, malnutrition, bowel hemorrhage, and perforation may occur; if radiation exposure is not exacerbated by other injury or pathology, patients will generally survive.
	Integument	■ Erythema or generalized reddening of the skin occurs when skin cells are damaged, with the appearance of a sunburn; more serious burns may occur with persistent exposure or extremely high radiation doses.
	Nervous and cardiovascular systems	■ With acute radiation exposure, blood vessel and nerve cells are damaged and the patient is incapacitated and experiences cardiovascular collapse, confusion, and even an "on fire" sensation throughout the body; symptoms this severe generally do not permit survival.
Chemical burns	Range from minor to life-threatening injuries	■ Remove clothing from injury site as well as any jewelry; flush chemical from skin with thorough decontamination; cover wounds loosely with a dry, sterile, or clean cloth.

Source: Adapted from CDC, 2018b.

mudslides, especially in mountainous regions. Flooding on rivers and streams may persist for several days or more after the storm (Department of Homeland Security, 2018b).

Common physical effects of hurricanes include asphyxia due to drowning; wounds; bone, joint, and muscle injuries; aggravation of chronic illnesses; stress-related symptoms; upper respiratory infections; gastrointestinal illnesses; cleanup injuries; animal, snake, and insect bites; skin irritations and infections; obstetric complications; and waterborne and insect-borne diseases from contaminated water supplies and insect breeding grounds (Veenema, 2018).

As a result of Hurricane Harvey in 2017, many people lost their homes, family members, friends, and the environment that supported their daily routines. Many basic physical needs in the aftermath of the hurricane could not be met, which put survivors at risk of dehydration, starvation or malnutrition, heat-related illnesses, and diseases and injuries related to lack of sanitation and safe housing.

Flying debris causes most fatalities and injuries in tornadoes. The physical effects include bone, muscle, and joint injuries; fractures; aggravation of chronic illnesses; obstetric complications; stress-related symptoms; upper respiratory infections and those associated with fiberglass; eye injuries; cleanup wounds; and gastrointestinal illnesses (Veenema, 2018).

Thunderstorms

Risk of a lightning strike is possible during a thunderstorm. The short duration of a lightning strike results in a very short flow of current internally, despite the high voltage of lightning. Additionally, the almost immediate flashover of current around the body usually results in very little, if any, skin breakdown or burning of muscle and tendon tissues (Veenema, 2018). However, the pathway that the current takes will determine the tissues at risk and the type of injury, as well as the duration of contact with the electrical current.

High electrolyte and water content in the body conduct the greatest electrical current. Hence, the greatest conductors of electrical current in the body are the nerves, muscles, and blood vessels. High resistors to electric current are bone, tendon, and fat, due to their tendency to heat up and coagulate instead of transmitting current. Much of the energy current may be dissipated at the skin surface. This may result in surface burns, especially in calloused areas (Veenema, 2018). Lightning strikes can also cause concussive blunt trauma, internal burns, cardiac or respiratory arrest, vascular spasm, and neurologic damage (Cooper, 2017).

Earthquakes and Tsunamis

Earthquakes have a high incidence of mortality and morbidity. The most common health effects experienced by victims of earthquakes include stress-related symptoms; wounds; bone, joint, and muscle injuries; burns from explosions; cleanup injuries; gastrointestinal and respiratory problems; aggravation of chronic illnesses; obstetric complications; and death (Veenema, 2018).

A *tsunami*, a seismic sea wave, is a series of ocean waves characterized by having a long period and wavelength and the ability to travel at speeds greater than 500 miles per hour. As a tsunami encounters shallow water, its height increases drastically, resulting in a sudden increase in sea level, thereby flooding low-lying coastal areas (**Figure 7.6** ■). Injuries are similar to those seen with hurricanes.

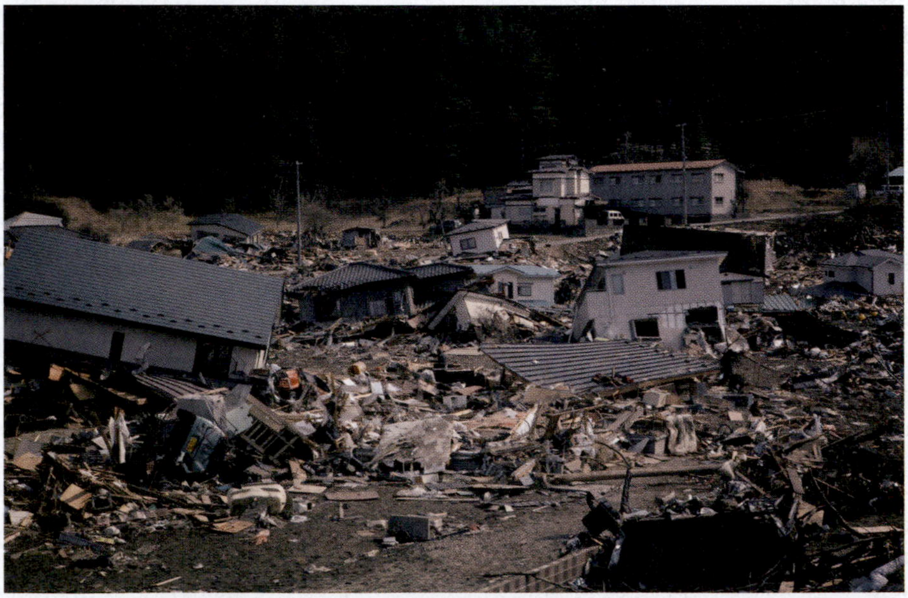

Figure 7.6 ■ Fukushima, Japan, the day after a tsunami inundated this coastal area, killing over 19,000 people. Three nuclear reactors were flooded, releasing radioactive material and causing 100,000 people to be evacuated (World Nuclear Association, 2017).

Snowstorms

Overexertion and exhaustion are major problems resulting from the snow shoveling that is done following a snowstorm. The exertion required to shovel heavy snow in the extreme cold may cause a myocardial infarction.

Hazardous Materials

Hazardous materials pose a potential risk to life, health, or property if they are released because of their chemical, biologic, or physical nature. The hazard exists during any stage of use, from the production and storage of these substances to their transportation, use, or disposal. Hazardous materials accidents range from the unintentional release of household hazardous materials, to chemical spills on highways, to groundwater contamination by naturally occurring methane gas (Veenema, 2018). Symptoms will vary depending on the type of hazardous material patients are exposed to. The nurse works closely with the intraprofessional team to identify the hazardous substance and develop a specific treatment plan.

Explosives

Blast injuries are the result of explosive munitions, often involving car or package bombs. Penetrating and blunt injuries are common following explosions. Care for individuals injured by blast injuries typically focuses on abdominal and lung injuries, penetrating wounds, traumatic amputations, and burns. There is high risk for hemorrhage so patients should be assessed and treated quickly (American College of Surgeons [ACS], 2018).

Radiologic Dispersion Bomb Blast

A radiologic dispersion bomb blast (dirty bomb) consists of a conventional explosive such as trinitrotoluene (TNT) packed with radioactive waste by-products from nuclear reactors. When the dirty bomb explodes, the radioactive material spreads in the wind like a dust cloud. In this way, it reaches far wider areas than the initial explosion (ACS, 2018). The long-term destructive force of the dirty bomb is caused by ionizing radiation from the radioactive material. In an individual's body, an ion's electrical charge may lead to unnatural chemical reactions inside the cells. The charge can break DNA chains. Cells with broken DNA strands either die or the DNA develops a mutation. Diseases develop as the result of widespread cell death. If the DNA mutates, a cell may become cancerous. The cancer may spread and the cells may malfunction. This series of events may result in a wide variety of symptoms collectively referred to as **radiation sickness**. Although this condition can be deadly, with stem cell transplantation it is survivable.

People are exposed to ionizing radiation frequently, but in small doses, with little if any ill effects. Some of the sources of this everyday exposure are outer space, stars, the sun, natural radioactive isotopes, and x-ray machines. The risk of cancer and radiation sickness is increased by exposure to a dirty bomb and the subsequent rise in radiation levels above normal. The fatal effects of the dirty bomb may not be apparent in the short term after exposure, but could kill people years later.

Nuclear Detonations

With a nuclear detonation, a thermal burn is the most common mechanism of injury and death. A tremendous amount of thermal energy is created by a nuclear reaction. This energy travels unimpeded through the air. The energy is absorbed by the contact surface where it may create burns or ignite combustibles. The burns may involve only the epidermis and upper layers of dermis because of the short duration of heat exposure; however, thermal burn injuries can be severe and are treated like any other burn. Radiation exposure results in injury from ionizing radiation, altering some cell structures. Cells are damaged from the changes in DNA in bone marrow, blood, bowel, skin, and nervous and cardiovascular systems. Radiation suppresses the immune system, so special care must be taken to reduce the potential infection often associated with full-thickness burns. More information on burn care can be found in Chapter 17.

The major activities performed for patients who have suffered a nuclear casualty are triage, evacuation or sheltering, search and rescue, radioactive monitoring, decontamination, and direct patient care. The patient will be assessed for injuries such as burns or blunt trauma. Pressure injuries such as lung injury, difficult breathing, or minor strokelike symptoms (air emboli) must be assessed quickly. Early complaints of radiation exposure may include nausea or fatigue. The manifestations of serious radiation exposure may not occur for several hours and do not suggest imminent death. Since radiation has a cumulative danger, shorter exposure times are less damaging. Flash blindness to the eyes caused by a detonation blast lasts only a few minutes during daylight and up to 30 minutes at night. Reassure patients that their eyesight will return, and have someone remain with them until their sight is restored.

The patient, along with the healthcare provider and first responders, should be evacuated from the exposure area. Wind shifts are monitored continuously to minimize exposure.

7.5 Care of Patients in a Disaster

Emergency preparedness and disaster response depend on the collaboration of an interprofessional healthcare team involving local, state, and federal governmental agencies. Training and participation in tabletop exercises, simulations, and mock incidents not only prepare the team members to assume their roles in case of disaster but also provide opportunities for frequent evaluations of the plan. These evaluations lead to more effective emergency plans and facilitate communications across the interprofessional team that is responsible for the development, implementation, and evaluation of an emergency response plan. Nurses often have contact with members of emergency medical services (EMS) in both emergency departments and disaster situations. A brief overview of the EMS system is presented in **Box 7.2**.

BOX 7.2
The Emergency Medical Services System

The emergency medical services (EMS) system is a network of resources that provides emergency care and transportation, that is, prehospital care, to victims of illness, injury, or disaster. EMS personnel, who must be trained and licensed, work under the auspices of a medical director, usually a hospital-based physician, who is consulted as needed. There are four levels of EMS professionals.

EMRs and EMTs provide basic life support:

- ***Emergency medical responders (EMRs)*** provide initial emergency care including assessment, opening airways, ventilating, controlling bleeding, performing CPR, stabilizing the spine and injured limbs, assisting with childbirth, and aiding other EMS personnel.
- ***Emergency medical technicians (EMTs)*** do everything EMRs do, but have received additional training and certification. This permits them to assist patients with prescribed medications and give aspirins, NSAIDs, oral glucose, and other medications when indicated.

AEMTs and paramedics are qualified to provide advanced life support:

- ***Advanced emergency medical technicians (AEMTs)*** have received advanced emergency training so they may start and administer IV fluids; give medications; and assess the need for and provide advanced airway procedures.
- ***Paramedics*** receive the most training and are qualified to do more in-depth assessments of patients, including the assessment of abnormal heart rhythms, and to perform some invasive procedures.

Interprofessional Care

Personal Protective Equipment and Isolation

All healthcare providers must apply clean or sterile gloves, gowns, masks, respirators, and protective eyewear according to the risk of exposure to potentially infective materials (National Institute for Occupational Safety and Health [NIOSH], 2018).

Gloves. Gloves are worn for three reasons:

1. Gloves protect the hands when the nurse is likely to handle any body substances.
2. Gloves reduce the likelihood of nurses' transmitting their own endogenous microorganisms to individuals receiving care. Nurses who have open sores or cuts on the hands must wear gloves for protection.
3. Gloves reduce the chance that the nurse's hands will transmit microorganisms or a fomite from one patient to another patient.

In all situations, nurses must change gloves between patient contacts. Nurses should clean their hands each time they remove gloves for two primary reasons: The gloves may have imperfections or may have been damaged during wearing, allowing microorganism entry, and the hands may become contaminated during glove removal.

Some of the gloves used in infection control are made of latex, as are various other items used in healthcare (e.g., catheters, blood pressure cuffs, rubber sheets, intravenous tubing, stockings and binders, adhesive bandages, and dental dams). Because of the frequent use of gloves, healthcare workers and some patients with chronic illnesses have increasingly reported allergic reactions to latex. Latex gloves that are lubricated by powder or cornstarch are particularly allergenic because the latex allergen adheres to the powder, which is aerosolized during glove use or removal of gloves and is then inhaled by the user. Latex gloves that are labeled "hypoallergenic" still contain measurable latex and should not be used by or on individuals with known latex sensitivity.

Gowns. The nurse wears a clean or disposable impervious (water-resistant) gown or plastic apron during procedures when the nurse's uniform is likely to become soiled. A sterile gown may be indicated when the nurse changes the dressings of a patient with extensive wounds (e.g., burns). *Single-use gown technique* (using a gown only once before it is discarded or laundered) is the usual practice in hospitals. After the gown has been worn, the nurse discards it (if it is paper) or places it in a laundry hamper. Before leaving the patient's room, the nurse cleanses his hands. An *isolation gown* is meant to be worn only one time. It is donned prior to entering the patient's room to provide bedside care and removed at the conclusion of care. The gown prevents contamination of the care provider's uniform by a patient's infection. It is important to review the agency's protocol for correct use of the type of isolation gown provided by the agency.

SAFETY ALERT: Wearing a patient hospital gown over your uniform does not serve any infection control purpose. Providers should wear isolation gowns to prevent contamination of their uniform or clothes and remove the gown at the end of the healthcare interaction. ■

Face Masks. Masks are worn to reduce the risk of transmitting organisms by the droplet contact and airborne routes and by splatters of body substances. Masks should be worn by the following individuals:

1. Individuals close to the patient if the infection (e.g., measles, mumps, or acute respiratory diseases in children) is transmitted by large-particle aerosols (droplets). Large-particle aerosols are transmitted by close contact and generally travel short distances (about 1 m or 3 feet).
2. All individuals entering the room if the infection (e.g., pulmonary tuberculosis and SARS-CoV) is transmitted by small-particle aerosols (droplet nuclei). Small-particle aerosols remain suspended in the air and thus travel greater distances by air. Special masks that provide a tighter face seal and better filtration may be used for these infections.

Various types of masks differ in their filtration effectiveness and fit. Single-use disposable surgical masks are effective for use while the nurse provides care to most patients, but they should be changed if they become wet or soiled. These masks are discarded in the waste container after use. Disposable particulate respirators of different types may be effective for droplet transmission, splatters, and airborne microorganisms.

During performance of certain techniques requiring surgical asepsis (sterile technique), masks are worn (a) to prevent droplet contact transmission of exhaled microorganisms to the sterile field or to a patient's open wound and (b) to protect the nurse from splashes of body substances from the patient.

Eyewear. Protective eyewear (goggles, glasses, or face shields) and masks are indicated in situations in which body substances may splatter the face. If the nurse wears prescription eyeglasses, goggles must be worn over the glasses to extend around the sides of the glasses.

Respirators. There are two basic types of respirators. The first type cleans the air to make it breathable. This type includes particulate respirators, which remove airborne particles, and gas masks, which remove chemicals and gases. The second type supplies clean air from another source. This type includes self-contained breathing apparatus (SCBA) (NIOSH, 2018). Gas masks are used in a broad range of military, industrial, and emergency situations to protect the user from hazardous dust, gas, or other aerosols. Biologic contaminants that are spread through aerosolized droplets create a threat to those not wearing personal protective equipment. A gas mask may be considered a high-performance respirator and is usually equipped with both eye protection and air supply protection or treatment. A hood, helmet, or headgear is generally worn to protect the skin, eyes, airway, and respiratory system.

Triage

During a disaster, healthcare providers are often required to perform triage. **Triage** means sorting. Nurses perform triage every day in every emergency department. Upon learning of a disaster, one of the most urgent unit-level priorities is triaging hospitalized patients to expedite the discharge or transfer of the lowest-acuity patients to free up resources for disaster victims. At the disaster site, a very basic triage system is to categorize or label victims needing the most support and emergency care as **red** (**Table 7.2**). Those less critical but still in need of transport to emergency centers for care are classified as **yellow**. Victims who have minor injuries and do not warrant transport to an emergency center are categorized as **green.** Victims who are least likely to survive or are already deceased are color coded as **black**. These are the triage levels given to patients under normal circumstances or when there are only a few victims.

However, when there is a mass casualty event with more than 100 patients, **reverse triage** may be instituted. Reverse triage works on the principle of the greatest good for the greatest number. For example, if there were a collision between a train full of railroad cars filled with toxic chemicals and a full tour bus in a highly populated area, this disaster would likely be called a mass casualty event. In this case, those persons who were the most ambulatory and least injured would be transported or instructed to move quickly to the warm zone, away from the immediate accident site to get decontaminated and processed first (**Box 7.3**). Those with minor injuries would be decontaminated next. Those with more severe to most severe injuries would be treated in that order. In this way, the most victims with the greatest chance of survival could be saved most efficiently with limited resources. Many emergency personnel will share the difficulty of making these decisions at disaster sites when the first inclination might be to rescue the most severely injured.

Triage is a continuous process in which priorities are reassigned as needed treatments, time, and the condition of the victims change. This process must balance human lives with the realities of the situation, such as supplies and personnel (**Box 7.4**). The triage role requires an individual who is able to rapidly assess patients' conditions under stressful, often adverse conditions and assign a category. Those assigned to triage are expected to function independently, yet as part of a coordinated team effort (ACS, 2018). It has been suggested that emergency personnel should triage/categorize the victims so that physicians and nurses can be

Table 7.2 Simple Triage and Rapid Transport (START) System

Red (emergent)	Critically injured, with problems that will require immediate intervention to correct. Patients with a respiratory rate above 30 are tagged *red*. If their respirations are below 30, assess their circulatory status. If capillary refill takes more than 2 seconds, tag them *red*. If it is below 2 seconds, assess mental status. Patients who cannot follow simple commands are tagged *red*.
Yellow (urgent)	Injured, and will require some medical attention, but will not die if care is delayed while you care for other patients; not ambulatory and will require a stretcher for transportation. Patients who can follow simple commands such as hand grips are tagged as *yellow*.
Green (ambulatory)	Not critically injured and can walk and care for themselves. Have them walk to a safe place, but do not lose track of them; every patient triaged at an incident is tracked to the best of the responder's ability.
Black (expectant)	Deceased, or have such catastrophic injuries that they are not expected to survive. If the patient is not breathing, open the airway manually. If the patient remains apneic, tag him or her *black*; if the patient begins breathing, he or she is tagged *red*.

Source: Adapted from ACS, 2018.

BOX 7.3 Hot, Warm, and Cold Zones

Hot zone: The site of a disaster where a weapon was released or where contamination occurred is called the *hot zone*. It is considered contaminated and only those persons in the appropriate **personal protective equipment (PPE)** may enter it. PPE is equipment used for the protection of personnel and includes gloves, masks, goggles, gowns, and biologic disposal bags. Typically, fire, police, and military personnel will collect evidence and begin their investigation in this zone.

Warm zone: The warm zone is adjacent to the hot zone. Another name for this area is the *control zone*. This area is where decontamination of victims or triage and emergency treatment take place. The level of PPE required is based on the dynamic risk assessment of the threat and agent involved.

Cold zone: The *cold zone* is considered to be the safe zone. It is adjacent to the warm zone and is the area where a more in-depth triage of victims would occur. Survivors may find shelter in this area, and the command and control vehicles would be found here as well as the emergency transport vehicles.

BOX 7.4
Key Triage Points to Remember

1. Use a triage system that is easy to learn, easy to implement in stressful conditions, and does not require advanced diagnostic skills yet allows for basic patient interventions.
2. Use the incident management system (defined by each facility and based on the area's civilian and military authorities) for every incident and wear personnel identification vests. Incident management systems use logical management structure, defined responsibilities, clear reporting channels, and a common language.
3. Get accurate preliminary and final patient counts and relay this information to the incident commander.
4. Use some type of visual color-coded identification system to indicate patient priority.
5. Do not fall into the trap of using your time to provide one-to-one patient care.
6. Retriage patients frequently, at the incident, on arrival at the treatment area, and periodically thereafter.
7. Make certain the walking-wounded are gathered and treated.
8. Preplan for potential incidents that may occur.
9. Be aware that emergency responders may be potential targets.
10. Practice, practice, practice.

best utilized in the treatment area, performing patient care. Advanced practice personnel will continue to triage and perform more complete assessments.

Crowd Control

When a disaster occurs, many people converge on the site. Those who come include the curious as well as those who truly mean to assist in the rescue and recovery of victims. This crowd of people needs to be controlled by authorities in charge of the site and rescue and recovery. Similarly, crowds may arrive at the hospital or healthcare delivery sites when injured or even when they think they may be injured or contaminated in some way. The job of crowd control is not under the auspices of nurses or other healthcare personnel. The agency's security personnel and/or the local police force must control these crowds. If control is not maintained, chaos ensues and those in greatest need of medical assistance may be unable to reach healthcare providers in order to avoid further declines in their health status. In fact, nurses, physicians, and other healthcare workers should not enter an area that has not been secured. To put one's safety at risk jeopardizes the potential treatment of many. Additionally, social services personnel or psychiatric service providers should be available to assist the worried to cope with the trauma they have experienced, witnessed, or heard about through the news media.

Psychosocial Needs

The importance of mental health services for victims, the public, first responders, and healthcare workers cannot be overstated. Both those individuals directly affected by the disaster as well as those indirectly affected will seek medical care and advice. Many who seek medical attention are simply anxious about the threat of injury. At times, reassurance is all that is necessary. However, with large numbers of people seeking healthcare, the system is quickly overwhelmed. Mental health experts may quickly assess individual needs, offer immediate advice, and refer for follow-up care if deemed appropriate.

People react to disasters in a variety of ways, both physically and behaviorally. Their reactions depend on the severity of the threat and their proximity to the area of direct impact. The closer the person is to the area of impact and the longer the exposure, the greater the likelihood of a more severe reaction to the event. **Table 7.3** summarizes the normal initial responses aimed at survival (CDC, 2018a; Potter & Moller, 2016).

Most people exhibit great coping mechanisms and resilience in the aftermath of a disaster. For those who do not, mechanisms should be developed for identifying and referring them to psychologic counseling. After the September 2001 terrorist attacks on the World Trade Center and the Pentagon, it was reported that 71% of people surveyed felt depressed, 49% had difficulty concentrating, and 33% had trouble sleeping at night. Most (92%) felt sad when watching news coverage of the event, yet 63% stated a compulsion to continue to watch the news (Pew Research Center for the People and the Press, 2001). Reactions to terrorist events and disasters in general are influenced by developmental level and maturity, prior experiences with disasters, and cultural background (Veenema, 2018).

Nursing Care

The Role of the Nurse in Disaster Relief

Nurses have roles in many facets of disaster management, including identifying the event, functioning as a first responder at the scene, working with a rapid needs assessment team to identify needed resources, and providing direct care to disaster victims in hospitals, federal medical stations, public health departments, or field medical teams. Nurses may be involved in managing communications and working with the media or assuming leadership roles in the coordination of multiple disaster response activities. Because nurses have an obligation to keep current in new and emerging trends in healthcare and threats to society, learning about the prevention and mitigation of disasters is essential. Nurses must first know how to take care of themselves in order to assist others. The Department of Homeland Security (2018a) suggests that everyone should have an emergency kit stocked with a 3-day supply food, water, and other necessities. This is often called a *go bag*. Instructions can be found at *www.ready.gov/build-a-kit*.

Nurses should remain aware of the roles they play in all aspects of disaster preparedness and response. By educating oneself and being proactive in regular drills and practice of skills, nurses take an active role in helping others to save

Table 7.3 Responses to Stress

Timing of Responses	Physical Responses	Behavioral Responses
Initial responses	■ Pupils dilate ■ Vision blurs ■ Hearing sharpens or diminishes	■ Misinterpret stimuli ■ Confusion ■ Poor concentration ■ Selective inattention ■ Need for assistance
Later responses	■ Stronger, faster heart rate ■ Stronger, faster respirations ■ Palpitations and arrhythmias ■ Elevated blood pressure ■ Increased muscle tension ■ Headaches ■ Increased basal metabolic rate ■ Increased temperature ■ Increased perspiration ■ Altered glucose, protein, and lipid metabolism ■ Hypoglycemia due to high energy demands ■ Increased blood clotting ■ Suppressed immune system ■ Fatigue ■ Weight loss ■ Altered digestion and elimination	■ Severe anxiety or panic ■ Increased startle response ■ Feeling of impending doom ■ Feelings of terror, fear, agitation ■ Excitability ■ Insomnia ■ Urgency of speech and movement
Delayed responses	■ Changes in appetite, energy, and activity levels ■ Difficulty sleeping ■ Difficulty concentrating ■ Headaches, body aches ■ Worsening of chronic health conditions ■ Anger ■ Increased use of alcohol, tobacco, and other substances	■ Nightmares ■ Grief ■ Survivor guilt ■ Posttraumatic stress disorder

lives and fulfill an important obligation to society. Roles of nurses in disasters include:

1. Prepare selves, families, friends, and communities for disasters in conjunction with the local disaster preparedness plan. Have a go bag packed and ready.
2. Continue educating self on various types of disasters and appropriate response.
3. Provide emergency services with consideration of victims' abilities, deficits, culture, language, or special needs.
4. Assist in the mobilization of healthcare personnel, food, water, shelter, medication, clothing, and other assistive devices.
5. Collaborate with agencies in authority including local, state, and federal representatives to deploy resources based on the greatest good for the greatest number.
6. Consider needs of victims including shelter both temporary and permanent, as well as psychologic, economic, legal, and spiritual factors.
7. Become involved with local, state, and national disaster planning agencies to schedule regular meetings to continually review and modify disaster plans.

Applying basic first aid skills can be very helpful in immediate disaster relief efforts until emergency help can be obtained. The American Red Cross invites nurse volunteers and will provide the necessary training. Many nurses have taken advantage of online disaster certificate programs, and efforts are being made to integrate disaster preparedness content into nursing courses.

In many different practice settings, nurses serve on disaster preparedness and response planning committees. Nurses are receiving in-service education on biologic, chemical, and radiologic threats to patient health as well as surveillance and reporting of suspicious activities. Although nursing professionals may not be asked to don decontamination gear to aid victims, nurses should be aware of decontamination procedures so that they will remain safe from exposure and be able to direct others when threatened with contamination. Some nurses choose to be actively involved with disaster medical assistance teams as part of the National Disaster Medical System (NDMS). The NDMS is a multiagency program (Department of Health and Human Services, Department of Defense, Veterans Administration, Department of Homeland Security) coordinated by the NRF that supplements an integrated national medical response to assisting states and local authorities in dealing with the medical aspects of peacetime disasters.

In a true mass casualty event, it is impossible to have physicians present at every station where they are needed. Nurses may have to assume expanded roles in making decisions for the most appropriate treatment of casualties. Discussions should take place among physicians, nurses, and policymakers regarding the necessity of the nurses' expanded roles in crisis situations. As noted earlier in the chapter, these agency policies must be documented in an agency-wide plan. Additionally, all healthcare personnel must receive specialized training required to be safe and competent practitioners of the expanded duties. This training must be practiced and updated, and those participating in the training must be tracked and notified of additional requirements as necessary. Refer to your state's nurse practice act or guidance on scope of practice issues related to disaster response.

Roles of Nurses Working with Victims of Disasters

The role of the nurse in a disaster depends on a number of variables, including the nature of the disaster, the number of victims and severity of injuries, the location of the disaster as well as the location of the nurse, and the availability of supplies, rescue and command personnel, and other necessary resources. The nurse must be able to perform under stressful conditions but will not be expected to endanger self, other nurses, or other rescuers.

If it is safe to do so, the nurse begins by triaging and assessing the victims for the best care and best use of available resources. Very quick, direct treatment may be given or the nurse may be involved in extended periods of time with a mobile surgical unit. Local authorities such as the police, fire, and emergency medical services will guide the nurse in securing the area and determining the safe zone for the nurse and others to work. The National Disaster Medical System is the agency responsible for coordinating disaster relief with local fire, police, and emergency medical services to provide overall disaster assistance. Victim assistance may be offered in the field in mobile shelters, in local clinics, in hospitals, or in makeshift buildings.

Nurses take on a variety of roles based on their expertise and the needs of the victims. Nurses are expected to follow the emergency preparedness plans outlined in their communities and in their agencies of employment. Communication and teamwork are essential when involved in disaster response. Moreover, individual nurses should be the leaders in their communities in discussing emergency preparedness and contingency plans.

Considerations for Patients with Special Needs

Older Adults. It is not appropriate to generalize the needs of all older adults. Many are quite independent and active into their 90s. However, some older persons lack the physical stamina to recover quickly from disastrous events. The nurse must assess the individual's ability to cope with and recover from unexpected events, socioeconomic factors, support systems, potential healthcare needs, and resources. See the accompanying Case Study & Nursing Care Plan.

Teaching about disaster preparedness is important in all communities. Older adults need to determine the appropriateness of sheltering in place should there be an environmental event outside of their homes. Evacuation plans for older adults who cannot care for themselves for prolonged periods of time should be addressed. Consideration should be given to additional factors such as the time of year and need for heating and cooling during an extended power outage. This becomes a very real issue when roads become impassable or usual modes of transportation and communication are disrupted.

Older adults should be encouraged to keep a current list of medications, doses, and times of administration in an easily accessible, secure place. The names and phone numbers of significant individuals, relatives, those with power of attorney, healthcare providers, or any others to be notified in case of emergency should also be kept in an easily accessible place. Additionally, the following materials should be considered essential to keep with the person should evacuation to a shelter be necessary: Eyeglasses and eyeglass prescriptions, style and serial numbers of medical devices such as pacemakers, healthcare policies and numbers, identification, list of allergies, blood type, checkbook, credit cards, insurance agent's name and number, driver's license, 72-hour supply of medications, dentures, list of special dietary needs, sturdy shoes, warm clothing, blankets, incontinence briefs, prostheses, hearing aids, hearing aid batteries, extra wheelchair batteries, oxygen, and other assistive devices.

Immunocompromised Patients. Patients who are immunocompromised pose special problems for the healthcare community, especially if access to healthcare is unavailable due to a disaster situation. A compromised immune system may be due to treatments such as chemotherapy or immunosuppressants or from an underlying disease such as HIV. The immunocompromised population would be at greater risk for complications and death than the general population should a bioterrorist attack occur.

An additional issue the nurse should discuss with this population is the patients' preparation for disaster events related to infection control. Patients should carry treatment calendars with them at all times so that any healthcare provider can determine where they are in their treatment program and disease process. Patients should plan a backup location to visit for chemotherapy if their usual office is inaccessible. Nurses should assess their patients' knowledge level regarding the avoidance of raw seafood or possibly contaminated water. Bottled water should be ready so the patient can avoid drinking water of questionable purity. Bone marrow and stem cell transplant patients are instructed not to eat fresh fruits and vegetables due to the risk of contamination and subsequent infection. It is safest for this population of patients to consume processed or canned foods if they can be heated to the proper temperatures.

Patients with Sensory, Speech, or Literacy Deficits. Persons who have sensory deficits, speech or language impairments, or low literacy levels must be assessed for the most effective means of communicating steps to be taken in the case of a disaster. Emergency personnel or rescue teams may need to learn a few basic phrases in American Sign Language. Something as simple as carrying a notepad and pencil or directions in large print may be what is necessary to share information with people who have hearing impairments or visual impairments, respectively. People with sensory or speech impairments will not all choose one particular means of communication; they will have individual preferences. A multitude of communication means are available through technologic support systems as well as written and visual cue boards. Public service announcements or reverse 9-1-1 calls may inform the general public about impending natural disasters and about proper steps to be taken to be safely rescued or sheltered. Nurses are in the position of alerting community leaders about special needs of members of their communities. Public service personnel, including fire, police, and emergency services, should be alerted to extenuating circumstances and needs of specific individuals in the community. The collaborative planning efforts of the individual, family members, caregivers, and emergency service personnel will help alleviate any undue pain and suffering caused by the lack of understanding of emergency messages and directives.

Patients with Mobility Deficits. As the U.S. population ages, many people require the use of assistive technology devices (ATDs) to accommodate mobility and other impairments. Careful planning must be in place in order to provide necessary support during and after a disaster. Arrangements should be made in advance to provide adequate numbers of volunteers or staff to assist when this group must be relocated or regrouped in a safe room or shelter. These individuals or their caregivers must provide input to service personnel to determine what kind of support services would be necessary in an emergency or disaster.

Patients with Limited Proficiency in English. It is ideal to obtain the assistance of an interpreter, preferably an interpreter with whom the patient is familiar (a family member or neighbor), to assist in translating information for the patient. Communication aids can be prepared in advance of disasters to be used during emergencies. The communication aids or disaster preparedness and response procedures should be practiced on a regular basis prior to an emergency. The use of visual aids is very helpful. Do not use children as interpreters if adults are available. The stress of interpretation can be overwhelming to the children and place an unnecessary burden on them.

Spiritual Considerations. Religion tends to be a source of comfort for those who are experiencing the threat of loss of life, property, or way of living. Churches, synagogues, mosques, and religious leaders become active in supporting their congregations in times of disaster. Religious leaders should be actively involved in community planning for disaster preparedness, especially if certain religious considerations should be strictly followed. For example, in some religions, the human body and all of its parts are considered sacred. To be sensitive to this religious belief, all tissues and blood would be collected at the site of a disaster by those trained to collect such material, as opposed to washing this matter away from the scene. In general, rescue personnel would need to be informed of specific religious obligations or rights in order to be sensitive to the individual's religious beliefs and practices.

Case Study & Nursing Care Plan

A Patient with Injuries from a Natural Disaster

Mr. Ed Jones, an 84-year-old widower, is retired from his job as a cabinetmaker. He continues to work with wood as a hobby in the basement of his home located on the banks of Deep River. He sells small toys at craft fairs and flea markets in nearby communities. His daughter lives approximately 20 minutes away and checks in on him at least every weekend. Mr. Jones is independent and sees his primary care provider occasionally for monitoring of his blood pressure, which is controlled with antihypertensive medications.

Following a week of heavy rainstorms, flash flooding occurred in the area and Mr. Jones's basement sustained much water damage and ruined most of his stored wood, wooden toy products, and the woodworking machinery. Mr. Jones waded through the waist-deep water to get to the rescue boat rather than wait for the boat to get to him. He is subsequently admitted to the medical-surgical unit due to concerns from the EMTs who triaged him at the fire station 5 miles inland from Mr. Jones's neighborhood.

ASSESSMENT	DIAGNOSES	EXPECTED OUTCOMES
Lisa Smith, RN, obtains a nursing assessment. Mr. Jones states that he has been on antihypertensive medications for "a few years" but only takes his medication "once in awhile" because it has been some time since his last office visit and he wants his remaining pills "to last" until he can get back to the doctor. He has had numerous cuts to his hands from his woodworking and has had a big ulcer on his right foot "for a few weeks" caused by a tool that fell on his foot. He did not seek medical care because he believed it would get better on its own. "It looks worse than it is. It really doesn't even hurt." When asked about his home, he states, "Everything is gone. My wife is gone, my wood, my tools . . . it's all over." Physical assessment findings include T 39.1°C (100.7°F) PO, P 96 bpm, R 20/min, and BP 178/100 mmHg. Skin cool and dry with multiple lesions on both hands and a stage II ulcer on his right dorsal foot with yellow-green exudate. Pain rated at a 2 on a 10-point scale, with 10 being the worst pain there could be. Lungs are clear, heart rate regular. No edema noted. Abdominal assessment is normal. Neurologically intact. Weight is normal for height and frame. A culture is ordered and taken of the yellow-green exudate of the right foot. Preliminary bloodwork results show WBCs at 15,000/mm^3. A peripheral IV is initiated with continuous fluids, and IV antibiotics are ordered every 6 hours. An antihypertensive medication is ordered on a regular schedule plus a prn antihypertensive for systolic >180 and diastolic >90.	■ Lacerations on the right foot and both hands and stage 2 ulcer with exudate on the right foot related to his woodworking hobby ■ Grief related to perceived loss of control over life situation ■ Fever related to infected skin lesions ■ Pain related to skin lesions	■ Patient will regain skin integrity—ulcer on right foot and lesions on hands will heal. ■ Patient will identify aspects of his life still under his control. ■ Patient will maintain body temperature at normothermic levels. ■ Patient will express feeling of comfort and relief from pain.

(continued)

PLANNING AND IMPLEMENTATION

- Assess skin every shift; describe and document skin condition; report changes.
- Clean lesions on hands and right foot every 8 hours and assess healing.
- Administer prescribed antibiotics and assess for effectiveness in treating infection.
- Arrange psychosocial consult(s).
- Guide Mr. Jones through a life review. Encourage reflection on past achievements.
- Help Mr. Jones identify the aspects of his life that are still under his control.
- Monitor temperature every 4 hours, more often if indicated.
- Monitor and record patient's heart rate and rhythm, blood pressure, and respiratory rate every 4 hours.
- Administer analgesics, antipyretics, and medications as indicated.
- Maintain hydration; monitor intake and output.
- Assess level of pain and administer pain medication as prescribed.

EVALUATION

Mr. Jones was hospitalized for 3 days, receiving intravenous antibiotic therapy, analgesics, an antidepressant, monitoring of his cardiac response to a new antihypertensive medication, wound care, and sessions with the social services representative and his daughter. His hand lesions are healed, the foot ulcer has developed new granulation tissue with no signs of infection, he is afebrile, and his blood pressure is maintained within normal limits. He will be discharged to his daughter's home until his home can be assessed for the extent of the water damage and feasibility of repair. He has agreed to visit a therapist to work through his feelings of grief and loss. He has expressed an interest in attending monthly support group meetings with his neighbors who also experienced losses in this disaster.

CLINICAL REASONING IN PATIENT CARE

1. What action did Mr. Jones take that probably exacerbated his skin lesions?
2. What other testing might you anticipate related to Mr. Jones's delayed healing?
3. What were the contributing factors to Mr. Jones's fever?
4. What life situations contributed to Mr. Jones's attitude about life?

See Evaluating Your Response in Appendix B.

CHAPTER HIGHLIGHTS

7.1 Disasters and Emergencies

Explain the difference between an emergency and a disaster.

- Disasters are destructive events that disrupt the normal functioning of a community. They can be natural or generated by humans.
- Emergencies are circumstances that require immediate action for one or more victims. Emergencies can usually be accommodated within the emergency management system.

7.2 The Disaster Continuum

Outline the five phases of the disaster continuum and discuss the nurse's role in each.

- The disaster continuum is a cycle that occurs before, during, and after a disaster.
- Preparedness, proactive planning and preparation while the threat of a disaster is still in the future, is the first phase of the disaster continuum.
- The mitigation phase includes measures to reduce the harmful effects of a disaster and occurs when there is knowledge about an impending disaster that has not yet occurred.
- The response phase happens after the disaster has occurred and includes the immediate response to the effects of the event.
- In the recovery phase, reconstruction, restoration, and reconstitution take place. This includes rebuilding, replacing lost or damaged property, returning to school and work, and continuing life without those who were killed in the disaster.
- Evaluation is the final phase, and it involves determining what worked and what didn't work.

7.3 Terrorism

Describe the types of injuries and manifestations associated with biologic, chemical, or radiologic terrorism.

- Terrorism is defined as the unlawful use of violence or the threat of violence, often motivated by religious, political, or other ideological beliefs, to instill fear and coerce governments or societies in pursuit of goals that are usually political.
- Conventional weapons of terror include guns and bombs. Nonconventional weapons of terror include chemical, biologic, and nuclear agents.

- Bioterrorism involves the use of etiologic agents (disease) with deliberate intent to cause illness or death in a population, food, and/or livestock.
- The nuclear category of nonconventional terrorist weapons encompasses the use of a nuclear device to cause mass murder and devastation.

7.4 Types of Disasters and Associated Common Injuries

Differentiate the common injuries associated with various types of disasters.

- Hurricanes are natural disasters that cause wind, rain, floods, and tornadoes. Injuries in hurricanes include asphyxia due to drowning; bone, joint, and muscle injuries; aggravation of chronic illnesses; stress-related symptoms; upper respiratory infections; gastrointestinal illnesses; cleanup injuries; animal, snake, and insect bites; skin irritations and infections; obstetric complications; and waterborne and insect-borne diseases.
- Tornadoes are wind storms that cause many fatalities and injuries primarily due to flying debris.
- Thunderstorms can generate lightning strikes resulting in surface burns, concussive blunt trauma, internal burns, cardiac or respiratory arrest, vascular spasm, and neurologic damage.
- Earthquakes are natural disasters that can cause bone, joint, and muscle injuries; burns from explosions; cleanup injuries; gastrointestinal and respiratory problems; aggravation of chronic illnesses; obstetric complications; and death. Tsunamis cause similar injuries.
- Hazardous materials pose a potential risk to life, health, or property if they are released because of their chemical, biologic, or physical nature. Symptoms will vary depending on the type of hazardous material patients are exposed to.
- Blast injuries from explosives cause penetrating and blunt injuries. Emergency care focuses on abdominal and lung injuries, penetrating wounds, traumatic amputations, and burns.
- Radiologic and nuclear blasts cause exposure to radiation, which has long-term consequences.

7.5 Care of Patients in a Disaster

Describe the interprofessional care and nursing care of patients in a disaster.

- Personal protective equipment, including gloves, gowns, masks, protective eyewear, and respirators, should be worn by all healthcare providers as needed in disaster situations.
- Triage is used to categorize or label victims needing the most support and emergency care. The principle in reverse disaster triage is to do the greatest good for the greatest number of people.
- Mental health services for victims, the community, and first responders is critical.
- Nurses have roles in many facets of disaster management, including identifying the event, functioning as a first responder at the scene, working with a rapid needs assessment team to identify needed resources, and providing direct care to disaster victims in hospitals, federal medical stations, public health departments, or field medical teams.
- Nurses should take into consideration the special needs of older adults, immunocompromised patients, and patients with communication or mobility issues.

TEST YOURSELF NCLEX-RN® REVIEW

1. The nurse has been asked to participate on the disaster planning committee. What should the nurse realize as being the difference between emergencies and disasters?
   A. Emergencies are controlled.
   B. Disasters result from human-generated errors.
   C. Emergencies can typically be handled by available emergency services.
   D. Disasters typically involve the local emergency services and no other agencies.
2. The nurse is reviewing the competencies needed when preparing and caring for victims of a disaster. In which activities is the nurse likely to participate? (Select all that apply.)
   A. Evaluating care provided during the disaster and fine-tuning disaster preparedness.
   B. Acting as incident commander at the site of a disaster.
   C. Participating in developing policies and planning for disasters.
   D. Educating the community about reducing human-generated disasters.
   E. Evaluating the impact of the disaster on vulnerable populations.
3. The nurse is using reverse triage with victims of a human-generated disaster. Which statement best describes the nurse's actions?
   A. Saving scarce resources for future use
   B. Saving those persons who are in the most critical condition
   C. Testing first responders on their triage classification categories
   D. Using limited resources to do the greatest good for the most people.

4. The nurse works with an interpreter when providing care to a victim of a disaster in a foreign country. Which assessment is primary?
   A. Does the patient speak any English
   B. Level of health literacy in the primary language
   C. Patient's comfort with using an interpreter
   D. Patient's ability to read instructions written in English
5. Prior to assessing a victim of a human-generated disaster, the nurse applies personal protective equipment. What is the best reason for this equipment to be used?
   A. It creates a barrier against hazards.
   B. Wearing PPE is an expectation for all healthcare personnel.
   C. It reduces the likelihood of occupational injury and/or illness.
   D. It prevents the need to follow universal precautions.
6. The charge nurse is discussing decontamination during disaster training. The charge nurse identifies that additional training is necessary when a nurse participant makes which statement?
   A. "Decontamination must be completed before the patient enters the hospital."
   B. "Decontamination is completed in the hot zone."
   C. "Decontamination may take place in the same area as initial emergency treatment."
   D. "Decontamination may be necessary for a variety of types of disasters."
7. The nurse is caring for a victim of a radiologic dispersion bomb. Which intervention would be most likely when caring for this victim?
   A. Apply sterile dressings over extensive burns.
   B. Assess for abdominal organ damage.
   C. Explain that eye injuries will heal in time.
   D. Assess for manifestations of radiation sickness.
8. The nurse is a member of a disaster response task force that is currently reviewing the reconstitution of a community after several tornadoes. What is the committee evaluating at this time?
   A. How the harmful effects of the disaster were reduced
   B. The extent to which the community has achieved a new normal
   C. What worked and what did not work when responding to the disaster
   D. The local healthcare organizations' abilities to respond beyond normal services
9. Why should the nurse assess the special needs of older adults as part of an emergency preparedness plan?
   A. All older adults will need some kind of special support.
   B. Some older adults will take the lead in evacuation efforts in nursing homes.
   C. Not all older adults need the same level of support in emergencies and disasters.
   D. Some older adults will be unable to evacuate even with multiple support systems.
10. After victims of a human-generated disaster are triaged and admitted to the hospital, the emergency department nurses are scheduled for appointments with a mental health professional. Why is this being done? (Select all that apply.)
   A. Determine which nurses need time off after the disaster.
   B. Problem-solve mental health issues of the patients admitted from the disaster.
   C. All nurses need the help of a mental health worker at some point in their careers.
   D. The nurses may feel overwhelmed by the disaster.
   E. The nurses may be traumatized similarly to direct victims of the disaster.

See Test Yourself answers in Appendix B.

REFERENCES

College of Surgeons, Committee on Trauma. (2018). *ATLS: Advanced Trauma Life Support* (10th ed.). Chicago: IL: American College of Surgeons.

Centers for Disease Control and Prevention (CDC). (2018a). *Coping with a disaster or traumatic event.* Retrieved from https://emergency.cdc.gov/coping/selfcare.asp.

Centers for Disease Control and Prevention (CDC). (2018b). *Emergency preparedness and response.* Retrieved from https://emergency.cdc.gov.

Centers for Disease Control and Prevention (CDC). (2018c). *Emergency preparedness and response: Bioterrorism.* Retrieved from https://emergency.cdc.gov/bioterrorism/index.asp.

Centers for Disease Control and Prevention (CDC). (2018d). *Emergency preparedness and response: Radiological terrorism planning and response toolkits.* Retrieved from https://emergency.cdc.gov/radiation/toolkits.asp.

Cooper, M. A. (2017). Lightning injuries. *Medscape.* Retrieved from https://emedicine.medscape.com/article/770642-overview.

Department of Homeland Security. (2016). *National response framework.* Retrieved from https://www.fema.gov/media-library-data/1466014682982-9bcf8245ba4c60c120aa915abe74e15d/National_Response_Framework3rd.pdf.

Department of Homeland Security. (2018a). *Build a kit.* Retrieved from https://www.ready.gov/build-a-kit.

Department of Homeland Security. (2018b). *Hurricanes. Ready.* Retrieved from https://www.ready.gov/hurricanes.

Ferreira, G. (2018, February 5). Officials release cause of the Whittier fire new Lake Cachuma. *The Tribune News.* Retrieved from www.sanluisobispo.com/news/state/california/fires/article198544179.html.

Holmes, R.C. (2018). Puerto Rico's recover, 7 months after Hurricane Maria. *PBS News Hour.* Retrieved from https://www.pbs.org/newshour/nation/puerto-ricos-recovery-7-months-after-hurricane-maria.

Hutton, A., Veenema, T., & Gebbie, K. (2016). Review of the International Council of Nurses (ICN) framework of disaster nursing competencies. *Prehospital and Disaster Medicine, 31*(6), 680–683.

Kishore, N., Marqués, D., Mahmud, A., Kiang, M. V., Rodriguez, I., Fuller, A., . . . Buckee, C. O. (2018, May 29). Mortality in Puerto Rico after Hurricane Maria. *New England Journal of Medicine.* Retrieved from https://www.nejm.org/doi/full/10.1056/NEJMsa1803972.

National Institute for Occupational Safety and Health (NIOSH). (2018). *Personal protective equipment.* Retrieved from https://www.cdc.gov/niosh/ppe/default.html.

Pew Research Center for the People and the Press. (2001). *American psyche reeling from terror attacks.* Retrieved from http://people-press.org/reports/display.php3?ReportID=3

Potter, M. L., & Moller, M. D. (2016). *Psychiatric-mental health nursing: From suffering to hope.* Hoboken, NJ: Pearson Education.

U.S. Department of Defense. (2018). *Dictionary of military and associated terms.* Retrieved from http://dtic.mil/doctrine/dod_dictionary.

Veenema, T. G.(2018). *Disaster nursing and emergency preparedness* (4th ed.). New York, NY: Springer.

Veenema, T. G., & Woolsey, C. (2013). Essentials of disaster planning. In T. G. Veenema (Ed.), *Disaster nursing and emergency preparedness* (3rd ed., pp. 1–20). New York, NY: Springer.

Wahedi, L. A. (2016). Does terrorism work?: The goals of violent actors, and how to avoid giving them what they want. *Global Policy.* Retrieved from https://www.globalpolicyjournal.com/blog/20/12/2016/does-terrorism-work-goals-violent-actors-and-how-avoid-giving-them-what-they-want.

World Health Organization (WHO) and International Council of Nurses (ICN). (2009). *ICN framework of disaster nursing competencies.* Geneva: International Council of Nurses.

World Nuclear Association. (2017). *Fukushima accident.* Retrieved from www.world-nuclear.org/information-library/safety-and-security/safety-of-plants/fukushima-accident.aspx.

ADDITIONAL RESOURCES

American Red Cross

www.redcross.org

ATLS: Advanced Trauma Life Support

https://www.facs.org/quality-programs/trauma/atls

Centers for Disease Control and Prevention (CDC)

https://emergency.cdc.gov

Federal Emergency Management Agency (FEMA)

https://www.fema.gov

National Incident Management System (NIMS)

https://www.fema.gov/national-incident-management-system

Unit

3

Pathophysiology and Patterns of Health

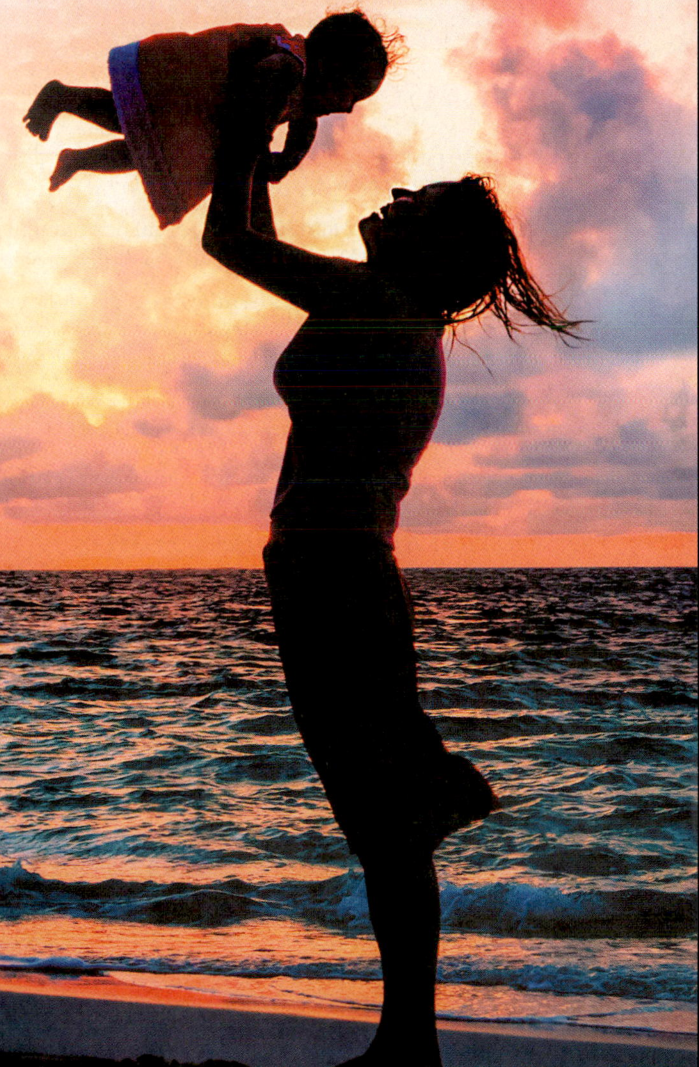

Chapter 8

Genetic Implications of Adult Health Nursing

Chapter Outline and Learning Outcomes

CLINICAL COMPETENCIES

- Integrate genetic assessment and the use of a pedigree family history into delivery of nursing care.
- Identify patients or families with actual or potential genetic conditions and initiate referrals to a genetics professional.
- Prepare patients and their families for a genetic evaluation and facilitate the genetic counseling process.
- Integrate basic genetic concepts into patient and family education with consideration of cultural and personal preferences and values of the family and the reinforcement of information provided to patients by genetic professionals.

KEY TERMS

alleles, 181
autosomal dominant, 182
autosomal recessive, 182
autosomes, 179
biologic markers, 182
chromosomes, 179
gene, 181
genotype, 181
heterozygous, 181
homozygous, 181
human genome, 179
meiosis, 180
mitosis, 179
penetrance, 184
phenotype, 181
polymorphisms, 182
sex chromosomes, 179
somatic cells, 179
translocation, 180
trisomy 21, 180
X-linked recessive, 182

Ongoing research in genetics has enhanced our understanding of the causes of disease, its natural course, and the factors that increase risk for the development of many diseases. Genetics research is focused not only on traditional genetic disorders, but also on common complex diseases such as heart disease, stroke, diabetes, and several kinds of cancer. The knowledge gained from the Human Genome Project (**Box 8.1**) and the continued efforts of scientists and clinicians has and will continue to have a profound impact on the prevention, diagnosis, and treatment of genetic disorders and complex diseases.

Genetic knowledge will continue to revolutionize how individuals perceive themselves, their health status, and their health potential. Therefore, nurses must integrate genetics into nursing practice. The book *Genetic/Genomics Nursing: Scope and Standards of Practice, Second Edition* (2016), from the American Nurses Association and the International Society of Nurses in Genetics (ANA/ISONG) defines the role of all nurses regardless of practice setting, thus emphasizing the importance of genetics for health promotion and treatment of disease.

BOX 8.1
Human Genome Project

In 1986, the U.S. Department of Energy announced the Human Genome Initiative and joined with the National Institutes of Health (NIH) to develop the Human Genome Project in 1990 (U.S. Department of Energy Genome Programs, 2008). Their goal was to sequence the **human genome**, a map to identify all human genes, which they accomplished in 2003 (National Human Genome Research Institute [NHGRI], 2015). The information obtained through the sequencing of the human genome has enabled researchers to identify genes associated with human disease. Current research involves understanding the complex functions of cellular regulation, human variation, and the interplay of genes and environment and how all the cell organelles, genes, and proteins work together in life's functions (NHGRI, 2015).

8.1 Genetic Basics

Life starts as a single cell, but the developed human body is made up of many cells. These cells share common features such as a nucleus that contains 46 chromosomes and organelles such as mitochondria (**Figure 8.1** ■). Many different types of specialized cells throughout the body function differently depending on their location. For example, pancreatic cells have a very different function than that of nerve cells.

All human cells, except mature red blood cells, contain a complete set of deoxyribonucleic acid (DNA) molecules. DNA molecules consist of long sequences of nucleotides or bases represented by the letters *A*, *T*, *G*, and *C*. The order of these bases gives the exact instructions for the functioning of that particular cell. Writing the correct order of the bases using the abbreviations represents the sequence of the bases in DNA. Together, the total sum of DNA in a human cell is referred to as the human *genome*, or the complete set of inheritance for an individual. The human genome includes the DNA in the cell nucleus as well as the DNA found in the mitochondria, which is discussed later in this section. Each individual's genome is unique. Identical (monozygotic) twins are the exception because they develop from only one fertilized ovum and share identical DNA.

The cell nucleus contains about 6 feet of DNA that is tightly wound and packaged into 23 pairs of chromosomes, making a complete set of 46 **chromosomes**. The structure and number of chromosomes can be shown by a karyotype, or picture, of an individual's chromosomes (**Figure 8.2** ■). There are two copies of each chromosome. One copy, or half of the complete set of these 46 chromosomes, is inherited from the mother and the other copy, or the other half of the 46 chromosomes, is inherited from the father. For example, an individual will have two copies of chromosome 1, one inherited from his or her mother and one inherited from his or her father. These two copies or pairs of inherited chromosomes are called *homologous* (the same) chromosomes. Chromosomes are numbered according to size (largest to smallest), with chromosome 1 being the largest. The first 22 pairs of chromosomes, known as **autosomes**, are alike in males and females. The 23rd pair, the **sex chromosomes**, determines an individual's gender. A female has two copies of the X chromosome (one copy inherited from each parent), and a male has one X chromosome (inherited from his mother) and one Y chromosome (inherited from his father).

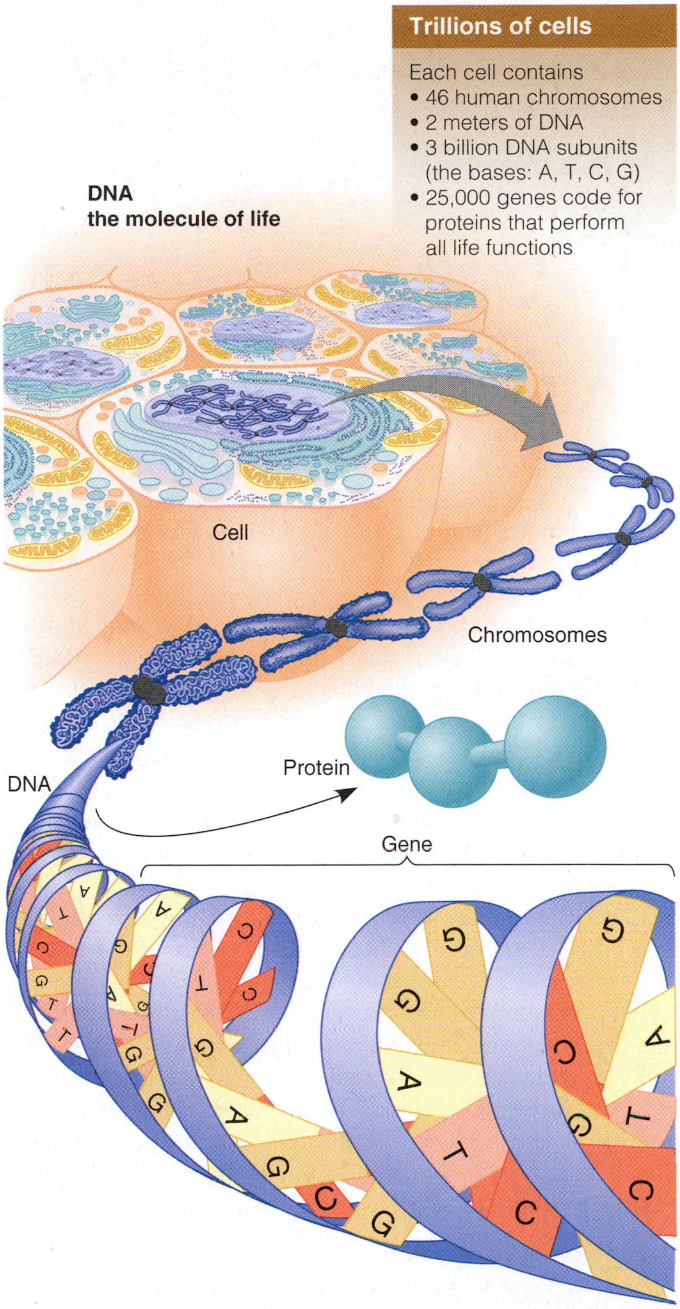
Trillions of cells
Each cell contains
• 46 human chromosomes
• 2 meters of DNA
• 3 billion DNA subunits (the bases: A, T, C, G)
• 25,000 genes code for proteins that perform all life functions
DNA
the molecule of life
Cell
Chromosomes
Protein
DNA
Gene

Figure 8.1 ■ Each cell nucleus throughout the body contains the genes, DNA, and chromosomes that make up the majority of an individual's genome. The remaining portion of the human genome is in the mitochondria.

Cell Division

Mitosis and meiosis are the two types of cell division in human cells. **Mitosis** is the process of making new cells and it takes place in the **somatic cells** (tissue cells) of the body. Cell division through mitosis results in two cells called

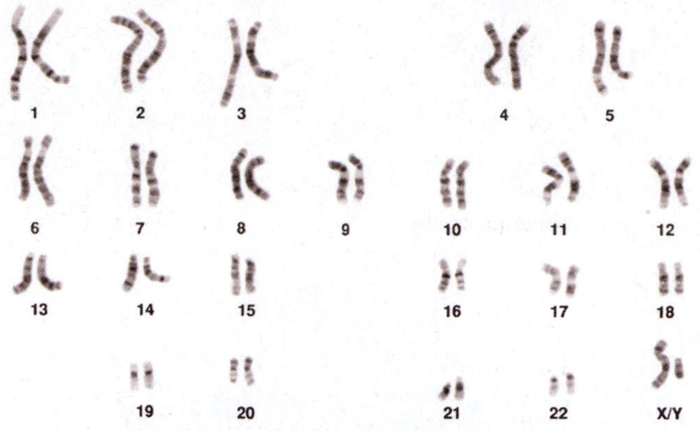
1
2
3
4
5
6
7
8
9
10
11
12
13
14
15
16
17
18
19
20
21
22
X/Y

Figure 8.2 ■ A karyotype is a picture of an individual's chromosomes. It shows the chromosomal structure and number of the 22 pairs of autosomes and the sex chromosomes.

> **BOX 8.2**
> **Terminology and Variations in Chromosomal Number**
>
> - ***Euploidy***—the presence of the normal number of 46 chromosomes
> - ***Aneuploidy***—the condition in which extra or missing chromosomes exist; in affected living individuals, physical abnormalities and/or intellectual disability are common
> - ***Monosomy***—the loss of a single chromosome from a pair; for example, Turner syndrome (45,XO)
> - ***Trisomy***—the gain of a single chromosome, making a total of three copies of a certain chromosome, for example, trisomy 21 or Down syndrome
> - ***Polyploidy***—the condition in which more than two pairs of all the chromosomes are present

daughter cells that are genetically identical to the original cell (*mother cell*), and to each other. Cell division through mitosis heals wounds and replaces cells lost daily on skin surfaces and in the lining of gastrointestinal and respiratory tracts. In addition, mitosis is responsible for human development. The mitotic activity of the zygote and its daughter cells is the foundation for a human's growth and development. The zygote undergoes mitosis to form a multicellular embryo, then fetus, and then infant.

Meiosis is also known as the reduction division of the cell. Meiosis occurs only in the sex cells of the testes and ovaries and results in the formation of the sperm and oocyte (gametes). Meiosis is very similar to mitosis in that it is a form of cell division; however, through a series of complex mechanisms, the amount of genetic material is reduced in half (23 chromosomes). This is very important because when the two sex cells combine during fertilization, the total number of chromosomes (46) is present in the offspring's cells. Meiosis has three purposes:

1. To produce gametes
2. To reduce the number of chromosomes by half
3. To make new combinations of genetic material from crossing over and independent assortment processes, which allows diversity in the human population.

Chromosomal Alterations

Alterations in chromosomes often occur during cell division and are classified as either alterations in the number of chromosomes or structural alterations. They involve either part of or the whole chromosome. The clinical consequences of number and structural changes in the chromosomes in an individual vary depending on the amount and type of DNA affected by the alterations.

Alterations in Chromosome Number

An increase or decrease in chromosomal numbers can occur during meiosis or mitosis (**Box 8.2**). Alterations occur often during meiosis because meiosis is a highly specific and complex process and each new daughter cell must contain exactly one chromosome from each pair of chromosomes. During meiosis, the paired chromosomes may fail to separate, resulting in an egg or sperm cell with either two copies or no copies of a particular chromosome. This is known as *nondisjunction*. When these egg or sperm cells are fertilized by a normal gamete that contains 23 copies of all of the chromosomes, a zygote that is monosomic (one member of the chromosome pair is missing) or trisomic (having three chromosomes instead of the usual two) results. These circumstances produce such conditions as *monosomy* of the sex chromosomes in a female (Turner syndrome) or *trisomy* of autosomes, of which **trisomy 21** (Down syndrome) is one of the more commonly known.

Alterations in Chromosome Structure

Alterations in chromosome structure include inversions, deletions, duplications, and translocations. In a chromosomal *inversion*, a segment of a chromosome is reversed, changing the DNA sequence for that portion of the chromosome. It occurs when a chromosome breaks in two places and the piece between the breaks turns upside down and reattaches within the same chromosome. The clinical consequences of an inversion depend on how much chromosomal material is involved, where the inversion occurs, and what type of inversion is present.

A chromosomal *alteration* that includes a missing (*deletion*) or additional (*duplication*) whole chromosome or segment of a chromosome is an unbalanced rearrangement. An unbalanced rearrangement can result in missing genes, confusing directions from the genes, or too much gene product, which often results in a condition that is not compatible with life or in altered physical and/or mental development. An example is cri-du-chat syndrome (intellectual disability, crying that sounds like a cat mewing, and low-set ears), which results from a large deletion on 5p (the short arm of chromosome 5).

Translocation (chromosomal reshuffling) occurs when a segment of a chromosome transfers or moves and attaches itself to another chromosome. An example is the reciprocal translocation that is found in 95% of patients with chronic myelogenous leukemia (CML) (National Cancer Institute, 2017). The contributing translocation occurs between chromosomes 9 and 22 and is known as the Philadelphia chromosome, which is not inheritable. However, this is not true for all translocations. About 4% of trisomy 21 cases are caused by a translocation; of these, half can be attributed to a translocation inherited from a parent (Mayo Clinic, 2018). The parent remains unaffected because although he or she has extra material, his or hers is a balanced chromosomal rearrangement.

Genes

A **gene** is a small portion (segment) of the nucleotide (base) sequence of a chromosome that provides specific directions for a particular function or characteristic. Each chromosome contains numerous genes arranged in a linear order. The specific sequence of nucleotides (the genes and the variations therein) is referred to as the individual's **genotype**. Researchers currently believe there are about 20,000 to 30,000 genes in the human genome (Genetics Home Reference, 2018g; Jameson & Kopp, 2015; Lister Hill National Center for Biomedical Communications, 2014).

With the exception of the genes on the sex chromosomes (X and Y) present in males, all genes come in pairs called **alleles**. All genes have a specific location on a specific chromosome. This is known as the *genetic locus*. For example, one of the many genes located on chromosome 19 is a gene for eye color. There may be slight variations or different forms of a gene, for instance, green versus blue eye color. When an individual has two identical forms (alleles) of a gene, they are said to be **homozygous** (*homo* = same). If an individual has two different forms (alleles) of the gene, they are said to be **heterozygous** (*hetero* = different). Genes can be described as *altered* or *mutated* when a change has taken place, or *expressed* when the gene has an impact on the outward appearance of an individual and/or the functioning of cells. The observable, outward expression of an individual's entire physical, biochemical, and physiologic makeup, as determined by his or her genotype (alleles) and environmental factors, is referred to as **phenotype**.

Function and Distribution of Genes

One function of genes is to provide directions for how to make proteins. These protein-directing genes are very important to life and functioning as a human. They are responsible for transmitting messages between cells, fighting infection, directing genes to turn "on" or "off," forming structures, and sensing light, taste, and smell (Genetics Home Reference, 2018d). Some gene activities change from moment to moment in response to tens of thousands of intra- and extracellular environmental signals. An example of this is the feedback mechanism that stimulates a cell to produce insulin after eating a candy bar. After eating, a gene on chromosome 11 directs pancreatic cells to produce, modify, and secrete insulin. Although the gene for producing insulin is present in all nucleated cells of the body, it is only functional in insulin-secreting pancreatic cells.

Mitochondrial Genes

Chromosomes in the cell nucleus are not the only site where genes reside. Several dozen that are involved in energy metabolism are located in the cell mitochondria (the powerhouse of the cell). *Mitochondria* are concerned with energy production and metabolism. Some cells contain more mitochondria than others, but each mitochondrion contains its own copies of DNA, identified as mitochondrial DNA (mtDNA). Because ova contain many mitochondria and sperm do not (most mitochondria are located in the tail of the sperm, which detaches after fertilization), mtDNA is primarily inherited from the mother. Therefore, mitochondrial genes and any diseases due to DNA alterations on those genes are transmitted through the mother in a matrilineal pattern. This pattern of inheritance is very different from the pattern of inheritance of genes found in the nucleus of the cell. Thus, an affected female will pass the mtDNA mutation to all of her children; however, an affected male will not pass the mtDNA mutation to any of his children (Carelli, 2015; John, Facucho-Oliveira, Jiang, Kelly, & Salah, 2010; Nussbaum, McInnes, & Willard, 2016). Manifestations of conditions due to mitochondrial gene alterations primarily involve high-energy tissues and organs such as skeletal muscle, heart muscle, the liver, the kidney, the brain, and nerve cells. The ears, eyes, and endocrine system are also affected. Symptoms develop over years as unhealthy or dying cells are not replaced. Hypertrophic cardiomyopathy, heart block, seizures, and deafness are associated with mtDNA gene alterations (John et al., 2010; Nussbaum et al., 2016).

Gene Alterations and Disease

Today, we know that gene alterations are responsible for approximately 6000 hereditary diseases (Nussbaum et al., 2016). However, different genetic alterations within a particular gene can result in a wide variety of signs and symptoms. For example, the *CFTR* gene for cystic fibrosis is a very large gene located on chromosome 7. More than 1000 different mutations of the *CFTR* gene have been reported to be associated with disease (Genetics Home Reference, 2018a). The area of the *CFTR* gene that controls mucus production can have more than 300 different alterations, resulting in a variety of symptoms ranging from no symptoms at all to mild or severe symptoms. Gene alterations, not the genes themselves, cause genetic diseases and conditions.

Gene Alterations that Decrease Risk of Disease

Although it is common to associate gene mutations with disease, it is important to remember that gene mutations can also be helpful in decreasing the risk of disease. Gene alterations and genetic variations may also have a protective role in the expression of diseases. A common example is the protective value of the gene alteration that causes sickle cell disease. Those individuals with this gene alteration have protection against malaria. Another example is the *APOE* gene. The *APOE* gene provides instructions for making the protein apolipoprotein E. This protein combines with fats (lipids) in the body to form molecules called *lipoproteins* that are responsible for packaging cholesterol and other fats and carrying them through the bloodstream. There are at least three slightly different versions (alleles) of the *APOE* gene. The major alleles are called e2, e3, and e4. Research has shown that a person who inherits at least one e4 allele will have a greater chance of developing Alzheimer disease. However, inheriting the e2 allele seems to indicate that a person is less likely to develop Alzheimer disease (Wu & Zhao, 2016).

Single-Nucleotide Polymorphisms

More than 99% of human DNA sequences are the same (Genetics Home Reference, 2018e). **Polymorphisms** are natural variations in gene DNA sequences in which each possible sequence is present in at least 1% of people, usually having no adverse effect on the individual.

Single-nucleotide polymorphisms (SNPs, or "snips") are the most common type of genetic variation among humans and are one-letter (base-pair) variations in the DNA sequence that serve as biologic markers. **Biologic markers** are important for the construction of chromosome maps and are easily tracked, stable segments of DNA. Scientists are hopeful that information gained from SNPs will provide information on how subtle differences in humans impact their response to drugs and the environment, thus making medical treatment and pharmacologic management more individualized.

8.2 Principles of Inheritance

Knowledge of inheritance allows the nurse to provide genetic information to patients and their families to assist them in managing their care and in making reproductive decisions. The basic underlying principles of inheritance that nurses can apply to inheritance risk assessment and teaching include (1) all genes are paired, (2) only one gene of each pair is transmitted (passed on) to an offspring, and (3) one copy of each gene in the offspring comes from the mother and the other copy comes from the father. Understanding the Mendelian patterns of inheritance is made easier by relating these principles.

Mendelian Pattern of Inheritance

Conditions that are caused by a mutation or alteration of a single gene are known as *monogenic* or *single-gene disorders*. The most common gene alterations that result in genetic disorders are predictably passed on from generation to generation following Mendelian inheritance patterns (Mendel's laws of inheritance). These single-gene mutations follow an **autosomal dominant, autosomal recessive, X-linked recessive**, or X-linked dominant inheritance pattern. The first three of these patterns are the most common. Modes of transmission or inheritance for thousands of conditions resulting from monogenic alterations have been identified (Genetics Home Reference, 2018c).

Autosomal Dominant

Autosomal dominant (AD) conditions are the result of an altered gene on any of the 22 autosomes or non–sex chromosomes (**Figure 8.3** ■). Examples of autosomal dominant disorders include neurofibromatosis, some breast and ovarian cancers, autosomal dominant polycystic kidney disease, Marfan syndrome (**Figure 8.4** ■), Huntington disease, and familial hypercholesterolemia. More than half of the known Mendelian conditions are autosomal dominant. In AD conditions, disease occurs in spite of the fact that one unaltered or normal gene exists. Homozygous dominant conditions (the individual has inherited dominant altered genes from both parents) are generally much more severe than heterozygous dominant conditions and are often lethal. Because homozygous dominant conditions are usually lethal and would result from both parents being affected, the nurse should consider an individual exhibiting an autosomal dominant condition as heterozygous. See **Box 8.3** for characteristics of an AD pattern of inheritance.

Autosomal Recessive

A gene or genetic condition is considered recessive when two copies of altered genes are needed to express the condition. Autosomal recessive (AR) conditions are the result of an altered gene on any of the 22 autosomes or non–sex chromosomes (**Figure 8.5** ■). Examples of autosomal recessive conditions include hemochromatosis type 1, cystic fibrosis, phenylketonuria, Tay-Sachs disease, and sickle cell disease. An individual with a recessive condition has inherited one altered gene from his or her mother and one from his or her father. In most cases, each of the parents has a single gene alteration on one chromosome of a pair and the normal, wild-type or unaltered form of the gene on the other

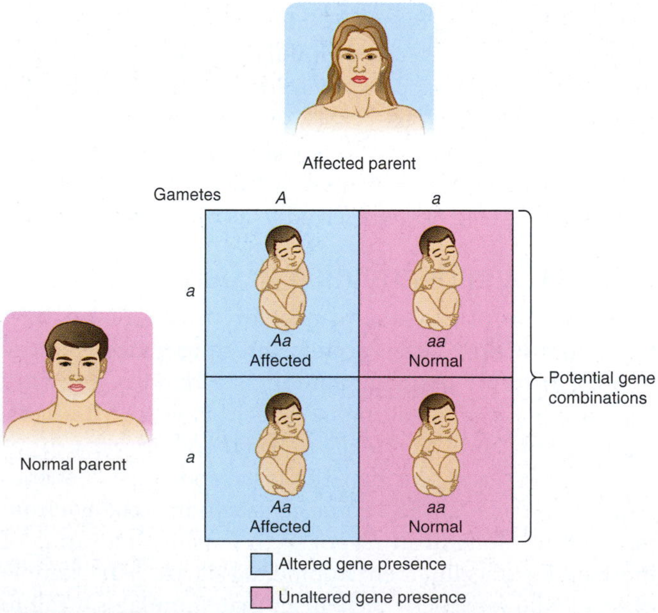
Affected parent
Gametes
A
a
a
a
Aa
Affected
aa
Normal
Aa
Affected
aa
Normal
Normal parent
Potential gene combinations
Altered gene presence
Unaltered gene presence

Figure 8.3 ■ This Punnett square shows potential gene combinations (genotypes) and resulting phenotypes of children from parent genotypes with an autosomal dominant altered gene. Phenotypes are expressed (affected) when a male *or* female has one copy of the gene alteration.

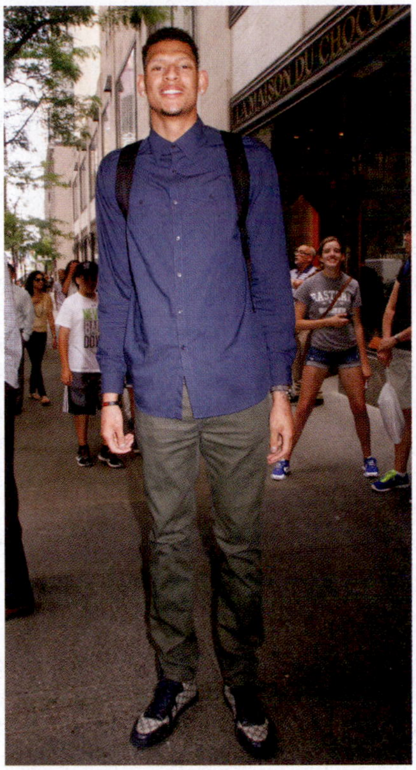

Figure 8.4 ■ Isaiah Austin, a 7-foot, 1-inch basketball player, was diagnosed with Marfan syndrome in 2014. After 2½ years of checkups and heart monitoring, he was cleared by his doctor to play again (NBA.com, 2016). He is currently playing for a professional team in Serbia.

chromosome. These parents would be known as *carriers* of the condition and they do not usually exhibit any manifestations of the condition. Because the gene alteration occurs on a non–sex chromosome, both males and females have an equal chance of inheriting the altered gene from their parent. See **Box 8.4** for characteristics of an AR pattern of inheritance.

X-Linked Recessive

X-linked conditions are the result of an altered gene on the X chromosome. Examples include hemophilia A and

BOX 8.3
Characteristics of Autosomal Dominant Pattern of Inheritance

When gathering a family history, the nurse should assess for any of the following characteristics of autosomal dominant inheritance:

1. Both males and females are affected.
2. Males and females are usually affected in equal numbers.
3. An affected child will have an affected parent and/or all generations will have an affected individual (appearing as a vertical pattern of affected individuals on the family pedigree).
4. Unaffected children of an affected parent will have unaffected offspring.
5. A significant proportion of isolated cases are due to a new mutation.

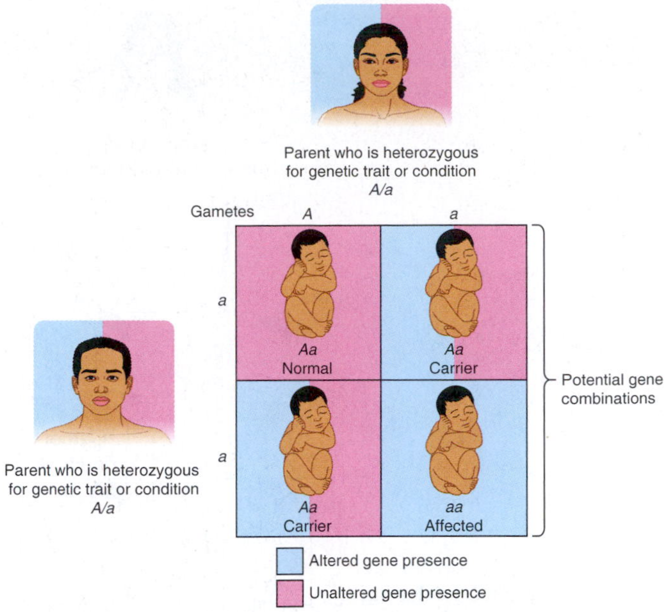
Parent who is heterozygous for genetic trait or condition
A/a
Gametes
A
a
a
a
Aa
Normal
Aa
Carrier
Aa
Carrier
aa
Affected
Potential gene combinations
Parent who is heterozygous for genetic trait or condition
A/a
Altered gene presence
Unaltered gene presence

Figure 8.5 ■ This Punnett square shows potential gene combinations (genotypes) and resulting phenotypes of children from parent genotypes with an autosomal recessive altered gene. Phenotypes are expressed (affected) when a male *or* female has two copies of the gene alteration.

Duchenne muscular dystrophy. Unlike the autosomes, the sex chromosome, X, is unevenly distributed to males and females. The female has two X chromosomes and the male has only one. If any of the genes on the X chromosome inherited by a male are altered, an unaltered counterpart is not present to override the altered functioning gene, and it becomes the copy that provides direction for those particular functions of these genes.

The family history and pattern of inheritance has a characteristic distribution pattern among the males and females in the family (**Figure 8.6** ■). The consequences of the altered

BOX 8.4
Characteristics of Autosomal Recessive Pattern of Inheritance

When gathering a family history, the nurse should assess for any of the following characteristics of autosomal recessive inheritance:

1. Both males and females are affected.
2. Males and females are usually affected in equal numbers.
3. An affected child will have an unaffected parent but may have affected siblings (appearing as a horizontal pattern of affected individuals on the family pedigree).
4. The condition may appear to skip a generation.
5. The parents of the affected child may be consanguineous (close blood relatives).
6. The family may be descendants of a certain ethnic group that is known to have a more frequent occurrence of a certain genetic condition. For example, Tay-Sachs disease is an autosomal recessive, progressive neurodegenerative disorder that is more common among Ashkenazi Jews than other ethnic groups.

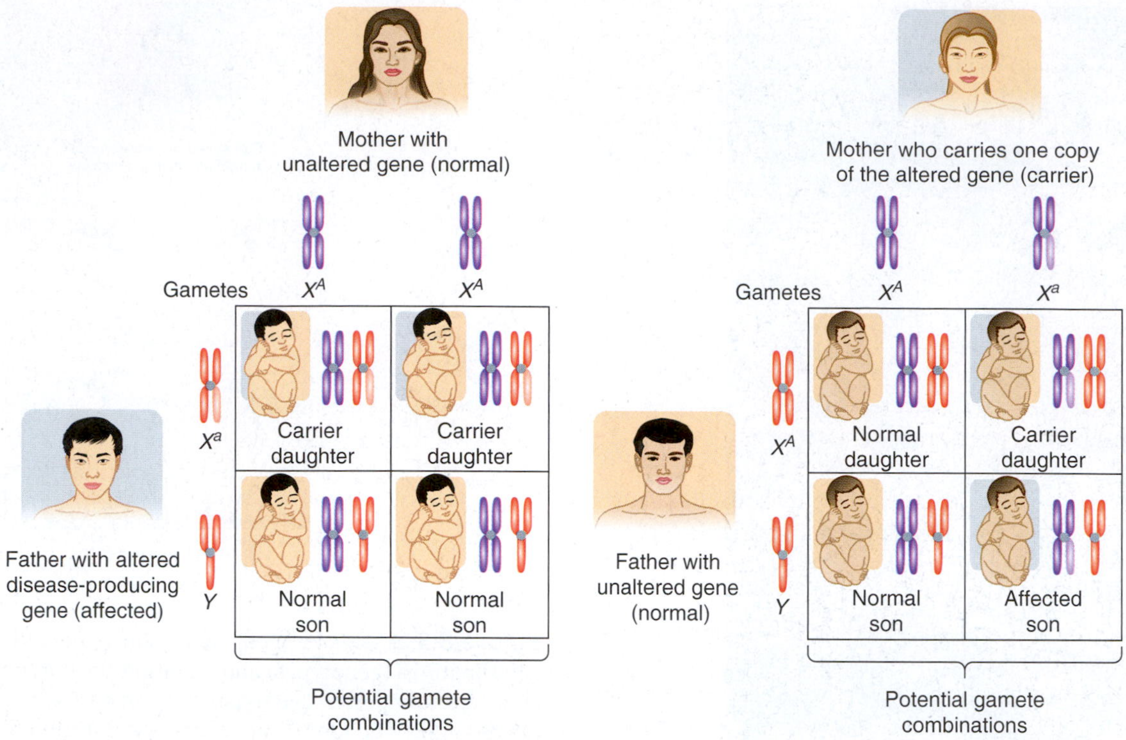
Mother with
unaltered gene (normal)
Gametes
X^A
X^A
X^a
Y
Carrier daughter
Carrier daughter
Normal son
Normal son
Father with altered disease-producing gene (affected)
Potential gamete combinations
Mother who carries one copy of the altered gene (carrier)
Gametes
X^A
X^a
X^A
Y
Normal daughter
Carrier daughter
Normal son
Affected son
Father with unaltered gene (normal)
Potential gamete combinations

Figure 8.6 ■ These Punnett squares show potential gene combinations (genotypes) and resulting phenotypes of children from different parent genotypes with an X-linked recessive altered gene. Phenotypes are expressed (affected) in a male with only one copy of the gene alteration and in a female with two copies of the altered gene.

gene on an X chromosome will be expressed in all males who receive that X chromosome from their mother. Females, on the other hand, will have two copies and the unaltered gene generally compensates for the altered gene, making the female a carrier. The male receives an X chromosome from his mother and his Y chromosome from his father. The female offspring receives an X chromosome from each of her parents. Thus, all affected males will pass on the altered X chromosome to all of their daughters who will be carriers of the altered gene. A male can never transmit an altered gene on the X chromosome to his sons because the male will transmit only the Y chromosome to his sons. Because of these transmission patterns, the most commonly occurring transmission of an X-linked condition is through a female who is a carrier of an altered gene. See **Box 8.5** for characteristics of an X-linked recessive pattern of inheritance.

X-Linked Dominant

X-linked dominant conditions also exist, but they are very rare. If a male is affected, the condition is severe and often lethal. A family history of multiple miscarriages of male fetuses may be a sign of an X-linked dominant condition. An example of a viable X-linked dominant condition is vitamin D–resistant rickets, also known as hypophosphatemic rickets.

Variability in Classic Mendelian Patterns of Inheritance

Along with understanding the classic Mendelian inheritance patterns, several other concepts are also important for families to understand when the nurse is assisting patients with or at risk for inheriting a genetic disorder. These include the following exceptions or variations to the traditional Mendelian patterns of inheritance.

BOX 8.5
Characteristics of X-Linked Recessive Pattern of Inheritance

When the nurse gathers a family history, he or she should assess for any of the following characteristics of X-linked recessive inheritance:

1. More males will be affected than females; rarely seen in females.
2. An affected male will have all carrier daughters.
3. There is no male-to-male inheritance.
4. Affected males are related by carrier females.
5. Females may report varying milder symptoms of the condition.
6. A new sporadic case could be due to a new mutation.

Penetrance

Penetrance is the probability that a gene will be expressed phenotypically. It is an "all-or-none" concept in that either the gene will be expressed (even if mildly expressed) or it will not be expressed at all. Penetrance can be measured in the following way. In a certain group of individuals with the same genotype, what percentage of them will exhibit at least some manifestations of the condition? If the number is less than 100%, then that condition is said to show reduced penetrance. For example, the gene alterations that cause achondroplasia (dwarfism) exhibit 100% penetrance and all individuals with one copy of the gene alteration will exhibit signs and symptoms of the condition (Nussbaum et al., 2016).

New Mutation

When there is no previous history of a condition including even subtle manifestations of the disease in any other immediate or distant family member, the disease may be caused by a spontaneous new mutation. This case is usually called a *de novo* mutation. New mutations of a gene are most frequently recognized in autosomal dominant conditions because one copy of an altered gene is all that is necessary to elicit a state of altered health. Autosomal dominant conditions known to have high mutation rates include neurofibromatosis, achondroplasia, and Marfan syndrome. New mutations are also possible in autosomal recessive diseases, although rarely expressed because two altered genes are necessary for signs and symptoms to appear. Finally, new mutations are often seen in X-linked recessive disorders, such as hemophilia A, because the male with just one altered gene will express the disease phenotype.

Anticipation

Anticipation occurs when successive generations of a family exhibit more severe manifestations of certain diseases and the disease often has an earlier onset. An example of a condition where this occurs is fragile X (**Figure 8.7** ■). Fragile X is the most common cause of inherited mental impairment, caused by a mutation in a gene known as *FMR-1*, which is located on the X chromosome. The mutation is a "genetic stutter" in which a small section within the gene is repeated too many times. A person who does not have fragile X has between 6 and 45 repeats (trinucleotide repeats). Individuals with 55 to 200 repeats have a premutation that can possibly expand when passed on to offspring. When this mutation is greater than 200 repeats, an individual has a full mutation. See **Box 8.6** for more information about fragile X.

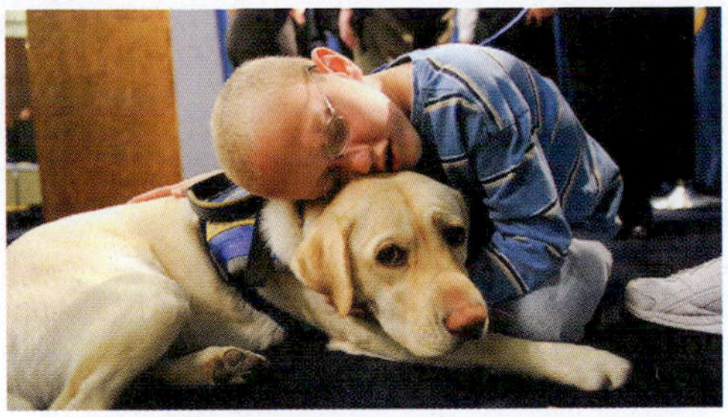

Figure 8.7 ■ A child with fragile X syndrome.

Variable Expressivity

The term *expressivity* is used to describe the severity of the *gene expression* of a phenotype. When people with the same genetic makeup (genotype) exhibit signs and/or symptoms with varying degrees of severity, the phenotype is described as *variable expression* (Nussbaum et al., 2016). Variable expression is common in the autosomal dominant condition neurofibromatosis. The diagnosis of neurofibromatosis is based on clinical criteria established by the 1987 Consensus Development Conference of the National Institutes of Health. Manifestations include café au lait spots,

BOX 8.6
Fragile X and Anticipation

Fragile X syndrome is transmitted in an X-linked dominant pattern (Genetics Home Reference, 2018b). This syndrome affects intellect, learning, behavior and social skills, speech and language, and sensory perception. It affects about 1 in 4000 males and 1 in 8000 females (Genetics Home Reference, 2018b). In general, boys with fragile X syndrome are more severely affected than girls. Physical manifestations of the disorder, which develop during puberty, include a narrow face, large head and ears, flexible joints, and flat feet.

Fragile X syndrome is caused by mutations in the *FMR1* gene on the X chromosome. In nearly all cases of fragile X syndrome, a certain DNA segment within this gene is repeated more than 200 times.

- ***Normal number of repeats:*** Individuals with a normal number of repeats (5 to 40) do not have fragile X syndrome and cannot pass it on to their offspring.
- ***Intermediate number of repeats or gray zone:*** Individuals who have between about 40 and 55 repeats are considered to be in a gray zone. The number of repeats can sometimes expand slightly when passed from parent to child.
- ***Premutation:*** Individuals with between 55 and 200 repeats have what is called a *premutation*. About 1 in 150 women and 1 in 450 men carry the premutation. Women with the premutation have a 50% chance of passing along the abnormal gene to her baby during each pregnancy and are at risk for having a child with fragile X syndrome (National Institute of Child Health and Human Development, 2017).
- Some children who inherit the abnormal gene have a permutation and no symptoms of fragile X syndrome. However, the number of repeats often expands when the gene is passed from mother to child. As a result, some children of carrier mothers inherit the full mutation (more than 200 repeats) and show symptoms of fragile X syndrome. A male with the premutation passes it on to all of his daughters but to none of his sons. The daughters are generally carriers of a premutation and may pass it on to their children. The premutation does not usually expand in size when passed from fathers to their daughters.
- ***Full mutation:*** Individuals with more than 200 repeats have the full mutation. A woman with a full fragile X mutation has a 50% chance of passing along the full mutation in each pregnancy. For reasons that are not understood, the full mutation shrinks back to a permutation in sperm. If a man with a full mutation has children, he will pass the permutation on to all of his daughters. His sons are not at risk because they do not inherit the X chromosome from their father (Online Mendelian Inheritance in Man, 2017).

optic gliomas, neurofibromas, and bone lesions, to name a few. Although neurofibromatosis has 100% penetrance, variable expressivity can occur within family members, meaning they all have the condition but not the same clinical manifestations.

Multifactorial (Polygenic or Complex) Disorders

Many birth defects such as cleft lip and palate, as well as many adult-onset conditions such as cancer, mental illness, asthma, diabetes, obesity, heart disease, and Alzheimer disease, have a multifactorial cause. *Multifactorial conditions* occur as a result of genetic variations and lifestyle and environmental influences that work together. Often, multiple genes contribute to the disorder (*polygenic*). The polygenic concept is illustrated with the multiple genes involved in an individual's susceptibility for breast cancer. These genes have been identified on chromosomes 6, 11, 13, 14, 15, 17, and 22. Exactly which genes interrelate and how many environmental influences are enough to cause the presentation of many of the common complex diseases or conditions is not known.

Multifactorial conditions do not follow the characteristic Mendelian patterns of inheritance seen with single-gene conditions. The risks of inheriting multifactorial conditions vary. Type 2 diabetes mellitus, for example, shows a strong inheritance pattern, with impaired glucose tolerance or diabetes present in 40% of an affected individual's siblings and 30% of that person's children. For diseases such as asthma, cardiovascular disease, and colon cancer, having two or more affected first-degree relatives is known to increase an individual's risk by two to five times that of someone without this strong family history (Nussbaum et al., 2016). A patient considered as high risk for an inheritable condition should be referred for a genetics consultation.

Some of the more common conditions caused by Mendelian patterns of inheritance are shown in **Table 8.1**.

Table 8.1 Selected Conditions Caused by Mendelian Patterns of Inheritance

Pattern of Inheritance	Selected Conditions
Autosomal dominant	Achondroplasia Autosomal dominant polycystic kidney disease Breast and ovarian cancer Familial hypercholesterolemia Huntington disease Marfan syndrome Neurofibromatosis
Autosomal recessive	Cystic fibrosis Hemochromatosis type 1 Phenylketonuria Sickle cell disease
X-linked recessive	Duchenne muscular dystrophy Hemophilia A
X-linked dominant	Hypophosphatemic rickets

8.3 Care of Patients with Genetic Disorders

Interprofessional Care

Many health professionals work together in the screening, diagnosis, identification, and treatment of genetic disorders. The goals of interprofessional care are early diagnosis through testing and assessment and development of an effective treatment plan. Psychosocial support to enhance coping and referral to a genetic specialist when needed are critical elements of the plan.

Genetic Testing

Genetic testing involves the analysis of DNA, RNA, chromosomes, and serum levels of specific enzymes or metabolites. Genetic tests can be classified into two categories: screening and diagnostic. A positive screening genetic test result indicates an increased risk or probability but must always be confirmed by diagnostic testing. Screening genetic tests are most commonly completed in prenatal, newborn, and carrier circumstances. In contrast, a diagnostic test can definitively validate or eliminate a genetic disorder in the symptomatic patient and then guide clinical management. **Box 8.7** lists some of the benefits and potential negative outcomes of genetic testing.

Although confidentiality and privacy are integral parts of delivery of care for all healthcare providers, this issue is of even more concern as it relates to genetic information (Brothers & Rothstein, 2015). Results of genetic tests can affect employment and insurance options. Will the results

BOX 8.7
Outcomes Related to Genetic Testing

BENEFITS OF GENETIC TESTING

- Early screening and preventive measures
- Future planning and life preparation
- Lifestyle adaptations
- Decreased confusion and anxiety
- Psychologic stress relief
- Reproductive choices
- Informed immediate/extended family members
- Early medical and/or surgical intervention
- Cost of medical follow-up potentially reduced with confirmation or refuting of a diagnosis

POSSIBLE NEGATIVE OUTCOMES OF GENETIC TESTING

- Survivor guilt
- Loss of identity
- No treatment may exist
- Employability and insurability affected
- Confusion about accessing healthcare and resources
- Risk for invasion of confidentiality and privacy
- Social stigmatization

affect the patient's ability to obtain and/or maintain insurance coverage? Can an employer refuse to hire or promote an individual because of genetic testing results? Can genetic information be released to the courts, military, schools, or adoption agencies? Would a patient with a known gene alteration for Huntington disease be offered a college scholarship to the best law school? There is debate over whether genetic privacy is different from medical privacy. The nurse should inform patients of their rights and responsibility to know who will have access to the genetic test results. Those providing the genetic tests must provide the patient with assurance that the results will be handled confidentially and that there will be no access to the genetic information by a third party without written permission of the individual being tested.

All genetic testing should be voluntary. It is the nurse's responsibility to ensure that the informed consent process includes discussion of the risks and benefits of the test, including any physical harm as well as potential psychologic and societal injury by stigmatization, discrimination, and emotional stress. Healthcare providers are legally liable to maintain that confidence. However, exceptions to the individual's privacy may be made when genetic test results indicate a significant probability of irreversible harm to a family member that can be prevented by knowledge of the threat (Brothers & Rothstein, 2015).

Diagnosis

Several categories of genetic tests are available and include the following (American Cancer Society, 2017; Genetics Home Reference, 2018f):

- ***Newborn screening*** can identify children who have an increased risk for a genetic disease such as phenylketonuria, sickle cell disease, or maple syrup urine disease. Several states now screen for more than 30 conditions (expanded newborn screen) as part of routine newborn care.
- ***Carrier testing*** is completed on asymptomatic individuals who may be carriers of a gene alteration that can be transmitted to offspring in an autosomal recessive or X-linked pattern of inheritance. This may be part of a couple's premarriage or preconception planning if they belong to an ethnic group with known risk for genetic disorders such as sickle cell disease and Tay-Sachs disease. It may be necessary to determine the exact gene mutation from an affected family member prior to carrier testing. This is often completed through lineage analysis.
- ***Preimplantation genetic diagnosis (PGD)*** allows detection of disease-causing gene alterations in human embryos before implantation in the uterus, thus providing an opportunity for preselection of unaffected embryos for implantation. This type of genetic testing is most often used by parents who are both carriers of a single-gene recessive disorder and who wish to implant into the uterus only the embryo(s) without the disease-causing gene alteration. It has also been used to determine tissue type for donation of tissue such as bone marrow to a sibling or parent. PGD is usually not covered by insurance, is very costly, and is available at only a small number of centers and for only a small number of disorders.
- ***Predictive genetic testing*** is usually made available to the asymptomatic individual and includes both predispositional and presymptomatic testing. A positive predispositional testing result indicates an increased risk that the individual might eventually develop the disease. Common examples include breast cancer and hereditary nonpolyposis colorectal cancer. A presymptomatic test is performed when development of the disease is certain if the gene alteration is present. These tests are medically indicated when the seriousness and mortality of the disease can be reduced with knowledge of the gene alteration. An example of this would be hereditary hemochromatosis or familial hypercholesterolemia. Life planning and lifestyle choices can be influenced by predictive testing.
- Other uses of genetic testing include organ transplantation tissue typing and pharmacogenetic testing. Pharmacogenetic testing involves predicting or studying the patient's response to particular medications. For example, 20% of Caucasians have a polymorphism on the cytochrome P450 *CYP2C9* gene and consequently metabolize warfarin more slowly and take longer to achieve therapeutic dosing (Dean, 2016). These patients require significantly less warfarin and are two to three times more likely to have an adverse hemorrhagic event. Controversy remains as to whether genetic testing should be undertaken for every patient prior to initiating warfarin therapy; however, the U.S. Food and Drug Administration has revised the product label for warfarin to include information on the benefits of genetic testing to guide warfarin treatment.

Chromosomal diagnostic examination can be accomplished with a blood, skin, or buccal cell sampling. A karyotype is completed in a cytogenetics laboratory. Chromosomes can be identified by their size and unique light and dark banding patterns. The pairs of autosomal chromosomes are arranged from 1 to 22 according to each chromosome's size, unique banding patterns, and *centromere* position. The sex chromosomes complete the picture, with the X chromosome(s) first, then the Y chromosome (if present). The karyotype shows all of the chromosome pairs lined up and positioned on a piece of paper, allowing for visual chromosomal analysis (refer to Figure 8.2). The final karyotype report contains numerical data that includes the total number of chromosomes present.

Guidelines for writing results of karyotyping are determined by the International System of Human Cytogenetic Nomenclature (ISCN). These guidelines allow for use of a standardized universal language by cytogenetic laboratories and in medical publications. For example, a normal female karyotype is written as 46, XX, whereas a karyotype of a female with trisomy 21 is written as 47, XX, +21. In the second example, the (+) symbol signifies an additional copy of chromosome 21, whereas a (–) would signify a deletion (Simons, Shaffer, & Hastings, 2016).

More than 1000 tests are available from several laboratories, with some tests available at only a small number of sites. *DNA-based tests* involve sophisticated technology that permits the examination of the DNA itself. DNA-based genetic testing can be performed on blood, bone marrow, amniotic fluid, fibroblast cells of the skin, or buccal cells from the mouth. These tests can look for common mutation(s) associated with a specific disorder or a mutation previously identified in a family member. Newborn screenings for conditions such as galactosemia are biochemical tests that look at enzyme levels. Genotyping must be done to confirm the diagnosis, identify the specific type of galactosemia, and provide more accurate genetic counseling for family planning. A third type of DNA-based test is a complete gene sequence that may be utilized when only one mutation can be found in a symptomatic patient or when none of the common mutations were found.

Nursing Care

Nurses must have basic genetic knowledge to care for the needs of patients and their families with known or suspected genetic disease. Basic interventions that meet the standards of genetic nursing include:

- Identify simple risk factors by completing a genetics-focused family history.
- Perform an accurate and thorough physical assessment.
- Apply concepts of health promotion and health maintenance to assist the patient and family in making informed decisions while facilitating autonomy.
- Be a patient advocate and provide patients with information about available resources and services.
- Provide patient education and make referrals when appropriate.
- Complete an evaluation of the plan of care for the patient.
- Apply knowledge of the ethical, legal, cultural, and social implications of genetic information.

Nurses can improve the nursing care provided to patients by applying fundamental genetic concepts to their practice. Psychosocial and economic issues need to be taken into consideration when caring for patients with the possibility of a genetic disorder.

- ***Psychosocial issues.*** Although family and individual anxiety may be decreased with a negative test result, the nurse must be prepared to address potential problems. Concerns about carrier status may interfere with development of intimacy and interpersonal relationships. Nonpaternity may be revealed through genetic testing. For example, the parents of a child born with an autosomal recessive condition will be considered carriers of the altered gene the majority of the time. To counsel the parents about future pregnancies, the parents would be tested to confirm their genotype, and nonpaternity may become an issue. A positive test result may lead to feelings of unworthiness, confusion, anger, depression, and self-image disturbance. Survivor guilt may affect adults with negative results if their siblings are positive. The individual carrying a gene alteration for a late-onset disease may have an increased tendency for risky behaviors and may choose not to be a positive member of society. Relatives of an individual affected with a genetic disorder may be very frightened when they realize what their own future might be. The individual who has inherited an altered disease-producing gene may foster deep resentment toward the parent who carries the altered gene. Parents and older generations may feel tremendous guilt for passing the altered gene to their children and grandchildren.
- ***Economic issues.*** The nurse should consider the cost of genetic tests, which can range from hundreds to thousands of dollars, depending on the size of the gene being tested. Most insurance companies do not cover genetic tests, but if there is insurance coverage the individual must weigh the cost of allowing the insurance company to have access to the genetic information (Genetics Home Reference, 2018h). Additionally, depending on the information that will be gained from obtaining the test, the family may wish to defer testing if it does not provide better outcomes or a change in treatment strategy for the patient.

Assessment

Patient Intake and History. Family history has long been a part of nursing assessment, but the relative importance of obtaining a family history has recently increased as our knowledge of the interaction of genes and the environment has expanded. In fact, it is an inexpensive first genetic screen, often underused by healthcare professionals. Professionals in primary care and other specialties share some of the responsibility for obtaining this information and making appropriate referrals.

Pedigrees. A *pedigree* is a pictorial representation or diagram of the medical history of a family (typically three generations). Multiple symbols are utilized to present this picture (**Figure 8.8** ■) and the finished pedigree presents a family's medical data and biologic relationship information at a glance (**Figure 8.9** ■). A pedigree provides the nurse, genetic counselor, or geneticist with a clear, visual representation of relationships of affected individuals to the immediate and extended family. It can identify other individuals in the family who might benefit from a genetic consultation. It can also identify a single-gene alteration pattern of inheritance or a cluster of multifactorial conditions. A referral and/or instruction on the reproductive risk for the individual and family can result. A family's learning can be enhanced by the visual teaching contribution a pedigree can provide. A pedigree can also clarify any inheritance misunderstandings or misconceptions.

By simply integrating into practice the genetic aspects of assessment, observation, and history gathering, the nurse can improve the standard of care delivered and have a positive effect on the patient. The nurse does not need to be a genetic

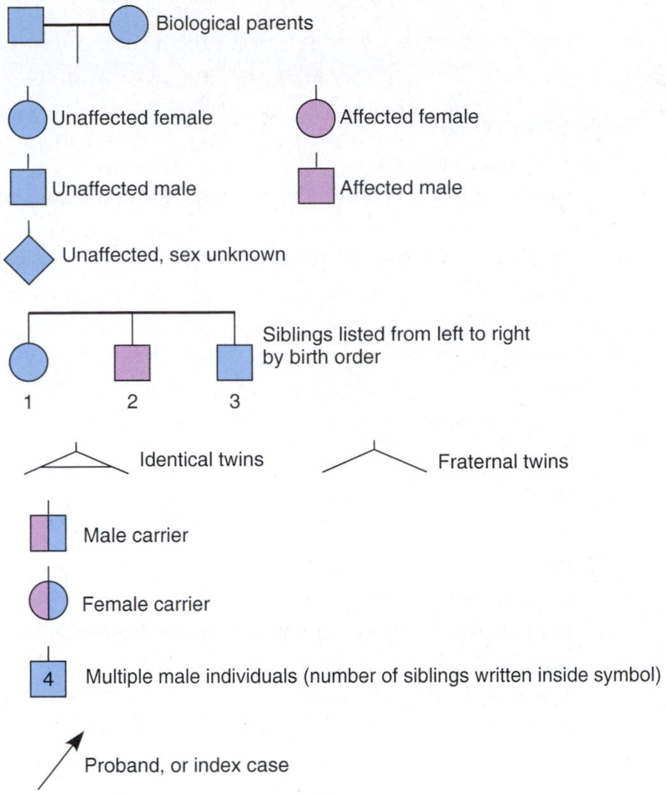

Biological parents
Unaffected female
Affected female
Unaffected male
Affected male
Unaffected, sex unknown
Siblings listed from left to right by birth order
1 2 3
Identical twins
Fraternal twins
Male carrier
Female carrier
4
Multiple male individuals (number of siblings written inside symbol)
Proband, or index case

Figure 8.8 ■ Selected standardized symbols for use in drawing a pedigree.

expert, but with heightened awareness, appropriate inquiries and referrals to genetic specialists can be completed.

Diagnoses, Outcomes, and Interventions

Nurses are responsible for comprehensively delivering the correct standard of care to patients, but must also be aware of the limitations of their own knowledge and expertise. In addition to integration of genetic aspects into assessments of the individual and family history, nurses are also responsible for carrying out interventions that include initiating referrals to genetic specialists and delivering care to the individual or family in any of the ways discussed in this section. Patients may be dealing with grief, anxiety, and poor coping skills. They may lack knowledge of genetic disorders, feel powerless, and have trouble making decisions.

Genetic Referrals and Counseling. Referral of a patient with a suspected genetic problem to a geneticist, genetic clinical nurse specialist, or genetic clinic is an expected nursing responsibility in the same way as referrals to a dietitian or a social worker are made. After gathering assessment data that incorporate genetic concepts, the nurse is able to initiate a referral to genetic specialists if there are indicators for a genetic referral (**Box 8.8**). The nurse should provide the patient with information about the advantages of a referral to genetic specialists, explain the disadvantages of not following through with the referral, and provide anticipatory guidance as to what to expect from his or her visit (**Box 8.9**).

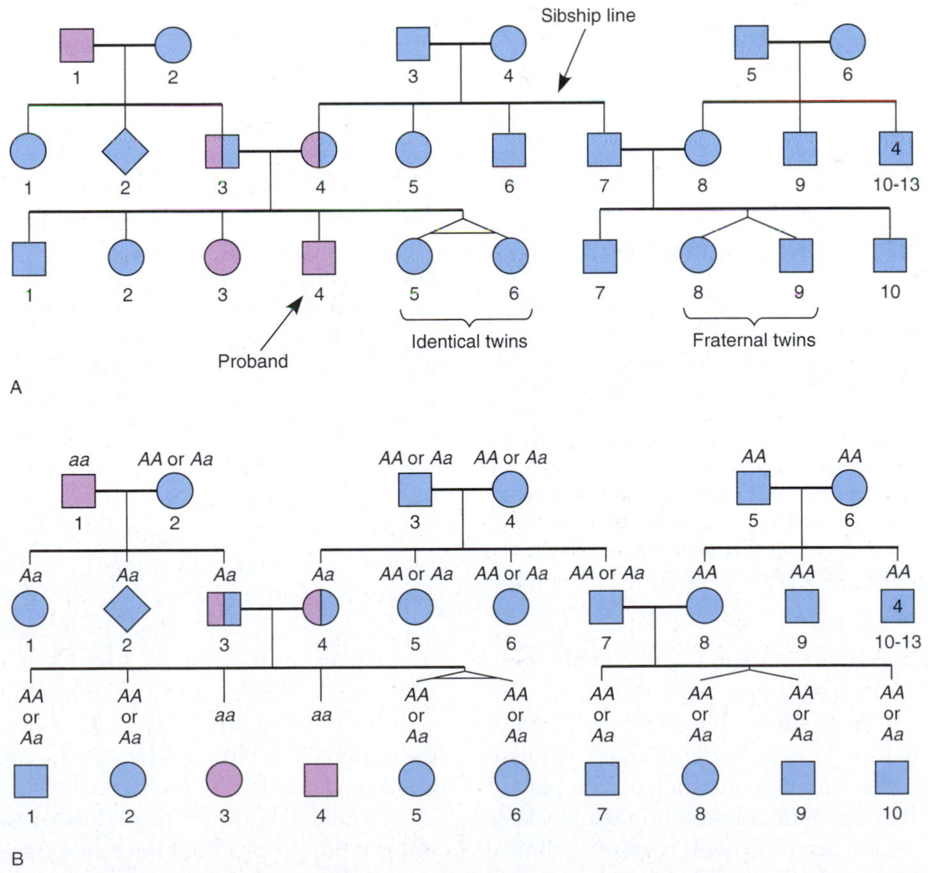

Sibship line
1 2 3 4 5 6
1 2 3 4 5 6 7 8 9 10-13
1 2 3 4 5 6 7 8 9 10
Proband
Identical twins
Fraternal twins
A
aa
AA or Aa
AA or Aa
AA or Aa
AA
AA
Aa Aa Aa Aa
AA or Aa
AA or Aa
AA or Aa
AA AA AA
AA or Aa
aa
aa
B

Figure 8.9 ■ Sample three-generation pedigree. **A,** A representative pedigree for a single character or genetic condition through three generations. **B,** The most probable genotypes of each individual in the pedigree for an autosomal recessive condition, represented by AA, Aa, or aa.

BOX 8.8
Indicators for a Referral to a Genetic Specialist

HISTORY ASSESSMENT DATA CONCERNS

- Several closely related individuals affected with the same or related conditions:
  a. Breast and ovarian cancer
  b. Colon and endometrial cancer
  c. Diabetes
  d. Hypertension
  e. Coronary heart disease
  f. Thyroid cancer
  g. Colon polyps
- A common disorder with earlier age of onset than typical (increase concern if it occurs in more than one family member):
  a. Breast cancer: <45–50 years of age or premenopausal
  b. Colon cancer: <45–50 years of age
  c. Prostate cancer: <45–60 years of age
  d. Vision loss: <55 years of age
  e. Hearing loss: <50–60 years of age
  f. Dementia: <60 years of age
  g. Heart disease: <40–60 years of age
  h. Stroke: <60 years of age
- A sudden or unexpected death in someone who seemed healthy:
  a. Renal disease
  b. Asthma
  c. Suicide

AN INDIVIDUAL WITH

- Two or more conditions
- A medical condition and *dysmorphic* (abnormal or misshapen) features
- Developmental delay with dysmorphic features and/or physical birth anomalies
- Learning disabilities
- Behavioral problems
- Unexplained:
  a. Movement disorders
  b. Seizures
  c. Hypotonia
  d. Ataxia
  e. Infertility
  f. Disproportionate tall or short stature
  g. Proportionate short stature with dysmorphic features
  h. Atypical sexual development
  i. Premature ovarian failure

BOX 8.9
Genetic Information Nondiscrimination Act of 2008

After 13 years of debate, on May 21, 2008, President George W. Bush signed into law the Genetic Information Nondiscrimination Act of 2008 (GINA) (National Human Genome Research Institute, 2012). The purpose of this federal law is to protect consumers from discrimination by employers and health insurance companies based on genetic information. Examples of protected tests are *BRCA1/BRCA2* (breast cancer), Huntington disease, and carrier screening for cystic fibrosis, sickle cell disease, and Tay-Sachs disease. GINA does not include considerations regarding life, disability, or long-term care insurance or members of the military.

Usually before the first visit for genetic evaluation, the patient will be contacted to provide a detailed medical and family history. The patient should be prepared to give as exact a family history as possible so that a detailed three-generation pedigree can be constructed. The patient should be informed that a genetic consultation usually lasts several hours. During the appointment, a genetic clinical nurse, genetic counselor, and/or physician will perform an initial interview with the patient. A geneticist will examine the patient in order to establish an accurate diagnosis. Tests may be ordered. These may include chromosome (cytogenetic) analysis, DNA-based testing, x-rays, biopsy, biochemical tests, and genome sequencing. After the exam and the completion of any applicable testing, the geneticist and/or genetic counselor will discuss the findings with the patient and make recommendations. The discussion will include the natural history of the condition, the inheritance patterns, the current preventative or treatment options, and the risks to the patient and/or family. The visit will also include opportunities for questions and answers as well as the assessment and evaluation of the patients' understanding. Poor retention of information is typical for a patient facing a new genetic diagnosis. This makes it imperative for the nurse to take advantage of opportunities to reinforce genetic concepts at a later time when the patient is ready.

As the visit concludes, the patient can expect appropriate referrals to be made, discussion of available services or research studies, and possible scheduling of a follow-up visit. A summary of the information is usually sent to the patient. The patient's healthcare provider will receive a report if requested by the patient.

Genetic healthcare providers present the patient with information to promote informed decisions. They are also sensitive to the importance of protecting the individual's autonomy. A challenge during any visit to a genetic specialist is providing nondirective counseling. Patients should be permitted to make decisions that are not influenced by any biases or values from the nurse, counselor, or geneticist. Many patients are accustomed to practitioners and nurses providing direction and guidance in their decision making. Patients may be uncomfortable with the nurse's approach to providing education; however, it is imperative for the nurse to remain unbiased and leave decision making to the patient. The patient may believe that the nurse or healthcare provider is withholding very bad news. The nurse should discuss the positives and negatives of each decision and present as many options as possible through the use of therapeutic listening and communication skills.

Patient Teaching and Support. The nurse must be aware of available genetic resources and participate in patient education about genetic disorders. The cultural and religious beliefs and values of patients must be assessed prior to teaching. Are the gene alterations viewed as uncontrollable and believed to be occurring secondary to cultural belief, such as a stranger looking at the patient? Or, are the gene alterations considered a form of punishment? Obtaining educational materials in the native language of the patient will also help facilitate the teaching–learning experience. Also, identifying and dealing with barriers to learning—such as denial, anxiety, or guilt—will enable teaching to be more useful and effective for the patient and family.

Nurses should encourage open discussions and the expression of fears and concerns with patients, reinforcing that genetic alterations are caused by changes within a gene and not by religious, superstitious, or cultural beliefs. However, it is important to remember that everyone has superstitions or beliefs and the nurse must remain nonjudgmental. The nurse is responsible for assessing the patient's coping mechanisms as well as available family, spiritual, cultural, and community support systems. Genetic conditions can cause a permanent strain on family dynamics and relationships. The nurse may need to help the patient reaffirm his or her self-worth and value.

Growth and development and meeting adult developmental milestones can be altered by actual or potential genetic disorders. Especially unique is the potential or actual inheritance of a late-onset condition such as Huntington disease. The patient with this altered gene may not achieve the developmental tasks in moving through adulthood. The patient may be worried about future goals and aspirations. The nurse must identify the impact of genetic knowledge on daily living activities but also achievement of developmental milestones. Both patient and family strengths need to be identified.

Useful resources for many families are support groups. Careful consideration must be made when utilizing support services and resources, The nurse can refer the patient to a support group. However, the nurse must have permission from the patient to provide a support group with the patient's name and contact information.

Another key role for the nurse is to help patients with the often difficult task of communicating genetic information such as inheritance patterns to extended family members. Cultural values of autonomy and privacy affect a patient's decision whether to communicate genetic information to extended family members who may also carry the altered gene. The history of a genetic alteration that may or may not cause disease can be extensive within a family, affecting multiple family members. Family members often have difficulty understanding that some genetic conditions have variable expressivity. Members of the extended family are often shocked and feel a profound sense of guilt that they are the one who has carried the gene alteration that caused their loved one to have a genetic condition.

Careful self-assessment of feelings is essential for the nurse. The nurse must continually advocate for patients and support their decisions even if the decisions conflict with the nurse's own ideals and morals. Coping with genetic revelations and making genetic-related treatment decisions are difficult. The nurse must remember that patients will need resources and support and also help in gathering information about reproductive options.

Evaluation

Expected outcomes of delivering nursing care with a genetic focus include:

- The patient will make informed and voluntary decisions related to genetic health issues.
- The patient will accurately identify the following:
    a. Basic genetic concepts and simple inheritance risk probabilities
    b. What to expect from a genetic referral
    c. The influence of genetic factors in health promotion and health maintenance
    d. Differences between medical and genetic tests
    e. Social, legal, and ethical issues related to genetic testing.

Transitions of Care

With knowledge of genetic conditions, the nurse can ensure health teaching and early detection of complications from genetic conditions with emphasis on primary and secondary care interventions. Consider the following examples:

- A woman with a strong family history and/or mutations in the *BRCA1* and *BRCA2* tumor suppressor genes should have screening clinical breast exams and mammography at an earlier age than the general population.
- A man with a strong family history and/or mutations in the *BRCA1* and *BRCA2* tumor suppressor genes should report any mass, tenderness, or swelling in the breast tissue and maintain early screening for prostate cancer.
- Colonoscopy screening every 1 to 2 years beginning at age 25 is important for the individual with a positive family history and/or mutations in the *MLH1/MSH2* gene, which increases the risk for hereditary nonpolyposis colorectal cancer.

Patients receiving early intervention and health promotion–focused care can live longer and with a much better quality of life than those who do not. The nurse must be able to identify both community-based and genetic-based resources that are available to assist the patient in strategies to support both health promotion and health maintenance activities. The following are reliable sources of information that can be used by professionals and consumers:

- U.S. Department of Health and Human Services, Surgeon General's Family Health History Initiative (www.hhs.gov/programs/prevention-and-wellness/family-health-history/index.html)
- Genetics Home Reference is a consumer-friendly website providing information on the effects of genetic variations on human health (ghr.nlm.nih.gov).

Nurses are often the primary caregivers to whom patients turn for information, guidance, and clarification of ideas. This nursing role is essential not only in providing direct nursing care but as a member of the community. As more information about the genetic revolution becomes available to consumers—in areas such as pharmacogenomics, gene transfer, ethics, genetic engineering, and stem cell research—the role of nurses remains not only vital but grows enormously. Nurses should remain educated, informed, knowledgeable, and ready to discuss trends and changes with patients and their families.

CHAPTER HIGHLIGHTS

8.1 Genetics Basics

Outline the basics of genetics including cell division, chromosomal alterations, and the role of genes.

- When cell division does not occur as expected, chromosomal alterations on the autosomes or sex chromosomes can result. Chromosomal alterations can be seen in a human karyotype.
- A gene is a small portion (segment) of the nucleotide (base) sequence of a chromosome that provides specific directions for a particular function or characteristic. Gene alterations are responsible for approximately 6000 hereditary diseases.

8.2 Principles of Inheritance

Describe the principles of inheritance.

- An individual may be identified as heterozygous or homozygous for a single gene. Some gene alterations cause disease and some are protective from disease. Multifactorial inheritance does not follow Mendelian inheritance patterns.
- Exceptions or variations to the traditional Mendelian patterns of inheritance include penetrance, new mutation, anticipation, and variable expressivity.

8.3 Care of Patients with Genetic Disorders

Describe the interprofessional care, nursing care, and transitions of care for patients with genetic disorders.

- Many types of genetic tests are available. All genetic tests have social, financial, ethical, and legal implications. Genetic healthcare providers are obligated to present the individual and his or her family with information to promote informed decisions.
- Nurses are responsible for basic genetic knowledge and for delivering the expected standard of genetic nursing care. Nurses must be aware of the social, ethical, cultural, and spiritual issues related to the delivery of genetic nursing care.
- Basic genetic nursing care involves assessing family risk through a detailed family history, integrating genetic concepts into a physical assessment, and initiating a referral to a genetic specialist.
- Genetic concepts can be applied to health promotion and health maintenance with the nurse taking into consideration cultural and spiritual influences on health decisions. Knowledge of the principles of inheritance allows the nurse to not only offer and reinforce genetic information to patients and their families but also to assist them in managing their care and in making reproductive decisions.

TEST YOURSELF NCLEX-RN® REVIEW

1. A patient learns that she has a health problem caused by an autosomal recessive gene. What should the nurse include when explaining the transmission of this disorder?
   A. The health problem can be lethal without adequate treatment.
   B. The health problem is transmitted through a sex chromosome.
   C. The health problem was inherited from both the mother and the father.
   D. The patient's parents have yet to be diagnosed with the same health problem.

2. A male patient is diagnosed with an X-linked recessive health problem. What should the nurse emphasize when teaching the patient about this health problem?
   A. All male offspring of the patient will be carriers of the disorder.
   B. All female offspring of the patient will be carriers of the disorder.
   C. All female offspring of the patient will be affected by the disorder.
   D. The health problem can only be transmitted through direct blood contact.
3. The nurse is providing information regarding genetic testing to a couple who believe they are carriers of an autosomal recessive gene alteration. Which statement by the nurse is appropriate?
   A. "Newborn screening will reveal if your child is affected."
   B. "Chromosomal studies will reveal if you are actually a carrier."
   C. "During the genetic evaluation, you will be asked to provide at least a three-generation family history."
   D. "If both of you are carriers, all of your sons will be affected and all of your daughters will be carriers."
4. When analyzing a family pedigree, the nurse notes the pedigree demonstrates that successive generations contain affected individuals, both males and females are affected, and there is no father-to-offspring inheritance. What is the most likely pattern of inheritance?
   A. Mitochondrial
   B. X-linked recessive
   C. Autosomal recessive
   D. Autosomal dominant
5. When beginning a health history, the patient questions the need to discuss family members' health problems. What should the nurse explain about the purpose of a family history?
   A. It is an inexpensive first genetic screen for the patient.
   B. It helps the nurse to focus on specific body systems to assess.
   C. It serves as a predictor of what health problems the patient will face in the future.
   D. It validates information collected by Health and Human Services on family health.
6. The nurse notes that a teaching session for a patient with a newly diagnosed genetic disorder has been scheduled for an hour. What is the purpose of this extra time?
   A. The information is complex and high level.
   B. Many patients do not want to know this information.
   C. Retention of information is typically low at this time.
   D. Genetic disorders are frequently accompanied by learning difficulty.
7. A patient scheduled for a genetic screening asks the nurse what will happen during the appointment. What should the nurse explain as likely to be included in a genetic referral? (Select all that apply.)
   A. Complete chromosomal studies.
   B. Ask to see photographs of relatives.
   C. Provide direction for important decision making.
   D. Prescribe medication to treat the genetic disorder.
   E. Provide information about the natural history of the condition.
8. After genetic testing a patient learns that she has the gene that causes breast cancer. The nurse will be alert for which problems common to this patient's care? (Select all that apply.)
   A. Difficulty coping with the information
   B. Lack of knowledge about the disease and prognosis
   C. Suicidal ideation
   D. Feeling powerless regarding personal health
   E. Anxiety regarding future health
9. A young male has a strong family history for coronary heart disease. What should the nurse recommend for this patient?
   A. Hematocrit levels every 3 months
   B. Genetic testing to identify the *MLH/MLH2* gene
   C. Lifestyle changes to reduce heart disease risk
   D. Statin therapy to reduce blood cholesterol levels
10. It protects against discrimination by health insurance companies based on genetic information.
   A. It mandates long-term care availability for those with genetic anomalies.
   B. It mandates genetic testing for all government employees and their children.
   C. It protects against discrimination by employers based on genetic information.
   D. It protects against discrimination by life insurance companies based on genetic information.

See Test Yourself answers in Appendix B.

REFERENCES

American Cancer Society. (2017). *Understanding genetic testing for cancer.* Retrieved from https://www.cancer.org/cancer/cancer-causes/genetics/understanding-genetic-testing-for-cancer.html.

American Nurses Association/International Society of Nurses in Genetics. (2016). *Genetics/genomics nursing: Scope and standards of practice* (2nd ed.). Washington DC: American Nurses Publishing.

Brothers, K. B., & Rothstein, M. A. (2015). Ethical, legal, and social implications of incorporating personalized medicine into healthcare. *Personalized Medicine, 12*(1), 43–51.

Carelli, V. (2015). Keeping in shape the dogma of mitochondrial DNA maternal inheritance. *PLoS Genetics.* Retrieved from https://doi.org/10.1371/journal.pgen.1005179.

Dean, L. (2016). Celecoxib therapy and *CYP2C9* genotype. *Medical Genetics Summaries.* Retrieved from https://www.ncbi.nlm.nih.gov/books/NBK379478/

Genetics Home Reference. (2018a). *Cystic fibrosis.* Retrieved from https://ghr.nlm.nih.gov/condition/cystic-fibrosis.

Genetics Home Reference. (2018b). *Fragile X syndrome.* Retrieved from https://ghr.nlm.nih.gov/condition/fragile-x-syndrome.

Genetics Home Reference. (2018c). *Health conditions.* Retrieved from https://ghr.nlm.nih.gov/condition.

Genetics Home Reference. (2018d). *How do genes direct the production of proteins?* Retrieved from https://ghr.nlm.nih.gov/primer/howgeneswork/makingprotein.

Genetics Home Reference. (2018e). *What are single nucleotide polymorphisms (SNPs).* Retrieved from https://ghr.nlm.nih.gov/primer/genomicresearch/snp.

Genetics Home Reference. (2018f). *What are the types of genetic tests?* Retrieved https://ghr.nlm.nih.gov/primer/testing/uses.

Genetics Home Reference. (2018g). *What is a gene?* Retrieved from https://ghr.nlm.nih.gov/primer/basics/gene.

Genetics Home Reference. (2018h). What is genetic discrimination? Retrieved from https://ghr.nlm.nih.gov/primer/testing/discrimination.

Jameson, J. L., & Kopp, P. (2015). Principles of human genetics. In D. Longo, A. Fauci, D. Kasper, S. Hauser, J. Jameson, & J. Loscalzo (Eds.), *Harrison's principles of internal medicine* (19th ed.), Chapter 82. New York, NY: McGraw-Hill.

John, J. C. S., Facucho-Oliveira, J., Jiang, Y., Kelly, R., & Salah, R. (2010). Mitochondrial DNA transmission, replication and inheritance: A journey from the gamete through the embryo and into offspring and embryonic stem cells. *Human Reproduction Update, 16*(5), 488–509.

Lister Hill National Center for Biomedical Communications. (2014). *Handbook: The Human Genome Project.* Retrieved from http://ghr.nlm.nih.gov/handbook/hgp.pdf.

Mayo Clinic. (2018). *The genetic basis of Down syndrome.* Retrieved from https://www.mayoclinic.org/diseases-conditions/down-syndrome/multimedia/the-genetic-basis-of-down-syndrome/img-20007912.

National Cancer Institute. (2017). *Chronic myelogenous leukemia.* Retrieved from https://www.cancer.gov/types/leukemia/hp/cml-treatment-pdq.

National Institute of Child Health and Human Development. (2017). Centers for collaborative research in fragile X. Retrieved from https://www.nichd.nih.gov/research/supported/ccrfx

National Human Genome Research Institute. (2012, March 16). *Genetic Information Nondiscrimination Act (GINA) of 2008.* Retrieved from www.genome.gov/24519851.

National Human Genome Research Institute. (2015). *GQT: Making the most of genomic big data.* Retrieved from http://ucgd.genetics.utah.edu/gqt-making-the-most-of-genomic-big-data/

NBA.com. (2016). *Isaiah Austin cleared to play after Marfan diagnosis.* Retrieved from www.nba.com/article/2016/12/01/isaiah-austin-cleared-play#/.

Nussbaum, R. L., McInnes, R. R., & Willard, H. F. (2016). *Thompson & Thompson genetics in medicine* (8th ed.). Philadelphia, PA: Saunders.

Online Mendelian Inheritance in Man (OMIM). (2017). McKusick-Nathans Institute for Genetics Medicine, Johns Hopkins University (Baltimore, MD) and National Center for Biotechnology Information Library of Medicine (Bethesda, MD). Retrieved from www.ncbi.nlm.nih.gov/omim.

Simons A., Shaffer, L. G., & Hastings, R. J. (2016). Cytogenetic nomenclature. *Cytogenetic and Genome Research, 149*, 1–2.

U.S. Department of Energy (USDOE) Genome Programs. (2008). *Genomics and its impact on science and society: The Human Genome Project and beyond.* Retrieved from www.ornl.gov/hgmis/publicat/primer.

Wu, L., & Zhao, L. (2016). ApoE2 and Alzheimers's disease: Time to take a closer look. *Neural Regeneration Research, 11*(3), 412–413.

ADDITIONAL RESOURCES

Genetics 101 for Health Care Professionals
www.genome.gov/27527637

Genetics Home Reference
https://ghr.nlm.nih.gov

National Human Genome Research Institute (NHGRI)
www.genome.gov

Chapter 9

Nursing Care of Patients in Pain

Chapter Outline and Learning Outcomes

CLINICAL COMPETENCIES

- Use clinical reasoning to provide individualized nursing care for patients experiencing pain.
- Assess patients' pain intensity, quality, location, pattern, intensifiers, relievers; side effects of analgesics; and effect on function and mood.
- Determine patient's expressed desire, values, preference, and support for pain management.
- In collaboration with the healthcare team, intervene with appropriate evidence-based nursing measures to promote patient comfort and include pharmacologic and nonpharmacologic methodologies.
- Revise plan of care according to patient's response to interventions and need for control.
- Use equianalgesia tables to select and transition among opioid analgesics.
- Teach patients about safe and effective self-management of pain.
- Evaluate effectiveness of interventions to relieve pain and promote comfort; retreat or adjust doses of medication and interventions as necessary.

KEY TERMS

acute pain, 200
addiction, 204
analgesic, 206
breakthrough pain, 203
chronic pain, 201
equianalgesic, 207
neuropathic pain, 203
nociceptive pain, 203
nociceptors, 198
pain, 196
pain tolerance, 204
titrate, 211

Pain is a subjective response to both physical and psychologic stressors. All people experience pain at some point during their lives. A seminal report on pain estimated that 100 million adult Americans live with chronic pain (Institute of Medicine, 2011). More current data from within the United States found that (Nahin, 2015):

- 23.4 million adults reported a lot of pain
- 126 million adults reported some type of pain in the 3 months prior to the survey.

Low back pain is one of the most common types of chronic pain, along with migraine and severe headache and joint pain. Eighty percent of patients undergoing surgery report experiencing postoperative pain and fewer than half indicate they experience adequate pain relief (Chou et al., 2016). Whether pain is acute, chronic, severe, or mild to moderate, the experience is pervasive and common in all healthcare settings and is associated with increased healthcare costs, loss of productivity, and an adverse effect on quality of life (Henschke, Kamper, & Maher, 2015).

9.1 The Concept of Pain

The Fifth Vital Sign

Although pain usually is experienced as uncomfortable and unwelcome, it also serves a protective role, warning of potentially health-threatening conditions. For this reason, pain is referred to as the *fifth vital sign*, with recommendations to assess pain with each vital sign assessment. Established standards have for many years identified the relief of pain as a patient right and required healthcare facilities to implement specific procedures for, and provider education on, pain assessment and management (Joint Commission, 2018). The Joint Commission's (2018) updated standards require healthcare facilities to:

- Establish a clinical leadership team for the treatment of pain
- Actively engage the interprofessional team in improving pain assessment and management, including strategies to decrease opioid use and minimize risks associated with opioid use
- Offer at least one complementary pain treatment modality
- Facilitate access to prescription drug monitoring programs
- Improve pain assessment by concentrating more on how pain is affecting patients' physical function
- Engage patients in treatment decisions about their pain management
- Educate patients on the topic of storage and disposal of opioids
- Provide referral of patients addicted to opioids to treatment programs.

Pain is a distinct and personal experience influenced by genetic, physiologic, psychologic, cognitive, sociocultural, cultural, and spiritual factors. It is the symptom most associated with describing oneself as ill, and it is the most common reason for seeking healthcare. The International Association for the Study of Pain (IASP; 2015) defines pain as an unpleasant sensory and emotional experience associated with actual or potential tissue damage, or described in terms of such damage. Although there are many definitions and descriptors of pain, the one most relevant for nurses is that pain is "whatever the person experiencing it says it is, and existing whenever the person says it does" (McCaffery, 1979, p. 11). This definition acknowledges the patient as the only person who can accurately define and describe his or her own pain and serves as the basis for nursing assessment and care of patients in pain. It also supports the values and beliefs about pain necessary for holistic nursing care, including:

- Only the person affected can experience pain; that is, pain has a personal meaning.
- If the patient says he or she has pain, the patient is in pain. All pain is real.
- Pain has physical, emotional, cognitive, sociocultural, and spiritual dimensions.
- Pain affects the whole body, usually negatively.
- Pain may serve as both a response to and a warning of actual or potential trauma.

Adverse Effects of Pain

Acute pain has a defined purpose: To warn of injury to body tissues. Although often attributable to a defined disorder (such as arthritis, migraine, or cancer), chronic pain often serves no useful purpose, becoming instead part of the problem. Physiologic responses to pain extend beyond the muscle spasm and fight-or-flight response (increased blood pressure, heart rate, and cardiac output, decreased gastric and intestinal motility) and can have adverse effects on the patient's health. Pain interferes with sleep quantity and quality, leading to exhaustion and possible disorientation. Metabolism and myocardial oxygen demand are increased. Catabolism (breakdown of body tissues) increases, and healing is impaired. Immune function is suppressed, increasing the risk for infection. Research shows a clear link between chronic pain and depression (Sorenson, Quinn, & Klein, 2019).

Myths and Misconceptions About Pain

Myths and misconceptions about pain and its management are common in both healthcare providers and patients. Some of the most common of these myths are below.

- ***Pain is a result, not a cause.*** According to the traditional view of pain, pain is a symptom, not a condition. Pain is now recognized as having both immediate and long-term effects, such as immobility, anger, and anxiety; pain may also delay healing and rehabilitation.
- ***Chronic pain is really a masked form of depression.*** Serotonin plays a chemical role in pain transmission and is the major modulator of depression. Therefore, pain and depression are chemically related, not mutually exclusive. It is common to find them coexisting.
- ***Narcotic medication is too risky to be used in chronic pain.*** This common misconception can deprive patients of the most effective source of pain relief. Opioid (narcotic) analgesics are recognized as an appropriate strategy for managing chronic pain unrelieved by other strategies.
- ***It is best to wait until a patient has pain before giving medication.*** Relieving pain before it escalates is widely accepted as having a noticeable effect on the amount of pain a patient experiences.
- ***Many patients lie about the existence or severity of their pain.*** Very few patients lie about their pain.
- ***Pain relief interferes with diagnosis.*** Effective pain management with analgesics in the emergency department (ED) has been shown to have no impact on physical assessment findings or diagnosis (Institute of Medicine [IOM], 2011).

9.2 Neurophysiology of Pain

The peripheral nervous system has two types of neurons: Sensory and motor. The pain experience involves both sensory stimulation and perception. Pain stimuli are generated and transmitted through the sensory neurons, perceived within the central nervous system (CNS), and responded to through the motor neurons. Connections or synapses occur within the spinal cord and again within the brain, where interpretation of the painful stimulus leads to a response. A pain stimulus may prompt an immediate reflex response that precedes awareness of the pain.

Pain Theories

Several theories explain the response to pain and the diversity of human experiences with pain. The meaning or perception of pain can be modified by past experiences, motivation, attention, suggestion, personality, and culture. *Specificity* and *pattern* theories describe nerve impulses of varying intensity terminating in pain centers in the forebrain. These theories provide explanations of the neurophysiologic basis of pain. In 1965, Melzack and Wall postulated the *gate-control theory* (Mendell, 2014). According to this theory, activation of large-diameter, faster-propagating fibers by a tactile stimulus (e.g., massaging the elbow after hitting it on a sharp object) activates a gating mechanism that then blocks impulses from smaller pain fibers (Sorenson et al., 2019). This mechanism was thought to exist at the segmental spinal cord level (**Figure 9.1** ■).

Ongoing research demonstrates that the control and modulation of pain is much more complex than the description in the gate-control theory, which served as a base for further research about pain-modulating systems. Tactile information is now known to be transmitted by both large- and small-diameter fibers, and interaction between sensory neurons is known to occur at multiple levels of the CNS. Melzack subsequently developed the *neuromatrix* theory of pain to integrate cultural and genetic factors with basic neurophysiologic function. This theory is consistent with, but more complex than, the gate-control theory. According to the neuromatrix theory, the brain contains a *body–self neuromatrix*, a widely distributed network of neurons that is affected by both genetic factors and sensory experiences. The neuromatrix integrates multiple sources of input in addition to the stimuli of pain and touch. The pain experience for the individual is affected by inputs from other sensory systems that help interpret the stimuli (e.g., seeing a wound); factors such as attention, expectation, personality, and culture; innate pain modulation systems; and components of stress-regulation systems (Sorenson et al., 2019).

One pain theory that is quite significant in clinical terms describes the effect of sensitizing the central and peripheral nervous system to painful stimuli. According to this theory, painful signals create a cascade of changes in the nervous system that increase the responsiveness of the peripheral and central neurons. These changes, in turn, increase the response to future signals and amplify pain. Sensitization occurs from nociceptive barrage and from the inflammation that follows an injury or incision. In adults this theory indicates the value of preventing sensitization as well as treating perceived pain with multimodal pain therapy. Local and regional anesthesia used in combination with central anesthesia prior to incision to diminish sensitization of these pathways results in significantly reduced consumption of intravenous morphine via patient-controlled analgesia (PCA) following surgery (Laufer, 2018).

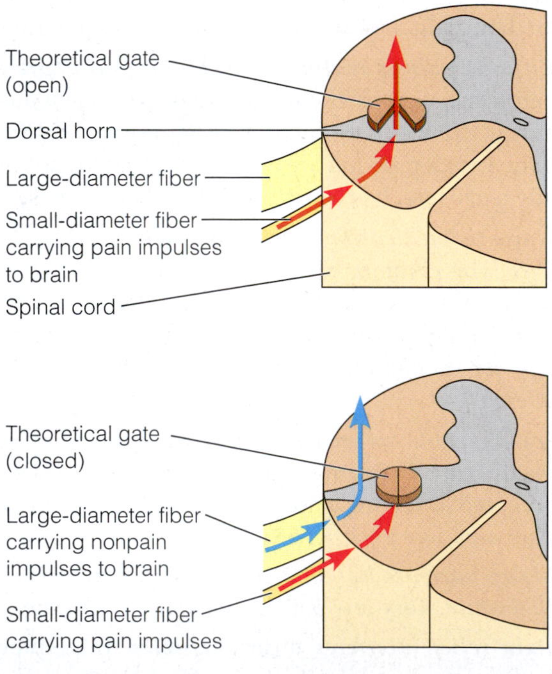
Theoretical gate
(open)
Dorsal horn
Large-diameter fiber
Small-diameter fiber
carrying pain impulses
to brain
Spinal cord
Theoretical gate
(closed)
Large-diameter fiber
carrying nonpain
impulses to brain
Small-diameter fiber
carrying pain impulses

Figure 9.1 ■ The spinal cord component of the gate-control theory. Pain transmission by small-diameter fibers is blocked when large-diameter fibers carrying touch impulses dominate, closing the gate in the dorsal horn of the spinal cord.

Physiology of Pain

Nerve receptors for pain are called **nociceptors**. These free nerve endings are woven throughout all the tissues of the body except the brain. Nociceptors are especially numerous in the skin and muscles. Pain occurs when the tissue containing nociceptors is subjected to a noxious insult. The intensity and duration of the stimuli determine the sensation. Long-lasting, intense stimulation produces greater pain than brief, mild stimulation (Sorenson et al., 2019).

Nociceptors respond to several different types of noxious stimuli: Chemical, mechanical, or thermal. Some nociceptors respond to only a single type of stimulus, whereas others respond to all three types of stimuli (**Table 9.1**). The perception of pain in different parts of the body is affected by this variation in sensitivity to type of stimulus and the distribution of nociceptors in various tissues.

Tissue trauma, inflammation, and ischemia prompt the release of a number of biochemicals. These biochemicals have several effects. Chemicals such as bradykinin, histamine, serotonin, and potassium ion directly stimulate

Table 9.1 Painful Stimuli

Stimulus	Examples
Chemical	■ Ischemia (e.g., angina, bowel infarct) ■ Tissue trauma ■ Inflammation, inflammatory mediators such as histamine, prostaglandins
Mechanical	■ Spasm (ureteral colic, gallstones) ■ Compression (e.g., mechanical or by a tumor, carpal tunnel syndrome, or compartment syndrome) ■ Extreme muscle stretch or contraction (e.g., following a fracture)
Thermal	■ Contact with extreme heat or cold

nociceptors, producing pain. These chemicals and others (such as ATP and prostaglandins) sensitize nociceptors, intensifying the pain response and causing normally innocuous stimuli (such as touch) to be perceived as pain. Chemical mediators act to perpetuate inflammation, which, in turn, causes release of additional chemicals that stimulate pain receptors. Furthermore, so-called *silent nociceptors* (e.g., sensory receptors that normally do not respond to mechanical or thermal stimuli) can become sensitive to mechanical stimuli in the presence of inflammatory mediators, leading to severe and debilitating pain and tenderness (Sorenson et al., 2019).

Pain Pathways

The neural pathways of pain, illustrated in **Figure 9.2** ■, can be summarized as:

1. A noxious stimulus is translated by nociceptors into an action potential that then is transmitted through small A-delta (Aδ) and even smaller C nerve fibers to the spinal cord. Aδ fibers are myelinated and transmit impulses rapidly. They produce what is called *fast pain* or first pain—sharp, well-defined pain sensations, such as those that result from cuts, electric shocks, or the impact of a blow. Aδ fibers are associated with acute pain from mechanical or thermal injury. C fibers are not myelinated and thus transmit pain impulses more slowly. Pain transmitted by C fibers may be described as *slow-wave pain* or second pain because it is slower to develop and lasts longer. This pain is more often prompted by chemical stimuli or persistent mechanical or thermal stimuli (Sorenson et al., 2019). The pain from deep body structures (such as muscles and viscera) is primarily transmitted by C fibers, producing diffuse burning or aching sensations. C fibers are associated with chronic pain. Both Aδ and C fibers are involved in most injuries. For example, if you bang your elbow, Aδ fibers transmit this pain stimulus within 0.1 second, and can actually prompt reflex withdrawal from the stimulus before pain is perceived. You feel this pain as a sharp, localized, smarting sensation. One or more seconds after the blow, you experience a duller, aching, diffuse sensation of pain impulses carried by the C fibers.
2. The sensory neuron enters the spinal cord via the dorsal root and terminates in the dorsal horn of the spinal cord. Here it synapses with spinal (or second-order) neurons that transmit the pain signal to the brain. Several chemical neurotransmitters, including glutamate, norepinephrine, and substance P, carry the pain signal from the sensory neuron to the spinal neurons. Each

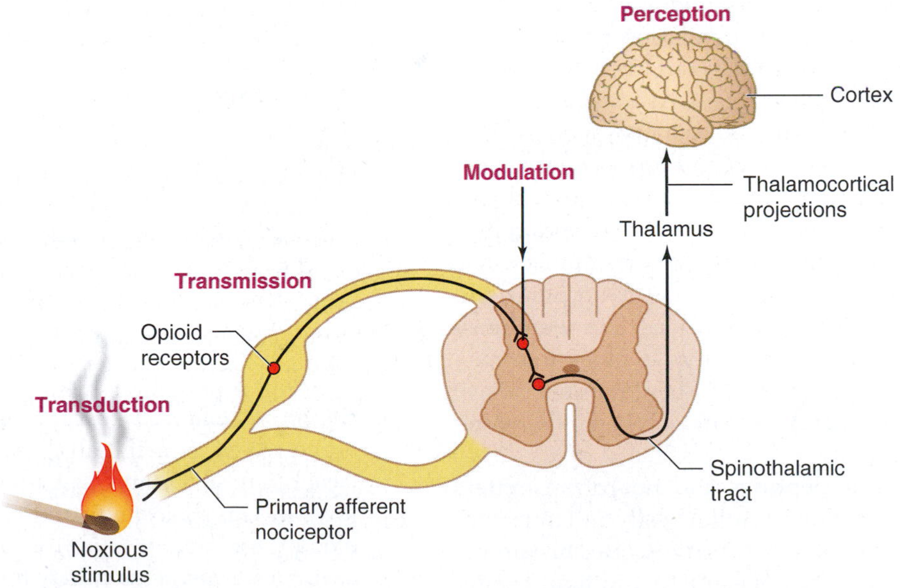
Perception
Cortex
Modulation
Thalamocortical
projections
Thalamus
Transmission
Opioid
receptors
Transduction
Spinothalamic
tract
Primary afferent
nociceptor
Noxious
stimulus

Figure 9.2 ■ Touching the flame activates nociceptors in the skin, generating pain impulses that travel via fast Aδ and slower C fibers to the spinal cord. Secondary neurons in the dorsal horn pass impulses across the spinal cord to the anterior spinothalamic tract. Pain impulses ascend to the thalamus and, from there, the impulses pass through the medulla and midbrain to the thalamus, and then to the cerebral cortex and the reticular and limbic systems in the brainstem, which integrate the emotional, cognitive, and autonomic responses to pain.

neuron contacts many spinal neurons, and each spinal neuron receives input from many peripheral neurons. This accounts for the phenomenon of referred pain (discussed under types of pain). Spinal neurons transmit the impulses via axons that cross over to the spinothalamic tract.

3. The impulses ascend the spinothalamic tracts and pass through the medulla and midbrain to the thalamus.
4. From the thalamus, the pain signal is distributed via third-order neurons to several areas of the cerebral cortex. The somatosensory area of the cerebral cortex localizes the pain and interprets its intensity and quality. Other thalamic neurons reach areas of the frontal lobe, generating an emotional or affective response to pain. Connections to the reticular and limbic systems of the brain are also involved in the emotional and autonomic responses to painful stimuli. Pain signals to these areas can activate the fight-or-flight response, stress responses, and cardiovascular changes. A noxious impulse becomes pain when the sensation reaches conscious levels and is perceived and evaluated by the person experiencing the sensation.

Modulation of Pain

No two people experience pain from an identical stimulus in the same way or at the same intensity; furthermore, the same person may perceive pain from the same stimulus differently on different occasions. A number of neural and chemical responses explain some of these differences.

Neural circuits that are thought to arise in the cerebral cortex link with the hypothalamus, midbrain, and medulla. These circuits interact with peripheral sensory axon terminals in the dorsal horn of the spinal cord to selectively control neurons that transmit pain signals. As a result, that pain response can be modified, that is, changed, increased, or dampened. Neurons within this circuit produce *endogenous opioids*, naturally occurring morphine-like neuropeptides. They also contain opioid receptors sensitive to endorphins and opioid drugs. Four types of endogenous opioids have been identified: Enkephalins, endorphins, dynorphins, and endomorphins. They are hormones that act like neurotransmitters, binding with opioid receptors to block transmission of painful stimuli (**Figure 9.3** ■). These substances have also been linked to a general sense of well-being (Sorenson et al., 2019).

Chemicals such as peptides and neurotransmitters also affect responses to pain stimuli. Locally, inflammatory mediators (e.g., prostaglandins, nitric oxide, histamine) lower the threshold for pain perception and tend to augment pain. ATP, substance P, and other peptides promote the local spread of pain and contribute to vasodilation and vascular permeability, increasing discomfort (Sorenson et al., 2019). In contrast, substances such as serotonin, norepinephrine, and others inhibit pain impulse transmission in the spinal cord and brain.

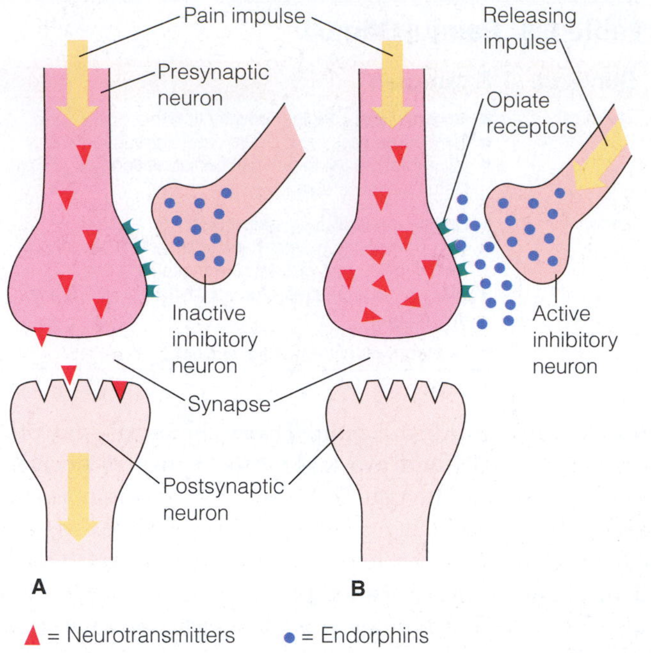

Pain impulse
Releasing impulse
Presynaptic neuron
Opiate receptors
Inactive inhibitory neuron
Active inhibitory neuron
Synapse
Postsynaptic neuron
A
B
▲ = Neurotransmitters
● = Endorphins

Figure 9.3 ■ **A**, Pain impulse causes presynaptic neuron to release burst of neurotransmitters across synapse. These bind to postsynaptic neuron and propagate impulse. **B**, Inhibitory neuron releases endorphins, which bind to presynaptic opiate receptors. Neurotransmitter release is inhibited, and pain impulse is interrupted.

9.3 Types and Characteristics of Pain

Pain typically is described and characterized in several ways: By its duration (acute or chronic), source or location, and referral. Various types of pain are summarized in **Table 9.2**.

Acute Pain

Acute pain has a sudden onset, is usually self-limited, and is localized. The cause of acute pain can generally be identified ("I tripped and twisted my ankle; now it really hurts"). The onset is usually sudden, most often resulting from tissue injury from trauma, surgery, or inflammation. The pain is usually sharp and localized, although it may radiate. Tissue healing relieves the pain. The three major types of acute pain are:

- ***Cutaneous and deep somatic pain***, which arises from nerve receptors originating in the skin (e.g., from a laceration), subcutaneous tissues, or deep body structures such as periosteum, muscles, tendons, joints, and blood vessels (acute pain from a fracture or sprain, for example). Somatic pain may be either sharp and well localized or dull and diffuse.
- ***Visceral pain***, which arises from body organs. Visceral pain is dull and poorly localized because of the low number of nociceptors. The viscera are sensitive to stretching, inflammation, and ischemia but relatively insensitive to cutting and temperature extremes.

Table 9.2 Types of Pain

Type of Pain	Description and Location	Examples
Central	Results from damage or injury to nerve conduction pathways within the central nervous system. Pain can appear in an area associated with the cause of injury, with a great deal of variance in severity and duration.	■ Epilepsy ■ Parkinson disease ■ Stroke
Myofascial	Pain of the skeletal muscle and surrounding fascia, usually a result of chronic overuse or acute muscle injury. Characterized by trigger points; highly sensitive areas within the muscle that are painful to touch, and referred pain. Myofascial pain affects the muscles of the head, neck, shoulder and arm, and back and hip.	■ Plantar fasciitis ■ Tension headache
Neuropathic	Pain without obvious injury or protracted pain that persists for months/years after the initial injury. Resulting from CNS or PNS dysfunction.	■ Carpal tunnel syndrome ■ Diabetic neuropathy ■ Postherpetic neuralgia ■ Trigeminal neuralgia
Phantom	Pain associated with a missing body part or surgically removed limb. Believed to result from damaged or dysfunctional nerve pathways at the site of injury.	■ Phantom limb pain ■ Pain after loss of an eye ■ Pain perceptions following a complete spinal cord injury
Psychogenic	Physical pain with psychological causes such as stress or anxiety.	■ Stress-induced headache ■ Facial or lower back pain following an emotional situation
Radicular pain	Pain caused by inflammation or compression of a spinal nerve root. The pain follows the sensory distribution of the affected nerve.	■ Cervical radicular pain ■ Lumbar radiculopathy
Somatic	Pain that rises from the skin, ligaments, muscles, bones, or joints, as a result of an acute injury or chronic degenerative disease.	■ Burns ■ Arthritis ■ Fracture
Vascular	Pain associated with dilation or constriction of blood vessels.	■ Chest pain as with angina or myocardial infarction ■ Lower extremity pain associated with peripheral artery disease ■ Migraine headache
Visceral	Pain originating from inflammation or obstruction of internal organs.	■ Appendicitis ■ Gallbladder disease ■ Kidney stones

Visceral pain often radiates or is referred. It may be described as deep cramping, splitting or stabbing pain, intermittent pain, or colicky pain. A kidney stone passing through the ureter to the bladder causes severe, acute visceral pain.

- *Referred pain* is pain that is perceived in an area distant from the site of the stimuli. It commonly occurs with pain that originates in thoracic or abdominal viscera. Visceral sensory fibers synapse at the level of the spinal cord, close to fibers innervating other subcutaneous tissue areas of the body (**Figure 9.4** ■). For example, the phrenic nerve, which innervates the central part of the diaphragm, enters the spinal cord at the C_3 to C_5 level; pain originating in the diaphragm or the parietal peritoneum lining it (e.g., peritonitis) may be perceived as shoulder pain. Sites of referred pain are determined during embryologic development.

Acute pain warns of actual or potential injury to tissues. As a stressor, it initiates the fight-or-flight autonomic stress response. Characteristic physical responses include tachycardia, rapid and shallow respirations, increased blood pressure, dilated pupils, sweating, and pallor. The pain may be accompanied by nausea and vomiting. Secondary reflex muscle spasms may develop, intensifying the pain. The person experiencing acute pain responds to this threat with anxiety and fear. This psychologic response may further increase the physical responses to acute pain.

Chronic Pain

Chronic pain is prolonged pain, or pain that persists after the condition causing it has resolved. Although the cause may be identifiable (e.g., arthritis, cancer, migraine headache, diabetic neuropathy), chronic pain does not always have an identifiable cause. In some cases, pain may be perpetuated by disease-caused damage that persists after the disease has resolved (e.g., sensory nerve damage or reflex muscle contraction). In others, an imbalance of pain modulation mechanisms is thought to cause the persistent pain. This imbalance may relate to changes in the peripheral nervous system such as increased neuronal sensitivity to stimuli (a lower pain threshold) or spontaneous impulse generation by damaged neurons. Changes in the dorsal root, spinal cord, and brain also affect pain modulation. Repeated stimulation of peripheral nerves leads to a progressive buildup of electrical response in the CNS, leading to more intense and prolonged pain.

Unlike acute pain, chronic pain has much more complex and poorly understood neurophysiology and purpose. Persistent chronic pain often serves no useful function. The pain itself becomes the problem, creating physical, psychosocial, and economic stresses on the affected individual and

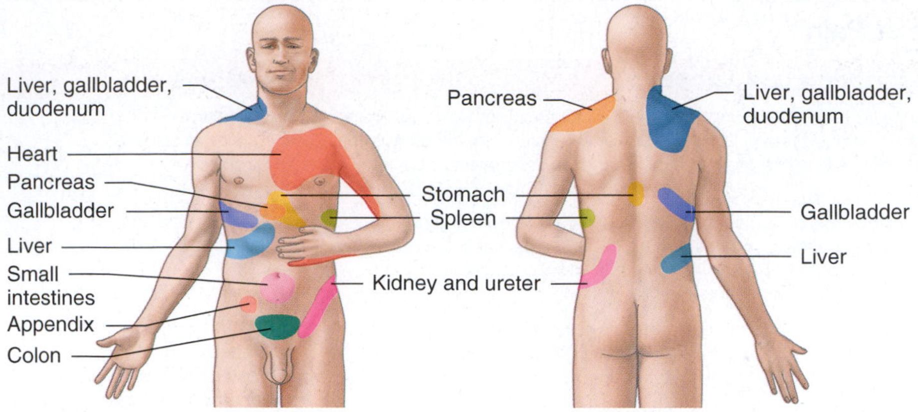
Liver, gallbladder, duodenum
Heart
Pancreas
Gallbladder
Liver
Small intestines
Appendix
Colon
Stomach
Spleen
Kidney and ureter
Pancreas
Liver, gallbladder, duodenum
Gallbladder
Liver

Figure 9.4 ■ Referred pain results from the convergence of sensory nerves from certain areas of the body within the spinal cord. For example, a toothache may be felt in the ear, pain from inflammation of the diaphragm may be felt in the shoulder, and pain from ischemia of the heart muscle (angina) may be felt in the left arm.

his or her family. Furthermore, emotional and psychologic factors can cause the pain itself or make it worse. There is a clear association between chronic pain and depression. Depletion of serotonin (a neurotransmitter) and endorphins, found in both chronic pain and in depression, suggest a common physiology in these disorders (Boakye et al., 2016).

Chronic pain can be subdivided into three categories:

- *Recurrent acute pain*, characterized by relatively well-defined episodes of pain interspersed with pain-free episodes. Migraine headache is an example of recurrent acute pain.
- *Chronic malignant pain*, caused by advance of a life-threatening disease or associated with treatment. Cancer pain is a type of chronic malignant pain.
- *Chronic nonmalignant pain*, non–life-threatening pain that nevertheless persists beyond the expected time for healing. Chronic lower back pain, a major cause of suffering and lost work time, falls into this category.

Patients with chronic pain often do not have the same physiologic responses to pain as are seen in acute pain. The heart and respiratory rates and blood pressure may remain within the normal range. Other autonomic nervous system responses such as nausea and vomiting, pallor, or sweating may not occur with persistent pain. The patient with chronic pain is often depressed, may have difficulty sleeping, and may be preoccupied with the pain. **Table 9.3** compares acute and chronic pain.

The most common chronic pain condition is lower back pain. Other common chronic pain conditions include the following (IOM, 2011):

- *Myofascial pain syndromes* are marked by injury to or disease of muscle and fascia. They include myositis, fibrositis, myofibrositis, myalgia, and muscle strain. Pain results from muscle spasm, stiffness, and collection of lactic acid in the muscle. The pain leads to *guarding* (a defensive tensing of the muscle) and limited motion, which, in turn, leads to weakness, stiffness, and spasm—and more pain.
- *Cancer* often produces chronic pain, usually due to factors such as a tumor growth that presses on nerves or other structures, stretching of viscera, obstruction of ducts, or metastasis to bones. The malignant tumor may mechanically stimulate pain or the production of biochemicals that cause pain. Pain may also be associated with treatments such as chemotherapy and radiation therapy.
- *Chronic postoperative pain* is uncommon, but may occur following incisions in the chest wall, radical mastectomy, radical neck dissection, and surgical amputation.

Table 9.3 Characteristics of Acute and Chronic Pain

Characteristic	Acute Pain	Chronic Pain
Purpose	Signals actual or potential tissue damage	May serve no useful function.
Onset and duration	Sudden; relieved by healing	Persists after acute problem is resolved.
Cause	Actual or potential tissue damage	May not be readily identifiable. May result from nerve damage or pain modulation mechanism imbalance.
Associated symptoms	Sympathetic nervous system responses (increased pulse and respiratory rates, increased blood pressure, sweating, nausea) Muscle spasms Anxiety, fear	Depression is common. Insomnia is present. Patient may experience a preoccupation with pain.

Breakthrough Pain

Breakthrough pain is pain that exceeds baseline chronic or persistent pain. It is often described as a sudden flare-up that exceeds the analgesic effect of long-acting pain medications. Whether the pain is malignant or nonmalignant in origin, treated or untreated, breakthrough pain is temporary and can be debilitating. The onset and intensity of breakthrough pain vary; its unpredictability and inconsistency are distressing to the patient and can make it difficult to manage.

Incident pain is a subtype of breakthrough pain. Incident or *episodic pain* is predictable, precipitated by an event or activity such as coughing, changing position, or being touched. Pain associated with a fractured bone is a good example of incident pain. When the patient remains still and the fracture is aligned and supported, little pain is experienced. Movement of the affected part, however, can precipitate sharp, intense pain.

Nociceptive Pain

Nociceptive pain is caused by stimulation of peripheral or visceral pain receptors. It is generally localized and responsive to treatment. Nociceptive pain may be either acute or chronic, resulting from disease processes (e.g., arthritis), tissue trauma, or medical treatment (e.g., surgery).

Neuropathic Pain

Neuropathic pain arises as a consequence of a lesion or disease affecting the somatosensory system (Finnerup et al., 2016). This definition better defines the origin of the pain as the result of disease instead of the result of hyperactive nociceptive stimulation (Finnerup et al., 2016). Although neuropathic pain may be acute (e.g., the pain associated with shingles [herpes zoster]), it is usually chronic, associated with conditions such as diabetic neuropathy or postherpetic neuralgia. The pain may be described as gnawing, electric shock–like, burning, shooting, or tingling. Pain may occur with a stimulus such as touch that normally does not produce pain (*allodynia*) or its intensity may be disproportionate to the stimulus (*hyperalgesia*) (Sorenson et al., 2019).

Central Pain

Central pain is caused by a lesion or damage in the brain or spinal cord. This damage leads to spontaneous generation of impulses that are perceived as pain. An infarction, tumor, trauma, or disorder such as multiple sclerosis or epilepsy may cause central pain. Central pain is constant, of moderate to severe intensity, and difficult to treat. The location of the pain depends on the area of the CNS affected. The pain may be described as burning, pressing, lacerating, or aching. Pins-and-needles sensations may be experienced along with the underlying pain. Affected areas may have decreased sensation (numbness). Thalamic pain, a type of central pain, may cause hyperesthesia (an abnormal sensitivity to touch, pain, or other sensory stimuli) on the side of the body opposite to the thalamic lesion.

Complex Regional Pain Syndromes

Complex regional pain syndromes (CRPS) cause extremity pain that is severe, diffuse, and burning. The pain is accompanied by vasomotor changes that affect skin color and temperature. Initially the affected extremity has typical inflammatory symptoms, with redness, warmth, and swelling. Later, it is cool, cyanotic, and edematous; skin and nail changes may be seen (Sorenson et al., 2019). The cause of CRPS is unclear; there may, in fact, be several causes, including damage to the central or peripheral nervous system or a disrupted healing or immune process. In CRPS, pain receptors in the affected part of the body become sensitized to catecholamines, neurotransmitters associated with sympathetic nervous system activity.

Phantom Limb Pain

Phantom limb pain is a pain syndrome that occurs following amputation of a body part. The patient experiences pain that may be described as burning, cramping, or shooting, in the missing body part. Phantom limb pain more frequently affects people who had pain in the amputated limb prior to its removal than those who did not. Several theories for phantom limb pain have been developed. These include regeneration of severed peripheral nerves and abnormal impulses generated by spinal cord neurons that no longer receive normal sensory input from the body (Sorenson et al., 2019). Adequate management of postoperative pain after an amputation will help prevent the development of phantom limb pain. Select medications shown to be effective for neuropathic pain are also used to treat phantom limb pain and include opioids, calcitonin/N-methyl-D-aspartate receptor antagonists, and ketamine, gabapentin, pregabalin, tricyclic antidepressants, and muscle relaxants. Encourage the patient to move the affected extremity, which helps the brain reconnect with the remaining portion of the limb. Movement will promote circulation and reduce edema, thereby reducing pain. Ongoing pain assessment is important to monitor the patient's pain status. Assist the patient in documenting ongoing pain assessment and encourage the patient to report his or her pain assessment to the healthcare provider.

While the available evidence is inconsistent as to effectiveness (Richardson & Kulkami, 2017), often a mirror box will be used for those with phantom pain (**Figure 9.5 ■**).

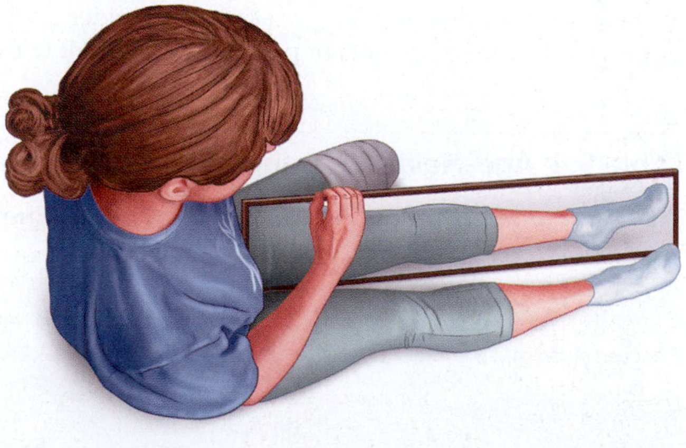

Figure 9.5 ■ Mirror box therapy for phantom limb pain.

Providing a mirror image of the remaining extremity appears to aid in inducing relaxation and reduction of pain.

9.4 Factors Affecting Responses to Pain

Responses to pain stimuli are as individualized as the person experiencing the stimulus. The previous discussion focused on types of pain and physiologic responses to pain stimuli. The individualized response to pain is shaped not only by physiologic responses, but by multiple and interacting factors, including genetics, age, gender, sociocultural influences, emotional state, past experiences with pain, the source and meaning of the pain, and knowledge base.

The *pain threshold* is the point at which a stimulus elicits a response. Although the pain threshold is relatively consistent, meaning that a given pain stimulus will elicit pain perception among most people, it can be affected by factors such as the presence of chronic pain (which tends to lower the threshold) or more intense pain at another site (which tends to raise the threshold).

Pain tolerance is the amount (duration, intensity) of pain an individual can endure before outwardly responding to it (Sorenson et al., 2019). Pain tolerance varies significantly among individuals and within an individual over time. It is influenced by culture, expectations, emotions, and psychosocial factors. The ability to tolerate pain may be decreased by repeated episodes of pain, fatigue, anger, anxiety, and sleep deprivation. Medications, alcohol, hypnosis, warmth, distraction, and spiritual practices may increase pain tolerance.

Age

Age influences a person's perception and expression of pain. There is, however, no evidence that nociception is altered by age. When compared with younger adults, pain stimulus transmission relies more on C fibers in older adults than on Aδ fibers. As a result, pain stimulus transmission is slower, and pain more frequently may be described as burning, dull, or aching. Central processing is often slowed, resulting in a slower response time to pain. Referred pain is less typical in older adults, and visceral pain may present as less severe than in younger adults. The older adult may report vague complaints of pain or may present with manifestations such as delirium rather than subjective reports of pain (Sorenson et al., 2019).

Many older adults experience both acute and chronic pain related to disorders such as arthritis or peripheral neuropathy. While peripheral vascular disease or diabetes may lead to neuropathy and interfere with normal nerve impulse transmission, neuropathy can manifest as hyperesthesias as well as hypoesthesias. Both of these manifestations cause discomfort. Pain tolerance decreases with aging, perhaps related to the prevalence of chronic pain in this population. Studies of older adults found that 45 to 85% of nursing home residents report daily persistent pain. Studies show that 25 to 50% of community-dwelling older adults experience persistent or frequent episodes of pain (Horgas, 2017a, 2017b). Effective assessment and management of pain in older adults can be challenging. Patients and healthcare professionals (including nurses) may believe that pain and discomfort are unavoidable aspects of aging. Individuals in this age group may fail to acknowledge pain, believing that pain is inevitable or fearing dependency if they alarm their loved ones. Patients and healthcare professionals may have misconceptions about the use of analgesics, including opioid medications, fearing adverse effects (such as respiratory depression) or **addiction**. Sensory impairments (e.g., impaired hearing) or cognitive impairments can interfere with the patient's ability to report pain and the healthcare professional's ability to assess pain. **Table 9.4** lists some age-related changes and their effects on pain in older adults.

Gender

Clinical and animal studies show that women have a lower pain threshold and experience higher intensity of pain than men (Fillingim, 2017). It has long been held that sociocultural factors account for these recognized differences in the pain experience. Research has recently provided evidence of physiologic differences in pain responses and the analgesic effect of opioid medications. These physiologic responses appear to be genetically encoded, involving the sex hormones and the activity of opioid receptors in the brain. Fluctuating estrogen levels associated with the menstrual cycle affect perceived pain intensity. The circuits that mediate the pain response differ in men and women, the opioid pain modulatory system in particular. Because of these differences, women and men may respond differently to opioid analgesics such as morphine (Fillingim, 2017).

Table 9.4 Age-Related Changes in Pain Perception and Response in Older Adults

Age-Related Factor	Effects
Decreased Aδ fiber transmission, greater reliance on C fiber transmission	Pain perceived as dull, aching, more diffuse rather than sharp, localized
Slowed central processing	Slower motor or avoidance responses
Reduced norepinephrine levels	Reduced sympathetic nervous system responses to pain (pulse, blood pressure, papillary dilation)
Decreased referred pain	May not exhibit classic manifestations of such disorders as myocardial infarction, acute abdomen
Reduced neurotransmitter levels	Increased risk of depression related to chronic pain

Sociocultural Influences

Each person's response to pain is strongly influenced by the family, community, and culture. Sociocultural influences affect pain behavior, dictating appropriate and inappropriate expressions of pain. People acquire beliefs about pain and norms for expressing response to pain over a lifetime of varying experiences that are influenced by social and culture factors. Whether they perceive pain as a sign of impending damage or disability, a short-term or permanent condition, or controllable or uncontrollable will influence their response (IOM, 2011). For example, if the patient's culture teaches that people should tolerate pain stoically, the patient may appear withdrawn and refuse (or not request) pain medication. If the cultural norm encourages open and intense emotional expression, the patient may cry freely and appear comfortable requesting pain medication.

Cultural standards also teach an individual how much pain to tolerate, what types of pain to report, to whom to report the pain, and what kind of treatment to seek. For example, some patients may value "being a good patient," which may cause them to avoid complaining about their pain, whereas others may value seeking information about their pain, which may cause them to discuss their pain often and in detail. Note, however, that behaviors vary greatly within a culture and from generation to generation. The nurse should approach each patient as an individual, observing the patient carefully, taking the time to ask questions, and avoiding assumptions. Although considering the meaning of pain and how a patient expresses pain from a cultural perspective is important, the nurse must avoid applying culturally based generalizations and instead treat the individual's response to pain from a patient-centered perspective.

The nurse also has a set of sociocultural values and beliefs about pain. If these values and beliefs differ from those of the patient, the assessment and management of pain may be based on the values of the nurse rather than on the needs of the patient. The nurse must be familiar with ethnic and cultural diversity in pain expression and management and respect cultural differences. It is particularly important to remember that pain behaviors are not an objective indicator of the amount of pain present for any individual. Most experts agree that cultural differences in the expression of, response to, and interpretation of the meaning of pain need further research.

Psychologic Influences

The intensity of perceived pain has been shown to be affected by psychologic variables such as attention, expectation, and suggestion. The sensation of pain may be blocked by intense concentration (during sports activities, for example) or may be increased by anxiety or fear. Pain is often increased when it occurs in conjunction with other illnesses or physical discomforts such as nausea and/or vomiting. The presence or absence of support people or caregivers that genuinely care about pain management may also alter emotional status and the perception of pain. The placebo effect, a positive patient response to an inactive substance, has been demonstrated through both observational studies and brain MRI studies (Kasper et al., 2016).

Anxiety may increase the perception of pain, and pain in turn may cause anxiety. In addition, the muscle tension common with anxiety can create its own source of pain. This association explains why nonpharmacologic interventions such as relaxation or guided imagery are helpful in relieving or decreasing pain.

Fatigue, lack of sleep, and depression are also related to pain experiences. Pain interferes with a person's ability to fall asleep and stay asleep and thus induces fatigue. In turn, fatigue can lower pain tolerance. Depression is clearly linked to pain: Serotonin, a neurotransmitter, is involved in the modulation of pain in the CNS. In clinically depressed people, serotonin is decreased, leading to an increase in pain sensations. The reverse is also true: In the presence of pain, depression is common.

The meaning associated with the pain influences the experience of pain. For example, the pain of labor to deliver a baby is experienced differently from the pain following removal of a cancerous organ. Because pain is the major signal for health problems, it is strongly linked to all associated meanings of health problems, such as disability, loss of role, and death. A lack of understanding of the source, outcome, and meaning of the pain can contribute negatively to the pain experience. For this reason, it is important to explain to patients the etiology and prognosis for the pain assessed.

If the patient perceives the pain as deserved (e.g., "just punishment for sins"), the patient may actually feel relief that the "punishment" has commenced. If the patient believes that the pain will relieve him or her of an unrewarding job, dangerous military service, or even stressful social obligations, there may similarly be a feeling of relief. In contrast, pain that is perceived as meaningless—for example, chronic low back pain or the unrelieved pain of arthritis—can cause anxiety and depression.

9.5 Care of the Patient in Pain

Interprofessional Care

Effective pain relief results from collaboration among the patient and all members of the healthcare team. Acute pain management may be straightforward, accomplished though short-term analgesia and management of the underlying problem. Chronic pain, on the other hand, frequently requires a multidisciplinary approach. Pain clinics are centers staffed by a team of healthcare professionals who use traditional pharmacologic agents and complementary therapies such as herbs, vitamins, and other dietary supplements; nutritional counseling; psychotherapy; biofeedback; hypnosis; acupuncture; massage; and other treatments. Hospices for dying patients also provide a multifaceted approach to pain management. Chapter 5 provides information about pain management during end-of-life care.

Medications

Medication is the most common approach to pain management. Management of acute pain is often relatively straightforward, relying on **analgesic** (pain-relieving) drugs such as acetaminophen, nonsteroidal anti-inflammatory drugs (NSAIDs), and opioid analgesics. Recent practice guidelines suggest using a multimodal approach to pain management for postoperative care (Chou et al., 2016). Multiple studies show that the use of adjuvant medications such as gabapentin and ketamine (administered IV) and regional pain management techniques such as peripheral nerve catheters improve postoperative pain control and reduce the use of opioids (Chou et al., 2016). Chronic pain presents additional challenges that may require use of a broader range of drug classes, including antidepressant medications, anticonvulsants, and long-term opioids.

In addition to administering the prescribed medications, the nurse may act interdependently in selecting the appropriate dosage and timing. The Joint Commission (2018) approves the use of range orders when appropriate policies and procedures are in place and nurses are educated in appropriate implementation. The nurse is also responsible for assessing the side effects of medications, evaluating medication effectiveness, and providing patient teaching. The nurse's role in pain relief is that of patient advocate as well as direct caregiver.

The World Health Organization's (WHO; 2013) "ladder of analgesia" effectively guides the use of medications for patients with malignant pain (**Figure 9.6** ■). Aspirin and NSAIDs are initially used, followed by the addition of mild opioid analgesics and then strong opioids until pain is relieved, reflecting the interactive nature of these two types of analgesics. Adjuvant drugs are used to manage fear and anxiety. This approach also emphasizes administering analgesics by the clock, rather than on demand, to maintain comfort.

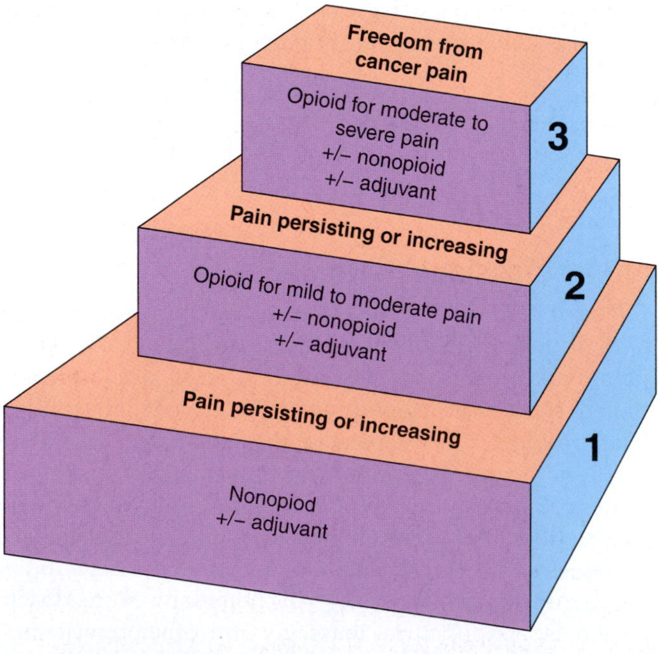
Freedom from cancer pain
Opioid for moderate to severe pain +/– nonopioid +/– adjuvant
3
Pain persisting or increasing
Opioid for mild to moderate pain +/– nonopioid +/– adjuvant
2
Pain persisting or increasing
1
Nonopiod +/– adjuvant

Figure 9.6 ■ The WHO analgesic ladder illustrates the process for selection of analgesic medications for pain management.

Aspirin, Acetaminophen, and NSAIDs. Nonopioid analgesics such as acetaminophen (Tylenol), aspirin, and NSAIDs produce analgesia and reduce fever. They are used to treat mild to moderate pain and are particularly effective for treating headache and musculoskeletal pain.

Acetaminophen appears to act on the CNS to relieve pain. Its exact mechanism of action is unknown, but it is believed to raise the pain threshold by acting on receptors in pain pathways. Acetaminophen is often combined with opioid analgesics to allow effective pain relief with a lower opioid dose (e.g., Percocet, Tylenol #3, Vicodin). It is important to remember that acetaminophen is toxic to the liver and is the number one cause of acute hepatic failure in the United States (Adams, Holland, & Urban, 2017). Hepatotoxicity is a particular risk in patients who are malnourished or who have a history of alcohol abuse or are immunosuppressed (Adams et al., 2017). As the patient develops tolerance to the opioid, increasing doses may be required to achieve effective analgesia, resulting in acetaminophen doses that increase the risk for hepatotoxicity.

Aspirin and NSAIDs act on peripheral nerve endings and minimize pain by interfering with two enzymes necessary for prostaglandin synthesis, cyclooxygenase type 1 (COX-1) and cyclooxygenase type 2 (COX-2). Examples include ibuprofen, indomethacin (Indocin), and ketorolac (Toradol). The NSAIDs have anti-inflammatory, analgesic, and antipyretic actions. NSAIDs are the treatment of choice for mild to moderate pain and continue to be effective when combined with narcotics for moderate to severe pain. NSAIDs are increasingly used in a *multimodal* approach to analgesic therapy; that is, in combination with opioid and adjunctive pain relief measures.

As a class, aspirin and NSAIDs are associated with gastric irritation. As cyclooxygenase (COX) inhibitors, they interfere with prostaglandin production. While this accounts for their anti-inflammatory effects, prostaglandins are necessary to maintain the gastric mucosal barrier. The gastric mucosal barrier (composed of mucus and bicarbonate) protects gastric mucosa from the irritating effects of ingested substances. NSAIDs, therefore, are not only irritating to gastric mucosa, they interfere with its protection as well. The risk for resultant gastrointestinal bleeding is greatest with aspirin because it interferes with platelets and blood clotting (Adams et al., 2017).

NSAIDs also increase blood pressure in many patients and, with long-term use, may be toxic to the kidneys. With the exception of aspirin, NSAIDs have been shown to have an associated increased cardiovascular risk (Duarte, Argoff, & Rubin, 2018). They are not recommended for use in people with kidney or liver disease, bleeding disorders, peptic ulcer disease, pregnancy, or a history of hypersensitivity to aspirin or other NSAIDs. Nursing implications for NSAIDs are found in **Medication Administration 9.A**. For more information about doses and precautions for specific NSAIDs, see Table 40.5 in Chapter 40, Nursing Care of Patients with Musculoskeletal Disorders.

Opioid Analgesics. *Opioid* (also called *narcotic*) analgesics are derivatives of the opium plant. These drugs (and their synthetic forms) are the most potent pain-relieving drugs available, and they are the treatment of choice for acute moderate-to-severe pain. Examples are morphine, codeine, and fentanyl (Duragesic, Actiq). Opioid analgesics produce analgesia by binding to opioid receptors both within and outside the CNS. They differ from one another in potency, speed of onset, duration of action, and preferred route of administration. Opioid *agonists* such as morphine produce their effect by stimulating the receptor they bind with. Drugs with a mixed *agonist–antagonist* effect block the activity of some receptors (mu receptors) while activating others (kappa receptors). This mixed agonist–antagonist activity can actually intensify pain responses in some patients. Buprenorphine (Buprenex), butorphanol (Stadol), nalbuphine (Nubain), and pentazocine (Talwin) are examples of opioids with mixed agonist–antagonist effects.

A summary of **equianalgesic** or approximate equivalent doses of selected opioid analgesics used to treat moderate to severe pain, their peak effect and duration, and nursing implications is provided in **Table 9.5**.

Opioid analgesics tend to have similar unintended effects. They are CNS and respiratory depressants. They commonly produce sedation, drowsiness, and dizziness. All should be avoided or used with caution in patients with chronic obstructive lung disease (COPD) or who are experiencing an acute asthma attack because these drugs can suppress respirations. Nausea and vomiting are common adverse effects, as is constipation. All opioid analgesics have the potential to cause physical and psychologic dependence, particularly when taken at high doses for an extended time (Dowell, Haegerich, & Chou, 2016).

A common concern among healthcare professionals is that using opioids for pain treatment poses a risk for addiction. When the medications are used as recommended, there is little to no risk of addiction. Rather, if pain is not adequately treated, the patient may seek more and more analgesic relief, thus increasing the risk of an adversarial relationship with the provider and a weakening of the trust relationship between patient and provider (**Box 9.1**).

Opioid analgesics commonly are used to treat chronic malignant pain (refer to Figure 9.6). Because of their potency and efficacy, they may also be used to treat chronic nonmalignant pain. Oral preparations of a fixed combination of an opioid and acetaminophen are used with caution. Tolerance can lead to higher required doses of the opioid, increasing the risk for hepatoxicity due to the increasing dose of acetaminophen. Nursing implications for opioid analgesics are found in **Medication Administration 9.B**.

Certain opioid analgesics, while still available, are not recommended for use because of toxic effects or their potential for abuse. As previously noted, the metabolite of meperidine (Demerol) is toxic to the CNS. While a single dose of meperidine may be used to relieve acute pain (e.g., migraine), it is not recommended for continued use (Lexicomp, 2018).

Medication Administration 9.A

Nonsteroidal Anti-Inflammatory Drugs

EXAMPLES OF NSAIDS

aspirin (acetylsalicylic acid)
celecoxib (Celebrex)
diflunisal (Dolobid)
fenoprofen calcium (Nalfon)
ibuprofen (Advil, Motrin)
indomethacin (Indocin)
ketoprofen (Orudis)
ketorolac tromethamine (Toradol)
nabumetone (Relafen)
naproxen (Aleve, Naprosyn)
piroxicam (Feldene)
sulindac (Clinoril)
tolmetin (Tolectin)

The NSAIDs have anti-inflammatory, analgesic, and antipyretic effects. It is believed that they inhibit the enzyme COX, thereby decreasing synthesis of prostaglandins. These drugs provide analgesic effects by reducing inflammation and by perhaps blocking the generation of noxious impulses.

Nursing Responsibilities

- Do not administer aspirin with other NSAIDs.
- Assess and document if the patient is taking a hypoglycemic agent or insulin; the NSAIDs may increase the hypoglycemic effect.
- Administer with meals, milk, or a full glass of water to decrease gastric irritation.
- Assess patients who are also taking anticoagulants for bleeding; the NSAIDs increase this risk.

Health Education for the Patient and Family

- Drugs may cause gastrointestinal bleeding (report nausea, vomiting of blood, dark stools), visual disturbances (report blurred or diminished vision), increased blood pressure, hearing problems, dizziness, skin rash, and kidney problems (report weight gain or edema).
- Take medications with meals to decrease gastric irritation.
- Avoid drinking alcohol or taking any over-the-counter drug unless approved by the healthcare provider.
- The desired effects may not appear for 3–5 days, and the full effects may not appear for 2–4 weeks.
- Maintain regular healthcare appointments.

Note: Drugs identified in blue are among the 200 most commonly prescribed medications in the United States.

Source: Data from Adams, Holland, & Urban, 2017.

Table 9.5 Opioid Effectiveness Equianalgesic Drug Chart

Analgesic	Dosage (mg)	Peak (min)	Duration (h)	Nursing Considerations
morphine sulfate	10 Subcut, IV 10–30 PO	30–60 min 60–90 min	3–4 h 3–6 h	PO dose is three to six times the IV dose. Oral modified release will have a longer peak time. A lower dose may be appropriate for older patients with chronic pain. Smaller doses (e.g., 2–5 mg) may be administered more frequently when using IV route.
codeine	15-60 PO	60–90 min	4–6 h	Analgesic potency about one-sixth that of morphine. Often given in combination with aspirin or acetaminophen for mild to moderate pain. Also used for its antitussive (cough suppressant) effect.
fentanyl (Duragesic, Sublimaze, Actiq)	50–100 mcg IV/IM 25 mcg/hour every 3 days transdermal 200 mcg stick lozenge (Actiq only) for breakthrough pain	3–5 min 24 h	2–5 h 48–72h	100 mcg/h parenteral or transdermal is equivalent to 4 mg/h of parenteral morphine. Rapid onset and short half-life; tissue storage can prolong half-life and effect with longer-term use. Transdermal fentanyl not recommended for acute pain management. Available by oral transmucosal route (lozenge on a stick).
hydrocodone (Vicodin, Lortab)	5–10 mg	60–90 min	4–6 h	Available PO only.
hydromorphone HCl (Dilaudid)	1–4 IM, Subcut, IV 7.5 PO, Rectal	30–90 min 10–20 min 30–90 min	3–4 h 3–4 h 3–4 h	PO dose is five times IM dose. Shorter acting than morphine.
levorphanol (Levo-Dromoran)	2 IM, Subcut, IV 4 PO	60–90 min 15–30 min 90–120 min	4–6 h 4–6 h 4–5 h	Longer acting than morphine when given in repeated, regular doses. Accumulates, so analgesic effect may increase over time.
meperidine (Demerol)	50–100 IM, Subcut, IV 50–100 PO	15–30 min 10–15 min 60–90 min	2–4 h 2–4 h	Not recommended as first-line opioid for acute or chronic pain. Metabolized to normeperidine, which is toxic to the CNS. Not recommended for older adults, patients with impaired kidney function, or for administration by continuous IV infusion.
methadone HCl (Dolophine)	2.5–10 IM, Subcut, Sublingual IV 10–30 PO	60–120 min 90–120 min	6–8 h 6–8 h	Initial PO dose is twice IM dose. Accumulates, so analgesic effect may increase over time. Initial doses lower in opioid-tolerant patients. Also used for heroin detoxification and maintenance.
oxycodone (Percocet, OxyContin)	5–20 PO (NA parenteral)	60–90 min	3–4 h	Used in combination with nonopioid analgesic (Percocet, Tylox) for moderate pain. Available as a single-entity product in immediate- or controlled-release forms (OxyContin) for severe pain. Has faster onset and higher peak effect than most PO narcotics, equivalent to oral morphine.
oxymorphone (Numorphan)	1–1.5 IM, Subcut, IV 10 PO or PR	30–90 min 15–30 min	3–6 h 3–4 h	Also available as rectal suppository (10 mg equianalgesic). Used for moderate to severe pain.
tramadol (Ultram, Zydol)	50–100 PO	120–180 min	3–6 h	Used for moderate to moderately severe pain. Causes less respiratory depression than morphine.

Note: Drugs identified in blue are among the 200 most commonly prescribed medications in the United States.

Note: Morphine sulfate 10 mg IM is the analgesic dose to which all other parenteral and PO doses in this table are considered equianalgesic.

Source: Data from Adams et al., 2017.

BOX 9.1
Pain Management, Addiction, and Regulation

The goals of pain control are to minimize discomfort and promote normal functioning. Although these goals can often be achieved through use of nonpharmacologic strategies and nonnarcotic analgesics, opioid medications currently provide the only effective option for pain associated with acute trauma, surgery, cancer, and some chronic conditions.

Crude opium has been available for thousands of years. Abuse of opium and its derivatives (e.g., heroin, morphine) increased dramatically with development of the hypodermic syringe. International efforts to control narcotic trafficking and abuse while ensuring availability for medical and scientific purposes began in the early 20th century.

The WHO estimates more than 80% of people with severe pain are inadequately treated (IOM, 2011). Despite significant data showing very little addiction as the result of treating pain with adequate analgesia, prescribers still tend to undertreat chronic nonmalignant pain (IOM, 2011). The American Society for Pain Management Nursing published its position statement on pain management in patients with substance abuse disorders in 2012 (Oliver et al., 2012). The position statement emphasizes every patient's right to be treated with dignity and respect and to receive high-quality pain assessment and management. Addiction is a neurophysiologic disease, separate and distinct from physical dependence and tolerance. See the following list for definitions of relevant terms.

Substance use is common in our society and illicit use of controlled substances is the leading category of medication misuse (Oliver et al., 2012). The development of highly effective oral opioid analgesics such as oxycodone (OxyContin) and hydrocodone (Vicodin) has resulted in increased reports of illicit substance use and an increase in individuals meeting diagnostic criteria for a drug use disorder. The abuse/misuse of prescribed medications occurs in all age groups and experts predict that as the population ages, drug abuse among older adults will rise significantly (Oliver et al., 2012). This has led to calls for legislation to limit the use and availability of these drugs, an option that concerns palliative care specialists.

Opioid analgesics are among the most effective, highly regulated, and significantly abused drugs available today. Treating patients in pain who have become addicted to drugs is complex and often involves an interprofessional approach that includes the expertise of a pain control specialist or pain treatment team. Patients with drug addictions frequently require large doses of medication to control their pain. Although addiction is a public health concern, so is undertreatment of pain (IOM, 2011; Oliver et al., 2012). Patients with substance use disorders must be treated with respect and dignity and their pain should be assessed and managed using the same standards as all other patients (Oliver et al., 2012). Clearly, there are no simple answers to the problems associated with drug trafficking, abuse, addiction, and adequate pain management for patients with substance abuse disorders.

The following list of definitions help to discern the difference between tolerance to opioids, physical dependence on opioids, and addiction to opioids. These three terms are sometimes confused and lead to poor patient outcomes.

- ***Addiction:*** A primary, chronic neurobiologic, treatable disease characterized by compulsive use of a substance despite negative consequences, such as health threats or legal problems.
- ***Drug abuse:*** The use of any chemical substance for other than a medical purpose.
- ***Physical drug dependence:*** Not the same as addiction; an expected physical response to a number of drug classes (such as opioids and benzodiazepines) that produces a drug class–specific withdrawal/abstinence syndrome with specific symptoms.
- ***Psychologic drug dependence:*** A psychologic need for a substance. If the substance is not supplied, psychologic withdrawal symptoms occur.
- ***Drug tolerance:*** Physical adaptation to the drug resulting in its diminished effects over time.
- ***Equianalgesic:*** Having the same pain-killing effect when administered to the same individual. Drug dosages are equianalgesic if they have the same effect as morphine sulfate 10 mg administered parenterally.
- ***Pseudoaddiction:*** An iatrogenic syndrome associated with undertreatment of pain and characterized by problematic behaviors that mimic abuse; can be distinguished from true addiction in that behaviors resolve when pain is adequately treated.

Medication Administration 9.B
Opioid Analgesics

EXAMPLES OF OPIOID ANALGESICS

buprenorphine HCl (Buprenex)
codeine
fentanyl (Duragesic)
hydrocodone (Hycodan, Norco, Vicodin)
hydromorphone HCl (Dilaudid)
levorphanol (Levo-Dromoran)
morphine sulfate
nalbuphine HCl (Nubain)
oxycodone (OxyContin)
oxymorphone HCl (Numorphan)
pentazocine (Talwin)

Opioid analgesics are used to treat severe pain. The drugs in this category include morphine, codeine, opium derivatives, and synthetic substances with activity similar to natural opioids. Morphine and codeine are pure chemical substances isolated from opium. These drugs decrease the awareness of the sensation of pain by binding to opiate receptors in the brain and spinal cord. It is also believed that they diminish the transmission of pain impulses by altering cell membrane permeability to sodium and by affecting the release of neurotransmitters for efferent nerves sensitive to noxious stimuli. Opioid analgesics affect the CNS, causing analgesia, euphoria, drowsiness, mental clouding, and lethargy. They have various other effects. Depending on the drug used, they can depress respirations, stimulate the vomiting center, suppress the cough reflex, induce peripheral vasodilation (resulting in hypotension), constrict the pupils, and decrease intestinal peristalsis (Adams et al., 2017). Opioid analgesics have the potential to cause tolerance and psychologic and physical dependence.

(continued)

Nursing Responsibilities

- Opioids are regulated by federal law; the nurse must record the date, time, patient name, type and amount of the drug used, and sign the entry in a narcotic inventory sheet or use an automated medication dispensing device such as Pyxis. If the drug must be wasted after it is signed out, the act must be witnessed and the nurse and the witness must both document. Computerized narcotic documentation methods are frequently integrated into the electronic health documentation system.
- Keep an opioid antagonist, such as naloxone, immediately available to treat respiratory depression.
- Assess allergies or adverse effects from opioids previously experienced by the patient.
- Assess for respiratory disorders (e.g., asthma or COPD), neuromuscular disorders (e.g., multiple sclerosis), and other conditions that might increase the risk associated with respiratory depression.
- Assess the characteristics of the pain and the effectiveness of drugs that have been previously used to treat the pain.
- Take and record baseline vital signs before administering the drug.
- Administer the drugs, following established guidelines.
- Monitor vital signs and respiratory status, level of consciousness, papillary response, nausea, bowel function, urinary function, and effectiveness of pain management at regular intervals and as indicated.
- Provide for patient safety.
- Report adverse effects such as continued nausea and vomiting or itching.
- Employ protocols or prn orders as needed to promote bowel function and prevent constipation.
- Meperidine (Demerol) is associated with CNS toxicity and thus involves significant patient risk (Lexicomp, 2018). Monitor any patient who is receiving more than one dose for nervousness, restlessness, tremors, twitching, shakiness, myoclonic jerks, diaphoresis, changes in level of awareness, agitation, disorientation, confusion, delirium, hallucinations, violent shivering, and/or seizures. Toxicity can occur with any route of administration or any dosing regimen. The risk is increased in patients with decreased renal function (including normal changes with aging). Report these manifestations to the physician. Oral administration is not recommended.
- Teach noninvasive methods of pain management for use in conjunction with opioid analgesics.

Health Education for the Patient and Family

- The use of opioid analgesics to treat severe pain is unlikely to cause addiction (IOM, 2011).
- Do not drink alcohol while taking these drugs.
- Do not take over-the-counter medications unless approved by the healthcare provider.
- Increase intake of fluids and fiber in the diet to prevent constipation. Contact your provider if additional measures (such as laxatives) are needed to manage constipation.
- The drugs often cause dizziness, drowsiness, and impaired thinking; use caution when driving or making decisions.
- Report adverse effects or decreasing effectiveness to the healthcare provider.

Note: Drugs identified in blue are among the 200 most commonly prescribed medications in the United States.

Source: Data from Adams, et al., 2017.

Antidepressants. Antidepressants, particularly those within the tricyclic and related chemical groups, are useful for treating chronic pain. Tricyclic antidepressants act on the production and retention of serotonin in the CNS, thus inhibiting pain sensation. The dose to provide analgesia is lower than that required to treat depression. These drugs potentiate the effects of opioid analgesics and may be used to help manage severe persistent or malignant pain. They also promote normal sleeping patterns, further alleviating the suffering of the patient in pain. They are particularly useful in treating neuropathic pain. Tricyclic antidepressants are not without adverse effects, however. They may cause orthostatic hypotension, drowsiness, urinary retention, constipation, and impaired memory. These effects can limit their usefulness in older adults in particular. Antidepressants from other classes such as serotonin norepinephrine reuptake inhibitors (venlafaxine [Effexor], duloxetine [Cymbalta]) appear to have an analgesic effect similar to that of tricyclic antidepressants with fewer adverse effects (Kasper et al., 2016).

Anticonvulsants. Similar to antidepressants, some seizure medications such as gabapentin (Neurontin), pregabalin (Lyrica), and topiramate (Topamax) are useful with neuropathic pain, including shingles (herpes zoster), migraine headaches, and diabetic neuropathy, and are frequently used with opioids in multimodal postoperative pain control (Chou et al., 2016). These drugs reduce pain and sleep disruption. Drugs that are primarily used to treat epilepsy (seizures) have been used to treat nerve pain conditions and migraine headache for several decades. Many anticonvulsant drugs have been shown in clinical studies to be effective in managing chronic pain (Argoff & Chen, 2018).

Local Anesthetics. Drugs such as benzocaine and lidocaine are part of a large group of substances that block the initiation and transmission of nerve impulses in a local area, thus blocking pain as well. Local anesthetics can be delivered by a variety of methods, including via transdermal patch to treat focal neuropathic pain (Collison & Argoff, 2018). They are sometimes used to enable a patient to begin moving and using a painful area to diminish long-term pain.

Local anesthetics can be delivered directly to the sheath of a nerve through a peripheral nerve catheter. During surgery, a soaker-type catheter can be inserted along a surgical incision to deliver local relief; this method may decrease the need for opioids and allow the patient to resume activity sooner (Fuzaylov et al., 2015).

Analgesic Administration

The ideal drug, route of administration, and dosing schedule to provide optimal pain relief vary, depending on such factors as the type of pain, its intensity and duration, and the individual patient. Each drug has a unique absorption and duration of action. The nurse must understand that no drug will have a totally predictable effect because each person absorbs, metabolizes, and excretes medications at different dosage levels. The only way to obtain reliable data about the effectiveness of the medication for the individual is to assess how that patient responds. Therefore, the best choice is to individualize the drug, route, and schedule.

Giving analgesics before the pain occurs or increases prevents some of the untoward effects of pain. This holds true for both acute and chronic pain: Poorly managed acute pain is one of the leading causes of persistent pain syndrome. Additional benefits of a preventive approach to pain can be summarized as follows:

- The patient may spend less time in pain. Pain has been shown to have a negative effect on healing; poorly relieved pain is associated with longer hospital stays.
- Inadequate relief of acute pain has been shown to be a significant contributing factor to chronic pain (Dowell et al., 2016).
- Frequent analgesic administration may allow for smaller doses and less analgesic administration.
- Smaller doses will in turn mean fewer side effects.
- The patient's fear and anxiety about the return of pain will decrease.
- Pain relief allows the patient to be more physically active and avoid complications of immobility.

Analgesics may be given either around-the-clock (ATC) or as necessary (prn, meaning *pro re nata*, Latin for "as circumstances may require"). ATC administration is recommended for the first 48 hours for acute pain related to surgery or traumatic injury. It is also appropriate for pain that has a predictable intensity and pattern. For pain that is not predictable or constant, prn administration is appropriate and should be given as soon as the pain begins. Breakthrough pain occurs in patients receiving long-acting analgesics for chronic pain. It is a transitory experience of moderate to severe pain often precipitated by coughing or movement but that may occur spontaneously. Breakthrough pain is managed using short-acting opioid analgesics in addition to ATC medications.

Maintaining effective pain relief while minimizing the adverse effects of a medication can be challenging. Within a prescribed range, the nurse can choose the correct dose according to the patient's response. It is the role of the nurse to notify the physician if the prescribed dosage does not meet the patient's needs or causes excessive drowsiness, unsteadiness, or significant adverse effects.

Routes of Administration

The route of administration significantly affects how much of a medication is needed to relieve pain. For example, because of differences in absorption and distribution, oral doses of some opioids must be up to five times greater than parenteral doses to achieve the same degree of pain relief. In addition, the potency of opioid analgesics varies. Consulting an equianalgesic chart when converting from one route of administration to another or from one drug to another helps ensure an equivalent effect for the patient. The analgesic effect of 10 mg of parenteral morphine is used as the base to which other opioids and routes of administration are compared. Table 9.4 earlier in this chapter is an example of an equianalgesic chart. Routes of administration include the following.

Oral. The simplest route for both patient and nurse is the oral (PO) route. Unless contraindicated, the oral route is preferred for most patients. Special nursing care is still required because some medications must be given with food, some are irritating to the gastrointestinal system, and some patients have trouble swallowing pills. Liquid and timed-release forms are available for special applications.

Some analgesics, such as fentanyl, are available in alternative forms, including a buccal tablet, a lozenge, or a lollipop. The buccal route provides a rapid onset of action because the medication is absorbed directly into the circulation, bypassing the gastrointestinal tract and first-pass liver metabolism. These delivery systems are particularly helpful for managing breakthrough pain. Special precautions must be taken in storing the lozenge and lollipop forms because children and pets may mistake these for candy.

Rectal. The rectal route is helpful for patients who are unable to swallow or who are experiencing nausea and vomiting. Acetaminophen, aspirin, and some NSAIDs and opioid analgesics are available in this form. The rectal route is effective and simple, but the patient and family may not accept it. To be effective, any rectal medication must be placed above the rectal sphincter.

Transdermal. The transdermal, or patch, form of medication is increasingly being used because it is simple, painless, and delivers a continuous level of medication. Transdermal medications are easy to store and apply. Reapplication every 72 hours enhances compliance. Additional short-acting medication may be needed for breakthrough pain. As with any route of administration, overdosage can occur. It is important to start with a low dose and **titrate** (increase or decrease a dose in small increments) to the effective level. Medication administered transdermally is in a lipid-soluble form and may be stored in fat cells longer than expected. Monitor level of sedation and respiratory effort.

A transdermal patch is applied to a clean, dry area on the upper torso. If hair is present, it should be clipped before applying the patch. Apply the patch immediately after opening the package, ensuring complete contact with the skin, especially around the edges. The patch is effective for about 72 hours. When replaced, the new patch should be applied on a different site. When transdermal therapy is initiated, approximately 12 to 24 hours is necessary for the therapeutic level to be absorbed. Similarly, when discontinuing, expect a gradual decline in level because of the medication reservoir in the skin. Fever or inflammation of the skin, exercise, and use of electric blankets or heating pads all increase or enhance absorption.

Parenteral. Once the most popular route for pain medication administration, the intramuscular (IM) route is no longer preferred. Its disadvantages include uneven absorption from the muscle, discomfort on administration, and time consumed to prepare and administer the medication. Subcutaneous administration may be used, primarily when continuous analgesic administration via a parenteral route is required.

Intravenous. The intravenous (IV) route provides the most rapid onset of effect, usually ranging from 1 to 15 minutes. Medication can be given by drip, bolus, or patient-controlled analgesia (PCA). PCA uses a pump with a control mechanism that allows the patient to self-manage pain (**Figure 9.7** ■). The advantages of PCA are dose precision, timeliness, and convenience. The patient does not have to wait for a nurse to assess the need for pain medication, then procure and deliver the analgesia. Respiratory depression and sedation are minimized when plasma levels of opioids are steady. PCA, especially with basal dosing (continuous infusion of a very small dose), facilitates frequent small dosing. Several drugs can be administered by this route. The disadvantages are the nursing care needed for any intravenous line, the potential for infection, and the cost of disposable supplies. In addition, the risk for a serious medication error requiring interventions in response has been shown to be greater with PCA than when other methods of analgesic delivery are used. Adverse events associated with PCA errors include depressed respirations, inadequate pain relief, and even patient death (McNicol, Ferguson, & Hudcova, 2015). Risk factors for respiratory depression include the use of basal infusion; age greater than 70; obesity; sleep apnea; concurrent use of CNS depressants; upper abdominal or thoracic surgery; renal hepatic, pulmonary, or cardiac impairment; and a PCA bolus of more than 1 mg morphine without a basal rate. Additionally, increased risk is attributed to the complexity of the systems involved when PCA is used to provide analgesia. The PCA method of administration requires close attention by the physician, pharmacist, and nurse, as well as careful patient teaching and monitoring.

SAFETY ALERT: Recommendations for nurses caring for at-risk patients on PCA include careful monitoring of respiratory rate and oxygen saturation and sedation levels. ■

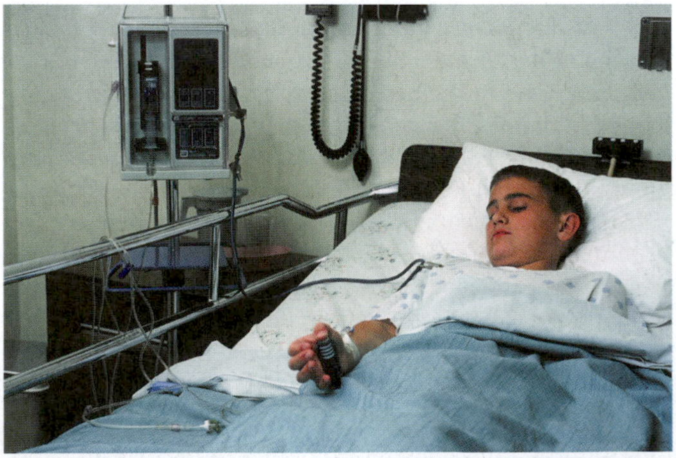

Figure 9.7 ■ PCA units allow the patient to self-manage acute pain. The units may be portable or mounted on intravenous poles.

Intraspinal. The intraspinal (intrathecal or epidural) route is invasive and requires more extensive nursing care. Intraspinal analgesia is used to manage chronic intractable malignant pain and postoperative pain. The use of the intraspinal route has decreased in acute care with improved peripheral nerve catheters that deliver local anesthesia postoperatively. However, intraspinal delivery may provide better analgesia and postoperative recovery than intravenous delivery for some patients. Many patients experience better pain relief, earlier bowel recovery, and earlier mobility when a combination of local anesthetics and opioids are infused by the epidural route. The risk for respiratory depression and failure is lower with epidural analgesia than with administration by other parenteral routes. Other complications can occur, however, including hypotension, development of an epidural hematoma or abscess, and neurologic damage.

Nerve Blocks. In a nerve block, a local anesthetic, sometimes in combination with steroidal anti-inflammatory drugs, is injected by a physician or nurse anesthetist into or near a nerve, usually in an area between the nociceptor and the dorsal root. The procedure may be performed to determine the precise location of the source of the pain: Pain relief indicates that the injection site is the site of the source of the pain.

Temporary (local) nerve blocks may give the patient enough relief to (1) develop a more hopeful attitude that pain relief is possible, (2) allow local procedures to be performed without causing discomfort, or (3) exercise and move the affected part. A temporary nerve block may be particularly useful for such painful conditions as fractured ribs, allowing the patient to deep-breathe, cough, and move with more ease during healing. Nerve blocks may also be performed to predict the results of neurosurgery. For long-term pain relief, a permanent neurolytic agent is used. Neurolytic blocks are usually reserved for terminally ill patients because of the risks of weakness, paralysis, and bowel and bladder dysfunction.

SAFETY ALERT: When you are caring for patients receiving frequent or continuous opioids, ensure that naloxone, an opioid antagonist, is immediately available to reverse respiratory depression, if necessary.

- Monitor the effectiveness of the pain management. Administer supplemental analgesics as ordered, and notify the healthcare provider if analgesia is inadequate (patient rates pain at 4 or higher on a scale of 0 to 10).
- Monitor intake and output. Narcotics may block the micturition reflex, causing urinary retention and necessitating intermittent catheterization or placement of an indwelling urinary catheter.
- Use sterile technique to care for the intraspinal catheter. ■

Surgery

As a pain relief measure, surgery is usually considered only after all other methods have failed. Surgical intervention is typically reserved for patients experiencing nerve pain, for example, the pain of trigeminal neuralgia, complex regional pain syndrome, or pain associated with spinal nerve or spinal cord injury. Patients need thorough knowledge of the implications of the use of surgery for pain relief. For example, motor function loss is an unwelcome side effect of some surgeries. Surgical procedures used to relieve pain are shown in **Figure 9.8** ■. Some surgical procedures can be accomplished through minimally invasive techniques (e.g., percutaneously); others require an open surgical procedure. Surgical approaches to pain relief may include:

Cordotomy. A *cordotomy* is an incision into the anterolateral tracts of the spinal cord to interrupt the transmission of pain. Because it is difficult to isolate the nerves responsible for upper body pain, this surgery is most often performed for pain in the abdominal region and legs, including severe pain from terminal cancer. A percutaneous cordotomy produces lesions of the anterolateral surface of the spinal cord by means of a radio-frequency current.

Neurectomy. A *neurectomy* is the removal or destruction of a nerve. It is sometimes used for pain relief, for example, to relieve the pain of trigeminal neuralgia. The nerve may be destroyed through several different methods, including injection of glycerol into the nerve, using radio-frequency-generated heat, or by compressing the nerve using a balloon. When an open approach is used, the nerve is exposed and severed. A peripheral neurectomy is the severing of a nerve at any point distal to the spinal cord.

Sympathectomy. The sympathetic nerves play an important role in producing and transmitting the sensation of pain. A *sympathectomy* involves destruction by injection or incision of the ganglia of sympathetic nerves, usually in the lumbar region or the cervicodorsal region at the base of the neck.

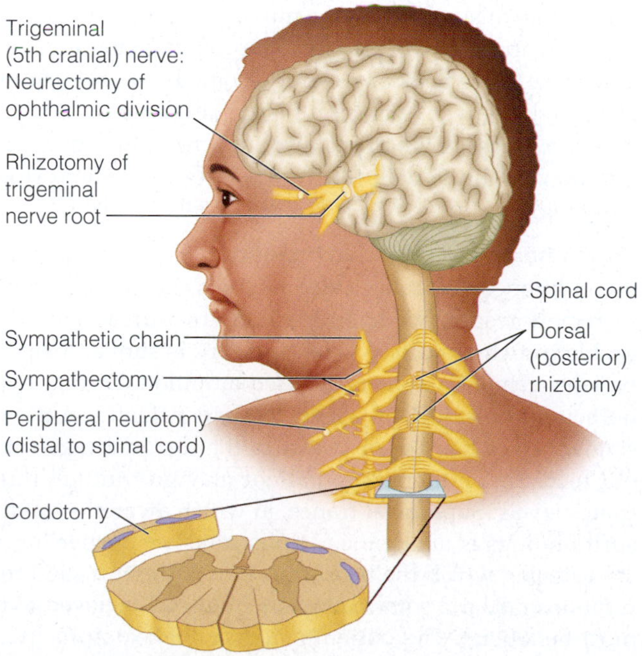
Trigeminal (5th cranial) nerve: Neurectomy of ophthalmic division
Rhizotomy of trigeminal nerve root
Spinal cord
Sympathetic chain
Sympathectomy
Dorsal (posterior) rhizotomy
Peripheral neurotomy (distal to spinal cord)
Cordotomy

Figure 9.8 ■ Surgical procedures may be used to treat severe pain that does not respond to other types of management. They include cordotomy, neurectomy, sympathectomy, and rhizotomy.

Rhizotomy. *Rhizotomy* is surgical severing of the dorsal spinal roots. It is most often performed to relieve the pain of cancer of the head, neck, or lungs. A rhizotomy may be performed by surgically cutting the nerve fibers, by injecting a chemical such as alcohol or phenol into the subarachnoid space, or by using a radio-frequency current to selectively destroy pain fibers.

Transcutaneous Electrical Nerve Stimulation

Transcutaneous electrical nerve stimulation (TENS) is the application of electrical current through the skin to control acute or chronic pain. A TENS unit consists of a battery-operated low-voltage transmitter connected to the skin using two or more electrodes (**Figure 9.9** ■). Electrodes may be placed by the patient or by the physical therapist. The TENS unit generates a high- or low-frequency electrical pulse. With high-frequency application, pulse intensity is low and does not cause muscle contraction; low-frequency applications produce an intensity that does produce muscle contraction. The patient experiences a gentle tapping or vibrating sensation over the electrodes. He or she can adjust the voltage to achieve maximum pain relief.

TENS controls pain in several ways. It activates opioid receptors in the spinal cord and medulla. It also affects release of both excitatory and inhibitory neurotransmitters, reducing the transmission of pain signals within the CNS. Furthermore, TENS stimulates large-diameter A-beta touch fibers to close the gate, controlling pain transmission within the spinal cord. Low-frequency TENS stimulates serotonin release, activates serotonin receptors, and prompts endorphin release.

A TENS unit is most commonly used to relieve chronic benign pain, neuropathic pain, and acute postoperative pain. Its use during obstetric care (labor in particular) is increasing, as is its use in treating orthopedic conditions. In

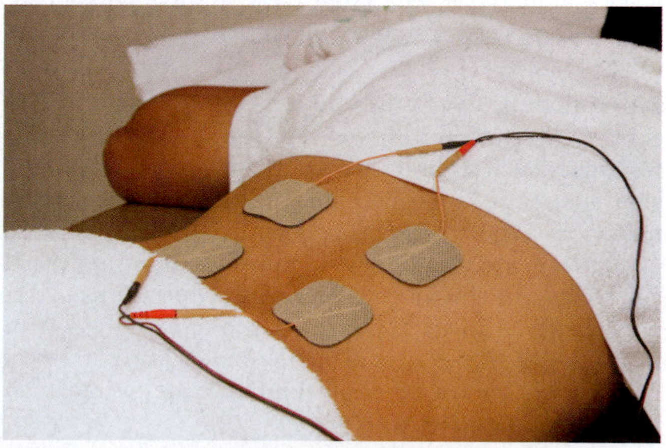

Figure 9.9 ■ The TENS unit is used to assist with acute and chronic pain management. Electrodes deliver low-voltage electrical stimuli through the skin to block transmission of pain stimuli.

any case, thorough patient teaching is essential, including an explanation of manufacturer's directions, instructions on where to place the electrodes, and the importance of placing the electrodes on clean, unbroken skin. The patient should assess the skin daily for signs of irritation. Patients who have a cardiac pacemaker or implanted cardioverter-defibrillator should not use TENS.

TENS offers several advantages: Avoidance of drug side effects, patient control, and good interaction with other therapies. Disadvantages are its cost and the need for expert training for initiation. Note also that TENS is not effective in relieving all types of pain or for all patients.

Integrative Therapies

The benefit of integrative therapies as part of a comprehensive pain management strategy is increasingly recognized. Around 44% of adults in the United States with pain or neurologic conditions are using some form of complementary or integrative medicine along with traditional medicine (Nahin, 2015).

Musculoskeletal aches and headaches are the most common conditions that prompt adults to use integrative therapies, a number of which are used to treat pain, including acupuncture, chiropractic and osteopathic medicine, massage, and relaxation. Discussion of some of the more commonly used therapies follows.

Acupuncture. *Acupuncture* is an ancient Chinese system involving the stimulation of certain specific points on the body to enhance the flow of vital energy (chi) along pathways called *meridians*. Acupuncture points can be stimulated by inserting and withdrawing needles, applying heat, massage, laser, electrical stimulation, or a combination of these methods. Only care providers with training in acupuncture techniques can use this method. Acupuncture is becoming a more widely accepted therapy, although evidence of its effectiveness in treating pain is mixed. Acupuncture has been shown to enhance traditional analgesia when used after abdominal surgery. The effectiveness of acupuncture in relieving chronic musculoskeletal pain has been extensively studied, with a beneficial effect shown in relieving chronic pain in the neck, lower back, or shoulder.

Biofeedback. *Biofeedback* is a method for learning to control physiologic responses of the body. Physiologic responses such as brain waves, muscle contraction, and skin temperature are measured electronically, "feeding" this information back to the patient. Biofeedback units use electrodes placed on the skin to transform data into visual cues, such as colored lights. The patient thus learns to recognize stress-related responses and to replace them with relaxation responses. Eventually, the patient learns to repeat independently those actions that produce the desired brain wave effect.

Biofeedback gives the patient a measure of control over the response to pain. It has been studied as an integrative therapy for migraine, fibromyalgia, traumatic brain injury, and temporomandibular disorder (TMD). In all studies, a beneficial effect was found, for example, reduced frequency of migraine headache or reduced intensity of pain associated with fibromyalgia and TMD (Fontaine, 2014).

Chiropractic. *Chiropractic* uses hands-on therapy, focusing on the relationship between body structure and function. This relationship between structure (primarily that of the spine) and function and its effect on health is a key concept of chiropractic medicine. Chiropractic therapy is directed at normalizing the relationship between structure and function to promote the body's innate ability to self-heal (Fontaine, 2014). The practice of chiropractic in the United States is limited to those who earn a doctor of chiropractic degree from an accredited college. Chiropractic is among the 10 most commonly used CAM procedures, with an estimated 20% of Americans receiving chiropractic care at some point during their lives. Most often, it is used in conjunction with conventional medical services.

Spinal manipulation has been demonstrated to be as effective for relieving mild-to-moderate low back pain as conventional treatments (National Center for Complementary and Integrative Health, 2016). Chiropractic is generally safe, with discomfort of the treated area, headache, and fatigue the most common adverse effects. Chiropractors may combine treatments such as application of heat or ice, electrical stimulation, exercise prescriptions, counseling, and dietary supplements with spinal manipulation.

Distraction. *Distraction* involves redirecting attention away from the pain and onto something that the patient finds more pleasant. Examples of distracting activities are practicing focused breathing, listening to music, or doing some form of rhythmic activity to music. For example, the patient using recorded music for distraction may sing along with the song, tap out the rhythm with the fingers or foot, clap to the music, conduct the music, or add harmony.

Participating in an activity that promotes laughter, such as reading a joke book or viewing a comedy, has been found to be highly effective in pain relief. Laughing for 20 minutes or more is known to produce an increase in endorphins that may continue pain relief even after the patient stops laughing.

Hypnotherapy and Guided Imagery. *Hypnotherapy* is the use of hypnosis, a trance state in which the mind becomes extremely responsive to suggestion, to address a specific problem such as pain. Guided imagery is similar, helping patients achieve a state of focused attention. During hypnotherapy or guided imagery, the patient enters a trance state in which he or she is aware of the surroundings without focusing on them. The patient may go through three trance levels: Superficial trance, in which awareness of the surroundings is maintained; alpha trance, a deeper trance state during which the heart rate, blood pressure, and respirations fall; and somnambulism, the level believed to be most beneficial. The patient's muscles relax, alpha brain waves predominate, and the patient experiences a sense of well-being and the ability to accept new ideas. During this state, the therapist may make suggestions to encourage pain relief. It is possible to achieve complete anesthesia or to modify pain in a variety of ways through hypnotism. For the technique to work, however, the patient must be fully relaxed and must want to be hypnotized.

Guided imagery, also called *creative visualization*, is use of the mind to create a scene or sensory experience that relaxes the muscles and moves the attention of the mind away from the pain experience. The therapist may create imagery to help the patient modify physical responses to stressors such as pain. To use guided imagery, the patient must be able to concentrate, use the imagination, and follow directions. The nurse can facilitate this technique by asking the patient for some descriptions of what the patient finds most relaxing. The nurse then speaks to the patient in a calm, soothing voice about those places or situations. Imagery can cause changes in vital signs, brain wave patterns, blood flow, and hormone and neurotransmitter levels (Fontaine, 2014).

Advantages of hypnotherapy and guided imagery include patient control and lack of side effects. Disadvantages include the need for a skilled practitioner and a willing patient. However, some patients can learn to enter into a trance state without assistance from a practitioner to achieve pain relief.

Massage. *Massage therapy* is often employed as a CAM therapy to relieve pain and promote relaxation. In massage therapy, muscles and soft tissues of the body are manipulated with the intent of relaxing them; increasing warmth, blood flow, and oxygen delivery to the area; and decreasing pain. There are over 80 different types of massage therapy. Among the most common are Swedish massage, deep tissue massage, trigger point massage, and shiatsu massage. Massage therapy carries very little risk, but should be used appropriately and performed by a licensed or certified massage professional.

Natural Products. *Natural products* are the most frequently employed CAM therapy overall, used by nearly 80% of the world's population (Fontaine, 2014). A number of products, including herbals, natural oils, and other natural substances, are available. Natural products have been studied for the relief of pain associated with migraine and other musculoskeletal conditions such as fibromyalgia and rheumatoid arthritis with mixed results (Fontaine, 2014).

Relaxation. *Relaxation* involves learning activities that deeply relax the body and mind. Relaxation distracts the patient's focus from the pain, lessens the effects of stress from pain, increases pain tolerance, increases the effectiveness of other pain relief measures, and increases perception of pain control. Examples of relaxation activities include:

- ***Diaphragmatic breathing*** can relax muscles, improve oxygen levels, and provide a feeling of release from tension. This technique is more effective when the patient either lies down or sits comfortably, remains in a quiet environment, and keeps the eyelids closed. Inhaling and exhaling slowly and regularly are also helpful.
- ***Progressive muscle relaxation*** may be used alone or in conjunction with deep breathing to help manage pain. The patient is taught to tighten one group of muscles (such as those of the face), hold the tension for a few seconds, and then relax the muscle group completely, repeating these actions for all parts of the body. This method is also more effective when the patient lies or sits comfortably, is in a quiet environment, and keeps the eyelids closed. Tapes are available to help the patient with this relaxation process.
- ***Meditation*** is a process whereby the patient empties the mind of all sensory data and, typically, concentrates on a single object, word, or idea. This activity produces a deeply relaxed state in which oxygen consumption decreases, muscles relax, and endorphins are produced. At its deepest level, the meditative state may resemble a trance state. A variety of exercises can induce the meditative state, and all are relatively easy to learn. Many books and tapes are available commercially.
- ***Music therapy*** uses music and the therapeutic relationship to reduce pain, anxiety, and depression. Music provides a familiar sensory stimulus that can provoke favorable responses such as muscle relaxation and reduced heart rate and blood pressure. Studies on the efficacy of music therapy to reduce pain perception in an acute care setting show a positive impact on pain. Music therapy is a simple and easy intervention that has minimal to no side effects and has been shown to be an effective adjuvant for pain control in multiple studies (Cole & LoBiondo-Wood, 2014).

Nursing Care

Nursing care of the patient with pain presents perhaps more of a challenge than almost any other type of illness or injury. Regardless of the type of pain, the goal of nursing care is to assist the patient to achieve optimal control of the pain.

Assessment

Pain assessment varies by the acuity of the pain and circumstances surrounding the patient's entry into the healthcare setting. Identifying the location, intensity, and triggering event may be the most appropriate initial assessment for a patient experiencing acute pain related to trauma. The approach to a patient experiencing acute pain without known trauma (e.g., acute chest, flank, or abdominal pain) may still be very focused due to the acuity of the situation. Additional information regarding the quality and timing of the pain and also the patient's health history often provide valuable clues about the underlying cause.

A common mnemonic that is useful for conducting a focused pain assessment is PQRST:

P = What **p**recipitated (triggered, stimulated) the pain? Has anything relieved the pain? What is the pattern of the pain (constant, episodic)?

Q = What are the **q**ualities of the pain? How would you describe the pain (sharp, stabbing, aching, burning, stinging, deep, crushing, viselike, gnawing)?

R = What is the **r**egion (location) of the pain? Can you put your finger on where the pain is? Does the pain radiate to other areas of the body?

S = What is the **s**everity or intensity of the pain?

T = What is the timing of the pain? When does it begin, how long does it last, and how is it related to other events in the patient's life?

When pain is chronic, a comprehensive approach to pain assessment is essential to ensure adequate and appropriate interventions. The four essential areas to assess are patient perceptions, physiologic responses, behavioral responses, and the patient's attempts to manage the pain, in addition to the effectiveness of these pain management strategies.

Patient Perceptions. The most reliable indicator of the presence and degree of pain is the patient's own statement about the pain.

The McGill Pain Questionnaire is a useful tool in assessing the subjective pain experience. It asks the patient to locate the pain and to describe its quality and intensity using terms that describe its sensory, affective, evaluative, and miscellaneous components. It is the nurse's responsibility to assess and document pain (**Figure 9.10** ■).

The most common method to assess the severity of pain is a pain rating scale. Pain rating scales can be used even in the most emergent situations. Two scales are illustrated in **Figure 9.11** ■. For patients who do not understand English or numerals, a scale using colors or the Wong-Baker FACES scale may be helpful. You can see the Wong-Baker FACES scale at wongbakerfaces.org. The following guidelines will help the nurse effectively use a pain rating scale:

- To ensure consistent communication, explain the specific pain rating scale being used. If a word descriptor scale is utilized, verify that the patient can read the language being used. If a numerical scale is used, be sure the patient can count to 10. Discuss the definition of the word *pain* to ensure that the patient and the provider are communicating on the same level. It is often helpful to use the patient's own words when describing the pain.
- Explain that the report of pain is important for promoting recovery, not just for achieving temporary comfort.
- Ask the patient to establish a comfort-function goal. This is a level of pain that does not interfere with or

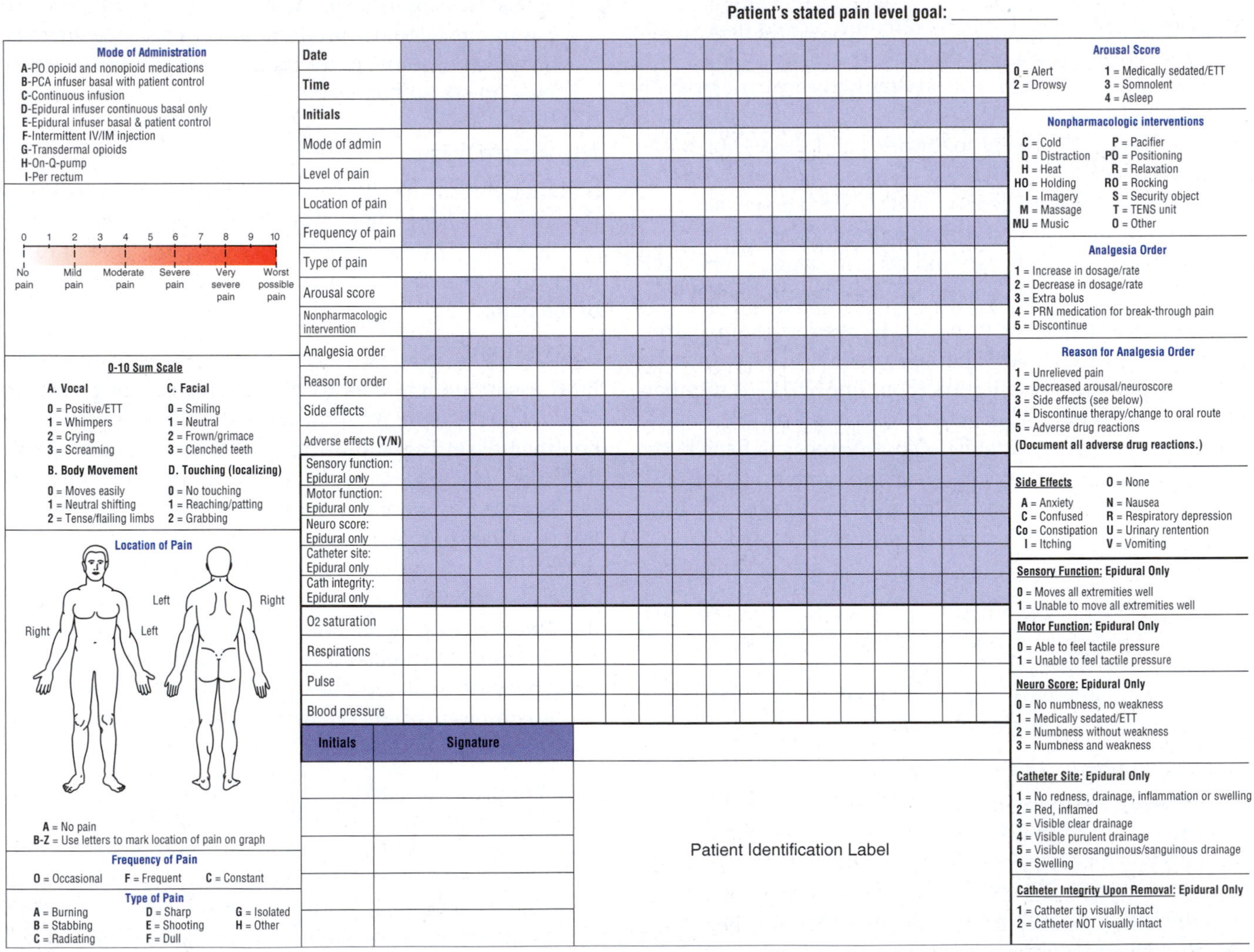
Patient's stated pain level goal: ____________

Mode of Administration
A-PO opioid and nonopioid medications
B-PCA infuser basal with patient control
C-Continuous infusion
D-Epidural infuser continuous basal only
E-Epidural infuser basal & patient control
F-Intermittent IV/IM injection
G-Transdermal opioids
H-On-Q-pump
I-Per rectum

0 1 2 3 4 5 6 7 8 9 10
No pain · Mild pain · Moderate pain · Severe pain · Very severe pain · Worst possible pain

0-10 Sum Scale

A. Vocal	C. Facial
0 = Positive/ETT	0 = Smiling
1 = Whimpers	1 = Neutral
2 = Crying	2 = Frown/grimace
3 = Screaming	3 = Clenched teeth
B. Body Movement	**D. Touching (localizing)**
0 = Moves easily	0 = No touching
1 = Neutral shifting	1 = Reaching/patting
2 = Tense/flailing limbs	2 = Grabbing

Location of Pain
Right · Left · Left · Right
A = No pain
B-Z = Use letters to mark location of pain on graph

Frequency of Pain
O = Occasional F = Frequent C = Constant

Type of Pain
A = Burning D = Sharp G = Isolated
B = Stabbing E = Shooting H = Other
C = Radiating F = Dull

Date																		
Time																		
Initials																		
Mode of admin																		
Level of pain																		
Location of pain																		
Frequency of pain																		
Type of pain																		
Arousal score																		
Nonpharmacologic intervention																		
Analgesia order																		
Reason for order																		
Side effects																		
Adverse effects (Y/N)																		
Sensory function: Epidural only																		
Motor function: Epidural only																		
Neuro score: Epidural only																		
Catheter site: Epidural only																		
Cath integrity: Epidural only																		
O2 saturation																		
Respirations																		
Pulse																		
Blood pressure																		

Initials	Signature

Patient Identification Label

Arousal Score
0 = Alert 1 = Medically sedated/ETT
2 = Drowsy 3 = Somnolent
4 = Asleep

Nonpharmacologic interventions
C = Cold P = Pacifier
D = Distraction PO = Positioning
H = Heat R = Relaxation
HO = Holding RO = Rocking
I = Imagery S = Security object
M = Massage T = TENS unit
MU = Music O = Other

Analgesia Order
1 = Increase in dosage/rate
2 = Decrease in dosage/rate
3 = Extra bolus
4 = PRN medication for break-through pain
5 = Discontinue

Reason for Analgesia Order
1 = Unrelieved pain
2 = Decreased arousal/neuroscore
3 = Side effects (see below)
4 = Discontinue therapy/change to oral route
5 = Adverse drug reactions
(Document all adverse drug reactions.)

Side Effects 0 = None
A = Anxiety N = Nausea
C = Confused R = Respiratory depression
Co = Constipation U = Urinary rentention
I = Itching V = Vomiting

Sensory Function: Epidural Only
0 = Moves all extremities well
1 = Unable to move all extremities well

Motor Function: Epidural Only
0 = Able to feel tactile pressure
1 = Unable to feel tactile pressure

Neuro Score: Epidural Only
0 = No numbness, no weakness
1 = Medically sedated/ETT
2 = Numbness without weakness
3 = Numbness and weakness

Catheter Site: Epidural Only
1 = No redness, drainage, inflammation or swelling
2 = Red, inflamed
3 = Visible clear drainage
4 = Visible purulent drainage
5 = Visible serosanguinous/sanguinous drainage
6 = Swelling

Catheter Integrity Upon Removal: Epidural Only
1 = Catheter tip visually intact
2 = Catheter NOT visually intact

Figure 9.10 ■ Sample pain management flow sheet for assessment and documentation.

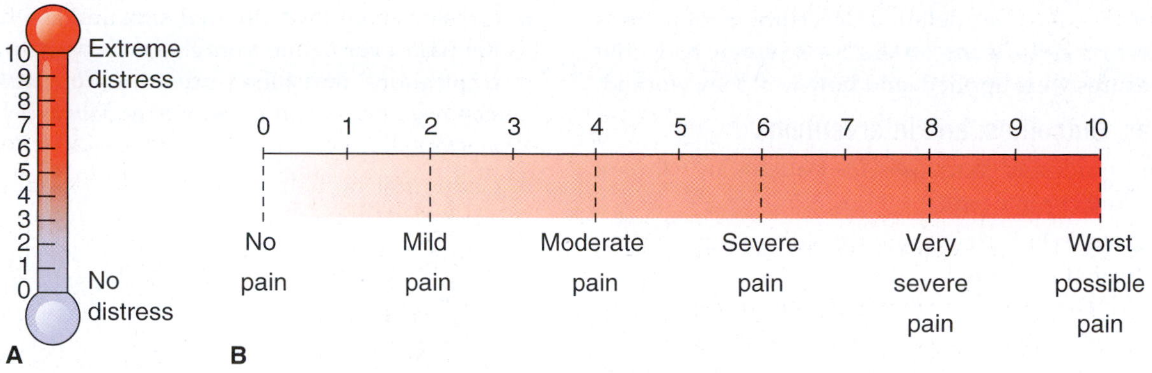
10
9
8
7
6
5
4
3
2
1
0
Extreme distress
No distress
A
0 1 2 3 4 5 6 7 8 9 10
No pain
Mild pain
Moderate pain
Severe pain
Very severe pain
Worst possible pain
B

Figure 9.11 ■ Examples of commonly used pain scales.

prevent the performance of essential activities of recovery or living. Often, pain assessment is made while a patient is sedentary. In this state the patient may experience less pain than when active and falsely estimate tolerable pain ratings. Provide guidelines for setting goals. Researchers found that pain ratings higher than 3 (scale of 0–10) interfered significantly with patients' activities, and scores of 6 and 7 decrease quality of life (IOM, 2011).

- Use the same scale across shifts and between institutions to promote accurate assessment in transitional care situations (Horgas, 2017a, 2017b).

Research has shown the numeric rating, verbal descriptor, and faces rating scales to be effective with young, middle, and older adults. Studies show that scales that use words as an indicator of pain such as the Verbal Descriptor Scale are more effective in assessing the pain of older adults (Horgas, 2017a). These scales are also more effective for use with older adults who have cognitive impairments. The Wong-Baker FACES scale is also effective in assessment of pain in older adults with cognitive difficulty (Horgas, 2017a).

Physiologic Responses. Predictable physiologic changes occur in the presence of acute pain. These may include muscle tension; tachycardia; rapid, shallow respirations; increased blood pressure; dilated pupils; sweating; and pallor. Over time, however, the pain stimulus triggers less of a sympathetic nervous system response, and these physiologic changes may be extinguished in patients with chronic pain.

Behavioral Responses. Some behaviors are so typical of people in pain that the behaviors are referred to as *pain behaviors*. They include facial grimacing, bracing or guarding the painful part, taking medication, crying, moaning, withdrawing from activity and socialization, becoming immobile, talking about pain, holding the painful area, breathing with increased effort, exhibiting a sad facial expression, and being restless.

Behavioral responses to pain may or may not coincide with the patient's report of pain and are not always reliable cues to the pain experience. Discrepancies between the patient's report of pain and behavioral responses may be the result of cultural factors, coping skills, fear, denial, or the utilization of relaxation or distraction techniques.

Behavior cues are critical for assessing pain intensity in patients with advanced dementia (unable to respond to simple yes or no questions) or who are nonverbal. The Pain Assessment in Advanced Dementia (PAINAD) scale uses five behavioral indicators of pain. Once trained, the nurse can use the scale by observing patient behaviors related to breathing (normal, labored, hyperventilation), vocalization (moaning, calling out, crying), facial expression (smiling or without expression, sad, frowning, grimacing), body language (relaxed, tense, rigid, or striking out), and consolability (distractible, reassured, or unable to console) (Horgas, 2017a).

Patients may deny pain for a variety of reasons, including fear of injections, fear of drug/narcotic addiction, misinterpretation of terms (the patient may not think that aching, soreness, or discomfort qualify as pain), or the misconception that healthcare providers know when patients experience pain. Some patients may deny pain as part of an attempt to deny that there is something wrong with them. Other patients, by contrast, may think that "as-needed" medications will be given only if their pain rating is high. Patients may also use pain as a mechanism to gain attention from family and healthcare providers.

Self-Management of Pain. The patient's attempts to manage pain are useful additions to the assessment database. This information is individualized and patient specific, including many factors such as culture, age, and patient knowledge. Get detailed descriptions of actions the patient or significant others took, when and how these measures were applied, and how well they worked.

Diagnoses, Outcomes, and Interventions

The primary nursing diagnoses for patients in pain are acute pain and chronic pain.

Relieve Acute Pain. Acute pain should be assessed regularly and treated as needed.

Expected Outcome: Patient will demonstrate pain control through appropriate assessment and treatment.

The nurse will assess the characteristics of the pain by asking the patient to:

- Point to the pain location or mark the pain location on a figure drawing. *Pain location provides information about the etiology of the pain and the type of pain experienced.*
- Rate the intensity of the pain by using an evidence-based pain scale (refer to Figure 9.11). Use the same scale with each assessment. *Pain and its intensity is a subjective experience. Consistently using the same scale to rate pain intensity allows evaluation of intervention effectiveness.*
- Describe the quality of the pain, saying, for example, "Describe what your pain feels like." If necessary, suggest word descriptors for the patient to select. *Descriptive terms provide insight into the nature and cause of the pain.*
- Describe the pattern of the pain, including time of onset, duration, persistence, and times without pain. Ask whether the pain is worse at regular times of the day and about its relationship to activity. *The pattern of pain provides clues about cause and location.*
- Describe any precipitating or relieving factors. *Precipitating factors provide clues to any underlying pathophysiology of the pain; relieving factors provide information that can be used when planning nursing interventions for pain management.*

The nurse will:

- Identify and use the most appropriate evidence-based pain scale based on patients' individual cognitive ability. *Do not assume that the older patient or the patient with a cognitive impairment is not having pain or is unable to identify its intensity. Many cognitively impaired patients are able to use a pain scale such as faces, numeric rating, or verbal descriptor.*
- Monitor manifestations of pain by taking vital signs; assessing skin temperature and moisture; observing pupils; observing facial expressions, position in bed, guarding of body parts; and noting restlessness. *Autonomic responses to pain may result in an increased blood pressure, tachycardia, rapid respirations, perspiration, and dilated pupils. Other responses to pain include grimacing, clenching the hands, muscle rigidity, guarding, restlessness, and nausea.*
- Consider pain the fifth vital sign and assess patients for pain every time you check temperature, pulse, respirations, and blood pressure. *The Joint Commission requires frequent assessment of pain as a standard of practice.*
- Communicate belief in the patient's pain. *Verbally acknowledge the presence of the pain, listen carefully to the description of pain, and act to help the patient manage the pain. Because pain is a personal, subjective experience, the nurse must convey belief in the patient's pain. By doing this, the nurse reduces anxiety and thereby lessens pain.*
- Administer prescribed analgesics, determining the preferred route of administration. Provide pain-relieving measures for severe pain on a regular around-the-clock basis or by self-administration (such as with a PCA pump). *The patient is a part of the decision-making process and can exert some control over the situation by choosing the administration route. Analgesics are usually most effective when they are administered before pain occurs or becomes severe. Around-the-clock administration has been proven to provide better pain management for both acute and chronic pain.*

SAFETY ALERT: Use extreme care to ensure the correct patient, medication, and dose when setting up and monitoring PCA for analgesia. Programming issues accounted for 71% of adverse events for patients with PCA. Consider PCA to be a process, not just a machine. ■

- To reduce the risk of medication errors associated with PCA, work with administration to develop the following strategies:
  a. Select patients who are good candidates for PCA. Confused patients are not good candidates.
  b. Use a single brand or type of pump within a facility to reduce programming and use complexity for caregivers.
  c. Use standard prescription sets and standard medication concentrations.
  d. Maintain proficiency with PCA machines, know how to enter a prescription correctly, and use independent nurse checks to confirm dosages.
  e. Use bar codes and electronic medical records to reduce errors that involve the wrong medication.
  f. Develop and use easily understood and standardized forms for PCA.

  The complexity of activities required to safely program PCA pumps, the use of different medications and concentrations, confusion of medical orders, and variations in documentation related to PCA are identified as contributing factors to PCA medication errors.
- Evaluate and monitor the effects of analgesics and other pain-relieving measures. Teach family members or significant others to be alert for adverse reactions to

pain medications. Sedation, constipation, nausea, and dizziness are common side effects of opioid analgesics. *Opioid analgesics stimulate mu receptors, leading to common adverse effects such as respiratory depression, nausea, and constipation.*

- Provide for safety of the patient receiving opioid analgesics:
  a. Check respiratory rate and oxygen saturation every 2 hours at the beginning of opioid therapy and after increasing dosage. Reduce the dose and notify the physician if the respiratory rate falls to eight per minute (or lower) or if the oxygen saturation falls. *Excessive sedation can progress to significant respiratory depression.*
  b. Use a sedation scale to monitor sedation levels consistently. *Using a scale will support a standardized approach to monitoring level of sedation.*
  c. Prevent falls that may result from sedation or dizziness. *Opioid analgesics can affect balance and judgment, increasing the risk for falls, particularly in older adults.*
  d. Administer an opioid antagonist such as naloxone (Narcan) if the patient develops symptoms of excessive opioid dosage. Administer prescribed dose (0.4 to 2 mg) by direct intravenous push over 10 to 15 seconds or by intravenous infusion. Titrate infusion or repeat direct IV push every 2 to 3 minutes (up to a total of 10 mg) to reverse respiratory depression or excessive sedation. Continue to monitor respiratory status and sedation, repeating naloxone as necessary. *The opioid agonist causing excessive sedation and respiratory depression may have a longer half-life than naloxone, leading to a fall in respiratory rate and decreased LOC after the initial dose of naloxone has been substantially eliminated. Administration of excessive naloxone may cause acute withdrawal and failure of pain relief. It may take considerable time to reestablish a therapeutic comfort level.*
- Teach the patient and family nonpharmacologic methods of pain management, such as relaxation, distraction, and cutaneous stimulation. *These techniques are especially useful when used in conjunction with pain medications. They can be beneficial for patients experiencing either acute or chronic pain.*
- Provide comfort measures, such as changing positions, back massage, oral care, skin care, and changing bed linens. *Basic comfort measures for personal cleanliness, skin care, and mobility promote physical and psychosocial well-being, lessening the perception of pain.*
- Provide patient and family teaching and make referrals, if necessary, to assist with coping, financial resources, and home care. *The patient (and family) with pain requires information about medications, noninvasive techniques for pain management, and sources of assistance with home-based care. The patient with acute pain requires information about the expected course of pain resolution.*

Manage Chronic Pain. The patient who has chronic pain may not demonstrate the same physiologic and behavioral responses to pain as are seen in the patient with acute pain. The intensity of the pain, however, may be as high or even higher than acute pain. Furthermore, chronic pain, whether of malignant or nonmalignant origin, has a negative effect on the patient's physical, psychosocial, emotional, and functional status. In addition to the nursing assessments and interventions identified for acute pain, consider the following interventions for the patient experiencing chronic pain.

Expected Outcome: Patient will verbalize pain at acceptable level using agency-specific pain scale, demonstrate ability to maintain optimal level of functioning, and report ability to maintain role performance and interpersonal relationships.

The nurse will:

- Ask the patient to describe the pain and its meaning, including its effects on lifestyle, self-concept, roles, and relationships. *Pain is a stressor that may affect the patient's coping ability. Chronic pain often interferes with sleep quality, job performance, personal relationships, and social interactions. The patient may have concerns about addiction to pain medication and costs as well.*
- Assess for depression using an accepted depression screening tool. *Chronic pain and depression commonly occur concurrently.*
- If the underlying cause of chronic pain has not been identified, advocate for consultations, diagnostic testing, or other means of establishing an accurate diagnosis. *Guidelines for chronic pain management call for treatment of the underlying cause whenever it can be identified.*
- Administer prescribed NSAIDs, opioid and nonopioid analgesics, and other medications around the clock and as ordered. Whenever possible, the oral or transdermal routes should be used. See **Table 9.6** for opioids used for long-term chronic pain. *Around-the-clock analgesic administration helps maintain pain within an acceptable range within which the patient remains comfortable and functional. As-needed medications may be required for breakthrough pain.*
- Not crush, break, or allow patients to chew controlled-release oral preparations. *Crushing, breaking, or chewing controlled-release oral preparations may lead to overdose. Capsules containing controlled-release pellets can be opened and sprinkled over soft food.*
- Teach the patient, family, and caregivers how to manage side and adverse effects of prescribed medications. Advise about the importance of taking NSAIDs with food to reduce the risk of gastrointestinal irritation and bleeding. Provide information about appropriate laxatives for the patient taking opioid analgesics. Instruct when to contact the prescribing care provider should adverse effects become problematic. *Many analgesics, while effective, have*

BOX 9.2
Nursing Care of the Older Adult in Pain

The nursing standard of care calls for older adults to be pain free or have their pain controlled to an acceptable level that allows the highest possible level of functioning (Horgas, 2017a). Achieving this standard requires comprehensive assessment of the patient, including the patient's history, subjective reports of pain, nonverbal and behavioral responses, and information from family members about the patient's pain experiences.

In addition to frequent and ongoing assessment, nursing care guidelines call for the nurse to anticipate and treat pain before, during, and after painful procedures and treatments. The nurse should educate the patient, family, and other clinicians about prophylactic analgesic use, using analgesics on a regular basis, and how to avoid allowing pain to escalate. Teaching must include information about the medications themselves, their side and adverse effects, and issues about addiction, dependence, and tolerance. Finally, the nurse teaches the patient, family, and other healthcare providers about nonpharmacologic pain management strategies such as relaxation, massage, and application of heat or cold (Horgas, 2017b).

adverse effects that may limit the patient's willingness to continue therapy. In most cases, appropriate management of these effects allows continued use of the medication.

- Encourage and advocate for a multimodal approach to pain management, teaching about the use of heat, cold, and integrative therapies, providing for referrals to healthcare providers (e.g., physical therapists, chiropractic physicians, massage therapists, acupuncturists) and chronic pain clinics as appropriate. *Using a multimodal approach to management of chronic pain improves the patient's perception of control over the pain and its effect on lifestyle. This also may result in less dependence on opioid and nonopioid analgesics.*
- Take special care of older adults in pain. See **Box 9.2**. *Older adults often have medical conditions associated with pain, such as arthritis, peripheral vascular disease, and diabetes. Many older adults have multiple health disorders causing them to experience both acute and chronic pain.*

Transitions of Care

Health promotion activities related to pain focus on providing effective relief of acute pain to avoid the negative consequences of inadequately managed pain. Evidence points to the existence of pain circuits established when acute pain is inadequately treated that perpetuate pain and contribute to chronic pain. Furthermore, pain has a negative effect on quality of life, resulting in decreased job performance, exercise, socialization, and activity-of-daily-living performance. Longer-term effects include depression, isolation, and loss of self-esteem (American Academy of Pain Medicine, 2018).

Caring for patients with acute or chronic pain requires educating the patient and family. Topics include:

- Specific drugs to be taken, including the frequency, potential side effects, possible drug interactions, and any special precautions to be taken (such as taking with food or avoiding alcohol)
- How to take or administer the drugs ordered for managing chronic malignant or nonmalignant pain (see Table 9.6)
- The importance of taking pain medications before the pain becomes severe
- An explanation that the risk of addiction to pain medications is very small when they are used for pain relief and management
- Discussion about physical tolerance and the importance of contacting the prescriber should medications become less effective
- The importance of scheduling periods of rest and sleep
- Use of integrative therapies to supplement or enhance traditional approaches to pain management.

Pain at the end of life is covered in Chapter 5, Palliative and End-of-Life Care.

Table 9.6 Opioids for Long-Term Analgesia for Chronic Pain

Drug	Route	Nursing Implications
oxycodone (OxyContin)	Oral	Available in a timed-release formulation for 12-hour dosing and as fast-acting formulations (OxyIR, OxyFAST) for breakthrough pain.
morphine (Kadian)	Oral	Formulated of timed-release particles in a capsule. If patient can't swallow the capsule, may be sprinkled over food or given by nasogastric or gastric tube.
fentanyl (Duragesic)	Transdermal	Absorbed slowly through the skin; allows 72-h dose schedule. Up to 14 h to achieve therapeutic level; when discontinued therapeutic effect will decay slowly.
fentanyl citrate (Actiq)	Transmucosal	A lozenge formulation used to treat breakthrough cancer pain in opioid-tolerant patients.

Note: Drugs identified in blue are among the 200 most commonly prescribed medications in the United States.

Source: Data from Adams, et al., 2017.

Case Study & Nursing Care Plan

A Patient Experiencing Chronic Pain

Susan Akers, age 37, is currently being seen at an outpatient clinic for chronic nonmalignant pain. She works at a local paper factory. She has a 3-year history of neck and shoulder pain that is usually accompanied by headaches. She believes the pain is related to lifting objects at work, but it is now precipitated by activities of daily living. Susan is absent from work approximately three times a month and states that the absences are due to her pain and headaches. She has been seeking care in the local emergency department on the average of twice monthly for injections for pain. She does not regularly use medications but does take Percocet-5 as needed (usually two to three times a day). Ms. Akers is divorced and has two children. She states that she has several friends in the area, but her parents and siblings live in another part of the United States.

ASSESSMENT	DIAGNOSES	EXPECTED OUTCOMES
During the nursing history, Ms. Akers rates her pain during an acute episode as a 7 on a scale of 1 to 10. She states that lifting objects and moving her hands and arms above shoulder level precipitate sharp pain. The pain never really goes away, but it does decrease with upper extremity rest. She says that when she lifts a lot at work, she has difficulty sleeping that night. She takes two Percocet-5 tablets every 6 hours when the pain is severe, but does not get complete relief.	■ Chronic pain related to muscle inflammation	■ Return for follow-up visits with a journal of activities and pain experiences. ■ After 3 to 5 days on regularly scheduled doses of pain medication, report a decrease in the level of pain from 7 to 3 or 4 on a scale of 1 to 10. ■ Decrease number of absences from work. ■ Modify activities at work and at home, especially when pain is intense.

PLANNING AND IMPLEMENTATION

- Encourage discussion of pain, and acknowledge belief in Ms. Akers's report of pain.
- Consult with a physician for an appropriate nonsteroidal anti-inflammatory analgesic with a minimum of side effects, and instruct in maintaining regular dosing schedules.
- For episodes of acute pain, take opioid analgesic as soon as the pain begins and every 6 hours while continuing the dosage of NSAID analgesic.
- Teach one relaxation technique that is personally useful.
- Explore distraction techniques such as listening to music, watching comedies, or reading.
- Provide clinic phone number and instruct to call if pain is unrelieved with opioid and NSAID analgesics.

EVALUATION

Ms. Akers returns for scheduled follow-up visits with a completed journal of her activities and associated pain. She reports that taking oral opioid analgesics has relieved her pain and that within 3 weeks of regular use, NSAID analgesics brought her pain under control. She also reports that her supervisor has reassigned her to a position that requires no lifting. She now rates her pain at 2 or 3 on a scale of 1 to 10. She has missed only 1 day of work in the last 3 months and reports that her children and friends have helped with her household tasks when she has requested they do so.

CLINICAL REASONING IN PATIENT CARE

1. Describe three factors that support the statement "Pain is a personal experience."
2. Ms. Akers asks you how often she should take her pain medications. You tell her to (a) take them on a regular basis or (b) wait until she experiences pain. Which action would you choose, and why?
3. Develop a care plan for Ms. Akers for the potential of developing constipation. Why is this necessary?

See Evaluating Your Response in Appendix B.

CHAPTER HIGHLIGHTS

9.1 The Concept of Pain

Define pain, why it is called the fifth vital sign, the adverse effects of it, and myths and misconceptions about it.

- Pain is a subjective response to both physical and psychologic stressors and all people experience pain at some point during their lives.
- Although pain is usually experienced as uncomfortable and unwelcome, it also serves a protective role, warning of potentially health-threatening conditions.
- Pain is a distinct and personal experience influenced by genetic, physiologic, psychologic, cognitive, sociocultural, cultural, and spiritual factors.
- Acute pain has a defined purpose: To warn of injury to body tissues.

9.2 Neurophysiology of Pain

Describe the theories about, physiology of, pathways of, and modulation of pain.

- Pain is transmitted by the peripheral and central nervous systems and perceived in the CNS. Opioids and other analgesics block the perception of pain; NSAIDs and most nonpharmacologic interventions block or decrease the transmission of pain from the periphery to the CNS.
- Pain occurs when the tissue containing nociceptors is subjected to a noxious insult; the intensity and duration of the stimuli determine the sensation.
- The pain pathway goes from transduction to transmission to modulation to perception.

9.3 Types and Characteristics of Pain

Differentiate definitions and characteristics of acute, chronic, breakthrough, nociceptive, and neuropathic pain.

- Acute pain, which may be cutaneous or deep somatic, visceral, or referred, usually decreases as healing progresses.
- Chronic pain may be episodic, experienced as recurrent acute pain, or may be persistent pain of either malignant or nonmalignant origin.
- Breakthrough pain is that which exceeds the baseline or persistent level of pain.
- Nociceptive pain is caused by stimulation of peripheral or visceral pain receptors. It is generally localized and responsive to treatment; it may be acute or chronic.
- Neuropathic pain arises as a consequence of a lesion or disease affecting the somatosensory system; it may be acute, but it is usually chronic. Examples include central pain, complex regional pain syndrome, and phantom limb pain.

9.4 Factors Affecting Responses to Pain

Outline factors affecting responses to pain.

- Age, gender, and culture impact pain perception and behavior.
- A patient's emotional state, past experiences with pain, and the underlying cause and meaning of the painful experience also affect responses to pain.
- Pain tolerance is the amount (duration, intensity) of pain an individual can endure before outwardly responding to it.
- The intensity of perceived pain has been shown to be affected by psychologic variables such as attention, expectation, and suggestion.

9.5 Care of the Patient in Pain

Describe interprofessional care, nursing care, and transitions of care for patients in pain.

- Nurses play a pivotal role in managing pain for patients in all healthcare settings.
- Completion of a comprehensive assessment and development of an individualized and patient-centered plan lead to effective pain management.
- Pain management involves pharmacologic and nonpharmacologic interventions.
- Behavioral assessment of pain intensity is less accurate than a patient's report of pain intensity, particularly when pain is chronic. Behavioral responses may be used to assess pain in patients who are significantly cognitively impaired. Older adults perceive pain as intensely as younger adults, but may hesitate to report pain for fear of losing independence. Physical tolerance develops with long-term opioid use, necessitating dose increases to achieve the same effect. Although patients who are addicted to opioids need greater doses of opioid analgesics to control pain because of tolerance, treating physicians and nurses providing care often withhold or use lower doses of opioid analgesics, leading to inadequate pain relief.
- Pain management includes assessment, intervention, and evaluation. It is important to verify that interventions have been effective. If not, interventions must be identified that bring pain down to a level of intensity with which the patient feels satisfied.

TEST YOURSELF NCLEX-RN® REVIEW

1. During an assessment, the nurse learns that a patient has had lower back pain for 9 months. For which type of pain will the nurse plan care?
   A. Chronic pain
   B. Somatic pain
   C. Visceral pain
   D. Neuropathic pain
2. A patient who smashed a finger in the car door relates that the pain initially was sharp but now it is dull and throbbing. What should the nurse recall as the reason for the current type of pain that the patient is experiencing?
   A. It is an example of the gate theory of pain transmission.
   B. Transmission of pain stimuli occurs via unmyelinated C fibers.
   C. Indicates that the injury is less severe than initially perceived.
   D. It is the result of interpretation of the pain stimulus by the thalamus.
3. A patient with arthritis has been taking over-the-counter NSAIDs for several years. Which questions should the nurse ask the patient while completing the health history? (Select all that apply.)
   A. "Tell me how and when you take this drug."
   B. "Do you have your blood pressure checked regularly?"
   C. "Have you noticed any problems with your breathing?"
   D. "Have you ever vomited blood or had very dark stools?"
   E. "Do you know that you may become addicted to this drug?"
4. What should the nurse include when teaching a patient about a transdermal pain medication? (Select all that apply.)
   A. When reapplying the patch, place it on the anterior thigh.
   B. Replace this patch every 24 hours, applying it to clean, dry skin.
   C. Contact the physician if this medication causes excessive sleepiness.
   D. This medication should be effective within 2 to 4 hours; contact the physician if the pain is not at an acceptable level after that.
   E. Place a heating pad over the patch to ensure adherence.
5. Which statement should the nurse use to determine the quality of a patient's pain?
   A. "Tell me where it hurts."
   B. "Rate the pain on a scale of 0 to 10."
   C. "Describe what the pain feels like."
   D. "Tell me how this pain affects sleeping."
6. A patient recovering from surgery rates pain as being 7 on a scale of 0 to 10 but the nurse notes the patient is relaxed, smiling, and visiting with friends. Which action should the nurse take?
   A. Administer the prescribed analgesic dose.
   B. Reassess the patient's pain after his friends have left.
   C. Document your assessment but take no further action.
   D. Note that the patient is developing tolerance to the prescribed opioid analgesic.
7. What information should the nurse include when teaching a patient with chronic malignant pain about opioid analgesics? (Select all that apply.)
   A. "This drug may cause itching and rash; take diphenhydramine (Benadryl) as needed."
   B. "This drug may interfere with urination; contact your physician if that becomes a problem."
   C. "Increase fluid and fiber intake; you may need a stool softener or laxative to prevent constipation."
   D. "There is a risk of addiction with this drug; stop the drug if you find that it no longer provides the degree of pain relief necessary."
   E. "Using techniques like relaxation or distraction may work with this medication to better control your pain."
8. What approach should the nurse use to assess pain in a patient who is moderately cognitively impaired?
   A. Ask the patient to rate the pain using the faces pain scale.
   B. Have the family evaluate the intensity of the patient's pain.
   C. Administer the prescribed analgesic on an around-the-clock basis.
   D. Use only behavioral cues such as grimacing, pacing, or agitation.
9. A patient who takes opioids has a respiratory rate of 6. Which nursing intervention is indicated?
   A. Administer naloxone by intravenous push.
   B. Hold the next dose of opioid.
   C. Continue to monitor as most opioids have a short half-life.
   D. Begin rescue breathing and chest compressions.

10. A patient recently took up meditation to counteract the stress of her job. She reports the added benefit of less pain from her chronic back condition. Which nursing response would be the most accurate?
    A. Natural narcotic-like substances are released during meditation.
    B. Activities such as meditation activate a natural "gate" in the spinal cord, blocking pain signals.
    C. Engaging in activities that reduce stress change pain circuits in the brain, reducing the perception of pain.
    D. With repeated stimulation through activities such as meditation, nociceptors in deep tissues become less sensitive to stimuli.

See Test Yourself answers in Appendix B.

REFERENCES

Adams, M. P., Holland, L. N., & Urban, C. (2017). *Pharmacology for nursing: A pathophysiologic approach* (5th ed.). Hoboken, NJ: Pearson Education.

Argoff, C. E., & Chen, N. (2018). Muscle relaxants, anticonvulsants as analgesics; antidepressants as analgesics. In C. E. Argoff, A. Dubin, & J. G. Pilitsis (Eds.), *Pain management secrets* (4th ed., pp. 224–227). St. Louis, MO: Elsevier.

American Academy of Pain Medicine (2018). *AAPN facts and figures on pain.* Retrieved from www.painmed.org/PatientCenter/Facts_on_Pain.aspx.

Boakye, P. A., Olechowski, C., Rashiq, S., Verrier, M., Kerr, B., Witmans, M., . . . Dick, B. (2016). A critical review of neurobiological factors involved in the interactions between chronic pain, depression, and sleep disruption. *Clinical Journal of Pain, 32*, 327–336.

Chou, R., Gordon, D. B., de Leon-Cassola, O. A., Rosenberg, J. M., Bickler, S., Brennan, T., . . . Wu, C. L. (2016). Management of postoperative pain: A clinical practice guideline from the American Pain Society, the American Society of Regional Anesthesia and Pain Medicine, and the American Society of Anesthesiologists' Committee on Regional Anesthesia, Executive Committee, and Administrative Council. *Journal of Pain, 17*(2), 131–157.

Cole, L. C., & LoBiondo-Wood, G. (2014). Music as an adjuvant therapy in control of pain and symptoms in hospitalized adults: A systematic review. *Pain Management Nursing, 15*(1), 137–142.

Collison, C., & Argoff, C. E. (2018). Topical analgesics. In C. E. Argoff, A. Dubin, & J. G. Pilitsis (Eds.), *Pain Management Secrets* (4th ed., pp. 197–205). St. Louis, MO: Elsevier.

Dowell, D., Haegerich, T. M., & Chou, R. (2016). CDC guideline for prescribing opioids for chronic pain – United States, 2016. *Journal of the American Medical Association, 315*(15), 1624–1645.

Duarte, R. A., Argoff, C. E., & Dubin, A. (2018). Postoperative pain management. In C. E. Argoff, A. Dubin, & J. G. Pilitsis (Eds.), *Pain management secrets* (4th ed., pp. 206–209). St. Louis, MO: Elsevier.

Fillingim, R. B. (2017). Sex, gender, and pain. In M. Legato (Ed.), *Principles of gender-specific medicine* (3rd ed., pp. 481–496). St. Louis, MO: Elsevier.

Finnerup, N. B., Haroutounian, S., Kamerman, P., Baron, R., Bennett, D. L. H., Bouhassira, D., . . . Jensen, T. S. (2016). Neuropathic pain: An updated grading system for research and clinical practice. *Pain, 157*(8), 1599–1606.

Fontaine, K. L. (2014). *Complementary and alternative therapies for nursing practice* (4th ed.). Upper Saddle River, NJ: Pearson Prentice Hall.

Fuzaylov, G., Kelly, K. L., Bline, C., Dunaev, A., Dylewski, M. L., & Driscoll, D. N. (2015). Post-operative pain control for burn reconstructive surgery in a resource-restricted country with subcutaneous infusion of local anesthetics through a soaker catheter to the surgical site: Preliminary results. *Burns, 41*, 1811–1815.

Henschke, N., Kamper, S, J., & Maher, C. G. (2015). The epidemiology and economic consequences of pain. *Mayo Clinic Proceedings, 90*(1), 139–147.

Horgas, A. L. (2017a). Pain assessment in older adults. *Nursing Clinics of North America, 52*(3), 375–385.

Horgas, A. L. (2017b). Pain management in older adults. *Nursing Clinics of North America, 52*(4), e1–e7.

Institute of Medicine (IOM). (2011). *Relieving pain in America: A blueprint for transforming prevention, care, education and research.* Washington, DC: National Academies Press.

International Association for the Study of Pain (IASP). (2015). *IASP taxonomy.* Retrieved from www.iasp-pain.org/Taxonomy.

The Joint Commission. (2018). *Pain management.* Retrieved from https://www.jointcommission.org/topics/pain_management.aspx,

Kasper, D. L., Fauci, A. S., Hauser, S. L., Longo, D. L., Jameson, L. J., & Loscalzo, J. (Eds.). (2016). *Harrison's manual of medicine* (19th ed.). New York, NY: McGraw-Hill.

Laufer, A. (2018). Postoperative pain management. In C. E. Argoff, A. Dubin, & J. G. Pilitsis (Eds.), *Pain management secrets* (4th ed., pp. 119–123). St. Louis, MO: Elsevier.

Lexicomp Online®. *Meperidine.* Hudson, OH: Lexi-Drugs.

McCaffery, M. (1979). *Nursing management of the patient with pain*. Philadelphia, PA: Lippincott.

McNicol, E. D., Ferguson, M. C., & Hudcova, J. (2015). Patient controlled opioid analgesia versus non-patient controlled opioid analgesia for postoperative pain. *Cochrane Database of Systematic Reviews*, Issue 6, Article No.: CD003348.

Mendell, L. M. (2014). Constructing and deconstructing the gate theory of pain. *Pain, 155*(2), 210–216.

Nahin, R. L. (2015). Estimates of pain prevalence and severity in adults: United States, 2012. *Journal of Pain, 16*(8), 769–780.

National Center for Complementary and Integrative Health. (2016). *Chiropractic: In depth.* Retrieved from https://nccih.nih.gov/health/chiropractic/introduction.htm.

Oliver, J., Cogging, C., Compton, P., Hagan, S., Matteliano, D., Stanton, M., . . . Turner, H. N. (2012). American Society for Pain Management Nursing position statement: Pain management in patients with substance use disorders. *Pain Management Nursing, 13*(3), 169–183.

Richardson, C., & Kulkami, J. (2017). A review of the management of phantom pain. *Journal of Pain Research, 10*, 1861–1870.

Sorenson, M., Quinn, L., & Klein, D. (2019). *Pathophysiology: Concepts of human disease.* Hoboken, NJ: Pearson Education.

World Health Organization (WHO). (2013). *WHO's pain ladder for adults.* Geneva: Author.

ADDITIONAL RESOURCES

American Academy of Pain Medicine
www.painmed.org

International Association for the Study of Pain
https://www.iasp-pain.org

Pain Management Nursing
www.painmanagementnursing.org

WHO's Cancer Pain Ladder for Adults
www.who.int/cancer/palliative/painladder/en

Chapter 10

Nursing Care of Patients with Altered Fluid, Electrolyte, and Acid–Base Balance

Chapter Outline and Learning Outcomes

CLINICAL COMPETENCIES

- Recognize patients at risk for fluid, electrolyte, or acid–base imbalances.
- Assess and monitor fluid, electrolyte, and acid–base balance, communicating findings with appropriate interprofessional team members.
- Demonstrate effective use of individualized and patient-centered strategies to reduce the risk of fluid, electrolyte, or acid–base imbalances.
- Effectively communicate and function within the interprofessional team to plan and provide care to patients with altered fluid, electrolyte, and acid–base balance.
- Administer fluids, medications, and other prescribed therapies knowledgeably and safely, using guidelines or protocols as appropriate.
- Adapt individual cultural values, expressed needs and preferences, and available evidence into the plan of care to provide knowledgeable and safe care to patients with fluid, electrolyte, or acid–base imbalances.
- Use assessed data, patient values, and evidence to provide patient and family teaching about strategies to promote, restore, and maintain fluid, electrolyte, and acid–base balance.
- Document care in the electronic medical record and use information management tools to monitor outcomes of care.
- Participate in studies and projects to improve the quality and safety of care for patients with fluid, electrolyte, or acid–base disorders.

KEY TERMS

acid, 265
acidosis, 266
alkalis, 265
alkalosis, 266
arterial blood gases (ABGs), 243
atrial natriuretic peptide (ANP), 233
base, 265
base excess (BE), 267
dehydration, 234
edema, 240
fluid volume deficit (FVD), 233
fluid volume excess (FVE), 240
homeostasis, 227
hypercapnia, 276
hypervolemia, 240
hypovolemia, 235
Kussmaul respirations, 272
second spacing, 235
serum bicarbonate, 267
tetany, 257
third spacing, 235

Normal physiologic processes depend on **homeostasis** (the ability to maintain internal equilibrium by adjusting physiologic processes) in the internal environment of the body. The fluid volume, electrolyte composition, and pH of both intracellular and extracellular spaces must remain constant within a relatively narrow range to maintain health and life. Changes in the normal distribution and composition of body fluids often occur in response to illness and trauma. These changes affect fluid balance of the intracellular and extracellular compartments of the body, the concentration of electrolytes within fluid compartments, and the body's hydrogen ion concentration (pH). Fluid and electrolyte imbalances occur in all adult age groups and in all healthcare settings.

Changes in the normal volume of fluids and their composition, distribution, and relative acidity or alkalinity have the potential to disrupt most functional health patterns. Imbalances of fluids, electrolytes, and pH affect the ability to maintain activities of daily living (activity–exercise), think clearly (cognitive–perceptual), and engage in self-care (health perception–health management). Conversely, alterations in a number of health patterns affect the ability to maintain homeostasis. Alterations in the nutritional–metabolic pattern affect the ability to consume adequate food and fluids. Disruptions of the elimination pattern may lead to retention or loss of excess amounts of fluids and electrolytes. Disrupted heart or respiratory function, which falls within the activity–exercise pattern, has the potential to affect fluid, electrolyte, and acid–base balance.

The goal in managing fluid, electrolyte, and acid–base imbalances is to reestablish and maintain homeostasis. Nursing care includes identifying and assessing patients who are likely to develop imbalances, monitoring patients for early manifestations, and implementing interprofessional and nursing interventions to prevent or correct imbalances. Effective nursing interventions require an understanding of the multiple processes that maintain fluid, electrolyte, and acid–base balance and an understanding of the causes and treatment of imbalances that occur. This chapter contains many references to disease processes that are discussed throughout the book and is most useful as a reference when learning about these disorders.

10.1 Overview of Fluid and Electrolyte Balance

Fluid and electrolyte balance in the body involves regulatory mechanisms that maintain the composition, distribution, and movement of fluids and electrolytes.

Body Fluid Composition

Body fluid is composed of water and various dissolved substances (solutes).

Water

Water is the primary component of body fluids and works in several ways to maintain normal cellular function. Water provides a medium for the transport and exchange of nutrients and other substances such as oxygen, carbon dioxide, and metabolic wastes to and from cells; provides a medium for metabolic reactions within cells; and assists in regulating body temperature through the evaporation of perspiration.

Total body water constitutes about 60% of the total body weight of a young adult male and 50% of that of a young adult female. The amount varies with age, gender, and the amount of body fat. Total body water decreases to about 45% of total body weight in older adults (Berman, Snyder, & Frandsen, 2016). Adipose tissue contains comparatively little water: In the person who is obese, the proportion of water to total body weight is less than in the person of average weight; an individual who is very thin has a higher proportion of water to total body weight. Adult females have a greater ratio of fat to lean tissue mass than adult males; therefore, they have a lower percentage of total body water.

To maintain normal fluid balance, body water intake and output should be approximately equal. The average fluid intake and output is about 2500 mL over a 24-hour period. Most water gain is from the intake of foods and fluids; carbohydrate metabolism and other metabolic processes produce an additional small amount. Urine production and excretion account for most water loss. The average daily urine output is 1200 to 1500 mL in adults (Berman et al., 2016). About 500 mL of urine per day is required to excrete metabolic wastes produced by the body. Insensible water loss occurs through the skin, lungs, and feces. These

Table 10.1 24-Hour Fluid Gain and Loss for an Adult

	Source	Amount (mL)
Gain	Fluids taken orally	1200
	Water in food	1000
	Water as by-product of food metabolism	300
		↓
	Total	**2500**
		↑
Loss	Urine	1500
	Feces	200
	Perspiration	500
	Respiration	300

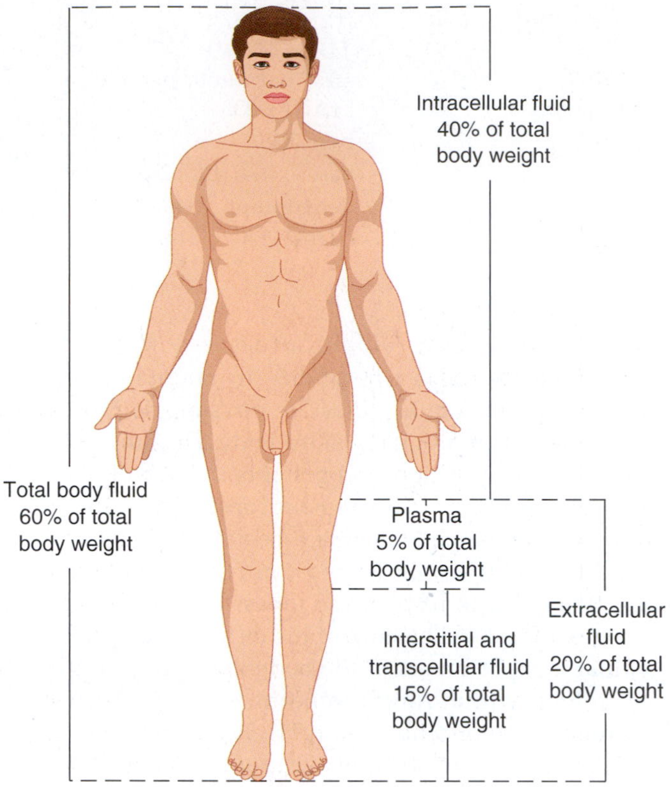
Intracellular fluid
40% of total
body weight
Total body fluid
60% of total
body weight
Plasma
5% of total
body weight
Extracellular
fluid
20% of total
body weight
Interstitial and
transcellular fluid
15% of total
body weight

Figure 10.1 ■ The major fluid compartments of the body.

losses, while normally small, can increase significantly during exercise, when environmental temperatures are high, and during illness that increases the respiratory rate, perspiration, or gastrointestinal (GI) losses (particularly diarrhea). **Table 10.1** shows the sources of fluid gain and loss.

Electrolytes

Body fluids contain both water molecules and chemical compounds. These chemical compounds can either remain intact in solution or dissociate into discrete particles. *Electrolytes* are substances that dissociate in solution to form charged particles called *ions*. *Cations* are positively charged electrolytes; *anions* are negatively charged electrolytes. Electrolytes have many functions, including assisting with the regulation of water balance, regulating and maintaining acid–base balance, and contributing to enzyme reactions. They are also essential for neuromuscular activity.

Body Fluid Distribution

Body fluid is classified by its location inside or outside of cells. *Intracellular fluid (ICF)* is found within cells (**Figure 10.1** ■). ICF is essential for normal cell function, providing a medium for metabolic processes. *Extracellular fluid (ECF)* is located outside of cells and is further classified by location:

- Interstitial fluid is located in the spaces between most of the cells of the body.
- Intravascular fluid, called *plasma*, is contained within the arteries, veins, and capillaries.
- Transcellular fluid includes urine; digestive secretions; perspiration; and cerebrospinal, pleural, synovial, intraocular, gonadal, and pericardial fluids.

Solutes

Although the overall concentration of solutes in ICF and ECF is nearly identical, the concentration of specific electrolytes differs significantly between these compartments, as shown in **Figure 10.2** ■. ICF contains high concentrations of potassium (K^+), magnesium (Mg^{2+}), and phosphate (PO_4^{2-}), as well as other solutes such as glucose and oxygen. Sodium (Na^+), chloride (Cl^-), and bicarbonate (HCO_3^-) are the principal extracellular electrolytes. The high sodium concentration in ECF is essential to regulating body fluid volume. The concentration of potassium in ECF is low. There is a minimal difference in electrolyte concentration between plasma and interstitial fluid. Normal values for electrolytes in plasma are shown in **Table 10.2**.

The body fluid compartments are separated by cell membranes and epithelial membranes. The cell membrane is selectively permeable; that is, it allows the passage of water, oxygen, carbon dioxide, and small water-soluble molecules, but bars proteins and other intracellular colloids (**Figure 10.3** ■). Capillary membranes separate plasma from interstitial fluid. The capillary membrane separating the plasma from the interstitial space is made of squamous epithelial cells. Pores in the membrane allow solute molecules (such as glucose and sodium), dissolved gases, and water to cross the membrane. Epithelial membranes separate transcellular fluid from interstitial fluid and plasma. These membranes include the mucosa of the stomach, intestines, and gallbladder; the pleural, peritoneal, and synovial membranes; and the tubules of the kidney.

Body Fluid Movement

Four chemical and physiologic processes control the movement of fluid, electrolytes, and other molecules across

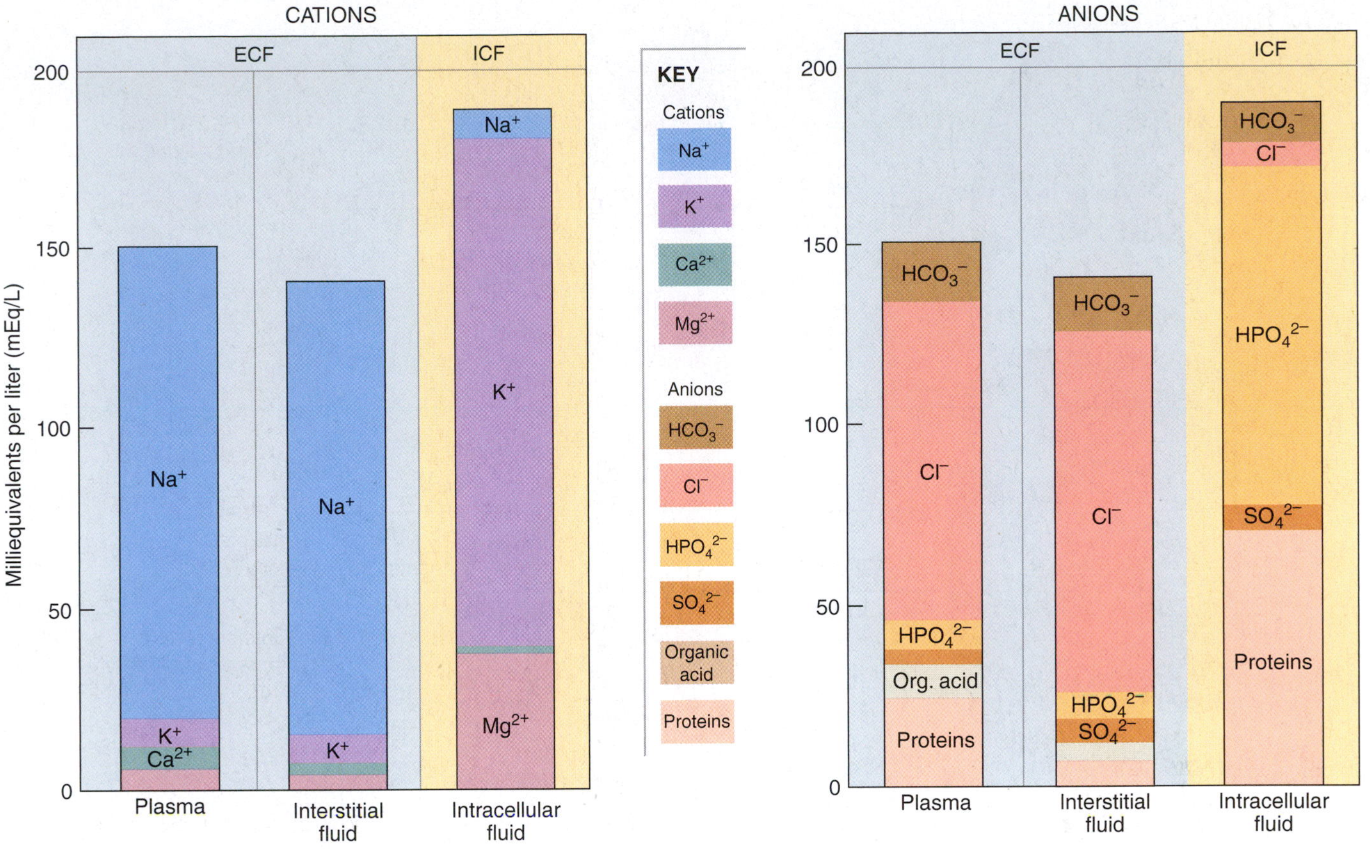

CATIONS
ECF
ICF
200
150
100
50
0
Milliequivalents per liter (mEq/L)
Na+
K+
Ca2+
Na+
K+
Na+
K+
Mg2+
Plasma
Interstitial fluid
Intracellular fluid
KEY
Cations
Na+
K+
Ca2+
Mg2+
Anions
HCO3−
Cl−
HPO42−
SO42−
Organic acid
Proteins
ANIONS
ECF
ICF
HCO3−
Cl−
HPO42−
Org. acid
Proteins
HCO3−
Cl−
HPO42−
SO42−
HCO3−
Cl−
HPO42−
SO42−
Proteins
Plasma
Interstitial fluid
Intracellular fluid

Figure 10.2 ■ Electrolyte composition (cations and anions) of body fluid compartments.

membranes between the intracellular and interstitial space and the interstitial space and plasma. These processes are osmosis, diffusion, filtration, and active transport.

Osmosis

Osmosis is the process by which water moves across a selectively permeable membrane from an area of lower solute concentration to an area of higher solute concentration (**Figure 10.4** ■). A selectively permeable membrane allows water molecules to cross but is relatively impermeable to dissolved substances (solutes). Osmosis continues until the solute concentration on both sides of the membrane is equal. For example, if pure water and a sodium chloride solution are separated by a selectively permeable membrane, then water molecules will move across the membrane to the sodium chloride solution. Osmosis is the primary process

Table 10.2 Normal Values for Electrolytes and Serum Osmolality

Serum Component	Values	
	Conventional	**SI**
Electrolytes		
Sodium (Na^+)	135–145 mEq/L	135–145 mmol/L
Chloride (Cl^-)	95–105 mEq/L	95–105 mmol/L
Bicarbonate (HCO_3^-, total carbon dioxide)	22–30 mEq/L	22–30 mmol/L
Calcium (Ca^{2+}) (total)	4.5–5.5 mEq/L (9–11 mg/dL)	2.3–2.8 mmol/L
Potassium (K^+)	3.5–5.3 mEq/L	3.5–5.0 mmol/L
Phosphate/inorganic phosphorus (PO_4^{2-})	1.7–2.6 mEq/L (2.5–4.5 mg/dL)	0.8–1.5 mmol/L
Magnesium (Mg^{2+})	1.5–2.5 mEq/L (1.8–3.0 mg/dL)	0.8–1.3 mmol/L
Serum osmolality	280–300 mOsm/kg	275–295 mmol/kg

Source: Kee, 2018.

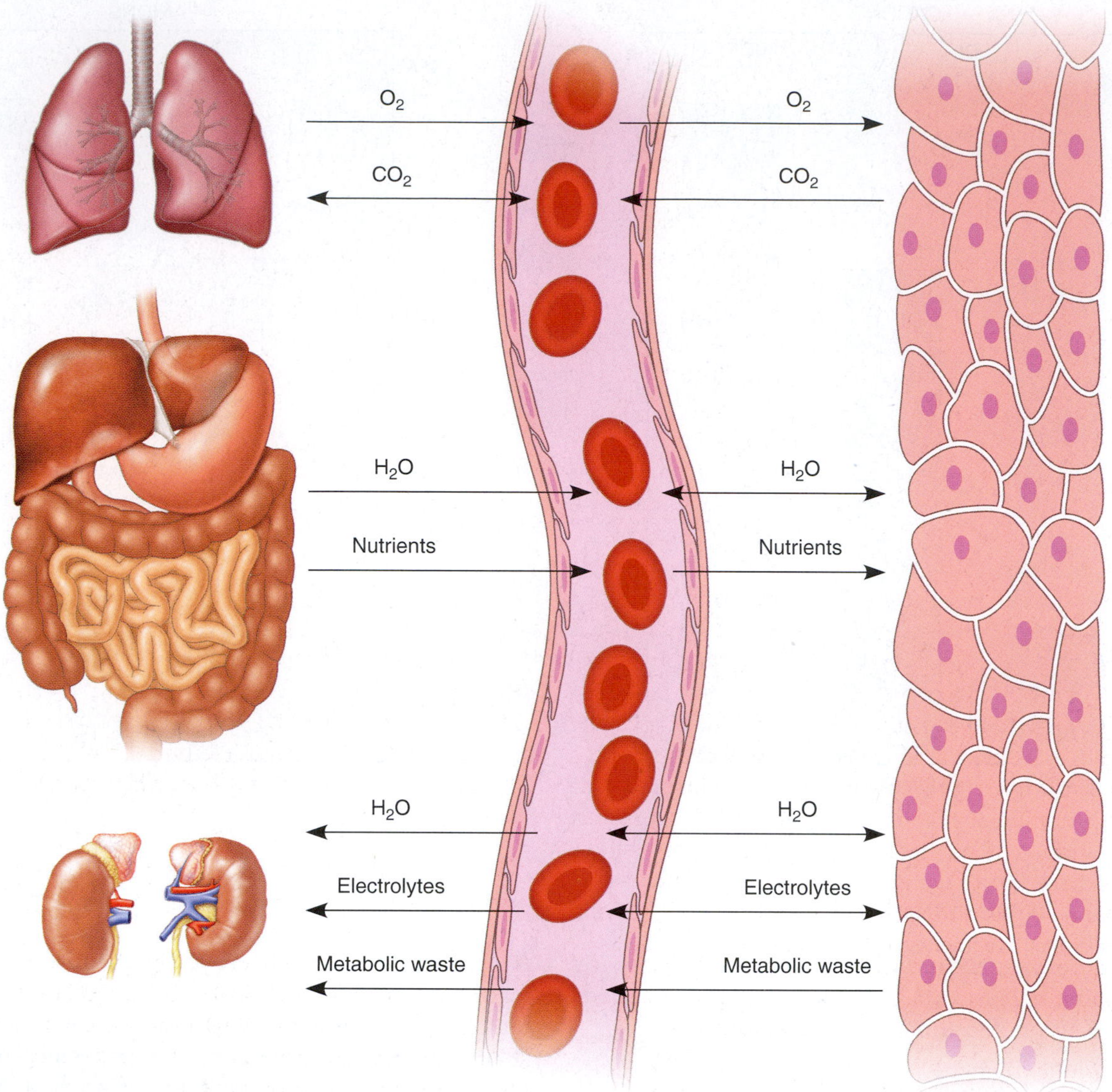
O_2
CO_2
O_2
CO_2
H_2O
Nutrients
H_2O
Nutrients
H_2O
Electrolytes
Metabolic waste
H_2O
Electrolytes
Metabolic waste

Figure 10.3 ■ Exchange of gases, nutrients, water, and wastes between the three fluid compartments of the body.

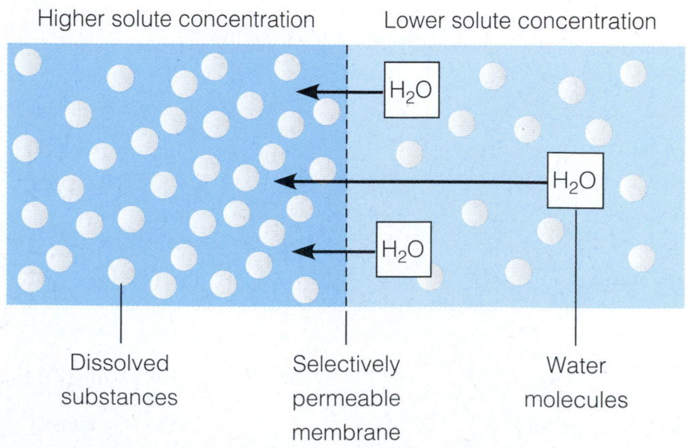
Higher solute concentration
Lower solute concentration
H_2O
H_2O
H_2O
Dissolved substances
Selectively permeable membrane
Water molecules

Figure 10.4 ■ Osmosis. Water molecules move through a selectively permeable membrane from an area of low solute concentration to an area of high solute concentration.

that controls body fluid movement between the ICF and ECF compartments.

Osmolality

Osmolality, or concentration of a solution, refers to the number of solutes per kilogram of water (by weight); it is reported in milliosmoles per kilogram (mOsm/kg). The osmolality of the ECF depends chiefly on sodium concentration. Serum osmolality may be estimated by doubling the serum sodium concentration (approximately 140 mEq/L). Glucose and urea contribute to the osmolality of ECF, although to a lesser extent than sodium.

Osmotic Pressure and Tonicity

The power of a solution to draw water across a membrane is known as the *osmotic pressure* of the solution. The composition of interstitial fluid and intravascular plasma is

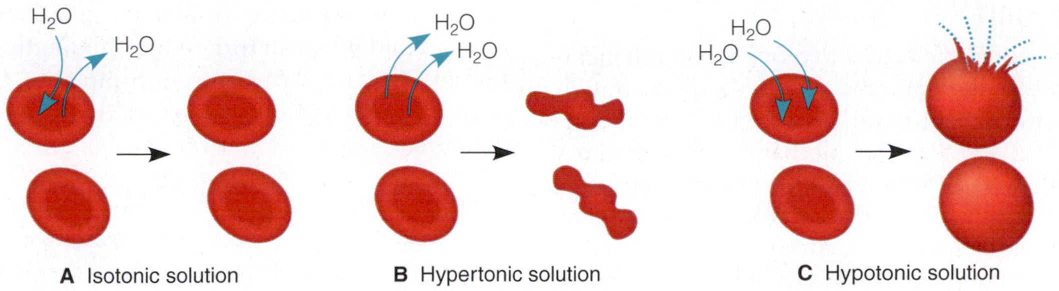

H_2O
H_2O
H_2O
H_2O
H_2O
H_2O
A Isotonic solution
B Hypertonic solution
C Hypotonic solution

Figure 10.5 ■ The effect of tonicity on red blood cells. **A**, In an isotonic solution, RBCs neither gain nor lose water, retaining their normal biconcave shape. **B**, In a hypertonic solution, cells lose water and shrink in size. **C**, In a hypotonic solution, cells absorb water and may burst (hemolysis).

essentially the same except for a higher concentration of proteins in the plasma. These proteins (especially albumin) exert *colloid osmotic pressure* (also called *oncotic pressure*), pulling fluid from the interstitial space into the intravascular compartment. Because the osmolalities of intravascular and interstitial fluid are essentially identical, the osmotic activity of plasma proteins is important in maintaining fluid balance between the interstitial and intravascular spaces, helping hold water within the vascular system.

Tonicity refers to the effect a solution's osmotic pressure has on water movement across the membrane of cells within that solution (**Figure 10.5** ■). Isotonic solutions have the same concentration of solutes as plasma. Cells placed in an isotonic solution will neither shrink nor swell because there is no net gain or loss of water within the cell and no change in cell volume (Figure 10.5A). Normal saline (0.9% sodium chloride solution) is an example of an isotonic solution.

Hypertonic solutions have a greater concentration of solutes than plasma. In their presence, water is drawn out of a cell, causing it to shrink (Figure 10.5B). A 3% sodium chloride solution is hypertonic. Hypotonic solutions (such as 0.45% sodium chloride) have a lower solute concentration than plasma (Figure 10.5C). When red blood cells are placed in a hypotonic solution, water moves into the cells, causing them to swell; rupture (hemolysis) of cells may occur with extremely hypotonic solutions.

The concepts of osmotic draw and tonicity are important in understanding the pathophysiologic changes that occur with fluid and electrolyte imbalances, as well as treatment measures. For example, an increased sodium concentration of extracellular fluid pulls water from the ICF compartment into the ECF compartment, causing cells to shrink. In this case, administering a hypotonic IV solution to reduce the sodium concentration and osmolality of ECF will facilitate water movement back into the cells.

Diffusion

Diffusion is the process by which solute molecules move from an area of high solute concentration to an area of low solute concentration to become evenly distributed. The two types of diffusion are simple and facilitated diffusion. *Simple diffusion* occurs by the random movement of particles through a solution. Water, carbon dioxide, oxygen, and solutes move between plasma and the interstitial space by simple diffusion through the capillary membrane. Water and solutes move into the cell by passing through protein channels or by dissolving in the lipid cell membrane. *Facilitated diffusion*, also called *carrier-mediated diffusion*, allows large water-soluble molecules, such as glucose and amino acids, to diffuse across cell membranes. Proteins embedded in the cell membrane function as carriers, helping large molecules cross the membrane. The rate of diffusion is influenced by a number of factors, such as the concentration of solute and the availability of carrier proteins in the cell membrane. The effect of both simple and facilitated diffusion is to establish equal concentrations of the molecules on both sides of a membrane.

Filtration

Filtration is the process by which water and dissolved substances (solutes) move from an area of high hydrostatic pressure to an area of low hydrostatic pressure. This usually occurs across capillary membranes. Hydrostatic pressure is created by the pumping action of the heart and gravity against the capillary wall. Filtration occurs in the glomerulus of the kidneys, as well as at the arterial end of capillaries.

A balance of hydrostatic (filtration) pressure and osmotic pressure regulates the movement of water between the intravascular and interstitial spaces in the capillary beds of the body. Hydrostatic pressure within the arterial end of the capillary pushes water into the interstitial space. At the venous end of the capillary, the osmotic force of plasma proteins draws fluid back into the capillary (**Figure 10.6** ■).

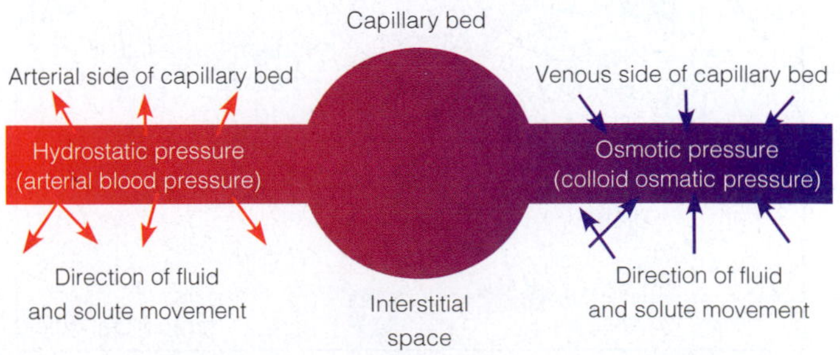

Capillary bed
Arterial side of capillary bed
Venous side of capillary bed
Hydrostatic pressure (arterial blood pressure)
Osmotic pressure (colloid osmatic pressure)
Direction of fluid and solute movement
Interstitial space
Direction of fluid and solute movement

Figure 10.6 ■ Fluid balance between the intravascular and interstitial spaces is maintained in the capillary beds by a balance of filtration at the arterial end and osmotic draw at the venous end.

Active Transport

Active transport allows molecules to move across cell membranes and epithelial membranes against a concentration gradient. This movement requires energy (adenosine triphosphate [ATP]) and a carrier mechanism to maintain a higher concentration of a substance on one side of the membrane than on the other. The sodium-potassium pump is an important example of active transport (**Figure 10.7** ■). High concentrations of potassium in intracellular fluids and of sodium in extracellular fluids are maintained because cells actively transport potassium from interstitial fluid into intracellular fluid.

Body Fluid Regulation

Homeostasis requires several regulatory mechanisms and processes to maintain the balance between fluid intake and excretion. These include thirst, the kidneys, the renin–angiotensin–aldosterone mechanism, antidiuretic hormone, and atrial natriuretic peptide. These mechanisms affect the volume, distribution, and composition of body fluids.

Thirst

Thirst is the primary regulator of water intake. Thirst plays an important role in maintaining fluid balance and preventing dehydration. The thirst center, located in the hypothalamus, is stimulated when the blood volume drops because of water losses or when serum osmolality increases. The thirst mechanism is highly effective in regulating extracellular sodium levels. Increased sodium in ECF increases serum osmolality, stimulating the thirst center. Fluid intake in turn reduces the sodium concentration of ECF and lowers serum osmolality. Conversely, a drop in serum sodium and low serum osmolality inhibit the thirst center.

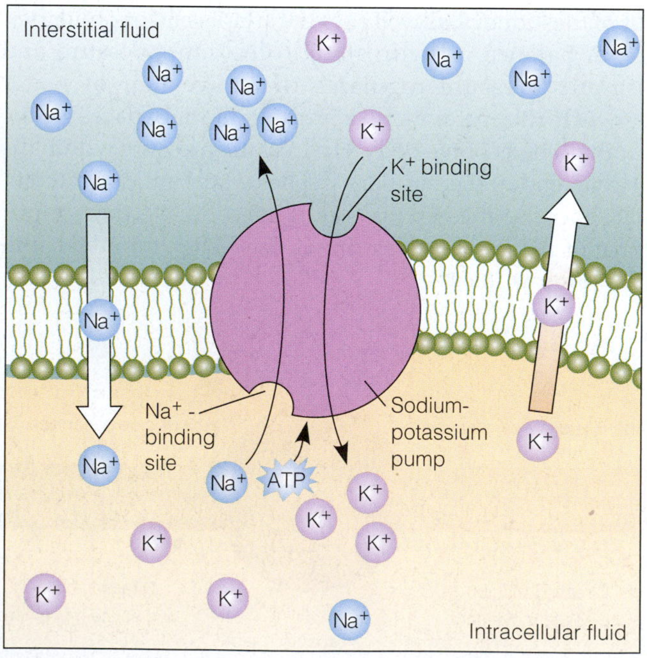
Interstitial fluid
Na^+
K^+
K^+ binding site
Na^+-binding site
ATP
Sodium-potassium pump
Intracellular fluid

Figure 10.7 ■ The sodium-potassium pump. Sodium and potassium ions are moved across the cell membranes against their concentration gradients. This active transport process is fueled by energy from ATP.

SAFETY ALERT: The thirst mechanism declines with aging, making older adults more vulnerable to dehydration and hyperosmolality. Patients with an altered level of consciousness or who are unable to respond to thirst, such as patients who are intubated or artificially fed, are also at risk. ■

Kidneys

The *kidneys* are primarily responsible for regulating fluid volume and electrolyte balance in the body. They regulate the volume and osmolality of body fluids by controlling the excretion of water and electrolytes. In adults, about 170 L of plasma are filtered through the glomeruli every day. By selectively reabsorbing water and electrolytes, the kidneys maintain the volume and osmolality of body fluids. About 99% of the glomerular filtrate is reabsorbed, and only about 1500 mL of urine is produced over a 24-hour period.

Renin–Angiotensin–Aldosterone System

The *renin–angiotensin–aldosterone system (RAAS)* helps to maintain intravascular fluid balance and blood pressure. A decrease in blood flow or blood pressure to the kidneys stimulates specialized receptors in the juxtaglomerular cells of the nephrons to produce renin, an enzyme. Renin converts angiotensinogen (a plasma protein) in the circulating blood into angiotensin I. Angiotensin I travels through the bloodstream to the lungs where it is converted to angiotensin II by angiotensin-converting enzyme (ACE). Angiotensin II is a potent vasoconstrictor; it raises the blood pressure. It also stimulates the thirst mechanism to promote fluid intake and acts directly on the kidneys, causing them to retain sodium and water. Angiotensin II stimulates the adrenal cortex to release aldosterone. Aldosterone promotes sodium and water retention in the distal nephron of the kidney, restoring blood volume (**Figure 10.8** ■).

Antidiuretic Hormone

Antidiuretic hormone (*ADH*; also known as *vasopressin*), released by the posterior pituitary gland, regulates water excretion from the kidneys. Osmoreceptors in the hypothalamus respond to increases in serum osmolality and decreases in blood volume, stimulating ADH production and release. ADH acts on the distal tubules of the kidney, making them more permeable to water and thus increasing water reabsorption. With increased water reabsorption, urine output falls, blood volume is restored, and serum osmolality drops as the water dilutes body fluids (**Figure 10.9** ■). Increased amounts of ADH are also released in response to stress situations such as nausea, pain, surgery and anesthesia, narcotics, and nicotine. Its release is inhibited

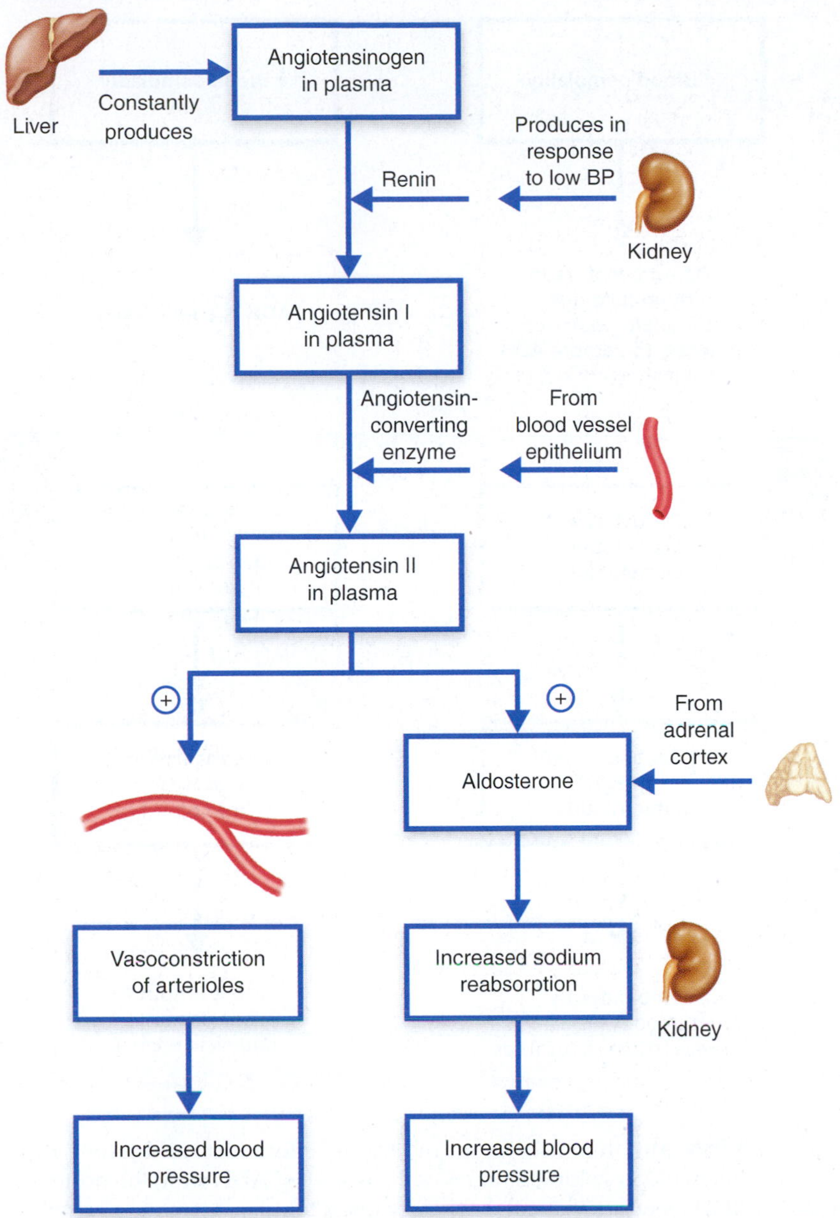
Liver
Constantly produces
Angiotensinogen in plasma
Renin
Produces in response to low BP
Kidney
Angiotensin I in plasma
Angiotensin-converting enzyme
From blood vessel epithelium
Angiotensin II in plasma
+
+
From adrenal cortex
Aldosterone
Vasoconstriction of arterioles
Increased sodium reabsorption
Kidney
Increased blood pressure
Increased blood pressure

Figure 10.8 ■ The RAAS. Decreased blood volume and renal perfusion set off a chain of reactions leading to release of aldosterone from the adrenal cortex. Increased levels of aldosterone regulate serum K^+ and Na^+, blood pressure, and water balance through effects on the kidney tubules.

by alcohol and medications such as phenytoin, as well as by increased blood volume and decreased serum osmolality.

Atrial Natriuretic Peptide

Atrial natriuretic peptide (ANP) is a hormone released by atrial muscle cells in response to distention from fluid overload. ANP affects several body systems, including the cardiovascular, renal, neural, GI, and endocrine systems, but it primarily opposes the RAAS by inhibiting renin secretion and blocking the secretion and sodium-retaining effects of aldosterone. As a result, ANP promotes sodium wasting and increased urine output.

10.2 Fluid and Electrolyte Imbalances

The Patient with a Fluid Volume Deficit

Fluid volume deficit (FVD) is a decrease in intravascular, interstitial, and/or intracellular fluid in the body. Fluid volume deficits may be the result of excessive fluid losses, insufficient fluid intake, or failure of regulatory mechanisms and fluid shifts within the body. FVD is a relatively common

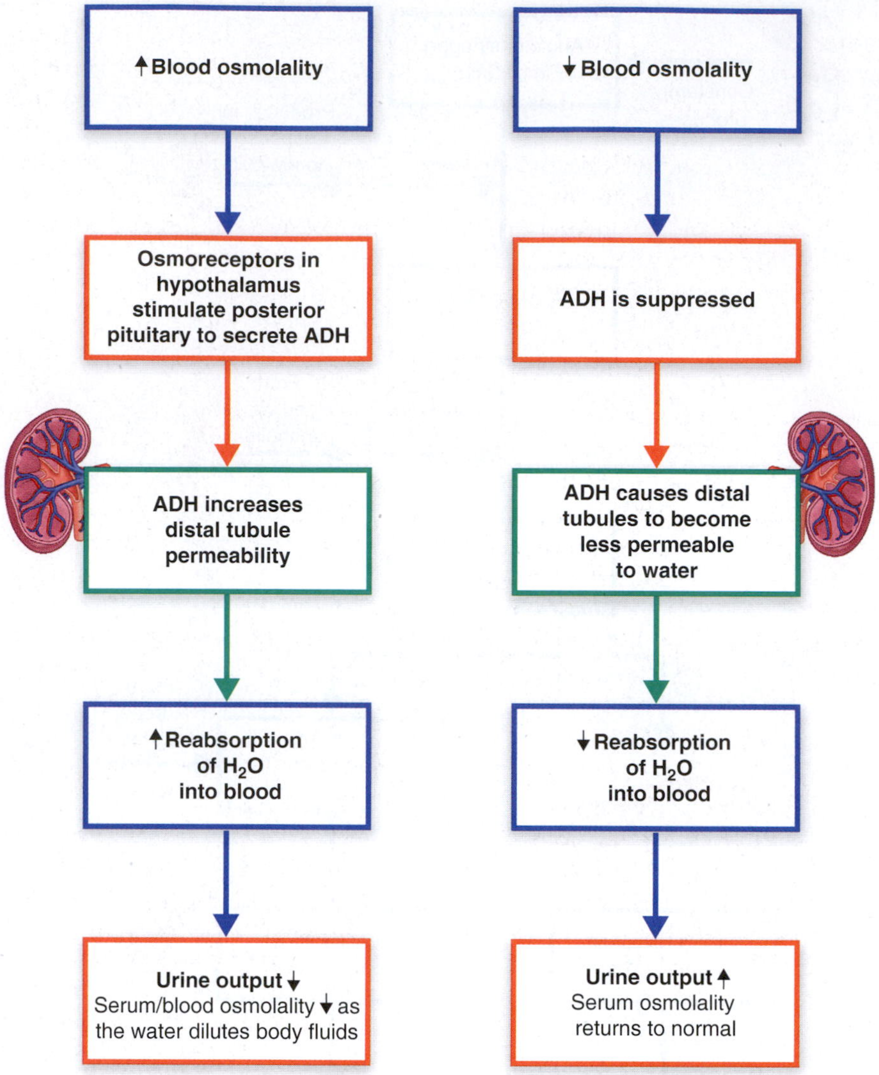
↑Blood osmolality
Osmoreceptors in hypothalamus stimulate posterior pituitary to secrete ADH
ADH increases distal tubule permeability
↑Reabsorption of H_2O into blood
Urine output ↓ Serum/blood osmolality ↓ as the water dilutes body fluids
↓Blood osmolality
ADH is suppressed
ADH causes distal tubules to become less permeable to water
↓Reabsorption of H_2O into blood
Urine output ↑ Serum osmolality returns to normal

Figure 10.9 ■ Antidiuretic hormone release and effect. Increased serum osmolality or a fall in blood volume stimulates the release of ADH from the posterior pituitary. ADH increases the permeability of distal tubules, promoting water reabsorption.

problem that may exist alone or in combination with other electrolyte or acid–base imbalances. The term **dehydration** refers to loss of water alone, even though it is often used interchangeably with fluid volume deficit.

Changes in the normal aging process affect homeostasis in several ways. In older adults, the percentage of total body water is about 10% lower than in younger or middle-aged adults, and thus they have less body reserve. Lean muscle mass is lower in older adults, and the percentage of body fat is higher; as a result, water accounts for about 50% of the total body weight (TBW) of an older man and about 45% TBW of an older woman. Sodium and water regulation become less efficient with aging. Renal blood flow and glomerular filtration decline with aging; the kidneys are less able to effectively concentrate the urine and conserve sodium and water. The perception of thirst decreases, interfering with the thirst mechanism. Consequently, the older adult may become dehydrated without being aware of the need to increase fluid intake.

Undetected fever in older adults can increase the total body need for water with every degree of temperature. Dehydration can cause a fever and further compound dehydration in the older adult. Older adults who have self-care deficits or who are confused, depressed, tube fed, on bedrest, or taking medications (such as sedatives, tranquilizers, diuretics, and laxatives) are at greatest risk for fluid volume imbalance. Older adults without air conditioning are at risk during extremely hot weather. In addition, functional changes and illnesses can affect fluid balance. For example, fear of incontinence can lead to self-limiting of fluid intake; physical disabilities associated with age-related illnesses, such as arthritis or stroke, may limit access to fluids; and cognitive impairments can interfere with recognition of thirst and the ability to respond to it.

Manifestations of FVD may be more difficult to recognize in the older adult. A change in mental status, memory, or attention may be an early manifestation. Skin turgor is less reliable as an indicator of dehydration, although assessing turgor over the sternum or on the inner aspect of the thigh may be more effective. Dry oral mucous membranes, increased tongue furrows, subnormal temperature, tachycardia, and a pinched facial expression are also indicative of dehydration. Orthostatic vital signs may not demonstrate typical changes in the dehydrated older adult.

Pathophysiology

The most common cause of FVD is excessive loss of GI fluids from vomiting, diarrhea, GI suctioning, intestinal fistulas, and intestinal drainage. Other causes of fluid losses include diuretics, renal disorders, endocrine disorders, excessive exercise, hot environment, hemorrhage, and chronic abuse of laxatives and/or enemas. Other factors involved in inadequate fluid intake include inability to access fluids, inability to request or to swallow fluids, oral trauma, or altered thirst mechanisms. Older adults are at particular risk for FVD.

Fluid volume deficit can develop slowly or rapidly, depending on the type of fluid loss. Loss of extracellular fluid volume can lead to **hypovolemia**, decreased circulating blood volume. Electrolytes are often lost along with fluid, resulting in an isotonic FVD. When both water and electrolytes are lost, the serum sodium level remains normal, although levels of other electrolytes such as potassium may fall. Fluid is drawn into the vascular compartment from the interstitial spaces as the body attempts to maintain tissue perfusion. This eventually depletes fluid in the intracellular compartment as well.

Hypovolemia stimulates regulatory mechanisms to maintain circulation. The sympathetic nervous system is stimulated, as is the thirst mechanism. ADH and aldosterone are released, prompting sodium and water retention by the kidneys. Severe fluid loss, as in hemorrhage, can lead to shock and cardiovascular collapse.

Second and Third Spacing

Second and third spacing are shifts of fluid from the vascular space into an area where it is not available to support normal physiologic processes. Fluid may be sequestered in the bowel, in a serous cavity such as the pleural or peritoneal space, or within soft tissues (e.g., interstitial) due to sepsis or following trauma or burns. **Second spacing** is when the fluid is in the interstitial space, and **third spacing** is when the fluid is in a transcellular space. The trapped fluid is unavailable to support cardiovascular or renal function; thus, it represents a volume loss.

Increased vascular permeability or decreased protein levels can trigger third spacing (Wagner & Hardin-Pierce, 2014). Stress hormones released in response to tissue trauma or sepsis (catecholamines in particular) promote redistribution of blood to vital organs (the heart and brain). Renal blood flow falls, stimulating the RAAS. This promotes sodium and water retention to maintain intravascular volume. The blood vessel and tissue damage caused by trauma or sepsis stimulate the release of inflammatory mediators such as histamine and prostaglandins. These substances lead to local vasodilation and increased capillary permeability, allowing fluid to accumulate in interstitial tissues. Hypoproteinemia (low plasma protein levels) affects the balance of hydrostatic pressure to osmotic pressure in capillary beds, allowing fluid to accumulate within serous cavities and interstitial tissues.

Assessing the extent of FVD resulting from second and third spacing is difficult. Fluid trapped within the body is not apparent as output. Some signs of second and third spacing are edema in dependent regions of the body, difficulty breathing (with edema in the pulmonary system), confusion, increased intracranial pressure (with edema in cranial space, usually brain tissue), and pleural effusions (with third spacing) (Wagner & Hardin-Pierce, 2014).

Manifestations

With a rapid fluid loss (such as hemorrhage or uncontrolled vomiting), manifestations of hypovolemia develop rapidly. When the loss of fluid occurs more gradually, the patient's fluid volume may fall to a very low level before manifestations develop. See the Multisystem Effects of Fluid Volume Deficit box on page 236.

Rapid weight loss is a good indicator of FVD. Each liter of body fluid weighs about 1 kg (2.2 lb). The severity of the FVD can be estimated by the percentage of rapid weight loss: A loss of 2% of body weight represents a mild FVD; 5%, moderate FVD; and 8% or greater, severe FVD (Metheny, 2012). Loss of interstitial fluid causes skin turgor to diminish. When pinched, the skin of a patient with FVD tents, remaining elevated in the pinched position. Postural or orthostatic hypotension is a sign of hypovolemia. A drop of more than 15 mmHg in systolic blood pressure when changing from a lying to a standing position often indicates loss of intravascular volume. Venous pressure falls as well, causing flat neck veins, even when the patient is recumbent. Compensatory mechanisms to conserve water and sodium and maintain circulation account for many of the manifestations of FVD, such as tachycardia; pale, cool skin (vasoconstriction); and decreased urine output. The specific gravity of urine increases as water is reabsorbed in the tubules. **Table 10.3** compares manifestations of fluid imbalances.

Interprofessional Care

The primary goals of care are to prevent deficits in patients at risk and to correct deficits and their underlying causes. Depending on the acuity of the imbalance, treatment may include replacement of fluids and electrolytes by the IV, oral, or enteral route. When possible, the oral or enteral route is preferred for administering fluids. In acute situations, however, IV fluid administration is necessary.

Diagnosis

Laboratory and diagnostic tests may be ordered when FVD is suspected. Such tests measure:

Multisystem Effects of
Fluid Volume Deficit

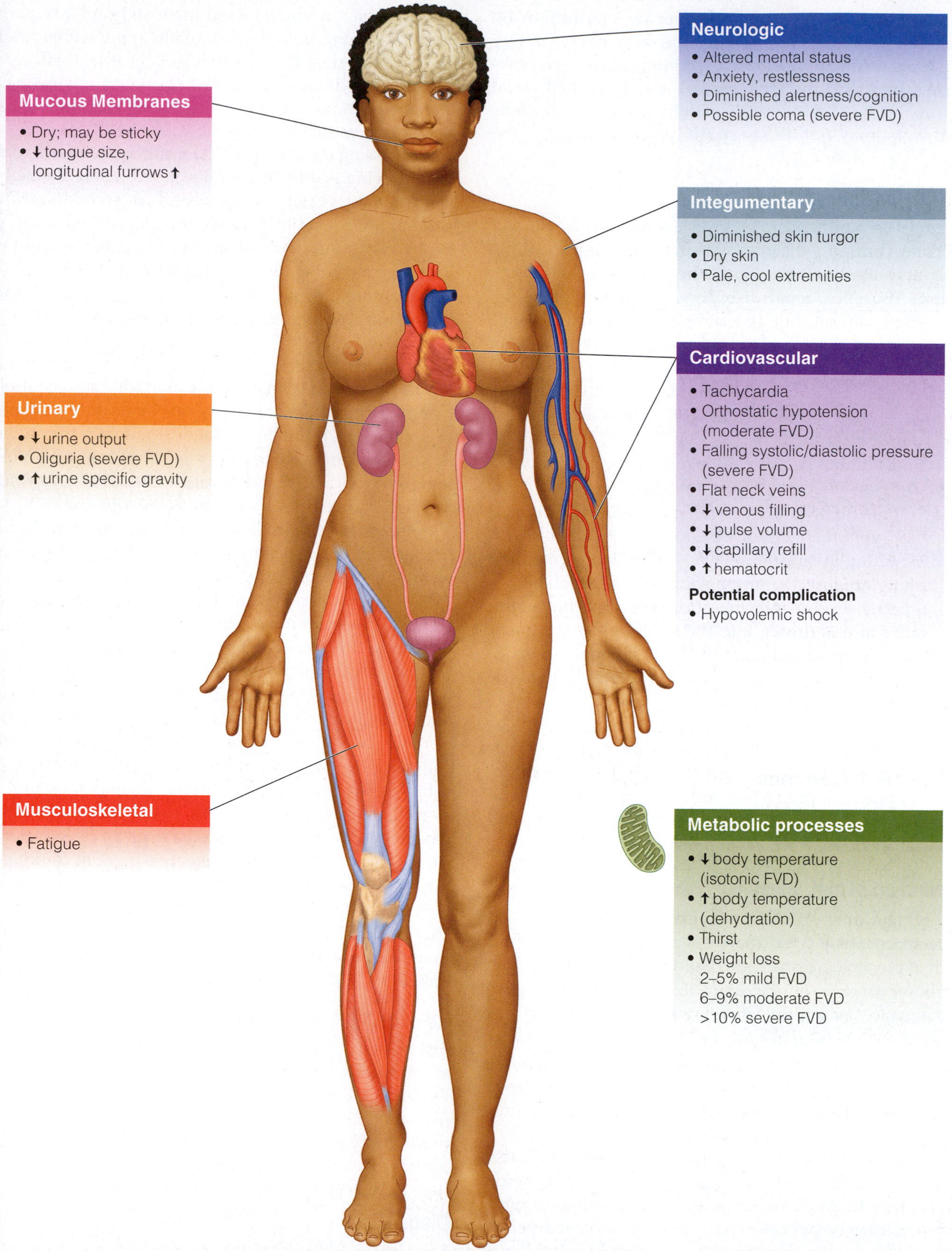
Neurologic
• Altered mental status
• Anxiety, restlessness
• Diminished alertness/cognition
• Possible coma (severe FVD)
Mucous Membranes
• Dry; may be sticky
• ↓ tongue size, longitudinal furrows ↑
Integumentary
• Diminished skin turgor
• Dry skin
• Pale, cool extremities
Cardiovascular
• Tachycardia
• Orthostatic hypotension (moderate FVD)
• Falling systolic/diastolic pressure (severe FVD)
• Flat neck veins
• ↓ venous filling
• ↓ pulse volume
• ↓ capillary refill
• ↑ hematocrit
Potential complication
• Hypovolemic shock
Urinary
• ↓ urine output
• Oliguria (severe FVD)
• ↑ urine specific gravity
Musculoskeletal
• Fatigue
Metabolic processes
• ↓ body temperature (isotonic FVD)
• ↑ body temperature (dehydration)
• Thirst
• Weight loss
2–5% mild FVD
6–9% moderate FVD
>10% severe FVD

Table 10.3 Comparison of the Manifestations of Fluid Imbalances

Assessment	Fluid Deficit	Fluid Excess
Blood pressure	Decreased systolic postural hypotension	Increased
Heart rate	Increased	Increased
Pulse amplitude	Decreased	Increased
Respirations	Normal	Moist crackles Wheezing
Jugular vein	Flat	Distended
Edema	Rare	Dependent
Skin turgor	Loose, poor turgor	Taut
Output	Low, concentrated	May be low or normal
Urine specific gravity	High	Low
Weight	Loss	Gain

- ***Serum electrolytes.*** In an isotonic fluid deficit, sodium levels are within normal limits; when the loss is water only, sodium levels are high. Decreases in potassium are common.
- ***Serum osmolality.*** Measurement of serum osmolality helps to differentiate isotonic fluid loss from water loss. With water loss, osmolality is high; it may be within normal limits with an isotonic fluid loss.
- ***Hemoglobin and hematocrit.*** The hematocrit is often elevated due to loss of intravascular volume and hemoconcentration.
- ***Urine specific gravity and osmolality.*** As the kidneys conserve water, both the specific gravity and osmolality of urine increase.
- ***Hemodynamic pressures.*** The mean arterial pressure (MAP), central venous pressure (CVP), right atrial pressure (RAP), and pulmonary artery wedge pressure (PAWP) are decreased in severe FVD (Perrin & MacLeod, 2018).

Fluid Management

Oral Rehydration. Oral rehydration is the safest and most effective treatment for FVD in alert patients who are able to take in and retain oral fluids. Adults require a minimum of 1500 mL of fluid per day or approximately 30 mL per kilogram of body weight (ideal body weight is used to calculate fluid requirements for patients who are obese) for maintenance. Fluids are replaced gradually, particularly in older adults, to prevent rapid rehydration of the cells.

For mild fluid deficits in which a loss of electrolytes has been minimal (e.g., moderate exercise in warm weather), water alone may be used for fluid replacement. When the fluid deficit is more severe and when electrolytes have also been lost (e.g., due to vomiting and/or diarrhea, strenuous exercise for longer than an hour or two), a carbohydrate/electrolyte solution such as a sports drink, ginger ale, or a rehydrating solution (e.g., Pedialyte or Rehydralyte) is more appropriate. These solutions provide sodium, potassium, chloride, and calories to help meet metabolic needs.

IV Rehydration. When the fluid deficit is severe or the patient is unable to ingest fluids, the IV route is used to administer replacement fluids. **Table 10.4** describes commonly administered IV fluids with nursing implications. Isotonic electrolyte solutions (0.9% NaCl or Ringer solution) are used to expand plasma volume in hypotensive patients or to replace abnormal losses, which are usually isotonic in nature. These solutions provide additional electrolytes

Table 10.4 Commonly Administered IV Fluids with Nursing Implications

Fluids	Nursing Implications
Isotonic Solutions	
0.9% sodium chloride (normal saline [NS]) Lactated Ringer solution Plasma-Lyte 148 5% dextrose in water (D_5W)	■ Monitor for fluid overload; if manifestations occur, discontinue fluids and notify the healthcare provider. ■ Do not administer lactated Ringer solution to patients with severe liver disease because the lactate may not convert to bicarbonate, leading to acidosis. Do not administer if the patient has a blood pH of more than 7.50. ■ If administering lactated Ringer solution, monitor potassium levels and cardiac rhythm; if abnormal, notify the healthcare provider. ■ D_5W should not be administered to patients at risk for cerebral edema.
Hypotonic Solutions	
0.45% sodium chloride (1/2NS) 0.225% sodium chloride (1/4NS)	■ Monitor for inflammation and infiltration at IV insertion site because hypotonic solutions may cause cell lysis, including at the insertion site. ■ Monitor plasma sodium levels. ■ Do not administer to patients at risk for increased intracranial pressure (e.g., head trauma, stroke, neurosurgery). ■ Do not administer to patients at risk for third-space shifts (burns, trauma, liver disease, malnutrition).
Hypertonic Solutions	
D_5 NS D_5 in lactated Ringer solution 10% dextrose in water ($D_{10}W$) 3% sodium chloride 5% sodium chloride Parenteral nutrition solutions	■ Monitor for inflammation and infiltration at IV insertion site because hypertonic solutions cause cells to shrink, exposing the basement membrane of the vein. ■ Monitor plasma sodium levels. ■ Monitor for circulatory overload. ■ Do not administer to patients with diabetic ketoacidosis or impaired cardiac or kidney function.
SAFETY ALERT: Hypertonic solutions should be administered through a central venous access device to reduce the risk of vessel damage. ■	

Sources: Data from Berman et al., 2016; Hogan, 2013; Perrin & MacLeod, 2018; Wagner & Hardin-Pierce, 2014.

such as potassium, a buffer (lactate or acetate) as needed, and water (Adams, Holland, & Urban, 2017). Normal saline (0.9% NaCl) tends to remain in the vascular compartment, increasing blood volume. When administered rapidly, however, this solution can precipitate acid–base imbalances, so balanced electrolyte solutions such as lactated Ringer solution are preferred to expand plasma volume.

Five percent dextrose in 0.45% saline (D_5 1/2NS) or 0.45% NaCl is given to provide water to treat total body water deficits. D_5W, although isotonic in the bag, is not used for fluid resuscitation because the dextrose is rapidly metabolized and the subsequent fluid is hypotonic. Saline solution (0.45% NaCl with or without added electrolytes) or 5% dextrose in 0.45% sodium chloride is used as a maintenance solution (Metheny, 2012). The addition of dextrose also provides a minimal number of calories.

Nursing Care

Nurses are responsible for identifying patients at risk for FVD, initiating and carrying out interventions to prevent and treat FVD, and monitoring the effects of therapy.

Assessment

Collect assessment data through the health history interview and physical examination:

- ***Health history:*** risk factors such as medications, acute or chronic renal or endocrine disease; precipitating factors such as hot weather, extensive exercise, lack of access to fluids, recent illness (especially if accompanied by fever, vomiting, and/or diarrhea); onset and duration of manifestations
- ***Physical assessment:*** weight; vital signs including orthostatic blood pressure and pulse; peripheral pulses and capillary refill; jugular neck vein distention; skin color, temperature, turgor; level of consciousness and mentation; urine output. Allow the older adult to stand quietly for a full minute before rechecking blood pressure and pulse when measuring orthostatic vital signs.

Priorities of Care

Restoration of adequate fluid volume is critical to support tissue perfusion and organ function. Concurrently, the nurse employs measures to prevent injury associated with FVD.

Diagnoses, Outcomes, and Interventions

Nursing diagnoses and interventions for the patient with FVD focus on managing the effects of the deficit and preventing complications.

Promote Adequate Fluid Volume. Patients with a FVD due to abnormal losses, inadequate intake, or impaired fluid regulation require close monitoring as well as immediate and ongoing fluid replacement.

Expected Outcome: Patient's fluid volume and balance will be restored as evidenced by weight within previous parameters and balanced intake and output.

The nurse will:

- Assess intake and output accurately, monitoring fluid balance. In acute situations, hourly intake and output may be indicated. *Urine output should normally be 30 to 60 mL per hour. Urine output of less than 0.5mL/kg/hr for more than 6 hours can indicate reduction in kidney function and a risk for acute renal injury* (Perrin & MacLeod, 2018). At the first sign of decreased urinary output, the healthcare provider should be notified.

SAFETY ALERT: Report a urine output of less than 30 mL per hour to the patient's healthcare provider. ■

- Assess vital signs, CVP, and peripheral pulse volume at least every 4 hours. *Hypotension, tachycardia, low CVP, and weak, easily obliterated peripheral pulses indicate hypovolemia.*
- Weigh daily under standard conditions (time of day, clothing, and scale). *In most instances (except third spacing), changes in weight accurately reflect fluid balance.*
- Administer and monitor the intake of oral fluids as prescribed. Identify beverage preferences and provide these on a schedule. *Oral fluid replacement is preferred when the patient is able to drink and retain fluids.*
- Administer IV fluids as prescribed using an infusion pump. Monitor for indicators of fluid overload if rapid fluid replacement is ordered: dyspnea, tachypnea, tachycardia, increased CVP, jugular vein distention, and edema. *Rapid fluid replacement may lead to hypervolemia, resulting in pulmonary edema and cardiac failure, particularly in patients with compromised cardiac and renal function.*
- Monitor laboratory values: electrolytes, serum osmolality, blood urea nitrogen (BUN), and hematocrit. *Rehydration may lead to changes in serum electrolytes, osmolality, BUN, and hematocrit. In some cases, electrolyte replacement may be necessary during rehydration.*

Promote Effective Tissue Perfusion. A FVD can lead to decreased perfusion of renal, cerebral, and peripheral tissues. Inadequate renal perfusion can lead to acute kidney injury. Decreased cerebral perfusion leads to changes in mental status and cognitive function, causing restlessness, anxiety, agitation, excitability, confusion, vertigo, fainting, and weakness.

Expected Outcome: Patient will not develop any manifestations of impaired tissue and organ perfusion.

The nurse will:

- Monitor for changes in level of consciousness and mental status. *Restlessness, anxiety, confusion, and agitation may indicate inadequate cerebral blood flow and circulatory collapse.*
- Monitor serum creatinine, BUN, and cardiac enzymes, reporting elevated levels to the physician. *Elevated levels may indicate impaired renal function or cardiac perfusion related to circulatory failure.*
- Turn at least every 2 hours. Provide good skin care and monitor for evidence of skin or tissue breakdown. *Impaired circulation to peripheral tissues increases the risk of skin breakdown. Turn frequently to relieve pressure over*

bony prominences. Keep skin clean, dry, and moisturized to help maintain integrity.

Reduce Risk for Injury. The patient with FVD is at risk for injury because of dizziness and loss of balance resulting from decreased cerebral perfusion secondary to hypovolemia.

Expected Outcome: Patient will be free of injury.

The nurse will:

- Institute safety precautions, including keeping the bed in a low position and slowly raising the patient from supine to sitting or sitting to standing position. *Using safety precautions and allowing time for the blood pressure to adjust to position changes reduce the risk of injury.*
- Teach patient and family members how to reduce orthostatic hypotension:
  a. Move from one position to another in stages; for example, sit on the side of the bed for a few minutes before standing.
  b. Avoid prolonged standing.
  c. Rest in a recliner rather than in bed during the day.
  d. Use assistive devices to pick up objects from the floor rather than stooping.

  Teaching measures to reduce orthostatic hypotension reduces the patient's risk for injury. Prolonged standing allows blood to pool in the legs, reducing venous return and cardiac output.

Delegating Nursing Care Activities

As appropriate and allowed by designated duties and responsibilities of assistive personnel, the nurse may delegate nursing care activities such as measuring fluid intake and output, collecting vital signs (including orthostatic vital signs), encouraging oral or enteral fluid intake, and skin care.

Transitions of Care

Preventing dehydration requires educating all age groups about the signs and symptoms of dehydration. This especially includes older adults, who may have changes in thirst patterns, and the young, who may not be able to obtain fluids on their own.

Discuss the importance of maintaining adequate fluid intake, particularly when exercising and during hot weather. Advise patients to use commercial sports drinks to replace both water and electrolytes when exercising during warm weather. Instruct patients to maintain fluid intake when ill, particularly during periods of fever or when diarrhea is a problem.

Depending on the severity and cause of the FVD, the acute patient may be managed in the home, hospital, or long-term care facility. For example, if the FVD is due to a gastrointestinal illness and the patient is able to retain small sips of fluids, then this can be managed at home under the guidance of the primary care provider. If the patient is older, confused, and unable to take in fluids, then this is managed best in an in-patient setting. Assess the patient's understanding of the cause of the deficit and the fluids necessary for providing replacement.

Carefully monitor the intake and output of patients at risk for abnormal fluid losses through vomiting, diarrhea, nasogastric suction, increased urine output, fever, or draining wounds. Monitor fluid intake in patients with decreased level of consciousness, disorientation, nausea, anorexia, and physical limitations.

When transitioning older adults from the acute care setting to a more long-term setting, it is important to provide information to the new facility concerning favorite fluids and any unusual signs and symptoms of dehydration that the patient has exhibited in the past.

See the accompanying Moving Evidence into Action box for a discussion about determining fluid intake requirements for residents of long-term care facilities.

Moving Evidence into Action

Determining Fluid Intake Requirements for Residents of Long-Term Care Facilities

Clinical Issue

Residents of long-term care facilities are at significant risk for developing FVD. Most are older adults, many have some degree of dementia, and a significant number are dependent on caregivers to provide fluids. Dehydration, when it occurs, can be a sentinel health event leading to serious and potentially life-threatening secondary problems.

External Evidence

A recent study examined fluid intake in a hospital setting, though the findings are applicable to a number of settings that care for older patients. The main issues discovered were the inability to open containers of different fluids *even for those who can eat without assistance*, incorrect preferred temperature, and the offering of limited types of fluids that are not preferred by the patient. Almost half of those in the study needed only limited or no assistance with feeding (49%), and no subject in the study received target fluid intake (250 mL) (McCrow, Morton, Travers, Harvey, & Eeles, 2016).

Internal Evidence

When examining internal evidence, one must consider what types of oral fluids are available to be offered. Taste buds change in older adults along with the ability to sense different temperatures. Something as simple as having nursing staff ask the following questions about fluids offered at mealtimes can lead to improvement in fluid intake:

- "Can I open up what you have to drink for you?"
- "Do you like what you have on your tray to drink?"
- "Would you like something else to drink?"
- "Do I need to warm up your beverage for you or add an ice cube to cool it down?"

This discussion, however, would take time, effort, and knowledge concerning which beverages are available. One would need to assess the cost of a nurse doing this or whether it can be delegated to unlicensed personnel.

(continued)

Patient Considerations

Patient input as to what fluids are consumed is important. Patients are more likely to drink if the fluids are liked and at the correct temperature. Not every facility will be able to offer every type of beverage, but a selection of different types should be available to the patients.

Putting the Pieces Together

Asking residents in nursing homes what type of fluids they wish to consume is important. Also, assisting with simple activities such as opening up the container can lead to increased fluid intake for those who eat independently. A plan should be in place on every floor to open up fluid containers and offer fluids between meals.

Reference

McCrow, J., Morton, M., Travers, C., Harvey K., and Eeles, E. (2016). Water, water everywhere: Dehydration in the midst of plenty—An observational study of barriers and enablers to adequate hydration in older hospitalized patients. *Clinical Nursing Studies*, 4(2); 1–7. http://dx.doi.org/10.5430/cns.v4n2p1

Address the following topics when preparing the patient and family for home care:

- The importance of maintaining adequate fluid intake (at least 1500 mL per day, more if extra fluid is being lost through perspiration, fever, or diarrhea)
- Manifestations of fluid imbalance, and how to monitor fluid balance
- How to prevent fluid deficit:
  a. Avoid exercising during extreme heat.
  b. Increase fluid intake during hot weather.
  c. If vomiting, take small frequent amounts of ice chips or clear liquids, such as weak tea, flat cola, or ginger ale.
  d. Reduce intake of coffee, tea, and alcohol, which increase urine output and can cause fluid loss.
- Replacement of fluids lost through diarrhea with fruit juices or bouillon, rather than large amounts of tap water
- Alternate sources of fluid (such as gelatin, frozen juices, or ice cream) for effective replacement of lost fluids.

At the end of life, dehydration is not painful and may convey some benefits such as less congestion in the lungs leading to less coughing. There can be less nausea and vomiting due to decreased fluids in the gastrointestinal tract, and less need to urinate. If the lips are dry and bothering the patient, then they can be moistened with a lubricant. Otherwise, fluids are not needed at the end of life unless requested by the patient.

The Patient with a Fluid Volume Excess

Fluid volume excess (FVE) results when both water and sodium are retained in the body. Fluid volume excess may be caused by fluid overload (excess water and sodium intake) or by impairment of the mechanisms that maintain homeostasis. The excess fluid can lead to **hypervolemia** (excess intravascular fluid) and **edema** (excess interstitial fluid).

Pathophysiology

Fluid volume excess usually results from conditions that cause retention of both sodium and water. These conditions include heart failure, cirrhosis of the liver, renal failure, adrenal gland disorders, corticosteroid administration, and stress conditions causing the release of ADH and aldosterone. Other causes include an excessive intake of sodium-containing foods, drugs that cause sodium retention, and the administration of excess amounts of sodium-containing IV fluids (such as 0.9% NaCl or Ringer solution). This *iatrogenic* (induced by the effects of treatment) cause of FVE primarily affects patients with impaired regulatory mechanisms.

In FVE, both water and sodium are gained in about the same proportions as normally exist in extracellular fluid. The total body sodium content is increased, which in turn causes an increase in total body water. Because the increase in sodium and water is isotonic, the serum sodium and osmolality remain normal, and the excess fluid remains in the extracellular space.

Stress responses activated before, during, and immediately after surgery commonly lead to increased ADH and aldosterone levels, leading to sodium and water retention. In the immediate postoperative period, however, this additional fluid tends to be sequestered in interstitial tissues and unavailable to support cardiovascular and renal function (see the earlier discussion on third spacing in this chapter). This sequestered fluid is reabsorbed into the circulation within about 48 to 72 hours after surgery. Although it is then normally eliminated through a process of diuresis, patients with heart or kidney failure are at risk for developing fluid overload.

Manifestations and Complications

Excess extracellular fluid leads to hypervolemia and circulatory overload. Excess fluid in the interstitial space causes peripheral or generalized edema. The manifestations of FVE relate to both the excess fluid and its effects on circulation.

Congestive heart failure (CHF) is not only a potential cause of FVE, but it is also a potential complication of the condition if the heart is unable to increase its workload to handle the excess blood volume. Severe fluid overload and CHF can lead to pulmonary edema, a medical emergency.

Interprofessional Care

Managing FVE focuses on prevention in patients at risk, treating its manifestations, and correcting the underlying cause. Management includes limiting sodium and water intake and administering diuretics.

Diagnosis

The following laboratory tests may be ordered:

- *Serum electrolytes* and *serum osmolality* are measured, but usually remain within normal limits.
- *Serum hematocrit* and *hemoglobin* are often decreased due to plasma dilution from excess extracellular fluid.
- *Renal* and *liver function* (such as serum creatinine, BUN, and liver enzymes) may be ordered to help determine the cause of FVE.

Medications

Diuretics are commonly used to treat FVE. They inhibit sodium and water reabsorption, increasing urine output. The three major classes of diuretics, each of which acts on a different part of the kidney tubule, are (1) loop diuretics act in the ascending loop of Henle, (2) thiazide-type diuretics act on the distal convoluted tubule, and (3) potassium-sparing diuretics affect the distal nephron. The nursing implications for diuretics are outlined in **Medication Administration 10.A**.

Treatments

Fluid Intake Restriction. Fluid intake may be restricted in patients who have FVE. The amount of fluid allowed per day is prescribed by the primary care provider. All fluid intake must be calculated, including meals and that used to administer medications orally or IV. **Box 10.1** provides guidelines for hospitalized patients with a fluid restriction.

BOX 10.1
Fluid Restriction Guidelines

- Subtract required fluids (e.g., ordered IV fluids, fluid used to dilute IV medications) from total daily allowance.
- Divide remaining fluid allowance—daytime: 50% of total; evening: 25% to 33% of total; nighttime: remainder.
- Explain the fluid restriction to the patient and family members.
- Identify preferred fluids and intake pattern of patient.
- Place allowed amounts of fluid in small glasses (gives perception of a full glass).
- Offer ice chips (when melted, ice chips are approximately half the frozen volume).
- Provide frequent oral care.
- Provide sugarless chewing gum (if allowed) to reduce thirst sensation.

Medication Administration 10.A
Diuretics for Fluid Volume Excess

Diuretics increase urinary excretion of water and sodium. They are used to enhance renal function and to treat vascular fluid overload and edema. Common side effects include orthostatic hypotension, dehydration, electrolyte imbalance, and possible hyperglycemia. Patient education is important to reduce the risk of these adverse effects (Adams et al., 2017). Diuretics should be used with caution in the older adult. Examples of each major type follow.

LOOP DIURETICS

bumetanide (Bumex)

ethacrynic acid (Edecrin)

furosemide (Lasix)

torsemide (Demadex)

Loop diuretics inhibit sodium and chloride reabsorption in the ascending loop of Henle. As a result, loop diuretics promote the excretion of sodium, chloride, potassium, and water.

THIAZIDE AND THIAZIDE-LIKE DIURETICS

bendroflumethiazide (Naturetin)

chlorothiazide (Diuril)

chlorthalidone (Hygroton)

hydrochlorothiazide (HydroDIURIL, Oretic)

indapamide (Lozol)

metolazone (Zaroxolyn)

polythiazide (Renese)

trichlormethiazide (Naqua)

Thiazide and thiazide-like diuretics promote the excretion of sodium, chloride, potassium, and water by decreasing absorption in the distal tubule.

POTASSIUM-SPARING DIURETICS

amiloride HCl (Midamor)

spironolactone (Aldactone)

triamterene (Dyrenium)

Potassium-sparing diuretics promote excretion of sodium and water by inhibiting sodium–potassium exchange in the distal tubule.

Health Education for the Patient and Family

- The drugs will increase the amount and frequency of urination.
- The drugs must be taken even when you feel well.
- Take the drugs in the morning and afternoon to avoid having to get up at night to urinate.
- Change position slowly to avoid dizziness.
- Report the following to your primary healthcare provider: dizziness; trouble breathing; or swelling of face, hands, or feet.
- Weigh yourself every day, and report sudden gains or losses.
- Avoid using the salt shaker when eating.
- If the drug increases potassium loss, consume foods high in potassium, such as orange juice and bananas.
- Do not use salt substitute if you are taking a potassium-sparing diuretic.

Note: Drugs identified in blue are among the 200 most commonly prescribed medications in the United States.

Source: Data from Adams et al., 2017.

SAFETY ALERT: Maintaining moisture of the oral cavity and lips is an important comfort measure for patients unable to provide self-care, particularly those on restricted fluids. Guidelines from the John A. Hartford Foundation Centers of Geriatric Nursing Excellence include the following recommendations for palliative oral care:

- Brush teeth, gums, and tongue with prescription-strength fluoridated toothpaste or gel to protect from caries.
- Use moisturizing products such as Biotine to reduce dryness and relieve oral discomfort. Use KY Jelly or Biotene gel on oral mucous membranes for lubrication and protection. Lanolin may be applied to the lips.
- Use an oral chlorhexidine gluconate (0.12%) rinse to prevent super-infection and help control plaque.
- Avoid hydrogen peroxide-, thymol-, and alcohol-containing products and lemon and glycerine swabs because they can further dry and damage oral tissues. ■

Dietary Management. The debate concerning sodium restriction in patients with heart failure and kidney failure is ongoing. Most patients are prescribed a lower-sodium diet with the planned outcome of a decrease in morbidity and mortality. Yet there is recent data that conflicts with this long-standing practice (see **Box 10.2**).

If a patient is prescribed a low-sodium diet, then the nurse must educate the patient on how to decrease sodium consumption (e.g., not adding salt to foods, how to read labels for sodium content, and what foods are high in sodium). Examples of foods high in sodium include lunch meat, bacon, cheese, dry cereal, canned soup, popcorn, ketchup, pickles, and seafood.

Nursing Care

Nursing care focuses on preventing FVE in patients at risk and on managing problems resulting from its effects.

Assessment

Collect assessment data through the health history interview and physical examination:

- ***Health history:*** risk factors such as medications; heart failure; acute or chronic renal or endocrine disease; precipitating factors such as a recent illness, change in diet, or change in medications; recent weight gain; complaints of persistent cough, shortness of breath, swelling of feet and ankles, or difficulty sleeping when lying down
- ***Physical assessment:*** weight; vital signs; peripheral pulses and capillary refill; jugular neck vein distention; edema; lung sounds (crackles or wheezes), dyspnea, cough, and sputum; urine output; mental status.

> **BOX 10.2**
> **Sodium Restriction**
>
> In a study by Doukky and colleagues (Doukky et al., 2016), patients with heart failure who had a dietary sodium restriction demonstrated an increased risk of death or hospitalization (42.3% vs. 26.2%; hazard ratio, 1.83; 95% confidence interval, 1.21 to 2.84; P = 0.004). A meta-analysis by Kelly and colleagues (Kelly et al., 2016) has demonstrated that for patients with chronic kidney disease, a healthy overall diet is better than simply restricting a few nutrients. The lack of agreement between some prescriptive practices (prescription of low-sodium diets) versus evidence against low-sodium diets presents a conundrum for the practicing nurse. Team conversations regarding current evidence and the therapeutic goal of specific interprofessional interventions (like a low-sodium diet) may be indicated.

Priorities of Care

Supporting cardiovascular and respiratory function are priority nursing responsibilities for the patient with FVE, particularly when severe or accompanied by heart failure or dyspnea.

Diagnoses, Outcomes, and Interventions

Manage Fluid Volume Excess. Nursing care for the patient with excess fluid volume includes collaborative interventions such as administering diuretics and maintaining fluid restriction and monitoring the status and effects of the excess fluid volume. This is particularly critical in older patients because of the age-related decline in cardiac and renal compensatory responses.

Expected Outcome: Patient will eliminate excess fluid volume as evidenced by weight within usual parameters, balanced fluid intake and output, and laboratory test results.

The nurse will:

- Assess vital signs, heart sounds, and peripheral pulse amplitude (strength). *Hypervolemia can cause hypertension, bounding peripheral pulses, and a third heart sound (S_3) due to the volume of blood flow through the heart.*
- Assess for the presence and extent of edema, particularly in the lower extremities and the back, sacral, and periorbital areas. *Initially, edema affects the dependent portions of the body—the lower extremities of ambulatory patients and the sacrum in bedridden patients. Periorbital edema indicates more generalized edema.*
- Assess urine output hourly. Maintain accurate intake and output records. Note urine output of less than 30 mL per hour or a positive fluid balance on 24-hour total intake and output calculations. *Heart failure and inadequate renal perfusion may result in decreased urine output and fluid retention.*
- Obtain daily weights at the same time of day, using approximately the same clothing and a balanced scale. *Daily weights are one of the most important gauges of fluid balance. Acute weight gain or loss represents fluid gain or loss. Weight gain of 2.2 lbs is equivalent to 1 L of fluid gain.*
- Administer oral and parenteral fluids cautiously, adhering to any prescribed fluid restriction. Discuss the restriction with the patient and significant others, including the total volume allowed, the rationale, and the importance of reporting all fluid taken. *All sources of fluid intake, including ice chips, are recorded to avoid excess fluid intake.*
- Provide oral hygiene at least every 2 hours. *Oral hygiene contributes to patient comfort and keeps mucous membranes intact; it also helps relieve thirst if fluids are restricted.*

BOX 10.3
Patient Teaching: Low-Sodium Diet

- Reducing sodium intake will help the body excrete excess sodium and water.
- The body needs less than one-tenth of a teaspoon of salt per day.
- Approximately one-third of sodium intake comes from salt added to foods during cooking and at the table; one-fourth to one-third comes from processed foods; and the rest comes from food and water naturally high in sodium.
- Read labels. Sodium compounds are used in foods as preservatives, leavening agents, and flavor enhancers.
- Many nonprescription drugs (such as analgesics, cough medicine, laxatives, and antacids) as well as toothpastes and mouthwashes contain high amounts of sodium.
- Low-sodium salt substitutes are not really sodium free and may contain half as much sodium as regular salt.
- Use salt substitutes sparingly; larger amounts often taste bitter instead of salty.
- The preference for salt will eventually diminish.
- Salt, monosodium glutamate, baking soda, and baking powder contain substantial amounts of sodium.
- In place of salt or salt substitutes, use herbs, spices, lemon juice, vinegar, and wine as flavoring when cooking.

- Teach patient and significant others about the sodium-restricted diet (see **Box 10.3**), and emphasize the importance of checking before bringing foods to the patient. *Excess sodium promotes water retention; a sodium-restricted diet is ordered to reduce water gain.*
- Administer prescribed diuretics as ordered, monitoring the patient's response to therapy. *Loop or high-ceiling diuretics such as furosemide can lead to rapid fluid loss and manifestations of hypovolemia and electrolyte imbalance.*
- Promptly report significant changes in serum electrolytes or osmolality or abnormal results of tests done to determine contributing factors to the FVE. *Gradual correction of serum electrolytes and osmolality is expected; however, aggressive diuretic therapy can lead to overcorrection.*

Reduce Risk for Skin Breakdown. Tissue edema decreases oxygen and nutrient delivery to the skin and subcutaneous tissues, increasing the risk of injury.

Expected Outcome: Patient's skin will remain intact without evidence of injury.

The nurse will:

- Frequently assess skin, particularly in pressure areas and over bony prominences. *Skin breakdown can progress rapidly when circulation is impaired.*
- Reposition the patient at least every 2 hours. Provide skin care with each position change. *Frequent position changes minimize tissue pressure and promote blood flow to tissues.*
- Provide an egg-crate mattress or alternating pressure mattress, foot cradle, heel protectors, and other devices to reduce pressure on tissues. *These devices, which distribute pressure away from bony prominences, reduce the risk of skin breakdown.*

Monitor Gas Exchange. With FVE, gas exchange may be impaired by edema of pulmonary interstitial tissues. Acute pulmonary edema is a serious and potentially life-threatening complication of pulmonary congestion.

Expected Outcome: Patient's gas exchange will not be compromised, as indicated by clear lung sounds and mental status, absence of dyspnea, and oxygen saturation and blood gas values within usual parameters.

The nurse will:

- Auscultate lungs for presence or worsening of crackles and wheezes; auscultate heart for extra heart sounds. *Crackles and wheezes indicate pulmonary congestion and edema. A gallop rhythm (S_3) may indicate diastolic overloading of the ventricles secondary to FVE.*

SAFETY ALERT: Place in Fowler position if dyspnea or orthopnea is present. Fowler position improves lung expansion by decreasing the pressure of abdominal contents on the diaphragm. ■

- Monitor oxygen saturation levels and **arterial blood gases (ABGs)** for evidence of impaired gas exchange ($SaO_2 < 92\%$ to 95%; $PaO_2 < 80$ mmHg). Administer oxygen as indicated. *Edema of interstitial lung tissues can interfere with gas exchange and delivery to body tissues. Supplemental oxygen promotes gas exchange across the alveolar-capillary membrane, improving tissue oxygenation.*

Delegating Nursing Care Activities

As appropriate, the nurse may delegate nursing care activities such as measuring intake and output, obtaining daily weights, and providing oral and skin care for the patient with excess fluid volume to assistive personnel.

Transitions of Care

Health promotion related to FVE focuses on teaching preventative measures to patients who are at risk (e.g., patients who have heart disease or kidney failure). Discuss the relationship between sodium intake and water retention. Provide guidelines for a low-sodium diet, and teach patients to carefully read food labels to identify sodium in processed foods. Instruct patients at risk to weigh themselves on a regular basis, using the same scale, and to notify their primary care provider if they gain more than 5 lb in a week or less.

Acute fluid overload usually occurs due to administration of excessive intravenous fluids in relation to the cardiovascular systems' ability to handle the fluid and the kidneys' ability to excrete the fluids. This can occur in the ICU or on a general medical-surgical floor. Accurate measurement of intake and output is important for preventing acute fluid overload. If there is an underlying medical condition (e.g., acute renal failure, myocardial infarction), the medical condition needs to be treated concurrently with the fluid overload.

Teaching for continuing care focuses on managing the underlying cause of FVE and preventing future episodes of excess fluid volume. Address the following topics when preparing the patient and family or caregivers for continuing care:

- Manifestations of excess fluid and when to contact the healthcare provider
- Prescribed medications: when and how to take, intended and adverse effects, what to report to healthcare provider
- Recommended or prescribed diet; ways to reduce sodium intake; how to read food labels for salt and sodium content; use of salt substitutes, if allowed
- If restricted, the amount and type of fluids to take each day; how to balance intake over 24 hours
- Monitoring weight; changes reported to healthcare provider
- Ways to decrease dependent edema:
  a. Change position frequently.
  b. Avoid restrictive clothing.
  c. Avoid crossing the legs when sitting.
  d. Wear support stockings or hose.
  e. Elevate feet and legs when sitting.
- How to protect edematous skin from injury:
  a. Do not walk barefoot.
  b. Buy properly fitted shoes; shop in the afternoon when feet are more likely to be swollen.
- Using additional pillows or a recliner to sleep to relieve orthopnea.

Symptomatic relief should be provided at the end of life with respect to fluid overload. This needs to take into account the wishes of the patient in relation to treating these symptoms, such as dyspnea secondary to pulmonary edema, discomfort due to ascites, or edema.

10.3 Sodium Imbalances

Sodium is the most plentiful electrolyte in ECF, with normal serum sodium levels ranging from 135 to 145 mEq/L. Sodium is the primary regulator of the volume, osmolality, and distribution of ECF. It is also important in maintaining neuromuscular activity. Due to the close interrelationship between sodium and water balance, disorders of fluid volume and sodium balance often occur together. Sodium imbalances affect the osmolality of ECF and water distribution between the fluid compartments. When sodium levels are low (hyponatremia), water is drawn into the cells of the body, causing them to swell. In contrast, high levels of sodium in ECF (hypernatremia) draw water out of body cells, causing them to shrink.

Most of the body's sodium comes from dietary intake. Although a sodium intake of 500 mg per day is usually sufficient to meet the body's needs and the American Heart Association recommends that all Americans limit their intake to no more than 2300 mg per day, with an ideal target of 1500 mg per day (about 3/4 teaspoon), the average intake of sodium by adults in the United States is about 3400 mg per day (American Heart Association, 2018; Centers for Disease Control and Prevention, 2017). Other sources of sodium include prescription drugs and some self-prescribed remedies.

The kidney is the primary regulator of sodium balance in the body. The kidney excretes or conserves sodium in response to changes in vascular volume. A fall in blood volume prompts several mechanisms that lead to sodium and water retention:

- The RAAS (refer to Figure 10.8) is stimulated. Angiotensin II prompts the renal tubules to reabsorb sodium. It also causes vasoconstriction, slowing blood flow through the kidney and reducing glomerular filtration. This further reduces the amount of sodium excreted. Angiotensin II promotes the release of aldosterone from the adrenal cortex. In the presence of aldosterone, more sodium is reabsorbed in the cortical collecting tubules of the kidney and more potassium is eliminated in the urine.
- ADH is released from the posterior pituitary (refer to Figure 10.9). ADH promotes sodium and water reabsorption in the distal tubules of the kidney, reducing urine output and expanding blood volume.

In contrast, when blood volume expands, more sodium and water are eliminated by the kidneys:

- The glomerular filtration rate increases, allowing more water and sodium to be filtered and excreted.
- The hormone ANP is released by cells in the atria of the heart. ANP increases renal blood flow and glomerular filtration rate and also inhibits the aldosterone secretion to increase sodium excretion by the kidneys.
- ADH release from the pituitary gland is inhibited by ANP. In the absence of ADH, the distal tubule is relatively impermeable to water, allowing more to be excreted in the urine.

Box 10.4 summarizes the manifestations of sodium imbalances.

The Patient with Hyponatremia

Hyponatremia is a serum sodium level of less than 135 mEq/L. Hyponatremia usually results from a loss of sodium from the body, but it may also be caused by water gains that dilute ECF.

Pathophysiology

Excess sodium loss can occur through the kidneys, GI tract, or skin. Diuretics, kidney diseases, or adrenal insufficiency with impaired aldosterone and cortisol production can lead to excessive sodium excretion in urine. Vomiting, diarrhea, and GI suction are common causes of excess sodium loss through the GI tract. Neurologic conditions, such as stroke, cerebral hemorrhage, trauma, or surgery can cause cerebral salt wasting (Hutto & French, 2017). Excessive sweating, loss of skin surface (as with an extensive burn), and third spacing can also cause excessive sodium loss.

BOX 10.4
Manifestations of Sodium Imbalances

Hyponatremia	Hypernatremia
■ Plasma sodium <135 mEq/L ■ Decreased serum osmolality ■ Muscle cramps, weakness ■ Headache ■ Irritability, lethargy ■ Hyperreflexia, seizures ■ Anorexia, nausea and vomiting ■ Hypotension, shock	■ Plasma sodium >145 mEq/L ■ Increased serum osmolality ■ Increased thirst, oliguria, increased urine specific gravity ■ Dry skin and mucous membranes, decreased skin turgor, furrowed tongue, dry mouth ■ Headache, restlessness ■ Seizures, coma ■ Tachycardia, hypotension, vascular collapse

Hyponatremia causes a decrease in serum osmolality. Water shifts from ECF into the intracellular space, causing cells to swell. Many of the manifestations of hyponatremia can be attributed to cellular edema, cerebral edema in particular. Water gains that can lead to hyponatremia may occur with systemic diseases such as heart failure, renal failure, or cirrhosis of the liver; syndrome of inappropriate secretion of antidiuretic hormone (SIADH); excessive administration of hypotonic IV fluids; and self-induced water intoxication.

Manifestations

The manifestations of hyponatremia depend on the rapidity of onset, the severity, and the cause of the imbalance. If the condition develops slowly, manifestations are usually not experienced until the serum sodium levels reach 125 mEq/L. In addition, the manifestations of hyponatremia vary, depending on extracellular fluid volume. Early manifestations of hyponatremia include muscle cramps, weakness, and fatigue from its effects on muscle cells. Gastrointestinal function is affected, causing anorexia, nausea and vomiting, and abdominal cramping.

As sodium levels continue to decrease, the brain and nervous system swell, causing cerebral edema. Neurologic manifestations progress rapidly when the serum sodium level falls below 120 mEq/L and include headache, depression, dulled sensorium, personality changes, irritability, lethargy, hyperreflexia, muscle twitching, and seizures. If serum sodium falls to very low levels, coma is likely to occur. When hyponatremia is associated with decreased ECF volume, the manifestations are those of hypovolemia (*hypovolemic hyponatremia*). In dilutional hyponatremia, associated with FVE, manifestations include those of hypervolemia.

Interprofessional Care

Interprofessional management of hyponatremia focuses on restoring normal blood volume and serum sodium levels.

Diagnosis

The following laboratory tests may be ordered:

- ***Serum sodium*** and ***osmolality*** are decreased in hyponatremia.
- A ***24-hour urine specimen*** is obtained to evaluate sodium excretion. In conditions associated with normal or increased extracellular volume (such as SIADH), urinary sodium is increased; in conditions resulting from losses of isotonic fluids (e.g., sweating, diarrhea, vomiting, and third-space fluid accumulation), by contrast, urinary sodium is decreased.

Medications

When both sodium and water have been lost (hyponatremia with hypovolemia), sodium-containing fluids are given to replace both water and sodium. Isotonic Ringer solution or isotonic saline (0.9% NaCl) solution may be administered. Cautious administration of IV 3% NaCl solution may be necessary in patients who have very low plasma sodium levels (110 to 115 mEq/L).

SAFETY ALERT: Carefully monitor patients receiving sodium-containing IV solutions for manifestations of hypervolemia (increased blood pressure, bounding pulses, tachypnea, tachycardia, gallop rhythm [S_3 and/or S_4 heart sounds], shortness of breath, crackles). Hypertonic saline solutions can lead to hypervolemia, particularly in patients with cardiovascular or renal disease. ■

Loop diuretics (e.g., furosemide) may be administered to patients who have hyponatremia with normal or excess ECF volume. Loop diuretics promote isotonic diuresis and fluid volume loss without hyponatremia. Oral salt tablets may be concurrently given to correct the sodium loss associated with diuresis (Mount, 2016). In addition, drugs to treat the underlying cause of hyponatremia may be administered, and newer medications are on the horizon (Hoorn & Zietse, 2017).

Fluid and Dietary Management

If hyponatremia is mild (serum sodium 130 mEq/L or higher), increasing the intake of foods high in sodium may restore normal sodium balance. Fluids are often restricted to help reduce ECF volume and correct hyponatremia (refer to **Box 10.1** for fluid restriction guidelines).

Nursing Care

Nursing care of the patient with hyponatremia focuses on identifying patients at risk and managing problems resulting from the systemic effects of the disorder.

Assessment

Assessment data related to hyponatremia include:

- ***Health history:*** current manifestations, including nausea and vomiting, abdominal discomfort, muscle weakness, headache, other manifestations; duration of manifestations and any precipitating factors such as heavy perspiration, vomiting, or diarrhea; chronic diseases such as heart or renal failure, cirrhosis of the liver, or endocrine disorders; current medications
- ***Physical assessment:*** mental status and level of consciousness; vital signs including orthostatic vital signs and peripheral pulses; presence of edema or weight gain.

Priorities of Care

Cerebral edema and impaired neurologic function present the greatest dangers in hyponatremia; thus, restoring sodium and water balance and preventing complications of cerebral edema are priority nursing actions.

Diagnoses, Outcomes, and Interventions

Reduce Risk for Imbalanced Fluid Volume. Because of its role in maintaining fluid balance, sodium imbalances are often accompanied by water imbalances. In addition, treatment of hyponatremia can affect the patient's fluid balance.

Expected Outcome: Patient's fluid and electrolyte balance will be restored without adverse effects of treatment.

The nurse will:

- Monitor intake and output, weigh daily, and calculate 24-hour fluid balance. *Fluid excess or deficit may occur with hyponatremia.*
- Use an infusion pump to administer hypertonic saline (3% NaCl) solutions; carefully monitor flow rate and response. *Hypertonic solutions can increase the risk of pulmonary and cerebral edema due to water retention. Careful monitoring is vital to prevent these complications and possible permanent damage.*
- If fluids are restricted, explain the reason for the restriction, the amount of fluid allowed, and how to calculate fluid intake. *Teaching increases the patient's sense of control and compliance.*

For additional nursing interventions that may apply to the patient with hyponatremia, review the discussions of FVD and FVE.

Reduce Risk for Ineffective Cerebral Tissue Perfusion. The patient with severe hyponatremia experiences fluid shifts that increase the intracellular fluid volume. This can cause brain cells to swell, increasing pressure within the cranial vault.

Expected Outcome: Patient's neurologic function will remain intact, as evidenced by level of consciousness (LOC), orientation, mental status, and muscle strength and tone.

The nurse will:

- Monitor serum electrolytes and serum osmolality. Report abnormal results to the healthcare provider. *As serum sodium and osmolality levels fall, the manifestations and neurologic effects of hyponatremia become increasingly severe.*
- Assess for neurologic changes, such as lethargy, altered LOC, confusion, and convulsions. Monitor mental status and orientation. Compare baseline data with continuing assessments. Institute seizure precautions as indicated. *If serum sodium levels continue to fall, the patient may become increasingly less responsive.*
- Assess muscle strength and tone and deep tendon reflexes. *Increased muscle weakness and decreased deep tendon reflexes are manifestations of increasing hyponatremia.*

Delegating Nursing Care Activities

As appropriate and allowed by the designated duties and responsibilities of assistive personnel, the nurse may delegate nursing care activities such as measuring intake and output and obtaining daily weights for the patient with hyponatremia.

Transitions of Care

People at risk for mild hyponatremia include those who participate in activities that increase fluid loss through excessive perspiration (diaphoresis) and then replace those losses by drinking large amounts of water or drinks with high sugar content. This includes athletes, people who do heavy labor in high environmental temperatures, and older adults living in non-air-conditioned settings during hot weather. Teach the following to patients who are at risk:

- Manifestations of mild hyponatremia, including headache, nausea, abdominal cramps, and muscle weakness
- The importance of drinking liquids containing sodium and other electrolytes at frequent intervals when perspiring heavily, when environmental temperatures are high, and/or if watery diarrhea persists for several days.

Acute hyponatremia will usually present suddenly with neurological symptoms (usually confusion) and possibly seizures. Acute hyponatremia can occur with some chemotherapeutics and oncological processes.

Teaching for home care focuses on the underlying cause of the sodium deficit and prevention. Teach patients about the following:

- Manifestations of mild and more severe hyponatremia to report to the primary care provider
- The importance of regular serum electrolyte monitoring if taking a potent diuretic or on a low-sodium diet
- Types of foods and fluids to replace sodium orally if dietary sodium is not restricted
- Older adults' increased risk for hyponatremia from the effects of medications and potential fluid imbalances.

The Patient with Hypernatremia

Hypernatremia is a serum sodium level greater than 145 mEq/L. It usually develops when water is lost in excess of sodium, but may also occur when excessive sodium is ingested or administered. Older adults with diminished thirst or who have limited access to water are at particular risk for hypernatremia (Mount, 2016).

Pathophysiology

Two regulatory mechanisms protect the body from hypernatremia: Excess sodium in ECF stimulates the release of ADH so more water is retained by the kidneys, and the thirst mechanism is stimulated to increase the intake of water. These two factors increase extracellular water, diluting the excess sodium and restoring normal levels.

Hypernatremia causes hyperosmolality of the ECF. As a result, water is drawn out of cells, leading to cellular dehydration. The most serious effects of cellular dehydration are seen in the brain. As brain cells contract, neurologic manifestations develop. The brain itself shrinks, causing mechanical traction on cerebral vessels. These vessels may tear and bleed. Although the brain rapidly adapts to hyperosmolality to minimize the water loss, acute hypernatremia can cause coma and seizures (Sorenson et al., 2019).

Water deprivation is a cause of hypernatremia in patients who are unable to respond to thirst due to altered mental status or physical disability. Excess water loss may also occur with watery diarrhea or increased water losses from fever, hyperventilation, or massive burns. Osmotic diuresis, such as that caused by hyperglycemia or an osmotic diuretic, can lead to excess water loss via the kidneys. Excess sodium intake can result from ingestion of excess salt or hypertonic IV solutions. Patients who experience near-drowning in seawater are at risk for hypernatremia, as are patients with heatstroke.

Manifestations

Thirst is the first manifestation of hypernatremia. If thirst is not relieved, the primary manifestations relate to altered neurologic function. Initial lethargy, weakness, and irritability can progress to seizures, coma, and death in severe hypernatremia. Both the severity of the sodium excess and the rapidity of its onset affect the manifestations of hypernatremia.

Interprofessional Care

Treatment of hypernatremia depends on its cause. Hypernatremia is corrected slowly (over a 48-hour period) to avoid development of cerebral edema secondary to a shift of water into the brain cells.

Diagnosis

The following laboratory and diagnostic tests may be ordered:

- ***Serum sodium levels*** are greater than 145 mEq/L in hypernatremia.
- ***Serum osmolality*** is greater than 295 mOsm/kg in hypernatremia.

Medications

The principal treatment for hypernatremia is oral, enteral, or IV water replacement. Hypotonic IV fluids such as 0.45% NaCl solution or 5% dextrose in water (which is isotonic when administered, but becomes hypotonic and provides pure water when the glucose is metabolized) may be administered to correct the water deficit. Diuretics may also be given to increase sodium excretion (Adams et al., 2017).

Nursing Care

The primary focus of nursing care related to hypernatremia is prevention. Measures to prevent hypernatremia include identifying risk factors, teaching patients and caregivers, monitoring laboratory test results, and collaborating with the interprofessional team to reduce the potential for hypernatremia.

Assessment

Assessment data related to hypernatremia include:

- ***Health history:*** duration of manifestations and any precipitating factors such as water deprivation, increased water loss due to heavy perspiration, temperature or rapid breathing, diarrhea, excess salt intake, diabetes mellitus or insipidus; current medications; perception of thirst
- ***Physical assessment:*** vital signs, mucous membranes; mental status or level of consciousness; manifestations of FVE or FVD.

Priorities of Care

Mental status and brain function may be affected by hypernatremia itself or by rapid correction of the condition that leads to cerebral edema. In either case, precautions to reduce the risk of injury are a priority.

Diagnoses, Outcomes, and Interventions

Reduce Risk for Injury. The patient with hypernatremia is at risk for bleeding and cerebral edema, changes in mental status, and seizure activity.

Expected Outcome: Patient will remain free of injury. The nurse will:

- Monitor and maintain fluid replacement to within the prescribed limits. Monitor serum sodium levels and osmolality; report rapid changes to the care provider. *Rapid water replacement or rapid changes in serum sodium or osmolality can increase the risk of bleeding or cerebral edema.*
- Monitor neurologic function, including mental status, level of consciousness, and other manifestations such as headache, nausea and vomiting, hypertension, and bradycardia. *Both hypernatremia and rapid correction of hypernatremia affect cerebral function. Careful monitoring is vital to detect changes in mental status that may indicate cerebral bleeding or edema.*
- Institute safety precautions as necessary: Keep the bed in its lowest position, side rails up and padded, and an airway at bedside. *Patients with sodium disorders are at risk for injury due to seizure activity and changes in mental status.*
- Orient to time, place, and circumstances as needed. Allow significant others to remain with the patient as much as possible. *An unfamiliar environment and altered thought processes can further increase the patient's risk for injury. Significant others provide a sense of security and reduce the patient's anxiety.*

Delegating Nursing Care Activities

As appropriate and allowed within the designated duties, the nurse may enlist assistive personnel in monitoring and recording vital signs and intake and output; obtaining daily weights; promoting safety; and providing oral and skin care for the patient with hypernatremia.

Transitions of Care

Patients at risk for hypernatremia, as well as their caregivers, need teaching to prevent this electrolyte disorder. Instruct caregivers of debilitated patients who are unable to perceive thirst or unable to respond to it to offer fluids at regular intervals. If the patient is unable to maintain adequate fluid intake, contact the healthcare provider about an alternate route for fluid intake (e.g., a feeding tube). Teach caregivers the importance of providing adequate water for patients receiving tube feedings (many of which are hypertonic).

Acute hypernatremia occurs when there is severe decrease in fluid intake and possibly an acute infection in older adults. Other than this population, acute hypernatremia is seen in the hospital setting related to treatment or iatrogenic cause.

When preparing the patient who has experienced hypernatremia for continuing care, discuss the following topics with the patient and caregivers:

- The importance of responding to thirst and consuming adequate fluids (If the patient is dependent on a caregiver, stress to the caregiver the importance of regularly offering fluids.)
- If prescribed, guidelines for following a low-sodium diet (refer to Box 10.3)
- The importance of following a schedule for regular monitoring of serum electrolyte levels and reporting manifestations of imbalance to healthcare provider.

10.4 Potassium Imbalances

Potassium, the primary intracellular cation, plays a vital role in cell metabolism and cardiac and neuromuscular function. The normal serum (ECF) potassium level is 3.5 to 5.0 mEq/L. To maintain balance, potassium must be replaced daily through diet. Virtually all foods contain potassium, although some foods and fluids are richer sources of this element than others.

Most potassium in the body is found within the ICF, which has a concentration of 140 to 150 mEq/L. This significant difference in the potassium concentrations of ICF and ECF helps maintain the resting membrane potential of nerve and muscle cells. Potassium imbalances affect transmission and conduction of nerve impulses, maintenance of normal cardiac rhythms, and contraction of skeletal and smooth muscle. The higher intracellular potassium concentration is maintained by the sodium-potassium pump. Potassium constantly shifts into and out of the cells. This movement between ICF and ECF can significantly affect the serum potassium level. For example, potassium shifts into or out of the cells in response to changes in hydrogen ion concentration (pH, discussed later in this chapter) as the body strives to maintain a stable acid–base balance.

Aldosterone helps regulate potassium elimination by the kidneys. An increased potassium concentration in ECF stimulates aldosterone production by the adrenal gland. The kidneys respond to aldosterone by increasing potassium excretion. Changes in aldosterone secretion can profoundly affect the serum potassium level.

The Patient with Hypokalemia

Hypokalemia is an abnormally low serum potassium level (less than 3.5 mEq/L). It usually results from excess potassium loss, although hospitalized patients may be at risk for hypokalemia because of inadequate potassium intake.

Pathophysiology

Hypokalemia may result from inadequate intake of potassium; excessive renal or intestinal losses; or redistribution between the ICF and ECF. An intake of a minimum of 40 to 50 mEq/day is needed to compensate for urinary losses (Sorenson et al., 2019). The kidneys are the main source of potassium excretion.

Renal and gastrointestinal losses deplete total potassium stores in the body, as can loss of potassium in perspiration.

- Excess potassium loss through the kidneys is often secondary to drugs such as potassium-wasting diuretics, corticosteroids, amphotericin B, and large doses of some antibiotics. Hyperaldosteronism, a condition in which the adrenal glands secrete excess aldosterone, also causes excess elimination of potassium through the kidneys. Renal losses of potassium also occur from stress, trauma, metabolic acidosis, and a magnesium deficit.
- Gastrointestinal losses of potassium are usually the result of loss of intestinal fluids through diarrhea or ileostomy drainage.

Transcellular potassium shifts (from the ECF to the ICF) occur in conditions such as metabolic alkalosis and treatment of diabetic ketoacidosis with insulin (insulin increases the movement of potassium into the cells).

Potassium intake may be inadequate in patients who are unable or unwilling to eat for prolonged periods. Hospitalized patients are at risk, especially those on extended parenteral fluid therapy with solutions that do not contain potassium. Patients with anorexia nervosa or alcoholism may develop hypokalemia due to both inadequate intake and loss of potassium through vomiting, diarrhea, or laxative or diuretic use.

Manifestations

Hypokalemia affects the transmission of nerve impulses, interfering with the contractility of smooth, skeletal, and cardiac muscle and as the regulation and transmission of cardiac impulses. Carbohydrate metabolism is affected by hypokalemia. Insulin secretion is suppressed, as is the synthesis of glycogen in skeletal muscle and the liver.

Manifestations of hypokalemia are more pronounced when potassium losses occur acutely. When hypokalemia develops gradually, potassium shifts out of the cells, helping maintain the ratio of intracellular to extracellular potassium. As a result, the neuromuscular manifestations of hypokalemia are less severe. See the Multisystem Effects of Hypokalemia box.

Multisystem Effects of Hypokalemia

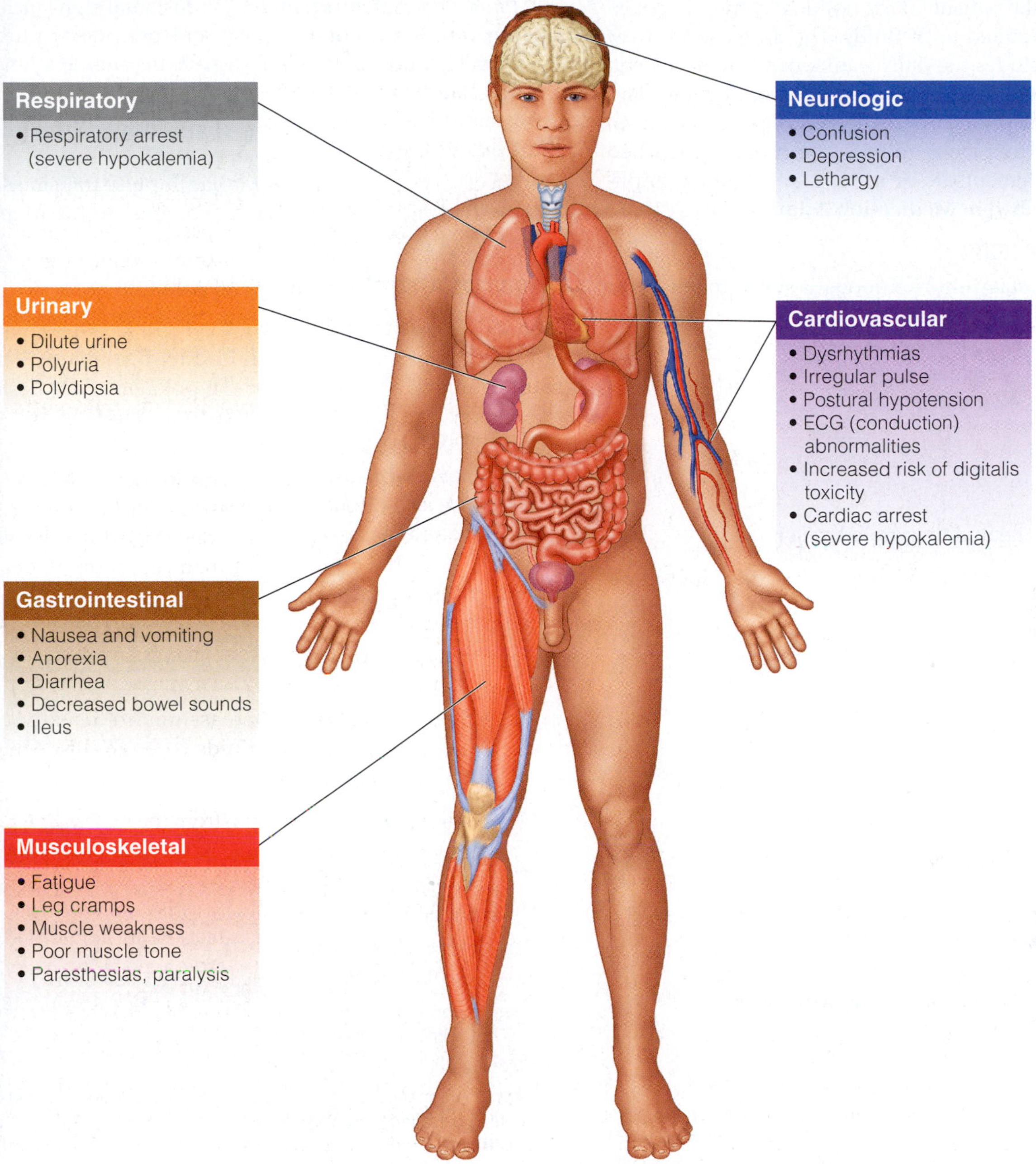
Respiratory
• Respiratory arrest (severe hypokalemia)
Urinary
• Dilute urine
• Polyuria
• Polydipsia
Gastrointestinal
• Nausea and vomiting
• Anorexia
• Diarrhea
• Decreased bowel sounds
• Ileus
Musculoskeletal
• Fatigue
• Leg cramps
• Muscle weakness
• Poor muscle tone
• Paresthesias, paralysis
Neurologic
• Confusion
• Depression
• Lethargy
Cardiovascular
• Dysrhythmias
• Irregular pulse
• Postural hypotension
• ECG (conduction) abnormalities
• Increased risk of digitalis toxicity
• Cardiac arrest (severe hypokalemia)

Interprofessional Care

The management of hypokalemia focuses on preventing a deficiency and treating imbalances.

Diagnosis

The following laboratory and diagnostic tests may be ordered:

- ***Serum potassium*** (K^+) is used to monitor potassium levels in patients who are at risk for or who are being treated for hypokalemia.
- ***Serum electrolytes*** *(Na^+, Ca^{2+}, HCO_3^-, and Mg^{2+})* are evaluated because imbalances often occur concurrently.
- ***Arterial blood gases (ABGs)*** are measured to determine acid–base status. An Increased pH (alkalosis) is often associated with hypokalemia. (See **Table 10.5** later in this chapter for normal ABG values.)
- ***Renal function studies,*** such as *serum creatinine* and *blood urea nitrogen (BUN),* may be ordered to evaluate for potential causes or effects of hypokalemia.
- ***ECG recordings*** are obtained to evaluate the effects of hypokalemia on the cardiac conduction system.

Medications

Oral and/or parenteral potassium supplements are given to prevent and, as needed, treat hypokalemia. To prevent hypokalemia in the patient taking nothing by mouth, potassium chloride is added to IV fluids. The dose used to treat hypokalemia includes the daily maintenance requirement, replacement of ongoing losses (e.g., gastric suction), and additional potassium to correct the existing deficit. Several days of therapy may be required. Commonly prescribed potassium supplements, their actions, and nursing implications are described in **Medication Administration 10.B**.

Dietary Management

A diet high in potassium-rich foods is recommended for patients at risk for developing hypokalemia or to supplement drug therapy. Examples of foods high in potassium include bananas, oranges, avocados, spinach, potatoes, tomatoes, meat, seafood, milk, and yogurt.

Nursing Care

Assessment

Assessment data related to hypokalemia include:

- *Health history:* current manifestations, including anorexia, nausea and vomiting, abdominal discomfort, muscle weakness or cramping, other manifestations; duration of manifestations and any precipitating factors such as diuretic use, prolonged vomiting or diarrhea; chronic diseases such as diabetes, hyperaldosteronism, or Cushing syndrome; current medications
- *Physical assessment:* mental status; vital signs including orthostatic vitals, apical and peripheral pulses; bowel sounds, abdominal distention; muscle strength and tone.

Priorities of Care

The effects of hypokalemia on cardiac impulse transmission and cardiac and skeletal muscle function are the highest priorities for nursing care.

Diagnoses, Outcomes, and Interventions

Monitor Cardiac Output. Hypokalemia affects the strength of cardiac contractions and can lead to dysrhythmias that further impair cardiac output. Hypokalemia also alters the response to cardiac drugs, such as digitalis and the antidysrhythmics.

Expected Outcome: Patient will maintain adequate cardiac output, as evidenced by clear mentation, stable vital signs, pink and warm skin, and urine output greater than 30 mL/h.

The nurse will:

- Monitor serum potassium levels in patients at risk for hypokalemia (those with excess losses due to drug

Medication Administration 10.B

Hypokalemia

POTASSIUM SOURCES

potassium acetate (Tri-K)

potassium bicarbonate (K + Care ET)

potassium citrate (K-Lyte)

potassium chloride (K-Lease, Micro-K 10, Apo-K)

potassium gluconate (Kaon Elixir, Royonate)

Potassium is rapidly absorbed from the GI tract; potassium chloride is the agent of choice because low chloride often accompanies low potassium. Potassium is used to prevent and/or treat hypokalemia (e.g., with parenteral nutrition and potassium-wasting diuretics, and prophylactically after major surgery).

Nursing Responsibilities

- When giving oral forms of potassium:
  a. Dilute or dissolve effervescent, soluble, or liquid potassium in fruit or vegetable juice or cold water.
  b. Chill to increase palatability.
  c. Give with food to minimize GI effects.
- When giving parenteral forms of potassium (KCl):
  a. Infuse at a rate not to exceed 10 mEq/h.
  b. Do *not* administer IV push, and do not add to fluids already hanging.
  c. Do *not* administer undiluted.
  d. Assess injection site frequently for manifestations of pain and inflammation. Discontinue and restart in another vein at first sign of infiltration.
  e. Use an infusion pump.
  f. Use cardiac monitoring if high doses are administered.
- Assess for abdominal pain, distention, GI bleeding; if present, do not administer medication. Notify healthcare provider.
- Monitor fluid intake and output.
- Assess for manifestations of hyperkalemia: weakness, feeling of heaviness in legs, mental confusion, hypotension, cardiac dysrhythmias, changes in ECG, increased serum potassium levels.

Health Education for the Patient and Family

- Do not take potassium supplements if you are also taking a potassium-sparing diuretic.
- When parenteral potassium is discontinued, eat potassium-rich foods.
- Do not chew enteric-coated tablets or allow them to dissolve in the mouth; this may affect the potency and action of the medications.
- Take potassium supplements with meals.
- Do not use salt substitutes when taking potassium (most salt substitutes are potassium based).

Note: Drugs identified in blue are among the 200 most commonly prescribed medications in the United States.

Source: Data from Adams et al., 2017.

therapy, GI losses, or who are unable to consume a normal diet). Report abnormal levels to the healthcare provider. *Potassium must be replaced daily because the body is unable to conserve it. Either lack of intake or abnormal losses of potassium in the urine or gastric fluids can lead to hypokalemia.*

- Monitor vital signs, including orthostatic vitals and peripheral pulses. *As cardiac output falls, the pulse becomes weak and thready. Orthostatic hypotension may be noted with decreased cardiac output.*

SAFETY ALERT: Severe hypokalemia (serum potassium < 2.5 mEq/L) can cause life-threatening dysrhythmias. Place a cardiac monitor on patients with severe hypokalemia and closely monitor cardiac rhythm. Observe for characteristic ECG changes of hypokalemia (ST segment depression, flattened T waves and U waves). Report rhythm changes immediately. ■

- Monitor patients taking digitalis for toxicity (such as fatigue, weakness, confusion, dizziness, hypotension, nausea). Monitor response to antidysrhythmic drugs. *Hypokalemia potentiates digitalis effects and increases resistance to certain antidysrhythmics.*
- Dilute IV potassium as prescribed and administer using an infusion pump. Closely Monitor IV flow rate and response to potassium replacement (Adams, Holland, & Urban, 2017). *Rapid potassium administration is dangerous and can lead to hyperkalemia and cardiac arrest.*

SAFETY ALERT: Never administer undiluted potassium directly into the vein. ■

Promote Activity Tolerance. Muscle cramping and weakness are common early manifestations of hypokalemia. The lower extremities are usually affected first. This muscle weakness can cause the patient to fatigue easily, particularly with activity.

Expected Outcome: Patient will resume and tolerate usual activities.

The nurse will:

- Monitor skeletal muscle strength and tone, which are affected by moderate hypokalemia. *Increasing weakness, paresthesias, or paralysis of muscles or progression of affected muscles to include the upper extremities or trunk can indicate a further drop in serum potassium levels.*
- Monitor respiratory rate, depth, and effort; heart rate and rhythm; and blood pressure at rest and following activity. *Tachypnea, dyspnea, tachycardia, and/or a change in blood pressure may indicate decreasing ability to tolerate activities. Report changes to the healthcare provider.*
- Assist with self-care activities as needed. *Increasing muscle weakness can lead to fatigue and affect the ability to meet self-care needs.*

Reduce Risk for Imbalanced Fluid Volume. Diarrhea and vomiting are common causes of fluid imbalance.

Expected Outcome: Patient will maintain fluid balance. The nurse will:

- Maintain accurate intake and output records. *Gastrointestinal fluid losses can lead to significant potassium losses.*
- Monitor bowel sounds and abdominal distention. *Hypokalemia affects smooth muscle function and can lead to slowed peristalsis and paralytic ileus.*

Delegating Nursing Care Activities

As appropriate, the nurse may delegate nursing care activities such as obtaining vital signs, measuring intake and output, and assisting the patient with self-care activities to assistive personnel.

Transitions of Care

When providing general health education, discuss using balanced electrolyte solutions (e.g., Pedialyte or sports drinks) to replace abnormal fluid losses (excess perspiration, vomiting, or severe diarrhea). Discuss the necessity of preventing hypokalemia with patients at risk. Provide diet teaching and refer patients with anorexia nervosa for counseling. Stress the potassium-losing effects of diuretics. Encourage a diet rich in high-potassium foods and regular monitoring of serum potassium levels.

Acute hypokalemia can be a medical emergency. With hypokalemia there is always a risk of dysrhythmia. Patients who are on any cardiac glycosides must be carefully observed when experiencing hypokalemia.

The focus in teaching the patient with or at risk for hypokalemia is prevention by self-care practices. Include the following topics when preparing the patient and family for home care:

- Recommended diet, including a list of potassium-rich foods
- Prescribed medications and potassium supplements, their use, and desired and unintended effects
- Using salt substitutes (if recommended) to increase potassium intake; avoiding substitutes if taking a potassium supplement or potassium-sparing diuretic
- Manifestations of potassium imbalance (hypokalemia or hyperkalemia) to report to healthcare provider
- Recommendations for monitoring serum potassium levels
- If taking digoxin, manifestations of digoxin toxicity to report to healthcare provider
- Managing GI disorders that cause potassium loss (vomiting, diarrhea, ileostomy drainage) to prevent hypokalemia.

The Patient with Hyperkalemia

Hyperkalemia is an abnormally high serum potassium (greater than 5.3 mEq/L). Hyperkalemia can result from inadequate excretion of potassium, excessively high intake of potassium, or a shift of potassium from the ICF to the ECF. Hyperkalemia affects neuromuscular and cardiac function.

Pathophysiology

Impaired renal excretion of potassium is a primary cause of hyperkalemia. Untreated renal failure, adrenal insufficiency (e.g., Addison disease or inadequate aldosterone production), and medications (such as potassium-sparing diuretics, ACE inhibitors, or angiotensin-receptor blockers [ARBs]) impair potassium excretion by the kidneys (Mount, 2016).

Rapid IV administration of potassium or transfusion of aged blood can lead to hyperkalemia. A shift of potassium ions from the ICF can occur in acidosis, with severe tissue trauma, during chemotherapy, and due to starvation. In acidosis, excess hydrogen ions enter the cells, displacing potassium and causing it to shift into the extracellular space. The extent of this shift is greater with metabolic acidosis than with respiratory acidosis (see the section "Acid–Base Imbalances").

Hyperkalemia alters the cell membrane potential, affecting the heart, skeletal muscle function, and the GI tract. The most harmful consequence of hyperkalemia is its effect on cardiac function. The cardiac conduction system is affected first, with slowing of the heart rate, possible heart blocks, and prolonged depolarization. ECG changes include peaked T waves, a prolonged PR interval, and widening of the QRS complex (**Figure 10.10** ■). Ventricular dysrhythmias develop, and cardiac arrest may occur, especially in severe hyperkalemia (serum K^+ greater than 8 mEq/L). Severe hyperkalemia decreases the strength of cardiac and skeletal muscle contractions.

Manifestations

The manifestations of hyperkalemia result from its effects on the heart, skeletal, and smooth muscles. Early manifestations include diarrhea, colic (abdominal cramping), anxiety, paresthesias, irritability, and muscle tremors and twitching. As serum potassium levels increase, muscle weakness develops, progressing to flaccid paralysis. The lower extremities are affected first, progressing to the trunk and upper extremities. The heart rate may be slow (bradycardia) and irregular.

Interprofessional Care

The management of hyperkalemia focuses on returning the serum potassium level to normal by treating the underlying cause and avoiding additional potassium intake. The choice of therapy for existing hyperkalemia is based on the severity of the hyperkalemia.

Diagnosis

The following laboratory and diagnostic tests may be ordered:

- ***Serum electrolytes*** show a serum potassium level greater than 5.3 mEq/L. Low calcium and sodium levels may increase the effects of hyperkalemia; therefore, these electrolytes are usually measured as well.
- ***ABGs*** are measured to determine if acidosis is present.
- An ***ECG*** is obtained and *continuous ECG monitoring* is instituted to evaluate the effects of hyperkalemia on cardiac conduction and rhythm.

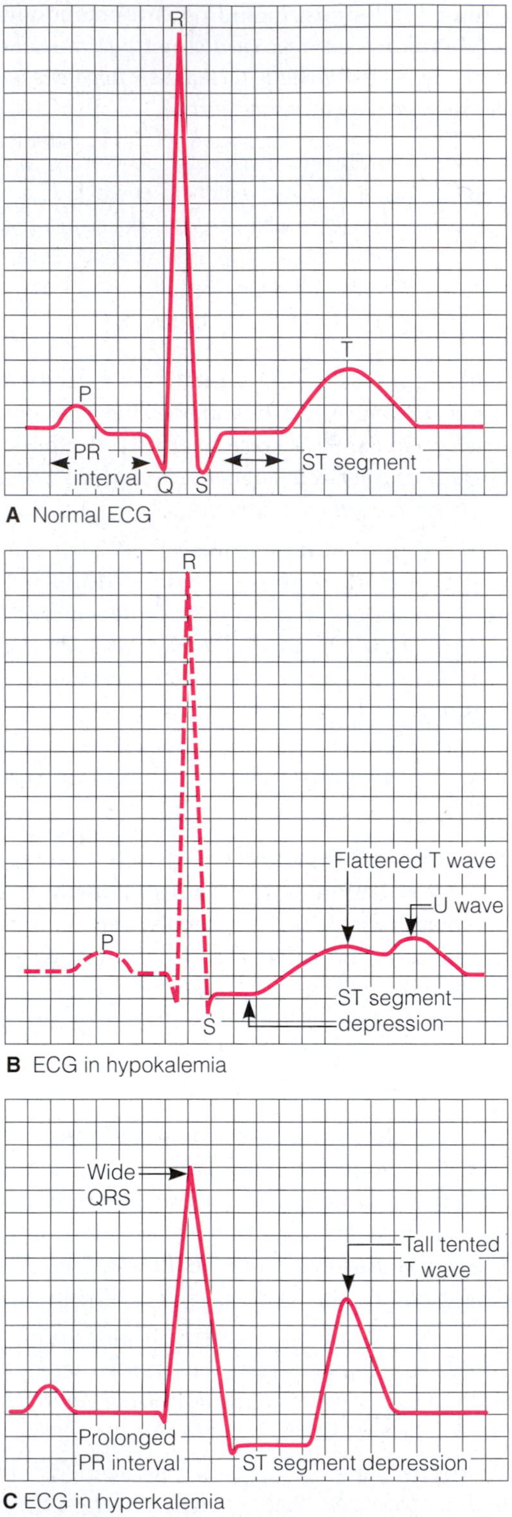
R
T
P
PR interval
Q
S
ST segment
A Normal ECG
R
Flattened T wave
U wave
P
ST segment depression
S
B ECG in hypokalemia
Wide QRS
Tall tented T wave
Prolonged PR interval
ST segment depression
C ECG in hyperkalemia

Figure 10.10 ■ The effects of changes in potassium levels on an ECG. **A**, Normal ECG. **B**, ECG in hypokalemia. **C**, ECG in hyperkalemia.

Medications

Medications are administered to lower the serum potassium and to stabilize the conduction system of the heart (Adams et al., 2017). If renal function is normal, diuretics such as furosemide are given to promote potassium excretion. For moderate to severe hyperkalemia, calcium gluconate is given IV to counter the effects of hyperkalemia on the cardiac conduction system. Although the effect of calcium gluconate lasts for only 1 hour, it allows time to initiate measures to lower serum potassium levels. To rapidly lower these levels, regular insulin and 50 g of glucose are administered. Insulin and glucose promote potassium uptake by the cells, shifting potassium out of ECF. In addition to insulin and glucose, a β_2-agonist such as albuterol may be given by nebulizer to enhance potassium movement into the cells.

To remove potassium from the body, sodium polystyrene sulfonate (SPS Suspension, Kayexalate), a resin that binds potassium in the GI tract, may be administered orally or rectally. Commonly prescribed drugs, their actions, and nursing implications are listed in **Medication Administration 10.C**.

Dialysis

When renal function is severely limited, either peritoneal dialysis or hemodialysis may be implemented to remove excess potassium. These measures are invasive and typically used only when other measures are ineffective.

Nursing Care

Nursing care interventions related to hyperkalemia include identifying patients at risk, preventing hyperkalemia, and addressing problems resulting from the systemic effects of hyperkalemia. See the Case Study & Nursing Care Plan for a patient with hyperkalemia on page 255.

Medication Administration 10.C

Hyperkalemia

DIURETICS

furosemide (Lasix)

Potassium-wasting diuretics, such as furosemide (Lasix), may be used to enhance renal excretion of potassium.

Nursing Responsibilities

- Monitor serum electrolytes.
- Monitor and record weight at regular intervals under standard conditions (same time of day, balanced scale, same clothing).
- Monitor intake and output.

INSULIN, HYPERTONIC DEXTROSE, AND SODIUM BICARBONATE

hypertonic dextrose

insulin

sodium bicarbonate

Insulin, hypertonic dextrose (10% to 50%), and possibly sodium bicarbonate are used in the emergency treatment of moderate to severe hyperkalemia (serum potassium $>$ 6.0 to 6.5 mEq/L). Insulin promotes the movement of potassium into the cell, and glucose prevents hypoglycemia. The onset of action of insulin and hypertonic dextrose occurs within 30 minutes and is effective for approximately 4 to 6 hours.

Sodium bicarbonate elevates the serum pH; potassium is moved into the cell in exchange for hydrogen ion. Sodium bicarbonate is used in the patient with metabolic acidosis (Perrin & MacLeod, 2018). Onset of effects occurs within 15 to 30 minutes and is effective for approximately 2 hours.

Nursing Responsibilities

- Administer IV insulin and dextrose over prescribed interval of time using an infusion pump.
- Administer sodium bicarbonate as prescribed. It may be administered as an IV bolus or added to a dextrose-in-water solution and given by infusion.
- In patients receiving sodium bicarbonate, monitor for sodium overload, particularly in patients with hypernatremia, heart failure, and renal failure.
- Monitor the ECG pattern closely.
- Monitor serum electrolytes (K^+, Na^+, Ca^{2+}, Mg^{2+}) frequently during treatment.

CALCIUM GLUCONATE AND CALCIUM CHLORIDE

IV calcium gluconate or calcium chloride is used as a temporary emergency measure to counter-act the toxic effects of potassium on myocardial conduction and function.

Nursing Responsibilities

- Closely monitor the ECG of the patient receiving IV calcium, particularly for bradycardia.
- Calcium should be used cautiously in patients receiving digitalis because calcium increases the cardiotonic effects of digitalis and may precipitate digitalis toxicity, leading to dysrhythmias.

SODIUM POLYSTYRENE SULFONATE (SPS, KAYEXALATE)

Sodium polystyrene sulfonate (SPS Suspension, Kayexalate) is used to treat moderate or severe hyperkalemia. Categorized as a cation exchange resin, SPS exchanges sodium or calcium for potassium in the large intestine. A laxative such as lactulose is given with SPS to promote bowel elimination. SPS may be administered orally, through a nasogastric tube, or rectally as a retention enema.

Nursing Responsibilities

- Because SPS contains sodium, monitor patients with heart failure and edema closely for water retention.
- Monitor serum electrolytes (K^+, Na^+, Ca^{2+}, Mg^{2+}) frequently during therapy.
- Restrict sodium intake in patients who are unable to tolerate increased sodium load (e.g., those with CHF or hypertension).
- SPS should not be given to patients at risk for intestinal necrosis, including patients who are postoperative, have a history of bowel obstruction, have ischemic bowel disease, or who have had a renal transplant.

Note: Drugs identified in blue are among the 200 most commonly prescribed medications in the United States.

Source: Data from Adams et al., 2017.

Assessment

Assessment data related to hyperkalemia include:

- ***Health history:*** current manifestations, including numbness and tingling, nausea and vomiting, abdominal cramping, muscle weakness, palpitations; duration of manifestations and any precipitating factors such as use of salt substitutes, potassium supplements, or reduced urine output; chronic diseases such as renal failure or endocrine disorders; current medications
- ***Physical assessment:*** apical and peripheral pulses; bowel sounds; muscle strength in upper and lower extremities; ECG pattern.

Priorities of Care

The effects of excess potassium on the electrical conduction and contractility of the heart are the highest priority for nursing care, particularly when the serum potassium level is 6.5 mEq/L or higher.

Diagnoses, Outcomes, and Interventions

Reduce Risk for Decreased Cardiac Output. Hyperkalemia affects depolarization of the atria and ventricles of the heart. Severe hyperkalemia can cause dysrhythmias with ventricular fibrillation and cardiac arrest. The cardiac effects of hyperkalemia are more pronounced when the serum potassium level rises rapidly. Low serum sodium and calcium levels, high serum magnesium levels, and acidosis contribute to the adverse effects of hyperkalemia on the heart muscle.

Expected Outcome: Patient's cardiac output will remain within expected range for patient, as evidenced by clear mentation; warm, dry skin; and stable vital signs and urine output consistent with patient norms.

The nurse will:

- Closely monitor the response to IV calcium gluconate, particularly in patients taking digitalis. *Calcium increases the risk of digitalis toxicity.*

SAFETY ALERT: Monitor the ECG pattern for development of peaked, narrow T waves, prolongation of the PR interval, depression of the ST segment, widened QRS interval, and loss of the P wave (refer to Figure 10.10). Notify the physician of changes. Progressive ECG changes from a peaked T wave to loss of the P wave and widening of the QRS complex indicate an increasing risk of dysrhythmias and cardiac arrest (Perrin & MacLeod, 2018). ■

Promote Activity Tolerance. Both hypokalemia (low serum potassium levels) and hyperkalemia (high serum potassium levels) affect neuromuscular activity and the function of cardiac, smooth, and skeletal muscles. Hyperkalemia can cause muscle weakness and even paralysis.

Expected Outcome: Patient will resume normal activity without evidence of weakness, fatigue, or shortness of breath.

The nurse will:

- Monitor skeletal muscle strength and tone.
- Monitor respiratory rate and depth. Regularly assess lung sounds. *Muscle weakness due to hyperkalemia can impair ventilation. In addition, medications such as sodium bicarbonate or sodium polystyrene sulfonate can cause fluid retention and pulmonary edema in patients with preexisting cardiovascular disease.*
- Assist with self-care activities as needed. *Increasing muscle weakness can lead to fatigue and affect the ability to meet self-care needs.*

Delegating Nursing Care Activities

As appropriate and allowed by the designated duties and responsibilities of assistive personnel, the nurse may delegate care activities such as measuring intake and output, obtaining daily weights, and assisting with self-care activities for the patient with hyperkalemia.

Transitions of Care

Patients at the greatest risk for developing hyperkalemia include those taking potassium supplements (prescribed or over the counter), using potassium-sparing diuretics or salt substitutes, and experiencing renal failure. Athletes participating in competition sports such as bodybuilding and those using anabolic steroids, muscle-building compounds, or energy drinks may also be at risk for hyperkalemia.

Teach all patients to carefully read food and dietary supplement labels. Discuss the importance of taking prescribed potassium supplements as ordered and not increasing the dose unless prescribed by the care provider. Advise patients taking a potassium supplement or potassium-sparing diuretic to avoid salt substitutes, which usually contain potassium. Discuss the importance of maintaining an adequate fluid intake (unless a fluid restriction has been prescribed) to maintain renal function to eliminate potassium from the body.

Acute symptoms of hyperkalemia are described above. Hyperkalemia is a medical emergency depending on the potassium level. Hyperkalemia can also be iatrogenic, which can be due to rapidly infused potassium and overadministration of multiple potassium-sparing diuretics without monitoring dietary intake.

Preventing future episodes of hyperkalemia is the focus when preparing the patient for home care. Include the family, a significant other, or a caregiver when teaching the following topics:

- Recommended diet and any restrictions including salt substitutes and foods high in potassium
- Medications to be avoided, including over-the-counter and fitness supplements
- Early manifestations of hyperkalemia to be reported to the care provider.

Case Study & Nursing Care Plan

A Patient with Hyperkalemia

Montigue Longacre, a 51-year-old male, has end-stage renal failure. He arrives at the emergency department complaining of shortness of breath on exertion and extreme weakness.

ASSESSMENT

Mr. Longacre tells the nurse, Janet Allen, RN, that he normally receives dialysis three times a week. He missed his last treatment, however, to attend his father's funeral. During the past several days, he has eaten a number of fresh oranges he received as a gift. Physical assessment findings include T 37.3°C (99.2°F), P 100 bpm, R 28/min, BP 168/96 mmHg, 2+ pretibial edema, and a 3.6-kg (6-lb) weight gain since his last hemodialysis treatment 4 days ago. Laboratory and diagnostic tests show the following abnormal results:

- K^+: 6.5 mEq/L (normal 3.5 to 5.3 mEq/L)
- BUN: 118 mg/dL (normal 7 to 18 mg/dL)
- Creatinine: 14 mg/dL (normal 0.7 to 1.3 mg/dL)
- HCO_3^-: 17 mEq/L (normal 22 to 30 mEq/L)
- Peaked T wave noted on ECG.

Mr. Longacre is placed on continuous ECG monitoring, and the physician prescribes hemodialysis. As an interim measure to lower the serum potassium, the physician prescribes $D_{50}W$ (25 g of dextrose), one ampule, to be administered IV with 10 units of regular insulin over 30 minutes.

DIAGNOSES

- Potential for decrease in cardiac output related to hypokalemia
- Inadequate knowledge of recommended diet for end-stage renal failure.
- Excessive fluid volume related to missing dialysis treatment.

EXPECTED OUTCOMES

- Patient will gradually resume usual physical activities.
- Patient will maintain serum potassium level within normal range.
- Patient will verbalize causes of hyperkalemia, the importance of having hemodialysis treatments as scheduled, and the role of diet in preventing hyperkalemia.

PLANNING AND IMPLEMENTATION

- Monitor intake and output.
- Monitor serum potassium and ECG closely during treatment.
- Teach causes of hyperkalemia and the relationship between hemodialysis and hyperkalemia.
- Discuss the importance of avoiding foods high in potassium to prevent or control hyperkalemia.

EVALUATION

Following treatment, Mr. Longacre's ECG and serum potassium level have returned to normal. His muscle strength has returned, and he verbalizes an understanding of his prescribed hemodialysis regimen. Janet Allen provides verbal and written information about hyperkalemia, the importance of complying with the hemodialysis regimen, and the importance of limiting intake of dietary sources of potassium in renal failure. She furnishes a list of foods high in potassium and cautions against using potassium-containing salt substitutes.

CLINICAL REASONING IN PATIENT CARE

1. What information given by Mr. Longacre indicated that he might be experiencing hyperkalemia?
2. Why was continuous ECG monitoring instituted as an emergency measure?
3. What additional emergency measures might have been instituted if Mr. Longacre's serum potassium level had been 8.5 mEq/L and his ECG had showed changes in impulse conduction?
4. Develop a plan of care related to increasing knowledge related to chronic illness.

See Evaluating Your Response in Appendix B.

10.5 Calcium Imbalances

Calcium is one of the most abundant ions in the body. The normal adult total serum calcium concentration is 9 to 11 mg/dL (4.5 to 5.5 mEq/L). Calcium is obtained from dietary sources, although only about 20% of the calcium ingested is absorbed into the blood. The remainder is excreted in feces. Extracellular calcium is excreted by the kidneys. Approximately 99% of the total calcium in the body is bound to phosphorus to form the minerals in bones and teeth. The remaining 1% is in extracellular fluid. About half of this extracellular calcium is ionized (free); it is this ionized calcium that is physiologically active. The remaining extracellular calcium is bound to protein or other ions. Ionized calcium is essential to a number of processes: stabilizing cell membranes, regulating muscle contraction and relaxation, maintaining cardiac function, and blood clotting (Sorenson et al., 2019).

Serum calcium levels are regulated by the interaction of three hormones: parathyroid hormone (PTH), calcitonin, and calcitriol (a metabolite of vitamin D). When serum calcium levels fall, the parathyroid glands secrete PTH, which mobilizes skeletal calcium stores, increases calcium absorption in the intestines, and promotes calcium reabsorption by the kidneys (**Figure 10.11** ■). Calcitriol facilitates this process by stimulating calcium release from the bones, absorption in the intestines, and reabsorption by the kidneys.

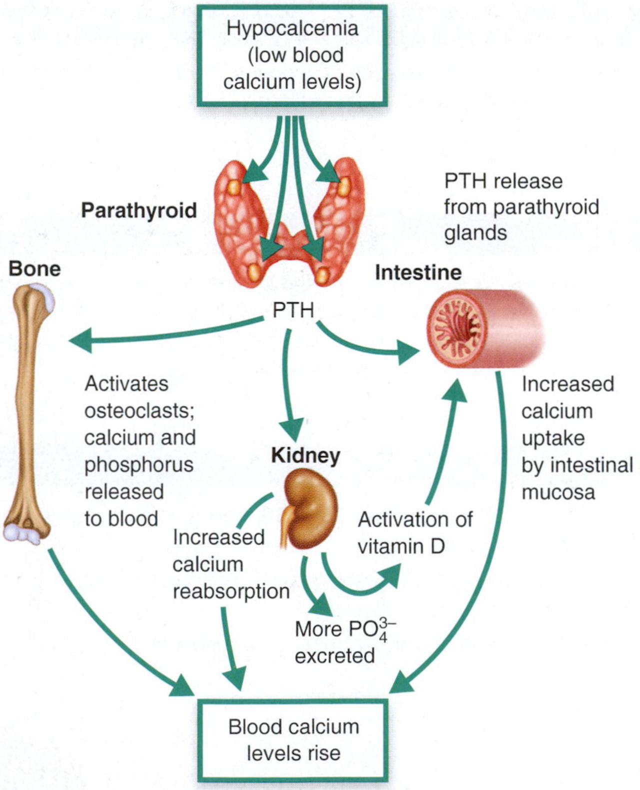

Hypocalcemia (low blood calcium levels)
Parathyroid
PTH release from parathyroid glands
Bone
Intestine
PTH
Activates osteoclasts; calcium and phosphorus released to blood
Increased calcium uptake by intestinal mucosa
Kidney
Increased calcium reabsorption
Activation of vitamin D
More PO_4^{3-} excreted
Blood calcium levels rise

Figure 10.11 ■ Low calcium levels (hypocalcemia) trigger the release of parathyroid hormone (PTH), increasing calcium ion levels through stimulation of bones, kidneys, and intestines.

Calcitonin is secreted by the thyroid gland in response to high serum calcium levels. Its effect on serum calcium levels is the opposite of PTH: It inhibits the movement of calcium out of bone, reduces intestinal absorption of calcium, and promotes calcium excretion by the kidneys.

Serum calcium levels are also affected by acid–base balance. When hydrogen ion concentration falls and the pH rises (alkalosis), more calcium binds with protein. While the total serum calcium remains unchanged, less calcium is available in the ionized, active form. Conversely, when hydrogen ion concentration increases and the pH falls (acidosis), calcium is released from protein, making more ionized calcium available.

Finally, the total amount of calcium in blood plasma fluctuates with plasma protein levels, particularly the albumin level. As the albumin level falls, the total amount of plasma calcium declines. **Box 10.5** summarizes the manifestations of calcium imbalances.

The Patient with Hypocalcemia

Hypocalcemia is a total serum calcium level of less than 9 mg/dL. Hypocalcemia can result from decreased total body calcium stores or low levels of extracellular calcium with normal amounts of calcium stored in bone. The systemic effects of hypocalcemia are caused by decreased levels of ionized calcium in extracellular fluid.

Risk Factors

Certain people are at greater risk for hypocalcemia: those who have had a parathyroidectomy (removal of the parathyroid glands), older adults (especially women), people with lactose intolerance, and those who have alcoholism. Patients who have undergone bariatric surgery for weight loss are at risk due to decreased food intake and malabsorption (Shah et al., 2017). Older adults often consume less milk and fewer milk products (good sources of calcium) and may have decreased exposure to the sun (a source of vitamin D). Older adults also may be less active, promoting calcium loss from bones. They are more likely to be taking drugs that interfere with calcium absorption or promote calcium excretion (e.g., furosemide). Older women are at particular

BOX 10.5
Manifestations of Calcium Imbalances

Hypocalcemia	Hypercalcemia
■ Serum calcium level < 9 mg/dL (<4.5 mEq/L)	■ Serum calcium level > 11.0 mg/dL (5.5 mEq/L)
■ Numbness and tingling	■ Increased thirst and urine output
■ Muscle cramping	■ Anorexia
■ Hyperactive reflexes	■ Nausea and vomiting
■ Tetany	■ Constipation
■ Carpopedal and laryngeal spasms	■ Muscle weakness
■ Positive Chvostek and Trousseau signs (see Figure 10.12)	■ Increased blood pressure
■ Decreased blood pressure	■ AV block
■ Ventricular dysrhythmias	■ Lethargy
■ Bone pain, fractures (chronic form)	■ Coma

risk after menopause because of reduced estrogen levels. Intolerance to lactose (found in milk and milk products) causes diarrhea and often limits the intake of milk and milk products, leading to possible calcium deficiency. Ethanol, or drinking alcohol, has a direct effect on calcium balance, reducing intestinal absorption and interfering with other processes involved in regulating serum calcium levels.

Pathophysiology

Common causes of hypocalcemia are hypoparathyroidism resulting from surgery (parathyroidectomy, thyroidectomy, radical neck dissection) and acute pancreatitis. In the patient who has undergone surgery, manifestations of hypocalcemia usually occur within the first 24 to 48 hours, but may be delayed.

SAFETY ALERT: Carefully monitor patients who have undergone neck surgery for manifestations of hypocalcemia. Check serum calcium levels, and document and report changes. ■

Additional causes of hypocalcemia include other electrolyte imbalances (such as hypomagnesemia or hyperphosphatemia), alkalosis, malabsorption disorders that interfere with calcium absorption in the bowel, and inadequate vitamin D (due to lack of sun exposure or malabsorption). Hyperphosphatemia often occurs in renal failure, with reciprocal hypocalcemia. Massive transfusion of banked blood can lead to hypocalcemia. Citrate is added to blood to prevent clotting and as a preservative. When blood is administered faster than the liver can metabolize the citrate, it can bind with calcium, temporarily removing ionized calcium from circulation. Many drugs increase the risk for hypocalcemia, including loop diuretics (such as furosemide [Lasix]), anticonvulsants (such as phenytoin [Dilantin] and phenobarbital), phosphates (including phosphate enemas), and drugs that lower serum magnesium levels (such as cisplatin [Platinol]).

Extracellular calcium acts to stabilize neuromuscular cell membranes. This effect is reduced in hypocalcemia, increasing neuromuscular irritability. The threshold of excitation of sensory nerve fibers is lowered as well, leading to paresthesias (altered sensation). The nervous system becomes more excitable, and muscle spasms develop. In the heart, this change in cell membranes can lead to dysrhythmias such as ventricular tachycardia and cardiac arrest. Hypocalcemia decreases the contractility of cardiac muscle fibers, leading to decreased cardiac output.

Manifestations and Complications

The most serious manifestations of hypocalcemia are **tetany** (tonic muscular spasms) and convulsions. Numbness and tingling around the mouth (circumoral) and in the hands and feet develop. Muscle spasms of the face and extremities occur, and deep tendon reflexes become hyperactive. Chvostek sign, contraction of the facial muscles produced by tapping the facial nerve in front of the ear, and Trousseau sign, carpal spasm induced by inflating a blood pressure cuff on the upper arm to above systolic blood pressure for 2 to 5 minutes, indicate increased neuromuscular excitability in patients without obvious manifestations (**Figure 10.12** ■), Tetany can also cause bronchial muscle spasms, simulating an asthma attack, and visceral muscle spasms, producing acute abdominal pain. Cardiovascular manifestations include hypotension, possible bradycardia (slow heart rate), and ventricular dysrhythmias.

Serious complications of hypocalcemia include airway obstruction and possible respiratory arrest from laryngospasm, ventricular dysrhythmias, prolonged QT intervals, cardiac arrest, heart failure, and convulsions.

Interprofessional Care

Management of hypocalcemia is directed toward restoring normal calcium balance and correcting the underlying cause.

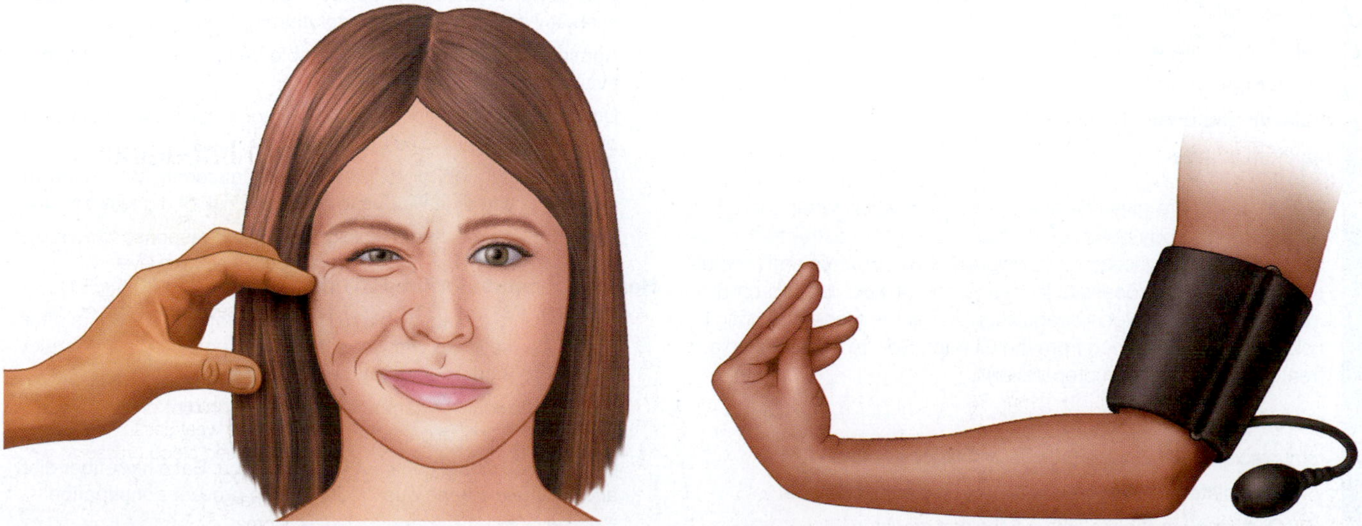

A Chvostek sign

B Trousseau sign

Figure 10.12 ■ **A**, Positive Chvostek sign. **B**, Positive Trousseau sign.

Diagnosis

The following laboratory and diagnostic tests may be ordered when hypocalcemia is known or suspected:

- ***Total serum calcium***, the amount of ionized (active) calcium available, usually is estimated. In critically ill patients, however, *ionized calcium* may be directly measured using ion-selective electrodes. Direct measurement of ionized calcium requires special handling of the blood specimen, including placing the specimen on ice and analyzing it immediately.
- ***Serum albumin*** because the albumin level affects serum calcium results. When the albumin level is low (hypoalbuminemia), the amount of ionized calcium may remain normal even though the total calcium level is low.
- ***Serum magnesium*** because hypocalcemia is often associated with hypomagnesemia (serum magnesium < 1.8 mg/dL). In this case, normal magnesium levels must be restored to correct the hypocalcemia.
- ***Serum phosphate*** because hyperphosphatemia (serum phosphate > 4.5 mg/dL) can lead to hypocalcemia due to the inverse relationship between phosphorus and calcium (as phosphate levels rise, calcium levels fall).
- ***Parathyroid hormone (PTH)***, to identify the possible diagnosis of hyperparathyroidism.
- An *ECG*, to evaluate the effects of hypocalcemia on the heart, such as a prolonged ST segment.

Medications

Hypocalcemia is treated with oral or IV calcium. The patient with severe hypocalcemia is treated with IV calcium to prevent life-threatening problems such as airway obstruction. The most common IV calcium preparations include calcium chloride and calcium gluconate (Adams et al., 2017). Although calcium chloride contains more elemental calcium than calcium gluconate, it is also more irritating to the veins and may cause venous sclerosis (hardening of the vein walls) if given into a peripheral vein. See **Medication Administration 10.D** for further information about calcium administration.

SAFETY ALERT: IV calcium preparations can cause necrosis and sloughing of tissue if they infiltrate into subcutaneous tissue. Rapid drug administration can lead to bradycardia and possible cardiac arrest due to overcorrection of hypocalcemia with resulting hypercalcemia. ■

Oral calcium preparations (calcium carbonate, calcium gluconate, or calcium lactate) are used to treat chronic, asymptomatic hypocalcemia. Calcium supplements may be combined with vitamin D, or vitamin D may be given alone to increase GI absorption of calcium.

Dietary Management

A diet high in calcium-rich foods may be recommended for patients with chronic hypocalcemia or with low total body stores of calcium. Foods high in calcium include dairy products, canned salmon, broccoli, spinach, and tofu.

Medication Administration 10.D

Calcium Salts

CALCIUM SALTS

calcium carbonate (BioCal, Calsan, Caltrate, Os-Cal, Tums, others)
calcium chloride
calcium citrate (Citracal)
calcium glubionate
calcium gluceptate
calcium gluconate (Kalcinate)
calcium lactate

Calcium salts are given to increase calcium levels when there is a deficit (a total body deficit or inadequate levels of extracellular calcium). Calcium is necessary to maintain bone structure and for multiple physiologic processes including neuromuscular and cardiac function as well as blood coagulation. In the presence of vitamin D, calcium is well absorbed from the GI tract. Severe hypocalcemia is treated with IV calcium preparations.

Nursing Responsibilities

Oral calcium salts:

- Administer 1 to 1.5 hours after meals and at bedtime.
- Give calcium tablets with a full glass of water.

IV calcium salts:

- Assess IV site for patency. Do not administer calcium if there is a risk of leakage into the tissues.
- May be given by slow IV push (dilute with sterile NS for injection prior to administering) or added to compatible parenteral fluids such as NS, lactated Ringer solution, or D_5W.
- Administer into the largest available vein; use a central line if available.
- Do not administer with bicarbonate or phosphate because a precipitate (insoluble salt) will form.
- Continuously monitor ECG when administering IV calcium to patients taking digitalis due to increased risk of digitalis toxicity.
- Frequently monitor serum calcium levels and response to therapy.

Health Education for the Patient and Family

- Take calcium tablets with a full glass of water 1 to 2 hours after meals. Do not take with food or milk. If possible, do not take within 1 to 2 hours of other medications.
- Maintain adequate vitamin D intake through diet or exposure to the sun to promote calcium absorption.
- Calcium carbonate can cause constipation. Eat a high-fiber diet and maintain a generous fluid intake to prevent constipation.

Note: Drugs identified in blue are among the 200 most commonly prescribed medications in the United States.

Source: Data from Adams et al., 2017.

Nursing Care

Assessment

Assessment data related to hypocalcemia include:

- ***Health history:*** current manifestations, including numbness and tingling around mouth and of hands and feet, abdominal pain, shortness of breath; acute or chronic diseases such as pancreatitis, liver or kidney disease; current medications
- ***Physical assessment:*** muscle spasms; deep tendon reflexes; Chvostek sign and Trousseau sign; vital signs and apical pulse; presence of convulsions.

Priorities of Care

The effect of hypocalcemia on neuromuscular irritability, with the risk for muscle spasm and convulsions, is the highest priority for nursing care of the patient.

Diagnoses, Outcomes, and Interventions

Reduce Risk for Injury. The patient with hypocalcemia is at risk for injury from possible laryngospasm, cardiac dysrhythmias, or convulsions. In addition, too rapid administration of IV calcium or infiltration of the medication into subcutaneous tissues can lead to injury.

Expected Outcome: Patient will remain free of injury or complications of hypocalcemia.

The nurse will:

- Frequently monitor airway and respiratory status, including oxygen saturation levels. Report changes such as respiratory stridor (a high-pitched, harsh inspiratory sound indicative of upper airway obstruction) or increased respiratory rate or effort to the physician. *These changes may indicate laryngeal spasm due to tetany.*

SAFETY ALERT: Laryngeal spasm is a respiratory emergency, requiring immediate intervention to maintain ventilation and gas exchange. ■

- Monitor cardiovascular status including heart rate and rhythm, blood pressure, and peripheral pulses. *Hypocalcemia decreases myocardial contractility, causing reduced cardiac output and hypotension. It can also cause bradycardia or ventricular dysrhythmias. Cardiac arrest may occur in severe hypocalcemia.*
- Continuously monitor ECG in patients receiving IV calcium preparations, especially if the patient is also taking digitalis. *Rapid administration of calcium salts can lead to hypercalcemia and cardiac dysrhythmias. Calcium administration increases the risk of digitalis toxicity and resultant dysrhythmias.*
- If the patient has tetany, provide a quiet environment and institute seizure precautions such as raising the side rails and keeping an airway at bedside. *A quiet environment reduces central nervous system stimuli and the risk of convulsions in the patient with tetany.*

Transitions of Care

Because of the large stores of calcium in bones, most healthy adults have a very low risk of developing hypocalcemia. However, a deficit of total body calcium is often associated with aging, increasing the risk of osteoporosis, fractures, and disability. Women have a higher risk for developing osteoporosis than men due to lower bone density and hormonal influences. Teach women of all ages the importance of maintaining adequate calcium intake through diet and, as needed, calcium supplements. Stress the relationship between weight-bearing exercise and bone density, and encourage women to engage in a regular aerobic and weight-training exercise regimen. Recommend screening for bone density in older women.

Acute hypocalcemia is described previously and usually occurs after neck surgery where the parathyroid gland can be damaged. Acute hypocalcemia can also occur with osteoblastic metastases and acute pancreatitis. The bedside nurse should always be on the lookout for the neurological changes of acute hypocalcemia.

In preparing the patient with hypocalcemia for home or continuing care, consider the circumstances leading to low serum calcium levels. Discuss risk factors for hypocalcemia specific to the patient, and provide information about managing these risk factors to avoid future episodes of hypocalcemia. Teach about prescribed medications, including calcium supplements. Provide a list of foods high in calcium, as well as sources of vitamin D if recommended. Discuss manifestations to report to the healthcare provider, and stress the importance of follow-up care as scheduled.

The Patient with Hypercalcemia

Hypercalcemia is a serum calcium value greater than 11.0 mg/dL. Excess ionized calcium in ECF can have serious widespread effects.

Pathophysiology

Hypercalcemia usually results from increased resorption of calcium from the bones. The two most common causes of bone resorption are hyperparathyroidism and malignancies (Sorenson et al., 2019). In hyperparathyroidism, excess PTH is produced. This causes calcium to be released from bones, as well as increased calcium absorption in the intestines and retention of calcium by the kidneys. Hypercalcemia is a common complication of malignancies. It may develop as a result of bone destruction by the tumor or due to hormone-like substances produced by the tumor itself. Prolonged immobility and lack of weight bearing also cause increased resorption of bone with calcium release into extracellular fluids. Self-limiting hypercalcemia may follow successful kidney transplant. Levels of parathyroid hormone may be altered in chronic renal failure, leading to increased serum calcium levels.

Increased intestinal absorption of calcium can also lead to hypercalcemia. This may result from excess vitamin D, overuse of calcium-containing antacids, or excessive milk ingestion. Renal failure and some drugs such as thiazide diuretics and lithium can interfere with elimination of calcium by the kidneys, causing high serum calcium levels.

The effects of hypercalcemia largely depend on the degree of serum calcium elevation and the length of time over which it develops. In general, higher serum calcium levels are associated with more serious effects. Calcium has a stabilizing effect on the neuromuscular junction; hypercalcemia decreases neuromuscular excitability, leading to muscle weakness and depressed deep tendon reflexes. Gastrointestinal motility is reduced as well. In the heart, calcium exerts an effect similar to digoxin, strengthening contractions and reducing the heart rate. Hypercalcemia affects the conduction system of the heart, leading to bradycardia and heart blocks. The ability of the kidneys to concentrate urine is impaired by hypercalcemia, causing excess sodium and water loss and increased thirst.

High serum calcium levels affect mental status. This is thought to be due to increased calcium in cerebrospinal fluid. Behavioral effects range from personality changes to confusion, impaired memory, and acute psychoses.

Manifestations and Complications

Manifestations of hypercalcemia may be subtle, particularly when it is mild and develops over time. Decreased neuromuscular excitability causes muscle weakness and fatigue, as well as GI manifestations such as anorexia, nausea and vomiting, and constipation. Central nervous system (CNS) effects may include difficulty concentrating, confusion, lethargy, behavior or personality changes, and coma. Cardiovascular effects include dysrhythmias, ECG changes, and possible hypertension. Hypercalcemia causes polyuria and, as a result, increased thirst.

Complications of hypercalcemia can affect several different organ systems. Peptic ulcer disease may develop due to increased gastric acid secretion. Pancreatitis can occur as a result of calcium deposits in pancreatic ducts. Excess calcium can precipitate out of urine to form kidney stones. Hypercalcemic crisis, an acute increase in the serum calcium level, can lead to cardiac arrest.

Interprofessional Care

The management of hypercalcemia focuses on correcting the underlying cause and reducing the serum calcium level. Treatment is particularly important in patients who have one or more of the following: serum calcium levels greater than 12 mg/dL, overt manifestations of hypercalcemia, compromised renal function, and inability to maintain an adequate fluid intake.

Diagnosis

The laboratory and diagnostic tests that may be ordered are:

- ***Serum electrolytes*** show a total serum calcium greater than 11.0 mg/dL.
- ***Serum PTH levels*** are measured to identify or rule out hyperparathyroidism as the cause of hypercalcemia.
- ***ECG*** changes in hypercalcemia include a shortened QT interval, shortened and depressed ST segment, and widened T wave. Bradycardia or heart block may be identified on the ECG.
- ***Bone density scans*** may be done to monitor bone resorption and the effects of treatment measures on mineralization of bone.

Medications

Measures to promote calcium elimination by the kidneys and reduce calcium resorption from bone are used to treat hypercalcemia. In acute hypercalcemia, IV fluids are given with a loop diuretic such as furosemide (Lasix) to promote elimination of excess calcium.

A number of drugs that inhibit bone resorption are available. The bisphosphonates (zoledronic acid [Reclast, Zometa], pamidronate [Aredia], and etidronate [Didronel]) are commonly used to treat hypercalcemia associated with malignancies. These drugs are also used to prevent and treat osteoporosis. (Nursing implications for bisphosphonate drugs are presented in the Medication Administration boxes in Chapter 40.) Rapid reversal of hypercalcemia in emergency situations may be accomplished by IV administration of sodium phosphate or potassium phosphate. Calcium binds to phosphate, thus decreasing serum calcium levels. Paradoxically, complications of this therapy can include fatal hypocalcemia resulting from binding of the ionized calcium and soft tissue calcifications.

Other drug therapies include the use of IV plicamycin (Mithramycin) to inhibit bone resorption. Glucocorticoids (cortisone), which compete with vitamin D, and a low-calcium diet may be prescribed to decrease GI absorption of calcium, to inhibit bone resorption, and to increase urinary calcium excretion. Also, calcitonin may be prescribed to decrease skeletal mobilization of calcium and phosphorus and to increase renal output of calcium and phosphorus. See Chapter 19 for more information about and nursing implications of glucocorticoid therapy.

Fluid Management

IV fluids, usually isotonic saline, are administered to patients with severe hypercalcemia to restore vascular volume and promote renal excretion of calcium. Isotonic saline is used because sodium excretion is accompanied by calcium excretion. Careful assessment of cardiovascular and renal function is done prior to fluid therapy; the patient is carefully monitored for evidence of fluid overload during treatment.

Nursing Care

Assessment

Assessment data related to hypercalcemia include:

- ***Health history:*** current manifestations, including weakness or fatigue, abdominal discomfort, nausea or vomiting, increased urination and thirst; changes in memory or thinking; duration of manifestations and any risk factors such as excess intake of milk or calcium products, prolonged immobility, malignancy, renal failure, or endocrine disorders; current medications
- ***Physical assessment:*** mental status and level of consciousness; vital signs including apical pulse; bowel

sounds; muscle strength of upper and lower extremities; deep tendon reflexes.

Priorities of Care

The patient with hypercalcemia is at risk for injury due to changes in mental status, muscle weakness, cardiac dysrhythmias, and loss of calcium from bones, making safety the priority of care.

Diagnoses, Outcomes, and Interventions

Reduce Risk for Injury. Monitor the patient with hypercalcemia carefully as risk for injury is high.

Expected Outcome: Patient will be free of injury, including complications of hypercalcemia.

The nurse will:

- Institute safety precautions if confusion or other changes in mental status are noted. *Changes in mental status may impair judgment and the patient's ability to maintain his or her own safety.*

SAFETY ALERT: Hypercalcemia can cause bradycardia, various heart blocks, and cardiac arrest. Immediate treatment may be necessary to preserve life. Monitor cardiac rate and rhythm, treating and/or reporting dysrhythmias as indicated. Prepare for possible cardiac arrest; keep emergency resuscitation equipment readily available. ■

- Observe for manifestations of digoxin toxicity (if administered), including vision changes, anorexia, and changes in heart rate and rhythm. Monitor serum digoxin levels. *Hypercalcemia increases the risk of digoxin toxicity.*
- Promote fluid intake to keep the patient well hydrated and maintain dilute urine. Encourage fluids such as prune or cranberry juice to help maintain acidic urine. *Acidic, dilute urine reduces the risk of calcium salts precipitating out to form kidney stones.*
- If excess bone reabsorption has occurred, use caution when turning, positioning, transferring, or ambulating. *Bones that have lost excess calcium may fracture with minimal stress or trauma (pathologic fractures).*

Monitor Fluid Volume. Large amounts of isotonic IV fluid are often administered to help correct acute hypercalcemia, leading to a risk for hypervolemia. Patients with preexisting cardiac or renal disease are at particular risk. Loop diuretics may be prescribed to help eliminate excess fluid and calcium.

Expected Outcome: Patient's fluid balance will be maintained.

The nurse will:

- Closely monitor intake and output. *A loop diuretic such as furosemide may be necessary if urinary output does not keep up with fluid administration.*
- Frequently assess vital signs, respiratory status, and heart sounds. *Increasing pulse rate, dyspnea, adventitious lung sounds, and an S_3 on auscultation of the heart may indicate excess fluid volume and potential heart failure.*
- Place in semi-Fowler or Fowler position. *Elevating the head of the bed improves lung expansion and reduces the work of breathing.*

Delegating Nursing Care Activities

Although the nurse retains responsibility for conducting initial and ongoing assessment of the patient, nursing care activities such as obtaining vital signs, measuring intake and output, helping promote fluid intake, and assisting with positioning and ambulation for the patient with hypercalcemia may be delegated to assistive personnel with appropriate education and documented competency.

Transitions of Care

Identify and monitor patients at risk for hypercalcemia. Promote mobility in patients when possible. Assist hospitalized patients to ambulate as soon as possible. In the home setting, discuss the benefits of regular weight-bearing activity with patients, families, and caregivers.

Encourage a generous fluid intake of up to 3 to 4 quarts per day. Encourage patients at risk to limit their intake of milk and milk products, as well as calcium-containing antacids and supplements. In addition, patients with prolonged immobility or hypercalcemia are encouraged to consume fluids that increase the acidity of urine (which inhibits calcium stone formation), such as cranberry or prune juice.

Discuss the following topics when preparing the patient for discharge:

- Avoid excess intake of calcium-rich foods and antacids.
- Use prescribed drugs to prevent excess calcium resorption. Discuss their dose, use, and desired and possible adverse effects.
- Increase fluid intake to 3 to 4 quarts per day; increase the intake of foods that help acidify urine (meats, fish, poultry, eggs, cranberries, plums, prunes); increase dietary fiber and fluid intake to prevent constipation.
- Maintain weight-bearing physical activity to prevent hypercalcemia.

10.6 Magnesium Imbalances

Only about 1% of the magnesium in the body is in extracellular fluid; the rest is found within the cells and in bone. The normal serum concentration of magnesium ranges from 1.8 to 3.0 mg/dL (1.5 to 2.5 mEq/L).

Magnesium is obtained through the diet (it is plentiful in green vegetables, grains, nuts, meats, and seafood) and excreted by the kidneys. Magnesium is vital to many intracellular processes, including enzyme reactions and synthesis of proteins and nucleic acids. Magnesium exerts a sedative effect on the neuromuscular junction, decreasing acetylcholine release. It is an essential ion for neuromuscular transmission and cardiovascular function. The physiologic effects of magnesium are affected by both potassium and calcium levels.

The Patient with Hypomagnesemia

Hypomagnesemia is a magnesium level of less than 1.8 mg/dL. It is a common problem in critically ill patients. Hypomagnesemia may be caused by deficient magnesium intake, excessive losses, or a shift between the intracellular and extracellular compartments.

Risk Factors

Loss of GI fluids, particularly from diarrhea, an ileostomy, or intestinal fistula, is a major risk factor for hypomagnesemia. Disruption of nutrient absorption in the small intestine also increases the risk. Multiple factors associated with alcoholism contribute to hypomagnesemia: deficient nutrient intake, increased GI losses, impaired absorption, and increased renal excretion (Sorenson et al., 2019). Other risk factors for hypomagnesemia include protein-calorie malnutrition or starvation; diabetic ketoacidosis; kidney disease; drugs such as loop or thiazide diuretics, aminoglycoside antibiotics, and cyclosporine; and rapid administration of citrated blood.

Pathophysiology

Magnesium deficiency usually occurs along with low serum potassium and calcium levels. The effects of hypomagnesemia relate not only to the magnesium deficiency but also to hypokalemia and hypocalcemia.

Hypomagnesemia causes increased neuromuscular excitability, with muscle weakness and tremors. The accompanying hypocalcemia contributes to this effect. In the central nervous system, this increased neural excitability can lead to seizures and changes in mental status. Deficient intracellular magnesium in the myocardium increases the risk of cardiac dysrhythmias and sudden death. Hypokalemia increases this risk. Hypomagnesemia also increases the risk of digoxin toxicity. Chronic hypomagnesemia may contribute to hypertension, probably due to increased vasoconstriction. Severe hypomagnesia is strongly linked to low serum calcium levels because both are associated with renal and GI losses.

Manifestations and Complications

Neuromuscular manifestations of hypomagnesemia include tremors, hyperreactive reflexes, positive Chvostek and Trousseau signs (refer to Figure 10.12), tetany, paresthesias, and seizures. CNS effects include confusion, mood changes (apathy, depression, agitation), hallucinations, and possible psychoses. An increased heart rate and ventricular dysrhythmias are common, especially when hypokalemia is present or the patient is taking digitalis. Cardiac arrest and sudden death may occur. **Box 10.6** summarizes manifestations of magnesium imbalances.

Interprofessional Care

Hypomagnesemia is diagnosed by measuring serum electrolyte levels. The ECG shows a pro-longed PR interval, widened QRS complex, and depression of the ST segment with T-wave in-version. Treatment is directed toward prevention and identification of an existing deficiency.

BOX 10.6 Manifestations of Magnesium Disorders

Hypomagnesemia	Hypermagnesemia
Serum magnesium level < 1.8 mg/dL (<1.5 mEq/L)	Serum magnesium level > 3.0 mg/dL (> 2.5 mEq/L)
Changes in personality	Confusion and lethargy
Nystagmus (lateral twitching of eyeballs)	Hypotension
Positive Babinski, Chvostek, and Trousseau signs	Cardiac dysrhythmias
Hypertension	Coma
Tachycardia	Cardiac arrest
Cardiac dysrhythmias	

Magnesium is added to parenteral nutrition solutions to prevent hypomagnesemia.

In patients able to eat, a mild deficiency may be corrected by increasing the intake of foods rich in magnesium (such as green leafy vegetables, seafood, milk, bananas, citrus fruits, and chocolate), or with oral magnesium supplements. Oral magnesium supplements may cause diarrhea, however, limiting their use.

Patients with manifestations of hypomagnesemia are treated with parenteral magnesium sulfate (Adams et al., 2017). Treatment is continued for several days to restore intracellular magnesium levels. Magnesium may be given IV or by deep IM injection. Renal function is evaluated prior to administration, and serum magnesium levels are monitored during treatment. The IV route is used for severe magnesium deficiency or if neurologic changes or cardiac dysrhythmias are present. See **Medication Administration 10.E** for the nursing implications of parenteral magnesium sulfate administration.

Nursing Care

Assessment

In addition to asking questions related to risk factors for hypomagnesemia, assess for manifestations of hypokalemia and hypocalcemia. Monitor diagnostic studies such as serum electrolytes, serum albumin levels, and the ECG. Monitor GI function, including bowel sounds and abdominal distention.

Priorities of Care

As is the case with many electrolyte imbalances, maintaining patient safety and preventing complications of the imbalance or its treatment are nursing care priorities.

Diagnoses, Outcomes, and Interventions

Nursing care for patients with hypomagnesemia focuses on careful monitoring of manifestations and responses to treatment, promoting safety, patient and family teaching, and administering prescribed medications. Monitor serum electrolytes, including magnesium, potassium, and calcium. Initiate cardiac monitoring, reporting and treating (as prescribed) ECG changes and dysrhythmias. In patients receiving digoxin, monitor for digoxin toxicity. Assess deep

Medication Administration 10.E

Magnesium Sulfate

Magnesium sulfate is used to prevent or treat hypomagnesemia. It may be given IV or by IM injection.

Nursing Responsibilities

- Assess serum magnesium levels and renal function tests (BUN and serum creatinine) prior to administering. Notify the care provider if magnesium levels are above normal limits or renal function is impaired.
- Frequently monitor neurologic status and deep tendon reflexes during therapy. Withhold magnesium and notify the care provider if deep tendon reflexes are hypoactive or absent.
- Monitor intake and output.
- Administer IM doses deep into the ventral or dorsal gluteal sites.
- IV magnesium sulfate may be given by direct IV push or by continuous infusion.
  a. Solutions with a concentration of 20% or lower may be administered undiluted by direct IV injection at a rate of no faster than 150 mg/min.
  b. When administering by infusion, give required dose over 4 hours, but no faster than 150 mg/min (Shields, Fox, & Liebrecht, 2018).

Health Education for the Patient and Family

- Explain purpose and duration of treatment.
- Discuss reason for frequent neurologic and reflex assessments.

Note: Drugs identified in blue are among the 200 most commonly prescribed medications in the United States.

Source: Data from Adams et al., 2017.

tendon reflexes frequently during IV magnesium infusions and prior to each IM dose. Depressed tendon reflexes indicate a high serum magnesium level. Institute seizure precautions and maintain a quiet, darkened environment to reduce neuromuscular and CNS irritability.

Transitions of Care

Discuss the importance of maintaining adequate magnesium intake through a well-balanced diet, particularly with patients at risk (people with alcoholism, malabsorption, or bowel surgery). Many hospitalized patients are at risk for hypomagnesemia due to protein-calorie malnutrition and other disorders. Monitor serum magnesium levels, reporting changes to the healthcare provider.

Prior to discharge, instruct the patient to increase dietary intake of foods high in magnesium and provide information about magnesium supplements. In addition, if alcohol abuse has precipitated a magnesium deficit, discuss alcohol treatment options, including support groups such as Alcoholics Anonymous, Al-Anon, and/or Alateen.

The Patient with Hypermagnesemia

Hypermagnesemia is a serum magnesium level greater than 3.0 mg/dL (2.5 mEq/L). It is much less common than hypomagnesemia. Hypermagnesemia can develop in renal failure, particularly if magnesium is administered parenterally or orally (e.g., magnesium-containing antacids or laxatives). Older adults are at risk for hypermagnesemia as renal function declines with age and they may be more likely to use over-the-counter laxatives and other preparations that contain magnesium.

Pathophysiology and Manifestations

Elevated serum magnesium levels interfere with neuromuscular transmission and depress the central nervous system (Sorenson et al., 2019). Hypermagnesemia also affects the cardiovascular system, potentially causing hypotension, flushing, sweating, and bradydysrhythmias.

Predictable manifestations occur with increasing serum magnesium levels. With lower levels, nausea and vomiting, hypotension, facial flushing, sweating, and a feeling of warmth occur. As levels increase, manifestations of CNS depression appear (weakness, lethargy, drowsiness, weak or absent deep tendon reflexes). Marked elevations cause respiratory depression, coma, and compromised cardiac function (ECG changes, bradycardia, heart block, and cardiac arrest).

Interprofessional Care

The management of hypermagnesemia focuses on identifying and treating the underlying cause. All medications or compounds containing magnesium (such as antacids, IV solutions, or enemas) are withheld. In the patient with renal failure, hemodialysis or peritoneal dialysis is instituted to remove the excess magnesium.

Calcium gluconate is administered IV to reverse the neuromuscular and cardiac effects of hypermagnesemia. The patient may require mechanical ventilation to support respiratory function and a pacemaker to maintain adequate cardiac output.

Nursing Care

Nursing care includes instituting measures to prevent and identify hypermagnesemia in patients at risk, monitoring for critical effects of hypermagnesemia, and providing measures to ensure the patient's safety. Nursing priorities include monitoring cardiac output and breathing patterns and reducing risk for injury.

Transitions of Care

The key to hypermagnesemia is to figure out the cause. Most causes are from inpatient administration of magnesium or in patients with kidney failure who are taking magnesium-containing antacids or laxatives. Educating patients on avoiding magnesium-containing products and foods is important.

10.7 Phosphate Imbalances

Although most phosphate (85%) is found in bones, it is the primary intracellular anion. About 14% is in intracellular fluid, and the remainder (1%) is in extracellular fluid. The normal serum phosphate (or phosphorus) level in adults is 2.5 to 4.5 mg/dL (1.7 to 2.6 mEq/L). Phosphorus levels vary with age, gender, and diet.

Phosphate is essential to intracellular processes such as the production of ATP, the fuel that supports muscle contraction, nerve cell transmission, and electrolyte transport. Phosphate is vital for red blood cell function and oxygen delivery to tissues; nervous system and muscle function; and the metabolism of fats, carbohydrates, and protein. It also assists in maintaining acid–base balance.

Phosphorus is ingested in the diet, absorbed in the jejunum, and primarily excreted by the kidneys. When phosphate intake is low, the kidneys conserve phosphorus, excreting less. An inverse relationship exists between phosphate and calcium levels: When one increases, the other decreases. Regulatory mechanisms for calcium levels (parathyroid hormone, calcitonin, and vitamin D) also influence phosphate levels. The manifestations of phosphate imbalances are summarized in **Box 10.7**.

The Patient with Hypophosphatemia

Hypophosphatemia is a serum phosphorus of less than 2.5 mg/dL. Low serum phosphate levels may indicate a total body deficit of phosphate or a shift of phosphate into the intracellular space, the most common cause of hypophosphatemia. Decreased GI absorption of phosphate or increased renal excretion of phosphate can also cause low phosphate levels. Hypophosphatemia is often iatrogenic (related to treatment). Selected causes of hypophosphatemia include:

- Refeeding syndrome can develop when malnourished patients are started on enteral or parenteral nutrition. Glucose in the formula or solution stimulates insulin release, which promotes the entry of glucose and phosphate into the cells, depleting extracellular phosphate levels.
- Medications frequently contribute to hypophosphatemia, including IV glucose solutions, antacids (aluminum- or magnesium-based antacids bind with phosphate), anabolic steroids, and diuretics.
- Alcoholism affects both the intake and absorption of phosphate.
- Hyperventilation and respiratory alkalosis cause phosphate to shift out of extracellular fluids into the intracellular space.
- Other causes include diabetic ketoacidosis with excess phosphate loss in the urine, stress responses, and extensive burns.

BOX 10.7
Manifestations of Phosphate Imbalances

Hypophosphatemia	Hyperphosphatemia
■ Serum phosphate level < 2.5 mg/dL (<1.7 mEq/L)	■ Serum phosphate level > 4.5 mg/dL (>2.6 mEq/L)
■ Intention tremor, paresthesias	■ Paresthesias
■ Confusion, stupor	■ Muscle weakness
■ Bone pain	■ Nausea and vomiting
■ Joint stiffness	■ Dysphagia
■ Bleeding disorders (platelet dysfunction)	■ Tetany
■ Impaired white blood cell function	■ Decreased blood pressure
■ Seizures	■ Cardiac dysrhythmias

Pathophysiology and Manifestations

Most effects of hypophosphatemia result from depletion of ATP and impaired oxygen delivery to the cells due to a deficiency of the red blood cell enzyme 2,3-DPG (Sorenson et al., 2019). Severe hypophosphatemia affects virtually every major organ system:

- ***Central nervous system:*** Reduced oxygen and ATP synthesis in the brain causes neurologic manifestations such as irritability, apprehension, weakness, paresthesias, lack of coordination, confusion, seizures, and coma.
- ***Hematologic:*** Oxygen delivery to the cells is reduced. Hemolytic anemia (excessive RBC destruction) may develop due to lack of ATP in red blood cells.
- ***Musculoskeletal:*** Decreased ATP causes muscle weakness and release of creatinine phosphokinase (CPK, a muscle enzyme); acute rhabdomyolysis (muscle cell break-down) can develop. Muscle cell destruction, in turn, can lead to acute kidney injury as myoglobin, a muscle cell protein, exerts a toxic effect on the kidney tubule.
- ***Cardiovascular:*** Hypophosphatemia decreases myocardial contractility; decreased oxygenation of the heart muscle can cause chest pain and dysrhythmias.
- ***Gastrointestinal:*** Anorexia can occur, as well as dysphagia (difficulty swallowing), nausea and vomiting, decreased bowel sounds, and possible ileus due to reduced GI motility.

Interprofessional Care

Treatment for hypophosphatemia is directed at prevention, treating the underlying cause of the disorder, and replacing phosphate. An improved diet and oral phosphate supplement (such as Neutra-Phos or Neutra-Phos K capsules) may restore normal phosphate levels in patients with a mild to moderate deficiency. IV phosphate (sodium phosphate or potassium phosphate) is given when serum phosphate levels are less than 1 mg/dL.

Nursing Care

Nurses can be instrumental in identifying patients at risk for phosphate deficiency and preventing it from developing. Nurses should closely monitor serum electrolyte values in patients at risk, including those who are malnourished, receiving IV glucose solutions or total parenteral nutrition, or being treated with diuretic therapy or antacids that bind with phosphate. Teach the patient and family about the causes and manifestations of hypophosphatemia. Discuss the importance of avoiding phosphorus-binding antacids, unless prescribed. Stress a well-balanced diet to maintain an adequate intake of phosphate.

The Patient with Hyperphosphatemia

Hyperphosphatemia is a serum phosphate level greater than 4.5 mg/dL. As with other electrolyte imbalances, it may be the result of impaired phosphate excretion, excess intake, or a shift of phosphate from the intracellular space into extracellular fluids.

- Acute or chronic renal failure is the primary cause of impaired phosphate excretion.
- Rapid administration of phosphate-containing solutions, including phosphate enemas, can increase serum phosphate levels. In addition, excess vitamin D increases phosphate absorption and can lead to hyperphosphatemia in patients with impaired renal function.
- A shift of phosphate from the intracellular to extracellular space can occur during chemotherapy, from sepsis or hypothermia, or because of extensive trauma or heat stroke.
- Because phosphate levels are affected by serum calcium concentrations, disruption of the mechanisms that regulate calcium levels (e.g., hypoparathyroidism, hyperthyroidism, or vitamin D intoxication) can lead to hyperphosphatemia.

Pathophysiology and Manifestations

Excessive serum phosphate levels cause few specific manifestations. The effects of high serum phosphate levels on nerves and muscles (muscle cramps and pain, paresthesias, tingling around the mouth, muscle spasms, tetany) are more the result of hypocalcemia that develops secondary to an elevated serum phosphorus level. The phosphate in the serum combines with ionized calcium, and the ionized serum calcium level falls (Sorenson et al., 2019).

Interprofessional Care

Treatment of the underlying disorder often corrects hyperphosphatemia. When this is not feasible, phosphate-containing drugs are eliminated and intake of phosphate-rich foods such as organ meats and milk and milk products is restricted. Agents that bind with phosphate in the GI tract (such as calcium-containing antacids) may be prescribed. If renal function is adequate, IV normal saline may be given to promote renal excretion of phosphate. Dialysis may be necessary to reduce phosphate levels in patients with renal failure.

Nursing Care

When providing nursing care for the patient with hyperphosphatemia, monitor the laboratory data for an excess of phosphorus and a deficit of calcium, as well as the manifestations of hypocalcemia. Discuss the risk of hyperphosphatemia related to using phosphate preparations as laxatives or enemas, particularly with patients who have other risk factors for the disorder (e.g., chronic kidney disease, endocrine disorders). When preparing the patient for discharge, teach about the use of phosphate-binding preparations as ordered and dietary phosphate restrictions.

10.8 Regulation of Acid–Base Balance

Homeostasis and optimal cellular function require maintenance of the hydrogen ion (H^+) concentration of body fluids within a relatively narrow range. Hydrogen ions determine the relative acidity of body fluids. **Acids** release hydrogen ions in solution; **bases** (or **alkalis**) accept hydrogen ions in solution. The hydrogen ion concentration of a solution is measured as its pH. The relationship between hydrogen ion concentration and pH is inverse; that is, as hydrogen ion concentration increases, the pH falls, and the solution becomes more acidic. As hydrogen ion concentration falls, the pH rises, and the solution becomes more alkaline or basic. The pH of body fluids is slightly basic, with the normal pH ranging from 7.35 to 7.45 (a pH of 7 is neutral).

A number of mechanisms work together to maintain the pH of the body within normal range. Metabolic processes in the body continuously produce acids, which fall into two categories: volatile acids and nonvolatile acids. Volatile acids can be eliminated from the body as a gas. Carbonic acid (H_2CO_3) is the only volatile acid produced in the body. It dissociates into carbon dioxide (CO_2) and water (H_2O); the carbon dioxide is then eliminated from the body through the lungs. All other acids produced in the body are nonvolatile acids that must be metabolized or excreted from the body in fluid. Lactic acid, hydrochloric acid, phosphoric acid, and sulfuric acid are examples of nonvolatile acids. Most acids and bases in the body are weak; that is, they neither release nor accept a significant amount of hydrogen ion.

Three systems work together in the body to maintain the pH despite continuous acid production: buffers, the respiratory system, and the renal system.

Buffer Systems

Buffers are substances that prevent major changes in pH by removing or releasing hydrogen ions. When excess acid is present in body fluid, buffers bind with hydrogen ions to minimize the change in pH. If body fluids become too basic or alkaline, buffers release hydrogen ions, restoring the pH. Although buffers act within a fraction of a second, their capacity to maintain pH is limited. The major buffer systems of the body are the bicarbonate–carbonic acid buffer system, phosphate buffer system, and protein buffers.

The bicarbonate–carbonic acid buffer system can be illustrated by the following equation:

$$CO_2 + H_2O \leftrightarrow H_2CO_3 \leftrightarrow H^+ + HCO_3^-$$

Bicarbonate (HCO_3^-) is a weak base; when an acid is added to the system, the hydrogen ion in the acid combines

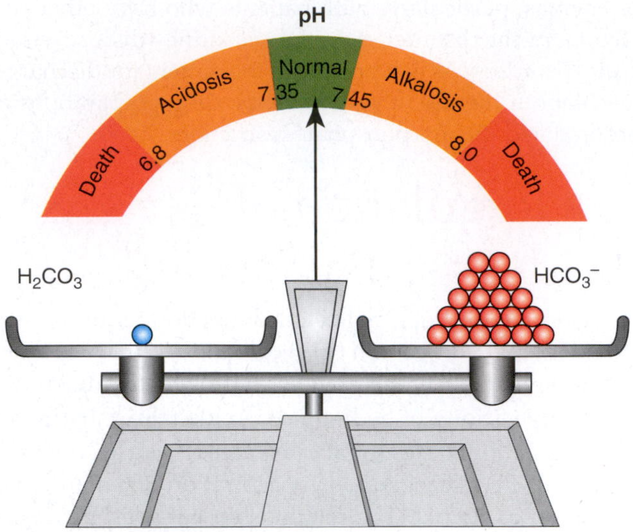
pH
Normal
7.35
7.45
Acidosis
Alkalosis
Death
6.8
8.0
Death
H_2CO_3
HCO_3^-

Figure 10.13 ■ The normal ratio of bicarbonate to carbonic acid is 20:1. As long as this ratio is maintained, the pH remains within the normal range of 7.35 to 7.45.

with bicarbonate, and the pH changes only slightly. Carbonic acid (H_2CO_3) is a weak acid produced when carbon dioxide dissolves in water. If a base is added to the system, it combines with carbonic acid, and the pH remains within the normal range. Although the amounts of bicarbonate and carbonic acid in the body vary to a certain extent, as long as a ratio of 20 parts bicarbonate (HCO_3^-) to 1 part carbonic acid (H_2CO_3) is maintained, the pH remains within the 7.35 to 7.45 range (**Figure 10.13** ■).

The normal serum bicarbonate level is 24 mEq/L, and that of carbonic acid is 1.2 mEq/L. Thus, the ratio of bicarbonate to carbonic acid is 20:1. It is this ratio that maintains the pH within the normal range. Adding a strong acid to extracellular fluid depletes bicarbonate, changing the 20:1 ratio and causing the pH to drop below 7.35. This is known as **acidosis**. The addition of a strong base depletes carbonic acid as it combines with the base. The 20:1 ratio again is disrupted and the pH rises above 7.45, a condition known as **alkalosis**.

Intracellular and plasma proteins also serve as buffers. Plasma proteins contribute to buffering of extracellular fluids. Proteins in intracellular fluid provide extensive buffering for organic acids produced by cellular metabolism. In red blood cells, hemoglobin acts as a buffer for hydrogen ions when carbonic acid dissociates. Inorganic phosphates also serve as extracellular buffers, although their roles are not as important as those of the bicarbonate–carbonic acid buffer system. Phosphates are, however, important intracellular buffers, helping to maintain a stable pH within the cells.

Respiratory System

The respiratory system (and the cerebral respiratory center) regulates carbonic acid in the body by eliminating or retaining carbon dioxide. Carbon dioxide is a potential acid; when combined with water, it forms carbonic acid (see the previous equation), a volatile acid. Acute increases in either carbon dioxide or hydrogen ions in the blood stimulate the respiratory center in the brain. As a result, both the rate and depth of respiration increase. The increased rate and depth of lung ventilation eliminate carbon dioxide from the body, and carbonic acid levels fall, bringing the pH to a more normal range. Although this compensation for increased hydrogen ion concentration occurs within minutes, it becomes less effective over time. Patients with chronic lung disease may have consistently high carbon dioxide levels in their blood.

Alkalosis, by contrast, depresses the respiratory center. Both the rate and depth of respiration decrease, and carbon dioxide is retained. The retained carbon dioxide then combines with water to restore carbonic acid levels and bring the pH back within the normal range.

Renal System

The *renal system* is responsible for the long-term regulation of acid–base balance in the body. The kidneys normally eliminate excess nonvolatile acids produced during metabolism. The kidneys also regulate bicarbonate levels in extracellular fluid by regenerating bicarbonate ions as well as reabsorbing them in the renal tubules. Although the kidneys respond more slowly to changes in pH (over hours to days), they can generate bicarbonate and selectively excrete or retain hydrogen ions as needed. In acidosis, when excess hydrogen ion is present and the pH falls, the kidneys excrete hydrogen ions and retain bicarbonate. In alkalosis, the kidneys retain hydrogen ions and excrete bicarbonate to restore acid–base balance.

Assessing Acid–Base Balance

Acid–base balance is evaluated primarily by measuring arterial blood gases. Arterial blood is used because it reflects acid–base balance throughout the entire body better than venous blood. Arterial blood also provides information about the effectiveness of the lungs in oxygenating blood. The elements measured are pH, the $PaCO_2$, the PaO_2, and bicarbonate level.

The abbreviations $PaCO_2$ and PaO_2 are used interchangeably with PCO_2 and PO_2. The *P* stands for partial pressure, the pressure exerted by the gas dissolved in the blood. The *a* indicates that the sample is arterial blood. Because these measurements are rarely done on venous blood, the *a* is often deleted from the abbreviation.

The $PaCO_2$ measures the pressure exerted by dissolved carbon dioxide in the blood. It reflects the respiratory component of acid–base regulation and balance and is regulated by the lungs. The normal value is 35 to 45 mmHg. A $PaCO_2$ of less than 35 mmHg is known as *hypocapnia*; a $PaCO_2$ greater than 45 mmHg is *hypercapnia*.

The PaO_2 is a measure of the pressure exerted by oxygen that is dissolved in the plasma. Only about 3% of oxygen in the blood is transported in solution; most is combined with hemoglobin. However, it is the dissolved oxygen that is available to the cells for metabolism. As dissolved oxygen diffuses out of plasma into the tissues, more is released from hemoglobin. The normal value for

Table 10.5 Normal Arterial Blood Gas Values

Value	Normal Range	Significance
pH	7.35–7.45	Reflects hydrogen ion (H^+) concentration ■ < 7.35 = acidosis ■ < 7.45 = alkalosis
$PaCO_2$	35–45 mmHg	Partial pressure of carbon dioxide (CO_2) in arterial blood ■ < 35 mmHg = hypocapnia ■ > 45 mmHg = hypercapnia
PaO_2	80–100 mmHg	Partial pressure of oxygen (O_2) in arterial blood ■ < 80 mmHg = hypoxemia
HCO_3^-	22–26 mEq/L	Bicarbonate concentration in plasma
BE	−3 to +3	Base excess; a measure of buffering capacity

PaO_2 is 80 to 100 mmHg. A PaO_2 of less than 80 mmHg is indicative of hypoxemia. The PaO_2 is valuable for evaluating respiratory function, but is not used as a primary measurement in determining acid–base status.

The **serum bicarbonate** (HCO_3^-) reflects the renal regulation of acid–base balance. It is often called the metabolic component of arterial blood gases. The normal HCO_3^- value is 22 to 26 mEq/L.

The **base excess (BE)** is a calculated value also known as *buffer base capacity*. The BE measures substances that can accept or combine with hydrogen ion. It reflects the degree of acid–base imbalance by indicating the status of the body's total buffering capacity. It represents the amount of acid or base that must be added to a blood sample to achieve a pH of 7.4. This is essentially a measure of increased or decreased bicarbonate. The normal value for BE for arterial blood is −3.0 to +3.0. Normal ABG values are summarized in **Table 10.5**.

ABGs are analyzed to identify acid–base disorders and their probable cause, to determine the extent of the imbalance, and to monitor treatment. When analyzing ABG results, it is important to use a systematic approach. First evaluate each individual measurement, then look at the interrelationships to determine the patient's acid–base status (see **Box 10.8**).

BOX 10.8
Interpreting Arterial Blood Gases

1. **Look at the pH.**
   - pH < 7.35 = acidosis
   - pH > 7.45 = alkalosis
2. **Look at the $PaCO_2$.**
   - $PaCO_2$ < 35 mmHg = hypocapnia; more carbon dioxide is being exhaled than normal
   - $PaCO_2$ > 45 mmHg = hypercapnia; carbon dioxide is being retained
3. **Evaluate the pH–$PaCO_2$ relationship for a possible respiratory problem.**
   - If the pH is < 7.35 (acidosis) and the $PaCO_2$ is > 45 mmHg (hypercapnia), retained carbon dioxide is causing increased H^+ concentration and *respiratory acidosis*.
   - If the pH is > 7.45 (alkalosis) and the $PaCO_2$ is < 35 mmHg (hypocapnia), low carbon dioxide levels and decreased H^+ concentration are causing *respiratory alkalosis*.
4. **Look at the bicarbonate.**
   - If the HCO_3^- is < 22 mEq/L, bicarbonate levels are lower than normal.
   - If the HCO_3^- is > 26 mEq/L, bicarbonate levels are higher than normal.
5. **Evaluate the pH, HCO_3^-, and BE for a possible metabolic problem.**
   - If the pH is < 7.35 (acidosis), the HCO_3^- is < 22 mEq/L, and the BE is <−3 mEq/L, then low bicarbonate levels and high H^+ concentrations are causing *metabolic acidosis*.
   - If the pH is > 7.45 (alkalosis), the HCO_3^- is > 26 mEq/L, and the BE is >+3 mEq/L, then high bicarbonate levels are causing *metabolic alkalosis*.
6. **Look for compensation.**
   - *Renal compensation:*
     a. In respiratory acidosis (pH < 7.35, $PaCO_2$ > 45 mmHg), the kidneys retain HCO_3^- to buffer the excess acid, so the HCO_3^- is > 26 mEq/L.
     b. In respiratory alkalosis (pH > 7.45, $PaCO_2$ < 35 mmHg), the kidneys excrete HO_3^- to minimize the alkalosis, so the HCO_3^- is < 22 mEq/L.
   - ***Respiratory compensation:***
     a. In metabolic acidosis (pH < 7.35, HCO_3^- < 22 mEq/L), the rate and depth of respirations increase, increasing carbon dioxide elimination, so the $PaCO_2$ is < 35 mmHg.
     b. In metabolic alkalosis (pH > 7.45, HCO_3^- > 26 mEq/L), respirations slow and carbon dioxide is retained, so the $PaCO_2$ is > 45 mmHg.
7. **Evaluate oxygenation.**
   - PaO_2 < 80 mmHg = hypoxemia; possible hypoventilation
   - PaO_2 > 100 mmHg = hyperventilation

10.9 Acid–Base Imbalances

Acid–base imbalances fall into two major categories: acidosis and alkalosis. *Acidosis* occurs when the hydrogen ion concentration increases above normal (pH below 7.35). *Alkalosis* occurs when the hydrogen ion concentration falls below normal (pH above 7.45).

Acid–base imbalances are further classified as metabolic or respiratory disorders. In metabolic disorders, the primary change is in the concentration of bicarbonate. In metabolic acidosis, the amount of bicarbonate is decreased in relation to the amount of acid in the body (**Figure 10.14** ■). It can develop as a result of abnormal bicarbonate losses or because of excess nonvolatile acids in the body. The pH falls below 7.35 and the bicarbonate concentration is less than 22 mEq/L. Metabolic alkalosis, by contrast, occurs when there is an excess of bicarbonate in relation to the amount of hydrogen ion (**Figure 10.15** ■). The pH is above 7.45 and the bicarbonate concentration is greater than 26 mEq/L.

In respiratory disorders, the primary change is in the concentration of carbonic acid. Respiratory acidosis occurs when carbon dioxide is retained, increasing the amount of carbonic acid in the body (**Figure 10.16** ■). As a result, the pH falls to less than 7.35, and the $PaCO_2$ is greater than 45 mmHg. When too much carbon dioxide is "blown off," carbonic acid levels fall and respiratory alkalosis develops (**Figure 10.17** ■). The pH rises to above 7.45 and the $PaCO_2$ is less than 35 mmHg.

Acid–base disorders are further defined as *primary* (simple) and *mixed*. Primary disorders are usually due to one cause. For example, respiratory failure often causes respiratory acidosis due to retained carbon dioxide; renal failure usually causes metabolic acidosis due to retained hydrogen ion and impaired bicarbonate production. **Table 10.6** summarizes primary acid–base imbalances with common causes of each. Mixed disorders occur from combinations of respiratory and metabolic disturbances. For example, a patient in cardiac arrest develops a mixed respiratory and metabolic acidosis due to lack of ventilation (and retained CO_2) and hypoxia of body tissues that leads to anaerobic metabolism and acid by-products (excess nonvolatile acids). Simple acid–base imbalances are more commonly seen than mixed imbalances. Common causes of simple acid–base imbalances include:

- Diabetic ketoacidosis (metabolic acidosis)
- Chronic obstructive lung disease (respiratory acidosis)
- Anxiety-related (psychogenic) hyperventilation (respiratory alkalosis)
- Critically ill patients are at higher risk for mixed acid–base imbalances.

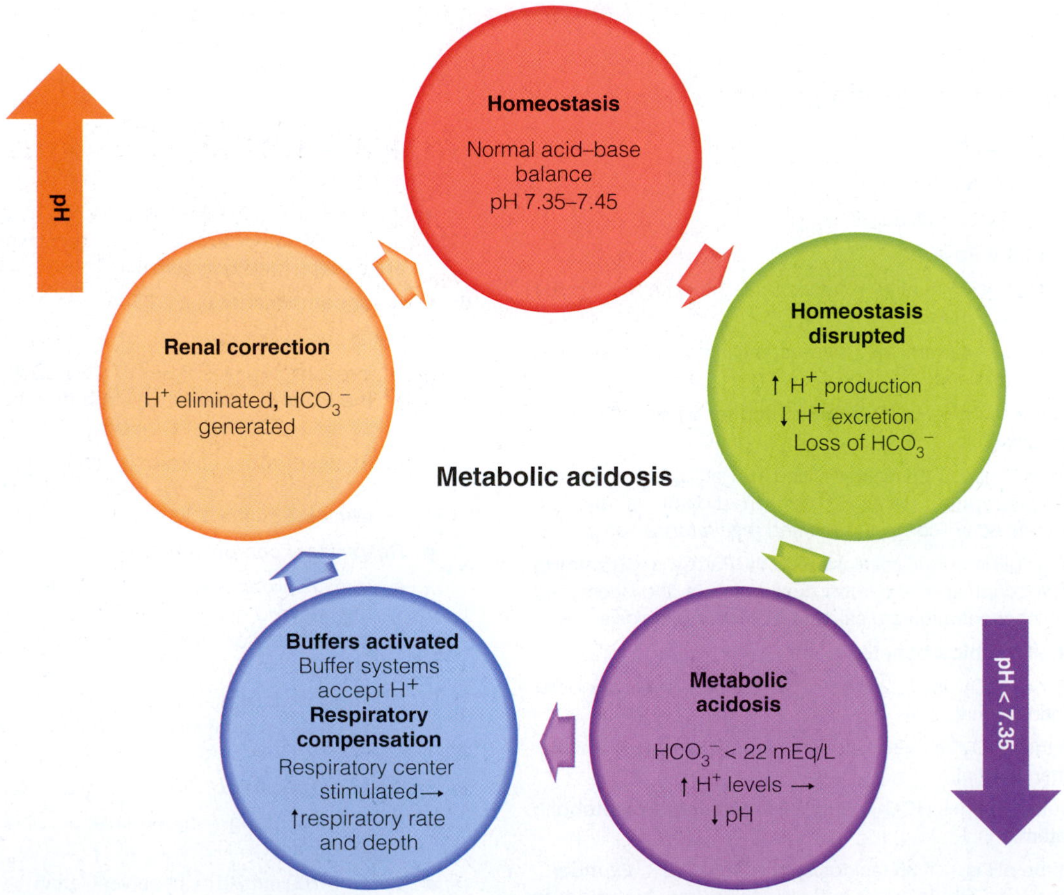
pH
Homeostasis
Normal acid–base balance
pH 7.35–7.45
Homeostasis disrupted
↑ H+ production
↓ H+ excretion
Loss of HCO3−
Metabolic acidosis
Metabolic acidosis
HCO3− < 22 mEq/L
↑ H+ levels →
↓ pH
pH < 7.35
Buffers activated
Buffer systems accept H+
Respiratory compensation
Respiratory center stimulated→
↑respiratory rate and depth
Renal correction
H+ eliminated, HCO3− generated

Figure 10.14 ■ Metabolic acidosis. Excess nonvolatile acids such as ketones or lactic acid or a loss of bicarbonate ions increases H^+ levels in body fluids, causing the pH to fall.

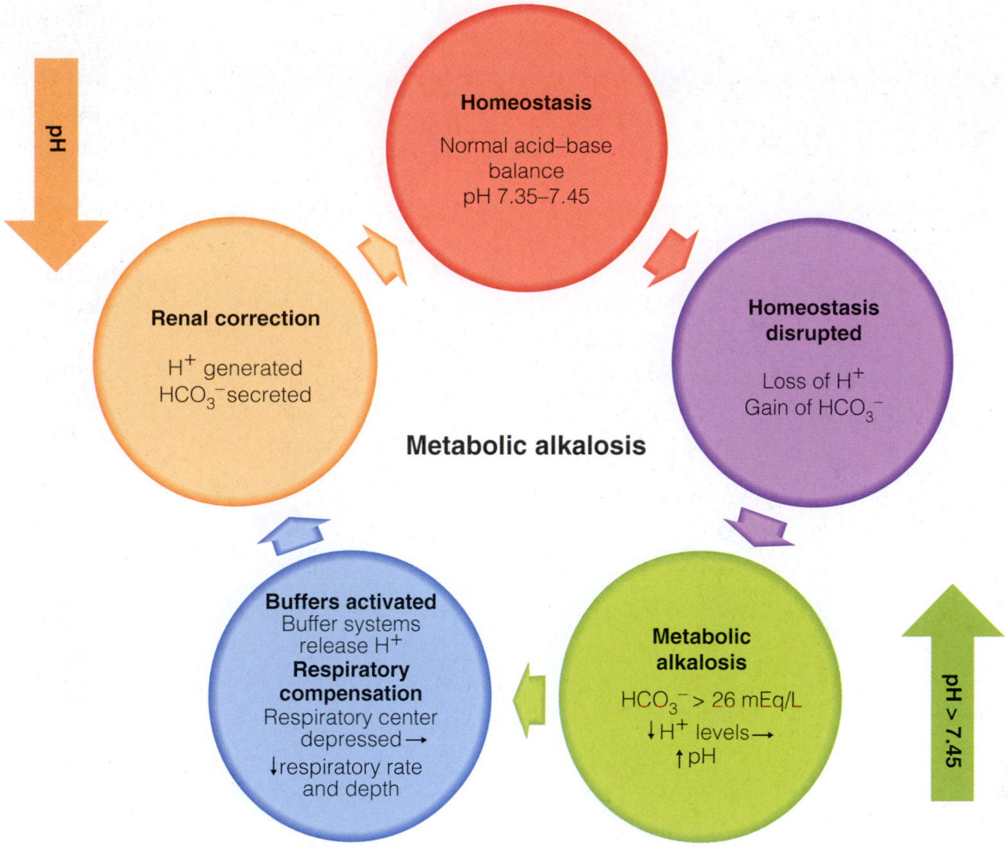

Homeostasis
Normal acid–base balance
pH 7.35–7.45
Homeostasis disrupted
Loss of H^+
Gain of HCO_3^-
Metabolic alkalosis
HCO_3^- > 26 mEq/L
↓H^+ levels→
↑pH
pH > 7.45
Buffers activated
Buffer systems release H^+
Respiratory compensation
Respiratory center depressed→
↓respiratory rate and depth
Renal correction
H^+ generated
HCO_3^- secreted
pH
Metabolic alkalosis

Figure 10.15 ■ Metabolic alkalosis. Loss of acids (e.g., loss of stomach acid with vomiting) or excess bicarbonate ingestion decreases H^+ levels in body fluids, causing the pH to rise.

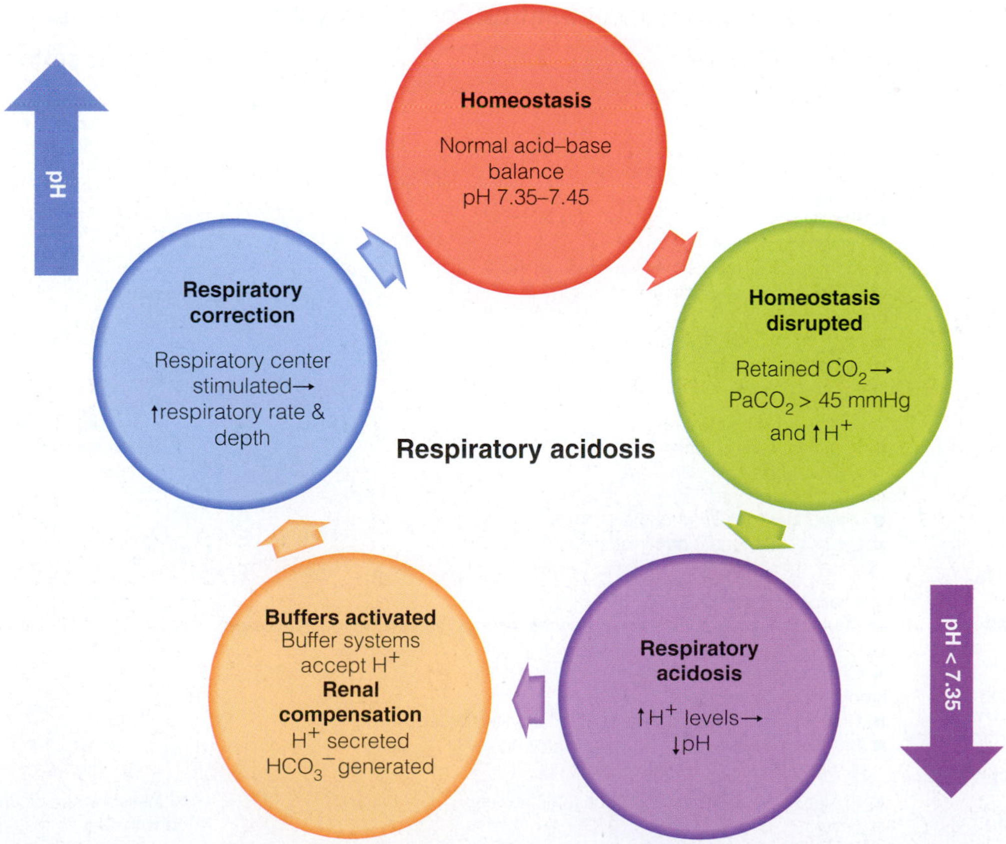

Homeostasis
Normal acid–base balance
pH 7.35–7.45
Homeostasis disrupted
Retained CO_2→
$PaCO_2$ > 45 mmHg
and ↑H^+
Respiratory acidosis
↑H^+ levels→
↓pH
pH < 7.35
Buffers activated
Buffer systems accept H^+
Renal compensation
H^+ secreted
HCO_3^- generated
Respiratory correction
Respiratory center stimulated→
↑respiratory rate & depth
pH
Respiratory acidosis

Figure 10.16 ■ Respiratory acidosis. Hypoventilation and retained CO_2 (increased $PaCO_2$) increase H^+ levels in body fluids, causing the pH to fall.

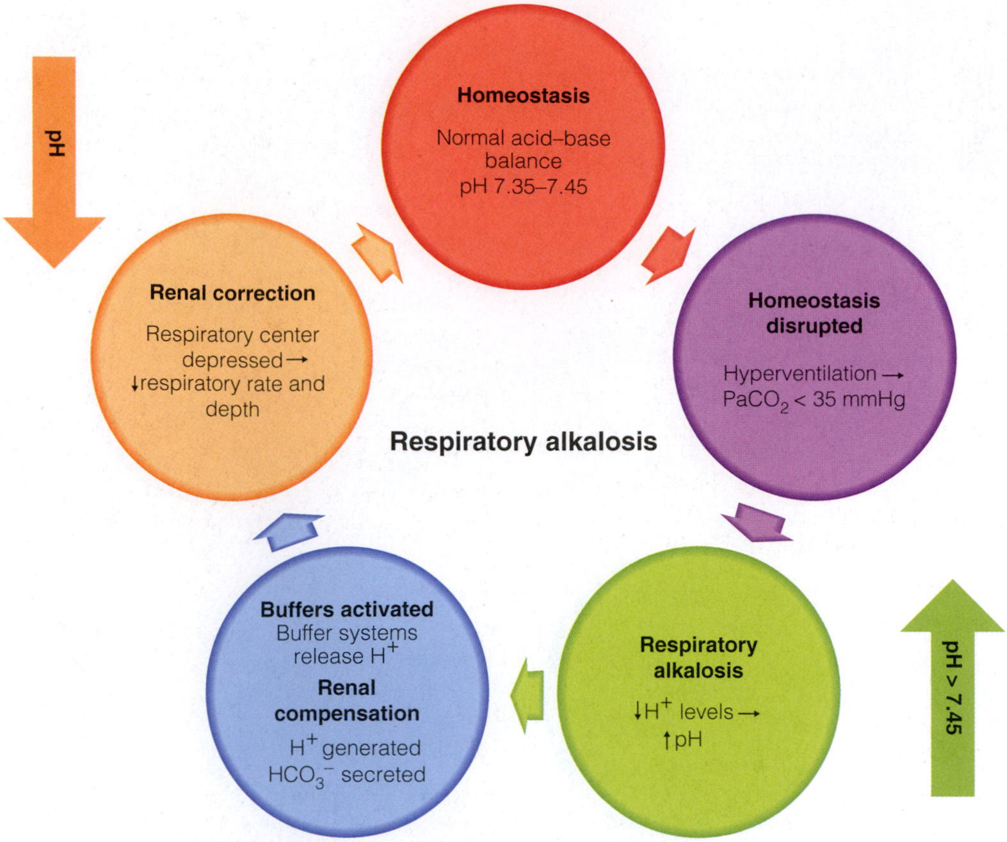

pH
Homeostasis
Normal acid–base balance
pH 7.35–7.45
Homeostasis disrupted
Hyperventilation →
PaCO2 < 35 mmHg
Respiratory alkalosis
↓H+ levels →
↑pH
pH > 7.45
Buffers activated
Buffer systems release H+
Renal compensation
H+ generated
HCO3− secreted
Renal correction
Respiratory center depressed →
↓respiratory rate and depth
Respiratory alkalosis

Figure 10.17 ■ Respiratory alkalosis. Hyperventilation and excess CO_2 elimination (decreased $PaCO_2$) decrease H^+ levels in body fluids, causing the pH to rise.

Table 10.6 Common Causes of and Compensation for Primary Acid–Base Imbalances

Imbalance	Common Causes	Compensation
Metabolic Acidosis		
pH < 7.35 **HCO_3^- < 22 mEq/L** *Critical values* pH < 7.20 HCO_3^- < 10 mEq/L	Increased acid production ■ Lactic acidosis ■ Ketoacidosis related to diabetes, starvation, or alcoholism Decreased acid excretion ■ Renal failure Increased bicarbonate loss ■ Diarrhea, ileostomy drainage, intestinal fistula ■ Biliary or pancreatic fistulas Increased chloride ■ Sodium chloride IV solutions ■ Renal tubular acidosis	Rate and depth of respirations increase, eliminating additional CO_2
Metabolic Alkalosis		
pH > 7.45 **HCO_3^- > 26 mEq/L** *Critical values* pH > 7.60 HCO_3^- > 40 mEq/L	Increased acid loss or excretion ■ Vomiting, gastric suction ■ Hypokalemia Increased bicarbonate ■ Alkali ingestion (bicarbonate of soda) ■ Excess bicarbonate administration	Rate and depth of respirations decrease, retaining CO_2
Respiratory Acidosis		
pH < 7.35 **$PaCO_2$ > 45 mmHg** *Critical values* pH < 7.2 $PaCO_2$ > 77 mmHg	Acute respiratory acidosis ■ Acute respiratory conditions (pulmonary edema, pneumonia, acute asthma) ■ Opiate overdose ■ Chest trauma Chronic respiratory acidosis ■ Chronic respiratory conditions (COPD, cystic fibrosis) ■ Multiple sclerosis, other neuromuscular diseases	Kidneys conserve bicarbonate to restore carbonic acid:bicarbonate ratio of 1:20
Respiratory Alkalosis		
pH > 7.45 **$PaCO_2$ < 35 mmHg** *Critical values* pH > 7.60 $PaCO_2$ < 20 mmHg	■ Anxiety-induced hyperventilation (e.g., anxiety) ■ Fever ■ Early salicylate intoxication ■ Hyperventilation with mechanical ventilator	Kidneys excrete bicarbonate and conserve H^+ to restore carbonic acid:bicarbonate ratio

Compensation

With primary acid–base disorders, compensatory changes in the other part of the regulatory system occur to restore a normal pH and homeostasis. In metabolic acid–base disorders, the change in pH affects the rate and depth of respirations. This, in turn, affects carbon dioxide elimination and the $PaCO_2$, helping restore the carbonic acid:bicarbonate ratio. The kidneys compensate for simple respiratory imbalances. The change in pH affects both bicarbonate conservation and hydrogen ion elimination (refer to Table 10.6).

Compensatory changes in respirations occur within minutes of a change in pH. These changes, however, become less effective over time. The renal response takes longer to restore the pH, but is a more effective long-term mechanism. If the pH is restored to within normal limits, the disorder is said to be fully compensated. When these changes are reflected in ABG values but the pH remains outside normal limits, the disorder is said to be partially compensated.

The Patient with Metabolic Acidosis

Metabolic acidosis (bicarbonate deficit) is characterized by low pH (< 7.35) and low bicarbonate (< 22 mEq/L) values. It may be caused by excess acid in the body or loss of bicarbonate from the body. When metabolic acidosis develops, the respiratory system attempts to return the pH to normal by increasing the rate and depth of respirations. Carbon dioxide elimination increases, and the $PaCO_2$ falls (< 35 mmHg) (refer to Figure 10.14).

Risk Factors

Metabolic acidosis is rarely a primary disorder; it usually develops during the course of another disease:

- Acute lactic acidosis usually results from tissue hypoxia due to shock or cardiac arrest.
- Patients with type 1 diabetes mellitus are at risk for developing diabetic ketoacidosis. (See Chapter 20 for more information about diabetes and its complications.)
- Acute or chronic renal failure impairs the excretion of metabolic acids.
- Diarrhea, intestinal suction, or abdominal fistulas increase the risk for excess bicarbonate loss.

Other common causes of metabolic acidosis are listed in Table 10.6.

Pathophysiology

Three basic mechanisms that can cause metabolic acidosis are (1) accumulation of metabolic acids, (2) excess loss of bicarbonate, and (3) an increase in chloride levels.

An accumulation of metabolic acids can result from excess acid production or impaired elimination of metabolic acids by the kidney. Lactic acidosis develops due to tissue hypoxia and a shift to anaerobic metabolism by the cells. Lactate and hydrogen ions are produced, forming lactic acid. Both oxygen and glucose are necessary for normal cell metabolism. When intracellular glucose is inadequate due to starvation or a lack of insulin to move it into cells, the body breaks down fatty tissue to meet its metabolic needs. In this process, fatty acids are released, which are converted to ketones; ketoacidosis develops. Substances such as aspirin, methanol (wood alcohol), and ethylene (contained in antifreeze and solvents) cause a toxic increase in body acids by either breaking down into acid products (salicylic acid) or stimulating metabolic acid production (Sorenson et al., 2019). Renal failure impairs the body's ability to excrete excess hydrogen ions and form bicarbonate.

Excess metabolic acids increase the hydrogen ion concentration of body fluids. The excess acid is buffered by bicarbonate, leading to what is known as a high anion gap acidosis (see **Box 10.9**).

The pancreas secretes bicarbonate-rich fluid into the small intestine. Intestinal suction, severe diarrhea, ileostomy drainage, or fistulas can lead to excess losses of bicarbonate. Hyperchloremic acidosis can develop when excess chloride solutions (such as NaCl or ammonium chloride) are infused, causing a rise in chloride concentrations. It may also be related to renal disease or administration of carbonic

BOX 10.9
Unraveling the Anion Gap

Calculation of the anion gap can help identify the underlying mechanism in metabolic acidosis if it is unclear.

The number of cations (positively charged ions) and anions (negatively charged ions) in ECF is normally equal (refer to Figure 10.2). Not all of these ions, however, are measured in laboratory testing (e.g., organic acids and proteins). The anion gap is calculated by subtracting the sum of two measured anions, chloride and bicarbonate, from the concentration of the major cation, sodium (see the accompanying figure). The normal anion gap is 8 to 12 mEq/L.

Excess acids in ECF are buffered by bicarbonate, reducing serum bicarbonate levels and the total measured concentration of anions. This increases the anion gap (**B** in figure). When bicarbonate is lost from the body or chloride levels increase, however, the anion gap remains within normal limits (**C** in figure). This occurs because an increase or decrease in one of these negatively charged ions causes a corresponding change in the other to maintain balance (e.g., $\downarrow HCO_3^- \leftrightarrow \uparrow Cl^-$), and there is no change in the amount of unmeasured anions.

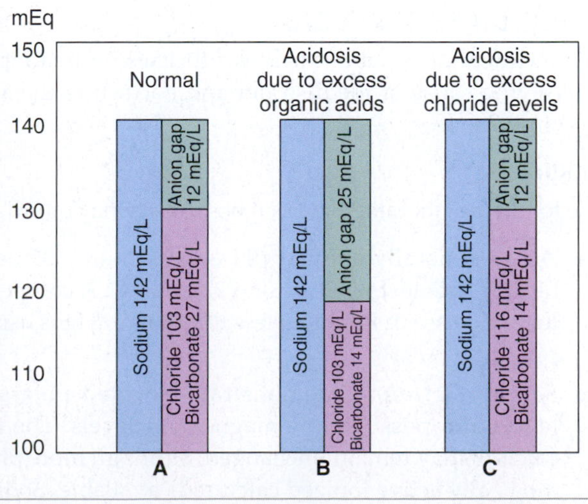
mEq
150
140
130
120
110
100
Normal
Acidosis due to excess organic acids
Acidosis due to excess chloride levels
Sodium 142 mEq/L
Anion gap 12 mEq/L
Chloride 103 mEq/L Bicarbonate 27 mEq/L
Sodium 142 mEq/L
Anion gap 25 mEq/L
Chloride 103 mEq/L Bicarbonate 14 mEq/L
Sodium 142 mEq/L
Anion gap 12 mEq/L
Chloride 116 mEq/L Bicarbonate 14 mEq/L
A
B
C

anhydrate inhibitor diuretics. The anion gap remains normal in metabolic acidosis due to bicarbonate loss or excess chloride.

Acidosis depresses cell membrane excitability, affecting neuromuscular function. It also increases the amount of free calcium in ECF by interfering with protein binding. Severe acidosis (pH of 7.0 or less) depresses myocardial contractility, leading to a fall in cardiac output. If kidney function is normal, acid excretion and ammonia production increase to eliminate excess hydrogen ions.

Acid–base imbalances also affect electrolyte balance. In acidosis, potassium is retained as the kidney excretes excess hydrogen ions. Excess hydrogen ions also enter the cells, displacing potassium from the intracellular space to maintain the balance of cations and anions within the cells. The effect of both processes is to increase serum potassium levels. Also, in acidosis, calcium is released from its bonds with plasma proteins, increasing the amount of ionized (free) calcium in the blood. Magnesium levels may fall in acidosis.

Manifestations

Metabolic acidosis affects the function of many body systems. Its general manifestations include:

- Anorexia, nausea and vomiting
- Abdominal pain
- Weakness and fatigue
- General malaise
- Decreasing levels of consciousness
- Dysrhythmias, bradycardia
- Warm, flushed skin
- Hyperventilation (Kussmaul respirations).

Gastrointestinal function is affected, causing anorexia, nausea and vomiting, and abdominal pain. The level of consciousness declines, leading to stupor and coma. Cardiac dysrhythmias develop, and cardiac arrest may occur. The skin is often warm and flushed. Manifestations of compensatory mechanisms are seen. The respirations, known as **Kussmaul respirations**, are labored, deep, and rapid. The patient may complain of shortness of breath or dyspnea.

Interprofessional Care

Management of metabolic acidosis focuses on treating the underlying cause of the disorder and correcting the acid–base imbalance.

Diagnosis

The following laboratory and diagnostic tests may be ordered:

- *ABGs* generally show a pH of less than 7.35 and a bicarbonate level of less than 22 mEq/L. A compensatory decrease in $PaCO_2$ to less than 35 mmHg is usually present.
- *Serum electrolytes* demonstrate elevated potassium levels and possible low magnesium levels. The total calcium may remain unchanged, although more physiologically active ionized calcium is available. Sodium, chloride, and bicarbonate levels are used to calculate the anion gap.
- *ECG* may show changes that reflect both the acidosis (particularly when severe) and the accompanying hyperkalemia.
- Other diagnostic studies such as blood glucose and renal function studies may be ordered to identify the underlying cause of metabolic acidosis.

Medications

An alkalinizing solution such as bicarbonate may be given for severe acidosis ($pH < 7.1$) to reduce the effects of the acidosis on cardiac function. Sodium bicarbonate is the most commonly used alkalinizing solution; others include lactate, citrate, and acetate solutions (which are metabolized to bicarbonate). Alkalinizing solutions are given IV for severe acute metabolic acidosis. In chronic metabolic acidosis, the oral route is used.

The patient treated with bicarbonate must be carefully monitored. Rapid correction of the acidosis may lead to metabolic alkalosis and hypokalemia. Hypernatremia and hyperosmolality may develop as well, leading to water retention and fluid overload.

SAFETY ALERT: As metabolic acidosis is corrected, potassium shifts back into the intracellular space. This can lead to hypokalemia and cardiac dysrhythmias. Carefully monitor serum potassium levels during treatment. ■

Treatment for diabetic ketoacidosis includes IV insulin and fluid. Alcoholic ketoacidosis is treated with saline solutions and glucose. Treatment for lactic acidosis from decreased tissue perfusion (e.g., shock or cardiac arrest) focuses on correcting the underlying problem and improving tissue perfusion. Patients with chronic renal failure and mild or moderate metabolic acidosis may or may not require treatment, depending on the pH and bicarbonate levels. When metabolic acidosis is due to diarrhea, treatment includes correcting the underlying cause and providing fluid and electrolyte replacement.

Nursing Care

Nurses frequently provide care for patients with metabolic acidosis, although the focus of care is often the disorder underlying the acidosis (e.g., diabetes mellitus, renal failure) rather than the acidosis itself. For this reason, it is vital for the nurse to be aware of the effects of the acidosis and its implications for nursing care.

Assessment

Assessment data related to metabolic acidosis include:

- *Health history:* current manifestations, including anorexia, nausea and vomiting, abdominal discomfort, fatigue, lethargy, other manifestations; duration of manifestations and any precipitating factors such as diarrhea, ingestion of a toxin such as aspirin, methanol, or ethylene; chronic diseases such as diabetes or renal failure, cirrhosis of the liver, or endocrine disorders; current medications

- *Physical assessment:* mental status and level of consciousness; vital signs; apical and peripheral pulses; skin color and temperature; abdominal contour and distention; bowel sounds; urine output.

Priorities of Care

While interprofessional management of the patient with metabolic acidosis focuses on correcting the imbalance and the underlying condition causing it, monitoring for adverse effects of the imbalance and treatment instituted is the priority for nursing management.

Diagnoses, Outcomes, and Interventions

Monitor Cardiac Output. Metabolic acidosis affects cardiac output by decreasing myocardial contractility, slowing the heart rate, and increasing the risk for dysrhythmias. The accompanying hyperkalemia increases the risk for decreased cardiac output as well (see the earlier discussion about hyperkalemia). As the acidosis is corrected, potassium shifts back into ICF, placing the patient at risk for hypokalemia.

Expected Outcome: Patient's cardiac output will remain within expected range as evidenced by clear mentation; normal color; warm, dry skin; stable vital signs; and urine output greater than 30 mL/h.

The nurse will:

- Monitor vital signs, including peripheral pulses and capillary refill. *Hypotension, diminished pulse strength, and slowed capillary refill may indicate decreased cardiac output and impaired tissue perfusion. Poor tissue perfusion can increase the risk for lactic acidosis.*
- Monitor the ECG pattern for dysrhythmias and changes characteristic of potassium imbalances (hyperkalemia or hypokalemia). Notify the physician of changes. *Progressive ECG changes such as widening of the QRS complex indicate an increasing risk of dysrhythmias and cardiac arrest. Dysrhythmias further decrease cardiac output, possibly intensifying the degree of acidosis.*
- Monitor laboratory values, including ABGs, serum electrolytes, and renal function studies (serum creatinine and BUN). *Frequent monitoring of laboratory values allows evaluation of the effectiveness of treatment as well as early identification of potential problems.*

SAFETY ALERT: Apply firm pressure to the puncture site for 2–5 minutes after the needle is withdrawn following aspiration of arterial blood to measure ABGs to prevent bleeding into the surrounding tissues. Pressure may need to be applied longer for patients receiving anticoagulation medications. ■

Monitor Fluid Volume. Administering bicarbonate to correct severe acidosis increases the risk for hypernatremia, hyperosmolality, and FVE.

Expected Outcome: Patient's fluid balance will be maintained as evidenced by balanced intake and output, stable weight and vital signs, and laboratory values within expected ranges.

The nurse will:

- Monitor and maintain fluid replacement as ordered. Monitor serum sodium levels and osmolality. *Bicarbonate administration can cause hypernatremia and hyperosmolality, leading to water retention.*
- Monitor heart and lung sounds, hemodynamic pressures, and respiratory status. *Increasing dyspnea, adventitious lung sounds and a high venous or atrial pressure reading, and a third heart sound (S_3) due to the volume of blood flow through the heart are indicative of hypervolemia and should be reported to the healthcare provider.*
- Assess for edema, particularly in the back, sacral, and periorbital areas. *Initially, edema affects dependent tissues—the back and sacrum in patients who are bedridden. Periorbital edema indicates more generalized edema.*
- Assess urine output hourly. Maintain accurate intake and output records. Note urine output less than 30 mL/h or a positive fluid balance on 24-hour total intake and output calculations. *Heart failure and inadequate renal perfusion may lead to decreased urine output.*
- Obtain daily weights using consistent conditions. *Daily weights are an accurate indicator of fluid balance.*
- Administer prescribed diuretics as ordered, monitoring the patient's response to therapy. *Loop or high-ceiling diuretics such as furosemide (Lasix) can lead to further electrolyte imbalances, especially hypokalemia. This is a significant risk like that seen during correction of metabolic acidosis.*

Reduce Risk for Injury. Mental status and brain function are affected by acidosis, increasing the risk for injury.

Expected Outcome: Patient will remain free of injury.

The nurse will:

- Monitor neurologic function, including mental status, level of consciousness, and muscle strength. *As the pH falls, mental functioning declines, leading to confusion, stupor, and a decreasing level of consciousness.*
- Institute safety precautions as necessary: Keep the bed in its lowest position, use a position alarm as needed. *These measures help protect the patient from injury resulting from confusion or disorientation.*
- Keep clocks, calendars, and familiar objects at bedside. Orient to time, place, and circumstances as needed. Allow significant others to remain with the patient as much as possible. *An unfamiliar environment and altered thought processes can further increase the risk for injury. Significant others provide a sense of security and reduce anxiety.*

Delegating Nursing Care Activities

As appropriate and allowed by the designated duties and responsibilities of assistive personnel, the nurse may delegate nursing care activities such as measuring intake and output, obtaining daily weights, and assisting with safety precautions and reorientation for the patient with metabolic acidosis.

Transitions of Care

To promote health in patients at risk for metabolic acidosis, discuss management of their underlying disease process (e.g., type 1 diabetes or renal failure) to prevent complications such as diabetic ketoacidosis and metabolic acidosis. Because early manifestations of metabolic acidosis (e.g., fatigue, general malaise, anorexia, nausea, abdominal pain) resemble those of common viral disorders such as the flu, stress the importance of promptly seeking treatment if these manifestations develop.

As described previously, acute metabolic disorder requires prompt action. Eliminating the underlying cause (if possible) and instituting appropriate treatment is required. Nursing care focuses on implementing the treatment and patient education of the treatment plan.

Discharge planning and teaching focus on the underlying cause of the imbalance. The patient who has developed ketoacidosis as a result of diabetes mellitus, starvation, or alcoholism needs interventions and teaching to prevent future episodes of acidosis. Diet, medication management, and alcohol dependency treatment are vital teaching areas. When metabolic acidosis is related to renal failure, the patient should be referred for management of the renal failure itself. Patients who have experienced diarrhea or excess ileostomy drainage leading to bicarbonate loss need information about appropriate diarrhea treatment strategies and when to call their primary care provider.

The Patient with Metabolic Alkalosis

Metabolic alkalosis (bicarbonate excess) is characterized by a high pH (>7.45) and a high bicarbonate ($>$ 26 mEq/L). It may be caused by loss of acid or excess bicarbonate in the body. When metabolic alkalosis develops, the respiratory system attempts to return the pH to normal by slowing the respiratory rate (refer to Figure 10.15). Carbon dioxide is retained, and the $PaCO_2$ increases ($>$ 45 mmHg).

Risk Factors

As is the case with other acid–base imbalances, metabolic alkalosis rarely occurs as a primary disorder. Risk factors include hospitalization, hypokalemia, and treatment with alkalinizing solutions (e.g., bicarbonate).

Pathophysiology

Hydrogen ions may be lost via gastric secretions, through the kidneys, or because of a shift of H^+ into the cells. Metabolic alkalosis due to loss of hydrogen ions usually occurs because of vomiting or gastric suction. Gastric secretions are highly acidic (pH 1 to 3). When these are lost through vomiting or gastric suction, both H^+ and chloride are lost. Chloride is the major anion in ECF; when it is lost, bicarbonate is retained as a replacement anion. As a result, the alkalinity of body fluids increases.

Increased renal excretion of hydrogen ions can be prompted by hypokalemia as the kidneys try to conserve potassium, excreting hydrogen ion instead. Hypokalemia contributes to metabolic alkalosis in another way as well. When potassium shifts out of cells to maintain extracellular potassium levels, hydrogen ions shift into the cells to maintain the balance between cations and anions within the cell.

Excess bicarbonate usually occurs as a result of ingesting antacids that contain bicarbonate (such as soda bicarbonate or Alka-Seltzer) or overzealous administration of bicarbonate to treat metabolic acidosis. Common causes of metabolic alkalosis are summarized in Table 10.6.

In alkalosis, more calcium combines with serum proteins, reducing the amount of ionized (physiologically active) calcium in the blood. This accounts for many of the common manifestations of metabolic alkalosis. Alkalosis also affects potassium balance: Hypokalemia not only can cause metabolic alkalosis (see the earlier discussion), but it also can result from metabolic alkalosis. Hydrogen ions shift out of the intracellular space to help restore the pH, prompting more potassium to enter the cells and depleting ECF potassium. The high pH depresses the respiratory system as the body retains carbon dioxide to restore the carbonic acid:bicarbonate ratio.

Manifestations and Complications

Manifestations of metabolic alkalosis occur as a result of decreased calcium ionization and are similar to those of hypocalcemia, including:

- Confusion
- Decreasing level of consciousness
- Hyperreflexia
- Tetany
- Dysrhythmias
- Hypotension
- Seizures
- Respiratory failure
- Numbness and tingling around the mouth, fingers, and toes
- Dizziness
- Trousseau sign
- Muscle spasms.

As the respiratory system compensates for metabolic alkalosis, respirations are depressed and respiratory failure with hypoxemia and respiratory acidosis may develop.

Interprofessional Care

Interprofessional management of metabolic alkalosis focuses on diagnosing and correcting the underlying cause.

Diagnosis

The following laboratory and diagnostic tests may be ordered:

- ***ABGs*** show a pH greater than 7.45 and bicarbonate level greater than 26 mEq/L. With compensatory hypoventilation, carbon dioxide is retained, and the $PaCO_2$ is greater than 45 mmHg.

- ***Serum electrolytes*** often demonstrate hypokalemia (serum $K^+ < 3.5$ mEq/L) and decreased chloride (< 95 mEq/L) levels. The serum bicarbonate level is high. Although the total serum calcium may be normal, the ionized fraction of calcium is low.
- ***Urine pH*** may be low (pH 1 to 3) if metabolic alkalosis is caused by hypokalemia. The kidneys selectively retain potassium and excrete hydrogen ion to restore ECF potassium levels. Urinary chloride levels may be normal or greater than 250 mEq/24 hours.
- ***ECG pattern*** shows changes similar to those seen with hypokalemia. These changes may be due to hypokalemia or to the alkalosis.

Medications

Treatment of metabolic alkalosis includes restoring normal fluid volume and administering potassium chloride and sodium chloride solution. The potassium restores serum and intracellular potassium levels, allowing the kidneys to more effectively conserve hydrogen ions. Chloride promotes renal excretion of bicarbonate. Sodium chloride solutions restore FVDs that can contribute to metabolic alkalosis. In severe alkalosis, an acidifying solution such as dilute hydrochloric acid or ammonium chloride may be administered. In addition, drugs may be used to treat the underlying cause of the alkalosis.

Nursing Care

Assessment

Focused assessment data related to metabolic alkalosis include:

- ***Health history:*** current manifestations, such as numbness and tingling, muscle spasms, dizziness, other manifestations; duration of manifestations and any precipitating factors such as bicarbonate ingestion, vomiting, diuretic therapy, or endocrine disorders; current medications
- ***Physical assessment:*** vital signs including apical pulse and rate and depth of respirations; muscle strength; deep tendon reflexes.

Priorities of Care

The risk for impaired gas exchange as a compensatory response to metabolic alkalosis is a priority problem, especially when the alkalosis is severe or when the patient's respiratory status is compromised by underlying lung disease.

Diagnoses, Outcomes, and Interventions

Monitor Gas Exchange. Respiratory compensation for metabolic alkalosis depresses the respiratory rate and reduces the depth of breathing to promote carbon dioxide retention. As a result, the patient is at risk for impaired gas exchange.

Expected Outcome: Patient's rate and depth of respirations and oxygen saturation levels will remain within normal range.

The nurse will:

- Monitor respiratory rate, depth, and effort. Monitor oxygen saturation continuously, reporting an oxygen saturation level of less than 95% (or as ordered). *The depressed respiratory drive associated with metabolic alkalosis can lead to hypoxemia and impaired oxygenation of tissues. Oxygen saturation levels of less than 90% indicate significant oxygenation problems.*
- Assess skin color; note and report cyanosis around the mouth. *Central cyanosis, seen around the mouth and oral mucous membranes, indicates significant hypoxia.*
- Monitor mental status and level of consciousness (LOC). Report decreasing LOC or behavior changes such as restlessness, agitation, or confusion. *Changes in mental status or behavior may be early manifestations of hypoxia.*
- Place in semi-Fowler or Fowler position as tolerated. *Elevating the head of the bed facilitates alveolar ventilation and gas exchange.*
- Schedule nursing care activities to allow rest periods. *The patient who is hypoxemic has limited energy reserves, necessitating frequent rest and limited activities.*
- Administer oxygen as ordered or necessary to maintain oxygen saturation levels. *Supplemental oxygen can help maintain blood and tissue oxygenation despite depressed respirations.*

Monitor Fluid Volume. Patients with metabolic alkalosis often have an accompanying FVD.

Expected Outcome: Patient's fluid balance will be maintained as evidenced by stable vital signs and weight, balanced intake and output, and laboratory values within expected ranges.

The nurse will:

- Assess vital signs, CVP, and peripheral pulse volume at least every 4 hours. *Hypotension, tachycardia, a low CVP, and weak, easily obliterated peripheral pulses indicate hypovolemia.*
- Weigh daily under standard conditions (time of day, clothing, and scale). *Rapid weight changes accurately reflect fluid balance.*
- Administer IV fluids as prescribed using an infusion pump. Monitor for indicators of fluid overload if rapid fluid replacement is ordered: dyspnea, tachypnea, tachycardia, Increased CVP, jugular vein distention, and edema. *Rapid fluid replacement may lead to hypervolemia, resulting in pulmonary edema and cardiac failure, particularly in patients with compromised cardiac and renal function.*
- Monitor serum electrolytes, osmolality, and ABG values. *Rehydration and administration of potassium chloride will affect both acid–base and fluid and electrolyte balance. Careful monitoring is important to identify changes.*

Delegating Nursing Care Activities

Under the direction of the nurse, nursing care activities such as positioning, measuring vital signs and intake and output, obtaining daily weights, and providing hygiene measures for the patient with metabolic alkalosis may be performed by assistive personnel.

Transitions of Care

Health promotion activities focus on teaching patients the risks of using sodium bicarbonate as an antacid to relieve heartburn or gastric distress. Stress the availability of other effective antacid preparations and the need to seek medical evaluation for persistent gastric manifestations. In the hospital setting, carefully monitor laboratory values for patients at risk for developing metabolic alkalosis, particularly patients undergoing continuous gastric suction.

Acute treatment of metabolic alkalosis includes the discussion above under treatment. During the acute treatment phase the nurse is responsible for assessment of the patient condition, carrying out the treatment regimen, and patient education concerning the treatment regimen.

When preparing the patient with metabolic alkalosis for discharge or continuing care, consider the cause of the alkalosis and any underlying factors. For example, provide teaching about:

- Using appropriate antacids for heartburn and gastric distress
- Using potassium supplements as ordered or eating high-potassium foods to avoid hypokalemia if taking a potassium-wasting diuretic or if aldosterone production is impaired
- Contacting the primary care provider if uncontrolled or extended vomiting develops.

The Patient with Respiratory Acidosis

Respiratory acidosis is caused by an excess of dissolved carbon dioxide or carbonic acid. It is characterized by a pH of < 7.35 and a $PaCO_2 > 45$ mmHg (refer to Figure 10.16). Respiratory acidosis may be either acute or chronic. In chronic respiratory acidosis, the bicarbonate is > 26 mEq/L as the kidneys compensate by retaining bicarbonate.

Risk Factors

Acute or chronic lung disease (e.g., pneumonia or chronic obstructive pulmonary disease [COPD]) is the primary risk factor for respiratory acidosis. Other conditions that depress or interfere with ventilation, such as opioid (narcotic) overdose, airway obstruction, or neuromuscular disease, are also risk factors for respiratory acidosis. Selected causes of respiratory acidosis are listed in Table 10.6.

Pathophysiology

Both acute and chronic respiratory acidosis result from carbon dioxide retention caused by alveolar hypoventilation. Hypoxemia (low oxygen in the arterial blood) frequently accompanies respiratory acidosis.

Acute Respiratory Acidosis

Acute respiratory acidosis occurs as the result of a sudden failure of ventilation. Chest trauma, aspiration of a foreign body, acute pneumonia, and overdoses of narcotic or sedative medications can lead to this condition. Because acute respiratory acidosis occurs with the sudden onset of hypoventilation—for example, with cardiac arrest—the $PaCO_2$ rises rapidly and the pH falls markedly. A pH of 7 or lower can occur within minutes (Sorenson et al., 2019). The serum bicarbonate level is initially unchanged because the compensatory response of the kidneys occurs over hours to days.

Hypercapnia (increased carbon dioxide levels) affects neurologic function and the cardiovascular system. Carbon dioxide rapidly crosses the blood–brain barrier. Cerebral blood vessels dilate and, if the condition continues, intracranial pressure increases and papilledema (swelling and inflammation of the optic nerve where it enters the retina) develops. Peripheral vasodilation also occurs, and the pulse rate increases to maintain cardiac output.

Chronic Respiratory Acidosis

Chronic respiratory acidosis is associated with chronic respiratory or neuromuscular conditions such as COPD, asthma, cystic fibrosis, or multiple sclerosis. These conditions affect alveolar ventilation because of airway obstruction, structural changes in the lung, or limited chest wall expansion. Most patients with chronic respiratory acidosis have COPD with chronic bronchitis and emphysema. In chronic respiratory acidosis, the $PaCO_2$ increases over time and remains elevated. The kidneys retain bicarbonate, increasing bicarbonate levels, and the pH often remains close to the normal range.

The acute effects of hypercapnia may not develop because carbon dioxide levels rise gradually, allowing compensatory changes to occur. When carbon dioxide levels are chronically elevated, the respiratory center becomes less sensitive to the gas as a stimulant of the respiratory drive. The PaO_2 provides the primary stimulus for respirations. Patients with chronic respiratory acidosis are at risk for developing carbon dioxide narcosis, with manifestations of acute respiratory acidosis, if the respiratory center is suppressed by administering excess supplemental oxygen.

SAFETY ALERT: Carefully monitor neurologic and respiratory status in patients with chronic respiratory acidosis who are receiving oxygen therapy. Immediately report a decreasing LOC or depressed respirations. ■

Manifestations

The manifestations of acute and chronic respiratory acidosis differ. In acute respiratory acidosis, the rapid rise in $PaCO_2$ levels causes manifestations of hypercapnia. Cerebral vasodilation causes manifestations such as headache, blurred vision, irritability, and mental cloudiness. If the condition continues, the level of consciousness progressively decreases. Rapid and dramatic changes in ABGs can lead to unconsciousness and ventricular fibrillation, a potentially lethal cardiac dysrhythmia. The skin of the patient with acute respiratory acidosis may be warm and flushed, and the pulse rate is elevated.

The manifestations of chronic respiratory acidosis include weakness and a dull headache. Sleep disturbances, daytime sleepiness, impaired memory, and personality changes may also be manifestations of chronic respiratory acidosis. The manifestations of acute and chronic respiratory acidosis are summarized in **Box 10.10**.

Interprofessional Care

Patients with acute respiratory failure usually require treatment in the emergency department or intensive care unit. The focus is on restoring adequate ventilation and gas exchange. Hypoxemia often accompanies acute respiratory acidosis, so oxygen is administered as well. Supplemental oxygen is administered with caution to patients with chronic respiratory acidosis.

Diagnosis

The following laboratory and diagnostic tests may be ordered:

- ***ABGs*** show a pH of less than 7.35 and a $PaCO_2$ of more than 45 mmHg. In acute respiratory acidosis, the bicarbonate level is initially within normal range but increases to greater than 26 mEq/L as the kidneys generate bicarbonate if the condition persists. In chronic respiratory acidosis, both the $PaCO_2$ and the HCO_3^- may be significantly elevated.
- ***Serum electrolytes*** may show hypochloremia (chloride level < 98 mEq/L) in chronic respiratory acidosis.

Additional diagnostic tests may be done to identify the underlying cause of the respiratory acidosis. *Chest x-ray* and *sputum studies* (cytology and culture) may be ordered to identify an acute or chronic lung disorder. If drug overdose is suspected, serum levels of the drug may be obtained. Pulmonary function tests may be done to determine if chronic lung disease is the cause of the respiratory acidosis.

Medications

Bronchodilator drugs may be administered to open the airways and antibiotics prescribed to treat respiratory infections. If excess narcotics or anesthetic has caused acute respiratory acidosis, drugs to reverse their effects (such as naloxone) may be given.

BOX 10.10

Differentiating Acute and Chronic Respiratory Acidosis

Acute Respiratory Acidosis	Chronic Respiratory Acidosis
■ Headache ■ Warm, flushed skin ■ Blurred vision ■ Irritability, altered mental status ■ Decreasing level of consciousness ■ Cardiac arrest	■ Weakness ■ Dull headache ■ Sleep disturbances with daytime sleepiness ■ Impaired memory ■ Personality changes

Respiratory Support

Treatment of respiratory acidosis, either acute or chronic, focuses on improving alveolar ventilation and gas exchange. Pulmonary hygiene measures, such as breathing treatments or percussion and drainage, may be instituted. Adequate hydration is important to promote removal of respiratory secretions. In patients with chronic respiratory acidosis, oxygen is administered cautiously to avoid carbon dioxide narcosis.

High-Acuity Care

Patients with severe respiratory acidosis and hypoxemia may require intubation and mechanical ventilation. The $PaCO_2$ level is lowered slowly to avoid complications such as cardiac dysrhythmias and decreased cerebral perfusion. In patients with chronic respiratory acidosis, mechanical ventilation allows administration of a higher percentage of oxygen because the ventilator can maintain adequate respirations should the respiratory center be depressed.

Nursing Care

Assessment

Assessment data related to respiratory acidosis include:

- ***Health history:*** current manifestations, including headache, irritability or lethargy, difficulty thinking, blurred vision, and other manifestations; duration of manifestations and any precipitating factors such as drug use or respiratory infection; chronic diseases such as cystic fibrosis or COPD; current medications
- ***Physical assessment:*** mental status and level of consciousness; vital signs; skin color and temperature; rate and depth of respirations, pulmonary excursion, lung sounds; examination of optic fundus for possible papilledema.

Priorities of Care

Restoring effective alveolar ventilation and gas exchange is the priority of interprofessional and nursing care for patients with respiratory acidosis.

Diagnoses, Outcomes, and Interventions

Monitor Gas Exchange. The patient in respiratory distress is at risk for carbon dioxide retention, resulting in respiratory acidosis.

Expected Outcome: Patient's gas exchange will be restored as evidenced by oxygen saturation and ABGs within normal ranges for patient.

The nurse will:

- Frequently assess respiratory status, including rate, depth, effort, and oxygen saturation levels. *Decreasing respiratory rate and effort along with decreasing oxygen saturation levels may signal worsening respiratory failure and respiratory acidosis.*
- Frequently assess level of consciousness. *A decline in LOC may indicate increasing hypercapnia and the need for increasing ventilatory support (such as intubation and mechanical ventilation).*

- Promptly evaluate and report ABG results to the physician and respiratory therapist. *Rapid changes in carbon dioxide or oxygen levels may necessitate modification of the treatment plan to prevent complications of overcorrection of respiratory acidosis.*
- Place in semi-Fowler to Fowler position as tolerated. *Elevating the head of the bed promotes lung expansion and gas exchange.*
- Administer oxygen as ordered. Carefully monitor response. Reduce the oxygen flow rate or percentage and immediately report increasing somnolence. *Supplemental oxygen can suppress the respiratory drive in patients with chronic respiratory acidosis.*

Maintain Effective Airway Clearance. The patient in respiratory distress is at risk for accumulation of respiratory secretions.

Expected Outcome: Effective ventilation will be restored as evidenced by clear lung sounds and a respiratory rate and depth that is normal for patient.

The nurse will:

- Frequently auscultate breath sounds (whether on or off a mechanical ventilator). *Increasing adventitious sounds or decreasing breath sounds (faint or absent) may indicate worsening airway clearance due to obstruction or fatigue.*
- Encourage the patient with chronic respiratory acidosis to use pursed-lip breathing. *Pursed-lip breathing helps maintain open airways throughout exhalation, promoting carbon dioxide elimination.*
- Frequently reposition and encourage ambulation as tolerated. *Repositioning, sitting at the bedside, and ambulation promote airway clearance and lung expansion.*
- Encourage fluid intake of up to 3000 mL per day as tolerated or allowed. *Fluids help liquefy secretions and hydrate respiratory mucous membranes, promoting airway clearance.*
- Administer medications such as inhaled bronchodilators as ordered. *Inhaled bronchodilators help relieve bronchial spasm, dilating airways.*
- Provide percussion, vibration, and postural drainage as ordered. *Pulmonary hygiene measures such as these help loosen respiratory secretions so they can be coughed out of airways.*

Delegating Nursing Care Activities

As appropriate and allowed by the designated duties and responsibilities of assistive personnel, the nurse may delegate nursing care activities such as measuring intake and output, obtaining vital signs and daily weights, repositioning and assisting with ambulation, and providing oral care.

See the Case Study & Nursing Care Plan for a patient with acute respiratory acidosis on page 279.

Transitions of Care

Health promotion activities related to respiratory acidosis focus on identifying, monitoring, and teaching patients at risk. Carefully monitor patients receiving anesthesia, narcotic analgesics, or sedatives for manifestations of respiratory depression. Monitor the response of patients with a history of chronic lung disease to oxygen therapy. Teach patients who have an identified risk for respiratory acidosis (such as people using narcotic analgesia for cancer pain and people with chronic lung disease) and their families about early manifestations of respiratory depression and acidosis, and instruct them to immediately contact their care provider if manifestations develop.

As described above, acute respiratory acidosis needs urgent medical attention. Acute respiratory acidosis can lead to respiratory failure and then ultimately death. The bedside nurse is in the position to assess and monitor for subtle changes in the patient that can indicate worsening respiratory acidosis, such as changes in mentation and respiratory rate.

Planning and teaching for home or continuing care focuses on the health problem that caused the patient to develop respiratory acidosis. The patient who developed acute respiratory acidosis as a result of acute pneumonia or chest trauma may only require teaching to prevent future problems. If acute respiratory acidosis occurred secondary to a narcotic overdose, determine if the drug was prescribed for pain or if it was an illicit street drug. Provide teaching to the patient who requires narcotic medication on a continuing basis. Refer the patient using illicit drugs to a substance abuse counselor, treatment center, or Narcotics Anonymous as appropriate.

For patients with chronic lung disease, discuss ways to avoid future episodes of acute respiratory failure. Encourage the patient to be immunized against pneumococcal pneumonia and influenza. Discuss ways to avoid acute respiratory infections and measures to take when respiratory status is further compromised.

The Patient with Respiratory Alkalosis

Respiratory alkalosis is characterized by a pH > 7.45 and a $PaCO_2 < 35$ mmHg. It is always caused by hyperventilation leading to a carbon dioxide deficit (refer to Figure 10.17).

Risk Factors

Anxiety with hyperventilation is the most common cause of respiratory alkalosis; therefore, anxiety disorders increase the risk for this acid–base imbalance. In the patient who is critically ill, mechanical ventilation is a risk factor for respiratory alkalosis.

Pathophysiology

In acute respiratory alkalosis, the pH rises rapidly as the $PaCO_2$ falls. Because the kidneys are unable to rapidly adapt to the change in pH, the bicarbonate level remains within normal limits. Anxiety-based hyperventilation is the most common cause of acute respiratory alkalosis. Other physiologic causes of hyperventilation

Case Study & Nursing Care Plan

A Patient with Acute Respiratory Acidosis

Marlene Hitz, age 76, is eating lunch when she suddenly begins to choke and is unable to breathe. After several minutes of trying, an attendant at the senior center successfully dislodges some meat caught in Ms. Hitz's throat by using the Heimlich maneuver. Ms. Hitz is taken by ambulance to the emergency department for follow-up.

ASSESSMENT

Ms. Hitz is placed in an observation room. Oxygen is started at 4 L/min per nasal cannula. David Love, the nurse admitting Ms. Hitz, makes the following assessments: T 38.8°C (98.2°F), P 102 bpm, R 36/min and shallow, BP 146/92 mmHg, O_2 sat 92%. Skin is warm and dry. Alert but restless and not oriented to time or place; responds slowly to questions. Stat ABGs are drawn, a chest x-ray is done, and D_5 1/2NS is started IV at 50 mL/h.

The chest x-ray shows no abnormality. ABG results are pH 7.32 (normal: 7.35 to 7.45), $PaCO_2$ 48 mmHg (normal: 35 to 45 mmHg), PaO_2 92 mmHg (normal: 80 to 100 mmHg), and HCO_3^- 24 mEq/L (normal: 22 to 26 mEq/L).

DIAGNOSES

- Impaired ventilation related to temporary airway obstruction.
- Anxiety and confusion related to emergent hospitalization and temporarily impaired ventilation.

EXPECTED OUTCOMES

- Patient will regain normal gas exchange and ABG values.
- Patient will be alert and oriented to time, place, and person.
- Patient will remain free of injury.

PLANNING AND IMPLEMENTATION

- Monitor ABGs, to be redrawn in 2 hours.
- Monitor vital signs and respiratory status (including oxygen saturation) every 15 minutes for the first hour, then every hour.
- Assess color of skin, nail beds, and oral mucous membranes every hour.
- Assess mental status and orientation every hour.
- Monitor anxiety level as evidenced by restlessness and agitation.
- Maintain a calm, quiet environment.
- Provide reorientation and explain all activities.

EVALUATION

Ms. Hitz remains in the emergency department for 6 hours. Her ABGs are still abnormal, and David now notes the presence of respiratory crackles and wheezes. She is less anxious and responds appropriately when asked who and where she is. Because she has not regained normal gas exchange, Ms. Hitz is admitted to the hospital for continued observation and treatment.

CLINICAL REASONING IN PATIENT CARE

1. Describe the pathophysiologic process that leads to acute respiratory acidosis in Ms. Hitz.
2. Describe the effect of acidosis on mental function.
3. The emergency department physician provides the following orders on Ms. Hitz's admission to the ED: continuous cardiac monitoring; O_2 at 4 L/min per nasal cannula; IV of D_5 1/2NS at 50 mL/h; stat chest x-ray, ABGs, CBC, and serum electrolytes; 12-lead ECG; NPO until fully alert; keep in Fowler position. How would you prioritize these orders for implementation?
4. What teaching would you provide to Ms. Hitz to prevent future episodes of choking?

See Evaluating Your Response in Appendix B.

include high fever, hypoxia, gram-negative bacteremia, and thyrotoxicosis. Early salicylate intoxication (aspirin overdose), encephalitis, and high progesterone levels in pregnancy directly stimulate the respiratory center, potentially leading to hyperventilation and respiratory alkalosis. Hyperventilation can also occur during anesthesia or mechanical ventilation if the rate and tidal volume (depth) of ventilations are excessive.

If hyperventilation continues, the kidneys compensate by eliminating bicarbonate to restore the carbonic acid:bicarbonate ratio. The bicarbonate level is lower than normal in chronic respiratory alkalosis, and the pH may be close to the normal range.

Alkalosis increases binding of extracellular calcium to albumin, reducing ionized calcium levels. As a result, neuromuscular excitability increases and manifestations similar to hypocalcemia develop. Low carbon dioxide levels in the blood cause vasoconstriction of cerebral vessels, increasing the neurologic manifestations of the disorder.

Manifestations

The manifestations of respiratory alkalosis include:

- Dizziness
- Lightheadedness
- Numbness and tingling around mouth, hands, and feet
- Difficulty concentrating
- Tinnitus
- Palpitations
- Dyspnea
- Chest tightness
- Anxiety/panic
- Circumoral and distal extremity paresthesias
- Positive Chvostek sign
- Positive Trousseau sign
- Tremors
- Tetany
- Seizures; loss of consciousness.

Interprofessional Care

Management of respiratory alkalosis focuses on correcting the imbalance and treating the underlying cause.

Diagnosis

ABGs generally show a pH > 7.45 and a $PaCO_2$ of < 35 mmHg. In chronic hyperventilation, there is a compensatory decrease in serum bicarbonate to < 22 mEq/L and the pH may be near normal.

Medications

A sedative or antianxiety agent may be necessary to relieve anxiety and restore a normal breathing pattern. Additional drugs to correct underlying problems other than anxiety-induced hyperventilation may be ordered.

Respiratory Therapy

The usual treatment for anxiety-related respiratory alkalosis involves instructing the patient to breathe more slowly and having the patient breathe into a paper bag or rebreather mask. This allows rebreathing of exhaled carbon dioxide, increasing $PaCO_2$ levels and reducing the pH. If excessive ventilation by a mechanical ventilator is the cause of respiratory alkalosis, ventilator settings are adjusted to reduce the respiratory rate and tidal volume as indicated. When hypoxia is the underlying cause of hyperventilation, oxygen is administered.

Nursing Care

Diagnoses, Outcomes, and Interventions

Maintain Effective Breathing Pattern. The usual cause of hyperventilation and respiratory alkalosis is psychologic, although physiologic disorders can also lead to hyperventilation. It is important to not only address the hyperventilation, but also to identify the underlying cause.

Expected Outcome: Patient's respiratory rate and depth and ABG values will be within normal ranges.

The nurse will:

- Assess respiratory rate, depth, and ease. Monitor vital signs (including temperature) and skin color. *Assessment data can help identify the underlying cause, such as a fever or hypoxia.*
- Obtain subjective assessment data such as circumstances leading up to the current situation, current health and recent illnesses or medication use, and current manifestations. *Subjective data provide cues to the cause and circumstances of the hyperventilation response.*
- Reassure the patient that he or she is not experiencing a heart attack and that manifestations will resolve when breathing returns to normal. *Manifestations of hyperventilation and respiratory alkalosis such as dyspnea, chest tightness or pain, and palpitations can mimic those of a heart attack.*
- Instruct the patient to maintain eye contact and breathe with you to slow the respiratory rate. *These measures help to make the patient aware of respirations and provide a sense of support and control.*
- Have the patient breathe into a paper bag or apply a rebreather mask. *This allows the patient to rebreathe exhaled carbon dioxide, increasing the* $PaCO_2$ *and decreasing the pH.*
- Protect the patient from injury. *If hyperventilation continues to the point at which the patient loses consciousness, respirations will return to normal, as will acid–base balance.*

Transitions of Care

Identify patients at risk in the hospital (e.g., patients on mechanical ventilation or who have a fever or infection), and monitor assessment data and ABGs to identify early manifestations of hyperventilation and respiratory alkalosis.

As stated above, acute respiratory acidosis is usually due to hyperventilation caused by anxiety. Providing a calm environment and reassurance along with any prescribed treatments will help the patient avoid anxiety.

Planning and teaching for home care is directed toward the underlying cause of hyperventilation. If anxiety precipitated the episode, discuss anxiety management strategies with the patient. Refer the patient and family to a counselor if appropriate. Teach the patient to identify a hyperventilation reaction and how to breathe into a paper bag to manage it at home.

CHAPTER HIGHLIGHTS

10.1 Overview of Fluid and Electrolyte Balance

Describe the functions and regulatory mechanisms that maintain water and electrolyte balance in the body.

- The volume and composition of body fluid is normally maintained by a balance of fluid and electrolyte intake; elimination of water, electrolytes, and acids by the kidneys; and hormonal influences.
- Changes in any of these factors can lead to a fluid, electrolyte, or acid–base imbalance that adversely affects health.

10.2 Fluid and Electrolyte Imbalances

Describe the pathophysiology and manifestations of fluid volume deficit and fluid volume excess, and outline the interprofessional care, nursing care, and transitions of care for patients with these disorders.

- Fluid, electrolyte, and acid–base imbalances can affect all body systems, especially the cardio vascular system, the central nervous system, and the transmission of nerve impulses.
- Conversely, primary disorders of the respiratory, renal, cardiovascular, endocrine, or other body systems can lead to an imbalance of fluids, electrolytes, or acid–base status.

10.3 Sodium Imbalances

Describe the pathophysiology and manifestations of hyponatremia and hypernatremia, and outline the interprofessional care, nursing care, and transitions of care for patients with these disorders.

- Fluid and sodium imbalances are related; both affect serum osmolality.
- Because of the effect on serum osmolality, correction of sodium levels should be done slowly. This is to prevent rapid fluid shifts in the brain. Careful monitoring of level of consciousness is required when treating hypo- or hypernatremia.

10.4 Potassium Imbalances

Describe the pathophysiology and manifestations of hypokalemia and hyperkalemia, and outline the interprofessional care, nursing care, and transitions of care for patients with these disorders.

- Potassium imbalances are commonly seen in patients with acute or chronic illnesses. Both hypokalemia and hyperkalemia affect cardiac conduction and function. Carefully monitor cardiac rhythm and status in patients with very low or very high potassium levels.
- Replacement of potassium requires careful monitoring. Reduction in high levels of potassium can be a medical emergency.

10.5 Calcium Imbalances

Describe the pathophysiology and manifestations of hypocalcemia and hypercalcemia, and outline the interprofessional care, nursing care, and transitions of care for patients with these disorders.

- Calcium imbalances primarily affect neuromuscular transmission: Hypocalcemia increases neuromuscular irritability; hypercalcemia depresses neuromuscular transmission. Magnesium imbalances have a similar effect.
- Hypocalcemia should always be suspected with surgery near or on the thyroid gland.
- With both hypo- and hypercalcemia, the nurse should monitor for dysrhythmias.

10.6 Magnesium Imbalances

Describe the pathophysiology and manifestations of hypomagnecemia and hypermagnecemia, and outline the interprofessional care, nursing care, and transitions of care for patients with these disorders.

- High levels of magnesium are usually seen in patients with renal failure, and adrenal insufficiency.
- Low levels of magnesium are usually seen in patients with pancreatitis and excessive loss from the gastrointestinal system.
- Careful monitoring is needed when replacing magnesium via intravenous route.

10.7 Phosphate Imbalances

Describe the pathophysiology and manifestations of hypophosphatemia and hyperphosphatemia, and outline the interprofessional care, nursing care, and transitions of care for patients with these disorders.

- Phosphate imbalances are usually iatrogenic in nature.
- When monitoring replacement of another electrolyte, phosphate should also be monitored.

10.8 Regulation of Acid–Base Balance

Describe the functions and regulatory mechanisms that maintain acid–base balance in the body.

- Buffers, lungs, and kidneys work together to maintain acid–base balance in the body.

- Buffers respond to changes almost immediately; the lungs respond within minutes; the kidneys require hours to days to restore normal acid–base balance.
- By assessing bloodwork including arterial blood gases, the nurse can determine the acid–base balance and compensatory mechanisms of the patient under treatment.

10.9 Acid–Base Imbalances

Describe the pathophysiology and manifestations of metabolic acidosis, metabolic alkalosis, respiratory acidosis, and respiratory alkalosis, and outline the interprofessional care, nursing care, and transitions of care for patients with these disorders.

- The lungs compensate for metabolic acid–base imbalances by excreting or retaining carbon dioxide. This is accomplished by increasing or decreasing the rate and depth of respirations.
- The kidneys compensate for respiratory acid–base imbalances by producing and retaining or excreting bicarbonate and by retaining or excreting hydrogen ions.
- Acid–base imbalances may be caused by either metabolic or respiratory health problems.
- Simple acid–base imbalances (respiratory or metabolic acidosis or alkalosis) are more commonly seen than mixed imbalances.

TEST YOURSELF NCLEX-RN® REVIEW

1. A patient is admitted to the emergency department with hypovolemia. Which IV solution should the nurse anticipate administering?
   A. 3% sodium chloride
   B. 10% dextrose in water
   C. 0.45% sodium chloride
   D. Lactated Ringer solution
2. Which manifestations should the nurse expect to assess in a patient with fluid volume deficit? (Select all that apply.)
   A. Dyspnea
   B. Respiratory crackles
   C. Increased pulse rate
   D. Orthostatic hypotension
   E. Flat neck veins
3. The nurse is planning care for a patient with acute hypernatremia. What should the nurse include in this patient's plan of care? (Select all that apply.)
   A. Maintain IV access.
   B. Limit length of visits.
   C. Restrict fluids to 1500 mL per day.
   D. Conduct frequent neurologic checks.
   E. Orient to time, place, and person every 2 hours.
4. A patient's serum potassium level is 2.2 mEq/L. Which nursing action is the highest priority for this patient?
   A. Start oxygen at 2 L/min.
   B. Initiate cardiac monitoring.
   C. Initiate seizure precautions.
   D. Keep the patient on bedrest.
5. The nurse instructs a patient on calcium supplement therapy. Which statement indicates that the patient understands how to take calcium supplementation? (Select all that apply.)
   A. "I will take the calcium with meals."
   B. "I will take the calcium with a full glass of water."
   C. "I will take these supplements as needed for tremulousness."
   D. "I should not take these supplements with milk."
   E. "I will wait at least an hour after taking my other medications before I take my calcium."
6. A patient is demonstrating confusion, hallucinations, and a positive Chvostek sign. Which medication(s) should the nurse prepare to provide to this patient?
   A. Calcium chloride
   B. Magnesium sulfate
   C. Insulin and glucose
   D. Sodium bicarbonate
7. A patient's arterial blood gas results are pH 7.21, PaO_2 98 mmHg, $PaCO_2$ 32 mmHg, and HCO_3^- 17 mEq/L. Which acid–base imbalance do these results indicate to the nurse?
   A. Metabolic acidosis
   B. Metabolic alkalosis
   C. Respiratory acidosis
   D. Respiratory alkalosis
8. A patient diagnosed with a suspected heroin overdose has a respiratory rate of 5 to 6 per minute. Which additional data should the nurse expect to collect on this patient? (Select all that apply.)
   A. pH 7.29
   B. $PaCO_2$ 54 mmHg
   C. HCO_3^- 32 mEq/L
   D. Alert and oriented
   E. Skin warm and flushed
9. The nurse is caring for a patient undergoing gastric decompression. This patient is at risk for which acid–base imbalance?
   A. Metabolic acidosis
   B. Metabolic alkalosis
   C. Respiratory acidosis
   D. Respiratory alkalosis

10. A patient being mechanically ventilated after a severe chest wall injury and flail chest complains of dizziness, tingling around the mouth, and anxiety. What should the nurse do first?
    A. Notify the physician.
    B. Obtain arterial blood gases.
    C. Administer prescribed analgesic.
    D. Contact respiratory therapy to evaluate ventilator settings.

See Test Yourself answers in Appendix B.

REFERENCES

Adams, M. P., Holland, L. N., & Urban, C. (2017). *Pharmacology for nursing: A pathophysiologic approach* (5th ed.). Hoboken, NJ: Pearson Education.

American Heart Association. (2018). *How much sodium should I eat per day? #BreakUpWithSalt*. Retrieved from https://sodiumbreakup.heart.org/how_much_sodium_should_i_eat?utm_source=SRI&utm_medium=HeartOrg&utm_term=Website&utm_content=SodiumAndSalt&utm_campaign=SodiumBreakup.

Berman, A.T., Snyder, S., & Frandsen, G. (2016). *Kozier & Erb's fundamentals of nursing* (10th ed.). Hoboken, NJ: Pearson Education.

Centers for Disease Control and Prevention (CDC). (2017). *Get the facts: Sodium and the dietary guidelines.* Retrieved from https://www.cdc.gov/salt/pdfs/sodium_dietary_guidelines.pdf.

Doukky, R., Avery, E., Mangla, A., Collado, F. M., Ibrahiam, Z., Poulin, M. F., . . . Powell, L. H. (2016). Impact of dietary sodium restriction on heart failure outcomes. *JACC Heart Failure, 4*(1), 24–35.

Hogan, M. (2013). *Fluids, electrolytes, and acid–base balance: Reviews and rationales* (3rd ed.). Hoboken, NJ: Pearson Education.

Hoorn, E. J., & Zietse, R. (2017). Diagnosis and treatment of hyponatremia: Compilation of the guidelines. *Journal of the American Society of Nephrology, 28*(5), 1340–1349.

Hutto, C., & French, M. (2017). Neurologic intensive care unit electrolyte management. *Nursing Clinics of North America, 52*(3), 321–329.

Kee, J. L. (2018). *Laboratory and diagnostic tests with nursing implications* (10th ed.). Hoboken, NJ: Pearson Education.

Kelly, J. T., Palmer, S. C., Wia, S. N., Ruospo, M., Carrerp, J. J., Campbell, K. L., & Strippoli, G. F. M. (2016). Healthy dietary patterns and risk of mortality and ESRD in CKC: A meta-analysis of cohort studies. *Clinical Journal of the American Society of Nephrology, 12*(2), 272–279.

McCrow, J., Morton, M., Travers, C., Harvey K., & Eeles, E. (2016). Water, water everywhere: Dehydration in the midst of plenty—An observational study of barriers and enablers to adequate hydration in older hospitalized patients. *Clinical Nursing Studies, 4*(2), 1–7.

Metheny, N. M. (2012). *Fluid and electrolyte balance: Nursing considerations* (5th ed.). Sudbury, MA: Jones & Bartlett Learning.

Mount, D. B. (2016). Fluid and electrolyte disturbances. In D. Longo, A. Fauci, D. Kasper, S. Hauser, J. Jameson, & J. Loscalzo (Eds.), *Harrison's principles of internal medicine, 63* (19th ed.). New York, NY: McGraw-Hill.

NANDA International. (2018). *NANDA International, Inc. Nursing diagnoses: Definitions and classification, 2018–2020* (11th ed.) (T. H. Herdman & S. Kamitsuru, Eds.). New York, NY: Thieme.

Perrin, K. O., & MacLeod, C. E. (2018). *Understanding the essentials of critical care nursing* (3rd ed.). Hoboken, NJ: Pearson Education.

Shah, M., Sharma, A., Wermers, R. A., Kennel, K. A., Kellopp, T. A., & Mundi, M. A. (2017). Hypocalcemia after bariatric surgery: Prevalence and associated risk factors. *Obesity Surgery, 27*(11), 2905–2911.

Shields, K. M., Fox, K. L., & Liebrecht, C. M. (2018). *Pearson nurse's drug guide: 2018*. Hoboken, NJ: Pearson Education.

Sorenson, M., Quinn, L., & Klein, D. (2019). *Pathophysiology: Concepts of human disease.* Hoboken, NJ: Pearson Education.

Wagner, K., & Hardin-Pierce, M. (2014). *High-acuity nursing* (6th ed.). Hoboken, NJ: Pearson Education.

ADDITIONAL RESOURCES

Alan Grogono of Tulane University Department of Anesthesiology: Acid–Base Tutorial

www.acid-base.com/index.php

Eric Strong, Stanford University: Online lectures on acid–base balances and imbalances:

- Normal acid–base regulation at:

  www.youtube.com/watch?v=CmQOtP3pFus&feature=related

- Elevated anion gap metabolic acidosis at:

  www.youtube.com/watch?v=CmQOtP3pFus&feature=related

- Six easy steps to acid–base interpretation at:

  www.youtube.com/watch?v=6stANI3zNA0&feature=related

Merck Manual: Acid–Base Balance

https://www.merckmanuals.com/professional/endocrine-and-metabolic-disorders/acid-base-regulation-and-disorders/acid-base-regulation

Merck Manual: Electrolyte Disorders

www.merckmanuals.com/professional/endocrine-and-metabolic-disorders/electrolyte-disorders

National Library of Medicine, MedLinePlus – Fluid and Electrolyte Balance

https://medlineplus.gov/fluidandelectrolytebalance.html#cat51

New England Journal of Medicine, Disorders of Fluids and Electrolytes

www.nejm.org/page/fluids-and-electrolytes

Nurses Labs, Fluid and Electrolytes

https://nurseslabs.com/fluid-and-electrolytes/

University of Connecticut: Acid–Base Tutorial

http://fitsweb.uchc.edu/student/selectives/TimurGraham/Welcome.html

Chapter 11

Nursing Care of Patients Experiencing Trauma and Shock

Chapter Outline and Learning Outcomes

CLINICAL COMPETENCIES

- Describe steps of the primary survey to diagnose and manage life-threatening injuries.
- Obtain initial subjective and objective data of the trauma patient to include history taking, assessment, review of past medical history, and communication with prehospital and other healthcare providers and family members.
- Evaluate patient response to medical and surgical interventions for patients sustaining multiple trauma and shock.
- Provide essential ongoing written communication for patient care and continuity of the trauma patient.
- Describe the role of the nurse in trauma prevention education and develop a plan of care to restore the functional health status of trauma patients.
- Communicate significant data and changes in the condition of the patient who has sustained trauma.
- Identify nursing diagnoses based on signs and symptoms recognized during the nursing assessment.
- Develop a plan of care for the trauma patient based on scientific knowledge and patient diversity that addresses the nursing diagnosis.
- Describe nursing monitoring of a patient at risk for or experiencing shock.
- Develop a plan of care for a patient experiencing the different types of shock.
- Advocate for the patient's rights as indicated by documentation for end-of-life care for a patient experiencing trauma or shock.

KEY TERMS

abrasion, 291
brain death criteria, 301
contusion, 291
intimate partner violence (IPV), 286
laceration, 291
pneumothorax, 289
puncture wound, 291
sepsis, 309
shock, 303
tension pneumothorax, 289
transfusion, 295
trauma, 285

11.1 Traumatic Injury

Trauma is defined as injury to human tissues and organs resulting from the transfer of energy from the environment. In the past the term *trauma* has been associated with the word *accident*. *Accident* means that the injury occurred without intent, a result of random chance. We now know that a considerable number of injuries are preventable and not of random chance. Intentional and nonintentional trauma encompasses a variety of injuries resulting from motor vehicle crashes, pedestrian injuries, gunshot wounds, falls, violence toward others, or self-inflicted violence. The injuries, disabilities, and deaths resulting from these acts constitute a major healthcare challenge.

Healthcare workers are at risk of trauma from patients and families. While the emergency department has some of the highest reported workplace violence to nurses, physicians, and other healthcare workers, violence can occur in other healthcare settings as well. Psychiatric settings are also high in rates of violence toward healthcare personnel. Finally, only three states (at the time of press, Wyoming, Montana, and South Carolina) have a law that enforces enhanced penalties for violence against healthcare workers (Phillips, 2016).

SAFETY ALERT: In situations where patients have the potential to become violent toward the healthcare providers working to treat their injuries, nurses should take appropriate precautions. In the clinical setting, security personnel or police officers should be present when needed. ■

Trauma usually occurs suddenly, leaving the patient and family with little time to prepare for its consequences. Nurses provide a vital link in providing both physical and psychosocial care to the injured patient and family. In caring for the patient who has experienced trauma, nurses must consider not only the initial physical injury, but also its long-term consequences, including rehabilitation. Trauma may alter the patient's previous way of life, potentially affecting independence, mobility, cognitive thinking, and appearance.

Components of Trauma

Trauma results from an abnormal exchange of energy between a host and a mechanism in a predisposing environment. The host is the person or group at risk of injury. Multiple factors influence the host's potential for injury: Age, sex, race, economic status, preexisting illnesses, and use of substances such as street drugs and alcohol.

The mechanism is the source of the energy transmitted to the host. The energy exchanged can be mechanical, gravitational, thermal, electrical, physical, or chemical. **Table 11.1** lists the most common mechanisms for each type of energy. Mechanical energy is the most common type of energy transferred to a host in trauma. The most common mechanical source of injury in all adult age groups is the motor vehicle.

Guns are another common mechanical source of injury. Trauma from gunshot wounds has steadily increased during the past 20 years and remains a major reason for emergency department and trauma center admissions, especially in large cities. As of the end of 2017, there were 12.4 gun-related deaths per 100,000 U.S. citizens, which shows a continual increase from the years before (Ahmad & Bastian, 2018).

When describing a traumatic injury, intention is included as a component. Most gunshot and stab wounds are examples of intentional injuries. It is important to remember, however, that some gunshot wounds are unintentional, such as those that occur when children play with their parents' guns. Other common unintentional injuries result from motor vehicle crashes, falls, drowning, fires, and hunting accidents.

The final component of trauma is the environment. For example, a road that has become slippery after a snowstorm is a physical environment that may contribute to an injury. Occupation is another important environmental factor to consider. Those in certain occupations face a high risk of trauma; examples include police officers, firefighters, professional athletes, racecar drivers, and taxi cab drivers. The social environment, such as the presence of gangs and neighborhood violence or violence within the home, also influences risk for injury.

Table 11.1 Common Mechanisms of Injury by Energy Source

Energy Source	Common Mechanisms of Injury
Mechanical	Motor vehicles Firearms Machines
Gravitational	Falls
Thermal	Heating appliances Fire Freezing temperatures
Electrical	Wires, sockets, and other electrical objects Lightning
Physical	Fists, feet, and other body parts (as in physical assault) Sharp objects, such as knives Ultraviolet radiation Ionizing radiation Water (drowning) Other submersion agents (e.g., grain) Explosions
Chemical	Drugs Poisons Industrial chemicals

Most incidents of **intimate partner violence (IPV)** are not reported, thus it is believed that the available data greatly underestimate the true magnitude of the problem. According to the National Coalition Against Domestic Violence, one in three women and one in four men have been physically abused by an intimate partner, with one in five women and one in seven men severely physically abused by an intimate partner. This victimization correlates with higher levels of depression and suicidal behavior, and only 34% of all victims who are injured receive medical care for their injuries. Finally, on average, every minute 20 people are physically abused by an intimate partner (National Coalition Against Domestic Violence, 2018).

Elder abuse has been defined in a number of ways, making comparisons difficult. In 2016, the Centers for Disease Control and Prevention (CDC), working with a number of other agencies and stakeholders, developed a consensus definition of *elder abuse*: "An intentional act or failure to act by a caregiver or another person in a relationship involving an expectation of trust that causes or creates a serious risk of harm to an older adult." This definition includes physical, sexual, emotional/psychological, neglect, and financial abuse. Finally, those with dementia experience some of the highest levels of abuse (National Center on Elder Abuse, 2018). See **Box 11.1** for a description steps in assessing interpersonal violence.

BOX 11.1
Assessing Intimate Partner Violence

The general approach to diagnosis in abuse situations is challenging and assessment is complex. The following are clues to identify violence-related injuries:

- Injuries that do not correlate with the history (e.g., bones that are not easily broken, older bruising, injuries that are more severe than the history states)
- Injuries that suggest a defensive posture (e.g., injuries on the tops of hands, sides of body, top aspects of arms)
- Injuries during pregnancy
- Pattern injuries
- Pattern burns
- Sexual abuse/rape
- Unusual or unexplained fractures
- Signs of confinement (e.g., weight loss, not sure of day/date, confusion concerning where the person is located; lack of knowledge of current events)
- Unusual interaction between patient and caregiver (e.g., patient will look to caregiver for the answer or for reassurance the answer is correct),
- Lack of medical attention (e.g., immunizations not up to date, poor dental health)
- Unexplained dehydration or malnutrition.

Types of Trauma

Minor trauma causes injury to a single part or system of the body and is usually treated in a physician's office or in the hospital emergency department. A fracture of the clavicle, a small second-degree burn, and a laceration requiring sutures are examples of minor trauma. Major or multiple trauma involves serious single-system injury (such as the traumatic amputation of a leg) or multiple-system injuries. Multiple trauma is most often the result of a motor vehicle crash.

Trauma is further classified as either blunt or penetrating. *Blunt trauma* occurs when there is no communication between the damaged tissues and the outside environment. Blunt trauma is the term for an injury caused by five types of force, including deceleration (a decrease in the speed of a moving object), acceleration (an increase in the speed of a moving object), shearing (forces occurring across a plane, with structures slipping across each other), compression (acute tissue pressure resulting in increased density), or crushing (high force that results in tissue destruction). Blunt forces often cause multiple injuries that may affect the head, spinal cord, bones, thorax, and abdomen. Blunt trauma is frequently caused by motor vehicle crashes, falls, assaults, and sports activities.

Penetrating trauma occurs when a foreign object enters the body, causing damage to body structures. Structures commonly affected include the brain, lungs, heart, liver, spleen, the intestines, and the vascular system. Examples of penetrating trauma are gunshot or stab wounds and impalement.

Other types of trauma include inhalation injuries from gases, smoke, or steam, burn or freezing injuries, and blast injuries from explosions. Blast injuries result from the temperature and velocity of air movement and the force of projectiles from an explosion. Blast injuries are more severe in water than in air since blast waves travel farther and faster in water. Trauma from blast injuries includes pulmonary edema and hemorrhage, damage to abdominal organs, burns, penetrating injuries, and ruptured tympanic membranes.

Outcome studies show a correlation between survival rates of multiple trauma victims and rapid response times by prehospital providers, coupled with appropriate decision making with regard to transporting victims to a facility capable of treating their injuries (Bledsoe & Cherry, 2017). As a result, a system was devised to assist prehospital providers to make the appropriate decisions. Trauma patients are classified as Class 1, 2, or 3 based on factors including mechanism of injury, vehicle speed, height of falls, and location of penetrating injuries. Class 3 trauma is the least severe. An example would be a same-level fall without loss of consciousness or significant injury. Class 1 trauma involves life-threatening injuries likely to require medical specialists or immediate surgical intervention. Although any hospital emergency department should be capable of caring for Class 3 trauma patients, patients meeting Class 1 or 2 criteria should be transported to a designated trauma center when possible. Facilities designated as trauma centers have medical specialists and surgical coverage available or on call 24 hours a day.

Effects of Traumatic Injury

Death is a common result of serious traumatic injury and falls into one of three categories related to the time span between injury and death, called the *trimodal distribution of trauma death* (**Figure 11.1** ■). Immediate death happens within minutes at the scene from such injuries as a torn thoracic aorta or decapitation. Early death occurs during the first few hours following the injury from major abdominal or thoracic injuries or progression of intracranial

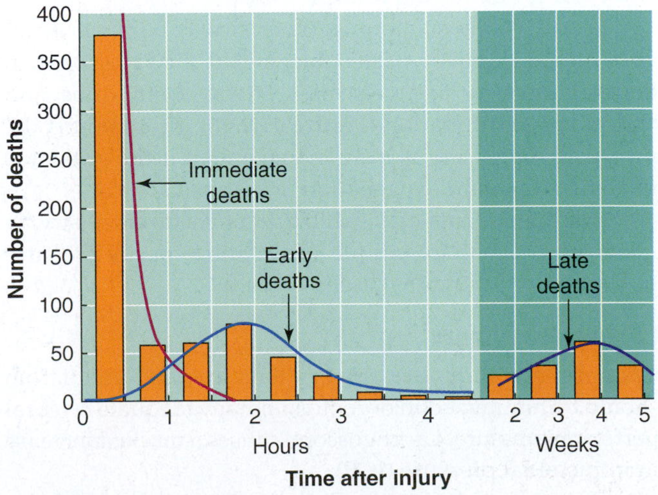

Number of deaths
400
350
300
250
200
150
100
50
0
Immediate deaths
Early deaths
Late deaths
0
1
2
3
4
2
3
4
5
Hours
Weeks
Time after injury

Figure 11.1 ■ Trimodal distribution of trauma deaths.

hemorrhage. Appropriate care during this time has been shown to improve survival. Late death generally occurs days or weeks after the injury and results from multiple organ failure, sepsis, and coagulopathies.

Because of the serious consequences of trauma, it is important to rapidly identify the patient's injuries and institute appropriate interventions quickly. Following are common results of trauma and interventions necessary for good outcomes.

Head and Neck Effects—Airway Obstruction

Maintenance of the airway and cervical spine are the highest priority in the trauma patient. Other distracting injuries may take the inexperienced practitioner away from the airway, but if the airway is not patent and the patient is unable to deliver oxygen to vital organs, all other interventions are futile.

Assessment includes determining airway patency. If the patient is unresponsive, manual opening of the airway using a jaw-thrust maneuver is necessary. The jaw-thrust is recommended in patients with actual and potential C-spine injury. Once the airway is opened, the practitioner must identify any potential obstruction from the tongue, loose teeth, foreign bodies, bleeding, secretions, vomitus, or edema. If the patient is responsive and can vocalize, that is a good indication that the airway is clear.

Any time the nurse performs an intervention it is important that you reassess the effectiveness of the intervention. For example, if you suction the airway to remove vomitus, you would reassess the airway after suctioning to determine if that intervention was successful or if you have to reintubate the airway a second time.

All trauma patients should receive high-flow oxygen until stabilized. Assessment of breathing effectiveness is paramount. Assessment should include determining if the patient has spontaneous breathing, good rise and fall of the chest, good skin color, general rate and depth of respirations, abdominal or accessory muscle use, position of the trachea, observation of chest wall integrity and presence of jugular vein distention, bilateral breath sounds, and the presence of any surface trauma. Consider pulse oximetry and cardiac monitoring as well.

In addition to suctioning, other airway adjuncts available include oral or nasal pharyngeal airways, oxygen delivery devices, laryngeal mask airway, Combitube, and endotracheal intubation (**Figure 11.2** ■). Intubation is the preferred method of airway management if the patient is unable to maintain oxygenation or an open airway.

Trauma patients may exhibit several aspects of airway management that are unique and require special preparation and precautions, as discussed next.

Closed Head Injury

Changes in hemodynamics, oxygenation, and ventilation should be minimized in order to maintain adequate cerebral perfusion pressure. Laryngoscopy causes a marked increase in intracranial pressure (ICP).

The goal is to maintain a $PaCO_2$ of 30 to 35 mmHg. Lidocaine administered 3 to 5 minutes prior to intubation can blunt an increase in ICP that is secondary to laryngeal stimulation. In a normotensive patient, beta blockers are given 2 to 3 minutes prior to intubation to attenuate the sympathetic response. Effective induction agents such as etomidate or thiopental can be used in this situation (Stollings, Diedrich, Oyen, & Brown, 2014).

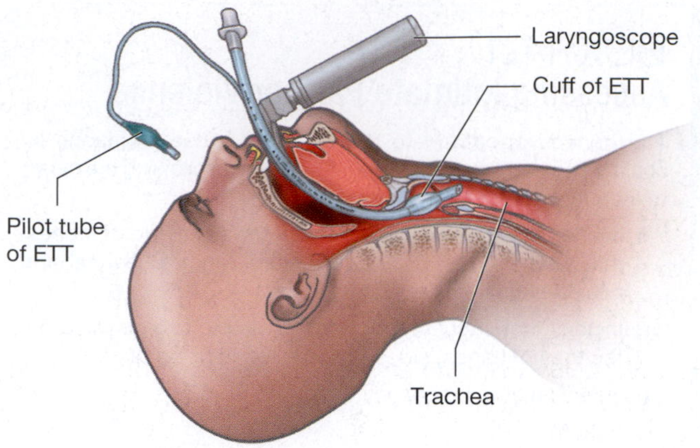
Laryngoscope
Cuff of ETT
Pilot tube of ETT
Trachea

Figure 11.2 ■ Placement of an oral endotracheal tube (ETT) for intubation. When the ETT is in place, air or oxygen can be blown into the external opening of the tube and enter the trachea.

Maxillofacial Trauma

Significant distortion of normal anatomy in facial trauma and respiratory compromise is not uncommon. Even in patients who present with mild respiratory compromise, rapid deterioration from edema or hemorrhage can occur. A surgical airway may be the only alternative.

Direct Airway Trauma

Penetrating trauma to the neck is associated with a high degree of morbidity and mortality. Airway involvement includes dyspnea, cyanosis, subcutaneous emphysema, hoarseness, or air bubbling from the wound. Orotracheal intubation with rapid sequence intubation is the technique of choice. The key is early identification of the need for intubation before the patient has no airway at all. Tracheobronchial injury occurs in approximately 10 to 20% of patients with penetrating neck injuries.

Cervical Spine Injury

In the presence of a presumed C-spine injury, precautions for securing an airway are consistently applied. Approximately 1.5 to 3% of major trauma victims have clinically significant C-spine injuries (Desjardins, 2013). Oral intubation with manual in-line stabilization (MILS) of the head and neck is a safe method for securing an airway. Rapid-sequence intubation protocol may be needed depending on the circumstances surrounding the oral intubation situation (Stollings et al., 2014). There is a decreased probability of C-spine injury if the following criteria are met:

- Absence of midline cervical spine tenderness
- Normal alertness
- Absence of intoxication

- Absence of a painful distracting injury
- No focal neurologic defects.

If the trauma patient is obtunded (diminished awareness), then a high-quality CT examination is needed before removal of a cervical spine collar (Patel et al., 2015).

Burns

Burn patients with airway compromise require aggressive management. Upper airway edema associated with inhalation or enclosed-space fires can progress during the postburn phase. Securing an airway sooner rather than later is the goal. See Chapter 17 for the nursing care of the patient with burns.

Thoracic Effects

Tension Pneumothorax

A **pneumothorax** results when air enters the potential space between the parietal and visceral pleura. The thorax is completely filled by the lungs. Surface tension between the pleural surfaces holds the lungs to the chest wall. Air present in the pleural space will eventually collapse the lungs. A **tension pneumothorax** is life-threatening and requires immediate intervention. On inspiration air enters the pleural space, does not escape on expiration, and increases the intrapleural pressure. This pressure collapses the injured lung and shifts the mediastinal contents, compressing the heart, great vessels, trachea, and eventually the uninjured lung. In turn, this causes the following signs and symptoms:

- Severe respiratory distress
- Hypotension
- Jugular vein distention
- Tracheal deviation toward the uninjured side
- Cyanosis.

If not treated immediately, then risk of shock and arrest with pulseless cardiac activity may occur.

The immediate short-term lifesaving intervention is a needle thoracostomy, inserting a large-bore over-the-needle catheter into the second intercostal space at the midclavicular line (MCL). See **Figure 11.3** ■.

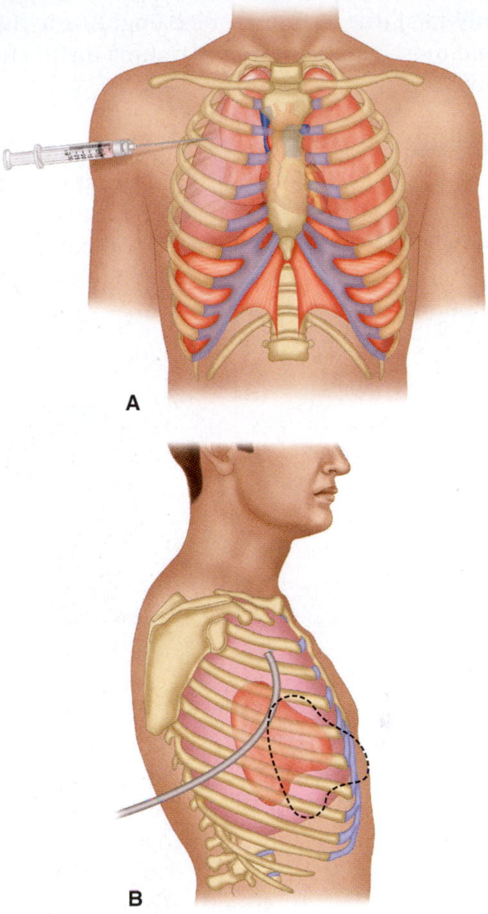
A
B

Figure 11.3 ■ A needle thoracostomy may be used in the emergency treatment of a tension pneumothorax. **A**, A large-gauge needle is introduced, and air and fluid are aspirated. **B**, Alternatively, a chest tube may be inserted and connected to a chest drainage system.

Flail Chest

Flail chest is the fracture of two or more ribs in two or more separate locations, leading to an unstable thoracic wall segment. Paradoxical movement of the chest wall is seen with the area sinking into the chest cavity with inspiration and protrusion with expiration. The area must be supported quickly to reestablish the thoracic bellows effect. The patient will exhibit dyspnea and pain at the fracture site. Depending on the severity, surgical intervention and/or mechanical ventilation will be needed. Pain control is a must to assist the patient in taking deep breaths. With a flailed chest there will almost always be a pulmonary contusion under the area of the fractures.

Thoracic Contusion and Rupture

Bruising of thoracic tissue is referred to as *contusion*. Pulmonary contusion is the most common traumatic chest injury. As a shock wave of force travels through the parenchyma, diffuse hemorrhage and alveolar edema develop, impairing gas exchange. Motor vehicle crashes are the most common cause of pulmonary contusions. Diaphragmatic rupture is a rare traumatic injury but can result in herniation of abdominal contents into the thoracic cavity, causing respiratory compromise.

Myocardial contusion results in extravasation of red blood cells into myocardial fibers. As myocardial cells are injured, it is believed that cardiac output diminishes due to reductions in contractile strength. Myocardial rupture is an acute traumatic tear of any structures of the heart. Although rare, myocardial rupture is usually fatal; atrial rupture has the best chance for survival.

Cardiac tamponade occurs when blood or fluid collects in the pericardial sac. Resulting in myocardial compression, this condition is potentially life-threatening and should be addressed immediately with pericardiocentesis. (See Chapter 31 for a discussion of nursing management of this condition.)

Aortic rupture (transection) can result in acceleration–deceleration injury or blunt chest trauma. This injury is commonly fatal due to profuse bleeding. Aortic rupture is the second most common cause of trauma death after traumatic brain injury.

Hemorrhage

When a patient has suffered an injury that causes external hemorrhage, such as severing of an artery, the bleeding must be controlled immediately. This may be done by applying direct pressure over the wound and over arterial pressure points (**Figure 11.4** ■).

Internal hemorrhage may result from either blunt or penetrating traumatic injury. Discovering the cause and location of the injury, as well as the extent of related blood loss, are the most important concerns. Several potential spaces in the body can accommodate large amounts of blood that may accumulate (called *third spacing*) following injury. For example, bleeding into the pleural space may occur with chest trauma (*hemothorax*), and bleeding into the abdominal cavity may occur with abdominal trauma. A pelvic fracture may cause massive hemorrhage in the retroperitoneal region. Once the source of internal hemorrhage has been recognized, interventions are initiated, including

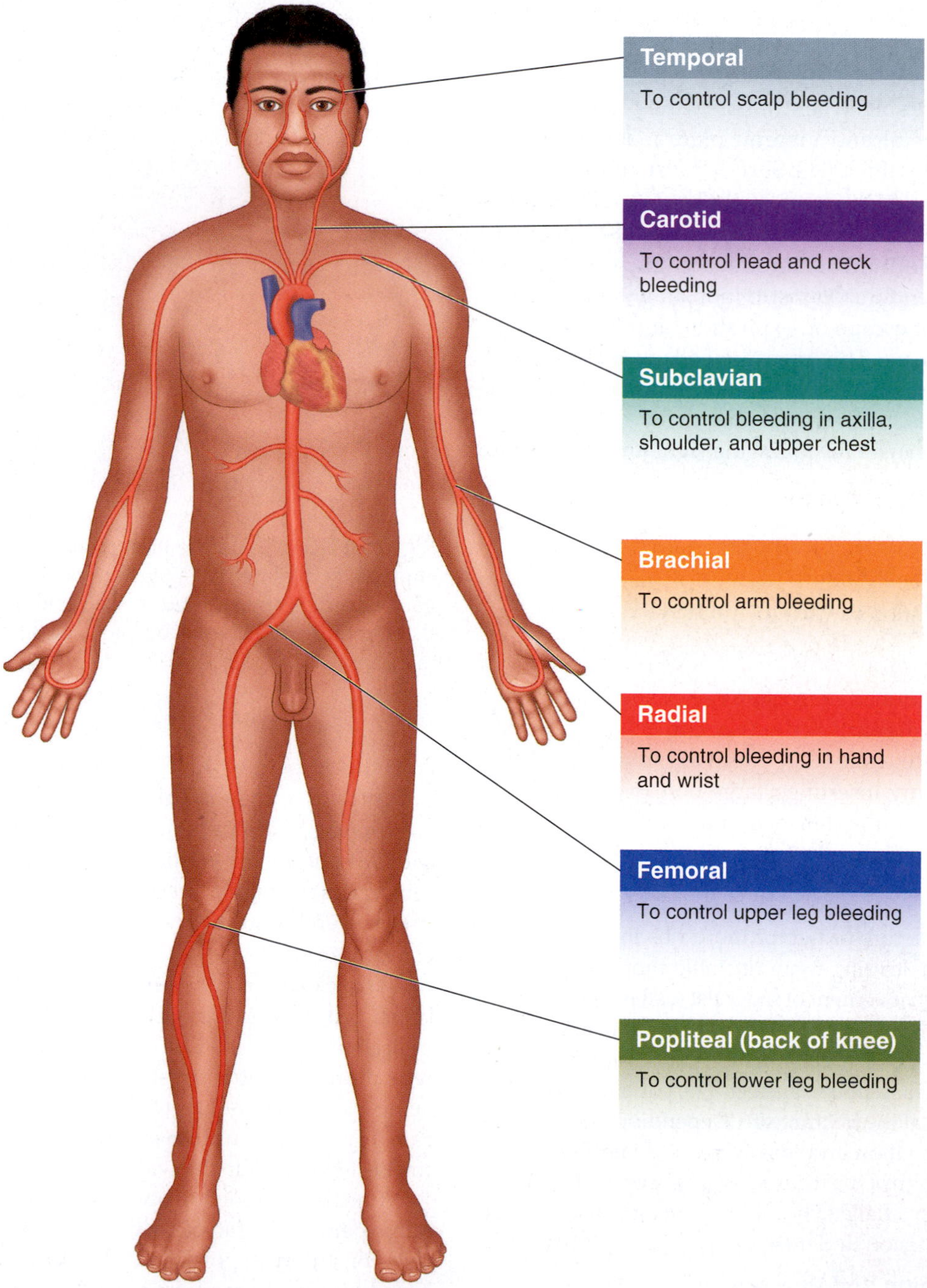
Temporal
To control scalp bleeding
Carotid
To control head and neck bleeding
Subclavian
To control bleeding in axilla, shoulder, and upper chest
Brachial
To control arm bleeding
Radial
To control bleeding in hand and wrist
Femoral
To control upper leg bleeding
Popliteal (back of knee)
To control lower leg bleeding

Figure 11.4 ■ The major pressure points used for the control of bleeding.

operative control of bleeding and continual assessment of the patient. Hemorrhage may result in hypovolemic shock (discussed later in the chapter).

Integumentary Effects

Injuries to the integument are generally not as serious as other injuries, with the exception of burns (see Chapter 17). The primary organ involved in integumentary trauma is the skin; however, underlying structures may also be injured. Injuries may result from either blunt or penetrating sources. It is important to evaluate all injuries to the integument because they may indicate a more serious injury such as an open fracture. Additionally, large wounds may contribute to significant blood loss.

Five specific injuries to the integument are contusions, abrasions, puncture wounds, lacerations, and full-thickness avulsion injuries (**Figure 11.5** ■). **Contusions**, or superficial tissue injuries, result from blunt trauma that causes the breakage of small blood vessels and bleeding into the surrounding tissue. **Abrasions**, or partial-thickness denudations of an area of integument, generally result from falls or scrapes. **Puncture wounds** occur when a sharp or blunt object penetrates the integument. **Lacerations** are open wounds that result from sharp cutting or tearing. Injuries to the integument are at risk for contamination from dirt, debris, or foreign objects. Infection may cause further physical stress to the patient with multiple injuries. Full-thickness avulsion injuries are injuries that result in loss of all of the layers of the skin, causing fat and muscle to be exposed. The size of the wound impacts both the length of time necessary for healing to take place as well as the risk for infection. These types of injuries are treated by allowing new skin to grow from the edges, by stitching the wound together, by reattaching avulsed skin, or by skin grafting.

Abdominal Effects

The abdomen contains both solid organs (liver, spleen, and pancreas) and hollow organs (stomach and intestines). Direct trauma to the abdomen can lacerate and compress the solid organs and cause burst injuries to the hollow organs. Blood vessels may be torn and organs may be displaced from their blood supply, producing life-threatening hemorrhage. Damage to the mesenteric vessels supplying the bowel can result in bowel ischemia and infarction. Injury to the stomach, pancreas, and small bowel may allow digestive enzymes to leak out into the abdominal cavity. Rupture of the large bowel results in escape of feces, which causes

A B

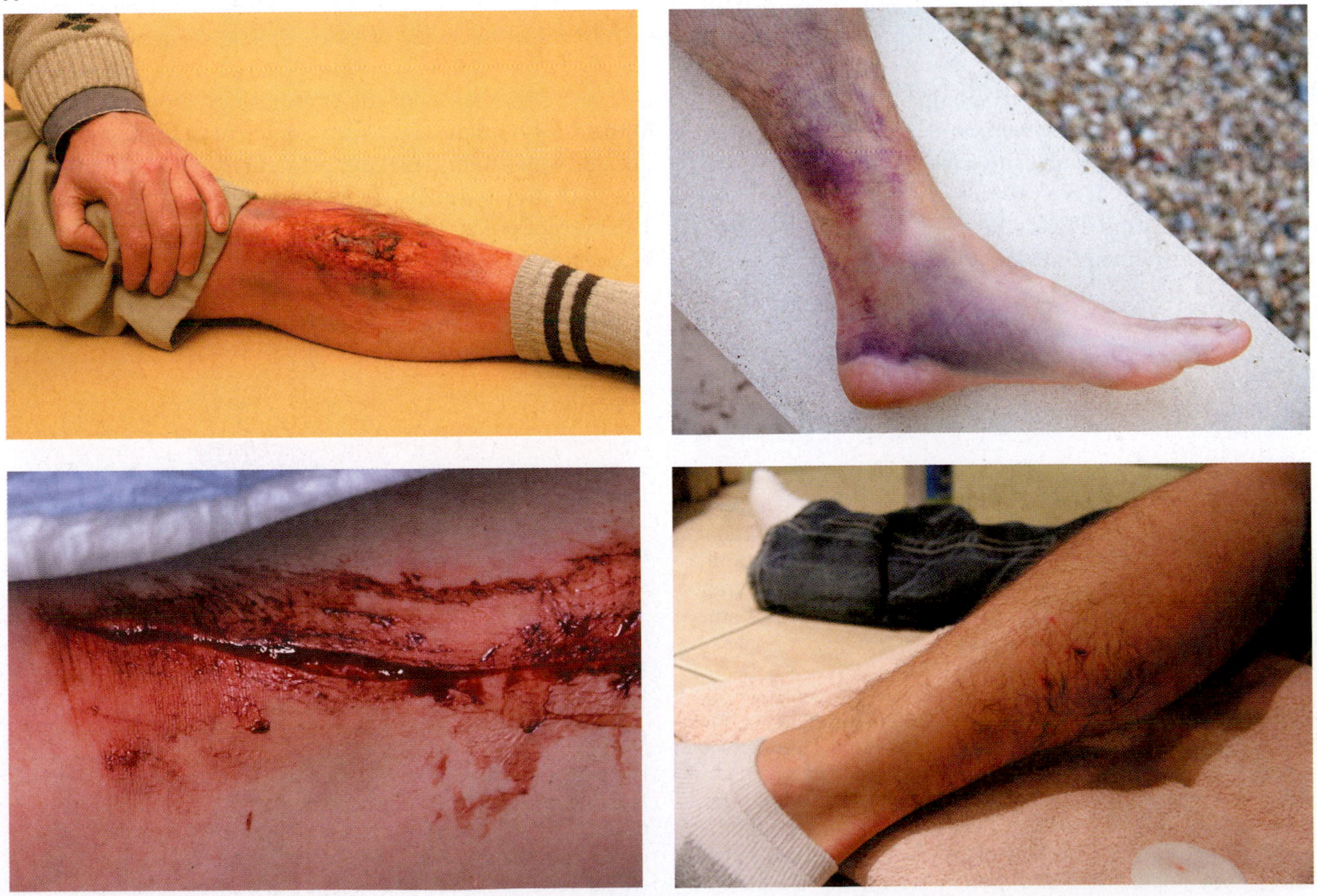

C D

Figure 11.5 ■ Traumatic injuries to the skin: **A**, Abrasion. **B**, Contusion. **C**, Laceration. **D**, Puncture wound (dog bite).

peritonitis. The immediate threat following abdominal trauma is hemorrhage; the later threat is peritonitis.

Musculoskeletal Effects

Musculoskeletal injuries may occur alone or with multiple injuries as the result of blunt or penetrating trauma. Musculoskeletal injuries are usually not considered a high priority in the care of the patient with multiple injuries. Exceptions are the life- or limb-threatening musculoskeletal injury, such as a dislocated hip, pulseless extremity, or significant blood loss such as from a femur or pelvic fracture. Other exceptions include fractures or dislocations with neurovascular compromise, open fractures, or compartment syndromes. Musculoskeletal injuries may provide clues to the presence of other serious injuries; for example, a fractured clavicle may indicate an associated thoracic injury. Care of the patient who has experienced a musculoskeletal injury is discussed in Chapter 39.

Neurologic Effects

Head injuries are a common type of injury sustained as the result of trauma. Injuries to the spinal cord, resulting in loss of neurologic function, are devastating outcomes of trauma, but they are much less common than head injuries. Most head and spinal cord injuries result from blunt trauma and are sustained in motor vehicle crashes. Falls, sports injuries, and assaults are other sources of neurologic injury. Care of the patient with a neurologic injury is discussed in Chapters 41, 42, and 43.

Multiple Organ Dysfunction Syndrome

Multiple organ dysfunction syndrome (MODS) is a common complication of severe injury and a frequent cause of death in intensive care units. It is a progressive impairment of two or more organ systems. This is the result of an uncontrolled inflammatory response to severe injury or illness.

Patients at risk for MODS are those with a disturbance in homeostasis resulting from one or a combination of the following conditions:

- Infection
- Injury
- Inflammation
- Ischemia
- Immune response
- Intoxication of substances
- Iatrogenic factors.

The primary organ systems involved in MODS are the respiratory, renal, hepatic, hematologic, cardiovascular, gastrointestinal, and neurologic systems. Supportive therapy depends on the identification of correctable causes and may involve one or a combination of several therapies. Surgical intervention, antibiotic administration, corticosteroid administration, or correction coagulopathies are some therapies used for this condition. If two organs have failed, the mortality rate is 67%, and if three or more organs have failed, the mortality rate is 100%. To help identify these at-risk patients earlier, a MODS prediction score for multitrauma patients has recently been developed (Rendy, Sapan, & Kalersaran, 2017).

Effects on the Family

Trauma usually occurs suddenly and with little warning. It may result in death or cause injury serious enough to alter both the patient's and the family's lives. The suddenness and seriousness of the event are precipitating factors in the development of a psychologic crisis. During the past decade, some emergency departments have instituted policies that allow families to be present during resuscitation. This type of policy is not without controversy, but it should be considered when appropriate.

Moving Evidence into Action

Caring for Families of Trauma Patients

Clinical Issue

Families of patients who have experienced trauma undergo psychological stress. While the care is focused on the trauma patient, the family can be forgotten. The family is important, though, as they will be the support for the patient once treatment is completed. Trauma can be disruptive to the family system.

External Evidence

Verharen et al. (2015) explored the needs of families whose relatives were undergoing trauma care and found that families need concrete information, assistance with communication with members of the treatment staff, and emotional support. One trauma center has developed an intervention to meet the needs of the families of trauma patients while in the emergency department and then in the intensive care unit. An interdisciplinary team headed by the chaplaincy department was developed as a method of providing information and support to families. They developed handouts on basic information such as roles and responsibilities of staff, guidelines of care of the trauma patient, and how family members can take care of themselves. An "orientation group" made up of a chaplain and a healthcare liaison meet with families to help orientate them to what is happening to their family member and what services are available. The group also provides psychological support as needed (Rutherford & von Wenckesternm, 2016).

Internal Evidence

It must be determined whether such an approach would be feasible in a given institution. Some institutions' emergency departments are not set up in a way where a chaplain could come in and start the process of the intervention. Also, nurses would need to be willing to "let go" of some of the support of families. Finally, the culture of the institution may not be one of patient- and family-centered care.

Patient Considerations

With an unconscious trauma patient, the nurse and interprofessional team may not know who the patient considers "family." There may be family dynamics that would not support the intervention. Also, there are privacy issues that must be addressed.

Putting the Pieces Together

When examining an intervention that includes the family, it is important to realize that one size will not fit all. Family dynamics, patient wishes (if known), and commitment of the staff to patient and family care must all be taken into account.

References

Rutherford, L. G., & von Wenckstternm, T. (2016). Trauma information groups: A level 1 trauma center's integrated approach to family support. *Journal of Trauma Nursing, 23*(6), 357–360.

Verharen, L., Mintjes, J., Kaljouw, M., Melief, W., Schilder, L., & van der Lann, G. (2015). Psychosocial needs of relatives of trauma patients. *Health and Social Work, 40*(3), 233–238.

11.2 The Patient Experiencing Trauma

Interprofessional Care

Interprofessional care of the trauma patient depends on a team approach. Providing trauma care with a team focus helps each team member know his or her role. Prompt delegation of tasks and responsibilities improves the patient's chances for survival and decreases the morbidity that may result from traumatic injuries.

Prehospital Care

The major functions of prehospital care include injury identification, critical interventions, and rapid transport. Early and effective care can help decrease the risk of hypothermia, coagulopathy, and acidosis, which are considered the lethal triad (**Figure 11.6** ■).

Injury Identification

Emergency care of the patient experiencing trauma is based on rapid assessment to identify injuries and begin appropriate interventions. Injuries that indicate the need for trauma center care include:

- Penetrating injuries to the abdomen, pelvis, chest, neck, or head
- Spinal cord injuries with deficit
- Crushing injuries to the abdomen, chest, or head
- Major burns
- Injuries leading to airway compromise or obstruction.

Many methods help healthcare providers determine the seriousness of patients' injuries and the potential for survival. Scoring systems such as the Trauma and Injury Severity Score (TRISS) can be helpful The TRISS score uses age, type of trauma (blunt vs. penetrating), systolic blood pressure, respiratory rate, injury severity score, and Glasgow Coma Scale score to predict survival based on a weighted algorithm that trauma centers input into a computer. There have been modifications to improve the predictability of the score, but most trauma centers still use the original (Schluter, 2011). A primary trauma assessment (also known as the primary survey) follows the **ABCDE** mnemonic:

Airway assessment (with C-spine immobilization) includes determining whether the airway is patent, maintainable, or nonmaintainable.

Breathing evaluation includes determining whether there are spontaneous respirations or ventilatory impedance such as by rib fractures or a collapsed lung.

Circulatory assessment includes palpating peripheral and central pulses; assessing capillary refill, skin color, and temperature; and identifying any external sources of bleeding.

Disability assessment of neurovascular status includes assessing level of consciousness, pupillary function, and response to verbal or painful stimuli. A mnemonic to assist with this is AVPU: A = Alert, V = responds to Voice, P = responds to Pain; U = Unresponsive.

Expose/environment includes a whole body assessment while ensuring that hypothermia does not occur.

After the primary survey is completed, then the secondary survey is started. This includes a careful head-to-toe assessment of the patient to determine whether other injuries are present. Along with this secondary survey, assessment of vital signs and, if possible, patient history should be obtained. To remember the important parts of the patients' history to obtain, the mnemonic **SAMPLE** can be used

- **S**igns/symptoms
- **A**llergies

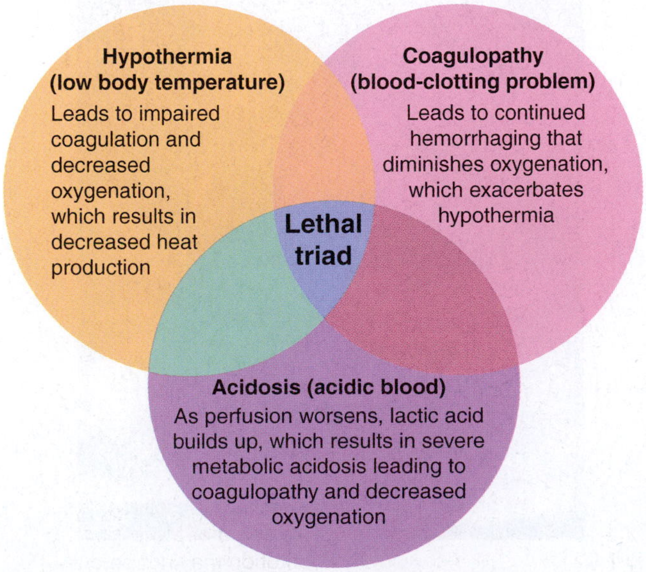
Hypothermia (low body temperature)
Leads to impaired coagulation and decreased oxygenation, which results in decreased heat production
Coagulopathy (blood-clotting problem)
Leads to continued hemorrhaging that diminishes oxygenation, which exacerbates hypothermia
Lethal triad
Acidosis (acidic blood)
As perfusion worsens, lactic acid builds up, which results in severe metabolic acidosis leading to coagulopathy and decreased oxygenation

Figure 11.6 ■ The lethal triad of trauma.

- **M**edications
- **P**ertinent past medical history
- **L**ast oral intake (and for women of childbearing age, last menstrual period)
- **E**vents leading up to the injury.

After the initial secondary survey, a tertiary survey is completed, which is a repeat of the secondary survey to look for missed injuries.

Critical Interventions

As life-threatening problems are identified during the primary assessment, appropriate on-the-scene interventions must be performed immediately. These include providing life support, immobilizing the cervical spine, managing the airway, and treating hemorrhage and shock.

Immobilization of the patient's cervical spine is a primary intervention. The patient is placed on a spine board and a cervical collar and head immobilizer applied (**Figure 11.7** ■). The cervical spine may also be immobilized by logrolling the patient onto a board, placing towel rolls or a head immobilizer along the sides of the patient's head, and securing the patient to the board. If the patient was wearing a helmet at the time of injury, the helmet should remain on until the patient arrives at the hospital, unless the patient's airway is at risk. If necessary, healthcare personnel at the scene will remove the helmet by manipulating it over the patient's nose and ears while holding the patient's head and neck immobile; safe removal requires at least two people. Improper removal of a helmet risks injury or additional injury to the spinal cord.

If the patient's airway is patent, oxygen is administered. Ventilations may be assisted with a bag–valve–mask resuscitator until airway management is achieved. Active external bleeding is controlled by direct pressure. Measures to reverse shock (discussed later in the chapter) are initiated.

Rapid Transport

Patients who have multiple injuries must be transported as soon as possible to a regional trauma center. The most common modes of rapid transport are ground ambulance and air ambulance, which includes specially staffed and equipped helicopters to care for trauma victims. **Figure 11.8** ■ shows a flight nurse assessing a patient. Stable patients within access of a ground ambulance are best transported by ground. Unstable patients and those injured in the wilderness or other areas in which ground access is difficult may best be transported by air. When these transport systems are unavailable, the patient is transported by any possible means. The goal is having the patient arrive to the emergency department as early as possible so definitive treatment can be provided. The ultimate goal is early treatment and prevention of the lethal triad.

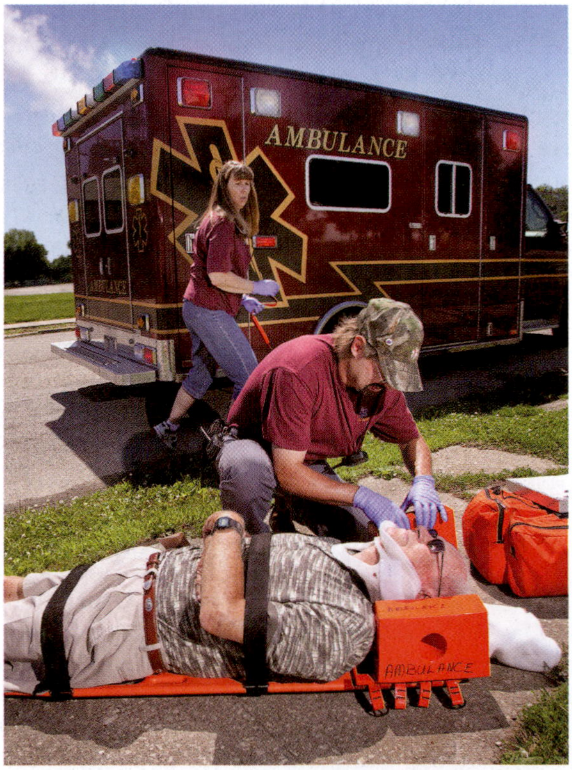
AMBULANCE

Figure 11.7 ■ Immobilization of the cervical spine at the scene of the accident is essential to preventing further injury to the spinal cord. The combined use of a hard cervical collar, head blocks, and tape best restricts flexion, extension, rotation, and lateral bending of the neck.

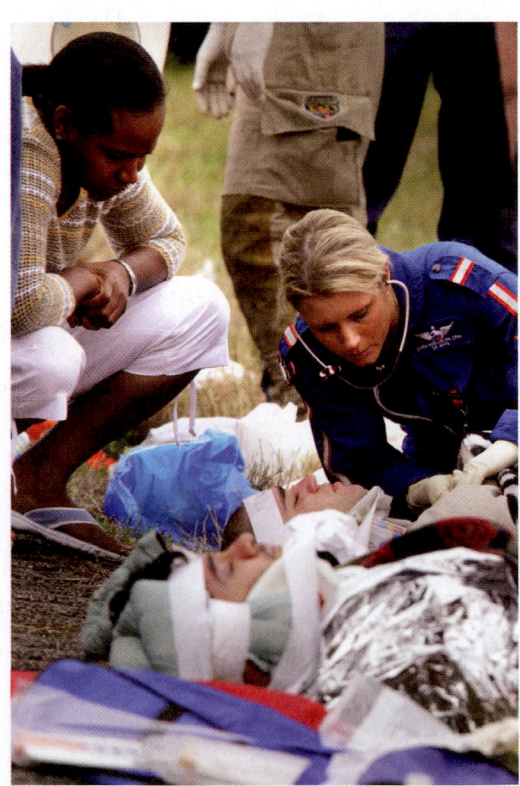

Figure 11.8 ■ Flight nurses provide initial assessment, stabilization, and support for patients with trauma.

Emergency Department Care

Diagnosis

The diagnostic tests ordered once the patient reaches the hospital depend on the type of injury the patient has sustained. Tests that may be ordered for victims of trauma include:

- ***Blood type and crossmatch*** involves typing the patient's blood for ABO antigens and Rh factor, screening the blood for antibodies, and crossmatching the patient's serum and donor red blood cells.
- ***Complete blood count*** evaluates the components of blood including red blood cell count and white blood cell count.
- ***Arterial blood gas*** evaluates oxygenation, acid–base balance, and the presence of metabolic or respiratory compensatory mechanisms.
- ***Blood alcohol level*** measures the amount of alcohol in a patient's blood. It has been found that between 20 and 50% of people who are injured may be intoxicated. Alcohol alters the patient's level of consciousness and response to pain.
- ***Urine drug screen*** may also be ordered. Like alcohol, such drugs as cocaine alter the patient's level of consciousness and overall response to the primary survey.
- ***Pregnancy test*** for any woman of childbearing age rules out the potential for pregnancy and fetal injury.
- ***Focused assessment by sonography in trauma (FAST)*** primarily focuses on evaluating the identification of blood in body cavities where it is not supposed to be. Primary focus is on the peritoneum. It is also helpful in identification of blood in the pleura and pericardium.
- ***Focused assessment with sonography in trauma (FAST) exam*** is a bedside ultrasound that can detect blood in the pericardial, peritoneal, or pleural spaces. The exam should be performed immediately after the primary survey and while the secondary survey is ongoing. The FAST exam can be performed while resuscitation efforts are ongoing.
- ***Computerized tomography (CT) scans*** can reveal injuries to the brain, skull, spine, spinal cord, chest, and abdomen.
- ***Magnetic resonance imaging (MRI) scans*** can reveal injuries to the brain and spinal cord.

Medications

Medications used to treat the patient who has experienced trauma depend on the type and severity of the injuries, as well as the degree of traumatic shock that is present. The following general categories of medications may be used:

- ***Blood components and crystalloids*** are administered intravenously in the initial treatment of traumatic shock to replace intravascular volume.
- ***Inotropic and vasopressive medications*** (medications that either increase myocardial contractility or cause vasoconstriction) are given to increase cardiac output and improve tissue perfusion. These medications should be *administered only after adequate fluid volume restoration*, as if there is not enough volume in the cardiovascular system, the medications will not work. These medications include dopamine (Dopastat, Intropin), dobutamine (Dobutrex), epinephrine (Adrenalin), norepinephrine (Levophed), vasopressin (Pitressin), and phenylephrine (Neo-synephrine). Some of these medications are used for other reasons of shock such as cardiac failure and postsurgery support.
- ***Opioids***, administered by bolus or continuous infusion, are used to treat pain as soon as possible. However, the effects of the pain medications may alter patient responses to injury, cause hypotension and respiratory depression, and mask potential injuries. If pain medications are administered, they must be carefully regulated and the patient must be closely monitored.
- ***Immunizations*** are given if the patient has penetrating and open wounds. Tetanus immunization status must be determined. If the patient is unable to remember when the last tetanus immunization was given, is unable to answer, or has not received a tetanus immunization within the past 5 years, then tetanus prophylaxis is given.

These medications and their administration are covered later in the chapter in the discussion of the collaborative care of the patient in shock.

Blood Transfusions

Blood and blood components are initially produced in the body and then donated for use by another person through a **transfusion** (an infusion of blood or blood components). A patient may be given whole blood, packed red blood cells (RBCs), platelets, plasma, albumin, clotting factors, prothrombin, or cryoprecipitate (**Table 11.2**). Blood and blood components increase the amount of hemoglobin available to carry oxygen to the cells, improve hemoglobin and hematocrit levels during active bleeding, increase intravascular volume, and replace deficient substances such as platelets and clotting factors (American Red Cross, 2017).

Each person has one of four blood types: A, B, AB, or O (American Red Cross, 2018). The blood group antigens A and B, present on RBC membranes, form the basis for the ABO blood categorization. The presence or absence of these inherited antigens determines one's blood type. People with blood type A have A antigens, those with type B have B antigens, those with type AB have both antigens, and those with neither antigen have blood type O (called a *universal donor*).

ABO antibodies develop in the serum of people whose RBCs lack the corresponding antigen; these antibodies are called anti-A and anti-B. The person with blood type B has A antibodies, the person with type A has B antibodies, the person with type O has both types of antibodies, and the person with blood type AB has no antibodies (called a *universal recipient*).

Table 11.2 Volume Resuscitation Therapies

Component	Indications	Advantages	Disadvantages
Ringer lactate	■ Restoration of circulating volume ■ Replacement of electrolyte deficits	■ Ready availability ■ Safe to use ■ Low cost ■ Aids in buffering acidosis	■ Rapid movement from the intravascular to the extravascular space, leading to three or more times requirement for replacement
Normal saline	■ Restoration of circulating volume ■ Vehicle compatible with administration of blood	■ Good availability ■ Low cost ■ Safe to use	■ Hyperchloremic acidosis associated with prolonged use of sodium solutions
Whole blood	■ Replaces blood volume and oxygen-carrying capacity in hemorrhage and shock	■ Contains RBCs, plasma proteins, clotting factors, and plasma	■ Contains few platelets or granulocytes; deficient in clotting factors V and VII ■ Greatest risks are for incompatibility or circulatory overload ■ Risk of transmitting bloodborne pathogens
Packed RBCs	■ Restoration of intravascular volume ■ Replacement of oxygen-carrying capacity	■ One unit of RBCs should increase the hemoglobin of a 70-kg (154-lb) adult by approximately 1 g/dL in the absence of volume overload or continuing blood loss	■ Red cells require compatibility testing ■ Risk of transmitting bloodborne pathogens ■ Should be warmed to prevent hypothermia ■ Contains little or no clotting factors
Platelets	■ Significant thrombocytopenia (platelet count <20,000–50,000 per mm^3) ■ Continued hemorrhage	■ Compatibility testing is not required ■ Typical platelet transfusion should raise the platelets of a 70-kg (154-lb) adult approximately 30,000–50,000/μL	■ Postexposure prophylaxis with anti-Rh immune globulin should be considered following Rh+ platelet transfusion to an Rh− woman ■ Risk of transmitting bloodborne pathogens
Albumin	■ Expands blood volume in shock and trauma	■ Good availability	■ Not a substitute for whole blood ■ Risk of hypersensitivity reactions ■ Risk of transmitting bloodborne pathogens
Fresh frozen plasma (FFP)	■ Documented coagulopathy ■ Restoration of clotting factors ■ Supplies plasma proteins	■ Crossmatching and Rh compatibility is not required	■ Must be thawed in a 37°C (98.6°F) water bath for approximately 30 min ■ Should be ABO compatible ■ Risk of transmitting bloodborne pathogens
Cryoprecipitate	■ Coagulopathy with low fibrinogen ■ Restoration of fibrinogen	■ Rh type not important	■ Risk of transmitting bloodborne pathogens ■ Contains hemagglutinins ■ If large volumes of ABO-incompatible cryoprecipitate are administered, intravascular hemolysis can occur

A third antigen on the RBC membrane is D. People who are Rh positive have the D antigen, whereas people who are Rh negative do not. These antigens and antibodies may cause ABO and Rh incompatibilities. Rh factor is referred to as positive (+) or negative (−) and is used as a descriptor with the blood type, for example, O+ or AB−.

A transfusion of incompatible blood causes hemolysis (breakdown) of the RBCs and agglutination of erythrocytes. (Agglutination is the clumping of cells that results from their interaction with specific antibodies.) The ABO blood group names and compatibilities are listed in **Table 11.3**.

Before RBCs or whole blood can be administered, a series of procedures determine donor and recipient ABO types and Rh groups. These procedures, called a *type and crossmatch*, are performed by mixing the donor cells with the recipient's serum and watching for agglutination. If none occurs, the blood is considered compatible.

Despite meticulous procedures for matching blood types and antigens, blood transfusion reactions may still occur. The most common is a febrile reaction. Antibodies within the patient receiving the blood are directed against the donor's white blood cells, causing fever and chills. Febrile reactions typically begin during the first 15 minutes of the transfusion. Using leukocyte-poor blood avoids future febrile reactions.

Hypersensitivity reactions result when antibodies in the patient's blood react against proteins, such as immunoglobulin A, in the donor blood. Hypersensitivity reactions may appear during or after the transfusion. The manifestations of hypersensitivity reaction include *urticaria* (the appearance of reddened wheals of various sizes on the skin) and itching.

Table 11.3 Blood Group Types and Compatibilities

Blood Group	RBC Agglutinogens	Serum Agglutinogens	Compatible Donor Blood Groups	Incompatible Donor Blood Groups
A	A	Anti-B	A, O	B, AB
B	B	Anti-A	B, O	A, AB
AB	A, B	None	A, B, AB, O	None
O	None	Anti-A, anti-B	O	A, B, AB

Hemolytic reactions, the most dangerous transfusion reactions, usually result from an ABO incompatibility. Clumping RBCs block capillaries, decreasing blood flow to vital organs. In addition, macrophages engulf the clumped RBCs, releasing free hemoglobin into the circulating blood; the hemoglobin is then filtered by the kidneys and may block the renal tubules, causing renal failure. Hemolytic reactions usually begin after infusion of 100 to 200 mL of incompatible blood. Manifestations of a hemolytic reaction include flushing of the face, a burning sensation along the vein, headache, urticaria, chills, fever, lumbar pain, abdominal pain, chest pain, nausea and vomiting, tachycardia, hypotension, and dyspnea. If any of these manifestations appear, the blood transfusion must be immediately discontinued.

Other risks to patients receiving blood include circulatory overload, electrolyte imbalances, and infectious diseases such as hepatitis or cytomegalovirus.

Patients who have experienced trauma of any severity have had substantial blood loss and are usually in hypovolemic shock. Blood replacement is the treatment of choice to restore oxygen-carrying capacity. Patients in severe shock with active bleeding are given universal, type O red blood cells immediately. Patients with less severe injuries or bleeding may be stabilized with other types of fluids until type-specific or crossmatched blood is available.

Some emergency departments and trauma centers use autotransfusion to provide blood for transfusions for a patient with multiple injuries and/or severe shock. Autotransfusion is a method of blood administration in which special equipment collects and returns the patient's own blood. The chest cavity is the typical source of blood to be autotransfused.

Nursing considerations for blood transfusion therapy are described in **Medication Administration 11.A**.

Medication Administration 11.A

Blood Transfusion

The risk for and seriousness of blood transfusion reactions require that extreme caution be taken when blood is administered. Most fatal transfusion reactions are the result of human error. Although general guidelines are provided here, each institution has specific policies and procedures that must be followed. Prior to beginning the transfusion, the nurse must determine that typed and crossmatched blood is available and collect the needed equipment: A Y-tubing blood administration set with a filter, a large-bore intravenous catheter (usually 18 or 19 gauge), and normal saline solution. Only normal saline is used with a blood transfusion. Dextrose causes clumping of RBCs, and distilled water causes hemolysis.

Nursing Responsibilities

- Obtain patient consent.
- Assess for any previous reactions to blood.
- Explain the procedure to the patient and answer any questions.
- Prepare the intravenous equipment. Shut off one side of the Y tubing, and attach the other side to the saline solution. Flush the tubing and filter with the saline.
- If venous access is not already in place, insert the intravenous needle (following body substance precautions), and begin administering the saline.
- Using institutional procedure, obtain the blood from the blood bank or laboratory. Administer the blood immediately; if this is not possible, return it to the blood bank or laboratory.
- Check and document that the donor and recipient blood have been tested and are compatible. This usually involves two nurses, each verifying the following:
  a. An order for blood has been written.
  b. A type and crossmatch has been done.
  c. The name of the patient and the name on the blood bag are identical.
  d. The number assigned to the unit of blood is identical to the one on the requisition for the blood.
  e. The blood type and Rh factor are compatible.
  f. The blood has not exceeded its expiration date.
  g. The unit of blood is intact and has no bubbles or discoloration.
- Identify the patient by reading the armband and asking the patient to tell you his or her name. Check the armband against the unit of blood.
- Gently invert the blood bag several times to mix the plasma and RBCs.
- Take and record vital signs as a baseline.
- Attach the open side of the Y tubing to the blood unit, and begin the transfusion at a slow rate of about 2 mL per minute. (Some trauma patients may have blood infused at a rapid rate. If blood is infused rapidly, it may need to be warmed prior to administration to prevent hypothermia.) Stay with the patient for at least the first 15 minutes of the transfusion, monitoring for manifestations of a reaction and taking the patient's vital signs.
- Continue to monitor the patient during the transfusion, assessing for manifestations of hypersensitivity or hemolytic reactions and taking and recording vital signs as directed by institutional policy.
- After the first 15 minutes, the rate of infusion is increased. If there is no danger of fluid volume overload, most patients can tolerate an infusion of a unit of blood (ranging from 250 to 500 mL, depending on the blood component administered) in 2 hours. The unit of blood should be administered within 3 to 4 hours; after this time, it has warmed and begins to deteriorate.
- Take the following actions if manifestations of a reaction occur:
  a. Stop the infusion of blood immediately, and notify the physician. Continue to infuse the saline.
  b. Take vital signs and assess manifestations.
  c. Compare the blood slip with the unit of blood to ensure that an identification error was not made.
  d. Save the blood bag and any remaining blood for return to the laboratory for further tests to determine the cause of the reaction.
  e. Follow institutional policy for collecting urine and venous blood samples.
  f. Continue to monitor the patient and provide prescribed interventions to treat hypersensitivity or hemolytic manifestations.

(continued)

Health Education for the Patient and Family

- The possible risks of blood transfusions include infectious diseases and acquired immune deficiency syndrome (AIDS). However, because of careful handling and storage of blood, bacterial contamination is rare. Although hepatitis may be transmitted by contaminated blood, new tests for hepatitis antibodies in the donor blood are reducing this risk. Many people are afraid of contracting AIDS from blood; however, donor screening and HIV-antibody testing of donor blood has virtually eliminated the transmission of HIV by blood transfusion. A new risk that has been identified is the transmission of West Nile virus through blood transfusions. Screening for this risk is asking potential donors about the presence of symptoms indicative of West Nile virus.
- During the transfusion, immediately report any warm feelings, chills, itching, feelings of weakness or fainting, or difficulty breathing.
- Report any signs of a delayed transfusion reaction—chills, fever, cough, difficulty breathing, hives, itching, or changes in circulation—and seek medical care immediately.
- Discuss any religious or cultural considerations related to blood transfusions.

Source: Data from Adams, Holland, & Urban, 2017.

Emergency Surgery

Immediate surgical intervention is indicated when the patient remains in shock despite resuscitation and there is no obvious external sign of blood loss. Abdominal and chest x-rays, ultrasound studies, FAST exam (or diagnostic peritoneal lavage if ultrasound is not available), or CT scan may be performed to help identify the potential source of the blood loss. It is important for the emergency or trauma nurse to speak with the family as soon as possible to keep everyone informed about what is happening to a family member. Unfortunately, the need for emergency surgery may not allow time for family members or significant others to see their loved one before transfer to the operating room.

Forensic Considerations

Injuries often happen under circumstances that require legal investigation. Many injuries, particularly penetrating trauma, may involve criminal activity. Therefore, the nurse must recognize the need to identify, store, and properly transfer potential evidence for medical–legal investigations.

Each item of clothing removed from a patient must be placed in a breathable container, such as a paper bag, and documented appropriately. Bullets or knives should be labeled, with their source specified, and given to the proper authorities. Holes found in clothing should not be disturbed. When it is necessary to cut off clothing, these areas should be avoided and never cut through if at all possible.

The patient's hands may yield important evidence, such as powder burns or residue on the skin or tissue or hair samples beneath the fingernails. In the case of death, it is recommended that paper bags be placed over the patient's hands if the presence of evidence is suspected; otherwise, the evidence should be collected by nail clippings.

Identify all wounds and document these findings with pictures, diagrams, or written descriptions. Once the evidence has been collected, identified, and properly stored, ensure that it is given to the appropriate authorities. A chain of custody needs to be maintained throughout the entire process. All evidence must be identified and labeled, and documentation procedures must chronicle where and in whose possession the evidence has been. For the chain of custody to remain intact, the evidence must remain in the continuous possession of identified people and be marked and sealed in tamper-proof containers.

Nursing Care

Nursing care of the patient who has been injured begins with a primary assessment and the initiation of collaborative interventions for any life-threatening injuries. Nursing care is directed toward the patient's specific responses to trauma.

Assessment

See the Interprofessional Care section for assessment of the patient experiencing trauma.

Priorities of Care

The nurse collaborates with the interprofessional team to ensure adequate treatment of the underlying injury while providing care that supports oxygenation and perfusion. Teaching the patient and, as appropriate, caregivers strategies to prevent injuries and optimize safe home and work environments should be considered priority nursing actions. The nurse also focuses on promoting comfort and maintaining asepsis for all interruptions of the integument.

Diagnoses, Outcomes, and Interventions

The trauma patient has many complex and interrelated actual or potential alterations in health. The nursing care in this section focuses on patient and family problems with respirations, infection, immobility, and spirituality. Nursing interventions for decreased cardiac output and altered perfusion are discussed in the section of the chapter on nursing care of the patient in shock. See the accompanying Case Study & Nursing Care Plan on page 302.

Manage Airway Clearance. The patient with multiple injuries is at great risk for developing airway obstruction and apnea. Facial injuries, loose teeth, blood, and vomitus increase the risk for aspiration and obstruction. Neurologic injuries and cerebral edema alter the patient's respiratory drive and ability to keep the airway clear.

Expected Outcome: Patient's airway will remain patent. The nurse will:

- Assess if airway is patent, maintainable, or unable to be maintained. Assess for manifestations of airway obstruction: Stridor, tachypnea, bradypnea, cough, cyanosis, dyspnea, decreased or absent breath sounds, changes in oxygen levels, and changes in level of consciousness. *Assessing the airway and initiating interventions are the first steps in managing the patient with multiple injuries.*

- Monitor oxygen saturation by applying a pulse oximeter. Adjust oxygen flow to maintain oxygen saturation from 94 to 100%. *Changes in oxygen saturation as measured by the pulse oximeter indicate the effectiveness of the patient's airway. Pulse oximetry in patients who have been exposed to carbon monoxide (i.e., house fires) is unreliable since it cannot differentiate carboxyhemoglobin from oxyhemoglobin.*
- Monitor level of consciousness. *An early sign of an ineffective airway is a change in the patient's behavior. If the patient becomes restless, anxious, combative, or unresponsive, the effectiveness of the airway needs to be immediately evaluated and appropriate interventions initiated.*

Reduce Risk for Infection. Traumatic injuries are considered dirty wounds. Projectiles enter the body through dirty surfaces and clothing, carrying dirt and debris into the wound. Open fractures provide a portal for the entry of bacteria and dirt. Even with surgical intervention, the wounds often remain contaminated.

Expected Outcome: Patient will avoid getting an infection as much as possible through careful hygiene and the use of correct aseptic technique and universal precautions.

The nurse will:

- Use careful hand hygiene practices. *Hand hygiene remains the single most important factor in preventing the spread of infection.*
- Use strict standard precautions and aseptic technique when caring for wounds. *Standard precautions are essential to protect the patient and the nurse from infection.* In addition:
    a. Monitor wounds for odor, redness, heat, swelling, and copious or purulent drainage.
    b. Monitor hidden wounds, such as those under casts, by asking the patient whether the pain has increased and observing for increased drainage and heat over the area of the wound.
- Ensure that cross-contamination between wounds does not occur. Collect drainage in ostomy bags if it is copious.*The skin is the first line of defense against infection. Wounds provide a portal of entry for organisms. Risk factors for wound infection include contamination, inadequate wound care, and the condition of the wound at the time of closure. Aseptic techniques used in applying and changing dressings reduce the entry of organisms.*
- Take and record vital signs, including temperature, every 2 to 4 hours. *Abnormal vital signs, particularly an elevated body temperature, can indicate the presence of an infection.*
- Provide adequate fluids and nutrition. *Adequate fluids, calories, and protein are essential to wound healing.*
- Assess for manifestations of gas gangrene: Fever, pain, and swelling in traumatized tissues; drainage with a foul odor. *Gas gangrene is usually caused by the organism* Clostridium perfringens. *This bacterium is found in the soil and can be introduced into the body during a traumatic injury. The organism grows in the tissues, causing necrosis; hydrogen and carbon dioxide are released, with resultant swelling of tissues. If the infection continues, tissues are progressively destroyed, and sepsis and death may result.*
- Assess for development of potentially life-threatening conditions such as necrotizing fasciitis where flesh-eating bacteria infect subcutaneous and dermal layers, spreading to the fascial plane. *Many types of bacteria can cause necrotizing fasciitis; however, methicillin-resistant* Staphylococcus aureus *is occurring with increasing frequency.*
- Assess the status of tetanus immunization and administer tetanus toxoid or human toxin-antitoxin (TAT) as prescribed. *Tetanus is caused by an exotoxin produced by* Clostridium tetani, *usually introduced through an open wound. The organism is commonly found in the soil.*
- Use strict aseptic technique when inserting catheters, suctioning, administering parenteral medications, or performing any other invasive procedure. *Using aseptic technique during invasive procedures reduces the risk of entry of organisms.*

Promote Physical Mobility. The patient with trauma injuries is often unable to change positions independently and is at risk for complications of the integumentary, cardiovascular, gastrointestinal, respiratory, musculoskeletal, and renal systems. Patients at greatest risk are those who have had multiple injuries, spinal cord injuries, peripheral nerve injuries, and traumatic amputations. Collaborate with the physical therapist and occupational therapist (if available) to determine the most effective types and schedule of exercises and assistive devices.

Expected Outcome: Patient will maintain joint range of motion, avoid development of contractures, and avoid pulmonary complications such as atelectasis with appropriate pulmonary hygiene.

The nurse will:

- Provide active or passive exercises, if active bleeding or edema is not present, to affected and unaffected extremities at least once every 8 hours. *Exercise improves muscle tone, maintains joint mobility, improves circulation, and prevents contractures.*
- Help the patient turn, cough, and deep-breathe and use the incentive spirometer at least every 2 hours. *Changing positions, coughing, deep breathing, and incentive spirometry reduce the risk of integumentary and respiratory complications.*
- Provide a specialty bed, such as the kinetic continuous rotation bed, if the patient is unable to be moved and positioned (**Figure 11.9** ■). *The kinetic continuous rotation bed allows continuous turning of the patient; the motion decreases pulmonary complications, venous stasis, postural hypotension, urinary stasis, muscle wasting, and bone demineralization.*
- Monitor the lower extremities each day for manifestations of deep venous thrombosis: Heat, swelling, and pain. Measure and record the circumference of the thigh

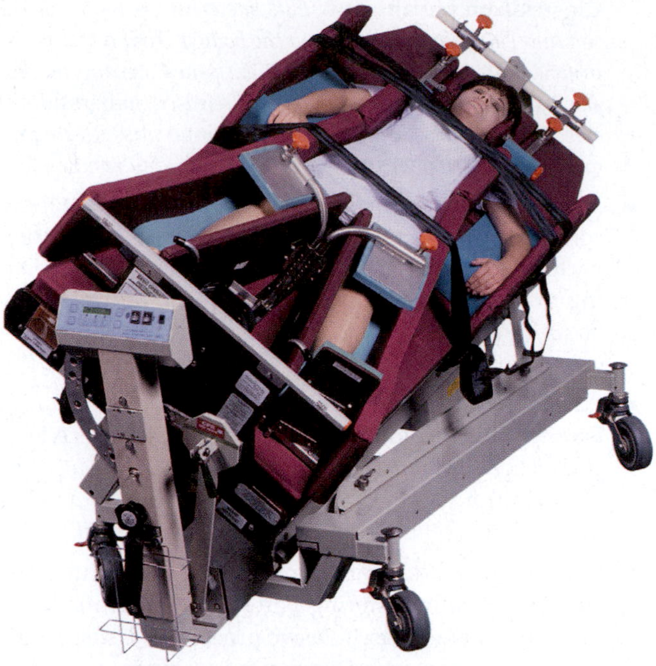

Figure 11.9 ■ A kinetic continuous rotation bed provides a means of turning the patient with multiple injuries to decrease the hazards of immobility.

and calf each day. If antiemboli stockings or intermittent compression stockings are used, remove them for 1 hour during each shift and assess the skin. *Venous stasis results when surrounding muscles are unable to contract and help move the blood through the veins. Thrombus (clot) formation in deep veins is a major risk for pulmonary embolism.*

Help Manage Feelings of Grief and Loss. Trauma generally strikes without warning and carries potentially devastating consequences, including severe alterations in the lives of the victim and family, and death. The traumatic death of a loved one may be the most difficult event a family will ever experience. The decision to cease life support systems or to donate organs challenges the family's belief systems and psychologic stability.

Expected Outcome: The patient and/or family, as appropriate, will express feelings of grief and lack of control over the traumatic situation.

Nursing care of the family (or patient) experiencing spiritual distress includes:

- Offer referral to a spiritual adviser, if needed. *Most hospitals have chaplain programs.*
- Give the family information about the option to donate the patient's organs. *The decision to donate organs needs to be based on information about the patient's condition, prognosis, and criteria by which brain death is determined. It is important to convey to family members that organ donation is only an option and that they should not feel they are obligated to consent or are doing something wrong if they do not consent.*
- Encourage the family to ask questions and express any feelings about the traumatic event and/or organ donation. *Allowing families to express their feelings may help prevent long-term consequences such as guilt.*
- Refer the family for follow-up care. Long-term follow-up is important for the family facing the sudden death of a loved one. *Grieving is not an overnight process, and providing the family with resources that may be used in the future may help prevent future crises and dysfunction.* (For more information, see Chapter 5.)

Teach Coping Strategies. Posttraumatic stress disorder is an intense, sustained emotional response to a disastrous event. It is also referred to as posttrauma syndrome. It is characterized by emotions that range from anger to fear and by flashbacks or psychic numbing. In the initial stage, the patient may be calm or may express feelings of anger, disbelief, terror, and shock. In the long-term phase, which begins anywhere from a few days to several months after the event, the patient often experiences flashbacks and nightmares of the traumatic event. The patient may call on ineffective coping mechanisms, such as alcohol or drugs, and withdraw from relationships.

Expected Outcome: Patient will verbalize feelings and fears as they move through the traumatic experience. Patient will report development or occurrence of flashbacks to appropriate healthcare personnel.

The nurse will:

- Assess emotional responses while providing physical care. Observe for crying, sleep problems, suspiciousness, and fear during the initial phase of treatment. If the patient is unconscious, encourage family members and friends to express their feelings. *These assessments provide valuable information about the patient's ability to cope with the trauma.*
- Be available if the patient wishes to talk about the trauma, and encourage expression of feelings. *The patient may initially deny negative feelings; this denial is a coping mechanism in the initial phase of recovery.*
- Teach relaxation techniques, such as deep breathing, progressive muscle relaxation, or imagery (see Chapter 4). *These techniques often help patients cope when thoughts of the trauma recur.*
- Refer the patient and family members for counseling, psychotherapy, or support groups as appropriate. *Continued therapy may be necessary in assisting the patient and family to resolve the acute and long-term effects of trauma.*

Delegating Nursing Care Activities

As appropriate and allowed by the designated duties and responsibilities of assistive personnel, the nurse may delegate nursing care activities such as measuring fluid intake and output, collecting vital signs (including orthostatic vital signs), encouraging oral or enteral fluid intake, and skin care.

Transitions of Care

Prevention efforts can reduce the incidence and severity of trauma. Areas of health promotion and trauma prevention interventions for individuals and communities include:

- ***Motor vehicle safety:*** Seat belts, air bags, helmets, driving under the influence of alcohol or drugs, reckless driving, visual or cognitive deficits in the older adult, cell phone use, driver fatigue
- ***Home safety:*** Snow and ice removal, electrical wiring, falls, burns, drowning
- ***Farm safety:*** Operating heavy equipment, safe storage of chemicals such as fertilizers
- ***Work safety:*** Operating work equipment, wearing safety equipment, removal of jewelry
- ***Relationships:*** Domestic violence, child abuse, older adult abuse, or neglect
- ***Communities:*** Gun control, gangs, condition of streets, neighborhood safety.

In providing information about trauma prevention to members of the community, the nurse serves as a healthcare educator, political activist, and safety advocate.

Address the following topics to prepare the patient and family for home care:

- The type of home environment to which the patient will be returning, including any changes that will be required to let the patient function in that environment
- Medications, dressings, wound care, equipment, and supplies
- Special diet, if needed
- Rehabilitation plan and its effect on the patient's family
- Follow-up appointments with the physician or at the trauma clinic
- Emotional changes that the patient may undergo as a result of the trauma
- Helpful resources:
    a. Home healthcare
    b. Community support groups
    c. National Institute of Neurological Disorders and Stroke.

Trauma resuscitation may not be successful or continued resuscitation may be stopped if care is futile. The family must be supported as the sudden realization their family member will die can be traumatic. A staff member should stay with the family as much as possible. The treating physician should be the person who tells the family of the death of their loved one. Like a death anywhere in the hospital, the family should be allowed time to be with their loved one. The trauma victim should be "cleaned up" as much as possible and anything that must stay in place for an autopsy should be explained to the family. If there are visible injuries or mutilations (such as major areas of skin removed that cannot be covered), this should be explained to the family. Time for questions should be provided along with information concerning release of the deceased family member's body and a phone number and information on who they could contact in case of questions after they leave. This information should be written down as the family may not remember what is told to them.

The Uniform Anatomical Gift Act (1968; amended 1987) requires that people be informed about their options for organ donation. Under this act, consent for organ donation may be given not only by the donor but also by a spouse, adult children, parents, adult siblings, guardian, or any adult authorized to do so. The act also encourages people to carry donor cards.

The increased success of organ transplantation has made it a more common and valuable method of prolonging and improving life; however, many people are still waiting for organs, and many people who may be suitable organ donors die each year from trauma. Organs and tissues that may be transplanted include bones, eyes, liver, lungs, skin, muscles and tendons, stomach, pancreas, intestines, kidneys, heart, and heart valves.

The organ donation process begins with identification of the potential organ donor. Most people are potential organ donors. Exceptions include those who:

- Currently abuse intravenous drugs
- Have preexisting untreated infections, such as septicemia
- Have any malignancy other than a primary brain tumor
- Have active tuberculosis.

In 2013, the HOPE Act (HIV Organ Policy Equity Act) became federal law. This means HIV-positive persons can sign up to donate their organs upon death. The organs would be transplanted into HIV-positive recipients.

The family needs to be made aware of the patient's prognosis and presented with the option of donating the patient's organs. Both the family's and the patient's feelings about organ donation must be explored. Even if the patient carries an organ donation card, many institutions will not remove any organs without a signature from a family member or other authorized person. The nurse must always respect the family's concerns and feelings in this process. Organ procurement agencies employ specially trained personnel who oversee organ donor identification and procurement. These professionals are trained to approach families regarding potential organ donation. **Box 11.2** lists **brain death criteria**. Once brain death has been confirmed, the family must also understand the diagnosis and be allowed time to accept the patient's death.

BOX 11.2
Brain Death Criteria

CLINICAL SIGNS

- Irreversible condition
- Apnea with a $PaCO_2$ greater than 60 mmHg
- No response to deep stimuli
- No spontaneous movement (some spinal cord reflexes may be present)
- No gag or corneal reflex
- No oculocephalic or oculovestibular reflex
- Absence of toxic or metabolic disorders

CONFIRMATORY TESTS

- Cerebral blood flow study
- Electroencephalogram

When caring for an adult patient who is an organ donor, the nurse carries out the following:

- Maintain systolic blood pressure of 90 mmHg to keep the patient's organs perfused until removal.
- Maintain urine output at more than 30 mL per hour. This is usually accomplished by administering fluids and/or inotropic agents such as dopamine.
- Maintain oxygen saturation at 90% or greater.

Case Study & Nursing Care Plan

A Patient with Multiple Injuries

Jane Souza is a 25-year-old married woman with two children who provides day care for preschool children in her home. As she is driving the interstate at 65 miles per hour, a car crosses the median and strikes her vehicle head-on. Mrs. Souza, who is not wearing a seat belt, is thrown forward against the steering wheel. Her lower extremities are entrapped by the dashboard structure of her car, which was crushed in by the car that struck hers.

After extensive efforts to extricate her from the car, Mrs. Souza is transported to the local trauma center. She is still conscious, is receiving high-flow oxygen by mask, and has one intravenous line in place. Her vital signs are a palpable systolic blood pressure of 80, a pulse rate of 120, and a respiratory rate of 36. On arrival, she states that she is having difficulty breathing.

ASSESSMENT

- Airway: Maintainable with high-flow oxygen in place.
- Breathing: Respiratory rate of 36, multiple bruising and abrasions on right side of her chest, decreased breath sounds on the right side.
- Circulation: No palpable radial pulses; palpable brachial pulses. Monitor shows sinus tachycardia. No active external bleeding noted. Skin color pale, cool to the touch, and diaphoretic. One intravenous line already established.
- Neurologic: Moved her fingers when asked; complains of difficulty breathing; denies that she is hurt. Pupils 4 mm, equal, and react to light. Has a broken right arm and an open fracture of the left ankle; because of these injuries, extremity movement is limited.

Because of Mrs. Souza's respiratory distress, she is intubated and ventilated with 100% oxygen. Another intravenous line is inserted and O-negative blood administered. It is determined that Mrs. Souza has sustained a pneumothorax in the right side and a chest tube is inserted.

DIAGNOSES

- Difficulty in breathing related to right chest trauma
- Decrease in perfusion due to presumed acute internal blood loss related to trauma

EXPECTED OUTCOMES

- Patient will maintain adequate oxygenation.
- Patient will maintain adequate circulating blood volume.

PLANNING AND IMPLEMENTATION

- Monitor airway and assist in any needed airway management.
- Explain all procedures.
- Monitor the effects of fluid and blood administration, including any changes in blood pressure and pulse.
- Prepare for transfer to the operating room for emergency surgery.
- Keep family informed about her condition.

EVALUATION

Mrs. Souza is transferred to the operating room, where it is determined that she has a ruptured spleen and a serious pelvic fracture. Her treatment continues in the operating room.

CLINICAL REASONING IN PATIENT CARE

1. Is the nursing diagnosis decreased perfusion appropriate for Mrs. Souza? Why or why not?
2. The assessment of a patient who has experienced trauma is, in order, A = airway, B = breathing, and C = circulation. What is the rationale for this sequence?
3. Following surgery, Mrs. Souza is moved to the surgical intensive care unit. She is very anxious and restless. What methods of assessments would help you identify the cause of her restlessness?
4. Infection is a common complication for the trauma patient. Describe five risks for infection that are present from the time of injury to the time of hospital discharge.

See Evaluating Your Response in Appendix B.

11.3 Shock

Shock is a clinical syndrome characterized by a systemic imbalance between oxygen supply and demand. This imbalance results in a state of inadequate blood flow to body organs and tissues, causing life-threatening cellular dysfunction.

Overview of Cellular Homeostasis and Hemodynamics

To maintain cellular metabolism, cells of all body organs and tissues require a regular and consistent supply of oxygen and the removal of metabolic wastes. This homeostatic regulation is maintained primarily by the cardiovascular system and depends on four physiologic components:

1. A cardiac output sufficient to meet bodily requirements
2. An uncompromised vascular system, in which the vessels have a diameter sufficient to allow unimpeded blood flow and have good tone (the ability to constrict or dilate to maintain normal pressure)
3. A volume of blood sufficient to fill the circulatory system, and a blood pressure adequate to maintain blood flow
4. Tissues that are able to extract and use the oxygen delivered through the capillaries.

In a healthy person, these components function as a system to maintain tissue perfusion. During shock, however, one or more of these components are disrupted. An understanding of basic hemodynamics is necessary to understand the pathophysiology of shock:

- ***Stroke volume (SV)*** is the amount of blood pumped into the aorta with each contraction of the left ventricle.
- ***Cardiac output (CO)*** is the amount of blood pumped per minute into the aorta by the left ventricle. CO is determined by multiplying the SV by the heart rate (HR): $CO = SV \times HR$.
- ***Systemic vascular resistance (SVR)*** is the resistance offered by the peripheral circulation.
- ***Mean arterial pressure (MAP)*** is the product of cardiac output and SVR: $MAP = CO \times SVR$. It can also be calculated as $MAP = [(2 \times \text{diastolic BP}) + \text{systolic BP}]/3$. When CO, SVR, or total blood volume rises, MAP and tissue perfusion increase. Conversely, when CO, SVR, or total blood volume falls, MAP and tissue perfusion decrease. A MAP of 70 to 110 is normal. A MAP of 60 mmHg is required to maintain adequate perfusion to the brain, heart, and kidneys.

The sympathetic nervous system maintains the smooth muscle surrounding the arteries and arterioles in a state of partial contraction called *sympathetic tone*. Increased sympathetic stimulation increases vasoconstriction and SVR; decreased sympathetic stimulation allows vasodilation, which decreases SVR.

Pathophysiology

When one or more cardiovascular components do not function properly, the body's hemodynamic properties are altered. Consequently, tissue perfusion may be inadequate to sustain normal cellular metabolism. The result is the clinical syndrome known as shock. The manifestations of shock result from the body's attempts to maintain vital organs (heart and brain) and to preserve life following a drop in cellular perfusion. However, if the injury or condition triggering shock is severe enough or of long enough duration, cellular hypoxia and cellular death occur.

Shock is triggered by a sustained drop in mean arterial pressure. This drop can occur after a decrease in cardiac output, a decrease in the circulating blood volume, or an increase in the size of the vascular bed due to peripheral vasodilation. If intervention is timely and effective, the physiologic events that characterize shock may be stopped; if not, shock may lead to death.

Stage 1: Early, Reversible, and Compensatory Shock

The initial stage of shock begins when baroreceptors in the aortic arch and the carotid sinus detect a sustained drop in MAP of less than 10 mmHg from normal levels. The circulating blood volume may decrease (usually to less than 500 mL), but not enough to cause serious effects.

The body reacts to the decrease in arterial pressure. The cerebral integration center initiates the body's response systems, causing the sympathetic nervous system to increase the heart rate and the force of cardiac contraction, thus increasing cardiac output. Sympathetic stimulation also causes peripheral vasoconstriction, resulting in increased systemic vascular resistance and a rise in arterial pressure. The net result is that the perfusion of cells, tissues, and organs is maintained. Symptoms are almost imperceptible during the early stage of shock. The pulse rate may be slightly elevated. If the injury is minor or of short duration, arterial pressure is usually maintained, and no further symptoms occur.

Compensatory shock begins after the MAP falls 10 to 15 mmHg below normal levels (Pollack, 2011). The circulating blood volume is reduced by 25 to 35% (1000 mL or more), but compensatory mechanisms are able to maintain blood pressure and tissue perfusion to vital organs, thereby preventing cell damage.

- Stimulation of the sympathetic nervous system results in the release of epinephrine from the adrenal medulla and the release of norepinephrine from the adrenal medulla and the sympathetic fibers. Both hormones rapidly stimulate the alpha- and beta-adrenergic fibers. Stimulated alpha-adrenergic fibers cause vasoconstriction in the blood vessels supplying the skin and most of the abdominal viscera. Perfusion of these areas decreases. Stimulated beta-adrenergic fibers cause vasodilation in vessels supplying the heart and skeletal muscles ($beta_1$ response) and increase the heart rate and force of cardiac contraction ($beta_2$ response). Furthermore, blood vessels in the respiratory system dilate, and the respiratory rate increases ($beta_2$ response). Thus, stimulation of the sympathetic nervous system results in increased cardiac output and oxygenation of these tissues.

- The renin–angiotensin response occurs as the blood flow to the kidneys decreases. Renin released from the kidneys acts on angiotensinogen to form angiotensin I. This is converted by angiotensin-converting enzyme in the lungs to angiotensin II, which causes vasoconstriction and stimulates the adrenal cortex to release aldosterone. Aldosterone causes the kidneys to reabsorb water and sodium and to lose potassium. The absorption of water maintains circulating blood volume, while increased vasoconstriction increases SVR, maintaining central vascular volume and raising blood pressure.
- The hypothalamus releases adrenocorticotropic hormone (ACTH), causing the adrenal glands to secrete aldosterone. Aldosterone promotes the reabsorption of water and sodium by the kidneys, preserving blood volume and pressure.
- The posterior pituitary gland releases antidiuretic hormone (ADH), which increases renal reabsorption of water to increase intravascular volume. The combined effects of hormones released by the hypothalamus and posterior pituitary glands work to conserve central vascular volume.
- As MAP falls in the compensatory stage of shock, decreased capillary hydrostatic pressure causes a fluid shift from the interstitial space into the capillaries. The net gain of fluid raises the blood volume.

Working together, these compensatory mechanisms can maintain MAP for only a short period of time. During this period, the perfusion and oxygenation of the heart and brain are adequate. If effective treatment is provided, the process is arrested, and no permanent damage occurs. However, unless the underlying cause of shock is reversed, these compensatory mechanisms soon become harmful, and shock perpetuates shock.

Stage 2: Intermediate or Progressive Shock

The progressive stage of shock occurs after a sustained decrease in MAP of 20 mmHg or more below normal levels and a fluid loss of 35 to 50% (1800 to 2500 mL of fluid) (Pollack, 2011). Although the compensatory mechanisms in the previous state remain activated, they are no longer able to maintain MAP at a level sufficient to ensure perfusion of vital organs.

The vasoconstriction response that first helped sustain MAP eventually limits blood flow to the point that cells become oxygen deficient. To remain alive, the affected cells switch from aerobic to anaerobic metabolism. The lactic acid formed as a by-product of anaerobic metabolism contributes to an acidotic state at the cellular level. As a result, adenosine triphosphate (ATP), the source of cellular energy, is produced inefficiently. Lacking energy, the sodium-potassium pump fails. Potassium moves out of the cell, while sodium and water move inward. As this process continues, the cell swells, cell membrane integrity is lost, and cell organelles are damaged. Lysosomes within the cell spill out their digestive enzymes, which disintegrate any remaining organelles. Some enzymes spread to adjacent cells, where they erode and rupture cell membranes.

The acid by-products of anaerobic metabolism dilate the precapillary arterioles and constrict the postcapillary venules. This causes increased hydrostatic pressure within the capillary, and fluid shifts back into the interstitial space. The capillaries also become increasingly permeable, allowing serum proteins to shift from the vascular space into the interstitium. The buildup of plasma proteins increases the osmotic pressure in the interstitium, further accelerating the fluid shift out of the capillaries.

Throughout this period, the heart rate and vasoconstriction increase; however, perfusion of the skin, skeletal muscles, kidneys, and gastrointestinal organs is greatly diminished. Cells in the heart and brain become hypoxic, while other body cells and tissues become ischemic and anoxic. A generalized state of acidosis and hyperkalemia ensues (see Chapter 10). Unless this stage of shock is treated rapidly, the patient's chances of survival are poor.

Stage 3: Refractory or Irreversible Shock

If shock progresses to the irreversible stage, tissue anoxia becomes so generalized and cellular death so widespread that no treatment can reverse the damage. Even if MAP is temporarily restored, too much cellular damage has occurred to maintain life. Death of cells is followed by death of tissues, which results in death of organs. Death of vital organs contributes to subsequent death of the body.

Effects of Shock on Body Systems

Whatever its causes, shock produces predictable effects on the body's organ systems. (See the Multisystem Effects of Shock feature.)

Cardiovascular System

The perfusion and oxygenation of the heart are adequate in the early stages of shock. As shock progresses, myocardial cells become hypoxic, and myocardial muscle function diminishes. Initially, the blood pressure may be normal or even slightly elevated (as a result of compensatory mechanisms) and the heart rate only slightly increased. Sympathetic stimulation increases the heart rate (a sinus tachycardia of 120 bpm is common) in an effort to increase cardiac output. As a result of vasoconstriction and decreased blood volume, the palpated pulse is rapid, weak, and thready; as shock progresses, peripheral pulses are usually nonpalpable.

Tachycardia reduces the time available for left-ventricular filling and coronary artery perfusion, further reducing cardiac output. With progressive shock, altered acid–base balance, hypoxia, and hyperkalemia damage the heart's electrical systems and contractility. Consequently, cardiac dysrhythmias may develop. Decreased blood volume with decreased venous return also decreases cardiac output, and blood pressure falls.

The blood pressure changes produced by shock are characterized by a progressive decrease in both systolic and

Multisystem Effects of Shock

Respiratory

- ↑ respiratory rate
- Respiratory acidosis

Potential complication

- ARDS

Urinary

- ↓ renal perfusion
- ↓ GFR

Late

- Oliguria

Potential complications

- Acute tubular necrosis
- Kidney failure

Hepatic

Early

- ↑ glucose production

Progressive

- ↓ glucose production = hypoglycemia
- ↓ lactic acid conversion = metabolic acidosis

Potential complication

- Destroyed Kupffer cells = systemic bacterial infections

Gastrointestinal

Early

- ↓ GI motility

Late

- Paralytic ileus
- Ulceration of GI mucosa

Potential complication

- Bowel necrosis

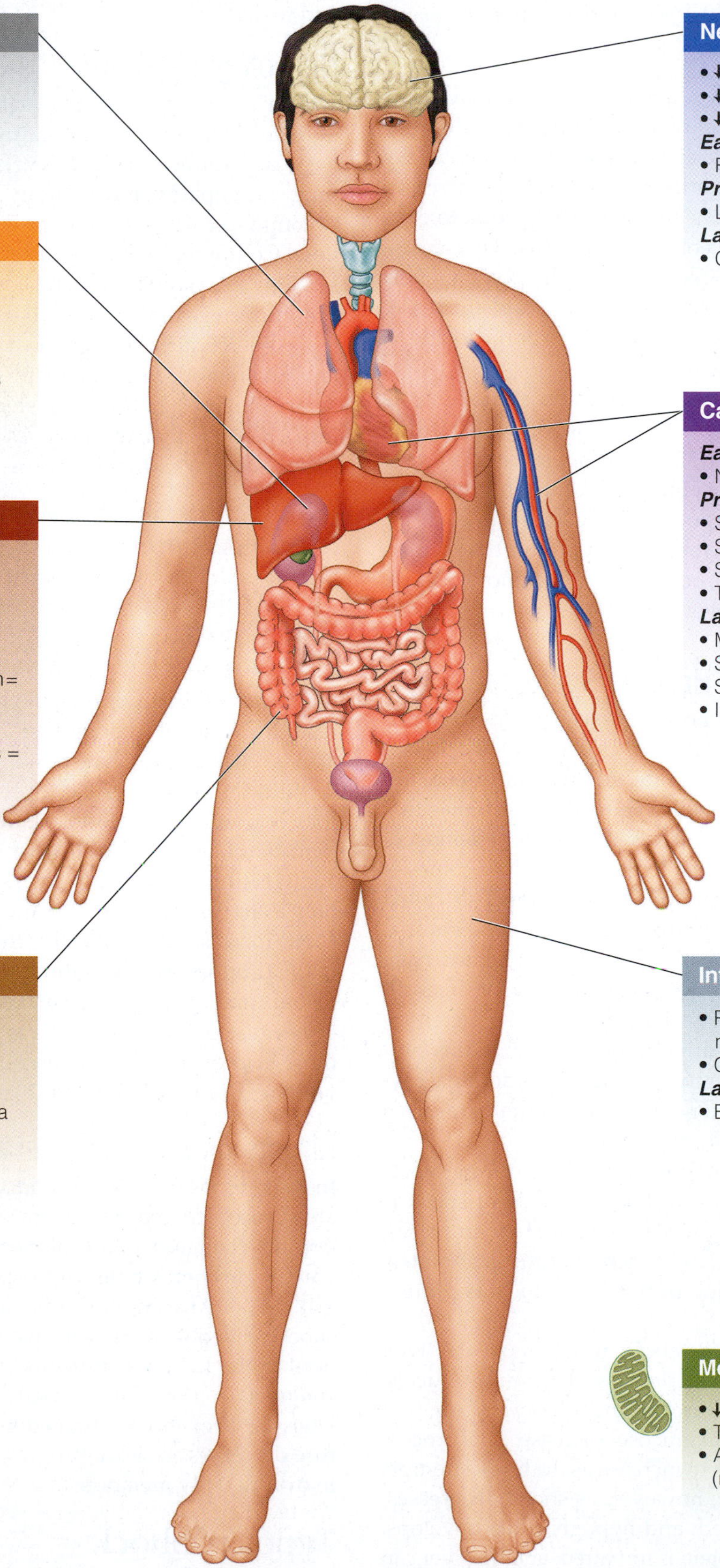

Neurologic

- ↓ cognition
- ↓ sympathetic activity
- ↓ consciousness

Early

- Restlessness, apathy

Progressive

- Lethargy

Late

- Coma

Cardiovascular

Early

- No change

Progressive

- Slightly ↑ BP
- Slowly ↑ HR
- Sinus tachycardia
- Thready pulse

Late

- MAP < 60 mmHg
- Steadily ↓ BP
- Steadily ↓ CO
- Imperceptible pulses

Integumentary

- Pallor (skin, lips, oral mucosa, nail beds, conjunctiva)
- Cool, moist skin

Late

- Edema

Metabolic Processes

- ↓ temperature
- Thirst
- Acidosis (metabolic and respiratory)

diastolic pressures and a narrowing pulse pressure. Auscultation of blood pressure is often difficult or impossible and is an inaccurate reflection of blood pressure status. For this reason, hemodynamic monitoring is usually instituted to follow the patient's cardiovascular status accurately.

Respiratory System

During shock, impaired oxygen delivery to cells may occur due to a drop in circulating blood volume or, in the case of blood loss, by an insufficient number of red blood cells that carry oxygen. Although the respiratory rate increases because of compensatory mechanisms that promote oxygenation, the number of alveoli that are perfused decreases, and gas exchange is impaired. As a result, oxygen levels in the blood decrease, and carbon dioxide levels increase. As perfusion of the lungs diminishes, carbon dioxide is retained, and respiratory acidosis occurs.

A complication of decreased perfusion of the lungs is acute respiratory distress syndrome (ARDS), which is discussed in detail in Chapter 37. The exact mechanism that produces ARDS is unknown, but some contributing factors have been identified. This potentially lethal form of respiratory failure may result from any condition that causes hypoperfusion of the lungs, but it is more common in shock caused by hemorrhage, severe allergic responses, trauma, and infection.

Gastrointestinal and Hepatic Systems

The gastrointestinal organs normally receive 25% of the cardiac output through the splanchnic circulation. Shock constricts the splanchnic arterioles and redirects arterial blood flow to the heart and brain. Consequently, gastrointestinal organs become ischemic and may be irreversibly damaged.

Gastric mucosa tends to ulcerate when it becomes is chemic. Lesions of the gastric and duodenal mucosa (called *stress ulcers*) can develop within hours of severe trauma, sepsis, or burns. Gastrointestinal ulcers may hemorrhage within 2 to 10 days following the original cause of shock. In addition, the permeability of damaged mucosa increases, allowing bacterial translocation to occur. During this process, enteric bacteria or their toxins enter the abdominal cavity, progress to the circulation, and can eventually result in sepsis (Wagner & Hardin-Pierce, 2014).

Gastric and intestinal motility is impaired during shock, and paralytic ileus may result. If the episode of shock is prolonged, necrosis of the bowel may occur. In many cases, alterations in the structure and function of the gastrointestinal tract impair absorption of nutrients, such as protein and glucose.

Shock also alters the metabolic functions of the liver. Initially, *gluconeogenesis* (the process of forming glucose from noncarbohydrate sources) and *glycogenolysis* (the breakdown of glycogen into glucose) increase. This process allows blood glucose levels to increase as the body attempts to respond to the stressor; however, as shock progresses, liver functions are impaired, and hypoglycemia develops. Metabolism of fats and protein is impaired, and the liver can no longer effectively remove lactic acid, contributing to the development of metabolic acidosis.

The destruction of the liver's reticuloendothelial Kupffer cells (phagocytes that destroy bacteria) causes a further problem. Bacteria may proliferate within the circulatory system, causing overwhelming bacterial infection and toxicity.

Neurologic System

The primary effects of shock on the neurologic system involve changes in mental status and orientation. Cerebral hypoxia produces altered levels of consciousness, beginning with apathy and lethargy and progressing to coma. A common early symptom of cerebral hypoxia is restlessness. Continued ischemia of brain cells eventually causes swelling, resulting in cerebral edema, neurotransmitter failure, and irreversible brain cell damage.

As cerebral ischemia worsens, the sympathetic activity and vasomotor centers are depressed. This leads to a loss of sympathetic tone, causing systemic vasodilation and pooling of blood in the periphery. As a result, venous return and cardiac output further decrease.

SAFETY ALERT: An early sign of shock is a change in the level of consciousness. Late signs of shock are mental status changes, hypotension, and marked tachycardia. ■

Renal System

Blood that normally perfuses the kidneys is shunted to the heart and brain during the progressive stage of shock, resulting in renal hypoperfusion. The drop in renal perfusion is reflected in a corresponding decrease in the glomerular filtration rate. Urine output is reduced, and the urine that is produced is highly concentrated. Oliguria of less than 20 mL per hour indicates progressive shock.

Healthy kidneys can tolerate a drop in perfusion for only a short time; thereafter, the risk of acute kidney injury (AKI) increases dramatically. This will be evident by a dramatic drop in urinary output (less than 0.5ml/kilo/hr for 6 hours and or an increase in creatinine of 0.3mg/dl within 48 hours. Recovery from AKI is variable and the best treatment is prevention by maintaining adequate circulatory volume (Perrin & MacLeod, 2018).

Effects on Skin, Temperature, and Thirst

In most types of shock, blood vessels supplying the skin are vasoconstricted, and the sweat glands are activated. As a result, changes in skin color occur. The skin of Caucasian patients becomes pale. In people with darker skin (such as those of African, Hispanic, or Mediterranean descent), shock-related skin color changes may be assessed as paleness of the lips, oral mucous membranes, nail beds, and conjunctiva. The skin is usually cool and moist and, in the later stages of shock, often edematous. The body temperature decreases as shock progresses, the result of a decrease in overall body metabolism.

Types of Shock

Shock is identified according to its underlying cause (**Figure 11.10** ■). All types of shock progress through the

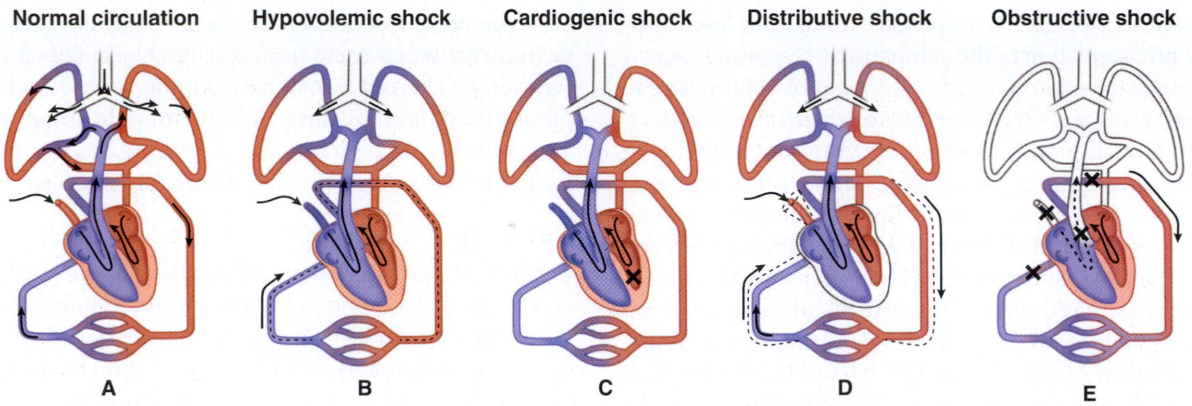
Normal circulation
Hypovolemic shock
Cardiogenic shock
Distributive shock
Obstructive shock
A
B
C
D
E

Figure 11.10 ■ Compare (**A**) normal circulation with (**B**) hypovolemic shock, (**C**) cardiogenic shock, (**D**) distributive shock, and (**E**) obstructive shock.

same stages and exert similar effects on body systems. Any differences are noted in the following discussion.

Hypovolemic Shock

Hypovolemic shock is caused by a decrease in intravascular volume of 15% or more (Perrin & MacLeod, 2018). In hypovolemic shock, the venous blood returning to the heart decreases, and ventricular filling drops. As a result, stroke volume and cardiac blood pressure decrease. Hypovolemic shock is the most common type of shock, and it often occurs simultaneously with other types.

The decrease in circulating blood volume that triggers hypovolemic shock may result from the following:

- Loss of blood volume from hemorrhage (from surgery, trauma, gastrointestinal bleeding, blood coagulation disorders, ruptured esophageal varices)
- Loss of intravascular fluid from the skin due to injuries such as burns (see Chapter 17)
- Loss of intravascular volume from severe dehydration
- Loss of body fluid from the gastrointestinal system due to persistent and severe vomiting or diarrhea or continuous nasogastric suctioning
- Renal losses of fluid due to the use of diuretics or to endocrine disorders such as diabetes insipidus
- Conditions causing fluid shifts from the intravascular compartment to the interstitial space
- Third spacing due to such disorders as liver diseases with ascites, pleural effusion, or intestinal obstruction.

Hypovolemic shock affects all body systems. Its effects vary depending on the patient's age, general state of health, extent of injury or severity of illness, length of time before treatment is provided, and the rate of volume loss.

The manifestations of hypovolemic shock result directly from the decrease in circulating blood volume and the initiation of compensatory mechanisms (**Figure 11.11** ■). The loss of circulating blood volume reduces cardiac output by decreasing venous return to the heart. As a result, blood pressure drops. The carotid and cardiac baroreceptors sense the decrease in blood pressure and communicate it to the vasomotor centers in the brainstem. The vasomotor centers then induce the

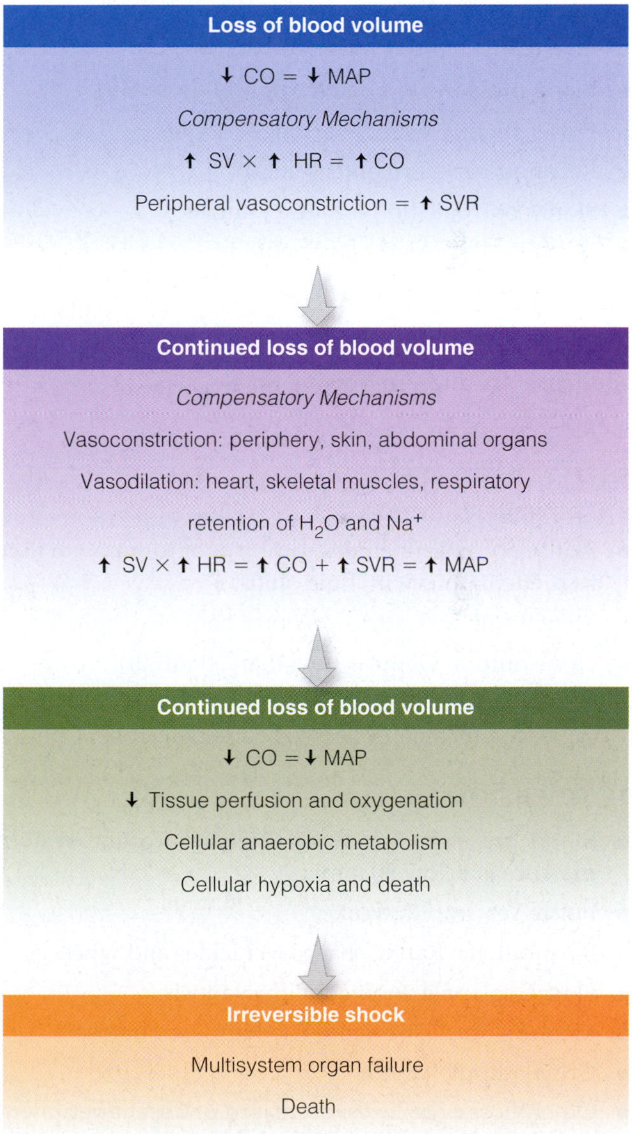
Loss of blood volume
↓ CO = ↓ MAP
Compensatory Mechanisms
↑ SV × ↑ HR = ↑ CO
Peripheral vasoconstriction = ↑ SVR
Continued loss of blood volume
Compensatory Mechanisms
Vasoconstriction: periphery, skin, abdominal organs
Vasodilation: heart, skeletal muscles, respiratory
retention of H2O and Na+
↑ SV × ↑ HR = ↑ CO + ↑ SVR = ↑ MAP
Continued loss of blood volume
↓ CO = ↓ MAP
↓ Tissue perfusion and oxygenation
Cellular anaerobic metabolism
Cellular hypoxia and death
Irreversible shock
Multisystem organ failure
Death

Key
CO: Cardiac output
HR: Heart rate
MAP: Mean arterial pressure
SV: Stroke volume
SVR: Systemic vascular resistance

Figure 11.11 ■ The stages of hypovolemic shock.

sympathetic compensatory responses. If the fluid loss is less than 500 mL, activation of the sympathetic response is generally adequate to restore cardiac output and blood pressure to near normal, although the heart rate may remain elevated.

With a sustained loss of blood volume (1000 mL or more), the shock stage progresses. Heart rate and vasoconstriction increase, and blood flow to the skin, skeletal muscles, kidneys, and abdominal organs decreases. Several renal mechanisms and a decline in capillary pressure help conserve blood volume. Eventually, the amount of blood flowing to cells is too low to oxygenate them and sustain production of cellular energy. Anaerobic metabolism begins, producing an acidotic environment for cells. As a result, cells lose their physical integrity. If untreated, shock causes multiple organ failure, and death results. Manifestations of various stages of hypovolemic shock include:

Initial Stage

- Blood pressure: Normal to slightly decreased
- Pulse: Slightly increased from baseline
- Respirations: Normal (baseline)
- Skin: Cool, pale (in periphery), moist
- Mental status: Alert and oriented
- Urine output: Slight decrease
- Other: Thirst, decreased capillary refill time.

Compensatory and Progressive Stages

- Blood pressure: Hypotension
- Pulse: Rapid, thready
- Respirations: Increased
- Skin: Cool, pale (includes trunk); poor turgor with fluid loss, edematous with fluid shift
- Mental status: Restless, anxious, confused, agitated
- Urine output: Oliguria (less than 30 mL/h)
- Other: Marked thirst, acidosis, hyperkalemia, decreased capillary refill time, decreased or absent peripheral pulses.

Irreversible Stage

- Blood pressure: Severe hypotension (often, systolic pressure is below 80 mmHg)
- Pulse: Very rapid, weak
- Respirations: Rapid, shallow; crackles and wheezes
- Skin: Cool, pale, mottled with cyanosis
- Mental status: Disoriented, lethargic, comatose
- Urine output: Anuria
- Other: Loss of reflexes, decreased or absent peripheral pulses.

With aging comes a relative decrease in sympathetic activity in relation to the cardiovascular system. Cardiac compliance also decreases with age. Atherosclerosis affects many vital organs' sensitivity to even the slightest reduction in blood flow. Many older patients experience secondary volume depletion due to chronic diuretic use or malnutrition. Also, patients prescribed beta-blockers may not present with tachycardia as an early indicator of shock. This important sign can be masked due to beta-adrenergic blockade. These patients will require early invasive monitoring in order to avoid excessive or inadequate volume restoration. This should be considered early in the treatment phase.

Cardiogenic Shock

Cardiogenic shock occurs when the heart's pumping ability is compromised to the point that it cannot maintain cardiac output and adequate tissue perfusion. Cardiac disorders are discussed in Chapters 30 and 31; this section focuses only on the effects of shock caused by these disorders.

The loss of the pumping action of the heart may be caused by the following conditions:

- Myocardial infarction
- Cardiac tamponade
- Restrictive pericarditis
- Cardiac arrest
- Dysrhythmias, such as fibrillation or ventricular tachycardia
- Pathologic changes in the valves
- Cardiomyopathies from hypertension, alcohol, bacterial or viral infections, or ischemia
- Complications of cardiac surgery
- Electrolyte imbalances (especially changes in normal potassium and calcium levels)
- Drugs affecting cardiac muscle contractility
- Head injuries causing damage to the cardioregulatory center.

Myocardial infarction is the most common cause of cardiogenic shock. Patients admitted to the hospital for treatment of myocardial infarction or cardiac surgery are at risk for cardiogenic shock. The severity and progression of shock are related to the amount of myocardial damage.

Whatever the cardiogenic cause, the decrease in cardiac output causes a decrease in MAP. Heart rate may increase in response to compensatory mechanisms. However, tachycardia increases myocardial oxygen consumption and decreases coronary perfusion. The myocardium becomes progressively depleted of oxygen, causing further myocardial ischemia and necrosis. The typical sequence of shock is essentially unchanged in cardiogenic shock.

Cyanosis, however, is more common in cardiogenic shock because stagnating blood increases extraction of oxygen from the hemoglobin at the capillary beds. As a result, the skin, lips, and nail beds may appear cyanotic. As cardiac failure (and cardiogenic shock) progresses, left-ventricular end-diastolic pressure increases. The increase is transmitted to the pulmonary capillary bed, and pulmonary edema may occur. Retention of blood in the right side of the heart increases right atrial pressure, which leads to jugular venous distention as a result of backflow through the vena cava. Manifestations of cardiogenic shock include:

- Blood pressure: Hypotension, possible narrowing pulse pressures
- Pulse: Rapid, thready; distention of veins of hands and neck
- Respirations: Increased, labored; crackles and wheezes; pulmonary edema
- Skin: Pale, cyanotic, cold, moist
- Mental status: Restless, anxious, lethargic progressing to comatose
- Urine output: Oliguria to anuria
- Other: Dependent edema; elevated CVP; elevated pulmonary capillary wedge pressure; arrhythmias.

Obstructive Shock

Obstructive shock is caused by an obstruction in the heart or great vessels that either impedes venous return or prevents effective cardiac pumping action. The causes of obstructive shock are impaired diastolic filling (e.g., pericardial tamponade or pneumothorax), increased right-ventricular afterload (e.g., pulmonary emboli), and increased left-ventricular afterload (e.g., aortic stenosis, abdominal distention). The manifestations are the result of decreased cardiac output and blood pressure, with reduced tissue perfusion and cellular metabolism.

Distributive Shock

Distributive shock (also called *vasogenic shock*) includes several types of shock that result from widespread vasodilation and decreased peripheral resistance. Because the blood volume does not change, relative hypovolemia results. Examples of distributive shock include septic, neurogenic, and anaphylactic shock. Treatment is based on the underlying pathogenesis.

Septic Shock

Sepsis is defined as life-threatening organ dysfunction caused by dysregulated host response to infection. Septic shock is a subset of sepsis where there are underlying circulatory and cellular/metabolic abnormalities that are profound enough to substantially increase mortality (Singer et al., 2016). A patient meets the criteria for septic shock when there is clinical evidence of sepsis and persistent hypotension requiring vasopressors to maintain a MAP 65 mmHg or greater and serum lactate levels greater than 2 mmols/dL despite adequate fluid volume resuscitation (Singer et al., 2016). At the bedside, a quick screen for those who are likely to have poorer outcomes related to sepsis (i.e., those who may be in septic shock) will have altered mentation, systolic blood pressure of 100 mmHg or less, and a respiratory rate of 22 breaths per minute or higher. This is helpful in areas where serum lactate levels are hard to obtain (Singer et al., 2016). This condition is most often the result of gram-negative bacterial infections (i.e., *Pseudomonas*, *E. coli*, *Klebsiella*), but may also follow gram-positive infections from *Staphylococcus* and *Streptococcus* bacteria. Gram-negative sepsis has a 38% mortality rate despite treatment (Moehring & Anderson, 2018). The pathophysiology of septic shock is complex and not completely understood.

Patients at risk for developing infections leading to septic shock include those who are hospitalized, have debilitating chronic illnesses, or have poor nutritional status. The risk is heightened after invasive procedures or surgery. Other patients at risk of septic shock include older adults and those who are immunocompromised. Portals of entry for infection that may lead to septic shock are:

- ***Urinary system:*** Catheterizations, suprapubic tubes, cystoscopy
- ***Respiratory system:*** Suctioning, aspiration, tracheostomy, endotracheal tubes, respiratory therapy, mechanical ventilators
- ***Gastrointestinal system:*** Peptic ulcers, ruptured appendix, peritonitis
- ***Integumentary system:*** Surgical wounds, intravenous catheters, intra-arterial catheters, invasive monitoring, decubitus ulcers, burns, trauma
- ***Female reproductive system:*** Elective surgical abortion, ascending infections from transmission of bacteria during the intrapartal and postpartal periods, tampon use, sexually transmitted infections.

Septic shock begins with *septicemia* (the presence of pathogens and their toxins in the blood). As pathogens are destroyed, their ruptured cell membranes allow endotoxins to leak into the plasma. The endotoxins disrupt the vascular system, coagulation mechanism, and immune system and trigger an immune and inflammatory response. For this reason, the initial effects of septic shock differ from those of hypovolemic and cardiogenic shock; cardiac output is high and systemic vascular resistance is low.

Endotoxins directly damage the endothelial lining of small blood vessels first; the small blood vessels of the kidneys and lungs are most susceptible. Cellular damage stimulates the release of vasoactive proteins and activates coagulation factor XII. The vasoactive proteins stimulate peripheral vasodilation and increase capillary permeability; the activation of coagulation factors results in the production of multiple intravascular blood clots.

As a result of the increased capillary permeability and vasodilation, fluid shifts from the intravascular space to the interstitial space. Hypovolemia results as fluid volume is lost from the circulating blood. Hypovolemia and intravascular coagulation alter oxygenation and cellular metabolism, leading to anaerobic metabolism, lactic acidosis, and cellular death.

Nurses caring for patients who may be at risk for sepsis and septic shock should be vigilant to the following changes (Perrin & MacLeod, 2018):

- Changes in respiratory function needing increase in FiO_2 requirements
- Decreases in blood pressure
- Decrease in urine output
- Changes in coagulation
- Changes in mentation

- Potential changes in liver function (changes in liver enzymes)
- Potential changes in GI function (e.g., decreased or absent bowl sounds).

Disseminated intravascular coagulation (DIC), a generalized response to injury, is a potential risk in septic shock. This condition is characterized by simultaneous bleeding and clotting throughout the vasculature. Sepsis injures blood cells, causing platelet aggregation and decreased blood flow. As a result, blood clots form throughout the microcirculation. The clotting slows circulation further while stimulating excess fibrinolysis. As the body's stores of clotting factors are depleted, generalized bleeding begins. DIC is further discussed in Chapter 13.

Neurogenic Shock

Neurogenic shock is the result of an imbalance between parasympathetic and sympathetic stimulation of vascular smooth muscle. If parasympathetic overstimulation or sympathetic understimulation persists, sustained vasodilation occurs, and blood pools in the venous and capillary beds.

Neurogenic shock causes a dramatic reduction in systemic vascular resistance as the size of the vascular compartment increases. As systemic vascular resistance decreases, pressure in the blood vessels becomes too low to drive nutrients across capillary membranes, and cellular metabolism is impaired.

The following conditions can cause neurogenic shock by increasing parasympathetic stimulation or inhibiting sympathetic stimulation of the smooth muscle of blood vessels:

- Head injury
- Trauma to the spinal cord (Spinal shock, a form of neurogenic shock, is described in Chapter 43.)
- Insulin reactions (which cause hypoglycemia, decreasing glucose to the medulla)
- Central nervous system depressant drugs (such as sedatives, barbiturates, or narcotics)
- Anesthesia (spinal and general)
- Severe pain
- Prolonged exposure to heat.

Bradycardia occurs early, but tachycardia begins as compensatory mechanisms are initiated. Central venous pressure drops as veins dilate, venous return to the heart decreases, stroke volume decreases, and MAP falls. In early stages, the extremities are warm and pink (from the pooling of blood), but as shock progresses, the skin becomes pale and cool. Manifestations of neurogenic shock include:

- Blood pressure: Hypotension
- Pulse: Slow and bounding
- Respirations: Vary
- Skin: Warm, dry
- Mental status: Anxious, restless, lethargic progressing to comatose
- Urine output: Oliguria to anuria
- Other: Lowered body temperature.

Anaphylactic Shock

Anaphylactic shock is the result of a widespread humorally mediated hypersensitivity reaction (called *anaphylaxis*). The pathophysiology in this type of shock includes vasodilation, pooling of blood in the periphery, and hypovolemia with altered cellular metabolism. These physiologic alterations occur when a sensitized person has contact with an *allergen* (a foreign substance to which an individual is hypersensitive). Many different allergens can cause anaphylactic shock, including medications, blood administration, latex, foods, snake venom, and insect stings.

Anaphylactic shock does not occur with the first exposure to an allergen. With the first exposure to a foreign substance (the *antigen*), the body produces specific immunoglobulin E (IgE) antibodies against this antigen. The person is thus sensitized to that specific antigen. With subsequent exposure, the antigen reacts with the already formed IgE antibodies, disrupting cellular integrity. In addition, large amounts of histamine and other vasoactive amines are released and distributed through the circulatory system. These substances cause increased capillary permeability and massive vasodilation, resulting in profound hypotension and eventual vascular collapse.

Histamine also causes constriction of smooth muscles in the bladder, uterus, intestines, and bronchioles. Respiratory distress, bronchospasm, laryngospasm, and severe abdominal cramping result. Serotonin (a neurotransmitter with vasoconstrictive properties) is released, further affecting respiratory status by increasing capillary permeability in the lungs. As a result, plasma leaks into the alveoli, gas exchange is impaired, and pulmonary edema may occur.

Anaphylactic shock begins and progresses rapidly. Manifestations may begin within 20 minutes of contact with an antigen. Unless appropriate intervention is provided, death can occur within a matter of minutes. Because anaphylaxis is rapid and potentially lethal, people with known allergies should carry some form of warning (such as a medical alert bracelet) informing others of their susceptibility. Some patients carry an *EpiPen* (epinephrine) to halt anaphylaxis. Healthcare providers should be extremely careful to assess and document allergies or previous drug reactions. Manifestations of anaphylactic shock include:

- Blood pressure: Hypotension
- Pulse: Increased, dysrhythmias
- Respirations: Dyspnea, stridor, wheezes, laryngospasm, bronchospasm, pulmonary edema
- Skin: Warm, edematous (lips, eyelids, tongue, hands, feet, genitals)
- Mental status: Restless, anxious, lethargic to comatose
- Urine output: Oliguria to anuria
- Other: Paresthesias; urticaria; pruritus; abdominal cramps, vomiting, diarrhea.

Similar, but not related, are anaphylactoid reactions that are not humorally mediated and do not require prior exposure to a trigger. These can have similar symptoms and are treated in a similar manner.

11.4 The Patient Experiencing Shock

For the patient with shock, the experience can be anxiety producing. All types of shock are medical emergencies. A number of members of the interprofessional team will be involved with the care of the patient, which can be confusing. Also, since decrease in cerebral perfusion is part of most types of shock, changes in mentation add to the disorientation of the patient. Finally, since there is a high mortality with shock, the patient and family may need emotional support.

Interprofessional Care

Medical care for the patient in shock focuses on treating the underlying cause, increasing arterial oxygenation, and improving tissue perfusion. Depending on the cause and type of shock, interventions include emergency care measures, oxygen therapy, fluid replacement, and medications. Emergency care is often the first course of collaborative action taken to arrest shock, as discussed earlier in this chapter. A *central venous catheter* may be used to aid in the differential diagnosis of shock and to provide information about the preload of the heart. A pulmonary artery catheter may be inserted to monitor cardiac dynamics, fluid balance, and the effects of vasoactive medications.

Diagnosis

The following diagnostic tests can help identify the type of shock and assess the patient's physical status:

- ***Blood hemoglobin* and *hematocrit*,** to detect the concentration that usually occurs in hypovolemic shock. These changes reflect the underlying etiology. In hypovolemic shock resulting from hemorrhage, the hemoglobin and hematocrit concentrations are lower than normal; in hypovolemic shock resulting from intravascular fluid loss, by contrast, the hemoglobin and hematocrit concentrations are higher than normal.
- ***Arterial blood gases (ABGs)*,** to determine oxygen and carbon dioxide levels and pH. The effects of shock and of the body's compensatory mechanisms cause a decrease in pH (indicating acidosis), a decrease in the partial pressure of oxygen (PaO_2) and in total oxygen saturation, and an increase in the partial pressure of carbon dioxide ($PaCO_2$).
- ***Serum electrolytes*,** to monitor the severity and progression of shock. As shock progresses, glucose levels decrease, sodium levels decrease, and potassium levels increase. Serum lactate is also important to obtain. Increase in serum lactate is an indicator of poor tissue perfusion.
- ***Blood urea nitrogen (BUN), serum creatinine levels, urine specific gravity,* and *osmolality*,** to check renal function. As perfusion of the kidneys is decreased and renal function is reduced, the BUN and creatinine levels increase as does urine specific gravity and osmolality.
- ***Blood cultures*,** to identify the causative organism in septic shock.
- ***White blood cell count* and *differential*,** in the patient with septic or anaphylactic shock. The total WBC count is increased in septic shock. Elevated neutrophils indicate acute infection, increased monocytes indicate a bacterial infection, and increased eosinophils indicate an allergic response.
- ***Serum cardiac enzymes*,** which are elevated in cardiogenic shock: Creatine kinase (CK), myoglobin, and C-reactive protein. Troponin can be elevated if the cause of cardiogenic shock is acute MI.

Other diagnostic tests may be ordered to determine the extent of injury or damage or to locate the site of internal hemorrhage. These tests might include x-ray studies, computerized tomography (CT) scans, magnetic resonance imaging (MRI), endoscopic examinations, and echocardiograms. Newer diagnostic methods for hypoperfusion include gastric tonometry and sublingual PCO_2. Gastric tonometry measures the partial pressure of carbon dioxide in the gastric lumen. The measurement of sublingual carbon dioxide correlates well with decreased MAP.

Medications

When fluid replacement alone is not sufficient to reverse shock, vasoactive drugs (drugs causing vasoconstriction or vasodilation) and inotropic drugs (drugs improving cardiac contractility) may be administered. When used to treat shock, these drugs increase venous return through vasoconstriction of peripheral vessels; they also improve the pumping ability of the heart by facilitating myocardial contractility and by dilating coronary arteries to increase perfusion of the myocardium.

Drugs used to treat shock are discussed in **Medication Administration 11.B**. Other drugs that may be administered to the patient in shock include:

- Diuretics to increase urine output after fluid replacement has been initiated
- Calcium to replace calcium lost as a result of blood transfusions
- Antiarrhythmic agents to stabilize heart rhythm
- Broad-spectrum antibiotics to suppress organisms responsible for septic shock
- Epinephrine, antihistamines, and inhaled $beta_2$-agonists to treat anaphylactic shock.

Oxygen Therapy

Establishing and maintaining a patent airway and ensuring adequate oxygenation are critical interventions in reversing shock. All patients in shock (even those with adequate respirations) should receive oxygen therapy (usually by mask or nasal cannula) to maintain the PaO_2 at greater than 80 mmHg during the first 4 to 6 hours of care. If the patient's unassisted respiration cannot maintain PaO_2 at this level, ventilatory assistance may be necessary. Care of the patient requiring ventilatory assistance is discussed in Chapter 37.

Medication Administration 11.B

The Patient in Shock

ADRENERGICS (SYMPATHOMIMETICS)

Vasoconstrictors

epinephrine (Adrenalin)
metaraminol (Aramine)
norepinephrine (Levophed)
vasopressin (Pitressin)

Inotropes

dopamine (Intropin)
dobutamine (Dobutrex)

Adrenergic drugs (also called *sympathomimetics*) mimic the fight-or-flight response of the sympathetic nervous system, selectively stimulating alpha-adrenergic and beta-adrenergic receptors. Many of these drugs have both vasopressor (vasoconstricting) effects and positive inotropic effects. Stimulation of alpha-adrenergic receptors results in vasoconstriction and increased systemic blood pressure. Stimulation of beta-adrenergic receptors increases the force and rate of myocardial contraction.

The physiologic effect of these drugs includes improved perfusion and oxygenation of the heart, with increased stroke volume and heart rate and increased cardiac output. Increased cardiac output in turn increases tissue perfusion and oxygenation. The major disadvantage is that increases in stroke volume and heart rate also increase the oxygen requirements of the myocardium. These drugs may be used in the early stages of shock, especially in types of shock characterized by vasodilation.

Nursing Responsibilities

- Carefully monitor responses in the older adult, who may be especially sensitive to sympathomimetics and require lower doses.
- When administering these drugs by the subcutaneous route, carefully aspirate the injection site to avoid injecting the drug directly into a blood vessel.
- Use the intravenous route only with continuous infusion pumps. Carefully adjust the dose to accommodate the patient's cardiovascular status (as ordered by the physician or by written protocol).
- Document lung sounds, vital signs, and hemodynamic parameters before starting the medication, and then according to institutional policy (usually every 5 to 15 minutes).
- Record and monitor urine output. Report output of less than 30 mL per hour.
- Be aware that the sympathomimetics are incompatible with sodium bicarbonate or alkaline solutions.
- When administering drugs that cause vasoconstriction, such as norepinephrine (Levophed) and metaraminol (Aramine), monitor the intravenous insertion site for infiltration. If infiltration does occur, stop the infusion and notify the physician immediately. (Infiltration may cause ischemia and necrosis of tissue.)

Health Education for the Patient and Family

- Because these drugs mimic a physiologic reaction to stress, they may cause feelings of anxiety.
- Close monitoring to adjust the dose will be carried out by qualified nurses using written protocols.
- Report heart palpitations or chest pain immediately.

VASODILATORS

amrinone (Inocor)
milrinone (Primicor)
nitroglycerin (Tridil)
nitroprusside (Nipride)

Drugs that cause vasodilation act directly on smooth muscle, affecting both arterioles and veins. Peripheral resistance, cardiac output, and pulmonary wedge pressure are all reduced as a result of the vasodilation. These effects decrease the oxygen need of the heart and decrease pulmonary congestion. Vasodilators are used primarily in the treatment of cardiogenic shock and may be combined with a sympathomimetic (e.g., dopamine).

Nursing Responsibilities

- Mix with D_5W or 0.9% saline.
- IV nitroglycerin must be mixed in glass bottles and infused through special, non-PVC tubing. Up to 40 to 80% of nitroglycerin can be absorbed by PVC bags or tubing.
- Infuse with an infusion pump, and use within 4 hours of reconstitution.
- Do not add other medications to the solution.
- Use cautiously in patients with increased intracranial pressure.
- Assess mental status, blood pressure, and pulse prior to initiating medication. Thereafter, assess blood pressure and pulse according to institutional policy (usually every 5 minutes initially, then every 15 minutes until stable, and then every hour).
- Monitor for confusion, dizziness, tachycardia, arrhythmias, hypotension, and adventitious breath sounds. Report these immediately if they occur, and slow infusion to a keep-open rate.
- Monitor patients receiving nitroprusside for signs of thiocyanate poisoning (nausea, disorientation, muscle spasms, decreased or absent reflexes) if infusion lasts longer than 72 hours.
- Keep patient in bed with side rails up.

Health Education for the Patient and Family

- It is important to stay in bed and change positions slowly to avoid dizziness.
- The blood pressure and pulse are taken frequently to adjust the dose of medication.
- Headache is a common side effect.

Note: Drugs identified in blue are among the 200 most commonly prescribed medications in the United States.

Source: Data from Adams et al., 2017.

Fluid Resuscitation

The most effective treatment for the patient in hypovolemic shock is the administration of intravenous fluids or blood. Fluids also treat septic and, more judiciously, neurogenic shock. However, the patient with cardiogenic shock may require either fluid replacement or restriction, depending on pulmonary artery pressure.

Various fluids may be administered alone or in combination as part of fluid replacement therapy in treating shock. Fluid replacements are administered in massive amounts through two large-bore peripheral lines or through a central line. Current fluid resuscitation protocols include rapid crystalloid infusion followed by blood transfusion. Fluid replacements, such as crystalloid and colloid solutions, increase circulating blood volume and tissue perfusion. Whole-blood or blood products increase the oxygen-carrying capacity of the blood and thus increase oxygenation of cells. However, these resuscitation fluids are not thought to minimize inflammation. Studies are under way to evaluate alternative resuscitation fluids such as an alternative colloid (hydroxyethyl starch [Hextend Biotime, Inc., Berkley, CA]), alternative crystalloid (Ringer's ethyl pyruvate), and hypertonic saline with dextran and polymerized hemoglobin.

Crystalloid Solutions. Crystalloid solutions contain dextrose or electrolytes dissolved in water; they are hypertonic, isotonic, or hypotonic. Hypertonic solutions include 3% saline. Isotonic solutions include normal saline (0.9%), lactated Ringer solution, and Ringer solution. Hypotonic solutions include one-half normal saline (0.45%) and 5% dextrose in water (D_5W).

Hypertonic crystalloid solutions pull fluid into the vascular space to promote excretion. Isotonic and hypotonic crystalloid solutions increase fluid volume in both the intravascular and the interstitial space. Of the total amount infused, only about 25% remains in the intravascular system; the remaining 75% moves into the interstitial space. Consequently, fluid volume is only minimally expanded and the potential for peripheral edema is increased when crystalloid solutions are used. However, Ringer lactate (an electrolyte solution) and 0.9% saline are the fluids of choice in treating hypovolemic shock, especially in the emergency phase of care while blood is being typed and crossmatched. Large amounts of these solutions may be infused rapidly, increasing blood volume and tissue perfusion.

Colloid Solutions. Colloid solutions contain substances (colloids) that should not diffuse through capillary walls. Hence, colloids tend to remain in the vascular system and increase the osmotic pressure of the serum, causing fluid to move into the vascular compartment from the interstitial space. As a result, plasma volume expands. Colloid solutions used to treat shock include 5% albumin, 25% albumin, hetastarch, plasma protein fraction, and dextran.

Colloid products reduce platelet adhesiveness and have been associated with reductions in blood coagulation. Consequently, the patient's prothrombin time (PT), INR, platelet count, and activated partial thromboplastin time (APTT) should be monitored when these solutions are administered. Normal values are as follows:

PT	10–15 seconds
INR	1–1.2 seconds
Platelets	150,000–400,000
APTT	<35 seconds

See **Medication Administration 11.C** for further information about colloid solutions and associated nursing responsibilities and patient teaching.

Medication Administration 11.C

Colloid Solutions (Plasma Expanders)

albumin 5% (Albuminar-5, Buminate 5%)

albumin 25% (Albuminar-25, Buminate 25%)

dextran 40 (Gentran 40)

dextran 70 (Gentran 70, Macrodex)

dextran 75 (Gentran 75)

hetastarch (Hespan [HES])

plasma protein fraction (Plasmanate, Plasma-Plex, Plasmatein, Protenate)

These solutions are blood volume expanders and are used to treat hypovolemic shock due to surgery, hemorrhage, burns, or other trauma. Albumin and plasma protein fraction are prepared from healthy blood donors. Dextran and hetastarch are synthetically prepared large molecules. The solutions promote circulatory volume and tissue perfusion by rapidly expanding plasma volume. Dextran solutions are infrequently used.

Nursing Responsibilities

- Before infusion begins, establish baseline for vital signs, lung sounds, heart sounds, and (if possible) CVP and pulmonary artery wedge pressure.
- Start administration of ordered intravenous fluids, using a large-gauge (18-gauge or larger) infusion needle.
- Obtain and record vital signs as required by institutional policy (usually every 15 to 60 minutes) and patient status.
- Obtain and record intake and output every 1 to 2 hours.
- Monitor for manifestations of congestive heart failure or pulmonary edema (dyspnea, cyanosis, cough, crackles, wheezes). If these manifestations appear, stop the fluids and notify the physician immediately.
- Monitor for bleeding from new sites; an increase in blood pressure may cause bleeding in severed vessels that did not bleed with decreased blood pressure.
- Monitor for manifestations of dehydration (dry lips; scant, dark-colored urine; loss of skin turgor). Increased intravenous fluids are usually ordered if the patient becomes dehydrated.
- Monitor for manifestations of circulatory overload (jugular vein distention, increase in CVP, increase in pulmonary capillary wedge pressure). If these manifestations occur, slow rate of infusion and notify physician.
- Monitor prothrombin time, partial thromboplastin time, and platelet counts.
- If administering dextran or plasma protein fraction, have epinephrine and antihistamines readily available for any manifestations of a hypersensitivity reaction (fever, chills, rash, headache, wheezing, flushing).
- Maintain patient on bedrest with side rails elevated.

Health Education for the Patient and Family

- The solutions are given to replace lost serum protein, which helps maintain the volume of blood.
- Vital signs are taken frequently to ensure the safety of the patient.

Source: Data from Adams et al., 2017.

Blood and Blood Products. If hypovolemic shock is due to hemorrhage, the infusion of blood and blood products may be indicated. Available blood and blood products include fresh whole blood, stored whole blood, packed RBCs, platelet concentrate, fresh frozen plasma, and cryoprecipitate. Often, packed RBCs are given to provide hemoglobin concentration and are supplemented with crystalloids to maintain an adequate circulatory volume (see the discussion of blood administration earlier in the chapter).

Nursing Care

Nursing assessments and interventions to prevent shock are an essential part of the nursing care of every patient. The primary nursing interventions to prevent shock are assessment and monitoring.

Assessment

Nursing assessments are critical in preventing shock. Identifying patients at risk and making focused assessments are essential. Although shock may occur at any age, physiologic changes with aging make the older adult a high-risk population.

- *Hypovolemic shock:* Patients who have undergone surgery, have sustained multiple traumatic injuries, or have been seriously burned are most likely to develop hypovolemic shock. Monitoring fluid status is essential in preventing shock and includes daily assessments of weight, fluid intake by all routes, measurable fluid loss (e.g., urine, vomitus, wound drainage, gastric drainage, and chest tube drainage), and fluid loss that must be estimated, such as profuse perspiration and wound drainage. Assessments for the critically ill patient are ongoing and include fluid balance, hemodynamic values, and vital signs.
- *Cardiogenic shock:* Patients with left anterior wall myocardial infarctions are at risk for developing cardiogenic shock. Nursing care to prevent the development of cardiogenic shock focuses on maintaining or improving myocardial oxygen supply by providing immediate pain relief, maintaining rest, and administering supplemental oxygen.
- *Neurogenic shock:* The risk of neurogenic shock is increased in patients who have spinal cord injuries and those who have received spinal anesthesia. Preventative nursing care includes maintaining immobility of patients with spinal cord trauma and elevating the head of the bed 15 to 20 degrees following spinal anesthesia. Elevations of more than 20 degrees, however, can potentiate headaches following spinal anesthesia and should be avoided.
- *Anaphylactic shock:* Prevent anaphylactic shock by collecting information about allergies and drug reactions during the health history. Note these allergies clearly on all documents and place a special armband on the patient. Careful and frequent assessments during blood administration may prevent serious reactions to blood or blood products.
- *Septic shock:* Patients who are hospitalized, debilitated, or chronically ill and those who have undergone invasive procedures or tube insertions are at high risk for septic shock. Nursing care to prevent septic shock includes careful and consistent hand hygiene, the use of aseptic techniques for procedures (e.g., catheterizations, suctioning, changing dressings, starting and maintaining intravenous fluids or medications), and monitoring for local and systemic manifestations (e.g., white blood cell and differential counts) of infection.

Priorities of Care

Supporting cardiovascular and respiratory function to maintain oxygenation and perfusion is the priority nursing responsibility for the patient in shock. Interprofessional interventions to ameliorate the precipitating injury are also care priorities.

Diagnoses, Outcomes, and Interventions

Nursing care for the patient in shock focuses on assessing and monitoring overall tissue perfusion and on meeting the psychosocial needs of the patient and the family. This section discusses nursing diagnoses that are appropriate for the patient with hypovolemic shock. See the accompanying Case Study & Nursing Care Plan on page 317.

Maintain Cardiac Output. Decreased cardiac output is the primary problem for the patient in shock. Although much of the care related to this diagnosis is collaborative, many independent nursing interventions are critical to the care of the patient in shock.

Expected Outcome: Patient will maintain adequate cardiac output.

The nurse will:

- Assess and monitor cardiovascular function via:
  a. Blood pressure
  b. Heart rate and rhythm
  c. Pulse oximetry
  d. Peripheral pulses
  e. Hemodynamic monitoring of arterial pressures, pulmonary artery pressures, and central venous pressures (CVPs).

  A baseline assessment is necessary to establish the stage of shock. If palpable peripheral pulses and audible (to auscultation) blood pressure are lost, inserting central arterial and venous catheters is essential to establish progression of shock accurately and to evaluate the patient's response to therapy.
- Measure and record intake and output (total output and urinary output) hourly. *A decrease in circulating blood volume with hypotension and the effect of the compensatory mechanisms associated with shock can cause renal failure. Urinary output of less than 30 mL per hour in an acutely ill adult indicates reduced renal blood flow.*
- Monitor bowel sounds, abdominal distention, and abdominal pain. *Decreased splanchnic blood flow reduces bowel motility and peristalsis; paralytic ileus may result.*

- Monitor for sudden, sharp chest pain, dyspnea, cyanosis, anxiety, and restlessness. *Hemoconcentration and increased platelet aggregation may result in pulmonary emboli.*
- Maintain bedrest and provide (to the extent possible) a calm, quiet environment. Place in a supine position with the legs elevated to about 20 degrees, trunk flat, and head and shoulders elevated higher than the chest (the semi-Fowler position can also be used with mechanically ventilated patients) (**Figure 11.12** ■). *Limiting activity and ensuring rest decreases the workload of the heart. The supine position with legs elevated increases venous return; however, this position should not be used for patients in cardiogenic shock. The Trendelenburg position is no longer recommended because it causes the abdominal organs to press against the diaphragm (limiting respirations), decreases filling of the coronary arteries, and initiates aortic and carotid sinus reflexes.*

Promote Adequate Tissue Perfusion. As shock progresses, diminished tissue perfusion causes ischemia and hypoxia of major organ systems. As shock worsens, blood flow and oxygenation of the lungs, heart, and brain are also impaired. Hypoxia and ischemia result from decreased tissue perfusion in the kidneys, brain, heart, lungs, gastrointestinal tract, and the periphery.

Expected Outcome: Patient will regain adequate tissue perfusion as evidenced by skin characteristics and vital signs within normal limits.

The nurse will:

- Monitor skin color, temperature, turgor, and moisture. *Decreased tissue perfusion is evidenced when the skin becomes pale, cool, and moist; as hemoglobin concentrations decrease, cyanosis occurs.*
- Monitor cardiopulmonary function by assessing/monitoring the following:
  a. Blood pressure (by auscultation or by hemodynamic monitoring)
  b. Rate and depth of respirations
  c. Lung sounds
  d. Pulse oximetry and arterial blood gases
  e. Peripheral pulses (brachial, radial, dorsalis pedis, and posterior tibial); include presence, equality, rate, rhythm, and quality (If unable to palpate pulses, use a device such as a Doppler ultrasound flowmeter to assess peripheral arterial blood flow.)
  f. Jugular vein distention
  g. CVP measurements

  Baseline vital signs are necessary to determine trends in subsequent findings. As shock progresses, the blood pressure decreases and the pulse becomes rapid, weak, and thready. As perfusion of the lungs decreases, crackles, wheezes, and dyspnea are commonly assessed. Capillary refill is prolonged, and peripheral pulses are weak or nonpalpable. Neck veins that cannot be seen when the patient is in the supine position indicate decreased intravascular volume. CVP is an accurate means of determining fluid status in the patient in shock; the findings will be low (5 to 15 cmH_2O or 2 to 6 mmHg is normal) in hypovolemic shock because of the decreased blood volume. (See Chapter 10 for a discussion of CVP.)

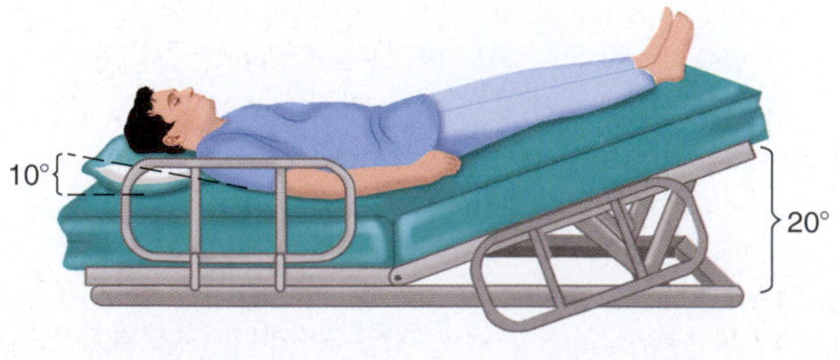
10°
20°

Figure 11.12 ■ The patient in shock should be positioned with the lower extremities elevated approximately 20 degrees (knees straight), trunk horizontal, and the head elevated about 10 degrees.

- Monitor body temperature. *An elevated body temperature increases metabolic demands, depleting reserves of bodily energy. It also increases myocardial oxygen demand and may place the patient with previous cardiac problems at even greater risk for hypoperfusion.*
- Monitor urinary output per Foley catheter hourly, using a urimeter. *Urine output is a reliable indicator of renal perfusion.*
- Assess mental status and level of consciousness. *The appropriateness of the patient's behavior and responses reflects the adequacy of cerebral circulation. Restlessness and anxiety are common early in shock; in later stages, the patient may become lethargic and progress to a comatose state. Altered levels of consciousness are the result of both cerebral hypoxia and the effects of acidosis on brain cells.*

Manage Anxiety. Many patients in hypovolemic shock have experienced some form of major trauma and may have multiple life-threatening injuries that result in emergency care and the potential for emergency surgery. Throughout this sequence of crisis events, treatment is invasive and contact with family is minimal. Patient and family responses to these situations of uncertainty, instability, and change include anxiety, fear, and powerlessness. These responses are affected by age, developmental level, cultural and ethnic group, combined with life experiences with illness and within the healthcare system, and support systems.

Expected Outcome: Patient and family, as appropriate, will identify anxiety-provoking situations and verbalize feelings related to such situations.

The nurse will:

- Assess the cause(s) of the anxiety, and manipulate the environment to provide periods of rest. *Reducing stimuli that cause anxiety is calming and facilitates rest, which is necessary in the patient at risk for bleeding.*

- Administer prescribed pain medications on a regular basis and implement any applicable nonpharmacologic comfort measures. *Pain precipitates and/or aggravates anxiety.*
- Provide interventions to increase comfort and reduce restlessness:
  a. Maintain a clean environment.
  b. Provide skin and oral care.
  c. Monitor the effectiveness of ventilation or oxygen therapy.
  d. Eliminate all nonessential activities.
  e. Remain with the patient during procedures.
  f. Speak slowly and calmly, using short sentences.
  g. Use touch to provide support.

  Unfamiliar sounds, sights, and odors can increase anxiety. Damp skin or a dry mouth increases discomfort. Inadequate gas exchange with a decrease in oxygen or an increase in carbon dioxide in the blood may cause the patient to experience a "feeling of doom." Activity increases the body's need for oxygen. Listening and touch provide support in an environment in which the patient often feels alone and abandoned. Severe anxiety interferes with the ability to understand others and to respond appropriately.
- Provide support for the patient and family:
  a. Provide time, space, and privacy for family members.
  b. Allow family members access to the patient when feasible.
  c. Encourage the expression of feelings and concerns. Provide anticipatory guidance to prepare for recovery or death and to support realistic hope.
  d. Acknowledge the beliefs, values, and expectations of the patient and family.

  Allowing the family access to the patient reduces anxiety and gives both the patient and the family some feeling of control. If prognosis is poor, access and involvement allow the family to begin the grieving process. If recovery is expected, contact provides the patient and family with a feeling of hope. Supporting the patient and family facilitates concrete problem solving, promotes acceptance of the illness and its implications, and helps them begin to establish ways of managing the illness experience.
- Provide information about the current setting to both the patient and family; give the family information about available resources (such as pastoral care, social services, temporary housing, meals). *Knowing what to expect and how to control the environment to meet basic needs reduces anxiety.*

Transitions of Care

In addition to the prevention of shock outlined above in the Assessment, it is important to note that assessment findings for shock vary in older adults:

- Cardiac changes may include a thickened left-ventricular wall, decreased elasticity of the myocardium, and more rigid valves. These changes result in a decreased stroke volume and cardiac output, thus decreasing responses to shock in general and increasing the risk of cardiogenic shock.
- Decreased arterial wall elasticity and vasomotor tone reduce the older adult's ability to respond to a decrease in oxygenation.
- Decreased elasticity and turgor of the skin make assessments of skin turgor more difficult.
- Previous medication and blood administration increase the risk of anaphylactic shock.
- Decreased immune system response increases the risk of septic shock.

Home care for the patient who has experienced shock is highly individualized, depending on the cause and the illness or injury that caused shock. The interprofessional team will create a discharge plan for the patient and family.

All types of shock have a high mortality risk. Families need to be kept informed as to the care and illness state of their loved one. Discussions of what the patient would want done in case of irreversible conditions should be discussed early in the care. When care is becoming futile, the family and the interprofessional team need to sit down and discuss the care of their loved ones.

Case Study & Nursing Care Plan

A Patient with Septic Shock

Huang Mei Lan is a 43-year-old unmarried female who lives alone in a major West Coast city. Ms. Huang came to America 15 years ago from China and now speaks English well. Her family still lives in China. She worked in a neighborhood sewing shop until 3 years ago, when she was diagnosed with breast cancer. Her treatment included mastectomy of the affected breast and follow-up chemotherapy.

Last month, Ms. Huang experienced a recurrence of cancer in the lymph glands of the affected side. Surgery to remove the glands was performed and chemotherapy started. Ms. Huang has a central line, a urinary catheter, and a surgical incision. She is underweight, weak, and depressed. Although she has multiple physical problems, she never complains or asks for any kind of medication.

ASSESSMENT

Ms. Huang's primary nurse, Robert O'Brien, enters her room early in the morning to make an initial assessment. He finds Ms. Huang huddled in the middle of the bed, shivering violently. Her vital signs are T 40°C (104°F), P 110 bpm, R 30/min, and BP 106/66 mmHg. Her skin is hot, dry, and flushed with poor turgor. She is alert and oriented, but is restless and appears anxious. Ms. Huang states she is nauseated and suddenly begins vomiting and is incontinent of liquid stool. Laboratory data indicate leukocytosis, respiratory alkalosis, increased lactate level, and reduced platelet count. Blood cultures, as well as cultures of Ms. Huang's sputum, urine, and wound drainage, are conducted. She is diagnosed as having septic shock.

Hetastarch is ordered per intravenous line and intravenous broad-spectrum antibiotics are begun until the organism and its portal of entry can be determined. Despite treatment, Ms. Huang's condition worsens. Her blood pressure continues to drop, her skin becomes cool and cyanotic, and she begins to have periods of disorientation. She is transferred to the critical care unit. As she is being prepared for the transfer, she begins to cry and asks, "Am I going to die?"

DIAGNOSES

- Decrease in gas exchange related to effects of sepsis
- Decrease in tissue perfusion related to body's response to sepsis
- Decrease in fluid volume related to body's response to sepsis
- Anxiety related to disease process and decreased perfusion

EXPECTED OUTCOMES

- Patient will regain and maintain blood gas parameters within normal limits.
- Patient will maintain adequate circulating blood volume.
- Patient will regain and maintain stable hemodynamic levels.
- Patient will verbalize increased ability to cope with stressors.

PLANNING AND IMPLEMENTATION

- Monitor results of arterial blood gases, blood counts, clotting times, and platelet counts.
- Monitor respiratory status, including respiratory rate, rhythm, and breath sounds.
- Monitor neurologic status, including mental status and level of consciousness.
- Monitor cardiovascular status, including arterial blood pressure; rate, rhythm, and quality of pulses; central venous pressure; pulmonary artery pressure; and cardiac output.
- Monitor body temperature every 2 hours.
- Monitor urinary output hourly, reporting any output of less than 30 mL per hour.
- Monitor color and character of skin.
- Explain procedures and provide comfort measures (oral care, skin care, turning, positioning).

EVALUATION

Despite intensive nursing and medical care, Ms. Huang's condition remains critical. The interventions are continued.

CLINICAL REASONING IN PATIENT CARE

1. Vasopressors may be used in the treatment of septic shock. Explain the rationale for their use.
2. While monitoring Ms. Huang's arterial blood gases, the nurse notes that her PaO_2 is < 60 mmHg and her $PaCO_2$ is > 50. What do these findings indicate, and why have they occurred?
3. Ms. Huang has been given large amounts of colloids intravenously. Hemodynamic monitoring indicates a higher than normal CVP and pulmonary artery pressure. What do these findings indicate? What physical assessments would you make to confirm the changes?

See Evaluating Your Response in Appendix B.

CHAPTER HIGHLIGHTS

11.1 Traumatic Injury

Outline the components and types of trauma and the effects of traumatic injury on the body.

- Trauma is defined as injury to human tissues and organs resulting from the transfer of energy from the environment. Energy sources can be mechanical, gravitational, thermal, electrical, physical, or chemical.
- Trauma types include minor trauma, which causes minimal damage to underlying tissues, or major/multiple trauma, which involves at minimum a serious single-system injury or multiple trauma. Trauma can also be categorized as blunt and penetrating trauma. Blunt trauma is caused by forces like deceleration, acceleration, shearing, compression, or crushing. Penetrating trauma is the entrance into the body of a foreign object.

11.2 The Patient Experiencing Trauma

Describe the pathophysiology and manifestations of traumatic injury, and outline the interprofessional care, nursing care, and transitions of care for patients experiencing trauma.

- Maintenance of the airway and cervical spine are the highest priority in the trauma patient, with airway assessment superseding all other interventions.
- The primary assessment conducted by the nurse identifies all life-threatening injuries and performance of appropriate interventions. The secondary assessment is when the nurse identifies all injuries in order to prioritize care.

11.3 Shock

Outline the pathophysiology of the different types of shock and the effects of shock on body systems.

- Shock is a clinical syndrome characterized by a systemic imbalance between oxygen supply and demand. This imbalance results in a state of inadequate blood flow to body organs and tissues, causing life-threatening cellular dysfunction.
- The symptoms of shock arise from the body's attempts to maintain vital organs (heart and brain) and to preserve life following a drop in oxygen delivery to the cells.
- An important early sign of shock is a change in the level of consciousness with restlessness a common symptom of cerebral hypoxia.
- Shock is defined in three stages: Compensatory (stage 1), an early and reversible stage; progressive (stage 2), where the affected cells switch from aerobic to anaerobic metabolism in order to stay alive; and the final stage, refractory/irreversible (stage 3), where tissue anoxia and death becomes widespread.
- Hypovolemic shock is the most common type of shock and is caused by a decrease in circulating blood volume.
- Cardiogenic shock is caused when the pumping ability of the heart is compromised to the point where adequate cardiac output cannot be maintained.
- Obstructive shock is caused by an obstruction in the heart or great vessels that either impedes venous return or prevents effective cardiac pumping action. Causes can include cardiac tamponade, pneumothorax, pulmonary embolism, and aortic stenosis.
- Distributive shock includes several types of shock that result from widespread vasodilation and decreased peripheral resistance. Because the blood volume does not change, relative hypovolemia results, leading to altered cellular metabolism. Examples of distributive shock include septic, neurogenic, and anaphylactic shock.
- Septic shock is a progression from sepsis and is a condition most commonly caused by gram-negative infections.
- Anaphylactic shock is caused by a fulminating hypersensitivity reaction to a foreign substance.

11.4 The Patient Experiencing Shock

Describe the pathophysiology and manifestations of shock, and outline the interprofessional care, nursing care, and transitions of care for patients with shock.

- Maintaining adequate intravascular volume is the most important aspect in the care of a patient who is experiencing shock.
- Supplemental oxygen is required.
- Monitoring of vital signs and patient condition for subtle changes is important.

TEST YOURSELF NCLEX-RN® REVIEW

1. A patient is brought to the emergency department after sustaining a mechanical trauma. What should the nurse remember as the most common mechanical source of injury in adults of all ages?
   A. Firearms
   B. Accidental fire
   C. Motor vehicles
   D. Swimming pools
2. The nurse is preparing to assess a patient with severe facial injuries caused by going through a windshield during a motor vehicle crash. For which complication should the nurse assess first?
   A. Fractures
   B. Hemorrhage
   C. Airway obstruction
   D. Shallow respirations
3. The nurse is caring for a 23-year-old female patient who sustained injuries after being thrown from a car during a motor vehicle crash. Which laboratory test should the nurse ensure is collected from this patient?
   A. Pregnancy test
   B. Serum electrolytes
   C. Complete blood count
   D. Blood type and crossmatch
4. The nurse is monitoring a blood transfusion being administered to a trauma patient experiencing shock. Which assessment findings best indicate a dangerous transfusion reaction? (Select all that apply.)
   A. Increasing dyspnea
   B. Increasing blood pressure
   C. Vomiting
   D. An increase in body temperature by 0.3 degree
   E. Facial flushing
5. A patient with traumatic injuries is experiencing widespread vasodilation and decreased peripheral resistance. For which type of shock should the nurse plan care for this patient?
   A. Septic shock
   B. Obstructive shock
   C. Cardiogenic shock
   D. Hypovolemic shock
6. A victim of multiple traumatic injuries is bleeding profusely from one arm and leg. What should the nurse use to help manage this bleeding?
   A. Vessel clamps
   B. Limb elevation
   C. Vasopressor application
   D. Direct pressure application
7. A patient is admitted with chest injuries from a motor vehicle crash. For what should the nurse assess to determine the patient's ultimate extent of the injury?
   A. Recreational activities
   B. Preexisting health problems
   C. Psychosocial status before the traumatic event
   D. Number and types of previous traumatic injuries
8. One week after a traumatic injury the patient's hemoglobin level begins to drop and temperature begins to rise. The nurse would conduct additional assessment for which complication?
   A. Liver lacerations
   B. Intracranial bleeding
   C. Gastrointestinal hemorrhage
   D. Postoperative internal bleeding
9. A patient experiencing cardiogenic shock is prescribed nitroprusside (Nipride). Which nursing interventions are indicated? (Select all that apply.)
   A. Monitor for thiocyanate poisoning.
   B. Report urine output of more than 150 mL per hour.
   C. Do not mix with other medications.
   D. Assess intravenous access site and apply ice if infiltration occurs.
   E. Report increased confusion.
10. The nurse is caring for a patient recovering from surgery. Which action should the nurse perform to prevent the onset of hypovolemic shock?
    A. Elevate the head of the bed.
    B. Provide immediate pain relief.
    C. Monitor strict intake and output.
    D. Practice careful and consistent hand hygiene.

See Test Yourself answers in Appendix B.

REFERENCES

Adams, M. P., Holland, L. N., & Urban, C. (2017). *Pharmacology for nursing: A pathophysiologic approach* (5th ed.). Hoboken, NJ: Pearson Education.

Ahmad, F. B., & Bastian, B. (2018). *Quarterly provisional estimates for selected indicators of mortality, 2016–Quarter 3, 2017.* Hyattsville, MD: National Center for Health Statistics. National Vital Statistics System, Vital Statistics Rapid Release Program.

American Red Cross. (2017). *A compendium of transfusion guidelines* (3rd ed.). Retrieved from http://success.redcross.org/success/file.php/1/TransfusionPractices-Compendium_3rdEdition.pdf.

American Red Cross. (2018). *Blood types.* Retrieved from http://www.redcrossblood.org/learn-about-blood/blood-types.

Bledsoe, B. E., & Cherry, R. A. (2017). *Paramedic care: Principles and practice* (5th ed.). Hoboken, NJ: Pearson Education.

Centers for Disease Control and Prevention (CDC). (2016). *Elder abuse surveillance: Uniform definitions and recommended core data elements.* Retrieved from https://www.cdc.gov/violenceprevention/pdf/EA_Book_Revised_2016.pdf.

Desjardins, G. (2013). *Injuries to the cervical spine.* Retrieved from www.trauma.org/archive/anaesthesia/cspineanaes.html.

Moehring, R., & Anderson, D. J. (2018). Gram-negative bacillary bacteremia in adults. *UpToDate.* Retrieved from https://www.uptodate.com/contents/gram-negative-bacillary-bacteremia-in-adults.

National Coalition Against Domestic Violence. (2018). *Statistics.* Retrieved from https://ncadv.org/statistics.

National Center on Elder Abuse. (2018). *Research.* Retrieved from https://ncea.acl.gov/whatwedo/research/statistics.html#prevalence.

Patel, M. B., Humbel, S. S., Cullinane, D. C., Day, M. A., Jawa, R. S., Devin, C. J., . . ., Como, J. J. (2015). Cervical spine collar clearance in the obtunded adult blunt trauma patients. *Journal of Trauma and Acute Care Surgery, 78*(2), 430–441.

Perrin, K. O., & MacLeod, C. E. (2018). *Understanding the essentials of critical care nursing* (3rd ed.). Upper Saddle River, NJ: Pearson Prentice-Hall.

Phillips, J. P. (2016). Workplace violence against health care workers in the United States. *New England Journal of Medicine, 374*, 1661–1669.

Pollack, A. N. (2011). *Critical care transport.* Sudbury, MA: Jones & Bartlett.

Rendy, L., Sapan, H. B., & Kalersaran, L. T. B. (2017). Multiorgan dysfunction syndrome (MODS) prediction score in multi-trauma patients. *International Journal of Surgery Open, 8*, 1–6.

Rutherford, L. G., & von Wencksternm, T. (2016). Trauma information groups: A level 1 trauma center's integrated approach to family support. *Journal of Trauma Nursing, 23*(6), 357–360.

Schluter, P. L. (2011). The Trauma and Injury Severity Score (TRISS) revised. *International Journal of the Care of the Injured, 42*, 90–96.

Singer, M., Deutschman, C. S., Seymour, C. W., Shankar-Hari, M., Annane, D., Bauer, M., . . ., Angus, D. C. (2016). The third international consensus definitions for sepsis and septic shock (Sepsis-3). *Journal of the American Medical Association, 315*(8), 801–810.

Stollings, J. L., Diedrich, D. A., Oyen, L. J., & Brown, D. R. (2014). Rapid sequence intubation: A review of the process and considerations when choosing medication. *Annals of Pharmacotherapy, 48*(1), 62–76.

Verharen, L., Mintjes, J., Kaljouw, M., Melief, W., Schilder, L., & van der Lann, G. (2015). Psychosocial needs of relatives of trauma patients. Health and Social Work, 40(3), 233–238.

Wagner, K., & Hardin-Pierce, M. (2014). *High-acuity nursing* (6th ed.). Hoboken, NJ: Pearson Education.

ADDITIONAL RESOURCES

American College of Emergency Physicians
www.acep.org

American Red Cross
http://redcross.org

Centers for Disease Control and Prevention, Violence Prevention
https://www.cdc.gov/violenceprevention/index.html

Society of Critical Care Medicine
www.sccm.org

Society of Trauma Nurses
www.traumanurses.org

Chapter 12

Nursing Care of Patients with Infections and Inflammation

Chapter Outline and Learning Outcomes

12.1 Overview of the Immune System and Inflammation 322

Explain the components and functions of the immune system and the immune response.

12.2 Acquired Immunity, Immunizations, and Precautions 334

Outline the process of acquired immunity and the importance of immunizations and isolation precautions in preventing disease.

12.3 Patients with Inflammation and Infection 340

Describe the pathophysiology and manifestations of inflammation and infection, and outline the interprofessional care, nursing care, and transitions of care for patients with these conditions.

CLINICAL COMPETENCIES

- Apply standard precautions and evidence-based practices to prevent the spread of infection within the patient, to other patients in the facility, and to members of the interprofessional team and visitors.
- Provide safe, effective, and respectful patient-centered care for patients with inflammation and infection.
- Collaborate with the interprofessional care team to integrate care of patients with infections.
- Promote therapeutic levels and complete dosage of anti-inflammatory and anti-infective medication through prompt administration and patient and family teaching.
- Assess for hypersensitivities to anti-inflammatory and anti-infective medication prior to and during administration.
- Participate in quality improvement processes to reduce the rates and risk of infection for a patient group or population.

KEY TERMS

abscess, 341
acquired immunity, 332
active immunity, 335
adaptive immune response, 322
anergy, 335
antibodies, 325
antibody-mediated (humoral) immune response, 325
antigens, 324
B lymphocytes (B cells), 324
cell-mediated (cellular) immune response, 325
cytokines, 333
endotoxins, 346
exotoxins, 346
healthcare-associated infections (HAIs), 348
immunity, 334
immunocompetent, 330
immunoglobulin (Ig), 330
infection, 346
inflammation, 327
innate immunity, 322
lymphocyte, 324
macrophages, 324
natural killer (NK) cells, 324
passive immunity, 335
pathogens, 346
phagocytosis, 329
septicemia, 348
T lymphocytes (T cells), 324
Vaccine, 336

The human body is continually threatened by foreign substances, infectious agents, and abnormal cells. The immune system is the body's major defense mechanism against these threats. Recent years have seen the emergence of resistant microorganisms such as methicillin-resistant *Staphylococcus aureus* (MRSA) and altered strains of familiar diseases, such as multiple-drug-resistant tuberculosis. Other diseases have also emerged, including severe acute respiratory syndrome (SARS), *Clostridium difficile*, and human immunodeficiency virus (HIV). The critical need to prevent healthcare-associated infections and their resulting impact on the patient and healthcare costs is an emerging theme as well.

A thorough knowledge of the immune system increases understanding of inflammatory responses, resistance to infectious disease, and the importance of immunization. This foundation can help the nurse promote patients' health by preventing and identifying infections and teaching patients and families about recommended treatment regimens.

12.1 Overview of the Immune System and Inflammation

The immune system is a complex and intricate network of specialized cells, tissues, and organs. Cells of the immune system seek out and destroy damaged cells and foreign tissue, yet recognize and preserve host cells. The immune system defends and protects the body from infection by pathogens; removes and destroys damaged or dead cells; and identifies and destroys malignant cells, thereby preventing their further development into tumors.

The immune system is activated by minor injuries, such as small lacerations or bruises, and by major insults, such as burns, surgeries, and systemic diseases (e.g., pneumonia). The immune response may be innate or adaptive. **Innate immunity** is considered the body's natural barriers to infection and injury. Innate immunity provides a nonspecific, generic response to harmful events. These responses prevent or limit the entry of invaders into the body, thereby limiting the extent of tissue damage and reducing the workload of the adaptive immune system. When innate immunity processes are unable to destroy invading organisms or toxins, a more specific response, called the **adaptive immune response**, is activated. Adaptive immunity develops over a person's lifetime and provides a response that is specific to unique organisms. Adaptive immunity includes memory, which hastens future responses to the organism.

Immune System Components

The immune system consists of molecules, cells, and organs that produce the immune response (**Table 12.1**). These components may be involved in the innate immunity response, the adaptive immune response, or both.

Leukocytes

Leukocytes (white blood cells [WBCs]) are the primary cells involved in both innate and adaptive immune system responses. Like all blood cells, leukocytes derive from stem cells, the hemocytoblasts, in the bone marrow (**Figure 12.1** ■). Leukocytes are not confined to circulation; instead, they use it for transport to the site of an inflammatory or immune response. As the mobile units of the immune system, leukocytes detect, attack, and destroy anything that is recognized as foreign. They are able to move through tissue spaces, locating damaged tissue and infection by responding to chemicals released by other leukocytes and damaged tissue.

The normal number of circulating leukocytes is 4,500 to 10,000 cells per cubic millimeter (mm^3) of blood. Many more leukocytes are marginated. *Margination* refers to adhesion of leukocytes to vascular epithelial cells along the vessel walls, in other tissue spaces, or in the lymph system. Marginated leukocytes migrate into injured areas or areas where pathogens infiltrate as part of the innate immune response. In the presence of an attack, such as an infection, additional WBCs are released from the bone marrow, leading to *leukocytosis*, a WBC count of greater than 10,000/mm^3. As WBCs move out of the bone marrow into the blood, the bone marrow increases its production of additional leukocytes. A decrease

Table 12.1 Cells and Tissues of the Immune System

Component	Location	Function
Leukocytes		
Granulocytes		
Neutrophils	Circulation	Phagocytosis and chemotaxis
Eosinophils	Circulation, respiratory tract, and gastrointestinal tract	Phagocytosis Protection against parasites Involved in allergic response
Basophils	Circulation	Release of chemotactic substances
Monocytes and macrophages	Circulation (monocytes) and body tissue, such as skin (histiocytes), liver (Kupffer cells), alveoli, spleen, tonsils, lymph nodes, bone, bone marrow, brain	Trapping and phagocytizing of foreign substances and cellular debris Secretion of interleukin-1 to stimulate lymphocyte growth Activation of T and B cells
Lymphocytes		
T cells (mature in thymus gland)	Circulation, lymph system, tissues	Control of viral infections and destruction of cancer cells Involved in hypersensitivity reactions and graft tissue rejection
B cells (mature in bone marrow)	Circulation, spleen	Production of antibodies (immunoglobulins) to specific antigens
Natural killer (NK) cells	Circulation	Cytotoxic; killing of tumor cells, fungi, viral-infected cells, and foreign tissue
Lymphoid Tissues		
Primary or central lymphoid structures	Bone marrow and thymus gland	Production of immune cells; sites for cell maturation
Secondary or peripheral lymphoid structures	Lymph nodes, spleen, tonsils, intestinal lymphoid tissue, lymphoid tissue in other organs	Sites for activation of immune cells by antigens

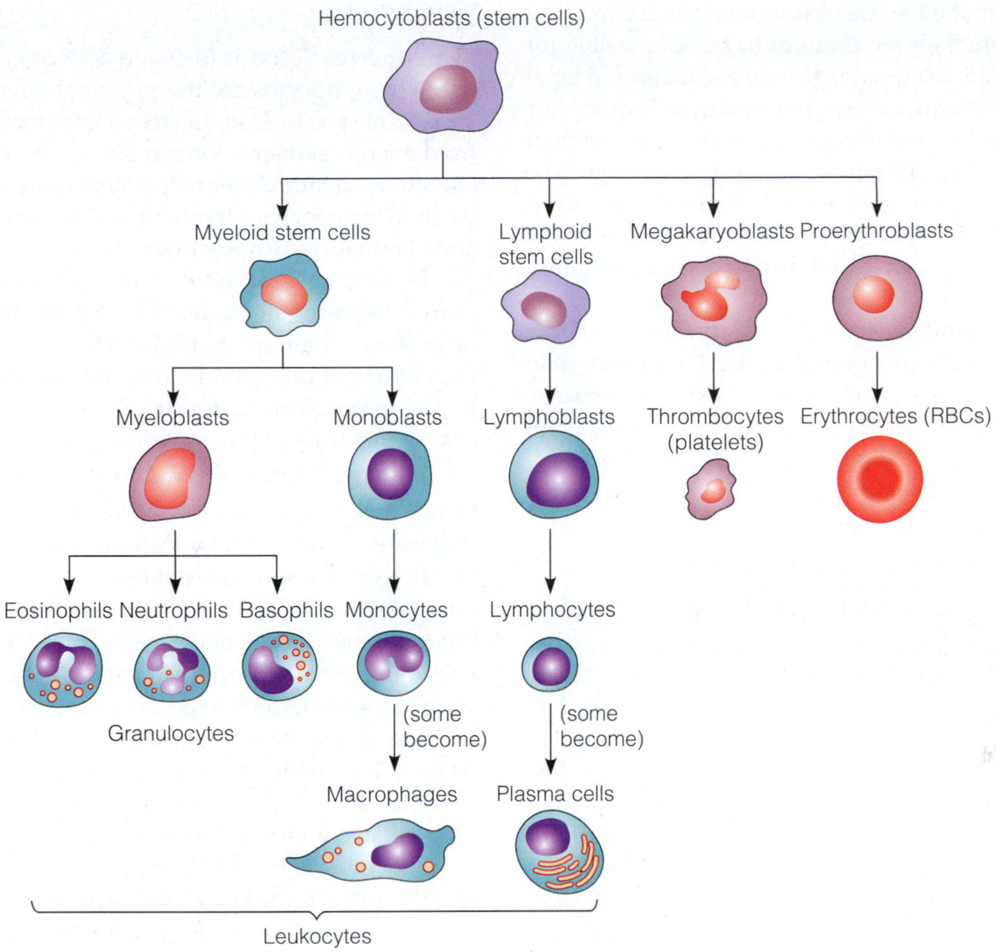

Hemocytoblasts (stem cells)
Myeloid stem cells
Lymphoid stem cells
Megakaryoblasts
Proerythroblasts
Myeloblasts
Monoblasts
Lymphoblasts
Thrombocytes (platelets)
Erythrocytes (RBCs)
Eosinophils
Neutrophils
Basophils
Monocytes
Lymphocytes
Granulocytes
(some become)
(some become)
Macrophages
Plasma cells
Leukocytes

Figure 12.1 ■ The development and differentiation of leukocytes from hemocytoblasts.

in the number of circulating leukocytes, known as *leukopenia*, occurs when bone marrow activity is suppressed or when leukocyte destruction increases.

Leukocytes are divided into three major groups: Granulocytes, monocytes, and lymphocytes. The granulocytes and monocytes derive from the myeloid stem cells of the bone marrow and are instrumental in the inflammatory response. Lymphocytes derive from the lymphoid stem cells of the bone marrow and are the primary cells involved in the specific immune response. In laboratory tests, the WBC count indicates the total number of circulating leukocytes. The WBC differential identifies the portion of the total represented by each type of leukocyte.

Granulocytes

Granulocytes constitute 60 to 80% of the total number of normal circulating leukocytes. Their cytoplasm has a granular appearance, and their nuclei are distinctively multilobular (refer to Figure 12.1). Granulocytes have a short lifespan, measured in hours to days. Granulocytes play a key role in protecting the body from harmful microorganisms during acute inflammation and infection. There are three types of granulocytes: Neutrophils, eosinophils, and basophils.

Neutrophils, also called *polymorphonuclear leukocytes* (*PMNs* or *polys*), are the most plentiful of the granulocytes, constituting 55 to 70% of the total number of circulating leukocytes. Neutrophils are *phagocytic* cells, responsible for engulfing and destroying foreign agents, particularly bacteria and small particles. Neutrophils are the first phagocytic cells to arrive at the site of invasion, drawn by chemicals released by damaged tissue and invading organisms.

Neutrophils are produced in the bone marrow and released into circulation when they mature. *Segmented* neutrophils (or *segs*) are mature forms, and usually account for about 55% of total leukocytes. *Bands* are immature neutrophils and usually comprise 5% of leukocytes. As neutrophils mature, their nucleus changes from round to kidney bean shaped (banded) and then the nucleus separates into small, attached segments, thus the designations *banded* versus *segmented* neutrophils. It takes about 10 days for a neutrophil to mature and be released into circulation. Once released, neutrophils have a circulating half-life of 6 to 10 hours. They cannot replicate and must be replaced constantly to maintain adequate numbers in the circulation. They do not return to the bone marrow.

Eosinophils account for 1 to 4% of the total number of circulating leukocytes. They mature in the bone marrow for 3 to 6 days before being released into circulation. Eosinophils have a circulating half-life of 30 minutes and a tissue half-life of 12 days. They are phagocytic cells, but are less efficient at this process than neutrophils. Eosinophils are found in large numbers in the respiratory and gastrointestinal tracts, where they are thought to be responsible for protecting the body from parasitic worms, including tapeworms, flukes, pinworms, and hookworms. Eosinophils surround the parasite and release toxic enzymes from their cytoplasmic granules. The parasite, although too large to be phagocytized, is destroyed. Eosinophils are also involved in a hypersensitivity response, inactivating some of the inflammatory chemicals released during the inflammatory response.

Basophils constitute about 0.5 to 1% of the circulating leukocytes. These cells are not phagocytic. Granules within basophils contain proteins and chemicals such as heparin, histamine, bradykinin, serotonin, and a slow-reacting substance of anaphylaxis (leukotrienes). These substances are released into the bloodstream during an acute hypersensitivity reaction or stress response.

Monocytes, Macrophages, and Dendritic Cells

Monocytes, macrophages, and dendritic cells are the mediators of immunity. They recognize foreign matter (from molecules to cells) and initiate immune responses. *Monocytes* are the largest of the leukocytes and constitute 2 to 3% of circulating leukocytes. After their release from the bone marrow, monocytes circulate in the serum for 1 to 2 days. They then migrate throughout the body, attaching themselves to various tissues, where they remain for months or even years until they are activated. Monocytes mature into **macrophages** after settling into the tissues. Once they have migrated and matured, macrophages are differentiated by the tissues in which they reside. *Histiocytes* are tissue macrophages in loose connective tissue, *Kupffer cells* are found in the liver, *alveolar macrophages* in the lungs, and *microglia* in the brain. Tissue macrophages are also found in the spleen, tonsils, lymph nodes, and bone marrow. Dendritic cells are star-shaped cells that serve as intermediaries between the innate and adaptive immune systems. Dendritic cells capture antigens, transporting them to lymphoid organs such as regional lymph nodes (Sorenson, Quinn, & Klein, 2019). Monocytes, macrophages, and dendritic cells are antigen-presenting cells (APCs), which activate immune responses in both B and T lymphocytes.

Monocytes, macrophages, and dendritic cells are actively phagocytic, with the capacity to phagocytize large foreign particles and cell debris. Like neutrophils, macrophages are drawn to an inflamed area by chemicals released from damaged tissue in a process known as *chemotaxis*. Once they are in the tissue, macrophages can multiply to encapsulate and trap foreign matter that cannot be phagocytized. Monocytes and macrophages activate the immune response against chronic infections such as tuberculosis, viral infections, and certain intracellular parasitic infections. Dendritic cells have long processes that can capture antigens and migrate to lymphoid tissue. They serve as sentinels for antigens in most organs including the heart, lungs, liver, kidney, and gastrointestinal tract. Dendritic cells activate T cells against cancer, assist B lymphocytes to produce antibodies, and downregulate the immune system.

Lymphocytes

Lymphocytes account for 20 to 40% of circulating leukocytes. Lymphocytes are the principal effector and regulator cells of specific immune responses that protect the body from microorganisms, foreign tissue, and cell mutations or alterations. Through a process known as immune surveillance, lymphocytes monitor the body for cancerous cells and eliminate or destroy them.

Like other leukocytes, lymphocytes derive from the stem cells in the bone marrow (**Figure 12.2** ■). Lymphocytes have "homing" patterns: They constantly circulate, then return to concentrate in lymphoid tissues (the lymph nodes, spleen, thymus, tonsils, Peyer patches in the submucosa of the distal ileum, and the appendix).

The three types of lymphocytes are **T lymphocytes (T cells)**, **B lymphocytes (B cells)**, and **natural killer cells (NK cells)**. None of these cells acts independently. Their functions are closely interrelated. T cells mature in the thymus gland, whereas B cells complete their maturation in the bone marrow. T cells and B cells are integral to the adaptive immune response. On contact with an antigen, B lymphocytes are activated and mature into either plasma cells, which secrete antibodies, or memory cells. On contact with APCs, T lymphocytes mature into active helper T (T_H) cells, cytotoxic T (T_C) cells, or memory T cells. Memory cells are inactive, sometimes for years, but activate immediately with subsequent exposure to the same antigen. They then proliferate rapidly, producing an intense immune response. Memory cells are responsible for providing acquired immunity.

NK cells are large, granular cells found in the spleen, lymph nodes, bone marrow, and blood. They constitute 15% of circulating lymphocytes. NK cells are part of the innate immune response. They provide immune surveillance, recognizing and destroying altered and abnormal host cells. Like B cells and T cells, NK cells are cytotoxic, but unlike T cells they do not require a specific antigen to become activated and kill cancer cells, virus-infected cells, and cells infected with microbes (Sorenson et al., 2019). Fortunately, NK cells are inhibited when contact is made with normal host cells.

Antigens

Substances the immune system recognizes as foreign or "nonself" are called **antigens**. Antigens provoke a specific immune response when introduced into the body. Typically, antigens are large protein molecules found on the cell membrane or cell wall of microorganisms or tissues such as transplanted tissue or organs. Other potentially antigenic substances include pollens, insect venom, and the resin of poison ivy (Braun & Anderson 2017; Sorenson et al., 2019).

Complete antigens, known as *immunogens*, have two characteristics: (1) *Immunogenicity*, the ability to stimulate a specific immune response, and (2) *specific reactivity*, the stimulation of specific immune system components. In contrast, *haptens* are small molecules (e.g., chemical toxins or dust) that must link with proteins to evoke an antigenic response.

When an antigen is encountered in the body, generation of an effective immune response involves two major groups of cells: Lymphocytes and antigen-presenting cells (APCs).

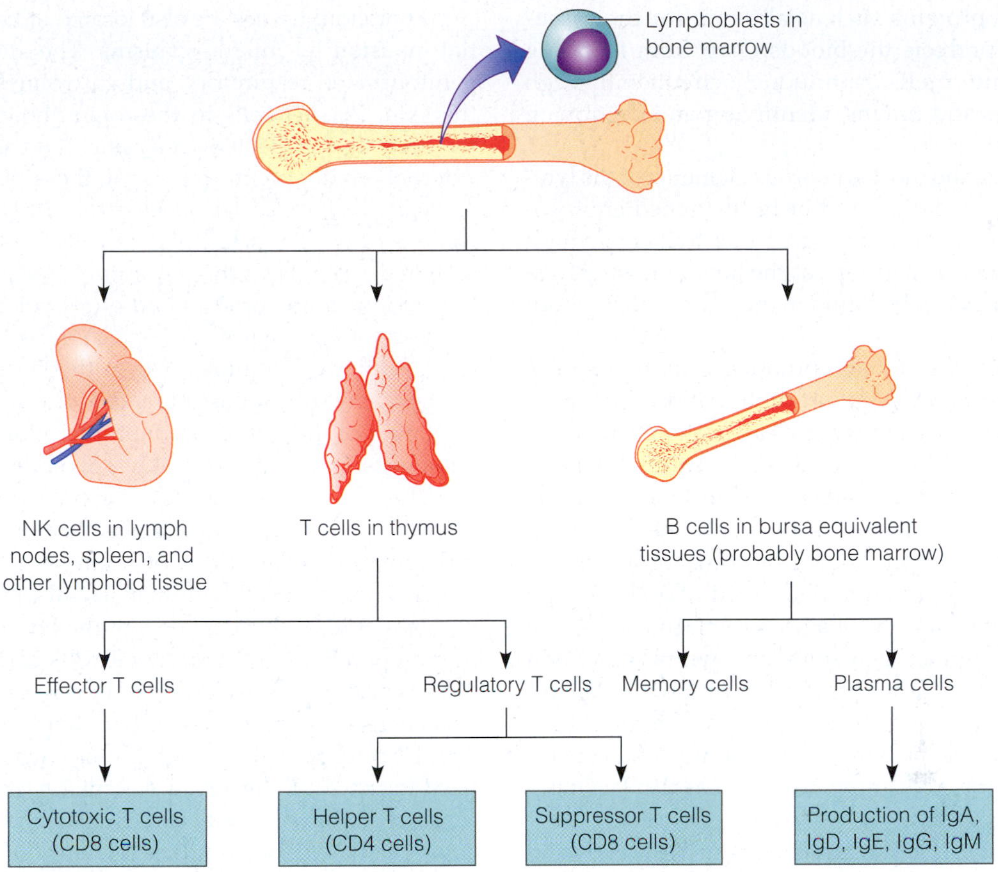
Lymphoblasts in bone marrow
NK cells in lymph nodes, spleen, and other lymphoid tissue
T cells in thymus
B cells in bursa equivalent tissues (probably bone marrow)
Effector T cells
Regulatory T cells
Memory cells
Plasma cells
Cytotoxic T cells (CD8 cells)
Helper T cells (CD4 cells)
Suppressor T cells (CD8 cells)
Production of IgA, IgD, IgE, IgG, IgM

Figure 12.2 ■ The development and differentiation of lymphocytes from the lymphoid stem cell (lymphoblasts).

Macrophages and dendritic cells function as APCs as they capture, process, and present antigens to the lymphocytes. Lymphocyte receptors recognize and respond to specific antigens, generating the immune response. Two separate, but overlapping, immune responses may occur, depending on the antigen itself and the type of immune cell activated by contact with the antigen. The B cell or humoral branch of the immune system mainly targets extracellular antigens such as bacteria, bacterial toxins, and free viruses through the production of **antibodies**, molecules that bind with the antigen and inactivate it. The five classes of antibodies are IgG, IgA, IgM, IgD, and IgE. These proteins make up the **antibody-mediated (humoral) immune response**. Intracellular pathogens, such as viral-infected cells, cancer cells, and foreign tissue, activate T lymphocytes, which are the primary agents of the **cell-mediated (cellular) immune response**. In this immune response, the lymphocytes themselves, in the form of helper T cells, cytotoxic T cells, and NK cells, inactivate the antigen, either directly or indirectly.

Lymphoid System

The *lymphoid system* consists of the lymph nodes, spleen, thymus, tonsils, lymphoid tissue scattered in connective tissues and mucosa, and bone marrow. The thymus and bone marrow, in which T cells and B cells mature, are considered central lymphoid organs. The spleen, lymph nodes, tonsils, and other peripheral lymphoid tissue are peripheral lymphoid organs (**Figure 12.3** ■). The lymphoid

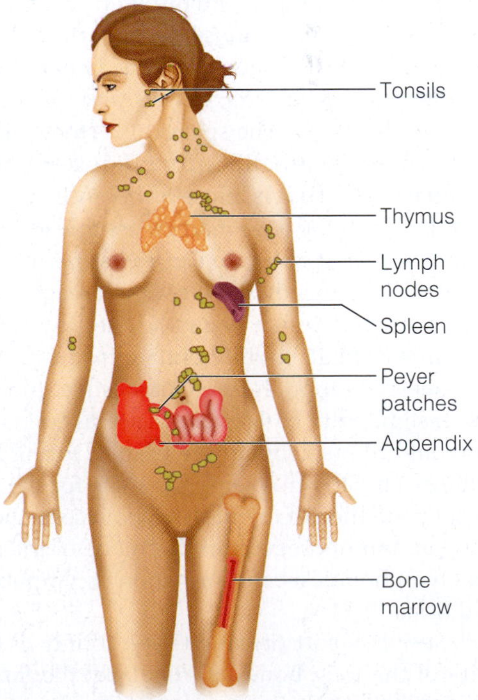
Tonsils
Thymus
Lymph nodes
Spleen
Peyer patches
Appendix
Bone marrow

Figure 12.3 ■ The lymphoid system: The central organs of the thymus and bone marrow, and the peripheral organs, including the spleen, tonsils, lymph nodes, and Peyer patches.

system recovers proteins such as albumin for the vascular system and protects the bloodstream from invading organisms. Immune cells continuously circulate through lymphoid tissues and organs, identifying and destroying foreign antigens.

Lymph nodes, the most numerous elements of the lymphoid system, are small, round or bean-shaped encapsulated bodies that vary in size from 1 mm to 2 cm. Lymph nodes generally occur in groups at the junction of the lymphatic vessels. They can be found in the neck, axillae, abdomen, and groin.

Lymph nodes filter foreign products or antigens from the lymph and house and support proliferation of lymphocytes and macrophages. Lymph, a clear, protein-containing fluid transported within lymph vessels, enters the node through afferent lymphatic vessels. Inside the node, the lymph flows through sinuses in the cortex of the lymph node where T and B lymphocytes and macrophages are abundant, then through sinuses of the medulla of the lymph node, which contains macrophages and plasma cells. The presence of a foreign antigen stimulates lymphocytes and macrophages to proliferate in the lymph nodes. Macrophages destroy the antigen by phagocytosis. Immune cells and lymph then leave the lymph node through efferent vessels. An abundant blood supply to the node also facilitates lymphocyte movement.

The *spleen* is the largest lymphoid organ in the body and the only lymphoid organ that can filter blood. The spleen is located in the upper left quadrant of the abdomen. The spleen has two kinds of tissue, white pulp and red pulp. White pulp is lymphoid tissue that serves as a site for lymphocyte proliferation and immune surveillance. B cells predominate in the white pulp. Blood filtration occurs in the red pulp. In blood-filled venous sinuses, phagocytic cells dispose of damaged or aged RBCs and platelets. Other debris and foreign matter, such as bacteria, viruses, and toxins, are also removed from the blood. The spleen also stores blood and the breakdown products of RBCs for future use. The spleen is not essential for life. If it is removed because of disease or trauma, the liver and the bone marrow assume its functions.

The *thymus gland* is located in the superior anterior mediastinal cavity beneath the sternum. It reaches its maximum size at puberty, then begins to atrophy slowly. By adulthood it is difficult to differentiate from surrounding adipose tissue even though it remains active. In the older adult, the vast majority of thymus tissue has been replaced by adipose and fibrous connective tissue. During fetal life and childhood, the thymus serves as a site for the maturation and differentiation of thymic lymphoid cells, the T cells. Thymosin, an immunoregulatory hormone of the thymus, stimulates lymphopoiesis, the formation of lymphocytes or lymphoid tissue.

Bone marrow is soft organic tissue found in the hollow cavity of the long bones, particularly the femur and humerus, as well as the flat bones of the pelvis, ribs, and sternum. Bone marrow produces and stores hematopoietic stem cells, from which all cellular components of the blood are derived (refer to Figure 12.1).

Lymphoid tissues are also located at key sites of potential invasion by microorganisms: The submucosa of the genitourinary, respiratory, and gastrointestinal tracts and the skin. Plasma cells in these lymphoid tissues defend the body against bacterial invasion at areas exposed to the external environment. In general, these tissues are known as *mucosa-associated lymphoid tissue (MALT)*. Diffuse collections of lymphocytes, plasma cells, and phagocytes are scattered throughout the respiratory tract, concentrating at bifurcations of the bronchi and bronchioles. Peyer patches, or *gut-associated lymphoid tissue (GALT)*, comprises the largest collection of immune cells in the body. Ingestion and absorption of solid foodstuffs and liquids continually expose the lining of the gut to resident microflora and infectious pathogens. Unlike peripheral lymph nodes, which respond to pathogens with acute inflammatory responses, GALT processes common intestinal antigens without producing acute inflammation. Collections of immune cells make up the GALT. Intraepithelial lymphocytes fill the spaces between mucosal epithelial cells. Beneath the basement membrane of gut epithelium lie abundant T cells and mature plasma cells, which are sources of IgA. Peyer patches hold dense collections of lymphocytes in lymphoid nodules. As naive B and T cells migrate through Peyer patches, they are sensitized to specific antigens. In mesenteric lymph nodes these sensitized cells proliferate and circulate throughout the vascular tree where they produce secretory IgA. Secretory IgA coats mucosal cells and prevents attachment of intraluminal bacteria in the intestine, upper respiratory tract, the bronchi, mammary ducts, and salivary glands. Thus, the GALT collection of immune cells effectively protects mucosa throughout the body that is exposed to resident and foreign pathogens.

Tonsils and adenoids protect the body from inhaled or ingested foreign agents. Skin-associated lymphoid tissue contains lymphocytes and dendritic cells such as Langerhans cells in the epidermis, which transport antigens to regional lymph nodes for destruction and development of specific immunity to the antigen.

Innate Immune Response and Inflammation

Innate or natural immunity is the first line of defense against infection. It is nonspecific and includes skin and mucosal barriers, vascular and cellular responses, and phagocytosis. Cells involved in innate immunity include phagocytic neutrophils and macrophages and NK cells, which target intracellular pathogens. Soluble molecules such as opsonins, cytokines, acute-phase proteins (such as C-reactive protein), and the complement system are also involved in innate immunity.

Barrier protection is the body's first defense against infection. Intact skin prevents invasion by external organisms. When the skin is damaged or lost (e.g., as a result of injury, surgery, or burns), infection is much more likely. A barrier of mucus, which traps microorganisms and other foreign substances, protects the membranes lining inner surfaces of the body. These can then be removed by other protective mechanisms, such as by ciliary movement or by the washing action of tears or urine. In addition, many body fluids contain bactericidal substances that provide barrier protection. These include acid in gastric fluid, zinc in prostatic fluid, and lysozyme in tears, nasal secretions, saliva, and sweat.

When these defenses are breached, the resulting tissue damage or foreign material entering the body induces inflammation, another innate defense mechanism. **Inflammation** is a response to injury that brings fluid, dissolved substances, and blood cells into the interstitial tissues where the invasion or damage has occurred. The response is nonspecific: The same events occur regardless of cause of the inflammatory process. Through the inflammatory reaction, the invader is neutralized and eliminated, destroyed tissue removed, and the process of healing and repair initiated. See **Pathophysiology Illustrated: Acute Inflammation.**

The inflammatory response has two stages: (1) A vascular response characterized by vasodilation and increased permeability of blood vessels and (2) a cellular response. Phagocytosis sets the stage for healing (tissue repair).

Vascular Response

After tissue cells are damaged, local blood vessels briefly constrict. Vasodilation of the capillary arterioles and venules follows almost immediately as inflammatory mediators such as histamine and kinins are released from damaged tissue (**Box 12.1**). Increased blood flow causes vasocongestion at the injury site with resultant redness and heat. The congestion also increases local hydrostatic pressure. This, along with the increased vessel permeability that results from chemical mediators, moves fluid out of the capillaries and into the interstitial spaces of the tissue. The escaping fluid, called *fluid exudate*, contains large amounts of protein. This protein increases osmotic pressure in the interstitial spaces, which draws water and causes local edema. Fluid exudate provides protection for the injured tissue by transporting to the tissue certain nutrients needed for tissue healing, diluting bacterial toxins, and transporting cells needed for phagocytosis. Exudate may range from *serous*, primarily plasma with some proteins, to *sanguineous*, containing large amounts of blood cells. *Fibrinous exudate* forms a thick, sticky meshwork of fibrinogen, in effect "walling off" inflamed tissues and preventing the spread of infection. In more severe or acute inflammation, the fluid contains fibrin, RBCs, and dead and live bacteria. This type of exudate, called *purulent exudate*, has an odor and color characteristic of the bacteria present.

Many of the outward manifestations of inflammation result from vasoactive substances such as *histamine*, *prostaglandins*, and *leukotrienes*. Stored in mast cells, basophils, and platelets, histamine is released when an injury occurs or with stimulation by the immune system. An important component of the early inflammatory response, histamine causes vasodilation and vascular permeability in the affected area. Histamine is also a key factor in many hypersensitivity reactions. The leukotrienes, collectively known as *slow-reacting substance of anaphylaxis (SRS-A)*, play a significant vasoactive role in the later stages of the inflammatory response.

Prostaglandins are chemotactic substances that draw leukocytes to the inflamed tissue. In addition, they play a vasoactive role and are pain and fever inducers. Aspirin and other nonsteroidal anti-inflammatory drugs (NSAIDs), as well as the glucocorticoids, inhibit prostaglandin synthesis, thereby reducing fever, pain, and inflammation.

Plasma proteases activate the clotting cascade, kinin system, and complement system. With activation of the clotting cascade, bacteria and other foreign substances are trapped in the area of tissue damage. Fibrin, which has vasoactive by-products, is also released. Activation of the complement system causes vasodilation, increases vessel permeability, and facilitates the phagocytic process. Through the release of bradykinin, the kinin system has similar effects. Bradykinin also stimulates pain receptors.

Major chemical mediators of inflammation are summarized in **Table 12.2**.

BOX 12.1
Inflammatory Mediators

Many of the manifestations of inflammation are produced by chemicals released as a result of immunologic processes or tissue injury or damage. These inflammatory mediators are broadly classified as follows:

- ***Vasoactive substances*** (e.g., histamine, prostaglandins, leukotrienes, and platelet-activating factor) produce smooth muscle constriction, vasodilation, and increased capillary permeability.
- ***Chemotactic factors*** (e.g., complement fragments and chemokines) attract leukocytes to the damaged tissue.
- ***Plasma enzymes*** (proteases) activate the complement system, the clotting cascade, and the vasoactive kinins system, contributing to the vascular phase of the inflammatory response.
- ***Miscellaneous cell products*** (e.g., oxygen metabolites and lysosomal enzymes) damage surrounding tissue.

Table 12.2 Major Chemical Mediators of Inflammation

Factor	Source	Effect
Histamine	Mast cells, basophils, and platelets	Vasodilation and increased capillary permeability, producing tissue redness, warmth, and edema
Kinins (bradykinin and others)	Plasma proteins	Histamine-like effects; chemotaxis and pain inducers
Prostaglandins	Formed from arachidonic acid found in cell membranes	Histamine-like effects; chemotaxis, pain, and fever inducers
Leukotrienes	Formed from arachidonic acid	Smooth muscle constriction (especially bronchoconstriction), increased vascular permeability, chemotaxis

Pathophysiology Illustrated

Acute Inflammation

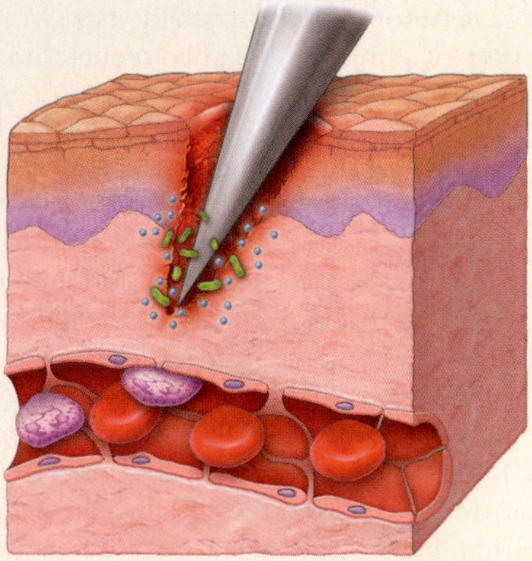

1. Inflammation is a key component of innate immunity, the body's immediate response to tissue damage or invasion of the body by foreign material. The inflammatory response serves to contain, control, and eliminate damaged cells and tissue, microorganisms, and antigens.

2. Vascular Response. Tissue damage causes brief, initial vasoconstriction which is rapidly followed by vasodilation, with resulting redness and warmth. Inflammatory mediators (e.g., histamine, prostaglandins, bradykinins) released in the innate immune response and by damaged tissue dilate local blood vessels and increase the permeability of capillaries in the area. Protein-rich fluid (exudate) accumulates in interstitial spaces, causing swelling and pain. Resulting edema slows blood flow, and together with activation of clotting in the area, helps localize and prevent microorganisms from spreading.

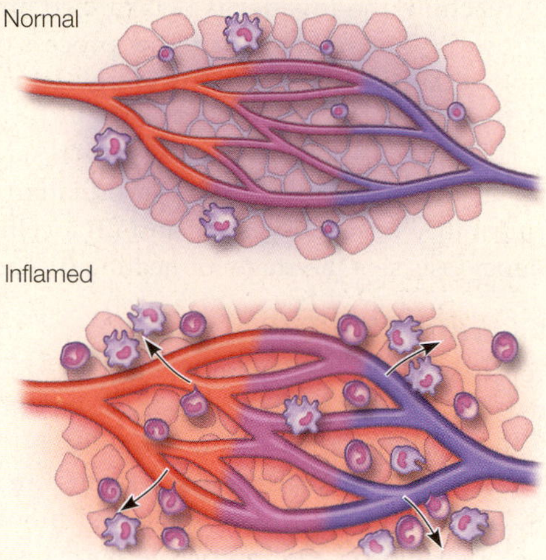
Normal
Inflamed

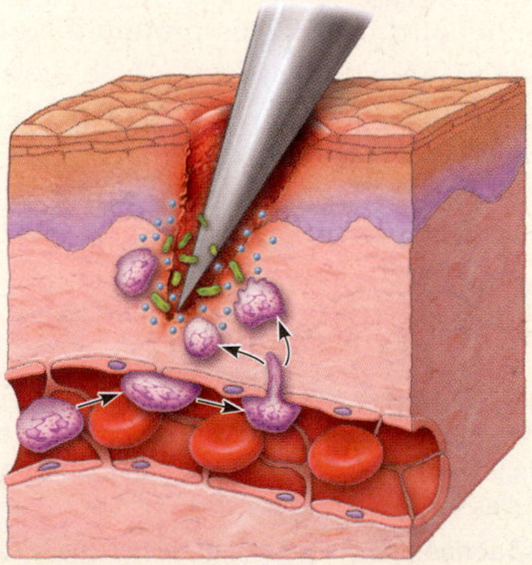

3. Cellular Response. Within less than an hour after the injury, the cellular stage of the inflammatory process brings phagocytic blood cells into the damaged tissue. Loss of serous fluid from capillaries increases blood viscosity in the area and slows its flow. Leukocytes marginate, moving to vessel periphery and adhering to the capillary endothelium. As a result, endothelial cells separate, allowing leukocytes to transmigrate through vessel walls into the tissue spaces. Chemotactic signals draw the leukocytes to the site of the injury or infection.

4. Phagocytosis. Once attracted to the inflammatory site, phagocytes engulf the foreign agent or target cell by projecting pseudopodia ("false feet") in all directions around it. This produces a phagosome containing the antigen, which is ingested into the cytoplasm. Once engulfed, lysosomes fuse with the phagosome, killing any live organism and releasing digestive enzymes, which destroy the antigen.

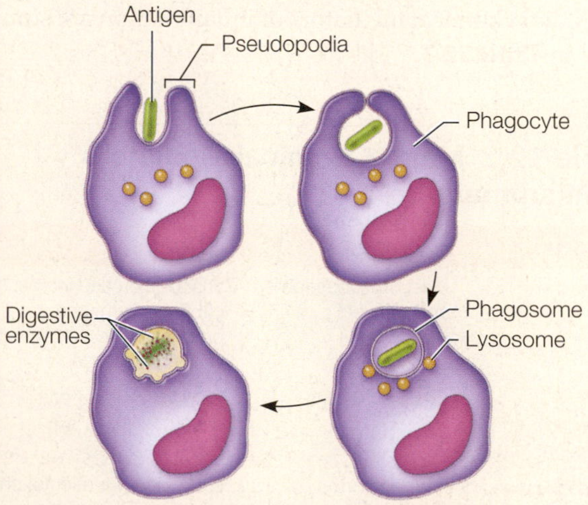
Antigen
Pseudopodia
Phagocyte
Phagosome
Lysosome
Digestive enzymes

The vascular response localizes invading bacteria and keeps them from spreading. Increased capillary permeability enhances the release of clotting factors such as fibrinogen, which converts to fibrin threads, entrapping the bacteria and walling them off from contact with the rest of the body.

Cellular Response

The cellular stage of the inflammatory process begins less than an hour after an injury. This stage is marked by changes in the lining of blood vessels and movement of phagocytic blood cells into the damaged tissue.

As serous fluid escapes the capillaries, the viscosity of blood in the area increases and its flow becomes more sluggish. Leukocytes move to the edges of the blood vessels where they accumulate, their movement slows, and they begin to adhere to the capillary endothelium. This process is known as *margination*. Leukocyte adhesion causes separation of endothelial cells, allowing leukocytes to transmigrate through the blood vessel wall into the tissue spaces. Within hours, millions of leukocytes emigrate into the area of inflammation.

Once leukocytes have emigrated, they are drawn to the damaged or inflamed tissues by chemotactic signals. Infectious agents, damaged tissues, and activated plasma substances such as complement fractions provide chemotactic signals that attract an army of neutrophils, monocytes, and macrophages to the injury site.

The number of neutrophils around the site increases to about 15,000 to 25,000/mm^3, and they begin their role in phagocytosis within a few hours. Monocytes become transient macrophages to augment the activity of the fixed macrophages and dendritic cells; together, they engulf dead cells, damaged tissue, nonfunctioning neutrophils, and invading bacteria.

Phagocytosis

Phagocytosis is a process by which a foreign agent or target cell is recognized, engulfed, and destroyed. Neutrophils, monocytes, and macrophages, known as *phagocytes*, are the primary cells involved in phagocytosis. Once attracted to the inflammatory site, phagocytes select and engulf foreign material.

The following factors or processes help phagocytes differentiate foreign tissue from normal cells:

- ***Smooth surface.*** Normal tissue has a smooth surface that is resistant to phagocytosis, whereas the rough surface of a foreign agent or target cell promotes phagocytosis.
- ***Surface charge.*** Healthy body cells present an electronegative surface charge that repels phagocytes. Cellular debris and foreign agents, by contrast, have an electropositive charge that attracts them.
- ***Opsonization.*** This immune process coats the surface of bacteria or target cells with soluble molecules (opsonins) such as complement, lectins, and other proteins. (See **Box 12.2** for more information about the complement system.) Opsonization enables the phagocyte to bind tightly with the foreign tissue, facilitating phagocytosis.

Phagocytes engulf the foreign agent or target cell by projecting pseudopodia (*false feet*) in all directions around it. This produces a chamber called a *phagosome* containing the antigen, which is ingested into the cytoplasm. Once the phagosome has been engulfed, lysosomes fuse with the phagosome, releasing antibacterial molecules and digestive enzymes that destroy the antigen.

Phagocytes produce bactericidal agents that kill most pathogens. These agents include toxic oxygen and nitrogen metabolites, such as nitric oxide, hydrogen peroxide, and superoxide, as well as digestive enzymes (e.g., lysozyme) that break down bacterial cell walls (Dieffenbach & Tramont, 2015). Some antigens, such as the tubercle bacillus, have coats or secrete substances that are resistant to lysosomal and bactericidal agents. To destroy such antigens, lysosomes release digestive enzymes into the phagosome. The lysosomes of neutrophils and macrophages contain an abundance of proteolytic (protein-destroying) enzymes that digest bacteria

BOX 12.2
The Complement System

The complement system consists of approximately 20 complex plasma proteins that are activated by a tissue injury or antigen–antibody reaction. The complement system is involved in both innate and adaptive immune responses. Its activation results in the production of effector molecules that are involved in the processes of inflammation, phagocytosis, and cell lysis or destruction (Sorenson et al., 2019). Specifically, complement activation leads to the following:

- *Mediation of the inflammatory response.* When the complement system is activated, chemical mediators such as histamine are released from mast cells and basophils, leading to smooth muscle contraction, increased vascular permeability and edema, and the attraction of leukocytes.
- *Opsonization (or coating) of microbes and antigen–antibody complexes.* Opsonization facilitates recognition of and binding to the antigen by the phagocyte and activation of phagocytosis.
- *Alteration of the cell membrane or viral capsule.* Complement can alter cell membranes, forming pores that cause cell lysis and death. Bacteria and viruses are destroyed; certain normal cells, such as RBCs, that are damaged or old may also be destroyed through this process.

The complement system has three arms, or pathways, of protein and enzyme reactions. The *classic pathway* is activated by antibody-containing immunoglobulins and other substances, such as DNA and C-reactive protein. The *alternate* and *lectin pathways* function in innate immunity; they do not require antibodies but are activated by tissue injury, properties of the microbial antigen, and proteins produced in response to injury (e.g., C-reactive protein) (Lubbers, van Essen, van Kooten, & Trouw, 2017; Mayer, 2017). Complement activation results in mediation of the inflammatory process, attraction of phagocytes, facilitation of phagocytosis, and lysis of microbes.

and other foreign protein components. The macrophage's lysosomes also contain lipases (fat-splitting enzymes) capable of digesting the thick lipid membranes of such bacteria as *Mycobacterium tuberculosis* and *Mycobacterium leprae*.

Once neutrophils have ingested toxic substances to their capacity, they in turn are destroyed. Neutrophils have the capacity to phagocytize 5 to 20 bacteria before they become inactive. Macrophages then digest the dead neutrophils. Monocytes or macrophages are capable of phagocytizing up to 100 bacteria. Because of their size, they can ingest larger particles than neutrophils can ingest, such as whole RBCs, necrotic tissue, cell fragments, malarial parasites, and dead neutrophils. Dendritic cells are also phagocytic and secrete IL-12, which is an important cytokine in the maturation of T_H cells. Macrophages have the ability to extrude (release) the toxic substances and lysosomal enzymes within their phagosomes. As a result, they can continue to function for months and even years.

Healing

During the initial inflammatory process, particulate matter, bacteria, damaged cells, and inflammatory exudate are removed by phagocytosis. This process, called *debridement*, prepares the wound for healing. Adequate nutrition is essential for inflammation and healing to proceed. Protein, glucose, and oxygen are needed by leukocytes for chemotaxis, phagocytosis, and intercellular killings.

The second phase of the healing process, known as *reconstruction*, may overlap the inflammatory phase. The ideal result of the healing process is *resolution*, the restoration of the original structure and function of the damaged tissue. Simple resolution occurs when there is no destruction of the normal tissue and the body is able to neutralize and remove the offending agent through the inflammatory process.

Resolution may also occur when the damaged tissue is capable of regeneration. The ability to regenerate, or replace lost *parenchyma* (functional tissue) with new, functional cells varies by tissue and cell type.

- ***Labile cells*** continue to regenerate throughout life. These cells are found in tissues where there is a daily turnover of cells—namely, bone marrow and the epithelial cells of the skin, mucous membranes, cervix, gastrointestinal tract, and genitourinary tract.
- ***Stable cells*** normally stop replicating when growth ceases, but are capable of regeneration when stimulated by an injury. Osteocytes (which are found in bone) and parenchymal cells of the kidneys, liver, and pancreas are stable cells.
- ***Permanent*** or ***fixed cells*** are unable to regenerate. When these cells are destroyed, they are replaced by fibrous scar tissue. Nerve cells, skeletal muscle cells, and cardiac muscle cells are fixed cells.

When regeneration and complete resolution are not possible, healing occurs by replacement of the destroyed tissue with collagen scar tissue. This process is known as *repair*. Although tissue that has undergone repair lacks the physiologic function of the destroyed tissue, the scar fills the lesion and provides tensile tissue strength.

Adaptive Immune Response

The *adaptive immune response* is a more specific reaction to the introduction of antigens into the body than innate immunity. On the first exposure to an antigen, a change occurs in the host, allowing a specific and rapid response following subsequent exposures.

The adaptive immune response has the following distinctive properties:

- The immune response is typically directed against materials recognized as foreign (i.e., from outside the body) and is not usually directed against the self (i.e., cells or structures produced by the body). This property is known as *self-recognition*.
- The immune response is *specific*. It is initiated by and directed against particular antigens (such as a specific virus, bacterium, or transplanted tissue).
- Unlike a localized inflammatory response, the immune response is *systemic*. Immunity is not restricted to the initial site of infection or entry of foreign tissue.
- The immune response has *memory*. Repeated exposures to an antigen produce a more rapid response.

A patient whose immune system is able to identify antigens and effectively destroy or remove them is said to be **immunocompetent**. There are two types of adaptive immune responses: Humoral or antibody-mediated immunity and cellular or cell-mediated immunity.

Antibody-Mediated Immune Response

The antibody-mediated (humoral) immune response is produced by B lymphocytes (B cells). B cells are constantly replaced through cell division and proliferation in the bone marrow. It is believed that B cells mature in the bone marrow and then migrate to the spleen to await activation. They normally constitute 10 to 15% of circulating lymphocytes.

B cells are activated by contact with an antigen and by T cells (discussed in the next section). Each B cell has receptor sites for a specific antigen or antigens. When the antigen is encountered, the activated B cell proliferates and differentiates into antibody-producing plasma cells and memory cells (**Figure 12.4** ■). Plasma cells are short lived, lasting only about 1 day. While alive they can produce thousands of antibody molecules per second. Memory cells retain antibody-producing information, allowing a rapid response if the antigen is again encountered.

An antibody is an **immunoglobulin (Ig)** molecule with the ability to bind to and inactivate a specific antigen. Immunoglobulins fall into five classes: IgG, IgA, IgM, IgD, and IgE. Each has a slightly different structure and function. Their roles are summarized in **Table 12.3**.

Antibodies are Y-shaped molecules with two light and two heavy polypeptide chains (**Figure 12.5** ■). The top portion of the Y, called the *Fab* or *antigen-binding fragment*, is chemically variable and specific to the antigen. The lower portion, the F_c, or *crystallized fragment*, is constant for its class of immunoglobulin and directs the biologic activity of the

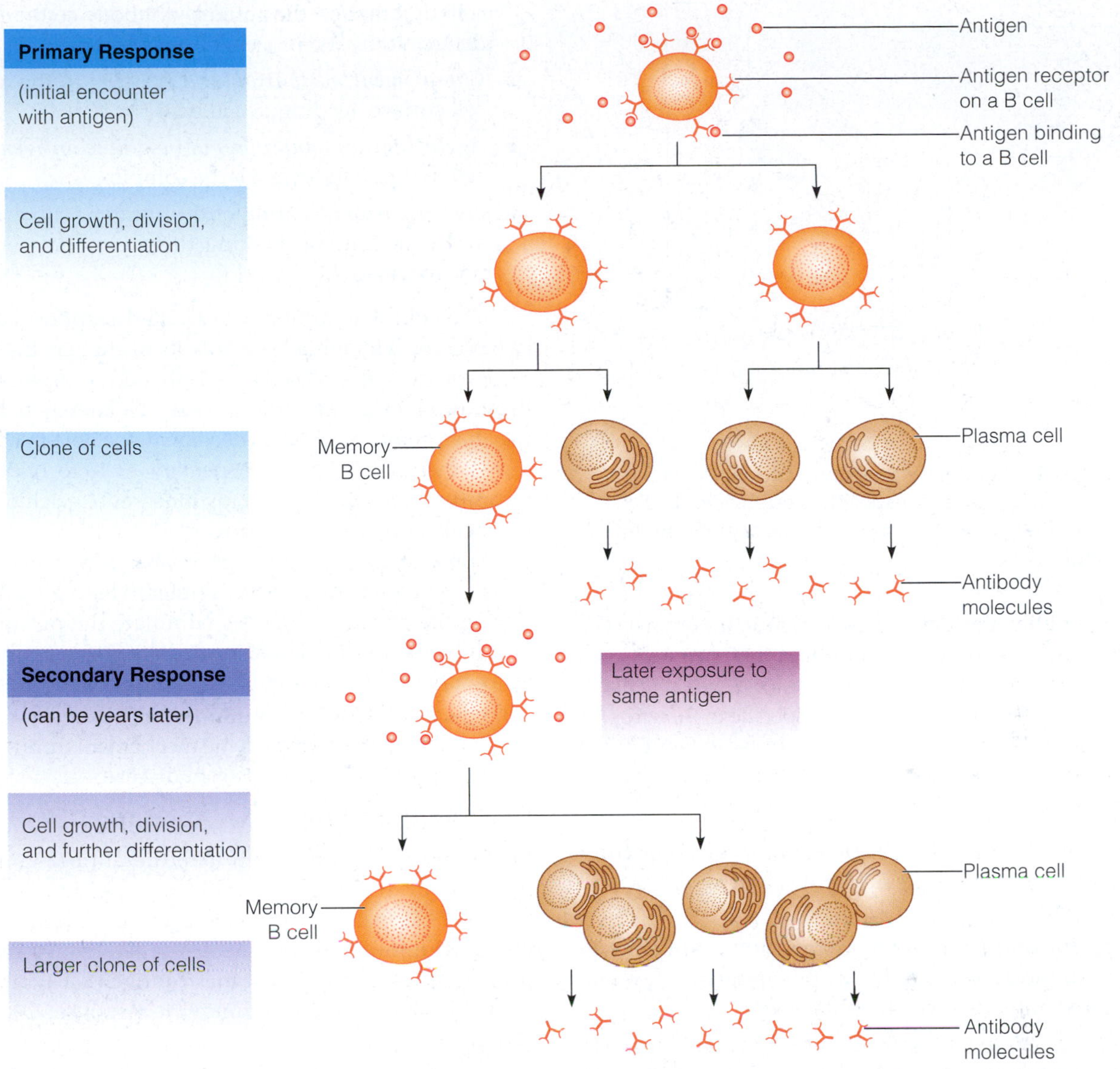
Primary Response
(initial encounter with antigen)
Cell growth, division, and differentiation
Clone of cells
Secondary Response
(can be years later)
Cell growth, division, and further differentiation
Larger clone of cells
Antigen
Antigen receptor on a B cell
Antigen binding to a B cell
Memory B cell
Plasma cell
Antibody molecules
Later exposure to same antigen
Memory B cell
Plasma cell
Antibody molecules

Figure 12.4 ■ Antibody-mediated (humoral) immunity. On initial exposure to the antigen, B cells with appropriate receptor sites are activated to become plasma cells, which produce antibodies or memory cells. This is known as the primary response. With subsequent exposures, memory cells respond rapidly with antibody production. This is known as the secondary response.

Table 12.3 Immunoglobulin Characteristics and Functions

Class	Percentage of Total	Characteristics and Function
IgG	75%	■ Most abundant Ig; also known as *gamma globulin*; found in blood, lymph, and intestines ■ Active against bacteria, bacterial toxins, and viruses ■ Activates complement and binds to macrophages ■ The only Ig to cross the placenta, providing immune protection to neonate
IgA	10–15%	■ Found in saliva; tears; and bronchial, gastrointestinal, prostatic, and vaginal secretions, as well as blood and lymph ■ Provides local protection on exposed mucous membrane surfaces and potent antiviral activity by preventing binding of the virus to epithelial cells ■ Levels decrease during stress
IgM	5–10%	■ Found in blood and lymph ■ First antibody produced with primary immune response ■ High concentrations early in infection, decreases within about a week ■ Mediates cytotoxic response and activates complement
IgD	< 1	■ Found in blood, lymph, and surfaces of B cells ■ Exact function unknown; may be receptor-binding antigens to B-cell surface
IgE	< 0.1	■ Found on mast cells and basophils ■ Involved in release of chemical mediators responsible for immediate hypersensitivity (allergic and anaphylactic) response and parasitic infections

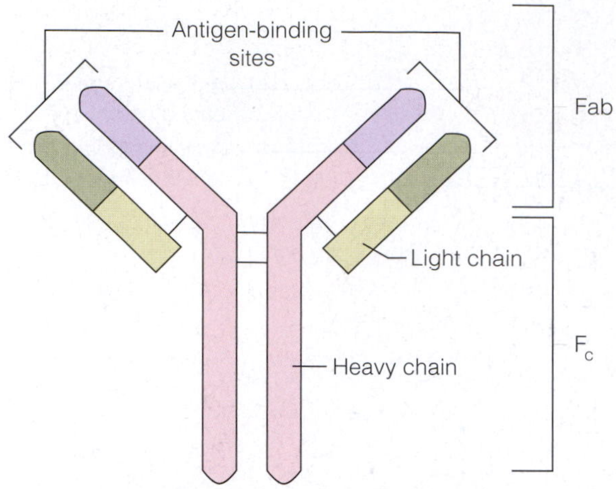
Antigen-binding sites
Fab
Light chain
F_c
Heavy chain

Figure 12.5 ■ An antibody molecule. The Fab section is unique, providing an antigen-specific binding site. The F_c section is common to each class of immunoglobulin (IgG, IgA, IgM, IgD, IgE).

immunoglobulin (the manner in which it functions). For example, the lower portion of immunoglobulin molecules produced against hepatitis A and hepatitis B is the same (IgG), but the upper portion is different and specific to the virus.

The antibodies produced by B cells (refer to Figure 12.4) link with the antigen (**Figure 12.6** ■) and inactivate it through one or more of the following processes:

- ***Covering the antigen with antibodies to attract phagocytes***, including neutrophils, macrophages, and eosinophils
- ***Precipitation:*** Combining with soluble antigens to form an insoluble complex or precipitate that can be captured and destroyed by phagocytes
- ***Neutralization:*** Combining with a virus or toxin to neutralize its effects by preventing it from attaching to cells and tissues; the antigen–antibody complex is then destroyed by the process of phagocytosis
- ***Complement activation and fixation*** to the antigenic cell surface, leading to cell lysis
- ***Agglutination (clumping) of insoluble antigens*** (e.g., a cell or virus) to form a large complex
- ***Opsonization:*** Coating of the antigen with antibodies and complement, making them more susceptible to phagocytosis.

The complete antibody-mediated response occurs in two phases. With initial exposure to an antigen, the primary response develops. B cells are activated to proliferate and begin producing antibodies. There is a latency period of 3 to 6 days before antibodies become detectable in the blood. Levels then continue to rise, peaking at 10 to 14 days after the initial exposure. With many illnesses (e.g., chickenpox), this peak correlates with recovery.

Subsequent exposure to the same antigen elicits a secondary response. Memory cells (refer to Figure 12.4) formed during the primary response stimulate the production of plasma cells, and an almost immediate rise in antibody levels occurs (**Figure 12.7** ■). This rapid secondary response is the basis of **acquired immunity** and is instrumental in preventing disease. It is also the mechanism through which vaccines provide protection from disease.

Cell-Mediated Immune Response

Many antigens cannot stimulate the antibody-mediated response or are hidden from it because they live inside the body's cells (e.g., viruses and mycobacteria). The cell-mediated immune response, also called *cellular immunity*, provides protection against these antigens. T lymphocytes (T cells) initiate this type of immune response.

T Cells

Approximately 70 to 80% of circulating lymphocytes are T cells. T cells migrate to the thymus during fetal and early life, establishing the lifetime pool of cells. T cells

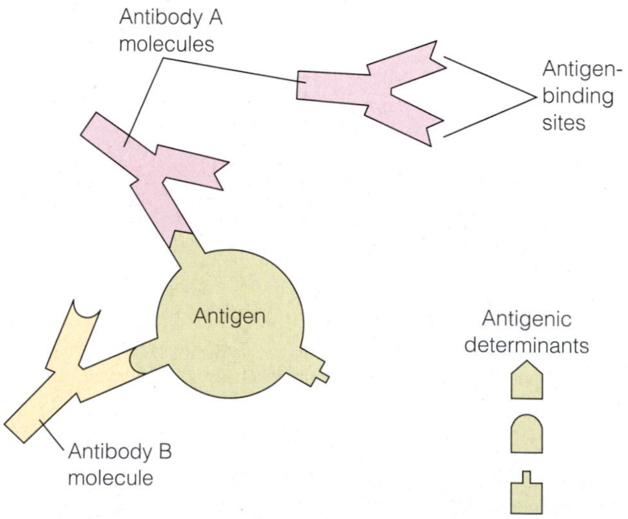
Antibody A
molecules
Antigen-
binding
sites
Antigen
Antigenic
determinants
Antibody B
molecule

Figure 12.6 ■ Antigen–antibody binding. The unique Fab site on the antibody binds with specific receptor sites on the antigen. As shown, more than one kind of antibody may be produced to an antigen.

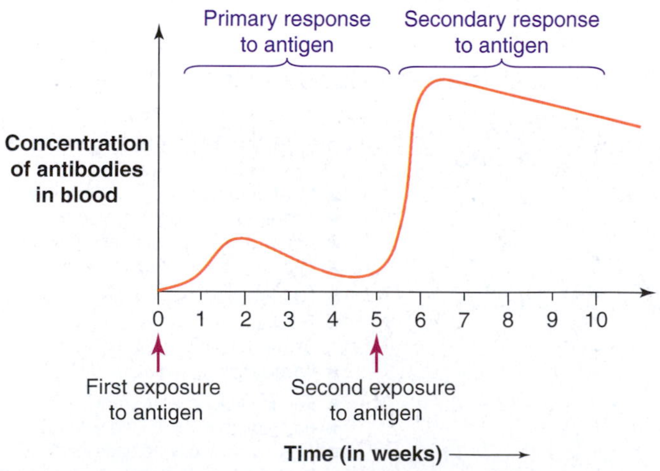
Primary response
to antigen
Secondary response
to antigen
Concentration
of antibodies
in blood
0 1 2 3 4 5 6 7 8 9 10
First exposure
to antigen
Second exposure
to antigen
Time (in weeks)

Figure 12.7 ■ Antibody production in the primary and secondary responses of the antibody-mediated immune response. Note the more rapid and effective production following subsequent exposure.

have a lifespan measured in years, maintaining their numbers through proliferation, primarily in the lymph nodes. T cells are much more complex than B cells. There are two major populations of T cells, CD4 cells and CD8 cells, differentiated by their cell surface proteins (or markers). T cells are antigen specific; that is, each subset is activated by a particular antigen. The antigens that activate T cells must be presented on another cell surface, such as pieces of virus presented on the surface of an infected cell or the histocompatibility locus antigen on a cell of transplanted tissue. When activated, T cells divide and proliferate, forming antigen-specific *clones* (**Figure 12.8** ■). Activated T cells further differentiate to become *cytotoxic cells*, *helper cells*, or *suppressor cells*. *Memory cells* are also formed; these remain in reserve for future encounters with the antigen.

- ***Cytotoxic T cells*** (*T_C* ***cells***), effector cells with the CD8 marker, seek out and destroy abnormal cells and cells harboring anything foreign (e.g., viruses). Cytotoxic T cells bind with cell surface antigens on virus-infected or foreign cells. T_C cells destroy the identified cell by combining with it and then either destroying its cell membrane or releasing cytotoxic substances into the cell. They are vital in the control of viral and bacterial infections.
- ***Helper T cells*** (*T_H* ***cells***) develop from T-cell populations with the CD4 marker. T_H cells coordinate immune responses to an antigen. They stimulate the proliferation of other T cells, amplify the cytotoxic activity of T_C cells, and amplify the innate immune response. T_H cells interact directly with B cells to promote their multiplication and conversion into plasma cells capable of producing antibodies.
- ***Suppressor T cells*** (*T_S* ***cells***), a much smaller subgroup of T cells, are important regulators of immune responses. Suppressor T cells release inhibitory cytokines, which inhibit the activity of other T cells and B cells and limit the extent of the immune response to an antigenic stimulus.

Cytokines

On activation, both effector and regulator T cells synthesize and release soluble proteins known as **cytokines**. Cytokines, essential components of an adequate immune response, are hormone-like polypeptides produced primarily by cells of the immune system. Cytokines are important in amplifying innate immunity and specific immune responses. They stimulate:

- B cells to become plasma cells and produce antibodies
- Attraction and activation of macrophages to become aggressive phagocytes
- Proliferation of cytotoxic T cells and memory helper T cells

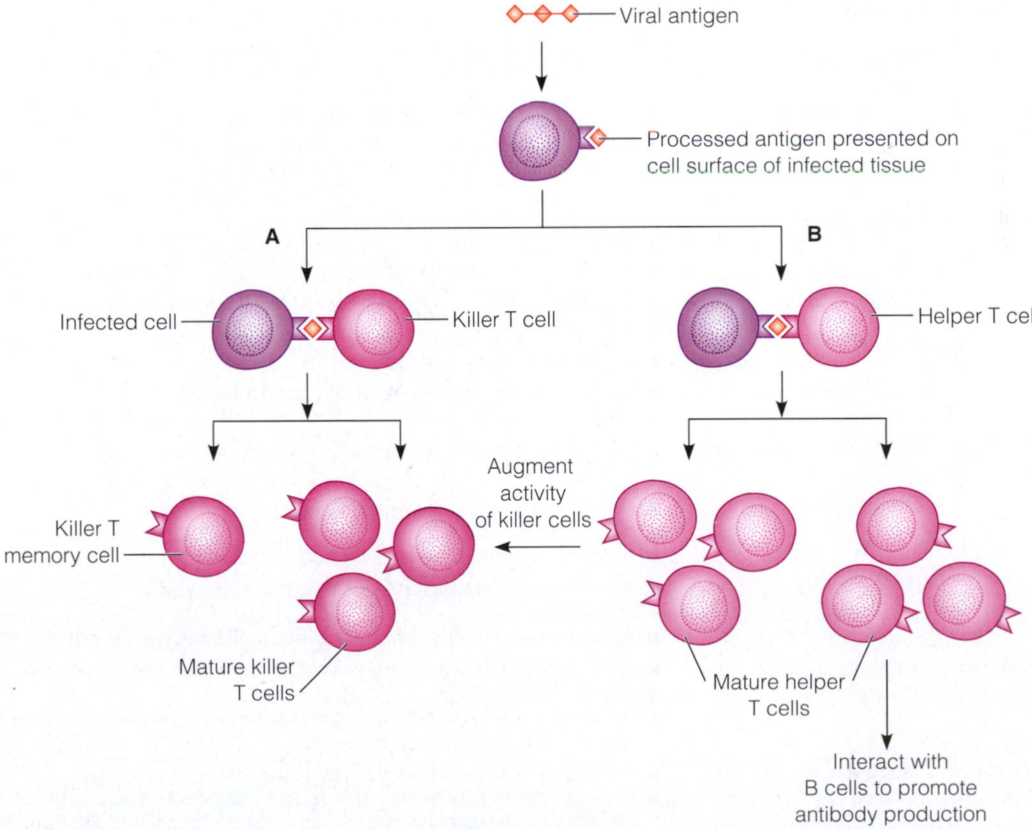

Viral antigen
Processed antigen presented on
cell surface of infected tissue
A
B
Infected cell
Killer T cell
Helper T cell
Augment
activity
of killer cells
Killer T
memory cell
Mature killer
T cells
Mature helper
T cells
Interact with
B cells to promote
antibody production

Figure 12.8 ■ Cellular immune response. **A**, An infected cell, abnormal cell, or phagocyte presents antigen on its surface that binds with a receptor site on a killer T cell or a helper T cell. The killer T cell is activated to proliferate into memory cells or mature cytotoxic cells. **B**, The helper T cell is activated to augment the cytotoxic response and stimulate the antibody-mediated immune response.

- Stimulation of cytotoxic T cells to destroy abnormal cells and pathogens.

Cytokines are also produced in small quantities in many different tissues throughout the body. Cytokines act as messengers of the immune system, facilitating communication between the cells to adjust or vary the inflammatory reaction or to initiate immune cell proliferation and differentiation. The major cytokines and their functions are summarized in **Table 12.4**.

The inflammatory cytokines contribute to illness behaviors. Patients respond to increases in these chemicals with increased sleep, a need to seek warmth, and reduced energy output. These are considered adaptive responses to illness. Interventions to reduce or eliminate the production of certain cytokines are common. Aspirin or NSAIDs to reduce pain and fever are commonly used. Because some cytokines cross the blood–brain barrier, their increase may explain depression and anxiety experienced during illness.

Interferons are a class of cytokine with broad antiviral and anticancer effects. A number of different forms of interferon exist, broadly grouped as alpha, beta, and gamma interferons. Interferon is synthesized by cells infected with a virus and secreted into extracellular fluid. It then binds to specific receptors on uninfected neighboring cells, protecting them from infection. The spread of the virus is thus inhibited and recovery from infection enhanced. It appears that interferons also moderate the activity of NK cells and may be involved in preventing the spread of abnormal malignant cells.

Although T cells are activated by specific antigens, much of the resulting effect is nonspecific—in other words, an enhanced inflammatory response. Like the antibody-mediated response, the cell-mediated response has memory. Subsequent exposures to an antigen result in a more rapid and effective inflammatory response and more effective phagocytosis by macrophages. This memory provides the basis for skin testing. For example, a patient previously exposed to tuberculosis develops a more pronounced inflammatory response when minute amounts of antigen are injected under the skin.

12.2 Acquired Immunity, Immunizations, and Precautions

Immunity

Immunity refers to the protection of the body from disease. Immunity to disease may be natural or acquired, active or passive.

Table 12.4 Major Cytokines and Their Functions

Cytokine	Where Produced	Primary Functions
Interleukin-1 (IL-1)	Monocytes, macrophages, and dendritic cells	■ Activates T and B cells ■ Induces fever and tissue catabolism ■ Enhances NK activity ■ Attracts neutrophils, macrophages, and lymphocytes ■ Stimulates bone marrow and endothelial cell growth, collagen, and collagenases
Interleukin-2 (IL-2)	Helper T cells	■ Stimulates T- and B-cell proliferation ■ Aids in discriminating between self and nonself ■ Activates killer T and NK cells
Interleukin-3 (IL-3)	T cells	■ Stimulates growth and differentiation of bone marrow stem cells
Interleukin-4 (IL-4)	T cells	■ Stimulates proliferation of T cells ■ Increases IgE secretion by B cells
Interleukin-5 (IL-5)	T cells and activated mast cells	■ Promotes differentiation of B cells and eosinophils ■ Stimulates production of IgA
Interleukin-6	T cells and macrophages	■ Pro-inflammatory and anti-inflammatory cytokine ■ Induces fever
Interleukin-8	Macrophages	■ Mediates the innate immune response ■ Induces fever ■ Angiogenic (stimulates vessel formation)
Gamma interferon	T and NK cells	■ Stimulates phagocytosis by neutrophils and macrocytes ■ Activates NK cells ■ Augments B-cell proliferation, enhancing both cellular and humoral immune responses
Alpha and beta interferons	Virus-infected cells; macrophages	■ Activate macrophages and endothelial cells; beta interferon induces fever ■ Augment NK cell activity ■ Act at gene level to protect neighboring cells from invasion by intracellular parasites, such as viruses, rickettsia, and malaria
Macrophage inflammatory proteins (MIP-1-4CC)	Macrophages, dendritic cells, and lymphocytes	■ Chemokines (CC), which are small cytokines ■ Promote inflammatory response, chemotaxis, and homeostasis (control migration of cells in maintenance and development)
Tumor necrosis factor (TNF)	Activated macrophages, T cells, and NK cells	■ Major chemical mediator of inflammatory response ■ Stimulates T-cell activation, antibody production, and accumulation of leukocytes at inflammatory site ■ Directly cytotoxic to some tumor cells ■ Induces fever

Immunity develops from the activation of the body's immune response. Depending on the antigen, antibody-mediated or cell-mediated responses are activated. The immune response typically involves components of both. In the *immunocompetent* (having an immune system capable of responding to pathogens and tissue damage) patient, these responses inactivate and remove the antigen, allowing recovery to occur or preventing the development of disease. Patients with suppressed or impaired immune function are more susceptible to disease and require protection from exposure to environmental elements. Isolation techniques are employed to prevent the spread of disease and to protect immune-suppressed patients.

The processes of antibody-mediated and cell-mediated immunity result in the development of **active immunity**. Active immunity occurs when the body produces antibodies or develops immune lymphocytes against specific antigens. Memory cells, which can produce an immediate immune response on reexposure to the antigen, provide long-term immunity. Active immunity can develop naturally, resulting from contact with the disease-producing antigen and subsequent development of the disease. For many diseases, however, the potential consequences of a single disease episode on the individual and society make prevention desirable, especially for highly contagious diseases capable of causing epidemics. In these instances, immunization or vaccination is used to provide artificially acquired active immunity. The purpose of vaccination is to establish adequate levels of antibody and/or memory cells to provide effective immunity. Vaccination introduces the disease-producing antigen into the body in a manner that will stimulate the immune system to form antibodies and memory cells but will not produce disease. Vaccines may be made of killed organisms or of live organisms that have been *attenuated* or modified to reduce their disease-producing capability. Typhoid is an example of a killed organism vaccine; measles–mumps–rubella (MMR) vaccine, by contrast, is made from attenuated organisms. Many newer vaccines use subunits of the antigen; these are portions of The organism that have antigenic properties but are unable to produce disease.

Passive immunity provides temporary protection against disease-producing antigens. Antibodies produced by other people or animals are the source of passive immunity. These acquired antibodies are used up; they either combine with the antigen or are naturally degraded by the body, and their protection is gradually lost. The transfer of maternal antibodies via the placenta and breast milk to the infant provides naturally acquired passive immunity. Rabies human immune globulin and hepatitis B immune globulin are examples of immunizations used to provide artificially acquired passive immunity. The types of active and passive immunity are summarized in **Table 12.5**.

A number of diagnostic tests can be performed to assess the patient's immune status:

- ***Serum protein*** measures the total protein in the blood, including albumin and globulins. Normal total protein levels for the adult are 6 to 8 g/dL. Total protein levels, albumin, and globulin are decreased in malnutrition and liver disease. Decreased globulin levels are noted with immunologic deficiencies.
- ***Protein electrophoresis*** analyzes protein content, especially for albumin and gamma globulin, and is used to assess immune function. Albumin is approximately 60% (3.2 to 4.5 g/dL) of the total serum protein, and globulins are normally 2.3 to 3.4 g/dL. Gamma globulins subjected to further electrophoresis separate into immunoglobulins: IgA, IgD, IgE, IgG, and IgM (refer to Table 12.3). Analysis of specific levels of each provides clues about the immune status of the patient. IgG levels are increased during acute infection. Decreased levels of IgG, IgA, and IgM are found in malignancies.
- ***Antibody testing*** is ordered to determine if a patient has developed antibodies in response to an infection or immunization. Antibodies for hepatitis, HIV, rubella, varicella (chickenpox), and certain other diseases can be identified. An elevated titer for varicella and rubella indicates immunity. Antibody testing may also be used to determine if the patient has the disease.
- ***Skin testing*** can assess cell-mediated immunity. A known antigen such as tuberculin purified protein derivative (PPD) or candida is injected intradermally. The site is then observed for induration and erythema, which typically peaks at 24 to 48 hours. An induration of at least 10 mm in diameter is a positive reaction indicating previous exposure and sensitization to the antigen. No reaction to common antigens, or **anergy**, indicates depressed cell-mediated immunity.

Table 12.5 Types of Acquired Immunity

Type of Immunity	How It Develops	Examples
Active Immunity		
Natural	Acquired by infection with a pathogen, resulting in the production of antibodies	Chickenpox
Artificial	Acquired by immunization with an antigen, such as an attenuated live virus vaccine	MMR, polio, DPT, hepatitis B vaccines
Passive Immunity		
Natural	Acquired by transfer of maternal antibodies to the fetus or neonate via the placenta or breast milk	Neonate initially protected against MMR if mother immune
Artificial	Acquired by administration of antibodies or antitoxins in immune globulin	Gamma globulin injection following hepatitis A exposure

Immunizations

Vaccines are suspensions of whole or fractionated bacteria or viruses that have been treated to make them nonpathogenic. Vaccines are given to induce an immune response and subsequent immunity. Although vaccine development has been a major factor in improving public health, no vaccine is completely effective or entirely safe. **Table 12.6** outlines the vaccines recommended for the adult patient to maintain optimal health and immune status (Centers for Disease Control and Prevention [CDC], 2018a).

Adults born before 1957 are generally considered to be immune to measles, mumps, and rubella by prior infection. Individuals born after 1956 should have documentation of one or more doses of MMR vaccine unless they have a medical contraindication to the vaccine or laboratory evidence of immunity to the three diseases (CDC, 2018). Adults who only received one dose of varicella (chickenpox) vaccine should receive a second dose. Adults ages 60 and older should receive zoster vaccine regardless of history of chickenpox or herpes zoster (shingles).

Tetanus and diphtheria (Td) toxoids are combined in a single immunization. The vaccine stimulates active immunity by inducing the production of antibodies and antitoxins. After an initial series of three immunizations, a booster injection is recommended every 10 years to maintain

Table 12.6 Recommended Immunizations for Adults

Vaccine	Type	Dose	Indications	Precautions and Nursing Implications
Influenza	Inactivated virus or viral components	0.5 mL IM	Yearly for all adults	Do not administer to acutely ill patients or patients with history of anaphylactic reaction to egg protein.
Tetanus and diphtheria toxoids (Td); pertussis (Tdap)	Inactivated toxins	0.5 mL IM	Initial series of three injections (two doses, 4–6 weeks apart; third dose 6–12 months after dose 2) if never immunized; booster every 10 years; following a major or contaminated wound if >5 years since last booster; replace one booster with Tdap	Should be administered during each pregnancy, preferably between weeks 27 and 36 gestation. Do not administer to patients with a history of anaphylactic reaction to horse serum; administer deep IM in deltoid of dominant arm.
Varicella	Live virus	0.5 mL subcutaneously (subcut)	All adults without evidence of immunity should receive two doses, 4–8 weeks apart, particularly people at high risk for exposure, transmission, or severe disease	Do not administer during pregnancy or to people with a history of life-threatening allergic reaction to the vaccine, gelatin, or neomycin. Use with caution in people who are immunocompromised (e.g., who have HIV or are taking immunosuppressant drugs).
Human papilloma virus (HPV)	Not a live virus	0.5 mL IM	Prior to exposure to HPV through sexual activity	Three doses for males and females ≤26 years; IM in deltoid.
Measles–mumps–rubella (MMR)	Live virus	0.5 mL subcut	All adults born after 1956, particularly those who are at risk for infection, such as college students, military recruits, and those working in a healthcare facility; rubella vaccination recommended for all seronegative females	As a live virus vaccine, should not be administered to pregnant women or immunocompromised patients. Do not administer to patients with a history of anaphylactic reaction to egg protein or neomycin. Give subcutaneously in fatty tissue over triceps.
Zoster (shingles)	Attenuated live virus (Zostavax®) Recombinant DNA (not live) (Shingrix®)	0.65 mL subcut	Adults 60 years or older including those who report having had shingles	Give Zostavax in fatty tissue over triceps. Give Singrix into deltoid muscle (IM). Do not administer during pregnancy or to immunocompromised or HIV-infected individuals. Cannot be used in children or in place of varicella vaccine.
Hepatitis A	Inactivated whole virus	1 mL IM	People with liver disease or who receive clotting factors; travel to areas with high endemicity; illicit drug use or men who have sex with men	Give IM in deltoid.
Hepatitis B (HB)	Inactive viral antigen	1.0 mL IM	Series of three doses: Initial and at 1 and 6 months; recommended for anyone at risk for exposure and for postexposure prophylaxis	Use with caution in pregnant or lactating females, older patients, and patients with active infection; have epinephrine 1:1000 available on unit in case of anaphylaxis and laryngospasm.
Pneumococcal	Bacterial polysaccharides	0.5 mL IM or subcut	One dose for patients over age 65 and those at risk for pneumococcal pneumonia, including patients with chronic lung disease or other chronic diseases	Do not administer to pregnant women.
Meningococcal vaccine	Inactive bacterial antigens	0.5 mL IM	College students living in dormitories and military recruits	Give in deltoid muscle; individuals previously diagnosed with Guillain-Barré syndrome should not receive this vaccine.

protection. Older patients, particularly those who never entered the workforce (e.g., older female adults), may have never received the initial series of Td vaccine. A resurgence of active cases of pertussis among adults and children has led the CDC to recommend that all adults under age 65 years and older adults (of any age) who have close contact with infants younger than 12 months receive one dose of tetanus/diphtheria/pertussis (Tdap) vaccine.

Hepatitis B (HB) vaccine is mandated by the Occupational Safety and Health Administration (OSHA) for healthcare workers and public safety workers. It is also recommended for people newly diagnosed with diabetes mellitus who are under age 60 years and for those in high-risk populations. High-risk populations include intravenous drug users, sexual partners of infected individuals, and patients on dialysis, have chronic liver disease, or are infected with HIV.

Influenza vaccine is now recommended annually for all adults. The antigenic strains included in the influenza vaccine vary each year, according to the predicted predominant strains affecting the population; therefore, yearly reimmunization is required. Pneumococcal vaccine is recommended for older adults, people living with chronic disease or who are immunosuppressed, and individuals who smoke cigarettes. Revaccination 5 years after the initial dose of pneumococcal vaccine may be recommended for some people. Pneumococcal vaccine for all senior citizens is a U.S. public health and Medicare goal. The purpose of immunization is to prevent respiratory infections and hospitalizations.

Human papillomavirus (HPV) vaccine has been shown to significantly reduce the risk for cervical and other cancers. HPV is recommended for all previously unvaccinated men and women through age 26 years. Other vaccines such as hepatitis A and meningococcal vaccine may be given if other risk factors are present, for example, occupational risk factors.

In addition to routine immunizations, people traveling outside the United States and Canada should receive vaccines against diseases that are endemic in certain regions of the world.

Other immunologic substances may be administered as indicated. Immune globulins provide passive immunity as protection against a known or potential exposure to an antigen. Standard immune globulin is given to household contacts of patients with hepatitis A and individuals traveling to areas in which hepatitis A is endemic. Hepatitis B immune globulin (HBIG) contains higher titers of antibody to hepatitis B virus and is used for individuals exposed by blood or sexual contact, providing immediate protection. HBIG does not provide the longer term protection of the hepatitis B vaccine. Following confirmed or suspected contact with a pathogen, selected vaccines may be administered to stimulate an immediate immune response.

For most vaccines, a sensitivity test should be performed prior to administration to detect sensitivity to substances such as horse serum or eggs. The substance is injected intradermally; if after 20 minutes there is no evidence of a reaction, the selected vaccine can be administered.

Moderate to severe local reactions may occur following administration of an immunization. Common reactions include redness, swelling, tenderness, and muscle ache. Administering the vaccine in the dominant arm of the patient helps minimize local reactions because use and movement of the arm facilitates absorption of the solution. Applying heat to the site is also beneficial. Occasionally local ulcerations occur; when they do, warm, wet pack, or sterile wet-to-dry dressings may be prescribed.

Nursing Care

Maintaining a population that is fully immunized against common, potentially epidemic, and devastating diseases is a major public health task for nursing. Nurses not only recommend and administer vaccines to individual patients and their families, but also plan and implement preventative care for whole communities.

Although this process may appear to be straightforward, multiple issues affect society's ability to immunize the entire population. For some people, for example, religious beliefs may preclude the use of immunizations to prevent disease. Also, people who are not citizens and the medically indigent population have difficulty accessing immunization services. Lack of immunization not only puts the individual at increased risk for infectious disease, but also increases the cost of medical services and the possibility of exposing immunocompromised people to disease.

In the public health setting, the nurse looks at the immunization needs and illness risk for an entire community. Communities include not only cities and localities but also groups of people, such as college populations and employees in a workplace. Public education needs may be met through presentations to groups of people, feature articles in newspapers and other local publications, advertising, radio presentations and public service announcements, and one-to-one discussion and teaching.

Assessment

Collect the following data through the health history and physical examination. Further focused assessments are described with nursing interventions in the next section.

- *Health history:* Age, medication use (corticosteroids and antibiotics) and blood transfusion, nutrition, known allergies, pregnancy status, infection, immunizations, autoimmune disorders, chronic diseases such as asthma, diabetes mellitus, cancer, smoking history
- *Physical assessment:* Skin lesions or rashes, breath sounds, respiratory rate.

Priorities of Care

Nursing care focuses on promoting immunity while preventing injury from the immunization and educating the patient. See the accompanying Case Study & Nursing Care Plan.

Diagnoses, Outcomes, and Interventions

Provide Education Regarding Vaccinations. For individual patients and their families, nurses promote immunocompetence by assessing immune status, recommending appropriate immunizations, and administering vaccines as ordered or indicated. Once an individual reaches adulthood, routine immunizations often become a neglected part of healthcare.

Expected Outcome: Verbalizes understanding of the purposes for, risks of, and schedules of recommended immunizations based on health needs.

The nurse will:

- Determine knowledge level, understanding, attitudes, and religious beliefs about immunization. *This provides a basis for further education and determines if religious beliefs may contraindicate immunization.*
- Discuss the value and reasons for recommended immunizations. *Understanding promotes adherence.*
- Reinforce positive health-seeking behaviors. *This will help promote future health maintenance activities.*
- Using recommended immunization schedules, develop a plan to attain optimal immunization status. *Adherence with recommended schedules for immunization is important in preventing disease and disability.*
- Do not administer influenza vaccine if the patient is allergic to eggs or tetanus antitoxin if sensitive to horse serum. *Vaccines prepared from chicken or duck embryos are contraindicated in patients who are allergic to eggs. Tetanus antitoxin is prepared from horse serum. Both will cause a severe allergic reaction.*
- Withhold administration of active immunologic products in the presence of an upper respiratory infection or other infection. *Active immunizations can cause a greater inflammatory reaction in the presence of infections.*
- Do not administer oral polio vaccine, MMR, or any live virus vaccine to immunosuppressed patients or to patients who are in close household contact with an immunosuppressed person. *Live virus vaccines can cause disease in the immunosuppressed patient. The virus may be transmitted from close household contacts during the initial postvaccination period.*
- Do not administer vaccines such as MMR, pneumococcal, or varicella to women who are pregnant. *Although the risk to the developing fetus is greatest during the first trimester, these vaccines are avoided throughout pregnancy.*
- Do not administer live attenuated virus vaccines and passive immunizations such as gamma globulin simultaneously. *Passive antibodies interfere with the response of the live attenuated virus.*
- Prior to administering the prescribed vaccine, check the expiration date and manufacturer's instructions. *Outdated vaccines cannot provide adequate immunization protection. Certain injection sites have better absorption than others.*
- Keep epinephrine 1:1000 readily available for subcutaneous injection when administering immunizations. *Epinephrine causes vasoconstriction and reduces laryngospasm; in acute anaphylaxis, it can be lifesaving.*

SAFETY ALERT: Observe the patient for 20 to 30 minutes following vaccine administration to monitor for possible adverse reactions. ■

Clinically important medical events including fever, injection-site hypersensitivity, unspecified rash, and injection-site edema that occur after vaccination should be reported to the Vaccine Adverse Event Reporting System (VAERS) by calling 1-800-822-7967 or by using the VAERS website. This report needs to be made even if the reporting person is not certain the event was caused by the vaccine. Approximately 85 to 90% of all reports describe mild side effects, with the remaining being serious adverse events, including life-threatening illness, hospitalization or prolongation of hospitalization, permanent disability, or death (CDC, 2017a).

Helpful resources include state and county health departments, the CDC, and the National Institute of Allergy and Infectious Diseases.

Case Study & Nursing Care Plan

A Patient with Acquired Immunity

Terry Adams is a 48-year-old executive who is planning a trip to Central Africa. In preparation, he contacts his local healthcare provider to obtain the necessary immunizations. Jane Wong, the registered nurse in the clinic, obtains a nursing history of Mr. Adams.

ASSESSMENT	DIAGNOSES	EXPECTED OUTCOMES
Mr. Adams's history reveals that he has always been very healthy and active, apart from mild asthma experienced during childhood. Mr. Adams has not seen a physician since recovering from an episode of hepatitis A more than 5 years ago and is unsure when he last received any immunizations. He does not know if he had all recommended childhood immunizations. His physical examination reveals an alert and healthy individual with no abnormalities noted. His vital signs are T 36.3°C (97.4°F), P 64 bpm, R 14/min, and BP 142/82 mmHg. The physician orders the following immunizations for Mr. Adams: ■ Measles–mumps–rubella (MMR) ■ Combined tetanus and diphtheria toxoids with pertussis (Tdap) ■ Yellow fever vaccine ■ Typhoid vaccine ■ Meningococcal meningitis vaccine.	■ Needs immunizations for international travel ■ Potential for adverse response to immunizations	■ Patient will obtain necessary immunizations. ■ Patient will verbalize a schedule for maintaining up-to-date immunization status. ■ Patient will experience no significant adverse effects from immunization.

PLANNING AND IMPLEMENTATION

- Administer MMR, Tdap, and meningococcal meningitis vaccines prior to discharge from clinic.
- Observe closely for 30 minutes following immunization for potential adverse responses.
- Schedule return visit in 1 week for typhoid vaccine.
- Provide referral to a registered vaccination center for yellow fever vaccine and documentation of vaccination.
- Provide instructions for comfort measures to relieve local and systemic adverse effects of vaccines.
- Provide written instructions on manifestations that should be reported to the physician.
- Document immunizations on a permanent record at the clinic and for the patient.

EVALUATION

Mr. Adams completes his prescribed immunizations without major adverse effects, although he does complain of mild fever, malaise, and general achiness for several days following the typhoid vaccination. His trip to Africa is successful, and he returns to the United States without contracting any infectious diseases.

CLINICAL REASONING IN PATIENT CARE

1. Explain the concept of *herd immunity* and why it is important for adults to continue receiving immunizations throughout their lifespan.
2. If a patient says to you, "I don't believe in immunizations; I hear they are dangerous and cause autism in children," how would you respond?
3. What manifestations would cause a patient to contact his or her primary caregiver after receiving an immunization? What is the rationale for the need to do this?

See Evaluating Your Response in Appendix B.

Isolation Precautions

Controlling the spread of infectious diseases in the hospital or long-term care setting is particularly important to preventing healthcare-associated infections. Hand hygiene remains the single most important factor in preventing the transmission of infections. Most infectious diseases are transmitted by either direct or indirect contact and their spread is prevented through the use of standard precautions. However, diseases such as chickenpox (varicella) are highly contagious and are spread by the airborne route, requiring special precautions to protect other hospitalized patients.

In determining the need for transmission-based precautions, healthcare personnel consider the usual reservoir or source of the microorganism, the mode of transmission, and the susceptibility of hospital staff and other patients. For example, patients with *P. jiroveci* pneumonia do not require isolation because immunocompetent individuals are not susceptible to this infection.

The CDC (2017d) has published guidelines for isolation precautions to be used in healthcare facilities. These guidelines include both *standard precautions* and *transmission-based* (or *category-specific*) *precautions*.

Standard Precautions

Standard precautions, published by the Hospital Infection Control Practices Advisory Committee of the Centers for Disease Control in 1996, provides guidelines for the handling of blood and other body fluids. These guidelines are used with all patients, regardless of whether they have a known infectious disease. The guidelines were developed in light of the realization that many patients with an infectious disease such as HIV or hepatitis B have no apparent manifestations, but can transmit the disease to others. Standard precautions are used by all healthcare workers who have direct or indirect contact with patients or with their body fluids. Activities involving indirect contact include such tasks as emptying trash, changing linens, or cleaning the room.

Standard precautions apply to the following:

- Blood
- All body fluids, secretions, and excretions, regardless of whether they contain visible blood
- Nonintact skin
- Mucous membranes.

Barrier protection is used to prevent exposing skin and mucous membrane surfaces to blood and body fluids. Barrier protection involves using gloves for touching or handling body fluids and adding other protection such as gowns, masks, and goggles if splashing or spraying is likely. Use of aseptic technique, sterile single-use disposable needles and syringes, and single-use vials for preparing and administering parenteral medications is emphasized. Needles and other sharp objects are not recapped or bent, but disposed of in puncture-proof containers to prevent inadvertent percutaneous (needlestick) exposure. Respiratory hygiene/cough etiquette is a recent addition to standard precautions (CDC, 2017d). Standard precautions are presented in Appendix A.

Transmission-Based Precautions

In addition to hand hygiene and standard precautions, the nature and spread of some infectious diseases require

Table 12.7 Transmission-Based Precautions

Infectious Diseases	Purpose	Precautions
Airborne Precautions		
Pulmonary tuberculosis, chickenpox (with contact precautions), measles	Reduce risk of airborne transmission of infectious agents. Airborne transmission occurs by dissemination of either airborne droplet nuclei or particles containing the infectious agent.	Private room with handwashing and toilet facilities and special ventilation that does not allow air to circulate to general facility ventilation; mask or special filter respirator for everyone entering room
Droplet Precautions		
Meningitis, pertussis, influenza	Reduce risk of droplet transmission of infectious agents. Droplet transmission involves contact of mucosal surfaces with respiratory droplets generated during coughing, sneezing, talking, or procedures such as suctioning.	Private room with handwashing and toilet facilities; mask, eye protection, and/or face shields worn by everyone entering room
Contact Precautions		
Acute diarrhea, chickenpox (with airborne precautions), respiratory syncytial virus (RSV); skin, wound, or urinary tract infection with multidrug-resistant organisms; *S. aureus* infections; scabies infestation	Reduce risk of transmission by direct or indirect contact. Direct contact transmission involves physical transfer of organisms from skin or blood. Indirect contact involves contact with a contaminated object.	Private room with handwashing and toilet facilities; gowns and protective apparel to provide barrier protection; disposable supplies or decontamination of all articles leaving room

that special techniques be used to protect uninfected patients and workers. The CDC identifies three types of transmission-based precautions: Airborne, droplet, and contact precautions. Transmission-based precautions may be combined for diseases that have multiple routes of transmission. Indications for the use of transmission-based isolation precautions and the specific measures to be taken are outlined in **Table 12.7**.

12.3 Patients with Inflammation and Infection

Inflammation is a nonspecific response to injury that serves to destroy, dilute, or contain the injurious agent or damaged tissue. Inflammation may be either acute or chronic. Acute inflammation is a short-term reaction of the body to all types of tissue damage. It is immediate and aimed at protecting the body and preventing further invasion or injury. Acute inflammation usually lasts less than 1 to 2 weeks. Once the injurious agent is removed, the inflammation subsides. Healing with tissue repair or scar formation occurs, and the body functions in normal or near-normal capacity.

Chronic inflammation is slower in onset and may not have an acute phase. Its clinical manifestations occur over months or years. While the effects of some chronic inflammatory processes may be evident (such as the joint damage and destruction associated with rheumatoid arthritis), the role chronic inflammation plays in diseases such as asthma, obesity, and heart disease has only recently been recognized.

The Patient with Tissue Inflammation

Pathophysiology and Manifestations

The tissue damage that evokes an inflammatory response may be caused by specific or nonspecific agents. These agents may be *exogenous*, from outside the body, or *endogenous*, from within the body. Causes of inflammation include:

- Mechanical injuries, such as cuts or surgical incisions
- Physical damage, such as burns
- Chemical injury from toxins or poisons
- Microorganisms, such as bacteria, viruses, or fungi
- Extremes of heat or cold
- Immunologic responses, such as hypersensitivity reactions
- Ischemic damage or trauma, such as a stroke or myocardial infarction.

Acute Inflammation

Regardless of the cause, location, or extent of the injury, the acute inflammatory response follows the previously outlined sequence of vascular response, cellular and phagocytic response, and healing.

Many of the manifestations of inflammation are produced by inflammatory mediators, such as histamine and prostaglandins, which are released when tissue is damaged (refer to Box 12.1). The primary manifestations of inflammation include:

- Erythema (redness)
- Local heat caused by increased blood flow to the injured area (hyperemia)
- Swelling due to accumulated fluid at the site
- Pain from tissue swelling and chemical irritation of nerve endings
- Loss of function caused by swelling and pain.

The degree of functional loss depends on the location and extent of the injury. With increased tissue damage, more fluid exudate is formed, resulting in increased swelling, pain, and functional impairment. Pain may be immediate or delayed. Prostaglandins intensify and prolong the pain. Kinins cause irritation to the nerve endings and contribute to the pain sensation.

Dead neutrophils, necrotic tissue, and (if the tissue is infected) digested bacteria accumulate as a result of inflammation and phagocytosis, forming *pus*. Pus usually forms and remains until after the infection subsides. Pus may push itself to the surface of the body or become internalized. In the latter case, pus is gradually autolyzed (self-digested) by enzymes over a period of days. The end product is then absorbed by the body. On occasion, pus may remain after the infection is resolved. An **abscess**, or localized collection of pus, may form, necessitating *incision and drainage (I&D)*, surgical removal of the pus.

Systemic responses to inflammation include lymph node swelling (*lymphadenopathy*) due to the proliferation of macrophages within the nodes in response to microorganisms in the lymph. Enlarged lymph nodes are usually noted in the groin, axillae, and neck. Fever, often precipitated by inflammatory mediators or bacterial toxins, inhibits the growth of many microorganisms and increases tissue repair functions. Loss of appetite and fatigue may occur in the effort to conserve energy during the inflammatory process. Leukocytosis occurs with increased WBC production to support inflammation and phagocytosis.

Chronic Inflammation

Whereas acute inflammation is a self-limiting process lasting less than 2 weeks, chronic inflammation tends to be self-perpetuating, lasting weeks to months or years. Chronic inflammation may develop when the acute inflammatory process has been ineffective in removing the offending agent. Persistent low-grade infection or irritation by chemicals, particulate matter, or physical irritants such as talc, asbestos, or silica may also result in chronic inflammation.

Granulomatous Inflammation. *Granulomatous inflammation* is characterized by dense infiltration of the site by lymphocytes and macrophages. The macrophages mass to surround the site; they in turn are surrounded by lymphocytes and other immune cells, forming a lesion called a *granuloma*. The granuloma isolates the offending agent from the rest of the body; however, the infectious agent or irritant may not be destroyed and can survive within the granuloma for a long period of time. Chronic inflammation and granuloma formation are common with *Mycobacterium tuberculosis* infection. The granuloma formed in tuberculosis is called a tubercle. *M. tuberculosis* can survive for many years within the tubercle, emerging when the patient's immune system is no longer able to contain it.

Nonspecific Chronic Inflammation. *Nonspecific chronic inflammation* is implicated in such disorders as pulmonary airway disease (asthma and chronic obstructive lung disease), cardiovascular disease, and autoimmune disorders such as inflammatory bowel disease (Garlough, 2017). This type of chronic inflammation is characterized by diffuse accumulation of macrophages and proliferation of fibroblasts in response to ongoing chemotaxis. The fibroblasts and fibrocytes, unique cells formed from monocytes, lead to formation of excessive fibrous connective tissue disrupting normal tissue function (Nasef, Mehta, & Ferguson, 2017). Inflammatory markers such as C-reactive protein, complement components, and inflammatory cytokines are present in chronic inflammation and associated disorders (Lubbers et al., 2017; Luo et al., 2017; Nasef et al., 2017; Wirtz & Kanel, 2017).

Complications

Inflammation and wound healing are highly metabolic processes that may be affected by a number of factors. Without adequate nutrition, blood supply, and oxygenation, tissues cannot effectively complete the process. Impaired inflammatory and immune processes can interfere with phagocytosis and preparation of the wound for healing. Infection prolongs the inflammatory process and delays healing.

Chronic diseases may also impair healing. High blood glucose levels and small blood vessel disease associated with diabetes mellitus impair chemotactic and phagocytic function. Collagen formation and tensile strength of the wound are also impaired. Arterial and venous disorders impair the delivery of oxygen and nutrients to healing tissues, as well as the removal of toxins, bacteria, and other waste products from the area. Drug therapy, particularly corticosteroid medications, may suppress the immune and inflammatory responses, delaying healing. Other external factors, such as exposure to ionizing radiation and wound cleansing agents, can also affect healing. **Table 12.8** summarizes major factors that affect the inflammatory process and wound healing.

Finally, there is growing evidence of the role chronic inflammation plays in diseases such as asthma, chronic obstructive lung disease, obesity, coronary heart disease, heart failure, and inflammatory bowel disease.

Interprofessional Care

Management of the patient with inflamed tissue focuses on promoting healing. Care is generally supportive, allowing the patient's own physiologic processes to remove foreign matter and damaged cells. Wound care may involve only

Table 12.8 Factors That May Impair Healing

Factor	Effect
Malnutrition	
Protein deficit	Prolongs inflammation and impairs healing process.
Carbohydrate and kilocalorie deficit	Impairs metabolic processes and promotes catabolism; proteins are used for energy rather than for healing.
Fat deficit	Impairs cell membrane synthesis in tissue repair.
Vitamin deficits	
Vitamin A	Limits epithelialization and capillary formation.
B-complex	Inhibits enzymatic reactions that contribute to wound healing.
Vitamin C	Impairs collagen synthesis.
Tissue hypoxia	Increases the risk of infection and impaired healing because oxygen is required to support cell function and collagen synthesis.
Impaired blood supply	Results in inadequate delivery of oxygen and nutrients to healing tissues and removal of waste products.
Impaired inflammatory and immune processes	Result in decreased phagocytosis and wound debridement; increased risk of infection; delayed healing.

simple cleaning or may require irrigations and debridement. The patient is encouraged to rest, to increase fluid intake, and to eat a well-balanced, nutritious diet. Antibiotics may be prescribed to help eliminate infectious causes of inflammation.

Diagnosis

The following diagnostic tests may be ordered to identify the source and extent of inflammation:

- *WBC with differential* provides information about the type and extent of inflammatory response. The differential count (the percentage of the total WBC made up by each type of leukocyte) provides further clues about inflammatory processes (**Table 12.9**).
- *Erythrocyte sedimentation rate (ESR)* is a nonspecific test to detect inflammation. The rate at which RBCs fall to the bottom of a vertical tube is an indicator of inflammation. An increased ESR may indicate acute or chronic inflammation.
- *C-reactive protein (CRP) test* is used to detect this glycoprotein produced by the liver and excreted into the bloodstream during the acute phase of an inflammatory process. The expected result of this test is negative for CRP. A positive result indicates an acute or chronic inflammatory process.

In addition, blood and other body fluids may be cultured to determine if infection is the cause of inflammation.

Medications

Although inflammation is a beneficial process to prepare acutely injured tissue for healing, its manifestations can be distressing. Chronic inflammation can lead to tissue damage and scarring, with resulting loss of function. Anti-inflammatory medications may be prescribed to manage these effects. Anti-inflammatory medications fall into three broad groups: Salicylates, such as aspirin; other NSAIDs; and corticosteroids.

Aspirin (acetylsalicylic acid, or ASA) has antipyretic, analgesic, and antiplatelet effects. Its beneficial effects are largely dose related. Low doses (as little as 81 mg/day) inhibit platelet aggregation and normal blood clotting. A 650-mg dose of aspirin is an effective analgesic and antipyretic. To relieve pain, aspirin acts primarily on peripheral sensory nerves by inhibiting the synthesis of prostaglandins and kinins, which are chemical stimuli of sensory nerves. As an antipyretic, aspirin acts both centrally and peripherally. It inhibits the formation of pyrogenic substances that raise the hypothalamic thermostat. It also dilates peripheral blood vessels and promotes diaphoresis, increasing the dissipation of heat (Adams, Holland, & Urban, 2017). Higher doses (650 to 1000 mg four to five times per day) are required to produce aspirin's anti-inflammatory effects. In therapeutic doses, aspirin mediates the inflammatory process by inhibiting the enzyme cyclooxygenase (COX) and preventing synthesis of prostaglandins. Inflammation is reduced, along with the swelling, redness, and impaired function that accompanies it.

The other NSAIDs have activity similar to that of aspirin. They inhibit COX and prostaglandin synthesis, reducing the inflammatory and pain response. Each NSAID has a slightly different mode of action; sometimes several different agents must be tried before the most effective is identified. Side effects also differ to a certain extent; however, all have a potential cross-sensitivity with aspirin, all irritate the gastrointestinal tract, and all are associated with an increased risk for cardiovascular events. NSAIDs are also more costly than aspirin, but they have a longer duration of action; therefore, fewer daily doses are required to achieve the desired effect.

For acute hypersensitivity reactions, such as reactions to poison ivy, or for inflammation that cannot be managed using NSAIDs, corticosteroid therapy may be prescribed. The glucocorticoids are hormones produced by the adrenal cortex that have widespread effects on metabolism and the immune response. Glucocorticoids inhibit inflammation and

Table 12.9 The White Blood Cell Count and Differential

Cell Type and Normal Value	Increased	Decreased
Total WBCs: 4,000 to 10,000 per mm^3	*Leukocytosis:* Infection or inflammation, leukemia, trauma or stress, tissue necrosis	*Leukopenia:* Bone marrow depression, overwhelming infection, viral infections, immunosuppression, autoimmune disease, dietary deficiency
Neutrophils (segs, PMNs, or polys): 55–70%	*Neutrophilia:* Acute infection or stress response, myelocytic leukemia, inflammatory or metabolic disorders	*Neutropenia:* Bone marrow depression, overwhelming bacterial infection, viral infection, Addison disease
Eosinophils (eos): 1–4%	*Eosinophilia:* Parasitic infections, hypersensitivity reactions, autoimmune disorders	*Eosinopenia:* Cushing syndrome, autoimmune disorders, stress, certain drugs
Basophils (basos): 0.5–1%	*Basophilia:* Hypersensitivity responses, chronic myelogenous leukemia, chickenpox or smallpox, splenectomy, hypothyroidism	*Basopenia:* Acute stress or hypersensitivity reactions, hyperthyroidism
Monocytes (monos): 2–8%	*Monocytosis:* Chronic inflammatory disorders, tuberculosis, viral infections, leukemia, Hodgkin lymphoma, multiple myeloma	*Monocytopenia:* Bone marrow depression, corticosteroid therapy
Lymphocytes (lymphs): 20–40%	*Lymphocytosis:* Chronic bacterial infection, viral infections, lymphocytic leukemia	*Lymphocytopenia:* Bone marrow depression, immunodeficiency, leukemia, Cushing syndrome, Hodgkin lymphoma, renal failure

may be lifesaving in acute or chronic progressive inflammation. When glucocorticoids are prescribed to manage inflammation, the smallest possible effective dose is used. Whenever possible, a local-acting preparation such as a topical agent, metered-dose inhaler, or intra-articular injection is prescribed to minimize systemic effects of the drug. The incidence of potentially harmful side effects increases with higher doses and prolonged therapy. Wound healing is impaired, and the metabolism of fats, proteins, and carbohydrates is altered. Blood glucose control is impaired. Fat distribution changes, producing a cushingoid appearance with a moon face, increased truncal fat, and "buffalo hump." Fluid retention and hypertension are potential problems, as are osteoporosis, gastrointestinal bleeding, and emotional disturbances.

Acetaminophen (Tylenol) may be administered to reduce the fever and pain associated with inflammation. It has no anti-inflammatory effect and will not reduce the inflammation, but can relieve associated manifestations such as fever and pain.

Antibiotics may be used either prophylactically to prevent infection from interfering with the healing process of damaged tissue or therapeutically to treat the infection. If infection is present, the organism and its response or sensitivity to various antibiotics is used to guide therapy. Antibiotic therapy is discussed in the section of this chapter on infectious diseases.

Nutrition

Healing depends on cell replication, protein synthesis, and the function of specific organs—the liver, heart, and lungs in particular. Malnutrition and protein depletion are risk factors for poor healing and wound complications. Illness produces protein catabolism resulting in a loss of up to 0.5 kg of lean muscle mass daily (Mason, 2016). The patient with an inflammatory process or healing wound requires a well-balanced diet of sufficient kilocalories to meet the metabolic needs of the body (refer to Table 12.8). Inflammation often produces catabolism, a state in which body tissues are broken down. By contrast, healing is a process of anabolism or building-up. Without sufficient kilocalories and nutrients, catabolism may dominate, impairing healing.

Adequate protein is necessary for tissue healing and the production of antibodies and WBCs. Lack of adequate protein increases the risk of infection. Complete protein sources, those that provide the essential amino acids, are preferred. Carbohydrates are important to meet energy demands, as well as to support leukocyte function. Care is taken to avoid hyperglycemia in patients with diabetes, however. Hyperglycemia interferes with oxygen delivery to the tissues as well as with the chemotactic and phagocytic function of neutrophils, impairing healing. Dietary fats are used in the synthesis of cell membranes.

Vitamins A, B complex, C, and K are also important to the healing process. Vitamin A is necessary for capillary formation and epithelialization. B-complex vitamins promote wound healing, and vitamin C is necessary for collagen synthesis. Vitamin K provides a vital component for the synthesis of clotting factors in the liver.

Although it has been established that minerals contribute to the inflammatory and healing processes, less is known about required amounts. Minerals serve important roles in maintaining normal cell function and as cofactors in enzyme reactions necessary for cell proliferation. Zinc is instrumental in protein and carbohydrate metabolism as well as maintaining the integrity of cell membranes (Jaffe & Wu, 2017).

Oxygen is another important element in healing. It is necessary for collagen synthesis. Phagocytes such as neutrophils and macrophages require oxygen to digest bacteria engulfed in the phagocytic process. Impaired oxygen delivery to the tissues slows healing and increases the risk for infection. Supplemental oxygen administered via nasal cannula or mask improves the oxygen saturation of hemoglobin and its availability to tissues. Hyperbaric oxygen delivery improves leukocyte and fibroblast function as well as the development of new blood vessels and may be beneficial to promote healing of inflamed ischemic tissues (Lam, Fontaine, Ross, & Chiu, 2017).

Nursing Care

Acute inflammation may be self-limiting or extensive and require hospitalization. Nursing care includes teaching patients with acute and chronic inflammatory conditions self-management at home.

Assessment

The following data are collected through the health history and physical examination. Further focused assessments are described with nursing interventions in the next section.

- *Health history:* Risk factors, nutrition, medication use (anti-inflammatory and corticosteroids), location, duration, and type (redness, heat, pain, swelling, and impaired function) of manifestations
- *Physical assessment:* Movement of injured area, pain, circulation, wounds, lymph nodes.

Priorities of Care

Nursing care priorities focus on relieving pain due to the inflammatory response, supporting tissue healing, and preventing infection.

Diagnoses, Outcomes, and Interventions

The nursing care needs of the patient with an inflammation are related to the manifestations of the inflammation and resulting altered tissue integrity.

Manage Pain. Along with redness, warmth, swelling, and impaired function, pain is one of the primary manifestations of inflammation. Depending on the cause, affected area, and degree of inflammation, pain may be acute and immobilizing or chronic and demoralizing. It is important to remember that pain is a subjective experience and that patient responses to pain vary.

Expected Outcome: Patient's pain will be alleviated to an acceptable level of comfort as defined by the patient.

The nurse will:

- Assess pain using a scale of 0 to 10, with 0 being no pain and 10 being the worst pain; note the character, location, and duration of the pain. *Because pain is subjective, the patient provides the most accurate information regarding his or her pain experience.*

- Use physical and nonverbal cues to further assess the level of pain. *This intervention is especially important if the patient is nonverbal or tends to underreport pain.*
- Administer anti-inflammatory medications as prescribed. *These medications help to reduce the pain resulting from acute inflammation. Most NSAIDs also have analgesic and antipyretic effects, further promoting comfort* (Adams et al., 2017).
- Administer analgesic medications as prescribed. *Moderate to severe pain may require treatment with an analgesic (e.g., an opioid drug). Acetaminophen and opioid analgesics act within the CNS to reduce pain. Opioids provide the most effective pain relief overall, activating pain-inhibitory neurons and inhibiting pain-transmission neurons* (Miner & Burton, 2018).

SAFETY ALERT: Because opioids can depress respirations, it is important to monitor oxygen saturation and encourage the patient to take deep breaths to keep oxygen saturation adequate. ■

- Provide comfort measures, such as back rubs, position changes, or relaxation techniques. *These measures reduce muscle tension, relieve areas of pressure, and provide distraction.*
- Encourage activities such as reading, watching television, and taking part in social interactions. *Such activities provide distraction from the pain experience.*
- Encourage rest. *Strenuous activity or exercising an inflamed body part may increase discomfort and tissue damage.*
- Provide cold or heat as pain relief measures, as ordered. *For an acute injury, cold reduces swelling and relieves pain; after the initial stage, heat increases blood flow to the affected tissue and relieves pain and swelling by promoting absorption of edema. Do not apply either heat or cold for more than 20 minutes at a time and ensure there is a covering between the patient and the application.*

SAFETY ALERT: Use heat or cold application cautiously in older patients who have fragile skin and are at risk for tissue injury. ■

- Elevate the inflamed area, if possible. *Elevation promotes venous return and reduces swelling.*
- Teach about the appropriate use and expected effects of anti-inflammatory medications. *If the patient's pain continues after the initial doses of anti-inflammatory medication, he or she may become discouraged and stop taking the medication before it becomes fully effective.*

Promote Good Tissue Integrity. The inflammatory response can either precipitate or result from impairment of the integrity of skin or other tissues.

Expected Outcome: Patient's tissue integrity will be maintained or restored.

The nurse will:

- Assess general health and nutritional status. *Poor general health or chronic diseases such as diabetes mellitus or renal failure interfere with the healing processes and increase the risk of infection.*
- Assess circulation to the affected area. *Adequate tissue perfusion and oxygenation are necessary for healing* (Sorenson et al., 2019).
- Monitor the skin and surrounding tissue for increased manifestations of inflammation. *Inflammation can spread to adjacent tissues, leading to conditions such as cellulitis.*
- Provide protection and support for inflamed tissue. *This reduces discomfort and decreases the risk of further tissue damage.*
- Clean inflamed tissue gently; if possible, use water, normal saline, or nontoxic wound cleansers. *Soap and harsh cleansers such as povidone-iodine (Betadine) and hydrogen peroxide can cause further drying and tissue damage. Granulation tissue in a healing wound is fragile and easily damaged.*
- Keep the inflamed area dry, and expose it to air as much as possible. *This promotes healing and helps prevent infection.*
- Balance rest with activity. *Rest decreases metabolic demands and allows for cell regeneration, while mobility helps to promote oxygenation and perfusion of the tissues.*
- Provide supplemental oxygen as ordered. *Supplemental oxygen improves tissue oxygenation and reduces hypoxia.*
- Provide a well-balanced diet with adequate kilocalories to meet the body's metabolic and healing needs. If the patient is allowed nothing by mouth (NPO), suggest parenteral or enteral nutrition. For the patient who is unable to consume an adequate diet, consult with a dietitian for between-meal supplements and/or multivitamin supplements. *Careful attention to diet and nutrient intake is important to provide the nutrients necessary for immune function and healing and to prevent catabolism* (Sorenson et al., 2019).

Reduce Risk for Infection. The inflammatory response often indicates that body defense mechanisms have been set in motion to protect against invading microorganisms. The patient with a healing wound is at particular risk for infection.

Expected Outcome: Patient will be free of manifestations of infection.

The nurse will:

- Assess the wound for specific manifestations of infection, including purulent drainage, foul odor, and delayed healing. *The normal inflammatory response can indicate infection and, on occasion, mask its presence.*
- Evaluate complete blood counts for adequate WBC response. *Leukocytosis may indicate infection or healthy response to injury and protection from infection. Immune-impaired patients may not respond with increased WBCs;*

manifestations of inflammation may be diminished in those individuals.

- Monitor vital signs at least every 4 hours. *In response to the inflammatory process the temperature rises, usually in the range of 37.2°C (99°F) to 38.2°C (100.9°F). A temperature of 38.3°C (101.0°F) or above indicates infection. Fever is usually accompanied by increased heart and respiratory rates.*
- Apply dry or moist heat to the affected area for no longer than 20 minutes several times a day. Monitor the temperature closely to prevent burns and further damage to the affected area. *Heat increases the circulation of blood to and from the inflamed tissue. Time is limited to prevent burns.*
- Provide and encourage fluid intake of 2500 mL/day as allowed. *Teach the purpose and importance of hydration to promote blood flow and nutrient supply to the tissues and also dilution and removal of waste products and heat from the body.*
- Ensure adequate nutrition. *Adequate nutrition enhances the function and production of T cells and B cells, which are important in the immune response.*
- Use good hand hygiene techniques consistently. *Hand hygiene removes transient microorganisms and is the best mechanism to prevent the spread of infection to a susceptible person.*
- Use aseptic technique when providing wound care. *Using sterile gloves and aseptic technique helps prevent further contamination of the wound and the spread of infection to other patients.*

Delegating Nursing Care Activities

As appropriate and allowed by the designated duties and responsibilities of assistive personnel, the nurse may delegate nursing care activities such as obtaining vital signs, assisting with positioning and activity, promoting food and fluid intake, and providing intact skin care for the patient with inflammation.

Transitions of Care

Health promotion activities to prevent inflammation focus on reducing the risk for accidents and exposure to harmful agents that can result in subsequent injury. It is important to educate the public about potential hazards in both the work and home environments. In addition, safety education guidelines such as not drinking and driving, wearing a protective helmet when riding a bicycle, and using a seat belt in the car are important areas for discussion. Because most injuries occur at home, it is also important to discuss ways to make the home safer.

Acute inflammation is usually self-limiting and should resolve within 1 to 10 days. Symptoms of swelling, pain, and redness should also resolve slowly within this time period. Teaching is important to prevent further compromise that could result in infection. Instructions, verbal and written, should include:

- Increase fluid intake to 2500 mL (approximately 2.5 quarts) per day.
- Eat a well-balanced diet high in vitamins and minerals and with adequate protein and kilocalories for healing.
- Use good hand hygiene, particularly when caring for wounds or inflamed tissue and after using the bathroom.
- Elevate the inflamed area to reduce swelling and pain.
- Apply heat or cold for no longer than 20 minutes at a time to reduce the risk of tissue damage from burns or frostbite.
- Take all medications as prescribed, notifying the physician if adverse effects or hypersensitivity responses are noted.
- Rest acutely inflamed tissue; do not engage in strenuous activity until the inflammation has subsided.

Chronic inflammation is considered an abnormal condition that results in persistent inflammation and destruction of tissue. Chronic inflammation can occur when acute phases of inflammation and immune functions are unsuccessful in generating complete healing of the affected body region and can persist for several weeks, months, or years.

- Chronic inflammation can also result from chronic injury such as infection or auto-immune conditions.
- Autoimmune diseases cause damage to joints, blood vessels, and the GI system.
- Treatment varies depending on the underlying condition but may include immunosuppressant therapy.
- Treatment may also involve attempts at removing the source of the injury such as antibiotics for chronic infection and long-term use of anti-inflammatory agents.
- Nonpharmacologic treatments may also be effective such as the use of heat, cold, and complementary therapies, including aromatherapy, acupuncture, and guided imagery. Inflammation is seen in many diseases and conditions contributing to death.
- Cancer cells increase immune responses as do chemotherapeutic agents. Inflammatory markers such as C-reactive protein and albumin are being used as prognostic markers in determining the severity of some forms of cancer and whether treatment is effective.
- Increases in inflammatory markers are seen at the end stages of life in patients with cancer.
- Loss of muscle mass in patients with cancer increases inflammation and causes further inflammation within the body, contributing to further declines in conditions.
- Inflammation is a factor leading to atherosclerosis and arterial wall thickening. In cardiovascular disease inflammation contributes to further immune responses and plaque buildup that eventually leads to myocardial infarctions and stroke.
- Chronic obstructive pulmonary disease is characterized by persistent airway limitation caused from damage and inflammation of pulmonary structures. Pulmonary as well as systemic inflammation is present due to immune responses. As the condition worsens,

inflammation causes an inability of ventilation and perfusion of oxygen, leading to death.

- Care of patients at the end of life includes antianxiety agents that decrease oxygen demands and may include steroid therapy to diminish further inflammatory processes.

The Patient with an Infection

Microorganisms—including bacteria, viruses, fungi, and parasites—often invade the human body and proliferate if undetected and controlled or eliminated by inflammatory and immune responses. In most cases, contact between humans and microorganisms is incidental and may even be beneficial to both organisms. Resident bacteria of the skin, mucous membranes, and gastrointestinal tract are an important part of the body's defense system. However, many microorganisms are virulent; that is, they have the ability to cause disease. **Pathogens** are virulent organisms rarely found in the absence of disease. Some microorganisms, known as opportunistic pathogens, rarely, if ever, cause harm to individuals with intact immune systems, but are capable of producing infectious disease in the immunocompromised host.

To a certain extent, modern medicine has contributed to the development of infectious diseases caused by antibiotic-resistant strains of microorganisms. Tuberculosis is on the rise in many countries, partially because organisms have become resistant to standard therapies. Patients receive immunosuppressive therapy following organ or tissue transplant or in the treatment of neoplasms, making them more susceptible to infection. Metal and plastic prosthetic devices are implanted, providing potential sites for colonization by disease-producing organisms. It has also become apparent that many diseases long considered unrelated to microorganisms may actually be infectious; for example, colonization of the gastric mucosa with *Helicobacter pylori* is the predominant cause of peptic ulcer disease, and oncogenic viruses have the ability to transform normal cells into malignant cells.

Pathophysiology

Infection occurs when an organism is able to colonize and multiply within a host. The host can be any organism capable of supporting the nutritional and physical growth requirements of the microorganism—for example, humans. When the host experiences injury, pathologic changes, inflammation, or organ dysfunction in response to an infection or from intoxication by cellular poisons produced by a pathogen, the host is said to have an infectious disease.

For a microorganism to cause infection, it must have disease-causing potential (virulence), be transmitted from its reservoir, and gain entry into a susceptible host. This is known as the *chain of infection* (**Figure 12.9** ■).

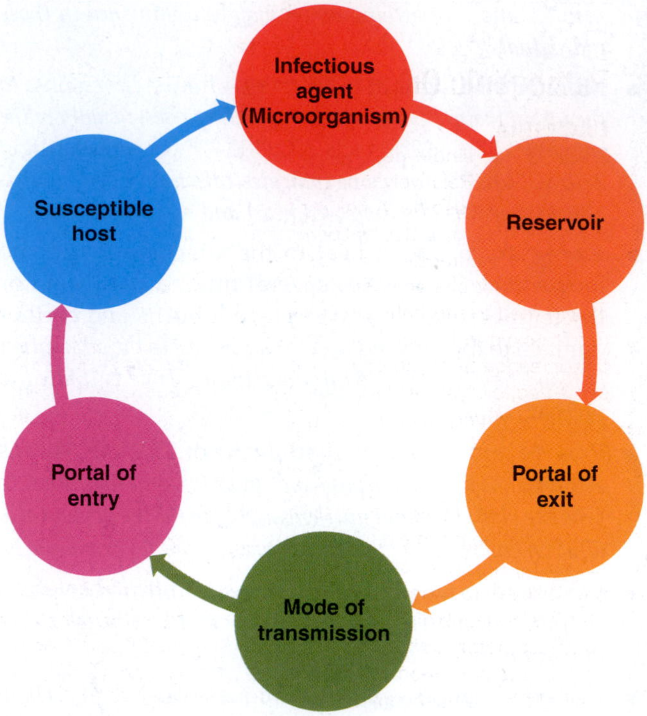
Infectious agent (Microorganism)
Reservoir
Portal of exit
Mode of transmission
Portal of entry
Susceptible host

Figure 12.9 ■ The chain of infection.

Pathogens

Pathogens capable of infecting and causing disease in a susceptible host include bacteria, viruses, mycoplasma, rickettsia, chlamydia, fungi, and parasites such as protozoa, helminths (worms), and arthropods (**Box 12.3**). Each organism causes a different specific reaction in the host.

A number of different mechanisms have evolved in pathogens to facilitate their transmission and increase their ability to invade the host and cause disease. Factors influencing the transmission of an organism include resistance to drying and to variations in environmental temperature. For example, spore-forming organisms are extremely resistant to drying.

Adhesion factors produced by or incorporated into the cell wall or membrane of the pathogen improve its ability to attach to and colonize the host. Pathogens may also produce enzymes to enhance their spread to local tissues, chemicals to block specific immune processes or deplete neutrophils and macrophages, or extracellular capsules to discourage phagocytosis.

Pathogens are often capable of producing toxins that affect the normal function of host cells and promote colonization, proliferation, and invasion by the pathogen. Toxins can increase the disease-producing capability of the pathogen and, in some cases, are totally responsible for it; for example, cholera, tetanus, and botulism result from bacterial toxins, not from the direct effects of the infection. **Exotoxins** are soluble proteins secreted into surrounding tissue by the microorganism. Exotoxins are highly poisonous, causing cell death or dysfunction. **Endotoxins** are found in the cell wall of gram-negative bacteria and are released only when the cell is disrupted. Endotoxins have less specific effects than exotoxins, but they act as activators of many human regulatory systems, producing fever; inflammation; and potentially clotting, bleeding, or hypotension when released in large quantities.

BOX 12.3
Pathogenic Organisms

BACTERIA

Bacteria are single-celled organisms capable of autonomous reproduction. Relatively small and simple organisms, they contain a single chromosome. A flexible cell membrane and rigid cell wall surround their cytoplasm, giving them a distinctive shape; some also have an extracellular capsule for additional protection. Bacteria have different characteristics and growth requirements; the colonies formed by replicating bacteria differ from one another. *Aerobes* require oxygen for survival, whereas *anaerobes* cannot survive in the presence of oxygen; *gram-positive* bacteria stain purple when subjected to crystal violet stain, whereas *gram-negative* bacteria do not stain with crystal violet but turn red when subjected to safranin stain.

PRIONS

Prions are not independent organisms but small molecules that can modify host proteins. They primarily affect the neurologic system, causing neurologic degeneration in diseases such as mad cow disease (bovine spongiform encephalopathy) in animals and Creutzfeldt-Jacob disease in humans. These are slowly progressive, noninflammatory conditions leading to dementia, lack of coordination, and death. Prion entry into the neurologic cells makes them resistant to the host immune system and antibacterial and antiviral medications. They enter the host by injection, transplantation of contaminated tissue or medical devices, and possibly food. They are very resistant to disinfection, requiring special procedures for sterilizing instruments, especially those used in CNS surgeries (Geschwind, 2016).

VIRUSES

Viruses are obligate intracellular parasites that are incapable of reproducing outside of a living cell. Viruses consist of a protein coat around a core of either DNA or RNA. Some viruses are shed continuously from infected cell surfaces; others, after inserting their genetic material into that of the infected cell, remain latent until they are stimulated to replicate. Viruses may or may not cause lysis and death of the host cell during replication. Oncogenic viruses are able to transform normal cells into malignant cells.

MYCOPLASMA

Although similar to bacteria, *mycoplasma* are smaller and have no cell wall, making them resistant to antibiotics that inhibit cell wall synthesis (e.g., penicillins).

RICKETTSIA AND CHLAMYDIA

As obligate intracellular parasites with a rigid cell wall, *rickettsia* and *Chlamydia* have some features of both bacteria and viruses. Rather than depending on the host cell for reproduction, they use vitamins, nutrients, or products of metabolism (e.g., ATP) from the host. *Chlamydia* are transmitted by direct contact, whereas many rickettsiae infect the cells of arthropods (e.g., fleas, ticks, and lice) and are transmitted from these vectors to humans.

FUNGI

Fungi are prevalent throughout the world, but few are capable of causing disease in humans. Most fungal infections are self-limited, affecting the skin and subcutaneous tissue. Some fungi, such as *Pneumocystis jiroveci*, can cause life-threatening opportunistic infections in the immunocompromised host.

PARASITES

The term *parasite* is typically applied to members of the animal kingdom that infect and cause disease in other animals. Protozoa, helminths, and arthropods are considered parasites. *Protozoa* are single-celled organisms (e.g., *Giardia lamblia* and *Trichomonas vaginalis*) transmitted via direct or indirect contact or an arthropod vector. *Helminths* are wormlike parasites; roundworms, tapeworms, and flukes are examples. They gain entry into humans primarily through ingestion of fertilized eggs or penetration of larvae through the skin or mucous membranes. *Arthropod* parasites, such as scabies (mites), lice, and fleas, typically infest external body surfaces, causing localized tissue damage and inflammation. Transmission is by direct contact with the arthropod or its eggs.

Reservoir and Transmission

The reservoir or source, where the pathogen lives and multiplies, may be either endogenous or exogenous. Organisms that reside on skin or mucosal surfaces of the host are endogenous. Exogenous sources can include other humans, animals, soil, water, an implanted device, or unclean equipment. Infectious diseases are usually transmitted from human sources, that is, people who have clinical disease or carriers with subclinical infection. Carriers harbor the pathogen without showing evidence of clinical disease. Pathogens exit human hosts via respiratory secretions, body fluids from the gastrointestinal and genitourinary tracts, skin or mucous membrane lesions, the placenta, and blood.

Organisms may be transmitted from the source to the susceptible host by direct or indirect contact, droplet or airborne transmission, or a vector. Direct contact includes person-to-person spread or contact with infected body fluids, as well as transmission from contaminated food or water. Indirect contact occurs when the infectious agent is contracted by use of inanimate objects, such as dirty eating utensils. Sneezing, talking, and coughing allow transmission by droplet contact when the host is within 2 to 3 feet of the source. Smaller respiratory particles that stay suspended in air and are carried via air currents allow airborne transmission. Vectors are insects and animals such as flies, mosquitoes, or rodents that act as intermediate hosts between the source and host. Microorganisms usually first colonize the portal of entry: Nonintact skin; wounds; mucous membranes; and the respiratory, gastrointestinal, or genitourinary tracts.

Host Factors

The susceptible host is the final link in the chain of infection. Exposure to pathogens does not automatically cause infection or infectious disease. The balance of microbial virulence and host resistance determines the outcome of contact with a pathogenic microorganism. Factors that can enable the host to resist infection include:

- Physical barriers, such as intact skin and mucous membranes
- The hostile environment created by acid stomach secretions, urine, and vaginal secretions
- Antimicrobial factors in saliva, tears, and prostatic fluid

- Respiratory defenses, including humidification, filtration, the mucociliary escalator, cough reflex, and alveolar macrophages
- Innate and adaptive immune responses to pathogenic invasion.

Stages of the Infectious Process

When infectious disease develops in the host, it typically follows a predictable course with stages based on the progression and intensity of manifestations.

The initial stage is the *incubation period*, during which the pathogen begins active replication but does not yet cause manifestations. Depending on the organism and host factors, the incubation period may last from hours, as with salmonella, to years, as with HIV infection.

The *prodromal stage* follows, during which manifestations first begin to appear. At this stage, manifestations are often nonspecific and include general malaise, fever, myalgias, headache, and fatigue.

Maximal impact of the infectious process is felt during the *acute phase* as the pathogen proliferates and disseminates rapidly. Toxic by-products of microorganism metabolism and cell lysis, along with the immune response, produce tissue damage and inflammation during this stage (Sorenson et al., 2019). Manifestations are more pronounced and specific to the infecting organism and site during the acute stage. Fever and chills may be significant during this phase. However, alcoholic patients and the very old may respond to severe infection by becoming hypothermic. The patient is often tachycardic and tachypneic because of increased metabolic demands. Localized manifestations include redness, heat, swelling, pain, and impaired function. When the infectious disease affects an internal organ, manifestations are related to inflammatory changes in that organ and surrounding tissue. The patient may experience tenderness to palpation over the site or show manifestations of impaired function, such as the hematuria and proteinuria characteristic of renal infections.

If the infectious process is prolonged, manifestations of the continuing immune response may become apparent. Catabolic and anorexic effects of the infection can lead to loss of body fat and muscle wasting. Immune complexes may be deposited at sites other than the primary infection, resulting in an inflammatory process. Glomerulonephritis (e.g., following strep throat) and vasculitis are possible results. Another possible consequence of prolonged infection and immune response is the triggering of an autoimmune disease process, such as rheumatic cardiomyopathy or celiac disease. As the infection is contained and the pathogen eliminated, the *convalescent stage* of the disease occurs. During this stage, affected tissues are repaired and manifestations resolve. Resolution of the infection is total elimination of the pathogen from the body without residual manifestations. If a balance between organism and host factors occurs with neither predominating, chronic disease may develop or the organism may be driven into a protected site, such as an abscess. A carrier state develops when host defenses eliminate the infectious disease but the organism continues to multiply on mucosal sites.

Complications

Multiple and varied complications are associated with infectious diseases. They are typically specific to the infecting organism and the body system affected.

Acute invasion of the blood by certain microorganisms or their toxins can result in septicemia and septic shock. Whereas *bacteremia*, the presence of bacteria in the blood, may not have serious effects, **septicemia** refers to systemic disease associated with their presence or toxins. Septic shock indicates a state of hypotension and impaired organ perfusion resulting from sepsis. Unless treated aggressively, septic shock leads to diffuse cell and tissue injury and potentially to organ failure.

Healthcare-Associated Infections

Healthcare-associated infections (HAIs) are acquired in a healthcare setting, such as a hospital or nursing home. Also called *nosocomial infections*, HAIs are estimated to occur in 1 of every 25 hospitalized patients in the United States, affecting 650,000 patients and contributing to an estimated 99,000 deaths annually (Agency for Healthcare Research and Quality [AHRQ], 2017; Rohde et al., 2016). It is estimated the annual direct medical costs of HAIs to be between $28 billion and $33 billion. Annually. HAIs add hospital days, reduce admissions by occupying available beds, and add to the cost of healthcare (AHRQ, 2017; Rohde et al., 2016). In an effort to reduce costs associated with HAIs, the Patient Protection and Affordable Care Act of 2010 limits or prohibits Medicare and Medicaid reimbursement to providers for treatment related to certain healthcare-associated conditions, including catheter-associated urinary tract infection (CAUTI) and surgical site infection following surgeries such as coronary artery bypass graft (CABG), bariatric surgery, and selected orthopedic procedures.

Many HAIs result from the use of invasive devices such as intravenous catheters, urinary catheters, and endotracheal tubes for ventilator support. Patients developing HAIs are often critically ill and among those least able to mount an effective immune defense against infection. Nosocomial infections also occur when antibiotic therapy has altered natural defenses and impaired resistance to harmful microorganisms. Endogenous organisms outside their normal habitats (such as in *Escherichia coli* in the urinary tract) become a threat to the patient. Other pharmacologic and therapeutic procedures such as chemotherapy, the use of corticosteroids, or radiation therapy also contribute to nosocomial infections. Surgical site infections are the most common HAI and may occur up to 30 days postoperatively (Anderson & Sexton, 2017). Superficial or deep wounds may be contaminated by endogenous or exogenous sources. Infections in body cavities or those associated with prosthetics are difficult to diagnose and may necessitate removal of the prosthetic device. **Box 12.4** lists interventions that should be used to prevent healthcare-associated infections.

Hospital-acquired pneumonia (HAP) is pneumonia that occurs in nonintubated patients more than 48 hours after discharge. Ventilator-associated pneumonia (VAP) is pneumonia occurring after 48 to 72 hours of mechanical

BOX 12.4

Interventions to Reduce Healthcare-Associated Infections

1. Central venous catheter infections have decreased by using chlorhexidine antiseptic for disinfection and maximal barrier precautions during insertion.
2. Ventilator-associated pneumonia is decreased by weaning patients off ventilators as soon as possible, limiting sedation of the patient, positioning patients with the head of the bed elevated to prevent gastric reflux and for maximal ventilation, and using proper hand hygiene and sterile technique for all ventilator-associated care.
3. Surgical site infections are reduced by administering a prophylactic antibiotic 1 hour before the incision and discontinuing it within 24 hours after surgery, limiting hair removal (no shaving), controlling perioperative glucose levels (especially in cardiac surgeries), and ensuring normothermia for the patient during the perioperative period (especially in colorectal surgeries).
4. Insert urinary catheters only when clearly indicated, using aseptic technique during insertion; minimize manipulation or opening of drainage systems (Schaeffer, 2017).

ventilation. Organisms causing the infection can be resistant to many drugs, not responding to antibiotics usually effective in treating infections acquired outside the hospital. More deaths are associated with HAP than any other site of infection (Micek, Chew, Hampton, & Kollef, 2016; Russell et al., 2016).

SAFETY ALERT: Hand hygiene is the most important practice in attempting to minimize HAIs. It is recommended that hands be washed with soap and water to remove the greatest number of microbes. If soap and water are not available, the use of alcohol-based hand sanitizers is recommended. Hand sanitizers should contain at least 60% alcohol. A soap-and-water wash is always recommended for visibly soiled hands (Booth, 2016; CDC, 2017b; Sickbert-Bennett et al., 2016). Wearing gloves does not eliminate the need to perform hand hygiene. ■

Effective hand hygiene is the single most important measure in infection control. Although infections may also be transmitted by the airborne route, from contaminated equipment, or from the environment, these are less significant causes. Invasive procedures and equipment should be used only when absolutely necessary; for example, it is not appropriate to insert an indwelling catheter when the only indication is incontinence. Peripheral intravenous equipment and sites must be kept clean and inspected regularly: Palpate the site for tenderness daily and visually inspect it if a transparent dressing is used. If the patient is not receiving blood, blood products, or fat emulsions, continuously used administration sets should be replaced no more frequently than every 96 hours, but at least every 7 days or per agency guidelines. Chlorhexidine-impregnated dressings are also recommended for adults age 18 and over (CDC, 2017c).

Antibiotic-Resistant Microorganisms

Antibiotic-resistant microorganisms are increasing at an alarming rate primarily due to prolonged or inappropriate use of antibiotic therapy. Although antibiotic therapy is expected to eradicate all targeted microorganisms, sometimes a few bacteria survive, leading to bacteria that reproduce with antibiotic resistance already encoded into their genetic makeup. Other bacteria produce enzymes that inactivate drugs, change drug binding sites, or alter their cell membranes to prevent drug absorption. It is important for infectious agents to be identified and treated with effective antibiotics; culture and sensitivity analysis guides prescription of effective antimicrobials. These reports need to be reviewed carefully and appropriate action taken if drug-resistant pathogens are found.

Standard precautions, most importantly hand hygiene and the use of carefully selected antibiotics, are critical actions for stopping the spread of these diseases. Equipment such as stethoscopes, blood pressure cuffs, and thermometers should be restricted to use by each patient identified with one of these diseases. Personal protective gear, used and disposed of appropriately, are important safeguards.

Interprofessional Care

The goals of care for the patient with an infection are to identify the organ system affected by the infection; to identify the causative agent; and to achieve a cure by the least toxic, least expensive, and most effective means. Fortunately, most infectious diseases are self-limiting and will resolve with little or no medical care. However, medical treatment can be lifesaving in an overwhelming infection or immunocompromised host.

The site of the infection is often obvious from the patient's history and presenting manifestations. Identifying the affected organ system allows the range of possible infecting organisms to be narrowed to those known to affect that system. Once the infecting agent has been identified, either positively or by probability, therapy can be specifically tailored to the patient's needs. Viral infections often resolve without treatment other than supportive care, such as providing rest and fluids. Skin infections may respond to a topical agent, avoiding the potential adverse effects of an agent administered systemically.

Immune function declines with age, placing older adults at greater risk of developing infections. Changes occur in both the innate and adaptive immune systems leading to increased levels of cytokines and chemokines, resulting in low-grade chronic inflammation. Infection risk increases at age 65 and those 80 years and older are at an even more increased risk (Yoshikawa & Norman, 2017). Physiologic changes that often occur with aging place the older adult at greater risk of acquiring an infection than younger people:

- *Cardiovascular changes:* Decreased tissue perfusion delays the inflammatory response and healing.
- *Respiratory system changes:* Decreased mucociliary clearance, decreased elastic recoil, and diminished

cough and laryngeal reflexes decrease the clearance of respiratory secretions and increase the risk for pneumonia. The older adult with pneumonia may not present with cough or sputum production due to decreased immune function. The leading causes of pneumonia in older adults include *S. pneumoniae*, *Haemophilus influenzae*, and *S. aureus*. Influenza A, a viral infection, is a significant risk factor for secondary bacterial pneumonia in older adults (Yoshikawa & Norman, 2017). Both pneumonia and influenza cause high mortality rates in the older person.

- ***Genitourinary changes:*** Loss of muscle tone, reduced bladder contractility, altered bladder reflexes, and prostatic hypertrophy in men increase the risk for incomplete bladder emptying, urinary incontinence, and urinary tract infection (UTI). UTI is the most common infection and the leading cause of bacteremia and sepsis in older adults, particularly those ages 85 and older.
- ***Gastrointestinal system changes:*** Impaired swallow reflex, decreased gastric acidity, and delayed gastric emptying increase the risk of aspiration with subsequent pneumonia.
- ***Skin and subcutaneous tissue changes:*** Thinning of skin, decreased cushioning, decreased sensation, and decreased vasculature increase the risk of injury, ulceration, and infection.
- ***Immune changes:*** Decreased phagocytosis, diminished antibody-mediated and cellular immune responses, and slowed or impaired healing processes increase the risk for infection. Immunoglobulin levels remain relatively stable, but primary and secondary antibody responses decline with age. T-cell and B-cell functions decline, which is felt to contribute to an inability to fight infections and control cancer-causing cells (Akhtar, 2018). Resistance to antigens such as *M. tuberculosis*, influenza and varicella-zoster viruses, malignant cells, and tissue grafts is reduced.

Other factors, such as a lower activity level, poor nutrition and an increased risk for dehydration, a higher prevalence of chronic diseases such as diabetes, use of multiple medications, and altered mentation contribute to the older adult's risk for infection.

Healthcare-associated infections are more common in older adults. The nurse must steadfastly adhere to principles of infection control. Nursing interventions to reduce the risk of HAI include (1) avoiding prolonged bedrest, (2) encouraging patients to take deep breaths, (3) providing adequate fluids, (4) providing regular toileting schedules with good hygiene, and (5) avoiding use of invasive devices such as indwelling catheters unless medically necessary.

The older adult may not exhibit the classic manifestations of inflammation and infection. The manifestations of inflammation—redness, heat, and swelling—tend to be diminished or absent in older adults. The classic manifestations of infection—fever and chills—may be absent altogether because of age-related changes in the immune system, loss of central temperature control mechanisms, decreased muscle mass, and loss of shivering ability. The older adult may have only subtle manifestations of infection or sepsis, including changes in mental status, disorientation, restlessness, and tachypnea.

Prompt identification and treatment of infection improves outcomes in the older adult. In addition to monitoring for changes in the patient's mental status or behavior, the nurse should assess fluid intake and urinary output, activity levels, complaints of fatigue, and respiratory status. Older adults are at increased risk for dehydration due to diminished thirst sensation and impaired water conservation by the kidneys. Carefully evaluate intake and output to determine if input is adequate.

Diagnosis

To assess the patient's response to infection, identify the infecting organism, and monitor the progress of therapy, the following diagnostic tests may be ordered:

- ***WBC count*** provides clues about the infecting organism and the body's immune response to it.
- ***WBC differential*** is also ordered (refer to Table 12.9). Neutrophilia, increased numbers of circulating neutrophils (or PMNs), is a common response with infection or inflammation as the bone marrow responds to an increased need for phagocytes. Along with neutrophilia, more immature neutrophils are present in circulation than normal, indicating an appropriate bone marrow response (**Figure 12.10** ■).
- ***Procalcitonin (CTpr) and C-reactive protein (CRP)*** are diagnostic markers of infection that can be measured in the blood. Blood levels of CTpr and CRP increase dramatically with serious bacterial infection and sepsis, making these markers useful early indicators of systemic infections.
- ***Cultures of the wound, blood, or other infected body fluids*** are used to identify probable microorganisms by their characteristics, such as shape, growth patterns, and Gram-staining qualities. After the organism is cultured, it is subjected to sensitivity testing using various antibiotics known to be effective against its particular strain to determine which antibiotic is likely to be most effective. Generally, 24 to 48 hours are required to grow the organism, potentially delaying the institution of therapy. Because antibiotics can alter the ability to culture an organism, specimens should be obtained before instituting therapy.
- ***Serologic testing*** provides an indirect means of identifying infecting agents by detecting antibodies to the suspected organism. When the antibody titer against a specific organism rises during the acute phase of an infectious disease and begins to fall during convalescence, the diagnosis is supported. Although it is not as accurate as culture, serology is particularly useful for organisms that cannot easily be cultured, such as hepatitis B or HIV.

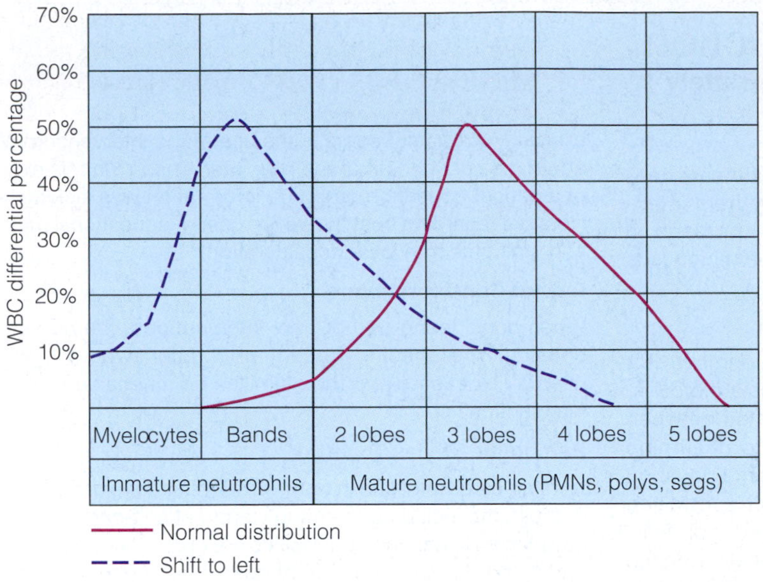
70%
60%
50%
40%
30%
20%
10%
WBC differential percentage
Myelocytes
Bands
2 lobes
3 lobes
4 lobes
5 lobes
Immature neutrophils
Mature neutrophils (PMNs, polys, segs)
Normal distribution
Shift to left

Type of WBC	Normal differential	Shift to left
Myelocytes	0%	Present
Banded neutrophils (bands)	3% to 5%	Increased
Segmented neutrophils (segs, polys, PMNs)	50% to 65%	May be stable, increased, or decreased

Figure 12.10 ■ Neutrophils by stage of maturity and normal distribution in the blood.

- ***Direct antigen detection methods*** use monoclonal antibodies (purified antibody forms) to detect antigens in specimens from the diseased host. These tests offer rapid and accurate identification of the offending microorganism.
- ***Antibiotic peak and trough levels*** monitor therapeutic blood levels of the prescribed medication(s). The therapeutic range, that is, the minimum and maximum blood levels at which the drug is effective, is known for a given drug. By measuring blood levels at the predicted peak (1 to 2 hours after oral administration, 1 hour after intramuscular administration, and 30 minutes after intravenous administration) and trough (lowest level, usually a few minutes before the next scheduled dose), healthcare personnel can determine that the patient is maintaining a level within the therapeutic range at all times, ensuring maximal effect from the drug. It is also possible to determine whether the drug is reaching a toxic or harmful level during therapy, increasing the likelihood of adverse effects.
- ***Radiologic examination of the chest, abdomen, or urinary system*** may be ordered to detect organ abnormalities, indicating an inflammatory response or tissue damage.
- ***Lumbar puncture*** is performed to obtain cerebrospinal fluid (CSF) for examination and culture if a CNS infection, such as meningitis or encephalitis, is suspected.
- ***Ultrasonic examination*** is a noninvasive diagnostic test such as an echocardiogram or renal ultrasonography to identify an infectious site or evaluate the effects of an infection on organ function.

Medications

After the infecting organism and affected body system have been identified, specific therapy to cure the infectious disease can be instituted. Antimicrobial preparations are broadly classified as bacteriostatic or bactericidal. *Bacteriostatic agents* inhibit the growth of the microorganism, leaving its destruction to the host's immune system. These agents are generally not indicated for the immunocompromised host. Tetracyclines, erythromycin, and chloramphenicol are bacteriostatic preparations. *Bactericidal agents*, including penicillins, cephalosporins, and aminoglycoside antibiotics, are capable of killing the organism without immune system intervention.

The activity of antimicrobial agents on bacteria, fungi, and viruses falls under five basic mechanisms:

- Impairing cell wall synthesis, leading to lysis and cell destruction
- Inhibiting protein synthesis, causing impaired microbial function
- Altering cell membrane permeability, causing intracellular contents to leak
- Inhibiting the synthesis of nucleic acids
- Inhibiting cell metabolism and growth.

Many microorganisms have the ability to develop resistance to an anti-infective agent; that is, the pathogen continues to live and grow in the presence of the anti-infective. Resistance develops as a result of a chance mutation by the pathogen, allowing a subpopulation of cells to survive. The chance of an organism becoming resistant to an agent is partially related to the dose delivered. Resistance is less likely to occur when a lethal dose is administered; therefore, it is vital that patients understand the need to take all doses of the prescribed drug as ordered. See the Moving Evidence into Action box.

Antibiotics. Medications used to treat bacterial infections are generally known as antibiotics. Most antibiotics

Moving Evidence into Action

Teaching to Take Antibiotics Appropriately

Clinical Issue

Antibiotic resistance is a growing public and healthcare concern leading to greater morbidity and mortality from infections. Antibiotic stewardship is a worldwide approach in ensuring appropriate prescribing and usage of antibiotics is performed.

External Evidence

A study was performed that involved the development of a program to enhance patient knowledge about antibiotics, The program was used to explore the association between antibiotic knowledge and health literacy and to determine the effect size for the association between patient education and improved antibiotic knowledge (David, O'Neal, Miller, Johnson, & Lloyd, 2017). Study results concluded that overall patients have a low-level knowledge of the differences between bacteria and viruses, along with treatments for them. Educational programs were shown to be beneficial in enhancing understanding of antibiotic use, and educational programs may be more effective in patients with higher educational backgrounds.

Internal Evidence

As part of the evaluation of internal evidence, one must consider the clinical feasibility (including access to appropriate patient educational materials), the outcome of interest (improving patient adherence with medication regimen), current policies/procedures in place for patient education including discharge teaching, and identification of stakeholders that influence uptake of the proposed intervention. One question to ask: Is the problem (patient knowledge of antibiotic use) significant in the population of your care environment? Does the clinical environment support the use of the intervention? What about the cost benefit of the new intervention? In this example of a patient education program, information was lacking in the literature regarding cost, however; cost of educational materials and staff time may be a consideration.

Patient Considerations

When considering use of new interventions, the nurse must consider the specific patient population where it will be used. Will patients and their families be amenable to the new intervention?

Putting the Pieces Together

Nursing care is holistic in nature and must consider all aspects of a patient, including their knowledge of self-care. Nurses are key players in ensuring antibiotics are prescribed, administered and taken following regulatory guidelines. Antibiotic stewardship includes questioning providers on prescribing antibiotics, reassessing the patient's response to the antibiotics, and ensuring discharge planning coincides with appropriate dose and route of administration. Nurses also must ensure patient understanding of all aspects of the medication (Manning, Pfeiffer, & Larson, 2016).

References

David, C., O'Neal, K., Miller, M., Johnson, J., & Lloyd, A. (2017). A literacy-sensitive approach to improving antibiotic understanding in a community-based setting. *International Journal of Pharmacy Practice, 25,* 394–398.

Manning, M. L., Pfeiffer, J., & Larson, E. (2016). Combating antibiotic resistance: The role of nursing in antibiotic stewardship. *American Journal of Infection Control, 44*, 1454–1457.

are biologic substances, that is, substances produced by other microorganisms. Antibiotics fall into classes of drugs with related chemical structure and activity. Some are effective against only gram-positive bacteria, and others are effective against only gram-negative organisms. Broad-spectrum antibiotics have activity against a wide variety of bacteria, including both gram-positive and gram-negative forms.

No antibiotic is totally safe. Hypersensitivity responses occur; always check for allergies before administering the first dose. Some drugs are toxic to organ systems, exhibiting hepatotoxicity, nephrotoxicity, ototoxicity, or bone marrow suppression. The antibiotics presented in **Medication Administration 12.A** are organized according to their antibacterial action.

Antivirals. Most antibiotics have little effect on viruses because the virus has no cell wall and no cytoplasm, produces no enzymes, and sequesters itself in a host cell to reproduce. Antiviral agents must be very selective in differentiating normal cellular activity from viral activity. In addition, the immune function of the host is a vital component in fighting viral infections; antiviral therapy may be relatively ineffective in the severely immunocompromised host. Timely diagnosis of viral infections can be an additional problem because viruses are less easily identified using laboratory techniques. Antiviral agents in common use are summarized in **Medication Administration 12.B**.

Antifungals. Antifungal agents are available in both topical and systemic forms. They act by interfering with the cytoplasmic membrane of the fungus. Topical agents include preparations for cutaneous use to treat candidiasis, tineas, and ringworm. Vaginal preparations to treat vulvovaginal candidiasis are also available, as are several nonprescription topical and vaginal antifungal agents.

Amphotericin B (Fungizone) is a systemic antifungal agent for parenteral administration. It is used to treat severe, life-threatening fungal infections including histoplasmosis, blastomycosis, and candidiasis. Another systemic antifungal in current use is flucytosine (Ancobon), which can be administered orally. It is used to treat severe candidiasis infections such as candida septicemia, endocarditis, pulmonary or urinary tract infections, and *Cryptococcus* meningitis.

Medication Administration 12.A

Antibiotic Therapy

I. Cell Wall Synthesis Inhibitors

PENICILLINS

amoxicillin (Amoxil)
ampicillin (Polycillin)
dicloxacillin (Dynapen)
nafcillin (Unipen)
oxacillin (Prostaphlin)
penicillin G
penicillin V
piperacillin (Pipracil)
ticarcillin (Ticar)

Combination Agents

amoxicillin and clavulanate (Augmentin)
ampicillin and sulbactam (Unasyn)
piperacillin and tazobactam (Zosyn)
ticarcillin and clavulanate (Timentin)

Penicillins are bactericidal and interfere with cell wall synthesis and the enzymes involved in cell division and synthesis. They are more effective on gram-positive than gram-negative organisms. Penicillins are considered to be safe, effective, and of low toxicity. Resistance is now more common among *Streptococci* and *Staphylococci*. Penicillins and related antibiotics such as the cephalosporins (see below) contain a molecular structure known as a beta-lactam ring. Some bacteria produce enzymes (beta-lactamases or penicillinases) that cleave (split or divide) this ring, making the antibiotics ineffective. To combat this resistance, beta-lactamase or penicillinase inhibitors such as sulbactam and clavulanate are combined with some antibiotics to create an antibiotic effective against drug-resistant bacterial strains.

Nursing Responsibilities

- Monitor for hypersensitivity responses such as local erythema and itching at the site of injection, skin rashes, urticaria (hives), itching, fever, chills, and anaphylaxis.
- Observe patients receiving parenteral penicillin for at least 30 minutes.
- Discontinue the drug immediately if any hypersensitivity response occurs. Be prepared to administer antihistamines or corticosteroids for a mild reaction. Anaphylaxis is treated with epinephrine subcutaneously or intravenously and with airway support.
- Do not administer penicillin to anyone with a history of a severe allergic reaction to any form of the drug; a cross-reactivity may occur in patients allergic to cephalosporin or carbapenem antibiotics.
- Assess for superinfection (vaginitis, stomatitis, or diarrhea) due to elimination of resident bacteria.

Health Education for the Patient and Family

- Notify the physician if you see white patches on the oral mucosa or if vaginitis develops. An antifungal drug may be prescribed and the antibiotic continued.
- Consuming yogurt or buttermilk may prevent superinfection. Do not take these products within 1 hour of taking the drug.

CEPHALOSPORINS

1st Generation

cefadroxil (Duricef)
cefazolin (Ancef)
cephalexin (Keflex)
cephradine (Velosef)

2nd Generation

cefaclor (Ceclor)
cefotetan (Cefotan)
cefoxitin (Mefoxin)
cefprozil (Cefzil)
cefuroxime (Ceftin)

3rd Generation

cefdinir (Omnicef)
cefditoren (Spectracef)
cefixime (Suprax)
cefotaxime (Claforan)
cefpodoxime (Vantin)
ceftazidime (Fortaz)
ceftibuten (Cedax)
ceftizoxime (Cefizox)
ceftriaxone (Rocephin)

4th Generation

cefepime(Maxipime)

Cephalosporins are structurally similar to the penicillins and also inhibit cell wall synthesis. They are divided into four groups, or generations. First-generation cephalosporins act primarily against gram-positive organisms. Second- and third-generation drugs are more effective against gram-negative organisms than against gram-positive ones. Fourth-generation cephalosporins act effectively against both gram-positive and gram-negative organisms.

Nursing Responsibilities

- Monitor for previous hypersensitivity response to cephalosporins or penicillins.
- Assess intravenous site for phlebitis; intramuscular injection may cause local pain.
- Monitor laboratory results for adverse response, such as leukopenia and thrombocytopenia, nephrotoxicity (elevated BUN and serum creatinine), or hepatotoxicity (elevated bilirubin, LDH, ALT, AST, and alkaline phosphatase).
- Assess for manifestations of superinfections.

Health Education for the Patient and Family

- Take the medication on an empty stomach, 1 hour before or 2 hours after meals.
- Avoid alcohol while using cefmetazole, cefoperazone, or cefotetan because alcohol intolerance can develop with these antibiotics. These same drugs intensify bleeding tendencies.
- Space doses of the medication relatively evenly throughout the day and evening hours.
- Increase consumption of buttermilk or yogurt to prevent intestinal superinfection.

CARBAPENEMS

ertapenem (Invanz)
imipenem (Primaxin)
meropenem (Merrem)

This newer class of antibiotics includes only three drugs and all must be given parenterally. Imipenem has the broadest antimicrobial spectrum of any drug. This makes it especially useful against mixed organism infections. These antibiotics cross the meninges and achieve therapeutic doses in CSF; they are effective against methicillin-resistant *Staphylococcus aureus* (MRSA). These antibiotics cause bacterial cell wall lysis and subsequent death of the bacteria. Side effects include nausea and vomiting, diarrhea, hypersensitivity reactions, occasional superinfections with bacteria or fungi, and, rarely, seizures.

(continued)

Nursing Responsibilities

- Ertapenem should not be mixed with dextrose or other drugs containing dextrose. IV infusions should be given over at least 30 minutes.
- Check for history of hypersensitivity to cephalosporins and penicillins and monitor for manifestations of reactions.
- Assess for manifestations of superinfection.
- Monitor laboratory indicators of renal function.

Health Education for the Patient and Family

- Report any manifestations of allergy such as skin rash, itching, or hives.

VANCOMYCIN

This antibiotic inhibits cell wall synthesis and is used for serious infections. It is only effective against gram-positive bacteria, especially *S. aureus* and *Staphylococcus epidermidis*, including the strains resistant to methicillin. *C. difficile* is also susceptible to this antibiotic, but infection with *C. difficile* is often treated first with metronidazole to delay emergence of resistance to vancomycin.

Nursing Responsibilities

- Infuse slowly over 60 minutes or more to avoid red man syndrome. The syndrome is characterized by erythematous rash, flushing, tachycardia, and hypotension. Patients may become dizzy and agitated. The occurrence is usually associated with a first dose of vancomycin and is seen within 4 to 6 minutes of the start of a dose or after completion.
- Ototoxicity is a serious adverse effect because hearing loss may be irreversible. Notify the physician immediately if the patient reports a sensation of fullness in the ears because this indicates ototoxicity.

II. Bacterial Protein Synthesis Inhibitors

TETRACYCLINES

demeclocycline (Declomycin)	minocycline HCl (Minocin)
doxycycline (Vibramycin)	tetracycline HCl (Sumycin)

Tetracyclines are active against many gram-positive and gram-negative bacteria, such as *Mycoplasma*, *Rickettsia*, and *Chlamydia*. They are bacteriostatic, interfering with microbial protein synthesis. Tetracycline binds readily with metal and solid elements in the bowel, limiting its absorption when administered with food; the other preparations are highly soluble in lipids and can be administered with food.

Nursing Responsibilities

- Schedule doses 1 hour before or 2 hours after meals. Do not give with milk or milk products or antacids.
- Monitor for manifestations of superinfection.
- If the patient is taking an anticoagulant, monitor prothrombin time and for manifestations of bleeding.

Health Education for the Patient and Family

- Avoid excessive sun exposure to reduce the risk of photosensitivity reactions.
- Tetracyclines can stain the enamel of developing teeth when taken during pregnancy; although deciduous (baby) teeth are affected, permanent teeth are not.

MACROLIDES

azithromycin (Zithromax)	erythromycin (E-Mycin, Erythrocin)
clarithromycin	troleandomycin (Tao)
dirithromycin (Dynabac)	

Macrolides are bacteriostatic and act effectively against gram-positive and gram-negative organisms. Erythromycin is used to treat streptococcal pharyngitis in patients who are allergic to penicillin and is the drug of choice for treating pertussis. Clarithromycin and azithromycin produce less nausea than erythromycin, increasing patient adherence.

Nursing Responsibilities

- Administer erythromycin on an empty stomach or immediately before meals.
- Give the drug with a full glass of water. Do not administer with acidic fruit juice.
- Intravenous doses are very irritating to veins; give slowly (20 to 60 minutes per gram).

Health Education for the Patient and Family

- Gastric distress is a common side effect with erythromycin.

AMINOGLYCOSIDES

amikacin (Amikin)	paromomycin (Humatin)
gentamicin (Garamycin)	streptomycin
kanamycin (Kantrex)	tobramycin (Nebcin)
neomycin (Mycifradin)	

Aminoglycosides are bactericidal, interfering with protein synthesis in the pathogen. They are especially effective against gram-negative organisms. To provide a broader spectrum of activity, they are often combined with other antibiotics, especially penicillins. Aminoglycosides can be administered in multiple or single daily doses. They are ototoxic and nephrotoxic; the risk is highest for older adults, patients with preexisting renal disease, and those receiving other ototoxic or nephrotoxic drugs. Use of paromomycin is limited to its local effects, treating intestinal parasites (amebiasis).

Nursing Responsibilities

- Assess renal function before and during aminoglycoside therapy. Monitor intake and output, daily weight, BUN, and serum creatinine.
- Assess for adverse effects on hearing such as loss of perception of high tones, tinnitus, and vertigo.
- Notify the physician if the patient is receiving other nephrotoxic or ototoxic drugs such as furosemide (Lasix) and ethacrynic acid (Edecrin).
- Administer intravenous preparations separately from other drugs; flush tubing before and after administration.

Health Education for the Patient and Family

- Monitor for a sudden weight gain that may indicate adverse effects on the kidney and report it to the physician.

OXAZOLIDINONES

Linezolid (Zyvox) is the first antibiotic in a class of antibiotics called oxazolidinones. This antibiotic inhibits protein synthesis and is effective against organisms that are resistant to both vancomycin and methicillin. Because of its usefulness against those organisms, its use should be reserved for infections caused by vancomycin-resistant enterococci (VRE) and MRSA.

Nursing Responsibilities

- Monitor for side effects including nausea, diarrhea, hypertension, and headache.
- Monitor platelets if patient is at risk for bleeding; this drug may cause thrombocytopenia.

Health Education for the Patient and Family

- It can be taken with or without food.
- Avoid taking ephedrine, pseudoephedrine, methylphenidate, or cocaine with this drug because high blood pressure may develop.

III. Bacterial Nucleic Acid Inhibitors

FLUOROQUINOLONES

ciprofloxacin (Cipro)	lomefloxacin (Maxaquin)
gatifloxacin (Zymar)	moxifloxacin (Avelox)
gemifloxacin (Factive)	norfloxacin (Noroxin)
levofloxacin (Levaquin)	ofloxacin (Floxin)

Fluoroquinolones are bactericidal and especially active against gram-negative and some gram-positive organisms. They are used to manage infections of the respiratory, gastrointestinal, and genitourinary tracts. Rarely, drugs in this class can cause tendon rupture, with the highest risk in people ages 60 and older and in those taking glucocorticoid medications.

Nursing Responsibilities

- Increase fluid intake to 2000 to 3000 mL/day unless contraindicated to prevent crystalluria.
- Monitor laboratory results for hepatotoxicity (elevated ALT, AST).

Health Education for the Patient and Family

- If tendon inflammation or pain develops, stop taking the drug and immediately report symptoms to your healthcare provider.
- Drink six to eight glasses of water per day.
- Avoid exposure to sunlight while taking these drugs.

SULFONAMIDES AND TRIMETHOPRIM

sulfadiazine (Coptin)
sulfamethoxazole (Gantanol)
sulfamethoxazole and trimethoprim (TMP-SMZ, Bactrim, Septra)
sulfisoxazole (Gantrisin)

Sulfonamides are bacteriostatic. Trimethoprim is an antibiotic effective against most gram-positive and many gram-negative organisms. It is often combined with sulfamethoxazole to manage urinary tract infections, *P. jiroveci* pneumonia, and otitis media. Skin rashes and pruritus are the most common hypersensitivity reactions. Severe reactions include exfoliative dermatitis and Stevens-Johnson syndrome.

Nursing Responsibilities

- Assess for history of hypersensitivity to sulfonamides and related medications, such as thiazide diuretics and sulfonylurea preparations.
- Monitor intake and output. Unless contraindicated, maintain a fluid intake of at least 1500 mL/day to prevent crystalluria.
- Assess for evidence of bleeding, easy bruising, or systemic infection, and monitor blood count for possible bone marrow depression.

Health Education for the Patient and Family

- Take medication on an empty stomach with a full glass of water. Maintain a fluid intake of at least 2 quarts per day.
- Protect the skin from excessive sun exposure with clothing and sunscreens to reduce the risk of photosensitivity.

METRONIDAZOLE (FLAGYL)

Metronidazole is effective against anaerobic gram-negative bacteria and protozoan infections caused by amebiasis, giardiasis, and trichomoniasis. It is commonly used to prevent and treat infections following intestinal surgery and is the drug of first choice with *C.difficile*.

Nursing Responsibilities

- Monitor for CNS effects of dizziness, headache, ataxia, confusion, depression, and peripheral neuropathy.
- Administer with food to minimize gastric distress and metallic taste. Infuse intravenous metronidazole over 60 minutes.
- Discontinue the medication and notify the physician if neurologic reactions occur.
- Increase fluid intake to 2500 mL/day to minimize the risk of nephrotoxicity.

Health Education for the Patient and Family

- This medication may turn urine reddish-brown; this is expected and not harmful.
- Stop taking the drug and notify the physician if hypersensitivity reaction or adverse effects occur, such as changes in mentation or coordination, painful or frequent urination, painful or difficult intercourse, and impotence.
- Do not drink alcohol while taking this medication; an Antabuse-type reaction (flushing, sweating, headache, vomiting, and abdominal cramps) may occur.
- Maintain a fluid intake of 2.5 to 3 quarts per day.
- When the drug is prescribed for *Trichomonas* infections, treatment of both partners is necessary. Use condoms to prevent cross-contamination during intercourse.

Note: Drugs, identified in blue, are among the 200 most commonly prescribed medications in the United States.

Source: Data from Adams et al., 2017.

Fluconazole (Diflucan) has the broadest use as an antifungal agent. It can be administered either orally or parenterally and is used to treat candidiasis infections as well as *Cryptococcus* meningitis. It is generally better tolerated than other systemic antifungal medications.

Antiparasitics. Drugs used to treat parasitic infections are as varied as the organisms that cause them. Parasites are organisms that invade a host insect or animal and can produce mild to severe consequences. Common parasites consist of protozoa (amebiasis, giardiasis, malaria, trichomoniasis), helminths (worms), and scabies and pediculi (lice), Generally, agents classified as antiparasitic are both expensive and likely to be toxic. Quinine was one of the first antiparasitic drugs developed in the treatment of malaria. Quinine is highly toxic, but newer forms such as chloroquine (Aralen, Chlorcon) and hydroxychloroquine (Plaquenil) are used widely as antimalarial drugs. Metronidazole (e.g., Flagyl) is used to treat infections of protozoan parasites (see **Medication Administration 12.C**).

Medication Administration 12.B

Antiviral Agents

NEURAMINIDASE INHIBITORS

Oseltamivir (Tamiflu) and zanamivir (Relenza) are used to prevent and treat influenza. They are active against both influenza A and B viruses. When given soon after symptoms develop, the duration and severity of manifestations are reduced. These drugs are generally well tolerated by healthy individuals, although zanamivir (administered as an inhaled powder) is not recommended for people with underlying lung disease.

ADAMANTANES

Amantadine (Symmetrel) and rimantadine (Flumadine) are used to prevent and treat influenza A. Although adamantanes can prevent the disease, viral resistance to these drugs develops rapidly. When administered within 48 hours after symptom onset, common manifestations of influenza are reduced. They are generally well tolerated; CNS side effects such as dizziness, anxiety, insomnia, and difficulty concentrating may occur.

ACYCLOVIR AND GANCICLOVIR

Acyclovir (Zovirax) and ganciclovir (Cytovene) are related compounds used primarily in the treatment of herpes viruses. Acyclovir and related drugs such as valacyclovir (Valtrex) and famciclovir (Famvir) are prescribed mainly to reduce the severity, duration, and frequency of recurrence of genital herpes manifestations. The use of ganciclovir, which profoundly suppresses bone marrow function, is limited primarily to the treatment of cytomegalovirus infection.

RIBAVIRIN

Ribavirin (Virazole) is a broad-spectrum antiviral medication used in combination with peginterferon alfa to treat hepatitis C. Ribavirin is a toxic drug, contraindicated for use during pregnancy. Hemolytic anemia can develop rapidly, necessitating periodic blood counts.

INTERFERONS

Interferons (IFN) are naturally produced cytokines that have antiviral activity. Pegylated interferon (peginterferon or PEG-IFN) is used to treat chronic hepatitis B and hepatitis C, often in combination therapy. Common adverse effects of PEG-IFN include fatigue, flu-like symptoms, muscle and joint pain, and possible depression and insomnia.

Source: Data from Adams et al., 2017; Aronson, 2016.

Medication Administration 12.C

Antifungal and Antiparasitic Agents

ANTIFUNGAL AGENTS

Systemic Antifungal Agents

Antifungal drugs work by either slowing the growth of the cell or by totally destroying it. Many of the antifungals disrupt cell membrane integrity or inhibit internal cellular metabolic processes. Medications that disrupt cell membranes permit fungal cell walls to become porous, allowing leakage and death to occur.

Common Antifungal Agents

amphotericin B (Abelcet, AmBisome, Amphtec, Fungizone)

anidulafungin (Eraxis)

caspofungin (Cancidas)

flucytosine (Ancobon)

micafungin (Mycamine)

Azoles

fluconazole (Diflucan)

itraconazole (Sporanox)

ketoconazole (Nizoral)

posaconazole (Noxafil)

voriconazole (Vfend)

Nursing Responsibilities

- Due to the body's normal defense mechanisms, fungal infections occur rarely in healthy individuals. Immunocompromised patients, such as those infected with HIV or undergoing chemotherapy, are at greater risk for fungal infections. Antifungal therapy may take several months to ensure the infection is completely eradicated.
- Ensure a complete health history is performed that includes neurologic, cardiac, respiratory, renal, and liver functions. Obtain any lab values that may be missing such as CBC, hepatic function studies, renal studies, and electrolytes.
- Amphotericin can be nephrotoxic, ototoxic, and hepatotoxic, so continuing surveillance of these systems is recommended.
- Obtain baseline vital signs, weight, and height.
- Throughout administration assess for desired therapeutic effects—diminished signs and symptoms of infection.
- Assess for adverse reactions such as nausea and vomiting, abdominal cramping, diarrhea, and electrolyte imbalances. Immediately report hypotension, tachycardia, arrhythmias, changes in level of consciousness, decreases in urine output, and seizures.

Health Education for Patient and Family

- Reproductive abnormalities may be present with administration of antifungals such as menstrual irregularities, gynecomastia, and drops in testosterone levels.
- Safety during pregnancy has not been established.
- Administration of aminoglycosides, cyclosporine, vancomycin and furosemide may interact with azoles and should be avoided during treatment.
- Avoid alcohol when taking antifungal medications to reduce the risk of increasing liver toxicity.

Topical Antifungal Agents

Topical antifungal agents are used for fungal infections of the skin and hair. Common fungal infections of the skin include tinea corporis (ringworm), tinea cruris (jock itch), tinea pedis (athlete's foot), and tinea capitis (scalp). These infections can cause redness, inflammation, and itching.

Onychomycosis or tinea unguium is a fungal infection of the finger or toe nail bed, which can cause brittle, thickened nails.

Candida is a fungal infection of the oropharyngeal and vulvovaginal areas of the body. Oralpharyngeal candidas is often called *thrush*.

Common Topical Antifungal Agents

clotrimazole (Lotrimin AF, Gyne-Lotrimin)

fluconazole (Diflucan)

itraconazole (Sporanox)

miconazole (Monistat)

nystatin (Mycostatin)
terbinafine (Lamisil)
tolnaftate (Tinactin)

Nursing Responsibilities

- Apply creams and lotions to clean, dry skin.
- Monitor for hypersensitivity responses including increased redness and itching at site.
- Discontinue drug if hypersensitivity occurs.
- Nystatin use for oral candida infection may cause diarrhea and nausea and vomiting.

Health Education for the Patient and Family

- Educate patient and family on proper application of medication to clean, dry tissues.
- Instruct that treatment to eradicate infection may require 1 to 2 weeks for skin infections.
- Instruct that treatment for nail bed infections may take anywhere from 1 week to 9 months.

ANTIPARASITIC AGENTS

The mechanism of action for antiparasitic drugs depends on the infecting organism. Side effects can range from mild rashes and nausea and vomiting to more severe conditions such as ototoxicity, neuropsychiatric symptoms, and liver disorders. Since effects vary, the nurse should research the specific drug to ensure understanding in order to monitor for side effects and perform patient teaching.

Common Amebiacide Drugs

iodoquinol (Aloquin)
metronidazole (Flagyl)
nitazoxanide (Alinia)
tinidazole (Tindamax)

Common Antimalarial Drugs

artemether (Coartem)
atovaquone (Malarone)
chloroquine phosphate (Aralen)
hydroxychloroquine (Plaquenil)
quinine

Common Antihelminthic Drugs

ivermectin (Stromectol)
mebendazole (Emverm)
pyrantel (Pin-X)

Common Scabicides/Pediculicides

lindane
malathion (Ovide)
permethrin (Elimite)
spinosad (Natroba)

Nursing Responsibilities

- Provide patient teaching on prevention of parasitic infections.
- Use parasitic drugs as prescribed and ensure that the full course of the medication is taken.
- Avoid alcoholic beverages while taking certain drugs such as metronidazole and tinidazole for 3 days after completion of prescription.
- Metronidazole may cause urine to darken and should not be prescribed to pregnant women.
- Pediculicide and scabicide agents vary in administration so specific product instructions should be followed carefully.
- Patients with pinworms, scabies, and pediculosis should wash bedding, clothes, and towels daily and follow strict handwashing practices.
- Chloroquine (and related drugs), oral metronidazole, and tinidazole should be administered with food to decrease gastrointestinal irritation.

Note: Drugs, identified in blue, are among the 200 most commonly prescribed medications in the United States.

Source: Data from Adams et al., 2017.

Nursing Care

Nursing management related to infectious disease focuses on health promotion, prevention, and prompt identification and treatment.

Assessment

The following data are collected through the health history and physical examination. Further focused assessments are described with nursing interventions in the next section.

- *Health history:* Current manifestations, age, medication use (antipyretics and anti-infectives), nutrition, exposure to infectious individuals, immunizations, invasive procedures and therapies, chronic diseases such as diabetes mellitus, cancer
- *Physical assessment:* Vital signs, body system(s) where infection is suspected, lymph node enlargement and tenderness.

Priorities of Care

Nursing care priorities related to infection focus on preventing spread of the infection to susceptible individuals and providing education and support for effective eradication of the pathogen.

Diagnoses, Outcomes, and Interventions

Patients with an infection may be managed in the hospital or at home, depending on the severity of the infection. During the acute phase, nursing care includes administering prescribed antibiotics, implementing and maintaining aseptic technique and infection control measures, and encouraging a balance of rest and activity, good nutritional intake, and other measures to support immunologic function and healing.

Reduce Risk for Infection. The spread of infection is a risk in any facility that houses many people. It is a particular risk in hospitals, where many patients have at least some degree of immunosuppression and many drug-resistant strains of pathogens are prevalent. It is vital that nurses use good hand hygiene techniques at all times, employ standard precautions with all patients, and use category-specific isolation techniques as indicated to prevent infectious spread to other patients, themselves, and their families.

Expected Outcome: Infection will be limited to involved patient without evidence of transmission to susceptible individuals.

The nurse will:

- Admit patients with known or suspected infections to a private room. *This is important to minimize the risk to other patients.*
- Perform hand hygiene using hand sanitizer on entering and leaving the patient's room. If visibly soiled, wash hands using a 10- to 15-second vigorous scrub with soap or antibacterial scrub solution. *A 10- to 15-second scrub removes transient microorganisms from the skin and helps prevent transmission of infection to or from the patient.*
- Use standard precautions and personal protective devices to reduce the risk of transmission. *Gloves, gowns, and masks are to be worn whenever there is a risk of skin or mucous membrane contamination by contact with infectious material, airborne spread of organisms, or droplet nuclei.*
- Explain the reasons for and importance of isolation procedures during hospitalization. *Patients with isolation precautions may feel neglected, dirty, or shunned. Explanation of reasons and procedures can enhance the patient's and family's understanding and acceptance.*
- Place a mask on the patient and/or cover all infectious lesions or wounds completely when transporting the patient for diagnostic or treatment procedures. *These measures help minimize air contamination and the risk to visitors and personnel.*
- Collect a culture and sensitivity (C&S) specimen as ordered or indicated by purulent drainage, pyuria, or other manifestations of infection. *C&S is performed to determine the presence and type of infectious organisms as well as antibiotics most likely to be effective in eradicating it.*

SAFETY ALERT: Collect the specimen for C&S before the first dose of antibiotics is administered to ensure adequate organisms for culture. ■

- Administer prescribed anti-infective agents. *Anti-infectives are used to destroy the invading microorganism.*
- Inform all personnel having contact with the patient of the diagnosis. *This is particularly important for a patient with a disease requiring category-specific isolation so that personnel can take appropriate precautions.*
- Ensure that visitors don appropriate protective wear before they enter the patient's room. *Protective wear reduces their risk of infection.*
- Use appropriate measures for disposing of contaminated tissues, dressings, or other material and for removing soiled linens and equipment from the patient's room. *Check hospital policy or published guidelines for category-specific isolation.*
- Teach the importance of complying with prescribed treatment for the entire course of the regimen. *Because anti-infective agents kill only a portion of the pathogen population with each dose, completion of the entire course of therapy is necessary to reduce the risk of relapse and of creating drug-resistant organisms.*

Reduce Anxiety. The patient with an infectious disease may experience anxiety related to his or her manifestations, treatment measures, the prognosis, and expected outcome of the disease. High levels of anxiety interfere with the ability to learn and to comprehend and follow directions.

Expected Outcome: Patient's anxiety level will not interfere with ability to understand and follow directions for treatment.

The nurse will:

- Assess level of anxiety. *The level of anxiety influences the patient's response to and interpretation of the situation and degree of threat it poses.*
- Discuss the infection, treatments, prognosis, and expected outcomes. *Discussions help to allay fears and misconceptions.*
- Support and enhance the patient's coping strategies. *An individual uses intrapersonal and interpersonal mechanisms to reduce or relieve anxiety.*
- Include significant others in the plan of care. *Inclusion of the patient and family members provides assurance and confidence, and promotes understanding of the unknown.*
- Explain isolation procedures, and answer any concerns. *Isolation may be necessary to prevent the spread of infection but can cause great anxiety for the patient and family members.*
- Provide referrals as needed for continuing care, for example, to home health agencies for dressing changes or periodic assessment. *Referrals are often necessary to provide ongoing interventions and maintain continuity of care.*

Manage Hyperthermia. Hyperthermia is an expected consequence of the infectious disease process. Fever may produce mild, short-term effects or, when prolonged, may cause serious life-threatening effects.

Expected Outcome: Patient's temperature will remain within defined limits.

The nurse will:

- Monitor temperature especially during episodes of chills; note heart rate and rhythm. *Chills indicate a rising temperature. Hyperthermia can cause dysrhythmias.*
- Administer prescribed antipyretic as indicated for elevated temperature. *Although antipyretics lower the temperature and enhance comfort for the patient, this benefit must be weighed against the possible beneficial effect of an elevated temperature in the immune response. Fever facilitates the immune response by increasing the motility and activity of neutrophils and stimulates the production of interferon. In addition, temperatures above the normal range inhibit the growth and reproduction of many microorganisms* (Sorenson et al., 2019).

- Promote body cooling through lowering the room temperature. *Rapid cooling stimulates the hypothalamus to increase the body's temperature; this increases both shivering and the metabolic rate.*

SAFETY ALERT: Use ice packs, cool/tepid baths, or a hypothermia blanket with caution to prevent unnecessary shivering. ■

- Monitor fluid loss; encourage increased fluid and electrolyte intake either orally or intravenously. *Hyperthermia causes fluid loss from evaporation and may result in dehydration and electrolyte imbalance.*
- If diaphoretic, bathe and provide dry clothing and bedding. *These measures increase patient comfort and decrease further water evaporation.*
- Promote rest periods. *Rest increases the energy reserve that is depleted by an increased metabolic, heart, and respiratory rate.*

Delegating Nursing Care Activities

As appropriate and allowed by the designated duties and responsibilities of assistive personnel, the nurse may delegate nursing care activities such as obtaining vital signs and temperature, measuring intake and output, promoting fluid intake, and providing oral and skin care for the patient with an infection. The nurse must verify caregivers' understanding of and ability to follow infection control and transmission precautions prior to delegating nursing care activities.

Transitions of Care

Preventing infection requires education of healthcare personnel and the general public. Education includes understanding the importance of immunizations, the guidelines for using antibiotics to prevent the development of drug-resistant microorganisms, and how to prevent the spread of infection. Check immunization records for all family members and encourage them to keep immunizations up to date. Increase public awareness regarding appropriate antibiotic use. Guidelines for preventing the spread of infection to others include:

- Avoid crowds and contact with susceptible individuals, especially those who are immunosuppressed (e.g., people who have HIV, who are undergoing therapy for cancer, or who have had an organ transplant).
- Use disposable tissues to contain respiratory secretions when coughing or sneezing. Cough into the elbow or upper arm instead of the hand if disposable tissues are not available.
- Use appropriate food-handling precautions for diseases spread via the fecal–oral route, such as hepatitis A.
- Avoid contact with or sharing of body fluids. For example, do not share needles or razors; use a condom during sexual activity, or abstain; have each person clean his or her own blood spills or wounds, if possible.

For patients with acute infections and their families, teaching is directed toward helping the patient recover from the infection or disease, preventing its spread to others, and preventing life-threatening complications. Instructions should include the following points:

- Use good hand hygiene techniques, particularly after touching infected wounds or lesions, coughing, sneezing, blowing the nose, or using the bathroom. Wash hands thoroughly before performing any procedures, such as dressing changes. Wash hands with soap and water before and after preparing food or eating and before and after using the toilet or handling diapers. Do not share eating utensils.
- Take all prescribed antibiotics as ordered even after manifestations have subsided. Take the prescription at prescribed intervals around the clock.
- Do not share your prescription or save medication in anticipation of future infection.
- Notify your healthcare provider in the following situations:
  a. Symptoms do not improve within 24 to 48 hours after antibiotic therapy is instituted or they worsen.
  b. Manifestations of antibiotic allergy (itching, rash, difficulty breathing or swallowing, swelling of the face or tongue) occur. Discontinue medication and contact prescriber.
  c. Adverse responses, such as gastrointestinal distress or diarrhea, interfere with completion of the prescription.
  d. Manifestations of infection recur after completing prescribed antibiotic.
- Report redness, swelling, or drainage around wounds or persistent high fever.
- Increase fluid intake to at least 2500 mL (2.5 quarts) per day.
- Report any manifestations of opportunistic infections: Loose, watery, and foul-smelling diarrhea; vaginal discharge or itching; fuzzy growth or white plaques in mouth or on tongue; blood in urine; chills; fever; or unusual cough.
- In addition, suggest the following resources: County or public health department, Centers for Disease Control and Prevention.

Chronic infections can be debilitating and may require ongoing care. These types of infections are commonly seen in older adults, in those who are immunocompromised, and in those who have a chronic viral disease. Common chronic infections include:

- Hepatitis B and C and HIV infections, which are caused by viruses. Treatment for these diseases has advanced and improved morbidity and mortality rates but patients often require continuous monitoring, pharmacologic treatments, and care to prevent complications and the development of other infections.
- Osteomyelitis, a chronic infection of the bone, is often seen in older patients due to decreases in immune responses. Blood supply to the bone is limited, which may prevent antibiotics from reaching the affected tissue. Antibiotic treatment is often augmented with

debridement, hyperbaric oxygen therapy, and nutritional supplementation.

- Chronic respiratory infections may be seen in patients with chronic obstructive pulmonary disorders such as emphysema and asthma. Patients with COPD have impaired respiratory immune responses that put them at greater risk of viral infections and bacterial and fungal colonization. Care should include:
  a. Counsel on smoking cessation
  b. Pulmonary rehabilitation
  c. Instruction on proper use of inhaled medication
  d. Teaching on hand hygiene and prevention of infection
  e. Ensuring the patient receives the influenza and pneumonia vaccines.

Individuals with diabetes are susceptible to chronic lower extremity wound infections due to effects of diabetes on blood vessels, nerves, and immune system.

- Prevention is the best method of care for the diabetic patient. Teaching should emphasize the need to inspect feet often and wear protective footwear.
- Wound care may include debridement of necrotic tissue, antibiotic therapy, and collagen-based dressings.

Septicemia is a term used for an infection of the blood. A release of cytokines takes place in response to infection in an attempt to control the infection and prevent further injury. Cytokines also increase the inflammatory process, which along with enzymatic activity cause damage to blood vessels, which in turn increases the inflammatory process. Other inflammatory processes result in alterations in clotting mechanisms producing the formation of blood clots interfering with circulation and perfusion. Often, the result of these metabolic processes results in multiorgan system failure and death. Immunocompromised individuals, older adults, and infants are at greatest risk.

CHAPTER HIGHLIGHTS

12.1 Overview of The Immune System and Inflammation

Explain the components and functions of the immune system and the immune response.

- Innate immunity, a nonspecific response to tissue injury, and the adaptive immune response, which directly targets invading microorganisms and abnormal cells, are critical components of the body's defenses. Supporting these defenses is a key nursing responsibility in promoting patient health.
- Both natural barriers and the immune system prevent the invasion and replication of pathogens.
- The adaptability and specificity of immune responses is possible because immune cells are genetically encoded to capture pathogens, move them to lymph nodes, and develop specific immune responses to destroy them.
- The inflammatory response serves to isolate invading antigens. When it occurs in response to acute injury, inflammation produces discomfort but serves a protective role. In contrast, chronic inflammation can damage affected tissue and may serve no protective function.
- Inflammation is a protective mechanism designed to prevent pathogens from entering the bloodstream and populating functional tissues such as heart, liver, and kidney. Pain acts as a signal that tissue has been damaged and stimulates protective responses such as limiting function while healing progresses. Healing occurs as the inflammatory process isolates the injury and repairs damaged tissue.

12.2 Acquired Immunity, Immunizations, and Precautions

Outline the process of acquired immunity and the importance of immunizations and isolation precautions in preventing disease.

- A fully immunized population is an important infection control strategy and a major factor in maintaining the health of individuals and the population as a whole.
- Nurses are instrumental in protecting vulnerable patients from infection, identifying early manifestations of infection, participating with the interprofessional team in treating infection, and educating patients and their families about effective treatment of infection.

12.3 Patients with Inflammation and Infection

Describe the pathophysiology and manifestations of inflammation and infection, and outline the interprofessional care, nursing care, and transitions of care for patients with these conditions.

- Localized infections may damage tissue and create pain, but systemic infections can be life-threatening. Unfortunately, hospitals are hazardous environments populated with collections of pathogens. Healthcare-associated infections are often introduced into the body by medical procedures. Isolation within healthcare organizations may be necessary to reduce the transmission of disease.
- Hygiene, protection from harm, and nutrition support the immune defenses. Antimicrobial medications limit the spread of pathogens, but can lose their effectiveness when microbes mutate and develop resistance.

TEST YOURSELF NCLEX-RN® REVIEW

1. A patient receives gamma globulin after being exposed to hepatitis A. Which type of immunity should the nurse expect the patient to develop?
   A. Natural active
   B. Natural passive
   C. Acquired active
   D. Acquired passive
2. The nurse is caring for a patient with an infection. Which nursing action is a priority when providing the prescribed treatment?
   A. Administer prescribed anti-infective.
   B. Obtain specimen for culture and sensitivity.
   C. Conduct initial assessment of hypersensitivities and allergies.
   D. Monitor for reaction to prescribed anti-infective.
3. The nurse is providing medications to a patient with an inflammation. Which medication provided by the nurse will inhibit prostaglandin synthesis?
   A. Aspirin
   B. Penicillin
   C. Morphine sulfate
   D. Warfarin (Coumadin)
4. While reviewing a patient's recent complete blood count, the nurse notes a large percentage of banded neutrophils. What does this finding indicate to the nurse?
   A. Renal failure
   B. Acute infection
   C. Hyperthyroidism
   D. Autoimmune disorder
5. A patient is admitted with methicillin-resistant *Staphylococcus aureus* cultured from a draining sacral wound. Which type of precaution should the nurse implement for this patient?
   A. Droplet
   B. Contact
   C. Airborne
   D. Protective
6. A patient with a systemic inflammation is resting in bed, periodically sleeping, and wants additional blankets. Which part of the immune system is responsible for this patient's illness behavior?
   A. Interferons
   B. Phagocytes
   C. Complement system
   D. Inflammatory cytokines
7. A patient is diagnosed with neutrophilia. What does this finding indicate to the nurse? (Select all that apply.)
   A. The patient has bone marrow depression.
   B. The patient may be experiencing a stressful response.
   C. There is an increase in circulating neutrophils
   D. The number of white blood cells is at the expected average.
   E. The patient may have an acute infection.
8. The nurse is preparing discharge instructions for a patient with an inflammation who is at risk for infection. What should the nurse include when teaching this patient? (Select all that apply.)
   A. Limit daily intake of calories.
   B. Apply heat for 20 minutes at a time.
   C. Resume normal activities of daily living.
   D. Take prescribed antibiotics until fever drops.
   E. Increase daily intake of fluids
9. The nurse is caring for an older patient recovering from an acute illness. Which intervention should the nurse implement to reduce the patient's risk of developing a healthcare-associated infection? (Select all that apply.)
   A. Teach the patient to restrict fluids throughout the day.
   B. Coach the patient to deep-breathe and cough frequently.
   C. Recommend placement of an indwelling urinary catheter.
   D. Wash hands with soap and water before entering the patient's room.
   E. Palpate intravenous site for tenderness daily
10. The nurse is instructing unlicensed assistive personnel (UAP) to use standard precautions when providing morning care to assigned patients. What should the nurse teach UAP to specifically do?
    A. Perform hand hygiene, wear masks, and recap needles.
    B. Apply a mask and gown, and prepare working surfaces by spraying with disinfectant.
    C. Apply gloves, gown, and goggles if splashing of body fluids is likely.
    D. Wash hands with alcohol-based hand rub for visibly dirty or blood-contaminated hands.

See Test Yourself answers in Appendix B.

REFERENCES

Adams, M. P., Holland, L. N., & Urban, C. (2017). *Pharmacology for nursing: A pathophysiologic approach* (5th ed.). Hoboken, NJ: Pearson Education.

Agency for Healthcare Research and Quality. (2017). *Health care–associated infections.* Retrieved from: https://psnet.ahrq.gov/primers/primer/7/health-care-associated-infections

Akhtar, S. (2018). Diseases of aging. In Hines & K. Marschall (Eds.) Stoeltings' Anesthesia and Co-existing Disease (7th ed.), pp. 327–343. Philadelphia, PA: Elsevier.

Anderson, D., & Sexton, D. (2017). Epidemiology of surgical site infection in adults. *UpToDate*. Retrieved from www.uptodate.com.

Aronson, J. K. (2016). *Meyler's side effects of drugs*. Waltham, MA: Elsevier.

Booth, K. (2016). Preventing healthcare-associated infections (HAIs). *Journal of Continuing Education Topics and Issues, 18*(1), 18–23.

Braun, C., & Anderson, C. (2017). *Applied pathophysiology a conceptual approach to the mechanisms of disease* (3rd ed.). Philadelphia, PA: Wolters Kluwer.

Centers for Disease Control and Prevention (CDC). (2017a). *Guideline for isolation precautions: Preventing transmission of infectious agents in healthcare settings.* Retrieved from https://www.cdc.gov/infectioncontrol/pdf/guidelines/isolation-guidelines.pdf.

Centers for Disease Control and Prevention. (2017d). *Vaccine safety: Vaccine adverse event reporting system (VAERS).* Retrieved from www.cdc.gov/vaccinesafety/Activities/vaers.html.

Centers for Disease Control and Prevention. (2017b). Handwashing: Clean hands save lives. Retrieved from https://www.cdc.gov/handwashing/show-me-the-science-hand-sanitizer.html.

Centers for Disease Control and Prevention.(2017c). Guidelines for the prevention of intravascular catheter-related infections, 2011. Retrieved from https://www.cdc.gov/infectioncontrol/pdf/guidelines/bsi-guidelines.pdf.

Centers for Disease Control and Prevention. (2018). *Recommended immunization schedule for adults aged 19 or older: United States 2017.* Retrieved from https://www.cdc.gov/vaccines/schedules/downloads/adult/adult-combined-schedule.pdf.

David, C., O'Neal, K., Miller, M., Johnson, J., & Lloyd, A. (2017). A literacy-sensitive approach to improving antibiotic understanding in a community-based setting. *International Journal of Pharmacy Practice, 25*, 394–398.

Dieffenbach, C., & Tramont, E. (2015). Innate (general or nonspecific) host defense mechanisms. In *Mandell, Douglas, and Bennett's principles and practice of infectious disease* (8th ed.), pp. 26–33. Philadelphia, PA: Elsevier Saunders.

Garlough, D. (2017, March 14). Turning the heat down: Solutions for reducing chronic inflammation in our patients' bodies. *RDH*. Retrieved from www.rdhmag.com/articles/print/volume-37/issue-3/contents/turning-the-heat-down-on-inflammation.html.

Geschwind, M. (2016). Prion diseases. In R. Daroff, J. Jankovic, J. Mazziotta, & S. Pomeroy (Eds.), *Bradley's neurology in clinical practice* (7th ed.), pp. 1365–1379. Philadelphia, PA: Elsevier Saunders.

Jaffe, L., & Wu, S. (2017). The role of nutrition in chronic wound care management: What patients eat affects how they heal. *Podiatry Management, 36*(9), 77–84.

Lam, G., Fontaine, R., Ross, F., & Chiu, E. (2017). Hyperbaric oxygen therapy: Exploring the clinical evidence. *Advances in Skin and Wound Care, 30*(4), 181–193.

Lubbers, R., van Essen, M. F., van Kooten, C., & Trouw, L. A. (2017). Production of complement components by cells of the immune system. *Clinical and Experimental Immunology, 188*(2), 183–194.

Luo, R., Liu, C., Elliott, S., Wang, W., Parchim, N., Iriyama, T., . . . Xia, Y. (2016). Transglutaminase is a critical link between inflammation and hypertension. *Journal of the American Heart Association, 5*, e003730.

Manning, M. L., Pfeiffer, J., & Larson, E. (2016). Combating antibiotic resistance: The role of nursing in antibiotic stewardship. *American Journal of Infection Control, 44*, 1454–1457.

Mayer, G. (2017). Innate (non-specific) immunity. *University of South Carolina School of Medicine's Microbiology and Immunology On-Line.* Retrieved from www.microbiologybook.org/ghaffar/innate.htm.

Mason, J. (2016). Nutritional principles and assessment of the gastroenterology patient. In *Sleisenger and Fordtran's gastrointestinal and liver disease* (10th ed.), pp. 57–82. Philadelphia, PA: Elsevier Saunders.

Micek, S., Chew, B., Hampton, N., & Kollef, M. (2016). A case-control study assessing the impact of nonventilated hospital-acquired pneumonia on patient outcomes. *Chest, 150*(5), 1008–1014.

Miner, J., & Burton, J. (2018). Pain management. In *Rosen's emergency medicine: Concepts and clinical practice* (9th ed.) Philadelphia, PA: Elsevier.

Nasef, N., Mehta, S., & Ferguson, L. (2017). Susceptibility to chronic inflammation: An update. *Archives of Toxicology, 91*(3), 1131–1141.

Rohde, R., Felkner, M., Reagan, J., Hogan Mitchell, A., & Tille, P. (2016). Healthcare-associated infections (HAI): The perfect storm has arrived! *Clinical Laboratory Science, 29*(1), 28–31.

Russell, C., Koch, O., Laurenson, I., O'Shea, D., Sutherland, R., & Mackintosh, C. (2016). Diagnosis and features of hospital-acquired pneumonia: A retrospective cohort study. *Journal of Hospital Infection, 92*(3), 273–279.

Schaeffer, A. (2017). Placement and management of urinary bladder catheters in adults. *UpToDate*. Retrieved from https://www.uptodate.com/contents/placement-and-management-of-urinary-bladder-catheters-in-adults.

Sickbert-Bennett, E., DiBiase, L., Schade, T., Wolak, E., Weber, D., & Rutala, W. (2016). Reduction of healthcare-associated infections by exceeding high compliance with hand hygiene practices. *Emerging Infectious Disease, 22*(9), 1628–1630.

Sorenson, M., Quinn, L., & Klein, D. (2019). *Pathophysiology: Concepts of human disease.* Hoboken, NJ: Pearson Education.

Wirtz, P., & Kanel, R. (2017). Psychological stress, inflammation, and coronary heart disease. *Current Cardiology Report,* 19, 111.

Yoshikawa, T., & Norman, D. (2017). Geriatric infectious diseases: Current concepts on diagnosis and management. *Journal of the American Geriatric Society, 65,* 631–641.

ADDITIONAL RESOURCES

AIDS.gov: Immune System 101

www.aids.gov/hiv-aids-basics/just-diagnosed-with-hiv-aids/hiv-in-your-body/immune-system-101/

American Academy of Allergy, Asthma and Immunology

www.aaaai.org/home.aspx

Centers for Disease Control and Prevention: Yearly Immunization Recommendations

www.cdc.gov/vaccines/schedules/downloads/adult/adult-combined-schedule.pdf

Center for Human Immunology, Autoimmunity, and Inflammation

http://chi.nhlbi.nih.gov/web/

National Institutes of Health: Understanding the Immune System

www.niaid.nih.gov/topics/immunesystem/Pages/default.aspx

Chapter 13

Nursing Care of Patients with Altered Immunity

Chapter Outline and Learning Outcomes

Review the normal immune system function, including self-recognition.

Compare and contrast the four types of hypersensitivity reactions.

Describe the pathophysiology and manifestations of autoimmune disorders and tissue transplant rejection, and outline the interprofessional care, nursing care, and transitions of care for patients with these disorders.

Describe the pathophysiology and manifestations of disorders of impaired immune response, and outline the interprofessional care, nursing care, and transitions of care for patients with these disorders.

CLINICAL COMPETENCIES

- Assess functional health of patients with altered immunity and monitor, document, and report unexpected manifestations and responses.
- Function competently within your own scope of practice as a member of the healthcare team caring for patients with altered immune function.
- Demonstrate sensitivity and respect for expressed values, culture, and preferences when planning and providing individualized and evidence-based care for individuals with altered immune responses.
- Apply quality measures and best practices in caring for patients with altered immune responses.
- Demonstrate effective strategies to reduce the risk of harm when caring for patients with altered immune responses.
- Apply technology and information management tools to support safe care for patients with altered immune responses.

KEY TERMS

acquired immunodeficiency syndrome (AIDS), 385
allergy, 366
allograft, 378
anaphylaxis, 366
antigenic substances, 365
autograft, 377
autoimmune disorder, 374
histocompatibility, 378
human immunodeficiency virus (HIV), 385
hypersensitivity, 366
immunosuppression, 377
Kaposi sarcoma (KS), 389
seroconversion, 387

Considering the complexity of the immune system, it is not surprising that abnormal or harmful responses occur. Altered immune system responses include those characterized by hyperresponsiveness of the immune system and those characterized by an impaired immune response. Allergies, autoimmune disorders, and reactions to organ or tissue transplants are all examples of hyperresponsive immune function. AIDS and other immunodeficiency disorders result from impairment of the immune system.

Our understanding of the components of the immune system and specific immune responses and their effects on health is rapidly increasing. Alterations of the immune system affect the functional health status of individuals in all areas; knowledge of the prevention and care of patients with disorders of the immune system is increasingly important in today's healthcare system.

13.1 Overview of the Altered Immune System

The immune system protects the body from invasion by foreign antigens, identifies and destroys potentially harmful cells, and removes cellular debris. The lymphoid organs and lymphocytes accomplish these functions through the processes of antibody-mediated immune response and cell-mediated immune response.

The effectiveness of the immune system depends on its ability to differentiate normal host tissue from abnormal or foreign tissue. Body cells, tissues, and fluids have unique antigenic properties recognized by the immune system as "self." **Antigenic substances** stimulate an immune system response, but when identified as "self," the competent immune system does not react. External agents, such as microorganisms, cells and tissues from other humans or animals, and some inorganic substances, have antigenic properties recognized by the immune system as "nonself."

Each body cell displays specific cell surface characteristics, or markers, that are unique to each individual. These are known as *human leukocyte antigens (HLAs)*. An individual's HLA characteristics are coded within a large cluster of genes known as the *major histocompatibility complex (MHC)* located on chromosome 6. Chromosomes are paired, with each individual inheriting one member of the pair from each parent. A chromosome pair contains multiple genes, each carrying instructions for production of one polypeptide chain. The number of genes in the MHC results in a multitude of HLA combinations. As a result, the possibility of two people having the same HLA type is extremely remote. Identical twins may be the exception, and some siblings have very similar HLA patterns. In tissue grafting and organ transplants, matching the HLA type as closely as possible tends to decrease rejection.

Immunocompetent people have an immune system that identifies antigens and effectively destroys or removes them. When the immune system functions improperly, the result may be an overreaction or a deficiency, resulting in health problems. Overreaction of the immune system leads to hypersensitivity disorders, such as allergies. When the immune system loses the ability to recognize self, autoimmune disorders may ensue. Immunodeficiency diseases or malignancies can develop when the immune system is incompetent or unable to respond effectively, as is the case with acquired immunodeficiency syndrome. These alterations in immunity are discussed later in this chapter.

The *antibody-mediated immune response* is accomplished by B lymphocytes (B cells) that are further divided into memory cells and plasma cells. They are activated by contact with an antigen and by T cells. B cells produce antibodies, also known as *immunoglobulins*, and serve to inactivate an invading antigen. Immunoglobulin M (or IgM) is formed early in nearly every immune response and is an important component of the immune system complexes seen in autoimmune disorders. The most prevalent immunoglobulin, IgG, is the major antibody protecting against bacterial and viral antigens. Memory cells remember an antigen and, when exposed to it a second time, immediately initiate the immune response. This action provides the foundation of acquired immunity.

The T-cell component of the immune system identifies cells containing antigens and signals B cells and other components of the immune system to attack infected cells. T lymphocytes are subdivided into effector cells and regulator cells. The cytotoxic T cell is the primary cell that responds to stimuli and is known as an effector cell. Regulator T cells are divided into two subsets known as helper T cells and suppressor T cells. In addition to destroying cells containing viruses, cytotoxic T lymphocytes also attack malignant cells and are responsible for the rejection of transplanted organs and grafted tissues.

Immune function tends to decline with age, a decline known as *immunosenescence* (Yoshikawa & Norman, 2017). External factors, such as nutritional status and the effects of chemical exposure, ultraviolet radiation, and environmental pollution, affect the older adult's immune status. Internal factors affect it as well, including genetics, the function of the neurologic and endocrine systems, chronic and prior illnesses, and individual anatomic and physiologic variations. These influences make it difficult to predict the effect of aging on the immune system. In some older individuals, the immune system is as effective as that of younger individuals.

Changes associated with immunosenescence include involution of the thymus with less competent T-cell maturation, diminished antibody production and adhesion, and decreased tolerance of self-antigens. As a result, the responsiveness, strength, and duration of immune responses decrease. Increased morbidity and mortality associated with infection and increases in cancer and autoimmune disorders are seen.

Assessing the Altered Immune System Response

Unlike body systems that are composed of closely related organs, the immune system is diverse and scattered.

Optimal immune function depends on intact skin and mucous membrane barriers, adequate blood cell production and differentiation, a functional system of lymphatics and the spleen, and the ability to differentiate foreign tissue and pathogens from normal body tissue and flora. Because of this diversity of organs and functions, assessment of the immune system is often integrated throughout the history and physical examination.

Health History

Before conducting the health history, review the biographic data, including age, gender, race, and ethnic background. Many autoimmune disorders are more prevalent in women than in men. Family history is also important because there is a genetic component in the etiology of many disorders affecting the immune system.

Many interview questions related to the immune system and disorders that affect it are of a sensitive nature. Be sure to provide privacy prior to the interview. If family members are present, request that they leave. Ask the least sensitive questions before moving into those that are more sensitive, such as those related to the use of illicit drugs or sexual activity. Cultural competence is necessary for effective communication.

Physical Assessment

The techniques of inspection and palpation are used to assess a patient's immune system.

- Assess the general appearance; evident fatigue or weakness may indicate acute or chronic illness or immunodeficiency. Note whether the stated and apparent age coincide. Assess height, weight, and body type for apparent weight loss or wasting. Observe ease of movement and note any evident stiffness or difficulty moving. Check vital signs. An elevated temperature may indicate an infection or inflammatory response.
- Inspect the mucous membranes of the nose and mouth for color and condition. Pale, boggy (edematous) nasal mucosa is often associated with chronic allergies. Note petechiae, white patches, or lacy white plaques in the oral mucosa; they may indicate hemolysis or immunodeficiency.
- Assess skin color, temperature, and moisture. Pale or jaundiced skin may indicate a hemolytic reaction. Pallor may also indicate bone marrow suppression with accompanying immunodeficiency. Inspect the skin for evidence of rashes or lesions, such as petechiae; numerous bruises; purple or blue patches or lesions indicative of Kaposi sarcoma; and wounds that are infected, inflamed, or unhealed. Note the location and distribution of any rashes or lesions.
- Inspect and palpate the cervical, axilla, and groin lymph nodes for evidence of lymphadenopathy (swelling) or tenderness.
- Inspect and palpate the joints for redness, swelling, tenderness, or deformity, which may indicate an autoimmune disorder such as rheumatoid arthritis or systemic lupus erythematosus. Assess joint range of motion, including the spine.

13.2 Hypersensitivity Reactions

Hypersensitivity is an altered immune response to an antigen that results in harm to the patient. When the antigen is environmental or exogenous, it is called an **allergy**, and the antigen is referred to as an *allergen*. The tissue response to a hypersensitivity reaction may be bothersome, causing a runny nose or itchy eyes, or it may be life-threatening, leading to blood cell hemolysis or laryngospasm, an involuntary tightening of the muscles of the larynx that causes difficulty inhaling.

Hypersensitivity reactions are primarily classified by the type of immune response that occurs on contact with the allergen. They may also be classified as immediate or delayed hypersensitivity responses. Anaphylaxis and transfusion reactions are examples of immediate hypersensitivity reactions; contact dermatitis is a typical delayed response. Allergies are sometimes referred to by the affected organ system (e.g., allergic rhinitis) or the allergen involved, as in hay fever. More than one type of reaction may occur simultaneously.

In a hypersensitivity reaction, an antigen–antibody or antigen–lymphocyte interaction causes a response that is damaging to body tissues. Antigen–antibody responses, or immediate hypersensitivity responses, are characterized as types I, II, and III. Type IV hypersensitivity is an antigen–lymphocyte reaction, resulting in a delayed hypersensitivity response.

Type I: Immediate Hypersensitivity

Common hypersensitivity reactions, such as allergic asthma, allergic rhinitis (hay fever), allergic conjunctivitis, hives (urticaria), and anaphylactic shock, are typical of type I immediate or IgE-mediated hypersensitivity. This type of hypersensitivity response is triggered when an allergen interacts with IgE bound to mast cells and basophils. The antigen–antibody complex prompts release of histamine and other chemical mediators, complement, acetylcholine, kinins, and chemotactic factors (**Figure 13.1** ■).

When a potent allergen such as bee or wasp venom or a drug is injected, resulting in widespread antibody–antigen reaction and response to these chemical mediators, a systemic response such as anaphylaxis, urticaria, or angioedema (localized, rapid swelling beneath the skin) results.

Anaphylaxis is an acute systemic type I response that occurs in highly sensitive individuals following injection of a specific antigen. Substances known to trigger anaphylaxis include:

- *Hormones:* Insulin, vasopressin, parathormone
- *Enzymes:* Trypsin, chymotrypsin, penicillinase

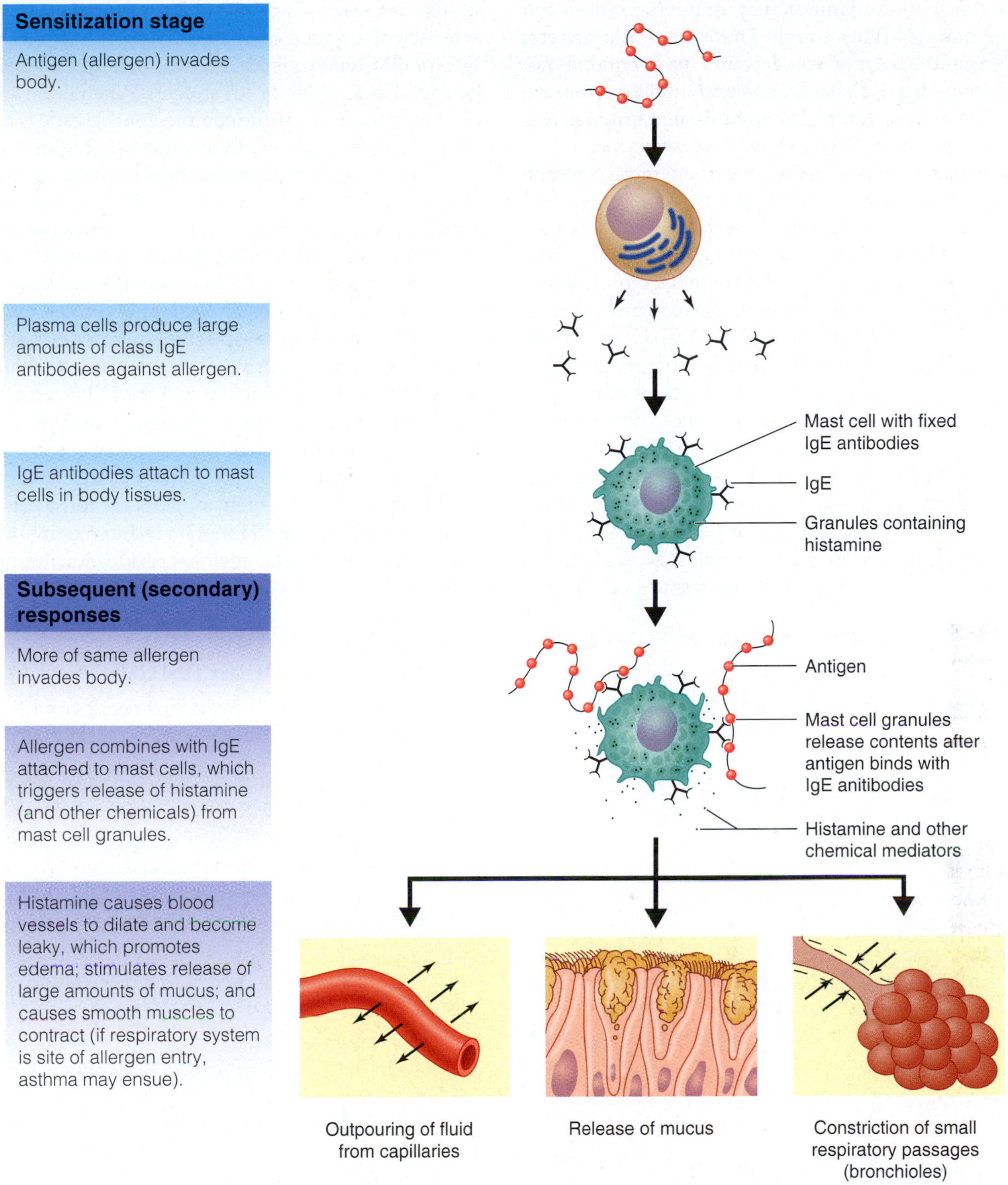
Sensitization stage
Antigen (allergen) invades body.
Plasma cells produce large amounts of class IgE antibodies against allergen.
IgE antibodies attach to mast cells in body tissues.
Mast cell with fixed IgE antibodies
IgE
Granules containing histamine
Subsequent (secondary) responses
More of same allergen invades body.
Antigen
Allergen combines with IgE attached to mast cells, which triggers release of histamine (and other chemicals) from mast cell granules.
Mast cell granules release contents after antigen binds with IgE anitibodies
Histamine and other chemical mediators
Histamine causes blood vessels to dilate and become leaky, which promotes edema; stimulates release of large amounts of mucus; and causes smooth muscles to contract (if respiratory system is site of allergen entry, asthma may ensue).
Outpouring of fluid from capillaries
Release of mucus
Constriction of small respiratory passages (bronchioles)

Figure 13.1 ■ Type I IgE-mediated hypersensitivity response.

- ***Pollens:*** Ragweed, grass, trees
- ***Foods:*** Eggs, seafood, peanuts, tree nuts, grains, beans, cottonseed oil, chocolate
- ***Vitamins:*** Thiamine, folic acid
- ***Insect venom:*** Yellow jacket, hornet, paper wasp, honey bee
- ***Occupational agents:*** Rubber, latex, industrial chemicals
- ***Antibiotics:*** Penicillins, cephalosporins, amphotericin B, nitrofurantoin
- ***Local anesthetics:*** Procaine, lidocaine.

The reaction begins within minutes of exposure to the allergen and may be almost instantaneous. The release of histamine and other mediators causes vasodilation and increased capillary permeability, smooth muscle contraction, and bronchial constriction. These chemical mediators cause the typical manifestations of anaphylaxis. Initially, a sense of foreboding or uneasiness, light-headedness, and itching palms and scalp may be noted. Hives may develop, along with angioedema of the eyelids, lips, tongue, hands, feet, and genitals. Swelling can also affect the uvula and larynx, impairing breathing. This is further complicated by bronchial constriction, manifested by air hunger, stridor and wheezing, and a barking cough. These respiratory effects can be lethal if the reaction is severe and intervention is not provided immediately. Vasodilation and fluid loss from the vascular system can lead to impaired tissue perfusion and hypotension, a condition known as *anaphylactic shock*.

Fortunately, localized responses are the more common manifestations of type I hypersensitivity. Atopic reactions, which have a genetic predisposition, are localized, rather than systemic, IgE-mediated responses to an allergen. They occur when an allergen contacts cell-bound IgE in the bronchial tree, nasal mucosa, and conjunctival tissues. Chemical mediators are released locally, producing symptoms such as asthma, allergic rhinitis (hay fever), conjunctivitis, or atopic dermatitis. Allergens commonly associated with atopic reactions of this type include pollens, fungal spores, house dust mites, animal dander, and feathers (Sorenson et al., 2019). When an allergic response to food occurs in the digestive system, nausea and vomiting, diarrhea, and cramping may develop. If the gastrointestinal mucosa is altered by a local allergic response, then the allergen may be absorbed, leading to a systemic reaction. Urticaria (hives) is the most common systemic response to food allergies.

Type II: Cytotoxic Hypersensitivity

Cytotoxic hypersensitivity reactions are characterized by formation of IgG or IgM antibodies against normal or foreign cells or tissues (Sorenson et al., 2019). A hemolytic transfusion reaction to blood of an incompatible type is characteristic of a type II or cytotoxic hypersensitivity reaction. IgG- or IgM-type antibodies are formed to a cell-bound antigen such as the ABO or Rh antigen. When these antibodies bind with the antigen, the complement cascade is activated, resulting in destruction of the target cell (**Figure 13.2** ■).

Type II reactions may be stimulated by an exogenous antigen, such as foreign tissue or cells, or a drug reaction in which the drug forms an antigenic complex on the surface of a blood cell, stimulating the production of antibodies. The affected cell is then destroyed in the resulting antigen–antibody reaction; for example, hemolytic anemia is sometimes associated with the administration of drugs such as penicillins, cephalosporins, and streptomycin. Withdrawal of the drug stops the reaction and the cell destruction.

Endogenous antigens can also stimulate a type II reaction, resulting in an autoimmune disorder such as Goodpasture syndrome (pulmonary hemorrhage and glomerulonephritis), in which antigens are formed to specific tissues in the lungs and kidneys. Hashimoto thyroiditis and autoimmune hemolytic anemia are additional examples of autoimmune type II reactions.

Type III: Immune Complex–Mediated Hypersensitivity

Type III hypersensitivity reactions result from the formation of IgG or IgM antibody–antigen immune complexes

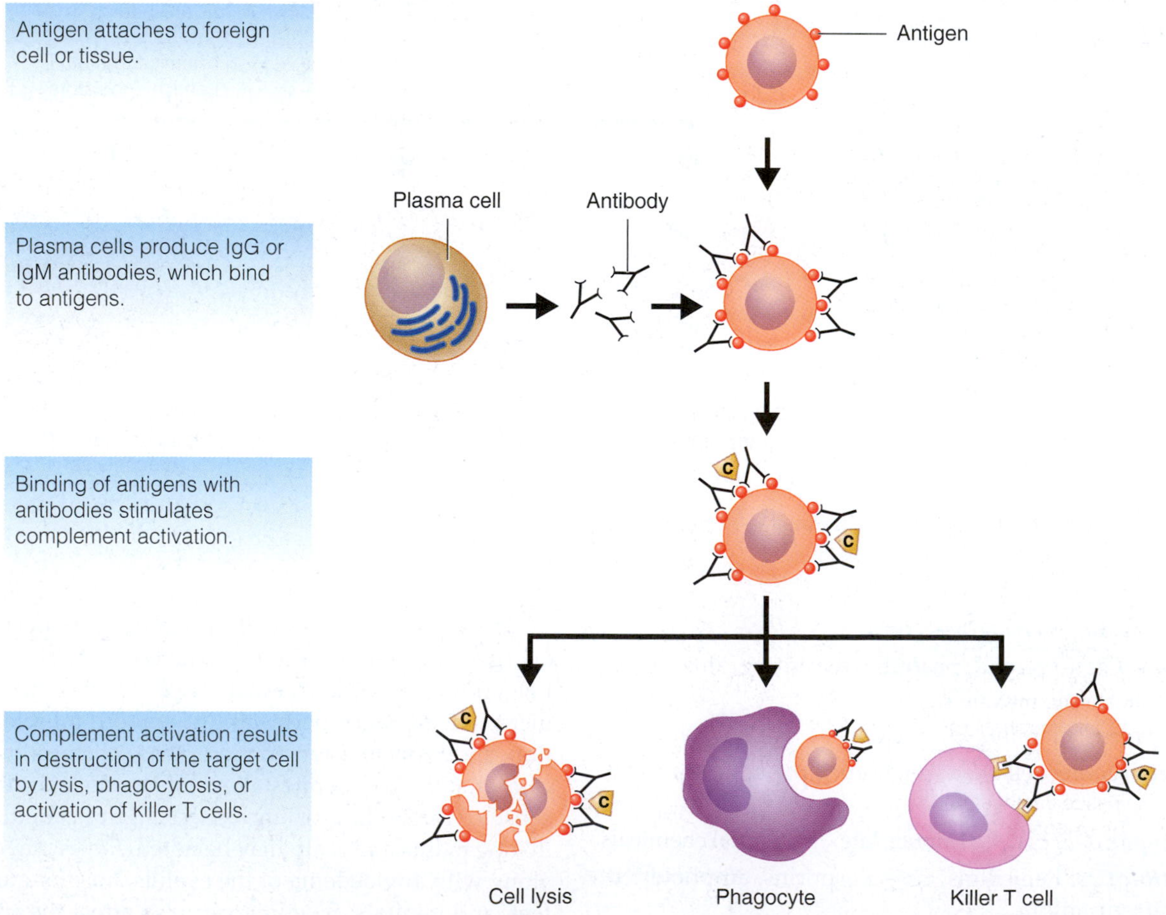
Antigen attaches to foreign cell or tissue.
Antigen
Plasma cells produce IgG or IgM antibodies, which bind to antigens.
Plasma cell
Antibody
Binding of antigens with antibodies stimulates complement activation.
C
Complement activation results in destruction of the target cell by lysis, phagocytosis, or activation of killer T cells.
Cell lysis
Phagocyte
Killer T cell

Figure 13.2 ■ Type II cytotoxic hypersensitivity response.

in the circulation. When these complexes are deposited in vessel walls and extravascular tissues, complement is activated and chemical mediators of inflammation such as histamine are released. Chemotactic factors attract neutrophils to the site of inflammation. When neutrophils attempt to phagocytize the immune complexes, lysosomal enzymes are released, increasing tissue damage (**Figure 13.3** ■).

Either systemic or local responses may be seen with type III reactions. For example, serum sickness is a systemic response, named because it was first identified after administration of foreign serum (e.g., horse antitetanus toxin). Although foreign serums are no longer administered, serum sickness still occurs in response to some drugs, such as penicillin and sulfonamides. Immune complexes are deposited in the walls of small blood vessels, the kidneys, and joints. Manifestations of serum sickness include fever, urticaria or rash, arthralgias, myalgias, and lymphadenopathy.

Localized responses may occur at a number of different sites. As immune complexes accumulate in the glomerular basement membrane of the kidneys—for example, following a streptococcal infection or with systemic lupus erythematosus—glomerulonephritis develops. An acute alveolar inflammatory response can occur when an antigen (such as dust from moldy hay) is inhaled by agricultural workers.

Type IV: Delayed Hypersensitivity

Type IV reactions differ from other hypersensitivity responses in two ways. First, these reactions are cell mediated rather than antibody mediated, involving T cells of the immune system. Second, type IV reactions are delayed rather than immediate, developing 24 to 48 hours after exposure to the antigen. Type IV hypersensitivity responses result from an exaggerated interaction between an antigen and normal cell-mediated mechanisms. This exaggerated interaction results in the release of soluble inflammatory

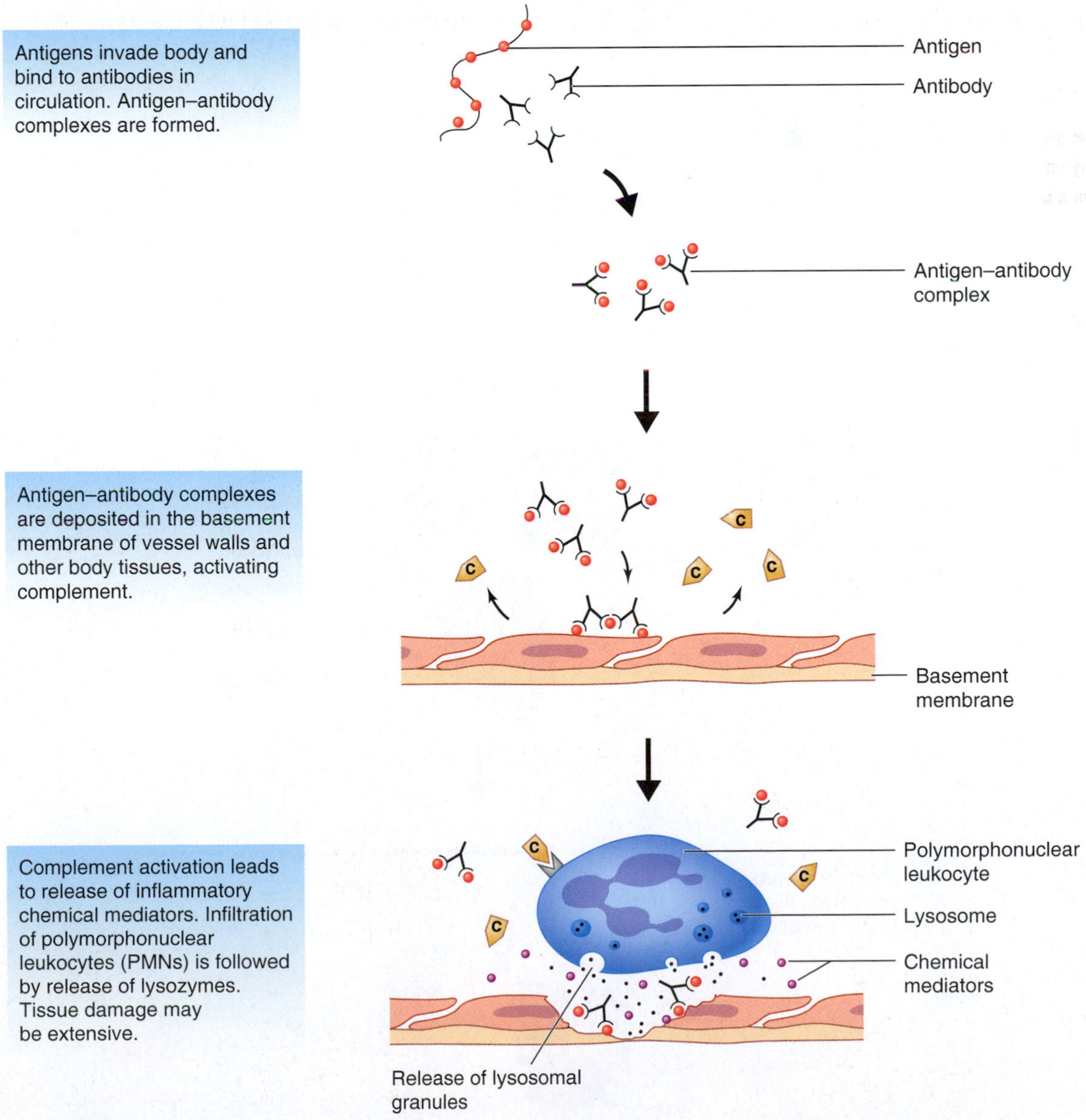
Antigens invade body and bind to antibodies in circulation. Antigen–antibody complexes are formed.
Antigen
Antibody
Antigen–antibody complex
Antigen–antibody complexes are deposited in the basement membrane of vessel walls and other body tissues, activating complement.
C
Basement membrane
Complement activation leads to release of inflammatory chemical mediators. Infiltration of polymorphonuclear leukocytes (PMNs) is followed by release of lysozymes. Tissue damage may be extensive.
Polymorphonuclear leukocyte
Lysosome
Chemical mediators
Release of lysosomal granules

Figure 13.3 ■ Type III immune complex–mediated hypersensitivity response.

and immune mediators (from the lysozymes within the macrophages) and recruitment of killer T cells, causing local tissue destruction (**Figure 13.4** ■).

Contact dermatitis is a classic example of a type IV reaction. Intense redness, itching, blister formation, and thickening affect the skin in the area exposed to the antigen. Many antigens can provoke this response; poison ivy is a prime example. In the healthcare setting, an allergic response to latex can produce contact dermatitis (see next section). Other examples of cell-mediated responses include a positive tuberculin test and graft rejection episodes.

Latex Allergy

Although protective against infection, the repetitive use of latex gloves creates a persistent exposure to latex for healthcare workers. When gloves are powdered with cornstarch to facilitate donning and removing gloves, the cornstarch particles aerosolize when the gloves are removed. The cornstarch includes latex particles. This creates respiratory exposure as well as dermal exposure to latex. In addition, chemicals used in the manufacture of latex products may be irritating. Many healthcare organizations are using synthetic latex–free gloves that is decreasing the incidence of latex allergies in healthcare workers (American Academy of Allergy, Asthma & Immunology, 2017). Products such as balloons, condoms, and rubber bands may be made of latex and cause allergic reactions.

Sensitivity to latex can present as a simple irritant dermatitis, the most common negative reaction to latex. Type IV hypersensitivity (contact dermatitis) typically presents 24 to 96 hours after contact. Type I systemic allergic reactions, including hives, itching, wheezing, or difficulty breathing, develop within minutes to hours after exposure (American Academy of Allergy, Asthma & Immunology, 2017). It is important to protect the patient and the healthcare worker who is allergic to latex. Employers can aid in prevention by selecting products free of latex. Nonlatex gloves are recommended for use where there is no contact with infectious materials or blood. Powder-free latex gloves reduce latex exposure, as does avoiding use of oil-based creams and lotions when using latex gloves. Hand hygiene after using latex products also limits exposure (National Institute of Occupational Safety and Health, 2014).

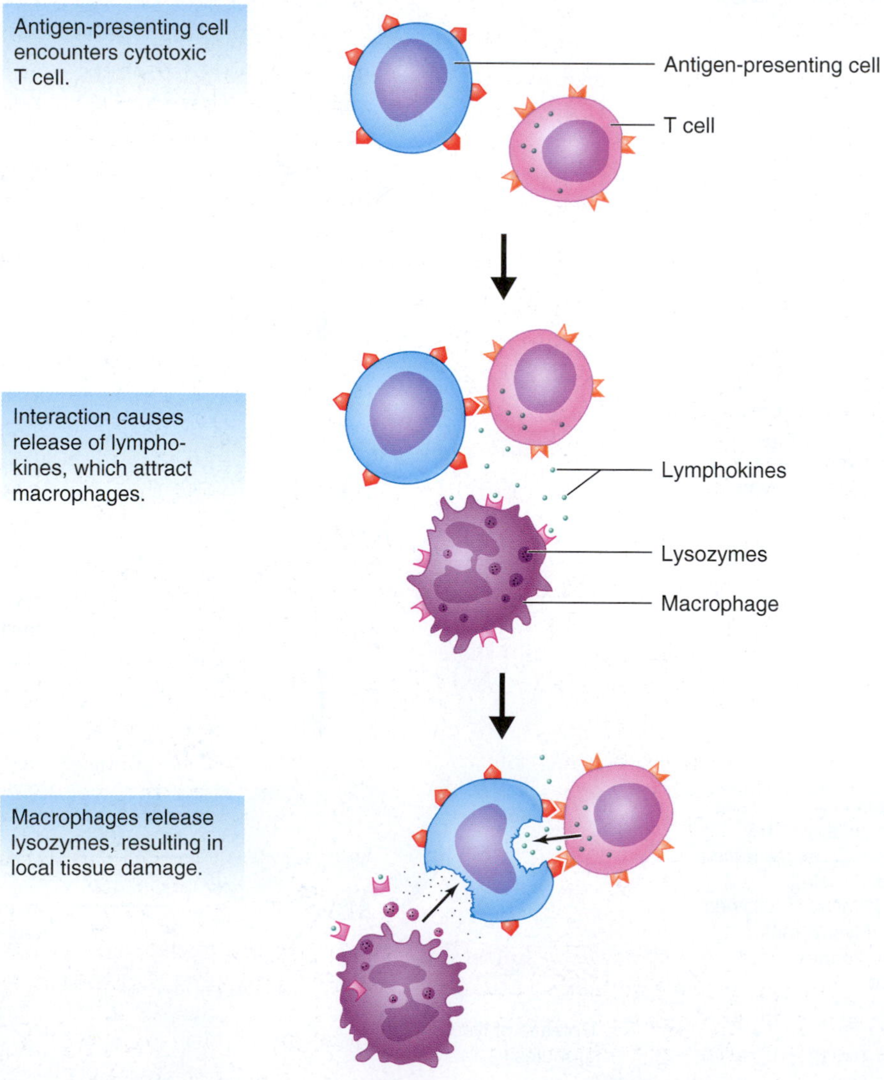
Antigen-presenting cell encounters cytotoxic T cell.
Antigen-presenting cell
T cell
Interaction causes release of lymphokines, which attract macrophages.
Lymphokines
Lysozymes
Macrophage
Macrophages release lysozymes, resulting in local tissue damage.

Figure 13.4 ■ Type IV delayed hypersensitivity response.

The Patient with a Hypersensitivity Reaction

The focus of care for patients with allergies is to minimize exposure to the allergen, prevent the hypersensitivity response, and provide prompt, effective interventions for allergic responses. Identifying allergens for the individual to reduce the likelihood of exposure is a key aspect of management. A complete history of the patient's allergies is obtained, including medications, foods, animals, plants, and other materials. The type of hypersensitivity response is documented, along with its onset, manifestations, and usual treatment.

Interprofessional Care

When a documented or suspected hypersensitivity reaction occurs, the allergen (e.g., intravenous medication or transfusion) is withdrawn immediately. With an acute systemic type I hypersensitivity response, managing the patient's airway takes highest priority, followed by maintaining cardiac output. Type II hypersensitivity responses may necessitate aggressive management of bleeding or renal failure. A type III (immune complex) reaction is treated by removing the offending antigen, thereby interrupting the inflammatory response.

With a hypersensitivity response, supportive care is important to relieve discomfort. This often involves the administration of selected antihistamine or anti-inflammatory medications. Other therapies may be prescribed in selected instances, such as plasmapheresis, a procedure that involves continually withdrawing and reinfusing blood from the patient while removing the allergic components from the plasma portion.

Diagnosis

To identify possible allergens or hypersensitivity reactions, the following laboratory tests may be ordered:

- ***White blood cell (WBC) count with differential*** can detect high levels of circulating eosinophils. Increased numbers of eosinophils are often present in patients with type I hypersensitivities.
- ***Radioallergosorbent test (RAST)*** is a blood test that measures the amount of IgE directed toward specific allergens. Test results are compared with control values and used to identify hypersensitivities. RAST is preferred to skin testing if a severe allergic response is suspected.
- ***Blood type and crossmatch*** are ordered prior to any anticipated transfusions. Other blood tests associated with blood transfusions are a *Coombs' direct* (to detect antibodies on red blood cells [RBCs]) and a *Coombs' indirect* (to check recipient's and donor's blood for antibodies before a blood transfusion).
- ***Immune complex assays*** may be performed to detect the presence of circulating immune complexes in suspected type III hypersensitivity responses. The normal result is a test negative for circulating immune complexes. A negative test does not, however, rule out an immune complex hypersensitivity response.
- ***Complement assay*** is also useful in detecting immune complex disorders. In these disorders, complement is, in effect, used up by the development of antigen–antibody complexes. Decreased levels are seen on examination. Both total complement level and amounts of individual components of the complement cascade can be determined.

Skin Tests for Allergies

Skin tests are also used to determine causes of hypersensitivity reactions. These tests are used to identify specific allergens to which an individual may be sensitive. Allergens for testing are selected according to the patient's history. Test solutions made from extracts of inhaled, ingested, or injected materials, such as pollens, mites, venoms, or some drugs, are used for the prick test and intradermal testing. Epicutaneous testing (prick testing) is generally done first to avoid a systemic reaction; it may be followed by intradermal testing of allergens with a negative response to prick testing.

- ***Prick (epicutaneous or puncture) test:*** A drop of diluted allergenic extract is placed on the skin, and the skin is then pricked or punctured through the drop. With a positive test, a localized pruritic (itchy) wheal and erythema occur. The response is maximal at 15 to 20 minutes.
- ***Intradermal:*** A small amount of allergen extract at a 1:500 or 1:1000 dilution is injected intradermally in the forearm or intrascapular area. If several allergens are being tested, injections are spaced 0.25 to 0.5 inch apart. As control measures, plain diluent (negative control) and histamine (positive control) are injected. If there is no response to a particular allergen at 15 to 20 minutes, the test is negative. The appearance of a wheal and erythema, with a wheal diameter at least 5 mm greater than that produced by the control, indicates a positive response (**Figure 13.5** ■).
- ***Patch:*** A 1-inch patch impregnated with the allergen (e.g., perfume, cosmetics, detergents, or clothing fibers) is applied to the skin for 48 hours. Absence of a response indicates a negative test result. Positive responses are graded from mild (erythema in the exposed area) to severe (erythema, papules, vesicles, or ulceration).

Food Allergy Testing

Food allergy testing is performed when a food allergy is suspected but the source or implicated food item has not been clearly identified. Food allergy symptoms are typically demonstrated within hours of eating. The patient is asked to keep a diary of foods consumed and allergic responses for a week. An elimination diet, excluding most common food allergens and all suspected foods, is then prescribed for 1 week. If symptoms do not improve, a different variation of the elimination diet is prescribed. If symptoms are relieved, foods are reintroduced to the diet one at a time until symptoms recur, indicating allergy to that food.

Medications

When it is impossible to avoid the offending allergen and allergic manifestations are severe or disrupt the patient's

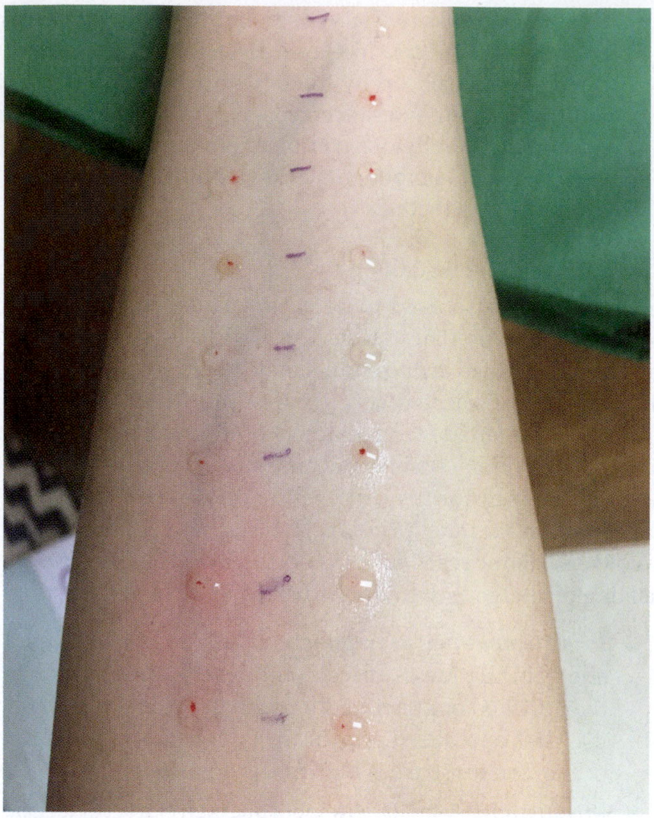

Figure 13.5 ■ Positive allergy skin test in a male patient.

activities of daily living (ADLs), medications may be prescribed. *Immunotherapy*, also called *hyposensitization* or *desensitization*, consists of injecting an extract of the allergen(s) in gradually increasing doses. Immunotherapy is used primarily for allergic rhinitis or asthma related to inhaled allergens. It has also been shown to be effective in preventing anaphylactic responses to insect venom. With weekly or biweekly subcutaneous injections of the allergen, the patient develops IgG antibodies to the allergen that appear to block effectively the allergic IgE-mediated response. Once a therapy plateau is reached, injections may be discontinued or continued indefinitely either monthly or bimonthly.

Antihistamines are the major class of drugs used in treating the symptoms of hypersensitivity responses, type I in particular. They are also useful to some extent in relieving manifestations (such as urticaria) of some type II and type III reactions. Antihistamines block H_1-histamine receptors, acting as a competitive antagonist to histamine, but they do not affect the production or release of histamine. The prototype antihistamine is diphenhydramine (Benadryl). It and other antihistamines alleviate the systemic effects of histamine such as urticaria and angioedema (localized tissue swelling). They are also useful in relieving allergic rhinitis, drying respiratory secretions through an anticholinergic effect. The preferred route of administration is oral, although diphenhydramine and others can be given parenterally, particularly when immediate action is needed, as in anaphylaxis. Side effects include drowsiness and dry mouth. Antihistamines are not effective in relieving asthmatic responses to allergens and may actually worsen symptoms by their drying effect on respiratory secretions. Antihistamines are often combined with a sympathomimetic agent such as pseudoephedrine to improve their decongestant activity and counteract their sedative effect.

Glucocorticoids (corticosteroids) are used in both systemic and topical forms for many types of hypersensitivity responses. Their anti-inflammatory effects, rather than their immunosuppressive effects, are of most benefit. A short course of corticosteroid therapy is often used for severe asthma, allergic contact dermatitis, and some immune complex disorders. Corticosteroids in topical forms or delivered by inhaler may be used for longer periods of time with few side effects; however, systemic absorption can occur.

Treatments

Other treatments used for hypersensitivity responses are generally dictated by the severity of the response and the organ system affected. Airway management takes highest priority for the patient with an acute anaphylactic reaction. Insertion of an endotracheal tube or emergency tracheostomy may be required to maintain airway patency with severe laryngospasm. Because anaphylaxis places the person at risk for vasomotor collapse and significant hypotension, it is necessary to insert an intravenous line and initiate fluid resuscitation with an isotonic solution such as Ringer lactate.

Plasmapheresis, removal of harmful components in the plasma (also known as *plasma exchange therapy*), may be used to treat immune complex responses such as glomerulonephritis and Goodpasture syndrome. Plasma and the glomerular-damaging antibody–antigen complexes are removed by passing the patient's blood through a blood cell separator. The RBCs are then returned to the patient along with an equal amount of albumin or human plasma. This procedure is usually done in a series rather than as a one-time treatment. It is not without risk, and informed consent is required. Potential complications of plasmapheresis include those associated with intravenous catheters, shifts in fluid balance, and alteration of blood clotting.

Anaphylaxis

The immediate treatment for anaphylaxis is parenteral epinephrine, an adrenergic agonist (sympathomimetic) drug that has both vasoconstricting and bronchodilating effects. These qualities, combined with its rapid action, make epinephrine ideal for treating an anaphylactic reaction. For mild reactions with wheezing, pruritus, urticaria, and angioedema, an intramuscular or subcutaneous injection of 0.3 to 0.5 mL of 1:1000 epinephrine is generally sufficient (Boyce & Austen, 2015). For patients with an injected toxin such as a bee sting, an additional amount equivalent to one-half the above may be injected directly into the site of the sting and a tourniquet applied above it to prevent further systemic absorption. Intravenous epinephrine diluted to a 1:100,000 concentration may be used in the patient with a more severe anaphylactic reaction.

Nursing Care

Nursing care related to hypersensitivity reactions is primarily directed toward prevention, early identification, and providing prompt, effective treatment.

Assessment

Collect the following data through the health history and physical examination. Further focused assessments are described with nursing interventions in the next section.

- ***Health history:*** Risk factors, hypersensitivities (medications, household dust, bee stings, etc.), reaction (rash, hives, difficulty breathing), type of treatment for hypersensitivity reactions; allergy skin testing; asthma, hay fever, or dermatitis
- ***Physical assessment:*** Mucous membranes of nose and mouth, skin for lesions or rashes, eyes (tearing and redness), respiratory rate, and adventitious breath sounds.

Priorities of Care

Airway, breathing, and circulation (the ABCs) are of greatest importance for the patient with an acute severe anaphylactic reaction.

Diagnoses, Outcomes, and Interventions

Priority nursing diagnoses will vary according to the type of hypersensitivity reaction experienced by the patient. Because nurses are most likely to become involved with a patient experiencing a type I or type II response, this section focuses on diagnoses for these patients.

Promote Effective Airway Clearance. In anaphylactic reactions, the airway may be obstructed due to facial angioedema, bronchospasm, or laryngeal edema. Establishing and maintaining a patent airway is of highest priority.

Expected Outcome: Patient's airway will remain open to allow adequate gas exchange.

The nurse will:

- Initiate oxygen per nasal cannula at a rate of 2 to 4 L/min. Apply oxygen emergently and obtain a physician order for oxygen administration, modifying flow rate and method of administration as ordered. *Providing external oxygen increases the alveolar oxygen and its availability to cells of the body.*
- Assess respiratory rate and pattern, level of consciousness and anxiety, nasal flaring, use of accessory muscles of respiration, chest wall movement, audible stridor, and oxygen saturation. Auscultate lung sounds and any adventitious sounds, such as wheezes. *Extreme anxiety or agitation, nasal flaring, stridor, and diminished lung sounds indicate air hunger and possible airway obstruction, necessitating immediate intervention.*
- Position in Fowler to high Fowler position *to promote optimal lung expansion and ease of breathing.*
- Insert a nasopharyngeal or oropharyngeal airway, and arrange for immediate intubation as indicated. *Ensuring an adequate airway is vital to preserve life.*
- Administer intramuscular or subcutaneous epinephrine 1:1000, 0.3 to 0.5 mL, as prescribed. This may be repeated in 20 to 30 minutes if necessary. Administer parenteral diphenhydramine (deep intramuscular or intravenous) as prescribed. *Epinephrine is a potent vasoconstrictor and bronchodilator, counteracting the effects of histamine. Effective plasma concentrations of epinephrine are achieved more rapidly when it is administered by IM injection into the vastus lateralis than when injected IM or subcutaneously into the arm* (Barksdale & Muelleman, 2018). *Diphenhydramine is an antihistamine that blocks histamine receptors and their effect. These medications can be effective in rapidly reversing manifestations of anaphylaxis.*
- Provide calm reassurance. *Hypoxemia and air hunger are terrifying for the patient. Anxiety can impair the patient's ability to cooperate with treatment and can increase the respiratory rate, making breathing less effective.*

Monitor Cardiac Output. Peripheral vasodilation and increased capillary permeability from the release of histamine can significantly impair cardiac output. When it falls to the degree that tissue perfusion becomes impaired and hypoxia results, a state of anaphylactic shock exists.

Expected Outcome: Patient's blood pressure, circulation, and effective tissue perfusion will be maintained.

The nurse will:

- Monitor vital signs frequently, noting fall in blood pressure, decreasing pulse pressure, tachycardia, and tachypnea. *These vital sign changes may indicate shock.*
- Assess skin color, temperature, capillary refill, edema, and other indicators of peripheral perfusion. *As cardiac output falls, peripheral vessels constrict and tissue perfusion is impaired.*
- Monitor level of consciousness. *A change in level of consciousness (lethargy, apprehension, or agitation) is often the first indicator of decreased cardiac output.*
- Insert one or more large-bore (18-gauge or larger) intravenous catheters as prescribed. *Intravenous catheters are inserted as soon as possible to provide sites for rapid fluid replacement.*
- Administer warmed intravenous solutions of lactated Ringer or normal saline, as prescribed. *These isotonic solutions help maintain intravascular volume. Warmed solutions are used to prevent hypothermia from the rapid administration of large amounts of fluid at room temperature (about 21°C, or 70°F).*
- Insert an indwelling catheter, and monitor urinary output frequently. *As the cardiac output drops, the glomerular filtration rate (GFR) falls. With an output of less than 30 mL/h, the patient is at risk for acute kidney injury from ischemia.*

SAFETY ALERT: Aggressive fluid therapy may lead to hypervolemia, resulting in pulmonary edema; assess for shortness of breath and crackles in the lungs. ■

Delegating Nursing Care Activities

As appropriate and allowed by the designated duties and responsibilities of assistive personnel, the nurse may delegate such nursing care activities as measuring intake and output, monitoring vital signs, and providing hygiene and physical comfort measures for the patient experiencing anaphylaxis.

Transitions of Care

Health promotion activities include helping patients identify possible allergens that prompt a hypersensitivity response and discussing strategies to avoid these allergens. Anyone with severe food allergies may need referral to a dietitian to discuss necessary dietary changes and ways to continue meeting nutrient needs. It is important for individuals with hypersensitivities to inform healthcare personnel of all allergens.

People who experience anaphylactic reactions should wear a medical alert bracelet or tag at all times to identify the substance(s) that provokes this response. Patients who have experienced an anaphylactic reaction to insect venom or other potentially unavoidable allergens should carry a kit (commonly called a *bee sting kit*) for immediate treatment of future exposures. This kit typically includes a prefilled syringe of epinephrine and an epinephrine nebulizer, allowing prompt self-treatment.

Most hypersensitivity responses are appropriately treated through self-care measures, by the patient or family members. Teaching is a vital component of care. If the patient is at risk for anaphylaxis, involving the family in teaching is essential because the response may occur with such rapidity that the patient will be unable to provide self-care. Include the following points in teaching the patient and family about managing hypersensitivities:

- When and how to use an anaphylaxis kit containing epinephrine and antihistamines in injectable, inhaler, and oral forms
- When to seek medical attention
- Use and adverse reactions of antihistamines and decongestants
- Advantages of autologous blood transfusion if future surgery is scheduled
- Skin care to prevent and care for contact dermatitis
- Helpful resources include:
    a. ALERT, Inc., Allergy to Latex Education and Resource Team (toll-free: 1-888-97-ALERT)
    b. Food Allergy and Anaphylaxis Network.

Anaphylactic reactions vary in severity but can rapidly progress, resulting in death. It is estimated that there are approximately 1500 fatalities related to anaphylaxis annually in the United States (Barksdale & Muelleman, 2018). It is important for healthcare personnel to know the signs and symptoms of anaphylaxis so early treatment with epinephrine antihistamines can be initiated. However, even with these treatments, worsening of condition and death can occur.

- Patients may progress from mild flushing and itching to cough, chest tightness, dyspnea, and wheezes.
- Worsening symptoms of laryngeal edema present as hoarseness and stridor, which is caused by tightening of musculature of the throat. If this occurs, intubation becomes difficult and surgical airway such as a tracheotomy may be necessary.
- Hypotension and dysrhythmias may lead to lightheadedness and syncope.
- Patients receiving early treatment are less likely to die from an acute anaphylactic reaction. However, within the community setting, lack of quick recognition and treatment for anaphylaxis does lead to death.

13.3 Autoimmune Disorders

Maintaining optimal health and preventing disease depend not only on the immune system's ability to recognize and destroy foreign tissues and other antigens, but also on the immune system's ability to recognize self. When self-recognition (also known as *self-tolerance*) is impaired and immune defenses are directed against normal host tissue, the result is an **autoimmune disorder**.

The Patient with an Autoimmune Disorder

Autoimmune disorders can affect any tissue in the body. Some are tissue or organ specific, affecting a particular tissue or a particular organ. Hashimoto thyroiditis is an example of an organ-specific autoimmune disorder. Circulating antibodies are formed to certain thyroid components, ultimately resulting in destruction of the gland. Diabetes mellitus can occur in genetically predisposed individuals from an immune-mediated response. In this type of diabetes, cytotoxic T cells and macrophages attack and destroy beta cells in pancreatic islets (Winter, Harris, Merkel, Collinsworth, & Clapp, 2017). Autoimmune disorders may also be systemic, with neither the immune response nor the resulting inflammatory lesions confined to any one organ. Rheumatologic disorders, such as rheumatoid arthritis and systemic lupus erythematosus (SLE), are characteristic of systemic autoimmune disorders.

Pathophysiology and Manifestations

The mechanism that causes the immune system to recognize host tissue as a foreign antigen is not clear. The following factors are under study as possible contributors to the development of autoimmune disorders:

- The release of previously "hidden" antigens into the circulation, such as DNA or other components of the cell nucleus, elicits an immune response.
- Chemical, physical, or biologic changes in host tissue cause self-antigens to stimulate the production of autoantibodies.
- The introduction of an antigen, such as a bacteria or virus, whose antigenic properties closely resemble those of host tissue, resulting in the production of antibodies that target not only the foreign antigen but also normal tissue. This is termed *molecular mimicry*. Heart damage in rheumatic fever and acute glomerulonephritis

following beta-hemolytic streptococcal infections are examples of the development of antibodies against normal tissue (Sorenson et al., 2019).

- A defect in normal cellular immune function that allows B cells to produce autoantibodies unchecked.

Although the exact mechanism producing autoimmunity is unclear, several characteristics of autoimmune diseases are known. It is apparent that genetics plays a role because a higher incidence is seen in family members of people with autoimmune disorders. More than one genetic change is likely occurring to cause development of these disorders. Additional factors believed to contribute to the development of autoimmune disorders include age, gender, and environmental factors such as exposure to infectious agents (Brooks, 2017).

The disorders tend to overlap, so that the patient with one autoimmune disorder may develop another or some manifestations of another. The onset of an autoimmune disorder is frequently associated with a physical or psychologic stressor. Autoimmune disorders are frequently characterized by periods of exacerbation and remission. See Multisystem Effects of Systemic Lupus Erythematosus for a list of common manifestations of autoimmune disorders.

Specific autoimmune disorders are discussed in the sections of this textbook related to the affected organ systems or functional disruption.

Interprofessional Care

For the most part, the diagnosis of an autoimmune disorder is based on the patient's manifestations. Although the manifestations of these disorders can often be managed, a cure is typically not possible unless the affected target tissue is removed (e.g., colectomy for the patient with ulcerative colitis).

Diagnosis

Serologic assays are used to identify and measure antibodies directed toward host tissue antigens or normal cellular components. Many detectable autoantibodies are not specific to a single autoimmune disorder and are used to establish the autoimmune process rather than the specific disorder. Although healthy people often have low levels of autoantibodies, levels are much higher in patients affected by an autoimmune disorder. The following serologic assays may be ordered:

- ***Antinuclear antibody (ANA)*** detects antibodies produced to DNA and other nuclear material. These antibodies can cause tissue damage characteristic of autoimmune disorders such as SLE. The patient's serum is combined with nuclear material and tagged antihuman antibody to detect ANA-antihuman antibody complexes. A negative, or normal, result is a titer of less than 1:40. When complexes are detected at higher levels (greater than 1:40), the test is positive for ANA (Bloch, Shmerling, & Curtis, 2017).
- ***Lupus erythematosus (LE) cell test*** is used to detect SLE and monitor its treatment. Neutrophils that contain large masses of phagocytized DNA from the nuclei of polymorphonuclear leukocytes (PMNs) are called *LE cells*. Like the ANA, the LE cell test is nonspecific for SLE. A positive result may also be seen in rheumatoid arthritis (RA) or with selected antibiotic and other medications such as phenytoin and oral contraceptives.
- ***Rheumatoid factor (RF)*** is an immunoglobulin present in the serum of approximately 80% of patients with rheumatoid arthritis. A titer of less than 1:80 (or less than 40 to 60 unit/mL) is considered normal. An RF titer of 1:80 or higher indicates RA. Titers between 1:20 and 1:80 may be present in other autoimmune disorders and diseases such as leukemia, liver cirrhosis, and renal disease.
- ***Complement assay*** may also be useful in identifying autoimmune disorders. In these disorders, complement may be consumed in the development of antigen–antibody complexes. Decreased levels are seen on examination. Both total complement level and amounts of individual components of the complement cascade can be determined.
- ***Anti-CCP antibody test*** is a blood test for RA. It measures anti–cyclic citrullinated peptide antibody in blood; the results are specific for RA. These antibodies replace normal protein in the joints of patients with RA.

Medications

Newer treatments for autoimmune disorders focus on suppressing autoimmune responses and restoring normal regulatory mechanisms to prevent target organ damage (Diamond & Lipsky, 2015). Therapy may be intermittent, used only during periods of exacerbation, or may be long term to prevent acute flare-ups. Because these drugs suppress the immune system, the patient taking them has an increased risk for infection.

- Immunosuppressive drugs such as azathioprine (Imuran), methotrexate (Rheumatrex, Trexall), abatacept (Orencia), etanercept (Enbrel), anakinra (Kineret), cyclophosphamide (Cytoxan), and cyclosporine (Sandimmune) may be used to inhibit immune responses in autoimmune disorders. These drugs may be cytotoxic, killing proliferating B cells and T cells, or may suppress the production of cytokines critical to the immune response (Adams, Holland, & Urban, 2017).
- Corticosteroids such as prednisone also suppress immune responses and have potent anti-inflammatory effects. Corticosteroids may be prescribed to reduce the inflammatory response and minimize tissue damage. Doses required for immunosuppression are large, increasing the risk for infection and cushingoid effects such as thin, fragile skin and osteoporosis-related fractures. These drugs are usually prescribed for acute

Multisystem Effects of Systemic Lupus Erythematosus

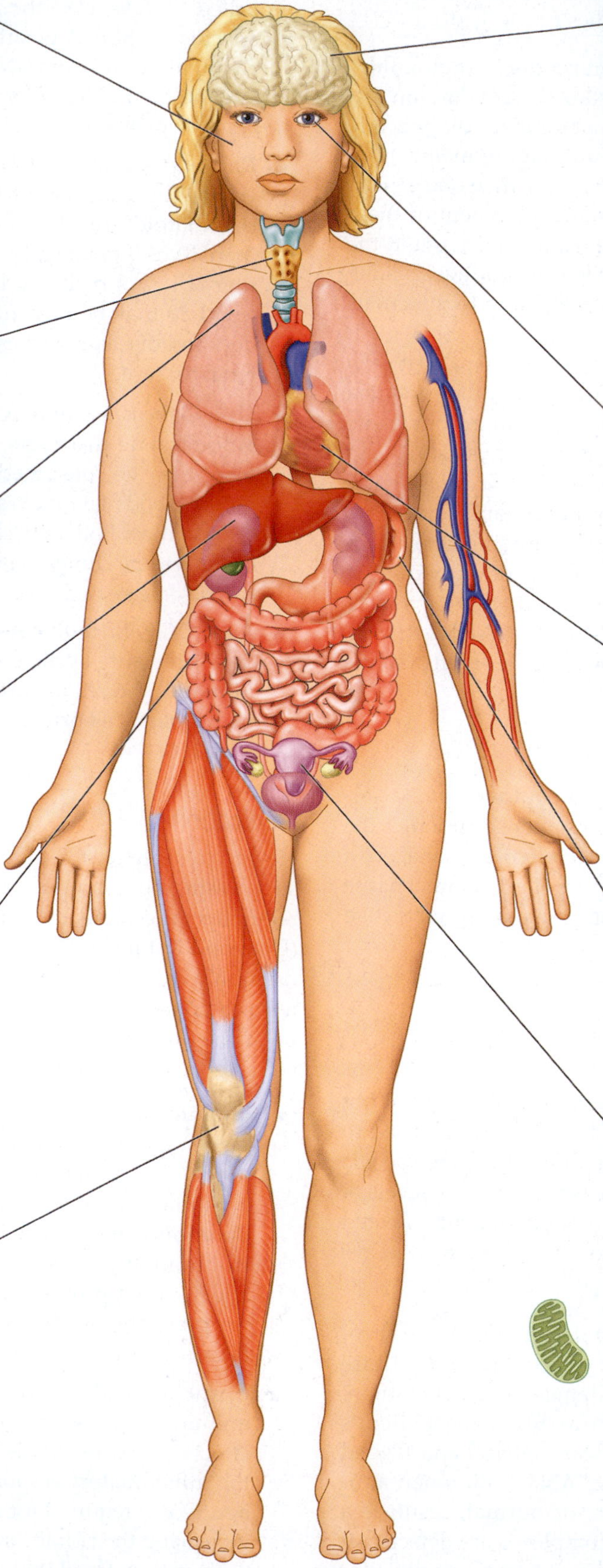

Integumentary
- Butterfly rash on face
- Photosensitivity
- Maculopapular rash on exposed body surfaces
- Discoid lesions
- Erythematous fingertip lesions
- Splinter hemorrhages
- Alopecia
- Ulcers (lip, mouth, nose)

Endocrine
- Thyroid abnormalities
- Hyperparathyroidism
- Glucose intolerance

Respiratory
- Pleurisy
- Pleural effusion
- Pneumonitis
- Interstitial fibrosis

Urinary
- Proteinuria
- Cellular casts

Potential complications
- Nephrotic syndrome
- Renal failure

Gastrointestinal
- Anorexia
- Nausea
- Abdominal pain
- Diarrhea
- Hepatomegaly

Musculoskeletal
- Arthralgias
- Symmetric polyarthritis
- Joint swelling and effusion
- Morning stiffness

Neurologic
- Neuropathies (peripheral and central)
- Seizures
- Depression
- Psychosis

Potential complications
- Stroke
- Organic brain syndrome
  - Intellectual impairment
  - Memory loss
  - Personality changes
  - Disorientation

Sensory
- Conjunctivitis
- Photophobia
- Retinal vasculitis with transient blindness
- Cotton-wool spots on retina

Cardiovascular
- Pericarditis
- Myocarditis
- Endocarditis
- Vasculitis
- Venous or arterial thrombosis

Hematologic
- Anemia
- Leukopenia
- Thrombocytopenia
- Splenomegaly

Reproductive
- Pregnancy-induced hypertension, edema, and proteinuria
- Fetal loss

Metabolic Processes
- Low-grade fever
- Malaise
- Weight loss

attacks and then tapered to reduce the risk of these issues (Frandsen & Pennington, 2018).

- Drugs known as *biologicals* are laboratory-produced antibodies that bind tumor necrosis factor alpha (TNF-α) and interleukin-1 (IL-1), both inflammatory elements. These medications decrease the inflammatory process in autoimmune disorders and include adalimumab (Humira), infliximab (Remicade), and Belatacept (Nulojix) (Adams et al., 2017).

Nursing Care

Nursing interventions for the patient with an autoimmune disorder are individualized and tailored to needs dictated by manifestations of the disorder. Nurses will often be involved with the patient in an outpatient setting, evaluating the patient's response to therapy and self-care management.

Consider the following nursing priorities in planning care for the patient with an autoimmune disorder:

- Promote activity tolerance related to fatigue caused by inflammatory effects of autoimmune disorder
- Teach effective coping strategies to help manage living with a chronic disease
- Educate family about autoimmune disorders and their effects
- Reduce risk of infection related to disordered immune function.

Transitions of Care

Because many autoimmune disorders are chronic, teaching the patient and family about the disorder and its management is a key nursing intervention. The patient may be taking drugs with multiple side effects or long-term effects, necessitating effective teaching. Patients with autoimmune disorders often do not appear to be ill, making it difficult for friends and families to understand their care needs. The chronicity of these disorders also puts the patient at high risk for unproven remedies and quackery. Provide psychologic support, listening, and teaching. In addition, suggest resources such as local support groups and the American Autoimmune Related Diseases Association.

The Patient with a Tissue Transplant

Since the first kidney transplant was performed from one identical twin to the other in 1954, organ and tissue transplantation have become increasingly popular, even preferred treatment options. The transplantation of avascular tissues, such as skin, cornea, bone, and heart valves, is considered routine, with little need for tissue matching and **immunosuppression** (the use of drugs to make the immune response less effective). Transplants of organs (e.g., the kidney, heart, heart and lung, liver, pancreas, and bone marrow) are increasingly common. More than 116,000 people are currently on a transplant waiting list (United Network for Organ Sharing, 2017). Commonly performed organ transplants are outlined in **Table 13.1**; success rates refer to survival of the transplant recipient.

Transplant success is closely tied to obtaining an organ with tissue antigens as close to those of the recipient as possible. Every body cell has cell surface antigens known as *human leukocyte antigens (HLAs)* that are unique to the individual. Even though identical twins may have the same HLA type, a few of their antigens may be dissimilar enough to cause a transplant between them to be rejected. Matching the HLA type of the donor and recipient as closely as possible decreases the potential for rejection of the transplanted organ or tissue but does not eliminate it.

Pathophysiology and Manifestations

An **autograft**, a transplant of the patient's own tissue, is the most successful type of tissue transplant. Skin grafts are the most common examples of autografts. Increasingly, autologous bone marrow or stem cell transplants and blood transfusions are being used to reduce immunologic responses. When the donor and recipient are identical twins, the term

Table 13.1 Organ Transplant Indications and Success Rate

Organ	Graft Type	Indications for Transplant	Survival Rate
Kidney	Allograft; may be isograft	End-stage renal disease	78.6% at 5 years
Heart	Allograft	End-stage cardiac disease refractory to medical management	77.7% at 5 years
Lung	Allograft	Pulmonary hypertension, cystic fibrosis, pulmonary fibrosis, chronic obstructive pulmonary disease	53.4% at 5 years
Liver	Allograft	Severe liver dysfunction due to chronic active hepatitis, primary biliary cirrhosis, sclerosing cholangitis	72.8% at 5 years
Intestine	Allograft	Intestinal failure (inability of intestine to absorb nutrients)	50.6% at 5 years
Bone marrow/stem cell	Autograft or allograft	Leukemia, aplastic anemia, congenital immunologic defects	30–70% cure
Skin	Autograft, allograft, or xenograft	Severe burns, plastic surgery	> 95% at 5 years
Cornea	Allograft	Corneal ulceration and opacification	> 95% at 5 years
Pancreas	Allograft	Pancreatic insufficiency, diabetes	81.5% at 5 years
Islet cells	Allograft (multiple donor)	Type 1 diabetes mellitus	100% > 2 years

Source: Organ Procurement and Transplantation Network (OPTN) and Scientific Registry of Transplant Recipients (SRTR) (2018) *Kaplan-Meier Graft Survival Rates for Transplants Performed: 2008–2015.* Retrieved from https://optn.transplant.hrsa.gov/data/view-data-reports/national-data/#.

isograft is used. Because of the high likelihood of an HLA match, the success of these grafts is good and rejection episodes are mild.

Few people, however, have an identical twin to provide tissue for donation, and when the need is for an organ such as the heart, liver, or lungs, a living-donor transplantation is not possible. Most often, organ and tissue transplants are **allografts**, which are grafts between members of the same species that have different genotypes and HLA. Allografts may come from living donors; examples are bone marrow, stem cells, blood, and a kidney. Most often, organs for transplantation are obtained from a cadaver. Donors are typically people who meet the criteria for brain death; are less than 65 years old; and are free of systemic disease, malignancy, or infection, including HIV, hepatitis B, or hepatitis C. The organ is removed immediately before or after cardiac arrest and preserved until it is transplanted into the waiting recipient. Finally, a *xenograft* is a transplant from an animal species to a human. These transplants are the least successful but may be used in selected instances, such as the use of pig skin as a temporary covering for a massive burn.

Histocompatibility, the ability of cells and tissues to survive transplantation without immunologic interference by the recipient, is determined by tissue typing. Tissue typing is performed in an attempt to match the donor and recipient as closely as possible for HLA type and blood type and to identify preformed antibodies to the donor's HLA.

Both antibody-mediated and cell-mediated immune responses are involved in the complex process of host-versus-graft transplant rejection. Host macrophages process donor antigen, presenting it to T and B lymphocytes. Activated lymphocytes (B and T cells) produce both antibody- and cell-mediated effects. Cytotoxic T cells bind with cells of the transplanted organ, resulting in cell lysis. Helper T cells stimulate the multiplication and differentiation of B cells, and antibodies are produced to graft endothelium. Complement activation or antibody-dependent cell-mediated cytotoxicity leads to transplant cell destruction. Rejection typically begins after the first 24 hours of the transplant, although it may present immediately. Rejection episodes are characterized as hyperacute, acute, or chronic, as summarized in **Table 13.2**.

- ***Hyperacute tissue rejection*** occurs immediately or up to 2 to 3 days after the transplant of new tissue. Hyperacute rejection is due to preformed antibodies and sensitized T cells to antigens in the donor organ. It is most likely to occur in patients who have had a previous organ or tissue transplant, such as a blood transfusion, and may be evident even before the transplant procedure is completed. The grafted organ initially appears pink and healthy, but soon becomes soft and cyanotic as blood flow is impaired. Organ function deteriorates rapidly, and manifestations of organ failure develop.
- ***Acute tissue rejection*** is the most common and treatable type of rejection episode. It occurs between 4 days and 3 months after the transplant. Acute rejection is mediated primarily by the cellular immune response, resulting in transplant cell destruction. The patient experiencing acute rejection demonstrates manifestations of inflammation, with fever, redness, swelling, and tenderness over the graft site. Signs of impaired function of the transplanted organ may be noted (e.g., elevated blood urea nitrogen [BUN] and creatinine, liver enzyme and bilirubin elevations, or elevated cardiac enzymes and signs of heart failure).
- ***Chronic tissue rejection*** occurs from 4 months to years after transplant of new tissue. Chronic rejection is most likely the result of antibody-mediated immune responses. Antibodies and complement are deposited in transplant vessel walls, causing narrowing and decreased function of the organ due to ischemia. The gradual deterioration of transplanted organ function is seen with chronic tissue rejection.
- ***Graft-versus-host disease (GVHD)*** is a potentially fatal complication of stem cell transplantation to immunocompromised patients (Reddy & Ferrara, 2018). In GVHD, immunocompetent cells in the grafted tissue recognize host tissue as foreign and mount a cell-mediated immune response. If the host is immunocompromised, as is often the case when a stem cell transplant is performed, host cells are unable to destroy the graft and instead become the targets of destruction. Three important strategies for preventing or decreasing the severity of GVHD include (1) deleting donor T cells in the tissue or organ prior to infusion into the patient (however, this may increase the

Table 13.2 Transplant Rejection Episodes

Type	Cause	Presentation	Treatment
Hyperacute	Preexisting antibodies to donor ABO or HLA antigens	Occurs within minutes to hours or days of the transplant Rapid deterioration of organ function	The transplant usually cannot be saved; prevent with crossmatch, and use antimetabolites or anti-inflammatory drugs before surgery.
Acute	Primarily a cell-mediated immune response to HLA antigens; antibody-mediated response may also contribute	Occurs within days to months after the transplant Signs of inflammation and impaired organ function	Increase immunosuppression using steroids, cyclosporine, monoclonal antibodies, or antilymphocyte globulins.
Chronic	Probably antibody-mediated response; may also involve inflammatory damage to vessel endothelium	Occurs 4 months to years after the transplant Gradual deterioration of organ function	None; loss of graft will occur, requiring retransplant.

risk of graft failure and infection), (2) using umbilical cord stem cells in adult patients, and (3) using closer HLA matching between donor and recipient. Acute GVHD occurs within the first 100 days following a transplant and primarily affects the skin, liver, and gastrointestinal tract. The patient develops a maculopapular pruritic rash beginning on the palms of the hands and soles of the feet. The rash may spread to involve the entire body and lead to desquamation. Gastrointestinal manifestations include abdominal pain, nausea, and bloody diarrhea. GVHD that begins after or lasts longer than 100 days is said to be chronic. If it is limited to the skin and liver, the prognosis is good. If multiple organs are involved, the prognosis is poor (Reddy & Ferrara, 2018).

Interprofessional Care

Care before and after tissue transplant is directed toward reducing the risk that transplanted tissue will be rejected or result in GVHD. Diagnostic studies are directed first at identifying the potential recipient's blood type and HLA profile. Potential donors are identified through diagnostic studies, and the recipient's immune response to the transplant is monitored. Immunosuppressive therapy with medications is a vital part of post-transplant care. The development of effective immunosuppressive drugs as well as improved methods of tissue typing are responsible for the success of organ transplants using allografts.

Diagnosis

Laboratories specializing in transplant procedures are equipped to make the following diagnostic tests prior to organ or tissue transplantation:

- ***Blood type*** of both the donor and recipient are determined and they must match.
- ***Crossmatching*** of the patient's serum against the donor's lymphocytes is performed to identify any preformed antibodies against antigens on donor tissues. If present, these antibodies would likely result in an immediate or hyperacute graft rejection with probable loss of the transplant.
- ***HLA testing*** of recipients and potential donors is performed. A close match of HLA antigens is most important to prevent bone marrow and kidney transplant rejection, but is less critical for heart, lung, and liver transplants. HLA tests are performed for six antigens important to transplant survival: Two each of HLA-A, HLA-B, and HLA-DR.
- ***Mixed lymphocyte culture (MLC) assay tests*** are also used to determine histocompatibility between the donor and the recipient. This test identifies whether lymphocytes of the recipient will react against the potential donor's HLA. When a pretransplant test reveals a high potential for reaction, potent immunosuppression may prevent rejection. If the intended recipient is severely immunocompromised, the results may be falsely negative.
- ***Panel reactive antibodies (PRA)*** are assessed to determine the patient's level of sensitization to donor antigens. High PRA levels indicate a greater risk for transplant rejection and increase the difficulty of finding a compatible donor organ.
- ***Ultrasonography*** or ***magnetic resonance imaging (MRI)*** of the transplanted organ may be performed to evaluate its size, perfusion, and function.
- ***Tissue biopsies*** of the transplanted organ are performed routinely to assess for evidence of tissue rejection.

Medications

The mainstays of drug therapy for patients following a tissue or organ transplant are immunosuppressive agents. See **Figure 13.6** ■ for an illustration of where various immunosuppressive drugs exert their effect on immune function. Varying regimens of these drugs are used, depending on the transplanted tissue and the medical center; however, a combination of corticosteroids and cyclosporine or tacrolimus is common for maintenance therapy. Antilymphocyte therapy and the use of monoclonal antibodies are increasingly common in the immediate post-transplant period and for treating steroid-resistant rejection episodes.

Corticosteroids, primarily prednisone (Deltasone, others) and methylprednisolone (Solu-Medrol, others), are important agents. Corticosteroids suppress production of IL-1 and IL-2, decrease monocyte migration, and suppress proliferative and cytotoxic T-cell activity. Although they are very effective, large doses of corticosteroids used post-transplant are associated with significant adverse effects. Wound healing is impaired, and the metabolism of fats, proteins, and carbohydrates is altered. Blood glucose increases with steroid use, impairing glucose control. Fat distribution changes, producing a cushingoid appearance with a moon face, increased truncal fat, and wasting of extremities. Fluid retention and hypertension are potential problems, as are osteoporosis, gastrointestinal bleeding, and emotional disturbances.

Cyclosporine and tacrolimus (Prograf) inhibit calcineurin, an enzyme necessary for the production of IL-2. As a result, B-cell and cytotoxic T-cell proliferation and the immune response are suppressed. The incidence of cyclosporine and tacrolimus toxicity and side effects is related to blood levels, so they are monitored closely. These drugs are nephrotoxic, especially at high doses. Observable toxic effects include hypertension and central nervous system (CNS) symptoms such as headache, tremor, and insomnia. An increased risk for malignancy is associated with long-term use. Hepatotoxicity can develop with high doses of cyclosporine, particularly when administered intramuscularly.

Azathioprine (Imuran) inhibits DNA synthesis and proliferation of T cells and B cells, thus suppressing both cell-mediated and antibody-mediated immunity. Because azathioprine is rapidly metabolized by the liver, it can be given to patients with impaired renal function, but may not be effective in patients with impaired hepatic function. Bone

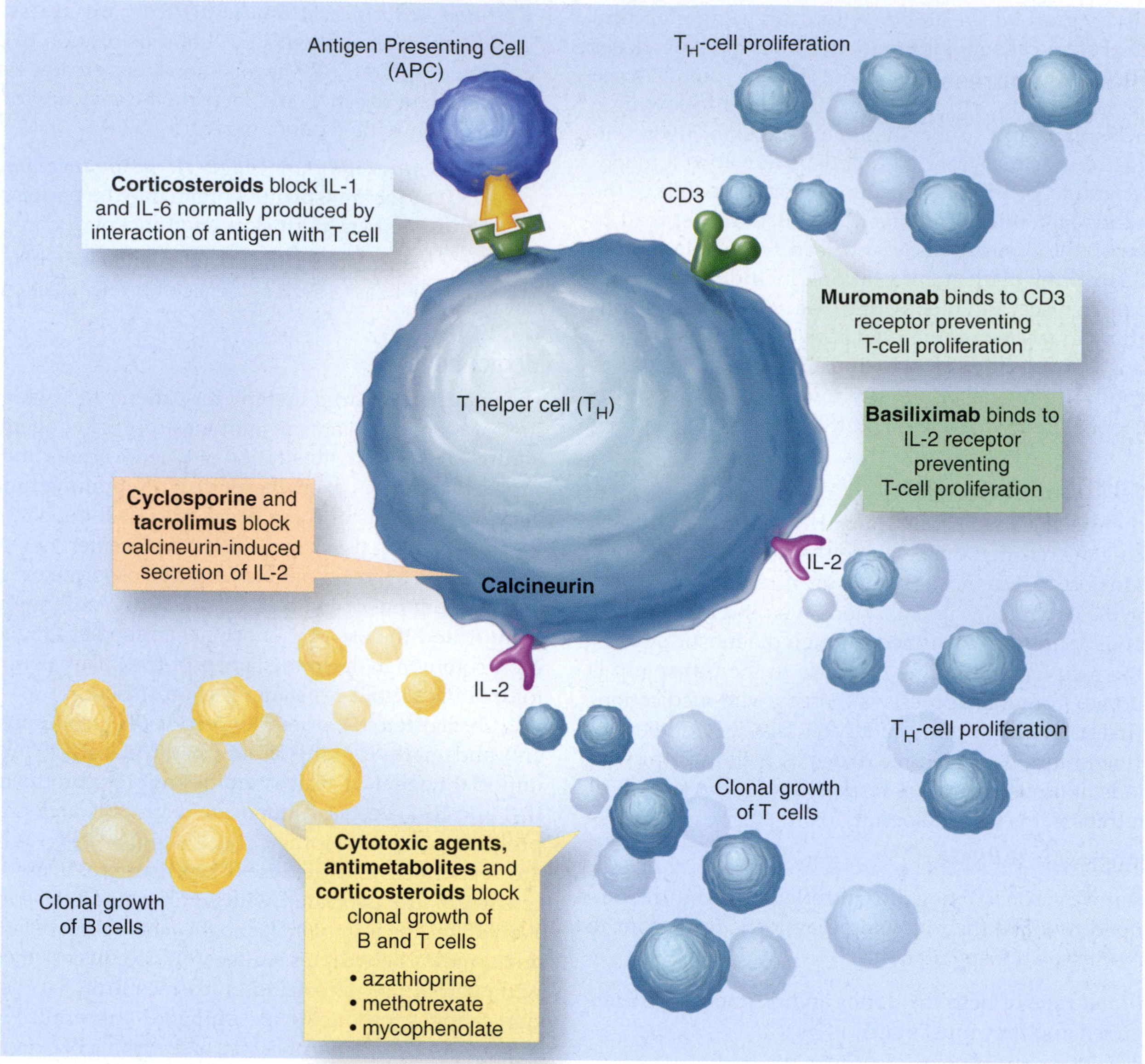
Antigen Presenting Cell (APC)
T_H-cell proliferation
Corticosteroids block IL-1 and IL-6 normally produced by interaction of antigen with T cell
CD3
Muromonab binds to CD3 receptor preventing T-cell proliferation
T helper cell (T_H)
Basiliximab binds to IL-2 receptor preventing T-cell proliferation
Cyclosporine and tacrolimus block calcineurin-induced secretion of IL-2
IL-2
Calcineurin
IL-2
T_H-cell proliferation
Clonal growth of T cells
Clonal growth of B cells
Cytotoxic agents, antimetabolites and corticosteroids block clonal growth of B and T cells
• azathioprine
• methotrexate
• mycophenolate

Figure 13.6 ■ Mechanism of action of immunosuppressive agents.

marrow suppression is the most common adverse effect of this drug, necessitating frequent evaluation of the complete blood count (CBC). Hepatotoxicity and increased risk of neoplasm are also associated with azathioprine administration. Nursing responsibilities related to azathioprine are listed in **Medication Administration 13.A**. Patients who cannot tolerate azathioprine may receive a newer immunosuppressant, mycophenolate mofetil (CellCept).

Muromonab-CD3, also known as OKT3 or Orthoclone, is the first monoclonal antibody produced for therapeutic use in humans. As a monoclonal antibody, OKT3 is specific to T cells, blocking their generation and function. It binds with a surface antigen on T cells, inactivating and removing them from circulation. It also blocks cytotoxic T cells attached to the graft. Because of significant side effects, the use of OKT3 is limited primarily to treatment of steroid-resistant rejection. Newer monoclonal antibodies such as basiliximab (Simulect) and daclizumab (Zenapax) cause fewer side effects and are more widely used.

Polyclonal antilymphocyte antibodies are also used as adjunctive immunosuppressant therapy. Lymphocyte immune globulin (Atgam) is usually used in combination with corticosteroids and a cytotoxic drug such as azathioprine to prevent rejection of a kidney transplant.

Nursing Care

The patient who has an organ or tissue transplant has both immediate and long-term nursing care needs. Both the patient and the family must be considered in providing nursing care.

Assessment

Assessment data collected following a tissue transplant focus on identifying potential rejection episodes. Further focused assessments are described with nursing interventions in the Diagnoses, Outcomes, and Interventions section.

Priorities of Care

Because of the continuing risk of transplant rejection and the need for immunosuppression, priorities for nursing care

Medication Administration 13.A

Immunosuppressive Agents

CALCINEURIN INHIBITORS AND RELATED DRUGS

cyclosporine (Gengraf, Neoral, Sandimmune)
sirolimus (Rapamune)
tacrolimus (Prograf)
temsirolimus (Torisel)

These drugs inhibit IL-2 production and B-cell and T-cell development and activation. They are given concurrently with a glucocorticoid and in combination with other immunosuppressants and inhibit immune system activity and organ rejection.

Nursing Responsibilities

- Monitor BUN and creatinine for evidence of nephrotoxicity.
- Teach the signs and symptoms of infection unique to immune-suppressed individuals. A temperature of 38.1°C (100.6°F) is significant evidence of infection. A sore throat may be a manifestation. Other signs and symptoms of inflammation and infection may be absent.
- Teach hygiene measures to avoid infection, with special emphasis on proper hand hygiene and avoidance of infected individuals.
- Monitor blood pressure and availability and use of antihypertensive medications.
- Teach to avoid grapefruit juice, which inhibits metabolism of these immunosuppressive drugs and increases the risk of toxicity. Lipid-lowering drugs may be necessary to prevent hyperlipidemias associated with these drugs.

CYTOTOXIC AGENTS

anakinra (Kineret)
azathioprine (Imuran)
cyclophosphamide (Cytoxan)
etanercept (Enbrel)
methotrexate (Rheumatrex, Trexall)
mycophenolate (CellCept)
thalidomide (Thalomid)

Cytotoxic agents act by decreasing the proliferation of cells within the immune system and are used widely to prevent rejection following a tissue or organ transplant. They are usually administered concurrently with corticosteroid therapy, allowing lower doses of both preparations and resulting in fewer side effects.

Nursing Responsibilities

- Monitor blood count, with particular attention to the WBC and platelet counts. Notify the healthcare provider if WBCs fall below 4000 or platelets below 75,000.
- Monitor renal and liver function studies, including creatinine, BUN, eGFR, creatinine clearance, and liver enzymes. Report abnormal levels to the healthcare provider.
- Administer the drug as ordered. Administer oral preparations with food to minimize gastrointestinal effects. Antacids may be ordered.
- Monitor intake and output.
- Monitor for signs of abnormal bleeding, bleeding gums, bruising, petechiae, joint pain, hematuria, and black or tarry stools.
- Use meticulous hand hygiene and other appropriate measures to protect the patient from infection. Assess for signs of infection.
- Pulmonary fibrosis is a rare (less than 1%) potential adverse effect of cyclophosphamides. Therefore, monitor respiratory function and for clinical signs of dyspnea or cough.

Health Education for the Patient and Family

- Increase fluids to maintain good hydration and urinary output; void frequently, and avoid taking the drug in the evening, which allows the drug to dwell in the bladder overnight.
- Avoid large crowds and situations where exposure to infection is probable.
- Report signs of infection, such as chills, fever, sore throat, fatigue, or malaise, to the healthcare provider.
- Use contraceptive measures to prevent pregnancy during treatment; these drugs are teratogenic.
- Avoid the use of aspirin or ibuprofen while taking these drugs. Report any signs of bleeding to the healthcare provider. Check labels: Many over-the-counter products contain aspirin.
- With cyclophosphamide, amenorrhea may occur.
- If taking cyclophosphamide, report difficulty breathing or cough to the healthcare provider.

KINASE IHIBITORS

everolimus (Zortress)
sirolimus (Rapamune)

Kinase inhibitors block kinase enzymes that activate B and T cells. They are often given along with other classification of immunosuppressant agents to prevent rejection and treat cancers. Siroliums is also being used with cardiac stents to prevent the development of tissue proliferation and blockage of the artery.

Nursing Responsibilities

- Observe closely for potential adverse effects, including chills and fever as sepsis is a potential life-threatening complication.
- Monitor CBC and platelet counts and note bruising, hematuria, and any other signs of bleeding due to thrombocytopenia.
- Assess BUN, creatinine, and urine output for potential kidney complications.
- These drugs may cause hyperlipidemia and hypercholesterolemia; patients with a history of cardiovascular disease may need careful monitoring.
- Assess for peripheral edema.
- Assess for infection.

MONOCLONAL ANTIBODIES

alemtuzumab (Campath)
basiliximab (Simulect)
belatacept (Nulojix, LEA 29Y)
daclizumab (Zenapax)
rituximab (Rituxan, MabThera)

Monoclonal antibodies (MAB) were previously formed in mice; however, human immune systems recognized them as foreign. They are now genetically engineered in an attempt to decrease complications. When injected into humans, monoclonal antibodies bind with a surface antigen on T cells, and, in some cases, B cells and NK cells, preventing their activation and immune functions. This classification of drug is primarily used in cancer therapy, treatment of rheumatoid arthritis (adalimumab, etanercept, certolizumab, infliximab), psoriasis (adalimumab, etanercept, infliximab), and asthma (omalizumab). Basiliximab (Simulect) is the only MAB approved for transplant recipients. Infusion reactions, acute hypersensitivity, and anaphylaxis may occur with these drugs. The patient should be closely observed for 2 hours following each dose. As with other immunosuppressive drugs, the risk for infection is increased.

(continued)

Nursing Responsibilities

- Premedicate as ordered with hydrocortisone, acetaminophen, and diphenhydramine to reduce potential adverse effects.
- Observe for signs of infusion reaction, including chills, fever, rash, and hypotension. Acute hypersensitivity responses also may occur; observe for evidence of urticaria, angioedema, laryngeal edema, wheezing, or other signs of anaphylactic reaction.
- Ensure that emergency medications for resuscitation are in the patient's room or in proximity to it.
- Observe closely for potential adverse effects, including chills and fever; tachycardia; headache and tremor; hypertension or hypotension; nausea and vomiting and diarrhea; chest pain, dyspnea, and wheezing.
- Monitor CBC for evidence of leukopenia or pancytopenia. Monitor kidney function (fluid balance, eGFR, BUN, creatinine) and liver function tests (alkaline phosphatase, ALT, AST, bilirubin). Monitor for signs of abnormal bleeding (easy bruising, bleeding gums, hematuria).
- Assess for infection.

Health Education for the Patient and Family

- Teach about the drug and its purpose.
- Discuss potential adverse and side effects, and emphasize the need to report symptoms promptly.
- Inform the patient that adverse effects are most likely to occur following initial doses, necessitating close observation at that time. Reassure the patient that this is standard protocol for this medication.

ANTILYMPHOCYTE GLOBULIN

lymphocyte immune globulin (Atgam, ATG)

Lymphocyte immune globulin contains antilymphocyte antibodies produced by immunizing rabbits and horses with human lymphocytes to stimulate antibody production (see the illustration). Rabbit preparations are more effective in decreasing the incidence of rejection and preferred in the United States (Adams, Ford, & Larsen, 2017). Once immunized, serum from the animal is then recovered, and the active IgG fraction is isolated, purified, and administered parenterally to the patient. It binds with peripheral lymphocytes and mononuclear cells, removing them from circulation. Lymphocyte immune globulin is used to prevent immediate transplant rejection and to treat steroid-resistant rejection episodes. As with monoclonal antibodies, multiple side effects and a risk for anaphylaxis are associated with ATG. A major side effect of these drugs is severe thrombocytopenia due to it targeting platelet-specific antibodies. Patients should be monitored closely with administration of lymphocyte immune globulin (Adams et al., 2017).

Nursing Responsibilities

- Premedicate as ordered with acetaminophen and diphenhydramine prior to each dose. Steroids may also be administered before the initial dose. Have epinephrine and hydrocortisone injections available at the bedside in case of anaphylactic reaction.
- Administer by intravenous infusion into a central line over 4 to 6 hours.
- Monitor vital signs hourly while medication is infusing.
- Assess for adverse effects, including chills and fever, erythema, and pruritus. Notify the healthcare provider; these may be treated symptomatically.
- Monitor CBC daily, notify the healthcare provider if WBC falls to less than 3000/mm^3 or platelet count to less than 100,000/mm^3. The medication may be stopped or reduced.
- Assess renal function studies to monitor for serum sickness. Report complaints of joint pain.

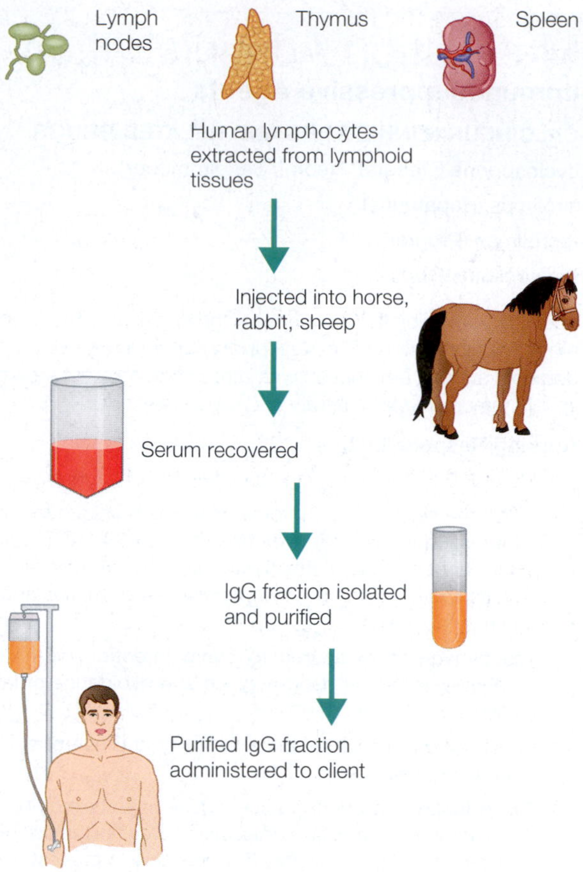
Lymph nodes
Thymus
Spleen
Human lymphocytes extracted from lymphoid tissues
Injected into horse, rabbit, sheep
Serum recovered
IgG fraction isolated and purified
Purified IgG fraction administered to client

A horse is inoculated with washed human lymphocytes, stimulating the production of immunoglobulin with poly antilymphocyte antibodies. These are then extracted from horse serum, purified, and administered intravenously to the patient.

- Monitor for signs of infection, and report any signs promptly. Patients are at an increased risk for developing viral infections.

CORTICOSTEROIDS

methylprednisolone (Medrol, Solu-Medrol)

prednisone

Corticosteroids suppress lymphocyte activity and proliferation. They are immunosuppressants when given in large doses, but have dangerous adverse effects when used for a prolonged time. These include increased risk for infection, thinning of the skin, and osteoporosis and pathologic fractures. Other adverse reactions include hypertension, hyperglycemia, and psychosis. A few months after transplantation, patients may be weaned off corticosteroids without increasing the frequency of rejection episodes.

Health Education for the Patient and Family

- Explain the need for special precautions and close monitoring while this drug is being administered.
- Instruct the patient to report any adverse effects, including malaise or joint pain, promptly.
- Ask the patient to report any evidence of easy bruising, bleeding gums, or black stools.
- Teach family members about the importance of not exposing the patient to individuals with infectious diseases.

Note: Medications identified in blue are among the 200 most frequently prescribed drugs in the United States.

Source: Data from Adams et al., 2017.

include reducing risk of infection and reducing risk of graft failure.

Diagnoses, Outcomes, and Interventions

Nursing care for the patient undergoing a tissue transplant must address the patient's underlying disease process as well as the transplant surgery. The continuing need for immunosuppressive drug therapy also has emotional and psychologic consequences.

Reduce Risk of Infection. Ineffective protection from infection is a problem for the transplant patient at all stages. Before the transplant occurs, failure of the affected organ may put the patient at risk for infection and other multisystemic problems. Incisions and invasive perioperative procedures impair skin and mucous membrane protection from infectious organisms and other antigens. Immunosuppressive drugs given postoperatively to prevent graft rejection disarm the immune response to a certain extent, increasing the risk of infections and malignant growths.

Expected Outcome: Patient will remain free of infection.

The nurse will:

- Wash hands and use hand sanitizer on entering room and before providing direct care. *Hand hygiene removes transient organisms from the skin, reducing the risk of transmission to the patient.*

SAFETY ALERT: Use strict aseptic technique when changing dressings and caring for invasive catheters such as intravenous lines and indwelling urinary catheters to protect against external and resident host microorganisms. ■

- Assess frequently for manifestations of infection. Monitor vital signs, including temperature, every 4 hours. Assess for evidence of inflammation, abnormal wound drainage, changes in urine or other body secretions, complaints of pain, or behavior changes that may indicate infection. Culture abnormal wound drainage. *The patient on immunosuppressive therapy is more susceptible to infection, and usual manifestations may not be evident. Both the body temperature and inflammatory response can be suppressed by therapy. Prompt identification and intervention for infection is important in the immunosuppressed patient.*
- Monitor laboratory values, including CBC and tests of organ function; report changes to the healthcare provider. *An elevation in the WBC count with increased numbers of immature cells (bands) or a decline in function of the transplanted organ (e.g., a rising BUN and creatinine in the patient with a kidney transplant) may be early indications of infection or transplant failure.*
- Initiate reverse or protective isolation procedures as indicated by the patient's immune status. *These procedures further protect the severely immunocompromised patient from infection.*
- Instruct ill family members and visitors to avoid contact with the patient. *A minor upper respiratory infection can be a significant illness in the immunocompromised host.*
- Help ensure adequate nutrient intake, offering supplementary feedings as indicated or maintaining enteral or parenteral nutrition, if necessary. *Adequate nutrition is important for healing and immune system function.*
- Change intravenous bags and tubing at least every 24 hours, and change peripheral intravenous sites every 72 to 96 hours, unless contraindicated. Remove invasive catheters and lines as soon as they are no longer necessary. *Changing lines and sites is important to reduce bacterial contamination. Fewer invasive lines provide fewer sites for bacterial invasion of the body.*
- Emphasize the importance of meticulous hand hygiene after using the bathroom and before eating. *This reduces the risk of infection with endogenous organisms.*
- Provide good mouth care. *Good mouth care reduces the population of oral microorganisms and helps maintain an intact mucous membrane lining.*
- Monitor for potential adverse effects of medications:
  a. Thrombocytopenia and possible bleeding
  b. Fluid retention with edema and possible hypertension
  c. Renal or hepatic toxicity
  d. Cardiac effects, particularly in the presence of fluid retention and hypervolemia.

  Medications used to maintain immunosuppression and preserve the allograft have many potential adverse effects that can alter normal protective and homeostatic mechanisms.

Reduce Risk for Graft Failure. The risk for transplant rejection is highest in the initial postoperative period, but it is never completely eliminated for the patient who has had an allograft. The patient who has had a stem cell (or bone marrow) transplant has the additional risk of developing GVHD, which can affect the integrity of skin, mucous membranes, and other organs.

Expected Outcome: Patient's episodes of rejection will be detected early and effectively managed to preserve the integrity of the transplant.

The nurse will:

- Administer immunosuppressive therapy as prescribed. *Suppression of the immune response is necessary to reduce the risk of graft destruction by normal immune responses and to preserve the graft's function.*
- Assess for evidence of graft rejection, including tenderness, erythema, and swelling over the site; sudden weight gain, edema, and hypertension; chills and fever; malaise; and an increased WBC count and sedimentation rate. Report any changes immediately. *Early identification of rejection allows adjustment of medication regimens and, possibly, preservation of the graft.*
- Monitor results of laboratory studies for function of the transplanted organ. *With a functional graft, results*

(e.g., renal or liver function studies) will improve; a functional decline may be an early indicator of rejection.

- Assess for and report signs of GVHD immediately, including maculopapular rash, erythema of the skin and possible desquamation, hair loss, abdominal cramping and diarrhea, or jaundice with elevated bilirubin and liver enzymes (AST, ALT). *GVHD is a potentially lethal complication in the immunosuppressed patient and necessitates immediate intervention.*
- Stress the importance of maintaining immunosuppressive therapy and reporting signs of graft rejection promptly to the healthcare provider. *Continued immunosuppression and prompt treatment of rejection are vital to preserving graft function.*

Reduce Anxiety. The patient who undergoes an organ or tissue transplant often faces the unwelcome choices of death from organ failure or receiving an organ that his or her body will likely attempt to reject. In most cases, the patient understands that to receive this transplant, someone else must die and be willing to give up an organ. When the transplant comes from a living donor (bone marrow or kidney), the patient may worry not only about him- or herself, but also about the condition of the donor. Fear of rejection and guilt may be even greater in this instance.

Expected Outcome: Patient will appropriately communicate needs, fears, and concerns.

The nurse will:

- Assess level of anxiety by noting such cues as expressions of apprehension, fear, or inadequacy; facial expression, tension, or shakiness; difficulty focusing; helplessness; poor eye contact; and restlessness. *Patients may have difficulty identifying or verbalizing feelings of fear and anxiety. Nonverbal cues are often useful in recognizing states of anxiety.*
- Provide opportunities to express feelings. Use opening statements such as "Facing an organ transplant must be very stressful" or "What concerns you most about this transplant?" Listen attentively. *Encouragement and active listening allow the patient to express feelings of anxiety or fear.*
- Arrange tasks to allow as much time with the patient as possible. When leaving, tell the patient when you will return. *Time spent with the patient facilitates the development of trust.*
- Provide clear, concise directions. *Highly anxious patients have difficulty focusing and retaining information.*
- Encourage involvement in care but do not request unnecessary decisions. *The patient needs to feel a sense of control, but may become irritated if asked to make decisions unrelated to the situation.*
- Encourage family members to remain with the patient as much as possible. *This can help reduce the patient's anxiety.*
- Encourage the use of coping behaviors that have been effective for the patient in the past. *Coping mechanisms and behaviors help lower anxiety to a more acceptable level.*
- Reduce or eliminate environmental stressors to the extent possible. *This gives the patient a better sense of control.*
- Assist with stress reduction and relaxation techniques, such as guided imagery, meditation, and muscle relaxation. *These techniques help the patient gain control over physical responses to anxiety.*
- Refer to a counselor, mental health specialist, or spiritual adviser as appropriate. *Counseling can help the patient identify and deal with his or her concerns and fears.*

Delegating Nursing Care Activities

As appropriate and allowed by the designated duties and responsibilities of assistive personnel, the nurse may delegate nursing care activities such as measuring intake and output, obtaining daily weights, and assisting with ADLs for the patient undergoing organ or tissue transplant.

Transitions of Care

Part of the health promotion activities focus on preventing the need for a tissue transplant. It is important to increase public awareness regarding unhealthy lifestyle behaviors, such as obesity and excessive alcohol consumption, and their relationship to chronic disease and organ failure. Patients with diabetes mellitus and hypertension must understand the importance of effectively managing these disorders to prevent end-stage renal disease. Other risk factors may simply relate to an individual's heredity; understanding how heredity could affect future health might influence the patient's lifestyle choices.

Teaching the patient and family about an organ or tissue transplant begins before the transplant and continues throughout hospitalization and follow-up treatment. Transplant coordinators are nurses specializing in the transplant process and are excellent resources for patients, families, and nursing staff.

Initial teaching focuses on the options, risks, and potential benefits of the transplant itself. Include the procedure by which the organ is selected and obtained, as well as the procedure by which it is transplanted into the patient. If a living related donor is an option, discuss the risks and benefits for both the patient and the donor. Outline the post-transplant treatment regimen, including any lifestyle changes that may be necessary. Being on a transplant registry is a tedious process; the patient must be ready to present for transplant when an organ is available. The transplant process is complex, expensive, and anxiety provoking.

Following the transplant, provide verbal and written instructions, including:

- Manifestations of transplant rejection and the importance of notifying the healthcare provider
- Immunosuppressive drug regimen and side effects
- Wound care
- Avoiding exposure to infectious diseases, particularly respiratory infections, and wearing a mask when going outside
- Meticulous personal hygiene, hand hygiene technique, and frequent mouth care
- Wearing a medical alert bracelet or tag

- Follow-up visits to the healthcare provider or clinic
- Helpful resources:
    a. American Council on Transplantation
    b. Local and state support groups related to specific organ transplant, such as the National Kidney Foundation.

Organ transplantation brings hope and possibility of lifesaving treatments for those facing organ failure. On the other hand, most organs used in transplantation become available through the death of other individuals. Ethical questions often arise as to the correct methods of approaching the family and when to harvest organs. Family and friends of the donor may need assistance in dealing with the death of a loved one, while at the same time being approached to approve organ donation. For some, the idea of providing life-sustaining organs to others eases the loss of their loved one. Multidisciplinary professionals assist in the communication with family members. Trained transplant nurses, chaplains, and physicians share in this responsibility. Recipients of transplantation also face challenges related to transplantation. The possibility of death prior to obtaining an organ and the possibility of rejection and possible death following the transplant are concerns. Medical teams must be available to answer questions and guide the patients through the complexities of decisions surrounding transplantation.

13.4 Impaired Immune Responses

Disorders of impaired immune responses may be either congenital or acquired. The function of either T or B cells may be impaired, reducing the body's ability to defend against foreign antigens or abnormal host tissue.

No matter what the cause, patients with immunodeficiency disorders demonstrate an unusual susceptibility to infection. When the antibody-mediated response is primarily affected, the patient is at particular risk for severe and chronic bacterial infections. These patients do not develop long-lasting immunity to such diseases as chickenpox and may experience recurrent episodes. Patients with a defect of cell-mediated immunity tend to develop disseminated viral infections such as herpes simplex and cytomegalovirus (CMV). Candidiasis (yeast) and other fungal infections are also common. Because T cells are involved with activating antibody-mediated immune responses as well, overwhelming bacterial infections may occur. Immunodeficiency in its most severe form occurs when both antibody-mediated and cell-mediated responses are impaired. Patients with combined immunodeficiency are susceptible to all varieties of infectious organisms, including those not normally considered to be pathogens.

Most immunodeficiency diseases are genetically determined and rare. They affect children more than adults. The noted exception is AIDS, an infectious disease caused by a virus.

The Patient with HIV Infection

In 1981, five cases of *Pneumocystis* pneumonia (PcP) and 26 cases of a rare cancer, Kaposi sarcoma, were diagnosed in young, previously healthy homosexual males in Los Angeles and New York City. The term **acquired immunodeficiency syndrome (AIDS)** was used to describe the immune system deficits associated with these opportunistic disorders. Prior to this time, both PcP and Kaposi had been seen only in older adults or debilitated or severely immunodeficient people. Other groups at risk for AIDS were soon identified: Injection drug users, individuals with hemophilia, recipients of blood transfusions, and immigrants from Haiti. Research to identify the cause of this apparently new disease progressed feverishly, and in 1983, a common antibody was identified in patients with AIDS. The **human immunodeficiency virus (HIV)** was isolated in 1984. It then became apparent that AIDS was the final, fatal stage of HIV infection. HIV is a retrovirus transmitted by direct contact with infected blood and body fluids. Significant concentrations of the virus are present in blood, semen, vaginal and cervical secretions, and cerebrospinal fluid (CSF) of infected individuals. It is also found in breast milk and saliva.

It began, like so many epidemics, with a few isolated cases, and has become a worldwide plague. An estimated 36 million people are infected with AIDS worldwide, with virtually every country in the world reporting cases (World Health Organization [WHO], 2017a). The highest incidence is found in sub-Saharan Africa, South and Southeast Asia, the United States, western Europe, South America, and Canada. Progression of HIV disease to AIDS has slowed because of the effectiveness of antiretroviral therapy (ART; or combination antiretroviral therapy [cART] or highly active antiretroviral therapy [HAART]). Without treatment, chronic HIV infection progresses to clinical disease (AIDS) in about 10 years; with the advent of ART, a young HIV-infected person in the United States can potentially expect to live another 50 years (Fauci & Lane, 2015).

Although the incidence of HIV has leveled and mortality due to AIDS has declined, the epidemic is far from over. The most common mode of transmission is sexual intercourse. The cofactors that increase the risk of HIV transmission include the presence of ulcerative or inflammatory sexually transmitted infections, trauma, and lack of male circumcision (Fauci & Lane, 2015). In the United States HIV infection continues to disproportionately affect African Americans, men who have sex with men (MSM), people who engage in high-risk heterosexual behavior (sex with individuals known to be infected with HIV or at high risk for having HIV), and injection drug users (Centers for Disease Control and Prevention [CDC], 2017b; Fauci & Lane, 2015).

Incidence and Prevalence

Through 2014, the CDC (2017a) estimated that 1.1 million people in the United States were living with HIV/AIDS, with 15% undiagnosed and unaware of their HIV infection. There were 37,600 new cases of AIDS in the United States in 2015, which is a 9% decline from 2010 to 2014. As of 2015, 39,513 people had the diagnosis of HIV/AIDS, which is a decline from 2010 to 2014. HIV/AIDs contributed to 6721 deaths in 2014 and was considered the eighth leading cause of death for people ages 25 to 34 and the ninth leading cause of death for those between 35 and 44 years of age. The decline in deaths is more than likely the result of improved treatments rather than a decline in spread of the disease. A continued decline in deaths is dependent on access to quality care and treatment and continued development of alternatives for those experiencing treatment failure.

The risk factors for HIV infection are behavioral. Among adults in the United States, 61% of reported new HIV infections are MSM. Unprotected anal intercourse is the major route of transmission in this group. Heterosexual intercourse is also a risk, accounting for an estimated 9339 of new HIV infections in 2015 (CDC, 2015). Injection drug use is another leading risk factor, accounting for approximately 17% of cases, with sharing of needles and other drug paraphernalia the primary route of transmission. Heterosexual intercourse with an infected drug user and exchanging sex for drugs are major risk factors for women.

Although HIV/AIDS is often thought of as a disease affecting young adults, adults over age 50 account for approximately 45% of individuals living with AIDS in the United States (CDC, 2017c). Survival of individuals infected earlier in their life accounts for a significant portion of these adults. Older adults, while continuing to be sexually active, may not see themselves as being at risk for HIV/AIDS and fail to use condoms or practice safer sex. In 2015, however, 17% of new HIV/AIDS diagnoses were in people ages 50 and older (CDC, 2017c). Manifestations may be overlooked by healthcare professionals, leading to a delayed diagnosis and increased severity of the disease.

It is clear that HIV is not transmitted by casual contact, nor is there any evidence of its transmission by vectors such as mosquitoes. Blood donation in developed countries poses little risk of contracting HIV to the donor, due to donor screening protocols and technologically advanced processing of blood products. A small but real occupational risk exists for healthcare workers. Percutaneous exposure to infected blood or body fluids through a needlestick injury or nonintact skin is the primary route of transmission (Fauci & Lane, 2015). Mucosal exposures,

Moving Evidence into Action

HIV/AIDS Prevention Strategies for Ethnically and Socioeconomically Diverse Women

Clinical Issue

Within the United States, populations comprised of ethnically diverse individuals with lower socioeconomic status have been significantly impacted by HIV infection. While the rate of HIV infection in African American women has fallen by 20% in recent years, these women still have a higher number of cases than women of other ethnicities and races (CDC, 2018), Socioeconomic status plays a role not only in contracting the disease but also in enacting methods of prevention.

External Evidence

A systematic review and meta-analysis was conducted to analyze prevention strategies directed toward economically diverse women. The study included 43 interventions in which 31 were considered effective, seven were partially effective and five were ineffective. Characteristics of effective interventions were cultural adaptation of methods, use of cognitive-behavioral approaches, and use of small groups with trained facilitators. The meta-analysis found that interventions that were culturally adapted and focused on the ethnicity and population improved knowledge of HIV transmission, elicited behavior changes such as increasing condom use, and reduced the risk of overall STI transmissions.

Internal Evidence

As part of the evaluation of internal evidence, one must consider the clinical feasibility (including access to prevention resources), the outcome of interest (decreasing incidence of HIV within diverse populations), current policies/procedures currently in place for HIV prevention, and identification of stakeholders that influence uptake of the proposed interventions. One question to ask: Is this problem (increased risk for contracting HIV in ethnically diverse women) significant in the population of your care environment? Does the clinical environment support the use of the intervention? What about the cost benefit of the new interventions? In this example of population-focused HIV prevention strategies, the lifetime cost of an HIV infection is $376,668 and the national total lifetime treatment cost of HIV was considered $16.6 billion in 2009 (CDC, 2017d).

Patient Considerations

When considering use of a new intervention, the nurse must consider the specific patient population where it will be used. Will patients and their families be amendable to the new intervention?

Putting the Pieces Together

The design and implementation of HIV prevention programs focused on ethnically and socioeconomically diverse women are essential for people at risk. To effectively implement a plan, it is important to evaluate the external evidence and consider the internal implications and patient/family issues. With the implementation of new prevention intervention, the outcome (decreased incidence of HIV in ethnically and socioeconomically diverse women) should be assessed in every patient and unit-level information should be collected and evaluated on a regular basis.

Reference

Centers for Disease Control and Prevention. (2018). *HIV/AIDS risk by racial ethnic groups.* Retrieved from https://www.cdc.gov/hiv/group/racialethnic/index.html; Ruiz-Perez, I., Murphy, M., Pastor-Moreno, G., Rojas-Garcia, A., & Rodriquez-Barranco, M. (2017). The effectiveness of HIV prevention interventions in socioeconomically disadvantaged ethnic minority women: A systematic review and meta-analysis. *American Journal of Public Health, 107*(12), e13–e21.

such as splashing in the eyes or mouth, pose a much smaller risk.

Pathophysiology

HIV is a retrovirus, meaning it carries its genetic information in RNA. On entry into the body, the virus infects cells that have the CD4 antigen (T lymphocytes). Once inside the cell, the virus sheds its protein coat and uses an enzyme called *reverse transcriptase* to convert the RNA to DNA (**Figure 13.7** ■). This viral DNA is then integrated into host cell DNA and duplicated during normal processes of cell division. Within the cell, the virus may remain latent or become activated to produce new RNA and to form *virions*. The virus then buds from the cell surface, disrupting its cell membrane and leading to destruction of the host cell.

Although the virus may remain inactive in infected cells for years, antibodies are produced to its proteins, a process known as **seroconversion**. These antibodies are usually detectable 6 weeks to 6 months after the initial infection. Helper T or CD4 cells are the primary cells infected by HIV, but it also infects macrophages, dendrites, and certain cells of the CNS. Helper T cells play a vital role in

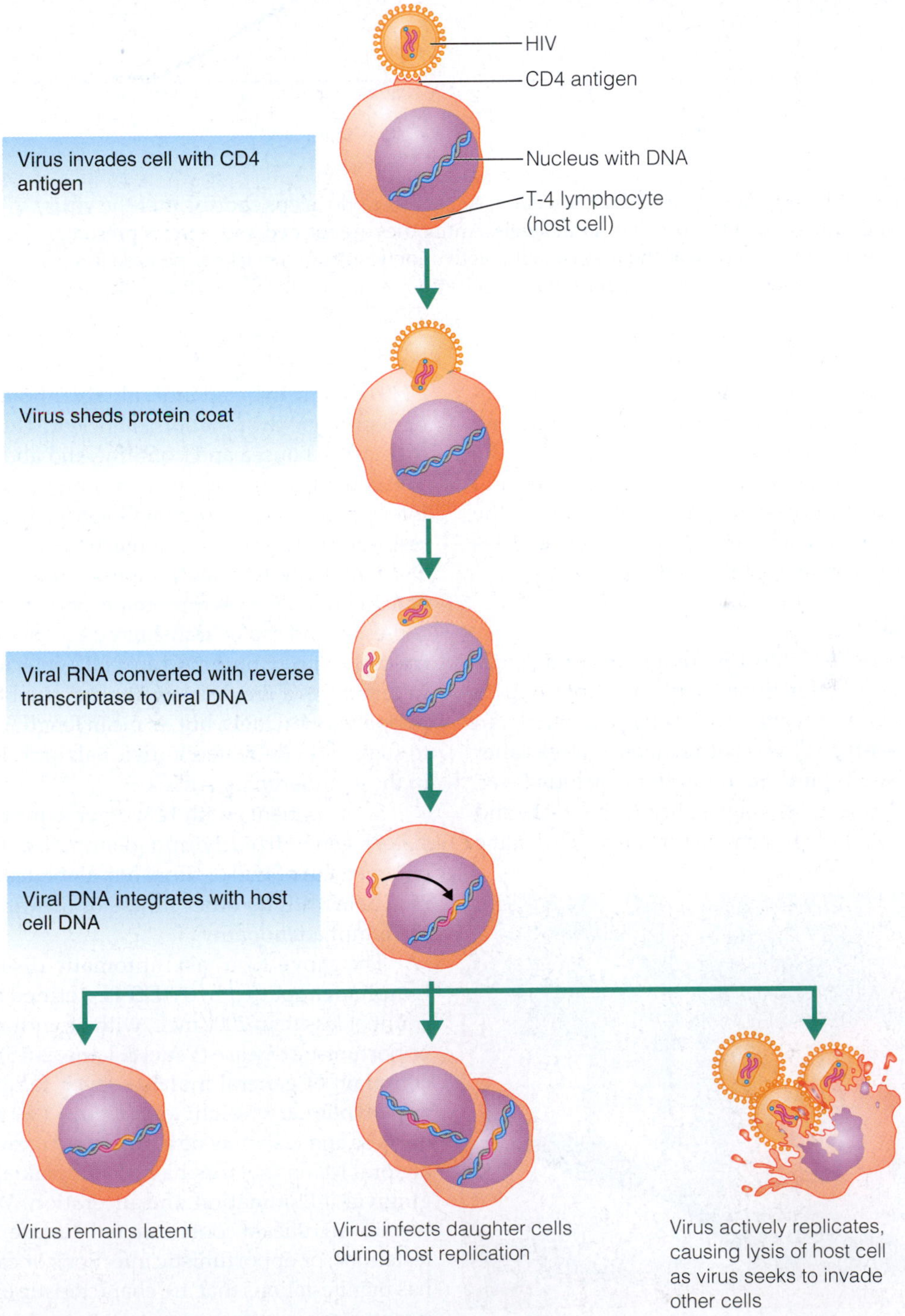
HIV
CD4 antigen
Nucleus with DNA
T-4 lymphocyte (host cell)
Virus invades cell with CD4 antigen
Virus sheds protein coat
Viral RNA converted with reverse transcriptase to viral DNA
Viral DNA integrates with host cell DNA
Virus remains latent
Virus infects daughter cells during host replication
Virus actively replicates, causing lysis of host cell as virus seeks to invade other cells

Figure 13.7 ■ How HIV infects and destroys CD4 cells.

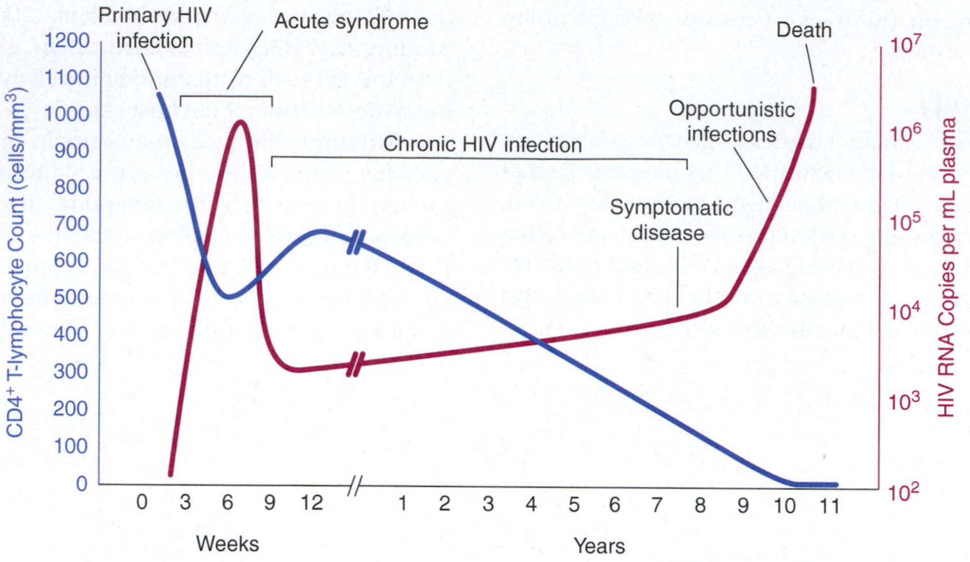
Primary HIV infection
Acute syndrome
Death
Opportunistic infections
Chronic HIV infection
Symptomatic disease
CD4+ T-lymphocyte Count (cells/mm3)
HIV RNA Copies per mL plasma
1200
1100
1000
900
800
700
600
500
400
300
200
100
0
10^7
10^6
10^5
10^4
10^3
10^2
0 3 6 9 12
1 2 3 4 5 6 7 8 9 10 11
Weeks
Years

Figure 13.8 ■ The progression of untreated HIV infection. Acute illness develops shortly after the virus is contracted, corresponding with a rapid rise in viral levels. Antibodies are formed and remain present throughout the course of infection. Late in the disease, viral activation results in a marked increase in virus, while CD4 cells diminish as they are destroyed with viral replication. Antibody levels gradually decrease as immune function is impaired.

normal immune system function, recognizing foreign antigens and infected cells and activating antibody-producing B cells. They also direct cell-mediated immune activity and influence the phagocytic activity of monocytes and macrophages. The loss of these helper T cells leads to the immunodeficiencies seen with HIV infection. **Figure 13.8** ■ illustrates the typical course of untreated HIV infection.

Manifestations

The manifestations of HIV infection range from no symptoms to severe immunodeficiency with multiple opportunistic infections and cancers. Most patients develop an acute mononucleosis-type illness within days to weeks after contracting the virus. Typical manifestations include fever, sore throat, arthralgias and myalgias, headache, rash, and lymphadenopathy. Pathologic changes are also noted in the CNS of many infected individuals although the mechanism of neurologic dysfunction is unclear. The patient may also experience nausea and vomiting and abdominal cramping. The patient often attributes this initial manifestation of HIV infection to a common viral illness such as influenza, upper respiratory infection, or stomach virus.

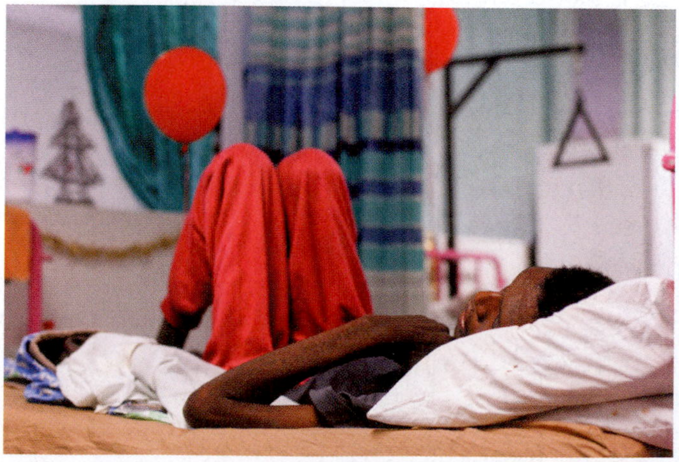

Figure 13.9 ■ Generalized wasting in a patient with AIDS.

Following this acute illness, patients who are treated enter a prolonged asymptomatic period. Although the virus is present and can be transmitted to others, the infected host has few or no symptoms. Most HIV-infected individuals are in this stage of the disease. The length of the asymptomatic period varies widely, but its mean length is estimated to be 8 to 10 years in untreated individuals and significantly longer in those undergoing ART.

Some patients with few other symptoms develop persistent generalized lymphadenopathy. This is defined as enlargement of two or more lymph nodes outside the inguinal chain with no other illness or condition to account for the lymphadenopathy.

The move from asymptomatic disease or persistent lymphadenopathy to AIDS is defined by a CD4 T-cell count of less than 200/mcL, with or without the presence of opportunistic disease (Fauci & Lane, 2015). The patient may complain of general malaise, fever, fatigue, night sweats, and involuntary weight loss (**Figure 13.9** ■). Persistent skin dryness and rash may be a problem. Diarrhea is common, as are oral lesions such as hairy leukoplakia, candidiasis, and gingival inflammation and ulceration. With the development of significant constitutional disease, neurologic manifestations, or opportunistic infections or cancers, the patient has manifestations that are characteristic of AIDS and a very poor prognosis. When manifestations develop, the outcome varies. Antiretroviral therapy is credited with prolonging the asymptomatic period of HIV disease, decreasing the incidence of opportunistic infections, and improving survival (Katz, 2017).

Neurologic Effects

Neurologic problems attributable to HIV include inflammatory, demyelinating, and degenerative changes (Fauci & Lane, 2015). They result from both the direct effects of the virus on the nervous system and opportunistic infections.

HIV-associated neurocognitive disorders (HAND) are a complex of neurologic manifestations of the HIV infection itself. These include disruptions of motor function as well as cognitive, behavioral, and psychosocial symptoms (Fauci & Lane, 2015). *HIV-associated dementia* (*HAD*; formerly called *AIDS dementia complex*), usually a late complication of HIV disease, is characterized by fluctuating memory loss, confusion, difficulty concentrating, lethargy, and diminished motor speed. Patients become apathetic, losing interest in work and social and recreational activities. As the complex progresses, the patient develops severe dementia with significant intellectual impairment and motor disturbances, ultimately entering a nearly vegetative state (Fauci & Lane, 2015).

Infections and lesions common with AIDS may also affect the CNS. Toxoplasmosis and non-Hodgkin lymphoma are space-occupying lesions that may cause headache, altered mental status, and neurologic deficits. Cryptococcal meningitis and CMV infection are also common in people with AIDS. CNS complications have declined with the use of ART (Katz, 2017).

Opportunistic Infections

Opportunistic infections are the most common manifestation of AIDS, often occurring simultaneously. The risk of opportunistic infections is predictable by the CD4 T-cell count. The normal CD4 T-cell count is greater than 1000/mcL. When the CD4 count falls to less than 500/mcL, manifestations of immunodeficiency are seen. With a count of less than 200/mcL, opportunistic infections and cancers are likely.

Pneumocystis Pneumonia. *Pneumocystis* pneumonia (PcP) is the most common pneumonia affecting patients with AIDS. PcP is an opportunistic infection; it rarely develops when the CD4 count is above 250/mcL (Katz, 2017). PcP is caused by *P. jiroveci*, a common environmental organism that is not pathogenic in patients with intact immune systems. Unlike many pneumonias, the manifestations of PcP are nonspecific and may progress insidiously. Patients often present with fever, cough, dyspnea, tachypnea, and tachycardia. Complaints of mild chest pain and sputum may also be present. Breath sounds may initially be normal. With severe disease, the patient may present with cyanosis and significant respiratory distress. The most common cause of pulmonary disease in individuals with HIV infection who have been treated with ART is community-acquired bacterial or viral pneumonia rather than PcP (Katz, 2017).

Tuberculosis. An estimated 4% of patients with AIDS develop tuberculosis (TB), contributing significantly to the rise in incidence of this disease in the United States (Katz, 2017). In some patients, active TB results from reactivation of a prior infection. In other patients, it is a new, primary disease facilitated by impaired immune function. Worldwide, TB is the leading cause of death among those with HIV infections (CDC, 2016). Rapid progression, diffuse pulmonary infiltrates, and disseminated disease occur more commonly in patients with AIDS. Multiple-drug-resistant strains of tuberculosis present a significant problem.

Patients with pulmonary TB present with a cough productive of purulent sputum, fever, fatigue, weight loss, and lymphadenopathy. Disseminated disease affects the bone marrow, bone, joints, liver, spleen, CSF, skin, kidneys, gastrointestinal tract, lymph nodes, brain, and other sites.

Other Infections. Herpes virus infections are common in patients with AIDS and may be severe. CMV can affect the retina, gastrointestinal tract, or lungs. Disseminated herpes simplex or herpes zoster may occur, although severe mucocutaneous manifestations are more common.

Even for patients receiving ART, sinusitis is common and often frustrating. It manifests as headache, fever, and sinus congestion and discharge. Treatment includes antibiotics and guaifenesin to reduce sinus congestion.

Parasitic infections with *Toxoplasma gondii* and *Cryptococcus neoformans* commonly affect the CNS. Toxoplasmosis occurs as encephalitis or an intracerebral mass lesion. Changes in mental status, focal neurologic signs, and seizures may result. *Cryptococcus* infection may present as either meningitis or disseminated disease, primarily affecting the lungs. *Cryptosporidium*, a protozoon affecting the gastrointestinal tract, is an important cause of prolonged diarrhea in patients with AIDS. Bacterial salmonella infections are also a relatively common cause of diarrhea.

Candida albicans infection is a common opportunistic infection in patients with AIDS. It is usually manifested as oral thrush or esophagitis. Oral thrush presents as white, friable plaques on the buccal mucosa or tongue and, in the patient with HIV infection, is often an early indication of progression to AIDS. Patients with esophagitis have difficulty swallowing and substernal pain or burning that increases with swallowing. Vaginal candidiasis is more common and more severe in women with HIV and is treated with topical or systemic medication.

Women with AIDS have a high incidence of pelvic inflammatory disease (PID). Although the pathogens appear to be the same as those in PID affecting non-HIV-infected women, the disease is more severe. Inpatient treatment with intravenous antibiotics is often necessary.

Secondary Cancers

As cell-mediated immune function declines, the risk of malignancy increases. The CDC classification of AIDS currently includes three cancers: Kaposi sarcoma, non-Hodgkin lymphoma, and invasive cervical carcinoma. Hodgkin lymphoma is also common (Fauci & Lane, 2015; Katz, 2017).

Kaposi Sarcoma. Early in the epidemic, **Kaposi sarcoma (KS)** was often the presenting symptom of AIDS. With the advent of ART, it is seen in fewer than 1% of patients with HIV. Kaposi sarcoma is caused by a herpes virus transmitted

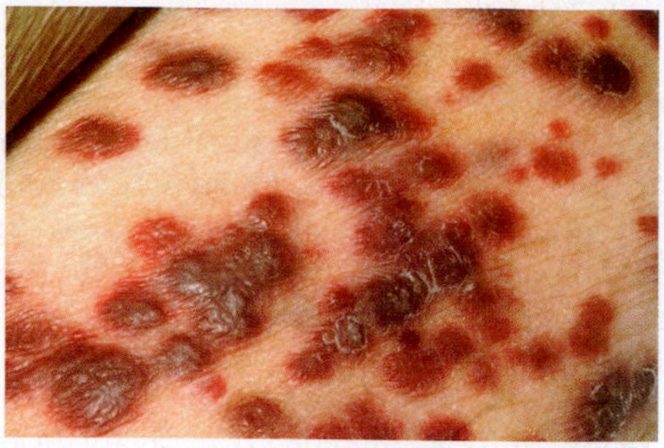

Figure 13.10 ■ Kaposi sarcoma lesions.

primarily through sexual contact; men who have sex with men are more likely to be infected with the virus responsible for KS. KS also may develop in people whose immune system is suppressed due to immunosuppressive medications.

A tumor of the endothelial cells lining small blood vessels, KS presents as vascular macules, papules, or violet lesions affecting the skin and viscera (**Figure 13.10** ■). The palate, toe webs, the face (especially the tip of the nose and pinnae of the ears), and visceral organs including the gastrointestinal tract, lungs, and lymphatic system are common sites for KS lesions.

The lesions of KS are initially painless, but may become painful as the disease progresses. Internally, the tumors may obstruct organ function or cause bleeding. When the lungs are involved, gas exchange may be severely impaired, resulting in pulmonary hemorrhage. Rapidly progressing KS is treated with chemotherapy; milder forms may improve with the initiation of ART (Katz, 2017).

Lymphomas. Lymphomas are malignancies of the lymphoid tissue, including lymphocytes, lymph nodes, and the lymphoid organs such as the spleen and bone marrow. Lymphomas are a late manifestation of HIV disease; the risk of lymphoma development increases with the duration of the disease, even with effective ART. The CNS is a common site for these lymphomas, although they may be found in the bone marrow, gastrointestinal tract, liver, skin, and mucous membranes. They are aggressive tumors, growing and spreading rapidly. Headache and changes in mental status are common early symptoms of lymphomas affecting the CNS. Hodgkin lymphoma also occurs more frequently in patients with HIV infection than in those without (CDC, 2017e).

Cervical Cancer. Cervical cancer develops frequently in women with HIV infection and tends to be aggressive. Women with concurrent HIV infection and cervical cancer usually die of the cervical cancer, not AIDS. Because of this, it is recommended that women with HIV infection have Papanicolaou (Pap) smears every 6 months and aggressive treatment of cervical dysplasia with colposcopic examination and cone biopsy.

Other HIV/AIDS-Associated Diseases

With the advances in ART, AIDS has become a chronic disease and patients face increased risk for developing cardiovascular and other diseases.

Cardiovascular Complications. Coronary heart disease (CHD), the leading cause of death in the United States, affects a significant percentage of patients with HIV infection. Dyslipidemia (high cholesterol, high triglycerides, low levels of high-density lipoproteins, high levels of low-density lipoproteins) and smoking, both major risk factors for CHD, are more common in patients with HIV infection than in those unaffected by HIV. CD4 counts lower than 500/mcL appear to be an independent risk factor for CHD, possibly due to the positive effect of viral replication on coagulation (Fauci & Lane, 2015).

Hepatic Complications. An estimated one-third of deaths in patients with HIV infection can be attributed to liver disease. As many as 90% of U.S. patients with HIV infection are also or have been infected with the hepatitis B virus; infection with HCV and other hepatitis viruses is common. Antiretroviral therapy can also have negative effects on the liver, resulting in injury (Fauci & Lane, 2015).

HIV-Associated Nephropathy. Nephropathy is a kidney disorder. HIV-associated nephropathy (HIVAN) is a complication of HIV infection that disproportionately affects African Americans and Hispanics/Latinos. It manifests as excessive protein in the urine, excessive nitrogen in the blood (azotemia), normal-to-large kidneys on ultrasound images, normal blood pressure, and glomerular lesions revealed by renal biopsy. Before ART, nephropathy rapidly progressed to renal failure and end-stage renal disease (ESRD), leading to the need for dialysis. HIVAN remains the leading cause of ESRD in patients with HIV infection (Fauci & Lane, 2015).

Interprofessional Care

Although multiple research studies to identify a cure for HIV infection and AIDS are under way, no cure is currently available. This makes prevention a vital strategy in HIV care. Search for a vaccine has not been successful to date. The FDA recently moved to approve daily use of an antiretroviral drug combination (Truvada, a combination of emtricitabine [Emtriva] and tenofovir disoproxil fumarate [Viread]) to prevent HIV infection in people at high risk, including gay and heterosexual partners of an individual with HIV infection. The drug is not a "magic bullet"; however, adherence to prescribed therapy along with safe sex practices remains a concern, especially in young MSM from ethnically diverse backgrounds. (Additional preventative measures are necessary to prevent contracting HIV [Hosek et al., 2017].)

The goals of care for the patient with HIV disease are as follows:

- Early identification of the infection and determination of appropriate treatment
- Promotion of health maintenance activities to prolong the asymptomatic period as long as possible
- Prevention of opportunistic infections
- Treatment of disease complications, such as cancers
- Provision of emotional and psychosocial support.

The number of older adults with HIV infection is increasing. Two factors contributing to this increase are that people with HIV infection are healthier and living longer, and older adults are less likely to use condoms, perceiving less risk of pregnancy and STIs. Consequently, the Panel on Antiretroviral Guidelines for Adults and Adolescents (2017) has provided guidelines for ART in older patients who have an HIV infection. These guidelines include the following recommendations:

- Use ART for patients over 50 years old, regardless of CD4 cell count, because older adults may have a less effective immunologic response to HIV.
- Closely monitor bone, kidney, metabolic, cardiovascular, and liver function in older adults on ART due to an increased risk for adverse effects of therapy.
- Regularly assess drug–drug interactions between antiretroviral drugs and other medications taken by the older adult.
- Collaborate with HIV specialists and primary care providers to optimize care for the older adult with complex comorbidities.
- Provide counseling to prevent secondary transmission of HIV.

BOX 13.1
Current Recommendations for HIV Testing of Adults and Adolescents

1. All HIV testing should be voluntary; verbal informed consent is sufficient. Testing is confidential and accompanied by appropriate pretest information and post-test counseling. Mechanisms should be in place to ensure correct, high-quality test results. Referral to appropriate prevention, care, and treatment services should be provided as indicated.
2. All individuals entering a healthcare setting—including primary and antenatal care, outpatient facilities, family planning, and sexually transmitted infection (STI) clinics—should receive routine, voluntary screening for HIV, regardless of risk.
3. All patients seeking treatment for STIs and all patients beginning treatment for TB should be screened for HIV.
4. Healthcare providers should encourage patients and their prospective sex partners to be tested before initiating a new sexual relationship or after a separation. Partners and family members of patients with HIV should be tested as soon as possible after the diagnosis.
5. Repeat HIV screening should be performed for patients with known risk at least annually. Individuals likely to be at high risk include injection drug users and their sex partners, individuals who exchange sex for money or drugs, sex partners of individuals with HIV infection, MSM, transgender people, and heterosexual individuals who themselves or whose sex partners have had more than one sex partner since their most recent HIV test.

Sources: Centers for Disease Control and Prevention. (2006). *Revised recommendations for HIV testing of adults, adolescents, and pregnant women in health-care settings.* Retrieved from www.cdc.gov/mmwr/preview/mmwrhtml; World Health Organization. (2017b). *HIV testing and counselling tool kit.* Retrieved from www.who.int/hiv/topics/vct/toolkit/introduction/en/index1.html.

Diagnosis

Diagnostic testing is used to screen for and identify the infection, as well as to monitor the patient's disease and immune status. When a preliminary, positive rapid test is explained to patients, phrases like "a possibility of being infected" or "false-positive results do occur" can be used to indicate the likelihood of HIV infection based on the HIV prevalence in the setting and the patient's individual risk. Confirmation of positive results is required with an ELISA or Western blot antibody test. See **Box 13.1** for current recommendations for HIV testing based on CDC and WHO guidelines.

- ***HIV rapid antibody test.*** The rapid tests consist of test strips with embedded HIV antigen. If antibodies to HIV are found in the patient's blood, the strip turns a color, indicating the test is positive. The results are interpreted visually and are used widely because results can be given immediately. Personnel without formal laboratory training (point-of-care testing) can perform rapid antibody tests. Although positive results must be confirmed with further testing, learning results immediately gives the patient important information to make wise choices about his or her behaviors and self-care.
- ***Enzyme-linked immunosorbent assay (ELISA)*** is the most widely used screening test for HIV infection. ELISA tests for HIV antibodies; it does not detect the virus. Therefore, a patient may have a negative ELISA test early in the course of infection, before detectable antibodies have developed. The test has a 99.5% or higher sensitivity when performed at least 13 weeks after infection (Fauci & Lane, 2015). This means that more than 99.5% of tests performed on blood containing HIV antibodies will show a positive result. False positives can occur; therefore, an initial positive result is always retested and confirmed using a different method of antibody detection, usually the Western blot.
- ***Western blot antibody testing*** is more reliable but more time consuming and more expensive than ELISA. When combined with ELISA, however, a specificity of greater than 99.9% is achieved. *Specificity* is a measure of the probability that a negative test result indicates that no antibodies are present. In this test, the patient's serum is mixed with HIV proteins to detect reaction. If antibodies to HIV are present, a detectable antigen–antibody response will occur.
- ***HIV viral load tests*** measure the amount of actively replicating HIV. Levels correlate with disease progression and response to antiretroviral medications. Several tests are available; the most commonly used are the RT-PCR assay and the bDNA assay to identify the number of HIV RNA copies in plasma or blood (Katz, 2017).
- ***CBC*** is performed to detect anemia, leukopenia, and thrombocytopenia, which are often present in HIV

infection. Lymphopenia (or low levels of lymphocytes) is especially common in this disease.

- ***Absolute CD4 lymphocyte count*** is the most widely used test to monitor the progress of the disease and guide therapy. The CD4 cell count correlates very closely with the immunodeficiency disorders seen in AIDS. AIDS is now defined not only by the presence of opportunistic infections and other diseases indicative of immunodeficiency, but also by HIV-seropositive status and a CD4 count of less than 200/mm^3 or a percentage of CD4 lymphocytes of less than 14%. CD4 counts are recommended every 3 to 6 months for all people with HIV disease.
- ***HIV drug-resistance testing*** is recommended when patients with HIV infection enter into care, regardless of when ART will be initiated (Panel on Antiretroviral Guidelines for Adults and Adolescents, 2017). HIV readily mutates to become resistant to antiretroviral drugs; the use of assays to determine antiretroviral drugs to which the virus is likely to be sensitive or resistant has become the standard of care helping guide ART.

Other diagnostic tests are used primarily to detect secondary cancers and opportunistic infections in the patient with HIV. Tests ordered are both general and specific to the patient's manifestations and may include:

- ***Tuberculin skin testing*** to detect possible tuberculosis infection
- ***MRI*** of the brain to identify lymphomas
- ***Specific cultures and serology examinations for opportunistic infections*** such as PcP, toxoplasmosis, and others
- ***Pap smears*** every 6 months for early detection of cervical cancer in women with cervical dysplasia.

MEDICATIONS

Pharmacologic management of the patient with HIV disease has three primary goals: (1) To suppress the infection itself, (2) to provide prophylaxis of opportunistic infections by preserving immunologic function, and (3) to reduce HIV morbidity, decreasing symptoms and prolonging life. Advances in drug therapy have decreased the HIV death rate, however; adherence to drug therapy is important. Even a short lapse in medication adherence can cause rapid acceleration of the HIV virus (Adams et al., 2017; Panel on Antiretroviral Guidelines for Adults and Adolescents, 2017).

The Panel on Antiretroviral Guidelines for Adults and Adolescents (2017) strongly recommends initiation of treatment when the CD4 count falls to 500/mm^3 or lower. Treatment should be initiated regardless of CD4 count in patients who are symptomatic (e.g., have an AIDS-defining disease), are co-infected with hepatitis B, have HIV-associated neuropathy, and in women who are pregnant. Effectiveness of treatment is monitored by viral load and CD4 cell counts; positive results are indicated by a reduction in viral load along with preserving the CD4 count above 350/mm^3. Starting treatment before immune failure, when the CD4 count is above 500 or 1000, may protect the immune system.

The action of antiretroviral drugs can be broadly classified as agents that inhibit replication of the virus and agents that block entry of the virus into cells. Nucleoside/nucleotide reverse transcriptase inhibitors (NRTIs), nonnucleoside reverse transcriptase inhibitors (NNRTIs), protease inhibitors (PIs), and integrase inhibitors (INSTIs) inhibit enzymes required for viral replication. Fusion inhibitors and CCR5 antagonists, in contrast, interfere with viral entry into cells. The current standard of treatment is a combination of three or more antiretroviral drugs from at least two different classes (Katz, 2017). Combination therapies increase the likelihood of decreasing viral load, and adherence to administration schedules has been eased by making various combinations available in one pill (Adams et al., 2017). Patients beginning the ART protocol must understand the benefits, risks, costs, and effects on daily life. ART does not eradicate HIV infection.

ART medications are expensive; the newer triple combinations such as Trizivir (one pill twice a day) and Atripla (one pill once a day) have a wholesale price of between $1931 and $3057 for a 30-day supply (Panel on Antiretroviral Guidelines for Adults and Adolescents, 2017). This cost does not include medications to prevent or treat opportunistic infections or cancer. In most cases, available fixed-dose combinations of ART drugs allow daily or twice-a-day dosing, simplifying treatment regimens. However, all ART medications cause significant adverse reactions leading to less than perfect adherence, as with most chronic diseases; in the case of HIV, however, the outcome could be fatal.

Each patient must be able to adhere to the treatment regimen. It may be preferable to delay initiating therapy until the patient is able to agree to adhere so irregular dosing does not lead to viral resistance. Some providers gauge patient ability to follow the ART regimen by the patient's success with prophylaxis for an opportunistic infection. Discontinuation or interruption of ART is considered dangerous; because of the burden of adverse reactions, patients may desire brief holidays from taking the medications. Counseling on the benefits of adhering versus the potential complications may be necessary.

Adherence to medication treatments can be difficult for HIV patients. Provider and nursing interventions that focus on individual patient characteristics can be very beneficial. Healthcare professionals who take the time to explain, one on one, the rationale for treatment, assist with personalizing how and when to take medications, and teach on potential problems of missed doses can be extremely helpful in gaining compliance (de Bruin et al., 2017). Building patients' idea of self-efficacy in being capable of caring for self has also been found to be of value in gaining adherence to medication regimens (Houston et al., 2016).

Nucleoside Reverse Transcriptase Inhibitors. The NRTIs (also called *nucleoside analogs*) are mainstays of ART. This class of drugs inhibits the action of viral reverse transcriptase, a retroviral enzyme that catalyzes the substrates for conversion and copying of viral RNA to DNA sequences. This enzyme is necessary for viral integration into cellular DNA and replication. The nucleoside analogs act as a chemical decoy for building blocks of the formation of the DNA copy, preventing the RNA from being copied into DNA. Each drug substitutes for a particular nucleoside base at different points on the chain. See **Medication Administration 13.B** for this group of drugs.

Zidovudine (Retrovir, AZT), the first antiretroviral agent approved for use with HIV infection, is now generally reserved for second- or third-line regimens because it causes anemia and neutropenia. Zidovudine is often given in combination with lamivudine (Combivir) or in combination with lamivudine and abacavir (Trizivir). Zidovudine may also be used prophylactically following a documented parenteral exposure to HIV.

Abacavir causes hypersensitivities in genetically predisposed individuals. Before prescribing this medication, HLA B*5701 testing should be done; if the test is positive, the patient will have a hypersensitivity reaction and should not take the medication.

Protease Inhibitors. Protease is a viral enzyme necessary for the formation of specific viral protein needed for viral assembly and maturation. PIs bond chemically with protease to block the function of the enzyme and result in the production of immature, noninfectious viral particles. When combined with other antiviral drugs, these chemicals increase the chance of eliminating the virus by interfering with different stages of its life cycle. However, viral resistance occurs rather quickly. PIs inhibit and induce metabolism of other drugs, so their use with other medications and the dose of those medications must be carefully planned. Some drugs will circulate longer because their metabolism is inhibited; others will be speedily metabolized and eliminated.

Protease inhibitors and nucleoside analogs are associated with serious metabolic derangements. These include elevated cholesterol and triglycerides, insulin resistance and diabetes mellitus, and changes in body fat composition, which are particularly distressing to the patients. These body fat changes are primarily abdominal obesity and skeletal wasting. This set of symptoms is referred to as lipodystrophy. Elevated cholesterol should be treated with pravastatin or atorvastatin. Lovastatin and simvastatin react with PIs, so they need to be avoided. Reduction of dietary sources of cholesterol should be made. Unlike most PIs, raltegravir (Ritonavir) has a beneficial effect on lipids, is effective in reducing viral load, and is usually well tolerated by patients (Ofotokun et al., 2015).

Nonnucleoside Reverse Transcriptase Inhibitors. Etravirine (Intelence), delavirdine (Rescriptor), efavirenz (Sustiva), and nevirapine (Viramune) are NNRTIs that may be used in combination with nucleoside analogs and protease inhibitors. However, one limitation to NNRTIs is the high incidence of cross-resistance to NRTIs. Some studies have shown that nevirapine and efavirenz may significantly reduce serum levels of the protease inhibitors. Only one NNRTI should be used at a time. Nevirapine has a reported risk for liver toxicity and severe rash, particularly when used in women with higher CD4 counts (Fauci & Lane, 2015).

Entry Inhibitors. These newer antiviral drugs act by binding to the virus or the host cells and preventing viral entry into the host cells. Enfuvirtide (Fuzeon) blocks the HIV virus from entering human cells. Unfortunately, it must be administered by injection twice a day and it is very expensive. Patients who develop resistance to ART regimens are candidates for this regimen. Side effects include injection site pain, itching, and hardening of the tissue; allergic reactions; peripheral neuropathy; insomnia; depression; dyspnea; anorexia; and arthralgia.

Maraviroc (Selzentry) is the first antiretroviral drug that targets the host cells rather than targeting the virus directly. CCR5 antagonists block certain HIV viruses from entry to host immune cells. Certain forms of HIV viruses (R5 tropic viruses) require a CCR5 receptor as a "co-receptor" to gain entry to the cell; with this entry inhibitor, the R5 tropic virus cannot interact with the receptor and therefore is blocked from entering human cells. Before prescribing, a blood test is done to identify the type of viruses the patient carries; if the R5 form of the virus is found, the patient may be a candidate for taking this drug. Preexisting cardiac and liver conditions are associated with adverse reactions.

HIV Integrase Strand Transfer Inhibitor. Raltegravir (Isentress) targets integrase, an HIV enzyme that integrates the viral genetic material into human DNA. Raltegravir is also called a *strand transfer inhibitor*, referring to the process of DNA strand transfer from the virus to the host. It is taken orally twice daily and side effects include nausea, diarrhea, and headache. It is approved only for individuals who have developed resistance to ART combinations, and it is not considered effective if used alone.

Other Drugs. The use of interferon-α, active immunotherapy with inactivated HIV, and other strategies such as bone marrow transplant and transfer of genetically modified lymphocytes are currently under investigation (Fauci & Lane, 2015). Patients who are coinfected with hepatitis B or C require drugs such as peginterferon-α or adefovir (Hepsera). As more drugs become available, the burden to choose the best regimen increases for the healthcare provider. Referral to a healthcare provider who specializes in care of patients with HIV/AIDS is recommended.

The most important limiting factor when choosing a regimen is patient adherence. Second to that is selecting an effective combination of drugs without overlapping toxicities or toxicities so debilitating that adherence will be further impaired. Interruption of ART is associated with rapid increases in viral load, a drop in CD4 cell counts, and an increased risk for disease progression (Fauci & Lane, 2015).

Body composition changes and metabolic abnormalities associated with ART include increased fat deposition to the midsection, breasts, and neck with atrophy in the face, buttocks, and extremities (**Figure 13.11** ■); increased low-density lipoprotein cholesterol and triglycerides; and insulin resistance. The combination of changes is

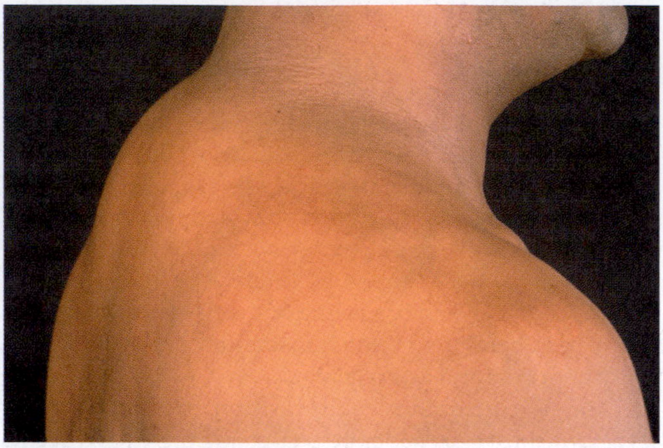

Figure 13.11 ■ Fat redistribution associated with protease inhibitors.

consistent with metabolic syndrome, which increases the risk of cardiovascular disease and diabetes. These conditions are commonly treated with medications. A number of pharmacologic agents are used to prevent and treat opportunistic infections and malignancies in the patient with HIV.

It is recommended that all patients with HIV infection receive pneumococcal, influenza, hepatitis A, hepatitis B, and *Haemophilus influenzae b* vaccines. Individuals with a positive PPD and negative chest x-ray are given prophylactic isoniazid. When the patient's CD4 cell count falls to less than 200/mm^3, prophylactic treatment for PcP is begun, usually with trimethoprim-sulfamethoxazole. As CD4 cell counts fall, prophylaxis against other opportunistic infections such as *Mycobacterium avium* complex (MAC) infection, toxoplasmosis, CMV infection, and endemic fungal diseases may be initiated (Katz, 2017).

Medication Administration 13.B

Antiretroviral Drugs

NUCLEOSIDE REVERSE TRANSCRIPTASE INHIBITORS (NRTIS)

delavirdine (Rescriptor)
efavirenz (Sustiva)
etravirine (Intelence)
nevirapine (Viramune)
rilpivirine (Edurant)

FUSION AND INTEGRASE INHIBITORS

dolutegravir (DTG, Tivicay)
elvitegravir (Vitekta)
enfuvirtide (Fuzeon)
maraviroc (Selzentry)
raltegravir (Isentress)

Nursing Responsibilities

- Assess for possible contraindications to therapy including allergic response, previous episodes of pancreatitis, and impaired renal or liver function.
- Abacavir sulfate causes allergic reactions in some patients. Prior to administering, HLA B*5701 testing is performed; if the test is positive, the patient should not take abacavir. Monitor for an allergic response: Sudden fever, skin rash, severe tiredness or achiness, diarrhea, nausea and vomiting, stomach pain, sore throat, shortness of breath, cough, or general ill feeling. Stop the medication and inform the healthcare provider immediately.
- Administer with caution to patients taking vincristine (cancer drug), rifampin (Tb), pentamidine (PcP), ethambutol (Tb), or metronidazole (bacterial and protozoal infections). Concurrent use may increase the risk of acute and fatal pancreatitis.
- Assess for adverse effects. Nausea and headache are common. They may be self-limiting, decreasing with time, or significant and continuing, necessitating a change of therapy. Peripheral neuropathies may develop; these manifest as a sharp, burning pain sensation in the hands and/or legs. Anemia and neutropenia are treated with erythropoietin (epoetin alpha) and G-CSF (filgrastim).
- Assess CBC with differential and serum chemistries for evidence of liver or pancreas changes. Lactic acidosis, an indication of liver disease, may develop; monitor lactate levels and pH. Notify the healthcare provider of significant changes.
- Didanosine interferes with the absorption of ketoconazole and dapsone (given for opportunistic infection prophylaxis or treatment). Doses of these drugs should be scheduled at least 2 hours apart from didanosine doses. Do not use alcohol while taking didanosine; alcohol may increase the risk of pancreatitis, which is a serious and common complication.

Health Education for the Patient and Family

- Antiretroviral medications will not cure HIV infection but rather slow its progress and reduce significant symptoms.
- Follow individual drug guidelines for administration with or without food, swallowing whole, and dissolving a powder or chewing a tablet.
- You are still infective and can pass the infection to others. Use safer sex practices and other measures to prevent transmission to partners. Do not donate blood or breast-feed.
- Notify the healthcare provider if signs of an infection or adverse response develop: Sore throat, swollen lymph glands, fever; unusual fatigue or weakness; easy bruising, bleeding gums, or an injury that will not heal; persistent or intractable nausea; muscle pain or wasting.
- Continue all scheduled follow-up visits and laboratory studies to monitor for drug toxicity.
- Check with the healthcare provider before taking any prescription or over-the-counter drug.

PROTEASE INHIBITORS

atazanavir (Reyataz)
darunavir (Prezista)
fosamprenavir (Lexiva)
indinavir (Crixivan)
lopinavir/ritonavir (Kaletra)
nelfinavir (Viracept)
ritonavir (Norvir)
saquinavir (Invairase)
tipranavir (Aptivus)

Nursing Responsibilities

- Assess for evidence of cardiovascular or liver disease and diabetes mellitus. Most PIs are associated with lipodystrophy (enlarged abdomen, loss of tissue from the face, arms, and legs) and diabetes mellitus (elevated blood glucose).
- The protease inhibitors are known to precipitate kidney stones. Monitor creatinine clearance and patient reports of colicky flank pain.
- Administer by mouth. Follow individual drug guidelines for administration with or without food, swallowing whole, and dissolving a powder or chewing a tablet.
- Assess for adverse effects. Nausea and intestinal distress are common. Headache and peripheral neuropathies are also common. Skin reactions may be severe in about 1% of patients. Side effects may be self-limiting, decreasing with time, or significant and necessitating a change of therapy.

NUCLEOSIDE AND NUCLEOTIDE REVERSE TRANSCRIPTASE INHIBITORS

abacavir (Ziagen)

didanosine (ddI, Videx)

emtricitabine (Emtriva, FTC)

lamivudine (Epivir, 3TC)

stavudine (d4T, Zerit)

tenofovir (TDF, Viread)

zidovudine (AZT, Retrovir)

Nursing Responsibilities

- Assess for history of liver disease before administering these drugs.
- Administer by mouth. Follow individual drug guidelines for administering with or without food, swallowing whole, dissolving a powder, or chewing a tablet.
- Assess for evidence of severe skin rash accompanied by blisters, fever, joint or muscle pain, redness and swelling of the eyes, sores in the mouth, and swelling; serious kidney problems; anemia; and liver and muscle problems. Individuals should tell their healthcare provider if they have any of these side effects.

MISCELLANEOUS ANTIRETROVIRALS

dolutegravir (Tivicay)

elvitegravir (Vitekta)

enfuvirtide (Fuzeon)

maraviroc (Selzentry)

raltegravir (Isentress)

Nursing Responsibilities

- Hypersensitivity may occur with these medications. Monitor patient closely for fever, skin rash, severe tiredness or achiness, diarrhea, nausea and vomiting, stomach pain, sore throat, shortness of breath, cough, or general ill feeling.
- Respiratory infections are a concern for patients taking maraviroc; monitor respiratory status carefully and encourage deep-breathing exercises or use of incentive spirometry. Ensure patient follows good hygiene such as washing hands; avoid people with respiratory infections.
- Both enfuvirtide and maraviroc must be given in combination with other antiviral drugs.
- Enfuvirtide is supplied as a powder and must be dissolved in water for injection. Roll but do not shake the mixture because excessive foam may form. Inject when completely dissolved or refrigerate up to 24 hours. Do not inject solution until it warms to room temperature. Rotate sites.
- Side effects may include cough, fever, upper respiratory tract infections, abdominal pain, dizziness, and rash. These may indicate allergy. Musculoskeletal aches, stiffness, or weakness may indicate bone necrosis caused by the drugs. Instruct patient to report these to the healthcare provider immediately.
- Monitor liver function (cirrhosis and hepatitis decrease liver function) tests including bilirubin, amylase, lipase, AST, and ALT.
- Administer by mouth except for Fuzeon, which is administered subcutaneously. Monitor injection site for site reactions.
- Assess for evidence of severe skin rash accompanied by blisters, fever, joint or muscle pain, redness and swelling of the eyes, sores in the mouth, and swelling; serious kidney problems; anemia; thrombocytopenia, neutropenia, and liver and muscle problems.
- Monitor kidney function (serum creatinine and BUN).

Source: Data from Adams et al., 2017.

Nursing Care

The patient with HIV and AIDS has many nursing care needs, including both physical and psychosocial support needs. Because there is as yet no cure for HIV, many of these needs fall within the realm of nursing to promote knowledge and understanding, self-care, comfort, and quality of life. Adherence to ART and the course of HIV infection may well be affected by the patient's social support systems, control, perceived self-efficacy in management, and coping mechanisms.

As the epidemic continues, nurses are providing care for increasing numbers of patients with HIV infection at various stages of disease including those who are undiagnosed. These patients are not only in special care settings, but also on general units, maternal–child units, hospice, and home settings. As patients with HIV live longer, nurses will increasingly encounter patients in whom HIV is a secondary diagnosis with another primary diagnosis, for example, seizures, heart disease, diabetes mellitus, or an operative procedure.

Assessment

Collect the following data through health history and physical examination. Further focused assessments are described with nursing interventions.

- *Health history:* Risk factors (transfusion, unprotected sex, needle exposure), infections (STIs, hepatitis, tuberculosis), medications, recreational drug use
- *Physical assessment:* Height, weight, nutrition, skin and mucous membranes, vision, lymph nodes, breath sounds, abdominal tenderness, motor strength, coordination, cranial nerves, gait, deep tendon reflexes, genitourinary examination, mental status.

Priorities of Care

Nursing care priorities for the patient with HIV infection change over the course of the disease. Health maintenance activities, education, and support of coping mechanisms are important in the early stages of the disease. As the disease progresses and the patient experiences more physical symptoms, direct care needs become more important while the need for psychosocial support continues.

Diagnoses, Outcomes, and Interventions

Teaching and counseling for health maintenance and prevention of the spread of HIV are important nursing roles for patients, people at high risk, and the general public. Counseling the patient with a new diagnosis of HIV infection is vital. HIV infection and AIDS continue to carry a social stigma that may interfere with the patient's usual support systems and coping mechanisms. Typically, the patient maintains self-care in the community, although acute opportunistic infections may necessitate hospitalization. See the accompanying Case Study & Nursing Care Plan.

Teach Coping Strategies. On receiving the test results indicating HIV seropositive status, the person with HIV infection is faced with multiple issues rarely affecting other patients. HIV is a chronic infection for which there currently is no known cure. Once the decision to initiate ART has been made, the patient faces a lifelong commitment to therapy that is expensive and associated with multiple adverse effects. Social support systems, family relationships, and the ability to obtain and retain useful work and health insurance may be disrupted by the disease. The patient may experience guilt about his or her lifestyle and how the disease was contracted. As the disease progresses, social isolation, fatigue, body image changes, medication side effects, and multiple other issues affect the patient's ability to cope.

Expected Outcome: Patient demonstrates acceptance of change in health status as evidenced by taking active role in healthcare decisions.

The nurse will:

- Assess social support network and usual methods of coping. *This will help both the nurse and the patient identify people and mechanisms that can help the patient cope more effectively with the disease.*
- Support the patient's social network. *Nontraditional families may offer more support than the traditional family. This in turn may necessitate a liberal interpretation of the term* family *in some healthcare settings.*
- Communication with HIV patients should focus on respect and concern. Respect has been shown to improve dialogue between the patient and clinician. Patients are more likely to feel comfortable in discussing psychosocial information that may impact their care. Respectful communication also fosters shared decision making, which improves continuation of treatment regimens (Flickinger et al., 2016; Fuller, Koester, Guinness, & Steward, 2017). *These are critical components of patient-centered care for the individual with HIV infection and his or her family.*
- Use short-term counseling to help the patient cope with the crisis presented by the diagnosis of HIV infection or by an AIDS-defining illness. *Short-term counseling can help the patient cope with the immediate crisis and return to a normal state of functioning.*
- Promote interaction between the patient, significant others, and family. *The diagnosis of HIV infection and manifestations of HIV disease may bring about isolation from others and decrease the patient's ability to cope.*
- Provide information, support, and, as appropriate, guidance for the patient in making decisions regarding care and treatment. *This gives the patient a greater sense of self-worth and control over the situation, increasing coping abilities.*
- Provide reassurance, acceptance, and encouragement during crisis episodes. *Providing consistent acceptance and support for the patient with HIV infection enhances coping during times of crisis.*
- Assist to accept responsibility for actions without blaming others. *Effective coping cannot occur without accepting responsibility for one's actions.*
- Support proactive coping behaviors as these behaviors have been shown to improve outcomes from greater adherence to treatment protocols. *Proactive coping includes resilience—resisting negative thoughts and concentrating on positive thinking about situations, reliance on religious beliefs, and support systems* (Pecoraro et al., 2016).

Reduce Risk-Prone Behaviors. The risk for contracting HIV infection is related to lifestyle and behaviors. Changing these unsafe behaviors, for example, engaging in unprotected sexual intercourse or sharing supplies for injection drug use, is critical to reducing an individual's risk. Once diagnosed with HIV, behavior modifications are important to prevent spread of the infection to others.

Expected Outcome: Patient will verbalize acceptance of health status changes and begin to make lifestyle and behavior changes to prevent disease spread to others.

The nurse will:

- Assist to accept responsibility for actions without blaming others. *Effective coping cannot occur without accepting responsibility for one's actions.*
- Provide positive reinforcement of self-directed lifestyle and behavior changes initiated by the patient. *Reinforcement of positive behaviors helps strengthen the patient's ability to maintain new ways of acting and develop behavioral habits to support a healthy lifestyle.*
- Assist the patient to clarify her or his own values and beliefs. *Identifying personal values and beliefs facilitates effective decision making.*
- Reinforce personal strengths that are identified. *Focusing on personal strengths enables movement away from negative thoughts.*
- Assist in setting realistic goals. *Establishing and meeting realistic short-term goals is helpful in increasing self-confidence and decreasing negative self-talk.*
- Refer to clergy, social worker, clinical specialist, and/or counselor as appropriate. *Individuals with expertise in counseling may be necessary to enable coping with current situation.*

Promote Good Skin Integrity. Dryness, malnutrition, immobility from fatigue, and skin lesions on pressure sites contribute to impaired integrity of the skin for the patient with HIV. Maintaining skin integrity is important as the first line of defense against infection in an immunosuppressed patient.

Expected Outcome: Patient's skin will remain intact without evidence of underlying tissue breakdown.

The nurse will:

- Assess the skin frequently for lesions and areas of breakdown. *Early identification of impaired skin integrity allows prompt intervention.*
- Monitor lesions for signs of infection or impaired healing. *Infection or poor tissue perfusion not only impairs healing but may lead to further skin breakdown.*
- Turn at least every 2 hours if unable to turn self, more frequently if necessary. Prevent skin shearing by using a turnsheet and adequate personnel when repositioning. *Turning decreases unrelieved pressure on bony prominences and improves circulation to the tissues. Shearing causes tissue trauma that can lead to decubitus ulcers.*
- Keep skin clean and dry using mild, nondrying soaps or oils for cleansing. *Night sweats and diarrhea, if present, can cause breakdown and damage to the skin. Frequent cleansing with nondrying products discourages bacterial growth, thus reducing the risk of infection.*

SAFETY ALERT: Applying protective creams to reddened areas in the rectal area protects skin from the caustic effects of diarrhea. ■

- If blisters are noted, leave intact and dress with a hydrocolloid (e.g., DuoDERM) dressing. *Blisters provide natural sterile coverings for damaged tissue, improving healing and preventing bacterial invasion.*
- Caution against scratching. If confused, trim fingernails and use mitts or soft restraints to prevent scratching. Check circulation of hands and fingers frequently if mitts or restraints are used. *Scratching and skin damage allow bacteria to be introduced into lesions, increasing the risk of infection. Tight or restrictive restraints or mitts may compromise circulation.*
- Encourage ambulation, if possible; if the patient is confined to bed, encourage active or passive range-of-motion exercises. *Activity increases circulation, decreases pressure and skin breakdown, and helps maintain muscle tone.*
- Monitor nutritional intake and albumin levels. *Maintenance of optimal nutrition decreases the risk of tissue breakdown and improves resistance to infection.*

Promote Adequate Weight and Nutrition. Many factors associated with HIV disease, including manifestations of the disease itself, put the patient at risk for altered nutrition and weight loss. Nausea and anorexia may be manifestations of the disease or the result of antiretroviral therapy. Chronic diarrhea is a common manifestation of HIV disease. Wasting syndrome is also common, manifested by involuntary weight loss of greater than 10 to 15% of baseline weight, severe diarrhea, fever, and chronic fatigue and weakness. The exact cause of wasting syndrome is unclear, but the diarrhea and fatigue contribute, as does the increased metabolic rate associated with fever. Oral and esophageal candidiasis and KS of the gastrointestinal tract may cause painful swallowing, making eating difficult and thereby contributing to anorexia. Poor nutritional status in the patient with HIV can ultimately result in altered comfort, a change in body image, muscle wasting, increased risk of infection, and higher mortality and morbidity.

Expected Outcome: Patient will maintain body weight appropriate for height and body mass index (BMI) and serum albumin within accepted ranges.

The nurse will:

- Assess nutritional status, including weight; BMI; caloric intake; and laboratory studies, such as total protein and albumin levels, hemoglobin, and hematocrit. *These factors provide a baseline to determine the effectiveness of interventions.*
- Identify possible causes of altered nutrition. *Identification of contributing factors provides direction for planned interventions.*
- Administer prescribed medications for candidiasis and other manifestations as prescribed. *Eliminating this opportunistic infection improves comfort and facilitates food intake. Topical viscous anesthetic can help reduce pain and improve oral intake.*
- Administer antidiarrheal medications after stools and antiemetics prior to meals. Provide antipyretics as needed to control fever. *Reducing diarrhea will improve nutrient absorption; preprandial medication with an antiemetic reduces nausea and improves food intake. Reduction of fever lowers the body's metabolic demands.*

SAFETY ALERT: High-fiber foods can increase intestinal motility and the incidence of diarrhea. ■

- Provide a diet high in protein and kilocalories. *A high-protein, high-kilocalorie diet provides the necessary nutrients to meet metabolic and tissue healing needs.*
- Offer soft foods and serve small portions. *Soft foods are easily digested. Small portions are more appealing to the anorectic or nauseated patient.*
- Involve in meal planning and encourage significant others to bring favorite foods from home. *The patient is more likely to consume adequate amounts of preferred foods. Allowing food choices enhances the patient's sense of control.*
- Assist with eating as needed. *Fatigue and weakness can prevent the patient from eating an adequate amount of food.*
- Provide supplementary vitamins and enteral feedings, such as Ensure. *This improves nutritional status and caloric intake.*
- Provide or assist with frequent oral hygiene. *Oral hygiene improves comfort and appetite and reduces the risk of mucosal lesions.*
- Administer appetite stimulants, such as megestrol (Megace) and dronabinol (Marinol), as ordered. *Both drugs may increase appetite and promote weight gain.*

Promote Sexual Function. The diagnosis of HIV infection can significantly alter the patient's expressions of sexuality. Guilt over the diagnosis may interfere with libido. The patient may be angry with a significant other or partner if that person was the probable source of infection. The patient may fear spreading the disease to others via sexual relations.

As the disease progresses, its manifestations can affect body image and self-esteem, impairing sexuality. Other symptoms, such as nausea, fatigue, and weakness, may also interfere with libido and sexual satisfaction. If nurses are not comfortable discussing sexuality, referral to a counselor is appropriate.

Expected Outcome: Patient and partner will demonstrate willingness to discuss impact of HIV infection on sexuality and sexual function.

The nurse will:

- Examine own feelings about sexuality, role in dealing with a patient's sexuality, the patient's lifestyle, and sexual preferences. *To deal effectively with the patient's concerns, the nurse must be comfortable with his or her own feelings of sexuality and be able to accept the patient's lifestyle. Referring the patient to another nurse or counselor may be necessary.*
- Establish a trusting, therapeutic relationship through the use of time, active listening, caring, and self-disclosure. Maintain a nonthreatening, nonjudgmental attitude toward the patient. *Sexuality is a private issue that will be uncomfortable or impossible for the nurse and patient to discuss without a mutually trusting relationship.*
- Provide factual information about HIV infection and its effects. *This helps the patient separate fears and myths from reality.*
- Discuss safer sex practices, including hugging, cuddling, nonsexual contact, the use of latex condoms and spermicidal lubricant, and mutual masturbation. *Alternative forms of sexual activity and expressing affection can allow the patient and significant other to remain close throughout the course of the disease.*
- Encourage discussion of fears and concerns with significant other. *Open communication helps the patient deal with issues related to sexuality.*
- For the patient without a significant other, stress the need to continue to meet people and develop social relationships while practicing safer sex. *The risk of isolation is high in the patient with HIV infection, and relationships with others help the patient to cope with the disease.*
- Refer the patient and significant other to local support groups for people and partners of people with HIV. *Support groups provide a social and support network of people facing the same issues.*

Delegating Nursing Care Activities

As appropriate and allowed by the designated duties and responsibilities of assistive personnel, the nurse may delegate nursing care activities such as measuring intake and output, obtaining daily weights, and assisting with activities and hygiene for the patient with HIV infection.

Case Study & Nursing Care Plan

A Patient with HIV Infection

Jeff Lu is a 36-year-old elementary school teacher who lives with two housemates. Mr. Lu sees his primary care physician, complaining of fatigue, persistent sore throat, intermittent bouts of diarrhea, and mild shortness of breath for about a month. He expresses fear that he has contracted HIV, and says he has avoided testing in the past because of the impact positive test results would have on his career, lifestyle, and family. Mr. Lu has been open about his homosexuality since his teens and is a vocal activist for gay, lesbian, and bisexual issues. He is not currently in a committed relationship and admits to using condoms "less than 100% of the time." The physician orders a mononucleosis test, ELISA, Western blot analysis, CD4 T-cell count, a p24 antigen test, and an erythrocyte sedimentation rate (ESR). Mr. Lu has a return appointment in 1 week for follow-up.

ASSESSMENT	DIAGNOSES	EXPECTED OUTCOMES
On Mr. Lu's follow-up visit, Carole Kee, RN, obtains a nursing history. Mr. Lu continues to have flulike symptoms and states that he just has not been as active as usual and is worried about his health. His appetite has decreased because of soreness in his mouth, and he has noted some whitish patches on his tongue and cheeks. A chest x-ray film reveals no abnormality. The results of laboratory tests are as follows: ▪ ELISA: Positive for antibodies against HIV ▪ Western blot analysis: Positive for antibodies against HIV ▪ p24 antigen test: Positive for circulating HIV antigens ▪ ESR: Increased to 25 mm/h (normal for men is 10 to 15 mm/h) ▪ CD4 T-cell count: 599/mm^3 (normal range is 600 to 1200 mm^3). Mr. Lu's physical examination reveals that he has enlarged lymph nodes in his neck and white patches on the oral mucosa. His skin is warm to the touch. Vital signs are T 37.7°C (99.9°F), P 84 bpm, R 20/min, and BP 120/78 mmHg. Mr. Lu is given the results of the laboratory tests and the medical diagnosis of HIV infection. He is obviously distressed but says that now that he has to face what he has avoided for so long, he needs to know "everything there is to know" about ART and how to live with HIV infection.	▪ Anxiety related to diagnosis and fear ▪ Education about the HIV disease process and self-care ▪ Weight loss related to soreness in mouth ▪ Potential for infection related to altered immune protection	▪ Patient will verbalize anxiety and use appropriate coping mechanisms. ▪ Patient will verbalize and demonstrate knowledge of HIV infection and its management. ▪ Patient will verbalize measures to prevent HIV transmission to others, including safer sex practices. ▪ Patient will maintain adequate nutrition for optimal body and cellular function. ▪ Patient will remain free of infections and their complications.

PLANNING AND IMPLEMENTATION

- Provide opportunities for Mr. Lu to verbalize his feelings.
- Avoid false reassurances.
- Provide appropriate and adequate information about HIV infection and ART.
- Coordinate referral to a healthcare provider who specializes in HIV infection management.
- Review safer sex practices and other measures to prevent HIV transmission.
- Teach anxiety-controlling techniques, such as deep breathing and meditation.
- Monitor weight and serum albumin levels at each visit until stabilized.
- Provide dietary consultation referral.
- Encourage oral care before and after meals.
- Assess bowel sounds and monitor elimination pattern.
- Teach Mr. Lu to avoid exposure to infection and people with known illnesses until his CD4 cell count returns to normal levels.
- Monitor response to prescribed medications.
- Encourage regular physical exercise.

EVALUATION

Mr. Lu receives a prescription for an antifungal medication and referral to a healthcare provider whose practice is limited to patients with HIV infection. When he meets with this healthcare provider, the decision is made to start ART based on his CD4 cell count and symptoms of HIV disease. Mr. Lu is initially started on combination ART with daily efavirenz, tenofovir, and emtricitabine (Atripla).

CRITICAL THINKING IN THE NURSING PROCESS

1. How does age affect the body's response to fighting HIV infection? What other factors affect the risk of HIV infection and its progression?
2. Which classes of antiretroviral drugs are found in the combination formula Atripla? What is the rationale for prescribing drugs from more than one class? What teaching regarding timing, interactions, and possible adverse reactions to the drugs does Mr. Lu need?
3. Although Mr. Lu has health insurance through his employer, he is concerned about the cost of the prescribed ART. How should the nurse respond? What resources are available to help with the cost burden of ART?
4. Mr. Lu tells the nurse that although he isn't ready to call it a committed relationship, he has been seeing one person exclusively for the past 3 months. He asks what his partner can do to minimize his risk of contracting HIV. How should the nurse respond?

See Evaluating Your Response in Appendix B.

Transitions of Care

To stop the spread of HIV, it is important to identify those who are infected but undiagnosed (approximately 21% of patients who are HIV positive). The CDC (2006) and WHO (2017b) recommend HIV testing for patients in all healthcare settings. The WHO also recommends that testing also be made available in community-based settings, particularly in HIV epidemic areas or settings. Informed consent is necessary for testing, although specific written consent is not required. In opt-out testing, consent for screening is part of the general consent for care, unless specifically declined by the patient. Current guidelines further recommend linking HIV testing and counseling with prevention, care, and treatment services (WHO, 2017a).

In the absence of an effective immunization to prevent HIV infection, education, counseling, and behavior modification are the primary tools for HIV/AIDS prevention. Nurses play a vital role in providing education about this epidemic and infection prevention for individuals and communities.

All sexually active individuals need to know how HIV is spread. Following are the only totally safe sex practices:

- No sex
- Long-term mutually monogamous sexual relations between two uninfected people
- Mutual masturbation without direct contact.

Patients who do engage in sexual activity need to know and practice safer sex. Reducing the number of sexual partners—for example, by entering into and remaining in a long-term, mutually monogamous relationship with an uninfected partner—reduces the risk. Patients should not engage in unprotected sex, especially if the HIV status of the partner is unknown. Latex condoms have been shown to reduce the risk of transmitting HIV. Their effectiveness is improved when nonoxynol-9, a spermicide, is used for lubrication; however, it may cause genital ulcers, which can facilitate HIV transmission. To be effective, condoms must be used with every sexual encounter involving vaginal, oral, or anal intercourse and they need to be applied and removed properly. A female condom is also available for use.

Healthy gay and bisexual men and heterosexual individuals whose partner has HIV infection may be able to further reduce the risk of contracting the infection by taking the combination antiretroviral medication Truvada (emtricitabine and tenofovir disoproxil fumarate) daily. Recent studies found the combination of condom use, counseling, and daily Truvada cut the risk of infection by 86% or more with strict adherence to treatment (Tetteh et al., 2017).

The most difficult group of high-risk people to reach and educate has been injection drug users. People in this group should never share needles, syringes, or other drug paraphernalia. Many cities have initiated needle exchange programs, providing a sterile needle and syringe in exchange for a used one. Undiluted household bleach is effective to clean paraphernalia when sterile supplies are not available. It is important to also teach people in this population about safer sex practices because most heterosexual HIV transmission occurs between injection drug users and their partners.

Screening of voluntary blood donors and donated blood supplies has reduced the risk of transmission by transfusion to 1 in 100,000. Because current blood-screening methods use antibody testing, receiving donated blood continues to carry a small risk. Patients in the *window period* between contraction of the virus and the development of detectable antibodies are able to transmit the virus to others, even though they do not yet test positive for HIV. This window period usually lasts from 6 weeks to 6 months; rarely, it lasts up to 1 year. When possible, encourage patients to use autologous transfusion, donating their own blood prior to an anticipated surgery.

Encourage patients who are HIV positive to abstain from donating blood, organs, or sperm. They should understand tactics to avoid exchange of body fluids by not sharing needles or other drug paraphernalia, not sharing razors, and not obtaining a tattoo. Stress the importance of informing all medical personnel providing direct care (especially anyone performing a dental, surgical, or obstetric procedure) about the diagnosis.

Healthcare workers can prevent most exposures to HIV by using standard precautions (see **Figure 13.12** ■ and Appendix A). Testing to determine HIV status remains voluntary and relies on the use of antibody-screening methods. It is therefore impossible to identify every patient who is HIV positive. With standard precautions, all patients are treated alike, eliminating the need to know the patient's HIV status. All high-risk body fluids are treated as if they are infectious, and barrier precautions are used to prevent skin, mucous membrane, or percutaneous exposure to them. Counseling, testing, and postexposure prophylaxis are provided to healthcare workers with a documented needlestick exposure to the blood of an individual with HIV infection.

Teaching needs for both patients with HIV and their significant others are extensive. The primary need is for information about the disease, its spread, and its expected course. The patient and family need current factual information to plan realistically and to combat myths, misperceptions, and prejudices. At the same time, it is important to include information about current research and progress in treating the disease to maintain a sense of hopefulness.

The following topics should be discussed with the patient and family to prepare for home care:

- Guidelines for safer sex practices
- Nutrition, rest and exercise, stress reduction, lifestyle changes, and maintaining a positive outlook
- Infection prevention and transmission including hand hygiene and wearing gloves when handling patients' secretions or excretions
- Importance of regular medical follow-up and monitoring of immune status

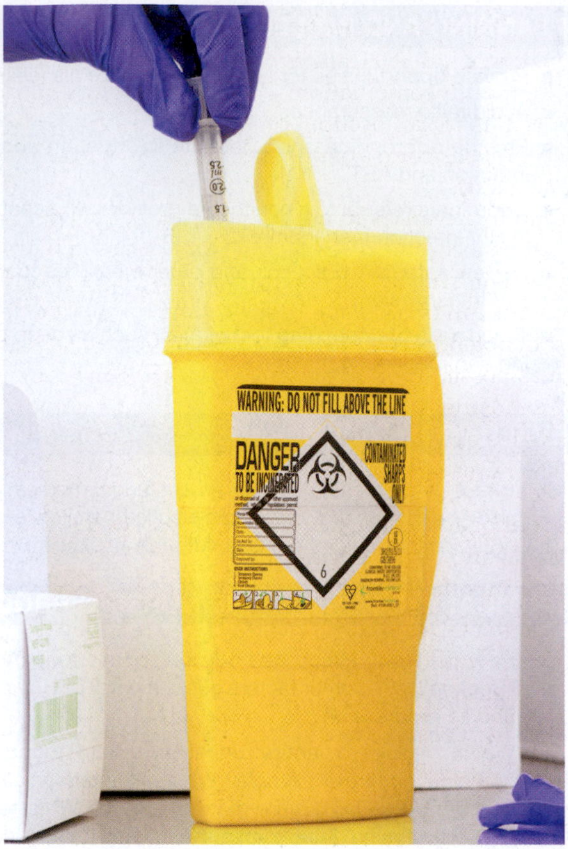
WARNING: DO NOT FILL ABOVE THE LINE
DANGER
TO BE INCINERATED
CONTAMINATED SHARPS ONLY

Figure 13.12 ■ This nurse is disposing of a needle and syringe in a special container, a necessary practice to avoid the transmission of HIV through needlesticks with contaminated needles.

- Signs and symptoms of opportunistic infections and malignancies, as well as other symptoms that should be reported
- Medications and adverse effects; the importance of adherence to prescribed ART once initiated
- Cessation of smoking, alcohol, and recreational or illicit drug use
- Home health, hospice, and respite care services as appropriate
- Community resources, such as support groups, social agencies, and counselors
- Helpful resources:
    a. CDC National AIDS Hotline
    b. Gay Men's Health Crisis Network
    c. National Association of People with AIDS
    d. National Organization on HIV over Fifty.

Healthcare workers exposed to HIV infection or adults who experience a high-risk exposure to HIV may choose postexposure prophylaxis. Risk of exposure for healthcare workers may occur via needlesticks or cuts with a sharp object or via mucous membrane or nonintact skin contact with semen, vaginal secretions, fluids contaminated with visible blood, and possibly CSF, synovial fluid, and pleural, peritoneal, pericardial, or amniotic fluids. CDC and National Public Health Service guidelines recommend treatment with combination ART, which includes three or more NRTIs for all occupational exposures (Kuhar et al., 2013). A 4-week course of treatment is recommended (Fauci & Lane, 2015).

Due to advances in antiretroviral drugs, HIV is now considered a chronic disease. Patients diagnosed with HIV are now living full lives. However, complications from these treatments can occur. Patients and their families should be aware of potential complications in order to prevent them as much as possible and to understand when to seek medical attention. Patients also need to understand the importance of adherence to drug therapy.

The nurse should:

- Monitor adherence to treatment plan and discuss emotional and psychosocial concerns with patient and significant others.
- Monitor CD4 response as drug resistance may develop, which would require reevaluation of drug therapy.
- Explain that due to metabolic changes, fat redistribution may occur, causing loss of adipose tissue in face, buttocks, arms, and legs and possible excess abdominal adipose tissue.
- Drug therapy side effects may include organ dysfunction (pancreas, liver, cardiovascular, kidney). Patients should be informed of symptoms (abdominal pain, diarrhea, nausea and vomiting, chest palpitations, dizziness, chest pain) of potential complications and understand the need to contact their medical provider without delay.
- Diligence is required by the patient to avoid opportunistic infections such as proper nutrition, good hygiene, and avoidance of those with current infectious illness. Instruct patient to monitor temperature and note any abnormal redness, discharge, and congestion.
- HIV patients are at an increased risk for developing cancers such as Kaposi sarcoma, lymphomas, and cervical cancer. Instruct patient on potential symptoms for early treatment of these conditions.
- Continued assessment of psychosocial needs and for any signs of isolation and depression is necessary, as depression can intensify any medical condition.

Even with the advances in treatment many deaths are due to the effects of the HIV virus, especially in certain populations such as those living in poverty and those without medical insurance. Patients within these populations are less likely to have advanced directives and participate in palliative and hospice care. Early initiation of palliative care can provide pain relief and alleviate symptoms associated with end-of-life conditions (Rhodes et al., 2016). End-of-life care also depends on the specific pathophysiologic problem since comorbidities such as liver failure, heart disease, cancers, and infections may be precipitating factors.

The role of the nurse in end-of-life care would include:

- Ensure patient wishes are outlined in advance directives.
- Encourage enrollment in palliative and hospice care.
- Ensure comfort by monitoring pain, anxiety, and depression levels and medicate as ordered.
- Promote skin integrity to avoid further problems and discomfort.
- Monitor albumin levels as this may indicate a poor prognosis (albumin levels of less than 2.5g indicate poorer prognosis).
- Respiratory depression can increase anxiety; perform nursing measures to improve respiratory status such as raising head of bed, apply oxygen as ordered, and administer pain medications.
- Provide emotional support to patient and significant others.

CHAPTER HIGHLIGHTS

13.1 Overview of the Altered Immune System

Review the normal immune system function, including self-recognition.

- Normal immune functioning is essential in protecting the body from internal and external threats. A hyperresponsive immune system, however, which overreacts to antigens or fails to distinguish self proteins from abnormal or nonself proteins, can threaten health and well-being.
- The immune system is a complex combination of cellular and humoral components that protect against disease. Immunity develops when the body recognizes foreign proteins as "nonself" and develops nonspecific inflammatory responses and specific cellular responses to each foreign antigen.
- With aging, there is a general decline in the sensitivity and regulation of the immune system, which may result in autoimmune disease.

13.2 Hypersensitivity Reactions

Compare and contrast the four types of hypersensitivity reactions.

- A type I IgE-mediated response is a rapidly occurring response to an antigen source where the antigen and mast cells bind with IgE cells. Mast cells contain histamine and are commonly found in the respiratory system. The response contributes to vasodilation, skin rash, nasal discharge, and bronchial constriction. Common sources are animal dander, pollen, dust, peanuts, shellfish, chocolate, and penicillin. Type I responses are the most common hypersensitivity reaction.

- In type II hypersensitivity response, Ig cell response to antigens originates on cell surfaces. The immune system targets these antigens and either destroys them by phagocytosis or through the complement system that actually attacks the cell membrane, causing lysis of the cell itself. The lysis causes further immune response. The most noted type II hypersensitivity reaction is a transfusion reaction where donor blood cells are incompatible with the recipient. Transfusion reactions can cause serious complications and require immediate attention.
- In type III immune complex-mediated reactions, this response is caused by antibody reactions to circulating antigens, which are then deposited within tissues such as joints and organs. The resulting deposits cause alterations in the structures. This reaction is common in rheumatoid arthritis and Raynaud disease. In Raynaud disease the immune response affects capillary circulation in the hands, feet, and nose, limiting blood flow and resulting in cyanosis of the affected area.
- Type IV delayed hypersensitivity reactions are caused by T lymphocytes rather than antibody–antigen reactions. Lymphocytes do not respond as quickly as antibodies to antigens; thus, a delay is seen in symptoms of the reaction. The body may take several days to respond to an antigen. A common example of this type of reaction is poison ivy where a person may have contact with the plant and not develop itching and rash until days later. Type IV reactions can also be seen in organ transplant patients.

13.3 Autoimmune Disorders

Describe the pathophysiology and manifestations of autoimmune disorders and tissue transplant rejection, and outline the interprofessional care, nursing care, and transitions of care for patients with these disorders.

- Immune function that targets normal cells and tissues (autoimmunity) or that leads to destruction of transplanted tissue or organs (transplant rejection) threatens the well-being of affected patients. Immunosuppressant therapy is used to prevent tissue and organ damage and maintain the function of transplanted tissue.
- Autoimmune disorders are diverse, ranging from damage limited to specific cells within an individual organ to systemic disorders with widespread effects, and characterized by an abnormal immune response to normal cells and tissues.
- Intentional immunosuppression is necessary to prevent initial rejection of a transplanted organ or tissue, to maintain the transplant, and to halt any rejection process that may develop. Most immunosuppressing drugs are nephrotoxic; immunosuppression places patients at greater risk for infection and cancers.

13.4 Impaired Immune Responses

Describe the pathophysiology and manifestations of disorders of impaired immune response, and outline the interprofessional care, nursing care, and transitions of care for patients with these disorders.

- Impaired immune function, whether congenital or acquired, threatens health and physiologic integrity because the patient cannot effectively respond to threats such as infection. Nurses play a major role in teaching behaviors to prevent HIV infection, the leading cause of acquired immunodeficiency, and in teaching health and disease management strategies to those affected.
- HIV infection continues to spread and many patients are unaware they have the virus. AIDS, the end stage of HIV infection, is profound immunosuppression that results from viral destruction of cellular components of host immunity.
- Although HIV infection cannot be cured, it can be treated with antiretroviral therapy (ART), a combination of drugs that limits viral replication and host susceptibility to opportunistic infections and cancer. Consistent adherence to the treatment regimen is critical to inhibiting viral replication. ART is, however, expensive and associated with significant adverse effects.
- Education, counseling, and psychosocial support are key components of care for the person with HIV infection and his or her significant others.

TEST YOURSELF NCLEX-RN® REVIEW

1. The nurse is caring for a patient experiencing a type I immediate hypersensitivity reaction. For which health problem is the nurse providing care to the patient?
   A. Anaphylaxis
   B. Graft rejection
   C. Hemolytic anemia
   D. Systemic lupus erythematosus
2. A patient received a liver transplant 1 day ago. If the patient were to develop an acute transplant rejection episode, when should the nurse expect to see the manifestations?
   A. Within the first 8 hours
   B. Within the first 24 hours
   C. Approximately 2 days later
   D. Approximately 4 days to 3 months later

3. The nurse notes a cough, shortness of breath, and tachypnea in a patient with AIDS. Which opportunistic infection is probably causing these manifestations?
   A. Cytomegalovirus
   B. *Toxoplasma gondii*
   C. *Pneumocystis jiroveci*
   D. *Cryptococcus neoformans*
4. Which explanation should the nurse provide to a patient who has a positive HIV rapid antibody test? (Select all that apply.)
   A. "You have been diagnosed with AIDS."
   B. "At this point, AIDS is not active in your blood."
   C. "Antibodies to the HIV may be present in your blood."
   D. "This means that you will not develop AIDS in the future."
   E. "Additional testing is necessary before a final diagnosis is made."
5. A patient is taking the nucleoside reverse transcriptase inhibitor zidovudine (Retrovir) for HIV. What should the nurse identify as an adverse reaction to this medication? (Select all that apply.)
   A. Neutropenia
   B. Polycythemia
   C. Cardiotoxicity
   D. Nephrotoxicity
   E. Anemia
6. A patient is being scheduled for allergy testing. Which method should a nurse expect to be used first?
   A. Prick test
   B. Inhalation
   C. Intradermal injection
   D. Subcutaneous injection
7. The nurse suspects a patient receiving a blood transfusion is experiencing a hypersensitivity reaction. What action should the nurse perform first?
   A. Administer oxygen.
   B. Replace all tubing and attach a new line with normal saline.
   C. Flush the line and run normal saline attached at the Y connection.
   D. Order a type and cross-match from the laboratory.
8. A patient diagnosed as being HIV positive is prescribed a protease inhibitor and nucleoside analog. For which metabolic abnormality should the nurse monitor in the patient?
   A. Diabetes mellitus
   B. Lactose intolerance
   C. Hashimoto thyroiditis
   D. Systemic lupus erythematosus
9. What should be the priority when initiating or changing the drug regimen in a patient who is HIV positive?
   A. Cost of therapy
   B. Access to dental care
   C. Toxicities associated with each drug
   D. Patient willingness to adhere to the drug regimen
10. A patient recovering from a kidney transplant is prescribed immunosuppressant therapy. Which agent should the nurse administer to induce immunosuppression immediately following the transplant?
   A. Azathioprine
   B. Corticosteroids
   C. Muromonab-cd3
   D. Lymphocyte immune globulin

See Test Yourself answers in Appendix B.

REFERENCES

Adams, A., Ford, M., & Larsen, C. (2017). Transplantation immunobiology and immunosuppression. In C. Townsend, D. Beauchamp, M. Evers, & K. Mattox (Eds.), *Sabiston textbook of surgery* (20th ed.), pp. 597–636. Philadelphia, PA: Elsevier.

Adams, M., Holland, N., & Urban, C. (2017). *Pharmacology for nurses a pathophysiologic approach* (5th ed.). Boston, MA: Pearson.

American Academy of Allergy, Asthma & Immunology. (2017). *Latex allergy.* Retrieved from https://www.aaaai.org/conditions-and-treatments/Library/At-a-Glance/Latex-Allergy.

Barksdale, A., & Muelleman, R. (2018). Allergy, hypersensitivity, and anaphylaxis. In *Rosen's emergency medicine: Concepts and clinical practice* (9th ed.), pp. 1418–1429. Philadelphia, PA: Elsevier.

Bloch, D., Shmerling, R., & Curtis, M. (2017). Measurement and clinical significance of antinuclear antibodies. *UpToDate*. Retrieved from www.uptodate.com.

Boyce, A. J., & Austen, K. F. (2015). Allergies, anaphylaxis, and systemic mastocytosis. In Kasper, D., Fauci, A., Houser, S., Longo, D., Jameson, J., & Loscalzo, J. (Eds.), *Harrison's principles of internal medicine, 376* (19th ed.). New York, NY: McGraw-Hill. Retrieved from https://accessmedicine.mhmedical.com/book.aspx?bookid=1130

Brooks, W. (2017). A review of autoimmune disease hypotheses with introduction of the "nucleolus" hypothesis. *Clinical Reviews in Allergy and Immunology, 52*(3), 333–350.

Centers for Disease and Prevention (CDC) (2015). *HIV surveillance report*. Retrieved from https://www.cdc.gov/

hiv/pdf/library/reports/surveillance/cdc-hiv-surveillance-report-2015-vol-27.pdf.

Centers for Disease Control and Prevention (CDC). (2016). *TB and HIV coinfection*. Retrieved from https://www.cdc.gov/tb/topic/basics/tbhivcoinfection.htm,

Centers for Disease Control and Prevention (CDC). (2017a). *HIV/AIDS basic statistics*. Retrieved from https://www.cdc.gov/hiv/basics/statistics.html.

Centers for Disease Control and Prevention (CDC). (2017b). *HIV among African Americans*. Retrieved from https://www.cdc.gov/hiv/group/racialethnic/africanamericans/index.html.

Centers for Disease Control and Prevention (CDC). (2017c). *HIV among people aged 50 and over.* Retrieved from https://www.cdc.gov/hiv/group/age/olderamericans/index.html.

Centers for Disease Control and Prevention (CDC). (2017d). *HIV cost effectiveness*. Retrieved from https://www.cdc.gov/hiv/programresources/guidance/costeffectiveness/index.html.

Centers for Disease Control and Prevention (CDC). (2017e). *Lymphoma*. Retrieved from https://www.cdc.gov/cancer/lymphoma/index.htm.

Centers for Disease Control and Prevention (CDC). (2018). *HIV/AIDS risk by racial/ethnic groups*. Retrieved from https://www.cdc.gov/hiv/group/racialethnic/index.html.

De Bruin, M., Oberje, E., Viechtbauer, W., Nobel, H., Hilligsmann, M., Nieuwkoop, C., . . . Prins, J. (2017). Effectiveness and cost-effectiveness of a nurse-delivered intervention to improve adherence to treatment for HIV: A pragmatic, multicenter, open-label, randomized clinical trial. *Lancet Infectious Diseases, 17*(6), 595–604.

Diamond, B., & Lipsky, P. (2015). Autoimmunity and autoimmune diseases. In D. Kasper, A, Fauci, S. Houser, D. Longo, L. Jameson, & J. Loscalzo (Eds.), *Harrison's principles of internal medicine, 377e* (19th ed.). New York, NY: McGraw-Hill Medical. Retrieved from https://accessmedicine.mhmedical.com/Content.aspx?bookId=1130&sectionId=79749895

Fauci, A., & Lane, H. (2015). Human immunodeficiency virus disease: AIDS and related disorders. In D. Kasper, A. Fauci, S. Houser, D. Longo, L. Jameson, & J. Loscalzo (Eds.), *Harrison's principles of internal medicine* (19th ed.). New York, NY: McGraw-Hill Medical.

Frandsen, G., & Pennington, S. (2018). *Abrams' clinical drug therapy rationales for nursing practice* (11th ed.). Philadelphia: Wolters Kluwer Health.

Flickinger, T., Saha, S., Roter, D., Korthuis, T., Sharp, V., Cohn, J., . . . Beach, M. (2016). Respecting patients is associated with more patient-centered communication behaviors in clinical encounters. *Patient Education and Counseling 99*. 250–255.

Fuller, S., Koester, K., Guinness, R., & Steward, W. (2017). Patients' perceptions and experiences of shared decision-making in primary HIV care clinics. *Journal of the Association of Nurses in AIDS Care, 28*(1), 75–84.

Hosek, S., Rudy, B., Landovits, R., Kapogiannis, B., Siberry, G., Rutledge, B., . . . Wilson, C. (2017). An HIV preexposure prophylaxis demonstration project and safety study for young MSM. *Acquired Immune Deficiency Syndrome, 74*(1), 21–29.

Houston, E., Mikrut, C., Guy, A., Fominaya, A., Tatum, A., Kim, J., & Brown, A. (2016). Another look at depressive symptoms and antiretroviral therapy adherence: The role of treatment self-efficacy. *Journal of Health Psychology, 21*(2), 2138–2147.

Katz, M. (2017). HIV infection and AIDS. In M. Papadaki, S. McPhee, & M. Rabow (Eds.), *Current medical diagnosis and treatment 2017* (56th ed.), pp. 1285–1315. New York, NY: McGraw-Hill Education.

Kuhar, D., Henderson, D., Struble, K., Heneine, W., Thomas, V., Cheever, L. et al. (2013). Updated U.S. Public Health Service guidelines for the management of occupational exposures to HIV and recommendations for postexposure prophylaxis. Atlanta, GA: Centers for Disease Control and Prevention. Retrieved from http://stacks.cdc.gov/view/cdc/20711.

National Institute for Occupational Safety and Health (NIOSH). (2014). *Latex allergy a prevention guide*. Retrieved from https://www.cdc.gov/niosh/docs/98-113/.

Ofotokun, I., Na, L. H., Landovitz, R. J., Ribaudo, H. J., McComsey, G. A., Godfrey, C., . . . Currier, J. S. (2015). Comparison of the metabolic effects of ritonavir-boosted darunavir or atazanavir versus raltegravir, and the impact of ritonavir plasma exposure: ACTG 5257. *Clinical Infectious Diseases: An Official Publication of the Infectious Diseases Society of America, 60*(12), 1842–1851.

Organ Procurement and Transplantation Network (OPTN) and Scientific Registry of Transplant Recipients (SRTR). (2018). *Kaplan-Meier Graft Survival Rates for Transplants Performed: 2008–2015.* Retrieved from https://optn.transplant.hrsa.gov/data/view-data-reports/national-data/#.

Panel on Antiretroviral Guidelines for Adults and Adolescents. (2017). *Guidelines for the use of antiretroviral agents in adults and adolescents living with HIV.* Retrieved from https://aidsinfo.nih.gov/contentfiles/lvguidelines/adultandadolescentgl.pdf.

Pecoraro, A., Pacciolla, A., O'Cleirigh, C., Mimiaga, M., Kwiatek, P., Blokhina, E., . . . Woody, G. (2016). Proactive coping and spirituality among patients who left or remained in antiretroviral treatment in St. Petersburg, Russian Federation. *AIDS Care, 28*(3), 334–338.

Reddy, P., & Ferrara, J. (2018). Graft-versus-host disease and graft-versus-leukemia responses. In R. Hoffman, E. Benz, L. Silberstein, H. Heslop, J. Weitz, J. Anastasi, M. Salama, & S. & Abutalib (Eds.), *Hematology:*

Basic principles and practice (7th ed.), pp. 1650–1668. Philadelphia, PA: Elsevier.

Rhodes, R., Nazir, F., Lopez, S., Xuan, L., Nijhawan, A., Alexander-Scott, N., & Halm, E. (2016). Use and predictors of end-of-life care among HIV patients in a safety net health system. *Journal of Pain and Symptom Management, 51*(1), 120–125.

Ruiz-Perez, I., Murphy, M., Pastor-Moreno, G., Rojas-Garcia, A., & Rodriquez-Barranco, M. (2017). The effectiveness of HIV prevention interventions in socioeconomically disadvantaged ethnic minority women: A systematic review and meta-analysis. *American Journal of Public Health, 107*(12), e13–e21.

Sorenson, M., Quinn, L., & Klein, D. (2019). *Pathophysiology: Concepts of human disease.* Hoboken, NJ: Pearson Education.

Tetteh, R., Yankey, B., Nartey, E., Lartey, M., Leufkens, & Dodoo, A. (2017). Pre-exposure prophylaxis for HIV prevention: Safety concerns. *Drug Safety, 40*(4), 273–283.

United Network for Organ Sharing. (2017). *National data.* Retrieved from https://optn.transplant.hrsa.gov/data/view-data-reports/national-data/#.

Winter, W., Harris, N., Merkel, K., Collinsworth, A., & Clapp, W. (2017). Organ-specific autoimmune diseases. In R. McPherson & M. Pincus (Eds.), *Henry's clinical diagnosis and management*, pp. 1032–1056. St. Louis, MO: Elsevier.

World Health Organization (WHO). (2017a). *HIV/AIDS* (Fact Sheet). Retrieved from www.who.int/mediacentre/factsheets/fs360/en/.

World Health Organization (WHO). (2017b). *HIV testing and counselling tool kit.* Retrieved from www.who.int/hiv/topics/vct/toolkit/introduction/en/index1.html.

Yoshikawa, T., & Norman, D. (2017). Geriatric infectious diseases: Current concepts on diagnosis and Management. *Journal of the American Geriatric Society, 65*, 631–641.

ADDITIONAL RESOURCES

AIDS.gov: Immune System 101

https://www.aids.gov/hiv-aids-basics/just-diagnosed-with-hiv-aids/hiv-in-your-body/immune-system-101/

American Academy of Allergy, Asthma and Immunology

www.aaaai.org/home.aspx

Immune Deficiency Foundation

www.primaryimmune.org

National Institutes of Health

http://aidsinfo.nih.gov

Organ Procurement and Transplantation Network

https://optn.transplant.hrsa.gov

Chapter 14

Nursing Care of Patients with Cancer

Chapter Outline and Learning Outcomes

CLINICAL COMPETENCIES

- Perform focused and comprehensive assessments of the patient with cancer, including functional status, physical and psychologic needs, as well as expressed values and preferences.
- Use assessed data to determine priority nursing diagnoses, select individualized nursing interventions, evaluate patient responses, and revise the plan of care as needed to promote, maintain, or restore functional health and to alleviate suffering.
- Provide effective care for patients with cancer, integrating planned nursing care with the interprofessional plan of care.
- Use current evidence and patient preferences to plan and implement optimal nursing care for patients with cancer.
- Plan and provide appropriate teaching for self-care of cancer-related and treatment-related symptoms, such as pain, nausea and vomiting, mucositis, fatigue, or anemia.
- Use quality measures, processes, and tools to improve outcomes for patients with cancer.
- Include cultural variation and diverse values in designing and implementing individualized plans of care for patients with cancer.
- Demonstrate effective use of technology, current evidence, and care standards to reduce the risk of harm for patients with cancer.
- Use technology to obtain high-quality healthcare information and plan, document, communicate, and coordinate care for patients with cancer.

KEY TERMS

anaplasia, 412
biotherapy, 430
brachytherapy, 432
cachexia, 417
cancer, 407
carcinogenesis, 412
carcinogens, 412
cell cycle, 411
chemotherapy, 425
differentiation, 411
dysplasia, 412
hyperplasia, 411
metaplasia, 411
metastasis, 414
neoplasm, 414
oncogene, 412
oncologic emergencies, 445
oncology, 407
proto-oncogenes, 412
radiation therapy, 432
tumor marker, 421
xerostomia, 442

Cancer is a group of complex diseases characterized by uncontrolled growth and spread of abnormal cells (American Cancer Society [ACS], 2018a). Cancer can manifest in different ways depending on which body system is affected and the type of tumor cells involved. Cancer can affect people of any age, gender, ethnicity, or geographic region. An estimated 15.5 million cancer survivors currently live in the United States. The cancer mortality rate has decreased by 26% since 1991 because of improved detection and treatment, as well as a decreased incidence of smoking (ACS, 2018a).

This chapter focuses on the general pathogenesis, pathophysiology, and etiology of cancer; identifies current diagnostic and treatment modalities; and discusses nursing care appropriate for patients with cancer. Discussions of cancers that affect specific body systems can be found in corresponding disorders chapters in the text.

Cancer occurs when normal cells mutate into abnormal cells with uncontrolled growth and spread in the body. Cancer can affect any body tissue. The nurse recognizes that cancer is a disruptive and life-threatening process affecting not only the person who is diagnosed with cancer, but also his or her significant others and family members. Nursing interventions are based on the understanding that cancer is a chronic disease with acute episodes and that the patient is often treated with a combination of treatment modalities. Equally important, the nurse recognizes that caring for the patient with cancer is multifaceted and involves patient education, delivery of accurate health information, symptom assessment and treatment, patient advocacy, and psychological support throughout the cancer continuum, including end-of-life care (Tariman & Szubski, 2015).

Oncology is the study of cancer. The term is derived from the Greek word *oncoma*, meaning "bulk." Oncologists specialize in caring for patients with cancer; they may be medical physicians, surgeons, radiologists, immunologists, or researchers. The oncology nurse is an important and significant member of the oncology team. Oncology nurses have received specialized training in cancer care and treatment. They have special skills in assisting the patient and family with physical and psychosocial issues associated with cancer, treatment, and palliation (Oncology Nursing Society [ONS], 2016). Collaboration among healthcare professionals (e.g., surgeons, oncologists, nurses, physical therapists, and social workers) ensures the most effective care and treatment for the patient with cancer.

14.1 Incidence and Mortality

In the United States, cancer is the second most common cause of death. There are approximately 1.7 million new cancer cases expected to be diagnosed and 609,640 expected deaths due to cancer in 2018 (ACS, 2018a). Approximately 40 out of 100 men and 38 out of 100 women will develop cancer in their lifetime (ACS, 2018a). Mortality rates for different cancers vary. Lung cancer remains the leading cause of cancer death in both men and women; prostate and breast cancer are the second leading causes of cancer death among men and women, respectively (ACS, 2018a). Due to advances in cancer prevention, early detection, and treatment, the 5-year survival rate for individuals with cancers continues to improve in the United States, increasing by 20% over the past 30 years (ACS, 2018a).

Socioeconomic Status

Individuals with a lower socioeconomic status are at higher risk of being both diagnosed with and dying of cancer compared to those with a higher socioeconomic status. Inadequate health insurance and limited access to healthcare, especially preventive screening and counseling, may be major factors (ACS, 2018a). Individuals with a lower socioeconomic status are also more likely to be diagnosed with more advanced stages of disease and may not receive standard treatments, including advancements in treatment. Although other factors that may be involved, such as diet and stress, usually come under the category of modifiable risks, these risks are frequently uncontrollable in this population, as these individuals may have less access to healthy foods and limited opportunities for physical activity. They are also at a higher risk of being diagnosed with cancer-causing infections and may have more exposure to occupational and environmental hazards (ACS, 2018a). See **Box 14.1** for more about cancer and social determinants of health.

BOX 14.1
Cancer and Social Determinants of Health

Despite overall improved cancer survival rates, African Americans have a disproportionate burden of cancer incidence. African American men have a 10% higher incidence of cancer and 23% higher mortality rate compared to non-Hispanic whites (ACS, 2018a). African American women have a 7% lower incidence of cancer compared to non-Hispanic whites, yet their mortality rate is 14% higher (ACS, 2018a). Although breast cancer is more common among non-Hispanic whites, the 5-year survival rate is 91% and 80% for non-Hispanic whites and African Americans, respectively (ACS, 2018a). It is important to note that even after controlling for age, tumor stage, grade, subtype, marital status, and tumor side (i.e., right/left), being African American remains an independent predictor for breast cancer (Wieder, Shafiq, & Adam, 2016). Apparently, differences in treatment, social barriers, tumor biology, comorbidities, and socioeconomic status (SES) may influence cancer mortality rates (Wieder et al., 2016).

The racial disparity persists across all stages of cancer diagnosis, with non-Hispanic whites doing better than African Americans regardless of disease severity (DeSantis et al., 2016). Disparities in access to resources—including employment, income, education, and housing—as well as barriers to cancer prevention, detection, and treatment likely contribute to these disparities (ACS, 2018a). African Americans and Hispanics are the most likely racial/ethnic groups to be uninsured, which increases the risk of being diagnosed with cancer at later stages (ACS, 2018a). In addition, these groups experience disproportionate poverty and discrimination and receive lower quality of care even when controlling for insurance, age, disease severity, or health status. Finally, racial and ethnic minorities may receive poor care or experience patient/provider miscommunication as a result of communication problems and/or patient/provider assumptions (ACS, 2018a). More research is needed to explore the relationship between social determinants of health and cancer rates.

Nonmodifiable Risk Factors

Risk factors make an individual or population vulnerable to a specific disease or other unhealthy outcome. They can be divided into risks that are modifiable and nonmodifiable. Knowledge and assessment of risk factors are especially important in counseling patients and families about strategies to prevent cancer. **Figure 14.1** ■ summarizes the interaction of factors that promote cancer.

Genetics and Heredity

Genetics is the study of genes. Genes encode for the growth and development of the body's cells. *Human genome* refers to the totality of human genes. *Genomics* is the study of all the genes in the human genome together, including the genes' interactions with each other, the environment, and the influence of other psychosocial and cultural factors (Jorde, Carey, & Bamshad, 2016). See Genetics Considerations for one way in which genomics can be used to help guide treatment decisions by patients and the interprofessional team.

Heredity is how genes are passed from generation to generation. In cancer, an estimated 5 to 10% of cancers have a hereditary component (ACS, 2018b; Jorde et al., 2016). Even though the majority of patients will not have an inherited cancer, it is important to determine which patients have a genetic predisposition. With the availability of cancer gene testing, such as for the breast cancer genes *BRCA1* and *BRC-2*, nurses need to understand the limitations of genetic testing. For example, when genetic testing is unable to identify a causative mutation, such as *BRCA1* and *BRCA2*, the testing result does not eliminate a risk for cancer in the patient or his or her family members (Jorde et al., 2016). Other examples of inherited syndromes that increase an individual's risk of developing cancer include Lynch syndrome and Li-Fraumeni syndrome.

Recurring patterns of cancer within a family are a risk factor for a hereditary component, but do not necessarily indicate that a specific gene or mutation is the cause. An increased rate of cancer between relatives can be due to genetics, as well as shared environmental exposures, lifestyle, and other nongenetic risk factors. Therefore, it is critical to elucidate other nongenetic risk factors. For example, consider a 65-year-old patient who never smoked and had no family history of lung cancer. For this patient, it is important to assess exposure to secondhand smoke, occupational exposures, and other potential inhaled toxins. Familial cancers generally occur

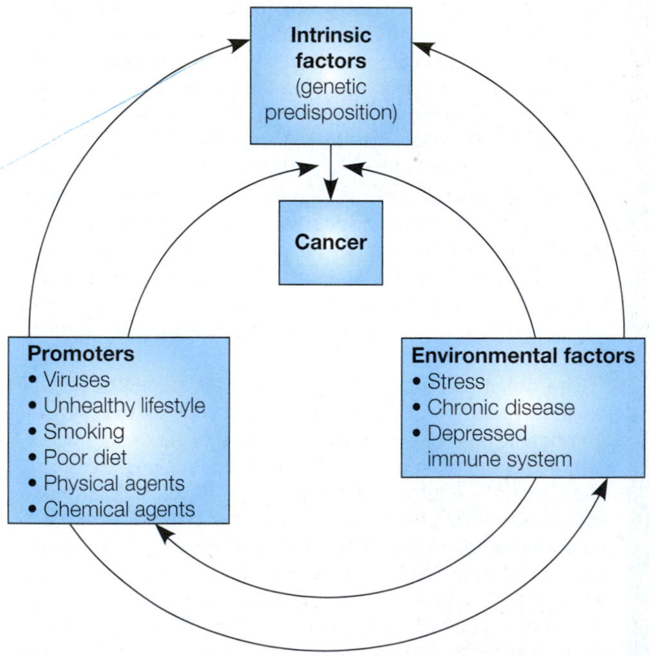
Intrinsic factors
(genetic predisposition)
Cancer
Promoters
• Viruses
• Unhealthy lifestyle
• Smoking
• Poor diet
• Physical agents
• Chemical agents
Environmental factors
• Stress
• Chronic disease
• Depressed immune system

Figure 14.1 ■ Interaction of factors that promote cancer. Most people have immune systems that are competent enough to resist the establishment of cancer from an initiated cell. Cancer can take hold, however, when a number of promotional factors occur together and over enough time to weaken immune resistance. Like factors are grouped together for ease of presentation but may occur in any combination.

Genetic Considerations

Genomics and Breast Cancer

Advances in genomics in diagnosing and treating cancer make it imperative for nurses to incorporate genomic competencies and skills into clinical practice. The Oncotype DX test for breast cancer is one example of how genomics can be used to help patients make informed and individualized treatment decisions. The Oncotype DX test analyzes the activity of a group of 21 genes in the patient's tumor that can affect how a cancer is likely to behave and respond to treatment. Nurses can use the knowledge of the Oncotype DX to help patients with early-stage invasive breast cancer to estimate the risk of cancer recurrence and make decisions about the risks and potential benefits of chemotherapy.

The Oncotype DX test assigns a recurrence score of 0 to 100 based on test results. Patients with early-stage invasive breast cancer are placed into three categories (i.e. low, intermediate, and high risk of recurrence).

- Recurrence score lower than 18: The cancer has a low risk of recurrence. The benefit of chemotherapy for early-stage breast cancer is likely to be small and will not outweigh the risks of side effects.
- Recurrence score between 18 and 31: The cancer has an intermediate risk of recurrence. It is unclear whether the benefits of chemotherapy for early-stage breast cancer outweigh the risks of side effects. However, current trials are ongoing to discern the benefit of chemotherapy in this group.
- Recurrence score greater than 31: The cancer has a high risk of recurrence, and the benefits of chemotherapy for early-stage breast cancer are likely to be greater than the risks of side effects.

Nurses can help patients by providing information regarding insurance coverage and financial assistance:

- The Medicare program and several other major insurance companies cover the Oncotype DX test.
- Genomic Health has the Genomic Access Program to assist the patient in verifying insurance coverage and obtaining reimbursement and to provide testing for the patient facing financial hardships or those who are uninsured or underinsured. The Oncotype DX test costs about $4,000. For insurance- and payment-related questions, call 866-ONCOTYPE (866-662-6897).

during old age, whereas hereditary cancers usually occur at a younger age. Other risk factors for inherited cancers include multiple cases of the same form of cancer, multiple types of cancer in the same individual, childhood cancer, and cancer occurring in multiple generations (ACS, 2018b). For most cancers, research has yet to distinguish true genetic transfer from environmental causes. Although further research is needed to identify cancers that are due to the inheritance of defective genes, familial predisposition to malignancies should be considered a risk factor so individuals can reduce behaviors that may promote cancer. For example, a patient with a family history of lung cancer should be counseled to avoid smoking, areas where smoking is allowed, and working in an occupation that may expose the patient to inhaled carcinogens.

Age

Cancer is a disease associated with aging—more than 87% of cancer diagnoses occur after age 50 (ACS, 2018a). A number of factors are associated with the increased risk of cancer among older adults. One of these factors is inflammation, which increases as individuals age and can contribute to DNA damage. In addition, *immunosenescence*, defined as the weakening of the immune system with age, increases an individual's susceptibility to cancer. The poor overall immune response that accompanies aging is a result of a diminution of the innate and adaptive immune system. For example, natural killer cells become less effective at removing cancerous cells (Fulop, Larbi, Kotb, de Angelis, & Pawelec, 2016). In addition, long-term exposure to high doses of promotional agents is usually necessary to allow the cancer to take hold, and this exposure increases with age. Hormonal changes that occur with aging can also be associated with cancer. For example, postmenopausal women receiving exogenous estrogen have an increased risk of breast and uterine cancers. However, it is important for the nurse to note that certain types of cancer typically present in specific age groups, such as neuroblastoma, osteosarcoma, and retinoblastoma in the pediatric population.

Gender

Gender is a risk factor for certain types of cancer. Breast cancer is the most frequently diagnosed cancer in women; prostate cancer in men. Thyroid cancer occurs more commonly among women, whereas the incidence of bladder cancer is about four times higher in men than in women (ACS, 2018a). See Chapters 48 and 49 for more information on gender-specific cancers.

Modifiable Risk Factors

While certain risk factors for cancer, such as age and gender, are nonmodifiable, there are various risk factors that are modifiable. Therefore, with proper education and counseling, modification of these risk factors could decrease an individual's risk of developing cancer. However, it is important for the nurse to note that while these risk factors are considered modifiable, factors such as socioeconomic status or geographic location could limit an individual's ability to modify his or her risk factors (e.g., occupation, exposure to stress).

Stress

Biobehavioral factors, such as stress, contribute to cancer through activation of the hypothalamic–pituitary–adrenocortical (HPA) axis and sympathetic nervous system (SNS). Activation of this system in response to psychological stress results in the release of corticotrophin-releasing hormone from the hypothalamus, which triggers release of the adrenocorticotrophic hormone, which ultimately stimulates the release of cortisol, a glucocorticoid, from the adrenal gland. Activation of the SNS results in secretion of epinephrine and norepinephrine, which are known to regulate the immune response. Combined, the production of glucocorticoids, catecholamines, and other neuroendocrine hormones alter immune function pertaining to tumor surveillance and contribute to other factors that contribute to cancer growth, including inflammation, tumor invasion, and angiogenesis (Lutgendorf & Andersen, 2015).

Diet

Dietary factors appear to be one of the most important factors for cancer risk. It is estimated that 20% of all cancers could be prevented by eating a healthy diet, managing weight, increasing physical activity, and limiting alcohol consumption (ACS, 2017). A diet that is high in red meat and saturated fat appears to increase risk. Evidence suggests that fruits and vegetables as well as a diet high in fiber may be protective (ACS, 2017). Some foods are considered genotoxic, such as the nitrosamines and nitrous indoles (a crystalline alkaloid compound) found in preserved meats and pickled, salted foods. Other foods, such as high-fat, low-fiber foods—the mainstay of many American diets—promote colon, breast, and sex-hormone-dependent tumors. When fish and meat are excessively fried or broiled, potent carcinogenic compounds can form that may cause tumors in the mammary glands, colon, liver, pancreas, and bladder. Repeatedly using fat to fry foods at high temperatures produces high levels of polycyclic hydrocarbons, which increase cancer risk considerably. Other food-related substances believed to increase cancer risk include sodium saccharine, red food dyes, and both regular and decaffeinated coffee.

Occupation

Occupational risk might be considered to be either modifiable or nonmodifiable. For some individuals, education may limit their choice of occupation; during times of high unemployment, moreover, changing one's occupation because it poses risk factors may not be a viable option. Federal standards are designed to protect workers from hazardous substances, but many believe that these standards are not strict enough and inspections are not frequent enough to prevent violations.

Specific risks vary according to the occupation. For example, outdoor workers such as farmers and construction workers are exposed to solar radiation, healthcare workers such as x-ray technicians and biomedical researchers are exposed to ionizing radiation and carcinogenic substances, and exposure to asbestos is a problem for people

Table 14.1 Chemical Carcinogens and Relationship to Occupation

Chemical Agent	Action	Occupation Affected
Polycyclic hydrocarbons (smoke, soot, tobacco, and smoked foods) and benzopyrene	Genotoxic	Miners, coal/gas workers, chimney sweeps, migrant workers, workers in offices where smoking is allowed in closed areas
Arsenic	Genotoxic	Pesticide manufacturers, miners
Vinyl chloride polymers	Promotional	Plastics workers, artists
Methylaminobenzine	Genotoxic	Fabric workers, rubber and glue workers
Asbestos	Promotional	Construction workers, workers in old, run-down buildings with asbestos insulation, insulation makers
Wood and leather dust	Promotional	Woodworkers, carpenters, leather toolers
Chemotherapy drugs	Genotoxic	Drug manufacturers, pharmacists, nurses

who work in old buildings with asbestos insulation in the walls. **Table 14.1** correlates known carcinogens and occupations.

Infection

A number of viruses have been linked to some cancers, such as hepatitis B and hepatitis C virus for liver and pancreatic cancer and the human papillomavirus (HPV) for cervical, anal, oral, and head and neck cancer (ACS, 2018a). Avoiding those specific infections will decrease risk. Although some infections may be unavoidable (Epstein-Barr, for example), others such as genital herpes and HPV-induced genital warts may often be avoided by following safer sex practices (e.g., the use of condoms) or obtaining the HPV vaccine.

Tobacco Use

Smoking-related diseases remain the world's most preventable cause of death and is attributed to approximately one-third of cancer-related deaths (ACS, 2018a). Lung cancer is considered highly preventable because of its relationship to smoking. The genotoxic carcinogenic substances in tobacco are considered weak; therefore, the damage may be reversed by stopping smoking. However, many other substances in tobacco are highly promotional, so that the larger the dose and longer the use, the higher the risk for developing cancer. Research has shown a significantly lower risk of lung cancer death for former smokers compared to current smokers.

Tobacco is related to other forms of cancer. Smokers face an increased risk of oropharyngeal, esophageal, laryngeal, gastric, pancreatic, kidney, liver, and bladder cancers (ACS, 2018a). Pipe and cigar smokers are especially susceptible to oropharyngeal and laryngeal cancers. Oral and esophageal cancers are more common among those who chew tobacco or use snuff. Smokers who have a genetic decrease in alpha$_1$-antitrypsin (an enzyme that protects lung tissue) that results in emphysema face an even higher cancer risk than smokers without this defect.

Secondhand smoke (SHS), or environmental tobacco smoke, contains 7000 chemicals, at least 70 of which are human carcinogens for which there is no safe level of exposure (U.S. Department of Health and Human Services, 2014). Approximately 5840 nonsmoking adults are diagnosed with lung cancer each year as a result of breathing SHS (Islami et al., 2017). In the United States, legislative efforts have been made to prevent SHS; for example, currently 900 municipalities and 25 states have passed smoke-free legislation.

Alcohol Use

Alcohol use is a risk factor for various types of cancers, including breast in females and oral, pharyngeal, laryngeal, esophageal, liver, and colorectal in both sexes. Individuals should be encouraged to limit alcohol consumption to two or fewer drinks per day for men and one per day for women (ACS, 2018a). People who both smoke and drink a considerable amount of alcohol daily have an increased risk for oral, esophageal, and laryngeal cancers (ACS, 2018a).

Recreational Drug Use

Recreational drug use often promotes an unhealthy lifestyle that increases general cancer risk; for example, drug users often do not maintain adequate nutrition. Furthermore, recreational drugs are implicated as promoters because of their suppressive effect on the immune system. Although it has not been directly implicated in cancer development, marijuana has been demonstrated to cause chromosomal damage that may over time result in cancer-causing deoxyribonucleic acid (DNA) damage and genetic mutations.

Obesity

Nutrition and physical activity play an important role in maintaining a healthy body weight. The combined effects of poor physical activity, weight, poor diet, and excess alcohol consumption have been attributed to approximately 18% of cancer cases and 16% of deaths (ACS, 2018a). Excessive body fat has been linked to an increased risk of hormone-dependent cancers. Because sex hormones are synthesized from fat, individuals who are considered obese often have excessive amounts of the hormones that feed hormone-dependent malignancies of the breast, bowel, ovary, endometrium, and prostate. Overweight and obesity are clearly associated with increased risk for developing many cancers, including cancers of the breast (in postmenopausal women), colon, pancreas, endometrium, liver, stomach, kidney, brain, thyroid, ovary, gallbladder, esophagus, and multiple myeloma (ACS, 2018a). Rates of obesity continue to increase, with the highest prevalence among Hispanic males and Hispanic and non-Hispanic black females (ACS, 2018a). Evidence suggests that physical activity may decrease the risk of cancers associated with obesity. Nurses should encourage patients to engage in physical activity, eat a healthy diet, and limit alcohol intake.

Sun Exposure

As the protective ozone layer thins, more of the sun's damaging ultraviolet radiation reaches the earth. As a consequence, the rate of skin cancers has increased. Sun-related skin cancers are now considered to be a problem for all people, regardless of skin color, but people of northern European descent with very fair skin, blue or green eyes, and light-colored hair are most vulnerable. Older adults with decreased pigment are more at risk, even those with darker skin. Sun exposure increases the risk of all skin cancers, the most commonly diagnosed cancer in the United States (ACS, 2018a). Nurses should educate patients to avoid sun exposure, wear protective clothing and sunscreen, avoid indoor tanning salons, and schedule routine appointments with a dermatologist for skin checks.

14.2 Pathophysiology

Cancer is a complex disease with hundreds of agents that can contribute to its pathogenesis. Advances in research have greatly increased the understanding of how cancer develops. We now know that the development of cancer is a process in which normal cells are changed and acquire malignant properties. Before a discussion of the various theories of the causes of cancer, a review of how normal cells divide and adapt to changing conditions will be useful.

Normal Cell Growth

Mature normal cells are uniform in size and have nuclei that are characteristic of the tissue to which the cells belong. Within the nucleus of normal cells, chromosomes containing DNA molecules carry the genetic information that controls the synthesis of polypeptides (proteins). Genes are subunits of chromosomes and consist of portions of DNA that specify the production of particular sets of proteins. Thus, genes control the development of specific traits. The genetic code in the DNA of every gene is translated into protein structures that determine the type, maturity, and function of a cell. Any change or disruption in a gene can result in an inaccurate "blueprint" that can produce an aberrant cell, which may then become cancerous. Some of the functions of DNA include:

- Determines protein production
- Instructs cells to produce specific chemicals
- Instructs cells to develop specific structures
- Determines individual traits and characteristics
- Controls other DNA by telling a cell to "switch on."

The Cell Cycle

Two coordinated events are responsible for cellular reproduction. Reproduction occurs as the result of replication of cellular DNA and mitosis, when the cell divides into two daughter cells with identical DNA.

The **cell cycle** consists of four phases. In the gap 1 or G_1 phase, the cell enlarges and synthesizes proteins to prepare for DNA replication. During this phase the cell prepares to replicate and enter into the synthesis phase. During the synthesis (S) phase, DNA is replicated and the chromosomes in the cell are duplicated. During the gap 2 or G_2 phase, the cell prepares itself for mitosis. Finally, with all preparation complete, the cell begins mitosis in the M phase. This phase culminates in the division of the parent cell into two exact copies called *daughter cells*, each having identical genetic material. The cells then immediately enter G_1 where they begin the cell cycle again, or divert into a resting phase, or G_0. The cell cycle is controlled by cyclins, which combine with and activate enzymes called *cyclin-dependent kinases*. Some cyclins cause a "braking" action and prevent the cycle from proceeding. Checkpoints in the cell cycle ensure that it proceeds in the correct order.

A malfunction of any of these regulators of cell growth and division can result in the rapid proliferation of immature cells. In some cases, these cells are considered cancerous (malignant). Knowledge of cell cycle events is used in the development of chemotherapeutic drugs, which are designed to disrupt the cancer cells during different stages of their cell cycle. These drugs and their use are discussed later in the chapter.

Differentiation

Differentiation is a normal process occurring over many cell cycles that allows cells to specialize in certain tasks. For example, some epithelial cells lining the lungs develop into tall columnar cells with cilia. These columnar cells sweep potentially dangerous debris out of the lungs. When adverse conditions occur in body tissues during differentiation, protective adaptations can produce alterations in cells. Some of these alterations are helpful, but in other cases the cells mutate beyond usefulness and become liabilities. Potentially unproductive cellular alterations that occur during cell differentiation include:

- **Hyperplasia** is an increase in the number or density of normal cells. Hyperplasia occurs in response to stress, increased metabolic demands, or elevated levels of hormones. Examples include the hyperplasia of myocardial cells in response to a prolonged increase in the body's demand for oxygen and hyperplasia of uterine cells in response to rising levels of estrogen during pregnancy. Hyperplastic cells are under normal DNA control.
- **Metaplasia** is a change in the normal pattern of differentiation such that dividing cells differentiate into cell types not normally found in that location in the body. The metaplastic cell is normal for its particular type, but it is not in its normal location. Some metaplastic cells are less functional than the cells they replace. Metaplasia is a protective response to adverse conditions. Metaplastic cells are under normal DNA control and are reversible when the stressor or other disruptive condition ceases.

- **Dysplasia** represents a loss of DNA control over differentiation occurring in response to adverse conditions. Dysplastic cells show abnormal variation in size, shape, and appearance and a disturbance in their usual arrangement. Examples of dysplasia include changes in the cervix in response to continued irritation, such as from HPV, or leukoplakia on oral mucous membranes in response to chronic irritation from smoking.
- **Anaplasia** is the regression of a cell to an immature or undifferentiated cell type. Anaplastic cell division is no longer under DNA control. Anaplasia usually occurs when a damaging or transforming event takes place inside the dividing, still undifferentiated cell, leading to loss of useful function. Anaplasia may occur in response to overwhelmingly destructive conditions inside the cell or in surrounding tissue.

Although hyperplasia, metaplasia, and dysplasia often reverse after the irritating factor is eliminated, they can lead to malignancy under certain conditions. This is especially true of dysplasia, which represents a loss of DNA control. Anaplasia is not reversible, but the degree of anaplasia determines the potential risk for cancer.

Theories of Carcinogenesis

Factors that cause cancer are both external (chemicals, radiation, and viruses) and internal (hormones, immune conditions, and inherited mutations). Causal factors may act together or in sequence to initiate or promote **carcinogenesis**, a process by which normal cells are transformed into cancer cells. Often, more than 10 years pass between exposures or mutations and detectable cancer.

Central to these theories are two important concepts about the etiology of cancer. First, damaged DNA, whether inherited or from external sources, sets up the necessary initial step for cancer to occur. Second, impairment of the human immune system, from whatever cause, lessens its ability to destroy abnormal cells.

Cellular Mutation

The theory of cellular mutation suggests that certain agents cause mutations in cellular DNA and transform cells into cancer cells. Such agents are called **carcinogens**. It is believed that the carcinogenic process has three stages: Initiation, promotion, and progression. The initiation stage involves permanent damage to the cellular DNA as a result of exposure to a carcinogen (e.g., radiation, chemicals) that was not repaired or had a defective repair. Promotion may last for years and includes conditions, such as smoking or alcohol use, that act repeatedly on the already affected cells. In the progression stage, further inherited changes acquired during cell replication develop into a cancer.

Oncogenes

Proto-oncogenes are normal genes that promote cell growth and repair. **Oncogenes** are abnormal genes that promote cell proliferation and are capable of triggering cancerous characteristics. Oncogenes can be classified according to their overall function. One classic example of an oncogene is BCR-ABL fusion protein, which results from a translocation between chromosomes 9 and 22, known as the Philadelphia chromosome. The increased expression of this protein allows for unregulated cell proliferation and is found in patients with chronic myelogenous leukemia (CML) and other leukemias (Soverini, De Benedittis, Mancini, & Martinelli, 2016).

A decrease in the body's immune surveillance may allow the expression of oncogenes; this can occur during times of stress or in response to certain carcinogens. For example, patients with AIDS, who have a decreased number of T-helper lymphocytes, have a much higher than normal incidence of certain cancers, including non-Hodgkin lymphoma and Kaposi sarcoma (Ji & Lu, 2017).

Tumor Suppressor Genes

Tumor suppressor genes normally block cell growth by suppressing oncogenes. They can become inactive by deletion or mutation. For example, inherited mutations in the *p53* gene are associated with sarcomas, breast cancer, leukemia, and renal tumors.

Known Carcinogens

A number of agents are known to cause cancer, or at least are strongly linked to certain kinds of cancers. These known carcinogens include viruses, drugs, hormones, and chemical and physical agents. The National Toxicology Program (NTP) and the International Agency for Research on Cancer (IARC) play an important role in the identification and evaluation of carcinogens. See their respective websites for a list of substances known or reasonably anticipated to be human carcinogens.

Carcinogens can be categorized into two groups: Genotoxic carcinogens directly alter DNA and cause mutations, and promoter substances cause other adverse biologic effects, such as cytotoxicity, hormonal imbalances, altered immunity, or chronic tissue damage. Promoter substances do not cause cancer in the absence of previous cell damage (initiation) and often require high-level and long-term contact with the altered cells (refer to Table 14.1). Although everyone comes in contact with a vast number of substances considered carcinogenic, not everyone develops cancer. Other factors, such as genetic predisposition, impairment of the immune response, and repeated exposure to the carcinogen, are necessary for a cancer to develop.

Viruses

Several viruses have been associated with the development of cancer. They damage cells and induce hyperplastic cell growth. Viral infection may play a role in cell mutation that can progress to malignant cells. Most people are able to suppress this progression. **Box 14.2** identifies these viruses and the cancers with which they are associated. In addition, viruses play a significant role in weakening immunologic defenses against neoplasms. For example, human immunodeficiency virus (HIV), which infects T-helper lymphocytes

BOX 14.2
Cancers Associated with Different Viruses

HERPES SIMPLEX VIRUS TYPES 1 AND 2 (HSV-1 AND HSV-2)

- Carcinoma of the lip
- Cervical carcinoma
- Kaposi sarcoma

HUMAN CYTOMEGALOVIRUS (HCMV)

- Kaposi sarcoma
- Prostate cancer

EPSTEIN-BARR VIRUS (EBV)

- Burkitt lymphoma

HUMAN HERPESVIRUS 6 (HHV-6)

- Lymphoma

HEPATITIS B VIRUS (HBV)

- Primary hepatocellular cancer

HUMAN PAPILLOMAVIRUS (HPV)

- Malignant melanoma
- Cervical, penile
- Head and neck (e.g., laryngeal cancers)

HUMAN T-LYMPHOTROPIC VIRUSES (HTLVS)

- Adult T-cell leukemia and lymphoma
- T-cell variant of hairy-cell leukemia
- Kaposi sarcoma

and monocytes, impairs an individual's protection against certain cancers such as non-Hodgkin lymphoma and Kaposi sarcoma (Ji & Lu, 2017).

Other viruses have been associated with human malignancies. Hepatitis B virus integrates its DNA with liver cell DNA and is believed to cause primary hepatocellular carcinoma. Papillomaviruses cause plantar, common, and flat warts, which are benign and usually regress spontaneously; however, they also cause genital warts and laryngeal papillomas, which are associated with malignant melanoma and cervical, penile, and laryngeal cancers.

Drugs and Hormones

Certain drugs can be either genotoxic or promotional. For example, chemotherapeutic drugs used to disrupt the cell cycle of malignant cells can be genotoxic for normal cells. They can also be promotional: By drastically reducing the number of leukocytes, they impair immune function, thus increasing the risk of cancer. Examples of these chemotherapeutic drugs include busulfan, chlorambucil, and cyclophosphamide. Some recreational drugs are implicated as carcinogens. These include the genotoxic betel nut chewed by many Pacific Islanders and the immunosuppressant promoters heroin and cocaine.

Hormones are also potential genotoxic carcinogens or promoters. Gonadotropic hormones often mediate cancers of the reproductive organs. Estrogen, both natural and synthetic, have been linked to cervical, endometrial, and breast cancers. Estrogen-containing contraceptive pills have been implicated in breast cancer, but they also have been shown to decrease the risk of ovarian cancer. Investigators have not reached a final conclusion about the cancer risk posed by contraceptives. Glucocorticosteroids (cortisone) and anabolic steroids may act as promoters by altering the immune response or endocrine balance.

Chemical Agents

Many chemicals are both genotoxic and promotional. Because many of these substances are encountered in the workplace, they constitute occupational hazards. Examples of industrial and environmental carcinogens include polycyclic hydrocarbons, found in soot; benzopyrene, found in cigarette smoke; and arsenic, found in pesticides. These chemicals have some genotoxic action; some alter DNA replication. Other industrial and environmental chemicals that are considered carcinogenic include wood dust, formaldehyde, diesel exhaust, carbon tetrachloride, and asbestos (National Toxicology Program [NTP], 2016). Polycyclic aromatic hydrocarbons, nitrosamines, phenols, and other chemicals in tobacco act as either carcinogens or promoters of cancer (refer to Table 14.1).

Natural substances in the body may also be carcinogenic or promotional. For example, end products of metabolism that are produced in excess amounts or are ineffectively eliminated, such as bile acids from a high-fat diet, may promote cancer.

Some foods contain carcinogens added during preparation or preservation. Examples include the sugar substitute sodium saccharine and nitrosamines and nitrous indoles, which are found in pickled, salted foods. In some cases, food contaminants produce carcinogenic chemicals. The *Aspergillus* fungi produce aflatoxin, a highly potent carcinogen. These organisms grow on improperly stored vegetable products, such as grains and peanuts.

Physical Agents

It has been well documented that excessive exposure to radiation causes increased rates of cancer by damaging the DNA in cells, by activating other oncogenic factors, or by suppressing antitumor activity (protein inhibitors). Both solar radiation from ultraviolet rays and ionizing radiation from industrial or medical sources are carcinogenic. This fact has implications for workers exposed to these agents and for the population in general. Radon, a naturally formed radioactive gas found in the basements of many homes, is a known carcinogen. People who have lived in areas where nuclear weapons have been tested or whose groundwater has been polluted by nuclear wastes are at risk for developing cancers. The effects of high-dose radiation exposure and subsequent cancer development have been demonstrated in the survivors of the atomic bombs at Nagasaki and Hiroshima and in workers exposed to radiation during the cleanup of nuclear disasters such as Chernobyl.

14.3 Characteristics and Behavior of Neoplasms

Types of Neoplasms

A **neoplasm** is a mass of new tissue (a collection of cells) that grows independently of its surrounding structures and has no physiologic purpose. The term *neoplasm* is often used interchangeably with *tumor*, from the Latin word meaning "swelling." Neoplasms are said to be autonomous because they grow at a rate uncoordinated with body needs, they share some of the properties of the parent cells but with altered size and shape, and they do not benefit the host and in some cases are harmful.

Neoplasms are not completely autonomous because they require a blood supply with nutrients and oxygen to sustain their growth. Neoplasms are typically classified as benign or malignant on the basis of their potential to damage the body and on their growth characteristics.

Benign Neoplasms

Benign neoplasms are localized growths. They form a solid mass, have well-defined borders, and are frequently encapsulated. Benign neoplasms tend to respond to the body's homeostatic controls. Thus, they often stop growing when they reach the boundaries of another tissue (a process called *contact inhibition*). They grow slowly and often remain stable in size. Because they are usually encapsulated, benign neoplasms are often easily removed and tend not to recur.

Although typically harmless, benign neoplasms nevertheless can be destructive if they crowd surrounding tissue and obstruct the function of organs. For example, a benign meningioma of the brain or spinal cord can cause increased intracranial pressure (IICP), which progressively impairs an individual's cerebral function. Unless the meningioma can be successfully removed, the steadily rising IICP will eventually lead to coma and death.

Malignant Neoplasms

In contrast to benign neoplasms, malignant neoplasms grow aggressively and do not respond to the body's homeostatic controls. Malignant neoplasms are not cohesive and present with an irregular shape. Instead of slowly crowding other tissues aside, malignant neoplasms cut through surrounding tissues, causing bleeding, inflammation, and necrosis (tissue death) as they grow. This invasive quality of malignant neoplasms is reflected in the word origin of *cancer*, from the Greek *karkinos*, meaning "crab."

Malignant cells from the primary tumor may travel through the blood or lymph to invade other tissues and organs of the body and form a secondary tumor called a **metastasis**. This term also refers to the process by which such spreading of malignant neoplasms—-perhaps their most destructive trait—occurs. Malignant neoplasms can recur after surgical removal of the primary and secondary tumors and after other treatments. **Table 14.2** compares benign and malignant neoplasms.

Table 14.2 Comparison of Benign and Malignant Neoplasms

Benign	Malignant
Local	Invasive
Cohesive	Noncohesive
Well-defined borders	Does not stop at tissue border
Pushes other tissues out of the way	Invades and destroys surrounding tissues
Slow growth	Rapid growth
Encapsulated	Metastasizes to distant sites
Easily removed	Not always easy to remove
Usually does not recur	Can recur

Malignant neoplasms vary in their degree of differentiation from the parent tissue. Highly differentiated cancer cells try to mimic the specialized function of the parent tissue, but undifferentiated cancers, consisting of immature cells, have almost no resemblance to the parent tissue and so perform no useful function. Undifferentiated cancers rob the body of its energy and nutrition as they grow. Undifferentiated anaplastic cells have little structural or functional relationship to the parent cells and are the basis of many malignant neoplasms. The degree of differentiation of anaplastic cells is a consideration in the classification and staging of neoplasms, discussed later in this chapter.

Characteristics of Malignant Cells

Malignant neoplasms may be identified by the following predictable cellular characteristics:

- ***Loss of regulation of the rate of mitosis***. This leads to rapid cell division and growth of the neoplasm.
- ***Loss of specialization and differentiation***. Malignant cells do not perform typical cellular functions. Many produce hormones and enzymes similar to those of the parent tissue, but usually in excessive amounts, possibly revealing their presence.
- ***Loss of contact inhibition***. Malignant cells do not respect other cellular boundaries. They easily invade and destroy other tissues.
- ***Progressive acquisition of a cancerous phenotype***. Cellular mutation seems to be a sequential process involving successive generations of cells, each generation becoming more deviant than the previous one. Additionally, malignant cells seem to be immortal; that is, they do not stop growing and die, as do normal cells, which have a genetically determined lifespan.
- ***Irreversibility***. The transformation into a malignant cell is irreversible. Rarely does a malignant neoplasm revert to a benign state.
- ***Altered cell structure***. Cytologic examination of malignant cells reveals distinct differences in the cell nucleus and cytoplasm as well as an overall cell shape that differs from that of normal cells of the particular tissue type.

- ***Simplified metabolic activities***. The work of malignant cells is simpler than that of normal cells; they show an increased synthesis of substances needed for cell division, and they have no need to create proteins for the specialized functions of the tissues they invade.
- ***Transplantability***. Malignant cells often break away from the primary tissue site and travel to other locations in the body, where they establish new growths.
- ***Ability to promote their own survival***. Malignant cells may create ectopic sites to produce the hormones they need for their growth. By their very presence and their ability to initiate vascular permeability, malignant cells promote the development of nonneoplastic stroma, a connective tissue framework consisting of collagen and other components, which then supports the neoplasm. They may create their own blood supply. Through a process called *angiogenesis*, tumor cells secrete a polypeptide angiogenic growth factor that stimulates blood vessels from surrounding normal tissue to grow into the tumor. Finally, malignant cells divert nutrition from the host to meet their own needs, by diffusion when the tumor is less than 1 mm, and thereafter by means of the newly formed blood vessels. If unchecked, malignant cells eventually destroy their host.

Tumor Invasion and Metastasis

Metastasis, the ability of cancer cells to invade adjacent tissues and travel to distant organs, is considered cancer cells' most ominous characteristic. This quality makes treatment a considerable challenge.

Invasion

Aggressive tumors possess several qualities that facilitate invasion (**Figure 14.2** ■):

- ***Ability to cause pressure atrophy***. The pressure of a growing tumor can cause atrophy and necrosis of adjacent tissues. The malignancy then moves into the vacated space.
- ***Ability to disrupt the basement membrane of normal cells***. Many cancer cells can bind to elements of the basement membrane and secrete enzymes that degrade that physical barrier, thus facilitating their movement into normal tissues, lymph, and blood circulation.
- ***Motility***. Because malignant cells are less tightly bound to each other than normal cells (reduced adhesiveness), they easily separate from the neoplasm and move into surrounding body fluids and tissues.
- ***Response to chemical signals from adjacent tissues***. Chemotaxis (the movement of cells in response to a chemical stimulus) calls the tumor cells into the normal tissues, possibly as a result of the degrading of the basement membranes of the normal cells. This breakdown of normal cellular membranes releases the chemical stimulus physiologically designed to draw normal phagocytic cells to clean up the debris. (Refer to Chapter 12 on the inflammatory response for more information on chemotaxis.) Malignant cells are known to respond chemotactically to the end product of cellular metabolism. Some cancer cells even produce a substance called autocrine motility factor, which calls other malignant cells to a normal tissue. The first invading cells produce this substance, which then actively draws other malignant cells from the primary tumor into the invaded normal tissue.

Metastasis

The factors that favor invasion also contribute to the process of metastasis. Metastasis can occur by means of one or more

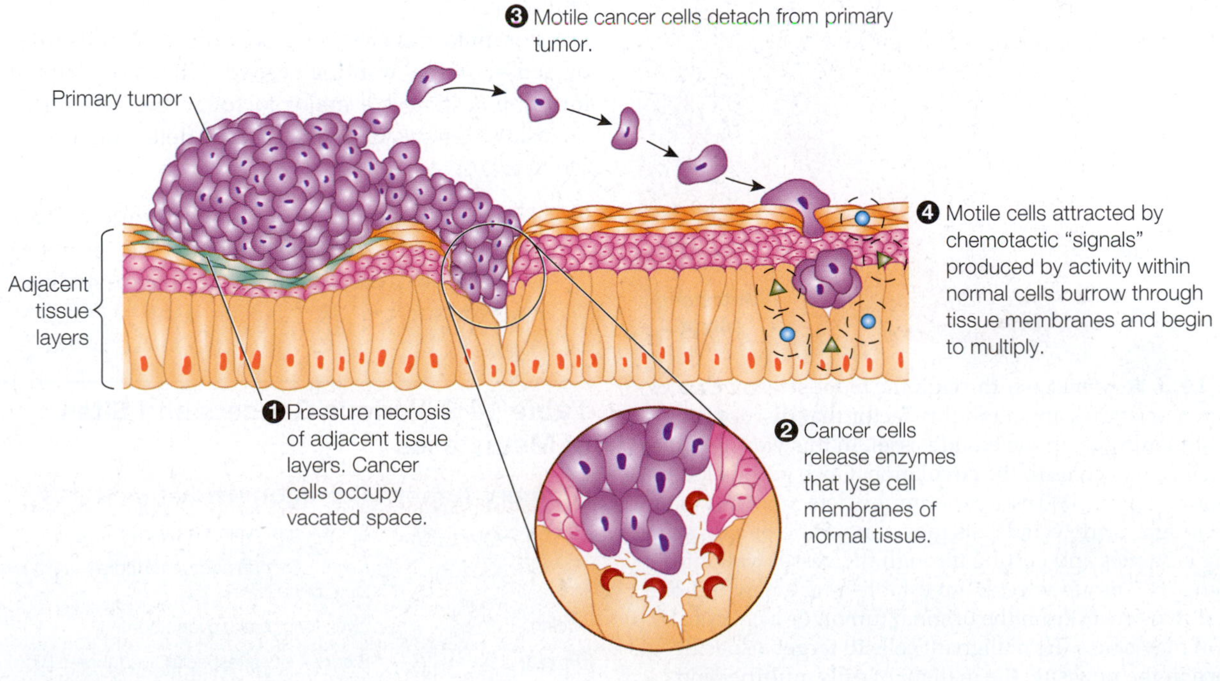

3 Motile cancer cells detach from primary tumor.
Primary tumor
Adjacent tissue layers
4 Motile cells attracted by chemotactic "signals" produced by activity within normal cells burrow through tissue membranes and begin to multiply.
1 Pressure necrosis of adjacent tissue layers. Cancer cells occupy vacated space.
2 Cancer cells release enzymes that lyse cell membranes of normal tissue.

Figure 14.2 ■ How cancer cells invade normal tissue.

mechanisms, including embolism in the blood or lymph, or spread by way of body cavities.

A blood- or lymph-borne metastasis allows a new tumor to be established in a distant organ. **Figure 14.3** ■ shows metastasis through the bloodstream. A tumor's ability to metastasize in this manner requires the following steps:

1. Intravasation of malignant cells through blood or lymphatic vessel walls and into the circulation
2. Survival of the malignant cells in the blood (to survive, the cells must escape the notice of the body's immune surveillance; only about 1 in 1000 cells does so).
3. Extravasation from the circulation and implantation in a new tissue.

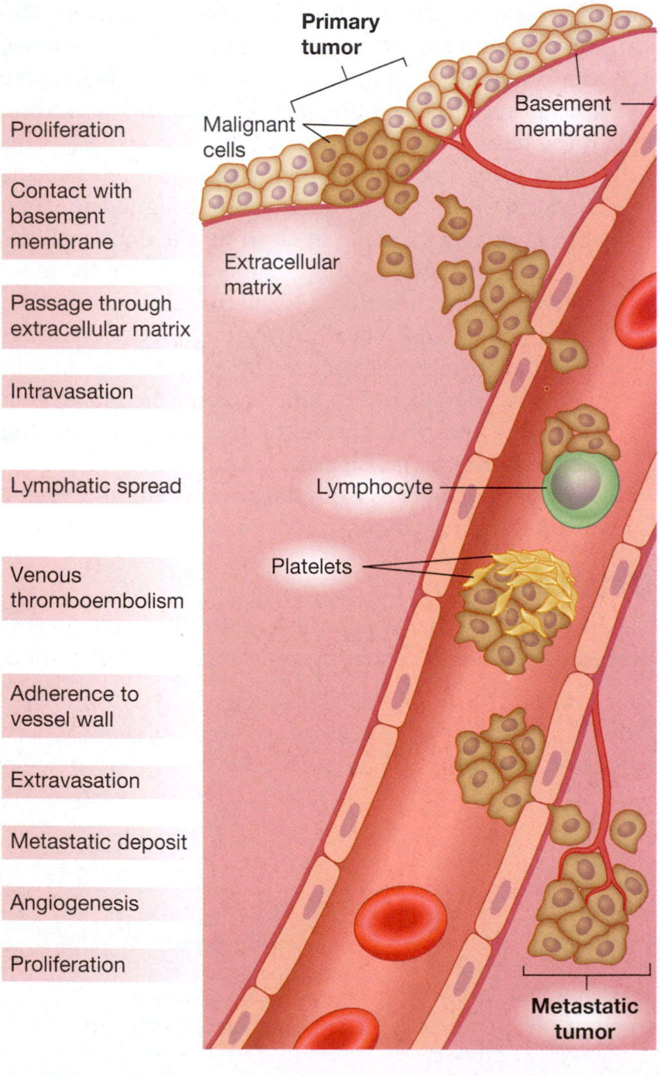
Primary tumor
Proliferation
Malignant cells
Basement membrane
Contact with basement membrane
Extracellular matrix
Passage through extracellular matrix
Intravasation
Lymphatic spread
Lymphocyte
Platelets
Venous thromboembolism
Adherence to vessel wall
Extravasation
Metastatic deposit
Angiogenesis
Proliferation
Metastatic tumor

Figure 14.3 ■ Metastasis through the bloodstream. Cancer cells secrete enzymes and a motility factor that disrupt the basement membrane in the blood vessel. In this way, the cancer cells gain access to the circulation. Once in the blood, only about 1 cell in 1000 escapes immune detection, but that can be enough. Undetected cells move out of the blood, again secreting enzymes and cutting through the vessel wall into new tissue. The tissue selected for establishing a new tumor may be downstream from the original tumor, or a chemical attraction may cause the malignant cells to target a specific site. Once in the new site, the malignant cells multiply and establish a metastatic tumor.

The tumor cells tend to clump together, forming an embolus, and continue growing until their size prevents further travel in the vessel or lymph channel. The growing neoplastic mass then uses its invasive abilities (secreting enzymes and motility factor) to move into the nearest organ.

About 60% of metastatic lesions tend to occur in a pattern that reflects blood or lymph circulation. However, it has been demonstrated that some malignant cells defy a bloodborne pattern and actually target specific organs to which they prefer to metastasize. For example, lung cancer frequently metastasizes to the adrenal glands, and breast cancer frequently metastasizes to bone. Malignant cells that gain access to lymph channels may travel to a preferred organ and then move into it the same way they move through blood vessels. Alternatively, the malignant cells may become trapped in the lymph node and continue to grow. Eventually, the malignant cells replace the node's tissues. At this point, emboli from the cancerous node disseminate to other nodes, creating a cascade reaction. The malignant cascade causes widespread transfer of the tumor to uncharacteristic sites.

A malignant tumor may break through the walls of the organ in which it is primarily housed, shedding cells into the nearby body cavity. The cells are then free to establish new tumors in a distant area of that cavity. For example, malignant cells from a colon cancer may be seeded into the peritoneal cavity, establishing a new tumor in the mesenteric epithelium.

Metastatic lesions are differentiated from primary neoplasms by cell morphology: Metastatic cells do not resemble the tissue in which they reside. The most common sites of metastasis are the lymph nodes, liver, lungs, bones, and brain. **Table 14.3** lists different cancers and common sites of metastasis.

For metastasis to occur, the cancerous cells must avoid detection by the immune system. Thus, impairment of the immune system is a major factor in the establishment of metastatic lesions. Cells may escape detection in several different ways:

- Aggressive cancer cells may compile a large mass (greater than 1 cm) so rapidly that the immune system is unable to overcome the tumor before it takes hold in a new tissue.

Table 14.3 Various Cancers and Sites of Metastases

Primary Tumor	Common Metastatic Sites
Bronchogenic (lung)	Spinal cord, brain, liver, bone
Breast	Regional lymph nodes, vertebrae, brain, liver, lung, bone
Colon	Liver, lung, brain, ovary, bone
Prostate	Bladder, bone (especially vertebrae), liver
Malignant melanoma	Lung, liver, spleen, regional lymph nodes, brain

- For tumor cells to be recognized as foreign by the immune system, they must display on their surface a special antigen called *tumor-associated antigen (TAA)*. TAA marks tumor cells for destruction by the lymphocytes. Some oncogenic viruses depress the expression of TAA on infected cells. Some tumors in advanced stages of growth no longer display TAA. Thus, such tumor cells escape detection as they travel through the blood or lymph.
- If an individual's immune response is weakened or altered, then a metastatic tumor may take hold with little opposition. Factors that may weaken or alter the immune response include:
    a. Accumulated stress
    b. Depression
    c. Increased age
    d. Pregnancy
    e. Chronic disease
    f. Chemotherapy treatment for the primary cancer.

Often, cancer has already metastasized by the time the primary tumor is identified. The time it takes for metastasis to occur is extremely variable and often difficult to predict. Some cancers, such as basal cell carcinomas, do not metastasize. The aggressiveness and location of the tumor, and the state of the person's immune system, determine whether and how rapidly metastasis takes place.

14.4 Physiologic and Psychologic Effects of Cancer

Much of the nursing care for patients with cancer is related to the effects of cancer disease and the side effects of cancer treatment.

Disruption of Function

Physiologic functioning can be upset by obstruction or pressure secondary to tumor growth. For example, a large tumor in the bowel can stop intestinal motility, resulting in a bowel obstruction. Prostatic tumors can obstruct the bladder neck or urethra, resulting in urine retention. Intracranial pressure can be dangerously increased by a glioma. Obstruction or pressure can cause anoxia and necrosis of surrounding tissues, which in turn cause a loss of function of the involved organ or tissue. For example, a kidney tumor may progress to renal failure. Pressure against the superior vena cava from an adjacent lung tumor or tumor-infiltrated lymph nodes can interrupt the blood flow to the heart.

In the liver, either a primary hepatocellular cancer or metastatic lesion can have several significant effects. In liver parenchymal tissue, it impairs the multiple life-sustaining functions of the liver, such as carbohydrate metabolism, synthesis of plasma proteins, detoxification, and immunologic functions. These functional impairments result in severe nutritional, hormonal, hematologic, and immunologic problems. (See Chapter 25 for a more complete discussion of liver functions and effects of disruption.) Because more than 1 L of blood per minute passes through the liver via the portal vein, obstruction to this flow by a tumor can cause portal hypertension. This results in backup of fluid and increased pressure in the splanchnic circulation. The end result is ascites (third-spaced fluid in the peritoneal cavity) and varices (friable, overdistended blood vessels) of the esophageal, gastric, mesenteric, and hemorrhoidal vessels.

Hematologic Alterations

Hematologic alterations can impair the normal function of blood cells. For example, in leukemia, a malignant proliferative disease of the hematopoietic (blood cell–producing) system, the immature leukocytes cannot perform the normal protective phagocytic functions, so immunity is compromised. The excessive numbers of immature leukocytes in the bone marrow diminish erythrocyte and thrombocyte (platelet) production, resulting in secondary anemia, neutropenia, and thrombocytopenia. In addition, gastrointestinal tumors disrupt the absorption of vitamin B_{12} and iron; growing tumors accumulate and store purines, depriving the bone marrow of substances needed for erythropoiesis (red blood cell production); and renal cell carcinoma produces its own erythropoietin hormone, resulting in production of an excessively large number of red blood cells and viscous blood, which impairs circulation, plugs small capillaries, and promotes thrombus formation (polycythemia).

Infection

If the tumor invades and connects two incompatible organs, such as the bowel and bladder, creating a fistula, infection becomes a serious problem. As they destroy viable tissue and thus their source of nutrition, tumors may become necrotic and septicemia may result. Some tumors are less efficient in creating capillaries; as a consequence, the center of the tumor may become necrotic and infected. When a tumor grows near the surface of the body, it may erode through to the surface, breaking down the natural defenses of intact skin and mucous membranes and providing a site for the entry of microorganisms. Any malignant involvement of the organs or tissues of immunity—such as the liver, bone marrow, Peyer patches in the small intestine, spleen, or lymph nodes—can seriously impair the immune response, allowing infections to develop in vulnerable tissues.

Hemorrhage

Tumor erosion through blood vessels can cause extensive bleeding, giving rise to severe anemia. Hemorrhage can be serious enough to cause life-threatening hypovolemic shock.

Anorexia-Cachexia Syndrome

Some individuals with cancer may develop a wasted appearance, called **cachexia**. In many cases, unexplained rapid weight loss is the first manifestation that brings the patient to a healthcare provider. This can be due to a variety of problems associated with cancer, such as pain, infection, depression, or the side effects of chemotherapy and radiation. Usually the emaciation, malnutrition, and loss of energy are attributed to anorexia-cachexia syndrome.

This syndrome is specific to cancer because of the effect of cancer cells on the host's metabolism. The neoplastic cells divert nutrition to their own use while causing changes that reduce the patient's appetite. Early in the disease, altered glucose metabolism leads to an increase in serum glucose levels, which creates negative feedback resulting in *anorexia* (loss of appetite). In addition, the tumor secretes substances that decrease appetite by altering taste and smell and producing early satiety. Pain, infection, and depression can contribute to anorexia. Some types of cancers cause specific food aversions, such as to red meat, coffee, or chocolate.

Avaricious cancer cells support their growth through widespread catabolism of the body's tissue and muscle proteins. This catabolism, coupled with inadequate nutrient intake, results in the typical cachexia. Normally, a starvation state reduces the body's basal metabolic rate. However, in many people with cancer, the metabolic rate is increased, probably because of the hyperactive metabolic and reproductive activities of the malignant cells. One theory suggests that cytokines that the body produces in response to the tumor are responsible for both early satiety and cachexia. One specific cytokine, called *tumor necrosis factor alpha* or *cachectin*, is believed to enhance the increased metabolic consumption of nutrients. Cancers of the gastrointestinal system further promote anorexia-cachexia by decreasing absorption and use of nutrients; the side effects of some treatment modalities enhance this effect. **Figure 14.4** ■ shows the characteristic appearance of a cachectic person.

Paraneoplastic Syndromes

Paraneoplastic syndromes are indirect effects of cancer. They may be early warning signs of cancer or indicate complications or return of a malignancy. The most frequently occurring paraneoplastic syndromes are endocrine, occurring when cancers set up ectopic sites of hormone production, and neurologic, occurring when cancer damages the nervous system (Grossman & Porth, 2014). **Table 14.4** lists laboratory indicators of ectopic functioning. These ectopic sites produce excessive amounts of the hormone, which harm the host. Consider the following examples:

- Breast, ovarian, and renal cancers may set up ectopic parathyroid hormone sites, causing severe hypercalcemia.
- Oat cell and other lung cancers may produce ectopic secretions of insulin (causing hypoglycemia), parathyroid hormone (PTH), antidiuretic hormone (ADH; causing excessive fluid retention, hypertension, and peripheral edema), and adrenocorticotropic hormone (ACTH). See Chapter 19 for a description of the multiple problems caused by excessive secretions of cortisone.

Other paraneoplastic syndromes include hematologic abnormalities such as anemia, thrombocytopenia, and coagulation abnormalities; nephrotic syndrome; cutaneous syndromes; and neurologic syndromes, such as distant tumors that produce IICP.

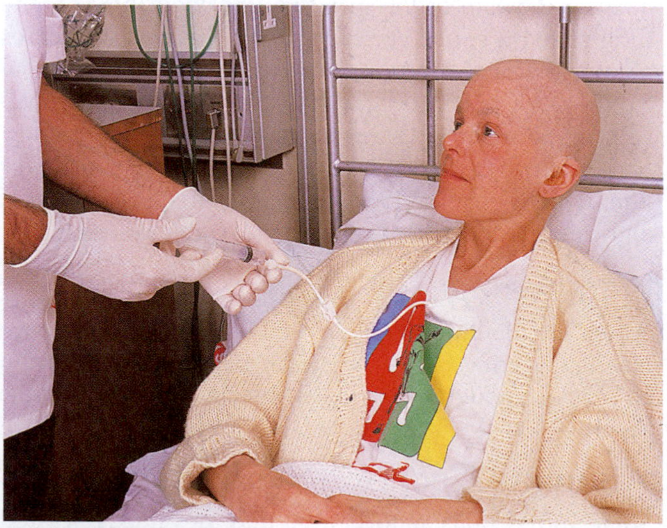

Figure 14.4 ■ Cachectic person. Cancer robs its host of nutrients and increases body catabolism of fat and muscle to meet its metabolic needs.

Pain

Pain is a major healthcare problem for patients with cancer. Despite extensive progress in the scientific understanding of pain, more than 70% of patients with cancer report cancer-related pain, with up to 50% of patients experiencing poorly controlled pain (Neufeld, Elnahal, & Alvarez, 2016). Undertreatment is usually attributed to both patient-related and healthcare provider–related factors such as failure to report pain, inadequate assessment of pain, lack of knowledge and training for healthcare providers, concerns related to side effects or potential for opioid addiction, cultural and religious beliefs, and cost of pain medication (Neufeld et al., 2016).

Types of Cancer Pain

Cancer pain can be divided into two main categories, acute and chronic, with subgroupings. These classifications serve

Table 14.4 Laboratory Indicators of Ectopic Functioning

Hormone	Specific Laboratory Test
Antidiuretic hormone (ADH)	Serum and urine osmolality
Adrenocorticotropic hormone (ACTH)	Plasma ACTH ACTH suppression test ACTH stimulation test Urine catecholamines
Calcitonin	Serum calcitonin
Insulin	Serum glucose Glucose tolerance test
Parathyroid hormone (PTH)	Serum PTH Serum calcium
Thyroxine	Serum thyroid-stimulating hormone (TSH), T_3, T_4

to indicate appropriate therapeutic approaches. Acute pain has a well-defined pattern of onset, exhibits common signs and symptoms, and is often identified with hyperactivity of the autonomic system. Chronic pain, which lasts more than 6 months, frequently lacks the objective manifestations of acute pain, primarily because the autonomic nervous system adapts to this chronic stress. Chronic pain often results in personality changes, alterations in functional abilities, and lifestyle disruptions that can seriously affect compliance with treatment and the quality of life.

Most cancer patients who report acute pain as the primary symptom that led to the diagnosis tend to associate pain with the introduction to their disease. Patients reporting pain after treatment may perceive the pain as a recurrence of the original cancer. In fact, adequate pain management has been shown to reduce patients' fear of cancer recurrence (Lopez et al., 2015).

Chronic pain may be related to treatment or may indicate progression of the disease. Identifying the pain as treatment related rather than tumor related is extremely important. For the patient whose pain is due to the advancement of the disease, psychologic factors play an even more important role. Hopelessness and fear of impending death intensify physiologic pain and contribute to overall suffering (which goes well beyond just physical pain).

Three other categories used to classify patients with cancer pain include patients with preexisting pain, those with a history of drug abuse, and hospice patients with cancer-related pain. The first two groups may have altered perceptions of pain and may not have the anticipated response to pain medication or other nonpharmacological interventions, such as meditation or music therapy. For the patient receiving hospice care, pain is strongly associated with both the patient's and family's confrontation of issues of hopelessness and death. Confronting these issues can intensify the perception of pain.

Causes of Cancer Pain

Direct tumor involvement is the primary cause of the pain experienced by people with cancer. This includes metastatic bone disease, nerve compression, and involvement of visceral organs. The pain from tumor involvement is believed to be mechanical, resulting from stretching of tissues and compression. Chemicals from ischemia or tumor metabolites and toxins that activate and sensitize nociceptors and mechanoreceptors are also responsible for tumor pain. Refer to Chapter 9 for a more complete discussion of the mechanics of pain.

Side effects or toxic effects of cancer therapies (e.g., surgery, radiation, and chemotherapy) may cause cancer pain. These are usually the result of traumatized tissue; one example of this is the oropharyngeal ulcerations that occur with some types of chemotherapy. However, these therapies may also be used to manage pain, such as radiation to decrease pain associated with bone metastasis.

Physical Stress

When the immune system discovers a neoplasm, it tries to destroy it using the resources of the body. The body mounts an all-out assault on the foreign invader, calling on many resources, including chemical mediators, hormones and enzymes, blood cells, antibodies, proteins, and inflammatory and immune responses. These protective responses mobilize fluid, electrolyte, and nutritional systems. This massive effort requires tremendous energy. If the neoplasm is small enough (i.e., microscopic), the immune system can destroy it, and a tumor will never manifest. A neoplasm of 1 cm is large enough to overwhelm most immune systems; however, the body will continue to try to fight it until it reaches the stage of exhaustion and is no longer capable (Selye, 1984). Thus, many patients with cancer present with fatigue, weight loss, anemia, dehydration, and altered blood chemistries (e.g., decreases in electrolytes).

Psychologic Stress

People confronted with the diagnosis of cancer exhibit a variety of psychologic and emotional responses. Some people see cancer as a death sentence and experience overwhelming grief and may feel like giving up. Others may feel guilt, considering the cancer a punishment for past behaviors, such as smoking, unhealthy eating habits, or delaying diagnosis or treatment. They may experience anger, especially if they believe that they had been practicing a healthy lifestyle; beneath that anger may reside feelings of powerlessness. Fear is common: Fear of the outcome of the illness, fear of the effects of treatment, fear of pain, fear of death, and fear of cancer recurrence. Some people feel isolated because of the stigma of cancer and old beliefs of contagion. Body image concerns and sexual dysfunction may be present but are often unexpressed, especially if the cancer is of the breast or sexual organs or causes visible body changes.

14.5 Care of the Patient with Cancer

Interprofessional Care

Interprofessional care for the patient with cancer begins with a variety of specialized laboratory and diagnostic tests.

Diagnosis

Several procedures are used to diagnose cancer. X-ray imaging, computed tomography (CT), ultrasonography, and magnetic resonance imaging (MRI) can locate abnormal tissues or tumors. However, only microscopic histologic examination of the tissue reveals the type of cell and its structural difference from the parent tissue. Tissue samples are acquired through biopsy, shed cells (e.g., Papanicolaou test), or collections of secretions (e.g., sputum). Lymph nodes are biopsied to determine whether metastasis has begun. Simple screening procedures can be used to identify substances secreted by the tumor (e.g., tumor markers), such as the prostatic-specific antigen (PSA) blood test used to identify early prostatic cancers. Increases in enzymes or hormones released by normal tissues when they are damaged can contribute to the diagnosis. For example, alkaline phosphatase noted in bone metastases and osteosarcoma is one example of an enzyme increase associated with cancer. Tumor markers are used for early diagnosis, tracking responses to therapy, and devising immunologic treatments.

Classification. To help standardize diagnosis and treatment protocols, an elaborate identification system has been developed. This consists of naming the tumor (classification) and describing its aggressiveness (grading) and spread within or beyond the tissue of origin (staging).

Tumors are classified and named based on the tissue or cell of origin. Tumor nomenclature often incorporates the Latin stem identifying the tissue from which the tumor arises. For example, a carcinoma arises from epithelial tissue; adjectives are added to further specify the location. Therefore, a glandular malignancy arising from epithelial tissue is classified as an adenocarcinoma; *adeno* denoting that the tumor is glandular and *carcinoma* that the cell of origin is epithelial. A tumor arising from supportive tissues is called a *sarcoma*; the specific type of tissue is added as a prefix. For example, a cancer of fibrous connective tissue is called *fibrosarcoma*, and a smooth muscle cancer is a *leiomyosarcoma*. A tumor from seminal or germ tissue is called a *seminoma*. **Table 14.5** compares the nomenclature of benign and malignant neoplasms.

Other names for tumors incorporate the name of the discoverer of that particular cancer, such as Burkitt lymphoma or Hodgkin lymphoma. Hematopoietic malignancies (known as *liquid tumors*) are usually named by the type of immature blood cell that dominates. An example is myelocytic leukemia, named for the immature form of the granulocyte (e.g., myelocyte) that is predominant in this malignancy.

Grading and Staging. Grading evaluates the degree of cell differentiation (level of functional maturity) and estimates the rate of growth based on the mitotic rate. Cells that are the most differentiated—that is, most like the parent tissue and therefore the least malignant—are classified as grade 1 and are associated with a better prognosis. Grade 4 is reserved for the least differentiated and most aggressively malignant cells. Because of the differences inherent in tumor appearance and biologic behavior, grading criteria may vary with different locations and types of tumors.

Staging is used to classify solid tumors and refers to the relative size of the tumor and extent of the disease to nearby tissues. The TNM classification system is an internationally recognized staging system: *T* stands for the relative tumor size, depth of invasion, and surface spread; *N* indicates the presence and extent of lymph node involvement; and *M* denotes the presence or absence of distant metastases. **Table 14.6** shows the basic outline of the TNM system; however, other systems are also used to differentiate types and locations of tumors (e.g., melanomas, cervical cancer, Hodgkin lymphoma).

Although the TNM staging system is most commonly used, other, more simplified staging categories may be used. Stage 0, also called *carcinoma in situ (CIS)*, denotes that abnormal cells are present, but have not spread. CIS is not cancer, but has the potential to develop into cancer. Stage I, II, and III denote ascending degrees of tumor size and spread into nearby tissues. Stage IV denotes that the cancer has spread to other parts of the body (e.g., breast cancer metastasized to the liver).

Cytologic Examination. For the malignant tissues to be identified by name, grade, and stage, they must first be subjected to histologic and cytologic examination by light or

Table 14.5 Nomenclature for Benign and Malignant Neoplasms

Tissue of Origin	Benign	Malignant
Ectoderm/Endoderm		
Epithelium	Papilloma	Carcinoma
Gland	Adenoma	Adenocarcinoma
Liver cells	Hepatocellular adenoma	Hepatocellular carcinoma
Neuroglia	Glioma	Glioma
Melanocytes	Melanoma	Malignant melanoma
Basal cells		Basal cell carcinoma
Germ cells	Tetroma	Seminoma
Mesoderm		
Connective tissue		
Adipose tissue	Lipoma	Liposarcoma
Fibrous tissue	Fibroma	Fibrosarcoma
Bone tissue	Osteoma	Osteosarcoma
Cartilage	Chondroma	Chondrosarcoma
Muscle		
Smooth muscle	Leiomyoma	Leiomyosarcoma
Striated muscle	Rhabdomyoma	Rhabdomyosarcoma
Neural tissue Nerve cells	Ganglioneuroma	Neuroblastoma
Endothelial tissues		
Blood vessels	Hemangioma	Angiosarcoma Kaposi sarcoma
Meninges	Meningioma	Malignant meningioma
Hematopoietic Tissues		
Granulocytes	Granulocytosis	Leukemia
Plasma cells		Multiple myeloma
Lymphocytes		Lymphomas

Table 14.6 TNM Staging Classification System

	Stage	Manifestations
Tumor	Tx	Tumor cannot be measured
	T_0	No evidence of primary tumor
	T_{IS}	Tumor *in situ*
	T_1, T_2, T_3, T_4	Ascending degrees of tumor size and involvement
Nodes	Nx	Cancer in lymph nodes cannot be measured
	N_0	No abnormal regional nodes
	N_{1a}, N_{2a}	Regional nodes—no metastasis
	N_{1b}, N_{2b}, N_{3b}	Regional lymph nodes—metastasis suspected
	N_x	Regional nodes cannot be assessed clinically
Metastasis	Mx	Metastasis cannot be measured
	M_0	No evidence of distant metastasis
	M_1, M_2, M_3	Ascending degrees of metastatic involvement of the host, including distant nodes

electron microscope. Specimens are collected by three basic methods:

1. *Exfoliation from an epithelial surface*. Examples include scraping cells from the cervix (Pap smear) or bronchial washings.
2. *Aspiration of fluid from body cavities or blood*. Examples include white blood cells for evaluation of hematopoietic (blood) cancers, pleural fluid, and cerebrospinal fluid.
3. *Needle aspiration of solid tumors*. This could include the breast, lung, or prostate.

Cytologic examination is also carried out on specimens from biopsied tissues or tumors and on collected body secretions, such as sputum or urine.

After collection, specimens are spread on a glass slide, fixed, and stained, if necessary. The morphologic features of the cells are examined, with special attention to the nucleus and cytoplasm. Other special pathologic procedures can be carried out on the specimen, but they must be ordered ahead of time if special preparations of the specimen are necessary. Several special diagnostic cytologic procedures, such as cytogenetics, are proving useful in diagnosing and monitoring patient response to treatment.

Tumor Markers. A **tumor marker** is a protein molecule detectable in serum or other body fluids. This marker is used as a biochemical indicator of the presence of a malignancy. Small amounts of tumor marker proteins are found in normal body tissues or benign tumors and are not specific for malignancy. However, high levels are suspicious and mandate follow-up diagnostic studies. Tumor marker tests are most useful for monitoring the patient's response to therapy and for detecting residual disease. For example, CA-125 is often used as an early marker for ovarian cancer recurrence. However, testing with CA-125 can result in false-positive findings and have not been shown to decrease overall mortality (Jin, 2018).

Tumor markers fall into two general categories: Those derived from the tumor itself and those associated with host (immune) response to the tumor. Examples of tumor markers include:

- *Antigens*. These are present in fetal tissue but are normally suppressed after birth. Thus, their presence in large amounts may reflect an anaplastic process in tumor cells. Alpha-fetoprotein (AFP) and carcinoembryonic antigen (CEA) are oncofetal antigens.
- *Hormones*. Hormones are present in considerable amounts in human blood and tissues, but very high levels not related to other conditions may signify the presence of a hormone-secreting malignancy. Some common hormones seen as tumor markers include human chorionic gonadotropin (HCG), ADH, PTH, calcitonin, and catecholamines.
- *Proteins*. These narrow down the type of tissue that may be malignant, although they can also be increased in hyperplastic disorders. Examples of tissue-specific proteins include serum immunoglobulin and beta$_2$ microglobulin.
- *Enzymes*. Rapid, excessive growth of a tissue may cause some of the enzymes and isoenzymes normally present in that particular tissue to spill into the bloodstream. Elevated levels can point to either hyperplasia of the tissue or cancer. Prostatic acid phosphatase (PAP) and neuron-specific enolase (NSE) are examples. **Table 14.7** compares selected tumor-derived markers with their presence in neoplasms and other conditions.

Oncologic Imaging. Because physical assessment usually does not detect cancer until the tumor has reached a size that poses a major risk for metastasis, radiologic examination is extremely important in early diagnosis. This diagnostic process may involve routine x-ray imaging (usually for screening only), CT, MRI, ultrasonography, nuclear imaging, angiography, and positron emission tomography. These diagnostic tests, including preparation and nursing implications, are discussed in the assessment chapters as well as with specific body system cancers throughout the book.

X-RAY Imaging. Standard x-ray imaging is the method of choice for screening such body areas as the breast (mammography), lung, and bone to identify changes in tissue density that may indicate malignancies. X-ray imaging is still the method of choice for lung cancer, but does not usually reveal tumors until late in their development when they have reached about 1 cm in size.

Computed Tomography. CT allows the visualization of cross-sections of the anatomy. Because CT scans reveal subtle differences in tissue densities, they are much more accurate than standard x-rays. CT scans can detect tumors in various locations to aid in the diagnosis and staging of the tumor and evaluate possible lymph node involvement.

Table 14.7 Tumor-Derived Markers Associated with Specific Neoplasms

	Tumor Marker	Associated Neoplasm
Oncofetal antigens	Carcinoembryonic antigen (CEA)	Adenocarcinomas of colon, lung, breast, ovary, stomach, pancreas
	Alpha-fetoprotein (AFP)	Hepatocellular carcinoma, gonadal germ cell tumors (seminoma)
Hormones	Human chorionic gonadotropin (HCG)	Gonadal germ cell tumors
	Calcitonin	Medullary cancer of thyroid
	Catecholamines/ metabolites	Pheochromocytoma
Isoenzymes	Prostatic acid phosphatase (PAP)	Adenocarcinoma of prostate
	Neuron-specific enolase (NSE)	Small-cell lung carcinoma, neuroblastoma
	Lactic dehydrogenase	Lymphoma, Ewing's sarcoma
Specific proteins	Prostate-specific antigen (PSA)	Adenocarcinoma of prostate
	Immunoglobin	Multiple myeloma
	CA 125	Epithelial ovarian cancer
	CA 19-9	Adenocarcinoma of pancreas, colon
	CA 15-3	Breast cancer

CT can also be used to guide biopsies and cancer treatments such as guiding radiation therapy. In addition, CT scans can be used to monitor cancer treatment response and determine if a tumor has recurred.

Magnetic Resonance Imaging. During an MRI, pulsed radio waves are directed at a patient within a strong magnetic field, and a computer analyzes the tissue characteristics based on the transmitted signals. MRI is the diagnostic tool of choice for both screening and follow-up of cranial and head and neck tumors. Similar to CT scans, an MRI produces cross-sections of the anatomy, but does not use radiation.

Ultrasonography. Ultrasonography can identify abnormalities that may indicate a tumor by measuring sound waves as they bounce off various body structures. For example, transrectal ultrasonography has provided excellent imaging of early prostate cancers and is used to guide needle biopsy. Ultrasound imaging is more useful for detecting masses in the denser breast tissue of young women.

Nuclear Imaging. Nuclear imaging is often used to check for possible bone or other organ metastasis. A scanner is used in conjunction with the ingestion or injection of specific radioactive isotopes, which are either absorbed more or less by cancer cells. Images that show where the radioactive isotope travels and collects will help to identify sites of potential organ metastasis.

Positron emission tomography (PET) and single-photon emission computed tomography (SPECT) are two examples of nuclear medicine. PET scans use a radioactive sugar that is taken up by rapidly dividing cells, such as cancer cells. Radiologists are then able to see areas that take up more sugar and, thus, may be cancerous. Newer tests are using monoclonal antibodies attached to radioactive substances. When monoclonal antibodies attached to radioactive substances are inserted into the bloodstream, they bind with cancerous cells and light up on an image. These tests are being used in prostate, colon, and ovarian cancer.

Angiography. Angiography is performed when the precise location of the tumor cannot be identified or there is a need to visualize the tumor's extent prior to surgery. The procedure involves injecting a radiopaque dye into a major blood vessel proximal to the organ or tissue to be examined. The movement of the dye through the vasculature of the organ or tissue is traced by means of fluoroscopy or serial x-ray films. Blockage to the flow of the dye indicates the tumor's location. Dye may be used to identify blood vessels supplying a tumor, allowing the surgeon to know where to safely ligate vessels.

Direct Visualization. Direct visualization procedures are invasive but do not require the use of radiography. Examples include sigmoidoscopy (viewing the sigmoid colon with a fiberoptic flexible sigmoidoscope), cystoscopy (viewing the urethra and bladder), endoscopy (viewing the upper gastrointestinal tract), and bronchoscopy (inspecting the tracheobronchial tree). These methods allow the visual identification of the organs within the limits of the scope and usually permit biopsy of suspicious lesions or masses (e.g., colon polyps). Flexible fiberoptic scopes may be more useful because they allow deeper penetration than do traditional scopes. These procedures all require some patient preparation, cause moderate to considerable discomfort, and may require sedation or anesthesia. Some procedures, such as sigmoidoscopy and cystoscopy, may be performed in the physician's office and therefore cost less, making them more accessible screening procedures. Of note, patients may elect a CT colonography in lieu of a colonoscopy, which uses CT imaging to assess for cancer or other diseases of the colon. While this test is less invasive and may be suitable for patients who cannot tolerate a colonoscopy, patients are exposed to radiation, so the risks and benefits should be weighed carefully.

When the tumor is exposed through direct visualization, a sample of tissue (biopsy) is sent to the pathology laboratory for a frozen-section histologic examination. This can be done rapidly while the patient remains on the operating table under anesthesia. If the initial report is negative, the benign mass is usually removed to prevent further symptoms. If the report is positive for cancer, the tumor, and often adjacent lymph nodes, are dissected, along with any other suspicious tissue. The tumor, nodes, and any other specimens are sent to the pathology laboratory for more in-depth analysis. The patient then receives the usual postoperative care.

Laboratory Tests. Most laboratory tests of blood, urine, and other body fluids are used to rule out nutritional disorders and other noncancerous conditions that may be causing the patient's symptoms. In conjunction with other diagnostic studies, some laboratory tests can be quite useful either in screening for other pathologic conditions or for validating the cancer diagnosis. **Table 14.8** identifies some useful laboratory tests, their normal values, and their possible indications.

Psychologic Support During Diagnosis. Preparing for and awaiting the results of diagnostic tests can create extreme anxiety. In addition to coping with the possibility of a life-threatening disease, or at least a life-altering one, patients often face the prospect of uncomfortable, even painful, diagnostic procedures. They have important decisions to make that depend on the outcome of those tests. Many unspoken questions may exist, including:

- Do I have cancer?
- If so, what kind, and how serious?
- Has it spread?
- Will I survive?
- What kind of treatment is needed?
- How will this affect my lifestyle?
- How will this affect family members and friends?

Denial or intellectualization can help some patients to cope with cancer, but others display signs of anxiety and stress as they attempt to cope. The nurse can provide valuable support during this very difficult stage by helping patients become actively involved in managing their life

Table 14.8 Laboratory Tests Used for Cancer Diagnosis*

Test	Reference Value	Abnormality Indicated
Acid phosphatase (ACP)	0.2–13 International Unit/L	Elevated in multiple myeloma and cancer of the prostate, breast, and bone
Adrenocorticotropic hormone (ACTH)	8–80 pg/mL (7:00–10:00 am) 5–50 pg/mL (4:00 pm) <10 pg/mL (10:00 pm–12:00 am)	Decreased in adrenal cancer Elevated in pituitary cancer
Alanine aminotransferase (ALT)	10–35 unit/L	Moderate elevation in liver cancer
Albumin	3.5–5.0 g/dL	Decreased in malnutrition and certain malignancies
Alkaline phosphatase (ALP)	42–136 unit/L	Elevated in cancer of liver, bone, breast, and prostate; in leukemia; and in multiple myeloma
Alpha-fetoprotein (AFP)	Male and nonpregnant female: <15 ng/mL	Elevated in germ cell tumors (e.g., seminoma), testicular cancer, liver metastasis
Aspartate aminotransferase (AST)	8–35 unit/mL	Elevated in liver cancer
Bilirubin	Total: 0.1–1.2 mg/dL Direct: 0.1–0.3 mg/dL	Elevated in liver metastasis
Bleeding time	Ivy method: 1–9 min	Prolonged in leukemia and decreased in Hodgkin disease
Calcitonin	Male: <40 pg/mL Female: <25 pg/mL	Elevated to >500 pg/mL in thyroid medullary cancer, breast cancer, and lung cancer
Calcium (Ca)	4.5–5.5 mEq/L 9.0–11.0 mg/Dl	Elevated in multiple myeloma and cancer of the bone, lung, breast, bladder, and kidney.
Carcinoembryonic antigen (CEA)	<2.5 ng/mL in nonsmokers <5 ng/mL in smokers >12 ng/mL neoplasms	Elevated with GI cancers, liver, lung, breast, bladder, kidney, pancreas, testicular, cervical, and leukemia Used to evaluate effectiveness of cancer treatment
Chloride (Cl)	95–105 mEq/L	Decreased in vomiting and diarrhea Elevated in stomach cancer and multiple myeloma
C-reactive protein	>1:2 titer is positive	Elevated in metastatic cancer
Creatinine	0.5–1.5 mg/dL	Elevated in cancer of the intestine, testes, bladder, uterus, and prostate; leukemia and Hodgkin disease
Estradiol-serum	Female: 20–500 pg/mL (depends on phase of menstrual cycle) Menopausal female: <30 pg/mL Male: 15–50 pg/mL	Elevated in ovarian, testicular, and adrenal cancer
Fibrinogen	200–400 mg/dL	Decreased in leukemia
Gamma glutamyltransferase (GGT)	Male: 4–23 International Unit/L Female: 3–13 International Unit/L	Elevated in cancer of liver, pancreas, prostate, breast, kidney, lung, and brain
Fasting blood sugar	70–110 mg/dL	Decreased in malnutrition, cancer of stomach, liver, and lung
Haptoglobin	60–270 mg/dL	Elevated in Hodgkin disease and cancer of lung, large intestine, stomach, breast, and liver
Hematocrit (Hct)	Male: 40–54% Female: 36–46%	Decreased in anemia, leukemia, Hodgkin disease, lymphosarcoma, multiple myeloma, and malnutrition and as a side effect of chemotherapy
Hemoglobin (Hgb)	Male: 13.5–18 g/dL Female: 12–15 g/dL 1:3 ratio of Hgb:Hct	Decreased in anemia; cancer of the GI tract, rectum, liver, and bone; Hodgkin disease; leukemia; malnutrition; and as a side effect of chemotherapy
Human chorionic gonadotropin (HCG)	Nonpregnant female <0.01 International Unit/L	Elevated in choriocarcinoma
Insulin	5–25 microunit/mL	Elevated in insulinoma (islet cell tumor)
Lactic dehydrogenase (LDH)	100–190 International Unit/L	Elevated in cancer of the liver, brain, kidney, cervix, testes, lung, intestines, stomach, and breast; acute leukemia; melanoma; and anemia
Occult blood	Negative	Positive in gastric and intestinal cancers
Parathyroid hormone (PTH-C terminal)	C terminal PTH: 50–330 pg/mL	Increased in PTH-secreting tumors
Platelet (thrombocyte) count	150,000–400,000/mm^3	Decreased in bone, GI tract, and brain cancer; leukemia; and as a side effect of chemotherapy
Potassium (K)	3.5–5.3 mEq/L	Decreased in vomiting and diarrhea and in malnutrition
Prostate-specific antigen (PSA)	0–4 ng/mL	Prostate cancer 10-20 ng/mL
Protein, total	6.0–8.0 g/dL	Decreased in malnutrition, gastrointestinal cancer, Hodgkin disease Elevated in vomiting, diarrhea, multiple myeloma

(continued)

Table 14.8 Laboratory Tests Used for Cancer Diagnosis*

Test	Reference Value	Abnormality Indicated
Red blood cells (RBCs)	Male: 4.6–6.0 million/μL × 10^{12}/L Female: 4.0–5.0 million/μL × 10^{12}/L	Decreased in anemia, leukemia, infection, multiple myeloma
Serum osmolality	280–300 mOsm/kg/H_2O	Decreased in SIADH and lung cancer
Sodium (Na)	135–145 mEq/L	Decreased in SIADH, vomiting Elevated in dehydration
Uric acid	Male: 3.5–8.0 mg/dL Female: 2.8–6.8 mg/dL	Increased in leukemia, metastatic cancer, multiple myeloma, and as a side effect of chemotherapy
Urine osmolality	50–1200 mOsm/kg/H_2O	Increased in SIADH
White blood cells (WBC)		
Total leukocytes	4,500–10,000/mm^3	Elevated in acute infection, leukemia, tissue necrosis; decreased as a side effect of chemotherapy
Neutrophils	50–70%	Elevated in bacterial infection and Hodgkin disease, myelocytic leukemia; decreased in leukemia (lymphocytic and monocytic) and as a side effect of chemotherapy
Eosinophils	1–3%	Elevated in cancer of bone, ovary, testes, and brain
Basophils	0.4–1.0%	Elevated in leukemia and healing stage of infection
Monocytes	4–6%	Elevated in infection, monocytic leukemia, and cancer; decreased in lymphocytic leukemia and as a side effect of chemotherapy
Lymphocytes	25–35%	Elevated in lymphocytic leukemia, Hodgkin disease, multiple myeloma, viral infections, and chronic infections; decreased in cancer and other leukemias and as a side effect of chemotherapy

Note: *All values refer to serum values unless otherwise indicated. Values are approximate; check the reference standards specified by your own agency's laboratory.

Source: Kee, 2018.

and disease. Talk with patients as soon as they enter the healthcare system, asking them about their understanding of what to expect and soliciting any questions from them. Taking this approach and encouraging patients to share what knowledge and experience they have allows them to maintain control. From there, the nurse can provide the information needed.

As patients begin to feel more comfortable with the nurse, they may express concerns, fears, and other emotions. The nurse should actively listen and be supportive, but avoid giving advice and false reassurance, providing appropriate information when needed. For patients who are not ready to discuss concerns or for those who appear angry, being nonjudgmental and providing nonverbal support may facilitate more open communication. An atmosphere of calmness, warmth, caring, and respect can ease the tension and often unspoken terror of this initial period.

Support of and communication with the patient's significant others is extremely important. Often they try to be strong for the patient but have many fears and emotional concerns that they do not feel comfortable expressing. The nurse needs to be available to the family while the patient is undergoing diagnostic procedures. Allowing them to talk without the need to edit for the patient's benefit can help them manage their own difficulties in coping with their loved one's potential cancer diagnosis.

Cancer Treatment

The goals of cancer treatment may overlap but are aimed at achieving remission or no evidence of disease (NED), control of disease, or palliation of symptoms. Cancer may be treated through surgery, chemotherapy, radiation therapy, biotherapy, bone marrow and stem cell transplants, and hormonal therapy. Once cancer is diagnosed, the initial focus is on treatment. The goals of treatment are:

- Eliminate the tumor or malignant cells (no evidence of disease).
- Prevent metastasis.
- Reduce cellular growth and the tumor burden.
- Promote functional abilities and provide pain relief to those whose disease has not responded to treatment.

Surgery

Surgery remains an important approach to the treatment of solid tumors. The goals of surgery have expanded to include prophylaxis, diagnosis, treatment, reconstruction, and palliation. Although surgery is usually the first intervention in the treatment of cancer, other interventions such as chemotherapy and/or radiation may be used if the tumor is too large and/or unable to be resected prior to surgery.

Prophylactic Surgery. Prophylactic surgery aims to remove tissues or organs that are likely to develop cancer. Advances in identification of genetic markers make prophylactic surgery an option for individuals with a strong family history and genetic predisposition for the development of cancer. For example, a woman with a strong history of breast cancer, positive findings of *BRCA1* or *BRCA2*, and an abnormal finding on mammography may consider prophylactic mastectomy as one of the selective options. Other examples of prophylactic operations include colectomy and oophorectomy. With limited research on the long-term physiologic and psychologic effects on individuals undergoing prophylactic surgery for cancer, it is vitally important for nurses and other healthcare professionals to discuss thoroughly with the patient and family potential risks and postoperative outcomes of the prophylactic surgery prior to the surgery. Nurses should respect the patient's decision to pursue the prophylactic surgery. For those patients who choose prophylactic surgery as a preventive measure for cancer, comprehensive preoperative teaching and counseling should be provided and long-term postoperative follow-up should be ensured to monitor the patient's physiologic and psychologic adjustment to the surgery.

Diagnostic Surgery. Diagnostic surgery aims to ensure histologic diagnosis and staging of cancer through biopsy, endoscopy, laparoscopy, and open surgical exploration. **Table 14.9** provides information about common surgical diagnostic procedures.

Tumor Removal. As a primary treatment for cancer, the goal of surgery is to remove the entire tumor and involved surrounding tissue and lymph nodes as much as possible. In addition, surgeons will remove a margin of normal tissue around the tumor to ensure that all malignant tissue has been removed. If the margin is not clear (i.e., when malignant cells are identified), further surgery or adjuvant treatment may be necessary.

Some surgeries may necessitate the creation of new structures to assume function of the lost structures. For example, removal of the distal sigmoid colon and rectum requires a new means of bowel elimination, so the remaining healthy segment of the bowel is brought out through a created opening (stoma) in the abdominal wall, resulting in a permanent colostomy (see Chapter 24). In like manner, when the bladder is removed, the ureters are transplanted into a created pouch just under the abdominal wall. This serves as a continent ileostomy, a substitute reservoir for urine (see Chapter 27). Surgery can destroy sensitive nerve plexuses, resulting in alteration or loss of normal functioning; for example, prostate surgery may result in incontinence and impotence. Surgical removal of involved regional lymph nodes can lead to chronic lymphedema (swelling in the affected area) that greatly impacts cancer survivors' quality of life. Nurses should assess symptoms related to lymphedema to promote early detection and quality of life among patients who develop the disorder (Cornelissen Anouk et al., 2018; Fu et al., 2018). Although the removal of any major body part has physiologic and psychologic consequences, the benefits often outweigh the risk when patients are faced with a potentially terminal disease.

Not all surgery results in such radical changes in functioning. The following surgeries can eliminate cancer successfully with less distressing results:

- Removing a nonessential portion of the organ or tissue containing the tumor, such as *in situ* small-bowel tumors
- Removing an organ whose function can be replaced chemically, such as the thyroid
- Resecting one of a pair of organs when the unaffected organ can take over the function of the missing one, such as a lung or kidney.

If a tumor is in a nonresectable location or deeply invaded with metastases, surgery may be done to reduce the bulk of the tumor and achieve palliation to promote organ function, relieve pain, provide comfort, or bypass an obstruction. In cases when extensive removal of tissue is contraindicated (e.g., surgical removal of a brain tumor), radiation may be used prior to surgery in an attempt to shrink the tumor before it is removed.

Surgical intervention may also be used for reconstruction and rehabilitation after curative or radical surgery. For example, a patient undergoing a mastectomy may elect to undergo reconstruction with saline or silicone implants or a procedure called an *autologous flap reconstruction* in which a portion of the patient's own tissue from an area of the body such as the thigh, buttocks, or abdomen is used to create a breast mound. Other examples of reconstruction include prosthetics for patients undergoing limb amputation for treatment of osteosarcoma.

Nursing responsibilities focus on preparing the patient physically and psychologically for surgery, as well as teaching routine postoperative care in which the patient is expected to participate (refer to Chapter 4). Before surgery, the nurse should give the patient the opportunity to ask questions and discuss concerns and fears. In some cases, the patient may want to discuss alternative treatment options. In the latter case, the nurse should contact the oncologist and the surgeon to set up a conference with the patient before surgery.

Table 14.9 Surgical Diagnostic Procedures

Procedure	Explanation
Fine-needle biopsy	Use of a very thin needle to aspirate a small amount of tissue from the tumors. May not be an adequate sample to establish a diagnosis.
Needle core biopsy	Use of a slightly larger needle than that used for a fine-needle biopsy to extract a small amount of tissue from tumors that cannot be aspirated by fine-needle aspiration. This procedure is done with local anesthesia.
Incisional biopsy	Removal of a portion of a larger tumor through incision. This procedure may involve local, regional, or general anesthesia.
Excisional biopsy	Removal of an entire tumor through operation. This procedure is used when above diagnostic measures confirm diagnosis and may involve local, regional, or general anesthesia.
Endoscopy	Use of a small viewing lens or video camera through a natural body opening to view tumors of the esophagus, stomach, or colon. Tissue samples may be removed, if indicated.
Laparoscopy	Use of a small viewing lens or video camera through a small incision in the abdominal wall. Tissue samples may be removed, if indicated.

Chemotherapy

Chemotherapy involves the use of cytotoxic medications to treat liquid and solid cancers, such as leukemias, lymphomas, breast, and prostate cancer; to decrease tumor size, adjunctive to surgery or radiation therapy; or to prevent or treat suspected metastases. All chemotherapy has side effects or toxic effects and the type and severity depend on the drugs used. Chemotherapy can be used in conjunction with other treatments such as surgery, radiation, biotherapy, bone marrow transplant, and hormonal therapy. Chemotherapy administered prior to surgery is neoadjuvant chemotherapy, aiming at decreasing the size of the tumor to enable dissection of the tumor. Chemotherapy administered after surgery is referred to as adjuvant chemotherapy, aiming at eliminating remaining cancerous cells that are not able to be surgically removed. Often, both neoadjuvant and adjuvant chemotherapy are used to ensure success of cancer treatment.

Chemotherapy disrupts the cell cycle in various phases by interrupting cell metabolism and replication. It also works by interfering with the ability of the malignant cell to synthesize vital enzymes and chemicals. Because cancer is a disease of rapidly growing abnormal cells, the goal of chemotherapy is to prevent cell replication (mitosis) by targeting DNA or RNA. Chemotherapy either works on cells that are actively dividing (cell-specific drugs) or on cells in any phase of the cell cycle (non–cell cycle specific). **Figure 14.5** ■ lists some of the drugs useful in each phase of the cell cycle.

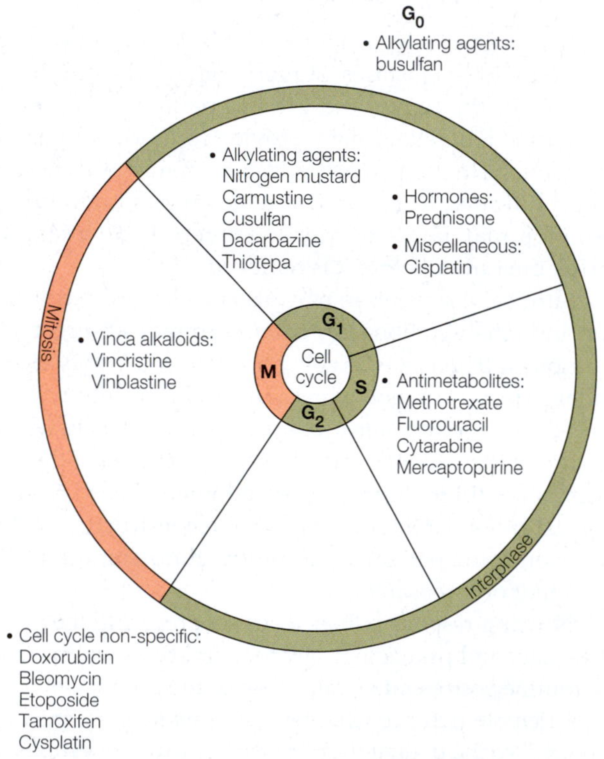
G_0
• Alkylating agents:
busulfan
• Alkylating agents:
Nitrogen mustard
Carmustine
Cusulfan
Dacarbazine
Thiotepa
• Hormones:
Prednisone
• Miscellaneous:
Cisplatin
Mitosis
• Vinca alkaloids:
Vincristine
Vinblastine
G_1
M
Cell cycle
S
G_2
• Antimetabolites:
Methotrexate
Fluorouracil
Cytarabine
Mercaptopurine
Interphase
• Cell cycle non-specific:
Doxorubicin
Bleomycin
Etoposide
Tamoxifen
Cysplatin

Figure 14.5 ■ Chemotherapeutic drugs useful in each phase of the cell cycle. Based on their chemical makeup and biologic activity, different drugs used for cancer treatment act in specific phases and subphases of the cell cycle. Some drugs, called non-phase-specific drugs, are generalized and act throughout the cycle. Chemotherapy often involves combinations of drugs designed to attack the cancer cells at many different times in the cycle to enhance effectiveness.

Most chemotherapy protocols involve combinations of drugs administered over varying periods of time. The combination of chemotherapeutic agents work synergistically to take advantage of multiple modes of action and avoid administering multiple agents with similar dose-limiting toxicities (e.g., nephrotoxicity, cardiotoxicity). For example, one protocol for Hodgkin lymphoma uses the acronym *ABVD*: Adriamycin (doxorubicin), bleomycin, vinblastine, and dacarbazine. Each chemotherapy agent is administered on day 1 and 15, which is considered one cycle. Because chemotherapy affects cancer cells as well as normal cells, such as those in the bone marrow, treatment regimens are administered in cycles with rest periods to maximize tumor-kill effect and allow bone marrow to regenerate normal cells (e.g., white blood cells, red blood cells, platelets). Rest periods are also important if toxic effects such as liver dysfunction or severe neutropenia (abnormally low amounts of neutrophils, a type of white blood cell) occur. Patients with Hodgkin lymphoma typically receive up to six cycles over approximately 6 months. If the cancer progresses, the particular protocol is abandoned and a new protocol may be tried. Additionally, patients may receive radiation therapy concurrently or after completion of chemotherapy.

Several courses of chemotherapy are necessary based on the hypothesis of cell killing. A 1-cm tumor contains about 10^9 (10 billion) total cells, most of which are viable. During each cell cycle, the chemotherapy kills a fixed percentage of cells, always leaving some behind. With each reduction, the tumor burden of cells decreases until the number of viable, clonogenic cells (i.e., those that are able to clone daughter cells) becomes small enough to allow the body's immune system to finish the job. For this reason, oncologists usually give the maximum amount of chemotherapy tolerated by the patient.

Classes of Chemotherapy Drugs. Chemotherapeutic agents can be classified either by the effects of the agent on the cell or by the pharmacologic properties of the agent. According to the effects of the agent on the cell, chemotherapeutic agents can be divided into cell cycle–specific and cell cycle–nonspecific agents. *Cell cycle–specific agents* are effective at a specific phase (e.g., S and M phases) in the cell cycle to prevent cell replication by damaging cellular DNA and blocking production of protein necessary for DNA and RNA synthesis. *Cell cycle–nonspecific agents* are effective throughout all the phases of the cell cycle, including the resting phase. Both cell cycle–specific and cell cycle–nonspecific agents are effective in rapidly dividing cells to prohibit the growth of fast-growing tumors.

The most common way of classifying chemotherapeutic agents is based on pharmacologic properties of the agent. Examples of chemotherapy classifications include alkylating agents, antimetabolites, antitumor antibiotics, and mitotic inhibitors. Each chemotherapy agent has toxic effects (also referred to as side effects).

- ***Alkylating agents*** are not phase specific and damage DNA to prevent cell replication. More specifically, they act on nucleic acids and cause cross-linking of DNA strands, which can permanently interfere with replication and transcription. Because they are not phase specific, alkylating agents work with both proliferating and nonproliferating cells (those in G_0 phase). Their toxicity relates to their ability to kill stem cells and manifests in delayed, prolonged, or permanent bone marrow failure. Toxicity can cause a mutagenic effect on bone marrow stem cells, culminating in a treatment-resistant form of acute myelogenous leukemia. Because of the alkylating agents' effect on stem cells, they may cause irreversible infertility. Other common adverse effects include nephrotoxicity (kidney damage) and hemorrhagic cystitis (bladder damage). The major toxicity factor is reversible impaired renal function.

Examples of alkylating agents include nitrogen mustard (mechlorethamine), nitrosoureas (carmustine), alkyl sulfonates (busulfan), triazines (dacarbazine), ethyleneamines (thiotepa), and cisplatin. Cisplatin is an alkylating agent containing platinum and chlorine atoms and is most active in the G_1 subphase.

- *Antimetabolites*. Antimetabolites are phase specific, working best in the S phase and having little effect in G_0. Most toxic effects relate to rapidly proliferating cells, such as cells in the gastrointestinal tract, hair, skin, and WBCs. The toxic effect of antimetabolites include nausea and vomiting, stomatitis, diarrhea, alopecia, and leukopenia. Some of the drugs can cause liver and lung toxicity.

  Examples of antimetabolites include folic acid analogues (methotrexate), pyrimidine analogues (5-fluorouracil), cytosine arabinoside (ARA-C), and purine analogues (6-mercaptopurine).

- *Antitumor antibiotics* are derived from natural sources that are generally too toxic to be used as antibacterial agents. They are not phase specific and act in several ways: They disrupt DNA replication and RNA transcription; create free radicals, which generate breaks in DNA and other forms of damage; and interfere with DNA repair. In addition, these drugs bind to cells and kill them, probably by damaging the cell membrane. Their main toxic effect is damage to the cardiac muscle. This limits the amount and duration of treatment.

  Examples of these antibiotics include actinomycin D, doxorubicin, bleomycin, mitomycin-C, and mithramycin.

- *Mitotic inhibitors* are drugs that act to prevent cell division during the M phase. Mitotic inhibitors include the plant alkaloids and taxoids. Plant alkaloids consist of medications extracted from plant sources: Vinca alkaloids (e.g., vincristine and vinblastine) and etoposide (called VP-16). The Vinca alkaloids are phase specific, acting during mitosis. They bind to a specific protein in tumor cells that promotes chromosome migration during mitosis and serves as a conduit for neurotransmitter transport along axons. The toxicity of these drugs is characterized by depression of deep tendon reflexes, paresthesias (pain and altered sensation, including jaw pain), motor weakness, cranial nerve disruptions, and paralytic ileus. Etoposide acts in all phases of the cell cycle, causing breaks in DNA and metaphase arrest. Although etoposide may cause bone marrow suppression and nausea and vomiting, the most common toxic effect is hypotension resulting from too-rapid intravenous administration. The taxoids act during the G_2 phase to inhibit cell division. Paclitaxel is used for the treatment of Kaposi sarcoma and metastatic breast and ovarian cancer. Taxotere is used for breast cancer. Toxicities associated with these drugs include alopecia, bone marrow depression, and severe hypersensitivity reactions (e.g., hypotension, dyspnea, and urticaria).

Effects of Chemotherapeutic Drugs. The toxic effects (also referred to as side effects) of chemotherapy vary with the type of drug and length of treatment. Because most of these drugs act on fast-growing cells, the side effects are manifestations of damage to normal rapidly dividing somatic cells. Normal tissues usually affected by cytotoxic drugs include:

- Mucous membranes of the mouth, tongue, esophagus, stomach, intestine, and rectum. This may result in anorexia, loss of taste, aversion to food, erythema and painful ulcerations in any portion of the gastrointestinal tract, nausea and vomiting, and diarrhea.
- Hair cells, resulting in alopecia.
- Bone marrow depression affecting most blood cells (e.g., granulocytes, lymphocytes, thrombocytes, and erythrocytes). This results in an impaired ability to respond to infection, a diminished ability to clot blood, and severe anemia.
- Organs, such as heart, lungs, bladder, kidneys. This kind of damage is related to specific agents, such as cardiac toxicity with doxorubicin or pneumonitis with bleomycin.
- Reproductive organs, resulting in impaired reproductive ability or altered fetal development.

Table 14.10 gives the classifications of chemotherapeutic drugs, common examples, target malignancies, adverse effects or side effects, and nursing implications. Consult current pharmacology textbooks for additional drugs and for new combination therapies as they are developed.

Chemotherapy Preparation and Administration. Many states and individual hospitals require that personnel be trained and certified to administer chemotherapy. Pharmacists in large hospitals and independent home care agencies usually prepare chemotherapeutic drugs for parenteral administration under specific safety guidelines established by the federal government or the Oncology Nursing Society. In some agencies, nurses both prepare and administer these drugs. Because of the potential carcinogenic effects of chemotherapy drugs, healthcare professionals should wear gloves, a mask, and a gown while preparing and administering the drug and disposing of equipment. The nurse must use care when handling excretory products (e.g., urine) of

Table 14.10 Classifications of Chemotherapeutic Drugs

Drug Classification	Common Drugs	Target Malignancies	Adverse Effects or Side Effects	Nursing Implications
Alkylating agents	Busulfan (Myleran)	Chronic myelogenous leukemia	Leukopenia Thrombocytopenia Renal failure Pulmonary fibrosis	Monitor WBCs, BUN. Maintain adequate fluid intake. Assess for infection. Assess lungs for fibrotic (coarse, loud) rales.
	Cyclophosphamide (Cytoxan)	Lymphomas Multiple myeloma Leukemias Adenocarcinoma of lung and breast	Hemorrhagic cystitis Renal failure Alopecia Stomatitis Liver dysfunction	Encourage daily fluid intake of 2–3 L during treatment. Monitor WBCs, BUN, liver enzymes. Teach care for hair loss.
	Cisplatin (CDDP) (Platinol)	Combination and single therapy for metastatic testicular and ovarian cancers, advanced bladder cancer, head and neck tumors, non–small cell lung carcinoma, osteogenic sarcoma, neuroblastoma	Bone marrow depression: Leukopenia and thrombocytopenia Renal tubular damage Deafness	Monitor WBCs with differential and platelets, BUN, creatinine, uric acid. Watch for bleeding. Monitor for signs of infection. Evaluate hearing; check for tinnitus. Ensure that patient is well hydrated before drug is administered. Encourage 2–3 L of fluid intake daily.
Antimetabolites	Methotrexate	Acute lymphoblastic leukemia Osteosarcoma Gestational trophoblastic carcinoma	Oral and gastrointestinal ulcerations Anorexia and nausea Leukopenia Thrombocytopenia Pancytopenia	Monitor CBC, WBC differential, BUN, uric acid, creatinine. Assess oral mucous membranes; treat ulcers prn. Assess for infection, bleeding.
	5-Fluorouracil (5-FU)	Colon carcinoma Rectal carcinoma Breast carcinoma Gastric carcinoma Pancreatic cancer	Stomatitis Alopecia Nausea and vomiting Gastritis Enteritis Diarrhea Anemia Leukopenia Thrombocytopenia	Monitor CBC with differential, BUN, uric acid. Administer antiemetics prn. Assess for bleeding; check stool occult blood. Evaluate hydration and nutrition status. Teach oral care for stomatitis. Assess for infection. Teach care for hair loss.
Antitumor antibiotics	Doxorubicin (Adriamycin)	Acute lymphoblastic leukemia (ALL) Acute myeloblastic leukemia Neuroblastoma Wilms' tumor Breast, ovarian, thyroid, lung cancer	Stomatitis Alopecia Nausea and vomiting Gastritis Enteritis Diarrhea Anemia Leukopenia Thrombocytopenia Cardiac toxicity	Monitor ECG; assess for arrhythmias, gallops, and congestive heart failure (CHF). Monitor CBC with differential, BUN, uric acid. Administer antiemetics prn. Assess for bleeding; check stool for occult blood. Evaluate hydration and nutrition status. Teach oral care for stomatitis. Assess for infection. Teach care for hair loss.
	Bleomycin (Blenoxane)	Squamous cell carcinoma Lymphosarcoma Reticulum cell sarcoma Testicular carcinoma Hodgkin lymphoma	Mucocutaneous ulcerations Alopecia Nausea and vomiting Chills and fever Pneumonitis and pulmonary fibrosis	Check for fever 3–6 hours after administration. Have chest x-ray films taken every 2–3 weeks. Assess respiratory status, and check for coarse rales. Evaluate hydration and nutrition status. Teach oral care for stomatitis. Assess for infection. Teach care for hair loss.
Plant alkaloids	Vincristine (Oncovin)	Combination therapy for acute leukemia, Hodgkin and non-Hodgkin lymphomas, rhabdomyosarcoma, neuroblastoma, Wilms' tumor	Areflexia Muscle weakness Peripheral neuritis Constipation Paralytic ileus Mild bone marrow depression	Assess neuromuscular function. Monitor CBC with differential. Evaluate gastrointestinal function. Manage constipation.
	Vinblastine (Velban)	Combination therapy for Hodgkin lymphoma, lymphocytic and histocytic lymphoma, Kaposi sarcoma, advanced testicular carcinoma, unresponsive breast cancer	Areflexia Alopecia Nausea and vomiting Bone marrow depression	Assess neuromuscular function. Monitor CBC with differential. Administer antiemetics prn. Teach care for hair loss.
	Etoposide, also called VP-16 (VePesid)	Nonresponsive testicular tumors Small-cell lung cancer	Alopecia Hypotension with rapid infusion	Hydrate adequately before administration. Administer over 60 min. Monitor vital signs every 15 min during administration and every 2–4 hours thereafter. Teach care for hair loss.

patients undergoing chemotherapy and teach patients to dispose of their own body fluids safely. Oral medications pose a lesser risk of exposure, but a risk nonetheless, primarily through excretion in the urine.

Most common administration is oral or intravenous. Chemotherapeutic drugs can be administered orally, such as cyclophosphamide (Cytoxan) and chlorambucil (Leukeran). Most often, chemotherapy is given via intravenous infusion or direct injection into intraperitoneal or intrapleural body cavities. Intravenous preparations can be given through large peripheral veins, but the risk of extravasation or irritation to the vein may preclude this method for long-term therapy. Many patients now receive vascular access devices (VADs), especially if their treatment requires several cycles over weeks or months, as these devices can be left in place for months to years. VADs are also useful for adjunctive parenteral nutrition in the patient who needs continuous intravenous infusions to manage pain or frequent blood drawing to monitor blood counts. Different types of VADs are available:

- Catheters that are inserted nonsurgically by threading them through a large peripheral vein into the vena cava. Called *peripherally inserted central catheters (PICCs)*, they have multiple lumens that facilitate blood drawing. Placement is usually monitored by fluoroscopy.
- Catheters tunneled under the skin on the chest into a major vein, such as the subclavian vein. Hickman or Groshong catheters may be used.
- Surgically implanted ports are placed under the skin with a connected catheter inserted into a major vein, often called a Port-A-Cath or Medi-Port. These are accessed by means of a special needle with a 90-degree angle inserted through the skin directly into the rubber dome of the port, which has a hard plastic back to prevent tissue damage. The benefit of this device in comparison to PICC lines or Hickman/Groshong catheters is that the port can stay in place for many years without a needle, so the port is concealed under the skin and patients are free to do activities such as bathing or swimming. **Figure 14.6** ■ shows examples of different catheters and vascular access ports.

Risk of infection, catheter obstruction, and extravasation are the main problems associated with VADs. Nurses must teach patients and family members to observe for redness, swelling, pain, or exudate at the insertion site, which may indicate infection; to observe for swelling of the neck or skin near the VAD for extravasation and infiltration; and to flush catheters and provide site care (cleaning and dressing changes) on a regular basis. During each encounter with the patient, the nurse always inspects the site; observes for infection, infiltration, and catheter occlusion; and provides site care when necessary. Patient education for those undergoing chemotherapy includes teaching the patient and family when to call for help, as outlined in **Box 14.3**, and nursing care for the patient undergoing chemotherapy, described in **Box 14.4**.

Hormonal Therapy

Corticosteroids (e.g., prednisone) are one example of hormones used to treat cancer. Corticosteroids are phase specific and work on the G_1 phase. These act by binding to specific intracellular receptors, repressing transcription of mRNA, and thereby altering cellular function and growth. Corticosteroids have multiple side effects such as impaired healing, hyperglycemia, hypertension, osteoporosis, and hirsutism.

Hormone antagonists are used to treat cancers that are fueled by hormones or hormone-binding tumors, usually those of the breast, prostate, and endometrium. They block the hormone's receptor site on the tumor and prevent it from receiving normal hormonal growth stimulation. Alternatively, they can prevent the production of the hormone.

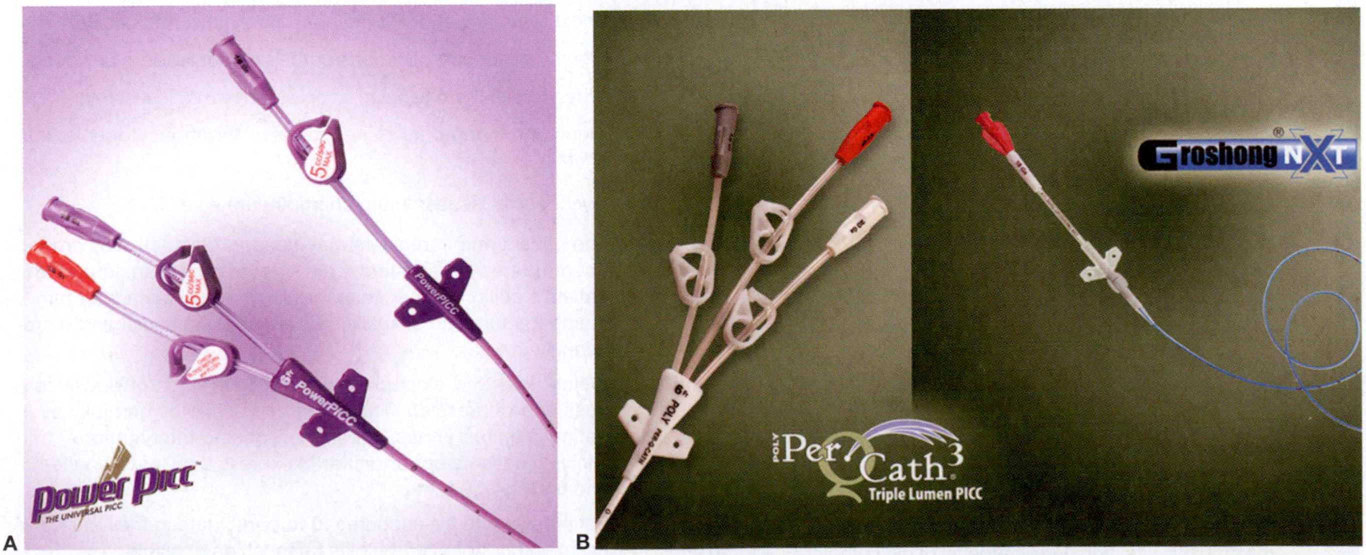
A
PowerPICC
PowerPICC
Power PICC
THE UNIVERSAL PICC
B
Groshong NXT
Per-Q-Cath 3
Triple Lumen PICC

Figure 14.6 ■ Vascular access devices. **A**, Single- and double-lumen catheters. **B**, Triple-lumen and groshong catheters.

BOX 14.3
When to Call for Help

CALL THE HEALTHCARE PROVIDER

Instruct the patient or family member to call the nurse or physician if any of the following manifestations are experienced:

- Oral temperature greater than 38.6°C (101.5°F)
- Severe headache; significant increase in pain at usual site, especially if the pain is not relieved by the medication regimen; or severe pain at a new site
- Difficulty breathing
- New bleeding from any site, such as rectal or vaginal bleeding
- Confusion, irritability, or restlessness
- Withdrawal, greatly decreased activity level, or frequent crying
- Verbalizations of deep sadness or a desire to end life
- Changes in body functioning, such as the inability to void or severe diarrhea or constipation
- Changes in eating patterns, such as refusal to eat, extreme hunger, or a significant increase in nausea and vomiting
- Appearance of edema in the extremities or significant increase in edema already present.

CALL 9-1-1

Instruct the patient or family member to call 9-1-1 in these situations:

- The patient is having difficulty breathing or if the patient's lips or face have a bluish tinge.
- The patient becomes unconscious or has a convulsion.
- The patient exhibits unmanageable behavior, such as being physically abusive, hurting self, or engaging in uncontrollable activity.

For example, Tamoxifen competes with estradiol receptors in breast tumors that are estrogen and progesterone receptor positive. Raloxifene blocks estrogen in the breast. Aromatase inhibitors (Arimidex, Femara, and Aromasin) reduce the amount of estrogen produced in postmenopausal women by blocking the conversion of androgens to estrogens. Antiandrogen (flutamide) and luteinizing hormone–releasing hormone block testosterone synthesis in patients with prostate cancer. The side effects of hormonal therapy are similar to the action of the hormone used or suppression of the normal hormone. For example, women may experience symptoms similar to menopause, including hot flashes, vaginal dryness, and weight gain. Other side effects include nausea, myalgia, arthralgia, and blood clots. Ultimately, patients are at a higher risk of osteoporosis secondary to decreased hormone levels.

Biotherapy

Biotherapy modifies the biologic processes that result in malignant cells primarily by targeting the cancer cells directly or, indirectly, by enhancing the person's own immune response against cancer. Treatment includes natural substances from organisms or laboratory-made versions of these substances. Immunotherapy enhances the individual's immune system response to cancer. Monoclonal antibodies target cancer cells by binding to a specific target antigen to inactivate or destroy cancer cells. Targeted therapies interfere with specific molecules that are involved in tumor growth and progression. Various types of biotherapies are discussed below.

The theory underlying tumor immunology is that most tumor cells have a structural appearance recognizable by the immune cells. *Tumor-associated antigens (TAAs)* exist on tumor cells but not on normal cells. TAAs elicit an immune

BOX 14.4
Nursing Care of Patients Receiving Chemotherapy

Careful assessment and monitoring of the patient receiving chemotherapy, including appropriate laboratory testing, alerts the nurse to the onset of adverse effects:

- Nausea and vomiting
- Diarrhea
- Mucositis and stomatitis (inflammation and ulceration of mucous membranes)
- Alopecia
- Skin changes
- Anorexia
- Fatigue

These side effects require specific medical and nursing actions (discussed later in this chapter under the appropriate nursing diagnoses). Indicators of organ toxicities, such as nephrotoxicity, neurotoxicity, or cardiac toxicity, must be reported to the physician immediately.

Patient education to manage side effects of chemotherapy should include:

- How to care for vascular access sites: Proper hand hygiene, sterile barriers to protect vascular access site, chlorhexidine to clean the insertion site, and timely removal of old catheters (ONS, 2018)
- How to dispose of used equipment and excretions safely
- Encourage the patient to increase fluid intake and get extra rest
- Identify major complications of their particular drug protocol
- When to call the physician or emergency medical services
- Signs and symptoms of neutropenia, thrombocytopenia, and anemia

Psychosocial issues during chemotherapy are:

- The patient and caregivers may need to plan activities around chemotherapy treatments as side effects can impair the patient's ability to work, manage a household or care for family members, function sexually, or participate in social and recreational activities
- Weight loss and alopecia may prompt feelings of powerlessness and depression. The nurse can assist by carefully evaluating manifestations, providing specific interventions, and allowing patients opportunities to express their fears, concerns, and feelings.
- Patients should be encouraged to participate in their care and maintain control over their life as much as possible.

response that, in an individual with a competent immune system, destroys or inhibits tumor growth. TAAs can be isolated from serum and used for both diagnosis and various treatment modalities. PSA is one such TAA currently used for the screening of prostate cancer.

As previously discussed, the immune system naturally protects individuals from the development of cancer. *Tumor-infiltrating lymphocytes (TILs)* indicate that there is an immune response to the tumor. However, tumors utilize various methods to avoid immune system detection, such as decreasing expression of tumor antigens and secreting substances that either inactivate or suppress the immune response and promote tumor cell growth.

Biotherapy is an example of precision medicine. Healthcare providers utilize precision medicine by examining the genetic changes of a tumor that allow it to grow and spread. In order to detect these genetic changes, the tumor is biopsied for DNA sequencing, genomic testing, molecular profiling, or tumor profiling. Once a genetic change is identified, healthcare providers determine if a treatment exists to target that change. Oftentimes, these treatments have less side effects than chemotherapy. One example of precision medicine is the identification of an *epidermal growth factor receptor (EGFR)* in non–small cell lung cancer (NSCLC). EGFR is a protein on cells involved in cell replication. Some individuals with NSCLC express higher amounts of EGFR, thus making the tumor more aggressive. Drugs that block EGFR can slow down cell growth. Because only individuals with NSCLC who express higher amounts of EGFR can be treated with EGFR, this treatment is an example of precision medicine.

Side effects of biotherapy are related to the stimulation of the immune system. The most common side effects are flulike symptoms (fever, myalgia, arthralgia, hypotension/hypertension, nausea and vomiting, chills, weakness, dizziness, fatigue, headache). The nurse must be aware that life-threatening hypersensitivity reactions may occur. Immune checkpoint inhibitors most often affect the skin, gastrointestinal tract, lungs, neuroendocrine system, musculoskeletal system, kidneys, blood, cardiovascular system, eyes, and nervous system (Brahmer et al., 2018). Adverse effects secondary to treatment should be ruled out for all patients who present with new signs and symptoms. Immune checkpoint inhibitors can cause autoimmune syndromes, so the risks and benefits should be carefully discussed with patients who have a history of autoimmune disorders (these patients have been excluded from clinical trials).

Monoclonal Antibodies

Monoclonal antibodies (MAbs) are a type of targeted therapy produced in the laboratory. MAbs are designed to recognize a specific antigen, ligand, or receptor that is involved in tumor cells growth, proliferation, or apoptosis and block signaling pathways (Hafeez, Gan, & Scott, 2018). One example of a monoclonal antibody is the use of trastuzumab (Herceptin) in patients with breast cancer. Approximately 15 to 30% of women diagnosed with breast cancer present with tumors that are associated with Her-2/neu receptor overexpression. Overexpression of Her-2/neu increases the risk of metastasis and is associated with a poor prognosis, which represents a target for selective monoclonal antibody therapy with trastuzumab (Maximiano, Magalhães, Guerreiro, & Morgado, 2016). Trastuzumab inhibits Her-2/neu by binding to the extracellular portion of the receptor to inhibit initial signal transduction, thus inhibiting growth, proliferation, and angiogenesis. Trastuzumab is considered the first-line therapy for patients with Her-2/neu positive breast cancer and is more effective when combined with chemotherapy (Maximiano et al., 2016). Side effects of trastuzumab include reversible cardiac toxicity and drug resistance.

Chimeric Antigen Receptor T-Cell Therapy

Chimeric antigen receptor T-cell (CART) therapy utilizes a chimeric antigen receptor, or a synthetic protein that directs a patient's own T cells to target cancerous cells. More specifically, the treatment genetically modifies a patient's T cells to express a chimeric antigen receptor that is designed to target a specific antigen on a malignant cell. These modified T cells trigger a cytotoxic reaction against the malignant cells. One example of this treatment that has been highly successful in the treatment of B-cell acute lymphoblastic leukemia (ALL) is CD19 CART therapy. CD19 is an antigen expressed on malignant B cells, thus T cells are genetically modified to target CD19.

Immune Checkpoint Inhibitors

Programmed death 1 (PD-1) is an immune checkpoint protein expressed on T cells. When PD-1 binds to its partner protein, programmed death ligand 1 (PD-L1), on both normal and abnormal tissue, the immune response is turned off. Under normal circumstances, this prevents an overly heightened T-cell response that can damage normal tissue. However, some cancer cells may overexpress PD-L1 to evade immune system detection. Therefore, by blocking the binding of PD-L1 (on tumor cells) to PD-1 (on T cells), T cells can detect cancerous cells, thus enhancing immune function against cancer. Nivolumab (Opdivo) and pembrolizumab (Keytruda) are two examples of PD-1 immune checkpoint inhibitors that are currently being used for NSCLC; melanoma; renal, bladder, and head and neck cancer; and Hodgkin lymphoma. Another example of an immune checkpoint protein is cytotoxic T-lymphocyte antigen-4 (CTLA-4). CTLA-4 binds with B7 proteins on antigen presenting cells and blocks the activation and proliferation of T cells (Cooper, Alrajhi, & Durand, 2017). Iplimumamb (Yervoy) is an example of a CTLA-4 inhibitor, which is currently being used to treat metastatic melanoma.

Immune Modulating Agents

Immune modulating agents enhance the body's immune system response. Cytokines are proteins that are naturally produced in the body and secreted by white blood cells to regulate immune function. Cytokines include interferons (INFs), interleukins (ILs), and hematopoietic growth factors (e.g., granulocyte macrophage colony-stimulating factor [GM-CSF] or granulocyte colony-stimulating factor

[G-CSF]). INFs activate natural killer and dendritic cells, while inhibiting cell proliferation and promoting apoptosis. Interleukin-2, a type of IL, enhances the immune response to cancer by increasing WBC proliferation (e.g., natural killer cells) and enhances antibody production by B cells to target malignant cells. GM-CSF and G-CSF treat the immune-depleting side effects of chemotherapy by increasing the production of WBCs, thus decreasing the risk of infection.

IFN–α may cause mental slowing, confusion, fatigue, and lethargy; combination therapy of 5-fluorouracil or IL-2 and IFN–α may cause severe flulike symptoms, with chills and fever of 39.4° to 41.1°C (103° to 106°F), nausea and vomiting, diarrhea, anorexia, severe fatigue, and stomatitis. The nurse should monitor enzymes and other appropriate biochemical indicators for acute alterations in renal, cardiac, liver, or gastrointestinal functioning, which can be side effects of IL-2.

Nursing care for patients receiving immunotherapy are outlined in **Box 14.5**.

Radiation Therapy

Still the treatment of choice for some tumors and of some oncologists, radiation may be used to kill the tumor, reduce its size, decrease pain, or relieve obstruction. Lymph nodes and adjacent tissues are irradiated when metastasis is suspected. **Radiation therapy** consists of delivering ionizing radiations of gamma and x-rays in one of two ways:

- ***External radiation***, also called *teletherapy*, involves delivery of radiation from a source at some distance from the patient. A relatively uniform dosage is delivered to the tumor.
- ***Internal radiation***, also called **brachytherapy**, is a process in which radiation is given inside the body by implanting small amounts of radioactive material directly into a tumor or body cavity while avoiding scattering radiation to the surrounding tissues or organs. This technique allows delivery of high doses of radiation to the tumor while sparing adjacent tissue. Brachytherapy is referred to as internal, interstitial, or intracavitary radiation. Among patients with breast cancer, the innovation of brachytherapy uses a MammoSite catheter to provide accelerated partial breast irradiation and holds the promise of reducing the risk of radiation-induced complications.

Another strategy is *intraoperative radiation therapy (IORT)*, in which radiation is administered while the patient is on the operating table and radiosensitive, nondiseased organs that may be damaged by radiation therapy are shielded from the radiation field. This technique allows a larger dose of penetrating radiation to be directed to the tumor bed with less trauma to vulnerable tissues or organs.

Intensity-modulated radiation therapy (IMRT) is an advanced radiotherapy that delivers a precise radiation dose to the tumor, while sparing normal surrounding tissue. IMRT uses multiple radiation beams; the dose and direction of these beams are determined with the use of imaging techniques (e.g., CT, MRI) and computerized calculations to direct the dose-intensity pattern. Most importantly the radiation dose is able to account for the tumor's three-dimensional shape and spare adjacent nonmalignant tissue. Radiation is delivered by computerized linear accelerators and the field of radiation comes from multiple directions to tailor radiotherapy delivery to the tumor shape.

Proton therapy is an emerging type of radiation therapy, often used in pediatric and young adults to protect vulnerable organs that are in close proximity to the tumor. Compared to conventional radiation therapy, which delivers energy through x-ray beams, proton therapy uses protons to deliver energy. The benefit of proton therapy is that the proton beams release their energy to the target tissue only and cause less damage to surrounding tissue. This is

BOX 14.5
Nursing Care of the Patient Receiving Immunotherapy

Nursing Responsibilities

- Evaluate response to therapy by conducting a thorough evaluation of patient's symptoms and provide interventions to manage symptoms as needed, such as fatigue and depression.
- Assess patient's coping behaviors and teach new strategies as needed.
- Encourage self-care and participation in decision making.
- If patient is unable to manage alone, teach medication administration and care of equipment to caregivers.
- The nurse should assess and document at each patient encounter.
- The American Society of Clinical Oncology has published guidelines on managing immune checkpoint inhibitor toxicities. Toxicities are reported as grade 1 to 4 for each organ system. Generally, therapy is continued for grade 1 toxicities and held for most grade 2 toxicities until symptoms/laboratory values improve to grade 1. High-dose corticosteroids are administered for grade 3 toxicities, and treatment is held until symptoms/laboratory values improve to grade 1. Grade 4 toxicities typically result in a permanent discontinuation of treatment.
- Nurses administering biotherapies need to receive chemotherapy and biotherapy certification and should review American Society of Clinical Oncology (ASCO) and institution guidelines.

Health Education for the Patient and Family

- Minimize symptoms by managing fever and flulike symptoms: Increase fluid intake, take analgesic and antipyretic medications, and maintain bedrest until symptoms abate.
- Seek help for serious problems not managed by usual means, such as dehydration from diarrhea.
- Identify how to work and care for ambulatory pumps when medication is administered through a vascular access device.

particularly beneficial for pediatric patients as their organs are rapidly developing and are in closer proximity.

Lethal injury to DNA is believed to be the primary mechanism by which radiation kills cells, especially cells in faster-growing tumors and tissues. As a result, when given over time, radiation can destroy not only rapidly multiplying cancer cells but also rapidly dividing normal cells, such as those of the skin and mucous membranes. A malignant tumor is considered cured when there are no surviving tumor stem cells. The goal of radiation therapy is to achieve maximum tumor control with minimum damage to normal tissue.

Implanted radiation can be dangerous for those living with, taking care of, or treating the patient. Caregivers must use protection by, for example, shielding themselves from the source of radiation, limiting the time of exposure to the patient, increasing the distance from the patient, and using specific safety procedures for handling secretions. **Box 14.6** identifies safety principles to be followed by those caring for patients undergoing internal radiation.

Tumors have different sensitivities to radiation. Tumors that have the greatest number of rapidly proliferating cancer cells usually exhibit the best early response to radiation. The decision to use radiation rather than other modalities is based on balancing the probability of controlling the tumor against the probability of causing complications, such as tissue damage. The decision is usually made via a risk–benefit analysis. In addition, healthcare providers will determine if radiation should be used in conjunction with other modalities such as surgery or chemotherapy. For patients with breast cancer, radiation therapy is often administered after surgery to treat remaining microscopic cells postsurgery. Planning for radiation therapy includes assessing the disease site, tumor size, and histologic findings. Treatment schedules vary based on these factors. The patient receiving external radiation may experience skin changes such as blanching, erythema, desquamation, sloughing, or hemorrhage. Ulcerations of mucous membranes may cause severe pain; in addition, oral secretions can decrease, making the patient more vulnerable to infection and dental caries. Gastrointestinal effects include nausea and vomiting, diarrhea, or bleeding. Lungs may develop interstitial exudate, a condition called *radiation pneumonia*. Occasionally, external radiation therapy may cause fistulas or necrosis of adjacent tissues. Implanted radioactive materials can lead to similar problems; moreover, the excretory products of these patients are usually considered dangerous and require special disposal.

Radiodermatitis secondary to ionizing radiation can result in erythematous rashes, desquamation, and even necrosis. The nurse should be aware that months to years after radiotherapy, patients may have delayed wound healing, fibrosis, and atrophy. Other changes that can occur include changes to the pigment of the skin, development of telangiectasia, and photosensitivity. Recall radiodermatitis is an acute inflammatory toxicity that occurs at the site of a previous radiation field in response to cytotoxic chemotherapy administration. Integumentary skin reactions can occur in 95% of patients receiving radiotherapy (ONS, 2017c).

See **Box 14.7** for nursing care of patients receiving radiation therapy.

BOX 14.6
Safety Principles for Radiation

These recommendations apply to caregivers working with patients receiving internal radiation (brachytherapy).

- Maintain the greatest possible distance from the source of radiation.
- Spend the minimum amount of time close to the radiation source.
- Shield yourself from the radiation with lead gloves and aprons when possible.
- If pregnant, avoid contact with radiation sources.
- If you work routinely near radiation, wear a monitoring device to measure whole-body exposure.
- Avoid direct exposure with radioisotope containers; for example, do not touch the container.
- Keep patients with implanted radioisotopes in a private room with a private bath and as far away from other hospitalized individuals as possible.
- Dispose of body fluids of patients with unsealed implanted radioisotopes with special care and in specially marked containers.
- Handle bed linens and clothing with care and according to agency protocol.
- Use long-handled forceps to place any dislodged implants into a lead container.
- Consult with the radiation therapy department for any questions or problems in caring for patients with radioactive implants.

Bone Marrow and Peripheral Blood Stem Cell Transplantations

Bone marrow transplantation (BMT), also called *hematopoietic stem cell transplantation (HSCT or SCT)*, is a treatment to stimulate nonfunctioning marrow or to replace marrow. BMT is given as an intravenous infusion of bone marrow cells from donor to patient. Most commonly used in leukemias, this therapy is being expanded to include treatment of other cancers including melanoma and testicular cancer. Chapter 33 provides an in-depth discussion of this procedure. *Peripheral blood stem cell transplantation (PBSCT)* is the process of removing circulating stem cells from the peripheral blood through apheresis and returning these cells to the patient after dose-intensive chemotherapy. PBSCT has fewer side effects, shorter hospitalization, and lower costs compared to BMT. The biggest risks with BMT are transplant rejection and infection.

Integrative Therapies

Although advances in cancer treatment have increased 5-year survival rates, cancer reoccurrence and the uncertainty about its cure compels some patients to look for complementary therapies. Complementary therapies are therapies that patients choose as a complement to medical treatment. Common complementary therapies for cancer can be categorized

BOX 14.7
Nursing Care of the Patient Receiving Radiation Therapy

There are several considerations for the nurse when caring for patients receiving radiotherapy.

- Assess and manage any complications, usually in collaboration with the radiation oncologist.
- Assist in documenting the results of the therapy; for example, patients receiving radiation for metastases to the spine will show improved neurologic functioning as tumor size diminishes.
- Provide emotional support, relief of physical and psychologic discomfort, and opportunities to talk about fears and concerns. For some patients, radiation therapy is a last chance for cure or even for relief of physical discomfort.

EXTERNAL RADIATION

Prior to the start of treatments, the treatment area will be specifically located by the radiation oncologist and marked with colored semipermanent ink or tattoos. Treatment is usually given 5 days per week for 15 to 30 minutes per day over 2 to 7 weeks.

Nursing Responsibilities

- Monitor for adverse effects: Skin changes, such as erythema, desquamation, necrosis, or hemorrhage; ulcerations of mucous membranes; nausea and vomiting, diarrhea, or gastrointestinal bleeding (ONS, 2017b, 2017c).
- Assess lungs for rales, which may indicate interstitial exudate. Observe for any dyspnea or changes in respiratory pattern.
- Identify and record any medications that the patient will be taking during the radiation treatment.
- Monitor for neutropenia and thrombocytopenia (ONS, 2018)

Health Education for the Patient and Family

- Wash the skin with a mild soap and apply moisturizer, especially for patients who have lymphedema. Maintaining clean and moisturized skin will help prevent skin breakdown and infection (ONS, 2017c). Choose a moisturizer without fragrance or lanolin.
- Avoid use of aluminum-containing deodorants to prevent any interaction with external-beam radiation treatment (ONS, 2017c).
- Be careful not rub, scratch, or scrub treated skin areas.
- Apply neither heat nor cold (e.g., heating pad or ice pack) to the treatment site.
- Inspect the skin for damage or serious changes, and report these to the radiologist or physician.
- Wear loose, soft clothing over the treated area.
- Protect skin from sun exposure during and after treatment. Cover skin with protective clothing and use sun-blocking agents that are PABA free with a sun protection factor (SPF) of at least 30.
- External radiation poses no risk to other people for radiation exposure, even with intimate physical contact.
- Be sure to get plenty of rest and eat a balanced diet.

INTERNAL RADIATION

The radiation source, called an *implant*, is placed into the affected tissue or body cavity and is sealed in tubes, containers, wires, seeds, capsules, or needles. An implant may be temporary or permanent. Internal radiation may be ingested or injected as a solution into the bloodstream or a body cavity or be introduced into the tumor through a catheter. The radioactive substance may transmit rays outside the body or be excreted in body fluids.

Nursing Responsibilities

- Place the patient in a private room.
- Limit visits to 10 to 30 minutes, and have visitors sit at least 6 feet from the patient.
- Monitor for side effects such as burning sensations, excessive perspiration, chills and fever, nausea and vomiting, or diarrhea.
- Assess for fistulas or necrosis of adjacent tissues.

Health Education for the Patient and Family

- While a temporary implant is in place, stay in bed and rest quietly to avoid dislodging the implant.
- For outpatient treatments, avoid close contact with others until treatment has been discontinued.
- If the radiologist indicates the need for such measures, dispose of excretory materials in special containers or in a toilet not used by others.
- Carry out daily activities as able; get extra rest if feeling fatigued.
- Eat a balanced diet; frequent, small meals are often better tolerated.
- Contact the nurse or physician for any concerns or questions after discharge.

into botanical agents, nutritional supplements, dietary regimens, mind–body modalities, energy healing, spiritual approaches, and miscellaneous therapies. **Box 14.8** provides information about complementary therapies.

To provide sensitive nursing care, nurses should be knowledgeable about common complementary therapies. It is important for nurses to provide truthful, nonjudgmental responses to patients' inquiries about complementary therapies. Nurses should encourage patients to report the use of any complementary therapies to their oncologist to prevent potential interactions of those therapies with their medical treatment.

Pain Management

Pain management is an important component of oncology care as adequate pain management is associated with improved quality of life (National Comprehensive Cancer Network [NCCN], 2018). Approximately 40% of patients with cancer report moderate to severe pain, with rates as high as 66% among patients with advanced or terminal disease (Van den Beuken-van Everdignen, Hochstenbach, Joosten, Tjan-Heijnen, & Janssen, 2016). There are three main categories of pain syndromes in patients with cancer, and the category influences the type of treatment:

- ***Pain associated with direct tumor involvement***. The most common causes are metastases to bone, nerve compression or infiltration, and involvement of hollow visceral organs.
- ***Pain associated with treatment***. This may include postsurgical incisional or wound pain; peripheral

BOX 14.8
Common Integrative Therapies for Cancer

TYPE	DESCRIPTION
Botanical agents	Many people believe that herbs are the most natural and safe plants that can be ingested with the hope that they will cure cancer. The safety for many of these botanical agents has not been proven, especially as a complement to medical treatment. Commonly used botanical agents include echinacea, Essiac, ginseng, green tea, pau d'arco, and Hoxsey.
Nutritional supplements	Chemical compounds that include vitamins, minerals, enzymes, amino acids, and essential fatty acids or proteins (such as shark cartilage) are believed to have the ability to promote health and help cure cancer. The safety of certain compounds such as vitamins has been established; however, in megadoses, many of the compounds can be toxic and have potential interactions with some therapeutic agents used for cancer such as chemotherapy.
Dietary regimens	The ingestion of only natural substances is believed to have the effect of purifying the body and slowing down the growth of cancer. Popular regimens include the grape diet, the carrot juice diet, and garlic, onion, and liver intake. The effectiveness of these dietary regimens remains to be established.
Mind–body modalities	The harmony of mind and body is believed to facilitate physiologic and psychologic healing. Such modalities include relaxation, yoga, hypnosis, tai chi, art therapy, meditation, or imagery. Recent research has shown that these modalities alleviate side effects such as nausea and vomiting and pain and improve psychosocial well-being and quality of life (Carlson et al., 2017).
Energy healing	The human body is believed to be an energy field and cancer might be the result of a disturbed energy field. Energy therapies, such as therapeutic touch and healing touch, can affect the energy field of the human body and promote physiologic healing. Therapeutic touch uses the hands on or near the body with the intent to promote healing. Healing touch uses energy healing techniques to heal by restoring the harmony and balance of the body. Clinical practice and research on energy healing have shown positive findings of energy healing in a variety of patients.
Spiritual approaches	Faith in God or a higher power of the universe is believed to help cancer healing. Spiritual approaches include faith healing, prayer to God, prayer groups, and chain prayer. Research has shown that faith in God or a higher power helped individuals with cancer to adjust to the experience of cancer.
Miscellaneous therapies	Aromatherapy has been used for patients with cancer to relieve nausea and vomiting or retching and to decrease anxiety. However, aromatherapy might not be appropriate for patients who are highly sensitive to strong fragrance. Music, art, and humor therapies have been used to help patients with cancer to reduce anxiety, express feelings of loss, and promote optimism.

neuropathy, ulceration of mucous membranes, and pain from herpes zoster outbreaks secondary to chemotherapy; and pain in nerve plexuses, muscles, and peripheral nerves from radiation therapy.

- ***Pain from a cause not related to either the cancer or therapy***, such as diabetic neuropathy.

The American Society of Clinical Oncology recommends screening patients for pain during each encounter to determine whether comprehensive pain management is needed for patients with complex needs (Paice et al., 2016). Assessment of pain must include tools that are evidence-based and allow for the nurse to document pain outcomes (Sundaramurthi, Gallagher, & Sterling, 2017). Pain management should be comprehensive, in that it addresses the complex biopsychosocial components of pain and incorporates both pharmacologic and nonpharmacologic modalities (NCCN, 2018).

According to the National Comprehensive Cancer Network (2018) guidelines, opioids may be prescribed to manage moderate to severe pain. They may also be prescribed to patients who do not respond to other, more conservative therapies or if patients experience distress or functional impairment (Paice et al., 2016). It is important for nurses to be aware of increased tolerance to ensure pain is adequately managed and carefully consider the risk of analgesic misuse. If patients are prescribed opioids, the nurse must ensure that educational materials are provided to the patient and family or caregiver in a format that is understandable (NCCN, 2018). This education must include the risks and benefits of opioid therapy and how to safely store and dispose of narcotics (Sundaramurthi et al., 2017).

According to NCCN (2018), there are five goals of pain management:

1. Provide/optimize analgesia
2. Optimize activities of daily living
3. Minimize adverse effects
4. Avoid aberrant drug use
5. Optimize patient affect.

To provide adequate pain management, a multidisciplinary team should be used that incorporates psychosocial support. The nurse must also assess for various barriers to adequate pain management including regulatory, legislative, or economic (Sundaramurthi et al., 2017). The healthcare system in which a nurse works is responsible for implementing institutional guidelines to adequately manage cancer pain.

Pharmacologic pain management follows these steps:

1. Conduct careful initial and ongoing assessment of the pain.
2. Evaluate the patient's functional goals.
3. Establish a plan that uses combinations of nonnarcotic drugs (such as aspirin or ibuprofen) with adjuvants (such as corticosteroids or antidepressants).
4. Evaluate the degree of pain relief.
5. Progress to stronger drugs as needed, from mild narcotics such as oxycodone (Percodan) or hydrocodone (Vicodan) to strong narcotics such as morphine or hydromorphone (Dilaudid), and monitor side effects.
6. Continue to try combinations and escalate dosages until maximal pain relief balanced with a patient's need to function is achieved.

Medication is usually administered by the oral route as long as this route continues to be effective. Medication is given on a regular time schedule (e.g., every 4 hours) with additional medication prescribed to cover breakthrough pain. When the oral route alone becomes inadequate, the primary narcotic can be administered intramuscularly, subcutaneously, or rectally on an intermittent schedule; continuously by transdermal patches; or intravenously by a continuous drip, usually controlled by an infusion pump. Some newer pumps are portable, deliver medication continuously, and allow patients to control their breakthrough pain with a limited number of boluses. Other therapies include injection of anesthetic drugs into spinal cord or specific nerve plexuses, surgical severing of nerves, radiation to reduce tumor size and pressure, and behavioral approaches.

Side effects of narcotics, such as constipation, nausea and vomiting, and itching, can be managed through the usual means and are discussed under the appropriate nursing diagnoses. If the patient has persistent untoward side effects that do not respond to treatment or if the patient does not get adequate relief from the narcotic, different narcotics and combinations are tried. Patients receiving high-dose narcotics should not have the medication abruptly stopped because withdrawal symptoms will occur. If the drug needs to be stopped, it must be tapered gradually. For more information on pain management, and on alternative therapies in particular, refer to Chapter 9.

Nursing Care

Nurses face a major challenge in educating patients about preventive measures and lifestyle changes to reduce the risk of cancer. At the same time, patients with cancer must be reassured that they are not responsible for having acquired cancer.

Once a cancer diagnosis is established, nurses help patients recover and support them during the rehabilitation phase. In cases of terminal cancer, nurses provide comfort and facilitate positive growth for the patient and significant others.

Assessment

The assessment chapters in this text contain questions about manifestations and risk factors for cancer that involves specific body systems.

Health History. Examples of appropriate questions to elicit information during a health history assessment follow. They are appropriate for use during the initial interview and at subsequent assessments:

- "What brought you in to see the doctor?" *Asking this question allows patients to tell their story in their own way, which may elicit more information than asking specific questions. The answer should elicit not only data about the signs and symptoms but also fears or concerns. If the cancer was discovered during a routine physical examination or checkup, the patient may have some difficulty accepting the disease, especially if there were no symptoms. For patients who offer insufficient information in response to this open-ended question, more specific questions may be necessary, such as "Did you have pain or any specific physical problems that caused you to seek healthcare?"*
- "Are any other medical conditions or problems troubling you at this time?" *It may be necessary to ask about specific diseases to help the patient focus. For example, "Do you have high blood pressure?" or "Are you having any problems with your lungs?" Information gained from these questions can help you anticipate problems and formulate potential nursing diagnoses related to other diseases that may interact with the cancer.*
- "Describe the kinds of physical problems you are having at this time. Do you have pain? How has your appetite and food intake been? Have you experienced a recent weight change? Tell me how well you are able to carry out your usual daily activities. How has your illness affected your mood or outlook on life?" *For each positive response, ask follow-up questions to narrow down or define the exact nature of the problem. These data help identify what nursing diagnoses should be included in the care plan.*
- "What options has your physician suggested for treating your cancer?" *The answer will indicate patients' knowledge about their treatment and, possibly, their communication with the physician. Often, under the stress of a cancer diagnosis, patients do not hear or understand what the physician is saying and are afraid to ask questions. Lack of knowledge indicates a need to collaborate with the physician to explain the information to the patient so that the patient can absorb and understand it.* If the patient has a good understanding of the treatment plan, discussing how he or she feels about it can be useful in exposing fears, concerns, and emotional responses.
- "What do you expect to happen as a result of this treatment?" *The answer may reveal unrealistic expectations or lack of understanding of consequences of the treatment.*
- "What effects are the disease and/or treatment having on your ability to carry on with your usual daily activities?" *Additional questions may be needed to pinpoint the types of limitations. The response to this question should provide information on the patient's functional status (see* **Box 14.9***). This information can be used to identify the need to collaborate with professionals from other disciplines. For example, if the patient is the sole financial support of the family and is unable to work, a social worker may be able to*

BOX 14.9
Example of an Instrument for Assessing Functional Status for Cancer Patients: Eastern Cooperative Oncology Group (ECOG) Scale

0 Fully active, able to carry out all predisease activities without restriction

1 Restricted in physically strenuous activity, but ambulatory and able to carry out work of a light or sedentary nature, for example, light housework or office work

2 Ambulatory and capable of all self-care, but unable to carry out work activities. Up and about more than 50% of waking hours

3 Capable of only limited self-care, confined to bed or chair 50% or more of waking hours

4 Completely disabled, cannot carry out any self-care, totally confined to bed or chair.

Source: Non-Small Cell Lung Cancer Collaborative Group, 1995.

help with resources; if the patient is extremely weak, referral to a physical therapist may help with energy conservation strategies and strengthening exercises.

- "Who is available to help you at home and run errands for you? Who can provide transportation for you to get to your appointments or treatments? Who can you rely on to be a good listener when you're sad or to be a comfortable companion? Have you identified someone to make healthcare decisions for you if there is a time when you are unable to make them for yourself?" *When the person with cancer is the one who usually takes care of everyone else, asking for help may be difficult for this person. This information can identify how much support and help the patient has access to. The last question introduces the concept of advanced directives and durable power of attorney regarding healthcare (refer to Chapter 5).*
- "How do you manage your stress or your feelings of discomfort? What helps you feel better? Do you think these measures work well for you?" *The responses to these questions provide information about the patient's coping strategies and may identify maladaptive strategies such as alcohol or drug use. Lack of appropriate coping methods can interfere with the patient's response to treatment and decrease overall quality of life.*

Physical Assessment. As soon as the patient is admitted to the healthcare service or agency, conduct a complete physical assessment to establish a baseline for subsequent evaluation of later changes. It is especially important to document the nutritional status of the patient using anthropomorphic measurements (i.e., height, weight, body fat, muscle mass, body mass index, and body composition) and to evaluate laboratory results and note any specific signs and symptoms. **Table 14.11** compares the manifestations of good nutrition with those of malnutrition.

It is important to assess the patient's hydration status, especially if the patient is not taking oral food and fluids well or is having bouts of vomiting. Specific assessments for hydration status include:

- Intake and output
- Rapid weight changes
- Skin turgor and moisture
- Venous filling
- Vital sign changes
- Tongue furrows and moisture
- Eyeball softness
- Lung sounds
- Laboratory values.

Other recommended assessments are discussed under the specific nursing diagnoses that follow. They can also be found in other chapters that address specific body systems affected by the cancer.

Table 14.11 Signs of Nutritional Status

System	Good Nutrition	Poor Nutrition
General	Alert, energetic, good endurance, psychologically stable Weight within range for height, age, body size	Withdrawn, apathetic, easily fatigued, irritable Over- or underweight
Integumentary	Skin glowing, good turgor, smooth, free of lesions Hair shiny, lustrous, minimal loss	Skin dull, pasty, scaly-dry, bruises, multiple lesions Hair brittle, dull, falls out easily
Head, eyes, ears, nose, and throat	Eyes bright, clear, no fatigue circles Oral mucous membranes pink-red and moist Gums pink, firm Tongue pink, moderately smooth, no swelling	Eyes dull, conjunctiva pale, discoloration under eyes Oral mucous membranes pale Gums red, spongy, and bleed easily Tongue bright to dark red, swollen
Abdomen	Abdomen flat, firm	Abdomen scaphoid (concave), flaccid, or distended (ascites)
Musculoskeletal	Firm, well-developed muscles Good posture No skeletal changes	Flaccid muscles, wasted appearance Stooped posture Skeletal malformations
Neurologic	Good attention span, good concentration, astute thought processes Good reflexes	Inattentive, easily distracted, impaired thought processes Paresthesias, reflexes diminished or hyperactive

Diagnoses, Outcomes, and Interventions

Nursing goals focus on supporting the whole person as well as their caregivers by providing interventions for specific problems such as pain, poor nutrition, dehydration, fatigue, poor psychosocial outcomes, altered individual and family coping, and the side effects of medical treatment. Ultimately, nursing care should focus on improving patient quality of life. Because cancer affects the whole family, nursing care includes everyone involved with the patient from the time of diagnosis through the entire disease and treatment process. Many diagnoses are pertinent to patients with cancer; this section addresses only the most common diagnoses. See the Case Study & Nursing Care Plan on page 442.

Relieve Anxiety. Early in the disease process (i.e., during diagnosis and treatment), patients may experience shock, denial, and despair, which can lead to anxiety, irritability, and changes in mood. This initial distress may be related to medical, patient, societal, or cultural factors. It is important for the nurse to evaluate the patient during this time and provide customized and appropriate support as needed (Mehta & Roth, 2015). Such psychologic and emotional disturbance may result from the anticipation of pain, disfigurement, or the threat of death. In particular, patients whose coping skills have been poor in the past may have a difficult time managing the diagnosis. The patient may manifest overt signs of anxiety: Trembling, restlessness, irritability, hyperactivity, stimulation of the sympathetic nervous system (increased blood pressure, pulse, respiration, excessive perspiration, pallor), withdrawal, worried facial expressions, and poor eye contact. The patient may report insomnia and feelings of tension and apprehension or express concerns regarding perceived changes brought about by the disease and fear of future events. The nurse should be aware that anxiety is often highest at the time of diagnosis and may improve with time (Smith, Cope, Sherner, & Walker, 2014).

Expected Outcome: Patient will be free of or have a decreased level of anxiety related to their cancer diagnosis and treatment.

The nurse will:

- Carefully assess the patient's level of anxiety, being mindful of patients with a lack of social support, advanced disease, functional limitations, or a history of trauma or anxiety disorders (Smith et al., 2014).
- When assessing patients for signs and symptoms of anxiety, ask about sleep habits and functional limitations (e.g., activities of daily living, ability to concentrate) (Smith et al., 2014).
- Assess level of anxiety with validated and approved tools (e.g., Distress Thermometer, General Anxiety Disorder–7 scale, Hospital Anxiety and Depression Scale [HADS], and State–Trait Anxiety Inventory [STAI]) (Smith et al., 2014).
- The nurse should work with the patient to determine appropriate interventions to manage anxiety. Activities that may help include yoga, art therapy, music therapy, massage, or mindfulness-based stress reduction (Smith et al., 2014). The nurse should provide an appropriate list of referrals for patients who may benefit from cognitive-behavioral therapy or pharmacologic interventions such as anxiolytics.
- The nurse is in a unique position to establish a therapeutic relationship by conveying warmth and empathy and listening in a nonjudgmental manner. This can often be done while patients are receiving their treatment. The nurse should also provide appropriate patient education materials and ensure that these are reviewed and understood by the patient.
- Review the coping strategies the patient has used in the past and build on past successful behaviors, introducing new strategies as appropriate. Explain why inappropriate strategies, such as repressing anger or turning to substances such as alcohol, are not helpful. *The patient will be more willing to make changes that build on what has already worked in the past and more likely to reject inappropriate strategies if he or she is educated about their use.*
- Identify resources in the community (such as crisis hotlines and support groups) that can help the patient manage anxiety-producing situations. *The patient may not have support systems available or the patient's significant others may be having their own difficulties in dealing with the cancer diagnosis. Programs such as "I Can Cope," sponsored by the American Cancer Society in most communities, provide education, counseling, and support in a group setting with other cancer patients.*
- Provide specific information for the patient about the disease, its treatment, and what may be expected, especially for those patients with obvious misinformation.
- Use crisis intervention theory to promote growth in the patient and significant others, regardless of the outcome of the disease. *During a major crisis, people can, with assistance, transform the experience from one that causes defeat and despair to one that enhances personal and spiritual growth. If you are not skilled in this area, a referral to an appropriate mental health professional may be helpful to the patient and family.*

Promote Acceptance of Changes to the Body. Cancer and cancer treatments frequently result in major physiologic and psychologic body image changes. Loss of a body part (e.g., amputation, prostatectomy, or mastectomy), skin changes and hair loss from chemotherapy or radiation therapy, disfigurement of a body part (e.g., lymphedema in the affected upper and lower extremities), or creation of unnatural openings on the body for elimination (e.g., colostomy or ileostomy) may have a major effect on the person's self-image. The gaunt, wasted appearance of the patient with cachexia or the draining, malodorous lesions that result when cancer breaks through the skin are other significant etiologies of body-image disturbance. This may give rise to fear of rejection, which plays a major role in sexual dysfunction and relationships. In addition to all of the other challenges the cancer brings about, the patient may undergo major changes in appearance and function. The patient may exhibit a visible physical alteration of some portion of the body, verbalize negative feelings about the body and/or fear of rejection by others, refuse to look at the affected site, and depersonalize the body change or lost part (e.g., by calling the colostomy "that thing").

Expected Outcome: Patient will accept the changes to their body after cancer treatment.

The nurse will:

- Discuss the meaning of the loss or change with the patient. *Doing so helps the nurse discover the best approach for this particular patient and involves the patient more actively in interventions. A small, seemingly trivial loss may have a big impact, especially when viewed in light of the other changes that are occurring in the patient's life. Likewise, a major loss may not be as important as the nurse might imagine. To ensure more appropriate and individualized care, evaluate each situation in terms of the reactions of the specific patient.*
- Observe and evaluate the patient's interaction with significant others. *People who are important to the patient may unintentionally reinforce negative feelings about body image; on the other hand, the patient may perceive rejection where none exists.*
- Allow denial, but do not participate in it; for example, if a patient does not want to look at the wound, the nurse may say, "I am going to change the dressing to your breast incision now." *During the initial stage of shock at the loss of a body part, denial is a protective mechanism and should not be challenged, nor should it be promoted. A matter-of-fact approach and an empathetic attitude will go far to facilitate the eventual acceptance of the change.*
- Assist the patient and significant others to cope with the changes in appearance:
  a. Provide a supportive environment.
  b. Encourage the patient and significant others to express feelings about the situation.
  c. Give matter-of-fact responses to questions and concerns.
  d. Identify new coping strategies to resolve feelings.
  e. Enlist family and friends in reaffirming the patient's worth.
- Teach the patient or significant others to participate in the care of the afflicted body area. Provide support and validation of their efforts. *Active involvement in providing care, such as changing a dressing or emptying a colostomy bag, empowers the patient and/or significant others. This intimate involvement also desensitizes feelings about disfigurement and promotes acceptance and closeness. Positive reinforcement from the nurse encourages them to continue these behaviors.*
- Teach strategies for minimizing physical changes, such as providing skin care during radiation therapy. *Early intervention can limit the negative side effects of treatment and actually promote recovery. Involving the patient provides an additional way for the patient to be in control of a difficult situation.*
- Provide anticipatory guidance regarding alopecia induced by chemotherapy:
  a. Discuss the pattern and timing of hair loss. *This allows the patient to cope with changes and incorporate them into daily activities.*
  b. Refer patient to a wig shop before hair loss is experienced. *Hair color and texture can be matched to minimize obvious changes in appearance. Some patients may prefer to purchase head coverings such as scarves and forgo the use of wigs.*
  c. Refer to support programs such as "Look Good . . . Feel Better," which is sponsored by the American Cancer Society and the Cosmetic, Toilet, and Fragrance Association Foundation. *A support group can diminish feelings of isolation and provide practical tips for managing problems. The American Cancer Society website is a great resource for patients and caregivers to search for local support groups.*
  d. Reassure the patient that hair will grow back after chemotherapy is discontinued, but also inform that the color and texture of the new hair may be different. Hair loss has been identified as one of the most distressing symptoms by many patients. *Interventions to reduce that loss can have a significant impact on body-image concerns. Moreover, knowing what to expect may decrease anxiety and distress.*

Promote Healthy Grieving. Grieving is a response to an actual, anticipated, or perceived loss (Herdman, 2018). Grieving can be a healthy response that allows the patient and family to accept the diagnosis or, when faced with a terminal disease, manage the dying process. Perceived changes in body image and lifestyle can prompt grieving. The patient or significant others may show sorrow, anger, depression, or withdrawal, expressing distress at the potential loss. (Refer to Chapter 5 for more on nursing care of the patient who is grieving or dying.)

Expected Outcome: Patient will use effective and healthy responses to actual, anticipated, or perceived cancer-related losses.

The nurse will:

- Use the therapeutic communication skills of active listening, silence, and nonverbal support to provide an open environment for the patient and significant others to discuss their feelings realistically and to express anger or other negative feelings appropriately. *This helps the patient and family to get in touch with feelings and confront the possibility of the loss or death.*
- Answer questions about illness and prognosis honestly, but always encourage hope. *This allows for realistic appraisal of the situation and planning and it helps combat feelings of hopelessness and depression.*
- Encourage the dying patient to make funeral and burial plans ahead of time and to be sure the will is in order.

Make sure the necessary phone numbers can be easily located. *This gives a sense of control and relieves family members of these concerns at a time when the patient is most in need of their support and when they themselves are extremely stressed.*

- Encourage the patient to continue taking part in activities he or she enjoys, including maintaining employment as long as possible. *This gives a sense of continuity of life even in the face of severe loss.*

Reduce Risk for Infection. Malnutrition, impaired skin and mucous membrane integrity, tumor necrosis, and suppression of the WBCs from chemotherapy or radiation may contribute to the risk for infection. Anorexia, as well as the disease itself, deprives the body of nutrients needed for healing, while impaired integrity of skin and mucous membranes (a result of chemotherapy and/or radiation therapy) compromises the first lines of defense against microbial invasion. Cells in the center of large or not very vascular tumors may die from malnutrition, eventually eroding through tissues to increase the risk of sepsis. Bone marrow depression due to the effects of certain types of cancers and chemotherapy impairs the body's ability to respond to infection. The patient may exhibit the classic signs of infection: Lassitude, fever, anorexia, pain in the affected area, and physical evidence of infection, such as a purulent, draining lesion or wound. If the bone marrow is compromised, the usual signs and symptoms of infection may be absent or reduced.

Expected Outcome: Patient will be free of infections related to cancer or treatment.

The nurse will:

- Monitor vital signs. *Fever and sympathetic nervous system responses, such as increased pulse and respiration, are usual early signs of infection. However, severely immunosuppressed patients may be unable to mount a fever; therefore, the absence of fever cannot rule out infection.*
- Maintain good hand hygiene; use alcohol-based sanitizer for caregivers and patient (ONS, 2018).
- Monitor WBC counts frequently, especially if the patient is receiving chemotherapy known to cause bone marrow suppression. *This allows the nurse to notify the physician at the first sign of diminishing WBC counts so that corrective action can be taken. Colony-stimulating factors (e.g., GM-CSF, G-CSF) may be started as either primary or secondary prophylaxis to prevent infection (ONS, 2018).*
- Teach the patient to avoid crowds, small children, and people with infections when WBC count is at nadir (lowest point during chemotherapy) and to practice scrupulous personal hygiene. *During periods of leukopenia, the patient may lose immunity to his or her own natural flora. Careful attention to hygiene reduces the risk of infection. Crowds, which promote contact with a greater variety of infectious agents, and friends with minor infections can be very dangerous to people who are immunosuppressed. Small children should be avoided because they often have microbes to which most people are usually immune but which the patient may not be able to resist.*
- Protect skin and mucous membranes from injury. Teach appropriate skin care measures, such as good hygiene, use of a moisturizing lotion to prevent dryness and cracking, frequent changes of position for the bed-bound, and immediate attention to skin breaks or lesions. *Ensuring intact skin strengthens the first line of defense against infection.*
- Encourage the patient to consume a diet high in protein, minerals, and vitamins, especially vitamin C. *Improving nutrition decreases the risk of infection. Vitamin C has been shown to help prevent certain types of infection, such as colds.*

Reduce Risk for Injury. In addition to infection, cancer can pose a risk for injury from, for example, obstruction by a large tumor or one located in a limited body space (e.g., in the brain, bowel, or bronchial airways). If the cancer is one that creates ectopic sites of hormones, elevated levels of hormones that are not under the control of the pituitary gland can injure the patient in a variety of ways. Signs of obstruction depend on the organ involved: Bowel obstruction presents with pain, distention, and cessation of bowel activities; obstruction in the brain gives signs of increased intracranial pressure or personality/behavioral change; bronchial obstruction manifests as respiratory distress, cyanosis, and altered arterial blood gases. Ectopic production of parathyroid hormone manifests as high serum calcium levels as well as signs of hypercalcemia; ectopic production of antidiuretic hormone causes fluid retention and manifests as hypertension and peripheral and pulmonary edema.

Expected Outcome: Patient will be free of injuries related to cancer or treatment.

The nurse will:

- Assess frequently for signs and symptoms indicating problems with organ obstruction. *Early detection of major problems allows the nurse to seek medical help before the problem evolves into a physiologic crisis.*
- Teach to differentiate minor problems from those of a serious nature. Encourage the patient to consult with the nurse or physician if in doubt or to call 911 if the patient becomes very ill.
- Monitor laboratory values that may indicate the presence of ectopic functioning and report abnormal findings to physicians immediately. (Refer to Table 14.4 for laboratory indicators of ectopic functions.) *Early detection promotes early medical intervention and prevents serious consequences from the ectopic secretion.* Refer to Chapters 10, 19, and 20 for specific signs and symptoms of electrolyte imbalances and endocrine disorders.

Restore and Promote Adequate Nutrition. Anorexia-cachexia syndrome (described earlier in this chapter) is a common cause of malnutrition in cancer patients. Metabolism increases in response to increased cancer cell production while the cancer's parasitic activity reduces the nutrients available to the body. Loss of appetite, food aversion, nausea and vomiting, and painful oral lesions from chemotherapy or radiation may contribute to impaired nutrition. Tumors of the gastrointestinal tract that affect absorption also contribute to the problem. Manifestations include wasted appearance, considerable weight loss over a relatively short period of time, anthropometric measurements below 85% of standard for fat and muscle tissue, decreases in serum proteins, and negative responses to antigen testing.

Expected Outcome: Patient will restore and maintain balanced nutrition.

The nurse will:

- Assess current eating patterns, including usual likes and dislikes, and identify factors that impair food intake. *This allows for a more individualized plan based on needs and preferences.*
- Evaluate degree of malnutrition:
  a. Check laboratory values for total serum protein, serum albumin and globins, total lymphocyte count, serum transferrin, hemoglobin, and hematocrit. *These values represent the laboratory values that are most likely to decrease with malnutrition.*
  b. Calculate nitrogen balance and creatinine-height index. Calculate skeletal muscle mass, and compare findings to normal ranges. *Urinary creatinine is an index of lean body mass and decreases in malnutrition. Lean muscle mass is catabolized for energy in patients with cancer.*
  c. Take anthropometric measurements and compare them to standards: Height, weight, elbow breadth, arm circumference, triceps skinfold thickness, and arm muscle mass. *This estimates the degree of wasting; findings below 85% of standard are considered malnutrition.*
- Teach the principles of maintaining good nutrition and adapting the diet to medical restrictions and current preferences. *This tailors the food plan to the patient's needs and thereby promotes compliance.*
- Manage problems that interfere with eating:
  a. Encourage eating whatever is appealing and consider adding nutritional supplements such as Ensure Plus or Isocal to diet. *It is better to eat something even if it is not nutritionally balanced.*
  b. Eat small, frequent meals. *These are more easily digested and absorbed and usually better tolerated by the patient with anorexia.*
  c. Encourage to try icy cold foods (such as ice cream) or those that are more highly seasoned if food has no taste. *Chemotherapy and radiation therapy may harm taste buds and prevent distinguishing the taste of foods. Strong seasonings and coldness make food more enjoyable to the patient with diminished taste. However, spicy foods are not recommended for patients with stomatitis.*
  d. Encourage cold and bland semisoft and liquid foods with painful oropharyngeal ulcers; use a nonalcohol anesthetic mouthwash prior to eating. *These foods are less irritating to sensitive mucous membranes; deadening the pain can make chewing and swallowing easier.*
  e. Manage nausea and vomiting by administering antiemetic drugs (around-the-clock medication may be an effective preventive measure). Encourage patient to eat small, frequent, low-fat meals with dry foods such as crackers and toast, to avoid liquids with meals, and to sit upright for an hour after meals. Remove emesis basins, and encourage oral hygiene before eating. *Dry, low-fat foods are more readily tolerated when nauseated. Removing vomiting cues, such as odor and supplies associated with vomiting, can reduce nausea.*
- Teach to supplement meals with nutritional supplements such as Ensure Plus or Isocal and to take multivitamin and mineral tablets with meals. Suggest increasing calories by adding ice cream or frozen yogurt to the liquid supplement or commercial protein-carbohydrate powders to milk or fruit juice. *Because the food intake is usually less than that needed to maintain or gain weight, these supplements can add calories in a manner often tolerated by patients who are ill.*
- Teach to keep a food diary to document daily intake. *If the patient can see how little is being consumed, he or she may eat more. A food diary helps the nurse keep a calorie count and alert the physician if more drastic nutritional measures, such as a feeding tube or parenteral nutrition, need to be instituted.*
- Teach to administer parenteral nutrition via a central line or other VAD. Teach safety measures and care of the VAD, and explain how the pump delivering the solution works. Provide an emergency phone number for help with administration problems. (See Chapter 22 for safety guidelines for administering parenteral nutrition.) *The patient with chronic or terminal cancer requiring parenteral nutrition is usually managed at home, so information on how to manage the entire process may be needed.*

Promote Integrity of Gastrointestinal Tissues. The most common impairment of tissue integrity occurs in the oral–pharyngeal–esophageal mucous membranes. Oral mucositis occurs secondary to the effects of some chemotherapeutic drugs and radiation treatment to the head and neck. The incidence of oral mucositis among patients treated with chemotherapy is approximately 40%, almost 100% among those treated with radiotherapy for head and neck cancer, and approximately 80% among those receiving a hematopoietic stem cell transplant (ONS, 2017b). The oral–pharyngeal–esophageal tissues are lined with cells with a high mitotic turnover rate and are therefore vulnerable to many chemotherapeutic drugs and the damaging effects of radiation. Some patients receiving biotherapies may have adverse effects to the oral cavity, so the nurse should ensure that the patient maintains adequate oral hygiene. Leukemias, bone marrow transplants, and herpes viral infections are other etiologic factors in the disruption of oral–pharyngeal–esophageal tissue.

Manifestations of this problem may include:

- Small ulcers occur on the tongue and mucous membranes in the mouth and throat (however, mucositis can occur anywhere along the gastrointestinal tract)
- Herpes simplex type 1 lesions or vesicles evolve into ulcerations
- Fungal infections, such as thrush (due to *Candida* infections), are manifested by a white, yellow, or tan coating with dry, red, fissured tissue underneath
- Red, swollen, friable gums bleed with minimal or no trauma
- Pain, ranging from mild to severe
- **Xerostomia** is excessive dryness of the mucous membranes (due to chemotherapy or radiation)
- Anorexia, dehydration, malnutrition, and weight loss may present secondary to poor dietary intake.

Expected Outcome: Tissue integrity will be restored and maintained.

The nurse will:

- Carefully assess and evaluate the type of tissue impairment present. Identify possible sources, such as chemotherapy or radiation therapy to head and neck. *This allows the nurse to implement corrective measures appropriate to the type of problem.*
- Implement and teach measures for preventing oropharyngeal infection (ONS, 2017b):
  a. Observe for systemic signs of infection. Be suspicious of any fever that has no apparent cause. *This facilitates early identification of an infection before it spreads.*
  b. Encourage cleaning teeth gently and using a non-alcohol mouthwash several times a day. This can be done after waking up in the morning, after any oral intake, and before bedtime. Soak dentures nightly in hydrogen peroxide and floss gently with waxed floss after meals and at bedtime; this measure may be contraindicated for people with leukemia or thrombocytopenia. *Disrupted mucous membranes allow the normal oral bacterial flora into the systemic circulation, which can result in sepsis in the immunocompromised person. Reducing the oral flora by frequent hygiene decreases the risk of infection.*
  c. Culture any oral lesions, and report the problem to the physician. Herpes lesions may not follow a typical pattern in immunosuppressed patients. *Identifying the cause of the infection, whether viral, fungal, or bacterial, allows the physician to prescribe the appropriate treatment.*
- Implement and teach measures for reducing trauma to delicate tissues:
  a. Counteract xerostomia with lubricating and moisturizing agents, such chewing sugarless gum or sucking on candy. The patient may also use saliva substitutes, mouth rinses, or medicines that can stimulate the salivary glands. *This protects mucous membranes from infection and trauma.*
  b. Avoid putting sharp instruments in the mouth. Use smooth plastic spoons and forks for eating, especially with a bleeding disorder. Dental work should be done by dental oncologists.
  c. Brush teeth with a very soft-bristle toothbrush and obtain a new toothbrush monthly. If gums are friable and bleeding, clean teeth with a soft cloth or toothpaste on finger. Chlorhexidine mouthwash (Peridex) may be used. *This protects gums from trauma and decreases risk of hemorrhage.*
- Administer specific medications as ordered to control infection and/or pain:
  a. Acyclovir is often used to treat viral infections.
  b. Systemic antibiotics are used to treat bacterial infections.
  c. Nystatin or clotrimazole solution for "swish and swallow" or lozenges that dissolve slowly in the mouth are used for fungal infections.
  d. Use viscous Xylocaine or various combination mouthwashes before meals and as needed. These agents reduce pain and inflammation.

Case Study & Nursing Care Plan

A Patient with Cancer

James Casey, age 72, has a history of chronic obstructive pulmonary disease, previous myocardial infarction, and type 1 diabetes mellitus. He reports that he lost his wife from lung cancer 5 years ago and still "misses her terribly." He describes his bad habits as smoking two packs of cigarettes a day for 52 years (a 104 pack/year smoking history), drinking one to two six-packs of beer a week and one "bourbon and water" a night, and eating "a lot of junk food, like French fries." He states that he quit smoking 2 years ago, when he could no longer walk a block without considerable shortness of breath, and just quit drinking alcohol a few weeks ago at his physician's insistence. Six months ago, he was diagnosed with bladder cancer and underwent two 6-week courses of BCG bladder instillations. His latest report indicates that the tumors have grown back and there is evidence of metastasis to pelvic lymph nodes and his spine. Mr. Casey decides to forego further treatment and to be managed at home with hospice care. He asks his daughter Mary to move in with him to provide care and support during his final months. The daughter accepts; she has been informed of the physical and emotional stress this will entail.

ASSESSMENT

Glynis Jackson, RN, Mr. Casey's hospice case manager, completes a health history and physical examination during her first two visits. She gathers this information over 2 days to conserve his strength and allow more time for Mr. Casey and his daughter to talk about their concerns.

Ms. Jackson notes that Mr. Casey is thin and pale, with a wasted appearance and a strained, worried facial expression. He complains of severe back pain no longer adequately relieved by oxycodone/aspirin (Percodan) and hydrocodone/acetaminophen (Vicodin) alternating every 2 to 4 hours. His vital signs are BP 90/50 mmHg, right arm sitting; apical pulse 102 bpm, regular; respirations 24/min and unlabored; breath sounds clear but diminished in the bases; oral temperature 36°C (96.8°F).

A tunneled Groshong catheter as a VAD is present in the right anterior chest. There is no drainage, redness, or swelling at the site. No medication is currently running via the VAD. Mary reports that his urinary output is adequate. Approximately 200 mL of yellow, cloudy, nonmalodorous urine is present in the urinal at the bedside.

Mr. Casey states that he spends most of his time either in bed or sitting up in a chair in his room. He reports that he has no energy and is unable to walk to the bathroom unassisted, dress himself, or manage his own personal hygiene. Ms. Jackson rates Mr. Casey's functional level at ECOG level 4: Capable of only limited self-care, confined to bed or chair 50% or more of waking hours. He tells the nurse that his daughter "is working day and night to help me and is looking awfully tired."

Mary reports that Mr. Casey is eating very poorly, usually eating a small bowl of oatmeal with milk for breakfast and vegetable soup and crackers for lunch, but he wants only fruit juice for dinner. Mr. Casey says that he has no appetite and eats just to please Mary. He does drink at least three to four glasses of water a day plus juice. His fingerstick blood sugars remain within normal range.

His current weight is 120 pounds at 67 inches tall, down from 180 pounds a year ago. He has lost about 30 pounds during the past 2 months.

Available laboratory values from his visit with the physician show the following:

Total protein: 4.1 g/dL (normal range: 6.0 to 8.0 g/dL)
Albumin: 2.2 g/dL (normal range: 3.5 to 5.0 g/dL)
Hemoglobin: 10.2 g/dL (normal range: 13.5 to 18.0 g/dL)
Hematocrit: 30.5% (normal range: 40.0 to 54.0%)
BUN: 30 mg/dL (normal range: 5 to 25 mg/dL, slightly higher in older people)
Creatinine: 2.2 mg/dL (normal range: 0.5 to 1.5 mg/dL).

DIAGNOSES

- Underweight related to anorexia and fatigue
- Chronic pain (malignant) related to progression of disease process
- Limited physical mobility related to pain, fatigue, and early neuromuscular impairment
- Potential for impaired skin integrity related to impaired physical mobility and undernutrition
- Potential for caregiver burnout due to severity of patient's illness and lack of help.

EXPECTED OUTCOMES

- Patient will increase oral intake.
- Patient will experience minimal pain for the rest of his life.
- Patient will continue his current activity level.
- Patient will maintain intact skin.
- Patient will continue receiving support and care from his daughter.

PLANNING AND IMPLEMENTATION

- Ask about favorite foods, and ask Mary to include these foods in meals and snacks. Encourage use of a nutritional supplement (e.g., Ensure).
- Collaborate with the interprofessional team to establish a pain control program, using the VAD and a CADD-PCA infusion pump with a continuous morphine infusion.
- Teach Mary how to manage the morphine infusion and pump, usual side effects of the morphine infusion and their management, and adverse effects that should be reported to the nurse.
- Instruct Mary to allow ample rest periods for Mr. Casey between activities.
- Order a hospital bed with electronic controls and a bedside commode for Mr. Casey.
- Refer to home health agency to provide a home health aide to assist with hygiene and household chores.
- Request a volunteer to stay with Mr. Casey twice a week, allowing Mary to attend to outside activities and chores. Encourage Mary to talk with family members about providing additional respite care for Mr. Casey.
- Instruct Mary and the home health aide to inspect skin daily, provide good skin care with emollient lotion after bathing, and report any lesions immediately to the nurse.

(continued)

EVALUATION

Mr. Casey did increase his oral intake a little, sometimes eating the special treats his daughter prepared and drinking one or two cans of liquid nutritional supplement a day. His daughter was very grateful for the extra help from the home health aide and the volunteer, though she could not bring herself to ask her family for help. She did become more rested and reported that "Dad and I had some wonderful 3:00 a.m. talks when he couldn't sleep."

Mr. Casey's pain was well controlled using the morphine infusion with boluses as needed for breakthrough pain. His skin remained intact and in good condition.

Mary reported that Mr. Casey died peacefully in his sleep, about 2 weeks after hospice care was started. She said spending the last weeks of his life together was a healing experience for both of them.

CLINICAL REASONING IN PATIENT CARE

1. What other tests could be done to evaluate Mr. Casey's nutritional status?
2. Mr. Casey had severe back pain. What were the possible pathophysiologic reasons for his pain?
3. What medications are available to improve Mr. Casey's appetite? What side effects might they have that would contraindicate these medications for him?
4. If Mr. Casey had developed sepsis, what manifestations would you expect to see? As the nurse making the home visits, what would be your nursing actions, and in what order of priority?

See Evaluating Your Response in Appendix B.

New self-help groups are emerging in many communities to support others through their "seasons of survival." Many cancer survivors speak to groups about assisting other cancer survivors. Patients and families need to be informed about the resources available through community agencies and survivor support groups.

Transitions of Care

Cancer prevention is the key to reduce the incidence and mortality of cancer. Strategies include smoking cessation, maintaining a healthy weight, and preventing infections (ACS, 2018a). Recent advances in cancer prevention through vaccines are promising. For example, human papillomavirus (HPV) vaccination holds the hope to prevent cervical and anal cancers.

Early detection and treatment are considered the most important factors influencing the prognosis of those who have cancer. However, many people do not seek early diagnosis and treatment because of denial, fear and anxiety, stigma, or the absence of specific signs such as pain or weight loss (which usually are late signs). For this reason, screening procedures such as mammograms, PSA tests, occult blood stool tests, and colonoscopies may be lifesaving.

The ACS promotes early cancer detection through promotion of cancer awareness and guidelines for screening procedures. See Table 3.5 in Chapter 3 for cancer screening recommendations by the ACS. Nurses have a special role in public education and should encourage patients to schedule cancer checkups and to seek medical attention when they discover signs and symptoms characteristic of cancer (**Box 14.10**). Some cancers may present with very few and vague symptoms. For example, only 20% of patients are diagnosed with ovarian cancer in the early stages. Symptoms include bloating, pelvic/abdominal pain, early satiety, trouble eating, and urinary urgency or frequency. These symptoms should not be dismissed in women who present with symptoms daily for more than a few weeks. Encourage people to report to the public health department any known leaking of chemicals or radioactive materials into the water or air and any noted increase in the incidence of cancer, especially of one specific type, in their communities.

For people without symptoms, the ACS recommends incorporating a cancer checkup into periodic health examinations. This general cancer checkup includes health counseling, teaching self-examination techniques when appropriate, and, depending on age and gender, screening for breast, colon, rectum, cervix, and lung cancer has been shown to reduce mortality (ACS, 2018a). If an individual is at increased risk due to heredity, ethnicity, environment, occupation, or lifestyle, special tests or more frequent examinations may be necessary. For example, the

BOX 14.10 Cancer Symptoms

Cancer can cause many different symptoms. Some of them are as follows:

- A thickening or lump in the breast or any other part of the body
- Changes in size, shape, or texture of breast skin or nipple
- A new mole or change in a preexisting mole
- A sore that does not heal
- Hoarseness or a cough that does not go away
- Changes in bowel or bladder habits (e.g., difficult/painful urination)
- Discomfort after eating or changes in appetite
- Dysphagia
- Weight gain or loss with no known reason
- Unusual bleeding or discharge (urine, vaginal, stool)
- Feeling weak or very tired
- Night sweats.

Source: National Cancer Institute, retrieved from https://www.cancer.gov/about-cancer/diagnosis-staging/symptoms.

ACS recommends that physicians discuss annual low-dose CT scans for lung cancer screening with current or former smokers who have a 30-pack/year or greater smoking history who are age 55 to 74 (e.g., people who smoked a pack of cigarettes/day for 30 years) (ACS, 2018a). Nurses must be familiar with the ACS guidelines so that they can advise patients, their families, and significant others.

In caring for patients with cancer, nurses may encounter a number of emergency situations in which their role may be pivotal to the patient's survival. Most of these emergencies require astute observations, accurate judgments, and rapid action once the problem has been identified. A brief description of the more common **oncologic emergencies** with nursing interventions is shown in **Box 14.11**. In all cases, immediate notification of the physician or emergency team is the first step.

Before the patient is discharged or transferred to a long-term care setting, teach both the patient and significant others or caregivers to manage the patient at home. Discuss problems that may result from the type of cancer and the treatment received, and provide information on how to manage these problems and when to call the physician.

BOX 14.11
Common Oncologic Emergencies

PERICARDIAL EFFUSION AND CARDIAC TAMPONADE

Malignant pericardial effusion is an accumulation of excess fluid in the pericardial sac that compresses the heart, restricts heart movement, and results in a cardiac tamponade. The signs of cardiac tamponade are caused by compression of the heart, which leads to decreased cardiac output and impaired cardiac function. Signs include hypotension, tachycardia, tachypnea, dyspnea, cyanosis, increased central venous pressure, anxiety, restlessness, and impaired consciousness.

Interventions include:

- Start oxygen and alert respiratory therapy for other respiratory support as needed.
- Insert an intravenous catheter if one is not already in place.
- Monitor vital signs and initiate hemodynamic monitoring.
- Prepare vasopressor drugs.
- Bring emergency cart to bedside.
- Set up for and assist the physician with a pericardiocentesis (pericardial tap).
- Reassure the patient.

SUPERIOR VENA CAVA SYNDROME

The superior vena cava can be compressed by mediastinal tumors or adjacent thoracic tumors. The most common cause is small-cell or squamous-cell lung cancers. Occasionally the problem is caused by thrombus around a central venous catheter that then occludes the vena cava, resulting in obstruction and backup of the blood flowing into the superior vena cava.

Obstruction of the vena cava causes increased venous pressure, venous stasis, and engorgement of veins that are drained by the superior vena cava. Signs and symptoms may develop slowly; facial, periorbital, and arm edema are early signs. As the problem progresses, respiratory distress, dyspnea, cyanosis, tachypnea, and altered consciousness and neurologic deficits may occur. **Figure 14.7** ■ illustrates superior vena cava syndrome.

Emergency measures include:

- Provide respiratory support with oxygen, and prepare for tracheostomy.
- Monitor vital signs.
- Administer corticosteroids (e.g., dexamethasone) to reduce edema.
- If the disorder is due to a clot, administer antifibrinolytic or anticoagulant drugs as ordered.
- Provide a safe environment, including seizure precautions.

After the emergency is managed, the patient often receives radiation or chemotherapy to reduce the tumor size.

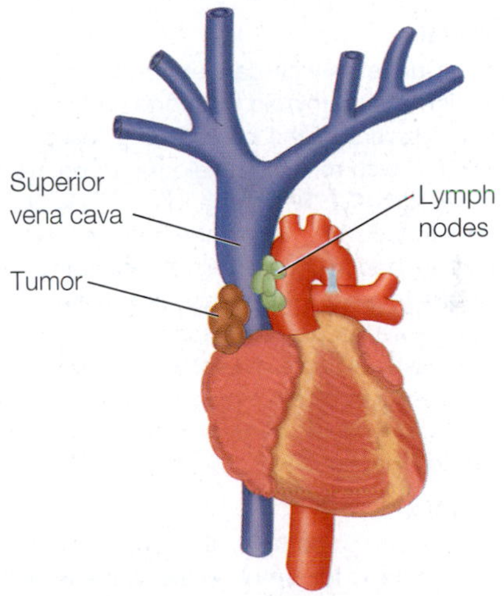
Superior vena cava
Lymph nodes
Tumor

Figure 14.7 ■ Superior vena cava syndrome. The enlargement of a tumor adjacent to the superior vena cava (usually in the lung or mediastinum) compresses that major blood vessel, which leads into the right atrium of the heart. As a result, blood backs up into the venous system behind the obstruction, diminishing blood flow into the heart.

SEPSIS AND SEPTIC SHOCK

Tumor necrosis, immune deficiency, antineoplastic therapy, malnutrition, and comorbid conditions can lead to the development of sepsis. Bacteria gain entrance to the blood, grow rapidly, and produce septicemia. Because malignant tumors are more likely to use anaerobic metabolic pathways, the bacteria of tumor sepsis are usually Gram negative and damage the body through a combination of bacterial endotoxins and an uncontrolled immune reaction. Gram-negative sepsis progresses to systemic shock and eventually results in multisystem failure.

Signs and symptoms appear in two phases. The first phase is characterized by vasodilation with hypovolemia, high fever, peripheral edema, hypotension, tachycardia, tachypnea, hot flushed skin with creeping mottling beginning in the lower extremities, and anxiety or restlessness. Without treatment, the shock progresses to the second phase, which shows the more classic signs of shock: Hypotension, rapid thready pulse, respiratory distress, cyanosis, subnormal temperature, cold and clammy skin, decreased urinary output, and altered mentation. Identifying the problem while the patient is still in the hyperdynamic state is crucial to the patient's survival. Refer to Chapter 11 for further discussion of septic shock.

(*continued*)

SPINAL CORD COMPRESSION

Spinal cord compression is most commonly associated with pressure from expanding tumors of the breast, lung, or prostate; lymphoma; or metastatic disease. Spinal cord compression constitutes an emergency because of the potential for irreversible paraplegia. Back pain is the initial symptom in almost all cases of spinal cord compression. This may progress to leg pain, numbness, paresthesias, and coldness. Later, bowel and bladder dysfunction occur and, finally, neurologic dysfunction progressing from weakness to paralysis. Treatment often consists of radiation or surgical decompression, but early detection is essential. See Chapter 43 for further discussion of spinal cord compression.

OBSTRUCTIVE UROPATHY

Patients with intra-abdominal, retroperitoneal, or pelvic malignancies, such as colorectal, prostate, cervical, or bladder cancers, may experience obstruction of the bladder neck or the ureters. Bladder neck obstruction usually manifests as urinary retention, flank pain, hematuria, or persistent urinary tract infections, but ureteral obstruction is not often evident until the patient is in renal failure. See Chapter 28 for further discussion of obstructive uropathy.

HYPERCALCEMIA

Hypercalcemia in patients with cancer results from the excessive ectopic production of parathyroid hormone and is most commonly associated with cancers of the breast, lung, esophagus, thyroid, head, and neck and with multiple myeloma. Bone metastases may also cause hypercalcemia. When the rate of calcium mobilization from the bone exceeds the renal threshold for excretion, serum calcium levels can become dangerously elevated. Patients with hypercalcemia often present with nonspecific symptoms of fatigue, anorexia, nausea, polyuria, and constipation. Neurologic symptoms include muscle weakness, lethargy, apathy, and diminished reflexes. Without treatment, hypercalcemia progresses to alterations in mental status, psychotic behavior, cardiac arrhythmias, seizures, coma, and death (refer to Chapter 10).

HYPERURICEMIA

Hyperuricemia is usually a complication of rapid necrosis of tumor cells after chemotherapy for lymphomas and leukemias. Hyperuricemia may be related to increased uric acid production or to the tumor lysis syndrome associated with Burkitt lymphoma and acute lymphoblastic leukemia (ALL). Uric acid crystals are deposited in the urinary tract, causing renal failure and uremia. Patients with hyperuricemia manifest with nausea and vomiting, lethargy, and oliguria.

TUMOR LYSIS SYNDROME

Tumor lysis syndrome (TLS) is a life-threatening emergency for patients with cancer. The syndrome develops secondary to massive and rapid destruction or death of cancer cells caused by cytotoxic treatment such as chemotherapy, radiation, biologic therapy, and hormonal therapy. It can occur spontaneously with sudden death of tumor cells. TLS is characterized by metabolic abnormalities, including hyperuricemia (as a result of nucleic acid breakdown), hyperphosphatemia, hyperkalemia, and hypocalcemia (Cheson et al., 2017; Howard, Trifilio, Gregory, Baxter, & McBride, 2016). A high incidence of TLS occurs in patients with high-grade lymphomas (Burkitt lymphoma) and ALL due to the high proliferation rate. Although the incidence of TLS in solid tumors is rare, cases of TLS following chemotherapy have been reported in patients with small-cell lung cancer, breast cancer, neuroblastoma, melanoma, and ovarian cancer.

The major cause of TLS is chemotherapy to tumors with a high proliferative rate, a relatively large tumor burden, and high sensitivity to cytotoxic agents, which leads to massive and rapid cell death. Once the body is no longer able to excrete the large amount of metabolic by-products from the cell death, intracellular contents and metabolic by-products (such as potassium, phosphorus, and nucleic acid) are released into the bloodstream (Howard et al., 2016). As a result, a combination of metabolic derangements occurs, including hyperkalemia, hyperuricemia, and hyperphosphatemia with secondary hypocalcemia (Howard et al., 2016). These metabolic abnormalities put patients at risk for cardiac dysfunction and renal failure.

Manifestations of TLS include nausea and vomiting, lethargy, edema, fluid overload, congestive heart failure, and sudden death (Cheson et al., 2017). Diagnosis of TLS mainly depends on laboratory tests and clinical signs and symptoms.

Prevention is crucial in management of TLS. Patients at risk for TLS include those with bulky chemosensitive cancer such as high-grade lymphomas and acute leukemia, elevated serum uric acid, potassium, phosphorus, and renal deficiency. Preventive and management measures include identifying patients at risk, promoting uric acid excretion, and managing electrolyte imbalances. Allopurinol is administered to inhibit the conversion of nucleic acid to uric acid, and hydration is used to promote uric acid and phosphate excretion. An oral phosphate binder is given to promote excretion of phosphate and potassium through the bowel. Hemodialysis may be required to manage electrolyte imbalances in patients with acute kidney injury or life-threatening electrolyte imbalances (Cheson et al., 2017).

- Teach wound care to the patient with an open wound or draining lesion, and provide a referral to a home health nurse to monitor progress.
- Explain special diets clearly, or refer the patient to a dietitian before discharge.
- Carefully review the physician's instructions with the patient and family, making sure they understand their medications and treatment plan, as well as when to see the physician for follow-up care.
- Provide or order equipment and supplies needed for home care, especially any specialized bed or equipment to aid mobility and ensure safety in the home.
- For the patient who will need complex care, such as parenteral nutrition, provide a referral to a home health nurse before discharge.

Because the hospital stay is often short, the patient and family will benefit from follow-up phone calls at home for several days. People do not learn well under the stress of going home; give the patient and family a number to call if they have concerns or questions.

Rehabilitation from cancer not only involves regaining strength, recovering from surgery or chemotherapy, and learning to live with an altered body part or appliance, but also entails recovering from associated psychologic and emotional turmoil.

Rehabilitation centers provide physical therapy, occupational therapy, speech therapy, job retraining, and an opportunity to recuperate before resuming full responsibilities. In addition, many patients go home to receive in-home support in the form of nursing supervision, direct care, and teaching. A certified home health aide can provide hygiene and home maintenance. Physical and occupational therapists provide muscle strengthening and mobility training (especially with prostheses) and home safety teaching.

Psychologic rehabilitation of cancer survivors addresses quality-of-life issues. Three "seasons of cancer survival" have been described (Mullan, 1985). The first starts with diagnosis but is dominated by treatment. The second stage is one of extended survival, which occurs when treatment ends and the watchful waiting period begins. This period is characterized by fear of recurrence. Permanent survival is said to begin when the survival period has gone on long enough that the risk of recurrence is small. In this period, the patient has to deal with secondary problems related to health and social issues resulting from the cancer experience. Employment may be a problem, health insurance may be canceled, and life insurance may be difficult to get. Relationships may have suffered from the strain of the illness on significant others and the essential self-focusing required for recovery. Both the patient and significant others may have undergone a personal and spiritual growth that ushers in a new and enriching period of their lives.

More and more patients with terminal cancer disease are electing to die at home. This decision has been made easier by the increased availability of hospice programs (see Chapter 5, Palliative and End-of-Life Care). When a patient and family or significant others elect hospice care, they are usually precluding additional hospitalizations other than those required to manage reversible problems.

Many hospice services are connected with an inpatient respite care unit, where the patient can receive 24-hour care for up to several weeks. This source provides the necessary care to the patient if a family member becomes ill or needs to be relieved temporarily of the tremendous burden of caring for a dying loved one.

CHAPTER HIGHLIGHTS

14.1 Incidence and Mortality

Differentiate the nonmodifiable and modifiable risk factors for cancer.

- Cancer is a life-threatening and complicated disease characterized by uncontrolled growth and spread of abnormal cells. Cancer can affect people of any age, gender, ethnicity, or geographic region.
- Cancer is the second leading cause of death in the United States. The incidence of cancer increases with advancing age. The most commonly seen cancers in women are breast, lung, colorectal, uterine, and thyroid. In men, prostate, lung, colorectal, bladder, and skin melanoma cancers occur most frequently.

14.2 Pathophysiology

Outline the process and theories of carcinogenesis, and list the known carcinogens.

- An estimated 5 to 10% of cancers have a hereditary component; therefore it is important to determine patients who have a genetic predisposition. Recurring patterns of cancer within a family may indicate a genetic component, as well as shared environmental exposures, lifestyle, and other nongenetic risk factors.

14.3 Characteristics and Behavior of Neoplasms

Describe the types and characteristics of neoplasms and the process of tumor invasion and metastasis.

- A neoplasm or tumor is a mass of new tissue that grows independently of its surrounding structures and has no physiologic purpose. Neoplasms are typically classified as benign or malignant on the basis of their potential to damage the body and on their growth characteristics.
- Malignant neoplasms (i.e., cancer) grow aggressively and do not respond to the body's homeostatic controls. Malignant cells from the primary tumor may travel through the blood or lymph to invade other tissues and organs of the body and form a secondary tumor called a metastasis.
- Metastasis, the ability of cancer cells to invade adjacent tissues and travel to distant organs, is considered cancer cells' most ominous characteristic. This quality makes treatment a considerable challenge.

14.4 Physiologic and Psychologic Effects of Cancer

Outline the physiologic and psychologic effects of cancer.

- The diagnosis and treatment of cancer is a pivotal, life-changing event that requires immediate and ongoing adjustment to this life-threatening illness. Effective physical and psychosocial adjustment to cancer diagnosis and treatment enhances patients' ability to cope and improves survival and quality of life.

14.5 Care of the Patient with Cancer

Describe the interprofessional care, nursing care, and transitions of care for patients with cancer.

- The goals of cancer treatment are aimed at cure and control of cancer as well as management of cancer-related and treatment-related symptoms.
- Cancer may be treated through surgery, chemotherapy, radiation therapy, biotherapy, photodynamic therapy, bone marrow and stem cell transplants, hormonal therapy, and complementary therapies. Chemotherapy uses cytotoxic medications to cure or control cancer by interrupting cell metabolism and replication and by

interfering with the ability of the malignant cell to synthesize vital enzymes and chemicals.

- Common complementary therapies for cancer include botanical agents, nutritional supplements, dietary regimens, mind–body modalities, spiritual approaches, and miscellaneous therapies.
- Nurses play a pivotal role in cancer prevention, providing quality patient-centered individualized care for patients with cancer.
- Managing cancer-related or treatment-related symptoms, such as pain, nausea and vomiting, mucositis, or fatigue, is a major nursing responsibility.
- Managing oncologic emergencies is an important nursing responsibility. Tumor lysis syndrome (TLS) is a life-threatening oncologic emergency for patients with cancer.

TEST YOURSELF NCLEX-RN® REVIEW

1. A patient with a history of colon cancer is informed that cells from the colon tumor have traveled to the liver. Which process should the nurse plan to explain to the patient?
   A. Mutation
   B. Dysplasia
   C. Metastasis
   D. Carcinogenesis
2. A patient diagnosed with lung cancer reports having difficulty sleeping and often feels tense. What would be the most appropriate initial nursing intervention?
   A. Offer an antianxiety drug such as Ativan (lorazepam).
   B. Obtain an order for medication for sleep from the physician.
   C. Encourage the patient to express feelings about the cancer diagnosis.
   D. Document the patient's report of difficulty sleeping and tenseness in the chart.
3. A patient is receiving external radiation for treatment of lung cancer. What should the nurse teach the patient to care for the skin in the marked area?
   A. Avoid contact with others.
   B. Cleanse the skin with soapy water.
   C. Apply antibacterial ointment daily.
   D. Avoid rubbing or scratching treated skin areas.
4. A patient is experiencing nausea and vomiting after daily chemotherapy treatments. What should the nurse do to help this patient?
   A. Schedule chemotherapy administration for bedtime.
   B. Provide clear liquids until the chemotherapy is completed.
   C. Keep the patient NPO until daily chemotherapy is completed.
   D. Provide antiemetic medication 30 to 40 minutes prior to each treatment.
5. A patient is experiencing bone marrow depression as a result of chemotherapy. Which assessment should the nurse expect because of this health problem?
   A. Alopecia
   B. Temperature 38.9°C (102°F)
   C. Nausea and vomiting
   D. Platelet count of 50,000
6. The nurse instructs a patient with cancer about chemotherapy. Which patient statement indicates that teaching has been effective?
   A. "Chemotherapy stops cancer cells from using body enzymes and chemicals."
   B. "Chemotherapy only uses a single drug to treat cancer because drug resistance is rare."
   C. "Chemotherapy uses drugs that promote the normal growth of cells while killing the cancer cells."
   D. "Chemotherapy is a preferred therapy because it has fewer adverse effects than radiation therapy."
7. A patient is going to begin a course of high-energy radiation to kill cancer cells through the use of a machine to focus a beam of radiation on the body. For which type of radiation therapy should the nurse instruct the patient?
   A. Brachytherapy
   B. Biochemotherapy
   C. External radiation therapy
   D. Internal-beam radiation therapy
8. The nurse is monitoring the uric acid, potassium, phosphorus, and calcium levels for a patient completing the first cycle of chemotherapy. For which complication is the nurse monitoring the patient?
   A. Septic shock
   B. Tumor lysis syndrome
   C. Spinal cord compression
   D. Superior vena cava syndrome

9. A patient is going to receive chemotherapeutic medication that affects DNA replication and chromosome duplication. Which phase of the cell cycle is this medication going to affect?
   A. S
   B. M
   C. G_1
   D. G_2

10. The nurse is preparing to instruct a group of patients newly diagnosed with cancer on the role of oncogenes. What should the nurse explain as a characteristic of oncogenes?
   A. They block cell growth.
   B. They are strictly regulated.
   C. They promote cell growth when activated.
   D. They stimulate a complex signaling process.

See Test Yourself answers in Appendix B.

REFERENCES

American Cancer Society (ACS). (2017). *ACS guidelines for nutrition and physical activity*. Retrieved from https://www.cancer.org/healthy/eat-healthy-get-active/acs-guidelines-nutrition-physical-activity-cancer-prevention/guidelines.html.

American Cancer Society (ACS). (2018a). *Cancer facts and figures—2018*. Atlanta, GA: Author.

American Cancer Society (ACS). (2018b). *Family cancer syndromes*. Atlanta, GA: Author.

Brahmer, J. R., Lacchetti C., Schneider, B. J., Atkins, M. B., Brassil, K. J., Caterino, J. M., . . . National Comprehensive Cancer Network. (2018). Management of immune-related adverse events in patients treated with immune checkpoint inhibitor therapy: American Society of Clinical Oncology Clinical Practice Guideline. *Journal of Clinical Oncology*, *36*(17), 1714–1768.

Carlson, L. E., Zelinski, E., Toivonen, K., Flynn, M., Qureshi, M., Piedalue, K. A., & Grant, R. (2017). Mind–body therapies in cancer: What is the latest evidence? *Current Oncology Reports*, *19*(10), 67.

Cheson, B. D., Enschede, S. H., Cerri, E., Desai, M., Potluri, J., Lamanna, N., & Tam, C. (2017). Tumor lysis syndrome in chronic lymphocytic leukemia with novel targeted agents. *The Oncologist*, *22*(11), 1283–1291.

Cooper, M. R., Alrajhi, A. M., & Durand, C. R. (2018). Role of immune checkpoint inhibitors in small cell lung cancer. *American Journal of Therapeutics*, *25*(3), e349–e356. Retrieved from https://www.ncbi.nlm.nih.gov/pubmed/29722737.

Cornelissen Anouk, J. M., Kool, M., Keuter Xavier, H. A., Heuts, E. M., Piatkowski de Grzymala, A. A., van der Hulst, R. W. J., & Shan Shan, Q. (2018). Quality of life questionnaires in breast cancer-related lymphedema patients: Review of the literature. *Lymphatic Research and Biology*, *16*(2), 134–139.

DeSantis, C. E., Siegel, R. L., Sauer, A. G., Miller, K. D., Fedewa, S. A., Alcaraz, K. I., & Jemal, A. (2016). Cancer statistics for African Americans, 2016: Progress and opportunities in reducing racial disparities. *CA: A Cancer Journal for Clinicians* , *66*(4), 290–308.

Fu, M. R., Wang, Y., Li, C., Qiu, Z., Axelrod, D., Guth, A. A., . . . Haber, J. (2018). Machine learning for detection of lymphedema among breast cancer survivors. *mHealth*, *4*(17), 1–11.

Fulop, T., Larbi, A., Kotb, R., de Angelis, F., & Pawelec, G. (2011). Aging, immunity, and cancer. *Discovery Medicine*, *11*(61), 537–550.

Grossman, S., & Porth, C. (2014). *Porth's pathophysiology: Concepts of altered health states* (9th ed.). Philadelphia, PA: Wolters Kluwer/Lippincott Williams & Wilkins.

Hafeez, U., Gan, H. K., & Scott, A. M. (2018). Monoclonal antibodies as immunomodulatory therapy against cancer and autoimmune diseases. *Current Opinion in Pharmacology*, *41*, 114–121.

Herdman, T. H. (Ed.). (2018). *NANDA International nursing diagnoses: Definitions and classification, 2018–2020*. Oxford, UK: Wiley-Blackwell.

Howard, S. C., Trifilio, S., Gregory, T. K., Baxter, N., & McBride, A. (2016). Tumor lysis syndrome in the era of novel and targeted agents in patients with hematologic malignancies: A systematic review. *Annals of Hematology*, *95*(4), 563–573.

Islami F., Goding Sauer, A., Miller, K. D., Siegel, R. L., Fedewa, S. A., Jacobs, E. J., . . . Jemal, A. (2017). Proportion and number of cancer cases and deaths attributable to potentially modifiable risk factors in the United States. *CA: A Cancer Journal for Clinicians*, *68*(1), 31–54.

Ji, Y., & Lu, H. (2017). Malignancies in HIV-infected and AIDS patients. *Advances in Experimental Medicine and Biology*, *1018*, 167–169.

Jin, J. (2018). Screening for ovarian cancer. *Journal of the American Medical Association*, *319*(6), 624.

Jorde, L. B., Carey, J. C., & Bamshad, M. J. (2016). *Medical genetics* (4th ed.). Philadelphia, PA: Mosby.

Kee, J. (2018). *Laboratory and diagnostic tests with nursing implications* (10th ed.). Upper Saddle River, NJ: Pearson.

Lopez, C., Charles, C., Rouby, P., Boinon, D., Laurent, S., Rey, A., . . . Dauchy, S. (2015). Relations between arthralgia and fear of cancer recurrence: Results of a cross-sectional study of breast cancer patients treated with adjuvant aromatase inhibitors therapy. *Supportive Care in Cancer*, *23*(12), 3581–3588.

Lutgendorf, S. K., & Andersen, B. L. (2015). Biobehavioral approaches to cancer progression and survival: Mechanisms and interventions. *American Psychologist*, *70*(2), 186–197.

Maximiano, S., Magalhães, P., Guerreiro, M. P., & Morgado, M. (2016). Trastuzumab in the treatment of breast cancer. *BioDrugs: Clinical Immunotherapeutics, Biopharmaceuticals and Gene Therapy*, *30*(2), 75–86.

Mehta, R. D., & Roth, A. J. (2015). Psychiatric considerations in the oncology setting. *CA: A Cancer Journal for Clinicians*, *65*(4), 299–314.

Mullan, F. (1985). Seasons of survival: Reflections of a physician with cancer. *New England Journal of Medicine*, *313*, 270–273.

National Comprehensive Cancer Network (NCCN). (2018). *Adult cancer pain*. Retrieved from https://www.nccn.org/professionals/physician_gls/pdf/pain.pdf.

National Toxicology Program. (2016). *Report on carcinogens, fourteenth edition*. Research Triangle Park, NC: U.S. Department of Health and Human Services, Public Health Service. Retrieved from https://ntp.niehs.nih.gov/go/roc14/.

Neufeld, N. J., Elnahal, S. M., & Alvarez, R. H. (2017). Cancer pain: A review of epidemiology, clinical quality and value impact. *Future Oncology*, *13*, 833–841.

Non-Small Cell Lung Cancer Collaborative Group. (1995). Chemotherapy in nonsmall cell lung cancer: A meta-analysis using updated data on individual patients from 52 randomised clinical trials. *British Medical Journal*, *311*(7010), 899–909.

Oncology Nursing Society (ONS). (2016). *Oncology nurse generalist competencies*. Retrieved from https://www.ons.org/sites/default/files/Oncology%20Nurse%20Generalist%20Competencies%202016.pdf.

Oncology Nursing Society (ONS). (2017a). *Anxiety: Putting evidence into practice (PEP card)*. Retrieved from https://www.ons.org/practice-resources/pep/anxiety.

Oncology Nursing Society (ONS). (2017b). *Mucositis: Putting evidence into practice (PEP card)*. Retrieved from https://www.ons.org/practice-resources/pep/mucositis.

Oncology Nursing Society (ONS). (2017c). *Radiodermatitis: Putting evidence into practice (PEP card)*. Retrieved from https://www.ons.org/practice-resources/pep/radiodermatitis.

Oncology Nursing Society (ONS). (2017d). *Skin reaction: Putting evidence into practice (PEP card)*. Retrieved from https://www.ons.org/practice-resources/pep/skin-reactions.

Oncology Nursing Society (ONS). (2018). *Prevention of infection: Putting evidence into practice (PEP card)*. Retrieved from https://www.ons.org/practice-resources/pep/prevention-infection.

Paice, J. A., Portenoy, R., Lacchetti, C., et al. (2016). Management of chronic pain in survivor of adult cancers: American Society of Clinical Oncology clinical practice guideline. *Journal of Clinical Oncology*, *34*(27), 3325–3345.

Selye, H. (1984). *The stress of life* (rev. 2nd ed.). New York, NY: McGraw-Hill.

Smith, P. R., Cope, D., Sherner, T. L., & Walker, D. K. (2014). Update on research-based interventions for anxiety in patients with cancer. *Clinical Journal of Oncology Nursing*, *18*(6), 5–16.

Soverini, S., De Benedittis, C., Mancini, M., & Martinelli, G. (2016). Best practices in chronic myeloid leukemia monitoring and management. *The Oncologist*, *21*(5), 626–633.

Sundaramurthi, T., Gallagher, N., & Sterling, B. (2017). Cancer-related acute pain: A systematic review of evidence-based interventions for putting evidence into practice. *Clinical Journal of Oncology Nursing*, *21*(3), 13–30.

Tariman, J. D., & Szubski, K. L. (2015). The evolving role of the nurse during the cancer treatment decision-making process: A literature review. *Clinical Journal of Oncology Nursing*, *19*(5), 548–556.

U.S. Department of Health and Human Services. (2014). *The health consequences of smoking—50 years of progress: A report of the Surgeon General*. Atlanta, GA: U.S. Department of Health and Human Services, Centers for Disease Control and Prevention, National Center for Chronic Disease Prevention and Health Promotion, Office on Smoking and Health.

van den Beuken-van Everdingen, M. H., Hochstenbach, L. M., Joosten, E. A., Tjan-Heijnen, V. C. & Janssen, D. J. (2016). Update on prevalence of pain in patients with cancer: Systematic review and meta-analysis. *Journal of Pain and Symptom Management*, *51*(6), 1070–1090.

Wieder, R., Shafiq, B., & Adam, N. (2016). African American race is an independent risk factor in survival from initially diagnosed localized breast cancer. *Journal of Cancer*, *18*(12), 1587–1598.

ADDITIONAL RESOURCES

American Cancer Society
www.cancer.org

Genes, Environment and Health Initiative
www.niehs.nih.gov/health/topics/science/gene-env/index.cfm/

NCI Cancer Mortality maps
http://ratecalc.cancer.gov

Survivor Link
www.cancersurvivorlink.org

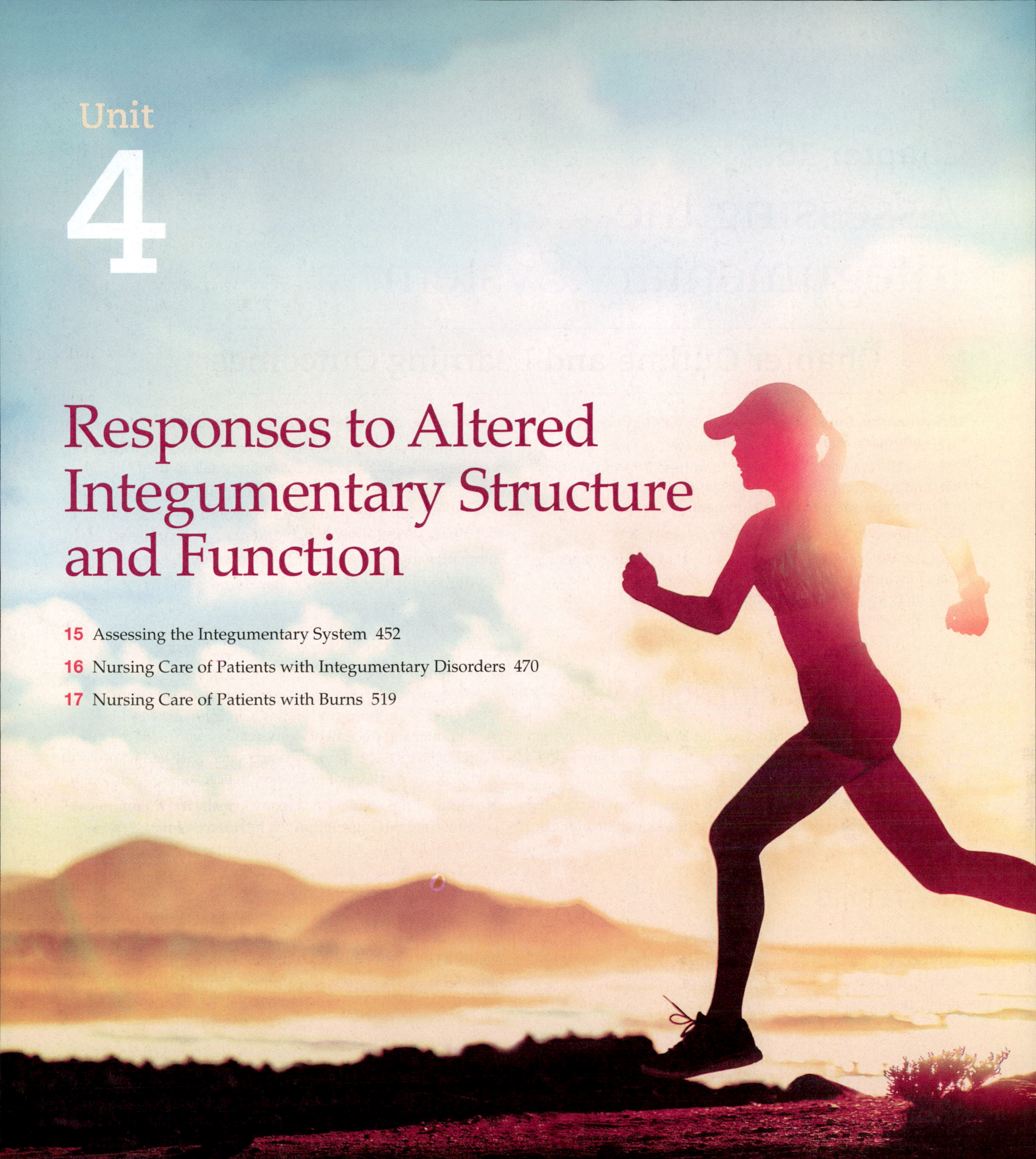

Unit

4

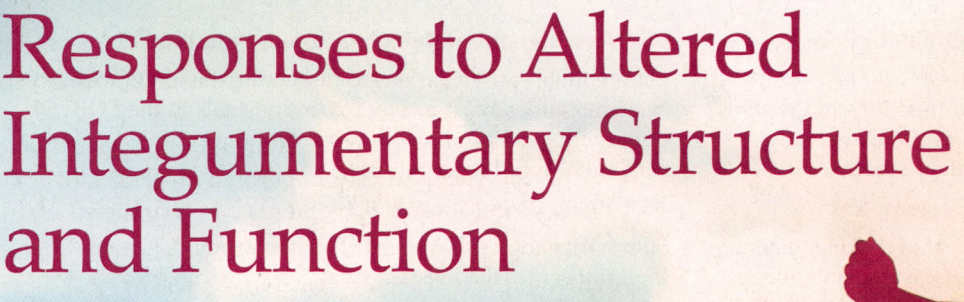

Responses to Altered Integumentary Structure and Function

Chapter 15

Assessing the Integumentary System

Chapter Outline and Learning Outcomes

Describe the anatomy, physiology, and functions of the skin, hair, and nails, and identify abnormal findings that may indicate impairment of the integumentary system.

Outline the components of the assessment of the integumentary system including topics for the health assessment interview, techniques for physical assessment, and the diagnostic tests used in the assessment.

Differentiate considerations for assessing the integumentary system of older adults, veterans, individuals in the LGBTQI population, and adults with sequelae from complex congenital conditions.

Summarize topics that nurses teach to promote healthy tissue integrity across the lifespan.

CLINICAL COMPETENCIES

- Complete a health history of the integumentary system incorporating an appraisal of psychosocial and physiologic issues.
- Conduct and document a health history for patients who have or are at risk for alterations in the skin, hair, or nails.
- Conduct and document a physical assessment of the integumentary system demonstrating sensitivity and respect for the diversity of the human experience.
- Monitor the results of diagnostic tests and communicate abnormal findings within the interprofessional team.

KEY TERMS

alopecia, 462
cyanosis, 455
ecchymosis, 461
edema, 462
erythema, 455
hirsutism, 462
jaundice, 455
keratin, 453
melanin, 453
pallor, 455
sebum, 454
urticaria, 461
vitiligo, 455

EQUIPMENT NEEDED

- Disposable gloves
- Ruler (metric to centimeters)
- Flashlight

15.1 Anatomy, Physiology, and Functions of the Integumentary System

The skin, hair, and nails make up the integumentary system. The skin, the largest organ of the body, provides an external covering for the body, separating and protecting the body's organs and tissues from the external environment (Sorenson, Quinn, & Klein, 2019). Functions of the skin, hair, and nails are summarized in **Table 15.1**.

The Skin

The skin has a total surface area of 15 to 20 square feet and weighs about 9 pounds. It has been estimated that each square inch of skin contains 15 feet of blood vessels, 4 yards of nerves, 650 sweat glands, 100 oil glands, 1500 sensory receptors, and more than 3 million cells that are constantly dying and being replaced. The skin is composed of two regions: the epidermis and the dermis (**Figure 15.1** ■). Alterations in the skin increase the risk for many physical and psychologic disorders, including fluid and electrolyte imbalance, altered temperature regulation, infection, delayed wound healing, and altered self-concept.

The Epidermis

The *epidermis*, which is the surface or outermost part of the skin, consists of epithelial cells. The epidermis has either four or five layers, depending on its location; there are five layers over the palms of the hands and the soles of the feet, and there are four layers over the rest of the body.

The *stratum basale* is the deepest layer of the epidermis. It contains *melanocytes*, cells that produce the pigment **melanin**, and *keratinocytes*, which produce **keratin**. Melanin forms a protective shield to protect the keratinocytes and the nerve endings in the dermis from the damaging effects of ultraviolet light. Melanocyte activity probably accounts for the difference in skin color in humans. Keratin is a fibrous, water-repellent protein that gives the epidermis its tough, protective quality. As keratinocytes mature, they move upward through the epidermal layers, eventually becoming dead cells at the surface of the skin. Millions of these cells are worn off by abrasion each day, but millions are simultaneously produced in the *stratum basale* (also known as *stratum germinativum*). The next layer of the epidermis is the *stratum spinosum*. Several cells thick, this layer contains abundant cells that arise from the bone marrow and migrate to the epidermis. Mitosis occurs at this layer, although not as abundantly as in the stratum basale.

The *stratum granulosum* is only two to three cells thick. The cells of the stratum granulosum contain a glycolipid that slows water loss across the epidermis. *Keratinization*, a thickening of the cells' plasma membranes, begins in the stratum granulosum. The *stratum lucidum* is present only in areas of thick skin; it is made up of flattened, dead keratinocytes. The outermost layer of the epidermis, the *stratum corneum*, is also the thickest, making up about 75% of the epidermis's total thickness. The stratum corneum consists of about 20 to 30 sheets of dead cells filled with keratin fragments arranged in shingles that flake off as dry skin.

The Dermis

The *dermis* is the second, deeper layer of skin. Made of flexible connective tissue, this layer is richly supplied with blood cells, nerve fibers, and lymphatic vessels. Most of the hair follicles, sebaceous glands, and sweat glands are located in the dermis. The dermis consists of a papillary and a reticular layer. The papillary layer contains capillaries and receptors for pain and touch. The deeper, reticular layer contains blood vessels, sweat and sebaceous glands, deep pressure receptors, and dense bundles of collagen fibers. The regions between these bundles form lines of cleavage in the skin. Surgical incisions parallel to these lines of cleavage heal more easily and with less scarring than incisions or traumatic wounds across cleavage lines.

Table 15.1 Functions of the Skin and Its Appendages

Structure	Functions
Epidermis	■ Protects tissues from physical, chemical, and biologic damage. ■ Prevents water loss and serves as a water-repellent layer. ■ Stores melanin, which protects tissues from the harmful effects of ultraviolet radiation in sunlight. ■ Converts cholesterol molecules to vitamin D when exposed to sunlight. ■ Contains phagocytes, which prevent bacteria from penetrating the skin.
Dermis	■ Regulates body temperature by dilating and constricting capillaries. ■ Transmits messages via nerve endings to the central nervous system.
Sebaceous (oil) glands	■ Secrete sebum, which lubricates skin and hair and plays a role in killing bacteria.
Eccrine sweat glands	■ Regulate body heat by excretion of perspiration.
Apocrine sweat glands	■ Remnants of sexual scent gland.
Hair	■ Cushions the scalp. ■ Eyelashes and cilia protect the body from foreign particles. ■ Provides insulation in cold weather.
Nails	■ Protect the fingers and toes, aid in grasping, and allow for various other activities, such as scratching the skin, picking up small items, peeling an orange, and so on.

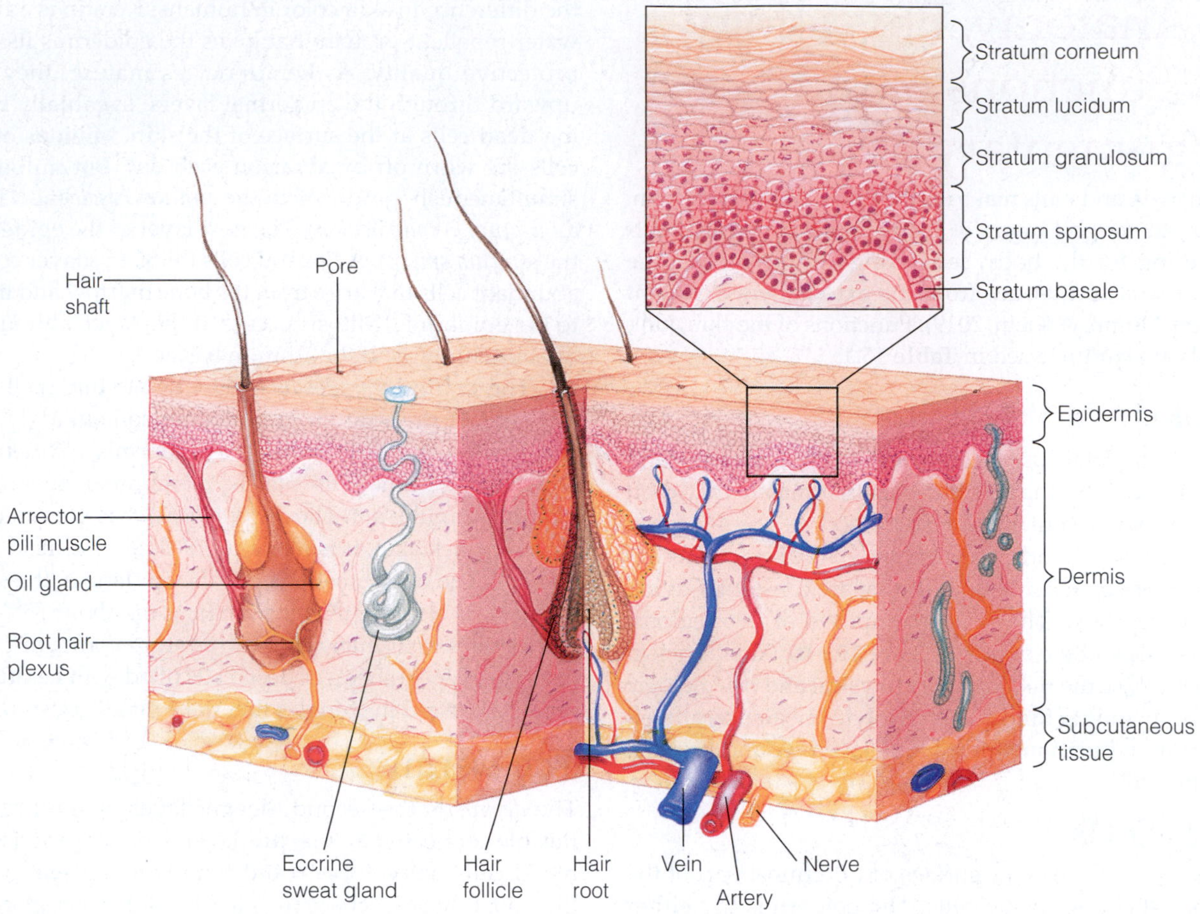
Stratum corneum
Stratum lucidum
Stratum granulosum
Stratum spinosum
Stratum basale
Hair shaft
Pore
Epidermis
Arrector pili muscle
Oil gland
Root hair plexus
Dermis
Subcutaneous tissue
Eccrine sweat gland
Hair follicle
Hair root
Vein
Artery
Nerve

Figure 15.1 ■ Anatomy of the skin.

Superficial Fascia

A layer of subcutaneous tissue called the *superficial fascia* lies under the dermis. It consists primarily of adipose (fat) tissue and helps the skin adhere to underlying structures.

Glands of the Skin

The skin contains *sebaceous* (oil) *glands*, *sudoriferous* (sweat) *glands*, and *ceruminous glands*. Each of these types of glands has a different function. Sebaceous glands are found all over the body except on the palms and soles. These glands secrete an oily substance called **sebum**, which is usually ducted into a hair follicle. Sebum softens and lubricates the skin and hair and decreases water loss from the skin in low humidity. Sebum protects the body from infection by killing bacteria. Hormones, especially androgens, stimulate the secretion of sebum. If a sebaceous gland becomes blocked, a pimple or whitehead appears on the surface of the skin; as the material oxidizes and dries, it forms a blackhead.

There are two types of sweat glands: *eccrine* and *apocrine*. Eccrine sweat glands are more numerous on the forehead, palms, and soles. The gland itself is located in the dermis; the duct to the skin rises through the epidermis to open in a pore at the surface. Sweat, the secretion of the eccrine glands, is composed mostly of water, combined with sodium, antibodies, small amounts of metabolic wastes, lactic acid, and vitamin C. The production of sweat is regulated by the sympathetic nervous system and serves to maintain normal body temperature and may occur in response to emotions.

Most apocrine sweat glands are located in the axillary, anal, and genital areas. The secretions from apocrine glands are similar to those of sweat glands, but they also contain fatty acids and proteins. Apocrine glands are a remnant of sexual scent glands. Ceruminous glands, located in the skin of the external ear, are modified apocrine sweat glands. They secrete yellow-brown, waxy cerumen that provides a sticky trap for foreign materials.

Skin Color

Skin color varies among individuals and among people of different races, ranging from a pinkish-white to various shades of brown and black. Areas of the skin that are normally exposed to the sun and environment, such as the face and hands, may have a slightly different color from areas that are usually covered with clothing. Special care must be taken when assessing changes in skin color in people who have darker skin, such as some African Americans, Latinos, Native Americans, Asian Americans, people of Mediterranean descent, and Caucasians who are deeply suntanned.

The color of the skin is the result of varying levels of pigmentation. *Melanin*, a yellow-to-brown pigment, is darker and is produced in greater amounts in individuals

Table 15.2 Skin Color Assessment Variations in People with Light and Dark Skin

Disorder and Cause	Change in Light Skin	Change in Dark Skin
Pallor: *A decrease or absence in skin color as the result of a decrease in tissue perfusion; a decrease in shape, size, or amount of RBCs; or an absence of melanin (local or generalized).*		
Anemia (decreased or abnormal size and shape of RBCs)	Generalized paleness	Brown skin is dull and has a yellow cast; black skin is dull and has an ashen gray cast
Hemorrhage (decreased amount of circulating RBCs)	Generalized paleness	Brown skin is dull and has a yellow cast; black skin is dull and has an ashen gray cast
Shock (decreased amount of circulating RBCs or decreased perfusion)	Generalized paleness	Brown skin is dull and has a yellow cast; black skin is dull and has an ashen gray cast
Arterial insufficiency (trauma, acute arterial occlusion, or arteriosclerosis)	Local paleness	Dull, ashen gray
Vitiligo (patchy loss of melanocytes)	Patches of white spots, most often found over the skin of the face, hands, or groin	Patches of white spots, most often found over the skin of the face, hands, or groin
Albinism (total absence of melanin)	White/pink	Tan, cream, or white
Cyanosis: *A bluish discoloration of the skin and mucous membranes resulting from a local or generalized excess of deoxygenated hemoglobin or a structural defect in the hemoglobin molecule.*		
Acute and chronic disorders of the structure and function of the heart and lungs (arterial insufficiency; exposure to cold, hypothermia)	Dusky blue; color may be generalized or local, depending on cause	Skin may appear darker, but will be dull; cyanosis is more readily assessed in the nail beds, oral mucous membranes, and conjunctivae
Erythema: *Redness of the skin or mucous membranes that is the result of dilation and congestion of superficial capillaries.*		
Hyperemia (inflammation, increased body temperature, hot environmental temperature, embarrassment, alcohol ingestion)	Red or bright pink	Difficult to assess; skin may have a dark red cast
Carbon monoxide poisoning (carbon monoxide displaces oxygen on the hemoglobin molecule, causing hypoxia, carboxyhemoglobinemia)	Cherry red in face and upper torso	Cherry red lips, oral mucous membranes, and nail beds
Venous stasis (inability of veins to return blood to heart; may result from edema, varicose veins, or pressure)	Dusky red	Difficult to assess
Jaundice: *Yellowish discoloration of the skin, mucous membranes, and sclerae of the eyes, caused by increased amounts of bilirubin or other pigments in the blood.*		
Increased serum bilirubin to > 2–3 mg/100 mL (liver disease, pancreatic disease, gallbladder disease, hemolysis such as following blood transfusion, severe burns or infections)	Yellowing of skin follows yellowing of sclerae and mucous membranes; may also be assessed in the fingernails and palms of the hands	Yellowing is best assessed at the junction of the hard palate and the soft palate or on the palms of the hands; sclerae may be yellow near the limbus (do not confuse with normal yellow eye pigmentation)
Uremia (retained urochrome pigments in the blood)	Orange-green or gray cast to skin	Difficult to assess; may appear as yellowish-green color in the sclera of the eye

with dark skin color than in those with light skin color. Exposure to the sun causes a buildup of melanin and a darkening or tanning of the skin in people with light skin. *Carotene*, a yellow-to-orange pigment, is found most in areas of the body where the stratum corneum is thickest, such as the palms of the hands. The epidermis in Caucasian skin has very little melanin and is almost transparent. Thus, the color of the hemoglobin found in red blood cells (RBCs) circulating through the dermis shows through, lending a pinkish skin tone.

Skin color is influenced by emotions and illnesses. **Erythema**, a reddening of the skin, may occur with embarrassment (blushing), fever, hypertension, or inflammation. Reddening may also result from a drug reaction, sunburn, acne rosacea, or other factors. A bluish discoloration of the skin and mucous membranes, called **cyanosis**, results from poor oxygenation of hemoglobin. **Pallor**, or paleness of skin, may occur with shock, fear, or anger or in anemia and hypoxia. **Jaundice** is a yellow-to-orange color visible in the skin and mucous membranes; it is most often the result of a hepatic disorder. **Table 15.2** further defines these terms and compares and contrasts skin color changes in people with light and dark skin.

The Hair

Hair is distributed all over the body, except the lips, nipples, parts of the external genitals, the palms of the hands, and the soles of the feet. Hair is produced by a hair bulb, and its root is enclosed in a hair follicle (**Figure 15.2** ■). The exposed part, called the *shaft*, consists mainly of dead cells. Hair follicles extend into the dermis and in some places, such as the scalp, below the dermis. Many factors, including nutrition and hormones, influence hair growth. Hair in various parts of the body has protective functions: The eyebrows and eyelashes protect the eyes, hair in the nose helps keep foreign materials out of the upper respiratory tract, and hair on the head protects the scalp from heat loss and sunlight.

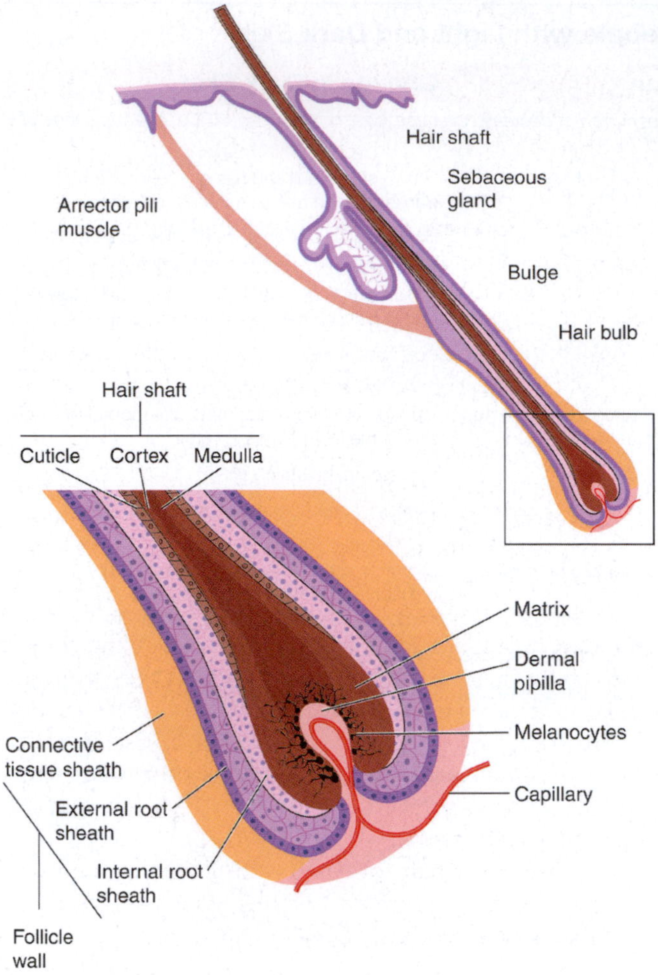

Hair shaft
Sebaceous gland
Arrector pili muscle
Bulge
Hair bulb
Hair shaft
Cuticle
Cortex
Medulla
Matrix
Dermal pipilla
Melanocytes
Capillary
Connective tissue sheath
External root sheath
Internal root sheath
Follicle wall

Figure 15.2 ■ Anatomy of a hair follicle.

The Nails

A nail is a modified scalelike epidermal structure. Like hair, nails consist mainly of dead cells. The body of the nail rests on the nail bed (**Figure 15.3** ■). The proximal visible end of the nail has a white crescent, called a *lunula*. The sides of the nail are overlapped by skin, called *nail folds*. The proximal nail fold is thickened and is called the *eponychium* or *cuticle*. Nails form a protective coating over the dorsum of each digit on the fingers and toes.

15.2 Assessing the Integumentary System

The structures of the integumentary system are assessed by findings from diagnostic tests, a health assessment interview to collect subjective data, and a physical assessment to collect objective data (Kottner & Surber, 2016).

Health Assessment Interview

A health assessment interview to determine problems with the integumentary system may be conducted as part of a health screening or complete health assessment, or it may focus on a chief complaint (such as itching or a rash). If the patient has a skin problem, analyze its onset, characteristics and course, severity, and precipitating and relieving factors, and note the timing and circumstances of any associated symptoms. For example, ask the patient the following:

- What type of itching have you experienced?
- When did you first notice a change in this mole?
- Did you change to any different kind of shampoo or other hair product just before you started to lose your hair?

Ask about any change in health, rashes, itching, color changes, dryness or oiliness, growth of or changes in warts or moles, and the presence of lesions. Precipitating causes—such as medications; the use of new soaps, skin care agents, or cosmetics; or pets, travel, stress, or dietary changes—must be explored. In assessing hair problems, ask about any thinning or baldness, excessive hair loss, change in the distribution of hair, use of hair care products, diet, and dieting. When assessing nail problems, ask about nail splitting or breakage, discoloration, infection, diet, and exposure to chemicals.

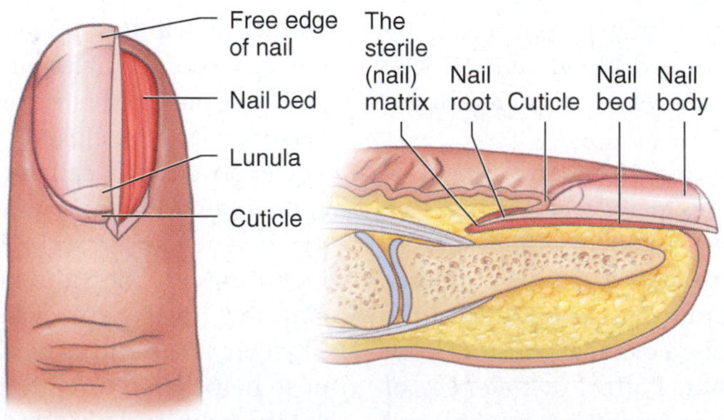

Free edge of nail
Nail bed
Lunula
Cuticle
The sterile (nail) matrix
Nail root
Cuticle
Nail bed
Nail body

Figure 15.3 ■ Anatomy of a nail.

The patient's medical history is important. Questions focus on previous problems, allergies, and lesions. Skin problems may be manifestations of other disorders, such as cardiovascular disease, endocrine disorders, hepatic disease, and hematologic disorders. Occupational and social history may provide cues to skin problems; ask the patient about travel, exposure to toxic substances at work, use of alcohol, and responses to stress. Responses should be documented in the patient's medical record.

Assess the presence of risk factors for skin cancer carefully. These include male gender; age over 50; family history of skin cancer; extended exposure to sunlight; tendency to sunburn; history of sunburn or other skin trauma; light-colored hair or eyes; residence in high altitudes or near the equator; and exposure to radiation, x-rays, coal, tar, or petroleum products. (Risks for skin cancer are further discussed in Chapter 16.) Include specific questions to identify risk factors for malignant melanoma. These include a large number of moles, the presence of atypical moles, a family history of melanoma, prior melanoma, repeated severe sunburns, ease of freckling and sunburning, or inability to tan.

When conducting a health assessment interview and physical assessment, the nurse should consider genetic influences on the health of the adult (National Institutes of Health, 2017). During the health assessment interview, ask about integumentary disorders or abnormalities in immediate family members and also inquire about their gender. During the physical assessment, assess for any manifestations that indicate a genetic disorder (see the Genetic Considerations box). If data are found that indicate genetic risk factors or alterations, ask about genetic testing and refer for appropriate genetic counseling and evaluation. Chapter 8 provides further information about genetic implications in medical-surgical nursing.

Physical Assessment

Physical assessment of the skin, hair, and nails may be performed either as part of a total assessment or may be a focused assessment of the integument for patients with known or suspected problems.

The examination should be conducted in a warm, private room. The patient removes all clothing and puts on a gown or drape. The areas to be examined should be fully exposed, but protect the patient's modesty by keeping other areas covered. The patient may be standing, sitting, or lying down at various times of the examination. Don disposable gloves when palpating open lesions, skin surfaces suspicious of infections or infestations, or discharge from lesions of the skin and mucous membranes. A ruler is used to measure the size of the lesions. A flashlight is used to better visualize lesions.

Physical assessment of the skin, hair, and nails is conducted by inspection and palpation. Assess the skin for color, presence of lesions (observable changes from normal skin structure), temperature, texture, moisture, turgor, and presence of edema. Characteristics of lesions to note include location and distribution, color, pattern, edges, size (measure with a ruler in centimeters), elevation, and type of exudate (if present).

Examine the hair for color, texture, quality, and scalp lesions. Determine the shape, color, contour, and condition of the nails. The terminology for skin lesions and associated disorders is outlined in **Table 15.3**. Primary, secondary, and vascular lesions are described and shown in **Tables 15.4, 15.5,** and **15.6**.

Genetic Considerations

Examples of Inherited Integumentary Disorders

- *Oculocutaneous albinism*, an autosomal recessive inheritance disorder, causes hypopigmentation (albinism or absence of color) of the skin, hair, and eyes as a result of an inability to synthesize melanin.
- *Keloids*, which are elevated scars, have a familial tendency and are more commonly found in Black individuals (Spector, 2017).
- *Vitiligo*, the sudden appearance of white patches on the skin, has a familial tendency.
- Male pattern baldness (the most common cause of baldness in men) is genetically predetermined.
- *Hirsutism* (excessive hair in women) may be genetically predetermined.
- Some Black individuals may have very dry scalps and dry, fragile hair of genetic origin (Spector, 2017).
- A family history of skin cancer is a risk factor for skin cancer.

Table 15.3 Terminology of Skin Lesions with Associated Disorders

Lesion	Examples of Disorders
Pigmented	Freckle, seborrheic keratosis, nevus, melanoma
Scaly	Psoriasis, dermatitis, xerosis, tinea, actinic keratoses
Pustular	Acne vulgaris, folliculitis, candidiasis
Vesicular	Herpes simplex, herpes zoster, scabies
Nodular	Warts, basal cell carcinoma, acne
Weepy, crusted	Acute contact allergic dermatitis, impetigo
Figurate (shaped) erythema	Urticaria, cellulites
Bullous	Pemphigus, toxic epidermal necrolysis
Pruritic	Xerosis, scabies, pediculosis
Ulcerated	Pressure ulcer, skin cancer, herpes simplex

Table 15.4 Primary Skin Lesions

Lesion	Description	Lesion	Description
Macule, patch 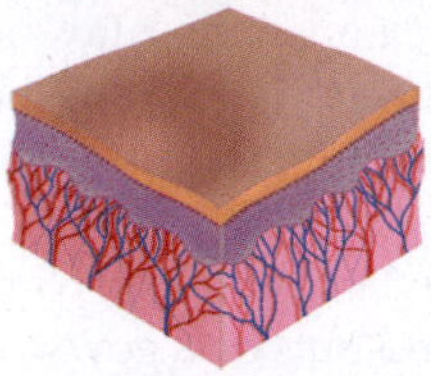	Flat, nonpalpable change in skin color. Macules are smaller than 1 cm, with a circumscribed border. Patches are larger than 1 cm and may have an irregular border. **Examples** Macules: freckles, measles, and petechiae Patches: Mongolian spots, port-wine stains, vitiligo, and chloasma	Vesicle, bulla 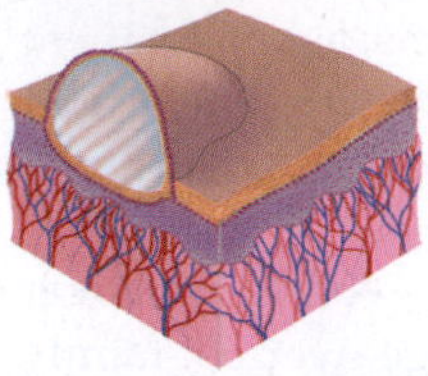	Elevated, fluid-filled, round- or oval-shaped palpable mass with thin, translucent walls and circumscribed borders. Vesicles are smaller than 0.5 cm; bullae are larger than 0.5 cm. **Examples** Vesicles: herpes simplex/zoster, early chickenpox, poison ivy, and small burn blisters Bullae: contact dermatitis, friction blisters, and large burn blisters
Papule, plaque 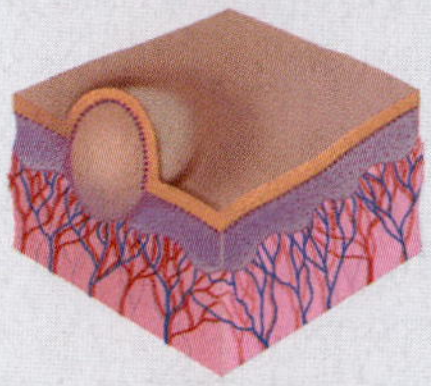	Elevated, solid, palpable mass with circumscribed border. Papules are smaller than 0.5 cm; plaques are groups of papules that form lesions larger than 0.5 cm. **Examples** Papules: elevated moles, warts, and lichen planus Plaques: psoriasis, actinic keratosis, and lichen planus	Wheal 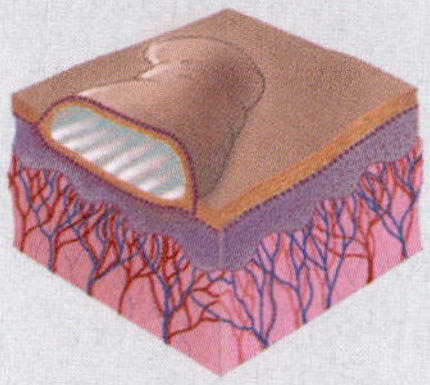	Elevated, often reddish area with irregular border caused by diffuse fluid in tissues rather than free fluid in a cavity, as in vesicles. Size varies. **Examples** Insect bites and hives (extensive wheals)
Nodule, tumor 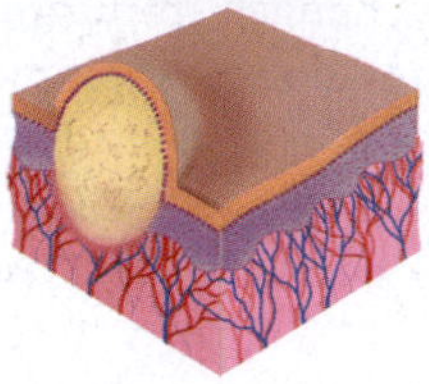	Elevated, solid, hard or soft palpable mass extending deeper into the dermis than a papule. Nodules have circumscribed borders and are 0.5 to 2 cm; tumors may have irregular borders and are larger than 2 cm. **Examples** Nodules: small lipoma, squamous cell carcinoma, fibroma, and intradermal nevi Tumors: large lipoma, carcinoma, and hemangioma	Pustule 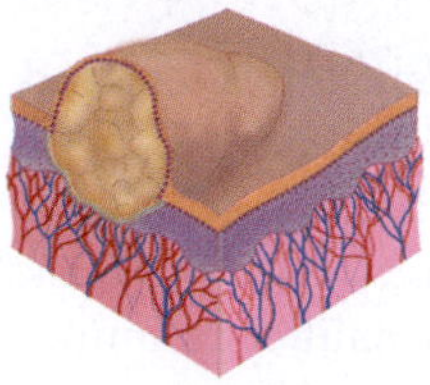	Elevated, pus-filled vesicle or bulla with circumscribed border. Size varies. **Examples** Acne, impetigo, and carbuncles (large boils)
		Cyst 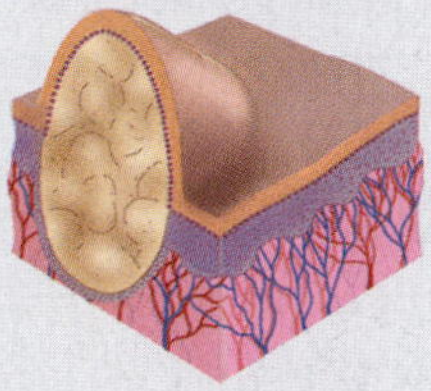	Elevated, encapsulated, fluid-filled or semisolid mass originating in the subcutaneous tissue or dermis, usually 1 cm or larger. **Examples** Varieties include sebaceous cysts and epidermoid cysts

Source: PEARSON EDUCATION, . ., NURSING: A CONCEPT-BASED APPROACH TO LEARNING, VOLUME I, 3rd Ed.,©2019. Reprinted and Electronically reproduced by permission of Pearson Education, Inc., New York, NY.

Table 15.5 Secondary Skin Lesions

Lesion	Description	Lesion	Description
Atrophy 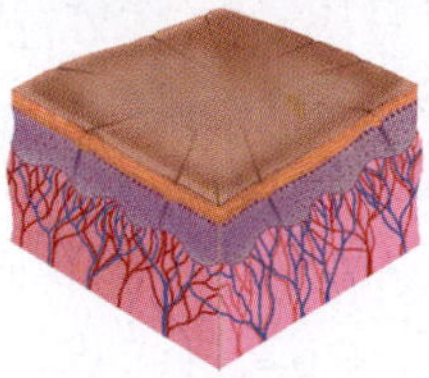	A translucent, dry, paper-like, sometimes wrinkled skin surface resulting from thinning or wasting of the skin due to loss of collagen and elastin. **Examples** Striae, aged skin	Ulcer 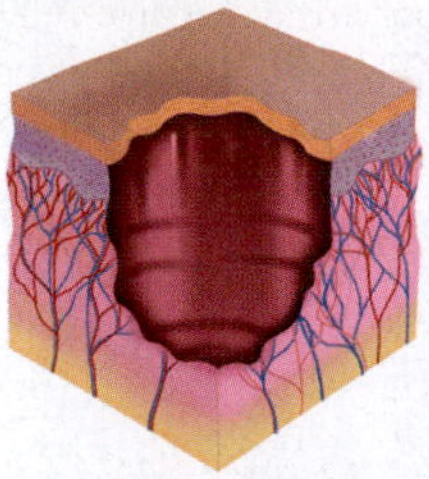	Deep, irregularly shaped area of skin loss extending into the dermis or subcutaneous tissue. May bleed. May leave scar. **Examples** Pressure injuries, stasis ulcers, chancres
Erosion 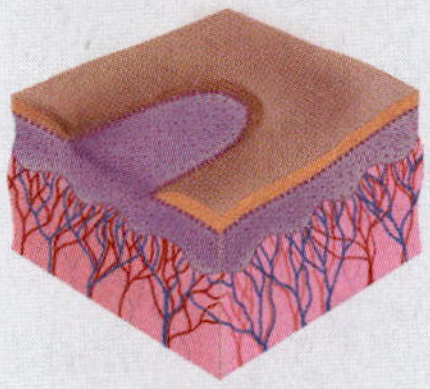	Wearing-away of the superficial epidermis causing a moist, shallow depression. Because erosions do not extend into the dermis, they heal without scarring. **Examples** Scratch marks, ruptured vesicles	Fissure 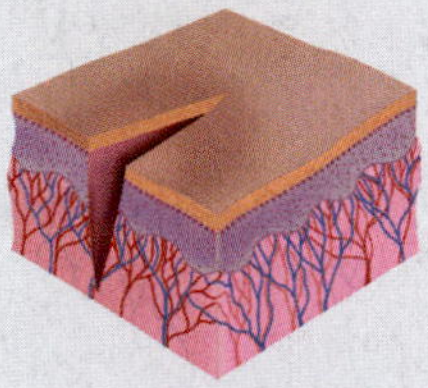	Linear crack with sharp edges, extending into the dermis. **Examples** Cracks at the corners of the mouth or in the hands, athlete's foot
Lichenification 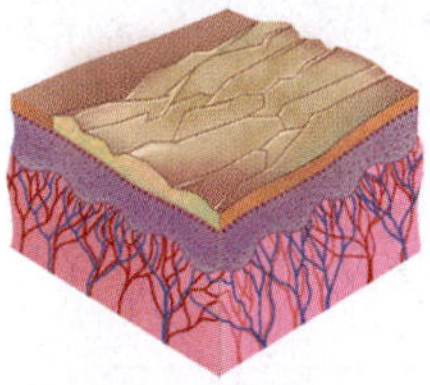	Rough, thickened, hardened area of epidermis resulting from chronic irritation such as scratching or rubbing. **Example** Chronic dermatitis	Scar 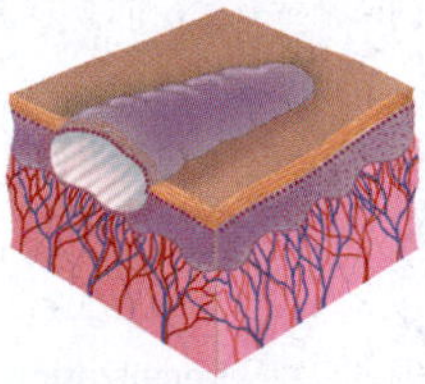	Flat, irregular area of connective tissue left after a lesion or wound has healed. New scars may be red or purple; older scars may be silvery or white. **Examples** Healed surgical wound or injury, healed acne
Scales 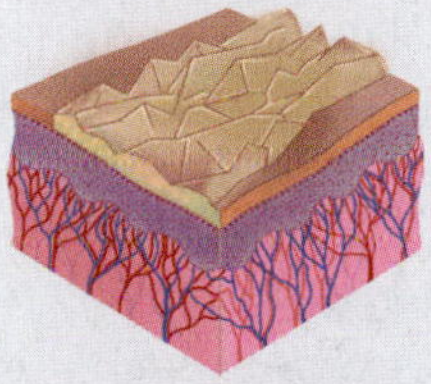	Shedding flakes of greasy, keratinized skin tissue. Color may be white, gray, or silver. Texture may vary from fine to thick. **Examples** Dry skin, dandruff, psoriasis, and eczema	Keloid 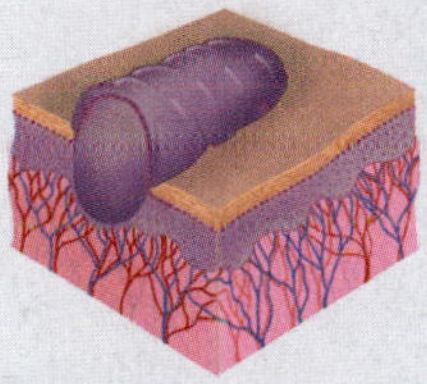	Elevated, irregular, darkened area of excess scar tissue caused by excessive collagen formation during healing. Extends beyond the site of the original injury. Higher incidence in people of African descent. **Example** Keloid from ear piercing or surgery
Crust 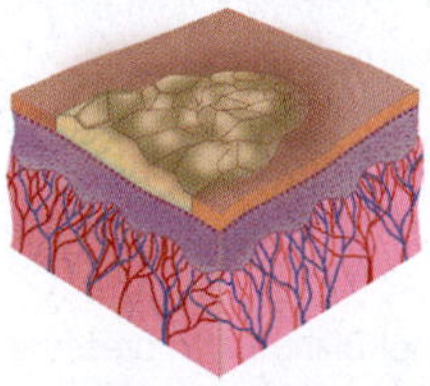	Dry blood, serum, or pus left on the skin surface when vesicles or pustules burst. Can be red-brown, orange, or yellow. Large crusts that adhere to the skin surface are called *scabs*. **Examples** Eczema, impetigo, herpes, or scabs following abrasion		

Table 15.6 Vascular Skin Lesions

Lesion	Description
Spider angioma 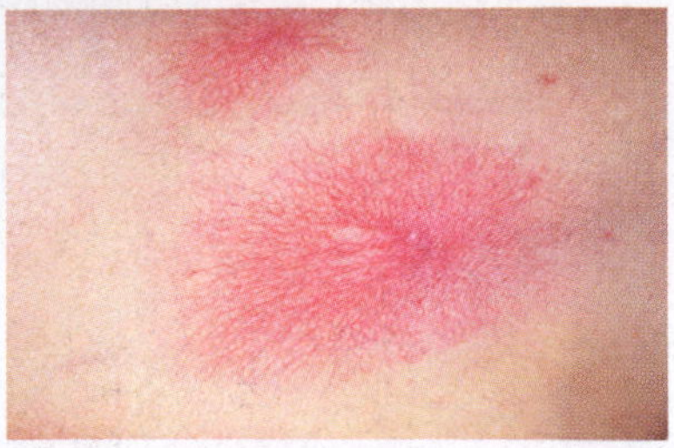	A flat, bright red dot with tiny radiating blood vessels ranging in size from a pinpoint to 2 cm. It blanches with pressure. **Cause** A type of telangiectasis (vascular dilation) caused by elevated estrogen levels, pregnancy, estrogen therapy, vitamin B deficiency, or liver disease, or may not be pathologic. **Localization/Distribution** Most commonly appears on the upper half of the body.
Venous star 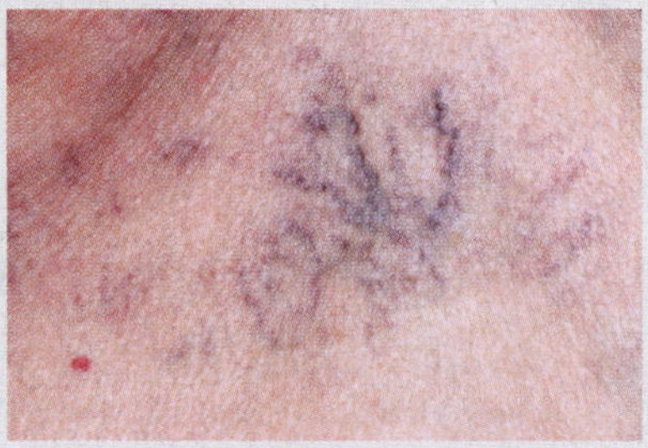	A flat blue lesion with radiating, cascading, or linear veins extending from the center. It ranges in size from 3 to 25 cm. **Cause** A type of telangiectasis (vascular dilation) caused by increased intravenous pressure in superficial veins. Standing for long periods and obesity can cause venous star lesions. **Localization/Distribution** Most commonly appears on the anterior chest and the lower legs near varicose veins.
Petechiae 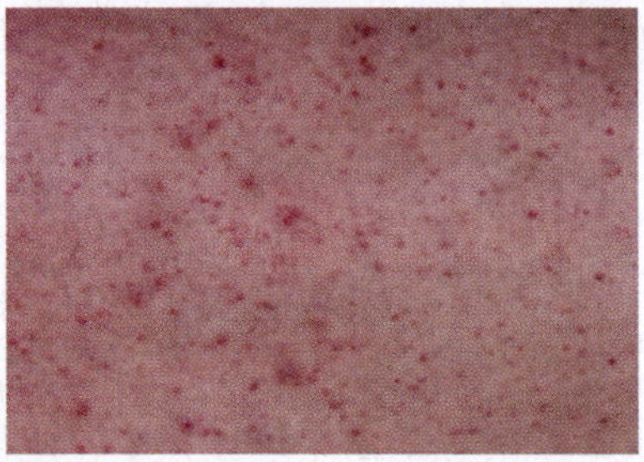	Flat red or purple rounded "freckles" approximately 1 to 3 mm in diameter. Difficult to detect in dark skin. Do not blanch. **Cause** Minute hemorrhages resulting from fragile capillaries, petechiae are caused by septicemias, liver disease, or vitamin C or K deficiency. They may also be caused by anticoagulant therapy. **Localization/Distribution** Most commonly appear on the dependent surfaces of the body (e.g., back, buttocks). In the patient with dark skin, look for them in the oral mucosa and conjunctivae.
Purpura 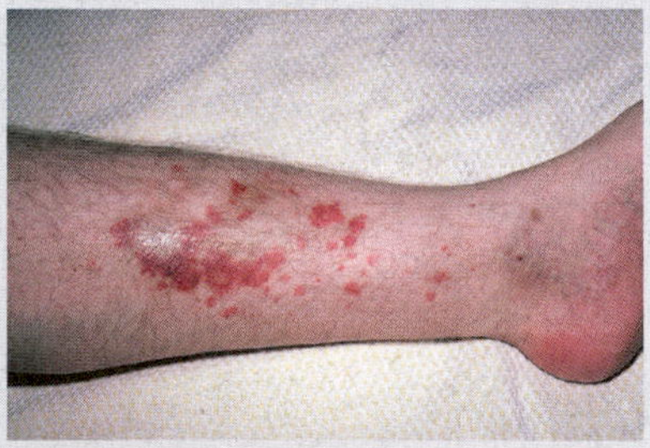	Flat, reddish-blue, irregularly shaped extensive patches of varying size. **Cause** Bleeding disorders, scurvy, and capillary fragility in the older adult (senile purpura). **Localization/Distribution** May appear anywhere on the body, but are most noticeable on the legs, arms, and backs of hands.
Ecchymosis 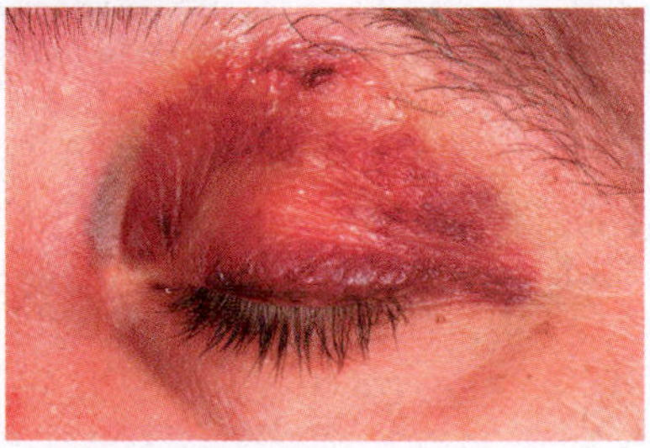	A flat, irregularly shaped lesion of varying size with no pulsation. Does not blanch with pressure. In light skin, it begins as bluish-purple mark that changes to greenish-yellow. In brown skin, it varies from blue to deep purple. In black skin, it appears as a darkened area. **Cause** Release of blood from superficial vessels into surrounding tissue due to trauma, hemophilia, liver disease, or deficiency of vitamin C or K. **Localization/Distribution** Occurs anywhere on the body at the site of trauma or pressure.

Integumentary Assessments

Technique and Normal Findings (*in italics*)	Abnormal Findings
Inspect skin color and note any odors coming from the skin. *Skin color should be even, appropriate to the age and race of the patient, without foul odors.*	■ A strong odor of perspiration may indicate poor hygiene and a need for patient teaching. A foul odor may indicate a disorder of the sweat glands. ■ Pallor and/or cyanosis are seen with exposure to cold and with decreased perfusion and oxygenation. In cyanotic dark-skinned patients, skin loses glow and appears dull. Cyanosis may be more visible in the mucous membranes and nail beds of these patients. ■ In dark-skinned patients, jaundice may be most apparent in the sclerae of the eyes. ■ Redness, swelling, and pain are seen with various rashes, inflammations, infections, and burns. First-degree (superficial) burns cause areas of painful erythema and swelling. Red, painful blisters appear in second-degree (partial-thickness) burns, whereas white or blackened areas are common in third-degree (full-thickness) burns. ■ Vitiligo, an abnormal loss of melanin in patches, typically occurs over the face, hands, or groin. Vitiligo is thought to be an autoimmune disorder.
Inspect the skin for lesions and alterations, including calluses, scars, tattoos, and piercings. Include inspection of skin creases and folds. *Skin should be intact without lesions.*	■ Primary, secondary, and vascular lesions are described and shown in Tables 15.4 through 15.6. ■ Pearly edged nodules with a central ulcer are seen in basal cell carcinoma. ■ Scaly, red, fast-growing papules are seen in squamous cell carcinoma. ■ Dark, asymmetric, multicolored patches (sometimes moles) with irregular edges appear in malignant melanoma. ■ Circular lesions are usually present in ringworm and in tinea versicolor. ■ Grouped vesicles may be seen in contact dermatitis. ■ Linear lesions appear in poison ivy and herpes zoster. ■ **Urticaria** (hives) appears as patches of pale, itchy wheals in an erythematous area. ■ In psoriasis, scaly red patches appear on the scalp, knees, back, and genitals. ■ In herpes zoster, vesicles appear along sensory nerve paths, turn into pustules, and then crust over. ■ Bruises (**ecchymosis**) are raised bluish or yellowish vascular lesions. Multiple bruises in various stages of healing suggest trauma or abuse.
Palpate skin temperature. *Skin should be warm.*	■ Skin is warm and red in inflammation and is generally warm with elevated body temperature. ■ Decreased blood flow decreases the skin temperature; this may be generalized, as in shock, or localized, as in arteriosclerosis.
Palpate skin texture. *Skin should be smooth.*	■ Changes in the texture of the skin may indicate irritation or trauma. ■ The skin is soft and smooth in hyperthyroidism and coarse in hypothyroidism.
Palpate skin moisture. *Skin should be dry.*	■ Excessively dry skin is often present in older adults and patients with hypothyroidism. ■ Oily skin is common in adolescents and young adults. Oily skin may be a normal finding, or it may accompany a skin disorder such as acne vulgaris. ■ Excessive perspiration may be associated with shock, fever, increased activity, or anxiety.
Palpate skin turgor. *Skinfold should return rapidly to normal position.*	■ Pinch the patient's skin gently over the back of the hand or collarbone. *Tenting*, in which the skin remains pinched for a few moments before resuming its normal position, is common in older patients who are thin (**Figure 15.4** ■). ■ Skin turgor is decreased in dehydration. It is increased in edema and scleroderma. 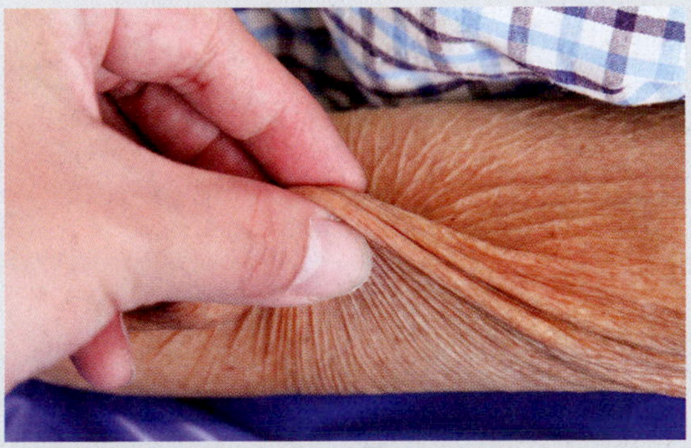 **Figure 15.4** ■ Tenting in an older patient.

(continued)

Integumentary Assessments (*continued*)

Technique and Normal Findings (*in italics*)	Abnormal Findings
Assess for edema. *No edema should be present.*	■ Assess **edema** (accumulation of fluid in the body's tissues) by depressing the patient's skin on the dependent extremities (**Figure 15.5** ■). Record findings as follows: ■ 1+ Slight pitting, no obvious distortion ■ 2+ Deeper pit, no obvious distortion ■ 3+ Pit is obvious; extremities are swollen ■ 4+ Pit remains with obvious distortion ■ Record depression rebound time in seconds if present. ■ Edema is common in cardiovascular disorders, renal failure, trauma, and cirrhosis of the liver. It also may be a side effect of certain drugs.

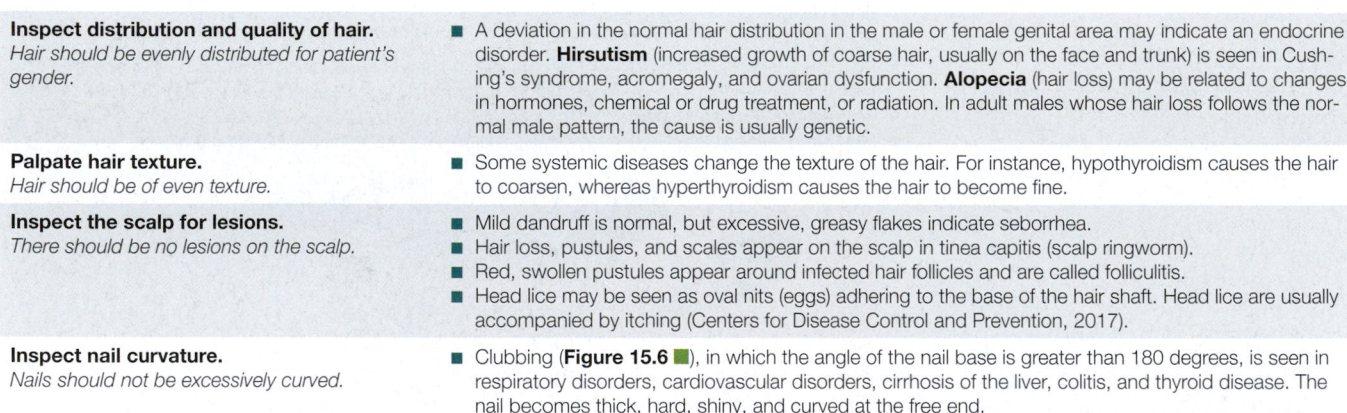

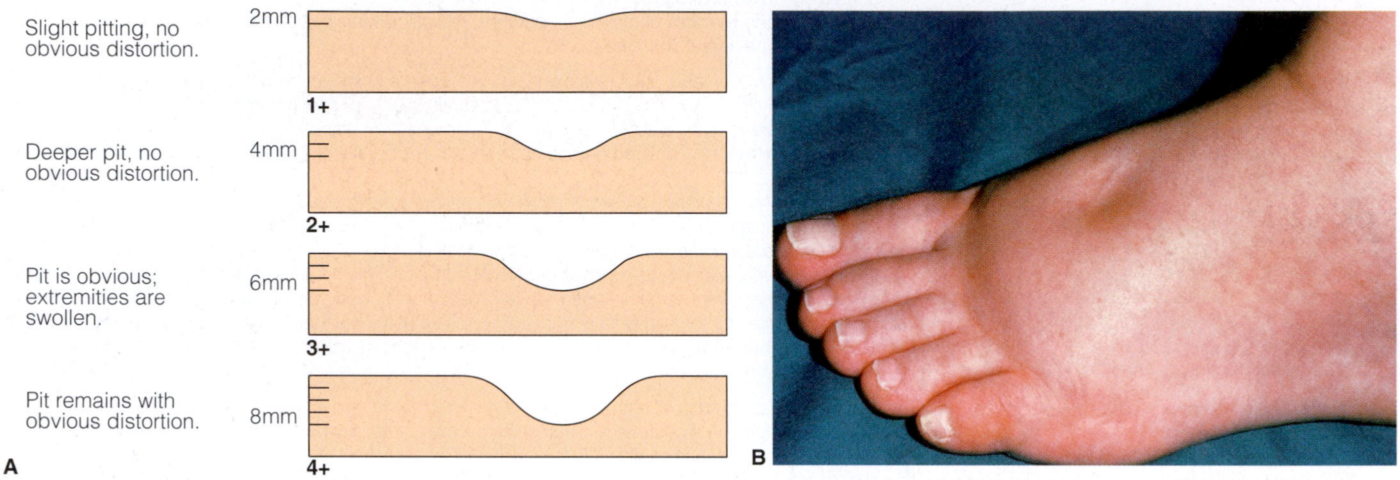
Slight pitting, no obvious distortion.
2mm
1+
Deeper pit, no obvious distortion.
4mm
2+
Pit is obvious; extremities are swollen.
6mm
3+
Pit remains with obvious distortion.
8mm
4+
A
B

Figure 15.5 ■ **A**, Degrees of pitting in edema. **B**, 4+ pitting.

Technique and Normal Findings (*in italics*)	Abnormal Findings
Inspect distribution and quality of hair. *Hair should be evenly distributed for patient's gender.*	■ A deviation in the normal hair distribution in the male or female genital area may indicate an endocrine disorder. **Hirsutism** (increased growth of coarse hair, usually on the face and trunk) is seen in Cushing's syndrome, acromegaly, and ovarian dysfunction. **Alopecia** (hair loss) may be related to changes in hormones, chemical or drug treatment, or radiation. In adult males whose hair loss follows the normal male pattern, the cause is usually genetic.
Palpate hair texture. *Hair should be of even texture.*	■ Some systemic diseases change the texture of the hair. For instance, hypothyroidism causes the hair to coarsen, whereas hyperthyroidism causes the hair to become fine.
Inspect the scalp for lesions. *There should be no lesions on the scalp.*	■ Mild dandruff is normal, but excessive, greasy flakes indicate seborrhea. ■ Hair loss, pustules, and scales appear on the scalp in tinea capitis (scalp ringworm). ■ Red, swollen pustules appear around infected hair follicles and are called folliculitis. ■ Head lice may be seen as oval nits (eggs) adhering to the base of the hair shaft. Head lice are usually accompanied by itching (Centers for Disease Control and Prevention, 2017).
Inspect nail curvature. *Nails should not be excessively curved.*	■ Clubbing (**Figure 15.6** ■), in which the angle of the nail base is greater than 180 degrees, is seen in respiratory disorders, cardiovascular disorders, cirrhosis of the liver, colitis, and thyroid disease. The nail becomes thick, hard, shiny, and curved at the free end.

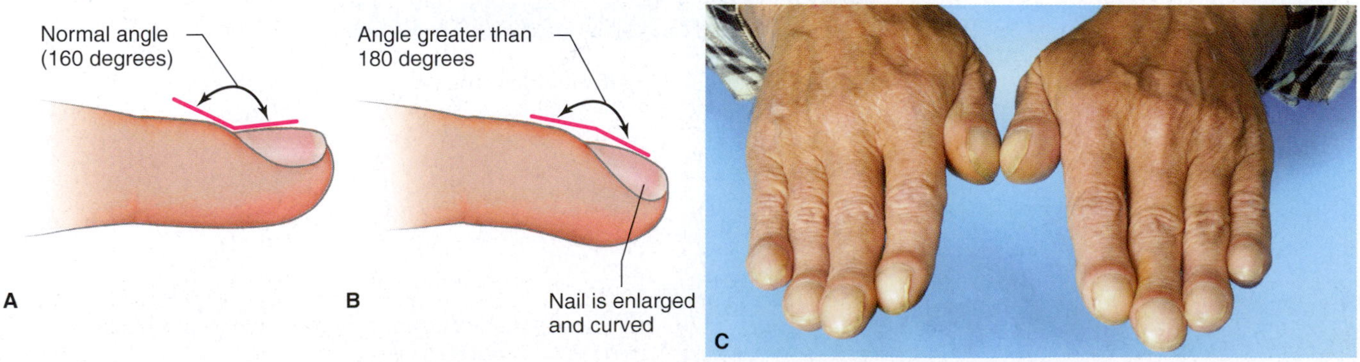
Normal angle (160 degrees)
Angle greater than 180 degrees
Nail is enlarged and curved
A
B
C

Figure 15.6 ■ **A**, Normal curvature of the nails. **B**, Clubbed fingernail. **C**, Hands with nail clubbing.

Technique and Normal Findings (*in italics*)	Abnormal Findings
Inspect the surface of the nails. *Nail surfaces should be smooth and nail folds firm, without redness.*	■ The nail folds become inflamed and swollen and the nail loosens in paronychia, an infection of the nails. ■ Inflammation and transverse rippling of the nail are associated with chronic paronychia and/or eczema. ■ The nail plate may separate from the nail bed in trauma, psoriasis, and *Pseudomonas* and *Candida* infections. This separation is called *onycholysis*. ■ Nail grooves may be caused by inflammation, by planus, or by nail biting. ■ Nail pitting may be seen with psoriasis. ■ A transverse groove (Beau's line) may be seen in trachoma and/or acute diseases. ■ Thin spoon-shaped nails (**Figure 15.7** ■) may be seen in anemia.
Inspect nail color. *Nail color should be even. Pigmented bands are normally found in more than 90% of African Americans.*	■ The sudden appearance of a pigmented band may indicate melanoma in people with light skin. ■ Yellowish nails are seen in psoriasis and fungal infections. ■ Dark nails occur with trauma, *Candida* infections, and hyperbilirubinemia. ■ Blackish-green nails are apparent in injury and in *Pseudomonas* infection. ■ Red splinter longitudinal hemorrhages may be seen in injury and/or psoriasis.
Inspect nail thickness. *Nails should not be excessively thick.*	■ Trauma to the nails usually causes thickening. Other causes of thick nails include psoriasis, fungal infections, and decreased peripheral vascular blood supply. ■ Thinning of the nails is seen in nutritional deficiencies.

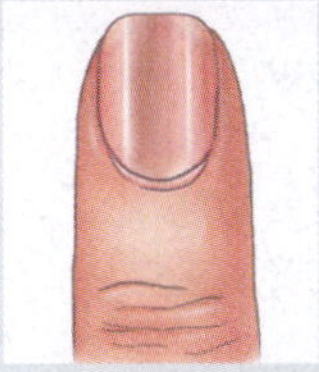

Figure 15.7 ■ Spoon-shaped nails.

Diagnosis

The results of diagnostic tests of the structure and function of the integumentary system are used to support the diagnosis of a specific injury or disease, to provide information to identify or modify the appropriate medication or treatments used to treat the disease, and to help the interprofessional team monitor a patient's responses to interventions (Kee, 2018). Some diagnostic tests are conducted to identify bacterial carriers. For example, if patients have repeated bacterial skin infections, or if a healthcare unit or agency experiences numerous bacterial infections of patients, nasal cultures may be performed to determine if the patients or the healthcare workers are carriers of the bacteria.

Regardless of the type of diagnostic test, the nurse is responsible for explaining the procedure and any special preparation needed, for assessing for medication use that may affect the outcome of the tests, for supporting the patient during the examination as necessary, for documenting the procedures as appropriate, and for monitoring the results of the tests.

Diagnostic tests to assess the integumentary system are described in the box below. More information is included in the discussion of specific health problems or injuries in Chapters 16 and 17.

Diagnostic Tests
Integumentary System

NAME OF TEST	PURPOSE AND DESCRIPTION	RELATED NURSING INTERVENTIONS
Biopsy	A punch biopsy is done to differentiate benign lesions from skin cancers. An instrument is used to remove a small section of dermis and subcutaneous fat. Depending on size, the incision may be sutured with a single suture. An incisional biopsy is done to differentiate benign lesions from skin cancers. An incision is made and the skin lesion or tumor is removed for analysis. The incision is closed with sutures.	Apply dressing and provide information about self-care and when to return for suture removal.
Culture	A culture of scrapings from a lesion, from drainage, or of exudate is done to identify fungal, bacterial, or viral skin infections.	Obtain the culture with a sterile Culturette swab and culture tubes. Maintain strict asepsis while obtaining the culture.

(continued)

Diagnostic Tests
of the Integumentary System (*continued*)

NAME OF TEST	PURPOSE AND DESCRIPTION	RELATED NURSING INTERVENTIONS
Immunofluorescent slides	Immunofluorescent studies of samples from skin and/or serum may be done to identify IgG antibodies (present in pemphigus vulgaris) and to identify varicella in skin cells (for herpes zoster). Skin or blood samples are placed on a slide and examined microscopically.	No special preparation is necessary.
Oil slides	Oil slides are used to determine the type of skin infestation present. Scrapings of the lesion are placed on a slide with mineral oil and examined microscopically.	No special preparation is necessary.
Patch test, scratch test	These tests are used to determine a specific allergen. In a patch test, a small amount of the suspected material is placed on the skin under an occlusive bandage. In a scratch test, a needle is used to "scratch" small amounts of potentially allergic materials on the skin surface.	Explain to the patient the need to return in 48 hours to have the patched or scratched areas evaluated.
Potassium hydroxide (KOH)	A specimen from hair or nails is examined for a fungal infection. The specimen is obtained by placing material from a scraping on a slide, adding a potassium hydroxide solution, and examining it microscopically.	No special preparation is necessary.
Tzanck smear	This test is used to diagnose herpes infections, but it does not differentiate herpes simplex from herpes zoster. Fluid and cells from the vesicles are obtained, put on a slide, stained, and examined microscopically.	Explain to the patient the need to collect fluid and cells from an open vesicle. Minor discomfort can occur during the incision to open the vesicle.
Wood lamp	This test uses an ultraviolet light that causes certain organisms to fluoresce (such as *Pseudomonas* organisms and fungi). The skin is examined under a special lamp.	Explain to the patient that the room is darkened to allow visualization of fluorescence.

15.3 Assessment of Selected Populations

Special consideration should be given to selected populations when assessing the integumentary system. For assessing patients with burns, refer to Chapter 17.

The skin of older adults undergoes changes due to aging (MedlinePlus, 2017a). Loss of structural thickness, fatty tissue, and elasticity result in the most visible changes. Age-related skin changes are outlined in **Table 15.7**. Common skin lesions of older adults include:

- *Skin tags:* Soft brown or flesh-colored benign papules
- *Keratoses:* Horny growths of keratinocytes; may be seborrheic (benign) or actinic (premalignant)
- *Lentigines (liver spots):* Brown or black benign macules with a defined border
- *Angiomas (hemangioma):* Benign vascular tumors with dilated blood vessels; found in the middle to upper dermis
- *Telangiectases:* Single dilated blood vessels, capillaries, or terminal arteries
- *Venous lakes:* Small, dark blue, slightly raised benign papules
- *Photoaging:* Wrinkling, mottling, pigmented areas, loss of elasticity, benign or malignant lesions.

In addition to the skin disorders seen in adults and older adults, veterans may have unusual presentations depending on their length of service, where they were stationed, and the

Table 15.7 Age-Related Skin Changes

Age-Related Change	Significance
Epidermis: ↓ thickness and miotic activity	■ Skin is more fragile and at greater risk for tears or injury ■ Delayed wound healing ■ Hyperkeratoses and skin cancers in sun-exposed areas are more evident
Epidermis: ↑ permeability, ↓ Langerhans cells	■ Increased risk of reactions to irritants ■ Decreased inflammatory response
Epidermis: ↓ number of active melanocytes	■ Increased susceptibility to sun exposure
Epidermis: hyperplasia of melanocytes, especially in sun-exposed areas	■ Small areas of hyperpigmentation (liver spots) and hypopigmentation (age spots), especially on the hands
Epidermis: ↓ vitamin D production	■ Increased risk of osteomalacia, osteoporosis
Epidermis: dermal–epidermal junction flattens	■ Increased risk of skin tears, purpura, and pressure ulcers
Dermis: ↓ perfusion	■ More susceptible to dry skin ■ Decreased sensation (pain, touch, temperature, and peripheral vibration) ■ Increased risk of injury
Dermis: ↓ vasomotor response	■ Greater risk of hyperthermia and hypothermia
Dermis: elastic fibers degenerate	■ Decreased tone and elasticity, with wrinkle formation
Dermis: proliferation of capillaries	■ Cherry hemangiomas are common
Subcutaneous skin layer: thins	■ Greater risk of hypothermia ■ Increased risk of pressure ulcers
Subcutaneous skin layer: adipose tissue is redistributed	■ Cellulite forms ■ Bags over and under the eyes ■ Double chin forms ■ Abdominal fat increases ■ Breasts sag ■ Skin returns to normal more slowly when pinched (called *tenting*)
Glands: ↓ eccrine and apocrine activity	■ Dry skin is common ■ Absent perspiration

chemicals or other substances to which they were exposed (Veterans Administration, 2015; Veterans Administration Public Health, 2015). Alterations to be aware of include:

- Chloracne (acneform disease) is the eruption of nodules, cysts, and blackheads that have been linked to contaminants found in herbicides like Agent Orange.
- Porphyria cutanea tarda (PCT) is the thinning/blistering of skin with sun exposure following hexachlorabenzene exposure in the presence of alcohol overuse. Skin irritation/chemical burns are secondary to industrial solvent exposure.

There are a few significant integumentary disorders that afflict the LGBTQI population more than the general population (MedlinePlus, 2017b). However, these are related to other primary disease processes. For example, tumors of Kaposi sarcoma (KS) are cancerous lesions arising from the cells lining lymph or blood vessels. One type of KS is related to HIV and is considered an AIDS-defining illness. With the advent of highly active antiretroviral therapy, onset of KS has declined.

15.4 Health Promotion

The nurse is instrumental in promoting health of the integumentary system throughout the lifespan. This includes careful self-surveillance and prevention of exposure to sun and environmental and occupational risks. First and foremost is promoting the use of sunscreen at all ages.

Use Sunscreen

It is well known that cumulative sun exposure positively correlates with nonmelanoma skin cancers (National Cancer Institute, 2017). Many skin cancers can be prevented by limiting exposure to risk factors. Primary prevention behaviors recommended by the American Cancer Society (2017) and the Skin Cancer Foundation (Moy & Famenini, 2017) include:

- Minimize sun exposure between the hours of 10:00 A.M. and 3:00 P.M., when ultraviolet rays are the strongest.
- Cover up with a wide-brimmed hat, sunglasses, long-sleeved shirt, and long pants made of tightly woven materials when in the sun.
- Apply a waterproof or water-resistant sunscreen with an SPF of 15 or more at least 30 minutes before every exposure to the sun. If swimming or sweating heavily, reapply every hour. Apply sunscreen not only on sunny days but also on cloudy days (when ultraviolet rays can penetrate 70% to 80% of the cloud cover).
- Apply adequate sunscreen to achieve SPF 15, which requires 2 mg of sunscreen per square centimeter of skin. This is about 2 tablespoons to exposed face and body, or about a nickel-sized amount for the face alone (Moy & Famenini, 2017).

- Use sunscreen and protective clothing when you are on or near sand, snow, concrete, or water (which can reflect more than 50% of the ultraviolet rays onto your skin).
- Avoid tanning booths; ultraviolet rays emitted by tanning booths damages the deep skin layers.

In addition to these preventative behaviors, the ACS recommends the Slip! Slop! Slap! Wrap! method:

Slip on a shirt

Slop on 15 SPF (or higher) sunscreen

Slap on a hat

Wrap on sunglasses before exposure to the sun.

Information about sunscreens is given in **Box 15.1**.

Nurses also provide patient and family education for early detection of nonmelanoma skin cancer. Numerous brochures describing the types of skin cancers, photographs of lesions, and prevention behaviors are available from the ACS, health education and support agencies, and pharmaceutical companies that manufacture sunscreen. Most of this literature is free.

The patient or family at risk for or diagnosed with a skin cancer must be taught how to conduct a self-examination of the skin, described in **Box 15.2**, as well as the importance of conducting the examination on the same day of each month. Family members can help with areas that are hard to examine, such as the ears, scalp, and back.

BOX 15.1
Sunscreen Information

TYPES OF SUNSCREEN

Chemical

Chemical sunscreens absorb ultraviolet light and act as a radiation filter. Examples are:

- *p*-Aminobenzoic acid (PABA)
- Benzophenones
- Anthranilates
- Salicylates.

Physical

Physical sunscreens reflect and scatter ultraviolet light. Examples are:

- Zinc oxide
- Titanium dioxide
- Magnesium silicate
- Ferric chloride
- Kaolin
- Ichthyol.

ADVERSE REACTIONS ASSOCIATED WITH SUNSCREENS

Adverse reactions associated with sunscreens include contact and photocontact dermatitis. People with previous hypersensitivity reactions to benzocaine, procaine, sulfonamides, or paraphenylenediamine may develop hypersensitivity responses to PABA. People who are also taking systemic thiazide diuretics or sulfonamides may develop eczematous dermatitis.

SUNSCREEN RATINGS

In the United States, the U.S. Food and Drug Administration (FDA, 2017) rates commercial sunscreens according to their sun protection factor, or SPF. The SPF value is the ratio of the time required to produce minimal skin redness through a sunscreen product to the time required to produce the same degree of redness without the sunscreen. A person who can tolerate 1/2 hour of sun without a sunscreen should be able to tolerate 3 hours of sun when a sunscreen of SPF 6 is applied to the skin. SPF values of sunscreens range from 2 to 100. An SPF of 15 or greater is recommended.

BOX 15.2
Skin Self-Examination

1. Choose the same day each month (such as the first day) to do the examination.
2. The best time to do the examination is after you take a bath or shower. Examine yourself in a well-lighted room in front of a full-length mirror. Have a hand mirror, a chair, and a hair dryer available. If you have difficulty seeing your back and scalp (or any other parts of your body), ask someone to help you.
3. Follow the same pattern with each examination:

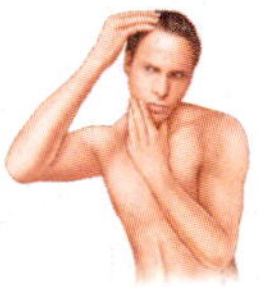

Examine head and face, using one or both mirrors. Use blow dryer to inspect scalp.

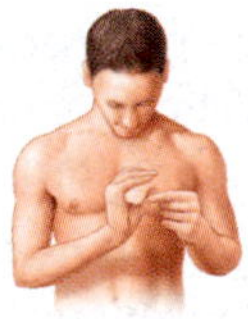

Check hands, including nails. In full-length mirror, examine elbows, arms, underarms.

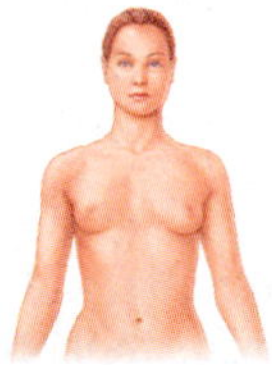

Focus on neck, chest, torso. Women: Check under breasts.

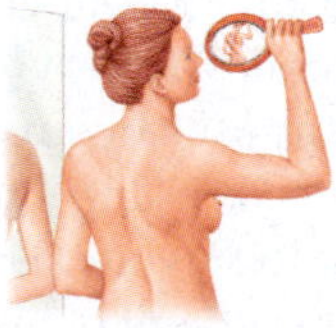

With back to the mirror, use hand mirror to inspect back of neck and back including buttocks.

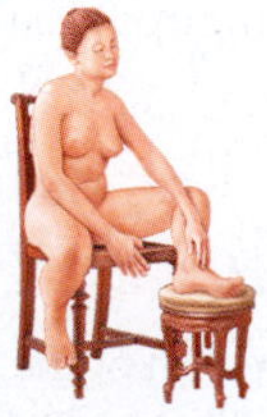

Sitting down, check legs and feet, including soles, heels, and nails. Use hand mirror to examine genitals.

Skin Self-Examination

Examining one's own skin is the first step in identifying concerns or changes (see Box 15.2 for patient teaching). All new changes in skin (new moles or other eruptions) or changes to existing skin features should be referred to the healthcare provider. According to the American Cancer Society (2017), the **ABCDE** rule provides a mnemonic for remembering the usual signs of melanoma:

Asymmetry: One half of a mole or birthmark does not match the other.

Border: The edges are irregular, ragged, notched, or blurred.

Color: The color is not the same all over and may include shades of brown or black, or sometimes with patches of pink, red, white, or blue.

Diameter: The spot is larger than 6 millimeters in diameter, although melanomas can sometimes be smaller than this.

Evolving: The mole is changing in size, shape, or color.

Prevention of Burns

Although treatments for burns have improved significantly during the past several decades, there is no cure for burns. Prevention remains the primary goal. With the public's increasing attention to health promotion and disease prevention, the nursing profession is currently well positioned to collaborate with other disciplines to develop initiatives to reduce the number of burn injuries. For example, as patient advocates, nurses can alert political leaders to the need to pass legislation aimed at reducing the incidence of burns. Appropriate legislative themes might center on safety in the workplace (e.g., requirements for smoke alarms and sprinkler systems), on the highways (e.g., regulations regarding the transportation of flammable liquids), and in the home (e.g., requirements for safety devices for water heaters and wood-burning stoves and for self-extinguishing cigarettes). As educators, nurses can develop teaching plans for families and communities to heighten awareness of the problem. As researchers, nurses can investigate conditions leading to burn injury and suggest methods to reduce its prevalence. Working together with healthcare policymakers and community leaders, nurses can join the effort to lower the number of annual burn cases.

CHAPTER HIGHLIGHTS

15.1 Anatomy, Physiology, and Function of the Integumentary System

Describe the anatomy, physiology, and functions of the skin, hair, and nails, and identify abnormal findings that may indicate impairment of the integumentary system.

- Intact structure and function of the integumentary system is vital to the protection of the body's organs from the external environment.
- The skin is the body's largest organ, providing protection of fluid–electrolyte balance, temperature regulation, and prevention of infection.
- The hair serves a protective function over the body, including temperature regulation and capture of foreign particles. Another function is to trap sweat, which contains pheromones, useful in attraction.
- The nails protect the tips of fingers and toes as well as the soft tissues of the distal ends of digits. The nails also enhance precise movements of the digits.

15.2 Assessing the Integumentary System

Outline the components of the assessment of the integumentary system including topics for the health assessment interview, techniques for physical assessment, and the diagnostic tests used in the assessment.

- Manifestations of dysfunction, injury, and disorders affecting the integumentary system may be detected during a general health assessment as well as during focused integumentary assessments.
- The health assessment interview determines the problems with the integumentary system as noted by the client.
- The physical assessment is conducted by inspection and palpation. Examination provides objective determination of integumentary issues.
- Diagnostic tests of the integumentary inform and support the diagnosis of specific injury or disease of the integumentary system.

15.3 Assessment of Selected Populations

Differentiate considerations for assessing the integumentary system of older adults, veterans, individuals in the LGBTQI population, and adults with sequelae from complex congenital conditions.

- Older adult integument commonly reveals expected age-related changes.

- Integumentary issues of veterans are commonly related to exposure to environmental, chemical, or other substances not experienced by the general population.
- While LGBTQI experience few primary integumentary conditions, those seen are usually related to other primary disease processes.
- Adults with a history of complex congenital conditions do not usually have significant integumentary disorders. Any disorders noted at birth are commonly addressed in infancy or childhood.

15.4 Health Promotion

Summarize topics that nurses teach to promote healthy tissue integrity across the lifespan.

- The use of sunscreen is the most important health-promoting action that patients can do to prevent long-term skin damage and reduce the risk of skin cancer.
- Skin self-examination is an underutilized, but important skill set for patients. Use of monthly self-examination provides early detection of skin changes.

TEST YOURSELF NCLEX-RN® REVIEW

1. Following a burn involving several layers of a patient's skin, the healed burn area does not grow hair or sweat. When teaching the patient, which layer of the skin should the nurse explain as being the deepest layer burned?
   A. Dermis
   B. Epidermis
   C. Stratum basale
   D. Stratum spinosum
2. During an assessment the nurse notes different areas of skin color over the back and chest of a patient who spends time in the sun. What is responsible for this change in skin color?
   A. Sebum
   B. Melanin
   C. Carotene
   D. Red blood cells
3. The nurse is preparing to assess a patient's integumentary status. Which technique will the nurse use first?
   A. Palpation
   B. Inspection
   C. Percussion
   D. Auscultation
4. A patient's oral body temperature is elevated by 3 degrees. What other assessment finding would be consistent with this body temperature?
   A. Pallor
   B. Jaundice
   C. Cyanosis
   D. Erythema
5. The nurse is assessing a patient who is complaining of severe itching. Which questions about the itching should the nurse ask the patient during the interview? (Select all that apply.)
   A. "Tell me how this itch feels."
   B. "Have you used a new soap?"
   C. "Why do you keep scratching it?"
   D. "When did you first notice the itch?"
   E. "Have you ever had itching like this before now?"
6. While conducting a skin assessment, the nurse suspects an older patient is experiencing dehydration. What did the nurse most likely assess in this patient?
   A. Decreased turgor
   B. Pallor or cyanosis
   C. Increased moisture
   D. Presence of lesions
7. The intravenous access site infiltrated in a patient's right hand. When assessing the degree of edema, the nurse finds obvious pitting and the entire hand is swollen. How should the nurse document this assessment finding?
   A. 1+
   B. 2+
   C. 3+
   D. 4+
8. The nurse assesses rough thickened areas on a patient with chronic dermatitis. What term should the nurse use to document this assessment finding?
   A. Ulcers
   B. Papules
   C. Atrophy
   D. Lichenification
9. The nurse notices multiple flat pinpoint red dots with tiny radiating blood vessels on the patient's skin. The lesions blanch with pressure. The nurse would conduct further assessment for which conditions? (Select all that apply.)
   A. Liver disease
   B. Poor hygiene
   C. Impaired immune system
   D. Vitamin B deficiency
   E. High sodium diet
10. The school nurse suspects an outbreak of head lice among children in a first grade classroom. The nurse would assess these children for the presence of which finding?
    A. Pustules behind the ears
    B. Greasy scaling
    C. Oval objects on the hair shafts
    D. White flakes throughout the hair

See Test Yourself answers in Appendix B.

REFERENCES

American Cancer Society. (2017). *What should I look for on a skin self-exam?* Retrieved from https://www.cancer.org/cancer/skin-cancer/prevention-and-early-detection/what-to-look-for.html.

Centers for Disease Control and Prevention. (2017). *Parasites—lice—head lice.* Retrieved from https://www.cdc.gov/parasites/lice/index.html.

Kee, J. L. (2018). *Laboratory and diagnostic tests with nursing implications.* (10th ed.). Hoboken, NJ: Pearson Education.

Kottner, J., & Surber, C. (2016). Skin care in nursing: A critical discussion of nursing practice and research. *International Journal of Nursing Studies 61*, 20–28.

MedlinePlus. (2017a). *Aging changes in skin*. Retrieved from https://medlineplus.gov/ency/article/004014.htm.

MedlinePlus. (2017b). *Gay, lesbian, bisexual, and transgender health.* Retrieved from https://medlineplus.gov/gaylesbianbisexualandtransgenderhealth.html#cat_79.

Moy, R. L., & Famenini, S. (2017). *Skin cancer prevention strategies: Tried, true, & new.* New York: Skin Cancer Foundation. Retrieved from http://www.skincancer.org/prevention/sun-protection/prevention-guidelines/new.

National Cancer Institute. (2017). *Skin cancer.* Retrieved from https://www.cancer.gov/types/skin/hp.

National Institutes of Health. (2017). *Genes and disease: Skin and connective tissue.* Retrieved from https://www.ncbi.nlm.nih.gov/books/NBK22247/pdf/Bookshelf_NBK22247.pdf.

Sorenson, M., Quinn, L., & Klein, D. (2019). *Pathophysiology: Concepts of human disease.* Hoboken, NJ: Pearson Education.

Spector, R. E. (2017). *Cultural diversity in health and illness* (9th ed.). Hoboken, NJ: Pearson Education.

U.S. Food and Drug Administration. (2017). Sunscreen: How to help protect your skin from the sun. Retrieved from https://www.fda.gov/Drugs/ResourcesForYou/Consumers/BuyingUsingMedicineSafely/UnderstandingOver-the-CounterMedicines/ucm239463.htm.

Veterans Administration. (2015). Disability compensation: "Presumptive" disability benefits. Retrieved from https://www.benefits.va.gov/BENEFITS/factsheets/serviceconnected/presumption.pdf.

Veterans Administration Public Health (VA Public Health). (2015). Veterans' diseases associated with Agent Orange. Retrieved from https://www.publichealth.va.gov/exposures/agentorange/conditions/.

ADDITIONAL RESOURCES

American Academy of Dermatology
https://www.aad.org/for-the-public

American Cancer Society: Skin Self-exam Gallery
https://www.cancer.org/cancer/skin-cancer/galleries/skin-self-exam-gallery.html

Livestrong: Crucial Tips to Guard Against Skin Cancer
https://www.livestrong.com/slideshow/1011066-crucial-tips-safeguard-against-skin-cancer/

Chapter 16

Nursing Care of Patients with Integumentary Disorders

Chapter Outline and Learning Outcomes

16.1 Common Skin Problems and Lesions 471

Describe the pathophysiology and manifestations of common skin problems and lesions, and outline the interprofessional care and nursing care of patients with these disorders.

16.2 Infections and Infestations of the Skin 477

Describe the pathophysiology and manifestations of infections and infestations of the skin, and outline the interprofessional care and nursing care of patients with these disorders.

16.3 Inflammatory Disorders of the Skin 488

Describe the pathophysiology and manifestations of inflammatory disorders of the skin, and outline the interprofessional care and nursing care of patients with these disorders.

16.4 Acute Skin Disorders 492

Describe the risk factors for and pathophysiology and manifestations of acute skin disorders, and outline the interprofessional care and nursing care of patients with these disorders.

16.5 Malignant Skin Disorders 493

Describe the risk factors for and pathophysiology and manifestations of malignant skin disorders, and outline the interprofessional care and nursing care of patients with these disorders.

16.6 Skin Trauma 503

Describe the pathophysiology and manifestations of skin trauma, and outline the interprofessional care and nursing care of patients with these disorders.

16.7 Hair and Nail Disorders 513

Describe the pathophysiology and manifestations of disorders of the hair and nails, and outline the interprofessional care and nursing care of patients with these disorders.

CLINICAL COMPETENCIES

- Assess functional health status of patients with integumentary disorders, and monitor, document, and report abnormal manifestations.
- Plan and implement evidence-based nursing interventions for patients with pressure injuries.
- Consider assessment findings, patient values and beliefs, cultural norms, best practices, and clinical expertise when developing and implementing an individualized plan of care.
- Apply safe practices during the administration of topical, oral, and injectable medications for the treatment of integumentary disorders.
- Collaborate with the interprofessional team in the planning and provision of care for patients with integumentary disorders.
- Implement patient teaching focused on prevention and management of integumentary disorders.
- Revise the plan of care as needed to provide effective interventions to promote, maintain, or restore functional health status to patients with disorders of the integument.

KEY TERMS

acne, 489
actinic keratosis, 493
angioma, 473
basal cell cancer, 494
carbuncle, 478
cellulitis, 478
comedones, 489
cyst, 472
dermatitis, 488
dermatophytoses, 481
folliculitis, 477
frostbite, 508
furuncle, 478
herpes simplex, 484
herpes zoster, 484
keloids, 473
keratosis, 474
lichen planus, 491
melanoma, 496
nevi, 473
paronychia, 514
pemphigus vulgaris, 491
pressure injury, 503
pruritus, 471
psoriasis, 474
rosacea, 490
scabies, 483
skin graft, 510
squamous cell cancer, 495
Stevens-Johnson syndrome, 492
warts, 483
xerosis, 471

The skin and its accessory structures (the integumentary system) enclose and cover the body, providing protection by serving as a barrier between the internal and external environments. The skin contains receptors for touch and sensation, helps regulate body temperature, and maintains fluid and electrolyte balance. The skin also provides cues to ethnic background and plays a major part in determining self-concept, roles, and relationships.

Disorders of the integument range from dry skin to life-threatening cancer. Many disorders are treated in an outpatient setting or by self-care. This chapter discusses disorders of the skin, hair, and nails. Chapter 17 discusses the patient with burns. Primary and secondary skin lesions are described and illustrated in Chapter 15, Tables 15.4 and 15.5. The terms introduced in those tables are used throughout this and the next chapter.

16.1 Common Skin Problems and Lesions

The disorders discussed in this section are those experienced by a large number of people. Although they are considered minor health problems in terms of healthcare, they may cause major problems for the person experiencing a high level of discomfort and/or chronicity.

The Patient with Pruritus

Pruritus is a subjective itching sensation that produces an urge to scratch. Pruritus may occur in a small, circumscribed area, or it may involve a widespread area; it may or may not be associated with a rash. The itch sensation begins in nerve endings in the skin, is carried to the dorsal horn of the spinal cord, and is then transmitted to the somatosensory cortex in the central nervous system (CNS). Itching may also be perceived by the brain, but not exist on the skin. Scratching is a neurologic reflex that can be controlled in varying degrees by the individual (Sorenson, Quinn, & Klein, 2019).

Almost anything in the internal or external environment can cause pruritus. Insects, animals, plants, fabrics, metals, medications, allergies, and emotional distress are among the most common causes. Pruritus may also occur as a secondary manifestation of systemic disorders, such as certain types of cancer, diabetes mellitus, liver disease, and renal failure. Although the exact physiology is unknown, heat and prostaglandins are known triggers of pruritus, and pruritus is increased by histamine and morphine.

The pathophysiologic response of pruritus to stimulation or irritation follows a similar pathway, regardless of cause. The irritating agent stimulates receptors in the junction between the epidermis and dermis and may also trigger the release of histamine and other chemical mediators that either further stimulate or mediate the itch response. The response of the person experiencing the itch is to scratch or rub the affected area. This may irritate the skin and cause further inflammation, which in turn sets off a cycle of increasingly intense itching and scratching, called the *itch–scratch–itch cycle.*

Secondary effects of scratching include skin excoriation, erythema (redness), wheals, changes in pigmentation, and infections. Persistent pruritus may interrupt sleep patterns because the itching sensation is often more intense at night. Long-term pruritus may be debilitating and increases the risk of infection as excoriation occurs.

Management of pruritus focuses on identifying and eliminating its cause and providing medications to relieve the itch. Antihistamines may relieve pruritus in some patients. Tranquilizers provide sedation, which may in turn relieve the emotional stress associated with pruritus; however, eliminating the stressors produces a more successful result. Topical or systemic antibiotics are used to treat the infection resulting from the scratching and excoriation. Topical medications that contain corticosteroids are often used to relieve the pruritus and inflammation. Topical medications may also be administered through therapeutic baths or soaks with agents that relieve pruritus, such as cornstarch and baking soda or coal tar concentrates. Creams containing a topical anesthetic or antibiotic may also be used. Therapeutic baths are discussed in **Medication Administration 16.A** on page 472. **Table 16.1** lists examples of topical agents used to treat skin disorders.

The Patient with Dry Skin (Xerosis)

Dry skin, also called **xerosis**, is most often a problem in the older adult. It is the result of a decrease in the activity of sebaceous and sweat glands, which reduces the skin's lubrication and moisture retention abilities. However, dry skin may occur at any age from exposure to environmental heat and low humidity, sunlight, excessive bathing, and a decreased intake of liquids.

Two types of severe dry skin are xeroderma and ichthyosis. *Xeroderma* is a chronic skin condition characterized by dry, rough skin. *Ichthyosis* is an inherited dermatologic condition in which the skin is dry, fissured, and hyperkeratotic; the surface of the skin has the appearance of fish scales.

Table 16.1 **Medications Used to Treat Skin Disorders**

Type	Use	Examples
Creams	Moisturize the skin	Aqua Care, Curel, Nutraderm
Ointments	Lubricate the skin and retard water loss	Aquaphor, Vaseline
Lotions	Moisturize and lubricate the skin	Alpha-Keri, Dermassage, Lubriderm
Anesthetics	Relieve itching	Xylocaine
Antibiotics	Treat infection	Bacitracin, Polysporin, Gentamicin, Silvadene
Corticosteroids	Suppress inflammation and relieve itching	Dexamethasone, Clocortolone, Desonide

Medication Administration 16.A

Therapeutic Baths

AGENTS USED IN THERAPEUTIC BATHS

Saline or tap water

Antibacterial agents: potassium permanganate, acetic acid, hexachlorophene

Colloid substances: oatmeal (Aveeno), cornstarch, sodium bicarbonate

Coal tar derivatives (Balnetar, Zetar, Polytar)

Emollients: Alpha Keri, Lubath, mineral oil

Therapeutic baths have a variety of uses in treating skin disorders. Depending on the agent used, therapeutic baths soothe the skin, lower the skin bacteria count, clean and hydrate the skin, loosen scales, and relieve itching.

Nursing Responsibilities

- Ensure that the bath water is at a comfortable temperature that is neither too hot nor too cool, usually 39°C (100°F) to 45°C (110°F); the ideal therapeutic bath is 100°F.
- Fill the tub one-third to one-half full.
- Mix the agent well with the water.
- Assist the patient into and out of the tub to prevent falls.
- Dry the patient's skin by blotting with the towel.

Health Education for the Patient and Family

- Use a bath mat in the tub because the medications may cause the tub to become slippery.
- Keep the bathroom warm but adequately ventilated.
- Follow directions carefully for the amount of medication to use in the bath.
- Fill the bath one-third to one-half full of water that is at a comfortable temperature.
- Stay in the bath for 20 to 30 minutes, and immerse the areas to be treated.
- Do not get the bath water in your eyes.
- Dry by blotting (not rubbing) with the towel.
- If the medications cause staining, use old towels or linens.
- If the itching is not relieved or the skin becomes excessively dry, call your healthcare provider.

Source: Data from Adams, Holland, & Urban, 2017.

The primary manifestation of dry skin is pruritus. Other manifestations include visible flaking of surface skin and an observable pattern of fine lines over the area. If the skin has been excessively dry and pruritic for a long period, the patient may have secondary skin lesions and lichenification (thickening).

Nursing care focuses on teaching the patient and family how to reduce the dry skin and relieve the pruritus, as follows:

- Wash clothing in a mild detergent and rinse twice; do not use fabric softeners.
- Avoid using perfumes and lotions containing alcohol.
- Apply skin lubricants after a bath to help retain moisture.
- Soaps and hot water are drying. Clean the skin with tepid water and either a mild soap or cleansing creams. If soap is used, rinse it off carefully.
- It is not necessary to take a bath every day.
- If bath oils are used, add them to the bath water at the end of the bath (the moist skin is more likely to retain the oil). Use care not to slip in the tub.
- Use a humidifier to humidify the air.
- Apply creams and lotions when the skin is slightly damp after bathing.
- Increase fluid intake.
- Keep nails trimmed short, wear loose clothing, and keep the environment cool.
- A brief application of pressure or cold may relieve pruritus.
- Cotton gloves may be worn at night if scratching during sleep causes skin excoriation.
- Distraction or relaxation techniques may prove helpful.

The Patient with Benign Skin Lesions

The skin is subject to many different types and kinds of benign skin lesions, including cysts, keloids, nevi, angiomas, skin tags, and keratoses. Although these benign lesions are often considered more of a nuisance than an illness, they do require monitoring for an increase in size that interferes with the skin's appearance or function. Most benign skin lesions do not require treatment, although excision or laser surgery may be desired or necessary. Cysts may enlarge, skin tags may become irritated and bleed, nevi may change in appearance, or any of the lesions may cause discomfort with appearance.

Cysts

Cysts of the skin are benign closed sacs in or under the skin surface that are lined with epithelium and contain fluid or a semisolid material. Epidermal inclusion cysts and pilar cysts are the most common types.

Epidermal inclusion cysts may occur anywhere on the body but are most often found on the head and trunk. Although they are painless, they may grow so large that they become irritated by contact with clothing (e.g., if located on the back of the neck) or cause obstruction (e.g., if located on the nose). The cysts contain a semisolid material consisting mainly of keratin. Pilar cysts are found on the scalp and originate from sebaceous glands. They are also painless. Both types of cysts rarely require treatment unless they become large and bothersome.

Keloids

Keloids are elevated, irregularly shaped, progressively enlarging scars. They arise from excessive amounts of collagen in the stratum corneum during scar formation in connective tissue repair. These lesions are more common in young adults and appear within 1 year of the initial trauma.

This response most often occurs in people of African and Asian descent who sustain burns of the skin, but even seemingly minor trauma can result in keloid formation. Certain skin surfaces are also more likely to develop keloids: the chin, ears, shoulders, back, and lower legs. There is a familial tendency to develop keloids.

Risk factors for keloid formation include:

- Being of African or Asian descent
- Having other family members with keloids
- Having excessive tension on a wound and poor alignment of skin edges following accidental or intentional skin trauma.

The excessive scar formation is associated with increased metabolic activity of fibroblasts and increased type III collagen (**Figure 16.1** ■). The swollen appearance of the keloids is the result of an excess of extracellular material. The keloids first appear as red, firm, rubbery plaques that persist for several months after the initial trauma. Uncontrolled overgrowth over time causes the keloids to extend beyond the original scar. Eventually, the keloid becomes smooth and hyperpigmented.

Nevi

Nevi, more commonly called *moles*, are flat or raised macules or papules with rounded, well-defined borders (**Figure 16.2** ■). Nevi arise from melanocytes during early childhood, with the cells initially accumulating at the junction of the dermis and epidermis. Over time, the cluster of cells moves into the dermis, and the lesion becomes visible. Nevi can occur on any skin surface of the body and may arise as single lesions or in groups. Almost all adults have nevi.

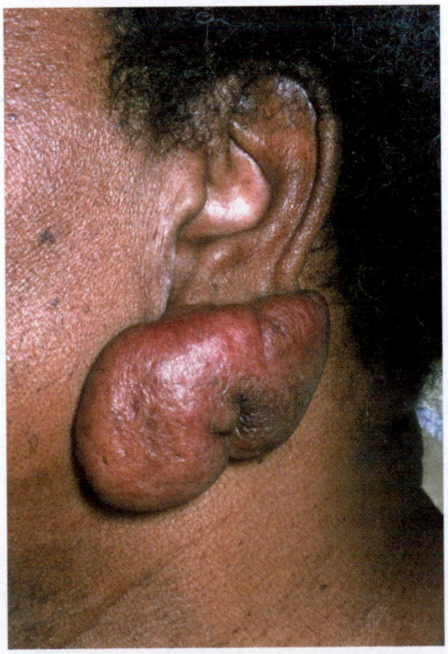

Figure 16.1 ■ Keloids form as a result of deposits of excessive amounts of collagen during scar formation.

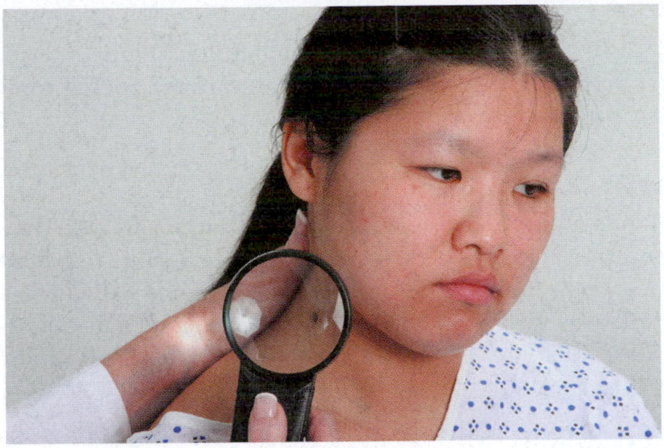

Figure 16.2 ■ Nevi (moles) arise from melanocytes and are common in all adults.

Nevocellular nevi are tan to deep brown, small in size, and grow in groups. *Dysplastic nevi* are larger than other nevi and may be flat, slightly raised, or appear as lesions with a darker, raised center and irregular border. Dysplastic nevi can transform into malignant lesions (see the later discussion about melanoma). It is important to monitor nevi for changes in size, thickness, color, bleeding, or itching. If any of these changes occur, the person should seek immediate professional assessment.

Angiomas

Angiomas, also called *hemangiomas*, are benign vascular tumors. They appear in the adult in different forms:

- ***Nevus flammeus*** (port-wine stain) is a congenital vascular lesion that involves the capillaries. The lesions tend to occur on the upper body or face as macular patches that range from light red to dark purple. These lesions are present at birth and grow proportionately with the child into adulthood.
- ***Cherry angiomas*** are small, rounded papules that may occur at any age, but they most commonly arise in the 40s and gradually increase in number. The lesions range in color from bright red to purple. These lesions are often found on the trunk.
- ***Spider angiomas*** are dilated superficial arteries. They are common in pregnant women and in patients with hepatic disease. Spider angiomas occur most often on the face, neck, and upper chest. The lesions are usually small, bright red papules with radiating lines.
- ***Telangiectases*** are single, dilated capillaries or terminal arteries that appear most often on the cheeks and nose. These lesions are more common in older adults and result from photoaged (aging, sun-damaged) skin. The lesions look like broken veins.

- *Venous lakes* are small, flat, blue blood vessels. They are seen on the exposed skin of the older adult: the ears, lips, and backs of the hands. They are considered compressible papules.

Skin Tags

Skin tags are soft papules on a pedicle (**Figure 16.3** ■). They can be as small as a pinhead or as large as a pea and are most often found on the front or side of the neck and in the axillae, as well as in areas where clothing (such as underwear) rubs the skin. These lesions have normal skin color and texture.

Keratoses

A **keratosis** is any skin condition in which there is a benign overgrowth and thickening of the cornified epithelium. These lesions most often appear in adults after age 50. *Seborrheic keratoses* appear as superficial flat, smooth, or warty-surfaced growths, 5 to 20 mm in diameter, most often on the face and trunk. The lesions may be tan, waxy yellow, dark brown, or flesh colored, and they often appear greasy. They are most often seen in the older adult and do not appear to be related to damage from sun exposure.

The Patient with Psoriasis

Psoriasis is a chronic immune skin disorder characterized by raised, reddened, round circumscribed (**Figure 16.4** ■). There are several different forms, but the most common is plaque psoriasis (psoriasis vulgaris), occurring in about 80% of cases (American Academy of Dermatology [AAD], 2017). As with any chronic illness, the skin manifestations may occur and disappear throughout life, with no discernible pattern to the recurrence.

As many as 7.5 million people in the United States have psoriasis; about 20% have moderate to severe forms (AAD, 2017). The incidence of psoriasis is lower in warm, sunny climates. The average age of onset is in the 30s, but it may occur at any age. Psoriasis occurs more often in Caucasians, and men and women are affected equally. Sunlight, stress, seasonal changes, hormone fluctuations, steroid withdrawal, and certain drugs (such as beta-blockers,

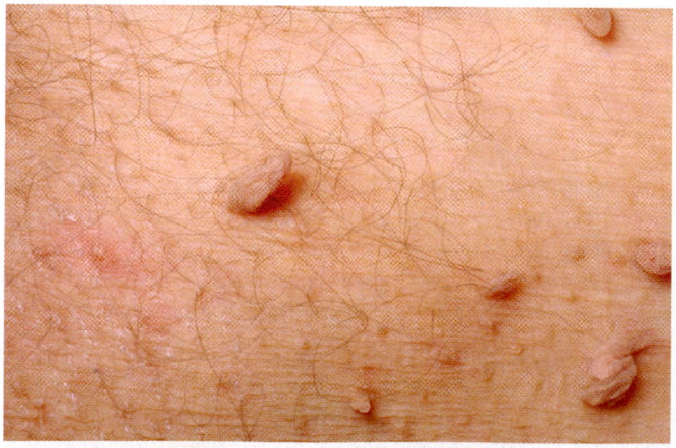

Figure 16.3 ■ Skin tags are soft papules.

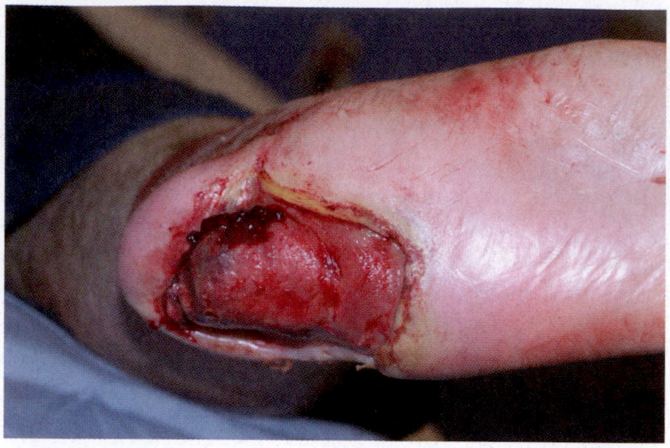

Figure 16.4 ■ The characteristic lesions of psoriasis are raised, red, round plaques covered with thick, silvery scales.

lithium, and chloroquine [an antimalarial]) appear to act as triggers to development of the disorder. About one-third of patients have a family history of psoriasis. Trauma to the skin from such events as surgery, sunburn, or excoriation is also a common precipitating factor; lesions that result from trauma are called *Koebner reaction* (Sorenson et al., 2019).

Pathophysiology and Manifestations

Normally, the keratinocyte (an epidermal cell making up 95% of the epidermis) migrates from the basal cell to the stratum corneum (the outer skin layer) in about 14 days and is sloughed off 14 days later. Psoriatic skin cells, by contrast, have a shorter cycle of growth, completing the journey to the stratum corneum in only 4 to 7 days, a condition called *hyperkeratosis*. These immature cells produce an abnormal keratin that forms thick, flaky scales at the surface of the skin. The increased cell metabolism stimulates increased vascularity, which contributes to the erythema of the lesions.

Although the exact cause is unknown, there is increasing evidence that a T-lymphocyte-mediated reaction results in the production of chemical messengers that stimulate the growth of keratinocytes and dermal blood vessels. The accompanying inflammation further contributes to plaque formation. The lesions can be found anywhere on the skin but most commonly involve the skin over the elbows, knees, and scalp. Lesions involving the hand and foot are especially problematic for the patient. Initially, the lesions are papules that form into well-defined erythematous plaques with thick, silvery scales. The plaques in darker-skinned people may appear purple.

Manifestations

The characteristic lesions in plaque psoriasis are well-demarcated regions of erythematous plaques that shed thick, silver-gray flakes. Pruritus is common over the psoriatic lesions. If the lesions are located in an intertriginous zone, such as between the toes, under the breasts, or in the perianal region, the psoriatic scales may soften, allowing painful fissures to form. When psoriasis affects the nails, pitting and a yellow or brown discoloration results. The nail may separate from the nail bed, thicken, and crumble. The involved nails, which are more often fingernails than toenails, are at high risk for infection. Psoriatic arthritis is a specific form of arthritis involving not only skin lesions but also inflammation of joints.

Interprofessional Care

Treatment is based on the type of psoriasis, the extent and location of the lesions, the age of the patient, and the degree of disfigurement or disability.

Diagnosis

Skin biopsy may be done if the patient presents with atypical manifestations or to differentiate psoriasis from other inflammatory or infectious skin disorders. In addition, an ultrasound may reveal typical psoriatic changes in the stratum corneum and inflammation of the dermis.

Medications

A variety of medications and treatments may be prescribed, including topical medications and photochemotherapy (Adams et al., 2017). Although there is no cure, treatment decreases the severity and pain of the lesions. Mild to moderate cases are commonly managed with topical agents. Corticosteroids, tar preparations (Balnetar), anthralin (Psoriatec), calcipotriene (Dovonex; a vitamin D derivative); and tazarotene (Tazorac; a synthetic retinoid) are typically used.

Topical corticosteroids decrease inflammation, suppress mitotic activity of psoriatic cells, and delay the movement of keratinocytes to the surface of the skin (thus giving them time to mature and decreasing hyperkeratosis). The most effective topical corticosteroids are potent preparations that are well absorbed through the skin and are used under an occlusive dressing. Corticosteroids may also be taken systemically or injected directly into the lesions. However, corticosteroids rarely cause a lasting remission and may cause the psoriasis to become unstable. They are therefore used for repeated short periods of treatment and combined with other measures, such as tar preparations, occlusion, or a topical retinoid.

Tar preparations (such as Estar, Psorigel, and Fototar) suppress mitotic activity and are also anti-inflammatory. Their exact mechanism of action is unknown, but they are effective in removing scales and increasing remission time. Preparations made of coal tar are messy, cause staining, and have an unpleasant odor, but they are an effective form of treatment. Salex shampoo is prescribed for patients with scalp psoriasis to remove plaques and scales. Psorent is a nonprescription cream that is made from coal tar but does not stain or have an odor.

Calcipotriene (Dovonex) has been effective and safe in both the short-term and long-term treatment of psoriasis. It inhibits cell proliferation in the epidermis and facilitates cell differentiation. Although more irritating than calcipotriene, tazarotene gel (Avage, Tazorac) is a topical retinoid that may also be used to treat mild to moderate psoriasis.

Severe cases usually involve systemic agents. Systemic therapy includes retinoids, methotrexate, cyclosporine (Neoral), or apremilast (Otezla). It also includes biological modifying agents such as anti-TNF agents adalimumab (Humira), etanercept (Enbrel), and infliximab (Remicade); the anti-interleukin (IL)-12/23 antibody ustekinumab (Stelara); and the anti-IL-17 antibody secukinumab (Cosentyx) (Feldman, 2017). These medications impact the inflammatory response as well as the immune response.

Treatments

Psoriasis that is generalized (i.e., involves more than 30% of the body surface) is difficult to treat with topical medications. Treatments for generalized psoriasis include ultraviolet light phototherapy and photochemotherapy.

Phototherapy. Ultraviolet-B (UVB) light or narrow-band UVB are treatments for generalized psoriasis. UVB light decreases the growth rate of epidermal cells, thereby decreasing hyperkeratosis. Mercury vapor lights or fluorescent ultraviolet tubes provide the UVB light; the latter are often arranged in a cabinet so the patient can stand and expose psoriatic lesions more easily. These units may be purchased or constructed, to be used in the patient's home. PUVA combines the oral or topical administration of psoralen (to make the skin more sensitive to light) with ultraviolet-A (UVA) light, which penetrates deeper into the skin than UVB. PUVA requires fewer treatments for remission of lesions, but has more side effects and long-term use increases the risk of skin cancers.

Light therapy is administered in gradually increasing exposure times, until the patient experiences a mild erythema, like mild sunburn. Treatments are given three times a week as an outpatient and are measured in seconds of exposure. The eyes are shielded during the treatment. The erythema response occurs in about 8 hours. Careful assessment is necessary to prevent more severe burning, which could exacerbate the psoriasis. In patients with extensive psoriasis, UVB treatments may be combined with tar preparations, which increase the photosensitivity of the skin.

Photochemotherapy. In photochemotherapy, a light-activated form of the drug methoxsalen is used. This drug is an antimetabolite that inhibits DNA synthesis and thereby prevents cell mitosis, decreasing hyperkeratosis. Exposure to UVA rays activates methoxsalen; it is administered orally, and the patient is exposed to UVA 2 hours later. Treatments are administered two to three times a week, for 10 to 20 total treatments. Treatment causes tanning, and direct sunlight must be avoided for 8 to 12 hours thereafter. Photochemotherapy has had a high success rate in achieving remission of psoriasis, but it can accelerate aging of exposed skin, induce cataract development, alter immune function, and increase the risk of melanoma.

Nursing Care

Assessment

Refer to the previous Manifestations and Interprofessional Care sections for assessment of the patient experiencing psoriasis.

Priorities of Care

Collaborating with the interprofessional team to ensure adequate treatment of the underlying process while providing care that supports the physical and psychologic responses to the disorder is a nursing priority. Teaching the patient and, as appropriate, caregivers strategies for self-care including the therapeutic regimen should also be considered a priority nursing action. The nurse also focuses on providing emotional support through nonjudgmental acceptance.

Diagnoses, Outcomes, and Interventions

Reduce Risk for Impaired Skin Integrity. Psoriatic lesions range from several scales to large, open areas. Typical psoriatic skin lesions increase the risk of infection, which can compromise healing. In addition, certain treatments (e.g., the use of UVA or retinoids) may cause erythema or peeling of the skin, further altering skin integrity.

Expected Outcome: Patient will experience lesion healing through primary intention as indicated by progressive reduction in lesion size and presence.

The nurse will:

- Teach methods to reduce injury to the skin when taking therapeutic baths or treatments: Use warm, not hot, water; gently rub lesions with a soft washcloth, using a circular motion; dry the skin with a soft towel, using a blotting or patting motion; and keep the skin lubricated at all times. *Hot water and dry skin increase pruritus, further stimulating the itch–scratch–itch cycle. Dry skin also worsens psoriasis. Washing or drying the skin with rough linens or pressure may excoriate the skin over the psoriatic lesions.*
- Teach how to apply topical medications (see **Box 16.1**). *Applying a thin layer of medication more frequently is often more effective than applying a single thick layer of medication. The medications used to treat psoriasis may irritate the eyes and mucous membranes; when applied in skinfolds, they may also cause maceration (skin breakdown due to prolonged exposure to moisture).*
- Teach manifestations of infection and how to contact the healthcare provider if these occur: elevated temperature, increased swelling, redness, pain, increase in drainage, and any change in the color of the drainage. *The patient with skin lesions is at high risk for infection, as the skin is the body's first line of defense.*
- Teach manifestations of the complications of treatment: excoriation, increased erythema, increased peeling, and blister formation. *The topical medications or treatments may damage cells through chemical burns or excessive exposure to ultraviolet light. Times and methods of treatment need to be adjusted if these manifestations occur.*

Address Disturbed Body Image. The chronic skin lesions of psoriasis may cause patients to isolate themselves from social contact, withdraw from normal roles and responsibilities, and feel helpless or powerless.

Expected Outcome: Patient will accept body appearance as evidenced by adjustment to changes in physical appearance.

The nurse will:

- Establish a trusting relationship by expressing acceptance of the patient, both verbally and nonverbally. For example, touch the patient during social communications, demonstrating that the lesions are not contagious or offensive. *One's body image is affected not only by self-perception but also by the responses of others. Nonjudgmental acceptance helps the patient adapt to the change in body image. By touching the patient during interactions, the nurse demonstrates acceptance.*
- Encourage expression of self-perception and the asking of questions about the disease and treatment in view of the chronic nature of psoriasis. *The patient adapts to a changed body image through a process of recognition, acceptance, and resolution. Each person responds individually to disfigurement and loss.*

BOX 16.1
General Guidelines for Applying Topical Medications

- Each time a medication is applied, the skin surface must be clean and dry. Remove the medication from the previous application. Remove creams by washing the skin with tap water; remove ointments by washing the skin first with mineral oil and then with a mild soap and water.
- ***To apply gels, creams, and pastes:*** Squeeze about 1/2 to 1 inch of the gel or cream into the palm of the hand. Rub the hands together until they are covered. Apply gels and creams to the affected areas with long strokes until the skin is thinly covered. Exceptions to these general guidelines follow:
  a. Corticosteroids are usually applied two to three times a day in small amounts and rubbed directly onto the lesions. Apply the medication after a bath and cover with an occlusive dressing.
  b. Apply medications containing tar in the direction of hair growth. Do not apply these medications to the face, to the genitals, or in skinfolds. If the tar is water based or oil based, it will stain clothing.
  c. Wear gloves when applying anthralin stains.
- ***To apply lotions:*** Shake the bottle of lotion well. Pour a small amount into the palm of the hand, and pat the medication onto the skin. If the lotion is thin, apply it with a gauze pad.
- ***To apply sprays:*** Hold the container about 6 inches from the skin and apply the medication in a short spray.
- ***To apply medicated shampoo:*** Rinse out medication from the previous application. Apply the shampoo, massage into the hair and over the scalp carefully, and allow it to remain for the prescribed time. Rinse.
- ***To apply pastes:*** Use enough paste on an applicator (such as a wooden tongue depressor) to cover the lesion thinly.

- Promote social interaction through family involvement in care and referral to support groups of people with psoriasis or other chronic skin conditions. *Acceptance by others is critical to acceptance of self. Psoriasis treatment is lifelong, time consuming, and often unappealing. By becoming involved in care, the family communicates acceptance. Sharing experiences with others who have the same health problem is a source of strength when adjusting to a visible, chronic illness.*

Delegating Nursing Care Activities

As appropriate and allowed by the designated duties and responsibilities of unlicensed assistive personnel, the nurse may delegate nursing care activities such as measuring fluid intake and output, collecting vital signs (including orthostatic vital signs), encouraging oral or enteral fluid intake, and nonpharmacologic skin care.

Transitions of Care

As psoriasis has a genetic component, the disease is not entirely preventable. However, weight maintenance, stress management, and reduction of alcohol intake can reduce flare-ups.

Psoriasis flare-up is the acute manifestation of the disease process. Topical and systemic treatments are indicated during flare-ups.

Patient and family teaching focuses on treatments and skin care needs. The following topics should be addressed:

- The chronic nature of the disease, factors that may precipitate an exacerbation, and methods to reduce stress.
- Interventions for pruritus and dry skin and specific care for psoriasis:
  a. Expose the skin to sunlight, but avoid sunburn.
  b. Avoid trauma to the skin (e.g., do not scrub off scales, and use only an electric razor).
  c. Avoid exposure to contagious illnesses such as influenza and colds.
  d. Discuss current medications with the healthcare provider. Certain drugs (such as indomethacin [Indocin], lithium, and beta-adrenergic blocking agents) are known to precipitate exacerbations of psoriasis.
- Suggest the National Psoriasis Foundation, the National Institutes of Health, or the American Academy of Dermatology as resources.

While psoriasis is a chronic condition with flare-ups and quiescent periods, the process is not life-threatening and does not have a terminal phase.

16.2 Infections and Infestations of the Skin

The skin's resistance to infections and infestations is provided by protective mechanisms, including skin flora, sebum, and the immune response. Although the skin is normally resistant to infections and infestations, these disorders may occur as a result of a break in the skin surface, a virulent agent, and/or decreased resistance due to a compromised immune system. This section discusses skin disorders resulting from bacterial infections, fungal infections, parasitic infestations, and viral infections.

The Patient with a Bacterial Infection of the Skin

A number of bacteria normally inhabit the skin and do not cause an infection. However, when a break in the skin allows invasion by pathogenic bacteria, an infection, called a *pyoderma*, may occur. The most common bacterial infections are caused by gram-positive *Staphylococcus aureus* and beta-hemolytic streptococci. Bacterial infections of the skin may be primary or secondary. Primary infections are caused by a single pathogen and arise from normal skin; secondary infections develop in traumatized or diseased skin.

Most bacterial infections are treated by a primary care provider, and the patient remains at home for care. If the infection becomes more serious, inpatient care may be required. In addition, nosocomial infections of wounds or open lesions in hospitalized patients are often the result of bacterial infections, especially by methicillin-resistant *Staphylococcus aureus* (MRSA) (**Figure 16.5** ■).

Pathophysiology and Manifestations

Bacterial infections of the skin arise from the hair follicle, where bacteria can accumulate and grow and cause a localized infection. However, the bacteria can also enter the body through open wounds, invade deeper tissues, and cause a systemic infection, a potentially life-threatening disorder. Various types of bacterial infections involve the skin, including folliculitis, furuncles and carbuncles, cellulitis, and MRSA.

Folliculitis

Folliculitis is a bacterial infection of the hair follicle, most commonly caused by *S. aureus*. The infection begins at the follicle opening and extends down into the follicle. The bacteria release enzymes and chemical agents that cause an inflammation. The lesions appear as pustules surrounded by an area of erythema on the surface of the skin (**Figure 16.6** ■). The lesions are accompanied by discomfort ranging from slight burning to intense itching. A major complication is abscess formation. Folliculitis is found most often on the scalp and extremities. It is also often seen on the face of bearded men (*sycosis barbae*), on the legs of women who shave, and on the eyelids (a *stye*). Although folliculitis may appear without any apparent cause, contributing factors include poor hygiene, poor nutrition, prolonged skin moisture, tight heavy fabrics on the upper legs, and trauma to the skin. A specific type of folliculitis, called "hot

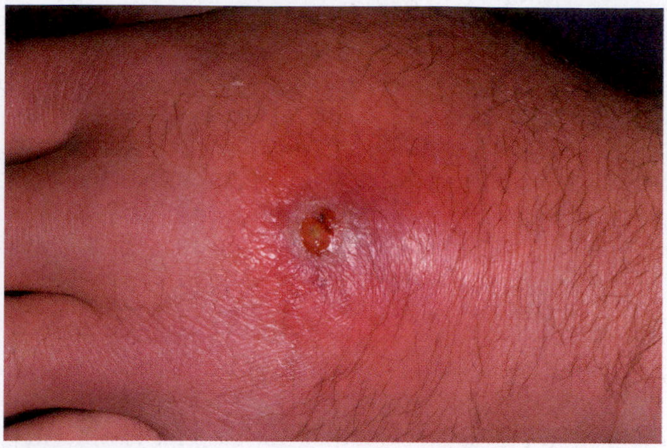

Figure 16.5 ■ Hand of a 52-year-old man with cellulitis and MRSA.

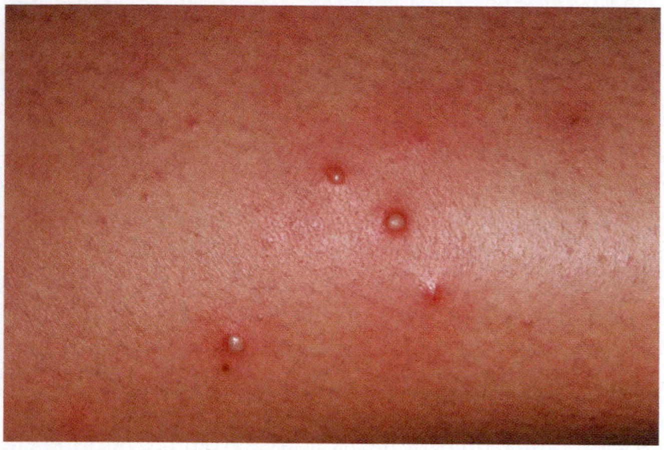

Figure 16.6 ■ The lesions of folliculitis are pustules surrounded by areas of erythema.

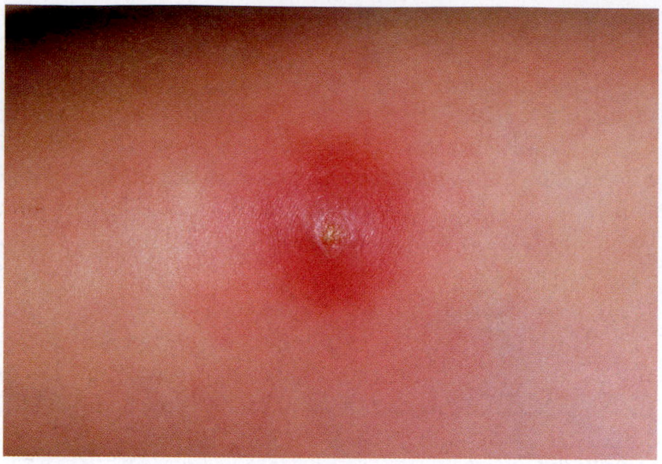

Figure 16.7 ■ A furuncle (boil) is a deep, firm, red, painful nodule.

tub folliculitis," is caused by *Pseudomonas aeruginosa* and is characterized by follicular or pustular lesions that occur 1 to 4 days after being in a hot tub, whirlpool, or public swimming pool.

Furuncles and Carbuncles

Furuncles, often called *boils*, are inflammations of the hair follicle. They often begin as folliculitis, but the infection spreads down the hair shaft, through the wall of the follicle, and into the dermis. The causative organism is commonly *S. aureus*. A furuncle is initially a deep, firm, red, painful nodule from 1 to 5 cm in diameter (**Figure 16.7** ■). After a few days, the nodule changes into a large, painful cystic nodule. The cysts may drain substantial amounts of purulent drainage. One or more furuncles may occur on any part of the body that has hair. Contributing factors include poor hygiene, trauma to the skin, areas of excessive moisture (including perspiration), and systemic diseases such as diabetes mellitus and hematologic malignancies.

A **carbuncle** is a group of infected hair follicles. The lesion begins as a firm mass located in the subcutaneous tissue and the lower dermis. This mass becomes swollen and painful and has multiple openings to the skin surface. Carbuncles are most frequently found on the back of the neck, the upper back, and the lateral thighs. In addition to the local manifestations, the patient may experience chills, fever, and malaise. The contributing factors for carbuncles are the same as for furuncles. Both infections are more common in hot, humid climates.

Cellulitis

Cellulitis is a localized infection of the dermis and subcutaneous tissue. Cellulitis can occur following a wound or skin ulcer or as an extension of furuncles or carbuncles. The infection spreads as a result of a substance produced by the causative organism, called *spreading factor* (hyaluronidase). This factor breaks down the fibrin network and other barriers that normally localize the infection. The area of cellulitis is red, swollen, and painful (**Figure 16.8** ■). In some cases, vesicles may form over the area of cellulitis. The patient may experience fever, chills, malaise, headache, and swollen lymph glands.

Methicillin-Resistant *Staphylococcus aureus* Infection

Methicillin-resistant *Staphylococcus aureus* (MRSA) infection is caused by the *S. aureus* bacteria, an organism resistant to the broad-spectrum antibiotics (such as methicillin, oxacillin, amoxicillin, and penicillin) usually used to treat it. This potentially fatal disease is divided into two types: *healthcare-associated infections* (HA-MRSA; acquired in hospitals and other healthcare settings) and *community-associated infections* (CA-MRSA; acquired in the community in otherwise healthy people). MRSA in hospitalized patients may lead to infections of wounds, skin around invasive tubes or catheters, the blood, the lungs, or the urinary system. MRSA in patients in the community is often manifested as skin infections and a potentially life-threatening pneumonia. CA-MRSA is an increasing healthcare problem resulting

from the inappropriate overuse or misuse of antibiotics such as antibiotic use to treat viral infections.

S. aureus are normally found on the skin and in the nose of about one-third of the population. If present, but not causing illness, the person is said to be colonized and capable of spreading the bacteria to other people. The bacteria are spread by direct contact with the bacteria or with contaminated equipment. The incidence of CA-MRSA is about 2 per 100,000 people (Centers for Disease Control and Prevention [CDC], 2018a). The rates of both types are highest in healthcare workers, in males, in those over age 65, and in those with HIV and AIDS. The risk for CA-MRSA is increased in those who participate in contact sports and in people sharing personal items and/or living in crowded or unsanitary conditions.

The infection usually begins as a small, raised, red nodule on the skin that resembles a pimple or spider bite. The nodule rapidly increases in size, becomes dark red, is painful, contains pus, and may become a deep abscess. Cellulitis involving the area containing the initial infection (such as an extremity) is common.

Interprofessional Care

The diagnosis of a bacterial infection of the skin is made by assessing the appearance of the lesion and by identifying the causative organism. Antibiotics effective against the organism are used in treatment.

Diagnosis

Drainage from a lesion or a blood culture may be ordered to identify the causative organism so that the most effective antibiotic can be chosen for treatment. People who experience repeated bacterial skin infections, or who provide care for others who exhibit infections, may have a culture taken from the external nares to determine whether they are carriers of bacteria (e.g., MRSA) and are reinfecting themselves or others.

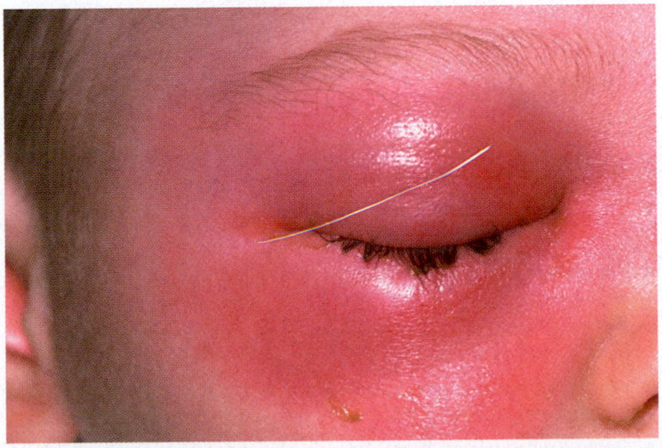

Figure 16.8 ■ Cellulitis is a bacterial infection localized in the dermis and subcutaneous tissue. The involved area is red, swollen, and painful.

Medications

The primary treatment for bacterial infections of the skin is an antibiotic specific to the organism (Adams et al., 2017). The antibiotic is usually taken orally, but may also be applied topically. Multiple furuncles and carbuncles may be treated with cloxacillin (a penicillinase-resistant penicillin); the cephalosporins are also often effective. MRSA infections may be treated with antimicrobial therapy, including trimethoprim-sulfamethoxazole (Bactrim), minocycline (Minocin), doxycycline (Vibramycin), or clindamycin (Cleocin). There are no recommended guidelines for treating colonization. Mupirocin ointment (Bactroban Nasal) and an antiseptic body wash should be limited to use in outbreaks or other high-prevalence situations (Sal, Laurent, Strale, Denis, & Byl, 2015).

Nursing Care

Nursing care focuses on preventing the spread of infection and restoring normal skin integrity. Many patients provide self-care at home, but need education about preventing CA-MRSA.

Assessment

Refer to the previous Manifestations and Interprofessional Care sections for assessment of the patient experiencing a bacterial infection of the skin.

Priorities of Care

Collaborating with the interprofessional team to ensure adequate treatment of the infection while providing care that supports infection control (including appropriate precautions) is a priority of care. Teaching the patient and, as appropriate, caregivers strategies to prevent spread of infection and optimize safe home and work environments should also be considered a priority nursing action. The nurse also focuses on promoting comfort and prevention of infection recurrence.

Diagnoses, Outcomes, and Interventions

Reduce the Risk for Infection. Infection risk for MRSA is based on hospital-based strains or community-based strains of the bacteria. Hospital-based risks include being hospitalized, undergoing an invasive medical procedure, or residing in a long-term care facility. Community-based risks include participating in contact sports or living in overcrowded conditions.

Expected Outcome: Patient's infection will be effectively managed as evidenced by skin integrity and body temperature within normal range.

The nurse will:

- Practice good hand hygiene and teach its importance. *Careful hand hygiene is one of the most effective methods to reduce the spread of infection both in and out of the hospital setting. Healthcare providers must wash their hands with soap and water before and after patient care and between each patient contact. All patients, family members, and visitors (both in the home and hospital setting) should be taught the importance of hand hygiene, but it is even more important for the patient with a bacterial infection.*

- Assess for and teach how to identify an increase in infection, which may be manifested systemically by fever, tachycardia, chills, and malaise. Local manifestations of the spread of the infection include an increase in erythema, the size of the lesion, and drainage. *This assessment is especially important for patients who are older, debilitated, or immunosuppressed and for those who have large or dirty wounds.*

SAFETY ALERT: If a patient with a bacterial skin infection is hospitalized, place him or her on isolation precautions to limit the spread of the organism to other patients. Depending on state nursing practice act and institutional rules, isolation may either require a provider order or may be instituted by the nurse. ■

- Cover draining lesions with a sterile dressing, and handle soiled dressings or linens according to standard precautions. When changing dressings, always wear disposable rubber gloves and masks. *These actions are necessary to prevent the spread of infection to other areas of the patient's body, to other patients, to visitors, and to the nurse providing care.*

Delegating Nursing Care Activities

As appropriate and allowed by the designated duties and responsibilities of unlicensed assistive personnel, the nurse may delegate nursing care activities such as measuring fluid intake and output, collecting vital signs (including orthostatic vital signs), encouraging oral or enteral fluid intake, and skin care.

Transitions of Care

The most important preventive action to reduce MRSA is good hand hygiene. Additional actions to prevent MRSA are outlined in **Box 16.2**.

In the hospital, MRSA is commonly spread to patients from the hands of healthcare workers. To minimize this risk, patients and family members can help to ensure that anyone who comes in contact with the patient washes their hands or uses an alcohol-based hand sanitizer before and after touching the patient. Patients with active infection should also wash their hands frequently.

Hospitalized patients who are colonized or infected with MRSA should be placed on "contact precautions." This means that healthcare workers entering the patient's room must wear gloves and a clean cover gown to prevent contamination of their clothing.

The increasing numbers of people with community-associated MRSA have resulted in state laws about reporting of or screening for MRSA. Many state public health departments have guidelines available about the manifestations, prevention, and treatment of CA-MRSA, and the CDC (2016) has issued treatment guidelines. Patient teaching for any bacterial infection focuses on facilitating tissue healing and eliminating the infection. Address the following topics:

- The importance of maintaining good nutrition
- The importance of maintaining cleanliness through careful hand hygiene and proper handling and disposal of dressings
- Preventing the spread of infection by not sharing linens and towels and washing clothing and linens in hot water
- The importance of not squeezing or trying to open a pimple or boil
- The importance of taking the full course of prescribed antibiotics.

If left untreated, MRSA can result in bacteremia and be fatal. The same precautions should be used as for patients whether managed in a hospital or at home.

The Patient with a Fungal Infection

Fungi are free-living, plantlike organisms that live in the soil, on animals, and on humans. The fungi that cause

BOX 16.2
Preventing MRSA in the Hospital and in the Community

IN THE HOSPITAL

- Wash your hands frequently.
- Ask all hospital staff to wash their hands or use an alcohol-based hand sanitizer every time before touching you or objects in your environment.
- Ensure all invasive tubes or needles are inserted under sterile conditions.

IN THE COMMUNITY

- Wash your hands often and for as long as it takes to hum the "Happy Birthday" song. Use a hand sanitizer with at least 60% alcohol for times when you can't wash your hands.
- Do not share personal items such as razors, towels, or athletic equipment.
- For athletes: Shower after practice or games with soap and water. Sit out practice or games if you have an infection of the skin. Wash towels and athletic clothing with hot water and bleach after every use.
- Keep cuts and scrapes covered with a dry sterile dressing until they are healed.
- Go to the physician if you have a skin infection that is painful and getting worse. Ask about being tested for MRSA.
- Use antibiotics appropriately. Take the full prescribed dose. Do not share.

superficial skin infections are called *dermatophytes*. In humans, the dermatophytes live on keratin in the stratum corneum, hair, and nails. Fungal disorders are also called *mycoses*.

Pathophysiology and Manifestations

Fungal infections include dermatophytoses (tinea or ringworm) and candidiasis (yeast) infections. The candidiasis infections may affect various parts of the body, but are more commonly seen in women as vaginal infections, discussed and illustrated in Chapter 50.

Dermatophytoses (Tinea)

Superficial fungal infections of the skin are called **dermatophytoses** or, more commonly, ringworm. Fungal infections occur when a susceptible host comes in contact with the organism. The organism may be transmitted by direct contact with animals or other infected individuals or by inanimate objects such as combs, pillowcases, towels, and hats. The most important factor in the development of the infection is moisture; the onset and spread of a fungal infection is greatest in areas where moisture content is high, such as within skinfolds, between the toes, and in the mouth. Other factors that increase the risk of a fungal infection include the use of broad-spectrum antibiotics that kill off normal flora and allow the fungi to grow, diabetes mellitus, immunodeficiencies, nutritional deficiencies, pregnancy, increasing age, and iron deficiency. Dermatophyte infections are named by the body part affected, for example:

- ***Tinea pedis*** is a fungal infection of the soles of the feet, the space between the toes, and/or the toenail (**Figure 16.9 ■**). More often called *athlete's foot*, it is the most common tinea infection. The lesions vary from mild scaliness to painful fissures with drainage, and they are usually accompanied by pruritus and a foul odor. The infection is often chronic, absent in winter but reappearing in hot weather when perspiring feet are encased in shoes.
- ***Tinea corporis*** is a fungal infection of the body. It can be caused by several different fungi, and the lesions vary according to the causative organism. The most common lesions are large circular patches with raised red borders of vesicles, papules, or pustules. Pruritus and erythema are also present.
- ***Tinea cruris*** is a fungal infection of the groin that may extend to the inner thighs and buttocks. Often called *jock itch*, it is often associated with tinea pedis and is more common in people who are physically active, are obese, and/or wear tight underclothing.

Interprofessional Care

Fungal infections are primarily diagnosed in outpatient settings and treated at home, but may also occur in hospitalized patients. The treatment is the same, regardless of the setting.

Diagnosis

Diagnostic tests are conducted to determine the causative fungi and may include cultures, microscopic examination

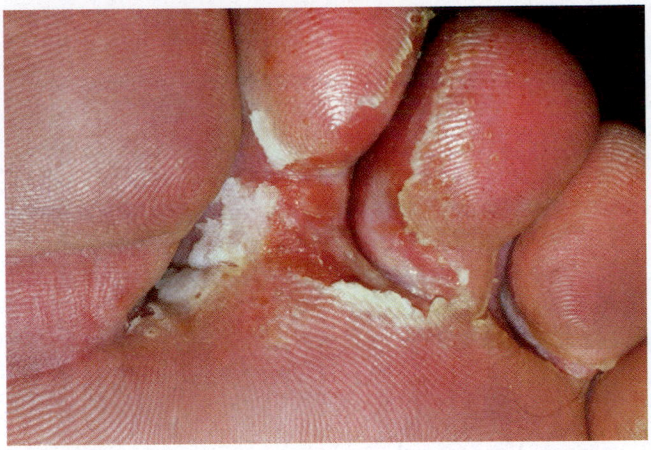

Figure 16.9 ■ Tinea pedis (athlete's foot) is a fungal infection that often occurs between the toes.

using KOH, and examination of the skin with ultraviolet light (Wood lamp), described in Chapter 15.

Medications

Fungal infections of the skin are treated by topical or systemic antifungal medications (Adams et al., 2017). The over-the-counter (OTC) medications (such as miconazole, clotrimazole, butenafine, and terbinafine) are often less expensive than prescription medications and are effective. Nursing implications for the antifungal medications are described in **Medication Administration 16.B**.

Nursing Care

Many people treat themselves with OTC antifungal medications. It is recommended, however, that the person be professionally diagnosed the first time the infection occurs. If symptoms reappear, self-treatment is usually satisfactory. The interventions discussed for nursing care of the patient with a bacterial infection are also appropriate for the patient with a fungal infection. Teaching topics specific to fungal infections are:

- Fungal diseases are contagious. Do not share linens or personal items with others.
- Use a clean towel and washcloth each day.
- Carefully dry all skinfolds, including those under the breasts, under the arms, and between the toes.
- Wear clean cotton underclothing each day.
- Fungi grow in moist environments, such as on sweaty feet. To prevent further infections, do not wear the same pair of shoes every day, wear socks that permit moisture to wick away from the skin surface, do not wear rubber- or plastic-soled shoes, and use talcum powder or an OTC antifungal powder twice a day.

The Patient with a Parasitic Infestation

Infestations of the skin by parasites are more common in developing countries but may occur in any geographic area of the world. They affect people of all social classes

Medication Administration 16.B

Antifungal Agents

EXAMPLES

amphotericin B (generic only)

Superficial

butenafine (Mentax)

nystatin (Mycostatin, Nilstat)

undecylenic acid (Desenex)

Azoles

clotrimazole (Mycelex)

econazole (generic only)

fluconazole (Diflucan)

ketoconazole (Nizoral)

miconazole (Monistat)

oxiconazole (Oxistat)

B-Glucan Synthesis Inhibitors

griseofulvin (generic only)

Antifungal medications are prepared in a variety of forms, depending on the specific drug: powders, creams, shampoos, suspensions, troches, vaginal suppositories, and oral tablets. Some drugs interfere with the permeability of the fungal cell membrane, others interfere with DNA synthesis. Most of these medications are fungistatic (inhibit fungal growth), but in large doses they may be fungicidal.

Nursing Responsibilities

- When taking the health history, ask about known hypersensitivity reactions to these agents; document carefully.
- Assess for side effects: skin rash, local irritation, gastrointestinal symptoms (if given PO), and mental status.
- Administer ketoconazole with food to minimize gastrointestinal irritation.
- Shake suspensions well before administration, and ask the patient to swish them around the mouth before swallowing.
- Tell the patient to allow oral tablets to dissolve in the mouth.

Health Education for the Patient and Family

- Therapy usually continues over a long period of time, but regular use of medications for the recommended period is necessary. Do not miss doses, and complete the full treatment.
- ***For griseofulvin:*** Take with meals or foods high in fat (such as ice cream) to avoid stomach upset and help with absorption. Avoid alcohol (which may cause rapid pulse and flushing) and exposure to sunlight (this drug causes increased sensitivity).
- ***For nystatin:*** Dissolve lozenges completely in the mouth. Hold suspensions in the mouth and swish throughout the mouth as long as possible before swallowing. Insert intravaginal medication high in the vagina. Continue with intravaginal applications throughout the menses.
- ***For antifungal shampoo:*** Use two times a week for 4 weeks, allowing at least 3 days between each shampoo. Wet hair, apply shampoo to produce lather, leave in place for 1 minute, and then rinse. Apply shampoo a second time, lather, leave in place for 3 minutes, and then rinse thoroughly.
- ***For topical application:*** Rub well into the affected areas, but do not get the medication in your eyes.
- ***For vaginal candidiasis infections:*** During therapy, refrain from sexual intercourse or advise partner to use a condom.
- Your sexual partner will need to be treated at the same time so that you do not pass the infection back and forth to each other.

Note: Medications identified in blue are among the 200 most frequently prescribed drugs in the United States.

Source: Data from Adams et al., 2017.

but are associated with crowded or unsanitary living conditions.

Pathophysiology and Manifestations

Two of the more common parasitic infestations of the skin are caused by lice and mites. These parasites do not normally live on the skin, but infest the skin through contact with an infested person or contact with clothing, linens, or objects infested with the parasites.

Pediculosis

Pediculosis is an infestation with lice, parasites that live on the blood of an animal or human host. The louse is a 2- to 4-mm oval organism with a stylet that pierces the skin; an anticoagulant in its saliva prevents host blood from clotting while it eats. The female louse lays its eggs (small pearl-gray or brown eggs, called nits) on hair shafts. The louse within the egg hatches, reaches the adult reproductive stage, and dies in 30 to 50 days (Sorenson et al., 2019).

Two common types of human pediculosis are:

- *Pediculosis corporis* is an infestation with body lice. This infestation is more common in people who do not have access to facilities for bathing or washing clothes, such as the homeless. The lice live in clothing fibers and are transmitted primarily by contact with infested clothing and bed linens. The skin lesions occur at the site of a louse bite; macules appear initially, followed by wheals and papules. Pruritus is common, and scratching often results in linear excoriations. The lesions are most often seen on the shoulders, trunk, and buttocks.
- *Pediculosis pubis* is an infestation with pubic lice (often called *crabs*). This infestation is spread through sexual activity with someone already infested or by contact with infested clothing or linens. The lice are found in the pubic region and occasionally spread to the axillae or men's beards. The lice cause skin irritation and intense itching.

Scabies

Scabies is a parasitic infestation caused by a mite (*Sarcoptes scabiei*). The pregnant female mite burrows into the skin and lays two to three eggs each day for about a month. The eggs hatch in 3 to 5 days, and the larvae migrate to the surface of the skin but burrow into the skin for food or protection. The larvae develop, and the cycle repeats. Scabies infestation affects people of all socioeconomic classes. The infestation is found in webs between the fingers, the inner surfaces of the wrist and elbow, the axillae, the female nipple, the penis, the belt line, and the gluteal crease. The lesions are a small red-brown burrow, about 2 mm in length, sometimes covered with vesicles, which appears as a rash. Pruritus in response to the mite or its feces is common, especially at night, and excoriations may develop. The excoriations predispose the person to secondary bacterial infections. The incidence of scabies in residents of nursing homes and extended care facilities has increased.

Interprofessional Care

Parasitic infestations are diagnosed by identifying the organism and are treated with medications that kill the lice or mites.

Diagnosis

When a patient has manifestations of pediculosis, the hair shaft and the clothing are examined to identify the lice or the nits. Microscopic examination of the parasite provides a positive diagnosis. Scabies is diagnosed by skin scrapings and microscopic examination for the mites or their feces.

Medications

Lice are eradicated with agents that kill the parasite (Adams et al., 2017). Infestations of the body and pubic area are treated with topical medications that contain gamma benzene hexachloride, malathion (Prioderm lotion), or permethrin (NIX).

Infestations of the hair are treated with shampoos containing lindane, such as Kwell. A fine-toothed comb can be used to comb the dead nits off the hair shaft. Scabies may be eradicated by a single treatment of lindane lotion or Kwell applied to the entire skin surface for 12 hours. The associated itching is treated with systemic or topical medications, including corticosteroids. Secondary bacterial infections are treated with the appropriate antibiotic.

Nursing Care

Nursing care for patients with a parasite infestation most often focuses on teaching to prevent infestation or to eradicate an existing infestation. For a hospitalized patient with pediculosis, isolation procedures are instituted until the patient no longer has the infestation.

Patient and family teaching is necessary to facilitate treatment at home, to prevent the spread of the infestation, and to dispel the myth that lice infest only people in dirty living conditions or with poor hygiene. Specific information includes:

- Wash clothing and linens in soap and hot water or have them dry cleaned.
- Ironing of clothes kills any lice eggs.
- All family members and sexual partners must also be treated.
- Lice and mites may infest anyone.

The Patient with a Viral Infection

Viruses are pathogens that consist of an RNA or DNA core surrounded by a protein coat. They depend on live cells for reproduction and so are classified as intracellular pathogens. The viruses that cause skin lesions invade the keratinocyte, reproduce, and either increase cellular growth or cause cellular death.

An increase in the incidence of viral skin disorders has been attributed to a variety of causes. Some commonly used drugs, such as birth control medications and corticosteroids, are known to have immunosuppressive properties that allow viruses to multiply. Other drugs, such as antibiotics, kill off normal skin bacteria that would otherwise serve as a defense against viral infections.

Pathophysiology and Manifestations

Viral infections cause many different kinds of skin disorders, including warts, herpes simplex infections, and herpes zoster infections.

Warts

Warts, or *verrucae*, are lesions of the skin caused by the human papillomavirus (HPV). Warts may be nongenital or genital. Nongenital warts are benign lesions; genital warts may be precancerous. Warts are transmitted through skin contact. Wart lesions may be flat, fusiform (tapered at both ends), or round, but most are round and raised and have a rough, gray surface. There are many different types of warts; location and appearance of the warts depend on the causative virus. (Genital warts are discussed in Chapter 50.) Commonly occurring warts are:

- ***Common warts*** (*verruca vulgaris*) may appear anywhere on the skin and mucous membranes of the body; they most commonly appear on the fingers. Common warts grow above the skin surface and may be dome shaped with ragged borders (**Figure 16.10** ■).
- ***Plantar warts*** occur at pressure points on the soles of the feet. The pressure of shoes and walking prevents these warts from growing outward, so they tend to extend deeper beneath the skin surface than do common warts. Plantar warts are often painful.
- ***Flat warts*** (*verruca plana*) are small, flat lesions, usually seen on the forehead or dorsum of the hand.

Depending on their size, location, and any associated discomfort, warts may be treated with medications, cryotherapy, or electrodesiccation and curettage. A common method of wart removal is acid therapy, using a colloidal solution of 16% salicylic acid and 16% lactic acid. The solution is applied to the wart every 12 to 24 hours; the wart disappears in 2 to 3 weeks. Other methods of eradicating

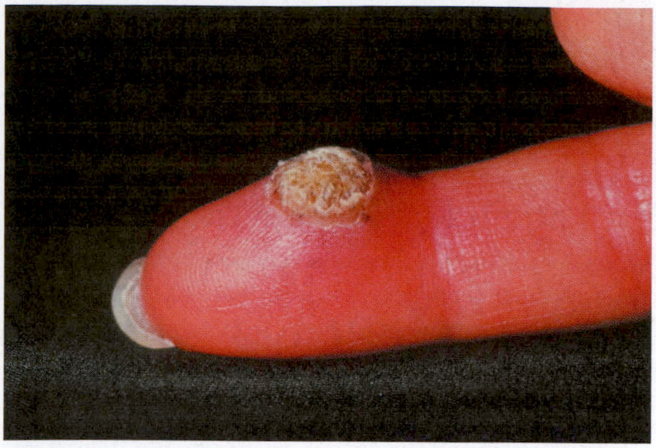

Figure 16.10 ■ The common wart, caused by a virus, appears as a raised, dome-shaped lesion.

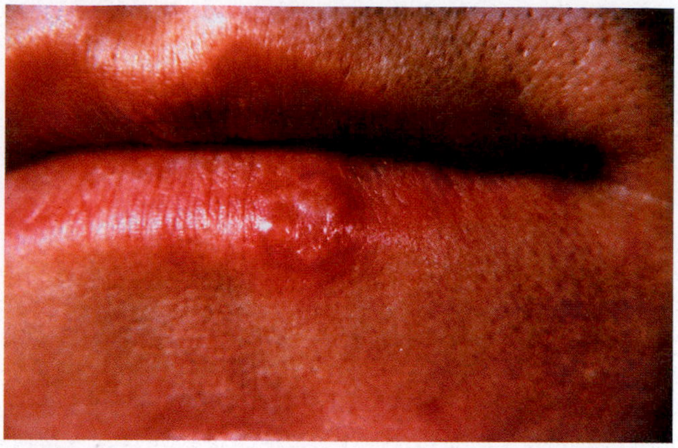

Figure 16.11 ■ Herpes simplex is a viral infection of the skin and mucous membranes.

warts are cryosurgery, freezing with liquid nitrogen, and electrodesiccation of the wart with an electric current followed by excision of the dead tissue. Warts may also resolve spontaneously when immunity to the virus develops. This response may take up to 5 years.

Herpes Simplex

Herpes simplex (*fever blister* or *cold sore*) virus infections of the skin and mucous membranes are caused by two types of herpesvirus: HSV-1 and HSV-2. Most infections above the waist are caused by HSV-1, with herpes simplex lesions most often found on the lips, face, and mouth. (Genital herpes infections, caused by HSV-2, are discussed in Chapter 50.) The virus may be transmitted by physical contact, oral sex, or kissing.

The infection begins with a burning or tingling sensation, followed by the development of erythema, vesicle formation, and pain (**Figure 16.11** ■). The vesicles progress through pustules, injuries, and crusting until healing occurs in 10 to 14 days.

The initial infection is often severe and accompanied by systemic manifestations, such as fever and sore throat; recurrences are more localized and less severe. The virus lives in nerve ganglia and may cause recurrent lesions in response to sunlight, menstruation, injury, or stress. Oral acyclovir may be used prophylactically to prevent reoccurrences and to treat recurrent outbreaks.

Herpes Zoster

Herpes zoster, also called *shingles*, is a viral infection of a dermatome section of the skin caused by varicella zoster (the herpes virus that causes chickenpox). The infection is believed to result from reactivation of a varicella virus remaining in the sensory dorsal ganglia after a childhood infection of chickenpox. When reactivated, the virus travels from the ganglia to the corresponding skin dermatome area.

Herpes zoster affects more than 1 million people in the United States each year, with more than half of the cases being in adults over the age of 60 (Sorenson et al., 2019). Patients with Hodgkin disease, certain types of leukemia, and lymphomas are more susceptible to an outbreak of the disease. Herpes zoster occurs more often in immunocompromised individuals, such as those with HIV infections, those receiving radiation therapy or chemotherapy, and those who have had major organ transplants. The appearance of the lesions in people with HIV infections may be one of the first manifestations of immune compromise. The herpes eruption lasts for about 2 to 3 weeks and usually does not recur.

Herpes zoster lesions are vesicles with an erythematous base. The vesicles appear on the skin area supplied by the neurons of a single or associated group of dorsal root ganglia (although they may occur beyond this area in immunosuppressed people). The lesions usually appear unilaterally on the face, trunk, and thorax (**Figure 16.12** ■). New lesions continue to erupt for 3 to 5 days, then crust and dry. Recovery occurs in 2 to 3 weeks. The patient often experiences severe pain for up to 48 hours before and during eruption of the lesions. The pain may continue for weeks to months after the lesions have disappeared. The older adult is especially sensitive to the pain

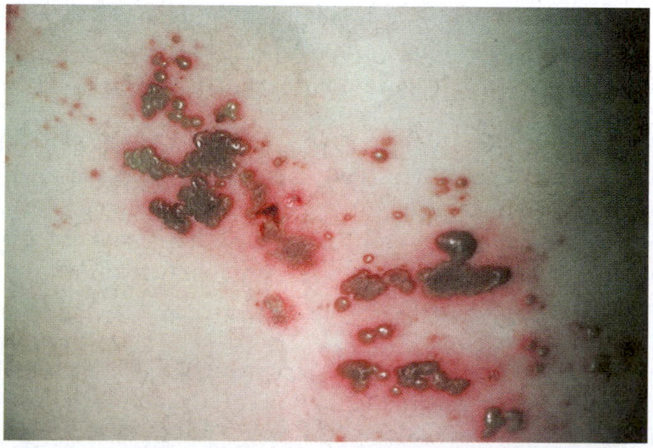

Figure 16.12 ■ Herpes zoster is a viral infection of a dermatome section of the skin. The typical lesions are painful vesicles lying along the path of the nerve.

and often experiences more severe outbreaks of herpes zoster lesions.

Eruption of vesicles over a single dermatome usually occurs only one time. Generalized herpes zoster may indicate that the patient has an associated immunocompromised disease, such as Hodgkin disease or HIV infection. Patients infected with HIV are 20 times more likely to develop herpes zoster.

Complications of herpes zoster include postherpetic neuralgia (a sharp, spasmodic pain along the course of one or more nerves) and visual loss. The neuralgia, described as burning or stabbing, results from inflammation of the root ganglia. Permanent loss of vision may follow occurrence of lesions that arise from the ophthalmic division of the trigeminal nerve. The disease may disseminate in immunocompromised patients, causing lesions beyond the dermatome, visceral lesions, and encephalitis. This serious complication may cause death (Sorenson et al., 2019).

Interprofessional Care

The treatment for viral skin infections focuses on stopping viral replication and treating patient responses, such as itching and pain.

Diagnosis

Although diagnosis is usually based on manifestations and appearance of the lesions, laboratory tests may be necessary to differentiate herpes zoster from contact dermatitis and herpes simplex. The laboratory tests include a Tzanck smear, which identifies the herpes virus but does not distinguish herpes zoster from herpes simplex. Cultures of fluid from the vesicles and antibody tests are used to make the differential diagnosis of herpes virus types. HIV testing should be considered if patients are under age 55 with a history of HIV risk factors. See Chapter 15 for more information about these tests.

Medications

Antiviral drugs are used to treat herpes zoster infections (Adams et al., 2017). Acyclovir (Zovirax) interferes with viral synthesis and replication. Although it does not cure herpes infections, it does decrease the severity of the illness and also decreases pain. It may be administered topically, orally, or parenterally. It is more effective if administration begins within the first 1 to 2 days after the first vesicles appear. Other antiviral medications include famciclovir (Famvir) and valacyclovir (Valtrex). Nerve blocks may be needed to treat initial pain. Narcotic and nonnarcotic analgesics are prescribed for pain management, and antihistamines may be administered for relief of pruritus. Patients with eye involvement are treated with topical steroid ophthalmic ointments and mydriatics.

Zostavax (a weakened form of varicella-zoster live virus) is a vaccine used for adults age 60 years or older to prevent herpes zoster. It works by increasing the immune system response; if the patient experiences an outbreak of blisters despite being vaccinated, the nerve pain that follows may be prevented. The vaccine should not be taken by people who are allergic to any of the ingredients, gelatin, or neomycin; those who have a weaker immune system (such as people with AIDS or leukemia); nor those taking steroids. Side effects include injection site manifestations (such as redness, itching, pain, bruising), headache, fever, hives at the injection site, joint or muscle pain, a rash, and swollen glands. A new vaccine was approved by the U.S. Food and Drug Administration (FDA) in 2017. Shingrix® is a recombinant zoster vaccine composed of lyophilized gE antigen. It is recommended for adults age 50 years and older to prevent shingles. Shingrix is recommended for persons who previously received the current shingles vaccine (Zostavax®) to prevent shingles and related complications. Once final recommendations from the CDC are approved, it will be the preferred vaccine for the prevention of shingles and related complications (CDC, 2018b).

Nursing Care

Patients with herpes zoster require nursing care for infection, pruritus, and pain. They also require teaching about preventing the spread of the virus to others. See the Case Study & Nursing Care Plan for the patient with herpes zoster.

Assessment

Refer to the earlier Interprofessional Care section for assessment of the patient with a viral skin infection.

Priorities of Care

Collaborating with the interprofessional team to ensure adequate treatment of a viral skin infection while providing care that promotes recovery and comfort is a nursing priority. Teaching the patient and, as appropriate, caregivers strategies to prevent infection, optimize comfort, and promote safe home and work environments should also be considered a priority nursing action. The nurse also focuses on promoting comfort and maintaining asepsis for all interruptions of the integument.

Diagnoses, Outcomes, and Interventions

Manage Acute Pain. The patient with herpes zoster often experiences severe pain over the entire dermatome supplied by the affected nerve root. The pain is described as burning, tearing, or stabbing. The patient may avoid movement and does not want clothing or bed linens to touch the affected area.

Expected Outcome: Patient will experience adequate pain control as evidenced by patient report of response to analgesics.

The nurse will:

- Monitor the location, duration, and intensity of the pain. *Each person experiences and expresses pain in his or her own manner. Pain tolerance is also individual. Accurate assessment of the patient's perception and tolerance of pain is essential in facilitating pain management.*
- Explain the rationale for taking prescribed medications on a regular schedule. *Delaying or withholding medications may allow the pain to reach an intensity at which the medication is less effective in promoting relief.*

Case Study & Nursing Care Plan

A Patient with Herpes Zoster

Jesus Rivera is a 34-year-old migrant farm worker who currently lives in temporary housing in a rural area of the southwestern United States. His family includes his wife, Marta, who is 3 months pregnant, and two children, ages 3 and 5. He takes his wife to a medical clinic staffed by volunteer nurses, physicians, and students from a nearby university for a prenatal checkup. The clinic is open only on Saturday and provides care on a sliding fee scale or for free if the family is unable to pay. While Mrs. Rivera is being examined, Mr. Rivera asks the nurse to have someone look at some very painful blisters on his chest that developed about a week ago. He is afraid that exposure to pesticides has caused the sores.

ASSESSMENT

Mr. Rivera speaks Spanish and is able to communicate only slightly in English. Anita Mendez, a student nurse fluent in Spanish, performs the initial assessment of Mr. Rivera. Mr. Rivera's history reveals problems with lower back pain but no significant past medical illnesses. He is not aware of any allergies and cannot remember having had chickenpox as a child. Two years ago, both children were sick and had blisters on their bodies, and a friend told them it was chickenpox. Mrs. Rivera thinks she had chickenpox as a child.

Because Mr. Rivera has not had any medical care for several years, baseline laboratory tests are ordered to screen for any other illnesses. The complete blood count (CBC), blood chemistry, and urinalysis are all within normal limits.

Mr. Rivera says that he did not feel well for several days before the blisters appeared, having experienced chills and general achiness. He had not taken his temperature because the family does not own a thermometer. Current vital signs are as follows: T 37.2°C (99°F), P 74 bpm, R 22/min, and BP 148/88 mmHg.

Physical examination of the trunk reveals a bandlike pattern of lesions across the left thorax. Some of the lesions are vesicles filled with serous fluid; others are darker in color and are oozing a light yellow drainage. The skin around the lesions is red and inflamed. Mr. Rivera complains of a severe, burning pain with itching across his chest. He is diagnosed with herpes zoster.

DIAGNOSIS

- Potential for infection related to open oozing areas on the left thorax
- Acute pain related to the presence of lesions and pruritus
- Lack of knowledge of the cause of the skin disorder and recommended treatment
- Anxiety related to need to work in areas of pesticide application
- Difficulty with health maintenance related to limited access to healthcare due to transitory work conditions and cultural and language barriers

EXPECTED OUTCOMES

- Patient's skin lesions will heal without evidence of a secondary infection.
- Patient will limit his exposure (as much as possible) to his wife and children and to individuals with debilitating illnesses to prevent the spread of the virus.
- Patient will obtain relief from pain and pruritus with the proper use of medications.
- Patient will verbalize an understanding of the disease process and participate in the treatment plan.
- Patient will obtain follow-up care.
- Patient will make an appointment for a referral for information about occupational hazards.

PLANNING AND IMPLEMENTATION

- Provide verbal and written instructions (in Spanish) for self-care:
  - a. Wear a clean cotton undershirt each day.
  - b. Trim the fingernails short, and keep the hands clean.
  - c. Wash hands each time the infected area is touched.
  - d. Wash any soiled clothes or linens in hot water and soap.
  - e. Do not allow other family members to use your towels.
  - f. Take medications as prescribed for itching and pain.
  - g. Take the medicine for your sores every 4 hours, even during nighttime hours, for 7 days.
  - h. As much as possible, do not touch your wife and children until the sores are covered with scabs.
  - i. Do not have sex with your wife while you have these sores.
- Teach how to take care of skin lesions:
  - a. Wear disposable gloves every time you do this treatment.
  - b. Wash the sores and the skin around them very gently with a soft washcloth and a mild soap.
  - c. Using your fingers, carefully rub the cream on the sores. Do this once every morning after breakfast and once every evening after supper.
  - d. Wash your hands carefully before and after each treatment.
- Make a follow-up appointment for the next week.
- Provide Mr. Rivera with the name and phone number of the Occupational Safety and Health Administration (OSHA) and recommend he call for an appointment to discuss his concerns about pesticides.

EVALUATION

Mrs. Rivera explains how she has taken care of her husband, and Mr. Rivera is careful to describe how he has followed the nurse's instructions. The skin lesions are dry and crusty, with no new blister formation. Mr. Rivera says he has not called OSHA and is not sure that he will, but he thanks Miss Mendez for the phone number. The nurses make an appointment in 1 month for a prenatal checkup for Mrs. Rivera and for follow-up of Mr. Rivera's herpes zoster. Mr. Rivera promises to return if they are still living close enough to keep the appointment.

CLINICAL REASONING IN PATIENT CARE

1. Identify barriers to care present in this case study. How may nursing interventions promote healthcare delivery to disadvantaged populations?
2. Although most cases of herpes zoster are self-limiting, what further assessments and interventions might have been indicated had the lesions shown little improvement over time and/or the pain remained severe?
3. If Mr. Rivera is advised not to work until his lesions heal, the family may face economic and sociocultural hardships. Develop a plan of care for Mr. Rivera that addresses his feelings about not being able to work.

See Evaluating Your Response in Appendix B.

- Teach measures to relieve pruritus: Take prescribed antipruritic medications, apply calamine lotion or wet compresses if prescribed, keep the room temperature cool, and use a bed cradle to keep sheets off affected areas of the body. *Pruritus is a common problem for patients with herpes zoster; scratching may excoriate the skin and increase the risk for secondary infections. Pruritus may intensify the experience of pain.*
- Encourage the use of distraction (such as music) or a specific relaxation technique (such as progressive muscle relaxation or deep breathing). *Noninvasive methods to relieve pain not only help the patient manage the pain experience but also increase the effectiveness of pain medications.*

Reduce the Risk for Infection. Patients with herpes zoster have impaired skin integrity and pruritus with scratching and possible excoriation. These factors contribute to a high risk for secondary bacterial infection. In addition, the patient is contagious to others who did not have chickenpox as children.

Expected Outcome: Patient's infection will be effectively managed as evidenced by skin integrity and body temperature within normal range.

The nurse will:

- If hospitalized, monitor white blood cell count and assess for lymph gland enlargement. *Secondary bacterial infections may occur in any patient with impaired skin integrity; if the patient is immunocompromised, the risk is even greater. Fever, changes in lesions or drainage, an increased white blood cell count, and lymph gland enlargement are manifestations of an infection.*
- Teach interventions to decrease the itch–scratch–itch cycle, thereby decreasing the possibility of excoriation (refer to the discussion about nursing care of patients with pruritus and psoriasis earlier in this chapter). *Excoriation from scratching provides an avenue for bacterial invasion.*
- Institute infection control procedures for patients who are hospitalized:

  a. Maintain strict isolation for immunocompromised patients.

  b. Wear gloves and gown if contact with lesions is likely.

  c. Instruct pregnant women to avoid exposure until lesions have crusted over.

  Isolation procedures are instituted for the immunocompromised patient to prevent patient infection. Wear gloves and gown to prevent spreading the infection to self or others. Pregnant women must avoid exposure to people with herpes zoster because the herpes virus can cross the placental barrier.

Delegating Nursing Care Activities

As appropriate and allowed by designated duties and responsibilities of unlicensed assistive personnel, the nurse may delegate nursing care activities such as measuring fluid intake and output, collecting vital signs (including orthostatic vital signs), encouraging oral or enteral fluid intake, and nonpharmacologic skin care.

Transitions of Care

Because most patients with viral infections provide self-care at home, the nurse focuses on teaching the patient and family how to provide the necessary care. With herpes zoster increasing in incidence in patients who are older or have a serious chronic illness, it may also be necessary to make a referral to a community health provider for continued support. Provide the following information and instructions:

- Vaccines are available to help prevent herpes zoster.
- The disease is usually self-limiting and heals completely. Second occurrences of herpes zoster are rare.
- Do not have social contact with children or pregnant women until crusts have formed over the blistered areas with herpes zoster because the disease is contagious to people who have not had chickenpox.
- Use pain medications regularly.
- Follow suggestions to help reduce itching, scratching, and pain: Use medications as prescribed, wear lightweight cotton clothing, keep room temperatures cool, wear cotton gloves at night if scratching is a problem, and practice relaxation and distraction activities.
- Report any increase in pain, fever, chills, drainage that smells bad and has pus, or a spread in the blisters to your healthcare provider.

16.3 Inflammatory Disorders of the Skin

The inflammatory skin disorders discussed in this section include dermatitis, acne, pemphigus, and lichen planus.

The Patient with Dermatitis

Dermatitis is an inflammation of the skin characterized by erythema and pain or pruritus. Dermatitis may be acute or chronic (Sorenson et al., 2019).

Pathophysiology and Manifestations

Various exogenous and endogenous agents can cause an inflammatory response of the skin. Different types of skin eruptions occur, that are often specific to the causative allergen, infection, or disease. The initial skin responses to these agents or illnesses include erythema, formation of vesicles and scales, and pruritus (**Figure 16.13** ■). Subsequently, irritation from scratching promotes edema, a serous discharge, and crusting. Long-term irritation in chronic dermatitis causes the skin to become thickened and leathery and darker in color.

Contact Dermatitis

Contact dermatitis is a type of dermatitis caused by a hypersensitivity response or chemical irritation. The major sources known to cause contact dermatitis are dyes, perfumes, poison plants (ivy, oak, sumac), chemicals, and metals. Common causes of contact dermatitis include:

- *Alkalis:* soaps, detergents, household ammonia, lye, cleaners
- *Cosmetics:* perfumes, dyes, oils
- *Hydrocarbons:* crude petroleum, lubricating oil, mineral oil, paraffin, asphalt, tar
- *Fabrics:* wool, polyester, dyes, sizing
- *Metal salts:* calcium chloride, zinc chloride, copper, mercury, nickel, silver
- *Plants:* ragweed, poison oak, poison sumac, poison ivy, pine.

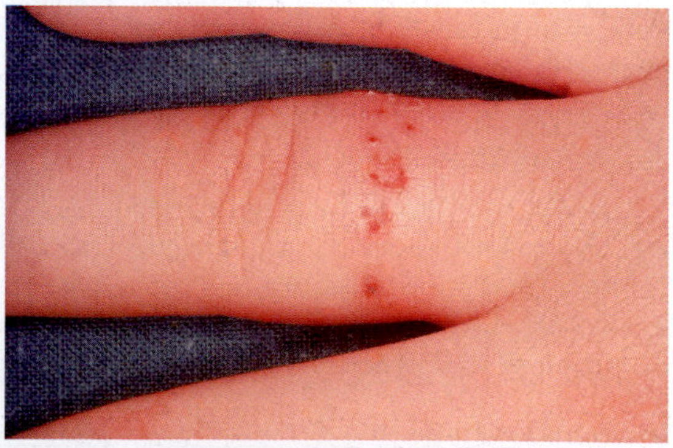

Figure 16.13 ■ Dermatitis may be a response to allergens, infections, or chemicals. This patient has contact dermatitis resulting from the metal salts in a ring.

A contact dermatitis common in the healthcare field is latex dermatitis. It is estimated that 8.7% of healthcare providers are allergic to latex (U.S. Food and Drug Administration, 2015). The most common type of allergic response to latex gloves is type IV, T-cell-mediated contact dermatitis. Type I IgE-mediated hypersensitivity, manifested by urticaria, rhinoconjunctivitis, asthma, or anaphylaxis, is far more serious than the T-cell-mediated type.

Allergic contact dermatitis is a cell-mediated or delayed hypersensitivity to a wide variety of allergens. Sensitizing antigens include microorganisms, plants, chemicals, drugs, metals, or foreign proteins. On initial contact with the skin, the allergen binds to a carrier protein, forming a sensitizing antigen. The antigen is processed and carried to the T cells, which in turn become sensitized to the antigen. The first exposure is the sensitizing contact and the person does not experience manifestations, which occur with subsequent exposures. The manifestations include erythema, swelling, and pruritic vesicles in the area of allergen contact. For example, a person hypersensitive to metal may have lesions under a ring or watch.

Irritant contact dermatitis is an inflammation of the skin from irritants; it is not a hypersensitivity response. Common sources of irritant contact dermatitis include chemicals (such as acids), soaps, and detergents. The skin lesions are similar to those seen in allergic contact dermatitis.

Atopic Dermatitis

Atopic dermatitis is an inflammatory skin disorder that is also called *eczema*. The exact cause is unknown, but related factors include depressed cell-mediated immunity, elevated IgE levels, and increased histamine sensitivity. Patients with atopic dermatitis have a family history of hypersensitivity reactions, such as dry skin, eczema, asthma, and allergic rhinitis. Although up to one-third of patients with atopic dermatitis also have food allergies, a positive correlation has not been found.

The dermatitis results from a type I hypersensitivity reaction (refer to Chapter 13). The immune response interacts with the allergen to create a chronic inflammatory condition. In the adult form of atopic dermatitis, characteristic lesions include chronic lichenification, erythema, and scaling, the result of pruritus and scratching. The lesions are usually found on the hands, feet, or flexor surfaces of the arms and legs. Scratching and excoriation increase the risk of secondary infections, as well as invasion of the skin by viruses such as herpes simplex. Serum studies may find elevated eosinophil and IgE levels.

Seborrheic Dermatitis

Seborrheic dermatitis is a chronic inflammatory disorder of the skin that involves the scalp, eyebrows, eyelids, ear canals, nasolabial folds, axillae, and trunk. The cause is unknown. Patients taking methyldopa (generic only) for hypertension occasionally develop this disorder, which is also a component of Parkinson disease. Seborrheic dermatitis is frequently seen in patients with AIDS.

The lesions are yellow or white plaques with scales and crusts. The scales are often yellow or orange and have a greasy appearance. Mild pruritus is also present. Diffuse dandruff with erythema of the scalp often accompanies the skin lesions.

Exfoliative Dermatitis

Exfoliative dermatitis is an inflammatory skin disorder characterized by excessive peeling or shedding of skin. The cause is unknown in about half of all cases, but a preexisting skin disorder (such as psoriasis, atopic dermatitis, contact dermatitis, or seborrheic dermatitis) is found in a majority of the cases. Reactions to medications, such as sulfonamides, account for less than half of all cases. Certain cancers (such as lymphoma) may also cause exfoliative dermatitis.

Both systemic and localized manifestations may appear. Systemic manifestations include weakness, malaise, fever, chills, and weight loss. Scaling, erythema, and pruritus may be localized or involve the entire body. In addition to peeling of skin, the patient may lose his or her hair and nails. Generalized exfoliative dermatitis may cause debility and dehydration. The impairment of skin integrity increases the risk for local and systemic infections.

Interprofessional Care

The patient with dermatitis is treated primarily with topical medications and therapeutic baths. If the dermatitis is due to hypersensitivity to an allergen, the patient avoids exposure to environmental irritants and suspected foods. The patient discontinues as many medications as possible to determine whether the dermatitis is the result of a drug allergy.

Diagnosis

The diagnosis is often based on the manifestations of the disorder and on a history of exposure to a known allergen. Scratch tests and intradermal tests are used to identify a specific allergen.

Medications

The medications used depend on the cause of the dermatitis and the severity of the manifestations. Minor cases are treated with antipruritic medications, whereas more severe cases are treated with oral antihistamines, oral and/or topical corticosteroids, and wet dressings for weeping lesions (Adams et al., 2017). Topical immunosuppressive modulators (tacrolimus and pimecrolimus) are effective, but the FDA has published an alert about a possible link with skin cancer and lymphoma. Topical anti-infectives may be prescribed if necessary.

Nursing Care

Nursing care of the patient with dermatitis focuses primarily on providing information for self-care at home. The patient is responsible for managing skin problems and requires education and support. Address the following topics:

- Medications and treatments do not cure the disease; they only relieve the symptoms.
- Dry skin increases pruritus, which stimulates scratching. Scratching may in turn cause excoriation, and excoriation increases the risk of infection.
- It may be necessary to change the diet or environment to avoid contact with allergens.
- When using steroid preparations, apply only a thin layer to slightly damp skin (e.g., after taking a bath).
- If occlusive dressings are necessary, a plastic suit may be used.
- When using oral corticosteroids, never abruptly stop taking the medication. Follow instructions to taper the dosage gradually.
- Advise to discuss use of topical steroids on the face for more than 2 weeks with healthcare provider to avoid adverse reactions.
- Antihistamines cause drowsiness. When using these medications, avoid alcohol and use caution when driving or working around machinery.

The Patient with Acne

Acne is a disorder of the pilosebaceous (hair and sebaceous gland) structure, which opens to the skin surface through a pore. The sebaceous glands, which empty directly into the hair follicle, produce sebum, a lipid substance. Sebum production is a response to direct hormonal stimulation by testicular androgens in men and adrenal and ovarian androgens in women.

Pathophysiology and Manifestations

Acne may be noninflammatory or inflammatory (Sorenson et al., 2019). Noninflammatory acne lesions are primarily **comedones**, more commonly called *pimples*, *whiteheads*, and *blackheads*. Whiteheads are pale, slightly elevated papules categorized as closed comedones. Blackheads are plugs of material that accumulate in the sebaceous glands. They are categorized as open comedones. The color is the result of the movement of melanin into the plug from surrounding epidermal cells. Inflammatory acne lesions include comedones, erythematous pustules, and cysts (**Figure 16.14** ■). Inflammation close to the skin surface results in pustules; deeper inflammation results in cysts. The inflammation is believed to result from irritation by fatty acid constituents of the sebum and by substances produced by *Propionibacterium acnes* bacteria, both of which escape into the dermis when the follicular wall of closed comedones ruptures. Several forms of acne occur at different periods of the lifespan. The most common are acne vulgaris, rosacea, and acne conglobata.

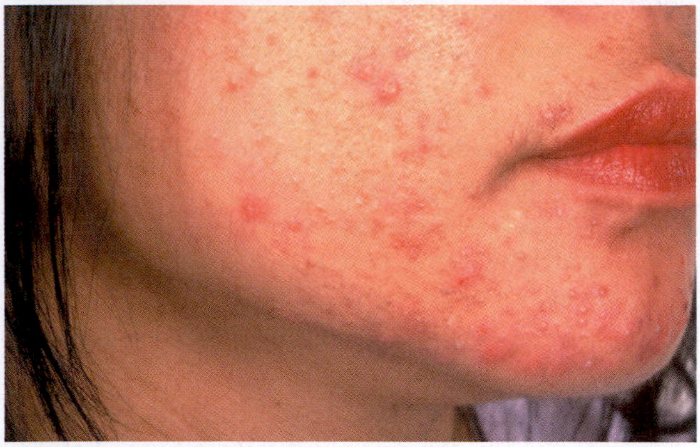

Figure 16.14 ■ Acne vulgaris lesions include comedones, erythematous pustules, and cysts.

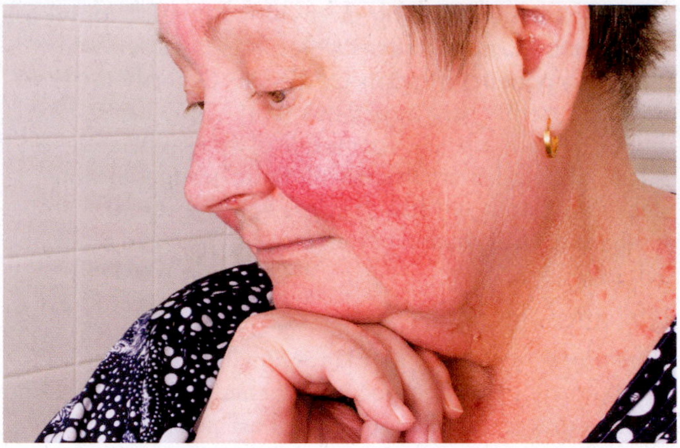

Figure 16.15 ■ Woman with a red rash characteristic of rosacea.

Acne Vulgaris

Acne vulgaris is the form of acne common in adolescents and young to middle adults. According to the Global Burden of Disease Study, approximately 85% of teenagers and young adults (ages 12 to 25) will have acne vulgaris at some point (Lynn, Umari, Dunnick, & Dellavalle, 2016). While the actual cause of acne vulgaris is unknown, possible causes include androgenic influence on the sebaceous glands, increased sebum production, and proliferation of the organism *Propionibacterium acnes*. Many factors once thought to cause acne vulgaris, including high-fat diets, chocolate, infections, and cosmetics, have been disproved.

Mild cases may involve only a few scattered comedones, but severe cases are manifested by multiple lesions of all types. Most acne vulgaris lesions form on the face and neck, but they also occur on the back, chest, and shoulders. Women in their 30s and 40s, often with no prior acne, may develop papular lesions on the chin and around the mouth. The lesions are usually mildly painful and may itch. The complications of severe acne vulgaris are formation of cysts, pigment changes in people with dark skin, severe scarring, and lowered self-concept from the skin eruptions. Scarring may be a sequelae of the disease or may result from the patient picking and manipulating the comedones.

Acne Conglobata

Acne conglobata is another chronic type of acne of unknown cause that begins in middle adulthood. This type causes serious skin lesions: Comedones, papules, pustules, nodules, cysts, and scars occur primarily on the back, buttocks, and chest but may occur on other body surfaces. The comedones have multiple openings and a discharge that ranges from serous to purulent with a foul odor.

Rosacea

Rosacea is a chronic facial condition that occurs more often in middle and older adults. The cause is unknown. The lesions of rosacea begin with erythema over the cheeks and nose (**Figure 16.15** ■). Other skin lesions may or may not appear. Over the years, the skin color changes to dark red, and the pores over the area become enlarged. The soft tissue of the nose may exhibit rhinophyma, an irregular bullous thickening. While no longer classified as a form of acne, it is treated in a similar manner to acne.

Interprofessional Care

The management of acne is similar, regardless of type. Because acne vulgaris is most common, the discussions of interprofessional and nursing care focus on that type. Treatment is based on the type and severity of the lesions.

Diagnosis

The disease is diagnosed by the typical location and appearance of lesions. If the patient has pustules, a culture of the drainage is performed to differentiate viral or bacterial dermatitis from acne.

Medications

The treatment of acne is tailored to the individual and is based on the severity of the lesions (Adams et al., 2017). For acne with comedones, tretinoin (retinoic acid, Retin-A) or benzoyl peroxide preparations are prescribed. Azelaic acid (Azelex) may also be used. The administration of these vitamin A analogues is discussed in **Medication Administration 16.C**. Benzoyl peroxide preparations are found in OTC medications such as Fostex, Acne-Dome, Desquam-X, Benzagel, Clear By Design, and Xerac BP. These products are keratolytic and loosen the comedones. Epiduo (a prescription gel) combines adapalene and benzoyl peroxide to treat acne vulgaris.

Mild forms of papular inflammatory acne are treated with topical clindamycin (Cleocin T), a bacteriostatic agent that decreases the amount of fatty acids on the skin surface. This medication may be combined with tretinoin therapy.

Moderate forms of papular inflammatory acne are treated with oral or topical antibiotics, such as tetracycline, erythromycin, and minocycline. These antibiotics are administered for 3 to 4 months; if the patient's skin is clear,

Medication Administration 16.C

Acne Medications

TRETINOIN (AVITA, RENOVA, RETIN-A)

- Use the cream in a test area twice at night to test for sensitivity; if no reaction occurs, increase applications gradually to the prescribed frequency.
- A pea-sized amount of the cream is enough to cover the entire face.
- Apply the cream to clean, dry skin.
- Do not apply the cream to the eyes, mouth, angles of the nose, or mucous membranes.
- Wash your face no more than two to three times a day, using a mild soap. Do not use skin preparations (such as aftershave lotion or perfumes) that contain alcohol, menthol, spice, or lime; they may irritate your skin.
- The medication may cause a temporary stinging or warm sensation but should not cause pain.
- The skin where you apply the cream will be mildly red and may peel; if you experience a more severe reaction, consult your healthcare provider.
- The medication may cause increased sensitivity to sunlight; use sunscreens and wear protective clothing when outdoors.
- Your acne may become worse during the first 2 weeks of treatment; this is an expected response.

Source: Data from Adams et al., 2017.

the dose is lowered gradually to a maintenance dose that will maintain clear skin.

Treatments

Acne scars may alter the individual's self-concept. The scars may be removed by dermabrasion and laser treatment. (Dermabrasion is discussed in greater detail later in this chapter.)

Nursing Care

Nursing care is individualized and is conducted primarily through teaching in clinics or healthcare provider offices. Regardless of the patient's age or gender, the nurse should remember that almost all patients with acne are embarrassed by and self-conscious of their appearance. Prior to teaching, establish rapport with the patient and clarify beliefs; for example, the patient may believe the lesions result from poor hygiene, masturbation, use of cosmetics, eating the wrong types of foods, or lack of sexual activity. It is critical to teach the patient about the causes of and factors involved in acne prior to teaching self-care.

The teaching plan for the patient with acne includes general guidelines for skin care and health as well as specific guidelines for care of the acne lesions. The following topics should be addressed:

- Wash the skin with a mild soap and water at least twice a day to remove accumulated oils.
- Shampoo the hair often enough to prevent oiliness.
- Eat a regular, well-balanced diet. Foods do not cause or increase acne.
- Expose the skin to sunlight, but avoid sunburn.
- Get regular exercise and sleep.
- Try to avoid putting your hands on your face.
- Do not squeeze a pimple. Squeezing forces the material of the pimple deeper into the skin and may cause the pimple to become larger and infected.
- The treatment for acne lasts months, in some cases for the rest of one's life. It is very important to take the medications each day for the prescribed length of time.

The Patient with Pemphigus Vulgaris

Pemphigus vulgaris is a chronic disorder of the skin and oral mucous membranes characterized by blister formation. The disease is caused by autoantibodies that cause acantholysis (the separation of epidermal cells from one another). The disorder is associated with IgG antibodies and HLA-A10 antigen. Septicemia from an infection of *Staphylococcus aureus* is the most common cause of death. The disease occurs in middle and older adults of all races and ethnic backgrounds. The disorder has been associated with other autoimmune disorders and with the administration of certain drugs, such as penicillamine and captopril.

The blisters that form in pemphigus vulgaris usually appear first in the mouth and on the scalp and then spread in crops or waves to involve large areas of the body, including the face, back, chest, umbilicus, and groin. The blisters form in the epidermis and cause the epidermal cells to separate above the basal layer. These blisters rupture, leaving denuded skin, crusting, and oozing of fluid with a musty odor. The lesions are painful. Pressure on a blister causes it to spread to adjacent skin (Nikolsky sign). The loss of fluid from the blisters may result in fluid and electrolyte imbalances. Secondary bacterial infections are a serious risk.

Plasmapheresis is occasionally used to treat pemphigus. In this procedure, the plasma is selectively removed from whole blood and donor plasma is reinfused into the patient. This decreases the serum level of antibodies for a period of time. Plasmapheresis with related nursing care is discussed in Chapter 44.

The Patient with Lichen Planus

Lichen planus is an inflammatory disorder of the mucous membranes and skin. It has no known cause but has been associated with exposure to drugs or to film processing chemicals. The disease affects adults of all ages.

The lesions first appear as violet papules, 2 to 10 mm in size, commonly occurring on the wrists, ankles, lower legs, and genitals. The lesions itch intensely. Over time, persistent lesions thicken and become dark red, forming hypertrophic lichen planus. Lesions on the oral mucous membranes appear as white, lacey rings; lesions may also appear on the mucous membranes of the vaginal area and the penis. The nails become thin and may shed.

Lichen planus lesions are self-limiting but last for an average of 12 to 18 months. The disorder is diagnosed by manifestations. Corticosteroids are used to control the inflammation, and antihistamines are used to control the pruritus.

16.4 Acute Skin Disorders

Skin disorders that arise suddenly are classified under acute skin disorders.

The Patient with Stevens-Johnson Syndrome

Stevens-Johnson syndrome is a rare condition. A worldwide-reported incidence is one to six cases per million people per year (Yang et al., 2016). In the United States, about 300 new diagnoses are made each year. The condition is more common in adults than in children.

Pathophysiology and Manifestations

Stevens-Johnson syndrome is a serious condition of the skin and mucus membranes usually caused by an unpredictable reaction to medications or an infection. In some cases, the underlying cause cannot be determined. The process is characterized by epidermal necrosis with minimal associated inflammation. Depending on the extent of the skin slough, it can be life-threatening.

Multiple risk factors have been described that increase the risk for developing Stevens-Johnson syndrome. These include:

- Immune system abnormalities related to organ transplant, autoimmune disease, or HIV/AIDS. Persons with HIV have approximately a 100 times greater risk than the general population.
- History of prior Stevens-Johnson syndrome, especially if medication related and the drug is taken again.
- Family history of Stevens-Johnson due to the potential genetic component of the *HLA-B*1502* gene. Expression of this gene increases risk for the syndrome. Persons of Chinese, Southeast Asian, or Indian descent are more likely to carry the gene.

The initial signs and symptoms can be general (fever) and integument specific (unexplained skin pain; red-purple spreading rash; development of skin and mucus membrane blisters, especially of mouth, nose, eyes, and/or genitals). Within days of blister formation, skin sloughing begins (Mayo Clinic, 2017).

Interprofessional Care

Due to the severity of the skin involvement, Stevens-Johnson syndrome requires hospitalization, often in an intensive care unit or a burn unit. Care focuses on stopping all nonessential medications to attempt to stop exposure to potential triggers.

If the underlying cause of Stevens-Johnson syndrome can be eliminated and the skin reaction stopped, new skin may begin to grow over the affected area within several days. In severe cases, full recovery may take several months.

Diagnosis

Diagnosis is made by careful history and physical examination. A skin biopsy may be used to confirm the diagnosis or rule out other causes of the presenting symptoms. Skin cultures may be used to confirm or rule out infection. The SCORTEN scale can provide a prognostic indicator of survival in severe cases (DermNet New Zealand, 2017b). This score should be calculated within 3 days of hospitalization.

The risk for death can be estimated using the SCORTEN scale, which takes seven prognostic indicators into account (over 40 years of age, presence of malignancy, tachycardia over 120 beats/minute, initial epidermal detachment over 10%, serum urea over 28mg/dL, serum glucose over 252 mg/dL, bicarbonate under 20 mmol/L). The more positive indicators, the higher the risk of death. It is helpful to calculate a SCORTEN within the first 3 days of hospitalization.

Medications

Medications used for treating patients with Stevens-Johnson syndrome focus on managing pain and reducing inflammation of the eyes and mucus membranes using topical steroids. When indicated, antibiotics may be used. Other immune-response modifiers or immunoglobulin, while controversial, may be indicated on a case-by-case basis (Mayo Clinic, 2017).

Treatments

Supportive care includes fluid replacement (intravenous) and nutrition (via nasogastric tube) and wound care of cool, wet compresses for blisters or burn-type dressings where sloughing has occurred. If the eyes are involved, opthalmology care may also be indicated.

Nursing Care

Nursing care focuses on skin care, reduction of discomfort, avoidance of fluid and electrolyte loss, and prevention of infection. For severe cases, nursing care is similar to care of the burn patient. See Chapter 17 for care of patients with burns.

Transitions of Care

Recovery after Stevens-Johnson syndrome can take weeks to months, depending on the severity of your condition. If it was caused by a medication, you'll need to permanently avoid that drug and others related closely to it.

Prevention may not be possible if no potential risk factors are present. However, if the patient is of Chinese, Southeast Asian, or Indian descent, discussions with his or her provider and consideration of genetic testing for presence of specific genes may be indicated prior to initiation of carbamazepine (Tegretol), a common drug used to treat epilepsy, bipolar disorders, and other conditions, because it is a known trigger for Stevens-Johnson syndrome. If a patient has had a prior bout of Stevens-Johnson syndrome and a medication trigger was identified, the patient must avoid the drug and other drugs in the same class. Recurrence of Stevens-Johnson syndrome is commonly more severe and potentially fatal. Family members of patients who have experienced medication-identified Stevens-Johnson syndrome should also avoid the drug involved as well as others in the same drug class due to the genetic risk factor (Mayo Clinic, 2017).

Stevens-Johnson syndrome requires hospitalization, often in an intensive care unit or a burn unit. In patients who have experienced Stevens-Johnson syndrome, the nurse should instruct them in the name of the causative drug and the drug class, including related medications to avoid. Patients should inform all healthcare providers of the history of Stevens-Johnson syndrome, including causative medications. Finally, the patient should be instructed and encouraged to wear a medical information bracelet or necklace in case of emergency (Mayo Clinic, 2017).

Depending on the severity of the syndrome, Stevens-Johnson can be life-threatening. A mortality rate of 5% has been reported in cases where less than 10% of the body surface is involved. Other outcomes include organ damage/failure, corneal damage, and blindness (Mayo Clinic, 2017).

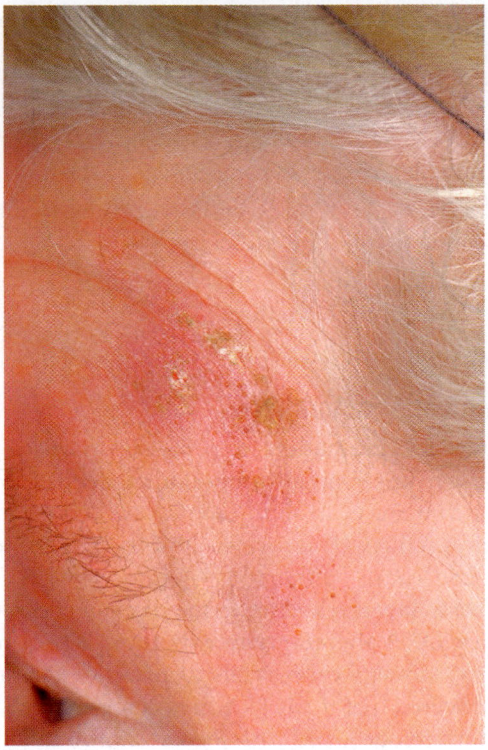

Figure 16.16 ■ The effects of long-term sun exposure are illustrated in this epidermal skin lesion, called *actinic keratosis*.

16.5 Malignant Skin Disorders

The skin, despite its ability to protect the internal body from external damage, is a fragile organ and is subject to damage from ultraviolet radiation and chemicals. Over time, this damage results in alterations in cellular structure and function, and malignancies of the skin occur. Many of these lesions are found on skin surfaces that have undergone long-term exposure to the sun or the environment. Up to 90% of skin changes visible with aging are caused by the sun. Malignant skin tumors are the most common of all cancers, and one in five Americans will develop skin cancer in the course of a lifetime.

The Patient with Actinic Keratosis

Actinic keratosis, also called *senile* or *solar keratosis*, is an epidermal skin lesion directly related to chronic sun exposure and photodamage. The prevalence is highest in people with light-colored skin; these lesions are rare in people with dark skin. About 10% of actinic keratoses convert to squamous cell carcinoma (Sorenson et al., 2019). However, there is some thought that the lesions are all premalignant.

The lesions are erythematous rough macules a few millimeters in diameter. They are often shiny but may be scaly; if the scales are removed, the underlying skin bleeds. They occur in multiple patches, primarily on the face, dorsa of the hands, the forearms, and sometimes on the upper trunk (**Figure 16.16** ■). Enlargement or ulceration of the lesions suggests transformation to malignancy. The lesions are usually treated by cryosurgery (freezing) or with 5-fluorouracil (5-FU) cream, which erodes the lesions.

The Patient with Nonmelanoma Skin Cancer

The nonmelanoma skin cancers are basal cell cancer and squamous cell cancer. Other types of nonmelanoma skin cancers, accounting for less than 1% of cases (American Cancer Society [ACS], 2017a), are Merkel cell carcinoma; Kaposi sarcoma; and lymphomas, sarcomas, and adnexal tumors of the skin. These uncommon tumors are not included in this discussion, but information can be found on the American Cancer Society website or the National Cancer Institute website.

Incidence and Risk Factors

Nonmelanoma skin cancer is the most common malignant neoplasm found in fair-skinned Americans. The ACS (2017b) estimates that more than 5.4 million new cases of nonmelanoma skin cancer are diagnosed in the United States each year. Of that number, about 80% are basal cell cancers and 20% are squamous cell cancers. Deaths from nonmelanoma skin cancer have dropped by 30% in the past 30 years. Men develop nonmelanoma skin cancer more often than do women, probably because of occupational exposures. Although nonmelanoma skin cancer may occur at any age, the incidence increases with each decade of life. Adults between the ages of 30 and 60 have the majority of these cancers.

Multiple etiologic factors are involved in the development of nonmelanoma skin cancer, including environmental factors and host factors. Risk factors for nonmelanoma skin cancer include:

- Fair skin, freckles, blue or green eyes, and blond or red hair
- Family history of skin cancer
- Unprotected and/or excessive exposure to ultraviolet radiation (natural or artificial)
- Occupational exposures to coal tar, pitch, creosote, arsenic compounds, or radium
- Severe sunburns as a child.

Environmental Factors

Ultraviolet (UV) radiation from the sun is believed to be the cause of most nonmelanoma skin cancers (ACS, 2017e). Sunlight contains both short-length rays (UVB) and long-length rays (UVA). UVB rays are absorbed by the top layer of skin and cause sunburn. UVA rays penetrate deeper into the skin layers, causing tissue damage. Both types of rays cause DNA alterations and suppress T-cell and B-cell immunity, allowing cancer cells to grow. Researchers have also discovered that many skin cancers contain changes in tumor suppressor genes (these genes normally help keep cells from growing out of control). The damaged gene found in basal cell cancer is *p53*, a gene that normally causes damaged cells to die. The damaged gene found in squamous cell cancer is the "patched" (*PTCH*) gene, which normally helps keep cell growth in check (ACS, 2017e).

The amount of ultraviolet radiation reaching the earth is increasing, most likely from depletion of the ozone layer surrounding the planet. The U.S. Environmental Protection Agency (2012) reported that for every 1% decrease in the ozone layer, a corresponding 1% to 3% increase per year in nonmelanoma skin cancer will occur.

Geographic, environmental, and lifestyle factors affect the amount of exposure to the sun and the risk for nonmelanoma skin cancer. People who live in latitudes close to the equator and those who live at higher altitudes receive greater ultraviolet radiation exposure. The amount of clothing worn, the time of day, and amount of time in the sun also determine the amount of exposure. Exposure to ultraviolet radiation in tanning booths is also implicated in the development of nonmelanoma skin cancer (ACS, 2017e).

Certain chemicals have long been associated with nonmelanoma skin cancer. Polycyclic aromatic hydrocarbons, found in mixtures of coal, tar, asphalt, soot, and mineral oils, have been linked with skin cancers. Psoralens, used in conjunction with UVA for treatment of psoriasis and cutaneous T-cell lymphoma, increase the risk of squamous cell cancer. Other factors associated with nonmelanoma skin cancer are the use of ionizing radiation, viruses, and physical trauma. X-ray therapy for tinea capitis and the use of radium to treat other malignancies are risk factors. Human papillomavirus is implicated in the development of squamous cell cancer, as is damage to the skin from burns. Organ transplant recipients who undergo immunosuppression to prevent rejection are also at risk for the development of squamous cell cancer.

Host Factors

Skin pigmentation is an important factor in the development of nonmelanoma skin cancer. The amount of melanin pigment produced by the melanocytes determines a person's skin color. The more melanin, the more the skin is protected from the damage produced by ultraviolet rays. Thus, Asians and people of African and Mediterranean descent have a much lower incidence of nonmelanoma skin cancer than do people who have fair complexions and tend to freckle or sunburn easily, such as people of Irish, Scandinavian, or English ancestry.

Although most people have numerous pigmented lesions on their body, almost all of these are normal. However, a major risk factor in the development of nonmelanoma skin cancer is a change in an existing lesion or the presence of a premalignant lesion, such as actinic keratosis.

Pathophysiology and Manifestations

Basal cell cancer and squamous cell cancer arise from epithelial tissue but have different pathophysiology, classifications, and manifestations. These cancers are classified as keratinocyte cancers; when viewed under a microscope they share some features with keratinocytes, the most abundant skin cell type.

Basal Cell Cancer

Basal cell cancer is an epithelial tumor believed to originate either from the basal layer of the epidermis or from cells in the surrounding dermal structures. These tumors are characterized by an impaired ability of the basal cells of the epidermis to mature into keratinocytes, with mitotic division beyond the basal layer. This results in a bulky tumor that grows by direct extension and, if untreated, destroys surrounding tissue, including healthy skin, nerves, blood vessels, lymphatic tissue, cartilage, and bone. Basal cell cancer is the most common but least aggressive type of skin cancer, rarely metastasizing. Although once seen only in middle to older adults, it is now being seen in younger people, probably due to increased sun exposure.

Basal cell cancers tend to recur. Tumors greater than 2 cm in diameter have a high recurrence rate. Predisposing factors for metastasis are the size of the tumor and the patient's resistance to treatment with surgery or chemotherapy. Even though they rarely metastasize, untreated basal cell cancers invade surrounding tissue and may destroy body parts, such as the nose or eyelid. Basal cell cancer is classified as nodular, superficial, pigmented, morpheaform, or keratotic.

Nodular basal cell cancer, the most common type of basal cell cancer, most often appears on the face, neck, and head. The tumor is made up of masses of cells that resemble epidermal basal cells and grow in a bulky, nodular form from lack of keratinization. In early stages, the tumor is a papule that looks like a smooth pimple. It is often pruritic and continues to grow at a steady rate, doubling in size every 6 to 12 months. As the tumor grows, the epidermis thins, but it remains intact. The skin over the tumor is shiny, pearly white, pink, or flesh colored. Telangiectasis may be visible over the area of the tumor. As the tumor continues to increase in size, the center or periphery may ulcerate, and the tumor develops well-circumscribed borders. It bleeds easily from mild injury.

Superficial basal cell cancer, found most often on the trunk and extremities, is the second most common type of basal cell cancer. This tumor is a proliferating tissue that attaches to the undersurface of the epithelium. The tumor is a flat papule or plaque, often erythematous, with well-defined borders. The tumor may ulcerate and be covered with crusts or shallow erosions (**Figure 16.17** ■).

Pigmented basal cell cancer, found on the head, neck, and face, is less common. This tumor concentrates melanin pigment in the center of the basal cancer cells, giving it a dark brown, blue, or black appearance. The border of the tumor is shiny and well defined.

Morpheaform basal cell cancer, the rarest form of basal cell cancer, usually develops on the head and neck. The tumor forms finger-like projections that extend in any direction along dermal tissue planes. The tumor resembles a flat ivory or flesh-colored scar. This form is more likely to extend into and destroy adjacent tissue, especially muscle, nerve, and bone. It is often more difficult to diagnose than other types of basal cell cancer because of its appearance.

Keratotic basal cell cancer (basosquamous) is found on the preauricular and postauricular groove. It contains both basal cells and squamoid-appearing cells that keratinize. Its appearance is much like that of nodular basal cell cancer. This type of basal cell cancer tends to recur locally and is also the type most likely to metastasize.

Squamous Cell Cancer

Squamous cell cancer is a malignant tumor of the squamous epithelium of the skin or mucous membranes. It occurs most often on areas of skin exposed to ultraviolet rays and weather, such as the forehead, helix of the ear, top of the nose, lower lip, and backs of the hands. Squamous cell cancer may also arise on skin that has been burned or has chronic inflammation. This is a much more aggressive cancer than basal cell cancer, with a faster growth rate and a much greater potential for metastasis if untreated. The tumors arise when the keratinizing cells of the squamous epithelium proliferate, producing a growth that eventually fills the epidermis and invades the dermal tissue planes. Keratinization of some cells is present, and the formation of keratin "pearls" is common. The keratin formation diminishes as the tumor grows. As the tumor grows, the tumor cells increase in number and rate of mitosis, forming odd shapes. An early form of squamous cell cancer is called *Bowen disease* or *cancer in situ*.

Squamous cell cancer begins as a small, firm red nodule. The tumor may be crusted with keratin products. As it grows, it may ulcerate, bleed, and become painful. As the tumor extends into the surrounding tissue and becomes a nodule, the area around the nodule becomes indurated (hardened) (**Figure 16.18** ■).

Recurrent squamous cell cancer can be invasive, increasing the risk of metastasis. Invasive squamous cell cancer may arise from preexisting skin lesions, such as scars and actinic keratosis, and extend into the dermis (called *intraepidermal squamous cell cancer*). This form appears as a slightly raised erythematous plaque with well-defined borders. Metastasis occurs most often via the lymphatics. The degree of risk for metastasis depends on the size and depth of penetration of the tumor.

Interprofessional Care

Treatment of nonmelanoma skin cancer focuses on removal of all malignant tissue using such methods as surgery, curettage and electrodesiccation, cryotherapy, or radiotherapy. These modalities offer a greater than 90% cure rate (National Cancer Institute, 2017). After the malignant tissue is removed, the patient should have regular examinations for recurrence.

Diagnosis

Nonmelanoma cancer is diagnosed by microscopic examination of tissue biopsied from the tumor. The biopsy is usually done as an office procedure under local anesthesia. The types of biopsy used are shave, punch, incisional, and excisional. Information about skin biopsy is provided in Chapter 15.

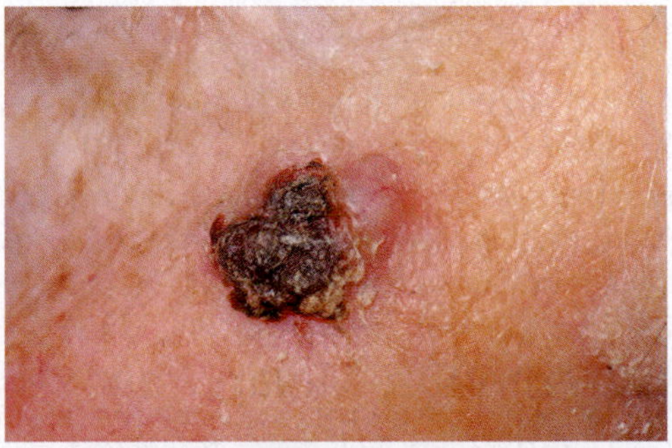

Figure 16.17 ■ A superficial basal cell cancer is characterized by erythema, ulcerations, and well-defined borders.

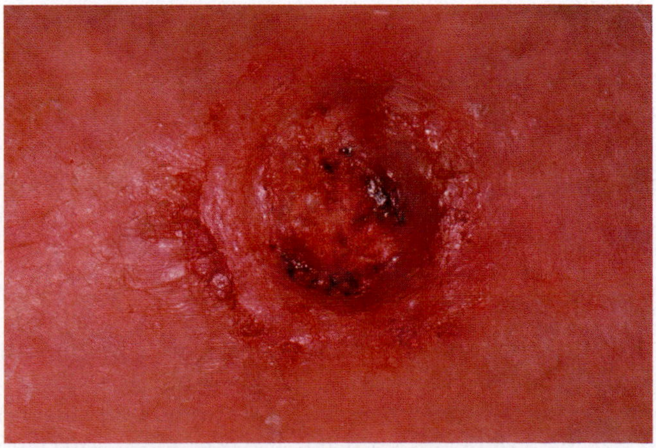

Figure 16.18 ■ As a squamous cell cancer grows, it tends to invade surrounding tissue. It also ulcerates, may bleed, and is painful.

Treatments

Depending on the stage, type, size, and location of a nonmelanoma cancer, it may be treated with surgical excision, Mohs surgery, curettage and electrodesiccation, radiation, or other forms of local therapy.

Surgical Excision. Both basal cell and squamous cell cancers are excised surgically. The surgery may be minor or major, depending on the size and location of the tumor. Surgery for small tumors is most often performed in the outpatient surgery department or in the surgeon's office. Surgical excision allows rapid healing and yields good cosmetic results.

The goal of surgical excision is to remove the tumor completely, so some surrounding tissue is excised along with the tumor. If the tumor is on the face, the incision is made along normal wrinkle or anatomic lines so that the scars will be less obvious. The incision is closed in layers to leave the smallest possible scar. A pressure dressing is usually applied over the incision to provide support. If a large tumor is removed, a skin graft or skin flap may be performed to cover the excised area. If grafting is necessary, the patient is hospitalized.

Mohs Surgery. In Mohs surgery, thin layers of the tumor are horizontally shaved off. A frozen section of the tissue is stained at each level to determine tumor margins. This method is the most accurate in assessing the extent of nonmelanoma skin cancer and the method that conserves the most normal tissue. It is often used in areas such as the nose, the nasolabial fold, the medial canthus, and the ear.

Curettage and Electrodesiccation. Curettage and electrodesiccation are used to treat basal cell cancers that are less than 2 cm in diameter, are superficial, or recur because of poor margin control. This treatment may also be used for primary squamous cell cancers that are less than 1 cm in diameter and have distinct borders. This type of treatment is most successful for tumors on anatomic sites over a fixed underlying surface, such as the ear, chest, and temple.

Abnormal tissue is scraped away (curettaged) within 1 to 2 mm of the margin and then a low-voltage electrode is used to abrade the tumor base (electrodesiccation). Curettage and electrodesiccation is not used for lesions where the dermis is thin (such as the eyelid) or where the tumor extends into the subcutaneous tissue. This treatment provides good cosmetic results and preserves normal tissue. However, healing time is longer, and it is difficult to ensure that all tumor margins have been removed.

Instead of a low-voltage electrode, some physicians use a carbon dioxide laser to vaporize the tumor. When used in conjunction with curettage, this treatment is effective on superficial basal cell cancers. Carbon dioxide vaporization results in minimal thermal injury to adjacent cells, less pain, and quicker healing.

Radiation. Radiation is most often used for lesions that are inoperable because of their location (such as tumors on the corner of the nose, the eyelid, the canthus, and the lip) or size (between 1 and 8 cm). It is also used for patients who are older and of poor surgical risk. Radiation is painless and can be used to treat areas surrounding the tumor if necessary. However, the treatment is given over 3 to 4 weeks in a clinical facility, does not allow control of tumor margins, and may itself cause skin cancer.

Other Forms of Local Therapy. Other forms of local therapy include:

- *Cryosurgery* involves applying liquid nitrogen to the tumor to freeze and kill abnormal cells.
- *Photodynamic therapy (PDT)* involves administering a topical or injectable chemical that collects in the tumor cells and makes them more sensitive to light. A light source is then focused on the tumor and the cells die.
- *Topical chemotherapy* involves an anticancer drug (usually 5-FU) that is applied as a cream directly on the skin to kill the tumor cells.
- *Immune response modifiers* cause an immune response to the cancer, causing it to decrease in size and die. The drugs used are imiquimod (Aldara; a topical cream) and interferon (injected directly into the tumor).
- *Laser surgery* uses laser light to vaporize cancer cells.
- *Vismodegib (Erivedge) and sonidegib (Odomzo)* are used to inhibit a target protein in the sonic hedgehog (SHH) pathway, which is necessary to the basal cell development cycle (Rimkus et al., 2016). The medications, which are taken orally once daily, can affect fetal development, so they should not be used by pregnant women.

Nursing Care

The increasing number of people with skin cancer means that nurses must be involved in prevention and early detection. Nurses have the opportunity to teach preventative behaviors in all settings, including the hospital, home, community, school, and clinic.

Nursing care for the patient with nonmelanoma skin cancer depends on the treatment used. Surgical excision is the most common form of treatment; nursing care depends on the extent of the procedure. However, regardless of the type of treatment, the patient will have impaired skin integrity, an increased risk for infection, and anxiety about the future following a diagnosis of cancer. Interventions with rationales for the patient with any type of skin cancer are discussed in the later section on melanoma.

Transitions of Care

Teach the patient and family specific measures for self-care following surgery, including the following information:

- How and when to change dressings
- The use of aseptic technique and careful hand hygiene when caring for the wound
- Symptoms to report (such as bleeding, fever, or signs of wound infection) and how to protect the operative site against trauma and irritations.

The Patient with Melanoma

Melanoma (also called *malignant melanoma*) arises from melanocytes. This serious skin cancer is increasing in incidence each year. Melanoma accounts for less than 5% of skin cancers, but it causes a large majority of skin cancer deaths (ACS, 2017c).

Incidence and Risk Factors

This disease is over 10 times more common in fair-skinned people than in dark-skinned people. It is slightly more common in men than in women. Melanoma occurs more often in people who live in sunny climates, burn easily, and patronize tanning salons. However, it may arise from already present lesions or from skin normally covered with clothing. Melanoma occurs in a wide age range, from adolescents to older adults, with the greatest rates in those over the age of 80 (ACS, 2017c).

Although the exact cause of melanoma is unknown, it is known that certain risk factors are associated with the disease. Risk factors for melanoma include:

- A high number of moles, or large moles
- Fair skin, freckling, blond hair, or blue eyes
- Close relative with the disease
- Men with gene changes from a family history of breast or ovarian cancer
- Treatment with medications that suppress the immune system
- Too much exposure to UV radiation from sunlight, tanning lamps, or tanning booths
- Over age 50
- Xeroderma pigmentosus, a rare inherited disease in which people are less able to repair damage caused by sunlight
- Past history of melanoma.

Pathophysiology and Manifestations

Melanomas arise from melanocytes, cells located at or near the basal layer (the deepest epidermal layer). These cells produce melanin, the dark skin pigment. Melanin is made in granules and transferred to keratinocytes, where it accumulates on the superficial side of each keratinocyte and forms a shield of pigment over the nucleus as protection against ultraviolet rays. Melanomas can develop wherever there is pigment, but about one-third of them originate in existing nevi (moles).

Almost all melanomas are more than 6 mm in diameter, are asymmetric, and initially develop within the epidermis over a long period. While they are still confined to the epidermis, the lesions (called *melanoma in situ*) are flat and relatively benign. However, when they penetrate the dermis, they mingle with blood and lymph vessels and are capable of metastasizing. At this latter stage, the tumors develop a raised or nodular appearance and often have smaller nodules, called *satellite lesions*, around the periphery.

The prognosis for survival for people diagnosed with melanoma is determined by several variables, including location of tumor, tumor thickness, ulceration, metastasis, site, age, and gender (ACS, 2017c). Younger patients and women have a somewhat better chance of survival. Patients with tumors on the scalp and neck have a lower survival rate.

Precursor Lesions

The three specific precursor lesions for the development of melanoma are congenital nevi, dysplastic nevi, and lentigo maligna. A precursor lesion is also called a *premalignant lesion*, a name that indicates that the lesion's risk of becoming malignant is greater than normal.

Congenital Nevi. *Congenital nevi* are present at birth. Some lesions are small; others are large enough to cover an entire body area. Their color can range from brown to black. They are often slightly raised, with an irregular surface and a fairly regular border.

Dysplastic Nevi. *Dysplastic nevi* are also called *atypical moles*. Although dysplastic nevi are not present at birth, they appear as normal nevi during childhood and become dysplastic (having abnormal development) after puberty. A patient with classic dysplastic nevi has more than 100 nevi, at least one of which is larger than 8 mm in diameter, and at least one of which has the characteristics of melanoma (asymmetry, irregular border, color variegation, and a diameter greater than 6 mm). A familial tendency to dysplastic nevi increases the risk for the development of melanoma. Having many moles, whether normal or atypical, is a risk factor for melanoma.

Dysplastic nevi most often appear on the face, trunk, and arms but are also seen on the scalp, female breast, groin, and buttocks. The pigmentation of the nevi is irregular, with mixtures of tan, brown, black, red, and pink, where an area of lighter pigmentation is surrounded by a papular area of deeper pigmentation (described as a "fried egg appearance"). The borders of the nevi are irregular.

Lentigo Maligna. *Lentigo maligna*, also called *Hutchinson freckle*, is a tan or black patch on the skin that looks like a freckle. It grows slowly, becoming mottled, dark, thick, and nodular. It is usually seen on one side of the face of an older adult who has had a large amount of sun exposure.

Classification

Melanomas are classified into different types. The major types are superficial spreading melanoma, lentigo maligna melanoma, nodular melanoma, and acral lentiginous melanoma. Each of these tumors is characterized by a radial and/or vertical growth phase. During the initial radial phase, which may last from 1 to 25 years (depending on the type), the melanoma grows parallel to the skin surface. During this phase, the tumor rarely metastasizes and is often curable by surgical excision. However, during the vertical growth phase, atypical melanocytes rapidly penetrate into the dermis and subcutaneous tissue, greatly increasing the risk for metastasis and death.

Superficial Spreading Melanoma. *Superficial spreading melanoma* is the most common type, comprising 70% to 80% of all melanomas (Sorenson et al., 2019). The lesions are usually flat and scaly or crusty and are about 2 cm in diameter. They often arise from a preexisting nevus. This type of melanoma is found on the trunk and back of men and on the legs of women. Superficial spreading melanomas occur more often in women than in men. The median age of occurrence is the 50s.

The radial growth phase lasts from 1 to 5 or more years. When the lesion enters the vertical growth phase, it grows rapidly, and its color changes from a mixture of tan, brown, and black to a characteristic red, white, and blue. The lesion also develops irregular borders and often has raised nodules and ulcerations (**Figure 16.19** ■).

Lentigo Maligna Melanoma. *Lentigo maligna melanoma* often arises from the precursor lesion, lentigo maligna. The lesions are large and tan with different shades of brown. This type of melanoma makes up 5% to 10% of malignant melanomas and is the least serious form (Sorenson et al., 2019). It occurs on skin that has had long-term sun exposure, such as the face, neck, and sometimes the dorsal surface of the hands and lower extremities. Lentigo maligna melanoma affects women more than men. It is typically diagnosed in people in their 60s and 70s.

Lentigo maligna melanoma is characterized by a proliferation of atypical melanocytes parallel to the basal layer of the epidermis. The radial growth phase may last from 10 to 25 years, with the lesion growing to as large as 10 cm. The lesion becomes malignant as soon as the melanocytes invade the dermis. In the vertical growth phase, raised nodules may appear on the surface of the lesion. The lesion tends to acquire a freckled or mottled appearance.

Nodular Melanoma. *Nodular melanoma* lesions are raised, dome-shaped, blue-black or red nodules on areas of the head, neck, and trunk that may or may not have been exposed to the sun. The lesions may look like a blood blister, or they may ulcerate and bleed. The lesions arise from unaffected skin rather than from a preexisting lesion. This type makes up 10% to 15% of malignant melanomas and is often diagnosed in people in their 50s (Sorenson et al., 2019).

Nodular melanoma has only a vertical growth phase, but it grows aggressively during that phase. However, the absence of a radial growth phase makes this type more difficult to diagnose before it metastasizes.

Acral Lentiginous Melanoma. *Acral lentiginous melanoma*, also called *mucocutaneous melanoma*, is less common in people with fair skin and more common in people with dark skin. The lesions progress from tan, brown, or black flat lesions to elevated nodules and are about 3 cm in diameter. The radial phase lasts from 2 to 5 years, and the lesions are found on the palms of the hands, soles of the feet, the mucous membranes, and the nail beds. Acral lentiginous melanoma affects both men and women equally and is most often diagnosed in people in their 50s and 60s (DermNet New Zealand, 2017a).

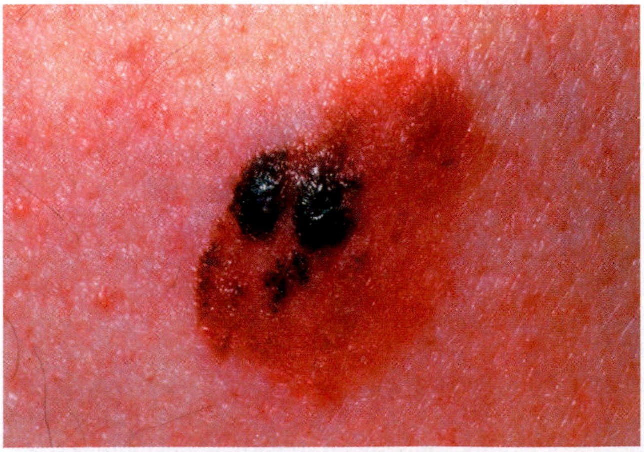

Figure 16.19 ■ Malignant melanoma is a serious skin cancer that arises from melanocytes.

Interprofessional Care

The management of the patient with melanoma begins with identification, diagnosis, and tumor staging. If treatable, the tumor is removed through surgical excision. Melanoma is also treated with chemotherapy, immunotherapy, and radiation therapy. Other therapies used with success include biologic therapies with interleukin-2 and interferon and therapeutic vaccines containing melanoma antigens.

Identification

Melanoma is most often found on the trunk of men and on the lower extremities of women. Nevertheless, it is important for the patient to have a complete physical examination and total skin assessment. In addition to a visual examination of all skin surfaces, palpation of regional lymph nodes, the liver, and the spleen is essential to assess for metastasis when a melanoma is suspected or found.

A change in the color or size of a nevus is reported in 70% of people diagnosed with a melanoma (ACS, 2016a). The ugly duckling sign (a mole that looks or feels different than other moles or changes differently over time than other moles) is often used in clinical practice. See Chapter 15 for the ABCDE rule used to assess suspicious lesions.

Diagnosis

In addition to biopsy of any suspicious lesion, diagnostic tests are conducted to determine whether the tumor has metastasized. Because malignant melanoma may metastasize to any organ or tissue of the body, a variety of tests may be conducted, including microscopic examination, biopsy, and tests for metastasis (liver function tests and CT scan of the liver, a complete blood count, serum blood chemistry profile, chest x-ray, bone scan, and CT scan or MRI of the brain).

Microstaging

The term *microstaging* describes the assessment of the level of invasion of a malignant melanoma and the maximum tumor thickness. In one method, the Clark system of microstaging, the vertical growth of the lesion is measured from the epidermis to the subcutaneous tissue to determine the level of invasion (**Figure 16.20** ■).

Treatments

Surgical excision is the preferred treatment for malignant melanoma. Other methods of treatment include chemotherapy (see Chapter 14), immunotherapy, radiation therapy, and biologic therapy.

Surgery. If a biopsy identifies the lesion as a melanoma, a wide excision is performed that includes the full thickness of the skin and subcutaneous tissue. Regional lymph nodes are the most common sites for metastasis of melanoma. Standard surgical treatment for clinically suspicious

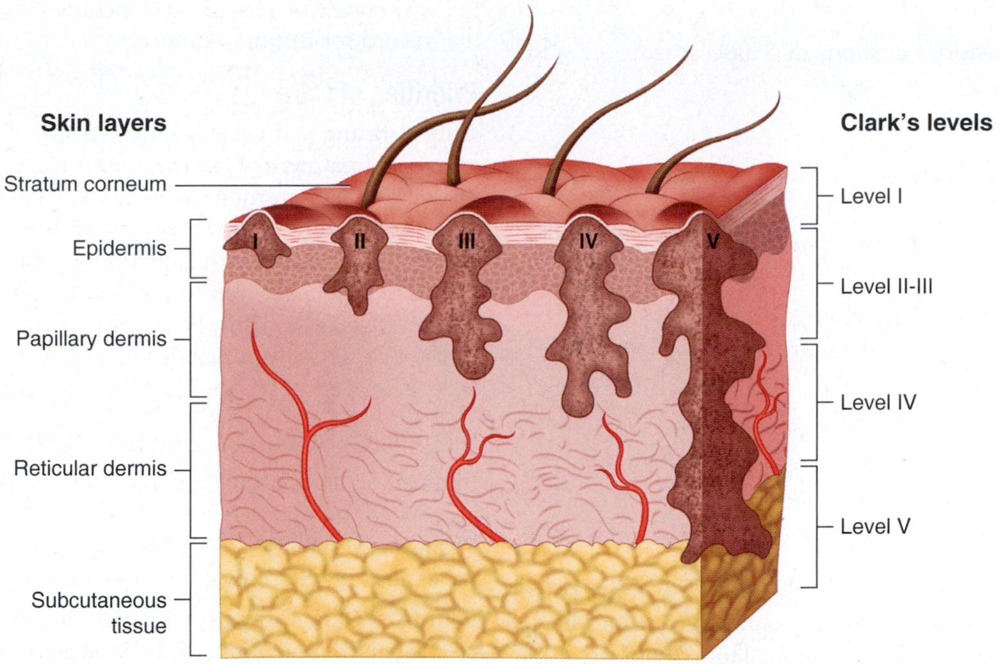
Skin layers
Clark's levels
Stratum corneum
Epidermis
Papillary dermis
Reticular dermis
Subcutaneous tissue
I
II
III
IV
V
Level I
Level II-III
Level IV
Level V

Figure 16.20 ■ The Clark levels for staging measure the invasion of a melanoma from the epidermis to the subcutaneous tissue.

lymph node involvement includes excision of the primary lesions as well as surgical dissection of the involved lymph nodes. Surgery is also indicated for palliative management of isolated metastasis. Removal of metastatic tumors in the brain, liver, lung, gastrointestinal tract, or subcutaneous tissue may relieve symptoms and prolong life. (See the Case Study & Nursing Care Plan on page 502.)

Immunotherapy. Immunotherapy is the use of medicines to stimulate the immune system to recognize and destroy cancer cells. The role of the immunologic response was initially recognized because of the numerous spontaneous remissions seen in patients with melanoma—a higher occurrence than with any other adult tumor. In addition, researchers have recently identified tumor-specific antigen–antibodies in patients with melanoma.

Agents such as interferons, interleukins, monoclonal antibodies, bacille Calmette-Guérin (BCG), levamisole, transfer factors, and tumor vaccines have shown activity in melanoma, with varying response rates. The effectiveness of these agents, used either alone, in combination with chemotherapy, or in combination with each other, is under investigation. The use of immunotherapy in the treatment of melanoma is still new and requires further investigation.

Radiation Therapy. Melanoma responds to higher-dose radiation, especially if the tumor is small. Response rates to radiation therapy depend on the site of the tumor, the thickness of the tumor, the type of melanoma, and the patient's general health, but may range from 0% to 71% (ACS, 2016c). Radiation is frequently used for palliation of symptoms resulting from metastasis to the brain, bone, lymph nodes, gastrointestinal tract, skin, or subcutaneous tissue. Liver and lung metastases are not treated with radiation therapy because a loss of organ function may result.

Biologic Therapy. Biologic therapy is used to boost or restore the ability of the immune system to fight the cancer. Agents used include the monoclonal antibodies, growth factors, and vaccines. These agents may also have a direct antitumor effect (National Cancer Institute, 2013).

New Methods of Treatment. Melanoma skin cancer research is ongoing and directed toward more specific methods of diagnosis and treatment. Examples are:

- *Gene therapy:* About 50% of melanomas have mutations in the *BRAF* gene (ACS, 2016b). Vemurafenib (Zelboraf) and dabrafenib (Tafinlar) are drugs that attack the BRAF protein directly and are taken orally twice daily. The *MEK* gene works in concert with the *BRAF* gene. The MEK inhibitors trametinib (Mekinist) and cobimetinib (Cotellic), pills that are taken once daily, have been shown to shrink some melanomas with *BRAF* changes.
- *Melanoma DNA research:* Genes such as *CDKN2A* (also known as *p16*) have been found to be mutated in some families with a high rate of melanoma.
- *Staging:* Very sensitive new tests can better detect the spread of melanoma to lymph nodes and can possibly better identify people who could be helped by a treatment such as immunotherapy after surgery.

Nursing Care

Nurses have the opportunity to assess the skin of patients requiring care for many different health problems and may be the first healthcare provider to identify suspicious lesions. Wide excision and the high risk of metastasis from melanoma usually requires inpatient surgical treatment, with the nurse providing care and teaching.

Assessment

Specific health history questions and assessments for skin cancer include:

Interview Questions.

- Have any members of your family ever been treated for skin cancer?
- Have you had a skin cancer removed from any part of your body?
- Have you noticed any change in the size, shape, or color of a mole, wart, birthmark, or scar?
- Do you have any moles, warts, birthmarks, or scars that itch, are painful, have crusting, or bleed?
- In what parts of the country or world have you lived?
- Have you ever been badly sunburned?
- Do you visit tanning salons?
- Are you exposed to any hazardous chemicals in your job?
- Have you been taught how to examine your skin? If so, how do you do this examination? How often?

Physical Assessment.

1. Ask the patient to remove all clothing and put on an examination gown. Ensure good light; natural, bright light is best for inspection of lesions. The patient may sit, stand, or lie down.
2. Inspect and palpate the skin. Stretching the skin tightly during assessment facilitates examination of nodular and scaly lesions and lesions in the dermis. Assess for the following:
   a. Obvious lesions
   b. Visible swellings
   c. Alterations in normal contour and borders of nevi
   d. Enlarged lymph glands
   e. Skin or mucosal discolorations
   f. Areas of ulceration, scaling, crusting, or erosion.
3. The order of assessment is:
   a. Head and neck: entire scalp, eyelids, external ear, auditory canals, external surface of the nose, internal surface of the nose, the oral cavity, facial skin, the facial glands (parotid, submaxillary, sublingual)
   b. Thyroid and neck, including lymph glands
   c. Chest and abdomen, with special attention under pendulous breasts, in skinfolds, and in areas covered with hair
   d. Back and buttocks, with special attention to the area between the buttocks
   e. Extremities, with special attention to the axillae, nail beds, webs between the fingers and toes, and soles of the feet
   f. External genitals, with special attention to skinfolds, mucous membranes, and areas covered with hair.
4. Measure and record a description of all skin lesions on an anatomic chart. Take photographs (if possible) of any suspicious lesion, and include them in the patient's record for future reference.

Priorities of Care

Collaborating with the interprofessional team to ensure adequate treatment of the melanoma skin cancer while providing care that promotes recovery and comfort is a nursing priority. Teaching the patient and, as appropriate, caregivers strategies to prevent infection, optimize comfort, and promote safe behaviors to prevent ongoing sun exposure should also be considered a priority nursing action. The nurse also focuses on promoting comfort and maintaining asepsis for all interruptions of the integument.

Diagnoses, Outcomes, and Interventions

In the patient with a melanoma, common patient responses are related to skin integrity and psychological impact (hopelessness and anxiety). These patient responses are also appropriate for use with patients with nonmelanoma skin cancer.

Promote Skin Integrity. Melanomas not only destroy skin layers but also invade body structures. Certain types of melanomas may ulcerate prior to diagnosis, and treatment typically involves some type of surgical biopsy and excision. Any open lesion or incision increases the risk for secondary infection.

Expected Outcome: Patient will experience effective wound healing through primary intention as indicated by progressive approximation of wound borders.

The nurse will:

- Monitor for manifestations of infection: fever, tachycardia, malaise, incisional erythema, swelling, pain, or drainage that increases or becomes purulent. *Intact skin is the first line of defense against infection; impaired skin integrity increases the risk for infection. If infection is present, the patient may have both systemic and local manifestations.*
- Keep the incision line clean and dry by changing dressings as necessary. *Moisture increases the risk of infection.*
- Follow principles of medical and surgical asepsis when caring for patient's incision. Teach family members and visitors the importance of careful hand hygiene. Maintain standard precautions if drainage is present. *Careful hand hygiene is essential in preventing the spread of infection. Aseptic techniques are necessary when caring for any surgical incision to prevent infection.*
- Encourage and maintain adequate caloric and protein intake in the diet. Suggest a consultation with a dietitian if the patient does not want to eat. *Adequate calories and protein are necessary for proper healing. The patient with cancer has increased metabolic needs; if these needs are not met, nutritional problems that impair healing may result.*

Promote Hopefulness. Hopelessness is an emotional state in which a person feels that there is no possibility that life will improve. Patients who experience hopelessness are often withdrawn, passive, and apathetic.

The diagnosis of melanoma threatens the quality and quantity of life as the patient faces the possibility or reality of metastasis; the possibility that the cancer may recur and cause death; and alterations in self-concept, roles, and relationships. Inspiring hope in patients during this health crisis is a legitimate nursing action.

Expected Outcome: Patient will express hope as evidenced by expectation of positive outcome.

The nurse will:

- Provide an environment that encourages the patient to identify and express feelings, concerns, and goals:
  a. Use active listening, ask open-ended questions, and reflect on the patient's statements.
  b. Acknowledge and respect feelings of apathy and/or anger as expressions of distress.
  c. Convey an empathetic understanding of fears and concerns.
  d. Provide opportunities to express positive emotions: hope, faith, a sense of purpose, and the will to live.
  e. Explore the patient's perceptions, and modify or clarify them if necessary by providing information and correcting misconceptions.
  f. Encourage the patient to identify support systems and sources of strength and coping in the past.

  Verbalizing feelings, concerns, and goals allows others to validate or correct them, promotes a therapeutic nurse–patient relationship, and fosters feelings of self-worth. Expressing positive emotions and calling on support systems and sources of strength that were effective in coping with past crises help the person resolve the crisis and develop hope.
- Encourage active participation in self-care as well as in mutual decision making and goal setting. *Meeting self-care needs and making decisions about care increase personal confidence in one's capacity for coping.*
- Encourage a focus not only on the present but also on the future: Review past occasions for hope, discuss the patient's personal meaning of hope, establish and evaluate short-term goals with the patient and family, and encourage them to express hope for the future. *The nurse mobilizes the patient's resources to strengthen motivation, hope, and the will to live.*

Reduce Anxiety. The intensity of anxiety, aroused by a perceived threat, depends on the severity of the present situation and the patient's ability to handle the threat. Anxiety is one of the most common psychosocial responses in patients with cancer. Anxiety increases at the time of diagnosis and remains a constant emotion throughout the course of treatment, regardless of treatment type or setting. Interventions center on helping the patient recognize the manifestations of anxiety, determining whether the patient wishes to do anything about the anxiety, and facilitating coping strategies.

Expected Outcome: Patient will exhibit self-control of anxiety through use of coping strategies.

The nurse will:

- Provide reassurance and comfort:
  a. Set aside time to sit quietly with the patient.
  b. Speak slowly and calmly.
  c. Convey empathetic understanding by touch and supporting present coping mechanisms, such as crying and talking.
  d. Do not make demands or expect the patient to make decisions.

  Coping behaviors differ from situation to situation and from person to person. Anxiety at moderate to severe levels narrows perceptions and the ability to function.
- Decrease sensory stimuli by using short, simple sentences; focusing on the here and now; and providing concise information. *Higher levels of anxiety result in a focus on the present, inability to concentrate, and difficulty in understanding verbal communications.*
- Provide interventions that decrease anxiety levels and increase coping:
  a. Provide accurate information about the illness, treatment, and expected length of recovery.
  b. Encourage discussion of expected physical changes and ways to minimize disfigurement through cosmetics and clothing.
  c. Include family members in teaching sessions.
  d. Encourage participation in care.

  Although the prognosis and treatment of melanoma depend on various factors, the prognosis of complete cure is decreased with metastasis. Surgical incisions include excision with wide margins, which may cause disfigurement. Active participation in care gives the patient some control over the future and is often an effective means of coping with anxiety.

Delegating Nursing Care Activities

As appropriate and allowed by the designated duties and responsibilities of unlicensed assistive personnel, the nurse may delegate nursing care activities such as measuring fluid intake and output, collecting vital signs (including orthostatic vital signs), encouraging oral or enteral fluid intake, and skin care.

Transitions of Care

Teaching for the patient and family experiencing the diagnosis and treatment of melanoma focuses on self-care and ongoing self-monitoring. Education for the patient and family is specific to the type of treatment.

The most important aspect of preventing melanoma is a health history and skin assessment. The ACS recommends that people between the ages of 20 and 40 see a skin specialist every 3 years and those over 40 have annual skin checkups. People with actinic keratoses should also have their skin checked regularly for any signs of change. Patients at risk (those with precancerous lesions and with personal risk factors), as well as those over the age of 40, should conduct a monthly skin self-examination (refer to Box 15.2 in Chapter 15).

Case Study & Nursing Care Plan

A Patient with Malignant Melanoma

Geoff Sanders, age 69, is retired from the postal service. He has always been an avid participant in outdoor sports: When he was younger he played baseball and tennis, and for the past 10 years he has played golf at least twice a week. He now lives in Connecticut, but as a younger man he lived in Florida for almost 15 years. Mr. Sanders has a variety of warts and moles and rarely pays attention to them. However, after taking a shower one day he noticed that a mole on his left lower leg looked bigger and darker. Mr. Sanders had just seen a public service announcement on television about the dangers of changes in moles, and he immediately called his primary care physician for an appointment at the dermatology clinic.

ASSESSMENT	DIAGNOSES	EXPECTED OUTCOMES
On arriving at the clinic, Mr. Sanders is interviewed and examined by Tom Hall, a clinical nurse specialist. Following the assessment, Mr. Hall documents the following information. Mr. Sanders has a family history of skin cancer; his father had several squamous cell cancers removed from his face. He has numerous nevi on his body; the one causing concern is located on the medial anterior left leg, 2 inches below the patella. Mr. Sanders states that the mole has been present for years but that he noticed just yesterday that it has become larger and darker. On further questioning, he states that the mole itches sometimes but has never hurt or bled. Mr. Sanders lived in Florida for 15 years and now experiences a sunburn early each summer before he tans. The sunburn involves the lower legs because Mr. Sanders wears shorts during his twice-weekly golf game. A complete skin assessment reveals various freckles, warts, and nevi. With the exception of the nevus that prompted Mr. Sanders to come to the clinic, all lesions appear normal. The nevus in question is raised, 3 cm in diameter, with irregular borders and a nodular surface. It is variegated in color, with various shades of brown. The skin surrounding the nevus is slightly erythematous. Inguinal lymph nodes are not enlarged or painful. Mr. Hall takes a photograph of the lesion with Mr. Sanders's permission. Following the assessment, Mr. Sanders discusses the lesion with a surgeon, who recommends excision. They discuss the possibility of skin cancer and the importance of early detection and treatment. Mr. Sanders is scheduled for a biopsy of the nevus under a local anesthetic the following morning. Following the biopsy, histologic examination reveals lentigo maligna melanoma. Staging of the tumor reveals that it is a melanoma in situ, with no metastasis to regional lymph nodes. Mr. Sanders undergoes a wide excision of the lesion the following afternoon.	■ Surgical wound related to excision of melanoma from the left lower leg ■ Potential for infection related to surgical wound on left lower leg ■ Acute pain related to wide excision of melanoma on left lower leg ■ Anxiety related to diagnosis of skin cancer	■ Patient will demonstrate complete healing of the incision without manifestations of infection. ■ Patient will verbalize relief of pain by the time the incision is healed. ■ Patient will verbalize fears and concerns about the diagnosis.

PLANNING AND IMPLEMENTATION

- Make the first dressing change, but ensure that Mr. Sanders can safely change the dressing himself prior to discharge the day after surgery.
- On discharge, provide adequate dressings and tape for the first home dressing change; include in discharge instructions necessary information about where to buy supplies and how many dressing supplies will be needed.
- Review and provide written instruction for prescribed systemic antibiotic and pain medication.
- Provide written instructions for dressing change, manifestations of infection, and phone number of clinic; stress importance of calling if any abnormal symptoms occur.
- Teach how to protect the incision from bumps and to protect the site from irritants.
- Discuss diagnosis, positive outlook for treatment of melanoma in situ, and the patient's concerns.
- Stress importance of lifelong regular healthcare evaluations to identify any recurrence or metastasis.

EVALUATION

Mr. Sanders returned to the dermatology clinic 1 week after his surgical incision. His incision is well approximated and shows no signs of infection. He is taking his antibiotic four times a day as prescribed and reports that his need for pain medications is decreasing. During his clinic visit the following week, Mr. Hall removes the sutures and assesses the wound as healed. Mr. Sanders completed his antibiotics and no longer requires pain medications. He says he is still "scared to death" about having cancer, but he has decided to join a local cancer support group. He also says he had gotten a list of skin safety rules from the American Cancer Society and will be sure to cover up and use sunscreen when he plays golf. Mr. Sanders makes an appointment for follow-up care in 3 months.

CLINICAL REASONING IN PATIENT CARE

1. Consider reasons why people who notice a change in a skin lesion put off seeking healthcare. What can nurses do to effect change?
2. Design a teaching plan for young adults for preventing skin cancers.
3. What would you say to Mr. Sanders if he called the clinic and said that the antibiotics were making him sick and he didn't think he needed them anyway?
4. Design a nursing care plan for Mr. Sanders for this feelings of powerlessness.

See Evaluating Your Response in Appendix B.

In addition to wound care, patients who have had a lymph node dissection need instructions in how to protect the extremity from bleeding, trauma, and infection. Address the following topics:

- Schedule regular medical checkups every 3 months for the first 2 years, every 6 months for the next 5 years, and yearly thereafter.
- Proper self-care combined with regular medical care can help the patient lead a fairly normal life.
- If assistance for home care is necessary, provide referrals to a community health agency or a home care agency. In addition, refer the patient to a local cancer support group if desired. Other resources are the ACS, the Skin Cancer Foundation, and the National Cancer Institute.

Postdiagnosis management is dependent on melanoma stage. For early-stage disease, excision with other treatment may suffice. In more severe stages, regular chemotherapy, immunotherapy or targeted therapy may be used to control the melanoma as long as possible. The nurse should work as part of the care team to develop a survivorship plan. This plan should include a suggested schedule of follow-up examinations and treatments, other tests to evaluate effects of melanoma treatment, a list of long-term side effects of treatment, and diet and activity suggestions.

Survival rates for melanoma range widely, from 97% 5-year survival for stage IA to 15% to 20% 5-year survival for stage IV (ACS, 2017d). For patients with a terminal diagnosis, care should focus on emotional support of the patient and family. Other important interventions are related to symptom management of pain, dyspnea, fatigue, and appetite changes. Of note, symptoms are dependent on the location of the tumor or metastasis. Comfort measures move to the forefront in treatment interventions.

16.6 Skin Trauma

Trauma to the skin can be unintentional or intentional (as in the case of surgery). Chemicals, radiation, pressure, or thermal changes cause skin trauma. This section discusses pressure injuries and frostbite, as well as intentional trauma from cutaneous and plastic surgery or treatment. Thermal injuries (burns) are discussed in Chapter 17.

The Patient with a Pressure Injury

Pressure injuries are ischemic lesions of the skin and underlying tissues caused by unrelieved pressure that impairs the flow of blood and lymph. The ischemia causes tissue necrosis and eventual ulceration. These injuries, also called *pressure ulcers*, *bed sores*, or *decubitus ulcers*, tend to develop over a bony prominence (such as the heels, greater trochanter, sacrum, and ischia), but they may appear on the skin of any part of the body subjected to external pressure, friction, or shearing forces.

Incidence and Risk Factors

The incidence of pressure injuries in hospitals is approximately 8%; the incidence in long-term care ranges from 2.4% to 23% (National Pressure Ulcer Advisory Panel, 2017). The increasing incidence of pressure injuries in all healthcare settings, but especially in hospitals and long-term care facilities, has resulted in infection, loss of function, and pain for patients. These complications, in turn, have caused increased lengths of stay and costs. As a result, the Centers for Medicare and Medicaid Services will no longer make additional reimbursement payments to hospitals to cover the cost of pressure injuries developed during a hospital stay.

The prevention and treatment of pressure injuries is a public health issue. An estimated 60,000 patients die each year from pressure injury complications, and the cost of treating these chronic wounds is about $11 billion a year. The national health policy statement *Healthy People 2020* (2017) set a target of a 10% improvement in the rate of pressure injury hospitalizations in older adults. Pressure injuries are preventable, with nursing care being a major part of prevention.

Although a pressure injury may develop in an adult of any age who has an impairment in mobility, those most at risk are older adults with limited mobility and fractured hips, people with quadriplegia, and patients in the critical care setting (Sorenson et al., 2019). Other patients prone to develop pressure injuries are those with fractures of large bones (e.g., hip or femur) or those who have undergone orthopedic surgery or sustained spinal cord injury. In addition to deficits in mobility and activity, incontinence and nutritional deficit also increase the risk of pressure injury development. Patients with chronic illnesses, such as renal failure and anemia, and those with edema or infection are also at increased risk.

Pathophysiology and Manifestations

Pressure injuries develop from external pressure that compresses blood vessels or from friction and shearing forces that tear and injure vessels. Both types of pressure cause traumatic injury and initiate the process of pressure injury development.

External pressure that is greater than capillary pressure and arteriolar pressure interrupts blood flow in capillary beds. When pressure is applied to skin over a bony prominence for 2 hours, tissue ischemia and hypoxia from external pressure cause irreversible tissue damage. For example, when the body is in the supine position, the body's weight applies pressure to the sacrum. The same amount of pressure causes more damage when it is applied to a small area than when it is distributed over a large surface.

Shearing forces result when one tissue layer slides over another. The stretching and bending of blood vessels cause injury and thrombosis. Patients in hospital beds are subject to shearing forces when the head of the bed is elevated and the torso slides down toward the foot of the bed. Pulling the patient up in bed also subjects the patient to shearing forces. (For this reason, always lift patients up in bed using a lift sheet.) In both cases, friction and moisture cause the skin and superficial fascia to remain fixed to the bed sheet, while the deep fascia and bony skeleton slides in the direction of body movement.

When a person lies or sits in one position for an extended length of time without moving, pressure on the tissue between a bony prominence and the external surface of the body distorts capillaries and interferes with normal blood flow. If the pressure is relieved, blood flow to the area increases, and a brief period of reactive hyperemia occurs without permanent damage. However, if the pressure continues, platelets aggregate in the endothelial cells surrounding the capillaries and form microthrombi. These microthrombi impede blood flow, resulting in ischemia and hypoxia of tissues. Eventually, the cells and tissues of the immediate area of pressure and of the surrounding area die and become necrotic.

Alterations in the involved tissue depend on the depth of the injury. Injury to superficial layers of skin results in blister formation, whereas injury to deeper structures causes the pressure injury area to appear dark reddish-blue. As the tissues die, the injury becomes an open wound that may be deep enough to expose the muscles and bone. The necrotic tissue elicits an inflammatory response, and the patient experiences increases in temperature, pain, and white blood cell count. Secondary bacterial invasion is common. Enzymes from bacteria and macrophages dissolve necrotic tissue, resulting in a foul-smelling drainage.

Pressure injuries are staged to classify the degree of tissue damage. The updated stages from the National Pressure Ulcer Advisory Panel (2016) are listed in **Box 16.3**.

Interprofessional Care

For the patient at risk for pressure injuries, the goal is prevention. Existing injuries require interprofessional treatment to promote healing and restore skin integrity.

Diagnosis

Diagnostic tests are conducted to determine the presence of a secondary infection and to differentiate the cause of the pressure injury. If the ulcer is deep or appears infected, drainage or biopsied tissue is cultured to determine the causative organism.

Medications

Topical and systemic antibiotics specific to the infectious organism eradicate any infection present (Adams et al., 2017). Additionally, a variety of products promote healing. Examples are listed in **Table 16.2**.

Treatments

Surgical debridement may be necessary if the pressure injury is deep, if subcutaneous tissues are involved, or if an eschar has formed over the ulcer, preventing healing by granulation. Large wounds may require skin grafting for complete closure.

Nursing Care

The patient with one or more pressure injuries not only has impaired skin integrity but also is at increased risk for infection, pain, and decreased mobility. Pressure injuries prolong treatment for other health problems, increase healthcare costs, and diminish the patient's quality of life. See the Moving Evidence into Action box below for information on evidence-based interventions.

Assessment

See the Risk Factors and Interprofessional Care sections for assessment of the patient with a pressure injury.

Priorities of Care

Collaborating with the interprofessional team to ensure adequate prevention for high-risk patients or treatment of the pressure injury while providing care that promotes healing and infection prevention is a priority. Teaching the patient and, as appropriate, caregivers strategies to prevent development or progression of pressure injuries should also be considered a priority nursing action. The nurse also focuses on promoting comfort and maintaining asepsis for all interruptions of the integument.

Diagnoses, Outcomes, and Interventions

The following interventions and rationales are adapted from the clinical guidelines developed and updated by the Agency for Health Care Research and Quality (2016) for identifying adults at risk and treating those with stage 1 pressure injuries.

Reduce the Risk for Impaired Skin Integrity.

Expected Outcome: Patient will experience wound healing through primary intention as indicated by progressive approximation of wound borders.

BOX 16.3
NPUAP's Updated Pressure Injury Staging

Stage 1

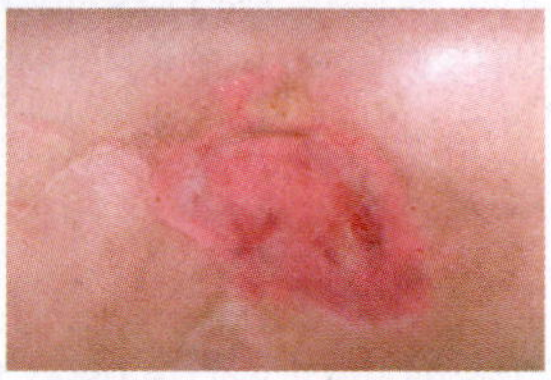

Nonblanchable redness of intact skin. Occurs in a localized area, usually over a bony prominence. The area may be painful, firm, soft, or warmer or cooler than adjacent tissue. May be difficult to detect in people with dark skin.

Stage 2

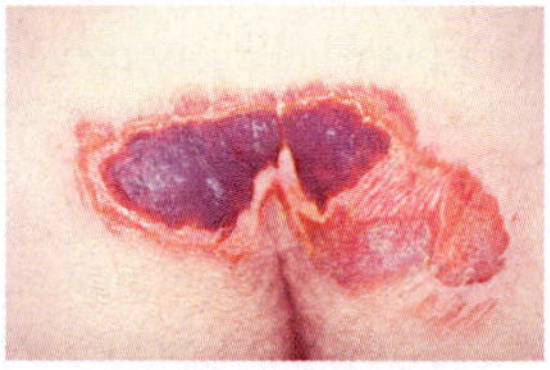

Partial-thickness skin loss with exposed dermis. This presents as a shallow open ulcer with a red or pink wound bed. May also present as an intact or open blister. The ulcer may be shiny or dry, without bruising or slough (loss of tissue).

Stage 3

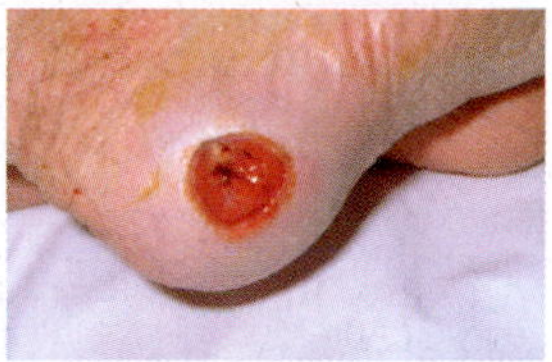

Full-thickness skin loss. Subcutaneous fat may be visible but bone, tendon, or muscle is *not* exposed. Slough may be present but does not obscure the depth of tissue loss. *May* include undermining and tunneling.

Stage 4

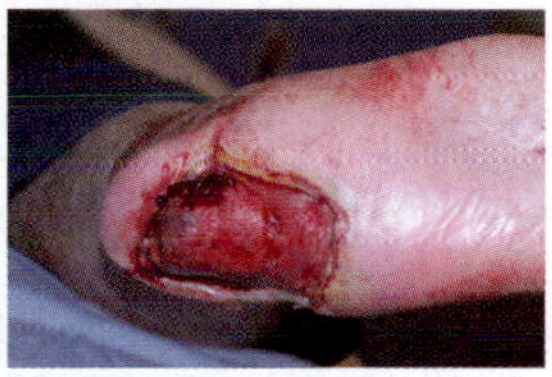

Full-thickness skin loss and tissue loss. The stage reveals exposed bone, tendon, or muscle. Slough or eschar (dead tissue such as a scab) may be present on some parts of the wound bed. Often includes undermining and tunneling.

Source: National Pressure Ulcer Advisory Panel, 2016.

Table 16.2 **Products Used to Treat Pressure Injuries**

Product	Purpose
Hydrocolloid dressing (such as DuoDERM)	May be used for stages 1, 2, 3, and 4 with minimal exudate. Forms a gel when it comes in contact with wound exudate. Forms an occlusive barrier over the ulcer while maintaining a moist environment and preventing infection. Helps prevent friction and shear.
Alginate dressing (such as SilvaSorb and Sorbsan)	May be used for stages 2, 3, and 4 with moderate to heavy drainage and in infected and noninfected wounds. Forms a gel when coming into contact with wound exudate. Should not be applied to dry or minimally draining wounds because dehydration and delay in healing may result.
Hydrofiber (such as Aquacel)	May be used for stages 2, 3, and 4 with moderate to heavy exudate. Can be used with actual or risk for infection. Combines the absorption of the hydrofiber with 1.2% silver as an antimicrobial agent.
Hydrogel dressing (such as IntraSite gel)	May be used for stages 2, 3, and 4. Rehydrates the wound bed and decreases pain. Promotes autolytic debridement.
Transparent adhesive dressing (such as OPSITE and Tegaderm)	May be used in shallow stage 1, 2, and 3 injuries. Provides a moist wound setting, prevents infection, and promotes reepithelialization. Minimizes friction and shear.
Wet-to-dry dressings	Provides mechanical debridement.
Vacuum-assisted closure (VAC) sponge	Stimulates wound contracture while removing the exudate and wound edema.

Moving Evidence into Action

Impact of Pressure Injury Prevention Strategies

Clinical Issue

Despite advances in healthcare, patients who are hospitalized continue to be at risk of developing pressure injuries. As part of international care standards, systematic risk assessment and use of pressure injury prevention strategies are recommended worldwide.

External Evidence

A systematic review of the literature was conducted to describe the evidence related to pressure injury prevention strategies for adult patients in intensive care units (ICUs) (Tayyib & Coyer, 2016). This systematic review included 25 studies. Meta-analysis revealed that a silicon foam dressing strategy was found to significantly reduce healthcare-associated pressure injuries (HAPUs) (effect size = 4.62; 95% CI: 0.05–0.29; $p < .00001$). While other interventions were also described (nutrition, skin-care regimen, positioning and repositioning schedule, support surfaces, and the role of education), the evidence was limited, so strong conclusions for these interventions could not be made.

Internal Evidence

As part of the evaluation of internal evidence, one must consider the clinical feasibility (including access to the proposed dressing for prophylactic use), the outcome of interest (reduction of pressure injury development), current policies/procedures in place for pressure injury prevention, and identification of stakeholders that influence uptake of the proposed intervention. One question to ask: Is this problem (increased risk for development of pressure injuries) significant in the population of your care environment? Does the clinical environment support the use of the intervention? What about the cost benefit of the new intervention? In this example of silicon dressings to reduce pressure injury development, Santamaria and colleagues (2015) reported average net cost for silicone dressing ($52.87) versus the care cost of controls ($107.91).

Patient Considerations

When considering use of a new intervention, the nurse must consider the specific patient population where it will be used. Will patients and their families be amenable to the new intervention?

Putting the Pieces Together

The design and implementation of a pressure injury prevention and treatment plan are essential for any person at risk. To effectively implement a plan, it is important to evaluate the external evidence and consider the internal implications and patient/family issues. With the implementation of a new prevention intervention, the outcome (occurrence of pressure injury development) should be assessed in every patient and unit-level information should be collected and evaluated on a regular basis.

References

Santamaria, N., Gerdtz, M., McCann, J., Freeman, A., Vassilou, T., DeVicentis, S., . . . Knott, J. (2015). A randomized controlled trial of the effectiveness of soft silicone multi-layered foam dressings in the prevention of sacral and heel pressure ulcers in trauma and critically ill patients: The border trial. *International Wound Journal, 12*(3), 302–308.

Tayyib, N., & Coyer, F. (2016). Effectiveness of pressure ulcer prevention strategies for adult patients in intensive care units; A systematic review. *Worldviews of Evidence Based Nursing, 13*(6), 432–444.

The nurse will:

- Identify at-risk individuals needing prevention and the specific factors placing them at risk.
- Assess bed- and chair-bound patients, as well as those who are unable to reposition themselves, for additional risk factors: immobility, incontinence, nutritional factors (such as inadequate dietary intake and impaired nutritional status), and altered level of consciousness.
- Assess patients on admission to acute care and rehabilitation hospitals, nursing homes, home care programs, and other healthcare facilities.
- Conduct a systematic risk assessment by using a validated risk assessment tool (such as the Braden scale; Braden & Bergstrom, 1988). See the information about predicting risk and using the Braden scale at the Nursing Center website.
- Document all assessments of risk. *Individuals at risk for pressure injuries must be identified so that risk factors can be reduced through intervention. The primary risk factors for pressure injuries are immobility and limited activity; therefore, assess patients who cannot reposition themselves or whose activity is limited to a bed or chair. Validated tools ensure systematic evaluation of individual risk factors. The patient requires periodic reassessment for pressure injuries. Accurate and complete documentation of all risk assessments ensures continuity of care and may be used as a foundation for the skin-care plan.*
- Conduct a systematic skin inspection at least once a day, paying particular attention to the bony prominences. Systematic, comprehensive, and routine skin care may decrease pressure ulcer incidence. Inspect the following to assess a pressure injury:
    - Location of any lesion or ulcer
    - Estimation of the stage
    - Dimensions of the ulcer: length, width, depth
    - Presence of any abnormal pathways in the wound
    - Sinus tract: a cavity or channel underneath the wound
    - Tunneling: a passageway or opening that may be visible at skin level, but with most of the tunnel under the surface of the skin
    - Undermining: areas of tissue destruction underneath intact skin along wound margins
    - Visible necrotic tissue (*Slough* is necrotic tissue that is in the process of separating from viable tissue.)
    - Presence of an exudate
    - Presence or absence of granulation tissue.

Skin inspection provides data the nurse uses in designing interventions to reduce risk and in evaluating outcomes of those interventions.

- Clean the skin at the time of soiling and at routine intervals, as frequently as the patient's need or preference dictates. Avoid hot water, use a mild cleansing agent, and clean the skin gently, applying as little force and friction as possible. *Metabolic wastes and environmental contaminants accumulate on the skin; these potentially irritating substances should be removed frequently. Feces and urine cause chemical irritation and should be removed as soon as possible. Hot water may cause skin injury. Mild cleansing agents are less likely to remove the skin's natural barrier.*
- Minimize environmental factors leading to skin drying, such as low humidity and exposure to cold. Treat dry skin with moisturizers. *Well-hydrated skin resists mechanical trauma. Hydration decreases as the ambient air temperature decreases, especially when the air humidity is low. Poorly hydrated skin is less pliable, and severe dryness is associated with fissuring and cracking of the stratum corneum. Moisturizers reduce dry skin.*
- Avoid massage over bony prominences. *Although massage has been practiced for years, evidence now suggests that massage over bony prominences may lead to deep tissue trauma in patients at risk for or with beginning skin manifestations of a pressure ulcer.*
- Minimize skin exposure to moisture due to incontinence, perspiration, or wound drainage. When these sources of moisture cannot be controlled, use breathable underpads or briefs made of materials that absorb moisture and present a quick-drying surface to the skin. Change underpads and briefs frequently. Do not place plastic directly against the skin. *Moisture from incontinence, perspiration, or wound drainage may contain factors that irritate the skin; moisture alone can increase the susceptibility of the skin to injury.*
- To minimize skin injury due to friction and shearing forces, use proper positioning, transferring, and turning techniques. Lubricants (such as cornstarch or creams), protective films (such as transparent dressings and skin sealants), protective dressings (such as hydrocolloids), and protective padding may also reduce friction injuries. *Shear injury occurs when skin remains stationary and the underlying tissue shifts. This shift diminishes the blood supply to the skin and results in ischemia and tissue damage. Proper positioning, however, can eliminate most shear injuries. Friction injuries to the skin occur when it moves across a coarse surface, such as bed linens. Most friction injuries can be avoided by using appropriate techniques to move patients so that their skin never drags across the linens. Any agent that eliminates contact or decreases the friction between the skin and the linens reduces the potential for injury.*
- Assess factors involved in inadequate dietary intake of protein or kilocalories. Offer nutritional supplements, and support the patient during mealtimes. If dietary intake remains inadequate, consult with a dietitian about other dietary interventions. *The role nutrition plays in the development of (and to a lesser degree, the healing of) pressure injuries is not understood, but poor dietary intake of kilocalories, protein, and iron has been associated with the development of pressure injuries.*
- Maintain the patient's current level of activity, mobility, and range of motion. *Frequent turning, repositioning, and movement are essential in reducing the risk of pressure injuries.*
- For the patient on bedrest or who is immobile, provide interventions against the adverse effects of the external mechanical forces of pressure, friction, and shear:
  a. Reposition all at-risk patients at least every 2 hours, using a written schedule for systematic turning and repositioning.
  b. For patients on bedrest, use positioning devices, such as pillows or foam wedges, to protect bony prominences.
- For completely immobile patients, use devices to totally relieve pressure on the heels (the most common method is to raise the heels off the bed). Do not use doughnut-type devices.
- Avoid placing patients in the side lying position directly on the trochanter.
- Maintain the head of the bed at the lowest degree of elevation consistent with the patient's medical condition and other restrictions. Limit the amount of time the head of the bed is elevated.
- Use assistive devices, such as a trapeze or bed linen, to move patients in bed who cannot assist during transfers and position changes.
- Place any at-risk patient on a pressure-reducing device, such as a foam, static air, alternating air, gel, or water mattress.

  Data indicate that the more spontaneous movements that bedridden, older adult patients make, the lower the incidence of pressure injuries and that fewer pressure injuries develop in at-risk patients who are turned every 2 to 3 hours. Proper positioning can reduce pressure on bony prominences. It is difficult to redistribute pressure under heels; suspending the heels is the best method. Doughnut cushions are more likely to cause than to prevent pressure injuries. Shearing forces are exerted on the body when the head of the bed is elevated. Lifting (rather than dragging) is less likely to cause injury from friction. Pressure-reducing devices and beds can decrease the incidence of pressure injuries.
- For chair-bound patients, use pressure-reducing devices. Consider postural alignment, distribution of weight, balance and stability, and pressure relief when positioning these patients. Avoid uninterrupted sitting in a chair or wheelchair. Reposition the patient every hour. Teach patients who can do so to shift their weight every 15 minutes. Use a written plan for positioning, movement, and the use of positioning devices. Do not use doughnut devices. *Prolonged, uninterrupted mechanical pressure results in tissue breakdown. The patient's weight should be shifted at least every hour.*

Delegating Nursing Care Activities

As appropriate and allowed by the designated duties and responsibilities of unlicensed assistive personnel, the nurse may delegate nursing care activities such as assisting the patient with position changes, fluid intake and output, collecting vital signs (including orthostatic vital signs), encouraging oral or enteral fluid intake, and nonpharmacologic skin care.

Transitions of Care

Prevention of pressure injuries is based on early identification of at-risk individuals and careful and thorough assessment upon admission using a validated risk assessment tool such as the Braden scale. These assessments drive use of interventions such as repositioning, careful and timely hygiene, and routine skin care.

Patient and family teaching for care of a pressure injury focuses on prevention and includes much of the same information presented in the preceding section. Because many patients with pressure injuries are older or have other serious illnesses, a caregiver may require teaching on such topics as:

- Definition and description of pressure injuries
- Common locations of pressure injuries
- Risk factors for the development of pressure injuries
- Skin care
- Ways to avoid injury
- Diet.

See **Box 16.4** for information about preventing pressure injuries in older adults.

When a patient has a pressure injury, careful assessment is important, including noting location, stage, dimensions, tract development, and presence of necrosis. Interventions focus on reducing pressure over the injury, repositioning, practicing pristine skin care, and dressing management as indicated. To minimize skin injury due to friction and shearing forces, use proper positioning, transferring, and turning techniques.

Chronic management of pressure injury continues with ongoing assessment, pressure reduction over the injury, dressing management, and careful infection control. Depending on the stage of the pressure injury, the nurse teaches the patient or caregiver how to care for injuries that are already present: how to change wet-to-dry dressings, apply skin barriers, and avoid injury and infection. Referrals to a home health agency or community health department can help the family through the lengthy healing process. Pain management may also be required.

Persons at end of life are especially vulnerable to pressure injuries. Even when pristine skin care and careful assessment and application of appropriate interventions have been provided, declines in nutritional intake, mobility, and cognition and development of incontinence may lead to the development of pressure injuries. While all pressure injuries should be managed, at end of life comfort is the overriding priority.

The Patient with Frostbite

Frostbite is an injury of the skin from freezing. If the exposure to freezing temperatures is limited, only the skin and subcutaneous tissues become involved. However, as exposure increases, deeper structures freeze. The skin freezes when the temperature drops to 21° to 24°C (14° to 24.8°F). Frostbite is most common on exposed or peripheral areas of the body, such as the nose, ears, feet, and hands (Sorenson et al., 2019).

As human tissues freeze, ice crystals form and increase intracellular sodium content. Small blood vessels initially vasoconstrict but then vasodilate and become more permeable, causing cellular and tissue swelling. With continued exposure, vasoconstriction and increased viscosity of the blood cause infarction and necrosis of the affected tissue.

Manifestations include:

- Superficial frostbite causes numbness, itching, and prickling.
- The skin appears cyanotic, reddened, or white.
- Deeper frostbite causes stiffness and paresthesia.
- As the skin and tissues thaw, the skin becomes white or yellow and loses its elasticity.
- The patient experiences burning pain. Edema, blisters, necrosis, and gangrene may appear.

BOX 16.4
Preventing Pressure Injuries in Older Adults

Older adults are at a greater risk than younger people for developing pressure injuries because of age-related changes in the integumentary system. Cell renewal slows, resulting in skin that has decreased elasticity. The margin between the epidermis and the dermis separates more easily, making the skin more prone to tearing. In addition, thinning subcutaneous tissue provides less cushioning over bony prominences. Water content decreases, and the skin becomes drier. These changes increase the older adult's susceptibility to skin trauma and prolong wound healing.

Chronic conditions associated with immobility and self-care deficit place older adults at risk of developing pressure injuries. For example, bowel or bladder incontinence can produce regions of wet skin that are prone to infections and breakdown. Furthermore, sensory-perceptual alterations and impaired cognitive functioning may reduce the frequency with which the older adult shifts position when sitting or lying in bed. Finally, undernutrition, which is often seen in older adults, heightens the risk for developing pressure injuries.

To prevent pressure injuries, the skin of older adults should be kept clean, dry, and well hydrated. Moisturizers are recommended to keep the skin free of excessive dryness. Older adults should be taught to avoid bumping into furniture and to wear long skirts or pants to help protect the lower extremities from trauma.

When hospitalized, older adults should have a validated risk assessment for pressure injuries completed on admission and as often as the tool suggests. A daily systematic skin inspection with particular attention to bony prominences should be completed.

Once pressure injuries develop in older adults, the treatment is the same as for younger patients. However, additional steps may need to be taken. Because local perfusion to tissues is compromised, steps should be taken to prevent under- or overhydration. It is essential for optimal nutritional status to be maintained. Also, keep in mind that it may take a longer time for the pressure ulcer to heal.

Rapid thawing may significantly decrease tissue necrosis. General guidelines for rewarming areas of frostbite are:

- If you are outdoors, treat superficial frostbite by applying firm pressure with a warm hand or by placing frostbitten hands in the axillae. If the feet are frostbitten, remove wet footwear, dry the feet, and put on dry footwear. Do not rub the areas with snow.
- In the hospital, rapidly rewarm affected areas in circulating warm water, 40° to 40.5°C (104° to 105°F), for 20 to 30 minutes. Do not rub or massage the areas.

Following rewarming, the patient is kept on bedrest with the affected parts elevated. Pain medications and anti-inflammatory agents are administered. Blisters are debrided. Whirlpool therapy may be used to clean the skin and debride necrotic tissue. Recovery from frostbite is usually complete if the involved area has not become necrotic. Necrotic tissue may require amputation.

The Patient Undergoing Cutaneous or Plastic Surgery

Although many skin disorders are so small and benign that no treatment is necessary, others require some type of surgery of the skin to remove the lesion. Other surgeries and treatments for skin lesions and deformities are used to restore function and change appearance. This section discusses both cutaneous and plastic surgery, as well as other types of treatment modalities used in the care of the patient with a skin disorder.

Interprofessional Care

Management of the patient undergoing plastic surgery is a team effort. As with all surgical patients, postoperative care focuses on pain management, prevention of infection, and reduction of other postoperative complications of anesthesia and immobility. These procedures can be provided in a multitude of settings such as acute care hospitals, outpatient surgical centers, or private surgical centers (American Society of Plastic Surgeons, 2016). Less invasive procedures may be carried out in office settings.

Cutaneous Surgery and Procedures

The basic types of cutaneous surgery described here are excision, electrosurgery, cryosurgery, curettage, and laser surgery. Two nonsurgical procedures, chemical destruction and sclerotherapy, are also discussed. Most of these procedures are performed in the office or outpatient clinic.

Fusiform Excision. *Fusiform excision* is the removal of a full thickness of the epidermis and dermis, usually with a thin layer of subcutaneous tissue. It is used to remove tissue for biopsies and for complete removal of benign and malignant lesions of the skin. Excision of small, superficial lesions is performed under a local anesthetic, and care is taken to place the incision in a way that will provide good cosmetic results.

Electrosurgery. *Electrosurgery* involves the destruction or removal of tissue with high-frequency alternating current. A variety of surgical procedures may be performed, including *electrodesiccation* (which produces superficial skin destruction), *electrocoagulation* (which produces deeper tissue destruction), and *electrosection* (which can cut through skin and tissue). Electrodesiccation is used to remove benign surface lesions, such as skin tags, keratoses, warts, and angiomas. It is also used to produce hemostasis for capillary bleeding. Electrocoagulation is used to remove telangiectases, warts, and superficial nonmelanoma skin cancers. Electrosection is used to make incisions, excise tissue, and perform biopsies.

Cryosurgery. *Cryosurgery* is the destruction of tissue by cold or freezing with agents such as fluorocarbon sprays, carbon dioxide snow, nitrous oxide, and liquid nitrogen. Cryosurgery is used to treat many skin lesions. The freezing agents are applied topically to the lesion. The effects depend on the degree of freeze. Light freezing causes damage to the epidermis with blistering or crusting that heals without scarring. Deeper freezes, used to treat malignant cells, cause edema, necrosis, and tissue slough. The effects of cryosurgery may not be obvious until 24 hours following the treatment. Postoperatively, infection is prevented by applying a topical antibiotic and keeping the treated areas clean. Healing occurs in 2 to 3 weeks.

Curettage. *Curettage* is the removal of lesions with a curette (a semi-sharp cutting instrument). It is used to remove benign and malignant superficial epidermal lesions. Benign lesions removed include keratoses, nevi, and angiomas. Nonmelanoma skin lesions are removed by curettage if they are small, well-defined, primary tumors. Curettage is also used to remove specimens of tissue for biopsy.

Following curettage, the wound may be treated with electrodesiccation to destroy any remaining malignant cells and to provide hemostasis. These wounds are not closed; rather, they are left open to heal by second intention. Topical antibiotic ointments and dressings may be used in the postoperative period.

Laser Surgery. *Laser surgery* is used to treat a variety of skin disorders. A *laser* is an intense light that produces a thermal injury on contact with tissue. The injury causes coagulation, vaporization, excision, and ablation (removal of a growth). Argon, pulsed dye, carbon dioxide, and Nd:YAG lasers are used in cutaneous and plastic surgery. A local anesthetic may be used, although a pulsed dye laser causes minimal pain and anesthesia is rarely required.

Chemical Destruction. *Chemical destruction* is the application of a specific chemical to produce destruction of skin lesions. Chemical destruction is used to treat both benign and premalignant lesions. The chemical is applied to the lesion or is used to cause peeling. After application, the treated area forms a thin crust that sloughs off in about a week.

Sclerotherapy. *Sclerotherapy* is the removal of benign skin lesions with a sclerosing agent that causes inflammation with fibrosis of tissue. Agents that cause therapeutic sclerosis include aethoxysklerol (Sclerodex) and hypertonic sodium chloride. This type of treatment is used for telangiectases and superficial spider veins of the lower extremities. The solution is injected into the affected veins, causing a reaction that closes the lumen of the vein.

Plastic Surgery

Plastic surgery is the alteration, replacement, or restoration of visible portions of the body, performed to correct a structural or cosmetic defect. The word *plastic* comes from the Greek word *plastikos*, which means "able to be molded."

Many skin disorders discussed in this chapter cause changes in appearance. For example, acne may leave deep pitting scars, nevi and keloids are often disfiguring, and skin cancers may require wide excision and skin grafting. These scars, lesions, and wounds often cause embarrassment and alterations in body image. In addition, the removal of lesions may leave unsightly scars or areas of obviously missing tissue.

Cosmetic surgery involves procedures to enhance the attractiveness of normal features. There were 17.1 million surgical cosmetic procedures performed in 2016, of which about 15.5 million were minimally invasive procedures (American Society of Plastic Surgeons, 2016). The most frequently performed procedures were Botox injections, liposuction, breast augmentation, and laser hair removal. Reconstructive surgery uses similar techniques; however, its purpose is to improve the function or appearance of parts of the body damaged by trauma, disease, or birth defects.

Many of the plastic surgeries permanently alter body image. To provide the patient with a preview of what surgery will accomplish, some surgeons integrate computer imaging into preoperative teaching. The computer projects a photograph of the targeted area onto a monitor and uses graphics to demonstrate how the size and/or shape of the body part or area will change as a result of the surgery.

Skin Grafts and Flaps. Skin grafts and flaps are used to restore function and an acceptable appearance. Both of these procedures involve the movement of skin from one part of the body to another part.

A **skin graft** is a surgical method of detaching skin from a donor site and placing it in a recipient site, where it develops a new blood supply from the base of the wound. Skin grafting is an effective way to cover wounds that have a good blood supply, that are not infected, and in which bleeding can be controlled.

Skin grafts may be either split thickness or full thickness. A split-thickness graft contains epidermis and only a portion of dermis of the donor site. A common donor site for a skin graft is the anterior thigh. Skin is removed in sheets from the donor site with a dermatome. A full-thickness graft contains both epidermis and dermis. These layers contain the greatest number of skin elements (sweat glands, sebaceous glands, or hair follicles) and are best able to withstand trauma. Areas of thin skin are the best donor sites for full-thickness skin grafts. The donor site must be surgically closed and will scar.

A *skin flap* is a piece of tissue whose free end is moved from a donor site to a recipient site while maintaining a continuous blood supply through its connection at the base or pedicle. Flaps carry their own blood supply and are therefore used to cover recipient sites that have a poor blood supply or have sustained a major tissue loss. They are often used for reconstruction or closure of large wounds. Microsurgical techniques, with anastomosis of small blood vessels and nerves, allow reconstruction with free flaps (in which the flap is completely removed from its donor site and moved to the recipient site).

Chemical Peeling. *Chemical peeling* is the application of a chemical to produce a controlled and predictable injury that alters the anatomy of the epidermis and superficial dermis. The result is skin that appears firmer, smoother, and less wrinkled. This form of cosmetic surgery is more useful in people who have fair, thin skin with fine wrinkling. Chemical agents used for peeling include phenol, trichloroacetic acid (TCA), and alpha-hydroxy acids (AHA).

Liposuction. *Liposuction* is a method of changing the contours of the body by aspirating fat from the subcutaneous layer of tissue. This treatment is used to remove excess fat from the buttocks, flanks, abdomen, thighs, upper arms, knees, ankles, and chin. It is not a cure for obesity and should not be used as a substitute for weight loss. The procedure is usually done for younger patients because their skin is more elastic. Liposuction may be performed on either an outpatient or inpatient basis.

To aspirate the fat, a small incision is made close to the area, and a suction cannula or curette is inserted and attached to a suction apparatus. The high vacuum pressure caused by the suction machine causes fat cells to emulsify, and they are aspirated out of the body. Following removal of the fat, a pressure dressing is applied to help the skin conform to the new tissue size.

Dermabrasion. *Dermabrasion* is a method of removing facial scars, severe acne, and pigment from unwanted tattoos. The area is sprayed with a chemical to cause light freezing and is then abraded with sandpaper or a revolving wire brush to remove the epidermis and a portion of the dermis.

Facial Cosmetic Surgery. Many different reconstructive surgeries may be performed to correct deformities or improve cosmetic appearance. Those discussed here are rhinoplasty, blepharoplasty, and rhytidectomy (facelift):

- *Rhinoplasty* is conducted to improve the appearance of the external nose. The nasal skeleton is reshaped, and the overlying skin and subcutaneous tissue are allowed to redrape over the new framework. A submucous resection of the nasal septum is often done at the same time; this surgery resects a segment of the septal cartilage to improve the nasal airway and also to alter the appearance of the nose. This surgery is done through incisions within the nose, so no visible scars remain after healing.
- *Blepharoplasty* is a cosmetic surgery in which loose skin and protruding periorbital fat are removed from the upper and lower eyelids. With aging, the eyelid skin sags, allowing the periorbital fat to bulge; the skin of the upper eyelid can be so lax that it partially obstructs vision. The procedure is performed under local anesthesia, and excess skin and fat are excised. The incision is made in the normal eyelid lines so that scars are not visible after healing.

- *Rhytidectomy*, or facelift, is a cosmetic surgery done to improve appearance by removing excess skin (and sometimes fat) from the face and neck. As one ages, the skin of the face and neck tends to become loose and wrinkled. The procedure is usually performed with local anesthesia. To perform the surgery, bilateral incisions are made from the scalp at the temple, in front of the ear in the natural skin line, around the earlobe, and to the occipital scalp. The skin is then elevated, fat is removed or suctioned, and excess skin is excised. The incision lines are sutured, and a pressure dressing is applied.

Nursing Care

Nursing care for the patient having cutaneous or plastic surgery is highly individualized. It depends on the type of surgery or procedure performed, the type of deficit treated, the reason for the surgery or procedure, the expected results of the treatment, and the response of the patient to the lesion or surgery. Although some surgeries, such as skin grafts and flaps, require in-hospital care, many of the surgeries are carried out in a primary care setting, and the patient provides self-care at home following or between treatments.

Assessment

Assessment is based on the extent of surgery and procedure performed.

Priorities of Care

Collaborating with the interprofessional team to ensure adequate treatment of the viral skin infection while providing care that promotes recovery and comfort is a nursing priority. Teaching the patient and, as appropriate, caregivers strategies to prevent infection, optimize comfort, and promote safe home and work environments should also be considered a priority nursing action. The nurse also focuses on promoting comfort and maintaining asepsis for all interruptions of the integument.

Diagnoses, Outcomes, and Interventions

For the patient having cutaneous or plastic surgery or procedures, common nursing considerations include addressing impaired skin integrity, management of acute pain, and supportive care to address disturbances in body image.

Address Impaired Skin Integrity. The patient having surgery of the skin has impaired skin integrity. Skin grafts and flaps are performed to repair large wounds, and it is necessary to inflict further wounds to collect the graft or flap from a donor site. Excisions and various cosmetic surgeries cause wounds. Skin is traumatized by freezing, chemicals, abrasion, sclerosing agents, electrical currents, and lasers. Although all of these treatment modalities are conducted to remove lesions, improve function, or improve appearance, they first impair the integrity of the skin. These impairments increase the risk for infection, which would further impair the skin integrity and may negate the benefits of surgery.

Expected Outcome: Patient will experience skin graft and flap healing as indicated by progressive approximation of wound borders.

Nurses provide preoperative care and teaching, intraoperative assistance, and postoperative care and teaching; in each case, care and teaching are specific to the type of surgical treatment and the individual patient. In all cases, the nurse provides appropriate preoperative interventions to prepare the patient physically and emotionally for surgery and the postoperative period. The following interventions are appropriate for the patient having inpatient skin grafts or flaps:

- Monitor incisions and graft, and flap donor and recipient sites, for manifestations of infection and necrosis:
  a. Take and record vital signs every 4 hours.
  b. Monitor all wounds for changes in color, consistency, amount, and odor of drainage every 4 to 8 hours.
  c. Monitor wounds for increased swelling, redness, and pain every 4 to 8 hours.
  d. Monitor and document assessment of graft every 4 hours.
  e. Monitor and document temperature, turgor, color, dermal bleeding, and capillary refill of flaps every 4 hours.

  When bacterial infection is present, the inflammatory phase of wound healing is prolonged, retarding healing. Increased body temperature and tachycardia are manifestations of infection. The drainage in wounds that become infected is often increased in amount, purulent, thicker, and has a musty or foul odor. Tissue response to infection includes edema, increased erythema, and pain. Grafts and flaps that do not have adequate blood supply will appear black instead of the normal pink-red color.
- Provide care for the donor site:
  a. Position the patient to minimize pressure on the donor site.
  b. Use a bed cradle to keep linens off the area.
  c. If the donor site is left open and a heat lamp is to be applied to the area, place the lamp no closer than 2 feet from the wound.
  d. Avoid moving the body part containing the donor site, if possible.
  e. If the donor site is on the posterior portion of the body, place the patient on a special bed (such as a low-pressure or fluidized bed) to decrease pressure and allow air circulation around the donor site.

  Minimizing trauma from pressure and movement facilitates healing of the donor site. Leaving the site open to the air and providing heat increase healing. Special beds minimize ischemia and allow donor sites on the posterior side of the body to dry.
- Encourage a diet high in protein, ascorbic acid, vitamins, and minerals. *An adequate protein intake is necessary to supply amino acids for tissue repair. Vitamin C is necessary for collagen formation and wound strength. Vitamins and minerals contribute to the healing process.*

- Change dressings as prescribed, or if the frequency is not indicated, as necessary. Determine which dressings are not to be removed during the healing process and which are to be changed and whether the wound is to be kept dry or moist. Use aseptic technique and follow standard precautions when changing dressings. Remove old dressings carefully and gently. *Donor sites may be covered with an adherent gauze dressing that is allowed to dry and remains adherent through the healing process. Aseptic techniques prevent secondary bacterial infections. Standard precautions protect the nurse from HIV infection. Unless care is taken, the removal of adherent old dressings may damage the wound by traumatizing granulation tissue or wound edges. The use of semipermeable transparent dressings provides an environment that optimizes wound healing by promoting collagen synthesis and the formation of granulation tissue; it also increases cell migration and epithelial resurfacing and prevents the formation of scabs, crusts, and eschar.*

Manage Acute Pain. The patient having a graft or flap has two wounds; in fact, the donor site may be more painful than the recipient site. Cutaneous surgeries, dermabrasions, and chemical treatments result in blistering, swelling, and loss of epidermal tissue. The patient having facial reconstructive surgery has edema, with resultant pain.

Expected Outcome: Patient will experience adequate pain relief and management as indicated by subjective report.

The nurse will:

- Administer pain medications on a regular basis, following guidelines for controlling pain in patients having operative procedures (refer to Chapter 9). *Established, severe pain is difficult to control and has negative physical and psychologic consequences.*
- Use alternative pain relief measures as appropriate and prescribed, such as ice bags or cold compresses. *Cold reduces swelling, acts as a local anesthetic, and decreases pain.*
- Teach noninvasive methods of pain relief, such as deep breathing, relaxation, and guided imagery. *Noninvasive methods of pain relief increase the effectiveness of pain medications and also allow the patient some control and self-management of pain.*

Promote a Healthy Body Image. Cosmetic surgery is performed for a variety of reasons in adult patients of all ages. Changes in appearance, especially in a society that values youth and beauty, affect one's self-perception. Lesions or scars, especially of the face, may decrease self-esteem and cause a person to avoid social interactions and relationships. With aging, the skin becomes looser and wrinkles appear; this can be a source of anxiety and despair, especially to the woman who has always prided herself on her youthful appearance. Most patients cite one reason for having plastic surgery: to "feel better about myself."

Expected Outcome: Patient's acceptance of body appearance as evidenced by adjustment to changes in physical appearance.

The nurse will:

- Provide preoperative teaching: Explain that bruising and swelling will be present and that it will be several weeks before these responses to surgery disappear. Explain that it may take a year for healing to be completed and the final results to appear. *Expectations differ; many people expect immediate results. Knowledge of postoperative responses is necessary for the patient to adapt to change. The patient may need to make arrangements to take time off from work during the initial healing stage.*
- Provide time for the patient to verbalize feelings and concerns. Be empathetic, and listen nonjudgmentally. *Such nurse–patient interaction facilitates acceptance of changes in body image.*
- Refer to a consultant who can provide information on the use of cosmetics and apparel to enhance personal appearance. *Knowledgeable use of cosmetics and clothing can make scars much less noticeable. If the patient feels better about appearance, body image is improved.*

Delegating Nursing Care Activities

Collaborating with the interprofessional team including unlicensed assistive personnel to promote postoperative progression while providing care that promotes recovery and comfort is a nursing priority. Teaching the patient and, as appropriate, caregivers strategies to prevent infection, optimize comfort, and promote safe behaviors to prevent postoperative infections or other complications should also be considered a priority nursing action. The nurse focuses on promoting comfort and maintaining asepsis for all interruptions of the integument.

Transitions of Care

In planned surgical procedures, there is no prevention of the surgery itself. Instead, prevention should focus on patient teaching of good skin and hand hygiene and early identification of signs and symptoms of infection.

The acute nursing care following surgical intervention focuses on pain control and prevention of postoperative complications. Pristine postoperative techniques for dressing changes, vascular access management, and management of drains or tubes are used to reduce postoperative infection. Early mobility while use of wound splinting reduces postoperative complications related to immobility.

As the patient moves beyond the acute postoperative phase, care focuses on continued wound or incision assessment and management, promotion of return to preoperative mobility/activity, and reduced need for pain management. The nurse teaches the patient and family to provide self-care at home after cutaneous and plastic surgery and procedures. The nurse asks about the patient's expectations and stresses that final results will not be seen for several months, providing written instructions about wound care and manifestations of infection. At this stage, patients express interest in developing new skills related to enhancing personal appearance.

16.7 Hair and Nail Disorders

Disorders of the hair and nails are not serious threats to health, but they may cause embarrassment and a negative body image. Changes in hair growth and pattern as well as in nail growth and character occur as secondary responses to other illnesses or treatments and are also a part of the aging process.

The Patient with a Disorder of the Hair

Gender and ethnic characteristics influence the amount and type of hair each individual has. Caucasians typically have more facial and body hair than do Asians. People of Mongolian or Native American descent usually have straight hair, those of African descent usually have wavy to curly hair, and Caucasians have straight or curly hair. In addition, male hair growth characteristics (such as facial hair and hair on the lower extremities) are normal in women in some families.

Pathophysiology and Manifestations

Hair color, growth, and pattern vary from person to person, and they are determined largely by genetic inheritance. Changes such as hair loss in men or excess facial hair in women may seem minor, but they may create psychosocial problems for the person experiencing the changes.

Hirsutism

Hirsutism (hypertrichosis) is the appearance of excessive hair in women. Hirsutism most often occurs in a male distribution (i.e., on the upper lip, chin, abdomen, and chest) in women. The excess hair is primarily the result of an increase in androgen levels (especially testosterone) that may be due to familial predisposition (considered normal); polycystic ovary syndrome; ovarian, adrenal, or pituitary tumors; Cushing syndrome (an adrenal disorder); some central nervous system disorders; and medications, such as minoxidil, cyclosporine, phenytoin, certain progestins, and anabolic steroids (Adams et al., 2017).

The manifestations of hirsutism include increased male pattern hair growth, acne, and menstrual irregularities. If the androgen excess is great, defeminization (a decrease in breast size and loss of normal adipose tissue) and virilization (frontal balding, increased muscle mass, deepening of the voice, and enlargement of the clitoris) may occur.

Alopecia

Alopecia is loss of hair, or baldness. Alopecia may result from scarring, various systemic diseases, or genetic predisposition. Scarring from trauma, radiation, and severe bacterial, fungal, or viral infections causes permanent and irreversible hair loss over the scarred area. Systemic diseases that may cause alopecia include systemic lupus erythematosus, thyroid disorders, and pituitary insufficiency. The hair loss from these disorders may be reversible. Hair loss from androgenic causes may also occur in the postmenopausal woman. Alopecia may be drug induced and is a side effect of a variety of medications (Adams et al., 2017). Check the patient's medication list for those that may cause alopecia.

Examples of types of alopecia are:

- *Male pattern baldness* is the most common cause of alopecia in men and is genetically predetermined. The hair loss begins at the temples, with recession of the hairline and baldness of the crown.
- *Female pattern alopecia* begins in women in their 20s and 30s, with progressive thinning and loss of hair over the central part of the scalp. Unlike men, women do not lose hair from the frontal hairline. Many of these women have elevated adrenal androgens.
- *Alopecia areata* is characterized by round or oval bald patches on the scalp as well as on other hairy parts of the body. The cause is unknown. This type of alopecia is usually self-limiting and reverses without treatment, although it often recurs.

Interprofessional Care

The patient with hirsutism is examined for hormone levels and indications of other systemic illnesses. Hirsutism is treated by addressing the underlying systemic disorder and stopping medications that may be causing the problem. Hirsutism is also treated using laser therapy, which reduces unwanted hair. Alopecia is diagnosed by assessing the appearance of the hair and hair loss and by assessing the patient for other systemic diseases and the use of medications that may cause hair loss. Various treatments are used to restore hair.

Diagnosis

Diagnostic tests that may be ordered for the woman with hirsutism include serum testosterone levels and an adrenal CT scan. Testosterone levels are measured and levels greater than 200 ng/dL indicate the need for further tests, such as a pelvic examination and tests of ovarian function (Kee, 2018). Adrenal tumors, a possible cause of hirsutism, are identified with an adrenal CT scan.

Medications

Hirsutism is treated with medications specific to the underlying cause (Adams et al., 2017). Oral contraceptives containing estrogen decrease ovarian androgen production and decrease free testosterone levels. Dexamethasone (Decadron) may be prescribed for people with high cortisol levels. Ketoconazole (Nizoral) inhibits androgen production. Antiandrogenic medications cause congenital abnormalities in male infants and are therefore given only to nonpregnant women, who are cautioned to avoid pregnancy while taking the medications.

Male pattern baldness has been successfully treated with topical minoxidil (Loniten) or Rogaine Extra Strength, a commercial product that contains minoxidil. These drugs, which are vasodilators, stimulate vertex hair growth, probably by stimulating the epithelium of the hair follicle.

Surgery

Hair transplant techniques are used to restore hair or reduce the size of areas of alopecia. Transplanting hairs as small hair plugs or single hairs taken from the back or sides of the scalp is an effective means of replacing hair to areas of alopecia. This procedure is done in an outpatient office or clinic. Other types of surgical procedures include scalp reduction and flaps.

Nursing Care

The patient with either hirsutism or alopecia is often self-conscious about appearance and tries a variety of OTC treatments before seeking medical care. Nursing care for the patient with hair disorders focuses on teaching the patient self-care and providing support during long-term care. Women with hirsutism are taught to use various means of removing unwanted hair, such as shaving, applying depilatories, waxing, or undergoing electrolysis. Women with mild hirsutism may bleach facial hair to make it less obvious. Patients with alopecia may wear hairpieces or wigs.

The Patient with a Disorder of the Nails

Nail disorders may be congenital or genetic, or they may be due to systemic diseases, trauma, allergies, or irritants. Nails may be discolored, multicolored, malformed, infected, or separated from underlying tissue.

Pathophysiology and Manifestations

The nail disorders discussed here are separation of the nail, infection, and ingrown toenails:

- ***Onycholysis*** is the separation of the distal nail plate from the nail bed. It occurs most often in the fingernails. This disorder may result from many different factors, including excessive or prolonged exposure to water, soaps, detergent, alkalies, and industrial keratolytic agents; *Candida* infections; nail hardeners; and thyroid disorders. Prolonged application of false fingernails may also cause this disorder.
- **Paronychia** is an infection of the cuticle of the fingernails or toenails. The disorder often follows a minor trauma and secondary infection with staphylococci, streptococci, or *Candida*. The acute form begins with a painful inflammation that may progress to an abscess. The chronic form is seen most often in people who have frequent exposure to water. In the chronic form, the skin around the nail is painful, edematous, and infected. The nail plate may become ridged and discolored.
- ***Onychomycosis*** is a fungal or dermatophyte infection of the nail plate. The nail plate elevates and becomes yellow or white. Psoriasis infections of the nail plate cause the nails to pit.
- ***Unguis incarnates*** (an ingrown toenail) results when the edge of the nail plate grows into the soft tissue of the toe. Pain and infection may occur. The infection, if untreated, may spread to the bone. This disorder is especially dangerous for the person with diabetes mellitus or peripheral vascular disease.

Interprofessional Care

The treatment of disorders of the nail varies from pharmacologic treatment to surgical removal. Infections of the nails are treated with antifungal or antibiotic medications. If the causative agent is a fungus or chronic dermatologic disorder, treatment is difficult and may not be effective. Persistently painful and/or infected nails are in some cases surgically removed.

Nursing Care

Nursing care of the patient with a disorder of the nail focuses on teaching self-care. Patients with nail disorders that are caused by frequent exposure to water are taught to protect the hands or feet by wearing rubber gloves or boots and to keep the nails as clean and dry as possible. Patients with ingrown toenails are cautioned not to cut into the lateral nail bed, but rather to soak the nail twice a day and insert a piece of cotton or gauze under the softened nail until the nail has grown out enough to trim.

CHAPTER HIGHLIGHTS

16.1 Common Skin Problems and Lesions

Describe the pathophysiology and manifestations of common skin problems and lesions, and outline the interprofessional care and nursing care of patients with these disorders.

- Pruritus (itching) accompanies dry skin (xerosis) and many skin disorders and may result in excoriation and infection as a result of scratching.
- Cysts, keloids, nevi, angiomas, skin tags, and keratoses are benign skin lesions. However, nevi should be monitored for changes indicating transformation into malignant lesions.
- Psoriasis is a chronic immune skin disorder arising from keratinocytes. A variety of medications and treatments are used, with ultraviolet light therapy being most effective for generalized lesions.

16.2 Infections and Infestations of the Skin

Describe the pathophysiology and manifestations of infections and infestations of the skin, and outline the interprofessional care and nursing care of patients with these disorders.

- Skin disorders may be caused by a variety of bacteria, fungi, parasites, and viruses. The disorders are treated with organism-specific antibiotics, fungicides, antiviral agents, or agents that kill the parasites.
- Methicillin-resistant *Staphylococcus aureus* (MRSA) infection is divided into two types: healthcare-associated infections (acquired in hospitals and other healthcare settings) and community-associated infections (acquired in the community in otherwise healthy people). MRSA causes significant impacts on care management, resource use, and costs.
- Herpes zoster, believed to follow a childhood infection with chickenpox, causes acute pain.

16.3 Inflammatory Disorders of the Skin

Describe the pathophysiology and manifestations of inflammatory disorders of the skin, and outline the interprofessional care and nursing care of patients with these disorders.

- Inflammatory disorders of the skin range from mild to potentially lethal.
- Acne, a disorder of the hair and sebaceous glands opening to the skin surface, is characterized by comedones, pustules, and cysts.
- Other inflammatory disorders include pemphigus vulgaris (chronic disorder of the skin and oral mucous membranes characterized by blister formation) and lichen planus (persistent thick, dark red lesions). Care focuses on reducing severity of the illness, symptom management, and prevention of infection.

16.4 Acute Skin Disorders

Describe the risk factors for and pathophysiology and manifestations of acute skin disorders, and outline the interprofessional care and nursing care of patients with these disorders.

- Stevens-Johnson syndrome, a rare and serious condition of the skin and mucus membranes, results as an immune response to medication or infection. The process is characterized by epidermal necrosis with minimal associated inflammation.
- Care focuses on skin care, reduction of discomfort, avoidance of fluid and electrolyte loss, and prevention of infection. For severe cases, nursing care is similar to care of the burn patient.

16.5 Malignant Skin Disorders

Describe the risk factors for and pathophysiology and manifestations of malignant skin disorders, and outline the interprofessional care and nursing care of patients with these disorders.

- Malignant skin disorders include actinic keratosis, non-melanoma skin cancer (basal cell cancer and squamous cell cancer), and malignant melanoma skin cancer. Skin cancer is the most common malignancy found in fair-skinned Americans.
- Avoiding sunburn, using sunscreen, and maintaining monthly skin self-examinations are critical in preventing loss of tissue or metastasis and death.

16.6 Skin Trauma

Describe the pathophysiology and manifestations of skin trauma, and outline the interprofessional care and nursing care of patients with these disorders.

- Skin trauma may be intentional (as in the case of cutaneous and plastic surgery) or unintentional (as from trauma, frostbite, and pressure injuries).
- Older adults with limited mobility, as well as patients who are unable to move or who are in critical care units, are at greater risk for pressure injuries. Prevention of pressure injuries is the goal of both interprofessional and nursing care.

16.7 Hair and Nail Disorders

Describe the pathophysiology and manifestations of disorders of the hair and nails, and outline the interprofessional care and nursing care of patients with these disorders.

- Disorders of the hair include hirsutism (excess hair in women) and alopecia (loss of hair).
- Nails may be discolored, multicolored, malformed, infected, or separated from underlying tissue.

TEST YOURSELF NCLEX-RN® REVIEW

1. An older patient has severe xerosis. What topic should the nurse include in a teaching plan for this patient? (Select all that apply.)
   A. Take a hot bath every day.
   B. Maintain a warm environment.
   C. Apply skin lotions after a bath.
   D. Use fabric softeners when laundering clothing.
   E. Add bath oils at the end of the bath.
2. The nurse is concerned that a patient's skin lesion with an irregular border could become malignant. Which lesion did the nurse assess in the patient?
   A. Nevi
   B. Keloid
   C. Skin tag
   D. Angioma
3. The nurse is teaching a patient with generalized psoriasis about ultraviolet light therapy (UVB). What should be included in this teaching? (Select all that apply.)
   A. "When combined with hot baths, UVB is very effective."
   B. "Treatments with UVB have to be given in the hospital to be safe."
   C. "UVB slows the growth of epidermal cells and decreases keratosis."
   D. "The exact effect of UVB is unknown, but it decreases severe itching."
   E. "You will wear eye shields during the treatment."
4. The nurse is preparing a teaching session for a group of community members on the dangers of skin cancer. Which skin lesion should the nurse emphasize as increasing the risk of developing skin cancer?
   A. Folliculitis
   B. Pressure ulcer
   C. Lice infestation
   D. Actinic keratosis
5. A patient is experiencing a rash of painful vesicles over the left thorax. What question should the nurse include when completing this patient's health history?
   A. "Have you ever been diagnosed with acne?"
   B. "Are you a regular patron of tanning salons?"
   C. "Do you remember being sunburned as a child?"
   D. "Did you have chickenpox when you were young?"
6. A patient is devastated after being diagnosed with body lice. What should the nurse remember about body lice to reassure this patient?
   A. "Lice are a form of fungus."
   B. "Only dirty people have lice."
   C. "Lice do not like to live on humans."
   D. "Lice are associated with crowded living conditions."
7. At the completion of an assessment the nurse determines that education on methods to reduce the patient's increased risk for developing nonmelanoma skin cancer is required. What did the nurse assess in this patient?
   A. Alopecia, thin hair, itching
   B. Blond hair, freckles, fair skin
   C. Dark hair, dark skin, dry skin
   D. Tanned skin, dark hair, edema
8. A patient is being assessed for a melanoma skin lesion. Which assessment finding suggests that further investigation for a melanoma is necessary?
   A. Change in the color or size of a nevus
   B. Dry, fissured, and hyperkeratotic skin
   C. Red circumscribed plaques covered by silvery white scales
   D. Firm mass located in the subcutaneous tissue and the lower dermis
9. When caring for a patient recovering from a stroke, the nurse coordinates a group of caregivers to help lift the patient up in bed. Why should the patient be lifted instead of pulled into position?
   A. Pulling a patient up in bed is hard on the patient's joints.
   B. Lifting a patient prevents tissue injury from shearing forces.
   C. Pulling a patient up in bed decreases tissue hypoxia.
   D. Lifting a patient allows a brief period of increased capillary circulation.
10. A young adult with acne scars asks the nurse what can be done to reduce the scarring. Which procedure should the nurse discuss with this patient?
    A. Skin flap
    B. Liposuction
    C. Dermabrasion
    D. Blepharoplasty

See Test Yourself answers in Appendix B.

REFERENCES

Adams, M. P., Holland, L. N., & Urban, C. (2017). *Pharmacology for nursing: A pathophysiologic approach* (5th ed.). Hoboken, NJ: Pearson Education.

Agency for Health Care Research and Quality. (2016). *AHRQ's safety program for nursing homes: On-time pressure ulcer prevention*. Retrieved from https://www.ahrq.gov/professionals/systems/long-term-care/resources/ontime/pruprev/index.html.

American Academy of Dermatology. (2017). *Psoriasis*. Retrieved from: https://www.aad.org/media/stats/conditions/psoriasis.

American Cancer Society. (2016a). *Melanoma skin cancer early detection, diagnosis, and staging*. Retrieved from https://www.cancer.org/content/dam/CRC/PDF/Public/8825.00.pdf.

American Cancer Society. (2016b). *Targeted therapy for melanoma skin cancers*. Retrieved from https://www.cancer.org/cancer/melanoma-skin-cancer/treating/targeted-therapy.html.

American Cancer Society. (2016c). *Treatment of melanoma skin cancer, by stage*. Retrieved from https://www.cancer.org/cancer/melanoma-skin-cancer/treating/by-stage.html.

American Cancer Society. (2017a). *Skin cancer*. Retrieved from www.cancer.org/cancer/skincancer/index.

American Cancer Society. (2017b). *Skin cancer: Basal and squamous cell*. Retrieved from www.cancer.org/cancer/skincancer-basalandsquamouscell/index.

American Cancer Society. (2017c). *Skin cancer: Melanoma*. Retrieved from https://www.cancer.org/cancer/melanoma-skin-cancer/treating/by-stage.html.

American Cancer Society. (2017d). *Survival rates for melanoma skin cancer, by stage*. Retrieved from https://www.cancer.org/cancer/melanoma-skin-cancer/detection-diagnosis-staging/survival-rates-for-melanoma-skin-cancer-by-stage.html.

American Cancer Society. (2017e). *UV radiation and cancer*. Retrieved from www.cancer.org/acs/groups/content/@nho/documents/document/uvradiationandcancerpdf.pdf.

American Society of Plastic Surgeons. (2016). *Plastic surgery statistics reveal focus on face and fat*. Retrieved from https://www.plasticsurgery.org/news/press-releases/new-plastic-surgery-statistics-reveal-focus-on-face-and-fat.

Braden, B., & Bergstrom, N. (1988). *Braden scale for predicting pressure sore risk*. Retrieved from www.bradenscale.com/images/bradenscale.pdf.

Centers for Disease Control and Prevention (CDC). (2016). *Methicillin resistant Staphylococcus aureus*. Retrieved from https://www.cdc.gov/mrsa/healthcare/clinicians/prevention/index.html.

Centers for Disease Control and Prevention (CDC). (2018a). *General information about MRSA in the community*. Retrieved from https://www.cdc.gov/mrsa/community/index.html.

Centers for Disease Control and Prevention (CDC). (2018b). *Shingles vaccination*. Retrieved from https://www.cdc.gov/shingles/vaccination.html.

DermNet New Zealand. (2017a). *Acral lentiginous melanoma*. Retrieved from https://www.dermnetnz.org/topics/acral-lentiginous-melanoma/.

DermNet New Zealand. (2017b). *Stevens-Johnson syndrome/toxic epidermal necrolysis*. Retrieved from https://www.dermnetnz.org/topics/stevens-johnson-syndrome-toxic-epidermal-necrolysis/.

Environmental Protection Agency. (2012). *Skin cancer is most common cancer in US, yet one of the most preventable/EPA, FDA, NPS, National Council on Skin Cancer Prevention highlight sun safety tips*. Retrieved from https://archive.epa.gov/epapages/newsroom_archive/newsreleases/73dd6944222cc12a85257a01005c1cf7.html.

Feldman, S. R. (2017). Treatment of psoriasis in adults. *Up to Date*. Retrieved from https://www.uptodate.com/contents/treatment-of-psoriasis-in-adults.

Food and Drug Administration. (2015). *Don't be misled by "latex free" claims*. Retrieved from www.fda.gov/ForConsumers/ConsumerUpdates/ucm342641.htm.

Healthy People 2020. (2017). *OA 10: Reduce the rate of pressure ulcer hospitalization among older adults*. Retrieved from https://www.healthypeople.gov/node/4970/data_details.

Kee, J. L. (2018). *Laboratory and diagnostic tests with nursing implications* (10th ed.). Boston, MA: Pearson.

Lynn, D. D., Umari, T., Dunnick, C. A., & Dellavalle, R. P. (2016). The epidemiology of acne vulgaris in late adolescence. *Adolescent Health and Medical Therapy, 7*, 13–25.

Mayo Clinic. (2017). *Stevens Johnson syndrome*. Retrieved from www.mayoclinic.org/diseases-conditions/stevens-johnson-syndrome/home/ovc-20317097.

NANDA International. (2018). *NANDA International, Inc. Nursing diagnoses: Definitions and classification, 2018–2020* (11th ed.) (T. H. Herdman & S. Kamitsuru, Eds.). New York, NY: Thieme.

National Cancer Institute. (2013). *Biological therapies for cancer*. Retrieved from https://www.cancer.gov/about-cancer/treatment/types/immunotherapy/bio-therapies-fact-sheet.

National Cancer Institute. (2017). *Skin cancer treatment*. Retrieved from https://www.cancer.gov/types/skin/hp/skin-treatment-pdq/.

National Pressure Ulcer Advisory Panel. (2016). *NPUAP pressure injury stages*. Retrieved from www.npuap

.org/resources/educational-and-clinical-resources/npuap-pressure-injury-stages/.

National Pressure Ulcer Advisory Panel. (2017). *NPUAP mission.* Retrieved from www.npuap.org/wp-content/uploads/2017/03/Padula-William-NPUAP-13FEB17.pdf.

Rimkus, T. K., Carpenter, R. L., Qasem, S., Chan, M., & Hui-Wen, L. (2016). Targeting the sonic hedgehog signaling pathway: Review of smoothened and GLI inhibitors. *Cancers (Basel), 8*(2). [Epub ahead of print]

Sal, N., Laurent, C., Strale, H., Denis, O., & Byl, B. (2015). Efficacy of decolonization of methicillin-resistant Staphylococcus aureus carriers in clinical practice. *Antimicrobial Resistance and Infection Control, 4.* [Epub ahead of print]

Santamaria, N., Gerdtz, M., McCann, J., Freeman, A., Vassilou, T., DeVicentis, S., ... Knott, J. (2015). A randomized controlled trial of the effectiveness of soft silicone multi-layered foam dressings in the prevention of sacral and heel pressure ulcers in trauma and critically ill patients: The border trial. *International Wound Journal, 12*(3), 302–308.

Sorenson, M., Quinn, L., & Klein, D. (2019). *Pathophysiology: Concepts of human disease.* Hoboken, NJ: Pearson Education.

Tayyib, N., & Coyer, F. (2016). Effectiveness of pressure ulcer prevention strategies for adult patients in intensive care units; A systematic review. *Worldviews of Evidence Based Nursing, 13*(6), 432–444.

Yang, M.-S., Lee, J. Y., Kim, J., Kim, G.-W., Kim, B.-K., Kim, J.-Y., ... Kang, H.-R. (2016). Incidence of Stevens-Johnson syndrome and toxic epidermal necrolysis: A nationwide population-based study using National Health Insurance Database in Korea. *PLOS ONE, 11*(11), e0165933.

ADDITIONAL RESOURCES

American Academy of Dermatology

www.aad.org/for-the-public

Centers for Disease Control and Prevention: Shingles (Herpes Zoster)

www.cdc.gov/shingles/

DermNet New Zealand

www.dermnetz.org

National Pressure Ulcer Advisory Panel

www.npuap.org

Wound Healing Society

www.woundheal.org

Chapter 17

Nursing Care of Patients with Burns

Chapter Outline and Learning Outcomes

CLINICAL COMPETENCIES

- Assess functional health status of patients with burns, and monitor, document, and report abnormal manifestations.
- Use evidence-based practice to plan and implement nursing care for patients with burns.
- Prioritize patient needs based on assessed data to select and implement individualized nursing interventions for patients with burns.
- Administer medications knowledgeably and safely to patients with burns.
- Integrate interprofessional care into the care of patients with burns.
- Provide teaching appropriate for prevention of burns.
- Revise plan of care as needed to provide effective interventions to promote, maintain, or restore functional health status to patients with burns.

KEY TERMS

A **burn** is an injury resulting from exposure to heat, chemicals, radiation, or electric current. A transfer of energy from a source of heat to the human body initiates a sequence of physiologic events that in the most severe cases leads to irreversible tissue destruction. Burns range in severity from a minor loss of small segments of the outermost layer of the skin to a complex injury involving all body systems. Treatments vary from simple application of a topical antiseptic agent in an outpatient clinic to an invasive, multisystem, interprofessional team approach in the aseptic environment of a burn center.

The American Burn Association (ABA, 2017) estimates that 486,000 burn injuries requiring medical intervention occurred in 2016 in the United States, and of those, about 40,000 required hospitalization, with approximately 3275 dying from burn or smoke inhalation injuries. The home is the most common site for fire-related burns (73%). Cooking accounted for 50.8% of residential fires in 2015 (U.S. Fire Administration, 2017b). A positive trend is the 22.7% decrease in fires, an 11.7% decrease in fire deaths, and a 7.9% decrease in burn injuries in the United States between 2005 and 2014 (U.S. Fire Administration, 2017a).

The most common factor associated with death from burns is age (adults greater than 85 years have the highest fire death rate, at 39.5%) (U.S. Fire Administration, 2017b). Common causes of burns that occur in the home include open flame, hot water/liquid or steam, hot metal or other objects, electrical current, or chemicals (Mayo Clinic, 2017). Fire injuries and deaths in college-age students most commonly occur off-campus and are related to cooking (National Fire Protection Association, 2017). Occupations involving work with chemicals, gasoline, or electricity pose another risk factor. Abuse is suspected when scald burns show a clear line of demarcation, indicating deliberate immersion. The presence of small, circular burns may be from cigarette burns inflicted by an abuser.

Older adults are more vulnerable to fire and burn injury because of decreased visual acuity, depth perception, and sense of smell and hearing, in addition to impaired mobility. All of these factors increase the risk for accidentally starting a fire and diminish the ability to survive it. More than 1332 deaths in adults ages 65 and older occurred in 2015 (U.S. Fire Administration, 2017a). Infants and older adults have a greater risk of mortality. Morbidity increases in patients with preexisting cardiac, pulmonary, or renal disorders, and diabetes mellitus. Patients with alcoholism have lower survival rates after a major burn injury due to the development of more complications. Men account for 68% of burn patients versus 32% for women (ABA, 2017).

17.1 Types of Burn Injury

The four types of burn injury are thermal, chemical, electrical, and radiation. Although all four types can lead to generalized tissue damage and multisystem involvement, the causative agents and priority treatment measures are unique to each (**Table 17.1**).

Table 17.1 Types of Burns, Their Causative Agents, and Priority Treatment Measures

Type and Causative Agents	Priority Treatment
Thermal ■ Open flame ■ Steam ■ Hot liquids (water, grease, tar, metal)	■ Extinguish flame (stop, drop, and roll). ■ Flush with cool water. ■ Consult fire department.
Chemical ■ Acids ■ Strong alkalis ■ Organic compounds	■ Neutralize or dilute chemical. ■ Remove clothing. ■ Consult poison control center.
Electrical ■ Direct current ■ Alternating current ■ Lightning	■ Disconnect source of current. ■ Initiate CPR if necessary. ■ Move to area of safety. ■ Consult electrical experts.
Radiation ■ Solar (ultraviolet) ■ X-rays ■ Radioactive agents	■ Shield the skin appropriately. ■ Limit time of exposure. ■ Move the patient away from the radiation source. ■ Consult a radiation expert.

Thermal Burns

Thermal burns result from exposure to dry heat (flames) or moist heat (steam and hot liquids). They are the most common burn injuries and occur most often in children and older adults. Direct exposure to the source of heat causes cellular destruction that can result in charring of vascular, bone, muscle, and nervous tissue.

Chemical Burns

Chemical burns are caused by direct skin contact with acids, alkaline agents, or organic compounds. These chemicals destroy tissue protein, leading to necrosis. More than 25,000 products found in the home or workplace can cause chemical burns. Some of these common household products include drain cleaners, lye, industrial-strength ammonia, household ammonia, oven cleaners, toilet bowl cleaners, dishwasher detergents, and bleach.

Burns caused by alkalis (such as lye) are more difficult to neutralize than are burns caused by acids. They also tend to have deeper penetration with a correspondingly more severe burn than from acid. Organic compound burns, such as those caused by petroleum distillates, result in cutaneous damage through fat solvent action and may also cause renal and liver failure if absorbed.

Chemical agents are further classified according to the manner by which they structurally alter proteins. Oxidizing agents, such as household bleach, alter protein configuration through the chemical process of reduction. Corrosives, such as lye, cause extensive protein denaturation. Protoplasmic poisons, such as organic compounds, form salts with proteins, inhibiting calcium and other ions needed for cell viability. The severity of the chemical burn is related to the type of agent, the concentration of the agent, the mechanism of action, the duration of contact, and the amount of body surface area exposed.

Electrical Burns

The severity of electrical burns depends on the type and duration of the current and the amount of voltage. It is particularly difficult to assess the extent of an electrical burn injury because the destructive processes initiated by the electrical insult are concealed and may persist for weeks beyond the time of the incident. It is challenging to assess the depth and extent of the burn because electricity follows the path of least resistance, which in the human body tends to lie along muscles, bone, blood vessels, and nerves. Entry and exit wounds tend to be small, masking widespread tissue damage underneath the wound. Tissue necrosis results from impaired blood flow, which is secondary to blood coagulation at the site of the electrical injury. Because electrical burn wounds of the extremities often cause severe tissue necrosis, they frequently develop gangrene that necessitates amputation.

Alternating current (AC), as is found in conventional households, produces repeated electrical surges that lead to tetanic muscle contractions. Such sustained muscle contractions inhibit respiratory efforts for the duration of contact and result in respiratory arrest. The contractions also cause the person to clamp down on the power source (such as an electrical cord) and thus may increase the duration of contact with the source. Direct current (DC), as in injury from a lightning bolt, exposes the body to very high voltage for an instantaneous period of time. A high-voltage (lightning) injury usually results in entry and exit wounds. The flashover effect, a phenomenon unique to lightning injury, actually saves the patient from death. It is seen in those instances in which the current travels over the moist surface of the skin rather than through deeper structures. Cardiopulmonary arrest is the most common cause of death from lightning.

Radiation Burns

Radiation burns are usually associated with sunburn or radiation treatment for cancer. These kinds of burns tend to be superficial, involving only the outermost layers of the epidermis. All functions of the skin remain intact. Symptoms are limited to mild systemic reactions: headache, chills, local discomfort, and nausea and vomiting. More extensive exposure to radiation or radioactive substances, as in nuclear power accidents, leads to the same degree of tissue damage and multisystem involvement associated with other types of burns.

17.2 Factors Affecting Burn Classification

Tissue damage following a burn is determined primarily by two factors: the depth of the burn (the layers of underlying tissue affected) and the extent of the burn (the percentage of body surface area involved).

Depth of the Burn

The depth of a burn injury is determined by the elements of the skin that have been damaged or destroyed. Burn depth results from a combination of the temperature of the burning agent and the length of contact. Burns are classified as either superficial, partial thickness, full thickness, or extension to deep tissue (International Society for Burn Injury (ISBI) Practice Guidelines Committee, 2016; Rice & Orgill, 2018). Characteristics of burns are described next, summarized in **Table 17.2** and illustrated in **Figure 17.1** ■.

Superficial Burns

A **superficial burn** involves only the epidermal layer of the skin. This type of burn most often results from a sunburn, ultraviolet light, a minor flash injury (from a sudden ignition or explosion), or a mild radiation burn associated with cancer treatment. Because the skin remains intact, this degree of burn is not part of a calculated burn injury estimate. The skin color ranges from pink to bright red, and

Table 17.2 Characteristics of Burns by Depth

Characteristic	Superficial	Partial Thickness (Superficial to Deep)	Full Thickness	Extension to Deep Tissue
Skin layers lost	Epidermis	Epidermis and dermis	Epidermis, dermis, and underlying tissues	All layers
Skin appearance over burn	Pink to red and dry; may have local edema	Fluid-filled blisters; bright pink or red with superficial partial-thickness burns Pale, mottled, waxy white with deep partial-thickness burns	Waxy white; dry, leathery, charred	Extends into fascia and/or muscle
Skin function	Present	Absent	Absent	Absent
Pain sensation	Present	Present	Absent	Absent
Manifestations at the burn site	Pain; local edema	Severe pain; edema; weeping of fluid	Little pain; edema	Deep pressure noted
Treatment	Regular cleaning Topical agent of choice	Regular cleaning Topical agent of choice May require skin grafting with deep partial-thickness burns	Regular cleaning Topical agent of choice Skin substitutes Excision of eschar Skin grafting	Requires surgical treatment Skin grafting
Scarring	None	May occur in deep burns	Of grafted area	Of grafted area
Time to heal	3–6 days	14–21+ days	Requires skin grafting to heal	Requires skin grafting to heal

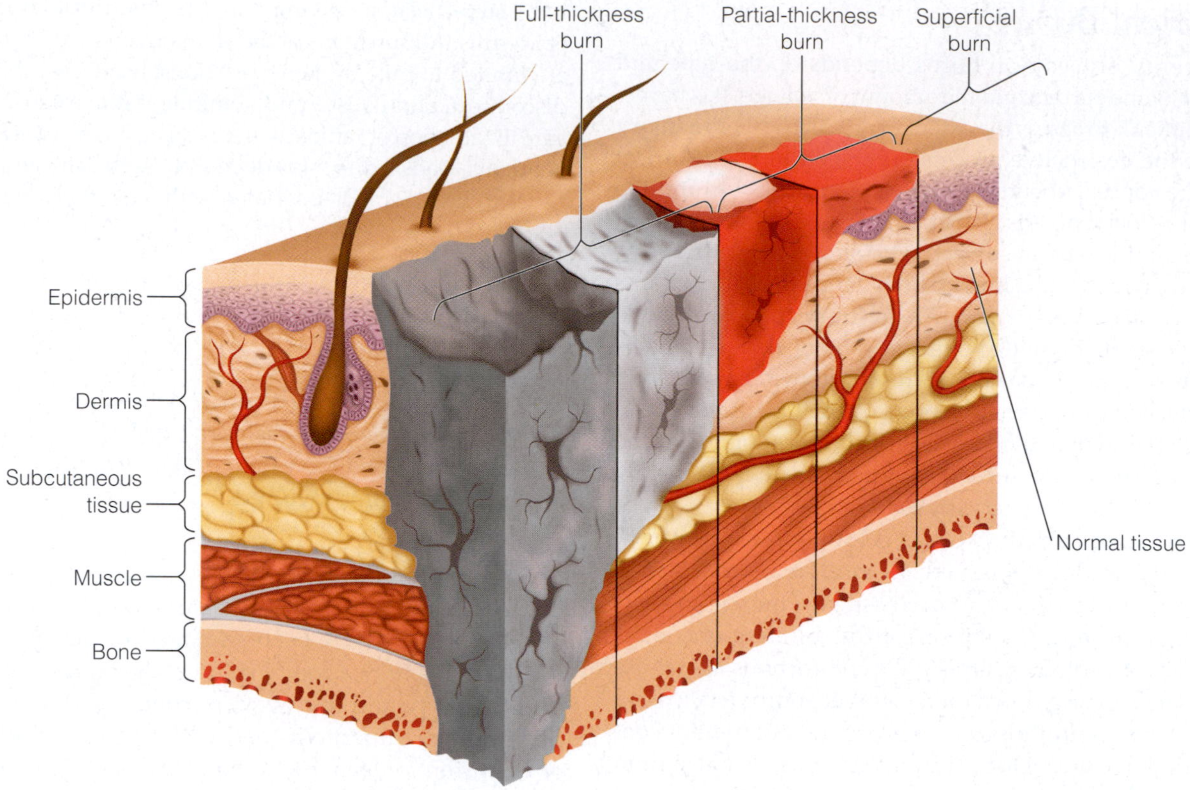
Full-thickness burn
Partial-thickness burn
Superficial burn
Epidermis
Dermis
Subcutaneous tissue
Muscle
Bone
Normal tissue

Figure 17.1 ■ Burn injury classification according to the depth of the burn.

there may be slight edema over the burned area. Superficial burns involving large body surface areas may be manifested by chills, headache, and nausea and vomiting. The injury usually heals in 3 to 6 days, with dryness and peeling of the outer layer of skin. There is no scar formation. Superficial burns are treated with mild analgesics and the application of water-soluble lotions. Extensive superficial burns, especially in older adults, may require intravenous fluid treatment.

Partial-Thickness Burns

Partial-thickness burns may be subdivided into superficial partial-thickness and deep dermal partial-thickness burns. The classification depends on the depth of the burn.

A *superficial partial-thickness burn* involves the epidermis and the papillae of the dermis. Causes may include such injuries as a brief exposure to flash flame or dilute chemical agents or contact with a hot surface. This burn is often bright red, but has a moist, glistening appearance with blister formation (**Figure 17.2** ■). The burned area will blanch on pressure, and touch and pain sensation remain intact. Pain in response to temperature and air is usually severe due to exposure of intact nerves. These injuries heal within 21 days with minimal or no scarring, but pigment changes are common. Analgesics are administered, and if large blistered areas are disrupted, skin substitutes may be used.

A *deep partial-thickness burn* also involves the entire epidermis but extends further into the dermis than a superficial partial-thickness burn. Hair follicles, sebaceous glands, and epidermal sweat glands remain intact (Sorenson, Quinn, & Klein, 2018). Hot liquids or solids, flash flame, direct flame, intense radiant energy, or chemical agents may cause this level of burn wound. The surface of the burn wound appears pale and waxy and may be moist or dry. Large, easily ruptured blisters may be present or the blisters may look like flat, dry tissue paper. Capillary refill is decreased, and sensation to deep pressure is present. The burn wound is less painful than a superficial partial-thickness burn due to more nerve destruction, reducing sensation, but areas of pain and areas of decreased sensation may be present. Deep partial-thickness burn wounds often require more than 21 days for healing and may convert to a full-thickness injury as necrosis extends the depth of the wound. Contractures are possible, as are hypertrophic scarring and functional impairment (**Figure 17.3** ■). Excision and grafting may be necessary to decrease scarring and loss of function.

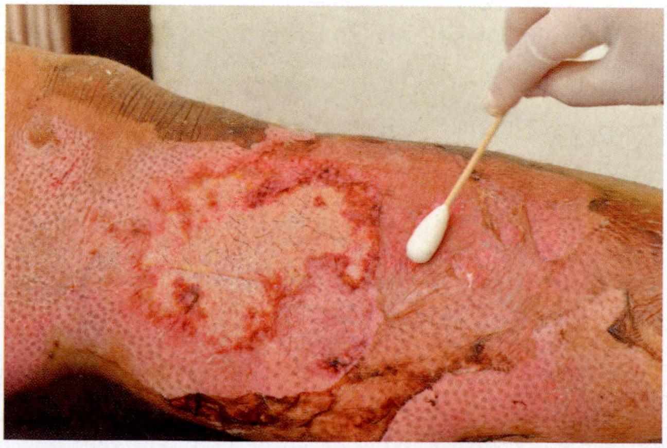

Figure 17.2 ■ Partial-thickness burn injury.

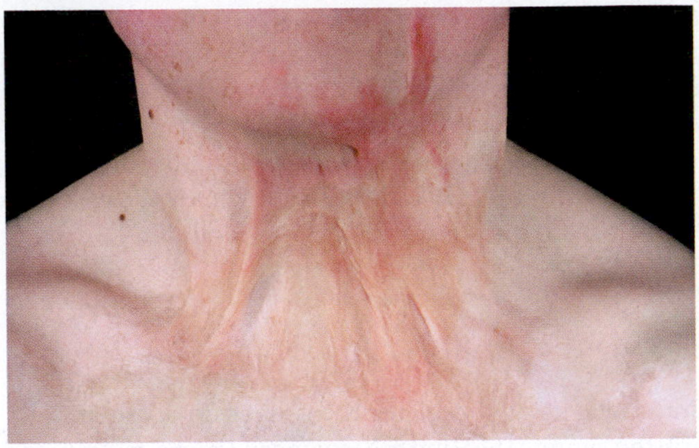

Figure 17.3 ■ Contractures from a burn wound.

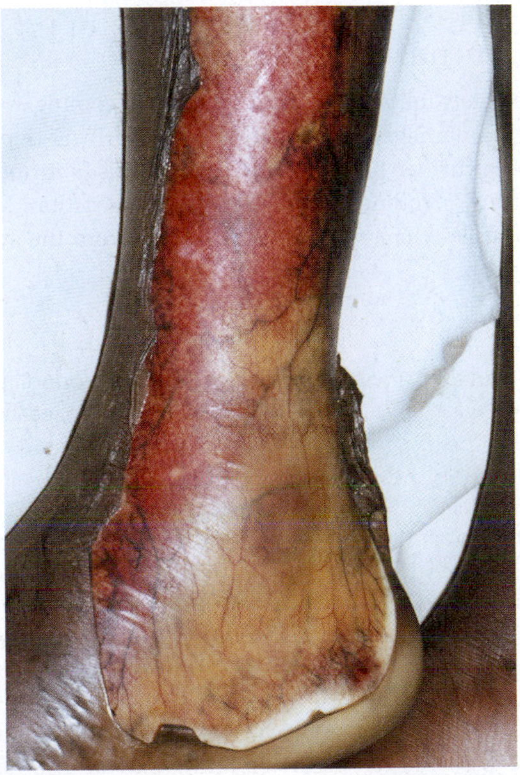

Figure 17.4 ■ Full-thickness burn injury.

Full-Thickness Burns

A **full-thickness burn** involves all layers of the skin, including the epidermis, the dermis, and the epidermal appendages (**Figure 17.4** ■). The burn wound may extend into the subcutaneous fat, connective tissue, muscle, and bone. Full-thickness burns are caused by prolonged contact with flames, steam, chemicals, or high-voltage electric current.

Depending on the cause of injury, the burn wound may appear pale, waxy, yellow, brown, mottled, charred, or nonblanching red. The wound surface is dry, leathery, and firm to the touch. Thrombosed blood vessels may be visible under the surface of the wound. There is no sensation of pain or light touch because pain and touch receptors have been destroyed. Full-thickness burns require skin grafting to heal.

Extension to Deep Tissue

Formerly called fourth degree, burns that extend to deep tissue (bone, fascia, muscle) are potentially life-threatening (Rice & Orgill, 2018). They are described in Table 17.2 and **Table 17.3**.

Extent of the Burn

The extent of the burn injury is expressed as a percentage of the *total body surface area (TBSA)*. Several methods are used to determine the extent of injury. The *"rule of nines"* is a rapid method of estimation used during the prehospital and emergency care phases. In this method, the body is divided into five surface areas—head and neck, trunk, arms, legs, and perineum—and percentages that equal or total a sum of nines are assigned to each body area (**Figure 17.5** ■). For example, a patient with burns of the face, anterior right arm, and anterior trunk has burn injury involving 27% of the TBSA (in this example, face = 4.5%, arm = 4.5%, and trunk = 18%, to total 27%). Only partial- and full-thickness burns are included in the estimation.

On the patient's admission to the hospital, critical care area, or burn center, more accurate methods for estimating the extent of injury are employed. For example, the *Lund*

Table 17.3 American Burn Association Classification of Burn Injury

Characteristics	Minor Burn Injury	Moderate Burn Injury	Major Burn Injury
Source and area of burns	Excludes electrical injury, inhalation injury, complicated injuries (such as multiple trauma), and all patients who are considered to be at high risk (such as older adults and those with chronic illnesses)	Excludes electrical injury, inhalation injury, complicated injuries (such as multiple trauma), and all patients who are considered to be at high risk (such as older adults and those with chronic illnesses)	Includes all burns of the hands, face, eyes, ears, feet, and perineum; all electrical injuries, inhalation injuries, multiple-trauma injuries, and all patients who are considered to be at high risk
Partial-thickness burns	Less than 15% of the total body surface area in adults	15 to 25% of the total body surface area in adults	Greater than 25% of the total body surface area in adults
Full-thickness burns and burns that extend to deep tissue	Less than 2% of the total body surface area not involving special care areas (eyes, ears, face, hands, feet, perineum)	Less than 10% of the total body surface area not involving special care areas (eyes, ears, face, hands, feet, perineum)	10% or greater of the total body surface area

Note: Burn injuries described in this table (except minor burns) should be treated in a specialized burn center. These criteria have been established by the American Burn Association.

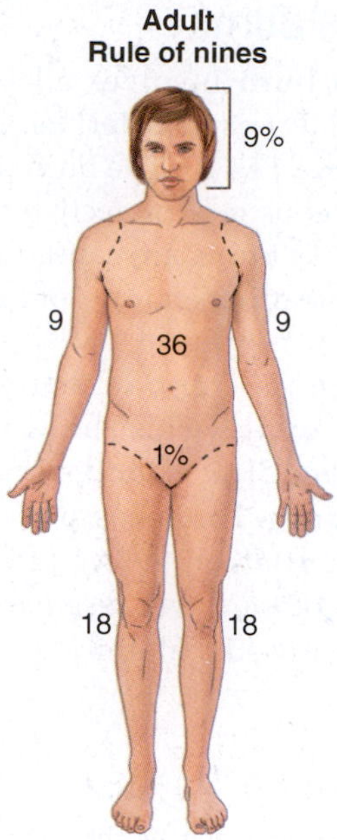
Adult
Rule of nines
9%
9
36
9
1%
18
18

Figure 17.5 ■ The "rule of nines" is a method for quickly estimating the percentage of TBSA affected by a burn injury. Although useful in emergency care situations, the rule of nines is not accurate for estimating TBSA for adults who are short, obese, or very thin.

and Browder method (**Figure 17.6** ■) determines surface area measurements for each body part according to the age of the patient and is considered the most accurate estimation of burn injury extent.

A recognized system for describing a burn injury, developed by the ABA, uses both the extent and depth of burn to classify burns as minor, moderate, or major (Table 17.3).

17.3 Burn Wound Healing

Burns heal using the same processes as do other wounds, but the wound healing phases occur more slowly and last longer. The healing process involves three phases: inflammation, proliferation, and remodeling (Sorenson et al., 2018).

Inflammation

Immediately following the injury, platelets coming in contact with the damaged tissue aggregate. Fibrin is deposited, trapping further platelets, and a thrombus is formed. The thrombus, combined with local vasoconstriction, leads to hemostasis, which walls off the wound from the systemic circulation.

Lund and Browder

Area	Age (years)					% 1°	% 2°	% 3°	% Total
	0–1	1–4	5–9	10–15	Adult				
Head	19	17	13	10	7				
Neck	2	2	2	2	2				
Ant. trunk	13	13	13	13	13				
Post. trunk	13	13	13	13	13				
R. buttock	2½	2½	2½	2½	2½				
L. buttock	2½	2½	2½	2½	2½				
Genitalia	1	1	1	1	1				
R.U. arm	4	4	4	4	4				
L.U. arm	4	4	4	4	4				
R.L. arm	3	3	3	3	3				
L.L. arm	3	3	3	3	3				
R. hand	2½	2½	2½	2½	2½				
L. hand	2½	2½	2½	2½	2½				
R. thigh	5½	6½	8½	8½	9½				
L. thigh	5½	6½	8½	8½	9½				
R. leg	5	5	5½	6	7				
L. leg	5	5	5½	6	7				
R. foot	3½	3½	3½	3½	3½				
L. foot	3½	3½	3½	3½	3½				
					Total				

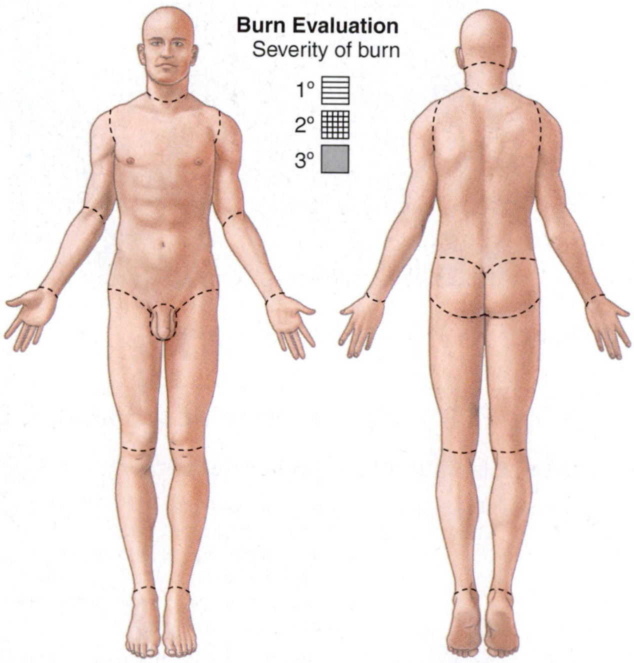
Burn Evaluation
Severity of burn
1°
2°
3°

Figure 17.6 ■ The Lund and Browder burn assessment chart. This method of estimating TBSA affected by a burn injury is more accurate than the "rule of nines" because it accounts for changes in body surface area across the lifespan.

Local vasodilation and an increase in capillary permeability follow hemostasis. Neutrophils infiltrate the wound and peak in about 24 hours, and then monocytes dominate. The monocytes are converted into macrophages, which consume pathogens and dead tissue and also secrete various growth factors. These growth factors stimulate the proliferation of fibroblasts and the deposit of a provisional wound matrix.

Proliferation

Within 2 to 3 days postburn, fibroblasts are the major cell within the wound. Their number peaks at about 14 days after the injury. Granulation tissue begins to form, with complete reepithelialization occurring during this stage. Epithelial cells cover the wound as each cell stretches across the wound surface to join with other epithelial cell sheets or the other side of the wound. The proliferation phase lasts until complete reepithelialization occurs, by epithelial cell migration, surgical intervention, or a combination of the two.

Remodeling

The remodeling phase may last for years. Collagen fibers, laid down during the proliferative phase, are reorganized into more compact areas. Scars contract and fade in color. In normal healing following a minor burn injury, the newly formed skin closely resembles its neighboring tissue. However, when a burn injury extends into the dermal layer of skin, two types of excessive scar may develop. A **hypertrophic scar** is an overgrowth of dermal tissue that remains within the boundaries of the wound. A **keloid** is a scar that extends beyond the boundaries of the original wound. People with dark skin are at greater risk for hypertrophic scars and keloids.

17.4 Minor Burns

Minor burn injuries consist of superficial burns that are not extensive, superficial partial-thickness burns that involve less than 15% of TBSA, and full-thickness burns that involve less than 2% of TBSA, excluding the special care areas (eyes, ears, face, hands, feet, perineum, and joints). Minor burn injuries are not associated with immunosuppression, hypermetabolism, or increased susceptibility to infection (Rowley-Conway, 2016).

A minor burn injury is usually treated in an outpatient facility. The goal of therapy is to promote wound healing, eliminate discomfort, maintain mobility, and prevent infection.

The Patient with a Minor Burn

Pathophysiology and Manifestations

Sunburn

Sunburns result from exposure to ultraviolet light. Such injuries, which tend to be superficial, are more commonly seen in patients with lighter skin. Because the skin remains intact, the manifestations in most cases are mild and are limited to pain, nausea and vomiting, skin redness, chills, and headache. Treatment is performed on an outpatient basis and generally consists of applying mild lotions, increasing liquid intake, administering mild analgesics, and maintaining warmth. Older adults should be monitored for evidence of dehydration. Proper use of sunscreen and limiting sun exposure to the less hazardous hours of the day (before 10:00 a.m. and after 3:00 p.m.) can prevent sunburn.

Scald Burn

Minor scald burns result from exposure to moist heat and involve superficial and superficial partial-thickness burns of less than 15% of TBSA. The goals of therapy are to prevent wound contamination and to promote healing. The nurse teaches the patient to apply antibiotic solutions and light dressings and to maintain adequate nutritional intake. Mild analgesics may be ordered to help the patient carry out activities of daily living.

Interprofessional Care

In the outpatient facility, the wound may be washed with mild soap and water. Tetanus toxoid booster is recommended for all patients whose immunization histories are in doubt. Minor burns with blisters may be left intact, or debrided. Follow-up care for a minor burn injury includes twice-daily wound cleansing with application of a topical ointment, range-of-motion (ROM) exercises to affected joints, and weekly clinic appointments until the wound heals completely.

Nursing Care

Although the nurse seldom treats minor burns in the acute care environment, the burn treatment methods used in the outpatient setting follow the same standard approaches to care. General nursing measures include taking the history, estimating the extent and depth of the injury, cleansing the wound, applying topical agents, dressing the wound, controlling pain, and establishing follow-up care.

Assessment

Assessment of minor burns includes health history and determining the extent and depth of the burn injury.

Priorities of Care

Collaborating with the interprofessional team to deliver adequate treatment of the underlying burn injury while providing care that supports the physical and psychologic responses to the injury is a nursing priority. Teaching the patient and, as appropriate, caregivers strategies for pain management, infection control, and self-care included in the therapeutic regimen should also be considered priority nursing actions. The nurse also focuses on providing emotional support throughout the patient's experience.

Transitions of Care

The nurse should address the following topics to facilitate self-care of minor burns at home:

- How to identify and report manifestations of impaired wound healing:
  a. Change in healthy appearance of the wound (altered skin integrity, swelling, blister formation, erythema)
  b. Signs of infection (fever, purulent drainage, foul odor).

- Wound care:
  a. Daily cleansing with mild soap and water
  b. Using sterile technique to change dressings
  c. Correct application of ordered topical agents.
- Pain management:
  a. Use mild analgesics as ordered
  b. Use alternative pain management therapies.

17.5 Major Burns

A major burn involves serious injury to the underlying layers of skin and covers a large body surface area. The ABA defines a major burn as one that involves:

- More than 25% TBSA in adults less than 40 years of age
- More than 20% TBSA in adults more than 40 years of age
- More than 10% TBSA full-thickness burn
- Injuries to the face, eyes, ears, hands, feet, or perineum
- High-voltage electrical injuries
- All burn injuries with inhalation injury or major trauma.

The Patient with a Major Burn

Pathophysiology

The pathophysiologic changes that result from major burn injuries involve all body systems. Extensive loss of skin (the body's protective barrier) can result in massive infection, fluid and electrolyte imbalances, and hypothermia (Sorenson et al., 2019). Often the person inhales the products of combustion, thus compromising respiratory function. Cardiac dysrhythmias and circulatory failure are common manifestations of serious burn injuries. A profound catabolic state dramatically increases caloric expenditure and nutritional deficiencies. An alteration in gastrointestinal motility predisposes the patient to developing paralytic ileus, and hyperacidity leads to gastric and duodenal ulcerations. Dehydration slows glomerular filtration rates and renal clearance of toxic wastes and may lead to acute tubular necrosis and renal failure (Sorenson et al., 2019). Overall body metabolism may be profoundly altered. Systemic responses to burns are shown in **Figure 17.7** ■ and are discussed in the following sections.

Integumentary System

The loss of skin in burn injuries interrupts normal skin functions and the skin's protective mechanisms (refer to Chapter 15). Key mechanisms lost in burn injuries include the prevention of evaporative water loss and bacteria entry, as well as the maintenance of body warmth.

Heat transfer to skin is a complex phenomenon. If the microcirculation of the skin remains intact during burning, it cools and protects the deeper portions of the skin and cools the outer surface once the heat source is removed. With extensive burn injury, the integrity of the microcirculation is lost, and the burning process continues even after the heat source is removed.

Burns have a characteristic skin surface appearance that resembles a bull's-eye, with the most severe burn located centrally and the lesser burns located along the peripheral wound edges. Depending on their intensity, burns consist of one, two, or three concentric three-dimensional zones closely corresponding on the skin surface to the depth of the burn (**Figure 17.8** ■):

- The outer zone of hyperemia is unburned tissue, blanches on pressure, and heals in 2 to 7 days postburn.

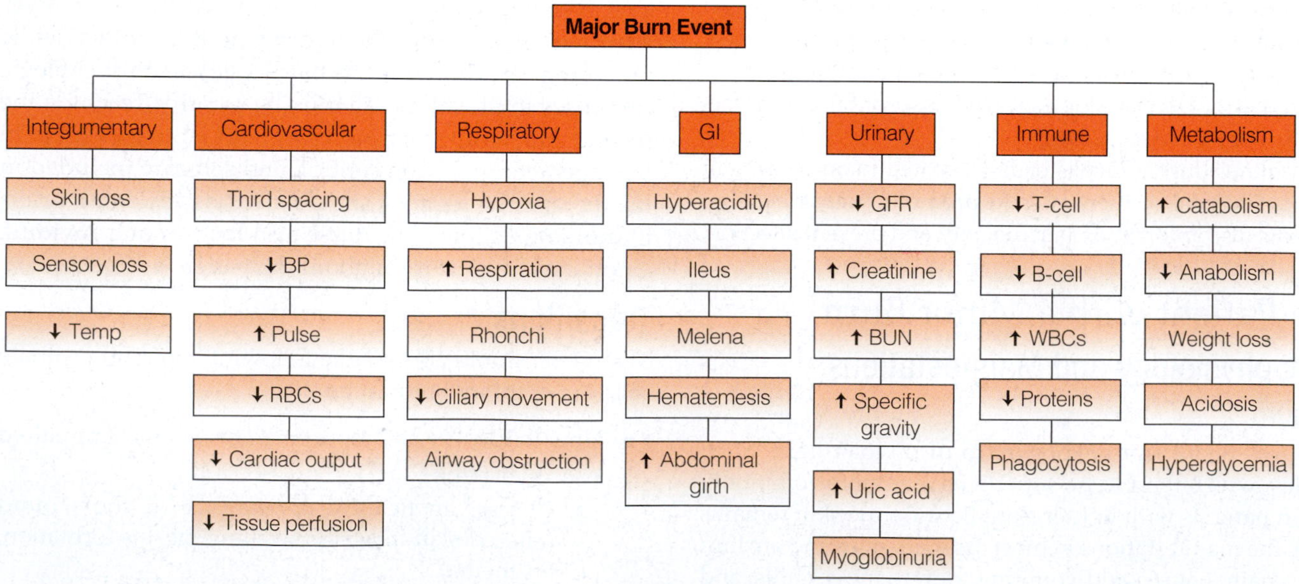

Major Burn Event
Integumentary
Skin loss
Sensory loss
↓ Temp
Cardiovascular
Third spacing
↓ BP
↑ Pulse
↓ RBCs
↓ Cardiac output
↓ Tissue perfusion
Respiratory
Hypoxia
↑ Respiration
Rhonchi
↓ Ciliary movement
Airway obstruction
GI
Hyperacidity
Ileus
Melena
Hematemesis
↑ Abdominal girth
Urinary
↓ GFR
↑ Creatinine
↑ BUN
↑ Specific gravity
↑ Uric acid
Myoglobinuria
Immune
↓ T-cell
↓ B-cell
↑ WBCs
↓ Proteins
Phagocytosis
Metabolism
↑ Catabolism
↓ Anabolism
Weight loss
Acidosis
Hyperglycemia

Figure 17.7 ■ Effects of a severe burn on major body systems and metabolism.

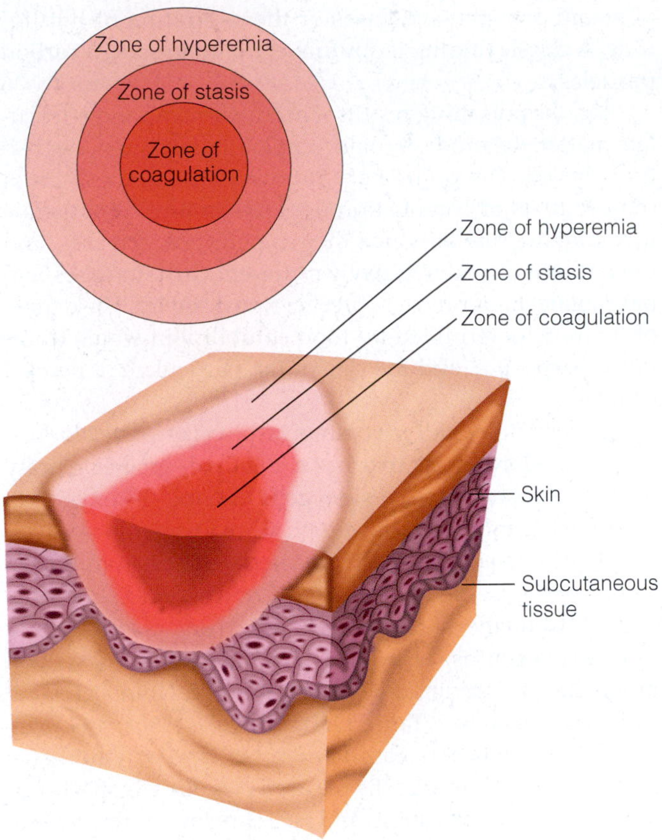
Zone of hyperemia
Zone of stasis
Zone of coagulation
Zone of hyperemia
Zone of stasis
Zone of coagulation
Skin
Subcutaneous tissue

Figure 17.8 ■ The zones of injury.

- The medial zone of stasis is initially moist, red, and blistered and blanches on pressure. It may recover or become pale and necrotic on days 3 to 7 postburn due to decreased perfusion or infection.
- The inner zone of coagulation immediately appears leathery and coagulated. It may merge with the zone of stasis in 3 to 7 days postburn.

The overall thickness of the dermis and epidermis varies considerably from one area of the body to another. Similar temperatures produce different depths of injury to different body parts. For example, in the adult, the skin covering the medial aspect of the forearm is thinner and more easily damaged than the skin covering the back of the same person. Skin dissipates heat maximally in areas of greatest vascularization. When heat absorption exceeds the rate of dissipation, cellular temperatures rise, and skin tissue is destroyed.

A burn injury results in the formation of necrotic skin and subcutaneous tissue. During the acute stage of the injury, a hard crust (**eschar**) forms, which covers the wound and harbors necrotic tissue. The eschar is characteristically leathery and rigid. Removal of the eschar facilitates healing.

Cardiovascular System

The effects of a major burn are manifested in all components of the vascular system and include hypovolemic shock (burn shock), cardiac dysrhythmias (such as ventricular fibrillation), cardiac arrest, and vascular compromise.

Hypovolemic Shock (Burn Shock). Within minutes of a burn injury, a cascade of cellular events is initiated, and a massive amount of fluid shifts from the intracellular and intravascular compartments into the interstitium (third spacing). This shift is a type of hypovolemic shock called **burn shock**, and it continues until capillary integrity is restored, usually within 24 to 36 hours of the injury. Although the pathophysiologic mechanisms of postburn vascular changes and fluid volume shifts are not clearly understood, three processes occur early in the postburn phase in patients with injury to more than 40% TBSA:

- Increase in microvascular permeability at the burn wound site
- Generalized impairment of cell wall function, resulting in intracellular edema
- Increase in osmotic pressure of the burned tissue, leading to extensive fluid accumulation.

During burn shock, the shifting of fluid is the direct result of a loss of cell wall integrity at the site of injury and in the capillary bed. Fluid leaks from the capillaries into interstitial compartments located at the burn wound site and throughout the body, resulting in a decrease in fluid volume within the intravascular space. Plasma proteins and sodium escape into the interstitium, enhancing edema formation. Blood pressure falls as cardiac output diminishes.

Vasoconstriction results as the vascular system attempts to compensate for fluid loss. Abnormal platelet aggregation and white blood cell (WBC) accumulation result in ischemia in the deeper tissue below the burn, leading to eventual thrombosis. Red blood cells (RBCs) and WBCs remain in the circulation, producing an elevation in erythrocyte and leukocyte counts secondary to hemoconcentration.

The leakage of fluid into the interstitium compromises the lymphatic system, resulting in intravascular hypovolemia and edema at the burn wound site. Edematous body surfaces impair peripheral circulation and result in necrosis of the underlying tissue. During burn shock, potassium ions leave the intracellular compartment, predisposing the patient to developing cardiac dysrhythmias. The process of burn shock continues until capillary integrity is restored, usually within 24 hours of the injury.

Burn shock reverses when fluid is reabsorbed from the interstitium into the intravascular compartment. The blood pressure rises as cardiac output increases, and urinary output improves. Diuresis continues from several days to 2 weeks postburn. During this phase, the extra cardiac workload may predispose the older patient, or the patient with cardiovascular disease, to fluid volume overload.

Cardiac Rhythm Alterations. Burns of more than 40% TBSA cause significant myocardial dysfunction, with a decrease in myocardial contractibility and cardiac output. These changes, which occur prior to a decrease in plasma volume, are believed to be due to the release of substances and oxygen-free radicals from the burn wound and from ischemic myocardial cells. Electrical burns often result in cardiac dysrhythmias or cardiopulmonary arrest caused by heat damage to the myocardium or electrical interference with cardiac electrical activity.

Peripheral Vascular Compromise. Direct heat damage to extremities, especially if circumferential burns are present, results in damage to blood vessels. Circulation to extremities may be further impaired by edema and by peripheral vasoconstriction that occurs during burn shock. In addition, **compartment syndrome** (in which the tissue pressure within a muscle compartment exceeds microvascular pressure, interrupting cellular perfusion) may result from circumferential burns and edema.

Respiratory System

Pulmonary damage may result from either direct inhalation injury or as part of the systemic response to the injury. Inhalation injury is a frequent and often lethal complication of burns. The injury may range from mild respiratory inflammation to massive pulmonary failure such as acute respiratory distress syndrome (ARDS). Exposure to heat, asphyxiants, and smoke initiates the pathophysiologic process associated with inhalation injury.

Inflammation occurs at localized sites within the airway and is manifested as hyperemia. As a result, cells are destroyed and the bronchial cilia are rendered inactive. Because the mucociliary transport mechanism no longer functions, the patient may develop bronchial congestion and infection.

Interstitial pulmonary edema develops secondary to the escape of fluid from the pulmonary vasculature into the interstitial compartment of the lung tissue. Surfactant is inactivated, resulting in atelectasis and alveolar collapse. Sloughing of the damaged and dead lung tissue occasionally produces debris that may lead to complete airway obstruction.

Upper airway (above the level of the glottis) thermal injury results from the inhalation of heated air or chemicals dissolved in water. Inhalation injury is suspected when the patient has singed facial, scalp, or nasal hair. Physical findings include the presence of soot, charring, edema, blisters, and ulcerations along the mucosal lining of the oropharynx and larynx. The resulting edema in the airway peaks within the first 24 to 48 hours of injury. Ominous signs of hoarseness, labored breathing, or stridor indicate possible airway obstruction due to edema. Lower airway thermal injury is a rare occurrence. Thermal injury below the vocal cords is seldom seen because the lower airway is protected by laryngeal reflexes. However, when it does occur, it is typically associated with the inhalation of steam or explosive gases or the aspiration of hot liquids. A classic finding is sputum containing soot or carbon particles.

Smoke poisoning results when toxic gases and particulate matter, the products of incomplete combustion, deposit directly onto the pulmonary mucosa. The composition of the products of combustion depends on the combustible material, the rate at which the temperature increases, and the amount of ambient oxygen present. Irritant gases and particulate matter have a direct cytotoxic effect. The degree of injury is determined by their solubility in water, duration of exposure, and the size of the particulate or aerosol droplet.

Carbon monoxide, a common asphyxiant, is a colorless, tasteless, odorless gas that has a 200 times greater affinity for hemoglobin than does oxygen. It displaces oxygen to bind with hemoglobin, forming carboxyhemoglobin. As a result, the decrease in arterial oxyhemoglobin produces tissue hypoxia (Centers for Disease Control and Prevention, 2017). Carbon monoxide impairs both oxygen delivery and cellular oxygen use. The clinical manifestations of carbon monoxide poisoning range from mild visual impairment to coma and death (see **Table 17.4**).

Cyanide gas is released when plastics, polyurethane, nylon, or silk is burned. The released cyanide gas affects cellular respiration. The brain and heart are most vulnerable to cyanide poisoning. Signs and symptoms of cyanide poisoning include headache, dizziness, seizures, tachycardia, and lethal dysrhythmias. Treatment addresses the inability of the body to use oxygen. Hyperbaric oxygen (oxygen delivery in a high-pressure chamber) may be used with inhalation of smoke. Hydroxocobalamin (Cyanokit) is a form of vitamin B_{12} that converts cyanide to a form that can be excreted from the body.

Gastrointestinal System

Dysfunction of the gastrointestinal system is directly related to the size of the burn wound. Patients with burns to 20% or more TBSA experience decreased peristalsis with resultant gastric distention and increased risk of aspiration. A decrease in or absence of bowel sounds is a manifestation of paralytic ileus (adynamic bowel) secondary to burn trauma. The resulting cessation of intestinal motility leads to gastric distention, nausea and vomiting, and hematemesis.

Curling ulcers (stress ulcers) are acute ulcerations of the stomach or duodenum that form following a burn injury. Abdominal pain, acidic gastric pH levels, hematemesis, and melena in the stool may indicate a gastric ulcer.

Table 17.4 Manifestations of Carbon Monoxide Poisoning

Level of Carbon Monoxide	Manifestations
10–20%	Headache, dizziness, nausea, abdominal pain
21–40%	Headache, nausea, drowsiness, dizziness, irritability, confusion, stupor, hypotension, bradycardia, skin color ranging from pale to dark red
41–60%	Convulsion, coma, hypotension, tachycardia
>60%	Death

In addition, ischemia of the intestine from splanchnic vasoconstriction increases the intestinal mucosal permeability. As a result, normal intestinal bacteria move from the lumen of the bowel to extraluminal sites, a process called *bacterial translocation*. This process is believed to be one of the mechanisms causing systemic sepsis and multiple organ dysfunction syndrome.

Urinary System

During the early stages of a burn injury, renal blood flow and glomerular filtration rates are greatly reduced from the decreased intravascular blood volume and the release of antidiuretic hormone (ADH) by the posterior pituitary. Urine output decreases, and serum creatinine and blood urea nitrogen levels increase.

Dark brown concentrated urine may indicate myoglobinuria or hemoglobinuria, the result of underlying muscle damage or the release of large amounts of dead or damaged erythrocytes after a major burn injury. When large amounts of these pigments are released, the liver cannot keep pace with conjugation and the pigments pass through the glomeruli. The pigments can occlude the renal tubules and cause renal failure, especially when dehydration, acidosis, or shock is also present.

Immune System

The function of the immune system is to protect the human body from invasion by foreign microorganisms. The capillary leak that occurs in the early stages of a burn injury continues throughout the burn shock phase and impairs the active components of both the cell-mediated and humoral immune systems.

The humoral immune system relies on B cells to produce antibodies or immunoglobulins (refer to Chapter 13). In the burn patient, the serum levels of all immunoglobulins are significantly diminished. Serum protein levels remain persistently low throughout the clinical course until wound closure is completed. A marked decrease in T-cell counts results in a reduction of cytotoxic activity and suppression of the cell-mediated immune system.

The compromise in the humoral and cell-mediated immune systems constitutes a state of acquired immunodeficiency, which places the burn patient at risk for infection. The period of vulnerability is transient and may last from 1 to 4 weeks following the onset of a burn injury. During this time frame, opportunistic infections can be fatal despite aggressive antimicrobial therapy.

Metabolism

Two distinct phases characterize the body's metabolic response to a burn injury. The ebb phase, occurring during the first 3 days of the injury, is manifested by decreased oxygen consumption, fluid imbalance, shock, and inadequate circulating volume. These responses protect the body from the initial impact of the injury.

A second phase, the flow phase, occurs when adequate burn resuscitation has been accomplished. This phase is characterized by increases in cellular activity and protein catabolism, lipolysis, and gluconeogenesis. The basal metabolic rate (BMR) significantly increases, reaching twice the normal rate. Body weight and heat drop dramatically. Total energy expenditure may exceed 100% of normal BMR. Hypermetabolism persists until after wound closure has been accomplished and may reappear if complications occur.

Interprofessional Care

The burn team is composed of an interprofessional group of healthcare professionals who together plan the care and treatment of the burn-injured patient during the acute and rehabilitative stages. The burn team consists of the nurse, physician, physical therapist, occupational therapist, nutritionist, psychiatrist/psychologist, and social worker. Team members meet regularly to discuss patient progress and to determine collaboratively the most effective regimen of care and psychosocial support.

Stages of Interprofessional Care

The clinical course of treatment for the burn patient is divided into three stages: the emergent/resuscitative stage, the acute stage, and the rehabilitative stage. Although these stages are useful predictors of the clinical needs of burn patients, it is important to recognize that the process of burn injury is dynamic and that, in many cases, the clinical stage may not be clearly delineated. Assessment and management of burn-injured patients are ongoing processes determined by the clinical picture; they last throughout the course of treatment. **Figure 17.9** ■ shows the burn patient's progression through the healthcare system during each clinical stage of burn care. During each stage, different groups of nurses, physicians, and other healthcare specialists collaborate to manage the patient's recovery.

The Emergent/Resuscitative Stage. The *emergent/resuscitative stage* lasts from the onset of injury through successful fluid resuscitation. During this stage, healthcare workers estimate the extent of burn injury, institute first-aid measures, and implement fluid resuscitation therapies. The patient is assessed for shock and evidence of respiratory distress. If indicated, intravenous lines are inserted, and the patient may be prophylactically intubated. During this stage, healthcare workers determine whether the patient needs to be transported to a burn center to take advantage of the complex intervention strategies offered by a specialized interprofessional burn team.

Although many burn injuries are treated in local tertiary care facilities, the ABA has developed guidelines for determining whether a patient should be transported to a burn center for interprofessional approaches to treatment and rehabilitation. Adult patients who should be treated at burn centers include those with:

- Second- or third-degree burns more than 10% TBSA in adults older than age 50
- Second- or third-degree burns more than 20% TBSA in adults younger than age 50
- Third-degree burns more than 5% TBSA in adults of any age

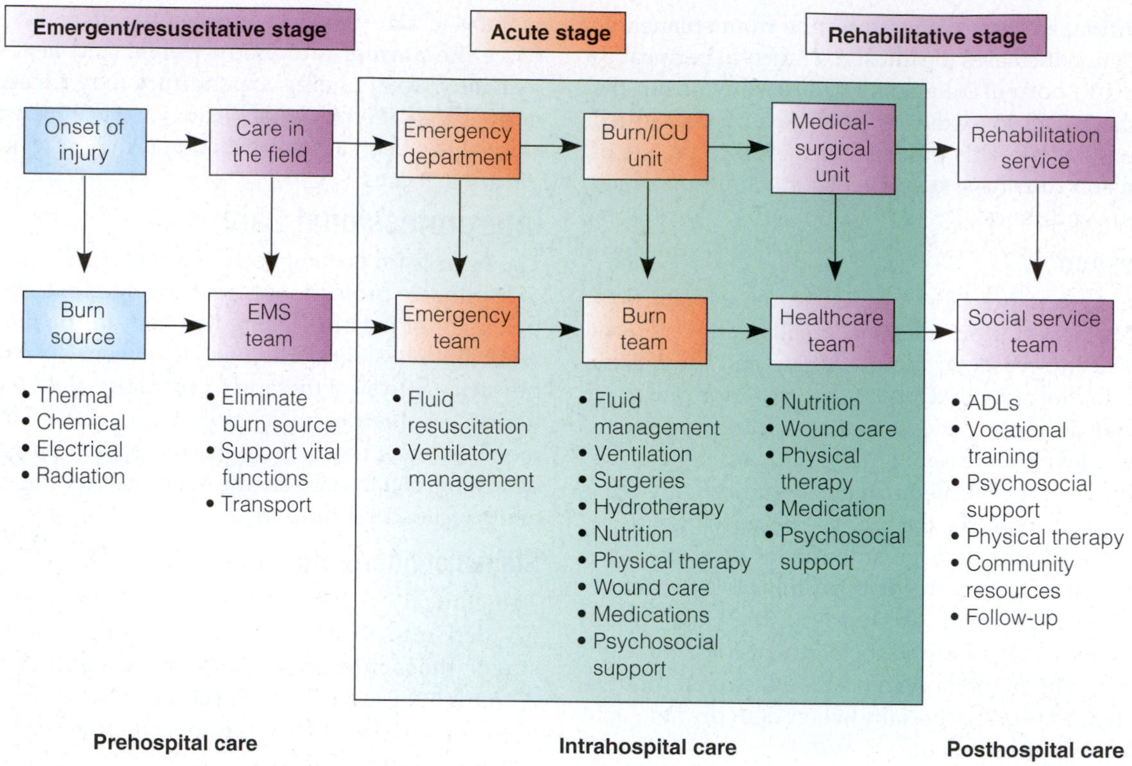

Emergent/resuscitative stage
Acute stage
Rehabilitative stage
Onset of injury
Care in the field
Emergency department
Burn/ICU unit
Medical-surgical unit
Rehabilitation service
Burn source
EMS team
Emergency team
Burn team
Healthcare team
Social service team
• Thermal
• Chemical
• Electrical
• Radiation
• Eliminate burn source
• Support vital functions
• Transport
• Fluid resuscitation
• Ventilatory management
• Fluid management
• Ventilation
• Surgeries
• Hydrotherapy
• Nutrition
• Physical therapy
• Wound care
• Medications
• Psychosocial support
• Nutrition
• Wound care
• Physical therapy
• Medication
• Psychosocial support
• ADLs
• Vocational training
• Psychosocial support
• Physical therapy
• Community resources
• Follow-up
Prehospital care
Intrahospital care
Posthospital care

Figure 17.9 ■ The patient's progression through the healthcare system during the emergent, acute, and rehabilitative stages of burn injury.

- Burns involving the hands, feet, face, eyes, ears, or perineum
- Electrical (including lightning), chemical, and inhalation injuries
- Circumferential burns of the extremities and/or chest
- Any burn associated with extenuating problems, preexisting illness, fractures, or other trauma.

The Acute Stage. The *acute stage* begins with the start of diuresis and ends with closure of the burn wound (either by natural healing or by using skin grafts). During this stage, wound care management, nutritional therapies, and measures to control infectious processes are initiated. Hydrotherapy and excision and grafting of full-thickness wounds are performed as soon as possible after injury. Enteral and parenteral nutritional interventions are started early in the treatment plan to address caloric needs resulting from extensive energy expenditure. Measures to combat infection are implemented during this stage, including the administration of topical and systemic antimicrobial agents. Tetanus toxoid booster is recommended for all patients whose immunization histories are in doubt. Pain management constitutes a significant segment of the nursing care plan throughout the clinical course of patients with burn injuries. The administration of narcotic pharmaceutical agents must precede all invasive procedures to maximize patient comfort and to reduce the anxieties associated with wound debridement and intensive physical therapy.

The Rehabilitative Stage. The *rehabilitative stage* begins with wound closure and ends when the patient returns to the highest level of health restoration, which may take years. During this stage, the primary focus is the biopsychosocial adjustment of the patient, specifically the prevention of contractures and scars and the patient's successful resumption of work, family, and social roles through physical, vocational, occupational, and psychosocial rehabilitation. The patient is taught to perform ROM exercises to enhance mobility and to support injured joints.

Prehospital Patient Management

Treatment at the injury scene includes measures to limit the severity of the burn and support vital functions. Before attempting to remove the patient from the source of burn injury, rescuers must ensure their own safety. Depending on the causative agent, rescuers may need to consult with experts to determine the best way to eliminate the source of the injury. Once the safety of the rescuers has been established, all prehospital interventions are aimed at eliminating the heat source, stabilizing the patient's condition, identifying the type of burn, preventing heat loss, reducing wound contamination, and preparing for emergency transport. Restrictive jewelry and clothing are removed at the scene to prevent circumferential constriction of the torso and extremities.

Stop the Burning Process. Emergency measures, by type of injury, include:

- ***Thermal burns:*** If the thermal injury has been caused by dry heat, smother inflamed clothing or lavage with water. Help the person "stop, drop, and roll" to extinguish the flame and limit the extent of burn. Once the flame has been extinguished, cover the body to prevent hypothermia. If the thermal injury has been caused by moist heat, lavage the area with cool water. Ice is not used for cooling because it causes vasoconstriction and may result in further injury. Tar and asphalt can be removed with Medisol, a citrus and petroleum distillate with a hydrocarbon structure.

- *Chemical burns:* For chemical burns, immediately remove the clothing and use a hose or shower to lavage the involved area thoroughly for a minimum of 20 minutes. Many chemicals are in powder form and as much dry chemical needs to be removed as possible before flushing the surface with water. Unusual chemicals may require consultation with the poison control center about appropriate treatment. Protective clothing should be worn during this process to protect the rescuer from chemical exposure. Chemical splashes in or near the eye require immediate eye irrigation with clean, cool water or saline.
- *Electrical burns:* Electrical injuries pose serious potential harm to both rescuer and burn victim. Ensure that the source of electrical current has been disconnected, or move the person to safety and away from the energy source using a nonconductive device such as an unpainted broomstick. If the person is unresponsive, assess for the presence of cardiac and respiratory function. If indicated, begin cardiopulmonary resuscitation (CPR). A spinal cord injury may be present secondary to the forceful contraction of the muscles of the neck and back during exposure to the current. If possible, place the person in a cervical collar and transport on a spinal board.
- *Radiation burns:* Radiation injuries are usually minor and involve only the epidermal layer of skin. Treatment focuses on helping normal body mechanisms promote wound healing. For severe radiation burns, such as those that result from industrial radiation accidents, trained personnel may need to render the area safe for entry prior to rescue. All interventions are aimed at shielding, establishing distance, and limiting the time of exposure to the radioactive source.

Support Vital Function. The initial assessment of the patient's respiratory and hemodynamic status begins with an evaluation of the patient's **ABCs**:

Airway
Breathing
Circulation.

- If the patient has no pulse and is not breathing, begin CPR. Establish an airway and start chest compressions. Continue CPR until spontaneous cardiopulmonary function returns or until the emergency management team takes over.
- Position the patient with the head elevated at greater than 30 degrees, and administer 100% humidified oxygen by face mask. Use nasotracheal suction as necessary to maintain a patent airway. Endotracheal intubation may be necessary if the patient has facial edema and inhalation injury. Auscultate the lungs often onsite to monitor respiratory status. Continuous pulse oximetry provides ongoing assessment of the patient's oxygen saturation levels.
- Monitor for cardiac dysrhythmias or arrest. When available, connect the patient to a cardiac monitor and observe for dysrhythmias. Elevate burned extremities above the level of the heart to facilitate circulation.
- Initiate fluid replacement therapy for burn wounds that involve more than 20% TBSA. Continuously assess heart and lung sounds and observe level of consciousness, cardiac rate and rhythm, blood pressure, and urine output.
- Cover the patient to maintain body temperature and to prevent further wound contamination and tissue damage.

Emergency and Acute Care

Prehospital personnel report to the emergency department staff all findings and medical interventions that occurred at the scene of the injury. The nurse obtains a history of the injury, estimates the depth and extent of the burn, begins fluid resuscitation, and maintains ventilation according to protocol (American College of Surgeons Committee on Trauma, 2018).

Fluid Resuscitation. **Fluid resuscitation** is the administration of intravenous fluids to restore the circulating blood volume during the acute period of increasing capillary permeability. To counteract the effects of burn shock, fluid resuscitation guidelines are used to replace the extensive fluid and electrolyte losses associated with major burn injuries. Fluid replacement is necessary in all burn wounds that involve 20% or more TBSA.

Crystalloid fluids are administered through two large-bore (14- to 16-gauge) catheters, preferably inserted through unburned skin. Warmed Ringer lactate solution is the intravenous fluid most widely used during the first 24 hours after burn injury because it most closely approximates the body's extracellular fluid composition. Several formulas may be used to replace fluid loss. The Consensus formula is the most commonly used:

- Lactated Ringer or other balanced saline solution is administered: 2 to 4 mL × kg × % TBSA burn.
- Half of the amount is infused during the first 8 hours. The remainder of the amount is infused during the next 16 hours.

Hourly urine output is often used as an indicator of effective fluid resuscitation, with about 0.5 mL/kg/hr for an adult considered adequate. Another indicator is heart rate; if fluid resuscitation is adequate, the rate should be fewer than 120 bpm or in the upper limits of normal for age. However, the fear, anxiety, and pain that accompany burn injuries often increase the heart rate. Blood pressure changes are less reliable because significant hypotension does not develop until volume losses exceed 30% due to the body's compensatory mechanisms. Assessment for narrowed pulse pressure, which indicates shock earlier, should be considered along with urine output to monitor adequate fluid resuscitation.

During the fluid resuscitation stage, the patient may require invasive hemodynamic monitoring (see Chapter 29). An arterial catheter cardiac output monitoring device can be used to monitor cardiac output and cardiac index. All measurements must be maintained within normal limits to effect adequate fluid resuscitation.

Respiratory Management. Upon the patient's admission to the emergency department, several baseline assessments of respiratory status must be obtained: chest x-ray study, arterial blood gases (ABGs), vital signs, and carboxyhemoglobin levels. Intubation is indicated for all patients with burns of the chest, face, or neck. The primary treatment plan is oriented toward preventing atelectasis and maintaining alveolar oxygen exchange. The following interventions should be initiated:

- Maintain the head of the bed at 30 degrees or greater to maximize the patient's ventilatory efforts. Turn the patient side to side every 2 hours to prevent hypostatic pneumonia.
- To keep airway passages clear, suction the patient frequently, encourage the patient to use incentive spirometry hourly, and help the patient perform coughing and deep-breathing exercises every 2 hours.
- In the face of impending airway obstruction, the patient will require immediate intubation. Orotracheal tube placement is the preferred route to reduce sinus infections seen with nasotracheal tubes. If the patient has suffered nasolabial burns, however, the orotracheal route is preferred. Nasotracheal and orotracheal intubation is reserved for short-term ventilatory management. For long-term ventilatory management (i.e., greater than 3 weeks), a tracheostomy is performed.
- Humidification of either room air or oxygen helps prevent the drying of tracheal secretions. Ambient air or oxygen flow is based on ABG results. The patient may be placed on a face mask, steam collar, T-piece, mechanical ventilation with positive end-expiratory pressure (PEEP), pressure support ventilation, or high-frequency jet ventilation. The goal of all therapies is to maintain adequate tissue oxygenation with the least amount of inspired oxygen flow necessary.
- Medications to dilate constricted bronchial passages are administered intravenously and as inhalants to control bronchospasms and wheezing. Mucolytic agents liquefy tenacious sputum and aid in expectoration.
- An arterial line is placed in the patient with major burn injury for continuous assessment of ABGs and blood pressure. Pulmonary artery pressure catheters may be inserted to measure pulmonary vascular resistance (PVR), pulmonary artery pressure (PAP), pulmonary artery wedge pressure (PAWP), and mixed venous oxygen saturation (SvO_2). The PVR and PAP rise in the presence of hypoxia. The SvO_2 is the average percentage of hemoglobin bound with oxygen in the venous blood and reflects overall tissue utilization of oxygen. Pulse oximetry monitors arterial oxygen saturation levels.
- In the presence of carbon monoxide (CO) poisoning, monitor carboxyhemoglobin (COHgb) levels. Pulse oximetry cannot distinguish between oxyhemoglobin and COHgb; thus, a false normal or high pulse oximetry reading is seen. High-flow 100% oxygen is given immediately by nonrebreather mask. Patients with COHgb greater than 15% may require hyperbaric oxygen therapy to replace the CO.
- Pain medications are administered if the patient is not in shock.

After stabilization in the emergency department, the patient is transferred to the critical care unit or a specialized burn center (a facility that has a burn physician as director of a specialized nursing unit with dedicated burn beds). In both settings, continuous monitoring of diagnostic tests, administration of medications, pain control, wound management, and nutrition support therapies constitute the initial plan of care.

Diagnosis

The following diagnostic tests are used to evaluate the patient's progress and to modify intervention strategies:

- ***Urinalysis*** indicates the adequacy of renal perfusion and the patient's nutritional status. In catabolic states, nitrogen is excreted in large amounts into the urine. Nitrogen loss is measured through 24-hour urine collections for total nitrogen, urea nitrogen, and amino acid nitrogen. *Myoglobinuria*, which manifests as a dark brown, wine-colored urine, signals the development of acute tubular necrosis. Loss of plasma protein and dehydration lead to proteinuria and elevated urine specific gravity. A fixed urine specific gravity of 1.010 can indicate renal failure even with normal volume. Glycosuria is a transient development following major burn injury; it indicates a need to adjust the nutritional program.
- ***Complete blood count*** is monitored regularly. Hematocrit is elevated secondary to hemoconcentration and fluid shifts from the intravascular compartment. Hemoglobin is decreased secondary to hemolysis. White blood cells are elevated if infection is present.
- ***Serum electrolytes*** are monitored regularly. Sodium levels are decreased secondary to massive fluid shifts into the interstitium. Potassium levels are initially elevated during burn shock, as a result of cell lysis and fluid shifts into the extracellular space. Potassium levels decrease after burn shock resolves, as fluid shifts back to intracellular and intravascular compartments.
- ***Renal function*** test results are closely monitored. Blood urea nitrogen (BUN) is elevated secondary to dehydration. Creatinine is elevated in the presence of renal insufficiency.
- ***Total protein, albumin, transferrin, prealbumin, retinol binding protein, alpha1-acid glycoprotein, and***

C-reactive protein levels indicate protein synthesis and nutritional status. Because of the fluid shifts that occur during the early stages of a burn injury, they are more useful as markers during the rehabilitative phase of care.

- ***Creatine phosphokinase (CPK)*** is elevated following an electrical burn, secondary to extensive muscle damage.
- ***Blood glucose*** is transiently elevated after major burn injury.
- ***Serial ABGs*** indicate the presence of hypoxia and acid–base disturbances and indicate patient responses to changes in oxygen therapies.
- ***Pulse oximetry*** allows continuous assessment of oxygen saturation levels. The burn-injured patient may have saturation levels below 95%.
- ***Serial chest x-ray studies*** document changes within the first 24 to 48 hours that may reflect the presence of atelectasis, pulmonary edema, or ARDS.
- ***Serial 12-lead electrocardiograms (ECGs)*** are necessary to monitor the development of dysrhythmias, especially those associated with hypokalemic and hyperkalemic states.

Medications

Pain Control. Burns often cause excruciating pain. In the emergent stages of care, intravenously administered narcotics such as morphine, hydromorphone, or fentanyl are the best means of managing pain (Adams, Holland, & Urban, 2017). Morphine is the drug of choice in a typical dosage of 3 to 5 mg intravenously every 5 to 10 minutes for an adult. Meperidine is avoided because of potential normeperidine accumulation, which can produce neurologic changes. Once the patient has been stabilized, it is appropriate to administer narcotics, especially intravenous fentanyl, prior to initiating hydrotherapy or intensive exercise routines. Burn treatments can also produce high levels of anxiety, necessitating the use of anxiolytic agents such as midazolam and lorazepam. Anxiolytics are especially useful when administered 1 hour before wound care. During the acute stage, opioids are administered around-the-clock to decrease pain that occurs at rest. Patient-controlled analgesia (PCA) enhances the patient's ability to cope with pain. The oral, subcutaneous, or intramuscular route of administration should be avoided until hemodynamic stability and unimpaired tissue perfusion returns.

As the patient enters the rehabilitative stage of care, alternative therapies for pain control may be added to the plan of care. Distraction, self-hypnosis, guided imagery, and relaxation techniques are helpful adjuncts in managing pain and coping with loss. Refer to Chapter 9 for a discussion of strategies for managing pain.

Antimicrobial Agents. Systemic infection is a leading cause of death in major burn patients. Gram-positive organisms such as *Staphylococcus* and *Streptococcus* colonize the burn surface during the first week postburn; gram-negative enteric organisms become more common with longer periods of hospitalization. Local signs of a burn wound infection include increased sloughing of burn tissue, increased edema around wound edges, partial-thickness wound converting to full-thickness wound, and black or brown areas of discoloration. Diagnosing infection is best done through a burn wound biopsy. To eliminate infection on the surface of the burn wound, topical antimicrobial therapy is used, depending on protocol. Generally, topical antimicrobials are not applied until the patient is admitted to a burn unit. Of the many antimicrobial agents available, the three most widely used are mafenide acetate (Sulfamylon) cream, silver sulfadiazine (Silvadene) cream, and silver nitrate 0.5% soaks. All three are broad-spectrum antibiotics. The choice of topical antibiotic is based on the extent of the burn wound, the presence of identified bacterial organisms, whether an open (exposing the wound to the air) or closed (using bulky dressings) method of treatment is used, and patient response. Despite antimicrobial therapy, patients with major burn assault have a greater risk for sepsis and septic shock.

Patients with major burns are usually given prophylactic antibiotics. Systemic antimicrobial therapy is indicated in the immediate preoperative and postoperative period associated with excision and autografting. Postoperatively, the therapy is discontinued as soon as the patient's hemodynamic status returns to normal, usually within the first 24 hours. In the long-term treatment of identified infectious processes, drug administration is limited to the least amount of time required to eradicate the infection. See **Medication Administration 17.A** for nursing implications when topical antimicrobial therapy is used with a burn patient.

Tetanus Prophylaxis. If the patient's immunization status is in doubt, tetanus toxoid is administered intramuscularly early in the acute phase of care to prevent *Clostridium tetani* infection.

Medication Administration 17.A

Topical Burn Medications

TOPICAL ANTIMICROBIAL AGENTS

mafenide acetate (Sulfamylon) [Antibiotic-sulfonamide]

silver nitrate [Topical antimicrobial]

silver sulfadiazine (Silvadene) [Topical anti-infective-sulfonamide]

Research shows that the most effective topical agents are those that (1) act against the major pathogens responsible for causing burn wound infection, (2) achieve levels of concentration sufficient to decrease microbial colonization, (3) are rapidly excreted or metabolized, (4) are nontoxic, and (5) are easy to use and inexpensive.

(continued)

Mafenide Acetate

Mafenide acetate is a synthetic antibiotic closely related chemically, but not pharmacologically, to the sulfonamides. Although the mechanism of action is unclear, the drug appears to interfere with the metabolism of bacterial cells. Mafenide acetate is a bacteriostatic agent effective against many gram-positive and gram-negative organisms.

For topical administration, mafenide acetate is used in an 8.5% cream in a water-miscible base. Following application, the drug is rapidly diffused through the burn eschar and absorbed systemically.

In the general circulation, mafenide acetate metabolizes to a weak carbonic anhydrase inhibitor known as *p*-carboxybenzenesulfonamide, a substance that impairs the renal mechanisms involved in the buffering of blood. Bicarbonate excretion in the urine increases, and ammonia and chloride excretion decreases. To maintain normal acid–base balance, the pulmonary system effects a compensatory hyperventilatory state. If the compensatory hyperventilation is insufficient, the patient develops metabolic acidosis.

Nursing Responsibilities

- Use mafenide acetate with caution in patients with renal or pulmonary disease.
- Approximately 3 to 5% of patients develop a hypersensitivity to mafenide acetate, resulting in a maculopapular rash on the unburned areas. Assess the patient for the following:
  - Pruritus
  - Facial edema
  - Swelling
  - Urticaria
  - Blisters
  - Eosinophilia

  If hypersensitivity reactions occur, discontinue the drug and administer antihistamines.
- Monitor the patient for superinfection within the burn eschar, in the subeschar tissue, or in viable tissue adjacent to the wound.

Health Education for the Patient and Family

- Expect intense pain, stinging, or a burning sensation following drug application. Take appropriate measures to control pain before applying the drug.
- Apply the drug to clean, debrided burn wounds once or twice daily. Continue applications until healing is apparent.
- If any signs of allergy develop, discontinue the drug and notify the physician.
- Report any sudden and prolonged increases in respiratory rate.

Silver Nitrate

Silver nitrate is a bacteriostatic agent that inhibits a wide variety of gram-positive and gram-negative organisms. Its antimicrobial effect is due to the actions of silver ions, which markedly alter the microbial cell wall and membrane. Additionally, the drug denatures bacterial protein, thereby inactivating and precipitating the microbes.

Nursing Responsibilities

- Silver nitrate is used as a 0.5% solution in distilled water. Apply the solution to bulky gauze dressings every 2 hours, and provide complete dressing changes twice daily.
- Silver nitrate has limited penetrating ability and is ineffective if used more than 72 hours following a burn injury.
- At the local tissue level, silver nitrate immediately interacts with chloride ions to form a black silver chloride precipitate that discolors both the burn wound and the adjacent tissues. The discoloration significantly hampers visual inspection of the wound.
- High concentrations of the drug result in cellular toxicity of surrounding healthy tissue.
- Because large amounts of water are systemically absorbed from the dressing site, the patient may demonstrate a hypotonic state. Hyponatremia and hypochloremic alkalosis are common manifestations in burn-injured patients treated with silver nitrate.

Health Education for the Patient and Family

- Watch for and report any signs and symptoms of hypotonicity: swelling, weight gain, difficulty in breathing.
- This drug causes a black discoloration on all skin surfaces and dressings with which it comes into contact.
- Because discoloration can conceal evidence of infection, watch for systemic manifestations of infection: fever, malaise, rapid pulse rate, and listlessness.
- Saturate the wound dressings every 2 hours with a 0.5% aqueous solution of the drug. Change the dressings completely twice daily.

Silver Sulfadiazine

Silver sulfadiazine, a sulfonamide, is the most commonly used topical agent. The drug acts on the cell membrane and cell wall of susceptible bacteria and binds to cellular DNA. The drug is bactericidal and effective against a wide variety of gram-negative and gram-positive organisms.

Nursing Responsibilities

- Many patients develop a marked leukopenia in response to this drug, which tends to improve spontaneously over the course of therapy. This finding does not contraindicate use of the drug.
- Hypersensitivity to silver sulfadiazine has been reported in a small number of cases. If the patient develops hypersensitivity, administer antihistamine and change the topical agent.
- If sulfa crystals form in the urine, keep the patient well hydrated.
- Treatment with this drug can cause systemic uptake of propylene glycol, which results in an elevated serum osmolality and high urine specific gravity in the patient who is not dehydrated. These findings tend to create confusion during the fluid resuscitative stage of care. Whenever the serum osmolality and urine specific gravity fail to correlate with a clinical picture that reflects fluid volume overload (elevated CVP/PCWP, rhonchi/wheezing, edema), suspect systemic propylene glycol uptake.

Health Education for the Patient and Family

- Apply the drug to clean, debrided wounds once or twice daily, completely covering the burn wound at all times.
- Continue applying the drug until healing is apparent.
- If any signs of allergy develop, discontinue the drug and notify the physician.
- Watch for evidence of concentrated urine, and notify the physician.
- If not contraindicated, drink large amounts of fluids to prevent sulfa crystals from forming in the urine.

Source: Data from Adams et al., 2017.

Preventing Gastric Hyperacidity. Hyperacidity must be controlled to prevent Curling ulcer. A nasogastric tube is placed during the emergent phase of care, and gastric aspirant is obtained hourly. The gastric pH should be assessed and maintained at levels above 5. To control gastric acid secretion during the acute phase of care, histamine H_2 blockers (e.g., famotidine [Pepcid]) or proton pump inhibitors (e.g., pantoprazole [Protonix]) can be administered intravenously, either intermittently or as continuous infusions. As soon as bowel sounds become audible, the patient is placed on an antacid regimen.

Treatments

Surgery. Three surgical interventions are commonly employed to manage the burn wound: escharotomy, surgical debridement, and autografting.

Escharotomy. When the burn eschar forms circumferentially around the torso or extremities, it acts as a tourniquet, impairing circulation. Left unchecked, the affected body part becomes gangrenous.

To prevent circumferential constriction of the torso or extremity, an **escharotomy** is performed by the physician with a scalpel or by electrocautery (**Figure 17.10** ■). A sterile surgical incision is made longitudinally along the extremity or the trunk to release taut skin and allow for expansion caused by edema formation. In the first 24 hours following the procedure, the incision should be gently packed with fine mesh gauze. After 24 hours, the site may be treated with a direct application of a topical antimicrobial agent. See **Box 17.1** for nursing implications for care of the patient undergoing escharotomy.

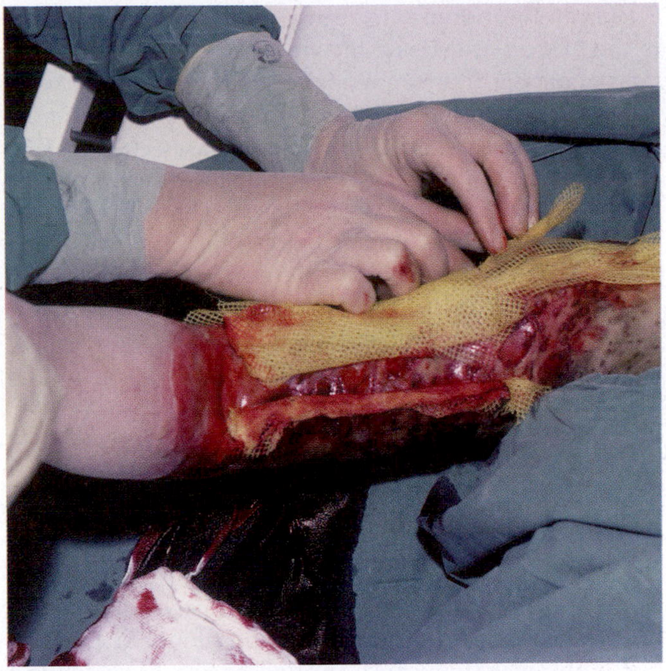

Figure 17.10 ■ Escharotomy. The surgical procedure consists of removing the eschar that forms on the skin and underlying tissue following severe burns. The procedure is particularly helpful in restoring circulation to the extremities of patients when scar tissue forms a tight, constrictive band around the circumference of a limb. For this patient, a longitudinal surgical incision has been made on the underside of the arm, and it has been packed with mesh gauze.

BOX 17.1
Nursing Implications for Circumferential Wound Management

ESCHAROTOMY

A circumferential burn wound increases the risk for impaired tissue perfusion of the involved area. To prevent arterial occlusion, an escharotomy is performed to release tension and permit unobstructed arterial blood flow. The nurse continuously assesses the involved area and notifies the physician of the need to perform this emergent procedure, which is done at the bedside. Because only the dead burn wound tissue is excised, the patient experiences very little pain.

NURSING RESPONSIBILITIES

- For circumferential burn wounds of the extremity, assess the extremity for absence of blood flow:
  a. Using a Doppler ultrasound stethoscope, check hourly for the presence of a pulse.
  b. Assess the extremity hourly for warmth, color, sensation, and capillary refill.
  c. Observe for evidence of numbness or tingling.
- For circumferential burn wounds of the torso, assess for evidence of respiratory distress:
  a. Obtain ABGs as needed.
  b. Auscultate lung sounds hourly.
  c. Observe for evidence of cyanosis, tachypnea, anxiety, or restlessness.
- For circumferential burn wounds of the neck, assess for evidence of respiratory distress. Prepare the patient for prophylactic intubation.
- Monitor for excessive blood loss, and transfuse the patient if indicated.
- Dress the open wound (escharotomy) with topical antimicrobial agents as ordered.

PATIENT TEACHING

- Teach the patient the importance of reporting any evidence of impaired circulation: numbness, tingling, blue color to the extremity, absence of sensation.
- Assure the patient that the procedure will not be painful and will provide immediate relief.
- Teach the patient the importance of protecting the open wound (escharotomy) from infection.
- Explain the rationale supporting prophylactic intubation for burn wounds involving the head and neck.
- Provide assurance that all blood loss will be replaced and that bleeding at the site will be controlled.

Surgical Debridement. **Surgical debridement** refers to the process of excising the wound to the level of fascia (fascial excision) or sequentially removing thin slices of the burn wound to the level of viable tissue (tangential excision). Because **fascial excision**, or **fasciectomy**, sacrifices potentially viable fat and lymphatic tissue, its use is reserved for patients with extensive or full-thickness burns. The most common technique is electrocautery with cutting and coagulating current capabilities. Tangential excision is performed with the use of a dermatome. Shallow burns and some of moderate depth bleed briskly after one slice. If bleeding does not occur, the procedure is repeated until a viable bed of dermis or subcutaneous fat is reached. Following surgical debridement, the patient is returned to the burn unit.

Autografting. A procedure performed in the surgical suite, **autografting** is used to effect permanent skin coverage. Early burn wound excision and skin grafting decrease the hospital stay and enhance rehabilitation. Skin is removed from healthy tissue (donor site) of the burn-injured patient and applied to the burn wound (**Figure 17.11** ■ and **Figure 17.12** ■). (Skin grafts and flaps are discussed in Chapter 16.) After the autograft is applied, the grafted area is immobilized. The site is assessed daily for evidence of adherence. The patient resumes ROM exercises 5 days postgraft. As the wound heals, the patient may complain of itching, which can be treated with mild lotions.

Cultured epithelial autografting is a technique in which skin cells are removed from unburned sites on the patient's body, then minced and placed in a culture medium for growth. Over a 5- to 7-day period, the cells expand to 50 to 70 times the size of the initial biopsies. The cells are again separated out and placed in a new culture medium for continued growth. With this technique, enough skin can be grown over a period of 3 to 4 weeks to cover an entire human body. The cells are prepared in sheets and attached to petroleum jelly gauze backing, which is applied to the burn wound site. Problems with infection and lack of attachment have occurred.

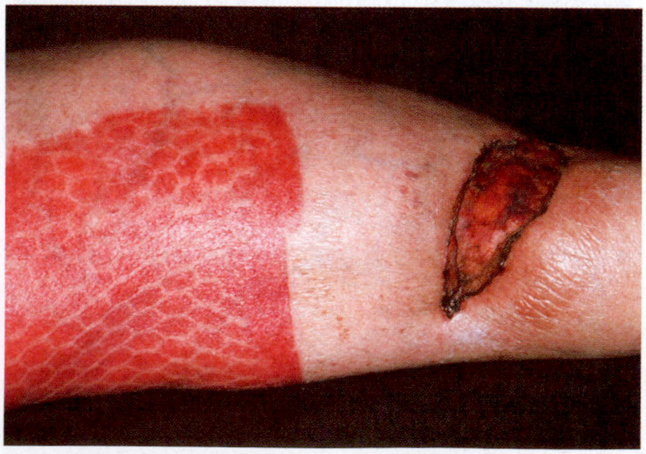

Figure 17.11 ■ Skin graft for burn injury (autograft).

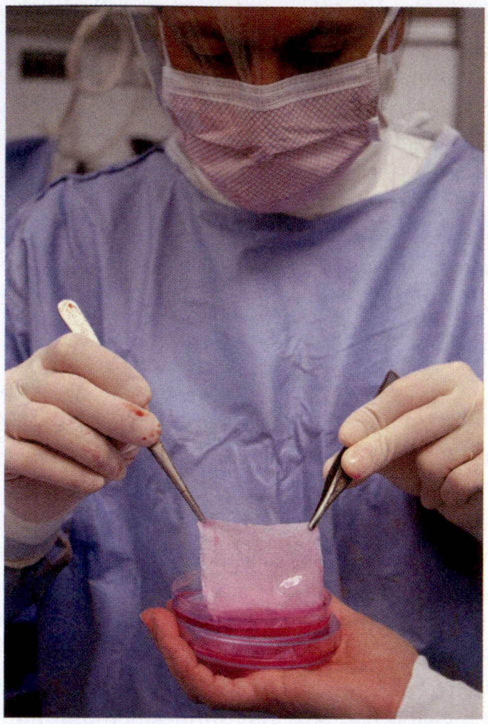

Figure 17.12 ■ Cultured epithelial autografting of a skin culture.

Biologic and Biosynthetic Dressings. The terms *biologic dressing* and *biosynthetic dressing* refer to any temporary material that rapidly adheres to the wound bed, promotes healing, and/or prepares the burn wound for permanent autograft coverage. Ideally, these kinds of dressings should be easy to apply and remove, inexpensive, nonantigenic, elastic, able to reduce pain, able to serve as a bacterial barrier, and able to enhance the natural healing process. The dressings are applied to the burn wound as soon as possible. Covering the wound eliminates the loss of water through evaporation, reduces infection, and promotes wound healing. Biologic and biosynthetic dressings that are currently in use include homograft (allograft), heterograft (xenograft), and synthetic materials.

Homograft, or **allograft**, is human skin that has been harvested from cadavers. It is stored in skin banks located throughout the nation. The development of methods to achieve prolonged storage of frozen, viable skin has increased the use of this dressing; however, its short supply and expense still pose problems. It is manufactured as strips cut to the pattern of the burn and applied using sterile technique. Under normal circumstances, a homograft provides effective temporary closure for 14 to 21 days following application.

Heterograft, or **xenograft**, is skin obtained from an animal, usually a pig. Although fresh porcine heterograft is available to some centers, frozen heterograft is much more commonly used. Once applied, heterograft appears to undergo early softening and lysis from enzymatic action from the wound. As a result, frequent changes of the heterograft dressing are necessary. Because of the high infection rates associated with this dressing, silver nitrate–treated porcine heterograft has been developed to retard microbial growth.

The multiple problems associated with the use of biologic dressings have driven the development of synthetic materials. One such material is Biobrane® (Smith & Nephew Global Products), a composite material consisting of nylon mesh bonded to silicone that has proved successful in the temporary coverage of second- and third-degree burns. Whereas Biobrane adheres well to moderately clean wounds, it cannot adhere to or lower bacterial counts in grossly contaminated wounds. Biobrane dressing is supplied in various sizes, cut to fit the wound site, and secured with tape or Steri-Strips. It spontaneously separates from the wound when the underlying tissue heals. Other biosynthetic wound dressings include Integra® (Integra Life Sciences Corp.) and Alloderm® (LifeCell Corp.). If dermal thickness is lost in deep partial-thickness or full-thickness burns, several products can serve as a dermal replacement. Integra is a synthetic dermal substitute, and Alloderm is human cadaver allograft dermis that is nonimmunogenic. These products are placed in the wound, and split-thickness autografts are then placed over the dermal replacement. These products are used to provide temporary wound coverage, reduce pain, and facilitate healing.

Two other temporary skin substitutes are TransCyte® (Advanced Biohealing) and Apligraf® (Organogenesis Inc.). TransCyte is a bioengineered substance, derived from human fibroblast cells grown within mesh. As the cells grow, they secrete human dermal collagen, matrix proteins, and growth factors. The product is produced, extensively tested for any infectious agents, and then frozen. It is used as a temporary covering for surgically debrided full-thickness and deep partial-thickness burn wounds and is an alternative to silver sulfadiazine and cadaver skin. TransCyte forms a transparent, protective barrier over the wound surface and is typically applied only once. The best results have been obtained when it was applied within 24 hours of injury. Apligraf is bilayered skin substitute cultured from neonatal foreskin.

Hydrocolloid dressings such as DuoDERM® (ConvaTec) are a type of synthetic material. They are occlusive wafers of gumlike materials that provide a water-resistant outer layer for coverage of the donor site. They protect healing tissue from excessive drying, liquefy necrotic tissue, and absorb wound drainage. Other synthetics are Aquacel® (ConvaTec), a temporary dressing (up to 14 days) that is impregnated with silver; Acticoat® (Smith & Nephew Inc.), an antimicrobial barrier dressing; and Calcium alginate [Kaltostat®] (ConvaTec), a calcium alginate absorptive dressing.

The newest treatment method uses a vacuum-assisted closure (VAC) device. VAC consists of a sponge placed over the wound and tubing that connects the sponge to a pump. An occlusive, adhesive dressing covers the wound and tubing, sealing the wound to create negative pressure. VAC has shown positive results in reducing wound edema, removing exudate, and improving wound healing in partial-thickness burns and deep hand burns.

Wound Management. The outcomes of care for the patient with a major burn depend on the prevention and treatment of infection through daily topical wound care, wound monitoring, and wound excision and closure. The goals of wound management are:

- Control microbial colonization and prevent wound infection.
- Prevent wound progression.
- Achieve wound coverage as early as possible.
- Promote function of healing skin.

Debriding the Wound. Burned tissue releases chemical mediators that stimulate phagocytosis in an attempt to digest debris left by decaying necrotic tissue. Necrotic tissue that remains despite phagocytic action retards healing and prolongs inflammation. **Debridement** is the process of removing all loose tissue, wound debris, and eschar (dead tissue) from the wound. Three methods of debridement are employed: mechanical, enzymatic, and surgical (surgical debridement was previously discussed).

A nurse may perform mechanical debridement by applying and removing gauze dressings (wet-to-dry or wet-to-moist), hydrotherapy, irrigation, or scissors and tweezers. However, removal of gauze dressings can cause pain and possibly damage granulation tissue. During hydrotherapy (in an immersion tank, a shower, or on a spray table) the burn injury may be gently washed with a mild, nonperfumed, antimicrobial soap or wound cleaner solution to remove dead skin and separate eschar. The solution is then rinsed off with warm saline or tap water. Body hair (except for eyebrows) should be shaved within the burn and to within 2.5 cm of the wound edges. Blistered skin is grasped with a dry gauze and gently removed. The edges of blisters or eschar are trimmed with blunt scissors. The wound is then covered with a topical antimicrobial agent.

Enzymatic debridement involves the use of a topical agent to dissolve and remove necrotic tissue, as well as lift eschar. An enzyme (such as Accuzyme, collagenase [Santyl], or fibrinolysis-deoxyribonuclease [Elase]) is applied in a thin layer only within the wound area and covered with one layer of fine mesh gauze. A topical antimicrobial agent is then applied and covered with a bulky wet dressing; the wound is immobilized with expandable mesh gauze. Enzymatic agents are discontinued once the eschar is removed and granulation tissue appears.

Dressing the Wound. Once the wound has been cleaned and debrided, it may be dressed using one of two methods. In the open method, the burn wound remains open to air, covered only by a topical antimicrobial agent. This method allows the wound to be easily assessed. Topical agents must be frequently reapplied because they tend to rub off onto the bedding. The open method also increases the risk for hypothermia.

In the closed method, a topical antimicrobial agent is applied to the wound site, which is covered with gauze or a nonadherent dressing and then gently wrapped with a gauze roll bandage (**Figure 17.13** ■). With the closed method, burn wounds are usually dressed twice daily and as needed. Dressings are applied circumferentially in a

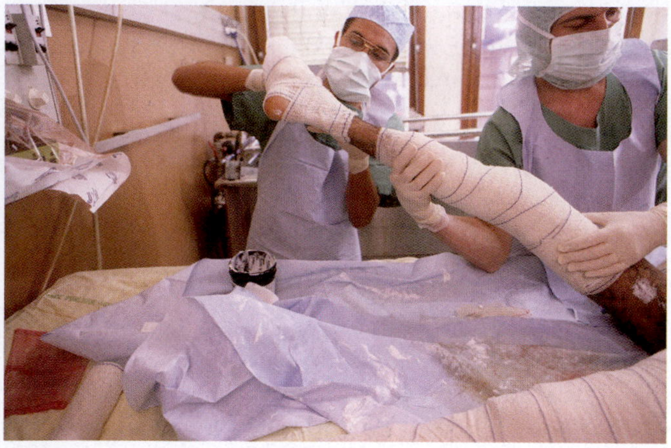

Figure 17.13 ■ Closed method of dressing a burn.

distal-to-proximal manner. All fingers and toes are wrapped separately. Dressings are held in place with stockinettes rather than tape to prevent further skin injury. The closed method decreases heat loss but may impair range of motion.

Positioning, Splints, and Exercise. **Contractures** are a common problem for patients with burn injuries. During therapy, the patient must be maintained in positions that prevent contractures from forming. Because flexion is the natural resting position of joints and extremities, early physical therapy includes maintaining antideformity positions. Splints immobilize body parts and prevent contractures of the joints. They are applied as soon as possible after the injury and removed according to schedules established by a physical therapist or occupational therapist.

Early in the acute phase of care, a physical therapist or occupational therapist prescribes active and passive ROM exercises, which are performed every 2 hours at the bedside, most often by physical therapy. Ideally an exercise program is initiated on admission and continued until wounds are healed. Early ambulation is also part of the plan of care once the patient's condition becomes stable.

Support Garments. Applying uniform pressure can prevent or reduce hypertrophic scarring. Tubular support bandages are applied 5 to 7 days postgraft to maintain a tension ranging from 10 to 20 mmHg to control scarring. The patient wears custom-made elastic pressure garments such as a Jobst garment for 6 months to a year postgraft. The garments are to be worn 7 days/week, 23 to 24 hours per day.

Nutritional Support. The patient with a major burn is in a hypermetabolic and catabolic state. The resting energy expenditure after severe burn injury can increase by as much as 100% above normal levels, depending on the extent of catabolism and the patient's physical activity, size, age, and gender. This increase is believed to be due to heat loss from the burn wound, an increase in beta-adrenergic activity, pain, and infection. As a result, total caloric needs may be as great as 4000 to 6000 kcal per day.

Traditional dietary management based on oral intake seldom meets the kcal requirements necessary to reverse negative nitrogen balance and begin the healing process. Enteral feedings with a nasointestinal feeding tube are therefore instituted within 24 to 48 hours of the burn injury to offset hypermetabolism, improve nitrogen balance, decrease sepsis, and decrease length of hospital stay. A nasointestinal feeding tube is placed under fluoroscopy, with the tip extending past the pylorus to prevent reflux and aspiration.

Although enteral feeding is the preferred nutritional therapy, it is contraindicated in Curling ulcer, bowel obstruction, feeding intolerance, pancreatitis, or septic ileus. When the enteral route cannot be used, a central venous catheter is inserted via the subclavian or jugular vein for the administration of total parenteral nutrition (TPN).

Nursing Care

The patient with a major burn has complex, multisystem needs. **Table 17.5** lists overall nursing interventions for the emergent, acute, and rehabilitative stages of burn injury. Also see the Case Study & Nursing Care Plan on page 543.

Assessment

Nursing assessment is continuous from the time of initial contact with a patient with a burn injury. This section describes the survey conducted when the patient arrives at the emergency department (ED).

Priorities of Care

Collaborating with the interprofessional team to deliver adequate treatment of the underlying burn injury while providing care that supports the physical and psychologic responses to the injury is a nursing priority. Once the patient arrives in the ED, the interprofessional team must act quickly to obtain the patient's history of the burn injury, including the time of injury, causative agents, early treatment, medical history, and patient's age and body weight. In most cases, the patient is awake and oriented and able to relate the information during the emergent phase of care. Because changes in sensorium will become evident within the first few hours following a major burn injury, the nurse obtains as much information as is possible immediately on the patient's arrival.

- ***Time of injury.*** In many cases, the patient is admitted to the ED an hour or more after the injury occurred. The time of the burn injury must be documented as precisely as possible at the scene because all fluid resuscitation calculations are based on the time of the burn injury, not on the patient's time of arrival at the ED.
- ***Cause of the injury.*** Because the type of burn injury determines which nursing measures take priority, identify the specific causative agent to establish the appropriate plan of care.
- ***First-aid treatment.*** Prior to the arrival of medical personnel, the patient or family may have applied home remedies to treat the burn wound. It is important for the nurse to ascertain and document the nature of all home treatment interventions, including the application of neutralizing agents, liquids, and immobilizing devices used to splint associated injuries.

Table 17.5 Interventions in Various Stages of Burn Injury

Stage of Burn Injury	Onset	End Point	Interventions
Emergent/resuscitative	Occurrence of burn injury	Successful fluid resuscitation	■ Remove patient from heat source. ■ Initiate first-aid. ■ Assess extent of burn injury. ■ Prevent hypothermia. ■ Assess for shock. ■ Determine need for intubation. ■ Determine need for intravenous therapy. ■ Follow protocol for fluid resuscitation. ■ Obtain history. ■ Transport to tertiary care facility.
Acute	Diuresis	Wound closure	■ Begin hydrotherapy. ■ Determine need for excision of burn wound. ■ Control spread of infection. ■ Institute wound care. ■ Start nutrition support. ■ Graft burn wound. ■ Initiate physical therapy. ■ Manage pain.
Rehabilitative	Wound closure	Return to highest level of health restoration	■ Prevent scar formation. ■ Continue physical therapy. ■ Address psychosocial, cultural, and spiritual needs. ■ Consider occupational therapy. ■ Consider vocational training. ■ Assess home maintenance management.

- ***Past medical history.*** Patients with histories of respiratory, cardiac, renal, metabolic, neurologic, gastrointestinal, or skin diseases; alcohol abuse; or altered immune states require more intense observation. Known allergies are obtained.
- ***Age.*** Older adults tend to require more supportive care and are at greater risk for burns of all degrees of severity. See Chapter 15.

  The care of the older adult with burns presents unique challenges. They may delay seeking treatment, thus increasing the risk of infection. Their care is often complicated by the presence of other chronic illnesses. They may live alone and have no one to care for them during rehabilitation. Even small burns have the potential to become lethal in older adults.

  Burn prevention topics for older adults are:

  a. Have a relative or neighbor routinely check for the odor of gas.
  b. Check the smoke detector battery once a month.
  c. Wear close-fitting clothing when cooking.
  d. Use a cooking timer with a loud alarm.
  e. Never lay anything over a heating device.
  f. Set the temperature of the hot water heater no higher than 120°F.
  g. Install antiscald devices in bathroom plumbing.
  h. Encourage no smoking in the house.
- ***Medications.*** Drugs, either prescribed or recreational, taken by the patient prior to the burn injury may further complicate the treatment regimen. Drugs that affect any of the major body systems or cause mood alterations will need to be factored into the treatment plan. As part of the early assessment, obtain and document blood levels of therapeutic pharmaceutical agents and mood-altering substances.
- ***Body weight.*** During the acute and rehabilitative phases of the burn injury, the patient will lose as much as 20% of preburn weight. This fact will have significant implications for all patients, especially for those who are underweight or cachectic at the time of the injury.

Diagnoses, Outcomes, and Interventions

A major burn affects virtually every body system, as well as social, cultural, economic, psychologic, and spiritual well-being. Immediate treatment in an intensive care setting is followed by years of rehabilitation and a lifetime of change in what was possible for an individual before the injury. Nursing care for the patient with a major burn injury includes maintaining skin integrity and fluid volume, managing pain, reducing risk for infection, assisting with physical mobility, promoting appropriate nutrition, and providing emotional support.

Maintain Skin Integrity. The burn injury significantly impairs skin integrity. The severity of wounds varies according to the depth and extent of the burn. General treatment measures are designed to restore normal skin function as quickly as possible. Nursing care focuses on assessing and cleansing the wound and controlling infection.

Expected Outcome: Patient will experience effective wound healing and infection management as evidenced by skin integrity and body temperature within normal range.

The nurse will:

- Estimate the extent and depth of the burn wound and recalculate extent of unhealed burns weekly. *The severity of the burn injury is the basis for determining which types of interventions are appropriate. Reassessment on a regular basis is necessary to monitor the healing process.*

- Provide daily wound care (including debridement method, dressing method, and medication administration) as prescribed *to remove dead tissue, control infection, and promote reepithelialization as soon as possible.*

SAFETY ALERT: When cleansing wounds, avoid cross-contamination of the patient's wounds. ■

- Elevate burned or newly skin-grafted extremities at or above heart level *to increase venous return and to prevent edema formation.*
- Immobilize skin graft sites for 3 to 5 days or as ordered *to promote graft adherence and to prevent loss of newly grafted skin.*

SAFETY ALERT: Move patients slowly and carefully across bed sheets to prevent shearing or dislodgement of the new skin grafts. ■

- Provide special skin care to sensitive body areas:
  a. Clean burns involving the eyes with normal saline or sterile water *to prevent corneal and conjunctival drying and adherence.* If contracture of the eyelid develops, apply drops or ointment to the eye *to prevent corneal abrasion.*
  b. Gently wipe burns of the lips with saline-soaked pads. Apply an antibiotic ointment as prescribed. Assess the mouth frequently, and perform mouth care routinely. If an oral endotracheal tube is in place, reposition it often *to prevent pressure ulcer formation.*
  c. Gently debride burns of the nose, and apply mafenide acetate (Sulfamylon) cream. Position nasogastric and nasotracheal tubes *to prevent excessive pressure.*
  d. Apply mafenide acetate (Sulfamylon) cream to burns of the ear. Gently debride and thoroughly clean the wound with a water spray. Do not cover ears with dressings. Do not use pillows; to reduce pressure to the area, use a foam doughnut instead. *Burns of the ears are prone to infection; special positioning devices are necessary to decrease pressure ulcer formation.*

Maintain Fluid Balance. Fluid resuscitation rates are adjusted periodically throughout the emergent stage of care. The nurse should be particularly aware of several situations that may warrant the administration of fluids at rates in excess of the calculations needed to maintain adequate urine output: initial underestimation of the burn size, sequestration of fluid into the lung tissue in inhalation injury, electrical injury (which tends to cause more extensive damage than is immediately visible), full-thickness burns, and inordinately delayed starts of fluid resuscitation.

Expected Outcome: Patient will achieve fluid balance as evidenced by blood pressure, pulse, and temperature readings within normal limits and adequate urine output.

The nurse will:

- Assess blood pressure and heart rate frequently. Note that tachycardia in the burn patient is not considered until the heart rate is greater than 120 bpm. *Vital signs rapidly deteriorate when fluid resuscitation is inadequate.*
- Monitor hemodynamic status, including CVP and PCWP. *Inadequate fluid resuscitation is manifested by a drop in the central venous pressure and pulmonary capillary wedge pressure.*
- Follow prescribed protocols for intravenous fluid resuscitation. *Therapy for burn shock is aimed at supporting the patient through the period of hypovolemic instability.*
- Monitor intake and output hourly. *Report urine outputs of less than 50 mL/h. Intake and output measurements indicate the adequacy of fluid resuscitation and should range from 30 to 50 mL/h in an adult.*
- Weigh daily. *Body weight is used to calculate fluid requirements.*
- Test all stools and emesis for the presence of blood. *Occult blood in emesis or stool indicates gastrointestinal bleeding.*
- Maintain a warm environment. *Hypothermia leads to shivering and further loss of body fluid through increased energy expenditure and catabolism.*
- Monitor for fluid volume overload. *Older patients and those with underlying cardiac disease may demonstrate symptoms of heart failure during the fluid resuscitation stage.*

SAFETY ALERT: Patients with major burns receive 10 or more liters of fluid and will gain weight with the fluid shifts. When capillary membrane integrity resumes, patients have a high CVP and urine output that necessitates monitoring urine electrolytes. ■

Manage Acute Pain. The patient experiences excruciating pain with extensive superficial and all partial-thickness burns. Intense pain is also experienced during wound care and physical therapy. In addition, increased levels of anxiety about treatments and outcomes may further increase the perception of pain.

Expected Outcome: Patient will achieve adequate pain control as evidenced by reduced pain-related behaviors and by effective patient rest and sleep behaviors.

The nurse will:

- Measure the patient's level of pain, using a consistent measurement tool. *Pain tolerance is the duration and intensity of pain that the patient is able to endure. Pain tolerance differs from one patient to the next and may vary in the same patient in different situations.*
- Medicate before painful procedures and determine when PCA is appropriate. *The inability to manage pain results in feelings of despair and frustration.*
- Administer intravenous narcotic analgesics as prescribed. *Nurses' fear of precipitating addiction often makes them reluctant to administer narcotics. During the acute*

stage of burn injury, however, invasive procedures and exposed neurosensory nerve endings dictate the need for narcotic pharmaceutical agents.

- Explain all procedures and expected levels of discomfort. *Patients who are prepared for painful procedures and know beforehand the actual sensations they will feel experience less stress.*
- Use methods of nonnarcotic pain control in combination with medications for pain. *Noninvasive pain relief measures (e.g., relaxation, massage, distraction) can enhance the therapeutic effects of pain relief medications.*
- Allow the patient to verbalize the pain experience. *Each person experiences and expresses pain in his or her own manner, using various sociocultural adaptation techniques.*

SAFETY ALERT: Narcotics are always administered intravenously rather than orally, subcutaneously, or intramuscularly in the emergent or acute stage of a burn due to decreased circulation and absorption of medications. ■

Reduce Risk of Infection. From the onset of the burn injury, loss of the body's natural barrier to the external environment increases the risk of infection. Nursing interventions focus on controlling infectious processes. Monitor the results of diagnostic tests, maintain nutritional therapies, and apply antimicrobial agents to monitor and prevent the spread of infection, a major complication of the burn injury.

Expected Outcome: Patient will experience effective infection management and control as evidenced by freedom from symptoms of infection, maintenance of WBC count and differential, and vital signs within normal limits.

The nurse will:

- Monitor daily for manifestations of wound infection. Remove topical medications and wound exudate and examine the entire wound. *Early manifestations of wound infection include swelling and inflammation in intact skin surrounding the wound; a change in the color, odor, or amount of exudate; increased pain; and loss of previously healed skin grafts.*
- Monitor for positive blood cultures, *which indicate bacteremia.*
- Monitor for hyperemia, cough, chest pain, wheezing, rhonchi, decreased oxygen saturation, and purulent sputum, *which are manifestations of pneumonia.*
- Monitor for the presence of bacteria in the urine, fever, urgency, frequency, dysuria, and superpubic pain, *which are manifestations of urinary tract infections.*
- Obtain daily WBC counts. *Leukocyte counts are indicators of immune system function; they increase in the presence of infection.*
- Determine tetanus immunization status. *Burn patients are at risk for anaerobic infection caused by* Clostridium tetani.
- Maintain high kilocalorie intake. *Nutritional support provides the nutrients needed to maintain the body's defense mechanisms.*
- Maintain an aseptic environment, using standard precautions (including gloving, gowning, and sterile procedures). *Strict isolation technique deters the development of a nosocomial infection.*
- Culture all wounds and body secretions per protocol. *Culture and sensitivity reports identify the presence of infectious microbes and indicate appropriate antimicrobial therapies.*
- Administer prescribed antimicrobial medications *to decrease invasive wound infections.*
- If the patient has an indwelling catheter, assess the urine for cloudiness and a foul odor, and obtain a urine culture and sensitivity at least weekly. *Urine culture and sensitivity reports identify presence of infectious microbes and indicate appropriate antimicrobial therapies.*

Assist with Physical Mobility. As the burn wound heals and new skin tissue forms, the involved area tends to shrink. Contractures form at the site and significantly limit mobility, especially when a joint is involved. Physical therapy is important, beginning in the early stages of treatment. The nurse institutes ambulation and planned exercise regimens as soon as the patient's condition stabilizes.

Expected Outcome: Maintenance of joint ROM with progression to transfers and ambulation.

The nurse will:

- Perform active or passive ROM exercises to all joints every 2 hours. Ambulate when stable. *Regular exercise prevents further loss of motion, restores movement, and improves functional status.*
- Apply splints as prescribed. Maintain antideformity positions, and reposition the patient hourly. *Splinting and positioning retard the formation of contractures.*
- Maintain limbs in functional alignment *to preserve joint mobility.*
- Anticipate the need for analgesia. *Administering analgesics promotes the patient's comfort during exercise sessions.*
- Assess all patients, but especially the older adult, for indications of pressure ulcer formation under a splint. *Careful integumentary assessment can prevent pressure ulcer formation by early detection of skin changes.*

Promote Appropriate Nutrition. The burn injury initiates a complex series of events that have a profound effect on the body's use of nutrients and expenditure of energy. Daily kilocalorie requirements are determined by the nutritionist, and enteral feedings are initiated as soon as possible. Nasointestinal tubes are placed to enhance intestinal absorption and retard gastric reflux. Parenteral nutrition is reserved for instances in which enteral feedings are contraindicated. Nursing measures focus on assessing feeding tolerance and use of nutrients.

Expected Outcome: Patient's nutritional intake will be adequate for meeting physiologic processes as evidenced by oral or enteral intake of a high-protein, high-nutrient diet.

Moving Evidence into Action

The Patient with a Major Burn

Clinical Issue

Due to the loss of the skin barrier and fluid shifts, patients with major burn injuries require fluid resuscitation to prevent onset of shock and to maintain cardiovascular stability. An ongoing discussion relates to the use of colloid versus crystalloid fluids.

External Evidence

Perel, Roberts, and Ker (2013) conducted a systematic review and meta-analysis comparing colloids versus crystalloids for fluid resuscitation in the critically ill patient, including burn patients. They identified 78 studies and included the 70 that reported mortality data. The authors found that colloids did not improve survival and, in fact, the use of hydroxyethyl starch was suspected of increasing mortality risk. Due to the combination of higher cost and lack of survival benefit, colloids are not supported by the evidence for use for fluid resuscitation in the critically ill patient.

Internal Evidence

As part of the evaluation of internal evidence, one must consider the clinical feasibility (including access to the appropriate resuscitative fluids), the outcome of interest (prevention of shock development), current policies/procedures in place for fluid resuscitation, and identification of stakeholders that influence uptake of the proposed intervention. One question to ask: Is this problem (increased risk for development of shock in the severe burn patient) significant in the population of your care environment? Does the clinical environment support the use of the intervention? What about the cost benefit of the new intervention? In this example of colloid solution versus crystalloid solution for fluid resuscitation, Bisonni, Holtgrave, Lawler, and Marley (1991) reported that per life saved cost for crystalloids was $45.13, while per life saved cost for colloidal solutions was $1493.60 (1990 dollars).

Patient Considerations

When considering use of a new intervention, the nurse must consider the specific patient population where it will be used. Will patients and their families be amenable to the new intervention?

Putting the Pieces Together

The design and implementation of a pressure ulcer prevention and treatment plan are essential for any person at risk. To effectively implement a plan, it is important to evaluate the external evidence and consider the internal implications and patient/family issues. With the implementation of a new prevention intervention, the outcome (occurrence of pressure ulcer development) should be assessed in every patient and unit-level information should be collected and evaluated on a regular basis.

References

Bisonni, R. S., Holtgrave, D. R., Lawler, F., & Marley, D. S. (1991). Colloids versus crystalloids in fluid resuscitation: An analysis of randomized controlled trials. *Journal of Family Practice*, *32*(4), 390–397.

Perel, R., Roberts, I., & Ker, K. (2013). Colloids versus crystalloids for fluid resuscitation in critically ill patients. *Cochrane Database of Systematic Reviews*, Issue 2. Article No.: CD000567. DOI: 10.1002/14651858.CD000567.pub6.

The nurse will:

- Maintain nasogastric/nasointestinal tube placement. *Correct tube placement ensures appropriate absorption of nutrients and prevents aspiration.*
- Maintain enteral/parenteral nutritional support as prescribed. Observe and report any evidence of feeding intolerance: diarrhea, vomiting, excessive gastric residual, abdominal distention, absent bowel sounds, and constipation. *The nutritionist, in collaboration with the physician, selects and individualizes the feeding formula according to the patient's daily energy expenditure requirements and feeding tolerance. Failure to maintain rates of infusion predisposes the patient to continued catabolism and negative nitrogen balance.*
- Weigh the patient daily. *Weight indicates the adequacy of nutritional support therapies.*
- Obtain daily laboratory values for protein, iron, CBC, glucose, and albumin. *Decreased serum values indicate inadequate nutritional intake.*

Provide Emotional Support. Usually, the patient with a major burn injury endures a lengthy hospital stay involving many treatments and care protocols that are beyond his or her control. During the early stages, much of the care regimen involves excruciating pain. Furthermore, the foreign environment of the burn unit makes it difficult for the patient to relate to the immediate surroundings. For example, the need to control infection in the burn unit requires hospital personnel and family members to don sterile clothing prior to coming to the patient's bedside. Family members and nursing personnel appear radically different when they are masked and gowned, and their odd appearance can add to the burn-injured patient's sense of alienation. The patient's body image is often altered, depending on the extent and location of the burn injury. Support and education should include the patient's family. See **Box 17.2** for detailed information regarding patient and family education.

Expected Outcome: Patient will resolve feelings of powerlessness and other related feelings as evidenced by participation in planning and implementation of care.

The nurse will:

- Allow the patient as much control over the surroundings and daily routine as possible. For example, allow the patient to choose times of dressing changes. *Powerlessness derives from the belief that one is unable to influence the outcome of a situation.*

- Keep needed items within reach, such as call bell, urinal, water pitcher, and tissues, *to reinforce the patient's feelings of control.*
- Encourage the patient to express feelings. *The nurse can help the patient cope by therapeutically listening, displaying a caring presence, clarifying misconceptions, and providing positive feedback.*
- Set short-term, realistic goals (e.g., set a goal for the patient to ambulate from bedside to chair twice daily). *Small incremental gains are easier to achieve than large ones and allow for frequent positive reinforcement.*

Box 17.2
Patient and Family Teaching

Patient and family teaching is an important component of all phases of burn care. As treatment progresses, the nurse encourages family members to assume more responsibility in providing care. From admission to discharge, the nurse teaches the patient and family to assess all findings, implement therapies, and evaluate progress. The following topics should be addressed in preparing the patient and family for home care:

- The long-term goals of rehabilitation care: to prevent soft tissue deformity, protect skin grafts, maintain physiologic function, manage scars, and return the patient to an optimal level of independence
- Avoiding exposure to people with colds or infections and following aseptic technique meticulously when caring for the wound
- The need for progressive physical activity
- How to apply splints, pressure support garments, and other assistive devices
- Dietary requirements with required kilocalories
- Alternative pain control therapies, such as guided imagery, relaxation techniques, and diversional activities
- Care of the graft and donor sites
- Referral for occupational therapy, social service, clergy, and/or psychiatric services as appropriate
- Helpful resources:
  a. American Burn Association
  b. International Society for Burn Injuries
  c. American Academy of Facial Plastic and Reconstructive Surgery.

Case Study & Nursing Care Plan
A Patient with a Major Burn

Craig Howard, a 39-year-old truck driver, is admitted to the hospital following an accident in which the cab of his truck caught on fire. He was freed from the truck by a passing motorist, who stayed with him until the rescue team arrived and transported him to a local emergency department (ED). Mr. Howard's wife, Mary, and twin daughters, Jessica and Jane, age 10, have been notified.

ASSESSMENT	DIAGNOSIS	EXPECTED OUTCOMES
On his admission to the ED, Mr. Howard is diagnosed with deep partial-thickness and full-thickness burns of the anterior chest, arms, and hands. A quick assessment based on the rule of nines estimates the extent of his burn injury at 36% TBSA. His vital signs are as follows: T 35.6°C (96.2°F), P 140 bpm, R 40/min, and BP 98/60 mmHg. In the field, the paramedics had inserted a large-bore central line into Mr. Howard's right subclavian vein and started the rapid infusion of lactated Ringer solution. Mr. Howard is receiving 40% humidified oxygen via face mask. Initial ABGs are pH 7.49, PO_2 60 mmHg, PCO_2 32 mmHg, and bicarbonate 22 mEq/L. Lung sounds indicate inspiratory and expiratory wheezing, and a persistent cough reveals sooty sputum production. A Foley catheter is inserted and initially drains a moderate amount of dark, concentrated urine. A nasogastric tube is connected to low-intermittent suction. Mr. Howard is alert and oriented and complains of severe pain associated with the burn injuries. The burn unit is notified, and Mr. Howard is transferred there.	■ Potential for impaired airway related to increasing lung congestion secondary to smoke inhalation ■ Fluid volume deficit related to abnormal fluid loss secondary to burn injury ■ Potential for inadequate peripheral tissue perfusion related to peripheral constriction secondary to circumferential burn wounds of the arms	■ Patient will demonstrate a patent airway, as evidenced by clear breath sounds; absence of cyanosis; and vital signs, chest x-ray findings, and ABGs within normal limits. ■ Patient will demonstrate adequate fluid volume and electrolyte balance, as evidenced by urine output, vital signs, mental status, and laboratory findings within normal limits (Kee, 2018). ■ Patient will demonstrate adequate tissue perfusion, as evidenced by palpable pulses, warm extremities, normal capillary refill, and absence of paresthesia.

(continued)

PLANNING AND IMPLEMENTATION

- Prepare for prophylactic nasotracheal intubation to maintain airway patency.
- Initiate fluid resuscitation therapy using the Consensus formula to calculate intravenous fluid rate for the first 24 hours postburn.
- Assist the physician to perform escharotomies of both upper extremities.

EVALUATION

The nurse anesthetist inserted a nasotracheal tube and connected Mr. Howard to a T-piece delivering 40% oxygen. Vigorous respiratory toileting has significantly improved his ABGs. Bronchodilators have been parenterally administered and mucolytic agents added to his respiratory treatments. His tracheal secretions have begun to show evidence of clearing. Hourly urine outputs indicate adequate fluid resuscitation. Urine output has been maintained at 50 mL/h, and color and concentration have improved. CVP readings have been maintained at 6 cm H_2O, and blood pressure has increased to 100/64 mmHg. The pulse rate has decreased to 100 bpm.

To improve tissue perfusion of both arms, the physician has performed bilateral escharotomies and the wounds are dressed, using sterile procedure. The extremities have demonstrated improved circulation.

CLINICAL REASONING IN PATIENT CARE

1. Explain the rationale for the immediate insertion of a Foley catheter and nasogastric tube.
2. An escharotomy was performed on both arms. Why was this procedure necessary in Mr. Howard's case?
3. What is the rationale supporting the intravenous administration of narcotics to control Mr. Howard's pain?
4. Explain the sequence of events that led to a fluid and electrolyte shift during the first 24 to 48 hours after Mr. Howard sustained his injury.

See Evaluating Your Response in Appendix B.

CHAPTER HIGHLIGHTS

17.1 Types of Burn Injury

Discuss the types and causative agents of burns.

- Four types of burn injuries are thermal, chemical, electrical, and radiation.

17.2 Factors Affecting Burn Classification

Explain burn classification by depth and extent of injury.

- The depth of the burn injury determines whether it is classified as a superficial, partial-thickness, or full-thickness burn.
- The "rule of nines" is a simple method to estimate the extent of a burn injury, but the Lund and Browder chart is considered the most accurate method as it compensates for changes in body shape with age.

17.3 Burn Wound Healing

Outline the three stages of burn wound healing.

- There are three stages to burn wound healing: inflammation, proliferation and remodeling. While the healing stages are similar to other wounds, in burns, these stages are longer in time.

17.4 Minor Burns

Describe the pathophysiology and manifestations of minor burns of the skin, and outline the interprofessional care and nursing care of patients with minor burns.

- Minor burn injuries consist of superficial burns that are not extensive. They involve less than 15% of the TBSA. Very limited full-thickness burns (less than 2% TBSA) are also considered minor burns.
- This type of burn injury has not been associated with significant systemic sequelae and are commonly treated in the outpatient setting.

17.5 Major Burns

Describe the pathophysiology and manifestations of major burns of the skin, and outline the interprofessional care and nursing care of patients with major burns.

- Major burns involve multiorgan pathophysiologic alterations. Most critical is the fluid shift from the intracellular and intravascular compartments into the interstitium, resulting in a type of hypovolemic shock called burn shock. Other pathologic processes include an impaired immune system, disturbed functions of the skin, inhalation injury, gastrointestinal ulcerations and ileus, renal failure, and hypermetabolism.

- Interprofessional care focuses on managing the patient during the emergent/resuscitative, acute, and rehabilitative stages. To counter the effects of burn shock, fluid resuscitation using guidelines such as the Consensus formula are initiated to replace fluid and electrolyte losses.
- Additional management for the patient with major burns includes preventing atelectasis, maintaining respiratory function, controlling pain, preventing infection and Curling ulcer, promoting nutrition, and providing wound care.
- Extensive eschar of an extremity or the torso, called circumferential wounds, can potentially occlude arterial flow or decrease respiratory function. An escharotomy is used to release tension, preventing additional complications.
- Surgical management of burn wounds include debridement and skin grafting. Biologic and biosynthetic dressings provide temporary covering and prepare the wound for permanent autografts.
- Continual psychologic support of the patient and family is essential throughout convalescence and rehabilitation.

TEST YOURSELF NCLEX-RN® REVIEW

1. The nurse is reviewing initial laboratory values for the patient who is in burn shock. Treatment had not been initiated prior to the laboratory being drawn. Which results should the nurse expect for the patient? (Select all that apply.)
   A. Increased hematocrit
   B. Increased serum albumin
   C. Decreased serum potassium
   D. Decreased blood urea nitrogen
   E. Decreased blood glucose
2. Which burn level is present if the skin is dry and leathery with no pain sensation present?
   A. Superficial
   B. Full thickness
   C. Deep partial thickness
   D. Superficial partial thickness
3. The nurse is triaging recent patients brought into the burn center. Which patient is most at risk for developing burn shock?
   A. 30-year-old with 10% TBSA from a gasoline explosion
   B. 21-year-old with 30% superficial burn from a tanning bed
   C. 39-year-old with radiation burns following treatment for cancer
   D. 48-year-old with more than 50% TBSA from a high-voltage electrical accident
4. A patient with a major burn is receiving silver sulfadiazine (Silvadene) treatment. What nursing action should be implemented when using this medication?
   A. Monitor WBC count daily.
   B. Monitor urine specific gravity for dehydration.
   C. Monitor serum electrolyte levels daily.
   D. Premedicate for pain prior to application.
5. A patient weighing 70 kg is being treated for full-thickness burns over 50% of the body. Using the Consensus formula, calculate the total amount of fluid replacement that the nurse should deliver in the first 8 hours.
   A. 3000 mL
   B. 7000 mL
   C. 10,500 mL
   D. 14,000 mL
6. The nurse is evaluating the effectiveness of fluid resuscitation provided to An 80-kg patient with a major burn. Which assessment finding indicates that fluid resuscitation has been effective during the first 24 hours of care?
   A. Blood pressure has been 90-96/65-70 mmHg since admission.
   B. Heart rate of 130-140 bpm since admission.
   C. Central venous pressure has been steadily decreasing central venous since fluids were initiated.
   D. Urine output has been 30 to 50 mL/hr for the last 4 hours.
7. The nurse is caring for a patient with deep partial-thickness burns to the entire left arm and left side of the back. After a routine assessment, what finding should be immediately reported to the physician?
   A. Pain in the left arm
   B. Decreased left radial pulse
   C. Fluid-filled vesicles on the left arm
   D. Blanching when pressure applied to the left hand
8. The nurse is calculating the percentage of total body surface area that has been burned for a patient with deep partial-thickness burns to the anterior trunk, perineum, and anterior and posterior left arm. Using the "rule of nines," what is the percent of TBSA that was burned?
   A. 18%
   B. 28%
   C. 36%
   D. 40%

9. The nurse is planning an educational program on burn prevention for residents of a senior citizen apartment complex. Which topics should the nurse include in this presentation? (Select all that apply.)
   A. Check smoke detectors annually.
   B. Set the water heater no higher than 120°F.
   C. Wear close-fitting clothing when cooking.
   D. Install antiscald devices in bathroom plumbing.
   E. Have a neighbor routinely check for the odor of gas.

10. The nurse is caring for a patient with possible carbon monoxide poisoning secondary to smoke inhalation. Which assessment findings are consistent with a 15% carbon monoxide level? (Select all the apply.)
    A. Dizziness
    B. Drowsiness
    C. Hypotension
    D. Dark red skin color
    E. Nausea

See Test Yourself answers in Appendix B.

REFERENCES

Adams, M., Holland, N., & Urban, C. (2017). *Pharmacology for nurses: A pathophysiologic approach* (5th ed.). Boston, MA: Pearson.

American Burn Association. (2017). *Burn incidence fact sheet*. Retrieved from http://ameriburn.org/who-we-are/media/burn-incidence-fact-sheet/.

American College of Surgeons Committee of Trauma. (2018). *ATLS: Advanced trauma life support* (10th ed.). Chicago, IL: American College of Surgeons.

Bisonni, R. S., Holtgrave, D. R., Lawler, F., & Marley, D. S. (1991). Colloids versus crystalloids in fluid resuscitation: An analysis of randomized controlled trials. *Journal of Family Practice*, *32*(4), 390–397.

Centers for Disease Control and Prevention. (2017). *Carbon monoxide poisoning*. Retrieved from https://www.cdc.gov/co/basics.htm.

International Society for Burn Injury (ISBI) Practice Guidelines Committee. (2016). ISBI practice guideline for burn care. *Burns*, *42*(5), 953–1021.

Kee, J. L. (2018). *Laboratory and diagnostic tests with nursing implications* (10th ed.). Boston, MA: Pearson.

Mayo Clinic. (2017). *Burns*. Retrieved from https://www.mayoclinic.org/diseases-conditions/burns/basics/causes/con-20035028.

NANDA International. (2018). *NANDA International, Inc. Nursing diagnoses: Definitions and classification, 2018–2020* (11th ed.) (T. H. Herdman & S. Kamitsuru, Eds.). New York, NY: Thieme.

National Fire Protection Association. (2017). *Campus and dorm fires*. Retrieved from http://www.nfpa.org/Public-Education/By-topic/Property-type-and-vehicles/Campus-and-dorm-fires.

Perel, R., Roberts, I., & Ker, K. (2013). Colloids versus crystalloids for fluid resuscitation in critically ill patients. *Cochrane Database of Systematic Reviews*, Issue 2. Article No.: CD000567. DOI: 10.1002/14651858.CD000567.pub6.

Rice, P. L., & Orgill, D. P. (2018). Classification of burn injury. *UpToDate*. Retrieved from https://www.uptodate.com/contents/classification-of-burn-injury.

Rowley-Conway, G. (2016). How to manage a minor burn. *Nursing Standard*, *30*(47), 53–57.

Sorenson, M., Quinn, L., & Klein, D. (2018). *Pathophysiology: Concepts of human disease*. New York: Pearson.

U.S. Fire Administration. (2017b). *U.S. fire statistics*. Retrieved from https://www.usfa.fema.gov/data/statistics/.

U.S. Fire Administration. (2017a). U.S. fire deaths, fire death rates, and risk of dying in a fire. Retrieved from https://www.usfa.fema.gov/data/statistics/fire_death_rates.html#tab-1b.

ADDITIONAL RESOURCES

Advanced Burn Life Support (ABLS)
ameriburn.org/education/abls-program/abls-now/

American Burn Association
ameriburn.org

Interview with a Burn Care Nurse
www.workingnurse.com/articles/Burn-Care-Nursing-Interview-with-Alison-Gavin-RN

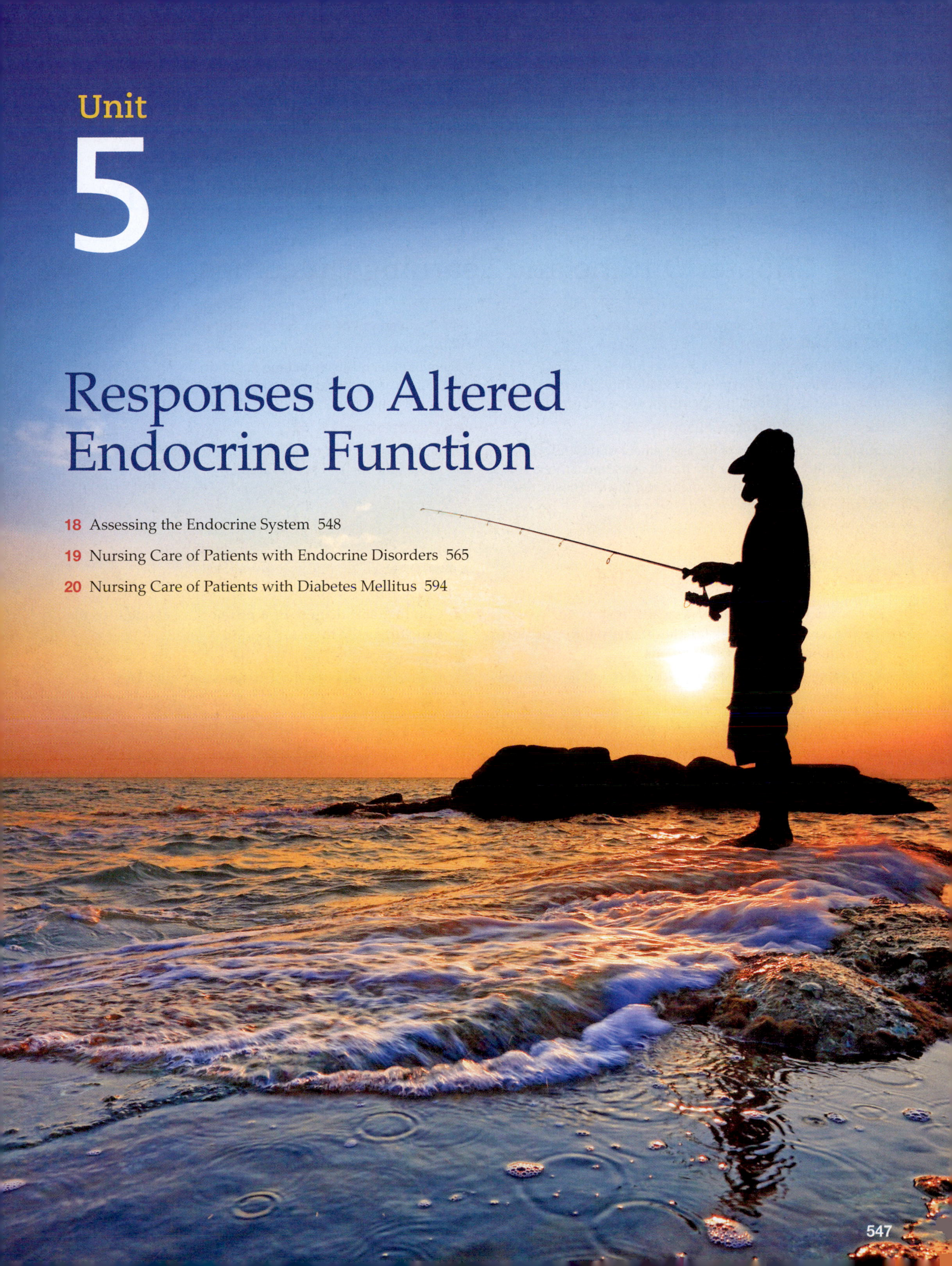

Unit 5

Responses to Altered Endocrine Function

Chapter 18

Assessing the Endocrine System

Chapter Outline and Learning Outcomes

18.1 Anatomy, Physiology, and Functions of the Endocrine System 549

Describe the anatomy, physiology, and functions of the endocrine glands and hormones, and identify abnormal findings that may indicate impairment of the endocrine system.

18.2 Assessing Endocrine Function 553

Outline the components of the assessment of the endocrine system including topics for the health assessment interview, techniques for physical assessment, and the diagnostic tests used in the assessment.

18.3 Assessment of Special Populations 561

Differentiate considerations for assessing the endocrine system of older adults, veterans, individuals in the LGBTQI population, and adults with sequelae of childhood/congenital conditions.

18.4 Health Promotion 562

Summarize topics that nurses teach to promote healthy endocrine function across the lifespan.

CLINICAL COMPETENCIES

- Conduct and document a health history for patients who have or are at risk for alterations in the structure or function of the endocrine glands.
- Monitor the results of diagnostic tests and report abnormal findings.
- Conduct and document a physical assessment of the structure of the thyroid gland.
- Assess and document the effects of altered endocrine function on other body structures and functions.

KEY TERMS

acromegaly, 555
carpal spasm, 555
Chvostek sign, 555
dwarfism, 555
exophthalmos, 555
goiter, 555
tetany, 555
Trousseau sign, 555

EQUIPMENT NEEDED

- Reflex hammer
- Safety pin, cotton ball, containers with hot and cold water, tuning fork
- Blood pressure cuff
- Stethoscope.

The endocrine system is essential to the regulation of the body's internal environment. Through hormones secreted by its glands, the endocrine system regulates such varied functions as growth, reproduction, metabolism, fluid and electrolyte balance, and gender differentiation. It also has a role in adapting to constant alterations in the internal and external environment. Disorders of the endocrine system primarily result from either too much or too little hormone production. These alterations in hormone levels affect a wide variety of human functions, including activity and exercise, nutrition and metabolism, elimination, self-perception and self-concept, sexuality and reproduction, coping with stress, and role-relationships.

18.1 Anatomy, Physiology, and Functions of the Endocrine System

The Glands of the Endocrine System

The endocrine system is comprised of the pituitary gland, thyroid gland, parathyroid glands, adrenal glands, pancreas, and gonads (reproductive glands). The locations of these glands are illustrated in **Figure 18.1** ■.

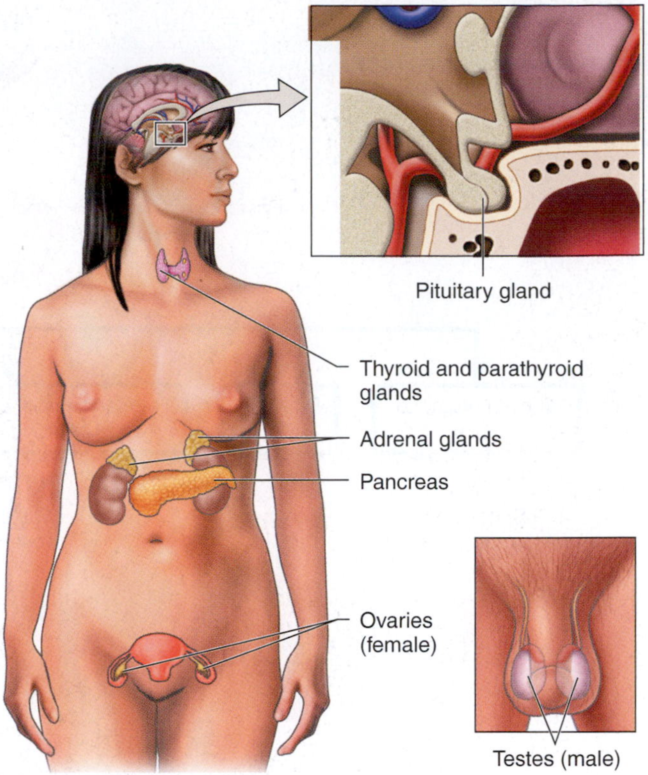
Pituitary gland
Thyroid and parathyroid glands
Adrenal glands
Pancreas
Ovaries (female)
Testes (male)

Figure 18.1 ■ Locations of the major endocrine glands.

Pituitary Gland

The *pituitary gland* (hypophysis) is located in the skull beneath the hypothalamus of the brain (**Figure 18.2** ■). It often is called the "master gland" because its hormones regulate many body functions. The pituitary gland has two parts: the anterior pituitary (or adenohypophysis) and the posterior pituitary (or neurohypophysis). The anterior pituitary is glandular tissue; the posterior pituitary is an extension of the hypothalamus.

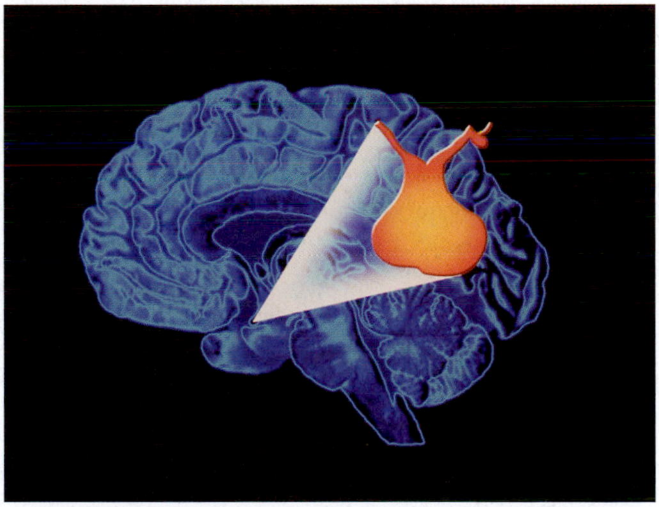

Figure 18.2 ■ Location of the pituitary gland.

Anterior Pituitary

The *anterior pituitary* has several types of endocrine cells and secretes at least six major hormones (**Figure 18.3** ■).

- Somatotropic cells secrete growth hormone (GH) (also called *somatotropin*). GH stimulates growth of the body by signaling cells to increase protein production and by stimulating the epiphyseal plates of the long bones.
- Lactotrophic cells secrete prolactin (PRL). Prolactin stimulates the production of breast milk.
- Gonadotropic cells secrete the gonadotropin hormones, follicle-stimulating hormone (FSH), and luteinizing hormone (LH). These hormones stimulate the ovaries and testes (the gonads).
- Thyrotropic cells secrete thyroid-stimulating hormone (TSH). TSH stimulates the synthesis and release of thyroid hormones from the thyroid gland.
- Corticotropic cells secrete adrenocorticotropic hormone (ACTH). ACTH stimulates release of hormones, especially glucocorticoids, from the adrenal cortex.

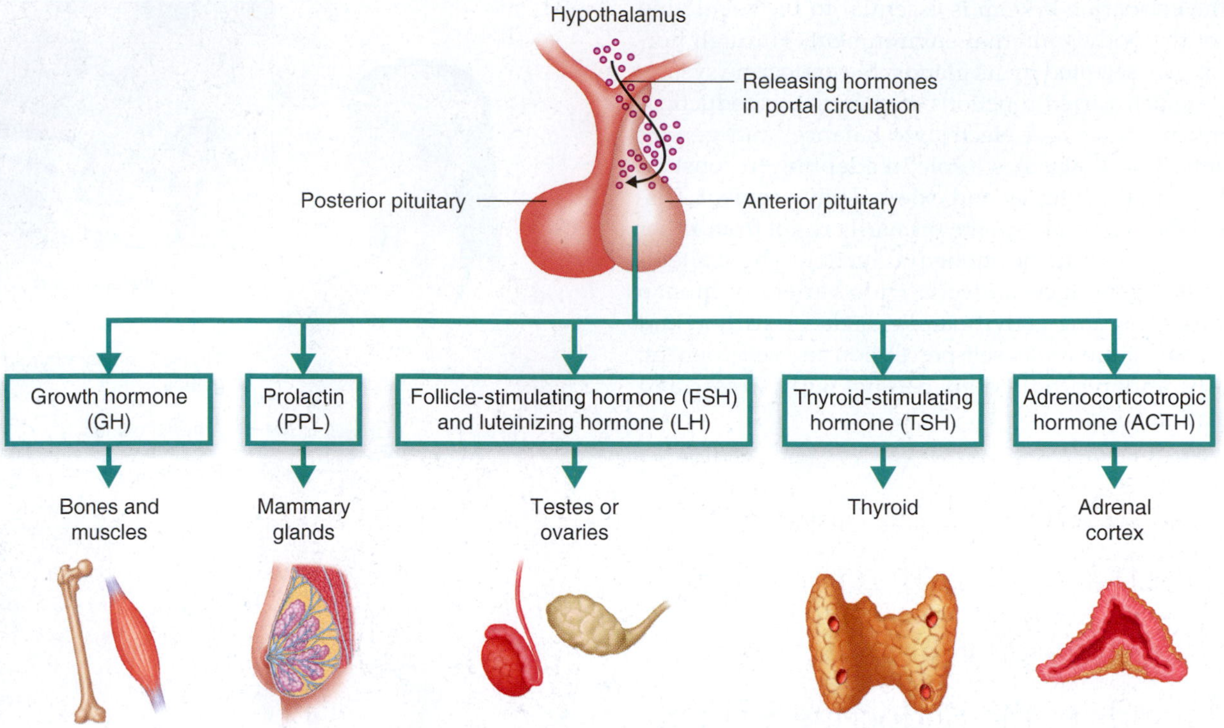
Hypothalamus
Releasing hormones in portal circulation
Posterior pituitary
Anterior pituitary
Growth hormone (GH)
Prolactin (PPL)
Follicle-stimulating hormone (FSH) and luteinizing hormone (LH)
Thyroid-stimulating hormone (TSH)
Adrenocorticotropic hormone (ACTH)
Bones and muscles
Mammary glands
Testes or ovaries
Thyroid
Adrenal cortex

Figure 18.3 ■ Actions of the major hormones of the anterior pituitary.

Posterior Pituitary

The *posterior pituitary* is made of nerve tissue. Its primary function is to store and release antidiuretic hormone and oxytocin, produced in the hypothalamus:

- *Antidiuretic hormone (ADH)*, also called *vasopressin*, decreases urine production by causing the renal tubules to reabsorb water from the urine and return it to the circulating blood.
- *Oxytocin* induces contraction of the smooth muscles in the reproductive organs. In women, oxytocin stimulates the myometrium of the uterus to contract during labor. It also induces milk ejection from the breasts.

Thyroid Gland

The *thyroid gland* (**Figure 18.4** ■) is anterior to the upper part of the trachea and just inferior to the larynx. This butterfly-shaped gland has two lobes connected by a structure called the *isthmus*.

The glandular tissue consists of follicles filled with a jelly-like colloid substance named *thyroglobulin*, a glycoprotein–iodine complex. Cells within the follicles secrete *thyroid hormone (TH)*, a general name for two similar hormones: thyroxine (T_4) and triiodothyronine (T_3). The primary role of thyroid hormones in adults is to increase metabolism. TH secretion is initiated by the release of TSH by the pituitary gland and is dependent on an adequate supply of iodine.

The thyroid gland also secretes *calcitonin*, a hormone that decreases excessive levels of calcium in the blood by slowing the calcium-releasing activity of bone cells, serves as a marker for sepsis, and is believed to be a mediator of inflammatory responses.

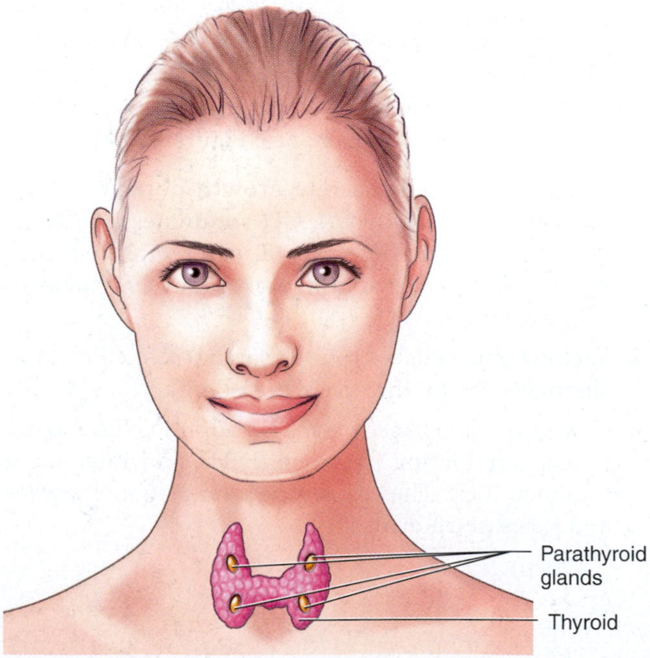
Parathyroid glands
Thyroid

Figure 18.4 ■ The thyroid gland.

Parathyroid Glands

The *parathyroid glands* (usually four to six in number) are embedded on the posterior surface of the lobes of the thyroid gland (see Figure 18.4). They secrete parathyroid hormone (PTH), or parathormone. When calcium levels in the plasma fall, PTH secretion increases. PTH also controls phosphate metabolism. It acts by increasing renal excretion of phosphate in the urine, by decreasing the excretion of calcium, and by increasing bone reabsorption to cause the release of calcium from bones. Normal levels of vitamin D are necessary for PTH to exert these effects on bone and kidneys.

Adrenal Glands

The two adrenal glands are pyramid-shaped organs that sit on top of the kidneys (**Figure 18.5** ■). Each gland consists of two parts, an inner medulla and an outer cortex.

The adrenal medulla produces two hormones (also called *catecholamines*): epinephrine (adrenalin) and norepinephrine (noradrenalin). These hormones are similar to substances also released by the sympathetic nervous system and thus are not essential to life. *Epinephrine* increases blood glucose levels and stimulates the release of ACTH from the pituitary; ACTH in turn stimulates the adrenal cortex to release glucocorticoids. Epinephrine also increases the rate and force of cardiac contractions; constricts blood vessels in the skin, mucous membranes, and kidneys; and dilates blood vessels in the skeletal muscles, coronary arteries, and pulmonary arteries. *Norepinephrine* increases heart rate, increases the force of cardiac contractions, and vasoconstricts blood vessels throughout the body.

The *adrenal cortex* secretes several hormones, all corticosteroids. They are classified into two groups: mineralocorticoids and glucocorticoids. These hormones are essential to life.

The release of the mineralocorticoids is controlled primarily by renin (an enzyme). When a decrease in blood pressure or sodium is detected, specialized kidney cells release renin to act on angiotensinogen, manufactured by the liver. Angiotensinogen is modified by renin and other enzymes to become angiotensin, which stimulates the release of aldosterone from the adrenal cortex. Aldosterone prompts the distal tubules of the kidneys to release increased amounts of water and sodium back into the circulating blood to increase circulating blood volume and pressure. This system (the renin–angiotensin–aldosterone system) is illustrated in Chapter 10 with the discussion of body fluid regulation.

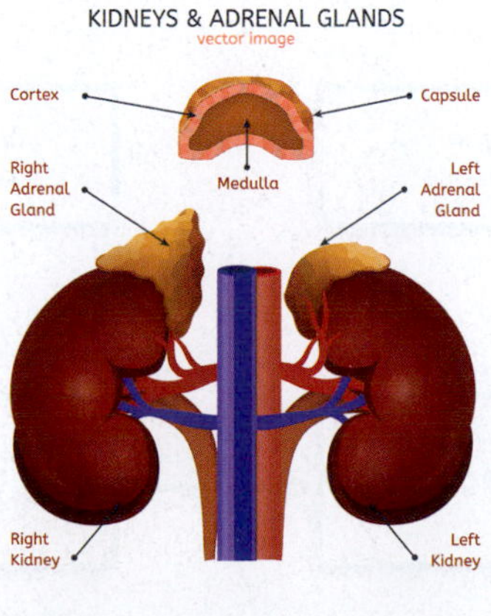
KIDNEYS & ADRENAL GLANDS
vector image
Cortex
Capsule
Medulla
Right
Adrenal
Gland
Left
Adrenal
Gland
Right
Kidney
Left
Kidney

Figure 18.5 ■ Location of the adrenal glands.

The glucocorticoids include cortisol and cortisone. These hormones affect carbohydrate metabolism by regulating glucose use in body tissues, mobilizing fatty acids from fatty tissue, and shifting the source of energy for muscle cells from glucose to fatty acids. Glucocorticoids are released in times of stress. An excess of glucocorticoids in the body depresses the inflammatory response and inhibits the effectiveness of the immune system.

Pancreas

The *pancreas*, located behind the stomach between the spleen and the duodenum, is both an endocrine gland (producing hormones) and an exocrine gland (producing digestive enzymes). The digestive enzymes produced by the pancreas are discussed in Chapter 21. The content in this chapter discusses the endocrine pancreatic hormones.

The endocrine cells of the pancreas produce hormones that regulate carbohydrate metabolism. They are clustered in structures called *pancreatic islets* (or *islets of Langerhans*) scattered throughout the pancreas. Pancreatic islets have at least four different cell types:

1. ***Alpha cells*** produce glucagon, which decreases glucose oxidation and promotes an increase in the blood glucose level by signaling the liver to release glucose from glycogen stores.
2. ***Beta cells*** produce insulin, which facilitates the uptake and use of glucose by muscle, liver, and fat cells and prevents an excessive breakdown of glycogen in the liver and muscle. In this way, insulin decreases blood glucose levels. Insulin also facilitates lipid formation, inhibits the breakdown and mobilization of stored fat, and helps amino acids move into cells to promote protein synthesis. In general, the actions of glucagon and insulin oppose one another, helping to maintain a stable blood glucose level.
3. ***Delta cells*** secrete somatostatin, which inhibits the secretion of glucagon and insulin by the alpha and beta cells.
4. ***F cells*** secrete pancreatic polypeptide, which is believed to inhibit the exocrine activity of the pancreas.

Gonads

The *gonads* are the testes in men and the ovaries in women. These organs are the primary source of steroid sex hormones in the body. The hormones of the gonads are important in regulating body growth and promoting the onset of puberty. The structure and functions of the gonads are discussed in Chapter 47.

An Overview of Hormones

Hormones are chemical messengers secreted by the endocrine organs and transported throughout the body, where they exert their action on specific cells called *target cells*.

Table 18.1 Organs, Hormones, Functions, and Feedback Mechanisms of the Endocrine System

Endocrine Gland	Hormone Secreted	Target Organ and Feedback Mechanism
Thyroid gland	Thyroid hormone (TH): thyroxine (T_4) is the major hormone secreted by the thyroid gland. It is converted to triiodothyronine (T_3) at the target tissues.	Maintains metabolic rate and growth and development of all tissues. T_3 and T_4 are secreted in response to TSH.
	Calcitonin	Maintains serum calcium levels by decreasing bone resorption and decreasing resorption of calcium in the kidneys in response to elevated levels of plasma calcium.
Parathyroid gland	Parathyroid hormone (PTH)	Maintains serum calcium levels by stimulating bone resorption and kidney resorption of calcium in response to falling levels of plasma calcium.
Adrenal cortex	Mineralocorticoids (e.g., aldosterone)	Promote reabsorption of sodium and water in kidney tubule and excretion of potassium in response to elevated levels of potassium and low levels of sodium, thereby increasing blood pressure and blood volume.
	Glucocorticoids (e.g., cortisol)	Help regulate metabolism of carbohydrates, fats, and proteins. Activate anti-inflammatory responses to stressors. Low cortisol levels stimulate hypothalamic secretion of corticotropin-releasing hormone (CRH), which stimulates the anterior pituitary gland to release ACTH, which in turn stimulates the adrenal cortex to secrete cortisol.
	Gonadocorticoids (androgens and small amounts of estrogen and progesterone)	The quantity of sex hormones produced here is small, and the mechanism is not well understood.
Adrenal medulla	Catecholamines (epinephrine and norepinephrine)	Stimulate the heart, constrict blood vessels, inhibit visceral muscles, dilate bronchioles, increase respiration and metabolism, increase blood glucose. Secreted in response to physical or psychologic stress.
Anterior pituitary (adenohypophysis)	Growth hormone (GH)	Promotes growth of body tissues by enhancing protein synthesis and promoting use of fat for energy and thus conserving glucose. Release is stimulated by growth hormone–releasing hormone (GHRH) in response to low GH levels, hypoglycemia, increased amino acids, low fatty acids, and stress.

Hormones do not cause reactions directly but rather regulate tissue responses. They may produce either generalized effects or local effects (Sorenson, Quinn, & Klein, 2019).

Table 18.1 summarizes the functions of the endocrine glands and their hormones. Specific information about the ovaries and testes is found in Chapters 47 through 49.

Hormones are transported from endocrine gland cells to target cells in the body in one of four ways:

1. Endocrine glands release most hormones, including TH and insulin, into the bloodstream. Some hormones require a protein carrier.
2. Neurons release some hormones, such as epinephrine, into the bloodstream. This is called the *neuroendocrine route*.
3. The hypothalamus releases its hormones directly to target cells in the posterior pituitary by nerve cell extension.
4. With the paracrine method, released messengers diffuse through the interstitial fluid. This method of transport involves a number of hormonal peptides that are released throughout various organs and cells and act locally. An example is endorphins, which act to relieve pain.

Hormone levels are controlled by the pituitary gland and by feedback mechanisms. Feedback is controlled much as the thermostat in a house regulates temperature. Sensors in the endocrine system detect changes in hormone levels and adjust hormone secretion to maintain normal levels. When the sensors detect a decrease in hormone levels, they start actions that cause an increase in hormone levels; when hormone levels rise above normal, the sensors cause a decrease in hormone production and release. For example, when thyroid hormone rises, the production of thyroid-stimulating hormone is inhibited, which results in a decrease in the output of TH by the thyroid gland. See **Figure 18.6** ■.

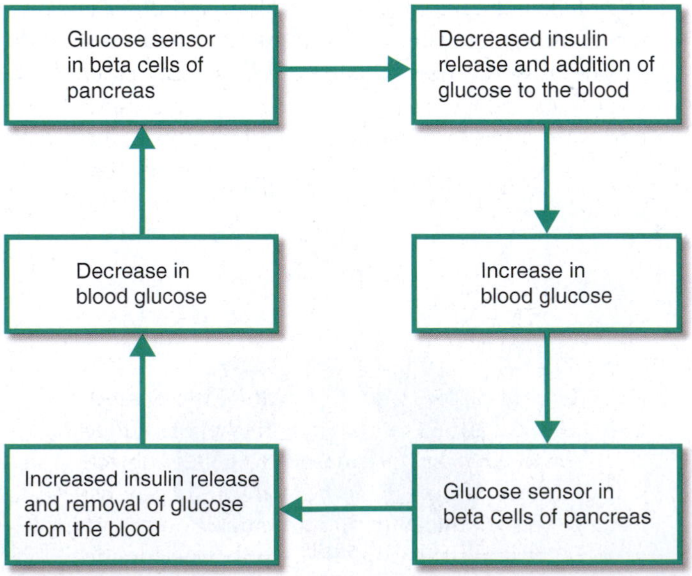
Glucose sensor in beta cells of pancreas
Decreased insulin release and addition of glucose to the blood
Decrease in blood glucose
Increase in blood glucose
Increased insulin release and removal of glucose from the blood
Glucose sensor in beta cells of pancreas

Figure 18.6 ■ Negative feedback.

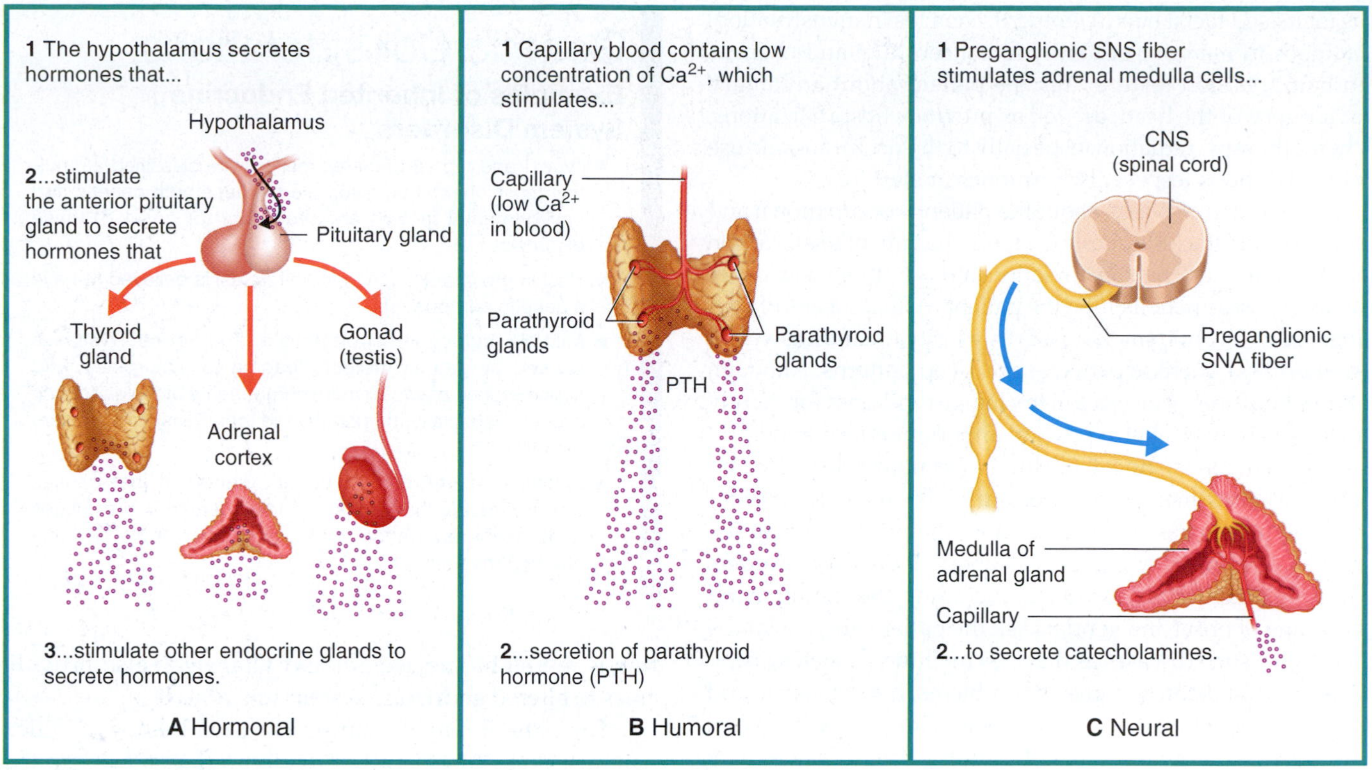
1 The hypothalamus secretes hormones that...
Hypothalamus
2...stimulate the anterior pituitary gland to secrete hormones that
Pituitary gland
Thyroid gland
Gonad (testis)
Adrenal cortex
3...stimulate other endocrine glands to secrete hormones.
A Hormonal
1 Capillary blood contains low concentration of Ca2+, which stimulates...
Capillary (low Ca2+ in blood)
Parathyroid glands
Parathyroid glands
PTH
2...secretion of parathyroid hormone (PTH)
B Humoral
1 Preganglionic SNS fiber stimulates adrenal medulla cells...
CNS (spinal cord)
Preganglionic SNA fiber
Medulla of adrenal gland
Capillary
2...to secrete catecholamines.
C Neural

Figure 18.7 ■ Examples of three mechanisms of hormone release: **A**, hormonal; **B**, humoral; or **C**, neural.

In positive feedback mechanisms, increasing levels of one hormone cause another gland to release a hormone. For example, the increased production of estradiol (a female ovarian hormone) during the follicular stage of the menstrual cycle in turn stimulates increased FSH production by the anterior pituitary gland. Estradiol levels continue to increase until the ovarian follicle disappears, eliminating the source of the stimulation for FSH, which then decreases.

Stimuli for hormone release may also be classified as hormonal, humoral, or neural (**Figure 18.7** ■). In *hormonal release*, hypothalamic hormones stimulate the anterior pituitary to release hormones. Fluctuations in the serum level of these hormones in turn prompt other endocrine glands to release hormones. In *humoral release*, fluctuations in the serum levels of certain ions and nutrients stimulate specific endocrine glands to release hormones to bring these levels back to normal. In *neural release*, nerve fibers stimulate the release of hormones.

18.2 Assessing Endocrine Function

The function of the endocrine glands is assessed by findings from a health assessment interview to collect subjective data, a physical assessment to collect objective data, and diagnostic tests. Hormones affect all body tissues and organs, and manifestations of dysfunction are often nonspecific, making assessment of endocrine function sometimes more difficult than assessment of other body systems (Bickley, 2017).

Health Assessment Interview

A health assessment interview to determine problems with the endocrine system may be part of a health screening or total health assessment, or it may focus on a chief complaint (such as increased urination or changes in energy levels). If the patient has a problem with endocrine function, the nurse analyzes its onset, characteristics and course, severity, precipitating and relieving factors, and any associated symptoms, noting the timing and circumstances. For example, the nurse may ask the patient:

- "Describe the swelling you noticed in the front of your neck. When did it begin? Have you noticed any changes in your energy level? If so, describe them."
- "When did you first notice that your hands and feet were getting larger?"
- "Have you noticed that your appetite has increased even though you have lost weight?"

The health history includes information about the patient's medical history, family history, and social and personal history. Ask the patient about any changes in normal growth and development as well as in height and weight. Changes in the size of extremities can often be detected by asking whether the patient has had to have rings enlarged or to buy increasingly larger gloves and shoes. Enlargement of the neck may be identified by asking whether the patient has difficulty finding shirts or blouses with a collar that fits. Also explore changes such as difficulty swallowing; increased or decreased thirst, appetite, and/or urination; visual changes; sleep disturbances; altered patterns of hair distribution (such as increased facial hair in women); changes in menstruation; changes in memory or ability to concentrate; and changes in hair and skin texture. Ask the patient about any injury or surgery of the head, as well as previous hospitalizations, chemotherapy, radiation (especially to the neck), and the use of medications (especially hormones or steroids).

The nurse also asks about the patient's occupational and social history. Include questions about the patient's satisfaction with occupation, personal relationships, and lifestyle. Other areas of assessment include the patient's usual means of coping; use of alcohol, smoking, or drugs; diet (including weight gain or loss); exercise patterns; and sleep patterns. Although the patient may not recognize changes in behavior, family members may be able to provide important information.

When conducting a health assessment interview and physical assessment, it is important for the nurse to consider genetic influences on the health of the adult. During the health assessment interview, ask about endocrine disorders in immediate family members, including the family members' age of onset and gender. Ask the patient about a family history of such diseases as diabetes mellitus, diabetes insipidus, thyroid disorders, growth problems, hypertension, and obesity. Ask women about problems with pregnancy, menstruation, and/or menopause. Examples of endocrine system disorders are presented in the Genetic Considerations box.

Genetic Considerations

Examples of Inherited Endocrine System Disorders

- Type 1 and type 2 diabetes mellitus are classified as multifactorial inheritance disorders because both genetic and environmental factors are necessary for onset of these disorders.
- Hashimoto disease (chronic thyroiditis) is believed to have a genetic component.
- Multiple endocrine neoplasia is a group of rare diseases caused by genetic defects leading to hyperplasia and hyperfunction of two or more components of the endocrine system (especially the parathyroid, pancreas, and pituitary glands).
- Fragile X syndrome is a genetic condition that causes developmental problems including learning disabilities and mental retardation. Males are usually more severely affected than females.

Physical Assessment

Physical assessment of the endocrine system may be performed as part of a total health assessment or it may be a focused assessment of patients with known or suspected problems with endocrine function.

The only endocrine organ that can be palpated is the thyroid gland; however, other assessments that provide information about endocrine pathophysiology include inspection of the skin, hair, nails, facial appearance, reflexes, and musculoskeletal system. Measuring and monitoring trends in height and weight and vital signs also provide clues to altered endocrine system function.

The patient may sit during the examination. A reflex hammer is used to test deep tendon reflexes. Prior to the examination, the nurse collects the necessary equipment and explains the techniques to the patient to decrease anxiety. Additional techniques for assessing hypocalcemic tetany, a complication of endocrine disorders or surgery, are included here in the examination sequence.

During the physical assessment, assess for any manifestations that might indicate a genetic disorder (see the Genetic Considerations box). If data are found to indicate genetic risk factors or alterations, ask about genetic testing and refer for appropriate genetic counseling and evaluation. Chapter 8 provides further information about genetics in medical-surgical nursing.

Endocrine Assessments

Technique/Normal Findings	Abnormal Findings
Skin Assessments	
Inspect skin color. *Skin color should be even and appropriate to age and race of the patient.* Palpate the skin, assessing texture, moisture, and the presence of lesions. *Skin color should be appropriate to the patient's race; smooth, warm, dry, and intact without lesions.*	■ Hyperpigmentation may be seen in patients with Addison disease or Cushing syndrome. ■ Acanthosis nigricans is a darkening of skinfolds seen especially at the nape of the neck, elbow folds, and under the arms. This condition has many causes, one of which is the hyperinsulinemia seen in prediabetes and type 2 diabetes. ■ A yellowish cast to the skin might indicate hypothyroidism. ■ Purple striae over the abdomen and bruising may be present in the patient with Cushing syndrome. ■ Rough, dry skin is often seen in patients with hypothyroidism, whereas smooth and flushed skin can be a sign of hyperthyroidism. ■ Lesions (such as ulcerations) on the lower extremities might indicate diabetes mellitus.
Nails and Hair Assessment	
Assess texture, distribution, and condition of nails and hair. *Hair should be of normal texture, appropriately distributed for gender; nail surfaces should have even color with smooth surfaces.*	■ Increased pigmentation of the nails is often seen in patients with Addison disease. ■ Dry, thick, brittle nails and hair may be apparent in hypothyroidism; thin, brittle nails and thin, soft hair may be apparent in hyperthyroidism. ■ Hirsutism (excessive facial, chest, or abdominal hair) may be seen in Cushing syndrome.

Technique/Normal Findings	Abnormal Findings
Facial Assessments	
Inspect the symmetry and form of the face. *Face should be bilaterally symmetrical.*	■ Variations of form and structure may indicate growth abnormalities such as **acromegaly** (continued growth of bone from growth hormone hypersecretion).
Inspect position of eyes. *Eyes should be equal in position on both sides of the face. Eyelids should close over eyes.*	■ **Exophthalmos** (protruding eyes) may be seen in hyperthyroidism.
Thyroid Gland Assessment	
Palpate the thyroid gland for size and consistency. Stand behind the patient and place your fingers on either side of the trachea below the thyroid cartilage (**Figure 18.8** ■). Ask the patient to tilt his or her head to the right. Now ask the patient to swallow. As the patient swallows, displace the left lobe while palpating the right lobe. Repeat to palpate the left lobe. *Thyroid gland is not usually palpable. If it is, lobes should feel smooth, rubbery, and free of nodules.*	■ The thyroid may be enlarged in patients with Graves disease or a **goiter** (enlarged thyroid gland). ■ Multiple nodules may be seen in metabolic disorders, whereas the presence of only one nodule may indicate a cyst or a benign or malignant tumor. ■ A single enlarged nodule suggests malignancy.
Motor Function Assessment	
Assess the deep tendon reflexes. Deep tendon reflexes are assessed with the reflex hammer and include the biceps reflex, brachioradialis reflex, triceps reflex, patellar reflex, and Achilles reflex. *Normal values range from 1+ (present, but decreased) to 2+ (normal) to 3+ (increased). See Chapter 41 for guidelines and illustrations of deep tendon reflex assessment.*	■ Increased reflexes may be seen in hyperthyroidism; decreased reflexes may be seen in hypothyroidism.
Sensory Function Assessment	
Test the patient's sensitivity to pain, temperature, vibration, light touch, and stereognosis (the ability to identify an object by touch). Compare symmetric areas on both sides of the body, and compare the distal to the proximal regions of the extremities. Ask the patient to close his or her eyes. *Sensory function should be bilaterally intact.* ■ To test pain, use the blunt and sharp ends of a new safety pin. Discard the pin after use. ■ To test temperature, use cups or other containers of cold and hot water. ■ To test vibration, use a tuning fork over one of the patient's finger or toe joints. ■ To test light touch, use a cotton wisp. ■ To test stereognosis, place in the patient's hand a simple, familiar object, such as a rubber band, cotton ball, or button. Ask the patient to identify the object.	■ Peripheral neuropathy and paresthesia (altered sensations) may occur in diabetes, hypothyroidism, or acromegaly.
Musculoskeletal Assessment	
Inspect the size and proportions of the patient's body structure. *Size and proportion of body structures should be bilaterally equal.*	■ Extremely short stature may indicate **dwarfism** (a condition characterized by short stature); insufficient pituitary growth hormone is one cause. ■ Extremely large bones may indicate acromegaly, caused by excessive growth hormone.
Assessing for Hypocalcemic Tetany	
Assess for **Trousseau sign** (a test for hypocalcemia) with resulting **tetany** (tonic muscle spasms) by inflating a blood pressure cuff above the antecubital space to a point greater than systolic blood pressure for 2–5 min. Trousseau sign is discussed in relation to hypocalcemia in Chapter 10. *A normal finding is no carpal spasm in response to compression of the arm by the blood pressure cuff.*	■ Decreased calcium levels cause the patient's hand and fingers to contract (**carpal spasm**).
Assess for **Chvostek sign** (a test for hypocalcemia) by tapping your finger in front of the patient's ear at the angle of the jaw. A positive Chvostek sign causes facial grimacing due to repeated contractions of the facial muscle. Chvostek sign is discussed and illustrated in relation to hypocalcemia in Chapter 10. *A normal finding is no facial grimacing in response to tapping the patient's face in front of the ear.*	■ Decreased calcium levels cause the patient's lateral facial muscles to contract.

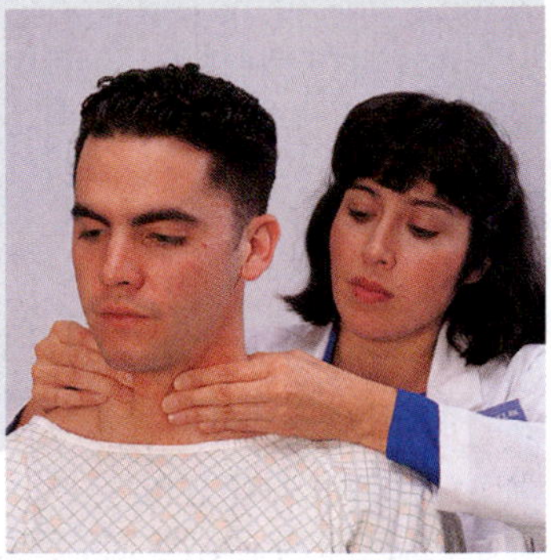

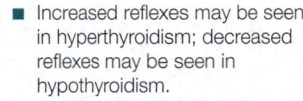

Figure 18.8 ■ Palpating the thyroid gland from behind the patient.

Diagnostic Tests

The results of diagnostic tests of the endocrine system are used to support the diagnosis of a specific disease, to provide information to identify or modify the appropriate medication or therapy used to treat the disease, and to help monitor the patient's responses to treatment and nursing care interventions (Kee, 2018). Diagnostic tests to assess the structure and function of the glands of the endocrine system are described in the following Diagnostic Tests feature. More information is included in the discussion of specific disorders in Chapters 19 and 20.

Regardless of the type of diagnostic test, the nurse is responsible for explaining the procedure and any special preparation needed, for assessing for medication use that may affect the outcome of the tests, for ensuring the consent form is signed (if necessary), for supporting the patient during the examination as necessary, for documenting the procedures as appropriate, and for monitoring the results of the tests. The nurse is also responsible for postprocedure care and patient teaching for self-care at home.

Diagnostic Tests of the Endocrine System

PITUITARY TESTS

NAME OF TEST	PURPOSE AND DESCRIPTION	RELATED NURSING INTERVENTIONS
Growth hormone (GH), human growth hormone (hGH)	In this blood test, GH levels (affected by food, stress, and activity) are measured to identify GH deficiency (dwarfism) or GH excess (gigantism, acromegaly). Normal value: Men: <5 ng/mL Women: <10 ng/mL	Tell patient not to eat or drink 8–10 h prior to having blood drawn. Have patient rest for 30–60 min before blood is drawn.
Magnetic resonance imaging (MRI)	This imaging study is done to identify tumors of the hypothalamus or pituitary gland.	Tell patient of need to lie still during the examination. Assess for any metallic implants (such as pacemakers, clips on brain aneurysms, body piercings, tattoos, shrapnel). If present, notify imaging physician. Remove transdermal medication patches unless otherwise ordered. Replace the patch following the procedure. Ask the patient to tell the staff about the patch when making the appointment and when completing the admission information. Ask if patient is pregnant; if so, the test is not performed. Ask about claustrophobia; if a problem, instruct patient to ask for a relaxing medication to take prior to the MRI.
Somatomedin C (insulin-like growth factor or IGF-1)	The results of this blood test are used to evaluate secretion of growth factor and to identify GH deficiency or excess (as discussed earlier). Normal value: 125–250 ng/mL	None; overnight fasting is preferred but not necessary.
Water deprivation test	This combination of blood and urine tests is used to identify causes of polyuria (increased urine output), including central diabetes insipidus, neurogenic diabetes insipidus, and psychogenic polydipsia (drinking excessive amounts of fluids). In patients without pathology, there is no change in urine and plasma osmolality. Urine osmolality increases in central diabetes insipidus and decreases in nephrogenic diabetes insipidus (Verbalis, 2016).	Tell patient not to smoke, eat, or drink as directed, and that the test will take up to 8 h. Assess weight, take postural BP (lying and standing measures separated by 2 min), assess urine volume and specific gravity, and send samples of urine to the lab for osmolality hourly during the test. Blood samples for osmolality are taken when urine samples are collected and when patient demonstrates orthostatic hypotension. Coordinate specimen collection with the laboratory (Verbalis, 2016).

THYROID TESTS		
NAME OF TEST	PURPOSE AND DESCRIPTION	RELATED NURSING INTERVENTIONS
Magnetic resonance imaging (MRI)—thyroid	This imaging study is done to identify tumors of the thyroid gland.	See information for MRI of the pituitary.
Radioactive iodine uptake (RIA)	This test provides a direct measure of thyroid activity and is useful in evaluating the activity of solitary thyroid nodules. Based on the rationale that the thyroid gland takes up iodine in any form, radioactive iodine is given orally or IV, and the thyroid gland uptake is measured with a scanner at several hourly intervals and at 24 h. Normal value for uptake: 2–4 h: 3%–19% 24 h: 11%–30%	The patient should not eat or drink for 6–8 h before the test, but can have food 1 h after the oral dose is given. Tell patients not to take supplemental iodine several weeks before the test and thyroid medications should be discontinued.
Thyroid antibodies (TA)	A blood test that is used to identify thyroid immune disease (Graves disease, chronic thyroiditis, Hashimoto thyroiditis). Normal values: Antithyroglobulin: negative to titer <1:20 Antimicrosomal: negative to titer <1:100	Assess for family history of thyroid disease and ask about recent viral infection (which could trigger autoimmune disease).
Thyroid scan	This nuclear scan evaluates thyroid nodules. Radioactive isotopes are given orally and a scanner is passed over the thyroid to make a graphic record of the radiation emitted. A normal thyroid scan has a homogeneous pattern of radiation with symmetric lobes. Benign lesions appear as warm spots (take up more radiation); malignant tumors appear as cold spots (less radiation taken up).	No special preparation is needed.
Thyroid-stimulating hormone (TSH)	In this blood test, levels of circulating TSH are measured, with levels above or below normal indicating thyroid disease. TSH levels are also compared with T_4 levels to differentiate between pituitary and thyroid dysfunction. A decreased T_4 level and a normal or increased TSH level can indicate a thyroid disorder. A decreased T_4 level and a decreased TSH level can indicate a pituitary disorder. Normal value: <3 ng/Ml	Tell patients to avoid shellfish for several days prior to the test. Assess medications: TSH value may be increased by aspirin, steroids, dopamine, and heparin and decreased by lithium and potassium iodide.
Thyroid suppression test	Triiodothyronine (T_3) is taken for 7–10 days, and a reduction of its uptake to less than half of the initial uptake after that time is considered normal. The test is used to diagnose hyperthyroidism and hypothyroidism.	Explain the importance of taking the triiodothyronine for the length of time prescribed.
Thyrotropin-releasing hormone (TRH) stimulation test	A baseline TSH is measured, followed by an injection of TRH to stimulate the pituitary to release TSH. A second blood sample is drawn 20–30 min later and the TSH level is again measured. Levels higher or lower than normal are indicative of thyroid disease.	No special preparation is needed.
Thyroxine (T_4)	The results of this blood test are used to determine thyroid function and aid in the diagnosis of hyperthyroidism and hypothyroidism. Normal value: Free T_4: 1.0–2.3 ng/dL	Assess medications: Value may be decreased by cortisone, chlorpromazine (Thorazine), phenytoin (Dilantin), heparin, lithium, sulfonamides, reserpine (Serpasil), testosterone, propranolol (Inderal), tolbutamide (Orinase), and salicylates in high doses. Values may be increased by oral contraceptives, estrogen, clofibrate, and perphenazine (Trilafon).

(continued)

Triiodothyronine (T_3)	The results of this blood test are used to diagnose hyperthyroidism and to compare T_3 with T_4 for diagnosis of thyroid disorder. Normal value: 80–200 ng/dL	Assess medications: Value can be decreased by propylthiouracil, methimazole (Tapazole), lithium, phenytoin (Dilantin), propranolol (Inderal), reserpine (Serpasil), large doses of aspirin, steroids, and sulfonamides. Value can be increased by estrogen, progestins, oral contraceptives, T_3, and methadone.
Triiodothyronine resin uptake (T_3RU)	This test is an indirect measure of free thyroxine (T_4). The patient's blood is mixed with radioactive T_3 and synthetic resin. The radioactive T_3 will bind with available thyroid-binding globulin sites. The unbound radioactive T_3 is added to resin for T_3 uptake. In hyperthyroidism, there are few binding sites left, more T_3 is taken up by the resin, and a high T_3 resin uptake results. The opposite occurs in hypothyroidism. Normal value: 25%–35% uptake	No special preparation is needed.
PARATHYROID TESTS		
NAME OF TEST	**PURPOSE AND DESCRIPTION**	**RELATED NURSING INTERVENTIONS**
Calcium (Ca)	This blood test is used to check for serum calcium excess or deficit in parathyroid and bone disorders and to monitor calcium levels. Normal value: 9.0–11.0 mg/dL, 4.5–5.5 mEq/L, or 2.3–2.8 mmol/L (SI units)	Assess for manifestations of tetany, including positive Chvostek and Trousseau signs, if hypocalcemia is present (see Chapter 10).
Magnetic resonance imaging (MRI)—parathyroid glands	This imaging study is done to identify tumors of the parathyroid glands.	See information for MRI of the pituitary for related nursing interventions.
Parathyroid hormone (PTH)	This blood test is used to identify hypoparathyroidism or hyperparathyroidism and is also used to monitor response to PTH therapy. Normal value: Intact PTH: 11–54 pg/mL C-terminal PTH: 50–330 pg/mL N-terminal PTH: 8–24 pg/mL	Tell patients not to eat or drink for 8 h before the test.
ADRENAL TESTS		
NAME OF TEST	**PURPOSE AND DESCRIPTION**	**RELATED NURSING INTERVENTIONS**
Adrenocorticotropic hormone (ACTH)	This blood test is used to determine if a decreased plasma level of cortisol is due to adrenal cortex hypofunction or pituitary hypofunction. Normal value: 7:00–10:00 a.m.: 8–80 pg/mL 4:00 p.m.: 5–30 pg/mL 10:00–12:00 p.m.: <10 pg/mL	Tell the patient that food and fluids may be restricted, and that stress and exercise may affect results. Assess medications: ACTH values may be increased by alcohol, amphetamines, estrogen, aldosterone, vasopressin, and insulin, and decreased by steroids, estrogen, and alcohol.
ACTH stimulation	This test is conducted to differentiate adrenal insufficiency from pituitary hypofunction. ACTH (cosyntropin) is administered; if the plasma cortisol level is unchanged in 1 h, adrenal insufficiency is the cause. To identify pituitary hypofunction, the drug metyrapone (Metopirone) is given to block the production of cortisol, thus causing increased ACTH secretion. If the ACTH level does not increase, the problem is pituitary insufficiency.	Assess medications and provide teaching as for ACTH test.

ACTH suppression	For the ACTH suppression test, the drug dexamethasone (Decadron) is given to suppress ACTH production. If an extremely high dose is needed, the cause is of pituitary origin; if the plasma cortisol remains high, the cause could be adrenal cortex hyperfunction (Cushing syndrome).	Provide teaching and assess medications as for ACTH test. If dexamethasone (Decadron) causes gastric irritation, milk or antacids may be required.
Aldosterone	This blood test is done to identify a deficit or an excess of aldosterone and to help determine the cause of overhydration. Normal value: <16 mcg/dL (fasting) A 24-h urine test is considered a more reliable measure of aldosterone than a random aldosterone test. Normal value: 6–25 mcg/24 h	Instruct patient to maintain usual diet prior to the test, avoiding excess salt or licorice, and to rest in the supine position for 1 h before blood is drawn as position changes affect the results. If a urine test is ordered, instruct patient to void, discarding urine and noting the time to start the test, then collect all urine in the designated container for 24 hours, including a final voiding when the test is to be concluded. Avoid feces or toilet paper in the urine. Results of serum or urine aldosterone tests may be altered by excess or low dietary sodium and antihypertensive drug therapy.
Computerized tomography (CT) of the abdomen	This radiologic study is used to assess the adrenal gland for tumors (including size and metastasis).	Determine if contrast medium will be used; if so, assess patient for allergy to iodine (shellfish) or radiologic contrast media.
Cortisol	This blood test is used to measure the total cortisol level in the serum and to evaluate adrenal cortex function. Values are decreased in Addison disease and hypothyroidism and increased in Cushing syndrome and hyperthyroidism. Normal value: 8:00–10:00 a.m.: 138–635 nmol 4:00–6:00 p.m.: 83–359 nmol A 24-h urine test may be conducted to measure free (unbound) cortisol Normal value: <100 mcg/24 h	Tell patient not to eat or drink and to rest for 2 h before the test. Evaluate medications: Cortisol is decreased by androgens and phenytoin (Dilantin) and increased by oral contraceptives, estrogen, and spironolactone (Aldactone). For a urine cortisol test, instruct patient to save urine for 24-h period (see urine aldosterone above) and to avoid stressful situations and physical activity for at least 24 h prior to the test.
Dexamethasone suppression test	This test is used to differentiate the cause of adrenal disorders. Baseline plasma cortisol and urine hydroxycorticosteroids (17-OHCS) are obtained. Dexamethasone 1 mg is administered orally at 11:00 p.m. A serum cortisol is collected at 8:00 a.m. the next morning. The dexamethasone suppresses ACTH. If an extremely high dose of dexamethasone is required to suppress ACTH, the primary disorder is adrenal cortex hyperplasia (Cushing disease). If ACTH is not suppressed with the synthetic cortisol, an adrenal tumor is suspected.	
17-Ketosteroids	This 24-hour urine test is done to measure metabolites in urine and evaluate adrenal cortex function. Normal value: Men: 5–25 mg in 24 h Women: 5–15 mg in 24 h	Instruct patient how to save urine (urine must contain a preservative and be refrigerated). Assess medications: Levels are affected by a variety of drugs; if possible, these should be discontinued for 48 h before the test (check with healthcare provider and agency protocol). Postpone the test for women who are menstruating because blood can cause a false-positive finding.

(continued)

Magnetic resonance imaging (MRI)—adrenal glands	This imaging study is done to identify tumors of the adrenal glands.	See information for MRI of the pituitary.
MIBG scan	This nuclear medicine scan is used to detect the presence and location of adrenal pheochromocytomas. A special radioactive dye is given and concentrates on the tumor in the adrenal gland; the tumor can then be seen on x-ray.	Explain that the test takes about an hour a day for 3 or 4 days.
PANCREATIC ENDOCRINE TESTS		
NAME OF TEST	PURPOSE AND DESCRIPTION	RELATED NURSING INTERVENTIONS
C-peptide	C-peptide has an essential function related to the synthesis of insulin in the beta cells. C-peptide is often used as a diagnostic test to prove that an individual with type 1 diabetes is not producing insulin and helps to differentiate between type 1 and type 2 diabetes.	Monitor results: A C-peptide level of zero means that the individual with diabetes produces no insulin and has type 1 diabetes. Individuals with type 2 diabetes produce insulin and will generally have positive C-peptide levels.
Computed tomography (CT) of the abdomen	This radiographic test is done to identify pancreatic tumors or cysts.	If contrast medium is used, assess for allergy to iodine (shellfish) or radiologic media.
Fasting blood sugar (FBS)	This blood test is used to identify or confirm a diagnosis of diabetes mellitus. It is also used to monitor treatment of diabetes mellitus. A finding of greater than 100 mg/dL, if confirmed with OGTT, and HbA1C is indicative of diabetes. Normal value: Serum/plasma: 70–110 mg/dL (value varies in individual laboratories)	Tell the patient not to eat or drink anything other than water for 6–8 h before the test. Do not administer insulin until blood specimen is taken. Assess medications: FBS may be increased by cortisone, diuretics, ACTH, levodopa, epinephrine, anesthetics, and phenytoin (Dilantin).
Oral glucose tolerance test (OGTT)	This blood and urine test is used to diagnose diabetes mellitus if prior fasting blood sugar (FBS) findings are increased or inconsistent. A solution of 75–100 g of glucose is administered and samples of blood and urine are taken immediately and at 30, 60, and 120 min (it may extend from 2 to 6 h). Values for 2-h plasma at 139 or below are considered normal; values at 200 or greater, if confirmed with a second test on a different day, are diagnostic of diabetes mellitus.	The tests will not be done if patient's FBS is consistently high. Tell the patient not to eat or drink (except water) for 6–8 h before the test. Assess medications: Drugs that may increase OGTT levels are steroids, oral contraceptives, estrogens, thiazide diuretics, and salicylates. Explain to the patient that he or she may feel weak and may perspire during the test and that these symptoms should be reported to the nurse. Although they usually are transitory, they may be manifestations of prediabetes.
Glycosylated hemoglobin (HbA1C or A1C)	This blood test is used as a diagnostic tool and to monitor diabetes mellitus management. The results represent an average blood glucose level during the life of the red blood cell (90–120 days); an elevated level indicates poorly controlled diabetes mellitus and increased risk for complications. Normal value: In most labs, the normal range is 2–5%. A glycosylated hemoglobin of 6.5% or higher is diagnostic for diabetes, and a level between 5.7% and 6.4% is indicative of impaired glucose tolerance or prediabetes. In individuals with well-controlled diabetes, it is less than 7.0%.	Monitor findings: Decreased levels can be caused by anemia, long-term blood loss, and chronic renal failure. Increased levels may result from hyperglycemia, alcohol ingestion, pregnancy, hemodialysis, prolonged cortisone intake, impaired glucose tolerance, or prediabetes.
Magnetic resonance imaging (MRI)—pancreas	This imaging study is done to identify tumors of the pancreas.	See information for MRI of the pituitary.

18.3 Assessment of Special Populations

A health assessment to determine problems with endocrine function in the older adult is an important aspect of a total assessment. Type 2 diabetes is the most common endocrine problem in older adults, affecting one in four Americans over the age of 65 (Centers for Disease Control and Prevention, 2017). The treatment of diabetes and prevention of hyperglycemia is important to decrease debilitating complications such as renal failure, stroke, heart disease, disability, and premature death (American Diabetes Association [ADA], 2018). In order to identify and treat diabetes early, the ADA (2018) recommends that all patients over the age of 45 be screened every 3 years for diabetes and those with prediabetes be screened annually. Diabetes is discussed further in Chapter 20.

Another potentially debilitating and common endocrine problem in older adults is low levels of vitamin D and deficient calcium. Deficient levels of vitamin D have been correlated with dementia and deterioration of cognitive abilities (Miller et al., 2015). Loss of calcium from bones puts older adults at risk for hip fractures which often lead to disability and increased mortality. Bliuc, Alarkawi, Nguyen, Eisman, and Center (2015) recommend treatment for osteopenia and osteoporosis to prevent complications and death in older adults. Age-related changes to the endocrine system are outlined in **Table 18.2**.

Disordered endocrine function also plays a significant role in posttraumatic stress disorder (PTSD). Many people suffer from PTSD, and veterans are particularly at risk as a result of traumatic experiences experienced during war. Intense, painful memories cause PTSD, and the endocrine system has a role in creating memories. Dysfunction of the hypothalamus–pituitary–adrenal axis (hormonal interaction between the hypothalamus, anterior pituitary, and adrenal cortex) results in decreased cortisol levels and increased catecholamines (epinephrine and norepinephrine). These endocrine changes increase the stress response and cause the brain to store vivid memories of traumatic events (Daskalakis, McGill, Lehrner, & Yehuda, 2016). Clinical manifestations that may signal PTSD include hyperarousal, high anxiety and fear, impaired memory and attention, and nightmares (Asalgoo, Jahromi, Meftahi, & Sahraeri 2015). PTSD can be very debilitating and treatment includes both physical and psychological approaches. The nurse can help to identify PTSD and communicate findings with the provider to initiate referral and therapy.

Recent endocrine research shows that gender identity is based on biologic and hormonal influences that often begin in childhood (Saraswat, Weinand, & Safer, 2015). Self-esteem is closely tied with gender identity, and the incidence of sexually transmitted diseases, drug abuse, and depression are significant in this population (Safer, 2016). Patients often seek treatment for hormone therapy that is very important to their gender identity and self-esteem. Analysis of steroid hormones such as androgen, testosterone, and estrogen also help to determine proper therapies. Neurotransmitters such as neurokinin B are being studied to determine their significance to gender identity (Saraswat et al., 2015). Further research in this new area of endocrine knowledge is ongoing.

This population has experienced discrimination and mistreatment not only from the public, but also from interactions with healthcare providers. It is important for the nurse to meet the healthcare needs of this population without judgment or discrimination (Safer, 2016). Potential healthcare needs of this population include education regarding the science of lesbian, gay, bisexual, transgender, queer or questioning, and intersex (LGBTQI), assessment for sexually transmitted diseases, assessment of depression, genetic and endocrine testing, hormonal therapies, and surgical correction of gender.

Table 18.2 Age-Related Endocrine Change

Age-Related Change	Significance
Pituitary: ↓ production of ACTH, TSH, FSH	■ Decreased secretion of glucocorticoids, 17-ketosteroids, progesterone, androgen, and estrogen (and thus lower levels on diagnostic tests)
Thyroid: ↑ in fibrosis and nodularity, ↓ in gland activity	■ Lower basal metabolic rate ■ Increased incidence of hypothyroidism ■ Palpable nodules on palpation
Adrenal medulla: ↑ secretion and level of norepinephrine, ↓ beta-adrenergic response to norepinephrine	■ Decreased response to beta-adrenergic receptor blockers (medications) ■ May contribute to increased incidence of hypertension
Pancreas: calcification of blood vessels and distention and dilation of pancreatic ducts	■ Decreased production of lipase with reduced fat absorption and digestion, leading to intolerance of fatty foods and indigestion ■ Decreased absorption of fat-soluble vitamins
Pancreas: delayed and decreased insulin release; believed accompanied by decreased sensitivity to circulating insulin	■ Decreased ability to metabolize glucose and increased insulin resistance with higher and more prolonged blood glucose levels may contribute to increased incidence of type 2 diabetes mellitus with aging (however, higher than normal blood glucose levels are not unusual in nondiabetic older adults)

18.4 Health Promotion

Endocrine dysfunction can have debilitating consequences and result in disability and even early mortality. The nurse can promote health at various levels—with an individual, within a family, and within a community to improve health and prevent specific disease complications.

There are many examples of health promotion to prevent type 2 diabetes. While working with an individual, the nurse may encourage the patient to develop goals related to control of weight and improved exercise to prevent type 2 diabetes (Handelsman, et al., 2015). At the family level, the nurse might encourage the family to work together on choosing healthy meals for the family. The nurse might do some community education related to the prevention of type 2 diabetes or participate in diabetes screening at a community health fair (American Association of Clinical Endocrinology / American College of Endocrinology et al., 2018).

Nursing care aimed at understanding toxic exposures and detecting sequelae is another area where health promotion is important (Gore, et al., 2015). The nurse might help the patient with Bisphenol A (BPA) exposure to understand its risk and how to prevent future exposures. The nurse could encourage the family to identify containers in the home that contain BPA and are used to store foods, and encourage them to dispose of the containers. Information regarding BPA exposure and its consequences could be presented at a community health fair. Health promotion that addresses the individual, the family, and the community may have more impact than health promotion aimed at just one of these groups.

CHAPTER HIGHLIGHTS

18.1 Anatomy, Physiology, and Functions of the Endocrine System

Describe the anatomy, physiology, and functions of the endocrine glands and hormones, and identify abnormal findings that may indicate impairment of the endocrine system.

- The endocrine system is comprised of several glands: the pituitary gland, thyroid gland, parathyroid glands, adrenal glands, pancreas, and gonads (reproductive glands).
- The endocrine system is essential to the regulation of the body's internal environment and affects a wide variety of human functions.
- Endocrine glands release most hormones, including thyroid hormone and insulin, into the bloodstream. Hormone receptors are located on or inside target cells. They recognize a specific hormone and translate the message into a cellular response.

18.2 Assessing Endocrine Function

Outline the components of the assessment of the endocrine system including topics for the health assessment interview, techniques for physical assessment, and the diagnostic tests used in the assessment.

- A targeted health history including genetic considerations and physical assessment will help to diagnose endocrine disorders.
- Various diagnostic tests are employed to diagnose endocrine disorders and to monitor treatments such as hormone replacement.

18.3 Assessment of Special Populations

Differentiate considerations for assessing the endocrine system of older adults, veterans, individuals in the LGBTQI population, and adults with sequelae of childhood/ congenital conditions.

- Identifying and treating endocrine disorders such as type 2 diabetes can have a huge impact on the older adult's quality and length of life.
- Veterans may have unique healthcare challenges such as PTSD. Understanding the endocrine component of PTSD is helpful in defining an effective plan of care.
- LGBTQI patients require a scientific approach to their treatment that is nonjudgmental and inclusive of their healthcare needs.

18.4 Health Promotion

Summarize topics that nurses teach to promote healthy endocrine function across the lifespan.

- Health promotion activities aimed at the individual, the family, and the community will be most effective in the prevention of endocrine dysfunction.

TEST YOURSELF NCLEX-RN® REVIEW

1. A patient is being treated for a condition where the pituitary gland is producing an increased amount of antidiuretic hormone. What finding would the nurse most likely assess in this patient?
   A. Increased output of urine
   B. Decreased output of urine
   C. Decreased production of testosterone
   D. Increased facial hair growth in women
2. During an assessment, the nurse decides to assess a patient's calcium level. Which action will the nurse take to identify a low calcium level?
   A. Palpate turgor of skin.
   B. Observe color of skin.
   C. Conduct a Trousseau sign test.
   D. Save urine to measure 17-ketosteroids.
3. A patient with adrenal cortex dysfunction is experiencing an increased amount of glucocorticoids being released into the general circulation. For which physiologic response should the nurse plan care for this patient?
   A. Delayed onset of puberty
   B. Decreased metabolic rate
   C. Inhibited immune response
   D. Increased response to glucagon
4. The nurse is conducting a health history with a patient that focuses on the endocrine system. Which question should the nurse include in this assessment? (Select all that apply.)
   A. "How did you get this scar on your leg?"
   B. "Have you noticed a change in your thirst?"
   C. "Do your children have problems with urination?"
   D. "When did you first notice the pain in your abdomen?"
   E. "Have you noticed that your rings feel tight?
5. The nurse is preparing to assess a patient's thyroid gland. For which criteria is the nurse assessing this gland?
   A. Pain and pulse rate
   B. Size and consistency
   C. Character and texture
   D. Edema and movement
6. The nurse notes that a patient has a low calcium level and plans to assess for Chvostek sign. How will the nurse conduct this assessment? (Select all that apply.)
   A. Depress the skin over the shin.
   B. Pinch a fold of skin over the sternum.
   C. Tap a finger in front of the patient's ear.
   D. Inflate a blood pressure cuff above the antecubital space.
   E. Observe for facial grimacing.
7. The nurse reviews the laboratory tests prescribed for a patient. Changes in which laboratory value would indicate a change in the patient's thyroid function?
   A. GH
   B. TSH
   C. FBS
   D. Aldosterone
8. The nurse is assessing the endocrine system of an older female patient. Which finding would the nurse attribute to aging?
   A. S1/S2heart tones
   B. Decreased facial hair
   C. Thyroid nodules present
   D. Pituitary enlarged and firm
9. The nurse is caring for a patient with newly diagnosed hypothyroidism. What should the nurse expect when assessing this patient's skin?
   A. Rough, dry skin
   B. Smooth, flushed skin
   C. Increased hair growth
   D. Cold and clammy skin
10. The nurse is assessing a patient's deep tendon reflexes. For which endocrine disorder is this nurse assessing?
    A. Tetany
    B. Acromegaly
    C. Hyperthyroidism
    D. Cushing syndrome

See Test Yourself answers in Appendix B.

REFERENCES

American Association of Clinical Endocrinology/ American College of Endocrinology (AACE/ACE), Garber, A. J., Abrahamson, M. J., Barzilay, J. I., Blonde, L., Bloomgarden, Z. T., . . . Umpierrez, G. E. (2018). *Consensus statement by the American Association of Clinical Endocrinology and American College of Endocrinology on the comprehensive type 2 diabetes algorithm – 2018 executive summary.* Retrieved from https://www.aace.com/sites/all/files/diabetes-algorithm-executive-summary.pdf.

American Diabetes Association (ADA). (2018). Standard of medical care in diabetes—2018. *Diabetes Care, 41*(Suppl.), S1–S159. Retrieved from http://care.diabetesjournals.org/content/diacare/suppl/2017/12/08/41.Supplement_1.DC1/DC_41_S1_Combined.pdf.

Asalgoo, S., Jahromi, G. P., Meftahi, G. H., & Sahraei, H. (2015). Posttraumatic stress disorder (PTSD): Mechanisms and possible treatments. *Neurophysiology, 47*(6), 482–489.

Bickley, L. (2017). *Bates' guide to physical examination and history taking* (12th ed.). Philadelphia, PA: Lippincott Williams & Wilkins.

Bliuc, D., Alarkawi, D., Nguyen, T. V., Eisman, J. A., & Center, J. R. (2015). Risk of subsequent fractures and mortality in elderly women and men with fragility fractures with and without osteoporotic bone density: The Dubbo Osteoporosis Epidemiology Study. *Journal of Bone and Mineral Research, 30*(4), 637–646.

Centers for Disease Control and Prevention (CDC). (2017). *Type 2 diabetes.* Retrieved from https://www.cdc.gov/diabetes/basics/type2.html.

Daskalakis, N. P., McGill, M. A., Lehrner, A., & Yehuda, R. (2016). Endocrine aspects of PTSD: Hypothalamic-pituitary-adrenal (HPA) axis and beyond. In C. R. Martin, V. R. Preedy, & V. B. Patel (Eds.), *Comprehensive guide to post-traumatic stress disorders* (pp. 245–260). Cham, Switzerland: Springer.

Gore, A. C., Chappell, V. A., Fenton, S. E., Flaws, J. A., Nadal, A., Prins, G. S., et al. . . . Zoeller, R. T. (2015). Executive summary to EDC-2: The Endocrine Society's second scientific statement on endocrine-disrupting chemicals. *Endocrine Reviews 36*(6), 593–602.

Handelsman, Y., Bloomgarden, Z. T., Grunberger, G., Umpierrez, G., Zimmerman, R. S., Bailey, T. S., . . . Zangeneh, F. (2015). American Association of Clinical Endocrinologists and American College of Endocrinology – Clinical practice guidelines for developing a diabetes mellitus comprehensive care plan – 2015 – Executive summary. *Endocrine Practice, 21*(4), 413–437.

Kee, J. L. (2018). *Laboratory and diagnostic tests with nursing implications* (10th ed.). Hoboken, NJ: Pearson Education.

Miller, J., Harvey, D., Beckett, L., Green, R., Tomaszewski Farias, S., Reed, B., . . . DeCarli, C. (2015). Vitamin D status and rates of cognitive decline in a multiethnic cohort of older adults. *JAMA Neurology, 72*(11), 1295–1303.

Safer, J. D. (2016). The large gaps in transgender medical knowledge among providers must be measured and addressed. *Endocrine Practice, 22*(7), 902–903.

Saraswat, A., Weinand, J., & Safer, J. D. (2015). Evidence supporting the biologic nature of gender identity. *Endocrine Practice, 21*(2), 199–204.

Sorenson, M., Quinn, L., & Klein, D. (2019). *Pathophysiology: Concepts of human disease.* Hoboken, NJ: Pearson Education.

Verbalis, J. G. (2016). *Diabetes insipidus: Principles of diagnosis and treatment.* Washington, DC: Endocrine Society.

ADDITIONAL RESOURCES

American Association of Diabetes Educators
www.aadenet.org

American Diabetes Association (ADA)
www.diabetes.org

American Thyroid Association
www.thyroid.org

National Institute of Diabetes and Digestive and Kidney Diseases
www.niddk.nih.gov/health-information/endocrine-diseases/adrenal-insufficiency-addisons-disease

Chapter 19

Nursing Care of Patients with Endocrine Disorders

Chapter Outline and Learning Outcomes

19.1 Disorders of the Thyroid Gland 566

Describe the pathophysiology and manifestations of disorders of the thyroid gland, and outline the interprofessional care and nursing care of patients with these disorders.

19.2 Disorders of the Parathyroid Glands 579

Describe the pathophysiology and manifestations of disorders of the parathyroid glands, and outline the interprofessional care and nursing care of patients with these disorders.

19.3 Disorders of the Adrenal Glands 580

Describe the pathophysiology and manifestations of disorders of the adrenal glands, and outline the interprofessional care and nursing care of patients with these disorders.

19.4 Disorders of the Pituitary Gland 589

Describe the pathophysiology and manifestations of disorders of the pituitary gland, and outline the interprofessional care and nursing care of patients with these disorders.

CLINICAL COMPETENCIES

- Assess health status of patients with endocrine disorders and monitor, document, and report unexpected or abnormal manifestations.
- Use assessed data, patient values, clinical expertise, and evidence to determine priority nursing diagnoses and select and implement nursing interventions.
- Effectively communicate with and function within the interprofessional team to plan and provide patient care.
- Administer medications knowledgeably and safely.
- Plan and provide patient and family teaching to promote, restore, and maintain health status.
- Monitor for respiratory problems and tetany in patients having a thyroidectomy.
- Adapt individual and cultural values and variations as well as expressed needs and preferences into each patient's plan of care.
- Evaluate responses to care and use data to revise plan as needed.

KEY TERMS

acromegaly, 589
Addison disease, 584
Addisonian crisis, 585
Cushing disease, 581
Cushing syndrome, 581
diabetes insipidus, 590
euthyroid, 568
exophthalmos, 566
gigantism, 589
goiter, 566
hyperparathyroidism, 579
hypoparathyroidism, 580
myxedema, 573
myxedema coma, 575
proptosis, 566
syndrome of inappropriate ADH secretion (SIADH), 590
tetany, 580
thyroid crisis or storm, 568
thyroidectomy, 569
thyroiditis, 568
thyrotoxicosis, 566

The thyroid, parathyroid, adrenal, and pituitary glands are part of the endocrine system. Disorders of the structure and function of these glands alter normal hormone levels and the way body tissues use those hormones. When hormone production increases or decreases, people experience alterations in health.

Patients with disorders of the glands discussed in this chapter require nursing care for multiple functional problems. They often face exhausting diagnostic tests, changes in physical appearance and emotional responses, and permanent alterations in lifestyle. Nursing care is directed toward meeting physiologic needs, providing education, and ensuring psychologic support for the patient and family. A holistic approach to the complex needs of patients with these endocrine disorders is an essential component of nursing care.

19.1 Disorders of the Thyroid Gland

Altered thyroid hormone (TH) production or use affects all major organ systems. In the adult, TH changes primarily affect metabolism, cardiovascular function, gastrointestinal function, and neuromuscular function. Thyroid disorders—both hyperthyroidism and hypothyroidism—are among the most common endocrine disorders.

The Patient with Hyperthyroidism

Hyperthyroidism (**thyrotoxicosis**) is a disorder caused by excessive delivery of TH to the tissues. Because the primary effect of TH is to increase metabolism and protein synthesis, hyperthyroidism affects all major organ systems of the body. The increase in metabolic rate and the alterations in cardiac output, peripheral blood flow, oxygen consumption, and body temperature are similar to those found in increased sympathetic nervous system activity (Sorenson, Quinn, & Klein, 2019).

Pathophysiology and Manifestations

The effects of hyperthyroidism are the result of increased circulating levels of TH. This hormonal excess increases the metabolic rate and heightens the sympathetic nervous system's physiologic response to stimulation. The sensitizing effect of abnormally elevated TH levels increases the cardiac rate and stroke volume. As a result, cardiac output and peripheral blood flow increase. Elevated TH levels increase carbohydrate, protein, and lipid metabolism. Lipids are depleted, and glucose tolerance decreases. Protein degradation increases, resulting in a negative nitrogen balance. Over time, the hypermetabolic effects of excess TH result in caloric and nutritional deficiencies.

Hyperthyroidism results from many different factors, including autoimmune stimulation (as in Graves disease), excess secretion of thyroid-stimulating hormone (TSH) by the pituitary gland, thyroiditis, neoplasms (such as toxic multinodular goiter), side effect of certain drugs, and an excessive intake of thyroid medications. The most common etiologies of hyperthyroidism are Graves disease and toxic multinodular goiter.

The patient with hyperthyroidism typically has an increased appetite and may gain weight, although weight loss is more typical, and may have hypermotile bowels and diarrhea. Additional manifestations related to hypermetabolism include emotional liability, heat intolerance, insomnia, palpitations, and increased sweating. The skin is smooth and warm, hair may become fine, and hair loss in the scalp, eyebrows, or axilla or pubic region is common. See Multisystem Effects of Hyperthyroidism page 567.

Graves Disease

Graves disease, the most common cause of hyperthyroidism, is an autoimmune disorder, sometimes associated with the presence of other autoimmune disorders such as myasthenia gravis, diabetes mellitus, celiac, and systemic lupus erythematosus (Yeung et al., 2016). The serum of patients with Graves disease has an antibody that binds to TSH receptors in the thyroid follicles and causes the thyroid cells to hyperfunction. When this antibody binds to the TSH receptors, it stimulates hormone synthesis and secretion, enlarging the gland. The cause is unknown, but there is a hereditary link. Graves disease is seen eight times more often in women than in men and occurs most frequently between the ages of 20 and 40 (Yeung et al., 2016).

Patients with Graves disease have a **goiter** (an enlarged thyroid gland) and manifestations of hyperthyroidism. The goiter can result from excess TSH stimulation (when the amount of circulating TH is deficient), abnormal growth-stimulating immunoglobulins, or substances that inhibit TH synthesis. A goiter may be present in hyperthyroidism or hypothyroidism.

The eye pathology of Graves disease is manifested as proptosis and visual dysfunction. **Proptosis** (forward displacement) of the eye occurs in about one-third of cases (Bickley, 2017). **Exophthalmos** (the forward protrusion of the eyeballs) results from an accumulation of inflammation by-products in the retro-orbital tissues. The sclera may be visible above the iris, the upper lids may be retracted, and the person has a characteristic unblinking stare (**Figure 19.1** ■). Exophthalmos is usually bilateral, but it may involve only one eye. The patient may experience blurred vision, diplopia, eye pain, lacrimation, and photophobia. The inability to close the eyelids completely over the protruding eyeballs increases the risk of corneal dryness, irritation, infection, and ulceration. Infiltration of the muscles that move the eye and of the optic nerve leads to paralysis and vision loss. The treatment of Graves disease may stabilize the manifestations but generally does not reverse these changes in the eyes.

Other manifestations include fatigue, difficulty sleeping, hand tremors, and changes in menstruation ranging from decreased flow to amenorrhea. Older patients may present with atrial fibrillation, angina, or congestive heart failure.

Multisystem Effects of
Hyperthyroidism

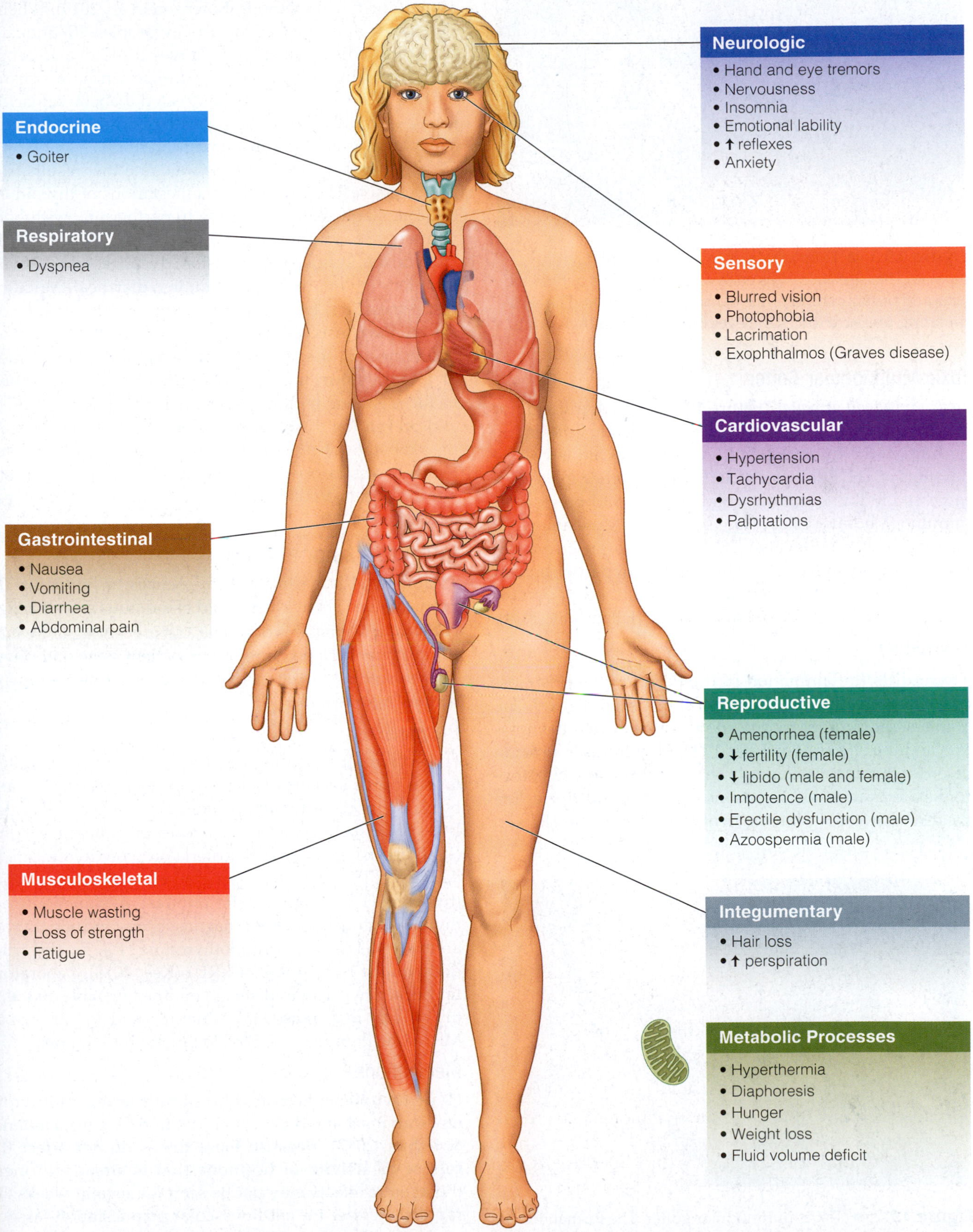
Neurologic
• Hand and eye tremors
• Nervousness
• Insomnia
• Emotional lability
• ↑ reflexes
• Anxiety
Endocrine
• Goiter
Respiratory
• Dyspnea
Sensory
• Blurred vision
• Photophobia
• Lacrimation
• Exophthalmos (Graves disease)
Cardiovascular
• Hypertension
• Tachycardia
• Dysrhythmias
• Palpitations
Gastrointestinal
• Nausea
• Vomiting
• Diarrhea
• Abdominal pain
Reproductive
• Amenorrhea (female)
• ↓ fertility (female)
• ↓ libido (male and female)
• Impotence (male)
• Erectile dysfunction (male)
• Azoospermia (male)
Musculoskeletal
• Muscle wasting
• Loss of strength
• Fatigue
Integumentary
• Hair loss
• ↑ perspiration
Metabolic Processes
• Hyperthermia
• Diaphoresis
• Hunger
• Weight loss
• Fluid volume deficit

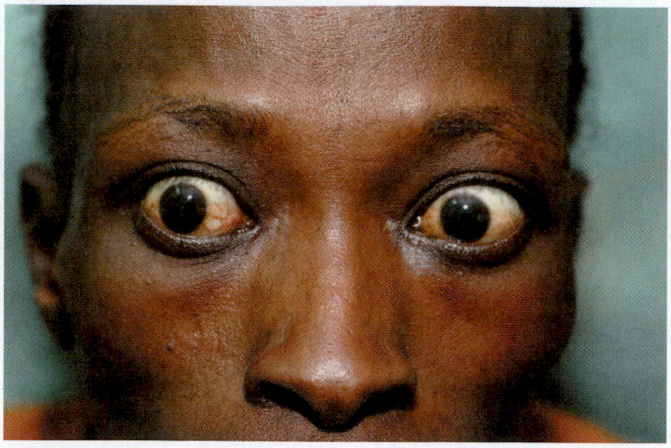

Figure 19.1 ■ Exophthalmos in a patient with Graves disease. The disease causes edema of fat deposits behind the eyes and inflammation of the extraocular muscles. The accumulating pressure forces the eyes outward from their orbits.

Toxic Multinodular Goiter

Toxic multinodular goiter (**Figure 19.2** ■) is a thyroid tumor characterized by small, discrete, independently functioning nodules in the thyroid gland tissue that secrete excessive amounts of TH. Etiologies include lack of iodine in the diet, increased iodide filtration in the kidneys, and presence of immunoglobulins (Ullah, Hafeez, Ahmad, Muahammal, & Gandapur, 2014). Elevated TH levels result in manifestations of hyperthyroidism. This type of hyperthyroidism usually affects older women. Toxic multinodular goiter increases the risk of thyroid malignancy (Ullah et al., 2014).

Thyroiditis

Thyroiditis (inflammation of the thyroid gland) is most often the result of a viral infection of the thyroid gland. The manifestations of thyroiditis are those of acute inflammation and the effects of increased TH. Thyroiditis is an acute disorder that may become chronic, resulting in a hypothyroid state as repeated infections destroy gland tissue. See the discussion of Hashimoto thyroiditis later in this chapter.

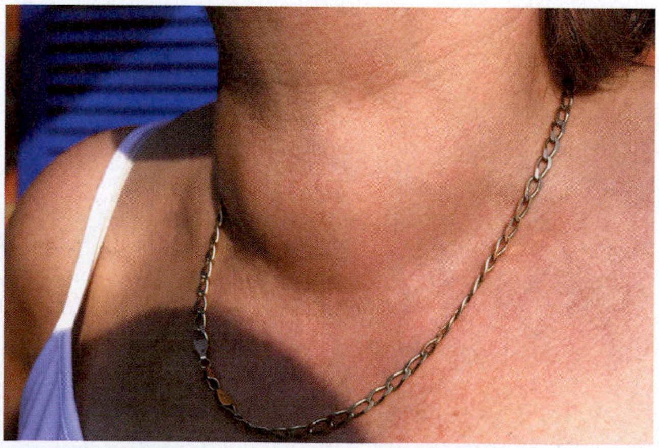

Figure 19.2 ■ Toxic multinodular goiter. The formation and growth of numerous nodules in the thyroid gland cause the characteristic massive enlargement of the neck.

Thyroid Crisis

Thyroid crisis (**thyroid storm**) is an extreme state of hyperthyroidism that is rare today because of improved diagnosis and treatment methods (Sorenson et al., 2019). When it does occur, those affected are usually people with untreated hyperthyroidism (most often Graves disease) and people with hyperthyroidism who have experienced a stressor, such as an infection, trauma, untreated diabetic ketoacidosis, or manipulation of the thyroid gland during surgery. Thyroid crisis is a life-threatening condition.

The rapid increase in metabolic rate that results from the excessive TH causes the manifestations of thyroid crisis. The manifestations include hyperthermia, with body temperatures ranging from 39° to 41°C (102° to 106°F), tachycardia, systolic hypertension, dyspnea, and GI manifestations (abdominal pain, vomiting, diarrhea). Agitation, restlessness, and tremors are common, progressing to confusion, psychosis, delirium, and seizures. Unrecognized and untreated, the mortality rate is high. Rapid treatment of thyroid storm is essential to preserve life. Treatment includes cooling without aspirin (which increases free TH) and prevention of shivering (which may further increase the temperature); replacing fluids, glucose, and electrolytes; relieving respiratory distress by administering oxygen; stabilizing cardiovascular function; and reducing TH synthesis and secretion.

Interprofessional Care

Treatment of hyperthyroidism focuses on reducing the production of TH by the thyroid gland, thus establishing a **euthyroid** (normal thyroid) state and preventing or treating complications. Depending on the patient's age and physical status, either medications, radioactive iodine therapy, or surgery may be used.

Diagnosis

Hyperthyroidism is diagnosed according to the manifestations of the specific disorders causing excessive TH and by the diagnostic test results described in Chapter 18. Elevated levels of TH (both T_3 and T_4) and increased radioactive iodine (RAI) uptake are diagnostic criteria of hyperthyroidism. In addition, a TSH level may be measured and compared with thyroxine (T_4) to differentiate pituitary dysfunction from thyroid dysfunction. Other diagnostic tests include thyroid antibodies (TA), TSH, triiodothyronine (T_3), T_4, and triiodothyronine resin uptake (T_3RU) (Kee, 2018). Laboratory findings in hyperthyroidism are outlined in **Table 19.1** ■. A thyroid scan may be used to evaluate thyroid nodules and an MRI of the thyroid is used to identify thyroid tumors.

Medications

Hyperthyroidism is treated by administering antithyroid medications that reduce TH production (Adams, Holland, & Urban, 2017). Because these drugs do not affect the release or activity of hormone that is already formed, therapeutic effects may not be seen for several weeks. To rapidly decrease the cardiovascular manifestations associated with hyperthyroidism, propranolol (Inderal), a beta-blocker, or esmolol, a rapid-acting parenteral beta-blocker,

Table 19.1 **Laboratory Findings in Thyroid Disorders**

Test	Normal Values	Hyperthyroidism	Hypothyroidism
Serum TA	Negative to 1:20	Increased	Normal
Serum TSH	<3 ng/mL	Decreased in primary hyperthyroidism	Increased in primary hypothyroidism
Serum T_4	5–12 mcg/dL	Increased	Decreased
Serum T_3	80–200 ng/dL	Increased	Decreased
T_3 uptake (T_3RU)	25–35 relative percentage	Increased	Decreased
Thyroid suppression		Increased RAI uptake and T_4 levels	No change

is part of initial treatment. Some commonly prescribed drugs, their actions, and nursing implications are shown in **Medication Administration 19.A**.

Radioactive Iodine Therapy

Because the thyroid gland takes up iodine in any form, radioactive iodine (^{131}I) concentrates in the thyroid gland and damages or destroys thyroid cells so that they produce less TH. Radioactive iodine is given orally. Results are typically seen in 6 to 8 weeks. In most instances, the patient is not hospitalized during treatment and does not require radiation precautions. This type of therapy is contraindicated in pregnant women because radioactive iodine crosses the placenta and can have negative effects on the developing fetal thyroid gland. Because the amount of gland destroyed is not readily controllable, the patient may develop hypothyroidism and require lifelong TH replacement. Adverse reactions include thyroiditis and cardiac instability due to liberation of stored thyroid hormone in the gland (Orlander et al., 2016).

Surgery

Some hyperthyroid patients have such enlarged thyroid glands that pressure on the esophagus or trachea causes breathing or swallowing problems. In these cases, removal of all or part of the gland (**thyroidectomy**) is indicated. A subtotal thyroidectomy is usually performed. This

Medication Administration 19.A

Hyperthyroidism

IODINE SOURCES

potassium iodide (SSKI, Thyro-Block, Pima)

strong iodine solution (Lugol solution)

Large doses of iodine for a short term inhibit TH synthesis and release. Iodine makes the hyperplastic thyroid less vascular prior to surgery and hastens the ability of other antithyroid drugs to reduce natural hormone output. It is also used in thyroid storm.

Nursing Responsibilities

- Assess for hypersensitivity to iodine before giving medication; for example, ask patient about allergies to shellfish.
- Dilute liquid iodine sources in water or orange juice to disguise bitter taste.
- Monitor for increased bleeding tendencies if the patient is also taking anticoagulants because iodine increases their effect.

Health Education for the Patient and Family

- The maximum effect of iodine in large doses usually occurs in 10 to 15 days.
- Long-term iodine therapy is not effective in controlling hyperthyroidism.

ANTITHYROID DRUGS

carbimazole (converted to methimazole when absorbed)

methimazole (Tapazole)

propylthiouracil (PTU, Propyl-Thyracil)

Antithyroid drugs inhibit TH production. They do not affect already formed hormones; thus, several weeks may elapse before the patient experiences therapeutic effects. Methimazole crosses the placenta and is not recommended during pregnancy (Wilson, Shannon, & Shields, 2017).

Nursing Responsibilities

- Monitor for side effects: Agranulocytosis (reduction in neutrophils, eosinophils, or basophils), hypothyroidism, pruritus, rash, elevated temperature, anorexia, loss of taste, hair loss, changes in menstruation.
- Administer drugs at the same time each day with meals to maintain stable blood levels.
- Monitor for manifestations of hypothyroidism: Fatigue, weight gain, periorbital edema.

Health Education for the Patient and Family

- Watch for unusual bleeding, redness, swelling, nausea, loss of taste, or epigastric pain. Report any such manifestations to the physician.
- Propylthiouracil is associated with weight changes; check weight daily when starting this medication to determine effect. Report significant changes to physician.
- If you are also taking warfarin, report any signs of bleeding.
- If you are taking lithium, be aware of manifestations of hypothyroidism.
- It may take up to 12 weeks before you experience the full effects of the drugs. Take the medication regularly and exactly as prescribed. Do not discontinue abruptly.

Note: Drugs identified in blue are among the 200 most commonly prescribed medications in the United States.

Source: Data from Adams et al., 2017.

procedure leaves enough of the gland in place to produce an adequate amount of TH. A total thyroidectomy is performed to treat cancer of the thyroid; the patient then requires lifelong hormone replacement (Yeung et al., 2016).

Before surgery, the patient should be in as nearly a euthyroid state as possible. The patient may be given antithyroid drugs to reduce hormone levels and iodine preparations to decrease the vascularity and size of the gland (which also reduces the risk of hemorrhage during and after surgery). Nursing care of the patient having a subtotal thyroidectomy is discussed in **Box 19.1**.

Nursing Care

Assessment

The following data are collected through the health history and physical examination. Further focused assessments are described with nursing interventions.

- ***Health history:*** Other diseases, family history of thyroid disease, when manifestations began, severity of manifestations, intake of thyroid medications, menstrual history, changes in weight, bowel elimination.
- ***Physical assessment:*** Muscle strength, tremors, vital signs, cardiovascular and peripheral vascular systems, integument, size of thyroid, presence of bruit over thyroid, eyes, and vision.

Priorities of Care

In planning and implementing nursing care for the patient with hyperthyroidism, the nurse considers the patient's responses to the systemic effects of the disorder. Although each patient may have different needs, diagnoses discussed in the next section focus on the most common health problems: Cardiovascular problems, visual deficits, weight loss, and mood disorders. See the accompanying Case Study & Nursing Care Plan on page 572.

Diagnoses, Outcomes, and Interventions

Reduce Risk for Heart Failure. The patient with hyperthyroidism is at risk for alterations in cardiac output. Excess TH directly affects the heart, resulting in increased rate and stroke volume. Increases in the metabolic demands and oxygen requirements of peripheral tissues increase the demands on the heart, and systolic hypertension, angina, dysrhythmias, or heart failure may occur. The patient often has palpitations and shortness of breath and is easily fatigued. The risk of complications is greater in patients with preexisting cardiovascular disorders.

BOX 19.1
Nursing Care of the Patient Having a Subtotal Thyroidectomy

PREOPERATIVE CARE

- Administer ordered antithyroid medications and iodine preparations, and monitor their effects. *Antithyroid drugs are given before surgery to promote a euthyroid state. Iodine preparations are given to the patient before surgery to decrease vascularity of the gland, thereby decreasing the risk of hemorrhage.*
- Teach the patient to support the neck by placing both hands behind the neck when sitting up in bed, while moving about, and while coughing. *Placing the hands behind the neck eases tension on the suture line in the front of the neck.*
- Answer questions, and allow time for the patient to verbalize concerns. *Because the incision is made at the base of the throat, patients (especially women) are often concerned about their appearance after surgery. Explain that the scar will eventually be only a thin line and that jewelry or scarves may be used to cover the scar.*
- Teach the patient to expect hoarseness due to generalized swelling at the suture line. *This is expected to diminish with healing and is not caused by laryngeal nerve damage.*

POSTOPERATIVE CARE

- Perform focused assessments to monitor for complications:
  a. ***Respiratory distress:*** Assess respiratory rate, rhythm, depth, and effort. Maintain humidification as ordered. Assist the patient with coughing and deep breathing. Have suction equipment, oxygen, and a tracheostomy set available for immediate use. *Respiratory distress may result from hemorrhage and edema, which may compress the trachea; from tetany and laryngeal spasms resulting from decreased hormones due to removal or damage to the parathyroid glands; and from damage to the laryngeal nerve, causing spasms of the vocal cords. Stridor is heard in acute obstructions. This is a high-pitched, squeaky sound and is a sign of airway obstruction. Equipment must be immediately available if the patient experiences respiratory distress that requires interventions and treatment.*
  b. ***Hemorrhage:*** Assess dressing (if present) and the area behind and under the patient's neck and shoulders for drainage. Monitor blood pressure and pulse for manifestations of hypovolemic shock. Assess tightness of dressing (if present). *The vascularity of the gland increases the risk of hemorrhage. The location of the incision and the position of the patient may cause the drainage to run back and under the patient. The danger of hemorrhage is greatest in the first 12 to 24 hours after surgery.*
  c. ***Laryngeal nerve damage:*** Assess for the ability to speak aloud, noting quality and tone of voice. *The location of the laryngeal nerve increases the risk of damage during thyroid surgery. Although hoarseness may be due to edema or use of an endotracheal tube during surgery and will subside, permanent hoarseness or loss of vocal volume is a potential danger.*
  d. ***Tetany:*** Assess for manifestations of latent tetany due to calcium deficiency, including tingling of toes, fingers, and lips; muscular twitches; positive Chvostek and Trousseau signs; and decreased serum calcium levels. Serum calcium levels will be monitored in the postoperative period. Keep calcium gluconate or calcium chloride available for immediate IV use, if necessary. *The parathyroid glands are located in and near the thyroid gland; surgery of the thyroid gland may injure or remove parathyroid glands, resulting in hypocalcemia and tetany. Tetany may occur in 1 to 7 days after thyroidectomy.*

Expected Outcome: Normal heart rate, blood pressure and pulse quality, and normal respiratory rate will be restored with treatment. Patient will experience no episodes of palpitations, fatigue with activity, and angina.

The nurse will:

- Monitor blood pressure, pulse rate and rhythm, respiratory rate, and breath sounds. Assess for peripheral edema, jugular vein distention, and increased activity intolerance. *Increased TH increases cardiac rate, stroke volume, and tissue demand for oxygen, causing stress on the heart. This may result in hypertension, arrhythmias, tachycardia, and congestive heart failure.*
- Suggest keeping the environment as cool and free of distraction as possible. Decrease stress by explaining interventions and teaching relaxation exercises. *A physically comfortable and psychologically calm environment can reduce stimuli and stressors. Stress increases circulating catecholamines, which further increase cardiac workload.*
- Encourage a balance of activity with rest periods. *Rest periods decrease energy expenditure and tissue requirements for oxygen, decreasing cardiac workload.*

Monitor Vision Changes. Visual changes that occur in patients with hyperthyroidism include difficulty focusing, diplopia (double vision), or visual loss. If the patient is unable to close the eyelids because of exophthalmos, the risk of corneal dryness with resultant infection or injury increases. Visual deficits may result from pressure on the optic nerve from retro-orbital edema. Although treatment of hyperthyroidism may stop the progression of eye changes, not all manifestations are reversible.

Expected Outcome: Patient should experience no worsening of visual acuity and the eyes will be moist at all times.

The nurse will:

- Monitor visual acuity, photophobia (excessive sensitivity to light), integrity of the cornea, and lid closure. *The cornea is at risk for dryness, injury, conjunctivitis, and corneal infections. Injury and infection of the cornea can result in further loss of visual acuity.*
- Teach measures for protecting the eye from injury and maintaining visual acuity:
  a. Use tinted glasses or shields as protection.
  b. Use artificial tears to moisten the eyes.
  c. Use cool, moist compresses to relieve irritation.
  d. Promptly report any pain or changes in vision.

  The measures outlined decrease the risk of injury, provide comfort, decrease periorbital edema that can further compromise vision, and ensure immediate care for problems, thereby minimizing the risk of further visual loss.

SAFETY ALERT: Teach the patient to cover the eyes at night if they do not close and to sleep with the head of the bed elevated 45 degrees to decrease periorbital fluid accumulation. ■

Limit Weight Loss. The hypermetabolic state that occurs in hyperthyroidism causes gastrointestinal hypermotility, with nausea and vomiting, diarrhea, and abdominal pain. Although the patient may have an increased appetite and eat more than usual, weight loss continues.

Expected Outcome: Patient's weight is appropriate for height and stable. Patient is free of nausea and vomiting, diarrhea, and abdominal pain.

The nurse will:

- Ask the patient to weigh daily (at the same time each day) and keep a record of results. *The inability to meet metabolic demands results in loss of body weight.*
- In collaboration with a dietitian, teach the patient the need for a diet high in carbohydrates and protein and including between-meal snacks. Six small meals a day may be more desirable than three large meals. *Increased nutrients as part of a well-balanced diet are necessary to meet metabolic demands. Patients are often better able to increase food intake by eating frequent, small meals. A 1-lb weight gain requires approximately 3500 extra kilocalories.*
- Monitor nutritional status through results of laboratory data. Serum albumin, transferrin, and total lymphocyte counts are commonly lower than normal in nutritional deficits. *A negative nitrogen balance signifies a catabolic state in which protein is lost and metabolic demands are not being met.*

Monitor Anxiety and Mood Disorders. Physical changes common in hyperthyroidism include exophthalmos, goiter, tremors, hair loss, increased perspiration, loss of strength, fatigue, weight loss, and changes in reproductive and sexual function (amenorrhea in women and impotence in men). In addition, the patient often has mood changes and insomnia and is constantly nervous and anxious. There may even be periods of psychosis. These changes are frightening not only for the patient but also for family members.

Expected Outcome: Patient's body image and anxiety are improved with resolution of symptoms of hyperthyroidism, decreased mood alterations, and normal sleep patterns.

The nurse will:

- Establish a trusting relationship; encourage the patient to verbalize feelings about self and to ask questions about the illness and treatment. Provide reliable information and clarify misconceptions. *Establishing trust facilitates open sharing of feelings and perceptions.*

Delegating Nursing Care Activities

The professional nurse may delegate nursing care activities such as repositioning and activity, providing hygiene, and assisting with feeding and dietary needs. The registered nurse assesses the patient on admission (or transfer of care), preoperatively, postoperatively, and upon discharge. The nurse provides teaching and develops the plan of care, coordinates the healthcare team, and evaluates the results of care provided. The nurse should be aware of individual state laws regarding delegation published in state board of nursing rules prior to delegating specific tasks.

- Provide comfort measures: Administer analgesic pain medications as ordered, and monitor their effectiveness; place the patient in a semi-Fowler position after recovery from anesthesia; support head and neck with pillows. *Analgesic medications reduce the perception of pain and reduce physical stress during the postoperative period. Positioning the patient in a semi-Fowler position and supporting the head and neck decrease strain on the suture line.*

Transitions of Care

Although hyperthyroidism is not preventable, nurses should teach patients the importance of regular healthcare provider visits and adherence to drug regimen. Thyroid hormone levels and TSH levels are assessed before beginning therapy and at regular intervals, usually several times per year. To evaluate the correct dosage of medication, the patient should be taught to monitor, record, and report to the provider weight, blood pressure, and heart rate trends at home and also be alert to signs of hyper- or hypothyroid.

Because hyperthyroid conditions cause a hypermetabolic state, patients are at risk for cardiovascular complications such as heart arrhythmias, acute myocardial infarction, and stroke. The increased heart rate and blood pressure result in increased myocardial oxygen demand, which can result in ischemia. The risk is especially high for those with atherosclerosis. Patients should be evaluated for signs of stroke and myocardial infarction, and if signs are present emergency evaluation is indicated (Biondi et al., 2015).

Patients with hyperthyroidism primarily provide self-care at home. Teaching is individualized to meet the patient's needs. Address the following topics:

- The patient taking oral medications must understand the need for lifelong treatment.
- The patient who has a thyroidectomy requires information about postoperative wound care.
- The patient having radioactive iodine therapy needs to know the manifestations of hypothyroidism.
- Depending on the age of the patient and the support systems available, referral to community healthcare agencies may be necessary.
- In addition, suggest the following resources: American Thyroid Association, Thyroid Foundation of Canada, and Endocrine Society.

Symptoms of hyperthyroid in older adults are sometimes mistaken for other problems. Cardiac arrhythmias and cardiovascular disease are often recognized and treated, though the cause, hyperthyroid, is missed. Another important effect of hyperthyroid in older adults is severe weight loss leading to weakness and even cachexia, increasing the risk for falls. Bone reabsorption is accelerated leading to osteoporosis and increased risk of fractures, including hip fractures. Palpitations, tremors, and anxiety that result from hyperthyroid can easily be mistaken for signs of dementia in the elderly population. These results of hyperthyroid severely limit the quality of life and increase morbidity and mortality. The nurse can intervene by recognizing signs of hyperthyroid such as palpitations, tremor, heat intolerance,

Case Study & Nursing Care Plan

A Patient with Graves Disease

Mrs. Juanita Manuel is a 33-year-old mother of four small children. She is a second-year student at the local community college, within one semester of completing the requirements for an associate's degree in early childhood education. For the past 3 months, Mrs. Manuel has been constantly hungry and has eaten more than usual, but she has still lost 6.8 kg (15 lb). She has repeated bouts of diarrhea and often feels nauseated. Her hands shake, she can feel her heart beating rapidly, and she finds herself laughing or crying for no apparent reason.

Mrs. Manuel makes an appointment with her family physician. The nurse at the office completes a health history and physical assessment. When asked how she has been feeling, Mrs. Manuel replies, "I don't know what's wrong with me—but I keep losing weight and I cry at the drop of a hat. I am so hot all the time, and I've never had that problem before."

ASSESSMENT	DIAGNOSES	EXPECTED OUTCOMES
The health history indicates that although her appetite has increased, Mrs. Manuel has lost 6.8 kg (15 lb). She states that she has had diarrhea, nausea, palpitations, heat intolerance, and mood changes. Physical assessment findings include T 38.3°C (101°F), P 110 bpm, R 24/min, and BP 162/86 mmHg. Her skin is moist and warm, her hair thin and fine. She has visible tremors in her hands. Her eyeballs protrude, and she is unable to close her eyelids completely. Her thyroid is enlarged and palpable. Diagnostic tests reveal the following abnormal results: T_3, 350 g/dL (normal range: 80 to 200 ng/dL); T_4, 15.1 mg/dL (normal range: 5 to 12 mg/dL). A thyroid scan demonstrates an enlarged thyroid with increased iodine uptake. After the medical diagnosis of Graves disease is made, Mrs. Manuel is started on the antithyroid medication propylthiouracil, 150 mg orally every 8 hours.	■ Weight loss of 6.8 kg (15 lb), with present weight 10% less than normal for height, related to inability to provide body requirements ■ Diarrhea related to increased peristalsis as evidenced by 8 to 10 liquid stools per day ■ Potential for vision damage related to an inability to close the eyelids completely ■ Anxiety related to thyroid hormone excess and lack of knowledge about disease process	■ Patient will gain at least 0.45 kg (1 lb) every 2 weeks. ■ Patient will regain normal bowel elimination patterns. ■ Patient will maintain normal vision (with no evidence of corneal damage) and verbalize measures to protect her eyes. ■ Patient will demonstrate self-monitoring of signs of hyperthyroid and follow up with medical treatment and self-care needs. ■ Patient will verbalize a decrease in anxiety.

PLANNING AND IMPLEMENTATION

- Request that she keep a record of daily weight.
- Discuss adopting a high-kilocalorie diet. Identify food likes and dislikes, as well as foods that increase diarrhea, before instituting a plan to increase food intake.
- Request that she keep a stool chart, noting the time, type, and precipitating factors for diarrhea stools. Teach comfort measures for irritated anal area (clean washcloth and soap, nonirritating ointment).
- Teach how to apply eyedrops (artificial tears).
- Explain the need to elevate the head of the bed to 45 degrees at night, and tape eye shields over eyes before sleep.
- Teach about Graves disease, the medication's effects and side effects, and the need for continued medical care.

EVALUATION

By her next office visit, Mrs. Manuel has gained 0.45 kg (1 lb) and has discussed her dietary needs with the nurse and her husband. She is having diarrhea less often. She has safely applied the eyedrops and states that she uses the eye shields and elevates the head of her bed at night. The office nurse reviewed the written and verbal information about Graves disease and the medication prescribed. Mrs. Manuel verbalizes her understanding, stating, "I'll always take my medicine—I never want to feel like that again!" She says that she feels much less anxious now that she understands what has happened.

CLINICAL REASONING IN PATIENT CARE

1. What is the pathophysiologic basis for Mrs. Manuel's abnormal vital signs?
2. What is the rationale for having the patient with exophthalmos elevate the head of the bed at night?
3. Outline a teaching plan that could be given to patients for home care following a subtotal thyroidectomy.

See Evaluating Your Response in Appendix B.

sweating, nervousness, and anxiety and reporting them to the provider. Evaluation and treatment of thyroid hormone excess in the elderly population can improve quality of life and limit severe complications and death (Biondi et al., 2016).

The Patient with Hypothyroidism

Hypothyroidism is a disorder that results when the thyroid gland produces an insufficient amount of TH. Because a decrease in TH levels decreases metabolic rate and heat production, hypothyroidism affects all body systems. Hypothyroidism is common in women between ages 30 and 60, with the incidence increasing after age 50. However, the disorder can occur at any stage of life. Careful evaluation of manifestations is important in the older adult because manifestations of hypothyroidism are often thought to be the result of aging instead of a pathologic process. The chronic, untreated hypothyroid state in adults is termed **myxedema**, with characteristic accumulation of nonpitting edema in the connective tissues throughout the body. The edema is the result of water retention in mucoprotein (hydrophilic proteoglycans) deposits in the interstitial spaces. The face of a patient with myxedema appears puffy, the tongue is enlarged, and the voice is hoarse and husky (Sorenson et al., 2019).

Pathophysiology and Manifestations

Hypothyroidism may be either primary or secondary. *Primary hypothyroidism* (which is more common) may be caused by congenital defects in the gland, loss of thyroid tissue following treatment for hyperthyroidism with surgery or radiation, antithyroid medications, Hashimoto thyroiditis, or endemic iodine deficiency. The cardiac drug amiodarone (Cordarone), which contains iodine, is increasingly being implicated in causing thyroid problems, especially hypothyroidism (Sorenson et al., 2019). Anabolic steroids, androgens, lithium, phenytoin, propranolol, interferon alpha, and interleukin-2 decrease T_4. The antithyroid drugs propylthiouracil and methimazole decrease T_4 level. *Secondary hypothyroidism* may result from pituitary TSH deficiency or peripheral resistance to thyroid hormones (Lee et al., 2016). Hypothyroidism has a slow onset, with manifestations occurring over months or even years. With treatment, the mental and physical manifestations rapidly reverse in patients of all ages.

When TH production decreases, the thyroid gland enlarges in a compensatory attempt to produce more hormone. The goiter that results is usually a simple or nontoxic form. People living in certain areas of the world where the soil is deficient in iodine, the substance necessary for TH synthesis and secretion, are more prone to become hypothyroid and develop simple goiter.

Patients with hypothyroidism characteristically have a goiter, fluid retention and edema, decreased appetite, weight gain, constipation, dry skin, dyspnea, pallor, hoarseness, and muscle stiffness. Many patients have a decreased sense of taste and smell, menstrual disorders, anemias, and cardiac enlargement. The pulse is typically slow. Deficient amounts of TH cause abnormalities in lipid metabolism, with elevated serum cholesterol and triglyceride levels. As a result, the patient is at increased risk for atherosclerosis and cardiac disorders. Decreased renal blood flow and glomerular filtration rate reduce the kidney's ability to excrete water, which may cause hyponatremia. Sleep apnea is more common in patients with hypothyroidism. The Multisystem Effects of Hypothyroidism are illustrated on page 574.

Multisystem Effects of
Hypothyroidism

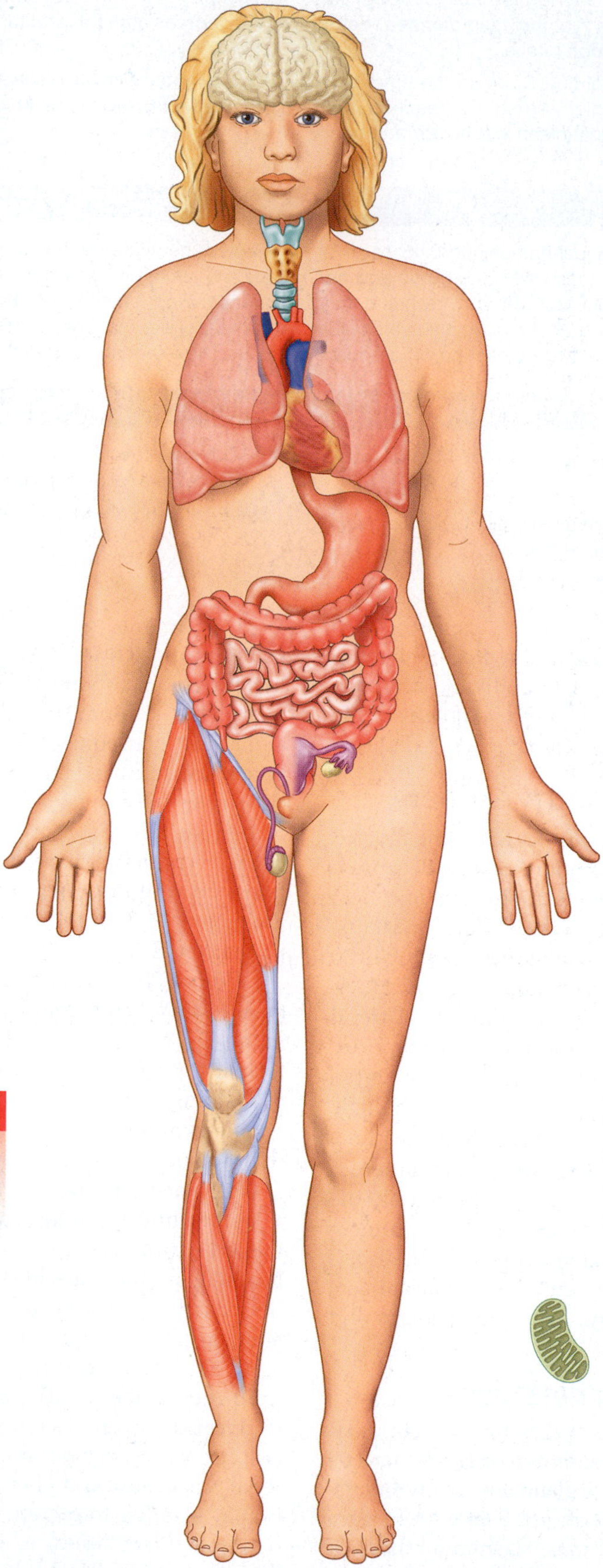

Endocrine
- Goiter

Respiratory
- Pleural effusion

Gastrointestinal
- Constipation

Musculoskeletal
- Muscle stiffness
- Weakness
- Fatigue

Neurologic
- Hand and foot paresthesias
- Lethargy
- Somnolence
- Confusion
- ↓ reflexes
- Slow speech
- Memory impairment

Sensory
- Periorbital edema

Cardiovascular
- Hypotension
- Bradycardia
- Dysrhythmias
- Enlarged heart
- Anemia

Reproductive
- Menorrhagia (female)
- Infertility (female)
- ↓ libido (male)

Integumentary
- Hair loss
- Brittle nails
- Coarse, dry skin
- Nonpitting edema

Metabolic Processes
- Hypothermia
- Anorexia
- Weight gain
- Systemic edema

Iodine Deficiency

Iodine is necessary for TH synthesis and secretion. Iodine deficiency may result from certain goitrogenic drugs (which block TH synthesis); lithium carbonate, used to treat bipolar mental disorders; and antithyroid drugs. Goitrogenic compounds in foods such as turnips, rutabagas, and soybeans may also block TH synthesis if consumed in sufficient quantities. In areas of the world where the soil is deficient in iodine, dietary intake of iodine may be inadequate. The use of iodized salt has reduced this risk in the United States (Sorenson et al., 2019).

Hashimoto Thyroiditis

Hashimoto thyroiditis is the most common cause of goiter and primary hypothyroidism. In this autoimmune disorder, antibodies develop that destroy thyroid tissue. Functional thyroid tissue is replaced with fibrous tissue, and TH levels decrease. In addition, decreasing levels of TH in the early stages of the disease prompt the gland to enlarge to compensate, causing a goiter. However, as the disease progresses, the thyroid gland becomes smaller. This disorder is more common in women and has a familial link (Sorenson et al., 2019).

Myxedema Coma

Myxedema coma is a life-threatening complication of long-standing, untreated hypothyroidism. It is characterized by severe metabolic disorders (hyponatremia, hypoglycemia, lactic acidosis), cardiovascular collapse, impaired cognition, and coma. Patients with myxedema coma are usually older adults and the condition may be precipitated by the use of central nervous system depressants or opioids, infections, stroke, trauma, or heart failure. Patients often present with severe hypothermia and severely slowed mental status. The treatment of myxedema coma addresses the precipitating factors and manifestations and involves maintaining a patent airway; maintaining fluid, electrolyte, and acid–base balance; maintaining cardiovascular status; increasing body temperature; and increasing TH levels. Even with intensive treatment, the mortality rate is high (Eledrisi, Griffing, Talavera, Khardori, & Lee, 2016).

Interprofessional Care

The treatment of the patient with hypothyroidism focuses on diagnosis, prevention or treatment of complications, and replacement of the deficient TH. With early and continued treatment, both appearance and mental function return to normal.

Diagnosis

Hypothyroidism is diagnosed by the clinical manifestations and by a decrease in TH, especially T_4. TSH concentration is often increased because the negative hormonal feedback from TH is lost. The same laboratory and diagnostic tests used to diagnose hyperthyroidism are also used to diagnose hypothyroidism, with opposite results in most cases (refer to Table 19.1). Refer to Chapter 18 for information on specific thyroid tests. Other laboratory tests associated with the diagnosis of hypothyroidism include elevated serum LDL cholesterol, triglycerides, and lipoproteins. Anemia, hypoglycemia, and hyponatremia are also common.

Medications

Hypothyroidism is treated with medications that replace TH. *Levothyroxine* (thyroxine, T_4) is the treatment of choice. Medications commonly used to treat hypothyroidism and their nursing implications are shown in **Medication Administration 19.B**. In the older adult, an age-related decrease in serum albumin and renal excretion can increase the amount of available drug and cause an exaggerated pharmacologic effect. Therefore, the older patient may require less thyroid medication than a younger patient.

Surgery

If a patient with hypothyroidism has a goiter large enough to cause respiratory difficulties or dysphagia, a subtotal thyroidectomy may be performed.

Medication Administration 19.B

Hypothyroidism

THYROID PREPARATIONS

levothyroxine sodium (T4) (Levoxyl, Levothroid, Synthroid)

liothyronine sodium (T_3) (Cytomel)

liotrix (T_3–T_4) (Euthyroid, Thyrolar)

Thyroid preparations increase blood levels of TH, thus raising the patient's metabolic rate. As a result, cardiac output, oxygen consumption, and body temperature increase. Levothyroxine speeds the elimination of vitamin K–dependent clotting factors, enhancing the effects of warfarin (Coumadin). Patients are at increased risk of bleeding if warfarin dosages are not appropriately reduced. The dosage depends on the drug chosen and the patient's degree of thyroid dysfunction, sensitivity to TH, age, body size, and health. The older adult may require lower doses.

Nursing Responsibilities

- Give 1 hour before meals or 2 hours after meals for best absorption.
- Thyroid preparations potentiate the effect of anticoagulant drugs. If the patient is also receiving an anticoagulant, monitor for bruising, bleeding gums, and blood in the urine.
- Thyroid medications potentiate the effect of digitalis. If the patient is also receiving a digitalis preparation, monitor for signs of digitalis toxicity.
- Monitor for manifestations of coronary insufficiency: Chest pain, dyspnea, tachycardia.

(continued)

- If the patient has insulin-dependent diabetes, monitor the effects of insulin. The effect of the insulin may change as thyroid function increases.
- During dose adjustment, take pulse before administering drug. Report pulse greater than 100 bpm.

Health Education for the Patient and Family

- Do not substitute brands of drugs or use generic equivalents without the physician's approval.
- The medications must be taken for the rest of your life.
- Report manifestations of excess thyroid hormone to the physician: Excess weight loss, palpitations, leg cramps, nervousness, or insomnia.
- If you have diabetes and use insulin, monitor blood glucose levels closely; the thyroid medications may alter the amount of insulin required.
- Thyroid preparations increase the risk of iodine toxicity. Do not use iodized salt or over-the-counter drugs containing iodine.
- If you are also taking an anticoagulant, report any signs of bleeding.
- Report any changes in menstrual periods.
- Take the thyroid preparation in the morning 30 minutes before eating to decrease the possibility of insomnia; take other medications such as calcium carbonate, iron, or antacids at least 4 hours before or after taking thyroid drugs; these medications may prevent absorption.
- Closely monitor blood pressure and pulse (older patients).
- Avoid excessive intake of foods that are known to inhibit TH utilization such as walnuts and high-fiber foods.

Note: Drugs identified in blue are among the 200 most commonly prescribed medications in the United States.

Source: Data from Adams et al., 2017.

Nursing Care

Assessment

Collect the following data through the health history and physical examination. Further focused assessments are described with nursing interventions that follow. When assessing the older patient, be aware of normal changes with aging, as described in Chapter 18.

- ***Health history:*** Pituitary diseases, history of hyperthyroidism and treatment with medications or radioactive iodine, thyroid surgery, treatment of head or neck cancer with radiation, diet, use of iodized salt, bowel elimination, depression, muscle or joint aching, cold intolerance, respiratory difficulties, heavy menstrual periods.
- ***Physical assessment:*** Muscle strength, deep tendon reflexes, vital signs, cardiovascular and peripheral vascular systems, integument, thyroid gland, weight.

Priorities of Care

In planning and implementing care for patients with hypothyroidism, the nurse takes into account that the disorder affects all organ systems. Although many diagnoses might be valid, the next section focuses on patient problems with cardiovascular function, elimination, and skin integrity. See the accompanying Case Study & Nursing Care Plan on page 578.

Diagnoses, Outcomes, and Interventions

Reduce Risk of Heart Failure. A TH deficit causes a reduction in heart rate and stroke volume, and additionally results in cardiac remodeling and heart failure. Hyperlipidemia and atherosclerosis results in coronary artery disease, further compromising cardiac function (Delitala, Fanciulli, Maioli, & Delitala, 2016). Decreased circulation exacerbates cold intolerance.

Expected Outcome: Patient's blood pressure and heart rate and rhythm will be within normal ranges. Patient's extremities will be warm.

The nurse will:

- Monitor blood pressure, heart rate and rhythm, apical and peripheral pulses. *Hypotension indicates decreasing peripheral blood flow. Weak pulses indicate decreased peripheral circulation. Decreased heart rate and stroke volume indicate heart failure.*
- Suggest the patient avoid chilling; increase room temperature, use additional bed covers, and avoid drafts. *Chilling increases metabolic rate and puts increased stress on the heart.*
- Explain the need to alternate activity with rest periods. Ask the patient to report any breathing difficulties, chest pain, heart palpitations, or dizziness. *Activity increases demands on the heart and should be balanced with rest. Manifestations of cardiac stress include dyspnea, chest pain, palpitations, and dizziness.*

Reduce Risk of Constipation. The hypothyroid patient is likely to have a reduced appetite and decreased metabolic rate, a diminished activity level, and reduced peristalsis to the point that fecal impactions may occur.

Expected Outcome: Patient's bowel sounds will be normal and usual bowel habits will be restored.

The nurse will:

- Encourage a fluid intake of up to 2000 mL/day. Discuss preferred liquids and the best times of day to drink fluids. If kilocalorie intake is restricted, ensure that liquids have no or low kilocalories. *Sufficient fluid intake is necessary to promote proper stool consistency.*
- Discuss ways to maintain a high-fiber diet. *Diets high in fiber and fluid produce soft stools. Fiber that is not digested absorbs water, which adds bulk to the stool and assists in the movement of fecal material through the intestines. High-fiber foods include beans, fruits, whole-grain breads, and unprocessed brown rice. Consult nutritional labels for fiber content. Instruct not to eat high-fiber foods within 4 hours of taking a thyroid hormone medication. These foods decrease absorption of thyroid hormone medications.*
- Encourage activity such as walking as tolerated. *Activity influences bowel elimination by improving muscle tone and stimulating peristalsis.*

Maintain Good Skin Integrity. The patient with hypothyroidism is at risk for poor skin integrity related to the accumulation of fluid in the interstitial spaces and to dry, rough skin. Decreased peripheral circulation, decreased activity levels, and slow wound healing further increase the risk.

Expected Outcome: Skin will be warm, moist, and intact without evidence of edema. Skin wounds will heal normally.

The nurse will:

- Monitor skin surfaces for redness or lesions, especially if the patient's activity is greatly reduced. Use a pressure ulcer risk assessment scale to identify patients at risk. *Hypothyroidism causes dry, rough, edematous skin conditions that increase the risk of skin breakdown.*
- Provide or teach immobile patient measures to promote optimal circulation:
  a. Use a turning schedule if the patient is on bedrest or teach the patient to change position every 2 hours.
  b. Limit the time for sitting in one position; shift weight or lift the body using arm rests every 20 to 30 minutes.
  c. Use pillows, pads, or sheepskin or foam cushions for bed and/or chair.
  d. Teach and implement a schedule of range-of-motion exercises.

  Prolonged pressure, especially in patients with edema and circulatory impairment, can occlude capillaries and cause hypoxic tissue damage.
- Provide or teach the patient measures to maintain skin integrity:
  a. Take baths only as necessary; use warm (not hot) water.
  b. Use gentle motions when washing and drying skin.
  c. Use alcohol-free skin oils and lotions.

  Dry skin and edema increase the risk of skin breakdown. Hot water, rough massage, and alcohol-based preparations may increase skin dryness, further impairing the body's ability to maintain skin integrity.

Delegating Nursing Care Activities

Often, dietary teaching is referred to the dietitian, and skin care and hygiene are delegated to assistive personnel. The professional nurse follows up on delegated activities. Assessments and evaluations of treatment are assessed by the nurse and communicated to other members of the healthcare team through documentation. Communication of assessments and collaboration of the healthcare team is essential to providing quality care to the patient.

Moving Evidence into Action
Hypothyroid

Subclinical hypothyroid (SCH) is positively associated with an increased risk for heart disease and type 2 diabetes (Jia et al., 2015). Based on this information, careful screening for hypothyroidism is indicated in susceptible patients. Nurses are an integral part of the evaluation team conducting screening.

External Evidence

Hypothyroid has been positively associated with heart disease and diabetes. SCH is present when there is elevated TSH with normal levels of thyroid hormone. SCH is quite common, occurring in 4% to 10% of the general population and 4% to 17% of those with type 2 diabetes (Jia et al., 2015). Research has found a positive correlation between SCH and both type 2 diabetes and heart disease. Additionally, there is a correlation between SCH and chronic kidney disease (Jia et al., 2015).

Internal Evidence

As part of the evaluation of internal evidence, one must consider the patient's response to the planned screening and the potential indicators that can be revealed. One question to ask: Are persons who are at risk for hypothyroidism confronted with positive screening and therefore increased risk for heart disease the population of your care environment? Does the clinical environment support the care needs related to positive screening results? How does providing more support for potential hypothyroid patients and their increased risk for heart disease in your environment impact costs?

Patient Considerations

When considering use of a new practice (like additional screening), the nurse must consider the specific patient population where it will be used. Will patients and their families be amenable to additional information related to results of screening?

Putting the Pieces Together

As the prevalence of heart disease and type 2 diabetes is increasing in the United States, there is more focus on prevention of each condition. Patients who present with SCH should also be screened for type 2 diabetes. Jia and colleagues (2015) suggest that patients with SCH be treated for hypothyroid. Appropriate treatment with levothyroxine (Synthroid) can improve the patient's outcome, so it is important to assess the patient's level of understanding and educate when necessary about the appropriate use and timing of Synthroid. Nurses can also help to educate the patient with SCH about the risk for heart disease and diabetes and prevention of these risk factors through lifestyle management. To effectively implement a plan, it is important to evaluate the external evidence and consider the internal implications and patient/family issues. With the use of decision-making themes, more effective patient decisions can be supported. This will lead to increased patient participation in his or her therapeutic plan and patient satisfaction.

Reference

Jia, F., Tian, J., Deng, F., Yang, G., Long, M., Cheng, W., . . . Liu, D. (2015). Subclinical hypothyroidism and the associations with macrovascular complications and chronic kidney disease in patients with Type 2 diabetes. *Diabetic Medicine, 32*(8), 1097–1103.

Transitions of Care

One of the most critical factors in preventing hypothyroidism is education of the public about the necessity of an adequate dietary intake of iodine. The use of iodized salt meets the requirements for hormone production. It is important to teach patients the importance of regular healthcare provider visits and medication intake.

Hypothyroid disease results in slowed metabolism and has multisystem effects. Many of the effects are chronic, though acute complications can result from the chronic sequelae of hypothyroidism. Cardiac ischemia results from heart failure. Hyperglycemia results from type 2 diabetes, and acute myocardial infarction results from cardiac atherosclerosis. The nurse should assess for acute complications and teach the patient to report and follow up on symptoms such as chest pain, shortness of breath, exercise intolerance, and frequent urination accompanied by thirst.

Patients with hypothyroidism require lifelong care, primarily at home. The nurse recognizes that the patient will need to take medication for the rest of one's life. Levothyroxine is the treatment of choice, and the patient will need information regarding how to take the medication correctly. If levothyroxine is taken with food or antacids, its absorption is reduced and can even be totally ineffective. Correct knowledge and adherence can greatly improve efficacy of the treatment.

Periodic follow-up with the healthcare provider is necessary. The provider will assess the patient and review measurements of serum hormone levels and TSH. The patient's reports of weight and blood pressure monitoring with signs of hypo- or hyperthyroid provide important data as to whether a medication dosage adjustment is necessary. Follow-up visits are recommended two to four times per year throughout therapy with levothyroxine, and 4 to 6 weeks after each dosage adjustment (Jonklaas et al., 2014).

If the patient is older or does not have a support system, helpful community resources include community support groups, senior centers, and home health nursing care. In addition, suggest the following resources: American Thyroid Association, Thyroid Foundation of Canada, and Endocrine Society.

Increasing the quality of life is a major goal of end-of-life care. Respiratory and heart failure are complications of hypothyroid that are managed through thyroid replacement and follow-up care. Screening and treatment of diabetes caused by hypothyroid is important, as it causes vascular complications and decreases life expectancy. Constipation can be severe, causing discomfort and bowel obstruction. Cold intolerance, especially in older adults, can cause discomfort and greatly reduce the quality of life. Thyroid replacement and careful management is important at the end of life to improve quality of life.

Case Study & Nursing Care Plan

A Patient with Hypothyroidism

Jane Lee is a 60-year-old retired nurse living with her husband and daughter on a farm that has been in the family for four generations. Mrs. Lee has gained 4.5 kg (10 lb) in the past few months, even though she is rarely hungry and eats much less than normal. She is always tired and weak—so tired that she has not even been able to help with the chores on the farm or do housework. She is concerned about her appearance and the way she sounds when she talks. Her face is puffy, and her tongue always feels thick.

ASSESSMENT

Brian Henning, RN, completes the health assessment for Mrs. Lee at the health center. He finds that she now weighs 68 kg (150 lb), an increase of 4.5 kg (10 lb) over her weight at her last visit 6 months earlier. Mrs. Lee states that she always feels cold, tired, and weak. She states that she is constipated, has difficulty remembering things, and looks different. Physical assessment findings include a palpable and bilaterally enlarged thyroid; dry, yellowish skin; nonpitting edema of the face and lower legs; and slow, slurred speech. Diagnostic tests revealed the following abnormal findings: T_3, 56 ng/dL (normal range: 80 to 200 ng/dL); T_4, 3.1 (normal range: 5 to 12 mg/dL); TSH increased. The medical diagnosis of hypothyroidism is made, and Mrs. Lee is started on levothyroxine 0.05 mg daily.

DIAGNOSES

- Constipation related to decreased peristalsis, as evidenced by hard, formed stools once per week.
- Difficulty with verbal communication related to changes in speech patterns and enlarged tongue
- Low self-esteem related to changes in physical appearance and activity intolerance

EXPECTED OUTCOMES

- Patient will regain normal bowel elimination patterns, having a soft, formed stool at least every other day.
- Patient will experience improvement in verbal communication.
- Patient will regain positive self-esteem as medication reduces physical changes and fatigue.

PLANNING AND IMPLEMENTATION

- Teach to increase fluids, bulk, and fiber in the diet to help regain a normal bowel elimination pattern of a soft, formed stool every other day.
- Take medication as prescribed and do not expect immediate reversal of manifestations affecting speech.
- Plan activities around rest periods. Encourage husband and daughter to help with housecleaning and cooking.

EVALUATION

On return to the health center 2 months later, Mrs. Lee reports that she is no longer constipated but that she is continuing to drink six glasses of water and eating oatmeal every day. She no longer feels cold, is regaining her normal energy, and even feels well enough to plant her garden. Her speech is clear and easy to understand.

CLINICAL REASONING IN PATIENT CARE

1. What physical changes that normally occur with aging are similar to the manifestations of hypothyroidism?
2. Describe the factors that put Mrs. Lee's safety at risk. What alterations in her home environment would you suggest to promote safety until the prescribed medication takes effect?
3. The patient taking oral thyroid medications may develop hyperthyroidism. List the manifestations you would include in a teaching plan to signal this condition.

See Evaluating Your Response in Appendix B.

The Patient with Cancer of the Thyroid

There were approximately 56,870 new cases of thyroid cancer diagnosed in 2017 and it accounted for about 2010 cancer deaths in 2017 (National Cancer Institute, 2017). The most consistent risk factor is exposure to ionizing radiation to the head and neck during childhood. For example, many adults in their 60s, 70s, and 80s received x-ray treatments for colds, tonsillitis, acne, and sinus infections during childhood.

Of the several types of thyroid cancer, the most common types are:

- ***Papillary thyroid carcinoma*** is the most common thyroid malignancy (National Cancer Institute, 2017). It is usually detected as a single nodule, but may arise from a multinodular goiter. It is most often diagnosed in women between ages 30 and 50. Risks for the development of this form are exposure to external x-ray treatments to the head or neck as a child, childhood exposure to radioactive isotopes of iodine in nuclear fallout, and a family history. Papillary thyroid carcinoma is the least aggressive type, but does metastasize to local and regional lymph nodes and lungs.
- ***Follicular thyroid cancer*** is the second most common thyroid malignancy. It is diagnosed at a slightly older age (40 to 60) than papillary and more commonly in women. This form is more aggressive than papillary, with potential for vascular invasion and spread to lung and bone. Exposure to radiation is not considered a risk factor for this type of thyroid cancer.
- ***Medullary thyroid cancer*** arises from the cells of the thyroid that produce the hormone calcitonin; these cells do not uptake iodine and, therefore, are not susceptible to treatment with radioactive iodine. Individuals with a family history of thyroid cancer have a change in a gene named *RET* and this can be passed from parent to child.

Thyroid cancer is manifested by a palpable, firm, nontender nodule in the thyroid. If undetected, the tumor may grow and impinge on the esophagus or trachea, causing difficulty with swallowing or breathing. Most people with thyroid cancer do not have elevated thyroid hormone levels. The diagnosis is made by measuring thyroid hormones, performing thyroid scans, and by fine-needle biopsy of the nodule. The usual treatment is subtotal or total thyroidectomy. TSH suppression therapy with levothyroxine may be conducted prior to surgery. Radioactive iodine therapy (^{131}I) and chemotherapy are additional therapeutic options. Although standard chemotherapy is not used often, new biologic chemotherapies offer promise of remission or cure for the more aggressive or refractory types of thyroid cancer (Konstantakos, Talavera, & Balducci, 2016). Nursing care for the patient with cancer is discussed in Chapter 14.

19.2 Disorders of the Parathyroid Glands

Disorders of the parathyroid glands, hyperparathyroidism, and hypoparathyroidism, are not as common as those of the thyroid gland. Hypercalcemia and hypocalcemia (the primary results of alterations in parathyroid function) are discussed in Chapter 10.

The Patient with Hyperparathyroidism

Hyperparathyroidism results from an increase in the secretion of parathyroid hormone (PTH), which regulates normal serum levels of calcium. The increase in PTH affects the kidneys and bones, resulting in increased resorption of calcium and excretion of phosphate by the kidneys (increasing the risk of hypercalcemia and hypophosphatemia), increased bicarbonate excretion and decreased acid excretion by the kidneys (increasing the risk of metabolic acidosis and hypokalemia), increased release of calcium and phosphorus by bones with resultant bone decalcification, and deposits of calcium in soft tissues and the formation of renal calculi.

Pathophysiology and Manifestations

Hyperparathyroidism occurs more often in older adults and is three times more common in women. The disorder itself is not common. *Primary hyperparathyroidism* occurs when there is hyperplasia or an adenoma in one of the parathyroid glands. *Secondary hyperparathyroidism* is a compensatory response to chronic hypocalcemia. The tertiary form is most often seen in patients with chronic renal failure.

Many patients with hyperparathyroidism are asymptomatic. When manifestations occur, they are related to hypercalcemia and various musculoskeletal, renal, and gastrointestinal manifestations. Bone reabsorption results in pathologic fractures, while elevated calcium levels alter neural and muscular activity, leading to muscle weakness and atrophy. Proximal renal tubule function is altered, and metabolic acidosis, renal calculi formation, and polyuria occur.

Manifestations of the effect of hypercalcemia on the gastrointestinal tract include abdominal pain, constipation, anorexia, and peptic ulcer formation. Hypercalcemia also affects the cardiovascular system, causing dysrhythmias, hypertension, and increased sensitivity to cardiotonic glycosides (e.g., digitalis preparations).

Interprofessional Care

Hyperparathyroidism is diagnosed by excluding all other possible causes of hypercalcemia, by at least a 6-month history of manifestations, and by laboratory analysis of levels of serum calcium and PTH levels (Kim, 2017).

Treatment of hyperparathyroidism focuses on decreasing the elevated serum calcium levels. Patients with mild hypercalcemia are urged to drink fluids and keep active. They should avoid immobilization, thiazide diuretics, large doses of vitamins A and D, antacids containing calcium, and calcium supplements. Severe hypercalcemia requires hospitalization and intensive treatment with intravenous saline. Medications to inhibit bone resorption and reduce hypercalcemia—such as pamidronate (Aredia), alendronate (Fosamax), and zoledronate (Zometa)—are used for short-term treatment, improve bone density, and may relieve bone pain. Calcitonin, a hormone produced by the thyroid gland, decreases plasma levels of calcium by inhibiting bone resorption and increasing calcium excretion by the kidney (Adams et al., 2017). A form of calcitonin from salmon is available as a nasal spray or by IM or subcutaneous injection. A medication for patients with hyperparathyroidism secondary to renal failure or parathyroid cancer is a calcimimetic. This drug increases the sensitivity of the calcium-sensing receptors of the parathyroid gland to serum calcium. The effect is decreased secretion of PTH and reduced serum calcium and phosphorus.

Surgical removal of the parathyroid glands affected by hyperplasia or adenoma treats primary hyperparathyroidism. The preoperative and postoperative nursing care of the patient having surgery of the parathyroids is essentially the same as that for the patient having a thyroidectomy. Manipulation of the thyroid while removing the parathyroids may result in TH release, causing increased cardiac rate and stroke volume.

Nursing Care

Nursing care of the patient with hyperparathyroidism focuses on its effects on calcium balance: Hypercalcemia and bone resorption with an increased risk for pathologic fractures. Nursing care of the patient with hypercalcemia is discussed in Chapter 10. The patient is also at risk for developing kidney stones; see Chapter 27 for nursing care for the patient with renal calculi.

The Patient with Hypoparathyroidism

Hypoparathyroidism results from abnormally low PTH levels. The most common cause is damage to or inadvertent removal of all of the parathyroid glands during thyroidectomy. The lack of circulating PTH causes hypocalcemia and an elevated blood phosphate level (Gonzalez-Campoy, Talavera, Shenker, Griffing, & Schade, 2016).

Pathophysiology and Manifestations

Reduced levels of PTH result in impaired renal tubular regulation of calcium and phosphate. In addition, decreased activation of vitamin D results in decreased absorption of calcium by the intestines. The low calcium levels cause changes in neuromuscular activity, affecting peripheral motor and sensory nerves. Hypocalcemia lowers the threshold for nerve and muscle excitability; a slight stimulus anywhere along a nerve or muscle fiber initiates an impulse (Sorenson et al., 2019).

The neuromuscular manifestations that result include numbness and tingling around the mouth and in the fingertips, muscle spasms of the hands and feet, convulsions, and laryngeal spasms. **Tetany**, a continuous spasm of muscles, is the primary symptom of hypocalcemia. In severe cases of tetany, death may occur. Assessments for tetany include Chvostek sign and Trousseau sign (refer to Chapter 18). Integumentary manifestations include brittle nails, hair loss, and dry, scaly skin. Gastrointestinal symptoms include abdominal cramps and malabsorption. CNS manifestations include paresthesias of the lips, hands, and feet; mood disorders such as irritability, depression, and anxiety; hyperactive reflexes, psychosis, and increased intracranial pressure. Dysrhythmias can also be present (Sorenson et al., 2019).

Interprofessional and Nursing Care

Hypoparathyroidism is diagnosed by low serum calcium levels and high phosphorous levels in the absence of renal failure, an absorption disorder, or a nutritional disorder.

Treatment of hypoparathyroidism focuses on increasing calcium levels. Intravenous calcium gluconate is given immediately to reduce tetany. Long-term therapy includes supplemental calcium, increased dietary calcium, and vitamin D therapy.

Calcium imbalance (hypocalcemia) is the primary manifestation of hypoparathyroidism and the nursing care focus. Nursing care for the patient with hypocalcemia is discussed in Chapter 10.

19.3 Disorders of the Adrenal Glands

The paired adrenal glands are made up of two distinct regions, the cortex (outer portion) and medulla (inner portion), each producing hormones with whole body effects.

Hormones of the adrenal cortex are essential to life. They maintain homeostasis in response to stressors. Disorders of the adrenal cortex result in complex physical, psychologic, and metabolic alterations that are potentially life-threatening. Hormones of the adrenal medulla are not essential to life because the sympathetic nervous system produces similar body responses. The primary adrenal disorders are hyperfunction and hypofunction of the adrenal cortex and hyperfunction of the adrenal medulla.

The Patient with Cushing Syndrome or Cushing Disease

Cushing syndrome (hypercortisolism) is a chronic disorder caused by excessive amounts of circulating cortisol. The most common cause of Cushing syndrome is pharmacologic therapy with corticosteroids. People who take corticosteroids for long periods of time (e.g., for the treatment of arthritis, after an organ transplant, or as an adjunct to chemotherapy) are at risk for developing the disorder (Sorenson et al., 2019). **Cushing disease** is caused by adenoma, a tumor on the pituitary gland that causes the overproduction of cortisol. Cushing disease is more common in women between the ages of 20 and 50 years (Endocrine Society, 2017).

Pathophysiology

The pituitary gland produces ACTH, and ACTH causes the adrenal glands to produce cortisol. Cushing adenomas, which are usually benign tumors, cause the pituitary gland to produce too much ACTH. The excess ACTH leads the adrenal glands to overproduce cortisol. The excess cortisol secretion suppresses pituitary ACTH production, resulting in atrophy of the uninvolved adrenal cortex (Endocrine Society, 2017). Cushing disease results from various causes. Research implicates proteins and genes in the etiology of Cushing disease. Two proteins, testicular orphan nuclear receptor 4 (TR4) and heat shock protein 90 (HSP90), may play a role in the development of the adenomas that result in Cushing disease (Sbiera et al., 2015). Mutation of the gene ubiquitin-specific peptidase 8 (USP8) is also implicated in many pituitary adenomas that increase levels of ACTH (Sbiera et al., 2015).

Manifestations

The manifestations of Cushing syndrome result from an excess of cortisol, which leads to exaggerated cortisol actions. Obesity and a redistribution of body fat result in fat deposits in the abdominal region (central obesity), fat pads under the clavicle, a "buffalo hump" over the upper back, and a round moon face (**Figure 19.3** ■). Changes in protein metabolism cause muscle weakness and wasting, especially in the extremities. Glucocorticoid excess inhibits fibroblasts, resulting in loss of collagen and connective tissue. Thinning of skin, abdominal striae (reddish purple stretch marks), easy bruising, poor wound healing, and frequent skin infections result. Glucose metabolism is altered in the majority of patients, and diabetes mellitus may occur. Electrolyte imbalances also occur with the increased hormone levels. Changes in calcium absorption result in osteoporosis, compression fractures of the vertebrae, fractures of the ribs, and renal calculi. Hypokalemia and hypertension occur as potassium is lost and sodium is retained. Inhibited immune responses increase the risk of infection, and increased gastric acid secretion increases the risk of peptic ulcers. Emotional changes range from depression to psychosis. In women, increasing androgen levels cause hirsutism (excessive facial hair in particular), acne, and menstrual irregularities.

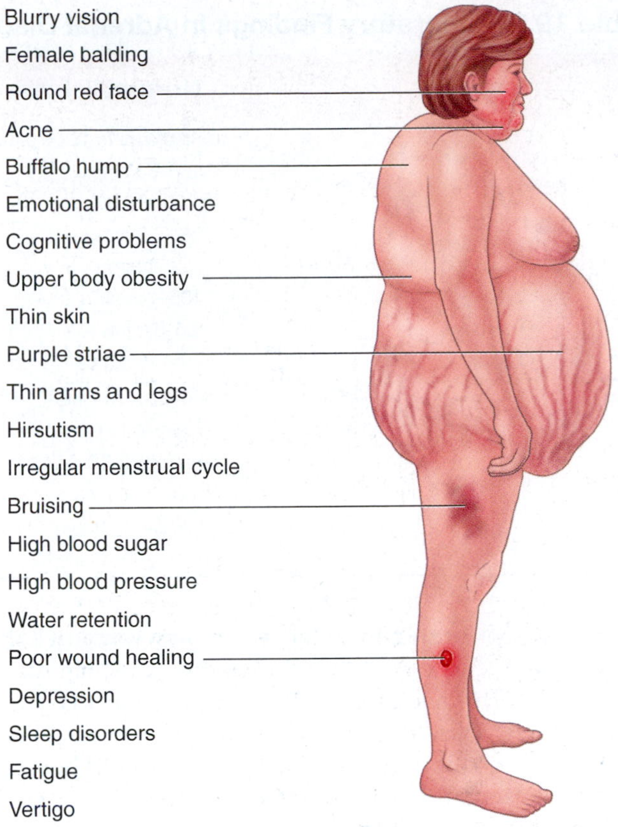
Blurry vision
Female balding
Round red face
Acne
Buffalo hump
Emotional disturbance
Cognitive problems
Upper body obesity
Thin skin
Purple striae
Thin arms and legs
Hirsutism
Irregular menstrual cycle
Bruising
High blood sugar
High blood pressure
Water retention
Poor wound healing
Depression
Sleep disorders
Fatigue
Vertigo

Figure 19.3 ■ Characteristic features of a patient with Cushing disease.

The complications of untreated Cushing syndrome include electrolyte imbalances (hyperglycemia, hypernatremia, and hypokalemia), hypertension, and emotional disturbances. Increased susceptibility to infections is also a factor. Compression fractures from osteoporosis and aseptic necrosis of the femoral head may result in serious disability. If the patient undergoes a bilateral adrenalectomy as a treatment for Cushing syndrome, an acute deficit of cortisol (Addisonian crisis) may result. Cushing disease results in medical complications and increased mortality.

Interprofessional Care

The treatment of Cushing syndrome includes medications, radiation therapy, or surgery, depending on the etiologic origin of the disorder.

Diagnosis

Cushing syndrome is diagnosed through a variety of diagnostic tests. In addition to the laboratory tests described in Chapter 18 and in **Table 19.2**, a dexamethasone suppression

Table 19.2 Laboratory Findings in Adrenal Disorders

	Test	Normal Values	Hyperfunction (Cushing Syndrome)	Hypofunction (Addison Disease)
Serum	Cortisol	8:00 a.m. to 10:00 p.m.: 138–635 mmol 4:00 to 6:00 p.m.: 83–359 mmol	Increased	Decreased
	Blood urea nitrogen (BUN)	5–25 mg/dL	Normal	Increased
	Sodium	135–145 mEq/L	Increased	Decreased
	Potassium	3.5–5.0 mEq/L	Decreased	Increased
	Glucose	70–110 mg/dL	Increased	Decreased
Urine	Urinary free cortisol (UFS)	10–50 mcg/24 h	Increased	Low/absent
	17-hydroxy-corticosteroids (17-OHCS)	Male: 3–12 mcg/24 h Female: 2–10 mg/24 h	Increased	Decreased
	17-ketosteroids (17-KS)	Male: 5–25 mg/24 h Female: 5–15 mg/24 h Age > 65: 4–8 mg/24 h	Increased	Decreased

test may be performed to differentiate between adrenal hyperplasia due to excess ACTH secretion (Cushing disease) and adrenal cancer (Kee, 2018). If the dexamethasone test is positive, a test for urinary-free cortisol is made. This measures the amount of cortisol in the urine over 24 hours. Other diagnostic studies, including a CT scan or MRI of the abdomen, may be conducted to assess the adrenal gland for tumors.

Medications

Cushing syndrome that results from a pituitary tumor is treated by medications as an adjunct to surgery or radiation. Medications are also used for patients with inoperable pituitary or adrenal malignancies (Adams et al., 2017). Although the drugs control manifestations, they do not effect a cure. Examples of some commonly prescribed drugs are:

- Mitotane directly suppresses activity of the adrenal cortex and decreases peripheral metabolism of corticosteroids. It is used to treat metastatic adrenal cancer.
- Aminoglutethimide or ketoconazole (or both) inhibit cortisol synthesis by the adrenal cortex and may be administered to patients with ectopic ACTH-secreting tumors that cannot be surgically removed.
- Somatostatin analog (octreotide) suppresses ACTH secretion in some patients.

Surgery

When Cushing syndrome is caused by an adrenal cortex tumor, an adrenalectomy may be performed to remove the tumor. Only one adrenal gland is usually involved; however, if an ACTH-producing ectopic tumor is involved, a bilateral adrenalectomy is performed. Lifelong hormone replacement is necessary if both adrenal glands are removed.

Surgical removal of the pituitary gland (hypophysectomy) is indicated when Cushing syndrome is the result of a pituitary disorder. The gland is removed either by a transsphenoidal route or by a craniotomy.

Nursing Care

Assessment

Collect the following data through the health history and physical examination. Further focused assessments are described with nursing interventions later.

- ***Health history:*** History of pituitary, adrenal, pancreatic, or pulmonary tumor; frequent infections; gastrointestinal bleeding; stress fractures; pain; changes in weight or fat distribution; change in height; fatigue; weakness; change in appearance; bruising; skin infections; menstrual history; sexual function
- ***Physical assessment:*** Vital signs, behavior, appearance, fat distribution, face, skin, hair quantity and distribution, muscle size and strength, gait.

Priorities of Care

The nurse caring for the patient with Cushing syndrome must take a holistic approach to plan and implement interventions for a wide variety of responses, including problems related to fluid and electrolyte balance, injury, infection, and body image. See the Case Study & Nursing Care Plan on page 588.

Diagnoses, Outcomes, and Interventions

Manage Fluid Volume. The excess cortisol secretion associated with Cushing syndrome results in sodium and water reabsorption, causing excess fluid volume (Sorenson et al., 2019). The patient will have weight gain, edema, and hypertension.

Expected Outcome: Patient's blood pressure and weight will be within normal limits; no jugular vein distention or edema will be present.

The nurse will:

- Ask the patient to weigh at the same time each day and maintain a record of results. *Body weight is an accurate indicator of fluid status. One liter of fluid retention corresponds to about 1 kg (2.2 lb) of body weight.*

- Monitor blood pressure, rate and rhythm of pulse, respiratory rate, and breath sounds. Assess for peripheral edema and jugular vein distention. *Extracellular fluid volume excess resulting from sodium and water retention is manifested by hypertension and a bounding, rapid pulse. There may also be crackles and wheezes, dependent edema, and venous distention.*
- Teach the patient and family the reasons for restricting fluid and the importance of limiting fluids if ordered. *Restricting fluid can help decrease the risk of fluid volume excess. Involving the patient and family in the plan of care and teaching the rationale for interventions help the patient achieve goals.*

Reduce Risk for Falls and Fractures. The patient with Cushing syndrome is at risk for injury from several causes. Excess cortisol causes increased absorption of calcium and demineralization of bones, resulting in risk of pathologic fractures. Muscle weakness and fatigue are common, increasing the potential for accidental falls.

Expected Outcome: Patient will be aware of accommodations to prevent injuries and will be free from injuries.

The nurse will teach the patient and caregivers the following:

- Keep unnecessary clutter and equipment out of the way and off the floor.
- Ensure adequate lighting, especially at night.
- Use assistive devices for ambulation or to ask for help if needed.
- Be sure corrective lenses are available and clean.
- Use nonskid slippers or shoes.
- Watch for signs of fatigue (increased pulse and respirations); plan rest periods.

A well-lighted environment free of clutter decreases the risk of falls and injury. Sensory and motor deficits increase the risk of falls; corrective lenses, assistive devices, and nonslip footwear can decrease this risk. Rest relieves fatigue. To reduce energy expenditure, include alternating periods of rest and activity in daily schedules.

Reduce Risk for Infection. Elevated cortisol levels impair the immune response and put the patient with Cushing syndrome at increased risk for infection. Increased cortisol also affects protein synthesis, causing delayed wound healing, and inhibits collagen formation, which results in epidermal atrophy, further inhibiting resistance to infection. In addition, impaired blood flow to edematous tissue results in altered cellular nutrition, which increases the potential for infection.

Expected Outcome: The patient will be aware of measures to prevent infections. The patient will be free from infections.

The nurse will:

- Monitor vital signs and verbalizations of subjective manifestations (e.g., the patient's response to "How do you feel?") every 4 hours. *Increased body temperature and pulse are systemic indicators of infection; however, because Cushing syndrome impairs the normal inflammatory response, the usual indicators of inflammation may not be present.*
- Monitor results of diagnostics such as white blood cell count and results of cultures. *Increased white blood cells are indicative of infection. Culture reports will specify the organism causing infection.*
- Use principles of medical and sterile asepsis when caring for the patient, conducting procedures, or providing wound care. *Impaired skin and tissues make aseptic techniques even more necessary to decrease the risk of infection. Intact skin is the first line of defense against infection; if invasive procedures are performed or a wound is present, this defense is lost.*
- If wounds are present, assess the color, odor, and consistency of wound drainage, and look for increased pain in and around the wound. *Cortisol excess delays wound healing and closure.*
- Teach the importance of increasing intake of protein and vitamins C and A. *Protein, vitamin C, and vitamin A are necessary to collagen formation; collagen helps support and repair body tissues.*
- Encourage recommended vaccinations.

SAFETY ALERT: A generalized feeling of malaise may be the primary manifestation of infection, especially in the older adult. ■

Discuss Coping Strategies. The patient with Cushing syndrome has obvious physical changes in appearance. The abnormal fat distribution, moon face, buffalo hump, striae, acne, and facial hair (in women) all contribute to disruptions in the way patients with this disorder perceive themselves.

Expected Outcome: Patient will discuss physical changes and ways to adapt to them. Patient will verbalize an understanding that physical changes are expected to improve with treatment of Cushing syndrome.

The nurse will:

- Encourage patients to express feelings and to ask questions about the disorder and its treatment. *The loss of one's normal body image may prompt feelings of hopelessness, powerlessness, anger, and depression. Understanding the disease and adapting to changes from that disease are the first steps in regaining control of one's own body.*
- Discuss strengths and previous coping strategies. Enlist the support of family or significant others in reaffirming the patient's worth. *Disturbances in body image are often accompanied by low self-esteem. Self-esteem derives from one's perception of competence and from appraisals of others.*
- Discuss signs of progress in controlling manifestations; for example, decreased facial edema or increased activity tolerance. *Many physical changes from cortisol excess disappear with treatment. Clearly communicate this fact because the patient may believe changes are permanent.*

Delegating Nursing Care Activities

The registered nurse performs the preoperative and postoperative assessments. These assessments are particularly important for identifying potential complications during and after surgery. Tasks that are often delegated include blood glucose measurements, toileting, and repositioning. The registered nurse develops the plan of care, provides teaching, coordinates the healthcare team, and evaluates the results of care provided. The nurse should be aware of individual state laws regarding delegation published in state board of nursing rules prior to delegating specific tasks.

Transitions of Care

Stress the importance of taking corticosteroid medications as ordered to reduce the risk of developing Cushing syndrome for patients with acute or chronic inflammation. The risk of abruptly discontinuing the medications is also an essential component of teaching.

The patient with Cushing syndrome requires education about self-care at home specific to the type of treatment given. Address the following topics:

- Safety measures to prevent falls if fatigue, weakness, and osteoporosis are present.
- Taking medications as prescribed, with information about side effects. Patients often require glucocorticoid medications for the rest of their lives, and dosage changes are highly likely.
- Having regular health assessments.

Some of the same issues that present in the acute treatment of Cushing syndrome continue throughout the patient's lifetime. Address the following topics:

- Wearing a medical alert ID indicating the patient has Cushing syndrome.
- Educate about cardiovascular risk and how to minimize it. *Patients taking glucocorticoids are at particularly high risk for cardiovascular events.*
- Monitor bone health. *Patients taking glucocorticoids are at particularly high risk for decreased bone mineral density.*
- Monitor for signs of infection and report early to healthcare provider.
- Educate about signs of diabetes such as thirst, frequent urination, weight loss, and hunger. *Patients taking glucocorticoids are at particularly high risk for diabetes.*
- Helping the patient with referrals to social services or community health services because of the complexity of the treatment and care required.
- Providing helpful resources: American Association of Clinical Endocrinologists and Endocrine Society.

The older individual with Cushing disease will need additional care and help to maximize the quality of life. Falls and fractures can be avoided by providing safeguards and assistive devices in the home. Medications and physical therapies aimed at improving bone mineral density will also be very helpful in preventing pathological fractures. Infections can be minimized by keeping the home environment clean and by limiting visitors with signs of illness. If the patient with Cushing disease gets sick, he or she should go to the doctor quickly as glucocorticoids decrease the patient's ability to fight infections. Depression is a common result of chronic disease. Depression can be successfully minimized at the end of life by encouraging the patient to be involved in healthcare decisions and solving problems and also through social involvement (Kim, Noh, & Chun, 2016).

The Patient with Chronic Adrenal Insufficiency

Chronic adrenal insufficiency is an uncommon disorder resulting from destruction or dysfunction of the adrenal cortex. The result is chronic deficiency of cortisol, aldosterone, and adrenal androgens, accompanied by skin pigmentation. It can occur at any age, although it is usually diagnosed in young adults (Griffing et al., 2016).

Pathophysiology

There are many possible causes of adrenal insufficiency. The etiologies include:

- Autoimmune destruction of the adrenals is the most common cause of primary adrenal insufficiency (**Addison disease**). It may occur alone or as part of a polyglandular autoimmune syndrome (PGA). Type 2 PGA is seen in adults (usually women), often associated with autoimmune thyroid disease (usually hypothyroidism), type 1 diabetes, primary ovarian or testicular failure, and pernicious anemia.
- The adrenal glands may also be destroyed by infection (tuberculosis is a common cause of Addison disease in developing countries), sepsis, metastatic cancer, hemorrhage, or heparin-induced thrombocytopenia (HIT).
- Adrenoleukodystrophy is an X-linked disorder characterized by an accumulation of very long-chain fatty acids in the adrenal cortex, testes, brain, and spinal cord.
- An ACTH deficit (secondary adrenal insufficiency) can result from pituitary tumors, pituitary surgery or irradiation, and the use of exogenous steroids.
- Abrupt withdrawal from long-term, high-dose steroid therapy can cause acute adrenal insufficiency.

Because the adrenal cortex has significant reserve capacity, initial manifestations may not be apparent. Basal glucocorticoid secretion is normal, but does not increase in response to stress and surgery. Trauma or infection can precipitate an adrenal crisis. As the destruction of the adrenal cortex continues, even basal secretion of glucocorticoids and mineralocorticoids is deficient. Decreasing plasma cortisol reduces the feedback inhibition of pituitary ACTH and, hence, plasma ACTH rises.

Acute secondary adrenocortical insufficiency occurs when either large doses or prolonged therapy with corticosteroids is abruptly withdrawn. Corticosteroids are used for their anti-inflammatory and immunosuppressive effects to treat diseases such as arthritis and asthma. High levels of circulating corticosteroids suppress the hypothalamic–pituitary–adrenal feedback mechanism and cause atrophy of the adrenal glands. If the steroid medications are suddenly discontinued, the glands cannot effectively respond to the reduced level of circulating glucocorticoids.

Manifestations

The onset of Addison disease is slow in most cases; the patient experiences manifestations after about 90% of the function of the gland is lost. The primary manifestations are the result of elevated ACTH levels and decreased aldosterone and cortisol. Aldosterone deficiency affects the ability of the distal tubules of the nephron to conserve sodium. Sodium is lost, potassium is retained, extracellular fluid is depleted, and the blood volume is decreased. Postural hypotension with tachycardia and syncope are common, and hypovolemic shock may occur. Hyponatremia causes dizziness, confusion, and neuromuscular irritability. Hyperkalemia causes cardiac dysrhythmias. The patient often experiences weakness and muscle pain (Sorenson et al., 2019).

Cortisol insufficiency also causes decreased hepatic gluconeogenesis with hypoglycemia. The patient tolerates stress poorly and experiences lethargy, weakness, anorexia, nausea and vomiting, and diarrhea. The increased ACTH levels stimulate pigmentation changes such as freckling; diffuse darkening of skin; and bluish-black patches on mucous membranes (Sorenson et al., 2019). Elevated ACTH levels and decreased aldosterone and cortisol also result in poor wound healing and menstrual changes in female patients.

Addisonian Crisis

Addisonian crisis is a life-threatening acute adrenal insufficiency. The disorder is chronic after the acute episode resolves.

Addisonian crisis is most commonly precipitated by major stressors, especially if the disease is poorly controlled. Triggers include surgery, acute systemic illness, and trauma. Addisonian crisis may occur in patients who are abruptly withdrawn from corticosteroid medications or who have hemorrhage into the adrenal glands from either septicemia or anticoagulant therapy.

The primary manifestations of the crisis develop rapidly and are a high fever; weakness; severe, penetrating pain in the abdomen, lower back, and legs; severe vomiting; diarrhea; hypotension; and circulatory collapse, shock, and coma. Treatment of the crisis is rapid intravenous replacement of fluids and glucocorticoids. Fluid balance is usually restored in 4 to 6 hours.

Interprofessional Care

The patient with Addison disease requires early diagnosis and treatment. Medical treatment includes glucocorticoid and mineralocorticoid replacement therapy.

Diagnostic Tests

Addison disease is diagnosed through findings of decreased levels of cortisol, aldosterone, and urinary 17-ketosteroids (17-KS). Dehydration may result in increased hematocrit and blood urea nitrogen (BUN). Blood glucose levels are decreased, and potassium is increased (Kee, 2018). A list of laboratory findings in Addison disease is shown in Table 19.2. The following diagnostic tests are used:

- *Serum cortisol levels*, which are decreased in adrenal insufficiency
- *Blood glucose levels*, which are decreased in adrenal insufficiency
- *Serum sodium levels*, which are decreased in adrenal insufficiency
- *Serum potassium levels*, which are increased in adrenal insufficiency
- *BUN levels*, which are increased in adrenal insufficiency
- *Urinary 17-hydroxycorticoids (17-OHCS)* and *17-KS levels*, which are decreased in adrenal insufficiency
- *Plasma ACTH levels*, which are increased in primary adrenal insufficiency (adrenal gland does not produce cortisol), but decreased in secondary adrenal insufficiency (ACTH not adequately produced by the pituitary)
- *ACTH stimulation test*, which is the most specific diagnostic test for Addison disease. (Cortisol levels rise with pituitary deficiency but do not rise in primary adrenal insufficiency.)
- *CT scans* of the head, which identify any intracranial lesion impinging on the pituitary gland.

Medications

The primary medical treatment of Addison disease is replacement of corticosteroids and mineralocorticoids, accompanied by increased sodium in the diet (Adams et al., 2017). Hydrocortisone (Cortef, others) is given orally to replace cortisol; fludrocortisone (Florinef) is given orally to replace mineralocorticoids. Nursing responsibilities in cortisol replacement are given in **Medication Administration 19.C**.

Nursing Care

Assessment

Collect the following data through the health history and physical examination. Further focused assessments are described with nursing interventions later in this chapter.

- *Health history:* Weight loss, changes in skin color, nausea and vomiting, anorexia, diarrhea, abdominal pain, weakness, amenorrhea, changes in sexual desire, confusion, and intolerance of stress
- *Physical assessment:* Height and weight, vital signs, skin, hair quality and distribution, muscle size and strength.

Priorities of Care

The patient with Addison disease requires nursing care for a wide variety of responses to the decrease in cortisol levels. Diagnoses discussed in the next section are directed toward

Medication Administration 19.C

Addison Disease

CORTICOSTEROID REPLACEMENTS

cortisone (Cortone, Cortogen)

dexamethasone (Decadron, Hexadrol, Dexasone)

fludrocortisone acetate (Florinef, F-Cortef)

hydrocortisone (Cortisol, Hydrocortone, Cortef)

methylprednisolone (Medrol, Solu-Medrol)

prednisolone (Meticortelone)

prednisone (Meticorten, Deltasone, Orasone)

Corticosteroids are used for replacement therapy in acute and chronic adrenal insufficiency. These drugs have anti-inflammatory and immunosuppressant effects. They also facilitate coping with stress.

Because corticosteroids are immunosuppressants, their use is contraindicated when an infection is suspected; they also mask the signs of infection. Immunizations with live vaccines should not be attempted. Corticosteroids are contraindicated in many other disorders, including peptic ulcer, Cushing syndrome, cardiac disease, hyperthyroidism, hypothyroidism, and tuberculosis. Concurrent use with NSAIDs is not recommended because of the combined effect on the gastrointestinal tract.

When these drugs are administered in small doses for replacement therapy, side effects are uncommon. Large doses or prolonged therapy may cause a Cushing-like syndrome, with atrophy of the adrenal cortex. Older patients, especially postmenopausal women, are more prone to develop hypertension and osteoporosis when undergoing glucocorticoid therapy. These drugs are used with caution in children and older adults and are not usually administered to pregnant women.

Nursing Responsibilities

- Establish baseline data, including mental status, neurologic function, vital signs, and weight.
- Identify medications that might interact with corticosteroids: Antidiabetic agents, cardiac glycosides, oral contraceptives, anticoagulants, NSAIDs.
- Document and report increased blood pressure, edema or weight gain, bleeding or bruising, weakness, or manifestations of Cushing syndrome.
- Administer oral forms of the drug with food to minimize its ulcerogenic effect.
- Monitor electrolyte levels for increased sodium and decreased potassium.
- Monitor capillary blood glucose for hyperglycemia in the patient with diabetes.

Health Education for the Patient and Family

- Take medications with food or milk, and report any gastric distress or dark stools.
- People with adrenal insufficiency need to take the medications for the rest of their lives.
- Consume a diet that is low in potassium and higher in sodium and protein.
- Weigh yourself each day at the same time, and report any consistent weight gain, which indicates fluid retention.
- Use safety measures in the home to prevent falls and injuries.
- Corticosteroids may impair the effectiveness of oral contraceptives.
- Take the medication regularly and continuously. *Abruptly discontinuing the medication is dangerous.*
- Obtain a medical alert bracelet.
- Monitor for increased stressors (infection, dental work, personal crisis) and increase the dose as indicated by the physician.
- Anticoagulant drugs or insulin may decrease the effectiveness of corticosteroids.
- Report the following to the physician: Dizziness on sitting or standing, nausea and vomiting, pain, thirst, feelings of anxiety, malaise, infections.

Note: Drugs identified in blue are among the 200 most commonly prescribed medications in the United States.

Source: Data from Adams et al., 2017.

problems with fluid and electrolyte balance and compliance with lifelong self-care. See the Case Study & Nursing Care Plan on page 588.

Diagnoses, Outcomes, and Interventions

Maintain Fluid Volume. Fluid volume deficit in the patient with Addison disease results from loss of water and sodium, as well as from vomiting and diarrhea. Extracellular fluid volume deficit, decreased cardiac output, hypotension, and hypovolemic shock may occur, especially in crisis situations. Interventions for this diagnosis are outlined for the patient who is hospitalized.

Expected Outcome: Patient's fluid balance will return to normal following treatment: Blood pressure will be normal, urine will be light amber with normal specific gravity, postural hypotension will be absent, and weight will return to baseline.

The nurse will:

- Monitor intake and output, and assess for signs of dehydration: dry mucous membranes; thirst; poor skin turgor; sunken eyeballs; scanty, dark urine; increased urine specific gravity; weight loss; and increased hemoconcentration (increased hematocrit and BUN). *Glucocorticoid and mineralocorticoid depletion causes fluid volume deficit. Fluid volume deficit may reach crisis levels if undetected, causing altered tissue perfusion and hypovolemic shock.*
- Monitor cardiovascular status: Take and record vital signs, assess character of pulses, and monitor potassium levels and ECGs. *Fluid volume deficit may lead to hypotension and a rapid, weak, or thready pulse. As aldosterone levels fall, renal excretion of potassium decreases, increasing blood levels of potassium.*
- Weigh the patient daily at the same time and in the same clothing. *Dehydration is manifested by weight loss.*
- Encourage increased oral fluid intake and an increased salt intake. *Cortisol deficiency increases fluid loss, leading to extracellular fluid volume depletion. Oral fluid*

replacement is necessary to balance this loss. An increase in dietary sodium can decrease the hyponatremia characteristic of adrenal insufficiency.

- Teach to sit and stand slowly, and provide assistance as necessary. *Extracellular fluid volume deficit causes orthostatic hypotension, dizziness, and possible loss of consciousness. These manifestations increase the risk of injury from falls.*

SAFETY ALERT: Hyperkalemia causes changes in cardiac muscle function, which are reflected in ECG changes. The patient should have heart monitoring and IV access in the hospital. The nurse recognizing ECG changes such as peaked T waves or ventricular arrhythmias would recommend emergency management of hyperkalemia. Management of hyperkalemia is accomplished through various medications and/or hemodialysis. Medications that may be chosen to decrease serum potassium include calcium, insulin administered with glucose, and Kayexalate. Hemodialysis normalizes serum potassium levels through the use of dialysate solution. ■

Delegating Nursing Care Activities

The registered nurse would monitor the unstable patient in Addisonian crisis. Once the patient is stabilized, activities such as vital signs, weight monitoring, blood glucose checks, and assisting with self-care activities could be delegated. The registered nurse develops the plan of care, develops the teaching plan, coordinates the healthcare team, and evaluates the results of care provided.

Transitions of Care

Health promotion related to adrenal insufficiency focuses on identifying situations in which emotional and physical stress require additional glucocorticoids. These situations should be avoided as much as possible. Also important is teaching patients about the risks associated with abruptly withdrawing prolonged or high-dose corticosteroid drugs. Interventions for the patient with Addison disease focus on careful assessments when the patient is under significant physiologic stress. Teaching to prevent or treat an Addisonian crisis is essential.

The patient with Addison disease provides self-care at home. One of the most important components of caring for the patient with Addison disease is teaching both the patient and family to provide care. Family stability, an awareness of the serious nature of the disease, and the effectiveness of treatment all promote adherence. The length of treatment and the side effects of medications, however, can discourage adherence. In addition to the information in the teaching topics included in the preceding section, include the following topics:

- Teach the effects of illness and treatment. Discuss patient and family concerns. *Lack of knowledge about the illness, as well as the possibility of complications from disregarding or altering the treatment, can negatively affect compliance.*
- Teach self-administration of steroids. *The patient should carry an emergency kit containing parenteral cortisone and a syringe/needle at all times.*
- Wear a medical alert bracelet that says "Adrenal insufficiency—takes hydrocortisone."
- Increase oral fluid intake and maintain a diet high in sodium and low in potassium.

Patients with Addison disease must learn to provide lifelong self-care that involves varied components: Medications, diet, and recognizing and responding to responses to stress. Changes in lifestyle are difficult to maintain permanently. The nurse needs to ensure that the patient and close family members will have the knowledge and resources necessary to manage Addison disease. In addition to the acute care topics, the patient will need to learn the management of chronic disease. Topics include:

- The importance of continuing healthcare. *One of the most important components of caring for the patient with Addison disease is teaching both the patient and family to provide care. The length of treatment and the side effects of medications can discourage adherence to the regimen.*
- Alter the medication dose when experiencing emotional or physical stressors. *An important aspect of therapy is preventing life-threatening Addison crisis. This is accomplished by taking additional glucocorticoids during times of emotional and physical stress.*
- Referral to social worker, if appropriate.
- Referral to community agencies for continued education and support.
- Helpful resources: National Institute of Diabetes and Digestive and Kidney Diseases (Addison disease), Endocrine Society, and American Association of Clinical Endocrinologists.

The Patient with Pheochromocytoma

Pheochromocytomas are tumors of the chromaffin tissues in the adrenal medulla (Blake, Sweeney, Griffing, Khardori, & Talavera, 2015; Sorenson et al., 2019). These tumors, which are usually benign, produce catecholamines (epinephrine or norepinephrine) that stimulate the sympathetic nervous system. Although many organs are affected, the most dangerous effects are peripheral vasoconstriction and increased cardiac rate and contractility with resultant paroxysmal hypertension. Systolic blood pressure may rise to 200 to 300 mmHg, the diastolic to 150 to 175 mmHg. Attacks are often precipitated by physical, emotional, or environmental stimuli. This condition, while rare, is life-threatening.

A pheochromocytoma is diagnosed by increased levels of catecholamines and their metabolites (metanephrines) in the blood or urine, by x-ray studies, and by surgical exploration. Removal of the tumor(s) by adrenalectomy is the treatment of choice.

Case Study & Nursing Care Plan

A Patient with Addison Disease

Addy, a 55-year-old professional, is brought to the emergency department (ED) by Emergency Medical Services with complaints of heart palpitations. Her husband reports that his wife is weak, dizzy, and has been experiencing nausea and vomiting and muscle weakness for several days. She was prescribed a cortisone drug for treatment of an autoimmune disease for the past 5 years. Because of family financial stress, the patient did not refill her medication.

ASSESSMENT

On admission to the ED, Addy is dehydrated, with dry skin and oral mucous membranes and decreased urine output. Her blood pressurev is 90/50, pulse is 105 and thready. She continues to feel weak and dizzy and is also confused about the day and time. Diagnostic tests reveal the following abnormal findings:

- ECG: elevated T wave and sinus tachycardia
- Sodium: 127 mEq/L (normal range: 135 to 145 mEq/L)
- Glucose: 63 mg/dL (normal range: 70 to 110 mg/dL)
- Potassium: 5.7 mEq/L (normal range: 3.5 to 5.3 mEq/L)
- Cortisol: 3 mg/dL (normal for a.m.: 5 to 23 mg/dL).

The physician's plan of care for Addy includes intravenous administration of normal saline (NS) at 250 mL/h and hydrocortisone (Solu-Cortef) 200 mg. Dextrose 50%, 12.5 grams, is administered intravenously. When Addy is stable, she is moved to a telemetry monitored in-patient bed.

DIAGNOSES

- Inadequate fluid volume related to adrenal insufficiency accompanied by nausea and vomiting.
- Poor tissue perfusion related to dehydration accompanied by low BP, high heart rate, and decreased urine output.
- Anxiety related to lack of knowledge about the cause and effects of adrenal insufficiency.

EXPECTED OUTCOMES

- Patient will regain normal fluid balance and return to baseline weight.
- Patient will regain normal perfusion with blood pressure, pulse, and urine output within normal ranges.
- Patient will demonstrate knowledge of the causes and effects of adrenal insufficiency.

PLANNING AND IMPLEMENTATION

- Seizure precautions until sodium is normal and stable.
- Cardiac monitoring.
- Monitor vital signs frequently until stable.
- Monitor electrolytes, and report abnormal results.
- Blood glucose monitoring.
- Monitor intake and output closely.
- Take and record daily weight in the morning before breakfast.
- Discuss a diet that is high in sodium, low in potassium, and has an increased fluid intake (3000 mL/day). Discuss the types of fluids desired and the best times for intake of increased fluids.
- Assist during activity to prevent falls.
- Provide verbal and written instructions, and encourage verbal feedback about the causes and effects of the disease, the effects of medications, the effects of not taking long-term cortisone drugs, the diet, and self-care at home.

EVALUATION

Following treatment for acute adrenal insufficiency, Addy is rehydrated and her blood pressure, pulse, and urine output have returned to normal. Seizure activity is avoided; she is no longer weak and dizzy and is reoriented. Cardiac events are avoided and blood glucose returns to normal levels. Addy understands how important glucocorticoids are following teaching and now knows how to monitor herself for signs of cortisol deficiency. A referral to the case manager will help Addy with her health-care costs and follow-up care.

CLINICAL REASONING IN PATIENT CARE

1. Adrenal insufficiency is often diagnosed only when the patient becomes seriously ill in response to a stressor. Explain why this statement is or is not true.
2. Describe the physical assessments that are found in the severely dehydrated patient.
3. Outline a teaching plan for Addy with foods for a high-sodium, low-potassium diet.

See Evaluating Your Response in Appendix B.

19.4 Disorders of the Pituitary Gland

The pituitary gland produces hormones that affect multiple body systems through regulation of endocrine function. Target tissues include the thyroid, adrenal cortex, ovary, uterus, mammary glands, testes, and kidneys. Disorders result from an excess or deficiency of one or more of the pituitary hormones due to a pathologic condition within the gland itself or to hypothalamic dysfunction.

Although disorders of the pituitary cause diverse and serious problems, they are not as common as disorders of other endocrine glands. Hyperpituitarism and hypopituitarism are discussed in this section.

The Patient with Disorders of the Anterior Pituitary Gland

Hyperfunction of the anterior pituitary gland, characterized by excess production and secretion of one or more trophic hormones, is usually the result of a pituitary tumor or pituitary hyperplasia. The most common cause of hyperpituitarism is a benign adenoma. The manifestations result from pressure on the optic nerve causing visual changes or an excess of growth hormone (GH), prolactin (PRL), ACTH, or TSH. Disorders related to excess growth hormone are discussed in the following.

Hypofunction of the anterior pituitary gland results in a deficiency of one or more of the gland's hormones. Conditions causing hypopituitarism include pituitary tumors; surgical removal of the pituitary gland; radiation; and pituitary infarction, infection, or trauma.

Pathophysiology and Manifestations

Growth hormone (somatotropin) is produced throughout life by cells in the anterior pituitary. GH stimulates the production of IGF-1 (an insulin-like growth factor) by the liver. GH is necessary for growth and also contributes to metabolic regulation. GH stimulates all aspects of cartilage growth, and one of its major effects is to stimulate the growth of the epiphyseal cartilage plates of long bones. In addition, other body tissues respond to the metabolic effect of GH and IGF-1 with increases in bone width and the growth of visceral and endocrine organs, skeletal and cardiac muscle, skin, and connective tissue. Gigantism and acromegaly result from overstimulation. Growth retardation and short stature result from deficient production of GH.

Gigantism

Gigantism occurs when GH hypersecretion begins before puberty and the closure of the epiphyseal plates. The person becomes abnormally tall, often exceeding 213 cm (7 ft) in height, but body proportions are relatively normal. Most often the result of a tumor, the condition is rare today as a result of improved diagnosis and treatment.

Acromegaly

Acromegaly, which literally means "enlarged extremities," occurs when sustained GH and IGF-1 hypersecretion begins during adulthood, most commonly because of pituitary tumors. When excess GH production develops in adulthood, the person does not grow taller because the long bone epiphyses are closed. As a result of excess GH, the small bones of the hands and feet, the membranous bones of the skull, connective tissue, and soft tissues continue to grow. The forehead enlarges, the maxilla lengthens, the tongue enlarges, and the voice deepens. Overgrowth of bone and soft tissue in the hands and feet causes patients to buy increasingly larger rings, gloves, and shoes. Other manifestations of acromegaly include peripheral nerve damage from entrapment of nerves, headache, hypertension, heart failure, skin thickening and copious sweating, seizures, and visual disturbances. Changes in appearance are subtle and diagnosis is usually made 10 years or more after onset of GH hypersecretion. Impaired glucose tolerance and diabetes may develop. Manifestations may be relieved by treatment that halts excessive GH and IGF-1 production.

Interprofessional and Nursing Care

Acromegaly is treated by surgical removal or irradiation of the pituitary tumor. A transsphenoidal or transfrontal surgical procedure is most commonly used. Somatostatin receptor binding drugs (SRBDs) suppress the anterior pituitary gland and decrease GH levels. These are administered by injection, and gastrointestinal side effects are common for the first couple of weeks. Gallstones may occur within a year of beginning treatment. Growth hormone receptor antagonists lower IGF-1 production and are used if manifestations persist with SRBDs. Radiation therapy is used when GH-producing tumors persist despite surgery or become resistant to medical therapies (Diaz-Thomas, Shim, & Schwartz, 2015).

Patients with anterior pituitary disorders require interventions to help in coping with physical and emotional changes, as well as to prevent complications involving other organs and functions of the endocrine system. Nursing care for the patient having cranial surgery is discussed in Chapter 42.

The Patient with Disorders of the Posterior Pituitary Gland

Disorders of the posterior pituitary are related primarily to excessive or deficient antidiuretic hormone (ADH) secretion. The disorders discussed here are the syndrome of inappropriate ADH secretion and diabetes insipidus.

Pathophysiology and Manifestations

Antidiuretic hormone, also known as *vasopressin*, regulates water excretion by the kidneys. ADH is secreted in response to increased serum osmolality and decreased circulatory volume, which are monitored by osmoreceptors in the hypothalamus. When hyperosmolality or a low circulating volume occur, ADH secretion increases and water is reabsorbed, thus restoring blood volume and reducing its osmolality. Hypo-osmolality suppresses ADH secretion, and renal water excretion increases.

Syndrome of Inappropriate ADH Secretion

The **syndrome of inappropriate ADH secretion (SIADH)** is characterized by high levels of ADH with water retention and small amounts of concentrated urine output. This disorder may be caused by the ectopic production of ADH by malignant tumors (e.g., oat cell carcinoma of the lung, pancreatic carcinoma, leukemia, and Hodgkin lymphoma). SIADH may occur with a head injury or CNS disorders such as stroke, pulmonary disease (including pneumonia or use of positive pressure ventilation), or as an adverse effect of medications such as selective serotonin reuptake inhibitors (SSRIs) used to treat depression, barbiturates, or anesthetics.

Manifestations of SIADH occur as a result of water retention causing hyponatremia and reduced serum osmolality. Water moves from the hypotonic plasma and the interstitial spaces into the cells. Despite fluid retention, the patient may experience thirst. Urinary output decreases and the urine becomes very concentrated. Changes in mental status or personality, lethargy, irritability, and seizures can follow if hyponatremia is significant, leading to cerebral edema. Weight gain may occur but usually no edema is present because water is distributed between the intracellular and extracellular spaces.

Treatment addresses the low serum sodium and cerebral edema. Fluid intake is restricted to gradually reduce total body water. Besides keeping the patient safe, nursing care involves teaching the patient about restricting fluids. Fluid restriction continues until the syndrome resolves or is corrected. Loop diuretics such as furosemide are used to decrease fluid volume. Demeclocycline (Declomycin) is a tetracycline antibiotic that suppresses ADH activity, resulting in increased urine production. Vasopressin receptor antagonists, such as Conivaptan and Tolvaptan, are especially beneficial to correct hyponatremia (Thomas et al., 2016).

An intravenous hypertonic solution of sodium chloride (3% saline) may be required if the sodium is critically low. IV replacement of sodium must be monitored carefully to prevent rapid infusion. Too rapid replacement of sodium can cause demyelination of the central nervous system, which results in permanent neurologic dysfunctions (Thomas et al., 2016).

Diabetes Insipidus

Diabetes insipidus is the result of ADH insufficiency. The two types are:

- ***Neurogenic diabetes insipidus*** can either result from a disruption of the hypothalamus and pituitary gland (as from trauma, irradiation, or cranial surgery) or be idiopathic.
- ***Nephrogenic diabetes insipidus*** is a disorder in which the renal tubules are not sensitive to ADH. This may be familial in origin or the result of renal failure.

Diabetes insipidus may result from brain tumors or infections, pituitary surgery, cerebrovascular accidents, and renal and organ failure. It is also a complication of closed head trauma with increased intracranial pressure (Khardori et al., 2016).

A deficit of ADH causes excretion of large amounts of dilute urine (*polyuria*), in some instances as much as 12 L/day. The patient has extreme thirst and drinks large volumes of water (*polydipsia*). If unable to replace the water loss, the patient becomes dehydrated and hypernatremic. Even though the serum osmolality is high, the urine is dilute and has a low specific gravity.

If this disorder is caused by cerebral injury, manifestations commonly appear 3 to 6 days after the initial injury and last for 7 to 10 days. Initial care of the patient is focused on correcting fluid deficits, normalizing the sodium levels, and replacing deficient ADH. Intake and output are measured carefully and fluid is often replaced based on a calculation that adds fluid losses from the prior hour to an hourly base rate of fluid. Rapid and careful fluid replacement is essential to prevent hypovolemia. Hypotonic solutions of sodium are used if the sodium level is high. High serum sodium can cause neurologic deficits and can result in seizures (refer to Chapter 10). Seizure precautions are indicated if serum sodium is critically high. ADH replacement is necessary and comes in a variety of preparations: Desmopressin (DDAVP) can be administered nasally or parenterally; vasopressin (Pitressin) can be administered as a titrated IV infusion (Thomas et al., 2016). Diabetes insipidus may also be a chronic illness requiring lifelong treatment and care. See **Table 19.3** for a comparison of posterior pituitary gland disorders.

Interprofessional and Nursing Care

SIADH is treated by correcting underlying causes, treating the hyponatremia with intravenous hypertonic saline, and restricting oral fluids to less than 800 mL/day.

Table 19.3 Comparison of Posterior Pituitary Gland Disorders

SIADH	Diabetes Insipidus
Excessive ADH	Deficient ADH
Fluid volume excess	Fluid volume deficit
Hyponatremia: Sodium < 135 mEq/L (low)	Hypernatremia: Sodium > 145 mEq/L (high)
Serum osmolality < 275 mOsm/kg (low)	Serum osmolality > 295 mOsm/kg (high)
Urinary specific gravity > 1.010 (concentrated, dark)	Urinary specific gravity < 1.005 (very dilute)
Restrict fluid intake	Encourage fluid intake
Slow sodium replacement	IV fluid replacement (replaced milliliter for milliliter) if necessary ADH replacement
Demeclocycline (Declomycin) (oral agent) to suppress ADH activity	Desmopressin (DDAVP) (nasal spray) to replace deficient ADH

Diabetes insipidus is treated by correcting underlying causes, if possible. Other medical interventions include administering intravenous hypotonic fluids, increasing oral fluids, and replacing ADH hormone. Nursing care for the patient with SIADH and diabetes insipidus focuses on patient problems with fluid and electrolyte balance. See Chapter 10 for specific nursing interventions for the patient with fluid volume excess or deficit, hyponatremia, or hypernatremia.

CHAPTER HIGHLIGHTS

19.1 Disorders of the Thyroid Gland

Describe the pathophysiology and manifestations of disorders of the thyroid gland, and outline the interprofessional care and nursing care of patients with these disorders.

- Thyroid disorders are the most common endocrine disorders. Occurring mainly among women, these diseases change body image and impose upsets to energy levels, creating fatigue and exhaustion.
- Graves disease, an autoimmune disorder of the thyroid gland, is the most common cause of hyperthyroid disease. This disease causes the thyroid gland to enlarge, manifested with a goiter. Older patients with hyperthyroid are at risk for acute life-threatening cardiovascular complications.
- Hypothyroidism results when thyroid hormone levels are insufficient. Myxedema coma is a life-threatening form of hypothyroidism that results in hyponatremia, hypoglycemia, hypothermia, and lactic acidosis.
- Diagnostic tests and therapies are available to identify and treat thyroid disorders. Surgery, radiation therapy, and medications support good quality of life, but the medications must be used throughout the lifetime.

19.2 Disorders of the Parathyroid Glands

Describe the pathophysiology and manifestations of disorders of the parathyroid glands, and outline the interprofessional care and nursing care of patients with these disorders.

- Hyperparathyroidism, though uncommon, usually occurs in older adults and results from increased parathyroid hormone (PTH). It manifests with hypercalcemia and hypophosphatemia. Metabolic acidosis and hypokalemia are complications.
- Hypoparathyroid results from low parathyroid hormone (PTH) and is often caused by damage or removal of the glands. It manifests with hypocalcemia and hyperphosphatemia.

19.3 Disorders of the Adrenal Glands

Describe the pathophysiology and manifestations of disorders of the adrenal glands, and outline the interprofessional care and nursing care of patients with these disorders.

- Cushing syndrome is caused by taking glucocorticoids, prescribed to treat chronic inflammatory conditions. Cushing disease is most commonly caused by adenomas (tumors) in the pituitary gland.
- Addison disease, insufficient cortisol, is caused by destruction of the adrenal glands through autoimmune disease or infection or destruction of the pituitary gland (ACTH deficit). Corticosteroid replacements are critical for these patients.

19.4 Disorders of the Pituitary Gland

Describe the pathophysiology and manifestations of disorders of the pituitary gland, and outline the interprofessional care and nursing care of patients with these disorders.

- The pituitary gland, in conjunction with the hypothalamus, is the master gland of the body. Pituitary disorders, therefore, can have wide-ranging effects.
- Disorders of the anterior pituitary are manifested by the effects of excess growth hormone. Gigantism occurs when excess growth hormone occurs before closure of the epiphyseal plates, resulting in tall stature, whereas acromegaly occurs with excess growth hormone after puberty, resulting in larger hands, feet, and skull.
- Disorders of the posterior pituitary include syndrome of inappropriate antidiuretic hormone (SIADH) and diabetes insipidus (DI). SIADH results from excess antidiuretic hormone (ADH), whereas DI results from inadequate ADH. Antidiuretic hormone affects fluid and electrolyte balance.

TEST YOURSELF NCLEX-RN® REVIEW

1. The nurse is preparing teaching for a patient diagnosed with Graves disease. What should the nurse explain about the etiology of this health problem?

   A. It is a genetic disorder.
   B. It is caused by an allergy.
   C. It occurs in response to an infection.
   D. It develops as an autoimmune response.

2. A patient with hyperthyroidism is scheduled to receive radioactive iodine. What should the nurse explain about the use of radioactive iodine in hyperthyroidism?
   A. The thyroid gland takes up iodine in any form.
   B. Radioactive iodine reduces the vascularity of the thyroid gland.
   C. Irradiation of the thyroid gland decreases the risk of hypothyroidism.
   D. Doses of radioactive iodine are too small to be hazardous to other body parts.
3. During a physical examination, the nurse assesses a patient with hypothyroidism as having a goiter. The nurse teaches the patient that which physiologic process caused the thyroid gland to enlarge?
   A. An increased dietary iodine intake
   B. A compensatory effort to produce more TH
   C. An excess of TH that stimulated thyroid follicles
   D. Tissue hypertrophy in response to increased TH
4. While reviewing a medication list, the nurse learns that a new patient has taken cortisone as treatment for rheumatoid arthritis for several years. The nurse increases assessment for which endocrine disorder?
   A. Acromegaly
   B. Hypothyroidism
   C. Hyperthyroidism
   D. Cushing syndrome
5. The nurse is teaching a patient with Addison disease about the disease process. Which statement illustrates that the patient understands the teaching?
   A. "I wonder why I look tan all the time."
   B. "I know I should never alter my dose of medications."
   C. "I have purchased an emergency kit and keep it with me all the time."
   D. "I will be sure to stop taking my medications when I have an infection."
6. The nurse suspects that a patient with syndrome of inappropriate antidiuretic hormone secretion is experiencing hyponatremia. Which manifestation of hyponatremia did the nurse most likely assess? (Select all that apply.)
   A. Irritability
   B. Weight loss
   C. Constipation
   D. Hyperkalemia
   E. Lethargy
7. The home health nurse is planning care for a patient with hyperparathyroidism and osteoporosis. Which patient problem is the priority in this situation?
   A. The patient is fearful.
   B. The patient is at risk for falls and other injury.
   C. The patient does not want to go out in public.
   D. The patient has low self-esteem.
8. A patient has been diagnosed with hypercalcemia. The nurse would attribute which finding to that diagnosis?
   A. Oliguria
   B. Positive Chvostek sign
   C. Constipation
   D. Hyperactive deep tendon reflexes
   E. Cardiac dysrhythmias
9. A patient recovering from a thyroidectomy is experiencing tingling around the mouth and fingertips. The nurse would assess for findings associated with which condition?
   A. Addisonian crisis
   B. Hypoparathyroidism
   C. Cushing syndrome
   D. Hyperparathyroidism
10. A female patient with Cushing syndrome is distressed because of the appearance of abdominal stretch marks. What should the nurse explain to the patient about this skin change?
   A. Excessive mineralocorticoids reduce the absorption of calcium.
   B. Excessive glucocorticoids affect normal carbohydrate metabolism.
   C. Excessive glucocorticoids cause a loss of collagen and connective tissue.
   D. Excessive cortisol results in changes in protein metabolism and protein catabolism.

See Test Yourself answers in Appendix B.

REFERENCES

Adams, M. P., Holland, L. N., & Urban, C. (2017). *Pharmacology for nursing: A pathophysiologic approach* (5th ed.). Hoboken, NJ: Pearson Education.

Biondi, B., Bartalena, L., Cooper, D. S., Hegedüs, L., Laurberg, P., & Kahaly, G. J. (2015). The 2015 European Thyroid Association guidelines on diagnosis and treatment of endogenous subclinical hyperthyroidism. *European Thyroid Journal*, *4*(3), 149–163.

Blake, M., Sweeney, A. T., Griffing, G., Khardori, R., & Talavera, F. (2016). Pheochromocytoma. *Medscape*. Retrieved from http://emedicine.medscape.com/article/124059-overview.

Bickley, L. (2017). *Bates' guide to physical examination and history taking* (12th ed.). Philadelphia, PA: Lippincott Williams & Wilkins.

Diaz-Thomas, A., Shim, M., & Schwartz, R. A. (2015). Gigantism and acromegaly. *Medscape*. Retrieved from http://emedicine.medscape.com/article/925446-overview.

Delitala, A. P., Fanciulli, G., Maioli, M., & Delitala, G. (2016). Subclinical hypothyroidism, lipid metabolism and cardiovascular disease. *European Journal of Internal Medicine, 38*, 17–24.

Eledrisi, M., Griffing, G., Talavera, F., Khardori, R., & Lee, S. (2016). Myxedema coma or crisis. *Medscape*. Retrieved from http://emedicine.medscape.com/article/123577-overview.

Endocrine Society, Hormone Health Network. (2017). *Cushing's disease*. Retrieved from www.hormone.org/diseases-and-conditions/pituitary/secretory-tumors/cushings-disease.

Gonzalez-Campoy, J. M., Talavera, F., Shenker, Y., Griffing, G., & Schade, D. (2016). Hypoparathyroidism. *Medscape*. Retrieved from http://emedicine.medscape.com/article/122207-overview.

Griffing, G., Odeke, S., Nagelberg, S., Talavera, F., Chausmer, A., & Khardori, R. (2016). Addison disease. *Medscape*. Retrieved from http://emedicine.medscape.com/article/116467-overview.

Jia, F., Tian, J., Deng, F., Yang, G., Long, M., Cheng, W., . . . Liu, D. (2015). Subclinical hypothyroidism and the associations with macrovascular complications and chronic kidney disease in patients with Type 2 diabetes. *Diabetic Medicine, 32*(8), 1097–1103.

Jonklaas, J., Bianco, A. C., Bauer, A. J., Burman, K. D., Cappola, A. R., & Celi, F. S. (2014). Guidelines for the treatment of hypothyroidism: Prepared by the American Thyroid Association task force on thyroid hormone replacement. *Thyroid: Official Journal of the American Thyroid Association, 24*(12), 1670–1751. Retrieved from http://online.liebertpub.com/doi/pdfplus/10.1089/thy.2014.0028.

Kee, J. L. (2018). *Laboratory and diagnostic tests with nursing implications* (10th ed.). Hoboken, NJ: Pearson Education.

Khardori, R., Ullal, J., Cooperman, M., Griffing, G., Talavera, F., & Ziel, F. (2016). Diabetes insipidus. *Medscape*. Retrieved from http://emedicine.medscape.com/article/117648-overview.

Kim, I. H., Noh, S., & Chun, H. (2016). Mediating and moderating effects in ageism and depression among the Korean elderly: The roles of emotional reactions and coping responses. *Osong Public Health and Research Perspectives, 7*(1), 3–11.

Kim, L. (2017). Hyperparathyroidism. *Medscape*. Retrieved from http://emedicine.medscape.com/article/127351-overview.

Konstantakos, A., Talavera, F., & Balducci, L., (2016). Medullary thyroid carcinoma. *Medscape*. Retrieved from http://reference.medscape.com/article/282084-overview.

Lee, S., Ananthakrishnan, S., Khardori, R., Allee, M., Aung, K., Baker, M. Z., et al. (2016). Subacute thyroiditis. *Medscape*. Retrieved from http://emedicine.medscape.com/article/125648-overview.

NANDA International. (2018). *NANDA International, Inc. Nursing diagnoses: Definitions and classification, 2018–2020* (11th ed.) (T. H. Herdman & S. Kamitsuru, Eds.). New York, NY: Thieme.

National Cancer Institute. (2017). *Thyroid cancer*. Retrieved from www.cancer.gov/canc ertopics/types/thyroid.

Orlander, P., Griffing, G., Talavera, F., Wehmeier, K., Gabbay, R., & Kermani, A. (2016). Toxic nodular goiter. *Medscape*. Retrieved from http://emedicine.medscape.com/article/120497-overview.

Sbiera, S., Deutschbein, T., Weigand, I., Reincke, M., Fassnacht, M., & Allolio, B. (2015). The new molecular landscape of Cushing's disease. *Trends in Endocrinology and Metabolism 26*(10), 573–583.

Sorenson, M., Quinn, L., & Klein, D. (2019). *Pathophysiology: Concepts of human disease.* Hoboken, NJ: Pearson Education.

Thomas, C., Batuman, V., Fraer, M., Lederer, E., Bessen, H., Bora, K., et al. (2016). Syndrome of inappropriate antidiuretic hormone secretion. *Medscape*. Retrieved from http://emedicine.medscape.com/article/246650-overview.

Ullah, I., Hafeez, M., Ahmad, N., Muahammad, G., & Gandapur, S. (2014). Incidence of thyroid malignancy in multinodular goiter. *Journal of Medical Science, 22*(4): 164–165.

Wilson, B., Shannon, M., & Shields, K. (2017). *Pearson nurse's drug guide 2017.* Hoboken, NJ: Pearson.

Yeung, S., Habra, M., Chiu, A., Talavera, F., Wehmeier, K., & Khardori, R. (2016). Graves disease. *Medscape*. Retrieved from http://emedicine.medscape.com/article/120619-overview.

ADDITIONAL RESOURCES

American Thyroid Association
www.thyroid.org

National Institute of Diabetes and Digestive and Kidney Diseases
www.niddk.nih.gov/health-information/endocrine-diseases/adrenal-insufficiency-addisons-disease

Chapter 20

Nursing Care of Patients with Diabetes Mellitus

Chapter Outline and Learning Outcomes

CLINICAL COMPETENCIES

- Use assessed data, patient values, clinical expertise, and evidence to determine priority nursing diagnoses and select and implement individualized nursing interventions.
- Adapt individual and cultural values and variations as well as expressed needs and preferences into the plan of care for patients with DM.
- Effectively communicate with and function within the interprofessional team to plan and provide patient care.
- Assess blood glucose levels and patterns of hyper- and hypoglycemia in patients with DM.
- Administer oral and injectable medications including mixing insulins, used to treat DM knowledgeably and safely.
- Provide individualized care to patients with hypoglycemia, hyperglycemia, diabetic ketoacidosis, and hyperosmolar hyperglycemic state.
- Provide appropriate teaching to facilitate blood glucose self-monitoring, administration of oral and injectable hypoglycemic medications, diabetic diet, appropriate exercise, and effective foot care.
- Revise plan of care as needed to provide effective interventions to promote, maintain, or restore normal glucose levels.

KEY TERMS

Diabetes mellitus (DM) is a common chronic disease of adults requiring continuing medical supervision and patient self-care education. However, depending on the type of DM and the age of the patient, both patient needs and nursing care may vary greatly.

20.1 Overview of Diabetes Mellitus

DM is not a single disorder but a group of chronic disorders of the endocrine pancreas, all categorized under a broad diagnostic label. The condition is characterized by inappropriate hyperglycemia caused by a relative or absolute deficiency of insulin or by cellular resistance to the action of insulin. Of the several classifications of DM, this chapter focuses on type 1 diabetes (T1D) and type 2 diabetes (T2D). T1D is the result of pancreatic islet cell destruction and a total deficit of circulating insulin; T2D results from insulin resistance with a defect in compensatory insulin secretion.

Consider the following examples:

- Cheryl Draheim is a 45-year-old schoolteacher. She developed T1D at age 14. Ms. Draheim has always been very careful about taking her insulin, following her diet, and exercising regularly. She uses a continuous glucose monitor to carefully regulate her blood glucose. Ms. Draheim says that sometimes she believes the disease controls her more than she controls it.
- Tom Chang is 53 years old. Early in his 30s, Tom was diagnosed with T2D. Although Mr. Chang was taught about the disease and the importance of taking his oral medications, following his diet plan, and getting exercise, he rarely did more than take the medication. Five years ago, he was hospitalized for hyperglycemia and started taking insulin. Last year, Mr. Chang had a stroke, leaving him unable to walk. Now, he has been admitted to the hospital for treatment of gangrene of the large toe on his left foot.
- Grace Staples is an independent 82-year-old woman who lives alone and happily takes care of her two dogs. She is slightly overweight. Last year, during Ms. Staples's annual eye examination, eye changes typical for DM were found. She was referred to her family physician, who diagnosed T2D and started her on oral medications. Ms. Staples sticks to her diet, walks a mile every day, and plans to live to be 100.

DM has been recognized as a disease for centuries, but it was not until 1921 that techniques were developed for extracting insulin from pancreatic tissue and for measuring blood glucose. At the same time, researchers discovered that insulin, when injected, produces a dramatic drop in blood glucose. This meant that DM was no longer a terminal illness because hyperglycemia could now be controlled. Since that time, oral hypoglycemic drugs, human insulin products, insulin pumps, intermittent and continuous blood glucose monitoring, and transplantation of the pancreas or of pancreatic islet or beta cells have advanced the treatment and care of people with DM.

Patients with DM face lifelong changes in lifestyle and health status. Nursing care is provided in many settings for the diagnosis and care of the disease and treatment of complications. A major role of the nurse is that of educator in both hospital and community settings.

Incidence and Prevalence

Approximately 30.3 million people, 9.4% of the population, in the United States have diabetes. Of that number, 23.1 million people have been diagnosed and an estimated 7.2 million are undiagnosed (Centers for Disease Control and Prevention [CDC], 2017b). Additionally, 84.1 million Americans over the age of 18 (33.9% of U.S. adults) have prediabetes (CDC, 2017b). The prevalence of DM (especially T2D) among American adults is increasing rapidly and younger adults are developing diabetes. Blacks and Native Americans are disproportionately affected by T2D. See the Focus on Cultural Diversity box.

DM is the seventh leading cause of death by disease in the United States, primarily because of the widespread cardiovascular effects that result in atherosclerosis, coronary heart disease, and stroke (CDC, 2017a). People with DM are two to four times more likely to have heart disease and two to four times more likely to have a stroke than people who do not have the disease. DM is the leading cause of end-stage renal disease (kidney failure) and the major cause of newly diagnosed blindness. DM is the most frequent cause of nontraumatic amputations (CDC, 2017a).

Diabetes is also costly. Approximately 20% of the nation's healthcare dollars go to the treatment of those with diabetes (CDC, 2017b). The cost of care for people with DM exceeded $245 billion in 2012, up from $174 billion in 2007 (CDC, 2017b). Because of the cost and the physical disability that results from diabetes, early diagnosis and careful management of the disease is paramount, and because of their close and extended contact with patients, nurses are ideally positioned to help in the identification and treatment of those with diabetes.

Focus on Cultural Diversity

Estimates of Prevalence of Diabetes Mellitus

- 15.1% of American Indians and Alaska Natives have DM. The rate varies; only 6% of Alaska natives have DM, whereas 22.2% of Native Americans in southern Arizona have DM.
- 12.7% of non-Hispanic Blacks ages 18 years or older have DM.
- 12.1% of Hispanic/Latino Americans ages 18 years or older have DM. Rates of diabetes are lower among Cuban Americans (9%) and Central and South Americans (8.5%) and higher for Mexican Americans (13.8%) and Puerto Rican Americans (12%).
- 8% of Asian Americans ages 18 years or older have DM.
- 7.4% of non-Hispanic Whites ages 18 years or older have DM (CDC, 2017b).

Blood Glucose Homeostasis

The hormones produced by several different cells of the endocrine pancreas, along with hormones produced by the small intestine, are responsible for glucose homeostasis in the body. The regulation of blood glucose levels by insulin and glucagon is illustrated in **Figure 20.1** ■.

The endocrine pancreas produces hormones necessary for the metabolism and cellular utilization of carbohydrates, proteins, and fats. The cells that produce these hormones are clustered in groups of cells called the *islets of Langerhans*. These islets have three different types of cells:

- ***Alpha cells*** produce the hormone *glucagon*, which stimulates the breakdown of glycogen and the formation of carbohydrates in the liver and the breakdown of lipids in both the liver and adipose tissue. The primary function of glucagon is to decrease glucose oxidation and to increase blood glucose levels. Through **glycogenolysis** (the breakdown of liver glycogen) and **gluconeogenesis** (the formation of glucose from fats and proteins), glucagon prevents blood glucose from decreasing below a certain level when the body is fasting or in between meals. The action of glucagon is initiated in most people when blood glucose falls below about 70 mg/dL.
- ***Beta cells*** secrete the hormone *insulin*, which facilitates the movement of glucose across cell membranes into cells, decreasing blood glucose levels. Insulin prevents the excessive breakdown of glycogen in the liver and in muscle, facilitates lipid formation while inhibiting the breakdown of stored fats, and helps move amino acids into cells for protein synthesis. After secretion by the beta cells, insulin enters the portal circulation, travels directly to the liver, and is then released into the general circulation. Circulating insulin is rapidly bound to receptor sites on peripheral tissues (especially muscle and fat cells) or is destroyed by the liver or kidneys. Insulin release is regulated by blood glucose; it increases when blood glucose levels increase, and it decreases when blood glucose levels decrease. When an individual eats food, insulin levels begin to rise in minutes, peak in 3 to 5 minutes, and return to baseline in 2 to 3 hours. *Amylin* is a glucose-regulating hormone secreted by the beta cells with insulin that affects postprandial (postmeal) glucose levels. It impairs glucagon secretion and slows the rate at which glucose travels to the small intestine for absorption.
- ***Delta cells*** produce *somatostatin*, which acts within the islets of Langerhans to inhibit the production of both glucagon and insulin. Somatostatin slows gastrointestinal motility, allowing more time for food to be absorbed.

In addition, the small intestine produces hormones that lower blood glucose following the intake of a meal. Glucagon-like peptide-1 (GLP-1) and glucose-dependent insulinotropic polypeptide (GIP) are secreted from the small intestine to increase insulin release after a meal has been ingested. This hormone-stimulated insulin increase following ingestion of food is called an *incretin effect*. An injectable form of these hormones, exenatide (Byetta), is an incretin mimetic used in the treatment of T2D.

All body tissues and organs require a constant supply of glucose; however, not all tissues require insulin for glucose uptake. The brain, liver, intestines, and renal tubules do not require insulin to transfer glucose into their cells. Skeletal muscle, cardiac muscle, and adipose tissue do require insulin for glucose movement into the cells.

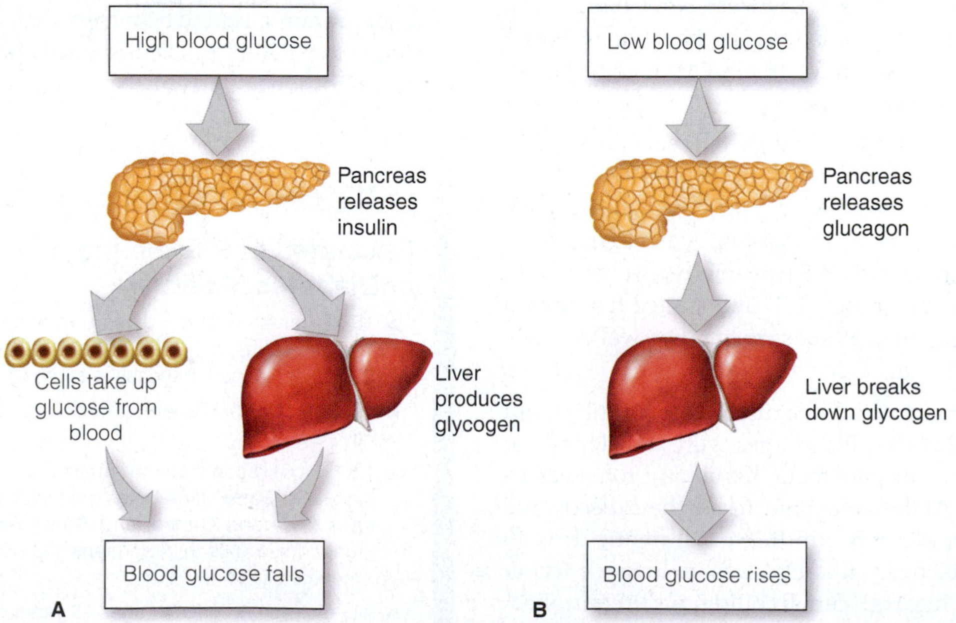
High blood glucose
Pancreas releases insulin
Cells take up glucose from blood
Liver produces glycogen
Blood glucose falls
A
Low blood glucose
Pancreas releases glucagon
Liver breaks down glycogen
Blood glucose rises
B

Figure 20.1 ■ Regulation (homeostasis) of blood glucose levels by insulin and glucagon. **A**, High blood glucose is lowered by insulin release. **B**, Low blood glucose is raised by glucagon release.

Normal blood glucose is maintained in healthy people primarily through the actions of insulin and glucagon. Increased blood glucose levels, amino acids, and fatty acids stimulate pancreatic beta cells to produce insulin. As cells of cardiac muscle, skeletal muscle, and adipose tissue take up glucose, plasma levels of nutrients decrease, suppressing the stimulus to produce insulin. If blood glucose falls, glucagon is released to raise hepatic glucose output, raising glucose levels. Catecholamines (epinephrine, norepinephrine, and dopamine), growth hormone, cortisol, and glucagon (collectively referred to as *glucose counterregulatory hormones*) also stimulate an increase in blood glucose in times of hypoglycemia, stress, growth, or increased metabolic demand.

20.2 Pathophysiology and Manifestations of Diabetes Mellitus

DM is a group of metabolic diseases characterized by hyperglycemia resulting from defects in the secretion of insulin, the action of insulin, or both. Carbohydrate, fat, and protein metabolism are affected by the imbalance between insulin availability and insulin need. Cellular starvation occurs as the body is unable to move glucose into fat and muscle cells (Sorenson, Quinn, & Klein, 2019).

There are four major types of DM:

1. T1D (5 to 10% of diagnosed cases)
2. T2D (90 to 95% of diagnosed cases)
3. Gestational diabetes mellitus (GDM) (2 to 5% of all pregnancies)
4. Other specific types of DM (1 to 2% of diagnosed cases).

The classification and characteristics of the four types are described in **Table 20.1**.

Type 1 Diabetes

Type 1 diabetes (T1D) most often occurs before the age of 30 years (often in childhood and adolescence), though it does occur in older people. This disorder is characterized by **hyperglycemia** (elevated blood glucose levels), a breakdown of body fats and proteins, and the development of **ketosis** (an accumulation of ketone bodies produced during the oxidation of fatty acids). T1D is the result of the destruction of the beta cells of the islets of Langerhans in the pancreas. When beta cells are destroyed, insulin is no longer produced. Five autoantibodies are thought to contribute to the destruction of the beta cells, including insulin autoantibodies, glutamate decarboxylase (GAD), IA-2, zinc transporter-8, and tetraspanin-7 (McLaughlin et al., 2016). It is now known that T1D has a prolonged onset that occurs in three stages (Insel et al., 2015). Stage one is defined by the presence of two or more autoantibodies with normal blood glucose levels. During stage two blood glucose levels start to rise, and in stage three the onset of T1D is unmistakable (Insel et al., 2015). Patients are often in diabetic ketoacidosis at the time of diagnosis.

Table 20.1 Classification and Characteristics of Diabetes Mellitus

	Classification	Characteristics
T1D	Immune mediated	Beta cells are destroyed, usually leading to absolute insulin deficiency. Markers to the immune destruction of the beta cells include insulin autoantibodies, glutamate decarboxylase (GAD), IA-2, zinc transporter-8, and tetraspanin-7. Destruction of the beta cells has genetic predispositions and is also related to environmental factors.
T2D		May range from predominantly insulin resistance with relative insulin deficiency to a predominantly secretory defect with insulin resistance. There is no immune destruction of beta cells. Most people with this form are obese or have an increased amount of abdominal fat. Risks for development include increasing age, obesity, and a sedentary lifestyle. Occurs more frequently in women who have had gestational DM and in people with lipid disorders or hypertension. There is a strong genetic predisposition.
Gestational diabetes mellitus (GDM)		Any degree of glucose intolerance with onset or first recognition during pregnancy.
Other specific types	**A.** Genetic defects of beta cell	Hyperglycemia occurs at an early age (usually before age 25). This type is referred to as *maturity-onset DM of the young (MODY)*.
	B. Genetic defects in insulin action	Genetically determined. Dysfunctions may range from hyperinsulinemia to severe DM.
	C. Diseases of the exocrine pancreas	Acquired processes causing DM include pancreatitis, trauma, infection, pancreatectomy, and pancreatic cancer. Severe forms of cystic fibrosis and hemochromatosis may damage beta cells and impair insulin secretion.
	D. Endocrine disorders	Excess amounts of counterregulatory hormones (e.g., growth hormone, cortisol, glucagon, and epinephrine) impair insulin secretion, resulting in DM in people with Cushing's syndrome, acromegaly, and pheochromocytoma.
	E. Drug or chemical induced	Many drugs impair insulin secretion, precipitating DM in people with predisposing insulin resistance. Examples are nicotinic acid, glucocorticoids, thyroid hormone, thiazides, and phenytoin.
	F. Infections	Certain viruses may cause beta-cell destruction, including congenital measles, cytomegalovirus, adenovirus, and mumps.

The disorder begins with *insulitis*, a chronic inflammatory process that occurs in response to the autoimmune destruction of islet cells. This process slowly destroys production of insulin, with the onset of hyperglycemia occurring when 80 to 90% of beta-cell function is lost. This process usually occurs over a long preclinical period. It is believed that both alpha-cell and beta-cell functions are abnormal, with a lack of insulin and a relative excess of glucagon resulting in hyperglycemia.

Risk Factors

Genetic predisposition plays a role in the development of T1D. Although the risk in the general population ranges from 1 in 400 to 1 in 1000, the child of an individual with DM has a 1 in 20 to 1 in 50 risk. Genetic markers that determine immune responses have been found in most people diagnosed with T1D. Although the presence of these markers does not guarantee that the individual will develop T1D, it does indicate increased susceptibility (Sorenson et al., 2019).

Environmental factors are believed to trigger the development of T1D. The trigger can be a viral infection (mumps, rubella, or coxsackievirus B4) or a chemical toxin, such as those found in smoked and cured meats. As a result of exposure to the virus or chemical, an abnormal autoimmune response occurs in which antibodies respond to normal islet beta cells as though they were foreign substances, destroying them. The manifestations of T1D appear when approximately 90% of the beta cells are destroyed. However, manifestations may appear at any time during the loss of beta cells if an acute illness or stress increases the demand for insulin beyond the reserves of the damaged cells.

Manifestations

The manifestations of T1D are the result of a lack of insulin to transport glucose across the cell membrane into the cells (**Figure 20.2** ■). Glucose molecules accumulate in the circulating blood, resulting in hyperglycemia. Hyperglycemia causes serum hyperosmolality, drawing water from the intracellular spaces into the vascular circulation. The increased blood volume increases renal blood flow, and the hyperglycemia acts as an osmotic diuretic. The resulting osmotic diuresis increases urine output and causes loss of electrolytes (sodium and potassium). This condition is called **polyuria**. When the blood glucose level exceeds the renal threshold for glucose—usually about 180 mg/dL—glucose is excreted in the urine, a condition called **glucosuria**. The decrease in interstitial and later intracellular volume and the increased urinary output cause dehydration. The mouth becomes dry and thirst sensors are activated, causing the person to drink increased amounts of fluid (**polydipsia**).

Because glucose cannot enter the cell without insulin, energy production decreases. This decrease in energy stimulates hunger, so the person eats more food (**polyphagia**). Despite increased food intake, the person loses weight as the body loses water and breaks down fats and later proteins in an attempt to restore energy sources. Malaise and fatigue accompany the decrease in energy. Blurred vision is common, resulting from osmotic effects that cause swelling of the lenses of the eyes.

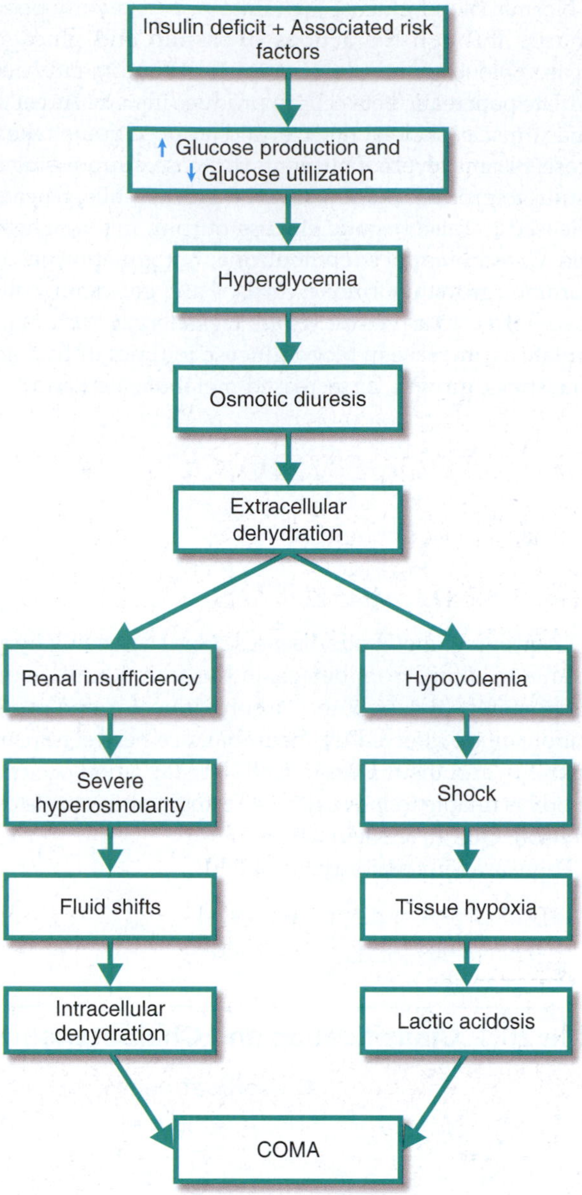
Insulin deficit + Associated risk factors
↑ Glucose production and
↓ Glucose utilization
Hyperglycemia
Osmotic diuresis
Extracellular dehydration
Renal insufficiency
Severe hyperosmolarity
Fluid shifts
Intracellular dehydration
Hypovolemia
Shock
Tissue hypoxia
Lactic acidosis
COMA

Figure 20.2 ■ Pathophysiologic results of T1D.

The classic manifestations are polyuria, polydipsia, and polyphagia, accompanied by weight loss, malaise, and fatigue, varying from slight to severe depending on the length of time the individual with T1D goes without insulin. People with T1D require an exogenous (external) source of insulin to maintain normal glucose metabolism. Without insulin, ketoacidosis rapidly threatens life. See the Multisystem Effects of Diabetes Mellitus illustration on page 600.

Type 2 Diabetes

Type 2 diabetes (T2D) is a condition of fasting hyperglycemia that occurs as a result of progressive insulin resistance. T2D is common in middle age and older people, though prevalence in younger adults and children is directly correlated to poor diet, obesity, and lack of exercise. It is the most common form of DM, and heredity plays a role in its transmission. The level of insulin produced varies in T2D, and despite its availability, insulin function is impaired by insulin resistance in peripheral tissues. The liver produces more glucose than normal, dietary carbohydrates are not metabolized well, and eventually the pancreas secretes less than adequate amounts of insulin (Sorenson et al., 2019). Insulin production is usually sufficient to prevent the breakdown of fats with resultant ketosis; thus, T2D is characterized as a nonketotic form of DM. However, the function of insulin available is not sufficient to lower blood glucose levels through the uptake of glucose by muscle and fat cells. Medications are begun when lifestyle changes such as diet and exercise are insufficient to maintain glycemic targets. Oral medication is often prescribed first, and treatment decisions are based on maintaining glycemic control and preventing complications (Handelsman et al., 2015).

Prediabetes and Metabolic Syndrome

A major factor in the development of T2D is cellular resistance to the effect of insulin. Insulin resistance occurs as much as 10 to 20 years before the onset of diabetes and is closely related to central obesity and lack of exercise. In obesity, insulin has a decreased ability to influence glucose absorption and metabolism by the liver, skeletal muscles, and adipose tissue. Increasing age, physiologic stress (as a result of illness and chronic stress), and some medications contribute to insulin resistance. **Metabolic syndrome** causes insulin resistance and leads to T2D. It is characterized by a group of abnormalities:

- Central obesity, defined as waist circumference larger than 40 inches in men or larger than 35 inches in women
- Hypertension, defined as blood pressure over 120/80 mmHg in adults
- Abnormal lipid panel with triglyceride levels over 150 mg/dL, high LDL, HDL less than 40 mg/dL in men or less than 50 mg/dL in women
- Fasting blood glucose greater than 100 mg/dL
- Hyperinsulinemia, which is often characterized by dark, thick, velvety skin in body folds and creases (*acanthosis nigricans*) commonly seen on the back of the neck and under the arms (American Heart Association, 2015).

Prediabetes is characterized by impaired glucose tolerance and is defined by an abnormal glucose tolerance test or elevated HbA1C. Insulin resistance coupled with impaired glucose tolerance leads to hyperglycemia, which is known to occur at short intervals and gradually increase in severity and duration many years before the diagnosis of diabetes. Hyperglycemia results in diabetes complications; thus, approximately half of those newly diagnosed with T2D already have complications (Handelsman et al., 2015).

Risk Factors

The major risk factors for T2D are:

- History of DM in parents or siblings. Although there is no identified HLA linkage, the children of an individual with T2D have a two- to four-fold increased risk of developing T2D and a 30% risk of developing glucose intolerance (the inability to metabolize carbohydrate normally)
- Obesity, defined as being at least 20% over desired body weight or having a body mass index (BMI) of at least 27
- Physical inactivity
- Race/ethnicity
- In women, a history of gestational DM, polycystic ovary syndrome, or delivering a baby weighing more than 9 lb
- Prediabetes and metabolic syndrome.

Manifestations

The person with T2D experiences a slow onset of manifestations and is often unaware of the disease until seeking healthcare for some other problem. The hyperglycemia in T2D is usually not as severe as in T1D because of the presence of insulin, but similar manifestations occur, especially polyuria and polydipsia. Polyphagia and weight loss are common, though the person is often obese at the time of diagnosis. Other manifestations are the result of hyperglycemia: Blurred vision, fatigue, paresthesias, and skin infections.

Diabetes Mellitus in the Older Adult

Older adults most often develop T2D as a result of increased insulin resistance and decreased production of insulin. The Centers for Disease Control and Prevention (2017b) estimates that 20.8% of the U.S. population over the age of 65 have DM. It is predicted that the number of older adults with DM will continue to increase because the incidence of the disease increases with age and because the number of older adults is increasing.

The normal physiologic changes of aging may mask manifestations of the onset of DM. Manifestations of DM in older adults may not include the classic symptoms of polyuria and thirst. Conditions that signal potential complications of hyperglycemia—such as hypertension, periodontal disease, frequent infections, central arterial disease (i.e., carotid, cerebral, or coronary), peripheral arterial disease (i.e., impotence), slow gastric emptying (gastroparesis), and neuropathy—warrant screening presence of diabetes (American Diabetes Association [ADA], 2018b; Handelsman et al., 2015). The older adult with DM also has a longer recovery period after surgery or serious illness. The benefits of tight glycemic control in an older adult with comorbid conditions versus the risks of hypoglycemia and decreased quality of life must be carefully balanced.

20.3 Complications of Diabetes Mellitus

The person with DM, regardless of type, is at increased risk for complications involving many different body systems. Alterations in blood glucose levels, alterations in the cardiovascular system, neuropathies, an increased susceptibility to infection, and periodontal disease are common. In addition, the interaction of several complications can cause

Multisystem Effects of
Diabetes Mellitus

Early manifestations

- T1D
  - Polyuria
  - Polydipsia
  - Polyphagia
  - Weight loss
  - Glycosuria
  - Fatigue
- T2D
  - Polyuria
  - Polydipsia
  - Blurred vision

Progressive complications

- Hyperglycemia
  - Diabetic ketoacidosis
  - Hyperglycemic hyperosmolar nonketotic coma
- Hypoglycemia

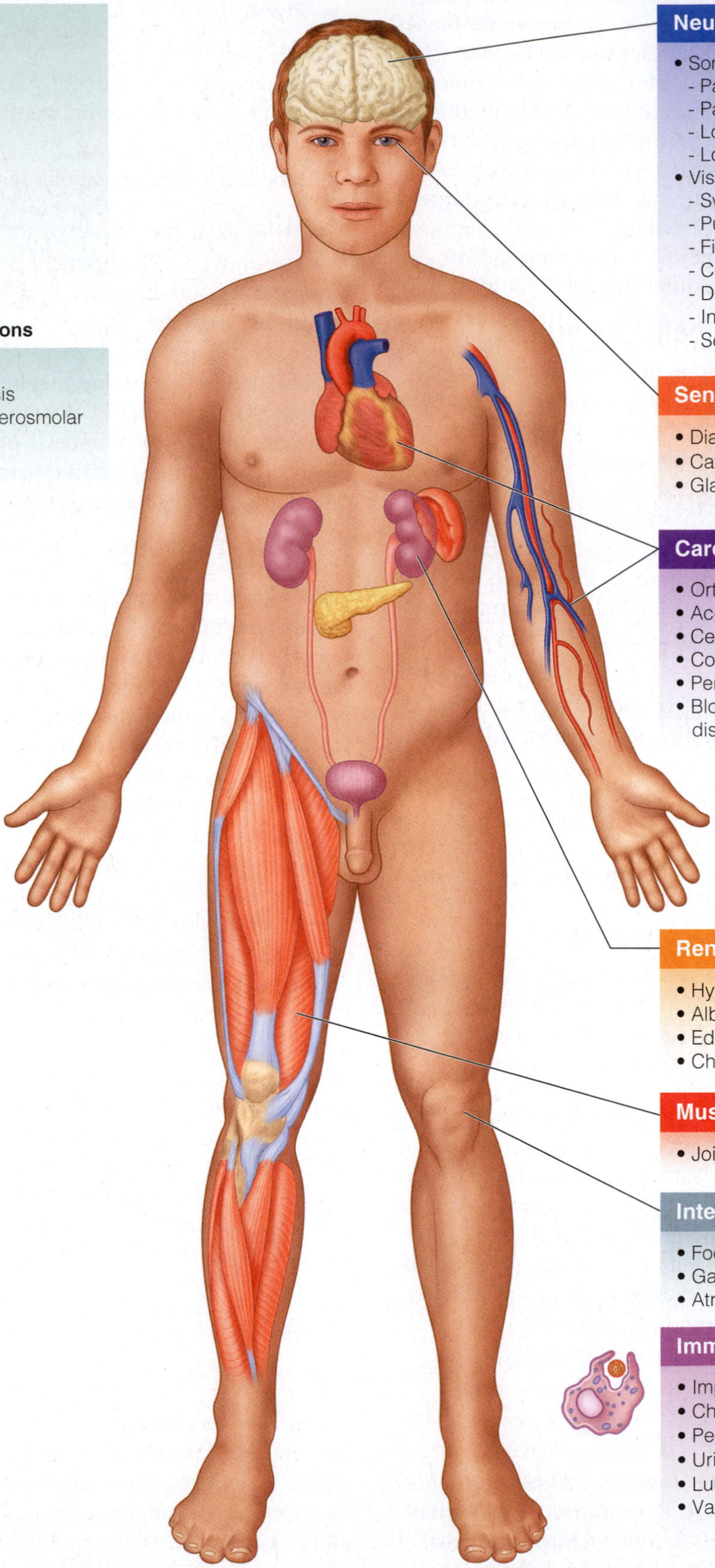

Late complications

Neurologic

- Somatic neuropathies
  - Paresthesias
  - Pain
  - Loss of cutaneous sensation
  - Loss of fine motor control
- Visceral neuropathies
  - Sweating dysfunction
  - Pupillary constriction
  - Fixed heart rate
  - Constipation
  - Diarrhea
  - Incomplete bladder emptying
  - Sexual dysfunction

Sensory

- Diabetic retinopathy
- Cataracts
- Glaucoma

Cardiovascular

- Orthostatic hypotension
- Accelerated atherosclerosis
- Cerebrovascular disease (stroke)
- Coronary artery disease (MI)
- Peripheral vascular disease
- Blood viscosity and platelet disorders

Renal

- Hypertension
- Albuminuria
- Edema
- Chronic renal failure

Musculoskeletal

- Joint contractures

Integumentary

- Foot ulcers
- Gangrene of the feet
- Atrophic changes

Immune System

- Impaired healing
- Chronic skin infections
- Periodontal disease
- Urinary tract infections
- Lung infections
- Vaginitis

problems of the feet. Periods of hyperglycemia lead to many of the chronic complications of diabetes. The Multisystem Effects of Diabetes Mellitus illustration on page 600 shows the progression from cardinal signs to acute and late complications for the patient with DM. A discussion of each of these complications follows; related interprofessional care and nursing care are discussed later in the chapter.

Acute Complications

The mechanisms maintaining normal blood glucose levels are impaired in the patient with diabetes. As a result, problems with either hyperglycemia or hypoglycemia can develop, often rapidly.

Hyperglycemia

The person with DM may experience relatively brief and transient episodes of hyperglycemia (the dawn phenomenon and the Somogyi phenomenon) as well as the acute complications of diabetic ketoacidosis (DKA) and hyperosmolar hyperglycemic state (HHS).

The Somogyi phenomenon is a combination of hypoglycemia during the night with a rebound morning rise in blood glucose to hyperglycemic levels. The hypoglycemia stimulates release of counterregulatory hormones (epinephrine, cortisol, glucagon, and growth hormone), which stimulate gluconeogenesis and glycogenolysis and inhibit peripheral glucose use, leading to hyperglycemia and insulin resistance. Using larger insulin doses to treat the hyperglycemia can induce a cycle of nocturnal hypoglycemia followed by early-morning hyperglycemia (Sorenson et al., 2019). Treatment includes prevention of severe hypoglycemic episodes.

The dawn phenomenon is a rise in blood glucose between 4:00 and 8:00 a.m. that is not a response to hypoglycemia. This condition occurs in people with both T1D and T2D. Nocturnal increases in growth hormone are believed to cause the dawn phenomenon.

Diabetic Ketoacidosis

Diabetic ketoacidosis (DKA) develops when there is a deficiency of insulin; this results in glucose deficiency at the cellular level. As the pathophysiology of untreated T1D continues, the glucose deficit causes fat stores to break down to provide energy, resulting in mobilization of fatty acids with a subsequent ketosis (refer to Figure 20.2). The lack of cellular glucose causes production of counterregulatory hormones (catecholamines, glucagon, cortisol, and growth hormone). Glucose production by the liver increases, peripheral glucose use decreases, fat mobilization increases, and ketogenesis (ketone formation) is stimulated. Increased glucagon levels activate the gluconeogenic and ketogenic pathways in the liver. In the presence of insulin deficiency, hepatic overproduction of beta-hydroxybutyrate and acetoacetic acids (ketone bodies) causes increased ketone concentrations and an increased release of free fatty acids. As a result of a loss of bicarbonate (which occurs when the ketone is formed), bicarbonate buffering does not occur and metabolic acidosis develops. Severe hyperglycemia results in osmotic diuresis, which leads to dehydration and loss of electrolytes. If left untreated, fluid volume deficit leads to poor tissue perfusion and lactic acidosis, further complicating the metabolic acidosis. Depression of the central nervous system (CNS) from the accumulation of ketones, the resulting acidosis, and severe dehydration may cause coma and death if left untreated (Adams, Holland, & Urban, 2017). The impact of DKA is illustrated in **Figure 20.3** ■.

DKA may also occur in an individual with diagnosed DM when energy requirements increase during physical or emotional stress. Stress states initiate the release of counterregulatory hormones (catecholamines, glucagon, cortisol, and growth hormone). The person who is sick, has an infection (the most frequent cause of DKA), or who decreases or omits insulin doses is at a greatly increased risk for developing DKA.

DKA involves four metabolic problems:

1. Hyperosmolarity from hyperglycemia and dehydration
2. Metabolic acidosis from an accumulation of ketoacids (and lactic acids if severe)
3. Extracellular volume depletion from osmotic diuresis
4. Electrolyte imbalances (such as loss of potassium and sodium) from osmotic diuresis.

Manifestations of DKA result from severe dehydration and acidosis. Manifestations from dehydration include thirst, dry mucous membranes, weakness, malaise, hypotension, rapid weak pulse, soft eyeballs, and warm, dry skin with poor turgor. Manifestations from metabolic acidosis (ketosis) include nausea and vomiting, lethargy, ketone breath odor (fruity, alcohol-like), and coma. Other manifestations include abdominal pain (cause unknown) and Kussmaul respirations (increased rate and depth of respirations with longer expiration to blow off carbon dioxide; a compensatory response to acidosis).

Laboratory findings include:

- Blood glucose levels higher than 250 mg/dL
- Plasma pH less than 7.3
- Plasma bicarbonate less than 15 mEq/L
- Presence of serum ketones
- Presence of urine ketones and glucose
- Abnormal levels of serum sodium, potassium, and chloride (Kee, 2018).

Interprofessional Care

DKA requires immediate medical attention. Admission to the hospital is appropriate when the person has a blood glucose of greater than 250 mg/dL, a decreasing pH, and ketones in the urine. If the patient is alert and conscious, fluids may be replaced orally. In the first 12 hours of treatment, adults usually require 8 to 10 L of fluid to replace losses from polyuria and vomiting. The initial fluid replacement may be accomplished by administering 0.9% saline solution at a rate of 500 to 1000 mL/h. After 2 to 3 hours (or when blood pressure is returning to normal), the administration of 0.45% saline at 200 to 500 mL/h may continue for several more hours. When the blood glucose levels reach 250 mg/dL, dextrose is added to IV solutions to prevent

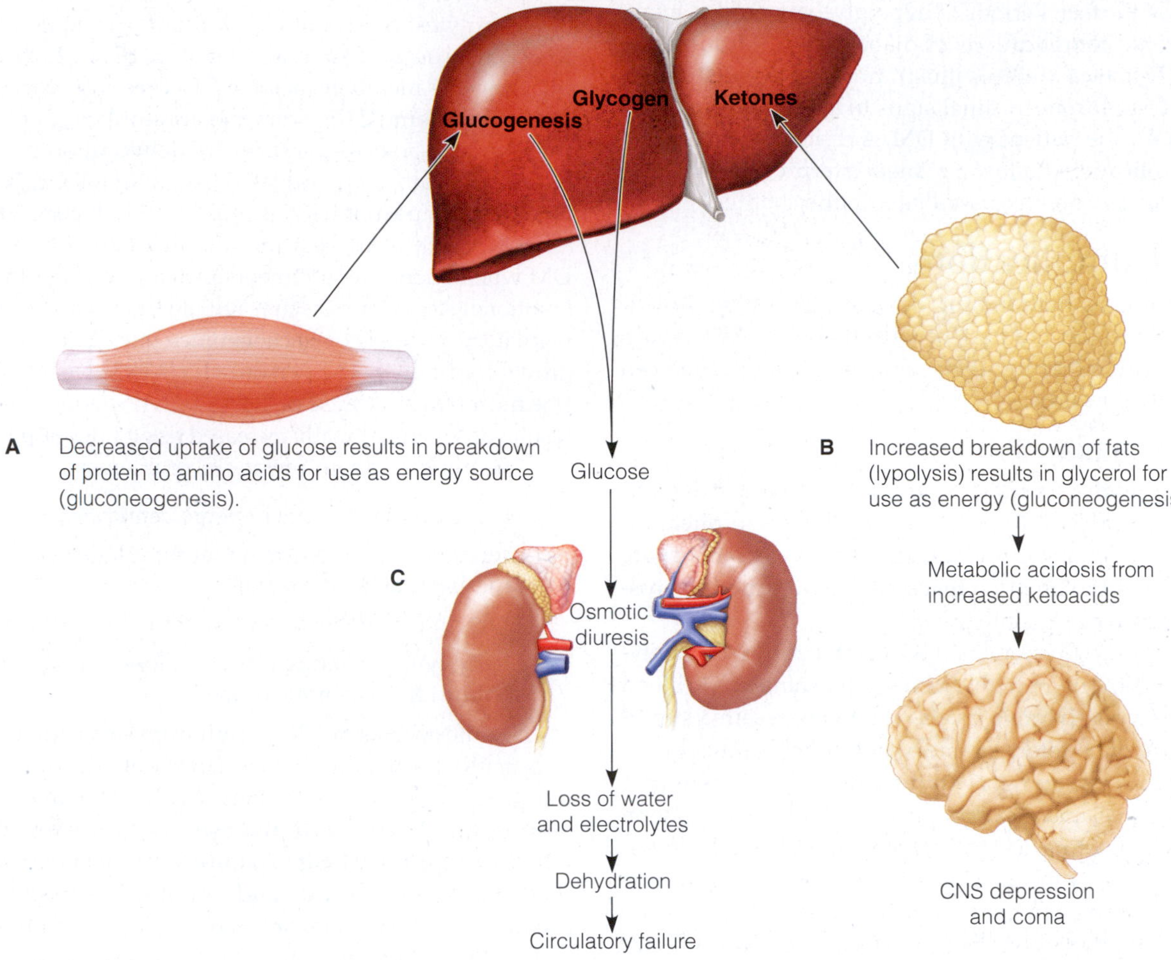
Glucogenesis
Glycogen
Ketones
A Decreased uptake of glucose results in breakdown of protein to amino acids for use as energy source (gluconeogenesis).
Glucose
B Increased breakdown of fats (lypolysis) results in glycerol for use as energy (gluconeogenesis).
Metabolic acidosis from increased ketoacids
C
Osmotic diuresis
Loss of water and electrolytes
Dehydration
Circulatory failure
CNS depression and coma

Figure 20.3 ■ DKA impact.

rapid decreases in glucose. There is a risk of fatal cerebral edema if the blood glucose is lowered too quickly or fluids are given too rapidly or excessively.

Regular intravenous insulin is used in the management of DKA. Nursing responsibilities for the patient receiving intravenous insulin are described in **Medication Administration 20.A**. When renal function and blood pressure are restored, potassium and sodium can be corrected. The electrolyte imbalance of primary concern is depletion of body stores of potassium. Initially, serum potassium levels may be normal, but they decrease during treatment as a result of intracellular potassium deficits. Insulin causes potassium to be shifted into the cells, causing serum hypokalemia. In DKA (and from rehydration), the body loses potassium from increased urinary output, acidosis, catabolic state, and vomiting or diarrhea. Potassium replacement is begun early in the course of treatment, usually by adding potassium to the rehydration fluids. Replacement is essential for preventing cardiac dysrhythmias secondary to hypokalemia. Cardiac rhythms are monitored continuously and potassium levels must be monitored every 2 to 4 hours.

Hyperosmolar Hyperglycemic State

The metabolic problem called **hyperosmolar hyperglycemic state (HHS)** occurs in people who have T2D. HHS is characterized by a plasma osmolarity of 320 mOsm/L or greater (the normal range is 280 to 300 mOsm/L), greatly elevated blood glucose levels (often over 600 mg/dL and sometimes over 1000 mg/dL), and altered levels of consciousness. HHS is a serious, life-threatening medical emergency and has a higher mortality rate than DKA. Mortality is high as a result of severe osmotic diuresis resulting in dehydration and electrolyte deficits. Additionally, patients with HHS are usually older and have other medical problems such as heart failure. The precipitating factors associated with HHS include infection, medications that cause hyperglycemia, therapeutic procedures, acute illness, and chronic illness (**Box 20.1**). The manifestations of this disorder may be slow to appear, with onset ranging from 24 hours to 2 weeks. The manifestations are initiated by hyperglycemia, which causes osmotic diuresis. With increased urine output, plasma volume decreases. The resulting decreased perfusion causes the glomerular filtration rate (GFR) to drop and can lead to acute kidney injury. Some patients with T2D have chronic HHS resulting from very poor control of hyperglycemia.

Serum hyperosmolarity results in severe dehydration, reducing intracellular water in all tissues, including the brain. The person has dry skin and mucous membranes, extreme thirst, and altered levels of consciousness

Medication Administration 20.A

Intravenous Insulin

General Guidelines

- Regular insulin may be given by bolus injection undiluted directly into the vein.
- Insulin infusions are diluted in 0.9% saline or 0.45% saline solution and are always administered using an IV pump to regulate the rate of infusion.
- Because glass or plastic infusion containers and plastic tubing may reduce insulin potency by at least 20% and possibly by up to 80% before the insulin reaches the venous system, 50 mL of the insulin solution should be flushed through the intravenous tubing prior to starting the infusion.

Nursing Responsibilities

- Monitor blood glucose levels at least hourly.
- Flush the intravenous tubing with 50 mL of insulin mixed with normal saline solution to saturate binding sites on the tubing before administering the insulin to the patient; this step increases the amount of insulin delivered during the first few hours.
- Do not discontinue the intravenous infusion until subcutaneous administration of insulin is resumed.
- Monitor for manifestations of hypoglycemia and hyperglycemia.
- Ensure that D_{50} is readily available as an antidote for hypoglycemia.

Source: Data from Adams et al., 2017.

BOX 20.1

Factors Associated with Hyperosmolar Hyperglycemic State

MEDICATIONS

- Glucocorticoids
- Diuretics
- Beta-adrenergic blocking agents
- Immunosuppressants
- Chlorpromazine
- Diazoxide.

THERAPEUTIC PROCEDURES

- Peritoneal dialysis
- Hemodialysis
- Hyperosmolar alimentation (oral or parenteral)
- Surgery.

ACUTE ILLNESS

- Infection
- Gangrene
- Urinary tract infection
- Burns
- Gastrointestinal bleeding
- Myocardial infarction
- Pancreatitis
- Stroke.

CHRONIC ILLNESS

- Kidney disease
- Cardiac disease
- Hypertension
- Previous stroke
- Alcoholism.

(progressing from lethargy to coma). Neurologic deficits may include hyperthermia, motor and sensory impairment, positive Babinski sign, and seizures. Metabolic acidosis is not usually part of the pathology; despite elevated blood glucose, sufficient insulin is present to prevent metabolism of fats. However, if dehydration is severe, it leads to decreased tissue perfusion and lactic acidosis will result. Treatment is directed toward correcting fluid and electrolyte imbalances, lowering blood glucose levels with insulin, and treating underlying conditions.

Interprofessional Care

HHS is a serious, life-threatening metabolic condition. The patient admitted to the intensive care unit for treatment typically manifests blood glucose levels over 600 mg/dL, dehydration with increased serum osmolarity, and altered levels of consciousness or seizures. Treatment is similar to that of DKA: Correcting fluid and electrolyte imbalances and providing insulin to lower hyperglycemia. In general, treatment modalities include:

- Establishing and maintaining adequate ventilation
- Correcting shock with adequate intravenous fluids
- Instituting nasogastric suction if comatose to prevent aspiration
- Maintaining fluid volume with intravenous isotonic or colloid solutions
- Administering potassium intravenously to replace losses
- Administering insulin to reduce blood glucose, usually discontinuing administration when blood glucose levels reach 250 mg/dL. (Because ketosis is not present, there is no need to continue insulin, as with DKA.)

Hypoglycemia

Hypoglycemia (low blood glucose levels) is common in people with T1D and occasionally occurs in people with T2D who are treated with certain oral hypoglycemic agents. This condition is sometimes referred to as insulin shock, insulin reaction, or "the lows" in patients with T1D. Hypoglycemia results primarily from a mismatch between insulin intake (e.g., an error in insulin dose), physical activity, and lack of carbohydrate availability (e.g., omitting a meal). The intake of alcohol and drugs such as chloramphenicol (Chloromycetin), Coumadin, monoamine oxidase inhibitors (MAOIs), probenecid (Benemid), salicylates, and sulfonamides can also cause hypoglycemia.

The manifestations of hypoglycemia result from a compensatory autonomic nervous system (ANS) response and from impaired cerebral function due to a decrease in glucose available for use by the brain. The manifestations vary, particularly in older adults. Manifestations caused by responses of the autonomic nervous system include:

- Hunger
- Nausea
- Anxiety
- Pale, cool skin
- Sweating
- Shakiness
- Irritability
- Rapid pulse
- Hypotension.

Manifestations caused by impaired cerebral function include:

- Strange or unusual feelings
- Headache
- Difficulty in thinking
- Inability to concentrate
- Change in emotional behavior
- Slurred speech
- Blurred vision
- Decreasing levels of consciousness
- Seizures
- Coma.

The onset is sudden, and blood glucose is usually less than 60 mg/dL. Severe hypoglycemia may cause death. **Table 20.2** compares DKA, HHS, and hypoglycemia.

People who have T1D for 4 or 5 years fail to secrete glucagon in response to a decrease in blood glucose. They then depend on epinephrine to serve as a counterregulatory response to hypoglycemia. However, this compensatory response can become absent or blunted. As a result, the person with T1D does not experience typical manifestations of hypoglycemia; the first symptoms include fatigue and inability to think followed by loss of consciousness and seizures. The individual with T1D should always have glucagon available and close family members (or significant others) and coworkers should be familiar with its administration.

Interprofessional Care

Mild Hypoglycemia. When mild hypoglycemia occurs, immediate treatment is necessary. People experiencing hypoglycemia should take about 15 g of a rapid-acting sugar. This amount of sugar is found, for example, in three glucose tablets, 1/2 cup (4 ounces) of fruit juice or regular soda, 8 oz of skim milk, five Life Savers candies, three large marshmallows, or 3 tsp of sugar or honey. Sugar should not be added to fruit juice. Adding sugar to the fruit sugar already in the juice could cause a rapid rise in blood glucose, with persistent hyperglycemia.

If the manifestations continue, the 15/15 rule should be followed: Wait 15 minutes, monitor blood glucose (BG), and, if it is low, eat another 15 g of carbohydrate. This procedure can be repeated until blood glucose levels return to normal (ADA, 2018a). People with DM should have some source of carbohydrate readily available at all times so that hypoglycemic manifestations can be quickly reversed. If hypoglycemia occurs more than two or three times a week, the DM management plan should be adjusted.

Severe Hypoglycemia. People with DM who have severe hypoglycemia should seek medical attention. The criteria for hospitalization are one or more of the following:

- Blood glucose is less than 50 mg/dL, and the prompt treatment of hypoglycemia has not resulted in recovery of sensorium.
- The patient has coma, seizures, or altered behavior.
- The hypoglycemia has been treated, but a responsible adult cannot be with the patient for the following 12 hours.
- The hypoglycemia was caused by a sulfonylurea drug (Adams et al., 2017).

If the patient is conscious and alert, 10 to 15 g of an oral carbohydrate may be given. If the patient has altered levels of consciousness, parenteral glucose or glucagon is administered. Fifty percent dextrose (D_{50}) is administered by intravenous push. This is the most rapid method of increasing BG levels. Glucagon is an antihypoglycemic agent that raises blood glucose by promoting the conversion of hepatic glycogen to glucose. It is used in severe insulin-induced hypoglycemia (usually outside of the hospital setting) and may be given in the recommended dose of 1 mg by the subcutaneous or intramuscular route. Glucagon has a short period of action. When the patient is conscious, an oral carbohydrate should be administered to prevent recurrence of hypoglycemia. A common side effect of glucagon is nausea and vomiting. Safety measures should be taken to prevent aspiration.

Chronic Complications

It is now clear that the level of chronic hyperglycemia correlates well with the development of chronic complications of diabetes. Increased intracellular glucose levels affect cell proteins and result in the release of abnormal metabolic end-products. The abnormal glycoproteins are believed to damage basement membranes, affecting the eyes, kidneys, and circulation (Sorenson et al., 2019).

Alterations in the Cardiovascular System

The relationship between hyperglycemia and vascular complications is now clear. The effect of hyperglycemia from impaired glucose tolerance and insulin resistance sets off an inflammatory process in the vascular endothelial lining. Proinflammatory cytokines are released in the presence of hyperglycemia, and they start a cascade that

Table 20.2 DKA, HHS, and Hypoglycemia Compared

		DKA	HHS	Hypoglycemia
DM type		Primarily T1D	T2D	Both
Onset		Acute	Chronic	Rapid
Cause		↓Insulin	↓Insulin Chronic hyperglycemia	↑Insulin Omitted meal/snack Error in insulin dose
Risk factors		Surgery Trauma Illness Omitted insulin Stress	Surgery Trauma Illness Dehydration Medications Dialysis Hyperalimentation	Surgery Trauma Illness Exercise Medications Lipodystrophy Renal failure Alcohol intake
Assessments	Skin	Flushed; dry; warm	Flushed; dry; warm	Pallor; moist; cool
	Perspiration	None	None	Profuse
	Breath	Fruity	Normal	Normal
	Vital signs	BP↓ ↑P R Kussmaul	BP↓ ↑P R normal	BP↓ ↑P R normal
	Mental status	Confused	Lethargic	Anxious; restless
	Thirst	Increased	Increased	Normal
	Fluid intake	Increased	Increased	Normal
	Gastrointestinal effects	Nausea and vomiting; abdominal pain	Nausea and vomiting; abdominal pain	Hunger
	Fluid loss	Moderate to severe	Profound	Normal
	Level of consciousness	Decreasing	Decreasing	Decreasing
	Energy level	Weak	Weak	Fatigue
	Other	Weight loss Blurred vision	Weight loss Malaise Extreme thirst Seizures	Headache Altered vision Mood changes Seizures
Laboratory findings	Blood glucose	>300 mg/dL	>400 dL	<70 mg/dL
	Plasma ketones	Increased	Normal	Normal
	Urine glucose	Increased	Increased	Normal
	Urine ketones	Increased	Normal	Normal
	Serum potassium	Abnormal	Abnormal	Normal
	Serum sodium	Abnormal	Abnormal	Normal
	Serum chloride	Abnormal	Abnormal	Normal
	Plasma pH	<7.3	Normal	Normal
	Osmolality	> 300 mOsm/L	> 320 mOsm/L	Normal
Treatment		Insulin Intravenous fluids Electrolytes	Insulin Intravenous fluids Electrolytes	Glucagon Rapid-acting carbohydrate Intravenous solution of 50% glucose

BP, blood pressure; P, pulse; R, respirations.

increases insulin resistance, increases hyperglycemia, and causes inflammatory damage in the endothelium. Polyol pathways are created, and oxidative stress at the cellular level occurs. Abnormal metabolic end products, vascular endothelial growth factor, and angiopoietin are also thought to contribute to vascular damage (Sorenson et al., 2019).

Macrovascular Complications

Macrovascular damage is manifested through atherosclerosis and often results in hypertension, coronary artery damage, cerebral artery and carotid artery damage, and peripheral arterial damage (Sorenson et al., 2019). People with undiagnosed diabetes often seek treatment for a vascular complication such as acute myocardial infarction or manifestations of peripheral vascular disease before the diagnosis of T2D. Metabolic syndrome, a known risk factor for diabetes, is a major risk factor for macrovascular disease as well.

Coronary Artery Disease

Coronary artery disease is a major risk factor in the development of myocardial infarction in people with DM, especially in the middle to older adult with T2D. Coronary artery disease is the most common cause of death in people with T2D (World Heart Federation, 2016). People with DM who have myocardial infarction are more prone to develop heart failure as a complication of the infarction and are also less likely to survive in the period immediately following the infarction.

Hypertension

Hypertension affects 75% of all people with DM and is a major risk factor for cardiovascular disease and microvascular complications such as retinopathy and nephropathy. Hypertension may be reduced by weight loss, exercise, avoiding or stopping smoking, and decreasing sodium intake and alcohol consumption. In addition, treatment with antihypertensive medications is necessary.

Stroke (Cerebrovascular Accident)

People with DM, especially older adults with T2D, are twice as likely to have a stroke than those who do not have DM (CDC, 2016). Atherosclerosis of the cerebral vessels develops at an earlier age and is more extensive in people with DM (Sorenson et al., 2019).

The manifestations of stroke or transient ischemic attacks are often similar to those of hypoglycemia or HHS: Blurred vision, slurred speech, weakness, and dizziness. Manifestations that are different with stroke include unilateral facial droop, weakness, or paralysis. People with these manifestations require immediate medical attention.

Peripheral Vascular Disease

Peripheral vascular disease of the lower extremities accompanies both types of DM and is related to hyperglycemia. Atherosclerosis of vessels in the legs of people with DM begins at an earlier age and advances more rapidly than in the general population. It is equally common in both men and women. Impaired peripheral arterial circulation impairs tissue perfusion and leads to intermittent claudication (pain) in the lower legs and ulcerations of the feet. Manifestations include:

- Loss of hair on lower leg, feet, and toes
- Atrophic skin changes: Shininess and thinning
- Cold feet
- Feet and ankles darker than leg
- Dependent rubor, blanching on elevation
- Thick toenails
- Diminished or absent pulses
- Nocturnal pain
- Pain at rest, relieved by standing or walking
- Intermittent claudication
- Patchy areas of gangrene on feet and toes.

Vascular damage, as well as alterations in neurologic function and increased risk of infection, can result in gangrene (*necrosis*, or the death of tissue). Gangrene from DM is the most common cause of nontraumatic amputations of the lower leg. In people with DM, dry gangrene is most common, manifested by cold, dry, shriveled, and black tissues of the toes and feet. The gangrene usually begins in the toes and moves proximally into the foot. (Peripheral vascular disease is discussed in Chapter 32.)

Microvascular Complications

Microvascular changes include capillary leak, microthromboses, and decreased transport of oxygen and glucose to the cells. The basement membrane of smaller blood vessels and capillaries thickens, eventually leading to decreased tissue perfusion. (The *basement membrane* is the structure that supports and serves as the boundary around the space occupied by epithelial cells.) Alterations in the microcirculation affect all body tissues.

Diabetic Retinopathy

Diabetic retinopathy is the name for the changes in the retina that occur in the person with DM. Microvascular damage and hemorrhages lead to scarring of the retina. Retinopathy is the leading cause of blindness in people with diabetes (CDC, 2017a). If exudate, edema, hemorrhage, or ischemia occurs near the fovea, the person experiences visual impairment. In addition, the person with DM is at increased risk for developing cataracts (opacity of the lens) as a result of increased glucose levels within the lens itself. Screening for retinopathy is important, as laser photocoagulation surgery has proven beneficial in preventing loss of vision.

Diabetic Nephropathy

Diabetic nephropathy results from microvascular disease of the kidneys and is characterized by the presence of albumin in the urine, hypertension, and progressive renal insufficiency. The most common cause of renal failure in the United States is diabetes (CDC, 2017a).

Microvascular damage results in thickening of the basement membrane of the glomeruli and eventually impairs renal function. Glomerulosclerosis thickens the basement membrane and simultaneously makes it functionally leaky, allowing large molecules such as protein to be lost in the urine. Kimmelstiel-Wilson syndrome is a type of glomerulosclerosis found only in people with DM. In advanced nephropathy, tubular atrophy occurs, and end-stage renal disease results. (Renal failure is discussed in Chapter 28.)

The first indication of nephropathy is *microalbuminuria*, an abnormal level of albumin in the urine. Without specific interventions, people with DM with sustained microalbuminuria will develop nephropathy, accompanied by hypertension. People with T2D often have microalbuminuria and nephropathy shortly after diagnosis of diabetes is made because prediabetes (or undiagnosed diabetes) with intermittent hyperglycemia has been present and untreated for many years. Because the hypertension accelerates the progress of diabetic nephropathy, aggressive antihypertensive management should be instituted. Management includes control of hypertension with ACE inhibitors, weight loss, reduced salt intake, and exercise.

Diabetic Neuropathies

Peripheral and visceral neuropathies are disorders of the peripheral nerves and the autonomic nervous system. In people with DM, these disorders are often called *diabetic neuropathies*. The etiology of diabetic neuropathies involves (1) a thickening of the walls of the blood vessels that supply nerves, causing a decrease in nutrients; (2) demyelinization of the Schwann cells that surround and insulate nerves, slowing nerve conduction; and (3) the formation and accumulation of sorbitol within the Schwann cells, impairing nerve conduction. The manifestations depend on the location of the lesions.

Peripheral Neuropathies

The *peripheral neuropathies* (also called *somatic neuropathies*) include polyneuropathies and mononeuropathies. *Polyneuropathies*, the most common type of neuropathy associated with DM, are bilateral sensory disorders. The manifestations appear first in the toes and feet and progress upward. The fingers and hands may be involved, but usually only in later stages of DM. The manifestations of polyneuropathy depend on the nerve fibers involved. The lack of sensation prevents awareness of injury and for this reason, people with diabetes must be taught to visually inspect their feet and legs daily, looking for evidence of injury.

The person with polyneuropathy commonly has distal paresthesias (a change in sensation, such as numbness or tingling); pain described as aching, burning, or shooting; and feelings of cold feet. Other manifestations may include impaired sensations of pain, light touch, two-point discrimination, and vibration. There is no specific treatment for polyneuropathy.

Mononeuropathies are isolated peripheral neuropathies that affect a single nerve. Depending on the nerve involved, manifestations may include:

- Palsy of the third cranial (oculomotor) nerve, with headache, eye pain, and an inability to move the eye up, down, or medially
- Radiculopathy, with pain over a dermatome and loss of cutaneous sensation, most often located in the chest
- Diabetic femoral neuropathy, with motor and sensory deficits (pain, weakness, areflexia) in the anterior thigh and medial calf
- Entrapment or compression of the medial nerve at the wrist, resulting in carpal tunnel syndrome with pain and weakness of the hand; the ulnar nerve at the elbow, with weakness and loss of sensation over the palmar surface of the fourth and fifth fingers; and the peroneal nerve at the head of the fibula, with foot drop.

Visceral Neuropathies

The *visceral neuropathies* (*autonomic neuropathies*) cause various manifestations, depending on the area of the ANS involved. These neuropathies may include:

- Sweating dysfunction, with an absence of sweating (anhidrosis) on the hands and feet and increased sweating on the face or trunk.
- Abnormal pupillary function, most commonly seen as constricted pupils that dilate slowly in the dark.
- Cardiovascular dysfunction, resulting in such abnormalities as a fixed cardiac rate that does not change with exercise, postural hypotension, and a failure to increase cardiac output or vascular tone with exercise.
- Gastrointestinal dysfunction, with changes in upper GI motility (**gastroparesis**) resulting in dysphagia, anorexia, heartburn, nausea and vomiting, and slowed digestion with altered blood glucose control. Constipation is one of the most common GI manifestations associated with DM, possibly a result of hypomotility of the bowel. Diabetic diarrhea is not as common, but it does occur and is often associated with fecal incontinence during sleep due to a defect in internal sphincter function.
- Genitourinary dysfunction, resulting in changes in bladder function and sexual function. Bladder function changes include an inability to empty the bladder completely, loss of sensation of bladder fullness, and an increased risk of urinary tract infections. Sexual dysfunctions in men include ejaculatory changes and impotence. Sexual dysfunctions in women include changes in arousal patterns, vaginal lubrication, and orgasm. Alterations in sexual function in people with DM are the result of both neurologic and vascular changes.

Mood Alterations

Individuals with DM, both type 1 and type 2, endure the chronic strains of living with complex self-care and are at increased risk for depression and DM-specific emotional distress. The management of diabetes can create financial, emotional, and social distress. Depression affects the ability to self-manage DM; depressed patients may forget to take their medications or run out of medications because they forget to refill their prescriptions in a timely manner. Treating depression has been associated with better control of serum glucose, so screening for depression is an important part of assessing the individual's ability to manage the disease (ADA, 2018b).

Interventions to help patients with depression include antidepressant medications and psychotherapy focused on restoring logical thinking and problem-solving skills. Nurses can assist depressed patients by correcting misconceptions about depression, identifying individual strengths in managing DM, acknowledging negative feelings that may be expressed, suggesting problem-solving behaviors to better manage the disease, and referring to appropriate resources.

Increased Susceptibility to Infection

The person with DM has an increased risk of developing infections. Vascular and neurologic impairments, hyperglycemia, inflammation, and altered neutrophil function are responsible for increased susceptibility to infections (Adams et al., 2017).

The person with DM may have sensory deficits resulting in inattention to trauma and vascular deficits that decrease circulation to the injured area; as a result, healing is slowed. Nephrosclerosis and inadequate bladder emptying with retention of urine predispose the person with DM to pyelonephritis and urinary tract infections. Surgical patients with hyperglycemia have higher infection rates (Martin et al., 2016).

Periodontal Disease

Although periodontal disease does not occur more often in people with DM, it does progress more rapidly, especially if the DM is poorly controlled. Vascular changes in the gums coupled with periods of hyperglycemia increase the risk of infection and decrease the localized response to infection. As a result, gingivitis (inflammation of the gums) and periodontitis (inflammation of the bone underlying the gums) occur.

Complications Involving the Feet

The high incidence of foot problems and amputations in people with DM is the result of angiopathy, neuropathy, and infection. People with DM, especially those who are not meeting recommended glycemic goals, are at high risk for amputation of a lower extremity.

Atherosclerosis and microvascular changes in the lower extremities of the person with DM impair tissue perfusion and oxygenation. The smaller blood vessels located below the knee are most affected with occlusions in the large, medium, and small arteries of the lower legs and feet. Multiple occlusions with decreased blood flow result in the manifestations of peripheral vascular disease.

Diabetic neuropathy impairs the sense of touch and perception of pain. As a result, the person with DM may experience foot trauma without being aware of it. Healing is impaired by the effects of DM and poor tissue perfusion, increasing the risk for ulceration and infection (see **Figure 20.4 ■**).

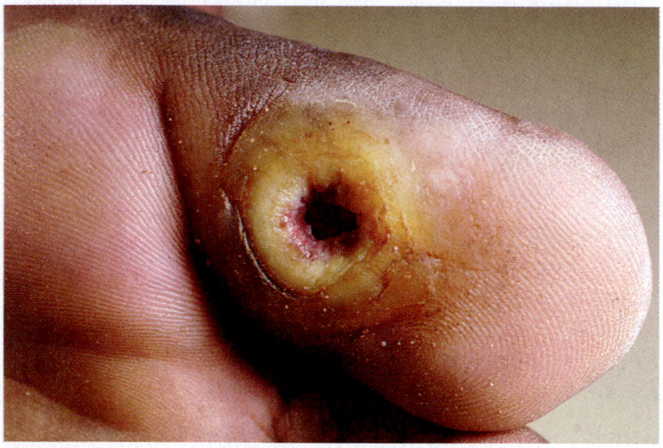

Figure 20.4 ■ Ulceration following trauma in the foot of an individual with diabetes.

The most common sources of foot trauma in the individual with DM are cracks and fissures caused by dry skin or infections such as athlete's foot, blisters caused by improperly fitting shoes, pressure from stockings or shoes, ingrown toenails, and direct trauma (cuts, bruises, or burns). An individual with diabetic neuropathy may not be aware that these injuries have occurred. In addition, when a part of the body loses sensation, the individual tends to dissociate from or ignore the part, so an injury may go unattended for days or weeks. The injury may even be forgotten entirely.

Foot lesions usually begin as a superficial skin ulcer. In time, the ulcer extends deeper into muscles and bone, leading to abscess or osteomyelitis. Gangrene can develop on one or more toes; if untreated, the whole foot eventually becomes gangrenous. (Care of the feet, an essential part of patient and family education, is discussed later in the chapter.)

Complications in Older Adults

The prevalence of both T1D and T2D in older adults is very common and people are living longer with the disease. There are unique challenges related to the management of diabetes and prevention of complications in this population. Problems such as frailty and disability, falls, mood disturbances such as depression, and cognitive impairment such as delirium are more common in the older patient with diabetes (Sinclair, Dunning, & Rodriguez-Mañas, 2015). A specific plan of care that is tailored to an older patient's functional abilities is important. Some older people are very functional and the plan of care many be similar to that of a younger person. However, the older person who is frail, has multiple disabilities, and may have depression or delirium will require a plan that enhances quality of life and functioning and also addresses safety issues to prevent injury and further complications (Sinclair et al., 2015). Complications of DM in older adults are summarized in **Table 20.3**.

Table 20.3 Complications in Older Adults with Diabetes Mellitus

Health Problem/ Complication	Implications for Nursing Care
Urinary incontinence	The older adult may assume urinary incontinence is a normal part of aging. Consequently, polyuria, a classic manifestation of DM, may be ignored.
Disability	It is important to assess and prevent disabilities. This is accomplished through coaching, caregiving, and appropriate changes to the plan of care as diabetes progresses.
Frailty	Loss of skeletal muscle mass and sarcopenia lead to lower limb dysfunction. Insulin resistance exacerbates this and may be helped somewhat with insulin sensitizers.
Falls	Disabilities such as neuropathy coupled with frailty lead to significant increased risk of falls. Fall precautions and assistive devices are important.
Depression	Mood disturbances such as depression are common and can result in poor management of diabetes. Identification and treatment of depression can decrease mortality.
Cognitive impairment	Delirium and dementia may be related to diabetes complications such as hypo- or hyperglycemia or side effects of medications (such as gabapentin). Sometimes a change in the treatment plan can help to relieve the debilitating effects of cognitive impairment.
Vascular disease	Older people are at increased risk for heart disease, chronic kidney disease, peripheral arterial disease, and stroke.

Sources: Data compiled from Sinclair et al., 2015; National Institute on Aging, 2018; Centers for Disease Control and Prevention, 2017a.

20.4 Interprofessional Care of the Patient with Diabetes Mellitus

Treatment of the patient with DM focuses on maintaining blood glucose at levels as nearly normal as possible through medications, dietary management, and exercise. The results of a landmark 10-year Diabetes Control and Complications Trial (DCCT), sponsored by the National Institutes of Health, had significant implications for the management of T1D (DCCT Research Group et al., 1993). People in the study who kept their blood glucose levels close to normal by frequent monitoring, several daily insulin injections, and lifestyle changes that included exercise and a healthier diet reduced their risk for the development and progression of complications involving the eyes, the kidneys, and the nervous system by 60%. Patients with either T1D or T2D benefit from similar levels of control.

Diagnosis

Diagnostic tests are conducted for screening purposes to diagnose DM, and ongoing laboratory tests are conducted to evaluate the effectiveness of diabetes management.

Diagnostic Screening

The diagnostic criteria recommended by the American Diabetes Association (2018b) have recently been updated and include:

1. A hemoglobin A1C greater than or equal to 6.5%. This test should be performed using a method that is both National Glycohemoglobin Standardization Program (NGSP) certified and standardized to the DCCT assay.
2. Fasting plasma glucose (FPG) greater than or equal to 126 mg/dL (7.0 mmol/L). Fasting is defined as no caloric intake for 8 hours.
3. Two-hour PG greater than or equal to 200 mg/dL (11.1 mmol/L) during an oral glucose tolerance test. The test should be performed with a glucose load containing the equivalent of 75 g anhydrous glucose dissolved in water.
4. A random plasma glucose greater than or equal to 200 mg/dL (11.1 mmol/L) in an individual with manifestations of hyperglycemia or hyperglycemic crisis.

When using these criteria, the following levels are used for the FPG:

- Normal fasting glucose ≤ 100 mg/dL (6.1 mmol/L)
- Impaired fasting glucose (IFG) = 100 to 126 mg/dL (6.1 to 7.0 mmol/L)
- Diagnosis of DM = > 126 mg/dL (7.0 mmol/L).

When using these criteria, the following levels are used for the OGTT:

- Normal glucose tolerance = 2-hr PG < 140 mg/dL (7.8 mmol/L)
- Impaired glucose tolerance (IGT) = 2-hr PG ≥ 140 (7.8 mmol/L) and < 200 mg/dL (11.1 mmol/L)
- Diagnosis of DM = 2-hr PG ≥ 200 mg/dL (11.1 mmol/L).

Prediabetes

A hemoglobin A1C level of 5.7% to 6.4% indicates a high risk for developing diabetes and vascular disease (peripheral vascular disease, acute myocardial infarction, and stroke) and is a marker for prediabetes. The ADA (2018b) and the American Association of Clinical Endocrinology/American College of Endocrinology (AACE/ACE; 2018) have issued specific recommendations to delay or prevent the onset of T2D. Weight loss and increased physical activity of at least 150 minutes per week are essential. In addition, annual monitoring for the onset of diabetes is suggested, and treatment with metformin to prevent or delay the onset of T2D should be considered.

DM Management

Tests used to monitor DM include a fasting blood glucose (FBG) and glycosylated hemoglobin (A1C). Normal values for these tests as well as nursing implications are described in Chapter 18.

Other tests that may be used are urine tests for glucose, ketones, and albumin. Urine analysis for increased glucose and ketones indicates hyperglycemia and ketosis. Urine tests for albumin are used to detect the early onset of kidney damage. Serum cholesterol and lipid levels identify those individuals at risk for cardiovascular disease.

Self-Monitoring

It is essential for patients with insulin-dependent diabetes to monitor their condition by testing glucose levels. Direct measurement of blood glucose is widely used in all types of healthcare settings and in the home. Urine tests for ketones are also recommended for patients with T1D and occasionally for those with T2D who no longer produce insulin. Ketone measurement is especially beneficial to determine whether ketosis (breakdown of fats) is occurring.

Urine Testing for Ketones

Urine ketone tests should be used by people with T1D, especially under times of physiologic stress (i.e., infections, disease) and emotional stress. During these times, an individual with T1D may become rapidly hyperglycemic with a relative insulin deficiency and switch to using fats for energy. This abnormal process can be measured with *ketones*, the by-product of fat metabolism. Positive urine ketone excretion is the beginning of diabetic ketoacidosis.

Self-Monitoring of Blood Glucose

Self-monitoring of blood glucose (SMBG) allows the individual with DM to monitor and achieve metabolic control and decrease the complications associated with both hypoglycemia and hyperglycemia. The ADA recommends that all patients with DM be taught some method of monitoring glycemic control. The timing of SMBG is highly individualized, depending on the person's diagnosis, general disease control, and physical state. SMBG is recommended three or more times a day for patients with T1D using multiple insulin injections or insulin pump therapy. Monitoring by patients with T2D who are not using insulin should be sufficient to help them reach glucose goals. Postprandial blood glucose is often the most useful information for evaluating level of glycemic control in the patient with T2D (ADA, 2018b). If patients were to check only their fasting glucose, they would be unaware of the postprandial results.

When adding or modifying therapy, patients with both types of DM should test more often than usual. SMBG is also useful when an individual is ill or pregnant or has manifestations of hypoglycemia or hyperglycemia. Both hypoglycemia and hyperglycemia may contribute to complications and decrease quality of life. With the information assessed with SMBG, patients can alter their diet, their physical activity, and even their medication to control blood glucose and the risk for complications.

The ADA publishes annually a comprehensive list of currently available blood glucose monitors and strips with approximate prices in *Diabetes Forecast*. Most medical insurance policies cover the cost of these monitors and the test strips. Many companies, however, provide a monitor free of cost, but the testing supplies are specific to each monitor, which obligates the recipient to purchase supplies for that monitor.

The following equipment is needed for SMBG:

- Some type of lancet device to perform a fingerstick for obtaining a drop of blood (such as an Autolet, Penlet, or Soft Touch).
- A blood glucose monitor (e.g., Glucometer, Accu-Chek, or One Touch). The manufacturer's instructions must be followed carefully even though the procedure for SMBG has been simplified such that most glucose monitors are very simple to use (**Figure 20.5** ■).
- Test strips that are specific to the glucose monitor being used (e.g., Accu-Chek Aviva).

A newer technology is continuous glucose monitoring (CGM). A CGM device has a sensor that is inserted under the skin and measures glucose readings every few minutes. This sensor provides a continuous glucose reading and warns the patient with diabetes with an alarm for when glucose levels are high or low (**Figure 20.6** ■). The CGM reveals patterns of glycemic control useful for the patient or healthcare provider to make treatment decisions. The data are downloaded to computer- or Internet-based applications and various reports such as daily trends, trends at a certain time of day, and long-term trends can be analyzed.

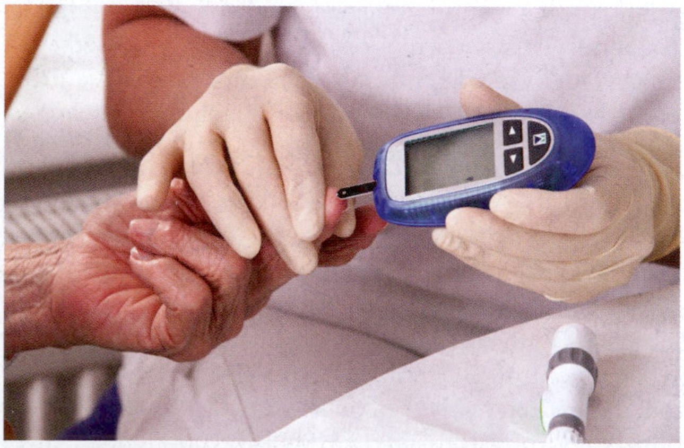

Figure 20.5 ■ A portable glucometer is used by the patient or caregivers to provide accurate blood glucose measurements.

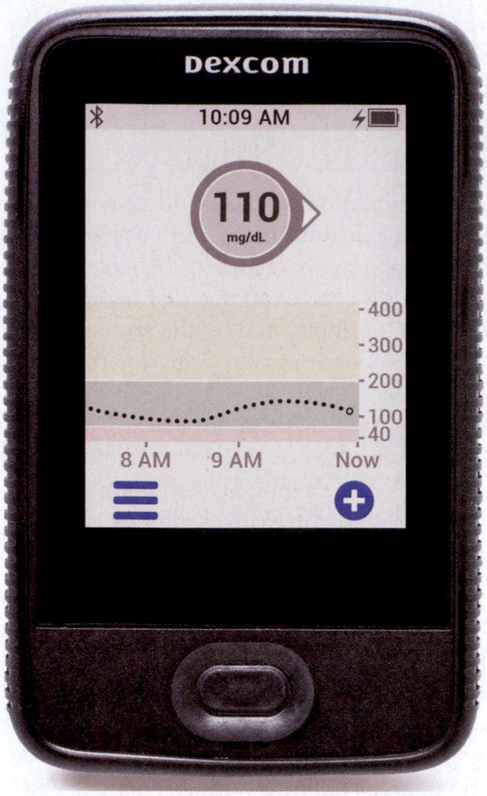
Dexcom
10:09 AM
110
mg/dL
400
300
200
100
40
8 AM
9 AM
Now

Figure 20.6 ■ Dexcom continuous glucose monitor showing a current glucose of 90 mg/dL and glucose trends during the preceding 3 hours.

Factors That Affect Glucose Meter Performance

According to the U.S. Food and Drug Administration (FDA; 2016), several factors affect the accuracy of blood glucose test results. The quality of the meter and test strips and the training on how to use the meter contribute to the degree of accuracy. Other factors can create falsely positive or negative readings.

Hematocrit

Patients with very high hematocrit values will usually test falsely low in blood glucose, and patients with very low hematocrit will test falsely higher. Anemia and sickle cell disease are two conditions that can affect hematocrit values.

Other Substances

Isopropyl alcohol, which is frequently used to clean the skin, will alter the results if it mixes with the blood sample, as will food residue on the skin and some lotions. Uric acid (a natural substance in the body that can be more concentrated in some people with DM), glutathione (an antioxidant also called *GSH*), and ascorbic acid (vitamin C) are known to interfere. Meters and supplies vary in sensitivity to medications.

Using Correct Supplies and Sample Volume

The test strips must be compatible with the glucose meter, not outdated, and stored according to directions.

Insufficient amounts of blood on the testing strip will cause a testing error.

Medications for Patients with Diabetes Mellitus

The pharmacologic treatment for DM depends on the type of DM. People with T1D must have insulin; those with T2D may be able to control glucose levels with an oral hypoglycemic medication, but they may require insulin if control is inadequate or if they are subjected to a stressor, such as surgery.

Insulin

The person with T1D requires a lifelong exogenous source of the insulin hormone to maintain life. Insulin is not a cure for DM; rather, it is a means of controlling hyperglycemia. People with T2D take insulin to control glucose levels when oral medications and/or diet and exercise are ineffective. Insulin needs are increased during times of increased metabolism, as can occur in the following situations:

- People who are experiencing physical stress (such as an infection or surgery) or who are taking corticosteroids
- Women with gestational DM
- People with diabetic ketoacidosis (DKA) or hyperosmolar hyperglycemic state (HHS)
- People who are ill and have an altered diet and exercise routine.

Sources of Insulin

Preparations of insulin are derived from recombinant DNA technology to form biosynthetic human insulin. Insulin analogs have been developed by modifying the amino acid sequence of the insulin molecule. Although pork- and beef-derived insulins were used in the past, today's insulin is derived from human DNA.

Insulin Preparations

Insulins are available in rapid-acting, short-acting, intermediate-acting, and long-acting preparations. Examples of various trade names and times of onset, peak, and duration of action are listed in **Table 20.4**.

Insulin lispro (Humalog) is a human insulin analog and is classified as a rapid-acting or ultra-short-acting insulin (Adams et al., 2017). Compared to regular insulin, lispro has a more rapid onset (less than 15 minutes), an earlier peak of glucose lowering (30 to 60 minutes), and a shorter duration of activity (3 to 4 hours). This means that lispro should be administered within 15 minutes before a meal (as compared to 30 minutes before as recommended for regular insulin). Because of its shorter duration, lispro is much less likely than regular insulin to cause nocturnal hypoglycemia. Patients using rapid-acting insulin usually also require concurrent use of a longer-acting insulin product.

Regular insulin is unmodified insulin, classified as a short-acting insulin. Regular insulin is clear in appearance and is used for subcutaneous injection as well as IV insulin therapy. While other insulins may also be clear, not all are appropriate for IV administration. Regular insulin is used in insulin infusions, as an IV bolus, or subcutaneously alone or in combination with intermediate-acting insulins to provide better glucose control. Only clear, short-acting insulins—regular, aspart, lispro, and glulisine—can be administered mixed with an intermediate- or long-acting insulin. Short- or rapid-acting insulins are used in insulin pumps so that if pump therapy is stopped the effect of the insulin rapidly declines.

The onset, peak, and duration of action of insulin can be changed by changing the insulin molecule or by adding protamine, a protein that slows insulin absorption. NPH insulin contains protamine to prolong its action, and it is classified as an intermediate-acting insulin. NPH insulin preparations appear cloudy when properly mixed prior to injection. Protamine is a foreign substance and may cause hypersensitivity reactions. Fixed-dose combinations of NPH insulin with a short-acting insulin are available to simplify administration.

Insulin detemir (Levemir) and insulin glargine (Lantus) are long-acting insulins, with a duration of action up to 24 hours. While these insulins are clear preparations, they must not be mixed with other insulins and cannot be used in insulin

Table 20.4 Insulin Preparations

Preparation	Name	Onset (h)	Peak (h)	Duration (h)
Rapid acting	lispro (Humalog)	0.25	1–1.5	3–4
	aspart (NovoLog)	0.25	40–50 min	3–5
	glulisine (Apidra)	0.25	1–1.5	3–5
Short acting	regular (Novolin-R, Humulin-R, Regular U-500)	0.5–1.0	2–3	4–6
Intermediate acting	NPH (Humulin N, Novolin N)	2	6–8	12–16
	detemir (Levemir)	Gradual	6–8	17–24
Long acting	glargine (Lantus, Toujeo)	1.1	3–4	10–24
Ultra-long acting (basal)	Degludec (Tresiba)	Gradual	6–12	42
	U-100 and U-200			
Combinations				
NPH and regular insulins	Humulin 50/50	0.5	3	22–24
	Humulin 70/30	0.5	4–8	24
	Novolin 70/30	0.5	4–8	24
Insulin aspart and insulin aspart protamine	Novolog Mix 70/30	0.25	4–8	24
Insulin lispro protamine and insulin lispro	Humalog Mix 75/25	0.25	4–8	24

pumps. Doses may be administered once or twice daily. Insulin glargine is used to treat patients with both T1D and T2D. It has a relatively constant effect (meaning it does not have a peak time of effect). It is not recommended for use in pregnancy.

SAFETY ALERT: Insulin glargine and insulin detemir are clear, unlike NPH insulins. Do not mistake these for regular insulin. Do not mix with any other insulins. Do not inject IV, only subcutaneously. ■

Concentrations of Insulin

Insulin is commonly dispensed as 100 units/mL (U-100), which means there are 100 units of insulin in 1 mL. Newer preparations of insulin are available in stronger concentrations such as 200 units/mL (U-200), 300 units/mL (U-300), and 500 units/mL (U-500). It is important for the nurse to verify the dose as well as the concentration of insulin prior to its administration. Regular insulin is now made in a 500 units/mL (U-500) concentration. It is important to check the concentration of the insulin administered as this insulin is five times as concentrated as the standard 100 units/mL (U-100) insulins.

Mixing Insulins

When an individual with DM requires more than one type of insulin, mixing is recommended to avoid administering two injections per dose. Two different types of insulin are administered because a single dose of intermediate-acting or long-acting insulin rarely provides adequate control of blood glucose levels. The procedure for mixing insulins is described in **Box 20.2**. Following are some general guidelines:

- Commercially mixed insulins are recommended if the insulin ratio is appropriate for the requirements of the patient.
- Glargine and detemir insulin cannot be mixed with other insulins.
- NPH insulin may be mixed with regular insulin or rapid-acting insulins (Humalog, Novalog).
- Always withdraw regular or rapid-acting insulin first to avoid contaminating the regular insulin with intermediate-acting insulin.

Insulin Administration

Nursing implications for administering insulin are outlined in **Medication Administration 20.B** and further discussion follows in the chapter. The considerations for administering

BOX 20.2
Mixing Insulins: 10 Units of Regular and 20 Units of NPH

1. Wash hands.
2. Inspect regular insulin for clarity.
3. Gently rotate NPH insulin to mix well.
4. Wipe off the top of both vials with an alcohol pad.
5. Draw 20 units of air into the syringe, and inject air into the NPH vial (Figure **A**). Withdraw needle. The vial should remain upright (not inverted) when adding air to the vial.
6. Draw 10 units of air into the syringe, and inject air into the regular vial (Figure **B**).
7. Invert the vial, and withdraw 10 units of regular insulin (Figure **C**). Withdraw the needle.
8. Insert the needle into the NPH vial, and carefully withdraw 20 units of NPH insulin (Figure **D**).
9. Don disposable gloves.
10. Administer the insulin.
11. Discard gloves, wash hands, and properly dispose of the syringe.
12. Document insulin administration.

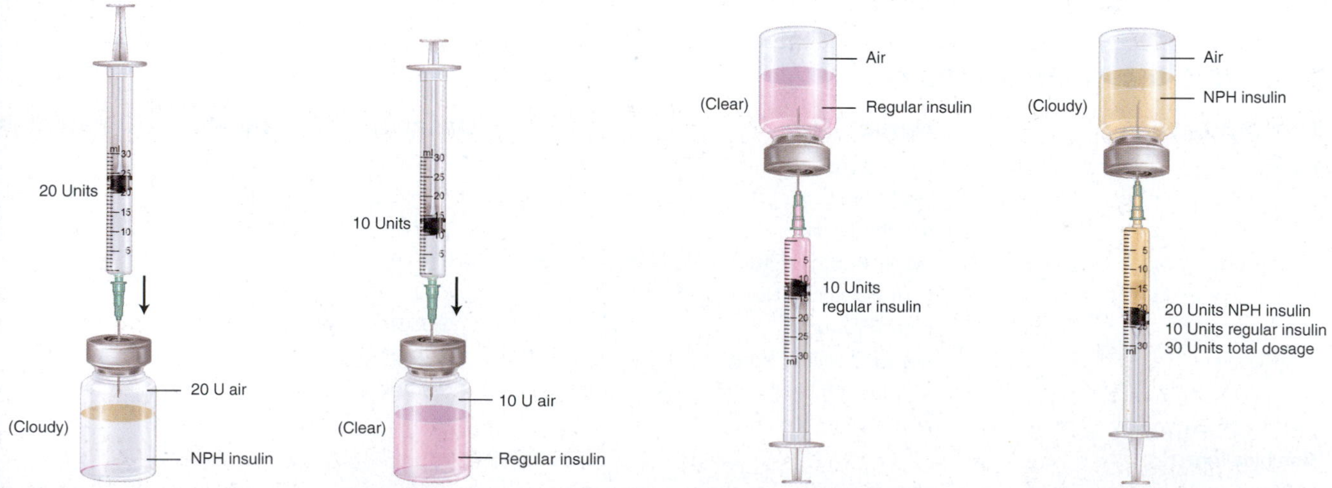

20 Units
20 U air
(Cloudy)
NPH insulin
10 Units
10 U air
(Clear)
Regular insulin
Air
(Clear)
Regular insulin
10 Units
regular insulin
Air
(Cloudy)
NPH insulin
20 Units NPH insulin
10 Units regular insulin
30 Units total dosage

A Injecting air into the NPH vial **B** Injecting air into the regular insulin vial **C** Withdrawing regular insulin **D** Withdrawing NPH insulin

Medication Administration 20.B

Insulin

Nursing Responsibilities

- Discard vials of insulin that have been open for more than 30 days or if expiration date has passed.
- Refrigerate extra insulin vials not currently in use (at about 4°C [40°F]), but do not freeze them.
- Store insulin in a cool place, and avoid exposure to temperature extremes or sunlight.
- Discard any vials with discoloration, clumping, granules, or solid deposits on the sides.
- If breakfast is delayed, also delay the administration of rapid-acting insulin.
- Monitor and maintain a record of blood glucose readings 30 minutes before each meal and bedtime (or as prescribed).
- Monitor food intake, and notify the healthcare provider if food is not being consumed.
- Monitor serum potassium and creatinine.
- Observe injection sites for manifestations of hypersensitivity, lipodystrophy, and lipoatrophy.
- If manifestations of hypoglycemia occur, confirm by testing blood glucose level, and administer an oral source of a fast-acting carbohydrate, such as 4 ounces of juice with six crackers or 8 ounces of skim milk. Hypoglycemic manifestations are described later under complications, but commonly include feelings of shakiness, hunger, and/or nervousness accompanied by sweating, tachycardia, or palpitations.
- If manifestations of hyperglycemia occur, confirm by testing blood glucose level, and notify the healthcare provider to obtain supplemental insulin or a change in oral medication therapy.

Health Education for the Patient and Family

- Demonstrate self-administration of insulin with a return demonstration:

  a. Wash hands carefully.
  b. Have a vial of insulin, the insulin syringe with needle, and alcohol pads ready to use.
  c. Remove the cover from the needle.
  d. Fill the syringe with an amount of air equal to the number of units of insulin, and insert the needle into the vial.
  e. Push air into the vial, invert the vial, and withdraw the prescribed units of insulin.
  f. Replace the cover over the needle.
  g. Wipe the selected site with alcohol. The injection is less likely to be painful if the alcohol is allowed to dry.
  h. Pinch up a fold of skin, and insert the needle into the tissue at the recommended angle.
  i. Administer the insulin.
  j. Withdraw the needle; if desired, apply firm pressure to the site for a few seconds.
  k. Discard the syringe in a needle disposal container.
  l. Insulin pens may be more convenient to use. The dose is selected with a dial on the pen. Needles should be changed with each use. Insulins, except for commercially mixed ones such as 70/30, cannot be mixed in a pen.

- Follow instructions for mixing insulins.
- Establish a plan for rotating injection sites, and observe closely for changes in tissues such as hardness, dimpling, or sunken areas.
- Always keep an extra vial or cartridge of insulin available; refrigerate insulins not in use. Discard insulin pens kept at room temperature for current use at 28 days. Discard vials of insulin kept at room temperature for 30 days. Stored, refrigerated vials and cartridges should be discarded if their expiration date is exceeded.
- Always have a vial of regular insulin available for emergencies.
- Be aware of the signs of hypersensitivity responses, hypoglycemia, and hyperglycemia.
- Keep a source of glucose available at all times to treat hypoglycemia if it occurs. Eat within 15 minutes of injecting rapid-acting insulins.
- Vision may be blurred during the first 6 to 8 weeks of insulin therapy; this is the result of fluid changes in the eye and should clear up in 8 weeks.
- Avoid alcoholic beverages, which may cause hypoglycemic unawareness.
- Follow these guidelines for sick days:

  a. Never omit insulin.
  b. Always monitor blood glucose and urine ketones at least every 2 to 4 hours.
  c. Always drink plenty of fluids; try to drink at least one glass of water or other calorie-free, caffeine-free liquid each hour.
  d. Get as much rest as possible.
  e. Contact the healthcare provider if there is persistent fever, vomiting, shortness of breath, severe pain in the abdomen, dehydration, loss of vision, chest pain, persistent diarrhea, blood glucose levels above 250 mg/dL, or ketones in the urine.

Source: Data from Adams et al., 2017.

insulin include routes of administration, syringe and needle selection, preparing the injection, sites of injection, mixing insulins, and insulin regimens.

Routes of Administration

All insulins are given parenterally. Regular insulin is given by both subcutaneous and IV routes; all others are given only subcutaneously. If the IV route is not available, regular insulin may also be administered IM in an emergency situation.

Continuous Subcutaneous Insulin Infusion

Regular or rapid-acting insulins are used in continuous subcutaneous insulin infusion (CSII) devices, often called *insulin pumps* (e.g., OmniPod, MiniMed, Tandem pumps). CSII devices have a small pump that holds a reservoir of insulin, connected to a subcutaneous needle. The pump is about the size of a small cell phone and can be worn on a belt or tucked into a pocket. The needle is placed in the skin, usually in the abdomen, and is changed routinely. This device delivers a constant amount of programmed insulin (basal dose) throughout each 24-hour period and also delivers a bolus of insulin before meals (ADA, 2015).

Programming the amount of insulin to be delivered with a pump is determined by frequent blood glucose monitoring. Several different pumps are available, and each has rechargeable batteries, a syringe, a programmable computer, and a motor and drive mechanism. The rapid-acting insulin analog lispro is an appropriate insulin for insulin pumps, or short-acting regular insulin may be used. Lispro is not approved for use during pregnancy.

Many people with DM believe the pump allows more normal regulation of blood glucose and provides greater lifestyle flexibility. Pumps are as safe as multiple-injection therapy when recommended procedures are followed. A potential complication is an undetected interruption in insulin delivery, which may result in the rapid onset of DKA. The needle site must be kept clean and changed on a regular basis (every 3 to 4 days) to prevent inflammation and infection. Although the patient who chooses an insulin pump has more to learn, many are very satisfied with having more normal glucose control (ADA, 2015).

Correctional Doses of Insulin

Maintaining normal blood glucose prior to and during hospitalization decreases the risk of postoperative infections and shortens hospital stays. Healing is impaired when hemoglobin is glycosylated (linked with a sugar molecule) because glycosylated Hgb has an increased affinity for oxygen, putting tissues at risk for ischemia, and decreases the effectiveness of white blood cells (increasing the risk of infection).

Treatment of hospitalized patients with T1D and T2D requires a medication regimen that is responsive to glycemic changes secondary to the admitting condition and its treatment, including surgery (Martin et al., 2016).

People with T2D may not be able to manage with oral medications during hospitalization because of the risk of hypoglycemia from not eating and the slow response of these medications to correct hyperglycemia. Significant hyperglycemia during hospitalization is common due to increased metabolic demand and stress hormones. The seminal work of the NICE-SUGAR Study Investigators (2009) found significantly reduced mortality and complications such as infections, acute kidney injury, decreased time on mechanical ventilation, and decreased length of ICU stays when glucose levels are maintained close to normal levels. Also, hypoglycemia (blood glucose less than 40 mg/dL) should be avoided as it increases mortality. Current recommendations for critically ill patients are to keep the blood glucose level close to normal limits (between 110 and 140 mg/dL) for patients who otherwise have good glycemic control if it is safe to do so without risk of significant hypoglycemia. In many critically ill patients with a history of poor glycemic control, a range of 140 to 180 mg/dL may be appropriate. For those who are not critically ill but hospitalized, pre-meal glucose levels should be less than 140 mg/dL and random levels should be below 180 mg/dL (ADA, 2018b).

The latest recommendations are to control hyperglycemia in hospitalized patients (including those taking oral medications at home) with insulin. Hyperglycemia is best managed with a basal dose of insulin, pre-meal insulin, and correctional doses. The basal dose is once- or twice-daily subcutaneous insulin such as insulin glargine (once daily) or NPH (twice daily). The prandial or mealtime dose is a short- or rapid-acting dose of insulin given before meals. Correctional doses are calculated based on food intake and prior hyperglycemia and hypoglycemia episodes. The mealtime short-acting insulin dose is corrected (either increased or decreased) to prevent hyperglycemic or hypoglycemic episodes (Handelsman et al., 2015). See **Box 20.3** for methods to calculate basal, prandial, and correction doses for hospitalized patients on scheduled subcutaneous insulin doses and patients with insulin pumps.

Syringe and Needle Selection

Insulin is administered by sterile, single-use needles and either disposable insulin syringes or a multiple-dose insulin pen (**Figure 20.7** ■), calibrated in units per milliliter. This means that in U-100 insulin, there are 100 units of insulin in 1 mL. Syringes for administering U-100 insulin can be purchased in either a 0.3-mL (30 U), 0.5-mL (50 U), or 1.0-mL (100 U) size. The advantage of the 0.3- and 0.5-mL sizes is that the distance between unit markings is greater, making it easier to see and measure the dose accurately.

Some hospitals and many patients are using insulin pens instead of insulin syringes to administer insulin. The pens, either reusable or disposable, contain prefilled cartridges of insulin; the desired dose is adjusted on the pen's dial prior to injection. A disposable needle is replaced for each injection. Insulin pens are convenient to use, eliminating the need to carry an insulin vial and fill a syringe. The prefilled syringe currently in use may be stored at room temperature and must be discarded at 28 days. Cartridges not in current use may be stored in the refrigerator. Prefilled syringes or pens are useful for people who are visually impaired or traveling (BD Diabetes, 2018).

Preparing the Injection

The vial of insulin currently being used may be kept at room temperature for up to 30 days. Stored vials should be kept in the refrigerator and brought to room temperature prior to administration.

Regular insulin does not require mixing. If the solution is cloudy or discolored, the vial should be discarded. Modified insulin such as NPH insulin must be mixed to disperse the particles evenly throughout the solution. Mix the vial by gently rolling it between the hands. It is critical that no air bubbles remain in the prepared dose because even a small bubble can displace several units of insulin.

Sites of Injection

Although in theory any area of the body with subcutaneous tissue may be used for injections of insulin, certain sites are recommended (**Figure 20.8** ■). The rate of

BOX 20.3
Methods for Calculating Basal, Prandial, and Correction Doses of Insulin

INSULIN TOTAL DAILY DOSE (ITDD)

1. The total amount of insulin that the patient administered daily by injection (rapid- or short-acting with intermediate- or long-acting); for example, 48 units (30 units NPH and 18 units regular insulin)

   OR

2. 0.5 to 1 unit/kg (normal kidney/liver function already on insulin); for example, 48 units for a 96-kg patient

   OR

3. 0.3–0.5 unit/kg (reduced kidney/liver function or initial insulin therapy); for example, 30 units for a 96-kg patient.

Test blood glucose with test strip before meals and at bedtime.

BASAL DOSE: 40–50% OF THE ITDD

1. ***Insulin pump:*** Multiply the ITDD by 50% (e.g., 48.0 × 0.5 = 24 units). The basal insulin pump dose for this patient is 24 units. Divide the basal insulin pump dose by 24 to get the hourly basal pump dose and rate (24/24 = 1.0 unit/hour). Use rapid-acting or regular insulin.
2. ***Subcutaneous insulin:*** Multiply the ITDD by 50% (e.g., 48.0 × 0.5 = 24 units). This will be administered as one insulin subcutaneous injection of long-acting insulin (e.g., insulin glargine) daily or twice-daily injections of 12 units each of intermediate-acting insulin (e.g., NPH).

Correction doses may be needed if the patient is hypoglycemic or hyperglycemic.

MEALTIME BOLUS DOSE

1. ***Insulin pump:*** To calculate bolus doses, the remaining 50% of the ITDD is divided by four doses according to the patient's meal plan for the day. To calculate the units for each of these four daily bolus doses, multiply the percent of each meal bolus times the total daily insulin pump dose. For example, for 48 units for a total daily dose:

   Breakfast dose is 20% (or 0.2) × 48 units = 10 units

   Lunch dose is 10% (or 0.1) × 48 units = 5 units

   Dinner dose is 15% (or 0.15) × 48 units = 8 units

   Bedtime snack dose is 5% (or 0.05) × 48 = 2 units

Correction doses may be needed if the patient is hypoglycemic or hyperglycemic.

2. ***Subcutaneous insulin mealtime dose:*** Divide half of the ITDD into three mealtime doses.

   Breakfast = 8 units; lunch = 8 units; dinner = 8 units. No bedtime dose is given.

   Rapid-acting insulin (regular or aspart) is given in conjunction with the meal.

MEALTIME CORRECTION DOSE

A mealtime correction dose of insulin may be given before hyperglycemia develops. It is given with the mealtime bolus dose of rapid-acting insulin.

1. Test blood glucose prior to each meal. If blood glucose level is less than 70 mg/dL or the patient is symptomatic for hypoglycemia, follow hypoglycemia protocol.

71–100	No correction dose needed.
101–150	Add 2 or 3 units if mealtime dose is greater than 20 units.
151–200	Add 4 units if mealtime dose is greater than 20 units.
201–250	Add 6 units if mealtime dose is greater than 20 units.
251–300	Add 8 units if mealtime dose is greater than 20 units.
> 300	Add 10 units if mealtime dose is greater than 20 units.

Note: When correction doses are needed, the scheduled doses of rapid-acting insulin need to be reordered at higher doses.

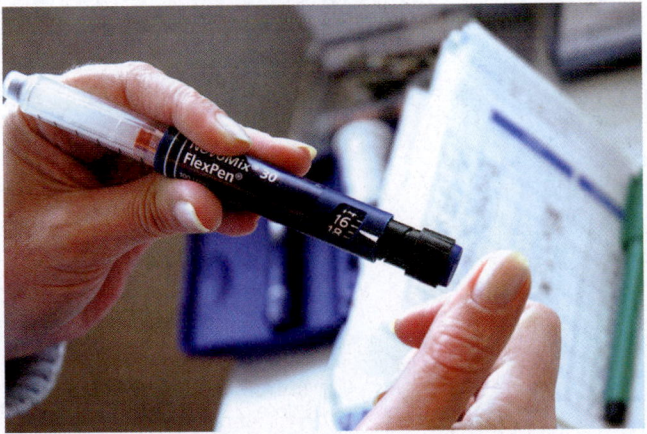
FlexPen

Figure 20.7 ■ Insulin pen with adjustable dose.

absorption and peak of action of insulin differ according to the site. The site that allows the most rapid absorption is the abdomen, followed by the subcutaneous tissue of the upper arm, thigh, and hip. Insulin sites are rotated with each injection. See **Box 20.4** for techniques to minimize painful injections.

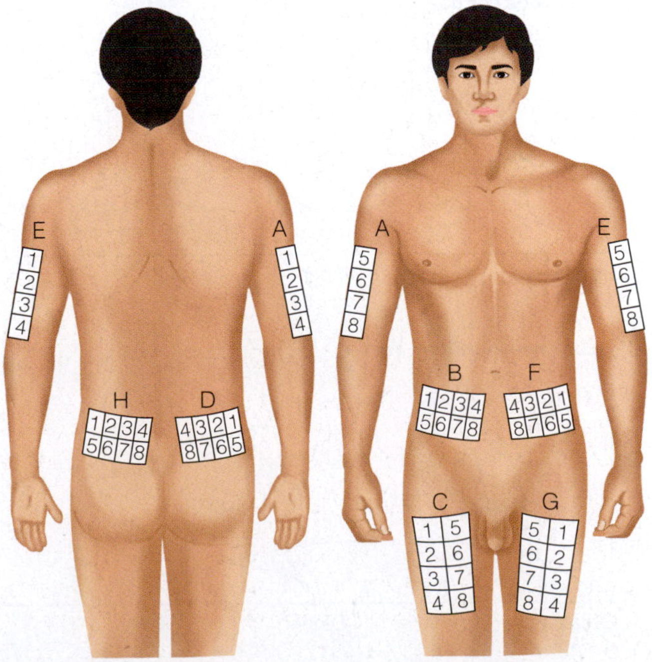
E
A
H
D
B
F
C
G

Figure 20.8 ■ Sites of insulin injection. The abdomen is the preferred site.

BOX 20.4
Techniques to Minimize Painful Injections

- Inject insulin that is at room temperature.
- Take care not to bend the needle before injection.
- Wait until alcohol on the skin completely dries before injecting the insulin.
- Quickly penetrate the skin with the needle.
- Don't change the direction of the needle during insertion or withdrawal.
- Don't reuse needles; they become dull with repeated use.

When administering insulin, gently pinch a fold of skin and inject the needle at a 90-degree angle. If the person is very thin, a 45-degree angle may be required to avoid injecting into muscle. Aspiration to check for blood is not necessary. Do not massage the site after administering the injection because this may interfere with absorption. Rotation of sites with body regions is recommended. The distance between injections should be about 1 inch (avoiding the area within a 2-inch radius around the umbilicus). Insulin should not be injected into an area to be exercised (such as the thigh before a vigorous walk) or to which heat will be applied; exercise or heat may increase the rate of absorption and cause a more rapid onset and peak of action.

Lipodystrophy (hypertrophy of subcutaneous tissue) or lipoatrophy (atrophy of subcutaneous tissue) may result if the same injection sites are used repeatedly. The tissues become hardened and have an orange-peel appearance. The use of refrigerated insulin may trigger the development of tissue atrophy or hypertrophy. These problems rarely occur, however, with the use of human insulins. Lipodystrophy and lipoatrophy alter insulin absorption, delaying its onset or retaining the insulin in the tissue for a period of time instead of allowing it to be absorbed into the body. Lipodystrophy usually resolves if the area is unused for a minimum of 6 months.

Insulin Regimens

Individualizing the appropriate insulin dosage is achieved through a balance among insulin, diet, and exercise. For most people with DM, the timing of insulin action requires two or more injections each day, often a mixture of rapid-acting and intermediate-acting insulins. Timing of the injections depends on blood glucose levels, food consumption, exercise, and types of insulin used. The objective is to avoid daytime and nighttime hypoglycemia while achieving adequate blood glucose control. Typical insulin regimens are outlined in **Table 20.5**.

Hypoglycemic Agents

Hypoglycemic agents are used to treat people with T2D. Nursing implications for this category of drugs are discussed in **Medication Administration 20.C**. These medications lower blood sugar by stimulating or increasing insulin secretion, preventing breakdown of glycogen to glucose by the liver, and increasing peripheral uptake of glucose by making cells less resistant to insulin. Peripheral uptake refers to uptake by muscles and fat in the arms and legs rather than in the trunk. Some hypoglycemic agents keep blood sugar low by blocking absorption of carbohydrates in the intestines. A hypoglycemic agent that is only available as an injectable is exenatide (Byetta). It has several modes of action: (1) It signals the pancreas to make insulin when nutrients are

Table 20.5 Insulin Regimens

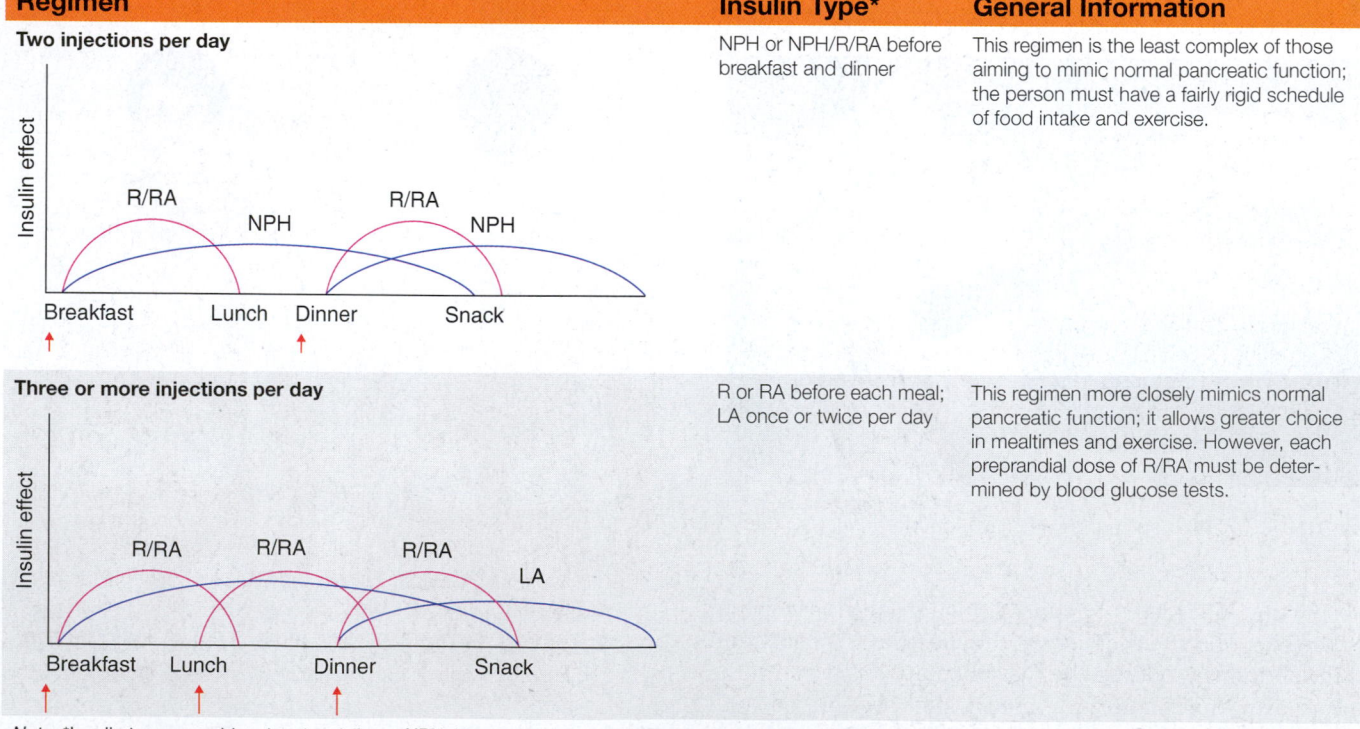

Regimen	Insulin Type*	General Information
Two injections per day 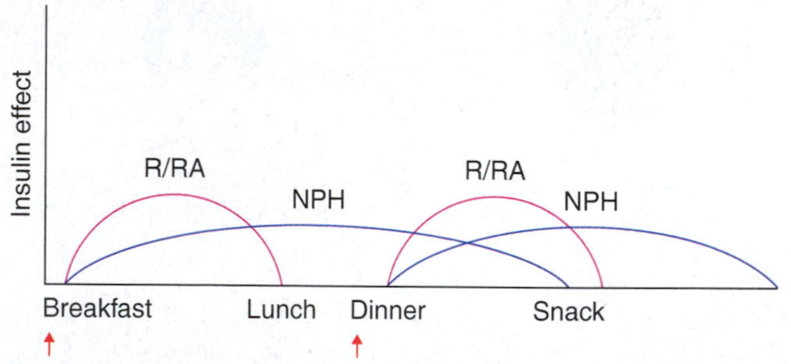 Insulin effect R/RA NPH R/RA NPH Breakfast Lunch Dinner Snack	NPH or NPH/R/RA before breakfast and dinner	This regimen is the least complex of those aiming to mimic normal pancreatic function; the person must have a fairly rigid schedule of food intake and exercise.
Three or more injections per day 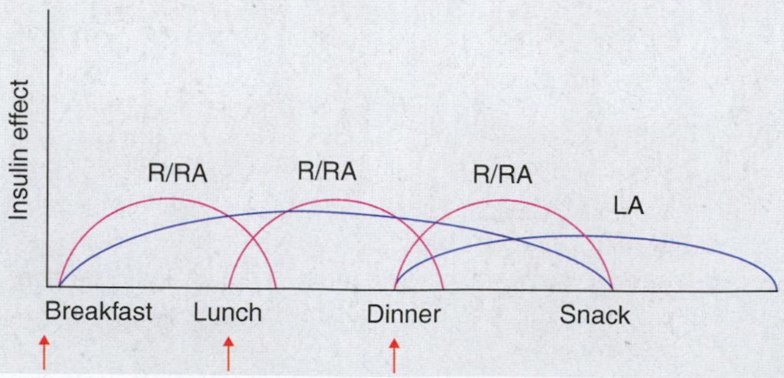 Insulin effect R/RA R/RA R/RA LA Breakfast Lunch Dinner Snack	R or RA before each meal; LA once or twice per day	This regimen more closely mimics normal pancreatic function; it allows greater choice in mealtimes and exercise. However, each preprandial dose of R/RA must be determined by blood glucose tests.

Note: *Insulin types are abbreviated as follows: NPH, intermediate acting; R, regular; RA, rapid acting; LA, long acting.

Medication Administration 20.C

Noninsulin Hypoglycemic Agents

SULFONYLUREAS

glimepiride (Amaryl)

glipizide (Glucotrol, Glucotrol XL)

glyburide (DiaBeta, Micronase)

tolazamide (Tolinase)

tolbutamide (Orinase)

These drugs are used primarily to treat mild, nonketotic T2D in people who are not obese. These patients cannot control the manifestations by diet alone, but they do not require insulin. Glyburide, glipizide, and glimepiride are 100 to 200 times more potent than tolbutamide. The drugs act by stimulating the pancreatic cells to secrete more insulin and by increasing the sensitivity of peripheral tissues to insulin. Dose adjustments must be made gradually and therefore these drugs are not useful for meeting acute changes that occur in illness or surgery. The most common side effect is hypoglycemia and this is exacerbated by NPO status. These drugs are also associated with weight gain. They are usually suspended during hospitalization (Adams et al., 2017).

BIGUANIDES

metformin (Glucophage)

Metformin reduces both the FBG and the degree of postprandial hyperglycemia in patients with T2D. It primarily decreases the overproduction of glucose by the liver and may also make insulin more effective in peripheral tissues. If renal insufficiency develops, metformin must be discontinued. It is used as an adjunct to diet, especially in patients who are obese or not responding to the sulfonylureas. Because of an increased risk of metformin-induced lactic acidosis, metformin is suspended during critical illness and in the presence of chronic kidney disease (DeFronzo, Fleming, Chen, & Bicsak, 2016). It should be discontinued temporarily before and for 48 hours after using intra-arterial iodinated contrast media for diagnostic imaging and anesthesia due to a small but significant risk of renal failure. In the Diabetes Prevention Program, some people treated with metformin reduced their risk of developing DM. An ADA panel recommends metformin for prevention for high-risk individuals (those with combined IGT and IFG, BMI greater than 30, and under 60 years of age with at least one other risk factor for DM). Lifestyle changes including diet and regular moderate exercise are part of preventing or delaying the onset of DM (ADA, 2018a).

ALPHA-GLUCOSIDE INHIBITORS

acarbose (Precose)

miglitol (Glyset)

These drugs work locally in the small intestine to slow carbohydrate digestion and delay glucose absorption. As a result, postprandial glucose and glycosylated hemoglobin are better controlled, reducing the risk of long-term complications. They do not cause hypoglycemia, but diminishing gastrointestinal side effects such as flatulence, diarrhea, and abdominal discomfort may occur.

MEGLITINIDES

nateglinide (Starlix)

repaglinide (Prandin)

This is a new class of oral medications for treatment of T2D. They stimulate rapid and short-duration insulin secretion from the pancreatic beta cells to decrease spikes in glucose following meals and also reduce the overall blood glucose level. They should be taken shortly before meals; without a meal, hypoglycemia is a risk. Side effects may occur and diminish with nateglinide; these include nausea and vomiting, diarrhea, joint pain, and flu-like symptoms. Repaglinide is associated with temporary weight gain, diarrhea, and joint pain.

INCRETIN MIMETICS

exenatide (Byetta), injectable only

This medication signals the pancreas to make the right amount of insulin after meals to help lower blood sugar closer to normal levels. It limits liver conversion of glycogen to glucose and slows the rate at which sugar enters the bloodstream, avoiding high blood sugar spikes.

DPP-4 INHIBITORS

sitagliptin (Januvia)

saxagliptin (Onglyza)

These drugs slow inactivation of incretin hormones and stabilize blood glucose levels by decreasing liver release of glucose and increasing insulin secretion. Side effects may include headache, nasopharyngitis, and urinary tract infections; there may also be allergic-like reactions such as rash and hives. They are taken once daily in combination with diet and exercise.

SYNTHETIC AMYLIN HORMONE

pramlintide (Symlin)

This medication is a synthetic form of amylin, a hormone cosecreted with insulin from the beta cells in the pancreas. It complements the role of insulin in limiting glucose levels by delaying gastric emptying and suppressing glucagon secretion after food intake. Patients with T1D almost totally lack this hormone. It is used with insulin as a subcutaneous injection at mealtime for type 1 and T2D and increases the risk of severe hypoglycemia.

Nursing Responsibilities

- Assess patients taking oral hypoglycemic agents closely for the first 7 days to determine therapeutic response.
- Alpha-glucosidase inhibitors should be administered with food. Most other oral hypoglycemic agents are taken 30 minutes before a meal.
- Teach the patient the importance of maintaining a prescribed diet and exercise program.
- Monitor for hypoglycemia if the patient is also taking nonsteroidal anti-inflammatory agents (NSAIDs), sulfonamide antibiotics, ranitidine, cimetidine, or beta-blockers; these drugs intensify the action of sulfonylureas.
- Monitor for hyperglycemia if the patient is also taking calcium channel blockers, oral contraceptives, glucocorticoids, phenothiazines, or thiazide diuretics; these drugs decrease the hypoglycemic responses to sulfonylureas.
- Assess for side effects: Nausea, heartburn, diarrhea, dizziness, fever, headache, jaundice, skin rash, urticaria, photophobia, thrombocytopenia, leukopenia, or anemia.
- If the patient is to have a thyroid test, determine whether the drug has been taken; sulfonylureas interfere with the uptake of radioactive iodine.
- Monitor for hypoglycemia with concurrent administration of an oral antidiabetic agent and insulin.
- Temporarily hold metformin for 2 days prior to injection of any radiocontrast agent to avoid potential lactic acidosis if renal failure occurs.

(continued)

Health Education for the Patient and Family

- Maintain prescribed diet and exercise regimen.
- You may need insulin if you have surgery, trauma, fever, or infection.
- Follow instructions to monitor blood glucose.
- Report illness or side effects to the healthcare provider.
- Undergo periodic laboratory evaluations as prescribed by your healthcare provider.
- Avoid alcohol intake, which may cause a reaction involving flushing, palpitations, and nausea.
- The medication interferes with the effectiveness of oral contraceptives; other birth control measures may be required.
- Mild manifestations of hyperglycemia may appear if a different agent is begun.
- Take medications as prescribed; for example, once a day at the same time each day. If you are taking acarbose, take the pill with the first bite of food at breakfast, lunch, and dinner.

Note: Drugs identified in blue are among the 200 most frequently prescribed medications in the United States.

Source: Data from Adams et al., 2017.

ingested and stop insulin release as blood sugar normalizes, (2) it stops liver conversion of glycogen to glucose, and (3) it decreases absorption of sugar from the intestines.

Aspirin Therapy

Cardiovascular disease is the most common cause of morbidity and mortality in people with DM (Handelsman et al., 2015). It is recommended that a once-daily dose of 81 to 160 mg of enteric-coated aspirin be considered as primary prevention for patients at risk for heart disease (Handelsman et al., 2015). Aspirin therapy is contraindicated for patients with aspirin allergy, bleeding tendency, anticoagulant therapy, recent gastrointestinal bleeding, or active liver disease.

Nutrition for Patients with Diabetes Mellitus

Nutrition therapy is an integral part of diabetes management and metabolic control in adults. The management of DM requires a balance between the intake of nutrients, the expenditure of energy, and the dose and timing of insulin or oral antidiabetic agents. The goals for dietary management for adults with DM, based on guidelines established by the American Association of Clinical Endocrinology (AACE/ACE, 2018), are:

- Promote and support healthy eating patterns that include a variety of nutrient-dense foods in appropriate portions.
- Achieve and maintain blood glucose levels with an HbA1C less than 7% or individualized for the patient based on age, duration of diabetes, health history, and other health conditions.
- Achieve and maintain optimal serum lipid levels to reduce the risk of vascular disease.
- Achieve and maintain blood pressure levels in the normal range.
- Achieve and maintain body weight goals.
- Prevent or at least slow the rate of development of complications of DM.
- Address individual nutrition needs, taking into account personal and cultural preferences, health literacy, access to healthful food choices, and willingness to change.
- Limit food choices only when research-based evidence supports doing so to maintain a positive outlook on food and the pleasure of eating.
- Provide practical tools for meal planning instead of focusing on individual nutrients (Handelsman et al., 2015).
- Meal planning should follow the recommended daily allowances of all nutrients. Monitoring carbohydrate intake is a key factor to maintaining glycemic control (ADA, 2018a, 2018b).

Recommended Intake of Specific Nutrients

Carbohydrates

The AACE (AACE/ACE, 2018) recommends that education be provided to help patients focus on healthful carbohydrates, those with higher fiber and nutrient value (Handelsman et al., 2015). This group of nutrients consists of plant foods such as grains, legumes, fruits, and vegetables. Carbohydrates can be divided into sugars, starch, and fiber, and carbohydrates with a lower glycemic index facilitate glycemic control (Handelsman et al., 2015). The glycemic index refers to the rate at which a food raises blood glucose, and determines the need for insulin. Proponents of low-carbohydrate diets use the glycemic index as the scientific foundation for decreasing intake of foods with a high glycemic index. However, many factors affect the digestion of carbohydrates; to date, research does not support using the glycemic index as a basis for therapy. The ADA recommends the majority of carbohydrate intake be from vegetables, fruits, whole grains, legumes, and dairy products (ADA, 2018a).

The use of sucrose as part of the total carbohydrate content in the diet does not impair blood glucose control in people with DM. Dietary fructose (from fruits and vegetables or from fructose-sweetened foods) produces a smaller rise in plasma glucose than sucrose and most starches, so it may offer an advantage as a sweetening agent. However, foods with added sugars often have less nutrient value than other carbohydrates, so amounts used should be limited.

Protein

As with carbohydrates, goals for dietary protein intake are individualized. Protein has 4 kcal per gram. Sources of protein should be low in saturated fat and cholesterol to reduce cardiovascular risk factors. Healthy proteins include fish, lean poultry, egg whites, and beans. Processed meats should be limited (Handelsman et al., 2015).

Fats

Dietary fats should be low in saturated fat, trans fatty acids, and cholesterol. Saturated and trans fatty acids are the principal dietary determinants of plasma LDL cholesterol. Saturated fats should be no higher than 10% of the total kilocalories allowed per day, intake of trans fatty acids should be minimal, and dietary cholesterol intake should be less than 300 mg per day. Fat has 9 kilocalories per gram. Recommendations of the different types of fat include:

- ***Limit saturated fat:*** Animal meats (butter fats, lard, bacon), cocoa butter, coconut oil, palm oil, and hydrogenated oils.
- ***Avoid trans fatty acids:*** Partially hydrogenated vegetable oils such as shortenings and animal fats. (Trans fats lower HDL cholesterol and increase LDL cholesterol, leading to coronary heart disease.)
- ***Consume healthful fat:*** Peanut oil, olive oil, and oils from other nuts and seeds, avocados, fish oils (Handelsman et al., 2015).

Limiting fat and cholesterol intake may help prevent or delay the onset of atherosclerosis, a common complication of DM. There is evidence to support recommending a Mediterranean-style diet, the DASH diet (which emphasizes fruits, vegetables, and low-fat dairy products), and vegetarian diets. Diets need to be tailored to patient preferences to be successful (Handelsman et al., 2015).

Fiber

Dietary fiber may be helpful in treating or preventing constipation and other gastrointestinal disorders, including colon cancer. It also helps provide a feeling of fullness, and large amounts of soluble fiber may be beneficial to serum lipids. Soluble fiber is found in dried beans, oats, barley, and in some vegetables and fruits (e.g., peas, corn, zucchini, cauliflower, broccoli, prunes, pears, apples, bananas, oranges). Insoluble fiber—which is found in wheat, corn, and in some vegetables and fruits (e.g., carrots, brussels sprouts, eggplant, green beans, pears, apples, strawberries)—does facilitate intestinal motility and give a feeling of fullness.

The ideal level of fiber has not been determined, but an intake of 14 g/1000 kcal per day is recommended (ADA, 2018a). An increase in fiber may cause nausea, diarrhea or constipation, and increased flatulence, especially if the person does not also increase fluid intake. Fiber should be increased gradually.

Sodium

Although the body requires sodium, most people consume much more than is needed each day, especially in processed foods. The recommended daily intake is 1000 mg of sodium per 1000 kcal, not to exceed 2000 mg per day, with lower levels (1500 mg) for people with hypertension. The primary concern with sodium is its association with hypertension, a common health problem in people with DM. It is suggested that table salt (which is 40% sodium) and processed foods high in sodium be avoided in the DM meal plan.

Sweeteners

The diet plan for people with DM restricts the amount of refined sugars. As a result, many people use noncaloric sweeteners and foods or drinks made with noncaloric sweeteners. The FDA has approved commercially produced nonnutritive sweeteners. Although questions have been raised about the safety of these substances in laboratory animal studies, they are considered safe for use by humans, when consumed in small amounts. Included in this category of sweeteners are saccharin (Sweet & Low), aspartame or neotame (NutraSweet, Equal), sucralose (Splenda), acesulfame potassium (Sunette), and stevia (Truvia). The nonnutritive sweeteners have negligible amounts of kilocalories and produce very little or no changes in blood glucose levels.

People with DM also use nutritive sweeteners, including fructose, sorbitol, and xylitol. The kilocalorie content of these substances is similar to that of table sugar (sucrose), but they cause less elevation in blood glucose. They are often included in foods labeled as "sugar free." Sorbitol may cause flatulence and diarrhea.

Researchers are continuing to study the safety and effectiveness of sweeteners. In addition, the FDA recommends that the food industry label products with the amount of each ingredient in milligrams per serving and the number of servings per container. When teaching patients about diet, the nurse should include information about the kilocalorie content of sweeteners and the meaning of such terms as *sugar free* and *dietetic* on labels.

Alcohol

Although drinking alcoholic beverages is not encouraged, neither is it totally prohibited for the patient with DM. Alcohol consumption may potentiate the hypoglycemic effects of insulin and oral agents. The ADA recommends that men with DM consume no more than two drinks and women with DM no more than one drink per day (ADA, 2018a). The following list provides guidelines for people who include alcohol in their diet plan:

- The signs of intoxication and hypoglycemia are similar; thus, the insulin-dependent diabetic is at increased risk for an insulin reaction.
- Two oral hypoglycemic agents (chlorpropamide and tolbutamide) may interact with the alcohol, causing headache, flushing, and nausea.
- Liqueurs, sweet wines, wine coolers, and sweet mixers contain large amounts of carbohydrate.
- Light beer is the recommended alcoholic drink.
- Alcohol should be consumed with meals and added to the daily food intake.

Meal Planning and Diet Plans

Meal Planning

Several different systems for meal planning are available to the person with DM. These systems include a consistent-carbohydrate DM meal plan, exchange lists, point systems, food groups, carbohydrate counting, and calorie counting. No matter what system is used, however, it must take into account the person's individualized eating habits, diet history, food values, and special needs. Altering eating patterns is often one of the most difficult tasks of DM management; careful consideration of individualized preferences enhances the ability of the patient with diabetes to manage glycemic control. Although the ADA recommends that a registered dietitian provide the nutrition prescription, nurses should know what is prescribed and be able to reinforce teaching and answer questions.

The Consistent-Carbohydrate DM Meal Plan

The consistent-carbohydrate DM meal plan, which is replacing the traditional exchange list plan, focuses on carbohydrate content. The patient eats a similar amount of carbohydrates at each meal or snack each day, based on an individual diet prescription and the United States Department of Agriculture's (2016) ChooseMyPlate recommendations (**Figure 20.9** ■).

Carbohydrates in a meal have the most effect on postprandial (after meals) blood glucose levels. They also determine, to a greater extent than do proteins and fats, insulin requirements before meals. Patients may be taught to count carbohydrates so they can administer 1 unit of regular insulin or insulin lispro for each 10 or 15 g of carbohydrate eaten at a meal. This method provides a better connection between food, medications, and exercise.

The Exchange Lists

The exchange list diet is based on an individual's ideal (or reasonable) weight, activity level, and age. These factors determine the total kilocalories that the person may consume each day. After the calories have been determined, the proportions of carbohydrates, proteins, and fats are calculated, using guidelines established by the American Diabetes Association and the American Dietetic Association.

The distribution of foods throughout the day is based on exchange lists. The name and quantity of food that make up one exchange (or serving) are listed; standard household measurements are used. One food portion on the list can be substituted (exchanged) for another with very little difference in calories or amount of carbohydrates, proteins, and fats. The meal plan prescribes how many exchanges are allowed for each food group per meal and snacks.

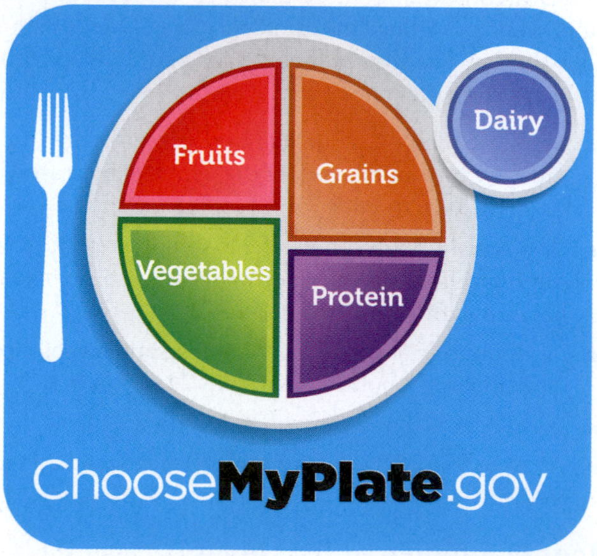
Fruits
Grains
Dairy
Vegetables
Protein
ChooseMyPlate.gov

Figure 20.9 ■ The United States Department of Agriculture's ChooseMyPlate program and website are excellent teaching tools to use with patients. Visit their website at www.choosemyplate.gov/MyPlate for more information.

Diet Plan for Insulin-Dependent DM

Diet and insulin prescriptions must be integrated for optimal energy metabolism and the prevention of hyperglycemia or hypoglycemia. The goals of the diet plan are to achieve optimal glucose and lipid levels and maintain overall health and a reasonable body weight. To meet these goals, the following strategies must be implemented:

- Glucose regulation requires correlating eating patterns with insulin onset and peak of action.
- Meals, snacks, and insulin regimens should be based on the person's lifestyle.
- Meal planning depends on the specific insulin regimen prescribed.
- Snacks are an important consideration in relation to the amount and timing of exercise.
- SMBG levels help the patient make adjustments for planned and unplanned changes in routines.

Diet Plan for T2D

The goals of the diet plan are to achieve glycemic targets, maintain overall health, prevent or delay complications, and attain or maintain reasonable body weight. Because the majority of these patients are overweight, weight loss is important and facilitates achieving the other goals.

In addition to decreasing kilocalories, it is recommended that the patient consume three small meals of equal size, evenly spaced approximately 4 to 5 hours apart, with one or two snacks. The person with T2D should also limit fat intake and consume many healthy vegetables and fruits, especially those that contain more fiber.

Diet Plan for the Older Adult

The majority of older adults with diabetes have T2D and should follow the general guidelines for that diet plan. However, special considerations for the older adult are important if the diet plan is to be followed, including dietary likes and dislikes, changes in taste perception, dental health, available income, and who prepares the food. Other factors to consider in planning the diet for the older adult include the age-related decline in kilocalorie requirements, decline in physical activity due to age and/or chronic illnesses, and the onset or progression of other chronic illnesses. The older adult who is overweight should reduce kilocalorie intake to ensure weight loss, but at the same time, careful monitoring for malnutrition is necessary.

Exercise for Patients with Diabetes Mellitus

The third component of DM management is a regular exercise program consisting of at least 150 minutes per week (ADA, 2018b). The benefits of exercise are the same for everyone, with or without DM: Improved physical fitness, improved emotional state, weight control, and improved work capacity. In people with DM, exercise increases the uptake of glucose by muscle cells, potentially reducing the need for insulin. Exercise decreases cholesterol and triglycerides, reducing the risk of cardiovascular disorders. People with DM should consult their primary healthcare provider before beginning or changing an exercise program. The ability to maintain an exercise program is affected by many different factors, including fatigue and glucose levels. It is as important to assess the person's usual lifestyle before establishing an exercise program as it is before planning a diet. Factors to consider include the patient's usual exercise habits, living environment, and community programs. The exercise that the person enjoys most is probably the one that he or she will continue throughout life. Instruct the patient to use proper footwear, inspect the feet daily and after exercise, avoid exercising in extreme heat or cold, and avoid exercising during periods of poor glucose control.

Patients with T1D

In the person with T1D, glycemic responses to exercise vary according to the type, intensity, and duration of the exercise. Other factors that influence responses include the timing of exercise in relation to meals and insulin injections and the time of day of the activity. Unless these factors are integrated into the exercise program, the person with T1D has an increased risk of hypoglycemia and hyperglycemia. General guidelines for an exercise program are:

- Patterns of hyperglycemia or hypoglycemia during exercise should be recognized and treated.
- The risk of exercise-induced hypoglycemia is lowest before breakfast, when free-insulin levels tend to be lower than they are before meals later in the day or at bedtime.
- Exercise should be moderate and regular; brief, intense exercise tends to cause hyperglycemia (due to release of stress hormones), and exercise can also lead to hypoglycemia.
- Exercising at a peak insulin action time may lead to hypoglycemia.
- SMBG is essential before, during, and after exercise.
- Food intake may need to be increased during exercise to treat hypoglycemia.
- Fluid intake, especially water, is essential.

Young adults are encouraged to participate in sports. Modifications in diet and insulin doses are expected during exercise. Athletes should begin training slowly and have a rapid carbohydrate source (such as juice or a snack) available during exercise to treat hypoglycemia.

Patients with T2D

An exercise program for the person with T2D is especially important. The benefits of regular exercise include weight loss in those who are overweight, improved glycemic control, increased well-being, socialization with others, and a reduction of cardiovascular risk factors. A combination of diet, exercise, and weight loss may decrease the need for oral hypoglycemic agents if it can be maintained. This decrease is due to an increased sensitivity to insulin, increased kilocalorie expenditure, and increased self-esteem.

General guidelines for an exercise program follow.

- Before beginning a program, have a medical screening.
- Begin the program slowly, and gradually increase intensity and duration.
- Exercise at least 150 minutes a week in regular sessions (30 minutes, five times per week).
- Include resistance exercise (muscle strengthening) and aerobic exercise in the program.

Surgery

Treating DM with Surgery

Surgical management of DM includes surgically revising the GI tract as well as replacing or transplanting the pancreas, pancreatic cells, or beta cells. Many researchers believe that transplantation of the tail of the pancreas or encapsulation of alpha and beta cells that produce insulin and glucagon is promising, and research is continuing. A patient with diabetes can receive a portion of a pancreas from a living relative, sometimes along with a kidney transplant. Transplants of more than one organ survive better than solo transplants (ADA, 2016b). Patients receiving organ transplants will receive medication for the rest of their lives to prevent immune rejection of the organ.

Studies of patients with DM who have gastrointestinal surgery for morbid obesity show improved insulin sensitivity and in some cases resolution of T2D. Roux-en-Y gastric bypass (RYGB) results in remarkable reductions in blood glucose levels and Hgb A1C. RYGB, which alters gastrointestinal anatomy, improves insulin sensitivity and is associated with remission of T2D in a significant percentage of patients (Coen et al., 2015). See Chapter 22 for more information about these procedures and related nursing care.

Managing DM in the Patient Having Surgery

Surgery is a stressor that often alters self-management and glycemic control in people with DM. In response to stress, levels of catecholamines, cortisol, glucagon, and growth hormones increase, as does insulin resistance. Hyperglycemia occurs, and protein stores are decreased. In addition, diet and activity patterns change, and medication types and dosages vary. Periods of hyperglycemia result in increased risk for postoperative infection, delayed wound healing, fluid and electrolyte imbalances, and DKA (Handelsman et al., 2015).

Preoperatively, all patients should be in the best possible metabolic state. Screening for complications and regular blood glucose monitoring are part of preoperative preparation. Oral hypoglycemic agents may be withheld for 1 or 2 days before surgery. Regular insulin is often administered to the patient with T2D and those with prediabetes (hyperglycemia but not diagnosed with DM) during the perioperative period. All patients with hyperglycemia follow a carefully prescribed insulin regimen individualized to specific needs.

Patients with diabetes who are critically ill in the perioperative period should receive IV glucose and insulin infusion in an intensive care unit. The target blood glucose level during surgery is between 110 and 140 mg/dL. This avoids hypoglycemia, which is difficult to detect under anesthesia, and prevents glycosuria, dehydration, and impaired wound healing (Handelsman et al., 2015).

The surgical procedure should be scheduled for as early as possible in the morning to minimize the duration of fasting. If food intake is restricted after surgery, intravenous dextrose is often prescribed, accompanied by subcutaneous regular insulin for the non critically ill surgical patient. Insulin doses are adjusted to blood glucose levels. Although kilocalorie intake is decreased postoperatively, physiologic stress can increase insulin requirements. Glucose control is also affected postoperatively by nausea and vomiting, anorexia, and gastrointestinal suction.

During the postoperative period, the patient with T2D may continue to require insulin or may resume oral medications, depending on glucose control. The patient with T1D may require reduced insulin as healing progresses and stress diminishes. Regular blood glucose monitoring is essential, as are assessments for hypoglycemia.

20.5 Nursing and Transition Care of the Patient with Diabetes Mellitus

Diabetes mellitus is a chronic condition and the plan of care is dedicated to preventing complications and maintaining or improving quality of life. The responses of the person with DM to the illness are often complex and individualized, involving multiple body systems. Assessments, planning, and implementation differ for the person with newly diagnosed DM, the person with long-term DM, and the person with acute complications of DM. The plan of care and content of teaching also differ according to the type of DM, the person's age and culture, and the person's intellectual, psychologic, and social resources. Nurses who are DM specialists and generalists are relied on to teach patients to successfully manage living with DM. To teach and support patients in their efforts to manage DM, all nurses need to understand DM, learn effective behavioral change strategies, and know appropriate interventions. The Moving Evidence into Action box on page 622 describes a nursing study of the effect of resilience in diabetes self-care.

Moving Evidence into Action

Nursing Management of Neuropathic Pain Through Massage and Aromatherapy

Clinical Issue

A common complication in diabetics is peripheral neuropathy with resulting neuropathic pain. The presence of neuropathic pain not only impairs function, but also quality of life. Addressing the patient experience with neuropathic pain using nonpharmacological interventions is within the purview of the nurse.

External Evidence

Gok-Metin, Donmez, Izgu, Ozdemir, and Arslan (2017) conducted an open-label randomized controlled trial comparing aromatherapy-enhanced massage three times a week to usual care (no massage or aromatherapy enhancement) for 8 weeks in 46 patients seen in a university hospital endocrine outpatient clinic in Turkey. Outcomes included a survey about neuropathic pain and a questionnaire of health-related quality of life in patients with neuropathic pain. The patients who received aromatherapy-enhanced massage reported significantly less neuropathic pain at week 4 as well as improvement in health-related quality of life.

Internal Evidence

As part of the evaluation of internal evidence, one must consider the patient's response to a novel intervention such as aromatherapy-enhanced massage and identification of stakeholders that impact uptake of new interventions. One question to ask: Are diabetic patients with neuropathic pain who would be offered a novel intervention like aromatherapy-enhanced massage the population of your care environment? Does the clinical environment support the use of novel nursing-independent interventions? How would the introduction of an independent nursing intervention that would require RN skill development impact costs?

Patient Considerations

When considering use of a new intervention practice (like aromatherapy-enhanced massage), the nurse must consider the specific patient population where it will be used. Will patients and their families be amenable to this new independent nursing intervention?

Putting the Pieces Together

In caring for patients with chronic illness, especially those with discomforting symptoms, the patient and family are partners with the healthcare team. Developing psychomotor skills to effectively deliver aromatherapy-enhanced massage is a critical skill in the uptake of this intervention. To effectively implement such a novel intervention, it is important to evaluate the external evidence and consider the internal implications and patient/family issues. The addition of independent nursing interventions may improve the patient experience and reduce neuropathic pain. This can lead to increased patient satisfaction and improve participation in their therapeutic plan.

Reference

Gok-Metin, Z., Donmez, A. A., Izgu, N., Ozdemir, L., & Arslan, I. E. (2017). Aromatherapy massage for neuropathic pain and quality of life in diabetic patients. *Journal of Nursing Scholarship, 49*(4), 370–388.

Nursing Care

Assessment

The following data are collected through the health history and physical examination. Further focused assessments are described in the following with nursing interventions. When assessing the older patient, be aware of normal aging changes in all body systems that may alter interpretation of findings.

- *Health history:* Family history of DM; history of hypertension or other cardiovascular problems; history of any change in vision (e.g., blurring) or speech, dizziness, numbness or tingling in hands or feet; pain when walking; frequent voiding; change in weight, appetite, infections, and healing; problems with gastrointestinal function or urination; or altered sexual function
- *Physical assessment:* Height/weight ratio, vital signs, visual acuity, cranial nerves, sensory ability (touch, hot/cold, vibration) of extremities, peripheral pulses, skin and mucous membranes (hair loss, appearance, lesions, rash, itching, vaginal discharge).

Priorities of Care

The priorities of care for the patient with DM are to maintain function, prevent complications, and teach self-management. Teaching the patient and significant others to manage the disease is vital to achieving long-term glycemic targets. Although the patient with an acute or chronic complication of DM may require focused nursing interventions to restore functional health, teaching to maintain health and prevent future complications remains a priority of nursing care.

Diagnoses, Outcomes, and Interventions

Although many different diagnoses are appropriate for the individual with DM, those discussed in this section address actual or potential problems with skin, infection, injury, sexuality, and coping. See the accompanying Case Study & Nursing Care Plan for more information.

Prevent Skin Breakdown. The person with DM is at increased risk for skin breakdown and wounds as a result of decreased sensation (if neuropathy is present) and decreased tissue perfusion. An open lesion is more prone to infection and delayed healing. Infection may lead to gangrene, especially in the feet and lower extremities.

Expected Outcomes: Patient's skin will remain intact without evidence of wounds or ulcers. Patient will demonstrate preventative foot care and will manage wounds as instructed. Patient will maintain glycemic control to promote healing and prevent complications. Wound care will be performed on open wounds.

The nurse will:

- Conduct baseline and ongoing assessments:
    a. Musculoskeletal assessment, including foot and ankle joint range of motion, bone abnormalities (bunions, hammertoes, overlapping digits), gait patterns, use of assistive devices for walking, and abnormal wear patterns on shoes
    b. Neurologic assessment, including sensations of touch and position, pain, and temperature
    c. Vascular assessment, including lower-extremity pulses, capillary refill, color and temperature of skin, lesions, and edema; checking hydration status, including dryness or excessive perspiration; checking for fissures between toes, corns, calluses, plantar warts, ingrown or overgrown toenails, redness over pressure points, blisters, cellulitis, or gangrene.

Peripheral neuropathies may result in altered pain perception, loss of deep tendon reflexes, loss of cutaneous pressure and position sensation, foot drop, changes in the shape of the foot, and changes in bones and joints. Peripheral vascular disease may cause intermittent claudication, absent pulses, delayed venous filling on elevation, dependent rubor, and gangrene. Injuries, lesions, and changes in skin hydration potentiate infections, delayed healing, and tissue loss in the person with DM.

- Teach foot hygiene. Use a variety of methods, including demonstration, return demonstration, audiovisual aids, and written lists. If the person is wearing shoes and socks, ask him or her to remove them to practice foot care effectively. *Foot care is a priority in DM management to prevent serious problems. Many people with DM are unaware of lesions or injury until infection and compromised circulation are far advanced.*
- Discuss the importance of not smoking if patient smokes. *Nicotine in tobacco causes vasoconstriction, further decreasing the blood supply to the feet.*
- Discuss the importance of maintaining blood glucose levels through diet, medication, and exercise. *Hyperglycemia is associated with a higher risk for the chronic complications of DM, including peripheral vascular disease and neuropathy.*

Prevent Infection. The person with DM is at increased risk for infection due to vascular insufficiency that limits tissue perfusion, an inhibited inflammatory response, neurologic abnormalities that limit the awareness of trauma, and increased growth of bacterial and fungal infections in the presence of hyperglycemia.

Expected Outcomes: Patient will be free from infection. Patient will treat infections per provider advice.

The nurse will:

- Use and teach meticulous hand hygiene. *Hand hygiene is the single most effective method for preventing the spread of infection.*
- Monitor for manifestations of infection: Increased temperature, pain, malaise, swelling, redness, discharge, cough. *Early diagnosis and treatment of infections can control their severity and decrease complications.*
- Discuss the importance of meticulous skin care. Keep the skin clean and dry, using lukewarm water and mild soap. *People with DM are more prone to develop furuncles and carbuncles; the infection often increases the need for insulin. Clean, intact skin and mucous membranes are the first line of defense against infection.*

- Teach dental health measures:
  a. Obtain a dental examination every 4 to 6 months.
  b. Maintain careful oral hygiene, which includes brushing the teeth with a soft toothbrush and fluoridated toothpaste at least twice a day and flossing as recommended.
  c. Be aware of the manifestations requiring dental care: Bad breath; unpleasant taste in the mouth; bleeding, red, or sore gums; and tooth pain.
- If dental surgery is necessary, monitor for need to make adjustments in insulin. *All people with DM need to be taught proper oral hygiene, the risk of periodontal disease, and the importance of obtaining dental care for manifestations of oral or dental problems.*
- Teach women about the manifestations and preventative measures for vaginitis caused by *Candida albicans*. The manifestations are an odorless, white or yellow cheeselike discharge and itching. *DM is a predisposing factor for* Candida albicans *vaginitis, the most common form of vaginitis. Poor personal hygiene and wearing clothing that keeps the vaginal area warm and moist increase the risk of vaginitis. The infection may spread to the urinary tract, resulting in urinary tract infections; preventing and treating vaginitis decrease this risk.*

Prevent Injury. The person with DM is at risk for injury from multiple factors. Neuropathies may alter sensation, gait, and muscle control. Cataracts or retinopathy may cause visual deficits. Hyperglycemia often causes osmotic changes in the lens of the eye, resulting in blurred vision. In addition, significant changes in blood glucose alter levels of consciousness and may cause seizures. The impaired mobility, sensory deficits, and neurologic effects of complications of DM increase the risk of accidents, burns, falls, and trauma.

Expected Outcomes: Patient will be free from injury. Patient will demonstrate an understanding of techniques to prevent injury and will implement safety measures in the home to prevent injury. The patient (and close caregivers) will demonstrate knowledge of diabetes, how to meet glycemic goals, and how to prevent diabetic emergencies.

The nurse will:

- Assess factors that increase the risk of injury: Blurred vision, cataracts, decreased adaptation to dark, decreased tactile sensitivity, hypoglycemia, hyperglycemia, dehydration, joint immobility, unstable gait. *A knowledge base is necessary to develop an individualized plan of care. The risk of injury increases with the number of factors identified.*
- Reduce environmental hazards in the healthcare facility, and teach the patient about safety in the home and in the community (see **Box 20.5**). *Strange environments and the presence of hazardous environmental factors increase the risk of falls or other accidents. Glare is often responsible for falls in people with visual deficits. The nurse can reduce factors that increase the risk of injury by implementing care and teaching safe practices during the activities of daily life.*
- Monitor for and teach the patient and family to recognize and seek care for the manifestations of DKA in the patient with T1D: Hyperglycemia, thirst, headaches, abdominal pain, nausea and vomiting, increased urine output, ketonuria, dehydration, and decreasing level of consciousness. *Blood glucose levels increase if the insulin need is unmet or insufficiently met; the cellular use of fats for fuel results in ketosis. Osmotic diuresis increases urinary output, resulting in thirst and dehydration.*
- Monitor for and teach the patient and family to recognize and seek care for the manifestations of HHS in the patient with T2D: Extreme hyperglycemia, increased urinary output, thirst, dehydration, hypotension, seizures, and decreasing level of consciousness. *HHS is a life-threatening condition requiring recognition and treatment.*
- Monitor for and teach the patient and family to recognize and treat the manifestations of hypoglycemia: Low blood glucose, anxiety, headache, uncoordinated movements, sweating, rapid pulse, drowsiness, and visual changes. Teach patient and family to carry some form of rapid-acting sugar source at all times. *Severe hypoglycemia causes a decrease in the level of consciousness. The decrease in blood glucose most often results from too much insulin, too little food, or too much exercise.*

BOX 20.5
Safety Considerations for the Patient with DM at Home and in the Community

IN THE HEALTHCARE FACILITY

- Orient the patient to new surroundings on admission.
- Keep the bed at the lowest level.
- Keep the floor free of objects.
- Use a nightlight.
- Use a thermometer to check the temperature of the bath or shower water before the patient uses it.
- Instruct the patient to wear shoes or slippers when out of bed.
- Monitor blood glucose levels regularly.
- Monitor for side effects of prescribed medications, such as dizziness or drowsiness.

IN THE HOME AND COMMUNITY

- Use a nightlight, preferably one with a soft, nonglare bulb.
- Use a thermometer to test the temperature of the bath or shower water before use.
- Wear shoes and slippers with nonskid soles.
- Do not use throw rugs.
- Install hand grips in the tub and shower and next to the toilet.

- Recommend that the patient wear a medical alert bracelet or necklace identifying self as an individual with DM. *In case of sudden, severe illness or accident, a medical alert bracelet can allow immediate medical attention for DM to be instituted.*

Promote Sexual Function. Sexuality is a complex and inseparable part of every person. It involves not only physical sexual activities but also an individual's self-perception as male or female, roles and relationships, and attractiveness and desirability. Changes in sexual function and in sexuality have been identified in both men and women with DM.

Alterations in erectile ability occur in approximately 50% of all men with DM. The incidence of impotence increases with the duration of the DM and is often associated with peripheral neuropathy and vascular disease. Libido is usually unaffected, even when impotence is present. Women with DM also have alterations in sexual function, although the reason is less clear. The problems reported by women involve decreased desire and decreased vaginal lubrication. Women with DM are also at increased risk for vaginitis and may avoid sexual intercourse in order to avoid pain.

Expected Outcome: The patient and his or her significant other will verbalize knowledge of sexual function, the potential effects of DM, and options if dysfunction is present.

The nurse will:

- Include a sexual history as part of the initial and ongoing assessment of the patient with DM. A specific history form may be used that addresses sexual development, personal and family values, current sexual practices and concerns, and changes desired. Ask a nonthreatening, open-ended question to elicit information, such as "Tell me about your experience with sexual function since you have been diagnosed with DM." *Obtaining accurate information to assess the sexual health of a patient is necessary before counseling can begin or referrals can be made. Patients may not discuss problems with sexual function unless the nurse initiates the conversation.*
- Provide information about the actual and potential physical effects of DM on sexual function. Discuss the effect of poor control of blood glucose on sexual function as part of any teaching plan. *Patients benefit from basic information about male and female anatomy, the sexual response cycle, and how DM can affect this part of the body. Changes in blood glucose levels not only may cause changes in desire and physical response but also may alter sexual responses as a result of vascular disease, depression, anxiety, and fatigue.*
- Provide counseling or make referrals as appropriate. The nurse is responsible for knowing about sexuality and sexual health throughout the lifespan and provides information based on knowledge of the effects of illness and treatment on sexual function. For example, men who are impotent may regain the ability to have sexual intercourse through penile implants, suction apparatus, the use of drugs that facilitate gaining and maintaining an erection such as sildenafil citrate (Viagra), or injections of medications (such as yohimbine, an alpha$_2$-adrenergic blocker) that increase vascular blood flow into the corpus of the penis. Women with decreased vaginal lubrication can decrease painful intercourse by using vaginal lubricants (such as K-Y Jelly) or estrogen creams. *The nurse may make specific suggestions to facilitate positive sexual functioning, referring the patient to the appropriate healthcare provider as necessary for intensive therapy.*

Promote Coping. Coping is the process of responding to internal or environmental stressors or potential stressors. The person diagnosed with DM is faced with lifelong changes in many parts of his or her life. Diet, exercise habits, and medications must be integrated into the person's lifestyle and be carefully controlled. Daily injections and fingersticks may be a reality. Fear of potential complications and of negative effects on the future is common.

If the person is unable to cope successfully with these changes, emotional stress can interfere with glycemic control. In addition, unsuccessful coping often results in noncompliance with prescribed treatment modalities, further impairing glycemic control and increasing the potential for acute and chronic complications.

Expected Outcome: Patient will follow the prescribed treatment plan, using available personal, family, and community resources as needed.

The nurse will:

- Assess the patient's psychosocial resources, including emotional resources, support resources, lifestyle, and communication skills. *Chronic illness affects all dimensions of an individual's life, as well as the lives of family members and significant others. A comprehensive assessment of strengths and weaknesses is the first step in developing an individualized plan of care to facilitate coping.*
- Explore with the patient and family the effects (actual and perceived) of the diagnosis and treatment of DM on finances, occupation, energy levels, and relationships. *Common frustrations associated with DM are the disease itself, the treatment modalities, and the healthcare system. Effective coping involves maintaining a healthy self-concept and satisfying relationships, emotional balance, and handling emotional stress.*
- Teach constructive problem-solving techniques. *Problem-focused behaviors include setting attainable and realistic goals, learning about all aspects of the problem, learning new procedures or skills that increase self-esteem, and reaching out to others for support.*
- Provide information about support groups and resources, such as suppliers of products, journals, books, and cookbooks for people with DM. *Sharing with others who have similar problems provides opportunities for mutual support and problem solving. Using available resources improves the ability to cope.*

Delegating Nursing Care Activities

The professional nurse may delegate nursing care activities such as doing blood glucose checks, providing hygiene, assisting with feeding, and assisting with physical activity. The professional nurse assesses the patient on admission (or transfer of care), preoperatively, postoperatively, and on discharge. The professional nurse also provides teaching and develops the plan of care, coordinates the healthcare team, and evaluates the results of care provided.

Transitions of Care

Health promotion activities primarily focus on preventing the onset and complications of DM. The prevention of type 2 diabetes has been shown in randomized controlled trials to be achievable in a significant number of individuals at risk. A combination of lifestyle changes (weight loss and increased physical activity) and medications (especially metformin) prevents or delays the onset of T2D (ADA, 2018b). Prevention of progression to DM is dependent on at-risk individuals accepting responsibility for learning and sustaining lifestyle changes through self-management education, counseling, and coaching. Blood glucose screening at 3-year intervals beginning at age 45 is recommended for those not in the high-risk group.

Care of the Newly Diagnosed Patient

Diabetes is a serious chronic disease and the diagnosis of diabetes can be overwhelming to the patient. Although the provider prescribes medications and treatments, the patient is responsible to implement those treatments and manage the day-to-day challenges of diabetes. Diabetes self-management education (DSME) and support from the healthcare team as the patient learns new skills will provide the patient with the tools necessary to manage the disease (Powers et al., 2015). Education and support of the patient with diabetes improves the quality of care provided and decreases the cost of healthcare as less complications occur. It is important that the patient knows that with careful planning the disease can be managed well and complications kept to a minimum (Powers et al., 2015). Topics that are important for the patient with newly diagnosed diabetes include:

- Information about the disease
- Diet information including foods that affect the blood glucose rapidly, and carbohydrate counting (if injecting insulin based on consumption of carbohydrates)
- Exercise including its importance and information tailored to the patient's current lifestyle and abilities
- Blood glucose monitoring and keeping a log of results
- Recognition of hypo- and hyperglycemia and treatment of each
- Insulin: Information about the medication prescribed and how to inject it
- Oral hypoglycemics: Information about new medications
- Other topics: Traveling with diabetes, alcohol use, smoking cessation, stress and illness, potential complications of diabetes and how to prevent them.

The patient will need education at each healthcare visit and support to successfully implement the plan of care to manage diabetes.

Care of the Patient with Diabetic Complications

The patient with diabetic complications often needs support in managing the disease. A careful assessment is the first step in identifying specific knowledge or motivational deficits. It is important to involve the patient in the plan of care and to tailor the plan to meet the patient's lifestyle. The nurse can encourage support from family and friends and can include significant others in education and teaching (AACE/ACE et al., 2018).

Nurses can foster resilience with four evidence-based skills. They include developing skills to manage stress successfully, goal setting and problem solving, positive evaluation of stressors, and making sense or finding advantages related to diabetes or its management (Rosenberg et al., 2015). The patient with improved resilience will have improved management of diabetes with less complications. The patient should also be assessed for the presence of depression or anxiety as these are common sequelae of chronic diseases such as diabetes. It is important to refer patients suffering from depression, anxiety, or other mood disorders for treatment, which can include medications as well as psychosocial interventions (AACE/ACE et al., 2018).

Sick Days

When an individual with DM is sick or has surgery, blood glucose level increases due to high metabolic needs. The person often mistakenly alters or omits the insulin dose in response to decreased food intake, causing hyperglycemia (sometimes severe). Guidelines for managing sick days are outlined in **Box 20.6**.

BOX 20.6
Sick-Day Management

When an individual with DM is sick or has surgery, blood glucose level increases due to high metabolic needs. The person often mistakenly alters or omits the insulin dose in response to decreased food intake, causing hyperglycemia (sometimes severe). The guidelines for dietary management during illness focus on preventing dehydration and providing nutrition to promote recovery (ADA, 2016a). In general, sick-day management includes:

- Monitoring blood glucose as much as every 2 to 3 hours
- Testing urine for ketones as often as every 4 hours
- Continuing to take insulin (may switch to sliding scale) or oral hypoglycemic agent and adding correctional insulin doses as prescribed by the healthcare provider
- Consuming many clear liquids (without caffeine)
- Calling the healthcare provider if the patient has had a fever for 2 days, if vomiting and diarrhea last for more than 6 hours or cannot keep any fluids down, if glucose is way out of range, if urine ketones are moderate or large, or if there are any signs of dehydration.

Teaching Self-Management

Teaching the patient and family to self-manage DM is a healthcare team responsibility. Nurses are very important resources and must be knowledgeable and up to date on their understanding of DM care. Even when a formal teaching plan is developed and implemented by diabetes nurse educators, all nurses must be able to reinforce knowledge and answer questions. Teaching is necessary for both the person who is newly diagnosed and for the person who has had DM for years. In fact, the latter may need almost as much teaching as the newly diagnosed person. Products for DM care, especially insulins, have changed dramatically and knowledge about risk reduction to prevent complications has increased.

The American Diabetes Association recommends that teaching be carried out on three levels. The first level focuses on survival skills, with the person learning basic knowledge and skills to be able to provide DM management for the first week or two while adjusting to the idea of having the disease. The second level focuses on home management, emphasizing self-reliance and independence in the daily management of DM. The third level aims at improving lifestyle and educating patients to individualize self-management of the illness.

Teaching may need to be adapted to the older adult. Because many patients with diabetes are older, considering the special needs of this population is essential. Uncontrolled DM in the older adult increases the potential for functional loss, social disengagement, and increased morbidity and mortality. Education for self-care allows the older adult to be more actively involved in his or her DM management and decreases the potential for acute and long-term complications from the disease. Considerations for teaching the older adult with DM include the following.

- Changes in diet may be difficult to implement for many reasons. Balanced meals at regular intervals may not have been part of the patient's lifestyle. Purchasing, storing, and preparing foods may be a problem. Changes in taste sensation may cause the patient to increase the use of salt and sugar.
- Exercise is important and must be individualized for any physical limitations imposed by other chronic illnesses, such as arthritis, Parkinson disease, chronic respiratory diseases, and/or cardiovascular diseases.
- The diagnosis of a chronic illness threatens independence and self-worth. The older adult with DM may now have to depend on others for help in meeting self-care needs.
- Money to purchase medications and supplies often must be taken out of a fixed income.
- Visual deficits may impair safe insulin administration. Visual deficits also interfere with blood glucose monitoring, food preparation, exercise, and foot care.

The nurse and patient should mutually establish goals based on the assessment data. Inquiries about patient and family priorities can be made effectively with the simple question "What concerns you most about having diabetes?" The topics of concern range from medications to economics. Addressing topics of greatest concern first increases the patient's and family's confidence that the information provided will be useful. It is equally important for family members to understand that the responsibility for daily management lies with the patient and that the primary role of the family is supportive. The patient is the person with the disease, and it is the patient who each day must take medications or inject insulin, test blood or urine, calculate and balance foods, exercise, adjust medications, inspect the body for injury, and determine whether and when medical assistance is needed. However, family members require the same knowledge so that they can provide emotional support as well as physical care if necessary.

The following should be included in teaching the patient and family about care at home:

- ***Metabolism:*** Information about normal metabolism and how DM changes it
- ***Diet plan:*** How diet helps keep blood glucose in normal range; number of kilocalories required and why; amount of carbohydrates, meats, and fats recommended and why; and how to calculate the diet, integrating personal food preferences
- ***Exercise:*** How it helps lower blood glucose, the importance of a regular program, types of exercise, integrating personal exercise preferences, how to handle increased activity
- ***Self-monitoring of blood glucose:*** How to perform the tests accurately, how to care for equipment, what to do for high or low blood glucose levels
- ***Medications:***
  a. *Insulin:* Type, dosage, mixing instructions (if necessary), times of onset and peak actions, how to get and care for equipment, how to give injections, where to give injections
  b. *Oral agents:* Type, dosage, side effects, interaction with other drugs
- ***Acute complications:*** Manifestations of acute complications of hypoglycemia and hyperglycemia; what to do when they occur
- ***Hygiene:*** Skin care, dental care, foot care
- ***Sick days***: What to do about food, fluids, and medications
- ***Helpful resources:*** American Diabetes Association, Juvenile Diabetes Research Foundation, American Dietetic Association, National Diabetes Information Clearinghouse, Indian Health Service, and National Council of La Raza.

Case Study & Nursing Care Plan

A Patient with T1D

Jim Meligrito, age 24, is a nursing student at a large university. Mr. Meligrito works 20 hours a week as a campus student security guard. His working hours are 8:00 p.m. to midnight, five nights a week. He lives with his father, who is also a student. Neither of the two men likes to cook, and they usually eat "whatever is handy." Mr. Meligrito has smoked 8 to 10 cigarettes a day for 5 years. He was diagnosed with T1D at age 12. Although his insulin dosage has varied, he currently takes a total of 32 units of insulin each day, 10 units of NPH, and 6 units of regular insulin each morning and evening. He monitors his blood glucose about three times a week. He feels that he is too busy for a regular exercise program and that he gets enough exercise in clinicals and in weekend sports activities. He has not seen a healthcare provider for over a year.

One day during a 6-hour clinical experience, Mr. Meligrito notices that he is urinating frequently, is thirsty, and has blurred vision. He is very tired but blames all his manifestations on drinking a couple of beers and having only 4 hours of sleep the night before while studying for an examination and also on the stress he has been under lately from school and work. When he remembers that he had forgotten to take his insulin that morning, he realizes he must have hyperglycemia but decides that he will be all right until he gets home in the afternoon. Around noon, he begins having abdominal pain, feels weak, has a rapid pulse, and vomits. When he reports his physical manifestations to his clinical instructor, she sends him immediately to the hospital emergency department, accompanied by another student.

ASSESSMENT

As soon as Mr. Meligrito arrives at the emergency department, his blood glucose level is measured at 400 mg/dL. Urine samples and additional blood samples are sent to the laboratory for analysis. Blood glucose is 430 mg/dL, Hgb A1C is 9.5%, urine shows the presence of ketones, electrolytes are normal, and pH is 7.1. His vital signs are T 37.2°C (99°F), P 140 bpm, R 28/min, and BP 102/52 mmHg. An intravenous infusion of 1000 mL normal (0.9%) saline with 20 mEq of KCl is started at a rate of 400 mL/h. Intravenous regular insulin at 5 units/h (diluted in 0.9% saline) is begun. Hourly blood glucose monitoring is initiated. Mr. Meligrito is nauseated and lethargic but remains oriented. Three hours later, he has a blood glucose level of 120 mg/dL, and his pulse and blood pressure are normal. He is dismissed from the emergency department after making an appointment for the next morning with the hospital's DM nurse educator. When he meets with the DM educator, he says that he no longer feels in control of the DM or his future goal to become a nurse anesthetist.

DIAGNOSIS

- Difficulty managing blood glucose levels as evidenced by recent episode of DKA and elevated Hgb A1C
- Feeling powerless due to a perceived lack of control of DM due to present demands on time
- Lack of knowledge related to self-management of DM

EXPECTED OUTCOMES

- Mr. Meligrito will identify those aspects of DM that can be controlled and participate in making decisions about self-managing care.
- Mr. Meligrito will explore his feelings about diabetes and his ability to control it.
- Mr. Meligrito will demonstrate an understanding of DM self-management through planned medication, diet, exercise, and blood glucose self-monitoring activities.

PLANNING AND IMPLEMENTATION

- Mutually establish specific and individualized short-term and long-term goals for self-management of blood glucose.
- Provide patient with opportunities to express feelings about himself and his illness.
- Explore perceptions of the patient's own ability to control his illness and his future, and clarify these perceptions by providing information about resources and support groups.
- Facilitate decision-making abilities in the patient for self-managing his prescribed treatment regimen.
- Provide positive reinforcement for increasing involvement in self-care activities.
- Provide relevant learning activities about insulin administration, dietary management, exercise, self-monitoring of blood glucose, and healthy lifestyle.

EVALUATION

After taking an active part in the weekly educational meetings for 2 months, Mr. Meligrito has greatly enhanced his understanding of and compliance with self-management of his DM. He states that he finally understands how insulin, food, and exercise affect his body, having previously thought they were "too hard to control." He decides to perform self-management activities one week at a time, rather than think too far into (and thereby feel overwhelmed by) the future. Both son and father have developed a workable meal schedule and weekly grocery list, and they have begun eating breakfast and dinner together. Mr. Meligrito and a friend have arranged to walk 2 to 3 miles three times a week on a community hiking trail. To gain a sense of control over his illness, he has worked out a schedule that allows time for school, healthcare, and himself.

CLINICAL REASONING IN PATIENT CARE

1. What is the pathophysiologic basis for the changes in temperature, pulse, respirations, and blood pressure that occurred on Mr. Meligrito's admission to the hospital emergency department?
2. How can smoking and poor self-management of DM increase the risk of long-term complications?
3. Is powerlessness a common response to a chronic illness? Why or why not?
4. Consider that you are teaching Mr. Meligrito and another patient, Mr. McDaniel (age 75, newly diagnosed with T2D). What components of your teaching plan would be the same and what components would be different?

See Evaluating Your Response in Appendix B.

CHAPTER HIGHLIGHTS

20.1 Overview of Diabetes Mellitus

Describe the prevalence and incidence of diabetes mellitus (DM).

- Diabetes mellitus is a very common condition with continued increased incidence and prevalence in the United States. The long-term complications of diabetes, including cardiovascular disease, stroke, and kidney failure, are among the leading causes of death in this country.
- Blood glucose homeostasis is maintained through constant feedback mechanisms that increase and decrease hormones. Insulin decreases blood glucose, whereas glucagon increases glucose. Stress hormones also increase blood glucose.

20.2 Pathophysiology and Manifestations of Diabetes Mellitus

Distinguish the pathophysiology, risk factors, manifestations, and complications of type 1 and type 2 DM.

- The onset, pathophysiology, and acute complications of T1D and T2D differ from one another. The development of T2D starts with insulin resistance (prediabetes) that may be asymptomatic for many years. The incidence of T2D is increasing in epidemic proportions in all racial and ethnic groups in the United States, often triggered by obesity and sedentary lifestyles.
- T1D is the result of pancreatic islet cell destruction and a total deficit of circulating insulin. The autoantibodies that cause T1D are present for many years before the onset of the disease.

20.3 Complications of Diabetes Mellitus

Differentiate the acute and chronic complications of DM and describe treatment plans for each.

- Acute complications of diabetes include hypoglycemia, hyperglycemia, and the hyperglycemic emergencies DKA and HHS.
- An estimated 50% of individuals newly diagnosed with T2D have already developed chronic complications secondary to hyperglycemia. Chronic complications are a result of vascular damage and hyperglycemia. They include retinopathy, nephropathy, wounds, infections, acute MI, stoke, and peripheral vascular disease, to name a few.
- Older adults with diabetes may experience urinary incontinence, disability, frailty, falls, depression, cognitive impairment, and vascular disease. It is important to assess the older adult and prevent these complications to improve safety and quality of life.

20.4 Interprofessional Care of the Patient with Diabetes Mellitus

Outline the diagnostic tests used for screening, diagnosing, and monitoring DM and the use of insulin and oral hypoglycemic agents to treat patients with DM.

- Early diagnosis and tighter, intensive glycemic control is increasingly the focus of care of patients with hyperglycemia (patients with diabetes and prediabetes).
- Self-monitoring blood glucose levels is an important aspect of care that results in better glucose control for the patient with diabetes.
- Products to manage DM include insulins, noninsulin hypoglycemics, and blood glucose monitoring devices. Nurses must be familiar with these products and help patients become proficient in their use.
- Nutrition, meal planning, and exercise are also important aspects of the management of diabetes and prevention of prolonged hyperglycemia.
- Weight loss surgeries are an effective measure to aid in the treatment of T2D. When the patient with diabetes is experiencing surgery, careful management of glucose is important to prevent complications such as infection.
- The nurse needs to understand sick-day management in order to teach the patient to prevent hyperglycemic emergencies during periods of illness.

20.5 Nursing and Transition Care of the Patient with Diabetes Mellitus

Design best practices of self-care management of DM related to diet planning, sick-day management, and exercise.

- Nursing care of the patient with diabetes is focused on assessment of problems and potential complications, developing accurate priorities of care, intervening and delegating care appropriately, and assessing outcomes.
- Nurses have a great impact in caring, guiding, and teaching the patient with diabetes during acute and chronic complications and at the end of life.

TEST YOURSELF NCLEX-RN® REVIEW

1. Through genetic testing a patient learns of having markers that indicate immune destruction of the beta cells. Which health problem is this patient prone to developing?
   A. Type 2 diabetes mellitus
   B. Maturity-onset diabetes mellitus
   C. Idiopathic type 1 diabetes mellitus
   D. Immune-mediated type 1 diabetes mellitus
2. The nurse is preparing to instruct a patient with type 1 diabetes mellitus on the complication of diabetic ketoacidosis. Which pathologic process should the nurse review with the patient about this complication?
   A. A decreased amount of glucagon causes low protein levels.
   B. An excess amount of insulin drives all glucose into the cells.
   C. A deficit of insulin causes fat stores to be used as an energy source.
   D. An increase occurs in the breakdown of glucose molecules with hypoglycemia.
3. The nurse is reviewing the health histories of newly admitted patients for the risk of developing endocrine disorders. Which patient would be most at risk for the development of type 2 diabetes mellitus?
   A. Middle-aged man who maintains normal weight
   B. Woman age 70 who is overweight and sedentary
   C. Young adult who is a professional basketball player
   D. Middle-aged woman who is the sole caretaker of her parents
4. The nurse identifies that a patient with type 2 diabetes mellitus is at risk for injury because of peripheral polyneuropathy involving both feet. Which assessments would support this concern? (Select all that apply.)
   A. Feet ache
   B. Feet feel hot
   C. Has lost two-point discrimination
   D. Increased sensation of vibration
   E. Shooting pain in feet
5. The nurse is providing discharge instructions to a patient with type 2 diabetes mellitus. Which patient statement indicates teaching about foot care at home has been successful?
   A. "I always buy my shoes as soon as the stores open."
   B. "I will walk barefooted as long as I am in the house."
   C. "I will check my feet for cuts and bruises every night."
   D. "If I get a blister, I will just put alcohol on it and bandage it."
6. The nurse is preparing a teaching session on insulin for a group of patients newly diagnosed with type 1 diabetes mellitus. Which safety feature should the nurse emphasize when discussing insulin glargine (Lantus) and insulin detemir (Levemir)? (Select all that apply.)
   A. These insulins are clear like regular insulin.
   B. These insulins are activated by vigorous agitation.
   C. These insulins are are given only subcutaneously.
   D. These insulins are subject to being inactivated by light.
   E. These insulins should not be mixed with any other insulins.
7. The nurse is preparing an insulin infusion for a patient in diabetic ketoacidosis (DKA). Which type of insulin can be given intravenously?
   A. NPH
   B. Regular
   C. Glargine
   D. Humalog
8. The nurse is reviewing laboratory values and notes that a patient will soon begin treatment for diabetes mellitus. Which glycosylated hemoglobin (A1C) level is on the patient's medical record?
   A. 1.7%
   B. 3.4%
   C. 5.2%
   D. 6.8%
9. A patient who is prescribed regular insulin for diabetes control is scheduled for surgery in the morning. What should the nurse anticipate regarding the prescribed morning regular insulin dose?
   A. It will be given intravenously.
   B. It should be chilled to slow absorption.
   C. It will be given at the usual prescribed dose.
   D. It should be combined with long-acting insulin.
10. The nurse is teaching a patient with type 1 diabetes mellitus how to self-administer the daily prescribed insulin. In which body area should the nurse teach that the most rapid absorption of the medication occurs?
    A. Hip
    B. Thigh
    C. Deltoid
    D. Abdomen

See Test Yourself answers in Appendix B.

REFERENCES

Adams, M. P., Holland, L. N., & Urban, C. (2017). *Pharmacology for nursing: A pathophysiologic approach* (5th ed.). Hoboken, NJ: Pearson Education.

American Association of Clinical Endocrinology/American College of Endocrinology (AACE/ACE), Garber, A. J., Abrahamson, M. J., Barzilay, J. I., Blonde, L., Bloomgarden, Z. T., . . . Umpierrez, G. E. (2018). *Consensus statement by the American Association of Clinical Endocrinology and American College of Endocrinology on the comprehensive type 2 diabetes algorithm – 2018 executive summary*. Retrieved from https://www.aace.com/sites/all/files/diabetes-algorithm-executive-summary.pdf.

American Diabetes Association (ADA). (2015). *Insulin pumps*. Retrieved from www.diabetes.org/living-with-diabetes/treatment-and-care/medication/insulin/insulin-pumps.html.

American Diabetes Association (ADA). (2016a). *Sick days*. Retrieved from www.diabetes.org/living-with-diabetes/parents-and-kids/everyday-life/sick-days.html.

American Diabetes Association (ADA). (2016b). *Transplantation*. Retrieved from www.diabetes.org/living-with-diabetes/treatment-and-care/transplantation/.

American Diabetes Association (ADA). (2018a). *Food and fitness*. Retrieved from www.diabetes.org/food-and-fitness/?gclid=EAIaIQobChMI-pPPy4rv2AIV1xyB-Ch3JUwmIEAAYASABEgKPJfD_BwE.

American Diabetes Association (ADA). (2018b). Standard of medical care in diabetes—2018. *Diabetes Care, 41*(Suppl.), S1–S159. Retrieved from http://care.diabetesjournals.org/content/diacare/suppl/2017/12/08/41.Supplement_1.DC1/DC_41_S1_Combined.pdf.

American Heart Association (AHA). (2015). *What is metabolic syndrome?* Retrieved from www.heart.org/idc/groups/heart-public/@wcm/@hcm/documents/downloadable/ucm_300322.pdf.

BD Diabetes. (2018). *Insulin pens and pen needles*. Retrieved from www.bd.com/us/diabetes/page.aspx?cat=7001&id=7254.

Centers for Disease Control and Prevention (CDC). (2016). *Diabetes at a glance, 2016: Working to reverse the US epidemic.* Retrieved from https://www.cdc.gov/chronicdisease/resources/publications/aag/diabetes.htm.

Centers for Disease Control and Prevention (CDC). (2017a). *Diabetes: Preventing complications.* Retrieved from https://www.cdc.gov/diabetes/managing/problems.html.

Centers for Disease Control and Prevention (CDC). (2017b). *National diabetes statistics report, 2017; Estimates of diabetes and its burden in the United States.* Retrieved from https://www.cdc.gov/diabetes/pdfs/data/statistics/national-diabetes-statistics-report.pdf.

Coen, P. M., Menshikova, E. V., Distefano, G., Zheng, D., Tanner, C. J., Standley, R. A., . . . Goodpaster, B. H. (2015). Exercise and weight loss improve muscle mitochondrial respiration, lipid partitioning, and insulin sensitivity after gastric bypass surgery. *Diabetes, 64*(11), 3737–3750.

DeFronzo, R., Fleming, G. A., Chen, K., & Bicsak, T. A. (2016). Metformin-associated lactic acidosis: Current perspectives on causes and risk. *Metabolism, 65*(9), 1432–1433.

Diabetes Control and Complications Trial Research Group, Nathan, D. M., Genuth, S., Lachin, J., Cleary, P., Crofford, O., . . . Siebert, C. (1993). The effect of intensive treatment of diabetes on the development and progression of long-term complications in insulin-dependent diabetes mellitus. *New England Journal of Medicine, 329*(14), 977–986.

Food and Drug Administration (FDA). (2016). *Self-monitoring blood glucose test systems for over-the-counter use*. Retrieved from https://www.fda.gov/downloads/MedicalDevices/DeviceRegulationandGuidance/GuidanceDocuments/UCM380327.pdf.

Gok-Metin, Z., Donmez, A. A., Izgu, N., Ozdemir, L., & Arslan, I. E. (2017). Aromatherapy massage for neuropathic pain and quality of life in diabetic patients. *Journal of Nursing Scholarship, 49*(4), 370–388.

Handelsman, Y., Bloomgarden, Z. T., Grunberger, G., Umpierrez, G., Zimmerman, R. S., Bailey, T. S., . . . Zangeneh, F. (2015). American Association of Clinical Endocrinologists and American College of Endocrinology – Clinical practice guidelines for developing a diabetes mellitus comprehensive care plan – 2015 – Executive summary. *Endocrine Practice, 21*(4), 413–437.

Insel, R. A., Dunne, J. L., Atkinson, M. A., Chiang, J. L., Dabelea, D., Gottlieb, P. A., . . . Ziegler, A. G. (2015). Staging presymptomatic type 1 diabetes: A scientific statement of JDRF, the Endocrine Society, and the American Diabetes Association. *Diabetes Care 38*(10), 1964–1974.

Kee, J. L. (2018). *Laboratory and diagnostic tests with nursing implications* (10th ed.). Hoboken, NJ: Pearson Education.

Martin, E., Kaye, K., Knott, C., Nguyen, H., Santarossa, M., Evans, R., . . . Jaber, L. (2016). Diabetes and risk of surgical site infection: A systematic review and meta-analysis. *Infection Control and Hospital Epidemiology*, 37(1), 88–99.

McLaughlin, K. A., Richardson, C. C., Ravishankar, A., Brigatti, C., Liberati, D., Lampasona, V., . . . Christie, M. R. (2016). Identification of tetraspanin-7 as a target of autoantibodies in type 1 diabetes. *Diabetes, 65*(6), 1690–1698.

NANDA International. (2018). *NANDA International, Inc. Nursing diagnoses: Definitions and classification,*

2018–2020 (11th ed.) (T. H. Herdman & S. Kamitsuru, Eds.). New York, NY: Thieme.

National Institute on Aging (NIA). (2018). *Diabetes in older adults.* Retrieved from https://www.nia.nih.gov/health/diabetes-older-people#managing.

NICE-SUGAR Study Investigators. (2009). Intensive versus conventional glucose control in critically ill patients. *New England Journal of Medicine, 360*(13), 1283–1297.

Powers, M. A., Bardsley, J., Cypress, M., Duker, P., Funnell, M. M., Hess-Fischl, A., . . . Vivian, E. (2015). Diabetes self-management education and support in type 2 diabetes: A joint position statement of the American Diabetes Association, the American Association of Diabetes Educators, and the Academy of Nutrition and Dietetics. *Diabetes Care 38*(7), 1372–1382.

Sinclair, A., Dunning, T., & Rodriguez-Mañas, L. (2015). Diabetes in older people: New insights and remaining challenges. *The Lancet Diabetes and Endocrinology 3*(4), 275–285.

Sorenson, M., Quinn, L., & Klein, D. (2019). *Pathophysiology: Concepts of human disease.* Hoboken, NJ: Pearson Education.

Tumminia, A., Sciacca, L., Frittitta, L., Squatrito, S., Vigneri, R., Le Moli, R., & Tomaselli, L. (2015). Integrated insulin pump therapy with continuous glucose monitoring for improved adherence: Technology update. *Patient Preference and Adherence, 9*, 1263–1270.

United States Department of Agriculture (USDA). (2016). *Choose My Plate. A snapshot of the 2015–2020 dietary guidelines for Americans.* Retrieved from https://www.choosemyplate.gov/snapshot-2015-2020-dietary-guidelines-americans.

World Heart Federation. (2016). *Diabetes as a risk factor for cardiovascular disease.* Retrieved from www.world-heart-federation.org/cardiovascular-health/cardiovascular-disease-risk-factors/diabetes/.

ADDITIONAL RESOURCES

American Association of Diabetes Educators
www.aadenet.org

American Diabetes Association (ADA)
www.diabetes.org

National Institute of Diabetes and Digestive and Kidney Diseases
www.niddk.nih.gov

United States Department of Agriculture
www.choosemyplate.gov

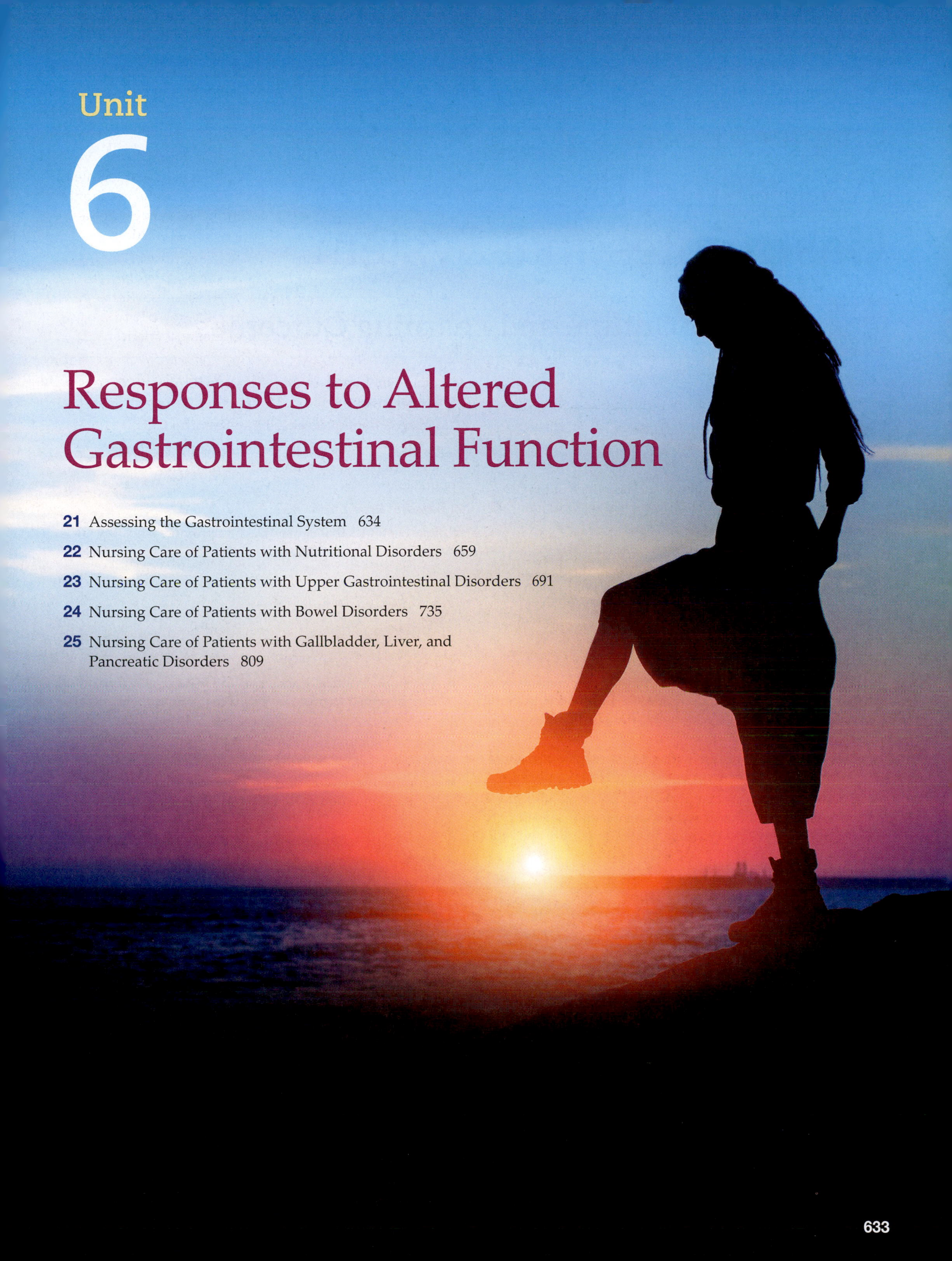

Unit 6

Responses to Altered Gastrointestinal Function

Chapter 21

Assessing the Gastrointestinal System

Chapter Outline and Learning Outcomes

21.1 Nutrients 635

Outline the nutrients absorbed in the gastrointestinal (GI) system.

21.2 Anatomy, Physiology, and Functions of the GI System 637

Describe the anatomy, physiology, and functions of the GI system and identify abnormal findings that may indicate impairment of the GI system.

21.3 Assessing Gastrointestinal Function 641

Outline the components of the assessment of the GI system including topics for the health assessment interview, techniques for physical assessment, and the diagnostic tests used in the assessment.

21.4 Assessment of Selected Populations 655

Differentiate considerations for assessing the GI system of older adults, veterans, and individuals in the LGBTQI population.

21.5 Health Promotion 655

Summarize topics that nurses teach to promote a healthy GI system across the lifespan.

CLINICAL COMPETENCIES

- Conduct and document a health history for patients who have or are at risk for alterations in GI function, eliciting patient values, preferences, and expressed needs as part of the interview.
- Individualize the health history to assess potential alterations of GI function experienced by special populations.
- Conduct and document a physical assessment of nutritional status and the GI system, demonstrating sensitivity and respect for dietary habits related to culture and individual belief systems.
- Develop a culturally sensitive and individualized plan of care designed to promote habits that support a healthy GI system.
- Provide supportive nursing care for patients undergoing invasive diagnostic procedures.
- Monitor the results of diagnostic tests, report abnormal findings and coordinate follow-up care.

KEY TERMS

bile, 639
borborygus, 645
bruit, 645
cheilosis, 644
dietary reference intakes (DRIs), 636
flatus, 642
gingivitis, 644
glossitis, 644
hernia, 647
leukoplakia, 644
melena, 648
microbiota, 640
nutrition, 635
ostomy, 642
steatorrhea, 648
striae, 645
tolerable upper intake level (UL), 636
Valsalva maneuver, 639

EQUIPMENT NEEDED

- Stethoscope
- Balance scale with height measuring attachment
- Tape measure
- Skinfold calipers
- Water-soluble lubricant
- Occult blood test, such as Occultest or Hemoccult II
- Disposable gloves

The GI system consists of the mouth, pharynx, esophagus, stomach, small intestine, and large intestine. The accessory digestive organs include the liver, gallbladder, and pancreas (**Figure 21.1** ■). **Nutrition** is the process by which the body, via the GI system and the accessory digestive organs, ingests, absorbs, transports, uses, and eliminates nutrients in food.

21.1 Nutrients

Nutrients are substances found in food that are used by the body to promote growth, maintenance, and repair. The categories of nutrients are carbohydrates, proteins, fats, vitamins, minerals, and water.

Carbohydrates

The primary sources of *carbohydrates* (sugars and starches) are plant foods. Monosaccharides and disaccharides come from milk, sugar cane, sugar beets, honey, and fruits. Polysaccharide starch is found in grains, legumes, and root vegetables. Following ingestion, digestion, and metabolism, carbohydrates are converted primarily to glucose, the molecule body cells use to make adenosine triphosphate (ATP). Excess glucose in the healthy person is converted to glycogen or fat. Glycogen is stored in the liver and muscles; fat is stored as adipose tissue.

Excess intake of carbohydrates over time can result in obesity, dental caries, and elevated plasma triglycerides. In comparison, long-standing carbohydrate deficiencies lead to

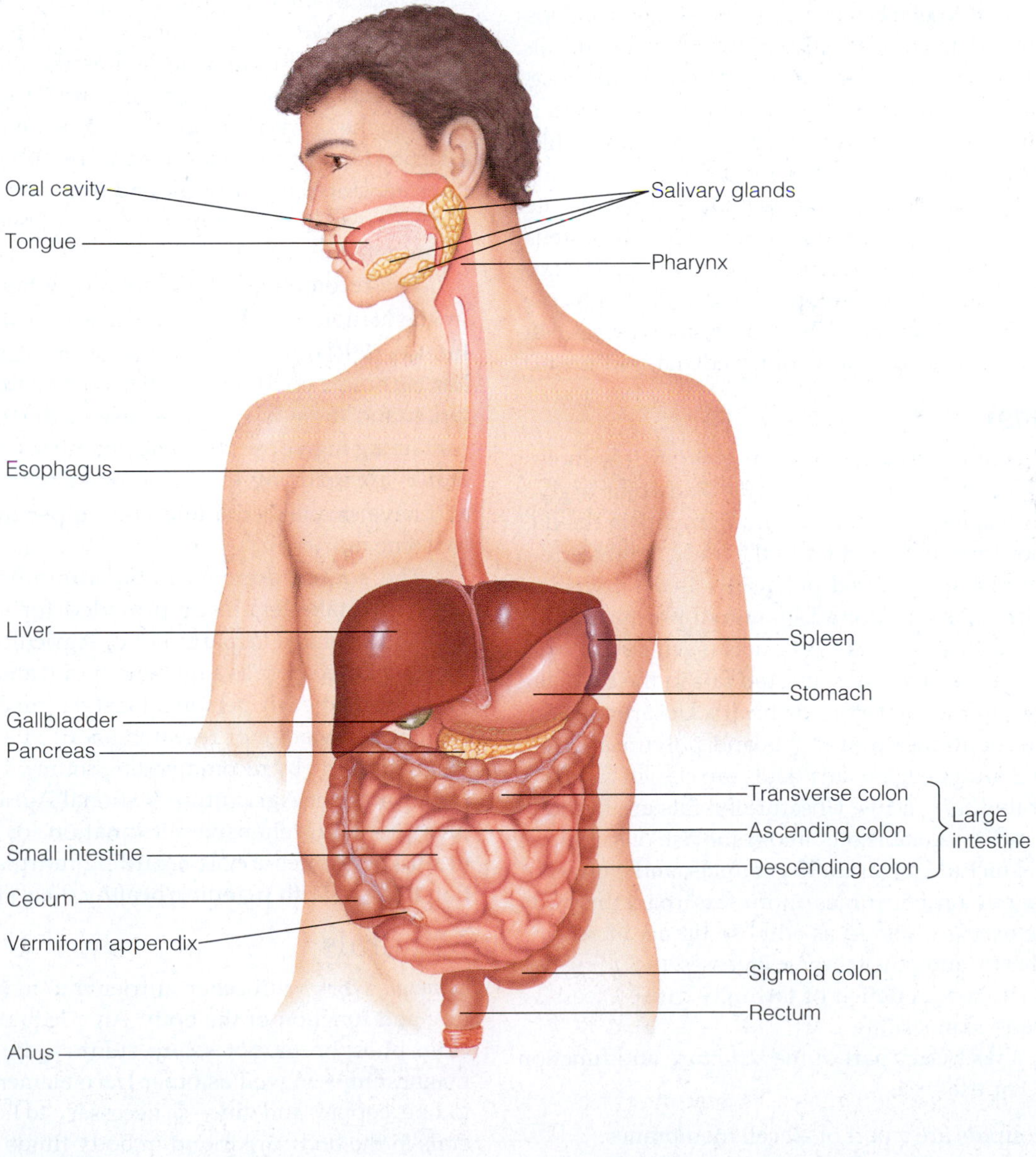
Oral cavity
Tongue
Salivary glands
Pharynx
Esophagus
Liver
Gallbladder
Pancreas
Spleen
Stomach
Transverse colon
Ascending colon
Descending colon
Large intestine
Small intestine
Cecum
Vermiform appendix
Sigmoid colon
Rectum
Anus

Figure 21.1 ■ Organs of the gastrointestinal system and accessory digestive organs.

tissue wasting from protein breakdown and metabolic acidosis from an excess of ketones as a by-product of fat breakdown.

Proteins

Proteins are classified as either complete (high value) or incomplete. Complete proteins are found in animal products such as eggs, milk, milk products, and meat. They contain the greatest amount of amino acids and meet the body's requirements for tissue growth and maintenance. Incomplete proteins are found in legumes, nuts, grains, cereals, and vegetables. These sources are low in or lack one or more of the amino acids essential for building complete proteins.

The body uses proteins to build many different structures, including skin keratin, the collagen and elastin in connective tissues, and muscles. They are also used to make enzymes, hemoglobin, plasma proteins, and some hormones.

Healthy people with adequate caloric intake have an equal rate of protein synthesis and protein breakdown and loss, reflected as nitrogen balance. If the breakdown and loss of proteins exceed intake, a negative nitrogen balance results. This may be due to starvation, altered physical states (e.g., from injury or illness), or altered emotional states (such as depression or anxiety). A positive nitrogen balance, which results when protein intake exceeds breakdown, is normal during growth, tissue repair, and pregnancy. Anabolic steroids affect the rate of protein use; for example, the adrenal corticosteroids are released in times of stress to increase protein breakdown and conversion of amino acids to glucose. Excessive intake of proteins may lead to obesity, whereas deficits cause weight loss and tissue wasting, edema, and anemia.

Fats (Lipids)

Fats (lipids) include phospholipids, steroids (such as cholesterol), and neutral fats, more commonly known as triglycerides. Triglycerides are the most abundant fats in the diet and the major form of stored fat in the body. Triglycerides exist with a mix of saturated or unsaturated fatty acids. Saturated fatty acids are found in animal products (milk and meats) and in some plant products (such as coconut). Trans fatty acids behave like saturated fats in the body but have a greater detrimental effect on health. Unsaturated fats include both monounsaturated fats and polyunsaturated fats. Omega-3 and omega-6 fatty acids are classifications of polyunsaturated fatty acids. Unsaturated fats are found in seeds, nuts, most vegetable oils, and some fish oils. Sources of cholesterol include meats, milk products, and egg yolks.

When a person consumes more fats than the body requires, the excess is stored as adipose tissue, increasing the risk of obesity and other chronic illnesses, including cardiovascular disease. A deficit of fats may cause excessive weight loss and skin lesions.

Fats are a necessary part of the structure and function of the body. For example:

- Phospholipids are a part of all cell membranes.
- Triglycerides are the major energy source for hepatocytes and skeletal muscle cells.
- Dietary fats facilitate absorption of fat-soluble vitamins.
- Linoleic acid, an essential fatty acid, helps form prostaglandins, regulatory molecules that assist in smooth muscle contraction, maintenance of blood pressure, and control of inflammatory responses.
- Cholesterol is the essential component of bile salts, steroid hormones, and vitamin D.
- Adipose tissue serves as a protection around body organs, as a layer of insulation under the skin, and as a concentrated source of fuel for cellular energy.

Vitamins

Vitamins are organic compounds that facilitate the body's use of carbohydrates, proteins, and fats. All of the vitamins except vitamins D and K must be ingested in foods or taken as supplements. Vitamin D is made by ultraviolet irradiation of cholesterol molecules in the skin. Vitamin K is synthesized by bacteria in the intestine.

Vitamins are categorized as either fat soluble or water soluble. The *fat-soluble vitamins* (A, D, E, and K) bind to ingested fats and are absorbed as the fats are absorbed. *Water-soluble vitamins* (B complex and C) are absorbed with water in the GI system (however, vitamin B_{12} must become attached to intrinsic factor to be absorbed). Fat-soluble vitamins are stored in the body, and excesses may cause toxicity; water-soluble vitamins in excess of body requirements are excreted in the urine.

The recommended amounts of vitamins are labeled by the National Academy of Sciences as **dietary reference intakes (DRIs)** per day. The use of supplemental nutrients has become a common practice among the general population and there is increased use of dietary supplements containing high doses of some vitamins. Consequently, scientists are realizing the potential toxicity of higher doses and have established a **tolerable upper intake level (UL)** for some nutrients.

The source, function, and minimum daily recommended intake levels are provided for each vitamin by the United States Department of Agriculture. The recommended DRIs serve as a reference point and should be individualized to each person's lifestyle, medical status, and current knowledge of research about vitamins. Note also that DRIs differ by recommending source. The United States Department of Agriculture National Agricultural Library provides comprehensive information for consumers and health care professionals regarding nutrition and information to assist with planning healthy diets (**Table 21.1**).

Minerals

Minerals work with other nutrients to maintain the structure and function of the body. An adequate supply of calcium, phosphorus, potassium, sulfur, sodium, chloride, and magnesium—as well as other trace elements such as iron, iodine, copper, and zinc—is necessary to health. Most minerals in the body are found in body fluids or are bound to organic compounds. The best sources of minerals are vegetables, legumes, milk, and some meats. The recommended

Table 21.1 Select Websites for Nutritional Information

Website Name	Purpose	URL
USDA National Agricultural Library	Provides comprehensive nutritional information for consumers and healthcare providers	www.nal.usda.gov/fnic
USDA Food Composition Databases	Allows for searches to identify food sources for specific nutrients	ndb.nal.usda.gov/ndb/nutrients/index
USDA Food and Nutrition Information Center	Allows healthcare professionals to calculate DRIs for individual patients	www.nal.usda.gov/fnic/interactiveDRI/

daily intake for minerals is provided by the United States Department of Agriculture (see Table 21.1).

21.2 Anatomy, Physiology, and Functions of the GI System

The GI system is a continuous hollow tube, extending from the mouth to the anus. Once foods are placed in the mouth, they are subjected to a variety of digestive processes that move them and break them down into end products that can be absorbed from the lumen of the small intestine into the blood or lymph. These processes are ingestion of food; movement of food and wastes; secretion of mucus, water, and enzymes; mechanical and chemical digestion of food; and absorption of digested food.

The Mouth

The *mouth*, also called the *oral* or *buccal cavity*, is lined with mucous membranes and is enclosed by the lips, cheeks, palate, and tongue (**Figure 21.2** ■).

The *lips* and *cheeks* are skeletal muscle covered externally by skin. Their function is to keep food in the mouth during chewing. The palate consists of the hard palate and the soft palate. The *hard palate* covers bone in the roof of the mouth and provides a hard surface against which the tongue forces food. The *soft palate*, extending from the hard palate and ending at the back of the mouth as a fold called the uvula, is primarily muscle. When food is swallowed, the soft palate rises as a reflex to close off the oropharynx.

The *tongue*, composed of skeletal muscle and connective tissue, contains mucous and serous glands, taste buds, and papillae. The tongue mixes food with saliva during chewing, forms the food into a bolus (a mass), and initiates swallowing. Some papillae provide surface roughness to facilitate licking and moving food; other papillae house the taste buds.

Saliva moistens food so it can be made into a bolus, dissolves food chemicals so they can be tasted, and provides enzymes (such as amylase) that begin the chemical breakdown of starches. Saliva is produced by salivary glands (parotid, submaxillary, and sublingual), most of which lie superior or inferior to the mouth and drain into it. Adults have 32 permanent teeth. The *teeth* chew (masticate) and grind food to break it down into smaller parts, mixed with saliva.

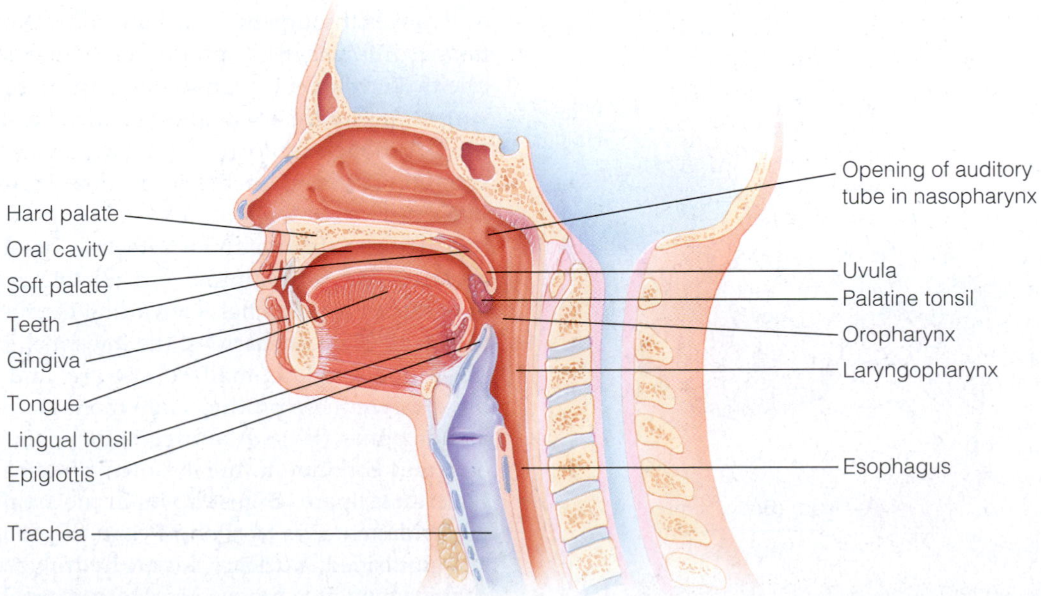

Hard palate
Oral cavity
Soft palate
Teeth
Gingiva
Tongue
Lingual tonsil
Epiglottis
Trachea
Opening of auditory tube in nasopharynx
Uvula
Palatine tonsil
Oropharynx
Laryngopharynx
Esophagus

Figure 21.2 ■ Structures of the mouth, the pharynx, and the esophagus.

The Pharynx

The *pharynx* consists of the oropharynx and the laryngopharynx (refer to Figure 21.2). Both structures provide passageways for food, fluids, and air. The pharynx is made of skeletal muscles and is lined with mucous membranes. The skeletal muscles move food to the esophagus via the pharynx through peristalsis (alternating waves of contraction and relaxation of involuntary muscle). The mucosa of the pharynx contains mucous-producing glands that provide fluid to facilitate the passage of the bolus of food as it is swallowed.

The Esophagus

The *esophagus*, a muscular tube about 25 cm (10 in.) long, serves as a passageway for food from the pharynx to the stomach (refer to Figures 21.1 and 21.2). The epiglottis, a flap of cartilage over the top of the larynx, keeps food out of the larynx during swallowing. The esophagus descends through the thorax and diaphragm, entering the stomach at the cardiac orifice. The gastroesophageal sphincter surrounds this opening. This sphincter, along with the diaphragm, keeps the orifice closed when food is not being swallowed.

The Stomach

The *stomach*, located high on the left side of the abdominal cavity, is connected to the esophagus at the upper end and to the small intestine at the lower end (**Figure 21.3** ■). Normally about 15 to 25 cm (10 to 15 in.) long, the stomach is a distensible organ that can expand to hold up to 4 L of food and fluid. The stomach may be divided into the cardiac region, fundus, body, and pylorus. The pyloric sphincter controls the emptying of the stomach into the duodenal portion of the small intestine. The stomach is a storage reservoir for food, continues the mechanical breakdown of food, begins the process of protein digestion, and mixes the food with gastric juices into a thick fluid called *chyme*.

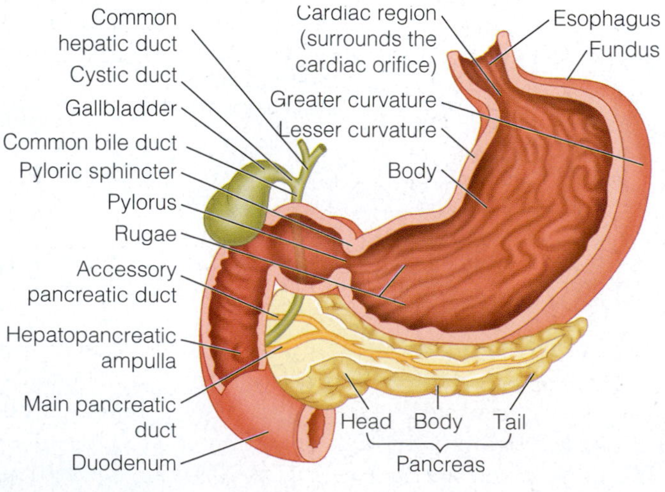
Common hepatic duct
Cystic duct
Gallbladder
Common bile duct
Pyloric sphincter
Pylorus
Rugae
Accessory pancreatic duct
Hepatopancreatic ampulla
Main pancreatic duct
Duodenum
Cardiac region (surrounds the cardiac orifice)
Greater curvature
Lesser curvature
Body
Esophagus
Fundus
Head
Body
Tail
Pancreas

Figure 21.3 ■ The internal anatomic structures of the stomach, including the pancreatic, cystic, and hepatic ducts; the pancreas; and the gallbladder.

The stomach is lined with columnar epithelial, mucous-producing cells. Millions of openings in the lining lead to gastric glands that can produce 4 to 5 L of gastric juice each day. The gastric glands contain a variety of secretory cells that produce substances to protect the stomach from being digested by gastric juice, secrete hydrochloric acid and intrinsic factor, and help regulate gastric motility.

The secretion of gastric juice is under both neural and endocrine control. Stimulation of the parasympathetic vagus nerve increases secretory activity; in contrast, stimulation of sympathetic nerves decreases secretions. Mechanical digestion is accomplished by peristaltic movements that churn and mix the food with the gastric juices to form chyme. After a person eats a well-balanced meal, the stomach empties completely in approximately 4 to 6 hours. Gastric emptying depends on the volume, chemical composition, and osmotic pressure of the gastric contents. The stomach empties large volumes of liquid content more rapidly, while gastric emptying is slowed by solids and fats.

The Small Intestine

The *small intestine* begins at the pyloric sphincter and ends at the ileocecal junction at the entrance of the large intestine (refer to Figure 21.1). The small intestine is about 6 m (20 ft) long but only about 2.5 cm (1 in.) in diameter. This long tube hangs in coils in the abdominal cavity, suspended by the mesentery and surrounded by the large intestine. The small intestine has three regions: The duodenum, the jejunum, and the ileum. The duodenum begins at the pyloric sphincter and extends around the head of the pancreas for about 25 cm (10 in.). Both pancreatic enzymes and bile from the liver enter the small intestine at the duodenum. The jejunum, the middle region of the small intestine, extends for about 2.4 m (8 ft). The ileum, the terminal end of the small intestine, is approximately 3.6 m (12 ft) long and meets the large intestine at the ileocecal valve.

Food is chemically digested and most of it absorbed as it moves through the small intestine. Circular folds containing villi (finger-like projections of the mucosa cells) and microvilli (tiny projections of the mucosa cells) increase the surface area of the small intestine to enhance absorption of food. Although up to 10 L of food, liquids, and secretions enter the GI system each day, less than 1 L reaches the large intestine.

Enzymes in the small intestine break down carbohydrates, proteins, lipids, and nucleic acids. Pancreatic amylase acts on starches, converting them to maltose, dextrins, and oligosaccharides; the intestinal enzymes dextrinase, glucoamylase, maltase, sucrase, and lactase further break down these products into monosaccharides. Pancreatic enzymes (trypsin and chymotrypsin) and intestinal enzymes continue to break down proteins into peptides. Pancreatic lipases digest lipids in the small intestine. Triglycerides enter as fat globules and are coated by bile salts and emulsified. Nucleic acids are hydrolyzed by pancreatic enzymes and then broken apart by intestinal enzymes. Both pancreatic enzymes and bile are excreted into the duodenum in response to the secretion of secretin and cholecystokinin, hormones produced by the intestinal mucosa cells when chyme enters the small intestine.

Nutrients are absorbed through the mucosa of the intestinal villi into the blood or lymph by active transport, facilitated transport, and passive diffusion. Almost all food products and water, as well as vitamins and most electrolytes, are absorbed in the small intestine, leaving only indigestible fibers, some water, and bacteria to enter the large intestine.

The Large Intestine

The *large intestine* (colon) begins at the ileocecal valve and terminates at the anus (**Figure 21.4** ■). It is about 1.5 m (5 ft) long. The large intestine includes the cecum, the appendix, the colon, the rectum, and the anal canal. The *colon* is divided into ascending, transverse, and descending segments. The *rectum* is a mucosa-lined tube approximately 12 cm (4.7 in.) in length (**Figure 21.5** ■). The rectum ends at the anal canal, which terminates at the *anus*, a hairless, dark-skinned area. The *anorectal junction* separates the rectum from the anal canal and may be the site of internal hemorrhoids (clusters of dilated veins in swollen anal tissue).

The major function of the large intestine is to eliminate indigestible food residue from the body. The large intestine absorbs water, salts, and vitamins formed by the food residue and bacteria. The semiliquid chyme that passes through the ileocecal valve is formed into feces as it moves through the large intestine by peristalsis. Goblet cells lining the large intestine secrete mucus to facilitate the lubrication and passage of feces.

The defecation reflex is initiated when feces enter the rectum and stretch the rectal wall. This spinal cord reflex causes the walls of the sigmoid colon to contract and the anal sphincters to relax. This reflex can be suppressed by voluntary control of the external sphincter. Closing the glottis and contracting the diaphragm and abdominal muscles to increase intra-abdominal pressure (**Valsalva maneuver**) facilitates expulsion of feces.

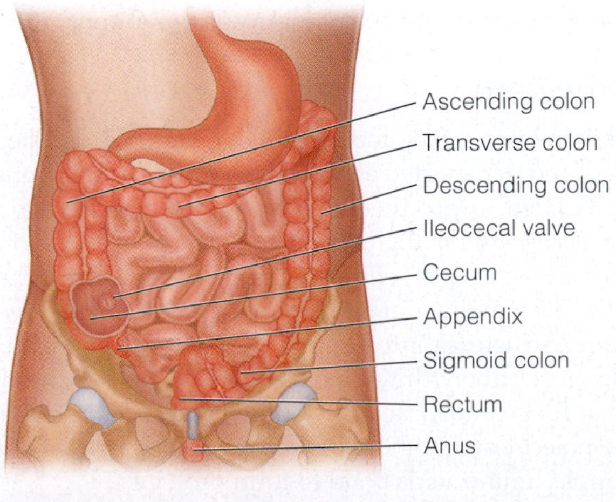
Ascending colon
Transverse colon
Descending colon
Ileocecal valve
Cecum
Appendix
Sigmoid colon
Rectum
Anus

Figure 21.4 ■ Anatomy of the large intestine.

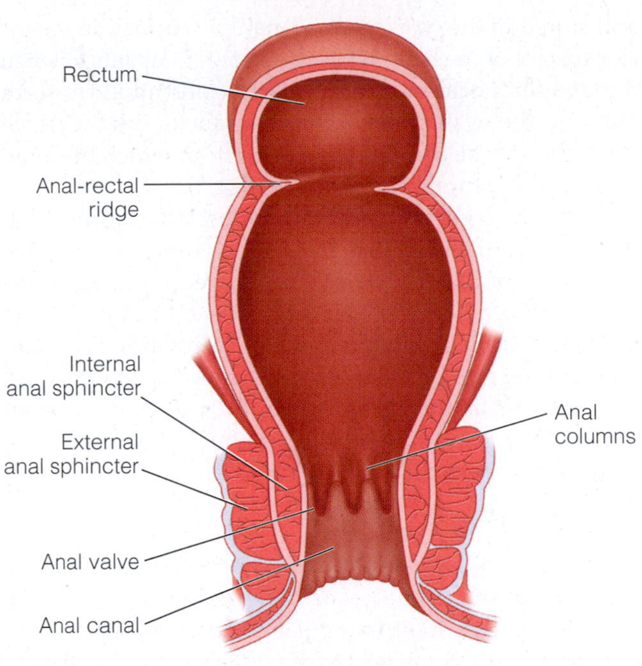
Rectum
Anal-rectal ridge
Internal anal sphincter
External anal sphincter
Anal valve
Anal canal
Anal columns

Figure 21.5 ■ Structure of the rectum and anus.

The Accessory Digestive Organs

The liver, gallbladder, and exocrine pancreas are accessory digestive organs. The liver produces bile, necessary for fat digestion and absorption, and stores it in the gallbladder. The liver also receives nutrients absorbed by the small intestine and metabolizes or synthesizes these nutrients so they are in a form that can be used by the cells of the body. The exocrine pancreas produces enzymes necessary for digestion of fats, proteins, and carbohydrates.

The Liver and Gallbladder

The *liver* weighs about 1.4 kg (3 lb) in the average-sized adult. It is located in the right side of the abdomen, inferior to the diaphragm and anterior to the stomach (refer to Figure 21.1). A mesenteric ligament separates the right and left lobes and suspends the liver from the diaphragm and anterior abdominal wall. The liver is encased in a fibroelastic capsule, called the *Glisson capsule*. This capsule contains blood vessels, lymphatics, and nerves.

Liver tissue consists of units called *lobules*, which are composed of plates of hepatocytes (liver cells). A branch of the hepatic artery, a branch of the hepatic portal vein, and a bile duct communicate with each lobule. *Sinusoids*, blood-filled spaces within the lobules, are lined with Kupffer cells. These phagocytic cells remove debris from the blood.

Bile production is the liver's primary digestive function. **Bile** is a greenish, watery solution containing bile salts, cholesterol, bilirubin, electrolytes, water, and phospholipids. These substances are necessary to emulsify and promote the absorption of fats. Liver cells make from 700 to 1200 mL of bile daily. When bile is not needed for digestion, the sphincter of Oddi (located at the point at which bile enters the duodenum) is closed, and the bile backs up the cystic duct into the gallbladder for storage. Bile is modified, concentrated, and stored in the *gallbladder*, a small sac cupped in the inferior surface of the liver. When food containing fats enters the duodenum, hormones stimulate the gallbladder to secrete bile into the cystic duct. The cystic duct joins the hepatic duct to form the common bile duct, from which bile enters into the duodenum (refer to Figure 21.3).

The major digestive and metabolic functions of the liver are outlined in **Box 21.1**. These functions require a large amount of blood, with the liver receiving blood from both venous and arterial blood vessels. The hepatic artery, branching from the abdominal aorta, provides oxygenated blood at the rate of 400 to 500 mL/min. The hepatic portal vein delivers about 1000 to 1200 mL/min of deoxygenated blood to the liver from the inferior and superior mesenteric veins and the splenic vein.

The Exocrine Pancreas

The *pancreas*, a gland located between the stomach and small intestine, is the primary enzyme-producing organ of the digestive system. It is a triangular gland extending across the abdomen, with its tail next to the spleen and its head next to the duodenum (refer to Figure 21.3). The body and tail of the pancreas are retroperitoneal, lying behind the greater curvature of the stomach. The pancreas is actually two organs in one, having both exocrine and endocrine structures and functions. The exocrine portion of the pancreas, through secretory units called *acini*, secretes alkaline pancreatic juice containing many different enzymes. The acini, clusters of secretory cells surrounding ducts, drain into the pancreatic duct. The pancreatic duct joins with the common bile duct just before it enters the duodenum (so that pancreatic juice and bile from the liver enter the small intestine together).

The pancreas produces from 1 to 1.5 L of pancreatic juice daily. Pancreatic juice is clear and has a high bicarbonate content. This alkaline fluid neutralizes the acidic chyme as it enters the duodenum, optimizing the pH for intestinal and pancreatic enzyme activity. The secretion of pancreatic juice is controlled by the vagus nerve and the intestinal hormones secretin and cholecystokinin. Pancreatic juice contains enzymes that aid in the digestion of all categories of foods: Lipase promotes fat breakdown and absorption; amylase completes starch digestion; and trypsin, chymotrypsin, and carboxypeptidase are responsible for half of all protein digestion. Nucleases break down nucleic acids.

BOX 21.1
Major Metabolic and Digestive Functions of the Liver

- Secretes bile
- Stores fat-soluble vitamins (A, D, E, and K)
- Metabolizes bilirubin
- Stores blood and releases blood into the general circulation during hemorrhage
- Synthesizes plasma proteins to maintain plasma oncotic pressure
- Synthesizes prothrombin, fibrinogen, and factors I, II, VII, IX, and X, which are necessary for blood clotting
- Synthesizes fats from carbohydrates and proteins to be used either for energy or stored as adipose tissue
- Synthesizes phospholipids and cholesterol necessary for the production of bile salts, steroid hormones, and plasma membranes
- Converts amino acids to carbohydrates through deamination
- Releases glucose during times of hypoglycemia
- Takes up glucose during times of hyperglycemia and stores it as glycogen or converts it to fat
- Alters chemicals, foreign molecules, and hormones to make them less toxic
- Inactivates drugs by removing and breaking down circulating drugs, thereby limiting the duration of their effects
- Stores iron as ferritin, which is released as needed for the production of red blood cells.

GI Microbiota

The entire GI tract from the oral cavity to the rectum is inhabited by a diverse collection of microbes called the human **microbiota**. Increasing evidence supports that colonization of the GI tract begins in utero and by adulthood, there are more than 1000 different species of bacteria in the GI tract (McElroy, Chung, & Regan, 2017). The GI microbiota is influenced by demographics, dietary intake, environmental exposures such as antibiotics, and physiologic maturation. Evidence suggests diet may have the most significant influence and the gut's response to changes is rapid. The colon or large bowel has a higher number of microbes because the digestive contents pass more slowly through this section of the system, allowing the microbes more time to multiply. Additionally, pH of the large intestine is more neutral to alkaline, thereby providing an environment where microbes can survive and multiply.

Microbes found in the GI tract can influence several physiologic functions related to digestion and immune system function. The normal microbe flora of a healthy large bowel promotes immune function, keeps the inflammatory process in check, and even effects mood regulation. The byproducts of healthy digestion help regulate the production of certain neurotransmitters (including serotonin), which influence mood, cognition and behavioral responses (Young, 2017).

Metabolism

After carbohydrates, fats, and proteins are ingested, digested, absorbed, and transported across cell membranes, they must be metabolized to produce and provide energy to maintain life. *Metabolism* is the process of biochemical reactions occurring in the body's cells. Metabolic processes are either catabolic or anabolic. *Catabolism* involves the breakdown of complex structures into simpler forms, for example, the breakdown of carbohydrates to produce ATP, an energy molecule that fuels cellular activity. In the process of *anabolism*, simpler molecules combine to build more complex structures; for example, amino acids bond to form proteins.

The biochemical reactions of metabolism produce water, carbon dioxide, and ATP. The energy value of foods is measured in kilocalories (kcal). A kilocalorie is defined as the amount of heat energy needed to raise the temperature of 1 kilogram (kg) of water 1 degree centigrade.

21.3 Assessing Gastrointestinal Function

The GI system is assessed by findings from a health assessment interview to collect subjective data, including information on diet and bowel elimination habits, consideration of a patient's genetics, diagnostic tests, and a physical assessment to collect objective data (D'Amico & Barbarito, 2016).

Health Assessment Interview

When conducting a health assessment interview and physical assessment, it is important for the nurse to consider genetic influences on the health of the adult. During the health assessment interview, ask about family members with known abnormalities of copper accumulation in the body, hypercholesterolemia, abnormal cholesterol or fat metabolism, obesity, or cancer of the pancreas, colon, or rectum. During the physical assessment, assess for any manifestations that might indicate a genetic disorder (see the Genetic Considerations box). If data are found to indicate genetic risk factors or alterations, ask about genetic testing and refer for appropriate genetic counseling and evaluation.

An interview to establish baseline dietary habits and preferences and to identify problems with nutrition and GI function may be conducted during a health screening. Including a dietitian in the nutrition interview has been shown to improve care planning related to nutritional needs (Quatrara, 2015). The interview may be part of a total health assessment or may focus on a chief complaint such as nausea or unexplained weight loss. A food frequency questionnaire can be used to assess usual intake of foods and food groups over time. If the patient has a health problem involving the GI system, analyze its onset, characteristics, and course; severity; precipitating and relieving factors; and any associated symptoms, noting the timing and circumstances. For example, the nurse may ask the patient:

- "What is your usual dietary intake pattern during a 24-hour period?"
- "Has your usual dietary intake pattern changed recently?"
- "Do you use vitamins or mineral supplements?" Determine dose, frequency, and constituents.
- "Do you use herbs or herbal medications?" Determine, dose, frequency and constituents.
- "Do you use over-the-counter weight loss or sports supplements?" Determine dose, frequency, and ingredients.
- "What over-the-counter and prescription medications are you taking?" Assess for drug–nutrient interactions or drug–herb interactions.
- "Have you had any episodes of indigestion, nausea and vomiting, diarrhea, or constipation? If so, describe the appearance of what was vomited or the stools and anything that makes these problems better or worse. How long have you had these problems?"
- "Have you ever had bleeding from your rectum? If so, describe the amount and color of the blood (e.g., was it bright red or dark red?)."

When collecting information about the patient's current health status, the nurse should inquire about the following:

- Have there been any changes in weight, appetite, and the ability to taste, chew, or swallow? What is the patient's perception of the role of nutrition in maintaining health?
- Who buys and prepares the food?
- What medications (prescribed, over-the-counter, or vitamins) is the patient currently taking? Does the patient take any vitamins, herbal supplements, or other "health food" items?

Genetic Considerations

Examples of Gastrointestinal Disorders

- An autosomal recessive disorder, Wilson disease is an abnormality of copper transport, resulting in copper accumulation and toxicity to the liver and brain. It causes neurologic disease in adults.
- Tangier disease is a disease of cholesterol transport, leading to characteristic orange tonsils, very low levels of high-density lipoprotein, and an enlarged liver and spleen.
- Hypercholesterolemia has a familial tendency.
- About 90% of human pancreatic cancers show a chromosome defect.
- Obesity is believed to result from a variety of factors, including genetics.
- Colon cancer is one of the most common inherited cancer syndromes.
- Familial adenomatous polyposis (FAP) and hereditary nonpolyposis colorectal cancer (HNPCC) are inherited disorders in which there is progressive development of colorectal adenomas. Unless treated, colorectal cancer inevitably occurs by the fourth or fifth decade of life.
- HNPCC, or Lynch syndrome, is a type of inherited cancer of the GI system, especially the colon and rectum. Colon polyps occur at an early age and are more likely to become malignant.
- In about 20% of cases, Crohn disease (an inflammatory bowel disease) appears to be familial in origin.
- Celiac disease (CD) is a genetic, inheritable disease responsible for the malabsorption of nutrients, resulting in malnutrition. If people with CD eat certain types of proteins (glutens, found in wheat, barley, rye, and oats), an autoimmune response causes damage to the small intestine, so that nutrients are not absorbed.
- Gaucher disease, more common in descendants of Jewish people from eastern Europe, results in lack of an enzyme to break down fats. Fats accumulate in the liver, spleen, and bone marrow, causing pain, fatigue, jaundice, bone damage, anemia, and even death.

- Does the patient consume alcohol (how much and what type)?
- Does the patient have braces, bridges, or dentures? If so, what self-care measures are used for such appliances?
- What are the patient's oral hygiene practices and frequency of dental visits?
- What is the patient's typical bowel elimination pattern?

If the patient has experienced nausea and/or vomiting, ask whether the vomitus contains bright red blood, dark (old) blood, bile, or fecal material. If the patient is very thin or verbalizes concerns about body size incongruent with the ratio of height to weight, ask whether the patient induces vomiting or uses laxatives to control weight. Ask about any medical conditions that may influence the patient's bowel elimination pattern, such as a stroke or spinal cord impairment, inflammatory GI diseases, endocrine disorders, and allergies. Note any recent travel to other countries. Assess the patient's lifestyle for any patterns of psychologic stress and/or depression, which may alter bowel elimination. Depression may be associated with constipation, whereas diarrhea (frequent passage of loose, watery stools) may occur in situations of high stress and anxiety. Explore the patient's activities of daily living (ADLs), including exercise, sleep–rest patterns, and dietary and fluid intake. Ask the patient to describe the frequency and character of stools. Ask about any history of diarrhea, constipation, or bleeding from the rectum, and collect information about the use of medications, laxatives, suppositories, or enemas. Anticholinergic drugs, antihistamines, tranquilizers, or narcotics may cause constipation.

Determine whether the patient has had any lower abdominal pain or rectal pain (Henderson et al., 2017). Crampy, colicky pains occur with diarrhea and/or constipation. A sudden onset of lower abdominal cramping occurs in obstruction of the colon. Left lower abdominal pain is associated with diverticulitis. Rectal pain may occur with stool retention and/or hemorrhoids.

If the patient has an **ostomy** (surgical opening into the bowel), ask about skin care problems, consistency of stool, foods that cause problems with diarrhea or **flatus** (intestinal gas), the number of times that the patient empties the appliance bag each day, and irrigation habits. It is also important to explore the patient's feelings about the appliance.

Explore any family history of colon cancer, colitis, gallbladder disease, or malabsorption syndromes, such as lactose intolerance and celiac sprue. Assess the patient's risk factors for cancer, including age greater than 50; family member with colon cancer; history of endometrial, ovarian, or breast cancer; and previous diagnoses of colon inflammation, polyps, or cancer.

Ask the patient to describe any heartburn, indigestion, abdominal discomfort, or pain. Explore the location of the pain, the type of pain, the time it occurs, foods that aggravate or relieve it, and how it is relieved. Abdominal pain is often referred to other sites. For example, a patient with a liver disorder may experience pain over the right shoulder (Kehr sign). Epigastric (middle upper abdominal) pain is experienced in cases of acute gastritis, obstruction of the small intestine, and acute pancreatitis. Pain in the right upper quadrant is associated with cholecystitis. Pain in the left upper quadrant may be related to a gastric ulcer.

The health history should include questions about any prior surgeries or trauma of the GI system. Explore the past history of any medical condition that may affect the patient's ingestion, digestion, and/or metabolism (e.g., Crohn disease or inflammatory bowel disease, diabetes mellitus, irritable bowel syndrome, peptic ulcers, or pancreatitis). Other areas significant to assessment are food allergies (especially to milk, which is evidenced as lactose intolerance with abdominal cramping, excessive flatus, and loose stools) and a family history that may provide clues to increased risk for health problems. The nurse should also ask about environmental exposures to parasites and microbes.

In addition to other factors assessed in the health history, culture and ethnicity are important components of nutritional status and GI health (Spector, 2017). Nutritional diversity is common among cultural and ethnic groups and questions should be included to identify specific customs, food likes and dislikes, and how foods are prepared and served. For example, in some ethnic groups, food is used to protect health, such as eating raw garlic or onions (Spector, 2017). In other cultures, dietary balance is believed to be necessary to keep the body in balance or harmony. Nurses need to know about specific culturally related nutritional values and practices and ask questions to identify health-related concerns specific to individualized dietary intake.

Fatigue is a frequent complaint of patients with gastrointestinal conditions. The nurse should assess the physical, cognitive, and psychosocial effects chronic GI disturbances are creating for the patient. Identifying the frequency, severity, and impact of fatigue on the patient's quality of life should be explored. Consider using an instrument designed to measure fatigue (Han, Heitkemper, & Jarrett, 2016) at each encounter with the patient to determine the ongoing effect of the GI disturbance.

Physical Assessment

Physical assessment of the GI system may be performed as part of a total health assessment, as a focused assessment of patients with known or suspected health problems, in combination with assessment of the urinary and reproductive systems (problems that may cause manifestations similar to those of the GI system), or alone for patients with known or suspected health problems. The techniques of inspection, auscultation, percussion, and palpation are used. Palpation is the last method used in assessing the abdomen because pressure on the abdominal wall and contents may interfere with bowel sound and cause pain, ending the examination. **Figure 21.6** ■ illustrates the four quadrants of the abdomen with the organs contained in each quadrant.

Collect objective data by obtaining anthropometric measurements (height, weight, triceps skinfolds, and midarm circumference) and by examining the mouth and abdomen. A thorough examination of the mouth should be completed on older adults who may have difficulties with oral self-care. Poor oral hygiene can compromise oral intake,

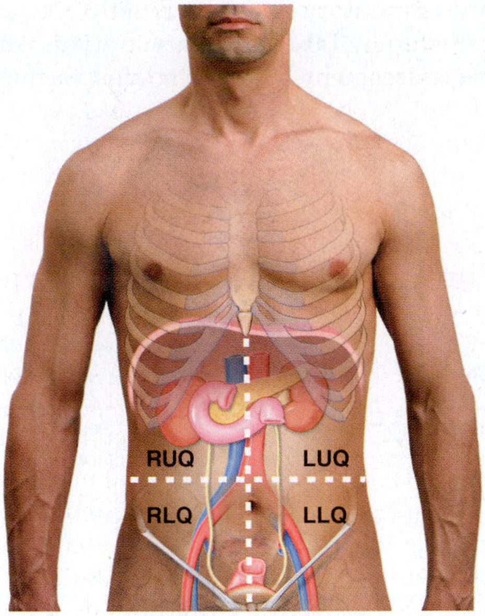
RUQ
LUQ
RLQ
LLQ

Right Upper Quadrant	Left Upper Quadrant
Liver and gallbladder	Left lobe of liver
Pylorus	Spleen
Duodenum	Stomach
Head of pancreas	Body of pancreas
Right adrenal gland	Left adrenal gland
Portion of right kidney	Portion of left kidney
Hepatic flexure of colon	Splenic flexure of colon
Portions of ascending and transverse colon	Portions of transverse and descending colon
Right Lower Quadrant	**Left Lower Quadrant**
Lower pole of right kidney	Lower pole of left kidney
Cecum and appendix	Sigmoid colon
Portion of ascending colon	Portion of descending colon
Bladder (if distended)	Bladder (if distended)
Right ovary and salpinx	Left ovary and salpinx
Right spermatic cord	Uterus (if enlarged)
Right ureter	Left spermatic cord
	Left ureter

Midline
Aorta
Umbilicus
Bladder
Uterus

Figure 21.6 ■ The four quadrants of the abdomen.

leading to nutritional deficits (Jennings, 2015). Prior to the examination, collect all necessary equipment and explain techniques to the patient to decrease anxiety.

The patient may be seated during assessment of the mouth, but is supine during the abdominal assessment. Ask the patient to empty the bladder before beginning the abdominal examination. Assist the patient to the dorsal recumbent (supine) position, with a small pillow under the head, a pillow under the knees (if desired), and the arms at the sides of the body. Warm the stethoscope before applying it to the patient's skin. Ask the patient to point to areas that are painful, and explain that those areas will be examined last. Expose the abdomen from below the breasts to the pubic symphysis, and drape the patient's thoracic and genital areas. When you document your findings, specify the location by abdominal quadrant.

General guidelines for abdominal assessment are:

1. Inspect the abdomen under a good light source that is shining across it. Sit at the right side of the patient, and note symmetry, distention, masses, visible peristalsis, and respiratory movements. If masses are detected, ask the patient to take a deep breath, which decreases the size of the abdominal cavity and makes any abnormality more visible.
2. Auscultate each quadrant of the abdomen, using the diaphragm of the stethoscope. Listen for bowel sounds, arterial bruits, venous hums, and friction rubs.
3. Percuss several areas within each quadrant of the abdomen, using a systematic path. (For example, always begin in the lower left quadrant, then proceed to the lower right quadrant, upper right quadrant, and upper left quadrant, respectively). The predominant percussion tones for the entire abdomen are tympany and dullness. Tympany is present over gas-filled intestines. Dullness is present over the liver, the spleen, an enlarged kidney, or a full stomach. Percuss for fluid, gaseous distention, and masses.
4. Palpate each quadrant of the abdomen for shape, position, mobility, size, consistency, and tenderness of the major abdominal organs. Begin this part of the assessment with light palpation, and increase the depth of palpation to elicit tenderness or better identify organ size and shape. Only nurses with considerable experience should conduct deep palpation. Remember to palpate areas of indicated tenderness last and to use gentle pressure. Palpation may be difficult or impossible if the patient exhibits muscle guarding from pain or is ticklish. The gallbladder and the spleen are normally not palpable.

Have the patient turn to the left lateral (Sims) position for the rectal examination. The older patient or the patient with limited mobility may need assistance in assuming this position. The patient should be standing to assess for an inguinal hernia.

Explain what will happen during the examination, and encourage the patient to take deep, regular breaths to increase relaxation. Explain that during the rectal examination, it may feel as though the patient is about to have a bowel movement and sometimes flatus (gas) is passed. Assure the patient that this is normal. Ensure that the examination area is private and the patient is draped properly to prevent unnecessary exposure.

Physical assessment of the integumentary system, nervous system, musculoskeletal system, cardiovascular system, and respiratory system may reflect the patient's nutritional status. **Table 21.2** summarizes abnormal nutritional assessment findings related to these body systems.

Table 21.2 Assessment Findings Due to Malnutrition

Body System	Assessment Findings
Nails	Soft and spoon shaped in iron deficiency. Splinter hemorrhages in vitamin C deficiency.
Hair	Dry, dull, and scarce in zinc, protein, and linoleic acid deficiencies.
Skin	Flaky and dry in vitamin A, vitamin B, and/or linoleic acid deficiency. Cracks and/or hyperpigmentation in niacin deficiency. Bruising in vitamin C or vitamin K deficiency. Poor wound healing.
Eyes	Eyes become dry and soft with decrease in vitamin A. Conjunctiva is pale with a decrease in iron, and red with a decrease in riboflavin.
Nervous system	Reflexes are decreased and patient may have peripheral neuropathies with thiamine deficiency. Patient may be irritable and/or disoriented with thiamine deficiency. Dementia, confusion, and ataxia may be seen.
Musculoskeletal system	Muscle wasting is seen with deficits in protein, carbohydrate, and fat metabolism. Calf pain occurs with thiamine deficiency; joint pain may occur with vitamin C deficiency.
Cardiovascular system	Heart size and rate may increase with thiamine deficiency. Diastolic blood pressure may be increased with a high intake of fat. Lowered cardiac output and decreased blood pressure may occur with caloric deficiencies over a long time period.
GI system	Cheilosis (sores at corner of mouth) seen in vitamin B complex deficiencies, especially riboflavin. Stomatitis and spongy, bleeding gums may also be seen in malnutrition.

Gastrointestinal Assessment

Technique/Normal Findings	Abnormal Findings
Anthropometric Assessment	
Weigh the patient and measure the patient's height. Compare the patient's actual weight to ideal body weight (IBW). *Weight should be appropriate to height as indicated on a standardized table.* (The National Institute of Health, National Heart, Lung and Blood Institute (NHLBI) provides height/weight tables at www.nhlbi.nih.gov/health/educational/lose_wt/BMI/bmi_tbl.htm.)	■ A weight 10 to 20% less than ideal body weight indicates malnutrition. ■ A weight 10% above ideal body weight is considered overweight. ■ A weight 20% above ideal body weight is considered obese.
Measure BMI. Determine BMI by using the accompanying formula. *BMI should be between 18.5 and 24.9.* (The NHLBI website provides resources for calculating BMI at www.nhlbi.nih.gov/health/educational/wecan/healthy-weight-basics/body-mass-index.htm.)	■ A BMI of 25–29.9 indicates overweight. $\frac{\text{Weight in kilograms} = \text{BMI}}{\text{Height in meters}}$
Determine waist-to-hip ratio. With the patient standing, measure the waist, and then measure the hips midway between the iliac crest and the greater trochanter. Use the accompanying formula to calculate the waist-to-hip ratio.	■ The NHLBI considers a waist circumference $>$ 102 cm (40.16 in.) in males and $>$ 88 cm (34.65 in.) in females as a risk for complications related to obesity. $\frac{\text{Waist circumference}}{\text{Hip circumference}} = \text{waist-to-hip ratio}$
Oral Assessment	
Inspect and palpate the lips. *Lips should be of normal color for race without lesions.*	■ **Cheilosis** (painful lesions at corners of mouth) is seen with riboflavin and/or niacin deficiency. ■ Cold sores or clear vesicles with a red base are seen in herpes simplex 1.
Inspect and palpate the tongue. *Tongue should be pink, smooth, and have good turgor.*	■ Atrophic smooth **glossitis** is characterized by a bright red tongue. It is seen in B_{12}, folic acid, and iron deficiencies. ■ Vertical fissures are seen in dehydration. ■ A black, hairy tongue may be seen following antibiotic therapy.
Inspect and palpate the buccal mucosa. *Mucosa should be moist, without lesions, and of appropriate color.*	■ **Leukoplakia** (small white patches) may be a sign of a premalignant condition. ■ A reddened, dry, swollen mucosa may be seen in stomatitis. ■ Candidiases (white cheesy patches that bleed when scraped) may be seen in immune-suppressed patients receiving antibiotics or chemotherapy and in terminally ill patients.
Inspect and palpate the teeth. *Teeth should be in a state of good hygiene without caries.*	■ Cavities and excessive plaque are seen with poor nutrition and/or poor oral hygiene.
Inspect and palpate the gums. *Gums should be of even color without swelling.*	■ Swollen, red gums that bleed easily (**gingivitis**) are seen in periodontal disease, vitamin C deficiencies, or with hormonal changes.
Inspect the throat and tonsils. *Tonsils (if present) should be of appropriate color and size.*	■ In acute infections, tonsils are red and swollen and may have white spots.
Note the patient's breath. *Breath should not have unusual or foul odors.*	■ Sweet, fruity breath is noted in diabetic ketoacidosis. ■ Acetone breath may be a sign of uremia. ■ Foul breath may result from liver disease, respiratory infections, and poor oral hygiene.

Abdominal Assessment

Technique/Normal Findings	Abnormal Findings
Assessment of the Abdomen	
Inspect abdominal contour, skin integrity, venous pattern, and aortic pulsation. *Abdomen should be slightly concave or rounded with intact skin. There should not be distended veins or obvious aortic pulsations.*	■ Generalized abdominal distention may be seen in gas retention or obesity. ■ Lower abdominal distention is seen in bladder distention, pregnancy, or ovarian mass. ■ General distention and an everted umbilicus are seen with ascites and/or tumors. ■ A scaphoid (sunken) abdomen is seen in malnutrition or when fat is replaced with muscle. ■ **Striae** (whitish-silver stretch marks) are seen in obesity and during or after pregnancy. ■ Spider angiomas may be seen in liver disease. ■ Dilated veins are prominent in cirrhosis of the liver, ascites, portal hypertension, or venocaval obstruction. ■ Pulsation is increased in aortic aneurysm.
Auscultate all four quadrants of the abdomen with the diaphragm of the stethoscope (**Figure 21.7** ■). Begin in the lower right quadrant, where bowel sounds are almost always present. If bowel sounds are not heard, ask a colleague to check your findings. *Normal bowel sounds (gurgling or clicking) occur every 5–15 seconds. Listen for at least 5 minutes in each of the four quadrants to confirm the absence of bowel sounds.*	■ **Borborygmus** (hyperactive high-pitched, tinkling, rushing, or growling bowel sounds) is heard in diarrhea or at the onset of bowel obstruction. ■ Bowel sounds may be absent later in bowel obstruction, with an inflamed peritoneum, and/or following surgery of the abdomen. 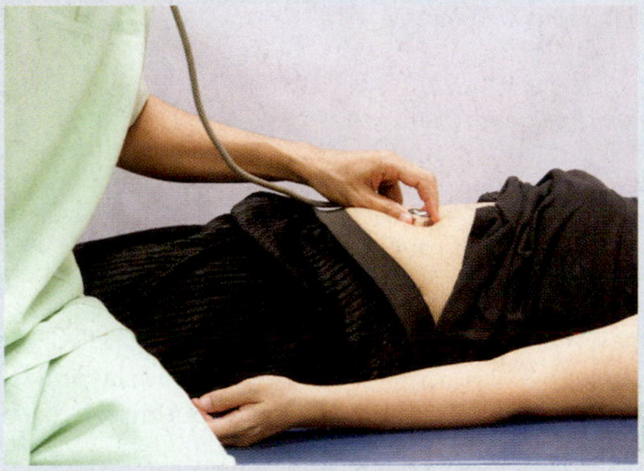 **Figure 21.7** ■ Auscultating the abdomen with the diaphragm of a stethoscope.
Auscultate the abdomen for vascular sounds with the bell of the stethoscope (**Figure 21.8** ■). *No sounds (bruits, venous hum, or friction rub) other than bowel sounds should be auscultated.*	■ **Bruits** (blowing sound due to restriction of blood flow through vessels) may be heard over constricted arteries. A bruit over the liver may be heard in hepatic carcinoma. ■ A venous hum (continuous medium-pitched sound) may be heard over a cirrhotic liver. ■ Friction rubs (rough grating sounds) may be heard over an inflamed liver or spleen. 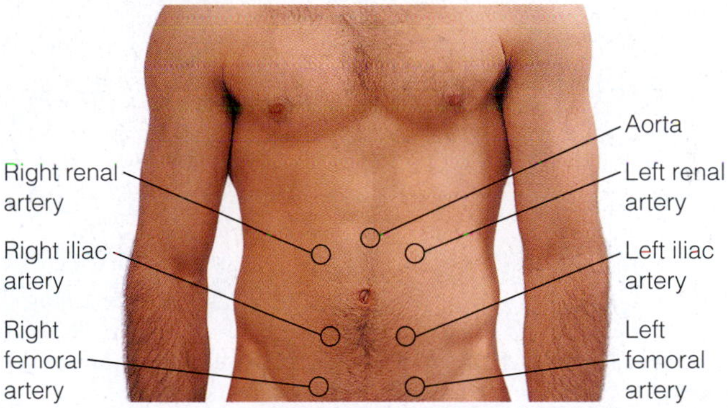 Aorta Right renal artery Left renal artery Right iliac artery Left iliac artery Right femoral artery Left femoral artery **Figure 21.8** ■ Location of placement of the stethoscope for auscultation of arteries of the abdomen.
Percuss the abdomen in all four quadrants (**Figure 21.9** ■). *Normally, tympany is heard over the stomach and gas-filled bowels.*	■ Dullness is heard when the bowel is displaced with fluid or tumors or filled with a fecal mass. 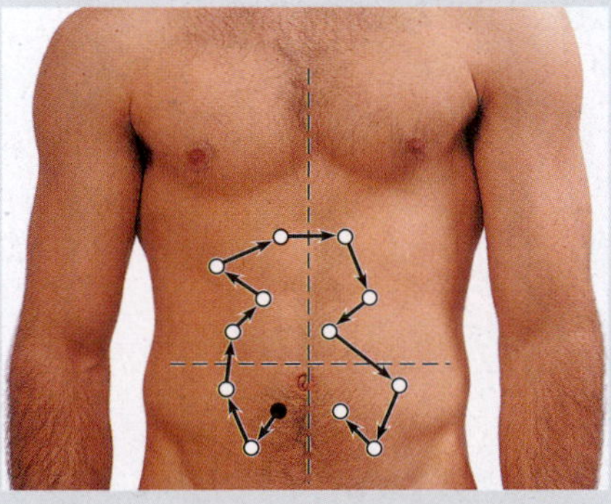 **Figure 21.9** ■ Location of sites for systematic percussion of all four quadrants.

(continued)

Abdominal Assessment (*continued*)

Technique/Normal Findings	Abnormal Findings

Percuss and palpate the liver to determine size.

1. Percuss in the midclavicular line (MCL), beginning below the umbilicus (see **Figure 21.10** ■ for landmarks). Begin to percuss over regions of tympany and move upward. The first dull percussion tone occurs at the lower boarder of the liver. Determine the upper liver border by beginning percussion over an area of lung resonance (in the MCL) and percussing downward to the first dull tone, usually at the 5th to 7th interspace. Mark each of these locations and measure the distance from one mark to the other to determine liver size.

   The normal liver size is 6 to 12 cm in the MLC; men have bigger livers than women.

2. Conduct bimanual palpation of the liver by placing your left hand under the patient at the level of the 11th to 12th ribs and applying upward pressure. Place your right hand below the costal margin, and palpate for the liver border.

   The liver is not normally palpable in a healthy adult, although it may be in very thin people.

■ In cirrhosis and/or hepatitis, the liver is greater than 6–10 cm in the MCL and greater than 4–8 cm in the midsternal line (MSL).

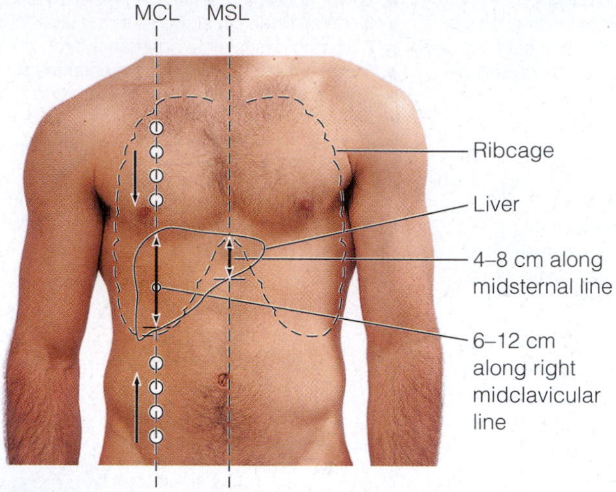
MCL
MSL
Ribcage
Liver
4–8 cm along midsternal line
6–12 cm along right midclavicular line

Figure 21.10 ■ Anatomic location of the liver, with the midclavicular line (MCL) and midsternal line (MSL) superimposed. The normal liver span is 6 to 12 cm.

Percuss the spleen for dullness posterior to the midaxillary line at the level of the 6th to 11th rib (**Figure 21.11** ■).
The spleen is percussed as an oval area of dullness approximately 7 cm wide near the left 10th rib and slightly posterior to the midaxillary line.

■ A large area of dullness that extends to the left anterior axillary line on inspiration is associated with an enlarged spleen and may be related to trauma, infection, or mononucleosis.

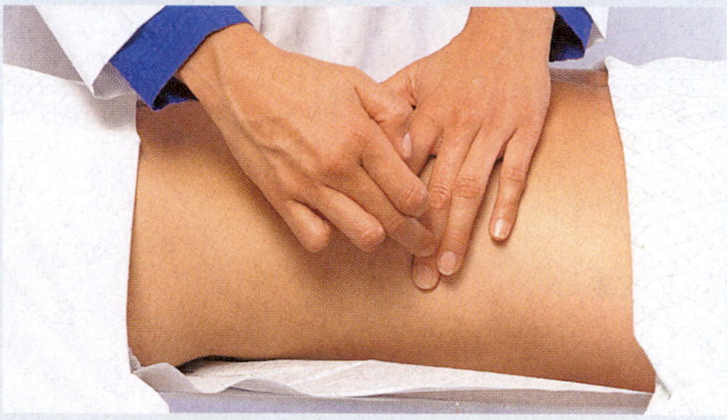

Figure 21.11 ■ Percussing the spleen.

Percuss for shifting dullness (**Figure 21.12** ■) *.If ascites is not present, the borders between tympany and dullness remain relatively constant despite position changes.*

■ In a patient with ascites, the level of dullness increases when the patient turns to the side.

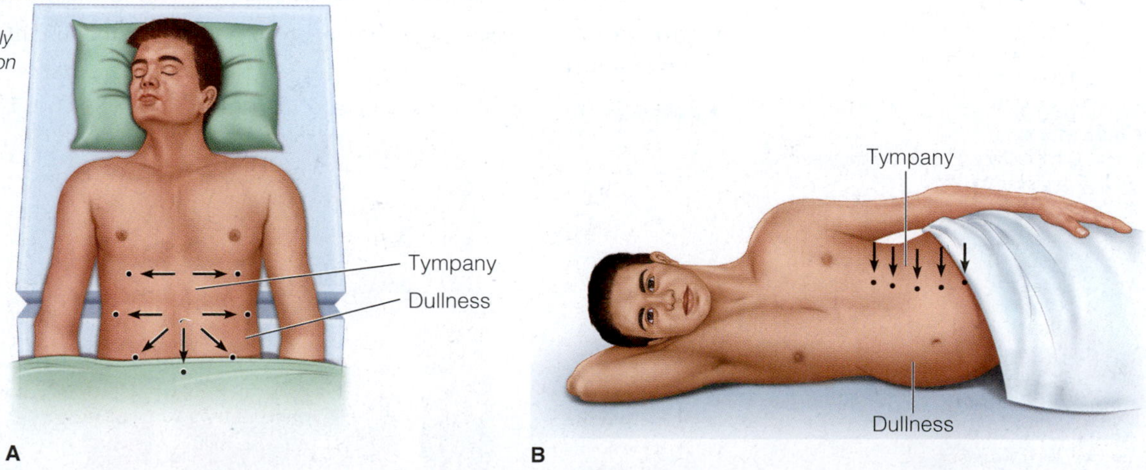
Tympany
Dullness
A
Tympany
Dullness
B

Figure 21.12 ■ Percussing for shifting dullness in ascites. **A,** Common percussion tones when the patient is lying supine; **B,** changes in percussion tones (shifting dullness) when the patient turns to the side.

Technique/Normal Findings	Abnormal Findings
Palpate the abdomen in all four quadrants (**Figure 21.13**). If the patient tightens the abdominal muscles (called "guarding"), flexing the knees may relax the muscles. *There should be no abdominal masses or pain on palpation.*	■ In cases of peritoneal inflammation, palpation causes abdominal pain and involuntary muscle spasms. ■ Abnormal masses include aortic aneurysms, neoplastic tumors of the colon or uterus, and a distended bladder or distended bowel due to obstruction. ■ A rigid, boardlike abdomen may be palpated when the patient has a perforated duodenal ulcer.

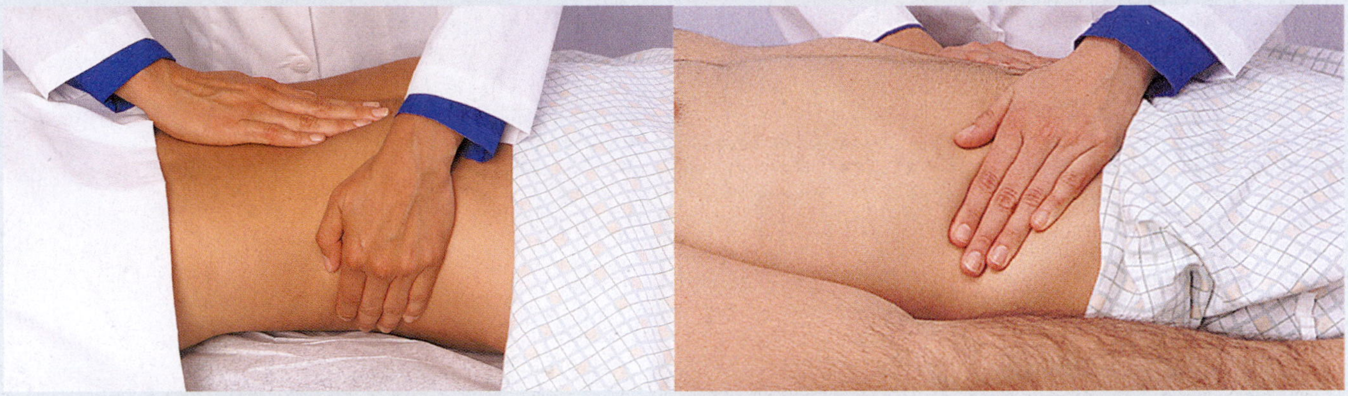

A B

Figure 21.13 ■ Light to moderate palpation of the abdomen. **A**, In light palpation, the examiner, keeping the fingers approximated, gently depresses the abdominal wall about 1 cm to assess for large masses, slight tenderness, and muscle guarding. **B**, The examiner performs moderate palpation by using the palm or the side of the hand to depress the abdominal wall to a slightly greater depth than in light palpation. This technique is useful for assessing abdominal organs that move with respiration (such as the liver and the spleen).

Technique/Normal Findings	Abnormal Findings
Use a circular motion to move the abdominal wall over underlying structures. Feel for masses and note any tenderness or pain the patient may have during this part of the exam. Palpate lightly at first (0.5 to 1.5 in.), then deeply (1.5 to 2 in.) with caution. If a mass is palpated, ask the patient to raise head and shoulders. A mass in the abdomen may become more prominent with this maneuver, as will a ventral abdominal wall hernia. If the mass is no longer palpable, it is deeper in the abdomen. *There should be no palpable masses or pain.*	
Palpate for rebound tenderness. Press the fingers into the abdomen slowly and release the pressure quickly. *Releasing pressure should not cause or increase pain.*	■ In peritoneal inflammation, pain occurs when the fingers are withdrawn. ■ Right upper quadrant pain occurs with acute cholecystitis. ■ Upper middle abdominal pain occurs with acute pancreatitis. ■ Right lower quadrant pain occurs with acute appendicitis. ■ Left lower quadrant pain is seen in acute diverticulitis.
Palpate the liver (see above and **Figure 21.14**). Note whether the patient guards the abdomen or reports any sharp pain, especially on inspiration. *The abdomen should be nontender, and the liver is usually nonpalpable.*	■ An enlarged liver with a smooth, tender edge may indicate hepatitis or venous congestion. ■ An enlarged, nontender liver may be felt in a malignant condition. ■ The patient with inflammation of the gallbladder feels sharp pain on inspiration and stops inspiring. This is called Murphy's sign.

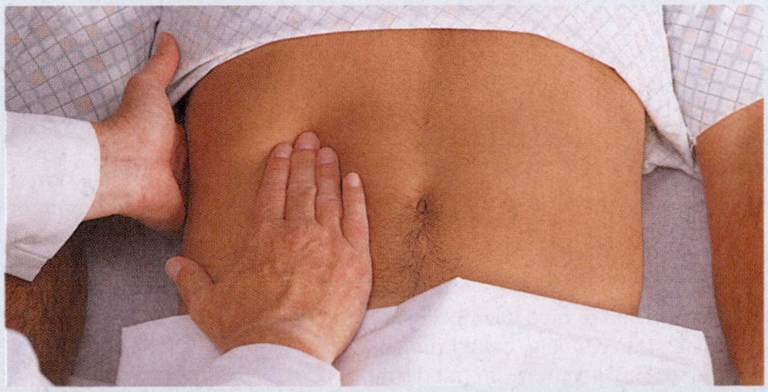

Figure 21.14 ■ Palpating the liver with the bimanual method.

Inguinal Area Assessment

Technique/Normal Findings	Abnormal Findings
Inspect the inguinal area for bulges after asking the patient to bear down. *The inguinal area is normally free of bulges.*	■ Bulges that appear in the inguinal area when the patient bears down may indicate a **hernia** (a defect in the abdominal wall that allows abdominal contents to protrude outward).

(continued)

Abdominal Assessment (*continued*)

Technique/Normal Findings	Abnormal Findings
Palpate the inguinal area with a gloved hand. Ask the patient to shift weight to the left to palpate the right inguinal area and vice versa. Place your right index finger upward into the inguinal area and ask the patient to bear down or cough. *Bulging or masses are normally not palpable.*	■ A bulge or mass may indicate a hernia.
Perianal Assessment	
Inspect the perianal area. Wearing gloves, spread the patient's buttocks apart. Observe the area, and ask the patient to bear down as if trying to have a bowel movement. *The perianal area should be intact, without obvious lesions.*	■ Swollen, painful, longitudinal breaks in the anal area may appear in patients with anal fissures. (These are caused by the passing of large, hard stools or by diarrhea.) ■ Dilated anal veins appear with hemorrhoids. ■ A red mass may appear with prolapsed internal hemorrhoids. ■ Doughnut-shaped red tissue at the anal area may appear with a prolapsed rectum.
Assessment of the Anus and Rectum Lubricate the gloved index finger and ask the patient to bear down. Touch the tip of your finger to the patient's anal opening. Flex the index finger, and slowly insert it into the anus, pointing the finger toward the umbilicus (**Figure 21.15** ■). Rotate the finger in both directions to palpate any lesions or masses. *There should be no masses in the anus or rectum.*	■ Movable, soft masses may be polyps. ■ Hard, firm, irregular embedded masses may indicate carcinoma.

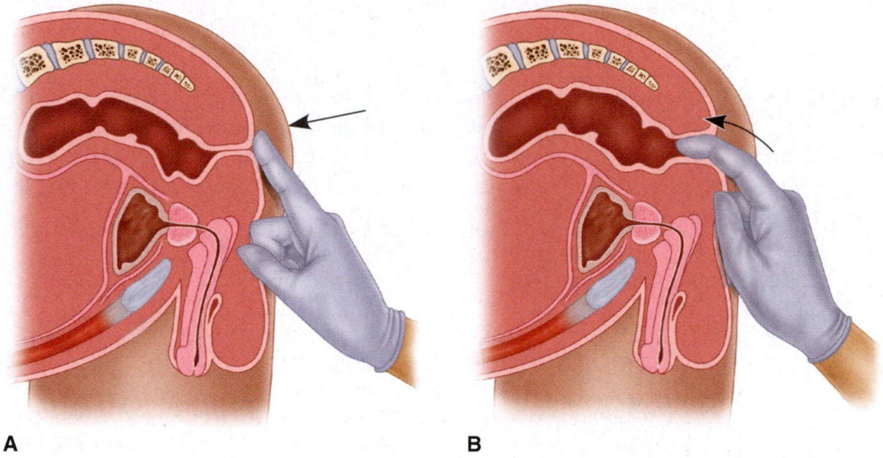
A
B

Figure 21.15 ■ Digital examination of the **A**, anus, and **B**, rectum.

Technique/Normal Findings	Abnormal Findings
Fecal Assessment	
Inspect the patient's feces. After palpating the rectum, withdraw your finger gently. Inspect any feces on the glove. Note color and/or presence of blood. Also use gloved fingers to note consistency. *Stool should be soft with no blood present.*	■ See Box 21.2 for information about stool characteristics.

BOX 21.2
Assessing Stool Characteristics

Inspect feces for color, odor, and consistency after the rectal exam or after defecation. Both hands should be gloved.

COLOR

- Blood *on* the stool results from bleeding from the sigmoid colon, anus, or rectum. Blood *within* the stool indicates bleeding from the colon due to ulcerative colitis, diverticulosis, or tumors. Black, tarry stools, called **melena**, occur with upper GI bleeding. Oral iron may turn stools black and mask melena.
- Grayish or whitish stools can result from biliary obstruction due to lack of bile in stool.
- Greasy, frothy, yellow stools, called **steatorrhea**, may appear with fat malabsorption.

ODOR

- Distinct, foul odors may be noted with stools containing blood or extra fat or in cases of colon cancer.

CONSISTENCY

- Hard stools or long, flat stools may result from a spastic colon or bowel obstruction due to a tumor or hemorrhoids. Hard stools may also result from ingestion of oral iron.
- Mucousy, slimy feces may indicate inflammation and occur in irritable bowel syndrome.
- Watery, diarrhea stools appear with malabsorption problems, irritable bowel syndrome, emotional or psychologic stress, ingestion of spoiled foods, or lactose intolerance.

Technique/Normal Findings	Abnormal Findings
Test the feces for occult blood. Use a testing kit such as Occultest or Hemoccult II. *There should be no occult blood in the feces.*	■ A positive occult blood test requires further testing for colon cancer or GI bleeding due to peptic ulcers, ulcerative colitis, or diverticulosis.
Note the odor of the feces. *No distinctly foul odors should be present.*	■ Distinctly foul odors may be noted with stools containing blood or extra fat or in cases of colon cancer.

SAFETY ALERT: A patient with abdominal pain may not tolerate any level of palpation. Never use deep palpation in a patient who has had a pulsatile abdominal mass, renal transplant, or polycystic kidneys or is at risk for hemorrhage. ■

Diagnosis

The results of diagnostic tests of nutritional status and GI function are used to support the diagnosis of a specific disease, to provide information to identify or modify the appropriate medication or therapy used to treat the disease, and to help nurses monitor the patient's responses to treatment and nursing care interventions. Diagnostic tests to assess nutritional status and function of the GI system and the accessory organs are described later in this chapter.

Regardless of the type of diagnostic test, the nurse is responsible for explaining the procedure and any special preparation needed, ensuring the consent form is signed (if necessary), supporting the patient during the examination as necessary, documenting the procedure as appropriate, and monitoring the results of the test. The nurse is also responsible for postprocedure care and patient teaching for self-care at home.

Diagnostic Tests
of the Gastrointestinal System

NAME OF TEST	PURPOSE AND DESCRIPTION	RELATED NURSING INTERVENTIONS
THE ESOPHAGUS AND STOMACH		
Barium swallow or upper GI series	These tests are conducted to diagnose esophageal varices, inflammation, ulcerations, hiatal hernia, foreign bodies, polyps, diverticula, and tumors of the esophagus, stomach, and duodenal bulb. The patient drinks 16–20 ounces of a chalky liquid (barium sulfate or meglumine diatrizoate [Gastrografin]) before the exam. These radiologic studies are done by observing the movement of a contrast medium with a fluoroscope (**Figure 21.16** ■).	Instruct the patient not to eat or drink fluids or smoke for 8–12 h before the test. A low-residue diet may be ordered 2–3 days before the test. Tell the patient not to take narcotics or anticholinergic medications for 24-h pretest and not to take any medications for 8-h pretest. Following the test, ensure the patient eliminates the barium by taking laxatives and forcing fluids as appropriate because barium can cause fecal impaction. Inform patient stools may be light colored for several days. 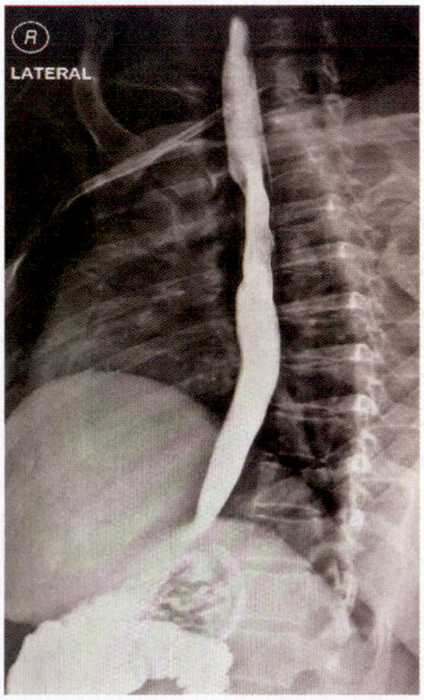 R LATERAL Figure 21.16 ■ A barium x-ray of a healthy stomach.

(continued)

NAME OF TEST	PURPOSE AND DESCRIPTION	RELATED NURSING INTERVENTIONS
Esophageal acidity, esophageal manometry, acid perfusion (Bernstein test) **Normal esophageal pH: 5–6**	Esophageal acidity is measured to diagnose problems of the lower esophageal sphincter and chronic reflux esophagitis. A catheter with a pH electrode is inserted into the esophagus through the mouth. The one-time measurement has been largely replaced by 24-h pH monitoring. Esophageal manometry is done to measure esophageal sphincter pressure and peristaltic contractions for diagnosis of esophageal motility problems, such as achalasia. A manometric catheter with a pressure transducer is inserted into the esophagus through the mouth, and esophageal pressure is measured before and after swallowing. Acid perfusion (Bernstein test) tests are done to distinguish between gastric acid reflux and cardiac involvement. A catheter is inserted through the nose into the esophagus. A saline solution, followed by a hydrochloric acid (HCl) solution, is dripped into the catheter and the patient is asked to indicate when pain occurs. HCl is turned off, and saline is started until symptoms have subsided.	Food and fluid will be restricted 8–12 h prior to test. Instruct patient to avoid alcohol intake for 24 h prior to the exam. Assess medications: Results of the tests may be affected by antacids, anticholinergics, and H_2 inhibitors, which increase the pH, reducing acidity and causing false test results. Alcohol, cholinergics, adrenergic blockers, and corticosteroids may increase acidity and relax the lower esophageal sphincter.
Gastric analysis **Normal values:** **Fasting: 1.0–5.0 mEq/L per hour** **Stimulation: 10–25 mEq/L per hour**	This test is used to evaluate gastric secretions for an increase or decrease of free hydrochloric acid by inserting a nasogastric tube into the stomach and aspirating stomach fluids. A stimulation gastric analysis may follow, with a gastric stimulant (such as Histalog or pentagastrin) administered and several gastric samples aspirated.	Instruct the patient to not smoke, eat, or drink fluids for 8–12 h prior to the test. Assess medications and fluid intake: Anticholinergics, cholinergics, adrenergic blockers, antacids, steroids, alcohol, and coffee can alter results. Obtain baseline vital signs. Remove loose dentures. Insert nasogastric tube. Aspirate gastric contents at 15- to 20-minute intervals as ordered.
Gastric emptying studies	To evaluate the ability of the stomach to empty liquids or solids. In this nuclear imaging study, the patient is asked to eat a cooked egg containing ^{99m}Tc (solids) or to drink orange juice with ^{99m}Tc (liquids). Sequential images are recorded with a gamma camera every 2 minutes for up to an hour.	Explain to the patient that the substances contain only very small amounts of radioactivity and are not hazardous.
Magnetic resonance imaging (MRI)—stomach	An MRI of the stomach may be conducted to identify the source of gastric bleeding.	Inform the patient of the need to lie still during the examination. Assess for any metallic implants (such as pacemakers, clips on brain aneurysms, body piercings, tattoos, shrapnel). If present, notify imaging physician. Remove transdermal medication patches (both OTC and prescribed) unless otherwise ordered. Replace the patch following the procedure. Tell the patient to inform the staff about the patch when making the appointment and when completing the admission information. Ask if the patient is pregnant; if so, the test is not performed. Ask about claustrophobia; if a problem, sedation may be required.

NAME OF TEST	PURPOSE AND DESCRIPTION	RELATED NURSING INTERVENTIONS
Upper GI endoscopy (esophagogastroduodenoscopy [EGD]), gastroscopy	These tests directly visualize the mucous membrane lining of the esophagus, stomach, and duodenum. A flexible fiberoptic endoscope is used to visualize inflammations, ulcerations, tumors, or varices, and video imaging may illustrate gastric motility. They may also be combined with an ultrasound examination by attaching an ultrasound transducer to the endoscope.	Schedule this test at least 2 days after a barium swallow or upper GI series. Remove dentures and eyeglasses. Inform the patient not to eat food or drink fluids for 6–8 h before the procedure. Tell the patient that the procedure takes about 20–30 minutes and that a local anesthetic will be administered to the throat to help prevent discomfort. A sedative/tranquilizer, a narcotic analgesic, and atropine may be given before the procedure and titrated intravenously during the procedure. After the procedure the patient is allowed to eat and drink as soon as he or she can swallow safely. Mild bloating, belching, or flatulence may occur after the procedure. Tell the patient to contact the physician postexamination for difficulty swallowing; epigastric, substernal, or shoulder pain; fever; vomiting blood; or having black tarry stools (Hay, Barnette, & Shaw, 2016).
THE INTESTINES		
Abdominal ultrasound	This test is used to identify abdominal masses, ascites, and disorders of the appendix. A lubricant gel is applied to the skin and a transducer is placed over the area of interest. High-frequency sound waves pass through the body structures and are recorded as they are reflected.	Tell the patient not to eat, drink, smoke, or chew gum for 6 h prior to the examination and to eat a fat-free meal the evening before the test. Ensure that the patient has not had any other tests that might interfere with results, such as an upper GI series.
Barium enema (Ba enema)	A barium enema is conducted to identify structural abnormalities of the colon and rectum. This fluoroscopic radiologic examination of the colon is done by administering a contrast medium rectally. Double-contrast or air-contrast studies are the examination of choice, with air being infused after the barium is evacuated.	The colon must be free from fecal material. Inform the patient to follow a clear liquid diet for 24 h and then to not eat or drink fluid for 8 h before the procedure. Instruct in the administration of the prescribed laxatives, enemas, or suppositories the evening before the procedure. Following the procedure, the patient should increase fluid intake and take a laxative, if prescribed. Stools may be white until all the barium is expelled.
Colonoscopy	A visual examination of the entire colon to the ileocecal valve is conducted to identify tumors, polyps, and inflammatory bowel disease and to dilate strictures. A flexible endoscope is inserted anally and advanced through the colon. Polyps are removed during the procedure to prevent future malignancies.	Tell the patient to follow the examining healthcare provider's order for preparation (this varies by provider or clinic), which may include a liquid diet the day prior to the examination, remaining NPO for 8 h before the procedure, and use of a bowel preparation, for example, citrate of magnesia, laxatives, or polyethylene glycol (Kunz & Gillespie, 2017). Oral phosphate used for test preparation may compromise kidney function, especially in older adults, or those who are dehydrated, have kidney disease or colitis, or are taking medications that affect kidney function. Explain that sedation is usually given during the procedure and that polyps (if present) will be removed. Instruct the patient to refrain from eating prepared foods that contain olestra (a synthetic fat additive used in products such as potato chips); the chemical may cover tissue lesions and also cause adhesive plaques to form on the colonoscopy instruments. Inform the patient that after the procedure increased flatus is common and to report to the healthcare provider any abdominal pain, chills, fever, rectal bleeding, or mucopurulent discharge. If polyps were removed, the patient should avoid high-fiber foods for 1–2 days and do no heavy lifting for 7 days.

(continued)

NAME OF TEST	PURPOSE AND DESCRIPTION	RELATED NURSING INTERVENTIONS
Guaiac fecal occult blood test (G-FOBT)	In this test, feces are tested for occult (hidden) blood. This is often done as a screening test for colon cancer. A stool specimen may be sent to the laboratory or the test may be done with a commercial kit such as Hemoccult II or Occultest.	When testing for occult blood with a commercial kit, place a smear of stool on the designated area and drop the reagent on the area. A blue color that develops in response to the reagent indicates the presence of blood. If the test is done at home, tell the patient to avoid (if recommended by the healthcare provider) taking aspirin, NSAIDs, anticoagulants, red meats, fish, broccoli and other high-fiber vegetables, mushrooms, vitamin C supplements, and iron supplements for 3 days prior to the stool collection.
Immunochemical fecal occult blood test (I-FOBT)	An I-FOBT is used to test for blood in the stool and is considered to be more effective in detecting colon cancer than is the guaiac fecal occult blood test. A brush is used to collect water drops around the surface of a stool while it is still in the toilet bowl. The sample is then sent to the laboratory for analysis.	No special preparation is necessary. The specimen is collected and sent to the laboratory.
Magnetic resonance imaging (MRI)—abdominal	An abdominal MRI may be done to identify sources of GI bleeding and to stage colon cancer.	See previous information about MRI of the stomach.
Sigmoidoscopy	A sigmoidoscopy is a visual examination of the anus, rectum, and sigmoid colon to identify tumors, polyps, infections, inflammations, hemorrhoids, and fissures. The test is done using a flexible sigmoidoscope. Specimens are obtained and polyps removed during the procedure.	Instruct the patient to eat a clear liquid or light diet the evening before the procedure and to take prescribed laxatives. An enema or rectal suppository may be required the morning of the procedure. Explain to the patient that after the procedure large amounts of flatus may be expelled if air was instilled into the bowel and to report any abdominal pain, fever, or rectal bleeding to the healthcare provider. If a polyp is removed, the patient should avoid heavy lifting for 7 days and avoid high-fiber foods for 1–2 days.
Small-bowel series	This radiologic examination is done to diagnose abnormalities of the esophagus, stomach, and small intestine. The patient drinks a contrast medium and films are taken every 20 minutes until the medium reaches the terminal ileum. It may also be done in conjunction with an upper GI series or barium swallow.	Inform the patient that a low-residue diet should be eaten as prescribed (usually up to 48 h preprocedure) and not to eat for 8 h or drink fluids for 4 h before the test. Tell the patient about the procedure: It takes several hours to complete, and barium may be given orally, into the bowel via an endoscope, or through a weighted tube. Following the procedure the patient should increase oral fluid intake and take a prescribed laxative to facilitate evacuation of the barium. The stools will be white for up to 72 h after the examination; normal color will return when all the barium has been evacuated.
Stool specimen, stool culture	A sample of stool is collected for gross and microscopic examination, as well as for form, consistency, and color. Gross examination includes volume and water content and the presence of any blood, pus, mucus, or excess fat. Microscopic examination identifies the presence of WBCs, unabsorbed fat, and parasites. When an enteric pathogen is suspected, a stool culture is done.	Ask the patient to provide a fresh stool sample. A sterile container should be used to collect a stool sample for a culture. Ask women of childbearing age if they are having their menstrual period; if so, note this on the laboratory request.
Stool DNA test (sDNA)	This test involves examining a stool specimen for DNA changes. Premalignant polyps and malignant lesions of the bowel shed cells that have been identified as DNA markers for bowel and rectal cancer. The patient uses a kit containing an ice pack (that must be frozen for several hours before use), collects one bowel movement in a special container, then mails or brings the container with the ice pack in a provided box to the laboratory.	No special preparation is needed. Explain the procedure to the patient.

NAME OF TEST	PURPOSE AND DESCRIPTION	RELATED NURSING INTERVENTIONS
Virtual colonography (VC)	A VC is used to diagnose polyps, diverticulosis, and cancer and may not be as accurate as the traditional colonoscopy. Computers are used to produce two- and three-dimensional images of the colon on a screen. If abnormalities are found, a conventional colonoscopy may be needed (such as to remove polyps or do a biopsy).	The preparation for virtual colonography is essentially the same as that used for traditional colonoscopy. Inform the patient that a tube is inserted into the rectum, air is instilled to inflate the colon, and scans are taken.
THE GALLBLADDER AND PANCREAS		
Abdominal ultrasound, hepatobiliary ultrasound, gallbladder ultrasound	Abdominal ultrasound is used to detect abdominal tumors, cysts, and ascites. Hepatobiliary ultrasound is used to visualize the biliary ducts and to detect subphrenic abscesses, cysts, tumors, and cirrhosis of the liver. Gallbladder ultrasound is used to detect gallstones. These noninvasive procedures record ultrasound waves as they are reflected off body structures. A conductive gel is applied to the skin and a transducer placed on the area of interest.	Instruct the patient to remain NPO for 8–12 h prior to the test.
Cholangiography ■ **Percutaneous transhepatic cholangiogram (PTC)** ■ **Surgical cholangiogram**	A PTC is done to evaluate filling of the hepatic and biliary ducts. Using local anesthesia, the liver and bile duct are entered with a long needle (using fluoroscopy), bile is withdrawn, and a contrast medium is injected into the bile duct. During a surgical cholangiogram with general anesthesia, contrast medium is injected into the common bile duct to evaluate filling of the duct.	Assess for allergy to iodine, seafood, or x-ray dye (many contain iodine). Assess medications: Oral hypoglycemic agents are contraindicated for use with iodinated contrast. Monitor for bile leakage or hemorrhage following the tests.
Cholecystography (oral) (GB series)	This test is used to detect gallbladder stones, inflammation, tumors, and obstruction of the cystic duct. Radiopaque tablets (e.g., iopanoic acid [Telepaque], sodium ipodate [Oragrafin], iodoalphionic acid [Priodax], or iodipamide meglumine [Cholografin]) are given the evening before the test; x-rays are taken the following morning. A high-fat meal may be given after the fasting x-rays are completed and further x-rays taken to determine how rapidly the GB expels the dye.	*If the patient is also having GI x-rays with barium, the GB tests should be done first because barium would interfere with the test.* Instruct the patient to eat a fat-free diet 24 h prior to test. No food or fluids except sips of water should be taken 12 h before the test. Radiopaque tablets are to be taken 2 h after the evening meal. Assess for allergy to iodine, seafood, or x-ray dye (many contain iodine). Assess medications: Oral hypoglycemic agents are contraindicated for use with iodinated contrast.
Computed tomography (CT)	The CT scan produces a narrow x-ray beam that examines the body sections from 360 degrees. CT of the abdomen is useful in visualizing many pathologic conditions of the liver, biliary tract, pancreas, spleen, GI tract, and gallbladder. Oral contrast media may be used.	No special preparation is needed. Observe for signs and symptoms of allergic reaction to contrast media. If contrast media is used, encourage patient to increase fluid after exam to enhance excretion of dye.
Endoscopic retrograde cholangiopancreatography (ERCP)	An ERCP is done to directly visualize GI structures and to retrieve gallstones from the distal common bile duct, dilate structures, and biopsy tumors. A fiberoptic endoscope is inserted through the mouth, esophagus, stomach, descending duodenum, and common bile ducts and pancreatic ducts. Contrast medium is injected into the ducts and structures are visualized.	Tell the patient not to drink fluids or eat for 8 h before the test. Assess patient for allergy to iodine, seafood, or x-ray dye (many contain iodine). Assess medications: Oral hypoglycemic agents are contraindicated for use with iodinated contrast. Assess gag reflex prior to giving food or fluids. If atropine was given, assess for manifestations of urinary retention. Tell the patient that a sore throat may be present for a few days after the test; suggest warm saline gargles to ease discomfort.
Magnetic resonance cholangiopancreatography (MRCP)	This noninvasive MRI study is done to evaluate the biliary and pancreatic ducts.	See previous information for MRI of the stomach.
Serum amylase **Normal value: 30–170 units/L**	This blood test is used to measure the secretion of amylase by the pancreas. It is used to diagnose acute pancreatitis, when amylase level peaks in 24 h and then drops to normal in 48–72 h.	No special preparation is needed.

(*continued*)

NAME OF TEST	PURPOSE AND DESCRIPTION	RELATED NURSING INTERVENTIONS
Serum lipase Normal value: 20–180 units/L (norms vary among laboratories)	This blood test is used to measure the secretion of lipase by the pancreas.	No special preparation is needed.
THE LIVER		
Liver biopsy	A liver biopsy is performed to rule out metastatic cancer or to detect a cyst or cirrhosis of the liver. The procedure is considered minor surgery and is done at a hospital. Using ultrasound, a biopsy needle is inserted into the liver and guided to the pathologic site. See **Figure 21.17** ■. A wide variety of blood tests are used to diagnose and monitor liver disease. See **Table 21.3**.	Inform the patient to tell the physician about any anticoagulants taken and to withhold aspirin and ibuprofen for a week before the procedure. Food and fluids are withheld for 4–6 h before the procedure. Assess and record baseline vital signs, and review prothrombin time and platelet count. Report abnormal findings. Administer vitamin K as prescribed. Ask the patient to void immediately before the procedure. After the needle is removed, pressure is applied; place the patient on the right side for 1–2 h to maintain pressure on the insertion site. Explain to the patient that pain may be experienced in the right shoulder as the local anesthetic loses effect, that the dressing will be assessed frequently, that food and fluids are withheld for 2 h after the biopsy, and that coughing, lifting, or straining should be avoided for 1–2 weeks. The patient will not be allowed to drive home and must go directly to bed for 8–10 h (or as prescribed by the physician).

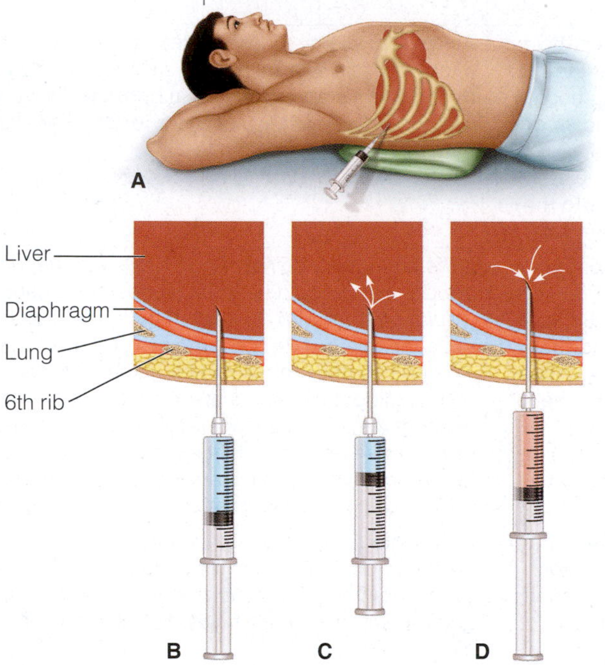
A
Liver
Diaphragm
Lung
6th rib
B
C
D

Figure 21.17 ■ Liver biopsy. **A**, The patient exhales completely, and then holds his or her breath. This brings the liver and diaphragm to their highest position. **B**, The biopsy needle is inserted into the liver. **C**, Approximately 1 mL of saline is injected to clear the needle of blood and tissue. **D**, The needle is advanced, and a tissue sample is aspirated. Pressure is applied to the site immediately after the needle is withdrawn. The specimen is sent to the laboratory for analysis.

Table 21.3 Liver Function Tests

Used to assess liver function, evaluate patients with jaundice, and detect liver disease such as hepatitis or alcoholic cirrhosis. Fasting is required for the bilirubin sample; samples for other liver function studies may be drawn without fasting. Water is permitted.

Note: All values are for adults.

Test	Normal Values
Alanine aminotransferase (ALT or SGPT)	10–35 units/L
Alkaline phosphatase (ALP)	42–136 units/L
Aspartate aminotransferase (AST or SGOT)	8–38 units/L
Gamma-glutamyltransferase (GGT)	Women: 3–13 units/L Men: 4–23 units/L
Serum bilirubin	Total: 0.1–1.2 mg/dL Conjugated (direct): 0.1–0.3 mg/dL

Source: Data from Kee, 2018.

21.4 Assessment of Selected Populations

Older adults are at greater risk for malnutrition than are younger people. Age-related changes that contribute to this problem include changes in taste and smell, poor oral health, loss of teeth or ill-fitting dentures, medication-related anorexia, and functional limitations that impair the ability to shop and cook (see **Table 21.4**). Older adults living on fixed incomes may not be able to afford well-balanced meals. Depression, social isolation, and loneliness often contribute to loss of appetite. Eating is a social event, and older adults who eat alone may not eat as well as those who share meals with companions.

Conduct a thorough assessment to determine nutritional status. Assess psychologic factors that influence eating habits, such as loneliness, isolation, and depression. Note the patient's general appearance and obtain a diet history, including information about foods and nutrients the patient consumes and recent weight loss or gain. Review laboratory values, including complete blood count, total protein, prealbumin, and albumin levels.

When evaluating a veteran who has served in the Persian Gulf, ask about diarrhea and constipation as about 20% of Iraq and Afghanistan veterans have a gastrointestinal disorder, the most common of which is irritable bowel syndrome (IBS). There is increased prevalence of primary liver cancer in Vietnam veterans, so include health assessment questions related to liver function. Older veterans have a higher prevalence of poor oral health and should receive comprehensive oral assessments in primary care and when hospitalized (Jennings, 2015).

Patients who identify as LGBTQI have higher prevalence of eating disorders (National Eating Disorders Association, 2018). Men who have sex with men (MSM) are 17 times more likely to develop anal cancer than heterosexual men and are at increased risk of acquiring sexually transmitted infections carrying viruses that cause hepatitis. The nurse should establish trust and carefully assess LGBTQI patients using culturally sensitive approaches when completing a health history

Adults with cystic fibrosis will need continued nutritional monitoring throughout their lifetime as this genetic disease affects secretion of the pancreatic enzymes critical to digestion. The nurse should monitor nutritional data, assist with adherence to dietary and medication regimens, and ensure care is coordinated among speciality providers involved in the patient's care.

21.5 Health Promotion

Maintaining a Healthy Weight

Maintaining a healthy weight throughout the lifespan begins in childhood. Children and teenagers who are obese continue to be so as adults. Promote healthy eating, including a diet rich in whole grains, fruits, and vegetables and low in fat. *Dietary Guidelines for Americans* are published jointly by the U.S. Department of Health and Human Services (USDHHS; n.d.) and the U.S. Department of Agriculture (USDA) and provide information and tools for establishing and maintain good dietary habits. Guidelines include specific dietary information for patients with select chronic illnesses and include documents to assist patients and families and health care providers. The MyPlate program published by

Table 21-4 Age-Related Gastrointestinal Changes

Age-Related Change	Significance
Teeth: ↑number of root cavities and cavities around existing dental work; tooth enamel harder and more brittle; dentin is more fibrous; tooth cusps flatten; root pulp shrinks; ↑ loss of bone supporting teeth	Increase in periodontal disease and tooth loss Increase in fractures of teeth Increased incidence of dentures
Gums: Gingiva retracts	Increase in periodontal disease
Taste: Less acute as tongue atrophies, especially for sweet sensations	Excessive seasoning of foods
Saliva: ↓amount is produced (one-third of that produced in younger years)	Decreased ability to break down starches Swallowing may take longer
Esophageal motility: ↓intensity of propulsive waves and slower emptying time, weaker gag reflex	Discomfort when swallowing food Increased risk of aspiration
Stomach: Mucosa atrophies, ↓production of hydrochloric acid and pepsin leading to higher pH in stomach	Increase in incidence of gastric irritation
Liver: Less efficient handling of cholesterol	Increased incidence of gallstones
Small intestine: ↓number of absorbing cells on intestinal wall, slowed fat absorption, faulty absorption of vitamin B_{12}, vitamin D, calcium, and iron	Decreased ability to absorb vitamins A, D, E, and K Increased risk of osteoporosis and fractures (↓calcium and vitamin D) Increased risk of iron-deficiency anemia (weakness, lassitude, pallor) (↓iron) Increased risk of pernicious anemia (weakness, dyspnea, glossitis, numbness, dementia, depression) (↓vitamin B_{12})
Large intestine: ↓mucous secretion and elasticity of the wall of the rectum, loss of tone in internal sphincter with decreased awareness of need to defecate	Increased tendency for constipation

the USDA (n.d.) provides visual guidance for appropriate food choices to maintain a healthy, well-balanced diet. In addition to promoting healthy dietary habits, encourage all children and adults to maintain an active lifestyle, balance calories with daily energy requirements, avoid oversized portions, and emphasize fruits, vegetables, whole grains, and low-fat dairy in the diet. Nurses should encourage all patients to engage in at least 30 minutes of aerobic activity daily. Encourage parents to limit time children spend watching television, using the computer, and playing video games. Discuss the effects of smoking and excess alcohol use on nutrition and activity. To reduce weight gain commonly associated with aging, encourage patients to gradually reduce the amount of calories consumed.

To maintain nutritional status, advise the older patient to do the following:

- Eat a well-balanced diet with fresh fruits and vegetables.
- Shop wisely to get the most value for the money.
- Avoid processed foods and foods high in fat.
- Drink adequate fluids.
- Exercise regularly.
- Contact local agencies for the availability of congregate meals (e.g., at local senior centers) or home-delivered meals (e.g., Meals on Wheels).

Reducing Risk of Cancer

Reducing or eliminating tobacco use (smoking and smokeless tobacco) and excess alcohol consumption can significantly reduce the incidence of oral cancer. Teach children and adolescents about the dangers of using tobacco and alcohol. Emphasize the relationship between smokeless tobacco and oral cancer. Discuss strategies to deal with peer pressure to use tobacco and alcohol.

To promote early identification of and intervention for oral cancer, teach patients about the risk factors for and manifestations of the disease. This is a particularly important nursing strategy in older men who have the highest incidence, and in populations in whom the disease often is advanced when detected (people of lower socioeconomic status, people who rarely see a dentist, and African American men). Encouraging and facilitating annual and biannual preventative dental care is an important nursing responsibility. Due to the increase in HPV, health teaching should include informing patients about the risk of infection from oral sex and instruction on preventative measures and safe sex practices.

Health promotion measures to reduce the risk for and incidence of esophageal cancer include educating people (especially young people) about the dangers of cigarette smoking and excess alcohol use. Refer to smoking cessation and alcohol treatment programs as indicated. Educate patients with GERD about the relationship between chronic damage to the esophagus due to reflux and esophageal cancer, and stress the importance of effective disease management. Provide education aimed to eliminate behavior leading to chronic liver disease including liver cancer, cirrhosis, and hepatitis (Gimenes et al., 2016). Encourage clients to avoid excessive alcohol intake, use of illegal IV drugs, and other behaviors leading to infection of bloodborne pathogens.

CHAPTER HIGHLIGHTS

21.1 Nutrients

Outline the nutrients absorbed in the gastrointestinal (GI) system.

- The categories of nutrients are carbohydrates, proteins, fats, vitamins, minerals, and water and are found in food.
- Overall health status is influenced by proper nutrition and a balanced diet.
- The etiology of many common illnesses is influenced by diet and nutrition, thereby making the nurse's role increasingly important in terms of conducting health assessments aimed at detecting early disease processes and teaching that promotes healthy dietary habits.

21.2 Anatomy, Physiology, and Functions of the GI System

Describe the anatomy, physiology, and functions of the GI system and identify abnormal findings that may indicate impairment of the GI system.

- The gastrointestinal system including the mouth, pharynx, esophagus, stomach, small intestine, large intestine, and the accessory digestive organs (liver, gallbladder, and pancreas) plays a critical role in providing nutrition to all other systems, thereby influencing homeostasis of the body.
- After carbohydrates, fats, and proteins are ingested and digested, absorbed and transported across cell membranes, they must be metabolized to provide energy required to maintain life.

21.3 Assessing Gastrointestinal Function

Outline the components of the assessment of the GI system including topics for the health assessment interview, techniques for physical assessment, and the diagnostic tests used in the assessment.

- Manifestations of dysfunctions and disorders affecting the gastrointestinal system may be detected during a general health assessment as well as during focused assessment of the gastrointestinal system.

- As a member of the interprofessional health care team, the nursing role involves preparing the patient for diagnostic tests and monitoring results.
- Patients who identify as LGBTQI should be assessed for eating disorders, as needed, and MSM should be assessed, as needed, for anal cancer and STIs.
- Adults with cystic fibrosis will need continued monitoring of their nutrition.

21.4 Assessment of Selected Populations

Differentiate considerations for assessing the GI system of older adults, veterans, and individuals in the LGBTQI population.

- Older adults can be at risk for malnutrition. Nurses should conduct a thorough assessment to determine nutritional status.
- Veterans of the Persian Gulf wars should be assessed for diarrhea, constipation, and IBS. Vietnam veterans should be assessed for liver disorders.

21.5 Health Promotion

Summarize topics that nurses teach to promote a healthy GI system across the lifespan.

- Interventions aimed at assisting patients to maintain a healthy weight through diet and exercise are primary nursing responsibilities.
- Health teaching should address behaviors and habits that increase the risk of esophageal cancer and chronic liver disease.

TEST YOURSELF NCLEX-RN® REVIEW

1. The nurse is preparing educational materials for a patient with a low serum albumin level. Which foods should the nurse instruct as being complete proteins? (Select all that apply.)
   A. Milk
   B. Eggs
   C. Fruits
   D. Butter
   E. Vegetables
2. The nurse suspects a patient recovering from surgery is deficient in vitamin K. What is a finding associated with vitamin K deficiency?
   A. Bruising
   B. Slow peristalsis
   C. Poor wound healing
   D. Surgical wound bleeding
3. The nurse notes that a patient's serum amylase level is elevated. For which health problem should the nurse plan patient care?
   A. Cheilosis
   B. Gallstones
   C. Gastric reflux
   D. Acute pancreatitis
4. While assessing the oral cavity, the nurse notes that an older patient has obvious caries and difficulty swallowing. When asked about eating, the patient mentions frequent issues with a dry mouth. Which health problem is this patient at most risk for developing?
   A. Acute pain
   B. Risk for infection
   C. Nutritional deficit
   D. Altered elimination
5. The nurse is conducting a physical examination of a patient with ascites. Which sound should the nurse expect to hear when percussing this patient's abdomen?
   A. Flatness
   B. Resonance
   C. Shifting dullness
   D. Alternating amplitude
6. A patient is upset to learn after a sigmoidoscopy that internal hemorrhoids were found. What should the nurse explain about this health problem? (Select all that apply.)
   A. "They are part of the lymphatic system."
   B. "They are part of the arteries of the body."
   C. "They are swollen veins in the anal canal."
   D. "They are just bits of tissue that occur for no reason."
   E. "Internal hemorrhoids may become external."
7. The nurse is completing an assessment for a patient with an ostomy. Which questions should the nurse include when conducting this assessment? (Select all that apply.)
   A. "Has your appetite changed lately?"
   B. "Do any particular foods cause flatus?"
   C. "What is the consistency of your stools?"
   D. "What does the skin around the stoma look like?"
   E. "Have you had any bleeding from your hemorrhoids?"

8. The healthcare provider suspects a patient is experiencing gastrointestinal effects from parasites. For which diagnostic test should the nurse prepare this patient to confirm the diagnosis?
   A. Colonoscopy
   B. Barium enema
   C. Stool specimen
   D. CT of the abdomen
9. A patient learns that during a colonoscopy two polyps were removed. Why is the removal of these structures important?
   A. Helps to identify genetic disorders.
   B. Prevents the development of cancer.
   C. Facilitates further examination of the bowel.
   D. Decreases future problems with constipation.
10. While conducting a health history, the nurse asks a patient if any family members had or have colon cancer. Which other questions help to assess increased risk for colon cancer? (Select all that apply.)
   A. "Have you ever been diagnosed with inflammation of the colon?"
   B. "Have you ever been diagnosed with breast or ovarian cancer?"
   C. "Have you ever been exposed to unpasteurized milk?"
   D. "Has anyone in your family been diagnosed with colon cancer."
   E. "Do you have asthma?"

See Test Yourself answers in Appendix B.

REFERENCES

D'Amico, D., & Barbarito, C. (2016). *Health and physical assessment in nursing* (2nd ed.). Upper Saddle River, NJ: Pearson Prentice Hall.

Gimenes, F. R. E., Reis, R. K., dos Santos da Silva, P. C., de Carmargo Silva, A. E. B., & Atila, E. (2016). Nursing assessment tool for people with liver cirrhosis. *Gastroenterology Nursing, 39*(4), 264–272.

Han, C. J., Heitkemper, M. M., & Jarrett, M. E. (2016). Fatigue measures in noncancer gastrointestinal disorders. *Gastroenterology Nursing, 39*(6), 443–454.

Hay, J. M., Barnette, W., & Shaw, S. E. (2016). Changing practice in gastrointestinal endoscopy. *Gastrointestinal Nursing, 39*(3), 181–185.

Henderson, W. A., Williams, B., Kim, K. H., Sherwin, L. B., Abey, S. K., Martino, A. C., . . . Zuccolotto, A. P. (2017). The gastrointestinal pain pointer: A valid and innovative method to assess gastrointestinal symptoms. *Gastroenterology Nursing, 40*(5), 357–362.

Jennings, A. (2015). Assessing oral hygiene in hospitalized older veterans. *MEDSURG Nursing, 24*(6), 420–424.

Kee, J. (2018). *Laboratory and diagnostic tests with nursing implications* (10th ed.). Upper Saddle River, NJ: Pearson Prentice Hall.

Kunz, L., & Gillespie, D. (2017). A comparison of bowel preparations for colonoscopy in constipated adults. *Gastroenterology Nursing, 40*(5), 364–374.

McElroy, K. G., Chung, S. Y., & Regan, M. (2017). Health and the human microbiome: A primer for nurses. *American Journal of Nursing, 117*(7), 24–30.

National Eating Disorders Association. (2018). *Suicidality and eating disorders among LGBTQ youth 2018: A national assessment.* Retrieved from https://www.nationaleatingdisorders.org/blog/eating-disorders-among-lgbtq-youth.

Quatrara, B. (2015, March/April). Nutrition to improve outcomes. *MEDSURG Nursing Newsletter*, pp. 2–15.

Spector, R. E. (2017). *Cultural diversity in health and illness* (9th ed.). Upper Saddle River, NJ: Pearson Education.

United States Department of Agriculture (USDA). (n.d.). *My Plate.* https://www.cnpp.usda.gov/MyPlate.

United States Department of Health and Human Services. (n.d.). *2015–2020 Dietary guidelines for Americans.* Retrieved from https://health.gov/dietaryguidelines/2015/guidelines/.

Young, V. B. (2017). The role of the microbiome in human health and disease: An introduction for clinicians. *British Medical Journal, 356*, j831.

ADDITIONAL RESOURCES

Alcoholics Anonymous
www.aa.org

American College of Gastroenterology (ACG)
http://patients.gi.org

American Liver Foundation
www.liverfoundation.org

Chronic Liver Disease Foundation
www.chronicliverdisease.org

The Society of Gastroenterology Nurses and Associates
www.sgna.org

Chapter 22

Nursing Care of Patients with Nutritional Disorders

Chapter Outline and Learning Outcomes

CLINICAL COMPETENCIES

- Assess and monitor the health status of patients with nutritional disorders, recognizing and reporting unexpected manifestations or responses to treatment.
- Using assessment data, research, and current standards of practice, plan and implement evidence-based nursing care for patients with nutritional disorders.
- Administer medications and enteral and parenteral nutrition knowledgeably and safely.
- Collaborate and coordinate with the patient and other members of the interprofessional care team to plan, prioritize, implement, and evaluate care.
- Incorporate cultural values and customs and personal preferences into the plan of care for patients with nutritional disorders.
- Use holistic data to plan and provide care and to evaluate care and responses to interventions focused on health teaching and health coaching.
- Use technology and information management tools to provide preventative interventions and health teaching for patients and populations at risk for developing complications resulting from nutritional disorders.

KEY TERMS

anorexia nervosa, 682
bariatrics, 660
basal metabolic rate (BMR), 661
binge-eating disorder, 682
body mass index (BMI), 660
bulimia nervosa, 682
catabolism, 674
enteral nutrition, 676
lower body obesity, 662
malnutrition, 673
metabolic syndrome, 662
nutrients, 661
obesity, 660
parenteral nutrition (PN), 678
protein-calorie malnutrition (PCM), 674
sarcopenic obesity, 662
starvation, 674
triglycerides, 661
upper body obesity, 661
very low calorie diet (VLCD), 665

22.1 Obesity

The World Health Organization (WHO; 2018) defines overweight and **obesity** as "abnormal or excessive fat accumulation that may impair health." Obesity is one of the most prevalent and preventable health problems in the United States and throughout the world (WHO, 2018). Obesity has serious physiologic and psychologic consequences and is associated with increased morbidity and mortality. It contributes to poor health-related quality of life to a greater extent than smoking, excess alcohol use, or poverty. The prevalence of obesity in the United States is high, with more than one in three in the adult population being obese (National Institute of Diabetes and Digestive and Kidney Diseases, 2018). The obesity epidemic has prompted rapid growth in **bariatrics**, the healthcare science that focuses on patients who are extremely obese. Obesity is associated with comorbid conditions such as coronary heart disease, type 2 diabetes mellitus, and various types of cancer, gallstones, and disability. These comorbid health problems are associated with higher use of healthcare services and costs among patients with obesity. Obesity is also associated with an increased risk for death, particularly in adults younger than 65 years of age (Kushner, 2015). Health-related problems associated with obesity are listed in **Table 22.1**.

Although obesity is often defined by weight, it is more accurately defined by the **body mass index (BMI)**, an indirect measure of the amount of body fat, or adipose tissue. Adipose tissue is created when energy consumption exceeds energy expenditure. A BMI of 25 to 29.9 is classified as *overweight*; obesity is a BMI of 30 or greater (CDC, 2015b). The terms *overweight* and *obese* are not mutually exclusive; a patient who is obese also is overweight.

Incidence and Prevalence

More than 39% of the adult population in the United States is obese and over two-thirds of all adults in the United States are overweight (National Center for Health Statistics, 2017). Approximately 1 in 20 Americans has a BMI greater than 40 (Centers for Disease Control and Prevention [CDC], 2015b). The prevalence of obesity is higher in women and in economically disadvantaged people of all races (National Center for Health Statistics, 2016). The prevalence of overweight has been increasing since 1960, and the prevalence of obesity is also increasing (CDC, 2015b). However, there are signs that the increasing prevalence is beginning to slow because of systematic strategies to education and available resources to the public (Budd & Peterson, 2014). Of particular concern is the increasing incidence of obesity in children and young adults. Adults of Asian heritage generally have a lower incidence of overweight and obesity compared with all other race and Hispanic-origin groups (CDC, 2017).

Table 22.1 Complications and Health-Related Problems Associated with Obesity

Body System	Obesity-Related Problems
Cardiovascular	■ Atherosclerosis ■ Congestive heart failure ■ Cor pulmonale ■ Coronary heart disease ■ Heart failure ■ Hypercholesterolemia ■ Hypertension ■ Pulmonary embolis ■ Stroke ■ Varicosities ■ Venous thrombosis
Respiratory	■ Asthma ■ Dyspnea ■ Hypoventilation syndrome ■ Obstructive sleep apnea ■ Pickwickian syndrome
Gastrointestinal	■ Cholelithiasis ■ Colon cancer ■ Gastroesophageal reflux disease ■ Hiatal hernia ■ Nonalcoholic fatty liver disease
Genitourinary	■ Obesity-related glomerulopathy ■ Prostate cancer ■ Urinary stress incontinence
Musculoskeletal	■ Hyperuricemia and gout ■ Immobility ■ Low back pain ■ Muscle strains and sprains ■ Osteoarthritis
Endocrine and reproductive	■ Breast and endometrial cancers ■ Diabetes mellitus, type 2 ■ Metabolic syndrome ■ Polycystic ovarian syndrome ■ Pregnancy complications
Integumentary	■ Cellulitis ■ Lymphedema ■ Straie distensae ■ Stasis pigmentation of legs
Other	■ Postoperative complications ■ Psychosocial ■ Depression/low self-esteem ■ Body image disturbance ■ Social stigmatization

According to the National Center for Health Statistics (Hales, Carroll, & Ogden, 2017), the prevalence of individuals who are obese in the United States is:

Women

- Non-Hispanic Black: 54.8%
- Hispanic: 50.6%
- Non-Hispanic White: 38%
- Non-Hispanic Asian: 14.8%

Men

- Hispanic: 43.1%
- Non-Hispanic White: 37.9%
- Non-Hispanic Black: 36.9%
- Non-Hispanic Asian: 10.1%

Risk Factors

Many factors contribute to obesity, including genetic, physiologic, metabolic, psychologic, behavioral, environmental, and sociocultural factors. Recent genetic research provides emerging understanding into the genesis of obesity. There is a strong correlation between the weight of adopted children and their biologic parents; in addition, identical twins tend to have similar BMIs, whether raised together or apart. Genetic influences contributing to obesity have been studied extensively over the past few decades and several genes that contribute to appetite and fat deposition have been identified (Sorenson, Quinn, & Klein, 2019).

Physical inactivity is a significant factor contributing to obesity. Inactive people may consume fewer calories than active people and continue to gain weight due to lack of energy expenditure. Social and environmental factors such as reliance on the automobile for transportation and increased time spent using the computer contribute to decreased energy expenditure among adults in the United States. Increased time spent watching television is seen as a major contributing factor to the increased incidence of obesity among children and adolescents (National Center for Health Statistics, 2017).

Environmental influences, such as an abundant and readily accessible food supply, fast-food restaurants, advertising, and vending machines, contribute to increased food intake. Sociocultural influences that contribute to obesity include increased consumption of restaurant meals, overeating at family meals, rewarding behavior with food, religious and family gatherings that promote food intake, and sedentary lifestyles. Socioeconomic status tends to correlate with the risk for overweight and obesity: In the United States, women with low incomes are more likely to be obese than those of higher socioeconomic status (National Center for Health Statistics, 2017). The association between socioeconomic status and obesity is less clear in men.

Psychologic factors, such as low self-esteem, also play a role in obesity. Low self-esteem may precipitate unhealthy eating behaviors, and the resulting weight gain in turn may diminish self-image even further. A person may overeat as a result of anxiety, depression, guilt, or boredom, or as a means of getting attention. Some experts characterize overeating as a food addiction and as a coping mechanism for stressful life events.

Overview of Normal Physiology

All body activities require energy, including activities of daily living, as well as those necessary to maintain cell and tissue function. **Nutrients** in food (or enteral or parenteral feedings) provide this energy and are the building blocks for growth and tissue repair. The body stores excess nutrients and energy (measured as kilocalories) to meet the body's needs when required nutrients are unavailable. This ability to store and release energy is important to maintaining body function. A significant portion of daily energy expenditure is fixed: More than 70% of the energy expended each day goes to maintaining the **basal metabolic rate (BMR)**, essentially the "cost" (in kilocalories) of being alive.

Energy is primarily stored as fat in adipose tissue. Although mature fat cells (adipocytes) do not multiply, the immature cells in adipose tissue can multiply, particularly when exposed to estrogen during puberty, in late adolescence, during breastfeeding, and in middle-aged adults who are overweight. Fat cells store excess energy as **triglycerides**, formed from dietary fats and carbohydrates. The body breaks down the triglycerides in fat cells when needed to provide energy (Sorenson et al., 2019).

The Patient with Obesity

Pathophysiology

Obesity occurs when excess calories are stored as fat. It can result from excess energy intake, decreased energy expenditure, or a combination of both. The etiology of obesity is not as simple as excess kilocalorie intake in relation to energy expenditure.

Energy intake and energy expenditure are regulated by a complex interaction of endocrine and neural signals. In the absence of external influences, these regulatory mechanisms increase appetite and reduce energy expenditure when weight loss occurs, and suppress appetite and increase energy expenditure after overfeeding. In a society where food is abundant and physical activity is limited, the latter is less effective.

Appetite, which affects food intake, is regulated by the central nervous system (CNS) and by emotional factors. The hunger center in the hypothalamus stimulates appetite in response to stimuli such as hypoglycemia and peptides produced in the gut. As nutrient levels rise, the satiety center (also in the hypothalamus) sends a message to stop eating. Gastrointestinal filling and hormonal factors also signal *satiety* (a sensation of fullness). Appetite may have little relationship to hunger or physical signals, however; some people eat to relieve depression or anxiety.

Several hormones are involved in regulating obesity, including thyroid hormone, insulin, and leptin (a peptide produced by fatty tissue that suppresses appetite and increases energy expenditure). Some studies suggest that leptin resistance is a cause of obesity. Insulin is associated with body fat distribution. The two major types of body fat distribution are upper body and lower body obesity (**Figure 22.1** ■).

Upper body obesity (*central obesity*) is identified by a waist-to-hip ratio of greater than 1 in men or 0.9 in women (Kushner, 2015). People with upper body obesity tend to have more intra-abdominal fat and higher levels of circulating free fatty acids (Sorenson et al., 2019). As a result, upper body obesity is associated with a greater risk of complications such as hypertension, abnormal blood lipid levels, heart disease, stroke, and elevated insulin levels. Men tend to have more intra-abdominal fat than women, although women develop a central fat distribution pattern after menopause.

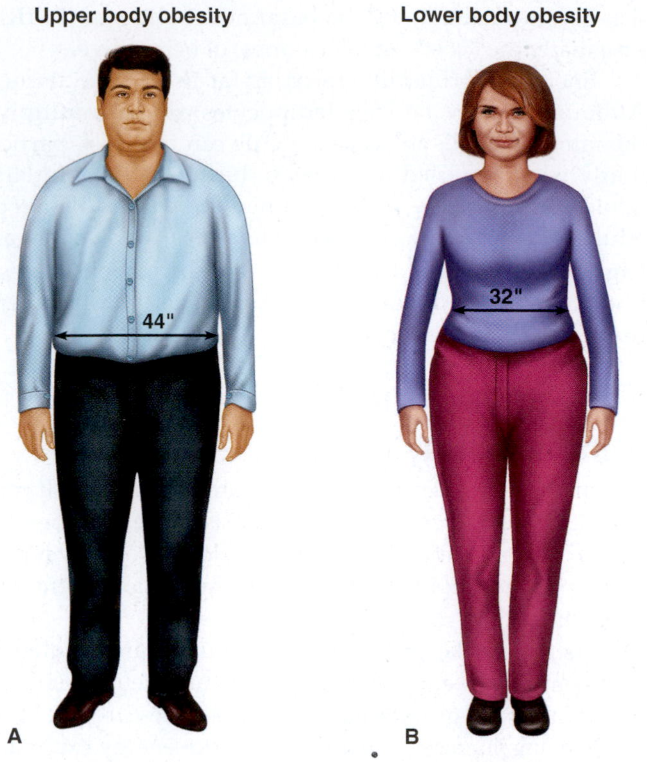
Upper body obesity
Lower body obesity
44"
32"
A
B

Figure 22.1 ■ Body fat distribution. **A**, upper body obesity. **B**, lower body obesity.

Lower body obesity (*peripheral obesity*), in which the waist-to-hip ratio is less than 0.9, is more commonly seen in women. The risk for hyperinsulinemia, abnormal lipids, and heart disease is lower in people with lower body obesity than in those with upper body obesity. Lower body obesity, however, may be more difficult to treat.

Sarcopenic obesity is associated with age-related loss of muscle mass and is described as the process of muscle loss combined with increased body fat (Laur & Keller, 2017). Sarcopenic obesity is more common in women and leads to loss of strength and function, reduced quality of life, and early death. Limited physical activity, disuse syndrome, decreased resting metabolic rate, and changes in dietary requirements are all variables that contribute to the increase in sarcopenic obesity in older adults.

Complications of Obesity

Obesity is a major health risk factor, increasing the risk of mortality from all causes over that of normal-weight people. As obesity increases, so does the risk of dying.

Cardiovascular Disease

Many obese individuals have **metabolic syndrome**, a constellation of cardiovascular risk factors, including increased waist circumference, hypertension, elevated blood triglycerides and fasting blood glucose, and low HDL cholesterol. Metabolic syndrome is an identified risk factor for atherosclerosis and coronary heart disease (CHD).

Obesity is a significant risk factor for cardiovascular disease, including hypertension, CHD, and heart failure. Several factors contribute to hypertension in individuals with obesity, increased vascular resistance, blood volume, and cardiac output. The increases in blood pressure seen with obesity increase the risk for CHD and stroke.

Patients who are obese, particularly those who have abdominal obesity, often have a lipid profile that promotes atherosclerosis. Levels of low-density lipoprotein (LDL) and very low-density lipoprotein (VLDL) cholesterol and triglycerides are increased, and levels of high-density lipoprotein (HDL or desirable) cholesterol are reduced. Furthermore, adipose tissue secretes cytokines that stimulate the liver to produce C-reactive protein (CRP), now recognized as a risk factor for CHD.

Obesity increases the risk for heart failure. Left-ventricular muscle mass increases, and the ventricle dilates in individuals with obesity, possibly related to increased blood volume and cardiac output.

Respiratory Disorders

Overweight and obesity increase the risk for developing asthma and COPD in adults. The relationship between obesity and asthma is not clear, but may be related to genetic factors and the connection between obesity and inflammation. Obesity is the major risk factor for obstructive *sleep apnea*, intermittent airflow obstruction due to upper airway collapse during sleep. Not only is obesity a risk factor for sleep apnea, the reverse also may be true: It may predispose patients for weight gain (Sorenson et al., 2019).

Diabetes Mellitus

Obesity increases the risk of insulin resistance and type 2 diabetes. While not all people who are obese develop diabetes, up to 80% of people with type 2 diabetes are obese. Both weight gain in adulthood and abdominal (central) obesity are positively correlated with the risk for developing type 2 diabetes (Sorenson et al., 2019).

Other Disorders

Obesity affects reproductive function in both men and women. Androgen (male sex hormone) levels are reduced in men with obesity; menstrual irregularities and polycystic ovarian syndrome (PCOS) are more common in women with obesity. PCOS is an additional risk factor for hyperinsulinemia and insulin resistance. Increased weight increases the risk for developing gallstones in both men and women. The risk for developing several types of cancer increases in obesity; these include colon, breast, and endometrial. Increased weight places abnormal stress on joints, increasing the prevalence of joint pain and osteoarthritis, particularly in weight-bearing joints (especially the knee joints). Refer to Table 22.1 for other health-related problems associated with obesity.

Interprofessional Care

The U.S. Preventative Services Task Force (USPSTF) recommends screening all adults for obesity and advocates for multicomponent behavioral interventions for adults with obesity (Moyer, 2012). Obesity treatment is far more complex than just reducing food consumption. Most experts recommend an individualized program of exercise, diet, and behavior modification designed to meet the patient's specific needs.

Diagnosis

Although body weight may be used to identify obesity, three key anthropometric measures should be considered in evaluating the degree of obesity: Weight, height, and waist circumference (Kushner, 2015). Males at ideal body weight have 10 to 20% body fat, whereas females at ideal body weight have 20 to 30% body fat.

- ***Body mass index*** is used to identify excess adipose tissue. BMI is calculated by dividing the weight (in kilograms) by the height in meters squared (m^2). BMI calculations may not as accurately reflect the extent of adipose tissue in people who are highly muscular (e.g., bodybuilders) or in those who have lost muscle mass (e.g., older adults). **Table 22.2** classifies overweight and obesity by BMI.
- ***Waist circumference*** measures excess abdominal fat and is assessed by measuring waste circumference or waist-to-hip ratio. Increased waist circumference indicates there is excess visceral adipose tissue, which is associated with higher risk for diabetes mellitus and cardiovascular disease (Kushner, 2015).
- ***Anthropometry*** includes measurements of height, weight, bone size, and skinfold to estimate subcutaneous fat. See Chapter 21 for more information about anthropometric measurements.
- ***Underwater weighing (hydrodensitometry)*** is considered the most accurate way to determine body fat. This technique involves submerging the whole body and then measuring the amount of displaced water.
- ***Bioelectrical impedance*** uses a low-energy electrical impulse to determine the percentage of body fat by measuring the electrical resistance of the body.

Other diagnostic tests may be done to help identify a physiologic cause of obesity, as well as complications of obesity:

- ***Thyroid profile*** is done to rule out thyroid disease.
- ***Serum glucose*** is measured to identify coexisting diabetes mellitus.
- ***Serum cholesterol*** is measured to assess for elevated levels.
- ***Lipid profile*** is ordered. HDL levels may be reduced in patients with obesity, whereas LDL levels are elevated.
- ***Electrocardiography (ECG)*** is performed to detect effects of obesity on the heart, such as rate or rhythm disruptions, myocardial infarction, or heart enlargement.

Table 22.2 Classification of Overweight and Obesity by Body Mass

Classification	Obesity Class	BMI	Risk of Disease
Underweight		< 18.5	
Normal		18.5–24.9	
Overweight		25–29.9	Increased
Obesity	I	30–34.9	High
Obesity	II	35–39.9	Very high
Obesity	III	≥ 40	Extremely high

Medications

The USPSTF suggests consideration of weight loss medications when the patient's BMI is 30 or greater than 27 with a comorbid condition. Drug therapy is not recommended for cosmetic weight loss. When used in combination with behavioral intervention that includes diet and exercise, drugs can help promote weight loss. The 2012 USPSTF clinical guidelines (Moyer, 2012) emphasize research that indicates the best outcomes are achieved when medication is combined with comprehensive treatment. Treatment includes 12 to 26 sessions a year in which progress is monitored and behavior modification is taught to develop healthy dietary habits and regular exercise.

Orlistat (Xenical) is a lipase inhibitor, reducing fat absorption from the GI tract and leading to weight loss. It reduces blood glucose and total and LDL cholesterol levels and lowers blood pressure. The adverse effects of orlistat relate to its inhibition of fat absorption: Oily stools, flatulence, and fecal urgency. These effects tend to diminish when dietary fat intake is limited.

Lorcaserin (Belviq) activates the serotonin 5-HT 2c receptor in the brain, causing an individual to feel full after eating smaller amounts and therefore eating less. Coadministration with other drugs that increase serotonin levels can lead to serotonin syndrome or even neuroleptic malignant syndrome. Consequently, lorcaserin should be avoided or used with extreme caution for patients taking selective serotonin reuptake inhibitors (SSRIs), serotonin-norepinephrine reuptake inhibitors (SNRIs), monoamine oxidase inhibitors (MAOIs), triptans, bupropion, dextromethorphan, or St. John's wort.

SAFETY ALERT: Lorcaserin should not be used with other medications that increase serotonin levels. ■

Qsymia is a combination of phentermine, a sympathomimetic amine anorectic, and topiramate extended release, an antiepileptic drug. This medication suppresses appetite and increases feelings of fullness, making food taste less appealing. It also increases calorie burning (Kushner, 2015).

Other drugs used as appetite suppressants include amphetamines and nonamphetamines and antidepressants such as bupropion (Wellbutrin, Zyban) and fluoxetine (Prozac). None of these drugs are approved for long-term use as appetite suppressants. Amphetamines carry a high abuse potential and are not approved for treating obesity. Nonamphetamines such as diethylpropion (Tenuate) and phentermine (Adipex-P) may be used, but these increase pulse rate and blood pressure.

Medication Administration 22.A

Drugs to Treat Obesity

APPETITE SUPPRESSANTS

phentermine (Adipex-P, Fastin, Ionamin, Obestin-30, Oby-Trim, others)

phentermine and topiramate extended release (Qsymia)

lorcaserin (Belviq)

Phentermine acts directly on the appetite-control center in the CNS to suppress the appetite and reduce hunger. Topiramate increases feelings of fullness and increases calorie burning.

Liraglutide (Saxenda, Victoza) is a glucagon-like peptide 1 (GLP-1) that causes increased insulin release and decreased glucagon release. Liraglutide is approved for the treatment of Type 2 diabetes but it also delays gastric emptying so has an independent weight loss effect.

Bupropion and naltrexone (Contrave) is a combination medication—a dopamine and norepinephrine reuptake inhibitor and opioid receptor antagonist. The combination decreases the motivation/reinforcement that food provides (dopamine effect) and the pleasure/palatability of eating (opioid effect).

Lorcaserin (Belviq) activates the serotonin 5-HT 2c receptor in the brain, which causes a person to feel full after eating smaller amounts of food.

These drugs may be used to treat obesity in patients with a BMI > 30 and patients with a BMI > 27 who have risk factors such as diabetes or hypertension.

Nursing Responsibilities

- Assess for contraindications, such as pregnancy or lactation, use of other appetite suppressants, impaired liver or kidney function, history of CHD, or alcohol abuse.
- Regularly monitor blood pressure and heart rate during treatment. Increases may indicate need to reduce dose or discontinue treatment.

Health Education for the Patient and Family

- Take as directed; do not exceed recommended dose. Do not take if you may be pregnant or are nursing.
- Take your last dose no later than 4:00 p.m. to avoid insomnia.
- You may experience difficulty sleeping, nervousness, or palpitations while taking this drug.
- Increase your fluid intake to reduce possible side effects of dry mouth and constipation.
- This drug does not replace diet and exercise for weight loss; continue to follow your prescribed regimen.

LIPASE INHIBITOR

orlistat (Alli, Xenical)

Orlistat inhibits lipases necessary for the breakdown and absorption of fat, thus decreasing the absorption of dietary fat. Its action is primarily local, within the GI tract, with few systemic effects.

Nursing Responsibilities

- Administer with meals or up to 1 hour following a meal.
- Provide a fat-soluble vitamin supplement (A, D, E, and K) daily. Separate administration time from orlistat by at least 2 hours.

Health Education for the Patient and Family

- Take as directed; do not increase dose. You may skip a dose if you do not consume a meal.
- Use in conjunction with a low-calorie, low-fat diet.
- Common gastrointestinal side effects include oily or fatty stools, flatulence, oily discharge, or frequent stools with difficulty controlling defecation. These side effects may diminish with time or increase if a meal high in fat is consumed.
- Notify your healthcare provider if you become pregnant while taking this medication.

Note: Drugs identified in *blue* are among the 200 most commonly prescribed medications in the U.S.

Source: Data from Adams, Holland, & Urban, 2017.

Treatment

Successful treatment of obesity (sustained achievement of normal body weight without adverse consequences) is challenging to achieve (Casazza et al., 2015). Research indicates most patients set unrealistic goals related to their ideal weight (Casazza et al., 2015). The nurse should assist the patient to create attainable goals that incorporate achievement of improved health outcomes. Studies indicate reducing body weight by 5 to 10% will result in positive health outcomes such as decreased blood pressure and improved glucose tolerance and cholesterol levels (Budd & Peterson, 2015). Treatment focuses on reducing the health risks associated with obesity by changing both eating and exercise habits (CDC, 2015a). A pound of body fat is equivalent to 3500 kcal. To lose 1 pound a person must reduce caloric intake by 500 kcal a day for 7 days or increase activity enough to burn the equivalent kilocalories. Research shows obese and overweight individuals may benefit from aggressive behavioral interventions aimed at reducing daily caloric intake and increasing physical activity (Budd & Peterson, 2015).

The USPSTF recommends screening all adults for obesity and patients with a BMI of 30 should be referred to intensive multicomponent behavioral interventions. A combination of physical activity, dietary therapy, behavior modification, pharmacology, and, in some cases, surgery is required to achieve and maintain weight loss.

See **Table 22.3** for treatment recommendations.

Exercise. Exercise is a critical element in weight loss and maintenance. Physical activity increases energy consumption and promotes weight loss while preserving lean body mass. Physical activity improves physical fitness, decreases appetite, promotes self-esteem, and increases the basal metabolic rate. The CDC recommends that all adults engage in both aerobic and muscle-strengthening activities each week and research indicates aerobic and resistance exercise combined with diet will yield greater outcomes in obese older adults and is more effective than diet and aerobic exercise only (Villareal et al., 2018). **Table 22.4** outlines CDC activity recommendations and gives example activities to achieve goals. Activities should be spread throughout the week and may be spread over the course of the day; however, it is

Table 22.3 Treatment Recommendations for Overweight and Obesity

Treatment	BMI				
	25–26.9	27–29.9	30–34.9	35–39.9	≥40
Diet, exercise, and behavior modification	With two or more comorbidities[1]	With two or more comorbidities[1]	Yes	Yes	Yes
Pharmacotherapy[2]		With two or more comorbidities[1]	Yes	Yes	Yes
Surgery			With two or more comorbidities[1]		

[1]For example, hypertension, hyperlipidemia, diabetes, and other obesity-related complications.
[2]Considered when 6 months of combined therapy has not produced a loss of 1 pound per week.
Source: Adapted from National Institutes of Health; National Heart, Lung, and Blood Institute; North American Association for the Study of Obesity. (2000). *The practical guide: Identification, evaluation, and treatment of overweight and obesity in adults.* Bethesda, MD: National Institutes of Health.

Table 22.4 CDC Physical Activity Recommendations for Adults

Activity	Recommendation	Examples
Aerobic activity	Engage in moderate- or vigorous-intensity activity for at least the recommended amount of time weekly, or in an equivalent combination of moderate- and vigorous-intensity activity.	
■ Moderate-intensity aerobic activity (target heart rate of 50 to 70% of maximum heart rate)	Two hours and 30 minutes (150 minutes) every week	■ Walking fast ■ Water aerobics ■ Bicycle riding on level ground ■ Doubles tennis ■ Ballroom dancing ■ Pushing a lawn mower ■ General gardening
■ Vigorous-intensity aerobic activity (target heart rate of 70 to 85% of maximum heart rate)	One hour and 15 minutes (75 minutes) every week	■ Race walking, jogging, running ■ Swimming laps ■ Singles tennis ■ Aerobic dancing ■ Bicycling 10 mph or faster ■ Heavy gardening (continuous hoeing or digging) ■ Hiking uphill
Muscle-strengthening activities	Two or more days per week: At least one set of 8 to 12 repetitions for all major muscle groups	■ Lifting weights ■ Using resistance bands ■ Exercises that use body weight for resistance (push-ups, sit-ups) ■ Heavy gardening ■ Yoga

Source: Data from CDC, 2015a.

important to expend moderate or vigorous effort for at least 10 minutes at a time when exercising (CDC, 2015a).

Because fitness levels differ, patients may be taught to use their target heart rate or perceived exertion to measure the vigor of activities. The *target heart rate* is calculated based on maximum heart rate; in turn, maximum heart rate is estimated using the formula 220 minus age in years. For example, while the maximum heart rate for a 35-year-old is 185 beats per minute (bpm), it would be 155 bpm for someone who is 65 years old. While the target heart rate for the 35-year-old engaging in vigorous, intense activity would be 130 to 157 bpm, it would be 108 to 132 bpm for the older adult. Perceived exertion is a subjective rating of activity intensity, using self-evaluation of factors such as heart and respiratory rate, sweating, and muscle fatigue (CDC, 2015a).

Nutrition. The diet is planned to create a daily 500- to 1000-kcal deficit. Ideally, the diet should be low in kilocalories and fat and contain adequate nutrients, minerals, and fiber. The patient should eat regular meals with small servings. A gradual, slow weight loss of no more than 1 to 2 pounds per week is recommended. This means a diet of 1000 to 1200 kcal/day for most women and 1200 to 1600 kcal/day for most men. Fewer than 1200 kcal each day may lead to loss of lean tissue and nutritional deficiencies. The recommended diet is generally low in fat and high in dietary fiber (**Table 22.5**). Excessive calorie restrictions can lead to failure to follow the prescribed diet, feelings of guilt, and overeating. Repeated cycles of weight loss and gain (sometimes called *yo-yo dieting*) may lead to a metabolic deficiency that makes subsequent weight loss efforts increasingly difficult.

Very low calorie diets (VLCD) are generally reserved for patients who have a BMI greater than 30 (Kushner, 2015). This type of program offers a protein-sparing modified fast (450 kcal/day) under close medical supervision (Kushner, 2015). VLCDs typically use commercially prepared formulas (liquid shakes or bars) to replace all food intake for several weeks or months, resulting in rapid weight loss while maintaining lean body mass. Exercise, nutrition, and behavior modification counseling should accompany the diet. Benefits include decreased blood pressure, blood glucose, and

Table 22.5 Recommended Nutrient Intake for Weight Loss

Nutrient	Recommended Intake
Calories	1000–1600 per day or approximately 500–1000 less than usual daily intake
Total fat	30% or less of total calories
Saturated fats	10% or less of total calories
Cholesterol	300 mg/day
Protein (from plant and lean animal sources)	Approximately 15% of total calories
Carbohydrate (complex carbohydrates from vegetables, fruits, and whole grains)	55% or more of total calories
Fiber (e.g., oat bran, legumes, barley, most fruits and vegetables)	20–30 g/day
Sodium chloride	< 2.4 g sodium or 6 g sodium chloride/day
Calcium	1000–1500 mg/day

Source: Adapted from National Institutes of Health; National Heart, Lung, and Blood Institute; North American Association for the Study of Obesity. (2000). *The practical guide: Identification, evaluation, and treatment of overweight and obesity in adults.* Bethesda, MD: National Institutes of Health.

cholesterol and triglyceride levels, along with improved exercise tolerance. VLCD may not be appropriate for use in people over age 50 due to normal loss of lean body mass and adverse effects such as fatigue, constipation, nausea, diarrhea, and gallstone formation. In the long term, weight gain is common, and VLCD may be no more effective for weight loss than a diet that includes 800 to 1000 daily kcal (Kushner, 2015).

Behavior Modification. Behavior modification is a critical component of successful weight management. Strategies such as keeping food records, eliminating cues that precipitate eating, and changing the act of eating are often helpful.

Recording food intake, amount, location of eating, and situations that induce eating often help the patient gain self-control. Researchers have found that most people who are overweight are stimulated to eat by external cues, such as the proximity to food and the time of day. In contrast, hunger and satiety are the cues that regulate eating in adults of normal weight. Strategies to control food cues include keeping food out of view, eliminating snack foods, and eating only in designated areas. See **Box 22.1** for a list of behavior modification strategies.

Other strategies focus on helping patients examine factors such as lifestyle, personality, and environment that affect eating behaviors. The goal is to empower the individual who is overweight to choose activities that are not related to food. Smartphone and computer technology offer access to free and low-cost applications that can assist patients to monitor caloric intake and physical activity. Several applications provide immediate feedback and generate individualized reminders and encouraging messages (Budd & Peterson, 2015). Wearable health monitoring technology allow patients to track activity, caloric expenditure, and physiological response such as heart rate, thereby providing immediate information and the ability to track progress toward exercise and weight loss goals over time. As nurses assume more roles in primary care (Bauer & Bodenheimer, 2017), becoming familiar with high impact weight-loss computer/smartphone resources and other wearable technology that can aid in monitoring diet and exercise is becoming increasingly important. When counseling patients with the uses of smartphone/computer applications the nurse should instruct them to look for an application with the following features (Budd & Peterson, 2015):

- An easy-to-use calorie tracker
- A high-capacity database of foods with nutritional information calculated according to serving size
- A bar scanner that allows the patient to upload information about prepared foods to the application database
- Interface with activity application and wearable technology.

BOX 22.1
Behavioral Change Strategies for the Patient with Obesity

CONTROLLING THE ENVIRONMENT

- Purchase low-calorie foods.
- Shop from a prepared list and on a full stomach.
- Keep all foods in the kitchen.
- Store all foods in the refrigerator or in the cabinets in opaque containers.
- Prepare exact portions of food to eliminate leftovers.
- Eat all foods in the same place.
- Avoid eating when watching television or reading.
- Develop behavioral strategies to maintain diet when eating out at restaurants, parties, and picnics.

CONTROLLING PHYSIOLOGIC RESPONSES TO FOOD

- Eat slowly by taking small bites, allowing 20 minutes for a meal.
- Eat a salad or drink a hot beverage before a meal.
- Chew each bite thoroughly and slowly.
- Put eating utensils or food down between bites.
- Concentrate on the eating process; savor the food.
- Stop eating with the first feelings of fullness.

CONTROLLING PSYCHOLOGIC RESPONSES TO FOOD

- Appreciate the aesthetic experience of eating.
- Use attractive dinnerware, and prepare a formal setting for eating.
- Use small plates and cups to make servings of food look larger.
- Concentrate on conversations and socialization during the meal.
- Use nonfood rewards for meeting a goal.
- Acknowledge small successes and improvements in all behavior.
- Substitute other activities for eating (e.g., reading, exercise, hobbies).

Social support and group programs such as Weight Watchers, Overeaters Anonymous, and Take Off Pounds Sensibly (TOPS) promote weight loss success through peer support. Most organized programs require participants to pay a fee, which may improve compliance.

Surgery. Surgical treatment of obesity (*bariatric surgery*) is generally limited to patients who are extremely obese (BMI over 40) who have had previous unsuccessful attempts at weight loss or those with a BMI greater than 35 who have serious obesity-related problems such as type 2 diabetes, CHD, poorly controlled hypertension, or severe sleep apnea (Schauer et al., 2017; Schiavon et al., 2017; Shukla, Buniak, & Aronne, 2015). In addition, patients must be able to tolerate surgery and be free of addiction to alcohol or other drugs. The benefits of surgery include major weight loss and improved blood pressure, plus a reduced risk of diabetes, sleep apnea, angina, heart failure, blood lipid levels, and venous disease. Bariatric surgery, however, is not without risk, and the decision to undergo surgery is a significant one.

The three major categories of bariatric surgery are classified as restrictive, malabsorptive, or a combination of both (Shukla et al., 2015). Restrictive procedures include vertical gastroplasty and adjustable gastric banding (AGB). Malabsorptive procedures with a restrictive component include Roux-en-Y gastric bypass, vertical sleeve gastrectomy, and biliopancreatic diversion with duodenal switch. Surgeons sometimes use a combination of both restrictive and malabsorptive procedures and, in general, more weight loss is achieved with more complex procedures.

The most common bariatric surgical procedures are AGB, gastric bypass, gastric sleeve, and biliopancreatic bypass with duodenal switch (**Figure 22.2** ■). These procedures restrict stomach capacity, limiting food intake, and, in most cases, bypass a portion of the small intestine to restrict absorption of calories and nutrients. In many cases, they can be performed laparoscopically.

The *Roux-en-Y gastric bypass* (Figure 22.2A), often called *gastric bypass*, creates a small stomach pouch to restrict food intake. A Y-shaped section of the jejunum is then attached to the pouch to allow food to bypass the lower stomach and duodenum. As a result, calorie and nutrient absorption is limited. The *vertical sleeve gastrectomy* (Figure 22.2B) was used as the first step in the biliopancreatic diversion with duodenal switch surgery but is often now used as a stand-alone procedure for high-risk patients with severe obesity. The surgery involves removal of a large portion of the stomach, leaving only a gastric sleeve. The procedure restricts intake and slows digestion. The *biliopancreatic diversion with duodenal switch surgery* (Figure 22.2C) is a more complex procedure and carries a higher risk of nutritional deficiencies and is usually performed for patients with severe obesity. This surgery, which is irreversible, may be performed in two stages, with the majority of the stomach removed and a gastric sleeve created during the first stage. Additionally, the duodenum and jejunum are bypassed by connecting the ileum directly to the stomach pouch or just distal to the pyloric valve. The surgery both restricts intake and slows digestion and absorption, and it has been shown to result in substantial weight loss and to significantly reduce the comorbidities associated with severe obesity (Budd & Peterson, 2015).

These surgeries that restrict nutrient intake and absorption produce rapid weight loss that is maintained over time. Many patients maintain a significant weight loss for 10 years or more, with improvement in obesity-associated health problems such as type 2 diabetes, hypertension, and sleep apnea. Because these procedures allow food to bypass the duodenum and jejunum, nutrient deficiencies are common, particularly of iron, calcium, vitamin B_{12}, and, possibly, the fat-soluble vitamins.

Restrictive procedures, such as *adjustable gastric banding* (*AGB*; Figure 22.2D), are safer and reversible, but generally less effective in the long term. In AGB, a hollow band of silicone rubber is placed around the upper (proximal) portion of the stomach. The band is inflated with saline solution to create a small stomach pouch with a narrow passage through to the rest of the stomach. The amount of band inflation can be adjusted using a port implanted under the skin. Few nutritional deficiencies are associated with restrictive bariatric procedures. Vomiting is a common postoperative risk with restrictive procedures. The band may slip or break, necessitating a return to surgery. Although patients typically lose about 50% of their excess body weight within the first year after these procedures, fewer maintain that weight loss over a 10-year period than those undergoing gastric bypass. The AGB is the safest of the available procedures and the FDA has approved the use of adjustable gastric bands for adults ages 18 and older with obesity. *Vertical-banded gastroplasty* (*VBG* Figure 22.2E) is a restrictive procedure sometimes referred to as *stomach stapling*. The surgeon cuts a small hole into the stomach a few inches below the esophagus and creates a small pouch by placing a line of staples to section off a small portion of the upper stomach. The pouch is anchored distally by a prosthetic band. The band slows digestion and the small stomach capacity gives the patient a feeling of early satiety.

Although the risk for postoperative complications is high, the mortality rate for bariatric procedures is low (less than 1% for restrictive surgeries and up to 5% for combination procedures). Possible postoperative complications include anastomosis leak with peritonitis, abdominal wall hernia, gallstones, wound infections, deep venous thrombosis and pulmonary embolism, nutritional deficiencies, and gastrointestinal symptoms. *Dumping syndrome*, a common complication that can be precipitated by a meal high in simple carbohydrates, may develop following gastric bypass surgeries. In dumping syndrome, stomach contents move rapidly through the small intestine, drawing fluid into the intestine by osmosis. Symptoms can arise 15 minutes to 2 hours after eating and generally last about 30 minutes. The patient experiences nausea, bloating, abdominal pain, diarrhea, weakness, sweating, tachycardia, and possibly syncope. Patients should be instructed to avoid foods high in simple carbohydrates. Meals should be small and

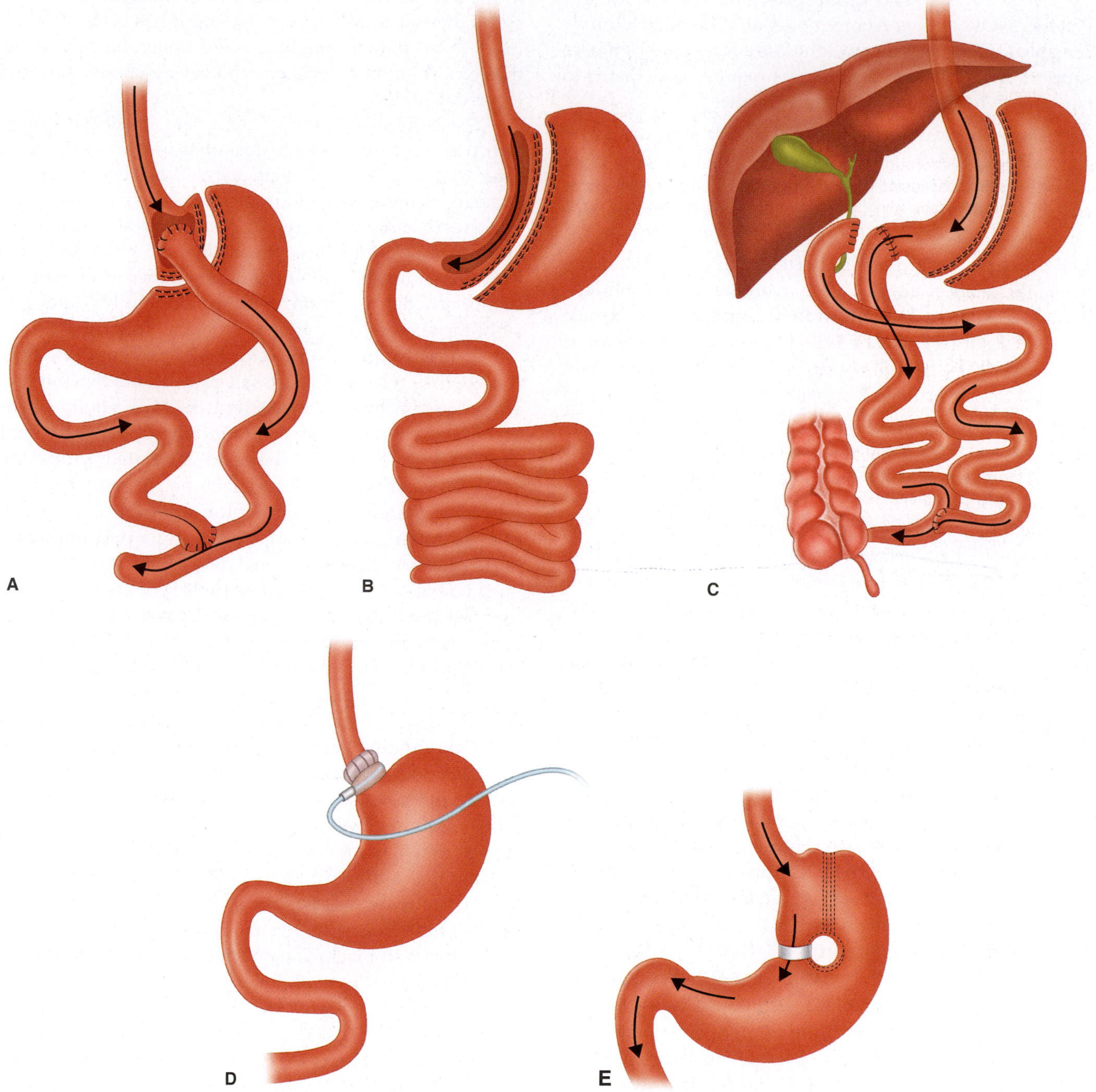
A
B
C
D
E

Figure 22.2 ■ Surgical procedures to treat obesity: **A**, Roux-en-Y gastric bypass. **B**, Vertical sleeve gastrectomy. **C**, Biliopancreatic diversion with duodenal switch. **D**, Adjustable gastric banding. **E**, Vertical-banded gastroplasty.

liquids and solids should not be taken together. Patients who undergo laparoscopic Roux-en-Y and patients with preexisting hyperlipidemia or gastroesophageal reflux disease are at high risk for dumping syndrome (Rodgers & Phillips, 2018).

Nursing care for the patient who has undergone bariatric surgery is outlined in **Box 22.2**. See also Chapter 23 for more information about gastric resection and associated nursing care. Bariatric patients have additional nursing care needs related to their obesity, as discussed in the Moving Evidence into Action box.

Maintaining Weight Loss

Losing weight and maintaining that loss are two separate but related issues. Most experts agree that the majority of dieters regain lost weight within a 2-year period. The potential risks associated with regaining weight make maintenance a critical issue. Patients are encouraged to continue exercise, self-monitoring, and treatment support. Long-term weight loss and maintenance mean a lifelong commitment to significant lifestyle changes, including food and eating habits, activity and exercise routines, and

BOX 22.2
Nursing Care of the Patient Undergoing Bariatric Surgery

Patients who are severely obese and who undergo bariatric or general surgery have unique nursing care needs to ensure personal and caregiver safety.

- Obtain a thorough preoperative health history and physical assessment (including skin assessment). Note any limitations of mobility or assistive devices used. *Bariatric patients often have multiple chronic health problems that may affect postoperative assessment and recovery. Skinfolds are at high risk for fungal infections that may compromise immune protection. Knowing about and providing assistive devices to accommodate mobility limitations will help promote early postoperative mobilization and reduce the risk for complications.*
- Obtain equipment of appropriate size and weight capacity, including bed, mechanical lifts, expanded-capacity wheelchair, walker, commode, bedside chair (without arms), sphygmomanometer, and scale. Clearly label any equipment provided by the patient. *Appropriately sized equipment is vital to promote the patient's comfort and safety. Equipment made to meet the needs of patients who are within normal weight and BMI measurements may fail or the patient may not be able to sit or recline without the risk of falling.*
- Provide friction-reducing devices such as sliders, foam, or pressure-reducing mattresses. *Following surgery, mobility may be limited. Special equipment facilitates skin care while helping maintain patient and caregiver safety.*
- Ensure training and availability of nursing staff in adequate numbers to ensure patient and caregiver safety during position changes, transfers, and caregiving activities such as hygiene. *Even with use of appropriate lifts, sliders, and other devices, as many as six to eight caregivers may be necessary to safely move and transfer the bariatric patient.*
- Elevate the head of the bed. Apply a continuous positive airway pressure (CPAP) device as ordered. *Thoracic and abdominal fat may restrict lung capacity, particularly when the patient is supine. Elevating the head of the bed reduces the pressure of abdominal fat on the diaphragm. Patients who are obese are at risk for obstructive sleep apnea due to upper airway collapse; CPAP helps maintain upper airway patency.*
- Frequently monitor level of consciousness and respiratory status (rate, breath sounds, and oxygen saturation). *The postsurgical bariatric patient may sequester anesthetic agents in fatty tissue, increasing the risk for respiratory depression after surgery.*
- Initiate cardiac monitoring and compare heart rhythm to preoperative ECG. Promptly report changes in rate or rhythm, such as frequent premature ventricular contractions. *The patient with obesity is at significant risk for CHD; surgery and anesthesia place an additional risk for cardiovascular complications. Development of dysrhythmias not seen preoperatively may indicate myocardial ischemia, hypoxia, or electrolyte imbalance.*
- Assess peripheral pulses, skin color, and temperature of extremities. Apply elastic compression stockings or sequential compression device of appropriate size for the patient. Teach and remind to perform foot and leg exercises. *The patient with obesity is at significant risk for developing deep venous thrombosis due to alterations in clotting and immobility. Furthermore, multiple risk factors for atherosclerosis increase the likelihood of peripheral vascular disease and impaired circulation.*
- Assess pain level and analgesic effectiveness frequently. *Maintaining adequate pain relief is important to promote lung expansion and prevent respiratory complications in the bariatric patient.*
- Regularly monitor blood glucose levels, administering insulin as ordered. *Surgery is a physiologic stressor that causes increased cortisol levels that, in turn, can increase blood glucose levels.*
- Provide meticulous wound care, using strict aseptic technique and frequently assessing for signs of infection. *Excess adipose tissue impairs healing and immune function. Wound infection further delays healing and can be difficult to eradicate.*

behavior modification. Failure to maintain weight loss can lead to feelings of inadequacy, powerlessness, and hopelessness.

Nursing Care

Assessment

Collect the following data through the health history and physical examination:

- ***Health history:*** Risk factors; current and usual weight; recent weight gains or losses; perception of weight and effect on health; usual diet and food intake; exercise/activity patterns; prior weight loss efforts and results; current medications; coexisting disorders such as cardiovascular disease and diabetes; tobacco use; family history of overweight, diabetes, and weight-related morbidity
- ***Physical examination:*** Vital signs; weight (use a scale of adequate capacity) and height; skinfold measurements; waist-to-hip ratio; BMI; inspect skin under the breasts and abdominal folds.

Priorities of Care

- Nursing care priorities for the patient seeking treatment for obesity must be patient centered and holistic, focusing on the physiologic, psychologic, and sociologic responses to weight and appearance.
- Ensuring that the patient maintains adequate nutrition and participates in supportive interventions required to make necessary diet and exercise habits permanent should be the focus of nursing care.
- The nurse collaborates with the interprofessional team in assisting the patient with various treatment options to include diet, exercise, medication, and possibly surgery.
- Monitor anthropometric measurements regularly during treatment to include weight and BMI. Assess general well-being with each patient encounter, including psychosocial status. Include diet recall, meat and snack patterns, food preparation methods, and dietary supplement use in assessment.

Moving Evidence into Action

Self-Care for Patients Undergoing Bariatric Surgery

Clinical Issue

Severe obesity is a chronic disease associated with adverse effects on quality of life, incurring significant health risks and increased risk for serious comorbid disease. Success with achieving desired weight loss and maintenance is dependent on adherence to a complex set of behaviors over time. Treatment of obesity and follow-up care after bariatric surgery encompasses a multitude of health-related issues. Patients need specialized resources and ongoing intraprofessional care for several years.

External Evidence

A comprehensive review of the literature was completed to achieve two aims: (1) To identify current evidence on adherence to pre- and postoperative self-management strategies aimed at increasing the success of bariatric surgery and (2) to make recommendations for improving adherence to treatment strategies identified as important to achieve positive post-surgical outcomes (Hood et al., 2016).

The authors reviewed and analyzed 79 studies and identified the following behaviors as significant for achieving and maintaining weight loss goals:

- Attending appointments
- Adhering to dietary recommendations
- Establishing and maintaining a postsurgical exercise regimen
- Adhering to recommendations for vitamin supplementation.

Continued encouragement to increase and maintain physical activity recommended during the preoperative period should be included in the postoperative plan of care. The authors conclude further nursing research is needed to identify which self-care activities are most important to implement postoperatively. Further studies should be conducted to determine which nursing interventions most effectively help patients to obtain and maintain their weight loss goals after surgery.

Internal Evidence

This analysis of the literature concludes individuals who undergo bariatric surgery need long-term follow-up utilizing the expertise of an intraprofessional team in order to maintain significant, permanent lifestyle changes.

Patient Considerations

Presurgical eating behaviors such as grazing and emotional eating and other behaviors associated with poor adherence to dietary advice must be addressed postoperatively. Barriers such as finances, time, home and work environment, and social situations should be assessed for all patients. Individual solutions should be developed using a variety of strategies such as increasing patient engagement, developing remotely delivered interventions, using smartphone apps, providing consistent and continuous screening, and using mobile health tools to facilitate patient self-monitoring of calorie intake, glucose level, physical activities, and other health variables through the use of technology.

Putting the Pieces Together

Achieving and maintaining significant weight loss is a struggle for most patients who are overweight and obese and these challenges persist after bariatric surgery. Current evidence points to the importance of using an interprofessional approach to behavior change and weight loss addressing teaching, coaching, and monitoring of reduced calorie intake and adherence to regular exercise. Engaging patients in an ongoing treatment plan using support groups or programs to help identify and maintain changes in eating behaviors yield positive outcomes. Patients frequently interact with nurses, which creates opportunity for providing health coaching and teaching on topics such as optimum diet, physical exercise, and adherence to vitamin supplementation. Nurses should be prepared to assist patients with strategies designed to meet their weight loss and health goals with every encounter.

References

Cooley, M. (2016). Preventing long-term poor outcomes in the bariatric patient postoperatively. *Dimensions of Critical Care Nursing*, *36*(1), 30–34.

Hood, M. M., Corsica, J., Bradley, L, Wilson, R., Chirinos, D., & Vivo, A. (2016). Managing severe obesity: Understanding and improving treatment adherence in bariatric surgery. *Journal of Behavioral Medicine*, *39*, 1092–1103.

- Monitor vital signs including blood pressure and blood glucose if patient has type 2 diabetes.
- Assess for clinical manifestations of nutritional deficiency.
- Monitor for side effects and drug interactions for patients using weight loss medications.

SAFETY ALERT: Use of an inappropriately sized sphygmomanometer is a common source of error in measuring blood pressure in patients with obesity. Choose a cuff on which the width of the bladder is 40% of the circumference of the arm and the length of the bladder is sufficient to cover at least 65% of the arm circumference. ■

Diagnoses, Outcomes, and Interventions

Support Weight Loss. Although many factors contribute to being overweight/obese, it always involves an imbalance of kilocalorie consumption to energy expenditure.

Expected Outcome: Patient will achieve weight loss goal through behaviors that promote optimal nutritional habits and exercise.

The nurse will:

- Encourage the patient to identify the factors that contribute to excess food intake. *Identification of cues to eating helps the patient eliminate or reduce these cues.*

- Establish realistic weight loss goals and exercise/activity objectives. *Small, reasonable goals, such as a loss of 1 to 2 pounds per week, increase the likelihood of success.*
- Assess the patient's knowledge and discuss diet plan options. Provide necessary teaching about diet. *Offering a selection of appropriate diet plans empowers the patient to choose a plan that best matches food preferences and lifestyle.*
- Discuss behavior modification strategies, such as self-monitoring and environmental management. *Behavior modification, diet, and exercise are critical to promoting successful, long-term weight loss.*
- Monitor weight loss, blood pressure, and laboratory data, including blood glucose and lipid levels. *Continuing assessment not only is important to evaluate the safety of weight loss strategies, but also to reinforce positive benefits of weight loss.* Refer to the Case Study and Nursing Care Plan.

Promote Activity Tolerance. Patients with obesity may experience excess fatigue, tachycardia, and shortness of breath with activity due to the physiologic effects of excess weight as well as a sedentary lifestyle. A medical evaluation may be needed before beginning an exercise program.

Expected Outcome: Patient will improve activity tolerance as demonstrated by decreased reports of activity-related fatigue and improved changes in heart rate, blood pressure, and breathing rate.

The nurse will:

- Assess current activity level and tolerance of that activity. Assess vital signs. *This provides baseline information when planning an activity program and assessing response to that activity.*
- After medical clearance, plan with the patient a program of regular, gradually increasing exercise. If desired, plan several 10- to 15-minute exercise periods over the course of the day. Develop plans for gradually increasing the duration and intensity of exercise. Consider a consultation with an exercise physiologist. *An individualized exercise program promotes activities within the patient's physical capabilities.*

Support Adherence to Treatment Plan. Most patients who are overweight or obese experience some difficulty integrating all the components of a weight loss program into a daily routine. To be successful, the patient who is overweight must modify dietary intake in a world of daily temptations. There may be many obstacles to exercise, including a busy schedule, activity intolerance, impaired physical mobility, lack of equipment, and the embarrassment of being fat.

Expected Outcome: Patient will implement resources to overcome barriers to incorporating healthy nutritional and exercise habits and will use identified behavioral and coping strategies to maintain dietary and exercise plan.

The nurse will:

- Discuss ability and willingness to incorporate changes into daily patterns of diet, exercise, and lifestyle. *This provides data from which to set realistic goals with the patient.*
- Help the patient identify behavior modification strategies and support systems for weight loss and maintenance. *Weight loss and maintenance are most successful if the patient establishes lifestyle patterns that promote interest and motivation and thus exercise and diet management. Family and social support is critical to successful adherence to the therapeutic regimen.*
- Have the patient establish strategies for dealing with "stress" eating or interruptions in the therapeutic regimen. *A sense of failure associated with overeating or lack of exercise can lead to further overeating. Identifying positive strategies to deal with these situations promotes self-acceptance and limits self-punishment through overeating.*

Promote Healthy Self-Esteem. Most individuals who are overweight or obese verbalize the experience of ridicule (sometimes called *fat prejudice*), embarrassment, and health problems attributed to being fat. These experiences, coupled with problems such as finding attractive clothing or a chair large enough to sit on, can affect self-esteem. Many patients report that fat jokes or comments contribute to a sense of negative self-worth.

Expected Outcome: Patient will demonstrate separation of self-perceptions from societal stigmas, describe personal strengths and attributes that will contribute to adhering to the weight loss plan, and identify positive coping skills to be used for achieving weight loss and exercise goals.

The nurse will:

- Encourage the patient to verbalize the experience of being overweight, and validate the patient's experience. *This provides baseline data to use in developing individualized interventions to address self-esteem issues.*
- Set small goals with the patient and offer positive feedback and encouragement. *Small goals provide more opportunities for success. Positive feedback and encouragement provide a comfortable environment in which to develop self-esteem.*
- Refer for counseling as appropriate. *Many patients benefit from counseling for issues related to self-esteem.*

Transitions of Care

Primary prevention interventions include nutritional assessment and health and lifestyle coaching which is likely to be addressed in the primary care setting. Secondary prevention strategies focused on frequent monitoring for the development of metabolic syndrome and other complications should be addressed in order initiate early treatment. Tertiary prevention includes monitoring for complications and the emergence of comorbidities associated with overweight/obesity.

The primary care nurse should document coaching sessions and health teaching provided to overweight and obese patients. The nurse should refer the patient to community-based weight loss programs when appropriate. Initiating referrals to clinics and providers specializing in caring for patients who are obese or overweight and experiencing complications is an important action in the primary care setting.

The acute care nurse must recognize obesity is a chronic condition and requires planning for continued treatment posthospitalization. Outcomes for bariatric patients are enhanced when the patient participates in postsurgical counseling and is monitored in a supportive postoperative clinical environment (Cooley, 2016). The acute care nurse should work with the interprofessional team to ensure the outpatient providers are aware of the patient's response to the bariatric surgery. Facilitating appropriate referrals and reinforcing the process for continued postoperative treatment should be included in the bariatric patient's discharge planning.

Obesity is a chronic disease that requires lifelong management. Chronic care is focused on managing the complications of obesity and related conditions such as metabolic syndrome. Many obese patients experience comorbidity such as heart disease and diabetes. The patient experiencing comorbidity related to the complications of obesity may require nurse case management to assist with coordinating, implementing, and evaluating complex treatment plans.

Weight reduction involves interprofessional care provided in a variety of settings. Continuity of care is essential for establishing and maintaining the treatment plan and necessary lifestyle changes. Weight loss and maintenance require a long-term commitment by the patient, family, and support systems. Address the following topics with the patient and family:

- Lifestyle changes are more effective than diets. Fad diets promote rapid weight loss but often are not nutritionally sound or may be difficult to maintain for a lifetime.
- All household members should consume a diet that is nutritionally sound, low in fat, and high in fiber.
- Establish realistic weight loss goals and a system of nonfood rewards for achieving each goal.
- Identify an exercise buddy or support system to promote continued physical activity.
- Expect occasional failures. Resume prescribed diet and exercise routine as soon as possible; the goal is long-term weight management.
- Community resources such as Weight Watchers, TOPS, or healthcare-based programs provide information, strategies, and support for successful weight management.

End-of-life care involves facilitating pain relief and symptom management. The nurse should monitor the effect of standard medications to relieve pain and other symptoms, noting the requirements for a therapeutic effect. The obese patient is at increased risk for respiratory distress and skin breakdown. The nurse should monitor respiratory status and initiate interventions focused on relieving the discomfort of dyspnea and initiate actions such as positioning and supplemental oxygen. The nurse should be vigilant in monitoring pressure points for the terminal bed-bound patient and promote frequent position changes to avoid pressure injuries.

End-of-life care will require the nurse to work with the interprofessional team to determine appropriate medication management aimed to promote optimum comfort.

Case Study & Nursing Care Plan

Patient with Obesity

Sam Elliott, age 57, has gained 30 pounds since his retirement 2 years ago. The most active thing he does each day is "puttering around" and "walking to the end of the driveway to get the mail." His 24-hour diet history includes juice, oatmeal, muffin, and coffee with cream for breakfast; doughnuts and coffee with friends midmorning; a bologna-and-cheese sandwich with chips and a root beer for lunch; and cheese, crackers, and wine before a dinner of meat, potatoes, vegetables, and dessert. He tells the nurse, "This is a pretty typical day. I have never had to diet. I just don't know how to get this weight off."

ASSESSMENT	DIAGNOSES	EXPECTED OUTCOMES
Mr. Elliott is 173 cm (5′ 8″) tall and weighs 91.2 kg (201 lb). His BMI is 30.1. His cholesterol is 240 mg/dL (normal 150 to 200 mg/dL) with an HDL of 37 mg/dL (normal male value > 45 mg/dL) and an LDL of 180 mg/dL (normal < 130 mg/dL). His BP is 138/90 mmHg. His fasting blood glucose is normal at 103 mg/dL. His ECG shows normal sinus rhythm. He reports fatigue and shortness of breath with activity. His healthcare provider has advised a weight loss of 30 pounds and a regular exercise program.	▪ Obesity related to food intake in excess of energy expenditure ▪ At risk for poor adherence to therapeutic regimen ▪ Difficulty with an exercise program due to sedentary lifestyle	▪ Patient will lose 1 pound each week. ▪ Patient will walk 30 minutes 5 days each week. ▪ Patient will verbalize an understanding of the relationship between weight loss, weight control, and exercise. ▪ Patient will identify behavior modification strategies to avoid overeating. ▪ Patient will identify support systems for behavior modification.

PLANNING AND IMPLEMENTATION

- Assess weight and blood pressure once or twice each week.
- Discuss current eating habits and strategies to reduce fat and calorie intake.
- Discuss cues that promote eating. Identify strategies to eliminate or reduce eating cues.
- Teach to keep a food diary to examine and change eating habits. Recommend smartphone applications to assist with monitoring daily fat, carbohydrate, and caloric intake. Instruct patient in how to use the application.
- Discuss the role of regular exercise in weight loss and weight control. Assist patient with setting realistic exercise goals. Instruct to maintain an exercise record to track the intensity and duration of activity. Encourage use of wearable health technology to monitor physical activity.
- Discuss lifestyle and behavior modification strategies to promote successful weight loss and control.

EVALUATION

Two weeks after changing his diet and beginning to exercise, Mr. Elliott has lost 2 pounds. He has maintained a food diary and monitored caloric intake using his smartphone app. He has identified boredom as a cue to eating. In light of that fact, he has started volunteering at the local hospital, where he is working with children. He is walking for 30 minutes 5 days a week and tracking his progress using wearable health technology. He plans to increase his activity periods to 45 minutes. He verbalizes commitment to a lifelong plan of exercising and eating a low-fat diet. His BP has ranged from 132/76 to 136/84 mmHg. He plans to have the employee health nurse at the hospital check his weight and BP each week and to join Weight Watchers for ongoing support.

CLINICAL REASONING IN PATIENT CARE

1. What are some possible pathophysiologic bases for Mr. Elliott's abnormal cholesterol, HDL, and LDL levels?
2. Develop a teaching plan for a group of men and women who are overweight.
3. Identify potential barriers to losing weight and strategies to reduce or eliminate these barriers.

See Evaluating Your Response in Appendix B.

22.2 Malnutrition

Malnutrition results from inadequate intake of nutrients. An individual may lack major nutrients (calories, carbohydrates, proteins, and fats) or micronutrients such as vitamins and minerals. Malnutrition may be caused by inadequate nutrient intake; impaired absorption and use of nutrients; loss of nutrients due to diarrhea, hemorrhage, or renal failure; or increased metabolic needs (e.g., infection or physiologic stressors).

Incidence and Prevalence

Malnutrition is a widespread cause of disease and mortality throughout the world. It is endemic in regions affected by famine. Groups at risk for malnutrition in the United States include the young, poor, older adults, homeless, low-income women, and ethnic minorities. The percentage of hospitalized patients with malnutrition is significant in Australia, Europe, the United Kingdom, and the United States. Malnutrition can increase complications, length of stay, mortality rates, and healthcare costs (Smith et al., 2017). Even when food is plentiful, patients may be undernourished because of poor food choices.

It is estimated that one-third to one-half of all hospitalized patients are malnourished (Smith et al., 2017). The costs associated with treating malnutrition and its underlying etiology and complications are estimated to be in excess of more than $11 billion annually in the United States (Smith et al., 2017). Malnutrition may be present on admission or develop as a result of surgery or serious illness. Malnutrition increases both mortality and the incidence of complications in both medical and surgical patients.

Risk Factors

Risk factors for malnutrition include:

- Age—older adults are at greater risk for malnutrition due to a variety of factors
- Poverty, homelessness, inadequate food storage and preparation facilities
- Functional health problems that limit mobility or vision
- History of weight loss of more than 20% of usual weight
- Oral or gastrointestinal problems that affect food intake, digestion, and absorption
- Inability to eat for 5 or more days
- Chronic pain or chronic diseases such as pulmonary, cardiovascular, renal, or endocrine disorders; cancer
- Dementia, mental health disorders, eating disorders
- Medications or treatments that affect appetite
- Alcohol or drug addiction
- Acute problems such as infection, surgery, or trauma.

The Patient with Malnutrition

Pathophysiology

Carbohydrates and fats in the diet are the body's primary energy source. Approximately 15 to 25% of the body is fat, the body's energy reservoir. The remainder (muscles, bones, other body tissues and organs) is lean body mass, metabolically active tissue. Proteins in the diet are primarily used to maintain this tissue. Glycogen and proteins in this lean body mass also act as energy stores.

When dietary intake of nutrients does not meet the body's energy needs, the body uses glycogen, body proteins, and lipids (fats) to support metabolism. In **starvation** (inadequate dietary intake), glycogen is initially used to provide energy. After the first 24 hours of starvation, gluconeogenesis (formation of glucose from proteins) is the major source of energy. As starvation continues, the body breaks down fats into free fatty acids and ketones, which provide energy for the brain. The size of all body compartments is reduced as body fats and muscle proteins are used to meet energy needs. As lean body mass is reduced, metabolically active tissue is lost, and energy expenditure decreases.

The stress of acute illness, surgery, or trauma produces a different response. The acute stress response produces a state of hypermetabolism and **catabolism** (cell and tissue breakdown). This hypermetabolic state increases energy expenditure and nutrient needs, resulting in **protein-calorie malnutrition (PCM)**. In PCM, both protein and calories are deficient. Lean body mass is broken down to meet these needs. If untreated, up to half of the body's protein stores can be used within 3 weeks. Visceral protein stores are also converted to energy, with loss of protein from organs such as the liver, gastrointestinal tract, kidneys, and heart. Loss of protein from the liver affects its ability to produce plasma proteins. Immune cells decrease, and wound healing is impaired. Atrophy of gastrointestinal mucosa leads to malabsorption, further compounding the protein deficit. Myocardial contractility and cardiac output decline, and respiratory function is compromised (Heimburger, 2015).

Two forms of severe malnutrition exist. Chronic protein deficiency with adequate calories to meet energy needs is called *kwashiorkor* and results from decreased protein intake and catabolism in acute and life-threatening illness. *Marasmus* refers to generalized starvation and occurs when both proteins and calories are insufficient to meet the body's needs. PCM is also known as marasmus.

Manifestations

The manifestations of malnutrition may vary among patients. Weight loss is the most apparent manifestation: The malnourished patient may have a body weight of less than 90% of ideal. Body mass is also reduced (refer to Table 22.2), as is skinfold thickness. Other manifestations include a wasted appearance, dry and brittle hair, and pale mucous membranes. Peripheral or abdominal edema may be present. Older adults may show general symptoms of frailty, including weakness, slow walking speed, low physical activity level, unintentional weight loss, and exhaustion. Manifestations of specific nutrient deficiencies may be present (see **Table 22.6**). See the Multisystem Effects of Malnutrition feature on page 677.

Subcutaneous fat and muscle proteins are broken down in PCM, impairing mobility and increasing the risk for skin and tissue breakdown (pressure ulcers). Protein synthesis is inhibited and wound healing delayed. Serum albumin levels fall, leading to abdominal edema, diarrhea, and impaired nutrient absorption. Immune function is impaired, increasing the risk of infection. Cardiac output falls, and the risk for postural hypotension increases.

Interprofessional Care

The goal of treatment for the patient who is malnourished is to restore ideal body weight while replacing and restoring depleted nutrients and minerals. The patient's age, severity of malnutrition, and coexisting health problems help determine interventions. Treatment may include oral supplementation, tube feedings, or parenteral nutrition.

Diagnosis

A nutrition screening tool can help identify patients at risk for malnutrition. Multiple valid and reliable screening and assessment tools have been developed and can assist with identifying patients at risk for malnutrition in community and acute care settings. Clinical practice guidelines provide evidence-based resources that can be used to develop an interprofessional plan of care (Anthony, 2008; Laur & Keller, 2017; McClave et al., 2016; Yordy, Roberts, & Taggart, 2017). The Joint Commission accreditation requires nutritional screening of patients within 24 hours of hospital admission

Table 22.6 Manifestations of Specific Nutrient Deficiencies

Deficiency	Assessment Data
Calorie	Weight loss Weakness, listlessness Loss of subcutaneous fat Muscle wasting
Protein	Thin or sparse hair Flaking skin Hepatomegaly
Vitamin A	Night blindness Altered taste and smell Dry, scaling, rough skin
Thiamine	Confusion, apathy Cardiomegaly, dyspnea Muscle cramping and wasting Paresthesias, neuropathy Ataxia
Riboflavin	Cheilosis, stomatitis, glossitis Neuropathy
Vitamin C	Swollen, bleeding gums Delayed wound healing Weakness Depression Easy bruising
Iron	Smooth tongue Listlessness, fatigue Dyspnea

Multisystem Effects of
Malnutrition

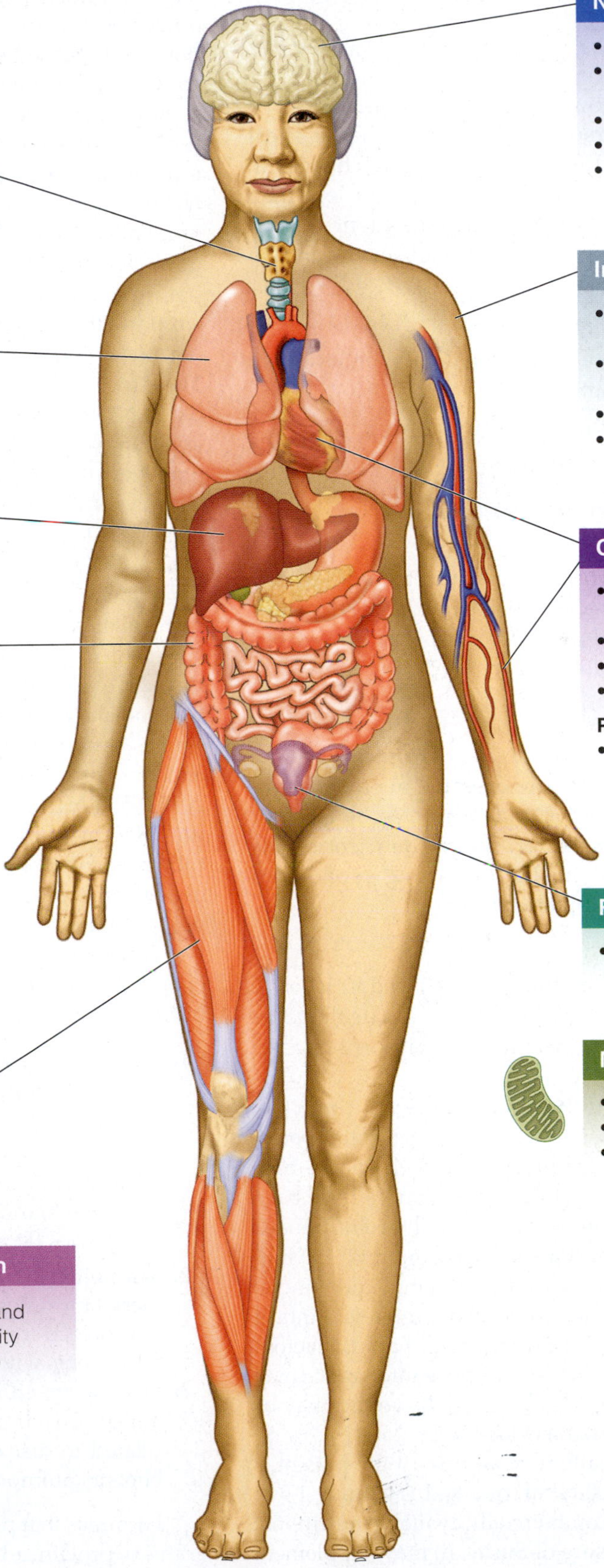

Neurologic
- ↓ Cognition
- ↓ Consciousness (drowsiness, lethargy)
- Tremors
- Paresthesias
- Impaired coordination

Endocrine
- ↓ Thyroid hormones
- ↓ Testosterone (male)
- ↓ Estrogen (female)

Respiratory
- ↓ Respiratory rate
- ↓ Vital capacity

Integumentary
- Hair: brittle, dull, dry, loss of color
- Nails: fragile, brittle, spoon-shaped
- Petechiae
- Poor wound healing

Hepatic
- Hepatomegaly
- ↓ Bile synthesis

Cardiovascular
- Dysrythmias and conduction disturbances
- ↓ HR
- ↓ BP
- Enlarged heart

Potential Complication
- Heart failure

Gastrointestinal
Oral/esophageal:
- Cheilosis
- Glossitis
- Gingivitis

Stomach/intestines:
- Ascites
- Constipation
- Intestinal atrophy
- Steatorrhea
- ↓ Gastric and pancreatic secretions

Potential Complication
- Malabsorption syndrome

Reproductive
- Amenorrhea

Musculoskeletal
- Muscle wasting
- Tenderness
- Impaired strength

Metabolic Processes
- ↓ Weight
- ↓ Core body temperature
- Edema

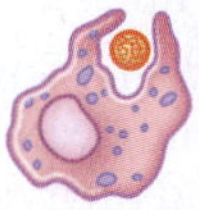

Immune System
- ↓ Cell-mediated and humoral immunity
- ↑ Susceptibility to infections

(Smith et al., 2017). As with obesity, the standard measurements to assess for malnutrition include height, weight, calculation of BMI, and skinfold measurements. A BMI of less than 18 to 20 may indicate malnutrition. The following laboratory studies also may be ordered:

- ***Serum albumin*** is reduced in PCM, and may be below 2.8 g/dL (Heimburger, 2015).
- ***Prealbumin*** (also known as *transthyretin*) is a transport protein and precursor to albumin. It has a short (2-day) half-life and is sensitive to acute changes in nutritional status. A prealbumin level of less than 10 mg/dL indicates severe nutritional deficiency; a level lower than 5 mg/dL is seen in severe protein depletion (Kee, 2018).
- ***Total lymphocyte count*** is reduced in PCM.
- ***Serum electrolytes*** are measured. Potassium levels are low in severe malnutrition.

The following specialized procedures to evaluate the extent of malnutrition may be ordered:

- ***Bioelectric impedance analysis*** measures body fat and total body water.
- ***Total daily energy expenditure*** (which includes resting energy expenditure, energy needed for digestion, plus physical activity needs) may be measured to help determine the patient's calorie intake needs.

Medications

Malnourished patients generally require supplemental vitamins and minerals to restore essential micronutrients. A multivitamin and mineral supplement may be given or therapy may be tailored to correct specific deficiencies. See **Medication Administration 22.B** for nursing implications of vitamin and mineral supplement use.

Treatment

Fluids and nutrients are carefully reintroduced in severely malnourished patients. Refeeding can precipitate fluid and electrolyte imbalances, heart failure, malabsorption, and diarrhea.

First, fluid and electrolyte imbalances are corrected, with particular attention paid to restoring normal potassium, magnesium, and calcium levels, as well as acid–base balance. Once fluid and electrolyte imbalances have been corrected, protein and calories are gradually reintroduced into the diet. Initial feedings are limited amounts (100 mL) of liquid formula to prevent diarrhea. Vitamin and mineral supplements at about twice the dietary reference intake (DRI) are provided along with refeeding. Fat and lactose are reintroduced into the diet last. Lactose intolerance may develop in severely malnourished patients; yogurt may be tolerated better than a milk-based formula.

Food intake is gradually increased until the patient is able to consume about 5000 kcal/day and is gaining 1.5 to 2.0 kg (3 to 5 lb) weekly. Commercially available nutritional supplements (such as Ensure or Sustacal) may supplement protein and calorie intake.

Enteral Nutrition. **Enteral nutrition**, or tube feeding, may be used to meet calorie and protein requirements in patients unable to consume adequate food. Significant evidence supports starting enteral nutrition rather than parental nutrition as early as possible to promote positive outcomes (O'Leary-Kelley & Bawel-Brinkley, 2017). Indications for tube feedings include difficulty swallowing, unresponsiveness, oral or neck surgery or trauma, anorexia, or serious illness. Most importantly, the patient must have a functioning gastrointestinal tract and is not able to meet nutritional needs through oral intake (Harvard Pilgrim Health Care, 2016). Tube feedings may provide part or all of a patient's nutritional needs. Enteral feedings provide nutrients directly to the gut and other digestive organs, support immune function, promote blood flow to the gut, and support other functions of the GI tract such as the release of hormones and epidermal growth factor (Smith et al., 2017). The American Society for Parental and Enteral Nutrition (ASPEN) identifies three methods of enteral nutrition delivery: Pump assisted, gravity assisted, and bolus. ASPEN recommends the use of infusion pumps with enteral nutrition because of the significant decrease in adverse events and complications correlated with the use of pumps (Pilgrim & Schub, 2017).

Tube feedings are usually administered through a soft, small-caliber nasogastric or nasoduodenal tube with a weighted tip. Tube feedings can also be administered through a gastrostomy tube (G-tube, PEG-tube), duodenal tube, or jejunostomy tube (J-tube). G-tubes, PEG-tubes, and J-tubes have a bumper or retention balloon that creates an anchor to prevent migration (Harvard Pilgrim Health Care, 2016). Feedings cannot begin until radiographic confirmation placement of tube has been established. Appropriate tube placement should be periodically checked by aspirating the tube and checking the pH of aspirated contents. A pH of 6 indicates the tube is in the jejunum.

Different types of formulas are available and can be categorized into three basic types based on the composition of nutrients (Harvard Pilgrim Health Care, 2016):

1. Standard polymeric formulas are isotonic (33 mOsm/L) and are formulated to match the nutritional requirements of a healthy individual. Standard formulas are available in a wide variety of energy, protein, complex carbohydrates, fat, vitamin, mineral, fiber, and water contents. Standard formulas typically provide 1.0 to 2.0 calories (Kcal) of nutrients per mL.
2. Semi-elemental (oligomeric) and elemental (monomeric) formulas contain one or more nutrients that are hydrolyzed for easier digestion and are typically used for patients with impaired GI digestion and absorption.
3. Disease-specific or specialized formulas have been developed for patients with specific nutritional needs related to disease. Examples include diabetes, renal, hepatic, pulmonary, and high fiber.

Formulas that provide more calories per milliliter, more grams of protein, added fiber, or lower fat are also available (**Table 22.7**). Commercial products provide instructions for

Medication Administration 22.B

Vitamin and Mineral Supplements

FAT-SOLUBLE VITAMINS

vitamin A

vitamin D

vitamin E

vitamin K

The fat-soluble vitamins are absorbed in the gastrointestinal tract. Vitamins A and D are stored in the liver. All fat-soluble vitamins may become toxic if taken in excess amounts.

Nursing Responsibilities

- Monitor for manifestations of vitamin excess as well as for adverse effects from vitamin administration.
- Monitor carefully for hypersensitivity reactions during the parenteral administration. Have emergency equipment available.
- Administer vitamin A with food.
- Do not administer vitamin K intravenously.

Health Education for the Patient and Family

- Teach the importance of eating a well-balanced diet. If indicated, provide a list of foods high in specific vitamins.
- Caution that excessive intake of these vitamins may lead to toxicity.

WATER-SOLUBLE VITAMINS

vitamin C (ascorbic acid)

vitamin B complex:

- thiamine (B_1)
- riboflavin (B_2)
- niacin (nicotinic acid)
- pyridoxine hydrochloride (B_6)
- pantothenic acid
- biotin

These vitamins are used to prevent or treat deficiency problems. If the diet is deficient in one vitamin, it is usually deficient in other vitamins as well; therefore, multivitamin preparations are often administered. Most of these vitamins are well absorbed from the gastrointestinal tract.

Nursing Responsibilities

- Monitor for responses to replacement therapy.
- Monitor for hypersensitivity reactions from parenteral administration. Have emergency equipment available.

Health Education for the Patient and Family

- Do not exceed the recommended daily intake for the specific vitamin.

MINERALS

calcium	manganese
chromium	potassium
copper	selenium
fluoride	sodium
iodine	zinc
magnesium	

Minerals are inorganic chemicals that are vital to a variety of physiologic functions. Also called *trace elements*, these minerals are part of a balanced diet. Recommended daily intakes have not been established for all mineral substances. The dosage of prescribed minerals depends on the specific deficiency, route of administration, and the patient's general health.

Nursing Responsibilities

- Monitor for manifestations of mineral imbalance.
- Prior to administration, dilute oral mineral preparations.
- Prior to the administration of iodine, assess for history of hypersensitivity to iodine or seafood; if hypersensitive, notify the physician.

Health Education for the Patient and Family

- Encourage the patient to avoid exceeding the known recommended daily intake of the mineral.
- Instruct the patient to take minerals other than fluoride and zinc with or after meals.

Note: Drugs identified in *blue* are among the 200 most commonly prescribed medications in the U.S.

Table 22.7 Selected Enteral Feeding Formulas

Formula Type	Contains	Examples
Standard —suitable for most patients requiring enteral feedings	■ 1 kcal/mL ■ Protein: ~14% total kcal ■ Fat: ~30% total kcal ■ Carbohydrate: ~60% total kcal ■ Recommended daily intake of all minerals and vitamins in 1500 mL/day	Compleat, Ensure, Isocal, Nutren, Isolan, Sustacal, Resource
Standard high-calorie complete—appropriate for patients on fluid restriction	As above; provides 1.5–2 kcal/Ml	Ensure Plus, Sustacal HC, Comply, Nutren 1.5, Resource Plus, Isocal HCN, Magnacal, TwoCal HN
Complete lactose-free, high-residue—used to prevent/treat diarrhea, constipation	As above; provides fiber	Jevity, Profiber, Nutren 1.0 with fiber, Fiberlan, Sustacal with fiber, Ultracal, Ensure with fiber, FiberSource, Accupep HPF, others
Disease-Specific Formulas		
Renal failure	Contain essential amino acids	Amin-Aid, Travasorb Renal, Aminess
Respiratory failure	Fat: >50% total kcal	Pulmocare, NutriVent
Liver failure with hepatic encephalopathy	High amounts of branched-chain amino acids	Hepatic-Aid II, Travasorb Hepatic

initiating therapy. Enteral feedings may initially be started with smaller volumes to prevent diarrhea, with the volume gradually increased to provide the required calories for maintenance and healing. Formulas may be administered as a bolus feeding or as a continuous-drip feeding regulated by a feeding pump.

Aspiration and diarrhea are the most common complications of enteral feedings. Continuous infusion of the formula reduces the risk of aspiration. The risk is reduced by placing the feeding tube in the jejunum rather than the stomach. To avoid aspiration, the nurse elevates the head of the bed at least 30 degrees during feeding and for at least 1 hour after feeding. Dual-lumen tubes that allow gastric suction with simultaneous instillation of an enteral feeding into the jejunum also reduce the risk for aspiration. Formulas that contain fiber can reduce the incidence of diarrhea. Fluid and electrolyte status is monitored carefully, and additional water is administered as needed. Check serum glucose every 6 hours or per order/facility policy and strive to maintain a serum blood glucose in the range of 140 to 180 mg/dL (Harvard Pilgrim Health Care, 2016).

Parenteral Nutrition. **Parenteral nutrition (PN)**, also known as *hyperalimentation, intravenous alimentation*, and *parenteral hyperalimentation* (Caple & DeVesty, 2017), is the intravenous administration of amino acids, often with added carbohydrates, fats, electrolytes, vitamins, and minerals. These hypertonic solutions are usually administered through a central vein, such as the subclavian vein (**Figure 22.3** ■), particularly when therapy may be prolonged. A peripherally inserted central catheter (PICC) line may be used for short-term PN.

Although oral intake or enteral feeding is preferred over parenteral nutrition, PN is initiated when a patient's nutritional requirements cannot be met through diet or enteral feedings. Increasingly, PN may be used concurrently with enteral nutrition. Patients who have undergone major surgery or trauma or are seriously undernourished are often candidates for PN. PN is used for both short- and long-term management of nutritional deficiencies and is increasingly being delivered in home-based settings (Kirby, Corrigan, Hendrickson, & Emery, 2017).

To begin therapy, a peripheral or central venous catheter is inserted under aseptic conditions. The location of the catheter tip is confirmed by x-ray. Parenteral nutrition solutions are mixed in the pharmacy and commonly contain 3 to 11.4% amino acids (a mixture of essential and nonessential amino acids), 10% or more dextrose, and added electrolytes, minerals, and vitamins. Fat emulsions (lipids) may be added to the solution, although they are often administered separately. The sterility of the solution is maintained, and no medication is added to the solution after it is mixed or to the lumen through which the PN is being administered. When given separately, fat emulsions may be administered either through a peripheral vein or via the same intravenous catheter as PN. PN solutions are always administered with an infusion pump to ensure the correct rate of infusion.

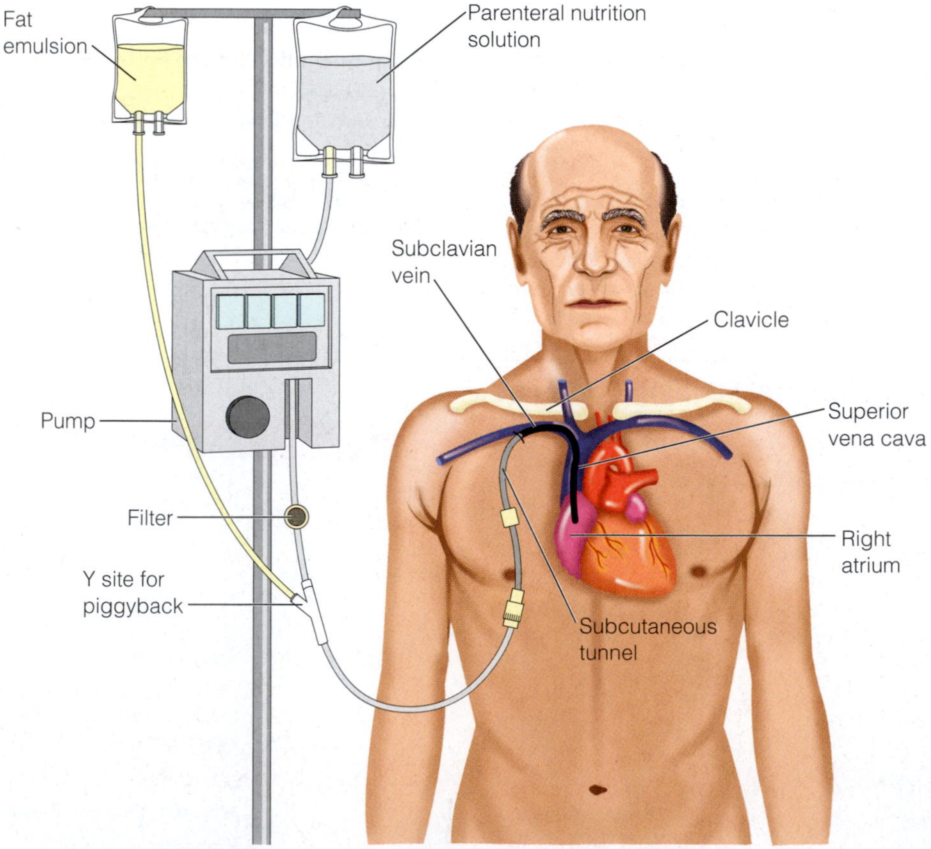
Fat emulsion
Parenteral nutrition solution
Subclavian vein
Clavicle
Superior vena cava
Pump
Filter
Right atrium
Y site for piggyback
Subcutaneous tunnel

Figure 22.3 ■ Parenteral nutrition infusing through a catheter in the right subclavian vein.

Complications. The patient receiving parenteral nutrition is at risk for fluid overload, infections, and metabolic and mechanical complications. Disruption of the skin barrier and administration of a solution high in glucose present a risk for infection in patients receiving PN. Infection may be local, limited to the insertion site or the catheter itself, or systemic. Meticulous sterile technique when inserting the catheter, preparing and administering PN solutions, and during site and catheter care reduces the risk for infection. Using a catheter impregnated with antiseptics and an in-line filter also reduce the risk for infection. The insertion site and the patient's temperature are monitored for evidence of infection. Cultures of the solution, catheter, and blood may be obtained if infection is suspected.

Glucose intolerance may develop, particularly early in the course of PN. The concentration of glucose in PN solutions may be gradually increased to reduce this risk. Blood and urine glucose levels are measured every 6 hours until insulin production adjusts to the increased glucose load. Patients with impaired kidney function or liver disease may develop excessively high blood urea nitrogen (BUN) levels or metabolic acidosis. Hyperlipidemia is a common complication of fat infusions; these solutions are given intermittently to allow fats to clear from the blood between infusions. Fluid overload or dehydration may develop, particularly in older adults. PN formulas can cause electrolyte shifts, with resulting imbalances.

Pneumothorax, brachial plexus injury, and improper position are possible mechanical complications of central venous catheter insertion. Once in place, a thrombus (clot) or fibrin sheath may form within or around the catheter. The catheter can also be mechanically occluded, or may dislodge, leak, or break and become an embolus.

Nursing Care

Assessment

Periodic nutritional-status assessment should be conducted for patients receiving nursing care in community-based settings. Nutritional status should be carefully assessed after hospitalization because multiple factors such as medications, functional limitations, and psychologic status can influence the intake, absorption, and digestion of nutrients. Community-dwelling older adults, homeless people, and other disadvantaged populations are at particular risk for being malnourished. Collect nutritional assessment data on admission and periodically (once or twice a week) during long-term institutionalization.

- *Health history:* Usual daily dietary pattern (type and amount of foods consumed); usual weight and recent changes; appetite and food tolerance; specific food likes and dislikes; difficulty swallowing; problems such as anorexia, nausea, diarrhea, or constipation; history of surgery and/or chronic diseases (e.g., chronic lung disease) and medications
- *Physical examination:* Height, weight, skinfold thickness, BMI; vital signs; general appearance, muscle wasting, mobility; skin and mucous membranes; bowel sounds; laboratory studies.

Use of a nutritional assessment tool is an increasingly expected practice that can help identify patients (older adults in particular) at risk for malnutrition (DiMaria-Ghalili et al., 2017).

Priorities of Care

Priorities of care include:

- Obtaining and documenting baseline indicators of nutritional status.
- Collaborating with physician, dietitian, and pharmacy to develop an interprofessional treatment plan designed to correct acute fluid and electrolyte imbalances.
- Ensuring patient is receiving supplemental nutritional support when appropriate.

Patients with malnutrition may be cared for at home or in the hospital with diet, enteral, or parenteral therapy. See the Moving Evidence into Action box.

Diagnoses, Outcomes, and Interventions

The complex effects of malnutrition on multiple body systems place the patient at high risk for a number of other problems. This section addresses problems with nutrition, infections, fluid volume, and skin integrity. See the Case Study & Nursing Care Plan on page 682 for the patient with malnutrition.

Promote Weight Gain and Well-Being. The nurse plays a critical role in the ongoing assessment of a patient who is malnourished, while collaborating with the interprofessional team to provide nutritional therapies.

Expected Outcome: Patient will achieve consistent weight gain by practicing nutritional habits that restore physical health and functional capacity, will improve indicators of nutritional status such as laboratory values, and will demonstrate improved functional status and describe general well-being.

The nurse will:

- Provide an environment and nursing measures that encourage eating, if the patient is able to eat; for example, adequate staff to assist with meals, sitting at the bedside or in a common area, and providing favorite foods. Avoid interrupting patients during mealtime and be sure the meal is in easy reach if the patient is self-feeding. *Measures to promote a more normal and social dining experience support the patient's intake* (Yordy et al., 2017).
- Eliminate foul odors, provide oral hygiene before and after meals, make meals appetizing, and offer frequent, small meals including preferred foods. Consult with the nutrition support team to provide adequate protein, calories, minerals, and vitamins. *Oral hygiene and a pleasant environment make food more appetizing. Frequent, small meals are generally more appealing and less overwhelming to a patient with anorexia. Many patients require complicated nutritional therapy such as enteral or parenteral therapy to meet nutritional needs.*
- Provide a rest period before and after meals. *Eating requires energy, and the malnourished patient may have decreased physical strength and energy.*

Moving Evidence into Action

Malnutrition in Hospitalized Adult Patients

Clinical Issue

Malnutrition is linked with a variety of hospital complications such as falls, pressure injuries, and catheter-associated urinary tract infections (National Association of Clinical Nurse Specialists, 2017; Yordy et al., 2017). Consequently, The Joint Commission (2018) mandates completion of a nutritional screening within 24 hours of admission to an acute care facility. However, no best tool for screening of malnutrition risk has been identified in hospitalized patients (Rabito, Marcadenti, da Silva Fink, Figueira, & Silva, 2017).

External Evidence

A questionnaire was developed to compare the accuracy of four commonly used assessment tools for malnutrition (Rabito et al., 2017). A total of 752 patients were included in the study. The Malnutrition Universal Screening Tool (MUST), Malnutrition Screening Tool (MST), and Short Nutritional Assessment Questionnaire (SNAQ) were compared with the Nutritional Risk Screening 2002 (NRS-2002). The tools were studied to determine (1) the best measure to identify patients at risk for malnutrition and (2) which tool best predicted morbidity and mortality. Outcomes measures included length of hospital stay, transfer to the intensive care unit, presence of infection, and incidence of mortality. All four tools demonstrated satisfactory performance to identify patients at nutritional risk and there was no significant statistical difference between them.

Internal Evidence

As part of the evaluation of internal evidence, one must consider the policy and procedure for ensuring comprehensive nutritional screening and assessment is completed on all patients. The outcome of interest (identifying patients at risk for malnutrition) and current policies/procedures in place for nutrition screening should be reviewed and revised using best evidence. The identification of stakeholders that influence the implementation of a comprehensive screening program must be included in using evidence to create policy and procedure. Educating the bedside nurse on best practices related to nutrition screening and mentoring on the use and adaptation of an agreed-upon tool is a critical consideration.

Patient Considerations

Patient demographics should be considered in the adaptation of the most feasible nutritional screening tool. Ensuring the adapted tool is culturally sensitive and the questions are easy for the patient to understand are important considerations.

Putting the Pieces Together

The design and implementation of a comprehensive nutritional screening plan are essential and a required activity in accredited acute care environments. To effectively implement a plan, the external evidence regarding validity and reliability of screening tools should be considered. Consider the internal implications for staff training, organizational work flow, and documentation systems. With implementation of a comprehensive nutritional screening plan, the outcome (fewer complications related to malnutrition) of every patient should be assessed, a nutritional treatment plan should be implemented, and unit-level information should be collected and evaluated on a regular basis.

References

National Association of Clinical Nurse Specialists. 2017. *Malnutrition in hospitalized adult patients: The role of the clinical nurse specialist.* https://nacns.org/professional-resources/toolkits-and-reports/malnutrition-in-hospitalized-adult-patients/

Rabito, E. I., Marcadenti, A., da Silva Fink, J., Figueira, L., & Silva, F. M. (2017). Nutritional Risk Screening 2002, Short Nutritional Assessment Questionnaire, Malnutrition Screening Tool, and Malnutrition Universal Screening Toll are good predictors of nutrition risk in and emergency service. *Nutrition in Clinical Practice*, *32*(4), 526–532.

The Joint Commission. *Nutrition and feeding standards*. Retrieved March 4, 2018 from www.jointcommission.org/standards_information/edition. aspx.

Yordy, B. M., Roberts, S., & Taggart, H. M. (2017). Quality improvement in clinical nutrition: Screening and mealtime protection for the hospitalized patient. *Clinical Nurse Specialist*, *31*(3), 149–156.

- Assess knowledge and provide appropriate teaching. *Lack of knowledge often contributes to undernutrition. Education empowers the patient to make healthy choices.*
- Start specialized nutritional support when a patient cannot, should not, or will not eat adequately and if the benefits of nutrition outweigh the associated risks. *Specialized nutritional support may be required to correct acute and life-threatening nutritional imbalances when malnourishment has been prolonged or during acute and critical illness.*

Reduce Risk for Infection. Patients who are malnourished have a much higher risk for infection than those who are well nourished. Malnutrition affects many components of the immune system, including the skin, mucous membranes, and lymph tissue and cells.

Expected Outcome: Patient will be free of signs and symptoms of infection.

The nurse will:

- Monitor temperature and assess for manifestations of infection every 4 hours. *Although the baseline temperature may be subnormal in malnourished patients, any elevation from baseline may indicate infection. Manifestations of infection may include chills, malaise, erythema, and leukocytosis. Early detection of infection may prevent complications.*
- Maintain medical asepsis when providing care and surgical asepsis when carrying out procedures. *Hand hygiene is the best strategy to prevent the spread of pathogens. Sterile technique is required for procedures such as inserting central lines and changing dressings.*

- Teach the signs and symptoms of infection, hand hygiene, and factors that increase the risk for infection. *Knowledge empowers the patient to participate in self-care, thus reducing exposure to infectious pathogens.*

Reduce Risk for Insufficient Fluid Volume. The patient with malnutrition may also have a fluid volume deficit. Difficulty swallowing food and fluids or administration of hyperosmolar nutritional solutions may lead to dehydration or electrolyte disturbances.

Expected Outcome: Patient will maintain adequate hydration status and will not develop complications related to compromised hydration status.

The nurse will:

- Monitor oral mucous membranes, urine specific gravity, level of consciousness, and laboratory findings every 4 to 8 hours. *Dry mucous membranes, increased urine specific gravity, decreased level of consciousness, and electrolyte imbalances may indicate dehydration.*
- Weigh daily and monitor intake and output. *Daily weights and intake and output measurements help monitor fluid balance.*
- Offer fluids frequently in small amounts, if allowed, considering the patient's preferences. *Frequent, small amounts of fluids are better tolerated and promote adequate intake.*

Reduce Risk for Skin Injury. Skin integrity depends on adequate nutrition. Loss of subcutaneous tissue and muscle increases the risk of pressure ulcers. In addition, healing is impaired in patients who are malnourished.

Expected Outcome: Patient will not exhibit signs of pressure injury.

The nurse will:

- Assess skin every 4 hours. *Baseline and ongoing assessments allow prompt identification of early manifestations of skin breakdown.*
- Turn and reposition at least every 2 hours. Encourage passive and active range-of-motion exercises. *These measures reduce pressure and promote oxygenation of cells.*
- Keep skin dry and clean, and minimize shearing forces. Keep linens smooth, clean, and dry. Provide therapeutic beds, mattresses, or pads. *These nursing measures promote comfort and reduce the risk of skin breakdown.*

Delegating Nursing Care Activities

- Conduct mealtime rounds to determine patients' needs for assistance with meals. *Identifying patients who need assistance with meals will ensure staff are available to help.*
- Ensure that unlicensed assistive personnel (UAP) keep fluids within patients' reach between mealtimes. *Medication and age can affect thirst sensation. Ensuring that fluids are accessible will remind the patient to sip fluids frequently.*
- Instruct UAP to enhance the environment by removing bedpans, urinals, and other equipment. *Ensuring that patients have pleasant surroundings at mealtime will increase the patient's appetite and improve nutritional intake.*
- Instruct and monitor UAP adherence to swallowing precautions. *Failure to follow swallowing precautions can lead to aspiration.*

Transitions of Care

Aggressive nursing assessment and interventions can help prevent malnutrition associated with hospitalization or long-term care. Nutrition screening using valid and reliable tools should be a regular assessment in primary care. Screening older adults for malnutrition should be done using a standardized process (Laur & Keller, 2017). In hospitalized patients, complete a nutritional assessment within 24 hours of hospitalization. Coordinate the implementation of an interprofessional plan to address nutritional needs for at-risk patients. Carefully monitor nutritional intake for all patients throughout their hospitalization. When a patient is placed on NPO status for surgery or tests, ask the care provider to restore diet orders as soon as possible. If allowed, encourage family members to provide favorite foods to promote intake. Each year, it is more common to see patients managing tube feeding or PN at home. Teaching for the patient and family includes the following topics:

- Diet recommendations and use of nutritional supplements
- Where to obtain recommended foods and nutritional supplements
- If continuing enteral or parenteral nutrition, (1) how to prepare and/or handle solutions, (2) how to add them to either the feeding tube or central line, (3) how to manage infusion pumps, (4) how to care for the feeding tube or central catheter, (5) how to recognize and manage problems and complications, and (6) how and when to notify the healthcare provider of problems.

In long-term care settings, promote socialization during meals. Assess food likes and dislikes for patients, and provide foods they are likely to eat. Monitor food intake. Perform regular comprehensive nutritional screening to detect early signs of malnutrition.

At the end of life, food preferences should be provided until patient can no longer chew or swallow. Family members may need to be reassured that loss of appetite is a normal physiologic response to the dying process.

Case Study & Nursing Care Plan

A Patient with Malnutrition

Kyo Morris is an 88-year-old widow who lives alone. She typically rises early and has a cup of tea before spending her morning puttering in her garden. She consumes her main meal of the day at lunch, which usually includes rice and some vegetables. For dinner, she generally eats a bowl of rice with "whatever is in the refrigerator." Mrs. Morris admits to little interest in cooking or eating since her husband died 10 years ago and her group of friends has been "dying off too."

ASSESSMENT	DIAGNOSES	EXPECTED OUTCOMES
Mrs. Morris weighs 43.1 kg (95 lb), is 160 cm (5′ 3″) tall, and has a BMI of 16.8. She reports weighing 53.5 kg (118 lb) 5 years ago. Her triceps skinfold thickness measurement is 11 mm (normal values for a female: >13 mm). Her skin is pale, and she appears thin and wasted. Her temperature is 36°C (97°F). Diagnostic test results include serum albumin 2.9 g/dL (normal 3.4 to 4.8 g/dL) and serum cholesterol 130 mg/dL (normal 150 to 200 mg/dL). A diagnosis of protein-calorie malnutrition is made, and a 1500-calorie-per-day diet is recommended.	▪ Underweight due to inadequate food consumption ▪ Potential for infection due to poor nutrition ▪ Decreased social support	▪ Patient will gain at least 1 pound per week. ▪ Patient will verbalize understanding of nutritional requirements and identify strategies to incorporate requirements into daily diet after discharge. ▪ Patient will remain infection free, evidenced by normal vital signs. ▪ Patient will identify strategies to increase social interaction, such as participating in senior citizens' lunches at local senior center.

PLANNING AND IMPLEMENTATION

- Weigh weekly at a consistent time of day.
- Refer to dietitian for evaluation of nutritional needs.
- Teach about nutritional requirements, and plan an eating program that includes high-calorie, high-protein foods and supplements and reflects her food preferences. Encourage frequent, small meals.
- Encourage to keep a food intake diary.
- Teach strategies to reduce risks for infection.
- Provide information about communal meals available to seniors in the community, and help Mrs. Morris develop a plan to participate.

EVALUATION

One month later, Mrs. Morris has gained 3 pounds and reports feeling "more energetic." A friend is helping her shop to ensure that she purchases foods to maintain her protein, calorie, and nutrient intake. She has begun attending senior lunches twice a week and is enjoying "being around people again." Although she still doesn't enjoy cooking like she used to, she is using prepared foods and supplements to maintain her nutrient intake.

CLINICAL REASONING IN PATIENT CARE

1. What is the physiologic basis for Mrs. Morris's low albumin and cholesterol levels?
2. Mrs. Morris asks, "Can I get better by just taking more vitamins?" How will you respond?
3. Design a teaching plan for a Hispanic patient with protein-calorie malnutrition.

See Evaluating Your Response in Appendix B.

22.3 Eating Disorders

Eating disorders are characterized by severely disturbed eating behavior and weight management. Eating disorders are more common in affluent societies where food is plentiful and occur in all socioeconomic and major ethnic groups. Eating disorders are manifested in both men and women. Women are slightly more affected than men (Ahacic, 2016). **Anorexia nervosa** is characterized by a refusal to maintain a minimally normal body weight, a distorted body image, and an intense fear of gaining weight or of loss of control over food intake. Anorexia nervosa affects about 1% of women in the United States at some time in their lives (Reus, 2015). **Bulimia nervosa**, which affects 1 to 3% of women in the United States, is characterized by recurring episodes of binge eating followed by purge behaviors such as self-induced vomiting, use of laxatives or diuretics, fasting, or excessive exercise. **Binge-eating disorder** is a subgroup believed to affect many more people than either anorexia or bulimia (Reus, 2015). Binge-eating disorder is characterized by recurrent episodes of binge eating—eating an excessive amount of food during a defined period of time and a sense of loss of control over eating during binge episodes (Reus, 2015).

The Patient with an Eating Disorder

Anorexia Nervosa

Anorexia nervosa typically begins during middle to late adolescence. Patients with anorexia nervosa have a distorted body image and irrational fear of gaining weight.

Refusal to maintain body weight at or above a minimally normal level for height and body type is a common manifestation of anorexia nervosa. Patients maintain weight loss by restricted calorie intake, often accompanied by excessive exercise. Some may exhibit binge–purge behavior.

Although its cause is unknown, psychologic, biologic, genetic, and cultural risk factors have been identified for anorexia nervosa. A history of sexual or physical abuse and family history of mood disorders are nonspecific risk factors. Abnormal levels of neurotransmitters and other hormones may play a role. Genetic factors are suggested by a higher incidence within families and in the monozygotic twin of an affected individual. Women who develop anorexia nervosa tend to be obsessive and perfectionistic and often feel inadequate or unable to maintain control in their lives. Family, social, or occupational (e.g., a career in modeling or ballet) pressures to maintain low body weight also contribute.

The manifestations of anorexia nervosa are shown in the Multisystem Effects feature. Patients who engage in binge–purge behavior have a higher risk for complications.

Bulimia Nervosa

Bulimia nervosa frequently develops in late adolescence or early adulthood. Unlike patients with anorexia nervosa, the weight of patients with bulimia may be within or above the normal range. Like anorexia nervosa, however, the cause is likely multifactorial, including cultural, psychosocial, and biologic factors. The patient with bulimia often restricts caloric intake, leading to increased hunger and overeating. Foods consumed during a binge are often high calorie, high fat, and sweet. After binge eating, the patient induces vomiting (usually by stimulating the gag reflex) or may take excessive quantities of laxatives or diuretics. Fluid and electrolyte balance may be severely disrupted by loss of fluid and gastrointestinal secretions. The complications of bulimia nervosa primarily result from the purging behavior.

Binge-Eating Disorder

Binge-eating disorder (BED) shares many of the characteristics of bulimia; however, patients with BED do not purge. BED commonly affects middle-aged adults who are obese. The cause of BED is unknown, although genetics may play a role in its development. Psychosocial factors contribute; people with BED are often depressed, anxious, or have a personality disorder. People with BED consume an excessive amount of food during binging episodes, eating even when not hungry and continuing to eat until uncomfortably full. Binging often occurs when the person is alone. After overeating, the patient may feel disgusted or guilty about the amount of food consumed and depressed about the inability to control eating.

Manifestations and complications of eating disorders are outlined in **Table 22.8**.

Table 22.8 Manifestations and Complications of Eating Disorders

Manifestations	Complications
Anorexia Nervosa	
■ Weight < 85% of normal, muscle wasting ■ Fear of weight gain, refusal to eat ■ Disturbed body image, excessive exercise ■ Amenorrhea ■ Skin and hair changes ■ Hypotension, bradycardia ■ Hypothermia, cold intolerance ■ Constipation ■ Insomnia	■ Electrolyte and acid–base disturbances ■ Reduced cardiac output, dysrhythmias ■ Elevated BUN, serum creatinine levels ■ Anemia ■ Hypoglycemia, elevated serum uric acid levels ■ Osteoporosis ■ Enlarged salivary glands ■ Delayed gastric emptying ■ Abnormal liver function ■ Lanugo (fine hair present over the face and body) ■ Dry, brittle hair ■ Dehydration ■ Sensitivity to noise and light ■ Inability to concentrate
Bulimia Nervosa	
■ Weight often normal; may be slightly overweight ■ Binge–purge behavior ■ Oligomenorrhea or amenorrhea ■ Lacerations of palate; callus on fingers or dorsum of hand	■ Enlarged salivary glands ■ Stomatitis, loss of dental enamel ■ Fluid, electrolyte, and acid–base imbalances ■ Dysrhythmias ■ Esophageal tears, stomach rupture, rectal tears
Binge-Eating Disorder	
■ Usually overweight or obese ■ Recurrent episodes of binge eating (2 or more days a week for 6 months) ■ Episodes characterized by: a. Eating more rapidly than usual b. Eating until uncomfortably full c. Eating large amounts of food when not physically hungry d. Eating alone due to embarrassment over quantity e. Disgust, depression, or guilt following a binge episode f. Marked distress about binging behavior	■ Type 2 diabetes ■ Hypertension, hyperlipidemia ■ Coronary heart disease, heart failure ■ Gallbladder disease ■ Depression, social isolation

Multisystem Effects of
Anorexia Nervosa

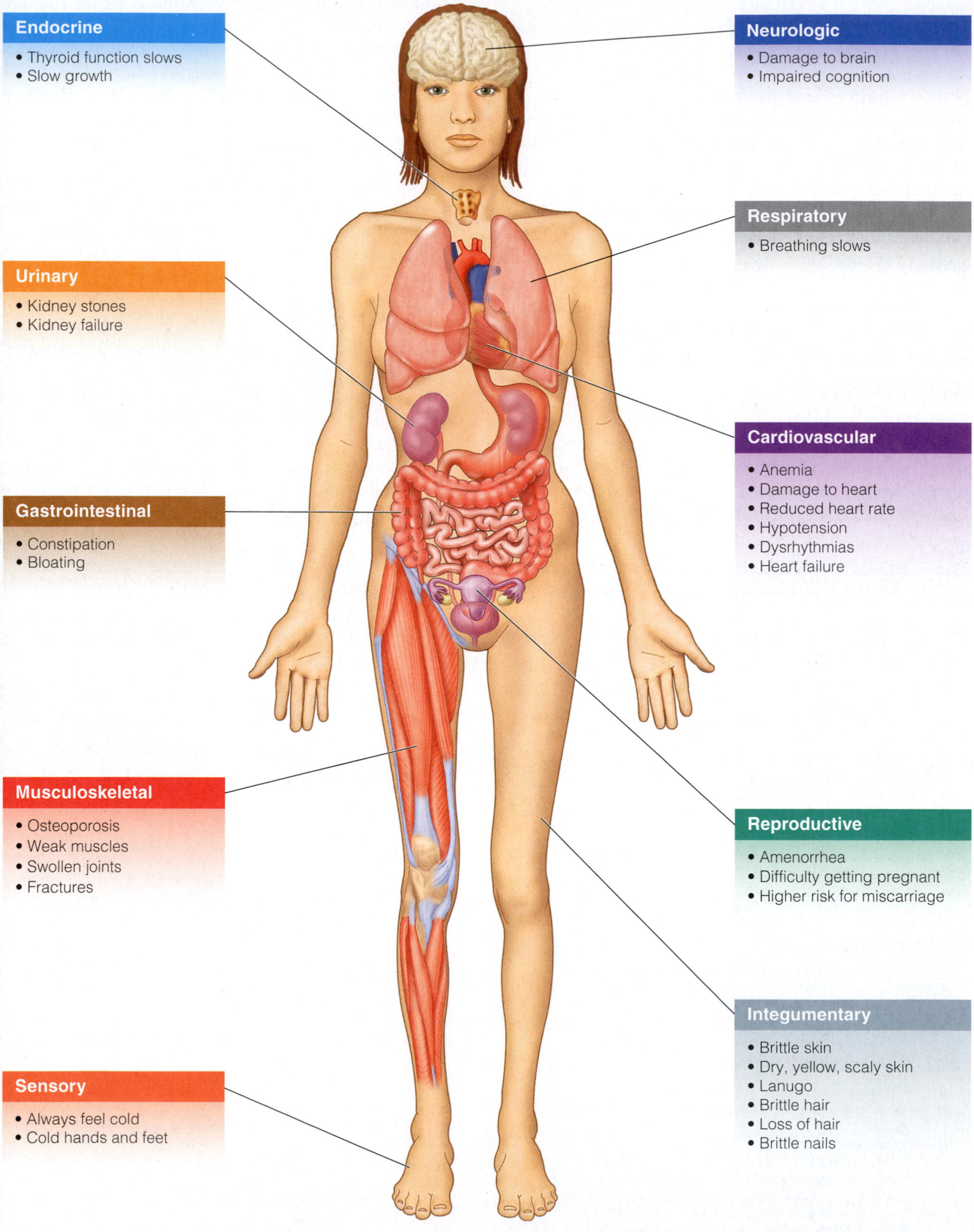
Endocrine
• Thyroid function slows
• Slow growth
Neurologic
• Damage to brain
• Impaired cognition
Respiratory
• Breathing slows
Urinary
• Kidney stones
• Kidney failure
Cardiovascular
• Anemia
• Damage to heart
• Reduced heart rate
• Hypotension
• Dysrhythmias
• Heart failure
Gastrointestinal
• Constipation
• Bloating
Musculoskeletal
• Osteoporosis
• Weak muscles
• Swollen joints
• Fractures
Reproductive
• Amenorrhea
• Difficulty getting pregnant
• Higher risk for miscarriage
Integumentary
• Brittle skin
• Dry, yellow, scaly skin
• Lanugo
• Brittle hair
• Loss of hair
• Brittle nails
Sensory
• Always feel cold
• Cold hands and feet

Interprofessional Care

Eating disorders, anorexia nervosa in particular, are difficult to treat effectively. Because of the intense fear of weight gain and the distorted body image of patients with anorexia, they strongly resist increasing food intake. While community-based care is appropriate for most patients with an eating disorder, complications of the disorder or resistance to treatment may necessitate hospitalization for some patients. In all cases, a comprehensive treatment plan for eating disorders includes medical care and monitoring, psychosocial interventions, and nutrition counseling.

Diagnosis

There is no specific diagnostic test for anorexia, bulimia, or binge-eating disorder. Laboratory studies in patients with anorexia or bulimia may show anemia and leukopenia on CBC, abnormal serum electrolyte levels, and elevated BUN and serum creatinine. In patients with BED, the blood glucose and lipid levels may be elevated. The BMI is usually above the normal range and may identify the patient as obese.

A mental health evaluation is indicated for patients with eating disorders to identify contributing factors and help direct treatment.

Treatment

Patients with anorexia nervosa may require hospitalization, particularly if their weight is less than 75% of normal. Refeeding is gradually introduced to avoid complications related to refeeding syndrome such as electrolyte and acid–base imbalance, respiratory distress, neurologic symptoms, cardiac dysrhythmia, hypotension, and congestive heart failure. Multivitamins are given along with calcium and vitamin D supplements to minimize bone loss. Meals must be supervised and a firm but empathetic attitude conveyed about the importance of adequate food intake. Intravenous feeding may be required in some cases. Psychologic treatment focuses on providing emotional support during weight gain and helping patients base their self-esteem on factors other than weight (e.g., personal relationships, satisfaction with achieving occupational goals) (Ahacic, 2016). Psychotherapy includes individual, group, and family therapy. Cognitive-behavioral therapy (CBT) or compassion-focused therapy may be used to monitor moods and develop problem-solving skills. Psychotherapy addresses shame, excessive self-criticism, and self-directed hostility. Antidepressants and antianxiety medications can be helpful to control moods and anxiety symptoms.

The goal of bulimia treatment is to reduce or eliminate binge eating and purging behavior. A combination of nutritional counseling and therapy, psychosocial interventions, and medications may be used. Nutritional counseling is directed at establishing a regular meal pattern and encouraging an appropriate amount of regular exercise. Fluoxetine is an FDA-approved medication used for treating bulimia nervosa. According to the National Institute of Mental Health, fluoxetine reduces binge-eating and purging behaviors and may reduce the chance of relapse and improve eating attitudes (Ahacic, 2016). CBT is also used to treat bulimia, focusing on excessive concerns about weight, persistent dieting, and binge–purge behaviors.

Treatment for patients with binge-eating disorder focuses on establishing healthy eating patterns, psychosocial therapy (including CBT and group counseling) to address underlying issues, and management of obesity and its complications. Patients with BED may also benefit from an SSRI or other antidepressant drug.

Nursing Care

Nurses can be instrumental in identifying patients with eating disorders and referring them for treatment. It is particularly important to identify these disorders early to prevent adverse effects on growth and increase the success of treatment. Nutritional education, promoting a healthy body image, and identification of risk factors and early signs of each disorder will increase the likelihood of successful treatment.

Assessment

In addition to the components of a standard nutritional assessment, a careful history related to weight loss patterns and descriptions of psychologic symptoms commonly associated with eating disorders should be explored. These symptoms include overvalued ideas about the importance of body shape and weight. Assess the patient for distractibility, depression, anxiety, agitation, sleep disturbance, obsessionality, and compulsivity.

Priorities of Care

Nursing priorities of care include monitoring indicators of nutritional status, including fluid and electrolyte status, establishing a therapeutic relationship with the patient, and supporting a psychosocial and behavioral treatment plan.

SAFETY ALERT: Refeeding syndrome is an uncommon but serious adverse effect associated with aggressive refeeding in the context of semistarvation. The nurse should monitor for fluid and electrolyte imbalance, hypophosphatemia, hypomagnesemia, rapid and significant peripheral edema, and signs and symptoms associated with heart failure when refeeding involves aggressive treatment such as enteral or parental feedings. ■

Diagnosis, Outcomes, and Interventions

The nurse is an integral part of the eating disorders treatment team. Promoting balanced nutrition is the focus of care for patients with anorexia or bulimia and with binge-eating disorder. The following patient and family issues should also be considered:

- Adherence to the therapeutic regimen
- Chronic low self-esteem
- Concerns with body image
- Dysfunctional family processes.

When planning and implementing care, consider the following nursing activities:

- Regularly monitor weight, using standard conditions. *Weight gain or loss provides information about the effectiveness of care, as well as the patient's risk for complications.*
- Monitor food intake during meals, recording percentage of meal and snack consumed. Maintain close observation for at least 1 hour following meals; do not allow patient alone in bathroom. *Observing the patient during and after meals helps prevent disposal of food and purging behavior after eating. Recording actual food intake allows accurate calculation of calorie intake.*
- Serve balanced meals, including all nutrient groups. Increase serving size gradually. *The patient may find normal food servings overwhelming, reducing the desire to eat. Calorie intake is initially limited to prevent complications associated with refeeding, then gradually increased.*
- Serve frequent, small feedings of cold or room-temperature foods. *Cool foods reduce sensations of early satiety, promoting greater food intake at a meal or snack.*
- Administer a multivitamin and mineral supplement to replace losses.

Patients with eating disorders require extended treatment of the disorder. Involvement of the family and social support persons is vital to success. Encourage family members to participate in teaching and nutritional counseling sessions. Discuss the value of family therapy to address issues that have contributed to the disorder. Emphasize the need to provide consistent messages of support for healthy eating habits. Discuss using rewards for food and calorie intake rather than weight gain. Provide referrals to a dietitian, nutritional support team, counseling, and support groups for people with eating disorders.

Transitions of Care

Primary prevention strategies focus on health promotion interventions that aim to address diet and nutrition status. Interventions include teaching patients and families about meal planning, food selection and preparation, and resources available to obtain a consistently healthy diet. Secondary prevention strategies include early identification of patients at risk for an eating disorder. The nurse should develop a trusting relationship with the at-risk patient and conduct a nutritional assessment using a nonjudgmental approach. The nurse should refer patients to a nutritionist and mental health provider once early signs of an eating disorder are identified.

Acute care management of a patient with an eating disorder will involve stabilizing fluid and electrolyte balance and monitoring for complications related to refeeding. The nurse should establish a trusting relationship and prepare the patient for the intensive follow-up treatment that will continue after being discharged from acute care. Introducing the patient to the members of the interprofessional team who will be involved in the outpatient treatment plan should be facilitated, if possible.

Eating disorders involve long-term outpatient care with possible exacerbations, and the nurse may assume a role as the patient's case manager, which will involve coordinating all aspects of care provided by each member of the interprofessional team. The nursing role will involve monitoring nutritional status, coordinating care with an interprofessional team, and maintaining a supportive and trusting relationship with the patient.

End-of-life care for the patient with an eating disorder will likely be an unexpected death and may involve resuscitation efforts and all postincident care, which will include supporting the patient's family and friends. Refer the family to support groups to assist with grieving.

CHAPTER HIGHLIGHTS

22.1 Obesity

Describe the pathophysiology, manifestations, and complications of obesity, and outline the interprofessional care and nursing care of patients with obesity.

- Obesity, defined as excess adipose tissue and a BMI greater than 30, is linked with many disorders, including type 2 diabetes, coronary heart disease, gallbladder disease, and osteoarthritis.
- Exercise and reduced kilocalorie intake are the mainstays of obesity treatment. Drugs that suppress the appetite or interfere with fat absorption in the gut may be used to facilitate weight loss in patients with multiple risk factors for obesity complications or people who have had difficulty achieving weight loss through diet and exercise.
- Bariatric surgery is a treatment option for patients who are morbidly obese. The primary types of bariatric surgery used in the United States are restrictive procedures that limit stomach capacity and food consumption, and combination restrictive/malabsorptive procedures that limit both capacity and nutrient absorption.
- Nursing care for patients with obesity focuses on health promotion, education, health coaching, and support of the prescribed treatment plan.

22.2 Malnutrition

Describe the pathophysiology and manifestations of malnutrition, and outline the interprofessional care and nursing care of patients with malnutrition.

- In the United States, protein-calorie malnutrition is a common problem among hospitalized patients. Malnutrition increases the risk for complications and impairs healing. Early identification and prevention are the primary focuses of treatment; nurses can be instrumental in identifying at-risk patients (e.g., older adults, patients living alone, people on extended NPO status).
- Refeeding of malnourished patients is a gradual process. Enteral feedings (oral or by feeding tube) are preferred whenever possible. Parenteral nutrition may be required when enteral feeding is not possible or not tolerated by the patient.

22.3 Eating Disorders

Describe the pathophysiology and manifestations of eating disorders, and outline the interprofessional care and nursing care of patients with these disorders.

- Eating disorders, including anorexia nervosa, bulimia nervosa, and binge-eating disorder, can be difficult to treat effectively and maintain in remission. While patients with anorexia are typically underweight and malnourished, resisting efforts to achieve a normal weight, patients with bulimia are more likely to be of normal weight and those with binge-eating disorder are more likely to be overweight or obese.
- Treatment for eating disorders is multifaceted, including physical care to restore electrolyte balance and treat complications, nutritional counseling and therapy, psychosocial therapy, family support, and possibly medication.

TEST YOURSELF NCLEX-RN® REVIEW

1. While reviewing the medical history, the nurse determines a patient is at risk for obesity.
   Which findings contribute to the nurse's assessment? (Select all that apply.)
   A. The patient's identical twin has a BMI of 27.8.
   B. The patient lists computer gaming as a major source of enjoyment.
   C. The patient takes medication for depression.
   D. The patient eats most meals at home.
   E. The patient rarely watches television.
2. A patient on a reduced-calorie diet asks the nurse what she can do to lose weight faster because most weeks she loses no more than 0.5 lb. "At this rate, it will take me years to get to my goal!" What should the nurse respond to this patient?
   A. "Let's reevaluate your long-term goal. Perhaps it was set too low for you."
   B. "You sound frustrated. Would you like to take some time off from your diet and exercise plan?"
   C. "Perhaps we should look into a diet supplement since you are unable to stick with your prescribed diet plan."
   D. "A pound of body fat equals 3500 calories. Let's reevaluate your diet and exercise plan for calorie intake and expenditure."
3. The nurse suspects a patient is experiencing protein-calorie malnutrition. What did the nurse assess to come to this conclusion? (Select all that apply.)
   A. Thin hair
   B. Dry, flaking skin
   C. Anxiety and agitation
   D. Recent 5-lb weight loss
   E. Hyperactive bowel sounds
4. The nurse is planning care for a patient scheduled for bariatric surgery. Which interventions should the nurse expect to be part of the patient's post-operative care? (Select all that apply.)
   A. Use of a continuous positive airway pressure (CPAP) device throughout the post-operative period
   B. Need to monitor effects of anesthesia for a shorter period of time than with patients of normal weight
   C. Continuation of cardiac monitor into the post-operative period
   D. Reduction of normal amounts of post-operative analgesics to reduce chance of respiratory depression
   E. Use of strict aseptic technique in all wound care activities
5. The nurse is negotiating goals of care with a patient being treated for anorexia nervosa. Which would be a realistic goal for this patient?
   A. Gain 2 pounds per week.
   B. Participate in family counseling.
   C. Rest alone in room following meals.
   D. Consume 100% of a 2500-calorie diet every day.
6. The nurse is identifying actual and potential problems for a patient with obesity. Which problem is the priority for a patient with a BMI of 30.4 and a waist-to-hip ratio of 1.1?
   A. Difficulty coping
   B. Insufficient knowledge regarding healthy diet choices
   C. Prior difficulty achieving weight loss goals
   D. Cardiac complications associated with obesity

7. The nurse is providing discharge instructions to a patient recovering from bariatric surgery. Which patient statements indicate diet teaching has been effective? (Select all that apply.)
   A. "I should drink fluids with meals to aid with digestion."
   B. "I should drink caffeinated carbonated liquids to aid with weight loss."
   C. "I can eat anything that I want because weight loss will occur regardless of food intake."
   D. "I should eat four to six small meals each day that are low in fat, high in complex carbohydrates, and high in protein."
   E. "I should avoid foods that are high in simple carbohydrates."
8. The home care nurse is planning care for a homebound older adult who is losing an unplanned 1 to 2 pounds each month. What should the nurse's plan of care for this patient include? (Select all that apply.)
   A. Referral for diagnostic studies
   B. Use of nutritional supplements
   C. Follow-up by primary care physician
   D. Placement in a residential care facility
   E. Transportation to congregate senior meals
9. The nurse is concerned that a postoperative patient is at risk for malnutrition. Which intervention would be a priority to prevent malnutrition in this patient?
   A. Measuring daily weights
   B. Maintaining aggressive pain management
   C. Maintaining intravenous flow
   D. Requesting early restoration of oral intake
10. Three days after gastric bypass surgery, a patient complains of increasing abdominal pain. Bowel sounds are absent and the abdomen is firm and very tender. What should the nurse do first?
   A. Discuss the findings with the surgeon.
   B. Evaluate the effectiveness of analgesia.
   C. Ambulate the patient to promote peristalsis.
   D. Chart assessment data and continue to monitor.

See Test Yourself answers in Appendix B.

REFERENCES

Adams, M. P., Holland, L. N., & Urban, C. (2017). *Pharmacology for nursing: A pathophysiologic approach* (5th ed.). Hoboken, NJ: Pearson Education.

Ahacic, J. A. (2016). A look at eating disorders. *Nursing Made Incredibly Easy, 14*(2), 28–36.

Anthony, P. S. (2008). Nutrition screen tools for hospitalized patients. *Nutrition in Clinical Practice, 23*(4), 373–382.

Bauer, L., & Bodenheimer, T. (2017). Expanded role of registered nurses in primary care delivery of the future. *Nursing Outlook, 65*, 624–632.

Budd, G. M., & Peterson, J. A. (2014). The obesity epidemic, part 1: Understanding the origins. *American Journal of Nursing, 114*(2), 40–46.

Budd, G. M., & Peterson, J. A. (2015). The obesity epidemic, part 2: Nursing assessment and intervention, a framework to guide patient care. *American Journal of Nursing, 115*(1), 38–46.

Caple, C., & DeVestry, G. (2017). *Parenteral nutrition: Assessing for and preventing complications.* Glendale, CA: Cinhal Information Systems.

Casazza, K., Brown, A., Astrup, A., Bertz, F., Baum, C., Brown, M. B., . . . Allison, D. B. (2015). Weighing the evidence of common belief in obesity research. *Critical Review Food, Science, Nutrition, 55*(14), 2014–2053.

Centers for Disease Control and Prevention (CDC). (2015a). *Physical activity basics*. Retrieved from www.cdc.gov/physicalactivity/basics/index.htm.

Centers for Disease Control and Prevention (CDC). (2015b). *Prevalence of obesity among adults and youth: United States, 2011–2014.* Retrieved from https://www.cdc.gov/nchs/data/databriefs/db219.pdf.

Centers for Disease Control and Prevention (CDC). (2015c). *Strategies to prevent obesity*. Retrieved from https://www.cdc.gov/obesity/strategies/index.html.

Centers for Disease Control and Prevention (CDC). (2017). *Overweight and obesity*. Retrieved from https://itunes.apple.com/us/app/pdf-reader-pro-free-edition/id919472673?mt=12.

Cooley, M. (2016). Preventing long-term poor outcomes in the bariatric patient postoperatively. *Dimensions of Critical Care Nursing, 36*(1), 30–34.

DiMaria-Ghalili, R. A., Gilbert., K., Lord, L., Neal, T., Richardson, D., Tyler, R., . . . American Society for Parenteral and Enteral Nutrition. (2016). Standards of nutrition care practice and professional performance for nutrition support and generalist nurses. *Nutrition in Clinical Practice*, *31*(4), 527–547.

Hales, C. M., Carroll, M. D., & Ogden, C. L. (2017). *Prevalence of obesity among adults and youth: United States, 2015–2016* [NCHS Data Brief No. 288]. Hyattsville, MD: National Center for Health Statistics.

Heimburger, D. C. (2015). Malnutrition and nutritional assessment. In D. Kasper, A. Fauci, S. Hauser, D. Longo, J. Jameson, & J. Loscalzo (Eds.), *Harrison's principles of internal medicine*, *97* (19th ed.). Retrieved from http://accessmedicine.mhmedical.com.liboff.ohsu.edu/content.aspx?bookid=1130&sectionid=79752839. New York: McGraw-Hill.

Hood, M. M., Corsica, J., Bradley, L, Wilson, R., Chirinos, D., & Vivo, A. (2016). Managing severe obesity: Understanding and improving treatment adherence in bariatric surgery. *Journal of Behavioral Medicine*, *39*, 1092–1103.

Kee, J. (2018). *Laboratory and diagnostic tests with nursing implications* (10th ed.). Upper Saddle River, NJ: Pearson Prentice Hall.

Kirby, D. F., Corrigan, M. L., Hendrickson, E., & Emery, D. M. (2017). Overview of home parenteral nutrition: An update. *Nutrition in Clinical Practice*, *32*(6), 739– 752.

Kushner, R. F. (2015). Evaluation and management of obesity. In D. Kasper, A. Fauci, S. Hauser, D. Longo, J. Jameson, & J. Loscalzo (Eds.), *Harrison's principles of internal medicine*, *416* (19th ed.). Retrieved from http://accessmedicine.mhmedical.com.liboff.ohsu.edu/content.aspx?bookid=1130&sectionid=79752839. New York: McGraw-Hill.

Laur, C., & Keller, H. (2017). Making the case for nutrition screening in older adults in primary care. *Nutrition Today*, *52*(3), 129–136.

McClave, S. A., Taylor, B. E., Martindale, R. G., Warren, M. M., Johnson, D. R., Braunschweig, C., . . . American Society of Parenteral and Enteral Nutrition (2016). Guidelines for the provision and assessment of nutrition support therapy in the adult critically ill patient. *Journal of Parenteral and Enteral Nutrition*, *40*(2), 159–211.

Moyer, V. A. (2012). Screening for and management of obesity in adults: U.S. Preventive Services Task Force recommendation statement. *Annals of Internal Medicine*, *157*(5), 373–378.

National Association of Clinical Nurse Specialists. (2017). *Malnutrition in hospitalized adult patients: The role of the clinical nurse specialist*. Retrieved from http://nacns.org/wp-content/uploads/2017/01/Malnutrition-Report.pdf.

National Center for Health Statistics. (2017). *National health and nutrition examination survey*. Retrieved from https://www.cdc.gov/nchs/data/factsheets/factsheet_nhanes.htm.

National Institute of Diabetes and Digestive and Kidney Diseases (NIDDK). (2018). *Overweight and obesity statistics*. Retrieved from https://www.niddk.nih.gov/health-information/health-statistics/overweight-obesity.

O'Leary-Kelley, C., & Bawel-Brinkley, K. (2017). Nutrition support protocols: Enhancing the delivery of enteral nutrition. *Critical Care Nurse*, *37*(2), e15–23.

Harvard Pilgrim Health Care. (2016). *Medical review criteria: Formulas and enteral nutrition: An overview*. Retrieved from https://www.harvardpilgrim.org/portal/page?_pageid=253,9729993&_dad=portal&_schema=PORTAL

Rabito, E. I., Marcadenti, A., da Silva Fink, J., Figueira, L., & Silva, F. M. (2017). Nutritional Risk Screening 2002, Short Nutritional Assessment Questionnaire, Malnutrition Screening Tool, and Malnutrition Universal Screening Toll are good predictors of nutrition risk in and emergency service. *Nutrition in Clinical Practice*, *32*(4), 526–532.

Reus, V. I. (2015). Mental disorders: Feeding and eating disorders (2015). In D. Kasper, A. Fauci, S. Hauser, D. Longo, J. Jameson, & J. Loscalzo (Eds.), *Harrison's principles of internal medicine*, *466* (19th ed.). Retrieved from http://accessmedicine.mhmedical.com.liboff.ohsu.edu/content.aspx?bookid=1130&sectionid=79752839. New York: McGraw-Hill.

Rodgers, L., & Phillips, C. A. (2018). Dumping syndrome: Causes, management, and patient education. *American Nurse Today*, *13*(1), 6–9.

Schauer, P. R., Bhatt, D. L., Kirwan, J. P., Wolski, K., Aminian, A., Brethauer, S. A., . . . STAMPEDE Investigators. (2017). Bariatric surgery versus intensive medical therapy for diabetes—5-year outcomes. *New England Journal of Medicine*, *376*(7), 641–651.

Schiavon, B. A., Bersch-Ferreira, A. C., Santucci, E. V., Oliveira, J. D., Torreglosa, C. R., Bueno, P. T., . . . Berwanger, O. (2017). Effects of bariatric surgery in obese patients with hypertension: The GATEWAY randomized trial Gastric Bypass to Treat Obese Patients with Steady Hypertension. *Circulation*, *137*, 1132–1142.

Shukla, A., Buniak, W. I., & Aronne, L. J. (2015). Treatment of obesity in 2015. *Journal of Cardiopulmonary Rehabilitation and Prevention*, *35*, 81–92.

Sorenson, M., Quinn, L., & Klein, D. (2019). *Pathophysiology: Concepts of human disease*. Hoboken, NJ: Pearson Education.

The Joint Commission. (2018). *Nutrition and Feeding Standards*. Retrieved March 4, 2018 from www.jointcommission.org/standards_information/edition.aspx.

Villareal, D. T., Acquirre, L., Gurney, A. B., Waters, D. L., Sinacore, D. R., Colombo, E., . . . Qualls, C. (2018). Aerobic or resistance exercise, or both, in dieting obese, older adults. *New England Journal of Medicine*, *365*(20), 1843–1955.

World Health Organization. (2018). *Obesity and overweight fact sheet.* Retrieved from http://www.who.int/mediacentre/factsheets/fs311/en/.

Yordy, B. M., Roberts, S., & Taggart, H. M. (2017). Quality improvement in clinical nutrition: Screening and mealtime protection for the hospitalized patient. *Clinical Nurse Specialist*, *31*(3), 149–156.

ADDITIONAL RESOURCES

National Institute of Diabetes and Digestive and Kidney Diseases
www.niddk.nih.gov

National Institute of Mental Health
www.nimh.nih.gov/health/publications/eating-disorders/index.shtml

The Joint Commission's *Nutrition and Feeding Standards* (2018)
www.jointcommission.org/standards_information/edition.aspx

Chapter 23

Nursing Care of Patients with Upper Gastrointestinal Disorders

Chapter Outline and Learning Outcomes

Describe the pathophysiology and manifestations of nausea and vomiting, and outline the interprofessional care and nursing care of patients with nausea and vomiting.

Describe the pathophysiology and manifestations of disorders of the mouth, and outline the interprofessional care and nursing care of patients with these disorders.

Describe the pathophysiology and manifestations of disorders of the esophagus, and outline the interprofessional care and nursing care of patients with these disorders.

Describe the pathophysiology and manifestations of disorders of the stomach and duodenum, and outline the interprofessional care and nursing care of patients with these disorders.

CLINICAL COMPETENCIES

- Assess the health status of patients with upper gastrointestinal disorders.
- Monitor, identify, document, and report significant manifestations of upper gastrointestinal disorders and their complications.
- Plan patient-centered nursing care using evidence-based practice guidelines, research, and, as appropriate, health information technology.
- Determine priority nursing diagnoses, problems, and interventions based on assessed data.
- Administer medications and prescribed care knowledgeably and safely.
- Integrate and coordinate interprofessional care into plan of care.
- Construct and revise individualized plans of care considering the culture and values of the patient.
- Plan and provide patient and family teaching to promote, maintain, and restore health.

KEY TERMS

achalasia, 710
anorexia, 725
Curling ulcers, 724
Cushing ulcers, 724
dumping syndrome, 728
dysphagia, 710
erosive (stress-induced) gastritis, 724
gastric mucosal barrier, 713
gastritis, 724
gastroesophageal reflux, 704
gastroesophageal reflux disease (GERD), 704
hematemesis, 713
hematochezia, 713
melena, 713
nausea, 692
occult bleeding, 714
partial gastrectomy, 728
peptic ulcer disease (PUD), 715
peptic ulcers, 715
steatorrhea, 719
stomatitis, 697
total gastrectomy, 728
ulcer, 716
vomiting, 692
Zollinger-Ellison syndrome, 719

The upper gastrointestinal tract includes the mouth, esophagus, stomach, and proximal small intestine (**Figure 23.1** ■). Food and fluids, ingested through the mouth, move through the esophagus to the stomach. The stomach and upper intestinal tract (duodenum and jejunum) are responsible for the majority of food digestion. When an acute or chronic condition or disease process interferes with the function of this portion of the gastrointestinal (GI) tract, nutritional status can be affected and the patient may experience symptoms that interfere with functional status and lifestyle.

Nurses provide acute care for the hospitalized patient, coordinate care in ambulatory and long-term care settings, and teach the skills and knowledge needed to manage these conditions at home.

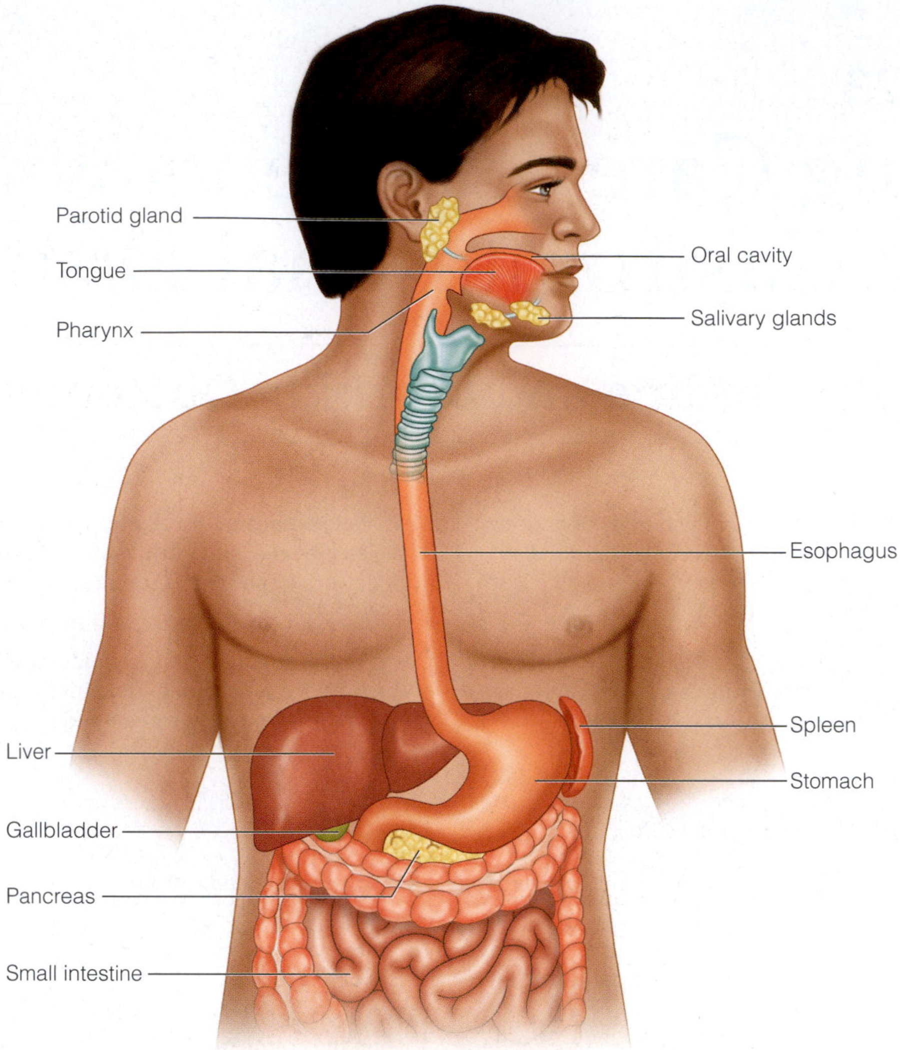
Parotid gland
Tongue
Pharynx
Oral cavity
Salivary glands
Esophagus
Spleen
Stomach
Liver
Gallbladder
Pancreas
Small intestine

Figure 23.1 ■ The upper gastrointestinal tract.

23.1 Nausea and Vomiting

Nausea and vomiting are common gastrointestinal symptoms. **Nausea** is a vague but unpleasant sensation of sickness or queasiness. It may or may not be accompanied by (and possibly relieved by) vomiting. **Vomiting** is the forceful expulsion of the contents of the upper GI tract resulting from contraction of muscles in the gut and abdominal wall. Nausea and vomiting without abdominal pain are commonly associated with food poisoning, infectious gastroenteritis (discussed in Chapter 24), gallbladder disease, or ingestion of toxins (drugs or alcohol). When associated with severe abdominal pain, they may indicate a serious disorder such as peritonitis, acute gastrointestinal obstruction, or pancreatitis.

The Patient with Nausea and Vomiting

Pathophysiology

Nausea, an unpleasant subjective sensation, occurs when the vomiting center in the medulla of the brain is stimulated. Distention of the duodenum is a common stimulus for nausea. The vomiting center can be stimulated by input from several different sources:

- The GI tract, produced by distention, irritation, or infection
- The vestibular system of the ear
- Higher central nervous system (CNS) centers in response to certain sights, smells, or emotional experiences
- Chemoreceptors outside the blood–brain barrier that are stimulated by drugs, chemotherapeutic agents, toxins, systemic disorders, and pregnancy
- Disorders such as acute myocardial infarction and heart failure commonly produce nausea and vomiting, possibly due to direct stimulation of the vomiting center by hypoxia
- Increased intracranial pressure (e.g., due to intracranial bleeding or a tumor) produces vomiting that may or may not be accompanied by nausea.

Anorexia (loss of appetite) commonly precedes nausea, just as nausea frequently precedes vomiting. Vomiting—a response that requires coordinated movements of the thorax and abdominal wall, the gut, the pharynx, and muscles of the mouth and face—is coordinated by the brainstem. *Emesis* (or *vomitus*) is produced when inspiratory muscles of the thorax (including the diaphragm) and abdomen contract, increasing intrathoracic and intra-abdominal pressures. The gastroesophageal sphincter relaxes, and the larynx moves upward to facilitate oral expulsion of gastric contents.

Manifestations

In addition to the subjective sensation of queasiness, nausea is frequently accompanied by autonomic nervous system manifestations such as pallor, sweating, tachycardia, and increased salivation (a reflex protecting the teeth from stomach acid). Vomiting, which stimulates the vagus nerve and parasympathetic nervous system, may be accompanied by dizziness, light-headedness, hypotension, and bradycardia.

Potential complications of vomiting include dehydration, hypokalemia, metabolic alkalosis (from loss of hydrochloric acid from the stomach), aspiration with resulting pneumonia, and rupture or tears of the esophagus.

In most cases, nausea and vomiting are self-limited and require no treatment. However, repeated studies show nausea is the most debilitating effect of chemotherapy for many patients (Vidall, Sharma, & Amlani, 2016) and is still a major problem for many surgical patients (Hasler, 2015). Moreover, evidence suggests healthcare professionals underestimate the occurrence of nausea in postoperative and chemotherapy patients and that it is often poorly assessed and underreported (Vidall et al., 2016). Identifying the etiology of nausea and vomiting will facilitate the development of an effective treatment plan.

Vomiting can have several potentially serious physical effects. Postoperative nausea and vomiting (PONV) can delay healing and postpone discharge. Strong contractions of the abdominal wall and thoracic skeletal muscles can increase postoperative pain. Pressure may burst wounds and increase stress on the eye following ophthalmic surgery and can dangerously increase intracranial pressure in cases of intracerebral hemorrhage or injury. Chronic and prolonged vomiting may cause fluid and electrolyte imbalance, disrupt acid–base balance, and lead to nutritional deficits. Prolonged vomiting can cause pitting and erosion of tooth enamel, causing dental decay. If vomiting is severe or accompanied by other symptoms, acute care may be required to determine the underlying problem and prevent or treat complications.

Interprofessional Care

Diagnostic tests may include serum electrolytes; pregnancy testing, if indicated; liver, pancreatic, and renal function studies; and imaging studies (flat plate of the abdomen, abdominal CT scan) to detect gastrointestinal obstruction. An upper endoscopy may be performed (see Chapter 21 for nursing care of the patient undergoing an upper endoscopy). A CT scan or MRI of the head may be ordered if an intracranial problem is suspected as the cause. Specialized testing such as gastrointestinal motility studies may be indicated when other diagnostic studies are negative for an anatomic cause of nausea and vomiting.

Food is initially withheld, although clear liquids in small quantities are encouraged to prevent dehydration. Dry foods such as soda crackers may reduce nausea and promote comfort.

Medications

Unless vomiting is associated with pregnancy, antiemetic medications may be prescribed to prevent or control nausea and vomiting. These drugs fall into a number of different classes and are often more effective when given in combination.

- Serotonin receptor antagonists are widely used drugs available for patients experiencing nausea and vomiting due to chemotherapy. They are effective when given only once or twice a day, an additional advantage. Palonosetron (Aloxi), with a half-life of 40 hours, is particularly effective for nausea and vomiting related to chemotherapy. Ondansetron (Zofran) is a commonly prescribed drug in this class.
- Phenothiazines and phenothiazine-like drugs (e.g., prochlorperazine [Compazine] and thiethylperazine [Torecan]), promethazine (Phenergan), trimethobenzamide (Tigan), and other drugs such as metoclopramide (Reglan), although effective, can produce extrapyramidal symptoms, sedation, and hypotension.
- Antihistamines such as meclizine (Antivert), hydroxyzine (Vistaril, Atarax), and dimenhydrinate (Dramamine) are primarily used to treat nausea and vomiting arising from vestibular center stimuli (e.g., motion sickness).
- Two drugs classed as cannabinoids, related to marijuana, are approved to treat nausea and vomiting associated with chemotherapy (Welliver, 2016). These drugs, dronabinol (Marinol) and nabilone (Cesamet), may produce unpleasant psychiatric effects such as dissociation and dysphoria and are contraindicated for patients with psychiatric disorders. Tachycardia and hypotension are additional possible side effects.
- Corticosteroids may be used in combination with other classes of antiemetics to treat nausea and vomiting associated with chemotherapy-induced nausea and vomiting (CINC). Methylprednisolone (Solu-Medrol) and dexamethasone (Decadron) may be used in combination to treat vomiting associated with cancer treatment.
- Lorazepam (Ativan) is a benzodiazepine drug approved for use as an antiemetic. It produces a degree of sedation, but can suppress anticipatory vomiting (e.g., before chemotherapy). It also helps control extrapyramidal symptoms associated with the phenothiazine antiemetics.
- Neurokinin receptor antagonists are used primarily to prevent nausea and vomiting associated with chemotherapy. Aprepitant (Emend) is a prototype of this class.

Nursing responsibilities and patient education for antiemetic drugs are outlined in **Medication Administration 23.A.**

Medication Administration 23.A

Drugs Used to Prevent and Treat Nausea and Vomiting

SEROTONIN RECEPTOR ANTAGONISTS

dolasetron (Anzemet)

granisetron (Kytril)

ondansetron (Zofran)

palonosetron (Aloxi)

The serotonin receptor antagonists suppress nausea and vomiting by blocking the effect of serotonin on vagal afferent nerves that stimulate the vomiting center. Their primary uses are to prevent and treat vomiting associated with chemotherapy, radiation therapy, and surgery.

Nursing Responsibilities

- Administer 30 to 60 minutes prior to chemotherapy or surgery as directed.
- May be given orally or intravenously (push or infusion; follow directions specific to the drug used).
- Monitor liver function and clotting studies; report abnormal levels to the physician.

Health Education for the Patient and Family

- Take this drug exactly as directed.
- This drug may be taken without regard to food intake.
- Headache is a common side effect of these drugs; use acetaminophen or another mild analgesic as directed by your physician.

PHENOTHIAZINE AND PHENOTHIAZINE-LIKE

chlorpromazine (Thorazine)

droperidol (Inapsine)

haloperidol (Haldol)

metoclopramide (Reglan)

prochlorperazine (Compazine)

promethazine (Phenergan)

thiethylperazine (Torecan)

These drugs act by blocking dopamine receptors in the chemoreceptor trigger zone (CTZ). Their primary use is to suppress the nausea and vomiting associated with surgery, cancer chemotherapy, and toxins. The major adverse effects associated with these drugs are sedation, hypotension, and extrapyramidal reactions. Older adults are more sensitive to the effects of these drugs; a lower dose is often indicated.

Nursing Responsibilities

- Administer orally or parenterally as ordered before surgery or before meals and procedures known to produce nausea and vomiting.
- These drugs may interact with a number of other medications, often increasing their sedative and hypotensive effects.
- Administer with caution to older adults, closely monitoring for adverse effects such as confusion, agitation, or changes in vital signs.
- Monitor for evidence of extrapyramidal symptoms, including tremor, restlessness, hyperactivity, anxiety, and impaired coordination; notify physician if symptoms develop.

Health Education for the Patient and Family

- Use the drug as ordered; do not increase your dose without consulting your primary care provider.
- These drugs may cause drowsiness. Avoid using other CNS depressants such as alcohol while taking these drugs.
- Change positions from lying to sitting and sitting to standing slowly because these drugs can cause light-headedness or dizziness.
- Promptly report changes in coordination, tremors, difficulty speaking or swallowing, or weakness to your physician.

NEUROKININ RECEPTOR ANTAGONIST

aprepitant (Emend)

Aprepitant is a new drug that can prevent both acute and delayed chemotherapy-induced nausea and vomiting when given in combination with other antiemetic drugs. It is well absorbed when given orally and has a prolonged duration of action.

Nursing Responsibilities

- Administer daily for 3 days, giving the first dose 1 hour before chemotherapy.
- Can be given with food or on an empty stomach.
- Monitor for toxic and desired effects of other drugs, including chemotherapy drugs, corticosteroids, and warfarin (Coumadin), because aprepitant can affect metabolism and blood levels.

Health Education for the Patient and Family

- Use barrier contraception while taking this drug because oral contraceptives will be less effective.
- Promptly contact your physician if you develop skin rash, difficulty breathing, changes in heartbeat or blood pressure, dizziness or confusion, leg or abdominal pain, or rectal bleeding.
- Contact your physician before taking any new prescription, over-the-counter, or herbal preparations.

ANTICHOLINERGICS AND ANTIHISTAMINES

buclizine (Bucladin-S)

cyclizine (Marezine)

dimenhydrinate (Dramamine)

diphenhydramine (Benadryl)

hydroxyzine (Vistaril, Atarax)

meclizine (Antivert)

Anticholinergics and antihistamines are primarily used to treat the nausea and vomiting associated with motion sickness. They act by blocking histamine and acetylcholine (muscarinic) receptors in the neural pathway from the inner ear to the vomiting center in the brainstem.

Nursing Responsibilities

- Do not administer these drugs to patients for whom anticholinergic drugs are contraindicated: People with narrow-angle glaucoma, urinary retention, or bowel obstruction.
- May be administered orally, parenterally, or rectally, depending on the preparation and the patient's ability to tolerate oral preparations.
- Use with caution in patients who are taking other CNS depressants or antihistamine preparations, tricyclic antidepressants, or monoamine oxidase inhibitors.

Health Education for the Patient and Family

- These drugs frequently cause drowsiness. Use caution when operating machinery or performing tasks requiring mental alertness.

- Avoid using alcohol or other substances that cause drowsiness or sedation while taking these drugs.
- The medication may cause dry mouth. Sips of water, ice chips, hard candies, and sugarless gum can be used for comfort.
- Use sunscreen and protective clothing to protect from sunburn while using these drugs.

CANNABINOIDS

dronabinol (Marinol)

nabilone (Cesamet)

Drugs in this class, which contain the same active ingredient as marijuana, are reserved for use to relieve nausea and vomiting associated with cancer chemotherapy in patients who have not responded to treatment with other antiemetics. Their action is thought to result from inhibition of the vomiting center in the medulla.

Nursing Responsibilities

- Use with caution in older adults and people with a history of cardiovascular disease or substance abuse. These drugs are contraindicated for patients with a history of psychiatric disorders.
- Monitor for adverse effects such as dizziness, tachycardia, hypotension, impaired thinking and judgment, incoordination, irritability, depersonalization, distorted vision, and hallucinations.

Health Education for the Patient and Family

- Take the drug 1 to 3 hours before chemotherapy.
- Change positions slowly after taking this drug to prevent dizziness.
- You may experience distorted thinking, visual disturbances, confusion, and other mental symptoms while taking this drug.
- Keep this and all drugs out of the reach of children. Do not share this drug with anyone else.

Note: Medications identified in blue are among the 200 most frequently prescribed drugs in the U.S.

Source: Data from Adams, Holland, & Urban, 2017.

Integrative Therapies

Mind–body interventions such as biofeedback, guided imagery, music therapy, and hypnosis may be effective for some patients with nausea. Biofeedback uses machinery to translate physiologic processes into audible or visible signals to teach the patient to exert conscious control over those processes. In guided imagery, the patient uses imagination to invoke specific images to modify physiologic responses. Music therapy involves creating or listening to music to affect physiologic and psychologic responses. In hypnosis, an altered mind state is induced to make the patient receptive to suggestions.

Ginger, an aromatic root frequently used in cooking, may be helpful in relieving nausea and vomiting (Arslan & Ozdemir, 2015). In limited clinical trials, it has been shown to be safe for reducing nausea associated with pregnancy. It may also help relieve nausea associated with cancer chemotherapy and can be used in combination with antiemetic medications.

Moving Evidence into Action

Integrative Therapy for Treating Nausea and Vomiting

Clinical Issues

Patients undergoing regimens for cancer treatment often experience treatment-related nausea and vomiting (Schub & Holle, 2018). Careful assessment will help the interprofessional team assess patients' risk for experiencing nausea and vomiting and plan interventions to prevent it. Newer antiemetic drugs are increasingly effective in preventing and treating radiation and chemotherapy-induced nausea and vomiting (CINV), but many patients still experience both acute and delayed nausea and vomiting. Integrative therapy may prevent delayed nausea and vomiting.

External Evidence

A study by Arslan and Ozdemir (2015) examined the effectiveness of ginger to prevent acute delayed nausea and vomiting for cancer patients receiving chemotherapy ($p > 0.0001$). Patients in the treatment group received 500 mg of powdered ginger twice a day during the first 3 days of chemotherapy. The study found that patients in the intervention group experienced less nausea and fewer episodes of vomiting than patients in the control group ($p < 0.001$).

Internal Evidence

As part of the evaluation of internal evidence, the feasibility of the intervention in relation to the outcome of interest (reduced nausea and vomiting) must be considered. Current standards of care and inclusion of the interprofessional team in the recommendation to include ginger as a component of the treatment plan must be considered. Several questions should be considered:

- Is the problem (CINV) significant in the population of your care environment?
- Does the interprofessional team support the use of the intervention?
- Are there any potential adverse interactions with other medications to consider?
- Are there any potential side effects related to the intervention?

Patient Considerations

When considering use of a new intervention, the nurse must consider the specific patient population where it will be used. Will patients and their caregivers be amenable to the new intervention?

Putting the Pieces Together

The design and implementation of a preventative plan to treat CINV is essential for any patient receiving chemotherapy. To

(continued)

effectively implement a plan, the external evidence must be evaluated and the internal implications for patient, caregivers, and family must be considered. With the implementation of integrative medicine interventions, the outcome (reduction in CINV) should be assessed in every patient and the aggregate data should be organized and evaluated on a regular basis to determine the best standards of care.

References

Arslan, M., & Ozdemir, L. (2015). Oral intake of ginger for chemotherapy-induced nausea and vomiting among women with breast cancer. *Clinical Journal of Oncology Nursing*, *19*(5), E92–E97.

Schub T., & Holle, M. (2018). *Chemotherapy-related nausea and vomiting*. Glendale, CA: Cinahl Information Systems.

Nursing Care

Assessment

Assessment of the patient is vital to help determine the cause of nausea and vomiting and to rule out underlying systemic disease or acute conditions that require immediate care (e.g., bowel obstruction). When the cause is known or no other acute symptoms are present, nursing interventions can promote comfort and prevent complications.

- ***Health history:*** Determine if the patient has a past history with nausea and vomiting. Personal or family history of PONV or motion sickness increases an individual's likelihood of experiencing both PONV and CINV. Establish onset and duration of nausea and frequency, quantity, and characteristics of emesis. Ask the patient what treatments he or she has used to control nausea and vomiting. Determine if the patient is experiencing signs and symptoms associated with dehydration or electrolyte imbalance.
- ***Physical assessment:*** Physical assessment should focus on signs and symptoms of dehydration and electrolyte imbalance and include vital signs, skin turgor, mucous membranes, and weight.

Priorities of Care

Prolonged nausea and vomiting can cause fluid, electrolyte, and nutritional deficits and can severely affect patients' health. Monitor carefully for these untoward effects.

Diagnosis, Outcomes, and Intervention

The diagnosis of nausea is defined as a subjective, unpleasant, wavelike sensation in the throat, epigastric region, or abdomen that may lead to vomiting (Sorenson, Quinn, & Klein, 2019).

Manage Nausea and Vomiting. Nursing care for the patient experiencing nausea and vomiting is supportive and educational. Both CINV and PONV should be treated aggressively with an aim toward preventing nausea and vomiting. CINV can result in an anticipatory response, which is nausea and vomiting occurring before drug administration due to a conditioned response to previous negative experience.

Expected Outcome: Patient's nausea will be relieved as evidenced by ample appetite, adequate hydration, absence of vomiting, and patient's reported relief from nausea.

The nurse will:

- Monitor subjective complaints of nausea. *Nausea is a subjective sensation best described by the patient.*
- Monitor vital signs, skin turgor and condition, and weight. Maintain accurate intake and output records. Monitor amount, color, and specific gravity of urine. *Nausea can cause aversion to food and fluids, leading to dehydration even when it is not accompanied by vomiting.*
- Administer antiemetic medication as prescribed, prior to meals and before treatments or procedures known to stimulate nausea. *Preventing nausea is particularly important for patients receiving chemotherapy, to avoid the association between the treatment and nausea. Preventing PONV is also important to expedite recovery and avoid prolonged hospitalization.*
- Instruct patient to deep breathe to voluntarily suppress the vomiting reflex. *Controlling vomiting helps prevent dehydration and other complications associated with prolonged or severe vomiting.*
- Instruct to consume small quantities of clear fluids and dry foods at separate times. *Separating the intake of dry foods and fluids helps reduce the nausea stimulus.*

Transitions of Care

Developing a patient-centered treatment plan in collaboration with the interprofessional team may prevent the nausea and vomiting associated with CINV and PONV. Completing a comprehensive assessment of each patient to assess personal characteristics and past experience with nausea and vomiting will create a personalized plan to prevent CINV and PONV (Schub & Holle, 2018). Support the patient in implementing nonpharmacologic treatment including behavioral therapy, hypnosis, guided imagery, and progressive muscle relaxation. Tertiary prevention includes monitoring for fluid and electrolyte imbalances when a patient experiences intractable nausea and vomiting over a prolonged period.

Administer antiemetics according to the interprofessional treatment plan for prevention and breakthrough nausea and vomiting. Advocate for a change in medications prescribed if medication is not preventing nausea and vomiting. Administer replacement IV fluids and electrolytes as ordered to correct the imbalances associated with intractable vomiting.

Studies indicate healthcare providers underestimate postdischarge nausea and vomiting and that up to one-third of ambulatory surgery patients experience PONV following discharge (Maurice, 2015). Providing thorough discharge teaching and ensuring patients have access to appropriate follow-up care will prevent unneeded rehospitalization.

Patients at risk for PONV or CINV should be contacted after discharge to determine if any nausea and vomiting was experienced and follow-up care should be initiated as needed.

Instruct the patient to restrict intake to small quantities of clear liquids (tea, apple juice, broth, Jell-O) and dry foods such as soda crackers to help reduce nausea and prevent vomiting. Teach to avoid food-preparation odors if they produce nausea. Advise to restrict fluid intake for 1 hour before and after meals. Stress the need to maintain fluid intake to prevent dehydration and the importance of seeking additional medical help if unable to take in fluids or keep food down. Provide information about electrolyte replacement solutions such as sports drinks and commercially available electrolyte replacement solutions.

Some chronic diseases such as heart, kidney, and neurologic conditions involve nausea and vomiting. Providing medications and nonpharmacological interventions should be included as part of the treatment plan, as nausea and vomiting adversely affect quality of life (Vidall et al., 2016). Teaching the patient to monitor symptoms and use medications for treatment is an essential nursing intervention for patients experiencing chronic nausea and vomiting.

Nausea and vomiting are often experienced at end of life and may be secondary to frequent administration of narcotics used to control pain and discomfort. Assessing the patient for nausea and vomiting should be an ongoing aspect of palliative care. Antiemetics and nonpharmacological interventions should be included in the plan of care.

23.2 Disorders of the Mouth

The health status of the oral cavity is linked to systemic diseases including cardiovascular disease and diabetes (Durso & Yellowitz, 2017). Inflammations, infections, and neoplastic lesions of the mouth affect food ingestion and nutrition. Oral lesions may have a variety of causes, including infection, trauma, irritants such as alcohol, and hypersensitivity. Appropriate treatment of the disorder, any underlying factors, and associated symptoms is essential.

The Patient with Stomatitis

Stomatitis, inflammation and ulcers of the oral mucosa, is a common disorder of the mouth (Schub & Heering, 2017). Viral infection is the most common cause. Other causes include bacterial or fungal infections, mechanical trauma (e.g., cheek biting), irritants (e.g., tobacco or ill-fitting dentures), nutritional deficiencies, and chemotherapeutic agents.

- Herpes simplex (cold sore) is the most frequent viral cause of stomatitis (**Figure 23.2** ■); others include primary varicella zoster (chickenpox), Epstein-Barr virus, influenza, cytomegalovirus, and HIV.
- Overgrowth of *Candida albicans* is the most frequent fungal cause of stomatitis, usually following antibiotic or corticosteroid therapy.
- About 40% of people undergoing chemotherapy to treat cancer experience *oral mucositis*, a type of stomatitis; 75% of those undergoing chemotherapy in preparation for bone marrow or stem cell transplant develop oral mucositis.
- Most patients undergoing radiation therapy of the head and neck develop oral mucositis.

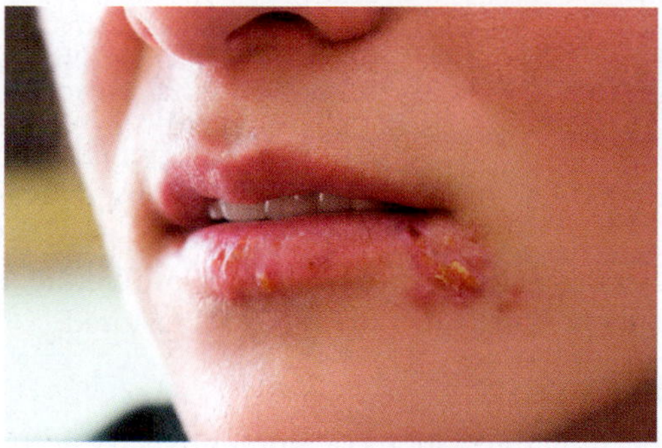

Figure 23.2 ■ Herpes simplex is the most frequent viral cause of stomatitis.

Stomatitis often affects people who are immunocompromised (e.g., patients with HIV disease or who have cancer and frail older adults). Common risk factors for stomatitis include:

- Age over 65 years
- Impaired immune status (HIV disease, cancer, diabetes)
- Chronic renal failure or heart failure
- Chemotherapy, radiation therapy, stem cell transplant
- Oxygen therapy, mouth breathing
- Medications (antibiotics, phenytoin, anticholinergics, corticosteroids)
- Poor oral hygiene, ill-fitting dentures
- Malnutrition and vitamin deficiencies
- Tobacco or alcohol use.

Pathophysiology

The oral mucosa, which lines the oral cavity, is a relatively thin, fragile layer of stratified squamous epithelial cells that is constantly being replaced. The blood supply to the oral mucosa is rich. As epithelial cells slough, stem cells in the submucosa develop into epithelial cells to replace those that are lost.

Frequent exposure to the environment, a rich blood supply, and the oral mucosa's delicate nature increase the risk of infection or inflammation, reaction to toxins, and trauma. Stomatitis results from persistent damage to oral mucosal cells. Damage is initially superficial, progressing to ulceration and involvement of the entire epithelium. Finally, healing begins within 2 to 4 weeks.

Oral mucositis progresses through identifiable stages. Radiotherapy and chemotherapy damage the DNA of epithelial cells, resulting in necrosis and death of some cells. This stimulates the release of inflammatory mediators that further damage tissues, causing additional epithelial cells to die. As a result, the oral mucosa thins. Tumor necrosis factor alpha (TNF-α) is released, which activates additional inflammatory cytokines. Tissues below the mucosa are damaged as well. In the ulcerative stage of oral mucositis, irregular ulcers that extend from the epithelium into the submucosa develop. As nerve endings are exposed, this stage is accompanied by significant pain. During the final healing stage, cells in the epithelium proliferate, and the normal thickness of the oral mucosa is restored.

Manifestations

The clinical manifestations of stomatitis vary according to its cause. **Table 23.1** outlines common causes of stomatitis with their manifestations and treatment. Chemotherapy or chemical irritation may result in initial generalized redness and swelling, followed by development of deep, irregular ulcerations. Ulcers may be covered with pseudomembranes. Oral pain associated with stomatitis can interfere with the ability to eat, drink, and swallow normally.

Potential complications of stomatitis include malnutrition, fluid and electrolyte imbalance, sepsis, and bacterial endocarditis.

Interprofessional Care

Stomatitis is diagnosed by direct physical examination and, if indicated, cultures, smears, and evaluation for systemic illness. Treatment addresses both the underlying cause and any coexisting illnesses (Critchlow, 2017). An undiagnosed oral lesion present for more than 1 week that does not respond to therapy must be evaluated for malignancy.

Direct smears and cultures of lesions may be obtained to identify causative organisms. If systemic illness is suspected, a variety of diagnostic tests may be ordered to identify the underlying cause.

General treatment measures include providing meticulous oral hygiene, with brushing using a soft brush and flossing (as tolerated). A solution of saline, sodium bicarbonate, or a combination of saline/bicarbonate promotes comfort and healing when used after and between meals.

Medications

Using a topical anesthetic, such as a mouthwash of 2% viscous lidocaine diluted with water, diphenhydramine (Benadryl) solution, or benzocaine spray or gel can promote comfort and the ability to consume oral food and fluids.

SAFETY ALERT: Instruct patients to expectorate lidocaine solution, not swallow it, to avoid impairment of swallowing. ■

Amlexanox (Aphthasol, OraDisc A) or Orabase, a protective paste, may be applied to oral ulcers to promote comfort. Amlexanox also speeds healing of aphthous ulcers. Triamcinolone acetonide may be mixed in Orabase to reduce inflammation and promote healing. Other coating agents include Amphojel or Kaopectate. Sodium bicarbonate mouthwashes may provide relief and promote cleansing, whereas alcohol-based mouthwashes may cause pain and burning and should be avoided. Agents that form a film over exposed nerve endings and deep ulcerations (e.g., Zilactin, Gelclair) may be used in patients with oral mucositis.

Fungal infections are often treated with a nystatin oral suspension; patients are instructed to "swish and swallow" the solution. Clotrimazole lozenges also treat oral fungal infections. If the infection does not resolve, oral antifungal medications such as fluconazole or ketoconazole may be used. Antifungals are usually continued for at least 3 days after symptoms disappear.

Table 23.1 Manifestations and Treatment of Common Stomatitis Conditions

Type	Cause	Manifestations	Treatment
Cold sore, fever blister	Herpes simplex virus	■ Initial burning at site ■ Clustered vesicular lesions on lip or oral mucosa	■ Self-limiting ■ Acyclovir, famciclovir, valacyclovir to shorten course
Aphthous ulcer (canker sore, ulcerative stomatitis)	Unknown; may be type of herpes virus	■ Well-circumscribed, shallow erosions with white or yellow center encircled by red ring ■ < 1 cm in diameter ■ Painful	■ Topical steroid ointment ■ Amlexanox oral paste (Aphthasol) ■ Oral prednisone
Candidiasis (thrush)	*Candida albicans*	■ Creamy white, curdlike patches ■ Red, erythematous mucosa	■ Fluconazole (Diflucan) ■ Ketoconazole (Nizoral) ■ Clotrimazole troches ■ Nystatin vaginal troches (dissolved orally) or mouth rinse
Necrotizing ulcerative gingivitis (trench mouth, Vincent infection)	Infection with spirochetes and bacilli or systemic infection	■ Acute gingival inflammation and necrosis ■ Bleeding, halitosis ■ Fever ■ Cervical lymphadenopathy	■ Correct any underlying disorders ■ Warm, half-strength peroxide mouthwashes ■ Oral penicillin
Oral mucositis	Damage to epithelial cells and stem cells in the submucosa caused by chemotherapy or radiation therapy	■ Erythema and inflammation of oral mucosa ■ Painful, irregularly shaped ulcerations, initially superficial, progressing to deep ulcers that may be confluent (overlapping with one another) ■ Pseudomembranes covering ulcers ■ Tissue necrosis with spontaneous bleeding, potential sepsis	■ Regular oral hygiene with brushing and flossing ■ Saline or sodium bicarbonate solution mouth rinses after and between meals ■ Gelclair mouth rinse before meals for analgesia ■ Palifermin, an epithelial cell growth factor per FDA, used preventatively ■ Low-level laser therapy

Herpetic lesions may be treated with topical or oral acyclovir (Zovirax), famciclovir (Famvir), or valacyclovir (Valtrex). Acyclovir ointment provides comfort and lubrication while limiting the spread of the virus. Oral preparations reduce the severity of symptoms and the duration of the lesions.

Bacterial infections are treated with antibiotics based on cultures and smears. Oral penicillin is the treatment of choice if the patient is not allergic and the cultured bacteria are sensitive. Nursing implications for selected drugs used to treat stomatitis are outlined in **Medication Administration 23.B.**

An epithelial cell growth-stimulating factor, palifermin (Kepivance), reduces the incidence and duration of oral mucositis in patients undergoing high-dose chemotherapy in preparation for bone marrow or stem cell transplant.

Nursing Care

Assessment

Oral assessment is important not only for patients who have been diagnosed with stomatitis, but also for those with risk factors, manifestations, or evidence of possible complications (e.g., recent weight loss).

- ***Health history:*** Ask about mouth pain, altered taste, lack of appetite, malaise; presence of dentures, oral care habits, regularity of dental care; current health status including chronic diseases; current medications; use of alcohol or tobacco
- ***Physical assessment:*** Inspect lips, gums, teeth, interior cheeks, tongue and base of tongue, soft and hard palate; tonsils; and oral pharynx. Inspect for evidence of dental caries, gingivitis, periodontitis, dental abscesses, tooth wear, and soft tissue lesions (Critchlow, 2016). Observe and assess general health status including temperature and weight. For patients undergoing chemotherapy and radiation therapy, consistent assessment of the oral cavity at regular intervals is important to identify early changes. Care of the hospitalized patient should include daily oral assessment. Document assessment findings, patient oral hygiene practices, and patient teaching provided (Coke, Otten, Staffileno, Minarich, & Nowiszewski, 2015).
- ***Diagnostic tests:*** Conduct WBC, sedimentation rate, and serum albumin tests.

Medication Administration 23.B

Drugs Used to Treat Stomatitis

TOPICAL ORAL ANESTHETICS

adrenal corticosteroid; glucocorticoid

benzocaine (Anbesol, Orajel)

local anesthetic (ester type)

triamcinolone acetonide

These drugs reduce the pain associated with mucous membrane lesions or stomatitis. They provide temporary relief of pain. Triamcinolone acetonide also reduces inflammation. Any oral lesion that persists longer than 1 week should be evaluated by an oral surgeon.

Nursing Responsibilities

- Instruct the patient to seek medical attention for any oral lesion that does not heal within 1 week.
- Monitor for local hypersensitivity reactions, and discontinue use if they occur.

Health Education for the Patient and Family

- Apply every 1 to 2 hours as needed.
- Perform oral hygiene after meals and at bedtime.

TOPICAL ANTIFUNGAL AGENT

clotrimazole

TOPICAL ANTIFUNGAL ANTIBIOTIC AGENT

nystatin

These products help in the topical treatment of candidiasis. Their effects are primarily local rather than systemic.

Nursing Responsibilities

- Instruct the patient to dissolve lozenges in the mouth.
- Instruct the patient to rinse mouth with oral suspension for at least 2 minutes and expectorate or swallow as directed.
- These drugs are contraindicated in pregnancy.

Health Education for the Patient and Family

- Take medication as prescribed.
- Do not eat or drink 30 minutes after medication.
- Contact physician if symptoms worsen.
- Perform good oral hygiene after meals and at bedtime; remove dentures at bedtime.

ANTIVIRAL AGENTS

acyclovir (Zovirax)

famciclovir (Famvir)

valacyclovir (Valtrex)

Acyclovir, famciclovir, and valacyclovir are useful in the treatment of oral herpes simplex virus. They help reduce the severity and frequency of infections. These antiviral agents interfere with the DNA synthesis of herpes simplex virus.

Nursing Responsibilities

- Start therapy as soon as herpetic lesions are noted.
- Administer with food or on an empty stomach.

Health Education for the Patient and Family

- The virus remains latent and can recur during stressful events, fever, trauma, sunlight exposure, and treatment with immunosuppressive drugs.
- Take the medication as ordered, and contact the physician if symptoms worsen.

Note: Medications identified in blue are among the 200 most frequently prescribed drugs in the U.S.

Source: Data from Adams et al., 2017.

Priorities of Care

Provide patient education focused on oral hygiene and frequently assess oral cavity of patients at risk for developing stomatitis and oral mucositis. Maintain adequate hydration and nutrition for patients experiencing stomatitis or oral mucositis.

SAFETY ALERT: Provide oral care twice daily for hospitalized patients. Routine oral care can reduce the risk of ventilator-acquired pneumonia (VAP) in critically ill patients (Caple & Mennella, 2016). ■

Diagnoses, Outcomes, and Interventions

Nursing care for the patient with stomatitis or oral mucositis focuses not only on the oral inflammation, but also on any underlying systemic diseases and the effects of the condition on the patient's comfort and nutrition.

Maintain Intact Oral Mucous Membrane. Stomatitis and oral mucositis disrupt the integrity of the oral mucous membrane. Regardless of cause, the pain and symptoms must be relieved to promote comfort as well as food and fluid intake.

Expected Outcome: Patient's mucous membranes will heal and be free from signs and symptoms of stomatitis or oral mucositis.

The nurse will:

- Assess and document oral mucous membranes and the character of any lesions every 4 to 8 hours. *Baseline and ongoing assessment data provide the basis for evaluation.*
- Assist with thorough mouth care after meals, at bedtime, and every 2 to 4 hours while awake. If unable to tolerate a toothbrush, offer sponge or gauze toothettes. Avoid using alcohol-based mouthwashes or lemon-glycerin swabs. Provide saline or sodium bicarbonate rinse or a combined saline/sodium bicarbonate rinse after every meal and between meals. *Mouth care promotes hygiene, comfort, and healing.*
- Assess knowledge and teach about condition, mouth care, and treatments. Instruct to avoid alcohol, tobacco, and spicy or irritating foods. *Knowledge promotes patient participation in the plan of care and compliance. Alcohol, tobacco, and hot, spicy, or rough foods may injure the inflamed mucous membranes.*

Promote Balanced Nutrition and Hydration. Oral lesions and pain may limit oral intake, which may in turn lead to nutritional deficits. Anorexia and general malaise may also contribute to decreased intake.

Expected Outcome: Patient will maintain adequate oral intake, report adequate energy levels, and maintain body mass and weight and normal lab values (transferrin, albumin, and electrolytes).

The nurse will:

- Assess food intake as well as the patient's ability to chew and swallow. Weigh daily. Provide appropriate assistive devices such as straws or feeding syringes. *Adequate nutrition is essential for healing. Daily weights allow monitoring of the adequacy of food intake. Assistive devices may allow food intake while avoiding irritation of ulcerations or lesions.*
- Encourage a high-calorie, high-protein diet considerate of food preferences. Offer soft, lukewarm, or cool foods or liquids such as eggnogs, milkshakes, nutritional supplements, popsicles, and puddings frequently in small amounts. Obtain nutritional consultation. *Oral intake may be limited, and enriched foods and liquids enhance nutrition. A nutritional consultation can help ensure an adequate diet and assist in meeting nutritional needs.*
- Provide analgesics for pain relief as needed. *Significant pain associated with stomatitis or oral mucositis can interfere with effective mouth care and food and fluid intake. Pain management is a vital part of nursing care.*

Delegating Nursing Care Activities

Nursing care activities such as providing or assisting the patient with oral care may be delegated to unlicensed assistive personnel. Instruct unlicensed assistive personnel in appropriate technique and use of preferred tool (toothbrush, sponge, gauze toothettes) for individual patient need and condition. The nurse may delegate nursing care activities such as obtaining daily weights, measuring intake and output, and assisting with meals. Ensure that unlicensed assistive personnel avoid feeding patient hot foods and provide oral hygiene after meals.

Transitions of Care

Nurses can help prevent stomatitis by identifying patients at risk and suggesting measures to reduce the likelihood that stomatitis will develop. Teach and encourage all patients to regularly perform mouth care, including toothbrushing and flossing. Provide frequent mouth care with nondrying agents for patients who are unable to provide self-care. Encourage patients with ill-fitting dentures or other dental prostheses (such as partial plates) to see a qualified dentist or denturist. Suggest patients taking an extended course of antibiotic therapy or who have impaired immune function consume 8 oz of yogurt containing live bacterial cultures or 8 oz of buttermilk daily unless contraindicated. Discuss dietary modifications, such as limiting consumption of highly spiced or acidic foods and avoiding very hot beverages. Patients undergoing chemotherapy or radiation therapy should avoid use of alcohol and tobacco because these substances further damage oral mucosa, increasing the risk for oral mucositis.

Aggressive oral care for the hospitalized patient includes daily oral assessment and provision of oral care at least twice a day. Patients should be assessed for the risk of developing mucositis/stomatitis. High-risk and critically ill patients should receive oral care more frequently.

Promoting ongoing oral health is important for patients with chronic illness and for older adults. Routine assessment of the oral cavity and encouraging regular oral hygiene should be encouraged. Patients with mild stomatitis generally provide self-care. Patients with cancer treatment–related oral mucositis may require more aggressive therapy. Coaching the patient and caregivers who are able to manage the regimen in home- or community-based settings should be part of routine care. Include the following topics in teaching for home care:

- Management of any underlying health conditions and ongoing treatments such as chemotherapy
- Inspection of the oral cavity at regular intervals; report early signs of oral mucositis
- The recommended diet and oral hygiene regimen, including foods and substances (e.g., alcohol, tobacco products) to avoid
- Nutritional supplements to help meet nutritional requirements
- Prescribed medication, its route, side effects, frequency of administration, and signs and symptoms to report
- The importance of completing the full course of antibiotic, antiviral, or antifungal treatment
- Manifestations to report and the importance of follow-up care.

At the end of life, the condition of the oral mucosa deteriorates due to changes in the patient's systemic conditions. The primary symptom causing discomfort is dry mouth. Terminal patients may also experience tongue inflammation and bleeding spots of the oral mucosa (Matsuo et al., 2016). Frequent oral care and the use of artificial saliva should be implemented to relieve symptoms related to dry mouth.

The Patient with Oral Cancer

Oral cancer (malignancy of the oral mucosa) may develop on the lips, tongue, floor of the mouth, or other oral tissues. Incidence rates are more than twice as high in men as in women. Recent studies have shown increases in cancers of the oropharynx associated with the human papillomavirus (HPV) infection among White men and women (National Cancer Institute, 2018b). It is seen more often in people over age 40. Although a lesion can develop in any area of the mouth, the most common sites are the lower lip, tongue, and floor of the mouth (National Cancer Institute, 2018a). The stage of an oral cancer determines the prognosis, treatment, and degree of disability. The primary risk factors for oral cancer are smoking, drinking alcohol, and chewing tobacco. Marijuana use, occupational exposures to chemicals, and viruses such as HPV may also contribute to the risk for oral cancer (National Cancer Institute, 2018b).

Pathophysiology

More than 90% of oral and oropharyngeal tumors are squamous cell carcinomas. Most early cancers present as inflamed areas with irregular, ill-defined borders. These lesions are typically not painful. More advanced cancers appear as deep ulcers that are fixed to deeper tissues. Early lesions involve the mucosa or submucosa, whereas more advanced tumors may invade and destroy underlying tissues, including muscles and bones of the face. Tumors frequently metastasize to regional lymph nodes. Other cancerous lesions, including lymphoma, malignant melanoma, and Kaposi sarcoma, may develop in the mouth, although less frequently than squamous cell carcinoma.

Manifestations

Manifestations of oral cancer include:

- White patches (leukoplakia)
- Red patches (erythroplakia)
- Ulcers
- Neck mass
- Pigmented areas (brownish or black)
- Fissures
- Lump or thickening in the throat or mouth
- Difficulty chewing, swallowing, or moving the tongue or jaws.

The earliest symptom of oral cancer is a painless oral ulceration or lesion (**Figure 23.3** ■). Later symptoms vary and may include difficulty speaking, swallowing, or chewing; swollen lymph nodes; and blood-tinged sputum. Any oral lesion that does not heal or respond to treatment within 1 to 2 weeks should be evaluated for malignancy.

Interprofessional Care

The first component of treatment is eliminating any causative factors such as chewing tobacco, smoking, or drinking alcohol. Tumor staging then determines therapy. The TNM (tumor, nodes, metastasis) classification is used to stage oral cancer (see **Table 23.2**). A biopsy of the oral lesion allows direct visualization of cells to determine the presence or absence of cancerous cells. Staging may require additional diagnostic studies such as computed tomography (CT) scans or magnetic resonance imaging (MRI).

Early cancers (stages I and II) are highly curable using surgery or radiation therapy. The treatment choice is based on the expected functional and cosmetic results of treatment. More advanced tumors (stages III and IV) generally require a treatment combination of surgery, radiation, and

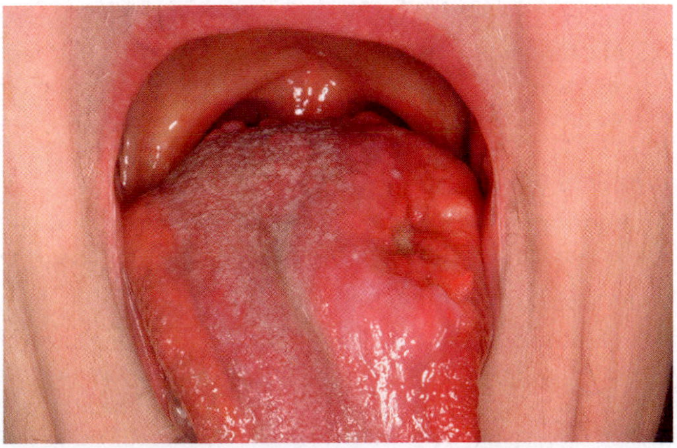

Figure 23.3 ■ Oral cancer.

Table 23.2 Oral Cancer Staging

Stage	Description
Stage 0	Carcinoma in situ
Stage I	Tumor ≤ 2 cm; no regional node involvement
Stage II	Tumor > 2 cm to ≤ 4 cm; no regional node involvement
Stage III	Tumor ≤ 2 cm to > 4 cm; one involved lymph node
Stages IVA and B	Tumor may invade adjacent structures; one or more nodes involved
Stage IVC	Distant metastasis present

possibly chemotherapy. See Chapter 14 for more information about radiation and chemotherapy to treat cancer.

Following biopsy and staging of the tumor, surgery is often indicated, although an advanced or extensive tumor may be considered unresectable. If the tumor involves surrounding tissues, the cosmetic effects of surgery are important considerations. The goal of surgery is removal of the lesion and potentially cancerous surrounding tissue or lymph nodes. Advanced carcinomas may require extensive excision or a *radical neck dissection*, a potentially disfiguring procedure in which the lymph nodes and muscles of the neck are removed. A tracheostomy is performed at the time of surgery. The tracheostomy may be temporary, but is often permanent. See Chapter 35 for more information about caring for a patient following radical neck dissection and a tracheostomy.

Nursing Care

Assessment

Early precancerous oral lesions are very treatable. Unfortunately, these lesions are usually painless, so diagnosis and treatment are often delayed. Assess the oral cavity of all patients, particularly those with risk factors for oral cancer.

- ***Health history:*** Ask about oral lesions that fail to heal; use (current or past) of tobacco products or excess alcohol.
- ***Physical assessment:*** Inspect and palpate lips and oral mucosa (including tongue and floor of mouth under the tongue) for tumors or lesions. Lesions may appear as velvety red or white patches that do not scrape off or as ulcers or areas of necrosis.

Priorities of Care

Monitoring airway clearance and maintaining adequate hydration and nutrition are key components of care.

Diagnoses, Outcomes, and Interventions

The mouth allows for food ingestion, and the lips are integral to verbal and nonverbal expression. The head, mouth, and lips are important to self-perception and body image. Diagnoses discussed in this section consider such problems as airway clearance, nutrition, communication, and body image. Also see the accompanying Case Study & Nursing Care Plan.

Manage Risk for Airway Obstruction and Problems with Oxygenation. The location and the extent of an oral cancer and its excision may compromise the airway. Swelling of adjacent tissues, increased oral secretions, or difficulty swallowing may contribute to respiratory distress. If extensive surgery is performed, a tracheostomy is usually done to maintain airway patency.

Expected Outcome: Patient's airway will remain patent as evidenced by ease of breathing, normal respiratory rate and rhythm, and $SpO_2 < 95$.

The nurse will:

- In the initial postoperative period, assess airway patency and respiratory status at least hourly. A patent airway is vital to maintain respirations and oxygenation of tissues. *Frequent assessment allows early identification of possible airway compromise.*
- Place patient in Fowler position, supporting the arms, unless contraindicated. Assist the patient to turn, cough, and deep breathe at least every 2 to 4 hours. *Fowler position promotes lung expansion. Turning, coughing, and deep breathing help maintain a patent airway by preventing pooling of secretions.*
- Maintain adequate hydration (2000 to 3000 mL per day unless contraindicated) and humidity of inspired air. *Adequate hydration helps thin and loosen secretions.*

Manage Nutritional and Fluid Requirements. Surgery affects oral food and fluid intake. Enteral feedings or parenteral nutrition may be required. A gastrostomy tube is usually inserted during surgery to maintain nutrition. If an oral diet is permitted, anorexia or pain may affect intake.

Expected Outcome: Patient will maintain adequate hydration and stable weight.

The nurse will:

- Weigh daily. Assess oral intake for adequacy of protein, calories, and nutrients. *Daily weights and nutritional assessments provide information about the adequacy of diet.*
- Offer soft, bland foods with supplements as indicated. Provide small, frequent feedings, making mealtimes pleasant. *Soft, bland foods may be better tolerated following oral surgery. Large meals may be overwhelming; small, frequent meals promote food and nutrient intake.*
- Provide enteral feedings per gastrostomy tube as ordered. Elevate the head of the bed 30 to 40 degrees. *Enteral feedings maintain nutritional status in the patient who is unable to consume foods orally. Elevating the head of the bed reduces the risk of regurgitation and aspiration of gastric contents.*
- Assess for gastric residual volume per facility protocol for the type of feeding (intermittent or continuous). Notify the physician of volumes greater than 200 mL or 50% of previous feeding if feeding is intermittent. *Excess residual volume may increase the risk for aspiration.*
- Consider a nutritional consultation to assess diet and plan appropriate supplements. *A registered dietitian can calculate energy requirements and develop an individualized diet plan to meet nutritional requirements.*

Promote Patient Communication. Oral surgery can interfere with communication. Effective communication is vital to postoperative recovery and prevention of complications.

Expected Outcome: Patient will accurately communicate status such as level of pain and comfort and respond to nurse's instructions. Patient will participate in speech therapy interventions.

The nurse will:

- Establish and practice a communication plan before surgery, such as using a white board or a text-to-speech app on a smartphone. *Practicing communication techniques reduces fear and anxiety while promoting communication.*
- Provide ample time for communication efforts and do not answer for the patient. Be alert for nonverbal communications. Use yes/no questions and simple phrases. *Providing adequate time allows the patient opportunity to express ideas and thoughts. Nonverbal communication provides cues regarding comfort or other needs. Simple yes/no questions are easily answered nonverbally.*
- Refer to or consult with a speech therapist, if indicated. *A speech therapist can help promote or restore effective communication.*

SAFETY ALERT: Provide an emergency call system and respond promptly. Make all staff aware that the patient cannot respond over an intercom system by posting an alert on the intercom. Nonverbal patients rely on an emergency call system to summon help. *Answering promptly reduces fear and anxiety and maintains safety.* ■

Manage Concerns with Body Image. Radical surgery of the head or neck seriously affects body image. An altered speech pattern and any disfigurement affect the ability to feel attractive or effective in work or social roles. Patients may defer lifesaving surgery to postpone disfiguring interventions or therapies.

Expected Outcome: Patient will identify personal strengths, acknowledge impact of situation on self-image, maintain close social interaction and personal interactions, and participate in self-care.

The nurse will:

- Assess coping style, self-perception, and responses to altered appearance or function. *This information can be used to identify appropriate interventions and care.*
- Encourage verbalization of feelings regarding perceived and actual changes. *Nonjudgmental acceptance of feelings and fears helps establish trust.*
- Provide emotional support, encourage self-care, and provide decision-making opportunities. *Self-care promotes self-acceptance and independence. Giving choices empowers the patient to participate in care.*

Plan Discharge. Discharge planning for the patient with oral cancer depends on the type of treatment planned and surgery performed. Depending on the patient's age, condition, and availability of support systems, referral to a rehabilitation center and community healthcare agencies may be an essential component of care. Visits from home care nurses can assist in meeting healthcare needs.

Expected Outcome: The patient and family will leave the hospital with the necessary knowledge, referrals, and instructions.

The nurse will discuss the following topics with the patient and family members or care providers:

- Diagnosis and prescribed care
- Monitoring for new lesions or recurrences
- Diet, nutrition, and activity
- Pain management
- Airway management, care of incision, and signs and symptoms to report.

Delegating Nursing Care Activities

As appropriate and allowed by the designated duties and responsibilities of unlicensed assistive personnel, the nurse may delegate nursing care activities such as measuring intake and output, obtaining daily weights, assisting with ADLs, and assisting with meals.

Ensuring that unlicensed assistive personnel are proficient in appropriate communication techniques and answer call lights promptly is important to promote patient-centered care.

Encourage unlicensed assistive personnel (UAP) to socialize and communicate frequently with the patient. Instruct UAP to encourage self-care while assisting patient with ADLs.

Transitions of Care

Preventing problems with the oral mucosa includes promoting oral hygiene and regular dental care. A balanced diet also promotes good oral health. Smoking cessation should be included in preventative health interventions. Use of oral tobacco products should be discouraged. See Chapter 21 for further information on assisting patient with smoking-cessation plans.

Secondary prevention strategies include aggressive screening for patients at risk for developing mucositis and other diseases of the mouth. Oral hygiene should be emphasized for patients receiving chemotherapy.

Patients experiencing acute conditions of the mouth should be treated aggressively. An interprofessional approach will include medication management, consultation with nutritionist, frequent oral care, and monitoring for changes in condition by the nurse.

Chronic conditions of the mouth require continuous attention to thorough oral hygiene practices. The nurse should coach and encourage the patient in optimum self-care practices. The nurse may need to coordinate care and ensure the patient has access to dental care.

Dry mouth is frequent and creates significant discomfort at the end of life. Frequent oral care and offering substitute saliva and moisture can alleviate discomfort.

Case Study & Nursing Care Plan

Patient with Oral Cancer

Juan Chavez, a married 44-year-old farmer, has two adult children. He and his wife raise and sell fruits and vegetables. Two months ago, Mr. Chavez developed a sore on his tongue that would not heal. Mr. Chavez tells his admission nurse, Sara Bucklin, "The doctor says he will have to remove part of my tongue," and anxiously asks, "Will I ever look the same? How will I be able to talk?"

ASSESSMENT	DIAGNOSES	EXPECTED OUTCOMES
Mr. Chavez's admission history reveals that he has been healthy, but has smoked two packs of cigarettes a day for more than 20 years and usually drinks two to four beers per day. He admits to being anxious and fearful of surgery and its outcomes. He says he quit smoking and drinking 2 weeks ago. The biopsy report is positive for squamous cell carcinoma of the tongue. Mr. Chavez has no enlarged cervical nodes and says he has no bloody sputum or saliva and no difficulty swallowing, chewing, or talking. His weight is in the normal range for his height. A wide excision of the oral lesion is planned.	▪ Risk for respiratory distress related to oral surgery ▪ Potential for weight loss and dehydration related to oral surgery ▪ Difficulty talking due to excision of a portion of the tongue ▪ Concerns about appearance related to oral surgery	▪ Patient will maintain a patent airway and remain free of respiratory distress. ▪ Patient will maintain a stable weight and level of hydration. ▪ Patient will effectively communicate with staff and family using a text-to-speech app on his smartphone. ▪ Patient will communicate an increased ability to accept changes in body image.

PLANNING AND IMPLEMENTATION

- Assess airway patency and respiratory status every hour until stable.
- Maintain semi-Fowler position, supporting arms. Encourage to turn, cough, and deep breathe every 2 to 4 hours.
- Teach the importance of activity, turning, coughing, and deep breathing.
- Monitor daily weights.
- Consult with dietitian to assess calorie needs and plan appropriate enteral feeding. Assess response to enteral feedings.
- Demonstrate and allow to practice using communication app prior to surgery.
- Allow adequate time for communication efforts.
- Keep emergency call system in reach at all times and answer light promptly. Alert all staff of inability to respond verbally.
- Encourage expression of feelings regarding perceived and actual changes.
- Provide emotional support and encourage self-care and participation in decision making.

EVALUATION

At the time of discharge, Mr. Chavez has maintained his weight and has started on oral liquids, including supplements and enriched liquids. His airway has remained clear, and he is effectively coughing and deep breathing. He has used the smartphone app to communicate throughout his hospital stay. He is regaining use of his tongue and can speak a few words. Although initially distressed, he is communicating an increased ability to cope with loss of part of his tongue. He and his wife say they understand his discharge instructions, including diet, activity, follow-up care, and signs and symptoms to report.

CLINICAL REASONING IN PATIENT CARE

1. What measures can you, as a nurse, implement to reduce the incidence of oral cancer?
2. Plan a health education program for young athletes who chew tobacco.
3. Mr. Chavez's wife calls you 2 weeks after discharge. She tells you that he refuses to try to talk and is relying on his smartphone app to communicate. How will you respond?

See Evaluating Your Response in Appendix B.

23.3 Disorders of the Esophagus

The esophagus plays an essential role in the ingestion of food and liquids. Disorders of the esophagus can be inflammatory, mechanical, or cancerous. Because of its location and neighboring organs, the symptoms of esophageal disorders may mimic those of a variety of other illnesses.

The Patient with Gastroesophageal Reflux Disease

Gastroesophageal reflux is the backward-flowing of gastric contents into the esophagus. When this occurs, the patient experiences heartburn. Many people with gastroesophageal reflux have few symptoms, whereas others develop inflammatory esophagitis as a result of exposure to gastric juices. **Gastroesophageal reflux disease (GERD)** is a common

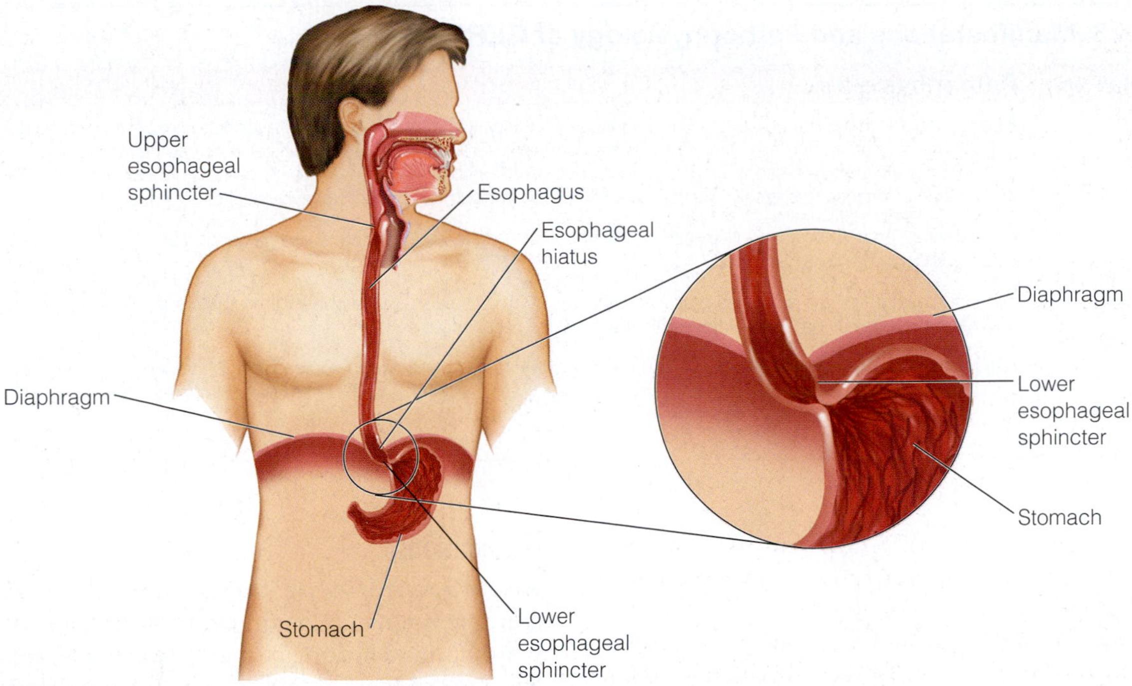
Upper
esophageal
sphincter
Esophagus
Esophageal
hiatus
Diaphragm
Diaphragm
Lower
esophageal
sphincter
Stomach
Stomach
Lower
esophageal
sphincter

Figure 23.4 ■ The esophagus. The inset shows a closer view of the lower esophageal sphincter.

gastrointestinal disorder. GERD affects 8.8 to 27% of adults, and up to 7% of them experience daily symptoms such as heartburn, regurgitation, and indigestion (Pilgrim & Parks-Chapman, 2018).

Pathophysiology

Normally, the lower esophageal sphincter remains closed except during swallowing. Reflux (backflow) of gastric contents into the esophagus is prevented by pressure differences between the stomach and the lower esophagus. The diaphragm, the lower esophageal sphincter, and the location of the gastroesophageal junction below the diaphragm help maintain this pressure difference (**Figure 23.4** ■).

Gastroesophageal reflux may result from transient relaxation of the lower esophageal sphincter, an incompetent lower esophageal sphincter, and/or increased pressure within the stomach. Factors contributing to gastroesophageal reflux include increased gastric volume (e.g., after meals), positioning that allows gastric contents to remain close to the gastroesophageal junction (e.g., bending over, lying down), and increased gastric pressure (e.g., obesity or wearing tight clothing). A hiatal hernia may contribute to GERD.

Gastric juices contain acid, pepsin, and bile, which are corrosive substances. Esophageal peristalsis and bicarbonate in salivary secretions normally clear and neutralize gastric juices in the esophagus. During sleep and in patients with impaired esophageal peristalsis or decreased salivation, the esophageal mucosa is damaged by gastric juices, causing an inflammatory response (**Figure 23.5** ■). With prolonged exposure, reflux esophagitis develops. In nonerosive reflux disease, the mucosa remains normal or mildly inflamed. Erosive esophagitis, however, is characterized by red, friable (easily torn) mucosa and superficial ulcers. If untreated, scarring occurs, and esophageal stricture may develop.

Manifestations

GERD causes heartburn, usually after meals, with bending over, or when reclining. Regurgitation of sour material into the mouth, or difficulty and pain with swallowing, may develop. Other manifestations may include atypical chest pain, sore throat, and hoarseness. See **Table 23.3**, which

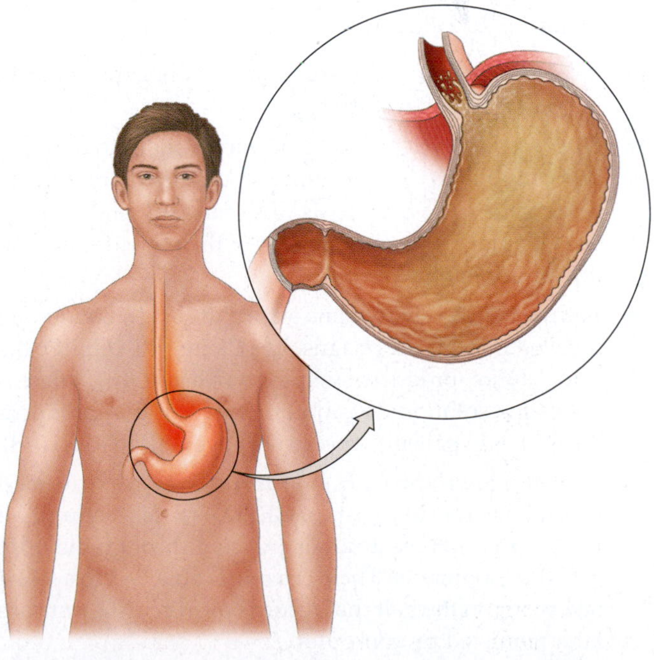

Figure 23.5 ■ In gastroesophageal reflux disease, reflux of corrosive gastric secretions into the lower esophagus causes inflammation of esophageal mucosa.

Table 23.3 Manifestations and Pathophysiology of GERD

Manifestation	Pathophysiology
Heartburn Chest pain Regurgitation Belching	Reflux of gastric juices through the lower esophageal (cardiac) sphincter into the lower esophagus exposes esophageal mucosa to corrosive pepsin, acid, and bile. Gastric juices are normally cleared by esophageal peristalsis or neutralized by saliva; when these mechanisms are impaired, esophageal mucosa becomes inflamed and eventually may ulcerate. Further exposure of the inflamed and ulcerated mucosa to corrosive gastric juices leads to heartburn or angina-like or atypical chest pain.
Dysphagia	Untreated esophagitis leads to inflammatory cell infiltrates, fibrosis, and scarring of esophageal tissue, constricting its lumen and causing difficult, painful swallowing.
Pain after eating	Increased gastric volume increases pressure within the stomach relative to the ability of the lower esophageal sphincter to prevent reflux into the esophagus. Reflux irritates already inflamed tissue, causing pain.
Chronic cough Hoarseness Laryngitis Pharyngitis	Reflux of gastric contents into the pharynx and mouth allows aspiration of gastric contents into the tracheobronchial tree. This usually occurs during sleep, when a recumbent position increases gastroesophageal reflux and relaxation of tissues and muscles in the oropharynx increases the risk of aspiration.

links the pathophysiology of GERD and its symptoms. Aspiration of gastric contents can cause hoarseness or respiratory symptoms.

Complications include esophageal strictures and Barrett's esophagus. Strictures, caused by scar tissue, edema, and spasm, can lead to dysphagia. Barrett's esophagus is characterized by changes in the cells lining the esophagus and an increased risk of developing esophageal cancer (McDevitt & Mason, 2018).

Interprofessional Care

Often the diagnosis of GERD is made by the history of symptoms and predisposing factors. Interprofessional care focuses on lifestyle changes, diet modification, and, for more severe cases, drug therapy. Surgery is reserved for patients who develop serious complications.

Diagnosis

Diagnostic tests that may be ordered for patients with manifestations of GERD include:

- ***Barium swallow*** to evaluate the esophagus, stomach, and upper small intestine.
- ***Upper endoscopy*** to permit direct visualization of the esophagus. Tissue may be obtained for biopsy to establish the diagnosis and rule out malignancy. See Chapter 21 for nursing care of the patient undergoing an upper endoscopy.
- ***Bernstein test***, where saline and dilute acid solutions are instilled into the esophagus. In patients with GERD, the acid solution produces symptoms of heartburn, whereas the saline solution does not; neither solution produces symptoms in patients who do not have GERD (Kee, 2018).
- ***24-hour ambulatory pH monitoring*** may be performed to establish the diagnosis of GERD. For this test, a small tube with a pH electrode is inserted through the nose into the esophagus. The electrode is attached to a small box worn on the belt that records the data. The data are later analyzed by computer.
- ***Esophageal manometry*** measures pressures of the esophageal sphincters and esophageal peristalsis.

Medications

Antacids, such as Mylanta or Maalox, relieve mild or moderate symptoms by neutralizing stomach acid. Gaviscon, which forms a floating barrier between the gastric contents and the esophageal mucosa when the patient is upright, may be used.

Proton-pump inhibitors (PPIs) such as omeprazole (Prilosec) and lansoprazole (Prevacid) reduce gastric secretions. PPIs promote healing of erosive esophagitis and relieve symptoms. An 8-week course of treatment is initially prescribed, although some patients may require 3 to 6 months of therapy. Relapse is common after PPI therapy is discontinued. Although these drugs have minimal side effects, they may interfere with absorption of calcium and other nutrients, which may cause osteopenia and osteoporosis. Research indicates there may be a link between PPI therapy and an increased the risk of hip fracture (Adams et al., 2017). Histamine$_2$-receptor (H_2-receptor) blockers reduce gastric acid production and are effective in treating GERD symptoms. When treating GERD, H_2-receptor blockers are usually given twice a day or more frequently for a prolonged period of time. Several H_2-receptor blockers approved by the FDA for the treatment of GERD are available over the counter. This class of drugs does not appear to increase hip-fracture risk (Adams et al., 2017). A promotility agent, such as metoclopramide (Reglan), may be ordered to enhance esophageal clearance and gastric emptying. Metoclopramide is used to treat patients with regurgitation, symptoms of indigestion, and nighttime symptoms. However, it is not recommended for long-time use. See **Medication Administration 23.C** for the nursing implications of drugs used to treat GERD.

Surgery

Surgery may be used for patients who do not respond to pharmacologic and lifestyle management. Antireflux surgeries increase pressure in the lower esophagus, inhibiting gastric content reflux. *Laparoscopic fundoplication*, a procedure in which the gastric fundus is wrapped around the distal esophagus, is the treatment of choice for GERD. An open surgical procedure known as *Nissen fundoplication* may

Medication Administration 23.C

Drugs Used to Treat GERD, Gastritis, and Peptic Ulcer Disease

PROTON-PUMP INHIBITORS

esomeprazole (Nexium)
lansoprazole (Prevacid)
omeprazole (Prilosec)
pantoprazole (Protonix)
rabeprazole (AcipHex)

Proton-pump inhibitors are the drugs of choice for severe GERD. PPIs inhibit the hydrogen–potassium–ATP pump, reducing gastric acid secretion. If the patient's symptoms do not improve with treatment, the dose may be increased.

Nursing Responsibilities

- Administer 30 minutes before breakfast (and at bedtime if ordered twice a day).
- Do not crush tablets.
- Monitor liver function tests for possible abnormal values, including increased AST, ALT, alkaline phosphatase, and bilirubin levels.

Health Education for the Patient and Family

- Take the drug as ordered for the full course of therapy, even if symptoms are relieved.
- Do not crush, break, or chew tablets.
- Increase your calcium intake or take a calcium supplement while using this drug because it can interfere with calcium absorption.
- Avoid cigarette smoking, alcohol, aspirin, and NSAIDs while taking this drug because these substances may interfere with healing.
- Report black tarry stools, diarrhea, or abdominal pain to your primary care provider.

H_2-RECEPTOR BLOCKERS

cimetidine (Tagamet)
famotidine (Pepcid)
nizatidine (Axid)
ranitidine (Zantac)

H_2-receptor blockers reduce acidity of gastric juices by blocking the ability of histamine to stimulate acid secretion by the gastric parietal cells. As a result, both the volume and concentration of hydrochloric acid in gastric juice are reduced. H_2-receptor blockers are given orally or intravenously. Both prescription and over-the-counter preparations are available.

Nursing Responsibilities

- To ensure absorption, do not give an antacid within 1 hour before or after giving an H_2-receptor blocker.
- When administered intravenously, do not mix with other drugs. Administer in 20 to 100 mL of solution over 15 to 30 minutes. Rapid intravenous injection as a bolus may cause dysrhythmias and hypotension.
- Monitor for interaction with such drugs as oral anticoagulants, beta-blockers, benzodiazepines, tricyclic antidepressants, and others. H_2-receptor blockers may inhibit the metabolism of other drugs, increasing the risk of toxicity.

Health Education for the Patient and Family

- Take the drug as directed, even if pain and gastric discomfort are relieved early in the course of therapy.
- Take at bedtime if once-a-day dosing is ordered. If spaced through the day, take before meals. Avoid taking antacids for 1 hour before and 1 hour after taking this drug.
- To promote healing, avoid cigarette smoking (which increases gastric acid secretion) and gastric mucosal irritants such as alcohol, aspirin, and NSAIDs.
- Long-term use of these drugs can lead to gynecomastia (breast enlargement) and impotence in men and breast tenderness in women. Discontinuing the drug will reverse these effects.
- Report possible adverse effects such as diarrhea, confusion, rash, fatigue, malaise, or bruising to your care provider.

ANTIULCER GASTRIADHESIVE AGENT

sucralfate (Carafate)

Sucralfate reacts with gastric acid to form a thick paste that adheres to damaged gastric mucosal tissue. It protects gastric mucosa and promotes healing through this local action.

Nursing Responsibilities

- Administer on an empty stomach, 1 hour before meals and at bedtime.
- Do not crush tablets.
- Separate administration time from antacids by at least 30 minutes and other medications (1 hour or longer).

Health Education for the Patient and Family

- Take as directed, even after symptoms have been relieved.
- Do not crush or chew tablets; shake suspension well.
- Increase your intake of fluids and dietary fiber to prevent constipation.

ANTACIDS

Antacids are alkaline, inorganic compounds of calcium, aluminum, magnesium, or sodium and buffer or neutralize gastric acid, usually acting locally. Antacids are used in GERD, gastritis, and peptic ulcer disease to relieve pain and prevent further damage to esophageal and gastric mucosa.

Nursing Responsibilities

- Antacids interfere with the absorption of many drugs given orally; separate administration times by at least 2 hours.
- Monitor for constipation or diarrhea resulting from antacid therapy. Notify the physician should either develop; a different antacid may be ordered.
- Although most antacids have little systemic effect, electrolyte imbalances can develop. Monitor serum electrolytes, particularly sodium, calcium, and magnesium levels.

Health Education for the Patient and Family

- Take your antacid frequently as prescribed, 1 to 3 hours after meals and at bedtime. To be effective, the antacid must be in contact with the lining of your stomach, so should be ingested on an empty stomach.
- Avoid taking an antacid for approximately 2 hours before and 1 hour after taking another medication.
- Shake suspensions well prior to administration.
- Chew tablets thoroughly, and follow with 4 to 6 ounces of water.
- Report worsening symptoms, diarrhea, or constipation to your primary care provider.

(continued)

- Continue taking the antacid for the duration prescribed. Although pain and discomfort often are relieved soon after treatment begins, healing takes 6 to 8 weeks.

GI STIMULANT

metoclopramide (Reglan)

By acting on the central nervous system, metoclopramide (Reglan) stimulates upper gastrointestinal motility and gastric emptying. As a result, nausea and vomiting and symptoms of GERD are reduced.

Nursing Implications

- Do not administer this drug to patients with possible gastrointestinal obstruction or bleeding or a history of seizure disorders, pheochromocytoma, or Parkinson disease.
- Monitor for extrapyramidal side effects (e.g., difficulty speaking or swallowing, loss of balance, gait disruptions, twitching or twisting movements, weakness of arms or legs) or manifestations of tardive dyskinesia (uncontrolled rhythmic facial movement, lip-smacking, tongue rolling). Report immediately.
- Give oral doses 30 minutes before meals and at bedtime.
- May be given by direct intravenous push over 1 to 2 minutes or diluted by slow infusion over 15 to 30 minutes.

Health Education for the Patient and Family

- Take this drug as directed. If you miss a dose, take as soon as you remember unless it is close to the time for the next dose.
- Do not drive or engage in other activities that require alertness if this drug makes you drowsy.
- Avoid using alcohol or other CNS depressants while you are taking this drug.
- Immediately contact your healthcare provider if you develop involuntary movements of your eyes, face, or limbs.

Note: Drugs identified in blue are among the 200 most frequently prescribed medications in the United States.

Source: Adams, et al., 2017.

also be done (**Figure 23.6** ■). Other laparoscopic procedures to tighten the lower esophageal sphincter may include use of an endoscopic suturing system or burning spots on the muscle surrounding the sphincter to create scar tissue. Surgery or ablation therapy is also recommended to reduce the risk of esophageal cancer in patients with persistent cell changes in the distal esophagus.

Nursing Care

Assessment

Assessment data related to GERD include:

- ***Health history:*** Manifestations such as frequent heartburn or atypical chest pain; intolerance of foods that are acidic, spicy, or fatty; regurgitation of acidic gastric juice; increased symptoms when bending over, lying down, or wearing tight clothing; difficulty swallowing; possible hoarseness
- ***Physical assessment:*** Epigastric tenderness.

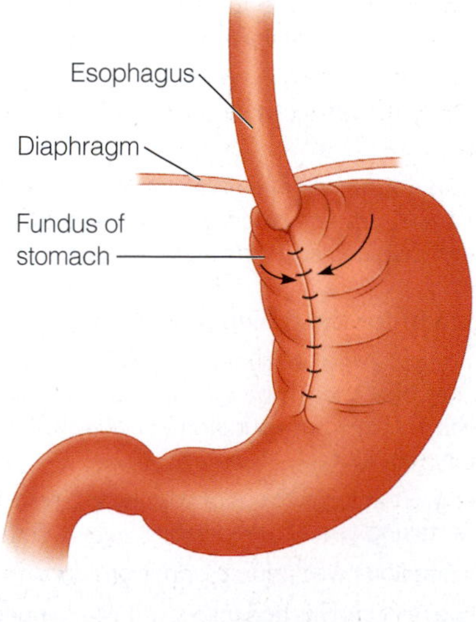
Esophagus
Diaphragm
Fundus of
stomach

Figure 23.6 ■ Nissen fundoplication. The fundus of the stomach is wrapped around the lower esophagus and the edges are sutured together.

Priorities of Care

Relieving the discomfort associated with GERD is the priority of nursing care. Teaching focuses on preventing symptoms and long-term consequences of the disorder.

Diagnoses, Outcomes, and Interventions

Nursing care for the patient with GERD focuses on symptom relief. Treatment involves medication management and nursing management that is supportive and educational. Left untreated, GERD can lead to serious complications so assisting the patient with needed lifestyle changes is important.

Manage Acute and Chronic Pain. The epigastric pain associated with GERD can be severe, interfering with rest and causing anxiety.

Expected Outcome: Patient will use preventative measures to control pain associated with GERD and will verbalize adequate pain control.

The nurse will:

- Provide frequent, small meals. Restrict intake of fat, acidic foods, coffee, and alcohol. *Limiting the size of meals reduces pressure in the stomach, reducing esophageal reflux. Fatty, acidic foods, coffee, and alcohol increase gastric acidity and interfere with gastric emptying, increasing the incidence of gastroesophageal reflux.*
- Instruct to stop smoking. Refer to a smoking cessation clinic or program as needed. *Cigarette smoking increases gastric acidity and interferes with healing of damaged mucosa.*
- Administer antacids, H_2-receptor blockers, and PPIs as prescribed. Instruct patient to continue therapy as prescribed, even after symptoms have been relieved. *These drugs neutralize or reduce gastric acid secretion, relieving symptoms and promoting healing.*
- Discuss the long-term nature of GERD and its management. *Lifestyle changes need to be continued after healing and symptom relief to manage the long-term effects of GERD.*

Transitions of Care

GERD is a chronic condition. Dietary and lifestyle changes are important to reduce symptoms and long-term effects of the disorder. Acidic foods such as tomato products, citrus fruits, spicy foods, and coffee are eliminated from the diet. Fatty foods, chocolate, peppermint, and alcohol relax the lower esophageal sphincter or delay gastric emptying, so they should be avoided. The patient is advised to maintain ideal body weight, eat smaller meals, refrain from eating for 3 hours before bedtime, and stay upright for 2 hours after meals. Elevating the head of the bed on 6- to 8-inch blocks is often beneficial. Stopping smoking and reducing alcohol consumption are necessary lifestyle changes. Avoiding tight clothing and avoiding bending may help to relieve symptoms.

Acute interventions include elevating the head of bed, administering medications including antacids for immediate relief of pain, and reassuring the patient the pain will decrease.

GERD is a lifelong condition best managed by the patient. Teach the patient and family about continuing management strategies, including dietary changes, remaining upright after meals, and avoiding eating for at least 3 hours before bedtime. Suggest elevating the head of the bed on 6- to 8-inch wooden blocks placed under the legs. Discuss the need for continued gastric acid reduction using antacids, H_2-receptor blockers, or PPIs. All are effective to reduce the acidity of gastric juices. Antacids are the most cost-effective measure, requiring frequent doses to neutralize gastric acid. H_2-receptor blockers, also available over the counter, are a cost-effective management strategy that requires only twice-a-day dosing. End-of-life care involves managing the acute symptoms associated with GERD to promote optimum comfort. Routine administration of medications to reduce gastric acid secretion may be needed. Interventions described above may also promote comfort.

The Patient with Hiatal Hernia

Pathophysiology and Manifestations

A *hiatal hernia* occurs when part of the stomach protrudes through the esophageal hiatus of the diaphragm into the thoracic cavity (**Figure 23.7** ■). Although hiatal hernia is thought to be a common problem, most affected individuals are asymptomatic. The incidence of hiatal hernia increases with age.

In a *sliding hiatal hernia*, the gastroesophageal junction and the fundus of the stomach slide upward through the esophageal hiatus. Several factors may contribute to a sliding hiatal hernia, including weakened anchors of the gastroesophageal junction to the diaphragm, shortening of the esophagus, or increased intra-abdominal pressure. Small sliding hiatal hernias produce few symptoms.

In a *paraesophageal hiatal hernia*, the junction between the esophagus and stomach remains in its normal position below the diaphragm while a part of the stomach herniates through the esophageal hiatus. A paraesophageal hernia can become incarcerated (constricted) and strangulate, impairing blood flow to the herniated tissue. Patients with paraesophageal hernia may develop gastritis or chronic or acute gastrointestinal bleeding. The manifestations of hiatal hernias include:

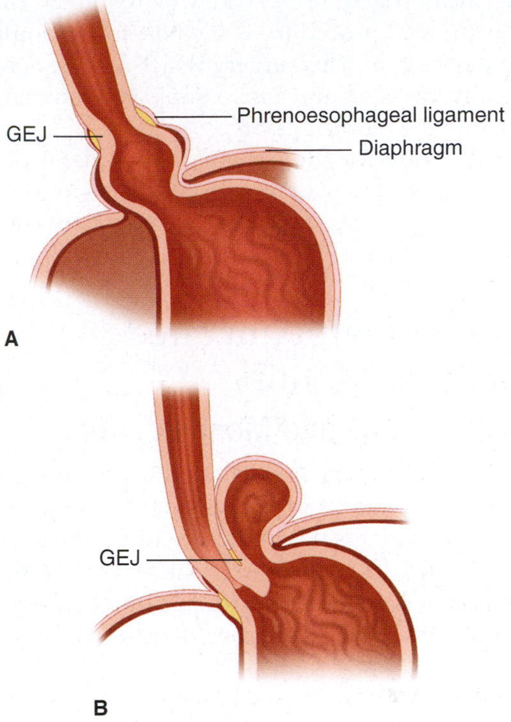
Phrenoesophageal ligament
GEJ
Diaphragm
A
GEJ
B

Figure 23.7 ■ Hiatal hernias. **A**, In a sliding hiatal hernia, the gastroesophageal junction (GEJ) and fundus of the stomach slide upward through the diaphragm, allowing gastric juices to reflux into the lower esophagus. **B**, In a paraesophageal hiatal hernia, the GEJ remains in the normal position, but a portion of the fundus herniates through the diaphragm.

- Reflux, heartburn
- Feeling of fullness
- Substernal chest pain
- Dysphagia
- Occult bleeding
- Belching, indigestion.

Interprofessional and Nursing Care

A barium swallow or an upper endoscopy may be done to diagnose hiatal hernia. Many patients with hiatal hernia have no or only mild symptoms and require no treatment. If symptoms are present, treatment measures such as those for patients with GERD may be ordered. Treatment begins with medications prescribed to address symptomatic gastric reflux (Sorenson et al., 2019). Large paraesophageal hernias may need to be surgically repaired due to risk of gastric volvulus or strangulation of the stomach (Kahrilas & Hirano, 2017).

If medical management is ineffective or the hernia becomes incarcerated, surgery may be required. The most common surgical procedure is the Nissen fundoplication (refer to Figure 23.6). This surgery, which may be done laparoscopically, prevents the gastroesophageal junction from slipping into the thoracic cavity.

Nursing care for the patient with a hiatal hernia is similar to that for the patient with GERD. If surgery is performed, nursing care is similar to that for patients undergoing gastric or thoracic surgery (see Chapter 4).

The Patient with Impaired Esophageal Motility

Pathophysiology and Manifestations

Disorders of esophageal motility can cause **dysphagia** (difficult or painful swallowing) or chest pain. It is estimated that nearly 65% of patients hospitalized with stroke experience dysphagia (American Stroke Association, 2013). Other neurologic disorders such as Parkinson disease, amyotrophic lateral sclerosis, and Alzheimer disease can also cause dysphagia.

Primary disorders of swallowing are less common. **Achalasia**, a disorder of unknown etiology, is characterized by impaired peristalsis of the smooth muscle of the esophagus and impaired relaxation of the lower esophageal sphincter (LES). The patient experiences gradually increasing dysphagia with both solid foods and liquids. Fullness in the chest during meals, chest pain, and nighttime cough are additional manifestations. Other patients may experience *diffuse esophageal spasm* that causes nonperistaltic contraction of esophageal smooth muscle. This disorder causes chest pain and/or dysphagia. The chest pain can be severe and usually occurs at rest.

Interprofessional and Nursing Care

Treatment of achalasia may include endoscopically guided injection of botulinum toxin into the lower esophageal sphincter or balloon dilation of the LES. Botulinum toxin injection lowers LES pressure, but may need to be repeated every 6 to 9 months. Balloon dilation tears muscle fibers in the LES, reducing its pressure (**Figure 23.8** ■). A laparoscopic myotomy (incision into the circular muscle layer of the LES) also reduces pressure and relieves symptoms.

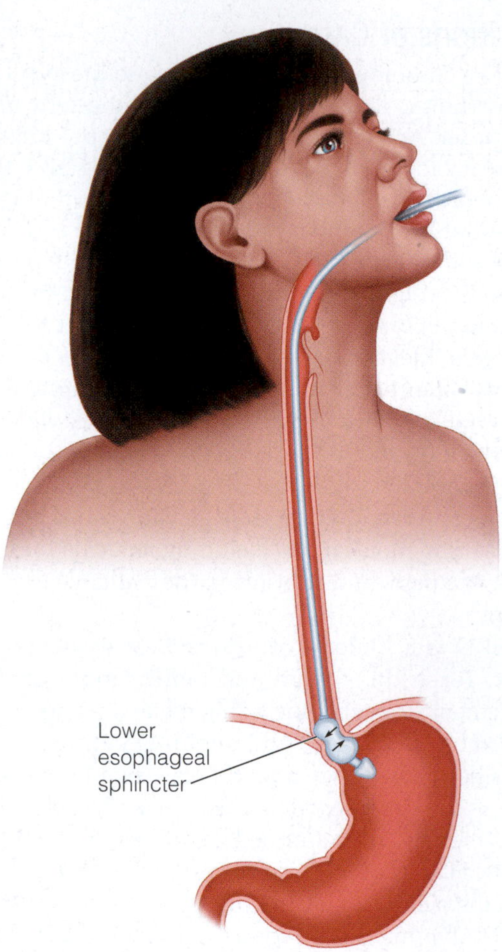
Lower
esophageal
sphincter

Figure 23.8 ■ Balloon dilation of the lower esophageal sphincter.

The Patient with Esophageal Cancer

Cancer of the esophagus is a relatively uncommon malignancy in the United States. It does, however, have a high mortality rate, primarily because symptoms are often not recognized until late in the course of the disease. Esophageal cancer is the seventh leading cause of cancer deaths in men and accounted for an estimated 13,480 deaths in 2018 (American Cancer Society [ACS], 2018). Esophageal cancer usually occurs after age 50; it is more common in men than in women and in Black populations than in White populations.

Pathophysiology

There are two types of esophageal tumors, adenocarcinoma and squamous cell carcinoma. During the past two decades, the incidence of squamous cell tumors of the esophagus has been decreasing, whereas the incidence of adenocarcinoma has increased dramatically. The increased rate has been linked to the increasing prevalence of GERD and obesity with GERD combined with a decrease in *Helicobacter pylori* infection (Sorenson et al., 2019). Cigarette smoking and chronic alcohol use are strong risk factors for squamous cell esophageal tumors and also appear to contribute to the risk of developing adenocarcinoma. Major identified risk factors for esophageal cancer include:

- Excess alcohol consumption
- Cigarette smoking
- Ingested carcinogens such as nitrates and industrial chemicals
- Smoked opiates
- Physical mucosal damage (e.g., hot tea, lye ingestion, radiation damage, chronic achalasia)
- Congenital disorders
- Chronic gastric reflux.

Adenocarcinomas tend to develop in dysplastic (abnormal) columnar epithelium in the distal esophagus. Squamous cell carcinoma (SCC) is more frequently found in the proximal to middle esophagus. Barrett esophagus is a premalignant condition that is associated with an increased risk of adenocarcinoma, and it is a possible complication of chronic GERD and achalasia (McDevitt & Mason, 2018).

The disease usually spreads to adjacent and supraclavicular lymph nodes and the liver, lungs, and pleura.

Manifestations

The most common symptoms of esophageal carcinoma are progressive dysphagia and recent weight loss. Other manifestations include:

- Dysphagia
- Anemia
- Weight loss
- GERD-like symptoms
- Regurgitation
- Anorexia
- Chest pain
- Persistent cough.

The cancer is often advanced and incurable by the time the disease is diagnosed because symptoms such as difficulty swallowing do not develop until more than 60% of the circumference of the esophagus is affected by tumor.

Tracheoesophageal fistulas may develop as the disease progresses, leading to aspiration and pneumonia. Paraneoplastic symptoms such as hypercalcemia may accompany advanced esophageal cancer.

Interprofessional Care

Controlling dysphagia and maintaining nutritional status are essential goals of therapy for patients with esophageal cancer, regardless of the stage of the disease. Treatment may involve surgery, radiation therapy, and/or chemotherapy.

Diagnosis

Diagnostic and staging procedures for esophageal cancer may include esophagography, bronchoscopy, and scans to detect metastasis. The following diagnostic tests may be performed (see Chapter 21):

- ***Barium swallow*** to identify irregular mucosal patterns or narrowing of the lumen, which suggests esophageal cancer
- ***Esophagoscopy*** to allow direct visualization of the tumor and obtain tissue for biopsy
- ***Chest x-ray, CT scans,*** or ***MRI*** to identify possible tumor metastases to other organs or tissues
- ***Complete blood count (CBC),*** which may indicate anemia due to chronic blood loss. Serum albumin levels may be low due to malnutrition, and liver function tests (ALT, alkaline phosphatase, AST, and bilirubin) are elevated if liver metastases are present.

Treatment

The treatment of esophageal cancer is challenging; fewer than 5% of patients survive 5 years after it is diagnosed (Mayer, 2014). A combination of chemotherapy and radiation, followed by surgery to resect the tumor, appears to be more effective than any single form of therapy.

Surgery involves resection of the affected portion of the esophagus (*esophagectomy*) and possible anastomosis of the stomach to the remaining esophagus. Mediastinal lymph nodes may be resected at the time of surgery. Esophagectomy is not without risk; potential surgical complications include anastomosis leak, respiratory complications such as pneumonia or acute respiratory distress syndrome, gastric necrosis or bleeding, cardiac dysrhythmias, and infection and sepsis. Intensive nursing care is required postoperatively to prevent and rapidly identify and treat complications that do develop.

The effectiveness of primary radiation therapy is similar to that with radical surgery. Complications associated with radiation therapy to the esophagus include perforation, hemorrhage, and strictures. When used, combination chemotherapy regimens are more effective in reducing tumor mass than single-drug regimens. When the tumor has spread locally or to distant sites, palliative therapy relieves dysphagia and pain (Mayer, 2014). Palliative therapy may include local treatments such as endoscopic dilation, wire stents or laser therapy to keep the esophagus patent, and placement of a gastrostomy or jejunostomy for enteral feeding and fluids.

Nursing Care

Assessment

Early diagnosis and treatment of esophageal cancer can make a difference in the patient's prognosis. Collect the following assessment data related to esophageal cancer:

- ***Health history:*** Current symptoms such as chest pain, dysphagia, odynophagia (pain with swallowing), coughing or hoarseness; duration of symptoms; recent weight loss; smoking history; current and past patterns of alcohol consumption
- ***Physical assessment:*** Weight; general health status; skin color; supraclavicular and cervical lymph nodes for lymphadenopathy.

Priorities of Care

Maintaining a patent airway is the primary priority of care. Ensuring the patient is comfortable is important, and maintaining adequate hydration and supporting nutritional intake are key areas of focus.

Diagnoses, Outcomes, and Interventions

Disruption of the integrity and function of the esophagus and the discomfort associated with swallowing in patients with esophageal cancer affect the patient's ability to maintain adequate nutritional status, and, potentially, a patent airway.

Promote Balanced Nutrition and Hydration. The patient diagnosed with esophageal cancer may already suffer from some degree of malnutrition because of difficulty and pain with swallowing. Enteral nutrition via nasogastric feeding tube or gastrostomy tube or parenteral nutrition maintains nutritional status after surgery or if the tumor is inoperable and obstruction occurs.

Expected Outcome: Patient will maintain body mass and weight within normal limits.

See Chapter 22 for nursing interventions related to enteral and parenteral feedings.

Manage Risk for Airway Obstruction and Promote Oxygenation. After surgery for esophageal cancer, the patient is at high risk for aspiration and difficulty maintaining a patent airway due to disruption of the esophagus and incision into the thoracic cavity.

Expected Outcome: Patient will maintain airway patency as evidenced by ease of breathing, normal respiratory rate and rhythm, and stated absence of dyspnea.

The nurse will:

- Assess mental and respiratory status (including rate, depth, breath sounds, and oxygen saturation levels) at least every hour during the initial postoperative period. *Altered mental status increases the risk for aspiration. An increased respiratory rate, dyspnea, diminished and/or abnormal breath sounds, or decreased oxygen saturation levels may indicate impaired airway clearance or possible aspiration pneumonia.*
- Provide aggressive pulmonary hygiene measures, including endotracheal suctioning and chest physiotherapy as indicated or ordered. Following extubation, encourage frequent coughing, deep breathing, and use of the incentive spirometer. *Respiratory complications are a frequent complication of esophagectomy. Aggressive nursing care helps mobilize secretions and prevent atelectasis and possible pneumonia.*
- Monitor chest tube function, if present, and drainage. Promptly report drainage that is bright red and excessive in amount (greater than 70 mL/h) or that is purulent. Maintain patency of chest tubes per unit protocol or physician's order. *If a thoracic incision has been used, chest tubes are placed to promote lung reinflation. Proper chest tube function is necessary to prevent pneumothorax and impaired lung inflation.*
- Monitor cardiopulmonary status and hemodynamic pressures. Administer intravenous fluids and fluid boluses as ordered. *Fluid volume imbalances that compromise cardiopulmonary status may develop following esophagectomy. Maintaining adequate fluid intake and preventing fluid overload are important postoperatively. The patient is also at risk for acute respiratory distress syndrome, a critical complication that can further compromise ventilation, gas exchange, and circulation.*
- Not move or manipulate the nasogastric tube. Maintain low gastric suction as ordered. *Manipulating or moving the nasogastric tube may disrupt suture lines, resulting in a leak into the mediastinum.*
- Verify enteral tube feeding placement by checking the pH of gastric aspirate. Stop enteral feedings if feelings of fullness or nausea occur. Suction gastrointestinal contents as needed, positioning the patient on the side. *Overdistention of the stomach or delayed gastric emptying may result in regurgitation of stomach contents. Nausea or a feeling of fullness may indicate stomach overdistention. Suctioning and positioning limit the risk of aspiration.*

Help Manage Feelings of Grief and Loss. Upon a diagnosis of cancer, the patient and family may experience a grief reaction. The pessimistic prognosis associated with esophageal cancer and the disruptions in relationships may result in an intense sense of loss. Chapter 5 discusses care for the patient experiencing grief and loss.

Delegating Nursing Care Activities

Nursing care activities such as providing or assisting the patient with oral care may be delegated to unlicensed assistive personnel. The nurse may delegate nursing care activities such as taking vital signs, measuring intake and output, and obtaining daily weights. Be sure to reinforce the need to be alert for signs and symptoms of respiratory distress.

Transitions of Care

Health promotion measures to reduce the risk for and incidence of esophageal cancer include educating people (especially young people) about the dangers of cigarette smoking and excess alcohol use. Refer to smoking cessation and alcohol treatment programs as indicated. Educate patients with GERD about the relationship between chronic damage to the esophagus due to reflux and esophageal cancer, and stress the importance of effective disease management.

Acute care will depend on the patient's individual problems presented. See Chapter 4 for care of the patient undergoing surgery. Patients may be hospitalized when receiving chemotherapy. See Chapter 14 for care of the patient with cancer.

Most care for patients with esophageal cancer is provided in community-based and home settings. Include the following topics in patient and family teaching for home care:

- Planned treatment options including the risks, benefits, and potential adverse effects of each option
- Wound and follow-up care following surgery
- Prevention and manifestations of complications such as wound or chest infection, anastomosis leak, deep venous thrombosis
- How to prepare, implement, and care for tube feedings or home parenteral nutrition.

Based on the patient's needs and prognosis, referral to a home health agency and/or hospice may be appropriate.

The patient with esophageal cancer will likely experience persistent and/or recurrent dysphagia throughout the course of the illness. Management includes stents, external beam radiation treatment, brachytherapy, chemoradiotherapy, laser treatment, and photodynamic therapy (Borrett, 2018). Additionally, the patient will receive care with speech and language therapy, clinical nutrition, and dietetic services (Borrett, 2018). Care coordination is an important nursing role throughout the chronic phase of the illness.

Supportive care at the end of life will focus on pain control. The client with esophageal cancer will likely be NPO. Care coordination as a member of the hospice team is an important nursing role at the end of life.

23.4 Disorders of the Stomach and Duodenum

The stomach and upper small intestine (duodenum and jejunum) are responsible for the majority of food digestion. The major disorders that affect digestion are nausea and vomiting, gastritis, peptic ulcer disease, and cancer of the stomach. Nursing roles in managing these disorders include both acute care for the hospitalized patient and teaching to give the patient the skills and knowledge to manage these conditions at home.

Overview of Normal Physiology

Normally, the stomach is protected from the digestive substances it secretes—namely, hydrochloric acid and pepsin—by the **gastric mucosal barrier**. The gastric mucosal barrier includes:

- An impermeable hydrophobic lipid layer that covers gastric epithelial cells. This lipid layer prevents diffusion of water-soluble molecules, but substances such as aspirin and alcohol can diffuse through it.
- Bicarbonate ions secreted in response to hydrochloric acid secretion by the parietal cells of the stomach. When bicarbonate (HCO_3^-) secretion is equal to hydrogen ion (H^+) secretion, the gastric mucosa remains intact. Prostaglandins, chemical messengers involved in the inflammatory response, support bicarbonate production and blood flow to the gastric mucosa.
- Mucous gel that protects the surface of the stomach lining from the damaging effects of pepsin and traps bicarbonate to neutralize hydrochloric acid. This gel also acts as a lubricant, preventing mechanical damage to the stomach lining from its contents.

When an acute or chronic irritant disrupts the mucosal barrier or when disease alters the processes that maintain the barrier, the gastric mucosa becomes irritated and inflamed. Lipid-soluble substances such as aspirin and alcohol penetrate the gastric mucosal barrier, leading to irritation and possible inflammation. Bile acids also break down the lipids in the mucosal barrier, increasing the potential for irritation (Sorenson et al., 2019). In addition, nonsteroidal anti-inflammatory drugs (NSAIDs) inhibit prostaglandins. NSAIDs alter the nature of gastric mucus, affecting its protective function.

The Patient with Gastrointestinal Bleeding

Pathophysiology

Because of its constant exposure to the environment, the gastrointestinal tract can be subjected to trauma, exposure to toxins, infection with pathogens such as *Helicobacter pylori*, inflammatory processes, and insults such as ischemia due to systemic diseases. While the mucosal lining of the GI tract is remarkably able to withstand these insults and heal rapidly, its rich supply of blood can result in significant bleeding when a vessel is eroded or abnormally distended (*varices*). Gastrointestinal hemorrhage is a relatively common admitting diagnosis and complication of critical illnesses. It is a medical emergency requiring aggressive medical and nursing care.

Although bleeding and hemorrhage can occur anywhere in the GI tract, the upper portion of the tract is more commonly affected. The three primary disorders leading to upper gastrointestinal (UGI) hemorrhage are erosive gastritis, peptic ulcer disease, and esophageal varices. Peptic ulcer disease and erosive gastritis are discussed in the following sections of this chapter; esophageal varices, usually seen as a complication of cirrhosis of the liver, are discussed in Chapter 25.

Blood in the GI tract has several effects. It is irritating to the stomach and typically leads to nausea and vomiting and sometimes **hematemesis** (vomiting blood). If the blood has been present in the stomach for a period of time and is partially digested, it may have a "coffee-grounds" appearance, rather than presenting as bright red blood. The accumulation of blood in the GI tract stimulates peristalsis, leading to hyperactive bowel sounds and diarrhea. Stools may be black and tarry (**melena**) or frankly bloody (**hematochezia**); stool containing partially digested blood has a foul characteristic odor. With significant upper GI bleeding, digestion of blood proteins increases blood urea nitrogen (BUN) levels.

GI hemorrhage, a medical emergency with loss of a significant amount of blood within a few hours, rapidly depletes blood volume, producing manifestations of decreased cardiac output: Tachycardia, hypotension, pallor, and decreased urine output. Peripheral blood vessels constrict to maintain perfusion of vital organs. Unless the blood volume is restored, hypovolemic shock progresses, leading to acidosis, renal failure, bowel infarction, acute coronary syndrome, coma, and death. See Chapter 11 for more information about shock and its management.

Manifestations

Physiologic responses to an upper GI bleed depend on the rapidity and magnitude of the blood loss. GI bleeding resulting from erosion of a small vessel is typically slow and may not be identified until the patient presents with manifestations of blood loss anemia due to depletion of iron stores. Although no visible blood may be visible in the stool, **occult (or hidden) bleeding** may be detected by chemical means.

Interprofessional Care

The acuity of the bleed and the patient's condition dictate the timing and extent of diagnostic testing and interventions. A patient with a massive GI hemorrhage is admitted to the critical care unit and aggressively treated to stem bleeding, restore blood volume, and stabilize the cardiovascular system. Identifying the cause of the bleeding is postponed in many cases until the patient's condition has been stabilized.

When the bleeding is slow or chronic, diagnostic testing and treatment may be managed in an ambulatory care setting.

Diagnosis

Diagnostic testing focuses on determining the extent and effects of the bleed, as well as its cause:

- *Complete blood count with hemoglobin and hematocrit* is obtained. In an acute bleed, the CBC, hemoglobin, and hematocrit may not initially indicate the extent of blood loss because plasma is lost along with blood cells.
- *Blood type and crossmatch* are performed to prepare for transfusion as necessary.
- *Serum electrolytes, osmolality,* and *BUN* are obtained to determine the effects of the blood loss and protein digestion on blood chemistries.
- *Liver function studies* and a *coagulation profile* may be obtained to help determine the cause of the bleeding.
- *Upper endoscopy* is performed as soon as possible to identify and, if possible, treat the source of bleeding. See Chapter 21 for nursing care of the patient undergoing an upper endoscopy.

Treatment

In acute GI hemorrhage, initial treatment focuses on stemming the bleeding and restoring cardiovascular stability. Oxygen should be administered to support myocardial oxygen demand. Fluid resuscitation is initiated. Intravenous fluids such as normal saline or a balanced electrolyte solution are administered through a large-bore intravenous catheter. Fresh whole blood, which contains clotting factors, is administered to restore blood volume and components in an acute hemorrhage. In less acute situations, packed red cells may be administered to restore the oxygen-carrying capacity of the blood.

Hemostasis is achieved using upper endoscopy whenever possible. A sclerosing agent may be injected into the bleeding vessel or the vessel may be sealed using a heated probe, electrocautery, or laser. Rarely, emergency surgery is required to stop hemorrhage.

Gastric lavage, washing-out of stomach contents, may be done in patients with upper GI hemorrhage to remove blood from the GI tract, prevent vomiting, and prepare for upper endoscopy.

Nursing Care

Assessment

Assessment of the patient experiencing an acute GI hemorrhage is very focused on the immediate crisis. The ability to obtain subjective information may be limited; however, it is important to identify possible contributing factors such as use of aspirin, other platelet inhibitors, or anticoagulant medications and the presence of any acute or chronic conditions that may contribute to bleeding (e.g., hypertension, a clotting disorder, peptic ulcer disease, chronic hepatitis, or cirrhosis of the liver). If possible, identify all current medications and their purpose, as well as any allergies to medications or other substances.

Physical examination focuses on the effect of the bleeding on cardiovascular status. Obtain vital signs and orthostatic vital signs (an early sign of hypovolemia). Place the acutely ill patient on a cardiac monitor and obtain a rhythm strip. Obtain oxygen saturation level. Assess peripheral pulse strength, as well as color, temperature, and capillary refill of extremities. Evaluate mental status, including level of consciousness and orientation. An indwelling catheter may be inserted to evaluate urine output.

Priorities of Care

Nursing care priorities for the patient with an acute GI bleed focus on restoring and maintaining an effective cardiac output and tissue perfusion, stopping the hemorrhage, and preventing further bleeding.

Diagnoses, Outcomes, and Interventions

Monitor for Early Signs of Shock. Significant amounts of blood may be lost in a very short time with an acute GI hemorrhage. Because some of the blood enters the bowel, it may be difficult to accurately estimate the amount of blood lost by measuring emesis, gastric suction return, and blood expelled as feces. As blood volume drops, venous return decreases. The heart rate increases to maintain the cardiac output, and peripheral blood vessels constrict to improve venous return and cardiac output.

Expected Outcome: Patient's stable hemodynamic status will be restored (i.e., vital signs within normal range with no evidence of decreased tissue perfusion).

The nurse will:

- Frequently assess and document vital signs, including blood pressure, pulse rate and cardiac rhythm, respiratory rate, and oxygen saturation levels. Obtain hemodynamic pressure measurements as ordered, reporting trends and changes. *The vital signs, oxygen saturation levels, and hemodynamic pressure values provide indicators of the effectiveness of peripheral tissue perfusion, oxygenation, and fluid replacement.*
- Monitor for and report changes in skin color, temperature, and moisture or slow capillary refill. *Peripheral vasoconstriction and activation of the sympathetic nervous system typically cause pale, cool, and moist or diaphoretic*

skin. Development of cyanosis or mottling indicates a further decrease in tissue perfusion and oxygenation.

- Insert an indwelling urinary catheter and measure urine output hourly. Report an output of less than 30 mL for 2 consecutive hours. *A fall in urine output may indicate further reduction in cardiac output. As cardiac output falls, the kidneys become ischemic and acute renal failure may develop.*
- Insert a nasogastric tube and connect to low suction, unless contraindicated. Measure gastric output hourly unless otherwise directed. *Measuring gastric output provides information about the amount of blood and fluid lost. This information helps determine fluid and blood replacement needs.*
- Maintain two peripheral intravenous lines with large-bore catheters or a central venous catheter for fluid and blood administration as ordered. Frequently monitor vital signs, respiratory status, and hemodynamic pressure measurements, reporting changes in status. *Rapid administration of isotonic intravenous fluids, blood, and blood products can lead to fluid overload and potential heart failure.*
- Replace gastric drainage with balanced electrolyte intravenous solutions as ordered. *GI losses are replaced in addition to fluids given to meet daily requirements to prevent fluid volume deficiency.*

Manage GI Bleeding. ***Expected Outcome:*** Patient will not experience recurrent episodes of GI bleeding (evidenced by lack of visible bleeding and negative evidence of occult bleeding).

The nurse will:

- Maintain gastric suction and drainage and patency of nasogastric tube. *Blood is irritating to the GI tract, precipitating vomiting and stimulating peristalsis, leading to diarrhea. In addition, digested blood can increase BUN levels, potentially leading to confusion and altered mental status.*
- Irrigate the nasogastric tube with room-temperature saline or tap water as ordered. Calculate intake and output, subtracting the amount of irrigant from gastric output. *Irrigation of the nasogastric tube helps remove irritating blood from the gut and produces a degree of vasoconstriction in the stomach mucosa, slowing bleeding.*
- Prepare for upper endoscopy or surgery as planned. *Endoscopy or emergency surgery may be performed to repair the bleeding site or sclerose bleeding vessels.*
- Monitor gastric pH, following an acute bleed and in patients at risk for GI bleeding, as ordered and check vomitus and feces for the presence of occult blood. Maintain infusions of drugs to reduce gastric acidity as ordered. *The patient remains at risk for GI bleeding. Monitoring for occult blood helps identify slow bleeding or recurrent hemorrhage. Reducing the acidity of gastric secretions reduces irritation of the gastric mucosa, reducing the risk of bleeding.*

Transitions of Care

Preventing GI bleeding is the most important step in reducing the mortality and morbidity associated with an acute GI hemorrhage. Identifying patients at risk and instituting regular gastric pH monitoring and maintenance of drug therapy to reduce gastric acidity are important preventative measures. All critically ill patients should be considered to be at risk for stress-related erosive gastritis, and proton pump inhibitors should be considered as a prophylactic intervention (Faust, Echevarria, Attridge, Sheperd, & Restrepo, 2017).

Following an acute GI hemorrhage, continuing care focuses on resolving the underlying disease process if possible and preventing future episodes of GI bleeding. If a bleeding gastric ulcer was identified, testing for *H. pylori* infection will be done and a treatment regimen prescribed to eradicate the infection (the section on peptic ulcer disease follows). The patient who experienced an episode of erosive stress gastritis will often be discharged with instructions to continue taking a gastric acid–reducing medication and avoid known gastric irritants such as aspirin and alcohol. The patient with esophageal varices due to cirrhosis or chronic hepatitis needs additional instructions (see Chapter 25).

Patients with minor or slow GI bleeding are often managed in the community. Provide teaching about the cause of the bleeding and measures to prevent future episodes. Provide verbal and written instructions for prescribed medications such as acid reducers and oral iron supplements. Discuss appropriate nutrition; although a special diet to "soothe the stomach" is rarely indicated, foods rich in iron may be recommended to treat the resulting anemia.

Ensure the patient can identify indicators of GI bleeding to be reported to the physician. If the source of bleeding has not been identified, provide instructions about prescribed follow-up diagnostic testing.

Patients with a terminal diagnosis related to the GI system may develop an acute GI bleed at the end of life. Family and caregivers should be made aware of the possibility and instructed to keep towels at the bedside to manage blood. An unexpected adult GI bleed can be fatal and family should be supported and offered assistance by social work and/or chaplain services.

The Patient with Peptic Ulcer Disease

Peptic ulcer disease (PUD), a break in the mucous lining of the gastrointestinal tract where it comes in contact with gastric juice, is a chronic health problem. PUD affects approximately 10 to 12% of the population, or 4 million people, in the United States every year, primarily those between ages 25 and 64 years (Del Valle, 2017). Furthermore, its complications account for an estimated 15,000 deaths annually (Del Valle, 2017).

Peptic ulcers occur in any area of the gastrointestinal tract exposed to acid-pepsin secretions, including the esophagus, stomach, or duodenum. *Duodenal ulcers* are the most common. They usually develop between the ages of 30 and 55 and are more common in men than in women. *Gastric ulcers* more often affect older patients between the ages of 55 and 70. Ulcers are more common in people who smoke and who are chronic users of NSAIDs. Alcohol and dietary intake do not seem to cause PUD, and the role of stress is uncertain. Although the incidence of PUD has dramatically decreased, the incidence of gastric ulcers is increasing and is believed to be due to the widespread use of NSAIDs (Del Valle, 2017).

Risk Factors

Chronic *H. pylori* infection and use of aspirin and NSAIDs are the major risk factors for PUD. Other contributing risk factors include:

- Older age
- Low socioeconomic status
- Birth in a developing country
- High congregate living conditions
- Unclean food or water
- History of ulcer
- Cigarette smoking
- Family history of PUD.

Overall, an estimated 10 to 15% of patients infected with *H. pylori* develop PUD. Of the NSAIDs, aspirin is the most ulcerogenic. A strong familial pattern suggests a genetic factor in the development of PUD. Cigarette smoking is a significant risk factor, doubling the risk of PUD. Cigarette smoking inhibits the secretion of bicarbonate by the pancreas and possibly causes more rapid transit of gastric acid into the duodenum.

Pathophysiology

The innermost layer of the stomach wall, the gastric mucosa, consists of columnar epithelial cells, supported by a middle layer of blood vessels and glands and a thin outer layer of smooth muscle. The mucosal barrier of the stomach, a thin coating of mucous gel and bicarbonate, protects the gastric mucosa. The mucosal barrier is maintained by bicarbonate secreted by the epithelial cells, by mucous gel production stimulated by prostaglandins, and by an adequate blood supply to the mucosa (see the overview of normal physiology earlier in this chapter).

An **ulcer**, or break in the gastrointestinal mucosa, develops when the mucosal barrier is unable to protect the mucosa from damage by hydrochloric acid and pepsin, the gastric digestive juices. See the accompanying Pathophysiology Illustrated: Peptic Ulcer Disease feature.

H. pylori infection is spread person to person (oral–oral or fecal–oral) and contributes to ulcer formation in several ways. The bacteria produce enzymes that reduce the efficacy of mucous gel in protecting the gastric mucosa. In addition, the host's inflammatory response to *H. pylori* contributes to gastric epithelial cell damage without producing immunity to the infection. Although the gastric mucosa is the usual site for *H. pylori* infection, this infection also contributes to duodenal ulcers. This is possibly related to an increase in gastric acid production associated with *H. pylori* infection.

NSAIDs contribute to PUD through both systemic and topical mechanisms. Prostaglandins are necessary for maintaining the gastric mucosal barrier. NSAIDs interrupt prostaglandin synthesis by disrupting the action of the enzyme cyclooxygenase (COX). The two forms of this enzyme are COX-1 and COX-2. The COX-1 enzyme is necessary to maintain the integrity of the gastric mucosa, but the anti-inflammatory effects of NSAIDs result from their ability to inhibit the COX-2 enzyme. The COX-2-selective NSAIDs may be less damaging to the gastric mucosa because they have less effect on the COX-1 enzyme. In addition to their systemic effect, aspirin and many NSAIDs cross the lipid membranes of gastric epithelial cells, damaging the cells themselves.

The ulcers of PUD may affect the esophagus, stomach, or duodenum. They may be superficial or deep, affecting all layers of the mucosa (see Pathophysiology Illustrated: Peptic Ulcer Disease). Duodenal ulcers, the most common, usually develop in the proximal portion of the duodenum, close to the pylorus (**Figure 23.9** ■). They are sharply demarcated and usually less than 1 cm in diameter (**Figure 23.10** ■). Gastric ulcers often are found on the lesser curvature and the area immediately proximal to the pylorus. Gastric ulcers are associated with an increased incidence of gastric cancer.

Peptic ulcer disease may be chronic, with spontaneous remissions and exacerbations. Exacerbations of the disease may be associated with trauma, infection, or other physical or psychologic stressors.

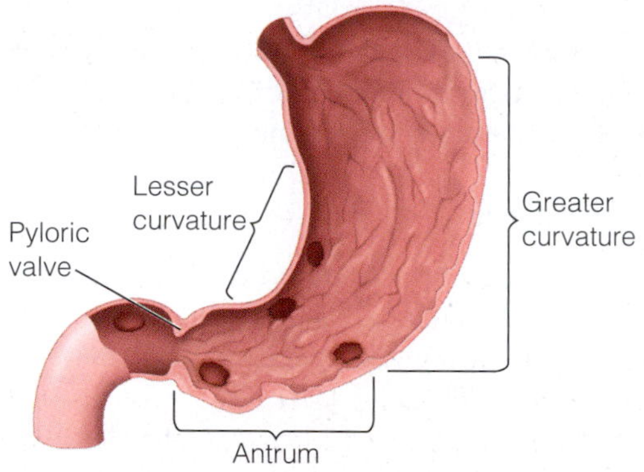
Lesser
curvature
Pyloric
valve
Greater
curvature
Antrum

Figure 23.9 ■ Common sites affected by peptic ulcer disease.

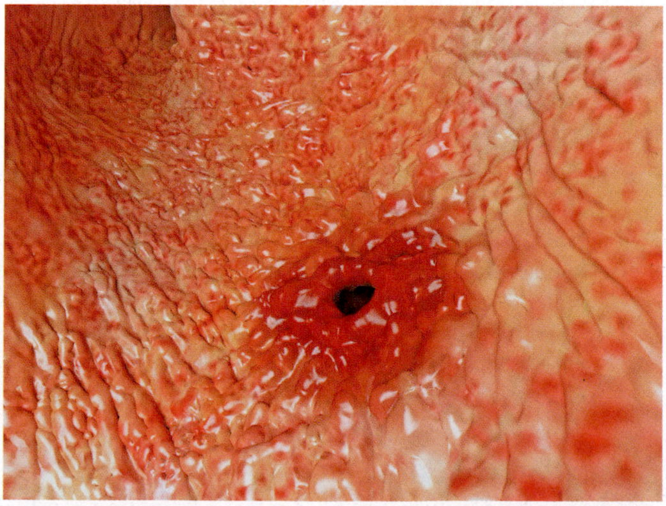

Figure 23.10 ■ A superficial peptic ulcer.

Pathophysiology Illustrated

Peptic Ulcer Disease

Normal gastric mucosa

In the stomach and duodenum, the mucosal barrier protects the gastric mucosa (including the epithelial, vascular, and smooth muscle layers) from damage. Specialized mucous cells throughout the gastric mucosa produce a mucus (a mixture of water, lipids, and glycoproteins) that serves as a barrier to the diffusion of ions (such as hydrogen ion) and molecules (such as pepsin). A thin layer of bicarbonate, secreted by surface epithelial cells, forms between the mucus and cell membranes. Blood flow to the gastric mucosa is vital to maintain this barrier. Prostaglandins and nitric oxide stimulate mucus and bicarbonate production, helping maintain it as well. The mucosal barrier constantly bathes surfaces of the gastric epithelial lining.

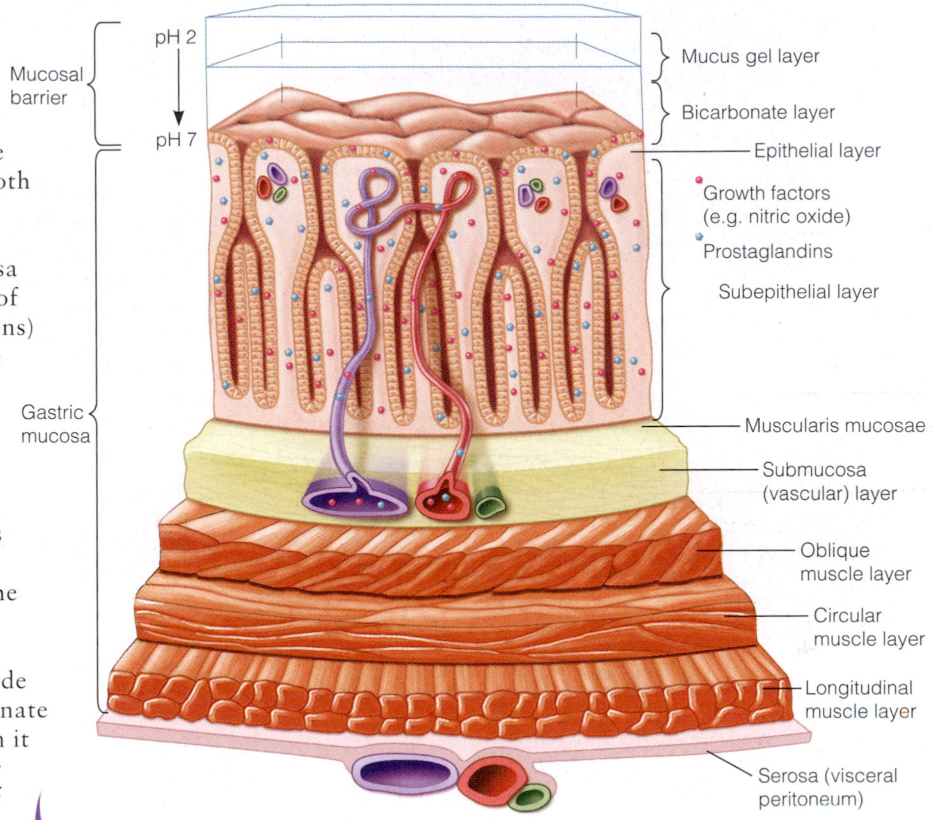

Mucosal barrier
pH 2
pH 7
Gastric mucosa
Mucus gel layer
Bicarbonate layer
Epithelial layer
Growth factors (e.g. nitric oxide)
Prostaglandins
Subepithelial layer
Muscularis mucosae
Submucosa (vascular) layer
Oblique muscle layer
Circular muscle layer
Longitudinal muscle layer
Serosa (visceral peritoneum)

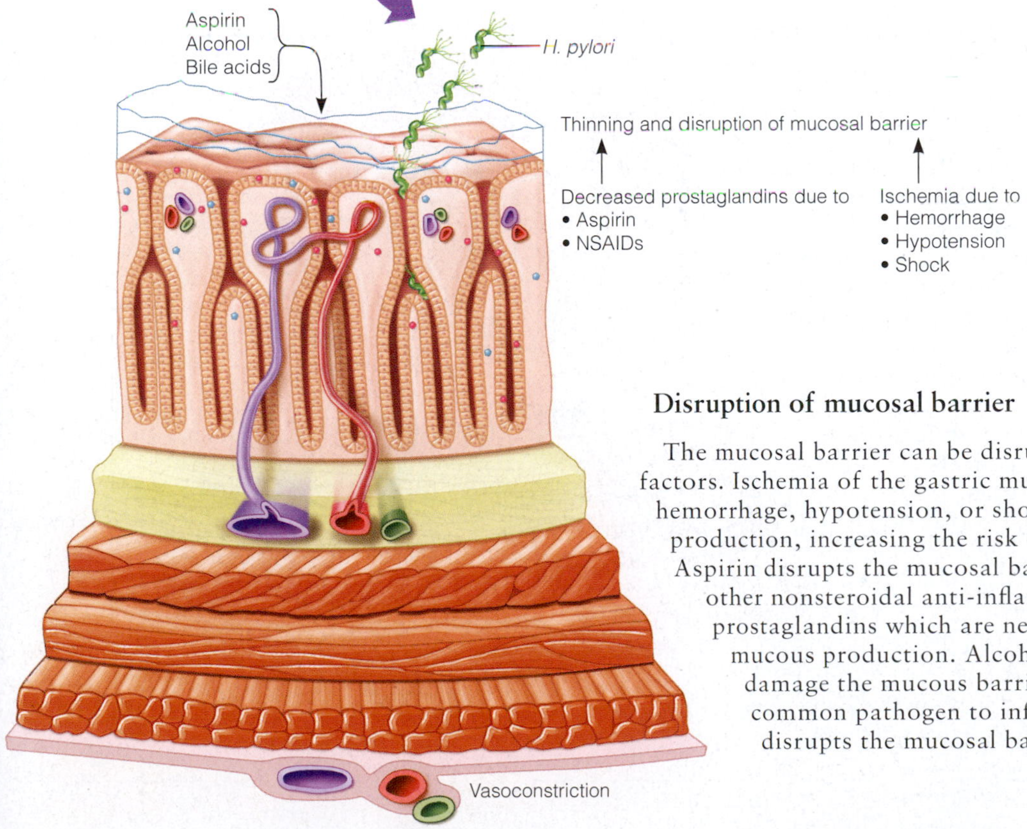

Aspirin
Alcohol
Bile acids
H. pylori
Thinning and disruption of mucosal barrier
Decreased prostaglandins due to
• Aspirin
• NSAIDs
Ischemia due to
• Hemorrhage
• Hypotension
• Shock
Vasoconstriction

Disruption of mucosal barrier

The mucosal barrier can be disrupted by a number of factors. Ischemia of the gastric mucosa (e.g., due to hemorrhage, hypotension, or shock) impairs mucous production, increasing the risk of damage to the mucosa. Aspirin disrupts the mucosal barrier, and, along with other nonsteroidal anti-inflammatory drugs, inhibits prostaglandins which are necessary to maintain mucous production. Alcohol and bile acids also damage the mucous barrier. *Helicobacter pylori*, a common pathogen to infect the gastric mucosa, disrupts the mucosal barrier.

(*continued*)

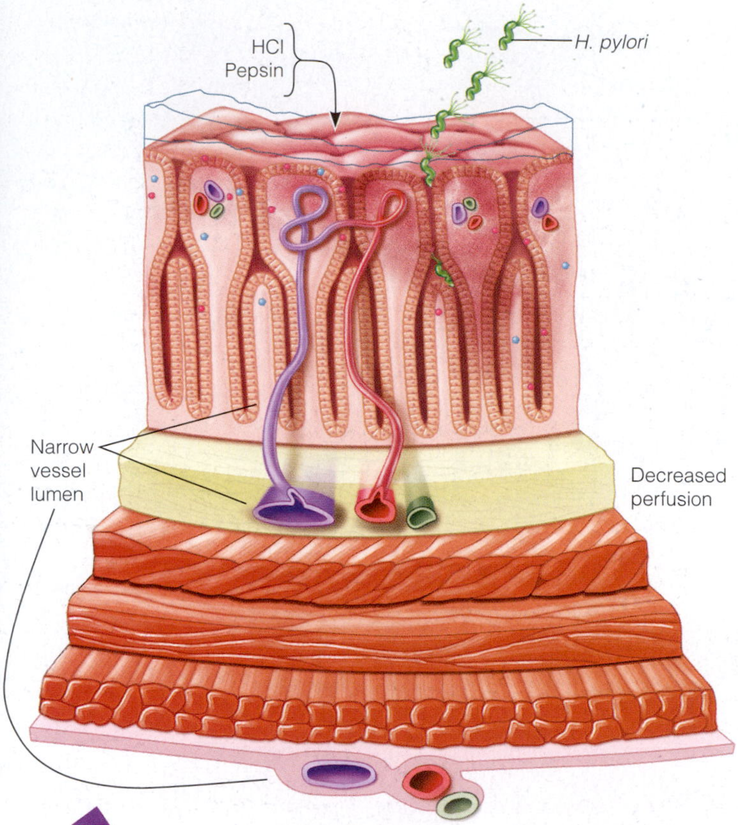
HCl
Pepsin
H. pylori
Narrow vessel lumen
Decreased perfusion

Inflammatory process

When the mucosal barrier is damaged, gastric acid and digestive juices disrupt the epithelial cell membranes, allowing acid to diffuse into cell walls. An acute inflammatory process results. Gastric epithelial cells migrate to the damaged area, a process known as restitution. Adequate blood flow and an alkaline environment are necessary for this repair process. Prostaglandins play an important role in epithelial repair. In the presence of *H. pylori* infection, excess acid production, inadequate blood flow, inhibition of prostaglandins, and other factors that are less clear, the inflammatory process further damages gastric and duodenal epithelial cells, leading to ulceration of the mucosa.

Erosion and ulcer formation

Superficial ulcers (erosions) erode the mucosa, but do not penetrate the muscularis mucosae. True ulcers extend through the muscularis mucosae and into deeper layers of the gastrointestinal wall, damaging blood vessels and potentially penetrating the entire wall. Hemorrhage and peritonitis are potential acute complications of peptic ulcers.

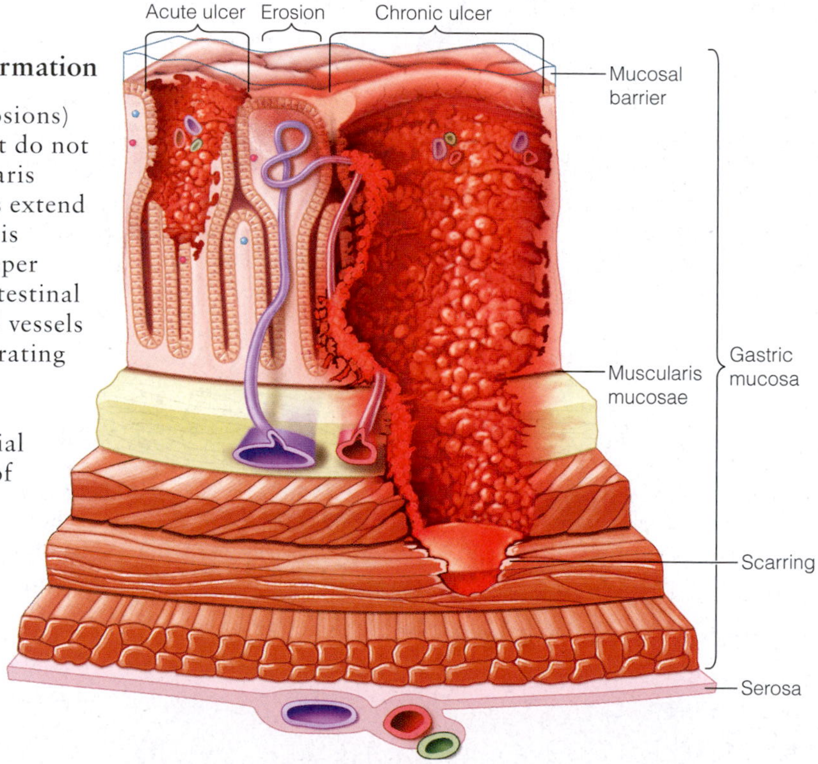
Acute ulcer
Erosion
Chronic ulcer
Mucosal barrier
Muscularis mucosae
Gastric mucosa
Scarring
Serosa

Manifestations

Pain is the classic symptom of peptic ulcer disease. The pain is typically described as gnawing, burning, aching, or hunger-like and is experienced in the epigastric region, sometimes radiating to the back. The pain occurs when the stomach is empty (2 to 3 hours after meals and in the middle of the night) and is relieved by eating with a classic "pain–food–relief" pattern. The patient may complain of heartburn or regurgitation and may vomit.

The presentation of peptic ulcer disease in the older adult is often less clear, with vague and poorly localized discomfort, perhaps chest pain or dysphagia, weight loss, or anemia. In the older adult, a complication of PUD such as upper GI hemorrhage or perforation of the stomach or duodenum may be the presenting symptom.

Complications

The complications associated with peptic ulcers include hemorrhage, obstruction, and perforation. See **Box 23.1** for the manifestations of these complications.

Among people with PUD, 10 to 20% experience hemorrhage as a result of ulceration and erosion into the blood vessels of the gastric mucosa. Bleeding is the most frequent complication in older adults. It is the presenting symptom in up to 20% of people with PUD (Del Valle, 2017). When small blood vessels erode, blood loss may be slow and insidious, with occult blood in the stool the only initial sign. If bleeding continues, the patient becomes anemic and experiences symptoms of weakness, fatigue, dizziness, and orthostatic hypotension. Erosion into a larger vessel can lead to sudden and severe bleeding with hematemesis, melena, or hematochezia (blood in the stool) and signs of hypovolemic shock.

Gastric outlet obstruction may result from edema surrounding the ulcer, smooth muscle spasm, or scar tissue. Generally, obstruction is a gradual rather than an acute process. Symptoms include a feeling of epigastric fullness, accentuated ulcer symptoms, and nausea. If the obstruction becomes complete, vomiting occurs. Hydrochloric acid, sodium, and potassium are lost in vomitus, potentially leading to fluid and electrolyte imbalance and metabolic alkalosis.

The most lethal complication of PUD is *perforation* of the ulcer through the mucosal wall. When perforation occurs, gastric or duodenal contents enter the peritoneum, causing an inflammatory process and peritonitis, which is a life-threatening condition. Chemical peritonitis from the hydrochloric acid, pepsin, bile, and pancreatic fluid is immediate; bacterial peritonitis follows within 6 to 12 hours from gastric contaminants entering the normally sterile peritoneal cavity. When an ulcer perforates, the patient has immediate, severe upper abdominal pain, radiating throughout the abdomen and possibly to the shoulder. The abdomen becomes rigid and boardlike, with absent bowel sounds. Signs of shock may be present, including diaphoresis, tachycardia, and rapid, shallow respirations.

SAFETY ALERT: Classic symptoms of perforation may not be present in an older adult. The older adult may instead present with mental confusion and other nonspecific symptoms. This atypical presentation can lead to delays in diagnosis and treatment, increasing the associated mortality rate. ■

BOX 23.1
Manifestations of PUD Complications

HEMORRHAGE

- Occult or obvious blood in the stool
- Hematemesis
- Fatigue
- Weakness, dizziness
- Orthostatic hypotension
- Hypovolemic shock

OBSTRUCTION

- Sensations of epigastric fullness
- Nausea and vomiting
- Electrolyte imbalances
- Metabolic alkalosis

PERFORATION

- Severe upper abdominal pain, radiating to the shoulder
- Rigid, boardlike abdomen
- Absence of bowel sounds
- Diaphoresis
- Tachycardia
- Rapid, shallow respirations
- Fever

Zollinger-Ellison Syndrome

Zollinger-Ellison syndrome is peptic ulcer disease caused by a gastrinoma, or gastrin-secreting tumor of the pancreas, stomach, or intestines. More than 60% of gastrinomas are malignant tumors. Gastrin is a hormone that stimulates the secretion of pepsin and hydrochloric acid. The increased gastrin levels associated with these tumors result in hypersecretion of gastric acid, which in turn causes mucosal ulceration.

The peptic ulcers of Zollinger-Ellison syndrome may affect any portion of the stomach or duodenum, as well as the esophagus or jejunum. Characteristic ulcer-like pain is common. The high levels of hydrochloric acid entering the duodenum may cause diarrhea and **steatorrhea** (excess fat in the feces) from impaired fat digestion and absorption. Complications of bleeding and perforation are often seen with Zollinger-Ellison syndrome. Fluid and electrolyte imbalances may result from persistent diarrhea with resultant losses of potassium and sodium in particular.

Interprofessional Care

Treatment for PUD focuses on eradicating *H. pylori* infection and treating or preventing ulcers related to use of NSAIDs.

Diagnosis

- ***Upper GI series*** using barium as a contrast medium can detect 80 to 90% of peptic ulcers. It commonly is the diagnostic procedure chosen first; it is less costly and less invasive than endoscopy. Small or very superficial ulcers may be missed, however.

- ***Endoscopy*** allows visualization of the esophageal, gastric, and duodenal mucosa and direct inspection of ulcers. Tissue can also be obtained for biopsy.
- ***Biopsy specimens*** obtained during an endoscopy can be tested for the presence of *H. pylori* using a *biopsy urease test*, which is more than 90% accurate in diagnosing the infection. It is, however, invasive and costly.
- Noninvasive methods of detecting *H. pylori* infection include fecal *H. pylori* antigen tests (to detect antigens to *H. pylori* in the feces) and the *urea breath test*. In this test, radiolabeled urea is given orally. The urease produced by *H. pylori* bacteria converts the urea to ammonia and radiolabeled carbon dioxide, which can then be measured as the patient exhales. These tests can also be used to evaluate the effectiveness of treatment to eradicate *H. pylori*. Treatment with PPIs interferes with urea breath test and fecal antigen test results, so these drugs should be discontinued for 7 or more days prior to testing.
- If Zollinger-Ellison syndrome is suspected, *gastric analysis* may be performed to evaluate gastric acid secretion. Stomach contents are aspirated through a nasogastric tube and analyzed. In Zollinger-Ellison syndrome, gastric acid levels are very high.

Medications

The medications used to treat PUD include agents to eradicate *H. pylori*, drugs to decrease gastric acid content, and agents that protect the mucosa. Nursing responsibilities related to selected drugs to treat GERD, gastritis, and PUD are found in Medication Administration 23.C.

Eradication of *H. pylori* generally requires 14 days of therapy using a combination of two antibiotics with a PPI or a bismuth compound (e.g., a PPI, clarithromycin, and amoxicillin or a PPI, bismuth subsalicylate, tetracycline, and metronidazole). With complete eradication of *H. pylori*, reinfection rates are less than 0.5% per year.

In patients who have NSAID-induced ulcers, the NSAID in use should be discontinued if at all possible. If this is not possible, twice-daily PPIs enable ulcer healing.

Medications that decrease gastric acid content include PPIs and the H_2-receptor antagonists:

- Proton-pump inhibitors bind the acid-secreting enzyme (H^+, K^+ ATPase) that functions as the proton pump, disabling it for up to 24 hours. These drugs are very effective, resulting in more than 90% ulcer healing after 4 weeks. Compared to the H_2-receptor blockers, the PPIs provide faster pain relief and more rapid ulcer healing.
- H_2-receptor blockers inhibit histamine binding to the receptors on the gastric parietal cells to reduce acid secretion. These drugs are very well tolerated and have few serious side effects; however, drug interactions can occur. These drugs must be continued for 8 weeks or longer for ulcer healing.

Agents that protect the mucosa include sucralfate, bismuth, antacids, and prostaglandin analogs:

- Sucralfate binds to proteins in the ulcer base, forming a protective barrier against acid, bile, and pepsin. Sucralfate also stimulates the secretion of mucus, bicarbonate, and prostaglandin.
- Bismuth compounds (e.g., Pepto-Bismol, CBS, BBS) stimulate mucosal bicarbonate and prostaglandin production to promote ulcer healing and likely provide a coating action that prevents further damage by HCl and pepsin. In addition, bismuth has an antibacterial action against *H. pylori*. There are very few side effects, other than constipation and a harmless darkening of stools and the tongue. When used in high doses for a prolonged period, bismuth compounds may be neurotoxic.
- Antacids stimulate gastric mucosal defenses, thereby aiding in ulcer healing. They provide rapid relief of ulcer symptoms and are often used as needed to supplement other antiulcer medications. Antacids are inexpensive, but patients often have difficulty with a regular regimen because the drugs must be taken frequently and may cause either constipation (from the aluminum-type antacids) or diarrhea (from the magnesium-based antacids). Antacids also interfere with the absorption of iron, digoxin, some antibiotics, and other drugs.
- Prostaglandin analogs (misoprostol) promote ulcer healing by stimulating mucus and bicarbonate secretions and by inhibiting acid secretion. Although not as effective as the other drugs discussed, misoprostol is used to prevent NSAID-induced ulcers.

Treatment

Nutrition. In addition to pharmacologic treatment, patients are encouraged to maintain good nutrition, consuming balanced meals at regular intervals. It is important to teach patients that bland or restrictive diets are unnecessary. Mild alcohol intake is not harmful. Smoking should be discouraged because it slows the rate of healing and increases the frequency of relapses.

Surgery. The identification of *H. pylori* as a cause of PUD and the availability of drugs to treat the infection and heal peptic ulcers has all but eliminated surgery as a primary treatment option for peptic ulcer disease. Surgery may be required to treat a complication of PUD, such as hemorrhage, perforation, or gastric outlet obstruction. See the section on gastric cancer for more information about gastric surgery and related nursing care.

Treatment of Complications. The patient hospitalized with a complication of PUD such as bleeding, gastrointestinal obstruction, or perforation and peritonitis requires additional interventions to restore homeostasis.

In hemorrhage associated with PUD, initial interventions focus on restoring and maintaining circulation. Normal saline, lactated Ringer, or other balanced electrolyte solutions are administered intravenously to restore intravascular volume if signs of shock (tachycardia, hypotension, pallor, low urine output, and anxiety) are present. Whole blood or packed red blood cells may be administered to restore hemoglobin and hematocrit levels. A nasogastric tube is inserted to prevent aspiration of vomited gastric contents.

Endoscopy with direct injection of a clotting or sclerosing agent into the bleeding vessel may be performed. Laser photocoagulation, using light energy, or electrocoagulation, which uses electric current to generate heat, can also be done via endoscopy to seal bleeding vessels.

The patient is kept NPO until bleeding is controlled. PPIs are administered intravenously (e.g., 40 mg of pantoprazole [Protonix] per intravenous push or admixture daily) to reduce the risk of rebleeding. Surgery may be necessary if medical measures are ineffective in controlling bleeding. Older adults who experience bleeding as a complication of PUD are more likely to rebleed or require surgery to control the hemorrhage. Nursing care of the patient having gastric surgery is discussed later in this chapter.

Repeated inflammation, healing, scarring, edema, and muscle spasm can lead to gastric outlet (pyloric) obstruction. Initial treatment includes gastric decompression with nasogastric suction and administration of intravenous normal saline and potassium chloride to correct fluid and electrolyte imbalance. H_2-receptor blockers are given intravenously as well. Balloon dilation of the gastric outlet may be done via upper endoscopy. If these measures are unsuccessful in relieving obstruction, surgery may be required.

Gastric or duodenal perforation resulting in contamination of the peritoneum with gastrointestinal contents often requires immediate intervention to restore homeostasis and minimize peritonitis. Intravenous fluids maintain fluid and electrolyte balance. Nasogastric suction removes gastric contents and minimizes peritoneal contamination. Placing the patient in Fowler or semi-Fowler position allows peritoneal contaminants to pool in the pelvis. Intravenous antibiotics aggressively treat bacterial infection from intestinal flora. Laparoscopic surgery or an open laparotomy may be performed to close the perforation.

Nursing Care

Assessment

Collect the following subjective and objective data when assessing the patient with peptic ulcer disease:

- *Health history:* Complaints of epigastric or left upper quadrant pain, heartburn, or discomfort; its character, severity, timing, and relationship to eating; measures used for relief; nausea or vomiting, presence of bright blood or "coffee-grounds" material in vomitus; current medications including use of aspirin or other NSAIDs; cigarette smoking and use of alcohol or other drugs
- *Physical assessment:* General appearance including height and weight relationship; vital signs including orthostatic measurements; abdominal examination including shape and contour, bowel sounds, and tenderness to palpation; presence of obvious or occult blood in vomitus and stool.

Priorities of Care

The priorities of nursing care for the patient with peptic ulcer disease are reducing discomfort, maintaining nutritional status, and preventing or rapidly identifying and intervening for potential complications. See the accompanying Case Study & Nursing Care Plan.

Diagnoses, Outcomes, and Interventions

Manage Acute and Chronic Pain. The pain of peptic ulcer disease is often predictable and preventable. Pain is typically experienced 2 to 4 hours after eating, as high levels of gastric acid and pepsin irritate the exposed mucosa. Measures to neutralize the acid, minimize its production, or protect the mucosa often relieve this pain, minimizing the need for analgesics.

Expected Outcome: Patient will identify pain triggers, use treatment plan (pharmacologic and nonpharmacologic) to prevent and alleviate discomfort, and report relief from pain.

The nurse will:

- Assess pain, including location, type, severity, frequency, and duration, and its relationship to food intake or other contributing factors. *Thorough pain assessment will aid in identifying triggers causing pain and help to determine preventative measures and best treatment options.*

SAFETY ALERT: Avoid making assumptions about pain. Acute pain may indicate a complication, such as perforation (often heralded by sudden, severe epigastric pain and a rigid, boardlike abdomen), or it may be totally unrelated to PUD (e.g., angina, gallbladder disease, pancreatitis). ■

- Administer PPIs, H_2-receptor antagonists, antacids, or mucosal protective agents as ordered. Monitor for effectiveness and side effects or adverse reactions. *The pain associated with PUD is generally caused by the effect of gastric juices on exposed mucosal tissue. These medications reduce pain and promote healing by reducing acid production, neutralizing acid, or providing a barrier for the damaged mucosa.*
- Teach relaxation, stress reduction, and lifestyle management techniques. Refer for stress management counseling or classes as indicated. *Although there is no clear relationship between stress and PUD, measures to relieve stress and promote physical and emotional rest help reduce the perception of pain and may reduce ulcer genesis.*

Promote Healthy Sleep Pattern. Nighttime ulcer pain, which typically occurs between 1:00 and 3:00 a.m., may disrupt the sleep cycle and result in inadequate rest. Anticipation of pain may lead to insomnia or other sleep disruptions.

Expected Outcome: Patient will report absence of symptoms of sleep disruption (anxiety, daytime drowsiness, tiredness).

The nurse will:

- Stress the importance of taking medications as prescribed. *The bedtime dose of PPI or H_2-receptor blocker minimizes hydrochloric acid production during the night, reducing nighttime pain.*

- Instruct to limit food intake after the evening meal, eliminating any bedtime snack. *Eating before bed can stimulate the production of gastric acid and pepsin, increasing the likelihood of nighttime pain.*
- Encourage use of relaxation techniques and comfort measures such as soft music as needed to promote sleep. *Once the pain associated with PUD has been controlled, these measures help reduce anxiety and reestablish a normal sleep pattern.*

Promote Balanced Nutrition. In an attempt to avoid discomfort, the patient with peptic ulcer disease may gradually reduce food intake, sometimes jeopardizing nutritional status. Anorexia and early satiety are additional problems associated with PUD.

Expected Outcome: Patient's weight and body mass index will stabilize and be within normal limits. Patient will describe intake of a well-balanced diet and normal eating patterns.

The nurse will:

- Assess current diet, including pattern of food intake, eating schedule, and foods that precipitate pain or are being avoided in anticipation of pain. *The patient may not realize the extent of self-imposed dietary limitations, especially if symptoms have persisted for an extended time. Assessment increases awareness and also helps identify the adequacy of nutrient intake.*
- Refer to a dietitian for meal planning to minimize PUD symptoms and meet nutritional needs. Consider normal eating patterns and preferences in meal planning. *Although no specific diet is recommended for PUD, patients should avoid foods that increase pain. Six small meals per day often help increase food tolerance and decrease postprandial discomfort.*
- Monitor for complaints of anorexia, fullness, and nausea and vomiting. Adjust dietary intake or medication schedule as indicated. *PUD and resultant scarring can lead to impaired gastric emptying, necessitating a treatment change.*
- Advise the patient to report increasing or persistent symptoms of anorexia, nausea and vomiting, or fullness to the healthcare provider. *These are symptoms of gastric outlet obstruction, which can lead to serious complications and nutritional deficiencies.*
- Monitor laboratory values for indications of anemia or other nutritional deficits. Monitor for therapeutic and side effects of treatment measures such as oral iron replacement. Instruct the patient taking oral iron replacement to avoid using an antacid within 1 to 2 hours of taking the iron preparation. *Anemia can result from poor nutrient absorption or chronic blood loss in patients with PUD. Oral iron supplements may cause GI distress, and nausea and vomiting; if these side effects are intolerable, notify the physician for a possible change of therapy. Antacids bind with oral iron preparations, blocking absorption.*

Monitor for Bleeding. Erosion of a blood vessel with resultant hemorrhage is a significant risk for the patient with peptic ulcer disease. Acute bleeding can lead to hypovolemia and fluid volume deficit, which can lead to a decrease in cardiac output and impaired tissue perfusion.

Expected Outcome: Patient will not exhibit signs of visible or occult blood. Hematocrit and hemoglobin will be maintained within normal limits. Vital signs will be maintained within normal limits and urine output will be greater than 30 mL/h.

The nurse will:

- Monitor and record blood pressure and apical pulse every 15 to 30 minutes until stable; monitor central venous pressure or pulmonary artery pressure as indicated. Insert a Foley catheter and monitor urinary output hourly. Weigh daily. *Continuous monitoring of cardiac output parameters is essential in patients with an acute hemorrhage to identify possible shock and assure interventions are initiated at an early stage.*

SAFETY ALERT: Erosion of a blood vessel with hemorrhage is a critical event. ■

- Monitor stools and gastric drainage for overt and occult blood. Assess gastric drainage (vomitus or from a nasogastric tube) to estimate the amount and rapidity of hemorrhage. *Drainage is bright red with possible clots in acute hemorrhage; dark red or the color of coffee grounds when blood has been in the stomach for a period of time.* Hematochezia *(stool containing red blood and clots) is present in acute hemorrhage;* melena *(black, tarry stool) is an indicator of less acute bleeding. When small vessels are disrupted, bleeding may be slow and not overtly evident. With chronic or slow gastrointestinal bleeding, the risk of a fluid volume deficit is minimal; anemia and activity intolerance are more likely.*
- Maintain intravenous therapy with fluid volume and electrolyte replacement solutions; administer whole blood or packed cells as ordered. *Both fluids and electrolytes are lost through vomiting, nasogastric drainage, and diarrhea in an episode of acute bleeding. To prevent shock, it is essential to maintain a blood volume and cardiac output sufficient to perfuse body tissues. Whole blood and packed cells replace both blood volume and red blood cells, providing additional oxygen-carrying capacity to meet cell needs.*
- Insert a nasogastric tube and maintain its position and patency according to agency policy and procedure. Initially, measure and record gastric output every hour, then every 4 to 8 hours. *Nasogastric suction removes blood from the gastrointestinal tract, preventing vomiting and possible aspiration. Gastric output is replaced milliliter for milliliter with a balanced electrolyte solution to maintain homeostasis.*
- Monitor hemoglobin and hematocrit, serum electrolytes, BUN, and creatinine values. Report abnormal findings. *Hemoglobin and hematocrit are lower than normal with acute or chronic GI bleeding. In acute hemorrhage, initial results may be within normal range because both cells and plasma are lost. Loss of fluids and electrolytes with*

gastric drainage and diarrhea will alter normal levels. Digestion and absorption of blood in the GI tract may result in elevated BUN and creatinine levels.

- Assess abdomen, including bowel sounds, distention, girth, and tenderness, every 4 hours and record findings. *Borborygmi or hyperactive bowel sounds with abdominal tenderness are common with acute GI bleeding. Increased distention, increasing abdominal girth, absent bowel sounds, or extreme tenderness with a rigid, boardlike abdomen may indicate perforation.*
- Maintain bedrest with the head of the bed elevated. Ensure safety. *Loss of blood volume may cause orthostatic hypotension with resultant syncope or dizziness upon standing.*

Transitions of Care

Although it is difficult to predict which patients will develop peptic ulcer disease, promote health by advising patients to avoid risk factors such as excessive aspirin or NSAID use and cigarette smoking. In addition, encourage patients to seek treatment for manifestations of GERD or chronic gastritis, both of which are associated with *H. pylori* infection.

The acutely ill patient due to peptic ulcer disease is experiencing acute blood loss and will require aggressive monitoring of vital signs, fluid volume replacement, administration of blood products, administration of PPI, and other supportive care.

Peptic ulcer disease is managed in home and community-based settings; only its complications typically require treatment in an acute care setting. Provide the following information when preparing the patient for home care:

- Prescribed medication regimen, including desired and potential adverse effects
- Importance of continuing therapy even when symptoms are relieved
- Relationship between peptic ulcers and factors such as NSAID use and smoking (If indicated, refer to a smoking cessation clinic or program.)
- Importance of avoiding use of aspirin and other NSAIDs; stress the necessity of reading the labels of over-the-counter medications for possible aspirin content
- Manifestations of complications that should be reported to the care provider, including increased abdominal pain or distention, vomiting, black or tarry stools, lightheadedness, or fainting
- Stress and lifestyle management techniques that may help prevent exacerbation. Refer to resources for stress management, such as classes, counseling, and formal or informal groups.

A patient with PUD may have an unexpected and sudden death. The nurse will participate in lifesaving interventions as a member of the interprofessional healthcare team. When a patient does not survive the event, the nurse provides comfort to the family and significant others and coordinates care provided by social work and chaplain services.

Case Study & Nursing Care Plan

A Patient with Peptic Ulcer Disease

Kamran Nassar is a 47-year-old police officer who lives and works in a metropolitan area. Mr. Nassar has had heartburn and abdominal discomfort for years, but thought it went along with his job. Last year, after becoming weak, light-headed, and short of breath, he was found to be anemic and was diagnosed as having a duodenal ulcer. He took omeprazole (Prilosec) and ferrous sulfate for 3 months before stopping both, saying he had "never felt better in his life." Mr. Nassar has now been admitted to the hospital with active upper GI bleeding.

ASSESSMENT	DIAGNOSES	EXPECTED OUTCOMES
Rachel Clark is Mr. Nassar's admitting nurse and case manager. On initial assessment, Mr. Nassar is alert and oriented, though apprehensive about his condition. Skin pale and cool; BP 136/78 mmHg, P 98/min; abdomen distended and tender with hyperactive bowel sounds; 200 mL bright red blood obtained on nasogastric tube insertion. Hemoglobin 8.2 g/dL and hematocrit 23% on admission. Mr. Nassar is taken to the endoscopy lab where his bleeding is controlled using laser photocoagulation. On his return to the nursing unit, he receives two units of packed RBCs and intravenous fluids to restore blood volume. A 5-day course of high-dose oral omeprazole (40 mg bid) is ordered to prevent rebleeding, and Mr. Nassar is allowed to begin a clear liquid diet 24 hours after his endoscopy. Tissue biopsy obtained during endoscopy confirms the presence of *H. pylori* infection.	▪ Decrease in fluid volume due to active bleeding ▪ Decrease in adherence to prescribed therapeutic regimen	▪ Patient will maintain normal blood pressure, pulse, and urine output (greater than 30 mL/h). ▪ Patient will seek information to reduce fear. ▪ Patient will describe prescribed therapeutic regimen. ▪ Patient will verbalize ability to manage prescribed regimen.

(continued)

PLANNING AND IMPLEMENTATION

- Place call light within reach and encourage to ask for help when getting up or ambulating. Remind to rise slowly from lying to sitting and sitting to standing.
- Discuss situation and provide information about all procedures and treatments.
- Reassure about the effectiveness of treatment in reducing the risk for further bleeding.
- Discuss current and planned treatment measures; stress the importance of completing the prescribed treatment to reduce the risk of further ulcer development.
- Encourage to avoid using aspirin or NSAIDs in the future; suggest alternative medications such as acetaminophen.
- Discuss stress reduction techniques and refer for stress reduction counseling or workshops as indicated.

EVALUATION

Mr. Nassar is discharged 48 hours after admission. He has had no further evidence of bleeding and has resumed a regular diet. His hemoglobin and hematocrit remain low, and he has a prescription for ferrous sulfate. He will complete the prescribed high-dose omeprazole regimen at home, then begin treatment with omeprazole, amoxicillin, and clarithromycin (Biaxin) to eradicate the *H. pylori* infection detected during endoscopy. After 2 weeks of this regimen, he will continue taking omeprazole at bedtime for 4 to 8 weeks. He verbalizes a good understanding of his treatment and the importance of completing the entire regimen. Mr. Nassar expresses concern about his ability to "keep his cool on the inside" when under stress. Ms. Clark, his case manager, gives him the names of several resources to help with stress management in case he wants help.

CLINICAL REASONING IN PATIENT CARE

1. How does *H. pylori* infection contribute to the development of peptic ulcers?
2. Describe the physiologic responses to fear and anxiety. Why is it important to alleviate fear and its physical consequences in patients with PUD?
3. What suggestions can you make to help Mr. Nassar manage his complex treatment regimen during the next 3 months?
4. Develop a teaching plan that includes stress-reduction techniques Mr. Nassar can use while performing his duties as a police officer.

See Evaluating Your Response in Appendix B.

The Patient with Gastritis

Gastritis, inflammation of the stomach lining, results from irritation of the gastric mucosa. Gastritis is common and may be caused by a variety of factors. The most common form of gastritis, *acute gastritis*, is generally a benign, self-limiting disorder associated with the ingestion of gastric irritants such as aspirin, alcohol, caffeine, or foods contaminated with certain bacteria. Manifestations of acute gastritis may range from asymptomatic to mild heartburn to severe gastric distress, vomiting, and bleeding with hematemesis (vomiting blood).

Chronic gastritis is a separate group of disorders characterized by progressive and irreversible changes in the gastric mucosa (Sorenson et al., 2019). Chronic gastritis is more common in older adults, individuals with alcoholism, and those who smoke cigarettes. When symptoms of chronic gastritis occur, they are often vague, ranging from a feeling of heaviness in the epigastric region after meals to gnawing, burning, ulcer-like epigastric pain unrelieved by antacids.

Pathophysiology

Acute Gastritis

Acute gastritis is characterized by disruption of the mucosal barrier by a local irritant. This disruption allows hydrochloric acid and pepsin to come into contact with the gastric tissue, resulting in irritation, inflammation, and superficial erosions. The gastric mucosa rapidly regenerates, generally making acute gastritis a self-limiting disorder, with resolution and healing occurring within several days.

The ingestion of aspirin or other NSAIDs, corticosteroids, alcohol, and caffeine is commonly associated with the development of acute gastritis. Accidental or purposeful ingestion of a corrosive alkali (such as ammonia, lye, Lysol, and other cleaning agents) or acid leads to severe inflammation and possible necrosis of the stomach. Gastric perforation, hemorrhage, and peritonitis are possible results. Iatrogenic causes of acute gastritis include radiation therapy and administration of certain chemotherapeutic agents.

A severe form of acute gastritis, **erosive (stress-induced) gastritis**, occurs as a complication of other life-threatening conditions such as shock, severe trauma, major surgery, sepsis, burns, or head injury. When these erosions follow a major burn, they are called **Curling ulcers**, after Thomas Curling, a British physician who first described them in 1842. When stress ulcers occur following head injury or CNS surgery, they are referred to as **Cushing ulcers**, after Harvey Cushing, a U.S. surgeon.

The primary mechanisms leading to erosive gastritis appear to be ischemia of the gastric mucosa resulting from sympathetic vasoconstriction and tissue injury due to gastric acid. As a result, multiple superficial erosions of the gastric mucosa develop. Maintaining the gastric pH at greater than 3.5 and inhibiting gastric acid secretion with medications help prevent erosive gastritis.

The patient with acute gastritis may have mild symptoms such as **anorexia** (loss of appetite) or mild epigastric discomfort relieved by belching or defecating. More severe manifestations include abdominal pain and nausea and vomiting. Gastric bleeding may occur, with hematemesis or melena (black, tarry stool that contains blood). Erosive gastritis is not typically associated with pain. The initial symptom is often painless gastric bleeding occurring 2 or more days after the initial stressor. Bleeding is typically minimal, but can be massive. Corrosive gastritis can cause severe bleeding, signs of shock, and an *acute abdomen* (severely painful, rigid, boardlike abdomen) if perforation occurs (see **Table 23.4**).

Chronic Gastritis

Unrelated to acute gastritis, *chronic gastritis* is a progressive disorder that begins with superficial inflammation and gradually leads to atrophy of gastric tissues. The initial stage is characterized by superficial changes in the gastric mucosa and a decrease in mucus. As the disease evolves, glands of the gastric mucosa are disrupted and destroyed. The inflammatory process involves deep portions of the mucosa, which thins and atrophies. There are several types of chronic gastritis; *H. pylori* gastritis and autoimmune gastritis are the most commonly seen.

H. pylori gastritis is the most common form of chronic gastritis. Its incidence increases with age and is significantly higher in developing countries than in industrialized countries (Del Valle, 2017). It is caused by chronic infection of the gastric mucosa by *H. pylori*, a gram-negative spiral bacterium. *H. pylori* infection causes inflammation of the gastric mucosa, with infiltration by neutrophils and lymphocytes. The outermost layer of gastric mucosa thins and atrophies, providing a less effective barrier against the autodigestive properties of hydrochloric acid and pepsin. Infection with *H. pylori* is also associated with peptic ulcer disease and an increased risk of developing gastric cancer.

Chronic gastritis is often asymptomatic until atrophy is sufficiently advanced to interfere with digestion and gastric emptying. The patient may complain of vague gastric distress, epigastric heaviness after meals, or ulcer-like symptoms. These symptoms are typically not relieved by antacids. In addition, the patient may experience fatigue and other symptoms of anemia. If intrinsic factor is lacking, paresthesias and other neurologic manifestations of vitamin B_{12} deficiency may be present. See Table 23.4.

Table 23.4 Manifestations of Acute and Chronic Gastritis

Gastrointestinal	Systemic
Acute Gastritis	
■ Anorexia ■ Nausea and vomiting ■ Hematemesis ■ Melena ■ Abdominal pain	■ Possible shock
Chronic Gastritis	
■ Vague discomfort after eating; may be asymptomatic	■ Anemia ■ Fatigue

Interprofessional Care

Acute gastritis is usually diagnosed by the history and clinical presentation. In contrast, the vague symptoms of chronic gastritis may require more extensive diagnostic testing.

Patients with acute and chronic gastritis are generally managed in community settings. The patient requires acute care only when nausea and vomiting are severe enough to interfere with normal fluid and electrolyte balance and nutritional status. If hemorrhage results, surgical intervention may be required.

Diagnosis

Diagnostic tests that may be ordered for the patient with gastritis include:

- ***Testing*** for ***H. pylori*** infection, including urea breath tests, serologic testing, and fecal antigen testing.
- ***Gastric analysis*** to assess hydrochloric acid secretion. Secretion may be decreased in patients with chronic gastritis.
- ***Hemoglobin***, ***hematocrit***, and ***red blood cell (RBC) indices*** are evaluated for evidence of anemia. The patient with gastritis may develop pernicious anemia because of parietal cell destruction or iron deficiency anemia because of chronic blood loss.
- ***Serum vitamin B_{12} levels*** are measured to evaluate for possible pernicious anemia. Normal values for vitamin B_{12} are 200 to 1000 pg/mL, with lower levels seen in older adults.
- ***Upper endoscopy*** may be done to inspect the gastric mucosa for changes, identify areas of bleeding, and obtain tissue for biopsy. Bleeding sites may be treated with electro- or laser coagulation or injected with a sclerosing agent during the procedure.

See Chapter 21 for patient preparation and teaching related to diagnostic tests for upper GI disorders.

Medications

Drugs such as a PPI, H_2-receptor blocker, or sucralfate may be ordered to prevent or treat acute stress gastritis. PPIs and H_2-receptor blockers reduce the amount or effects of hydrochloric acid on the gastric mucosa. Lansoprazole (Prevacid), esomeprazole (Nexium), and omeprazole (Prilosec) are examples of PPIs. H_2-receptor blockers include cimetidine (Tagamet), ranitidine (Zantac), famotidine (Pepcid), and nizatidine (Axid). These drugs are also available in nonprescription strength. Sucralfate (Carafate) works locally to prevent the damaging effects of acid and pepsin on gastric tissue. It does not neutralize or reduce acid secretion. Nursing implications for drugs commonly used in managing gastritis are included in Medication Administration 23.C earlier in this chapter.

Chronic *H. pylori* infection may be treated using combination therapy that includes two antibiotics (such as metronidazole, amoxicillin, clarithromycin, or tetracycline), a bismuth compound, and possibly a PPI. In some cases, eradication of the infection is not warranted and the patient is treated symptomatically.

Treatment

In acute gastritis, gastrointestinal tract rest is provided by 6 to 12 hours of NPO status, then slow reintroduction of clear liquids (broth, tea, gelatin, carbonated beverages), followed by ingestion of heavier liquids (cream soups, puddings, milk), and finally a gradual reintroduction of solid food.

If nausea and vomiting threaten fluid and electrolyte balance, intravenous fluids and electrolytes are ordered.

Acute gastritis resulting from ingestion of a poisonous or corrosive substance (acid or strong alkali) is treated with immediate dilution and removal of the substance. Vomiting is not induced because it might further damage the esophagus and possibly the trachea; instead, gastric lavage (washing-out of the stomach contents) is performed.

Integrative Therapies

Complementary health approaches such as herbal remedies or aromatherapy may be appropriate to recommend for patients with gastritis. Refer the patient to a healthcare provider trained in natural and herbal remedies or to an aromatherapist for an individualized treatment plan. Recommendations may include:

- Chamomile tea or the essential oil used in aromatherapy
- Garlic; one clove chopped fine and taken daily at bedtime
- Ginger, powdered or in capsules or made into a tea taken before or after meals
- Mint oil aromatherapy via a diffuser, in a bath, or diluted with a carrier oil and used for a soothing massage.

Nursing Care

Assessment

Assessment data to collect for patients with acute or chronic gastritis include:

- ***Health history:*** Current symptoms and their duration; relieving and aggravating factors; history of ingestion of toxins, contaminated food, alcohol, aspirin, or NSAIDs; other medications
- ***Physical assessment:*** Vital signs including orthostatic vitals, if indicated; peripheral pulses; general appearance; abdominal assessment including appearance, bowel sounds, and tenderness.

Priorities of Care

Managing pain and other symptoms associated with gastritis is the key to promoting healing of tissue damage related to gastritis. Ensuring the patient's nutritional status is adequate is also a priority.

Diagnoses, Outcomes, and Interventions

In planning and implementing nursing care for the patient with acute or chronic gastritis, consider both the direct effects of the disorder on the gastrointestinal system and nutritional status as well as its effects on lifestyle and psychosocial integrity. This section focuses on problems related to nausea and anorexia associated with gastritis.

Manage Nausea. Nausea and vomiting and abdominal distress are the primary manifestations of acute gastritis. Patients with chronic gastritis often experience anorexia and nausea that can interfere with food intake and nutritional status.

Expected Outcome: Patient will express relief from nausea and be free from emesis. Patient's fluid intake will be adequate to establish and maintain an adequate fluid balance as evidenced by stable vital signs and urine output greater than 30 mL/h.

The nurse will:

- Monitor subjective complaints of nausea. *Nausea is a subjective sensation best described by the patient.*
- Monitor vital signs, skin turgor and condition, and weight for the patient with acute gastritis. Maintain accurate intake and output records. Monitor amount, color, and specific gravity of urine. *Nausea and vomiting associated with acute gastritis can significantly affect food and fluid intake, leading to dehydration.*
- Administer antiemetic medication, as ordered, prior to meals and before treatments or procedures known to stimulate nausea. *Preventing nausea is particularly important to ensure the patient can resume a nutritional diet that will facilitate healing of damaged tissue.*
- Instruct to consume small quantities of clear fluids and dry foods at separate times. *Separating the intake of dry foods and fluids helps reduce the nausea stimulus.*

Promote Balanced Nutrition and Hydration. Manifestations of chronic gastritis may lead to reduced food intake and malnutrition. The patient often associates these unpleasant sensations with eating and may gradually reduce food intake. Associated anorexia also contributes to poor food intake.

Expected Outcome: Patient's food intake will meet caloric and nutritional demand required to meet metabolic needs and promote healing of damaged tissue.

The nurse will:

- Monitor and record food and fluid intake and any abnormal losses (such as vomiting). *Careful monitoring can help in developing a dietary plan to meet the caloric needs of the patient.*
- Monitor weight and laboratory studies such as serum albumin, hemoglobin, and RBC indices. *Weights and laboratory values provide data regarding nutritional status and the effectiveness of interventions.*
- Arrange for a dietary consultation to determine caloric and nutrient needs and develop a dietary plan. Consider food preferences and tolerances in menu planning. *A diet high in protein, vitamins, and minerals may be prescribed to meet nutritional needs of the patient with chronic gastritis. In addition, specific food intolerances may need to be considered. Planning to include preferred foods in the diet helps ensure consumption of the prescribed diet.*

- Provide nutritional supplements between meals or frequent, small feedings as needed. *Many patients with chronic gastritis tolerate frequent, small feedings better than three large meals per day.*
- Maintain tube feedings or parenteral nutrition as ordered. Refer to Chapter 22 for further information on enteral and parenteral feedings.

Delegating Nursing Care Activities

As appropriate and allowed by the designated duties and responsibilities of unlicensed assistive personnel, the nurse may delegate nursing care activities such as measuring intake and output, obtaining daily weights, and assisting with meals.

Transitions of Care

Teach all patients and community members about measures to prevent acute gastritis. Food contaminated with bacteria is a significant cause of acute gastritis. Discuss food safety measures such as fully cooking meats and egg products and promptly refrigerating foods after cooking to avoid bacterial growth. Stress that food contaminated with potential pathogens often looks, smells, and tastes good, making it difficult to identify. Teach patients to abstain from eating or drinking anything during an acute episode of vomiting, then reintroduce clear liquids gradually once vomiting has stopped (2 to 4 hours after the last episode of vomiting). Suggest using liquids such as Pedialyte or a sports drink to replace lost electrolytes and fluid. Instruct patients to avoid milk and milk products until they easily tolerate clear liquids and solid foods such as dry toast or saltine crackers.

Because acute or chronic gastritis is usually managed in community-based settings, teaching is vital. For the patient with acute gastritis, teaching focuses on managing acute symptoms, reintroducing fluids and solid foods, identifying indicators of possible complications (e.g., continued vomiting, signs of fluid and electrolyte imbalance), and preventing future episodes.

Provide the following information for patients with chronic gastritis:

- How to maintain optimal nutrition
- Helpful dietary modifications
- Use of prescribed medications
- How to avoid known gastric irritants, such as aspirin, alcohol, and cigarette smoking. Referral to smoking-cessation classes or programs to treat alcohol abuse may be necessary.

The Patient with Cancer of the Stomach

Worldwide, cancer of the stomach is the most common cancer (after skin cancer), but it is less common in the United States. An estimated 26,240 new cases of stomach cancer are diagnosed annually in the United States (ACS, 2018). Its incidence is highest in Hispanics, African Americans, and Asian Americans. Men are affected nearly twice as often as women. Older adults are more likely to develop gastric cancer. The mean age at time of diagnosis is 63. People in lower socioeconomic groups are more often affected by gastric cancer.

Risk Factors

H. pylori infection is a major risk factor for cancer of the distal portion of the stomach; 60 to 90% of cases can be attributed to this infection. Other risk factors are a genetic predisposition, chronic gastritis, pernicious anemia, gastric polyps, smoking, or carcinogenic factors in the diet (such as smoked foods and nitrates). Achlorhydria, a lack of hydrochloric acid in the stomach, is a known risk factor. The risk for gastric cancer is also increased in people who have had a partial gastric resection.

Pathophysiology

Adenocarcinoma, which involves the mucus-producing cells of the stomach, is the most common form of gastric cancer. These carcinomas may arise anywhere on the mucosal surface of the stomach but are most frequently found in the distal portion. More than half of all gastric cancers occur in the antrum or pyloric region. Gastric cancer begins as a localized lesion (*in situ*), then progresses to involve the mucosa or submucosa (early gastric carcinoma). Lesions may spread by direct extension to tissues surrounding the stomach, the liver in particular. The lesion may ulcerate or appear as a polypoid (polyp-like) mass (**Figure 23.11 ■**). Lymph node involvement and metastasis occur early due to the rich blood and lymphatic supply to the stomach. Metastatic lesions are often found in the liver, lungs, ovaries, and peritoneum.

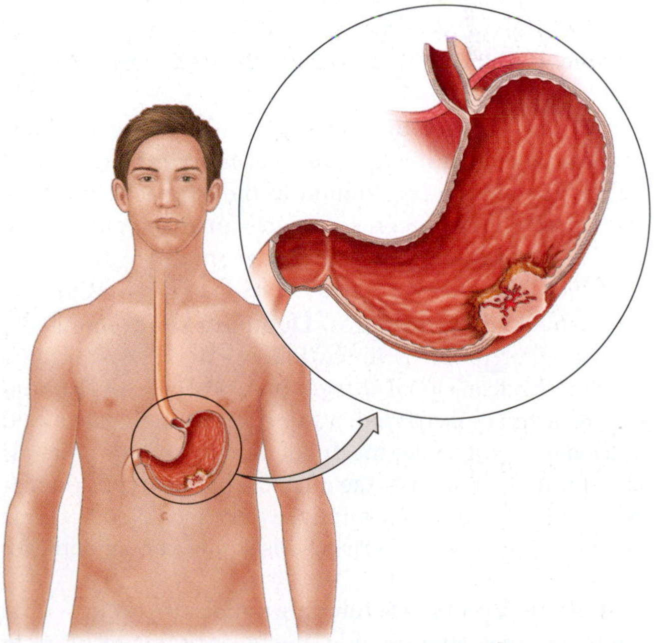

Figure 23.11 ■ Gastric cancer affecting the antrum of the stomach.

Manifestations

Gastric cancer has few manifestations. Unfortunately, the disease is often quite advanced and metastases are usually present at the time of diagnosis. Early symptoms are vague, including feelings of early satiety, anorexia, indigestion, and possibly vomiting. The patient may experience ulcer-like pain unrelieved by antacids, typically occurring after meals. As the disease progresses, weight loss occurs, and the patient may be *cachectic* (in very poor health and malnourished) at the time of diagnosis. An abdominal mass may be palpable, and occult blood may be present in the stool, indicating gastrointestinal bleeding.

Interprofessional Care

Diagnosis

Anemia detected by a CBC is often the first indication of gastric cancer. Upper endoscopy should be performed on patients over age 55 with new onset of epigastric symptoms and in anyone with persistent dyspepsia. An upper GI x-ray with barium swallow is an acceptable alternative to identify lesions, and ultrasound or other radiologic techniques may identify a mass. Upper endoscopy with visualization and biopsy of the lesion provides a definitive diagnosis of gastric cancer.

Surgery

When gastric cancer is identified prior to the development of metastasis, surgical removal of part or all of the stomach and regional lymph nodes is the treatment of choice. **Partial gastrectomy** involves removal of a portion of the stomach, usually the distal half to two-thirds. In partial gastrectomy, the surgeon constructs an anastomosis from the remainder of the stomach directly to the duodenum or to the proximal jejunum. The *gastroduodenostomy* (Billroth I) and the *gastrojejunostomy* (Billroth II) are commonly used partial gastrectomy procedures.

A **total gastrectomy**, removal of the entire stomach, may be done for diffuse cancer that is spread throughout the gastric mucosa but limited to the stomach. In a total gastrectomy, the surgeon constructs an anastomosis from the esophagus to the duodenum or jejunum.

Several long-term complications may develop following gastrectomy procedures. **Dumping syndrome** is the most common problem. It may follow a partial gastrectomy with duodenal or jejunal anastomosis. When the pylorus has been resected or bypassed, a hypertonic, undigested food bolus may rapidly enter the duodenum or jejunum. Water is pulled into the lumen of the intestine by the hyperosmolar character of the chyme, resulting in decreased blood volume and intestinal dilation. Peristalsis is stimulated, and intestinal motility is increased.

Early symptoms of dumping syndrome occur within 5 to 30 minutes after eating. These symptoms result from intestinal dilation, peristaltic stimulation, and hypovolemia caused by undigested food in the proximal small intestine. Manifestations include nausea with possible vomiting, epigastric pain with cramping and *borborygmi* (loud, hyperactive bowel sounds), and diarrhea. Systemic symptoms from the hypovolemia and reflex sympathetic stimulation include tachycardia, orthostatic hypotension, dizziness, flushing, and diaphoresis.

The entry of hyperosmolar chyme into the jejunum also causes a rapid rise in the blood glucose. This stimulates the release of an excessive amount of insulin, leading to hypoglycemic symptoms 2 to 3 hours after a meal. Dumping syndrome is typically self-limiting, lasting 6 to 12 months after surgery; however, a small percentage of people continue to experience long-term symptoms.

Dumping syndrome is managed primarily by a dietary pattern that delays gastric emptying and allows smaller boluses of undigested food to enter the intestine. Meals should be small and more frequent. Liquids and solids are taken at separate times instead of together during a meal. The amount of proteins and fats in the diet is increased because they exit the stomach more slowly than carbohydrates. Carbohydrates, especially simple sugars, are reduced. The patient is instructed to rest in a recumbent or semirecumbent position for 30 to 60 minutes after meals. Anticholinergics, sedatives, and antispasmodics may be prescribed.

Anemia may be a chronic problem after a major gastric resection. Iron is absorbed primarily in the duodenum and proximal jejunum; rapid gastric emptying or a gastrojejunostomy may interfere with adequate absorption.

The cells of the stomach produce intrinsic factor, required for the absorption of vitamin B_{12}. Vitamin B_{12} deficiency leads to pernicious anemia. Because of hepatic stores of vitamin B_{12}, symptoms of anemia may not be seen for 1 to 2 years after surgery. Vitamin B_{12} levels are routinely monitored following extensive gastric resections.

Other nutritional problems seen following surgery include folic acid deficiency and decreased absorption of calcium and vitamin D. Poor absorption of nutrients, combined with the inability to eat large meals, puts the patient at risk for weight loss in addition to the more specific nutrient deficiencies. Nearly 50% of patients who have gastric surgery experience significant weight loss, primarily because of insufficient calorie intake. Factors contributing to insufficient intake of calories include early satiety (feeling of fullness), decreased stomach size, and altered emptying patterns.

Other Therapies

Combination chemotherapy administered before surgery and in combination with radiation therapy after surgery has been found to reduce tumor recurrence and prolong survival. For the patient with more advanced disease, treatment is palliative and may include surgery, radiation therapy, and chemotherapy. These patients may require a gastrostomy or jejunostomy feeding tube.

Because gastric cancer is generally advanced by the time of diagnosis, the prognosis is poor. The 5-year survival rate of all patients treated for gastric carcinoma is 10%.

Nursing Care

Assessment

Assessment data related to gastric cancer include:

- ***Health history:*** Manifestations such as anorexia, early satiety, indigestion, or vomiting; epigastric pain after meals; recent unintentional weight loss
- ***Physical assessment:*** General appearance, weight for height; abdominal distention or a palpable upper abdominal mass; occult blood in stool or vomitus.

Priorities of Care

Priorities of nursing care for the patient with gastric cancer focus on effects of the disease and its treatment on nutritional status and on the implications of a potentially fatal disease on the patient and family. See the accompanying Case Study & Nursing Care Plan.

Diagnoses, Outcomes, and Interventions

Promote Balanced Nutrition and Hydration. The patient with gastric cancer may be malnourished because of anorexia, early satiety, and increased metabolic needs related to the tumor. Extensive gastric resection also makes it difficult to consume an adequate diet. Malnourishment, in turn, impairs healing and the patient's ability to tolerate cancer treatment.

Expected Outcome: Patient will maintain adequate oral intake; report adequate energy levels; maintain body mass and weight and normal lab values (transferrin, albumin, and electrolytes); and will describe intake of a well-balanced diet and normal eating patterns.

The nurse will:

- Consult with dietitian for a complete nutrition assessment and diet planning. *The patient is at risk for protein-calorie malnutrition, which impairs the ability to heal and recover from extensive surgery.*
- Weigh daily. Monitor laboratory values such as hemoglobin, hematocrit, and serum albumin levels. *Daily weights are a valuable measurement of both fluid and nutritional status. Laboratory values provide further evidence of nutritional status.*
- Provide preferred foods; have family prepare meals when possible. Provide supplemental feedings between meals. *Frequent, small feedings and preferred foods encourage intake of nutrients.*
- Assess ability to consume adequate nutrients. *Nausea and feelings of early satiety may impair nutrient consumption, indicating a need to institute enteral or parenteral feedings.*
- Arrange for visitors to be present during meals. *Eating is a social function as well as a physiologic one. Companionship often improves food intake.*
- Administer pain and antiemetic medications as needed before meals. *Pain and nausea suppress the appetite; relief promotes food intake.*

Support the Grieving Patient and Family. Gastric cancer is a potentially fatal disease.

Expected Outcome: Patient and family will express thoughts, feelings, and spiritual beliefs about loss and progress through the stages of grief.

The nurse will:

- Encourage family members to spend as much time as possible with the patient. *The family may feel helpless and ineffectual. Supporting family members' presence can encourage this vital interaction.*
- Encourage acceptance if denial is present. *Denial is a coping mechanism that protects the patient from hopelessness.*
- Allow the patient to talk openly if desired about the condition and the prognosis. *Acceptance of the patient's fears helps reduce anxiety and promote coping behaviors.*
- Actively listen to the patient's and family's expressions of grieving. Avoid interrupting or offering meaningless words of consolation. *Being present and listening actively are often the most effective interventions for the grieving patient.*

Transitions of Care

Although the exact causes of gastric cancer are unknown, contributing factors such as *H. pylori* infection and consumption of foods preserved with nitrates have been identified. History of smoking is also a significant risk factor. To reduce their risk of developing gastric cancer, encourage patients with known *H. pylori* infection to complete the prescribed course of treatment and verify that it has eradicated the infection. With all patients, discuss the relationship between gastric cancer and consumption of foods preserved with nitrates (such as bacon and other processed meats) and encourage limited consumption of these products. Encourage patients to stop smoking and assist them with accessing smoking-cessation resources.

Acute care will involve perioperative care. See Chapter 4 for care of the patient undergoing surgery.

Although the patient with gastric cancer may be hospitalized for surgery, most care is provided in the home and community-based settings such as hospice care. When preparing the patient and family for home care, discuss the following topics:

- Care of incision and feeding tube (if present) or central venous line
- Maintaining nutrition and preventing complications of surgery such as dumping syndrome
- Pain management
- Referrals to home care agencies, hospice, and cancer support groups as appropriate
- Information about services available through the local chapter of the American Cancer Society.

Prognosis will be primarily determined by the presence of metastases at the time of diagnosis. Metastases to the liver indicate a poor prognosis. Developing a caring relation with the patient and family is a priority. Consultation with hospice services should be considered in collaboration with the patient, the patient's family, and the interprofessional healthcare team.

Case Study & Nursing Care Plan

A Patient with Gastric Cancer

George Harvey is a 61-year-old estate attorney who lives with his wife, Harriet. For the last 3 months, Mr. Harvey has had increasing anorexia and difficulty eating. He has lost 10 pounds. His physician has diagnosed gastric cancer, and Mr. Harvey is admitted for a partial gastrectomy and gastrojejunostomy. The oncologist has recommended postoperative chemotherapy and radiation. Mr. Harvey reports that the physician told him "that will give me the best chance for cure."

ASSESSMENT

On admission before surgery, Mr. Harvey tells his nurse, Lauren Walsh, that he has eaten very little in the past few weeks. He asks, "What will happen to my wife if something happens to me? I'm afraid this cancer will get me." Mr. Harvey weighs 67 kg (147 lb) and is 183 cm (72 in.) tall. He is pale and thin; his vital signs are BP 148/86 mmHg, P 92 bpm, R 18/min, and T 36.6°C (97.8°F) PO. A firm mass is palpable in the left epigastric region. The rest of his physical assessment data is within normal limits. Mr. Harvey's hemoglobin is 12.8 g/dL, hematocrit is 39%, and serum albumin level is 3.2 g/dL, indicating that he is mildly malnourished. All other preoperative laboratory and diagnostic studies are within normal limits.

DIAGNOSES

- Weight loss related to anorexia and difficulty eating
- Potential for pain related to surgery
- Potential for respiratory difficulties related to upper abdominal surgery
- Anxiety related to recent diagnosis of cancer

EXPECTED OUTCOMES

- Patient will maintain present weight during hospitalization.
- Patient will resume a high-calorie, high-protein diet by time of discharge.
- Patient will verbalize effective pain management, maintaining a reported pain level of 3 or less on a scale of 1 to 10.
- Patient will maintain a patent airway and clear breath sounds.
- Patient will verbalize feelings regarding diagnosis and participate in decision making.

PLANNING AND IMPLEMENTATION

- Weigh daily.
- Maintain nasogastric tube placement, patency, and suction as ordered.
- Maintain intravenous fluids and parenteral nutrition as ordered until oral food intake is resumed.
- Arrange for diet teaching, including strategies to prevent dumping syndrome, before discharge.
- Maintain patient-controlled analgesia until able to take oral analgesics.
- Assess respiratory status including rate, depth, and breath sounds every hour initially, then every 4 hours.
- Assist to cough, deep breathe, and use incentive spirometer every 2 to 4 hours and as needed. Splint abdomen during coughing.
- Encourage verbalization of feelings about diagnosis and perceived losses.
- Encourage participation in decision making.

EVALUATION

Mr. Harvey's weight remained stable through his hospitalization. On discharge he is taking a high-protein, high-calorie diet in six small feedings per day. He and his wife have reviewed his diet with the dietitian and are planning on using some dietary supplements at home to meet protein needs. He verbalizes an understanding of measures to prevent dumping syndrome, including separating his intake of solid foods and liquids. Mr. Harvey is using oral analgesics in the morning and at bedtime to control his pain. He and his wife have begun to discuss the meaning of his diagnosis. Mrs. Harvey tells the discharge nurse, "We are going to go to a support group called 'Coping with Cancer' when George is stronger."

CLINICAL REASONING IN PATIENT CARE

1. What is the rationale for maintaining nasogastric suction after gastrojejunostomy?
2. Develop a preoperative teaching plan for a patient undergoing a partial gastrectomy.
3. Mr. Harvey calls you just before the initial dose of chemotherapy and says, "Everyone tells me that chemotherapy will cause vomiting, and I don't think I can take being sick again." How would you respond?
4. Design interventions to ensure adequate nutrition for people with advanced gastric cancer.

See Evaluating Your Response in Appendix B.

CHAPTER HIGHLIGHTS

23.1 The Patient with Nausea and Vomiting

Describe the pathophysiology and manifestations of nausea and vomiting, and outline the interprofessional care and nursing care of patients with nausea and vomiting.

- Nausea and vomiting, common GI symptoms, may be indicative of disorders affecting many organ systems, including the GI tract, inner ear, CNS, or heart. Nausea and vomiting are also frequently related to medical interventions, such as drugs and cancer therapies. Complications such as dehydration, electrolyte imbalance, and aspiration of gastric contents are primary concerns when treating nausea and vomiting.

23.2 Disorders of the Mouth

Describe the pathophysiology and manifestations of disorders of the mouth, and outline the interprofessional care and nursing care of patients with these disorders.

- Stomatitis and oral mucositis are common disorders of the mouth, potentially having a significant effect on comfort and nutrition. In most cases, management is symptomatic and supportive, directed toward promoting comfort and maintaining nutritional status.
- Oral cancer is treatable when diagnosed in the early stages. Treatment can affect nutrition and body image. Management includes teaching the patient to alter diet to meet nutritional needs. Nursing interventions involve coordinating care and supporting the patient through the treatment phase.

23.3 Disorders of the Esophagus

Describe the pathophysiology and manifestations of disorders of the esophagus, and outline the interprofessional care and nursing care of patients with these disorders.

- GERD is common. While it is often considered to be a benign condition, prolonged exposure of the lower esophagus to gastric juices can lead to esophagitis, hemorrhage, and scarring. Treatment begins with pharmacologic agents for symptoms of gastric reflux.
- Hiatal hernia and impaired esophageal motility create discomfort and lead to compromised nutritional status.
- Both esophageal and gastric cancer are often diagnosed late in the disease because their symptoms may be vague. Cancers of the upper GI tract are serious and require multiple treatment and coordinated interprofessional care. Encourage patients with complaints of dysphagia, a sensation of gastric fullness, or heartburn to seek medical evaluation. Surgical resection of the cancerous portion of the esophagus or stomach is the treatment of choice when the tumor is diagnosed early.

23.4 Disorders of the Stomach and Duodenum

Describe the pathophysiology and manifestations of the stomach and duodenum, and outline the interprofessional care and nursing care of patients with these disorders.

- Upper gastrointestinal bleeding can lead to significant blood loss and shock. Peptic ulcer disease accounts for the majority of UGI hemorrhage, although erosive gastritis and esophageal varices are also common causes. Nursing care focuses on monitoring and promoting cardiovascular stability and preventing further hemorrhage.
- Peptic ulcer disease is chronic erosion, destruction, and ulceration in the lining of the stomach and duodenum. The primary etiologies for PUD are *H. pylori* infection and use of NSAIDs. Proton-pump inhibitors or H_2-receptor blockers are used to heal the damaged tissue. Antacids are used for symptom relief. Antibiotics are used to treat *H. pylori*.
- Acute gastritis, often associated with aspirin or NSAID use, is generally benign and self-limited. Erosive gastritis, a complication of critical conditions such as shock, trauma, a major burn, or head injury, can lead to unexpected gastric hemorrhage. Prophylactic therapy with proton-pump inhibitors or H_2-receptor blockers is important to prevent erosive gastritis in at-risk patients. Chronic gastritis is an unrelated disorder usually associated with *H. pylori* infection.
- *H. pylori* infection is also a major risk factor for peptic ulcer disease and gastric cancer. Effectively treating the infection can reduce or eliminate the risk of future exacerbations of PUD.
- An acute change in the nature of abdominal pain in a patient with PUD, especially when accompanied by vomiting, guarding of the abdomen, or a change in bowel sounds, could indicate an obstruction or perforation and release of gastric contents into the peritoneal cavity.

TEST YOURSELF NCLEX-RN® REVIEW

1. The nurse is assessing a patient with a persistent sore on the tongue. For which oral cancer risk factors should the nurse assess this patient? (Select all that apply.)
   A. Tobacco use in any form
   B. Drinking alcohol
   C. Consumption of highly spiced foods
   D. Thumbsucking or pacifier use as a child
   E. Infection with human papilloma virus
2. The nurse is preparing teaching for a patient with gastroesophageal reflux disease. What should this teaching include? (Select all that apply.)
   A. There is no treatment for this disease.
   B. Avoid lying down immediately after eating.
   C. Elevate the head of the bed on 6- to 8-inch blocks.
   D. Peppermint and chocolate candies can help relieve symptoms.
   E. Stop taking the prescribed proton-pump inhibitor once symptoms are relieved.
3. The nurse provides discharge teaching to a patient with acute gastritis. Which patient statement indicates that teaching has been effective? (Select all that apply.)
   A. "I will eat only bland foods."
   B. "I will have yearly upper endoscopy exams."
   C. "I will fully cook all meat, poultry, and egg products."
   D. "I will avoid using aspirin or NSAIDs for routine pain relief."
   E. "If I begin to vomit again, I will wait 24 hours before I eat or drink anything."
4. The nurse is identifying interventions appropriate for a patient with a possible perforation from peptic ulcer disease. Interventions to address which patient problem are apriority for this patient?
   A. Nausea
   B. Acute pain
   C. Risk for acute bleeding
   D. Inability to provide self-care
5. The nurse is concerned that a patient recovering from a partial gastrectomy for stomach cancer is at risk for nutritional deficiencies. For which nutritional deficiencies should the nurse focus care? (Select all that apply.)
   A. Red blood cells
   B. Calcium
   C. Folic acid
   D. Vitamin C
   E. Vitamin B_{12}
6. The nurse is caring for a patient receiving radiation therapy for esophageal cancer. Which manifestation should the nurse immediately report to the healthcare provider?
   A. Weight loss
   B. Bright bleeding from the mouth
   C. Difficulty swallowing solid foods
   D. Crackles in the base of the right lung
7. A patient is prescribed omeprazole 20 mg twice daily, clarithromycin 500 mg twice daily, and amoxicillin 1 g daily for treatment of peptic ulcer disease caused by *H. pylori*. What is the most important instruction for the nurse to give the patient about these medications?
   A. Take the drugs with a full glass of water.
   B. Complete the full course of all medications as prescribed.
   C. Consume 8 oz of yogurt or buttermilk daily while taking these drugs.
   D. Take the drugs on an empty stomach, 1 hour before breakfast and at least 2 hours after dinner.
8. A patient receiving chemotherapy is experiencing stomatitis. Which intervention should be a priority for this patient?
   A. Refer the patient to a smoking-cessation program.
   B. Allow patient to select appealing foods from a menu.
   C. Assist patient to cleanse mouth with mouthwash following meals.
   D. Provide viscous lidocaine to relieve mouth pain before meals.
9. The evening following surgery for esophageal cancer, the nurse notes that there has been no drainage from the nasogastric tube for the past 3 hours. What should the nurse do first?
   A. Chart the finding.
   B. Notify the surgeon.
   C. Reposition the nasogastric tube.
   D. Gently irrigate the tube with normal saline.
10. A patient with a history of peptic ulcer disease suddenly begins to complain of severe abdominal pain. Which actions should the nurse take at this time? (Select all that apply.)
    A. Notify the physician.
    B. Withhold oral food and fluids.
    C. Place the patient in Fowler position.
    D. Obtain an order for a narcotic analgesic.
    E. Administer the prescribed proton-pump inhibitor.

See Test Yourself answers in Appendix B.

REFERENCES

Adams, M. P., Holland, L. N., & Urban, C. Q. (2017). *Pharmacology for nurses: A pathophysiologic approach* (5th ed.). New York, NY: Pearson.

Arslan, M., & Ozdemir, L. (2015). Oral intake of ginger for chemotherapy-induced nausea and vomiting among women with breast cancer. *Clinical Journal of Oncology Nursing, 19*(5), E92–E97.

American Cancer Society. (2018). *Cancer facts and figures 2018*. Atlanta, GA: Author.

American Stroke Association. (2013). *Difficulty swallowing after stroke (dysphagia)*. Retrieved from www.strokeassociation.org/STROKEORG/LifeAfterStroke/RegainingIndependence/CommunicationChallenges/Difficulty-Swallowing-After-Stroke-Dysphagia_UCM_310084_Article.jsp#.WsVCDi7waUk.

Borrett, K. (2018). Interventions for dysphagia in esophageal cancer. *Gastroenterology Nursing, 41*(1), 73–75.

Caple, C., & Mennella, H. (2016). *Oral care of the hospitalized patient*. Glendale, CA: Cinahl Information Systems, Division of EBSCO Information Systems.

Coke, L., Otten, K., Staffileno, B., Minarich, L., & Nowiszewski, C. (2015). The impact of an oral hygiene education module on patient practices and nursing documentation. *Clinical Journal of Oncology Nursing 19*(1), 75–79.

Critchlow, D. (2016). Diagnosis of oral diseases in the housebound patient. *British Journal of Community Nursing, 21*(12), 623–627.

Critchlow, D. (2017). Part 3: Impact of systemic conditions and medications on oral health. *British Journal of Community Nursing, 22*(4), 181–190.

Del Valle, J. (2017). Peptic ulcer disease and related disorders. In D. Kasper, A. Fauci, S. Hauser, D. Longo, J. Jameson, & J. Loscalzo (Eds.), *Harrison's principles of internal medicine, 348* (19th ed.). Retrieved from http://accessmedicine.mhmedical.com.liboff.ohsu.edu/content.aspx?bookid=1130&sectionid=79747602. New York, NY: McGraw-Hill.

Durso, S. C., & Yellowitz, J. (2017). Atlas of oral manifestations of disease. In D. Kasper, A. Fauci, S. Hauser, D. Longo, J. Jameson, & J. Loscalzo (Eds.), *Harrison's principles of internal medicine, Atlas 46e* (19th ed.). Retrieved from https://accessmedicine.mhmedical.com/content.aspx?bookid=1130&sectionid=66487517&jumpsectionID=98705281. New York, NY: McGraw-Hill.

Faust, A. C., Echevarria, K., Attridge, R., Sheperd, L., & Restrepo, M. (2017). Prophylactic acid-suppressive therapy in hospitalized adults: Indications, benefits, and infectious complications. *Critical Care Nurse, 37*(3), 18–28.

Hasler. W. L. (2015). Nausea, vomiting and indigestion. In D. Kasper, A. Fauci, S. Hauser, D. Longo, J. Jameson, & J. Loscalzo (Eds.), *Harrison's principles of internal medicine, 54* (19th ed.). New York, NY: McGraw-Hill.

Kahrilas, P. J., & Hirano, I. (2017). Diseases of the esophagus. In D. Kasper, A. Fauci, S. Hauser, D. Longo, J. Jameson, & J. Loscalzo (Eds.), *Harrison's principles of internal medicine, 347* (19th ed.). New York, NY: McGraw-Hill.

Kee, J. L. (2018). *Handbook of laboratory and diagnostic tests with nursing implications* (10th ed.). New York, NY: Pearson.

Matsuo, K., Watanabe, R., Kanamori, D., Nakagawa, K., Fujii, W., Urasaki, Y., . . . Higashiguchi, T. (2016). Associations between oral complications and days to death in palliative care patients. *Support Care Cancer, 24*, 157–164.

Maurice, E. (2015). Timely patient discharge from the ambulatory surgical setting. *AORN Journal, 102*(2), 185–187.

Mayer, R., J. (2017). Upper gastrointestinal tract cancers. In D. Kasper, A. Fauci, S. Hauser, D. Longo, J. Jameson, & J. Loscalzo (Eds.), *Harrison's principles of internal medicine* (19th ed.). New York, NY: McGraw-Hill.

McDevitt, D., & Mason, A., (2018). Treating Barrett esophagus with radiofrequency ablation. *Nursing 2018, 49*(1), 26–32.

National Cancer Institute. (2018a). *Lip and oral cavity cancer treatment (PDQ®)* (Health professional version). Retrieved from www.cancer.gov/cancertopics/pdq/treatment/lip-and-oral-cavity/HealthProfessional.

National Cancer Institute. (2018b). *Oral cancer prevention (PDQ®)* (Health professional version). Retrieved from www.cancer.gov/cancertopics/pdq/prevention/oral/HealthProfessional/page1/AllPages.

Pilgrim, J., & Parks-Chapman, J. (2018). Gastroesophageal reflux disease. Glendale, CA: Cinahl Information Systems, Division of EBSCO Information Systems.

Schub, T., & Heering., H. (2017). Stomatitis (oral mucositis). Glendale, CA: Cinahl Information Systems, Division of EBSCO Information Systems.

Schub T., & Holle, M. (2018). *Chemotherapy-related nausea and vomiting*. Glendale, CA: Cinahl Information Systems.

Sorenson, M., Quinn, L., & Klein, D. (2019). *Pathophysiology: Concepts of human disease*. Hoboken, NJ: Pearson Education.

Vidall, C., Sharma, S., & Amlani, B. (2016). Patient–practitioner perception gap in treatment-induced nausea and vomiting. *British Journal of Nursing, 25*(16), S4–S11.

Welliver, M. (2016). Cannabinoid agonists for nausea and vomiting. *Gastroenterology Nursing*, 39(2), 137–139.

ADDITIONAL RESOURCES

Society of Gastroenterology Nurses and Associates
http://www.sgna.org

American College of Gastroenterology (ACG)
http://patients.gi.org

Chapter 24

Nursing Care of Patients with Bowel Disorders

Chapter Outline and Learning Outcomes

CLINICAL COMPETENCIES

- Assess the functional status of patients with bowel disorders, and recognize, document, and report unexpected or abnormal findings.
- Use assessment data to determine priority nursing diagnoses, identify and implement patient-centered evidence-based nursing interventions, and revise the plan of care for patients with bowel disorders.
- Integrate interprofessional care and administer medications knowledgeably and safely for patients with bowel disorders.
- Provide skilled care to patients having bowel surgery, an ostomy, or perianal surgery.
- Provide culturally appropriate teaching to promote nutrition, encourage screening, and prevention interventions for acute and chronic bowel disorders.
- Plan and provide patient and family-centered care to facilitate transitions between care settings.
- Promote continuity of care by providing patient and family teaching aimed to promote, maintain, and restore health.

KEY TERMS

appendicitis, 749
borborygmi, 739
celiac disease, 780
colectomy, 771
colorectal cancer, 786
colostomy, 788
constipation, 740
diarrhea, 736
diverticulitis, 778
diverticulosis, 776
fecal incontinence, 747
gastroenteritis, 757
hematochezia, 772
hemorrhoid, 801
hernia, 794
ileostomy, 771
inflammatory bowel disease (IBD), 764
intestinal obstruction, 797
irritable bowel syndrome (IBS), 745
lactase deficiency, 783
malabsorption, 780
paralytic ileus, 754
peritonitis, 752
polyps, 785
short bowel syndrome, 784
steatorrhea, 739
stoma, 771

Few body functions respond as readily to internal and external influences as the process of defecation. Factors affecting the gastrointestinal (GI) tract directly, such as food intake and bacterial population, affect the number and consistency of stools. Indirect factors, such as psychologic stress or voluntary postponement of defecation, also affect elimination.

In modern society, normal bowel elimination patterns vary widely. For some patients, two to three stools per day is the usual pattern. Others may normally have as few as three stools per week. It is important to evaluate each patient's bowel elimination against his or her own normal pattern.

Food and fluids enter the small intestine, which forms the middle portion of the digestive tract and consists of three subdivisions—the duodenum, jejunum, and ilium. The length of the small intestine is nearly 10 feet long. Food is digested and absorbed as it travels through the small intestine to the large intestine. The large intestine forms the lower GI tract and is approximately 4.5 to 5 feet long. The lower GI tract is divided into the cecum, colon, rectum, and anal canal. The appendix arises from the cecum approximately 1.5 cm from the ileocecal valve, which prevents the return of feces from the cecum to the small intestine. The colon is divided into the ascending, transverse, descending, and sigmoid portions. The descending colon extends from the colic flexure to the rectum. The rectum extends from the sigmoid colon to the anus.

24.1 Disorders of Intestinal Motility

The Patient with Diarrhea

Diarrhea is an increase in the frequency, volume, and fluid content of a stool. In diarrhea, the water content of feces is increased, usually due to either malabsorption or water secretion in the bowel. It is a manifestation rather than a primary disorder.

Diarrhea may be acute or chronic. Acute diarrhea, which lasts less than a week, is usually due to an infectious agent. Chronic diarrhea (diarrhea that persists longer than 3 to 4 weeks) may be caused by inflammatory bowel disorders, malabsorption, or endocrine disorders.

Pathophysiology

About 1500 mL of digested material enters the large intestine daily. Normally, most of the water and some of the solutes are reabsorbed in the bowel, leaving only about 200 mL of feces to be eliminated.

Large-volume diarrhea, characterized by both increased numbers and volume of stools, is caused by increased water content of the stool. This increased water content may result from either osmotic or secretory processes. Water may be pulled into the bowel lumen by osmosis when the feces contain osmotically active molecules. Some stool softeners and laxatives work on this principle. When the lactose in milk is not broken down and absorbed, the lactose molecules exert an osmotic pull, causing diarrhea. The diarrhea associated with cholera and *Escherichia coli* infection is caused by increased water secretion in the small and large intestines. Unabsorbed dietary fat, some cathartics and other drugs, and other factors can cause secretory diarrhea.

Small-volume diarrhea, characterized by frequent small stools, is usually caused by inflammation or disease of the colon. Diseases that affect the intestinal mucosa, such as inflammatory bowel disease, cause an exudative diarrhea. The mucosal inflammation causes plasma, serum proteins, blood, and mucus to accumulate in the bowel, increasing fecal bulk and fluidity. An increased rate of propulsion within the bowel can also decrease the amount of water normally absorbed from the chyme, leading to diarrhea. For this reason, laxatives that increase bowel motility and bowel resection or bypass can lead to diarrhea.

Antibiotic-associated diarrhea may occur as a result of disruption of normal intestinal flora by antibiotic therapy. Loss of normal flora can affect food digestion, leading to diarrhea, or can allow overgrowth of pathogens such as *Clostridium difficile* (see the section on gastroenteritis for more information about *C. difficile*).

Manifestations

The manifestations of diarrhea depend on its cause, duration, and severity, as well as the area of bowel affected and the patient's general health. Diarrhea can present as several large, watery stools daily or very frequent, small stools that contain blood, mucus, or exudate.

Complications

Diarrhea can have devastating effects. Water and electrolytes are lost in diarrheal stool. This can lead to dehydration, particularly in the very young, the older adult, or the debilitated patient unable to respond to thirst. With severe diarrhea, vascular collapse and hypovolemic shock may occur. Potassium and magnesium are lost, potentially leading to hypokalemia and hypomagnesemia. The loss of bicarbonate in the stool can lead to metabolic acidosis. See Chapter 10 for further discussion of the effects of these imbalances.

SAFETY ALERT: Monitor orthostatic vital signs, skin turgor, serum electrolytes and osmolality, and urinalysis to identify and respond to possible adverse effects of diarrhea. ■

Interprofessional Care

Management of diarrhea focuses on identifying and treating the underlying cause. In addition, the diarrhea itself may need to be treated to promote comfort and to prevent complications. The history (including the onset and associated circumstances of the diarrhea) and physical examination often provide enough information to identify its cause.

Diagnosis

Diagnostic tests that may be ordered to help identify the cause of diarrhea include a stool specimen analysis and culture. A sigmoidoscopy may be conducted to directly visualize the bowel mucosa. (See Chapter 21 for further information on diagnostic tests.) Tissue biopsy may be performed to identify chronic inflammatory processes, infection, and other causes of diarrhea. In addition, laboratory tests of serum electrolytes, serum osmolality, and arterial blood gases (ABGs) may be ordered to assess for adverse effects of diarrhea. Increased serum osmolality indicates water loss and dehydration.

Medications

Antidiarrheal medications are used sparingly or not at all until the cause of diarrhea has been identified. In diarrhea associated with botulism or bacillary dysentery, giving an antidiarrheal agent can worsen or prolong the disease by slowing elimination of the toxin from the bowel. Once the underlying cause for diarrhea has been established, specific medications may be ordered to treat the cause. Antibiotics are used with caution because they alter the normal bacterial population of the bowel and may actually worsen diarrhea. A balanced electrolyte solution may be required to replace fluid losses. Intravenous or oral potassium preparations may be prescribed.

Opium and some of its derivatives, anticholinergics, absorbents, and demulcents are commonly used as antidiarrheal preparations. Specific preparations, their method of action, and the nursing implications for these medications are outlined in **Medication Administration 24.A**.

Medication Administration 24.A

Antidiarrheal Preparations

OPIOIDS

camphorated opium tincture (Paregoric)
cifenoxin with atropine (Motofen)
ciphenoxylate with atropine (Lomotil)
loperamide (Imodium)

Opium and its derivatives act on the central nervous system (CNS) to decrease the motility of the ileum and colon, slowing transit time and promoting more water absorption. They also decrease the sensation of a full rectum and increase anal sphincter tone. Paregoric and tincture of opium have a greater potential for abuse and are prescription drugs subject to controls under the federal Controlled Substances Act of 1970. Difenoxin, diphenoxylate, and loperamide are derivatives of opium with few analgesic, euphoric, or abuse-promoting effects and are in more common use today.

Nursing Responsibilities

- Assess for contraindications to antidiarrheal or narcotic medications prior to giving these drugs.
- Administer paregoric undiluted with water.
- Do not administer difenoxin and diphenoxylate to patients receiving monoamine oxidase inhibitors (MAOIs); hypertensive crises may occur.
- Observe closely for increased effects of other CNS depressants, such as alcohol, narcotic analgesics, or barbiturate sedatives.
- Observe for abdominal distention; toxic megacolon may occur if these drugs are given to the patient with ulcerative colitis.

Health Education for the Patient and Family

- Take the medication as recommended at the onset of diarrhea and after each loose stool.
- These drugs may be habit forming; use for no more than 48 hours.
- Avoid using alcohol and OTC cold preparations while taking these drugs.
- These preparations may cause drowsiness; avoid driving or operating machinery while taking them.

MISCELLANEOUS DRUGS

bismuth salts (Pepto-Bismol)
lactobacillus acidophilus
octreotide (Sandostatin)

Nursing Responsibilities

- Bismuth subsalicylate, available without a prescription, has antisecretory, anti-inflammatory, and antibacterial effects. It is widely used to control traveler's diarrhea. Although it is generally safe at recommended doses, bismuth subsalicylate has potential toxic effects and interacts with drugs such as aspirin and oral anticoagulants.
- Assess for contraindications to antidiarrheal therapy, such as some infections or chronic inflammatory bowel disease, including ulcerative colitis.
- Administer as ordered.
- Do not administer within 1 hour of other drugs because it may interfere with their absorption.
- Monitor for increased anticoagulant effect when given with warfarin (Coumadin) or aspirin.
- If fever is present, check with physician before giving the medication.
- Administer these medications at least 1 hour before or 2 hours after other oral medications; they may interfere with the absorption of other drugs.
- Observe the patient's response to the medication. Constipation is a potential problem.

Health Education for the Patient and Family

- Take the recommended dosage at the onset of diarrhea and after each loose stool.
- Do not take any of these preparations for more than 48 hours. If diarrhea persists, notify the physician.
- Do not give antidiarrheal medications to debilitated older patients without physician supervision.
- Chew bismuth subsalicylate tablets, rather than swallowing them whole, for maximal effectiveness.
- This drug may cause harmless darkening of your tongue and stools.
- If you are allergic to aspirin, use bismuth subsalicylate with caution. Do not use aspirin while you are taking this drug unless directed to do so by your physician. Contact your physician if diarrhea persists for more than 2 days.

Source: Data from Adams, Holland, & Urban, 2017.

Nutrition

Fluid replacement is of primary importance in managing the patient with diarrhea. If the patient is able to tolerate oral fluids (i.e., if the patient is not experiencing nausea and vomiting), an oral glucose/balanced electrolyte solution provides the best fluid replacement. Commercial preparations such as Gatorade and other sports drinks are available, as are pediatric solutions (e.g., Pedialyte), which can be used for adults as well as children. Oral rehydration mixtures may be made at home. Several recipes are available; one example is mixing 1 teaspoon of salt and 8 teaspoons of sugar into 1 liter of water, along with 4 ounces of orange juice. Another common solution of 5 mL (1 teaspoon) each of table salt and baking soda and 20 mL (4 teaspoons) of granulated sugar added with desired flavoring (such as lemon extract or juice) to 1 L (1 quart) of water can be made at home to replace water and electrolytes.

Solid food is withheld in the first 24 hours of acute diarrhea to rest the bowel. After that time, frequent, small, soft feedings can be added. The BRAT diet (bananas, rice, applesauce, and toast) is frequently recommended as a good start to beginning solid foods. Milk and milk products are added last because the lactose they contain frequently aggravates diarrhea. Raw fruits and vegetables, fried foods, bran, whole-grain cereals, condiments, spices, coffee, and alcoholic beverages are avoided during the recovery period.

Patients with chronic diarrhea may benefit by eliminating specific foods from the diet. Foods and nonfood substances that may aggravate diarrhea are outlined in **Table 24.1**. The diet should be high in calories and nutritional value. Vitamin supplements may be necessary, particularly the fat-soluble vitamins (A, D, E, and K). Patients with severe chronic diarrhea may require parenteral nutrition(see Chapter 22).

Integrative Therapies

Herbal or homeopathic therapies may be used to help relieve diarrhea. Patients who are lactose intolerant may use lactase enzyme tablets or drops when consuming milk products. Herbal treatments may include a strong tea of peppermint, chamomile, coriander, rosemary, sandalwood, or thyme. Ginger in the form of tea or capsules can be helpful in reducing intestinal inflammation and lessening the effects of food poisoning. Homeopathic practitioners may use podophyllum tablets to treat diarrhea. Probiotics, live microorganisms similar to those normally found in the gut, may be used to prevent or treat antibiotic-associated diarrhea (National Center for Complementary and Integrative Health, 2012). Probiotics are available as dietary supplements and foods (e.g., yogurt, yogurt drinks). Refer the patient to a qualified practitioner for more information about using complementary and integrative therapies to treat diarrhea.

Fecal Microbiota Transplant

Fecal bacteriotherapy treatment is gaining acceptance for patients who experience chronic diarrhea related to various etiologies (e.g., *Clostridium difficile* infection [CDI], irritable bowel syndrome). Fecal microbiota transplant is a process that restores the colon's homeostasis by instilling normal bacterial flora from a healthy person (donor) into the GI tract of the affected patient and is becoming more common for treatment of recurrent *Clostridium difficile* infection (Kelly et al., 2015; Walton, Burns, & Gaehle, 2017). The donor screening process usually begins with the patient's spouse/significant other or a household family member. Potential donors are screened for overall health, exposure to infectious disease, recent receipt of systemic antibiotics, CDI, ova, parasites, and enteric bacterial pathogens.

Once the donor has been selected and sufficiently screened, the instillation process can begin. The donor stool is broken down into a liquid suspension. Most patients receive their fecal bacteriotherapy through a retention enema or colonoscopy in an outpatient setting. The recipient of the fecal transplant is pretreated with oral antibiotics (vancomycin) for several days. Fecal bacteriotherapy is considered safe and effective, with a success rate of treating CDI of 81 to 100%. This treatment is considered cost effective, breaks the cycle of repeated antibiotic use, prevents the emergence of antibiotic-resistant strains of bacteria, avoids the risk of allergic reactions, and is considered a low-risk procedure (Kelly et al., 2015).

Nursing Care

Diarrhea is a common problem that may complicate patient care.

Table 24.1 Foods That May Aggravate Chronic Diarrhea

Foods	Reason
Milk, ice cream, yogurt, soft cheeses, cottage cheese	Contain lactose; not tolerated by patients with lactase deficiency who cannot digest lactose.
Apple juice, pear juice, grapes, honey, dates, nuts, figs, fruit-flavored soft drinks	Contain fructose; when consumed in large quantities, fructose may not be totally absorbed, causing an osmotic pull of fluid into the bowel.
Table sugar	Contains sucrose; not tolerated by patients with sucrase deficiency.
Apple juice, pear juice, sugarless gums, and mints	May contain sorbitol or mannitol, sugars that are not absorbed and can cause osmotic draw.
Antacids	Magnesium-containing antacids decrease bowel transit time and contain poorly absorbed salts that can exert an osmotic draw.
Coffee, tea, cola drinks, over-the-counter (OTC) analgesics	Contain caffeine, which can increase bowel transit time.

Assessment

The nursing assessment can help identify the cause of a patient's diarrhea, as well as early signs of complications. Collect the following assessment data:

- ***Health history:*** Duration and extent of diarrhea; associated manifestations; dietary intake; recent travel out of the country or to wilderness areas; previous history of diarrhea; chronic diseases; prescription and nonprescription medications
- ***Physical assessment:*** Vital signs (including orthostatic blood pressure); peripheral pulses; skin temperature, moisture, turgor; color and moisture of mucous membranes; abdominal contour and girth; bowel sounds; stool for obvious or occult blood, pus, mucus, or **steatorrhea** (bulky, foul-smelling stool containing fat/grease).

Priorities of Care

The primary priority of care is ensuring that the patient is monitoring and maintaining fluid and electrolyte balance. Managing nutritional intake is a key component of care for patients experiencing chronic diarrhea.

Diagnoses, Outcomes, and Interventions

Nursing care of the patient with diarrhea focuses on identifying the cause, relieving the manifestations, preventing complications, and preventing the potential spread of infection to others.

Control Diarrhea. Nursing interventions for diarrhea are provided to help the patient recover a normal elimination pattern without adverse consequences.

Expected Outcome: Patient's diarrhea will be controlled or eliminated as demonstrated by resumption of normal bowel elimination patterns.

The nurse will:

- Monitor and record the frequency and characteristics of bowel movements. *This provides a measure of the effectiveness of treatment.*
- Establish and document patient's normal bowel elimination pattern. *Individual bowel elimination patterns vary widely. Establishing the patient's baseline pattern is necessary to measure progress toward meeting desired outcome.*
- Measure abdominal girth and auscultate bowel sounds every 8 hours as indicated. Loud, rushing bowel sounds (**borborygmi**) indicate increased peristalsis and may be heard in patients with acute diarrhea. *Diminished or absent bowel sounds may indicate a complication of treatment, such as constipation or toxic megacolon.*
- Use standard precautions and contact precautions as needed, including gloves and hand hygiene. *Standard precautions help prevent the spread of infection to others. Contact precautions in the acute and long-term care environments are recommended to prevent the spread of infectious diarrhea* (Berman, Snyder, & Frandsen, 2016).
- Provide ready access to bathroom, commode, or bedpan. *The patient may have little warning of the need to defecate. Easily accessed toileting facilities reduce the risk for soiling or injury.*
- Administer antidiarrheal medications as prescribed. *This promotes comfort and prevents excess fluid loss.*
- Limit food intake if the diarrhea is acute, reintroducing solid foods slowly and in small amounts. *This allows the bowel to rest and mucosa to heal in acute diarrhea states.*

Promote Balanced Fluid and Electrolyte Status. The increased water content of diarrheal stool places the patient at risk for fluid deficit.

Expected Outcome: Deficient fluid volume in the patient will be prevented as evidenced by normal vital signs, lab values, and absence of physical signs of dehydration (e.g., thirst, change in mental status, decreased urine output, dry skin and mucous membrane, weakness, sudden weight loss).

The nurse will:

- Record intake and output; weigh daily; assess skin turgor, mucous membranes, and urine specific gravity every 8 hours. *These assessments are used to monitor fluid volume.*
- Assess skin turgor over the sternum in the older adult. Loss of subcutaneous fat associated with aging makes skin turgor assessment on the arms or hands less reliable.
- Monitor vital signs, including orthostatic blood pressures (BP). *Orthostatic hypotension is identified by a drop in BP of more than 10 mmHg and pulse increase of 10 bpm when changing from a lying to a sitting position or from a sitting to a standing position. It is an indicator of fluid volume deficit.*
- Institute safety precautions such as providing assistance when ambulating the patient with orthostatic hypotension. *The fall in blood pressure with position changes can cause light-headedness and syncope.*
- Provide fluid and electrolyte replacement solutions as indicated. Ensure ready access to fluids; assist the debilitated patient with fluid intake. Notify the care provider if the patient is unable to tolerate oral fluids. *Oral fluids are encouraged as tolerated to prevent dehydration. Intravenous fluids are necessary if oral fluids are not tolerated. An intake of 3000 mL/day or more is often needed to replace fluid losses.*

Prevent Injury to Skin Integrity. Decreased extracellular fluid volume and the irritating effects of diarrheal stool increase the risk for skin breakdown.

Expected Outcome: Patient's skin will remain intact and will not show redness or excoriation.

The nurse will:

- Assist with cleaning the perianal area as needed. Use warm water, a gentle cleanser, and soft cloths. *Cleansing removes irritating substances in the stool. Gentle cleansing helps maintain the integrity of dehydrated skin.*
- Apply protective ointment to the perianal area. *Moisture-barrier ointments or creams protect the skin from excoriation and help prevent tissue breakdown.*

Transitions of Care

Teach all patients about the importance of proper hand hygiene as a measure to prevent the spread of infectious diseases, including those that cause diarrhea. Teach safe food-handling techniques to prevent bacterial contamination, and discuss measures to ensure safe drinking water. For patients planning to travel outside the United States or to wilderness areas, teach measures to purify water for drinking and cooking.

Acute and chronic diarrhea are generally managed by the patient in the home. Teach the patient and family members about the following subjects:

- Causes of diarrhea (as directed by the diagnosis)
- Importance of hand hygiene and other hygiene measures
- Importance of maintaining adequate fluid intake to replace lost water and electrolytes
- Use of a balanced electrolyte solution such as Gatorade or a similar product (purchased or home prepared) for fluid replacement
- Recommendations to limit food intake during acute diarrhea, and resume gradually with small feedings of foods that have a constipating effect: Applesauce, bananas, crackers, rice, potatoes
- To avoid foods high in fiber, milk products, and caffeine
- Ways to maintain nutrition if chronic diarrhea is a problem: Frequent, small meals; nutritional supplements; vitamin supplements
- Precautions and limitations of antidiarrheal preparations
- Importance of seeking medical intervention if diarrhea continues or recurs.

Patients often lose their thirst mechanism at the end of life and may be unable to swallow or will refuse oral fluids. The nurse should explain to the family that this is a normal response to the dying process and reassure caregivers the patient is not experiencing the untoward effects of dehydration.

The Patient with Constipation

There is not universal agreement on the definition of constipation (Holroyd, 2015) and is typically described as the infrequent passage of hard, dry stool (Sorenson, Quinn, & Klein, 2019). Chronic **constipation** is defined as including two of the following symptoms for at least 12 weeks in the past 12 months: Fewer than three bowel movements (BMs) per week, straining, hard stools, incomplete evacuation, or manual evacuation required for 25% of BMs (Holroyd, 2015). Constipation affects older adults more frequently than younger people and occurs 2.5 times more frequently in women than in men. Although fecal transit in the large intestine slows with aging, the increased incidence of constipation is thought to relate more to impaired general health status, increased medication use, and decreased physical activity in the older adult.

Pathophysiology

Constipation may be a primary problem or a manifestation secondary to another disease or condition. Acute constipation, a definite change in the bowel elimination pattern, is often caused by an organic process. A change in bowel patterns that persists or becomes more frequent or severe may be due to a tumor or other partial bowel obstruction. With chronic constipation, functional causes that impair storage, transport, and evacuation mechanisms impede the normal passage of stools. Common causes of constipation are listed in **Table 24.2**.

Psychogenic factors are frequently associated with causes of chronic constipation. These factors include postponing defecation when the urge is felt, and the perception of satisfaction with defecation. Patients often use laxatives and enemas to stimulate a bowel movement when constipation is perceived. Overuse of these measures can lead to real intestinal problems that worsen the condition. For example, *cathartic colon* (impaired colonic motility and changes in bowel structure) mimics ulcerative colitis in that the normal pouchlike or saccular appearance of the colon is lost. *Melanosis coli* is a brownish-black discoloration of the colon mucosa. Both conditions may be caused by long-term laxative use.

Manifestations and Complications

The manifestations of constipation include having bowel movements less often than the usual pattern, frequent flatus, abdominal discomfort, anorexia, straining to have a bowel movement, and the passage of hard, dry stools.

With significant constipation or long-term dependence on laxatives or enemas, fecal impaction may develop.

Table 24.2 Selected Causes of Constipation

Factor	Related Cause
Activity	Lack of exercise; bedrest
Dietary	Highly refined, low-fiber foods; inadequate fluid intake
Drugs	Antacids containing aluminum or calcium salts; narcotic analgesics; anticholinergics; many antidepressants, tranquilizers, and sedatives; antihypertensives, such as ganglionic blockers, calcium-channel blockers, beta-adrenergic blockers, and diuretics; iron salts
Large bowel	Diverticular disease, inflammatory disease, tumor, obstruction; changes in rectal or anal structure or function
Psychogenic	Voluntary suppression of urge; perceived need to defecate on schedule; depression
Systemic	Advanced age; pregnancy; neurologic conditions (trauma, multiple sclerosis, tumors, cerebrovascular accident, parkinsonism); endocrine and metabolic disorders (hypothyroidism, hypercalcemia, uremia, porphyria)
Other	Chronic laxative or enema use

Impaction may also occur following barium administration for radiologic exam. The impaction is felt as a rock-hard or putty-like mass of feces in the rectum. Abdominal cramping and a full sensation in the rectal area may be manifestations of impaction. Watery mucus or foul-smelling liquid stool may be passed around the impaction, causing the patient to complain of diarrhea.

Interprofessional Care

Initial evaluation of constipation is based on the history and physical examination. The abdomen may appear somewhat distended, and bowel sounds may be reduced. If an impaction is present, digital examination of the rectum reveals a palpable, hard, or putty-like fecal mass.

Simple or chronic constipation is treated with education (a daily bowel movement is not necessary for health) and modification of diet and exercise routines. If the problem is acute or does not resolve, further diagnostic examination may be ordered.

Diagnosis

A barium enema may be ordered to identify bowel structure, tumors, or diverticula. If the problem is acute, a sigmoidoscopy or colonoscopy may be used for evaluation and biopsy. Computed tomography colonography (CTC) may be ordered instead of barium enema. CTC may be preferred because of the increased sensitivity to detection of polyps and cancer. (See Chapter 21 for nursing implications of these tests.)

Medications

Laxative and cathartic preparations are used to promote stool evacuation. Milder preparations are generally known as laxatives; cathartics have a stronger effect. Most laxatives are appropriate only for short-term use. Cathartics and enemas interfere with normal bowel reflexes and should not be used for simple constipation. Laxatives should not be given if a patient has an undiagnosed intestinal obstruction, abdominal pain, fecal impaction, rectal fissures, ulcerated hemorrhoids, Crohn disease, ulcerative colitis, or chronic inflammatory bowel disease. When the bowel is obstructed, laxatives or cathartics may cause serious mechanical damage and perforate the bowel.

The only laxatives that are appropriate and safe for long-term use are bulking agents, such as psyllium seed, calcium polycarbophil, and methylcellulose. These agents act by increasing the bulk of the feces and drawing water into the bowel to soften it. Commonly prescribed laxatives and cathartics are discussed in **Medication Administration 24.B**.

Medication Administration 24.B

Laxatives and Cathartics

BULK-FORMING AGENTS

calcium polycarbophil (Fibercon, others)

methylcellulose (Citrucel)

psyllium (Metamucil, others)

Bulk-forming agents contain vegetable fiber, which is not digested or absorbed in the gut. This natural fiber creates bulk and draws water into the intestine, softening the stool mass.

Nursing Responsibilities

- Mix the agent with a full glass of cool liquid just prior to administering.
- Do not administer to patients with possible stool impaction or bowel obstruction.

Health Education for the Patient and Family

- Drink at least six to eight full glasses of nonalcoholic fluid per day. Adequate hydration is necessary to produce the medication's laxative effect.
- These agents may be mixed with water, milk, or fruit juice.
- Take the drug in the morning or with meals. To reduce the risk of impaction, do not take at bedtime.
- Because of the increased risk of impaction, check with the physician before increasing dietary fiber while you are taking these agents.

STOOL SOFTENER/SURFACTANT

docusate (Colace, Surfak, Doxidan, others)

Wetting agents reduce stool surface tension and form an emulsion of fat and water, softening the stool. They are used primarily to prevent straining and reduce the discomfort of expelling hard stools.

Nursing Responsibilities

- Administer with ample fluids to promote softening effect.
- Wetting agents may alter the absorption of other drugs. Do not administer within 1 hour of other oral medications.
- Do not attempt to crush or open caplets; a liquid form is available for patients who cannot swallow pills or capsules.

Health Education for the Patient and Family

- Do not use for more than 1 week unless specifically recommended by the physician.
- Take the medication in the morning or evening, but avoid taking it with other medications.
- Adequate fluid is necessary to obtain the beneficial effect of the drug. Drink six to eight glasses of nonalcoholic fluid per day.

SALINE AND OSMOTIC

lactulose (Chronulac)

magnesium hydroxide (Milk of Magnesia)

polyethylene glycol (Miralax)

sodium biphosphate (Fleet Phospho-Soda)

Laxatives in this group contain poorly absorbed salts or carbohydrates that remain in the bowel, increasing osmotic pressure and drawing water into the intestine. Stool volume increases, consistency decreases, and peristalsis is stimulated. Many of these agents also have an irritant effect on the bowel, further stimulating peristalsis. They are used to stimulate rapid or complete bowel evacuation

(*continued*)

Medication Administration 24.B

Laxatives and Cathartics (*continued*)

to relieve constipation and to prepare the bowel for diagnostic and surgical procedures. They should be limited to acute, short-term use; chronic use may suppress normal bowel reflexes.

Nursing Responsibilities

- Assess for possible contraindications to osmotic or saline laxatives, including bowel ulceration or obstruction, dehydration, electrolyte imbalances, heart failure (which may be aggravated by the sodium content), or renal failure.
- Administer with a full glass of liquid, preferably in the morning to avoid sleep disturbance.
- Monitor fluid and electrolyte status: Skin turgor, mucous membranes; intake and output; daily weight; and laboratory studies, such as hemoglobin and hematocrit levels, serum osmolality and electrolytes, and urine specific gravity.

Health Education for the Patient and Family

- Do not use these agents on a routine basis to treat or prevent constipation.
- Chill the solution to increase its palatability.
- Expect some abdominal cramping.
- Use only as directed. Increase fluid intake to at least 6 to 8 glasses of nonalcoholic fluid daily.
- Notify the physician if adverse effects occur, including abdominal pain, bloody stool, excessive skin or mucous membrane dryness, rapid weight loss, dizziness, or other unusual symptoms.
- These agents work in 3 to 6 hours; take them in the morning or early evening to avoid sleep disturbance.

STIMULANT LAXATIVES

bisacodyl (Dulcolax, Bisco-Lax, Carter's Liver Pills, Codylax, others)

Stimulant laxatives work by stimulating the motility and secretion of intestinal mucosa. Their use results in watery stool, often accompanied by abdominal cramping and pain. They are used to relieve constipation, although they should not be used as the initial treatment. Stimulant laxatives are also used for preparing the bowel for diagnostic testing.

Nursing Responsibilities

- Assess for potential contraindications to these laxatives, including abdominal pain and cramping, nausea and vomiting, and anal or rectal fissures.
- Administer on an empty stomach to minimize the effects of food on its dissolution and absorption.
- Do not crush enteric-coated bisacodyl tablets or administer with alkaline products. This may hasten their dissolution in the stomach, leading to gastric distress.

Health Education for the Patient and Family

- Discourage the use of this type of laxative, even in OTC preparations, for the initial or continuing relief of constipation.
- Do not use the laxative for more than 1 week; chronic use can be habit forming and may suppress normal bowel reflexes.
- These laxatives are excreted in breast milk and should not be used by lactating women.
- Phenolphthalein-containing products may discolor the urine pink or red. Report possible hypersensitivity manifestations, such as difficulty breathing, dizziness or light-headedness, or skin rashes, to the primary care provider, and stop taking the medication.

HERBAL AGENTS

senna (Senna laxative, Fletcher's Castoria)

castor oil

Herbal agents are natural products and are available OTC. Senna is a common herbal laxative and irritates the bowel, which increases peristalsis.

Nursing Responsibility

- Assess for potential contraindications to these laxatives, including abdominal pain and cramping, nausea and vomiting, and anal or rectal fissures.
- Use only as directed. Increase fluid intake to at least six to eight glasses of nonalcoholic fluid daily.

Health Education for Patient and Family

- Encourage dietary modifications such as increasing fiber and decreasing high-fat foods.
- Increase fluid intake to at least six to eight glasses of nonalcoholic fluid daily.

MISCELLANEOUS DRUGS

mineral oil

Mineral oil acts by forming an oily coat on the fecal mass, preventing the reabsorption of water, and resulting in softer stool. Problems associated with the use of mineral oil as a laxative include reduced absorption of the fat-soluble vitamins A, D, E, and K; possible damage to the liver and spleen due to systemic absorption; and potential pneumonitis from aspiration of oil droplets into the lungs.

Nursing Responsibilities

- Assess for possible contraindications to use of mineral oil, including advanced age, preexisting lung disease, and hemorrhoids or other rectal lesions.
- Do not give mineral oil concurrently with wetting agents or stool softeners because these increase the potential for systemic absorption and increase the effects of the mineral oil.
- Administer mineral oil in the evening before bedtime to reduce the effect on the absorption of fat-soluble vitamins and minimize the risk of aspiration.
- Assess for manifestations of vitamin deficiency. Monitor the patient taking oral anticoagulants for evidence of increased bleeding, such as bleeding gums, easy bruising, or melena.

Health Education for the Patient and Family

- Long-term use of mineral oil is not recommended because of its risks and adverse effects.
- Do not use mineral oil if hemorrhoids or rectal lesions are present; leakage of the oil through the anal sphincter may cause itching and interfere with healing.
- Suck on a lemon or orange slice after taking oral mineral oil to reduce the oily aftertaste.

Note: Drugs identified in *blue* are among the 200 most commonly prescribed medications in the United States.

Source: Data from Adams et al., 2017.

Nutrition

Foods that have high fiber content are recommended. Vegetable fiber is largely indigestible and unabsorbable, so it increases stool bulk. Fiber helps draw water into the fecal mass, softening the stool and making defecation easier. Raw fruits and vegetables are good sources of dietary fiber, as is cereal bran. Use 2 to 3 teaspoons of unprocessed bran with meals (sprinkled on fruit or cereal) or up to 1/4 cup daily to supply adequate fiber.

Fluids are important to maintain bowel motility and soft stools. The patient should drink six to eight glasses of fluid per day. It is important to advise the patient to increase fluid intake when dietary fiber is initially increased to decrease flatus and help maintain softer stools.

In older adults, constipation may be due to inadequate food intake. Carefully evaluate diet history and usual daily intake.

Enemas

Significant or chronic constipation or a fecal impaction may require the administration of an enema. As a general rule, enemas are used only in acute situations and only on a short-term basis. They may be ordered to prepare the bowel for diagnostic testing or examination. The following types of enemas may be prescribed:

- ***Saline enemas*** of 500 to 2000 mL of warmed physiologic saline solution are the least irritating to the bowel.
- ***Tap-water enemas*** use 500 to 1000 mL of water to soften feces and irritate the bowel mucosa, stimulating peristalsis and evacuation.
- ***Soap-solution enemas*** consist of a tap-water solution to which soap is added as a further irritant.
- ***Phosphate enemas*** (e.g., Fleet) use a hypertonic saline solution to draw fluid into the bowel and irritate the mucosa, leading to evacuation.
- ***Oil retention enemas*** instill mineral or vegetable oil into the bowel to soften the fecal mass. The instilled oil is retained overnight or for several hours before evacuation.

The repeated use of enemas can lead not only to impaired bowel function, but also to fluid and electrolyte imbalances. Tap-water and phosphate enemas are particularly likely to cause these problems. In acute conditions with risk of bowel obstruction, perforation, ulceration, or other problems, enemas should not be administered until their safe use can be established.

Integrative Therapies

Herbal or homeopathic therapies may be used to help relieve constipation. Flaxseed oil lubricates the colon for easier passage of stool. Patients are instructed to take 1 to 2 tablespoons daily. Flax seeds are a lesser known but highly concentrated source of fiber, and 1 to 2 tablespoons of ground flaxseeds can be sprinkled on cereals or salads daily, followed by 10 ounces of water. Acupressure, massage, reflexology, aromatherapy, and stress management therapies can be beneficial in relieving constipation. Other recommendations include exercise to stimulate intestinal contractions.

Nursing Care

Assessment

To assess the patient with real or perceived constipation, collect the following data:

- ***Health history:*** Usual and current pattern of defecation, including time of day, amount, and stool consistency; usual diet, fluid intake, and activity pattern; possible contributing factors such as opioid analgesics, activity limitations, painful hemorrhoids, perianal surgery; chronic diseases such as endocrine or neurologic disorders; prescription and nonprescription medications. Determine patients' perspectives on their bowel function and establish toilet accessibility.
- ***Physical assessment:*** Abdominal girth and shape, bowel sounds, tenderness, and percussion tone; digital exam of the rectum if impaction is suspected. An oral examination should be included to identify any difficulty with chewing or swallowing that can lead to a decrease in fiber intake. Assess musculoskeletal and functional level to determine patient's capacity for accessing toileting facilities.

Priorities of Care

Educate the patient and caregivers as appropriate to ensure that the patient establishes regular elimination habits, hydration, an exercise or mobility plan, and a high-fiber diet. Preventing constipation associated with other diagnoses, medical procedures, and medications is a key nursing responsibility.

Diagnoses, Outcomes, and Interventions

Nursing interventions for the patient with constipation focus chiefly on education.

Resolve Constipation. Whether real or perceived, constipation is disruptive to the patient's activities of daily living (ADLs) and life satisfaction. Constipation is a common problem in older adults (see **Box 24.1**).

BOX 24.1
Constipation and the Older Adult

Constipation and perceived constipation are common problems in older adults. Although constipation is not a normal consequence of aging, factors such as slowed peristalsis, lowered activity levels, reduced food and fluid intake, and decreased sensory perception contribute to the higher incidence of constipation seen in older adults. Chronic diseases such as diabetes, mobility problems, and medications also increase the risk of constipation in older adults.

Cultural influences and advertising lead many older adults to believe that a daily bowel movement is important for health. This belief contributes to an increased incidence of perceived constipation in older adults. Because of this perception, the older adult may come to rely on laxatives, suppositories, or enemas to facilitate regular bowel movements. These external aids to defecation can further impair the ability to maintain normal bowel habits.

Expected Outcome: Patient will report passage of stool with reduction of straining and pain and verbalize knowledge of bowel regimen necessary to avoid the constipating side effects of medication.

The nurse will:

- Monitor pattern of defecation and stool consistency. *This information helps establish the patient's usual pattern of defecation and differentiate between actual and perceived constipation.*
- Provide additional fluids to maintain an intake of at least 2500 mL per day. *A generous fluid intake helps maintain soft stool consistency and promote intestinal motility.*
- Encourage drinking a glass of warm water before breakfast. Provide time and privacy following breakfast for bowel elimination. *This helps develop a pattern of natural elimination; the warm water provides mild stimulation of bowel peristalsis.*
- Consult with the dietitian to provide a diet high in natural fiber unless contraindicated. Provide foods such as natural bran, prunes, or prune juice. *Natural fiber adds bulk to the stool and has a mild stimulant effect.*
- Encourage activities such as ambulation or chair exercises (e.g., range of motion, stretching, wheelchair lifts) as tolerated. *Activity stimulates peristalsis and strengthens abdominal muscles, facilitating elimination.*
- If indicated, consult with primary care provider about the use of bulk laxatives, stool softeners, or other laxatives as needed. *Laxatives may be necessary to relieve acute constipation. Patients with long-term activity or diet restrictions or impaired abdominal muscle strength may need a bulk-forming laxative to maintain normal elimination patterns and prevent constipation.*

Transitions of Care

Constipation is a common complaint after discharge from a hospitalization (Konradsen, Rasmussen, Noisesen, & Trosborg, 2017). Assessing for constipation and monitoring bowel habit as the patient transitions from one care setting to another should be a priority (Holroyd, 2015). Providing education at discharge and at home visits can prevent constipation. Teach patients the importance of maintaining a diet high in natural fiber. Foods such as fresh fruits, vegetables, whole-grain products, and bran provide natural fiber. Encourage reducing consumption of meats and refined foods, which are low in fiber and can be constipating. Emphasize the need to maintain a high fluid intake every day, particularly during hot weather and exercise. Discuss the relationship between exercise and bowel regularity. Encourage patients to engage in some form of exercise, such as walking daily.

Discuss normal bowel habits, and explain that a daily bowel movement is not the norm for all people. Encourage patients to respond to the urge to defecate when it occurs. Suggest setting aside a time, usually following a meal, for elimination.

The acute care nurse should monitor bowel movements daily. If there is early indication the patient is becoming constipated, the nurse should advocate to begin medication or treatment. The nurse should instruct unlicensed assistive personnel who assist patients with toileting to monitor bowel movements and report any concerns to the nurse.

Chronic constipation is a common condition accompanying other chronic conditions that inhibit mobility and a healthy dietary intake. Managing chronic constipation requires constant monitoring and teaching. Conservative management involves promoting lifestyle changes such as exercise and increased fluid intake. Medication can be used and some patients may require a combination of medications to achieve results. Regulating a patient's bowel habit may involve titrating two or three medications to achieve desired results.

Constipation is frequently a challenging problem for patients and caregivers at the end of life. Constipation is primarily the result of opioid treatment (Prichard & Bharucha, 2015). Additionally, bowel motility slows at the end of life and bowel movements may decrease or cease with limited oral intake. The nurse should assess for signs of constipation and work with the hospice/palliative care team to determine appropriate treatment if the patient becomes constipated and is uncomfortable. Monitoring for constipation should be an ongoing assessment during the dying process and medications may need to be adjusted to promote optimum patient comfort (Pitlick & Fritz, 2013).

Include the following topics when teaching self-care measures to prevent and treat constipation:

- Increasing dietary fiber intake by including fresh fruits and vegetables, whole grains, high-fiber breakfast cereals, and unprocessed bran in the diet (Bran can be sprinkled on cereals, mixed into bread or muffin recipes, or mixed with fruit juice to increase its palatability.)
- Maintaining fluid intake of six to eight glasses of water per day (unless contraindicated)
- Suggestions for remaining physically active to promote bowel function and maintain muscle tone
- Responding to the urge to defecate when perceived
- Appropriate use of laxatives:
    a. Do not use laxatives, suppositories, or enemas on a regular basis.
    b. Bulk-forming agents provide insoluble fiber and are safe for long-term use; it is important to drink at least 6 to 8 glasses of water daily when using these (or any) laxatives.
    c. Other laxatives such as milk of magnesia, docusate (Colace, DSS), bisacodyl (Dulcolax), cascara, or castor oil should be used only occasionally to relieve constipation.
- Reporting any change in bowel habits such as new or persistent constipation or diarrhea, abdominal pain, black or bloody stools, nausea or anorexia, weakness, or unexplained weight loss to the primary care provider.

The Patient with Irritable Bowel Syndrome

Irritable bowel syndrome (IBS), also known as *spastic bowel* or *mucous colitis*, is a motility disorder of the lower GI tract. It is a functional and chronic disorder with no identifiable organic causes characterized by abdominal pain and bloating with constipation, diarrhea, or both.

Irritable bowel syndrome is common, affecting 10 to 15% of the adult population of both developed and developing countries (Ghiyasvandian, Ghorbani, Zakerimoghadam, Prufarzad, & Kazemnejad, 2016). It usually affects young people, with about 50% of patients diagnosed before age 35. There is a higher prevalence of IBS in women than in men (McQuaid, 2018).

Pathophysiology

In IBS, it appears that CNS regulation of the motor and sensory functions of the bowel is altered. Patients with IBS often experience increased motor reactivity of the small bowel and colon in response to stimuli such as food intake, hormonal influences, and physiologic or psychologic stress. IBS is characterized by visceral hypersensitivity and hyperactivity of the GI tract. Hypersecretion of colonic mucus is a common feature of the syndrome.

A lower visceral pain threshold is often found in patients with IBS. Patients may complain of pain, bloating, and distention when intestinal gas levels are normal. Psychologic factors such as depression or anxiety have been linked to IBS; however, they have not been identified as causes of the disorder. Recent research does indicate a correlation between emotional, physical, and early childhood trauma and IBS (Weaver, Melkus, & Henderson, 2017).

Manifestations

IBS is characterized by abdominal pain that often is relieved by defecation and a change in bowel habits. The pain may either be colicky, occurring in spasms, or dull and continuous. Altered patterns of defecation may include:

- A change in frequency
- Abnormal stool form (hard or lumpy, loose or watery)
- Altered stool passage (straining, urgency, or a sensation of incomplete evacuation)
- Passage of mucus.

The patient may also complain of abdominal bloating and excess gas. Other manifestations include nausea and vomiting, anorexia, fatigue, headache, depression, or anxiety. The abdomen is often tender to palpation, particularly over the sigmoid colon.

Interprofessional Care

Irritable bowel syndrome is diagnosed based on the presence of abdominal pain or discomfort at least 3 days per month in the past 3 months that has at least two of the following characteristics: (1) Improved with defecation, (2) associated with a change in frequency of elimination, or (3) associated with a change in stool form (Weaver et al., 2017). Management is directed toward relieving manifestations and reducing or eliminating precipitating factors. Many patients benefit from cognitive-behavioral strategies (Weaver et al., 2017).

Diagnosis

The primary purpose of diagnostic testing is to rule out other causes of abdominal pain and altered fecal elimination. The stools may be examined for occult blood, ova and parasites, and white blood cells (WBCs). A sigmoidoscopy, colonoscopy, and/or a small-bowel series (upper GI series with small-bowel follow-through) and barium enema may be performed to visually examine the bowel mucosa, measure intraluminal pressures, and biopsy suspicious lesions. However, serious organic disease is often not present, so overtesting should be avoided (McQuaid, 2018). Nursing care for these procedures is outlined in Chapter 21. Laboratory tests include a complete blood count (CBC) with differential and erythrocyte sedimentation rate to evaluate for anemia from bleeding or a possible tumor. An increased WBC count indicates a bacterial infection.

Medications

Although not curative, medications may be prescribed to manage the manifestations of IBS. Pharmacologic management of IBS targets the predominant bowel malady (diarrhea or constipation) and addresses abdominal pain (Weaver et al., 2017). Antispasmodic agents are sometimes used for treatment of acute episodes characterized by significant pain or bloating. Cyoscyamine, dicylomine, or methscopolamine may be used for short-term treatment of severe symptoms. The nurse should teach the patient to monitor for anticholinergic side effects including urinary retention, constipation, and dry mouth. Loreramide may be used for patients with diarrhea and oral osmotic laxatives may be used for patients experiencing constipation (McQuaid, 2018).

Antidepressant drugs, including tricyclics and selective serotonin reuptake inhibitors (SSRIs), may help relieve abdominal pain associated with IBS (McQuaid, 2018). Although the anticholinergic side effects of the tricyclics (such as desipramine [Norpramin] and imipramine [Tofranil]) may help decrease diarrhea, they have more adverse effects than SSRIs such as sertraline (Zoloft) and fluoxetine (Prozac). Alosetron (Lotronex) is a serotonin receptor antagonist that reduces abdominal pain and diarrhea in patients with IBS. Its use is limited, however, by its association with ischemic colitis.

Nutrition

Many patients with IBS benefit from additional dietary fiber. Adding bran to meals provides added bulk and water content to the stool, reducing the incidence of both loose diarrheal stools and hard, constipated stools. Other dietary changes are specific to individual triggers for IBS manifestations. Some patients may benefit from limiting lactose, fructose, or sorbitol intake (refer to **Table 24.1**). When excess gas and flatulence are problems, reducing the intake of gas-forming foods, such as beans, cabbage, apple and grape juices, nuts, and raisins, may be helpful. Caffeinated drinks, such as coffee, tea, and soft drinks, act as gastrointestinal stimulants; limiting intake of these fluids may prove beneficial.

Integrative Therapies

Herbal preparations may provide some benefit for patients with IBS. Herbs with an antispasmodic effect, such as anise, chamomile, peppermint, and sage, may be used to reduce the manifestations of IBS. Ginger root can be consumed as a tea or capsule to assist with reduction of gas, bloating, and diarrhea and to improve the functioning of the stomach. Probiotic therapies (such as yogurt with active bacterial cultures) have been shown to benefit patients with IBS, as has hypnosis (Weaver et al., 2017). Many patients use complementary and alternative medicine in addition to traditional medicine in the treatment of IBS. The accompanying Moving Evidence into Action box illustrates the importance of providing patient-centered care for patients experiencing chronic illness like IBS.

Nursing Care

Assessment

Careful assessment is important to help identify the effects of IBS on the patient. Collect the following assessment data:

- ***Health history:*** Current manifestations, their onset and duration; current treatment measures; effect of manifestations on lifestyle; careful exploration of history of emotional, physical, or sexual abuse
- ***Physical assessment:*** Apparent general state of health; abdominal shape and contour, bowel sounds, tenderness.

Priorities of Care

Managing symptoms of IBS through dietary modification and stress reduction is the focus of nursing care. Monitoring the patient's nutritional status is a key component of ongoing care. Cognitive-behavioral strategies focused on education and relaxation improves anxiety and depression.

Moving Evidence into Action

Irritable Bowel Syndrome

Clinical Issue

Irritable bowel syndrome is a functional disorder characterized by abdominal pain and discomfort, alterations in bowel function presenting as constipation, diarrhea, or alternating episodes of both. The patient's symptoms are real, however, the physical findings are often absent or limited. The development and trajectory of IBS symptoms are described as multifactorial, making diagnosis and treatment complicated. Stress has been identified as one of the many mechanisms that contribute to the development and persistence of IBS. Treatment is focused on reducing patient symptoms and decreasing the occurrences of alterations in bowel dysfunction (Weaver et al., 2017).

External Evidence

Nurse researchers Ghiyasvandian et al. (2016) conducted a study to determine the effects of a self-care program on the severity of symptoms and quality for patients with IBS. This quasi-experimental study used pre and post surveys to evaluate an intervention focused on self-management strategies that can be used to reduce symptoms. All study subjects received standard medical care through a gastroenterology practice. The experimental group of patients received written and digital information about IBS, several follow-up phone calls by a nurse, an individual teaching session, and group training that focused on progressive muscle relaxation and abdominal breathing exercises with 10 to 15 other patients. The control group received one phone call to address the potential Hawthorne effect in research. Pre and post data included evaluating patients' quality of life using the IBS-Quality of Life questionnaire. The severity of symptoms was evaluated by the IBS-Symptom Severity Scale. Both measures showed significant improvement for patients in the experimental group, demonstrating that a self-care program can improve quality of life and reduce symptoms for patients with IBS.

Internal Evidence

Because IBS is a multifactorial illness with varying physical symptoms that can be associated with psychological concerns, each patient's treatment plan must be individualized. Determining the most appropriate self-care strategy that will likely address the patient's stress and physical symptoms should be assessed and then used to develop an individual teaching and stress management plan.

Patient Considerations

Determining each patient's preferred approach to learning new knowledge and skills should be incorporated into the plan. Group training may be effective for some patients. The entire education and stress reduction training program should be created in partnership with each individual patient. The IBS-Quality of Life questionnaire and the IBS-Symptom Severity Scale can be used to monitor response to individualized self-care treatment plans.

Putting the Pieces Together

IBS can potentially be a debilitating chronic condition affecting quality of life. Comprehensive self-management combined with medical management can effectively improve quality of life and decrease the severity of symptoms. Thorough assessment using validated questionnaires provide data used to objectively monitor the patient's response to intervention. Nurses should develop, facilitate, and evaluate individualized education plans and group training focused on adapting self-management strategies.

References

Ghiyasvandian, S., Ghorbanic, M., Zakerimoghadam, M., Purfoarzad, Z., & Kazemnejad, A. (2016). The effects of a self-care program on the severity of symptoms and quality of life of patients with irritable bowel syndrome. *Gastroenterology Nursing*, *39*(5), 359–365.

Weaver, K. R., Melkus, G. D., & Henderson, W. (2017). Irritable bowel syndrome: An evidence-based review of new diagnostic criteria and treatment recommendations. *American Journal of Nursing*, *117*(6), 48–55.

Diagnoses, Outcomes, and Intervention

The primary nursing responsibility to patients with IBS is education; providing referrals and counseling are additional nursing responsibilities. See the previous sections on diarrhea and constipation for selected nursing interventions.

Transitions of Care

There is no cure for IBS and current treatment focuses on managing symptoms through lifestyle and dietary modifications. Patient education and exercise are important aspects of managing this chronic illness.

Patients with IBS rarely require acute care for it as a primary problem. However, nurses frequently interact with these patients in clinics and other community settings.

Include the following topics in teaching for the patient with IBS:

- The nature of the disorder and the reality of the patient's manifestations
- Stress and anxiety reduction techniques, such as meditation, visualization, exercise, "time-out," and progressive relaxation
- Dietary influences that may contribute to IBS and suggested dietary changes, such as additional fiber and water intake
- The use and role of prescribed medications, their adverse effects, and when to contact the physician
- The importance of routine follow-up appointments and of notifying the primary care provider if manifestations change (such as blood in the stool, significant constipation or diarrhea, increasing abdominal pain, or weight loss).
- Fecal microbiota transplantation may improve IBS symptoms. Providing patient education on this emerging treatment may need to be provided
- Increased physical activity reduces the severity of IBS symptoms. The nurse should assist the patient in developing a plan for participating in consistent physical activity.

If needed, refer the patient to a counselor or other mental health professional for assistance in dealing with psychologic factors.

The Patient with Fecal Incontinence

Fecal incontinence, also known as *bowel incontinence*, is the loss of voluntary control of defecation. It occurs less frequently than urinary incontinence but is no less distressing to the patient. Multiple factors may contribute to fecal incontinence (see **Box 24.2**). Bowel incontinence is usually considered a symptom, not a disease or disorder. Patients often do not reveal fecal incontinence in discussing health concerns. Little information is available about its incidence and prevalence. Because many of the etiologic factors are more prevalent in the older adult, older patients are more often affected.

Pathophysiology

To understand the pathophysiology of fecal incontinence, it is necessary to understand the normal mechanisms of defecation. The rectum is normally empty. The defecation reflex is stimulated when the rectum is distended by feces entering from the sigmoid colon. This reflex causes involuntary relaxation of the internal sphincter and stimulates the urge to defecate. When the external sphincter, which is under both somatic (voluntary) and autonomic (involuntary) control, relaxes, defecation occurs. Adults can normally override the defecation reflex by voluntary contraction of the external sphincter and pelvic floor muscles. The wall of the rectum gradually relaxes, and the urge to defecate subsides.

BOX 24.2
Selected Causes of Fecal Incontinence

NEUROLOGIC CAUSES

- Spinal cord injury or disease
- Head injury, stroke, or brain tumor
- Degenerative neurologic disease, such as multiple sclerosis, amyotrophic lateral sclerosis (ALS), dementia
- Diabetic neuropathy

LOCAL TRAUMA

- Obstetric tears
- Anorectal injury
- Anorectal surgery with sphincter damage

INFLAMMATORY PROCESSES

- Infection
- Radiation

OTHER CAUSES

- Diarrhea
- Stool impaction
- Pelvic floor relaxation or loss of sphincter tone
- Tumors

The most common causes of fecal incontinence are those that interfere with either sensory or motor control of the rectum and anal sphincters. If the external sphincter is paralyzed as a result of spinal cord injury or disease, defecation occurs automatically when the internal sphincter relaxes with the defecation reflex. If sphincter muscles have been damaged or excessive pelvic floor relaxation has occurred, it may not be possible to override the defecation reflex with voluntary control.

Age-related changes in anal sphincter tone and response to rectal distention increase the risk for fecal incontinence in older adults. Resting and maximal anal sphincter pressures are decreased, particularly in older women. In addition, less rectal distention is needed to produce sustained relaxation of the anal sphincter in older females.

Manifestations

Fecal incontinence is characterized by inability to respond normally to the urge to defecate, resulting in soiling oneself with stool (Gump & Schmelzer, 2016). Incontinent stools are difficult to contain, create unpleasant odor, and are difficult to clean. Fecal incontinence interferes with all aspects of life and can be an embarrassment, making it difficult for the patient to talk about it.

Interprofessional Care

The diagnosis of fecal incontinence is based on the patient's history. Physical examination of the pelvic floor and anus is performed to evaluate muscle tone and rule out a fecal impaction. Impaired sphincter muscle may be palpable on digital exam. Anorectal manometry or a rectal motility test may be used to evaluate the functional ability of the sphincter muscles. In this test, a small, flexible balloon catheter is introduced into the rectum, and pressures are measured in the rectum and internal and external sphincters. Normally, rectal dilation causes the internal sphincter to relax and the external sphincter to contract. Sigmoidoscopy may be used to examine the rectum and anal canal.

Management of fecal incontinence is directed toward the identified cause. Medications to relieve diarrhea or constipation may be prescribed. A high-fiber diet, ample fluids, and regular exercise are helpful for many patients. Exercises to improve sphincter and pelvic floor muscle tone (Kegel exercises) may be of long-term benefit. Patients may benefit from using loperamide before meals and prophylactically before running errands or leaving the house. Research shows biofeedback therapy is helpful for mentally alert patients with intact sphincter muscles but low muscle tone (Gump & Schmelzer, 2016). With motivation and reinforcement, patients achieve improved sphincter control in response to a stimulus. The goal of biofeedback is to improve sensation, coordination, and strength of the sphincter muscle.

When damage to the sphincter or rectal prolapse (protrusion of rectal mucous membrane through the anus) is the cause of fecal incontinence, surgical repair is the treatment of choice. Surgery may be indicated when conservative measures have not been effective. Permanent colostomy, the creation of an opening from the large bowel on the abdominal wall, is a last-choice option for some patients, but it can control fecal output when other measures fail.

Nursing Care

Managing fecal incontinence is a challenging problem for the patient and family caregivers. For the patient with intact cognition, it can be psychologically devastating. The patient may become socially isolated from fear of odor or soiling clothing. Self-esteem may suffer from a sense of lost control over body functions and the inability to provide self-care. It is important to stress that incontinence is never normal (i.e., aging alone is not a cause of incontinence) and is often treatable. Encourage the patient to seek medical evaluation of the problem.

Topics of patient and family education include:

- Recommended dietary measures such as consuming a high-fiber diet and ample fluids to maintain soft, formed stool or a low-residue diet to reduce the number of stools. See Tables 24.8 and 24.9 later in the chapter for details regarding a high-fiber and low-residue diet.
- Suggestions for regular exercise to stimulate bowel peristalsis and regular evacuation.
- Use of bulk-forming laxatives, such as psyllium seed (Metamucil), to provide stool bulk and reduce the number of small, liquid stools.
- Prescribed medications (such as loperamide to reduce the number of stools), their appropriate use, and management of adverse effects (such as constipation).
- Bowel training program instructions, including techniques for digital anal stimulation, inserting suppositories, or administering enemas as recommended. For digital anal simulation, teach to insert a lubricated gloved finger through the anal sphincter into the rectum 1.5 to 2 inches while seated on the toilet or commode, then use a circular side-to-side movement to gently stretch the rectal wall until the internal sphincter relaxes.
- The importance of good skin care, particularly if neurologic impairment is present.
- The potential benefits and associated risks of biofeedback and surgical treatment, if recommended.
- Provide referrals for home care or community health services as indicated.

Assessment

- ***Health history:*** Extent, onset, and duration of incontinence; identified contributing factors; history of spinal cord or anorectal injury or surgery; chronic diseases such as diabetes, multiple sclerosis, or other neurologic disorders
- ***Physical assessment:*** Mental status; general health; examination of perianal tissues; digital rectal examination.

Priorities of Care

Studies reveal fecal incontinence has a significant impact on quality of life. Many patients experience anxiety about possible embarrassment from visible soiling or fecal odor. Assessing for depression, social isolation, and anxiety is important, as is assessing skin integrity.

Diagnoses, Outcomes, and Interventions

Manage Bowel Incontinence. Nurses are often responsible for instituting bowel training programs and other measures to manage fecal incontinence.

Expected Outcome: Patient will control stool passage by establishing routine bowel habits, recognizing the urge to defecate, and responding to urge in a timely manner.

The nurse will:

- Teach caregivers to place the patient on a toilet or commode and provide for privacy at a certain time of day. *Placing the patient in a normal position to defecate at a consistent time of day stimulates the defecation reflex and helps reestablish a pattern of stool evacuation.*
- If necessary, insert a glycerin or bisacodyl (Dulcolax) suppository 15 to 20 minutes before positioning on the

toilet or commode. *This helps to stimulate evacuation. Once a regular elimination pattern has been established, it may be possible to discontinue suppository use.*

- Maintain a caring, nonjudgmental manner in providing care. *This promotes a feeling of acceptance when the patient may feel unacceptable.*

Promote Self-Care and Socialization. The patient may develop negative feelings about self or self-care capabilities due to long-standing and frequent inability to control bowel evacuation. This may lead to social isolation due to fear of soiling and foul odor.

Expected Outcome: Patient will demonstrate self-esteem as evidenced by maintaining grooming and hygiene and participation in social situations such as work, school, or social groups.

The nurse will:

- Provide room odor control with deodorizer tablets, sprays, or other devices. *Controlling odor is important to preserve the patient's self-esteem.*
- Assist patient with hygiene and grooming quickly when fecal incontinence occurs. *Helping patient maintain personal hygiene and a pleasant environment will promote feelings of well-being and control.*

Promote Good Skin Care. Good skin care is vital for the patient with fecal incontinence. Stool contains enzymes and other irritating substances that promote skin breakdown when they are not promptly removed. This can lead to pressure injury, particularly when a neurologic disorder (such as spinal cord injury, dementia, or stroke) impairs mobility.

Expected Outcome: Patient's skin will remain intact with no evidence of redness or breakdown.

The nurse will:

- Clean the skin thoroughly with mild soap and water after each bowel movement. *Toilet tissue may be more irritating to the skin and less effective in removing fecal material.*
- Apply a skin barrier cream or ointment after each bowel movement. *These help protect the skin from irritating substances in the feces.*
- If incontinence pads or briefs are used, check frequently for soiling and change when feces are noted. *Although these help protect bedding and clothing from soiling, they can contribute to skin breakdown if they are not checked and changed frequently.*

Transitions of Care

A bowel training program to establish a regular pattern of elimination is often effective in relieving fecal incontinence. Teach the patient to establish a regular time of day for elimination, usually 15 to 30 minutes after breakfast. A stimulant, such as a cup of coffee, a rectal suppository, or even a phosphate enema, may be given to prompt defecation. Patients with neurologic incontinence may learn to stimulate the anal canal digitally to initiate defecation.

Dietary changes may be useful in managing fecal incontinence. If incontinence occurs only with mild loose or liquid stools, increasing dietary fiber or using a bulking agent to increase stool bulk and solidity may be effective. The majority of the fiber should come from a fiber-rich diet because fiber supplements provide only a limited amount of additional fiber. When incontinence of solid stool occurs, a low-residue diet of foods that are easily digested and absorbed may be prescribed to reduce the frequency of defecation. See Table 24.8 later in this chapter for a list of foods from a low-residue diet.

Fecal incontinence is experienced frequently by acute and critically ill patients because of cognitive deficits, enteral tube feedings, and medications. Keeping the patient clean, observing for skin breakdown, and using barrier cream to protect the skin are priority nursing actions.

Whenever possible the nurse should work with the interprofessional team to eliminate the etiology of fecal incontinence. Often the cause of chronic fecal incontinence cannot be eliminated. The nurse should provide strategies aimed at improving fecal consistency, promoting regular defecation, and containing stool. Helping the patient identify bathrooms that are readily accessible and encouraging use of disposable undergarments can reduce the embarrassment and potential for social isolation.

Patients may experience fecal incontinence at the end of life due to medication and changes in cognitive function. Prompt cleaning and measures to protect skin integrity to promote comfort are priorities. The nurse may need to teach family caregivers how to bathe and change linens for dying patients that are bedbound.

24.2 Acute Inflammatory and Infectious Bowel Disorders

The GI tract is particularly vulnerable to inflammation and infection because of its continual exposure to the external environment. Although most pathogens affecting the GI tract are ingested in food or water, infection may be spread by direct contact, possibly by the respiratory route. Pathogens may also be transmitted sexually through anal intercourse.

Acute disease of the GI tract may be caused by the pathogen itself or by a bacterial or other toxin. Acute inflammatory disorders such as appendicitis and peritonitis result from contamination of damaged or normally sterile tissue by the patient's own endogenous or resident bacteria.

The Patient with Appendicitis

Appendicitis, inflammation of the vermiform appendix, is a common cause of acute abdominal pain. Appendicitis can occur at any age, but is more common in adolescents and young adults and slightly more common in males than in females.

Pathophysiology

The *appendix* is a tubelike pouch attached to the cecum just below the ileocecal valve. It is usually located in the right iliac region, at an area designated as McBurney point (**Figure 24.1** ■). The function of the appendix is not fully understood, although it may serve as a type of reservoir for beneficial intestinal bacteria.

Obstruction of the proximal lumen of the appendix is apparent in most acutely inflamed appendices. The obstruction is often caused by a *fecalith*, or a hard mass of feces. Other obstructive causes include a calculus or stone, a foreign body, inflammation, a tumor, parasites (e.g., pinworms), or edema of lymphoid tissue. Following obstruction, the appendix becomes distended with fluid secreted by its mucosa. Pressure within the lumen of the appendix increases, impairing its blood supply and leading to inflammation, edema, ulceration, and infection. Purulent exudate forms, further distending the appendix. Within 24 to 36 hours, tissue necrosis and gangrene result, leading to perforation if treatment is not initiated. Perforation results in bacterial peritonitis.

Appendicitis can be classified as simple, gangrenous, or perforated, depending on the stage of the process. In simple appendicitis, the appendix is inflamed but intact. When areas of tissue necrosis and microscopic perforations are present in the appendix, the disorder is called *gangrenous appendicitis*. A perforated appendix shows evidence of gross perforation and contamination of the peritoneal cavity.

Manifestations

Continuous mild generalized or upper abdominal pain is the initial characteristic manifestation of acute appendicitis. During the next 4 hours, the pain intensifies and localizes in the right lower quadrant of the abdomen, aggravated by moving, walking, or coughing. On palpation, localized and rebound tenderness are noted at McBurney point. *Rebound tenderness* is demonstrated by relief of pain with direct palpation of McBurney point followed by pain on release of pressure. Extension or internal rotation of the right hip increases the pain. In addition to pain, a low-grade temperature, anorexia, and nausea and vomiting are often present.

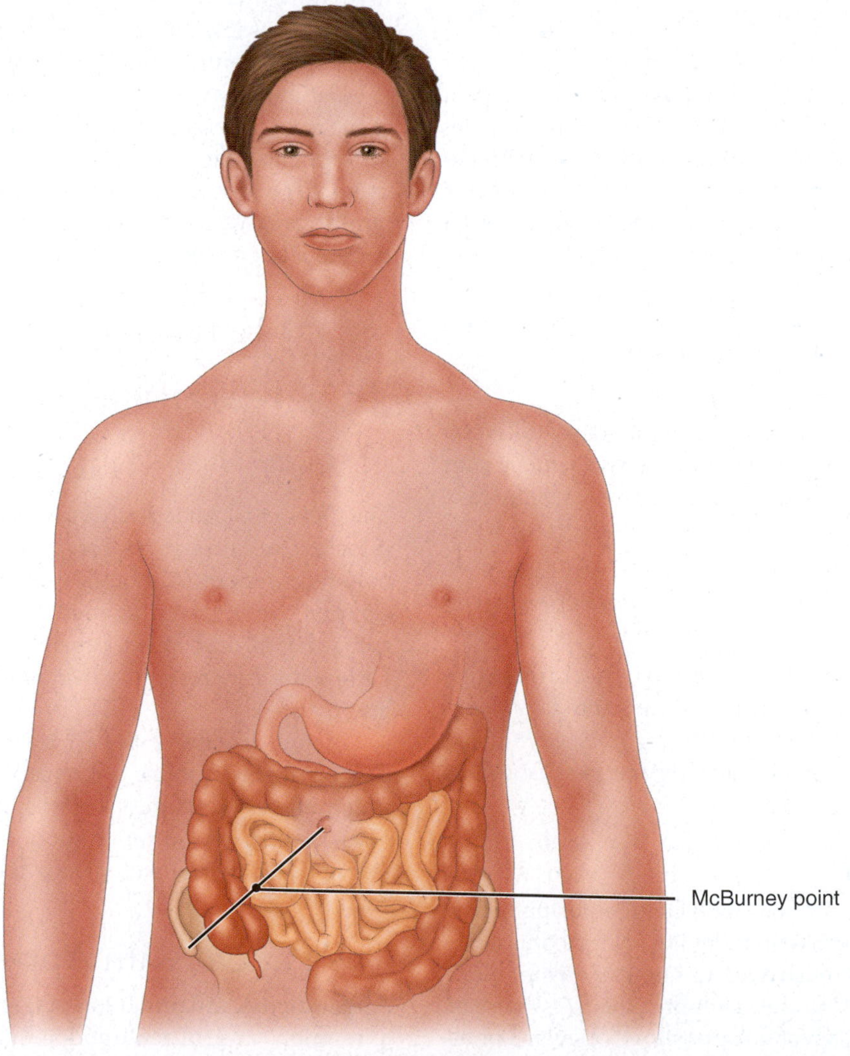
McBurney point

Figure 24.1 ■ McBurney point, located midway between the umbilicus and the anterior iliac crest in the right lower quadrant. It is the usual site for localized pain and rebound tenderness due to appendicitis.

Pain and local tenderness may be less acute in older adults, delaying the diagnosis. This can present a significant problem; the course of acute appendicitis in older adults is more virulent and complications develop sooner. Pregnant women may develop right lower quadrant, periumbilical, or right subcostal (under the rib cage) pain due to possible displacement of the appendix by the distended uterus. Appendicitis can be difficult to diagnose (Sorenson et al., 2019).

Complications

Perforation, peritonitis, and abscess are possible complications of acute appendicitis. Perforation is manifested by increased pain and a high fever. It can lead to a small, localized abscess, local peritonitis, or significant generalized peritonitis. (Peritonitis is discussed in the next section of this chapter.)

A less common disorder is chronic appendicitis, characterized by chronic abdominal pain and recurrent acute attacks at intervals of several months or more. Other conditions, such as inflammatory bowel disease and renal disorders, often cause manifestations attributed to chronic appendicitis.

Interprofessional Care

The acutely inflamed appendix can perforate within 24 hours, so rapid diagnosis and treatment are important. Because of this urgency and the low incidence of surgical complications, diagnostic testing and preoperative treatment may be limited. The patient is admitted to the hospital, and intravenous fluids and antibiotics are initiated. Oral food and fluids are withheld until a diagnosis is confirmed. Once the diagnosis is established, an appendectomy is performed.

Diagnosis

Diagnostic and laboratory tests are used to help confirm the diagnosis and rule out other possible causes for the manifestations. Abdominal ultrasound is the most effective test for diagnosing acute appendicitis. Ultrasound examination has reduced the incidence of exploratory surgery and is particularly useful for patients with atypical symptoms, such as older adults. Other diagnostic tests used to accurately diagnose appendicitis include abdominal x-rays, an intravenous pyelogram, a urinalysis, and a pelvic examination. In addition, a WBC count with differential is obtained. With appendicitis, the total white count is elevated (10,000 to 20,000/mm^3), with an increased number of immature WBC (bands).

Medications

Prior to surgery, intravenous fluids are given to restore or maintain vascular volume and prevent electrolyte imbalance. Antibiotic therapy with a third-generation cephalosporin effective against many Gram-negative bacteria—such as cefoperazone (Cefobid), cefotaxime (Claforan), ceftazidime (Fortaz), or ceftriaxone (Rocephin)—is initiated prior to surgery. The antibiotic is repeated during surgery and continued for at least 48 hours postoperatively. (The nursing implications for cephalosporin antibiotics are discussed in Chapter 12.) Pain medications are administered as prescribed.

Surgery

The treatment of choice for acute appendicitis is an *appendectomy*, surgical removal of the appendix. Either a laparoscopic approach (insertion of a laparoscope to view abdominal contents) or laparotomy (surgical opening of the abdomen) may be used for appendectomy. A laparoscopic appendectomy is generally preferred because this procedure requires a very small incision through which the laparoscope is inserted. This procedure has several advantages: (1) Direct visualization of the appendix allows definitive diagnosis without laparotomy; (2) postoperative hospitalization is short; (3) postoperative complications are infrequent; and (4) recovery and resumption of normal activities is rapid. Disadvantages include increased cost and longer operating time (about 20 minutes longer than an open appendectomy).

A needle appendectomy is a newer type of laparoscopic procedure and is comparable to a traditional laparoscopic appendectomy in terms of complications and hospital length of stay (Donmez et al., 2016). A needle appendectomy is associated with a longer operative time but significantly less postoperative pain.

An open appendectomy is performed by laparotomy. A small transverse incision is made at McBurney point (refer to Figure 24.1); the appendix is isolated and ligated (tied off) to prevent contamination of the site with bowel contents, and then removed. Laparotomy is generally used when the appendix has ruptured. It allows removal of contaminants from the peritoneal cavity by irrigation with sterile normal saline. Occasionally the wound may be left unsutured for periodic irrigation. Recovery is generally uneventful. Refer to Chapter 4 for a discussion of preoperative and postoperative nursing care.

Surgery remains the common treatment for appendicitis and has long been considered the only treatment for appendicitis. However, medical management is sometimes used for cases of simple appendicitis (Sorenson et al., 2019).

Nursing Care

See the Case Study & Nursing Care Plan for a patient with appendicitis.

Assessment

Because appendicitis can rapidly progress from inflammation to perforation, prompt assessment is vital. Obtain the following assessment data:

- ***Health history:*** Current manifestations, including onset, duration, progression, and aggravating or relieving factors; most recent food or fluid intake; known medication or other allergies; current medications; history of chronic diseases
- ***Physical assessment:*** Vital signs including temperature; apparent general health; abdominal shape and contour, bowel sounds, tenderness to light palpation.

Priorities of Care

Assessing patient for signs and symptoms of ruptured appendix is the priority focus of care. Prevention of dehydration and correction of fluid and electrolyte imbalance are also of key importance. Administration of prescribed antibiotics should be a priority nursing action. Managing the patient's pain pre- and postoperatively is an important component of care.

Diagnoses, Outcomes, and Interventions

Preoperative nursing care is directed toward preparing the patient physically and psychologically for emergency surgery. Limited time is available for preoperative teaching.

Monitor for signs and Complications of Infection. Preventing complications during the preoperative and postoperative periods is a primary nursing care goal. Perforation and peritonitis are the most likely preoperative complications; postoperative complications include wound infection, abscess, and possible peritonitis.

Expected Outcome: Patient will not exhibit signs and symptoms of perforation and peritonitis. Patient will remain afebrile, and WBC will decrease or remain at baseline. Patient will remain free of pain associated with perforation and peritonitis.

The nurse will:

- Monitor vital signs, including temperature. *Tachycardia and rapid shallow respirations may indicate perforation of the appendix with resulting peritonitis. Fever may develop as well, and the blood pressure may fall if sepsis is present.*

SAFETY ALERT: Assess abdominal status frequently, including distention, bowel sounds, and tenderness. Increasing generalized pain, a rigid, boardlike abdomen, and abdominal distention may indicate developing peritonitis. ■

- Maintain intravenous infusion until oral intake is adequate. *Intravenous fluids are given to maintain vascular volume and to provide a route for antibiotic administration.*
- Assess wound, abdominal girth, and postoperative pain. *Swelling of the wound, increased abdominal girth, or an increase in pain may indicate infection or peritonitis.*
- Keep the patient with suspected appendicitis NPO, and do not administer laxatives or enemas. *Laxatives or enemas may cause perforation of the appendix.*
- No heat should be applied to the abdomen. *Heat may increase circulation to the appendix and also cause perforation.*

Manage Acute Pain. The patient with appendicitis experiences pain before and after surgery. Analgesia is limited until the diagnosis is established. Postoperative pain is controlled by narcotic or nonnarcotic analgesics.

Expected Outcome: Patient will express tolerable preoperative pain using pain scale. Patient will report adequate pain control postoperatively.

The nurse will:

- Assess pain, including its character, location, severity, and duration. Report any unexpected changes in the nature of pain. *Both preoperatively and postoperatively, the patient's pain provides important clues about the diagnosis and possible complications such as rupture of the appendix or peritonitis.*

SAFETY ALERT: Sudden relief of preoperative pain may signal rupture of the distended and edematous appendix. ■

- Administer analgesics as ordered. *Preoperatively, pain medication may be given cautiously until a diagnosis is established. Postoperatively, provide analgesics to maintain comfort and enhance mobility.*
- Assess effectiveness of medication 30 minutes after administration. Report unrelieved pain. *Pain unrelieved by prescribed analgesic may indicate a complication or the need for further assessment. For example, continued abdominal discomfort and distention may indicate excess intestinal gas that may be better relieved by ambulation.*

Transitions of Care

The incidence of appendicitis is lower in cultures where higher fiber intake is common. Encouraging a diet high in fiber and low in animal fats may prevent the development of appendicitis.

Preoperative teaching may be limited by pain and the urgent nature of surgery. Explain why food and fluids are not permitted during this time. If time allows, teach postoperative turning, coughing, deep breathing, and pain management.

With uncomplicated appendectomy, the patient is often discharged either the day of surgery or the day following surgery. Postoperative teaching includes:

- Wound or incision care, including hand hygiene and dressing change procedures as indicated
- Instructions to report fever, increased abdominal pain, swelling, redness, drainage, bleeding, or warmth of the operative site to the physician
- Activity limitations (e.g., lifting, driving), if any
- Returning to work, if appropriate.

The Patient with Peritonitis

Peritonitis, inflammation of the peritoneum, is a serious complication of many acute abdominal disorders. Peritonitis is usually caused by enteric bacteria entering the peritoneal cavity through a perforated ulcer, ruptured appendix, perforated diverticulum (discussed later in this chapter), necrotic bowel, or during abdominal surgery. Pelvic inflammatory disease, gallbladder rupture, abdominal trauma, or peritoneal dialysis can also lead to peritonitis.

Pathophysiology

The *peritoneum* is a double-layered serous membrane lining the walls (parietal peritoneum) and organs (visceral peritoneum) of the abdominal cavity. There is a potential space between the parietal and visceral layers of the peritoneum that contains a small amount of serous fluid.

Peritonitis results from contamination of the normally sterile peritoneal cavity by infection or a chemical irritant. Chemical peritonitis often precedes bacterial peritonitis.

Case Study & Nursing Care Plan

A Patient with Acute Appendicitis

Jamie Lynn is a 19-year-old college student majoring in physical therapy. Ms. Lynn arrives at the emergency department at 1:00 a.m. complaining of general lower abdominal pain that had started the previous evening. By midnight, the pain was more localized over the right lower quadrant. She also reports nausea and vomiting.

ASSESSMENT

Sue Grady, RN, completes the admission assessment in the emergency department. Ms. Lynn is complaining of nausea and severe abdominal pain, stating, "Walking makes my stomach hurt worse." Physical assessment findings include T 37.8°C (100.2°F), P 84 bpm, R 16/min, and BP 110/70 mmHg; skin warm to touch; abdomen flat and guarded, with marked tenderness in right lower quadrant. Ms. Lynn's CBC shows WBC 14,000/mm^3; neutrophils 81.1%; lymphocytes 12.5%. The diagnosis of acute appendicitis is made, and Ms. Lynn is transferred to surgery for a laparoscopic appendectomy.

DIAGNOSES

- Potential for surgical incision complications
- Acute pain related to surgery
- Anxiety related to surgery

EXPECTED OUTCOMES

- Patient's incision will heal without infection or complications.
- Patient will verbalize adequate pain relief.
- Patient will verbalize decreased anxiety.
- Patient will return to preoperative activities.

PLANNING AND IMPLEMENTATION

- Assess pain using a pain scale; provide analgesics as needed.
- Teach pain management following discharge.
- Teach abdominal splinting during coughing, turning, or ambulating as needed.
- Teach home care of incision.
- Discuss activity limitations as ordered.
- Instruct to report fever or warmth, redness, or drainage from the incision.

EVALUATION

On discharge the following evening, Ms. Lynn is fully ambulatory. Her appetite has returned, and she is tolerating food and fluids well. Her temperature is normal. The nurse provides Ms. Lynn with written and verbal information on postoperative care following an appendectomy.

CLINICAL REASONING IN PATIENT CARE

1. What is the pathophysiologic basis for Ms. Lynn's elevated WBC on admission?
2. How would Ms. Lynn's postoperative care and teaching differ if she had undergone a laparotomy instead of a laparoscopic appendectomy?
3. Outline a teaching plan to give to patients for home care following an appendectomy.
4. Develop a care plan for Ms. Lynn for the nursing diagnosis of anxiety related to surgery.

See Evaluating Your Response in Appendix B.

Perforation of a peptic ulcer or rupture of the gallbladder releases gastric juices (hydrochloric acid and pepsin) or bile into the peritoneal cavity, causing an acute inflammatory response.

Bacterial peritonitis is usually caused by infection by *Escherichia coli*, *Klebsiella*, *Proteus*, or *Pseudomonas* bacteria, which normally inhabit the bowel. Inflammatory and immune defense mechanisms are activated when bacteria enter the peritoneal space. These defenses can effectively eliminate small numbers of bacteria, but may be overwhelmed by massive or continued contamination. When this occurs, mast cells release histamine and other vasoactive substances, causing local vasodilation and increased capillary permeability. Polymorphonuclear leukocytes (a type of WBC) infiltrate the peritoneum to phagocytize bacteria and foreign matter. Fibrinogen-rich plasma exudate promotes bacterial destruction and forms fibrin clots to seal off and segregate the bacteria. This process helps limit and localize the infection, allowing host defenses to eradicate it. Continued contamination, however, leads to generalized inflammation of the peritoneal cavity. The inflammatory process causes fluid to shift into the peritoneal space (third spacing). Circulating blood volume is depleted, leading to hypovolemia. *Septicemia*, a systemic disease caused by pathogens or their toxins in the blood, may follow.

Manifestations

Manifestations of peritonitis depend on the severity and extent of the infection, as well as the age and general health of the patient. Both local and systemic manifestations are present. The patient often presents with evidence of an *acute abdomen*, an abrupt onset of diffuse, severe abdominal pain.

The pain may localize and intensify near the area of infection. Movement may intensify the pain. The entire abdomen is tender, with guarding or rigidity of abdominal muscles. The acute abdomen is often described as boardlike. Rebound tenderness may be present over the area of inflammation. Peritoneal inflammation inhibits peristalsis, resulting in a **paralytic ileus** (impaired propulsion or forward movement of bowel contents). Bowel sounds are markedly diminished or absent, and progressive abdominal distention is noted. Pooling of GI secretions may cause nausea and vomiting. Systemic manifestations of peritonitis include fever, malaise, tachycardia and tachypnea, restlessness, and possible disorientation. The patient may be oliguric (having little urine output) and show signs of dehydration and shock.

Patients who are older, chronically debilitated, or immunosuppressed may present with few of the classic signs of peritonitis. Increased confusion and restlessness, decreased urinary output, and vague abdominal complaints may be the only manifestations present. These patients are at increased risk for delayed diagnosis, contributing to a higher mortality rate.

Complications

Complications of peritonitis may be life-threatening. Abscess formation is common. This defense mechanism is designed to isolate and localize the infection, but it can also prevent immune responses and systemic antibiotics from reaching the source of the infection. Fibrous adhesions in the abdominal cavity are a late complication and may lead to subsequent obstruction. Patients with other medical conditions, older patients, and those with greater bacterial contamination have a higher risk of dying.

Without prompt and effective treatment, septicemia and septic shock can develop. Fluid loss into the abdominal cavity may lead to hypovolemic shock. These potentially lethal complications require immediate, aggressive intervention to prevent multiple organ failure and death. Septicemia, shock, and its management are discussed in Chapter 11.

Interprofessional Care

Care of the patient with peritonitis focuses on establishing the diagnosis and identifying and treating its cause as well as the peritonitis. Preventing complications is an important aspect of care.

Diagnosis

Diagnostic tests are performed to establish the diagnosis of peritonitis, rule out other disorders, and help identify the cause. The tests that may be ordered include a WBC (elevated to approximately 20,000/mm^3 in peritonitis), blood cultures, abdominal CT scan, liver and renal function studies, serum electrolytes, and a paracentesis (in peritonitis, peritoneal fluid will contain increased protein and WBCs). Increased numbers of immature blood cells are present as the bone marrow releases them in response to the infection.

Medications

Until the infecting organism has been identified, a broad-spectrum antibiotic effective against organisms commonly implicated in peritonitis is prescribed. A beta-lactam antibiotic such as imipenem (Primaxin) or meropenem (Merrem), which has a very broad spectrum of action, may be used. Once culture results have been obtained, antibiotic therapy is modified to the specific organism(s) responsible. Antibiotics that may be ordered include ampicillin (e.g., Omnipen, Polycillin), metronidazole (Flagyl), ciprofloxacin (Cipro), clindamycin (Cleocin), a cephalosporin such as ceftriaxone (Rocephin), or an aminoglycoside antibiotic such as gentamicin (Garamycin) or amikacin (Amikin). Nursing implications for antibiotic therapy are discussed in Chapter 12. Analgesics are prescribed to promote comfort.

Surgery

If the cause of peritonitis is a perforation, gangrenous bowel, or inflamed appendix, a laparotomy is done to close the perforation or remove the damaged and inflamed tissue. If an abscess is present, it may be surgically drained or removed.

Peritoneal lavage, washing of the peritoneal cavity with copious amounts of warm isotonic fluid, may be done during surgery. This procedure dilutes residual bacteria and removes gross contaminants, blood, and fibrin clots. In rare instances, peritoneal lavage may be continued for several days following surgery. The solution is infused into the upper portion of the peritoneal cavity and removed via drains in the pelvic cul-de-sac. Careful attention to fluid and electrolyte status and strict aseptic technique are necessary.

Patients who have had a laparotomy for peritonitis often return from surgery with either a Penrose or closed drain system such as a Jackson-Pratt drain. In some cases, the incision may be left unsutured. With severe and long-standing peritonitis, the abdomen may be closed temporarily with polypropylene mesh containing a nylon zipper or Velcro to allow repeated exploration of the abdomen and drainage of infectious sites.

Nutrition

Intravenous fluids and electrolyte replacements are administered to maintain vascular volume and fluid and electrolyte balance. Parenteral nutrition is given until adequate oral intake resumes.

Intestinal Decompression

The inflammatory process of peritonitis often draws large amounts of fluid into the abdominal cavity and the bowel. In addition, peristaltic activity of the bowel is slowed or halted by the inflammation, causing paralytic ileus (or *ileus*). Intestinal decompression is used to relieve abdominal distention, facilitate closure, and minimize postoperative respiratory problems. A nasogastric or long intestinal tube is inserted and connected to continuous drainage (**Figure 24.2 ■**). If prolonged intestinal decompression is anticipated, a jejunostomy may be performed for comfort. Suction is maintained until peristalsis resumes, bowel sounds are present, and the patient is passing flatus. Food and fluids are withheld until intestinal motility has returned and suction is discontinued.

Moving Evidence into Action

Enterally Fed, Seriously Ill Patient

Clinical Issue

A vital component of the treatment and care of seriously ill patients (such as those with peritonitis) is providing nutritional support, primarily through enteral feedings. Enteral feeding involves the placement of a tube in the stomach or small intestine. A variety of formulas are available and are infused intermittently or continuously through the gastric or enteral feeding tube. Although this remains the method of choice for the seriously ill population and has many advantages, enteral feeding also comes with the risk of malposition of the feeding tube, resulting in pulmonary injury associated with aspiration, pneumothorax, atelectasis, and pleural effusion. Not much information has been published about how to assess for misplacement and migration of the tube in enterally fed patients.

External Evidence

Stepter (2012) conducted a systematic review of the literature to identify recommendations to improve the quality and safety of administering enteral nutrition to seriously ill patients. This systematic review found that nurses frequently use methods to care for patients that are not supported by evidence. Leckey, Davis, and Raphael-Grimm (2017) surveyed patients receiving gastric and enteral feeding in an outpatient setting and found patients and caregivers need ongoing education and support to safely manage tube feedings. Recommended techniques to prevent complications associated with enteral tube feedings included:

- Prevent aspiration with feeding tube placement by verifying placement via radiologic confirmation. After verifying the placement, the tube should be securely taped and the external tube length should be measured, noted, and marked on the tube as a reference point for further tube placement checks. If the position of the tube is questioned, the x-ray should be repeated.
- Maintain the head of the bed at an angle of at least 30 degrees, with 45 degrees being ideal. Stop feedings 30 to 60 minutes before placing the patient in the supine position.
- Flush with water only (no juice, soda, or meat tenderizer).
- Eliminate the use of blue dye in feedings.
- Maintain cuff pressure in patients with artificial airways at 20 to 30 cm H_2O.
- Administer medications separately, flushing with water before and after each drug is administered.

Internal Evidence

As part of the evaluation of internal evidence the nurse must consider this type of enteral feeding tube (gastrostomy tube, percutaneous endoscopic gastrostomy tube, jejunostomy tube), the underlying reason tube feeding was initiated, medications that will be administered via the tube, the outcome of interest (improved nutritional status), current policies/procedures and potential complications. The patient's response to tube feedings should be assessed throughout the treatment period. The patient and family caregivers must be taught to recognize signs of incorrect tube placement (Leckey et al., 2017).

Patient Considerations

During hospitalization daily assessments of the patient and the feeding tube using multiple methods (including x-ray, external length marking, pH testing, aspirate characteristics, or trypsin/pepsin levels) should be conducted by caregivers who have the knowledge to accurately interpret the results. Careful and continuous monitoring for signs of incorrect enteral tube placement such as aspiration, pneumothorax, atelectasis, and pleural effusion is an essential aspect of nursing care. Patients may be discharged with gastric and enteral tube feedings. Nurses should ensure transitional care is in place to provide ongoing assessment and teaching for the patient once at home (Leckey et al., 2017).

Putting the Pieces Together

Using best practice when administering tube feedings via gastric and enteral feeding tubes will decrease the incidence of complications. Using agency policy and external evidence, traditional habits can be replaced with evidence-based practice that will minimize the risk of complications and assure the patient attains nutritional goals (Leckey et al., 2017; Stepter, 2012).

References

Leckey, J., Davis, S., & Raphael-Grimm, T. (2017). Nursing assessment of patients requiring enteral and gastric feeding tubes. *Gastroenterology Nursing*, *40*(6), 469–483.

Stepter, C. (2012). Maintaining placement of temporary enteral feeding tubes in adults: A critical appraisal of the evidence. *Medsurg Nursing*, *21*(2), 61–68.

Nursing Care

Assessment

- *Health history:* Pain, its onset, character, severity, location, aggravating and relieving factors; associated symptoms such as anorexia, nausea and vomiting; current and previous history of peptic ulcer disease, gallbladder disease, chronic diseases; current medications
- *Physical assessment:* Vital signs including temperature; level of consciousness; skin color, temperature, warmth, capillary refill, and turgor; abdominal shape, contour, bowel sounds, tenderness, tympany, and guarding.

Priorities of Care

Patients with peritonitis require intensive nursing and medical care to prevent complications and recover fully. Nursing care priorities include interventions to manage pain, altered fluid balance, infection, and anxiety. The patient is placed on bedrest in Fowler position to help localize the infection and promote lung ventilation. Oxygen is often administered to facilitate cellular metabolism and healing.

Diagnoses, Outcomes, and Interventions

Relieve Acute Pain. Abdominal distention and acute inflammation contribute to the pain associated with peritonitis. Surgery further disrupts abdominal muscles and other tissues, causing pain. Effective pain management promotes immune function, healing, mobility, and recovery.

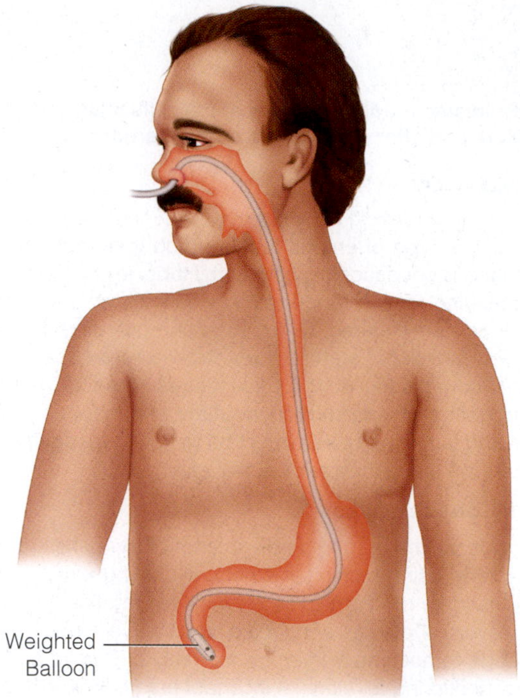
Weighted
Balloon

Figure 24.2 ■ The weighted tip or inflated balloon at the end of an intestinal tube is drawn into the intestine by gravity and peristalsis.

Expected Outcome: Patient will identify early escalation of pain, will use treatment plan (pharmacologic and nonpharmacologic) to prevent and alleviate discomfort, and will report relief from pain.

The nurse will:

- Assess pain, including its location, severity (using a standard pain scale), and type. Monitor analgesic effectiveness. Report changes to the primary care provider. *A change in pain may indicate the patient's condition is worsening.*

SAFETY ALERT: Unrelieved pain or a change in the location, severity, or type of pain may indicate spread of infection, abscess formation, or other complications of peritonitis. ■

- Place in Fowler or semi-Fowler position with the knees and feet elevated. *This position reduces stress on abdominal structures and facilitates respirations, promoting comfort.*
- Administer analgesics as ordered on a routine basis or using patient-controlled analgesia (PCA). *Routine analgesic administration maintains a therapeutic blood level and helps maintain comfort, facilitating healing and movement.*
- Teach and assist with adjunctive pain management techniques such as meditation, visualization, massage, and progressive relaxation. *Adjunctive measures augment analgesics and help promote a sense of control over pain.*

Restore Vascular Fluid Volume. In peritonitis, significant amounts of fluid are drawn into the abdominal cavity and bowel, reducing vascular volume and cardiac output. This fluid may also be lost from the body by intestinal suction or through drains placed in the abdomen during surgery. An unsutured incision causes additional significant fluid loss.

Expected Outcome: Deficient fluid volume in the patient will be prevented as evidenced by normal vital signs, lab values, and absence of physical signs of dehydration (e.g., thirst, change in mental status, decreased urine output, dry skin and mucous membrane, weakness, sudden weight loss).

The nurse will:

- Maintain accurate intake and output records. Measure urine output every 1 to 2 hours; report output of less than 30 mL/h. Measure gastrointestinal output at least every 4 hours. *Intake and output records provide valuable information about fluid volume status.*

SAFETY ALERT: Urine output of less than 30 mL/h may indicate hypovolemia, decreased cardiac output, and impaired tissue perfusion. ■

- Monitor vital signs and hemodynamic parameters such as central venous pressure, cardiac output, and pulmonary artery pressures every hour or as indicated. *These measurements provide important information about fluid and vascular volumes as well as cardiovascular status.*
- Weigh daily. *Weight is an accurate indicator of fluid status. Rapid weight gains or losses reflect changes in fluid volume.*
- Assess skin turgor, color, temperature, and mucous membranes at least every 8 hours. *Warm, dry skin with poor turgor and dry, shiny mucous membranes indicate dehydration.*
- Measure or estimate fluid losses through abdominal drains and on dressings. *Significant amounts of exudative fluid may be lost.*
- Monitor laboratory values, including hemoglobin and hematocrit, urine specific gravity, serum osmolality and electrolytes, and ABGs. Report changes to the physician. *Laboratory results provide information about fluid and electrolyte status and acid–base balance.*
- Administer intravenous fluids and electrolytes as ordered. Gastrointestinal drainage may be replaced milliliter for milliliter with a balanced electrolyte solution. *Intravenous fluids are necessary to meet daily fluid intake needs, as well as replace continuing losses of water and electrolytes.*
- Provide good skin care and frequent oral hygiene. *Fluid deficit increases the risk of skin breakdown and ulceration of mucous membranes.*

Promote Surgical Recovery. Repeated surgeries, an unsutured incision, and the presence of drains interrupt skin integrity and the body's first line of defense against microorganisms. In addition, immune defenses are stressed by the infection and potential malnutrition. An acute infection such as peritonitis causes a stress response with excess energy expenditure and loss of body proteins and cell mass. Glycogen stores are rapidly depleted, and body proteins are used to meet energy needs. Withholding food further complicates this process, leading to rapid development of protein-calorie malnutrition (PCM). PCM impairs the immune response and slows healing. As a result, the risk for impaired healing and further infection is increased.

Expected Outcome: Patient will experience regeneration of cells and tissue without signs of infection (e.g., redness, swelling, purulent drainage, fever).

The nurse will:

- Monitor temperature, pulse rate, and for localized signs of infection such as redness and swelling around incisions and drain sites, increased or purulent drainage, and cloudy or malodorous urine. *Impaired defenses increase the risk for extension of the infection or unrelated infections.*
- Obtain cultures of purulent drainage from any site. *Early identification of any additional infection allows timely intervention.*
- Monitor WBC and differential, serum protein, and albumin. *An increased WBC with a higher percentage of immature cells present in the blood is an indicator of infection and normal immune response. Serum albumin and protein levels are indicators of nutritional status as well as immune function.*
- Practice meticulous hand hygiene and use standard precautions at all times. *Hand hygiene reduces transient bacteria on the skin and remains the most important method of controlling infection. Standard precautions reduce the risk of spreading infection to or from the patient.*
- Use strict aseptic technique for dressing changes, wound care, and irrigations. *Disruption of the protective barrier of the skin increases the risk of contamination and further infection.*
- Maintain fluid balance and nutritional status through enteral or parenteral feedings, as indicated. See the Moving Evidence into Action box for evidence-based recommendations for care of enterally fed patients. *Adequate nutrition and fluid balance are necessary for optimal immune system function.*

Provide Discharge Teaching and Planning. Teaching for home care includes the following topics:

- Wound care procedures, including dressing changes or irrigations. Provide verbal and written instructions on how to change dressings or do irrigations as well as where to obtain supplies, and allow opportunities to practice and demonstrate the procedure prior to discharge.
- Prescribed medications, including name and purpose of the drug, potential adverse effects, and their management
- Manifestations of further infection (redness, heat, swelling, purulent drainage, chills, and fever) and potential complications to be reported to the care provider
- Prescribed activity restrictions
- Instructions for a high-calorie, high-protein diet for healing and optimal immune function.

Provide a referral to home health services for assessment, wound care, and further teaching, as needed.

Transitions of Care

Peritonitis is a serious illness. Early recognition and treatment are important to minimize the risk of complications.

Acute peritonitis requires ongoing assessment and management by the nurse as a member of the interprofessional healthcare team. Stabilizing vital signs, obtaining hemodynamic homeostasis, and aggressive treatment of the infection is the focus of care.

Primary bacterial peritonitis associated with chronic disease such as cirrhosis of the liver, metastatic malignancy, congestive heart failure, and other chronic conditions has a high rate of reoccurrence. Use of prophylactic antibiotics is recommended (Barshak & Kasper, 2018). The nurse managing patients in the outpatient setting should teach patients the early signs of infection, monitor the administration of antibiotics, and coordinate ongoing care.

Death due to peritonitis will likely be unexpected and associated with a critical condition. The nurse should support the family and assist with preparing the body for viewing. Collaborating with the interprofessional team including social work and spiritual care will be the focus of end-of-life care.

The Patient with Gastroenteritis

Gastroenteritis, or *enteritis*, is an inflammation of the stomach and small intestine. Enteritis may be caused by bacteria, viruses, parasites, or toxins. Upper GI manifestations such as anorexia and nausea and vomiting are common. Diarrhea of varying intensity and abdominal discomfort are nearly universal features of gastroenteritis.

The infectious organism usually enters the body in contaminated water or food. For this reason, gastroenteritis is often called *food poisoning*. Viruses commonly cause acute diarrheal illness. Diarrhea due to rotaviruses or the Norwalk virus occurs year-round in both adults and children. These illnesses are generally mild and self-limited, and reinfections are progressively less severe. However, rotaviruses can have severe consequences in the very young, the very old, or in people with impaired immune function.

Pathophysiology

Bacterial or viral infection of the GI tract produces inflammation, tissue damage, and manifestations by two primary mechanisms:

- ***Production of exotoxins:*** A number of bacteria produce and excrete an exotoxin that enters the surrounding environment (intestinal lumen), causing damage and inflammation. Exotoxins in the GI tract are often referred to as *enterotoxins*. They impair intestinal absorption and can cause secretion of significant amounts of electrolytes and water into the bowel, resulting in diarrhea and fluid loss. Common bacterial enterotoxins include those produced by *Staphylococcus*, *Clostridium perfringens*, *Clostridium botulinum*, some strains of *Escherichia coli*, *Vibrio cholera*, and *C. difficile*.

- *Invasion and ulceration of the mucosa:* Other bacteria, including some *Shigella*, *Salmonella*, and *E. coli* species, damage tissue more directly. They invade the intestinal mucosa of the small bowel or colon, producing microscopic ulceration, bleeding, fluid exudate, and water and electrolyte secretion.

In some cases, the mechanism of injury is unclear. It may be a combination of direct and toxic damage. For example, the Norwalk virus damages the mucosa of the jejunum.

Manifestations

Although the manifestations of bacterial and viral enteritis vary according to the organism involved, several features are common. Anorexia and nausea and vomiting are caused by distention of the upper GI tract by unabsorbed chyme and excess water. Bowel distention, along with irritation of the bowel mucosa and gas production due to fermentation of undigested food, leads to abdominal pain and cramping. Borborygmi, excessively loud and hyperactive bowel sounds, are another result. The abdomen is often distended and tender.

Diarrhea is usually predominant with enteritis. Fluid is secreted into the bowel lumen, and the unabsorbed chyme and electrolytes create an osmotic pull of fluid into the bowel. Motility is stimulated, and stools become watery and frequent. Loss of fluids and electrolytes through diarrhea can lead to the most serious manifestations of enteritis. Refer to Chapter 10 for manifestations related to fluid and electrolyte loss. Fluid volume can be rapidly depleted, leading to dehydration and hypovolemia. Orthostatic hypotension and fever may be noted initially. If fluid loss continues, hypovolemic shock may develop.

Complications

Electrolyte and acid–base imbalances may result from gastroenteritis. Extensive vomiting can lead to metabolic alkalosis due to the loss of hydrochloric acid from the stomach. When diarrhea dominates, metabolic acidosis is more likely. Potassium is lost in either case, leading to hypokalemia. Hyponatremia may develop if fluids are replaced with pure water. Headache, cardiac irregularities, changes in respiratory rate and pattern, malaise and weakness, muscle aching, and signs of neuromuscular irritability are the possible manifestations of these disturbances in homeostasis.

Several gastrointestinal infections produce specific effects that are summarized in **Table 24.3**.

Interprofessional Care

The goals of care for gastroenteritis are to manage the manifestations, prevent complications, identify the cause of the

Table 24.3 Selected Bacterial Infections of the Bowel

Disease and Organism	Incubation	Pathogenesis	Manifestations	Management
Traveler's diarrhea: *Escherichia coli*	24.172 hours	Enterotoxin causes hypersecretion of the small intestine.	Abrupt onset of diarrhea; vomiting rare	Prophylactic bismuth subsalicylate; antidiarrheal such as loperamide; 3-day course of norfloxacin, ciprofloxacin, or azithromycin
Hemorrhagic colitis: *E. coli* O157:H7	1–3 days	Enterotoxin causes direct mucosal damage in large intestine; also toxic to vascular endothelial cells.	Severe abdominal cramping, watery diarrhea that becomes grossly bloody; fever; possible complications: Hemolytic uremic syndrome and thrombotic thrombocytopenic purpura	Supportive care with fluid replacement and bland diet; may require dialysis or plasmapheresis for complications
Staphylococcal food poisoning	2–8 hours	Enterotoxin impairs intestinal absorption and affects vomiting centers in the brain.	Severe nausea and vomiting; abdominal cramping and diarrhea; headache and fever	Fluid and electrolyte replacement as needed
Cholera: *Vibrio cholerae*	1–3 days	Enterotoxin affects entire small intestine, causing secretion of water and electrolytes into bowel lumen.	Severe diarrhea with "rice water stool," gray, cloudy, odorless, with no blood or pus; vomiting; thirst, oliguria, muscle cramps, weakness; dehydration and vascular collapse	Oral or intravenous rehydration; possible antimicrobial therapy with tetracycline, doxycycline, ciprofloxacin, others
Salmonellosis: *Salmonella*	8–48 hours	Superficial infection of the GI tract without invasion or production of toxins.	Diarrhea with abdominal cramping and nausea and vomiting; low-grade fever, chills, weakness	Treatment of symptoms; a third-generation cephalosporin or a fluoroquinolone antibiotic for severe illness
Shigellosis (bacillary dysentery): *Shigella*	1–4 days	Local tissue invasion, primarily involving large intestine and distal ileum; endotoxin causes fluid and electrolyte secretion into bowel lumen.	Watery diarrhea with severe abdominal cramping and tenesmus; lethargy	Fluid and electrolyte replacement; correction of acidosis; antibiotic therapy with ciprofloxacin, ceftriaxone, others
Clostridium difficile colitis: *C. difficile*	1–2 weeks	Antibiotic therapy interferes with normal protective bacteria in the colon; *C. difficile* colonizes and releases toxins that cause mucosal inflammation and damage.	Diarrhea, abdominal cramps, malaise, fever, anorexia	Cessation of the causative antibiotic; antibiotic therapy with metronidazole (specific for *C. difficile*)—possibly vancomycin for resistant strains

Moving Evidence into Action

Decreasing *Clostridium difficile* Infections

Clinical Issue

Clostridium difficile is a severe infection of the colon that occurs after normal flora of the gut is eliminated through the use of antibiotics. The incidence of *C. difficile* infection (CDI) is increasing in hospitals and is the most common cause of antibiotic-associated infection. CDI is listed as an epidemiologically significant organism in The Joint Commission's National Safety Goal and an estimated 7178 inpatients are infected with CDI in the U.S. hospitals in any one day. The estimated cost of CDI in the United States is approximately $32.1 billion per year (Pokrywka et al., 2014).

External Evidence

Numerous studies have shown that hand hygiene using soap and water is significantly more effective at removing *C. difficile* spores than are alcohol-based hand rubs. Edmonds et al. (2013) compared use of soap and water with several hand hygiene preparations. Results showed commonly used alcohol-based hand hygiene preparations used in hospitals did not aid in spore removal. Preparations more effective than soap and water were too harsh for the skin given the frequency of handwashing required. The researchers confirmed the recommendation for hand hygiene practice with antimicrobial soap and water using friction for a minimum of 15 seconds. Another study demonstrated the importance of ensuring patients' handwashing is included in strategies aimed to reduce *C. difficile* hospital-acquired infection (Haverstick et al., 2017). Ensuring that hospital staff and visitors comply with contact precautions was also confirmed as an important standard of care to implement for patients with CDI (O'Connor, 2017).

Internal Evidence

As part of the evaluation of internal evidence, one must consider the incidence of *C. difficile* in the facility. Correctly identifying a new case as a community-acquired infection or one that was acquired in the facility is important to prevent the spread of disease in the setting. Identifying whether a transmission is occurring in an organization or in the community helps the facility determine whether practices need to be changed.

Patient Considerations

Patients are getting sicker and pathogens continue to evolve as the prevalence of healthcare-associated infections increases. In addition to assuming responsibility for creating, implementing, and evaluating plans of care for individual patients with CDI, nurses must participate in developing a plan of care for the environment to prevent transmission to other patients and staff (O'Connor, 2017).

Putting the Pieces Together

In summary, hand hygiene using soap and water along with contact precautions is necessary to prevent the spread of CDI. Contaminated medical equipment such as stethoscopes, commodes, and bathtubs contribute to the transmission of CD. Ensuring that the environmental services department uses appropriate disinfectants to eradicate CDI spores is essential. Educating unlicensed assistive personnel (UAP) on precautions to prevent transmission of CDI among patients should be included in planned nursing interventions (O'Connor, 2017).

References

Edmonds, S. L., Zapka, C. Kasper, D., Gerber, R., McCormack, R., Macinga, D., . . . Gerding, D.N. (2013); Effectiveness of hand hygiene for removal of *Clostridium difficile* spores from hands. *Infection Control and Hospital Epidemiology*, *14*(3), 302–305.

Haverstick, S., Goodrich, C., Freeman, R., James, S., Kullar, R., & Ahrens, M. (2017). Patients' hand washing and reducing hospital-acquired infection. *Critical Care Nurse*, *37*(3), e1–e8.

O'Connor, N. (2017). Six things you can do to today to prevent hospital-onset *C. difficile* tomorrow. *American Journal of Nursing*, *117*(9), 47–49.

Pokrywka, M., Feigel, J., Douglas, B., Grossberger, S., Hensler, A., & Weber, D. (2014). A bundle strategy including patient hand hygiene to decrease *clostridium difficile* infections. *Medsurg Nursing*, *23*(3), 145–148.

infection, and prevent its spread. The history and manifestations provide valuable cues about the cause. Diagnostic testing is used to identify the pathogen and evaluate its effects. In most cases, treatment is supportive, directed toward relieving manifestations, restoring fluid and electrolyte balance, and maintaining function.

Diagnosis

If manifestations are severe or do not resolve within about 48 hours, laboratory testing is used to identify the causative organism and to assess fluid, electrolyte, and acid–base balance. A stool specimen for culture, ova and parasites, and fecal leukocytes usually reveals the infective organism, but may require up to 6 weeks to identify some bacteria. In infections such as botulism, the toxin itself may be isolated in the stool. Contamination of the stool by urine or treatment with antibiotics, bismuth subsalicylate (Pepto-Bismol), or mineral oil may interfere with pathogen growth, altering stool culture results. Use a clean bedpan or collection device to obtain the stool specimen, and instruct the patient to avoid mixing the stool with urine or toilet tissue.

A sigmoidoscopy may be done to differentiate inflammatory bowel disease from infectious processes. It does not replace stool cultures because the lesions associated with some infectious processes are indistinguishable from those of ulcerative colitis. (Nursing care of the patient having a sigmoidoscopy is discussed in Chapter 21.)

Serum osmolality and electrolytes and ABGs are done to assess and monitor fluid, electrolyte, and acid–base balance. Common imbalances associated with enteritis and diarrhea are outlined in **Table 24.4**.

Medications

Acute enteritis usually resolves spontaneously, and no drug treatment is required. If the patient is severely ill and manifestations are prolonged, medications may be prescribed.

Antibiotic therapy specific to the organism may be used to treat bacterial colitis, cholera, salmonellosis, or shigellosis. Ciprofloxacin (Cipro), clarithromycin (Biaxin), erythromycin, amoxicillin–clavulanate (Augmentin), or another antibiotic may be prescribed. Stool culture is obtained prior to starting antibiotics, but treatment may begin before

Table 24.4 Laboratory Values Associated with Enteritis and Diarrhea

Test	Normal Value	Change with Significant Diarrhea
Serum osmolality	280–300 mOsm/kg	Increased; levels above 320 mOsm/kg indicate significant dehydration.
Serum potassium	3.5–5.3 mEq/L	Decreased due to loss through stool and vomitus; levels below 2.5 mEq/L are critical.
Serum sodium	135–145 mEq/L	Decreased due to loss through stool and vomitus; may be significant when fluid losses are replaced with pure water; levels below 120 mEq/L may be critical.
Serum chloride	95–105 mEq/L	Increased when sodium loss is greater than chloride loss; decreased with severe diarrhea and with vomiting; possible critical values are below 80 mEq/L or above 115 mEq/L.
Blood gases		
▪ pH	Arterial: 7.35–7.45	Decreased in metabolic acidosis, a possible result of severe diarrhea; increased in metabolic alkalosis, a possible result of severe vomiting and chloride loss; values below 7.25 or above 7.55 are critical.
▪ $PaCO_2$	Arterial: 35–45 mmHg	Typically decreased in metabolic acidosis as the body attempts to eliminate excess acid by "blowing off" CO_2; increased with metabolic alkalosis as the body retains CO_2 in an attempt to normalize pH.
▪ Bicarbonate	24.128 mEq/L	Decreased in metabolic acidosis; increased in metabolic alkalosis.
Hematocrit	Males: 40–54% Females: 36–46%	Increased with dehydration and hypovolemia as a result of concentration of blood cells.
Urine specific gravity	1.005–1.030	Increased with dehydration and hypovolemia as kidneys attempt to conserve fluid.

culture results are available. A presumptive diagnosis based on history and presenting manifestations guides the choice of antibiotic.

An antidiarrheal drug may be prescribed to promote comfort and reduce fluid loss. Nursing measures related to antidiarrheal medications are outlined in Medication Administration 24.A.

Use of antidiarrheal preparations prolongs the course and increases risk for complications in some types of gastroenteritis, and therefore is contraindicated. Obtain a careful history before recommending these agents to the patient.

Nutrition and Fluids

Replacing lost fluids and electrolytes is vital when vomiting and/or diarrhea are severe or prolonged. In many cases of enteritis, fluid and electrolyte replacement are all that is required until the infection resolves.

Oral rehydration is preferred for replacing physiologic fluids. An oral glucose-electrolyte solution is often well tolerated in sips, even when vomiting is present. Intravenous rehydration may be necessary with severe diarrhea and fluid loss. In some cases, a combination of oral and intravenous fluids may be used to replace lost fluids and maintain vascular volume. Balanced electrolyte solutions, such as glucose in normal saline and Ringer solution, are used. Lactated Ringer solution or another alkalinizing solution may be ordered if metabolic acidosis is present.

Gastric Lavage

Gastric lavage and catharsis—in effect, "washing out" the stomach and intestines—may be performed to remove unabsorbed toxin from the GI tract if botulism is suspected.

Plasmapheresis

Plasmapheresis (plasma exchange therapy) may be performed to remove circulating toxins for hemorrhagic colitis caused by *E. coli*. See Chapter 44 for the nursing care of a patient having this procedure. Potential complications include those associated with intravenous catheters, shifts in fluid balance, and altered blood clotting.

Dialysis

Acute tubular necrosis and renal failure associated with hemorrhagic colitis may necessitate dialysis to remove wastes and prevent severe fluid and electrolyte imbalances and metabolic acidosis. Although acute renal failure often resolves spontaneously and renal function resumes, dialysis can be lifesaving. Either hemodialysis or peritoneal dialysis may be used, generally as a temporary measure. Nursing care related to acute renal failure and dialysis is discussed in Chapter 28.

Nursing Care

Most patients are treated in community settings. Assessment, education, and support of self-care measures are major nursing responsibilities.

Assessment

- *Health history:* Onset, duration, and severity of manifestations; recent activities such as attending a picnic or potluck, international travel, or camping; other affected members of the household; measures taken to relieve manifestations or replace fluids
- *Physical assessment:* Vital signs including temperature and orthostatic blood pressure; skin color, temperature, moisture, and turgor; peripheral pulses and capillary refill; abdominal shape, contour, bowel sounds, tenderness.

Priorities of Care

Diarrhea and dehydration are priority nursing diagnoses. See the earlier section of this chapter on diarrhea for specific nursing interventions related to these diagnoses. Nausea and vomiting frequently accompany the diarrhea associated with gastroenteritis. Nursing care of the patient experiencing nausea and vomiting is detailed in Chapter 23.

Diagnoses, Outcomes, and Interventions

Nursing care for the patient with diarrhea is supportive and educational. Manifestations of diarrhea can interfere with the patient's ability to maintain normal roles and responsibilities.

Transitions of Care

Nurses play significant roles in preventing enteritis as educators, community health providers, and advocates for environmental safety.

Teach the importance of proper food handling and maintaining appropriate temperatures. Raw fruits and vegetables should be thoroughly washed before consuming. Adequate cooking of meat products is vital to prevent disorders such as staphylococcal food poisoning, *E. coli* hemorrhagic colitis, and salmonellosis. Emphasize the importance of not consuming raw meat products, and cooking hamburger, in particular, to the point that no redness is noted in the meat. The highly pathogenic *E. coli* serotype O157:H7 is present in the gut of infected animals. Meats from the animal may be contaminated with bowel contents. The organism is readily destroyed by heat, so cuts of meat such as steaks or roasts are less likely to cause infection, since the organism is on the outside of the meat. However, the process of grinding hamburger allows *E. coli* to be mixed throughout the meat. Thorough cooking destroys the organism. This pathogen (and others) may be spread through unpasteurized milk. Discuss the dangers of consuming milk that has not been pasteurized and encourage patients to avoid it.

Dairy products, eggs, and egg products left at room temperature provide a good growth medium for bacteria. Discuss the importance of prompt refrigeration of meats and these products to minimize this risk. Many gastrointestinal infections are spread through contaminated water. Encourage travelers to consume only bottled water unless local water supplies are clearly safe. Water purification tablets are available for hikers and campers, and may be used when traveling abroad.

Acute care of the patient with gastroenteritis will focus on providing IV therapy to restore fluid and electrolyte balance. Antibiotic therapy will be initiated for the patient requiring hospitalization. The patient will be placed in isolation and nursing responsibilities include strict handwashing and environmental control to prevent the spread of infection in the facility.

Discuss the following self-care topics with the patient:

- The importance of good hand hygiene, particularly before handling food and after each bowel movement
- The need to wash clothing and linens contaminated with feces separately in hot water and detergent
- Oral solutions to replace lost fluids and electrolytes
- Appropriate use of antidiarrheal medications, if recommended
- Manifestations of complications to report to the healthcare provider.

The Patient with a Protozoal Bowel Infection

Parasites live within, on, or at the expense of other organisms. Parasitic intestinal infections are common in developing countries. They include both protozoal and helminthic (parasitic worm) infections. Parasites that infect the bowel usually enter the GI tract through the mouth by the fecal–oral route; some are spread by direct contact or through sexual activity.

Of the protozoal bowel infections, only giardiasis is common in the United States. Amebiasis is found chiefly in the tropics and where sanitation is poor. Cryptosporidiosis, a form of coccidiosis, is an important worldwide cause of sporadic mild diarrhea, traveler's diarrhea, and severe diarrhea in people who are immunocompromised.

Pathophysiology and Manifestations

The most common protozoal infections of the bowel are summarized in **Table 24.5**.

Interprofessional Care

Management of protozoal bowel infections includes identifying the causative organism and administering medications.

Diagnosis

Diagnostic testing includes a stool examination for ova and parasites and possibly for their antigens. Many protozoa are shed intermittently rather than continuously; stools are collected sequentially (e.g., every other day for a total of three specimens). These organisms are often fragile, requiring a fresh stool specimen. Serology testing for an immune response to the suspected parasite may be performed. A sigmoidoscopy may be done to examine the bowel mucosa and collect a stool specimen for examination (in this case, no bowel prep is done prior to the test). When giardiasis is suspected, duodenal aspirate may be stained and examined microscopically for the protozoa. Small-bowel biopsy can identify giardiasis or *Cryptosporidium* infection.

Medications

Pharmacologic treatment includes both local and systemic antiparasitic drugs, such as iodoquinol (Amebaquin), paromomycin (Humatin), metronidazole (Flagyl), tinidazole (Tindamax), or nitazoxanide (Alinia). Treatment is usually provided on an outpatient basis. Severe amebic dysentery may require hospitalization for intravenous fluid and electrolyte replacements. Nursing care related to common antiprotozoal drugs is outlined in **Medication Administration 24.C**.

Nursing Care

Nursing assessment, diagnoses, and interventions for the patient with a protozoal GI infection are similar to those indicated for patients with bacterial or viral infections. Diarrhea and potential for dehydration are priority nursing diagnoses. See previous sections of this chapter for specific nursing interventions related to these diagnoses.

Table 24.5 Common Protozoal Infections of the Bowel

Disease and Organism	Incubation	Pathogenesis	Manifestations	Management
Giardiasis: *Giardia lamblia*	1–3 weeks or more	Trophozoite attaches to mucosa in duodenum and jejunum, causing superficial invasion, inflammation, and tissue destruction.	Diarrhea, mild or severe, daily or intermittent; anorexia, nausea and vomiting; epigastric pain, cramping, distention; flatulence and belching; may be asymptomatic	Metronidazole (Flagyl, others), tinidazole (Tindamax), nitazoxanide (Alinia)
Amebiasis: *Entamoeba histolytica*	2–4 weeks	Organisms may reside in large intestine without causing disease or can invade colon wall, causing ulceration; may be carried via blood to liver to produce abscess.	Usually asymptomatic; diarrhea may be mild, with few semiformed mucus-containing stools per day, or severe, with 10–20 blood-streaked liquid stools per day; abdominal cramps and flatulence; colic, tenesmus, vomiting, tenderness; fatigue, weight loss; prostration and toxicity	Metronidazole and paromomycin (Humatin) or iodoquinol (Diiodohydroxyquin, Yodoxin); metronidazole or tinidazole for hepatic abscess
Cryptosporidiosis: *Cryptosporidium*	2–10 days	Organisms attach to epithelial surface of small bowel (jejunum), causing villous atrophy and mild inflammatory changes; may secrete enterotoxin.	In immunocompetent patients: Asymptomatic to profuse, watery diarrhea of sudden onset, abdominal cramping; malaise, fever; anorexia, nausea and vomiting. In immunodeficient patients: Profuse watery diarrhea with loss of up to 15–20 L/day; severe malabsorption, electrolyte imbalance; weight loss; lymphadenopathy	Self-limiting in immunocompetent patients. For immunodeficient patients: Spiramycin, zidovudine (AZT), paromomycin (Humatin), octreotide, eflornithine; fluid and electrolyte replacement; parenteral nutrition as needed

Medication Administration 24.C

Antiprotozoal Agents

ANTI-INFECTIVE, ANTIPROTOZOAN MEDICATIONS

Amebicides

iodoquinol (Yodoxin, Amebaquin)

metronidazole (Flagyl, Metazol, others)

paromomycin (Humatin)

Antiprotozoal

nitrazoxanide (Alina)

tinidazole (Tindamax)

Patients with symptomatic protozoal infections are generally treated with a systemic antiprotozoal agent. Metronidazole is the most widely used of these antiprotozoal agents and is the drug of choice for treating amebiasis.

Nursing Responsibilities

- Assess for possible contraindications to therapy:
  a. Hypersensitivity to the prescribed agent or related drugs
  b. Liver dysfunction or blood dyscrasias
  c. Concurrent use of alcohol or an MAOI
  d. Pregnancy
- Administer as ordered:
  a. Metronidazole may be given orally after meals or as a continuous or intermittent intravenous infusion.
  b. Administer furazolidone and albendazole orally with meals to minimize gastric distress.
- Observe for possible adverse effects; notify the physician if significant. Gastrointestinal effects are common.
  a. Peripheral neuropathy and CNS effects may occur with metronidazole.
  b. Blood dyscrasias may develop with furazolidone or albendazole; monitor CBC and report abnormal results.
  c. Furazolidone can cause hypoglycemia; carefully monitor blood glucose in patients with diabetes.
  d. Report abnormal liver function test results.
- Monitor the character and number of stools; obtain specimens as ordered to evaluate the effectiveness of therapy.

Health Education for the Patient and Family

- Take the drug as prescribed for the full duration of the prescription.
- Taking oral preparations after meals helps minimize gastrointestinal side effects. Notify the physician if nausea and vomiting continue.
- Do not use alcohol while taking these drugs. An Antabuse-type response with severe headache, flushing, and vomiting may occur.
- Report adverse effects to the physician, including dizziness and other nervous system changes, sore throats, fatigue, bruising, or infection.
- Candidiasis of the mouth or vagina may occur with metronidazole therapy. Report symptoms to the physician.
- A harmless change in urine color to deep yellow (quinacrine) or rust or brown (metronidazole or chloroquine) may occur while taking these drugs.
- If you have diabetes and are taking furazolidone, carefully monitor blood glucose levels because hypoglycemia may develop.
- Practice good hand hygiene, particularly after using the toilet, to prevent transmitting the protozoa to others.

Note: Drugs identified in *blue* are among the 200 most commonly prescribed medications in the United States.

Source: Data from Adams et al., 2017.

Transitions of Care

Nurses need to teach the public how parasitic diseases are transmitted and how to avoid spreading the infection. Prevention of amebiasis and giardiasis involves:

- Provision of safe water supplies
- Appropriate disposal of human feces
- Safe food storage, handling, and preparation
- Adequate hand hygiene after defecating and before handling food.

Instruct people living in high-risk areas (e.g., tropical climates, areas with untreated water supplies) to boil, filter, or treat water supplies with iodine to eliminate protozoal contamination. Instruct them to avoid foods that cannot be peeled or cooked. Teach the manifestations of protozoal infections and where to obtain treatment.

Emphasize the importance of keeping toilet areas clean and maintaining good personal hygiene. Advise the patient to avoid rectal contact during sexual activity. Other household members should have stool specimens examined for parasites. Contaminated recreational water (swimming pools, water slides) is increasingly recognized as a potential source of cryptosporidiosis; advise immunocompromised individuals to avoid this exposure.

Patients with diarrhea related to bowel infection will likely receive care in a community-based setting. Treatment for fluid and electrolyte imbalances may require intravenous therapy and will likely be administered in an outpatient setting such as an ambulatory care clinic or emergency department.

Treatment may include long-term antibiotic therapy for bowel infections that are difficult to treat. *Clostridium difficile* infections can become long-standing and recurring infections. Nutrition, fluid and electrolyte, and quality of life assessments and interventions should be the focus of care.

Bowel infections in developed countries are treatable and should not result in unexpected death. However, communicable bowel infections are a major cause of morbidity and mortality in developing and third-world countries. Life-threatening diarrhea causing severe dehydration is also a major concern in disasters. Infants and the frail elderly are at most risk. The nurse's actions should focus on preventing disease, providing safe food and water, accessing medications, comforting family, and other responsibilities assigned as a member of a disaster team.

The Patient with a Helminthic Disorder

Helminths are parasitic worms, capable of causing infectious diseases in humans. Helminths are subclassified as round worms (nematodes), flukes (trematodes), or tapeworms (cestodes).

Pathophysiology and Manifestations

Although all helminths can infect humans, the definitive host and intermediate hosts vary with each organism. In nearly all instances of helminthic disorders, the organism enters the body through the GI tract in contaminated and inadequately cooked foods. Some of these organisms remain in the intestinal tract; others migrate to infect the liver, lungs, or other structures. **Table 24.6** summarizes the most common helminths and their effects.

Table 24.6 Selected Helminthic Diseases

Infection	Host	Area	Pathogenesis	Manifestations
Nematode Infections				
Ascariasis	Humans	Worldwide, cosmopolitan; warm, moist climates	Eggs are ingested in fecally contaminated food and drink; motile larvae migrate to lungs and back to small intestine, where they mature to produce more eggs.	Pulmonary: Low-grade fever, cough, blood-tinged sputum, wheezing, dyspnea, substernal chest pain GI: Ulcer-like epigastric pain, vomiting, abdominal distention
Enterobiasis (pinworm infection)	Humans	Worldwide, cosmopolitan	Infect cecum; eggs deposit on perianal skin, organisms may be transmitted to others or reinfect host by oral ingestion.	Nocturnal perianal and perineal pruritus; insomnia, irritability, restlessness
Hookworm disease	Humans	Tropics and subtropics	Larvae enter through skin or by ingestion and migrate to lungs, up bronchial tree, and down esophagus to mature in upper small bowel, where they attach and suck blood.	Skin: Pruritic dermatitis at site of entry Pulmonary: Dry cough, wheezing, blood-tinged sputum GI: Anorexia, diarrhea, abdominal pain Systemic: Anemia, pallor, cardiac insufficiency
Trichinosis	Pigs, dogs, cats, rats, many wild animals	Temperate areas where pork is consumed	Larvae are ingested in undercooked meat; adult female burrows into mucosa of small intestine to produce larvae tthat disseminate via blood and lymphatic system to body tissues and become encysted in striated muscle.	GI: Diarrhea, abdominal cramps, malaise Muscle: Fever; muscle pain, tenderness, edema, and spasm Systemic: Periorbital and facial edema, sweating; photophobia and conjunctivitis; manifestations of inflammation in tissues invaded by larvae
Cestode Infections				
Fasciolopsiasis (intestinal fluke) Tapeworm	Humans; other mammals and fish	Worldwide	Organism is ingested by eating uncooked fish or meat containing embryo cysts, by fecal contamination, or by swallowing infected intermediate hosts, such as arthropods, fleas, or lice; head (scolex) of adult worm attaches in upper small intestine, and eggs form in individual segments.	Large tapeworms: Often asymptomatic; infection may cause mild nausea, diarrhea, abdominal pain; anemia, thrombocytopenia, and mild leukopenia Small tapeworms: May be asymptomatic; diarrhea, abdominal pain, anorexia, vomiting, weight loss, and irritability

Interprofessional Care

The management of helminthic disorders includes diagnostic testing and medications.

Diagnosis

The primary means of diagnosing helminthic disorders is examination of the stool for ova and parasites. Enterobiasis is diagnosed by the presence of the parasite's eggs on the perianal skin or on cellulose tape placed over the anus. A CBC may also be ordered. Anemia may be present, particularly with hookworm disease. *Eosinophilia* (an increased percentage of eosinophils in the blood) is common in helminthic disorders. With trichinosis, serum muscle enzymes such as creatinine kinase (CK) and aspartate aminotransferase (AST) are typically elevated. Serologic testing for antibodies to the worm may be performed. Blood, duodenal washings, and cerebrospinal fluid (CSF) may be examined for the presence of the trichinosis larvae. Inflamed muscle may be biopsied.

Medications

Helminthic infections are often treated with a single oral dose or 3-day course of pyrantel pamoate (Antiminth), albendazole (Albenza), or mebendazole (Vermox). Doses may need to be repeated every 2 weeks for patients with heavy infections. These drugs are generally safe, requiring few precautions. Giving the drug after meals minimizes GI side effects. Treatment is followed by a stool culture at 2 weeks to evaluate effectiveness. If necessary, an additional course of the drug is prescribed. Other members of the household are generally also treated.

Nursing Care

Because many patients with these disorders are asymptomatic, nurses need to be alert for histories that indicate risk and subtle manifestations of the disorder. The patient with a helminthic disorder may feel dirty or be ashamed of the disease. Emphasize the prevalence of these disorders and ensure the patient that infection can occur despite good health practices when the eggs or larva of the organism are prevalent.

Use standard precautions to minimize the risk of spreading these infections to other patients. Wear gloves and gowns as necessary to prevent fecal contamination of hands and clothing. On rare occasions, parasites may be present in the sputum or vomitus, so handle these secretions with care. Disinfect toilets, toilet seats, and commodes after use. Teach the patient the importance of hand hygiene after using the toilet and before handling food to prevent reinfection.

Transitions of Care

Discuss measures to prevent spread of the disease in the household. Emphasize the importance of hygiene measures including changing bedding, daily cleaning of toilets with disinfectant, and hand hygiene.

Many helminthic disorders are acquired by consuming food that has been fecally contaminated or contains larvae of the organism. Explain the importance of not fertilizing food or grain crops with fecal material, particularly human feces. Teach patients to cook all meats and fish adequately to destroy possible larvae. In general, pickled or salt-preserved meats and fish are no safer than raw. Smoking, another means of preserving fish and meat, may not achieve temperatures high enough to destroy the organisms. Vegetables grown in soil that may be contaminated with eggs or larvae should be peeled or cooked prior to eating.

Emphasize the importance of safe water supplies. Encourage people traveling to areas in which water supplies are questionable to drink only bottled water or carry purification tablets. Work with patients who have private water systems to protect water from fecal contamination by either humans or animals.

24.3 Chronic Inflammatory Bowel Disorders

The Patient with Inflammatory Bowel Disease

Chronic **inflammatory bowel disease (IBD)** includes two separate but closely related conditions: Ulcerative colitis and Crohn disease. These conditions have a number of similarities. The etiology of both illnesses is unknown, although current evidence implicates both genetic and environmental factors. In 2015, as estimated 3 million Americans have IBD (Centers for Disease Control and Prevention, 2018); that number is divided about equally between ulcerative colitis and Crohn disease (Crohn & Colitis Foundation of America [CCFA], 2018). It tends to run in families, with 15 to 25% of patients having a close relative with one of the types of IBD (CCFA, 2018). Factors such as an abnormal immune response to microorganisms normally found in the gut are thought to play a role in the development of IBD. Factors such as smoking and oral contraceptive use also affect the risk for IBD.

The peak incidence of IBD is in adolescents and young adults between the ages of 15 and 30 years, but it also affects older adults (Dudley-Brown, 2017). IBD is a chronic and recurrent disease process. Responses to physiologic or psychologic stresses do not cause IBD, but often play a role in exacerbations of the disease.

Despite the similarities, ulcerative colitis and Crohn disease have distinct differences (**Figure 24.3** ■). Ulcerative colitis primarily affects the large bowel in a continuous pattern, progressing distally to proximally. In Crohn disease, a patchy pattern of involvement is seen, affecting primarily the small intestine. Ulcerative colitis shows mainly mucosal involvement; in Crohn disease, the submucosal layers of the bowel are affected. A comparison of ulcerative colitis and Crohn disease is given in **Table 24.7**. See the Multisystem Effects of Inflammatory Bowel Disease feature on page 767.

Ulcerative Colitis

Ulcerative colitis is a chronic inflammatory bowel disorder that affects the mucosa and submucosa of the colon and

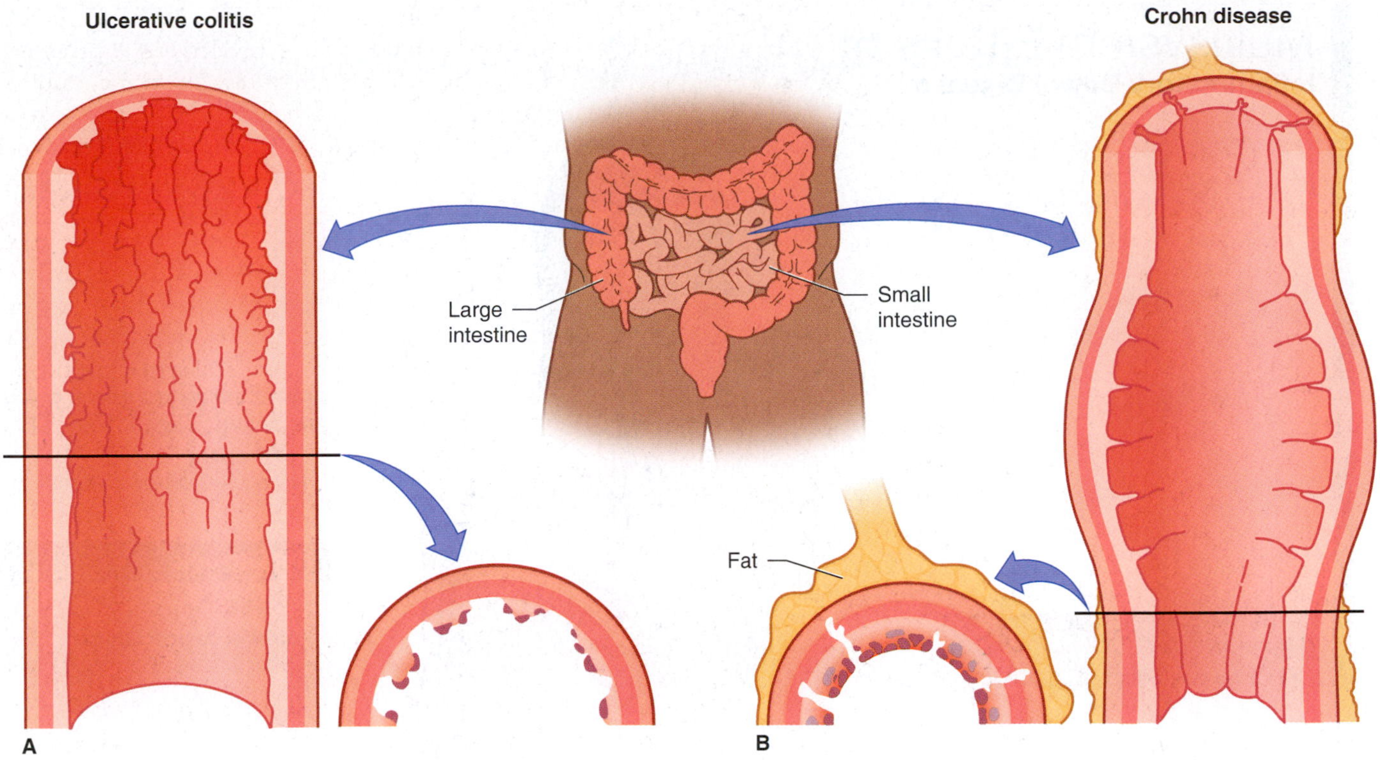
Ulcerative colitis
Crohn disease
Large intestine
Small intestine
Fat
A
B

Figure 24.3 ■ Comparison of **A**, ulcerative colitis, and **B**, Crohn disease.

rectum. Most people with ulcerative colitis have mild or moderate disease, with six or fewer stools per day. Its onset is usually insidious, with attacks that last 1 to 3 months occurring at intervals of months to years. Typically, only the distal colon is affected, with few systemic manifestations of the disease. Approximately 15% of people with ulcerative colitis develop *fulminant colitis*, with involvement of the entire colon, severe bloody diarrhea, acute abdominal pain, and fever. Patients with fulminant disease are at high risk for complications.

Table 24.7 Characteristics of Ulcerative Colitis and Crohn Disease

Characteristic	Ulcerative Colitis	Crohn Disease
Clinical		
Gender	Equal	Equal
Age at onset	15–30 years; secondary peak 60–80 years	15–30 years; secondary peak 60–80 years
Course of disease	Typically chronic and intermittent	Slowly progressive, relapsing
Diarrhea	5–30 stools per day with blood and mucus	Common, usually less severe than colitis, with no obvious blood or mucus in stool
Abdominal pain	Cramping in left lower quadrant; relieved by defecation	Cramping or steady right lower quadrant or periumbilical pain; tenderness and mass noted in right lower quadrant
Nutritional deficit	Common; involves anemia, hypoalbuminemia, and weight loss	Common and significant; involves anemia, weight loss, and multiple vitamin and mineral deficits
Constitutional manifestations	Fever rare; may have associated arthritic, skin, or other organ involvement, such as erythema nodosum or uveitis	Fever, malaise, fatigue; may have some associated conditions plus urinary complications
Pathologic		
Depth of involvement	Mucosa and submucosa	Transmural (entire bowel wall)
Portion of bowel involved	Typically rectum and sigmoid colon; may extend to involve entire large bowel	Any portion of GI tract; terminal ileum and ascending colon involvement predominates
Distribution	Continuous from rectum	Patchy; skip lesions
Appearance of mucosa	Granular, dull, hyperemic, friable; disease uniform in affected bowel; pseudopolyps may be seen	Cobblestone appearance, with areas of normal tissue surrounded by ulceration and fissures
Complications		
Acute	Toxic megacolon, perforation, massive hemorrhage	Obstruction, fistulization, abscess formation, malabsorption
Long term	Colorectal cancer	Colon cancer

Multisystem Effects of
Inflammatory Bowel Disease

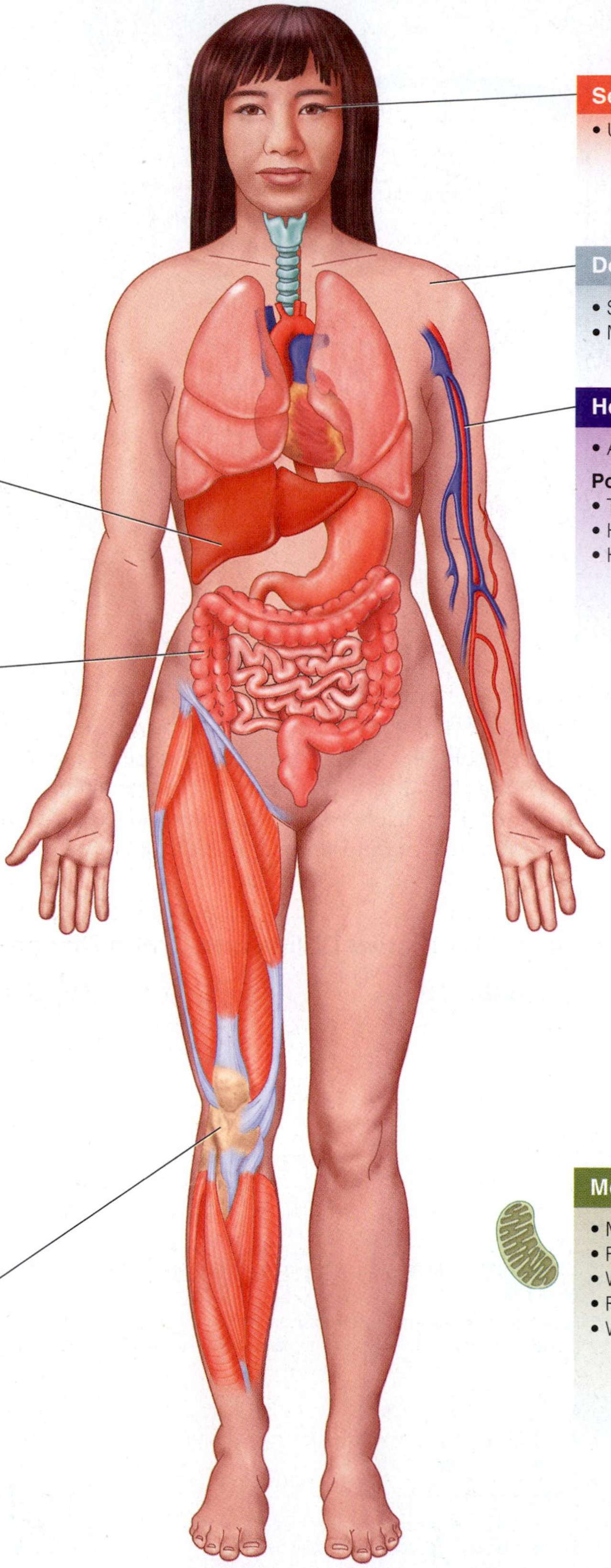

Sensory
- Uveitis

Dermatologic
- Skin lesions
- Mucous membrane lesions

Hematologic
- Anemia

Potential complications
- Thromboemboli
- Hemorrhage
- Hypovolemia

Hepatic
- Risk for sclerosing cholangitis

Gastrointestinal
- Diarrhea
- Blood and mucous in stool
- Intermittent rectal bleeding and mucous
- Fecal urgency
- Tenesmus
- Abdominal pain, tenderness, cramping, often relieved by defecation
- Anorexia
- Nausea, vomiting, epigastric pain
- Palpable right lower quadrant mass
- Anorectal lesions

Potential complications
- Toxic megacolon
- Perforation with peritonitis
- Obstruction
- Abscess
- Fistula formation

Musculoskeletal
- Arthritis of one or more joints
- Ankylosing spondylitis

Metabolic Processes
- Malnutrition
- Fatigue
- Weakness
- Fever
- Weight loss

Pathophysiology

The inflammatory process of ulcerative colitis begins at the rectosigmoid area of the anal canal and progresses proximally. In most patients, the disease is confined to the rectum and sigmoid colon. It may progress to involve the entire colon, stopping at the ileocecal junction.

Ulcerative colitis begins with inflammation at the base of the crypts of Lieberkühn in the distal large intestine and rectum (**Figure 24.4** ■). Microscopic, pinpoint mucosal hemorrhages occur, and crypt abscesses develop. These abscesses penetrate the superficial submucosa and spread laterally, leading to necrosis and sloughing of bowel mucosa. Further tissue damage is caused by inflammatory exudates and the release of inflammatory mediators, such as prostaglandins and other cytokines (see Chapter 12 for further discussion of the inflammatory process). The mucosa is red and edematous due to vascular congestion, friable (easily broken), and ulcerated. It bleeds easily, and hemorrhage is common. Edema creates a granular appearance. Pseudopolyps, tonguelike projections of bowel mucosa into the lumen, may develop as the epithelial lining of the bowel regenerates. Chronic inflammation leads to atrophy, narrowing, and shortening of the colon, with loss of its normal haustra (series of pouches producing a series of internal folds).

Manifestations

Diarrhea is the predominant manifestation of ulcerative colitis. Stools contain both blood and mucus. Nocturnal diarrhea may occur. Mild ulcerative colitis is characterized by fewer than four stools per day, intermittent rectal bleeding and mucus, and few systemic manifestations. Severe ulcerative colitis can lead to more than 5 to 30 bloody stools per day, extensive colon involvement, anemia, hypovolemia, and malnutrition. Rectal inflammation causes fecal urgency and tenesmus. Left lower quadrant cramping relieved by defecation is common. Other manifestations include fatigue, anorexia, and weakness.

Patients with severe disease may also have systemic manifestations such as arthritis involving one or several joints, skin and mucous membrane lesions, or *uveitis* (inflammation of the uvea, the vascular layer of the eye, which may also involve the sclera and cornea). Some patients develop thromboemboli, with blood vessel obstruction due to clots carried from the site of their formation. The liver and biliary system may be affected by the disease, as may the kidneys, with an increased risk for gallstones, cirrhosis, kidney stones, and ureteral obstruction (McQuaid, 2018).

Complications

Acute complications of ulcerative colitis include hemorrhage, toxic megacolon, and colon perforation. Massive hemorrhage may occur with severe attacks of the disease. *Toxic megacolon*, a condition characterized by acute motor paralysis and dilation of the colon to greater than 6 cm (2.4 in.), may affect part or all of the colon. The transverse segment of the bowel is most often affected. Toxic megacolon may be triggered by the use of laxatives or narcotics and by electrolyte imbalances (McQuaid, 2018). Manifestations of toxic megacolon include fever, tachycardia, hypotension, dehydration, abdominal tenderness and cramping, and a change in the number of stools per day. Perforation is rare, but the risk of this dangerous complication is increased with toxic megacolon. Perforation leads to peritonitis.

The risk for colorectal cancer is increased in patients with ulcerative colitis. Beginning 8 to 15 years after the diagnosis, annual or biennial colonoscopies with biopsy to detect masses or cell dysplasia are recommended for patients who have extensive ulcerative colitis (McQuaid, 2018).

Crohn Disease

Like ulcerative colitis, *Crohn disease*, also known as *regional enteritis*, is a chronic, relapsing inflammatory disorder affecting the gastrointestinal tract. Crohn disease can affect any portion of the GI tract from the mouth to the anus, but usually affects the terminal ileum and ascending colon. Only the small bowel is involved in nearly 40% of patients with Crohn disease. The disease is limited to the colon only in 30% of those affected. Both the small and large intestine are involved in the remaining 30% of patients (McQuaid, 2018).

Pathophysiology

Crohn disease typically begins as a small inflammatory *aphthoid lesion* (shallow ulcers with a white base and elevated margin, similar to a canker sore) of the mucosa and submucosa of the bowel (**Figure 24.5** ■). These initial lesions may regress, or the inflammatory process can progress to involve all layers of the intestinal wall. Deeper ulcerations,

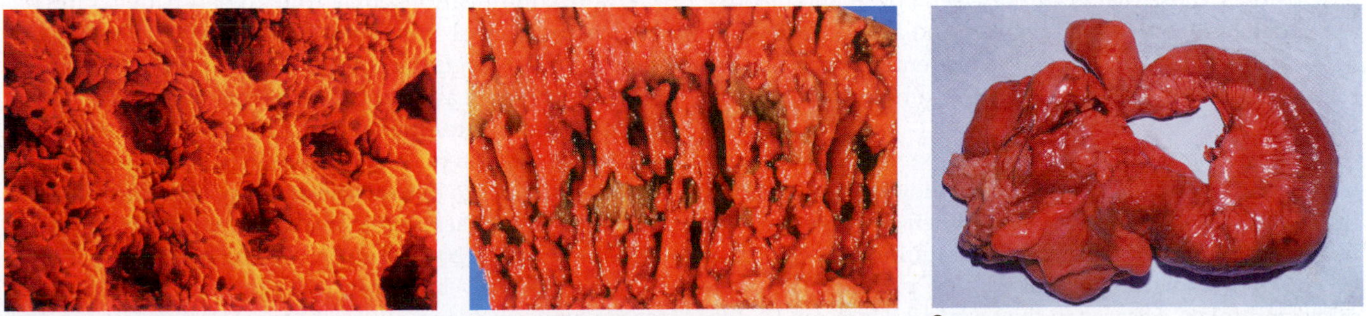

A B C

Figure 24.4 ■ **A**, Photomicrograph of the mucosa of the large intestine showing the entrances to the crypts of Lieberkühn. The crypts are the focal points for **B**, ulcerative colitis, and **C**, Crohn disease.

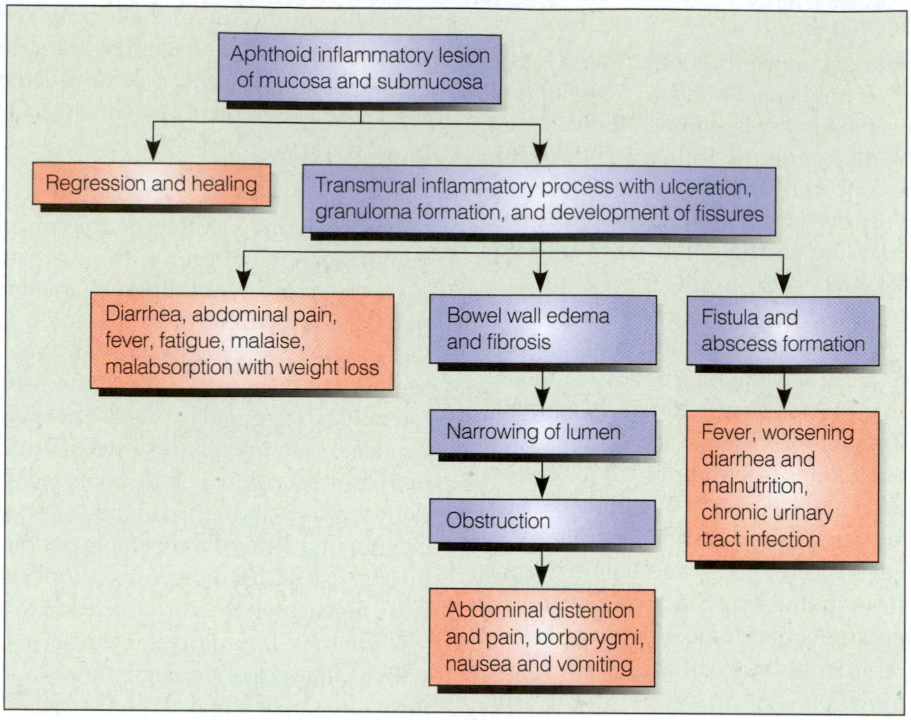
Aphthoid inflammatory lesion of mucosa and submucosa
Regression and healing
Transmural inflammatory process with ulceration, granuloma formation, and development of fissures
Diarrhea, abdominal pain, fever, fatigue, malaise, malabsorption with weight loss
Bowel wall edema and fibrosis
Fistula and abscess formation
Narrowing of lumen
Obstruction
Abdominal distention and pain, borborygmi, nausea and vomiting
Fever, worsening diarrhea and malnutrition, chronic urinary tract infection

Figure 24.5 ■ The progression of Crohn disease.

granulomatous lesions, and fissures (knifelike clefts that extend deeply into the bowel wall) develop. The inflammatory process involves the entire bowel wall (transmural).

The lumen of the affected bowel assumes a cobblestone appearance as fissures and ulcers surround islands of intact mucosa over edematous submucosa. The inflammatory lesions of Crohn disease are not continuous; rather, they often occur as skip lesions with intervening areas of normal-appearing bowel. Some evidence suggests that despite its normal appearance, the entire bowel is affected by this disorder.

As the disease progresses, fibrotic changes in the bowel wall cause thickening and loss of flexibility; the bowel wall takes on an appearance that has been likened to rubber hosing. The inflammation, edema, and fibrosis can lead to local obstruction, abscess development, and the formation of fistulas between loops of bowel or bowel and other organs. Fistulas between loops of bowel are known as enteroenteric fistulas; those that occur between bowel and bladder are known as enterovesical fistulas; and fistulas that occur between bowel and skin are known as enterocutaneous fistulas. Perineal fistulas are relatively common, originating in the ileum.

Depending on the severity and extent of the disease, malabsorption and malnutrition may develop as the ulcers prevent absorption of nutrients. When the jejunum and ileum are affected, the absorption of multiple nutrients may be impaired, including carbohydrates, proteins, fats, vitamins, and folate. Disease in the terminal ileum can lead to vitamin B_{12} malabsorption and bile salt reabsorption. The ulcerations can also lead to protein loss and chronic, slow blood loss with consequent anemia.

Manifestations

Because the GI system involvement in Crohn disease can be so diverse, manifestations vary among patients. The majority of people with Crohn disease experience persistent diarrhea. Stools are liquid or semiformed and typically do not contain blood, although blood may be passed if the colon is involved. Abdominal pain and tenderness are also common. The pain may be located in the right lower quadrant and relieved by defecation. A palpable right lower quadrant mass is often present. Systemic manifestations such as fever, fatigue, malaise, weight loss, and anemia are common. Anorectal lesions such as fissures, ulcers, fistulas, and abscesses are also common and may occur years before intestinal disease is apparent. If the stomach and duodenum are involved, nausea and vomiting and epigastric pain may occur.

Complications

Certain complications of Crohn disease (e.g., intestinal obstruction, abscess, and fistula) are so common that they are considered part of the disease process. For many patients, the disease initially presents with one of these complications. Intestinal obstruction is a common complication caused by repeated inflammation and scarring of the bowel that leads to fibrosis and stricture. Obstruction of the bowel lumen causes abdominal distention, cramping pain, and borborygmi. Nausea and vomiting may occur.

Fistulas may be asymptomatic, particularly if they occur between loops of small bowel. When fistulization causes an abscess, chills and fever, a tender abdominal mass, and leukocytosis develop. A fistula between the small bowel and colon may exacerbate diarrhea, weight loss, and malnutrition. When the bladder is involved, recurrent urinary tract infections occur.

Perforation of the bowel is uncommon, but can lead to generalized peritonitis. Massive hemorrhage is also an uncommon complication of Crohn disease. Long-standing Crohn disease increases the risk of cancer of the small intestine or colon by five to six times. This cancer risk, however, is significantly lower than the risk associated with ulcerative colitis.

Interprofessional Care

Interprofessional care for inflammatory bowel disease begins by establishing the diagnosis and the extent and severity of the disease. Treatment is supportive, including medications and dietary measures to decrease inflammation, promote intestinal rest and healing, and reduce intestinal motility. Many patients with IBD require surgery at some point to manage the disease or its complications.

Diagnosis

Diagnostic testing is used to establish the diagnosis of IBD, assess the extent of the disease, and evaluate the effects of the disorder. A sigmoidoscopy, colonoscopy, or a barium upper and lower x-ray series is performed to inspect the bowel mucosa for the characteristic changes of IBD. (Nursing implications for these tests are outlined in Chapter 21.)

Laboratory tests to differentiate IBD and to identify effects and complications of the disease include a stool examination for blood and mucus and stool cultures to rule out infectious causes of bowel inflammation and diarrhea. CBC with hemoglobin and hematocrit shows anemia from chronic inflammation, blood loss, and malnutrition and leukocytosis due to inflammation and possible abscess formation. The sedimentation rate and levels of C-reactive protein are typically elevated during periods of acute inflammation. Serum albumin may be decreased because of malabsorption, malnutrition, protein loss through intestinal lesions, and chronic inflammation. Folic acid and serum levels of most vitamins—including A, B complex, C, and the fat-soluble vitamins—are often decreased due to malabsorption. Additional tests for renal and hepatic function may be done if the patient has significant systemic manifestations of the disease.

Medications

The ultimate goal of care is to achieve and maintain remission of the disease and its symptoms. Drug therapy plays a key role in achieving this goal. Locally acting and systemic anti-inflammatory drugs are the primary medications used to manage mild to moderate IBD. Drugs to suppress the immune response may be used to treat patients with severe disease.

Sulfasalazine (Azulfidine) is a sulfonamide antibiotic and anti-inflammatory that is poorly absorbed from the gastrointestinal tract and acts topically on the colonic mucosa to inhibit the inflammatory process. The active anti-inflammatory ingredient in sulfasalazine, 5-aminosalicylic acid (5-ASA), is also available in preparations that do not contain sulfa, such as olsalazine and mesalamine. They have the advantage of causing fewer adverse effects than sulfasalazine. Azo compounds, such as balsalazide and olsalazine, are 5-ASA compounds that are released in the colon and are especially useful for treating ulcerative colitis. Mesalamine (Asacol, Canasa, Rowasa) is an orally or rectally administered 5-ASA compound that provides topical anti-inflammatory action in the colon of patients with ulcerative colitis. Specific preparations, their method of action, and nursing implications for these medications are outlined in **Medication Administration 24.D**.

For acute exacerbations of IBD, corticosteroids are given to reduce inflammation and induce remission. For ulcerative colitis, the drug may be administered rectally for its local effect and to minimize systemic effects. Hydrocortisone can be administered rectally. Intravenous corticosteroids may be required to treat severe disease; oral preparations are used for less severe manifestations and long-term therapy. Budesonide (Entocort-EC, Uceris) is a corticosteroid that can be used as a first-line therapy for IBD as the drug is released slowly and reaches high concentration in the terminal ileium and proximal colon (Adams et al., 2017). This medication shows fewer long-term effects than frequently seen with long-term use of other corticosteroids (Adams et al., 2017). Corticosteroids are tapered off once remission has been achieved.

Mercaptopurine (6-MP, Purinethol) and other immunosuppressive agents such as azathioprine (Imuran) and methotrexate (MTX, Rhematrex, Trexal) can be used to treat patients who have not responded to other treatments or who require chronic steroid therapy. These drugs may allow withdrawal from corticosteroids, maintain remission, and facilitate healing. Long-term therapy may be required to produce a beneficial effect. For more information about immunosuppressive drugs, see Chapter 13.

Biologic therapies are newer treatments for IBD and employ other immune response modifiers, such as the monoclonal antibodies infliximab (Remicade) and adalimumab (Humira), to suppress tumor necrosis factor (TNF; an inflammatory mediator substance) in patients who have not responded to standard therapies. Natatlizumab (Tysabri) is approved for treating Crohn disease but has potentially serious side effects (Adams et al., 2017). Vedoizuman (Entyvio) is another new medication used to treat IB and is given intravenously. Patients experience a high rate of serious infection when taking biologic therapies and the cost of these medications is significant. (For more information about biologic therapies, see Chapter 13.)

Although antibiotic therapy is generally not indicated in IBD, metronidazole (Flagyl) has active anti-inflammatory effects. It may be prescribed to help prevent remission after ileal resection in Crohn disease. Ciprofloxacin (Cipro) is an alternative to metronidazole.

Antidiarrheal agents, such as loperamide and diphenoxylate, may be given to slow gastrointestinal motility and reduce diarrhea. These drugs are safe for patients with mild, chronic manifestations, but they are not given during acute attacks because they may precipitate toxic dilation of the colon.

Medication Administration 24.D

Inflammatory Bowel Disease

SULFASALAZINE (AZULFIDINE)

Sulfasalazine is an anti-inflammatory drug used for its local effect on the intestinal mucosa in inflammatory bowel disease. The active part of the drug is 5-ASA, which inhibits prostaglandin production in the bowel. Prostaglandin is an important mediator of the inflammatory process; blocking its production reduces inflammation.

Nursing Responsibilities

- Assess for contraindications, including pregnancy or a history of hypersensitivity to sulfonamides or salicylates.
- Assess baseline values for renal function tests (serum creatinine, BUN, urinalysis), liver function tests, and CBC.
- Administer as ordered. Suppositories or retention enemas may be administered at bedtime. Administer oral forms with a full glass of water.
- Have resuscitation equipment available; anaphylactic responses may occur.
- Evaluate for therapeutic response, including reduced number of stools, reduced mucus and blood, and improved stool consistency.
- Monitor for possible adverse responses:
  a. Headache, anorexia, or nausea and vomiting
  b. Skin rash, dermatitis, urticaria, or pruritus
  c. Evidence of blood dyscrasias, such as bleeding, easy bruising, fever
  d. Leukopenia, thrombocytopenia, hemolytic anemia, or agranulocytosis
  e. Changes in urinary output or renal function studies
  f. Evidence of hepatitis or myocarditis.

Health Education for the Patient and Family

- Take oral preparations after meals to decrease gastric distress.
- Drink at least 2 quarts of fluid per day to reduce the risk of kidney damage.
- Use sunscreen to prevent burns; this drug increases sensitivity to the sun.
- Do not take aspirin, vitamin C, or any other OTC medications containing aspirin or vitamin C without consulting your doctor.
- This medication may interfere with the effectiveness of oral contraceptives; use alternative methods of contraception.
- Notify your doctor if you develop headache, anorexia, nausea and vomiting, skin rash or hives, sore throat or mouth, bleeding gums, joint pain, easy bruising, or fever.

MESALAMINE (ASACOL, CANASA, ROWASA) AND OLSALAZINE (DIPENTUM)

Mesalamine and olsalazine contain the same active ingredient, 5-ASA, as sulfasalazine, but cause fewer adverse effects. Their mechanism of action is the same as that of sulfasalazine. These drugs are available as suppositories, suspension for enema, or oral tablets.

Nursing Responsibilities

- Assess for possible contraindications such as pregnancy, lactation, or hypersensitivity to these drugs or aspirin.
- Administer as ordered. If more than one dose per day is ordered, space doses evenly over the 24-hour period.
- Evaluate for desired effects (as for sulfasalazine) and potential adverse effects:
  a. Nausea, diarrhea, abdominal cramps, or flatulence
  b. CNS effects including headache, dizziness, insomnia, weakness, or fatigue
  c. Rash or itching
  d. Flulike symptoms, general malaise.

Health Education for the Patient and Family

- Teach the recommended method of administration, including how to insert rectal suppositories or administer a retention enema.
- Shake suspension forms well prior to using.
- Diarrhea is the most common side effect of these drugs. Notify your doctor if adverse effects occur.

CORTICOSTEROIDS

methylprednisolone (Medrol, Solu-Medrol)
prednisolone (Delta-Cortel)
prednisone

Glucocorticoids are hormones produced by the adrenal cortex. These hormones are necessary for the stress response. Cortisol, the main glucocorticoid, has potent anti-inflammatory effects. Corticosteroids are used to treat acute episodes of IBD. Because of their multiple and significant side effects, they are not used to maintain remission.

Nursing Responsibilities

- Assess for conditions that may be adversely affected by corticosteroid drugs: Peptic ulcer disease, glaucoma or cataracts, diabetes, or psychiatric disorders.
- Obtain baseline vital signs and weight; monitor both routinely during therapy. Hypertension and weight gain may result from salt and water retention.
- Monitor for edema.
- Administer as ordered. For daily or alternate-day dosing, administer in the morning, when physiologic glucocorticoid levels are highest, to reduce adrenal cortisone suppression.
- Administer oral preparations with food to decrease gastrointestinal side effects. Antacids or histamine H_2-receptor blocking agents, such as cimetidine (Tagamet), may be prescribed during corticosteroid therapy.
- Monitor for desired effects: Reduced diarrhea, less blood and mucus in the stool, and less abdominal cramping.
- Monitor for adverse effects:
  a. Increased susceptibility to infection and masking of early signs of infection
  b. Hyperglycemia
  c. Hypokalemia, as manifested by muscle weakness, nausea and vomiting, and cardiac rhythm disturbances
  d. Edema, hypertension, and signs of heart failure
  e. Peptic ulcer formation and possible gastrointestinal hemorrhage (abdominal pain, black or tarry stools, and signs of bleeding)
  f. Changes in mental status, including depression, euphoria, aggression, and behavioral changes

g. With long-term use, cushingoid effects, such as abnormal fat deposits in the face (moon faces) and trunk (buffalo hump), muscle wasting and thin extremities, thinning of the skin, and osteoporosis.

Health Education for the Patient and Family

- Take as prescribed; do not change the dose or time of day. Do not stop the medication abruptly. The dose will be tapered down gradually when the drug is discontinued.
- Notify the physician if adverse or cushingoid effects occur.
- Take with food or at mealtimes to decrease the gastrointestinal effects.
- Monitor weight. If a gain of more than 5 pounds is noted, notify the physician.
- Moderate salt intake and avoid foods and snacks high in sodium, such as processed meats and potato chips. Increase intake of foods high in potassium, such as fruits, vegetables, and lean meats.
- Carry a card or wear a bracelet or tag at all times identifying corticosteroid use.

Note: Drugs identified in blue are among the 200 most commonly prescribed medications in the United States.

Sources: Data from Adams et al, 2017; Dudley-Brown, 2017.

Nutrition

Antigens in the diet may stimulate the immune response in the bowel, exacerbating IBD. As a result, dietary management for inflammatory bowel disease is individualized. Some patients benefit from eliminating all milk and milk products from the diet. Increased dietary fiber may help reduce diarrhea and relieve rectal manifestations, but is contraindicated for patients with intestinal strictures caused by repeated inflammation and scarring.

All food may be withheld to promote bowel rest during an acute exacerbation of Crohn disease. Nutritional status is maintained using enteral nutrition or TPN. An elemental diet such as Ensure, which contains all essential nutrients in a residue-free formula, may be prescribed. Elemental diets provide essential nutrients to the small intestine to support cell growth, but are not always palatable. TPN carries a higher risk of complications than does enteral nutrition.

Surgery

Surgical interventions for IBD differ, depending on the primary disease process and the portion of the bowel affected. Generally, surgery is performed only when necessitated by complications of the disease or failure of conservative treatment measures.

Bowel obstruction is the leading indication for surgery in Crohn disease. Other complications that may require surgical intervention include perforation, internal or external fistula, abscess, and perianal complications. Resection of the affected portion of bowel with an end-to-end anastomosis to preserve as much bowel as possible is the usual treatment. The disease process tends to recur in other areas following removal of affected bowel segments. There is an increased risk of fistula formation following surgery. Bowel strictures may be treated with a strictureplasty. In this procedure, longitudinal incisions are made in the narrowed segment to relieve the stricture while preserving bowel.

Colectomy. Patients with extensive chronic ulcerative colitis may require a total **colectomy** (surgical resection and removal of the colon) to treat the disease itself; for complications such as toxic megacolon, perforation, or hemorrhage; or as a prophylactic measure due to the high colon cancer risk associated with extensive ulcerative colitis.

The surgical procedure of choice for extensive ulcerative colitis is a *total colectomy with an ileal pouch–anal anastomosis (IPAA)*. In this procedure, the entire colon and rectum are removed; a pouch is formed from the terminal ileum; and the pouch is brought into the pelvis and anastomosed to the anal canal (**Figure 24.6** ■). A temporary or loop ileostomy (described in the next section) is generally performed at the same time and is maintained for 2 to 3 months to allow the anal anastomosis to heal. When the healing is complete, the ileostomy is closed and the patient evacuates through the anus. Six to eight daily bowel movements through the anus may occur due to the liquid nature of the ileal contents. Advanced age, obesity, or other factors may preclude an IPAA. For these patients, a permanent ileostomy or continent ileostomy may be created.

Ostomy. An intestinal ostomy is a surgically created opening between the intestine and the abdominal wall that allows the passage of fecal material. The surface opening is called a **stoma** (**Figure 24.7** ■). The precise name of the ostomy depends on the location of the stoma. An **ileostomy** is an ostomy made in the ileum of the small intestine. In an ileostomy, the colon, rectum, and anus are usually completely removed (*total proctocolectomy with permanent ileostomy*). The anal canal is closed, and the end of the terminal

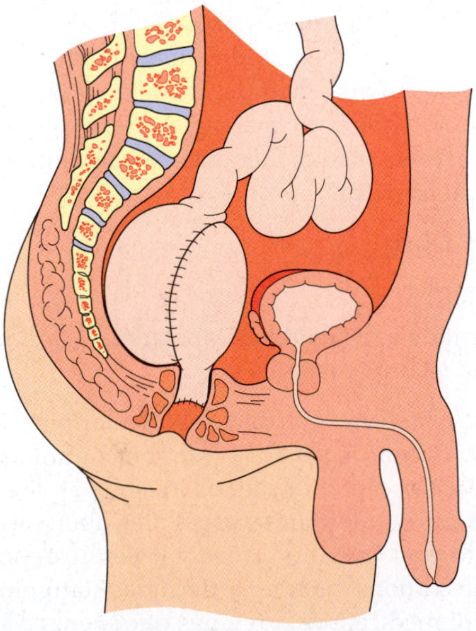

Figure 24.6 ■ Ileal pouch–anal anastomosis (IPAA).

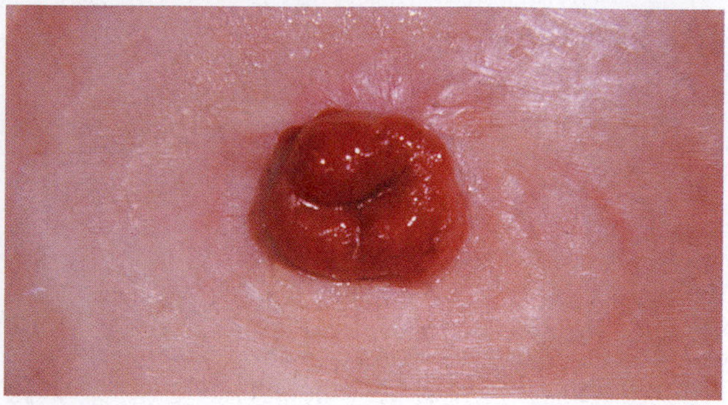

Figure 24.7 ■ A healthy-appearing stoma.

ileum is brought to the body surface through the right abdominal wall to form the stoma and allow stool drainage into an external pouch. A temporary or *loop ileostomy* may be formed to eliminate feces and allow tissue healing for 2 to 3 months following an IPAA. When the ileostomy is no longer necessary, a second surgery is performed to close the stoma and repair the bowel, restoring fecal elimination through the anus.

In a *continent ileostomy* an intra-abdominal reservoir is constructed and a nipple valve formed (the ileum folded back on itself) from the terminal ileum before it is brought to the surface of the abdominal wall. Stool collects in the internal pouch; the nipple valve prevents it from leaking through the stoma. A catheter is inserted into the pouch to drain the stool.

Nursing care of the patient with an ileostomy is outlined in **Box 24.3**.

Integrative Therapies

The chronic nature of IBD and adverse effects of many prescribed treatments lead up to 50% of patients with IBD to seek or use complementary and alternative therapies. Peppermint tea is an excellent tonic for reducing nausea, relieving abdominal pain, and providing a calming effect. Many complementary and alternative therapies for IBD may interact with prescribed medications; instruct the patient to discuss all potential therapies with the primary care provider. Acupressure, body massage, reflexology, aromatherapy, and stress reduction therapies can also aid in reducing manifestations of IBD.

Nursing Care

Assessment

Assessment data related to IBD includes the following subjective and objective data:

- ***Health history:*** Current manifestations, including onset, duration, severity (number of stools per day, presence of blood or mucus in stool, abdominal pain or cramping, tenesmus); usual diet, ability to maintain weight and nutrition, food intolerances; associated manifestations such as arthralgias, fatigue, malaise; current medications; previous treatment and diagnostic tests
- ***Physical assessment:*** General appearance; weight; vital signs including orthostatic vitals and temperature; abdominal assessment including shape, contour, bowel sounds, palpation for tenderness and masses, presence of stoma or scars.

Priorities of Care

Teaching is a major aspect of care. Diarrhea and disturbed body image are significant nursing care problems for the patient with IBD. With severe disease, impaired nutrition must be considered a priority problem as well. See the accompanying Case Study & Nursing Care Plan for a patient with ulcerative colitis.

Diagnoses, Outcomes, and Interventions

When planning nursing care for the patient with IBD, it is vital to consider the chronic, recurrent nature of the disorder. Living with a chronic disease such as IBD requires nursing care to help the patient adapt and effectively cope with symptoms of the disease such as pain, fatigue, diarrhea, anxiety, and depression.

Control Diarrhea. During an acute exacerbation of IBD, diarrhea can be frequent and painful. The frequency of defecation and associated abdominal pain and cramping may interfere with ADLs and increase the risk for fluid volume deficit and impaired skin integrity.

Expected Outcome: Patient's diarrhea will be controlled as demonstrated by stable fluid and electrolyte balance, successful self-care of ostomy, and reduction in symptom severity.

The nurse will:

- Record the frequency, amount, and color of stools using a stool chart. Measure and record liquid stool as output. *The severity of diarrhea is an indicator of the severity of the disease and helps determine the need for fluid replacement.*
- Observe stools for obvious blood and test for occult blood as indicated. Report grossly bloody stools (**hematochezia**), which may indicate hemorrhage and necessitate emergency surgery.
- Monitor vital signs every 4 hours. *Tachycardia, tachypnea, and fever may be indicators of fluid volume deficit.*
- Weigh daily and record. *Rapid weight loss (over days to a week) usually indicates fluid loss, whereas weight loss over weeks to months may indicate malnutrition.*
- Assess for other indications of fluid deficit: Warm, dry skin; poor skin turgor; dry, shiny mucous membranes; weakness; lethargy; complaints of thirst. *The extent of fluid loss may not be readily evident with diarrhea, particularly if the patient uses the bathroom without assistance. Systemic manifestations of fluid volume deficit may be the first indicators of the problem.*
- Maintain bowel rest by keeping NPO or limiting oral intake to elemental feedings as indicated. *Bowel rest during an acute exacerbation of IBD promotes healing and reduces diarrhea and other manifestations.*
- Administer prescribed anti-inflammatory and antidiarrheal medications as indicated. *Anti-inflammatory*

BOX 24.3
Nursing Care of the Patient Having an Ileostomy

PREOPERATIVE CARE

The patient preoperative care for a patient having an ileostomy includes routine preoperative care and teaching, as outlined in Chapter 4. It will be important to facilitate a referral to an enterostomal therapist for making and teaching about the stoma location, preparing for ostomy care, and options for ostomy appliances.

- Begin teaching prior to surgery will help the patient be prepared for postoperative self-care required and facilitate the acceptance of the ostomy after surgery. Include information about the local United Ostomy Association chapter and provide a referral, if desired by the patient and family. Local chapters have members with ostomies who can provide information and support.
- Preoperative care will likely involve cleansing the bowel. Cathartics, enemas, and preoperative antibiotics are often ordered to reduce the risk of abdominal contamination and infection after surgery.

POSTOPERATIVE CARE

In addition to providing routine postoperative care and teaching, as outlined in Chapter 4, nursing care will include assessment, management, and teaching the patient about caring for the stoma.

- Monitor the stool from the ileostomy. Stool from an ileostomy is expressed continuously or irregularly, and it is liquid in nature; continuous use of a pouch to collect the drainage is necessary. The patient will likely return to the unit from surgery with an appliance in place. Reapply an ostomy pouch over the stoma if the seal is disrupted. Be sure to consult with the enterostomal therapist if the seal is becoming disrupted as there may need to be a change in the appliance.
- Assess the stoma frequently for bleeding, stoma viability, and function. In the early postoperative period, small amounts of blood in the pouch are expected. A healthy stoma appears pink or red and moist as a result of mucus production (refer to Figure 24.7). It should protrude approximately 2 cm from the abdominal wall. Frequent assessment is particularly important in the initial postoperative period to ensure stoma health and monitor for possible complications. A dusky, brown, black, or white stoma indicates circulatory compromise. Other possible stoma complications include retraction (indentation or loss of the external portion of the stoma) or prolapse (outward telescoping of the stoma, that is, an abnormally long stoma).
- As the stoma starts to function, empty the pouch, explaining the procedure to the patient. Initial drainage is dark green, viscid, and usually odorless. Drainage gradually thickens and becomes yellow-brown. Empty the pouch when it is one-third full. Measure drainage, and include it as output on intake-and-output records. Rinse the pouch and reapply the clamp. Emptying the pouch when it is no more than one-third full helps prevent the skin seal from breaking as a result of the weight of the pouch. Because of the potential for excess fluid loss through ileostomy drainage, it is important to include it as fluid output.
- Assess the peristomal skin. Skin around the stoma should remain clean and pink and free of irritation, rashes, inflammation, or excoriation. Skin complications may arise from appliance irritation or hypersensitivity, excoriation from a leaking appliance, or *Candida albicans*, a yeast infection. Excoriation of skin surrounding the stoma impairs the first line of defense against microorganisms and can interfere with the ability to achieve a tight skin seal and prevent pouch leakage.
- Protecting peristomal skin from enzymes and bile salts in the ileostomy effluent requires using a skin barrier on the pouch; be sure to change the pouch if leakage occurs or if the patient complains of burning or itching skin.
- Report the following abnormal assessment findings to the enterostomal nurse therapist or physician:
  a. Allergic or contact dermatitis.
  b. Purulent ulcerated areas surrounding the stoma.
  c. A red, bumpy, itchy rash or white-coated area (a manifestation of *Candida albicans*, a yeast infection).
  d. Bulging around the stoma (may indicate herniation, caused by loops of intestine protruding through the abdominal wall).
- Apply protective ointments to the perirectal area of patients with newly functioning ileoanal reservoirs and anastomoses. This helps protect the skin from the initial stools. As stools thicken and become fewer per day, the patient experiences less perirectal irritation.

Health Education for the Patient and Family

- While caring for the ostomy, explain procedures to the patient. Teach the patient how to manage the pouch clamp and to empty, rinse, and perform pouch changes. Ongoing assessment is important for optimal health and function of the stoma and surrounding skin so teach the patient and caregiver to check the stoma regularly. Chronic skin irritation by ileostomy effluent may lead to pseudoverrucous lesions or wartlike nodules, so teach the patient to avoid stripping of tape or excessively frequent pouch removal may cause mechanical trauma to peristomal skin.
- Instruct the patient and caregiver to report abnormal appearance of the stoma or surrounding skin to the physician. Abnormal appearance of the stoma to be reported includes:
  a. Narrowing of the stoma lumen. This indicates stenosis and may interfere with fecal elimination.
  b. Lacerations or cuts in the stoma. The stoma contains no nerves, so trauma may occur without pain.
  c. Separation of the stoma from the abdominal surface. This potential complication may require surgical repair.
- Emphasize the importance of adequate fluid and salt intake; the risk for dehydration and hyponatremia is increased particularly during hot weather, when fluid is lost through perspiration as well as ileostomy drainage. Water intake should be sufficient to maintain pale urine and an output of at least 1 quart per day. When exercising in hot weather, the patient should consume extra water and salt. High-potassium foods, such as bananas and oranges, may be recommended. Loss of the reabsorptive surface of the large bowel increases the amount of water and sodium loss in the stool. If the ileostomy is high (more proximal in the ileum), additional potassium losses may also occur.
- Discuss dietary concerns. A low-residue diet is recommended initially (see **Table 24.8**). Foods that may cause excessive odor or gas are typically avoided as well. Because food blockage is a potential problem, high-fiber foods are limited, and foods that may cause blockage—such as popcorn, corn, nuts, cucumbers, celery, fresh tomatoes, figs, strawberries, blackberries, and caraway seeds—are avoided. Symptoms of food blockage include abdominal cramping, swelling of the stoma, and absence of ileostomy output for over 4 to 6 hours.
- Food blockage can usually be managed at home so provide the patient with strategies to try and encourage early intervention. Strategies to address food blockage are:
  a. Take a warm shower or tub bath. This can help relax the abdominal muscles.

(continued)

BOX 24.3
Nursing Care of the Patient Having An Ileostomy *(continued)*

b. Assume a knee–chest position. The knee–chest position reduces intra-abdominal pressure.

c. Drink warm fluids or grape juice if not vomiting. This provides a mild cathartic effect.

d. Massage peristomal area. Massage may stimulate peristalsis and fecal elimination.

e. Remove pouch if the stoma is swollen, and apply a pouch with a larger opening. If the stoma swells, the pouch may create a mechanical obstruction to output.

- Notify the physician or enterostomal therapy nurse if:
  a. The measures listed above fail to relieve the obstruction.
  b. Signs of a partial obstruction persist, including high-volume odorous fluid output, abdominal cramps, and nausea and vomiting.
  c. There is no ileostomy output for 4 to 6 hours.
  d. Signs of fluid and electrolyte imbalance occur, such as weakness, dizziness, light-headedness, or headache.

Table 24.8 Low-Residue Diet

Food Group	Allowed	Avoid
Beverages	Coffee, teas, juices, carbonated beverages; milk limited to 2 cups per day	Alcohol, prune juice
Breads and cereals	Products made from refined flours (white bread, crackers) or finely milled grains (e.g., corn flakes, crisp rice cereal, puffed wheat)	Whole-grain breads, rolls, or cereal; breads or rolls with seeds, nuts, or bran
Desserts	Gelatins, tapioca, plain custards, or puddings; angel food or sponge cake; ice cream or frozen desserts without fruit or nuts	Any desserts containing dried fruits, nuts, seeds, or coconut; rich pastries, pies
Fruits	Fruit juices and strained fruits; cooked or canned apples, apricots, cherries, peaches, pears; bananas	All other raw or cooked fruits
Meats and other protein sources	Roasted, baked, or broiled tender or ground beef, veal, pork, lamb, poultry, or fish; smooth peanut butter; cottage, cream, American, or mild cheddar cheeses in small amounts	Tough or spiced meats and those prepared by frying; highly flavored cheeses; nuts
Potatoes, rice, and pasta	Peeled potatoes; white rice; most pasta products	Potato skins, potato chips, or fried potatoes; brown rice; whole-grain pasta products
Sweets	Sugar, honey, jelly, hard candy and gumdrops, plain chocolates	Jam, marmalade; candy made with seeds, nuts, coconut
Vegetables	Vegetable juices and strained vegetables; cooked or canned vegetables	Raw or whole cooked vegetables
Other	Salt, ground seasonings; cream sauce and plain gravy	Chili sauce, horseradish; popcorn, seeds of any kind; whole spices, olives, vinegar

medications reduce the extent of bowel inflammation and diarrhea. Unless contraindicated, antidiarrheal medications help reduce fluid loss and increase comfort.

SAFETY ALERT: When giving antidiarrheal medications to a patient with ulcerative colitis, closely observe for manifestations of toxic megacolon: Fever, tachycardia, hypotension, dehydration, abdominal pain and cramping, and an abrupt relief of diarrhea. ■

- Maintain fluid intake by mouth or intravenously as indicated. *The patient with IBD requires fluid to replace ongoing losses, as well as fluid to meet the usual daily needs of the body. If an elemental diet or TPN is prescribed, additional fluids may be required to meet fluid intake needs.*
- Provide good skin care. *Fluid deficit and tissue dehydration increase the risk for skin excoriations or breakdown.*
- Assess perianal area for irritation or denuded skin from the diarrhea. Use gentle cleansing agents, such as a peri-wash or Tucks, diaper wipes, or cotton balls saturated with witch hazel. Apply a protective cream, such as zinc oxide–based preparations, to protect skin from the irritating effects of diarrheal stool. *Digestive enzymes in the stool are very corrosive, increasing the risk of skin breakdown where exposed to diarrheal stool.*

Promote Self-Care and Acceptance of Change in Body Image. The patient with IBD may experience frustration at not being able to control, or even predict, fecal elimination, particularly when the disease is severe. Diarrhea can interfere with the ability to complete tasks, maintain employment or engage in social activities, and even meet basic needs such as eating, sleeping, and sexual activity. Body image can suffer as a result. Treatment of IBD, be it total colectomy with IPAA, ileostomy, or chronic corticosteroid therapy, can affect the view of self.

Expected Outcome: Patient will consistently demonstrate satisfaction with body appearance and function and willingly manage required self-care activities.

The nurse will:

- Accept feelings and perception of self. *Negating or denying the reality of the patient's perception impairs trust.*
- Encourage discussion of physical changes and their consequences as they relate to self-concept. *This demonstrates acceptance and provides an opportunity to express the impact of the disease and its treatment on the patient's life.*
- Encourage discussion about concerns regarding the effect of the disease or treatment on close personal relationships. *This demonstrates understanding and provides an opportunity for the patient to express feelings about the impact of the disease on relationships and significant others.*
- Encourage the patient to make choices and decisions regarding care. *This increases the patient's sense of control over the disease and his or her future.*
- Discuss possible treatment options and their effects openly and honestly. *Open discussion allows more informed decisions.*
- Involve the patient in care, teaching and demonstrating as needed. *This encourages and facilitates independence and decision making.*
- Provide care in an accepting, nonjudgmental manner. *Acceptance of the patient despite potential embarrassment about odors or diarrhea enhances self-esteem.*
- Arrange for interaction with other patients or groups of people with IBD or ostomies. *The patient may feel that only someone who has experienced a similar problem can understand his or her feelings.*
- Teach coping strategies (odor control, dietary modifications, and so on), and support their use. *This facilitates healthy adaptation to the disease.*

Maintain Adequate Nutrition. Crohn disease can significantly alter the bowel's ability to absorb nutrients. In both forms of IBD, blood and protein-rich fluid may be lost in diarrheal stools. With malabsorption and continuing nutrient losses, multiple nutrient deficits can develop, affecting growth and development, healing, muscle mass, bone density, and electrolyte balances.

Expected Outcome: Patient will maintain adequate oral intake, report adequate energy levels, and maintain body mass and weight and normal lab values (hemoglobin and hematocrit, albumin, and electrolytes).

The nurse will:

- Monitor laboratory results, including hemoglobin and hematocrit, serum electrolytes, and total serum protein and albumin levels. *These studies provide an indicator of nutritional status.*
- Provide the prescribed diet: High-kilocalorie, high-protein, low-fat diet with restricted milk and milk products if lactose intolerance is present. *Calories and protein are important to replace lost nutrients. Fat restriction helps reduce diarrhea and nutrient loss, particularly when significant portions of the terminal ileum have been resected.*
- Provide parenteral nutrition as necessary if the patient is unable to absorb enteral nutrients. *Parenteral nutrition can help reverse nutritional deficits and promote weight gain and healing in the patient with acute manifestations.*
- Arrange for dietary consultation. Consider food preferences as allowed. *Providing preferred foods in the prescribed diet increases intake and supports nutritional status.*
- Provide or administer elemental enteral nutrition and supplements as ordered. *Elemental enteral nutritional supplements support healing while providing for bowel rest. They can replace losses and improve nutritional status more rapidly than diet alone.*
- Include family members, the primary food preparer in particular, in teaching and dietary discussions. *Families can reinforce teaching and help the patient maintain required restrictions or kilocalorie intake.*

Transitions of Care

Although IBD cannot be predicted or prevented, effective management may help the patient avoid complications of the disease. Stress the importance of complying with the prescribed treatment regimen and promptly reporting manifestations of exacerbations to the physician.

If surgery is planned or has been done, include the following topics in home care instructions:

- Ileal pouch–anal anastomosis or ileostomy care as indicated
- Where to obtain ostomy supplies
- Use of nonprescription drugs, such as enteric-coated and timed-release capsules, that may not be adequately absorbed before elimination through the ileostomy
- Community and national ostomy support groups.

Provide referrals to a dietary consultant or nutritionist, a community healthcare agency, home care services, and home intravenous care services as indicated. In addition, suggest the following resources:

- Crohn's and Colitis Foundation of America, Inc.
- The Israel Foundation for Crohn's Disease and Ulcerative Colitis
- United Ostomy Association, Inc.

IBD is a chronic condition for which the patient provides daily self-management. For this reason, teaching is a vital component of care. Teach the patient and family about the following topics:

- The type of IBD affecting the patient, including the disease process, short- and long-term effects, the relationship of stress to disease exacerbations, and the manifestations of complications
- Prescribed medications, including drug names, desired effects, schedules for tapering the doses if ordered

(as with corticosteroids), and possible side effects or adverse reactions and their management

- The recommended diet and the rationale for any specific restrictions
- Use of nutritional supplements such as Ensure to maintain weight and nutritional status
- Indicators of malabsorption and impaired nutrition; recommendations for self-care and when to seek medical intervention
- If discharged with a central catheter and home parenteral nutrition, written and verbal instructions on catheter care, troubleshooting, and parenteral nutrition administration (have the patient and a family member demonstrate catheter care and parenteral nutrition maintenance).
- The importance of maintaining a fluid intake of at least 2 to 3 quarts per day, increasing fluid intake during warm weather, exercise, or strenuous work and when fever is present
- The increased risk for colorectal cancer and importance of regular bowel exams
- Risks and benefits of various treatment options
- Importance of informing interprofessional care team of complementary and alternative therapy use.

The Patient with Diverticular Disease

Diverticula are small (0.5- to 1.0-cm) outpouchings of the colon that occur in rows. Diverticula may occur anywhere in the intestinal tract, excluding the rectum. The vast majority affect the large intestine, with 85 to 95% occurring in the sigmoid colon (Sorenson et al., 2019).

People in the United States, Australia, the United Kingdom, and France have high and increasing incidence rates of diverticular disease. The incidence of diverticula increases with age, with 5 to 10% of the population older than 45 years of age and almost 80% of those older than 85 years of age having them. Most of the people diagnosed with diverticular disease remain asymptomatic. Men and women are equally affected.

Cultural factors, particularly diet, are thought to play an important role in the development of diverticula. A diet consisting of highly refined and fiber-deficient foods is believed to be the major factor contributing to the disease. Decreased activity levels and delaying defecation have been suggested as contributing factors. The increasing incidence of diverticula with aging suggests that dietary factors (lack of fiber), a decrease in physical activity, poor bowel habits (neglecting the urge to defecate), and the effects of aging contribute to development of the disease (Sorenson et al., 2019).

Pathophysiology

Diverticula form when increased pressure within the bowel lumen causes bowel mucosa to herniate through defects in the colon wall. The circular and longitudinal muscles often thicken or hypertrophy in the area affected by diverticula. This narrows the bowel lumen, increasing intraluminal pressure. Deficient dietary fiber and a lack of fecal bulk contribute to muscle hypertrophy and narrowing of the bowel. Contraction of the muscles in response to normal stimuli such as meals may occlude the narrowed lumen, further increasing intraluminal pressure. The high pressure causes mucosa to herniate through the muscle wall, forming a diverticulum. Areas where nutrient blood vessels penetrate the circular muscle layer are the most common sites for diverticula formation.

Diverticulosis indicates the presence of diverticula (**Figure 24.8** ■). More than two-thirds of patients with diverticulosis are asymptomatic. When manifestations such as episodic pain (usually left-sided), constipation, and diarrhea occur, they can often be attributed to IBS, which commonly accompanies diverticular disease. As the disease progresses, abdominal cramping, narrow stools (decrease in caliber), increased constipation, bleeding in the stools, weakness, and fatigue may develop.

Complications of diverticulosis include hemorrhage and diverticulitis. A diverticulum may bleed, whether it

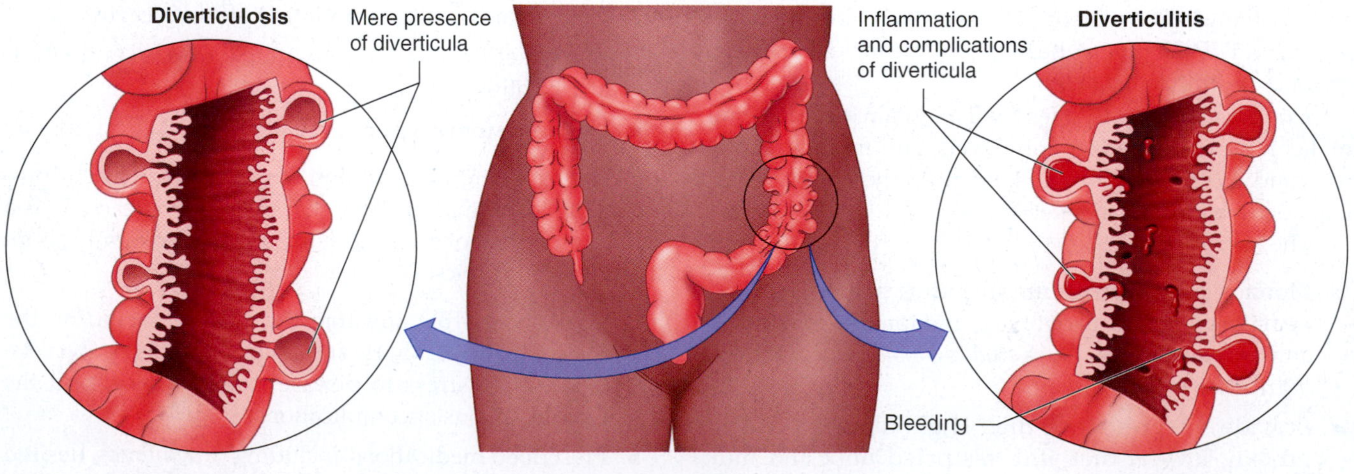
Diverticulosis
Mere presence of diverticula
Inflammation and complications of diverticula
Diverticulitis
Bleeding

Figure 24.8 ■ Diverticulitis and diverticulosis of the bowel.

Case Study & Nursing Care Plan

A Patient with Ulcerative Colitis

Cortez Lewis is a 42-year-old real estate agent and mother of three school-age children. She has had ulcerative colitis for 18 years and has been treated with prednisone and sulfasalazine. She did not tolerate treatment with biologic therapies and experienced side effects requiring her to discontinue the medications. During the past 4 months she has been having abdominal pain and cramping and frequent bloody, diarrheal stools. During the same period, she has lost 9 kg (20 lb) and has had difficulty maintaining her career. She recently developed several lesions of the lower leg identified as erythema nodosum. A recent colonoscopy revealed extensive involvement of the entire colon. On admission, Mrs. Lewis states, "I'm tired of fighting this disease. I am a prisoner in my home because of the diarrhea." She is admitted for a total proctocolectomy and ileal pouch–anal anastomosis.

ASSESSMENT

Janet Wheeler, RN, completes the admission assessment. Mrs. Lewis now weighs 52.2 kg (115 lb). She complains of abdominal cramping, pain, and frequent bloody, diarrheal stools. Several reddened lesions are noted on her lower legs. Physical assessment findings include T 36.6°C (98°F), P 72 bpm, R 20/min, and BP 104/72 mmHg. Skin cool and pale. Abnormal laboratory findings include hemoglobin 7.3 g/dL (normal 11.7 to 15.7 g/dL); hematocrit 23.3% (normal 35 to 47%); WBC 15,580/mm^3 (normal 3500 to 11,000/mm^3); platelet count 995,000/mm^3 (normal 150,000 to 450,000/mm^3); serum protein 4.6 g/dL (normal 6 to 8 g/dL); serum albumin 2.4 g/dL (normal 3.5 to 5 g/dL). Preparation for surgery is begun.

DIAGNOSES

- Weight loss due to impaired absorption
- Diarrhea related to inflammation of bowel
- Dehydration related to excessive fluid loss
- Anemia related to low hemoglobin
- Potential skin damage due to drainage from temporary ileostomy
- Acute pain related to surgical intervention
- Potential problems with sexual activity related to temporary ileostomy

EXPECTED OUTCOMES

- Patient will resume prescribed diet within 5 days after surgery.
- Patient will demonstrate normal fecal elimination through the temporary ileostomy.
- Patient will maintain adequate tissue perfusion
- Patient will maintain adequate fluid balance.
- Patient will demonstrate appropriate ostomy care prior to discharge.
- Patient will report a tolerable level of discomfort.
- Patient will verbalize feelings about sexuality and acknowledge importance of discussing sexual issues with husband.

PLANNING AND IMPLEMENTATION

- Discuss dietary modifications related to nutritional status and presence of ileostomy. Provide referral to dietitian for diet planning and teaching.
- Teach importance of maintaining a high fluid intake and manifestations of dehydration.
- Teach activity conservation and importance of maintaining balance of rest with progressive activity.
- Teach to empty and change ostomy pouch of choice.
- Teach stoma and peristomal skin assessment with each pouch change.
- Teach food blockage management.
- Refer to local United Ostomy Association.
- Provide list of local medical suppliers for ostomy appliances.

EVALUATION

On discharge, Mrs. Lewis is caring for her ileostomy by demonstrating her ability to empty, rinse, and change the pouch. The enterostomal therapy (ET) nurse has provided written and verbal instructions on ileostomy care. Mrs. Lewis verbalizes her understanding of the recommended diet and the need to limit high-fiber food intake and avoid enteric-coated and timed-release medications. The ET nurse has discussed sexual aspects of having an ileostomy and has given Mrs. Lewis a booklet, "Sex and the Female Ostomate," available through the United Ostomy Association. Mrs. Lewis is looking forward to the planned surgery to close the temporary ileostomy.

CLINICAL REASONING IN PATIENT CARE

1. Why is the patient with an ileostomy at risk for dehydration? How can Mrs. Lewis monitor her fluid status at home?
2. Why were Mrs. Lewis's hemoglobin and hematocrit values low on admission? If her hemoglobin had been low but her hematocrit normal on admission, what might be the explanation?
3. Outline a teaching plan that could be given to patients for home care of an ileostomy.
4. Develop a care plan for Mrs. Lewis for the nursing priority of potential for impaired skin integrity.

See Evaluating Your Response in Appendix B.

is inflamed or not, possibly due to erosion of an adjacent blood vessel by a fecalith (hard mass) in the diverticulum.

Diverticulitis is inflammation in and around the diverticular sac (see Figure 24.8). It typically affects only one diverticulum, usually in the sigmoid colon. Undigested food and bacteria collect in the diverticula, forming a hard mass that impairs the mucosal blood supply, allowing bacterial invasion. Mucosal ischemia leads to perforation. With microscopic perforation, inflammation is localized. Gross perforation of a diverticulum results in more extensive bacterial contamination and can lead to abscess formation or peritonitis.

Manifestations

Pain is a common manifestation of diverticulitis. It is usually left-sided and may be mild to severe and either steady or cramping. The patient may also experience either constipation or increased frequency of defecation. Depending on the location and severity of the inflammation, nausea and vomiting and a low-grade fever may occur. On examination, the abdomen may be distended, with tenderness and a palpable mass in the left lower quadrant resulting from the inflammatory response.

The older adult may have less specific manifestations, complaining of vague abdominal pain. A palpable mass and signs of a large-bowel obstruction may be present.

Complications

Complications associated with diverticulitis (in addition to peritonitis and abscess formation) include bowel obstruction, fistula formation, and hemorrhage. Severe or repeated episodes of diverticulitis may lead to scarring and fibrosis of the bowel wall, further narrowing the bowel lumen. This increases the risk for obstruction of the large bowel. Acutely inflamed tissue may adhere to the small bowel, increasing the potential for small-bowel obstruction as well. Fistulas may form, usually between the sigmoid colon and the bladder. Urinary tract infection is the usual sign of a colovesical fistula. Fistulas may also perforate into the small intestine, ureter, vagina, perineum, or abdominal wall. Bleeding from perforation of a vessel wall can occur with diverticulitis. Although it may be significant, bleeding usually stops spontaneously.

Interprofessional Care

Management of diverticular disease varies from no prescribed treatment to surgical resection of affected colon, depending on the severity of the disease and its complications.

Diagnosis

Diagnostic testing is used to identify diverticular disease when the disease is symptomatic or complications develop. In addition to illustrating diverticula, a colonoscopy may be done to detect diverticulosis, assess for strictures or bleeding, and rule out tumor as the cause of the patient's manifestations. CT scan will be done to confirm diagnosis, grade severity, detect abscess of fistula, and guide treatment (Lamanna & Moran, 2018).

Laboratory tests include Hemoccult or guaiac testing of stool to identify the presence of occult blood and a WBC count, which may show leukocytosis with a left shift (an increased number of immature WBCs) due to inflammation in diverticulitis.

Medications

Systemic broad-spectrum antibiotics effective against usual bowel flora are prescribed to treat acute diverticulitis. Oral antibiotics such as metronidazole (Flagyl) and ciprofloxacin (Cipro) or trimethoprim-sulfamethoxazole (Septra, Bactrim) may be prescribed if manifestations are mild. Severe, acute attacks often necessitate hospitalization and treatment with intravenous fluids and antibiotics effective against anaerobic and Gram-negative bacteria. Therapy may include a second-generation cephalosporin such as cefoxitin (Mefoxin), or another antibiotic such as piperacillin-tazobactam (Zosyn) or ticarcillin-clavulanate (Timentin). Antibiotics and their nursing implications are discussed in Chapter 12.

Although a stool softener such as docusate sodium (Colace) may be prescribed, it is important to note that laxatives (which can further increase intraluminal pressure in the colon) are avoided for the patient with diverticular disease.

Nutrition

Dietary modification is central to the management of diverticular disease. It appears that dietary changes can reduce the risk of complications of diverticulosis. A high-fiber diet is recommended; it increases stool bulk, decreases intraluminal pressures, and may reduce spasm (**Table 24.9**). Bran is a low-cost fiber supplement that can be added to cereal, soups, salads, or other foods. Commercial bulk-forming products, such as psyllium seed (Metamucil) or methylcellulose, also may be recommended. These products are discussed in Medication Administration 24.B. The patient is often advised to avoid foods with small seeds (such as popcorn, caraway seeds, figs, or berries), which could obstruct diverticula, but these traditional dietary restrictions are not based on rigorous evidence-based research (Lamanna & Moran, 2019).

Bowel rest is prescribed during an acute episode of diverticulitis. Most patients can be treated as outpatients and will be instructed to maintain a clear liquid diet until

Table 24.9 Foods Recommended in a High-Fiber, High-Residue Diet

Food Group	Recommended Foods
Cereals and grains	Wheat or oat bran; cooked cereals, such as oatmeal; dry cereals, such as bran buds or flakes, corn flakes, shredded wheat; whole-grain breads or crackers; brown rice
Fruits	Unpeeled raw apples, peaches, and pears; oranges; blackberries, raspberries, strawberries (may be restricted for the patient with diverticulosis)
Vegetables	Dried beans (navy, kidney, pinto), lima beans; broccoli; peas; corn; squash; raw vegetables, such as carrots, celery, and tomatoes; potatoes (with skins)

symptoms subside. The patient with complicated diverticulitis may be hospitalized and initially may be NPO with intravenous fluids and IV medication for pain control. Feeding is resumed gradually in both the outpatient and inpatient setting. Initially, a clear liquid diet is prescribed with gradual advancement to a soft, low-roughage diet (i.e., a diet low in insoluble fiber) with daily added psyllium seed to soften stool and increase its bulk. Among the foods the patient should avoid are wheat and corn bran, vegetable and fruit skins, nuts, and dry beans. The high-fiber diet is resumed following full recovery.

Surgery

Patients with acute diverticulitis may require surgery, usually to treat generalized peritonitis or an abscess that fails to respond to medical treatment. Hemorrhage that recurs or cannot be controlled may also necessitate surgery. Elective surgery may be performed for recurrent episodes of diverticulitis or persistent diverticulitis with continuing pain, tenderness, and a palpable mass. However, surgery for recurrent episodes of diverticulitis is less prevalent than in the past (Lamanna & Moran, 2019).

The affected bowel segment is resected, and if possible an anastomosis of the proximal and distal portions is performed. When an acute infection and diverticulitis are present, a two-stage Hartmann procedure is required. A temporary colostomy is created and anastomosis delayed until the inflammation has subsided. A second surgery is performed 2 to 3 months later to reconnect the bowel and close the temporary colostomy.

Nursing Care

Assessment

Because most patients with diverticular disease have few or no manifestations, nursing assessment focuses on manifestations of complications.

- ***Health history:*** Abdominal pain or cramping, chronic constipation or irregular bowel habits; nausea and vomiting; history of diverticular disease or irritable bowel syndrome
- ***Physical assessment:*** Bowel sounds, presence of abdominal tenderness of masses and location; stool for occult blood.

Priorities of Care

Priority care focuses on preventing complications of diverticulitis and managing pain and anxiety related to the possibility of a significant complication or possible surgery. Refer to Chapter 4 and Chapter 9 for nursing care related to acute pain and anxiety.

Diagnoses, Outcomes, and Interventions

Patients with acute diverticulitis are acutely ill and have multiple nursing care needs. The risk of perforation and resulting peritonitis or abscess formation is high.

Reduce Risk of Complication. During an acute attack of diverticulitis, inflammation and mucosal ischemia place the patient at risk for perforation and peritonitis. In addition to maintaining bowel rest to reduce the risk of perforation, the nurse monitors for manifestations of perforation and possible sepsis.

Expected Outcome: Patient will remain free from exhibiting signs and symptoms of complications related to diverticulitis. Patient will remain afebrile, maintain heart and respiratory rate within normal limits, maintain normal abdominal girth, have normal bowel patterns, and test negative for occult blood on a guaiac test.

The nurse will:

- Monitor vital signs including temperature at least every 4 hours. *Tachycardia and tachypnea may be early indications of increased inflammation and resulting fluid shift. Fever greater than 38.3°C (101°F) may indicate increased inflammation or spread of inflammation. Note, however, that little temperature elevation may occur in the older patient. A change in behavior or increasing lethargy may be subtle indications of infection in the older adult.*
- Assess abdomen every 4 to 8 hours or more often as indicated, including observing for distention, auscultating bowel sounds, and palpating for tenderness. Promptly report significant changes to the physician. *Increasing abdominal distention, a decrease or change in the quality of bowel sounds, and/or increasing tenderness or guarding may indicate spread of the infectious process or peritonitis.*
- Assess for evidence of lower intestinal bleeding by visual examination and guaiac testing of stools for occult blood. *Perforation of a diverticulum may produce either intestinal or intra-abdominal bleeding and require immediate treatment such as surgery.*
- Maintain intravenous fluids, TPN, and accurate intake and output records. *During acute diverticulitis, oral intake is usually prohibited or restricted. Intravenous fluids are given to maintain fluid and electrolyte balance; TPN is used to maintain nutritional status, facilitating healing and recovery.*

Transitions of Care

Teaching patients about the benefits of a high-fiber diet is an important primary prevention for diverticular disease. Nurses working with groups and individuals in the community should emphasize the importance of a high-fiber diet and its benefits in preventing diverticular disease and other disorders. In facilities such as residential settings, the nurse can work with dietary staff and care providers to increase the amount of fiber in residents' diets, unless this is contraindicated by a preexisting condition.

Provide a referral to a dietitian for teaching as indicated. Prior to discharge of the patient with acute diverticulitis, discuss the following:

- Food and fluid limitations, including recommendations for a low-residue diet during the initial period of healing
- Colostomy management (if a temporary colostomy has been created), including where to obtain supplies and dietary management

- Planned procedure to reanastomose the colon and revise the colostomy. Refer to community healthcare agencies as indicated.

The patient with diverticular disease is responsible for self-care. Discuss the following topics for home care:

- Prescribed high-fiber diet and the need to maintain the diet for life to reduce the incidence of complications, including ways to increase dietary fiber
- Complications of diverticular disease and its manifestations.

24.4 Malabsorption Syndromes

Malabsorption is a condition in which the intestinal mucosa ineffectively absorbs nutrients—including carbohydrates, proteins, fats, water, electrolytes, minerals, and vitamins—resulting in their excretion in the stool. Many bowel disorders can lead to malabsorption.

Diseases of the small intestine often cause malabsorption. Other medical and/or surgical conditions can result in malabsorption if they affect digestion or the intestinal mucosa. Primary diseases of the small-bowel mucosa, such as sprue, Crohn disease, and acute infections, can lead to malabsorption. It can also result from *maldigestion*, inadequate preparation of chyme for absorption. For example, major gastric resections, pancreatic disorders with impaired pancreatic enzyme secretion, and biliary disorders that affect bile secretion can impair digestion and absorption of chyme. Selected causes of impaired absorption and digestion are listed in **Box 24.4**.

BOX 24.4
Selected Causes of Malabsorption

IMPAIRED ABSORPTION

- Celiac disease
- Short bowel syndrome
- Gastric bypass surgeries
- Acute enteritis and other bowel infections or infestations
- AIDS-related opportunistic infections and Kaposi sarcoma
- Crohn disease
- Intestinal ischemia or infarction
- Scleroderma.

IMPAIRED DIGESTION

- Biliary obstruction
- Chronic pancreatitis, cancer of the pancreas
- Cirrhosis, hepatitis, or liver failure
- Cystic fibrosis
- Gastrectomy
- Lactose intolerance
- Zollinger-Ellison syndrome.

Regardless of the cause, malabsorption causes common manifestations resulting from impaired absorption of chyme and the nutrients it contains. Predominant GI manifestations include anorexia; abdominal bloating; diarrhea with loose, bulky, foul-smelling stools; and steatorrhea (fatty stools). Weight loss, weakness, general malaise, muscle cramps, bone pain, abnormal bleeding, and anemia are common systemic manifestations of malabsorption. These manifestations result from malnutrition and fluid loss due to poor absorption.

Three common malabsorption disorders in adults are celiac disease, lactose intolerance, and short bowel syndrome.

The Patient with Celiac Disease

Celiac disease (known as *cèliac sprue* or *nontropical sprue*) is a chronic T-cell-mediated autoimmune genetic disorder of the small intestine in which the absorption of nutrients, particularly fats, is impaired. It is characterized by sensitivity to the gliadin fraction of gluten, a cereal protein. Gluten is found in wheat, rye, barley, oats, and as a filler in many prepared foods and medications.

The cause of celiac disease is a genetic illness that affects the small intestine; in most people the duodenum is affected first, and the jejunum may also be involved. Caucasian Americans of European descent are most commonly affected (Peterson & Grossman, 2016). Having a first-degree relative with celiac disease significantly increases the risk. Nearly all people with celiac disease share the HAL-DQ2 allele, although only a small percentage of people with this allele actually have celiac disease (Peterson & Grossman, 2016). Celiac disease affects 0.5 to 1% of the U.S. population and, according to a consensus statement by the National Institutes of Health, it is a disease that is widely underrecognized (Peterson & Grossman, 2016).

Manifestations of celiac disease often develop in childhood, but may develop at any age. The average time from onset of symptoms to diagnosis of celiac disease in adults in the United States is 10 years (McCabe et al., 2012). Celiac disease is one of the most commonly diagnosed genetic diseases in Europe. The severity of the disease depends on the extent of mucosal involvement in the intestine and the duration of the disease. Three factors—immunology, genetics, and environment—contribute to the pathogenesis of celiac disease (McCabe et al., 2012).

Pathophysiology

Most absorption of nutrients occurs in the small intestine. The mucosa of the small intestine is arranged in microscopic folds, which in turn contain even smaller finger-like projections called *villi*. The cells of the villi are covered with microscopic hairs, microvilli, projecting from the cell membrane. The folds, villi, and microvilli of the intestinal mucosa provide a huge surface area for nutrient absorption. Cells of the intestines are specialized to absorb different nutrients. Readily digested nutrients are absorbed in the proximal intestine; others are absorbed more distally in the intestines. Nutrients are absorbed by the processes of simple diffusion (water and small lipids), facilitated diffusion (water-soluble vitamins), and active transport (glucose and amino acids). Once absorbed into the cells of the villi, nutrients enter the blood or lymph for systemic distribution.

Celiac disease is provoked by the ingestion of gluten and affects an individual who has a genetic predisposition for the disease. The intestinal mucosa is damaged by an immunologic response. Gliadin acts as an antigen (a substance that induces the formation of antibodies that interact specifically with it), prompting an inappropriate T-cell-mediated immune response. People with celiac disease have increased antibodies to other antigens as well. The immune response prompts an inflammatory response in the small bowel, resulting in loss of villi and microvilli. The villi shorten and atrophy, resulting in loss of intestinal folds and absorptive surface. Digestive enzyme production, including disaccharidase and particularly lactase, is reduced as well. The proximal small bowel is affected to the greatest extent, likely due to its greater exposure to dietary gluten.

Manifestations

Manifestations of celiac disease may develop at any age and recent studies show increased incidence after age 55. Researchers are unsure whether this reflects diagnosis or late emergence of the condition (Peterson & Grossman, 2016). Local manifestations include abdominal bloating and cramps, diarrhea, and steatorrhea. Systemic manifestations result from the effects of malabsorption and resulting deficiencies (see **Table 24.10**). Anemia is common. Patients are often small in stature and may have delayed maturity. Other signs of nutrient deficiencies include tetany, vitamin deficiencies, muscle wasting, and rickets (impaired bone development). When gluten is removed from the diet, the manifestations resolve.

Presentation of celiac disease can be highly variable. The symptoms may be severe and include the typical sequelae of GI malabsorption syndromes. Patients with severe celiac disease experience diarrhea, abdominal pain, bloating and distention, constipation, and reflux. Mild cases involve only the duodenum and is characterized by minimal or mild GI symptoms. Some patients are asymptomatic and remain undiagnosed throughout most of their lives (Peterson & Grossman, 2016). Patients learn they have the disease when it is discovered through serologic screening or when villous atrophy is found during endoscopy or biopsy performed for other reasons.

Some experts purport there is a spectrum of gluten disorders that distinguishes between celiac disease, wheat allergy, and gluten sensitivity. Wheat allergy is defined as an adverse immunologic response to wheat proteins, and IGE antibodies play a central role in the body's response to exposure to gluten.

Gastrointestinal malignancies and intestinal lymphoma are potential complications of celiac disease. Other complications include intestinal ulceration and development of refractory disease or disease that no longer responds to a gluten-free diet (Peterson & Grossman, 2016).

Interprofessional Care

With any malabsorptive disorder, the initial focus of management is to identify the cause. Once this has been determined, specific therapy can be prescribed.

Diagnosis

Physical exam and laboratory and diagnostic testing are used to make the differential diagnosis for various causes of malabsorption syndromes and to determine the severity of nutrient deficiencies.

An enteroscopy permits direct examination of intestinal mucosa and collection of a tissue specimen for biopsy. Tissue biopsy is necessary to establish the diagnosis of celiac disease.

Genetic testing for the presence of HLA genes is available and testing is recommended for patients who are symptomatic and have a first- or second-degree relative with celiac disease (McCabe et al., 2012). Serologic testing for IgA endomysial antibodies and IgG and IgA antigliadin antibodies is used to diagnose celiac disease and evaluate

Table 24.10 Local and Systemic Manifestations of Malabsorption

Manifestation	Cause
Local	
Diarrhea	Disruption of bowel mucosa impairs absorption of fluid and electrolytes, leading to excess water in the stool
Abdominal distention	Gas formation from fermentation of undigested carbohydrates
Steatorrhea	Impaired fat absorption leading to excess fat in feces
Systemic	
Weight loss	Carbohydrate, protein, and fat deficit
Weakness and malaise	Kilocalorie deficit; impaired absorption of micronutrients (vitamins and minerals), leading to nutrient deficiencies, anemia; fluid and electrolyte losses
Anemia	Vitamin B_{12}, folic acid, and iron deficits impair erythropoiesis
Bone pain	Calcium and vitamin D deficits lead to bone demineralization
Muscle cramps, paresthesias	Protein wasting and vitamin B_{12} and electrolyte deficits impair neuromuscular function
Easy bruising and bleeding	Vitamin K deficit
Glossitis, cheilosis	Iron, folic acid, and vitamin B_{12} deficits

compliance with the prescribed gluten-free diet. Biopsy of the jejunum is the gold standard for diagnosis (McCabe et al., 2012). Laboratory tests are used to identify pathophysiologic effects of the disease. Fecal fat is measured to document the presence of steatorrhea. The fat content of stool is increased in many malabsorptive disorders, including celiac disease. Serum levels of protein, albumin, cholesterol, electrolytes, and iron may be ordered to evaluate for nutrient deficiencies. The hemoglobin, hematocrit, and RBC indices are used to evaluate anemia. Prothrombin time is increased in vitamin K deficiency.

Medications

Patients with severe nutritional deficits may require vitamin and mineral supplements, as well as iron and folic acid to correct anemia. Vitamin K may be administered parenterally if the prothrombin time is prolonged. In patients whose disease fails to respond to dietary management, corticosteroids may be ordered to suppress the inflammatory response.

Nutrition

The patient with celiac disease is placed on a gluten-free diet. This treatment is generally successful, as long as the patient avoids gluten totally. Gluten is so widely used in prepared foods that this may be no easy task. Consultation with a dietitian and detailed dietary instructions are necessary. Patients need to become aware of hidden sources of gluten and to analyze dietary labels. Common sources of gluten and foods to be avoided are indicated in **Table 24.11**.

The prescribed diet is high in calories and protein to correct nutrient deficits. Fat content is restricted to minimize steatorrhea. The diet is usually restricted in lactose as well to compensate for the loss of lactase-containing microvilli. Foods containing lactose may be reintroduced once remission has occurred.

Nursing Care

Nursing care for the patient with celiac disease focuses on the effects of the disorder on health and nutrition, as well as the patient's ability to manage the disease.

Assessment

- ***Health history:*** Onset, duration, and severity of manifestations; number and character of stools; previous teaching related to disorder; current treatment and diet
- ***Physical assessment:*** Vital signs; abdominal shape, contour, bowel sounds; manifestations of malnutrition (e.g., anemia, small stature, muscle wasting, signs of other nutrient deficiencies).

Priorities of Care

Diarrhea and malnutrition are significant problems for the patient with celiac disease and are priorities for nursing intervention.

Diagnoses, Outcomes, and Interventions

Control Diarrhea. Steatorrhea and diarrhea typically occur with celiac disease because fat, water, and other nutrients are poorly absorbed, remaining in the bowel to be eliminated in the stool. Diarrhea can interfere with lifestyle, ADLs, skin integrity, and fluid and electrolyte balance.

Expected Outcome: Patient's diarrhea will be controlled or eliminated as demonstrated by resumption of normal bowel elimination patterns.

The nurse will:

- Assess and document the frequency and nature of stools. *Bowel elimination reflects the severity of the disease and efficacy of treatment. With effective treatment, stools become less frequent and more normal in color and appearance.*
- Weigh daily, monitor intake and output, and assess skin turgor and mucous membranes for indications of fluid balance. *Diarrhea increases the risk for hypovolemia and dehydration resulting from excess fluid loss in the stool.*
- Assess and document perianal skin condition. *Frequent defecation can irritate skin and mucous membranes, increasing the risk of breakdown.*
- Encourage a liberal fluid intake. *Oral fluids help replace fluid lost through diarrheal stool.*

Table 24.11 Dietary Sources of Gluten

Food Group	Contains Gluten	May Contain Gluten
Cereals, grains, and grain products	Bread, crackers, cereal, and pasta containing wheat, rye, or barley grain or flour	Seasoned rice and potato mixes
Beverages	Malt, Postum, Ovaltine, beers, and ales	Commercial chocolate milk, cocoa, and other beverage mixes, such as instant tea mix, dietary supplements
Desserts	Cakes, cookies, and pastries made with wheat, rye, or barley flour	Commercial ice cream and sherbet
Meats and other protein sources		Meat loaf, cold cuts and prepared meats, breaded meats; cheese products; soy protein meat substitutes; commercial egg products
Fruits and vegetables		Commercial seasoned vegetable mixes or vegetables with sauce; canned baked beans; commercial pie fillings
Miscellaneous		Commercial salad dressings and mayonnaise; ketchup and prepared mustard; gravy, white sauce; nondairy creamer; syrups; commercial pickles; fillers used in prescription and OTC medications

Promote Adequate Nutrition. Celiac disease is a chronic condition. With continuing malabsorption, multiple nutrient deficits may occur, resulting in impaired growth and development, impaired healing, muscle wasting, bone disease, and electrolyte imbalances.

Expected Outcome: Patient will maintain adequate oral intake, report adequate energy levels, and maintain body mass, weight, and normal lab values (hemoglobin and hematocrit, albumin, and electrolytes).

The nurse will:

- Maintain accurate dietary intake records. *Assessment of dietary intake provides information about compliance with the prescribed diet as well as the adequacy of nutrient intake.*
- Monitor laboratory results, including hemoglobin and hematocrit, serum electrolytes, total serum protein, and albumin levels. *These studies provide information about nutritional status.*
- Arrange for dietary consultation. Provide for food preferences as allowed. *An individualized diet developed to address the patient's food preferences as well as nutrient needs will promote appetite and food intake.*
- Provide the prescribed high-kilocalorie, high-protein, low-fat, gluten-free diet for the patient with celiac sprue. Restrict lactose (dairy product) intake as indicated. *Calories and protein are important to replace lost nutrients. Fat restriction helps reduce diarrhea and nutrient loss. Lactose may be restricted during initial treatment, then slowly reintroduced into the diet as the gut heals and its normal structure is restored.*
- Provide parenteral nutrition as ordered if the patient is unable to absorb enteral nutrients. *Parenteral nutrition can help reverse nutritional deficits and promote weight gain when manifestations are acute.*
- Encourage nutritional supplements. *Nutritional supplements are often necessary to replace losses and restore nutrient levels to normal more rapidly than diet alone can achieve.*
- Include family members, the primary food preparer in particular, in teaching and dietary discussions. *Families can reinforce teaching and help the patient maintain required restrictions or kilocalorie intake.*

Transitions of Care

Celiac disease cannot be prevented as it is an autoimmune disorder with genetic predisposition triggered by an environmental variable (gluten) (Peterson & Grossman, 2016). Secondary prevention involves screening patients with a familial history. Tertiary strategies to prevent complications of the disease are critical for patients with a diagnosis of celiac disease.

If corticosteroids have been prescribed, stress the importance of taking the medication as ordered. Emphasize the need to avoid stopping the medication abruptly and to notify all caregivers that a corticosteroid is part of the patient's medication regimen. Instruct patient to frequently monitor weight. A weight gain of 2.3 kg (5 lb) or more in less than a week usually reflects fluid gain, a possible adverse effect of corticosteroids. Other potential effects include decreased resistance to infection, an impaired inflammatory response, and changes in the metabolism of carbohydrates, proteins, and fats.

The patient with celiac disease has a chronic condition that requires continual dietary management.

Provide a detailed list of foods containing gluten. Identify foods that need to be eliminated from the diet, as well as foods that are allowed. Teach the patient and family how to identify gluten-containing commercial products by reading labels and lists of ingredients. Encourage the purchase and use of a gluten-free cookbook. Discuss potential long-term complications of the disorder and manifestations to be reported to the primary care provider. Infertility may be a complication of celiac disease. Strict adherence to a gluten-free diet may have a positive impact on fertility and improve pregnancy outcomes (Peterson & Grossman, 2016).

The Patient with Lactase Deficiency

Pathophysiology and Manifestations

For carbohydrates to be absorbed from the small intestine, they first must be broken down into simple sugars, or monosaccharides. *Lactose* is the primary carbohydrate in milk and milk products. Lactose is a disaccharide, requiring the enzyme lactase for digestion and absorption. **Lactase deficiency** can lead to *lactose intolerance* and manifestations of malabsorption. Lactase deficiency is usually genetic in origin, but also occurs secondarily to celiac disease, Crohn disease, and other disorders affecting the mucosa of the small intestine.

Many people with lactase deficiency are asymptomatic. Small to moderate amounts of milk (one to two 8-ounce glasses) may be well tolerated. Manifestations of lactose intolerance include lower abdominal cramping, pain, and diarrhea following milk ingestion. Undigested lactose ferments in the intestine, forming gases that contribute to bloating and flatus. Lactic and fatty acids produced by this fermentation irritate the bowel, leading to increased motility and abdominal cramping. The undigested lactose draws water into the intestine, which contributes to increased motility and diarrhea. The diarrhea associated with lactose intolerance may be explosive.

Interprofessional Care

The diagnosis of lactase deficiency is usually based on a history of intolerance to milk and milk products and a trial of a lactose-free diet. If manifestations resolve when lactose intake is eliminated, the diagnosis of lactase deficiency is confirmed.

Diagnosis

The lactose breath test is a noninvasive test that may be used to diagnose lactase deficiency. Expired hydrogen gas (H_2) is measured following oral administration of 50 g of lactose. If lactose is digested and absorbed normally, then little change occurs in the amount of exhaled H_2 from fasting to postlactose administration. With lactose intolerance, exhaled H_2 increases following lactose administration as the sugar ferments in the bowel.

For the lactose tolerance test, 50 to 100 g of lactose solution is orally administered, followed by measurement of blood glucose levels at intervals of 30 minutes and 1, 2, and 3 hours. If lactose is digested and absorbed normally, the blood glucose rises more than 20 mg/dL. The expected blood glucose elevation does not occur in lactase deficiency.

Nutrition

A lactose-free or reduced-lactose diet relieves the manifestations of the disorder. Some patients require total elimination of milk and milk products from the diet. Many can tolerate limited amounts of lactose. Milk pretreated with lactase is readily available. Nonprescription lactase enzyme preparations are available to improve milk tolerance. Yogurt containing bacterial lactases may be well tolerated. Calcium supplements are often recommended, particularly for women on a reduced-lactose or lactose-free diet.

Nursing Care

Nursing care for the patient with lactose intolerance focuses on providing education and support. Discuss sources of lactose: Milk, ice cream, and cottage cheese are high in lactose; aged cheese and yogurt contain much smaller amounts. Potential hidden sources of lactose include sherbets, desserts made from milk and milk chocolate, sauces and gravies, and cream soups. Suggest a trial of lactase-treated milk or lactase enzyme supplements. Emphasize the importance of obtaining nutrients contained in dairy products from other sources. Proteins may be obtained from meats, eggs, legumes, and grains. Other sources of calcium include sardines, oysters, and salmon, as well as plant sources such as beans, cauliflower, rhubarb, and green leafy vegetables.

The Patient with Short Bowel Syndrome

Pathophysiology and Manifestations

The small bowel may be resected due to tumors, infarction of bowel mucosa, incarcerated hernias, Crohn disease, bariatric surgery, trauma, and enteropathy resulting from radiation therapy. Resection of significant portions of the small intestine may result in a condition known as **short bowel syndrome**. The severity of the disorder depends on the total amount of bowel resected, as well as the portions of bowel removed. Removal of the proximal portions—including the duodenum, jejunum, proximal ileum, and the distal portion of the ileum—is associated with more severe malabsorption and manifestations than is resection of midportions of the ileum.

Resection of the small intestine affects the absorption of water, nutrients, vitamins, and minerals. Transit time of ingested foods and fluids is reduced, and digestive processes are impaired. The bowel undergoes an adaptive process in which the remaining villi enlarge and lengthen to increase absorptive surface following resection. For many patients, absorption and bowel function return to preoperative or near-normal levels. Others have continued significant impairment of digestion and absorption, leading to nutrient deficiencies, weight loss, and diarrhea. Short bowel syndrome is associated with an increased risk for kidney stones and gallstones.

Interprofessional and Nursing Care

Management of short bowel syndrome focuses on alleviating manifestations. Patients often simply require frequent, small, high-kilocalorie, high-protein feedings.

Diagnosis

Laboratory and diagnostic studies are used to evaluate nutrient deficiencies. Total serum proteins and albumin are reduced, as are serum levels of folate, iron, vitamins, minerals, and electrolytes. Anemia and a prolonged prothrombin time (indicative of vitamin K deficiency) may develop.

Medications

Multivitamin and mineral supplementation is frequently necessary. Antidiarrheal medications are used to reduce bowel motility, allowing a greater amount of time for nutrient absorption. Some patients are affected by gastric hypersecretion following bowel resection. For these patients, a proton-pump inhibitor such as omeprazole (Prilosec) may be ordered. Patients with severe manifestations of short bowel syndrome may require parenteral nutrition (PN).

Transition of Care

Prevention involves tertiary strategies aimed to prevent complications of short-bowel syndrome. Most complications are related to nutrient deficiencies.

Nursing care for the patient with short bowel syndrome focuses on the problems of potential fluid volume deficit, malnutrition, and diarrhea.

Fluid losses are generally greatest in the initial periods following surgery, warranting the closest attention at that time. Close monitoring of vital signs, intake and output, daily weights, skin turgor, and condition of mucous membranes is vital. It is important to remember that the risk is also high when other abnormal fluid losses occur through, for example, fever, draining wounds, or excess perspiration.

Document nutritional status, including weight, anthropometric measurements, laboratory values, and kilocalorie intake. Provide nutritional supplementation with enteral feedings as needed. Maintain central lines and PN, using aseptic technique.

For diarrhea, document the number and character of stools. Administer antidiarrheal medications as ordered. If the patient is lactose intolerant, limit intake of milk and milk products. Provide good skin care of the perianal region to prevent breakdown from frequent bowel movements. Refer to the discussion of nursing care for the patient with celiac disease for other measures for altered nutrition and diarrhea.

The patient and family affected by this condition require extensive education. Because there is no way to cure or replace the lost bowel at this time, the patient must manage the disorder on a day-to-day basis. Provide instructions about the recommended diet and medication regimen. Emphasize the importance of maintaining an adequate fluid intake, particularly in hot weather or during strenuous exercise. Teach the patient to monitor his or her weight frequently and report changes. Include teaching about possible manifestations of dehydration and nutrient deficiencies that should be reported to the physician. Referring the patient to a dietitian or counselor can help the person cope with what may be a lifelong problem. See Chapter 23 for discussion and treatment of dumping syndrome, which is a possible complication of bowel surgery.

24.5 Neoplastic Disorders

Cancer remains the second leading cause of death in the United States, preceded only by heart disease. Although cancer may affect any portion of the digestive tract, the large intestine and rectum are the most common sites. Malignant neoplasms of the lower bowel are the second leading cause of death from cancer (after lung cancer), making this a significant healthcare concern.

The Patient with Polyps

A **polyp** is a mass of tissue that arises from the bowel wall and protrudes into the lumen. Polyps may develop in any portion of the bowel, but they occur most often in the sigmoid colon and rectum. They vary considerably in size and may be single or multiple. It is estimated that approximately 30% of people over the age of 50 have polyps. Although most polyps are benign, some have the potential to become malignant. *Familial adenomatous polyposis (FAP)* is a syndrome with a dominant inheritance pattern that leads to the development of hundreds to thousands of adenomatous polyps. Some of these polyps will inevitably become malignant.

Pathophysiology

Polyps are identified by their structure and tissue type. Most polyps are *adenomas*, benign epithelial tumors that are considered premalignant lesions. More than 95% of adenocarcinomas arise from adenomas. Of polyps that are removed during colonoscopy, more than 70% are adenomatous (Cornett & Dea, 2018).

Adenomatous polyps represent disruption of the normal process of cell proliferation to replace epithelial cells lining the intestine. Cells are constantly being reproduced to replace those shed as feces move through the colon. Disruption of the normal process of cell division and maturation can lead to formation of a polyp composed of tightly packed epithelial cells. The cells may appear grossly normal or show signs of dysplasia. Polyps may develop as tubular, villous, or tubulovillous adenomas. Polyps may be named by the way they are attached to the bowel wall as either sessile (raised nodules) or pedunculated (attached by a stalk) (**Figure 24.9** ■).

Tubular adenomas (also called *pedunculated polyps*) are more common than sessile polyps and account for about 20 to 53% of benign polyps of the large intestine (Sorenson et al., 2019) (Figure 24.9A). A tubular adenoma is a globelike structure attached to the intestinal wall by a thin, stalklike stem. The incidence of this type of polyp increases with age, although it occurs in all age groups and in both genders. Most are small, 1 cm or less in diameter, although they may be as large as 4 to 5 cm. The malignant potential of these polyps seems to be related to their size. Small adenomas less than 1 cm have a low risk of being malignant, but larger adenomas (>1 cm) have a much higher risk of harboring malignancy or a high-grade dysplasia.

Villous adenomas (also called *sessile polyps*) have a broad base and an elevated, cauliflower-like surface (Figure 24.9B). They typically develop in the rectosigmoid colon. This type of polyp is often larger than a tubular adenoma, usually more than 5 cm. Villous adenomas are not common, accounting for about 10% of colon polyps. They have a higher malignant potential than tubular adenomas. Some adenomatous polyps contain both tubular epithelium and villi and are known as *tubulovillous adenomas*.

Manifestations

Most polyps are asymptomatic, found coincidentally during routine examination or diagnostic testing. Intermittent painless rectal bleeding, bright or dark red, is the most common presenting complaint. A large polyp may cause abdominal cramping, pain, or manifestations of obstruction. Diarrhea and mucous discharge may be associated with a large villous adenoma.

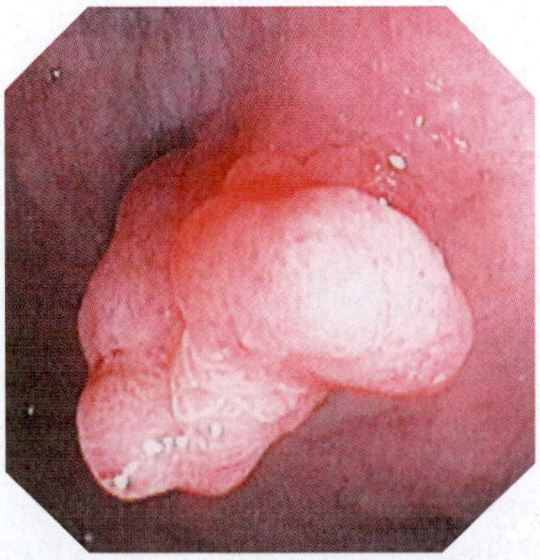

A

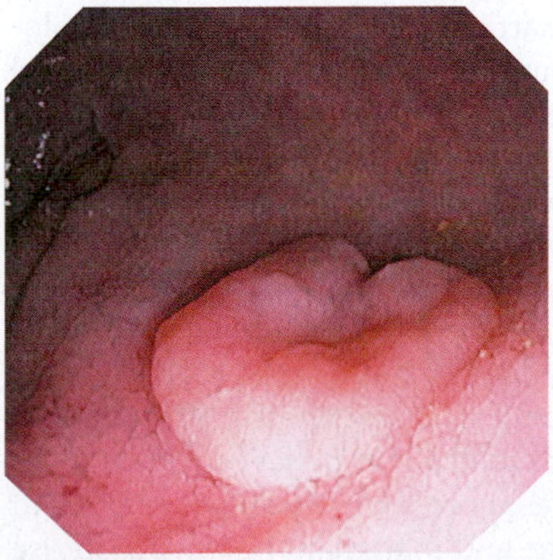

B

Figure 24.9 ■ **A**, Tubular (or pedunculated) and **B**, villous (or sessile) polyps.

Interprofessional Care

The diagnosis of intestinal polyps is generally based on diagnostic studies such as sigmoidoscopy or colonoscopy. A rectal polyp may be palpable on digital examination, but further studies are necessary to determine its size and type and the extent of colon involvement and to assess for malignancy. Genetic testing and counseling are offered to patients with a family history of FAP. First-degree relatives of a patient with FAP undergo annual sigmoidoscopy beginning at age 10 years.

Once identified, polyps are removed because of the risk of malignancy. Pedunculated polyps and small villous lesions may be removed during colonoscopy using an electrocautery snare or hot biopsy forceps passed through the scope. This relatively safe procedure has less than a 2% risk of complications such as perforation or hemorrhage. Large villous adenomas are completely excised and examined histologically for evidence of malignancy. In some cases, the colon segment containing the polyp is resected. Patients with FAP usually undergo a total colectomy with ileorectal anastomosis before age 30 years to significantly reduce their risk for developing colon cancer.

Treatment following polypectomy depends on histologic examination of the excised tissue. Because polyps tend to recur, follow-up colonoscopy is recommended in 3 years and then every 5 years if no further polyps are detected. When the polyp is found to be malignant, follow-up care is determined by the tissue type and degree of invasion.

Nursing Care

Assessment

Polyps are a silent disease, with few or no manifestations.

- *Health history:* Rectal bleeding; personal or family history of intestinal polyps or colorectal cancer.

Diagnoses, Outcomes, and Interventions

Nursing care for the patient with polyps focuses on education and assisting the patient through diagnostic testing and polyp removal. Before and after colonoscopy and polypectomy, provide direct care and teaching about the procedure, expected sensations during the procedure, and anticipated postoperative care. Cathartics are prescribed prior to colonoscopy; cleansing enemas may be ordered. Observe for evidence of fluid and electrolyte imbalance during preoperative preparation. If enemas are ordered, use normal saline (not tap water) to reduce the risk of electrolyte imbalances. Following polypectomy, observe closely for possible complications such as hemorrhage.

Transitions of Care

The incidence of intestinal polyps increases with age. They affect men and women equally. It is believed that an adenomatous polyp requires more than 5 years of growth to become significant in size and malignant potential. Advise all patients to have a screening for colorectal cancer at age 50 and as recommended thereafter for early detection of polyps (American Cancer Society [ACS], 2013).

Include the following topics when teaching for home care:

- The significance of polyps and their relationship to colorectal cancer
- The importance of keeping follow-up appointments and undergoing repeat colonoscopy as recommended: At 3 years following polypectomy, then every 5 to 10 years unless additional polyps are found
- Manifestations to report to the physician include diarrhea, pain, rectal bleeding, light-headedness, or other indications of possible blood loss.

The Patient with Colorectal Cancer

Colorectal cancer (cancer of the colon or rectum) is the third most common cancer diagnosed in the United States. The incidence of colorectal cancer has been decreasing since 1980 because of adaptation of modifiable risk factors and increases in routine screening for adults beginning at age 50 (Sorenson et al., 2019). Additionally, earlier diagnosis and better treatment have improved the survival rate for colorectal cancer. The incidence of colorectal cancer varies among race and ethnic groups. It is higher among African Americans when compared to all other races and ethnicities, and Hispanic and Asian/Pacific Islanders have the lowest rates (ACS, 2018). Colorectal cancer occurs most frequently after age 50. The incidence continues to rise with increasing age. With early diagnosis and treatment, the 5-year survival rate for colorectal cancer is 90%; however, only 39% of colorectal cancers are diagnosed at this early stage.

Risk Factors

Although the specific cause of colorectal cancer is unknown, a number of risk factors have been identified, including:

- Age over 50 years
- Polyps of the colon and/or rectum
- Family history of colorectal cancer
- Personal history of colorectal, ovarian, endometrial, or breast cancer
- Inflammatory bowel disease
- Exposure to radiation
- Diet: High animal fat and kilocalorie intake
- Obesity, smoking, and alcohol use.

Genetic factors are linked to the risk for colorectal cancer. Individuals with familial adenomatous polyposis inevitably will develop colon cancer unless the colon is removed. Hereditary nonpolyposis colorectal cancer (also known as Lynch syndrome) is an autosomal dominant disorder that significantly increases the risk for developing colorectal and other cancers. Tumors associated with Lynch syndrome often affect the ascending colon and tend to occur at an earlier age. Inflammatory bowel diseases increase the risk of colorectal cancer. Studies indicate individuals with type 2 diabetes are at higher risk for developing cancer (ACS, 2018).

Diet plays a role in the development of colorectal cancer. The disease is prevalent in economically prosperous countries where people consume diets high in calories, meat proteins, and fats. This dietary pattern, common in the United States, is thought to increase the population of anaerobic bacteria in the gut. These anaerobes convert bile acids into carcinogens. Diets high in fruits and vegetables, folic acid, and calcium appear to reduce the risk of colorectal cancer. Other factors that may reduce the risk of colorectal cancer include regular exercise, taking a daily multivitamin, and the use of aspirin and other NSAIDs.

Pathophysiology

Nearly all colorectal cancers that begin as adenomatous polyps are adenocarcinomas. Most tumors develop in the rectum and sigmoid colon, although any portion of the colon may be affected (**Figure 24.10** ■). The tumor typically grows undetected, producing few manifestations. By the time manifestations occur, the disease may have spread into deeper layers of the bowel tissue and adjacent organs. Colorectal cancer spreads by direct extension to involve the entire bowel circumference, the submucosa, and outer bowel wall layers. Neighboring structures such as the liver, greater curvature of the stomach, duodenum, small intestine, pancreas, spleen, genitourinary tract, and abdominal wall may also be involved by direct extension. Metastasis to regional lymph nodes is the most common form of tumor spread. This is not always an orderly process; distal nodes may contain cancer cells while regional nodes remain normal. Cancerous cells from the primary tumor may spread by way of the lymphatic system or circulatory system to secondary sites such as the liver, lungs, brain, bones, and kidneys. "Seeding" of the tumor to other areas of the peritoneal cavity can occur when the tumor extends through the serosa or during surgical resection.

Manifestations

Bowel cancer often produces no manifestations until it is advanced. Because it grows slowly, 5 to 15 years of growth may occur before manifestations develop. The manifestations depend on its location, type and extent, and complications. Rectal bleeding is often the initial manifestation that prompts patients to seek medical care. Other common early manifestations include a change in bowel habits, either diarrhea or constipation. Pain, anorexia, and weight loss are characteristic in advanced disease. A palpable abdominal or rectal mass may be present. Occasionally the patient presents with anemia from occult bleeding.

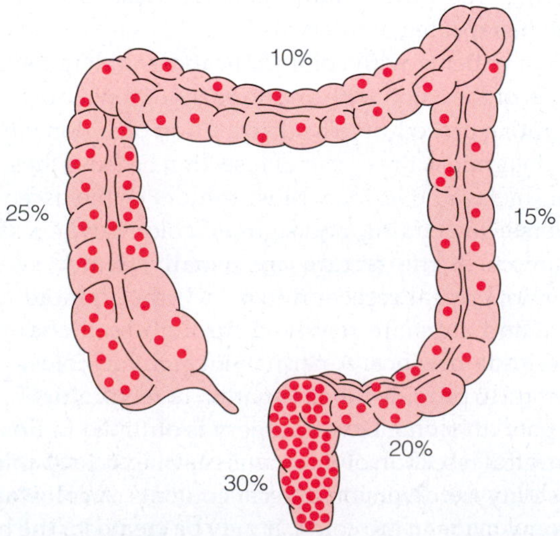
10%
25%
15%
20%
30%

Figure 24.10 ■ The distribution and frequency of cancer of the colon and rectum.

Complications

The primary complications associated with colorectal cancer are (1) bowel obstruction due to narrowing of the bowel lumen by the lesion; (2) perforation of the bowel wall by the tumor, allowing contamination of the peritoneal cavity by bowel contents; and (3) direct extension of the tumor to involve adjacent organs.

Most recurrences of colorectal cancer after tumor removal occur within the first 4 years. The size of the primary tumor does not necessarily relate to long-term survival. The number of involved lymph nodes, penetration of the tumor through the bowel wall, and tumor adherence to adjacent organs are better predictors of the prognosis for the disease.

Interprofessional Care

The focus of interprofessional care for colorectal cancer is prevention, early detection, and intervention. Colorectal cancer is always treated by surgical resection, with chemotherapy and radiation therapy used as adjuncts.

Screening

The ACS (2018) recommends one of the following testing schedules for the early detection of colorectal cancer, beginning at age 50. These options are acceptable choices for average-risk adults.

- Yearly fecal occult blood test (FOBT) or fecal immunochemical test (FIT) or stool DNA test (sDNA)
- Flexible sigmoidoscopy every 5 years, *or*
- Double-contrast barium enema every 5 years, *or*
- CT colonography (virtual colonoscopy) every 5 years, *or*
- Colonoscopy every 10 years.

Diagnosis

Diagnostic and laboratory tests are used for screening, diagnosis, and monitoring purposes. Diagnostic tests include a sigmoidoscopy or colonoscopy as the primary diagnostic test used to detect and visualize tumors. While flexible sigmoidoscopy can detect 50 to 65% of colorectal cancers, many clinicians recommend colonoscopy. Tissue for biopsy is obtained at the time of endoscopy to confirm cancerous tissue and evaluate cell differentiation. Current staging methods primarily use the TNM system, as outlined in **Table 24.12** and shown in **Figure 24.11** ■. Radiologic examinations may include a chest x-ray to detect tumor metastasis to the lung. Computed tomography (CT) scan, magnetic resonance imaging (MRI), or ultrasonic examination may be used to assess tumor depth and involvement of other organs by direct extension or metastasis.

Table 24.12 The TNM Classification for Colorectal Cancer

Stage	Primary Tumor (T)	Regional Lymph Nodes (N)	Distant Metastasis (M)
	TX—Primary tumor cannot be assessed TO—No evidence of primary tumor	NX—Regional lymph nodes cannot be assessed	MX—Presence of distant metastasis cannot be assessed
Stage 0	Tis—Carcinoma *in situ*	NO—No regional lymph node metastasis	MO—No distant metastasis
Stage I	T1—Tumor invades submucosa		
	T2—Tumor invades muscularis propria		
Stage II	T3—Tumor invades through muscularis propria into subserosa or into nonperitonealized pericolic or perirectal tissues		
	T4—Tumor perforates visceral peritoneum or directly invades other organs or structures		
Stage III	Any T	N1—Metastasis in one to three pericolic or perirectal lymph nodes	
		N2—Metastasis in four or more pericolic or perirectal lymph nodes	
Stage IV	Any T	Any N	M1—Distant metastasis

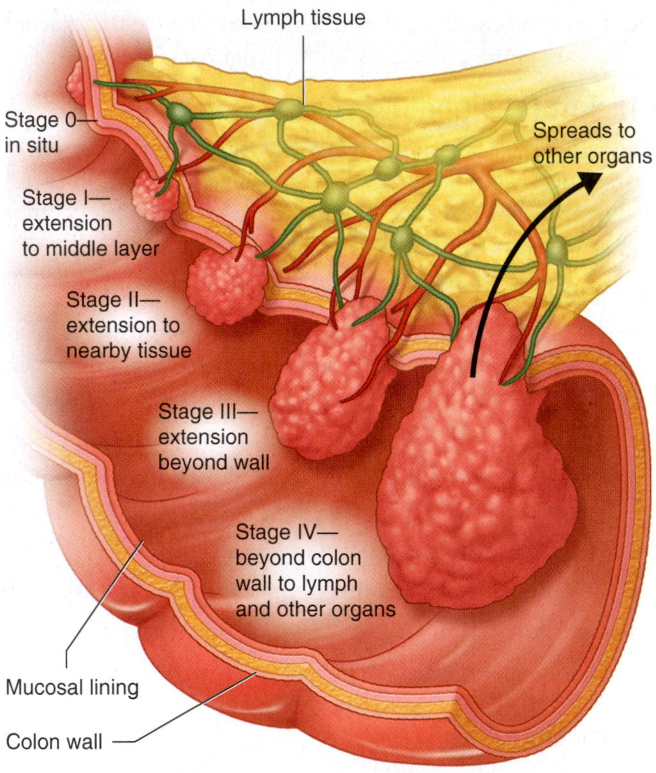
Lymph tissue
Stage 0—
in situ
Spreads to
other organs
Stage I—
extension
to middle layer
Stage II—
extension to
nearby tissue
Stage III—
extension
beyond wall
Stage IV—
beyond colon
wall to lymph
and other organs
Mucosal lining
Colon wall

Figure 24.11 ■ Staging of colorectal cancer.

Laboratory tests used are a fecal occult blood test (by guaiac or Hemoccult testing) to detect blood in the feces and a CBC to detect anemia resulting from chronic blood loss and tumor growth. Carcinoembryonic antigen (CEA) is a tumor marker that can be detected in the blood of patients with colorectal cancer. CEA levels are used to estimate prognosis, monitor treatment, and detect cancer recurrence.

Surgery

Surgical resection of the tumor, adjacent colon, and regional lymph nodes is the treatment of choice for colorectal cancer. Options for surgical treatment vary from destruction of the tumor by laser photocoagulation performed during endoscopy to abdominoperineal resection with permanent colostomy. When possible, the anal sphincter is preserved and colostomy avoided.

Laser photocoagulation uses a very small, intense beam of light to generate heat in tissues toward which it is directed. The heat generated by the laser beam can be used to destroy small tumors. It is also used for palliative surgery of advanced tumors to remove obstruction. Laser photocoagulation can be performed endoscopically and is useful for patients who cannot tolerate major surgery.

Other surgical treatment options for small, localized tumors include local excision and fulguration. These procedures may be performed during endoscopy, eliminating the need for abdominal surgery. Local excision may be used to remove a disk of rectum containing a tumor in patients with a small, well-differentiated, mobile polypoid lesion. *Fulguration* or electrocoagulation is used to reduce the size of some large tumors for patients who are poor surgical risks. This procedure requires general anesthesia and may need to be repeated at intervals.

Most patients with colorectal cancer undergo surgical resection of the colon with anastomosis of remaining bowel as a curative procedure. The distribution of regional lymph nodes determines the extent of resection because these may contain metastatic lesions. Most tumors of the ascending, transverse, descending, and sigmoid colon can be resected.

Tumors of the rectum are usually treated with an abdominoperineal resection in which the sigmoid colon, rectum, and anus are removed through both abdominal and perineal incisions. A permanent sigmoid colostomy is performed to provide for elimination of feces. Nursing care of the patient having bowel surgery is outlined in **Box 24.5**.

Surgical resection of the bowel may be accompanied by a colostomy for diversion of fecal contents. A **colostomy** is an ostomy made in the colon. It may be created if the bowel is obstructed by the tumor, as a temporary measure to promote healing of anastomoses, or as a permanent means

BOX 24.5
Nursing Care of the Patient Having Bowel Surgery

PREOPERATIVE NURSING CARE

Provide routine preoperative care for the surgical patient, as outlined in Chapter 4. If the patient is likely to have a colostomy, arrange for consultation with an enterostomal therapy (ET) nurse specialist, if appropriate. The ET nurse will provide initial ostomy teaching and identify and mark an appropriate stoma location. Occasionally the surgeon will order insertion of a nasogastric tube preoperatively to remove secretions. The nasogastric tube is usually inserted in the surgical suite just prior to surgery. The patient will typically require bowel preparation procedures to reduce the risk of peritoneal contamination by bowel contents during surgery.

Cleansing enemas can often be delegated to nonlicensed assistive personnel. Oral and parenteral antibiotics may need to be administered as prescribed to reduce the risk of infection.

POSTOPERATIVE NURSING CARE

Provide routine care for the surgical patient, as outlined in Chapter 4. Regular focused assessment will include monitoring bowel sounds, the passage of flatus, and the degree of abdominal distention. Bowel surgery can often result in an ileus, so monitoring for the return of peristalsis is important and the surgeon should be notified if abdominal distention becomes extreme. Assisting the patient with mobility will aid in preventing and treating an ileus. The patient will return from surgery with a nasogastric tube. Assess the position and patency and ensure the tube is connected to low or intermittent suction as ordered. Monitor the characteristics and volume of nasogastric tube drainage. Initial drainage may be bright red and then become dark and finally clear or greenish yellow over the first 2 to 3 days. A change in the color, amount, or odor of the drainage may indicate a complication such as hemorrhage, intestinal obstruction, or infection. Assess color, amount, and odor of drainage from surgical drains and the colostomy (if present), noting any changes or the presence of clots or bright bleeding. Alert all personnel caring for the patient with an abdominoperineal resection to avoid rectal temperatures, suppositories, or other rectal procedures. These procedures could disrupt the anal suture line, causing bleeding, infection, or impaired healing. Maintain intravenous fluids while nasogastric suction is in place. The patient on nasogastric suction is unable to take oral food and fluids and, moreover, is losing electrolyte-rich fluid through the nasogastric tube. If replacement fluid and electrolytes are not maintained, the patient is at risk for dehydration; sodium, potassium, and chloride imbalance; and metabolic alkalosis. Provide antacids, H_2-receptor antagonists, proton-pump inhibitors, and antibiotic therapy as ordered. These medications may be ordered for the postoperative patient, depending on the procedure performed. Antibiotic therapy is a common measure to prevent infection resulting from contamination of the abdominal cavity with gastric contents.

Oral feedings are reintroduced slowly to minimize abdominal distention and trauma to the suture lines. Initial feedings may be clear liquids, progressing to full liquids, and then frequent small feedings of regular foods. Monitor bowel sounds and monitor for abdominal distention frequently during this period.

Discharge planning and teaching should be initiated early, especially if the patient has a new colostomy. Reinforcement of self-care teaching may need to be instituted over several sessions to ensure the patient and/or caregiver can manage the colostomy. Dietary considerations should be included in the discharge plan. Consult with a dietitian for instructions and menu planning; reinforce teaching. Teach about potential postoperative complications such as abdominal abscess or bowel obstruction, their signs and symptoms, and preventive measures.

---

of fecal evacuation when the distal colon and rectum are removed. Colostomies take the name of the portion of the colon from which they are formed: Ascending colostomy, transverse colostomy, descending colostomy, and sigmoid colostomy (**Figure 24.12 ■**).

A *sigmoid colostomy* is the most common permanent colostomy performed, particularly for cancer of the rectum. It is usually created during an abdominoperineal resection. This procedure involves the removal of the sigmoid colon, rectum, and anus through abdominal and perineal incisions. The anal canal is closed, and a stoma formed from the proximal sigmoid colon. The stoma is usually located on the lower left quadrant of the abdomen.

When a *double-barrel colostomy* is performed, two separate stomas are created (**Figure 24.13 ■**). The distal colon is not removed, but bypassed. The *proximal stoma,* which is functional, diverts feces to the abdominal wall. The *distal stoma,* also called the *mucous fistula,* expels mucus from the distal colon. It may be pouched or dressed with a 4 × 4 gauge dressing. A double-barrel colostomy may be created for cases of trauma, tumor, or inflammation, and it may be temporary or permanent.

An emergency procedure used to relieve an intestinal obstruction or perforation is called a *transverse loop colostomy.* During this procedure, a loop of the transverse colon is brought out from the abdominal wall and suspended over a plastic rod or bridge, which prevents the loop from slipping back into the abdominal cavity. The loop stoma may be opened at the time of surgery or a few days later at the patient's bedside. The bridge may be removed in 1 to 2 weeks. Transverse loop colostomies are typically temporary.

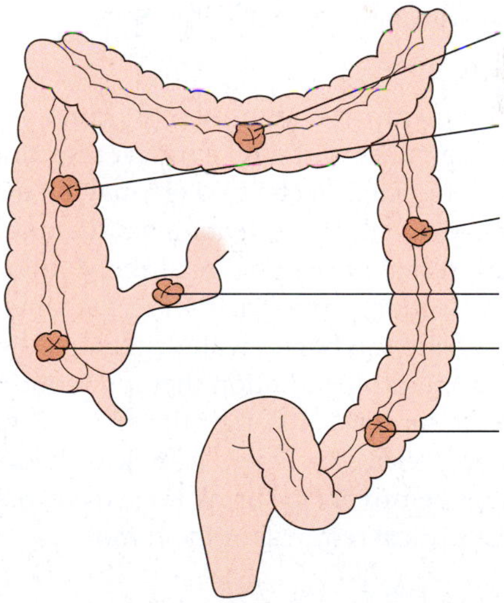
Transverse colostomy
Ascending colostomy
Descending colostomy
Ileostomy
Cecostomy
Sigmoid colostomy

Figure 24.12 ■ Various ostomy levels and sites.

In a *Hartmann procedure,* a common temporary colostomy procedure, the distal portion of the colon is left in

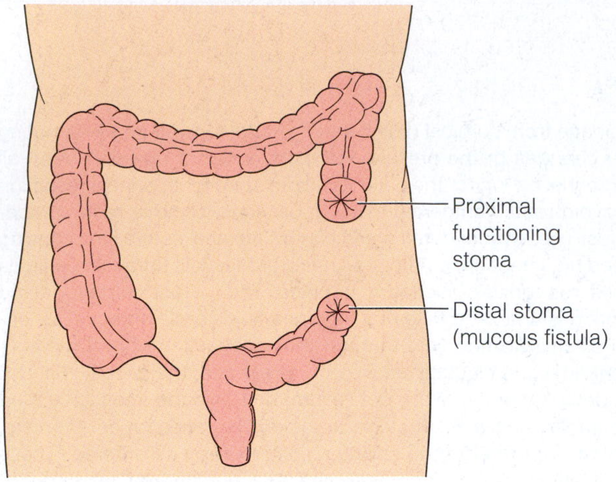
Proximal
functioning
stoma
Distal stoma
(mucous fistula)

Figure 24.13 ■ A double-barrel colostomy. The proximal stoma is the functioning stoma; the distal stoma expels mucus from the distal colon.

place and is oversewn for closure. A temporary colostomy may be done to allow bowel rest or healing, such as following tumor resection or inflammation of the bowel. It may also be created following traumatic injury to the colon, such as a gunshot wound. Anastomosis of the severed portions of the colon is delayed because bacterial colonization of the colon would prevent proper healing of the anastomosis. About 3 to 6 months following a temporary colostomy, the colostomy is closed and the colon is reconnected. Patients with temporary colostomies require the same care as patients with permanent colostomies. See **Box 24.6**, Nursing Care of a Patient with a Colostomy.

Radiation Therapy

Although radiation therapy is not used as a primary treatment for colon cancer, it is used with surgical resection for treating rectal tumors. Small rectal cancers may be treated with intracavitary, external, or implantation radiation. Rectal cancer has a high rate of regional recurrence following complete surgical resection, particularly when the tumor has invaded tissues outside the bowel wall or regional lymph nodes. Pre- or postoperative radiation therapy reduces the recurrence of pelvic tumors, although the effect of radiation therapy on long-term survival is less clear. Radiation therapy is used preoperatively to shrink large rectal tumors enough to permit surgical removal of the tumor.

Chemotherapy

Chemotherapeutic agents, such as intravenous fluorouracil (5-FU) and folinic acid (leucovorin), are used postoperatively as adjunctive therapy for colorectal cancer. When combined with radiation therapy, chemotherapy reduces the rate of tumor recurrence and prolongs survival for patients with stage II and stage III rectal tumors. The benefit for colon cancers is less clear, but chemotherapy may be used to reduce its spread to the liver and prevent recurrence. Irinotecan (CPT-11) or oxaliplatin may be used in chemotherapy regimens for colorectal cancer. Further discussion about chemotherapy and nursing implications is included in Chapter 14.

Nursing Care

Assessment

- *Health history:* Usual bowel patterns and any recent changes; weight loss, fatigue, decreased activity tolerance; presence of blood in the stool; pain with defecation, abdominal discomfort, perineal pain; usual diet; family history of colon cancer; other specific risk factors such as inflammatory bowel disease or colon polyps
- *Physical assessment:* General appearance; weight; abdominal shape, contour; bowel sounds, abdominal tenderness; stool Hemoccult or guaiac.

Priorities of Care

Nursing care includes providing emotional support, teaching, and direct care before and after diagnostic procedures and surgery and during adjunctive treatments. Priority nursing care includes relieving pain, ensuring adequate nutrition, managing grief, and discussing sexual function.

Diagnoses, Outcomes, and Interventions

In planning and implementing care, consider both physical care needs and emotional response to the diagnosis. Because colorectal cancer is often advanced at the time of diagnosis, the prognosis, even with treatment, may be poor. Denial and anger are common. Extensive abdominal surgery and potentially a colostomy may be necessary, and the effects of chemotherapy and radiation therapy can leave the patient fatigued and discouraged. A Case Study & Nursing Care Plan for a patient with colorectal cancer is provided on page 796.

SAFETY ALERT: If an abdominoperineal resection has been performed, alert all care personnel to avoid rectal temperatures, suppository use, or other procedures that could damage sutures. ■

Relieve Acute Pain. Surgery for colorectal cancer is a major procedure and will require aggressive postoperative pain management.

Expected Outcome: Patient will use treatment plan (pharmacologic and nonpharmacologic) to prevent and alleviate discomfort. Patient will consistently verbalize a pain level of 3 or less on a pain scale of 1 to 10 and will not exhibit nonverbal signs associated with uncontrolled pain. Patient will participate in postoperative care such as ambulation, coughing, deep breathing, and use of an incentive spirometer.

The nurse will:

- Monitor for adequate pain relief. Use subjective and objective information, including the location, intensity, and character of pain, as well as nonverbal signs, such as grimacing; muscle tension; apparent dozing; changes in pulse or blood pressure; or rapid, shallow respirations. *The patient may assume that pain is to be expected or tolerated or may fear becoming addicted to analgesic medications. Careful questioning and assessment can provide*

BOX 24.6
Nursing Care of the Patient with a Colostomy

Care of the Patient with a New Colostomy

- Assess the stoma, monitoring the output, and providing ostomy care will be a priority nursing action for the patient with a new colostomy.
- Provide teaching and coaching when caring for the colostomy will help the patient and caregivers learn the procedures they will need to perform after discharge. The enterostomal therapy (ET) nurse will typically prescribe the type of appliance and develop the teaching plan. The ET nurse is an important resource to assist with challenging situations.
- When completing the first postoperative assessment, determine the location of the stoma and the type of colostomy performed. Assess stoma appearance and surrounding skin condition frequently so emerging complications are predicted and early treatment can be initiated. Regular assessment of colostomy draining is important. Reassure the patient the drainage will change over time. Initial drainage may contain more mucus and serosanguineous fluid than fecal material. As the bowel starts to resume function, drainage becomes fecal in nature and the consistency of drainage depends on the stoma location in the bowel.
- Be sure to keep the stoma free from irritants by positioning a collection bag or drainable pouch over the stoma. If there are problems refer to the ET nurse for a change in procedure or appliance. Empty a drainable pouch or replace the colostomy bag as needed or when it is no more than one-third full. If the pouch is allowed to overfill, its weight may impair the seal and cause leakage.
- Provide stomal and skin care for the patient with a colostomy as for the patient with an ileostomy (see Box 24.1). Use caulking agents, such as Stomahesive or karaya paste, and a skin barrier wafer as needed to maintain a secure ostomy pouch. This may be particularly important for the patient with a loop colostomy. A small needle hole high on the colostomy pouch will allow flatus to escape. This hole may be closed with a bandage and opened only while the patient is in the bathroom for odor control. If gas collects, ostomy bags may "balloon" out, disrupting the skin seal.

Health Education for the Patient and Family

- Prior to discharge, provide written, verbal, and psychomotor instruction on colostomy care, pouch management, skin care, and irrigation for the patient. Allow ample time for the patient (and family, if necessary) to practice changing the pouch, either on the patient or a model.
- If an abdominoperineal resection has been performed, emphasize the importance of using no rectal suppositories, rectal temperatures, or enemas. These measures are important to prevent trauma to the tissues when the rectum has been removed. Suggest that the patient carry medical identification or wear a medical alert tag or bracelet.
- The diet for a patient with a colostomy is individualized and may require no alteration from that consumed preoperatively. Dietary teaching should, however, include information on foods that cause stool odor and gas and foods that thicken and loosen stools. Foods that cause these effects on ostomy output are listed next.

Foods That Increase Stool Odor

- Asparagus
- Beans
- Cabbage
- Eggs
- Fish
- Garlic
- Onions
- Some spices

Foods That Increase Intestinal Gas

- Beer
- Broccoli
- Brussels sprouts
- Cabbage
- Carbonated drinks
- Cauliflower
- Corn
- Cucumbers
- Dairy products
- Dried beans
- Peas
- Radishes
- Spinach

Foods That Thicken Stools

- Applesauce
- Bananas
- Bread
- Cheese
- Creamy peanut butter
- Pasta
- Pretzels
- Rice
- Tapioca

Foods That Loosen Stools

- Chocolate
- Dried beans
- Fried foods
- Greasy foods
- Highly spiced foods
- Green leafy vegetables
- Raw fruits and juices
- Raw vegetables

Foods That Color Stools

- Beets
- Red gelatin

Care of the Patient with an Established Colostomy

- Some patients irrigate their colostomy routinely because water stimulates the colon to empty. Patients who routinely irrigate their colostomy will likely have an established procedure they prefer to use and the nurse should encourage the patient to lead the procedure through verbal instructions and maintain the routine. When a colostomy irrigation is ordered for a patient with a double-barrel or loop colostomy, irrigate the proximal stoma as the distal bowel carries no fecal contents and does not need irrigation. It may be irrigated for cleansing just prior to reanastomosis.

accurate information about pain status, allowing better control of discomfort.

- Ask patient to rate pain using a 0 to 10 pain scale. Document the level of pain. *Pain is a subjective experience. Patients perceive and respond to pain differently. Religion and ethnic background may affect the response to pain.*
- Monitor analgesic effectiveness 30 minutes after administration. Monitor for pain relief and adverse effects. *The method of delivery, dosage, or medication itself may need to be adjusted to provide adequate pain relief.*
- Assess the incision for inflammation or swelling; assess drainage catheters and tubes for patency. *Poorly controlled pain or pain that changes may be related to organ distention from an obstructed nasogastric tube, urinary catheter, or wound drain or may indicate an infection.*
- Assess the abdomen for distention, tenderness, and bowel sounds. *Intra-abdominal bleeding, peritonitis, or paralytic ileus can cause pain that may be confused with incisional pain.*
- Administer analgesia prior to an activity or procedure. *Adequate pain relief reduces muscle tension, allowing for more comfortable participation in activities.*
- Assist with adjunctive comfort measures, such as positioning, diversional activities, management of environmental stimuli, guided imagery, and relaxation techniques. *These measures enhance the effects of analgesia by reducing muscle tension.*
- Splint incision with a pillow, and teach the patient how to self-splint when coughing and deep breathing. *This prevents respiratory complications related to fear of pain.*

Ensure Adequate Nutrition. Bowel preparation for diagnostic procedures, surgery, radiation therapy, and chemotherapy place the patient with colorectal cancer at risk for nutritional deficiencies. Fluid and electrolyte replacement is provided following surgery, along with possible parental nutrition (PN) (see Chapter 22). Adequate kilocalorie and nutrient intake are necessary for healing after surgery. Additionally, if the tumor is advanced, metabolic needs may be increased and the appetite decreased.

Expected Outcomes: Patient will maintain fluid and electrolyte balance, avoid complications associated with parenteral nutrition, maintain body mass and weight and normal lab values (transferrin, albumin, and electrolytes), and resume a healthy diet.

The nurse will:

- Assess nutritional status, using data such as height and weight, skinfold measurements, a body mass index (BMI) calculation (see Chapter 21), and laboratory data including serum albumin level. Refer to a dietitian or nutritionist for dietary management. *The patient who is malnourished before beginning aggressive cancer treatment requires vigorous nutrition management to promote healing.*
- Assess readiness for resumption of oral intake after surgery or procedures using data such as statements of hunger, presence of bowel sounds, passage of flatus, and minimal abdominal distention. *Manipulation of the bowel interrupts peristalsis of the GI tract. It is important to ensure that peristalsis has resumed prior to resumption of oral intake.*
- Monitor and document food and fluid intake. *Documentation helps identify the adequacy of kilocalories and other nutrient intake.*
- Weigh daily. *Weight fluctuation may indicate adequate or inadequate dietary intake.*
- Maintain PN and central intravenous lines as ordered. *Parenteral nutrition prevents tissue catabolism and promotes healing when food intake is disrupted for more than 2 to 3 days.*
- When oral intake resumes, help the patient develop a meal plan that incorporates food preferences and considers the patient's schedule and environment. *Consideration of likes, dislikes, and circumstances in meal planning promotes adequate intake.*

Support Adjustment to Change in Health Status. When a bowel resection is performed for colorectal cancer, the patient needs to adjust to the loss of a major body part as well as to the diagnosis of cancer. Even when the prognosis for recovery is good, many people perceive cancer as fatal. Supporting the patient and family during the initial stages of grieving can improve physical recovery as well as psychologic coping and eventual adaptation.

Expected Outcome: Patient and family will express thoughts and feelings about fears and perceived losses related to diagnosis and treatments (colostomy) and progress through the stages of grief to acceptance.

The nurse will:

- Work to develop a trusting relationship with the patient and family. *This increases the nurse's effectiveness in helping them work through the grieving process.*
- Listen actively, encouraging the patient and family to express their fears and concerns. Assist to identify strengths, past experiences, and support systems.
- Demonstrate respect for cultural, spiritual, and religious values and beliefs; encourage use of these resources to cope with losses.
- Encourage discussion of the potential impact of loss on individual family members, family structure, and family function. Assist family members to share concerns with one another.
- Refer to cancer support groups, social services, or counseling as appropriate. *These resources can be used throughout the grieving process.*

Discuss Changes in Sexuality Self-Image and Function. Colorectal cancer and ostomy surgery increase the risk for sexual dysfunction, defined as a change in sexual function so that it becomes unsatisfying, unrewarding, or inadequate. Physical factors that can lead to sexual dysfunction include disruption of nerves and blood vessels that supply the genitals, radiation therapy, chemotherapy, and other medications prescribed after surgery.

Psychologically, an *ostomate* (patient with an ostomy) experiences an altered body image and may develop low self-esteem. The patient may feel undesirable and fear rejection. He or she may be concerned about odors or pouch leakage during sexual activity. This emotional stress can contribute to sexual dysfunction.

Expected Outcome: Patient and family will express thoughts, feelings, and concerns regarding actual and perceived changes in sexual function. Patient will identify resources available for ongoing support and information related to changes in sexual function.

The nurse will:

- Provide opportunities for the patient and family to express feelings about the cancer diagnosis, ostomy, and effects of other treatments. *Encouraging verbalization of feelings about the diagnosis, ostomy, and treatments provides an opportunity to validate that feelings of anger and depression are normal responses to the diagnosis and change in body function.*
- Provide consistent colostomy care. *An accepting attitude and consistent care that provides a secure appliance and controls odor and leakage instill a sense of confidence in the patient.*
- Encourage expression of sexual concerns. Provide privacy and caregivers who have established trust with the patient and family and are comfortable with discussions about sexual concerns. *Sexuality is a very private concern to most people. The patient and family are not likely to express their concerns openly unless trust has been established.*
- Reassure the patient and significant other that the effect of physical illness and prescribed interventions on sexuality usually is temporary. *The patient and partner may misinterpret an initial decrease in libido as evidence that sexual activity will not be possible or resume following recovery.*
- Refer the patient and partner to social services or a family counselor for further interventions. *Patients are often discharged from acute care settings well before concerns about sexual activity surface. Ongoing counseling provides a continuing resource.*
- Arrange for a visit from a member of the United Ostomy Association. *People who are living and coping with an ostomy can provide information and support, helping the new ostomate overcome feelings of isolation and rejection.*

Transitions of Care

Primary prevention of colorectal cancer is a significant nursing care issue. Teach patients the importance of maintaining an optimal weight and staying physically active. Discuss dietary recommendations provided by the ACS for the prevention of colorectal cancer. These recommendations include decreasing the amount of fat, refined sugar, and red meat in the diet while increasing intake of dietary fiber. Foods that contain high amounts of fiber include raw fruits and vegetables, legumes, and whole-grain products.

Stress the importance of regular health examinations, including digital rectal exams. Discuss recommendations for regular Hemoccult testing of stool after age 40. Include the importance of seeking medical treatment if blood is noted in or on the stool. Teach patients the warning signs for cancer, including those specific to bowel cancer, such as a change in bowel habits.

Measures to prevent colon cancer that are considered to be effective and safe include consuming a diet high in fruits and vegetables and low in saturated fat and red meat, regular exercise, maintaining a healthy weight, limiting alcohol consumption, and quitting smoking. Consuming fiber supplements, minerals such as calcium, vitamins, and NSAIDs may help prevent colorectal cancer (ACS, 2018). Although considered safe, these measures are the subject of further research to demonstrate conclusive proof of effectiveness.

During the diagnostic and preoperative periods, provide instruction regarding anticipated postoperative care. Priority nursing care focuses on pain management, focused assessment to monitor GI function, and assisting with ostomy care as appropriate. The patient's care will be complex in the early postoperative care and the nurse will need to coordinate care between specialties and disciplines. Supporting the patient and family if there is new cancer diagnosis is an important nursing role.

Once treatment has been initiated, include the following topics (as appropriate) in teaching for home care:

- Pain management
- Skin care and management of potential adverse effects of radiation therapy and/or chemotherapy (Refer to Chapter 14 for further discussion of teaching needs related to these therapies.)
- Incision and ostomy care
- Recommended diet
- Follow-up appointments and care
- Community resources such as the American Cancer Society or ostomy support services.

If the tumor is inoperable or a cure is not anticipated, provide information about pain and symptom management. Discuss the hospice philosophy and available services. Provide a referral to a local hospice or home health department.

Case Study & Nursing Care Plan

A Patient with Colorectal Cancer

William Cunningham is a 65-year-old retired railroad employee, husband, and father of three grown children. For the past 3 months, Mr. Cunningham has noticed small amounts of blood and occasional mucus in his stools. He has a sensation of pressure in the rectum and notices that his stools are smaller in diameter, about the size of pencil. After palpating a mass on digital examination of the rectum, the physician orders a colonoscopy. A large sessile lesion is found in the rectum and biopsied. The pathology report shows the lesion to be adenocarcinoma. Mr. Cunningham is scheduled for an abdominoperineal resection and sigmoid colostomy.

ASSESSMENT

Madonna Hart, RN, completes the admission assessment. Mr. Cunningham states that his bowel habits have recently changed, but denies pain or other symptoms. Physical assessment findings include T 36.9°C (98.4°F), P 82 bpm, R 18/min, and BP 118/78 mmHg. He is 178 cm (70 in.) tall and weighs 84 kg (185 lb). Laboratory findings are normal except for the previous pathology report of adenocarcinoma of rectal lesion.

Mr. Cunningham states, "I really don't want a colostomy, but if that is what it takes to get rid of this, I'm ready to get it over with."

DIAGNOSES

- Acute pain related to surgical intervention
- Potential skin damage related to fecal drainage and pouch adhesive
- Potential constipation/diarrhea related to effects of surgery on bowel function
- Potential for poor body image related to colostomy
- Potential disruption of sexual function related to wide rectal incision, radiation therapy, and colostomy

EXPECTED OUTCOMES

- Patient will report pain is within an acceptable range that allows ease of movement and ambulation.
- Patient will perform colostomy care using correct technique.
- Patient will demonstrate willingness to discuss changes in sexual function.
- Patient will wear clothing to enhance physical and emotional self-esteem.

PLANNING AND IMPLEMENTATION

- Provide analgesia as ordered, evaluating its effectiveness.
- Discuss foods that cause odor and gas.
- Teach colostomy care.
- Maintain consistent nursing personnel assignment to facilitate trust.
- Refer to the local United Ostomy Association.
- Provide a list of local medical supply companies for ostomy supplies.
- Provide for privacy when teaching and discussing concerns about ostomy.

EVALUATION

On discharge, Mr. Cunningham is able to empty and rinse out his colostomy pouch. He is changing the pouch and caring for surrounding skin appropriately. Ms. Hart has given him verbal and written instructions on colostomy care. He verbalizes understanding of phantom rectal pain and the importance of avoiding rectal suppositories. He expresses an understanding of the need to avoid heavy lifting and the importance of follow-up care. Ms. Hart has referred Mr. Cunningham to a home health agency in his community for further questions and follow-up care.

CLINICAL REASONING IN PATIENT CARE

1. What is the cause of phantom rectal pain?
2. Why is it important to discuss dietary concerns with a patient with a colostomy, especially odor- and gas-forming foods?
3. Outline a plan to teach Mr. Cunningham how to irrigate a colostomy.
4. Develop a care plan for Mr. Cunningham for the nursing diagnosis potential for poor body image related to colostomy.

See Evaluating Your Response in Appendix B.

24.6 Structural and Obstructive Bowel Disorders

Any portion of the intestines may be affected by a structural or obstructive disorder. Defects in the abdominal wall may allow intra-abdominal contents (such as loops of bowel) to protrude, indirectly affecting bowel function. Likewise, obstructions may result from disease of the bowel itself or from obstruction of the bowel lumen by an external force.

The Patient with a Hernia

A **hernia** is a defect in the abdominal wall that allows abdominal contents to protrude out of the abdominal cavity. Trauma, surgery, and increased intra-abdominal pressure caused by such conditions as pregnancy, obesity, weightlifting, or tumors are risk factors for hernia formation.

Pathophysiology

Hernias are classified by location (**Figure 24.14** ■) and may be congenital or acquired. Most hernias occur in the

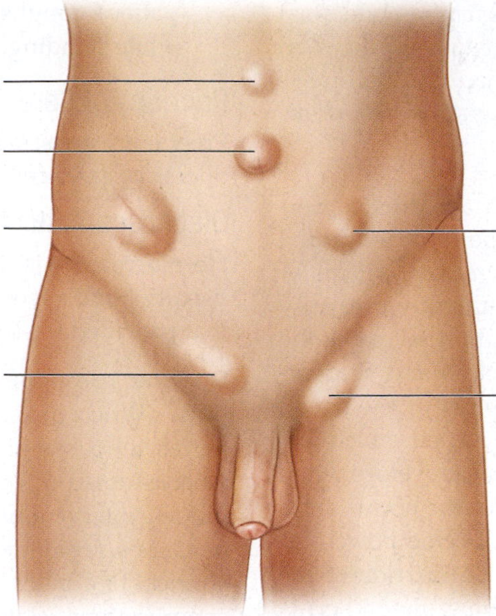
Epigastric hernia
Umbilical hernia
Incisional hernia
Spigelian hernia
Inguinal hernia
Femoral hernia

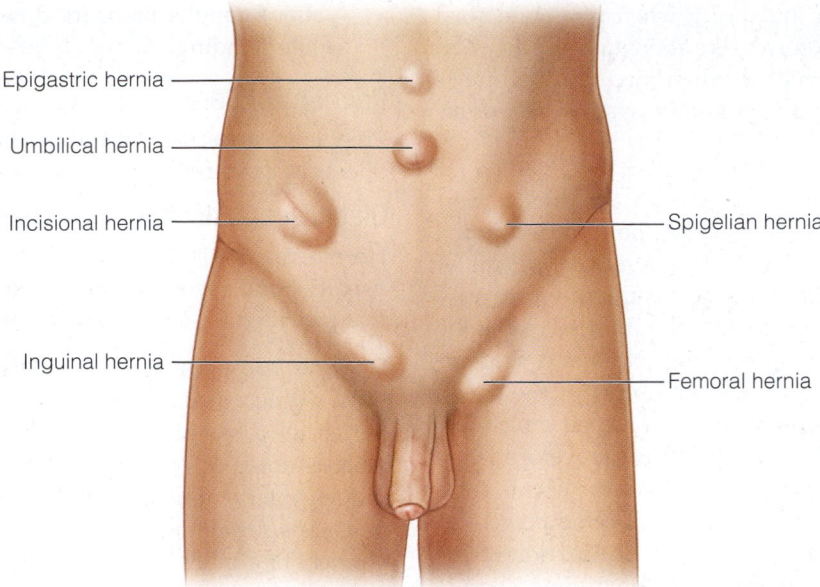

Figure 24.14 ■ Types of hernias are named for their location.

groin (inguinal or femoral hernias). Inguinal hernias are often congenital, caused by improper closure of the tract that develops as the testes descend into the scrotum during fetal development. Groin hernias may be acquired, resulting from weakness of fascia in a region called *Hesselbach area* or from dilation of the femoral ring (e.g., during pregnancy and childbirth). Ventral or incisional hernias of the abdominal wall are generally acquired, caused by weakening of normal abdominal wall musculature. Umbilical hernias are also congenital and are usually detected in infancy. Hiatal hernias develop in the diaphragm (see Chapter 23).

Inguinal Hernia

Inguinal hernias usually affect males and may be classified as indirect or direct inguinal hernias. *Indirect inguinal hernias* are caused by improper closure of the tract that develops as the testes descend into the scrotum before birth. A sac of abdominal contents protrudes through the internal inguinal ring into the inguinal canal. It often descends into the scrotum. Although indirect inguinal hernias are congenital defects, they are often not evident until adulthood, when increased intra-abdominal pressure and dilation of the inguinal ring allow abdominal contents to enter the channel.

Direct inguinal hernias are acquired defects that result from weakness of the posterior inguinal wall. Direct inguinal hernias usually affect older adults. *Femoral hernias* are acquired defects in which a peritoneal sac protrudes through the femoral ring. These hernias usually affect women who are pregnant or obese.

Inguinal hernias may produce no symptoms and are discovered during routine physical examination. They may cause a lump, swelling, or bulge in the groin, particularly with lifting or straining. An inguinal hernia may cause sharp pain or a dull ache that radiates into the scrotum. A palpable mass may be present in the groin, although it may be felt only with increased intra-abdominal pressure (as occurs during coughing) and invagination of the scrotum toward the inguinal ring.

Umbilical Hernia

Pregnancy and obesity contribute to the development of umbilical hernias in adults. *Umbilical hernias* may be congenital and evident during infancy or acquired as the tissue closing the umbilical ring weakens, allowing protrusion of abdominal contents. These hernias are more common in women. Other predisposing factors include multiple pregnancies with prolonged labor, ascites, and large intra-abdominal tumors.

Umbilical hernias tend to enlarge steadily and contain omentum, although they may also contain small or large bowel. The hernia may cause sharp pain on coughing or straining or a dull, aching sensation. Strangulation is a common complication of umbilical hernias.

Incisional or Ventral Hernia

Incisional or *ventral hernias* occur at a previous surgical incision or following abdominal muscle tears. Inadequate healing of the incision or tear can lead to hernia development. Contributing factors include poor wound closure, postoperative infection, age or debility, obesity, inadequate nutrition, and excess incisional stress caused by vigorous coughing.

Ventral hernias are characterized by a bulge at the incisional site, often noted when the patient pulls to a sitting position from a lying position. Ventral hernias are often asymptomatic, and the risk of incarceration is low because of the size of the defect (see the following section on complications).

Manifestations

Abdominal contents (peritoneum, bowel, and other abdominal organs) can protrude through the abdominal wall to form a sac covered by skin and subcutaneous tissues. In most cases, abdominal contents move into the sac when intra-abdominal pressure increases, then return to the abdominal cavity when pressure returns to normal or when manual pressure is placed on the bulging sac. This is known as a *reducible hernia*.

Complications

The risk for complications is low with a reducible hernia. If the contents of a hernia cannot be returned to the abdominal cavity, it is said to be *incarcerated*. Contents of an incarcerated hernia are trapped, usually by a narrow neck or opening to the hernia. Incarceration increases the risk of complications, including obstruction and strangulation. Obstruction occurs when the lumen of the bowel contained within the hernia becomes occluded, much like the crimping of a hose. A *strangulated hernia* develops when blood supply to bowel and other tissues in the hernia sac is compromised, leading to necrosis. The affected bowel can infarct, leading to perforation with contamination of the peritoneal cavity. Manifestations of a strangulated hernia include severe abdominal pain and distention, nausea and vomiting, tachycardia, and fever.

Interprofessional Care

The diagnosis of a hernia is made by a physical examination. The patient is examined in a supine or standing position. A bulge may be seen or felt when the patient coughs or bears down. No laboratory or diagnostic testing is usually required, unless bowel obstruction or strangulation is suspected.

Following inguinal hernia diagnosis there will likely be a trial of nonsurgical treatment. The patient will be instructed to modify activity for 6 to 8 weeks and prescribed anti-inflammatory medication, stool softeners, and physical therapy focused on core strengthening and stretching. Surgical exploration and repair will be pursued if the patient remains symptomatic (Vacca, 2017).

Surgical repair, or *herniorrhaphy*, is a frequent treatment of hernia. Surgery is generally well tolerated by people of all ages and carries a much lower risk than the complications of incarceration, obstruction, and strangulation. Emergency surgery is indicated for a hernia that is incarcerated, painful, or tender. In a herniorrhaphy, the abdominal wall defect is closed by suturing or with wire or mesh over the defect. If incarceration has occurred or strangulation is suspected, the abdomen is explored at the time of surgery and any infarcted bowel resected. Heavy lifting and heavy manual labor are restricted for approximately 3 weeks after surgery.

Nursing Care

Assessment

- ***Health history:*** Ask about manifestations of hernia, such as bulging in the groin or of the abdominal wall when coughing, straining, or moving from lying to standing; pain (abdominal, groin, or scrotal); history of hernia or abdominal surgery
- ***Physical assessment:*** Observe for bulging of the abdominal wall or around the umbilicus when raising head and shoulders from supine position; wearing gloves, palpate inguinal region for bulges when the patient coughs or bears down (Valsalva maneuver) while standing.

Priorities of Care

Preoperative assessment and teaching and immediate postoperative care are the primary nursing care needs.

Diagnoses, Outcomes, and Interventions

Herniorrhaphy is generally an uncomplicated procedure, usually performed as same-day surgery. Care is similar to that provided for a patient with an appendectomy.

Reduce Risk for Lack of Blood Supply and Infection. When providing care for a patient with a known hernia, the possibility of obstruction and strangulation must be considered throughout nursing assessments. Although nursing interventions may not be able to prevent these complications, rapid identification of the problem allows timely surgical treatment. Prompt treatment may prevent major complications related to infection and peritoneal contamination by bowel contents.

Expected Outcome: Patient will resume normal bowel sounds within 8 hours after surgery and be free from unusual pain and abdominal distention.

The nurse will:

- Assess bowel sounds and abdominal distention at least every 8 hours. *A change in bowel sounds—either cessation of sounds or an onset of hyperactive, high-pitched sounds—may indicate obstruction. With obstruction, abdominal girth may increase.*

SAFETY ALERT: Promptly report any acute increase in abdominal, groin, perineal, or scrotal pain. An abrupt increase in the intensity of pain may indicate bowel ischemia due to strangulation. ■

- Notify primary care provider if the hernia becomes painful or tender. *Pain and tenderness may indicate incarceration and increased risk for strangulation.*
- If signs of possible obstruction or strangulation occur, notify the physician. Place patient in supine position with the hips elevated and knees slightly bent. Withhold all food and fluids (NPO), and begin preparations for surgery. *This position helps relax abdominal muscles and may facilitate reduction of the hernia. Strangulation or obstruction requires immediate surgical intervention.*

Transitions of Care

Maintaining a healthy weight and active lifestyle may prevent hernias. Exercises to improve core muscle strength and using proper body mechanics when lifting heavy objects may prevent development of hernias.

Most hernia repair will involve same-day surgery, requiring the nurse to manage the pre- and postoperative period and provide home care instructions in a compressed period of time. Include the following topics when teaching patients about hernias and home care:

- Rationale for examining the groin and abdomen for bulges

- The nature of hernias, risk factors, and manifestations
- Surgical intervention for hernias
- The importance of seeking immediate medical intervention for signs of strangulation or obstruction
- The need to notify the physician if upper respiratory infection and cough develop preoperatively (forceful coughing is not recommended postoperatively)
- Postoperative pain management and activity restrictions.

Symptomatic hernias will be repaired, eliminating hernias as a chronic health condition. However, if the patient does not have surgery chronic care focuses on many of the same strategies as prevention. The patient should exercise to improve core muscle strength, use assistive devices, and use proper body mechanics when lifting and moving heavy objects.

The Patient with Intestinal Obstruction

Intestinal obstruction is failure of intestinal contents to move through the bowel lumen. Intestinal obstructions may affect either the large or small bowel. The small intestine is more commonly affected; however, bowel obstructions may also occur in the large intestine. Obstruction is the most common reason for small-bowel surgery.

Pathophysiology

Intestinal obstructions may be either mechanical or functional in nature. *Mechanical* obstructions may be caused by (1) problems outside the intestine, such as bands of scar tissue (adhesions) or hernias; (2) problems within the intestine, such as tumors or inflammatory bowel disease; or (3) obstruction of the intestinal lumen (**Figure 24.15** ■). The obstruction may be partial or complete. In some mechanical obstructions, such as a strangulated hernia, blood supply to the affected portion of bowel is also impaired, resulting in necrosis of the affected segment. *Functional* obstruction occurs when peristalsis fails to propel intestinal contents, although there is no mechanical obstruction. *Adynamic ileus* (also called *paralytic ileus* or simply *ileus*) is the most common functional obstruction after abdominal surgery. Obstructions are further classified by the portion of intestine affected.

When the intestine is obstructed, gas and fluid accumulate proximal to and within the obstructed segment, distending the bowel. Swallowed air accounts for most of the gas. Ingested fluid, saliva, gastric juice, and pancreatic secretions contribute to accumulated fluid. Water and sodium are drawn into the bowel lumen, contributing to fluid accumulation, distention, and vascular fluid losses. Distention of the bowel lumen interferes with peristaltic movement, leading to atony and further distention. Significant distention of the bowel lumen compromises blood flow to mucosa, eventually leading to necrosis. Gangrenous bowel may perforate with resulting peritonitis. Rapid bacterial growth in the obstructed bowel can lead to sepsis and death.

Significant bowel distention, vomiting, and third spacing of fluids in the bowel and peritoneal cavity can lead to massive loss of fluids and electrolytes with resulting hypovolemia, hypokalemia, renal insufficiency, and shock.

Small-Bowel Obstruction

Adhesions, or bands of scar tissue, and hernias account for most mechanical small-bowel obstructions. In adults, adhesions develop following abdominal surgery or inflammatory processes. Adhesions usually produce a *simple obstruction*, or single blockage in one portion of the intestine (Figure 24.15A). The obstruction produced by an incarcerated hernia is a *closed-loop obstruction*, with two different portions of the bowel lumen obstructed (Figure 24.15B).

Tumors, either intrinsic (of the bowel itself) or extrinsic (of another organ but affecting the bowel because of their size), can progressively occlude the bowel lumen and eventually obstruct it. Other, less common causes of bowel obstruction include intussusception (rare in adults) (Figure 24.15C); volvulus, which is the rotation of loops of bowel about a fixed point (Figure 24.15D); foreign bodies; stricture; and inflammatory bowel disease.

Both volvulus and an incarcerated hernia can cause a *strangulated obstruction*. In a strangulated obstruction, not only is the lumen of the bowel obstructed, but the blood supply to the affected portion is also compromised.

In a functional obstruction or adynamic ileus, peristalsis stops due to either neurogenic or muscular impairment. The bowel lumen remains patent, but contents are

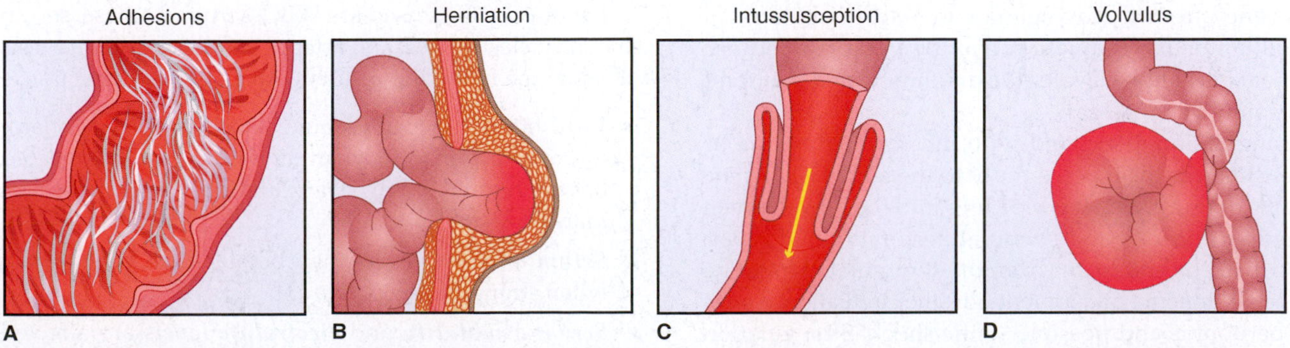
Adhesions
Herniation
Intussusception
Volvulus
A
B
C
D

Figure 24.15 ■ Types of bowel obstruction. **A**, Adhesions; **B**, herniation; **C**, Intussusception; and **D**, Volvulus.

not propelled forward. Temporary ileus commonly follows gastrointestinal surgery. It may result from tissue anoxia or peritoneal irritation due to hemorrhage, peritonitis, or perforation of an organ. Other conditions that can precipitate paralytic ileus include renal colic, spinal cord injuries, uremia, and electrolyte imbalances, hypokalemia in particular. In addition, the effects of some narcotics, anticholinergic drugs, and antidiarrheal medications such as diphenoxylate can produce a functional obstruction.

Manifestations. The manifestations of a small-bowel obstruction vary, depending on the type and level of obstruction and how rapidly it develops. Cramping or colicky abdominal pain that may be intermittent or increasing in intensity is common. Vomiting is common, particularly in high or proximal obstructions, because distention of the lumen stimulates the vomiting center. In a high obstruction, vomitus contains bile and mucus. As bacterial fermentation occurs, vomitus often contains fecal matter, particularly with a low or distal obstruction. Flatus and feces already present in the lower bowel may be expelled early in the obstructive process, but this expulsion ceases as the obstruction continues.

Early in the course of a mechanical obstruction, borborygmi and high-pitched tinkling bowel sounds are often present. Borborygmi may coincide with waves of colicky abdominal pain as the intestine attempts to propel contents past the obstruction. Visible peristaltic waves may be noted in the distended loops of bowel in thin patients. In the later stages, the bowel becomes silent. With a paralytic ileus, bowel sounds are greatly diminished or absent throughout the process. Abdominal distention is minimal with proximal obstructions, but may be pronounced with distal obstruction and paralytic ileus. The abdomen may be tender to palpation as well.

In addition to abdominal and gastrointestinal manifestations, signs of fluid and electrolyte imbalance develop. Hypovolemia can develop rapidly as extracellular fluid is sequestered in the bowel and vomiting occurs. Although early vital signs may be normal, changes are noted as dehydration and hypovolemia develop. The patient becomes tachycardic and tachypneic, and blood pressure falls. Temperature may be elevated. Urine output drops, and signs of hypovolemic shock may be seen.

Complications. Hypovolemia and hypovolemic shock with multiple organ dysfunction are significant complications of bowel obstruction and can lead to death. Renal insufficiency from hypovolemia can lead to acute renal failure. Pulmonary ventilation may be impaired because abdominal distention elevates the diaphragm and interferes with respiratory processes.

Strangulation associated with incarcerated hernia or volvulus impairs the blood supply to the bowel. Gangrene may rapidly result, causing bleeding into the bowel lumen and peritoneal cavity and eventual perforation. With perforation, bacteria and toxins from the strangulated intestine enter the peritoneum and, potentially, the circulation, resulting in peritonitis and possible septic shock. Strangulation greatly increases the risk of mortality.

Large-Bowel Obstruction

Obstruction of the large intestine occurs much less frequently than small-bowel obstruction. Although any portion of the colon may be affected, obstruction usually occurs in the sigmoid segment. Cancer of the bowel is the most common cause; other causes include volvulus, diverticular disease, inflammatory disorders, and fecal impaction.

Manifestations. Constipation and colicky abdominal pain are usual manifestations of large-bowel obstruction. The pain is often deep and cramping; severe, continuous pain may signal bowel ischemia and possible perforation. Vomiting is a late sign, if it occurs at all. The abdomen is distended, with high-pitched, tinkling bowel sounds with rushes and gurgles. On palpation, localized tenderness or a mass may be noted.

Complications. If the ileocecal valve between the small and large intestines is competent, distention proximal to the obstruction is limited to the colon itself. This is known as a *closed-loop obstruction*. It can lead to massive colon dilation as the ileum continues to empty gas and fluid into the colon. Increasing pressure within the obstructed colon impairs circulation to the bowel wall. Gangrene, perforation, and peritonitis are potential complications. Massive distention can impair function of the diaphragm, leading to atelectasis. Pressure on the inferior vena cava may impair venous return.

Interprofessional Care

The management of a bowel obstruction focuses on relieving the pressure and obstruction and providing supportive care. The intestine is decompressed, and fluid and electrolyte balance is restored. Surgery may be necessary to relieve a mechanical obstruction or if strangulation is suspected.

Diagnosis

Radiologic studies (x-rays and CT scan) are used to confirm the diagnosis of bowel obstruction. Laboratory testing is used to evaluate for the presence of infection and fluid and electrolyte imbalances.

An abdominal x-ray often shows distended loops of intestine with fluid and gas in a small-bowel obstruction. Free air under the diaphragm indicates a perforation. X-ray or CT scan with contrast media may be required to confirm a mechanical obstruction and assess the completeness of the obstruction. Gastrografin is often used to provide contrast rather than barium when a bowel obstruction is suspected.

Laboratory tests used are WBC, serum amylase, serum osmolality, electrolytes, and arterial blood gases. These tests will show the following results with a bowel obstruction:

- *WBC* often shows mild leukocytosis due to an inflammatory response to changes within the obstructed bowel lumen. With strangulation, leukocytosis is marked.
- *Serum amylase levels* may be elevated, particularly when strangulation is present.
- *Serum osmolality* and *electrolyte levels* are affected by fluid and electrolyte losses from vomiting and

fluid sequestering in the bowel lumen. With hypovolemia, the serum osmolality and urine specific gravity increase. Potassium and chloride are lost through vomiting, leading to hypokalemia and hypochloremia.

- *ABGs* may reveal metabolic alkalosis (pH > 7.45, bicarbonate > 24 mEq/L, PCO_2 > 45 mmHg) with small-bowel obstruction due to loss of hydrochloric acid from the stomach.

Gastrointestinal Decompression

Most partial small-bowel obstructions are successfully treated with gastrointestinal decompression using a nasogastric tube. Functional obstructions respond to treatment with bowel rest and intestinal decompression as well. Current evidence indicates that a standard nasogastric tube is as effective for gastrointestinal decompression as a longer intestinal tube. Collected fluid and gas are removed using low suction until peristalsis resumes or the obstruction is relieved.

Surgery

Surgical intervention is required for complete mechanical obstructions as well as for strangulated or incarcerated obstructions of the small intestine. Patients with incomplete mechanical obstruction may also require surgery if the obstruction persists.

Prior to surgery, a nasogastric tube is inserted to relieve vomiting and abdominal distention and to prevent aspiration of intestinal contents. Fluid and electrolyte balance must be restored before surgery. Isotonic intravenous fluids, such as normal (physiologic) saline, Ringer solution, or other balanced electrolyte solutions, are used. Additional electrolytes may be added to the solution to correct low levels. It is particularly important to correct hypokalemia prior to surgery. Acid–base imbalances are also addressed, often using intravenous acidifiers or alkalinizing agents. If strangulation has occurred, the patient may require plasma or blood replacement. Intravenous broad-spectrum antibiotics are administered prophylactically (see the section on peritonitis).

Simple mechanical obstruction due to adhesions may be relieved using laparoscopic surgery to remove or lyse the scar tissue. A laparotomy may be performed to allow inspection of the small intestine and removal of infarcted or gangrenous tissue. Obstructing tumors are resected, and foreign bodies are removed. Any bowel that appears to be gangrenous is resected, usually followed by an end-to-end anastomosis of remaining intestine. If a large tumor mass or dense adhesions are found, the area of obstruction may be bypassed by anastomosis of proximal small bowel to the small or large intestine distal to the obstruction. Nursing care of the patient having bowel surgery is provided in Box 24.5.

Obstructions of the large intestine usually necessitate surgery. The primary goal is to relieve colonic distention and prevent perforation; the secondary goal is to remove the obstructing lesion. In some cases, colonoscopy may be used to relieve the distention. If the patient's condition prohibits major surgery or the obstructing tumor is advanced, laser photocoagulation may be used to enlarge the bowel lumen and a stent inserted to reduce the risk of reobstruction. Removal of the obstructing lesion is the preferred treatment. The proximal and distal bowel segments may be anastomosed, or a permanent colostomy or ileostomy may be required.

Nursing Care

Assessment

Nurses may be instrumental in the early identification of intestinal obstructions in older adults, the homebound patient, or the institutionalized patient. Early identification and intervention significantly reduce morbidity from bowel obstruction.

- *Health history:* Complaints of abdominal pain and bloating, constipation; previous history of bowel obstruction or risk factors such as hernia, inflammatory bowel disease, diverticulosis, or previous abdominal surgery; current medications
- *Physical assessment:* Vital signs including orthostatic blood pressure, temperature; skin color, temperature, texture, and turgor; color and moisture of mucous membranes; abdominal shape, contour, bowel sounds, presence of tenderness or masses on palpation.

Priorities of Care

Monitoring for fluid and electrolyte imbalance, acid–base imbalances, hypovolemic shock, perforation, and peritonitis is the focus of care. Managing pain and discomfort before and after surgery for bowel obstruction is a priority.

Diagnoses, Outcomes, and Interventions

In patients with a suspected or confirmed bowel obstruction, frequent assessment for complications is necessary.

Ensure Adequate Hydration. Because of the large collection of fluid in the bowel proximal to an obstruction, the accompanying vomiting, and nasogastric suction, the patient with an intestinal obstruction often has a fluid volume deficit. If not corrected promptly, hypovolemic shock, acute renal failure, and multiple organ system dysfunction from poor tissue perfusion may result.

Expected Outcome: Deficient fluid volume in the patient will be prevented as evidenced by normal vital signs, lab values, and absence of physical signs of dehydration (e.g., thirst, change in mental status, decreased urine output, dry skin and mucous membranes, low pulmonary artery pressures, cardiac output, and central venous pressure).

The nurse will:

- Monitor vital signs, pulmonary artery pressures, cardiac output (CO), and central venous pressure (CVP) hourly. *A decrease in blood pressure, tachycardia, and tachypnea may indicate hypovolemia. Although invasive, hemodynamic parameters such as pulmonary artery pressures, CO, and CVP allow accurate assessment of fluid volume status.*
- Measure urinary output hourly and nasogastric drainage every 2 to 4 hours. *A urinary output of 30 mL/h or*

more usually indicates an adequate glomerular filtration rate (GFR), another indicator of fluid volume. Nasogastric output provides a tool for evaluating fluid replacement needs.

SAFETY ALERT: Promptly report urine output of less than 30 mL/h. This often indicates hypovolemia and an increased risk for shock and acute renal failure. ■

- Maintain intravenous fluids and blood volume expanders as ordered. The amount of fluid administered is calculated to meet ongoing fluid needs and replace previous and current losses. *Restoration and maintenance of blood volume are necessary to maintain cardiac output and tissue and organ perfusion.*
- Evaluate for distention every 4 to 8 hours. Mark the level of measurement on the abdomen. *An increase in abdominal girth indicates increasing intestinal distention.*
- Notify the physician of changes in status. *Changes in vital signs, pain, and signs of increasing distention can indicate the need for immediate surgical intervention.*

Promote Adequate Blood and Oxygen Supply. Perfusion of the intestinal wall and mucosa may be impaired by the obstructive process itself (e.g., strangulation or volvulus) or by significant intestinal distention. The goal is to maintain tissue perfusion and promote normal peristalsis and bowel elimination.

Expected Outcome: Stable perfusion of the patient's intestinal wall will be restored and demonstrated by vital signs within normal range, hourly urine output of 30 mL or greater, resumption of bowel sounds, and a soft, nontender abdomen without distention.

The nurse will:

- Monitor vital signs hourly. Assess peripheral pulses, skin color, temperature, and capillary refill. *Cardiovascular assessment is vital to detect early signs of hypovolemic shock resulting from sequestering large volumes of fluid in the intestines. Hypovolemia and shock can convert mild bowel ischemia to infarction as the blood supply to the tissue falls.*
- Monitor urine output hourly. Report output of less than 30 mL/h. *Urine output is a good indicator of the GFR and tissue perfusion. The urine output often falls before vital sign changes are apparent in hypovolemia.*
- Monitor temperature at least every 4 hours. *An elevated temperature may be an early indication of sepsis from bowel perforation as a result of gangrene.*
- Frequently assess pain. *A change in the character of pain or a rapid increase in its intensity may signal bowel infarction or perforation.*
- Maintain NPO status until peristalsis resumes. *Enteral food or fluids may increase distention and bowel ischemia. They are also restricted until the possibility of perforation is eliminated.*

Maintain Effective Breathing. Significant abdominal distention from a bowel obstruction can cause the diaphragm to flatten, impairing pulmonary ventilation. Following surgery, splinting of abdominal muscles to avoid pain can lead to shallow respirations. These factors, plus the risk of aspiration of gastrointestinal contents during vomiting, place the patient at high risk for respiratory complications, particularly with a small-bowel obstruction.

Expected Outcome: Patient will maintain airway patency and adequate gas exchange as evidenced by ease of breathing, normal respiratory rate and rhythm, normal lung sounds on auscultation, pulse oximetry at patient's baseline, arterial blood gases within normal limits, and stated absence of dyspnea.

The nurse will:

- Assess respiratory rate, pattern, and lung sounds at least every 2 to 4 hours. *Tachypnea, shortness of breath, or apparent dyspnea may be early signs of respiratory compromise. Diminished breath sounds, particularly in the bases of the lungs, or crackles indicate poor lung expansion and possible impaired ventilation.*
- Monitor ABG results for possible effects of altered respiratory status. *Tachypnea may lead to respiratory alkalosis as excess carbon dioxide is eliminated. Conversely, impaired chest expansion can lead to respiratory acidosis because of alveolar hypoventilation.*
- Elevate the head of the bed. *Elevating the head of the bed reduces the work of breathing and improves alveolar ventilation by reducing the pressure of abdominal distention on the diaphragm.*
- Provide a pillow or folded bath blanket to use in splinting the abdomen while coughing postoperatively. *Splinting abdominal muscles and incisions improves the ease and effectiveness of coughing postoperatively.*
- Maintain nasogastric or intestinal tube patency. *Maintaining gastrointestinal suction helps reduce abdominal distention and prevent aspiration associated with vomiting.*
- Encourage use of incentive spirometer or other assistive device hourly. *These devices encourage deep breathing, opening distal airways and preventing atelectasis.*
- Contact respiratory therapy as indicated. *The respiratory therapist may suggest or perform additional measures to maintain effective pulmonary ventilation.*
- Provide good oral care at least every 4 hours. *Dehydration and nasogastric suction dry the mucous membranes of the mouth and throat, increasing the risk of bacterial growth. Many respiratory infections result from aspirated organisms.*

Transitions of Care

Teach health promotion activities, such as increasing dietary fiber intake, maintaining a generous fluid intake, and exercising daily to help prevent constipation and possible large-bowel obstruction, particularly in the older adult. Stress the importance of complying with dietary restrictions (such as avoiding popcorn) for patients who experience repeated small-bowel obstructions.

Include the following topics when teaching the patient with intestinal obstruction in preparation for home care:

- Wound care
- Activity level, return to work, and any other recommended restrictions

- Recommended follow-up care
- Care of temporary colostomy (if appropriate) and planned reanastomosis
- For recurrent obstructions, their cause, early identification of manifestations, and possible preventive measures.

Bowel resections may result in changes in bowel function. The patient may experience diarrhea or possible constipation and may need to adapt dietary habits. Death resulting from a bowel resection would be sudden and related to an unexpected complication. Nursing care would focus on providing support for the family and facilitating consultation with a social worker or chaplain.

24.7 Anorectal Disorders

Anorectal lesions include hemorrhoids, a normal condition common to many adults, that may become enlarged and painful; anal fissure; anorectal abscess; anorectal fistulas; and pilonidal disease.

The Patient with Hemorrhoids

Rectal bleeding is a common symptom for referral to colorectal clinics and in all cases requires examination, diagnosis, and treatment but is most commonly associated with anorectal conditions such as hemorrhoids. The anus and anal canal contain two superficial venous plexuses with the hemorrhoidal veins. When pressure on these veins is increased or venous return impeded, they can develop *varices*, or varicosities, becoming weak and distended. This condition is commonly known as **hemorrhoids**, or *piles*. When asymptomatic, hemorrhoids are considered to be a normal condition found in all adults.

Pathophysiology and Manifestations

Hemorrhoids develop when venous return from the anal canal is impaired. Straining to defecate increases venous pressure and is the most common cause of distended hemorrhoids. Pregnancy increases intra-abdominal pressure, raising venous pressure, and is another cause of hemorrhoids. Other factors that may contribute to symptomatic hemorrhoids include prolonged sitting, obesity, chronic constipation, and a low-fiber diet.

Hemorrhoids are classed as either internal or external. *Internal* hemorrhoids affect the venous plexus above the mucocutaneous junction of the anus (**Figure 24.16** ■). Internal hemorrhoids rarely cause pain, usually presenting with bleeding. Bleeding from internal hemorrhoids is bright red and unmixed with the stool. It can vary in quantity from streaks on toilet tissue to enough to color the water in the toilet. Recurrent bleeding of internal hemorrhoids may be sufficient to cause anemia. Mucous discharge and a feeling of incomplete evacuation of stool may also be manifestations of internal hemorrhoids.

External hemorrhoids affect the inferior hemorrhoidal plexus below the mucocutaneous junction. Bleeding is rare with external hemorrhoids. Anal irritation, a feeling of pressure, and difficulty cleaning the anal region may be manifestations of external hemorrhoids.

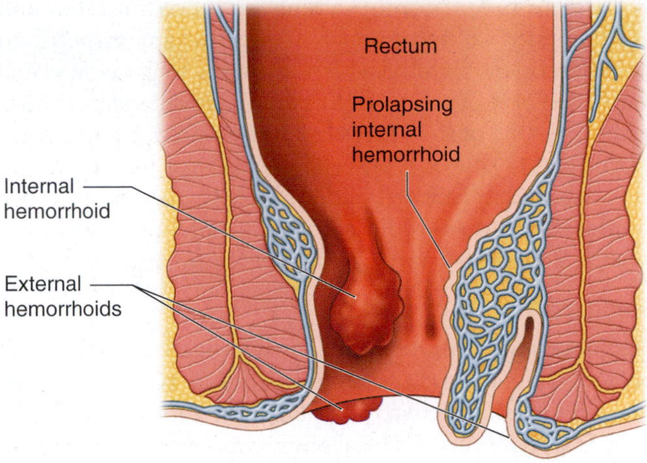
Rectum
Prolapsing internal hemorrhoid
Internal hemorrhoid
External hemorrhoids

Figure 24.16 ■ The location of internal and external hemorrhoids.

As they enlarge, hemorrhoids may prolapse or protrude through the anus. Initially, prolapse occurs only with defecation and the hemorrhoids spontaneously regress back into the anal canal. Eventually, the patient may need to manually replace internal hemorrhoids after defecation, or they may become permanently prolapsed, in which case replacement is not possible. Manifestations of permanently prolapsed hemorrhoids include mucous discharge and clothing soilage.

Normal hemorrhoids are not painful. Prolapsed hemorrhoids may become strangulated as a result of congestion and edema, leading to thrombosis. Hemorrhoidal thrombosis causes extreme pain and may lead to infarction of skin and mucosa overlying the hemorrhoid. Internal hemorrhoids associated with portal hypertension in liver disease may bleed profusely if ruptured.

A *thrombosed external hemorrhoid* is a thrombosis of the subcutaneous external hemorrhoidal veins of the anal canal, rather than a true hemorrhoid. It appears as a painful bluish hematoma beneath the skin and typically occurs following a sudden increase in venous pressure, for example, heavy lifting, coughing, or straining. Pain is significant at onset but gradually subsides. Spontaneous rupture with bleeding may occur. Thrombosed external hemorrhoids resolve without intervention.

Interprofessional Care

Because hemorrhoids are a normal condition, management is conservative unless complications such as permanent prolapse or thrombosis occur.

Diagnosis

Hemorrhoids are diagnosed by the patient's history and by examination of the anorectal area. External hemorrhoids can be seen on visual inspection, especially if thrombosed. The patient is asked to strain (Valsalva's maneuver) during the examination to detect prolapse. Internal hemorrhoids are usually not palpable or tender on digital examination of the rectum. Anoscopic examination is used to detect and evaluate internal hemorrhoids. For this exam, a speculum or endoscope is introduced into the anus to provide visual inspection of the tissues. Additional diagnostic examinations include testing of stool for occult blood and sigmoidoscopy, performed to rule out cancer of the colon or rectum, which may aggravate hemorrhoidal manifestations or produce similar manifestations. If liver disease with portal hypertension is suspected, liver function studies are ordered.

Medications

Bulk-forming laxatives such as psyllium seed (Metamucil) or stool softeners such as docusate sodium (Colace) may be prescribed to improve constipation and reduce straining as well. Suppositories and local ointments such as Preparation H or Nupercaine have an anesthetic and astringent effect, reducing discomfort and irritation of surrounding tissues. They have little or no effect on the hemorrhoid itself. Warm sitz baths, bedrest, and local astringent compresses may be recommended to reduce the swelling of edematous prolapsed hemorrhoids after digital reduction.

Nutrition

Hemorrhoids that are not permanently prolapsed or acutely thrombosed are generally treated conservatively. A high-fiber diet and increased water intake to increase stool bulk, improve its softness, and reduce straining are effective for most patients with internal or external hemorrhoids.

Sclerotherapy

Hemorrhoids that are permanently prolapsed, are thrombosed, or produce significant manifestations may be treated more aggressively. *Sclerotherapy* involves injecting a chemical irritant into tissues surrounding the hemorrhoid to induce inflammation and eventual fibrosis and scarring. It is used to treat recurrent bleeding and early prolapse of internal hemorrhoids. The treatment produces minimal pain. Enlarged or prolapsing hemorrhoids may also be treated with rubber band ligation. A rubber band is placed snugly around the hemorrhoidal plexus and surrounding mucosa, causing the tissue to necrose and slough within 7 to 10 days. Treatment is limited to one hemorrhoidal complex at a time, so repeat treatments may be necessary. Pain should be minimal if the band is placed appropriately; persistent pain following band ligation may signal an infection. Bleeding can occur as the hemorrhoid sloughs. Other procedures used to treat hemorrhoids include cryosurgery, in which hemorrhoids are necrosed by freezing with a cryoprobe; infrared photocoagulation; or electrocoagulation.

Hemorrhoidectomy

Patients with chronic manifestations, permanent prolapse, chronic bleeding and anemia, or painful thrombosed hemorrhoids may be treated surgically with a *hemorrhoidectomy*. In this procedure, hemorrhoids are surgically excised, leaving normal skin and surrounding tissues. This procedure may use conventional techniques or a laser to remove both internal and external hemorrhoids. Few complications are associated with hemorrhoidectomy.

Diagnoses, Outcomes, and Interventions

Whether caring for a patient with hemorrhoids or a hemorrhoidectomy, priorities of care will include:

- Relieving pain related to inflamed anal tissues
- Preventing constipation related to dietary habits and/or delay of defecation
- Reducing risk of infection related to disruption of anal tissue.

When a hemorrhoidectomy is performed, it is same-day surgery that requires more direct nursing intervention in the time that the patient is recovering from the procedure. Anal packing may be in place for the first 24 hours following the procedure. Inspect the rectal dressing every 2 to 3 hours and remove the dressing an hour or so before the patient is discharged. The patient may be instructed to return to a clinic to have the packing removed the day after surgery. When removed, observe the patient closely for bleeding. Pain is a common postoperative problem. Although the operative procedure is minor, postoperative discomfort can be significant because the anal region is richly innervated and muscle spasms may occur. In addition to systemic analgesics, sitz baths are usually ordered. These not only help promote relaxation and reduce discomfort but also clean the anal area. Use of a rubber ring or doughnut device minimizes pressure on the surgical site while the patient sits in the bath. Provide home care instructions regarding sitz bath procedures, ensuring the patient cleans the tub and rubber ring after each use to prevent infection. Ice packs can be applied to the rectal area to treat pain. The patient will need stool softeners for several days and should be instructed to avoid becoming constipated. Using an analgesic before the first bowel movement is recommended, if possible. Teach the patient to drink at least 2000 mL/day. Encourage a diet high in fiber and teach the patient to exercise moderately to promote normal bowel movements. Instruct the patient to report the following symptoms to the physician: Rectal bleeding, continued pain on defecation, fever greater than 38.3°C (101°F), or purulent rectal drainage.

Transitions of Care

Primary prevention of symptomatic hemorrhoids involves education of patients of all ages. Stress the importance of maintaining an adequate intake of dietary fiber, a liberal fluid intake, and regular exercise to maintain stool bulk, softness, and regularity. Discuss the need to respond to the urge to defecate rather than postponing defecation. Teach appropriate constipation management, including the use of bulk-forming laxatives.

Most patients with hemorrhoids are treated in community settings where the primary nursing focus is educational. Discuss the appropriate use of OTC preparations and sitz baths for the relief of minor hemorrhoidal manifestations. If necessary, teach patients how to reduce prolapsed hemorrhoids digitally.

Teach manifestations of possible hemorrhoidal complications, such as chronic bleeding, prolapse, and thrombosis.

Stress the need to seek medical evaluation if manifestations persist. Discuss the link between manifestations of hemorrhoids and colorectal cancer, and urge the patient to seek medical intervention for persistent, unresolved, or progressive manifestations.

Stool softeners, adequate fluids, and analgesia before defecation can reduce anxiety and discomfort. Adequate cleaning following defecation, usually with a sitz bath, is vital.

The Patient with an Anorectal Lesion

Unlike the rectum, which is relatively insensitive to pain, the anal canal is richly supplied with sensory nerves and highly sensitive to painful stimuli. Lesions of the anorectal area may cause significant pain, particularly with defecation. Infection is a potential complication of anorectal lesions because of contamination by fecal bacteria. The superior boundary of the anal canal (the anorectal juncture or pectinate line) contains 8 to 12 anal crypts where anorectal abscesses or fistulas can form. Lesions of the anorectal area include fissures, abscesses, fistulas, and pilonidal disease.

Pathophysiology and Manifestations

Anal Fissure

Anal fissures or ulcers occur when the epithelium of the anal canal over the internal sphincter becomes denuded or abraded. Irritating diarrheal stools and tightening of the anal canal with increased sphincter tension are frequent causes of anal fissures. Other factors that may contribute to their development include childbirth trauma, habitual cathartic use, laceration by a foreign body, and anal intercourse. Chronic inflammation and infection of surrounding tissues accompanies an anal fissure.

Patients with anal fissures typically have periods of exacerbation and remission. Because they occur below the mucocutaneous line, anal fissures are painful. The pain occurs with defecation and may be described as tearing, burning, or cutting. Bright red bleeding is noted with a bowel movement. Bleeding is typically minor and noted on toilet tissue. Because of fear of defecation, the patient may develop constipation, which further disrupts normal bowel habits and aggravates manifestations.

The diagnosis of anal fissure is made on gentle digital examination of the anal canal and anoscopy using a small anoscope. Treatment is usually conservative, involving dietary changes to increase fiber intake and stool bulk, increased fluid intake, and use of bulk-forming laxatives. A topical agent such as hydrocortisone cream may be prescribed. Surgical intervention with an internal sphincterotomy, an incision into the internal sphincter to increase its diameter, is considered when the fissure does not heal with medical intervention.

Anorectal Abscess

Invasion of the pararectal spaces by pathogenic bacteria can lead to an *anorectal abscess*. Commonly caused by infection that extends from the anal crypt into a pararectal space, the abscess may appear small but often contains a large amount of pus. Multiple pathogens may be present, including *Escherichia coli*, *Proteus*, streptococci, and staphylococci. Other factors that may contribute to the development of an anorectal abscess include infection of a hair follicle, sebaceous gland, or sweat gland and abrasions, fissures, or anal trauma. The incidence of anorectal abscess is higher in men.

Pain is the primary manifestation of an anorectal abscess. Sitting or walking may aggravate the pain, but it is unrelated to defecation. External swelling, redness, heat, and tenderness are apparent on examination. With a deeper abscess, swelling may not be visible, but the abscess is palpable on digital examination.

If the abscess either does not drain spontaneously or is not drained surgically, adjacent anatomic spaces will be affected. Systemic sepsis is also a potential complication.

Incision and drainage is the treatment of choice for an anorectal abscess because it rarely resolves with antibiotic therapy alone. This treatment often leads to a persistent fistula, which is surgically closed after the infection has cleared.

Anorectal Fistula

A *fistula* is a tunnel or tubelike tract with openings at each end. *Anorectal fistulas* have one opening in the anal canal with the other usually found in perianal skin. Most occur spontaneously or as a result of anorectal abscess drainage. Crohn disease is a predisposing factor to fistula development.

The primary manifestation of an anorectal fistula is intermittent or constant drainage or discharge, which may be purulent. This may be accompanied by local itching, tenderness, and pain associated with defecation.

Digital and anoscopic examination with gentle probing of the fistula tract are used to establish the diagnosis. Although some fistulas may heal spontaneously, the treatment of choice is a fistulotomy. The primary opening of the fistula is removed, and the tract is opened to allow it to heal by secondary intention, from the inside outward. If the sphincter is involved, a two-stage operation may be done to preserve the muscle and prevent fecal incontinence.

Pilonidal Disease

The patient with *pilonidal disease* has an acute abscess or chronic draining sinus in the sacrococcygeal area. Underlying the abscess or sinus is a cyst with granulation tissue, fibrosis, and, often, hair tufts. This disease usually affects young hirsute (hairy) males and is probably due to hair entrapment in deep tissues of the sacrococcygeal area. Some researchers believe that it is a congenital disorder.

The lesion of pilonidal disease is generally asymptomatic unless it becomes acutely infected. Manifestations of acute inflammation accompany infection, including pain, tenderness, redness, heat, and swelling of the affected area. Purulent discharge may be noted from one or more sinuses or openings in the midline.

The preferred treatment option for pilonidal disease is incision and drainage. The sinus tract and underlying cyst are excised and closed by either primary- or secondary-intention healing. The patient may be instructed to remove hair from the area routinely by shaving or using a depilatory to prevent further hair entrapment and recurrence of the problem.

Nursing Care

Patients with anorectal disorders are often treated in the community, and the primary nursing responsibility is education. Teach the importance of maintaining a high-fiber diet and liberal fluid intake to increase stool bulk and softness and thereby decrease discomfort with defecation. Stress the importance of responding to the urge to defecate to prevent constipation.

Following surgical treatment of any of these disorders, teach the patient to keep the perianal region clean and dry. If a dressing is in place, instruct to avoid soiling it with urine or feces during elimination. Following removal of the dressing, teach to clean the area gently with soap and water following a bowel movement. Discuss the use of sitz baths for cleaning and comfort. Suggest taking an analgesic, if necessary, prior to defecation, but caution that some analgesics may promote constipation. Teach manifestations of infection or other possible complications to report to the physician. If an antibiotic has been prescribed, provide written and verbal instructions about its use, its desired and possible adverse effects, and their management.

CHAPTER HIGHLIGHTS

24.1 Disorders of Intestinal Motility

Describe the pathophysiology and manifestations of disorders of motility, and outline the interprofessional care and nursing care of patients with these disorders.

- Disorders of intestinal motility include diarrhea, constipation, irritable bowel syndrome, and fecal incontinence. Diarrhea is a manifestation of many other bowel disorders, including lactose intolerance, infections, and inflammatory diseases of the bowel. Constipation may be a primary problem (especially for the older adult) or a manifestation of another disorder. Irritable bowel syndrome (IBS) is a functional disorder without any identifiable organic cause. Fecal incontinence is usually considered to be the manifestation of a disorder rather than a disorder itself.
- Nursing care involves treating the underlying etiology of problems with intestinal mobility in collaboration with the interprofessional healthcare team. Managing symptoms is the focus of nursing care and assisting the patient to adapt to chronic symptoms while promoting self-care and strategies that enhance quality of life are important nursing interventions.

24.2 Acute Inflammatory and Infectious Bowel Disorders

Describe the pathophysiology and manifestations of acute inflammatory and infectious bowel disorders, and outline the interprofessional care and nursing care of patients with these disorders.

- Appendicitis is an acute inflammation of the vermiform appendix, manifested by abdominal pain that localizes in the right lower quadrant of the abdomen. On palpation, localized and rebound tenderness is present at McBurney point. It is treated most often with an appendectomy.
- Peritonitis (inflammation of the peritoneum from infection or chemical irritant) is a serious complication of a wide variety of acute abdominal disorders, including perforated ulcer, ruptured appendix, abdominal trauma or surgery, or necrotic bowel. Complications may be life-threatening; without prompt and effective treatment, septicemia and septic shock may occur.
- Gastroenteritis, which may result from bacterial or viral infections, parasites, or toxins, is often the result of consuming contaminated water or food. Manifestations include nausea and vomiting, diarrhea, and abdominal discomfort.
- Nurses provide education to help prevent protozoal infections (such as giardiasis, amebiasis, and coccidiosis) and helminthic infestations (roundworms, flukes, or tapeworms). Both types of bowel disorders are treated with medications.

24.3 Chronic Inflammatory Bowel Disorders

Describe the pathophysiology and manifestations of chronic inflammatory bowel disorders, and outline the interprofessional care and nursing care of patients with these disorders.

- Chronic inflammatory bowel disease (IBD) includes two separate but closely related conditions: Ulcerative colitis and Crohn disease. Ulcerative colitis affects the mucosa and submucosa of the colon and rectum. Crohn disease can affect any part of the GI tract, but usually involves the terminal ilium and ascending colon. Diarrhea is common to both disorders. A colectomy (removal of the large colon) may be performed to treat ulcerative colitis; an ileostomy (artificial opening from the abdomen to the ileum) may be performed to treat Crohn disease.

- Diverticula are saclike projections of mucosa through the muscular layer of the colon. When these sacs become inflamed, the condition is labeled diverticulitis. A diet high in fiber is recommended for self-care.
- Nursing care related to inflammatory bowel disease focuses on symptom management and adapting to issues related to chronic illness. Teaching the patient and family about medications, dietary modifications, and activity is an important role. Providing nursing actions in the acute care setting for patients with IBD includes postoperative care or actions that aim to restore fluide, electrolyte, and nutritional status. Pain control is a focus of care for the patient with IBD. IBD is a complex disease and likely involves multiple providers. The nursing role often involves coordinating care between providers and settings.

24.4 Malabsorption Syndromes

Describe the pathophysiology and manifestations of malabsorption disorders, and outline the interprofessional care and nursing care of patients with these disorders.

- Malabsorption syndromes, in which the intestinal mucosa ineffectively absorbs nutrients, may be caused by a wide variety of diseases. However, three common malabsorption disorders in adults are celiac disease, lactase deficiency with resulting lactose intolerance of milk and milk products, and short bowel syndrome (a condition that can develop following resection of the small bowel).
- Nursing care involves focus on promoting adequate nutrition and hydration. Interprofessional care frequently involves working closely with a dietitian and reinforcing prescribed dietary teaching. Care coordination as a member of the interprofessional team is an important nursing role for many patients with malabsorption syndromes.

24.5 Neoplastic Disorders

Describe the pathophysiology and manifestations of neoplastic disorders, and outline the interprofessional care and nursing care of patients with these disorders.

- Malignant tumors of the lower bowel are the second leading cause of death from cancer. The risk of colon cancer may be reduced through health-related screenings and a diet high in fruits, vegetables, folic acid, and calcium. Rectal bleeding is the most common initial manifestation but may not occur until the cancer is well advanced. Surgical treatment is through resection of the bowel, accompanied by a colostomy for diversion of fecal contents.
- Care of the patient with cancer will involve multiple disciplines and care will likely be delivered across settings. Care will also be complex and may include many forms of treatment including chemotherapy and radiation. Nursing actions include promoting adequate nutrition, hydration, and symptom control related to the disease and possible treatment. Coordinating care is an essential nursing role for patients with cancer of the GI tract.

24.6 Structural and Obstructive Bowel Disorders

Describe the pathophysiology and manifestations of structural and obstructive bowel disorders, and outline the interprofessional care and nursing care of patients with these disorders.

- A hernia is a defect in the abdominal wall that allows intra-abdominal contents to protrude out of the abdominal cavity. Hernias may follow trauma, surgery, and increased intra-abdominal pressure (e.g., from pregnancy or obesity). Hernias may be congenital or acquired and may be inguinal, umbilical, incisional, or ventral.
- Intestinal obstructions occur when intestinal contents cannot move through the lumen of the bowel. They may occur in either the large or small intestine, may be partial or complete, and are caused by many factors, ranging from surgical ileus following abdominal surgery to adhesions or tumors.
- Assessing general health and GI status, managing pain, and supporting fluid and electrolyte balance are priorities when caring for patients with structural and obstructive disorders. Post-operative care, nutritional and activity instructions, and teaching signs and symptoms of complications should also be included.

24.7 Anorectal Disorders

Describe the pathophysiology and manifestations of anorectal disorders, and outline the interprofessional care and nursing care of patients with these disorders.

- Anorectal disorders include hemorrhoids, anorectal lesions (fissures, abscess, and fistula), and pilonidal disease. These disorders are painful and pose a risk for bleeding and infection.
- Nursing care involves providing pharmacological and nonpharmacological strategies to reduce pain and reestablishment of normal bowel habits.

TEST YOURSELF NCLEX-RN® REVIEW

1. A patient has been experiencing diarrhea for the past week. What should the nurse do first when caring for this patient?
   A. Ask the patient to describe the number and character of daily stools.
   B. Advise the patient to abstain from all oral intake until the diarrhea subsides.
   C. Recommend an over-the-counter antidiarrheal preparation such as Pepto-Bismol.
   D. Question the patient about possible exposure to an enterotoxin or protozoal infection.
2. A patient comes into the emergency department with manifestations of appendicitis. What is the highest priority when caring for this patient?
   A. Withhold all food and fluids.
   B. Perform preoperative skin preparation.
   C. Insert saline lock for intravenous pain medication.
   D. Teach postoperative deep breathing, coughing, and leg exercises.
3. A patient with inflammatory bowel disease is prescribed sulfasalazine (Azulfidine). What should the nurse teach the patient about taking this medication? (Select all that apply.)
   A. Take vitamin C while on the drug.
   B. Take the drug after a meal.
   C. Use a sunscreen while taking the drug.
   D. Limit fluid intake to 1500 mL per day or less.
   E. Use aspirin rather than NSAIDs for minor pain.
4. A patient is experiencing frequent large, fatty, foul-smelling stools. What additional information should the nurse obtain from the patient?
   A. Known family history of colorectal cancer
   B. The relationship of episodes to particular foods
   C. History of alternating diarrhea and constipation
   D. Possible exposure to enterotoxins in food or water
5. A patient has heard of several friends being diagnosed with colon cancer and does not want to develop the same health problem. What should the nurse recommend to this patient? (Select all that apply.)
   A. Exercise regularly.
   B. Maintain a healthy weight.
   C. Ingest two servings of red wine every day.
   D. Obtain recommended screening after age 50.
   E. Consume a diet high in fruits and vegetables.
6. A patient with a bowel obstruction has a nasogastric tube in place for gastric decompression. The nurse will perform which interventions associated with this treatment? (Select all that apply.)
   A. Measure abdominal girth every 4 to 8 hours.
   B. Provide the patient with generous amounts of oral fluids.
   C. Keep an accurate record of intake and output every 2 to 4 hours.
   D. Document the amount and color of nasogastric tube drainage every shift.
   E. Monitor mental status at each patient encounter.
7. A patient has developed a paralytic ileus following recent abdominal surgery. What is the most important nursing action when caring for this patient?
   A. Monitor bowel sounds every hour.
   B. Maintain the patient on strict bedrest.
   C. Ensure nasogastric tube is functioning.
   D. Ensure that the patient is given a clear liquid diet.
8. The nurse is preparing discharge diet teaching for a patient with diverticulosis. The nurse evaluates that teaching has been effective when the patient lists which foods to include in the diet? (Select all that apply.)
   A. Soup
   B. Salad
   C. Raspberries
   D. Whole-wheat bread
   E. Popcorn
9. An older patient is experiencing constipation. What should the nurse teach this patient to help with this health problem? (Select all that apply.)
   A. Eat a bran cereal for breakfast.
   B. Take bisacodyl (Dulcolax) daily.
   C. Eat plenty of fresh fruits and vegetables daily.
   D. Eat whole-wheat bread instead of white bread.
   E. Drink six to eight glasses of nonalcoholic fluid daily.
10. A patient with a severe *Clostridium difficile* infection is to be treated with fecal microbiota transplant. The nurse evaluates that teaching about this treatment is understood when the patient makes which statements? (Select all that apply.)
    A. "My wife is not a good donor because she is over 45 years old."
    B. "I can expect the transplanted material to be administered by enema."
    C. "I will need to take an antibiotic for several days before the transplant."
    D. "I will be hospitalized for at least a month following this transplant."
    E. "This is a rare and dangerous treatment and I am at risk for developing HIV as a result."

See Test Yourself answers in Appendix B.

REFERENCES

Adams, M., Holland, N., & Urban, C. (2017). *Pharmacology for nurses: A pathophysiologic approach* (5th ed.). Upper Saddle River, NJ: Prentice Hall.

American Cancer Society. (2018). *Cancer facts & figures 2018.* Atlanta, GA: Author.

Barshak, M., & Kasper, D. L. Intraabdominal infections and abscesses. In J. Jameson, A. S. Fauci, D. L. Kasper, S. L. Hauser, D. L. Longo, & J. Loscalzo (Eds.), *Harrison's principles of internal medicine* (20th ed.). New York, NY: McGraw-Hill. http://accessmedicine.mhmedical.com.liboff.ohsu.edu/content.aspx?bookid=2129&sectionid=186949739. Accessed May 06, 2018.

Berman, A. T., Snyder, S., Frandsen, G. (2016). *Kozier & Erb's Fundamentals of Nursing,* 10th ed. Hoboken, NJ: Pearson Education.

Centers for Disease Control and Prevention. (2018). Inflammatory bowel disease prevalence (IBD) in the United States. *Data and Statistics.* Retrieved from https://www.cdc.gov/ibd/data-statistics.htm.

Cornett, P. A., & Dea, T. O. (2018). Cancer. In M. A. Papakakis, S. J. McPhee, & M. W. Rabow (Eds.), *Current medical diagnosis and treatment 2018.* New York, NY: McGraw-Hill.

Crohn & Colitis Foundation of America (CCFA). (2018). *What are Crohn and colitis?* Retrieved from www.ccfa.org/info/about/crohns.

Donmez, T., Hut, A., Avaroglu, H., Uzman, S., Yildirim, D., Ferahman, S., & Cekic, E. (2016). Two-port laparoscopic appendectomy assisted with needle grasper comparison with conventional laparoscopic appendectomy. *Annals of Surgical Treatment and Research, 91*(2), 59–65.

Dudley-Brown, S. (2017). Optimizing inflammatory bowel disease. *Gastroenterology Nursing, 40*(15), S1–S14.

Edmonds, S. L., Zapka, C., Kasper, D., Gerber, R., McCormack, R., Macinga, D., . . . Gerding, D. N. (2013). Effectiveness of hand hygiene for removal of *Clostridium difficile* spores from hands. *Infection Control and Hospital Epidemiology, 14*(3), 302–305.

Ghiyasvandian, S., Ghorbani, M., Zakerimoghadam, M., Prufarzad, Z., & Kazemnejad, A. (2016). The effects of a self-care program on the severity of symptoms and quality of life of patients with irritable bowel syndrome. *Gastroenterology Nursing, 39*(5), 359–365.

Gump, K. & Schmelzer, M. (2016). Gaining control over fecal continence. *Medsurg Nursing, 25*(2), 97–102.

Haverstick S., Goodrich, C., Freeman, R., James., S., Kullar, R., & Ahrens, M. (2017). Patients' hand washing and reducing hospital-acquired infection. *Critical Care Nurse, 37*(3), e1–e8.

Holroyd, S. (2015). How can community nurses manage chronic constipation? *Journal of Community Nursing, 29*(5), 74–82.

Kelly, C. R., Kahn, S., Kashyap, P., Laine, L., Rubin, D., Atreja, A., . . . Wu, G. (2015). Update on fecal microbiota transplantation 2015: Indications, mechanisms, and outlook. *Gastroenterology 149*(1), 223–237.

Konradsen, H., Rasmussen, M. L. T., Noisesen, E., & Trosborg, I. (2017). Effect of home care nursing on patients discharged from hospital with self-reported signs of constipation. *Gastroenterology Nursing, 40*(6), 463–468.

Lamanna, L., & Moran, P. (2018). Diverticular disease. *Gastroenterology Nursing, 41*(2), 111–119.

Leckey, J., Davis, S., & Raphael-Grimm, T. (2017). Nursing assessment of patients requiring enternal and gastric feeding tubes. *Gastroenterology Nursing, 40*(6), 469–483.

McCabe, M. A., Toughill, E. H., Parkhill, A. M., Bossett, M. S., Jevic, M. S., & Nye, M. L. (2012). Celiac disease: A medical puzzle. *American Journal of Nursing, 112*(10), 34–44.

McQuaid, K. R. (2018). Gastrointestinal disorders. In M. A. Papakakis, S. J. McPhee, & M. W. Rabow (Eds.), *Current medical diagnosis and treatment 2018.* New York, NY, McGraw-Hill. http://accessmedicine.mhmedical.com.liboff.ohsu.edu/content.aspx?bookid=2192$sectionid=168013478. Accessed May 08, 2018.

National Center for Complementary and Integrative Health. (2012). *An introduction to probiotics.* Retrieved from http://nccam.nih.gov/health/probiotics.

O'Connor, N. (2017). Six things you can do to today to prevent hospital-onset *C. difficile* tomorrow. *American Journal of Nursing, 117*(9), 47–49.

Peterson, M., & Grossman, S. (2016). Managing celiac disease for women. *Gastroenterology Nursing, 39*(3), 186–194.

Pitlick, M., & Fritz, D. (2013). Evidence about the pharmacological management of constipation. Part 2: Implications for palliative care. *Home Healthcare Nurse, 31*(4), 207–216.

Pokrywka, M., Feigel, J., Douglas., B., Grossberger, S., Hensler, A., & Weber, D. (2014). A bundle strategy including patient hand hygiene to decrease *Clostridium difficile* infections. *Medsurg Nursing, 23*(3), 145–148.

Prichard, D., & Bharucha, A. (2015). Management of opioid-induced constipation for people in palliative care. *International Journal of Palliative Nursing, 21*(6), 272–279.

Sorenson, M., Quinn, L., & Klein, D. (2019). *Pathophysiology: Concepts of human disease.* Hoboken, NJ: Pearson Education.

Stepter, C. (2012). Maintaining placement of temporary enteral feeding tubes in adults: A critical appraisal of evidence. *Medsurg Nursing, 21*(2), 61–68.

Vacca. V. M. (2017). Inguinal hernia: A battle of the bulge. *Nursing 2017, 47*(8), 28–35.

Walton, J., Burns, D., & Gaehle, K. (2017). Process and outcome of fecal microbiota transplants in patients with recurrent *Clostridium difficile* infection. *Gastroenterology Nursing, 40*(5), 411–419.

Weaver, K. R., Melkus, G. D., & Henderson, W. (2017). Irritable bowel syndrome: An evidence-based review of new diagnostic criteria and treatment recommendations. *American Journal of Nursing, 117*(6), 48–55.

ADDITIONAL RESOURCES

Beyond Celiac (formerly National Foundation for Celiac Awareness)

www.beyondceliac.org

Crohn's & Colitis Foundation of America

www.ccfa.org

National Center for Complementary and Integrative Health

https://nccih.nih

National Institute of Diabetes and Digestive Diseases and Kidney Diseases

www.niddk.nih.gov/health-information/digestive-diseases

U.S. Food and Drug Administration. Gluten and food labeling.

www.fda.gov/Food/GuidanceRegulation/G GuidanceDocumentsRegulatoryInformation/Allergens/ucm367654.htm.

Chapter 25

Nursing Care of Patients with Gallbladder, Liver, and Pancreatic Disorders

Chapter Outline and Learning Outcomes

Describe the pathophysiology and manifestations of gallbladder disorders, and outline the interprofessional care and nursing care of patients with these disorders.

Describe the pathophysiology and manifestations of liver disorders, and outline the interprofessional care and nursing care of patients with these disorders.

Describe the pathophysiology and manifestations of exocrine pancreas disorders, and outline the interprofessional care and nursing care of patients with these disorders.

CLINICAL COMPETENCIES

- Assess health status of patients with gallbladder, liver, or pancreatic disease, eliciting patient values, preferences, and expressed needs when assessing, planning, and implementing care.
- Monitor for, recognize, document, and report expected and unexpected manifestations in patients with gallbladder, liver, or pancreatic disease.
- Integrate interprofessional measures into nursing care and teaching of the patient with a gallbladder, liver, or pancreatic disorder.
- Provide safe, patient-centered nursing care for the patient who has surgery of the gallbladder, liver, or pancreas.
- Integrate psychosocial, cultural, and spiritual considerations into the plan of care for a patient with a gallbladder, liver, or pancreatic disorder.
- Use evidence-based practice, technology, and information management tools to develop, implement, evaluate, and, as needed, revise the plan of care for patients with disorders of the gallbladder, liver, or pancreas.
- Provide appropriate evidence-based patient and family teaching to promote, maintain, and restore functional health status for patients with gallbladder, liver, and pancreatic disorders.

KEY TERMS

ascites, 817
biliary colic, 811
cholecystitis, 811
cholelithiasis, 811
cirrhosis, 825
esophageal varices, 818
hepatitis, 818
jaundice, 817
pancreatitis, 841
paracentesis, 832
portal hypertension, 818
portal systemic encephalopathy, 818
steatorrhea, 842

The pancreas, liver, and gallbladder are considered accessory organs to the gastrointestinal system and aid in digestion and metabolism of nutrients during phases of gastric activity (**Figure 25.1** ■). The pancreas lies posterior to the stomach and is primarily an exocrine organ producing digestive enzymes and buffers. The large pancreatic duct reaches the duodenum where it meets the common bile duct from the liver and the gallbladder. The liver is a large visceral organ and is the center for the body's metabolic regulation. The liver lies in the right hypochondriac and epigastric regions and has a complex circulatory system. The liver secretes bile into a network of channels that eventually unite to form the common hepatic duct. The bile in the hepatic duct flows into the common bile duct, which empties into the duodenum or enters the cystic duct, which leads to the gallbladder. The common bile duct is formed by the unions of the common hepatic duct and the cystic duct. The gallbladder is located near the liver and the major function is bile storage. Bile is released from the gallbladder into the duodenum when stimulated by the intestinal hormone CCK.

25.1 Gallbladder Disorders

Altered bile flow through the hepatic, cystic, or common bile duct is a common problem and a frequent cause of hospitalization. It often leads to inflammation and other

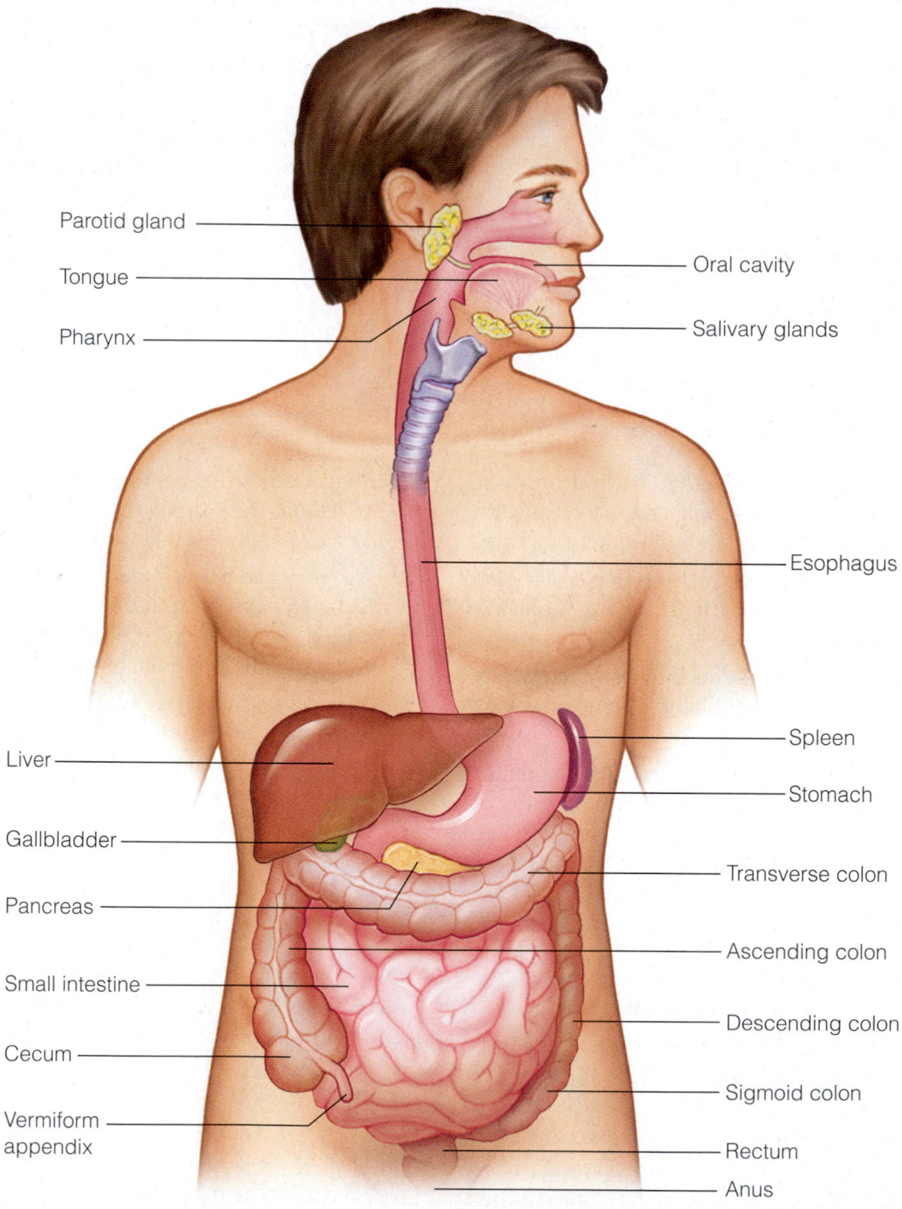
Parotid gland
Tongue
Pharynx
Oral cavity
Salivary glands
Esophagus
Liver
Gallbladder
Pancreas
Small intestine
Cecum
Vermiform appendix
Spleen
Stomach
Transverse colon
Ascending colon
Descending colon
Sigmoid colon
Rectum
Anus

Figure 25.1 ■ Accessory organs of the gastrointestinal system.

complications. Gallstones are the most common cause of obstructed flow. Tumors and abscesses can also obstruct bile flow.

The Patient with Gallstones

Cholelithiasis is the formation of stones (*calculi* or *gallstones*) within the gallbladder or biliary duct system. Cholelithiasis is a common problem in the United States, affecting 10 to 15% of the population in the United States, and represents the second most common discharge diagnosis in U.S. hospitalizations (Pak & Lindseth, 2016). Risk factors for gallstones include age, family history, obesity, hyperlipidemia, rapid weight loss, being female, using hormonal contraceptives, biliary stasis, and presence of certain disorders such as diabetes, cirrhosis, ileal disease, or sickle cell disease.

Gender is one of the most significant risk factors for gallbladder disease. Women of all ages have a higher risk of cholelithiasis due to higher estrogen levels (Pak & Lindseth, 2016). Incidence of gallbladder disease is higher for Native Americans in both the Northern and Southern Hemispheres. North American Indians have a particularly high rate of gallstone disease and are more likely to experience complications (Pak & Lindseth, 2016). Many studies suggest there is a strong correlation between high cholesterol levels and the development of cholesterol-laden gallstone development. The western diet has been identified as one of the strongest predictors for developing cholesterol gallstones. Obesity, especially central adiposity, increases risk for developing gallbladder disease. Physical activity appears to decrease the likelihood of developing gallbladder disease (Pak & Lindseth, 2016).

Physiology Review

Normally, bile is formed by the liver and stored in the gallbladder. Bile contains bile salts, bilirubin, water, electrolytes, cholesterol, fatty acids, and lecithin. In the gallbladder, some of the water and electrolytes are absorbed, further concentrating the bile. Food entering the intestine stimulates the gallbladder to contract and release bile through the common bile duct and sphincter of Oddi into the intestine. The bile salts in bile increase the solubility and absorption of dietary fats.

Pathophysiology and Manifestations

Cholelithiasis

Gallstones form when several factors interact: Abnormal bile composition, biliary stasis, and inflammation of the gallbladder. Most gallstones (80%) consist primarily of cholesterol; the rest contain a mixture of bile components. Excess cholesterol in bile is associated with obesity, a high-calorie and high-cholesterol diet, and drugs that lower serum cholesterol levels. When bile is supersaturated with cholesterol, it can precipitate out to form stones. Biliary stasis, or slowed emptying of the gallbladder, contributes to cholelithiasis. Stones do not form when the gallbladder empties completely in response to hormonal stimulation. Slowed or incomplete emptying allows cholesterol to concentrate and increases the risk of stone formation. Finally, inflammation of the gallbladder allows excess water and bile salt reabsorption, increasing the risk for lithiasis. Certain very-low-calorie diets are associated with a high risk of cholelithiasis. Increased cholesterol concentration in the bile and decreased gallbladder contractions associated with fasting increase the risk of gallstone formation.

Most gallstones are formed in the gallbladder. They then may migrate into the ducts (**Figure 25.2 ■**), leading to *cholangitis* (duct inflammation). Although some people with cholelithiasis are asymptomatic, many develop manifestations. Early manifestations of gallstones may be vague: Epigastric fullness or mild gastric distress after eating a large or fatty meal. Stones that obstruct the cystic duct or common bile duct lead to distention and increased pressure behind the stone. This causes **biliary colic**, a severe, steady pain in the epigastric region or right upper quadrant of the abdomen. The pain may radiate to the back, right scapula, or shoulder. The pain often begins suddenly following a meal and may last as long as 5 hours. It is often accompanied by nausea and vomiting.

Obstruction of the common bile duct may cause bile reflux into the liver, leading to jaundice, pain, and possible liver damage. If the common duct is obstructed, pancreatic enzymes will be unable to enter the small intestine, and pancreatitis (discussed later in this chapter) becomes a potential complication.

Cholecystitis

Cholecystitis is inflammation of the gallbladder. *Acute cholecystitis* usually follows obstruction of the cystic duct by a stone. The obstruction increases pressure within the gallbladder, leading to ischemia of the gallbladder wall and mucosa. Retained bile causes chemical irritation, and bacterial inflammation often follows. The ischemia can lead to necrosis and perforation of the gallbladder wall.

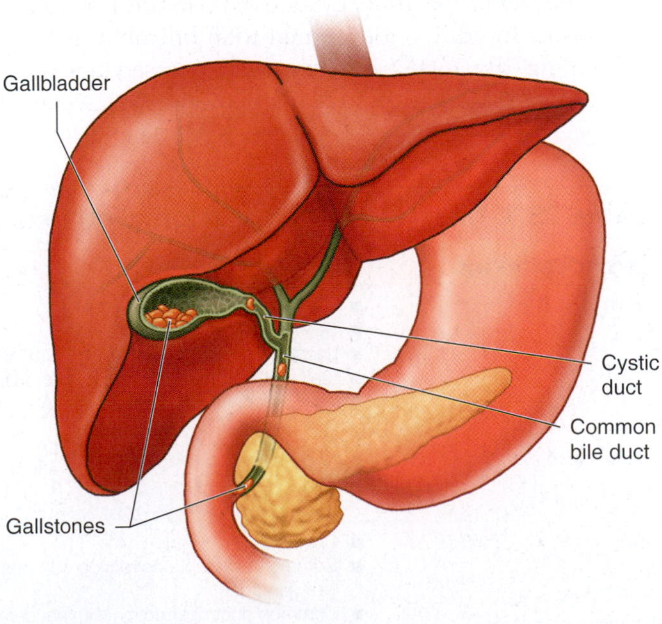
Gallbladder
Cystic duct
Common bile duct
Gallstones

Figure 25.2 ■ Common locations of gallstones.

Acute cholecystitis usually begins with an attack of biliary colic. The pain involves the entire right upper quadrant (RUQ) and may radiate to the back, right scapula, or shoulder. Movement or deep breathing may aggravate the pain. The pain usually lasts longer than biliary colic, continuing for 12 to 18 hours. Anorexia and nausea and vomiting are common. Fever is often present and may be accompanied by chills. The RUQ is tender to palpation.

Chronic cholecystitis may result from repeated bouts of acute cholecystitis or from persistent irritation of the gallbladder wall by stones. Bacteria may be present in the bile as well. Chronic cholecystitis is often asymptomatic.

Complications of cholecystitis include *empyema*, a collection of infected fluid within the gallbladder; gangrene and perforation with resulting peritonitis or abscess formation; formation of a fistula into an adjacent organ (such as the duodenum, colon, or stomach); or obstruction of the small intestine by a large gallstone (*gallstone ileus*). **Table 25.1** compares the manifestations and complications of acute cholelithiasis with those of cholecystitis.

Interprofessional Care

Treatment of the patient with gallstones depends on the acuity of the condition and the patient's overall health status. When gallstones are present but asymptomatic and the patient has a low risk for complications, conservative treatment is indicated. However, when the patient experiences frequent symptoms, has acute cholecystitis, or has very large stones, the gallbladder and stones are usually surgically removed.

Diagnosis

Diagnostic tests are ordered to identify the presence and location of stones, identify possible complications, and help differentiate gallbladder disease from other disorders.

- ***Serum bilirubin*** is measured. Elevated direct (conjugated) bilirubin may indicate obstructed bile flow in the biliary duct system (**Box 25.1**).
- ***Total (serum) bilirubin*** includes both indirect and direct forms. In adults, the normal total bilirubin is 0.1 to 1.2 mg/dL. Total bilirubin levels increase when more is being produced (e.g., RBC hemolysis) or when its metabolism or excretion is impaired (e.g., liver disease or biliary obstruction).
- ***Direct (conjugated) bilirubin levels***, normally 0.1 to 0.3 mg/dL in adults, rise when its excretion is impaired by obstruction within the liver (e.g., in cirrhosis, hepatitis, exposure to hepatotoxins) or in the biliary system.
- ***Indirect (unconjugated) bilirubin levels***, normally <1.0 mg/dL in adults, rise in RBC hemolysis (e.g., sickle cell disease or transfusion reaction).
- ***Complete blood count (CBC)*** may show an elevated WBC count in the presence of inflammation and infection.
- ***Alkaline phosphate levels*** may be elevated and may indicate blockage of the common bile duct caused by a gallstone (Devendorf, Murray, & Sharp, 2018).
- ***Ultrasonography of the gallbladder*** is a noninvasive exam that can accurately diagnose cholelithiasis with more than 95% accuracy (Devendorf et al., 2018). It can also be used to assess emptying of the gallbladder.
- ***Gallbladder scans*** (e.g., HIDA, DIDA, or DISIDA scans) use an intravenous radioactive solution that is rapidly extracted from the blood and excreted into the biliary tree to diagnose cystic duct obstruction and acute or chronic cholecystitis.

See Chapter 21 for more information about and the nursing implications of these diagnostic tests.

BOX 25.1
Sorting Out Total, Direct, and Indirect Bilirubin Levels

When serum bilirubin levels are drawn, the results are usually reported as the total bilirubin, direct bilirubin, and indirect bilirubin levels. Most bilirubin is formed from hemoglobin, as aging or abnormal RBCs are removed from circulation and destroyed. It is then bound to protein and transported to the liver. This protein-bound bilirubin is called *indirect* or *unconjugated* bilirubin. Once in the liver, bilirubin is separated from the protein and converted to a soluble form, *direct* or *conjugated* bilirubin. Conjugated bilirubin is then excreted in the bile.

Table 25.1 Manifestations and Complications of Cholelithiasis and Cholecystitis

Manifestations	Cholelithiasis	Cholecystitis
Pain	■ Abrupt onset ■ Severe, steady ■ Localized to epigastrium and RUQ of abdomen ■ May radiate to back, right scapula, and shoulder ■ Lasts 30 minutes to 5 hours	■ Abrupt onset ■ Severe, steady ■ Generalized in RUQ of abdomen ■ May radiate to back, right scapula, and shoulder ■ Lasts 12 to 18 hours ■ Aggravated by movement, breathing
Associated symptoms	■ Nausea and vomiting	■ Anorexia, nausea and vomiting ■ RUQ tenderness and guarding ■ Chills and fever
Complications	■ Cholecystitis ■ Common bile duct obstruction with possible jaundice and liver damage ■ Common duct obstruction with pancreatitis	■ Gangrene and perforation with peritonitis ■ Chronic cholecystitis ■ Empyema ■ Fistula formation ■ Gallstone ileus

Medications

Patients who refuse surgery or for whom surgery is inappropriate may be treated with a medication to dissolve the gallstones. Ursodeoxycholic acid is a bile salt and can be given orally for up to 2 years. Statins are used to lower cholesterol and reduce the development of gallstones with high cholesterol content. The primary disadvantages of pharmacologic treatment for gallstones include long duration (2 years or more) and the high incidence of recurrent stone formation when treatment is discontinued.

If infection is suspected, antibiotics may be ordered to cure the infection and reduce associated inflammation and edema. Patients with pruritus (itching) due to severe obstructive jaundice and an accumulation of bile salts on the skin may be given cholestyramine (Questran). This drug binds with bile salts to promote their excretion in the feces. Ketorolac or an opioid analgesic such as morphine may be required for pain relief during an acute attack of cholecystitis. Antiemetics such as *ondansetron* (Zofran) or *prochlorperazine* (Compazine) may be given to reduce nausea and vomiting (Devendorf et al., 2018).

Nutrition

Food intake may be eliminated during an acute attack of cholecystitis, and a nasogastric tube may be inserted to relieve nausea and vomiting. Dietary fat intake may be limited, especially if the patient is obese. If bile flow is obstructed, fat-soluble vitamins (A, D, E, and K) and bile salts may need to be administered.

Surgery

Laparoscopic cholecystectomy (removal of the gallbladder) is the treatment of choice for symptomatic cholelithiasis or cholecystitis. This minimally invasive procedure has a low risk of complications and generally requires a hospital stay of less than 24 hours. Not all patients are candidates for laparoscopic cholecystectomy, and there is a risk that it may be converted to a *laparotomy* (surgical opening into the abdomen) during the procedure. See the **Box 25.2** for nursing care of a patient having a laparoscopic cholecystectomy.

When stones are lodged within the ducts, a cholecystectomy with common bile duct exploration may be done. A T-tube (**Figure 25.3** ■) is inserted to maintain patency of the duct and promote bile passage while the edema decreases. Excess bile is collected in a drainage bag secured below the surgical site. If it is suspected that a stone has been retained following surgery, a postoperative cholangiogram via the T-tube or direct visualization of the duct with an endoscope may be performed. Some patients who are poor surgical risks and for whom laparoscopic cholecystectomy is inappropriate may have either a *cholecystostomy* to drain the gallbladder or a *choledochostomy* to remove stones and position a T-tube in the common bile duct.

Nursing Care

In addition to the nursing care discussed in this section, see the Case Study & Nursing Care Plan for a patient with cholelithiasis on page 817.

BOX 25.2
Nursing Care of the Patient Having a Laparoscopic Cholecystectomy

PREOPERATIVE CARE

- Provide routine preoperative care as ordered (see Chapter 4).
- Assess for manifestations of cholecystitis and other complications of gallstones. *An acutely inflamed gallbladder and ductal system increase surgical complexity and may necessitate open cholecystectomy.*
- Reinforce teaching about the procedure and postoperative expectations, including pain management, deep breathing, and mobilization. *Preoperative teaching reduces anxiety and promotes rapid postoperative recovery.*

POSTOPERATIVE CARE

- Provide routine postoperative recovery care as ordered (see Chapter 4).
- Treat postoperative pain and nausea and vomiting prophylactically and as needed to relieve symptoms. *Postoperative pain is common during the first 24 to 48 hours after surgery. Manipulation of the bowel and insufflation of the abdomen with gas commonly lead to postoperative nausea.*
- Assist to chair at bedside as allowed. *Early mobilization promotes lung ventilation and circulation, reducing the potential for postoperative complications.*
- Advance oral intake from ice chips to regular diet as tolerated. *Oral intake can be rapidly resumed due to minimal disruption of the gastrointestinal tract during surgery.*
- Provide and reinforce teaching: Pain management, incision care, activity level, postoperative follow-up appointments. *With early discharge, the patient and family assume responsibility for the majority of postoperative care. A clear understanding of this care and expected needs reduces anxiety and the risk of postoperative complications.*
- Initiate follow-up contact 24 to 48 hours after discharge to evaluate adequacy of pain control, incision management, and discharge understanding. *Contact following discharge provides an opportunity to evaluate care and reinforce teaching.*

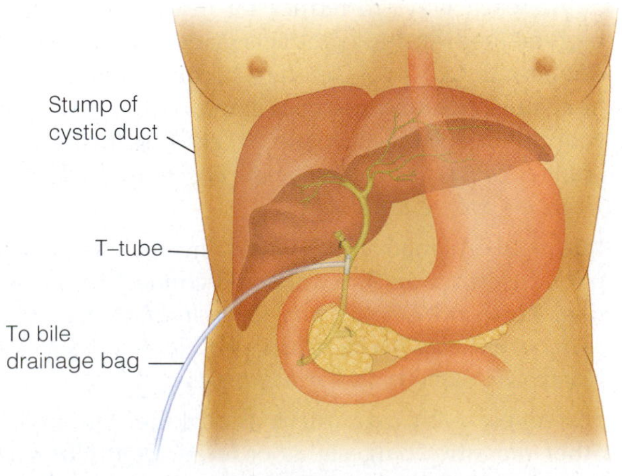
Stump of
cystic duct
T–tube
To bile
drainage bag

Figure 25.3 ■ T-tube placement in the common bile duct. Bile fluid flows with gravity into a drainage collection device below the level of the common bile duct.

Assessment

Assessment data related to cholelithiasis and cholecystitis include:

- ***Health history:*** Current manifestations, including RUQ pain, its character and relationship to meals, duration, and radiation, nausea and vomiting, or other symptoms; duration of symptoms; risk factors or previous history of symptoms; chronic diseases such as diabetes, cirrhosis, or inflammatory bowel disease; current diet; use of oral contraceptives or possibility of pregnancy
- ***Physical assessment:*** Current weight; color of skin and sclera; abdominal assessment including light palpation for tenderness; color of urine and stool
- ***Diagnostic tests:*** WBC, serum bilirubin, liver enzymes, and pancreatic enzyme (amylase and lipase) results.

Priorities of Care

Priority nursing care for the patient with cholelithiasis or cholecystitis often includes managing pain related to biliary colic or surgery, addressing the nutritional imbalance related to the effects of altered bile flow, nausea and anorexia, and treating infection related to potential rupture of an acutely inflamed gallbladder. Nursing interventions for the patient who has undergone a laparoscopic or open cholecystectomy are similar to those for other patients having abdominal surgery.

Diagnoses, Outcomes, and Interventions

Relieve Pain. The pain associated with cholelithiasis can be severe. Sometimes a combination of interventions is indicated.

Expected Outcome: Patient will identify pain triggers, use treatment plan (pharmacologic and nonpharmacologic) to prevent and alleviate discomfort, and report relief from pain.

The nurse will:

- Discuss the relationship between fat intake and the pain. Teach ways to reduce fat intake. Examples of high-fat foods include products made with whole milk, doughnuts, avocados, sausage, bacon, hot dogs, gravy, most nuts, potato chips, corn chips, butter, fried foods, peanut butter, and chocolate. *Fat entering the duodenum initiates gallbladder contractions, causing pain when gallstones are present in the ducts.*
- Withhold oral food and fluids during episodes of acute pain. Insert nasogastric tube and connect to low suction, if ordered. *Emptying the stomach reduces the amount of chyme entering the duodenum and the stimulus for gallbladder contractions, thus reducing pain.*
- For severe pain, administer morphine, fentanyl, or other narcotic analgesia as ordered. *Controlling pain prevents pain-related complications such as atelectasis and thrombosis.*
- Place in Fowler position. *Fowler position decreases pressure on the inflamed gallbladder.*

Promote Balanced Nutrition and Hydration. The patient with severe gallbladder disease may develop nutritional imbalances related to anorexia, pain, and nausea following meals and to impaired bile flow that alters absorption of fat and fat-soluble vitamins (A, D, E, and K) from the gut.

Expected Outcome: Patient will maintain adequate oral intake, report adequate energy levels, and maintain body mass and weight and normal lab values (transferrin, albumin, and electrolytes).

The nurse will:

- Assess nutritional status, including diet history, height and weight, and skinfold measurements. *Even though often obese, patients with gallbladder disease may have an imbalanced diet or may have specific vitamin deficiencies, particularly of the fat-soluble vitamins.*
- Evaluate laboratory results, including serum bilirubin, serum transferrin, serum albumin, glucose, electrolytes, and cholesterol levels. Report abnormal results to the primary care provider. *Elevated serum bilirubin may indicate impaired bilirubin excretion due to obstructed bile flow. A low serum albumin may indicate poor nutritional status. Glucose intolerance and hypercholesterolemia are risk factors for cholelithiasis.*
- Refer to a dietitian or nutritionist for diet counseling to promote healthy weight loss and reduce pain episodes. *A low-carbohydrate, low-fat, higher-protein diet reduces symptoms of cholecystitis. Although fasting and very-low-calorie diets are contraindicated, a moderate reduction in calorie intake and increased activity levels promote weight loss.*
- Administer vitamin supplements as ordered. *Patients who do not absorb fat well due to obstructed bile flow may require supplements of the fat-soluble vitamins.*

Monitor for Infection. An acutely inflamed gallbladder may become necrotic and rupture, releasing its contents into the abdominal cavity. While the resulting infection often remains localized, peritonitis can result from chemical irritation and bacterial contamination of the peritoneal cavity.

SAFETY ALERT: Rupture of an acutely inflamed gallbladder may be heralded by abrupt but transient pain relief as contents are released from the distended gallbladder into the abdomen. Promptly report this change to the physician. ■

Following open cholecystectomy (*laparotomy*), the risk for pulmonary infection is significant due to the high abdominal incision.

Expected Outcome: Patient will be free from signs and symptoms of infection including vital signs within normal limits, clear lung sounds, and incision without redness, tenderness, drainage, or swelling.

The nurse will:

- Monitor vital signs including temperature every 4 hours. Promptly report vital sign changes or temperature elevation. *Tachycardia, increased respiratory rate, or an elevated temperature may indicate an infectious process.*

- Assess abdomen every 4 hours and as indicated (e.g., when pain level changes abruptly). *Increasing abdominal tenderness or a rigid, boardlike abdomen may indicate rupture of the gallbladder with peritonitis.*
- Assist to cough and deep-breathe or use incentive spirometer every 1 to 2 hours while awake. Splint abdominal incision with a blanket or pillow during coughing. *The high abdominal incision of an open cholecystectomy interferes with effective coughing and deep breathing, increasing the risk of atelectasis and respiratory infections such as pneumonia.*
- Place in Fowler position and encourage ambulation as allowed. *Fowler position and ambulating promote lung expansion and airway clearance, reducing the risk of respiratory infections.*
- Administer antibiotics as ordered. *Antibiotics may be given preoperatively to reduce the risk of infection from infected gallbladder contents and may be continued postoperatively to prevent infection.*

Transitions of Care

Although not all risk factors for cholelithiasis can be controlled or modified, several can. Modifiable risk factors include obesity, hyperlipidemia, extremely low-calorie diets, and diets high in cholesterol. By contrast, physical activity, a high-fiber and low-carbohydrate diet, and consumption of unsaturated fats all appear to have a protective effect, reducing the incidence of gallstones and cholecystitis. Discuss the dangers of "yo-yo" dieting, with cycles of weight loss followed by weight gain, and of extremely low-calorie diets. Encourage patients with high serum cholesterol levels to discuss using cholesterol-lowering drugs with their primary care provider.

Teaching varies for patients with acute gallbladder disease, depending on the choice of treatment options for cholelithiasis and cholecystitis. If surgery is not an option, teach about medications that dissolve stones, their use and adverse effects (diarrhea is a common side effect), and the importance of maintaining a low-fat and low-carbohydrate diet, if indicated. Include an explanation about the role of bile and the function of the gallbladder in terms that the patient and family can understand.

Provide appropriate preoperative teaching for the planned procedure. Discuss the possibility of open cholecystectomy even when a laparoscopic procedure is planned. Teach postoperative self-care measures to manage pain and prevent complications. If the patient will be discharged with a T-tube, provide instructions about its care. Discuss manifestations of complications to report to the physician. Stress the importance of follow-up appointments.

Following cholecystectomy, a low-fat diet may initially be recommended. Refer the patient and food preparer to a dietitian to review low-fat foods. Higher-fat foods may be gradually added to the diet as tolerated.

Management of chronic gallbladder disease primarily involves altering diet. A balanced, low-fat diet should be promoted. Teach the patient to consume healthy fats such as olive oil and cannola oil. Encourage the patient to increase dietary fiber and decrease simple carbohydrates. Regular physical activity should be promoted to promote stable weight control.

Case Study & Nursing Care Plan

A Patient with Cholelithiasis

Joyce Colbert is a 44-year-old married mother of three children. A member of the Chickasaw tribe, she is active in tribal activities and works part time as a cook at a community kitchen. Recently Mrs. Colbert has noticed a dull pain in her upper abdomen that gets worse after eating fatty foods; nausea and sometimes vomiting accompany the pain. She had a similar pain after the birth of her last child. She is diagnosed with cholelithiasis and is admitted for a laparoscopic cholecystectomy.

ASSESSMENT	DIAGNOSES	EXPECTED OUTCOMES
David Corbin, RN, takes Mrs. Colbert's admission history. It includes intolerance to fatty foods and intermittent "stabbing" abdominal pain that radiates to her back. Her usual diet includes tacos or fried bread and biscuits with gravy for breakfast. She reports "not wanting to eat much of anything lately." She states she has never had surgery before and hopes "everything goes well." Physical assessment includes T 37.7°C (100°F), P 88 bpm, R 20/min, and BP 130/84 mmHg. She has had a recent 2.3-kg (5-lb) weight loss, currently weighing 59 kg (130 lb). She is 160 cm (63 in.) tall. Abdominal examination elicits tenderness in the right upper abdominal quadrant. She has no jaundice, chills, or evidence of complications.	▪ Poor nutrition related to anorexia and recent weight loss ▪ Acute pain related to inflamed gallbladder and surgical incisions ▪ Risk of infection related to potential bacterial contamination of abdominal cavity ▪ Anxiety related to lack of information about perioperative experience	▪ Patient will maintain present weight within 2.3 kg (5 lb) during the next 3 weeks. ▪ Patient will resume regular diet, decreasing intake of foods high in fat. ▪ Patient will verbalize adequate pain control after surgery and with activity resumption. ▪ Patient will remain free of infection. ▪ Patient will verbalize a decrease in anxiety before surgery.

(continued)

PLANNING AND IMPLEMENTATION

- Teach about the gallbladder and the function of bile.
- Discuss pre- and postoperative care, including self-care following discharge.
- Promote mobility as soon as allowed after surgery.
- Teach home care of incisions and recognition of signs of infection.
- Review specific high-fat foods to avoid and ways to maintain her weight.
- Provide analgesia as needed postoperatively. Teach appropriate analgesic use after discharge.

EVALUATION

Mrs. Colbert is discharged the morning after her surgery. She is afebrile, has no signs of infection, and is able to appropriately care for her incisions. She identifies signs of infection and talks about ways to reduce her fat intake while keeping her weight stable. She verbalizes understanding of initial activity restrictions and resumption of normal activities. Mrs. Colbert states, "It wasn't as bad as I thought it would be at first." She has an appointment to see her surgeon in 1 week.

CLINICAL REASONING IN PATIENT CARE

1. What is the rationale for a low-fat diet with cholelithiasis? Discuss nutritional practices as they relate to the medical problem and Mrs. Colbert's culture.
2. How would your discharge teaching for Mrs. Colbert differ if she had had an open cholecystectomy instead of a laparoscopic cholecystectomy?
3. Design a nursing care plan for Mrs. Colbert addressing difficulty performing ADLs due to fatigue.

See Evaluating Your Response in Appendix B.

The Patient with Cancer of the Gallbladder

Cancer of the gallbladder is rare, primarily affecting people over age 65, and diagnosis is typically delayed, as early symptoms are subtle and mimic other gastrointestinal disorders (Sorenson, Quinn, & Klein, 2019). Women are more likely to develop the disorder. Manifestations of gallbladder cancer include intense pain and a palpable mass in the RUQ of the abdomen. Jaundice and weight loss are common. Gallbladder cancers spread by direct extension to the liver, and metastasize via the blood and lymph system.

At the time of diagnosis, the cancer is usually too advanced to treat surgically. Survival depends on the stage of the cancer at the time of diagnosis. Radical and extensive surgical interventions may be performed, but the prognosis is poor regardless of treatment. Nursing care is palliative, focusing on maintaining comfort and independence to the extent possible.

25.2 Liver Disorders

The liver is a complex organ with multiple metabolic and regulatory functions (**Figure 25.4** ■). Optimal liver function is essential to health. Because of the significant amount of blood in the liver at all times, it is exposed to the effects of pathogens, drugs, toxins, and possibly malignant cells. As a result, liver cells may become inflamed or damaged or cancerous tumors may develop.

The essential functions of the liver include the metabolism of proteins, carbohydrates, and fats. It is also responsible for the metabolism of steroid hormones and most drugs. It synthesizes essential blood proteins, including albumin and clotting factors in particular. The liver detoxifies alcohol and other toxic substances. Ammonia, a toxic by-product of protein metabolism, is converted to urea in the liver for elimination by the kidneys. The liver produces bile, an essential substance for absorbing fats and eliminating bilirubin from the body. Minerals and fat-soluble vitamins are stored in the liver, as is glycogen (stored carbohydrate for energy reserves). The Kupffer cells that line the sinusoids phagocytize foreign cells and damaged blood cells. See Chapter 21 for more information about the liver.

Common Manifestations of Liver Disorders

Although many different disorders can disrupt liver function, their manifestations relate to three primary effects: Disrupted liver cell function, impaired bilirubin conversion

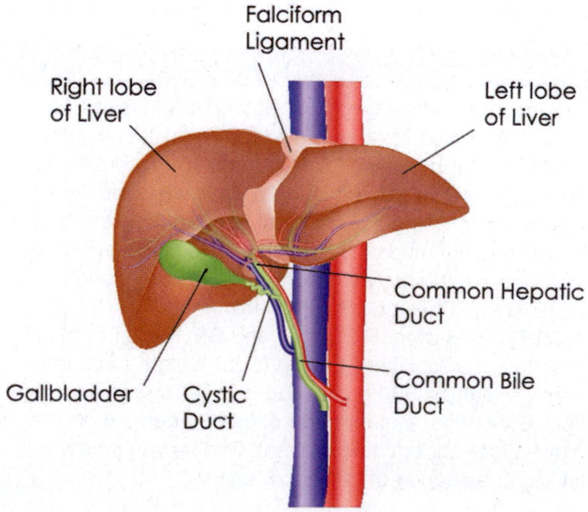
Falciform Ligament
Right lobe of Liver
Left lobe of Liver
Common Hepatic Duct
Gallbladder
Cystic Duct
Common Bile Duct

Figure 25.4 ■ Anatomy of the liver.

and excretion leading to jaundice, and disrupted blood flow through the liver, with resulting portal hypertension.

Hepatocellular Failure

The liver is vital to digestion and metabolism of nutrients; the production of plasma proteins, including those involved in clotting, and the metabolism and excretion of compounds such as bilirubin, steroid hormones, and ammonia, as well as toxins (such as alcohol) and drugs. Impaired function of liver cells has multiple effects, including:

- Impaired protein metabolism with decreased production of albumin and clotting factors. Low albumin levels contribute to edema in peripheral tissues and **ascites**, accumulation of fluid in the abdomen (**Figure 25.5** ■), as plasma oncotic pressure is reduced. Impaired clotting factor production increases the risk for bleeding.
- Disrupted glucose metabolism and storage with resulting alterations in blood glucose levels (either hyperglycemia or hypoglycemia).
- Reduced bile production that impairs the absorption of lipids and fat-soluble vitamins. Inadequate vitamin K, a fat-soluble vitamin, affects the production of clotting factors, leading to a bleeding tendency.
- Impaired metabolism of steroid hormones (including estrogen and testosterone) leads to feminization in men and irregular menses in women.

Jaundice

Disrupted metabolism and excretion of bilirubin allows it to accumulate in tissues, leading to **jaundice**, yellow staining of tissues (**Figure 25.6** ■). Jaundice (*icterus*) is often first noticeable in the sclera of the eyes, then the skin.

When RBCs are destroyed (due to cell aging or disease), hemoglobin is released. The hemoglobin molecule breaks up into globin, a protein, and heme, the iron-containing portion of the molecule. In this process, biliverdin, later converted to fat-soluble bilirubin (*unconjugated bilirubin*), is released. The bilirubin binds with albumin to be transported to the liver. In the liver, it is converted to a water-soluble form (*conjugated bilirubin*) to be excreted in the bile. Refer to **Box 25.1** for more information about bilirubin metabolism.

Jaundice can result from disruptions at any point in the production and metabolism of bilirubin:

- ***Prehepatic/hemolytic jaundice*** develops when excess RBC destruction (hemolysis) releases more bilirubin into circulation than the liver is able to process. High blood levels of unconjugated bilirubin are seen.
- ***Intrahepatic/hepatic jaundice*** occurs when impaired liver cell (*hepatocyte*) function disrupts the conversion and excretion of bilirubin. Blood levels of both conjugated and unconjugated bilirubin may be elevated. Stools may appear normal or clay colored, and urine is dark because the conjugated bilirubin is excreted by the kidneys.
- ***Posthepatic/obstructive jaundice*** is caused by obstruction of bile flow within the biliary system (the gallbladder and bile ducts), which impairs bilirubin excretion. Levels of conjugated bilirubin are elevated. Stools are light or clay colored due to lack of bile pigment and urine is dark because the kidneys excrete bilirubin.

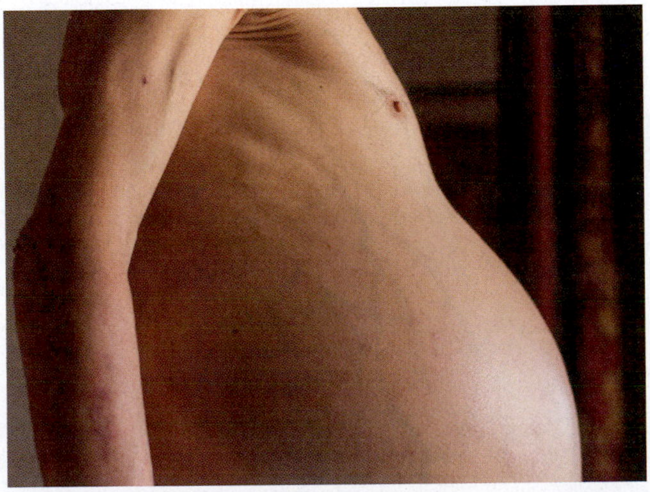

Figure 25.5 ■ In ascites, serous fluid collects in the abdominal cavity, causing uniform distention.

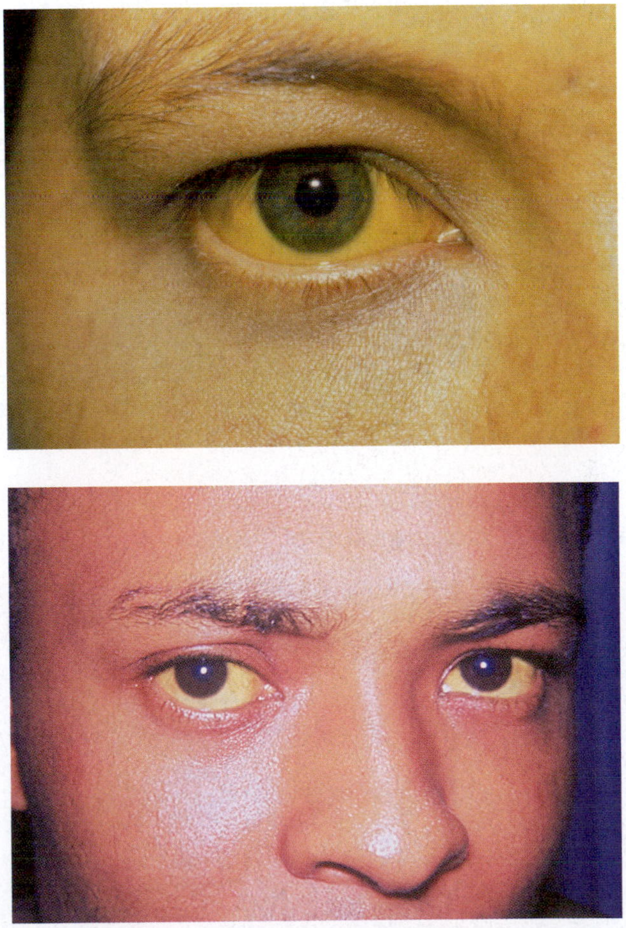

B

Figure 25.6 ■ Jaundice. Note the yellowing of the white (sclera) of the eye and of the surrounding facial skin.

Portal Hypertension

Impaired blood flow through the liver increases pressure in the portal venous system that drains the gastrointestinal tract, the spleen, and surface veins of the abdomen. **Portal hypertension**, increased pressure in the portal system, has several effects when it is prolonged:

- Veins in the gastrointestinal tract and the abdominal wall dilate. This congestion tends to suppress the appetite and lead to formation of collateral vessels in the distal esophagus, stomach, and rectum. The dilated, congested vessels in the esophagus are known as **esophageal varices**; in the rectum, they lead to the development of hemorrhoids. In advanced liver failure, superficial varices may develop around the umbilicus, a feature known as *caput medusae*.
- The spleen enlarges (*splenomegaly*).
- Fluid accumulates in the peritoneal cavity, a condition called *ascites*. Increased hydrostatic pressure in abdominal vessels forces fluid out of the vessels and into the peritoneal cavity. Low serum albumin levels (*hypoalbuminemia*) contribute to fluid accumulation by reducing the osmotic draw of fluid back into vessels.
- **Portal systemic encephalopathy** (or *hepatic encephalopathy*), impaired consciousness and mental status, results from the accumulation of toxic waste products in the blood (ammonia in particular) as blood bypasses the congested liver. It appears that factors other than elevated ammonia levels contribute, including the presence of toxic fatty acids and altered neurotransmitters and an imbalance of plasma amino acid ratios. Cerebral edema develops late in the course of liver failure, resulting from both the accumulation of toxins and vascular mechanisms. As cerebral edema progresses, intracranial pressure increases, cerebral perfusion decreases, and brain cells become hypoxic.
- *Hepatorenal syndrome* is acute kidney failure due to disrupted blood flow to the kidneys. See Chapter 28 for more information about kidney failure.

The Patient with Hepatitis

Hepatitis is inflammation of the liver. It is usually caused by a virus, although it may result from exposure to alcohol, drugs, toxins, or other pathogens and sometimes develops secondary to other viral infections such as those caused by Epstein-Barr, herpes simplex, varicella-zoster, and cytomegalovirus. Hepatitis may be acute or chronic in nature. Cirrhosis, discussed in the next section, is a potential consequence of severe hepatocellular damage. Chronic hepatitis also increases the risk for developing liver cancer.

Pathophysiology and Manifestations

The inflammatory process of hepatitis, whether caused by a virus, toxin, or other mechanism, damages hepatic cells and disrupts liver function. Cell-mediated immune responses damage hepatocytes and Kupffer cells, leading to hyperplasia, necrosis, and cellular regeneration. The flow of bile through bile canaliculi and into the biliary system can be impaired by the inflammatory process, leading to jaundice. When the inflammatory process is mild (e.g., hepatitis A), the liver parenchyma is not significantly damaged. The inflammatory processes associated with hepatitis B and hepatitis C, however, can lead to severe liver damage. The metabolism of nutrients, drugs, alcohol, and toxins and the process of bile elimination are disrupted by the inflammation of hepatitis. See Chapter 21 for more information about the liver and the preceding section for more information about the effects of disrupted liver function.

Viral Hepatitis

Viral hepatitis is nearly always caused by one of five viruses: Hepatitis A virus (HAV), hepatitis B virus (HBV), hepatitis C virus (HCV), the hepatitis B–associated delta virus (HDV), and hepatitis E virus (HEV). With the exception of HBV, all of the hepatitis viruses are RNA viruses; HBV is a DNA virus. The viruses differ from one another in mode of transmission, incubation period, the severity and type of liver damage they cause, and their ability to become chronic or develop a carrier (asymptomatic) state. The illnesses they cause, however, are clinically very similar. **Table 25.2** identifies unique features of the primary hepatitis viruses.

Table 25.2 Comparison of Types of Viral Hepatitis

Virus	Hepatitis A (HAV)	Hepatitis B (HBV)	Hepatitis C (HCV)	Hepatitis D (HDV)	Hepatitis E (HEV)
Mode of transmission	Fecal–oral	Blood and body fluids; perinatal	Blood and body fluids	Blood and body fluids; perinatal	Fecal–oral
Incubation (in weeks)	2–6	6–24	5–12	3–13	3–6
Onset	Abrupt	Slow	Slow	Abrupt	Abrupt
Carrier state	No	Yes	Yes	Yes	Yes
Possible complications	Rare	Chronic hepatitis	Cirrhosis	Liver cancer	Chronic hepatitis
Cirrhosis	Liver cancer	Chronic hepatitis	Cirrhosis	Fulminant hepatitis	May be severe in pregnant women
Laboratory findings	Anti-HAV antibodies present	Positive HBsAg (HBV surface antigen); anti-HBV antibodies present	Anti-HCV antibodies present	Positive HDVAg (delta antigen) early; anti-HDV antibodies later	Anti-HEV antibodies present

In the United States:

- Hepatitis A is less common than hepatitis B and the incidence continues to decline, with a reported 1808 acute cases in 2016 in the U.S. (Walker, 2018). The rate of hepatitis A infections per 100,000 population fell steadily since the introduction of hepatitis A vaccine to the lowest ever reported rate of 0.5 in 2014.
- Reported cases of hepatitis B in 2016 numbered 3218 in the U.S. The rate of reported hepatitis B infections peaked at 11.5 per 100,000 population in 1985, then fell to 1.1 in 2010 and have been fluctuating around 3000 cases annually.
- In 2016, 2967 cases of hepatitis C were reported in the U.S. and cases have been increasing beginning in 2012. The increased rate reflects new infections associated with rising rates of injection drug use and to a lesser extent to improved early detection. The Centers for Disease Control and Prevention (CDC; 2016a) recommends one-time testing for HCV infection for adults born between 1945 and 1965 and among others with increased risk.

Hepatitis viruses replicate in the liver, indirectly damaging liver cells (hepatocytes). The viruses provoke an immune response that causes inflammation and necrosis of hepatocytes, leading to the clinical presentation of acute disease. Although the extent of damage and the immune response vary among the different hepatitis viruses, the disease itself usually follows a predictable pattern.

No manifestations are present during the incubation period after exposure to the virus. The *prodromal* or *preicteric* (before jaundice) *phase* may begin abruptly or insidiously, with general malaise, anorexia, fatigue, and muscle and body aches. These manifestations are often mistaken for the flu. Nausea and vomiting, diarrhea, or constipation may develop, as well as mild RUQ abdominal pain. Chills and fever may be present.

The *icteric* (jaundiced) *phase* usually begins 5 to 10 days after the onset of symptoms. It is heralded by jaundice of the sclera, skin, and mucous membranes. Inflammation of the liver and bile ducts prevents bilirubin from being excreted into the small intestine. As a result, the serum bilirubin levels are elevated, causing yellowing of the skin and mucous membranes. Pruritus may develop due to deposition of bile salts on the skin. The stools are light brown or clay colored because bile pigment is not excreted through the normal fecal pathway. Instead, the pigment is excreted by the kidneys, causing the urine to turn brown. Whereas patients with acute hepatitis A or B are likely to develop jaundice, many people with hepatitis C do not develop jaundice. As a result, the infection may go undiagnosed for an extended period of time.

During the icteric phase, the initial prodromal manifestations usually diminish even though the serum bilirubin increases. The appetite increases, and the temperature returns to normal. When uncomplicated, spontaneous recovery usually begins within 2 weeks of the onset of jaundice.

The final phase is referred to as the recovery phase or posticteric phase and typically follows the beginning resolution of jaundice. The recovery phase can last several weeks after exposure (Sorenson et al., 2019). During this time, manifestations gradually improve: Serum enzymes decrease, liver pain decreases, and gastrointestinal symptoms and weakness subside.

Hepatitis A. Hepatitis A, or *infectious hepatitis*, is transmitted by the fecal–oral route via contaminated food, water, shellfish, or direct contact with an infected person. International travel is the primary risk factor for developing hepatitis A; others include close household or sexual contact with an infected partner (CDC, 2016a). The virus is in the stool of infected individuals up to 2 weeks before symptoms develop. Once jaundice develops, the amount of virus in the stool and the risk of spreading the disease decrease significantly. Although hepatitis A usually has an abrupt onset, it is typically a benign and self-limited disease with few long-term consequences. Symptoms last up to 2 months.

Hepatitis B. HBV infection has phases that reflect the immune status of the host and the degree of viral replications. The *immune tolerant or prodromal phase* can be 10 to 30 years in individuals infected perinatally. The prodromal phase is short for those infected as children or adults and typically begins about 2 weeks after being exposed. Symptoms are vague and nonspecific and continues until jaundice develops. Liver damage is often minimal because the immune system develops a tolerance to the virus. The *icteric or immune active phase* begins about 2 weeks after the prodromal phase because the immune system ceases to tolerate the virus and attacks the liver cell. Most individuals become symptomatic and seek treatment during this phase. The risk for developing progressive liver disease such as cirrhosis, liver failure, and liver cancer is highest during this phase. The final phase is called the *recovery or inactive carrier phase* and seroconversion occurs when the virus is no longer detected in the blood (Branstetter-Hall & Felicilda-Reynaldo, 2017; Sorenson et al., 2019).

This virus is spread through contact with infected blood and body fluids. High-risk groups for hepatitis B include injection drug users, people with multiple sex partners, men who have sex with other men, and people frequently exposed to blood products (such as people on hemodialysis). Healthcare workers are at risk through exposure to blood and needlestick injuries (Branstetter-Hall & Felicilda-Reynaldo, 2017).

In hepatitis B, liver cells are damaged by the immune response to this antigen. Damage may affect only portions or the majority of the liver. The liver shows evidence of injury and scarring, regeneration, and proliferation of inflammatory cells. During the prodromal period, patients with HBV may experience such immune-mediated manifestations as urticaria and other rashes, arthralgias, serum sickness, or glomerulonephritis (Sorenson et al., 2019). The disease itself may be asymptomatic.

Hepatitis C. Hepatitis C affects 185 million people worldwide and without treatment causes progressive liver disease such as cirrhosis and hepatocellular carcinoma (Felicilda-Reynaldo & Patterson, 2018). It is transmitted through infected blood and body fluids and is more common than HBV. About 70% of patients progress to develop chronic hepatitis and up to 30% have cirrhosis of the liver (Adams, Holland, & Urban, 2017). Injection drug use is the primary risk factor for HCV infection, accounting for nearly half of all new infections (CDC, 2016a). Acute hepatitis C is usually asymptomatic; if symptoms do develop, they are often mild and nonspecific. The disease is often recognized long after exposure occurred, when secondary effects of the disease (such as chronic hepatitis or cirrhosis) develop. Prognosis and treatment is dependent on the HCV genotype, severity of liver fibrosis or cirrhosis, patient comorbidities, and previous treatment (Felicilda-Reynaldo & Patterson, 2018).

Nurses frequently care for patients whose hepatitis antigen status is unknown or who have a secondary diagnosis of chronic hepatitis B or C. Exercise standard precautions including hand hygiene and personal protective equipment use with all patients to reduce the risk of exposure to these bloodborne pathogens.

Hepatitis Delta. Hepatitis delta only causes infection in people who are also infected with hepatitis B. It can cause acute or chronic infection and can increase the severity of HBV infection (Sorenson et al., 2019). It is transmitted in the same manner as HBV; as the number of people with immunity to HBV has increased, the incidence of hepatitis delta has decreased (Sorenson et al., 2019).

Hepatitis E. Hepatitis E is rare in the United States. It is transmitted by fecal contamination of water supplies in developing areas such as Southeast Asia, parts of Africa, and Central America. Person-to-person transmission is rare. It primarily affects young adults. It can cause fulminant, fatal hepatitis in pregnant women.

Chronic Hepatitis

Chronic hepatitis is chronic infection of the liver. Although it may cause few symptoms, it is the primary cause of liver damage leading to cirrhosis, liver cancer, and liver transplantation. Three of the known hepatitis viruses cause chronic hepatitis: HBV, HCV, and HDV. Patients with chronic hepatitis may have periods of active liver disease interspersed with periods of inactivity. Liver damage and fibrosis variably progress during periods of disease activity. Manifestations of chronic hepatitis include malaise, fatigue, and hepatomegaly. Occasional icteric (jaundiced) periods may occur. Liver enzymes, particularly serum aminotransferase levels, are typically elevated.

In chronic active hepatitis, inflammation extends to involve entire hepatic lobules. Chronic active hepatitis often leads to cirrhosis and sometimes leads to end-stage liver disease. Complications of end-stage liver disease include ascites, variceal hemorrhage, hepatic encephalopathy, hepatocellular carcinoma, and renal impairment (Cox-North, Doorenbos, Shannon, Scott, & Curtis, 2013).

Fulminant Hepatitis

Fulminant hepatitis is a rapidly progressive disease, with liver failure developing within 2 to 3 weeks after the onset of symptoms. Although uncommon, it is usually related to HBV with concurrent HDV infection.

Toxic Hepatitis

Many substances, including alcohol, certain drugs, and other toxins, can directly damage liver cells. Alcoholic hepatitis can result from chronic alcohol abuse or from an acute toxic reaction to alcohol. Alcoholic hepatitis causes necrosis of hepatocytes and inflammation of the liver parenchyma (functional tissue). Unless alcohol intake is avoided, progression to cirrhosis is common.

Other potential hepatotoxins include acetaminophen, benzene, carbon tetrachloride, halothane, chloroform, and poisonous mushrooms. These substances directly damage liver cells, leading to necrosis. The degree of damage often depends on age and the extent of exposure (dose) to the hepatotoxin. Acetaminophen overdose is the leading cause of acute liver failure.

Autoimmune Hepatitis

Autoimmune hepatitis is a progressive inflammatory disorder in which a cell-mediated immune response directed against liver cells causes persistent inflammation and necrosis with fibrosis and scarring (Sorenson et al., 2019). Circulating autoantibodies such as antinuclear antibody (ANA) are usually present. Many affected individuals have a personal or family history of other autoimmune disorders, such as rheumatoid arthritis or thyroiditis, suggesting a genetic link to the disorder. Chronic autoimmune hepatitis can ultimately lead to cirrhosis and liver failure.

Interprofessional Care

Management of hepatitis focuses on determining its cause, providing appropriate treatment and support, and teaching strategies to prevent further liver damage. Effective management begins with thorough assessment of diagnostic and laboratory data.

Diagnosis

Liver function tests, such as blood levels of bilirubin and enzymes commonly released when liver cells are damaged, are obtained. These include:

- ***Alanine aminotransferase (ALT)*** is an enzyme contained within each liver cell. When liver cells are damaged, ALT is released into the blood. Levels may exceed 1000 units/L or more in acute hepatitis.
- ***Aspartate aminotransferase (AST)*** is an enzyme found predominantly in heart and liver cells. AST levels rise when liver cells are damaged; with severe damage, blood levels may be 20 to 100 times normal values.
- ***Alkaline phosphatase (ALP)*** is an enzyme present in liver cells and bone. Serum ALP levels often are elevated in hepatitis, and may remain elevated after ALT and AST levels have returned to normal ranges.
- ***Serum bilirubin*** levels, including *conjugated* and *unconjugated*, are elevated in viral hepatitis due to impaired bilirubin metabolism and obstruction of the hepatobiliary ducts by inflammation and edema. The bilirubin level decreases as inflammation and edema subside.

- Laboratory tests for viral antigens and their specific antibodies may be done to identify the infecting virus and its state of activity. These tests are summarized in **Table 25.2**.
- ***Liver biopsy*** may be done to detect and evaluate chronic hepatitis. (Nursing implications for this test are outlined in Chapter 21.)

Medications

Prevention. Hepatitis A and hepatitis B are preventable diseases. Vaccines are available, as are preparations to prevent the disease following known or suspected exposure.

Hepatitis A vaccine provides long-term protection against HAV infection. It is an inactivated whole-virus vaccine available in pediatric and adult formulations. Two doses are recommended for full protection. See **Table 25.3**.

Three doses of hepatitis B vaccine provide immunity to HBV infection in 90% of healthy adults. Because the hepatitis delta virus requires the presence of the hepatitis B virus, hepatitis B vaccine also protects against HDV. Hepatitis B vaccine is a recombinant vaccine. Vaccines produced by different manufacturers may be used interchangeably, although their dosages differ. Older adults are less likely to achieve immunity than younger adults. Patients on hemodialysis and people who are immunocompromised may need larger or more doses of the vaccine to achieve adequate protection. Serologic testing for immunity is recommended on completion of the series for people in these high-risk groups.

A combined hepatitis A and hepatitis B vaccine is available for use. It is recommended for the same high-risk populations as the single vaccines. Three doses are given: The initial dose, followed by doses no sooner than 4 weeks and 6 months later.

Postexposure Prophylaxis. Postexposure prophylaxis may be recommended for household or sexual contacts of people with HAV or HBV and other people who are known to have been exposed to these viruses. It is not necessary if the exposed individual has been vaccinated and is known to be immune.

Hepatitis A prophylaxis is provided by a single dose of immune globulin (IG) given within 2 weeks after exposure. IG is recommended for all people with household or sexual contact with an individual known to be infected with hepatitis A. See **Table 25.3** for current recommendations, and nurses should check the CDC website regularly for updates.

Hepatitis B postexposure prophylaxis is indicated for people exposed to the hepatitis B virus. Hepatitis B immune globulin (HBIG) is given to provide for short-term

Table 25.3 CDC Recommendations for Hepatitis Prevention in Adults*

Disease/Strategy	Immunization	Adverse Reactions	Population Recommendations
Hepatitis A			
Prevention	Hepatitis A vaccine (Havrix; VAQTA), two doses with at least 6 months between doses Injected IM into deltoid muscle Combined hepatitis A and hepatitis B vaccine (Twinrix), three doses (initial dose followed by doses 4 weeks and 6 months later) given IM into deltoid muscle	Pain at injection site	■ Everyone who desires protection from HAV infection ■ International travelers ■ Men who have sex with men ■ Injection drug users ■ Individuals with clotting-factor disorders, chronic liver disease ■ Individuals with occupational risk ■ Close contacts of newly adopted non-U.S. children
Postexposure prophylaxis	Standard immune globulin IM into large muscle mass within 2 weeks of exposure Hepatitis A vaccine may be used in healthy people age 40 and younger	Rare; risk of anaphylaxis in people with IgA deficiency	■ Close contacts of people with known hepatitis A ■ People potentially exposed to hepatitis A at child care center or restaurant with infected food handler
Hepatitis B			
Prevention	Recombinant hepatitis B vaccine (Recombivax HB; Engerix-B), three doses (minimum of 16 weeks between dose #1 and #3) given IM into deltoid muscle Combined hepatitis A and hepatitis B vaccine (Twinrix), three doses (initial dose followed by doses 4 weeks and 6 months later) given IM into deltoid muscle	Pain at injection site; fatigue, headache	■ Infants and adolescents ■ Adults seeking protection from HBV infection ■ People with chronic liver disease ■ Men who have sex with men ■ Prostitutes; heterosexuals with multiple sexual partners ■ People with an STI ■ Injection drug users ■ Long-term male prisoners ■ People on hemodialysis ■ Healthcare workers
Postexposure prophylaxis	Hepatitis B immune globulin (HBIG) given IM into large muscle mass within 24 hours of exposure; concurrent initiation of hepatitis B vaccine series	Infrequent; muscle stiffness, pain	■ Infants born to women with HBV infection ■ Percutaneous or permucosal exposure to HBV when unvaccinated or antibody response is negative or unknown

*Nurses should check the CDC website regularly for updates to these recommendations.

Source: CDC, 2016a.

immunity. HBV vaccine may be given concurrently. Candidates for postexposure prophylaxis include those with known or suspected percutaneous or permucosal contact with infected blood, sexual partners of patients with acute HBV or who are HBV carriers, and household contacts of patients with acute HBV infection (CDC, 2016b).

Disease Treatment. The goals of treatment for hepatitis are to decrease the viral load, reduce the risk of transmission, and reduce liver damage (Branstetter-Hall & Felicidla-Reynaldo, 2017). The American Association for Study of Liver Disease (AASLD) provides recommendations for treatment and monitoring of liver function based on the phase of the disease (Terrault et al., 2016). Adults with immune-active hepatitis B should initially be treated with pegylated inferon (Pegasys), entecavir (Baraclude), or tenofovir disopoxil furmarate (Viread) (Branstetter-Hall & Felicilda-Reynaldo, 2017). Using an antiviral drug in combination with an interferon reduces liver inflammation and fibrosis. Although side effects are minimal, patients may become resistant to the beneficial effects of these drugs. Entecavir is the most potent of the HBV antivirals and may be used as an alternate to lamivudine or adefovir.

Combination therapy with peginterferon and ribavirin has been the treatment of choice for chronic hepatitis C. Acute hepatitis C is generally treated with interferon alpha, an antiviral agent, to reduce the risk of chronic hepatitis C. Typically, a long-acting interferon (peginterferon [Pegasys]) may be combined with the antiviral drug ribavirin (Rebetol, Virazole). Recently, new antiviral pharmacologic therapy has been approved and shows promise in treating hepatitis C with up to 90% efficacy (Felicilda-Reynaldo & Patterson, 2017; Sorenson et al., 2019). The addition of one of the newer antiviral medications (boceprivir, simeprevir, sofosbuvir, telaprivir) to a regimen of interferon and ribavirin is becoming the standard of care (Adams et al., 2017). In addition, combination fixed-dose medications have recently been approved (Harvoni, Viekira Pak) (Adams et al., 2017), which allows the patient to take one tablet a day, improving compliance with treatment (Polis, Zablostska-Manos, Zekry, & Maher, 2017). See **Medication Administration 25.A** for nursing responsibilities related to interferons and antiviral drugs.

IFN–α interferes with viral replication, reducing the viral load. It is given by intramuscular or subcutaneous injection. Virtually all patients treated with interferon develop a flulike syndrome with fever, fatigue, muscle aches, headache, and chills. Acetaminophen helps alleviate some of these adverse effects, which tend to decrease over time. Depression is a common adverse effect of this drug. Instruct patients to contact their physician if suicidal thoughts or manifestations of depression develop. Ribavirin has two major adverse effects: Hemolytic anemia and birth defects. Blood counts are obtained before and during treatment to detect early signs of hemolytic anemia. Because of the risk for birth defects, this drug is contraindicated for use during pregnancy, and two reliable methods of birth control must be used by women taking the drug and female sexual partners of men taking the drug. New antiviral agents have been approved for treating hepatitis C and are associated with fewer side effects. Treatment is informed by the HCV genotype so a priority nursing consideration is to ensure the HCV genotype testing is completed for the patient (Felicilda-Reynaldo & Patterson, 2017).

Treatment of acute hepatitis also includes as-needed bedrest, adequate nutrition as tolerated, and avoidance of strenuous activity, alcohol, and agents that are toxic to the liver. In most cases, clinical recovery takes 3 to 16 weeks.

Medication Administration 25.A

Drugs to Treat Chronic Hepatitis

INTERFERON

Conventional Interferons

interferon alfa-2a (Roferon-A)

interferon alfa-2b (Intron A)

interferon alfacon-1 (Infergen)

Long-Acting Interferons

peginterferon alfa-2a (Pegasys)

peginterferon alfa-2b (PEG-Intron)

Human interferons have antiviral, immunosuppressive, and antineoplastic activity. IFN–α interferes with viral replication by blocking the virus from entering host cells, inhibiting syntheses of viral RNA and proteins, and viral release from host cells. Conventional interferons have a short half-life and must be administered several times weekly; long-acting preparations can be given once weekly. Long-acting preparations have a higher incidence of adverse effects, however.

Nursing Responsibilities

- Administer by subcutaneous injection. Do not use if solution is discolored or contains visible particulates.
- Monitor for manifestations of hypersensitivity (e.g., angioedema or bronchoconstriction); immediately notify physician and administer emergency treatment as needed to maintain cardiorespiratory status.
- Monitor CBC, platelet count, and renal and liver function studies. Frequently assess mental status. Withhold the drug and notify the physician of significant changes in lab values, manifestations of neuropsychiatric effects, severe abdominal pain, or changes in vision.

Patient Education

- This drug may cause flulike symptoms with fever, fatigue, body aches, headache, and chills. These symptoms tend to diminish over time with continued use of the drug. If approved by your physician, acetaminophen may be used to promote comfort.
- Notify your physician immediately if you become severely depressed or develop thoughts of suicide, have severe chest

pain or difficulty breathing, notice unusual bleeding or bruising or have bloody diarrhea, notice a change in your vision, develop severe stomach or lower back pain, or notice a new or worsening skin condition.

- Keep all appointments for lab tests and follow-up visits to your physician.
- Women: Use a reliable means of birth control and notify your physician immediately if you become pregnant.

ANTIRETROVIRAL DRUGS

adefovir dipovoxil (Hepsera)
aoceprivir (Victrelis)
daclatasir (Daklinza)
entecavir (Baraclude)
lamivudine (Epivir)
ribavirin (Copegus, Rebetrol, others)
simeprevir (Olsyio)
sofobusvir (Sovaldi)
telaprevir (Incivek)
telbivudine (Tyzeka)
tenoforvir (Viread)

The nucleoside/nucleotide analog antiretroviral drugs were originally developed for treating HIV infection and now also are approved for HBV treatment, although the recommended doses differ for these two uses. Protease inhibitors are the new group of antiviral medications used to treat hepatitis C. Antiviral drugs inhibit synthesis of viral DNA. Therapy with antiretroviral drugs may be prolonged as relapse is common when the drug is stopped. Viral resistance to the drug is also a concern.

Nursing Responsibilities

- Administer PO as ordered.
- Monitor baseline and periodic renal and liver function tests, CBC with differential, blood chemistries, and serum electrolytes. Notify the physician of significant changes.
- Lactic acidosis is a risk with these drugs; monitor for manifestations such as hyperventilation, lethargy, and ABG values indicative of metabolic acidosis. Withhold the drug and notify the physician if manifestations of lactic acidosis develop.

Patient Teaching

- Take the drug as prescribed.
- Notify your physician if you develop severe abdominal pain, nausea and vomiting, or anorexia or if you become jaundiced.
- Symptoms of recurrent hepatitis B may develop after you stop taking this drug; notify your physician if this occurs.

Source: Adams et al., 2017.

Integrative Therapies

Milk thistle, with its active ingredient silymarin, has been used by herbalists to treat liver disease for over 2000 years. Clinical evidence indicate that milk thistle is no better than placebo for treating hepatitis C (National Center for Complementary and Integrative Health, 2018).

Herbalists may use licorice root to treat hepatitis. It has both antiviral and anti-inflammatory effects. Long-term use of licorice root, however, can lead to hypertension and affect fluid and electrolyte balance.

Herbal preparations may be used to relieve the adverse effects of IFN–α Ginger may help relieve nausea for some patients, and St. John's wort is used for the depression associated with IFN–α use.

Patients should be instructed to communicate with the provider prescribing medications regarding the use of integrative therapies. The nurse should stay up to date on clinical trials for integrative therapies and work with patients to address their desire to use integrative therapy as part of the treatment plan for hepatitis. Lack of adherence to the medication regimen for hepatitis is a challenge and the nurse must reinforce the importance of taking prescribed medications as directed for optimum outcomes (Phillips & Barnes, 2016; Polis et al., 2017; Redulla, Rajender, Faust, & Dudley-Brown, 2015).

Nursing Care

Assessment

Collect assessment data related to hepatitis, such as:

- *Health history:* Current manifestations, including anorexia, nausea and vomiting, abdominal discomfort, changes in bowel elimination or color of stools; muscle or joint pain, fatigue; changes in color of skin or sclera; duration of symptoms; known exposure to hepatitis; high-risk behaviors such as injection drug use or multiple sexual partners; previous history of liver disorders; current medications, prescription and over the counter
- *Physical assessment:* Vital signs including temperature; color of sclera and mucous membranes; skin color and condition; abdominal contour and tenderness; color of stool and urine
- *Diagnostic tests:* Serum bilirubin, liver function tests, serologic antibody–antigen levels.

Priorities of Care

Nursing care focuses on preventing spread of the infection to others, promoting the patient's comfort, helping with energy conservation, supporting the ability to provide self-care, and promoting adherence with the prescribed medication regimen. Jaundice and associated rashes and itching can affect a patient's body image and increase the risk of skin breakdown. Nursing measures to prevent skin breakdown and address body image are discussed in the following section on cirrhosis.

Diagnoses, Outcomes, and Interventions

Patients with acute or chronic hepatitis usually are treated in community settings; hospitalization is rarely required.

Prevent Transmission of the Disease. An important goal when caring for patients with acute viral hepatitis is preventing spread of the infection.

Expected Outcome: Eliminate or reduce the spread of hepatitis viruses in the patient's home, community, and in the healthcare setting where patient is seeking treatment and care.

The nurse will:

- Use standard precautions. Practice meticulous hand hygiene. *The hepatitis viruses are spread by direct contact with feces or blood and body fluids. The use of standard precautions and good hand hygiene protect both healthcare workers and other patients from exposure to the virus.*
- For patients with HAV or HEV, use standard precautions and contact isolation if fecal incontinence is present. *The fecal–oral route is the primary mode of transmission of these viruses. Other hepatitis viruses are transmitted through blood and other body fluids.*
- Encourage prophylactic treatment of all members of household and intimate sexual contacts. *Prophylactic treatment of people in close contact with the patient decreases their risk of contacting the disease or, if already infected, the severity of the disease.*
- If the patient diagnosed with hepatitis A is employed as a food handler or child care worker, contact the local health department to report possible exposure of patrons. Maintain confidentiality. *Prophylactic treatment of people who have possibly been exposed to the virus can prevent a local epidemic of the disease.*

Teach Energy Conservation Strategies. Fatigue and possible weakness are common in acute hepatitis. Although bedrest is rarely indicated, adequate rest periods and limitation of activities may be necessary. Many patients with acute hepatitis may be unable to resume normal activity levels for 4 or more weeks.

Expected Outcome: Patient will use energy conservation strategies to adapt to fatigue as evidenced by balancing rest and activity, maintaining adequate nutrition intake, and maintaining social interactions.

The nurse will:

- Encourage planned rest periods throughout the day. *Adequate rest is necessary for optimal immune function.*
- Assist to identify essential activities and those that can be deferred or delegated to others. *Identifying essential and nonessential activities promotes the patient's sense of control.*
- Suggest using level of fatigue to determine activity level, with gradual resumption of activities as fatigue is reduced and a sense of well-being improves. *Fatigue associated with activity is an indicator of appropriate and inappropriate activity levels. As recovery progresses, increasing activity levels are tolerated with less fatigue.*

Promote Adequate Nutrition. Adequate nutrition is important for immune function and healing in patients with acute or chronic hepatitis.

Expected Outcome: Patient's food intake will meet caloric and nutritional demand required to meet metabolic needs and promote healing of damaged tissue.

The nurse will:

- Help plan a diet of appealing foods that provides a high-kilocalorie intake of approximately 16 carbohydrate kilocalories per kilogram of ideal body weight. *Sufficient energy is required for healing; adequate carbohydrate intake can spare protein.*
- Encourage planning food intake according to symptoms of the disease. Discuss eating smaller meals and using between-meal snacks to maintain nutrient and calorie intake. *Patients with acute hepatitis are often more anorexic and nauseated in the afternoon and evening; planning the majority of calorie intake in the morning helps maintain adequate intake. Limiting fat intake and the size of meals may reduce the incidence of nausea.*
- Instruct to avoid alcohol intake and diet drinks. *Alcohol avoidance is vital to prevent further liver damage and promote healing. Diet drinks (e.g., diet sodas or juice drinks) provide few calories when an increased calorie intake is needed for healing.*
- Encourage use of nutritional supplements such as Ensure or instant breakfast drinks to maintain calorie and nutrient intake. *Nutritional supplement drinks are an additional source of concentrated calories and nutrients.*

Transitions of Care

Nurses play an instrumental role in preventing the spread of hepatitis. Stress the importance of hygiene measures such as hand hygiene after toileting and before all food handling. Discuss the dangers of injection drug use and, with drug users, of sharing needles or other equipment. Encourage all sexually active patients to use safer sexual practices such as abstinence, mutual monogamy, and barrier protection (such as male or female condoms).

Discuss recommendations for hepatitis A and hepatitis B vaccine with people in moderate- or high-risk groups for these infections. Ensure that nurses and other healthcare workers at risk for exposure to blood and body fluids are effectively vaccinated against hepatitis A and B. Encourage all people with known or probable exposure to HAV or HBV to obtain postexposure prophylaxis. Facilitate screening for Hepatitis C for people born between 1945 and 1964. See the accompanying Moving Evidence into Action feature for a study of promoting therapy adherence for veterans infected with hepatitis C.

For patients recovering from an acute infection, the nurse will provide discharge teaching to patients and their families for home care including the following topics:

- Recommended prophylactic treatment
- Infection control measures such as frequent hand hygiene; not sharing eating utensils; avoiding food handling or preparation activities by the patient with hepatitis A; abstaining from sexual relations during acute infection; and using barrier protection if a carrier or for chronic infection
- Managing fatigue and limited activity

Moving Evidence into Action

Adherence to Hepatitis C Treatment in Military Veterans

Clinical Issue

The prevalence of hepatitis C in the veteran population is about three times the rate of that in the U. S. general population. The Veterans Administration health system is the nation's largest provider of care for patients with HCV. Consequently, the prevalence of liver failure among the veteran population is projected to escalate. The VA system has launched a major healthcare initiative aimed to address the multifactorial burden of this chronic disease. The standard of therapy now includes triple HCV pharmacological therapy, which involves complicated schedules of self-medication regimens, frequent laboratory tests, and clinic visits (Sebhatu & Martin, 2016). Additionally, the side effects of medications can be debilitating making it difficult to adhere to the prescribed medication. Side effects must be managed. The goal of therapy is eradication of the virus and adherence to taking the medication as prescribed, which is crucial for success.

External Evidence

The researchers sought to understand patient adherence through the lived experience of U.S. military veterans undergoing treatment for hepatitis C. Specifically, this qualitative study identified the factors influencing the choice to remain adherent or nonadherent. Results suggest obtaining a commitment to stay on the medication, reinforcing the military culture of discipline and the ideation of "not ready to leave this world," as the study identified these were the primary motivators for behaviors associated with adherence. Staying busy, conserving energy, looking forward, and the opportunity to start over related to past risky behaviors were identified as cognitive strategies used to support adherence. This research concludes ongoing education and focus on side effect management is needed throughout the treatment period and suggests incorporating psychological support aimed to support the veteran's motivation should be addressed through all phases of disease management (Phillips & Barnes, 2016).

Internal Evidence

As part of the evaluation of internal evidence, the nurse must consider the options for providing needed education and support. The patient's access to clinic visits, current resources available for ongoing patient education, psychological support, and medication management should be considered.

Patient Considerations

The patient's preferred approach to patient education and support should be incorporated into the plan. Including the individuals involved in the patient's support system should be considered when planning patient education (Koman, 2018; Redulla et al., 2015).

Putting the Pieces Together

The design and implementation of a patient education plan for veteran patients undergoing treatment for hepatitis C is essential. To effectively implement a plan, it's important to incorporate external evidence addressing strategies that promote adherence to complex treatment and medication regimens. Consideration of the preferences for patient/family education and psychological support should be incorporated into plans. With implementation of a plan to support adherence, the desired outcome to eradicate the virus and decrease progression of fibrosis or liver scarring will be enhanced.

References

Koman, D. (2018). Increasing hepatitis C virus knowledge through an evidence-based educational intervention. *Gastroenterology Nursing, 41*(2), 95–101.

Phillips, F. H., & Barnes, D. M. (2016). Meaning of adherence in hepatitis C-infected military veterans. *Gastroenterology Nursing, 39*(1), 17–23.

Redulla, R. R., Rajender, K., Faust, T. W., & Dudley-Brown, S. (2015). Project P.E.A.C.H. (Pathway and Education toward Adherence and Completion in Hepatitis C Therapy): A nurse-driven evidence-based protocol. *Gastroenterology Nursing, 38*(5), 369–378.

Sebuhatu, P., & Martin, M. M. (2016). Genotype 1 hepatitis C virus and the pharmacist's role in treatment. *American Journal of Health-System Pharmacists, 73*(11), 764–744.

- Managing pruritus and maintaining skin integrity: Use warm, not hot, water when bathing; use mild or no soap; limit duration of baths and showers; pat dry, do not rub, apply an alcohol-free lotion soon after bathing to retain skin moisture; wear loose cotton garments that allow moisture to evaporate from skin; reduce room temperature, especially at night, to prevent overheating; keep fingernails short, and wear cotton mittens or gloves as needed to prevent scratching during sleep
- Promoting nutrient intake
- Avoiding hepatic toxins such as alcohol, acetaminophen, and selected other drugs; encourage to alert all care providers to presence of infection
- Recommended follow-up.

If a patient with chronic hepatitis B or C is being treated with medications, teach how to administer the drug, its dosing schedule, precautions, and management of adverse effects. Stress the importance of keeping follow-up appointments, including recommended laboratory testing.

Hepatitis may progress to the development of incurable cirrhosis of the liver and focus of care will be on symptom management. See specific information related to providing end-of-life care in the following section.

The Patient with Cirrhosis

Cirrhosis is characterized by fibrosis of liver tissue leading to decreased mass, impaired liver function, and altered blood flow. Cirrhosis is the 12th leading cause of death in the United States overall (Murphy, Xu, Kochanek, Curtin, & Arias, 2017).

Alcoholic cirrhosis is the most common type of cirrhosis in the United States. Chronic hepatitis B or C are leading causes of cirrhosis, particularly in people who consume alcohol excessively. Other causes include prolonged obstruction of the biliary (bile drainage) system; long-term, severe right heart failure; and uncommon liver disorders. The incidence and mortality attributable to cirrhosis and chronic liver disease vary significantly among populations (Murphy et al., 2017).

Overall, the death rate due to cirrhosis and chronic liver disease in men is more than twice that of women. Although cirrhosis/chronic liver disease is the 12th leading cause of death overall in the United States, it is the sixth leading cause of death for people of Native American (including Alaska Natives) and Hispanic (or Latino) origin. Native American men have the highest incidence and mortality rate from cirrhosis and chronic liver disease, followed by Native American women, Hispanic men, and women of Hispanic or Latino origin (Murphy et al., 2017).

Pathophysiology

In cirrhosis, functional liver tissue is gradually destroyed and replaced by fibrous scar tissue. As hepatocytes and liver lobules are destroyed, the metabolic functions of the liver are lost. Structurally abnormal nodules encircled by connective tissue develop. This fibrous connective tissue forms constrictive bands that disrupt blood and bile flow within liver lobules. Blood no longer flows freely through the liver to the inferior vena cava. This restricted blood flow leads to portal hypertension, increased pressure in the portal venous system.

Alcoholic Cirrhosis

Alcoholic cirrhosis is the end result of alcoholic liver disease. Its development is directly related to alcohol consumption: Total amount of alcohol consumed, number of years of excessive alcohol consumption, and blood alcohol levels. Women develop cirrhosis at lower overall levels of alcohol use than men. This may relate to the effects of estrogen and less effective metabolism of alcohol in women, resulting in higher blood alcohol levels.

Alcohol causes metabolic changes in the liver: Triglyceride and fatty acid synthesis increases, and the formation and release of lipoproteins decrease, leading to fatty infiltration of hepatocytes (fatty liver). At this stage, abstinence from alcohol can allow the liver to heal; however, with continued alcohol abuse, the disease progresses. Inflammatory cells infiltrate the liver (alcoholic hepatitis), causing necrosis, fibrosis, and destruction of functional liver tissue. In the final stage of alcoholic cirrhosis, regenerative nodules form, and the liver shrinks and develops a nodular appearance. Malnutrition commonly accompanies alcoholic cirrhosis. See the Pathophysiology Illustrated feature on the following pages.

Posthepatic Cirrhosis

Advanced progressive liver disease resulting from chronic hepatitis B or C, autoimmune hepatitis, or nonalcoholic fatty liver disease is known as *posthepatic* or *postnecrotic* cirrhosis. Chronic viral hepatitis is the leading cause of posthepatic cirrhosis in the United States. About 25% of persons with chronic hepatitis B or C will eventually develop cirrhosis. The immune response is responsible for producing liver damage and fibrosis in chronic and autoimmune hepatitis. The liver is shrunken and nodular, with extensive liver cell loss and fibrosis. The obesity epidemic is seen as a major factor contributing to an increased incidence of cirrhosis due to nonalcoholic fatty liver disease.

Biliary Cirrhosis

When bile flow is obstructed within the liver or in the biliary system, retained bile damages and destroys liver cells close to the interlobular bile ducts. This leads to inflammation, fibrosis, and formation of regenerative nodules. Within the liver, bile ducts are narrowed or obstructed, leading to elevated bilirubin levels and progressive liver failure.

Manifestations and Complications

Early in the course of cirrhosis, few manifestations may be present. The liver is usually enlarged and may be tender. A dull, aching pain in the epigastric area or RUQ may be present. Other early signs include weight loss, weakness, and anorexia. Bowel function is disrupted with diarrhea or constipation.

As the disease progresses, manifestations related to liver cell failure and portal hypertension develop. Impaired metabolism causes such manifestations as bleeding, ascites, gynecomastia (breast enlargement) in men and infertility in women, jaundice, and neurologic changes. Portal hypertension accounts for such manifestations as ascites, peripheral edema, anemia, and low WBC and platelet counts. See the Multisystem Effects feature on page 831.

Portal Hypertension

Increased pressure in the portal system causes blood to be rerouted to adjoining lower pressure vessels. This *shunting* of blood involves collateral vessels. Affected veins, which become engorged and congested, are located in the esophagus, rectum, and abdomen. Portal hypertension increases the hydrostatic pressure in vessels of the portal system. Increased hydrostatic pressure in the capillaries pushes fluid out, contributing to ascites formation.

Splenomegaly

The spleen enlarges (splenomegaly) because portal hypertension causes blood to be shunted into the splenic vein. Splenomegaly increases the rate at which red and white blood cells and platelets are removed from circulation and destroyed. This increased blood cell destruction leads to anemia, leukopenia, and thrombocytopenia.

Ascites *Ascites* is the accumulation of plasma-rich fluid in the abdominal cavity. Although portal hypertension is the primary cause of ascites, decreased serum proteins and increased aldosterone also contribute to the fluid accumulation. *Hypoalbuminemia*, low serum albumin, decreases the colloidal osmotic pressure of plasma. This pressure normally holds fluid in the intravascular compartment; when plasma colloidal osmotic pressure decreases, fluid escapes into extravascular compartments. *Hyperaldosteronism*, an increase in aldosterone levels, causes sodium and water retention, contributing to ascites and generalized edema.

Pathophysiology Illustrated

Cirrhosis and Portal Hypertension

Normal liver

The liver contains multiple lobules made up of plates of hepatocytes, the functional cells of the liver, surrounded by small capillaries called sinusoids. These sinusoids receive a mixture of venous and arterial blood from branches of the portal vein and hepatic artery. Blood from the sinusoids drains into the central vein of the lobule. Hepatocytes produce bile, which drains outward to bile ducts.

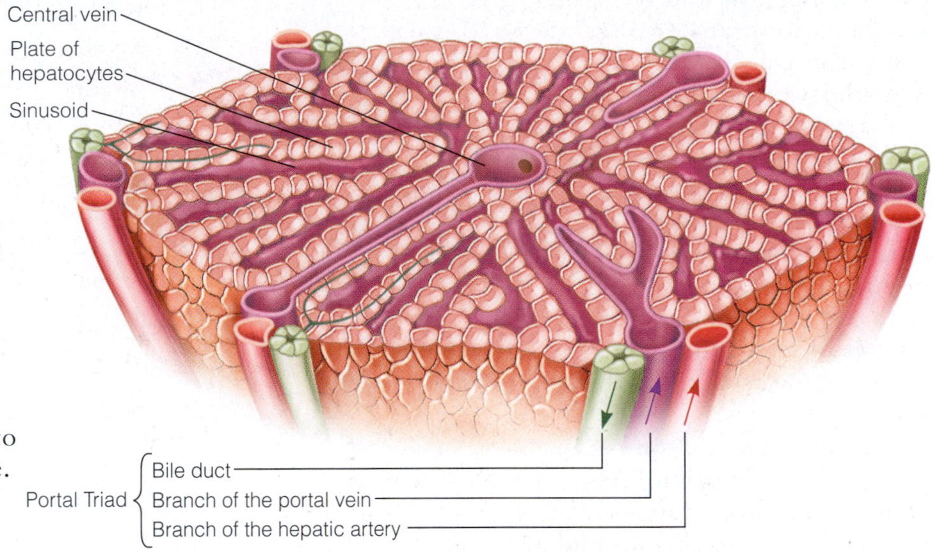

Central vein
Plate of hepatocytes
Sinusoid
Portal Triad
Bile duct
Branch of the portal vein
Branch of the hepatic artery

Fatty liver

Ingested alcohol is primarily metabolized in the liver. Acetaldehyde, formed when alcohol is metabolized, damages hepatocytes and impairs the oxidation of fatty acids. As a result, fat accumulates within hepatocytes and liver lobules. Other alcohol metabolism by-products, including oxygen free radicals, promote inflammation and may stimulate autoantibody production.

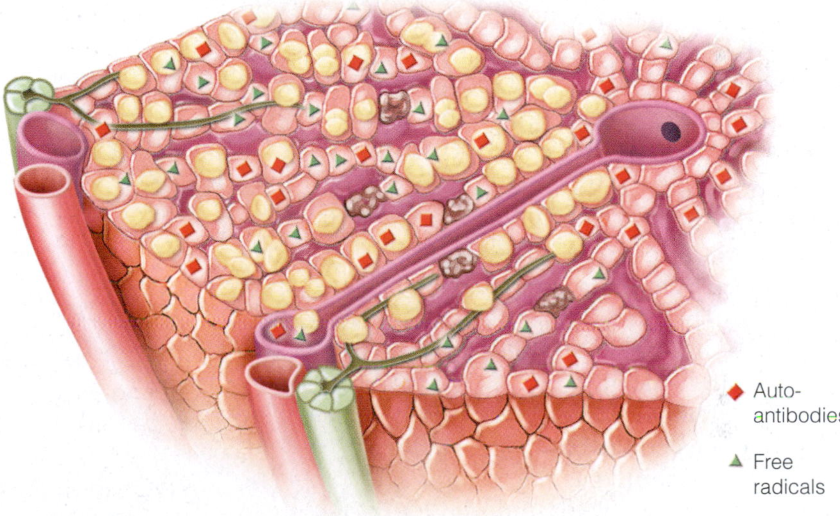

Auto-antibodies
Free radicals

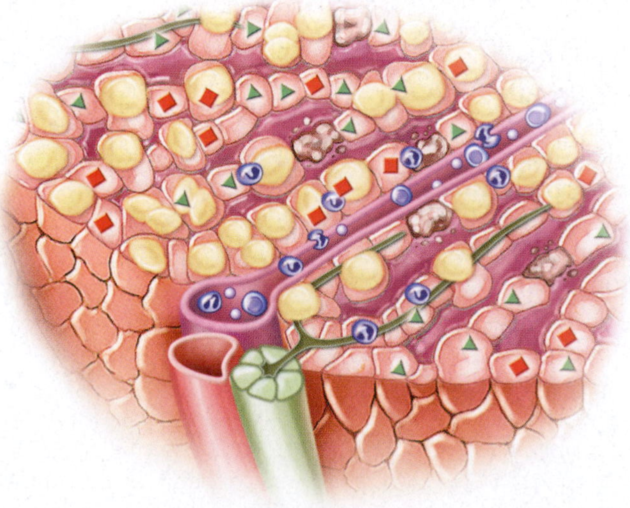

Alcoholic hepatitis

With continued alcohol intake, liver cells degenerate and spotty cellular necrosis occurs. Inflammatory cells such as polymorphonuclear leukocytes and lymphocytes infiltrate the lobule.

Alcoholic cirrhosis

Cellular necrosis and inflammation transform some liver cells into fibroblasts that produce and deposit collagen. Weblike bands of connective tissue develop around the portal triads and central vein, eventually connecting with one another. Small islands of liver cells continue to regenerate, forming nodules. Hepatocyte destruction outpaces regeneration. As a result of cell loss, fibrosis, and scarring, the liver shrinks and becomes hard and nodular.

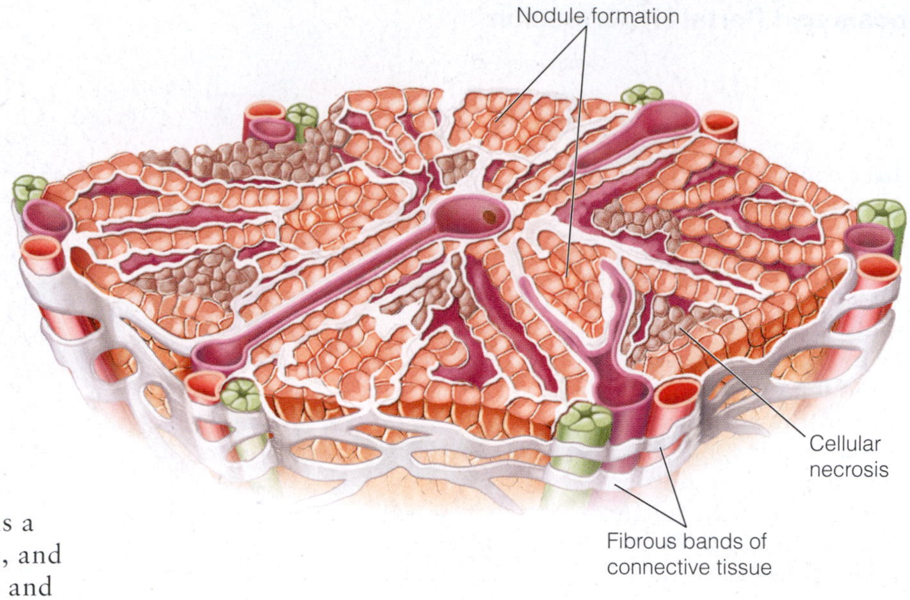
Nodule formation
Cellular necrosis
Fibrous bands of connective tissue

Portal hypertension

Bands of fibrotic scar tissue obstruct the sinusoids and blood flow from the portal vein to the hepatic vein. Pressure in the portal venous system, which drains the gastrointestinal tract, pancreas, and spleen, increases. This increased pressure opens collateral vessels in the esophagus, anterior abdominal wall, and rectum, allowing blood to bypass the obstructed portal vessels. Prolonged portal hypertension leads to the development of (1) varices (fragile, distended veins) in the lower esophagus, stomach, and rectum; (2) splenomegaly (an enlarged spleen); (3) ascites (accumulation of fluid in the abdomen); and (4) portal systemic encephalopathy (disrupted CNS function with altered consciousness).

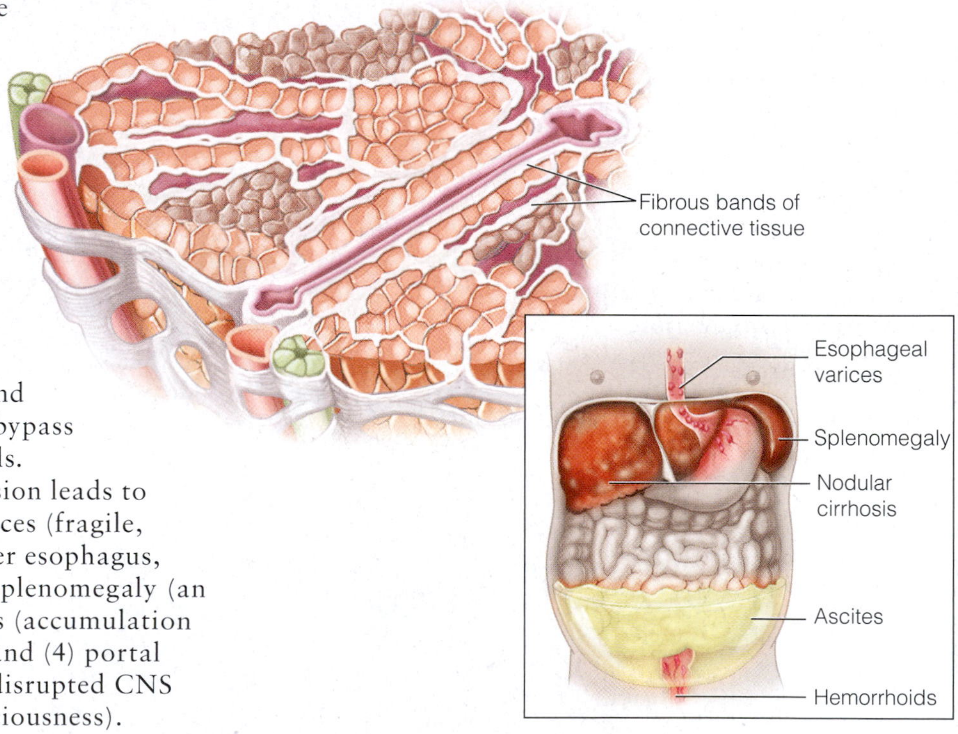
Fibrous bands of connective tissue
Esophageal varices
Splenomegaly
Nodular cirrhosis
Ascites
Hemorrhoids

Multisystem Effects of CIRRHOSIS

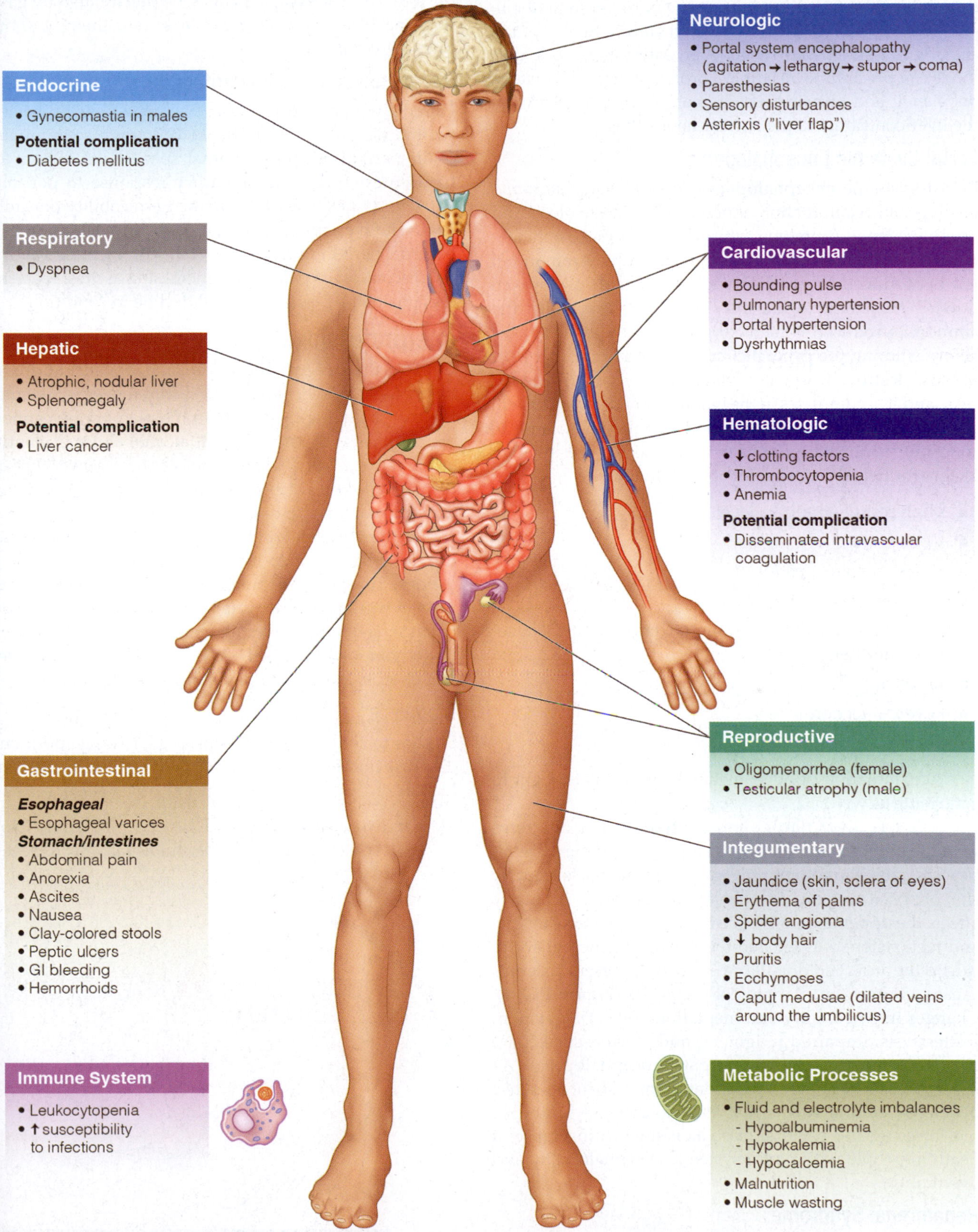
Neurologic
• Portal system encephalopathy (agitation → lethargy → stupor → coma)
• Paresthesias
• Sensory disturbances
• Asterixis ("liver flap")
Endocrine
• Gynecomastia in males
Potential complication
• Diabetes mellitus
Respiratory
• Dyspnea
Cardiovascular
• Bounding pulse
• Pulmonary hypertension
• Portal hypertension
• Dysrhythmias
Hepatic
• Atrophic, nodular liver
• Splenomegaly
Potential complication
• Liver cancer
Hematologic
• ↓ clotting factors
• Thrombocytopenia
• Anemia
Potential complication
• Disseminated intravascular coagulation
Reproductive
• Oligomenorrhea (female)
• Testicular atrophy (male)
Gastrointestinal
Esophageal
• Esophageal varices
Stomach/intestines
• Abdominal pain
• Anorexia
• Ascites
• Nausea
• Clay-colored stools
• Peptic ulcers
• GI bleeding
• Hemorrhoids
Integumentary
• Jaundice (skin, sclera of eyes)
• Erythema of palms
• Spider angioma
• ↓ body hair
• Pruritis
• Ecchymoses
• Caput medusae (dilated veins around the umbilicus)
Immune System
• Leukocytopenia
• ↑ susceptibility to infections
Metabolic Processes
• Fluid and electrolyte imbalances
- Hypoalbuminemia
- Hypokalemia
- Hypocalcemia
• Malnutrition
• Muscle wasting

Esophageal Varices

Esophageal varices are enlarged, thin-walled veins that form in the submucosa of the esophagus. These collateral vessels form when blood is shunted from the portal system due to portal hypertension. The thin-walled varices may rupture, causing massive hemorrhage; even eating high-roughage foods can precipitate bleeding. Thrombocytopenia, platelet deficiency, and impaired production of clotting factors by the liver contribute to the risk for hemorrhage.

Portal Systemic Encephalopathy

Portal systemic encephalopathy (*hepatic encephalopathy*) results from accumulation of neurotoxins in the blood and cerebral edema. Ammonia, a by-product of protein metabolism, contributes to hepatic encephalopathy. Ammonium ion is produced as proteins and amino acids are broken down by bacteria in the intestinal tract. Normally, the ammonia produced is then converted by the liver to urea before entering the general circulation. As functional liver tissue is destroyed, ammonia can no longer be converted to urea, and it accumulates in the blood. Other nervous system depressants, such as narcotics and tranquilizers, can also contribute to hepatic encephalopathy. Selected precipitating factors for hepatic encephalopathy include:

- High serum ammonia level
- Constipation
- Blood transfusions
- Gastrointestinal bleeding
- Medications: Sedatives, tranquilizers, narcotic analgesics, anesthetics
- Hypoxia
- Severe infection
- Surgery.

Accumulation of other metabolic toxins is thought to contribute as well.

Asterixis (liver flap), a muscle tremor that interferes with the ability to maintain a fixed position of the extremities and causes involuntary jerking movements, is an early sign of portal systemic encephalopathy. Asterixis primarily affects the upper extremities, but also may affect the tongue and feet. Asterixis is elicited by instructing the patient to extend the arms and dorsiflex the wrists. If present, asterixis causes a downward flapping of the hands (**Figure 25.7** ■). Changes in personality and mentation develop; agitation, restlessness, impaired judgment, and slurred speech are also early manifestations of hepatic encephalopathy. As it progresses, confusion, disorientation, and incoherence develop. Cerebral edema that leads to increased intracranial pressure and cerebral hypoxia is the leading cause of death in people with portal systemic encephalopathy and liver failure.

Hepatorenal Syndrome

Although the cause is unclear, renal failure with azotemia (excess nitrogenous waste products in the blood), sodium retention, oliguria, and hypotension may develop in patients with advanced cirrhosis and ascites. Hepatorenal syndrome appears to be the result of imbalanced blood flow, leading to constriction of vessels leading to and within the kidneys. The syndrome may be precipitated by gastrointestinal bleeding, by aggressive diuretic therapy, or by an unknown cause.

Spontaneous Bacterial Peritonitis

Patients with cirrhosis and ascites may develop bacterial peritonitis, even in the absence of known contamination of the peritoneal cavity or other specific risk factors (e.g., paracentesis). The inflammatory response to peritonitis worsens ascites by increasing the permeability of capillaries in the mesentery. The manifestations of spontaneous bacterial peritonitis may be subtle, with increased abdominal discomfort or pain, fever, increasing ascites, worsening encephalopathy, and an overall decline in condition.

Interprofessional Care

Care for the patient with cirrhosis is holistic, addressing physiologic, psychosocial, and spiritual needs. The importance of including the family in the plan of care cannot be overemphasized, particularly if alcohol abuse is identified as the cause. Alcohol abstinence is critical: Fewer than 50% of patients who have experienced complications of cirrhosis and who continue to drink will survive for 5 years.

Treatment of cirrhosis is supportive, directed at slowing the progression to liver failure and reducing complications. Treatment includes medications to help regulate protein metabolism, maintenance of fluid and electrolyte balance, and supportive therapies, including treatment of underlying problems, such as malnutrition, anemia, bleeding, encephalopathy, renal failure, and infections.

Diagnosis

Studies to confirm the diagnosis of cirrhosis and identify its cause and effects are performed. Diagnostic tests may include:

- ***Liver function studies*** include *ALT*, *AST*, and *ALP*. All may be elevated in cirrhosis, but usually not as severely

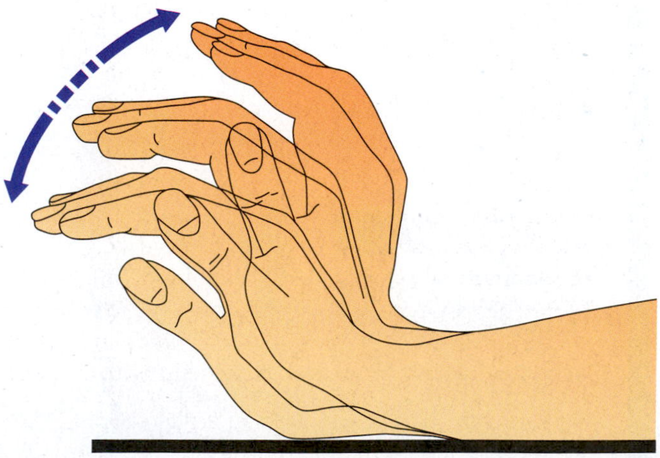

Figure 25.7 ■ Asterixis. Note the downward tremor of the hand on dorsiflexion of the wrist.

as in acute hepatitis. Elevations in these enzymes may not correlate well with the extent of liver damage in cirrhosis.

- ***CBC with platelets*** is done. A low RBC count, hemoglobin, and hematocrit demonstrate anemia related to bone marrow suppression, increased RBC destruction, bleeding, and deficiencies of folic acid and vitamin B_{12}. Platelets are low, related to increased destruction by the spleen. Leukopenia (low WBC count) also relates to splenomegaly.
- ***Coagulation studies*** show a prolonged prothrombin time due to impaired production of coagulation proteins and lack of vitamin K.
- ***Serum electrolytes*** are measured. Hyponatremia is common, due to hemodilution. Hypokalemia, hypophosphatemia, and hypomagnesemia are also frequently seen, related to malnutrition and altered renal excretion of these electrolytes.
- ***Bilirubin*** levels are usually elevated in severe cirrhosis, including both direct (conjugated) and indirect (unconjugated) bilirubin.
- ***Serum albumin*** levels show hypoalbuminemia due to impaired liver production.
- ***Serum ammonia*** levels are elevated because the liver fails to effectively convert ammonia to urea for renal excretion.
- ***Serum glucose*** and ***cholesterol*** levels are frequently abnormal in patients with cirrhosis.
- ***Abdominal ultrasound*** is performed to evaluate liver size, detect ascites, and identify liver nodules. Ultrasound may be used in conjunction with *Doppler studies* to evaluate blood flow through the liver and spleen.
- ***Esophagoscopy*** (upper endoscopy) may be done to determine the presence of esophageal varices.
- ***Liver biopsy*** is not always necessary to diagnose cirrhosis, but may be done to distinguish cirrhosis from other forms of liver disease. Biopsy may be deferred if the bleeding time is prolonged (such as a prothrombin time [PT] greater than 3 seconds over the control).

See Chapter 21 for more information about the nursing implications of the aforementioned diagnostic tests.

Medications

Medications are used to treat the complications and effects of cirrhosis; they do not reverse or slow the process of cirrhosis itself. Known hepatotoxic drugs and alcohol are avoided, as are drugs metabolized by the liver (e.g., barbiturates, sedatives, hypnotics, and acetaminophen). Several groups of drugs are commonly prescribed. See **Medication Administration 25.B** for nursing responsibilities and patient teaching for commonly used drugs in patients with cirrhosis.

- Diuretics reduce fluid retention and ascites. Spironolactone (Aldactone) is frequently the drug of first choice because it addresses one of the causes of ascites—increased aldosterone levels. If additional diuresis is necessary, a loop diuretic such as furosemide (Lasix) may be added to the regimen.
- Medications to reduce the nitrogenous load and lower serum ammonia levels are added when manifestations of hepatic encephalopathy develop. Commonly administered medications are lactulose and antibiotics such as neomycin, metronidazole, or rifaximin. Lactulose reduces the number of ammonia-forming organisms in the bowel and increases the acidity of colon contents, converting ammonia into ammonium ion. Ammonium ion is not absorbable and is excreted in the feces. Neomycin sulfate is a locally acting antibiotic that also reduces the number of ammonia-forming bacteria in the bowel. Because it is toxic to the kidneys and auditory system, it is alternated with metronidazole. Metronidazole is a systemic antibiotic effective against common Gram-negative bacteria that inhabit the bowel. Peripheral neuropathy is a potential toxic effect of metronidazole. Rifaximin, a poorly absorbed antibiotic, acts locally within the bowel and has few adverse or toxic effects.
- A beta-blocker such as nadolol (Corgard) or propranolol (Inderal) may be given to reduce portal hypertension and prevent bleeding of esophageal varices.
- Ferrous sulfate and folic acid are given as indicated to treat anemia. Vitamin K may be ordered to reduce the risk of bleeding. When bleeding is acute, packed RBCs, fresh frozen plasma, or platelets may be administered to restore blood components and promote hemostasis.
- Antacids are prescribed as indicated. A drug regimen to treat *Helicobacter pylori* infection may also be effective (see Chapter 23).
- Oxazepam (Serax), a benzodiazepine antianxiety/sedative drug, is not metabolized by the liver and may be used to treat acute agitation.

Nutrition and Fluid Management

Dietary support is an essential part of care for the patient with cirrhosis. Dietary needs change as hepatic function fluctuates.

- Sodium intake is restricted to less than 2 g/day, and fluids are restricted as necessary to reduce ascites and generalized edema. Fluids are often limited to 1500 mL/day. Fluid needs are calculated based on response to diuretic therapy, urine output, and serum electrolyte values.
- Unless serum ammonia levels are high, a palatable diet with adequate calories and protein is recommended. Although dietary protein restriction has previously been recommended for patients with cirrhosis and hepatic encephalopathy, it is now recognized that the effects of protein-calorie malnutrition are more damaging than protein consumption (McClain, 2016). Vegetable proteins may be recommended along with restricted red meat consumption. Parenteral nutrition is used as needed to maintain nutritional status when food intake is limited.

Medication Administration 25.B

The Patient with Cirrhosis

DIURETICS

furosemide (Lasix)

spironolactone (Aldactone)

Spironolactone is a potassium-sparing diuretic that competes with aldosterone. It reduces ascites by increasing renal excretion of fluid and decreasing aldosterone levels. Furosemide is a loop diuretic that promotes the excretion of potassium. Drugs may be given in combination if serum potassium level permits.

Nursing Responsibilities

- Monitor ECG, serum potassium, BUN, creatinine levels, and hydration status.
- Weigh daily.
- Carefully monitor intake and output.
- Monitor for signs of hyperkalemia if taking spironolactone alone: Bradycardia; widening QRS, spiking T waves, or ST segment depression on ECG; diarrhea; and muscle twitching.
- Assess for hyponatremia: Confusion, lethargy, apprehension.

Health Education for the Patient and Family

- Maintain diet and fluid restrictions as prescribed.
- Report increases in weight or edema.
- Immediately report signs of hyponatremia, hyperkalemia, or hypokalemia.
- Expect increased urinary output; take medications in morning hours to avoid nocturia.

LAXATIVES

lactulose (Cephulac, Chronulac)

Lactulose is a disaccharide laxative that is not absorbed by the gastrointestinal tract. It reduces the number of ammonia-producing bacteria and lowers the pH in the colon. The lower pH (increased acidity) converts ammonia to ammonium ion, a nonabsorbable form that is excreted in the feces. Lactulose also pulls water into the bowel lumen, increasing the number of daily stools.

Nursing Responsibilities

- Assess bowel sounds and abdominal girth.
- Maintain accurate stool chart.
- Adjust dose to achieve two to four soft stools per day.
- Monitor electrolytes and hydration.

Health Education for the Patient and Family

- Drink adequate fluids.
- Report diarrhea; if present, decrease dose. You should have an average of two to four stools per day.
- This drug may cause nausea. Continue taking the drug; taking it with crackers or a soft drink may reduce nausea.

ANTIBIOTICS

metronidazole (Flagyl)

neomycin sulfate (Neo Tabs)

rifaximin (Xifaxan)

These antibiotics act in the gut to reduce intestinal bacteria and decrease ammonia production in the bowel lumen. Neomycin may be administered as an oral or rectal preparation; metronidazole and rifaximin are administered orally.

Nursing Responsibilities

- Monitor hearing, renal, and neurologic functions. Neomycin is ototoxic, nephrotoxic, and neurotoxic. Metronidazole is neurotoxic.
- Prior to administration, check for previous hypersensitivity reaction.
- Monitor intake and output.
- Monitor BUN and creatinine levels.

Health Education for the Patient and Family

- Report dizziness, tinnitus (ringing in ears), hearing loss, headaches, tremors, vision changes, or extremity numbness and tingling immediately.
- Keep follow-up appointments.
- Maintain fluids; avoid dehydration. (Teach signs of dehydration.)

Note: Drugs identified in blue are among the 200 most commonly prescribed medications in the United States.

Source: Data from Adams et al., 2017.

- Vitamin and mineral supplements are ordered based on laboratory values. Deficiencies in the B-complex vitamins—particularly thiamin, folate, and B_{12}—and the fat-soluble vitamins A, D, and E are common. These vitamins may need to be administered in a water-soluble form. Patients with alcohol-induced cirrhosis are at high risk for magnesium deficiency, which needs to be replaced.

Management of Complications

Ascites. **Paracentesis**, aspiration of fluid from the peritoneal cavity, may be a diagnostic or a therapeutic procedure. It may be done therapeutically to relieve severe ascites that does not respond to diuretic therapy. The goal of paracentesis is to relieve respiratory distress caused by excess fluid in the abdomen. Ascites fluid may be withdrawn in moderate amounts of 500 mL to 1 L daily to reduce the risk of fluid and electrolyte imbalances. Large-volume paracentesis, withdrawal of 4 to 6 L of fluid at one time, may be used. Albumin is often administered intravenously during large-volume paracentesis to maintain intravascular volume as the pressure of the ascites fluid in the abdomen is relieved. Nursing care of the patient undergoing paracentesis is outlined in **Box 25.3**.

Esophageal Varices. Primary care for esophageal varices involves screening with endoscopy. When varices are identified, beta-blocker therapy may be initiated to lower portal venous pressure, or endoscopic variceal ligation or sclerotherapy may be performed. In *variceal ligation* or *banding*, small rubber bands are placed on varices to occlude blood flow. *Endoscopic sclerosis* involves injecting a sclerosing agent directly into the varices to induce inflammation and clotting. See Chapter 21 for the nursing implications of endoscopy.

BOX 25.3
Nursing Care of the Patient Undergoing Paracentesis

PREPARATION

- Verify presence of an informed consent. *Paracentesis is an invasive procedure requiring informed consent.*
- Describe what to expect during paracentesis. Following cleansing and local anesthesia, a small incision may be made and a needle or trocar inserted to withdraw fluid. The trocar is connected to tubing and a collection bottle; specimens may be sent to a laboratory. Blood pressure is monitored during the procedure. *A clear understanding of the procedure and its purpose reduces anxiety and facilitates cooperation during the procedure.*
- Weigh prior to paracentesis. Measure abdominal girth at the level of the umbilicus. *Weight is an accurate means of determining fluid balance, particularly in patients with edema. Abdominal girth provides an additional measure of the effectiveness of paracentesis.*
- Assess vital signs for baseline. *Fluid shifts during and after paracentesis can affect cardiovascular stability. Baseline vital signs provide a reference for subsequent measurements.*
- Have patient void immediately prior to the test. *The bladder must be empty prior to paracentesis to reduce the risk for bladder puncture.*
- Position seated, either on the side of the bed or in a chair, with feet supported. *The sitting position allows ascites fluid to collect in the lower abdomen, facilitating its removal.*

DURING THE PROCEDURE

- Responsibilities during the procedure include assisting the practitioner and reassuring/coaching the patient.
- The procedure should be done using sterile technique, so help the practitioner maintain the sterile field.

  Following cleansing and local anesthesia, a small incision may be made and a needle or trocar inserted to withdraw fluid. The trocar is connected to tubing and a collection bottle; specimens may be sent to a laboratory. Blood pressure is monitored during the procedure.

AFTER THE PROCEDURE

- A small dressing is placed over the puncture site after the needle is withdrawn. There may be some fluid leakage from the site. *Depending on the size of the trocar inserted and the amount of remaining ascites fluid, the insertion puncture may not immediately seal, allowing fluid to escape.*
- Monitor vital signs every 15 minutes for 1 hour, every 30 minutes for 1 hour, then every 4 hours. Measure abdominal girth and obtain weight. *Removal of large amounts of fluid from the abdominal cavity can cause significant fluid shifts with resulting vascular instability. Weight and abdominal girth measurements provide information about fluid balance.*
- Salt-poor albumin may be given after the procedure to replace lost protein. *Removing ascites fluid reduces pressure within the peritoneal cavity. In the patient with hypoalbuminemia and portal hypertension, a significant amount of vascular fluid can escape as a result, leading to hypovolemia. Albumin is given to increase plasma oncotic pressure, helping retain fluid within the vascular system.*

Bleeding esophageal varices are life-threatening and require intensive care management. Restoration of hemodynamic stability is the first priority. A central line is inserted and central venous and pulmonary artery pressures are monitored. Blood is given to restore blood volume, and fresh frozen plasma may be administered to restore clotting factors. Somatostatin or octreotide, drugs that constrict blood vessels in the gut, are given intravenously to reduce blood flow in the portal venous system.

When the blood pressure and cardiac output have stabilized, upper endoscopy is performed to evaluate and treat the varices. A large nasogastric tube is inserted prior to endoscopy, and gastric lavage (irrigation of the stomach with large quantities of normal saline) is performed to improve visualization. During endoscopy, the varices may be banded or sclerosed to reduce the risk of recurrent bleeding. *Balloon tamponade* of bleeding varices may be used if bleeding cannot be controlled through vasoconstriction or if endoscopy is unavailable or contraindicated by the patient's condition. A multiple-lumen nasogastric (NG) tube (such as a Sengstaken-Blakemore tube or a Minnesota tube) is inserted, and the gastric and esophageal balloons are inflated to apply direct pressure on the bleeding varices (**Figure 25.8** ■). Tension is applied to the tube to further compress the varices. Balloon tamponade carries a number of risks, including aspiration, airway obstruction, and tissue ischemia and necrosis. An endotracheal tube is inserted prior to nasogastric intubation to support the airway and reduce the risk of aspiration. This short-term measure is used only until more definitive treatment can be done. Without definitive treatment, rebleeding is common when balloon tamponade is discontinued.

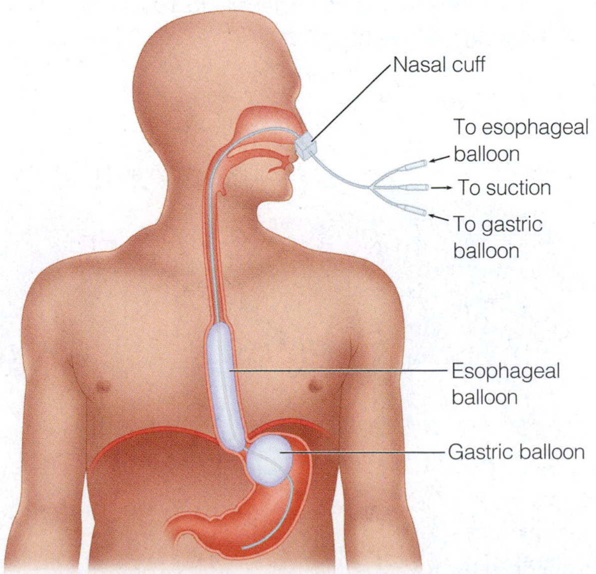
Nasal cuff
To esophageal balloon
To suction
To gastric balloon
Esophageal balloon
Gastric balloon

Figure 25.8 ■ Triple-lumen nasogastric tube (Sengstaken-Blakemore) used to control bleeding esophageal varices.

SAFETY ALERT: When caring for a patient with a multiple-lumen NG tube, always deflate the esophageal balloon before the gastric balloon. This practice prevents the balloon from becoming misplaced and occluding the airway. Always keep an appropriate syringe at the bedside to deflate the esophageal balloon should the patient develop respiratory distress. ■

Portal Hypertension. *Transjugular intrahepatic portosystemic shunt (TIPS)* may be used as an emergency measure to relieve portal hypertension and its complications of esophageal varices and ascites. A channel is created through the liver tissue using a needle inserted transcutaneously (**Figure 25.9** ■). An expandable metal stent is inserted into this channel to allow blood to flow directly from the portal vein into the hepatic vein, bypassing the cirrhotic liver. The shunt relieves pressure in esophageal varices and allows better control of fluid retention with diuretic therapy. Stenosis and occlusion of the shunt are frequent complications. TIPS increases the risk of developing hepatic encephalopathy (due to decreased perfusion of the liver and impaired ammonia metabolism) and may reduce long-term survival. It is generally used as a short-term measure until liver transplant is performed.

Surgery

Liver transplantation is indicated for some patients with irreversible, progressive cirrhosis. A decline in functional status, increasing bilirubin levels, falling albumin levels, and increasing problems with complications that respond poorly to treatment are indications for liver transplantation. Malignancy, active alcohol or drug abuse, and poor surgical risk are contraindications for the surgery. See **Box 25.4** for nursing care of the patient undergoing a liver transplant.

SAFETY ALERT: Carefully monitor the respiratory status of the patient with a Sengstaken-Blakemore or Minnesota tube. Displacement of the tube can obstruct the airway unless an endotracheal tube is in place. The esophageal balloon prevents the patient from swallowing oral secretions, increasing the risk for aspiration. Keep the head of the bed elevated to 45 degrees to reduce the risk of aspiration and promote gas exchange. ■

Nursing Care

In addition to the nursing care discussed in this section, see the Case Study & Nursing Care Plan for a patient with alcoholic cirrhosis on page 848.

Assessment

Assessment data related to cirrhosis include:

- ***Health history:*** Current manifestations, including abdominal pain or discomfort, recent weight loss, weakness, and anorexia; altered bowel elimination; excess bleeding or bruising; abdominal distention; jaundice, pruritus; altered libido or impotence; duration of symptoms; history of liver or gallbladder disease; pattern and extent of alcohol or injection drug use; use of other prescription and nonprescription drugs
- ***Physical assessment:*** Vital signs; mental status; color and condition of skin and mucous membranes; peripheral pulses and presence of peripheral edema; abdominal assessment including appearance, shape and contour, bowel sounds, abdominal girth, percussion for liver borders, and palpation for tenderness and liver size.

Priorities of Care

Nursing care for the patient with cirrhosis focuses on problems with fluid and electrolyte balance, disturbed thought processes, risk for bleeding, skin integrity, and nutrition.

Diagnoses, Outcomes, and Interventions

Nursing care of the patient with cirrhosis presents many challenges because liver function affects all body systems. The nurse is responsible for coordinating care among healthcare providers. Many nursing diagnoses may apply.

Monitor and Restore Normal Fluid Volume. Cirrhosis affects water and salt regulation due to portal hypertension, hypoalbuminemia, and hyperaldosteronism. Signs of fluid volume overload and portal hypertension may develop: Ascites, peripheral edema, internal hemorrhoids and varices, and prominent abdominal wall veins. Careful

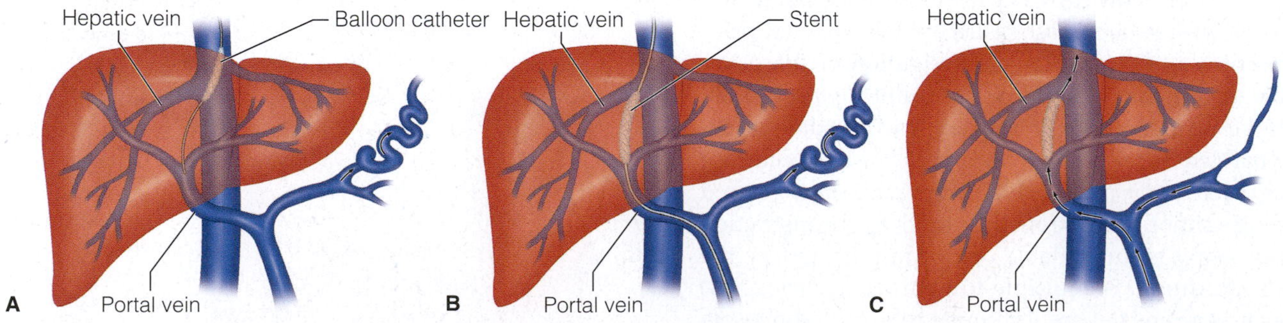
Hepatic vein
Balloon catheter
Portal vein
A
Hepatic vein
Stent
Portal vein
B
Hepatic vein
Portal vein
C

Figure 25.9 ■ Transjugular intrahepatic portosystemic shunt (TIPS). **A**, Guided by angiography, a balloon catheter inserted via the jugular vein is advanced to the hepatic veins and through the substance of the liver to create a portacaval (portal vein-to-vena cava) channel. **B**, A metal stent is positioned into the channel and expanded by inflating the balloon. **C**, The stent remains in place after the catheter is removed, creating a shunt for blood to flow directly from the portal vein into the hepatic vein.

BOX 25.4
Nursing Care of the Patient Undergoing Liver Transplantation

PREOPERATIVE CARE

- Obtain a complete nursing history and physical examination. *A complete preoperative nursing assessment provides baseline data for comparison after surgery.*
- Provide routine preoperative care as ordered. *Preoperative care is similar to that provided for other patients undergoing major surgery.*
- Discuss preoperative and postoperative expectations with the patient and family. Introduce to the intensive care unit, and discuss anticipated drainage tubes and supportive measures in the immediate postoperative period. Provide information about visiting policies and family accommodations (if available). *Preoperative teaching helps relieve anxiety in the patient and family members. Patients return from surgery to an intensive care or specialized care unit. Restrictions on the number of visitors and the time they may spend with the patient are common.*
- Once a donor liver is located, check for evidence of infection; if no infection is present, begin preoperative antibiotics as ordered. *An acute or chronic infection may contraindicate liver transplantation as drugs given postoperatively to suppress rejection of the transplanted organ also impair the ability to fight infection.*

POSTOPERATIVE CARE

- Provide routine postoperative care as ordered (see Chapter 4).
- Maintain airway and ventilatory support until awake and alert. *Until the new liver clears the anesthesia, the patient requires measures to support respirations and ventilation.*
- Monitor temperature and implement rewarming measures (such as warming blankets, heating lamps, and head covers) as indicated. *The patient is often hypothermic after liver transplant, necessitating careful rewarming while maintaining hemodynamic stability.*
- Frequently monitor hemodynamic pressures, including arterial blood pressure, central venous pressure, and pulmonary artery pressure. *Postoperative fluid volume status may be difficult to determine without careful pressure measurements. The rate and type of fluids administered are determined by hemodynamic status.*
- Monitor urine output hourly; maintain careful intake and output records. Weigh daily. *Urine output and weight provide additional information about fluid volume status. In addition, renal function may be altered after liver transplant; acute renal failure is a significant risk. See* Chapter 28 *for more information about acute renal failure and its management.*
- Monitor for signs of active bleeding, including excess drainage, increasing abdominal girth, bloody nasogastric drainage, black tarry stools, tachypnea, tachycardia, diminished peripheral pulses, or pallor. Report immediately. *Altered coagulation in the early postoperative period increases the risk for bleeding. Blood products to replace volume and clotting factors may be necessary.*
- Monitor serum electrolytes and laboratory values related to blood coagulation, liver function, and renal function. Report abnormal results or significant changes immediately. *Electrolyte imbalances are common postoperatively. Altered liver or renal function tests may indicate rejection of the transplanted liver or acute renal failure. Other early signs of transplant rejection include fever, a drop in bile output, or a change in bile color and viscosity.*
- Monitor neurologic status. *With good function of the transplanted organ, mental status should clear within days of the transplant.*
- Provide discharge teaching:
  a. Teach how to reduce risk of infection and signs of infection to report.
  b. Instruct how to recognize and report signs of organ rejection.
  c. Discuss all medications, including their purpose, schedule, adverse effects, and potential long-term effects. Stress the importance of complying with all prescribed medications and postoperative precautions for the remainder of the patient's life.
  d. Discuss possible changes in body image and psychologic responses to receiving a transplanted organ. Refer to a counselor or support group as indicated.
  e. Refer to home health services for continued assessment and teaching.
  f. Stress importance of continued follow-up with transplant team and primary care provider.

monitoring is necessary because treatment measures can lead to further fluid and electrolyte imbalances.

Expected Outcome: Patient's fluid balance will not be compromised as evidenced by 24-hour intake and output balance, stable body weight, and absence of worsening ascites and peripheral edema.

The nurse will:

- Weigh daily. Assess for jugular vein distention, measure abdominal girth daily, and check for peripheral edema. Monitor intake and output. *Careful assessment is important to detect fluid shifts.*
- Assess urine specific gravity. *Specific gravity measures the concentration of urine, an indicator of hydration.*
- Monitor the patient with cirrhosis for signs of impaired renal function, such as oliguria, a fixed specific gravity of about 1.012, central edema (around the eyes and of the face), and increasing serum creatinine and BUN levels. *Such signs may indicate hepatorenal syndrome or acute renal failure from another cause.*
- Provide a low-sodium diet (500 to 2000 mg/day) and restrict fluids as ordered. *Excess sodium leads to water retention and can increase fluid volume, ascites, and portal hypertension.*

Monitor Mentation and Respond to Confusion. Accumulated nitrogenous waste products and other metabolites affect mental status and thought processes. Effects of portal systemic encephalopathy can range from mild confusion to agitation to coma.

Expected Outcome: Patient will demonstrate cognitive orientation as demonstrated by accurate identification of self, significant other, current location, current date and time, recollection of recent significant events, and appropriate behavioral response to situation.

The nurse will:

- Assess neurologic status, including level of consciousness and mental status. Observe for signs of early encephalopathy: Changes in handwriting, speech, and asterixis. *Early identification of evidence of encephalopathy allows prompt intervention—subtle changes in neurologic functioning are important!*
- Closely monitor patients who have experienced gastrointestinal bleeding for signs of portal systemic encephalopathy. *Blood in the intestinal tract is digested as a protein, increasing serum ammonia levels and the risk for portal systemic encephalopathy.*
- Avoid factors that may precipitate portal systemic encephalopathy. Avoid hepatotoxic medications and CNS depressant drugs. *Cautious use of medications and close monitoring can eliminate iatrogenic causes of encephalopathy.*
- If possible, plan for consistent nursing care assignments. *Consistent care providers facilitate early identification of subtle neurologic changes indicative of portal systemic encephalopathy.*
- Administer medications or enemas as ordered to reduce nitrogenous products. Monitor bowel function and provide measures to promote regular elimination and prevent constipation. *Oral or rectally administered (per enema) medications are ordered to reduce intestinal bacteria and the ammonia they produce. Regular bowel elimination promotes protein and ammonia elimination in the feces.*
- Orient to surroundings, person, and place; provide simple explanations and reassurance. *Modification of verbal interactions to level of understanding and mental status may reduce anxiety and agitation.*

Prevent Hypovolemia Due to Initial and Recurrent Bleeding. Impaired coagulation, esophageal varices, and possible acute gastritis place the patient with cirrhosis at significant risk for hemorrhage. Clotting is altered by vitamin K deficiency; impaired manufacture of coagulation Factors II, VII, IX, and X; and increased platelet destruction due to splenomegaly.

Expected Outcome: Patient will not exhibit signs of visible or occult blood, and hematocrit and hemoglobin will be maintained within normal limits. Vital signs will be maintained within normal limits and urine output will be greater than 30 mL/hr.

The nurse will:

- Monitor vital signs; report tachycardia or hypotension. *Increased pulse and decreasing blood pressure may indicate hypovolemia due to hemorrhage.*
- Institute bleeding precautions as outlined in **Box 25.5**. *Preventive measures can decrease the risk for active bleeding.*
- Monitor coagulation studies and platelet count. Report abnormal results. *Coagulation studies help determine the risk for bleeding and the need for treatment.*
- Carefully monitor the patient who has had bleeding esophageal varices for evidence of rebleeding: Hematemesis, hematochezia (bright blood in the stool) or tarry stools, signs of hypovolemia or shock. *Rebleeding is common following variceal hemorrhage, especially within the first week.*

SAFETY ALERT: Carefully monitor the respiratory status of the patient with a Sengstaken-Blakemore or Minnesota tube. Displacement of the tube can obstruct the airway unless an endotracheal tube is in place. The esophageal balloon prevents the patient from swallowing oral secretions, increasing the risk for aspiration. Keep the head of the bed elevated to 45 degrees to reduce the risk of aspiration and promote gas exchange. ■

Prevent Skin Breakdown. Severe jaundice with bile salt deposits on the skin may cause pruritus. Scratching related to the pruritus damages the skin and impairs its integrity. Malnutrition, particularly protein deficiency, and edema also increase the risk for tissue breakdown and impaired skin integrity.

Expected Outcome: Patient's skin will remain intact and will not show redness or excoriation. Patient will not scratch skin or complain of itching.

The nurse will:

- Use warm water rather than hot water when bathing. *Hot water increases pruritus.*
- Use measures to prevent dry skin. Apply an emollient or lubricant as needed to keep skin moist, avoid soap or preparations with alcohol, and do not rub the skin. *Dry skin contributes to pruritus.*
- If indicated, apply mittens to the hands to prevent scratching. *Patients with encephalopathy may not understand the need to refrain from scratching.*
- Institute measures to prevent skin and tissue breakdown. Turn at least every 2 hours, use an alternating pressure mattress, and frequently assess skin condition. *Frequent position changes relieve pressure and promote circulation and tissue oxygenation.*
- Administer prescribed antihistamine (to relieve pruritus) cautiously. *Decreased liver function increases the risk for altered drug responses.*

Promote Adequate Nutrition. The patient with cirrhosis is at risk for malnutrition for a number of reasons: Possible chronic alcohol use, anorexia, impaired vitamin and mineral absorption, and impaired protein metabolism. In addition, salt restrictions may make the diet less palatable and appealing to the patient.

Expected Outcome: Patient will maintain adequate oral intake, report adequate energy levels, and maintain body mass and weight and normal lab values (transferrin, albumin, and electrolytes).

The nurse will:

- Weigh daily. Instruct to weigh at least weekly at home. *Weight is a good indicator of both nutritional status and fluid balance. Short-term weight fluctuations tend to reflect fluid balance, whereas longer-term changes in weight are more reflective of nutritional status.*
- Provide small meals with between-meal snacks. *A small meal is more appealing for an anorexic patient. Between-meal snacks help maintain adequate calorie and nutrient intake.*
- Unless protein is restricted due to impending portal systemic encephalopathy, promote protein and nutrient intake by providing nutritional supplements such

as Ensure or instant breakfasts. *The sodium and protein content of all meals and snacks must be calculated when maintaining restrictions of these nutrients.*

- Arrange for consultation with a dietitian for diet planning while hospitalized and at home. *The dietitian can provide detailed instructions, sample menus, and suggestions for improving the palatability of the diet and promoting intake.*

Transitions of Care

For most patients, high-risk behaviors are the risk factors for cirrhosis. With all patients (including children and young adults), stress the relationship between alcohol and drug abuse and liver disorders. Although many patients tolerate alcohol use in moderation with no adverse effects on the liver, excess alcohol use is the leading cause of cirrhosis. Injection drug use is also a significant risk factor, increasing the risk for contracting bloodborne hepatitis (B, C, or D). These types of viral hepatitis can lead to chronic hepatitis and, ultimately, to cirrhosis. Provide information and referral as appropriate for hepatitis B immunization. Discuss abstinence or safer sex practices as another measure to prevent viral hepatitis and potential liver damage.

Patients hospitalized for liver failure and cirrhosis will be experiencing acute liver failure, will be very ill, and are likely to be cared for in the critical care unit. The focus of care will address complications related to acute liver failure. Priorities of care will focus on support of the respiratory, circulatory, and neurological systems. The patient may require mechanical ventilation, hemodynamic monitoring, and vasopressor support. Neurological involvement is a major complication of acute liver failure and care will focus on decreasing ammonia levels and monitoring intracranial pressure. The patient may be agitated and can require sedation. Patients with liver failure are at increased risk for falls (Yildirim, 2017), so instituting strict fall precautions should be considered. Complications include renal failure, increased risk for infection, and fluid and electrolyte imbalances. See the illustration on page 831 for the multisystem effects of cirrhosis. The patient with liver failure causing hospitalization will likely have more than one major system involved.

Cirrhosis is a chronic, progressive disease. As such, the patient and family assume major roles in managing the disease and its manifestations and in preventing complications. Teaching topics for home care include:

- The absolute necessity of avoiding alcohol and other hepatotoxic drugs. Suggest inpatient or community-based alcohol treatment programs and Alcoholics Anonymous as indicated.
- Diet and fluid intake restrictions and recommendations. Include suggestions to promote nutritional intake and increase the flavor of food when sodium is restricted.
- Prescribed medications, their timing, intended and adverse effects, and manifestations to report to the primary care provider.
- Bleeding precautions (refer to **Box 25.5**).
- Manifestations of potential complications to be reported to the primary care provider. Stress the importance of promptly reporting evidence of gastrointestinal bleeding for prompt intervention for potential hemorrhage.
- Skin care techniques to reduce pruritus and the risk of damage.
- Ways to manage fatigue and conserve energy.

Provide referrals for home health services, dietary consultation, social services, and counseling as needed by the patient and family. Suggest local support groups where available.

If appropriate, suggest hospice services for the patient with end-stage liver disease. The focus of end-of-life care will address reducing multisystem symptom burden (Cox-North et al., 2013). The patient's condition will deteriorate over time, requiring complete care by a caregiver. Common symptoms that will need to be managed include:

- ***Mild to severe pain:*** Avoid acetaminophen for mild pain, administer low-dose opioids, hydromorphone, oxycodone, or fentanyl as ordered by the practitioner.
- ***Itching:*** Can be a debilitating symptom and may need to be medicated. Cholestyramine, colestipol, or naloxone may be ordered.
- ***Ascites:*** The patient will receive diuretic therapy and therapeutic paracentesis may be performed to relieve symptoms.
- ***Hepatic encephalophathy:*** The patient's neurological and mentation will deteriorate as the liver failure progresses. Lactulose may be administered to control symptoms, which will cause loose stools to diarrhea. Ensuring the patient's skin is clean and dry and supporting the caregivers will be a priority. The patient may become comatose. Prepare the family and caregivers for this likely change.
- ***Functional limitations:*** The patient will be very weak and require increasing assistance for activities of daily living. Teaching the caregiver and family to provide supportive care related to all activities will be a priority. Providing emotional support to the family and caregiver will be a significant part of the ongoing phase throughout the dying process.

BOX 25.5
Bleeding Precautions

- Prevent constipation.
- Avoid rectal temperatures or enemas.
- Avoid injections; if needed, use small-gauge needle and apply gentle pressure.
- Monitor platelet count, PT, and aPPT.
- Assess for ecchymotic areas and areas of purpura.
- Apply pressure to bleeding sites. After venipuncture, apply direct pressure for at least 5 minutes.
- Use only a soft-bristle toothbrush.
- Avoid blowing nose.
- Assess oral cavity for bleeding gums.

Case Study & Nursing Care Plan

A Patient with Alcoholic Cirrhosis

Richard Wright is a 48-year-old divorced father of two teenagers. Mr. Wright has been admitted to the community hospital with ascites and malnutrition. He has had three previous hospital stays for cirrhosis, the most recent being 6 months ago.

ASSESSMENT

Mr. Wright is lethargic but responds appropriately to verbal stimuli. He complains of "spitting up blood the past week or so" and says, "I'm just not hungry." He has lost 9 kg (20 lb) since his previous admission. He is jaundiced and has petechiae and ecchymoses on his arms and legs. Liz Mowdi, Mr. Wright's nurse, notes pitting pretibial edema. Abdominal assessment reveals a tight, protuberant abdomen with caput medusae. The liver margin is not palpable; the spleen is enlarged. Vital signs are T 37.7°C (100°F), P 110 bpm, R 25/min, and BP 110/70 mmHg.

Abnormal laboratory results include WBC 3700/mm^3 (normal 4300 to 10,800/mm^3); RBC 4.0 million/mm^3 (normal 4.6 to 5.9 million/mm^3); platelets 75,000/mm^3 (normal 150,000 to 350,000/mm^3); serum ammonia 105 μm/dL (normal 35 to 65 μm/dL); total bilirubin 4.9 mcg/dL (normal 0.1 to 1.0 mcg/dL); and serum sodium 150 mEq/L (normal 135 to 145 mEq/L). Potassium, hemoglobin, hematocrit, total protein, and albumin levels are markedly decreased. Hepatic enzymes are elevated. Blood urea nitrogen and creatinine levels are marginally elevated. Oxygen saturation (O_2 sat) is 88% (normal range: 96 to 100%) per pulse oximetry.

Endoscopy shows bleeding from gastric ulcer and the diagnosis of alcoholic cirrhosis with gastritis is made. Mr. Wright is started on Aldactone, 25 mg PO q8h; Riopan, 30 mL 2 h p.c. and at bedtime; lactulose, 30 mL every hour until onset of diarrhea, then 15 mL tid; and 800 mg sodium diet; fluid restriction of 1500 mL/day.

DIAGNOSES

- Difficulty breathing related to pressure of ascites fluid on the diaphragm as manifested by tachypnea and decreased oxygen saturation
- Edema and fluid volume overload related to electrolyte imbalance and hypoalbuminemia as manifested by ascites and peripheral edema
- Inadequate nutritional intake related to anorexia and possible alcohol abuse as manifested by weight loss and low serum protein levels
- Alterations in mentation related to effects of high ammonia levels as manifested by lethargy
- Potential hemorrhage related to impaired platelet formation and portal hypertension

EXPECTED OUTCOMES

- Patient's respiratory rate and O_2 saturation will be within normal limits.
- Patient's abdominal girth will decrease by 1 to 2 cm per day; peripheral edema will decrease.
- Patient will gain 0.45 kg (1 lb) per week without evidence of increased fluid retention. Serum albumin levels will return to normal range.
- Patient will be alert and oriented; serum ammonia levels will be within normal range.
- Patient will demonstrate no further evidence of active bleeding.
- Patient will verbalize willingness to join a community support group.

PLANNING AND IMPLEMENTATION

- Weigh daily.
- Provide high-calorie, low-salt, low-protein diet with between-meal snacks.
- Maintain stool chart.
- Assign same nurses to care as much as possible to facilitate evaluation of mental status. Promptly report changes in status or laboratory values.
- Measure abdominal girth every 8 hours, marking level of measurement.
- Institute bleeding precautions.
- Elevate head of bed; assist to chair with legs elevated tid as tolerated.
- Include significant others in care and teaching; refer to community agencies for discharge follow-up.

EVALUATION

A week after admission, Mr. Wright's ascites has decreased and no further active bleeding is noted. His serum protein levels have increased, and his laboratory values are improving. No further bruising is noted during hospitalization. Although he shows a 2.3-kg (5-lb) weight loss as excess water is eliminated, he is consuming 100% of his diet. His serum ammonia levels have returned to normal. On discharge, O_2 sat is 96%; respirations are 18. Lactulose will be continued on discharge.

Ms. Mowdi provides both written and verbal information about the medication and cirrhosis, including measures to prevent complications. Mr. Wright and his children express interest in Alcoholics Anonymous and Al-Anon and are referred to those agencies. Prior to discharge, follow-up appointments are made with a psychiatric social worker and a primary caregiver.

CLINICAL REASONING IN PATIENT CARE

1. Describe the relationship between portal hypertension, liver dysfunction, and ascites.
2. Outline a 1-day menu for a low-protein, low-sodium, high-calorie diet.
3. What is the pathophysiologic basis for portal systemic encephalopathy? What are the nursing responsibilities related to lactulose and neomycin?
4. Design a nursing care plan for Mr. Wright for supporting self-care and adherence to medication management.

See Evaluating Your Response in Appendix B.

The Patient with Cancer of the Liver

Primary liver cancer is uncommon in the United States, accounting for only 0.5 to 3% of all cancers (American Cancer Society [ACS], 2017). It is, however, a common malignancy worldwide. Hepatocellular carcinoma is common in parts of Asia and Africa, where the incidence is as high as 500 cases per 100,000 people. This higher incidence is linked to chronic hepatitis B or C infection.

The incidence of liver cancer is higher in Hispanics than it is in Black and non-Hispanic Whites; Blacks have a higher incidence than Whites (ACS, 2017). The prognosis for primary liver cancer is poor, in part because the disease is often advanced at the time of diagnosis. Metastasis to the liver from primary tumors of the lung, breast, and gastrointestinal tract are relatively common.

Pathophysiology

More than 80% of primary hepatic cancers arise from the liver's parenchymal cells (hepatocellular carcinoma); the remainder form in the bile ducts (cholangiocarcinoma). Regardless of the origin, the progress of the disease is similar. Several etiologic factors have been identified:

- Chronic hepatitis C infection
- Chronic hepatitis B infection
- Cirrhosis, regardless of type
- Aflatoxin (a toxin produced by *Aspergillus* molds) exposure
- Chronic ethanol consumption
- Nonalcoholic fatty liver (steatohepatitis or NASH)

Most primary liver cancer in the United States is related to alcoholic cirrhosis, HBV, or HCV.

The underlying pathophysiology of primary liver cancer is damage to hepatocellular DNA. This damage may be caused by integration of HBV or HCV into the DNA or by repeated cycles of cell necrosis and regeneration that facilitate DNA mutations. HBV and aflatoxins damage a specific tumor suppressor gene. Tumors may be limited to one specific area, may occur as nodules throughout the liver, or may develop as surface infiltrates. The tumor interferes with normal hepatic function, leading to biliary obstruction and jaundice, portal hypertension, and metabolic disruptions (hypoalbuminemia, hypoglycemia, and bleeding disorders). It also may secrete bile products and produce hormones (paraneoplastic syndrome) that may lead to polycythemia, hypoglycemia, and hypercalcemia. Tumors usually grow rapidly and metastasize early.

Manifestations

Initial manifestations of liver cancer develop insidiously and are often masked by the presence of cirrhosis or chronic hepatitis. Weakness, anorexia, weight loss, fatigue, and malaise are common early manifestations. Abdominal pain and a palpable mass in the right upper quadrant are common presenting symptoms. Ascites and jaundice may be present at diagnosis. Signs of liver failure with portal hypertension, splenomegaly, and altered metabolism develop as the tumor progresses.

Interprofessional Care and Nursing Care

Ultrasound of the liver is used as a screening tool for liver cancer. CT scan with contrast and MRI are used to determine tumor size and extent. A liver biopsy is done to confirm the diagnosis and identify the tumor type or origin. Serum alpha-fetoprotein (AFP) levels, normally low in nonpregnant adults, rise in most patients with hepatocellular cancer.

Small, localized tumors may be surgically resected or destroyed using radio-frequency ablation or injection of an agent such as ethanol directly into the tumor. Most tumors, however, have spread extensively or have distant metastasis at the time of diagnosis, so this is frequently not an option. Additionally, patients with underlying liver disease such as cirrhosis may not tolerate loss of additional functional liver tissue. Liver transplantation may be done for stage I or II tumors (no apparent lymph node involvement or distant metastasis). Liver transplantation is limited as a treatment option by the availability of donor organs.

Radiation therapy may be used to shrink the tumor, decreasing pressure on surrounding organs and reducing pain. Chemotherapy may be used as primary treatment for advanced tumors. Direct continuous hepatic arterial infusion with an implanted pump has shown promise in prolonging survival rates. See Chapter 14 for nursing care of patients receiving radiation therapy or chemotherapy.

Nursing diagnoses, interventions, and teaching for the patient with liver cancer are similar to those for patients with cirrhosis (see pages 825–838).

Transitions of Care

Encourage patients with risk factors for primary liver cancer to avoid alcohol and other substances that may further damage the liver. Urge them to discuss regular screening for liver tumors (such as serum AFP levels) with their primary care physician.

Both the patient and the family need extensive nursing support. Controlling pain is a priority. Because of the poor prognosis, early referral for hospice services may be appropriate.

The Patient with Liver Trauma

Blunt or penetrating trauma to the abdomen can damage the liver. Liver trauma is frequently seen in combination with injuries to other abdominal organs. Motor vehicle crashes, stab or gunshot wounds, and iatrogenic sources such as liver biopsy are among the causes of these injuries.

Pathophysiology and Manifestations

Liver trauma generally causes bleeding due to the vascularity of the organ. Liver injury may cause a surface hematoma, hematoma within the liver parenchyma, laceration of liver tissue, or disruption of vessels leading to or from the liver. Severe bleeding can rapidly disrupt hemodynamic stability and lead to shock.

SAFETY ALERT: Bleeding due to liver trauma may not be immediately apparent. Instruct the patient with apparent or potential liver trauma to immediately report light-headedness, rapid heart rate, shortness of breath, thirst, or increasing abdominal pain. ■

Interprofessional Care

Diagnostic peritoneal lavage is often used along with CT scan to diagnose liver trauma. The procedure is performed by making a small abdominal incision into the peritoneum (after the bladder has been emptied) and inserting a small catheter into the peritoneal cavity. If blood is immediately detected, the patient is taken directly to surgery for abdominal exploration. If frank bleeding is not apparent, a liter of isotonic fluid is instilled into the abdomen, then drained and sent for laboratory analysis.

Intravenous fluids, fresh frozen plasma, platelets, and other clotting factors are administered to restore blood volume and promote hemostasis. Hemodynamic status is closely monitored; continued instability may indicate a need for surgical intervention to control hemorrhage. Postoperative nursing care focuses on preventing pulmonary complications, such as atelectasis, and detecting and preventing infection.

Nursing Care

Nursing care of the patient with liver trauma focuses on fluid management and other supportive care related to shock. Keeping family members informed is an important aspect of care, especially during the period of patient instability. Diagnoses include:

- Manage hypovolemia related to hemorrhage
- Prevent infection related to wound or abdominal contamination
- Monitor for hemorrhage related to impaired coagulation.

The Patient with Liver Abscess

Liver abscesses are usually bacterial or amoebic (protozoal) in origin. Bacterial abscesses may follow trauma or surgical procedures, including biopsy. Multiple or single abscesses occur most commonly in the right lobe. Amoebic abscesses most frequently occur following infestation of the liver by *Entamoeba histolytica*. Amoebic infestation is associated with poor hygiene, unsafe sexual practices, or travel in areas where drinking water is contaminated.

Pathophysiology and Manifestations

Following bacterial or amoebic invasion of the liver, healthy tissue is destroyed, leaving an area of necrosis, inflammatory exudate, and blood. This damaged region becomes walled off from the healthy liver tissue. Pyogenic (bacterial) liver abscess may be caused by cholangitis or distant or intra-abdominal infections, such as peritonitis or diverticulitis. *Escherichia coli* is the most frequently identified causative organism. The onset of pyogenic abscess is usually sudden, causing acute symptoms such as fever, malaise, vomiting, hyperbilirubinemia, and pain in the right upper abdomen.

The infection pathway for amoebic hepatic abscesses is usually the portal venous circulation from the right colon. Generally, the onset of amoebic abscess is insidious.

Interprofessional Care

Hepatic abscess is diagnosed through biopsy, hepatic aspirate, blood and fecal cultures, and CT scan and ultrasound studies. Therapy is based on identifying the causative organism through laboratory cultures. Pyogenic abscesses are treated with antibiotics to which the causative organism is sensitive.

Pharmacologic agents used for amebic hepatic abscess are the same as those used for intestinal amebic infestation (see Chapter 24); combination therapy is commonly used. Two commonly used drugs for treating amebic liver abscesses are metronidazole (Flagyl) and iodoquinol (Diquinol). Both medications can cause gastrointestinal symptoms. Bone marrow suppression is a risk with metronidazole.

If the abscess does not respond to antibiotic therapy, percutaneous aspiration or surgical drainage may be done. In these procedures, a *percutaneous closed-catheter drain* is placed in the abscess to promote drainage of purulent material.

Nursing Care

A major aspect of nursing care is prevention; teaching patients to avoid contaminated water and foods is especially important. Nursing interventions include teaching hikers to treat water and food handlers to wash hands thoroughly.

Patients who have a liver abscess require supportive care to prevent dehydration from the accompanying fever, nausea and vomiting, and anorexia. Careful monitoring of fluid and electrolyte status is indicated, as are comfort measures for abdominal pain. Possible nursing problems include:

- Prevent hypovolemia due to effects of prolonged fever and vomiting
- Provide patient education related to transmission of amebic abscess
- Support activities of daily living due to pain and weakness.

25.3 Exocrine Pancreas Disorders

The pancreas is both an exocrine and an endocrine gland. It is made up of two basic cell types, each having different functions. The exocrine cells produce enzymes that empty through ducts into the small intestine, whereas the endocrine cells produce hormones that enter the bloodstream directly. Disorders of the exocrine pancreas affect the secretion and glandular control of digestive enzymes, whereas disorders of the endocrine pancreas affect the production of hormones necessary for normal carbohydrate, protein, and fat metabolism (Conwell, Banks, & Greenberger, 2014). Disorders of the exocrine pancreas are discussed in this section of the chapter; diabetes mellitus, a disorder of the endocrine pancreas, is discussed in Chapter 20.

The Patient with Pancreatitis

Pancreatitis, or inflammation of the pancreas, is characterized by the release of pancreatic enzymes into the tissue of the pancreas itself, leading to hemorrhage and necrosis. Pancreatitis may be either acute or chronic. About 5000 new cases of acute pancreatitis are diagnosed every year in the United States. It is a serious disease, with a mortality rate of approximately 10% (Longo et al., 2013). Hospitalizations for acute pancreatitis have increased during the past 15 years. Alcoholism and gallstones are the primary risk factors for acute pancreatitis, however, the etiology of about 30% of cases is unclear.

The incidence of chronic pancreatitis is less clear because many people with chronic pancreatitis do not have classic manifestations of the disease. Patients with chronic pancreatitis may have long-term effects of the disease, with chronic changes in enzyme and hormone production.

Physiology Review

Knowledge of the normal structure and functions of the exocrine pancreas is important to understand how inflammation affects it and the patient. The exocrine pancreas consists of lobules of acinar cells. The acinar cells secrete digestive enzymes and fluids (pancreatic juices) into ducts that empty into the main pancreatic duct (the duct of Wirsung). The pancreatic duct joins the common bile duct and empties into the duodenum through the ampulla of Vater (in some people the main pancreatic duct empties directly into the duodenum). The epithelial lining of the pancreatic ducts secretes water and bicarbonate to modify the composition of the pancreatic secretions. Pancreatic enzymes are secreted primarily in an inactive form and are activated in the intestine, a modification that prevents digestion of pancreatic tissue by its own enzymes (Sorenson et al., 2019). The pancreatic enzymes, with related functions, are:

- Proteolytic enzymes, including trypsin, chymotrypsin, carboxypolypeptidase, ribonuclease, and deoxyribonuclease, which break down dietary proteins
- Pancreatic amylase, which breaks down starch
- Lipase, which breaks down fats into glycerol and fatty acids.

Pathophysiology and Manifestations

Acute Pancreatitis

Acute pancreatitis is an inflammatory disorder that involves self-destruction of the pancreas by its own enzymes through autodigestion (Krenzer, 2016). The milder form of acute pancreatitis, *interstitial edematous pancreatitis*, leads to inflammation and edema of pancreatic tissue. It is often self-limiting. The more severe form, *necrotizing pancreatitis*, is characterized by inflammation, hemorrhage, and ultimately necrosis of pancreatic tissue.

Acute pancreatitis is more common in middle-aged adults; its incidence is higher in men than in women. Gallstones are the leading cause of acute pancreatitis, with alcohol being the second leading cause (Sorenson et al., 2019). Some patients recover completely, others experience recurring attacks, and still others develop chronic pancreatitis. The mortality and symptoms depend on the severity and type of pancreatitis, as well as the patient's age and general health. Organ failure (respiratory failure in particular) is the leading cause of death in acute pancreatitis (Perrin & MacLeod, 2018; Sorenson et al., 2019).

Although the exact cause of pancreatitis is not known, the following factors may activate pancreatic enzymes within the pancreas, leading to autodigestion, inflammation, edema, and/or necrosis:

- Gallstones may obstruct the pancreatic duct or cause bile reflux, activating pancreatic enzymes in the pancreatic duct system
- Alcohol causes duodenal edema and may increase pressure and spasm in the sphincter of Oddi, obstructing pancreatic outflow. It also stimulates pancreatic enzyme production, thus raising pressure within the pancreas.

Other factors associated with acute pancreatitis include tissue ischemia or anoxia, trauma or surgery, pancreatic tumors, third-trimester pregnancy, infectious agents (viral, bacterial, or parasitic), elevated calcium levels, and hyperlipidemia. Some medications have been linked with this disorder, including thiazide diuretics, estrogen, steroids, salicylates, and NSAIDs.

Regardless of the precipitating factor, the pathophysiologic process begins with the release of activated pancreatic enzymes into pancreatic tissue. Activated proteolytic enzymes, trypsin in particular, digest pancreatic tissue and activate other enzymes such as phospholipase A, which digests cell membrane phospholipids, and elastase, which digests the elastic tissue of blood vessel walls. This leads to proteolysis, edema, vascular damage and hemorrhage, and necrosis of parenchymal cells. Cellular damage and necrosis release activated enzymes and vasoactive substances that produce vasodilation, increase vascular permeability, and cause edema. A large volume of fluid may shift from circulating blood into the retroperitoneal space, the peripancreatic spaces, and the abdominal cavity.

Manifestations. Acute pancreatitis develops suddenly, typically with an abrupt onset of continuous severe epigastric and abdominal pain. This pain commonly radiates to the back and is relieved somewhat by sitting up and leaning forward. The pain is often initiated by a fatty meal or excessive alcohol intake.

Other manifestations include nausea and vomiting; abdominal distention and rigidity; decreased bowel sounds; tachycardia; hypotension; elevated temperature; and cold, clammy skin. Within 24 hours, mild jaundice may appear. Retroperitoneal bleeding may occur 3 to 6 days after the onset of acute pancreatitis; signs of bleeding include bruising in the flanks (Turner sign) or around the umbilicus (Cullen sign).

Complications. Systemic complications of acute pancreatitis include intravascular volume depletion with shock, acute tubular necrosis and renal failure (see Chapter 28 for more information about acute kidney injury), and acute respiratory distress syndrome (ARDS). Hypovolemic shock and acute renal failure usually develop within 24 hours after the onset of acute pancreatitis. Manifestations of ARDS may be seen 3 to 7 days after its onset, particularly in patients who have experienced severe volume depletion.

Upon diagnosis of acute pancreatitis, the health-care team will determine the severity of disease to determine if the patient is likely to develop severe disease. Determining the severity of disease is critical to ensuring positive outcomes. The grading system includes mild, moderately severe, and severe. The characteristics of each category are:

- ***Mild acute pancreatitis:*** Absence of organ failure, local or minor systemic complications; most patients do not require pancreatic imaging and are discharged in 3 to 5 days
- ***Moderately severe acute pancreatitis:*** Characterized by either no organ failure or transient failure and local complications
- ***Severe acute pancreatitis:*** Characterized by persistent organ failure for more than 48 hours and imaging shows pancreatic necrosis (Perrin & MacLeod, 2018).

Identifying organ failure is critical when determining severity of disease so the patient can be triaged to the appropriate level of care. Patients with severe acute pancreatitis will be cared for in the critical care unit (Perrin & MacLeod, 2018).

Localized complications include pancreatic necrosis, abscess, pseudocysts, and pancreatic ascites. Pancreatic necrosis causes an inflammatory mass that may be infected. It may lead to shock and multiple-organ failure. A pancreatic abscess may form late in the course of the disease (6 or more weeks after its onset), causing an epigastric mass and tenderness (Perrin & MacLeod, 2018). Pancreatic pseudocysts, encapsulated collections of fluid, may develop both within the pancreas itself and in the abdominal cavity (**Figure 25.10** ■). They may impinge on other structures, or may rupture, causing generalized peritonitis. Rupture of a pseudocyst or of the pancreatic duct can lead to pancreatic ascites. Pancreatic ascites is recognized by gradually increasing abdominal girth and persistent elevation of the serum amylase level without abdominal pain.

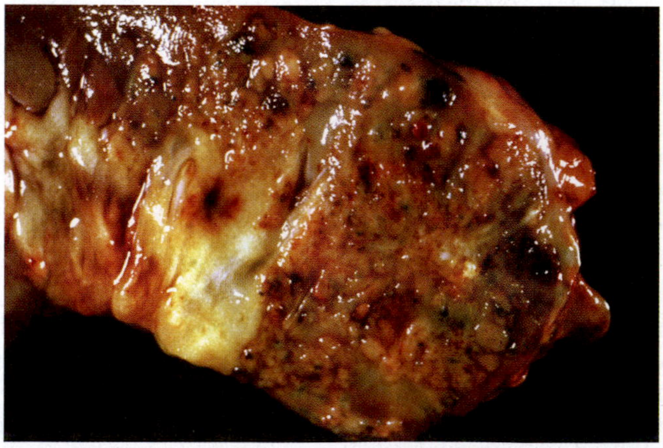

Figure 25.10 ■ Acute pancreatitis. Gross clinical specimen of a pancreas affected by acute pancreatitis. Pseudocyst, a pus-filled bleb seen as the yellow area (lower left center), is a potential complication of acute pancreatitis.

Chronic Pancreatitis

Chronic pancreatitis is characterized by chronic inflammation, fibrosis, and gradual destruction of functional pancreatic tissue. In contrast to acute pancreatitis, which is reversible, chronic pancreatitis is an irreversible process that eventually leads to pancreatic insufficiency. Alcoholism is the primary risk factor for chronic pancreatitis in the United States. Malnutrition is a major worldwide risk factor. About 10 to 20% of chronic pancreatitis is idiopathic, with no identified cause. A genetic mutation on a gene associated with cystic fibrosis may play a role in these cases. Children or young adults with cystic fibrosis may develop chronic pancreatitis as well.

In chronic pancreatitis related to alcoholism, pancreatic secretions have an increased concentration of insoluble proteins. These proteins calcify, forming plugs that block pancreatic ducts and the flow of pancreatic juices. This blockage leads to inflammation and fibrosis of pancreatic tissue. In other cases, a stricture or stone may block pancreatic outflow, causing chronic obstructive pancreatitis. In chronic pancreatitis, recurrent episodes of inflammation eventually lead to fibrotic changes in the parenchyma of the pancreas, with loss of exocrine function. This leads to malabsorption from pancreatic insufficiency. If endocrine function is disrupted as well, clinical diabetes mellitus may develop.

Manifestations. Chronic pancreatitis typically causes recurrent episodes of epigastric and left upper abdominal pain that radiates to the back. This pain may last for days to weeks. As the disease progresses, the interval between episodes of pain becomes shorter. Other manifestations include anorexia, nausea and vomiting, weight loss, flatulence, constipation, and **steatorrhea** (fatty, frothy, foul-smelling stools caused by a decrease in pancreatic enzyme secretion).

Complications. Complications of chronic pancreatitis include malabsorption, malnutrition, and possible peptic ulcer disease. Pancreatic pseudocyst or abscess may form or stricture of the common bile duct may develop. Diabetes mellitus may develop, and there is an increased risk for pancreatic cancer. Opioid addiction related to frequent, severe pain episodes is common.

Interprofessional Care

Acute pancreatitis is often a mild, self-limiting disease. Treatment focuses on reducing pancreatic secretions and providing supportive care. Treatment to eliminate the causative factor is begun after the acute inflammatory process resolves. Severe necrotizing pancreatitis may require intensive care management. Treatment for chronic pancreatitis often focuses on managing pain and treating malabsorption and malnutrition.

Diagnosis

The laboratory tests that may be ordered when pancreatitis is suspected are summarized in **Table 25.4**. Diagnostic studies include:

- *Ultrasonography* can identify gallstones, a pancreatic mass, or pseudocyst.
- *Endoscopic ultrasonography* can detect changes indicative of chronic pancreatitis in the pancreatic duct and parenchyma.
- *Contrast-enhanced CT scan* may be ordered to identify pancreatic enlargement, ductal calcifications, fluid collections in or around the pancreas, and perfusion deficits in areas of necrosis.
- *Magnetic resonance cholangiopancreatography (MRCP)* is a noninvasive test that allows visualization of the bile and pancreatic ducts.
- *Endoscopic retrograde cholangiopancreatography (ERCP)* may be performed to diagnose chronic pancreatitis and to differentiate inflammation and fibrosis from carcinoma.
- *Percutaneous fine-needle aspiration biopsy* may be performed to differentiate chronic pancreatitis from cancer of the pancreas; the cells that are aspirated are examined for malignancy.

More information about these tests and their nursing implications can be found in Chapter 21.

Medications

The treatment of acute pancreatitis is largely supportive. Opioid analgesics such as morphine sulfate or hydromorphone (Dilaudid) are used as needed to control pain. Prophylactic antibiotics are prescribed for patients with severe or necrotizing pancreatitis to prevent infection.

Patients with chronic pancreatitis may also require analgesics, but are closely monitored to prevent drug dependence. Pancreatic enzyme supplements are given to manage abdominal pain and reduce steatorrhea (see **Medication Administration 25.C**). Patients with chronic pancreatitis may need to remain on pancreatic enzyme supplements for life. H_2-blockers, such as cimetidine (Tagamet) and ranitidine (Zantac), and proton-pump inhibitors such as omeprazole (Prilosec) may be given to neutralize or decrease gastric secretions. Octreotide (Sandostatin), a synthetic hormone, suppresses pancreatic enzyme secretion and may also be used to relieve pain in chronic pancreatitis.

Nutrition

Oral food and fluids are generally withheld during acute episodes of pancreatitis to reduce pancreatic secretions and promote rest of the organ. A nasogastric tube may be inserted and connected to suction. Intravenous fluids are administered to maintain vascular volume, and total parenteral nutrition (TPN) is initiated. Oral food and fluids are begun once the serum amylase levels have returned to normal, bowel sounds are present, and pain disappears. A low-fat diet is ordered, and alcohol intake is strictly prohibited.

Surgery

If the pancreatitis is the result of a gallstone lodged in the sphincter of Oddi, an *endoscopic transduodenal sphincterotomy* may be performed to remove the stone. When cholelithiasis is identified as a causative factor, a cholecystectomy is performed once the acute pancreatitis has resolved. Surgical procedures to promote drainage of pancreatic enzymes into the duodenum or resection of all or part of the pancreas may be done to provide pain relief in patients with chronic pancreatitis. Large pancreatic pseudocysts may be drained endoscopically or surgically.

Integrative Therapies

Several complementary therapies may be used in conjunction with traditional treatments for patients with acute or chronic pancreatitis. Fasting or use of low-salt, low-fat vegetarian diets may reduce episodes of recurrent pain. Qigong, a system of gentle exercise, meditation, and controlled breathing, is believed to balance the flow of qi (a vital life force) through the body. Qigong lowers the metabolic rate and may reduce the stimulation of pancreatic enzyme secretion (Putiri, Close, Lilly, Guillaume, & Sun, 2017). All integrative therapies should be prescribed by a trained and competent practitioner.

Table 25.4 Laboratory Tests in Exocrine Pancreatic Disorders

Test	Normal Value	Significance
Serum amylase	30–170 units/L	Rises within 2–12 hours of onset of acute pancreatitis to two to three times normal. Returns to normal in 3–4 days.
Serum lipase	14–280 units/L	Levels rise in acute pancreatitis; remain elevated for 7–14 days.
Urine amylase	4–37 units/L/2h	Urine amylase levels rise in acute pancreatitis.
Serum glucose	70–110 mg/dL	May be transient elevation in acute pancreatitis.
Serum bilirubin	0.1–1.2 mg/dL	Compression of the common duct may increase bilirubin levels in acute pancreatitis.
Serum alkaline phosphatase (ALP)	42–136 units/L	Compression of the common duct may increase levels in acute pancreatitis.
Serum calcium	9–11 mg/dL or 4.5–5.5 mEq/L	Hypocalcemia develops in up to 25% of patients with acute pancreatitis.
White blood cells	4500–10,000/mm^3	Leukocytosis indicates inflammation and is usually present in acute pancreatitis.

Medication Administration 25.C

The Patient with Chronic Pancreatitis

PANCREATIC ENZYMES

pancrelipase (Creon, Pacreaze, others)

Pancrelipase enhances the digestion of starches and fats in the gastrointestinal tract by supplying an exogenous source of the enzymes protease, amylase, and lipase. The drug promotes nutrition and decreases the number of bowel movements.

Nursing Responsibilities

- Assess for allergy to pork protein.
- Monitor frequency and consistency of stools.
- Weigh every other day. Record weights.
- Give with meals; if not enteric coated, H_2 antagonists or antacids may be given concurrently to prevent destruction of the enzymes by hydrochloric acid.
- Monitor for side effects: Rash, hives, respiratory difficulty, hematuria, hyperuricemia, or joint pain.

Health Education for the Patient and Family

- Take with meals or snacks.
- If medicine is enteric coated, do not crush, chew, or mix with alkaline foods (e.g., milk, ice cream).
- Be sure to follow prescribed diet.
- Continue taking this drug until or unless advised by physician that it is no longer necessary.

Sources: Data from Adams, et al., 2017; Felicilda-Reynaldo & Kenneally, 2016.

Nursing Care

In addition to the nursing care discussed in this section, see the Case Study & Nursing Care Plan for a patient with acute pancreatitis on page 848.

Assessment

Assessment data related to acute or chronic pancreatitis include:

- ***Health history:*** Current manifestations; abdominal pain (location, nature, onset and duration, identified precipitating factors); anorexia, nausea and vomiting; flatulence, diarrhea, constipation, or stool changes; recent weight loss; history of previous episodes or gallstones; alcohol use (extent and duration); current medications
- ***Physical assessment:*** Vital signs including orthostatic vitals and peripheral pulses; temperature; skin temperature and color, presence of any flank or periumbilical ecchymoses; abdominal assessment including bowel sounds, presence of distention, tenderness, or guarding.

Priorities of Care

Nursing care for the patient with acute pancreatitis focuses on managing pain, promoting nutrition, and maintaining fluid balance.

Diagnoses, Outcomes, and Interventions

Relieve Acute Pain. Obstruction of pancreatic ducts and inflammation, edema, and swelling of the pancreas caused by pancreatic autodigestion cause severe epigastric, left upper abdominal, or midscapular back pain. The pain is often accompanied by nausea and vomiting, abdominal tenderness, and muscle guarding.

Expected Outcome: Patient will identify pain triggers, use treatment plan (pharmacologic and nonpharmacologic) to prevent and alleviate discomfort, and report relief from pain.

The nurse will:

- Using a standard pain scale (see Chapter 9), assess pain, including location, radiation, duration, and character. Note nonverbal cues of pain: Restlessness or remaining rigidly still; tense facial features; clenched fists; rapid, shallow respirations; tachycardia; and diaphoresis. Administer analgesics on a regular schedule. *Pain assessment before and after analgesic administration measures its effectiveness. Administering analgesics on a regular schedule prevents pain from becoming established, severe, and difficult to control. Unrelieved pain has negative consequences; for example, pain, anxiety, and restlessness may increase pancreatic enzyme secretion.*
- Regularly assess respiratory status (at least every 4 to 8 hours), including respiratory rate, depth, and pattern; breath sounds; oxygen saturation; and arterial blood gas results. Report tachypnea, adventitious or absent breath sounds, oxygen saturation levels below 92%, $PaO_2 < 70$ mmHg or $PaCO_2 > 45$ mmHg. *Severe abdominal pain causes shallow respirations and hypoventilation and suppresses cough effectiveness, which can lead to pooling of secretions, atelectasis, and pneumonia.*
- Maintain NPO status and nasogastric tube patency as ordered. *Gastric secretions stimulate hormones that cause pancreatic secretion, aggravating pain. Eliminating oral intake and maintaining gastric suction reduce gastric secretions. Nasogastric suction also decreases nausea and vomiting, and intestinal distention.*
- Maintain bedrest in a calm, quiet environment. Encourage use of nonpharmacologic pain management techniques such as meditation and guided imagery. *Decreasing physical movement and mental stimulation decreases the metabolic rate, gastrointestinal secretion, pancreatic secretions, and resulting pain. Adjunctive pain relief measures enhance the effectiveness of analgesics* (see Chapter 9).
- Assist to a comfortable position, such as a side-lying position with knees flexed and head elevated

45 degrees. *Sitting up, leaning forward, or lying in a fetal position tends to decrease pain caused by stretching of the peritoneum by edema and swelling.*

- Remind family and visitors to avoid bringing food into the patient's room. *The sight or smell of food may stimulate secretory activity of the pancreas through the cephalic phase of digestion.*

Support Adequate Nutrition. The effects of pancreatitis and its treatment may result in malnutrition. Inflammation increases metabolic demand and frequently causes nausea and vomiting and diarrhea. At a time of increased metabolic demand, NPO status and gastric suction further decrease available nutrients. In the patient with chronic pancreatitis, loss of digestive enzymes affects the digestion and use of nutrients.

Expected Outcome: Patient's weight and body mass index and lab values (transferrin, albumin, hemoglobin, hematocrit, and electrolytes) will stabilize and be within normal limits. Patient will describe intake of a low-fat, well-balanced diet and will report normal eating patterns.

The nurse will:

- Monitor laboratory values: Serum transferrin, serum albumin, electrolytes, hemoglobin, and hematocrit. *Serum albumin, serum transferrin (which transports iron in the blood), hemoglobin, and hematocrit levels are decreased in malnutrition. Decreased pancreatic enzymes affect protein catabolism and absorption; decreased transferrin affects iron absorption and transport, thereby decreasing hematocrit and hemoglobin levels. Prolonged poor nutrition may cause electrolyte imbalance.*
- Weigh daily or every other day. *Short-term weight changes (over hours to days) accurately reflect fluid balance, whereas weight changes over days to weeks reflect nutritional status.*
- Maintain stool chart; note frequency, color, odor, and consistency of stools. *Protein and fat metabolism are impaired in pancreatitis; undigested fats are excreted in the stool. Steatorrhea indicates impaired digestion and, possibly, an increase in the severity of pancreatitis.*
- Monitor bowel sounds. *The return of bowel sounds indicates return of peristalsis; nasogastric suction is usually discontinued within 24 to 48 hours thereafter.*
- Administer prescribed intravenous fluids and/or TPN. *Intravenous fluids are given to maintain hydration. TPN is used to provide fluids, electrolytes, and kilocalories when fasting is prolonged (more than 2 to 3 days).*
- Provide oral and nasal care every 1 to 2 hours. *Fasting and nasogastric suction increase the risk for mucous membrane irritation and breakdown.*
- When oral intake resumes, offer small, frequent feedings. Provide oral hygiene before and after meals. *Small, frequent feedings reduce pancreatic enzyme secretion and are more easily digested and absorbed. Oral hygiene decreases oral microorganisms that can cause foul odor and taste, decreasing appetite.*

Promote Adequate Fluid Balance. Acute pancreatitis can lead to a fluid shift from the intravascular space into the abdominal cavity (third spacing). Third spacing of fluid may cause hypovolemic shock, affecting cardiovascular function, respiratory function, renal function, and mental status.

Expected Outcome: Deficient fluid volume will be prevented as evidenced by normal vital signs, normal hemodynamic parameters, normal lab values, and absence of physical signs of dehydration (e.g., thirst, change in mental status, decreased urine output, dry skin and mucous membranes, weakness).

The nurse will:

- Assess cardiovascular status every 4 hours or as indicated, including vital signs, cardiac rhythm, hemodynamic parameters (central venous and pulmonary artery pressures); peripheral pulses and capillary refill; and skin color, temperature, moisture, and turgor. *These measurements are indicative of fluid volume status and are used to monitor response to treatment. Stable values are as follows: Heart rate less than 100 bpm; blood pressure within 10 mmHg of baseline; central venous pressure 0 to 8 mmHg; pulmonary wedge pressure 8 to 12 mmHg; cardiac output approximately 5 L/min; and skin warm and dry, with good turgor and color.*
- Monitor renal function. Obtain hourly urine output; report if less than 30 mL/hr. Weigh daily. *Urine output of less than 30 mL/hr indicates decreased renal perfusion or acute renal failure, a major complication of acute pancreatitis. Weight changes are an effective indicator of fluid volume status.*
- Monitor neurologic function, including mental status, level of consciousness, and behavior. *Hypotension and hypoxemia may decrease cerebral perfusion, causing changes in mental status, decreased level of consciousness, and changes in behavior. In addition, alcohol withdrawal is a risk in the patient with acute pancreatitis.*

Transitions of Care

Teach patients who abuse alcohol about the risk for developing pancreatitis. Advise abstinence to reduce this risk and refer to an alcohol treatment program or Alcoholics Anonymous.

The patient with acute pancreatitis is often very ill. The patient and family members need information about hospital procedures and probable self-care requirements to be implemented following discharge. During the acute stage, keep explanations brief and simple.

Prior to discharge, teach the patient and family about the disease and how to prevent further attacks of inflammation. Include the following topics as appropriate:

- Alcohol can cause stones to form, blocking pancreatic ducts and the outflow of pancreatic juice. Continued alcohol intake is likely to cause further inflammation and destruction of the pancreas. Avoid alcohol entirely.
- Smoking and stress stimulate the pancreas and should be avoided.
- If pancreatic function has been severely impaired, discuss appropriate use of pancreatic enzymes, including

timing, dose, potential side effects, and monitoring of effectiveness.

- A low-fat diet is recommended. Provide a list of high-fat foods to avoid. Crash dieting and binge eating should also be avoided as they may sometimes precipitate attacks. Spicy foods, coffee, tea, or colas, and gas-forming foods stimulate gastric and pancreatic secretions and may precipitate pain. Avoid them if this occurs.
- Report symptoms of infection (fever of 38.8°C [102°F] or more, pain, rapid pulse, malaise) because a pancreatic abscess can develop after initial recovery.

Refer to a dietitian or nutritionist for diet teaching as needed. If appropriate, refer to community agencies, such as Alcoholics Anonymous, or to an alcohol treatment program. Provide referrals to community or home health agencies as needed for continued monitoring and teaching at home.

Management of chronic pancreatitis focuses on management of symptoms related to irreversible damage to the pancreas. Patients typically present with complaints of pain and weight loss. Many of the interventions used for acute pancreatitis apply to chronic pancreatitis. The nursing role will focus on assisting the patient and caregiver to address nutrition and pain management. Pancreatic enzymes may be prescribed and typically restores reabsorption of fat and leads to weight gain. Pain management is a major focus of care in chronic pancreatitis. The patient may require referral to a pain specialist.

Case Study & Nursing Care Plan

A Patient with Acute Pancreatitis

Rose Schliefer is a 59-year-old wife, mother of three, and grandmother of four. She has been hospitalized for the past 6 weeks for acute hemorrhagic pancreatitis and pseudocyst. The pancreatitis was caused by gallstones. Mrs. Schliefer spent 3 weeks in intensive care and then underwent surgery to remove the gallstones and to insert drains into the pseudocyst. Prior to discharge, she had progressed to a soft, high-carbohydrate, low-fat diet; had all drains removed; and was able to walk in the hall. Mrs. Schliefer was referred to a community health agency in her hometown for continued follow-up.

ASSESSMENT

Lee Quinn, the community health nurse, assesses Mrs. Schliefer at home after discharge. Mrs. Schliefer is thin and appears anxious and tired. She states that she lost 13.6 kg (30 lb) in the hospital and now weighs only 46 kg (102 lb). She is 168 cm (66 in.) tall. Her vital signs are within normal limits. Mrs. Schliefer has a well-healed upper abdominal scar and two small wounds (from drains) on each side of her abdomen. The wounds are closed but still have scabs. Her skin is cool and dry, and turgor is poor. She is alert and oriented and responds appropriately to questions. Blood glucose levels are normal. Mrs. Schliefer states that her main problems are lack of energy and lack of appetite for the low-fat diet that has been ordered. Mrs. Schliefer's husband and daughters express concern about their ability to provide care. Although they have been taught all about the disease and how to provide care, they are still not sure they know exactly what should be done now that Mrs. Schliefer is at home.

DIAGNOSES

- Fatigue related to decreased metabolic energy production
- Promote adequate nutrition related to prolonged hospitalization, dietary restrictions, and impaired digestion
- Challenges performing ADLs related to decreased strength and endurance
- Support and teach the caregiver appropriate tasks

EXPECTED OUTCOMES

- Patient will set priorities for daily and weekly activities, and incorporate a rest period into daily activity.
- Patient will gain 0.5 to 1 kg (1 to 2 lb) per week.
- Patient will bathe and maintain personal hygiene without assistance.
- Family members will verbalize comfort with providing necessary care.

PLANNING AND IMPLEMENTATION

- Explain causes of fatigue. Review effects of pancreatitis, surgery, and acute illness on energy levels.
- Develop activity goals, incorporating small, incremental steps toward achieving goals. Mrs. Schliefer indicates that she wants to cook a meal for the whole family. To reach this goal, she will do the following:
  a. Schedule the meal when her energy level is highest.
  b. List actions necessary to prepare the meal and delegate difficult tasks to family members.
  c. Ask daughters to reorganize the kitchen to avoid unnecessary steps.
  d. Plan the meal no sooner than the third week after being home.
- Instruct her to do the following:
  a. Rest in bed each day from 1:00 p.m. to 3:00 p.m.
  b. Eat six small meals a day with family members or friends.
  c. Sit and rest quietly for 15 minutes before eating.
- Discuss dietary restrictions and how to adapt them to usual diet.
- Advise to use shower chair and develop self-care goals for bathing and hygiene in small steps. Add self-care tasks gradually as tolerated.
- Discuss division of responsibilities for physical care, home maintenance, and medical care with family members.
- Encourage family discussion of concerns about future; acknowledge family strengths.

EVALUATION

One month after discharge, Mrs. Schliefer and her family have established new routines based on her energy levels. Mrs. Schliefer now fixes lunch because she feels best during midday. She and her husband share this time together without interruption. Mrs. Schliefer still rests during the day but can now provide self-care. She has gained only 1 kg (2 lb), but states that she is getting used to the new diet and that "things are even starting to taste good without butter." She says that sitting quietly before meals is helpful and that she prefers eating six small meals a day. Mr. and Mrs. Schliefer and their daughters agree that their initial worries about Mrs. Schliefer's care have been resolved; now they all know what they must do, and the future looks much brighter.

CLINICAL REASONING IN PATIENT CARE

1. Your patient with acute pancreatitis also abuses alcohol. Describe assessments that indicate the beginnings of withdrawal.
2. Discuss the pathophysiologic basis of hypovolemic shock in acute necrotic pancreatitis.
3. Outline a teaching plan that includes specific foods to omit and to include in a high-carbohydrate, low-protein, low-fat diet.
4. Develop a plan of care for the problem with weakness/fatigue and inability to perform self-care activities.

See Evaluating Your Response in Appendix B.

The Patient with Pancreatic Cancer

Cancer is the fourth leading cause of cancer deaths in the United States and is one of the most lethal cancers: The 5-year survival rate is only about 6%. The prevalence of new cases occurring in the United States has been increasing by 1% per year, with approximately 43,090 deaths from cancer of the pancreas in 2017 (ACS, 2017). The incidence of pancreatic cancer increases after age 50. The incidence is higher in Blacks than in Whites.

Risk Factors

Identified risk factors for pancreatic cancer include:

- Cigarette smoking—the incidence is twice as high in smokers as in nonsmokers
- Chronic pancreatitis
- Diabetes mellitus
- Cirrhosis
- Obesity; high-fat diet, possibly red meat consumption
- Genetic predisposition.

In contrast to acute and chronic pancreatitis, alcohol abuse and gallstones are not identified risk factors for pancreatic cancer.

Pathophysiology and Manifestations

Most cancers of the pancreas occur in the exocrine pancreas, are adenocarcinomas, and are fatal within 1 to 3 years after diagnosis.

Cancer of the pancreas often causes few symptoms until advanced. Early manifestations are nonspecific, including anorexia, nausea, weight loss, flatulence, and dull epigastric pain. The pain increases in severity as the tumor grows. Other manifestations depend on the location of the tumor. Cancer of the head of the pancreas, which is the most common site, often obstructs bile flow through the common bile duct and the ampulla of Vater, resulting in jaundice, clay-colored stools, dark urine, and pruritus. Cancer of the body of the pancreas presses on the celiac ganglion, causing pain that increases when the person eats or lies supine. Cancer of the tail of the pancreas often causes no symptoms until it has metastasized. Other late manifestations include a palpable abdominal mass and ascites. Because the manifestations are nonspecific, up to 85% of patients with cancer of the pancreas do not seek healthcare until the cancer becomes too far advanced for a cure.

Interprofessional and Nursing Care

Early cancers of the head of the pancreas may be resectable. A *pancreatoduodenectomy* (commonly called *Whipple procedure*) is performed to remove the head of the pancreas, the entire duodenum, the distal third of the stomach, a portion of the jejunum, and the lower half of the common bile duct. The common bile duct is then sutured to the end of the jejunum, and the remaining pancreas and stomach are sutured to the side of the jejunum (**Figure 25.11** ■). Radiation and chemotherapy are often used in addition to surgery.

Preoperative care involves routine preoperative nursing care as ordered (see Chapter 4).

Be sure to clarify teaching and learning as needed and provide psychologic support for patient and family. The patient and family faced with a diagnosis of pancreatic cancer may require reinforcement of teaching because anxiety, fear, and possible denial can interfere with learning. Use agency standards and provide postoperative care as ordered (see Chapter 4).

The patient is at risk for respiratory complications because of the high abdominal surgical incision. The patient should be maintained in semi-Fowler position. The semi-Fowler position facilitates lung expansion and reduces stress on the anastomosis and suture line. The patient will return from the operating room with a nasogastric tube. Maintain low gastrointestinal suction and monitor the amount of drainage every 4 to 8 hours. If drainage is not adequate, obtain an order to irrigate, using minimal pressure. Do not reposition nasogastric tube as pressure within the operative area from retained secretions increases intraluminal

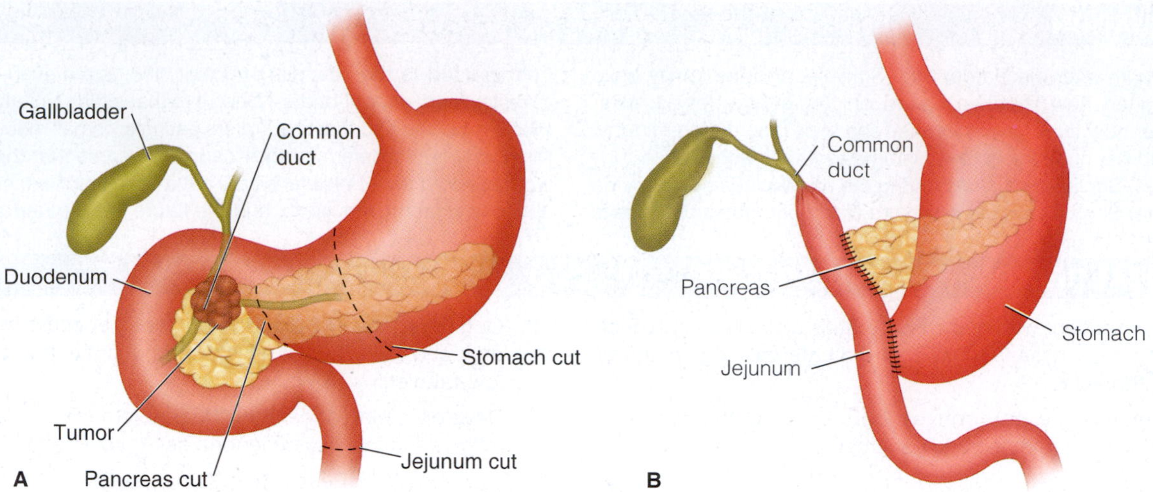
Gallbladder
Common duct
Duodenum
Stomach cut
Tumor
Pancreas cut
Jejunum cut
A
Common duct
Pancreas
Stomach
Jejunum
B

Figure 25.11 ■ Pancreatoduodenectomy (Whipple procedure). **A**, Areas of resection. **B**, Appearance following resection.

pressure and places stress on the suture line. Forceful irrigations and repositioning of the nasogastric tube may disrupt the suture line. Pain control will be a significant focus of care.

Maintain pain control using analgesics as prescribed (PCA, infusion, or given on a regular basis) and assess effectiveness of pain management. Doses higher than normal may be required if narcotic analgesics have been used prior to surgery to manage pain. Increased pain may indicate complications such as disruption of suture line, leakage from anastomosis, or peritonitis. Adequate pain management increases resistance to stress, facilitates healing, and increases the ability to cough, deep-breathe, and change position.

Promoting oxygenation is another focus of care. Assist with coughing, deep breathing, and changing position every 1 to 2 hours. Splint incision during coughing and deep breathing. The location of the incision makes coughing and deep breathing more painful. The prolonged surgical procedure, anesthesia, location of incision, and immobility increase the risk of retained secretions, atelectasis, and pneumonia. Changing position facilitates drainage of secretions; effective coughing and deep breathing remove secretions and open distal alveoli.

The major complications following Whipple's procedure are hemorrhage, bile leak, hypovolemic shock, and hepatorenal failure. The assessments listed provide information about the patient's status and alert the nurse to abnormal findings that signal the onset of these complications.

The patient with pancreatic cancer has multiple problems requiring nursing care. Chapter 14 provides a discussion of care of the patient with cancer; the nursing diagnoses and interventions discussed for the patient with pancreatitis are also appropriate for the patient with pancreatic cancer.

CHAPTER HIGHLIGHTS

25.1 Gallbladder Disorders

Describe the pathophysiology and manifestations of gallbladder disorders, and outline the interprofessional care and nursing care of patients with these disorders.

- Gallstones (cholelithiasis) are common and are often unrecognized until the patient develops manifestations of biliary colic or acute cholecystitis. Laparoscopic cholecystectomy is the treatment of choice for symptomatic gallbladder disease.
- Cancer of the gallbladder is rare and mimics the signs and symptoms associated with liver and pancreatic cancer. Survival rate depends on the stage of cancer at diagnosis.

25.2 Liver Disorders

Describe the pathophysiology and manifestations of liver disorders, and outline the interprofessional care and nursing care of patients with these disorders.

- Common manifestations of liver disorders are jaundice, malnutrition, weakness and fatigue, neurological changes, abnormal coagulation of the blood, and portal hypertension.
- Hepatitis, inflammation of functional liver tissue, is usually a viral disease and requires long-term treatment and monitoring. Preventing the spread of hepatitis through use of standard and body substance precautions is an important nursing responsibility.

- Hepatitis A, commonly transmitted via the fecal–oral route, is generally a self-limiting disease with few long-term sequelae. Some types of viral hepatitis, most notably hepatitis B and C, can become chronic and ultimately lead to liver failure and an increased risk for liver cancer. Hepatitis B and C can result in a carrier state in which the infected patient has no symptoms of the disease, but can spread it to others.
- Alcohol abuse is a significant risk factor for liver and pancreatic disorders. Prevention, early identification, and treatment of alcohol abuse reduce the risk of these disorders. Absolute abstinence from alcohol is an important part of the treatment plan for patients with liver and pancreatic disorders.
- Cirrhosis leads to portal hypertension and liver failure, which, in turn, account for most of the manifestations and complications of the disorder. Complications such as ascites, splenomegaly, esophageal varices, and portal systemic encephalopathy affect multiple body systems and significantly contribute to the mortality and morbidity associated with cirrhosis.
- Bleeding from esophageal varices may be massive, resulting in a medical emergency and requiring prompt control to maintain cardiac output.
- Liver cancer has a poor survival rate; early symptoms are often vague, delaying diagnosis. Weakness, weight loss, and abdominal bloating are early signs that are often ignored. Treatment depends of the size of the tumor and stage of the cancer.

25.3 Exocrine Pancreas Disorders

Describe the pathophysiology and manifestations of exocrine pancreas disorders, and outline the interprofessional care and nursing care of patients with these disorders.

- Acute pancreatitis often develops as a complication of gallstones. Acute pancreatitis often resolves with no long-term consequences. Chronic pancreatitis is more frequently related to alcohol abuse and can lead to continuing pain and digestive disruptions.
- All of the accessory organs of digestion (the gallbladder, liver, and pancreas) can be primary sites of malignancy. Cancer of the gallbladder is uncommon; hepatocellular and pancreatic cancers are more common and their incidence is increasing. These cancers are often advanced when diagnosed, reducing treatment options and the chance for cure.

TEST YOURSELF NCLEX-RN® REVIEW

1. A patient has been diagnosed with cholelithiasis. What should the nurse expect to assess in this patient? (Select all that apply.)
   A. A history of abrupt onset right upper quadrant pain
   B. Pain for the last 18 hours
   C. Chills and fever
   D. Recurrent heartburn and acid reflux
   E. Nausea and vomiting
2. The nurse is planning instruction for a patient with acute cholecystitis. What should this teaching include? (Select all that apply.)
   A. Surgery cannot be done if infection is present.
   B. Follow a low-carbohydrate diet for weight loss.
   C. Call the physician if severe abdominal pain and a temperature occur.
   D. Avoid consumption of foods high in fat such as gravies and peanut butter.
   E. Limit intake to dry crackers and clear liquids during episodes of acute pain.
3. The community health nurse has been asked to provide teaching to employees of a local restaurant about ways to reduce the incidence of hepatitis A after an outbreak of the disease was traced back to the restaurant. What should the nurse teach these employees to eliminate future outbreaks of the disease?
   A. Test all new employees for hepatitis A antigen.
   B. Use gloves for handling food if any cuts or scrapes are on hands.
   C. Wash hands thoroughly before handling food and after using the bathroom.
   D. Emphasize the need for all food handlers to be immunized against hepatitis A.
4. The nurse instructs a patient with chronic hepatitis C about the disease process. Which patient statement indicates that teaching has been effective?
   A. "I will avoid donating blood and will use barrier protection during sex."
   B. "I will reduce my alcohol intake and use only acetaminophen for pain relief."
   C. "Even though no treatment is available for this disease, I plan to live a long life."
   D. "I understand that I must return to the doctor every year for a follow-up liver biopsy."
5. The nurse is interviewing a patient with hepatitis A. The nurse will ask assessment questions about which priority concerns? (Select all that apply.)
   A. Immunization status
   B. Sexual partners
   C. Close household contacts
   D. Food preparation activities
   E. Presence of blood in feces

6. A patient with cirrhosis and esophageal varices vomits 200 mL of bright red blood. What should the nurse do first?
   A. Insert a nasogastric tube.
   B. Lower the head of the bed.
   C. Check stool for occult blood.
   D. Prepare for central line insertion.
7. A patient is having an abdominal paracentesis as an outpatient procedure. The nurse will provide which instruction?
   A. Empty the bladder before the procedure.
   B. Report excess flatus after the procedure to the physician.
   C. Scrub the abdomen with antiseptic soap before the procedure.
   D. Avoid eating or drinking fluid for 6 hours after the procedure.
8. A patient with cirrhosis and severe ascites develops a fever and confusion. What action will the nurse take?
   A. Inquire about headache and check for nuchal rigidity.
   B. Measure abdominal girth and percuss for shifting dullness.
   C. Observe for neck vein distention and auscultate lung sounds.
   D. Auscultate breath sounds and measure diaphragmatic excursion.
9. A patient is surprised to be diagnosed with acute pancreatitis because the patient reports no history of alcohol intake. How will the nurse respond to this patient?
   A. "Was there a time in your life that you did drink heavily?"
   B. "It is also prevalent in smokers; do you smoke cigarettes?"
   C. "Gallstones are also a risk factor. We'll evaluate for them."
   D. "Intravenous drug use is a risk factor. Do you use drugs by injection?"
10. The nurse is caring for a patient who just had a Whipple procedure. The nurse prioritizes which care? (Select all that apply.)
    A. Provide pain control.
    B. Stabilize the nasogastric tube.
    C. Ambulate within the first 6 hours following surgery.
    D. Maintain in semi-Fowler position.
    E. Turn frequently, encourage deep-breathing and coughing exercises.

See Test Yourself answers in Appendix B.

REFERENCES

Adams, M., Holland, N., & Urban, C. (2017). *Pharmacology for nurses: A pathophysiologic approach* (5th ed.). Hoboken, NJ: Pearson Education.

American Cancer Society. (2017). *Cancer facts and figures 2017*. Atlanta, GA: Author. Retrieved from https://www.cancer.org/content/dam/cancer-org/research/cancer-facts-and-statistics/annual-cancer-facts-and-figures/2017/cancer-facts-and-figures-2017.pdf.

Branstetter-Hall, J. E., & Felicilda-Reynaldo, R. F. (2017). Antiviral medication, Part 3: Evidence-based treatment of hepatitis B. *Medsurg Nursing, 26*(6), 393–398.

Centers for Disease Control and Prevention (CDC). (2016a). *Epidemiology and prevention of vaccine-preventable diseases* (12th ed.). Washington, DC: Public Health Foundation.

Centers for Disease Control and Prevention (CDC). (2016b). *Viral hepatitis surveillance, 2016.* Retrieved from https://www.cdc.gov/hepatitis/statistics/2016surveillance/index.htm.

Conwell, D. L., Banks, P., & Greenberger, N. J. (2014). Acute and chronic pancreatitis. In D. Kasper, A. Fauci, S. Hauser, D. Longo, J. Jameson, & J. Loscalzo (Eds.), *Harrison's principles of internal medicine* (19th ed.). New York, NY: McGraw-Hill. 2014. http://accessmedicine.mhmedical.com.liboff.ohsu.edu/content.aspx?bookid=1130&sectionid=79749276. Accessed May 21, 2018.

Cox-North, P., Doorenbos, A., Shannon, S. E., Scott, J., & Curtis, R. (2013). The transition to end-of-life care in end-stage liver disease. *Journal of Hospice and Palliative Care Nursing, 15*(3), 209–215.

Devendorf, C., Murray, C. & Sharp, M. (2018, March/April). What do you know about cholecystitis. *Nursing Made Incredibly Easy, 16*(2), 16–18.

Felicilda-Reynaldo, R. F. & Kenneally, M. (2016). Digestive enzyme replacement therapy: Pancreatic enzymes and lactase. *MedSurg Nursing, 25*(3), 182-185.

Felicilda-Reynaldo, R. F., & Patterson, K. A. (2018). Antiviral medications, part 4: Evidence-based treatment of hepatitis C. *Medsurg Nursing, 26*(6), 49–52.

Koman, D. (2018). Increasing hepatitis C virus knowledge through an evidence-based educational intervention. *Gastroenterology Nursing, 41*(2), 95–101.

Krenzer, M. E. (2016). Understanding acute pancreatitis. *Nursing, 45*(6), 35–40.

McClain, C. J. (2016). Nutrition in patients with cirrhosis. *Gastroenterology & Hepatology, 12*(8), 507–510.

Murphy, S. L., Xu, J. Q., Kochanek, K. D., Curtin, C. C., & Arias, D. (2017). Deaths: Final data for 2010. *National Vital Statistics Reports, 66*(6). Hyattsville, MD: National Center for Health Statistics.

National Center for Complementary and Integrative Health. (2018). *Hepatitis C and dietary supplements.* Retrieved from https://nccih.nih.gov/health/hepatitisc/hepatitiscfacts.htm.

Pak, M., & Lindseth, G. (2016). Risk factors for cholelithiasis. *Gastroenterology Nursing, 39*(4), 297–309.

Perrin, K. O., & MacLeod, C. E. (2018). *Understanding the essentials of critical care nursing* (3rd ed.). Hoboken, NJ: Pearson Education.

Phillips, F. H., & Barnes, D. M. (2016). Meaning of adherence in hepatitis C-infected military veterans. *Gastroenterology Nursing, 39*(1), 17–23.

Polis, S., Zablotska-Manos, I., Zekry, A., & Maher, L. (2017). Adherence to hepatitis B antiviral therapy. *Gastroenterology Nursing, 40*(3), 239–245.

Putiri, A. L., Close, J. R., Lilly, H. R., Guillaume, N., & Sun, G.-C. (2017). Qigong exercises for the management of type 2 diabetes mellitus. *Medicines, 4*(3), 59.

Redulla, R. R., Rajender, K. Faust, T. W., & Dudley-Brown, S. (2015). Project P.E.A.C.H. (Pathway and Education toward Adherence and Completion in Hepatitis C Therapy): A nurse-driven evidence-based protocol. *Gastroenterology Nursing, 38*(5), 369–378.

Sebhatu, P., & Martin, M. (2016). Genotype 1 hepatitis C virus and the pharmacist's role in treatment. *American Journal of Health System Pharmacists, 73*(11), 764–774.

Sorenson, M., Quinn, L., & Klein, D. (2019). *Pathophysiology: Concepts of human disease.* Hoboken, NJ: Pearson Education.

Terrault, N. A., Bzowej, N. H., Chang, K. M., Hwang, J., & Murad, M. (2016). AASLD guidelines for treating hepatitis B: Practice guidelines. *Hepatology 63*(1), 261–283.

Walker, B. W. (2018). Hepatitis A infections: On alert for outbreaks. *Nursing 2018, 48*(4), 66–69.

Yildirim, M. (2017). Falls in patients with liver cirrhosis. *Gastroenterology Nursing, 105*(4), 306–310.

ADDITIONAL RESOURCES

Alcoholics Anonymous
www.aa.org

American Gastroenterological Association
www.gastro.org

American Liver Foundation
www.liverfoundation.org

Cancer Treatment Centers of America, Pancreatic Cancer
www.cancercenter.com/pancreatic-cancer/risk-factors

Chronic Liver Disease Foundation
www.chronicliverdisease.org

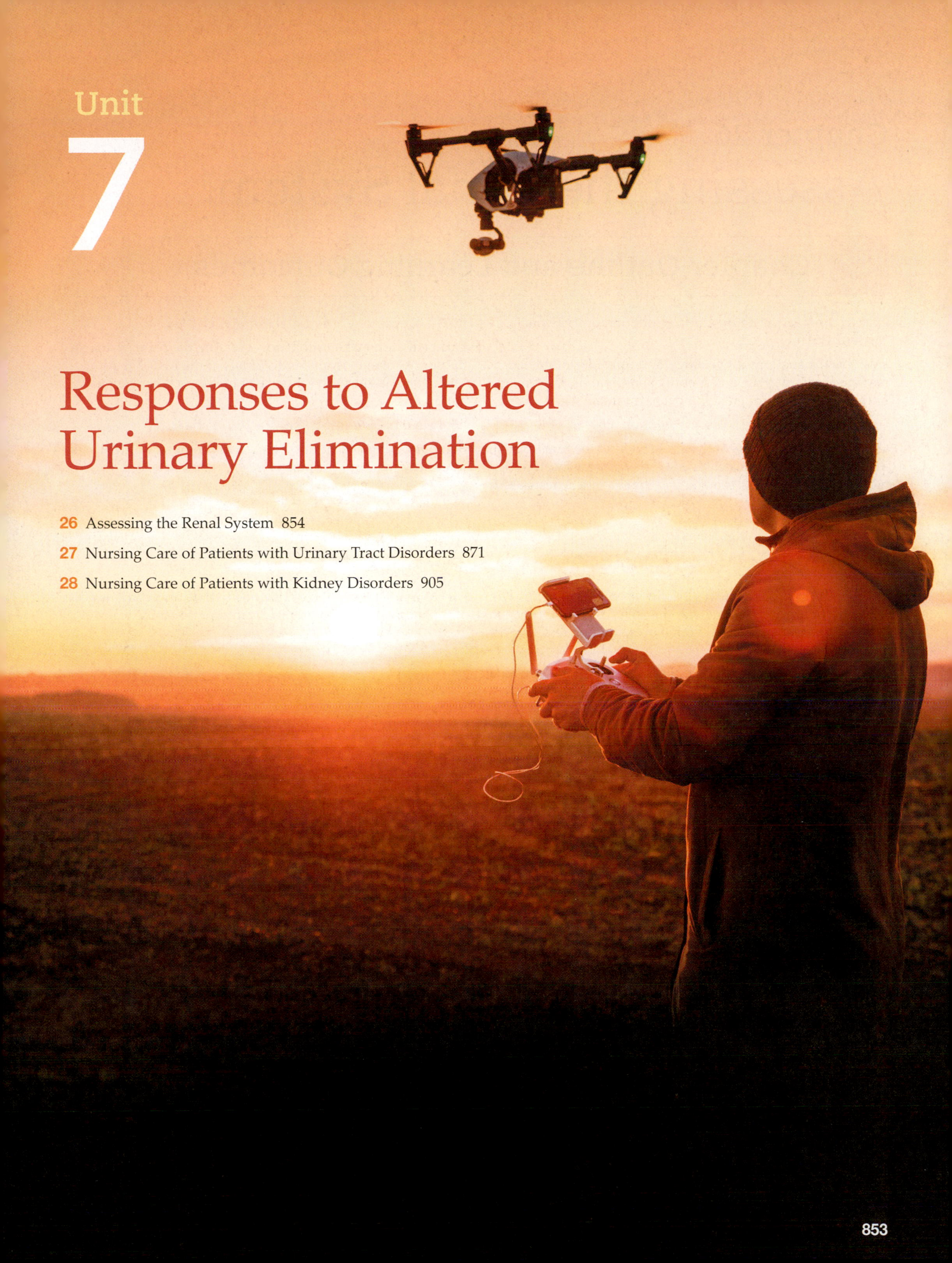

Unit

7

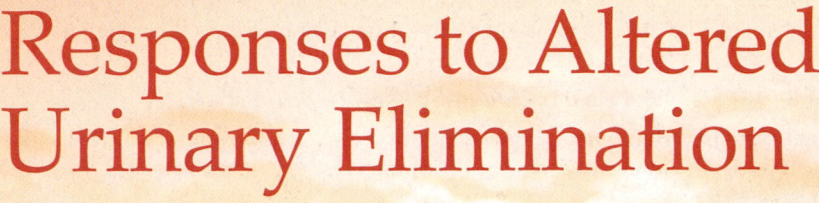

Responses to Altered Urinary Elimination

Chapter 26

Assessing the Renal System

Chapter Outline and Learning Outcomes

CLINICAL COMPETENCIES

- Conduct and document a health history for patients who have or are at risk for alterations in renal system function, eliciting patient values, preferences, and expressed needs as part of the interview.
- Conduct and document a physical assessment of the renal system, demonstrating sensitivity and respect for the diversity of human experience.
- Monitor the results of diagnostic tests and communicate abnormal findings within the interprofessional team.

KEY TERMS

dysuria, 860
glomerular filtration rate (GFR), 857
hematuria, 857
micturition, 859
nocturia, 867
urea, 858

EQUIPMENT NEEDED

- Urine specimen container
- Disposable gloves
- Stethoscope.

The functions of the *renal system*, or *urinary system*, are to regulate body fluids, to filter metabolic wastes from the bloodstream, to reabsorb needed substances and water into the bloodstream, and to eliminate metabolic wastes and water as urine. Disorders of the renal system affect the whole body and may result in alterations in fluid and electrolyte balance, cardiovascular function, and nutritional status. In turn, healthy renal system function depends on the health of other body systems, especially the circulatory, endocrine, and nervous systems.

26.1 Anatomy, Physiology, and Functions of the Renal System

The organs of the renal system are the paired kidneys, the paired ureters, the urinary bladder, and the urethra (**Figure 26.1** ■). Each structure is essential to the total functioning of the renal system.

The Kidneys

The two *kidneys* are located outside the peritoneal cavity and on either side of the vertebral column at the levels of T_{12} through L_3. These highly vascular, bean-shaped organs are approximately 11.4 cm (4.5 in.) long and 6.4 cm (2.5 in.) wide. The lateral surface of the kidney is convex; the medial surface is concave and forms a vertical cleft, the *hilum*. The ureter, renal artery, renal vein, lymphatic vessels, and nerves enter or exit the kidney at the level of the hilum.

Internally, each kidney has three distinct regions: The cortex, medulla, and pelvis. The outer region, or *renal cortex*, is light in color and has a granular appearance (**Figure 26.2** ■). This region of the kidney contains the *nephrons*, the functional units of the kidney.

The *renal medulla*, just below the cortex, contains cone-shaped tissue masses called *renal pyramids*, formed almost entirely of bundles of collecting tubules. The collecting tubules that make up the pyramids channel urine into the calyces and the innermost region, the *renal pelvis*. The renal pelvis is continuous with the ureter as it leaves the hilum. The *calyces* serve to collect urine and empty it into the pelvis. From the pelvis, urine is channeled through the ureter and into the bladder for storage. The walls of the calyces, the renal pelvis, and the ureter contain smooth muscle that moves urine along by peristalsis.

Formation of Urine

Each kidney contains approximately 1 million *nephrons*, which process the blood to make urine (**Figure 26.3** ■). Each nephron consists of a glomerulus, a tuft of capillaries,

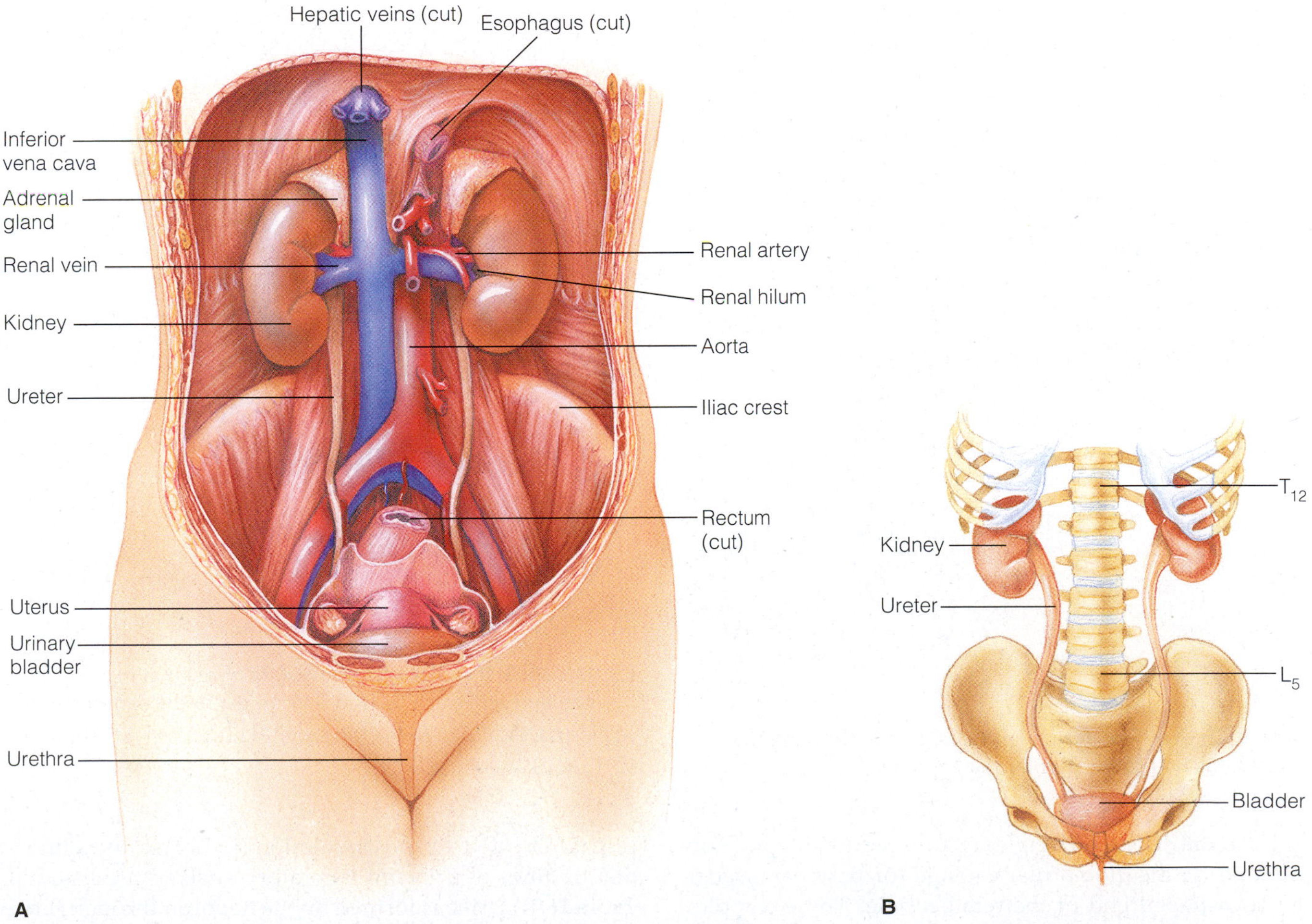
Hepatic veins (cut)
Esophagus (cut)
Inferior vena cava
Adrenal gland
Renal vein
Kidney
Ureter
Renal artery
Renal hilum
Aorta
Iliac crest
Rectum (cut)
Uterus
Urinary bladder
Urethra
A
T12
Kidney
Ureter
L5
Bladder
Urethra
B

Figure 26.1 ■ The renal system. **A**, Anterior view of the renal system in a female. **B**, The kidneys are shown in relation to the vertebrae and ribs.

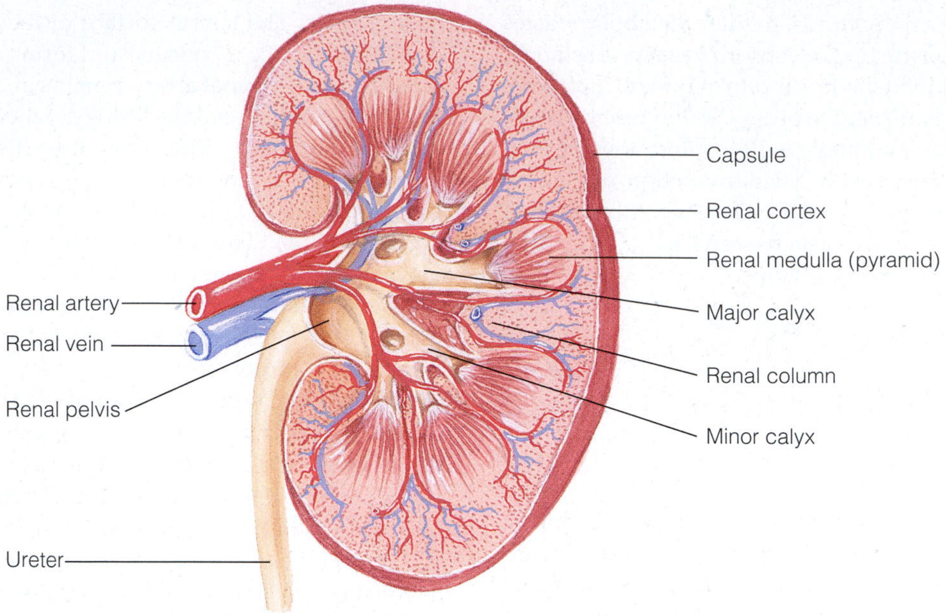
Capsule
Renal cortex
Renal medulla (pyramid)
Major calyx
Renal column
Minor calyx
Renal artery
Renal vein
Renal pelvis
Ureter

Figure 26.2 ■ Internal anatomy of the kidney.

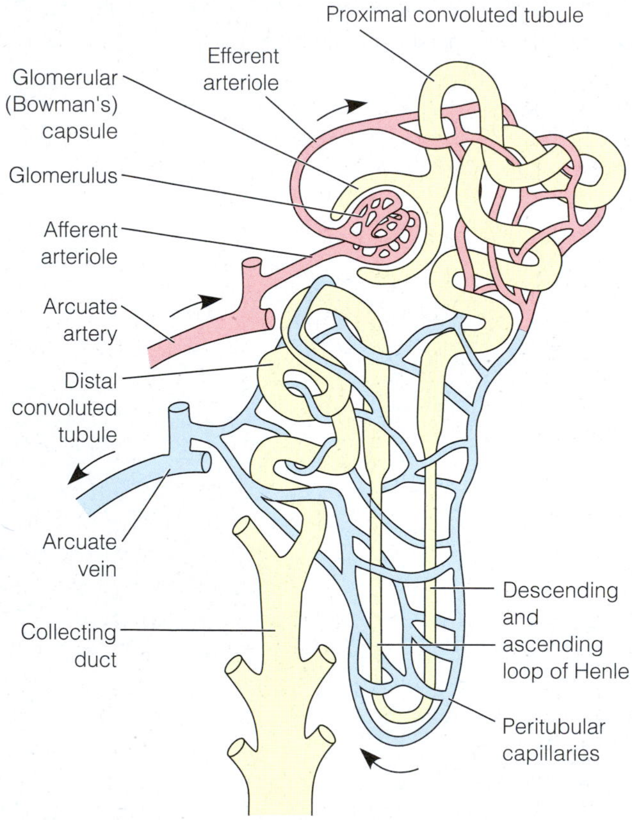
Proximal convoluted tubule
Efferent arteriole
Glomerular (Bowman's) capsule
Glomerulus
Afferent arteriole
Arcuate artery
Distal convoluted tubule
Arcuate vein
Collecting duct
Descending and ascending loop of Henle
Peritubular capillaries

Figure 26.3 ■ The structure of a nephron, showing the glomerulus within the glomerular capsule.

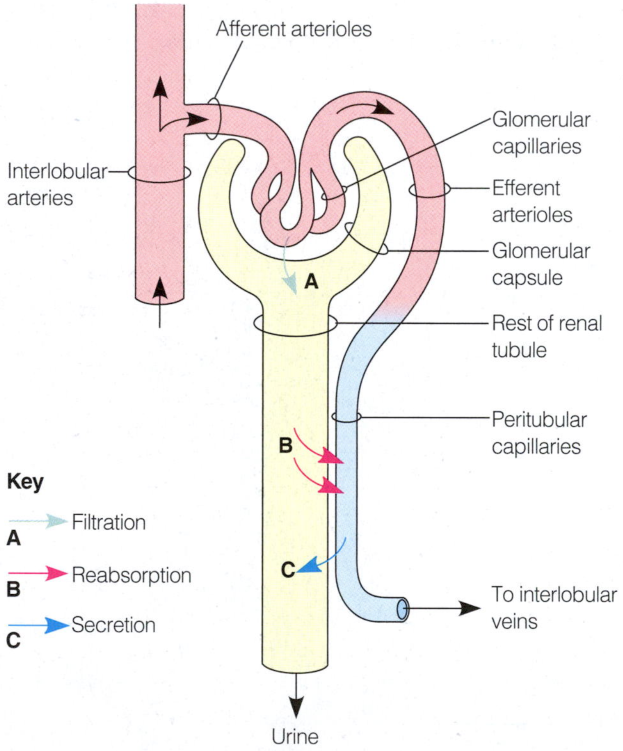
Afferent arterioles
Interlobular arteries
Glomerular capillaries
Efferent arterioles
Glomerular capsule
Rest of renal tubule
Peritubular capillaries
A
B
C
Key
A Filtration
B Reabsorption
C Secretion
To interlobular veins
Urine

Figure 26.4 ■ Schematic view of the three major mechanisms by which the kidneys adjust to the composition of plasma. **A.** Glomerular filtration. **B.** Tubular reabsorption. **C.** Tubular secretion.

and a renal tubule. The glomerulus is completely surrounded by the glomerular capsule (or Bowman space), the cup-shaped end of the renal tubule. These complex structures process about 180 L (47 gal) of filtrate each day. Of this amount, only 1% is excreted as urine; the rest is returned to the circulation. (Normal and abnormal findings of urine on laboratory analysis are listed in **Table 26.1**.) Urine is formed by the nephron through three processes: Glomerular filtration, tubular reabsorption, and tubular secretion (**Figure 26.4** ■).

Table 26.1 Normal Results and Abnormal Findings: Urinalysis

Characteristic or Component	Normal Results	Abnormal Findings with Possible Cause
Color	Light straw to amber yellow	■ Red, dark, smoky color may be the result of blood in the urine (**hematuria** or menstrual blood). ■ Cloudy urine occurs from infection (pyuria). ■ Colorless indicates very dilute urine, such as in overhydration, kidney disease, alcohol ingestion, or diabetes insipidus. ■ Very dark yellow urine indicates dehydration and/or fever. ■ Red or red brown urine may be caused by sulfisoxazole-phenazopyridine (Azo Gantrisin), phenytoin (Dilantin), cascara, chlorpromazine (Thorazine), docusate calcium, and phenolphthalein (Doxidan) and by carrots, rhubarb, and food coloring. ■ Orange urine is caused by fever, urobilin, phenazopyridine (Pyridium), amidopyrine, nitrofurantoin, and sulfonamides and carrots, beets, and food coloring. ■ Blue or green urine is caused by *Pseudomonas*, amitriptyline (Elavil), methylene blue, methocarbamol (Robaxin), and yeast concentrate. ■ Brown or black urine is caused by Lysol poisoning, melanin, bilirubin, methemoglobin, porphyrin, cascara, and injectable iron.
Appearance	Clear	■ Hazy or cloudy urine indicates bacteria, pus, RBCs, WBCs, phosphates, prostatic fluid spermatozoa, or urates. ■ Milky urine is the result of fats or pyuria. ■ Yellow foam results from bilirubin, bile, or severe cirrhosis of the liver. ■ A dark yellow to brownish color is seen with deficient fluid volume.
Odor	Aromatic	■ Ammonia smell increases as urine stands outside the body. ■ Urinary tract infection (UTI) causes a foul or unpleasant odor, depending on the causative organism. ■ Asparagus causes a distinctive odor. ■ Mousy odors result from phenylketonuria. ■ Sweet or fruity odors occur in starvation and diabetic ketoacidosis.
pH	4.5–8.0	■ Less than 4.5: Metabolic acidosis, respiratory acidosis, diet high in meat protein, ammonium chloride, and mandelic acid ■ More than 8.0: Bacteriuria, UTI, antibiotics (neomycin, kanamycin), sulfonamides, sodium bicarbonate, acetazolamide (Diamox), potassium citrate
Specific gravity	1.005–1.030	■ Less than 1.005: Diabetes insipidus, overhydration, renal disease, severe potassium deficit ■ More than 1.030: Dehydration, fever, diabetes mellitus, vomiting, diarrhea, contrast media
Protein	0–5 mg/dL	■ More than 5 mg/dL: Proteinuria, exercise, fever, stress, acute infection, kidney disease, lupus erythematosus, leukemia, multiple myeloma, cardiac disease, toxemia of pregnancy, septicemia, lead, mercury, neomycin, barbiturates, sulfonamides
Glucose	Negative	■ More than 15 mg/dL or +4: Diabetes mellitus, stroke, Cushing syndrome, anesthesia, glucose infusions, severe stress, infections, ascorbic acid, aspirin, cephalosporins, and epinephrine
Ketones	Negative	■ +1 to 3: Ketoacidosis, starvation, high-protein diet
RBCs	Rare	■ More than 2 per low-power field: Kidney trauma, kidney diseases, renal calculi, cystitis, excess aspirin, anticoagulants, sulfonamides, menstrual contamination
WBCs	3–4	■ More than 4 per low-power field: UTI, fever, strenuous exercise, kidney diseases
Casts	Occasional hyaline	■ Fever, kidney diseases, heart failure

Glomerular Filtration

Glomerular filtration is a passive process in which hydrostatic pressure forces fluid and solutes out of glomerular capillaries and into the surrounding capsule. The amount of filtrate produced by the kidneys per minute is called the **glomerular filtration rate (GFR)**. Three factors influence this rate: The number of functional nephrons, the permeability of the filtration membrane (composed of capillary endothelium, basement membrane, and capsular epithelium), and the net filtration pressure.

Two forces determine net filtration pressure: Hydrostatic pressure (push) and osmotic pressure (pull). Glomerular hydrostatic pressure pushes water and solutes across the filtration membrane. This pressure is opposed by the osmotic pressure in the glomerulus (primarily the colloid osmotic pressure of plasma proteins in the blood) and the capsular hydrostatic pressure exerted by fluids within the glomerular capsule. The difference between these forces determines the net filtration pressure, which is directly proportional to the GFR.

The normal GFR in adults is 120 to 125 mL/min. This rate is held constant under normal conditions by renal autoregulation. The myogenic mechanism, one factor in renal autoregulation, responds to pressure changes in the renal blood vessels, controlling the diameter of afferent arterioles. An increase in systemic blood pressure causes the renal vessels to constrict, whereas a decrease in blood pressure causes the afferent arterioles to dilate. These changes adjust glomerular hydrostatic pressure and, indirectly, maintain the GFR.

Hormones of the renin–angiotensin–aldosterone system also regulate the GFR (Sorenson, Quinn, & Klein, 2019). The juxtaglomerular apparatus, located in the distal tubules, responds to stimuli such as the systemic blood pressure and the flow and NaCl concentration of filtrate. A sustained drop in systemic blood pressure triggers the juxtaglomerular cells to release renin. Renin acts on a plasma globulin, angiotensinogen, to release angiotensin I, which is in turn converted to angiotensin II. As a vasoconstrictor, angiotensin II activates vascular smooth muscle throughout the body, causing systemic blood pressure to rise.

Glomerular filtration is also controlled by the sympathetic nervous system (SNS). During periods of stress or emergency, SNS stimulation constricts the afferent arterioles and inhibits filtrate formation. The SNS also stimulates the juxtaglomerular cells to release renin, increasing systemic blood pressure.

Tubular Reabsorption

Tubular reabsorption occurs as the filtrate moves through the tubules and into the collecting ducts. In healthy kidneys, almost all organic nutrients such as glucose and amino acids are reabsorbed. However, the tubules constantly regulate and adjust the rate and degree of water and ion reabsorption in response to hormonal signals. Reabsorption may be active or passive. Substances reclaimed through active tubular reabsorption are usually moving against electrical and/or chemical gradients. These substances, including glucose, amino acids, lactate, vitamins, and most ions, require an ATP-dependent carrier to be transported into the interstitial space. In passive tubular reabsorption, which includes diffusion and osmosis, substances move along their gradient without expenditure of energy.

Tubular Secretion

The final process in urine formation is tubular secretion, which is essentially reabsorption in reverse. Substances such as hydrogen and potassium ions, creatinine, ammonia, and organic acids move from the blood of the peritubular capillaries into the tubules themselves. Thus, urine consists of both filtered and secreted substances. Tubular secretion is important for disposing of substances not already in the filtrate, such as medications. This process eliminates undesirable substances that have been reabsorbed by passive processes and rids the body of excessive potassium ions. It is also a vital force in the regulation of blood pH.

Maintaining Normal Composition and Volume of Urine

Urine is composed, by volume, of about 95% water and 5% solutes. The largest component of urine by weight is **urea** (a nitrogenous waste product formed in the liver from the breakdown of amino acids). Other solutes normally excreted in the urine include sodium, potassium, phosphate, sulfate, creatinine, uric acid, calcium, magnesium, and bicarbonate.

Maintaining the normal composition and volume of urine involves a countercurrent exchange system. In this system, fluid flows in opposite directions through the parallel tubes of the loop of Henle and the vasa recta, tiny capillaries that run along the loop of Henle. Fluid and solutes are exchanged across these parallel membranes in response to a concentration gradient (**Figure 26.5** ■). As the filtrate then flows through the collecting ducts and deep medullary

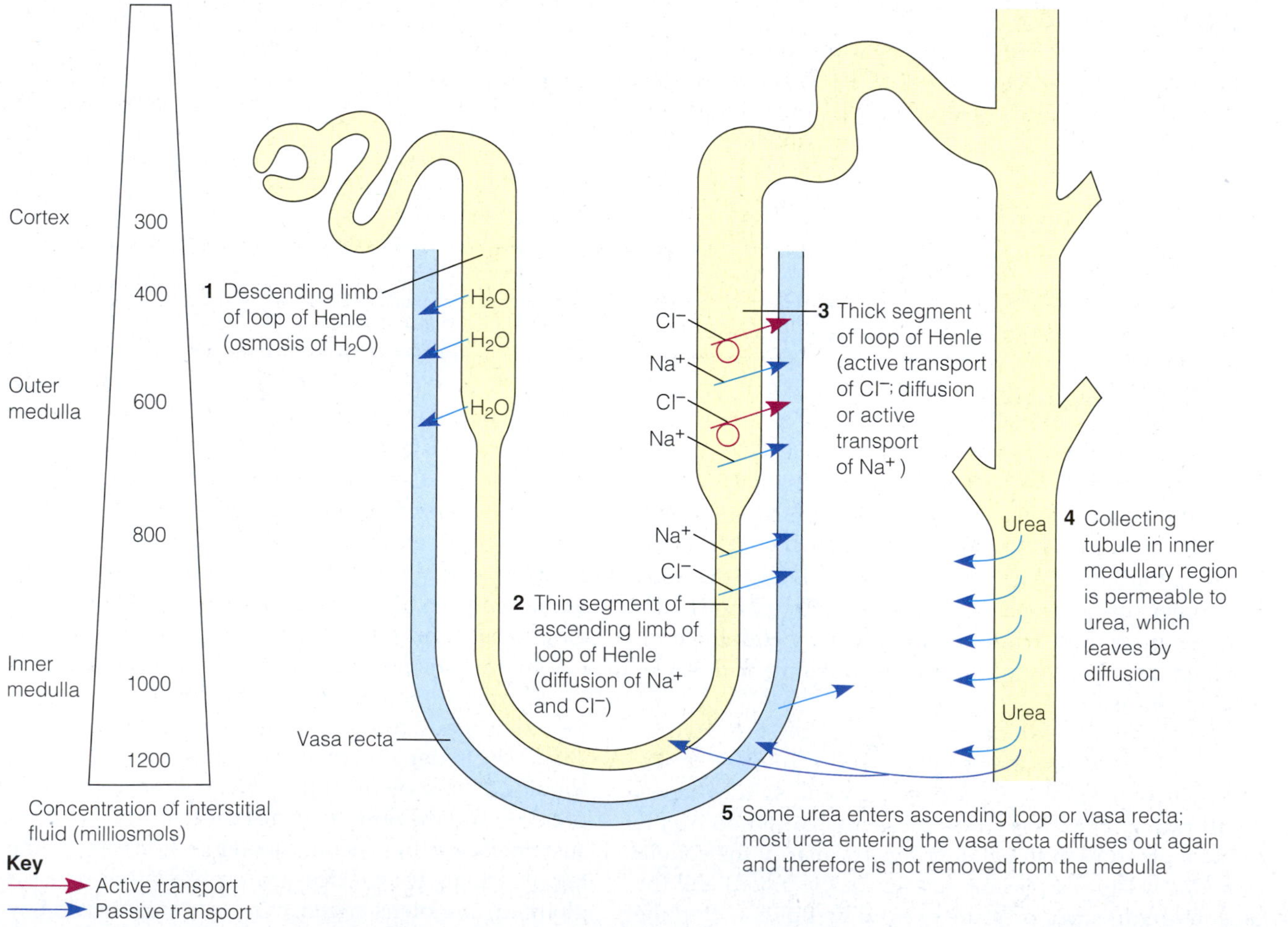
Cortex
300
400
Outer medulla
600
800
Inner medulla
1000
1200
Concentration of interstitial fluid (milliosmols)
1 Descending limb of loop of Henle (osmosis of H_2O)
H_2O
H_2O
H_2O
Cl^-
Na^+
Cl^-
Na^+
3 Thick segment of loop of Henle (active transport of Cl^-; diffusion or active transport of Na^+)
Na^+
Cl^-
2 Thin segment of ascending limb of loop of Henle (diffusion of Na^+ and Cl^-)
Vasa recta
Urea
Urea
4 Collecting tubule in inner medullary region is permeable to urea, which leaves by diffusion
5 Some urea enters ascending loop or vasa recta; most urea entering the vasa recta diffuses out again and therefore is not removed from the medulla
Key
Active transport
Passive transport

Figure 26.5 ■ The countercurrent exchange system is responsible for establishing and maintaining the osmotic gradient necessary for the composition, volume, and pH of urine.

regions of the kidney, water and urea are reabsorbed. The dilution or concentration of urine is largely determined by antidiuretic hormone (ADH), secreted by the posterior pituitary gland in response to blood volume and serum osmolality. When serum osmolality increases or blood volume falls, ADH is secreted. Pores of the collecting tubules enlarge in response, and more water is reabsorbed. When serum osmolality falls, ADH is not secreted and the filtrate passes through the system without further water reabsorption, and urine is more dilute.

Renal Clearance

The kidneys excrete water-soluble waste products and other chemicals or substances from the body. This process is called *renal clearance*, which refers to the volume of plasma that is cleared (or cleansed) of a particular substance in a given time (usually 1 minute). The kidneys clear 25 to 30 g of urea each day. They also clear creatinine (an end product of creatine phosphate, found in skeletal muscle), uric acid (a metabolite of nucleic acid metabolism), and ammonia as well as bacterial toxins and water-soluble drugs. Tests of renal clearance are done to determine the GFR and kidney function.

Renal Hormones

Hormones either activated or synthesized by the kidneys include the active form of vitamin D, erythropoietin, and natriuretic hormone.

Vitamin D is necessary for the absorption of calcium and phosphate by the small intestine. In an inactive form, vitamin D enters the body either by dietary intake or through the action of ultraviolet rays on cholesterol in the skin. Activation occurs in two steps, the first in the liver and the second in the kidneys. The renal step is stimulated by parathyroid hormone, which in turn responds to a decreased plasma calcium level.

Erythropoietin stimulates the bone marrow to produce red blood cells in response to tissue hypoxia. The stimulus for the production of erythropoietin by the kidneys is decreased oxygen delivery to kidney cells.

The right atria of the heart releases natriuretic hormone in response to increased volume and stretch, as occurs in increased extracellular volume. This hormone inhibits ADH secretion, so that the collecting tubules are less porous and a large amount of dilute urine is produced.

The Ureters, Urinary Bladder, and Urethra

The ureters are bilateral tubes approximately 26 to 30 cm (10 to 12 in.) long. They transport urine from the kidney to the bladder through peristaltic waves originating in the renal pelvis. The wall of the ureter has three layers: An inner epithelial mucosa, a middle layer of smooth muscle, and an outer layer of fibrous connective tissue. The urinary bladder is posterior to the symphysis pubis and serves as a storage site for urine. In males, the bladder lies immediately in front of the rectum; in females, the bladder lies in front of the vagina and the uterus. Openings for the ureters and the urethra are inside the bladder. The *trigone* is the smooth triangular portion of the base of the bladder outlined by the openings for the ureters and urethra (**Figure 26.6** ■).

The size of the bladder varies with the amount of urine it contains. In healthy adults, the bladder holds about 300 to 500 mL of urine before internal pressure rises and signals the need to empty the bladder through **micturition** (urination or voiding). However, the bladder can hold more than twice that amount if necessary. The bladder has an internal urethral sphincter that relaxes in response to a full bladder and signals the need to urinate. A second external urethral sphincter is formed by skeletal muscle and is under voluntary control.

The urethra is a thin-walled muscular tube that channels urine to the outside of the body. It extends from the base of the bladder to the external urinary meatus. In males, the urethra is approximately 20 cm (8 in.) long and serves as a channel for semen as well as urine (refer to Figure 26.6A). The prostate gland encircles the urethra at the base of the bladder in males. The male urinary meatus is located at the end of the glans penis. In females, the urethra is approximately 3 to 5 cm (1.5 in.) long, and the urinary meatus is anterior to the vaginal orifice (refer to Figure 26.6B).

26.2 Assessing Renal System Function

Renal system function is assessed by a health assessment interview to collect subjective data and identify genetic considerations, a physical assessment to collect objective data, and findings from diagnostic tests.

Health Assessment Interview

A health assessment interview to determine problems with renal system structure and function may be conducted during a health screening, may focus on a chief complaint (such as burning on urination or difficulty starting the stream when urinating), or may be part of a total health assessment (Bickley, 2016). Patients with problems affecting renal system function may be embarrassed to talk about urinary elimination patterns. It is often helpful to discuss less personal information first.

Assess the patient's current urinary elimination status. Focus questions on changes in patterns of urination, changes in the urine, and pain. Assess changes in patterns of urination by asking the patient questions such as:

- Have you noticed any changes from your normal urination problems?
- "How many times a day do you urinate?"
- "Do you feel that you empty your bladder each time?"
- "How many times do you get up at night to urinate?"
- "Do you experience a very strong desire to urinate and feel that you just cannot wait?"
- "Have you noticed that you urinate small amounts of dark, strong-smelling urine?"

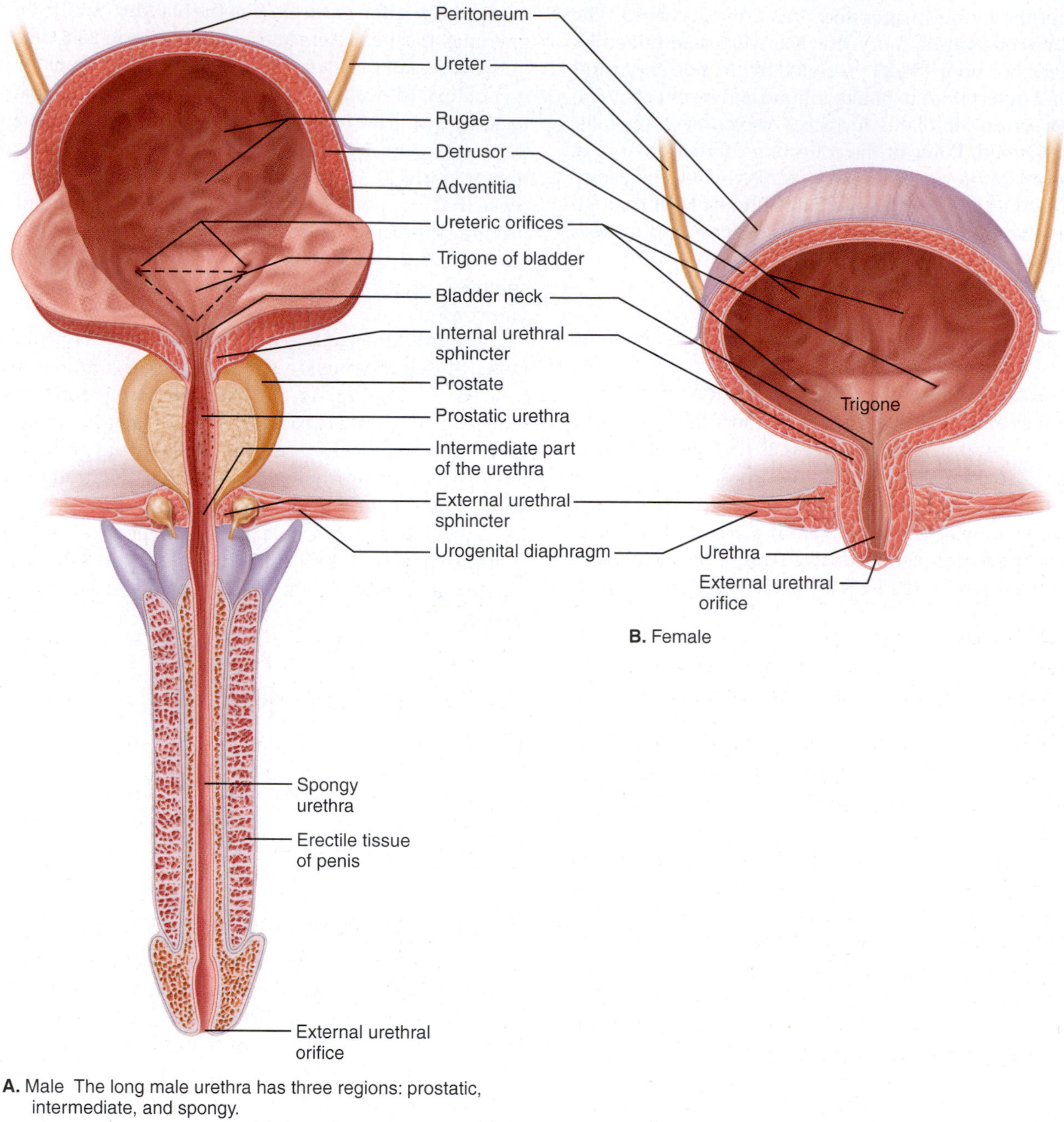
Peritoneum
Ureter
Rugae
Detrusor
Adventitia
Ureteric orifices
Trigone of bladder
Bladder neck
Internal urethral sphincter
Prostate
Prostatic urethra
Intermediate part of the urethra
External urethral sphincter
Urogenital diaphragm
Spongy urethra
Erectile tissue of penis
External urethral orifice
A. Male The long male urethra has three regions: prostatic, intermediate, and spongy.
Trigone
Urethra
External urethral orifice
B. Female

Figure 26.6 ■ The urinary bladder, trigone, urethra, and surrounding structures of **A**, the male, and **B**, the female. The long male urethra has three regions: Prostatic, intermediate, and spongy.

- Has anyone in your family had a kidney disease or urinary problem?
- Have you ever been diagnosed with a disease or illness of the kidney or bladder?

Changes in the urine that should be explored include the presence of blood or a cloudy appearance. If the patient has noticed blood, explore the use of medications (such as anticoagulants or dye-containing drugs) or bleeding problems. Cloudy, foul-smelling urine often indicates infection (pyuria); ask the patient about temperature elevations, chills, and general malaise. Cloudy urine in men may result from retrograde ejaculation (when semen is discharged into the bladder instead of from the penis) during intercourse.

If the patient reports pain, explore its location, duration, and intensity. Kidney pain is experienced in the back and the costovertebral angle (the angle between the lower ribs and adjacent vertebrae) and may spread toward the umbilicus. Renal colic (pain in response to renal calculi moving through the ureter) is severe, sharp, stabbing, and excruciating; it is often felt in the flank, bladder, urethra, testes, or ovaries. Bladder and urethral pain is usually dull and continuous but may be experienced as spasms. The patient with a distended bladder experiences constant pain increased by any pressure over the bladder. Pain experienced during voiding (**dysuria**) is often associated with urinary tract infection.

Information about surgeries or other treatment of previous renal problems is essential to the health history, as is a family history of altered structure or function. Explore information regarding family occurrence of chronic kidney disease, renal calculi, and frequent infections as well as related problems such as hypertension and diabetes mellitus.

Questions about lifestyle, diet, and work history should explore cigarette smoking and/or exposure to toxic industrial or environmental chemicals (to identify risks for cancer), usual amount and type of fluid intake, and self-care measures to replace fluids lost during work or physical activity. Examples of renal system disorders are identified in the Genetic Considerations box.

Genetic Considerations

When conducting a health assessment interview and physical assessment, it is important to consider genetic influences on adult health. During the health assessment interview, ask about family members with health problems affecting kidney function or those diagnosed with polycystic disease or diabetes mellitus. During the physical assessment, assess for manifestations that might indicate a genetic disorder. If data indicate the presence of genetic risk factors or alterations, ask about genetic testing and refer for appropriate genetic counseling and evaluation.

Examples of Renal System Disorders

- Adult polycystic kidney disease (APKD) is linked to a familial chromosome 16 disorder. The disease is characterized by large cysts in one or both kidneys and a gradual loss of kidney tissue with resultant chronic kidney disease.
- Chronic kidney disease may be a complication of type 1 and type 2 diabetes mellitus (DM), but is seen more often in patients with type 1 DM. Type 1 and type 2 DM are classified as multifactorial inheritance disorders because both genetic and environmental factors are necessary for onset of the disorder.
- Bladder cancer is the fourth most common type of cancer in men. Genetic factors related to chromosome 9 are interrelated with risk factors such as smoking and exposure to industrial chemicals to cause bladder cancer.

Physical Assessment

The renal system is assessed by examining the skin, abdomen, kidneys, bladder, and urinary meatus. Guidelines for abdominal assessment are outlined in Chapter 21. Normal age-related findings for the older adult are summarized in the Assessment of Special Populations section, later in this chapter.

Physical assessment of the renal system may be performed as part of a total health assessment, as part of an abdominal assessment, or as part of the back examination (for the kidneys). The techniques of inspection, auscultation, palpation, and percussion are used.

Before beginning the assessment, ask the patient to provide a clean-catch urine specimen (if ordered) and give the patient a specimen cup. Assess the specimen for color, odor, and clarity before you send it to the laboratory.

At the beginning of the assessment, the patient may be sitting or lying supine. Prior to the examination, collect all necessary equipment and explain the techniques to the patient to decrease anxiety. Because the examination involves exposure of the genital area, give the patient a gown and drape the patient appropriately to minimize exposure.

SAFETY ALERT: Auscultate immediately after inspection to avoid interference by bowel sounds stimulated by palpation and percussion. ■

Guidelines for percussion and palpation of the kidneys are outlined in **Box 26.1**, and urinary assessments are outlined in the assessment feature.

BOX 26.1
Guidelines for Physical Assessment of the Kidneys

PERCUSSION OF THE KIDNEYS

Percussion helps assess pain or tenderness. Assist the patient to a sitting position, and stand behind the patient. Use the ulnar surface of your dominant hand, curled into a fist, for percussing the kidneys. For direct percussion, strike the area over the costovertebral angle with only enough force so the patient feels a gentle thud. For indirect percussion, place the palm of your nondominant hand over the costovertebral angle (see figure A). Strike the back of your hand with your dominant hand (see figure B). Repeat the technique for the other kidney. Percussion is usually done at the end of the assessment.

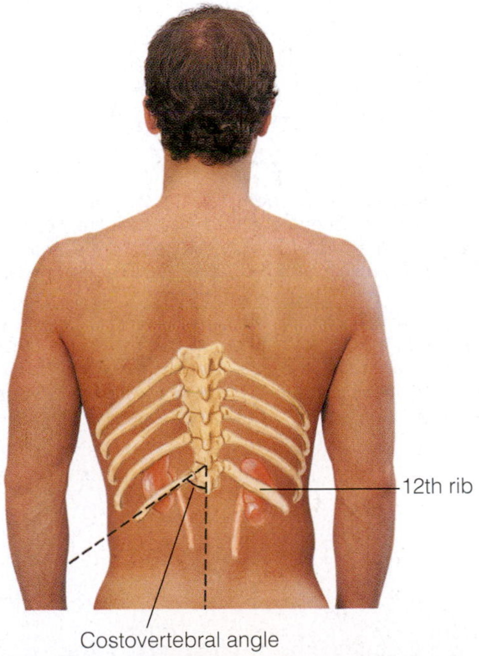
12th rib
Costovertebral angle

A

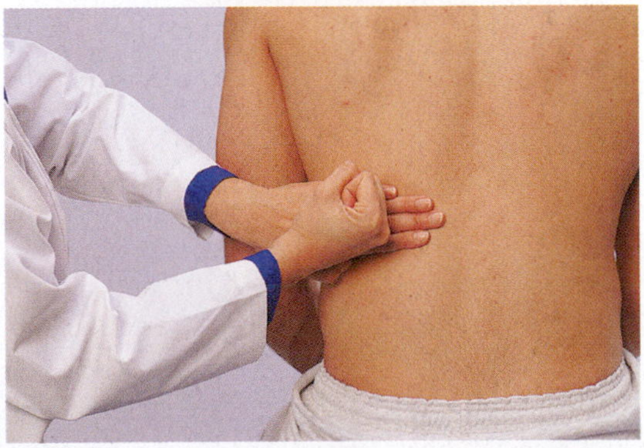

B

(continued)

PALPATION OF THE KIDNEYS

Although the technique of palpation of the kidneys is outlined here, this technique is best performed by an advanced practitioner because it involves deep palpation and can cause tissue trauma.

Assist the patient to the supine position and stand at the right side of the patient. To palpate the left kidney, reach across the patient and place your left hand under the patient's left flank with your palm upward. Elevate the left flank with your fingers, displacing the kidney upward. Ask the patient to take a deep breath and use the palmer surface of your right hand to palpate the kidney (figure C). Repeat the technique for the right kidney.

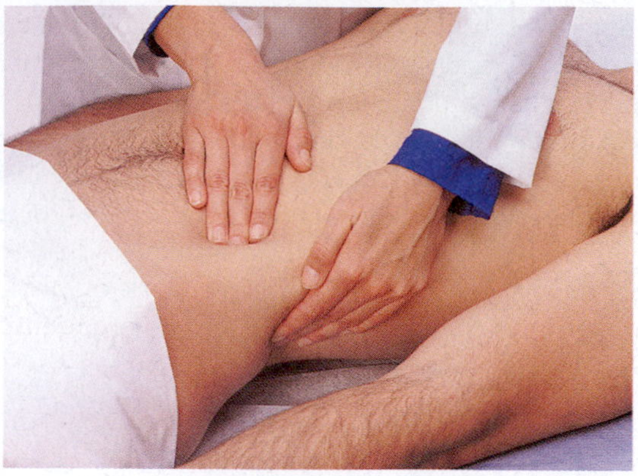
C

Urinary System Assessments

Technique/Normal Findings	Abnormal Findings
Skin Assessment Inspect the skin and mucous membranes, noting color, turgor, edema, and excretions. *The color of skin and mucous membranes should be even and appropriate to the age and race of the patient; skin should be dry with no visible excretions.*	■ Pallor may indicate anemia secondary to kidney disease. ■ Decreased skin turgor may indicate dehydration. ■ Edema (generalized or in the lower extremities) may indicate fluid volume excess. (Changes in skin turgor may indicate renal insufficiency with either excess fluid loss or retention.) ■ An accumulation of uric acid crystals, called *uremic frost*, may be seen on the skin of the patient with end-stage renal disease.
Abdominal Assessment Inspect the abdomen, noting size, symmetry, masses or lumps, swelling, distention, glistening, or skin tightness. *The abdomen should be slightly concave, symmetric, and without distention or masses.*	■ Swellings or asymmetry may indicate a hernia or superficial mass. ■ If the urinary bladder is distended, it rises above the symphysis pubis as a rounded mass. ■ Distention, glistening, or skin tightness may be associated with fluid retention. ■ Ascites is an accumulation of fluid in the peritoneal cavity.
Urinary Meatus Assessment This technique is not part of a routine assessment, but it is an important component in patients with health problems of the renal system. *For the male patient:* With the patient in a sitting or standing position, compress the tip of the glans penis with the gloved hand to open the urinary meatus (**Figure 26.7** ■). *For the female patient:* With the patient in the dorsal lithotomy position, spread the labia with your gloved hand to expose the urinary meatus. *The urinary meatus should be midline and free of redness, lesions, or discharge.*	■ Increased redness, swelling, or discharge from the urinary meatus may indicate UTI or sexually transmitted infection. ■ Ulceration of the urinary meatus may indicate a sexually transmitted infection. ■ Hypospadias is displacement of the urinary meatus to the ventral surface of the penis. ■ Epispadias is displacement of the urinary meatus to the dorsal surface of the penis.

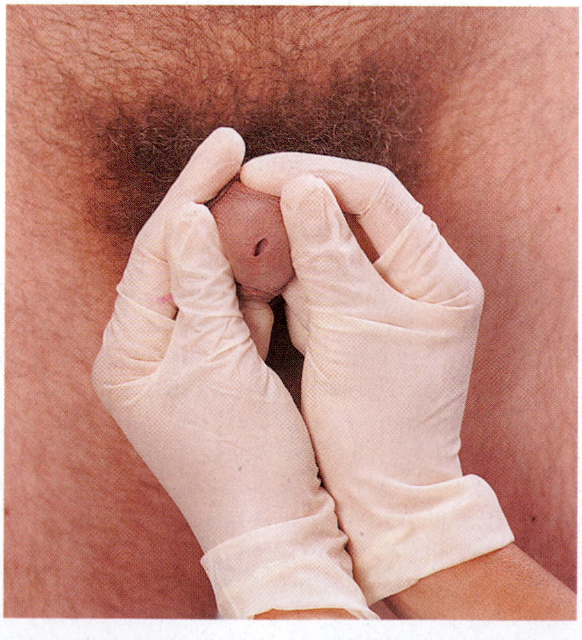

Figure 26.7 ■ Inspecting the urinary meatus of the male.

Technique/Normal Findings	Abnormal Findings
Kidney Assessment Refer to **Box 26.1** for guidelines for percussion and palpation of the kidneys. Auscultate the renal arteries by placing the bell of the stethoscope lightly in the areas of the renal arteries, located in the left and right upper abdominal quadrants. *Bruits are not normally heard over the renal arteries.*	■ Systolic bruits ("whooshing" sounds) may indicate renal artery stenosis.
Percuss the kidneys for tenderness or pain. *No tenderness or pain should be elicited.* Palpate the kidneys. The lower pole of the right kidney may be palpable with deep palpation; the remaining right kidney and the left kidney are normally not palpable. *If palpable, they should be nontender, bilaterally of appropriate size and density, and without palpable masses.*	■ Tenderness and pain on percussion of the costovertebral angle suggests kidney disease. ■ A painful or enlarged palpable kidney may suggest a tumor, cyst, or hydronephrosis.
Bladder Assessment Percuss the bladder for tone and position. *The bladder should be midline without dullness.*	■ A dull percussion tone over the bladder of a patient who has just urinated may indicate urinary retention. ■ A distended bladder may be palpated at any point from the symphysis pubis to the umbilicus and is felt as a firm, rounded organ. It indicates urinary retention.

Diagnostic Tests

The results of diagnostic tests of renal system function are used to support the diagnosis of a specific disease or condition, to provide information to identify or modify appropriate treatment, and to help monitor the patient's responses to treatment and nursing care interventions. Diagnostic tests to assess the structures and functions of the renal system are described in the Diagnostic Tests feature.

Regardless of the type of diagnostic test, the nurse is responsible for explaining the procedure and any special preparation needed, assessing for medication use that may affect the outcome of the tests, ensuring the consent form is signed (if necessary), supporting the patient during the examination as necessary, documenting procedures as appropriate, and monitoring the results of tests. The nurse is responsible for postprocedure care and patient teaching for self-care at home.

Diagnostic Tests of the Renal System

NAME OF TEST	PURPOSE AND DESCRIPTION	RELATED NURSING INTERVENTIONS
Blood urea nitrogen (BUN)	This blood test measures urea, a by-product of protein metabolism. It is used to determine renal function and the elimination of nitrogenous waste products. Urea levels rise in acute kidney injury and chronic kidney disease. Normal values: 5–25 mg/dL	Assess hydration status, medications, and for other factors (such as critical illness, trauma, gastrointestinal bleeding, sepsis, or liver disease) that may affect results (Kee, 2018). If BUN is mildly elevated, encourage increased fluid intake as allowed.
Creatinine (serum)	This blood test is used to evaluate kidney function. Creatinine is a by-product of the breakdown of muscle and is excreted by the kidneys. Serum creatinine levels rise as the GFR decreases. Normal BUN/creatine ratio is 10:1 Normal value: Serum: 0.5–1.5 mg/dL (Older adults and women may have decreased values due to decreased muscle mass.)	Assess hydration; fluid overload can result in falsely low serum creatinine levels, delaying diagnosis of acute kidney injury (Kee, 2018). Assess medications; values may be affected by some antibiotics (cephalosporins, aminoglycosides, kanamycin), ascorbic acid, cimetidine, L-dopa, methyldopa (Aldomet), and lithium carbonate. Suggest not eating red meat the evening before the test (red meat can increase the value).
Creatinine clearance	A blood sample and 24-hour urine test to evaluate GFR and renal function. Normal value: 85–135/min (Women and older adults may have slightly lower values.)	Assess medications: Phenacetin, steroids, and thiazides may decrease creatinine clearance; ascorbic acid, cimetidine, steroids, L-dopa, methyldopa (Aldomet), and cefoxitin may increase creatinine clearance. Ask the patient to void and discard first voiding. Instruct patient, family, and staff (if hospitalized) to save all urine for a clearly designated 24-hour period, maintaining the specimen in the container on ice or in the refrigerator.

(continued)

NAME OF TEST	PURPOSE AND DESCRIPTION	RELATED NURSING INTERVENTIONS
CT scan of kidneys	Allows evaluation of kidney size, tumors, abscesses, suprarenal masses, and obstructions. A contrast dye may be administered orally or injected IV, allowing improved visualization of the density of renal tissue and masses in comparison to an ultrasound.	Assess the patient for allergies to iodine, x-ray contrast dye, and seafood. Assess medications: Oral hypoglycemic agents are contraindicated for use with iodinated contrast. Ensure that serum creatinine and BUN levels are available. Tell the patient to remain NPO for 4 hours prior to the test and that laxatives or enemas may be ordered to remove gas or fecal material from the bowel. Post-test, monitor for and tell the patient to report allergic reactions to the dye (rash, itching, headache, vomiting) and to increase fluid intake to help excrete the dye.
Cystatin C	This blood test may be used to evaluate kidney function. Cystatin C is a protein that is produced at a constant rate and filtered by the kidneys; increased concentrations in the blood indicate a decrease in GFR and kidney dysfunction. Normal value: <0.70 mg/mL	No special preparation is required. Results of the test are not significantly affected by muscle mass, gender, age, or race.
Cystometrogram (CMG) (voiding cystogram)	This test is conducted to evaluate bladder capacity and neuromuscular functions of the bladder, urethral pressures, and causes of bladder dysfunction. A measured quantity of fluid is instilled into the bladder, and the filling capacity and voiding pressures are measured. Normal value: Urine stream strong and uninterrupted, normal filling pattern and sensation of fullness; bladder capacity: 300–600 mL; urge to void: >150 mL; fullness felt: 300 mL	Tell patient that the bladder will be filled and during filling he or she will be asked to describe the first urge to void and the sensation of being unable to delay urination any longer.
Cystoscopy, cystography	Direct visualization of the bladder wall and urethra is accomplished by using a cystoscope. During the procedure small calculi can be removed from the ureter, bladder, or urethra, and tissue biopsy can be done. It also permits determination of the cause of hematuria or UTI. A stent may be inserted during the procedure to facilitate urinary drainage past an obstruction. A retrograde pyelogram may be done during the cystoscopy. By instilling a contrast dye into the bladder (cystography), neurogenic bladder, fistulas, tumors, or ruptures can be identified. The test may be done with either local or general anesthesia.	Assess history of cystitis or prostatitis (these disorders could result in sepsis after the procedure), hypersensitivity to anesthetics, and urinary patterns (amount, color, odor). Take and record vital signs. Following the procedure, assess for complications (hemorrhage, bladder perforation, urinary retention) and report gross hematuria (blood in the urine). Apply heat to the lower abdomen or assist with sitz bath, if ordered, to relieve pain and muscle spasms. Tell the patient to avoid alcoholic drinks for 2 days, to increase fluid intake, and that a slight burning sensation with voiding may occur for a day or two. Instruct the patient to immediately notify the physician if the urine remains bloody for more than three voidings after the procedure or if bright bleeding, low urine output, abdominal or flank pain, chills, or fever develop.
Estimated GFR (eGFR)	Calculated based on the serum creatinine, age, gender, and (in some instances) racial origin. It is widely used in lieu of the measured GFR, a complicated and expensive diagnostic test. Normal value: 90–120 mL/min	No special preparation is necessary.

NAME OF TEST	PURPOSE AND DESCRIPTION	RELATED NURSING INTERVENTIONS
Intravenous pyelogram (IVP), retrograde pyelogram	A radiologic examination to visualize the entire urinary tract to diagnose kidney disorders or to detect calculi (stones), tumors, or cysts. A radiopaque substance is injected IV and a series of x-rays taken. If the patient is allergic to iodine or radiologic dyes or has kidney disease, a retrograde pyelogram, in which radiopaque dye is instilled directly into the ureter, may be done. It may be performed alone or in conjunction with a cystoscopy.	Schedule IVP prior to any ordered barium or gallbladder studies using contrast material. Ask about allergy to seafood, iodine, or radiologic contrast dye. Notify physician or radiologist if allergies are known. Assess medications: Oral hypoglycemic agents are contraindicated for use with iodinated contrast. Assess renal and fluid status, including serum osmolality, creatinine, and BUN levels. Notify the physician of any abnormal values. Instruct the patient to complete ordered pretest bowel preparation, including prescribed laxative or cathartic the evening before the test, and an enema or suppository the morning of the test. Tell the patient not to eat food for 8–12 hr prior to the test; clear liquids are allowed. Take and record vital signs. Instruct the patient to contact the healthcare provider for any delayed reactions to the dye (breathing difficulty, rash, itching, rapid heartbeat).
MRI of the kidneys	Used to visualize the kidneys by assessing computer-generated films of radio-frequency waves and changes in magnetic fields.	Inform patient of need to lie still during the examination. Assess for any metallic implants (such as pacemakers, clips on brain aneurysms, body piercings, tattoos, shrapnel). If present, notify imaging physician. Remove transdermal medication patches (both OTC and prescribed) unless otherwise ordered. Replace the patch following the procedure. Tell the patient to inform the staff about the patch when making the appointment and when completing the admission information. Ask if patient is pregnant; if so, the test is not performed. Ask about claustrophobia; if this is a problem, ask the patient to request a relaxing medication to take prior to the MRI.
Portable ultrasonic bladder scan	This test is used to obtain information about residual urine. Warmed ultrasound gel is applied over the lower abdomen, and the ultrasound probe is placed just above the pubic bone. The scanner shows an outline of the bladder and displays the amount of urine in the bladder in milliliters.	No special preparation is needed, but the test is usually not used for pregnant women. Report a residual amount of more than 100 mL.
Renal arteriogram or angiogram	This radiologic test is done to visualize renal blood vessels to detect renal artery stenosis, renal thrombosis or embolism, tumors, cysts, or aneurysm; to evaluate a possible causative factor for hypertension; and to evaluate renal circulation. A contrast medium is injected into the femoral artery.	Assess for allergy to iodine, seafood, or other contrast dye from other x-ray procedures. Assess medications: Oral hypoglycemic agents are contraindicated for use with iodinated contrast; anticoagulants should be discontinued. Instruct the patient to take a laxative or cleansing enema the night before the test (if ordered) and to remain NPO for 8–12 hr prior to the test. Take and record vital signs. Ask the patient to void and remove dentures and jewelry before the test. After the test, monitor for bleeding from the femoral artery, restrict activity for a day, assess peripheral pulses, and monitor urine output. Instruct the patient to contact the healthcare provider for any delayed reactions to the dye (such as breathing difficulty, rash, itching, rapid heartbeat, decreased urine output).

(continued)

NAME OF TEST	PURPOSE AND DESCRIPTION	RELATED NURSING INTERVENTIONS
Renal biopsy	Determines the cause of renal disease, to rule out cancer metastasis to the kidney, or if rejection is occurring with a kidney transplant. It is performed by using a cystoscope, excising a wedge of kidney tissue, or through the skin with a biopsy needle (percutaneous route).	If a general anesthetic is used, ask the patient not to eat or drink fluids for 8–12 hr before the biopsy. Take and record vital signs. Note hemoglobin and hematocrit values and report abnormal findings. After the biopsy, if the percutaneous route was used, apply pressure to the site for about 20 min to prevent bleeding. Assess bowel sounds if surgical interventions were used. Tell the patient to increase oral fluid intake and to report decreased urination or burning on urination.
Renal scan	This test is done to evaluate kidney blood flow, location, size, and shape and to assess kidney perfusion and urine production. Radioactive isotopes are injected IV and radiation detector probes are placed over the kidneys to monitor activity in the kidneys. Radioisotope distribution in the kidneys is scanned and graphed. Nonfunctioning tissue, such as in tumors and cysts, appears as cold spots.	Ask patient to drink several glasses of water prior to the test. Obtain weight and have patient void. After the procedure, increase fluid intake.
Renal ultrasound	This noninvasive test is conducted to detect renal or perirenal masses, identify obstructions, and diagnose renal cysts and solid masses. It is done by applying a conductive gel to the skin and placing a small external ultrasound probe on the patient's skin. Sound waves are recorded on a computer as they are reflected off tissues.	No special preparation is needed.
Residual urine (postvoiding residual urine)	Residual urine is measured to determine the amount of urine left in the bladder after voiding. Normal value: < 50 mL	Ask the patient to void in a collection device and measure the amount. Immediately after voiding, catheterize using sterile technique and a straight catheter. Drain bladder completely. Document time, amount voided, amount obtained on catheterization, color, clarity, odor, and any other significant data. Report amount of residual urine if it is more than 100 mL.
Urinalysis (UA)	This test examines the constituents of a urine sample to establish a baseline, provide data for diagnosis, or monitor treatment results. Expected findings and abnormal findings with causes are outlined in **Table 26.1**.	Provide a clean specimen cup for a urine sample. An early-morning specimen is preferred. Note on the laboratory slip if the patient is menstruating (if so, some menstrual blood may be present in the urine sample). Assess medications, fluid status, and foods that might affect urinalysis results. Tell the patient to refrigerate the specimen until it can be taken for analysis.
Urine culture (midstream, clean-catch)	A urine culture is conducted to identify the causative organism of a UTI. Normal value: $< 10{,}000$ organisms/mL (urine is sterile but urethra contains bacteria and a few WBCs); values of $>100{,}000$ organisms/mL indicate UTI	Provide a sterile container for the urine sample. Instruct the patient to wash and dry the genitals and perineal area with soap and water. Ask women to separate labia with one hand and clean labia with other hand, using two or three disposable antiseptic towelettes, wiping once front to back with each towelette. Ask men to retract the foreskin and cleanse glans with antiseptic towelettes, using a circular motion. After cleaning, tell patient to begin voiding and then collect specimen in the container (initial voiding will contain urethral contaminants). If patient is unable to void, it may be necessary to obtain a specimen by urinary catheterization. Instruct the patient to avoid taking antibiotics or sulfonamides until after the specimen is collected and to refrigerate the specimen until it can be taken for testing. If the patient is taking antibiotics, it should be noted on the laboratory slip.
Uroflowmetry	This test measures the volume of urine voided per second.	Ask the patient to increase fluid intake and refrain from voiding for several hours before the test to ensure a full bladder and a strong urge to void during testing. Tell the patient he or she will be asked to urinate into a funnel.

26.3 Assessment of Special Populations

Age-Related Changes in Kidney Function

Glomeruli in the renal cortex are lost with aging, reducing kidney mass. Because of the large functional reserve of the kidneys, however, renal function remains adequate unless additional stressors affect the renal system. The glomerular filtration rate (GFR), the amount of filtrate made by the kidneys per minute, declines due to age-related factors affecting the renovascular system (such as arteriosclerosis, decreased renal vascularity, and decreased cardiac output). By age 80, the GFR may be less than half of what it was at age 30.

Age-related changes in renal function have significant implications. The kidneys are less able to concentrate urine and compensate for increased or decreased salt intake. When combined with diminished effectiveness of antidiuretic hormone (ADH) and a reduced thirst response, both common in aging, this decreased ability to concentrate urine increases the risk for dehydration. Potassium excretion may be decreased because of lower aldosterone levels. As a result, fluid and electrolyte imbalances are more common and potentially critical in the older patient.

Decreased GFR in the older adult also reduces the clearance of drugs excreted through the kidneys. This reduced clearance prolongs the half-life of drugs and may necessitate lower drug doses and longer dosing intervals. Common medications affected by decreased GFR include:

- Cardiac drugs: Digoxin, procainamide
- Antibiotics: Aminoglycosides, tetracyclines, cephalosporins
- Histamine H_2 antagonists: Cimetidine
- Antidiabetic agents: Chlorpropamide.

When caring for older adults, it is especially important to monitor drugs that are toxic to the renal tubules. Radiologic dyes and aminoglycoside, tetracycline, and the cephalosporin antibiotics are part of this group.

Age-related changes in renal function are outlined in **Table 26.2**, and nursing care of older adults with age-related changes in kidney function and related nursing implications are summarized in **Table 26.3**.

Chronic Kidney Disease in Older Adults

Structural and functional changes occur in the aging kidney. Structurally, the number of nephrons decreases. The GFR declines, resulting in decreased renal clearance of

Table 26.2 Age-Related Renal System Changes

Age-Related Change	Significance
Kidneys	
↓ size of renal cortex and number of nephrons ↓ growth of renal tissue ↑ risk of atherosclerosis, all of which may result in atrophy of the kidneys	■ Decreased renal blood flow. ■ GFR decreases by about 50% between ages 20 and 90.
Renal Tubules	
↓ function, with less effective exchange of substances, water and sodium conservation, and suppression of ADH secretion in presence of hypo-osmolality	■ Risk of hyponatremia and **nocturia** (voiding more often at night). ■ Effects of medications may be altered (with decreased filtration). ■ Decreased reabsorption of glucose may result in 1+ proteinuria and glycosuria, which are not of major clinical significance.
Bladder	
■ Muscles weaken and bladder capacity decreases. ■ More difficult to empty bladder. ■ Delayed micturition reflex.	■ Urinary retention is more common. ■ Urinary frequency, urgency, and nocturia are more common with aging. ■ Larger amounts of residual urine present after voiding. ■ Some stress incontinence may occur, especially in multiparous women. ■ Urinary incontinence is not a normal outcome of aging.

Table 26.3 Nursing Implications of Age-Related Changes in Kidney Function

Functional Change	Effect	Nursing Implications
Decreased GFR	Decreased clearance of drugs excreted primarily through the kidneys increases drug half-life and blood levels and risk of drug toxicity.	Monitor carefully for signs of toxicity, especially when administering digoxin, aminoglycoside antibiotics, tetracycline, vancomycin, chlorpropamide, procainamide, cimetidine, and cephalosporin antibiotics.
Decreased number of functional nephrons; lower levels of aldosterone; increased resistance to ADH	Ability to conserve water and sodium is decreased; potassium excretion is impaired; and hydrogen ion excretion is decreased, resulting in reduced ability to compensate for acidosis.	Monitor for dehydration and hyponatremia. Maintain fluid intake of 1500–2500 mL/day unless contraindicated. Monitor for hyperkalemia, especially if taking a potassium-sparing diuretic, heparin, angiotensin-converting enzyme (ACE) inhibitor, angiotensin receptor blocker (ARB), beta-blocker, or NSAID; increased risk for acidosis.
Reduced numbers of functional nephrons	Renal reserve is decreased, leading to increased risk of failure.	Avoid giving nephrotoxic drugs, if possible. Monitor urine output and blood chemistries for early signs of renal failure.

drugs. Urine-concentrating ability decreases, and the kidney is less able to conserve sodium. Renal compensation for acid–base imbalances takes longer. Despite these changes, the kidney retains its ability to regulate fluid and electrolyte homeostasis remarkably well unless additional stresses are added. Any additional stressors such as hypotension, exposure to nephrotoxic drugs, or an inflammatory process such as glomerulonephritis may precipitate renal failure in the older adult.

The manifestations of chronic kidney disease are often missed in aging patients (e.g., edema may be attributed to heart failure or high blood pressure to preexisting hypertension). Serum creatinine levels may rise slowly. Because older adults have less muscle mass, they produce less creatinine, a by-product of muscle cell metabolism. Likewise, the BUN may remain within normal limits.

The same measures are used to treat end-stage renal disease in older adults as in younger people. Hemodialysis, peritoneal dialysis, and renal transplantation are appropriate, if necessary. Treatment options (including conservative treatment or no treatment) and their potential benefits and ramifications should be clearly explained.

Assessing for Home Care

A number of factors should be considered in assessing the older adult's ability to manage treatment such as dialysis at home:

- Does the patient have reasonable access to a dialysis center or outpatient unit? Is transportation available?
- Would home hemodialysis be appropriate? Is a caregiver available to be trained to manage dialysis? Does the patient's home have appropriate electrical and plumbing fixtures?
- Would continuous ambulatory peritoneal dialysis be appropriate? Does the patient have the manual dexterity, will, and cognitive ability to manage dialysis infusions? If not, would intermittent peritoneal dialysis using a dialyzing machine be more appropriate?
- Are family members or other support persons available to provide assistance to the patient as needed?

Resources for Home Care

The following resources may be useful for patients with kidney disease:

- American Association of Kidney Patients (www.aakp.org) 800-749-2257
- American Kidney Fund (www.kidneyfund.org) 866-300-2900 (Help Line) (Also available for Spanish)
- National Kidney Foundation (www.kidney.org) 800-622-9010

26.4 Health Promotion

Health promotion of the urinary system focuses on maintaining optimal function and reducing risk for infections. According to the Society of Urologic Nurses and Associates (SUNA; 2018), bladder health promotion focuses on prevention of urinary tract infections (UTIs), urinary incontinence, and bladder cancer (see also Society of Urologic Nurses, 2018).

Prevention of UTIs focuses on teaching measures to prevent UTI in all patients, particularly young, sexually active women, and includes:

- Encouraging patients to maintain a generous fluid intake of 2.0 to 2.5 quarts per day, increasing intake during hot weather or strenuous activity.
- Discussing the need to avoid voluntary urinary retention, emptying the bladder every 3 to 4 hours.
- Instructing women to cleanse the perineal area from front to back after voiding and defecating.
- Teaching women to void before and after sexual intercourse to flush out bacteria introduced into the urethra and bladder.
- Teaching measures to maintain the integrity of perineal tissues: Avoid bubble baths, feminine hygiene sprays, and vaginal douches; wear cotton briefs, avoid synthetic materials; if postmenopausal, use hormone replacement therapy or estrogen cream.
- Suggesting measures to maintain acid urine (unless contraindicated): Drink two glasses of low-sugar cranberry juice daily; take ascorbic acid (vitamin C); and avoid excess intake of milk and milk products, other fruit juices, and sodium bicarbonate (baking soda).

Teaching measures related to prevention of urinary incontinence include:

- Developing an appropriate voiding schedule
- Teaching the importance of completely emptying the bladder when voiding
- Teaching about medications that affect bladder control.

Health promotion teaching for preventing bladder cancer focuses on avoiding exposure to cancer-causing chemicals. Most important is smoking cessation—smokers are four to seven times more likely to develop bladder cancer than nonsmokers (American Society of Clinical Oncologists, 2017). Drinking plenty of water and eating lots of fruits and vegetables also might help protect against bladder cancer (American Cancer Society, 2016).

CHAPTER HIGHLIGHTS

26.1 Anatomy, Physiology, and Functions of the Renal System

Describe the anatomy, physiology, and functions of the kidneys and urinary tract, and identify abnormal findings that may indicate impairments of the renal system.

- The renal system, including the kidneys, ureters, urinary bladder, and urethra, plays a critical role in maintaining homeostasis of the body.

26.2 Assessing Renal System Function

Outline the components of the assessment of the renal system, including topics for the health assessment interview, techniques for physical assessment, and the diagnostic tests used in the assessment.

- Manifestations of dysfunction and disorders affecting the renal system may be detected during a general health assessment as well as during focused assessment of renal system organs.

26.3 Assessment of Special Populations

Differentiate considerations for assessing the renal systems of older adults, veterans, individuals in the LGBTQI population, and adults with sequelae of childhood/congenital conditions.

- Older adults have increased risk for urinary dysfunction related to age-related changes of the urinary system.

26.4 Health Promotion

Summarize topics that nurses teach to promote healthy tissue integrity across the lifespan.

- Health promotion of the urinary system focuses on patient teaching to promote normal function and to reduce risk of infection. Health promotion includes teaching good hygiene, teaching women to void before and after sex, encouraging consumption of lots of fruits and vegetables, and encouraging smoking cessation.

TEST YOURSELF NCLEX-RN® REVIEW

1. The nurse suspects that an older female patient has a health problem affecting the renal system. Which statement did the patient make that caused the nurse to come to this conclusion?
   A. "I leak urine all the time."
   B. "I sometimes have to get up at night to urinate."
   C. "When I have to urinate, I really feel an urge to go."
   D. "My doctor told me I have a slight amount of protein in my urine."
2. A patient has been vomiting for 4 hours. Which hormone will increase secretion in response to the physiologic changes caused by the vomiting?
   A. ADH
   B. Renin
   C. Thyroxin
   D. Aldosterone
3. A patient is experiencing changes in the renal system. What diagnostic test will help the nurse determine this patient's glomerular filtration rate and glomerular damage?
   A. Renal scan
   B. Renal biopsy
   C. Routine urinalysis
   D. Creatinine clearance
4. During the health history of an older male patient, the nurse focuses on the gland that encircles the male urethra at the base of the bladder. Which organ is this?
   A. Spleen
   B. Prostate
   C. Adrenal
   D. Pancreas
5. During a health history interview, a patient reports having to get up to void several times during the night and there is burning when passing urine. Which terms should the nurse use when documenting this patient's manifestations? (Select all that apply.)
   A. Pyuria
   B. Dysuria
   C. Polyuria
   D. Nocturia
   E. Hematuria

6. The nurse is preparing a patient for an intravenous pyelogram. What should be a part of the patient's care at this time? (Select all that apply.)
   A. Assess for allergies to seafood or iodine.
   B. Instruct on preprocedure bowel preparation.
   C. Teach to eat a soft diet the morning of the test.
   D. Remind to withhold taking diuretics the day of the test.
   E. Check prescribed medications for oral hypoglycemic agents.
7. The nurse is beginning to assess a patient's renal system. What should the nurse ask the patient to do before this examination? (Select all that apply.)
   A. Assume the lithotomy position.
   B. Provide a urine specimen if prescribed.
   C. Take several deep breaths.
   D. Drink several glasses of water.
   E. Change into a gown.
8. A patient has undergone cystoscopy and is being prepared for discharge. Which teaching will the nurse provide? (Select all that apply.)
   A. Do not drink alcohol for at least 2 days.
   B. Expect significant burning to occur during the first several voidings.
   C. Increase your fluid intake.
   D. Urine may be slightly bloody for two or three voidings.
   E. You will not void as much as normal for the next few days.
9. A patient is diagnosed with a renal system disorder that is believed to be the result of genetic and environmental factors. Which health problem is the patient most likely experiencing?
   A. Hematuria
   B. Incontinence
   C. Bladder cancer
   D. Kidney infection
10. The nurse is conducting a physical examination of a patient's renal system. What assessment would the nurse use to assess the hydration status of a patient?
   A. Palpation for skin turgor
   B. Palpation of both kidneys
   C. Auscultation of renal arteries
   D. Percussion for dullness over bladder

See Test Yourself answers in Appendix B.

REFERENCES

American Cancer Society. (2016). *Can bladder cancer be prevented?* Retrieved from https://www.cancer.org/cancer/bladder-cancer/causes-risks-prevention/prevention.html.

American Society of Clinical Oncologists. (2017). Bladder cancer: Risk factors. Cancer.net, Retrieved from https://www.cancer.net/cancer-types/bladder-cancer/risk-factors.

Bickley, L. (2016). *Bates' guide to physical examination and history taking* (12th ed.). Philadelphia, PA: Lippincott Williams & Wilkins.

Kee, J. L. (2018). *Laboratory and diagnostic tests with nursing implications* (10th ed.). Hoboken, NJ: Pearson Education.

Society of Urologic Nurses and Associates. (2018). *Patient education.* Retrieved from https://www.suna.org/resource/patient-education.

Sorenson, M., Quinn, L., & Klein, D. (2019). *Pathophysiology: Concepts of human disease.* Hoboken, NJ: Pearson Education.

ADDITIONAL RESOURCES

American Cancer Society
www.cancer.org

National Kidney Foundation
www.kidney.org

Society of Urologic Nurses and Associates (SUNA)
www.suna.org

Chapter 27

Nursing Care of Patients with Urinary Tract Disorders

Chapter Outline and Learning Outcomes

Describe the pathophysiology and manifestations of a urinary tract infection, and outline the interprofessional care and nursing care of patients with this disorder.

Describe the pathophysiology and manifestations of urinary calculi, and outline the interprofessional care and nursing care of patients with this disorder.

Describe the pathophysiology and manifestations of urinary tract tumors, and outline the interprofessional care and nursing care of patients with such disorders.

Describe the pathophysiology and manifestations of disorders of urinary elimination (urinary retention, neurogenic bladder, and urinary incontinence), and outline the interprofessional care and nursing care of patients with these disorders.

CLINICAL COMPETENCIES

- Assess the functional health status of patients with urinary tract disorders, using data and expressed needs, values, and preferences to determine priority nursing diagnoses and select individualized nursing interventions.
- Identify, document, and monitor abnormal or unexpected changes in patient status, communicating information within the interprofessional team as appropriate.
- Use evidence-based research to plan and implement nursing care for patients with urinary tract disorders.
- Integrate the interprofessional plan of care into care for patients with urinary tract disorders.
- Knowledgeably and safely administer prescribed medications and treatments for patients with urinary tract disorders.
- Provide safe and effective nursing care for patients undergoing invasive procedures or surgery of the urinary tract.
- Plan and provide appropriate teaching for prevention of and self-care of urinary tract disorders.
- Use evidence-based care guidelines to reduce the incidence of healthcare-associated urinary tract infections.
- Participate in studies and projects to improve the quality and safety of care for patients with urinary tract disorders.
- Document care in the electronic medical record and use information management tools to monitor outcomes of care.

KEY TERMS

cystectomy, 887
cystitis, 873
dysuria, 873
hematuria, 873
hydronephrosis, 882
lithiasis, 880
lithotripsy, 883
neurogenic bladder, 894
nocturia, 873
pyelonephritis, 873
renal colic, 882
ureteral stent, 876
ureteroplasty, 876
urgency, 873
urinary calculi, 880
urinary diversion, 888
urinary incontinence (UI), 896

The urinary system includes the kidneys, ureters, urinary bladder, and urethra. This organ system can be affected by a variety of disorders, including urinary tract infections, renal calculi, tumors, and neurologic conditions. Any portion of the system—from the kidney through the urethra—can be affected with serious or even life-threatening consequences unless the problem is appropriately diagnosed and treated. Kidney disorders can affect urine production and waste elimination directly and are discussed in Chapter 28. Disorders of the urinary drainage system (the kidney pelvis, ureters, bladder, and urethra) may obstruct urine flow or spread to the kidneys, affecting urine production and elimination.

When caring for patients with urinary tract disorders, it is important to consider the patient's modesty in voiding, possible difficulty in discussing the genitals, embarrassment about being exposed for examination and testing, and fear of changes in body image or function. These psychosocial issues may interfere with the patient's willingness to seek help, discuss treatment, and learn about preventive measures.

Nursing interventions for patients with urinary tract disorders are directed toward primary prevention, early detection, and management of the disorder through health teaching and nursing care.

27.1 Urinary Tract Infection

Bacterial infections of the urinary tract are a common reason for seeking health services, second only to upper respiratory infections. Community-acquired urinary tract infections (UTIs) are common in young women and unusual in men under the age of 50. Out of 100 women, 50 will suffer from a UTI at some point in their life (Office of Population Affairs, 2018). Worldwide, 150 million UTIs occur yearly, incurring $6 billion in healthcare expenditures (American Urological Society, 2018). In healthcare settings, 40% of healthcare-associated infections (HAIs) are UTIs (American Urological Society, 2018).

Pathophysiology

The urinary tract is normally sterile above the urethra. Adequate urine volume, a free flow from the kidneys through the urinary meatus, and complete bladder emptying are the most important mechanisms maintaining sterility. Pathogens that enter and contaminate the distal urethra are washed out during voiding. Other defenses for maintaining sterile urine include its normal acidity and bacteriostatic properties of the bladder and urethral cells. The peristaltic activity of the ureters and a competent vesicoureteral junction help maintain sterility of the upper urinary tract. As the ureter enters the bladder, its distal portion tunnels between the mucosa and muscle layers of the bladder wall (**Figure 27.1** ■). During voiding, increased intravesicular pressure compresses the ureter, preventing reflux (backflow of urine) toward the kidneys. In males, a long urethra and the antibacterial effect of zinc in prostatic fluid also help prevent contamination of this normally sterile environment.

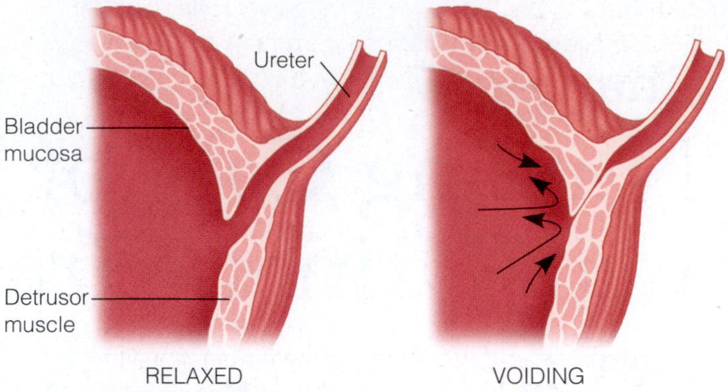
Ureter
Bladder mucosa
Detrusor muscle
RELAXED
VOIDING

Figure 27.1 ■ A competent vesicoureteral junction. Note how increased intravesicular pressure during voiding occludes the distal portion of the ureter, preventing reflux.

Risk Factors

Patients can be predisposed to UTI by a variety of factors. Some risk factors cannot be changed (e.g., aging and the female anatomy). Congenital or acquired factors contributing to the risk of infection include urinary tract obstruction by tumors or calculi, structural abnormalities such as strictures, impaired bladder innervation, bowel incontinence, and chronic diseases such as diabetes mellitus.

In women, sexual activity increases the risk for UTI, thought to result from bacteria introduced into the bladder via the urethra during sexual intercourse. Use of spermicidal compounds with a diaphragm, cervical cap, or condom alters the normal bacterial flora of the vagina and perineal tissues and further increases the risk for UTI. Some females lack a normally protective mucosal enzyme and have decreased levels of cervicovaginal antibodies to enterobacteria, further increasing their risk. Pregnancy increases the risk of UTI and asymptomatic bacteriuria due to hormonal effects, physical compression by the expanding uterus, and pregnancy-related changes in the bladder mucosa.

In men, prostatic hypertrophy and bacterial prostatitis are risk factors. Unprotected anal intercourse is a risk factor. Circumcision appears to have a protective effect.

Instrumentation of the urinary tract (e.g., catheterization or cystoscopy) is a major risk factor for UTI. Even when performed under strict aseptic conditions, catheterization can result in bladder infection. The placement of the catheter prevents the flushing action of voiding, and bacteria may ascend to the bladder either through the catheter lumen or via exudate between the urethral mucosa and the catheter.

Older patients have an increased incidence of UTI. The greatest degree of increase is seen in men, as the ratio of female-to-male UTI in older adults changes from 50:1 to less than 5:1. An increased risk of urinary stasis, chronic disease states (such as diabetes mellitus), and an impaired immune response contribute to the higher incidence of UTI in the older adult. In men, the prostate typically enlarges with aging, potentially resulting in urinary retention as the urethra narrows. Prostatic secretions are lessened, diminishing their protective, antibacterial effect. In older women, loss of tissue elasticity and weakening of perineal muscles often contribute to the development of a cystocele or rectocele. Resulting changes in bladder and urethral position increase the risk of incomplete bladder emptying.

Manifestations

Pathogens usually enter the urinary tract by ascending from the mucous membranes of the perineal area into the lower urinary tract. Bacteria that have colonized the urethra, vagina, or perineal tissues are the usual source of infection (Sorenson, Quinn, & Klein, 2019). From the bladder, bacteria may continue to ascend the urinary tract, eventually infecting the parenchyma (functional tissue) of the kidneys. Hematogenous spread of infection to the urinary tract is rare. Infections introduced in this manner are usually associated with previous damage or scarring of the urinary tract. Bacteria introduced into the urinary tract may cause asymptomatic bacteriuria or an inflammatory response with manifestations of UTI. Asymptomatic bacteriuria is commonly found in pregnant women, older adults, and patients with diabetes mellitus or who have an indwelling urinary catheter.

UTIs can be categorized in several ways. Anatomically, they may affect the lower or the upper urinary tract. Lower urinary tract infections include *urethritis*, inflammation of the urethra; *prostatitis*, inflammation of the prostate gland; and **cystitis**, inflammation of the urinary bladder. The most common upper urinary tract infection is **pyelonephritis**, inflammation of the kidney and renal pelvis. The infection may involve superficial tissues such as the bladder mucosa or may invade other tissues such as prostate or renal tissues. Epidemiologically, UTIs are identified as community acquired or catheter associated.

Cystitis

Cystitis, inflammation of the urinary bladder, is the most common UTI. It usually results from colonization of the bladder by bacteria normally found in the lower gastrointestinal tract. The infection tends to remain superficial, involving the bladder mucosa. The mucosa becomes hyperemic (red) and may hemorrhage, and the inflammatory response causes pus to form (**Figure 27.2** ■). This process causes the classic manifestations associated with cystitis, including **dysuria** (painful or difficult urination), urinary frequency and **urgency** (a sudden, compelling need to urinate), and **nocturia** (voiding two or more times at night). In addition, the urine may have a foul odor and appear cloudy (*pyuria*) or bloody (**hematuria**) because of mucus, excess white cells in the urine, and bleeding of the inflamed bladder wall. Suprapubic pain and tenderness also may be present.

Older patients may not experience the classic symptoms of cystitis. Instead, they often present with nonspecific manifestations such as nocturia, incontinence, confusion, behavior change, lethargy, and anorexia. Fever may be present; however, hypothermia may also develop in an older adult.

Although the bacteriostatic effect of prostatic fluid and a longer urethra provide an effective barrier to bladder infection for adult males, in older men an enlarged prostate can impede urine flow, leading to incomplete bladder emptying and urinary stasis. Bacteria are not completely flushed with voiding, allowing colonization of the bladder.

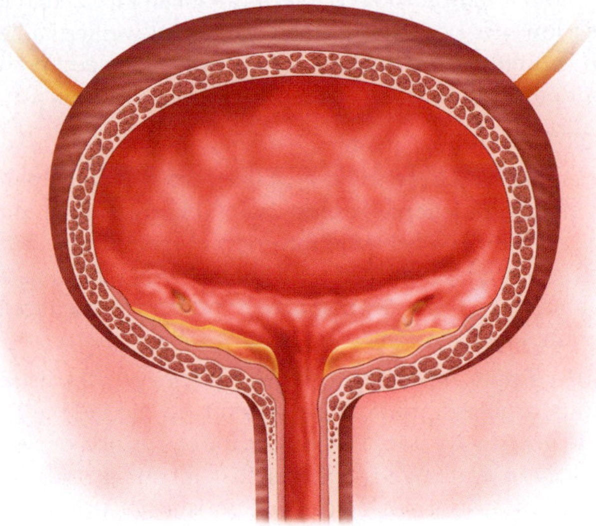

Figure 27.2 ■ Appearance of the bladder wall affected by cystitis.

Cystitis is usually uncomplicated and readily responds to treatment. When left untreated, the infection can ascend to involve the kidneys. Severe or prolonged infection may lead to sloughing of bladder mucosa and ulcer formation. Chronic cystitis can lead to bladder stones (discussed later in this chapter).

Complications

Urinary tract infections can result in the following complications. These complications are related to medical devices (urinary catheters), and inflammatory processes. Management of these complications is imperative to urinary tract health.

Catheter-Associated Urinary Tract Infections

Catheter-associated urinary tract infections (CAUTIs) are the most commonly reported healthcare-associated infection; about 80% of hospital-acquired UTIs are associated with a urinary catheter (Centers for Medicare and Medicaid Services, 2018). The longer the catheter remains in place, the greater the risk for infection. Bacteria, including *E. coli*, *Proteus*, *Pseudomonas*, and *Klebsiella*, reach the bladder by either migrating through the column of urine within the catheter or by moving up the mucous sheath of the urethra outside the catheter. These pathogens are relatively resistant to antibiotics, making catheter removal necessary to remove the source of the infection (American Nurses Association [ANA], 2018). Causative organisms associated with CAUTI are more likely to demonstrate antibiotic resistance than those found in community-acquired UTI.

CAUTIs, including pyelonephritis, are often asymptomatic. Gram-negative bacteremia is the most significant complication associated with these UTIs. Most CAUTIs resolve when the catheter is removed and a 7- to 14-day course of antibiotic is administered. Intermittent catheterization carries a lower risk of infection than does an indwelling catheter and is preferred for patients who are unable to empty their bladder by voiding (e.g., patients with spinal cord injury).

Pyelonephritis

Pyelonephritis is inflammation of the renal pelvis and parenchyma, the functional kidney tissue (**Figure 27.3** ■). *Acute pyelonephritis* is a bacterial infection of the kidney; *chronic pyelonephritis* is associated with nonbacterial infections and inflammatory processes that may be metabolic, chemical, or immunologic in origin.

Acute Pyelonephritis. Acute pyelonephritis usually results from an infection that ascends to the kidney from the lower urinary tract. Asymptomatic bacteriuria or cystitis can lead to acute pyelonephritis. Risk factors include pregnancy (because of slowed ureteral peristalsis), urinary tract obstruction, and congenital malformation. Urinary tract trauma, scarring, calculi (stones), kidney disorders such as polycystic or hypertensive kidney disease, and chronic diseases such as diabetes may also contribute to pyelonephritis. *Vesicoureteral reflux*, a condition in which urine moves from the bladder back toward the kidney, is a common risk factor in children who develop pyelonephritis and is also seen in adults when bladder outflow is obstructed.

The infection spreads from the renal pelvis to the renal cortex. The pelvis, calyces, and medulla of the kidney are primarily affected, with white blood cell (WBC) infiltration and inflammation. The kidney becomes grossly edematous. Localized abscesses may develop on the cortical surface of the kidney. As with cystitis, *E. coli* is the organism responsible for 85% of the cases of acute pyelonephritis. Other organisms commonly found include *Proteus* and *Klebsiella*, bacteria that normally inhabit the intestinal tract.

The onset of acute pyelonephritis is typically rapid, with chills and fever, malaise, vomiting, flank pain, costovertebral tenderness, urinary frequency, and dysuria. Symptoms of cystitis may also be present. The older adult may present with a change in behavior, acute confusion, incontinence, or a general deterioration in condition.

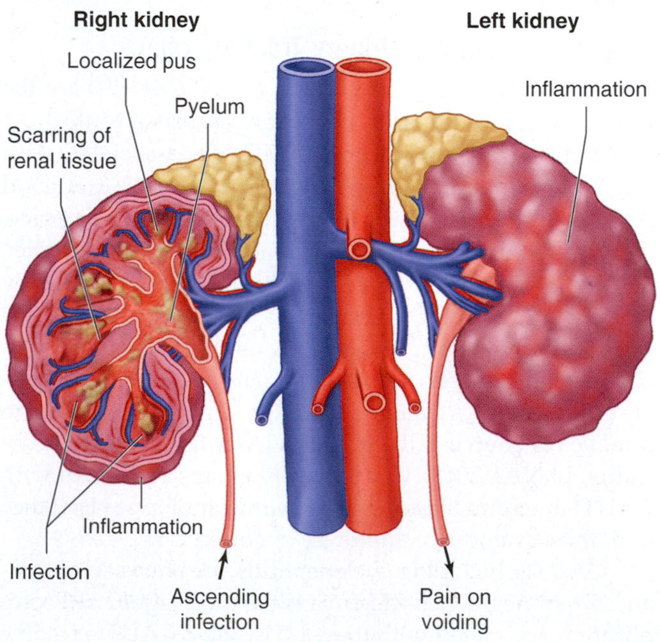
Right kidney
Left kidney
Localized pus
Pyelum
Scarring of renal tissue
Inflammation
Inflammation
Infection
Ascending infection
Pain on voiding

Figure 27.3 ■ Pyelonephritis.

Chronic Pyelonephritis. Chronic pyelonephritis involves chronic inflammation and scarring of the tubules and interstitial tissues of the kidney. It is a common cause of chronic kidney disease. It may develop as a result of UTIs or other conditions that damage the kidneys, such as hypertension or vascular conditions, severe vesicoureteral reflux, or obstruction of the urinary tract.

The patient with chronic pyelonephritis may be asymptomatic or have mild manifestations such as urinary frequency, dysuria, and flank pain. Hypertension can develop as kidney tissue is destroyed.

Interprofessional Care

Treatment of UTI focuses on eliminating the causative organism, preventing relapse or reinfection, and identifying and correcting any contributing factors. Drug treatment with antibiotics and urinary anti-infectives is commonly used. In some cases, surgery may be indicated to correct contributing factors.

Diagnosis

Laboratory testing for UTI includes:

- ***Urinalysis*** to assess for pyuria, bacteria, and blood cells in the urine. A bacteria count greater than 100,000 (10^5) per milliliter is indicative of infection. Rapid tests for bacteria in the urine include using a *nitrite dipstick* (which turns pink in the presence of bacteria) and the *leukocyte esterase test*, an indirect method of detecting bacteria by identifying lysed or intact WBCs in the urine. Urine should be collected via suprapubic aspiration or by midstream clean-catch specimen; if necessary, straight catheterization or "mini-cath," with strict aseptic technique, may be used. Catheterization is avoided, if possible, to reduce the risk of further infection.
- ***Gram stain of the urine*** may be done to identify the infecting organism by shape and characteristic (Gram-positive or Gram-negative).
- ***Urine culture and sensitivity*** tests may be ordered to identify the infecting organism and the most effective antibiotic. Culture requires 24 to 72 hours, so treatment to eliminate the most common organisms is often initiated without culture.
- ***WBC with differential*** may be done to detect typical changes associated with infection, such as *leukocytosis* (elevated WBC) and increased numbers of neutrophils.

SAFETY ALERT: Obtain urine specimens from a patient with an indwelling urinary catheter by briefly (15 minutes or less) clamping the proximal drainage tubing, then withdrawing urine directly from the port using sterile technique. Sterile technique is necessary to reduce the risk of catheter-associated UTI. ■

In men and in adult women with recurrent infections or persistent bacteriuria, additional diagnostic testing may be ordered to evaluate for structural abnormalities and other contributing factors:

- ***Intravenous pyelography (IVP)*** or ***CT scan*** are used to evaluate for structural or functional abnormalities, such as vesicoureteral reflux, of the kidneys, ureters, and bladder.
- ***Voiding cystourethrography*** may be ordered to detect structural or functional abnormalities of the bladder and urethral strictures.
- ***Cystoscopy*** may be used to diagnose conditions such as prostatic hypertrophy, urethral strictures, bladder calculi, tumors, polyps or diverticula, and congenital abnormalities. A tissue biopsy may be obtained during the procedure and other interventions performed (e.g., stone removal or stricture dilation).
- ***Manual pelvic*** or ***prostate examinations*** are done to assess for structural changes of the genitourinary tract, such as prostatic enlargement, cystocele, or rectocele.

Medications

Most acute uncomplicated infections of the lower urinary tract in women can be treated with a short course of antibiotic therapy. In contrast, upper UTIs and those occurring in men usually require longer treatment to eradicate the infecting organism and prevent recurrence.

Short-course therapy (a 3-day course of treatment) reduces treatment cost, increases compliance, and has a lower rate of side effects. Oral *trimethoprim-sulfamethoxazole (TMP-SMX)*, SMX, TMP, or a quinolone antibiotic such as *ciprofloxacin* (Cipro), ofloxacin (Floxin), or levofloxacin (Levaquin, Quixin) may be ordered. Rates of bacterial resistance to TMP-SMX and ciprofloxacin are increasing in some regions; a 5- to 7-day course of nitrofurantoin (Furadantin, Macrobid, Macrodantin) is an effective alternative. Sulfonamides and quinolone antibiotics are avoided during pregnancy. Ampicillin and cephalosporin antibiotics have been shown to be safe and are the drugs of choice for treating UTI during pregnancy (Johnson, 2017).

Men and women with pyelonephritis, urinary tract abnormalities or stones, or a history of previous infections with antibiotic-resistant infections require a 7- to 10-day antibiotic course. The patient with severe illness may need hospitalization and intravenous antibiotic therapy. An antibiotic combination such as IV ampicillin and gentamicin or ceftriaxone (Rocephin) may be prescribed for severe illness or sepsis associated with UTI. The nursing implications for antibiotic therapy can be found in Chapter 12.

SAFETY ALERT: Follow-up urine culture is scheduled 10 days to 2 weeks following completion of antibiotic therapy for UTI to ensure that bacteria have been eradicated from the urinary tract. ■

The outcome of treatment for UTI is determined by follow-up urinalysis and culture. *Cure*, as evidenced by no pathogens present in the urine, is the desired outcome. Treatment *failure* occurs when therapy fails to eradicate bacteria in the urine. *Recurrent infection* occurs when a persistent source of infection causes repeated infection after initial cure. *Reinfection* is the development of a new infection with a different pathogen following successful UTI treatment.

Patients who experience frequent symptomatic UTIs may be treated prophylactically with a drug such as TMP-SMZ, TMP, nitrofurantoin, or methenamine (Hiprex, Urex). TMP and nitrofurantoin do not achieve effective plasma concentrations at recommended doses, but do reach effective concentrations in the urine. Nursing implications for these urinary anti-infectives and for phenazopyridine (Pyridium), a urinary analgesic, are outlined in **Medication Administration 27.A.**

Antibiotics and urinary anti-infectives are not generally recommended to treat asymptomatic bacteriuria except

Medication Administration 27.A

Urinary Anti-Infectives and Analgesics

URINARY ANTI-INFECTIVES

methenamine (Hiprex, Urex)

nitrofurantoin (Furadantin, Macrobid, Macrodantin)

trimethoprim (Proloprim, Trimpex)

Urinary anti-infectives are usually used prophylactically to prevent recurrence of UTI in patients with frequent symptomatic infections. Nitrofurantoin may also be used to treat UTI.

Nursing Responsibilities

- These drugs are contraindicated for patients with impaired renal function; methenamine and trimethoprim are also contraindicated for patients with impaired liver function. Report abnormal laboratory values such as elevated creatinine or BUN, bilirubin, alanine aminotransferase (ALT), aspartate aminotransferase (AST), and lactic dehydrogenase (LDH).
- Use with caution in older or chronically ill patients. Monitor closely for adverse effects.
- Do not administer trimethoprim to pregnant women because of possible adverse effects on the fetus.
- Monitor the patient taking nitrofurantoin for manifestations of pulmonary sensitivity or peripheral neuropathy. Discontinue the drug and notify the physician.
- Monitor for signs of phenytoin toxicity (sedation, ataxia, and increased blood levels) if trimethoprim is given concurrently. Phenytoin doses may need to be reduced.

Health Education for the Patient and Family

- These drugs are used along with hygiene practices to prevent recurrent UTI. Take as directed, even when no symptoms are present.
- Drink six to eight glasses of water or fluid per day while taking these drugs.
- Take the drug with meals or food to reduce gastric effects; however, avoid milk products because they may interfere with absorption.

(continued)

- Trimethoprim should not be taken during pregnancy. Contact your physician before attempting to become pregnant.
- Contact your doctor if you develop any of the following: Chest pain, difficulty breathing, cough, chills, and fever; numbness and tingling or weakness of the extremities; rash or pruritus (itching).
- Nitrofurantoin turns the urine brown. This is not harmful and subsides when the drug is discontinued.

URINARY ANALGESIC

phenazopyridine (Pyridium)

Phenazopyridine is a urinary tract analgesic that may be used for symptomatic relief of the pain, burning, frequency, and urgency associated with UTI during the first 24 to 48 hours of therapy. Its use is somewhat controversial because it does not treat the infection and may delay effective treatment in the patient with recurrent UTI who saves a dose or two "for the next time."

Nursing Responsibilities

- Monitor renal function (urine output, weight, serum creatinine, and BUN) during treatment; report changes.

Health Education for the Patient and Family

- Take with meals to minimize gastric upset.
- Consume 2 to 3 quarts of fluid daily while taking this drug.
- If you have diabetes, check your blood sugar regularly while taking this drug.
- This drug turns urine orange or red. Protect your clothing from staining.
- Contact lenses may become stained if worn while taking this drug.
- Promptly contact your doctor if symptoms of UTI recur; do not take phenazopyridine before you seek medical treatment.
- If you develop itching or notice a yellow tinge to your skin or eyes, stop taking the drug and notify the physician.

Note: Drugs identified in blue are among the 200 most commonly prescribed medications in the United States.

Source: Data from Adams, Holland, & Urban, 2017.

in pregnant women. The preferred treatment for catheter-associated UTI is removal of the indwelling catheter followed by a 10- to 14-day course of antibiotic therapy to eliminate the infection.

Surgery

Surgery may be indicated for recurrent UTI if diagnostic testing indicates calculi, structural anomalies, or strictures that contribute to the risk of infection. Stones, or *calculi*, in the renal pelvis or in the bladder are an irritant and provide a matrix for bacterial colonization. Treatment may include surgical removal of a large calculus from the renal pelvis or cystoscopic removal of bladder calculi. *Percutaneous ultrasonic pyelolithotomy* or *extracorporeal shock wave lithotripsy* (described later in this chapter) may be used instead of surgery to crush and remove stones. **Ureteroplasty**, surgical repair of a ureter, may be indicated for structural abnormality or stricture of a ureter. This may be combined with a ureteral reimplantation if vesicoureteral reflux is present. The patient returns from these surgeries with an indwelling urinary catheter (Foley or suprapubic) and a **ureteral stent** (a thin catheter inserted into the ureter to provide for urine flow and ureteral support), which remains in place for 3 to 5 days. See **Box 27.1** for nursing care of the patient with a ureteral stent.

Integrative Therapies

Integrative therapies such as homeopathy, aromatherapy, or herbal preparations may be used in conjunction with antibiotics to treat UTI. Cranberry products may help prevent UTIs in women with recurrent symptomatic infections (National Center for Complementary and Integrative Health [NCCIH], 2016). Adding bergamot, sandalwood, lavender, or juniper oil to bath water helps relieve the discomfort of UTI. Consult a qualified herbologist for recommended doses and appropriate use.

Nursing Care

Assessment

Focused assessment data for the patient with a UTI includes:

- *Health history:* Current symptoms, including frequency, urgency, burning on urination, voidings per night; color, clarity, and odor of urine; other manifestations such as lower abdominal, back, or flank pain; nausea and/or vomiting; fever; duration of symptoms and any treatment attempted; history of previous UTIs and their frequency; possibility of pregnancy and type of birth control used; chronic diseases such as diabetes; current medications and any known allergies
- *Physical assessment:* General health; vital signs including temperature; abdominal shape, contour, tenderness to palpation (especially suprapubic); percuss for costovertebral tenderness; observe color, clarity, and odor of urine.

Note that the older adult with a UTI may not complain of dysuria. Be alert for other manifestations of UTI such as incontinence or cloudy or malodorous urine. Inflammatory and immune responses tend to diminish with age, reducing the irritative symptoms of UTI.

Priorities of Care

Collaborating with the interprofessional team to ensure adequate treatment and eradication of the infection is the priority for nursing care. Teaching the patient and caregivers (as appropriate) strategies to prevent future UTIs should also be considered priority nursing actions. The nurse also focuses on promoting comfort and maintaining urinary elimination.

Diagnoses, Outcomes, and Interventions

The patient's general health, abilities for self-care, and risk factors that may contribute to UTI are considered when planning and implementing nursing care for the patient

BOX 27.1
Nursing Care of the Patient with a Ureteral Stent

Ureteral stents are used to maintain patency and promote healing of the ureters. A stent may be temporary, used during and after a surgical procedure, or it may be used for longer periods in patients with ureteral obstruction due to tumors, strictures, or other causes.

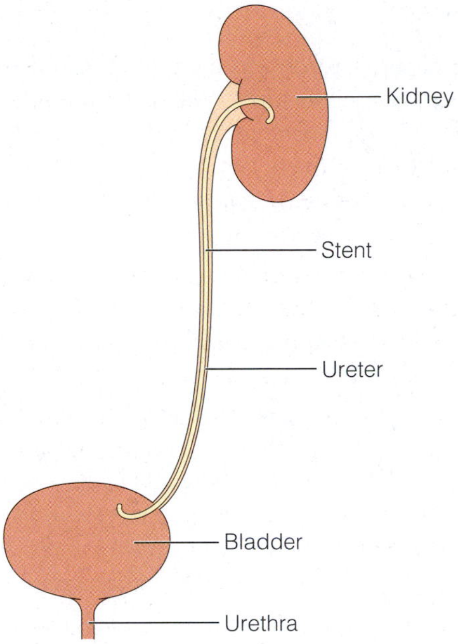
Kidney
Stent
Ureter
Bladder
Urethra

Stents made of a nontoxic material such as silicone or polyurethane may be positioned during surgery or cystoscopy. They are radiopaque with side drainage holes placed along the length of the stent. One or both ends of the stent may be pigtail or J shaped to prevent migration.

- Label all drainage tubes including stents for easy identification. Attach each catheter and stent to a separate closed drainage system. *Careful labeling allows close monitoring of output from all sources and reservoirs. The use of separate drainage systems minimizes the risk of infection.*
- If the stent has been brought to the surface, secure it and maintain its position. *The stent is usually placed in the renal pelvis. It is important to secure it well to prevent trauma to the kidney, inadvertent removal of the stent, and ureter obstruction.*
- Monitor urine output, including color, consistency, and odor. Monitor for signs of infection or bleeding: Fever, tachycardia, pain, hematuria, and cloudy or malodorous urine. *The stent facilitates urine flow but may become obstructed because of bleeding, calculi, or sediment. Obstruction may result in hydronephrosis and kidney damage. The stent itself is a foreign body in the urinary tract and can increase the risk of UTI.*
- Maintain fluid intake, encouraging fluids that acidify urine, such as cranberry juice. *The stent can precipitate calculus formation as well as UTI. Increasing fluid intake and acidifying the urine help prevent these complications.*
- For an indwelling stent, stress the need for regular follow-up to monitor for and prevent complications such as UTI and calculi. *The patient with an indwelling stent may tend to forget that the stent is in place and become lax in compliance with follow-up and preventive measures.*

with a UTI. See the Case Study & Nursing Care Plan for the patient with cystitis on page 879.

Relieve Acute Pain. Pain is a common manifestation of both lower and upper UTI. Urinary tract pain is caused primarily by distention and increased pressure within the tract. The severity of the pain is related to the rate at which inflammation and distention develop, not their degree.

In cystitis, inflammation causes a sensation of fullness; dull, constant suprapubic pain; and possibly low back pain. The inflamed bladder wall and urethra cause dysuria, pain, and burning on urination. Bladder spasms may develop, causing periodic severe, stabbing discomfort. Pain associated with pyelonephritis is often steady and dull, localized to the outer abdomen or flank region. Urologic disorders rarely cause central abdominal pain.

Expected Outcome: Patient will express improved comfort and rate pain at an acceptable level.

The nurse will:

- Assess the timing, quality, intensity, location, duration, and aggravating and alleviating factors of pain. *A change in the nature, location, or intensity of the pain could indicate an extension of the infection or a related but separate problem.*
- Teach or provide comfort measures such as warm sitz baths, warm packs or heating pads, and balanced rest and activity. Systemic analgesics, urinary analgesics, or antispasmodic medication may be used as ordered. *Warmth relaxes muscles, relieves spasms, and increases local blood supply. Because pain can stimulate a stress response and delay healing, it should be relieved when possible.*
- Encourage increased fluid intake unless contraindicated. *Increased fluid dilutes urine, reducing irritation of the inflamed bladder and urethral mucosa.*
- Instruct to notify primary care provider if pain and discomfort continue or intensify after therapy is initiated. *Pain and discomfort in voiding are typically relieved within 24 hours of the initiation of antibiotic therapy. Continued discomfort may indicate a complicated UTI or other urinary tract disorder.*

Restore Normal Urinary Elimination. Inflammation of the bladder and urethral mucosa affects the normal process and patterns of voiding, causing frequency, urgency, and burning on urination, as well as nocturia. Urine may be blood tinged, cloudy, and malodorous. The patient with short- or long-term urinary retention requires additional measures to assess for and prevent UTI.

Expected Outcome: The patient's usual patterns of urinary elimination will be restored.

The nurse will:

- Monitor (or instruct the patient to monitor) color, clarity, and odor of urine. *Urine should return to clear yellow within 48 hours, unless drug therapy causes a change in the color of urine. If clarity does not return, further investigation may be necessary.*

- Instruct to avoid caffeinated drinks, including coffee, tea, and cola; citrus juices; drinks containing artificial sweeteners; and alcoholic beverages. *Caffeine, citrus juices, and artificial sweeteners irritate bladder mucosa and the detrusor muscle and can increase urgency and bladder spasms.*
- Use strict aseptic technique and a closed urinary drainage system when inserting a straight or indwelling urinary catheter. Unless contraindicated, instill anesthetic lubricating gel into the urethra (10 mL for a male and 6 mL for a female) prior to catheter insertion. Insert indwelling catheters to the full recommended length (4 or more inches in women and to the bifurcation in men) before inflating the balloon. *Bacteria colonizing the perineal tissues or on the nurse's hands can be introduced into the bladder during catheterization. Aseptic technique reduces this risk. Anesthetic gel promotes comfort, protects fragile urethral tissues from trauma, and reduces the risk for CAUTI. Inflation of the balloon while in the urethra damages urethral tissues and can cause significant discomfort for the patient.*
- When possible, use intermittent straight catheterization to relieve urinary retention. Remove indwelling urinary catheters as soon as possible. *Using intermittent straight catheterization allows the bladder to fill and completely empty in a more normal manner, maintaining physiologic function and reducing the risk of infection (Agency for Healthcare Research and Quality [AHRQ], 2015). See the accompanying Moving Evidence into Action box for evidence-based practice aimed at reducing the risk of catheter-associated UTI.*
- Maintain the closed urinary drainage system, and use aseptic technique when emptying the catheter drainage bag. Maintain gravity flow, preventing reflux of urine into the bladder from the drainage system. *Bacteria can enter the drainage system when its integrity is interrupted (e.g., disconnecting the catheter from the drainage system) or during emptying of the drainage bag. These bacteria can ascend the column of urine to the bladder, causing UTI.*
- Provide perineal care on a regular basis and following defecation. Use antiseptic preparations only as ordered. *Regular cleansing of perineal tissues reduces the risk of colonization by bowel or other bacteria. While antiseptic solutions may be ordered for catheter care, they can dry perineal tissues and reduce normal flora, increasing the risk of colonization by pathogens, and should not routinely be used.*

SAFETY ALERT: Provide for easy access to toileting. Make sure that lighting is adequate and that pathways are free of obstacles. Frequency, urgency, and nocturia increase the risk of urinary incontinence and of injury due to falls, particularly in a patient who is older or debilitated. ■

Promote Self-Management Through Education. The patient with a urinary tract infection is at an increased risk for future UTI and needs to understand risk factors and measures to prevent recurrent infection. In addition, once the manifestations of UTI are relieved, motivation to continue the treatment plan declines. Failure to complete the full course of therapy and recommended follow-up can lead to continued bacteriuria, recurrent infections, and the development of antibiotic-resistant bacteria.

Expected Outcome: Patient will verbalize understanding of the infectious process and its treatment and ways to reduce risk for future UTIs.

The nurse will:

- Teach how to obtain a midstream clean-catch urine specimen. *Cleansing of the urinary meatus and perineal area reduces contamination of the specimen by external cells and bacteria. Ninety percent of urethral bacteria are cleared in the first 10 mL of voided urine; a midstream specimen is representative of urine in the bladder.*
- Assess knowledge about the disease process, risk factors, and preventive measures. *The patient may have little understanding of UTI, its causes, and contributing factors.*
- Discuss the prescribed treatment plan and the importance of taking all prescribed antibiotics. *Symptoms are largely relieved within 24 to 48 hours of starting antibiotic therapy; however, bacteria may remain in the urinary tract. Completing the prescribed regimen is important to prevent recurrent infections and resistant bacteria.*
- Help the patient develop a plan for taking medications. *Missed doses of antibiotic can result in subtherapeutic blood levels and reduced effectiveness. Taking medication in association with a regular daily activity such as meals helps patients remember doses.*
- Instruct to keep appointments for follow-up and urine culture. *Follow-up urine culture, often scheduled 7 to 14 days after completion of antibiotic therapy, is vital to ensure complete eradication of bacteria and prevent relapse or recurrence.*
- Teach measures to prevent future UTI (see Section 26.4, Health Promotion, in Chapter 26). *A history of UTI is an independent risk factor for future infections. Teaching measures to manage other risk factors can reduce the patient's risk for future UTIs.*

Delegating Nursing Care Activities

As appropriate and allowed within the designated duties and responsibilities of assistive personnel, the nurse may delegate nursing care activities such as obtaining a clean-catch urine specimen, assisting with toileting and hygiene, and providing urinary catheter care for the patient with UTI.

Transitions of Care

Because both upper and lower urinary tract infections are usually managed in the community, teaching is the most important nursing intervention. See Section 26.4, Health Promotion, in Chapter 26 for UTI prevention. Provide instruction on the following topics:

Case Study & Nursing Care Plan

A Patient with Cystitis

Miija Waisanen is a 25-year-old second-year nursing student who recently got married. Mrs. Waisanen has never been pregnant, and she is using a diaphragm for birth control. She presents at the local urgent care clinic complaining of low back pain, frequency, urgency, and burning on urination that began the day before.

ASSESSMENT

Patrice Ramiros, RN, admits Mrs. Waisanen to the clinic. Mrs. Waisanen denies having had similar symptoms in the past or ever having been diagnosed with a UTI. She describes her pain as a constant, dull ache that does not change with movement. She feels the need to urinate almost constantly, but experiences difficulty in starting her stream and burning pain and cramping when voiding. She reports getting up four times the night before to urinate. She denies painful intercourse and states that her last menstrual period began only 2 weeks ago. Physical examination reveals BP 112/68 mmHg; P 90 bpm and regular, afebrile. Suprapubic tenderness noted but no flank or costovertebral angle tenderness. Clean-catch urine specimen shows hematuria, multiple WBCs, and a bacteria count greater than 10^5 per milliliter.

The nurse practitioner prescribes trimethoprim-sulfamethoxazole (TMP-SMZ) 160 mg/800 mg PO bid for 3 days and aspirin or acetaminophen 650 mg PO every 4 hours as needed for pain. Mrs. Waisanen is instructed to return to the clinic in 7 days for a follow-up urine culture, or sooner if her symptoms do not improve.

DIAGNOSES

- Acute pain related to infection and inflammatory process in the urinary tract
- Abnormal urinary elimination related to inflammation as evidenced by frequency, urgency, nocturia, and dysuria
- Needs education related to risk factors for and treatment of UTI

EXPECTED OUTCOMES

- Patient will report relief of low back pain and burning on urination.
- Patient will regain a normal voiding pattern without frequency, urgency, nocturia, and abnormal urine characteristics.
- Patient will verbalize understanding of the disease process, related risk factors, follow-up instructions, and symptoms of recurrence indicating the need for medical attention.

PLANNING AND IMPLEMENTATION

- Teach comfort measures: Warm sitz baths, a heating pad on low heat applied to her lower back or abdomen, rest, increased fluid intake, avoiding caffeinated beverages, and taking aspirin or acetaminophen as ordered.
- Advise to refrain from sexual intercourse until infection and inflammation have cleared to avoid further irritation of inflamed tissues.
- Discuss the possible relationship between using a diaphragm for birth control and UTI in women.
- Discuss dietary and hygiene practices to prevent UTI, symptoms indicating the need for further intervention, and the risks of undertreatment.

EVALUATION

Six months later, Mrs. Waisanen rotates through the urgent care clinic for her community-based nursing experience. Ms. Ramiros asks how she is doing. Mrs. Waisanen reports that her symptoms and urine cleared within about a day after starting the antibiotic and she has had no further problems. She has seen her women's healthcare nurse practitioner to change her birth control to oral contraceptives, increased her intake of fluid and vitamin C, and no longer puts off urinating until she "has time to go."

CLINICAL REASONING IN PATIENT CARE

1. What additional information should you obtain from Mrs. Waisanen prior to her discharge from the clinic?
2. Identify important teaching related to Mrs. Waisanen's prescribed antibiotic therapy and recommended follow-up care.
3. What physiologic and psychosocial factors put Mrs. Waisanen at risk for developing a UTI?
4. Compare and contrast the benefits and drawbacks to short-course therapy versus conventional therapy for UTI.
5. Develop a care plan for Mrs. Waisanen for educating her about managing her health.

See Evaluating Your Response in Appendix B.

- Risk factors for UTI and how to minimize or eliminate these factors through increased fluid intake, regular elimination, and personal hygiene measures
- Early manifestations of UTI and the importance of seeking medical intervention promptly
- Maintaining optimal immune system function by attending to physical and psychosocial stressors, such as inadequate rest, poor nutrition, and high levels of emotional stress
- The importance of completing the prescribed treatment and keeping follow-up appointments.

Moving Evidence into Action

Preventing Catheter-Associated Urinary Tract Infections Using the ANA CAUTI Prevention Tool

Clinical Issue

CAUTI infections are the most common healthcare-acquired infection. Due to overwhelming numbers as well as CAUTI prevention techniques, the Centers for Medicare and Medicaid Services (CMS) suspended reimbursement for CAUTI infections in 2009 (McNeill, 2017; Panchisin, 2016). In light of these combined pressures, prevention of CAUTIs is a critical nursing responsibility.

External Evidence

The American Nurses Association (2018) developed a CAUTI prevention tool focusing on three important concepts: (1) Use of fewer indwelling catheters; (2) catheter removal as soon as feasible; and (3) recommendations for insertion, maintenance of the indwelling catheter, and postremoval care. The preventive algorithm begins with the Centers for Disease Control and Prevention criteria for indwelling catheters. If the criteria are met, insertion is recommended. The following steps reflect evidence-based instructions for insertion, catheter management, and postremoval patient care.

Internal Evidence

As part of the evaluation of internal evidence, one must consider the impact of the external evidence findings on how healthcare providers implement indwelling catheter use and management. As CAUTI is an identified nonreimbursable expense by CMS, most healthcare organizations now include CAUTI and indwelling catheter use within quality initiatives. The nurse should investigate organizational policies regarding indwelling catheter use.

Patient Considerations

The determination of use of indwelling catheters is based on medical need (see the CDC indications on the tool). When considering the initiation of an indwelling catheter, the nurse must consider the specific patient population and the individual indication(s) for use.

Putting the Pieces Together

The incidence of CAUTIs and cost of treatment has led to suspension of reimbursement for treatment of CAUTIs. Management of indwelling catheters is a nursing responsibility. The publication by the American Nurses Association provides a user-friendly tool for use by nurses. The use of this prevention tool should be the standard in caring for persons requiring indwelling catheters.

References

American Nurses Association (ANA). (2018). *ANA CAUTI Prevention Tool*. Retrieved from https://www.nursingworld.org/practice-policy/innovation-evidence/clinical-practice-material/ana-cauti-prevention-tool/.

McNeill, L. (2017). Back to basics: How evidence-based nursing practice can prevent catheter-associated urinary tract infections. *Urologic Nursing, 37*(4), 204–206.

Panchisin, T. L. (2016). Improving outcomes with the ANA CAUTI prevention tool. *Nursing, 46*(3), 55–59.

Acute management of UTI focuses on early diagnosis and determination of the underlying organism. Based on the etiology of the infection, patients should be instructed to complete all pharmacologic treatment as indicated. Residents of long-term care facilities, people with impaired cognition, and those who require an indwelling urinary catheter or intermittent catheterization have a significant risk of reinfection. Teach caregivers to recognize subtle signs of infection such as increased urinary incontinence, a change in behavior, or increasing frailty. In addition, include the following topics:

- Use alternatives to an indwelling catheter when possible. For urinary incontinence, try scheduled toileting, incontinence pads or diapers, and external catheters, if possible. For urinary retention, teach the patient or caregiver to perform straight catheterization every 3 to 4 hours using clean technique.
- When an indwelling catheter is necessary, teach measures such as perineal care, managing and emptying the collection chamber, maintaining a closed system, and bladder irrigation or flushing, if ordered.

27.2 Urinary Calculi

Obstruction of urine flow impairs renal function and is a common cause of acute and chronic kidney disease (Sorenson et al., 2019). See **Table 27.1** for common causes of urinary tract obstruction. **Urinary calculi**, stones in the urinary tract, are the most common cause of upper urinary tract obstruction. The term **lithiasis** means stone formation. When the stones form in the kidney, it is known as *nephrolithiasis*; when they form elsewhere in the urinary tract (for example, the bladder), it is called *urolithiasis*. Stones may form and obstruct the urinary tract at any point (**Figure 27.4** ■); however, in the United States and other industrialized countries, renal or kidney stones are the most common.

Pathophysiology

Normally, a balance exists in the kidneys between the need to conserve water and the need to eliminate poorly soluble materials such as calcium salts. This balance is affected by factors such as diet, environmental temperature, and activity. Protective inorganic and organic substances in the urine, such as pyrophosphate, citrate, and glycoproteins, normally inhibit stone formation.

Three factors contribute to urolithiasis: Supersaturation, nucleation, and lack of inhibitory substances in the urine.

When the concentration of an insoluble salt in the urine is very high, that is, when the urine is supersaturated, crystals may form. Usually, these crystals disperse and are

Table 27.1 Major Causes of Urinary Tract Obstruction by Location

Location	Obstructive Process
Kidney pelvis	■ Calculi (stones) ■ Polycystic kidney disease ■ Infection and scarring
Ureters	■ Calculi ■ Scarring and stricture ■ Congenital defects or strictures ■ External processes such as pregnancy, tumors, lymph node enlargement
Bladder	■ Neurogenic bladder ■ Tumors ■ Calculi and other foreign bodies
Urethra	■ Benign prostatic hypertrophy ■ Tumors ■ Scarring and stricture ■ Trauma

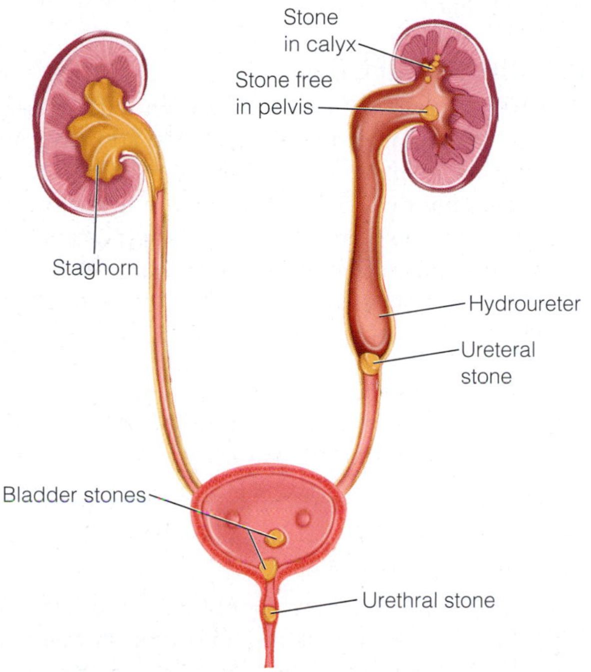
Stone
in calyx
Stone free
in pelvis
Staghorn
Hydroureter
Ureteral
stone
Bladder stones
Urethral stone

Figure 27.4 ■ Development and location of calculi within the urinary tract.

eliminated because the bonds holding them together are weak. However, a nucleus of crystals may develop stable bonds to form a stone. More often, crystals form around an organic matrix or mucoprotein nucleus to become a stone. The stimulus required to initiate crystallization in supersaturated urine may be minimal. Ingesting a meal high in insoluble salt, or decreased fluid intake as occurs during sleep, allows the concentration to increase to the point where precipitation occurs and stones are formed and grow. When fluid intake is adequate, no stone growth occurs. The acidity or alkalinity of the urine and the presence or absence of calculus-inhibiting compounds also affects lithiasis.

The majority of kidney stones are *calcium stones*, composed of calcium oxalate and/or calcium phosphate (Sorenson et al., 2019). These stones are generally associated with high concentrations of calcium in the blood or urine. *Uric acid stones* develop when the urine concentration of uric acid is high. They are more common in men and may be associated with gout. Genetic factors contribute to the development of uric acid stones and calcium stones. *Struvite* (magnesium-ammonium phosphate) *stones* are associated with UTI caused by urease-producing bacteria such as *Proteus*. These stones can grow to become very large, filling the renal pelvis and calyces. They are often called *staghorn stones* because of their shape (refer to Figure 27.4). *Cystine stones* are rare and are associated with a genetic defect. The types of renal calculi, contributing factors, and recommended dietary modifications are listed in **Table 27.2**.

Risk Factors

Urolithiasis is common; about 1 in 11 people in the United States will develop urinary stones at some point during their lifetime (Scales, Smith, Hanley, & Saigal, 2012). In the United States, the incidence varies by region, with the highest frequency in the southern and midwestern states. Calculi are more common among White populations than other ethnicities. Most people affected are in young or middle adulthood.

Table 27.2 Renal Calculi: Types, Contributing Factors, and Interventions

Stone Type and Incidence	Risk Factors	Management
Calcium phosphate and/or oxalate 70%	Hypercalciuria and hypercalcemia: Hyperparathyroidism, immobility, bone disease, vitamin D intoxication, multiple myeloma, renal tubular acidosis, prolonged steroid intake Alkaline urine Dehydration Inflammatory bowel disease	***Pharmacology:*** Thiazide diuretics, phosphates ***Dietary:*** Limit foods high in sodium and protein, maintain calcium intake, increase foods that acidify urine ***Other:*** Increase hydration, exercise
Uric acid 5–10%	Gout, increased purine intake, acid urine	***Pharmacology:*** Potassium citrate (to alkalinize urine), allopurinol ***Dietary:*** Avoid foods that are high in purines ***Other:*** Increase hydration
Struvite 10–12%	UTIs, especially *Proteus* infections	***Pharmacology:*** Antibiotic therapy for UTI ***Other:*** Surgical intervention or a lithotripsy is performed to remove stone
Cystine 1%	Genetic defect, acid urine	***Pharmacology:*** Penicillamine, sodium bicarbonate ***Dietary:*** Restrict sodium ***Other:*** Increase hydration

Source: Hall, 2010.

Although the majority of stones are idiopathic (having no demonstrable cause), a number of risk factors have been identified. The greatest risk factor for stone formation is a prior personal or family history of urinary calculi. A genetic predisposition toward the accumulation of certain mineral substances in the urine or a congenital lack of protective factors may explain the familial link. Other identified risk factors include dehydration with resultant increased urine concentration, immobility, and excess dietary intake of calcium, oxalate, or proteins. Gout, hyperparathyroidism, and urinary stasis or repeated infections also contribute to calculus formation.

Manifestations

The symptoms caused by urinary calculi vary with their size and location. Manifestations develop as a result of obstructed urine flow with resulting distention and tissue trauma caused by passage of the rough-edged, crystalline stone.

Calculi affecting the kidney calyces and pelvis may cause few symptoms. If the stone has gradually or partially obstructed urinary flow, dull, aching flank pain may be present, but renal calculi are often silent, without symptoms. Bladder calculi may cause few symptoms other than dull suprapubic pain with exercise or after voiding.

Renal colic, acute, severe flank pain on the affected side, develops when a stone obstructs the ureter, causing ureteral spasm. The pain of renal colic may radiate to the suprapubic region, groin, and external genitals (the scrotum or labia). The severity of the pain often causes a sympathetic response with associated nausea and vomiting, pallor, and cool, clammy skin.

Manifestations of UTI, including chills and fever, frequency, urgency, and dysuria, may accompany urinary calculi at any level. Trauma to the urinary tract by the calculi may cause gross or microscopic hematuria. Gross hematuria is often the only sign of bladder stones.

Complications

Urinary stones may obstruct urine flow, leading to complications such as hydronephrosis and urinary stasis with subsequent infection.

Obstruction

Stones can obstruct the urinary tract at any point from the calyces of the kidney to the distal urethra, impeding the outflow of urine. If the obstruction develops slowly, there may be few or no symptoms, whereas sudden obstruction (e.g., blockage of a ureter by a passing stone) may cause severe manifestations. Urinary tract obstruction can ultimately lead to renal failure. The degree of obstruction, its location, and the duration of impaired urine flow determine the effect on renal function.

Hydronephrosis

The kidneys continue to produce urine, causing increased pressure and distention of the urinary tract behind the obstruction. **Hydronephrosis**, distention of the renal pelvis and calyces, and *hydroureter*, distention of the ureter, are possible results. If the pressure is unrelieved, the collecting tubules, proximal tubules, and glomeruli of the kidney are damaged, causing a gradual loss of renal function.

Acute hydronephrosis typically causes colicky pain on the affected side. The pain may radiate into the groin. Chronic hydronephrosis develops slowly and may have few manifestations other than dull, aching back or flank pain. When hydronephrosis is significant, a palpable mass may be felt in the flank region. Hematuria and signs of UTI such as pyuria, fever, and discomfort may occur. Gastrointestinal symptoms such as nausea and vomiting and abdominal pain may accompany hydronephrosis.

Infection

Urinary stasis associated with partial or complete obstruction increases the risk of urinary tract infection. Either upper or lower UTI may develop.

Interprofessional Care

Management of urinary calculi focuses on relieving acute symptoms, destroying or removing stones, and preventing further stone formation. Asymptomatic stones (those not causing pain, infection, or obstruction) are treated conservatively. Kidney stones are commonly asymptomatic while ureteral stones cause much more severe symptoms including flank and radiating pain, nausea and vomiting, and cool, clammy skin.

Diagnosis

Laboratory and diagnostic tests that may be ordered when urinary calculi are suspected include:

- ***Urinalysis*** to assess for hematuria and the presence of WBCs and crystal fragments. The urine pH is helpful in identifying the type of stone.
- ***Chemical analysis*** of any stones passed in the urine determines the type of stone and suggests measures to prevent further stone formation. Retrieving stones or teaching the patient to do so is a nursing responsibility. All urine is strained and may be saved. Any visible stones or sediment is sent for analysis.
- ***Urine calcium, uric acid***, and ***oxalate*** levels measure the amount of these substances excreted over a 24-hour period and may be assessed to help identify possible causes of lithiasis. Elevated calcium levels occur in hyperparathyroidism, Cushing syndrome, and osteoporosis, all of which may contribute to lithiasis. Uric acid levels may be elevated in patients with gout and those at risk for forming uric acid calculi. Urine oxalate excretion may help to differentiate calcium oxalate from calcium phosphate stones.
- ***Serum calcium, phosphorus***, and ***uric acid*** levels may be obtained to help identify factors contributing to calculus formation.
- *KUB* (kidneys, ureters, and bladder) x-ray of the lower abdomen may show calculi as opacities in the kidneys, ureters, and bladder.

- *Renal ultrasonography* uses reflected sound waves to detect stones and evaluate the kidneys for possible hydronephrosis.
- *Spiral computed tomography (CT) scan* of the kidney, with or without contrast medium, shows calculi, ureteral obstruction, and other renal disorders.
- *Cystoscopy* is used to visualize and possibly remove calculi from the urinary bladder and distal ureters.

Medications

An acute episode of renal colic is treated with analgesia, medications to promote stone passage, and hydration. A narcotic analgesic such as morphine sulfate is given, often intravenously, to relieve pain and reduce ureteral spasm. Indomethacin, a nonsteroidal anti-inflammatory drug (NSAID) given as a suppository, may reduce the amount of narcotic analgesia required for acute renal colic. An oral alpha-adrenergic blocker such as tamsulosin (Flomax) is prescribed to relax ureteral muscle and promote passage of the stone. Oral or intravenous fluids reduce the risk of further stone formation and promote urine output.

After analysis of the calculus, various medications may be ordered to inhibit or prevent further lithiasis. A thiazide diuretic, frequently prescribed for calcium calculi, acts to reduce urinary calcium excretion and is very effective in preventing further stones. Potassium citrate alkalinizes urine (raises the pH) and is often prescribed to prevent stones that tend to form in acidic urine (uric acid, cystine, and some forms of calcium stones). Refer to Table 27.2 for other preparations related to types of stones. Nursing responsibilities focus on teaching the patient about the prescribed medication, its importance in preventing further stone formation, and potential adverse effects.

Nutrition

Diet modifications may be prescribed to address factors found to contribute to lithiasis (National Institute of Diabetes and Digestive and Kidney Diseases [NIDDK], 2017). Increased fluid intake of 2.5 to 3.0 L/day is recommended, regardless of stone composition. A fluid intake to ensure the production of approximately 2.0 to 2.5 L of urine a day prevents the stone-forming salts from becoming concentrated enough to precipitate. Fluid intake should be spaced throughout the day and evening. Some authorities recommend that patients drink one to two glasses of water at night to prevent concentration of urine during sleep.

Recommended dietary changes may include reduced intake of the primary substance forming the calculi. For calcium stones, however, restricting dietary calcium may actually increase the risk of stone formation while promoting bone loss. A low-sodium, restricted-protein diet has been shown to be more effective in preventing the recurrence of calcium stones. Dietary sodium is also restricted in patients who form cystine stones (NIDDK, 2017). Oxalate may be limited in patients found to have calcium oxalate stones and high levels of oxalate in their urine. Foods high in oxalate include asparagus, beer and colas, beets, cabbage, celery, spinach, chocolate and cocoa, fruits, green beans, nuts, tea, and tomatoes.

The patient with uric acid stones requires a diet low in purines. Purine-rich foods, which should be avoided, include organ meats, goose, sardines, and herring. Foods with moderate levels of purines, such as red and white meats, crab, and salmon, should be limited.

Treatment

Treatment of existing calculi depends on the location of the stone, the extent of obstruction, renal function, the presence or absence of UTI, and the patient's general state of health. In general, the stone is removed if it is causing obstruction, infection, unrelieved pain, or serious bleeding.

Lithotripsy, using sound or shock waves to crush a stone, is the preferred treatment for urinary calculi. Several techniques are available. *Extracorporeal shock wave lithotripsy (ESWL)* is a noninvasive technique for fragmenting kidney stones using shock waves generated outside the body. Acoustic shock waves are aimed under fluoroscopic guidance at the stone (**Figure 27.5** ■). These shock waves travel through soft tissue without causing damage, but shatter the stone as its greater density stops their progress. Repeated shock waves pulverize the stone into fragments small enough to be eliminated in the urine. The procedure may require 30 minutes to 2 hours to complete. Intravenous sedation is generally adequate to maintain comfort during the procedure. Pregnancy is an absolute contraindication for lithotripsy procedures, and, because its effects on the ovary are unknown, it is relatively contraindicated for women of childbearing age. Lithotripsy also may be performed using a percutaneous ultrasonic or laser technique.

Percutaneous nephrolithotomy uses a nephroscope inserted into the kidney pelvis through a small flank incision (**Figure 27.6** ■). The stone is fragmented using a small ultrasonic transducer or laser, and the fragments are removed through the nephroscope. In a *ureteroscopy* procedure, laser beams are used to disintegrate the stone, without damaging soft tissue. A ureteroscope (passed up the ureter from the bladder during cystoscopy) is used to guide the laser probe into direct contact with the stone.

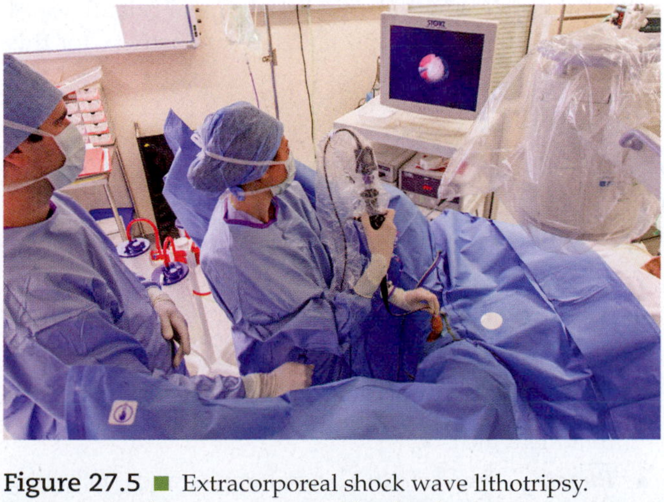

Figure 27.5 ■ Extracorporeal shock wave lithotripsy. Acoustic shock waves generated by the shock wave generator travel through soft tissue to shatter the urinary stone into fragments, which are then eliminated in the urine.

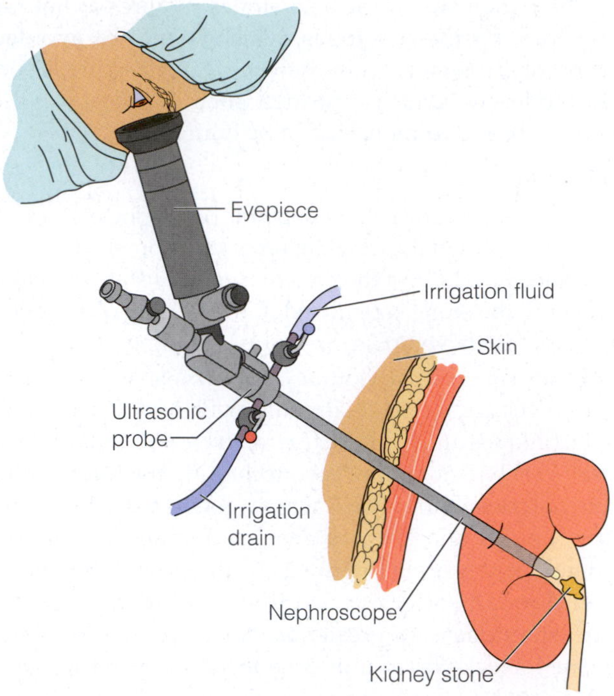
Eyepiece
Irrigation fluid
Skin
Ultrasonic probe
Irrigation drain
Nephroscope
Kidney stone

Figure 27.6 ■ Percutaneous ultrasonic lithotripsy. A nephroscope is inserted into the renal pelvis, and ultrasonic waves are used to fragment the stone. The fragments are then removed through the nephroscope.

A double-J stent may be inserted into the affected ureter to maintain its patency following ESWL or other lithotripsy procedures. Bladder stones may be removed using an instrument passed through a cystoscope to crush the stones. The remaining stone fragments are then irrigated out of the bladder using an acid solution to counteract the alkalinity that precipitated stone formation. See **Box 27.2** for nursing care of the patient having lithotripsy.

Integrative Therapy Nonpharmacologic measures such as positioning, moist heat, relaxation techniques, guided imagery, and diversion as adjunctive therapy for pain relief. There have been no specific evidence-based integrative therapies that directly impact renal calculi. Good hydration is the most important self-care activity for this disorder.

Nursing Care

Assessment

Obtain subjective and objective assessment data specific to urolithiasis:

- *Health history:* Complaints of flank, back, or abdominal pain, radiation, characteristics and timing, aggravating or relieving factors; nausea and vomiting; possible contributing factors such as dehydration; previous or family history of kidney stones; current or previous treatment measures
- *Physical assessment:* General appearance including position, vital signs; skin color, temperature, moisture, turgor; abdominal, flank, or costovertebral tenderness; amount, color, and characteristics of urine (presence of hematuria, bacteria, pyuria, pH).

BOX 27.2
Nursing Care of the Patient Having Lithotripsy

PREOPERATIVE CARE

- Assess knowledge and understanding of the procedure, providing information as needed. *Anxiety is reduced, and recovery is enhanced and hastened when the patient is fully prepared for surgery.*
- Follow directions from the radiology department, physician, or anesthetist for withholding food and fluids and for bowel preparation prior to surgery. *Conscious sedation, general anesthesia, or spinal anesthesia may be required, depending on the procedure. Fecal material in the bowel may impede fluoroscopic visualization of the kidney and stone.*

POSTOPERATIVE CARE

- In the initial period, monitor vital signs frequently. *The kidney is highly vascular; therefore, hemorrhage and resulting shock are potential complications of lithotripsy. Bleeding may be internal or retroperitoneal and difficult to detect.*
- Monitor amount, color, and clarity of urine output. *Urine is often bright red initially, but bleeding should diminish within 48 to 72 hours. Cloudy urine may indicate the presence of an infection.*
- Maintain placement and patency of urinary catheters, if present. Anchor ureteral catheters or nephrostomy tubes securely. Irrigate gently, if ordered. *A kinked or plugged catheter may result in hydroureter, hydronephrosis, and kidney damage. Decreased urinary output and flank pain are possible symptoms of obstructed urine flow. Excessive force in irrigation may cause trauma and bleeding.*
- Prepare for discharge by teaching care of the indwelling catheter, urine-collection device, and incision site (if present). Teach signs and symptoms to report: Urine leakage from incision for more than 4 days, symptoms of infection, pain, and bright hematuria. *Many patients are discharged with dressings and catheters in place. The patient and family need necessary information to provide self-care.*
- Teach measures to reduce the risk of further lithiasis. *Many patients have repeated episodes of lithiasis and renal colic. Prevention of stone formation is important to preserve renal function.*

Priorities of Care

Maintaining unobstructed urine flow from the kidneys through the urinary meatus is the interprofessional care priority. The nurse assesses urinary output and monitors for complications such as hydronephrosis or acute kidney injury. Promoting comfort is also a nursing care priority, particularly in the patient with renal colic.

Diagnoses, Outcomes, and Interventions

Relieve Acute Pain. Pain is the primary outward manifestation of urolithiasis, particularly when a stone lodges within a ureter, causing acute obstruction and distention. Invasive and noninvasive procedures to remove or crush stones may also be painful.

Expected Outcome: Patient will report pain at a level of 2 or lower on a scale of 0 to 10.

The nurse will:

- Assess pain using a standard pain scale and its characteristics. Administer analgesia as ordered and monitor its effectiveness. *The intensity, type of pain, and its responsiveness to analgesia provide valuable clues as to its cause. Regular administration of prescribed analgesics controls pain more effectively than waiting until pain becomes intolerable. Administering an ordered NSAID on a routine schedule may significantly reduce the need for narcotic analgesia in patients with renal colic.*

- Encourage fluid intake and ambulation in the patient with renal colic unless contraindicated. *Increased fluids and ambulation increase urinary output, facilitating movement of the calculus through the ureter and decreasing pain.*
- Use nonpharmacologic measures such as positioning, moist heat, relaxation techniques, guided imagery, and diversion as adjunctive therapy for pain relief. *Adjunctive pain relief measures can enhance the effectiveness of analgesics and other prescribed treatment.*

SAFETY ALERT: The intensity of renal colic pain can cause a vasovagal response with resulting hypotension and syncope. Always provide for the patient's safety. ■

Promote Normal Urinary Elimination. Obstruction of the urinary tract is the primary complication associated with urolithiasis. Obstruction can ultimately lead to stasis, infection, or irreversible renal damage.

Expected Outcome: Patient's urinary output and renal function studies will remain within expected parameters.

The nurse will:

- Monitor amount and character of urine output. If catheterized, measure output hourly. Document any hematuria, dysuria, frequency, urgency, and pyuria. Strain all urine for stones, saving any recovered stones for laboratory analysis. *The amount of urine output helps determine urinary tract patency and adequacy of hydration. Hematuria, gross or microscopic, is often associated with calculi and with procedures used to remove stones, such as cystoscopy or lithotripsy. A change in the amount of hematuria may indicate stone passage or a complication. Dysuria, frequency, urgency, and cloudy urine are symptoms of UTI, often associated with urolithiasis. Antibiotic therapy may be required. Analysis of stones recovered from the urine can direct measures to prevent further lithiasis.*
- Maintain patency and integrity of all catheter systems. Secure catheters well, label as indicated, and use sterile technique for all ordered irrigations or other procedures. *A kinked or plugged catheter, particularly a ureteral catheter or nephrostomy tube, may damage the urinary system. Labeling catheters can prevent mistakes, such as inappropriate irrigation or clamping. Any catheter increases the risk of infection; use of aseptic technique in all procedures reduces this risk.*

SAFETY ALERT: A stone that completely obstructs the ureter can lead to hydronephrosis and acute kidney injury on the affected side. Report symptoms such as dull flank pain or aching and changes in renal function studies (BUN, serum creatinine, and eGFR). Because the other kidney continues to function, urine output may not fall significantly with obstruction of one ureter. A drop in eGFR or rising BUN and serum creatinine levels may be early signs of renal failure. ■

Teach Self-Care. When pain can be managed with oral analgesics, urinary stones are managed in the community. The patient needs to know how and why to collect the calculus and indicators of complications, such as reduced urine output and cloudy or bloody urine. The patient with urolithiasis needs information about the disease and its possible consequences, any diagnostic or therapeutic procedures performed, and strategies to prevent future lithiasis.

Expected Outcome: Patient will verbalize an understanding of the disease, factors contributing to its development, recommended treatment, and self-care strategies to prevent future episodes of stone development.

The nurse will:

- Assess understanding and previous learning. *Relating information to previously learned material enhances retention and understanding.*
- Present all material in a manner appropriate to knowledge base, developmental and educational level, and current needs. *Learning is an active process that requires the patient's participation. Tailoring teaching to the individual increases involvement.*
- Teach about all diagnostic and treatment procedures. *Knowing what to expect reduces anxiety, enhances compliance, and hastens recovery.*
- If the patient will be managed in the community, teach to:
  a. Collect and strain all urine, saving any stones.
  b. Report stone passage to the physician and bring the stone in for analysis.
  c. Report any changes in the amount or character of urine output to physician.
- Teach measures to prevent further urolithiasis:
  a. Increase fluid intake to 2500 to 3500 mL/day.
  b. Follow recommended dietary guidelines.
  c. Maintain activity level to prevent urinary stasis and bone resorption.
- Take medications as prescribed. *The risk of recurrent lithiasis is approximately 50%; however, this risk can be reduced by following measures to prevent conditions favoring stone formation.*
- Teach about the relationship between urinary calculi and UTI, emphasizing preventive measures and the importance of prompt treatment. *Urinary tract infection promotes urolithiasis and thus requires prompt treatment to reduce this risk.*

Delegating Nursing Care Activities

As appropriate and allowed within the designated duties and responsibilities of assistive personnel, the nurse may delegate nursing care activities such as measuring intake and output, straining all urine, and assisting with ADLs for the patient with urinary calculi.

Transitions of Care

The patient with urinary calculi needs to know how to manage existing stones and what to do to reduce the risk of future stone formation. Discuss the following topics to prepare the patient and family for home care:

- Importance of maintaining a fluid intake adequate to produce 2.0 to 2.5 quarts of urine per day
- Prescribed medications, their management, and potential adverse effects
- Dietary recommendations
- Prevention, recognition, and management of UTI
- Any further diagnostic or treatment measures planned.

When the patient is to be discharged with dressings, a nephrostomy tube, or a catheter, teach the patient and family about the following:

- How to change dressings, maintaining aseptic technique
- Assessment of the wound and skin for healing and possible complications such as infection or skin breakdown
- How to manage drainage systems and maintain their patency
- Emptying drainage bags and assessing urine output
- When to contact the physician and recommendations for follow-up care.

Acute management of urinary calculi focuses on early diagnosis and determination of the underlying cause. Treatment focuses on pain alleviation, reduction of complications and resolution of the calculi by passage, or removal. All pharmacologic treatments should be completed as ordered. Patient education regarding diet to manage uric acid can reduce recurrence of urinary calculi formation. Patients should be instructed that development of urinary calculi increases the risk for future urinary calculi formation (National Kidney Foundation, 2016).

27.3 Urinary Tract Tumors

A malignancy can develop in any part of the urinary tract from the kidney pelvis to the urinary meatus. According to the American Cancer Society (2018), more than 81,000 cases of bladder cancer, 63,000 cases of kidney cancer, and 3800 cases of uteral cancer are estimated. When diagnosed early, the 5-year survival rate for bladder cancer is 96% (ACS, 2018).

Pathophysiology

Most urinary tract malignancies arise from epithelial tissue. Transitional epithelium lines the entire tract from the renal pelvis through the urethra. Carcinogenic breakdown products of certain chemicals and from cigarette smoke are excreted in the urine and stored in the bladder, possibly causing a local influence on abnormal cell development. Squamous cell carcinoma of the urinary tract occurs less frequently than transitional epithelial cell tumors.

Urinary tract tumors begin as nonspecific cellular alterations that develop into either flat or papillary lesions. These lesions may be either superficial or invasive. Most bladder tumors are papillary lesions (*papillomas*), a polyp-like structure attached by a stalk to the bladder mucosa. Papillomas are generally superficial, noninvasive tumors that bleed easily and frequently recur. They rarely progress to become invasive, and the prognosis for recovery is good.

Carcinoma in situ (CIS), which occurs less frequently, is a poorly differentiated flat tumor that invades directly and is associated with a poorer prognosis. These tumors often initially present as superficial lesions, later progressing to become invasive (**Figure 27.7** ■). Grade I tumors are highly differentiated and rarely progress to become invasive, whereas grade III tumors are poorly differentiated and usually progress. The tumor, node, metastasis (TNM) system, outlined in **Table 27.3**, is used to stage bladder tumors. When metastasis occurs, the pelvic lymph nodes, lungs, bones, and liver are most commonly involved. More information about tumor grading and staging can be found in Chapter 14, which discusses cancer physiology, treatment, and nursing care of the patient with cancer.

Risk Factors

Two major factors are implicated in the development of bladder cancer: The presence of carcinogens in the urine and chronic inflammation or infection of bladder mucosa. Cigarette smoking is the primary risk factor for bladder cancer. The risk in smokers is twice that of nonsmokers (ACS, 2018). The chemicals and dyes used in the plastics, rubber, and cable industries; substances in the work environment of textile workers, leather finishers, spray painters, and petroleum workers; and high levels of arsenic in drinking water are also associated with a higher risk of bladder cancer. Additional risk factors for bladder cancer include residence in an urban area, chronic UTIs, and bladder calculi. The risk for bladder cancer appears to be reduced by increasing the intake of fluids and vegetables.

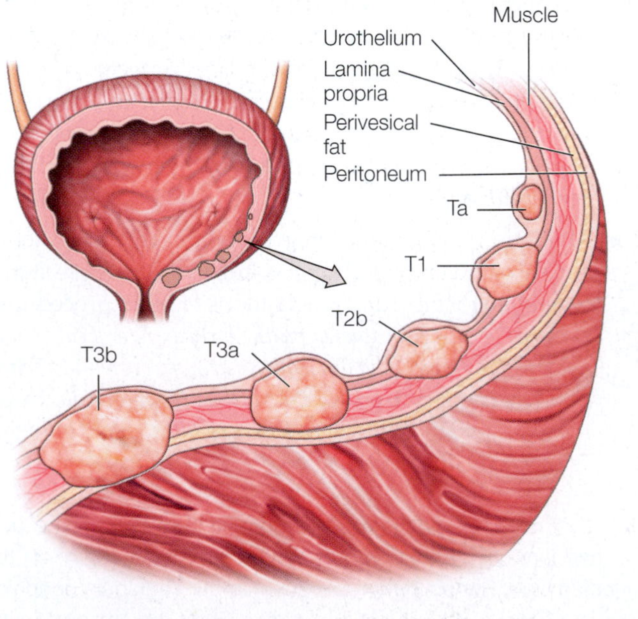
Muscle
Urothelium
Lamina propria
Perivesical fat
Peritoneum
Ta
T1
T2b
T3a
T3b

Figure 27.7 ■ Stages of bladder tumor development and invasiveness, beginning at the 3 o'clock position of the bladder and continuing in a clockwise manner.

Table 27.3 Bladder Tumor Staging

Depth of Involvement	Stage	TNM (Tumor, Node, Metastasis) Stage	Tumor Involvement
Superficial	C_{IS}	T_a	Limited to the bladder mucosa
	I	T_1	Involvement of the bladder mucosa and submucosal layers
Invasive	II	T_2	Invasion of superficial muscle of bladder wall
		T_{3a}	Deep muscle invasion
	III	T_{3b}	Involvement of perivesicular fat
	IV	$T_{3-4}N_+$	Regional (pelvic) lymph node involvement
		$T_{3-4}M_1$	Metastasis to distant lymph nodes or organs

Manifestations

Painless hematuria is the presenting sign in 75% of urinary tract tumors (ACS, 2018). Hematuria may be gross or microscopic and is often intermittent, causing delay in seeking treatment. Inflammation surrounding the tumor occasionally causes manifestations of a UTI, including frequency, urgency, and dysuria. Ureteral tumors may cause colicky pain from obstruction. Tumors of the urinary tract typically cause few outward signs and may not be discovered until obstructed urine flow causes flank pain or renal failure.

SAFETY ALERT: Intermittent painless hematuria is the most common presenting symptom of bladder cancer. Instruct all patients with painless hematuria to contact their physician for follow-up testing. ■

Interprofessional Care

Treatment of the patient with a tumor of the urinary tract focuses on removing or destroying the cancerous tissue, preventing further invasion or metastasis, and maintaining renal and urinary function.

Diagnosis

When a urinary tract tumor is suspected, the following diagnostic tests may be ordered:

- ***Urinalysis*** is done to evaluate for hematuria. Gross or microscopic hematuria is often the first indicator of a neoplasm in the urinary tract.
- ***Urine cytology***, microscopic examination of cells in the urine, is performed to identify abnormal cells (tumor or pretumor cells). Periodic urine cytology is recommended for patients at high risk for bladder cancer or its recurrence due to carcinogen exposure.
- ***Ultrasound of the bladder*** is a noninvasive test to detect bladder tumors. *Intravenous pyelography* may reveal a rigid deformity of the bladder wall, obstruction of urine flow at the point of the tumor, or bladder filling or emptying defects.
- ***Cystoscopy*** and ***ureteroscopy*** allow direct visualization, assessment, and biopsy of lesions of the urethra, bladder, or ureters to provide definitive diagnosis of urinary tract tumors.
- ***CT scan*** or ***MRI*** is primarily used to evaluate tumor invasion or metastasis.

Medications

Immunologic or chemotherapeutic agents administered by intravesical instillation (into the bladder) may be used either as the primary treatment for bladder cancer when multiple early lesions are present or to prevent recurrence following endoscopic tumor removal. Bacille Calmette-Guérin (BCG; BCG Live, TheraCys) is a suspension of attenuated *Mycobacterium bovis* used to treat CIS and recurrent bladder tumors. Instillation into the bladder causes a local inflammatory reaction that eliminates or reduces superficial tumors. Systemic mycobacterial infection is a rare complication of intravesical BCG therapy that may require antituberculin treatment. Other chemotherapeutic agents may be administered intravesically, including thiotepa, mitomycin C, and interferon. Bladder irritation, frequency, dysuria, and contact dermatitis are possible adverse reactions to intravesical chemotherapy. Suppression of bone marrow function can occur as a result of intravesical treatment.

Radiation Therapy

Radiation therapy is primarily used as a palliative treatment for inoperable tumors and patients who cannot tolerate surgery. Radiation therapy may be used in combination with systemic chemotherapy to improve local and distant relapse rates.

Surgery

A number of surgical procedures, ranging from simple resection of noninvasive tumors to removal of the bladder and surrounding structures, are used to treat urinary tract tumors. Indications for each procedure and specific nursing implications are outlined in **Table 27.4**.

Transurethral tumor resection may be performed by excision, *fulguration* (destruction of tissue using electric sparks generated by high-frequency current), or *laser photocoagulation* (use of light energy to destroy abnormal tissue). Laser surgery carries the lowest risk of bleeding and perforation of the bladder wall. Following cystoscopic tumor resection, patients are followed at 3-month intervals for tumor recurrence. Recurrences may develop anywhere in the urinary tract, including the renal pelvis, ureter, or urethra.

Cystectomy, surgical removal of the bladder, is necessary to treat invasive cancers. Partial cystectomy may be done to remove a solitary lesion; however,

Table 27.4 Surgical Procedures to Treat Bladder Tumors

Procedure	Indications	Nursing Implications
Transurethral resection of bladder tumor	Diagnose and resect superficial bladder tumors; control bleeding	Maintain continuous bladder irrigation postoperatively; monitor for excessive bleeding; ensure catheter patency. Increase fluids to 2500–3000 mL/day. Give stool softeners to prevent straining.
Partial cystectomy	Resect solitary, isolated tumor at stage T_2 or T_3 not involving trigone	Maintain patency of urethral and/or suprapubic catheter to make sure suture lines are free of pressure. Monitor for excess bleeding.
Complete or radical cystectomy	Remove large, invasive tumors; involvement of trigone	Permanent urinary diversion is required. Maintain patency and position of stents; urethral catheter may be in place to drain pelvic cavity.

radical cystectomy is the standard treatment for invasive tumors. The bladder and adjacent muscles and tissues are removed. In men, the prostate and seminal vessels are also removed, resulting in impotence. In women, a total hysterectomy and bilateral salpingo-oophorectomy (removal of the uterus, fallopian tubes, and ovaries) accompanies the procedure, causing sterility. At the time of surgery, a **urinary diversion** is created to provide for urine collection and drainage (**Figure 27.8** ■). An ileal conduit, bilateral cutaneous urostomy, or a continent urinary diversion is created to collect and drain urine. **Table 27.5** describes the most frequently used urinary diversion techniques.

Surgical procedures to remove tumors involving other portions of the urinary tract vary according to the site and stage of the tumor. When the distal ureter is involved, the tumor may be resected and the ureter implanted into the opposite ureter to provide for drainage. A proximal ureteral tumor necessitates removal of the ureter and kidney on the affected side. **Box 27.3** outlines the nursing care of the patient having a cystectomy and urinary diversion and **Box 27.4** describes self-care instructions for the patient with a urinary stoma.

Nursing Care

The patient who undergoes treatment for a tumor of the urinary tract has many nursing care needs because of alterations in the elimination, health perception–health management, cognitive-perceptual, self-perception–self-concept, role-relationships, and coping–stress tolerance health patterns.

Assessment

Nursing assessment related to urinary tract cancer includes both subjective and objective information:

- ***Health history:*** Risk factors; history of hematuria or manifestations of UTI (dysuria, frequency, urgency, pyuria); lower abdominal discomfort or flank pain
- ***Physical assessment:*** General health; abdominal tenderness; urine for analysis.

Priorities of Care

Maintaining urinary output is the priority nursing care focus for the patient with a bladder tumor. Priority needs for the patient who has undergone a urinary diversion procedure also include maintaining skin integrity, preventing infection, and helping restore a healthy body image.

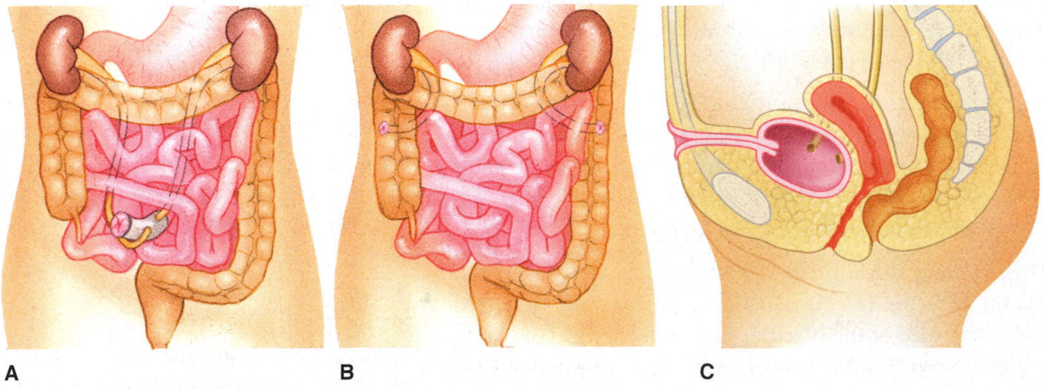
A
B
C

Figure 27.8 ■ Common urinary diversion procedures. **A**, Ileal conduit. A segment of ileum is separated from the small intestine and formed into a tubular pouch with the open end brought to the skin surface to form a stoma. The ureters are connected to the pouch. **B**, Bilateral cutaneous urostomy. The ureters are brought to the surface of the abdomen to form individual stomas. **C**, Continent urinary diversion. A segment of ileum is separated from the small intestine and formed into a pouch. Nipple valves are formed at each end of the pouch by intussuscepting tissue backward into the reservoir to prevent leakage.

Table 27.5 Urinary Diversion Procedures

Procedure	Description	Nursing Considerations
Ileal conduit	Portion of ileum is isolated from small intestine, leaving vascular, lymphatic, and neural connections intact; ileum is formed into pouch with the open end brought to surface to form a stoma; ureters are inserted into pouch.	Most common urinary diversion. Continuous urine drainage necessitates appliance. Postoperative edema may interfere with urine output. Risk of infection is less than for cutaneous ureterostomy, but potential for reflux is high. Good skin care is vital because of constant contact with urine.
Cutaneous ureterostomy	Each ureter is brought to the surface of the abdomen to form a stoma.	Continuous urine drainage requires dual appliances. Risk of infection is high due to direct route from the skin to the kidneys. Good skin care is vital because of constant contact with urine.
Continent urinary reservoir	A portion of the stomach, colon, or small intestine is used to form a reservoir to which the ureters are attached. Nipple valves are formed to prevent reflux. A nipple valve and stoma may be formed or the pouch may be attached to the urethral stump, avoiding creation of a stoma.	Drainage collection device not necessary. Patient must be able and motivated to manage self-catheterization. Reservoir may absorb urea and electrolytes, resulting in imbalances. Significant portion of bowel is required to form pouch and stoma.

BOX 27.3
Nursing Care of the Patient Having a Cystectomy and Urinary Diversion

PREOPERATIVE CARE

- Provide routine preoperative care.
- Assess knowledge of the proposed surgery and its long-term implications, clarifying misunderstandings and discussing concerns. *Patients having surgery for cancer of the urinary tract are trying to cope with the diagnosis of cancer and may not fully understand the surgery and its potential effects. Open discussion can facilitate postoperative recovery and adjustment.*
- Begin teaching about postoperative tubes and drains, self-care of stoma, and control of drainage and odor. *Postoperative physiologic and psychologic stressors may interfere with learning. A basic understanding of what to expect in the way of tubes, drains, and procedures reduces stress in the immediate postoperative period. Preoperative teaching can enhance recall and postoperative learning.*
- Assist in identifying stoma site, avoiding folds of skin, bones, scar tissue, and the waistline or belt area. Be sure to consider the patient's occupation and style of clothing. The site should be visible to the patient and accessible for manipulation. *Stoma placement is a vital component of adjustment and self-care. Care is taken to place the stoma away from areas of constant irritation by clothing or movement. It should be located so that the patient can cover and disguise the collecting device, maintain the seal to prevent leakage, and effectively cleanse and maintain the site.*
- Perform bowel-preparation activities as ordered. *Bowel preparation is done to prevent fecal contamination of the peritoneal cavity and to decompress the bowel during surgery.*

POSTOPERATIVE CARE

- Provide routine postoperative care.
- Monitor intake and output carefully, assessing urine output every hour for the first 24 hours, then every 4 hours or as ordered. Call the physician if urine output is less than 30 mL/hr. *Tissue edema and bleeding may interfere with urinary output from stoma, catheters, or drains. Maintenance of urine outflow is vital to prevent hydronephrosis and possible renal damage. A urine output of at least 30 mL/hr is necessary for effective renal function.*
- Assess color and consistency of urine. Expect pink or bright red urine fading to pink and then clearing by the third postoperative day. Urine may be cloudy due to mucus production by bowel mucosa. *Bright red blood in the urine from a urinary diversion may indicate hemorrhage, necessitating further surgery. Excessive cloudiness or malodorous urine may indicate infection.*
- Assess size, color, and condition of the stoma and surrounding skin every 2 hours for the first 24 hours, then every 4 hours for 48 to 72 hours. Expect the stoma to appear bright red and slightly edematous initially. Slight bleeding during cleansing is normal. *Compromised circulation causes the stoma to appear pale, gray, or cyanotic or blanch when touched. Other complications, such as infection or impaired healing, may be evidenced by a change in the appearance of the stoma or incision.*
- Irrigate the ileal diversion catheter with 30 to 60 mL of normal saline every 4 hours or as ordered. *Mucus produced by the bowel wall may accumulate in the newly devised reservoir or obstruct catheters.*
- Monitor serum electrolyte values, acid–base balance, and renal function tests such as BUN and serum creatinine. *Reabsorption of electrolytes from reservoirs created by portions of bowel may result in electrolyte imbalance and metabolic acidosis. Optimal renal function is necessary to maintain a normal state of homeostasis.*
- Teach the patient and family about stoma and urinary diversion care, including odor management, skin care, increased fluid intake, pouch application and leakage prevention (refer to Box 27.1), self-catheterization for patients with continent reservoirs, and signs of infection and other complications. *The ability to provide self-care is a significant factor in the adjustment to a changed body image. Teaching family members facilitates acceptance and adjustment. The family also needs this knowledge in case illness or disability interferes with the self-care capacity.*

BOX 27.4
Teaching for Self-Care: Urinary Stoma Care

- Assess knowledge, learning needs, and ability and willingness to assist with procedure. Explain the procedure and respond to questions as needed.
- Instruct to gather all supplies prior to starting procedure: A clean, disposable pouch; liquid skin barrier or barrier ring; 4 × 4 gauze squares; stoma guide; adhesive solvent; clean gloves; and a clean washcloth.

Provide the following instructions:

- Wash hands prior to starting procedure; gloves may be worn if desired.
- Remove old pouch, pulling gently away from skin. Warm water or adhesive solvent may be used to loosen the seal, if necessary.
- Assess stoma. Normally the stoma is bright red and appears moist. Report a dark purple, black, or very pale stoma to the physician. Slight bleeding with cleansing is normal, especially in the immediate postoperative period.
- Prevent urine flow during cleaning by placing a rolled gauze square or tampon over the stoma opening.
- Cleanse skin around the stoma with soap and water, rinse, and pat or air dry.
- Use the stoma guide to determine correct size for the bag opening and/or protective ring seal. Trim the bag or seal as needed.
- Apply skin barrier; allow to dry.
- Apply the bag with an opening no more than 1 to 2 mm wider than outside of stoma. Allow no wrinkles or creases where the bag contacts the skin.
- Connect bag to the urine-collection device. Dispose of old pouch, used supplies, and gloves appropriately. Wash hands.

Document teaching, ability to follow directions and perform the procedure, and response of the patient.

Diagnoses, Outcomes, and Interventions

For additional potential nursing priorities and interventions for the patient with a bladder tumor, see the Case Study & Nursing Care Plan on page 892.

Promote Normal Urinary Elimination. Whether the patient has undergone transurethral resection of a bladder tumor or radical cystectomy with urinary diversion, urinary elimination is altered at least temporarily.

Expected Outcome: Patient's urine output will remain within expected parameters for amount, color, clarity, and odor.

The nurse will:

- Monitor urine output from all catheters, stents, and tubes for amount, color, and clarity hourly for the first 24 hours postoperatively, then every 4 to 8 hours. *Decreased urine output may indicate impaired catheter or drainage system patency. Prompt intervention is necessary to prevent hydronephrosis. A change in color or clarity may indicate a complication such as hemorrhage or infection.*

SAFETY ALERT: Promptly report urine output of less than 30 mL/hr, which may indicate low vascular volume or renal insufficiency. Prompt intervention is vital to restore cardiac output and prevent acute kidney injury. ■

- Label all catheters, stents, and their drainage containers. Maintain separate closed gravity drainage systems for each. *Clear identification of each tube can prevent errors in irrigating and calculating outputs. Separate closed systems minimize the risk and extent of potential bacterial contamination and resultant infection.*
- Secure ureteral catheters and stents with tape; prevent kinking or occlusion; and maintain gravity flow by keeping drainage bag below level of kidneys. *Impaired urine flow can lead to urinary retention and distention of the bladder, a newly created reservoir, or the renal pelvis (hydronephrosis).*

SAFETY ALERT: Use aseptic techniques and strictly follow guidelines for irrigating catheters. Catheters placed in the kidney pelvis are irrigated using gentle pressure and small amounts of fluid (10 to 15 mL) to avoid damaging renal tissues. ■

Encourage fluid intake of 3000 mL/day. *Increased fluid intake maintains a high urinary output, reducing the risk of infection. Dilute urine is less irritating to the skin surrounding the stoma site. Electrolyte reabsorption from reservoirs may increase risk of calculi; high fluid intake and urine output reduce this risk.*

- Monitor urine output closely for first 24 hours after stents or ureteral catheters are removed. *Edema or stricture of ureters may impede output, leading to hydronephrosis and kidney damage.*
- Encourage activity to tolerance. *Ambulation promotes drainage of urine from reservoirs and helps prevent calcium loss from bones, which could precipitate calculus formation.*

Reduce Risk for Impaired Skin Integrity. The skin surrounding the stoma site of an ileal conduit is at risk for irritation and breakdown. Because urine is acidic and contains high concentrations of electrolytes, it has a corrosive effect on skin. In addition, adhesives and sealants used to prevent pouch leakage may irritate the skin.

Expected Outcome: Patient's peristomal skin will remain intact without evidence of irritation or impending breakdown.

The nurse will:

- Assess peristomal skin for redness, excoriation, or signs of breakdown. Assess for urine leakage from catheters, stents, or drains. Keep the skin clean and dry. Change wet dressings. *Intact skin is the first line of defense against infection. Impaired skin integrity may lead to local or systemic infection and impaired healing.*
- Ensure gravity drainage of urine collection device or empty bag every 2 hours. *Overfilling of the collection bag may damage the seal, allowing leakage and contact of urine with skin.*
- Change urine collection appliance as needed, removing any mucus from stoma. *Meticulous care and protection of skin surrounding stoma can maintain integrity and prevent breakdown.*

Promote Healthy Body Image. A radical cystectomy and urinary diversion affect the patient's body image. In most cases, an abdominal stoma is created, requiring either a drainage appliance or regular catheterization of the stoma to drain urine. Removal of the prostate and seminal vesicles or the uterus and ovaries leaves the patient sterile. If radiation or chemotherapy is planned as adjunctive therapy, the patient may experience hair loss, stomatitis, nausea and vomiting, or other disturbing side effects of therapy.

Expected Outcome: Patient will acknowledge impact of bladder cancer treatment or surgery on personal roles and relationships.

The nurse will:

- Use therapeutic communication techniques, actively listening and responding to the patient's and family's concerns. *Patients must know their feelings and concerns are respected and valued. Denial, anger, guilt, bargaining, or depression are common during grieving and normal for a patient undergoing a significant change in body image.*
- Recognize and accept behaviors that indicate use of coping mechanisms, encouraging adaptive mechanisms. *The patient may initially use defensive coping mechanisms such as denial, minimization, and dissociation from the immediate situation to reduce anxiety and maintain psychologic integrity. Adaptive mechanisms include learning as much as possible about the surgery and its effects, practicing procedures, setting realistic goals, and rehearsing various alternative outcomes.*
- Encourage looking at, touching, and caring for the stoma and appliance as soon as possible. Allow the patient to proceed gradually, providing support and encouragement. *Accepting the stoma as part of the self is vital to adapting to the changed body image and is indicated by a willingness to provide self-care.*
- Discuss concerns about returning to usual activities, perceived relationship changes, and resumption of sexual relations. Provide referral to support group or contact with someone who has successfully adjusted to a urinary diversion. *Patients and families may be reluctant to discuss topics of concern. An atmosphere of openness and acceptance facilitates expression of concerns and anxieties related to the changed body image.*

Reduce Risk for Infection. Diagnostic instrumentation procedures, surgical manipulation, and disruption of normal urinary tract defense mechanisms increase the risk of ascending urinary tract infection. When an ileal conduit or artificial bladder is created using bowel tissue, the normal bacteriostatic activity of bladder mucosa is lost. In addition, the peristaltic action of the ureters may be disrupted, and the vesicoureteral junction no longer prevents urine reflux. Adjunctive chemotherapy or radiation treatments may impair normal immune function and further increase the risk of infection.

Expected Outcome: Patient will remain free of urinary tract infection.

The nurse will:

- Maintain separate closed drainage systems, keeping drainage bags lower than the kidney, and prevent loops or kinks in drainage tubing, which impede urine flow. *Although urine is sterile when it leaves the kidney, bacteria grow rapidly in urine. Prevention of urine reflux is essential to preventing UTI.*
- Monitor for signs of infection: Elevated temperature, cloudy or foul-smelling urine, hematuria, general malaise, back or abdominal pain, and nausea and vomiting. *Infection undermines the healing process. Early detection and treatment help prevent long-term consequences such as chronic pyelonephritis.*
- Teach signs and symptoms of infection and self-care measures to prevent UTI. *The patient with a cystectomy and ileal diversion, urostomy, or continent reservoir is at risk of UTI for life because of impaired urinary defense mechanisms. Using clean or aseptic technique in providing care, increasing fluid intake, and using measures to acidify urine minimize this risk to a certain degree but do not eliminate it.*
- Teach about impaired immune function (due to aging or the effects of chemotherapy) and urine cloudiness (related to the effects of urine on ileal mucosa). *This can mask usual signs of UTI such as fever and altered urine clarity. Be alert for more generalized manifestations such as increased fatigue and malaise.*

Delegating Nursing Care Activities

As appropriate and allowed by the designated duties and responsibilities of unlicensed assistive personnel, the nurse may delegate nursing care activities such as recording intake and output and assisting with ambulation and hygiene for the patient with a urinary tract tumor.

Transitions of Care

The need for individual and family teaching for the patient who has had surgery to treat a urinary tract tumor is significant. For many patients, surgery means a lifelong change in urinary elimination. Even the patient who has undergone transurethral excision of bladder tumors requires follow-up cystoscopy on a regular basis and needs to be alert for signs of tumor recurrence.

The patient who has had a urinary diversion needs teaching about care of the stoma and surrounding skin, prevention of urine reflux and infection, signs and symptoms of UTI and renal calculi, and, in some cases, self-catheterization using clean technique.

A primary teaching need to prepare the patient and family affected by a urinary tract tumor resulting in a urinary diversion is information about the disease itself, expected prognosis, and planned treatment strategies. Provide honest information; do not promote false hope. Include the following additional topics in teaching for home care:

- Planned treatments such as chemotherapy or radiation therapy, including expected effects and usual side effects of each
- Strategies to cope with noxious effects of radiation or chemotherapy
- Activities and exercises to improve strength and regain function for the postoperative patient

Case Study & Nursing Care Plan

A Patient with a Bladder Tumor

Ben Hussain is a 61-year-old married man with five adult children. One week ago, Mr. Hussain became alarmed when his urine became bright red. Even though he had no other symptoms, he called his physician. The physician ordered a urinalysis and urine cytology, revealing gross hematuria and poorly differentiated abnormal cells. Cystoscopy and tissue biopsy confirm a stage C tumor involving the bladder trigone. Mr. Hussain is admitted for a radical cystectomy and continent urinary diversion.

ASSESSMENT

Mr. Hussain's admission history, obtained by Tara Mills, RN, indicates that he has lost 4.5 to 7 kg (10 to 15 lb) during the past few months. He smoked two to three packs of cigarettes per day for 40 years, but cut back to a pack a day about a year ago. He says he could not quit smoking entirely. He drinks five to six cups of coffee daily and consumes an average of three to four alcoholic drinks a day. Mr. Hussain says that he is "a little nervous about surgery and what they're going to find." Ms. Mills notes that he fidgets and talks rapidly throughout their interview. He expresses concern about how he will handle the pain after surgery because he had never been hospitalized before his cystoscopy. Physical assessment findings include T 36.7°C (98.2°F) PO, P 84 bpm, R 18/min, and BP 154/86 mmHg. Examinations of the skin, neuromuscular, and cardiac systems are within normal limits. Scattered expiratory crackles are noted on auscultation of lung fields. Bowel sounds are very active; Mr. Hussain explains that he began taking his bowel-preparation laxative the day before admission. Slight tenderness is noted in the suprapubic region. Mr. Hussain's urine is clear and bright pink. CBC and chemistry screening results are within normal limits. Surgery is planned for 9:00 a.m. the following day.

DIAGNOSES

- Anxiety related to undetermined extent of disease and fear of pain
- Needs education related to care and management of cystectomy and urinary diversion
- Inadequate gas exchange related to smoking history and effects of anesthesia

EXPECTED OUTCOMES

- Patient will verbalize decreased feelings of anxiety.
- Patient will demonstrate appropriate postoperative pain relief through subjective reports of pain severity and objective findings.
- Patient will be able to care for urinary diversion and surrounding skin prior to discharge.
- Patient will demonstrate self-catheterization of stoma using appropriate technique prior to discharge.
- Patient will maintain normal urine output with acceptable color and clarity and no signs of infection.
- Patient will maintain adequate gas exchange as evidenced by good skin color, O_2 saturation greater than 95%, and clear lung sounds on auscultation.

PLANNING AND IMPLEMENTATION

- Orient Mr. Hussain and his family to care unit preoperatively, answering questions fully and encouraging expression of fears.
- Provide written and verbal explanations when feasible.
- Administer analgesia around the clock for the first 48 to 72 hours. Monitor for signs of unrelieved pain.
- Explain all procedures related to stoma and diversion care as they are being performed.
- Encourage Mr. Hussain to look at stoma and touch it when ready.
- Teach stoma and skin care, as well as self-catheterization, emphasizing measures to prevent skin irritation and urinary tract infection.
- Monitor urine output, color, clarity, and consistency every hour for first 24 hours, then every 4 hours for 24 hours, then every 8 hours. Report output of less than 30 mL/hr, bright bleeding, or excessively cloudy or malodorous urine.
- Assist with use of incentive spirometer every hour while awake. Ambulate as soon as possible. Assess lung sounds every 4 hours, reporting increased crackles or diminished breath sounds.
- Refer Mr. and Mrs. Hussain to local stoma group on discharge.

EVALUATION

On discharge, Mr. Hussain has performed self-catheterization and stoma and skin care several times. His wife is able to catheterize the stoma and demonstrate skin care. His urine is pale yellow and slightly cloudy. Mr. Hussain is ambulating independently and using hydrocodone with acetaminophen (Vicodin) twice a day for pain relief. His lungs are clear, and he is very proud of having "survived" 7 days without a cigarette. He says, "Now I'm going to shoot for 7 weeks, then 7 months, then 7 years without a smoke!" A home health referral is made to continue teaching Mr. Hussain to care for his diversion and appliance.

CLINICAL REASONING IN PATIENT CARE

1. Review Mr. Hussain's assessment (above). Do you think any additional priority nursing diagnoses should be included in his plan of care? If so, identify them.
2. How does cigarette smoking contribute to the increased risk of urinary tract tumors?
3. Mr. Hussain expresses fear of becoming addicted to hydrocodone and says he does not intend to take the prescription once he gets home. How should you respond?
4. Suppose Mr. Hussain had become confused, disoriented, and tremorous and had begun to experience visual hallucinations 2 to 3 days postoperatively. What would you suspect the cause to be? What would be the appropriate response?
5. Develop a care plan for Mr. Hussain for the potential for sexual dysfunction.

See Evaluating Your Response in Appendix B.

- The need to continue coughing and deep-breathing exercises at home
- Symptoms to report to the healthcare provider: Fever, changes in urine volume, consistency, swelling, or incisional drainage
- Use of prescribed medications, including desired and potential side effects and interactions with other drugs or foods
- Use of analgesics and other pain relief measures for postoperative or cancer pain.

Information about hospice services and local cancer support groups should be provided for patients and caregivers. Refer the patient and family for home health services including nursing care, assistance with ADLs, respiratory care, and respite care as needed.

27.4 Disorders of Urinary Elimination

The Patient with Urinary Retention

Urinary retention, incomplete emptying of the bladder, can lead to overdistention of the bladder, poor detrusor muscle contractility, and inability to urinate. If the problem persists, hydroureter and hydronephrosis can result.

Pathophysiology

Normally, bladder emptying is controlled by the interaction of muscle tone and the autonomic nervous system. The sympathetic nervous system (SNS) relaxes the detrusor muscle, allowing the bladder to fill with urine. The internal sphincter, a continuation of the detrusor muscle, remains closed during filling. Pressures within the bladder remain low during filling, in contrast to high sphincter and urethral pressures. Voluntary muscles of the external sphincter and pelvic floor help maintain these high pressures. When the bladder contains 150 to 300 mL of urine, signals from stretch receptors in the bladder wall are transmitted to the spinal cord and cerebral cortex. Reflexive bladder emptying can be consciously inhibited. During *micturition* (bladder emptying), parasympathetic stimulation causes the detrusor muscle of the bladder fundus to contract, opening the internal sphincter. The external sphincter then relaxes, allowing urine to flow out.

Either mechanical obstruction of the bladder outlet or a functional problem can cause urinary retention. *Benign prostatic hypertrophy (BPH)* is a common cause; difficulty initiating and maintaining urine flow is often the presenting complaint in men with BPH. Fecal impaction may be a contributing factor in urinary retention, particularly in older adults or immobile patients. Acute inflammation associated with infection or trauma of the bladder, urethra, or perineal tissues may also interfere with micturition. Scarring due to repeated UTI can lead to urethral stricture and a mechanical obstruction. Bladder calculi may also obstruct the urethral opening from the bladder.

Surgery may disrupt detrusor muscle function, leading to urine retention. Abdominal or pelvic surgery, use of spinal anesthesia, and surgeries of long duration carry the highest risk for disrupting bladder function (NIDDK, 2018). Long-standing diabetes and drugs may also interfere with its function. Anticholinergic medications such as atropine, glycopyrrolate (Robinul), propantheline bromide (Pro-Banthine), scopolamine hydrochloride (Transderm-Scop), and others can lead to acute urinary retention and bladder distention. Many other drug groups have anticholinergic side effects and may cause urinary retention. Among these are antianxiety agents such as diazepam (Valium), antidepressant and tricyclic drugs such as imipramine (Tofranil), antiparkinsonian drugs, antipsychotic agents, and some sedative/hypnotic drugs. In addition, antihistamines common in over-the-counter (OTC) cough, cold, allergy, and sleep-promoting drugs have anticholinergic effects and may interfere with bladder emptying. Diphenhydramine (Benadryl) is an example of a nonprescription antihistamine.

Voluntary urinary retention (particularly common among nurses) may lead to overfilling of the bladder and a loss of detrusor muscle tone.

Manifestations

The patient with urinary retention is unable to empty the bladder completely. Overflow voiding or incontinence may occur, with 25 to 50 mL of urine eliminated at frequent intervals. Assessment reveals a firm, distended bladder that may be displaced to one side of midline. Percussion of the lower abdomen reveals a dull tone, reflective of fluid in the bladder.

Severe urinary retention with resulting bladder distention impairs the ability of the vesicoureteral junction to prevent backflow of urine into the ureters (refer to Figure 27.1 on page 872). Reflux of urine from the distended bladder distends the ureters (hydroureter) and kidneys (hydronephrosis). Hydronephrosis impairs renal function, and acute kidney injury can result.

Interprofessional Care

Urinary retention is confirmed using a bladder scan or by inserting a urinary catheter (if possible) and measuring the urine output. Use of a bladder scan is preferred to reduce the risk of UTI.

An indwelling urinary catheter or intermittent straight catheterization can prevent urinary retention and overdistention of the bladder. In acute situations, patients treated with intermittent catheterization may regain normal voiding patterns sooner than those in whom an indwelling urinary catheter is used (NIDDK, 2018). Cholinergic medications such as bethanechol chloride (Urecholine), which promote detrusor muscle contraction and bladder emptying, may be used. A medication with no anticholinergic side effects may be substituted when urinary retention is related to drug therapy.

Mechanical obstructions are treated by removing or repairing the obstruction, when possible. Resection of the prostate gland may be done for urinary retention related to BPH. Bladder calculi are removed, and measures to prevent their formation are instituted.

Nursing Care

Nursing measures to promote urination include placing the patient in normal voiding position and providing for privacy. Additional measures include running water, placing the patient's hands in warm water, pouring warm water over the perineum, or taking a warm sitz bath.

In acute urinary retention, catheterization may be necessary to relieve bladder distention and prevent hydronephrosis. Use a relatively small catheter (16 Fr. for a man, 14 Fr. for a woman). A coudé-tipped catheter is passed more easily in the older man with an enlarged prostate. Use of 2% lidocaine gel (10 mL injected into the male urethra or 6 mL injected into the female urethra) reduces discomfort during catheterization and the risk of catheter-associated infection and promotes pelvic muscle relaxation (Mu et al., 2017). Carefully observe the patient as the distended bladder drains.

Continuing care for the patient with urinary retention varies, depending on the cause. Some patients may be taught intermittent self-catheterization. Instruct all patients who have experienced urinary retention to avoid OTC drugs that affect micturition, especially those with an anticholinergic effect (allergy and cold medications, many nonprescription sleep aids). Other measures include double-voiding (urinate, remain on the toilet for 2 to 5 minutes, then urinate again), scheduled voiding, or, when other measures fail, an indwelling catheter. When an indwelling catheter is necessary, teach the patient and family to use clean technique when changing from overnight bag to leg bag and to promptly report signs of UTI to the primary care provider.

SAFETY ALERT: Some patients may experience a vasovagal response, becoming pale, sweaty, and hypotensive, if the bladder is rapidly drained. Draining urine in 500-mL increments and clamping the catheter for 5 to 10 minutes between increments may prevent this response. Hematuria may also occur with rapid bladder decompression. Promptly notify the physician if hematuria develops. ■

Transitions of Care

Health promotion measures to prevent urinary retention include monitoring urine output and performing repeated bladder scans in at-risk patients and evaluating drug regimens for medications known to interfere with detrusor muscle function. Pay particular attention to elimination when these drugs are ordered for (or used by) a patient with BPH or other mechanical obstruction of urine flow.

Nursing care focuses on promoting urination. Teaching self-catheterization is a primary nursing responsibility. Other interprofessional care focuses on addressing the underlying cause of retention such as urethral blockage or prostate enlargement.

The Patient with Neurogenic Bladder

The neurologic connections influencing bladder filling, the perception of fullness and the need to void, and bladder emptying are complex. Disruption of the central or peripheral nervous systems may interfere with normal mechanisms, causing **neurogenic bladder**.

Pathophysiology, Risk Factors, and Manifestations

As noted in the physiology section on urinary retention, bladder filling and emptying are controlled by the central nervous system (CNS). This neurologic control can be disrupted at any level: The cerebral cortex (voluntary impulses), the micturition center of the midbrain, the spinal cord tracts, or the peripheral nerves of the bladder itself.

Spastic Bladder Dysfunction

A simple reflex arc exists between the bladder and the spinal cord at levels S_2 through S_4. The stimulus of more than 400 mL of urine in the bladder causes reflex contraction of the detrusor muscle and bladder emptying unless voluntary control (cerebral input) is used to suppress it. Disruption of CNS transmission above the sacral spinal cord segment typically leads to *spastic neurogenic bladder*. Both sensory and voluntary control of urination are interrupted partially or totally, while the sacral reflex arc remains intact. The stimuli generated by bladder filling cause frequent spontaneous detrusor muscle contraction and involuntary bladder emptying. Spinal cord injury above the sacral segment is the most common cause of a spastic bladder. Other causes include stroke, multiple sclerosis, and other CNS lesions.

Flaccid Bladder Dysfunction

Damage to the sacral spinal cord at the level of the reflex arc, the cauda equina, or the sacral nerve roots causes loss of detrusor muscle tone and a *flaccid neurogenic bladder*. The perception of bladder fullness is lost, and the bladder becomes overdistended, with weak and ineffective detrusor muscle contractions. Flaccid neurogenic bladder is seen with myelomeningocele and during the spinal shock phase of a spinal cord injury above the sacral region. During the spinal shock phase, all reflex activity below the level of spinal cord injury is suppressed.

Peripheral neuropathies may cause bladder atony and overfilling. Either sensory or motor pathways (or both) may be disrupted, leading to incomplete bladder emptying and large residual volumes after voiding. Diabetes mellitus is the most common cause of peripheral bladder neuropathy. Other causes include multiple sclerosis, chronic alcoholism, and prolonged overdistention of the bladder.

The patient with a flaccid bladder may require catheterization to completely empty the bladder. An indwelling catheter may be used initially, but intermittent catheterization is preferred (NIDDK, 2017). Clean intermittent self-catheterization is performed every 3 to 4 hours to prevent overdistention of the bladder.

Interprofessional Care

Management of neurogenic bladder focuses on maintaining continence and avoiding complications associated with overfilling or incomplete emptying of the bladder. Because self-care is the goal, teaching is a primary intervention for the healthcare team.

Diagnosis

The following diagnostic tests may be ordered for the patient with a neurogenic bladder:

- ***Urine culture*** to detect possible UTI related to impaired bladder function.
- ***Urinalysis*** and ***eGFR***, ***serum creatinine*** and ***BUN*** to evaluate renal function. Ascending infection or hydronephrosis resulting from bladder overfilling and vesicoureteral reflux can damage the kidneys. Impaired

renal function may lead to blood cells or protein in the urine and elevated BUN and creatinine levels.

- *Postvoid bladder scan* to measure residual urine. Amounts greater than 50 mL may indicate ineffective detrusor muscle contractions, common in neurogenic bladder.
- *Cystometrography* to evaluate bladder filling and the detrusor muscle tone and function.

Medications

Medications may be prescribed to increase or decrease the contractility of the detrusor muscle, to increase or decrease the tone of the internal sphincter, or to relax the external urethral sphincter.

Bethanechol, a cholinergic drug, stimulates detrusor muscle contraction in flaccid neurogenic bladder. It is generally used to manage short-term urinary retention (e.g., following surgery or childbirth). It may be used in combination with bladder-training techniques to promote complete emptying of a neurogenic bladder. Anticholinesterase drugs such as neostigmine (Prostigmin) and pyridostigmine (Mestinon) may also be used to increase detrusor muscle tone.

Anticholinergic drugs (parasympathetic blockers) relax the detrusor muscle and contract the internal sphincter, increasing bladder capacity in patients with spastic bladder dysfunction. *Oxybutynin (Ditropan)*, tolterodine (Detrol), darifenacin (Enablex), solifenacin succinate (VESIcare), and trospium (Sanctura) inhibit the muscarinic effects of acetylcholine on smooth muscle, reducing detrusor muscle spasticity and promoting bladder filling. Other anticholinergic drugs may also be used, including propantheline (Pro-Banthine) or flavoxate (Urispas). Dry mouth, blurred vision, and constipation are potential adverse effects of anticholinergic medications. See **Medication Administration 27.B** for drugs used to modify detrusor muscle activity.

Medication Administration 27.B

The Patient with Neurogenic Bladder

ANTICHOLINERGIC DRUGS TO TREAT SPASTIC BLADDER

darifenacin (Enablex)
flavoxate hydrochloride (Urispas)
oxybutynin (Ditropan, Ditropan XL)
propantheline bromide (Pro-Banthine)
solifenacin succinate (VESIcare)
tolterodine (Detrol, Detrol LA)
trospium (Sanctura)

Anticholinergic drugs inhibit the response to acetylcholine, relaxing the detrusor muscle and increasing internal sphincter tone. The combination of detrusor relaxation and internal sphincter contraction increases the bladder capacity of patients with spastic or hyperreflexive neurogenic bladder. Of these medications, darifenacin, solifenacin succinate, and tolterodine have the most specific effects on the detrusor muscle with fewer anticholinergic side effects.

Nursing Responsibilities

- Assess for contraindications, such as glaucoma, gastrointestinal or urinary tract obstruction, severe ulcerative colitis or toxic megacolon, unstable cardiovascular status, or myasthenia gravis.
- Observe for the desired effect of increased bladder capacity with decreased incontinence and spasm.
- Monitor for possible interaction with other drugs such as narcotic analgesics, antidysrhythmic medications, antihistamines, antidepressants, or psychoactive drugs.
- Monitor heart rate and blood pressure, especially when given to patients with known cardiovascular disease.
- Assess for adverse effects such as urinary hesitancy or retention, dysrhythmias, mental status changes, and gastrointestinal disturbances.

Health Education for the Patient and Family

- Take the drug as ordered. Some of these drugs (e.g., trospium) need to be taken on an empty stomach for optimal absorption; others may be taken irrespective of food intake.
- Promptly report eye pain, rapid heartbeat, difficulty breathing, rash or hives, or changes in mental function to your primary care provider.
- These drugs may cause drowsiness or blurred vision. Use caution when driving, operating machinery, or performing other tasks requiring mental acuity.
- Hard candies help relieve dry mouth associated with these drugs.
- Do not use alcohol or nonprescription antihistamines while taking these drugs.

CHOLINERGIC DRUGS TO STIMULATE MICTURITION

bethanechol chloride (Urecholine)

Bethanechol stimulates the parasympathetic nervous system, increasing detrusor muscle tone and producing a contraction strong enough to initiate micturition. It is used primarily to treat acute postoperative and postpartum urinary retention.

Nursing Responsibilities

- Assess for contraindications, including hypersensitivity, hyperthyroidism, peptic ulcer disease, asthma, significant bradycardia or hypotension, coronary heart disease, epilepsy, and parkinsonism.
- Do not give to patients who have had recent gastrointestinal or bladder surgery or those with possible gastrointestinal or urinary tract obstruction.
- Give oral forms on an empty stomach to reduce the risk of nausea and vomiting.
- Administer parenteral bethanechol subcutaneously. Keep atropine, the antidote for bethanechol overdose or toxicity, available.
- Observe for desired effect within 30 to 60 minutes after oral administration, 5 to 15 minutes after injection.
- Assess for adverse effects such as malaise, headache, abdominal cramping, nausea, hypotension with reflex tachycardia, wheezing, and dyspnea.

Health Education for the Patient and Family

- Take the medication 1 hour before or 2 hours after meals.
- Use caution when rising from a recumbent or sitting position; you may feel dizzy or lightheaded.

Note: Drugs identified in blue are among the 200 most commonly prescribed medications in the United States.

Source: Data from Adams et al., 2017.

Nutrition

Dietary measures to reduce the risk for UTI and urinary calculi may be suggested for the patient with neurogenic bladder. A moderate to high fluid intake and a diet that acidifies the urine are helpful. Cranberry juice is recommended to maintain urine acidity (NCCIH, 2016). The patient may be advised to avoid foods high in oxalate or purine to help prevent urolithiasis. The timing of fluid intake may be regulated to promote continence.

Bladder Retraining

Patients with spastic neurogenic bladder may use measures to stimulate reflex voiding, allowing scheduled toileting. Techniques include using trigger points, for example, stroking or pinching the abdomen, inner thigh, or glans penis. Pulling pubic hairs, tapping the suprapubic region, or inserting a gloved finger into the rectum and gently stretching the anal sphincter can also stimulate urination.

The *Credé method* (applying pressure to the suprapubic region with the fingers of one or both hands), manual pressure on the abdomen, and the Valsalva maneuver (bearing down while holding one's breath) promote bladder emptying for the patient with a spastic or flaccid bladder.

SAFETY ALERT: Increasing lower abdominal and bladder pressure with the Credé method can stimulate autonomic dysreflexia in some patients with spinal cord injuries. Autonomic dysreflexia is a medical emergency in which the blood pressure rises rapidly due to SNS stimulation. ■

Surgery

Surgery may be required when urination cannot be effectively managed using more conservative measures. Injection of botulinum toxin A into the detrusor muscle via cystoscopy has been shown to improve bladder capacity (Weckx, Tutolo, De Ridder, & Van Der Aa, 2016). *Rhizotomy*, or destruction of the nerve supply to the detrusor muscle or the external sphincter, may be used for patients with hyperreflexia or spasticity. Urinary diversion is another surgical technique used when conservative management fails. Implantation of an artificial sphincter may be useful for some patients with neurogenic bladder. Refer to Table 27.5 for urinary diversion techniques and **Box 27.3** for nursing care of the patient undergoing a urinary diversion.

Nursing Care

Nursing care of the patient with a neurogenic bladder is directed toward promoting urinary drainage and continence, preventing complications, and teaching the patient and family self-care techniques.

Assessment

Nursing assessment for neurogenic bladder includes obtaining a complete nursing history and focusing on information related to CNS or spinal cord injury or disease, as well as disorders that affect the peripheral nervous system (e.g., diabetes). Ask about measures used to stimulate or control urination. Inspect and palpate the lower abdomen and suprapubic region for tenderness or bladder distention. If available, evaluate the volume of urine in the bladder using a portable bladder scanner. Alternately, percuss the suprapubic region for a dull percussion tone indicative of a full bladder. Dullness up to the level of the umbilicus indicates at least 500 mL of urine in the bladder. Assess urine for color, clarity, and odor. Collect a specimen for analysis as indicated.

Priorities of Care

Although each patient has individual nursing care needs, priorities of care for the patient with a neurogenic bladder include:

- Teach methods of urinary elimination related to impaired bladder innervation
- Provide instruction on self-care toileting related to neurologic injury
- Reduce risk for impaired skin integrity related to urinary incontinence
- Reduce risk for infection related to impaired urination reflex.

Include the following in teaching for the patient with neurogenic bladder and family members:

- Measures to stimulate reflex voiding and promote bladder emptying
- Use of prescribed medications, including desired and adverse effects and interactions with other drugs
- Manifestations of UTI or urolithiasis and measures to reduce the risk of these complications.

Transitions of Care

Acute management of neurogenic bladder is based on the underlying etiology. For the flaccid bladder, the nurse should promote increased fluid intake and intermittent self-catheterization. For the spastic bladder, the nurse will promote measures that trigger urination and treat urge incontinence.

The Patient with Urinary Incontinence

The most common manifestation of impaired bladder control is **urinary incontinence (UI)**, or involuntary urination. UI can have a significant impact on patients, leading to physical problems such as skin breakdown, infection, and rashes. Psychosocial consequences include embarrassment, isolation and withdrawal, feelings of worthlessness and helplessness, and depression.

An estimated 25 million people in the United States have some degree of urinary incontinence, with urinary incontinence affecting 200 million worldwide (National Association for Continence, 2017). The actual prevalence of urinary incontinence is nearly impossible to determine. Embarrassment and the availability of products to protect clothing and prevent detection contribute to patients' not seeking evaluation of and treatment for incontinence. In women, 1 in

4 women over age 18 have some degree of involuntary urine leakage (National Association for Continence, 2017).

Urinary incontinence is a common problem in older adults. Although UI should never be considered a normal consequence of aging, age-related changes contribute to its development. Bladder capacity tends to decline with age and involuntary bladder muscle contractions are more common. Fluid ingested during the day tends to be excreted later in the day and into the night. In women, decreased estrogen levels and pelvic muscle relaxation decrease bladder outlet and urethral resistance pressures. Decreased estrogen also causes atrophic vaginitis and urethritis, with manifestations of dysuria and urgency. In men, the prostate enlarges with aging. Other risk factors for UI in older adults include impaired mobility and chronic degenerative diseases, impaired cognition, medications, low fluid intake, diabetes, and stroke.

Pathophysiology

Urinary continence requires input from the CNS, a bladder able to expand and contract, and sphincters that can maintain a urethral pressure higher than that in the bladder. Intact cognition, mobility, motivation, and manual dexterity are also necessary to maintain continence. Mechanically, incontinence results when the pressure within the urinary bladder exceeds urethral resistance, allowing urine to escape. Any condition causing higher than normal bladder pressures or reduced urethral resistance can potentially result in incontinence. Relaxation of the pelvic musculature, disruption of cerebral and nervous system control, and disturbances of the bladder and its musculature are common contributing factors.

Incontinence may be an acute, self-limited disorder or it may be chronic (Bardsley, 2016). The causes may be congenital or acquired, reversible or irreversible. Congenital disorders associated with incontinence include epispadias (absence of the upper wall of the urethra) and meningomyelocele (a neural tube defect in which a portion of the spinal cord and its surrounding meninges protrude through the vertebral column). CNS or spinal cord trauma, stroke, and chronic neurologic disorders such as multiple sclerosis and Parkinson disease are examples of acquired, irreversible causes of incontinence. Reversible causes include acute confusion, medications such as diuretics or sedatives, prostatic enlargement, vaginal and urethral atrophy, UTI, and fecal impaction.

Incontinence is commonly categorized as stress incontinence, urge incontinence (or overactive bladder), overflow incontinence, and functional incontinence. **Table 27.6** summarizes each type of incontinence and its physiologic cause and associated factors. *Mixed incontinence*, with elements of both stress and urge incontinence, is common. *Total incontinence* is loss of all voluntary control over urination, with urine loss occurring without stimulus and in all positions.

Incontinence is associated with an increased risk for falls, fractures, pressure ulcers, urinary tract infection, and depression. It contributes to the stress of caregivers, and often is a factor in institutionalizing a patient.

Interprofessional Care

UI management is directed at identifying and correcting the cause, if possible. If the underlying disorder cannot be corrected, techniques to manage urine output can often be

Table 27.6 Types of Urinary Incontinence

Description	Pathophysiology	Contributing Factors
Stress		
Loss of urine associated with increased intra-abdominal pressure during sneezing, coughing, lifting. Quantity of urine lost is usually small.	Relaxation of pelvic musculature and weakness of urethra and surrounding muscles and tissues lead to decreased urethral resistance.	■ Multiple pregnancies ■ Decreased estrogen levels ■ Short urethra, change in angle between bladder and urethra ■ Abdominal wall weakness ■ Prostate surgery ■ Increased intra-abdominal pressure due to tumor, ascites, obesity
Urge		
Involuntary loss of urine associated with a strong urge to void	Hypertonic or overactive detrusor muscle leads to increased pressure within bladder and inability to inhibit voiding.	■ Neurologic disorders such as stroke, Parkinson disease, multiple sclerosis; peripheral nervous system disorders ■ Detrusor muscle overactivity associated with bladder outlet obstruction, aging, or disorders such as diabetes
Overflow		
Inability to empty bladder, resulting in overdistention and frequent loss of small amounts of urine	Outlet obstruction or lack of normal detrusor activity leads to overfilling of bladder and increased pressure.	■ Spinal cord injuries below S_2 ■ Diabetic neuropathy ■ Prostatic hypertrophy ■ Fecal impaction ■ Drugs, especially those with anticholinergic effect
Functional		
Incontinence resulting from physical, environmental, or psychosocial causes	Ability to respond to the need to urinate is impaired.	■ Confusion or dementia ■ Physical disability or impaired mobility ■ Therapy or sedation ■ Depression ■ Regression

taught. For stress, urge, or mixed UI, evidence-based treatment guidelines support use of conservative measures such as pelvic floor muscle training (Kegel exercises, as described in **Box 27.5**) and bladder training for a minimum of 3 months in women before considering use of medications or surgery (National Association for Continence, 2017).

Evaluation for incontinence begins with a complete history, including specific questions about lower urinary tract symptoms and the duration, frequency, volume, and associated circumstances of urine loss. A voiding diary (**Figure 27.9** ■) is often used to collect detailed information. The history also includes information about chronic or acute illnesses, previous surgeries, and current medication use, both prescription and OTC.

Physical assessment includes abdominal, rectal, and pelvic assessment as well as evaluation of mental and neurologic status, mobility, and dexterity. Findings often associated with incontinence in women include weak abdominal and pelvic muscle tone, cystocele or urethrocele, and atrophic vaginitis. In men, an enlarged prostate gland is the physical finding most commonly associated with incontinence.

BOX 27.5
Pelvic Floor Muscle (Kegel) Exercises

- Identify the pelvic muscles with these techniques:
  a. Stop the flow of urine during voiding and hold for a few seconds.
  b. Tighten the muscles at the vaginal entrance around a gloved finger or tampon.
  c. Tighten the muscles around the anus as though resisting defecation.
- Perform exercises by tightening pelvic muscles, holding for 10 seconds, and relaxing for 10 seconds. Continue the sequence (tighten, hold, relax) for 25 repetitions.
- Keep abdominal muscles and breathing relaxed while performing exercises.
- Perform 25 repetitions twice per day.
- Encourage exercising at a specific time each day or in conjunction with another daily activity (such as bathing or watching the news). Establish a routine because these exercises should be continued for life.
- Assistive devices, such as vaginal cones and biofeedback, may be useful for patients who have difficulty identifying appropriate muscle groups.

Your Daily Voiding Diary **Date** ________________

This diary will help you and your healthcare team identify factors causing bladder control problems. Choose a 24-hour period when you can record your fluid intake (type and amount), urine output and episodes of urine leakage, any strong urge to void just prior to leaking, and your activity when leak episodes occur. The line below illustrates how to use your diary.

Time 	Fluid Intake 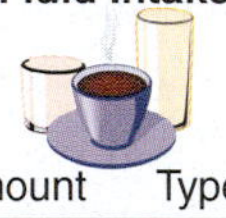 Amount	 Type	Urine Output 	Leaks 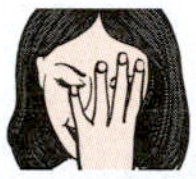	Urge 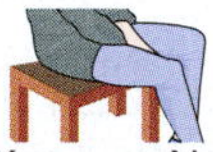 Yes No	Activity 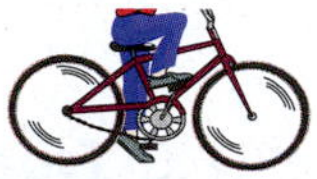
7 am	2 cups	coffee	sm (med) lg	(sm) med lg	Yes	walking
			sm med lg	sm med lg		
			sm med lg	sm med lg		
			sm med lg	sm med lg		
			sm med lg	sm med lg		
			sm med lg	sm med lg		
			sm med lg	sm med lg		
			sm med lg	sm med lg		
			sm med lg	sm med lg		
			sm med lg	sm med lg		
			sm med lg	sm med lg		
			sm med lg	sm med lg		
			sm med lg	sm med lg		
			sm med lg	sm med lg		
			sm med lg	sm med lg		
			sm med lg	sm med lg		
			sm med lg	sm med lg		
			sm med lg	sm med lg		

I used___pads today. I used___diapers today.

Questions to ask my healthcare team: ____________________

____

____

Figure 27.9 ■ A sample voiding diary.

Diagnosis

With an appropriate history and physical examination, diagnostic testing is rarely required. Certain tests may, however, be done to rule out UTI or to guide treatment:

- ***Urinalysis*** and ***urine culture*** using a clean-catch specimen are done to rule out infection and other acute causes of incontinence.
- ***Postvoiding residual (PVR) volume*** may be measured to determine how completely the bladder empties with voiding. Less than 50 mL PVR is expected; when 100 mL or more is obtained, further testing is indicated.
- ***Bladder stress testing*** may be performed. In this test, a measured amount of fluid is instilled into the bladder and the patient observed for urine leakage during coughing in both the supine and standing positions.

If conservative treatment measures have failed to correct UI, the following diagnostic tests may be considered:

- ***Cystometrography*** is used to assess neuromuscular function of the bladder by evaluating detrusor muscle function, pressure within the bladder, and the filling pattern of the bladder.
- ***Uroflowmetry*** is a noninvasive test used to evaluate voiding patterns.
- ***Cystoscopy*** or ***ultrasonography*** may be ordered to identify structural disorders contributing to incontinence, such as an enlarged prostate or a tumor.

Medications

Both stress and urge incontinence may improve with drug treatment.

Drugs that contract the smooth muscles of the bladder neck may reduce episodes of mild stress incontinence. Duloxetine (Cymbalta), a drug that inhibits the uptake of both norepinephrine and serotonin, is the drug of choice for treating stress UI that is not fully controlled with nonpharmacologic treatment (e.g., teaching, pelvic muscle exercise). In clinical trials, this drug reduced the frequency of UI and the number of voidings per day, particularly when combined with pelvic floor muscle training. Adverse effects such as nausea, headache, insomnia, and constipation are common with duloxetine; for most patients, however, these effects diminish over time (Shields, Fox, & Liebrecht, 2018).

When incontinence is associated with postmenopausal atrophic vaginitis, estrogen therapy may be effective. Both systemic estrogens and local creams are used. Results are improved with the addition of an α-adrenergic receptor agonist such as pseudoephedrine or phenylephrine unless contraindicated by a preexisting condition such as hypertension (Shields et al., 2018).

Patients with urge incontinence may be treated with preparations that increase bladder capacity. Anticholinergic drugs inhibit muscarinic receptors of the parasympathetic nervous system, reducing detrusor muscle contractions. A number of drugs have been approved to treat urge UI, including *oxybutynin* (Ditropan and the extended-release form, Ditropan XL), tolterodine (Detrol and its longer-acting form, Detrol LA), trospium (Sanctura), darifenacin (Enablex), and solifenacin (VESIcare). These drugs can be taken once or twice a day and have fewer side effects than less specific anticholinergic drugs. These drugs are contraindicated for the patient with acute glaucoma. Urinary retention is a potential side effect that must be considered when these drugs are used (see Medication Administration 27.B). Studies about the use and effectiveness of botulinum toxin A to control detrusor muscle overactivity are currently underway in the United States and Europe. Botulinum toxin A is injected directly into the muscle; its effects last for a period of 3 to 9 months, necessitating repeated injections.

Surgery

Surgery may be used to treat stress incontinence associated with cystocele or urethrocele and overflow incontinence associated with an enlarged prostate gland.

Suspension of the bladder neck, a technique that brings the angle between the bladder and urethra closer to normal, is effective in treating stress incontinence associated with urethrocele. A laparoscopic, vaginal, or abdominal approach may be used to perform this surgery.

Prostatectomy, using either the transurethral or suprapubic approach, is indicated for the patient who is experiencing overflow incontinence as a result of an enlarged prostate gland and urethral obstruction. Other surgical procedures of potential benefit in the treatment of incontinence include implantation of an artificial sphincter, formation of a urethral sling to elevate and compress the urethra, and augmentation of the bladder with bowel segments to increase bladder capacity.

Integrative Therapies

Biofeedback and relaxation techniques may help reduce episodes of UI (Mayo Clinic, 2018). Biofeedback uses electronic monitors to teach conscious control over physiologic responses of which the individual is not normally aware. Developing awareness of perceptible information allows the patient to gain voluntary control over urination. Biofeedback is widely used to manage urinary incontinence.

Nursing Care

Assessment

Nursing assessment for the patient with UI includes both subjective and objective data:

- ***Health history:*** Voiding diary; frequency of incontinent episodes, amount of urine loss and activities associated with incontinence; methods used to deal with incontinence; use of Kegel exercises or medications; any chronic diseases, related surgeries, and so on; effects of incontinence on usual activities, including social activities
- ***Physical assessment:*** Physical and mental status, including any physical limitations or impaired cognition; inspect, palpate, and percuss abdomen for bladder distention; inspect perineal tissues for redness, irritation, or tissue breakdown; observe for bulging of

bladder into vagina when bearing down; assess pelvic muscle tone as indicated.

Assessment for UI in the older adult focuses on risk factors, the extent and manifestations of the disorder, and contributing factors. Using clear language, ask about problems with urine loss, its frequency, and any contributing factors. Inquire about frequency, urgency, and burning on urination. Identify current medications and the time of day each is taken. Assess patterns of fluid intake and output. Assess the abdomen for evidence of bladder distention or tenderness. Perform a mental status examination, if indicated.

Assess the home environment (whether in the community or a residential living facility) for possible barriers to urinary elimination:

- Inadequate lighting, particularly at night
- Narrow doorways that may interfere with access to the toilet
- Inadequate toilet facilities
- The need for mobility aids such as safety bars, a raised toilet seat, or a bedside commode.

Discuss the following points to help prevent UI in the older adult:

- Maintain a generous fluid intake. Reduce or eliminate fluid intake after the evening meal to reduce nocturia.
- Wear comfortable clothing that is easy to remove for toileting.
- Maintain good hygiene, but do not bathe more often than necessary; frequent bathing and feminine hygiene sprays or douches may dry perineal tissues, increasing the risk of UI.
- Perform pelvic muscle exercises (Kegel exercises) several times a day to increase perineal muscle tone.
- Reduce consumption of caffeine-containing beverages (coffee, tea, colas), citrus juices, and artificially sweetened beverages containing NutraSweet.
- Use behavioral techniques such as scheduled toileting, habit training, and bladder training to reduce the frequency of incontinence. *Scheduled toileting* is toileting at regular intervals (e.g., every 2 to 4 hours). *Habit training* is toileting the patient on a schedule that corresponds with the normal pattern. *Bladder training* gradually increases the bladder capacity by increasing the intervals between voidings and resisting the urge to void.
- See your primary care provider regularly for a pelvic or prostate exam.
- For women, discuss possible benefits and risks of hormone replacement therapy, physical therapy, or surgery to treat incontinence.
- Report a change in urine color, odor, or clarity or symptoms such as burning, frequency, or urgency to your primary care provider.

Priorities of Care

Although the priority of specific interventions depends on the patient's mental and physical status, teaching to manage symptoms and prevent complications associated with urinary incontinence is always a priority. Teaching is directed toward the patient whenever possible and toward caregivers (personal or institutional) when the patient must depend on others for toileting assistance.

Diagnoses, Interventions, and Outcomes

In planning nursing care, consider the patient's mental status, mobility, and motivation. Behavioral techniques can be effective, but require long-term commitment and the physical and mental capability to use them.

Nursing care and modification of routines can restore continence fully or partially even in a patient who is institutionalized. Scheduled toileting, bladder training, and prompted voiding combined with positive reinforcement such as praise can reduce the need for diapers, incontinence pads, and indwelling catheters.

Enhance Urinary Elimination. Dietary modifications, exercises to strengthen pelvic floor muscles, and bladder training programs are often effective to restore and maintain continence.

Expected Outcome: Patient will demonstrate a normal pattern of urinary elimination without episodes of urinary incontinence.

The nurse will:

- Instruct the patient to keep a voiding diary, recording the time and amount of all fluid intake and urinary output, status at the time of voiding (dry or wet) and on arising from sleep, and activities. *Voiding diaries provide valuable information for identifying the type of incontinence and possible measures to reduce or eliminate incontinent episodes.*
- Teach pelvic floor muscle exercises (refer to Box 27.5). Instruct to consciously tighten pelvic muscles when the need to void is perceived and to relax the abdomen while walking to the bathroom. *Improved pelvic muscle strength helps retain urine and prevent stress incontinence by increasing urethral pressure. Exercises also decrease abnormal detrusor muscle contractions, decreasing pressure within the bladder.*
- Using the patient's voiding diary, suggest dietary and fluid intake modifications to reduce stress and urge incontinence. Include the potential benefits of limiting caffeine, alcohol, citrus juice, and artificial sweetener consumption; limiting fluid intake to no less than 1.5 to 2.0 L/day; and limiting evening fluid intake. *Caffeine, alcohol, and citrus juices are bladder irritants and may promote detrusor instability, increasing the risk of urge incontinence. Artificial sweeteners may also irritate the bladder. Fluid intake of 1.5 to 2.0 L/day is adequate to maintain health for most patients; excess fluid may increase stress incontinence if bathroom facilities are not readily available.*

Promote Self-Care Toileting. Functional incontinence may be the predominant problem in an older adult who is institutionalized. Limited mobility, impaired vision, dementia, lack of access to facilities and privacy, and tight staffing patterns increase the risk for incontinence in previously continent residents. The primary problem in functional incontinence is an outside factor that interferes with the ability to respond normally to the urge to void. An immobilized patient may wet the bed if a call light is not within reach; a patient with Alzheimer disease may perceive the urge to void but be unable to interpret its meaning or respond by seeking a bathroom. For these patients, self-care deficit in toileting is a primary problem.

Expected Outcome: Patient will recognize and respond to urge to urinate or will recognize and acknowledge need for help with toileting.

The nurse will:

- Assess physical and mental abilities and limitations, usual voiding pattern, and ability to assist with toileting. *A thorough assessment allows planned interventions to address specific needs and promote independence.*
- Provide assistive devices as needed to facilitate independence, such as raised toilet seats, grab bars, a bedside commode, or nightlights. *Fostering independence in toileting bolsters self-concept and maintains a positive body image.*
- Plan a toileting schedule based on the patient's normal elimination patterns to achieve approximately 300 mL of urine output with each voiding. *Allowing the bladder to fill to a point at which the urge to void is experienced and then emptying it completely helps maintain normal bladder capacity and bacteriostatic functions.*
- Position for ease of voiding—sitting for females, standing for males—and provide privacy. *Normal positioning, usual toileting facilities, and privacy enhance the ability to void on schedule and empty the bladder completely.*
- Adjust fluid intake so that the majority of fluids are consumed during times of the day when the patient is most able to remain continent. Unless fluids are restricted, maintain a fluid intake of at least 1.5 to 2.0 L/day. *An adequate fluid intake is vital to promote hydration and urinary function. Overly concentrated urine can irritate the bladder, increasing incontinence.*
- Assist with clothing that is easily removed (e.g., elastic-waist pants or loose dresses). Velcro and zipper fasteners may be easier to use than snaps and buttons. *Clothing that is difficult to remove can increase the risk of incontinence in the patient with mobility problems or impaired dexterity.*

Reduced Social Isolation Due to Urinary Demands. Urinary incontinence increases the risk for social isolation due to embarrassment, fear of not having ready access to a bathroom, body odor, or other factors. Social isolation, in turn, can increase problems of incontinence because normal cues and relationships are lost and the need to remain dry is less strongly felt.

Expected Outcome: Patient will resume previous pattern of social interactions.

The nurse will:

- Assess reasons for and extent of social isolation. Verify the degree of social isolation with the patient or significant other. *Do not assume that social isolation is only related to urinary incontinence. Other problems frequently associated with aging (such as a hearing deficit) may be primary or contributing factors.*
- Refer patient for urologic examination and incontinence evaluation. *Patients who assume that urinary incontinence is a normal part of the aging process may not be aware of treatment options.*
- Explore alternative coping strategies with patient, significant other, staff, and other healthcare team members. *Protective pads or shields, good perineal hygiene, scheduled voiding, and clothing that does not interfere with toileting can enhance continence.*

Delegating Nursing Care Activities

As appropriate and allowed by the designated duties and responsibilities of unlicensed assistive personnel, the nurse may delegate nursing care activities such as assisting to obtain a clean-catch urine specimen, maintaining a voiding diary for the patient who is unable to do so, and using a bladder scanner to determine postvoid residual urine. Many nursing care activities to reduce incontinent episodes are appropriate for delegation to unlicensed caregivers, particularly for residents of long-term care facilities. These activities include scheduled toileting, positioning the patient for ease of voiding, adjusting the schedule of fluid intake, and encouraging clothing that is easy to remove for toileting.

Transitions of Care

Because UI is a contributing factor in the institutionalization of many older people, patient and family teaching can have a significant impact on maintaining independence and residence in the community. Address possible causes of incontinence and appropriate treatment measures. Refer for urologic examination if not already completed. Discuss fluid intake management, perineal care, and products for clothing protection.

Preventive strategies for UI include good bladder hygiene with regular bathroom use, adequate fluid intake, and teaching related to underlying conditions that result in UI. Management of acute episodes of UI includes bladder management program with frequent toileting. An important focus for teaching and nursing care is pristine skin care to reduce skin contact with urine-soaked clothing, bedding, or furniture.

CHAPTER HIGHLIGHTS

27.1 Urinary Tract Infection

Describe the pathophysiology and manifestations of a urinary tract infection, and outline the interprofessional care and nursing care of patients with this disorder.

- Urinary tract infections (UTIs) are common among adult women and patients in hospitals and long-term care facilities. In the untreated or immunocompromised patient, UTI can lead to sepsis or chronic kidney disease. Preventing UTI through patient and caregiver teaching and use of evidence-based guidelines is a major nursing responsibility.
- Short-course antibiotic therapy is appropriate for uncomplicated infections of the lower urinary tract that are not associated with the presence of an indwelling urinary catheter.
- Teach patients about perineal hygiene and the importance of maintaining adequate fluid intake as measures to help prevent UTI.

27.2 Urinary Calculi

Describe the pathophysiology and manifestations of urinary calculi, and outline the interprofessional care and nursing care of patients with this disorder.

- The urinary tract can be affected by obstructive processes such as stones and tumors. Early recognition of obstructive processes and maintaining unobstructed urinary output are critical to maintain kidney function.
- Urinary stones (most commonly kidney stones in the United States) can obstruct the urinary tract at any level and cause significant pain as they move from the kidney through the ureter. Instruct patients who have had a kidney stone to maintain a generous fluid intake, particularly during exercise and warm weather, to reduce the risk of further stone formation.

27.3 Urinary Tract Tumors

Describe the pathophysiology and manifestations of urinary tract tumors, and outline the interprofessional care and nursing care of patients with such disorders.

- Bladder cancer is the most commonly occurring malignancy of the urinary tract. When identified and treated early, bladder function can be preserved and the prognosis is good. Invasive bladder cancer may necessitate removal of the bladder and urinary diversion, altering patterns of urinary elimination and body image.
- The risk for bladder cancer is greater among men than women, and cigarette smoking is the most significant risk factor for bladder cancer. Most tumors can be resected transurethrally if diagnosed early, before spreading to deeper layers of the bladder wall, the lymph nodes, and adjacent tissue.
- When resection of the urinary bladder is necessary, a urinary diversion is created to collect urine. A collection appliance must be worn constantly on an ileal conduit; when a continent urinary diversion is created, the pouch is emptied by intermittent catheterization of the stoma.

27.4 Disorders of Urinary Elimination

Describe the pathophysiology and manifestations of disorders of urinary elimination (urinary retention, neurogenic bladder, and urinary incontinence), and outline the interprofessional care and nursing care of patients with these disorders.

- Changes in muscle tone can affect the ability to effectively empty the urinary bladder and/or maintain urinary continence. Urinary incontinence, while treatable and rarely life-threatening, can lead to embarrassment, social isolation, and institutionalization.
- Urinary retention may occur as a result of some medications, neurologic damage or disease, or obstruction (e.g., an enlarged prostate gland). If the underlying condition cannot be treated, medications or intermittent catheterization are used to promote bladder emptying.
- Older adults in particular are at risk for urinary incontinence, a treatable condition. A health history, voiding diary, and diagnostic testing are used to establish the type of urinary incontinence and direct treatments such as surgery, pelvic floor muscle exercises, medications, and scheduled toileting.

TEST YOURSELF NCLEX-RN® REVIEW

1. A female patient who was treated 3 months ago for a urinary tract infection is experiencing the same symptoms now. What should the nurse ask the patient during the health assessment?

   A. "How much milk do you drink each day?"
   B. "What form of birth control are you using?"
   C. "Does your partner have similar symptoms?"
   D. "Did you complete the antibiotic prescribed for the first infection?"

2. A perimenopausal patient is experiencing frequency, urgency, nocturia, dysuria, and cloudy, rust-colored urine for the third time in the past 2 years. What should the nurse include when teaching this patient? (Select all that apply.)
   A. Preprocedure instruction for an IVP
   B. Recommendations for perineal cleansing
   C. Recommendations for screening cystoscopy
   D. Potential benefits of estrogen vaginal cream
   E. Return to the office in 10 days for follow-up culture
3. The nurse identifies that a patient with immobility is at risk for the development of urolithiasis. What should the nurse include when planning this patient's care?
   A. Monitor urine pH.
   B. Administer calcium supplements.
   C. Maintain an indwelling urinary catheter.
   D. Increase fluid intake to 3000 mL/day.
4. A patient with a history of kidney stones suddenly experiences acute crampy pain on the left side that radiates into the groin. The patient is nauseated, vomits clear fluid, and voids pink urine. What should the nurse do first?
   A. Strain all urine.
   B. Notify the physician.
   C. Administer the prescribed narcotic analgesic.
   D. Obtain a bladder scan to assess for residual urine.
5. The nurse is teaching a group of community members about measures to reduce the risk for bladder cancer. What should the nurse include when providing these instructions? (Select all that apply.)
   A. Empty the bladder every 2 hours.
   B. Do not start smoking; if you smoke, stop.
   C. Increase the intake of fluids and vegetables.
   D. Avoid using hair dyes and pesticides in the home.
   E. Limit the intake of coffee and other caffeinated beverages.
6. At a local health fair, a male participant remarks to the nurse about urine occasionally being pink and wonders if this should be a concern. How should the nurse respond?
   A. Advise to make an appointment to see a physician.
   B. Teach to increase fluid intake to 2.5 to 3 quarts per day.
   C. Instruct to track the relationship between urine color and activities.
   D. Instruct to notify the physician if pain or difficulty voiding develops.
7. The nurse evaluates teaching provided to a patient with a newly created ileal diversion with a continent reservoir. Which patient behaviors indicate teaching has been effective? (Select all that apply.)
   A. Demonstrates care for the collection device.
   B. Demonstrates self-catheterization of the stoma.
   C. Identifies factors contributing to the risk for bladder cancer.
   D. States the importance of promptly reporting cloudy urine to the physician.
   E. Identifies symptoms of electrolyte imbalance
8. The nurse is identifying goals of care for a patient with stress incontinence. Which goal would be a priority for this patient?
   A. States chronic and benign nature of the disorder.
   B. Identifies products for protecting clothing and furniture.
   C. Limits intake of high-fluid fruits and vegetables.
   D. Performs pelvic floor muscle exercises as taught several a day.
9. A patient has been diagnosed with urinary incontinence. What should the nurse teach this patient? (Select all that apply.)
   A. Wear clothing that is easily removed for toileting.
   B. Establish a voiding schedule that includes emptying the bladder at least every 2 hours.
   C. Reduce fluid intake after the evening meal.
   D. Use a feminine hygiene spray to control odor.
   E. Drink at least 6 ounces of orange juice daily.
10. The nurse is caring for a patient in the spinal shock phase following spinal cord injury. Which action is the most appropriate to maintain this patient's bladder functioning?
   A. Stimulate voiding using the Credé method.
   B. Assess for urinary retention following each voiding.
   C. Catheterize with straight catheter every 3 to 4 hours.
   D. Insert an indwelling urinary catheter to accurately measure output.

See Test Yourself answers in Appendix B.

REFERENCES

Adams, M. P., Holland, L. N., & Urban, C. (2017). *Pharmacology for nursing: A pathophysiologic approach* (5th ed.). Hoboken, NJ: Pearson Education.

Agency for Healthcare Research and Quality. (2015). *Toolkit for reducing catheter-associated urinary tract infections in hospital units: Implementation guide.* Retrieved from https://www.ahrq.gov/professionals/quality-patient-safety/hais/cauti-tools/guides/implguide-pt3.html.

American Cancer Society. (2018). *Cancer facts and figures 2018.* Atlanta, GA: Author. Retrieved from https://www.cancer.org/content/dam/cancer-org/research/cancer-facts-and-statistics/

annual-cancer-facts-and-figures/2018/cancer-facts-and-figures-2018.pdf.

American Nurses Association (ANA). (2018). *ANA CAUTI Prevention Tool*. Retrieved from https://www.nursingworld.org/practice-policy/innovation-evidence/clinical-practice-material/ana-cauti-prevention-tool/.

American Urological Society. (2018). *UTI epidemiologic and socioeconomics education*. Retrieved from www.auanet.org/education/auauniversity/medical-student-education/medical-student-curriculum/adult-uti.

Bardsley, A. (2016). An overview of urinary incontinence. *British Journal of Nursing*, *25*(18), S14–S21.

Centers for Medicare and Medicaid Services (CMS). (2018). *Catheter-associated urinary tract infections (CAUTI)*. Retrieved from https://partnershipforpatients.cms.gov/p4p_resources/tsp-catheterassociatedurinarytractinfections/toolcatheter-associatedurinarytractinfectionscauti.html.

Hall, P. (2010). *Nephrolithiasis*. Cleveland Clinic: Center for Continuing Education. Retrieved from www.clevelandclinicmeded.com/medicalpubs/diseasemanagement/nephrology/nephrolithiasis/.

Johnson, E. K. (2017). Urinary tract infections in pregnancy: Treatment and management. *Medscape*. Retrieved from https://emedicine.medscape.com/article/452604-treatment.

Mayo Clinic. (2018). *Overactive bladder*. Retrieved from https://www.mayoclinic.org/diseases-conditions/overactive-bladder/diagnosis-treatment/drc-20355721.

McNeill, L. (2017). Back to basics: How evidence-based nursing practice can prevent catheter-associated urinary tract infections. *Urologic Nursing*, *37*(4), 204–206.

Mu, L., Geng, L.-S., Xu, H., Luo, M., Geng, M.-J., & Li, L. (2017). Lidocaine-prilocaine cream reduces catheter-related bladder discomfort in male patients during the general anesthesia recovery period: A prospective, randomized, case-control STROBE study. *Medicine*, *96*(14), e6494.

National Association for Continence. (2017). *Health care professional overview*. Retrieved from https://www.nafc.org/providers-1/.

National Center for Complementary and Integrative Health (NCCIH). (2016). *Cranberry*. Retrieved from https://nccih.nih.gov/health/cranberry.

National Institute of Diabetes and Digestive and Kidney Disorders (NIDDK). (2017). *Eating, diet, and nutrition for kidney stones*. Retrieved from https://www.niddk.nih.gov/health-information/urologic-diseases/kidney-stones/eating-diet-nutrition.

National Institute of Diabetes and Digestive and Kidney Disorders (NIDDK). (2018). *Urinary retention*. Retrieved from https://www.niddk.nih.gov/health-information/urologic-diseases/urinary-retention.

National Kidney Foundation. (2016). *Kidney stones*. Retrieved from https://www.kidney.org/atoz/content/kidneystones.

Office of Population Affairs. (2018). *Urinary tract infection (UTI)*. Retrieved from https://www.hhs.gov/opa/reproductive-health/fact-sheets/urinary-tract-infections/index.html.

Panchisin, T. L. (2016). Improving outcomes with the ANA CAUTI prevention tool. *Nursing*, *46*(3), 55–59.

Scales, C. D., Smith, A. C., Hanley, J. M., & Saigal, C. S. (2012). Prevalence of kidney stones in the United States. *European Urology*, *62*(1), 160–165.

Shields, K. M., Fox, K. L., & Liebrecht, C. (2018). *Pearson nurse's drug guide*. Boston, MA: Pearson.

Sorenson, M., Quinn, L., & Klein, D. (2019). *Pathophysiology: Concepts of human disease*. Hoboken, NJ: Pearson Education.

Weckx, F., Tutulo, M., DeRidder, D., & Van Der Aa, F. (2016). The role of botulinum toxin A in treating neurogenic bladder. *Translational Andrology and Urology*, *5*(1), 63–71.

ADDITIONAL RESOURCES

American Cancer Society, Bladder Cancer

www.cancer.org/cancer/bladder-cancer.html

National Institute of Diabetes and Digestive and Kidney Diseases

www.niddk.nih.gov/

Urology Care Foundation

www.urologyhealth.org

Chapter 28

Nursing Care of Patients with Kidney Disorders

Chapter Outline and Learning Outcomes

28.1 Kidney Disorders 906

Describe the pathophysiology and manifestations of kidney disorders, including polycystic kidney disease, glomerular disorder, vascular kidney disorder, kidney trauma, and renal tumor, and outline the interprofessional care and nursing care of patients with these disorders.

28.2 Kidney Failure 921

Describe the pathophysiology and manifestations of kidney failure (i.e., acute kidney injury and chronic kidney disease), and outline the interprofessional care and nursing care of patients with these disorders.

CLINICAL COMPETENCIES

- Assess and monitor the health status of patients with kidney disorders, recognizing and reporting unexpected manifestations or status changes.
- Provide safe and effective nursing care for patients undergoing renal replacement therapies, surgery involving the kidneys, or renal transplant, respecting the patient's expressed needs, values, and preferences.
- Using assessed data and current standards of practice, plan and implement evidence-based nursing care for patients with renal disorders using research and best practices.
- Collaborate and coordinate with the patient and other members of the interprofessional team to prioritize and implement care.
- Provide teaching appropriate to the individual and situation for patients with kidney disorders.
- Evaluate patient responses to care, revising the plan of care as needed to promote, maintain, or restore functional health status for patients with renal disorders.
- Participate in studies and projects to improve outcomes for patients with acute or chronic kidney disorders.
- Apply technology and information management tools to support safe processes of care for patients with kidney disorders.

KEY TERMS

acute kidney injury (AKI), 921
acute tubular necrosis (ATN), 923
azotemia, 907
chronic kidney disease (CKD), 934
dialysis, 926
glomerulonephritis, 908
hematuria, 907
hemodialysis, 928
kidney failure, 921
nephrectomy, 917
nephrotic syndrome, 909
oliguria, 908
peritoneal dialysis, 928
proteinuria, 907
ultrafiltration, 928
uremia, 935

The internal environment of the body normally remains in a relatively constant or *homeostatic* state. The kidneys help maintain homeostasis by regulating the composition and volume of extracellular fluid. They excrete excess water and solutes and can conserve water and solutes when deficits occur. In addition, the kidneys help regulate acid–base balance and excrete metabolic wastes. Regulation of blood pressure is another key function of the kidneys. Both primary kidney disorders (such as glomerulonephritis) and systemic diseases (such as diabetes mellitus) can affect renal function. In the United States, about 14% of adults have chronic kidney disease. More than 661,000 Americans have kidney failure. Of these, 468,000 are on dialysis and 193,000 are living with a kidney transplant (National Institute of Diabetes, Digestive and Kidney Diseases [NIDDK], 2016). In 2016, 4.9 million Americans were diagnosed with kidney disease (Centers for Disease Control and Prevention, 2017). Kidney disease accounted for more than 49,959 deaths in 2016 (NIDDK, 2016). Diabetes is the leading cause of end-stage renal disease (ESRD) in the United States; hypertension is the second leading cause (NIDDK, 2016). The incidence of chronic kidney disease is growing most rapidly among people ages 65 and older, whereas it remains stable in younger adults.

28.1 Kidney Disorders

The Patient with Polycystic Kidney Disease

Polycystic kidney disease, a hereditary disease characterized by formation of fluid-filled cysts and massive kidney enlargement, affects both children and adults. This disease has two forms: The autosomal dominant form primarily affects adults; the autosomal recessive form is present at birth (Sorenson, Quinn, & Klein, 2019). Autosomal recessive polycystic kidney disease is rare. It is usually diagnosed prenatally or in infancy. Renal failure generally develops during childhood, necessitating kidney transplant or dialysis. Autosomal dominant polycystic kidney disease (ADPKD) is relatively common, affecting 1 in every 400 to 1000 people and accounting for approximately 4% of patients with ESRD in the United States (NIDDK, 2018). This section focuses on autosomal dominant polycystic kidney disease, the more common form of the disorder.

Pathophysiology

Renal cysts are fluid-filled sacs affecting the nephron, the functional unit of the kidneys. The cysts, which arise from tubular epithelial cells, may range in size from microscopic to several centimeters in diameter and affect the renal cortex and medulla of both kidneys. Cysts may detach from the tubule, continuing to enlarge by active fluid secretion. As the cysts enlarge and multiply, the kidneys also enlarge. Although only a small percentage of nephrons are involved, the cysts compress adjacent renal parenchyma. Renal blood vessels and nephrons are compressed and obstructed, leading to tissue ischemia. This activates the renin–angiotensin–aldosterone system within the kidney. Functional tissue is destroyed, with compression, ischemia, and accumulation of inflammatory mediators likely playing a role (**Figure 28.1** ■).

People affected by polycystic kidney disease often develop cysts elsewhere in the body, including the liver, spleen, pancreas, lungs, and reproductive organs. Up to 83% of people with ADPKD develop liver cysts, which may bleed or become infected. Diverticular disease of the colon is common and may lead to perforation of the bowel. About 25% of people with polycystic kidney disease have cardiac valve abnormalities, including mitral valve prolapse ("floppy" mitral valves) and aortic valve insufficiency. The risk of subarachnoid or cerebral hemorrhage from a ruptured cerebral aneurysm is significantly increased in patients with ADPKD (NIDDK, 2018).

Risk Factors

ADPKD is primarily a genetic disease. See the Genetics Considerations feature.

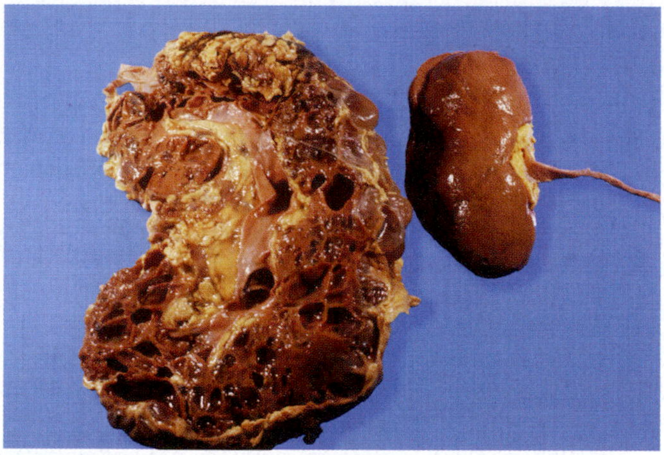

Figure 28.1 ■ A polycystic kidney. The functional tissue of the kidneys is gradually destroyed and replaced with fluid-filled cysts.

Genetic Considerations

Adult Polycystic Kidney Disease

- Approximately 90% of cases are inherited as an autosomal dominant trait; the remaining 10% are due to spontaneous mutations.
- ADPKD type 1, due to mutation of a gene on chromosome 16, accounts for approximately 85% of cases. It tends to have an earlier onset of symptoms and renal failure.
- ADPKD type 2, due to gene mutation on chromosome 4, is responsible for most remaining cases. The onset of manifestations and renal failure is later with this form of the disease.
- In both types of ADPKD, the genetic mutation affects production of *polycystin* membrane proteins and tubular epithelial cell growth and differentiation (Genetics Home Reference, 2018).

Manifestations

Polycystic kidney disease is slowly progressive. Symptoms usually develop by age 40 to 50. Common manifestations include flank pain, microscopic or gross **hematuria** (blood in the urine), **proteinuria** (proteins in the urine), and *polyuria* and *nocturia*, as the concentrating ability of the kidney is impaired. Urinary tract infection and renal calculi are common, as cysts interfere with normal urine drainage. Most patients develop hypertension from disruption of renal vessels. The kidneys become palpable, enlarged, and knobby. Symptoms of renal insufficiency and chronic renal failure typically develop by age 60 to 70. The progression to ESRD tends to occur more rapidly in Blacks and in men.

Interprofessional Care

Diagnostic tests used to determine the extent of polycystic kidney disease include:

- ***Renal ultrasonography*** is the diagnostic procedure of choice for polycystic kidney disease.
- ***Computed tomography (CT) scan*** or ***MRI*** of the kidney may be used to detect cystic disease at an earlier stage when there is a positive family history.
- ***Genetic testing*** for ADPKD type 1 and type 2 is available and is particularly important when a family member is being considered as a potential kidney donor.

Management of adult polycystic kidney disease is largely supportive. Care is taken to avoid further renal damage by nephrotoxic substances, UTI, obstruction, or hypertension. A fluid intake of 2000 to 2500 mL/day is encouraged to help prevent UTI and lithiasis. Hypertension associated with polycystic disease is generally controlled using a multidrug regimen to achieve a target blood pressure of 130/80 mmHg. Angiotensin-converting enzyme (ACE) inhibitors and angiotensin receptor blockers (ARBs) may slow the expansion of renal cysts and help preserve glomerular filtration rate (GFR). Ultimately, dialysis or renal transplantation is required. Patients with polycystic kidney disease are typically good candidates for transplantation because of the absence of associated systemic disease, but may still experience effects of the extrarenal elements of the disease.

Nursing Care

For those with adult polycystic kidney disease, an autosomal dominant disorder, discuss genetic counseling and screening of family members for evidence of the disease.

Teach the patient with polycystic kidney disease about the disease, its genetic nature, and its usual course. Discuss measures to maintain optimal renal function. Instruct to maintain a fluid intake of at least 2500 mL/day. Include additional information about preventing UTI (such as hygiene measures) and early manifestations of UTI. Stress the importance of seeking treatment to prevent further kidney damage. Advise to avoid drugs that are potentially toxic to the kidneys and to check with the primary care provider before taking any new drug. Discuss the potential benefits of genetic counseling with the patient and family.

Transitions of Care

There are no known preventive measures for polycystic kidney disease, as it is a genetic disease. Upon diagnosis of polycystic kidney disease, lifestyle changes should be instituted. Moderate daily exercise, maintaining weight within normal range, adequate sleep, and smoking cessation are all encouraged. Depending on renal function, dietary recommendations to reduce phosphorus and potassium may be indicated. Dietary and fluid management may include careful protein intake, balanced fluids, and reductions in sodium.

The Patient with a Glomerular Disorder

Disorders and diseases involving the glomerulus are the leading cause of chronic kidney disease in the United States. They are the underlying disease process for more than half of those people needing dialysis and result in a significant number of deaths per year.

Glomerular disorders may be either primary, involving mainly the kidney, or secondary to a multisystem disease or hereditary condition. Primary glomerular disease is often immunologic or idiopathic in origin. The most common primary glomerular disorder is acute *poststreptococcal glomerulonephritis* (also called *acute proliferative glomerulonephritis*). Diabetes mellitus, undiagnosed or inadequately treated hypertension, and systemic lupus erythematosus (SLE) are frequently implicated in secondary glomerular disorders. Early manifestations include hematuria, proteinuria, and hypertension.

Pathophysiology

The *glomerulus* is a tuft of capillaries surrounded by a thin, double-walled capsule (Bowman capsule). About 20% of the resting cardiac output flows through the glomeruli of the kidneys, forming approximately 180 L of plasma filtrate. More than 99% of this filtrate is reabsorbed in the renal tubules. The rate of glomerular filtration is controlled by opposing forces: The pressure and amount of blood flowing through the glomeruli promote filtration, whereas the pressure in Bowman capsule and the colloid osmotic (*oncotic*) pressure of the blood oppose it. The total surface area of glomerular capillaries also affects the GFR. The glomerular capillary membrane has three layers: The capillary endothelial layer, the basement membrane, and the capsule epithelial layer. Water and the smallest solutes (such as electrolytes) pass freely across this membrane, whereas larger molecules (such as plasma proteins) are retained in the blood.

Glomerular disease affects both the structure and function of the glomerulus, disrupting glomerular filtration. The capillary membrane becomes more permeable to plasma proteins and blood cells. This increased permeability in the glomerulus causes the manifestations common to glomerular disorders: Hematuria, proteinuria, and edema. The GFR falls, leading to **azotemia** (increased blood levels of nitrogenous waste products) and hypertension. Glomerular involvement may be diffuse (involving all glomeruli) or focal (involving some glomeruli, while others remain essentially normal).

Both hematuria and proteinuria are caused by glomerular capillary membrane damage, which allows blood cells and proteins to escape from the blood into the glomerular filtrate. Hematuria may be either gross or microscopic. Proteinuria is considered to be the most important indicator of glomerular injury because it increases progressively with increased glomerular damage. Loss of plasma proteins leads to *hypoalbuminemia* (low serum albumin levels), which in turn reduces the plasma oncotic pressure (osmotic pressure created by plasma proteins), leading to edema.

As plasma proteins are lost, the forces opposing filtration diminish and the amount of filtrate increases. The increased flow of filtrate stimulates the renin–angiotensin–aldosterone mechanism, producing vasoconstriction and a resulting fall in GFR. Increased aldosterone production causes salt and water retention, which further contribute to edema. As the GFR falls, filtration and elimination of nitrogenous wastes, including urea, decrease, causing azotemia. **Oliguria**, urine output of less than 400 mL in 24 hours, may result from the decreased GFR. Hypertension results from fluid retention and disruption of the renin–angiotensin system, a key regulator of blood pressure.

The major primary glomerular disorders include acute glomerulonephritis, rapidly progressive glomerulonephritis, nephrotic syndrome, and chronic glomerulonephritis. Diabetic nephropathy and lupus nephritis are the most common secondary forms of glomerular disease.

Acute Postinfectious Glomerulonephritis

Glomerulonephritis is inflammation of the glomerular capillary membrane. Acute glomerulonephritis can result from systemic diseases or primary glomerular diseases, but *acute postinfectious glomerulonephritis* (also known as *acute poststreptococcal glomerulonephritis*) is the most common form. The usual initiating event for this disorder is infection of the pharynx or skin with group A beta-hemolytic streptococci. Staphylococcal or viral infections, such as hepatitis B, mumps, or varicella (chickenpox), can lead to a similar postinfectious acute glomerulonephritis. Acute postinfectious glomerulonephritis is primarily a disease of childhood that can also affect adults.

In acute postinfectious glomerulonephritis, circulating antigen–antibody immune complexes formed during the primary infection become trapped in the glomerular membrane, leading to an inflammatory response. The complement system is activated, and vasoactive substances and inflammatory mediators are released. Endothelial cells proliferate, and the glomerular membrane swells and becomes permeable to plasma proteins and blood cells. Renal involvement is diffuse, spread throughout the kidneys. See the Pathophysiology Illustrated: Acute Postinfectious Glomerulonephritis feature.

Manifestations and Complications

Acute postinfectious glomerulonephritis is characterized by an abrupt onset of hematuria, proteinuria, salt and water retention, and evidence of azotemia occurring 10 to 14 days after the initial infection. The urine often appears brown or cola colored. Salt and water retention increase extracellular fluid volume, leading to hypertension and edema. The edema is primarily noted in the face, particularly around the eyes (*periorbital edema*) (**Figure 28.2** ■). Dependent edema, affecting the hands and upper extremities in particular, may be noted. Other manifestations may include fatigue, anorexia, nausea and vomiting, and headache.

The older adult may have less apparent symptoms. Nausea, malaise, arthralgias, and proteinuria are common manifestations; hypertension and edema are seen less often. Pulmonary infiltrates may occur early in the disorder, often due to worsening of a preexisting condition such as heart failure.

The prognosis for adults with acute glomerulonephritis is less favorable than it is for children. The symptoms may resolve spontaneously within 10 to 14 days. Full recovery is usual in children, whereas only 60% or more of affected adults recover completely. The remaining patients have persistent symptoms, and some have permanent kidney damage.

Antiglomerular Basement Membrane Glomerulonephritis

Antiglomerular basement membrane (anti-GBM) glomerulonephritis is characterized by autoantibodies to antigens in the glomerular basement membrane and manifestations of severe glomerular injury. Anti-GBM glomerulonephritis often progresses to renal failure within months. When lung hemorrhage accompanies the disorder, it is called *Goodpasture syndrome*. Although people of all ages can be affected, Goodpasture syndrome is primarily seen in young men under the age of 30 and in older adults in their 60s and 70s (Sorenson et al., 2019).

In anti-GBM glomerulonephritis, glomerular cells proliferate and, together with macrophages, form crescent-shaped lesions that obliterate Bowman space. Glomerular damage is diffuse, leading to a rapid, progressive decline

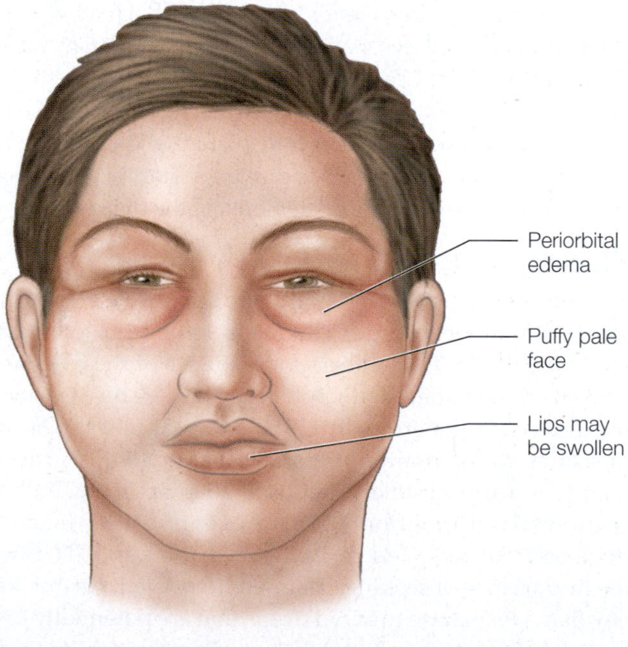
Periorbital edema
Puffy pale face
Lips may be swollen

Figure 28.2 ■ Severe edema characteristic of nephrotic syndrome.

Pathophysiology Illustrated

Acute Postinfectious Glomerulonephritis

Infection from group A beta-hemolytic streptococci causes an immune response that results in inflammation and damage to the glomeruli. Protein and red blood cells are allowed to pass through the glomeruli. Blood flow to the glomeruli is reduced due to obstruction with damaged cells and renal insufficiency results, leading to the retention of sodium, water, and waste.

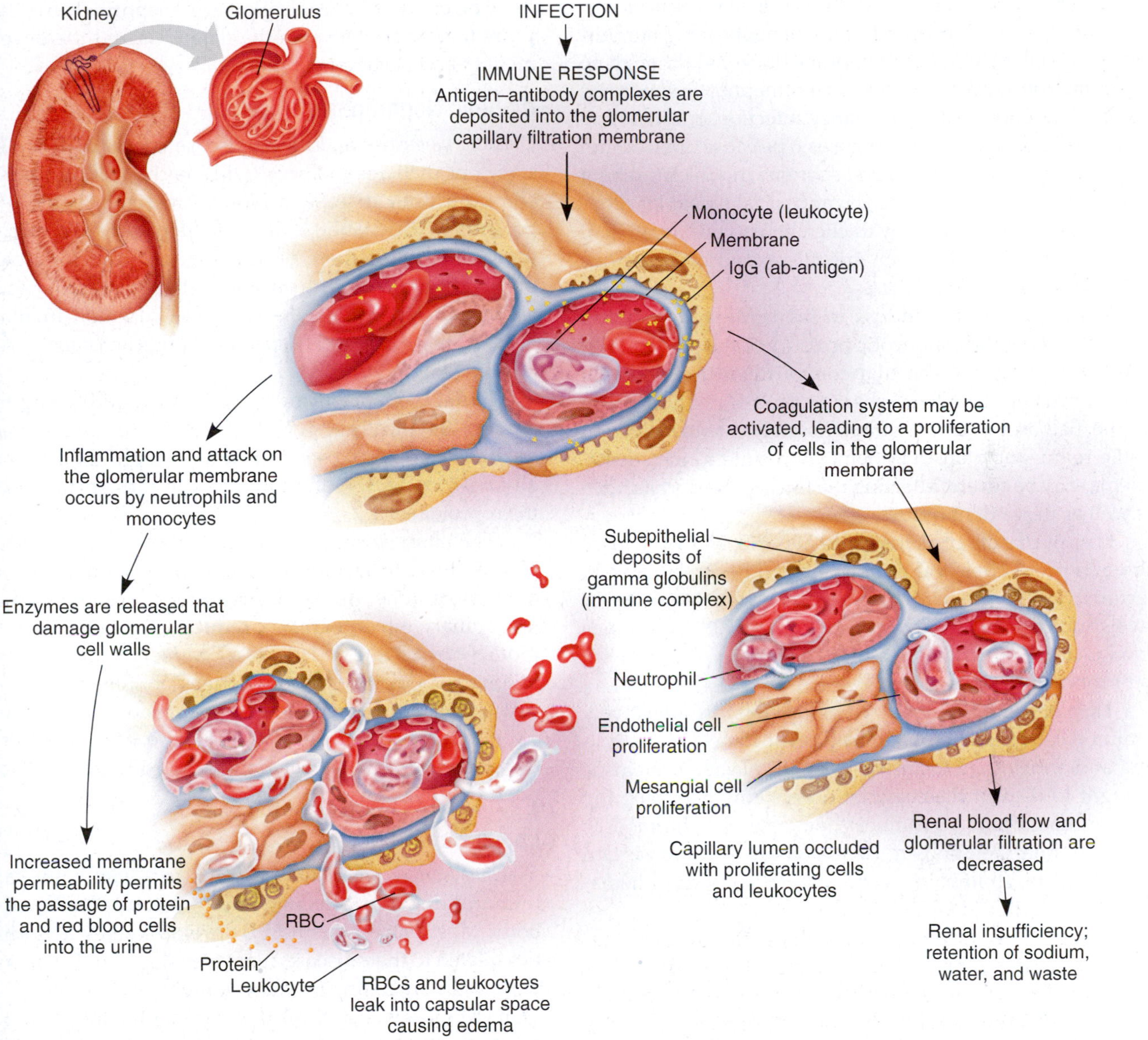
Kidney
Glomerulus
INFECTION
IMMUNE RESPONSE
Antigen–antibody complexes are deposited into the glomerular capillary filtration membrane
Monocyte (leukocyte)
Membrane
IgG (ab-antigen)
Coagulation system may be activated, leading to a proliferation of cells in the glomerular membrane
Inflammation and attack on the glomerular membrane occurs by neutrophils and monocytes
Enzymes are released that damage glomerular cell walls
Subepithelial deposits of gamma globulins (immune complex)
Neutrophil
Endothelial cell proliferation
Mesangial cell proliferation
Capillary lumen occluded with proliferating cells and leukocytes
Renal blood flow and glomerular filtration are decreased
Renal insufficiency; retention of sodium, water, and waste
Increased membrane permeability permits the passage of protein and red blood cells into the urine
RBC
Protein
Leukocyte
RBCs and leukocytes leak into capsular space causing edema

in renal function. In Goodpasture syndrome, antibodies may also bind to alveolar basement membranes, damaging alveoli and causing pulmonary hemorrhage.

Patients with anti-GBM glomerulonephritis often present with complaints of weakness, nausea and vomiting, and possible abdominal or flank pain. Some may relate a history of an upper respiratory tract infection preceding the onset of the glomerulonephritis. Renal manifestations include hematuria, proteinuria, and edema. Moderate hypertension may develop. On urinalysis, hematuria and massive proteinuria are noted. Presentation with oliguria is an ominous sign; rapid progression to renal failure may occur. Alveolar membrane damage can lead to mild or life-threatening pulmonary hemorrhage. Cough, shortness of breath, and hemoptysis (bloody sputum) are early respiratory manifestations.

Nephrotic Syndrome

Nephrotic syndrome is a group of clinical findings as opposed to a specific disorder. It is characterized by massive proteinuria, hypoalbuminemia, hyperlipidemia, and edema. A number of disorders can affect the glomerular capillary membrane, changing its porosity and allowing plasma proteins to escape into the urine.

Minimal change disease (MCD) is the most common cause of nephrotic syndrome in children but accounts for only 10 to 15% of adults with nephrotic syndrome. In MCD, the size and form of glomeruli appear normal by light microscopy. Relapse, common in children, occurs less frequently in adults. When it occurs, however, relapse can be resistant to effective treatment.

In White, non-Hispanic adults, *membranous glomerulonephropathy* is the most common cause of nephrotic syndrome. The glomerular basement membrane thickens, although no inflammation is present. This form of nephrotic syndrome develops secondarily to malignancy, infection, or an autoimmune disorder in up to 30% of cases. The cause often cannot be identified (idiopathic). *Focal sclerosis*, in which scarring (sclerosis) of glomeruli occurs, and *membranoproliferative glomerulonephritis*, caused by thickening and proliferation of glomerular basement membrane cells, are additional forms of nephrotic syndrome.

With plasma protein loss in the urine and resulting hypoalbuminemia, the oncotic pressure of the plasma falls. Fluid shifts from the vascular compartment to interstitial spaces, causing the edema characteristic of nephrotic syndrome. Salt and water retention, possibly due to activation of the renin–angiotensin system, contribute to the edema. Edema may be severe, affecting the face and periorbital area as well as dependent tissues.

Loss of plasma proteins stimulates the liver to increase albumin production and lipoprotein synthesis. As a result, serum triglyceride and low-density lipoprotein (LDL) levels increase, as do urine lipids (*lipiduria*). Hyperlipidemia increases the risk for atherosclerosis in patients with nephrotic syndrome.

Thromboemboli (mobilized blood clots) are a relatively common complication of nephrotic syndrome. Loss of clotting and anticlotting factors along with plasma proteins is thought to disrupt the coagulation system, increasing the risk for renal venous thrombosis, deep venous thrombosis, and pulmonary embolism. Renal venous thrombosis can cause flank or groin pain on one or both sides, gross hematuria, and a reduced GFR.

Nephrotic syndrome usually resolves without long-term effects in children. The prognosis for adults is less optimistic because the syndrome often occurs secondarily to another disorder. Many adults do not recover completely, experiencing persistent proteinuria and, potentially, progressive renal impairment.

Chronic Glomerulonephritis

Chronic glomerulonephritis is typically the result of progressive glomerular disorders such as anti-GBM glomerulonephritis, lupus nephritis, or diabetic nephropathy. In many cases, however, no previous glomerular disease has been identified.

Slow, progressive destruction of the glomeruli and a gradual decline in renal function are characteristic of chronic glomerulonephritis. The kidneys decrease in size symmetrically, and their surfaces become granular or roughened. Eventually, entire nephrons are lost.

Symptoms develop insidiously, and the disease is often not recognized until signs of renal failure develop. Chronic glomerulonephritis may be diagnosed when hypertension and impaired renal function are found coincidentally during a routine physical examination or treatment for an unrelated disorder. Viral or bacterial infectious diseases can exacerbate the disorder, prompting its diagnosis.

The course of chronic glomerulonephritis varies, with years to decades between the diagnosis and the development of end-stage renal failure.

Diabetic Nephropathy

Diabetic nephropathy, kidney disease common in the later stages of diabetes mellitus (DM), is the leading cause of chronic kidney disease in North America. About 40% of patients with diabetes develop nephropathy; because type 2 diabetes is more prevalent, it accounts for a higher portion of patients with chronic kidney disease. Diabetes-associated kidney lesions are more common in Blacks, Native Americans, and Hispanics (American Diabetes Association, [ADA], 2018).

Initial evidence of microproteinuria indicating renal damage is typically seen within 5 to 10 years after the onset of diabetes. Overt proteinuria and nephropathy generally develop within another 5 to 10 years of the onset of microproteinuria.

The characteristic lesion of diabetic nephropathy is glomerulosclerosis and thickening of the glomerular basement membrane. As the disease progresses, the glomerular capillary lumen narrows, reducing the surface area for glomerular filtration. Arteriosclerosis, a common feature of long-term diabetes and hypertension, contributes to the disease, as do nephritis and tubular lesions. Pyelonephritis, inflammation of the kidney, is also implicated in the development of diabetic nephropathy. More about diabetic nephropathy is found in Chapter 20.

Lupus Nephritis

Systemic lupus erythematosus (SLE) is an inflammatory autoimmune disorder affecting the connective tissue of the body. Most patients with SLE develop kidney abnormalities related to their disease; many develop manifestations of nephritis. Circulating immune complexes deposited in the glomerulus as well as those that form within the glomerular capillary wall trigger an inflammatory response leading to glomerular injury in SLE. Manifestations of lupus nephritis range from microscopic hematuria to massive proteinuria. Its progression may be slow and chronic or *fulminant*, with a sudden onset and the rapid development of renal failure. End-stage kidney disease eventually develops in about 20% of patients with lupus nephritis. Improved management of the underlying disease, immunotherapy, dialysis, and renal transplantation have significantly improved the prognosis in recent years.

Interprofessional Care

Management of all types of glomerulonephritis—acute and chronic, primary and secondary—focuses on identifying the underlying disease process and preserving kidney function. In most glomerular disorders, there is no specific treatment to achieve a cure. Treatment goals are to maintain renal function, prevent complications, and support the healing process.

Diagnosis

Laboratory and diagnostic testing are valuable to evaluate kidney function and identify the cause of glomerulonephritis.

The following studies are used to evaluate kidney function:

- ***Urinalysis*** often shows red blood cells (RBCs) and proteins in the urine of patients with a glomerular disorder and may be the first indication of the disease. These substances, normally too large to enter glomerular filtrate, escape due to increased porosity of glomerular capillaries in glomerular disorders.
- ***Blood urea nitrogen (BUN)*** is measured. Urea is eliminated from the body by filtration in the glomerulus; minimal amounts are reabsorbed in the renal tubules. Glomerular diseases interfere with filtration and elimination of urea nitrogen, causing blood levels to rise. Normal BUN values are listed in **Table 28.1**. Levels up to 50 mg/dL or 17.7 mmol/L indicate mild azotemia, and levels higher than 100 mg/dL or 35.7 mmol/L indicate severe renal impairment.
- ***Serum creatinine*** is a good indicator of kidney function. Levels greater than 4 mg/dL indicate serious renal impairment.
- ***Urine creatinine*** levels decrease when renal function is impaired because creatinine is not effectively eliminated from the body.
- ***Estimated GFR (eGFR)*** is a calculated value used to evaluate renal function. Four variables are used to calculate the eGFR: Serum creatinine, age in years, gender, and race (African American or other). Values of 60 mL/min/1.73 m^2 body surface area (BSA) are within the normal range for adults (20 years old and above) and may simply be reported as >60 mL/min/1.73 m^2.
- ***Creatinine clearance*** may be used to evaluate the GFR. The *clearance*, or amount of blood cleared of creatinine in 1 minute, depends on the amount and pressure of blood being filtered and the filtering ability of the glomeruli. Disorders such as glomerulonephritis affect glomerular filtration, decreasing the creatinine clearance.
- ***Serum electrolytes*** are evaluated because impaired kidney function alters their excretion.

The following studies may be ordered to help identify the underlying cause or etiology:

- ***Antistreptolysin O (ASO) titer*** and other tests detect antigenic proteins or antibodies (such as anti-dsDNA, anti-DNA, and others) to help determine the underlying cause of glomerular dysfunction.
- ***Renal ultrasound*** may show enlarged kidneys in acute glomerulonephritis, whereas bilateral small kidneys are typical of late chronic glomerulonephritis.
- ***Kidney scan*** demonstrates delayed uptake and excretion of the radioactive material in glomerular diseases.
- ***Biopsy*** is the most reliable diagnostic procedure for glomerular disorders. Biopsy helps determine the type of glomerulonephritis, the prognosis, and appropriate treatment.

Table 28.1 Changes in Laboratory Values Associated with Kidney Disease

Test	Normal Value	Value in Renal Disease
Blood urea nitrogen (BUN)	5–25 mg/dL Slightly higher in older adults	25–50 mg/dL or higher
BUN:creatinine ratio	10:1 to 20:1	Decreased ratio in acute tubular necrosis; increased in glomerular disease, azotemia
Creatinine, serum	0.5–1.2 mg/dL; 45–106 mmol/L (SI units) Slightly lower in females, older adults	Elevated; levels >4 mg/dL indicate severe impairment of renal function
Creatinine clearance	85–135 mL/min Slightly lower in females Values decline in older adults	Reduced renal reserve: 32.5–85.0 mL/min Renal insufficiency: 6.5–32.5 mL/min Renal failure: <6.5 mL/min
eGFR	≥ 60 mL/min/1.73 m^2	Decreased in renal impairment
Serum albumin	3.5–5 g/dL; 52–68% of total protein; lower in older adults	Decreased in nephrotic syndrome
Serum electrolytes	Potassium: 3.5–5.3 mEq/L; 3.5–5.3 mmol/L Sodium: 135–145 mEq/L; 135–145 mmol/L Calcium: 4.5–5.5 mEq/L; 9–11 mg/dL; 2.3–2.8 mmol/L Phosphorus: 1.7–2.6 mEq/L; 2.5–4.5 mg/dL; 0.78–1.52 mmol/L	Increased in renal insufficiency Decreased in nephrotic syndrome Decreased in renal failure Increased in renal failure
Red blood cell count	Female: 4.0–5.0 million/mm^3 Male: 4.6–6.0 million/mm^3	Decreased in chronic kidney disease
Urine creatinine	1–2 g/24 h	Decreased in disorders of impaired renal function
Urine protein	25–150 mg/24 h	Increased in disorders of impaired renal function
Urine red blood cells	<2/HPF; no RBC casts	Present in glomerular disorders

Medications

Although no drugs are available to cure glomerular disorders, medications are used to treat underlying disorders, reduce inflammation, and manage the symptoms.

Antibiotics are prescribed for the patient with poststreptococcal glomerulonephritis to eradicate any remaining bacteria, removing the stimulus for antibody production. Nephrotoxic antibiotics, such as the aminoglycoside antibiotics, streptomycin, and some cephalosporins, are avoided.

Aggressive immunosuppressive therapy is used to treat acute inflammatory processes such as anti-GBM glomerulonephritis, Goodpasture syndrome, and exacerbations of SLE. When begun early, immunosuppressive therapy significantly reduces the risk of ESRD and renal failure. Prednisone, a glucocorticoid, is prescribed in relatively large doses of 1 mg per kilogram of body weight per day; for example, a 73-kg (160-lb) man would receive 70 to 75 mg per day. Other immunosuppressive agents such as cyclophosphamide (Cytoxan), azathioprine (Imuran), or cyclosporine (Sandimmune, Restasis, others) are prescribed in conjunction with corticosteroids. Corticosteroid use in poststreptococcal glomerulonephritis may actually worsen the condition, so it is avoided.

Oral glucocorticoids such as prednisone are also used in high doses to induce remission of nephrotic syndrome. When glucocorticoids alone are ineffective, other immunosuppressive agents such as cyclophosphamide or chlorambucil (Leukeran) may be used to induce or maintain remission.

ACE inhibitors or ARBs may be ordered to reduce protein loss associated with nephrotic syndrome and slow the progression of renal failure. They have a protective effect on the kidney in patients with diabetic nephropathy and other glomerular disorders.

Antihypertensives are prescribed to maintain the blood pressure within normal levels. Blood pressure management is important because systemic and renal hypertension are associated with a poorer prognosis in patients with glomerular disorders.

Treatment

Restricted activity may be recommended during the acute phase of poststreptococcal glomerulonephritis. When the edema of nephrotic syndrome is significant or the patient is hypertensive, sodium intake may be restricted to 1 to 2 g/day. Dietary protein may be restricted if azotemia is present. When proteins are restricted, those included in the diet should be complete or high-value proteins. Complete proteins supply the essential amino acids required for growth and tissue maintenance. Complete and incomplete (low-quality) proteins are compared in **Table 28.2**.

Plasma exchange therapy (also called *plasmapheresis*), a procedure to remove damaging antibodies from the plasma, is used in conjunction with immunosuppressive therapy to treat anti-GBM glomerulonephritis and Goodpasture syndrome. Plasma and glomerular-damaging antibodies are removed using a blood cell separator. The RBCs are then returned to the patient along with albumin or human plasma to replace the plasma removed. This procedure is usually done in a series of treatments. It is not without risk, and informed consent is required. Potential complications of plasma exchange therapy include those associated with intravenous catheters, fluid volume shifts, and altered coagulation.

Renal failure resulting from a glomerular disorder may necessitate dialysis to restore fluid and electrolyte balance and remove waste products from the body. Dialysis procedures and related nursing care are explained in the acute kidney injury section later in this chapter.

Nursing Care

Assessment

Focused assessment data related to glomerular disorders include:

- ***Health history:*** Complaints of facial or peripheral edema or weight gain, fatigue, nausea and vomiting, headache, general malaise, abdominal or flank pain; cough or shortness of breath; changes in amount, color, or character of urine (e.g., frothy urine); history of skin or pharyngeal streptococcal infection, diabetes, SLE, or kidney disease; current medications
- ***Physical assessment:*** General appearance; vital signs; weight; presence of periorbital, facial, or peripheral edema; inspect skin for lesions, infection; inspect throat, obtain culture as indicated; obtain urine specimen for color, character, odor.

Priorities of Care

Monitoring renal function and fluid volume status are key components of care, as is protecting the patient from infection.

Diagnoses, Outcomes, and Interventions

Nursing care for the patient with a glomerular disorder is supportive and educational. Both manifestations of glomerular disorders and their treatment can interfere with a patient's ability to maintain usual roles and responsibilities. For additional potential nursing diagnoses and interventions, see the Case Study & Nursing Care Plan on page 63.

Table 28.2 Complete and Incomplete Protein Sources

	Complete Proteins	Incomplete Proteins
Definition	Provide all essential amino acids needed for growth and tissue maintenance	Lack one or more essential amino acids or contain inadequate proportions
Examples	Milk, eggs, cheese, meats, poultry, fish, and soy	Vegetables, breads, cereals and grains, legumes, seeds, and nuts

Balance Fluid Volume. Excessive fluid volume and resulting edema are common manifestations of glomerular disorders. When proteins are lost in the urine, the oncotic pressure of plasma falls and fluid shifts into the interstitial spaces. The body responds to this fluid shift by retaining sodium and water to maintain intravascular volume, leading to excess fluid volume.

Expected Outcome: Patient's fluid balance will be restored (weight within expected range for individual, no evidence of central or peripheral edema).

The nurse will:

- Monitor vital signs, including blood pressure, apical pulse, respirations, and breath sounds, at least every 4 hours. Report significant changes and unexpected results. *Excess fluid increases the cardiac workload and the blood pressure. Tachycardia may result. Associated electrolyte imbalances can cause dysrhythmias. Increased pulmonary vascular pressure can lead to pulmonary edema, tachypnea, dyspnea, and crackles (rales) in the lungs.*
- Record intake and output every 4 to 8 hours, or more frequently as indicated. *Accurate intake and output records help determine fluid volume status.*
- Weigh daily, using consistent technique (time of day, scale, and clothing). *Accurate daily weights are the best indicator of approximate fluid balance.*
- Monitor serum electrolytes, hemoglobin and hematocrit, BUN, creatinine, and eGFR. *Glomerular disorders affect fluid balance and may alter electrolyte balance as well, potentially leading to complications such as cardiac dysrhythmias. Increased intravascular volume can result in low hemoglobin and hematocrit values. BUN, creatinine, and eGFR provide information about renal function.*
- Maintain fluid restriction as ordered. Offer ice chips (in limited and measured amounts) and frequent mouth care to relieve thirst. With the patient, develop a fluid intake schedule. *Fluids may be restricted to reduce fluid overload, edema, and hypertension. Ice chips and frequent mouth care moisten mucous membranes and help relieve thirst while maintaining oral tissue integrity. Including the patient in planning fluid intake promotes a sense of control and understanding of the treatment regimen.*
- Arrange dietary consultation regarding sodium- or protein-restricted diets. *Including the patient and dietitian in planning allows individualization of the diet to patient preferences. The glomerular disorder may reduce appetite; considering food preferences can help maintain adequate nutrition.*
- Monitor for desired and adverse effects of prescribed medications. *Diuretic therapy helps reduce excess fluid volume; however, glomerular disorders can affect the patient's response to treatment. In addition, diuretics can exacerbate the electrolyte imbalances and muscle weakness often associated with glomerular disorders.*
- Provide frequent position changes and good skin care. *Perfusion may be altered by tissue edema, increasing the risk of breakdown.*

SAFETY ALERT: Carefully monitor and regulate intravenous infusions; include fluid used to dilute IV medications as intake. Significant "hidden" fluid intake can occur with intravenous medication administration. ■

Manage Fatigue. Fatigue is a common manifestation of glomerular disorders. Anemia, loss of plasma proteins, headache, anorexia, and nausea compound this fatigue. The ability to maintain usual physical and mental activities may be impaired.

Expected Outcome: Patient will use energy conservation techniques to allow effective ADL maintenance and role performance.

The nurse will:

- Document energy level. *As glomerular function improves, fatigue begins to resolve and energy increases.*
- Schedule activities and procedures to provide adequate rest and energy conservation. Prevent unnecessary fatigue. *Adequate rest and energy conservation reduce fatigue and improve the patient's ability to tolerate and cope with required treatments and activities.*
- Assist with ADLs as needed. *The goal is to conserve limited energy reserves.*
- Discuss the relationship between fatigue and the disease process with patient and family. *Understanding the nature of the disease and associated fatigue helps the patient and family cope with reduced energy and comply with prescribed rest.*
- Reduce energy demands with frequent, small meals and short periods of activity. Limit the number of visitors and visit length. *Small, frequent meals reduce the energy needed for eating and digestion. Limiting visitors and visit length helps conserve energy. In addition, nurses can assist the fatigued patient who may be reluctant to ask visitors to leave.*

Reduce Risk for Infection. The effects of both the glomerular disorder and treatment with anti-inflammatory and cytotoxic drugs can depress the immune system, increasing the risk for infection. The anti-inflammatory effect of corticosteroids may mask early manifestations of infection.

Expected Outcome: Patient will remain free of infection.

The nurse will:

- Monitor vital signs, temperature, and mental status every 4 hours. *An elevated temperature may indicate infection; anti-inflammatory drugs may moderate this response, however. Tachycardia, increasing lethargy, or confusion may be the initial signs of infection.*
- Assess frequently for signs of infection such as purulent wound drainage, productive cough, adventitious breath sounds, and red or inflamed lesions. Monitor for manifestations of UTI, such as dysuria, frequency and urgency, and cloudy, foul-smelling urine. *Early identification and treatment of infection is important to prevent systemic complications in the susceptible patient.*

- Monitor CBC, focusing on the WBC and differential. *An elevated WBC and increased numbers of immature WBCs in the blood (left shift) may be early indicators of infection.*
- Perform effective hand hygiene. Protect from cross-infection by providing a private room and restricting ill visitors. *Patients with decreased resistance to infection need increased protection.*
- Avoid or minimize invasive procedures. *Maintaining the protective skin barrier is especially important for the patient with altered immune status.*
- If catheterization is required, use sterile intermittent straight catheterization or maintain a closed drainage system for an indwelling catheter. Prevent urine reflux from the drainage system to the bladder or the bladder to the kidneys by ensuring a patent, gravity flow system. *The urinary tract is a frequent entry point for infection, particularly in the hospitalized or institutionalized patient. Maintaining strict asepsis during catheterization is vital. Intermittent catheterization is associated with a lower risk of UTI than an indwelling catheter.*
- Provide a nutritionally sound diet with complete proteins. *A well-balanced, nutritionally sound diet is important to maintain nutritional status and support immune function.*
- Teach measures to prevent infection. *Care is often provided in the home, requiring the patient and family to use appropriate infection control measures.*

Support the Need to Modify Responsibilities. The manifestations and treatment of glomerular disorders can affect the ability to maintain usual roles and activities. Fatigue and muscle weakness may limit physical and social activities. Activity limitations may be ordered to minimize the degree of proteinuria. If azotemia is present, malaise, nausea, and mental status changes can interfere with role function. Facial and periorbital edema affect the patient's self-esteem and may lead to isolation.

Expected Outcome: Patient will acknowledge impact of the disorder and its manifestations on ability to maintain current roles and identify strategies to meet or modify responsibilities.

The nurse will:

- Encourage self-care and active participation in decision making. *Increased autonomy helps restore self-confidence and reduce powerlessness.*
- Provide time for verbalization of thoughts and feelings; listen actively, acknowledging and accepting fears and concerns. *Adequate time and active listening encourage expression of concerns and the effect of the disease or treatments on daily life. This helps the patient deal with the illness, its treatment, and associated losses.*
- Teach coping skills and help the patient identify personal strengths. *This support helps the patient gain confidence.*
- When possible, enlist the support of family, other patients, and friends. *These people can provide physical, psychologic, emotional, and social support.*
- Discuss the effect of the disease and treatments on roles and relationships, helping identify potential changes in roles, relationships, and lifestyle. Help the patient and family develop a plan for alternative behaviors and relationships, encouraging the patient to maintain usual roles to the extent possible. *Developing a plan helps reduce the strain of role changes and maintain a sense of dignity and control.*
- Evaluate the need for additional support and social services for the patient and family. Provide referrals as indicated. *Depending on patient and family strengths, the severity of the disorder, and its treatment and prognosis, ongoing social support services may be necessary to facilitate coping and adaptation.*

Delegating Nursing Care Activities

As appropriate and allowed by the designated duties and responsibilities of unlicensed assistive personnel, the nurse may delegate nursing care activities such as measuring intake and output, obtaining daily weights, assisting with ADLs, and providing for distraction and socialization for the patient with a glomerular disorder.

Transitions of Care

Glomerular disorders may be self-limited or progressive. In either case, the course is lengthy, ranging from months to years. Self-management is essential.

Discuss the importance of effectively treating streptococcal infections in all age groups to help reduce the risk for acute glomerulonephritis. Stress the importance of completing the full course of antibiotic therapy to eradicate the infecting bacteria. Teach patients with diabetes mellitus and SLE about potential renal effects of their disease. Discuss measures to reduce the risk of associated nephritis, such as effectively managing the disease, treating hypertension, and avoiding drugs and substances that are potentially toxic to the kidneys.

Provide instructions for the patient and family who will be providing care at home, including the following topics:

- Information about the disease and the prognosis
- Prescribed treatment, including activity and diet restrictions; the use and potential effects, both beneficial and adverse, of all medications
- Risks, manifestations, prevention, and management of complications such as edema and infection
- Signs, symptoms, and implications of improving or declining renal function
- Measures to prevent further kidney damage, such as nephrotoxic drugs to avoid
- Community resources, such as home care providers and support groups.

Case Study & Nursing Care Plan

A Patient with Acute Glomerulonephritis

Jung-Lin Chang is a 23-year-old graduate student who presents at the university health center with brown and foamy urine. The physician admits him to the infirmary and orders a throat culture, ASO titer, CBC, BUN, serum creatinine, eGFR, and urinalysis.

ASSESSMENT

Connie King, the nurse admitting Mr. Chang, notes that his history is essentially negative for past kidney or urinary problems. He relates having had a "pretty bad" sore throat a couple of weeks before admission, which he self-treated with a few leftover antibiotics. The sore throat resolved, and he felt well until noticing the change in his urine. He has eaten little the past 2 days, but was not alarmed because his food intake is irregular most of the time.

Physical assessment findings include T 37.1°C (98.8°F) PO, P 98 bpm, R 18/min, and BP 136/90 mmHg. Weight 75 kg (165 lb), up from his normal of 72.5 kg (160 lb). Moderate periorbital edema and edema of hands and fingers noted.

Throat culture is negative, but the ASO titer is high. CBC essentially normal. BUN 42 mg/dL, serum creatinine 2.1 mg/dL. Urinalysis reveals the presence of protein, red blood cells, and RBC casts. A subsequent 24-hour urine protein analysis shows 1025 mg of protein (normal 30 to 150 mg/24 h).

The physician diagnoses acute poststreptococcal glomerulonephritis and places Mr. Chang on limited activities, a fluid restriction (1200 mL/day), and a restricted sodium and protein diet.

DIAGNOSES

- Fluid volume imbalance related to loss of plasma protein and retention of sodium and water
- Weight loss related to anorexia
- Lack of knowledge of glomerulonephritis and treatment

EXPECTED OUTCOMES

- Patient will maintain blood pressure within normal limits.
- Patient will return to usual weight with no evidence of edema.
- Patient will consume adequate calories following prescribed dietary limitations.
- Patient will demonstrate an understanding of acute glomerulonephritis and prescribed treatment regimen.

PLANNING AND IMPLEMENTATION

- Take vital signs every 4 hours; notify physician of significant changes.
- Weigh daily; intake and output every 8 hours.
- Assist to develop a plan for consuming allowed fluids throughout the day.
- Arrange dietary consultation to plan a diet that includes preferred foods as allowed.
- Provide small meals with high-carbohydrate between-meal snacks.
- Teach Mr. Chang and his family about acute glomerulonephritis and prescribed treatment.
- Instruct in appropriate antibiotic use.

EVALUATION

Mr. Chang decides to return to his parents' home for the 6 to 12 weeks of convalescence prescribed by his physician. His renal function gradually returns to normal with no further azotemia and minimal proteinuria after 4 months. He verbalizes understanding of the relationship between the strep throat, his inappropriate use of antibiotics, and the glomerulonephritis. He says, "I may not always remember to take every pill on time in the future, but I sure won't save them for the next time again!"

CLINICAL REASONING IN PATIENT CARE

1. How did Mr. Chang's self-treatment with antibiotics from a previous infection potentially contribute to his current situation?
2. In addition to acute glomerulonephritis, what other abnormal immune responses may develop as a consequence of group A beta-hemolytic streptococcal infection?
3. What teaching should the nurse provide to reduce Mr. Chang's risk of future infection-related problems?
4. What additional diagnostic studies would you anticipate should Mr. Chang's symptoms, BUN, serum creatinine, and urinalysis fail to resolve?
5. Identify important nursing responsibilities and patient teaching related to these studies.
6. The initial manifestations of acute poststreptococcal glomerulonephritis and anti-GBM glomerulonephritis are very similar. What diagnostic test would the physician use to make the differential diagnosis? Develop a plan of care for a patient undergoing this examination.

See Evaluating Your Response in Appendix B.

The Patient with a Vascular Kidney Disorder

Renal function is dependent on an adequate supply of blood. Blood supports renal cell metabolism and is vital to kidney function, the nephron in particular. The kidney can regulate fluid, electrolyte, and acid–base balance and serve as a major organ of excretion only when its blood supply is sufficient.

Hypertension

Hypertension, sustained elevation of the systemic blood pressure, can result from or cause kidney disease.

Prolonged hypertension damages the walls of arterioles and accelerates the process of atherosclerosis. This damage primarily affects the heart, brain, kidneys, eyes, and major blood vessels. In the kidney, arteriosclerotic lesions develop in the *afferent* (leading into) and *efferent* (going out of) arterioles and the glomerular capillaries. The glomerular filtration rate declines and tubular function is affected, resulting in proteinuria and microscopic hematuria. In the United States, an estimated 20% of adults with hypertension have chronic kidney disease, and uncontrolled or poorly controlled hypertension is the second leading cause of chronic kidney disease (Inker et al., 2014).

Malignant hypertension is a rapidly progressive form of hypertension that can develop in patients with untreated primary hypertension or in people with no prior history of hypertension. The diastolic pressure is in excess of 120 mmHg and may be as high as 150 to 170 mmHg. Malignant hypertension affects less than 1% of hypertensive patients; it is more common in African Americans than in people of European ancestry. Untreated, malignant hypertension causes a rapid decline in renal function due to vessel changes, renal ischemia, and infarction.

Approximately 5 to 10% of hypertensive patients have *secondary hypertension*, which is actually a manifestation of an underlying disease. Renal vascular disease and diseases of the renal parenchyma, such as diabetic nephropathy, are commonly associated with secondary hypertension.

Management of hypertension to maintain the blood pressure within an optimal range is vital to prevent kidney damage. When hypertension is secondary to kidney disease, adequate blood pressure control can slow the decline in renal function. See Chapter 32 for more information about hypertension and its management.

Renal Artery Stenosis

Renal artery stenosis (RAS), which causes between 1 and 10% of all cases of hypertension, can affect one or both kidneys (Spinowitz, 2017). It is most often caused by atherosclerosis, particularly in older adults. The lumen of the renal artery is gradually occluded by plaque, affecting blood flow to the kidney. Atherosclerotic renovascular disease is more commonly found in people with evidence of coronary heart disease or peripheral vascular disease. In younger women, RAS is usually due to fibromuscular dysplasia, structural abnormalities of the arterial wall.

Renal artery stenosis stimulates the renin–angiotensin system as well as the sympathetic nervous system. Hypertension develops, along with flushing and significant blood pressure variations. Most patients have evidence of chronic kidney disease and significant cardiovascular risk by the time RAS is diagnosed. An epigastric bruit (murmur) and other manifestations of vascular insufficiency may also be present.

Doppler ultrasonography is used to screen for RAS. The affected kidney appears small and atrophied on renal ultrasound. Magnetic resonance angiography (MRA) and computed tomography (CT) angiography with contrast allow visualization of renal blood vessels and are used to diagnose RAS.

Conservative therapy is used for most patients with RAS. ACE inhibitors or ARBs are used along with other antihypertensive drugs to control blood pressure. Statins may be prescribed to slow atherosclerotic plaque deposition, and low-dose aspirin is used to prevent clotting within partially occluded vessels. In some cases, percutaneous transluminal angioplasty is performed to dilate the affected vessel and position a stent to maintain patency. In this procedure, a balloon-tipped catheter is inserted via the femoral artery and aorta to dilate the renal artery. While this procedure is often effective, particularly in fibromuscular dysplasia, it is not without risk, including loss of renal function.

Nursing care of the patient with RAS focuses on collaborating with the interprofessional team to achieve target blood pressures, monitoring renal function, implementing measures to preserve remaining renal function (e.g., ensuring adequate hydration, preventing urinary tract infection, and avoiding nephrotoxic medications), and teaching the patient and family about the prescribed treatment.

Renal Artery Occlusion

Renal arteries can be occluded by either a primary process affecting the renal vessels or by emboli, clots, or other foreign material. Risk factors for acute renal artery thrombosis (formation of a blood clot in the renal artery) include severe abdominal trauma, vessel trauma from surgery or angiography, aortic or renal artery aneurysms, and severe aortic or renal artery atherosclerosis. Emboli from the left side of the heart can travel via the aorta to occlude the renal artery. Emboli may form as a result of atrial fibrillation (irregular and uncoordinated electrical activity of the atria), following myocardial infarction, as vegetative growths on heart valves associated with bacterial endocarditis, or from fatty plaque in the aorta.

Renal arterial occlusion may be asymptomatic when the occlusion develops slowly and the affected vessels are small. Acute occlusion leading to ischemia and infarction typically causes sudden, severe localized flank pain, nausea and vomiting, fever, and hypertension. Hematuria and oliguria may occur. In the older patient, the new onset of hypertension or worsening of previously controlled hypertension may signal renal artery thrombosis.

Laboratory studies reveal leukocytosis (elevated WBC), and elevated renal enzyme levels, including aspartate transaminase (AST) and lactic dehydrogenase (LDH). These enzymes, normally present in renal cells, are released into the circulation when cells necrose and die. With bilateral arterial occlusion and infarction, renal function deteriorates rapidly, leading to acute kidney injury.

Surgery to restore blood flow to the affected kidney may be indicated for acute occlusion. Management is usually more conservative, using anticoagulant therapy, intrarenal fibrinolysis, hypertension control, and supportive treatment.

Renal Vein Occlusion

A thrombus (clot) formed in a renal vein can occlude the vessel. The cause of the thrombus is often unclear. In adults, renal venous thrombosis usually occurs with nephrotic syndrome. Other predisposing factors include pregnancy, oral contraceptive use, and certain malignancies.

Gradual or acute deterioration of renal function may be the only manifestation of renal vein occlusion. If the thrombus breaks loose, it can become a pulmonary embolism. The definitive diagnosis is made by visualizing the thrombus through renal venography.

Fibrinolytic drugs such as streptokinase or tissue plasminogen activator (tPA) may be given to dissolve or break up the thrombus. Anticoagulant therapy is used to prevent further clotting and pulmonary emboli. Renal function often improves with treatment.

The Patient with Kidney Trauma

The kidneys are relatively well protected by the rib cage, back muscles, and abdominal contents, but trauma due to blunt force or penetrating injury may inflict damage. Many renal injuries heal uneventfully, but prompt diagnosis and immediate treatment can be lifesaving in the event of major damage.

Pathophysiology

Blunt force is the most common cause of kidney injury. Falls, motor vehicle crashes, and sports injuries can damage the kidney. Damage may occur from a direct blow, as a result of rapid acceleration/deceleration injury, or a combination. The injury may be minor, causing a contusion or small hematoma, or more serious, resulting in laceration or other damage. The kidney may fragment or "shatter," causing significant blood loss and urine extravasation. Tearing of the renal artery or vein may cause rapid hemorrhage, with shock and possible death.

Gunshot wounds, knife wounds, impalement injuries, and fractured ribs can penetrate the kidney. Minor penetrating injuries may lacerate the capsule or renal cortex. Major injuries include laceration or destruction of renal parenchyma or the vascular supply. Renal artery, renal vein, and renal pelvis lacerations are critical injuries.

Manifestations

The primary manifestations of kidney trauma are hematuria (gross or microscopic), flank or abdominal pain, and oliguria or anuria. There may be localized swelling, tenderness, or ecchymoses in the flank region. Retroperitoneal bleeding from the kidney may cause Turner's sign, a bluish discoloration of the flank. Signs of shock may be present, including hypotension, tachycardia, tachypnea, cool and pale skin, and an altered level of consciousness.

Interprofessional Care

Diagnosis

Hemoglobin and hematocrit levels fall in significant renal injury with hemorrhage. Hematuria is typically noted on urinalysis. AST levels rise within 12 hours of significant renal trauma. Renal ultrasonography is used to diagnose bleeding and kidney damage. A CT scan with contrast may be performed to visualize renal structures and establish a definitive diagnosis.

Treatment

Treatment of minor kidney injuries is generally conservative, including bedrest and observation. In these injuries, bleeding is typically minor and self-limiting. With major or critical trauma, immediate treatment focuses on controlling hemorrhage and treating or preventing shock. Surgery may be required to stop the bleeding. Major lacerations may require surgical repair or partial or total **nephrectomy** (removal) of the damaged kidney (Lusaya, 2017).

Nursing Care

Nursing care for the patient who has experienced renal trauma focuses on timely and accurate assessment, close observation, and appropriate intervention to preserve life and prevent complications (Lusaya, 2017). Obtain a urine specimen for analysis when kidney trauma is suspected. Monitor level of consciousness, vital signs, skin color and temperature, and urine output for possible signs of shock.

Transitions of Care

Prevention focuses on trauma and sports injury prevention. Using seat belts in vehicles and appropriate safety equipment when playing sports is important. Acute care often takes place in emergency departments followed by surgery or observation. Home care following discharge includes assessment and management of convalescence from injuries.

The Patient with a Renal Tumor

Renal tumors may be benign or malignant, primary or metastatic. Benign renal tumors are infrequent and are often found only on autopsy. Primary renal malignancies account for about 4% of adult cancers and approximately 10,010 deaths per year (American Cancer Society [ACS], 2018). Most primary renal tumors arise from renal cells; a primary tumor may develop in the renal pelvis, although less frequently. Wilms tumor is kidney cancer of childhood, accounting for about 4% of childhood cancers (ACS, 2018). Metastatic lesions to the kidney are associated with lung and breast cancer, melanoma, and malignant lymphoma.

Renal tumors may present with hematuria, flank pain, and a palpable abdominal mass. Less specific signs include fever, fatigue, weight loss, and/or anemia.

Pathophysiology

Most (92%) primary renal tumors are renal cell carcinomas (ACS, 2018). These tumors arise from tubular epithelium and can occur anywhere in the kidney. The tumor, which can range in size up to several centimeters, has clearly defined margins and contains areas of ischemia, necrosis, and hemorrhage. Renal tumors tend to invade the renal vein and often have metastasized when first identified. Metastases tend to occur in the lungs, bone, lymph nodes, liver, and brain.

Risk Factors

Males are affected by renal cancer more than females by a 2:1 ratio. The highest incidence is seen in people over the age of 55. Smoking and obesity are risk factors, as are hypertension and occupational exposure to certain chemicals. Some renal cancers are associated with genetic factors. Patients with ESRD may also develop renal cancer.

Manifestations

Renal tumors are often silent, with few manifestations. The classic triad of symptoms—gross hematuria, flank pain, and a palpable abdominal mass—is seen in only about 10% of people with renal cell carcinoma. Hematuria, often microscopic, is the most consistent symptom. Systemic manifestations include fever without infection, fatigue, and weight loss.

The tumor may produce hormones or hormone-like substances, including parathyroid hormone, prostaglandins, prolactin, renin, gonadotropins, and glucocorticoids. These substances produce *paraneoplastic syndromes*, with additional manifestations such as hypercalcemia, hypertension, and hyperglycemia. The progression of renal cell carcinomas varies from prolonged periods of stable disease to very aggressive. **Table 28.3** outlines the staging and prognosis for renal cell cancers.

Interprofessional Care

Diagnosis

Hematuria is often the only initial manifestation of renal cancer; its presence indicates a need for further diagnostic studies, including:

- *Renal ultrasonography* to detect renal masses and differentiate cystic kidney disease from renal carcinoma.
- *CT scan* of the abdomen and pelvis to determine tumor density, local extension of the tumor, and regional lymph node or vascular involvement (**Figure 28.3** ■).
- *Chest x-ray, bone scan, MRI,* and *liver function studies* to identify potential metastases.

Table 28.3 Renal Cell Cancer Staging

Stage	Extent of Tumor
I	Confined to the kidney capsule
II	Invasion through the capsule but confined to local fascia
III	Regional lymph node, ipsilateral renal vein, or inferior vena cava involvement
IV	Locally invasive or distant metastases

Source: Adapted from ACS, 2018.

Medications

No chemotherapy drug consistently causes tumor regression in patients with advanced renal carcinoma. Sunitinib (Sutent), sorafenib (Nexavar), and pazopanib (Votrient) are orally administered antiangiogenesis agents (drugs that inhibit new blood vessel formation) used as first-line treatment for advanced renal cancer. Interferon-α and interleukin-2 have led to prolonged remission in a small proportion of patients and may be used. Targeted therapy with monoclonal antibodies may be used, but is associated with significant adverse effects (Shields, Fox, & Liebrecht, 2018).

Surgery

Surgical intervention may be a component of the treatment plan for the patient with a renal tumor. *Radical nephrectomy* is the treatment of choice for stage I or II kidney tumors. In a radical nephrectomy, the adrenal gland, upper ureter, fat and fascia surrounding the kidney, and the entire kidney are removed. Regional lymph nodes may also be resected. Although nephrectomy can be done using a laparoscopic approach, laparotomy is primarily used for radical nephrectomy. See **Box 28.1** for nursing care of the patient having a nephrectomy.

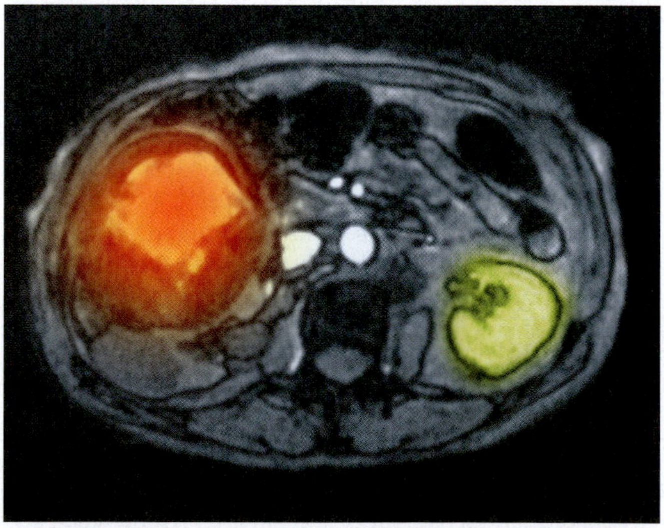

Figure 28.3 ■ CT scan of the abdomen shows a tumor of the right kidney (shown in red). Note that CT scans are read looking up from the feet; so the red kidney on the left of the image is the patient's right kidney. The tumor distorts the shape of the right kidney (shown in red) compared with the health kidney (shown in green).

BOX 28.1
Nursing Care of the Patient Having a Nephrectomy

PREOPERATIVE CARE

- Provide routine preoperative care.
- Report abnormal laboratory values to the surgeon. *Bacteriuria, blood coagulation abnormalities, or other significant abnormal values may affect surgery and postoperative care.*
- Discuss operative and postoperative expectations as indicated, including the location of the incision (refer to Figure 28.4) and anticipated tubes, stents, and drains. *Preoperative teaching about postoperative expectations reduces anxiety for the patient and family during the early postoperative period.*

POSTOPERATIVE CARE

- Provide routine postoperative care.
- Frequently assess urine color, amount, and character, noting any hematuria, pyuria, or sediment. Promptly report oliguria or anuria, as well as changes in urine color or clarity. *Preserving function of the remaining kidney is critical; frequent assessment allows early intervention for potential problems.*
- Note the placement, status, and drainage from ureteral catheters, stents, nephrostomy tubes, or drains. Label each clearly. Maintain gravity drainage; irrigate only as ordered. *Maintaining drainage tube patency is vital to prevent potential hydronephrosis. Bright bleeding or unexpected drainage may indicate a surgical complication.*
- Support the grieving process and adjustment to the loss of a kidney. *Loss of a major organ leads to a body image change and grief response. When renal cancer is the underlying diagnosis, the patient may also grieve the loss of health and potential loss of life.*
- Provide the following home care instructions for the patient and family:
  a. The importance of protecting the remaining kidney by preventing UTI, renal calculi, and trauma. See Chapter 27 for measures to prevent UTI and calculi. *Damage to the remaining kidney by UTI, renal calculi, or trauma can lead to renal failure.*
  b. Maintain a fluid intake of 2000 to 2500 mL/day. *This important measure helps prevent dehydration and maintain good urine flow.*
  c. Gradually increase exercise to tolerance, avoiding heavy lifting for a year after surgery. Participation in contact sports is not recommended to reduce the risk of injury to the remaining kidney. *Lifting is avoided to allow full tissue healing. Trauma to the remaining kidney could seriously jeopardize renal function.*
  d. Care of the incision and any remaining drainage tubes, catheters, or stents. *This routine postoperative instruction is vital to prepare the patient for self-care and prevent complications.*
  e. Report unexpected signs and symptoms to the physician, including manifestations of UTI (dysuria, frequency, urgency, nocturia, or cloudy, malodorous urine) or systemic infection (fever, general malaise, or fatigue), redness, swelling, pain, or drainage from the incision or any catheter or drain tube site. *Prompt treatment of postoperative infection is vital to allow continued healing and prevent compromise of the remaining kidney.*

Nursing Care

Assessment

Nursing assessment includes focused assessment of renal function and determination of tumor type, size, and location. If surgery is planned, a detailed preoperative assessment is indicated.

Diagnoses, Outcomes, and Interventions

Nursing care for the patient with renal cancer focuses on needs related to the cancer diagnosis and to the surgical intervention. Postoperative pain may be significant and the risk for respiratory complications is high. The remaining kidney must be protected from damage to preserve renal function. Psychologically, the patient may grieve the loss of a major organ and the diagnosis of cancer.

Relieve Surgical Pain. The size and location of the incision used for a radical nephrectomy (**Figure 28.4** ■) make pain management a challenge. Intercostal blocks, patient-controlled analgesia (PCA), or routine analgesic administration can effectively relieve the discomfort. Nursing care focuses on assessing pain relief, providing supportive measures to enhance analgesia, and ensuring that pain or the fear of pain does not lead to respiratory complications.

Expected Outcome: Patient will report and manage pain within an acceptable range.

The nurse will:

- Assess frequently for adequate pain relief. Use a standard pain scale and nonverbal signs such as grimacing, tense body position, apparent dozing, elevated pulse, change of blood pressure, or rapid, shallow respirations. Notify the physician of inadequate pain relief. *The patient may assume that pain is to be expected or may fear becoming addicted to analgesics. Careful questioning and assessment allow effective pain management. Responses to analgesics are individual, and the prescribed dose may need to be adjusted.*
- Assess the incision for inflammation or swelling and drainage catheters and tubes for patency. *An obstructed catheter can lead to hydronephrosis, hematoma, or abscess, increasing incisional pain.*
- Assess for abdominal distention, tenderness, and bowel sounds. *Intra-abdominal bleeding, peritonitis, or paralytic ileus can cause pain that may be confused with incisional pain.*
- Use adjunctive pain relief measures such as positioning, diversional activities, management of environmental stimuli, guided imagery, and relaxation techniques. *These can enhance the effects of analgesia.*

Reduce Risk of Breathing Pattern that Increases Risk for Postoperative Respiratory Complications. The location of the incision combined with the respiratory depressant effects of narcotic analgesics increases the risk

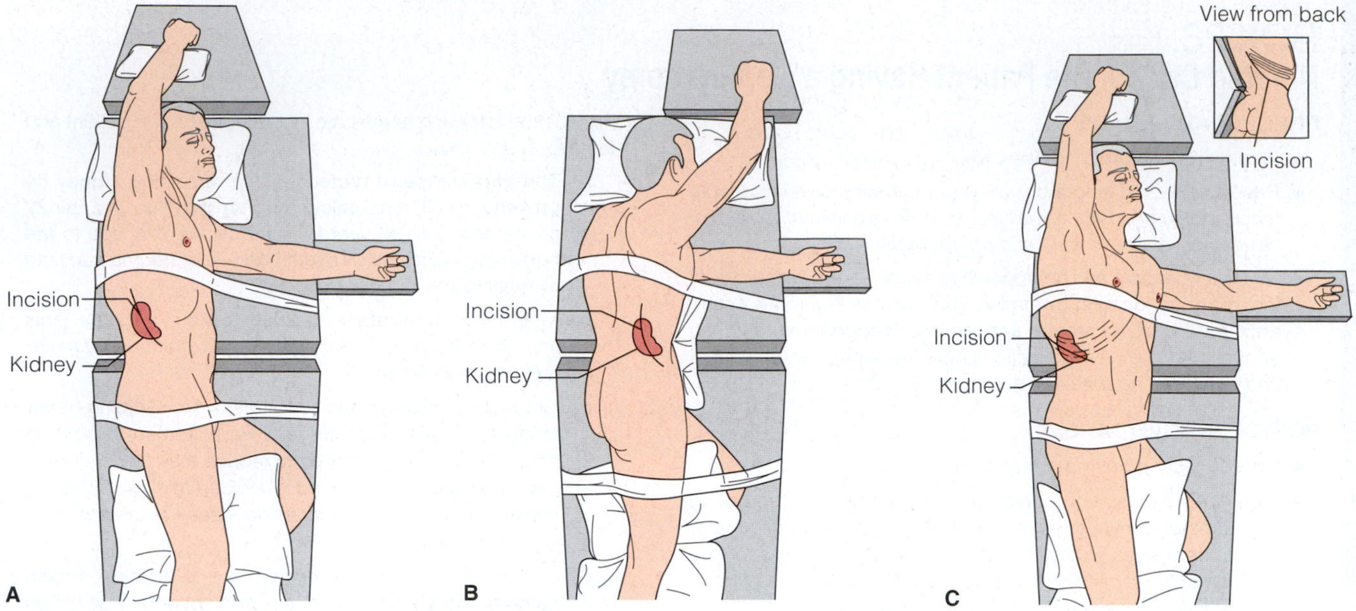
View from back
Incision
Incision
Kidney
A
Incision
Kidney
B
Incision
Kidney
C

Figure 28.4 ■ Incisions used for kidney surgery. **A**, Flank. **B**, Lumbar. **C**, Thoracoabdominal.

for respiratory complications in the patient who has had a nephrectomy.

Expected Outcome: Patient will maintain open airways and effective ventilation.

The nurse will:

- Position to promote respiratory excursion, using semi-Fowler position and sidelying positions as allowed and tolerated. *Lung expansion is improved in semi-Fowler and Fowler positions.*
- Change position frequently; ambulate as soon as possible. *These measures promote lung expansion and the movement of mucus out of airways.*
- Encourage frequent (every 1 to 2 hours) deep breathing, spirometer use, and coughing. Assist to splint the incision. *These measures promote alveolar ventilation, gas exchange, and airway clearance.*

SAFETY ALERT: Pneumothorax on the operative side is common. Assess respiratory status frequently, including rate and depth, cough, breath sounds, oxygen saturation, and temperature. Early identification and intervention can prevent major respiratory complications. ■

Maintain Fluid Balance. Surgery involving the urinary tract increases the risk for altered renal function and urine elimination. In addition, removal of one kidney dictates extra caution to maintain renal circulation, a sterile urinary tract, and free urine flow.

Expected Outcome: Patient's urinary output and fluid balance will remain within normal ranges without evidence of infection or compromised renal function.

The nurse will:

- Monitor vital signs, central venous pressure (CVP), and urine output every 1 to 2 hours initially, then every 4 hours. *Hypovolemia due to hemorrhage, diuresis, or fluid sequestering (third spacing) reduces blood flow to the kidney and increases the risk of renal ischemia with possible acute tubular necrosis and acute kidney injury.*
- Frequently assess the amount and nature of drainage on surgical dressings and from drainage tubes, stents, and catheters. Measure and record output from each drain or catheter separately. *Frequent and accurate assessment of drainage helps to identify excess bleeding, abnormal fluid loss, infection, or other potential surgical complications.*
- Maintain fluid intake with intravenous fluids until oral intake is resumed. Encourage an intake of 2000 to 2500 mL/day as soon as the patient tolerates oral liquids. *A liberal fluid intake prevents dehydration, helps to dilute any nephrotoxic substances, and promotes good urinary output.*
- Use strict aseptic technique in caring for all urinary catheters, tubes, stents, drains, and incisions. *Asepsis is vital to prevent infection and possible compromise of the remaining kidney.*
- Following catheter removal, assess frequently for urinary retention. Notify the physician if the patient is unable to void within 4 to 6 hours or if manifestations of retention (distended bladder, discomfort, urinary dribbling) develop. *Maintenance of urine output is vital to prevent stasis and possible complications such as infection and hydronephrosis.*
- Monitor laboratory results, including urinalysis, BUN, serum creatinine, and serum electrolytes. Report abnormal findings to the physician. *Abnormal values may indicate early acute renal failure; prompt intervention is necessary to preserve renal function.*

SAFETY ALERT: Prevent kinking, twisting, or tension on drains and tubes. Do not clamp. Irrigate carefully and only with a physician's order. Notify the physician immediately if any tube becomes dislodged. It is vital to maintain the patency of drains, particularly any affecting the remaining kidney, to prevent the excess pressure of hydronephrosis. ■

Support Grieving Patient and Family. The patient having a radical nephrectomy for renal cancer not only loses a major organ but also has to adjust to the diagnosis of cancer. Although the prognosis for recovery may be good, many people perceive cancer as always fatal. Providing support for the patient and family during the initial stages of grieving can improve physical recovery, psychologic coping, and eventual adaptation.

Expected Outcome: Patient will verbalize thoughts, feelings, fears, and concerns about loss.

The nurse will:

- Work to develop a trusting relationship with the patient and family members. *Trust increases the nurse's effectiveness in helping them work through the process of grieving.*
- Listen actively, encouraging the patient and family to express fears and concerns. *As they begin to express their concerns, patient and family members can begin to deal more effectively with them.*
- Assist the patient and family members to identify strengths, past experiences, and support systems. *These resources can be employed when working through the grieving process.*
- Demonstrate respect for cultural, spiritual, and religious values and beliefs; encourage use of these resources to cope with losses. *Value and belief systems can provide a structure and form for dealing with the grieving process.*
- Encourage discussion of the potential impact of loss on the patient and the family structure and function. Assist family members to share concerns with one another. *Sharing of fears and concerns among family members promotes involvement and support of the entire family unit so that the individual is not left to cope alone.*
- Refer to cancer support groups, social services, or counseling as appropriate. *Support groups and counseling services provide additional resources for coping.*

Delegating Nursing Care Activities

As appropriate and allowed by the designated duties and responsibilities of unlicensed assistive personnel, the nurse may delegate nursing care activities such as measuring intake and output, obtaining vital signs, encouraging use of an incentive spirometer, and assisting with ambulation and ADLs for the patient with renal cancer.

Transitions of Care

If renal cancer was detected at an early stage and cure is anticipated, teaching for home care focuses on protecting the remaining kidney. Acute nursing care of the patient undergoing a nephrectomy focuses on close postoperative supervision, pain management, and urinary elimination. Most patients will have an indwelling urinary catheter in the early postoperative period. See Chapter 27 for indwelling catheter management information.

Teaching for home care should include the following measures to prevent infection, renal calculi, hydronephrosis, and trauma:

- Maintain a fluid intake of 2000 to 2500 mL/day, increasing the amount during hot weather or strenuous exercise.
- Urinate when the urge is perceived and before and after sexual intercourse.
- Properly clean the perineal area.
- Watch for manifestations of UTI and understand the importance of early and appropriate evaluation and intervention.
- If the patient is an older adult male, he should watch for manifestations of prostatic hypertrophy, a major cause of urinary tract obstruction. Stress the importance of routine screening examinations.
- Avoid contact sports such as football or hockey; use measures to prevent motor vehicle crashes and falls, which could damage the remaining kidney.

28.2 Kidney Failure

Kidney failure is a condition in which the kidneys are unable to effectively remove accumulated metabolites from the blood, leading to altered fluid, electrolyte, and acid–base balance. The cause may be a primary kidney disorder or it may occur secondary to a systemic disease or other urologic defects. The onset of kidney failure may be either acute or chronic. Acute kidney injury has an abrupt onset and with prompt intervention is often reversible. *Chronic kidney disease (CKD)*, which may culminate in kidney failure, develops slowly and insidiously, often producing few symptoms until the kidneys are severely damaged and unable to meet the excretory needs of the body. Acute kidney injury and the final stages of chronic kidney disease are characterized by azotemia, increased levels of nitrogenous wastes in the blood. Kidney failure is also called *end-stage renal disease (ESRD)*. ESRD is irreversible and requires renal replacement (transplant or dialysis). Kidney failure is common and costly. In 2016, more than 468,000 patients with ESRD were being treated with dialysis and approximately 193,000 had a functioning kidney transplant. The annual cost of ESRD treatment (in 2013 dollars) is over $50 billion. The cost is also measured in lives and lifestyle. The 5-year survival rate for patients undergoing dialysis is 35%. Although many patients report satisfaction with their quality of life, patients on dialysis are often unable to work, and the family structure may disintegrate under the strain of treatment. Kidney transplant improves both survival (84.6% at 5 years) and quality of life (NIDDK, 2016).

The Patient with Acute Kidney Injury

Acute kidney injury (AKI), previously known as *acute renal failure (ARF)*, is a rapid decline in renal function with azotemia and fluid and electrolyte imbalances. Serum creatinine and/or BUN values significantly increase over hours to days in AKI, and the urine output often falls (Sorenson et al., 2019). The most common causes of acute kidney injury are ischemia, sepsis, and nephrotoxins. The kidney is particularly vulnerable because of the amount of blood that passes through it. A fall in blood pressure or volume can cause ischemia of kidney tissues. Sepsis also produces hemodynamic effects with generalized vasodilation and a fall in GFR. Nephrotoxins in the blood damage renal tissue directly.

Pathophysiology

The functional unit of the kidneys, the nephron, produces urine through three processes: Glomerular filtration, tubular reabsorption, and tubular secretion. In the glomerulus, a filtrate of water and small solutes is formed. The solute concentration of this filtrate is equal to that of plasma, with the exception of large molecules such as plasma proteins and blood cells. The GFR, the amount of filtrate formed per minute, is affected by blood volume and pressure, the autonomic nervous system, and other factors. From the glomerulus, the filtrate flows into the tubules, where the processes of tubular reabsorption and tubular secretion change its composition. Most water and many filtered solutes such as electrolytes and glucose are reabsorbed. Metabolic waste products such as urea, hydrogen ion, ammonia, and some creatinine are secreted into the tubule for elimination. By the time urine exits the collecting duct into the renal pelvis, 99% of the filtrate has been reabsorbed.

The causes and pathophysiology of acute kidney injury are commonly categorized as prerenal, intrinsic kidney injury, and postrenal obstruction (**Figure 28.5** ■). Prerenal AKI is the most common, accounting for about 21% of the total. In *prerenal AKI*, hypoperfusion and ischemia lead to an acute increase in serum creatinine or BUN without directly affecting the integrity of kidney tissues. *Intrinsic AKI*, due to direct damage to functional kidney tissue, is responsible for another 40%. Urinary tract obstruction with resulting kidney damage is the precipitating factor for *postrenal AKI*, the least common form (10%). Intrinsic AKI accounts for 69% of total acute kidney injuries and serves as the diagnosis when prerenal and postrenal AKI are ruled out (NIDDK, 2016). **Table 28.4** summarizes the causes of acute kidney injury. See also Pathophysiology Illustrated: Acute Kidney Injury on page 71.

Prerenal AKI

Prerenal AKI results from conditions that affect renal blood flow and perfusion. Any disorder that significantly decreases vascular volume, cardiac output, or systemic vascular resistance can affect renal blood flow. The kidneys normally receive 20 to 25% of the cardiac output to maintain the GFR. A drop in renal blood flow to less than 20% of normal causes the GFR to fall. As the filtration of substances by the glomeruli is reduced, less reabsorption of substances in the tubule is required. As a result, kidney cells require less energy and oxygen and their metabolism slows. Prerenal AKI is rapidly reversed when blood flow is restored and the renal parenchyma remains undamaged. Continued ischemia can lead to tubular cell necrosis and significant nephron damage. Intrinsic AKI due to ischemic injury may result.

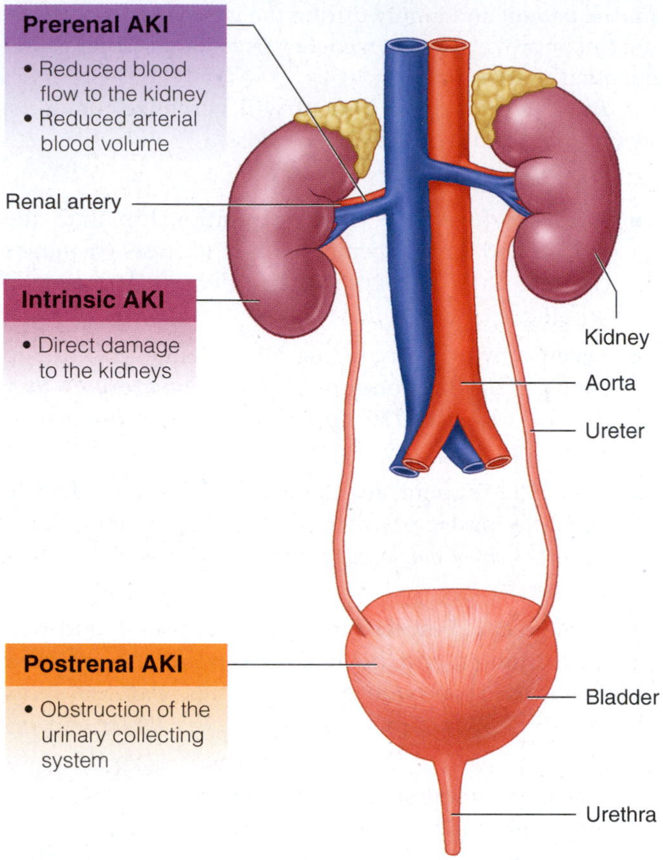
Prerenal AKI
• Reduced blood flow to the kidney
• Reduced arterial blood volume
Renal artery
Intrinsic AKI
• Direct damage to the kidneys
Postrenal AKI
• Obstruction of the urinary collecting system
Kidney
Aorta
Ureter
Bladder
Urethra

Figure 28.5 ■ AKI is classified into prerenal, intrinsic, and postrenal causes. Renal causes of AKI should be considered under the different anatomic components of the kidney (vascular supply; glomerular, tubular, and interstitial disease).

Table 28.4 Causes of Acute Kidney Injury

Cause	Examples
Prerenal	
Hypovolemia	Hemorrhage, dehydration, excess fluid loss from GI tract, burns, wounds
Low cardiac output	Heart failure, cardiogenic shock
Altered vascular resistance	Sepsis, anaphylaxis, vasoactive drugs
Intrarenal	
Glomerular/microvascular injury	Glomerulonephritis, disseminated intravascular coagulation (DIC), vasculitis, hypertension, toxemia of pregnancy, hemolytic uremic syndrome
Acute tubular necrosis	Ischemia due to conditions associated with prerenal AKI; toxins such as drugs, heavy metals; hemolysis, rhabdomyolysis (muscle cell breakdown)
Interstitial nephritis	Nephrotoxic drugs, infectious diseases, immunologic disorders, idiopathic
Postrenal	
Ureteral obstruction	Calculi, cancer, external compression
Urethral obstruction	Prostatic enlargement, calculi, cancer, stricture, blood clot

Pathophysiology Illustrated

Acute Kidney Injury

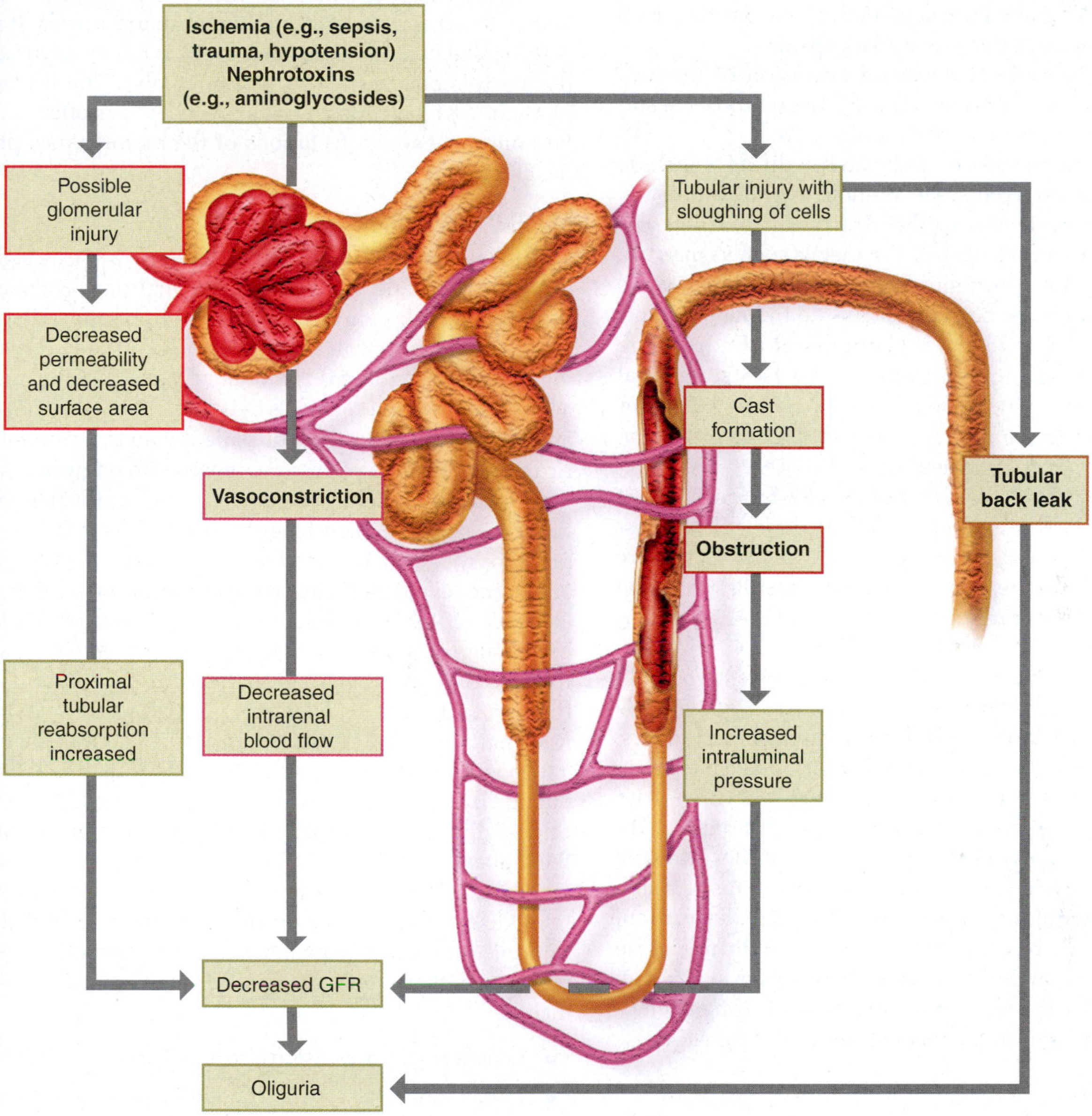
Ischemia (e.g., sepsis, trauma, hypotension) Nephrotoxins (e.g., aminoglycosides)
Possible glomerular injury
Decreased permeability and decreased surface area
Proximal tubular reabsorption increased
Vasoconstriction
Decreased intrarenal blood flow
Tubular injury with sloughing of cells
Cast formation
Obstruction
Increased intraluminal pressure
Tubular back leak
Decreased GFR
Oliguria

Postrenal AKI

Obstructive causes of acute renal failure are classified as postrenal. Any condition that prevents urine excretion can lead to postrenal AKI. Benign prostatic hypertrophy is the most common precipitating factor. Others include renal or urinary tract calculi and tumors. See Chapter 27 for more information about kidney stones.

Intrinsic AKI

Intrinsic acute kidney injury is characterized by acute damage to the renal parenchyma and nephrons. Sepsis, ischemia, and nephrotoxins are the most common causes of intrinsic AKI. Less commonly, infectious diseases or immunologic disorders can cause intrinsic AKI. In acute glomerulonephritis, glomerular inflammation can reduce renal blood flow and cause AKI.

Nephrons are especially susceptible to injury from ischemia or exposure to nephrotoxins. **Acute tubular necrosis (ATN)**, destruction of tubular epithelial cells, causes an abrupt and progressive decline of renal function. Prolonged ischemia is the primary cause of ATN. When ischemia and nephrotoxin exposure occur concurrently, the risk for ATN and tubular dysfunction is especially high. Risk factors for ischemic ATN include major surgery, severe hypovolemia, sepsis, trauma, and burns. The impact of ischemia resulting from vasodilation and fluid loss in sepsis, trauma, and burns is often compounded by toxins released by bacteria or from damaged tissue.

Ischemia lasting more than 2 hours causes severe and irreversible damage to kidney tubules with patchy cellular necrosis and sloughing. The GFR is significantly reduced as a result of (1) ischemia, (2) activation of the renin–angiotensin system, and (3) tubular obstruction by cellular debris, which raises the pressure in the glomerular capsule.

Sepsis affects blood flow and perfusion of the kidneys. Furthermore, sepsis may cause interstitial edema and inflammatory damage to renal tubular cells.

Common nephrotoxins associated with ATN include radiologic contrast agents, the aminoglycoside antibiotics, and amphotericin B. Many other drugs (e.g., NSAIDs and some chemotherapy drugs), heavy metals such as mercury and gold, and some common chemicals such as ethylene glycol (antifreeze) are potentially toxic to the renal tubule. The risk for ATN is higher when nephrotoxic drugs are given to older patients or patients with preexisting renal insufficiency and when used in combination with other nephrotoxins. Dehydration increases the risk by increasing the toxin concentration in nephrons.

Nephrotoxins destroy tubular cells by both direct and indirect effects. As tubular cells are damaged and lost through necrosis and sloughing, the tubule becomes more permeable. This increased permeability results in filtrate reabsorption, further reducing the ability of the nephron to eliminate wastes.

Rhabdomyolysis caused by release of excess myoglobin from injured skeletal muscles can cause ATN. Myoglobin is a protein that acts as the oxygen reservoir for muscle fibers, much as hemoglobin does for the blood. Muscle trauma, strenuous exercise, hyperthermia or hypothermia, drug overdose, infection, and other factors can precipitate rhabdomyolysis. The myoglobin clogs renal tubules, causing ischemic injury, and contains an iron pigment that directly damages the tubules. *Hemolysis*, red blood cell destruction, releases hemoglobin into the circulation with much the same effect as rhabdomyolysis. In tumor lysis syndrome, uric acid released from tumor cells destroyed by chemotherapy precipitates in the renal tubules, causing AKI.

Risk Factors

The mortality rate for AKI in seriously ill patients is as high as 62% (Doyle & Forni, 2016). This high death rate is probably more related to the populations affected by AKI—older patients and the critically ill—than to the disorder itself (Sorenson et al., 2019).

Major trauma or surgery, infection and sepsis, hemorrhage, severe heart failure, severe liver disease, and urinary tract obstruction are risk factors for AKI. Drugs and radiologic contrast media that are toxic to the kidney (*nephrotoxic*) also increase the risk for AKI. Older adults develop AKI more frequently due to their higher incidence of serious illness, major surgeries, and treatment with nephrotoxic drugs. The older adult may also have some degree of preexisting renal insufficiency associated with aging.

Manifestations

The course of acute kidney injury due to ATN typically includes three phases: Initiation, maintenance, and recovery.

Initiation Phase

The initiation phase may last hours to days and may be seen as a continuum from prerenal azotemia to intrinsic AKI (NIDDK, 2016). It begins with the initiating event (e.g., hemorrhage) and ends when tubular injury occurs. If AKI is recognized and the initiating event is effectively treated during this phase, the prognosis is good. The initiation phase of AKI has few symptoms; in fact, it is often identified only when manifestations of the maintenance phase develop.

Maintenance Phase

The maintenance phase of AKI is characterized by a significant fall in GFR and tubular necrosis. Oliguria may develop, and the kidney cannot efficiently eliminate metabolic wastes, water, electrolytes, and acids from the body during this phase. Azotemia, fluid retention, electrolyte imbalances, and metabolic acidosis develop. These abnormalities are more severe in the oliguric patient than in the nonoliguric one, leading to a poorer prognosis with oliguria.

During the maintenance phase, salt and water retention cause edema, increasing the risk for heart failure and pulmonary edema. Retained fluid can result in lower serum creatinine levels, delaying recognition of worsening AKI (NIDDK, 2016). Impaired potassium excretion leads to hyperkalemia. When the serum potassium level is greater than 6.0 to 6.5 mEq/L, manifestations of its effect on neuromuscular function develop. These include muscle weakness, nausea and diarrhea, electrocardiographic changes, and possible cardiac arrest. Other electrolyte imbalances include hyperphosphatemia and hypocalcemia. Metabolic acidosis results from impaired hydrogen ion elimination by the kidneys.

Erythropoietin secretion by the kidneys is suppressed in AKI, causing anemia to develop after several days. Immune function may be impaired, increasing the risk for infection. Other manifestations of the maintenance phase include:

- Edema and hypertension due to salt and water retention
- Confusion, disorientation, agitation or lethargy, hyperreflexia, and possible seizures or coma due to azotemia and electrolyte and acid–base imbalances
- Anorexia, nausea and vomiting, and decreased or absent bowel sounds
- Uremic syndrome if AKI is prolonged (see the section on chronic kidney disease later in this chapter).

Recovery Phase

The recovery phase of ATN is characterized by a process of tubule cell repair and regeneration and gradual return of the GFR to normal or pre-AKI levels. Diuresis may occur as the nephrons and GFR recover and retained salt, water, and solutes are excreted. Serum creatinine, BUN, potassium, and phosphate levels remain high and may continue to rise in spite of increasing urine output. Renal function improves rapidly during the first 5 to 25 days of the recovery phase and continues to improve for up to 1 year.

Complications

Although mild AKI may be asymptomatic, AKI can have significant effects on the kidneys' excretory and regulatory functions. Uremia, accumulation of toxic waste products in the body, affects multiple organs and body functions, including mental status. Uremia is discussed in depth in a later section on chronic kidney disease. Fluid, electrolyte, and acid–base balance are disrupted, with initial hypervolemia, hyperkalemia, and metabolic acidosis. Hypovolemia may develop during the diuretic phase of AKI. Other potential complications include infections, bleeding, cardiac complications (such as dysrhythmias and pericarditis), and malnutrition (Doyle & Forni, 2016).

Interprofessional Care

Preventing acute kidney injury is a goal in caring for all patients, especially those in high-risk groups. Maintaining an adequate vascular volume, cardiac output, and blood pressure is vital to preserve kidney perfusion. Nephrotoxic drugs are avoided whenever possible. When a nephrotoxic drug or substance must be used, the risk of AKI can be reduced by using the minimum effective dose, maintaining hydration, and eliminating other known nephrotoxins from the medication regimen.

Treatment goals for acute kidney injury are to (1) identify and correct the underlying cause, (2) prevent additional kidney damage, (3) restore the urine output and kidney function, and (4) compensate for renal impairment until kidney function is restored.

Staging

Staging is used to guide treatment decisions for patients with AKI. Two systems are currently in use for staging AKI: The RIFLE and AKIN criteria (Inker et al., 2014; Kidney Disease: Improving Global Outcomes [KDIGO] Acute Kidney Injury Work Group, 2012). Both systems use serum creatinine and urine output to determine the severity of AKI; the GFR may be used to determine the RIFLE class (**Table 28.5**).

Diagnosis

Diagnostic tests are used to identify the cause of acute kidney injury and monitor its effects on homeostasis:

- ***Urinalysis*** often shows the following abnormal findings in acute kidney injury:
  a. A fixed specific gravity of 1.010 (equal to the specific gravity of plasma) because the tubules are unable to concentrate the filtrate
  b. Proteinuria, which may be significant if glomerular damage is the cause of AKI
  c. The presence of RBCs (due to glomerular dysfunction), WBCs (related to inflammation), and renal tubular epithelial cells (indicating ATN)
  d. Cell casts, which are protein and cellular debris molded in the shape of the tubular lumen. In AKI, red and white blood cells and renal tubular epithelial casts may be present. Brownish pigmented casts and positive tests for occult blood indicate hemoglobinuria or myoglobinuria.
- ***Serum creatinine, BUN, BUN/creatinine ratio,*** and ***eGFR*** are used to evaluate renal function. In AKI, serum creatinine levels increase rapidly, within 24 to 48 hours of the onset. The BUN/creatinine ratio is reduced, and the eGFR falls in AKI. Creatinine levels generally peak within 5 to 10 days. Creatinine and BUN levels tend to increase more slowly when urine output is maintained. The onset of recovery is marked by a halt in the rise of the serum creatinine and BUN.
- ***Serum electrolytes*** are monitored to evaluate the fluid and electrolyte status. The serum potassium rises at a moderate rate and is often used to indicate the need for dialysis. Hyponatremia is common, due to the water excess associated with AKI.
- ***Arterial blood gases*** often show a metabolic acidosis due to the kidneys' inability to adequately eliminate metabolic wastes and hydrogen ions.
- ***CBC*** shows reduced RBCs, moderate anemia, and a low hematocrit. AKI affects erythropoietin secretion and RBC production. Iron and folate absorption may also be impaired, further contributing to anemia.

Laboratory findings associated with kidney disease are summarized in Table 28.1 earlier in this chapter.

- ***Renal ultrasonography*** is used to identify obstructive causes of renal failure and to differentiate acute kidney injury from end-stage chronic kidney disease. In AKI, the kidneys may be enlarged, whereas they typically appear small and shrunken in chronic kidney disease.
- ***CT scan*** or ***MRI*** may be done to evaluate kidney size and identify possible obstructions.
- ***Kidney biopsy*** may be necessary to differentiate between AKI and chronic renal failure.

Table 28.5 Acute Kidney Injury Staging Criteria

AKIN Stage	RIFLE Class	Serum Creatinine	Urine Output
Stage 1	Risk	Increased 1.5 × (150%) from baseline	Less than 0.5 mL/kg/h for more than 6 h
Stage 2	Injury	Increased 2 × (200%) from baseline	Less than 0.5 mL/kg/h for more than 12 h
Stage 3	Failure	Increased 3 × (300%) from baseline	Less than 0.3 mL/kg/h for 24 h or anuria for 12 h
	Loss		Persistent acute renal failure: Complete loss of kidney function for more than 4 weeks
	End-stage kidney disease		Complete loss of kidney function for more than 3 months

Source: Adapted from Inker et al., 2014; KDIGO, 2012.

Medications

The primary focus in drug management for acute kidney injury is to restore and maintain renal perfusion and to eliminate drugs that are nephrotoxic from the treatment regimen.

Intravenous fluids and blood volume expanders are given as needed to restore renal perfusion. Dopamine (Intropin) may be administered in low doses by intravenous infusion, to increase renal blood flow. Alternately, norepinephrine (Levarterenol, Noradrenaline), a vasopressor and cardiac inotrope, may be used. Fenoldopam (Corlopam), a rapid-acting vasodilator that increases renal blood flow, may be used to prevent AKI in critically ill patients (Doyle & Forni, 2016). Atrial natriuretic peptide (ANP) in low doses has been shown to reduce the need for dialysis and shorten the length of hospitalization in patients with AKI (Doyle & Forni, 2016).

If restoration of renal blood flow does not improve urinary output, a loop diuretic such as furosemide (Lasix) or an osmotic diuretic such as mannitol may be given with intravenous fluids to help manage fluid overload. A combination of a loop diuretic and a thiazide diuretic may be used in patients who fail to respond to a loop or osmotic diuretic.

Aggressive hypertension management limits renal injury when AKI is associated with disorders such as toxemia and pregnancy-induced hypertension. ACE inhibitors, ARBs, or other antihypertensive medications are used to control arterial pressures.

All drugs that are either directly nephrotoxic or that may interfere with renal perfusion (such as potent vasoconstrictors) are discontinued. NSAIDs, nephrotoxic antibiotics such as the aminoglycosides, and other potentially harmful drugs (e.g., contrast media) are avoided throughout the course of acute kidney injury.

The patient with AKI has an increased risk of gastrointestinal bleeding, probably related to the stress response and impaired platelet function. Regular doses of antacids, histamine H_2-receptor antagonists (e.g., famotidine or ranitidine), or a proton-pump inhibitor such as omeprazole (Prilosec) are often ordered to prevent GI hemorrhage.

Hyperkalemia may require active intervention as well as restricted potassium intake. Serum levels greater than 6.5 mEq/L are treated to prevent cardiac effects of hyperkalemia. With significant hyperkalemia, calcium chloride, bicarbonate, and insulin and glucose may be given intravenously to reduce serum potassium levels by moving potassium into the cells. Nebulized albuterol, a β_2-agonist, may be used in combination with insulin and glucose to reduce serum potassium levels. A potassium-binding exchange resin such as sodium polystyrene sulfonate (Kayexalate, SPS Suspension) may be given orally or by enema. This agent removes potassium from the body by exchanging sodium for potassium, primarily in the large intestine. Aluminum hydroxide (AlternaGEL, Amphojel, Nephrox), an antacid, is used to control hyperphosphatemia in renal failure. It binds with phosphates in the GI tract, which are then excreted in the feces.

Because many drugs are eliminated from the body by the kidney, drug dosages may need to be adjusted. Doses within the usual range can lead to potentially toxic blood levels because their elimination is slowed and half-life prolonged. Nursing implications for medications commonly prescribed for the patient with AKI are summarized in **Medication Administration 28.A**.

Fluid Management

Once vascular volume and renal perfusion are restored, fluid intake is usually restricted. The allowed daily fluid intake is calculated by allowing 500 to 800 mL for insensible losses (respiration, perspiration, bowel losses) and adding the amount excreted as urine (or lost in vomitus) during the previous 24 hours. For example, if a patient with AKI excretes 325 mL of urine in 24 hours, the patient is allowed a fluid intake (including oral and intravenous fluids) of 825 to 1125 mL for the next 24 hours. Fluid balance is carefully monitored, using accurate weight measurements and the serum sodium as the primary indicators. Hemodynamic monitoring may be initiated to aid in fluid management of the critically ill patient.

Nutrition

Renal insufficiency and the underlying disease process increase the rate of *catabolism* (the breakdown of body proteins) and decrease the rate of *anabolism* (body tissue repair). The patient with AKI needs adequate nutrients and calories (between 25 and 45 calories/kg/day) to prevent catabolism. Proteins may be limited to minimize the degree of azotemia; however, current evidence supports protein intake adequate to prevent protein malnutrition (1 or more grams per kilogram per day). Dietary proteins should be of high biologic value (rich in essential amino acids). Carbohydrates and fats are increased to maintain adequate calorie intake and provide a protein-sparing effect. Oral or enteral nutrition is provided whenever possible to support gastrointestinal integrity (Inker et al., 2014; KDIGO, 2012). Parenteral nutrition may be instituted if enteral nutrition fails to meet the patient's needs or results in additional problems. The disadvantages of parenteral nutrition in the patient with AKI are the high volume of fluid required and the risk for infection through the venous line.

Renal Replacement Therapy

Manifestations of *uremia*, organ dysfunction due to accumulated metabolic wastes, severe fluid overload, hyperkalemia, or metabolic acidosis in a patient with renal failure, indicate a need to replace renal function. **Dialysis** is the diffusion of solute molecules across a semipermeable membrane from an area of higher solute concentration to one of lower concentration. It is used to remove excess fluid and metabolic waste products in acute kidney injury and renal failure. Early use of dialysis can reduce the rate of complications. Dialysis may be used to rapidly remove nephrotoxins in acute tubular necrosis. While dialysis compensates for lost renal elimination functions, it does not replace lost erythropoietin production. Anemia is a continuing problem for the patient receiving dialysis.

Medication Administration 28.A

The Patient with Acute Kidney Injury

LOOP DIURETICS

bumetanide (Bumex)

ethacrynic acid (Edecrin)

furosemide (Lasix)

torsemide (Demadex)

The loop diuretics, named for their primary site of action in the loop of Henle, are highly effective diuretics used to manage hypervolemia in AKI. Loop diuretics may be given with intravenous dopamine to promote renal blood flow. In ATN due to a nephrotoxin, loop diuretics are used to clear the toxin from the nephrons more rapidly. Loop diuretics cause potassium wasting, which is generally not a concern in AKI because renal failure impairs normal potassium elimination.

Nursing Responsibilities

- Monitor intake and output, daily weight (or more frequently as ordered), vital signs, skin turgor, and other indicators of fluid volume status frequently.
- Assess for orthostatic hypotension because these potent diuretics can lead to hypovolemia.
- Monitor laboratory results, especially serum electrolyte, glucose, BUN, and creatinine levels.
- Administer by mouth or, if ordered, by intravenous injection or infusion.
- Assess response. Urine output typically increases within 10 minutes after intravenous administration.
- Monitor hearing and for complaints such as tinnitus. High doses of loop diuretics increase the risk of ototoxicity, especially with ethacrynic acid. These effects may be reversible if detected early and the drug is discontinued.
- Avoid administering concurrently with other ototoxic agents, such as aminoglycoside antibiotics and cisplatin.

Health Education for the Patient and Family

- Maintain fluid intake or restriction as ordered.
- Rise slowly from lying or sitting positions because a fall in blood pressure may cause light-headedness.
- Take in the morning and, if ordered twice a day, late afternoon to avoid sleep disturbance.
- Take with food or milk to prevent gastric distress.
- NSAIDs interfere with the effectiveness of loop diuretics and should be avoided.

OSMOTIC DIURETICS

mannitol (Osmitrol, Isotol)

Osmotic diuretics act by increasing the osmotic draw in the blood and urine. In the blood, the effect is to pull extracellular water into the vascular system, increasing the GFR. These substances are then freely filtered in the glomerulus and increase the osmotic draw of the urine, inhibiting water reabsorption. The effect is to increase urine volume and flow. In addition, osmotic diuretics dilute waste products in the urine, decreasing the risk of renal damage due to excess concentrations.

Nursing Responsibilities

- Assess urine output. Osmotic diuretics are contraindicated in anuria. A test dose may be administered; urine output of 30 mL/h following the test dose shows an adequate response.
- Do not give these diuretics to patients who have heart failure or who are severely dehydrated. They increase vascular volume and may worsen heart failure. These drugs are not effective unless extracellular volume is adequate.
- Administer mannitol intravenously as ordered, using a 5-micron in-line filter.
- Monitor vital signs, breath sounds, and urinary output.
- Discontinue the drug if signs of heart failure or pulmonary edema develop or if renal function continues to decline.

Health Education for the Patient and Family

- Report shortness of breath, headache, chest pain, or dizziness immediately.

ELECTROLYTES AND ELECTROLYTE MODIFIERS

calcium chloride

calcium gluconate

sodium bicarbonate

sodium polystyrene sulfonate (Kayexalate)

Calcium chloride or gluconate is administered intravenously in the initial management of hyperkalemia. Calcium is administered to correct hypocalcemia and reduce hyperphosphatemia. (Calcium and phosphate have a reciprocal relationship in the body: As the level of one rises, the level of the other falls.) Sodium bicarbonate helps correct acidosis and move potassium back into the intracellular space. Sodium polystyrene sulfonate is not used to replace an electrolyte, but to remove excess potassium from the body by exchanging sodium for potassium in the large intestine.

Nursing Responsibilities

- Assess serum electrolyte levels prior to and during therapy. Report rapid shifts or adverse responses to the physician.
- Administer as appropriate and prescribed:
  a. Intravenous calcium chloride or calcium gluconate into a large vein through a small-bore needle; avoid infiltration because extravasation of intravenous solution will cause tissue necrosis.
  b. Intravenous sodium bicarbonate per infusion or as oral tablets.
  c. Sodium polystyrene sulfonate as an oral solution or as a retention enema.
- Monitor for adverse reactions, such as dysrhythmias, electrolyte imbalances, and metabolic alkalosis.

Health Education for the Patient and Family

- Intravenous calcium may make you light-headed; remain in bed for at least 30 minutes after administration.
- Chew sodium bicarbonate tablets and follow with 8 ounces of water. Do not take with milk.
- Retain the sodium polystyrene sulfonate enema as long as possible.

Note: Drugs identified in blue are among the 200 most commonly prescribed medications in the United States.

Source: Data from Adams, Holland, & Urban, 2017.

In dialysis, blood is separated from a dialysis solution (*dialysate*) by a semipermeable membrane. Either **hemodialysis**, a procedure in which blood passes through a semipermeable membrane filter outside the body, or **peritoneal dialysis**, which uses the peritoneum surrounding the abdominal cavity as the dialyzing membrane, may be used. Intermittent hemodialysis is most commonly used for the patient with AKI in the United States (Inker et al., 2014; NIDDK, 2016).

Intermittent Hemodialysis. Hemodialysis uses the principles of diffusion and ultrafiltration to remove electrolytes, waste products, and excess water from the body. Blood is taken from the patient via a vascular access and pumped to the dialyzer (**Figure 28.6** ■). The porous membranes of the dialyzer unit allow small molecules such as water, glucose, and electrolytes to pass through, but block larger molecules such as serum proteins and blood cells. The dialysate, a solution of approximately the same composition and temperature as normal extracellular fluid, passes along the other side of the membrane. Small solute molecules move freely across the membrane by diffusion. The direction of movement for any substance is determined by the concentrations of that substance in the blood and the dialysate. Electrolytes and waste products such as urea and creatinine diffuse from the blood into the dialysate. If it is necessary to add something to the blood, such as calcium to replace depleted stores, it can be added to the dialysate to diffuse into the blood. Excess water is removed by creating a higher hydrostatic pressure of the blood moving through the dialyzer than of the dialysate, which flows in the opposite direction. This process is known as **ultrafiltration**. Solute is carried in solution across the membrane in a process known as *convection*.

Initially, patients with AKI typically undergo hemodialysis for 3 to 4 hours per day for three to four times per week as indicated. Hemodialysis is not used if the patient is hemodynamically unstable (e.g., with hypotension or low cardiac output). The following complications are associated with hemodialysis:

- Hypotension, the most frequent complication during hemodialysis, due to changes in serum osmolality, rapid removal of fluid from the vascular compartment, vasodilation, and other factors
- Bleeding related to altered platelet function associated with uremia and the use of heparin during dialysis
- Infection (local or systemic) related to WBC damage and immune system suppression. *Staphylococcus aureus*

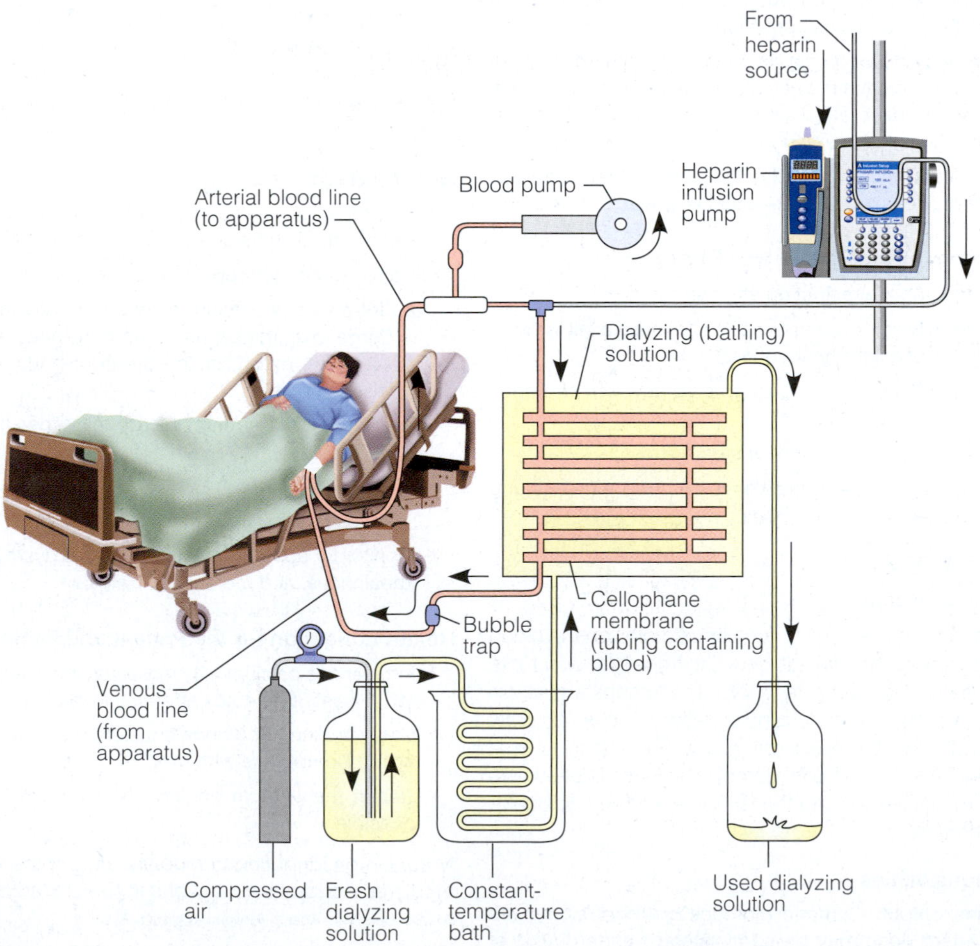
From heparin source
Heparin infusion pump
Blood pump
Arterial blood line (to apparatus)
Dialyzing (bathing) solution
Cellophane membrane (tubing containing blood)
Bubble trap
Venous blood line (from apparatus)
Compressed air
Fresh dialyzing solution
Constant-temperature bath
Used dialyzing solution

Figure 28.6 ■ The components of a hemodialysis system.

septicemia is commonly associated with contamination of the vascular access site. Patients on chronic hemodialysis have higher rates of hepatitis B, hepatitis C, cytomegalovirus, and HIV infection than the general population.

See **Box 28.2** for nursing care of the patient undergoing hemodialysis.

Continuous Renal Replacement Therapy. Patients with acute kidney injury may be unable to tolerate hemodialysis and rapid fluid removal if their cardiovascular status is unstable (e.g., due to trauma, major surgery, heart failure). *Continuous renal replacement therapy (CRRT)* is a procedure that allows more gradual fluid and solute removal. In CRRT, blood is continuously circulated through a highly porous hemofilter for a period of 8 to 12 or more hours (**Figure 28.7** ■). Excess water and solutes such as electrolytes, urea, creatinine, uric acid, and glucose drain into a collection device. Fluid is replaced with normal saline or a balanced electrolyte solution as needed during CRRT. This slower process helps maintain hemodynamic stability and avoid complications associated with rapid changes in ECF composition. The most common CRRT techniques are outlined in **Table 28.6**.

CRRT is typically performed in an intensive care unit or specialized nephrology unit. A double-lumen venous catheter is used for most types of CRRT. Strict aseptic technique is vital in caring for vascular access sites to reduce the risk of infection.

SAFETY ALERT: When longer-term dialysis is anticipated, arteriovenous fistula (AVF) is preferred for vascular access. Complications related to vascular access, such as infection and clotting, occur at a significantly lower rate with AVF than with catheters. ■

Vascular Access. Acute or temporary vascular access for hemodialysis or CRRT usually is gained by inserting a double-lumen catheter into the subclavian, jugular, or femoral vein. The double-lumen catheter has a central partition separating the blood withdrawal side of the catheter from the return side. Blood is drawn into the catheter through small openings in the proximal portion of the catheter and returned to the circulation through an opening in the distal end of the catheter to avoid withdrawing the blood that has just been dialyzed.

For longer-term vascular access, an *arteriovenous fistula (AVF)* (**Figure 28.8** ■) is created. In preparation for fistula formation, the nondominant arm is not used for

BOX 28.2
Nursing Care of the Patient Undergoing Hemodialysis

PREDIALYSIS CARE

- Assess vital signs, including orthostatic blood pressures (lying, sitting, and standing), apical pulse, respirations, and lung sounds. *These data provide baseline information to help evaluate the effects of hemodialysis. The patient who is hypotensive may not tolerate rapid fluid volume changes during dialysis.*
- Record weight. *Weight changes are an effective indicator of fluid volume.*
- Assess vascular access site for a palpable pulsation or vibration and an audible bruit and for inflammation. *Infection and thrombus formation are the most common problems affecting the access site in patients undergoing hemodialysis.*
- Use strict aseptic technique when accessing the AV fistula or graft and during the dialysis procedure. *Preventing infection, a major complication of hemodialysis and vascular access, is a critical nursing responsibility.*
- Alert all personnel to avoid using the extremity with the vascular access site (or the nondominant arm, if long-term access has not been established) for blood pressures or venipuncture. *These procedures may damage vessels and lead to failure of the arteriovenous fistula.*

POSTDIALYSIS CARE

- Assess and document vital signs, weight, and vascular access site condition. *Rapid fluid and solute removal during dialysis may lead to hypotension, the most acute complication of hemodialysis.*
- Monitor BUN, serum creatinine, serum electrolyte, and hematocrit levels between dialysis treatments. *These values help determine the effectiveness of the treatment and the timing of future dialysis sessions. Significant anemia may necessitate iron and folate supplements or periodic blood transfusions.*
- Assess for dialysis disequilibrium syndrome, with headache, nausea and vomiting, altered level of consciousness, and hypertension. *Rapid changes in BUN, pH, and electrolyte levels during dialysis may lead to cerebral edema and increased intracranial pressure.*
- Assess for other adverse responses to dialysis, such as dehydration, muscle cramps, or seizure activity. Treat as ordered. *Excess fluid removal and rapid changes in electrolyte balance can cause fluid deficit, muscle cramps, and seizure activity.*
- Assess for bleeding at the access site or elsewhere. Use standard precautions at all times. *Renal failure and heparinization during dialysis increase the risk for bleeding. Frequent exposure to blood and blood products increases the risk for hepatitis B or C or other bloodborne diseases.*
- If a transfusion is given during dialysis, monitor for possible transfusion reaction (e.g., chills and fever; dyspnea; chest, back, or arm pain; and urticaria or itching). *Patients in renal failure may receive multiple transfusions, increasing the risk of transfusion reaction. Close monitoring during and after the transfusion is important to identify early signs of a reaction.*
- Provide psychologic support and listen actively. Address concerns and accept responses such as anger, depression, and noncompliance. Reinforce patient and family strengths in coping with renal failure and hemodialysis. *Grieving is a normal response to loss of organ function. The patient may feel hopeless or helpless and resent dependence on a machine. The nurse can help the patient and family work through these responses and focus on positive aspects of living.*
- Refer to social services and counseling as indicated. *Patients with renal failure may need additional support services to help them adapt to and live with their disease.*

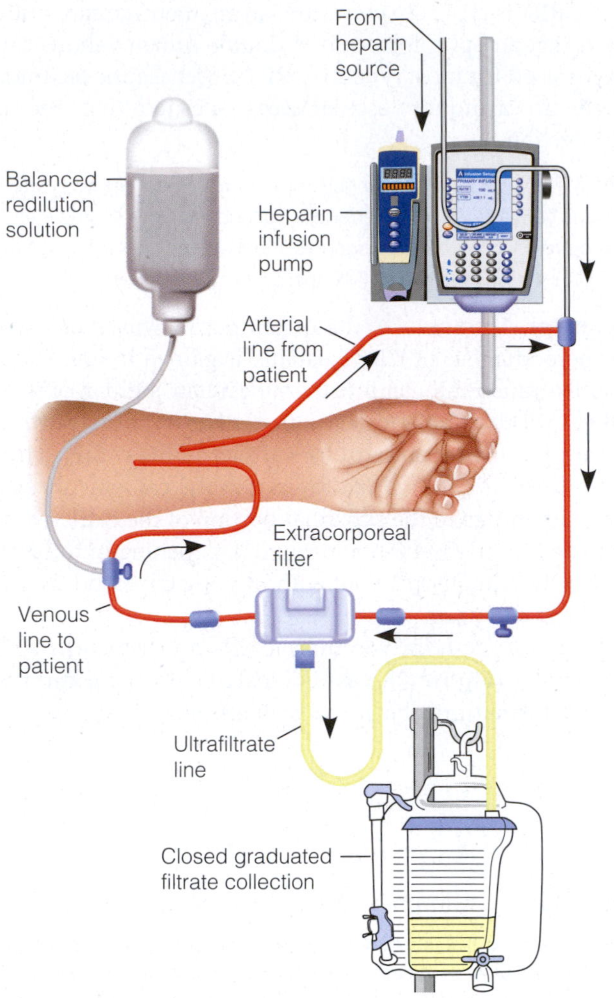

From heparin source
Balanced redilution solution
Heparin infusion pump
Arterial line from patient
Extracorporeal filter
Venous line to patient
Ultrafiltrate line
Closed graduated filtrate collection

Figure 28.7 ■ Continuous renal replacement therapy (CRRT).

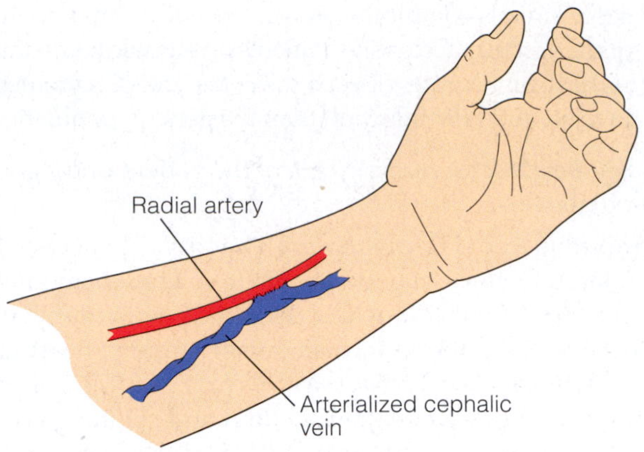

Radial artery
Arterialized cephalic vein

Figure 28.8 ■ An arteriovenous fistula.

venipuncture or blood pressure measurement during renal failure. The fistula is created by surgical anastomosis of an artery and vein, usually the radial artery and cephalic vein. It takes about a month for the fistula to mature so that it can be used for taking and replacing blood during dialysis. A functional AVF has a palpable pulsation and a bruit on auscultation. Venipunctures and blood pressures are avoided on the arm with the fistula.

An *arteriovenous graft* may also be used for vascular access. The graft, a tube made of Gore-Tex, is surgically implanted and connects the artery and the vein. Blood flows through the graft from the artery to the vein. The rate of complications and mortality associated with catheter access is higher than with AV fistulas or grafts. Ideally, an AV fistula is created as soon as the potential need for long-term renal replacement therapies is identified. Localized AV fistula or graft problems can occur, however. Infection and clotting or thrombosis is the most common shunt problem. Aneurysms may also develop. Both infection and thrombosis can lead to systemic complications such as septicemia and embolization. These local complications may cause the fistula or graft to fail, necessitating development of a new site. The psychologic impact of AV fistula or graft failure is significant, often causing depression and low self-esteem.

Peritoneal Dialysis. In peritoneal dialysis, the highly vascular peritoneal membrane serves as the dialyzing surface (**Figure 28.9** ■). Warmed sterile dialysate is instilled (either manually or using an automated peritoneal dialysis cycler) into the peritoneal cavity through a catheter inserted into the peritoneal cavity. Metabolic waste products and excess electrolytes diffuse into the dialysate while it remains in the abdomen. Water movement is controlled using dextrose as an osmotic agent to draw it into the dialysate. The fluid is then drained by gravity out of the peritoneal cavity into a sterile bag. This process of dialysate infusion, dwell time of the solution in the abdomen, and drainage is repeated at prescribed intervals.

Because excess fluid and solutes are removed more gradually in peritoneal dialysis, it poses less risk for the

Table 28.6 Continuous Renal Replacement Therapies

Type	Indications	Description
Continuous venovenous hemofiltration (CVVH)	Removes fluid and some solutes.	Convective dialysis: Venous blood circulates through a hemofilter, where fluid and small-to-midsized solutes are removed by ultrafiltration and convection; crystalloid replacement fluid is required.
Continuous venovenous hemodialysis (CVVHD)	Removes fluid and waste products.	Diffusive dialysis: Venous blood circulates through a hemofilter surrounded by dialysate where mostly small molecules are removed by diffusion; blood and dialysate flow rates are slower than for hemodialysis; replacement fluid is not required.
Continuous venovenous hemodiafiltration (CVVHDF)	Removes fluid and waste products.	Convective and diffusive clearance: Venous blood circulates through a hemofilter surrounded by dialysate, replacement fluid is added; effective in clearing small and midsize molecules and urea.

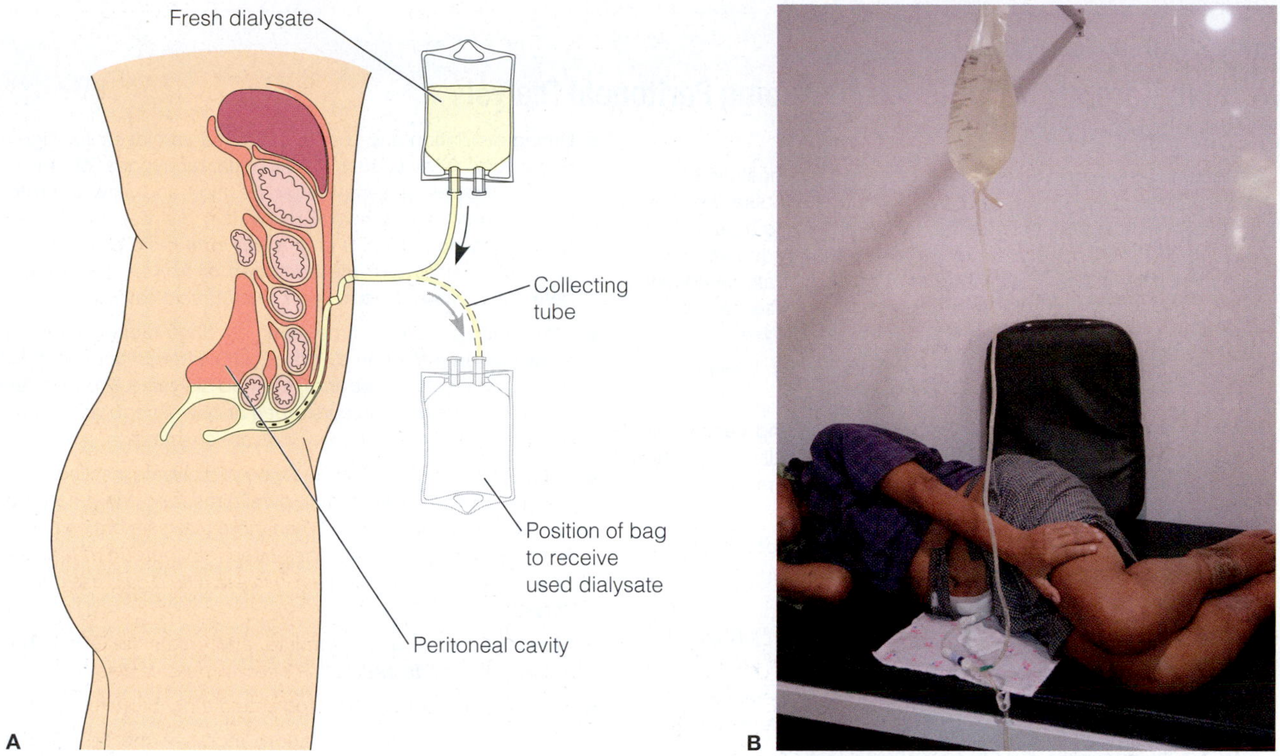
Fresh dialysate
Collecting tube
Position of bag to receive used dialysate
Peritoneal cavity
A
B

Figure 28.9 ■ **A**, The components of peritoneal dialysis. **B**, A patient receiving peritoneal dialysis.

unstable patient; however, this slower rate of metabolite removal can be a disadvantage in AKI. Peritoneal dialysis increases the risk for developing peritonitis. It is contraindicated for patients who have had recent abdominal surgery, significant lung disease, or peritonitis. See **Box 28.3** for nursing care of the patient having peritoneal dialysis.

Nursing Care

Assessment

Both subjective and objective data are useful when assessing the patient with acute kidney injury:

- ***Health history:*** Complaints of anorexia, nausea, weight gain, or edema; recent exposure to a nephrotoxin such as an aminoglycoside antibiotic or radiologic procedure using an injected contrast medium; previous transfusion reaction; chronic diseases such as diabetes, heart failure, or kidney disease
- ***Physical assessment:*** Vital signs including temperature; urine output (amount, color, clarity, specific gravity, presence of blood cells or protein); weight; skin color, peripheral pulses; presence of edema (periorbital or dependent); lung sounds, heart sounds, and bowel tones.

Priorities of Care

Priority nursing care needs for the patient with AKI relate to addressing alterations in fluid and electrolyte balance, supporting nutritional status, and teaching/learning.

Diagnoses, Outcomes, and Interventions

The patient with acute kidney injury has numerous nursing care needs related not only to the renal failure but also to the underlying condition that precipitated it.

SAFETY ALERT: Frequently assess breath and heart sounds, neck veins for distention, and back and extremities for edema. Report abnormal findings. Adventitious breath sounds (crackles), abnormal heart sounds such as an S_3 or S_4 gallop, distended neck veins, and peripheral edema may indicate hypervolemia, heart failure, or pulmonary edema. ■

Restore Fluid and Electrolyte Balance. In acute kidney injury, the kidneys often cannot excrete adequate urine to maintain a normal extracellular fluid balance. Metabolic waste products are retained, and electrolyte homeostasis is disrupted.

Expected Outcome: Patient's fluid and electrolyte balance will be restored, and patient will experience no adverse effects of altered homeostasis.

The nurse will:

- Maintain hourly intake and output records. *Accurate intake and output records help guide therapy, especially fluid restrictions.*
- Weigh daily or more frequently, as ordered. Use standard technique (same scale, clothing, or coverings) to ensure accuracy. *Rapid weight changes are an accurate indicator of fluid volume status, particularly in the patient with oliguria.*

BOX 28.3
Nursing Care of the Patient Undergoing Peritoneal Dialysis

PREDIALYSIS CARE

- Document vital signs including temperature, orthostatic blood pressures (lying, sitting, and standing), apical pulse, respirations, and lung sounds. *These baseline data help assess fluid volume status and tolerance of the dialysis procedure. Poor respiratory function may affect the ability to tolerate peritoneal dialysis. Temperature measurement is vital because infection is the most common complication of peritoneal dialysis.*
- Weigh daily or between dialysis runs as indicated. *Weight is an accurate indicator of fluid volume status.*
- Note BUN, serum electrolyte, creatinine, pH, and hematocrit levels prior to peritoneal dialysis and periodically during the procedure. *These values are used to assess the efficacy of treatment.*
- Measure and record abdominal girth. *Increasing abdominal girth may indicate retained dialysate, excess fluid volume, or early peritonitis.*
- Maintain fluid and dietary restrictions as ordered. *Fluid and diet restrictions help reduce hypervolemia and control azotemia.*
- Have the patient empty the bladder prior to catheter insertion. *Emptying the bladder reduces the risk of inadvertent puncture.*
- Warm the prescribed dialysate solution to body temperature (37°C [98.6°F]) if the procedure is being performed manually. *Dialysate is warmed to prevent hypothermia; an automated cycler will warm the dialysate prior to instillation.*
- Explain all procedures and expected sensations. *Knowledge helps reduce anxiety and elicit cooperation.*

INTRADIALYSIS CARE

- Use strict aseptic technique during the dialysis procedure and when caring for the peritoneal catheter. *Peritonitis is a common complication of peritoneal dialysis; sterile technique reduces the risk.*
- Add prescribed medications to the appropriate dialysate; prime the tubing with solution and connect it to the peritoneal catheter, securing connections and avoiding kinks. *This allows dialysate to flow freely into the abdominal cavity and prevents leaking or contamination.*
- Instill dialysate into the abdominal cavity over a period of approximately 10 minutes. Clamp tubing and allow the dialysate to remain in the abdomen for the prescribed dwell time. Keep drainage tubing clamped at all times during instillation and dwell time. *Dialysate should flow freely into the abdomen if the peritoneal catheter is patent. Dialysis, the exchange of solutes and water between the blood and dialysate, occurs across the peritoneal membrane during the dwell time.*
- During instillation and dwell time, observe closely for signs of respiratory distress, such as dyspnea, tachypnea, or crackles. Place in Fowler or semi-Fowler position and slow the rate of instillation slightly to relieve respiratory distress if it develops. *Respiratory compromise may result from rapid dialysate instillation or overfilling of the abdomen or from a diaphragmatic defect that allows fluid to enter the thoracic cavity.*
- After prescribed dwell time, open drainage tubing clamps and allow dialysate to drain by gravity into a sterile container. Note the clarity, color, and odor of returned dialysate. *Blood or feces in the dialysate may indicate organ or bowel perforation; cloudy or malodorous dialysate may indicate an infection.*
- Accurately record amount and type of dialysate instilled (including any added medications), dwell time, and the amount and character of the drainage. *When more dialysate drains than has been instilled, excess fluid has been lost (output). If less dialysate is returned than has been instilled, a fluid gain has occurred (intake).*
- Monitor BUN, serum electrolyte, and creatinine levels. *These values are used to assess the effectiveness of dialysis.*
- Troubleshoot for possible problems during dialysis:
  a. Slow dialysate instillation. Increase the height of the container and reposition the patient. Check tubing and catheter for kinks. Check abdominal dressing for wetness, indicating leakage around the catheter. *Slow dialysate flow may be related to a partially obstructed tube or catheter.*
  b. Excess dwell time. *Prolonged dwell time may lead to water depletion or hyperglycemia.*
  c. Poor dialysate drainage. Lower the drainage container, reposition, check for tubing kinks. Check abdominal dressing. *Tubing or catheter obstruction can interfere with dialysate drainage.*

POSTDIALYSIS CARE

- Assess vital signs, including temperature. *Comparison of pre- and postdialysis vital signs helps identify beneficial and adverse effects of the procedure.*
- Time meals to correspond with dialysis outflow. *Scheduling meals while the abdomen is empty of dialysate enhances intake and reduces nausea.*
- Teach the patient and family about the procedure. *The patient may elect to use peritoneal dialysis at home to manage end-stage renal disease and prevent uremia.*

- Assess vital signs at least every 4 hours. *Hypertension, tachycardia, and tachypnea may indicate excess fluid volume.*
- If not contraindicated, place in semi-Fowler position. *This enhances cardiac and respiratory function.*
- Report abnormal serum electrolyte values and manifestations of electrolyte imbalance. The patient with AKI is at particular risk for the following electrolyte imbalances:
  a. *Hyperkalemia* due to impaired potassium excretion. Manifestations include irritability, nausea, diarrhea, abdominal cramping, cardiac dysrhythmias, and ECG changes.
  b. *Hyponatremia* due to water retention. Manifestations include nausea and vomiting and headache, with possible central nervous system (CNS) manifestations of lethargy, confusion, seizures, and coma.
  c. *Hyperphosphatemia* due to decreased phosphate excretion. Manifestations include hyperreflexia, paresthesias, and possible tetany.

  AKI impairs electrolyte and water excretion, causing multiple electrolyte imbalances.

- Restrict fluids as ordered. Provide frequent mouth care and encourage using hard candies to decrease thirst. If ice chips are allowed, include the water content (approximately one-half of the total volume) as intake. *Fluids are restricted to minimize fluid retention and complications of fluid volume excess.*
- Administer medications with meals. *Giving oral medications with meals minimizes ingestion of excess fluids.*
- Turn frequently and provide good skin care. *Edema decreases tissue perfusion and increases the risk of skin breakdown, especially in the older or debilitated patient.*

Maintain Adequate Nutrition. Anorexia and nausea associated with renal failure often interfere with food intake and nutrition. In addition, patients experiencing AKI are at risk for protein-energy malnutrition related to their disease process (Inker et al., 2014; KDIGO, 2012).

Expected Outcome: Patient will maintain adequate nutritional status as evidenced by stable weight and serum albumin levels within expected parameters.

The nurse will:

- Monitor and record food intake, including the amount and type of food consumed. *A detailed intake record helps guide decisions about nutritional status and necessary supplements.*
- Weigh daily. *Weight changes over time (days to weeks) reflect nutritional status, while rapid weight changes are more reflective of fluid volume status. In AKI, weight may remain stable or increase due to fluid retention even though tissue mass is being lost.*
- Arrange for dietary consultation to plan meals within prescribed limitations that consider the patient's food preferences. *Diets restricted in protein, salt, and potassium can be unpalatable; intake and appetite improve when preferred foods are included as allowed.*
- Engage the patient in planning daily menus. *Participation in meal planning increases the patient's sense of control and autonomy.*
- Allow family members to prepare meals within dietary restrictions. Encourage family members to eat with the patient. *Familiar foods and social interaction encourage eating and increase enjoyment of meals.*
- Provide frequent, small meals or between-meal snacks. *These measures promote food intake in patients who are fatigued or anorectic.*
- Administer antiemetics as ordered and provide mouth care prior to meals. *Nausea and a metallic taste in the mouth, common manifestations of uremia, can decrease food intake.*
- Administer parenteral nutrition as ordered if the patient is unable to eat or tolerate enteral nutrition. *Preventing or slowing tissue catabolism is important for the patient with AKI.*

SAFETY ALERT: Intravenous lines and parenteral nutrition solutions can increase the risk for infection. Monitor sites carefully for signs of infection or inflammation. ■

Promote Patient Learning. The patient with AKI has multiple learning needs. These include information about AKI, diagnostic and laboratory studies, management strategies, and implications for the recovery period.

Expected Outcome: Patient will express an understanding of condition and its management.

The nurse will:

- Assess anxiety level and ability to comprehend instruction. Tailor information and presentation to developmental level and physical, mental, and emotional status. *The patient with AKI may be critically ill or have uremic effects that hinder learning. During the initial stages of AKI, it may be necessary to limit information to immediate concerns.*
- Assess knowledge and understanding. *To enhance understanding and retention, relate information presented to previous learning.*
- Teach about diagnostic tests and therapeutic procedures. *Teaching reduces anxiety and improves understanding and cooperation.*
- Discuss dietary and fluid restrictions. *These measures may be continued after discharge.*
- If the patient is discharged prior to the recovery phase of AKI, teach the signs and symptoms of complications, such as fluid volume excess or deficit, heart failure, and electrolyte imbalances. *As kidney function returns, urine output increases, but the concentrating ability of the nephrons and electrolyte excretion remain impaired. This impaired function increases the risk of excess fluid loss, possible dehydration, orthostatic hypotension, and electrolyte imbalance.*
- Teach how to monitor weight, blood pressure, and pulse. *These are important means of assessing fluid status.*
- Instruct to avoid nephrotoxic drugs and chemicals for up to 1 year following an episode of AKI. *During recovery, nephrons are vulnerable to damage by nephrotoxins such as NSAIDs, some antibiotics, radiologic contrast media, and heavy metals. Because alcohol can increase the nephrotoxicity of some materials, discourage alcohol ingestion.*

Delegating Nursing Care Activities

As appropriate and allowed by the designated duties and responsibilities of unlicensed assistive personnel (UAP), the nurse may delegate nursing care activities such as measuring vital signs and intake and output, obtaining daily weights, and assisting with hygiene and activities for the patient with AKI. When delegating care, ensure UAP have a clear understanding of fluid restrictions, the necessity of accuracy when measuring fluid intake and output, and restrictions on use of the designated extremity for measuring blood pressure.

Transitions of Care

Care of the patient with AKI occurs across therapeutic environments. Patient care and teaching should be provided when appropriate based on the clinical presentation.

Acute kidney injury can often be prevented by measures that maintain fluid volume and cardiac output and reduce the risk of exposure to nephrotoxins. Carefully monitor critically ill, postoperative, and other at-risk patients for early signs of hypovolemia (low urine output; altered mental status; changes in vital signs, skin color, or temperature) or infection. Promptly report a fall in urine output to less than 30 mL/h and other evidence of decreased cardiac output. Maintain intravenous fluids as ordered. Alert the physician if the patient is receiving more than one nephrotoxic drug or if a nephrotoxic drug is ordered for a dehydrated patient. Closely observe patients receiving blood or blood cells for early signs of transfusion reaction and intervene appropriately.

Often the patient is critically ill when AKI develops. Critical illness and the resulting state of the patient and family crisis can impair learning and retention of information. Include family members in teaching during the initial stages to promote understanding of what is happening and the reasons for specific treatment measures. Inclusion of the family reduces their anxiety and provides a valuable resource for reinforcing patient teaching about care after discharge.

Patient teaching needs for home care include:

- Avoiding exposure to nephrotoxins, particularly those in over-the-counter products
- Preventing infection and other major stressors that can slow healing
- Monitoring weight, blood pressure, and pulse
- Manifestations of relapse
- Continuing dietary restrictions
- Knowing when to contact the physician.

The Patient with Chronic Kidney Disease

Although the kidneys often recover from acute injury, many chronic conditions can lead to progressive destruction of kidney tissue and loss of function. Nephron units are lost and kidney mass decreases, with progressive deterioration of glomerular filtration, tubular secretion, and reabsorption. This process may progress slowly for many years without being recognized. **Chronic kidney disease (CKD)** is defined as kidney damage with resulting dysfunction (GFR less than 60 mL/min) that persists for three or more months (NIDDK, 2016). Eventually, the kidneys are unable to excrete metabolic wastes and regulate fluid and electrolyte balance adequately, a condition known as kidney failure or ESRD, the final stage of CKD.

The incidence of CKD and ESRD is increasing, particularly in older adults. The incidence of recognized CKD among people ages 65 and older more than doubled from 2000 to 2008 (Inker et al., 2014; NDIGO, 2012).

Pathophysiology

The pathophysiology of CKD varies, depending on the underlying disease process. **Table 28.7** outlines the pathologic processes leading to nephron destruction, CKD, and kidney failure for the most common causes. Regardless of the initiating cause, glomerulosclerosis and interstitial inflammation and fibrosis are characteristic of CKD and contribute to declining renal function (Sorenson et al., 2019). Entire nephron units are gradually destroyed. In the early stages, as nephrons are lost, remaining functional nephrons hypertrophy. Glomerular capillary flow and pressure increase in these nephrons, and more solute particles are filtered to compensate for lost renal mass. This increased demand predisposes the remaining nephrons to glomerulosclerosis (scarring), resulting in their eventual destruction. Proteinuria resulting from glomerular damage is thought to contribute to tubular injury. This process of continued loss of nephron function may continue even after the initial disease process has resolved (Sorenson et al., 2019).

The course of CKD is variable, progressing over a period of months to many years. In the early stages, unaffected nephrons compensate for the lost nephrons. The GFR is normal or slightly decreased, and the patient is asymptomatic with normal BUN and serum creatinine levels. As the disease progresses and the GFR falls further, hypertension and some manifestations of renal insufficiency such as fatigue, anemia, and fluid and electrolyte imbalances may be seen. Any further insult to the kidneys at this stage (such as infection, dehydration, exposure to nephrotoxins, or urinary tract obstruction) can further reduce function and precipitate the onset of renal failure and uremic syndrome. The serum creatinine and BUN levels rise sharply, the patient becomes oliguric, and manifestations of uremia are seen. In ESRD, the final stage of CKD, the GFR is less

Table 28.7 Pathophysiology of Chronic Kidney Disease

Cause	Pathophysiology
Diabetic nephropathy	Initial increases in glomerular flow rate lead to hyperfiltration with eventual glomerular damage and thickening and sclerosis of the glomerular basement membrane and the glomerulus. Gradual destruction of nephrons leads to a fall in the GFR.
Hypertensive nephrosclerosis	Long-standing hypertension leads to sclerosis and narrowing of renal arterioles and small arteries with subsequent reduction of blood flow, leading to ischemia, glomerular destruction, and tubular atrophy.
Chronic glomerulonephritis	Chronic interstitial inflammation of renal parenchyma leads to obstruction and damage to the tubules and capillaries that surround them, affecting glomerular filtration and tubular secretion and reabsorption, with gradual loss of entire nephrons.
Polycystic kidney disease	Multiple bilateral cysts compress renal tissue, impairing renal perfusion and leading to ischemia, renal vascular remodeling, and release of inflammatory mediators, which damage and destroy normal kidney tissue.

than 15 mL/min and renal replacement therapy is necessary to sustain life. **Table 28.8** summarizes the stages of chronic kidney disease.

Risk Factors

Conditions causing CKD typically involve diffuse, bilateral disease of the kidneys with progressive destruction and scarring of the entire nephron. Acute kidney injury significantly increases the risk for CKD. Other known risk factors include autoimmune disease, proteinuria, or a family history of kidney disease (NIDDK, 2016).

Manifestations

Chronic kidney disease may not be identified until its final, uremic stage is reached. **Uremia** (or *uremic syndrome*), which means "urine in the blood," refers to the syndrome or group of symptoms associated with ESRD. In uremia, fluid and electrolyte balance is altered, the regulatory and endocrine functions of the kidney are impaired, and accumulated metabolic waste products affect essentially every other organ system. Declining renal function is associated with progressive systemic inflammation and elevated levels of C-reactive protein and other inflammatory substances. This inflammatory response contributes to accelerated cardiovascular disease and the negative nutritional impact of CKD (Sorenson, et al., 2019).

Early manifestations of uremia include nausea, apathy, weakness, and fatigue, symptoms that are often dismissed as a viral infection or influenza.

Complications

As the condition progresses, frequent vomiting, increasing weakness, lethargy, and confusion develop. See the Multisystem Effects of Uremia feature on page 936.

Fluid and Electrolyte Effects

Loss of functional kidney tissue impairs its ability to regulate fluid, electrolyte, and acid–base balance. In the early stages of CKD, impaired filtration and reabsorption lead to proteinuria, hematuria, and decreased urine-concentrating ability. Salt and water are poorly conserved, and risk for dehydration increases. Polyuria, nocturia, and a fixed specific gravity of 1.008 to 1.012 are common. As the GFR decreases and renal function deteriorates further, sodium and water retention are common, necessitating salt and water restrictions.

Hyperkalemia develops as renal failure progresses. Manifestations of hyperkalemia, such as muscle weakness, paresthesias, and ECG changes, are not usually seen until the GFR is less than 5 mL/min. Phosphate excretion is impaired, leading to hyperphosphatemia and hypocalcemia. Reduced calcium absorption due to impaired vitamin D activation also contributes to hypocalcemia. Hypermagnesemia develops with advancing renal failure; magnesium-containing antacids are avoided for this reason.

As renal failure advances, hydrogen ion excretion and buffer production are impaired, leading to metabolic acidosis. Respiratory rate and depth increase (Kussmaul's respirations) to compensate for metabolic acidosis. Although metabolic acidosis is often asymptomatic, other possible manifestations include general malaise, weakness, headache, nausea and vomiting, and abdominal pain.

Cardiovascular Effects

Cardiovascular disease is the leading cause of death in patients with CKD. It results from accelerated atherosclerosis. Hypertension, hyperlipidemia, and inflammation all contribute to the process. Cerebral and peripheral vascular manifestations of atherosclerosis are also seen.

Systemic hypertension is a common manifestation of CKD. Hypertension results from excess fluid volume, increased renin–angiotensin activity, increased peripheral vascular resistance, and decreased prostaglandins. Increased extracellular fluid volume can lead to edema and heart failure. Pulmonary edema may result from heart failure and increased permeability of the alveolar capillary membrane.

Retained metabolic toxins can irritate the pericardial sac, causing an inflammatory response and signs of pericarditis. *Cardiac tamponade*, a potential complication of pericarditis, occurs when inflammatory fluid in the pericardial sac interferes with ventricular filling and cardiac output. Once a common complication of uremia, pericarditis is less common when dialysis is initiated early.

Table 28.8 Stages of Chronic Kidney Disease

Stage	Glomerular Filtration Rate	Description and Manifestations
Stage 1	>90 mL/min/1.73 m^2	Kidney damage with normal or increased GFR Asymptomatic; normal BUN and creatinine
Stage 2	60–89 mL/min/1.73 m^2	Mildly decreased GFR Asymptomatic, possible hypertension; bloodwork generally within normal limits
Stage 3	30–59 mL/min/1.73 m^2	Moderate GFR decrease Hypertension; possible anemia and fatigue, anorexia, possible malnutrition, bone pain; slight elevation of BUN and serum creatinine
Stage 4	15–29 mL/min/1.73 m^2	Severely decreased GFR Hypertension, anemia, malnutrition, altered bone metabolism; edema, metabolic acidosis, hypercalcemia; possible uremia; azotemia with increasing BUN and serum creatinine levels
Stage 5	<15 mL/min/1.73 m^2	End-stage renal disease Kidney failure with azotemia and overt uremia

Source: Adapted from NIDDK, 2016.

Multisystem Effects of Uremia

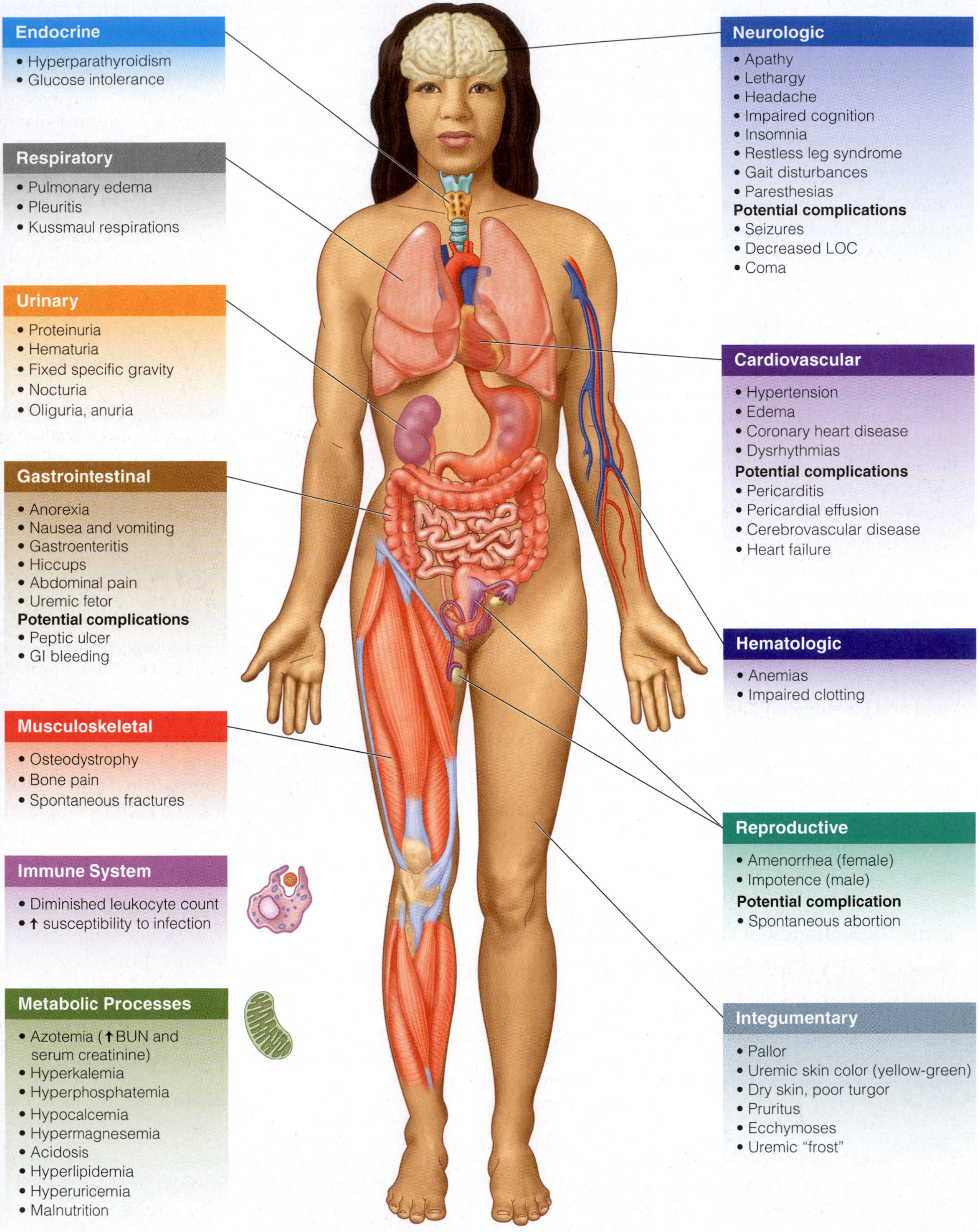
Endocrine
• Hyperparathyroidism
• Glucose intolerance
Respiratory
• Pulmonary edema
• Pleuritis
• Kussmaul respirations
Urinary
• Proteinuria
• Hematuria
• Fixed specific gravity
• Nocturia
• Oliguria, anuria
Gastrointestinal
• Anorexia
• Nausea and vomiting
• Gastroenteritis
• Hiccups
• Abdominal pain
• Uremic fetor
Potential complications
• Peptic ulcer
• GI bleeding
Musculoskeletal
• Osteodystrophy
• Bone pain
• Spontaneous fractures
Immune System
• Diminished leukocyte count
• ↑ susceptibility to infection
Metabolic Processes
• Azotemia (↑BUN and serum creatinine)
• Hyperkalemia
• Hyperphosphatemia
• Hypocalcemia
• Hypermagnesemia
• Acidosis
• Hyperlipidemia
• Hyperuricemia
• Malnutrition
Neurologic
• Apathy
• Lethargy
• Headache
• Impaired cognition
• Insomnia
• Restless leg syndrome
• Gait disturbances
• Paresthesias
Potential complications
• Seizures
• Decreased LOC
• Coma
Cardiovascular
• Hypertension
• Edema
• Coronary heart disease
• Dysrhythmias
Potential complications
• Pericarditis
• Pericardial effusion
• Cerebrovascular disease
• Heart failure
Hematologic
• Anemias
• Impaired clotting
Reproductive
• Amenorrhea (female)
• Impotence (male)
Potential complication
• Spontaneous abortion
Integumentary
• Pallor
• Uremic skin color (yellow-green)
• Dry skin, poor turgor
• Pruritus
• Ecchymoses
• Uremic "frost"

Hematologic Effects

Anemia is common in CKD, caused by multiple factors. The kidneys produce erythropoietin, a hormone that controls RBC production. In renal failure, erythropoietin production declines. Retained metabolic toxins further suppress RBC production and contribute to a shortened RBC lifespan. Nutritional deficiencies (iron and folate) and inflammation with impaired iron utilization also contribute to anemia.

Anemia contributes to manifestations such as fatigue, weakness, depression, and impaired cognition. It affects cardiovascular function and may be a major contributing factor to coronary heart disease and heart failure associated with ESRD.

Renal failure impairs platelet function, increasing the risk of bleeding disorders such as epistaxis and GI bleeding. The mechanism of impaired platelet function associated with renal failure is poorly understood.

Immune System Effects

Uremia increases the risk for infection. High levels of urea and retained metabolic wastes impair all aspects of inflammation and immune function. The WBC declines, humoral and cell-mediated immunity are impaired, and phagocyte function is defective. Both the acute inflammatory response and delayed hypersensitivity responses are affected (Sorenson et al., 2019). Fever is suppressed, often delaying the diagnosis of infection.

Gastrointestinal Effects

Anorexia and nausea and vomiting are the most common early symptoms of uremia. Hiccups are also commonly experienced. Gastroenteritis is frequent. Ulcerations may affect any level of the GI tract and contribute to an increased risk of GI bleeding. Peptic ulcer disease is particularly common in patients with uremia. *Uremic fetor*, a urine-like breath odor often associated with a metallic taste in the mouth, may develop. Uremic fetor can further contribute to anorexia.

Neurologic Effects

Uremia alters both central and peripheral nervous system function. CNS manifestations occur early and include changes in mentation, difficulty concentrating, fatigue, and insomnia. Psychotic symptoms, seizures, and coma are associated with advanced uremic encephalopathy.

Peripheral neuropathy is common in advanced uremia. Both the sensory and motor tracts are involved. The lower limbs are initially affected. *Restless legs syndrome*, sensations of crawling or creeping, prickling, or itching of the lower legs with frequent leg movement, increases during rest. Paresthesias and sensory loss typically occur in a "stocking-glove" pattern. As uremia progresses, motor function is impaired, causing muscle weakness, decreased deep tendon reflexes, and gait disturbances.

Musculoskeletal Effects

Hyperphosphatemia and hypocalcemia associated with uremia stimulate parathyroid hormone secretion. Parathyroid hormone causes increased calcium resorption from bone. In addition, osteoblast (bone-forming) and osteoclast (bone-dissolving) cell activities are affected. This bone resorption and remodeling, combined with decreased vitamin D synthesis and decreased calcium absorption from the GI tract, lead to *renal osteodystrophy*, also known as renal rickets. Osteodystrophy is characterized by osteomalacia, softening of the bones, and osteoporosis, decreased bone mass. Bone cysts may develop. Manifestations of osteodystrophy include bone tenderness, pain, and muscle weakness. The patient is at increased risk for spontaneous fractures.

Endocrine and Metabolic Effects

Accumulated waste products of protein metabolism are a primary factor involved in the effects and manifestations of uremia. Serum creatinine and BUN levels are significantly elevated. Uric acid levels are increased, contributing to an increased risk of gout.

Tissues become resistant to the effects of insulin in uremia, leading to glucose intolerance. High blood triglyceride levels and lower than normal high-density lipoprotein (HDL) levels contribute to the accelerated atherosclerotic process.

Reproductive function is affected. Pregnancies are rarely carried to term, and menstrual irregularities are common. Reduced testosterone levels, low sperm counts, and impotence affect the male patient with ESRD.

Dermatologic Effects

Anemia and retained pigmented metabolites cause pallor and a yellowish hue to the skin in uremia. Dry skin with poor turgor, a result of dehydration and sweat gland atrophy, is common. Bruising and excoriations are frequently seen. Metabolic wastes not eliminated by the kidneys may be deposited in the skin, contributing to itching or pruritus. In advanced uremia, high levels of urea in the sweat may result in *uremic frost*, crystallized deposits of urea on the skin.

Interprofessional Care

Early management of CKD focuses on eliminating or controlling factors that may cause additional kidney damage and further decrease renal function. Included are measures to slow the progression of the disease to ESRD. Additional treatment goals include:

- Maintain nutritional status while minimizing the accumulation of toxic waste products and manifestations of uremia.
- Prevent and treat cardiovascular disease.
- Identify and treat complications of CKD.
- Prepare for renal replacement therapies such as dialysis or renal transplant.

Diagnosis

Diagnostic testing is used both to identify CKD and to monitor kidney function. A number of tests may be performed to determine the underlying renal disorder. Once the diagnosis is established, renal function is monitored primarily through blood levels of metabolic wastes and electrolytes.

- ***Urinalysis*** is done to detect abnormal urine components. In CKD, the specific gravity may be fixed at approximately 1.010 due to impaired tubular secretion, reabsorption, and urine concentrating ability. Abnormal proteins, blood cells, and cellular casts may be noted in the urine.
- ***Urine culture*** is ordered to identify any urinary tract infection that may hasten the progress of CKD.
- ***BUN* and *serum creatinine*** are obtained to evaluate kidney function and assess the progress of renal failure. A BUN of 20 to 50 mg/dL signals mild azotemia; levels greater than 100 mg/dL indicate severe renal impairment. Uremic symptoms are seen when the BUN is around 200 mg/dL or higher. Serum creatinine levels of greater than 4 mg/dL indicate serious renal impairment.
- ***eGFR*** is used to evaluate the GFR and stage of chronic kidney disease. The eGFR is a calculated value determined using a formula that includes the serum creatinine, patient's age, gender, and race (African American or non–African American).
- ***Serum electrolytes*** are monitored throughout the course of CKD. The serum sodium may be within normal limits or low because of water retention or impaired sodium conservation. Potassium levels are elevated but usually remain below 6.5 mEq/L. Serum phosphate is elevated, and the calcium level is decreased. Metabolic acidosis is identified by a low pH, low CO_2, and low bicarbonate levels.
- ***CBC*** reveals moderately severe anemia with a hematocrit of 20 to 30% and low hemoglobin. The number of RBCs and platelets is reduced.
- ***Renal ultrasonography*** is done to evaluate kidney size. In long-standing CRF, kidney size decreases as nephrons are destroyed and kidney mass is reduced.
- ***Kidney biopsy*** may be done to identify the underlying disease process if this is unclear. It is also used to identify an acute process from chronic failure. Kidney biopsy may be performed in surgery or done percutaneously using needle biopsy.

Medications

Chronic kidney disease affects both the pharmacokinetic and pharmacodynamic effects of drug therapy. Most medications are excreted primarily by the kidney. The half-life and plasma levels of many drugs increase in chronic kidney disease. Drug absorption may be decreased when phosphate-binding agents are administered concurrently. Proteinuria can significantly reduce plasma protein levels, leading to manifestations of toxicity when highly protein-bound drugs are given. In addition, any potentially nephrotoxic agent is avoided or used with extreme caution. Drugs such as meperidine, metformin (Glucophage), and other oral hypoglycemic agents eliminated by the kidney are avoided entirely. NSAIDs, which may cause a further decline in kidney function, are avoided (Shields et al., 2018). Because the kidneys are the primary route of magnesium excretion, magnesium-containing antacids and laxatives are avoided in CKD (Shields et al., 2018).

ACE inhibitors and ARBs have been shown to reduce proteinuria and slow the progression of CKD (Shields et al., 2018) and are often used for this purpose. Diuretics such as furosemide or other loop diuretics may be prescribed to reduce extracellular fluid volume and edema. Diuretic therapy can reduce hypertension and cause potassium wasting, lowering serum potassium levels. Other antihypertensive agents, particularly the calcium channel blockers diltiazem (Cardizem, others) and verapamil (Calan, Isoptin, others), are used to maintain the blood pressure within normal levels, slow the progress of renal failure, and prevent complications of coronary heart disease and cerebrovascular disease.

Patients with CKD have a significantly increased risk for cardiovascular disease and premature death. Numerous randomized controlled trials have demonstrated the benefit of statin drugs in reducing cardiovascular mortality in patients with CKD (Shields et al., 2018).

Other drugs may be used to manage electrolyte imbalances and acidosis. Sodium bicarbonate or calcium carbonate may be used to correct mild acidosis. Oral phosphorus binding agents such as calcium carbonate or calcium acetate are given to lower serum phosphate levels and normalize serum calcium levels. Phosphate binders such as lanthanum (Fosrenol) or sevelamer (Renagel) may be used as alternates to calcium-containing products. Drugs that can promote potassium retention (such as potassium-sparing diuretics, NSAIDs, ACE inhibitors, and ARBs) are eliminated if measures such as dietary potassium restriction fail to prevent hyperkalemia (Shields et al., 2018). If the serum potassium rises to dangerously high levels, a combination of bicarbonate, insulin, and glucose may be given intravenously to promote potassium movement into the cells. Sodium polystyrene sulfonate (Kayexalate), a potassium–ion exchange resin, can be given either orally or rectally (as an enema).

Folic acid and iron supplements are given to combat anemia associated with chronic renal failure. A multiple vitamin preparation is often prescribed because anorexia, nausea, and dietary restrictions may limit nutrient intake. Epoetin alfa (Epogen, Procrit, human recombinant erythropoietin) or darbepoetin (Aranesp) is used to stimulate red blood cell production in patients with CKD who are severely anemic. These drugs are not without risk: Hypertension is a common adverse effect, and adverse cardiovascular events such as stroke and thromboembolism have occurred (Shields et al., 2018).

Nutrition

Maintaining adequate nutrition and preventing protein-calorie malnutrition are the focus of nutritional management during early stages of CKD. As renal function declines, the elimination of water, solutes, and metabolic wastes is impaired. Accumulation of these wastes in the body leads to uremic symptoms. Dietary modifications can slow the progress of nephron destruction, reduce uremic symptoms, and help prevent complications.

Unlike carbohydrates and fats, the body is unable to store excess proteins. Unused dietary proteins are degraded into urea and other nitrogenous wastes, which are then eliminated by the kidneys. Protein-rich foods contain inorganic ions such as hydrogen ion, phosphate, and sulfites that are eliminated by the kidneys. A daily protein intake of 0.6 to 0.75 g/kg of body weight, or approximately 40 to 50 g/day for an average male patient, provides the amino acids necessary for tissue repair. The majority of proteins should be of high biologic value, rich in the essential amino acids. Carbohydrate and fat intake is increased to maintain energy requirements and provide approximately 35 kcal/kg per day.

Sodium intake is regulated to help manage hypertension and maintain the extracellular fluid volume at normal levels. Sodium is restricted to 3 g/day initially (mild restriction) or to 2 g/day if necessary to control hypertension and prevent heart failure (Sorenson et al., 2019). More stringent sodium restriction may be necessary as renal failure progresses. Unless hyponatremia is present, the patient is instructed to drink adequate water to prevent thirst. The patient is instructed to monitor weight daily and report any weight gain in excess of 2.3 kg (5 lb) over a 2-day period.

In stages 4 and 5, intake of potassium and phosphorus is restricted. Potassium intake is limited to less than 2 g/day (normal intake is about 3 g/day). The patient is cautioned to avoid using salt substitutes, which typically contain high levels of potassium chloride. Intake of phosphorus is limited to 800 to 1000 mg/day (the usual daily intake is 1000 to 1200 mg/day). Foods high in phosphorus include eggs, dairy products, and meat.

Renal Replacement Therapies

When pharmacologic and dietary management strategies are no longer effective to maintain fluid and electrolyte balance and prevent uremia, dialysis or kidney transplantation is considered.

A number of considerations affect the choice of long-term treatment. Hemodialysis and peritoneal dialysis each have advantages and disadvantages. Establishing vascular access for hemodialysis may take several months. Planning ahead to develop the access before dialysis is necessary can ease the transition to dialysis. Established access is not a consideration for peritoneal dialysis. The peritoneal catheter can be placed and treatment initiated as soon as it is indicated. When dialysis treatments will be performed at home, initiating instruction before it is required can result in more effective learning. If a family member will serve as a dialysis helper, training begins prior to the onset of uremia.

If transplantation is considered, tissue typing and identification of potential living related donors can be done prior to the onset of ESRD. To make an informed decision, both the patient and the potential donor need to understand the risks, benefits, and options available. If the decision for transplant is made early, dialysis can potentially be avoided. The patient's age, concurrent health problems, donor availability, and personal preference influence the choice of renal replacement therapy.

Dialysis. Approximately 70% of all people being treated for ESRD in the United States are receiving dialysis at an average maintenance cost of about $87,945 per year for hemodialysis patients and $71,630 for patients using peritoneal dialysis (United States Renal Data System [USRDS], 2013). For the patient who is not a candidate for renal transplantation or who has had a transplant failure, dialysis is life-sustaining.

The most common therapies for ESRD in the United States are hemodialysis performed in a dialysis center, followed by kidney transplant and peritoneal dialysis (USRDS, 2013). Both hemodialysis and peritoneal dialysis can be done in the home, but few patients use home hemodialysis. Of the two, peritoneal dialysis is typically the choice for at-home treatment. Because the morbidity and mortality for each are comparable, factors such as the desire and ability to manage home care, employment, and availability of a dialysis center become the primary factors influencing the choice of hemodialysis or peritoneal dialysis.

Patients on long-term dialysis have a higher risk for complications and death than the general population. Many have other chronic diseases along with ESRD. Infection and cardiovascular disease are common causes of illness and death. The 1-year survival rate for patients receiving dialysis is nearly 80%; long-term survival, however, falls to 35.8% at 5 years (Inker et al., 2014).

The decision to initiate dialysis is not easy. Like insulin therapy for people with diabetes, dialysis manages the symptoms of ESRD but does not cure it. Dialysis is a constant factor of life, requiring thinking and planning ahead at all times. Patients on dialysis may not be able to maintain a job. Families often fall apart with the day-to-day stress. Even with dialysis, the patient may have constant flulike symptoms, never feeling truly well. Patients on hemodialysis may feel powerless because of their dependence on others for treatment. On the other hand, home peritoneal dialysis places a continuing burden on the patient to maintain treatment. In the end, the patient may choose to discontinue treatment, preferring death over continued dialysis.

Hemodialysis for ESRD is typically done three times a week for a total of 9 to 12 hours per week. The amount of dialysis needed (or *dialysis dose*) is individually determined by factors such as body size, residual renal function, dietary intake, and concurrent illness. Hypotension and muscle cramps are common complications during hemodialysis treatments. Infection and vascular access problems are common long-term complications of hemodialysis. Cardiovascular disease is the leading cause of death for patients receiving hemodialysis. The death rate from cardiovascular disease is higher in patients on hemodialysis than those on peritoneal dialysis or who have had a kidney transplant for reasons that are unclear (NIDDK, 2016). See the previous section on AKI and Box 28.2 for more information about hemodialysis and related nursing care.

Peritoneal dialysis is currently used by approximately 5% of people who require long-term dialysis in the United States. In Canada and Europe, 35 to 45% of patients with ESRD are treated with peritoneal dialysis.

In underdeveloped countries, peritoneal dialysis is used to treat the majority of patients with ESRD (USRDS, 2013).

Continuous ambulatory peritoneal dialysis (CAPD) is the most common form of peritoneal dialysis used. Dialysate (2 L) is instilled into the peritoneal cavity, and the catheter is sealed. The patient can then continue normal daily activities, emptying the peritoneal cavity and replacing the dialysate three to five times per day. No special equipment is needed. A variation of CAPD is *continuous cyclic peritoneal dialysis (CCPD)*, which uses a delivery device during nighttime hours and a continuous dwell (dialysate retained in the peritoneal cavity) during the day. CAPD can be performed anywhere, and CCPD allows for home treatment at night, leaving the patient free during the day.

Peritoneal dialysis has several advantages over hemodialysis. Heparinization and vascular complications associated with an AV fistula are avoided. The clearance of metabolic wastes is slower but more continuous, avoiding rapid fluctuations in extracellular fluid composition and associated symptoms. More liberal intake of fluids and nutrients is often allowed for the patient on CAPD. While glucose absorbed from dialysate can increase blood glucose levels in an individual with diabetes, regular insulin can be added to the infusion to manage hyperglycemia. The patient on peritoneal dialysis is better able to self-manage the treatment regimen, reducing feelings of helplessness.

The major disadvantages of peritoneal dialysis include less effective metabolite elimination and risk of infection (peritonitis). Peritoneal dialysis may not be effective for large patients with no residual kidney function. Metabolic complications of peritoneal dialysis are common, including weight gain, hyperglycemia, and hypoproteinemia. Absorption of dextrose from the dialysate can add several hundred calories daily, while albumin and other proteins are lost across the peritoneal membrane. Finally, the presence of an indwelling peritoneal catheter may cause a body image disturbance. See Box 28.2 and Box 28.3 for more information about nursing care for patients undergoing hemodialysis and peritoneal dialysis.

Kidney Transplantation. Kidney transplantation has become the treatment of choice for many patients with ESRD. Kidneys are the solid organs most commonly transplanted, and to date kidney transplantation is the most successful of transplantation procedures. The first kidney transplant was performed in 1954; the donor and recipient were identical twins. Kidney transplantation as a treatment for ESRD is limited primarily by availability of organs. In 2016, over 19,000 people received a kidney transplant; however, based on Organ Procurement and Transportation Network (OPTN) data as of December 2016, more than 93,000 people are currently awaiting a transplant (Hart et al., 2018).

Kidney transplant improves both survival and quality of life for the patient with ESRD. The patient on dialysis has an 80% probability of surviving after a year of dialysis; the transplant recipient has a greater than 91.7% probability of survival after a year. At 5 years, the difference is even greater: 35.8% for dialysis compared with more than 84.6% for transplant (NIDDK, 2016). The transplant patient is no longer tethered to a dialysis catheter, machine, or center. Dietary and fluid restrictions are reduced, and the body image is more whole.

Most transplanted kidneys are obtained from deceased donors (70.7% in 2017); however, transplants from living donors are increasing. In 2017, of transplanted kidneys, 29.3% came from living donors, most of whom were related to the recipient (United Network for Organ Sharing [UNOS], 2018). With both deceased- and living-donor transplants, a close match between blood and tissue type is desired. In general, a match of ABO blood group is necessary; that is, the donor and recipient must share the same blood group (A, B, or O). Human leukocyte antigens (HLAs) are compared between the donor and recipient; six antigens in common are considered to be a "perfect" match. The success of well-matched living-donor transplants is better than for deceased donor organ transplants, with a 1-year graft survival of 95.1% compared to 89% for deceased-donor transplants (Hart et al., 2018). Close tissue matching probably accounts for the better outcome with living donors. People with normal kidneys who are in good physical health may donate a kidney. Predonation counseling is vital: Although a laparoscopic approach may be used to remove the donor's kidney, there is a risk that trauma or disease may damage the remaining kidney in the future. If the transplant fails, the psychologic impact on the donor can be significant. See Box 28.1 for nursing care of the patient having a nephrectomy.

Ideally, deceased donor kidneys are obtained from people who meet the criteria for brain death, are less than 60 years old, and are free of systemic disease, malignancy, or infection, including HIV and hepatitis B or C. Expanded deceased donor criteria may allow donation of a kidney from a deceased donor who is older than 60 years or who has cardiovascular disease (hypertension or stroke) or an elevated serum creatinine (OPTN, 2018). Kidneys are removed after brain death has been determined and are preserved by hypothermia or a technique called *continuous hypothermic pulsatile perfusion*. A kidney preserved by hypothermia is transplanted within 24 to 48 hours. Continuous pulsatile perfusion allows up to 3 days before transplantation. The system used to allocate deceased donor kidneys for transplantation is outlined in **Box 28.4**.

The donor kidney is placed in the lower abdominal cavity of the recipient, and the renal artery, vein, and ureter are anastomosed (**Figure 28.10** ■). The renal artery of the donor kidney is connected to the hypogastric artery and the renal vein to the iliac vein. The ureter is connected to one of the recipient's ureters or directly to the bladder, using a tunnel technique to prevent reflux.

Unless the donor and recipient are identical twins, the grafted organ stimulates an immune response to reject the transplanted organ. Immunosuppressive drugs minimize this response. Azathioprine or mycophenolate mofetil are commonly used, often in combination with prednisone, a corticosteroid. Cyclosporine, a potent immunosuppressive, may also be used. These drugs suppress a portion of the immune system and the inflammatory response, increasing the risk for infections and cancers with long-term

BOX 28.4
How Deceased Donor Kidneys Are Allocated for Transplant

The scarcity of organs for transplant raises questions about how deceased donor kidneys are allocated—who receives a kidney and who does not. Past inequities in the allocation process (e.g., more men than women, more Caucasians than people of other ethnicities, more rich than poor, and more young than old) led to the development of the United Network for Organ Sharing (UNOS) in 1986. UNOS has policies for organ distribution, including kidneys, hearts, livers, and other transplanted organs. In 2014, UNOS developed a new kidney allocation system. The new allocation system has multiple components including expanded donor quality metrics, a recipient predictive score for post-transplant survival, adjustments for patients with positive tissue typing (HLA antigens), and expansion of priority for pediatric candidates. In addition, modifications to variances related to rare blood types has also been incorporated (Organ Procurement and Transplantation Network [OPTN], 2018).

UNOS maintains national, regional, and local lists of patients awaiting transplants. When an organ becomes available, donor information is entered into the UNOS computer. The computer then runs a match program, generating a list of patients ranked by criteria such as blood and tissue type, organ size, and medical urgency of the patient. Factors such as time on the waiting list and distance between the donor and the transplant center are also considered. A candidate with a perfect match (six HLAs in common) and compatible blood type gets priority for the kidney, regardless of region or geographic area. Otherwise, the list of patients in the local area is checked first, then the regional list of patients awaiting transplant. If no match is found in the region, the organ becomes available to patients nationwide.

The UNOS allocation system, standardized fees, and Medicare coverage for transplantation have done much to ensure equitable access to available kidneys. Still, controversy exists. Patients with resources for travel may register in several different regions for an organ. A transplantation center can accept or reject a candidate for transplant who has lost a kidney because of noncompliance.

As long as the demand for kidneys exceeds the supply of donor organs, it is likely that controversy will exist regarding their allocation. Nurses can help by identifying potential donors and contacting the transplant coordinator. In addition, nurses can inform the public about organ donation and the allocation system and encourage donation.

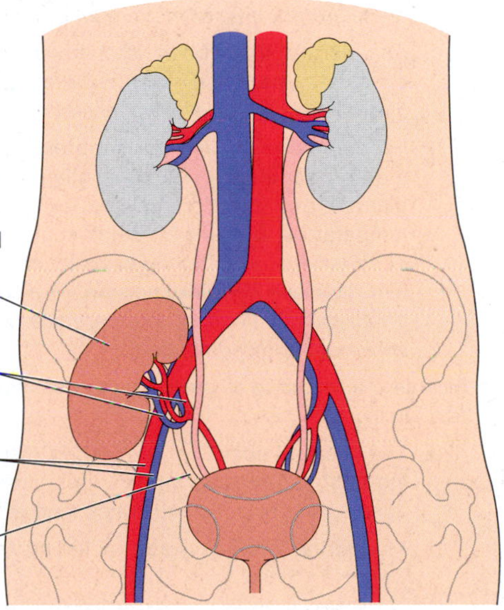
Transplanted kidney
Internal iliac artery and vein
External iliac artery and vein
Grafted ureter

Figure 28.10 ■ Placement of a transplanted kidney in the iliac fossa with anastomosis to the hypogastric artery, iliac vein, and bladder.

therapy. Glucocorticoids such as prednisone and methylprednisolone are used for both maintenance of immunosuppression and to treat acute rejection episodes. Side effects of long-term corticosteroid use include impaired wound healing, emotional disturbances, osteoporosis, and cushingoid effects on glucose, protein, and fat metabolism.

Azathioprine inhibits both cellular and humoral immunity. Because the liver rapidly metabolizes this drug, the dose may not need to be altered in the presence of renal failure. Bone marrow suppression, abnormalities of liver function, and alopecia are the primary significant adverse effects for azathioprine. The action of mycophenolate mofetil is similar to that of azathioprine. Its advantages are minimal bone marrow suppression and increased potency in preventing or reversing rejection of the transplanted organ (Shields et al., 2018).

Cyclosporine primarily affects cellular immunity, the helper T cells in particular. Among its many adverse effects, which include hepatotoxicity and hirsutism, nephrotoxicity is a primary concern for the patient undergoing a kidney transplant.

Even with immunosuppressive therapy, the transplanted kidney can be rejected at any time. Either acute or chronic rejection may develop. *Acute rejection* develops within months of the transplant. It is caused by a cellular immune response with T-lymphocyte proliferation (Sorenson et al., 2019). Few manifestations may be apparent other than a rise in serum creatinine and possible oliguria. Methylprednisolone, a glucocorticoid, and OKT3 monoclonal antibody are used to manage acute rejection episodes. OKT3 can cause severe systemic reactions, including chills, fever, hypotension, headache, and possible pulmonary edema. *Chronic rejection*, which may develop months to years following the transplant, is a major cause of graft loss. Both humoral and cellular immune responses are involved in chronic rejection. It does not respond to increased immunosuppression. The presenting manifestations of chronic rejection—progressive azotemia, proteinuria, and hypertension—are those of progressive renal failure.

Hypertension is a possible complication of kidney transplant, resulting from graft rejection, renal artery stenosis, or renal vasoconstriction. Patients may develop glomerular lesions and manifestations of nephrosis. Hypertension and altered blood lipids (increased LDLs and decreased HDLs) increase the risk of death from myocardial infarction and stroke following transplant.

Long-term immunosuppression has adverse effects as well. Infection is a continuing threat. Bacterial and viral infections may develop, as well as fungal infections of the blood, lungs, and CNS. Tumors are common, with carcinoma in situ of the cervix, lymphomas, and skin cancers most prevalent. The risk of congenital anomalies is increased in infants whose mothers have undergone immunosuppressive therapy. Corticosteroid use may lead to bone problems, gastrointestinal disorders such as peptic ulcer disease, and cataract formation. **Box 28.5** outlines the nursing care of the patient having kidney transplantation.

Nursing Care

Assessment

Both subjective and objective data are used to assess the patient with CKD:

- ***Health history:*** Complaints of anorexia, nausea, weight gain, or edema; current treatment (if any), including type and frequency of dialysis or previous kidney

BOX 28.5
Nursing Care of the Patient Having Kidney Transplantation

PREOPERATIVE CARE

- Provide routine preoperative care.
- Assess knowledge and feelings about the procedure, answering questions and clarifying information as needed. Listen and address concerns about surgery, the source of the donor organ, and possible complications. *Addressing concerns and reducing preoperative anxiety improve postoperative recovery.*
- Continue dialysis as ordered. *Continued renal replacement therapy is necessary to manage fluid and electrolyte balance and prevent uremia prior to surgery.*
- Administer immunosuppressive drugs as ordered before surgery. *Immunosuppression is initiated before transplantation to prevent immediate graft rejection.*
- Report abnormal or unexpected laboratory values to the surgical team. *Significant hyperkalemia increases the risk for intraoperative cardiac dysrhythmias (National Kidney Foundation, 2017).*

POSTOPERATIVE CARE

- Provide routine postoperative care.
- Maintain urinary catheter patency and a closed system. *Catheter patency is vital to keep the bladder decompressed and prevent pressure on suture lines. A closed drainage system minimizes the risk for urinary tract infection.*
- Measure urine output every 30 to 60 minutes initially. *Careful assessment of urine output helps determine fluid balance and transplant function. Acute tubular necrosis is a common early complication, usually due to tissue ischemia during the period between removal of the kidney from the donor and transplantation. Oliguria is an early sign.*
- Monitor vital signs and hemodynamic pressures closely. *Diuresis may occur immediately, resulting in hypovolemia, low cardiac output, and impaired perfusion of the transplanted kidney.*
- Maintain fluid replacement, generally calculated to replace urine output over the previous 30 or 60 minutes, milliliter for milliliter. *Fluid replacement is vital to maintain vascular volume and tissue perfusion.*
- Administer diuretics as ordered. *Loop and/or osmotic diuretics such as furosemide or mannitol may be used to promote postoperative diuresis.*
- Remove the catheter within 2 to 3 days or as ordered. Encourage to void every 1 to 2 hours and assess frequently for signs of urinary retention following catheter removal. *The bladder may have atrophied prior to surgery, reducing its capacity. Urinary retention places stress on suture lines and increases the risk of infection.*
- Monitor serum electrolytes and renal function tests. *These tests are used to monitor graft function and fluid and electrolyte status. Electrolyte imbalances may develop as the transplanted kidney begins to function and diuresis occurs. Elevated serum creatinine and BUN levels may be early signs of rejection or graft failure.*
- Monitor for possible complications:
    a. *Hemorrhage* from an arterial or venous anastomosis can be either acute or insidious. Indicators include swelling at the operative site, increased abdominal girth, and signs of shock, including changes in vital signs and level of consciousness. *Hemorrhage is a surgical emergency, requiring prompt recognition and treatment to preserve the graft.*
    b. *Ureteral anastomosis failure* causes urine leakage into the peritoneal cavity. It may be marked by decreased urine output with abdominal swelling and tenderness. *Failure of the ureteral anastomosis requires surgical intervention.*
    c. *Renal artery thrombosis* is characterized by an abrupt onset of hypertension and reduced GFR. *Renal artery thrombosis can result in transplant failure.*
    d. *Infection* due to immunosuppression is an immediate and continuing risk. The inflammatory response is blunted, and infection may not significantly elevate the temperature. Monitor for signs such as change in level of consciousness, cloudy or malodorous urine, or purulent drainage from the incision. *Prevention and prompt treatment of infections are particularly important in the immunosuppressed patient.*
- Include the following in predischarge teaching for the patient and family:
    a. The use and effects of prescribed medications, including antihypertensive medications, immunosuppressive agents, prophylactic antibiotics, and others as ordered.
    b. Monitoring of vital signs (including temperature) and weight.
    c. Manifestations of organ rejection, such as swelling and tenderness over the graft site, fever, joint aches, weight gain, and decreased urinary output. Stress the importance of promptly reporting signs and symptoms to the physician.
    d. Ordered or recommended dietary restrictions such as restricted carbohydrate and sodium intake and increased protein intake.
    e. Measures to prevent infection, such as avoiding crowds and obviously ill individuals.

  The patient and family will manage care after discharge, and therefore need a good understanding of what to expect, how to monitor graft status, and measures to reduce the adverse effects of medications.
- Provide psychologic support, address concerns, and provide information as needed. *The patient knows that transplant success is not guaranteed. In addition, the patient has often been managing a chronic disease independently and is used to having a degree of control. Providing information and allowing the patient to retain control relieves anxiety and improves recovery.*

transplant; chronic diseases such as diabetes, heart failure, or kidney disease

- ***Physical assessment:*** Mental status; vital signs including temperature, heart and lung sounds, and peripheral pulses; urine output (if any); weight; skin color, moisture, condition; presence of edema (periorbital or dependent); bowel tones; presence and location of an AV fistula, shunt, graft, or peritoneal catheter.

Priorities of Care

Nursing care priorities for the patient with chronic kidney disease change over time. During stages 1 through 3, measures to support kidney function and prevent further damage are of highest priority. Maintaining fluid balance, preventing urinary tract infection, effectively managing diabetes and hypertension, and avoiding exposure to nephrotoxins are important nursing care priorities. With the onset of ESRD, the nurse collaborates with the interprofessional team in managing renal replacement therapies and patient responses to declining kidney function.

Diagnoses, Outcomes, and Interventions

Whether the patient with CKD and ESRD is facing long-term dialysis or renal transplantation, a number of nursing care needs can be identified. This section focuses on nursing care related to impaired renal function, nutritional deficits due to dietary restrictions and nausea, increased risk for infection, and changes in body image. See the Case Study & Nursing Care Plan on page 946 for additional potential nursing diagnoses and interventions for the patient with chronic kidney disease.

Monitor and Support Kidney Function. Chronic diseases such as diabetes mellitus and hypertension are the leading causes of CKD. As kidney and nephron function declines, the kidney is less able to maintain fluid and electrolyte balance and eliminate waste products from the body.

Expected Outcome: Patient will not experience adverse effects of declining kidney function.

The nurse will:

- Monitor intake and output, vital signs including orthostatic blood pressures, and weight. *These provide important data to identify changes in fluid volume. Weight changes are a more accurate indicator of fluid volume status in the oliguric or anuric patient than intake and output measurements.*
- Monitor respiratory status, including lung sounds, every 4 to 8 hours. *Fluid volume overload may lead to heart failure and possible pulmonary edema.*
- Monitor BUN, serum creatinine, eGFR, pH, electrolytes, and CBC. Report significant changes. *As renal function declines, the GFR falls and progressive azotemia with increasing BUN and serum creatinine is seen. Metabolic acidosis develops as the kidney is unable to eliminate hydrogen ions and conserve bicarbonate. Hyponatremia, hyperkalemia, hyperphosphatemia, and hypocalcemia are associated with renal failure. The RBC count, hemoglobin, and hematocrit decline due to deficient erythropoietin to stimulate cell production in the bone marrow. An acute fall in hemoglobin and hematocrit may indicate GI bleeding, a risk in patients with ESRD.*
- Report manifestations of electrolyte imbalances, such as cardiac dysrhythmias and other ECG changes, muscle tremors and possible tetany, and Kussmaul's respirations. *Manifestations of electrolyte imbalance may indicate the need for intervention.*
- Administer medications to treat electrolyte imbalances as ordered. *Medications may be prescribed to help maintain electrolyte and acid–base balance and prevent adverse effects of imbalances.*
- Collaborate with the patient who has diabetes to maintain the blood glucose within a range of 90 to 130 mg/dL. As appropriate, discuss the selection and use of oral hypoglycemic medications with the interprofessional team. *Evidence supports preventing hyperglycemia as a strategy to slow the progression of CKD (Neumiller & Hirsch, 2015). Selected oral hypoglycemic drugs may increase the risk for complications such as hypoglycemia, fluid and electrolyte imbalances, and metabolic acidosis.*
- Administer antihypertensive medications as ordered. *Hypertension management is an important factor in slowing the progression of CKD.*
- Time activities and procedures to allow rest periods. *The anemia associated with CKD may cause significant fatigue and activity intolerance.*

SAFETY ALERT: Monitor carefully for desired and adverse effects of all medications. Impaired renal function affects drug elimination and increases the risk for toxic effects. ■

Maintain Adequate Nutritional Intake. Anorexia and nausea and vomiting are common manifestations of ESRD and uremia. The patient often has a metallic taste and bad breath, which also diminish appetite. A diet restricted in protein and sodium will compound these problems. Food intake may be insufficient to meet metabolic needs. Catabolism, the breakdown of body proteins to meet energy needs, exacerbates azotemia and uremia.

Expected Outcome: Patient will maintain adequate nutritional status as evidenced by stable weight, body mass index (BMI), and laboratory values.

The patient will:

- Monitor food and nutrient intake as well as episodes of vomiting. *Careful monitoring helps determine the adequacy of intake.*
- Weigh daily before breakfast. *This provides the most accurate measurement. Remember that a gain of 1 kg (2.2 lb) or more over a 24-hour period is more likely to reflect fluid retention than a gain in body mass.*
- Administer antiemetic agents 30 to 60 minutes before eating. *Antiemetics reduce nausea and the risk of vomiting with food intake.*
- Assist with mouth care prior to meals and at bedtime. *Mouth care improves taste, stimulates the appetite, and maintains the integrity of oral mucous membranes.*

- Serve small meals and provide between-meal snacks. *Small meals are less likely to prompt nausea and help improve food intake.*
- Arrange for a dietary consultation. Provide preferred foods to the extent possible, and involve the patient in planning daily menus. Encourage family members to bring food as dietary restrictions allow. *Providing preferred foods within restrictions promotes intake.*
- Monitor nutritional status by tracking weight, laboratory values such as serum albumin and BUN, and anthropometric measurements. *Indicators of impaired nutrition develop gradually and may be subtle. Careful assessment is important.*
- Administer enteral or parenteral nutrition as prescribed. Routinely monitor blood glucose levels, and use strict aseptic technique when handling parenteral nutrition solutions and the venous access site. *When the patient is unable to consume adequate nutrients, enteral nutritional support is preferred. Parenteral nutrition may be necessary to prevent catabolism and increasing azotemia. Hyperglycemia and infection are risks associated with parenteral nutrition. Immune system suppression associated with renal failure further increases the risk for infection.*

Reduce Risk for Infection. Chronic kidney disease affects the immune system and leukocyte function, increasing susceptibility to infection. Invasive devices required for hemodialysis or peritoneal dialysis add to this risk. The patient who has had a kidney transplant remains on immunosuppressive therapy for life, further depressing the immune system and increasing the risk for infection.

Expected Outcome: Patient will remain free of infection or sepsis.

The nurse will:

- Use standard precautions and good hand hygiene technique at all times. *Hand hygiene is a primary means of preventing the transfer of organisms. Patients who are on hemodialysis or who have had blood transfusions to treat anemia have an increased risk for hepatitis B, hepatitis C, and HIV infection.*
- Monitor temperature and vital signs at least every 4 hours. *A low-grade fever or increased pulse rate may indicate an infection in the immunosuppressed patient.*
- Monitor WBC count and differential. *Increased WBCs may indicate a bacterial infection; decreased WBCs may indicate viral infection. A shift in the differential showing more immature WBCs (bands) in circulation is another indicator of infection.*
- Culture urine, peritoneal dialysis fluid, and other drainage as indicated. *Culture is done to verify the presence of pathogens.*
- Monitor clarity of dialysate return. *Dialysate should return clear in the patient undergoing peritoneal dialysis. Cloudy dialysate may indicate peritonitis, the most common complication of peritoneal dialysis, and should be reported and cultured.*
- Provide good respiratory hygiene including position changes, coughing, and deep breathing. *These measures improve clearance of respiratory secretions, reducing the risk for infection.*
- Restrict visits from obviously ill people. Teach the patient and family about the risk for infection and measures to reduce the spread of infection. *The patient's resistance to infection is impaired, necessitating extra caution in preventing unnecessary exposures.*

Moving Evidence into Action

Physical Activity in Patients with ESRD

Clinical Issue

Following kidney transplant, few interventions have been found to be effective in promoting and maintaining physical activity.

External Evidence

O'Brien, Hathaway, Russell, and Moore (2017) proposed use of the theory-based SystemCHANGE™ + Activity Tracker framework. The SystemCHANGE + Activity Tracker approach combines small, individual-driven exercise sessions for increasing physical activity with visual feedback from the wireless activity tracker. This feedback helps the kidney transplant recipient to evaluate their physical activity progress.

Internal Evidence

As part of the evaluation of internal evidence, one must consider the feasibility of implementing an innovative program such as SystemCHANGE™ to promote physical activity in the kidney transplant recipient population. Determining organizational buy-in is also an important consideration. The nurse should investigate organizational policies regarding innovative strategies and proprietary tools to promote physical activity.

Patient Considerations

The determination of use of proprietary tools to promote physical activity requires patient consideration. When planning for the use of equipment such as the described system, the nurse must consider the specific patient population and the individual willingness to use the equipment.

Putting the Pieces Together

Physical activity after kidney transplant is an important, but undersupported, lifestyle modification that helps to promote maximal function. Previous interventions to promote physical activity in this population have not been widely successful. Promoting physical activity in the kidney transplant recipient is a nursing responsibility. The SystemCHANGE + Activity Tracker approach may be an innovative strategy to get the kidney transplant recipient moving.

Reference

O'Brien, T., Hathaway, D., Russell, C. L., & Moore, S. (2017). Merging an activity tracker with SystemCHANGE™ to improve physical activity in older kidney transplant recipients. *Nephrology Nursing Journal, 44*(2), 153–157.

Promote Healthy Body Image. Chronic disease and impaired kidney function can affect a patient's body image. Hemodialysis requires an arteriovenous fistula or shunt; a permanent peritoneal catheter is required for peritoneal dialysis. Although kidney transplant can restore an image of wholeness, a visible scar remains and the organ may be perceived as "foreign."

Expected Outcome: Patient will acknowledge impact of CKD and treatment on roles, relationships, and lifestyle and express willingness to use available resources in developing an adaptive response to changes.

The nurse will:

- Involve the patient in care, including meal planning, dialysis, and catheter, port, or incision care to the extent possible. *Involvement improves acceptance and stimulates discussion about the effect of the disease and treatment measures on the patient's life.*
- Encourage expression of feelings and concerns, accepting perceptions and feelings without criticism. *Self-expression enhances the patient's self-worth and acceptance.*
- Include the patient in decision making and encourage self-care. *Increased autonomy enhances the patient's sense of control, independence, and self-worth.*
- Support positive gains, but do not support denial. *The patient may have difficulty accepting the renal failure, but adaptation to the loss is important.*
- Help the patient develop and achieve realistic goals. *Realistic goals allow the patient to see progress.*
- Provide positive reinforcement and feedback. *These measures support growth and adaptation.*
- Reinforce effective coping strategies. *Reinforcement helps the patient develop positive versus negative strategies for coping.*
- Facilitate contact with a support group or other community members affected by renal failure. *The patient benefits by providing and receiving support in a group of people going through similar circumstances.*
- Refer for mental health counseling as indicated or desired. *Counseling can help the patient develop effective coping and adaptation strategies.*

Delegating Nursing Care Activities

As appropriate and allowed by the designated duties and responsibilities of unlicensed assistive personnel, the nurse may delegate nursing care activities such as obtaining vital signs and daily weights and assisting with ambulation and ADLs for a patient with chronic kidney disease.

Transitions of Care

Chronic kidney disease and ESRD are long-term processes that require patient management. No matter what treatment option is chosen (hemodialysis, peritoneal dialysis, or renal transplantation), day-to-day management falls to the patient and family.

Measures to reduce the risk of CKD focus on preventing kidney disease and appropriately managing diabetes and hypertension. Promote early and effective treatment of all infections, particularly skin and pharyngeal infections caused by streptococcal bacteria. Discuss measures to reduce the risk for urinary tract infections, and stress the importance of prompt treatment to eradicate the infecting organism. Discuss the relationship among diabetes, hypertension, and kidney disease. Emphasize that maintaining blood glucose levels and blood pressure within the recommended ranges reduces the risk of adverse effects on the kidneys. Ensure that all patients with less than optimal renal function are well hydrated, particularly when a nephrotoxic drug is prescribed or anticipated. Finally, encourage the patient with CKD to investigate options for early transplantation to avoid long-term dialysis.

Teaching for home care includes the following topics:

- Nature of chronic kidney disease and renal failure, including expected progression and effects
- Monitoring of weight, vital signs, and temperature
- Prescribed medications, including purpose, intended effect, and potential adverse effects and their management
- Prescribed dietary restrictions (involve the patient, a dietitian, and the family member usually responsible for cooking. Include strategies to manage nausea and prevent thirst within allowed limits.)
- How to assess and protect a fistula or shunt for hemodialysis (or the extremity to be used if one is anticipated)
- Peritoneal catheter care and the procedure for peritoneal dialysis as indicated (include a family member or significant other, in case the patient is unable to perform the procedure independently at some time.)
- Following kidney transplant, prescribed medications, adverse effects and their management, infection prevention, graft protection, and manifestations of organ rejection
- The benefits of and strategies for incorporating physical activity into daily life and the treatment plan.

Refer to a dietitian for diet planning and counseling. If home hemodialysis is planned, refer the designated dialysis helper for formal training. Both the National Kidney Foundation and the American Association of Kidney Patients may be able to provide support and educational materials for the patient with ESRD. Local and state chapters of these organizations can provide additional support.

Case Study & Nursing Care Plan

A Patient with End-Stage Renal Disease

Walter Cohen, 45 years old, has had type 1 diabetes since the age of 20. He was diagnosed with diabetic nephropathy 10 years ago. Despite ACE inhibitor therapy, blood pressure control with antihypertensive medications, and frequent blood glucose monitoring with insulin coverage, he developed overt proteinuria 5 years ago and has now progressed to end-stage renal disease. He enters the nephrology unit for temporary hemodialysis and to prepare for home peritoneal dialysis.

ASSESSMENT

Mr. Cohen states that his diabetes has always been difficult to control. He has had numerous hypoglycemic episodes and has been hospitalized "several times" for ketoacidosis. Recently he has developed symptoms of peripheral neuropathy and increasing retinopathy. He attributed his lack of appetite, nausea and vomiting, and fatigue during the past month to "a touch of the flu." His weight remained stable, so he did not worry about not eating much.

Physical assessment findings include T 36.5°C (97.8°F) PO, P 96 bpm, R 20/min, and BP 178/100 mmHg. Skin cool and dry. Breath odor fetid. Scattered fine rales noted in bilateral lung bases. Soft S_3 gallop noted at cardiac apex. Bilateral pitting edema of lower extremities to just below the knees; fingers and hands edematous. Abdominal assessment essentially normal, with hypoactive bowel sounds. Urinalysis shows a specific gravity of 1.011, gross proteinuria, and multiple cell casts. CBC results: RBC 2.9 million/mm^3; hemoglobin 9.4 g/dL; hematocrit 28%. Blood chemistry abnormalities include BUN 198 mg/dL; creatinine 18.5 mg/dL; sodium 125 mEq/L; potassium 5.7 mEq/L; calcium 7.1 mg/dL; phosphate 6.8 mg/dL. A temporary jugular venous catheter will be placed for hemodialysis the next day, followed by peritoneal catheter insertion later in the week.

DIAGNOSES

- Imbalanced fluid volume related to failure of kidneys to eliminate excess body fluid
- Weight loss related to effects of uremia
- Infection due to invasive catheters and impaired immune function

EXPECTED OUTCOMES

- Patient will adhere to the prescribed fluid restriction of 900 mL/day.
- Patient will demonstrate reduced extracellular fluid volume by weight loss, decreased peripheral edema, clear lung sounds, and normal heart sounds.
- Patient will consume and retain 100% of prescribed diet, including snacks.
- Patient will remain free of infection.
- Patient will demonstrate appropriate peritoneal catheter care and CAPD.

PLANNING AND IMPLEMENTATION

- Collaborate with Mr. Cohen to distribute allowed fluids throughout the day.
- Provide mouth care at least every 4 hours and before every meal.
- Keep sugarless hard candy and ice chips at the bedside; include ice consumed as fluid intake.
- Weigh daily before breakfast; monitor vital signs, and heart and lung sounds, every 4 hours.
- Document intake and output every 4 hours.
- Arrange dietary consultation for menu planning.
- Administer prescribed antiemetic 1 hour before meals.
- Monitor food intake, noting percentage and types of food consumed.
- Teach CAPD procedure and peritoneal catheter care.
- Assist to identify strengths and needs in health regimen management.

EVALUATION

Mr. Cohen was hospitalized for 2 weeks, undergoing four hemodialysis sessions to reduce uremic symptoms. An arteriovenous fistula has been created in his left arm in case he should need hemodialysis in the future. He begins peritoneal dialysis the second week, and by discharge he is able to manage the catheter care and dialysis runs with the help of his wife. His heart and lung sounds are normal, and he has minimal peripheral edema on discharge. His temperature is normal, and no evidence of infection is noted. Mr. Cohen remains anorectic and slightly nauseated, but is eating most of his prescribed diet and snacks. He has lost 4.5 kg (10 lb) with excess fluid removal by dialysis, but his weight remains stable during the second week. Mr. Cohen and his wife have been introduced to another patient who has been on CAPD for several years and promises to help them with problem solving.

CLINICAL REASONING IN PATIENT CARE

1. Compare Mr. Cohen's CBC and chemistry values with normal ranges for these tests. Explain the pathologic processes contributing to changes from the normal. What nursing processes should you initiate to help ensure Mr. Cohen's safety and abilities to carry out his ADLs?
2. What are the safety implications of Mr. Cohen's peripheral neuropathy and increasing retinopathy? Identify nursing care measures to reduce his risk for injury.
3. How does diabetes mellitus damage the kidneys and lead to CKD? Why is this more significant for a patient with type 1 diabetes than for someone with type 2 diabetes?
4. Why do high levels of urea in the blood often cause changes in cognition and mental status? What manifestations of encephalopathy would you expect to see?
5. How might Mr. Cohen's insulin dosage and diet need to be changed with the institution of peritoneal dialysis? Why?

See Evaluating Your Response in Appendix B.

CHAPTER HIGHLIGHTS

28.1 Kidney Disorders

Describe the pathophysiology and manifestations of kidney disorders, including polycystic kidney disease, glomerular disorder, vascular kidney disorder, kidney trauma, and renal tumor, and outline the interprofessional care and nursing care of patients with these disorders.

- Congenital and acquired disorders of the kidneys can profoundly affect urinary elimination and ultimately all body systems.
- Glomerulonephritis, inflammation of the glomerulus of the kidney, leads to loss of proteins and blood cells in the urine, a decrease in the glomerular filtration rate, and severe edema.
- The renal and cardiovascular systems are closely interrelated. Vascular disorders, such as hypertension, renal artery stenosis, or obstruction of the renal artery or vein, can have serious consequences in terms of renal function.
- Renal cell malignancies, while uncommon, are often not evident until the cancer is advanced and has metastasized to other sites.

28.2 Kidney Failure

Describe the pathophysiology and manifestations of kidney failure (i.e., acute kidney injury and chronic kidney disease), and outline the interprofessional care and nursing care of patients with these disorders.

- Acute kidney injury is a frequent complication of hospitalization and critical illness that increases mortality, length of stay, costs, and the risk for subsequent chronic kidney disease. Nurses play a key role in preventing and recognizing acute kidney injury, thus minimizing its negative consequences.
- Ischemic and nephrotoxic damage to the kidney are the most common precipitating factors for AKI.
- Diabetes mellitus and hypertension are the leading causes of chronic kidney disease and kidney failure. Aggressive glycemic control and blood pressure management reduce the risk of kidney disease; likewise, early identification and effective management of chronic kidney disease can delay the onset of kidney failure.
- When the kidneys fail, renal replacement therapies are necessary to eliminate metabolic waste products and sustain life. Dialysis and kidney transplant are the primary renal replacement therapies used.

TEST YOURSELF NCLEX-RN® REVIEW

1. The community health nurse is presenting a seminar on "Keeping Your Kidneys Healthy." The nurse evaluates that a participant has achieved learning when which statement is made? (Select all that apply.)
   A. My kidneys help to regulate my blood pressure.
   B. If I develop diabetes my risk for kidney problems increases.
   C. Since I am under age 65, I don't yet need to be concerned about kidney problems.
   D. Since dialysis is widely available, I don't have to worry about developing kidney problems.
   E. Kidney disease is very rare among adults in the United States.
2. After being diagnosed with polycystic kidney disease, an adult patient asks if current children are at risk for developing the disorder. How should the nurse respond?
   A. The adult form of this disorder is rare and should not affect grown children.
   B. The children should undergo genetic testing and screening for evidence of the disease.
   C. Because the condition was just diagnosed, there is no risk of passing the condition on to any children.
   D. The children would have developed symptoms of the disorder in utero or shortly after birth if they had inherited the defective gene.
3. The nurse is completing a health history with a young adult patient diagnosed with acute postinfectious glomerulonephritis. When focusing on recent health problems, about which disease process should the nurse ask the patient? (Select all that apply.)
   A. Strep throat
   B. Urinary tract infection
   C. Gastrointestinal disorder
   D. Fractures or other musculoskeletal trauma
   E. Skin infection
4. The nurse is evaluating teaching provided to a patient with acute glomerulonephritis. Which patient action indicates that additional teaching is not necessary?
   A. Limits fluid intake to less than 1500 mL/day.
   B. Demonstrates care of the vascular access device for dialysis.
   C. Selects soy or animal proteins for allowed grams of protein in diet.
   D. States the need to remain on bedrest until urine returns to clear yellow.

5. A patient recovering from a partial nephrectomy is in the postanesthesia care unit. Which interventions would be a priority for this patient? (Select all that apply.)
   A. Irrigate all catheters with sterile normal saline.
   B. Label and secure all catheters, tubes, and drains.
   C. Administer cough suppressant medication as needed.
   D. Report the onset of bright red bleeding to the surgeon.
   E. Connect all catheters and drains to a single collection device.
6. The nurse is planning care to reduce the risk of a patient in the intensive care unit from developing acute kidney injury. Which intervention should the nurse implement for this patient?
   A. Administer antihypertensive drugs.
   B. Avoid all potentially nephrotoxic drugs.
   C. Maintain fluid volume and cardiac output.
   D. Assess for a history of diabetes or hypertension.
7. During a home visit the nurse evaluates discharge teaching provided to a patient recovering from an acute kidney injury. Which patient statement indicates that teaching has been effective?
   A. "I will eat only vegetable proteins."
   B. "I will avoid taking drugs that may harm my kidneys."
   C. "I will limit my fluid intake to 1500 mL or less per day."
   D. "I will catheterize myself for residual urine at least once a week."
8. The nurse is planning care for a patient beginning hemodialysis. What should be included in this patient's plan of care? (Select all that apply.)
   A. Restrict fluid and protein intake.
   B. Obtain weight and orthostatic vital signs.
   C. Determine urine specific gravity and pH.
   D. Monitor serum creatinine, BUN, and hematocrit levels.
   E. Assess blood pressure of extremity where fistula has been created.
9. The nurse is discussing the goals of treatment with a patient experiencing end-stage renal disease. Which goal should the nurse identify as being appropriate for this patient?
   A. Identify a live-in caregiver.
   B. Demonstrate the ability to independently perform hemodialysis in the home.
   C. State the advantages and disadvantages of types of renal replacement therapies.
   D. Relate the hospice philosophy and identify indicators of the need for hospice care.
10. Following a kidney transplant, the nurse notes that a patient's urine is cloudy. What should the nurse do about this finding?
   A. Record the finding.
   B. Notify the physician.
   C. Irrigate the urinary catheter.
   D. Increase the intravenous flow rate.

REFERENCES

Adams, M. P., Holland, L. N., & Urban, C. (2017). *Pharmacology for nursing: A pathophysiologic approach.* (5th ed.). Hoboken, NJ: Pearson Education.

American Cancer Society. (2018). *Cancer facts and figures 2018.* Atlanta, GA: Author. Retrieved from https://www.cancer.org/content/dam/cancer-org/research/cancer-facts-and-statistics/annual-cancer-facts-and-figures/2018/cancer-facts-and-figures-2018.pdf.

American Diabetes Association (ADA). (2018). *Kidney disease: Nephropathy.* Retrieved from www.diabetes.org/living-with-diabetes/complications/kidney-disease-nephropathy.html.

Centers for Disease Control and Prevention (CDC). (2017). *Kidney disease.* Retrieved from https://www.cdc.gov/nchs/fastats/kidney-disease.htm.

Doyle, J. F., & Forni, L. G. (2016). Acute kidney injury: Short-term and long-term effects. *Critical Care, 20,* 188. Retrieved from https://ccforum.biomedcentral.com/track/pdf/10.1186/s13054-016-1353-y.

Genetics Home Reference. (2018). *Polycystic kidney disease.* Retrieved from https://ghr.nlm.nih.gov/condition/polycystic-kidney-disease#statistics.

Hart, A., Smith, J. M., Skeans, M. A., Gustafson, S. K., Wilk, A. R., Robinson, A., . . . Israni, A. K. (2018). OPTN/SRTR 2016 Annual Data Report: Kidney. *American Journal of Transplantation, 18*(Suppl. 1), 18–113.

Inker, L. A., Astor, B. C., Fox, C. H., Iaskova, T., Lash, J. P., Peralta, C. A., . . . & Feldman, H. I. (2014). KDOQI US Commentary on the 2012 KDIGO Clinical Practice Guideline for the Evaluation and Management of CKD. *American Journal of Kidney Disease, 63*(5), 713–735. Retrieved from https://www.ajkd.org/article/S0272-6386(14)00491-0/pdf.

Kidney Disease: Improving Global Outcomes (KDIGO) Acute Kidney Injury Work Group. (2012). KDIGO Clinical Practice Guideline for Acute Kidney Injury. *Kidney International,* 2(Suppl. 2012), 1–138.

Lusaya, D. G. (2017). Renal trauma. *Medscape.* Retrieved from https://emedicine.medscape.com/article/440811-overview.

National Institute of Diabetes and Digestive and Kidney Disorders (NIDDK). (2016). *Kidney disease statistics for the United States.* Retrieved from https://www.niddk.nih.gov/health-information/health-statistics/kidney-disease.

National Institute of Diabetes and Digestive and Kidney Disorders (NIDDK). (2018). *Autosomal dominant polycystic kidney disease.* Retrieved from https://www.niddk.nih.gov/health-information/kidney-disease/polycystic-kidney-disease/autosomal-dominant-pkd.

National Kidney Foundation. (2017). Facts about high potassium in patients with kidney disease. Retrieved from https://www.kidney.org/atoz/content/hyperkalemia/facts.

Neumiller, J. J., & Hirsch, I. B. (2015). Management of hyperglycemia in diabetic kidney disease. *Diabetes Spectrum, 28*(3), 214–219.

O'Brien, T., Hathaway, D., Russell, C. L., & Moore, S. (2017). Merging an activity tracker with SystemCHANGE™ to improve physical activity in older kidney transplant recipients. *Nephrology Nursing Journal, 44*(2), 153–157.

Organ Procurement and Transplantation Network (OPTN). (2018). *Kidney Allocation System.* Retrieved from https://optn.transplant.hrsa.gov/learn/professional-education/kidney-allocation-system/.

Shields, K. M., Fox, K. L., & Liebrecht, C. (2018). *Pearson nurse's drug guide*. Boston, MA: Pearson.

Sorenson, M., Quinn, L., & Klein, D. (2019). *Pathophysiology: Concepts of human disease.* New York, NY: Pearson.

Spinowitz, B. S. (2017). Renal artery stenosis. *Medscape.* Retrieved from https://emedicine.medscape.com/article/245023-overview.

United Network for Organ Sharing (UNOS). (2018). Transplant trends. Retrieved from https://unos.org/data/transplant-trends/#transplants_by_donor_type+organ+Kidney

U.S. Renal Data System (USRDS). (2013). *USRDS 2013 annual data report: Atlas of chronic kidney disease and end-stage renal disease in the United States*. Bethesda, MD: National Institutes of Health, National Institute of Diabetes and Digestive and Kidney Diseases. Retrieved from https://www.usrds.org/2013/view/v2_11.aspx.

ADDITIONAL RESOURCES

American Nephrology Nurses Association
www.annanurse.org

The National Kidney Foundation
www.kidney.org

The National Kidney Foundation Kidney Disease Outcomes Quality Initiative (NKF KDOQI)
www.kidney.org/professionals/kdoqi/index.cfm

Kidney Early Evaluation Program (KEEP)
www.kidney.org/news/keep/index.cfm

Acute Kidney Injury Network
www.akinet.org

The Nephron Information Center
http://nephron.com

Kidney Disease/Improving Global Outcomes at
www.kdigo.org

Unit 8

Responses to Altered Cardiovascular Function

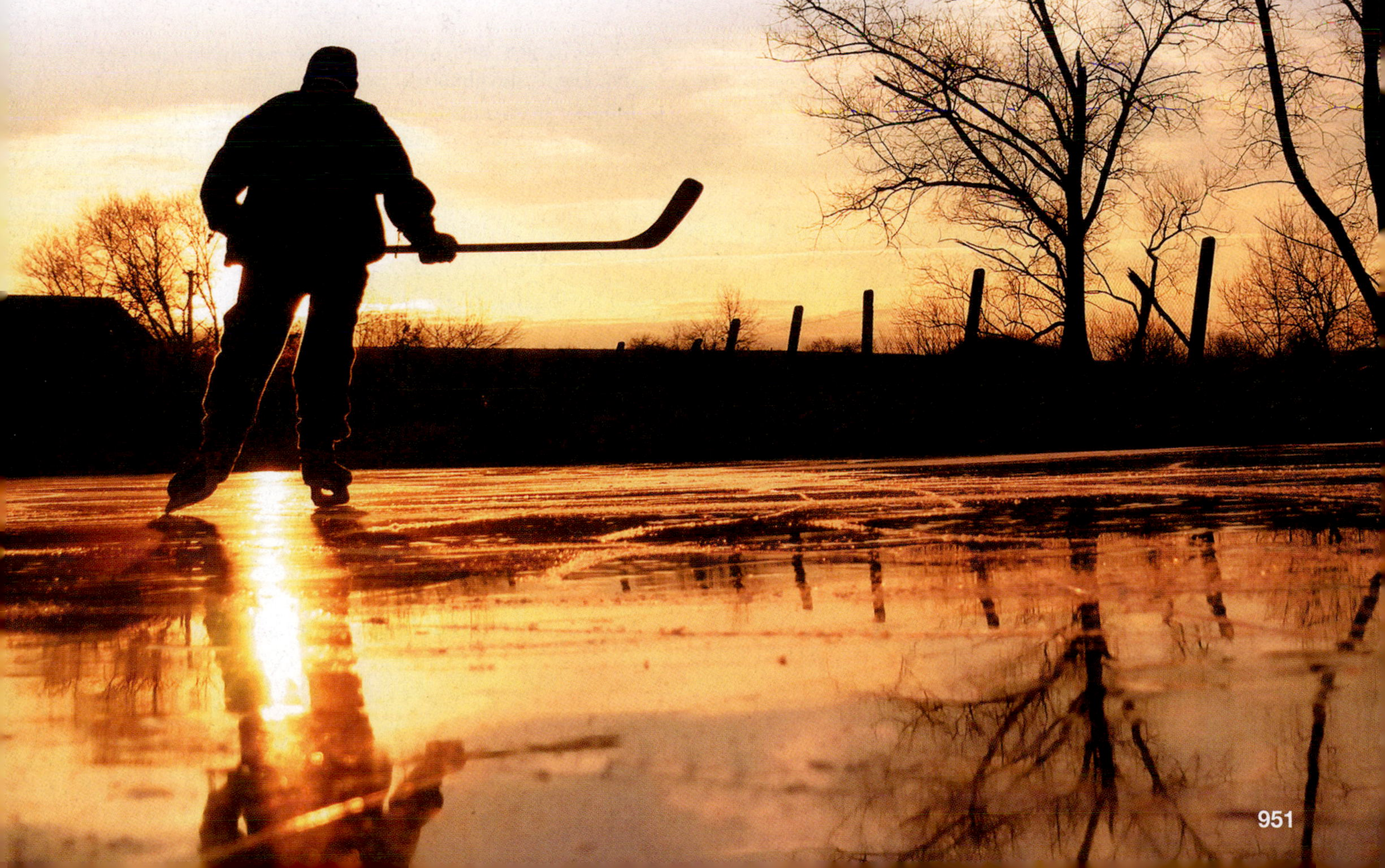

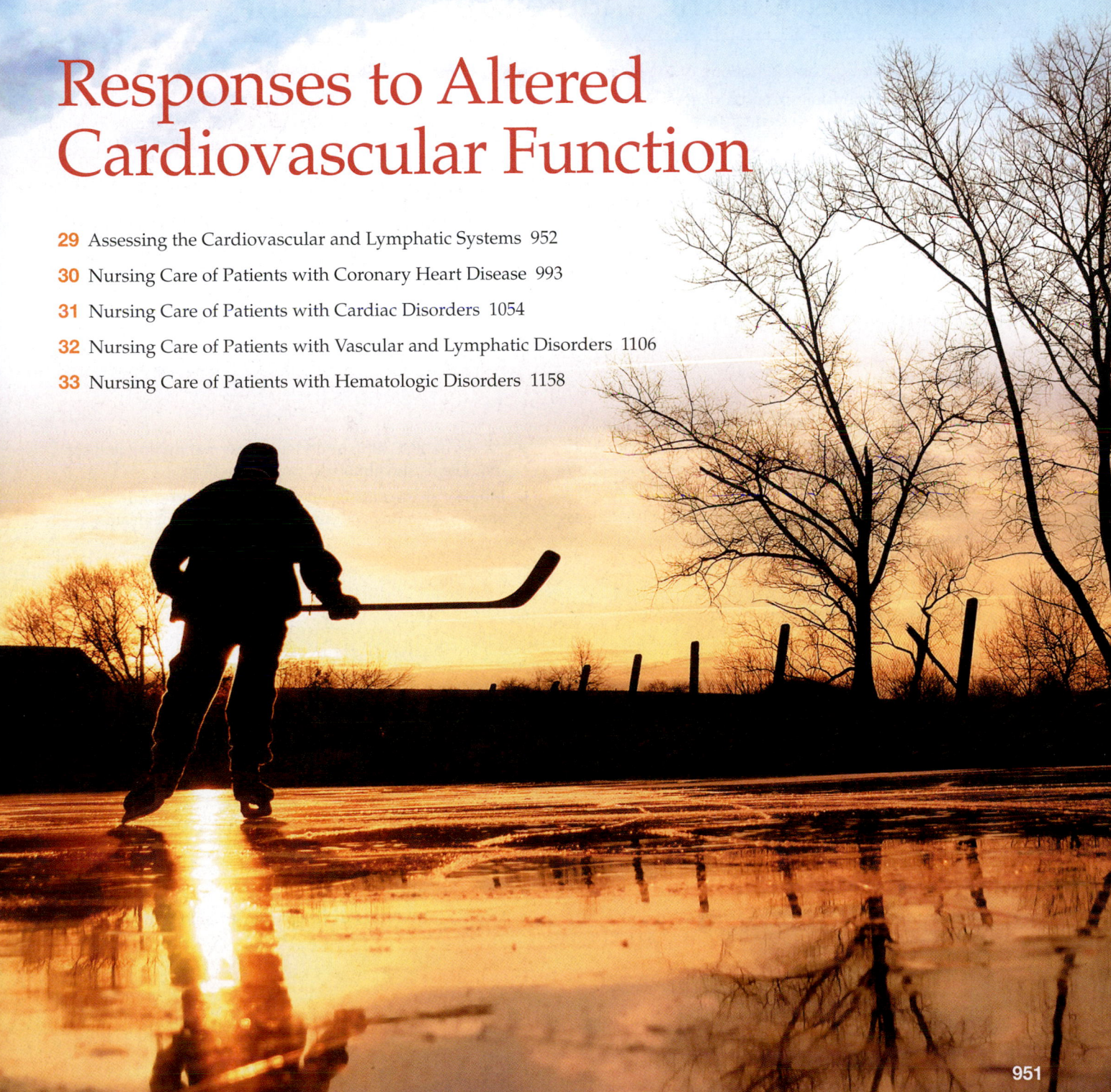

Chapter 29

Assessing the Cardiovascular and Lymphatic Systems

Chapter Outline and Learning Outcomes

CLINICAL COMPETENCIES

- Complete a health history for patients having alterations in the structure and functions of the cardiovascular or lymphatic systems.
- Conduct and document a physical assessment of cardiovascular and lymphatic status.
- Assess an ECG strip and identify normal rhythm and cardiac events and abnormal cardiac rhythm.
- Monitor the results of diagnostic tests and communicate abnormal findings within the interprofessional team.

KEY TERMS

apical impulse, 969
cardiac index (CI), 957
cardiac output (CO), 956
dysrhythmia, 971
heave, 969
hemostasis, 966
ischemic, 956
Korotkoff sounds, 973
lift, 969
lymphadenopathy, 977
lymphedema, 974
orthostatic hypotension, 973
retraction, 969
thrill, 970
thrust, 969

EQUIPMENT NEEDED

- Stethoscope with a diaphragm and a bell
- Blood pressure cuff
- Good light source
- Watch with a second hand
- Centimeter ruler
- Tape measure
- Doppler ultrasound device (if needed) and transducer gel

The cardiovascular system is comprised of the heart (the system's pump), the peripheral vascular system (a network of arteries, veins, and capillaries), and the hematologic system (blood and blood components). The lymphatic system (the lymph, lymph nodes, and spleen) is a special vascular system that helps maintain sufficient blood volume in the cardiovascular system by picking up excess tissue fluid and returning it to the bloodstream.

The heart beats an average of 80 times per minute, or once every 0.86 seconds, every minute of an individual's life. As the heart ejects blood with each beat, a closed system of blood vessels transports oxygenated blood to all body organs and tissues and then returns deoxygenated blood to the heart for reoxygenation in the lungs. Deficits in the structure or function of the cardiovascular and lymphatic system may adversely affect all body tissues and may affect self-care, mobility, comfort, self-concept, sexuality, and role performance.

29.1 Anatomy, Physiology, and Functions of the Heart

The *heart* is a hollow, cone-shaped organ approximately the size of an adult man's fist. Beating from 60 to 100 beats each minute for a lifetime, it moves more than 1800 gallons of blood each day (Sorenson, Quinn, & Klein, 2018). Located in the mediastinum of the thoracic cavity, between the vertebral column and the sternum, the heart is flanked laterally by the lungs. The heart weighs < 0.5 kg (1 lb) in a normal healthy adult. Two-thirds of the heart mass lies to the left of the sternum; the upper base lies beneath the second rib, and the pointed apex is approximate with the fifth intercostal space, midpoint to the clavicle (**Figure 29.1** ■).

The heart is covered by the *pericardium*, a double layer of fibroserous membrane (**Figure 29.2** ■). The pericardium encases the heart and anchors it to surrounding structures, forming the pericardial sac. The snug fit of the pericardium prevents the heart from overfilling with blood. The outermost layer is the parietal pericardium; the visceral pericardium (or epicardium) adheres to the heart surface. The small space between the visceral and parietal layers of the pericardium is called the *pericardial cavity*, and 10 to 30 mL of a serous lubricating fluid produced in this space cushions the heart as it beats.

The heart wall consists of three layers of tissue: The epicardium, the myocardium, and the endocardium (see Figure 29.2). The *epicardium* covers the entire heart and great vessels, and then folds over to form the parietal layer that lines the pericardium and adheres to the heart surface. The *myocardium*, the middle layer of the heart wall, consists of specialized cardiac muscle cells (myofibrils) that provide the bulk of contractile heart muscle. The *endocardium* is a thin three-layer membrane that lines the inside of the heart's chambers and great vessels.

Chambers and Valves of the Heart

The heart has two upper atria and two lower ventricles. They are separated longitudinally by the interventricular septum (**Figure 29.3** ■). The *right atrium* receives

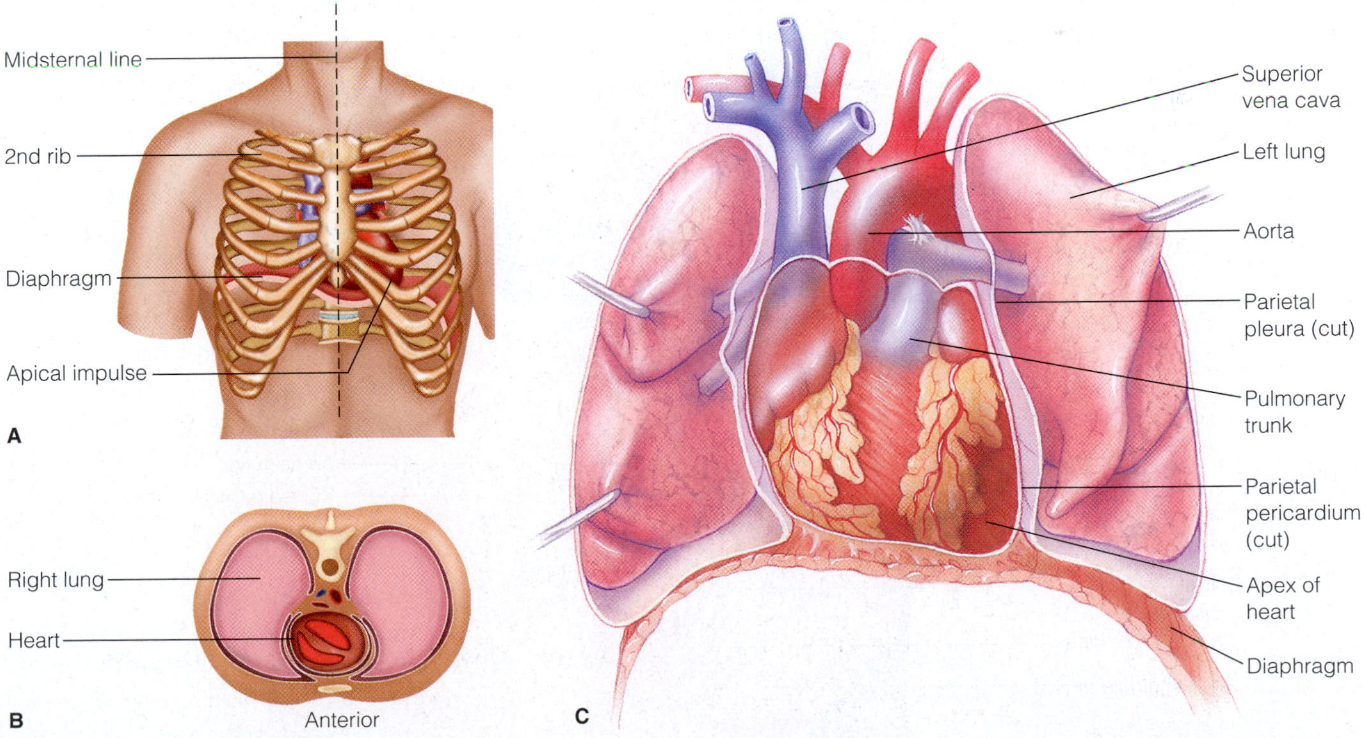
Midsternal line
2nd rib
Diaphragm
Apical impulse
A
Right lung
Heart
Anterior
B
C
Superior vena cava
Left lung
Aorta
Parietal pleura (cut)
Pulmonary trunk
Parietal pericardium (cut)
Apex of heart
Diaphragm

Figure 29.1 ■ Location of the heart in the mediastinum of the thorax. **A**, Relationship of the heart to the sternum, ribs, and diaphragm. **B**, Cross-sectional view showing relative position of the heart in the thorax. **C**, Relationship of the heart and great vessels to the lungs.

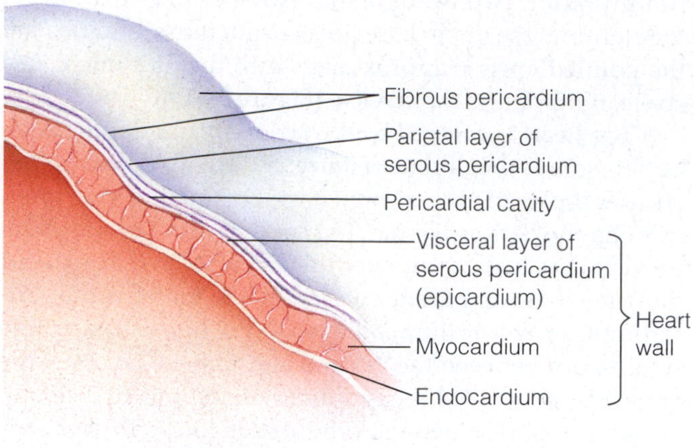
Fibrous pericardium
Parietal layer of serous pericardium
Pericardial cavity
Visceral layer of serous pericardium (epicardium)
Myocardium
Endocardium
Heart wall

Figure 29.2 ■ Coverings and layers of the heart.

deoxygenated blood from the veins of the body: The *superior vena cava* returns blood from the body area above the diaphragm, the *inferior vena cava* returns blood from the body below the diaphragm, and the coronary sinus drains blood from the heart. The *left atrium* receives freshly oxygenated blood from the lungs through the pulmonary veins. The *right ventricle* receives deoxygenated blood from the right atrium and pumps it through the pulmonary artery to the pulmonary capillary bed for oxygenation. The newly oxygenated blood then travels through the pulmonary veins to the left atrium. Blood enters the left atrium and crosses the mitral (bicuspid) valve into the *left ventricle*. Blood is then pumped out of the aorta to the arterial circulation.

The heart's chambers are each separated by a valve that allows unidirectional blood flow to the next chamber or great vessel (see Figure 29.3). The atria are separated from the ventricles by the two *atrioventricular (AV) valves*; the tricuspid valve is on the right side, and the bicuspid (or mitral) valve is on the left. The flaps of each of these valves are anchored to the papillary muscles of the ventricles by the *chordae tendineae*. These structures control the movement of the AV valves to prevent backflow of blood. The ventricles are connected to their great vessels by the *semilunar valves*. On the right, the pulmonary (pulmonic) valve joins the right ventricle with the pulmonary artery. On the left, the aortic valve joins the left ventricle to the aorta. Closure of the AV valves at the onset of contraction (systole) produces the first heart sound, or S_1 (characterized by the syllable *lub*); closure of the semilunar valves at the onset of relaxation (diastole) produces the second heart sound, or S_2 (characterized by the syllable *dub*).

Systemic, Pulmonary, and Coronary Circulation

Because each side of the heart both receives and ejects blood, the heart is often described as a double pump. Blood enters the right atrium and moves to the pulmonary bed at almost the exact same time that blood is entering the left atrium. The circulatory system has two parts: The systemic circulation (a high-pressure system), which supplies blood to all other body tissues, and the pulmonary circulation (a low-pressure system). The *systemic circulation* consists

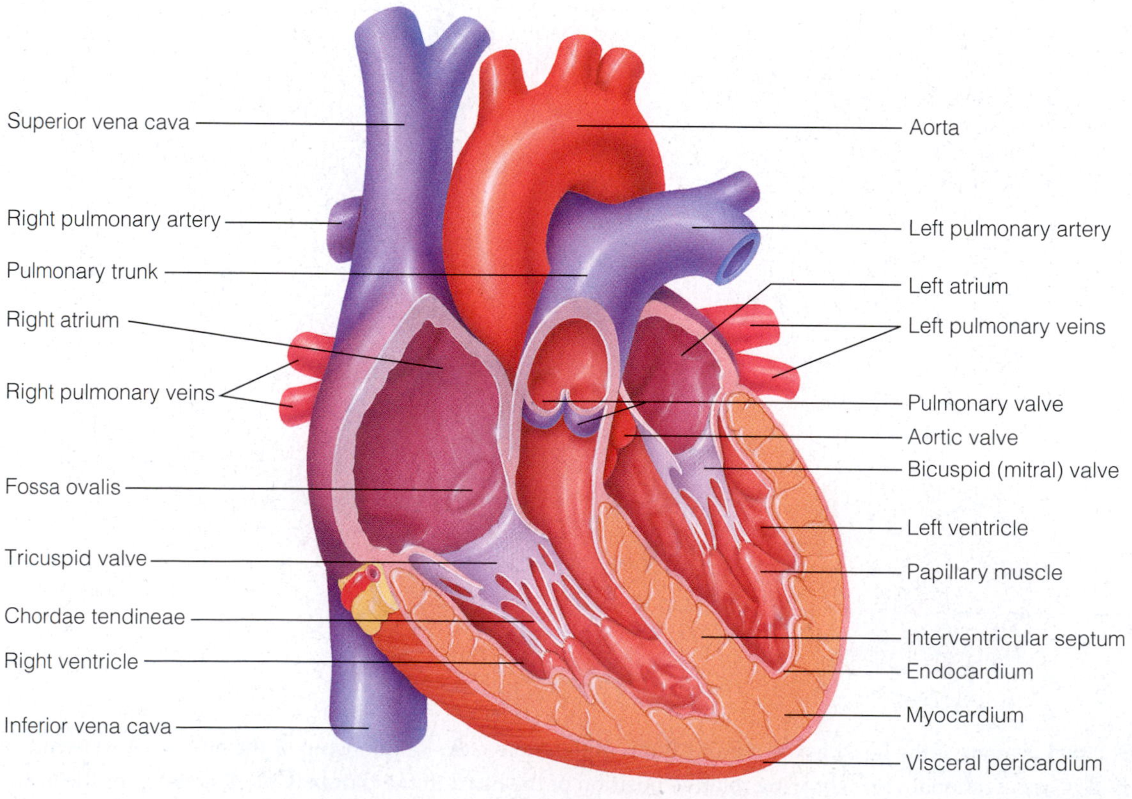
Superior vena cava
Right pulmonary artery
Pulmonary trunk
Right atrium
Right pulmonary veins
Fossa ovalis
Tricuspid valve
Chordae tendineae
Right ventricle
Inferior vena cava
Aorta
Left pulmonary artery
Left atrium
Left pulmonary veins
Pulmonary valve
Aortic valve
Bicuspid (mitral) valve
Left ventricle
Papillary muscle
Interventricular septum
Endocardium
Myocardium
Visceral pericardium

Figure 29.3 ■ The internal anatomy of the heart, frontal section.

of the left side of the heart, the aorta and its branches, the capillaries that supply the brain and peripheral tissues, the systemic venous system, and the vena cava. The *pulmonary circulation* consists of the right side of the heart, the pulmonary artery, the pulmonary capillaries, and the pulmonary vein. Pulmonary circulation begins with the right side of the heart. Deoxygenated blood from the venous system enters the right atrium through two large veins, the superior and inferior venae cavae, and is transported to the lungs via the pulmonary artery and its branches (**Figure 29.4** ■). After oxygen and carbon dioxide are exchanged in the pulmonary capillaries, oxygen-rich blood returns to the left atrium through several pulmonary veins. Blood is then pumped out of the left ventricle through the aorta and its major branches to supply all body tissues by the systemic circulation.

Oxygen is supplied to the heart muscle by its own network of vessels through the coronary circulation (**Figure 29.5** ■). The left and right coronary arteries originate at the base of the aorta and branch out to encircle the myocardium (Figure 29.5A), supplying it with blood, oxygen, and nutrients. The left main coronary artery divides to form the anterior descending and circumflex arteries. The anterior descending artery supplies the anterior interventricular septum and the left ventricle. The circumflex branch supplies the left lateral wall of the left ventricle. The right coronary artery supplies the right ventricle and forms the posterior descending artery. The posterior descending artery supplies the posterior portion of the heart. While ventricular contraction delivers blood through the pulmonary circulation and the systemic circulation, it is during ventricular relaxation that the coronary arteries fill with oxygenated blood. After the blood perfuses the heart muscle, the cardiac veins drain the blood into the coronary sinus, which empties into the right atrium of the heart (Figure 29.5B).

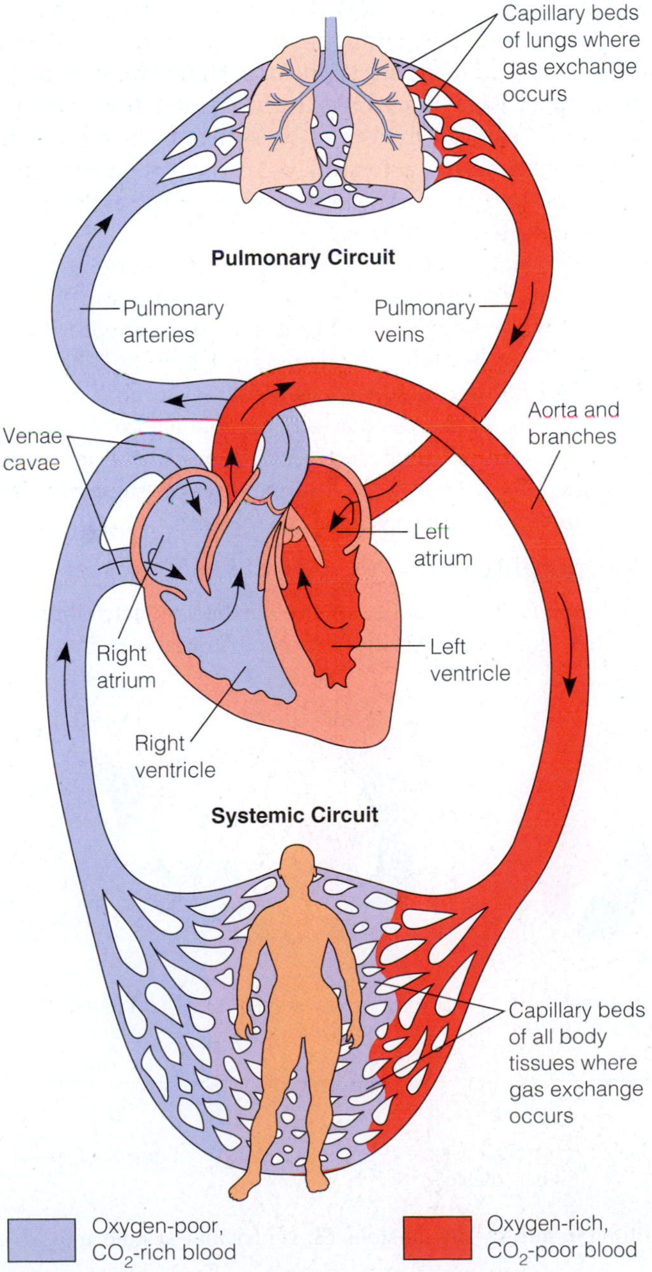
Capillary beds of lungs where gas exchange occurs
Pulmonary Circuit
Pulmonary arteries
Pulmonary veins
Aorta and branches
Venae cavae
Left atrium
Right atrium
Left ventricle
Right ventricle
Systemic Circuit
Capillary beds of all body tissues where gas exchange occurs
Oxygen-poor, CO2-rich blood
Oxygen-rich, CO2-poor blood

Figure 29.4 ■ Pulmonary and systemic circulation.

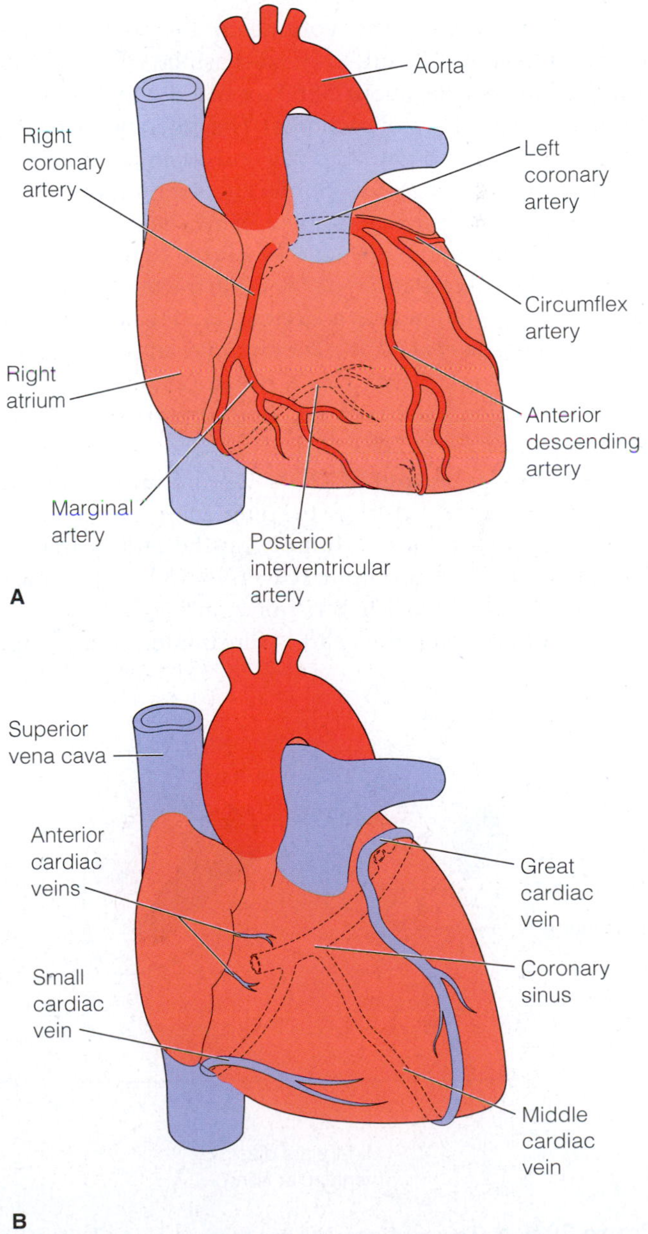
Aorta
Right coronary artery
Left coronary artery
Circumflex artery
Right atrium
Anterior descending artery
Marginal artery
Posterior interventricular artery
A
Superior vena cava
Anterior cardiac veins
Great cardiac vein
Coronary sinus
Small cardiac vein
Middle cardiac vein
B

Figure 29.5 ■ Coronary circulation. **A**, Coronary arteries. **B**, Coronary veins.

Blood flow through the coronary arteries is regulated by several factors. Aortic pressure is the primary factor. Other factors include the heart rate (most flow occurs during diastole, when the muscle is relaxed), metabolic activity of the heart, and blood vessel tone (constriction).

The Cardiac Cycle and Cardiac Output

The contraction and relaxation of the heart constitute one heartbeat, and this process is called the *cardiac cycle* (**Figure 29.6** ■). Ventricular filling is followed by ventricular *systole*, a phase during which the ventricles contract and eject blood into the pulmonary and systemic circuits. Systole is followed by a relaxation phase known as *diastole*, during which the ventricles refill, the atria contract, and the myocardium is perfused. Normally, the complete cardiac cycle occurs about 70 to 80 times per minute, measured as the *heart rate (HR)*.

During diastole, the volume in the ventricles is increased to about 120 mL (the end-diastolic volume), and at the end of systole, about 50 mL of blood remains in the ventricles (the end-systolic volume). The difference between the end-diastolic volume and the end-systolic volume is called the *stroke volume (SV)*. Stroke volume ranges from 60 to 100 mL/beat and averages about 70 mL/beat in an adult. The ejection fraction is the stroke volume divided by the end-diastolic volume and represents the fraction or percent of the diastolic volume that is ejected from the heart during systole (Sorenson et al., 2018). For example, an end-diastolic volume of 120 mL divided by a stroke volume of 80 mL equals an ejection fraction of 66%. The normal ejection fraction ranges from 50 to 70%.

The **cardiac output (CO)** is the amount of blood pumped by the ventricles into the pulmonary and systemic circulations in 1 minute. Multiplying the HR by the SV determines the cardiac output: HR × SV = CO. The average adult CO ranges from 4 to 8 L/min. Cardiac output is an indicator of how well the heart is functioning as a pump. If the heart cannot pump effectively, CO and tissue perfusion are decreased. Body tissues that do not receive enough blood and oxygen (carried in the blood on hemoglobin) become **ischemic** (deprived of oxygen). If the tissues do not receive enough blood flow to maintain the functions of the cells, the cells die, resulting in necrosis (infarction).

Activity level, metabolic rate, physiologic and psychologic stress responses, age, and body size all influence CO. In addition, CO is determined by the interaction of four major factors: Heart rate, contractility, preload, and afterload. Changes in each of these variables influence CO intrinsically, and each can be manipulated to affect CO. The heart's ability to respond to the body's changing need for CO is called *cardiac reserve*.

Heart Rate

Heart rate is affected by both direct and indirect autonomic nervous system stimulation. Direct stimulation is accomplished through the innervation of the heart muscle by sympathetic and parasympathetic nerves. The sympathetic nervous system increases the heart rate, whereas the parasympathetic vagal tone slows the heart rate. Reflex regulation of the heart rate in response to systemic blood pressure also occurs through activation of baroreceptors (pressure receptors) located in the carotid sinus, aortic arch, venae cavae, and pulmonary veins.

If heart rate increases, CO increases (up to a point), even if there is no change in stroke volume. However, rapid heart rates decrease the amount of time available for ventricular filling during diastole. Cardiac output then falls because decreased filling time decreases stroke volume. Coronary artery perfusion also decreases because the coronary arteries fill primarily during diastole. Cardiac output decreases during bradycardia if stroke volume stays the same because the number of cardiac cycles is decreased.

Contractility

Contractility is the ability of the cardiac muscle fibers to shorten. Poor contractility of the heart muscle reduces the

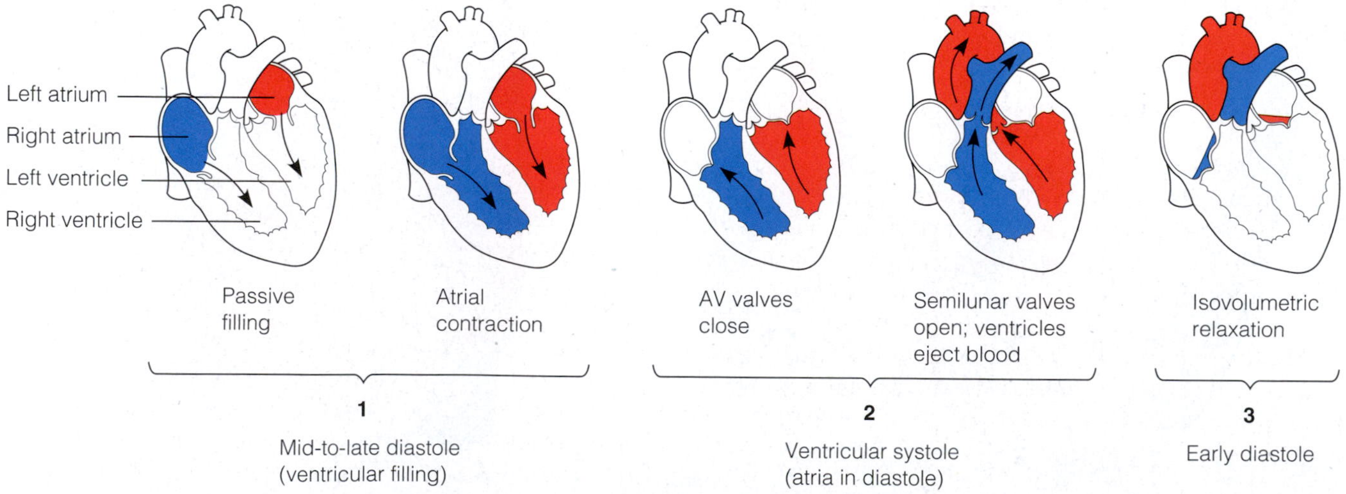
Left atrium
Right atrium
Left ventricle
Right ventricle
Passive filling
Atrial contraction
AV valves close
Semilunar valves open; ventricles eject blood
Isovolumetric relaxation
1
Mid-to-late diastole (ventricular filling)
2
Ventricular systole (atria in diastole)
3
Early diastole

Figure 29.6 ■ The cardiac cycle has three events: (**1**) Ventricular filling in mid-to-late diastole, (**2**) ventricular systole, and (**3**) isovolumetric relaxation in early diastole.

forward flow of blood from the heart, increases the ventricular pressures from accumulation of blood volume, and reduces CO. Increased contractility may stress the heart by increasing the SV in pathologic conditions.

Preload

Preload is the amount of cardiac muscle fiber tension, or stretch, that exists at the end of diastole, just before contraction of the ventricles. Preload is influenced by venous return (volume) and the compliance of the ventricles (resulting pressure). Preload is based on *ventricular end-diastolic volume (VEDV)* and *ventricular end-diastolic pressure (VEDP)*. It is related to the total volume of blood in the ventricles: The greater the volume, the greater the stretch of the cardiac muscle fibers, and the greater the force with which the fibers contract to accomplish emptying. This principle is called the *Starling law of the heart*. Disorders such as renal disease and congestive heart failure result in sodium and water retention and increased preload. Vasoconstriction also increases venous return and preload. This mechanism has a physiologic limit. Just as continuous overstretching of a rubber band causes the band to relax and lose its ability to recoil, overstretching of the cardiac muscle fibers eventually results in ineffective contraction.

Too little circulating blood volume results in a decreased venous return and therefore a decreased preload. A decreased preload reduces stroke volume and thus cardiac output. Decreased preload may result from hemorrhage or misdistribution of blood volume, as occurs in third spacing (see Chapter 11).

Afterload

Afterload is the force the ventricles must overcome to eject their blood volume. It is the pressure in the arterial system ahead of the ventricles. The right ventricle must generate enough tension to open the pulmonary valve and eject its volume into the low-pressure pulmonary arteries. Right ventricle afterload is measured as *pulmonary vascular resistance (PVR)*. The left ventricle, in contrast, ejects its load by overcoming the pressure behind the aortic valve. Afterload of the left ventricle is measured as *systemic vascular resistance (SVR)*. Arterial pressures are much higher than pulmonary pressures; thus, the left ventricle has to work much harder than the right ventricle.

Alterations in vascular tone affect afterload and ventricular work. As the pulmonary or arterial blood pressure increases (e.g., through vasoconstriction), PVR and/or SVR increases, and the work of the ventricles increases. As workload increases, consumption of myocardial oxygen also increases. A compromised heart cannot effectively meet this increased oxygen demand, and a vicious cycle ensues. By contrast, a very low afterload decreases the forward flow of blood into the systemic circulation and the coronary arteries.

Clinical Indicators of Cardiac Output

For many critically ill patients, invasive hemodynamic monitoring catheters are used to measure CO in quantifiable numbers. However, advanced technology is not the only way to identify and assess compromised blood flow. Because CO perfuses the body's tissues, clinical indicators of low CO may be manifested by changes in organ function that result from compromised blood flow. For example, a decrease in blood flow to the brain presents as a change in level of consciousness. Other manifestations of decreased CO are discussed in Chapter 11 and 30.

Cardiac index (CI) is the CO adjusted for the patient's body size, also called the patient's *body surface area (BSA)*. Because it takes into account the patient's BSA, the cardiac index provides more meaningful data about the heart's ability to perfuse the tissues and therefore is a more accurate indicator of the effectiveness of the circulation than the CO.

BSA is stated in square meters (m^2), and cardiac index is calculated as CO divided by BSA. Cardiac measurements are considered adequate when they fall within the range of 2.5 to 4.2 $L/min/m^2$. For example, two patients have a CO of 4 L/min. This parameter is within normal limits. However, one patient is 157 cm (5 ft, 2 in.) tall and weighs 54.5 kg (120 lb), with a BSA of 1.54 m^2. This patient's cardiac index is 4 ÷ 1.54, or 2.6 $L/min/m^2$. The second patient is 188 cm (6 ft, 2 in.) tall and weighs 81.7 kg (280 lb), with a BSA of 2.52 m^2. This patient's cardiac index is 4 ÷ 2.52, or 1.6 $L/min/m^2$. The cardiac index results show that the same CO of 4 L/min is adequate for the first patient but grossly inadequate for the second patient.

The Conduction System of the Heart

The cardiac cycle is perpetuated by a complex electrical circuit commonly known as the *intrinsic conduction system of the heart*. Cardiac muscle cells possess an inherent characteristic of self-excitation, which enables them to initiate and transmit impulses independent of a stimulus. However, specialized areas of myocardial cells typically exert a controlling influence in this electrical pathway.

One of these specialized areas is the *sinoatrial (SA) node*, located at the junction of the superior vena cava and right atrium (**Figure 29.7** ■). The SA node acts as the normal "pacemaker" of the heart, usually generating an impulse 60 to 100 times per minute. This impulse travels across the atria via internodal pathways to the AV node, in the floor of the interatrial septum. The very small junctional fibers of the AV node slow the impulse, slightly delaying its transmission to the ventricles. It then passes through the bundle of His at the atrioventricular junction and continues down the interventricular septum through the right and left bundle branches and out to the Purkinje fibers in the ventricular muscle walls.

This path of electrical transmission produces a series of changes in ion concentration across the membrane of each cardiac muscle cell. The electrical stimulus increases the permeability of the cell membrane, creating an action potential (electrical potential). The result is an exchange of sodium, potassium, and calcium ions across the cell membrane, which changes the intracellular electrical charge to a positive state. This process of depolarization results in myocardial contraction. As the ion exchange reverses and

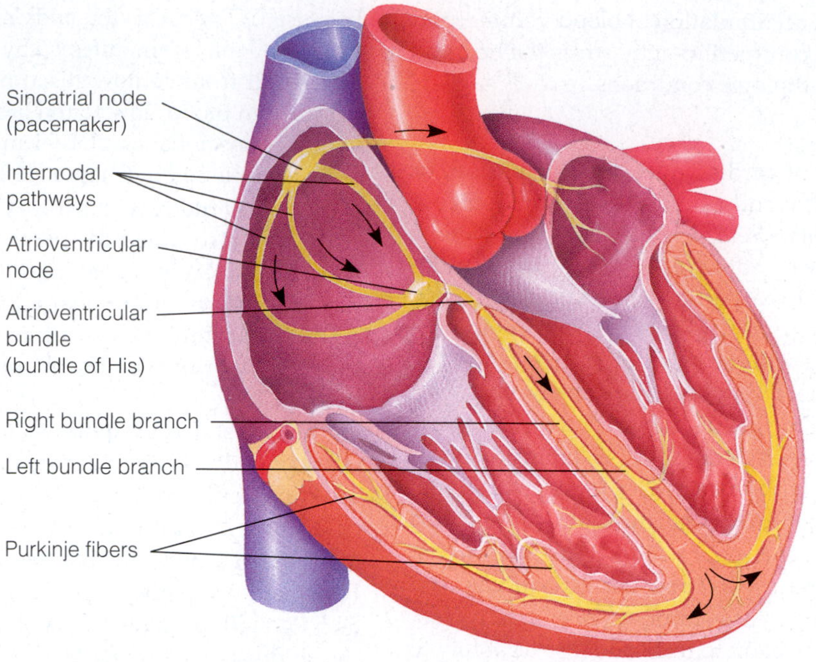
Sinoatrial node
(pacemaker)
Internodal
pathways
Atrioventricular
node
Atrioventricular
bundle
(bundle of His)
Right bundle branch
Left bundle branch
Purkinje fibers

Figure 29.7 ■ The intrinsic conduction system of the heart.

the cell returns to its resting state of electronegativity, the cell is repolarized, and cardiac muscle relaxes. The cellular action potential serves as the basis for *electrocardiography*, a diagnostic test of cardiac function.

29.2 The Peripheral Vascular System

The two components of the peripheral vascular system are the arterial network and the venous network. The *arterial network* begins with the major arteries that branch from the aorta. The major arteries of the systemic circulation are illustrated in **Figure 29.8** ■. These major arteries branch into successively smaller arteries, which in turn subdivide into the smallest of the arterial vessels, called *arterioles*. The smallest arterioles feed into beds of hairlike capillaries in the body's organs and tissues.

In the capillary beds, oxygen and nutrients are exchanged for metabolic wastes, and deoxygenated blood moves back to the heart through *venules*, the smallest vessels of the venous network. Venules join the smallest of veins, which in turn join larger and larger veins, comprising the *venous network*. The blood transported by the veins empties into the superior and inferior venae cavae entering the right side of the heart. The major veins of the systemic circulation are shown in **Figure 29.9** ■.

Structure of Blood Vessels

The structure of blood vessels reflects their different functions within the circulatory system (**Figure 29.10** ■). Except for the tiniest vessels, blood vessel walls have three layers: The tunica intima, the tunica media, and the tunica adventitia. The *tunica intima*, the innermost layer, is made of endothelium that provides a slick surface to facilitate the flow of blood. In arteries, the middle layer, or *tunica media*, is made of smooth muscle and is thicker than the tunica media of veins. This makes arteries more elastic than veins and allows the arteries to alternately expand and recoil as the heart contracts and relaxes with each beat, producing a pressure wave that can be felt as a pulse over an artery. The smaller arterioles are less elastic than arteries but contain more smooth muscle, which promotes their constriction and dilation. In fact, arterioles exert the major control over arterial blood pressure. The *tunica adventitia*, or outermost layer, is made of connective tissue and serves to protect and anchor the vessel. Veins have a thicker tunica adventitia than do arteries.

Blood in the veins travels at a much lower pressure than does blood in the arteries. Veins have thinner walls, a larger lumen, and greater capacity, and many are supplied with valves that help blood flow against gravity back to the heart. The "milking" action of skeletal muscle contraction supports venous return. When skeletal muscles contract against veins, the valves proximal to the contraction open, and blood is propelled toward the heart. The abdominal and thoracic pressure changes that occur with breathing also propel blood toward the heart.

The tiny capillaries, which connect the arterioles and venules, contain only one thin layer of tunica intima that is permeable to the gases and molecules exchanged between blood and tissue cells. Capillaries are typically found in interwoven networks. They filter and shunt blood from precapillary arterioles to postcapillary venules.

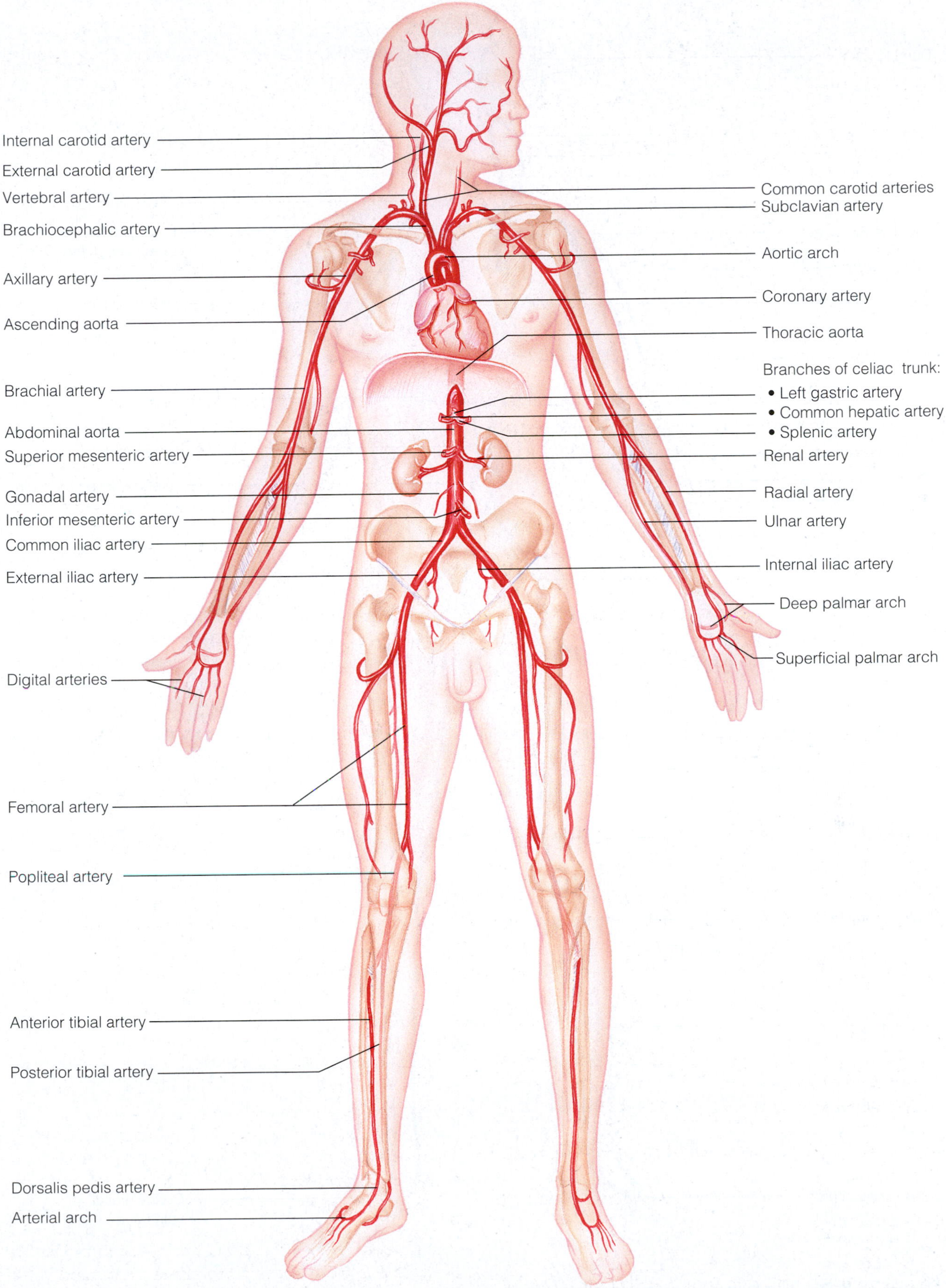
Internal carotid artery
External carotid artery
Vertebral artery
Brachiocephalic artery
Axillary artery
Ascending aorta
Brachial artery
Abdominal aorta
Superior mesenteric artery
Gonadal artery
Inferior mesenteric artery
Common iliac artery
External iliac artery
Digital arteries
Femoral artery
Popliteal artery
Anterior tibial artery
Posterior tibial artery
Dorsalis pedis artery
Arterial arch
Common carotid arteries
Subclavian artery
Aortic arch
Coronary artery
Thoracic aorta
Branches of celiac trunk:
• Left gastric artery
• Common hepatic artery
• Splenic artery
Renal artery
Radial artery
Ulnar artery
Internal iliac artery
Deep palmar arch
Superficial palmar arch

Figure 29.8 ■ Major arteries of the systemic circulation.

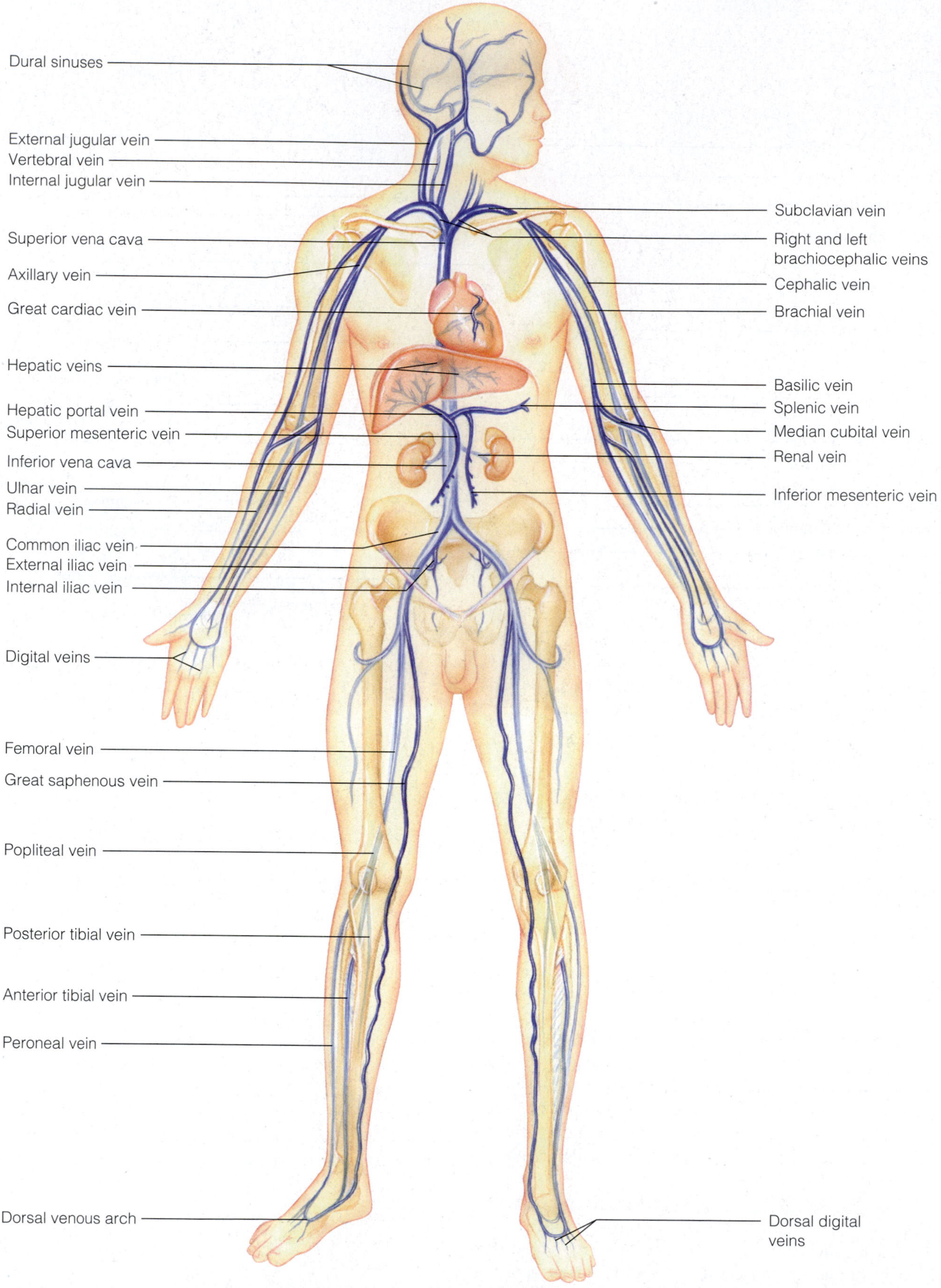

Dural sinuses
External jugular vein
Vertebral vein
Internal jugular vein
Superior vena cava
Axillary vein
Great cardiac vein
Hepatic veins
Hepatic portal vein
Superior mesenteric vein
Inferior vena cava
Ulnar vein
Radial vein
Common iliac vein
External iliac vein
Internal iliac vein
Digital veins
Femoral vein
Great saphenous vein
Popliteal vein
Posterior tibial vein
Anterior tibial vein
Peroneal vein
Dorsal venous arch
Subclavian vein
Right and left brachiocephalic veins
Cephalic vein
Brachial vein
Basilic vein
Splenic vein
Median cubital vein
Renal vein
Inferior mesenteric vein
Dorsal digital veins

Figure 29.9 ■ Major veins of the systemic circulation.

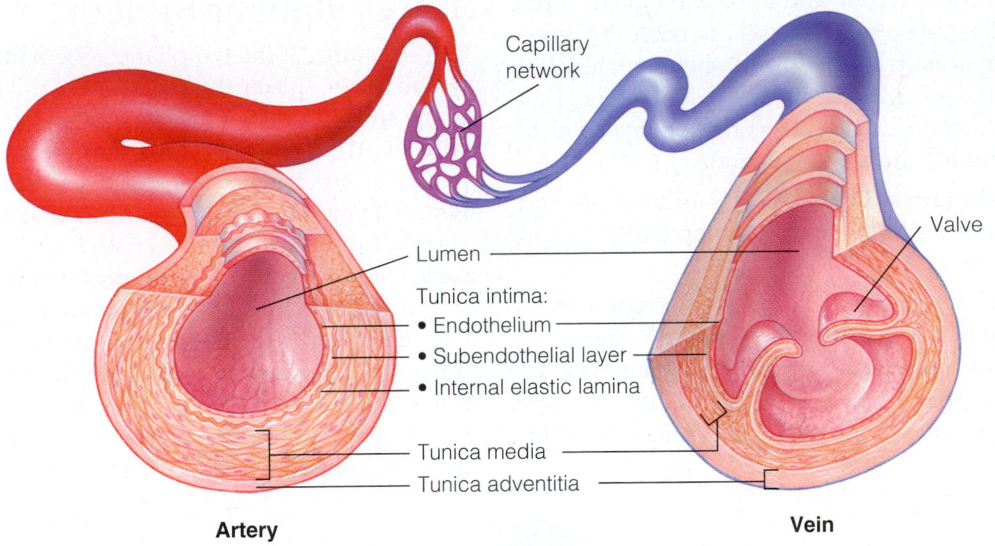
Capillary network
Valve
Lumen
Tunica intima:
• Endothelium
• Subendothelial layer
• Internal elastic lamina
Tunica media
Tunica adventitia
Artery
Vein

Figure 29.10 ■ Structure of arteries, veins, and capillaries. Capillaries are composed of only a fine tunica intima. Notice that the tunica media is thicker in arteries than in veins.

Arterial Circulation

The factors that affect arterial circulation are blood flow, peripheral vascular resistance, and blood pressure. *Blood flow* refers to the volume of blood transported in a vessel, in an organ, or throughout the entire circulation over a given period of time. It is commonly expressed as liters or milliliters per minute or cubic centimeters per second.

Peripheral vascular resistance (PVR) refers to the opposing forces or impedance to blood flow as the arterial channels become more and more distant from the heart. PVR is determined by three factors:

- ***Blood viscosity:*** The greater the viscosity, or thickness, of the blood, the greater its resistance to moving and flowing.
- ***Length of the vessel:*** The longer the vessel, the greater the resistance to blood flow.
- ***Diameter of the vessel:*** The smaller the diameter of a vessel, the greater the friction against the walls of the vessel and, thus, the greater the impedance to blood flow.

Blood pressure (BP) is the force exerted against the walls of the arteries by the blood as it is pumped from the heart. It is most accurately referred to as *mean arterial pressure (MAP)*. The highest pressure exerted against the arterial walls at the peak of ventricular contraction (systole) is called the *systolic BP*. The lowest pressure exerted during ventricular relaxation (diastole) is the *diastolic BP*.

MAP is regulated mainly by cardiac output and peripheral vascular resistance, as represented in this formula: MAP = CO × PVR. For clinical use, the MAP may be estimated by calculating the diastolic blood pressure plus one-third of the pulse pressure (the difference between the systolic and diastolic blood pressure).

Factors Influencing Arterial Blood Pressure

Blood flow, peripheral vascular resistance, and BP, which influence arterial circulation, are in turn influenced by various factors:

- The sympathetic and parasympathetic nervous systems are the primary mechanisms that regulate BP. Stimulation of the sympathetic nervous system exerts a major effect on peripheral resistance by causing vasoconstriction of the arterioles, thereby increasing BP. Parasympathetic stimulation causes vasodilation of the arterioles, lowering BP.
- Baroreceptors and chemoreceptors in the aortic arch, carotid sinus, and other large vessels are sensitive to pressure and chemical changes and cause reflex sympathetic stimulation, resulting in vasoconstriction, increased heart rate, and increased BP.
- The kidneys help maintain BP by excreting or conserving sodium and water. When BP decreases, the kidneys initiate the renin–angiotensin mechanism. This stimulates vasoconstriction, resulting in the release of the hormone aldosterone from the adrenal cortex, increasing sodium ion reabsorption and water retention. In addition, pituitary release of antidiuretic hormone (ADH) promotes renal reabsorption of water. The net result is an increase in blood volume and a consequent increase in CO and BP.
- Temperatures may affect peripheral resistance: Cold causes vasoconstriction, whereas warmth produces vasodilation.
- Many chemicals, hormones, and drugs influence BP by affecting CO and/or PVR. For example, epinephrine

causes vasoconstriction and increased heart rate; prostaglandins dilate blood vessel diameter (by relaxing vascular smooth muscle); endothelin, a chemical released by the inner lining of vessels, is a potent vasoconstrictor; nicotine causes vasoconstriction; and alcohol and histamine cause vasodilation.

- Dietary factors such as intake of salt, saturated fats, and cholesterol elevate BP by affecting blood volume and vessel diameter.
- Race, gender, age, weight, time of day, position, exercise, and emotional state may also affect BP. These factors influence the arterial pressure. Systemic venous pressure, though it is much lower, is also influenced by such factors as blood volume, venous tone, and right-atrial pressure.

The Lymphatic System

The structures of the lymphatic system include the lymph, lymph nodes, spleen, thymus, tonsils, and the Peyer patches of the small intestine. *Lymph nodes* are small aggregates of specialized cells that assist the immune system by removing foreign material, infectious organisms, and tumor cells from lymph. Lymph nodes are distributed along the lymphatic vessels, forming clusters in certain body regions such as the neck, axilla, and groin (see **Figure 29.11** ■).

The *spleen*, the largest lymphoid organ, is in the upper left quadrant of the abdomen under the thorax. The main function of the spleen is to filter the blood by breaking down old red blood cells and storing or releasing to the liver their by-products (such as iron). The spleen also synthesizes lymphocytes, stores platelets for blood clotting,

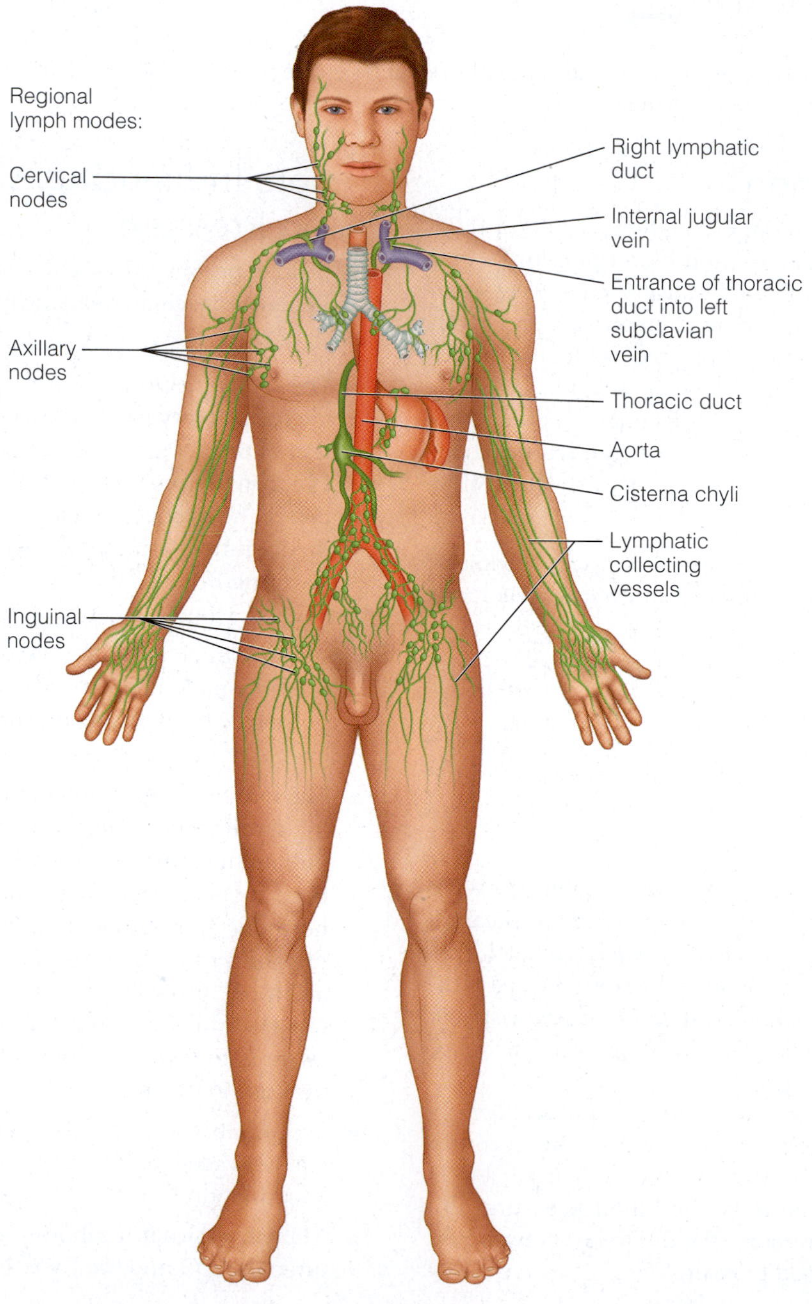
Regional
lymph modes:
Cervical
nodes
Axillary
nodes
Inguinal
nodes
Right lymphatic
duct
Internal jugular
vein
Entrance of thoracic
duct into left
subclavian
vein
Thoracic duct
Aorta
Cisterna chyli
Lymphatic
collecting
vessels

Figure 29.11 ■ The lymphatic system.

and serves as a reservoir of blood. The thymus gland is in the lower throat and is most active in childhood, producing hormones (such as thymosin) that facilitate the immune action of lymphocytes. The tonsils of the pharynx and Peyer patches of the small intestine are lymphoid organs that protect the upper respiratory and digestive tracts from foreign pathogens.

The *lymphatic vessels*, or *lymphatics*, form a network around the arterial and venous channels and interweave at the capillary beds. They collect and drain excess tissue fluid, called *lymph*, that leaks from the cardiovascular system and accumulates at the venous end of the capillary bed. The lymphatics return this fluid to the heart through a one-way system of lymphatic venules and veins that eventually drain into the right lymphatic duct and left thoracic duct, both of which empty into their respective subclavian veins. Lymphatics are a low-pressure system without a pump; their fluid transport depends on the rhythmic contraction of their smooth muscle and the muscular and respiratory movements that assist venous circulation.

The Hematologic System

Blood consists of plasma, solutes (e.g., proteins, electrolytes, and organic constituents), red blood cells, white blood cells, and platelets (which are fragments of cells). The hematopoietic (blood-forming) system includes the bone marrow (myeloid) tissues, where blood cells form, and the lymphoid tissues of the lymph nodes, where white blood cells mature and circulate. All blood cells originate from cells in the bone marrow called *stem cells*, or *hemocytoblasts*. The origin of the cellular components of blood is illustrated in **Figure 29.12 ■**. Normal laboratory values for blood components are found in **Table 29.1**.

Regulatory mechanisms cause stem cells to differentiate into families of parent cells, each of which gives rise to one of the formed elements of the blood (red blood cells, platelets, and white blood cells). The functions of blood include transporting oxygen, nutrients, hormones, and metabolic wastes; protecting against invasion of pathogens; maintaining blood coagulation; and regulating fluids, electrolytes, acids, bases, and body temperature.

Red Blood Cells

Red blood cells (RBCs), or *erythrocytes*, are the most common type of blood cell. They are shaped like biconcave disks (**Figure 29.13 ■**). This unique shape increases the surface area of the cell and allows the cell to pass through very small capillaries without disrupting the cell membrane. RBCs and the hemoglobin molecules they contain transport oxygen to body tissues. Hemoglobin also binds with some carbon dioxide, carrying it to the lungs for excretion. Abnormal numbers of RBCs, changes in their size and shape, or altered hemoglobin content or structure can adversely affect health. *Anemia*, the most common RBC disorder, is an abnormally low RBC count or reduced hemoglobin content; *polycythemia* is an abnormally high RBC count.

Hemoglobin, synthesized within the RBC, is the oxygen-carrying protein. It consists of the heme molecule and globin, a protein molecule. Globin is made of four polypeptide chains—two alpha chains and two beta chains (**Figure 29.14 ■**). Each of the four polypeptide chains has a heme unit that contains an iron atom. The iron atom binds reversibly with oxygen, allowing it to transport oxygen as oxyhemoglobin to the cells. The rate of synthesis depends on the availability of iron. The size, color, and shape of stained RBCs may also be analyzed. RBCs may be normocytic (normal size), smaller than normal (microcytic), or larger than normal (macrocytic). Their color may be normal (normochromic) or diminished (hypochromic).

Red Blood Cell Production and Regulation

In adults, RBC production (erythropoiesis) (**Figure 29.15 ■**) begins in the red bone marrow of the vertebrae, sternum, ribs, and pelvis and is completed in the blood or spleen. Erythroblasts begin forming hemoglobin while they are in the bone marrow, a process that continues throughout the RBC lifespan. The cells enter the circulation as reticulocytes, which fully mature in about 48 hours. The complete sequence from stem cell to RBC takes 3 to 5 days.

The stimulus for increased RBC production is tissue hypoxia. The hormone *erythropoietin* is released by the kidneys in response to hypoxia. It stimulates the bone marrow to produce RBCs. However, the process of RBC production takes about 5 days to maximize. During periods of increased RBC production, the percentage of reticulocytes (immature RBCs) in the blood exceeds that of mature cells.

Red Blood Cell Destruction

RBCs have a lifespan of about 120 days. Old or damaged RBCs are lysed (destroyed) by phagocytes in the spleen, liver, bone marrow, and lymph nodes. The process of RBC destruction is called *hemolysis*. Phagocytes save and reuse amino acids and iron from heme units in the lysed RBCs. Most of the heme unit is converted to *bilirubin*, an orange-yellow pigment that is removed from the blood by the liver and excreted in the bile. During disease processes causing increased hemolysis or impaired liver function, bilirubin accumulates in the serum, causing *jaundice*, a yellowish appearance of the skin and sclera.

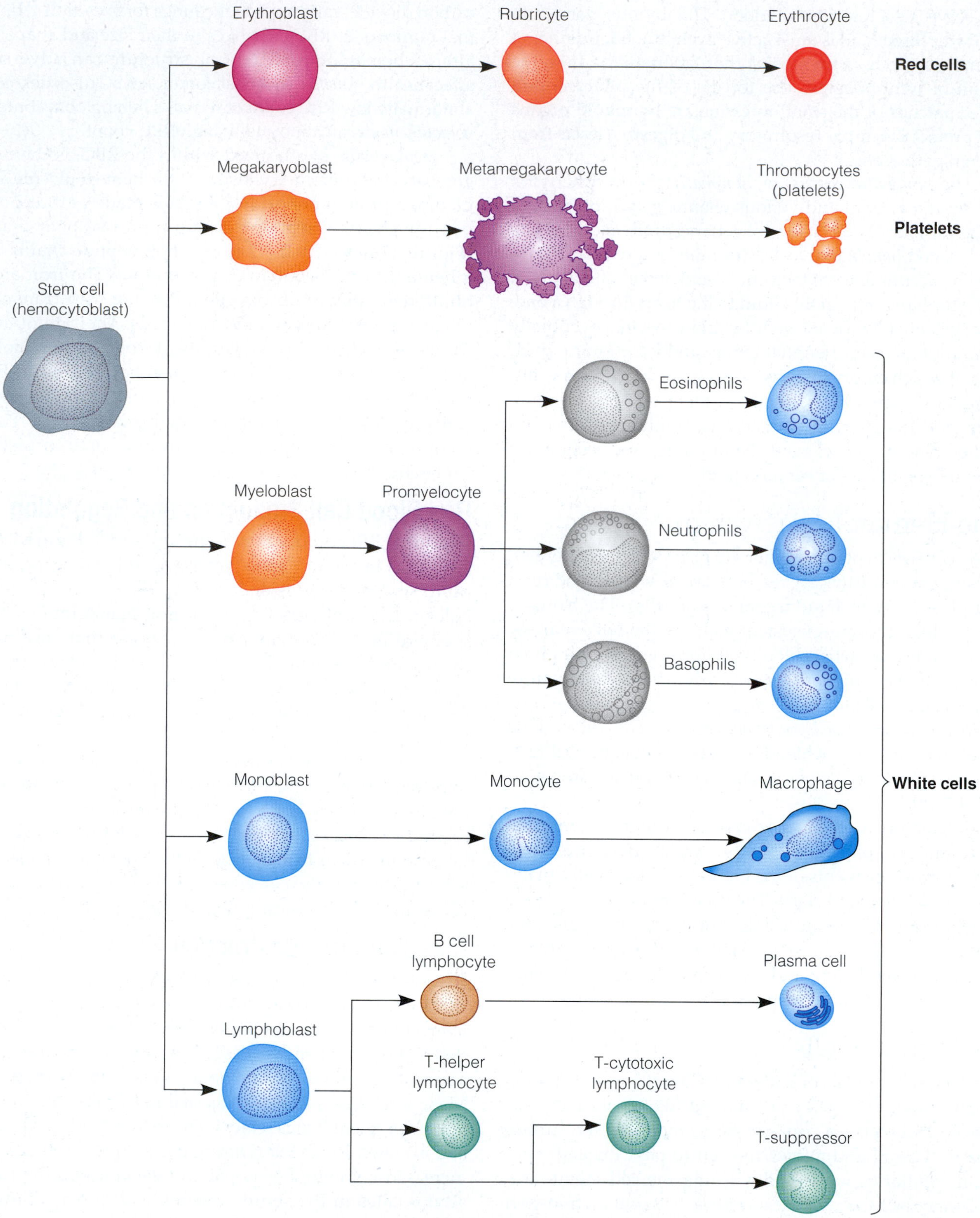
Erythroblast
Rubricyte
Erythrocyte
Red cells
Megakaryoblast
Metamegakaryocyte
Thrombocytes (platelets)
Platelets
Stem cell (hemocytoblast)
Eosinophils
Myeloblast
Promyelocyte
Neutrophils
Basophils
Monoblast
Monocyte
Macrophage
White cells
B cell lymphocyte
Plasma cell
Lymphoblast
T-helper lymphocyte
T-cytotoxic lymphocyte
T-suppressor

Figure 29.12 ■ Blood cell formation from stem cells. Regulatory factors control the differentiation of stem cells into blasts. Each of the five kinds of blasts is committed to producing one type of mature blood cell. Erythroblasts, for example, can differentiate only into RBCs; megakaryoblasts can differentiate only into platelets.

Table 29.1 Complete Blood Count (CBC)

Component	Purpose	Normal Values
Hemoglobin (Hb)	Measures the capacity of the hemoglobin to carry gases.	Women: 12–16 g/dL Men: 13.5–18 g/dL
Hematocrit (Hct)	Measures packed cell volume of RBCs, expressed as a percent of the total blood volume.	Women: 38–47% Men: 40–54%
Total RBC count	Counts number of circulating RBCs.	Women: 4–5 × 10^6/μL Men: 4.5–6 × 10^6/μL
Red cell indices: MCV 10^6MCH	Determines relative size of MCV (mean corpuscular volume). Measures average weight of Hb/RBC.	82–98 fL 27–29 pg
MCHC	Evaluates RBC saturation with Hb.	32–36%
WBC count	Measures total number of leukocytes (total count) and whether each kind of WBC is present in proper proportion (differential).	Total WBC count: 4000–11,000/μL (4–11 × 10^9/L) WBC differential: neutrophils: 50–70%; eosinophils: 2–4%; basophils: 0–2%; lymphocytes: 20–40%; monocytes: 4–8%
Platelets	Measures number of platelets available to maintain clotting functions.	150,000–400,000/μL (150–400 × 10^9/L)

Note: MCH, mean corpuscular hemoglobin; MCHC, mean corpuscular hemoglobin concentration.

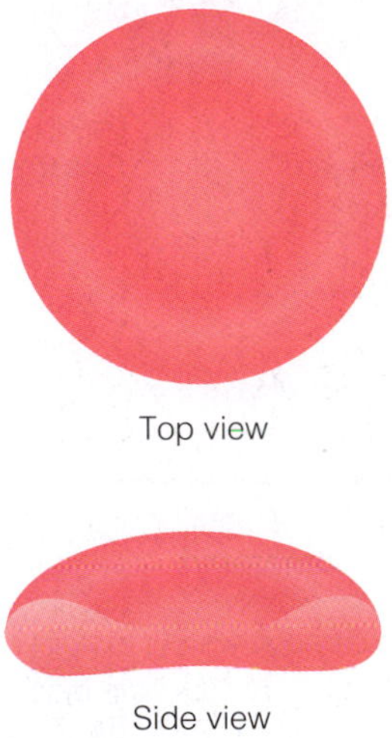

Top view
Side view

Figure 29.13 ■ Top and side view of a red blood cell (erythrocyte). Note the distinctive biconcave shape.

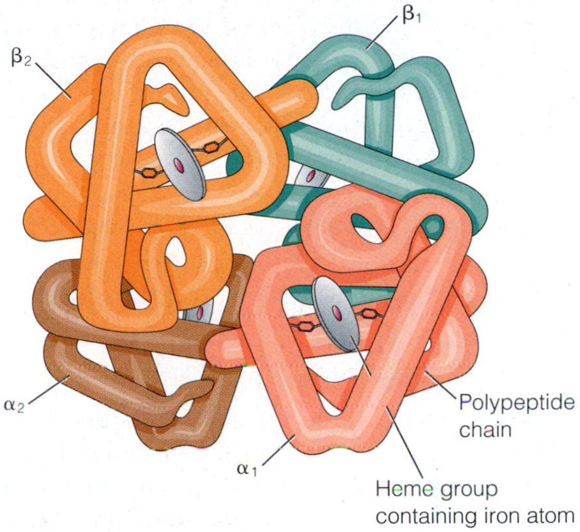

β1
β2
α2
α1
Polypeptide chain
Heme group containing iron atom

Figure 29.14 ■ The hemoglobin molecule includes globin (a protein) and heme, which contains iron. Globin is made of four subunits, two alpha and two beta polypeptide chains. A heme disk containing an iron atom (red dot) nests within the folds of each protein subunit. The iron atoms combine reversibly with oxygen, transporting it to the cells.

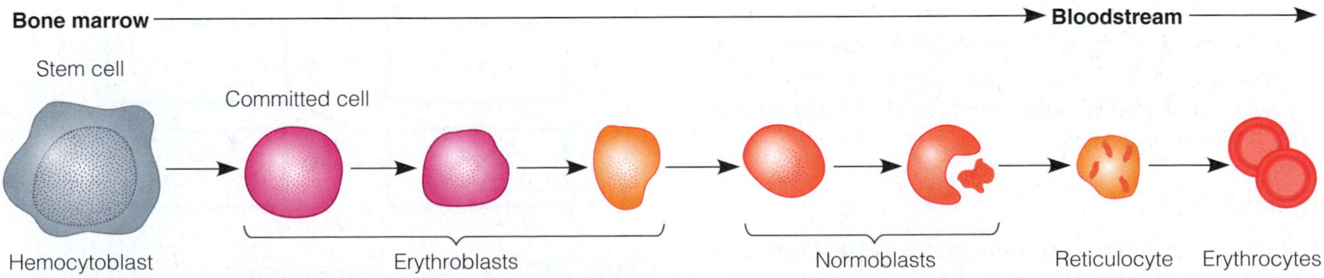

Bone marrow
Bloodstream
Stem cell
Committed cell
Hemocytoblast
Erythroblasts
Normoblasts
Reticulocyte
Erythrocytes

Figure 29.15 ■ Erythropoiesis. RBCs begin as erythroblasts within the bone marrow, maturing into normoblasts, which eventually eject their nucleus and organelles to become reticulocytes. Reticulocytes mature within the blood or spleen to become erythrocytes.

White Blood Cells

White blood cells (WBCs), or *leukocytes*, originate from hemopoietic stem cells in the bone marrow and differentiate into the various types of white blood cells. They are a part of the body's defense against microorganisms. *Leukocytosis* is a higher-than-normal WBC count; *leukopenia* is a WBC count that is lower than normal.

The two basic types of WBCs are *granular leukocytes* (or *granulocytes*) and *nongranular leukocytes* (or *agranulocytes*). Stimulated by granulocyte-macrophage colony-stimulating factor (GM-CSF) and granulocyte colony-stimulating factor (G-CSF), granulocytes mature fully in the bone marrow before being released into the bloodstream. The three types of granulocytes are:

- ***Neutrophils*** (also called *polymorphonuclear [PMN]* or *segmented [segs] leukocytes*) are active phagocytes, the first cells to arrive at a site of injury. Their numbers increase during inflammation. Immature forms of neutrophils (bands) are released during inflammation or infections, and are referred to as having a shift to the left (so named because immature cell frequencies appear on the left side of the graph) on a differential blood count. Neutrophils have a lifespan of only about 10 hours and are constantly being replaced.
- ***Eosinophils*** are found in large numbers in the mucosa of the intestines and lungs. Their numbers increase during allergic reactions and parasitic infestations.
- ***Basophils*** contain histamine, heparin, and other inflammatory mediators. Basophils increase in numbers during allergic and inflammatory reactions.

Agranulocytes include the monocytes and lymphocytes. They enter the bloodstream before final maturation. These cells are an active part of the inflammatory and immune responses and are discussed in Chapter 12 and 13.

Platelets

Platelets (thrombocytes) produce ATP and release mediators required for clotting. Platelets are formed in the bone marrow as pinched-off portions of large megakaryocytes. Platelet production is controlled by *thrombopoietin*, a protein produced by the liver, kidney, smooth muscle, and bone marrow. The number of circulating platelets controls thrombopoietin release. Platelets live up to 10 days in circulation. An excess of platelets is called *thrombocytosis*; a deficit of platelets is *thrombocytopenia*.

Hemostasis

Platelet and coagulation disorders affect **hemostasis** (control of bleeding). Hemostasis is a series of complex interactions between platelets and clotting mechanisms that maintain a relatively steady state of blood volume, BP, and blood flow through injured vessels. The five stages of hemostasis are (1) vessel spasm, (2) formation of the platelet plug, (3) development of an insoluble fibrin clot, (4) clot retraction, and (5) clot dissolution.

Vessel Spasm

When a blood vessel is damaged, thromboxane A_2 (TXA_2) is released from platelets and cells, causing vessel spasm. This spasm constricts the damaged vessel for about 1 minute, reducing blood flow.

Formation of the Platelet Plug

Platelets attracted to the damaged vessel wall change from smooth disks to spiny spheres. Receptors on the activated platelets bind with von Willebrand factor (a protein molecule) and exposed collagen fibers at the site of injury to form the platelet plug (**Figure 29.16** ■). The platelets release

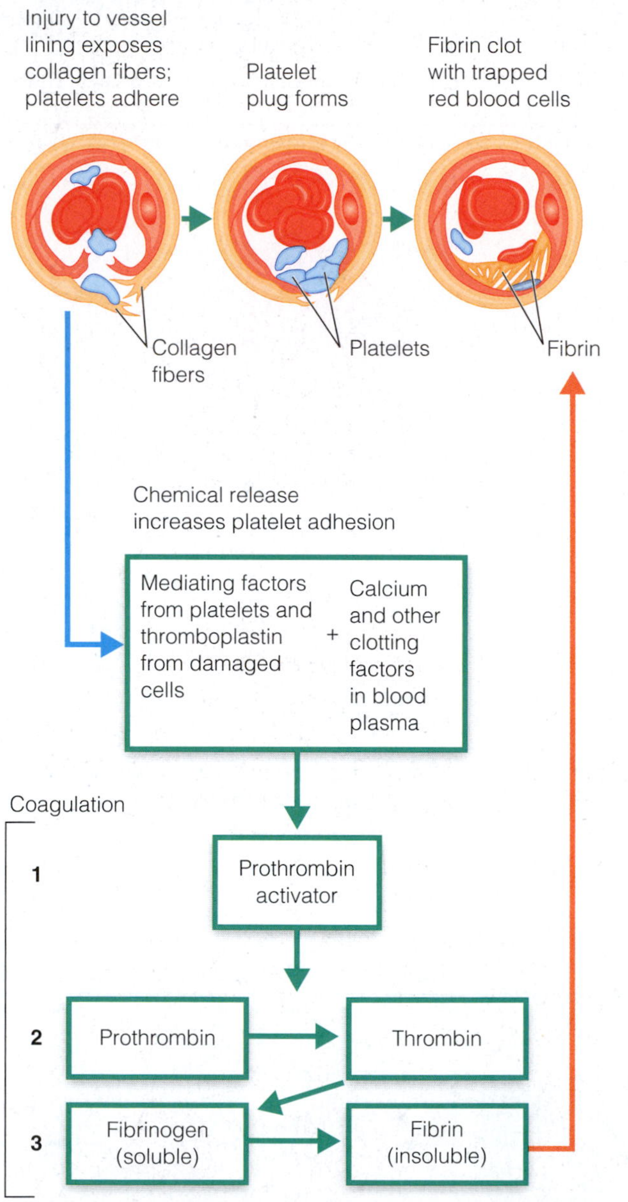
Injury to vessel lining exposes collagen fibers; platelets adhere
Platelet plug forms
Fibrin clot with trapped red blood cells
Collagen fibers
Platelets
Fibrin
Chemical release increases platelet adhesion
Mediating factors from platelets and thromboplastin from damaged cells
+
Calcium and other clotting factors in blood plasma
Coagulation
1
Prothrombin activator
2
Prothrombin
Thrombin
3
Fibrinogen (soluble)
Fibrin (insoluble)

Figure 29.16 ■ Platelet plug formation and blood clotting. This flow diagram summarizes the events leading to fibrin clot formation. PF_3 (blue arrow) released from damaged tissue combines with other clotting factors to release prothrombin activator, the first step of coagulation. Second, prothrombin is converted into thrombin. Finally, thrombin transforms soluble fibrinogen into insoluble fibrin (red arrow) to form a clot.

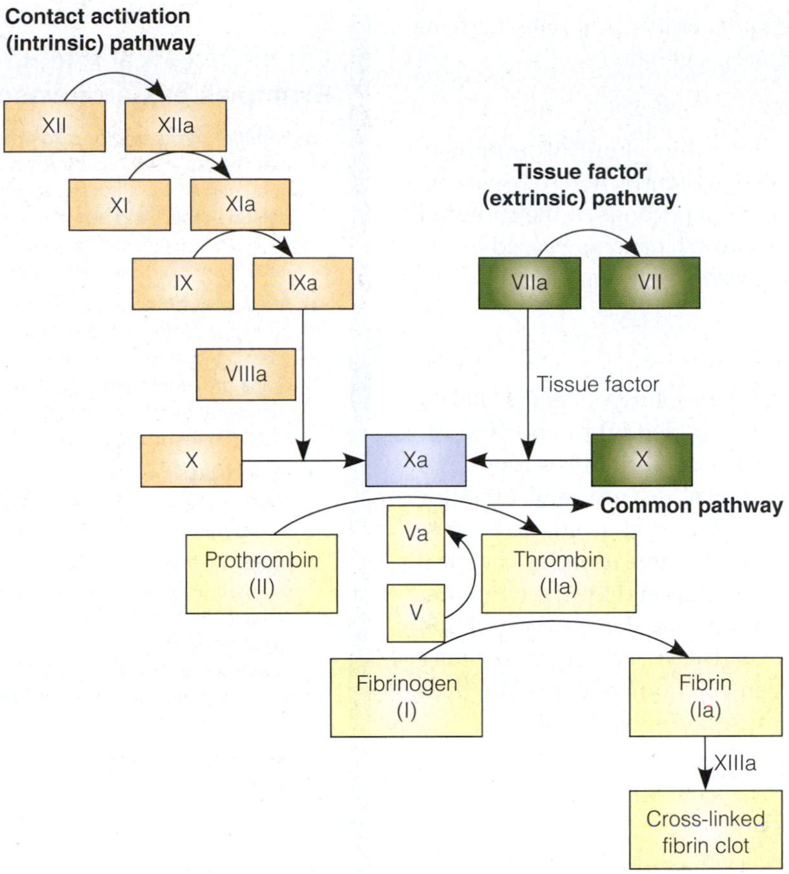
Contact activation (intrinsic) pathway
XII
XIIa
XI
XIa
IX
IXa
VIIIa
X
Xa
Tissue factor (extrinsic) pathway
VIIa
VII
Tissue factor
X
Common pathway
Prothrombin (II)
Va
V
Thrombin (IIa)
Fibrinogen (I)
Fibrin (Ia)
XIIIa
Cross-linked fibrin clot

Figure 29.17 ■ Clot formation. Both the slower intrinsic pathway and the more rapid extrinsic pathway activate Factor X. Factor X then combines with other factors to form prothrombin activator. Prothrombin activator transforms prothrombin into thrombin, which then transforms fibrinogen into long fibrin strands. Thrombin also activates Factor XIII, which draws the fibrin strands together into a dense meshwork. The complete process of clot formation occurs within 3 to 6 minutes after blood vessel damage.

adenosine diphosphate (ADP) and TXA_2 to activate nearby platelets, adhering them to the developing plug. Activation of the clotting pathway on the platelet surface converts fibrinogen to fibrin. Fibrin, in turn, forms a meshwork that binds the platelets and other blood cells to form a stable plug.

Development of the Fibrin Clot

The process of coagulation creates a meshwork of fibrin strands that cements the blood components to form an insoluble clot. Coagulation requires many interactive reactions and two clotting pathways (**Figure 29.17** ■). The slower intrinsic pathway is activated when blood contacts collagen in the injured vessel wall; the faster extrinsic pathway is activated when blood is exposed to tissues. The final outcome of both pathways is fibrin clot formation. Each procoagulation substance is activated in sequence; the activation of one coagulation factor activates another in turn. **Table 29.2** lists known factors, their origin, and their function or pathway. A

Table 29.2 Blood Coagulation Factors

Factor	Name	Function or Pathway
I	Fibrinogen	Converted to fibrin strands
II	Prothrombin	Converted to thrombin
III	Thromboplastin	Catalyzes conversion of thrombin
IV	Calcium ions	Needed for all steps of coagulation
V	Proaccelerin	Extrinsic/intrinsic pathways
VII	Serum prothrombin conversion accelerator	Extrinsic pathway
VIII	Antihemophilic factor	Intrinsic pathway
IX	Plasma prothrombin component	Intrinsic pathway
X	Stuart factor	Extrinsic/intrinsic pathways
XI	Plasma prothrombin antecedent	Intrinsic pathway
XII	Hageman factor	Intrinsic pathway
XIII	Fibrin stabilizing factor	Cross-links fibrin strands to form insoluble clot

deficiency of one or more factors or inappropriate inactivation of any factor alters normal coagulation.

Clot Retraction

After the clot is stabilized (within about 30 minutes), trapped platelets contract. Platelet contraction squeezes the fibrin strands, pulling the broken portions of the ruptured blood vessel closer together. Growth factors released by the platelets stimulate cell division and tissue repair of the damaged vessel.

Clot Dissolution

Fibrinolysis, the process of clot dissolution, begins shortly after the clot has formed, restoring blood flow and promoting tissue repair. Like coagulation, fibrinolysis requires a sequence of interactions between activator and inhibitor substances. *Plasminogen*, an enzyme that promotes fibrinolysis, is converted into *plasmin*, its active form, by chemical mediators released from vessel walls and the liver. Plasmin dissolves the clot's fibrin strands and certain coagulation factors. Stimuli such as exercise, fever, and vasoactive drugs promote plasminogen activator release. The liver and endothelium also produce fibrinolytic inhibitors.

29.3 Assessing Cardiovascular and Lymphatic Function

Cardiovascular function is assessed by findings from diagnostic tests, a health assessment interview to collect subjective data, and a physical assessment to collect objective data.

Health Assessment Interview

A health assessment interview to determine problems with cardiovascular or lymphatic structure and function may be conducted during a health screening, may focus on a chief complaint (such as chest pain or leg pain when walking), or may be part of a complete health assessment (Bickley, 2016). If the patient has a problem with cardiovascular or lymphatic function, analyze its onset, characteristics, course, severity, precipitating and relieving factors, and any associated symptoms, noting the timing and circumstances. For example, ask the patient:

- "What is the location of the chest pain you experienced? Did it move up to your jaw or into your left arm?"
- "Describe the type of activity that brings on your chest pain."
- "Does the leg pain occur only with activities such as walking, or during rest or sleep?"
- "Have you felt light-headed during the times your heart is racing?"

When conducting a health assessment interview and physical assessment, it is important for the nurse to consider genetic influences on the health of the adult. Ask about family members with health problems affecting the cardiovascular system, such as high BP, high cholesterol levels, leukemia, or early-onset CAD. Depending on the racial and ethnic background of the patient, ask about any family members with sickle cell disease or thalassemia. During the physical assessment, assess for any manifestations that might indicate a genetic disorder (see the Genetic Considerations box on page 970). If data are found to indicate genetic risk factors or alterations, ask about genetic testing and refer for appropriate genetic counseling and evaluation. Chapter 8 provides further information about genetics in medical-surgical nursing.

Genetic Considerations

Examples of Cardiovascular Disorders

- ***Familial hypercholesterolemia*** is a single-gene disorder that results in atherosclerosis and CAD, which may occur at an earlier age than in the general population (i.e., before age 55 in men and age 65 in women). However, increased cholesterol levels may also be inherited and are a risk factor for CAD in both men and women.
- ***Marfan syndrome*** is an autosomal-dominant inherited disorder that affects the skeleton, the eyes, and the cardiovascular system. The cardiovascular effects are a dilation of the proximal aorta and aortic dissection associated with degeneration of the elastic fibers in the tunica media of the aorta. There may also be thoracic aortic aneurysms.
- ***Hypertrophic cardiomyopathy*** is a disease of the sarcomere proteins. More than 100 different mutations in 10 genes encoding contractile sarcomeres have been identified.
- ***Long QT syndrome (LQTS)*** is an inherited genetic disorder that results from structural abnormalities of the sodium, potassium, and calcium channels in the heart, leading to dysrhythmias. This can result in unconsciousness and may cause sudden cardiac death in teenagers and young adults when exposed to stressors ranging from exercise to loud sounds.
- ***Sickle cell disease*** is the most common inherited blood disorder in the United States, affecting 1 in 500 people of African descent. It is characterized by episodes of pain, chronic hemolytic anemia, and severe infections.
- ***Gaucher disease***, more common in descendants of Eastern European Jewish people, is an inherited illness caused by a gene mutation. The gene is responsible for an enzyme that breaks down a specific fat. When the fat is not broken down, it accumulates in the liver, spleen, and bone marrow, causing pain, fatigue, jaundice, bone damage, anemia, and even death.
- ***Hemophilia A*** is a hereditary blood disorder, primarily affecting males, characterized by a deficiency of Factor VIII, a blood clotting factor. Abnormal bleeding results.
- ***Chronic myeloid leukemia (CML)***, a cancer of blood cells, is characterized by replacement of bone marrow with malignant, leukemic cells. Leukemic cells also circulate in the blood, causing enlargement of the spleen, liver, and other organs. This leukemia is the result of a chromosomal abnormality called the *Philadelphia chromosome*.
- ***Thalassemia***, an inherited disease of faulty hemoglobin synthesis, is more often found in descendants of people living near the Mediterranean Sea, Africa, the Middle East, and Asia. It comprises a group of disorders that range from very mild blood abnormalities to severe or fatal anemia.

Table 29.3 Assessing Chest Pain

Characteristic	Examples
Location	Substernal, precordial, jaw (more common in women), back (more common in women) Localized or diffuse Radiation to neck, jaw, shoulder, arm, back between the shoulders
Character/quality	Pressure; tightness; crushing, burning, or aching quality; heaviness; dullness; "heartburn" or indigestion
Timing: Onset, duration, and frequency	Onset: Sudden or gradual? Duration: How many minutes does the pain last? Frequency: Is the pain continuous or periodic?
Setting/precipitating factors	Awake, at rest, sleep interrupted? With activity? With eating, exertion, exercise, elimination, emotional upset?
Intensity/severity	Can range from 0 (no pain) to 10 (worst pain ever felt)
Aggravating factors	Activity, breathing, temperature
Relieving factors	Medication (nitroglycerin, antacid), rest; there may be no relieving factors
Associated symptoms	Fatigue, shortness of breath (more common in women), palpitations, nausea and vomiting (more common in women), sweating, anxiety, light-headedness or dizziness

The interview begins by exploring the patient's chief complaint (e.g., chest pain, leg pain, or fatigue). Describe the patient's chest pain or leg pain in terms of location, quality or character, timing, setting or precipitating factors, severity, aggravating and relieving factors, and associated symptoms (**Table 29.3**).

Explore the patient's medical history for any cardiovascular disorders such as angina, heart attack, congestive heart failure (CHF), stroke, hypertension (HTN), peripheral vascular disease (PVD), or other chronic illnesses (such as diabetes or bleeding disorders). Ask the patient about previous heart surgery or illnesses—such as rheumatic fever, scarlet fever, or recurrent streptococcal throat infections—and radiation treatment for breast cancer. Review the patient's family history for CAD, HTN, stroke, hyperlipidemia, diabetes, congenital heart disease, or sudden death.

Ask the patient about past or present occurrence of cardiovascular symptoms, such as chest pain, shortness of breath, difficulty breathing, cough, palpitations, fatigue, light-headedness or dizziness, fainting, heart murmur, blood clots, leg cramps or swelling, changes in skin color or temperature, varicose veins, or edema. Because cardiovascular function affects all other body systems, a full history may need to explore other related systems, such as respiratory function. Ask about past or present bleeding (from the nose, gums or mouth, or rectum) as well as associated symptoms (such as pallor, dizziness, fatigue), lymph node changes (swelling, pain, heat), swelling of extremities, and recurrent infections.

Review the patient's personal habits and nutritional history, including body weight; eating patterns; dietary intake of fats, salt, fluids; dietary restrictions; hypersensitivities or intolerances to food or medication; and the use of caffeine and alcohol. If the patient uses tobacco products, ask about type (cigarettes, pipe, cigars, snuff), duration, amount, and efforts to quit. If the patient uses street drugs, ask about type, method of intake (e.g., inhaled or injected), duration of use, and efforts to quit. Include questions about the patient's activity level and tolerance, recreational activities, and relaxation habits. Assess the patient's sleep patterns for interruptions in sleep due to dyspnea, cough, discomfort, urination, or stress. Ask how many pillows the patient uses when sleeping.

It is important to consider socioeconomic factors that may precipitate or aggravate circulatory problems, such as inadequate clothing, shoes, or shelter; and occupational levels such as prolonged sitting or standing, exposure to radiation, or extremes of temperature. Lifestyle, including intravenous drug use or sexual practices, may be significant in determining the risk for diseases associated with bleeding and impaired lymphatic function.

Physical Assessment

Physical assessment of cardiovascular function may be performed either as part of a total assessment or alone for patients with suspected or known problems with heart, peripheral vascular, lymphatic, or hematologic function (Bickley, 2016). The patient may sit or lie in the supine position. Before beginning the assessment, collect all required equipment and explain the techniques to the patient to decrease anxiety.

Assess the heart through inspection, palpation, and auscultation over the precordium (the area of the chest wall overlying the heart) (**Figure 29.18** ■). Movements over the precordium may be more easily seen with tangential lighting (in which the light is directed at a right angle to the area being observed, producing shadows). A quiet environment is essential to hear and assess heart sounds accurately. Assess the heart and thorax for the following:

- The **apical impulse** is a normal, visible pulsation (**thrust**) in the area of the midclavicular line in the left fifth intercostal space. It can be seen on inspection in about half of the adult population. (The apical impulse was previously called the *point of maximal impulse [PMI]*, but this term is no longer used because a maximal impulse may occur in other areas of the precordium as a result of abnormal conditions.)
- **Retraction** is a pulling-in of the tissue of the precordium; a slight retraction just medial to the midclavicular line at the area of the apical impulse is normal and is more likely to be visible in thin patients.
- *Pulsations* (other than the normal apical pulsations), which may be called **heaves** or **lifts**, are considered abnormal. They may occur as the result of an enlarged ventricle.

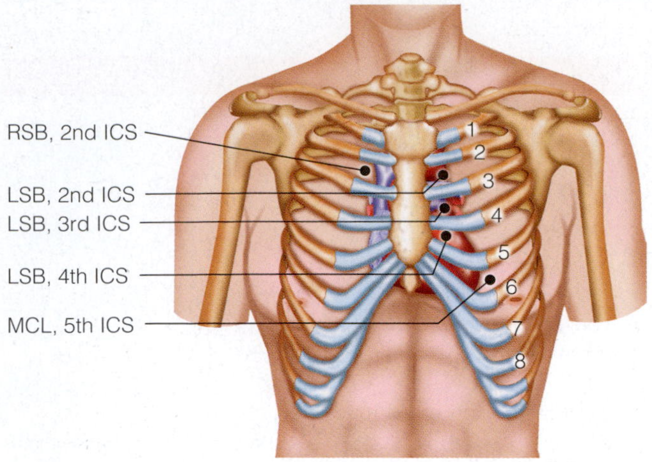
RSB, 2nd ICS
LSB, 2nd ICS
LSB, 3rd ICS
LSB, 4th ICS
MCL, 5th ICS
1
2
3
4
5
6
7
8

Figure 29.18 ■ Areas for inspection and palpation of the precordium, indicating the sequence for palpation.

The techniques used to assess the peripheral vascular and lymphatic systems include inspecting the skin for such changes as edema, ulcerations, or alterations in color and temperature; auscultating BP; and palpating the major pulse points of the body (**Figure 29.19** ■) and lymph nodes. The 5 Ps of peripheral vascular disease include pulselessness, pallor, pain, paresthesias, and paralysis. The patient may be assessed in the supine, sitting, and standing positions. Physical assessment of the lymphatic system, using inspection and palpation, is usually integrated into the assessment of other body systems. For example, the tonsils are inspected with the pharynx during the head and neck assessment; the regional lymph nodes are evaluated with corresponding body regions (e.g., occipital, auricular, and cervical nodes are evaluated with assessment of the head and neck, axillary nodes with assessment of the breast or thorax, epitrochlear node with assessment of the peripheral vascular exam of the arms, and inguinal nodes with assessment of the abdomen); and the spleen can be palpated during the abdominal assessment.

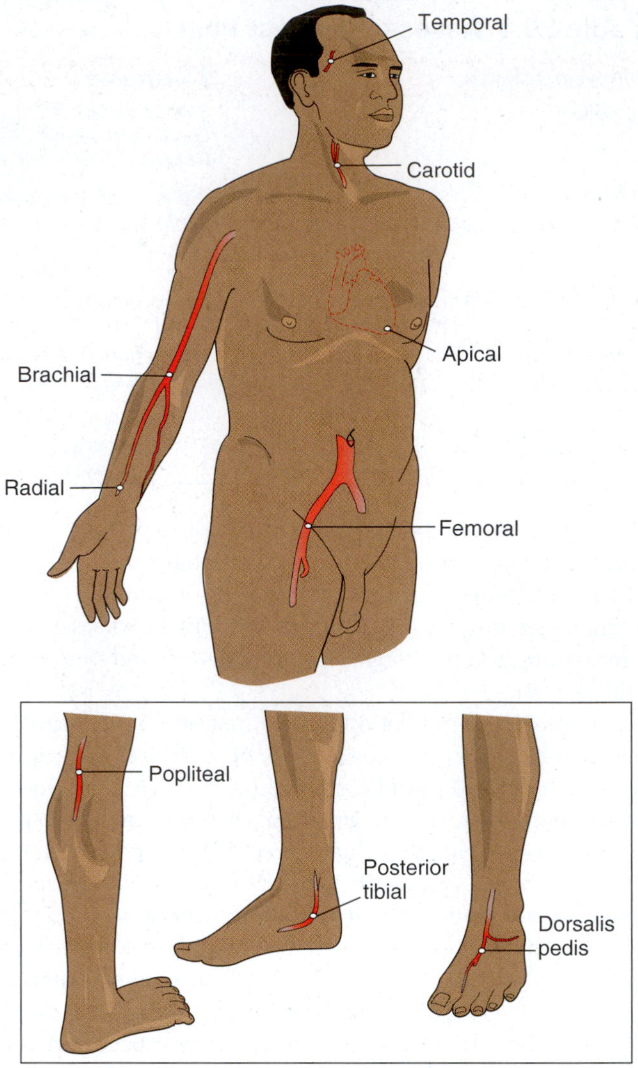
Temporal
Carotid
Apical
Brachial
Radial
Femoral
Popliteal
Posterior tibial
Dorsalis pedis

Figure 29.19 ■ Body sites at which peripheral pulses are most easily palpated.

Cardiovascular Assessments

Technique/Normal Findings	Abnormal Findings
Apical Impulse Assessment	
First using the palmar surface and then repeating with finger pads, palpate the precordium for symmetry of movement and the apical impulse for location, size, amplitude, and duration. Refer to Figure 29.19 for the sequence for palpation. To locate the apical impulse, ask the patient to assume a left lateral recumbent position. Simultaneous palpation of the carotid pulse may also be helpful. *The apical impulse is not palpable in all patients. The apical impulse may be palpated in the mitral area, and has only a brief small amplitude.*	■ An enlarged or displaced heart is associated with an apical impulse lateral to the midclavicular line (MCL) or below the fifth left intercostal space (ICS). ■ Increased size, amplitude, and duration of the apical impulse are associated with left-ventricular volume overload (increased afterload) in conditions such as HTN and aortic stenosis and with pressure overload (increased preload) in conditions such as aortic or mitral regurgitation. ■ Increased amplitude alone may occur with hyperkinetic states, such as anxiety, hyperthyroidism, and anemia. ■ Decreased amplitude is associated with a dilated heart in cardiomyopathy. ■ Displacement alone may also occur with dextrocardia, diaphragmatic hernia, gastric distention, or chronic lung disease. ■ A **thrill** (a palpable vibration over the precordium or an artery) may accompany severe valve stenosis. ■ A marked increase in amplitude of the apical impulse at the right-ventricular area occurs with right-ventricular volume overload in atrial septal defect. ■ An increase in amplitude and duration occurs with right-ventricular pressure overload in pulmonic stenosis and pulmonary hypertension. A lift or heave may also be seen in these conditions (and in chronic lung disease). ■ A palpable thrill in this area occurs with ventricular septal defect.

Technique/Normal Findings	Abnormal Findings
Palpate the subxiphoid area with the index and middle finger. *No pulsations or vibrations should be palpated.*	■ Right-ventricular enlargement may produce a downward pulsation against the fingertips. ■ An accentuated pulsation at the pulmonary area may be present in hyperkinetic states. ■ A prominent pulsation reflects increased flow or dilation of the pulmonary artery. ■ A thrill may be associated with aortic or pulmonary stenosis, aortic stenosis, pulmonary HTN, or atrial septal defect. ■ Increased pulsation at the aortic area may suggest aortic aneurysm. ■ A palpable second heart sound (S_2) may be noted with systemic HTN.
Cardiac Rate and Rhythm Assessment	
Auscultate heart rate (**Figure 29.20** ■). *The heart rate should be 60 to 100 beats per minute (bpm) with regular rhythm.*	■ A heart rate greater than 100 bpm is tachycardia. A heart rate less than 60 bpm is bradycardia. 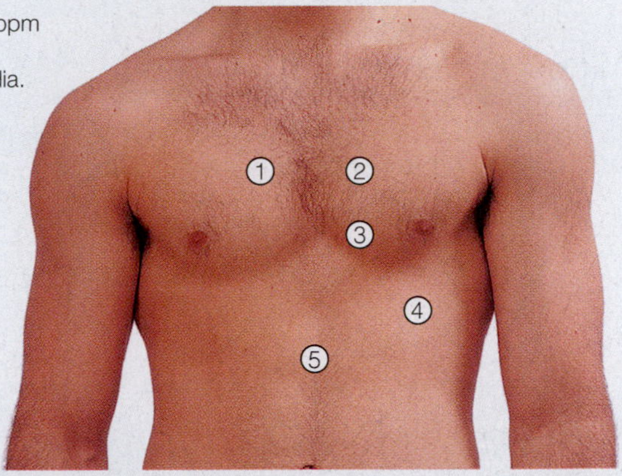 **Figure 29.20** ■ Areas for auscultation of the heart.
Simultaneously palpate the radial pulse while listening to the apical pulse. *The radial and apical pulses should be equal.*	■ If the radial pulse falls behind the apical rate, the patient has a pulse deficit, indicating weak, ineffective contractions of the left ventricle.
Auscultate heart rhythm. *The heart rhythm should be regular.*	■ **Dysrhythmias** (abnormal heart rate or rhythm) may be regular or irregular in rhythm; their rates may be slow or fast. Irregular rhythms may occur in a pattern (e.g., an early beat every second beat, called *bigeminy*), sporadically, or with frequency and disorganization (e.g., atrial fibrillation). A pattern of gradual increase and decrease in heart rate that is within the normal heart rate and that correlates with inspiration and expiration is called *sinus arrhythmia*.
Heart Sounds Assessment	
See guidelines for cardiac auscultation in **Box 29.1**.	
Identify S_1 (first heart sound) and note its intensity. At each auscultatory area, listen for several cardiac cycles. *S_1 is loudest at the apex of the heart.*	■ An accentuated S_1 occurs with tachycardia, states in which CO is high (fever, anxiety, exercise, anemia, hyperthyroidism), complete heart block, and mitral stenosis. ■ A diminished S_1 occurs with first-degree heart block, mitral regurgitation, CHF, CAD, and pulmonary or systemic HTN. The intensity is also decreased with obesity, emphysema, and pericardial effusion. Varying intensity of S_1 occurs with complete heart block and grossly irregular rhythms.
Listen for splitting of S_1. *Splitting of S_1 may occur during inspiration.*	■ Abnormal splitting of S_1 may be heard with right bundle branch block and premature ventricular contractions.
Identify S_2 (second heart sound) and note its intensity. *S_2 immediately follows S_1 and is loudest at the base of the heart.*	■ An accentuated S_2 may be heard with HTN, exercise, excitement, and conditions of pulmonary HTN such as CHF and cor pulmonale. ■ A diminished S_2 occurs with aortic stenosis, a fall in systolic BP (shock), and increased anteroposterior chest diameter.

(continued)

BOX 29.1
Guidelines for Cardiac Auscultation

1. Locate the major auscultatory areas on the precordium (refer to Figure 29.20).
2. Choose a sequence of listening. Either begin from the apex and move upward along the sternal border to the base or begin at the base and move downward to the apex. One suggested sequence is shown in Figure 29.20.
3. Listen first with the patient in the sitting or supine position. Then ask the patient to lie on the left side. Lastly, ask the patient to sit up and lean forward. These position changes bring the heart closer to the chest wall and enhance auscultation. Carry out the following steps when the patient assumes each of these positions:
   a. First, auscultate each area with the diaphragm of the stethoscope to listen for high-pitched sounds: S_1, S_2, murmurs, pericardial friction rubs.
   b. Next, auscultate each area with the bell of the stethoscope to listen for lower-pitched sounds: S_3, S_4, murmurs.
   c. Listen for the effect of respirations on each sound; while the patient is sitting up and leaning forward, ask him or her to exhale and hold the breath while you listen to heart sounds.

Cardiovascular Assessments (*continued*)

Technique/Normal Findings	Abnormal Findings
Listen for splitting of S_2. *No splitting of S_2 should be heard.*	■ Wide splitting of S_2 is associated with delayed emptying of the right ventricle, resulting in delayed pulmonary valve closure (e.g., mitral regurgitation, pulmonary stenosis, and right bundle branch block). ■ Fixed splitting occurs when right-ventricular output is greater than left-ventricular output and pulmonary valve closure is delayed (e.g., with atrial septal defect and right-ventricular failure). ■ Paradoxical splitting occurs when closure of the aortic valve is delayed (e.g., left bundle branch block).
Identify extra heart sounds in systole. *Extra heart sounds are not present in systole.*	■ Ejection sounds (or clicks) result from the opening of deformed semilunar valves (e.g., aortic and pulmonary stenosis). ■ A midsystolic click is heard with mitral valve prolapse (MVP).
Identify the presence of extra heart sounds in diastole. *Extra heart sounds are not present in diastole.*	■ An opening snap results from the opening sound of a stenotic mitral valve. ■ A pathologic S_3 (a third heart sound that immediately follows S_2, called a *ventricular gallop*) results from myocardial failure and ventricular volume overload (e.g., CHF, mitral or tricuspid regurgitation). ■ An S_4 (a fourth heart sound that immediately precedes S_1, called an *atrial gallop*) results from increased resistance to ventricular filling after atrial contraction (e.g., HTN, CAD, aortic stenosis, and cardiomyopathy). ■ A combined S_3 and S_4 is called a *summation gallop* and occurs with severe CHF. ■ A pericardial friction rub results from inflammation of the pericardial sac, as with pericarditis.
Murmur Assessment	
Identify any murmurs. Note location, timing, presence during systole or diastole, and intensity. Use the following scale to grade murmurs: I = Barely heard II = Quietly heard III = Clearly heard IV = Loud V = Very loud VI = Loudest; may be heard with stethoscope off the chest. A thrill may accompany murmurs of grade IV to grade VI. Note pitch (low, medium, or high) and quality (harsh, blowing, or musical). Note pattern/shape, crescendo, decrescendo, and radiation/transmission (to axilla, neck). *No murmurs should be heard.*	■ Midsystolic murmurs are heard with semilunar valve disease (e.g., aortic and pulmonary stenosis) and with hypertrophic cardiomyopathy. ■ Pansystolic (holosystolic) murmurs are heard with AV valve disease (e.g., mitral and tricuspid regurgitation, ventricular septal defect). ■ A late systolic murmur is heard with MVP. ■ Early diastolic murmurs occur with regurgitant flow across incompetent semilunar valves (e.g., aortic regurgitation). ■ Mid-diastolic and presystolic murmurs, such as with mitral stenosis, occur with turbulent flow across the AV valves. ■ Continuous murmurs throughout systole and all or part of diastole occur with patent ductus arteriosus.
Blood Pressure and Pulse Pressure Assessment	
See **Box 29.2** for blood pressure measurement guidelines.	

BOX 29.2
Guidelines for Blood Pressure Assessment

REVIEW OF KOROTKOFF SOUNDS

The first sound heard is the systolic pressure; at least two consecutive sounds should be clear. If the sound disappears and then is heard again 10 to 15 mm later, an auscultatory gap is present; this may be a normal variant or it may be associated with hypertension. The first diastolic sound is heard as a muffling of the Korotkoff sound and is considered the best approximation of the true diastolic pressure. The second diastolic sound is the level at which sounds are no longer heard.

The American Heart Association recommends documenting all three readings when measuring BP, for example, 120/72/64 mmHg. If only two readings are documented, the systolic and the second diastolic pressure are taken, for example, 120/64 mmHg.

TECHNIQUE REMINDERS

- Choose a cuff of an appropriate size: The cuff should snugly cover two-thirds of the upper arm, and the bladder should completely encircle the arm. The bladder should be centered over the brachial artery, with the lower edge 2 to 3 cm above the antecubital space.
- The patient's arm should be slightly flexed and supported (on a table or by the examiner) at heart level.
- To determine how high to inflate the cuff, palpate the brachial pulse, and inflate the cuff to the point on the manometer at which the pulse is no longer felt; then, add 30 mmHg to this reading, and use the sum as the target for inflation. Wait 15 seconds before reinflating the cuff to auscultate the BP.
- To recheck a BP, wait at least 30 seconds before attempting another inflation.
- Always inflate the cuff completely, and then deflate it. Once deflation begins, allow it to continue; do not try to reinflate the cuff if the first systolic sound is not heard or if the cuff inadvertently deflates.
- The bell of the stethoscope more effectively transmits the low-pitched sounds of BP.

SOURCES OF ERROR

- Falsely high readings can occur if the cuff is too small, too loose, or if the patient supports his or her own arm.
- Falsely low readings can occur if a standard cuff is used on a patient with thin arms.
- Inadequate inflation may result in underestimation of the systolic pressure or overestimation of the diastolic pressure if an auscultatory gap is present.
- Rapid deflation and repeated or slow inflations (causing venous congestion) can lead to underestimation of the systolic BP and overestimation of the diastolic BP.

Technique/Normal Findings	Abnormal Findings

FACTORS ALTERING BLOOD PRESSURE

- A change from the horizontal to upright position causes a slight decrease (5 to 10 mm) in systolic BP; the diastolic BP remains unchanged or rises slightly.
- BP taken in the arm is lower when the patient is standing.
- If the BP is taken with the patient in the lateral recumbent position, a lower BP reading may be obtained in both arms; this is especially apparent in the right arm with the patient in the left lateral position.
- Factors that increase BP include exercise, caffeine, tobacco use, cold environment, eating a large meal, painful stimuli, and emotions.
- Factors that lower BP include sleep (by 20 mmHg) and very fast, slow, or irregular heart rates.
- BP tends to be higher in taller or heavier patients.
- Legs should not be crossed when sitting, lying, or standing during BP measurement.

ALTERNATIVE METHODS OF BLOOD PRESSURE MEASUREMENT

- The palpatory method may be necessary if severe hypotension is present and the BP is inaudible. Palpate the brachial pulse, and inflate the cuff 30 mm above the point where the pulse disappears; deflate the cuff, and note the point on the manometer where the pulse becomes palpable again. Record this as the palpatory systolic BP.
- Leg BP measurement may be needed when there is injury of the arms or to rule out coarctation of the aorta or aortic insufficiency when arm diastolic BP is over 90 mmHg. Place the patient in the prone or supine position with the leg slightly flexed. Place a large leg cuff on the thigh with the bladder centered over the popliteal artery. Place the bell of the stethoscope over the popliteal space. Normal leg systolic BP is higher than arm BP; diastolic BP should be equal to or lower than arm BP. Abnormally low leg BP occurs with aortic insufficiency and coarctation of the aorta.

Auscultate BP in each arm with the patient seated.
The normal BP is considered to be ≤120/≤80 mmHg (American College of Cardiology, 2017).

- Consistent BP readings over 130/80 in adults is considered hypertension.
- BP 120–129 *and* diastolic ≤ 80 is considered elevated.
- Stage 1: Systolic between 130 and 139 *or* diastolic between 80 and 89
- Stage 2: Systolic at least 140 *or* diastolic at least 90 mm Hg
- Hypertensive crisis: Systolic over 180 and/or diastolic over 120
- BP under 90/60 is considered hypotension
- An auscultatory gap—a temporary disappearance of sound between the systolic and diastolic BP—may be a normal variation, or it may be associated with systolic HTN or a drop in diastolic BP due to aortic stenosis.
- **Korotkoff sounds** (refer to Box 29.2) may be heard down to zero with cardiac valve replacements, hyperkinetic states, thyrotoxicosis, and severe anemia, as well as after vigorous exercise.
- The sounds of aortic regurgitation may obscure the diastolic BP.
- A difference of > 10 mmHg between arms suggests arterial compression on the side of the lower reading, aortic dissection, or coarctation of the aorta.

Auscultate BP in each arm with the patient standing. If orthostatic changes occur, measure the BP with the patient supine, legs dangling, and again with the patient standing, 1–3 min apart.
A decrease of systolic BP is expected, but should be <10 mmHg; diastolic BP should not drop on standing.
Observe the pulse pressure. The pulse pressure is the difference between the systolic and diastolic BP. For example, if the BP is 140/80 mmHg, the pulse pressure is 60.
A normal pulse pressure is one-third the systolic measurement.

- A decrease in systolic BP of > 10–15 mmHg and a drop in diastolic BP on standing are called **orthostatic hypotension**. Causes include antihypertensive medications, volume depletion, PVD, prolonged bedrest, and aging.
- A widened pulse pressure with an elevated systolic BP occurs with exercise, arteriosclerosis, severe anemia, thyrotoxicosis, and increased intracranial pressure.
- A narrowed pulse pressure with a decreased systolic BP occurs with shock, cardiac failure, and pulmonary embolus.

SAFETY ALERT: If unable to auscultate BP or palpate pulses, a Doppler ultrasound device may be used to evaluate blood flow. Apply a dime-sized amount of gel over the blood vessel to be assessed and lightly place the probe over the gel. Listen for a whooshing (artery) or rushing (vein) sound. ■

Skin Assessment

Inspect the color of the skin.
The skin color should be appropriate to the patient's age and race.

- Pallor reflects constriction of peripheral blood flow (e.g., due to syncope or shock) or decreased circulating oxyhemoglobin (e.g., due to hemorrhage or anemia).
- Central cyanosis of the lips, earlobes, oral mucosa, and tongue suggests chronic cardiopulmonary disease. (See **Box 29.3** for abnormal findings associated with peripheral vascular and lymphatic assessment.)

BOX 29.3
Abnormal Findings Associated with Peripheral Vascular and Lymphatic Assessment

- ***Pallor*** is an absence of color of the skin. The degree of pallor depends on the patient's normal skin color and health status. Dark skin may appear ashen or have a yellowish tinge.
- ***Cyanosis*** is a bluish discoloration of the skin and mucous membranes in people with light skin. In people with dark skin, cyanosis may be difficult to observe. Inspect the nail beds and conjunctiva.
- ***Edema*** is an abnormal accumulation of fluid in the interstitial spaces of body tissues. It is often most apparent in the lower extremities.
- ***Varicose veins*** are tortuous and dilated veins that have incompetent valves. The saphenous veins of the legs are most commonly affected.
- ***Enlarged lymph nodes*** result from infection or malignancy.
- ***Atrophic changes*** are changes in the size or activity of body tissues as a result of pathology or injury. Decreased blood flow and oxygenation of the lower extremities often cause atrophic changes of loss of hair, thickened toenails, changes in pigmentation, and ulcerations.
- ***Gangrene*** is the necrosis (or death) of tissue, most often the result of loss of blood supply and infection. Gangrene often begins in the most distal of the tissues of the extremities.
- ***Pressure injuries***, also called *decubitus ulcers* or *bedsores*, are the result of ischemia and hypoxia of tissue following prolonged pressure. These ulcers are often located over bony prominences. If untreated, the tissue changes proceed from red skin to deep, crater-like ulcers.

(continued)

Cardiovascular Assessments (*continued*)

Technique/Normal Findings	Abnormal Findings
Inspect the skin of the extremities and over the regional lymph nodes, noting any edema, erythema, red streaks, or skin lesions. *There should be no edema, redness, or lesions over the regional lymph nodes.*	■ Lymphangitis (inflammation of a lymphatic vessel) may produce a red streak with induration (hardness) following the course of the lymphatic collecting duct; infected skin lesions may be present, particularly between the digits. ■ **Lymphedema** (swelling due to lymphatic obstruction) occurs with congenital lymphatic anomaly (Milroy disease) or with trauma to the regional lymphatic ducts from surgery or metastasis (e.g., arm lymphedema after radical mastectomy with axillary node removal). ■ Edema of lymphatic origin is usually not pitting, and the skin may be thickened; one example is the taut swelling of the face and body that occurs with myxedema, associated with hypothyroidism.
Artery and Vein Assessment	
Palpate the temporal arteries. *There should be no redness, swelling, nodules, or variations in pulse amplitude.*	■ Redness, swelling, nodularity, and variations in pulse amplitude may occur with temporal arteritis.
Inspect and palpate the carotid arteries. Note symmetry and the pulse rate, rhythm, volume, and amplitude. *Note any variation with respiration. Describe all pulses as increased, normal, diminished, or absent. Scales ranging from 0 to 4+ are sometimes used as follows:* 0 = Absent 1+ = Diminished 2+ = Normal 3+ = Increased 4+ = Bounding	
Pulse waveforms are shown in **Figure 29.21** ■. *The carotid pulses should be bilaterally equal in rate, rhythm, volume, and amplitude.*	■ A unilateral pulsating bulge is seen with a tortuous or kinked carotid artery. ■ Alterations in pulse rate or rhythm are due to cardiac dysrhythmias. ■ An absent pulse indicates arterial occlusion. ■ A hypokinetic (weak) pulse is associated with decreased stroke volume (Figure 29.21B). This may be due to congestive heart failure (CHF), aortic stenosis, or hypovolemia; to increased peripheral resistance, which may result from cold temperatures; or to arterial narrowing, commonly found with atherosclerosis. ■ A hyperkinetic (bounding) pulse occurs with increased stroke volume and/or decreased peripheral resistance (Figure 29.21C). This may result from states in which CO is high or from aortic regurgitation. It also may occur with anemia, hyperthyroidism, bradycardia, or reduced compliance, as with atherosclerosis. ■ A bigeminal pulse is marked by decreased amplitude of every second beat (Figure 29.21D). This may be due to premature contractions (usually ventricular). ■ Pulsus alternans is a regular pulse with alternating strong and weak beats (Figure 29.21E). This may be due to left-ventricular failure and severe HTN.

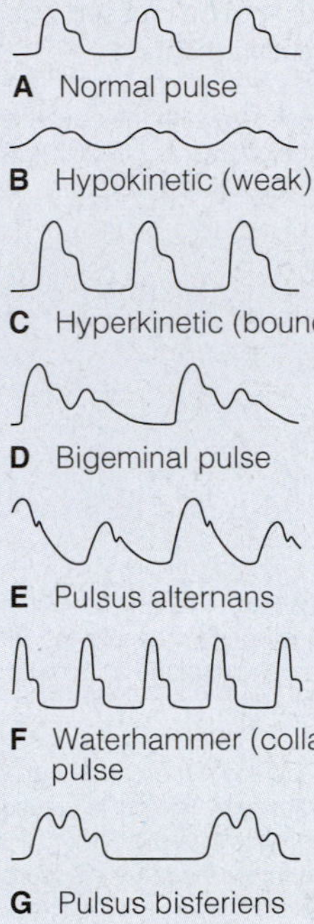
A Normal pulse
B Hypokinetic (weak) pulse
C Hyperkinetic (bounding) pulse
D Bigeminal pulse
E Pulsus alternans
F Waterhammer (collapsing) pulse
G Pulsus bisferiens

Figure 29.21 ■ Types of pulse patterns.

Technique/Normal Findings	Abnormal Findings
Auscultate the carotid arteries, using the bell of the stethoscope. *No bruits should be heard.*	■ A murmuring or blowing sound heard over stenosed peripheral vessels is known as a *bruit*. A bruit heard over the middle to upper carotid artery suggests atherosclerosis.
Inspect and palpate the internal and external jugular veins for venous pressure. *See* **Box 29.4** *for guidelines for assessing jugular venous pressure.*	■ An increase in jugular venous pressure (JVP) over 3 cm and located above the sternal angle reflects increased right-atrial pressure. This occurs with right-ventricular failure or, less commonly, with constrictive pericarditis, tricuspid stenosis, and superior venae cavae obstruction.
If venous pressure is elevated, assess the hepatojugular reflex. (Compress the liver in the right upper abdominal quadrant with the palm of the hand for 30–60 sec while observing the jugular veins.)	■ A decrease in venous pressure reflects reduced left-ventricular output or blood volume. ■ Unilateral neck vein distention suggests local compression or anatomic anomaly. ■ A rise in the column of neck vein distention over 1 cm with liver compression indicates right heart failure.
Upper Extremity Assessment	
Inspect and palpate the arms and hands, noting size and symmetry, skin color, and temperature. *Arms and hands should be symmetrical in size and shape, warm, and of appropriate skin color.*	■ Unilateral swelling with venous prominence occurs with venous obstruction. ■ Cyanosis of the nail beds reflects chronic cardiopulmonary disease. ■ Unilateral swelling with venous prominence occurs with venous obstruction. ■ Cold temperature of the hands and fingers occurs with vasoconstriction.

Technique/Normal Findings	Abnormal Findings

BOX 29.4
Assessing Jugular Venous Pressure

When a patient with normal venous pressure lies in the supine position, full neck veins are normally visible, but as the head of the bed is elevated, the pulsations disappear. In the patient with greatly elevated venous pressure, visible pulsations of the jugular vein are present even in the upright position. To conduct the inspection, do the following:

1. Remove clothing from the patient's neck and chest. Elevate the head of the bed 30 to 45 degrees, and turn the patient's head to the opposite side. Shine a light tangentially across the neck to increase shadows. If the external jugular veins are distended, they will be visible vertically between the mandible and outer clavicle.
2. If jugular distention is present, assess the jugular venous pressure by measuring from the highest point of visible distention to the sternal angle (the point at which the clavicles meet) on both sides of the neck (see the accompanying figure). Bilateral measurements above 3 cm are considered elevated and indicate increased venous pressure; distention on only one side may indicate obstruction.

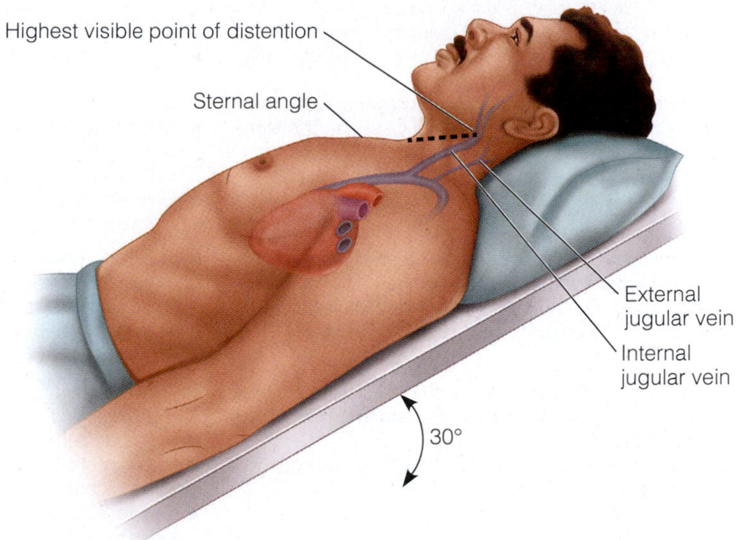
Highest visible point of distention
Sternal angle
External jugular vein
Internal jugular vein
30°
Assessment of the highest point of jugular vein distention.

Technique/Normal Findings	Abnormal Findings
Palpate the nail beds for capillary refill. (Apply pressure to the patient's fingertips. Watch for blanching of the nail beds. Release the pressure. Note the time it takes for capillary refill, indicated by the return of pink color on release of pressure.) *Capillary refill should be < 2 seconds (i.e., immediate).*	■ Capillary refill that takes < 3 sec reflects circulatory compromise, such as hypovolemia or anemia.
Assess venous pattern and pressure. (Elevate one of the patient's arms over the head for a few seconds. Slowly lower the arm. Observe the filling of the patient's hand veins.) *Hand veins should fill equally and immediately.*	■ Distention of hand veins at elevations over 9 cm above heart level reflects an increase in systemic venous pressure.
Palpate the radial and brachial pulses. Note rate, rhythm, volume amplitude, symmetry, and variations with respiration. (Refer to Figure 29.21 for pulse patterns.) *Radial and brachial pulses should have equal and normal rate, be strong, and not vary with respirations.*	■ Alterations in pulse rate or rhythm are due to cardiac dysrhythmias (such as atrial fibrillation, atrial flutter, and premature ventricular contractions). A pulse rate over 100 bpm is tachycardia; a pulse rate below 60 bpm is bradycardia. ■ A pulse deficit (slower radial rate than apical rate) occurs with dysrhythmias and CHF. ■ Irregularities of rhythm produce early beats and pauses (skipped beats) in the pulse, which may be regular, sporadic, or grossly irregular in pattern. ■ Diminished or absent radial pulses may be due to thromboangiitis obliterans (Buerger disease) or acute arterial occlusion. ■ A weak and thready pulse, often with tachycardia, reflects decreased CO. ■ A bounding pulse occurs with hyperkinetic states and atherosclerosis. ■ Unequal pulses between extremities suggest arterial narrowing or obstruction on one side. ■ In sinus dysrhythmia (a normal variant, especially in young adults), the pulse rate increases with inspiration and decreases with expiration.
If arterial insufficiency is suspected, palpate the ulnar pulse and perform the Allen test: ■ Have the patient make a tight fist. ■ Compress both the radial and ulnar arteries. ■ Have the patient open the hand to a slightly flexed position. ■ Observe for pallor and manifestations of pain. ■ Release the ulnar artery and observe for the return of pink color within 3–5 sec. ■ Repeat the procedure on the radial artery. *Color should return within 3–5 sec in both the ulnar and the radial arteries.*	■ The normal ulnar artery may or may not have a palpable pulse. ■ Persistent pallor with the Allen test suggests ulnar artery occlusion.

(continued)

Cardiovascular Assessments (*continued*)

Technique/Normal Findings	Abnormal Findings
Lower Extremity Assessment	
Inspect and palpate each leg, noting size, shape, and symmetry; arterial pattern; skin color, temperature, and texture; hair pattern; pigmentation; rashes; ulcers, sensation; and capillary refill. *Legs should be symmetric in size and shape, arterial pattern, appropriate color, warm, without lesions. Capillary refill on toenails should be immediate.*	■ Chronic arterial insufficiency may be due to arteriosclerosis or autonomic dysfunction or to acute occlusion resulting from thrombosis, embolus, or aneurysm. ■ Signs of arterial disruption include pallor, dependent rubor (dusky redness); cool to cold temperature; and atrophic changes, such as hair loss with shiny and smooth texture, thickened nails, sensory loss, slow capillary refill, and muscle atrophy. ■ Ulcers with symmetric margins, a deep base, black or necrotic tissue, and absence of bleeding may occur at pressure points on or between the toes, on the heel, on the lateral malleolar or tibial area, over the metatarsal heads, or along the side or sole of the foot. ■ Gangrene due to complete arterial occlusion presents as black, dry, hard skin; pregangrenous color changes include deep cyanosis and purple-black discoloration.
With the patient supine, assess the venous pattern of the legs. Repeat with the patient standing. *Venous pattern on both legs should be symmetric, and there should be no edema, cyanosis, or lesions.*	■ Signs of venous insufficiency include swelling, thickened skin, cyanosis, stasis dermatitis (brown pigmentation, erythema, and scaling), and superficial ankle ulcers located predominantly at the medial malleolus with uneven margins, ruddy granulation tissue, and bleeding. ■ Varicose veins appear as dilated, tortuous, and thickened veins, which are more prominent in a dependent position.
Palpate the femoral, popliteal, posterior tibial, and dorsalis pedis pulses for volume, amplitude, and symmetry (refer to Figure 29.19). *All lower extremity pulses should be strong and equal in amplitude.*	■ Diminished or absent leg pulses suggest partial or complete arterial occlusion of the proximal vessel and are often due to arteriosclerosis obliterans. ■ Increased and widened femoral and popliteal pulsations suggest aneurysm. ■ Absence of a posterior tibial pulse with signs and symptoms of arterial insufficiency is usually due to acute occlusion by thrombosis or embolus. ■ Diminished or absent pedal pulses are often due to popliteal occlusion associated with diabetes mellitus.
If pulses are diminished, observe for postural color changes. Elevate both legs 60 degrees, and observe the color of the soles of the feet. Have the patient sit and dangle the legs; note the return of color to the feet.	■ Extensive pallor on elevation is suggestive of arterial insufficiency. ■ Rubor (dusky redness) of the toes and feet along with delayed venous return (over 45 sec) suggests arterial insufficiency.
If arterial insufficiency is suspected, auscultate the femoral arteries. *No bruits should be heard.*	■ Femoral bruits suggest arterial narrowing due to arteriosclerosis.
Inspect and gently palpate the calves. *There should be no redness or swelling, heat, or pain in the calves of the legs.*	■ Redness, warmth, swelling, tenderness, and cords along a superficial vein suggest thrombophlebitis or deep venous thrombosis.
Inspect and palpate for edema (**Figure 29.22** ■). Use your thumb to compress the dorsum of the patient's foot, around the ankles, and along the tibia (Figure 29.22A). A depression in the skin that does not immediately refill is called *pitting edema*. *Normally, there is no edema.*	Edema can be graded on a scale from 1+ to 4+ (Figure 29.22B): 1+ (–2-mm depression): No visible change in the leg; slight pitting 2+ (–4-mm depression): No marked change in the shape of the leg; pitting slightly deeper 3+ (–6-mm depression): Leg visibly swollen; pitting deep 4+ (–8-mm depression): Leg very swollen; pitting very deep ■ Edema may be caused by disease of the cardiovascular system such as CHF; by renal, hepatic, or lymphatic problems; or by infection. ■ Venous distention suggests venous insufficiency or incompetence.

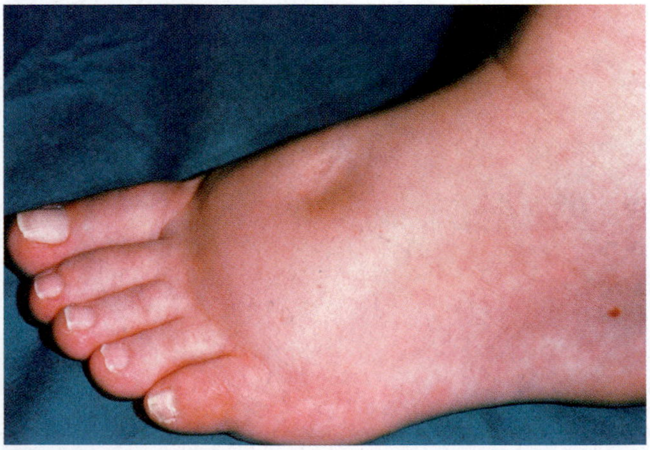

A

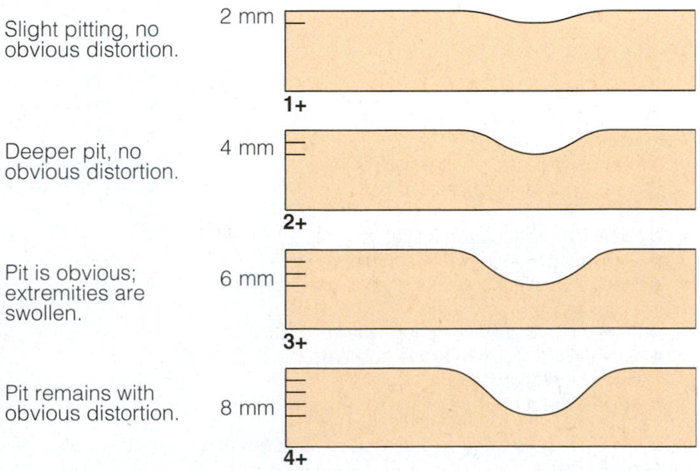
Slight pitting, no obvious distortion.
2 mm
1+
Deeper pit, no obvious distortion.
4 mm
2+
Pit is obvious; extremities are swollen.
6 mm
3+
Pit remains with obvious distortion.
8 mm
4+

B

Figure 29.22 ■ Evaluation of edema. **A**, Palpating for edema over the dorsum of the foot. **B**, Four-point scale for grading edema.

Technique/Normal Findings	Abnormal Findings
Abdominal Assessment	
Inspect and palpate the abdominal aorta. Note size, width, and any visible pulsations or bulging. *Abdominal aorta should be of appropriate size without visible pulsations or bulging.*	■ A pulsating mass in the upper abdomen suggests an aortic aneurysm, particularly in the older adult. ■ An aorta > 2.5–3 cm in width reflects pathologic dilation, most likely due to arteriosclerosis.
Auscultate the epigastrium and each abdominal quadrant, using the bell of the stethoscope (**Figure 29.23** ■). *No bruits should be heard over the abdominal aorta.*	■ Abdominal bruits reflect turbulent blood flow associated with partial arterial occlusion. ■ A bruit heard over the aorta suggests an aneurysm. ■ A bruit heard over the epigastrium and radiating laterally, especially with HTN, suggests renal artery stenosis. ■ Bruits heard in the lower abdominal quadrants suggest partial occlusion of the iliac arteries.

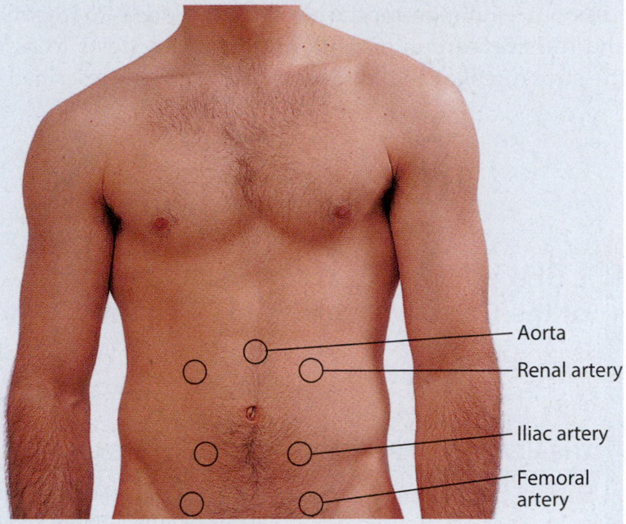
Aorta
Renal artery
Iliac artery
Femoral artery
Figure 29.23 ■ Auscultation sites of the abdominal aorta and its branches.

Technique/Normal Findings	Abnormal Findings
Lymph Node Assessment	
Palpate the regional lymph nodes of the head and neck, axillae, arms, and groin. Use firm, circular movements of the finger pads and note size, shape, symmetry, consistency, delineation, mobility, tenderness, sensation, and condition of overlying skin. *Nodes should not be enlarged or painful.*	■ **Lymphadenopathy** refers to the enlargement of lymph nodes (over 1 cm) with or without tenderness. It may be caused by inflammation, infection, or malignancy of the nodes or the regions drained by the nodes. ■ Lymph node enlargement with tenderness suggests inflammation (*lymphadenitis*). With bacterial infection, the nodes may be warm and matted with localized swelling. ■ Malignant or metastatic nodes may be hard, indicating lymphoma; rubbery, indicating Hodgkin's disease; or fixed to adjacent structures. They are usually not tender. ■ Ear infections and scalp and facial lesions, such as acne, may cause enlargement of the preauricular and cervical nodes. ■ Anterior cervical nodes are enlarged and infected with streptococcal pharyngitis and mononucleosis. ■ Lymphadenitis of the cervical and submandibular nodes occurs with herpes simplex lesions. ■ Enlargement of supraclavicular nodes, especially the left, is highly suggestive of metastatic disease from abdominal and thoracic cancer. ■ Axillary lymphadenopathy is associated with breast cancer. ■ Lesions of the genitals may produce enlargement of the inguinal nodes. ■ Persistent generalized lymphadenopathy is associated with acquired immunodeficiency syndrome (AIDS) and AIDS-related complex.
Spleen Assessment	
Palpate for the spleen, in the upper left quadrant of the abdomen. *The spleen is normally not palpable.*	A palpable spleen in the left upper abdominal quadrant of an adult may indicate abnormal enlargement (splenomegaly) and may be associated with cancer, blood dyscrasias, and viral infection, such as mononucleosis.
Percuss for splenic dullness in the lowest left intercostal space (ICS) at the anterior axillary line or in the 9th to 10th ICS at the midaxillary line (**Figure 29.24** ■). *Normally, tympany is heard.*	A dull percussion note in the lowest left ICS at the anterior axillary line or below the 10th rib at the midaxillary line suggests splenic enlargement.

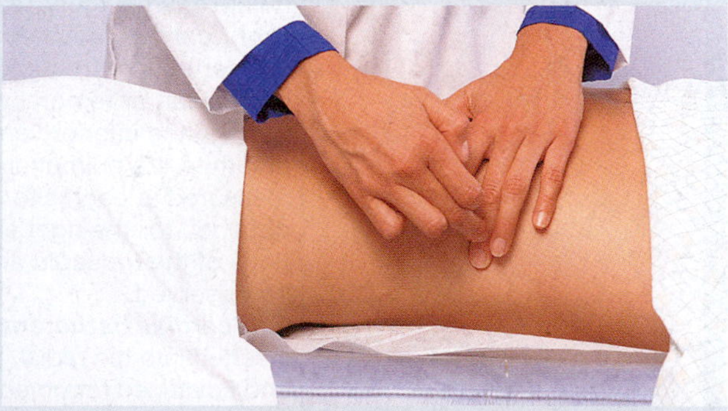
Figure 29.24 ■ Percussing the spleen.

Diagnosis

The results of diagnostic tests of cardiac function are used to support the diagnosis of a specific disease, to provide information to identify or modify the appropriate medications or therapy used to treat the disease, and to help the interprofessional team monitor the patient's responses to treatment and nursing care interventions. Diagnostic tests to assess the structures and functions of the heart are described on page 980. More information is included in the discussion of specific disorders in Chapter 30 through 33.

Regardless of the type of diagnostic test, the nurse is responsible for explaining the procedure and any special preparation needed, ensuring the consent form is signed (if necessary), supporting the patient during the examination as necessary, documenting the procedure as appropriate, and monitoring the results of the test. The nurse is responsible for postprocedure care and patient teaching for self-care at home.

Diagnostic Tests
of the Cardiovascular and Lymphatic System

NAME OF TEST	PURPOSE AND DESCRIPTION	RELATED NURSING INTERVENTIONS
THE HEART AND PERIPHERAL VASCULAR SYSTEM		
Blood pool imaging (gated scan or multigated acquisition scan [MUGA])	This test is useful for evaluation of cardiac status following myocardial infarction and congestive heart failure and effectiveness of cardiac medications. Also used to evaluate left-ventricular function during rest and exercise. Following IV injection of technetium-99m pertechnetate, sequential evaluation of the heart can be performed for several hours. It can be done at the patient's bedside.	No special preparation is needed.
Cardiac catheterization (coronary angiography, coronary arteriography)	A cardiac catheterization may be performed to identify coronary artery disease (CAD) or cardiac valvular disease, to determine pulmonary artery or heart chamber pressures, to obtain a myocardial biopsy, to evaluate artificial valves, or to perform angioplasty or stent an area of CAD. The test is performed by inserting a long catheter into a vein or artery (depending on whether the right side or the left side of the heart is being examined) in the arm or leg. Using fluoroscopy, the catheter is then threaded to the heart chambers or coronary arteries or both. Contrast dye is injected and heart structures are visualized and heart activity filmed. The test is done in the hospital for diagnosis and before heart surgery. ***Right cardiac catheterization:*** The catheter is inserted into the brachial, subclavian, internal jugular, or femoral vein and then threaded through the inferior vena cava into the right atrium to the pulmonary artery. Pressures are measured at each site and blood samples can be obtained for the right side of the heart. The functions of the tricuspid and pulmonary valves can be observed. ***Left cardiac catheterization:*** The catheter is inserted into the radial, brachial, or femoral artery and advanced retrograde through the aorta to the coronary arteries and/or left ventricle. The patency of the coronary arteries and/or functions of the aortic and mitral valves and left ventricle can be observed.	Inform the patient that food and fluids should not be taken for 6–8 h before the test. Assess for allergies to seafood, iodine, or iodine contrast dyes. If an allergic response to the dye is possible, antihistamines (such as Benadryl) or steroids may be administered the evening before and the morning of the test. Assess for use of aspirin or NSAIDs (risk of bleeding), Viagra (risk of heart problems), or history of kidney disease (dye used may be toxic to the kidneys). Take and record vital signs, including peripheral pulses. Explain that the patient is positioned on a padded table that tilts. A local anesthetic is used at the site of catheter insertion. ECG leads are applied and vital signs are monitored during the procedure. The patient lies supine and is asked to cough and deep-breathe frequently. The procedure takes 0.5–3 h. After the procedure, monitor vital signs every 15 min for the first hour and then every 30 min until stable. Assess cardiac rhythm and rate for alterations. Assess peripheral pulses distal to the insertion site. Assess for chest heaviness, dyspnea, level of consciousness, and abdominal or groin pain. Monitor catheter insertion site for bleeding or hematoma. Administer pain medications as prescribed. Instruct patient to increase fluid intake and restrict activity as ordered.

NAME OF TEST	PURPOSE AND DESCRIPTION	RELATED NURSING INTERVENTIONS
Cardiolite scan	This test is used to evaluate blood flow in different parts of the heart. Cardiolite (technetium-99m sestamibi) is injected IV. In pharmacologic stress scans, dipyridamole (Persantine) or adenosine is injected to increase blood flow to coronary arteries. Additional pharmacologic stress scans can use dobutamine or arbutamine for their positive inotropic properties. These scans may be done in conjunction with a treadmill test.	See information in this table for treadmill test. Instruct the patient to avoid intake of caffeine (including chocolate) for 12–24 h before having a test with dipyridamole Cardiolite.
Cardiac computed tomography (CT) scan	A cardiac CT scan may be conducted to visualize the heart anatomy or coronary circulation or to quantify early calcium deposits in coronary arteries. The calcium score screening heart scan is used to evaluate risk for future coronary artery disease and coronary artery bypass graft patency. It does not require injection of IV iodine. If calcium is present, a score is generated that estimates the extent of coronary artery disease. A negative test does not rule out the potential for soft plaque atherosclerosis.	Assess for allergy to iodine or seafood if contrast medium is to be administered. If allergy exists, follow orders for times and types of medications. For IV contrast studies, instruct patient not to eat or drink for 4 h prior to the test. Assess medications: Oral hypoglycemic agents are contraindicated for use with iodinated contrast. Request patient remove hairpins, earrings, and dentures.
Chest x-ray	An x-ray of the thorax can illustrate the contours, placement, and chambers of the heart. It may be done to identify heart displacement or hypertrophy or fluid in the pericardial sac.	No special preparation is needed.
Echocardiogram ■ M-mode ■ Two-dimensional (2-D) ■ Spectral Doppler ■ Color Doppler ■ Three-dimensional (3-D) ■ Four-dimensional (4-D) ■ Stress echocardiogram	Echocardiograms use a transducer to record waves that are bounced off the heart and to record the direction and flow of blood through the heart in audio and graphic data. An *M (motion)-mode echocardiogram* records the motion, wall thickness, and chamber size of the heart. A *2-D echocardiogram* provides a cross-sectional view of the heart. *Spectral Doppler* records blood flow through the chambers and septal wall defects. *Color Doppler* detects blood flow through the heart, valve function, and presence of shunting. *Three-dimensional echocardiography* combines 2-D echocardiography and ultrasound technology to evaluate the speed and direction of blood flow through the heart, which can identify pathology such as leaky valves. *Four-dimensional echocardiography* provides a moving picture of the 3D echo. *Stress echocardiography* combines a treadmill test with ultrasound images to evaluate segmental function and wall motion. If the patient is not physically able to exercise, IV dobutamine may be administered and ultrasound images taken.	No special preparation is needed; see related nursing care for the patient having a treadmill test for a stress echocardiogram.
Electrocardiogram (ECG)	See **Boxes 29.5** and **29.6**.	No special preparation is needed.
Lipids	Blood lipids are cholesterol, triglycerides, and phospholipids. They circulate bound to proteins, and so are known as *lipoproteins*. Lipids are measured to evaluate risk for CAD and to monitor effectiveness of anticholesterol medications (Nayor & Vasan, 2016). Normal values: Cholesterol: < 200 mg/dL Triglycerides: < 150 mg/dL HDL: Optimal: > 60 mg/dL Men: > 40 mg/dL Women: > 50 mg/dL LDL: < 100 mg/dL (*Note:* Normal values may vary by laboratory.)	Recommend a low-fat meal the evening prior to the test, then no food for 8–12 h. Instruct the patient to have no alcohol intake for 24 h prior to the test. Assess medications. Blood lipids may be increased by thyroxine, estrogens, aspirin, antibiotics (tetracycline and neomycin), nicotinic acid, heparin, and colchicine.

(*continued*)

Diagnostic Tests
of the Cardiovascular and Lymphatic System (*continued*)

NAME OF TEST	PURPOSE AND DESCRIPTION	RELATED NURSING INTERVENTIONS
Magnetic resonance imaging (MRI)	An MRI may be used to identify and locate areas of myocardial infarction, perfusion of the heart, and patency of coronary arteries after coronary grafts and to evaluate pericarditis and cardiac tumors.	Assess for any metallic implants (such as clips on brain aneurysms, pacemaker, body piercing, tattoos, and shrapnel). If present, notify physician. Remove transdermal medication patches (both OTC and prescribed) unless otherwise ordered. Replace the patch following the procedure. Tell the patient to inform the staff about the patch when making the appointment and when completing the admission information. Ask if patient is pregnant; if so, the test is not performed. Ask about claustrophobia; if a problem exists, request patient to ask the referring physician for a relaxing medication prior to the MRI. If the patient is very claustrophobic, obese, or confused, an open MRI may be used. A contrast agent (gadolinium) may be used, especially in those allergic to dyes used in CT scanning.
Nuclear dobutamine stress test	Dobutamine is an adrenergic drug that increases myocardial contractility, heart rate, and systolic BP, which increases coronary oxygen consumption and thus increases coronary blood flow. The test is conducted in two parts: Resting and stress. The test usually takes about 3.5–4 h.	Instruct the patient to not eat food or drink fluids other than water after midnight or during the test. Tell the patient to discontinue beta-blockers, calcium channel blockers, and ACE inhibitors for 36 h prior to the test. If hospitalized, do not administer nitrates for 6 h prior to the test.
Nuclear dipyridamole (Persantine) stress test	This test is used when the patient is not physically able to walk on a treadmill. Dipyridamole (Persantine), given IV, dilates the coronary arteries and increases myocardial blood flow. Coronary arteries that are narrowed from CAD cannot dilate to increase myocardial perfusion.	Patient is NPO after midnight except for water. Food, fluids, and drugs that contain caffeine should be avoided for 24 h prior to the test, as should decaffeinated fluids. Some drugs, such as theophylline preparations, are discontinued for 36 h prior to the test.
Pericardiocentesis	This procedure is performed in the hospital to remove fluid from the pericardial sac for diagnostic or therapeutic purposes. It may also be done as an emergency procedure for the patient with cardiac tamponade (which may result in death). After local anesthetic, a large-gauge (16–18) needle is inserted to the left of the xiphoid process into the pericardial sac and excess fluid is withdrawn (**Figure 29.25** ■).	Take and record baseline vital signs. Assess for history of cardiac problems. Explain to patient the need to remain still during the procedure, that the procedure takes about 30 min, and that a local anesthetic will be used at the needle insertion site. Monitor the ECG during and after the procedure and report abnormal findings to the physician. Monitor vital signs after the procedure as ordered. Notify the physician of changes in cardiac rhythm, BP, heart rate, or level of consciousness. If the procedure is to treat an emergency, monitor central venous pressure (CVP) and BP closely. As the effusion is relieved, CVP will decrease and BP will increase.

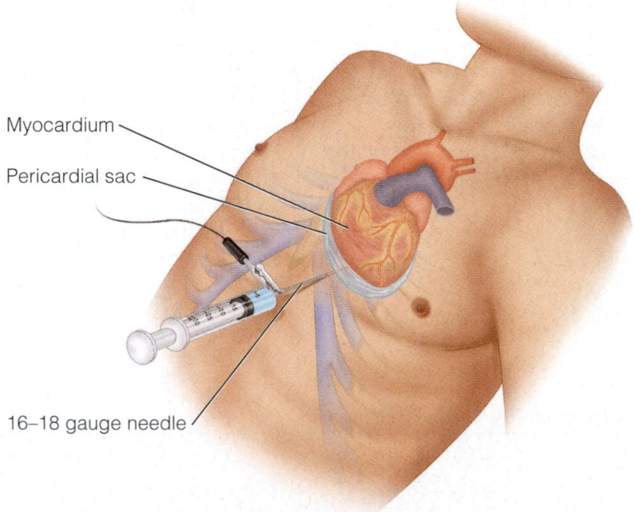
Myocardium
Pericardial sac
16–18 gauge needle

Figure 29.25 ■ Pericardiocentesis.

NAME OF TEST	PURPOSE AND DESCRIPTION	RELATED NURSING INTERVENTIONS
Positron emission tomography (PET)	Following injection of a radionuclide, two scans are performed (resting and chemically induced stress) and the resulting images are compared for myocardial perfusion and myocardial metabolic function. A stress test (treadmill) may be a part of the test. If the myocardium is ischemic or damaged, the images will be different. Normally, the images will be the same.	Assess the patient's blood glucose: For accurate metabolic activity images, the blood glucose level must be between 60 and 140 mg/dL. If exercise is included in the test, instruct the patient to be NPO and avoid smoking and caffeine for 24 h prior to the test.
Thallium/technetium stress test (myocardial imaging perfusion test, cardiac blood pool imaging)	*Thallium stress test:* Thallium-201, a radioisotope that accumulates in myocardial cells, is used during the stress test to evaluate myocardial perfusion. Second scans are done 2–3 h later when the heart is at rest; this is to differentiate between an ischemic area and an infarcted or scarred area of myocardium. *Exercise technetium perfusion test:* Technetium-99m-laced compounds are administered and a scan is done to evaluate cardiac perfusion, wall motion, and ejection fraction. This is probably the most useful noninvasive test to diagnose and monitor CAD.	Assess medications; those that affect the BP or heart rate should be discontinued for 24–36 h prior to the test (unless the test is being done to monitor the effectiveness of the medications). See treadmill test for other interventions.
Treadmill test (stress test)	Stress testing is based on the theory that coronary artery disease results in depression of the ST segment with exercise. Depression of the ST segment and depression or inversion of the T wave indicates myocardial ischemia. When the patient is walking on a treadmill machine, the work rate of the heart is changed every 3 min for 15 min by increasing the speed and degree of incline by 3% each time. Patients exercise until they are fatigued, develop symptoms, or reach their maximum predicted heart rate.	Ask the patient to wear comfortable shoes and to avoid food, fluids, and smoking for 2–3 h before the test. Assess for events that contraindicate the tests: Recent myocardial infarction; severe, unstable angina; controlled dysrhythmias; congestive heart failure; or recent pulmonary embolism.
Transesophageal echocardiography (TEE)	A TEE allows visualization of adjacent cardiac and extracardiac structures to identify or monitor mitral and aortic valve pathology, left atrium intracardiac thrombus, acute dissection of the aorta, endocarditis, perioperative left-ventricular function, and intracardiac repairs during surgery. A transducer (probe) attached to an endoscope is inserted into the esophagus, and images are taken. Concurrent IV contrast medium, Doppler ultrasound, and color flow imaging may be used.	Instruct the patient to not eat or drink fluids for 4 h before the test. Explain that a sedative will be given before the test. Take and record vital signs.
THE LYMPHATIC SYSTEM		
Abdominal or thoracic CT scan	A radiologic study used to assess the liver or spleen and enlarged lymph nodes in the mediastinum.	Tell the patient not to eat or drink for 4 h before the test. Oral hypoglycemic agents should not be taken if iodinated contrast is used. Assess for allergy to iodine products and notify physician if allergy is found. Administer oral contrast as prescribed. Following the test, tell the patient to increase oral intake of fluids to help flush out the dye and to report any allergic reactions to the dye (such as skin rash, headache, vomiting, or kidney dysfunction).

(*continued*)

Diagnostic Tests
of the Cardiovascular and Lymphatic System (*continued*)

NAME OF TEST	PURPOSE AND DESCRIPTION	RELATED NURSING INTERVENTIONS
Lymph node biopsy	A lymph node biopsy is done to obtain tissue for histologic examination for diagnosis and treatment. It may be open (performed in the operating room) or closed (needle) by needle aspiration of tissue from a lymph node.	Use sterile technique when changing dressings.
Lymphangiography (lymphangiogram)	This is an x-ray examination of the lymphatic vessels and lymph nodes, used to assess metastasis of the lymph nodes, to identify malignant lymphoma, and to identify the cause of lymphedema. An iodine contrast substance is injected at various sites and fluoroscopy is used to visualize lymphatic filling.	Ask the patient about allergies to seafood, iodine, or contrast medium used in a previous x-ray test. Tell the patient that the blue contrast dye discolors the urine and possibly the skin for a few days. Take and record vital signs. Ask patient to void before the test. After the test, monitor for dyspnea, pain, and hypotension; assess incision sites for manifestations of infection, and assess for leg edema. Elevate lower extremities as indicated.
Magnetic resonance imaging (MRI)—liver, spleen, lymph nodes	A radiologic study used to visualize the liver, spleen, and lymph nodes. It does not require injection of contrast medium.	Assess for any metallic implants (such as clips on brain aneurysms, pacemaker, body piercing, tattoos, and shrapnel). If present, notify physician. Remove transdermal medication patches (both OTC and prescribed) unless otherwise ordered. Replace the patch following the procedure. Tell the patient to inform the staff about the patch when making the appointment and when completing the admission information. Ask if patient is pregnant; if so, the test is not performed. Ask about claustrophobia; if a problem exists, request patient to ask the referring physician for a relaxing medication prior to the MRI. If the patient is very claustrophobic, obese, or confused, an open MRI may be used.
THE HEMATOLOGIC SYSTEM		
Bone marrow examination	A bone marrow examination is conducted to evaluate blood-forming tissue; to diagnose multiple myeloma, leukemia, and some lymphomas; and to assess effectiveness of therapy for leukemia. Bone marrow specimens are obtained by either aspiration or biopsy. The preferred site for bone marrow aspiration is the posterior iliac crest; the sternum may also be used. The procedure is performed by inserting a needle into the bone and drawing out a sample of the blood in the marrow. A bone marrow biopsy is performed by making a small incision over the bone and screwing a core biopsy instrument into the bone to obtain a specimen. Bone marrow studies are used to diagnose leukemias, metastatic cancer, lymphoma, aplastic anemia, and Hodgkin disease.	Explain that the procedure (either aspiration or biopsy) takes about 20 min, a sedative may be given prior to the procedure, and that it is important to remain very still during the procedure to prevent accidental injury. Tell the patient that although the area will be anesthetized with a local anesthetic, insertion of the needle will be painful for a short time. Taking deep breaths may make this part of the procedure less painful. The aspiration site may ache for 1 or 2 days. Take and record vital signs and ask the patient to void. If specimen is taken from the sternum or iliac crest, place patient in the supine position; if the posterior iliac crest is used, place patient in the prone position. After the procedure apply pressure to the puncture site for 5–10 min. Apply a sterile dressing to the puncture site and monitor for bleeding for 24 h.
Complete blood count (CBC)	This is a blood test that measures blood components. Refer to Table 29.1.	None

NAME OF TEST	PURPOSE AND DESCRIPTION	RELATED NURSING INTERVENTIONS
Erythrocyte sedimentation rate (ESR)	This blood test is done as a measure of inflammation and is increased in many illnesses, including cancer, heart disease, and kidney disease. Normal values: Women: 1–20 mm/h Men: 1–15 mm/h	None
Magnetic resonance angiography (MRA)	An MRA is used to visualize vascular occlusive disease and aneurysms of the abdominal aorta. The procedure is done by using a non-iodine-based contrast medium injected IV.	See MRI entry earlier in this table

BOX 29.5
Electrocardiogram

The *electrocardiogram (ECG)* is a graphic record of the heart's activity. Electrodes applied to the body surface are used to obtain a graphic representation of cardiac electrical activity. These electrodes detect the magnitude and direction of electrical currents produced in the heart. They attach to the electrocardiograph by an insulated wire called a *lead*. The electrocardiograph converts the electrical impulses it receives into a series of waveforms that represent cardiac depolarization and repolarization. Placement of electrodes on different parts of the body allows different views of this electrical activity, much like turning the head while holding a camera provides different views of the scenery. ECG waveforms and patterns are examined to detect dysrhythmias as well as myocardial damage, the effects of drugs, and electrolyte imbalances.

ECG waveforms reflect the direction of electrical flow in relation to a positive electrode. Current flowing toward the positive electrode produces an upward (positive) waveform; current flowing away from the positive electrode produces a downward (negative) waveform. Current flowing perpendicular to the positive pole produces a biphasic (both positive and negative) waveform. Absence of electrical activity, called the *isoelectric line*, is represented by a straight line.

ECG waveforms are recorded by a heated stylus on heat-sensitive paper. The paper is marked at standard intervals that represent time and voltage or amplitude (see **Figure 1**). Each small box is 1 mm^2. The recording speed of the standard ECG is 25 mm/second, so each small box represents 0.04 second. Five small boxes horizontally and vertically make one large box, equivalent to 0.20 second. Five large boxes represent 1 full second. Measured vertically, each small box represents 0.1 mV.

Both bipolar and unipolar leads are used in recording the ECG. A bipolar lead uses two electrodes of opposite polarity (negative and positive). In a *unipolar* lead, one positive electrode and a negative reference point at the center of the heart are used. The electrical potential between the two monitoring points is graphically recorded as the ECG waveform.

The heart can be viewed from both the frontal plane and the horizontal plane (see **Figure 2**). Each plane provides a unique perspective of

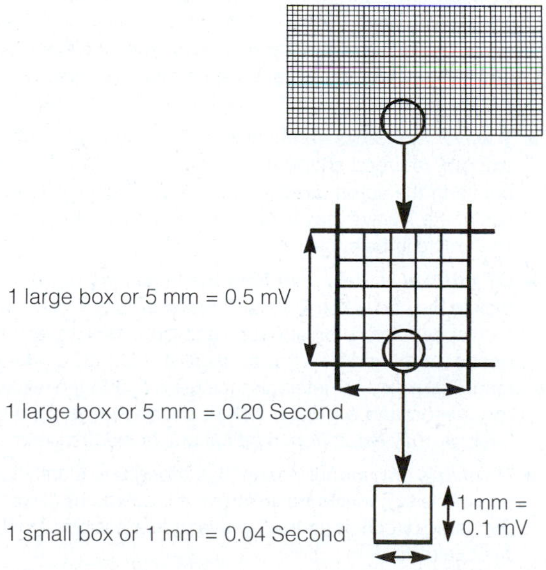
1 large box or 5 mm = 0.5 mV
1 large box or 5 mm = 0.20 Second
1 small box or 1 mm = 0.04 Second
1 mm =
0.1 mV

Figure 1 ■ Time and speed voltage measurements on ECG paper at a recording speed of 25 mm/second.

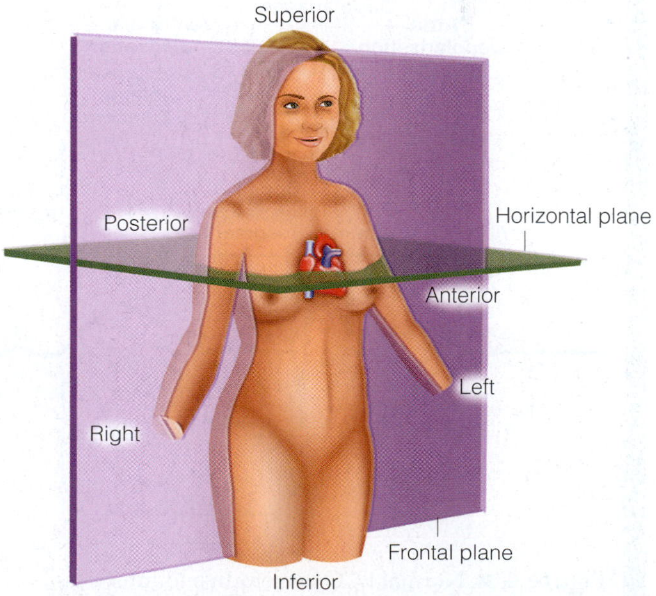
Superior
Posterior
Horizontal plane
Anterior
Left
Right
Frontal plane
Inferior

Figure 2 ■ Planes of the heart: Frontal and horizontal.

(continued)

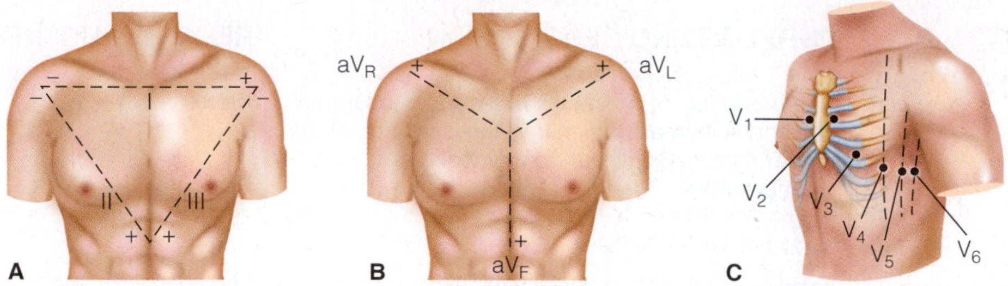
I
II
III
A
aV_R
aV_L
aV_F
B
V_1
V_2
V_3
V_4
V_5
V_6
C

Figure 3 ■ Leads of the 12-lead ECG. **A**, Bipolar limb leads I, II, III. **B**, Unipolar limb leads aV_R, aV_L, aV_F. **C**, Unipolar precordial leads V_1 to V_6.

the heart muscle. The *frontal plane* is an imaginary cut through the body that views the heart from top to bottom (superior–inferior) and side to side (right–left). This perspective of the heart is analogous to a paper doll cutout. It provides information about the inferior and lateral walls of the heart. The *horizontal plane* is a cross-sectional view of the heart from front to back (anterior–posterior) and side to side (right–left). Information regarding the anterior, septal, and lateral walls of the heart, as well as the posterior wall, is obtained from this view.

A standard 12-lead ECG provides a simultaneous recording of six limb leads and six precordial leads (see **Figure 3**). The limb leads provide information about the heart in the frontal plane and include three bipolar leads (I, II, III) and three unipolar leads (aV_R, aV_L, and aV_F). The bipolar limb leads measure electrical activity between a negative lead on one extremity and a positive lead on another. The *unipolar limb leads* (also called *augmented leads*) measure the electrical activity between a single positive electrode on a limb (right arm [R], left arm [L], or left leg [F for foot]) and the center of the heart.

The *precordial leads*, also known as *chest leads* or *V leads*, view the heart in the horizontal plane. They include six unipolar leads (V_1, V_2, V_3, V_4, V_5, and V_6), which measure electrical activity between the center of the heart and a positive electrode on the chest wall.

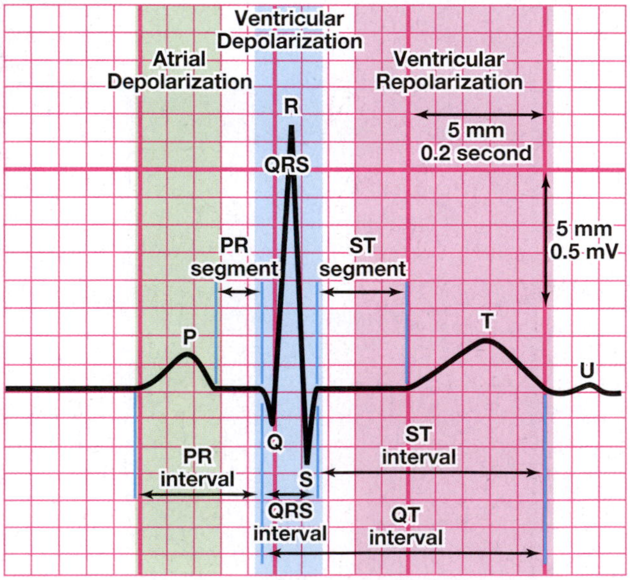
Ventricular Depolarization
Atrial Depolarization
Ventricular Repolarization
R
QRS
5 mm
0.2 second
5 mm
0.5 mV
PR segment
ST segment
P
T
U
Q
S
PR interval
ST interval
QRS interval
QT interval

Figure 4 ■ Normal ECG waveform and intervals.

The cardiac cycle is depicted as a series of waveforms, the P, Q, R, S, and T waves (see **Figure 4**).

- ***P wave*** represents atrial depolarization and contraction. The impulse is from the sinus node. The P wave precedes the QRS complex and is normally smooth, round, and upright. P waves may be absent when the SA node is not acting as the pacemaker. Atrial repolarization occurs during ventricular depolarization and is usually not seen on the ECG.
- ***PR interval*** represents the time required for the sinus impulse to travel to the AV node and into the Purkinje fibers. This interval is measured from beginning of the P wave to beginning of the QRS complex. If no Q wave is seen, the beginning of the R wave is used. The PR interval is normally 0.12 to 0.20 second (up to 0.24 second is considered normal in patients over age 65). PR intervals > 0.20 second indicate a delay in conduction from the SA node to the ventricles.
- ***QRS complex*** represents ventricular depolarization and contraction. The QRS complex includes three separate waves: The Q wave is the first negative deflection, the R wave is the positive or upright deflection, and the S wave is the first negative deflection after the R wave. Not all QRS complexes have all three waves; nonetheless, the complex is called a *QRS complex*. The normal duration of a QRS complex is from 0.06 to 0.10 second. QRS complexes > 0.10 second indicate delays in transmitting the impulse through the ventricular conduction system.
- ***ST segment*** signifies the beginning of ventricular repolarization. The ST segment, the period from the end of the QRS complex to the beginning of the T wave, should be isoelectric. An abnormal ST segment is displaced (elevated or depressed) from the isoelectric line.
- ***T wave*** represents ventricular repolarization. It normally has a smooth, rounded shape that is usually < 10 mm tall. It usually points in the same direction as the QRS complex. Abnormalities of the T wave may indicate myocardial ischemia or injury or electrolyte imbalances.
- ***QT interval*** is measured from the beginning of the QRS complex to the end of the T wave. It represents the total time of ventricular depolarization and repolarization. Its duration varies with gender, age, and heart rate; usually, it is 0.32 to 0.44 second long. Prolonged QT intervals indicate a prolonged relative refractory period and a greater risk of dysrhythmias. Shortened QT intervals may result from medications or electrolyte imbalances.
- ***U wave*** is not normally seen. It is thought to signify repolarization of the terminal Purkinje fibers. If present, the U wave follows the same direction as the T wave. It is most commonly seen in hypokalemia.

BOX 29.6
Interpreting an ECG

Interpreting an ECG strip to determine the cardiac rhythm is a skill that takes practice to learn and master. Many methods are used to analyze ECGs. It is important to use a consistent method for ECG analysis. Identifying and interpreting complex dysrhythmias requires advanced skills and knowledge obtained through further education. One method follows.

STEP 1: DETERMINE RATE

Assess heart rate. Use P waves to determine the atrial rate and R waves for the ventricular rate. Several approaches can determine the heart rate:

- Count the number of complexes in a 6-second rhythm strip (the top margin of ECG paper is marked at 3-second intervals), and multiply by 10. This provides an estimate of the rate and is particularly valuable if rhythms are irregular.
- Count the number of large boxes between two consecutive complexes, and divide by 300 (the number of large boxes in 1 minute). For example, there are six large boxes between two R waves; 300 divided by 6 equals a ventricular rate of 50 bpm. Memorize the following sequence for rapid rate determination: 300, 150, 100, 75, 60, 50, 43. One large box between complexes equals a rate of 300; two, a rate of 150; three, a rate of 100; and so on.
- Count the number of small boxes between two consecutive complexes, and divide 1500 (the number of small boxes in 1 minute) by this number. For example, there are 19 small boxes between two R waves; 1500 divided by 19 equals a ventricular rate of 79 bpm. This is the most precise measurement of heart rate.

STEP 2: DETERMINE REGULARITY

Regularity is the consistency with which the P waves or QRS complexes occur. In a regular rhythm, all waves occur at a consistent rate. Rhythm regularity is determined by measuring the interval between consecutive waves. Place one point of an ECG caliper (a measuring device) on the peak of the P wave (for atrial rhythm) or the R wave (for ventricular rhythm). Adjust the other point to the peak of the next wave, P to P or R to R. Keeping the calipers set at this distance, evaluate intervals between consecutive waves. The rhythm is *regular* if all caliper points fall on succeeding wave peaks. Alternately, use a strip of blank paper on top of the ECG strip, marking the peaks of two or three consecutive waves. Then move the paper along the strip to consecutive waves. Wave peaks that vary by more than one to three small boxes (depending on the rate) are *irregular*. Irregular rhythms may be *irregularly irregular* (if the intervals have no pattern) or *regularly irregular* (if a consistent pattern to the irregularity can be identified).

STEP 3: ASSESS P WAVE

The presence or absence of P waves helps determine the origin of the rhythm. All the P waves should be alike in size and shape (*morphology*). If P waves are not seen or they differ in shape, the rhythm may not originate in the sinus node.

STEP 4: ASSESS P TO QRS RELATIONSHIP

Determine the relationship between P waves and QRS complexes. There should be one and only one P wave for every QRS complex because the normal stimulus for ventricular contraction originates in the sinus node.

STEP 5: DETERMINE INTERVAL DURATIONS

To evaluate impulse transmission through the cardiac conduction system, measure the PR interval, QRS duration, and QT interval. To measure, count the number of small boxes from the beginning of the interval to the end, and multiply by 0.04 second. Then determine whether the interval duration is within its normal limits. For example, the PR interval is 3.5 small boxes wide, or 0.14 second. This is within the normal limits of 0.12 to 0.20 second. This interval should be consistent, not varying from beat to beat. A PR interval > 0.20 second or one that varies from beat to beat is abnormal.

The QRS complex duration is normally between 0.06 and 0.10 second. A QRS complex > 0.12 second indicates delayed ventricular conduction.

The QT interval is normally 0.32 to 0.44 second. It varies inversely with the heart rate: The faster the heart rate, the shorter the QT interval. As a general rule, the QT interval should be no more than half the previous R–R interval. A prolonged QT interval indicates a prolonged relative refractory period of the heart.

STEP 6: IDENTIFY ABNORMALITIES

Note the presence and frequency of *ectopic* (extra) beats, deviation of the ST segment above or below the baseline, and abnormalities in waveform shape and duration.

29.4 Assessment of Special Populations

Normal age-related findings for the older adult are summarized in **Table 29.4**.

According to the Department of Veterans Affairs, research has reported relationships between cardiac disease and both posttraumatic stress disorder (PTSD). Several studies reported that in veterans with PTSD, premature development of cardiovascular disease, especially ischemic changes, was seen. Additionally, PTSD severity appeared to be related to severity of ischemic changes (Turner, Neylan, Schiller, Li, & Cohen, 2013; Wentworth, Foraker, Girton, & Mansfield, 2013). In another study, a relationship between PTSD and heart failure was noted (Roy, et al., 2015). A relationship was also noted in the development of cardiac disease and combat deployment believed to be related to intense stress of the experience of deployment (Crum-Cianflone et al., 2014).

No differences have been noted for LGBTQI persons related to cardiovascular disease and risk. All persons should be screened and treated based on physiologic findings. Patients born with congenital conditions may have significant risk for comorbidities including anemia and vascular disorders, in addition to development of coronary artery disease and hypertension related to aging. Some patients are at risk for development of pathology of the aorta. Increased risk is also seen for thromboembolism. History of congenital conditions should trigger careful assessment for these comorbidities (Lui et al. 2017).

29.5 Health Promotion

Preventing Heart Disease

Modifiable risk factors include lifestyle factors and pathologic conditions that predispose the patient to developing cardiac disease. Disease conditions that contribute to heart disease

Table 29.4 Age-Related Cardiovascular Changes

Age-Related Change	Significance
Myocardium: ↓ efficiency and contractibility Sinus node: ↑ in thickness of shell surrounding the node, and ↓ in the number of pacemaker cells throughout the conduction system	■ Decreased CO when under physiologic stress with resulting tachycardia that lasts longer. The person may require rest time between physical activities.
Left ventricle: Slight hypertrophy, prolonged isometric contraction phase and relaxation time; ↑ time for diastolic filling and systolic emptying cycle	■ Stroke volume may increase to compensate for tachycardia, leading to increased BP.
Valves and blood vessels: Aorta is elongated and dilated, valves are thicker and more rigid, and resistance to peripheral blood flow increases by 1% per year	■ BP increases to compensate for increased peripheral resistance and decreased CO. ■ Baroreceptor response decreases.
Bone marrow: ↓ ability of bone marrow to respond to need for increased RBCs, WBCs, and platelets	■ Anemia may result.
Blood vessels Tunica intima: Fibrosis, calcium and lipid accumulation, cellular proliferation	■ As a result of age-related changes, the systolic BP rises. Decreased arterial elasticity results in vascular changes in the heart, kidneys, and pituitary gland. Decreased baroreceptor function results in postural hypotension. Vessels in the head, neck, and extremities are more prominent.
Tunica media: Thins, elastin fibers calcify; increase in calcium results in stiffening Baroreceptor function is impaired and peripheral resistance increases	■ Inefficient vasoconstriction, decreased CO, and reduced muscle mass and subcutaneous tissue lead to a reduced ability to respond to cold temperatures. ■ With a decrease in BP and changes in blood vessel walls, tissue perfusion may be inadequate, leading to edema, inflammation, pressure ulcers, and changes in effects of medications.
Immune system	■ Increased risk for infection, with decreased manifestations of an actual infection.
Impaired function of B and T lymphocytes: ↓ production of antibodies	■ Increased incidence of cancers.

include hypertension, diabetes mellitus, and hyperlipidemia. Although these conditions are not a matter of choice, they are modifiable risk factors that can often be controlled through medication, weight control, diet, and exercise.

Behavioral or lifestyle factors can be controlled or completely eliminated. Smoking, physical inactivity, and an unhealthy diet are modifiable lifestyle factors (National Heart, Lung, and Blood Institute [NHLBI], 2017b). Behavioral factors such as underlying anxiety have been identified as an independent risk factor for heart disease. Lifestyle changes require significant commitment by the patient; ongoing support from the healthcare team is vital for success.

Hypertension

Hypertension is consistent blood pressure readings > 130 mmHg systolic or 80 mmHg diastolic. Hypertension is common, affecting more than one-third of people over age 50 in the United States. Its prevalence is higher in African Americans than in Hispanics and higher in Hispanics than in Caucasian Americans. Hypertension damages the endothelial cells of arteries, possibly by excess pressure and altered characteristics of blood flow. This damage can stimulate the development of atherosclerotic plaque. Hypertension can be managed with medication in concert with lifestyle changes. Teaching patients the importance of adhering to their medication regimen for hypertension is an important nursing task.

Diabetes

Diabetes mellitus contributes to CHD in several ways. Diabetes is associated with higher blood lipid levels, a higher incidence of hypertension, and obesity—all risk factors in their own right. Nurses can help identify risk factors for diabetes and encourage patients to eat a balanced diet and exercise. In addition, diabetes affects the endothelium of blood vessels, contributing to the process of atherosclerosis. Hyperglycemia and hyperinsulinemia, altered platelet function, elevated fibrinogen levels, and inflammation are also thought to play a role in the development of atherosclerosis in people with diabetes. Helping patients with diabetes with the physical and emotional components of managing their disease will help to preserve and promote health.

Abnormal Blood Lipids

Hyperlipidemia is an abnormally high level of blood lipids and lipoproteins. Lipoproteins carry cholesterol in the blood. *Low-density lipoproteins (LDLs)* are the primary carriers of cholesterol. High levels of LDL promote atherosclerosis because LDL deposits cholesterol on artery walls. **Table 29.5** lists desirable and high-risk levels for total and LDL cholesterol. In contrast, *high-density lipoproteins (HDLs)* help clear cholesterol from the arteries, transporting it to the liver for excretion. HDL levels above 35 mg/dL have a protective effect, reducing the risk of CHD; in contrast, HDL levels lower than 35 mg/dL are associated with an increased risk for CHD. Triglycerides, compounds of fatty acids bound to glycerol and used for fat storage by the body, are carried on *very-low-density lipoprotein (VLDL)* molecules. Elevated triglycerides also contribute to the risk for CHD. Any easy way to distinguish between LDLs and HDLs is:

LDLs = Less desirable lipoproteins

HDLs = Highly desirable lipoproteins.

Table 29.5 Classification of Serum Cholesterol and Triglyceride Values*

	Total Cholesterol (mg/dL)	LDL Cholesterol (mg/dL)	Triglyceride (mg/dL)
Optimal		< 100	
Desirable	< 200	100–129	< 150
Borderline	200–239	130–159	150–199
High	≥ 240	160–189	200–499
Very high		≥ 190	≥ 500

Note: *As defined by the National Blood, Lung, and Heart Institute's National Cholesterol Education Program (2017a).

Hyperlipidemia can be managed with medication and lifestyle changes, and nurses can promote health by encouraging patients to take their medications regularly (Jellinger et al., 2017; Lloyd-Jones et al., 2017).

Cigarette Smoking

Cigarette smoking is the leading independent risk factor for CHD. It is responsible for more deaths from CHD than from lung cancer or pulmonary disease. The effects of smoking on the cardiovascular system are dose dependent. The male cigarette smoker has two to three times the risk of developing heart disease than the nonsmoker; the female who smokes has up to four times the risk. The risk of mortality from CHD is reduced by half for both men and women who stop smoking. Secondhand (or environmental) tobacco smoke also increases the risk of death from CHD by as much as 30%. Tobacco smoke promotes CHD in several ways. Carbon monoxide damages vascular endothelium, promoting cholesterol deposition. Nicotine stimulates catecholamine release, increasing blood pressure, heart rate, and myocardial oxygen use. Nicotine also constricts arteries, limiting tissue perfusion (blood flow and oxygen delivery). Furthermore, nicotine reduces HDL levels and increases platelet aggregation, increasing the risk of thrombus formation. Nurses should educate patients about the dangers of smoking, encourage them to quit, and support their efforts to do so.

Obesity

Obesity (excess adipose tissue), generally defined as a body mass index (BMI) of 30 or greater, and fat distribution affect the risk for CHD. People with obesity have higher rates of hypertension, diabetes, and hyperlipidemia. As shown in the classic Framingham Heart Study, men over age 50 who were obese had twice the incidence of CHD and acute MI of those who were within 10% of their ideal weight (Hubert, Feinleib, McNamara, & Castelli, 1983). Central obesity, or intra-abdominal fat, is associated with an increased risk for CHD. The best indicator of central obesity is the waist circumference. A waist-to-hip ratio of > 0.8 (women) or 0.9 (men) increases the risk for CHD. Nurses should promote a healthy weight for all patients, but they should be mindful that the topic of weight can have cultural implications. The nurse must be sensitive to the role weight carries for the patient and his or her self-image.

Physical Inactivity

Physical inactivity is associated with higher risk of CHD. Research data indicate that people who maintain a regular program of physical activity are less prone to developing CHD than sedentary people. Cardiovascular benefits of exercise include increased availability of oxygen to the heart muscle, decreased oxygen demand and cardiac workload, and increased myocardial function and electrical stability. Other positive effects of regular physical activity include decreased blood pressure, blood lipids, insulin levels, platelet aggregation, and weight. Nurses should encourage all patients to exercise regularly. Walking just 30 minutes a day, 5 days a week, can bring enormous benefit to patients (American Heart Association [AHA], 2017).

Diet

Diet is a risk factor for cardiac disease, independent of fat and cholesterol intake. Diets high in fruits, vegetables, whole grains, and unsaturated fatty acids appear to have a protective effect. The underlying factors are not clear, but probably relate to nutrients such as antioxidants, folic acid, other B vitamins, omega-3 fatty acids, and other unidentified micronutrients (AHA, 2017). Nurses should encourage patients to eat a healthy, balanced diet. Directing patients to ChooseMyPlate.gov is a great place to start.

Other Risk Factors

Research has demonstrated a link between elevated serum *homocysteine levels* and CHD. Until menopause, women have lower homocysteine levels than men, which may partially explain their lower risk for CHD. Homocysteine levels are negatively correlated with serum folate and dietary folate intake; that is, increasing folate intake lowers homocysteine levels.

Based on evidence that aspirin and antiplatelet therapies reduce the risk for myocardial infarction, *clot-promoting factors* are identified as CHD risk factors. Inflammation has also recently been identified as a risk factor. Inflammatory processes may increase the development of atherosclerotic plaque and are implicated in plaque rupture. Inflammation also promotes clot formation at the site of ruptured plaque. Although identified as risk factors, it is not generally recommended that patients routinely be tested for these factors.

Metabolic Syndrome

Metabolic syndrome, a group of metabolic risk factors occurring in an individual, is a strong risk factor for CHD (**Box 29.7**). Metabolic syndrome has emerged as a risk factor for premature CHD that is equal to that of cigarette smoking. Three underlying causes of metabolic syndrome have been identified: Overweight/obesity, physical inactivity,

BOX 29.7
Characteristics of Metabolic Syndrome

- Abdominal obesity
- Abnormal blood lipids (low HDL, high triglycerides)
- Hypertension
- Elevated fasting blood glucose
- Clotting tendency
- Inflammatory factors

and genetic factors. It is closely associated with *insulin resistance*, impaired tissue responses to insulin. Genetic factors play a role in insulin resistance, as do the acquired factors of abdominal obesity and physical inactivity.

Risk Factors Unique to Women

Risk factors unique to women include *premature menopause*, *oral contraceptive use*, and *hormone replacement therapy (HRT)* (National Heart, Lung, and Blood Institute [NHLBI], 2017b). At menopause, serum HDL levels drop and LDL levels rise, increasing the risk of CHD. Early menopause (natural or surgically induced) increases the risk of CHD and MI. Women who have a bilateral oophorectomy before age 35 without hormone replacement are eight times more likely to have an MI than women experiencing natural menopause. Estrogen replacement therapy reduces the risk of CHD and MI in these women. Oral contraceptives, by contrast, increase the risk for MI, particularly in women who also smoke. This increased risk is due to the tendency of oral contraceptives to promote clotting and to increase blood pressure, serum lipids, and glucose tolerance. The Women's Health Initiative randomized trial of HRT showed an increased risk for CHD in previously healthy women taking a commonly prescribed combination of estrogen and progestin. This well-controlled research study was terminated early when it showed a small but significant increased risk for CHD, stroke, pulmonary embolism, and invasive breast cancer in women taking HRT (NHLBI, 2018).

Maintaining Appropriate Blood Pressure

In 2017, the American College of Cardiology published new guidelines for the prevention, detection, evaluation, and treatment of high blood pressure (Whelton et al., 2017). This guideline provides the update to the seventh report of the Joint National Committee on Prevention, Detection, Evaluation and Treatment of High Blood Pressure (JNC-7). A significant change from prior guidelines is the identification of a lower threshold to define hypertension. Hypertension is now defined as a blood pressure equal to or > 130/80 mmHg. Prior guidelines set the threshold at 140/90 mmHg (Whelton et al., 2017). According to the authors, about half of U.S. adults (46%) are considered to have hypertension now. The largest increase in prevalence is expected in men and women

Moving Evidence into Action
Will More Intensive Therapy Lead to More Adverse Reactions?

Clinical Issue

With the changes in the hypertension guidelines, there is some concern that more intensive antihypertensive therapy may lead to more adverse reactions to medications.

External Evidence

Berlowitz and colleagues (2017) recently published a randomized controlled trial of more than 9000 patients with hypertension, randomizing to either intensive control (BP < 120/80) or routine care (BP < 140/90). Outcomes measured included physical and mental scores, adherence to medications, and satisfaction with treatment. Findings revealed no significant differences between the groups, with high satisfaction for blood pressure care in both groups. Patients in the intensive management group averaged one additional medication compared to the routine management group. No untoward effects were seen with either intensive therapy or routine care.

Internal Evidence

As part of the evaluation of internal evidence, one must consider the clinical feasibility of intensive hypertensive management, the outcome of interest (reduction of blood pressure), current policies/procedures in place for blood pressure management, and identification of stakeholders that influence uptake of the proposed intervention. Some questions to ask: Is this problem (increased risk for morbidity/mortality related to elevated hypertension) significant in the population of your care environment? Does the clinical environment support the use of the intervention? What about the cost benefit of the new intervention? In the use of intensive antihypertensive therapy, Berlowitz and colleagues (2017) reported no significant differences in patient-reported outcomes between intensive therapy and routine management.

Patient Considerations

When considering use of a new intervention, the nurse must consider the specific patient population where it will be used. Will patients and their families be amenable to the new intervention?

Putting the Pieces Together

The use of intensive hypertensive management will continue to be of clinical interest as the latest guidelines are recommending a broadened definition of hypertension. To effectively implement a plan, it is important to evaluate the external evidence and consider the internal implications and patient/family issues. With the implementation of a new, more intensive hypertension management program, patient-centered outcomes are also important to consider.

References

Berlowitz, D. R., Kazis, L. E., Bolin, L. P., Conroy, M. B., Fitzpatrick, P., Gure, T. R., . . . Whittle, J. (2017). Effect of intensive blood-pressure treatment on patient-reported outcomes. *New England Journal of Medicine, 377*(8), 733–744.

less than 45 years of age. While there will be more persons diagnosed with hypertension, only a small increase in persons on antihypertensive medications is expected (Whelton et al., 2017).

Lifestyle Modifications

Lifestyle modifications are recommended for all patients whose blood pressure falls outside the normal range of less than or equal to 120/80 mmHg. The stage of "prehypertension" has been eliminated. These modifications, all of which can be recommended by nurses, include weight loss, dietary changes, restricted alcohol use and cigarette smoking, increased physical activity, and stress reduction (**Box 29.8**).

BOX 29.8
Lifestyle Modifications for Hypertension

- Maintain normal body weight; lose weight if overweight.
- Make dietary modifications:
  a. Eat a diet rich in fruits, vegetables, and low-fat dairy products.
  b. Reduce sodium intake.
  c. Reduce intake of cholesterol and total and saturated fat.
- Limit alcohol intake to no more than 1 oz of ethanol (1/2 oz for women and lighter-weight people) per day.
- Engage in aerobic exercise for 30 minutes most days of the week (5 to 6).
- Stop smoking.
- Use stress management techniques such as relaxation therapy.

Diet

Dietary approaches to managing hypertension focus on reducing sodium intake, maintaining adequate potassium and calcium intakes, and reducing total and saturated fat intake. A mild to moderate sodium restriction (no added salt) lowers blood pressure and potentiates the effect of antihypertensive drugs for most hypertensive patients. The DASH (Dietary Approaches to Stop Hypertension) diet has proven beneficial effects in lowering blood pressure. This diet (**Box 29.9**) focuses on whole foods rather than individual nutrients. It is rich in fruits and vegetables (up to 10 servings per day) and low in total and saturated fats.

Weight loss is recommended for patients who are obese. Loss of as little as 4.5 kg (10 lb) reduces blood pressure in many people. A balanced diet such as the DASH diet is recommended for weight loss.

Physical Activity

Regular exercise (such as walking, cycling, jogging, or swimming) reduces blood pressure and contributes to weight loss, stress reduction, and feelings of overall well-being. Previously sedentary patients are encouraged to engage in aerobic exercise for 30 to 45 minutes per day most days of the week (5 to 6 days). Isometric exercise (such as weight training) may not be appropriate because it can raise the systolic blood pressure.

BOX 29.9
DASH Diet Recommendations

- Grains—seven to eight servings per day
- Vegetables—four to five servings per day
- Fruits—four to five servings per day
- Nonfat/low-fat dairy products—two to three servings per day
- Meats, poultry, and fish—two or fewer 3-oz servings per day
- Nuts, seeds, and dry beans—four to five servings per week
- Fats and oils—two to three servings per day
- Sweets—five servings per week (should be low in fat)

Alcohol and Tobacco Use

The recommended alcohol intake for patients with hypertension is no more than 1 oz of ethanol or two drinks per day. A drink is 12 oz of beer, 5 oz of wine, or 1.5 oz of 80-proof whiskey. Women and lighter-weight people should reduce this limit by half. Although alcohol withdrawal may increase blood pressure, this is usually temporary and diminishes as abstinence or restricted intake continues.

Although nicotine is a vasoconstrictor, substantial data linking smoking to hypertension are lacking. A definitive link exists between smoking and heart disease, however. Patients who smoke are strongly urged to quit. Smoking reduces the effect of some antihypertensive medications such as propranolol (Inderal). Smoking cessation aids such as nicotine patches and gum contain lower amounts of nicotine and usually do not raise blood pressure.

Stress Reduction

Stress stimulates the sympathetic nervous system, increasing vasoconstriction, systemic vascular resistance, cardiac output, and blood pressure. Regular, moderate exercise is the treatment of choice for reducing stress in hypertensive patients. Relaxation techniques such as biofeedback, therapeutic touch, yoga, and meditation to relax both mind and body may also lower blood pressure, although their effect has not been proven in hypertension management.

CHAPTER HIGHLIGHTS

29.1 Anatomy, Physiology, and Functions of the Heart

Describe the anatomy, physiology, and functions of the cardiovascular and lymphatic systems.

- Normal anatomy, physiology, and functions of the heart, blood vessels, and lymphatic system are the basis for assessment.

29.2 The Peripheral Vascular System

Describe the anatomy, physiology, and functions of the peripheral vascular system.

- The peripheral vascular system includes arteries, veins, and the capillary beds.
- Factors that affect arterial circulation are blood flow, peripheral vascular resistance, and blood pressure.
- The lymph system is made up of small aggregates of specialized cells that assist the immune system by removing foreign material, infectious organisms, and tumor cells via lymph nodes and lymphatic vessels. The blood consists of plasma, solutes (e.g., proteins, electrolytes, and organic constituents), red blood cells, white blood cells, and platelets (which are fragments of cells).

29.3 Assessing Cardiovascular and Lymphatic Function

Outline the components of the assessment of the cardiovascular and lymphatic systems including topics for the health assessment interview, techniques for physical assessment, and the diagnostic tests used in the assessment.

- Both general health and focused cardiovascular and lymphatic system assessments can detect dysfunction, injury, and disorders.
- Assessment of the cardiovascular and lymphatic systems includes diagnostic tests, genetic considerations, a health interview, and a physical assessment.

29.4 Assessment of Special Populations

Differentiate considerations for assessing the cardiovascular and lymphatic systems of older adults, veterans, individuals in the LGBTQI population, and adults with sequelae of childhood/congenital conditions.

- Veterans who have developed PTSD are at higher risk for developing heart disease.

Patients with sequelae from childhood congenital conditions are at increased risk for hematologic or vascular comorbidities.

29.5 Health Promotion

Summarize topics that nurses teach to promote cardiovascular and lymphatic health across the lifespan.

- Management of modifiable risk factors can prevent the development of heart disease.
- Maintaining normal blood pressure is essential to cardiovascular health. Based on the latest guidelines, hypertension is now considered when blood pressure measures 130/80 mmHg and higher.

TEST YOURSELF NCLEX-RN® REVIEW

1. A patient who is hemorrhaging has decreased preload. What physiologic effect should the nurse expect to occur with this patient?
   A. Increased afterload
   B. Decreased cardiac output
   C. Decreased action potential
   D. Increased ejection fraction
2. The nurse is preparing to assess a patient who is experiencing chest pain. Which question should the nurse ask to learn more information about the intensity of the pain?
   A. "Did the pain move into your left arm?"
   B. "Was the pain a pressure, a burning, or tightness?"
   C. "Was your pain relieved by resting or worse when you were busy?"
   D. "On a scale of 0 (no pain) to 10 (worst pain), what number is your pain?"
3. The nurse is preparing to assess a patient's apical impulse. Which anatomic location should the nurse use to make this assessment?
   A. Right nipple line, any intercostal space
   B. Left substernal line, sixth intercostal space
   C. Left midclavicular line, fifth intercostal space
   D. Right midaxillary line, second intercostal space
4. The nurse assesses a patient's heart rate as being 50 beats per minute. How should the nurse document this finding?
   A. Bradycardia
   B. Tachycardia
   C. Dysrhythmic
   D. Apical

5. A patient has a low red blood cell count secondary to chronic gastrointestinal bleeding. What subjective data should the nurse expect to assess that is consistent with this data? (Select all that apply.)
   A. Fatigue
   B. Nausea
   C. Chest pain
   D. Pallor
   E. Dizziness
6. A patient is being admitted for a low platelet count. Which finding should the nurse expect when conducting a physical assessment of this patient? (Select all that apply.)
   A. Varicose veins
   B. Excessive bruising
   C. Enlarged lymph nodes
   D. Changes in pulse pressure
   E. Bleeding gums
7. The nurse determines that an older patient would benefit from interventions to address peripheral vascular resistance. What manifestations did the nurse assess in this patient? (Select all that apply.)
   A. Joint pain
   B. Sunken eyeballs
   C. Distant bowel sounds
   D. Elevated blood pressure
   E. Lower extremity fatigue
8. The nurse is preparing to assess a patient's carotid arteries. Which techniques should the nurse use for this assessment? (Select all that apply.)
   A. Palpate for pulse rate.
   B. Inspect for pulsations.
   C. Auscultate for rhythm.
   D. Percuss for arterial wall density.
   E. Palpate deeply for arterial wall integrity.
9. During the physical examination of a patient's abdomen, the nurse auscultates a blowing sound over the aorta. How should the nurse document this finding?
   A. Bruit
   B. Dysrhythmia
   C. Bigeminal pulse
   D. Hypokinetic pulse
10. A patient has been admitted with severe leg pain. The limb is cyanotic, cool to the touch, and peripheral pulses are absent. What should the nurse do first after this assessment?
   A. Document the findings.
   B. Teach relaxation techniques.
   C. Notify the physician immediately.
   D. Ask how long the limb has been hurting.

See Test Yourself answers in Appendix B.

REFERENCES

American College of Cardiology. (2017). *New ACC/AHA high blood pressure guidelines lower definition of hypertension*. Retrieved from www.acc.org/latest-in-cardiology/articles/2017/11/08/11/47/mon-5pm-bp-guideline-aha-2017.

American Heart Association (AHA). (2017). *Diet and lifestyle recommendations*. Retrieved from www.heart.org/HEARTORG/HealthyLiving/HealthyEating/Nutrition/The-American-Heart-Associations-Diet-and-Lifestyle-Recommendations_UCM_305855_Article.jsp#.

Berlowitz, D. R., Kazis, L. E., Bolin, L. P., Conroy, M. B., Fitzpatrick, P., Gure, T. R., . . . Whittle, J. (2017). Effect of intensive blood-pressure treatment on patient-reported outcomes. *New England Journal of Medicine, 377*(8), 733–744.

Bickley, L. (2016). *Bates' guide to physical examination and history taking* (12th ed.). Philadelphia, PA: Lippincott Williams & Wilkins.

Crum-Cianflone, N. F., Gagnell, M. E., Schaller, E., Boyko, E. J., Smith, B., Maynard, C., . . . Smith, T. C. (2014). Impact of combat deployment and post-traumatic stress disorder on newly reported coronary heart disease among US active duty and reserve forces. *Circulation, 129*(18), 1813–1820.

Hubert, H. B., Feinleib, P. M., McNamara, P. M., & Castelli, W. P. (1983). Obesity as an independent risk factor for cardiovascular disease: A 26-year follow-up of participants in the Framingham Heart Study. *Circulation*, 67, 968–977.

Jellinger, P. S., Handelsman, Y., Rosenblit, P. D., Bloomgarden, Z. T., Fonseca, V. A., Garber, A. J., . . . Bush, M. A. (2017). American Association of Clinical Endocrinologists and American College of Endocrinology guidelines for management of dyslipidemia and prevention of cardiovascular disease. *Endocrine Practice, 23*(Suppl. 2), 1–87.

Lloyd-Jones, D. M., Morris, P. B., Ballantyne, C. M., Birtcher, K. K., Daly, D. D. Jr., DePalma, S. M., . . . Smith, S. C. Jr. (2017). 2017 focused update of the 2016 ACC Expert Consensus Decision Pathway on the role of non-statin therapies for LDL-cholesterol lowering in the management of atherosclerotic cardiovascular disease risk. *Journal of the American College of Cardiology, 70*(14), 1785–1822.

Lui, G. K., Saidi, A., Bhatt, A. B., Burchill, L. J., Deen, J. F., Earing, M. G., & Gewitz, M. (2017). Diagnosis and management of noncardiac complications in adults with congenital heart disease: A scientific statement from the American Heart Association. *Circulation, 136.* [Epub ahead of print]

National Heart, Lung, and Blood Institute (NHLBI), National Institutes of Health. (2018). *Women's Health Initiative (WHI).* Retrieved from https://www.nhlbi.nih.gov/science/womens-health-initiative-whi.

National Heart, Lung, and Blood Institute (NHLBI), National Institutes of Health. (2017a). *High blood cholesterol. What you need to know.* Retrieved from https://www.nhlbi.nih.gov/health/resources/heart/heart-cholesterol-hbc-what-html.

National Heart, Lung, and Blood Institute (NHLBI), National Institutes of Health. (2017b). *What are the risk factors for heart disease?* Retrieved from https://www.nhlbi.nih.gov/health/educational/hearttruth/lower-risk/risk-factors.htm.

Nayor, M., & Vasan, R. S. (2016). Recent update to the US Cholesterol Treatment Guidelines: A comparison with international guidelines. *Circulation, 133,* 1795–1806.

Roy, S. S., Foraker, R. E., Girton, R. A., & Mansfield, A. J. (2015). Post-traumatic stress disorder and incident heart failure among a community-based sample of US veterans. *American Journal of Public Health, 105*(4), 757–763.

Sorenson, M., Quinn, L., & Klein, D. (2018). *Pathophysiology: Concepts of human disease.* New York: Pearson.

Turner, J. H., Neylan, T. C., Schiller, N. B., Li, Y., & Cohen, B. E. (2013). Objective evidence of myocardial ischemia in patients with post-traumatic stress disorder. *Biological Psychiatry, 74*(11), 861–866.

Wentworth, B. A., Stein, M. B., Redwine, L. S., Xue, Y., Taub, P. R., Clopton, P., . . . & Maisel, A. S. (2013). Post-traumatic stress disorder: A fast track to premature cardiovascular disease? *Cardiology Review, 21*(1), 16–22.

Whelton, P. K., Carey, R. M., Aronow, W. S., Casey, D, E. Jr., Collins, K. J., Dennison Himmelfarb, C., . . . Wright, J. T. Jr. (2017). ACC/AHA/AAPA/ABC/ACPM/AGS/APhA/ASH/ASPC/NMA/PCNA guideline for the prevention, detection, evaluation, and management of high blood pressure in adults. *Hypertension.* [Epub ahead of print].

ADDITIONAL RESOURCES

Mahmood, S. S., Levy, D., Vasan, R. S., & Wang, T. J. (2014). The Framingham Heart Study and the epidemiology of cardiovascular disease: A historical perspective. *Lancet, 383* (9921), 999–1008.

Mended Hearts. (2018). *Homepage.*

mendedhearts.org.

National Heart, Lung, and Blood Institute (NHLBI), National Institutes of Health. (2018). *American Heart Month #Move with Heart.*

www.nhlbi.nih.gov/health-topics/education-and-awareness/heart-month.

U.S. Department of Health and Human Services (DHHS). (2018). *Million Hearts.*

millionhearts.hhs.gov.

Chapter 30

Nursing Care of Patients with Coronary Heart Disease

Chapter Outline and Learning Outcomes

30.1 Disorders of Myocardial Perfusion 994

Describe the pathophysiology and manifestations of disorders of myocardial perfusion, and outline the interprofessional care and nursing care of patients with these disorders.

30.2 Cardiac Rhythm Disorders 1029

Describe the pathophysiology and manifestations of cardiac dysrhythmias, and outline the interprofessional care and nursing care of patients with these disorders.

CLINICAL COMPETENCIES

- Assess functional health status of patients with coronary heart disease and/or a dysrhythmia, including the impact of the disorder on the patient's ability to perform activities of daily living and usual tasks.
- Use knowledge of the normal anatomy and physiology of the heart in caring for patients with coronary heart disease.
- Monitor patients with coronary heart disease or dysrhythmias for expected and unexpected manifestations, reporting and recording findings as indicated.
- Use assessed data to select nursing diagnoses, determine priorities of care, and develop and implement individualized nursing interventions for patients with coronary heart disease and dysrhythmias.
- Administer medications and treatments for patients with coronary heart disease and dysrhythmias safely and knowledgably.
- Integrate interprofessional care into nursing care planning and implementation for patients with coronary heart disease and dysrhythmias.
- Provide appropriate teaching for prevention, health promotion, and self-care related to coronary heart disease and dysrhythmias.
- Evaluate the effectiveness of nursing interventions, revising or modifying the plan of care as needed to promote, maintain, or restore functional health for patients with coronary heart disease or dysrhythmias.

KEY TERMS

acute coronary syndrome (ACS), 1009
acute myocardial infarction (AMI), 1018
angina pectoris, 1003
atherosclerosis, 994
atrial kick, 1030
cardiac arrest, 1036
cardiac rehabilitation, 1025
cardiovascular disease (CVD), 994
collateral channel, 994
coronary heart disease (CHD), 994
dysrhythmia, 1020
ectopic beat, 1030
heart block, 1030
ischemia, 1004
pacemaker, 1040
paroxysmal, 1034
sudden cardiac death (SCD), 1047

Impaired blood flow to the myocardium, changes in the conduction of electrical impulses through the heart, and structural changes in the heart itself affect the heart's ability to fulfill its major purpose: To pump enough blood to meet the body's demand for oxygen and nutrients. Impaired cardiac function, no matter what the underlying cause, affects the patient's ability to participate in exercise and activities and to fulfill life roles. Disruptions in cardiac function affect other organ systems as well, potentially leading to organ system failure and death.

Cardiovascular disease (CVD) is a generic term for disorders of the heart and blood vessels. CVD is the leading cause of death and disability in the United States. About 92.1 million people (or one in three) have some type of cardiovascular disease (Benjamin et al., 2017). Heart disease accounts for over 2200 deaths each day. In 2016, more women in the United States died of CVD than cancer, chronic lung diseases, and Alzheimer disease combined. The direct CVD costs in 2016 were estimated to be $316 billion (Benjamin et al., 2017). Because heart disease is the leading cause of death in the United States, *Healthy People 2020* included Heart Disease and Stroke as one of its topics (U.S. Department of Health and Human Services [USDHHS], 2018).

This chapter focuses on disorders of myocardial blood flow (coronary heart disease) and cardiac rhythm. Disorders of cardiac structure and function are discussed in Chapter 31. Review the normal anatomy and physiology and nursing assessment of the heart in Chapter 29 before proceeding with this chapter.

30.1 Disorders of Myocardial Perfusion

The Patient with Coronary Heart Disease

Coronary heart disease (CHD), or *coronary artery disease (CAD)*, is the cause of more than 370,000 deaths annually in the United States (Benjamin et al., 2017). CHD is caused by impaired blood flow to the myocardium. Accumulation of atherosclerotic plaque in the coronary arteries is the usual cause. CHD may be asymptomatic or may lead to angina pectoris, acute coronary syndrome, myocardial infarction (MI or heart attack), dysrhythmias, heart failure, and even sudden death.

The two main coronary arteries, the left and the right, supply blood, oxygen, and nutrients to the myocardium. They originate in the root of the aorta, just outside the aortic valve. The *left main coronary artery* divides to form the anterior descending and circumflex arteries. The *anterior descending artery* supplies the anterior interventricular septum and the left ventricle, including the apex of the heart. The *circumflex* branch supplies the lateral wall of the left ventricle. The *right coronary artery* supplies the right ventricle and forms the posterior descending artery. The *posterior descending artery* supplies the posterior portion of the heart (refer to Figure 29.5).

Blood flow through the coronary arteries is primarily regulated by aortic pressure. Other factors include the heart rate (most flow occurs during diastole, when the muscle is relaxed), metabolic activity of the heart, blood vessel tone (constriction), and collateral circulation. Although there are no connections between the large coronary arteries, small arteries are joined by **collateral channels**. If large vessels are gradually occluded, these channels enlarge, providing alternative routes for blood flow (Sorenson, Quinn, & Klein, 2019).

Pathophysiology

Coronary atherosclerosis is the most common cause of reduced coronary blood flow (see Pathophysiology Illustrated on page 997).

Atherosclerosis

Atherosclerosis is a progressive disease characterized by *atheroma* (plaque) formation, which affects the intimal and medial layers of large and midsize arteries. See the Pathophysiology Illustrated feature.

Atherosclerosis is initiated by unknown precipitating factors that cause lipoproteins and fibrous tissue to accumulate in the arterial wall. Although the precise mechanisms are unknown, abnormal lipid metabolism and injury to or inflammation of endothelial cells lining the artery appear to be key to its development (National Heart, Lung, and Blood Institute [NHLBI], 2017a).

In the bloodstream, lipids are transported attached to proteins called *apoproteins*. High levels of certain *lipoproteins*, a type of apoprotein, increase the risk of atherosclerosis. *Low-density lipoproteins*, which are high in cholesterol, carry cholesterol to peripheral tissues, where some of it is released to be taken up and incorporated into cells for use in producing energy. *Very-low-density lipoproteins*, large molecules primarily composed of triglycerides and cholesterol, carry triglycerides to muscle and fat cells. When the triglycerides are released into these tissues, the remainder of the molecule is a low-density lipoprotein. *High-density lipoproteins*, in contrast, attract cholesterol, returning it from peripheral tissues to the liver.

Hyperlipidemia itself may damage arterial endothelium. Other potential mechanisms of vessel injury include excessive pressures within the arterial system (hypertension), toxins found in cigarette smoke, infections, and inflammation. Endothelial damage promotes platelet adhesion and aggregation and attracts leukocytes to the area.

At the site of injury, *atherogenic* (atherosclerosis-promoting) lipoproteins collect in the intimal lining of the artery, binding to the extracellular portion of the vessel endothelium. Macrophages migrate to the injured site as part of the inflammatory process. Contact with platelets, cholesterol, and other blood components stimulates abnormal proliferation of smooth muscle cells and connective tissue within the vessel wall. Although blood flow is not affected at this stage, this early lesion appears as

Pathophysiology Illustrated
Coronary Heart Disease

Coronary heart disease usually is due to *atherosclerosis*, occlusion of the coronary arteries by fibrous, fatty plaque. Coronary heart disease is manifested by ***angina pectoris, acute coronary syndrome,*** and/or ***myocardial infarction***. Risk factors for coronary heart disease include age (over 50 years), heredity, smoking, obesity, high serum cholesterol levels, hypertension, and diabetes mellitus. Other factors, such as diet and lack of exercise, also contribute to the risk of CHD.

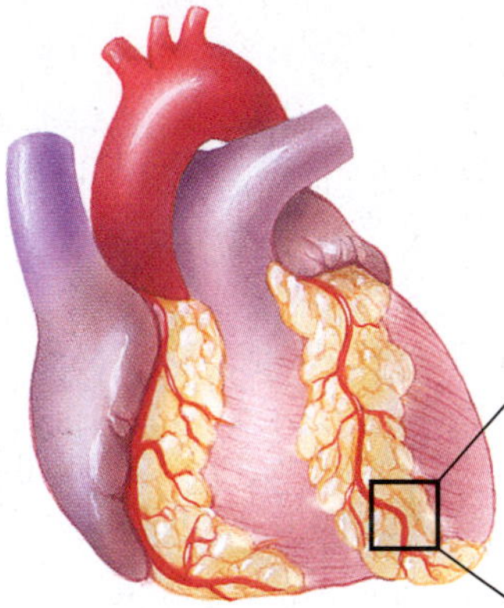

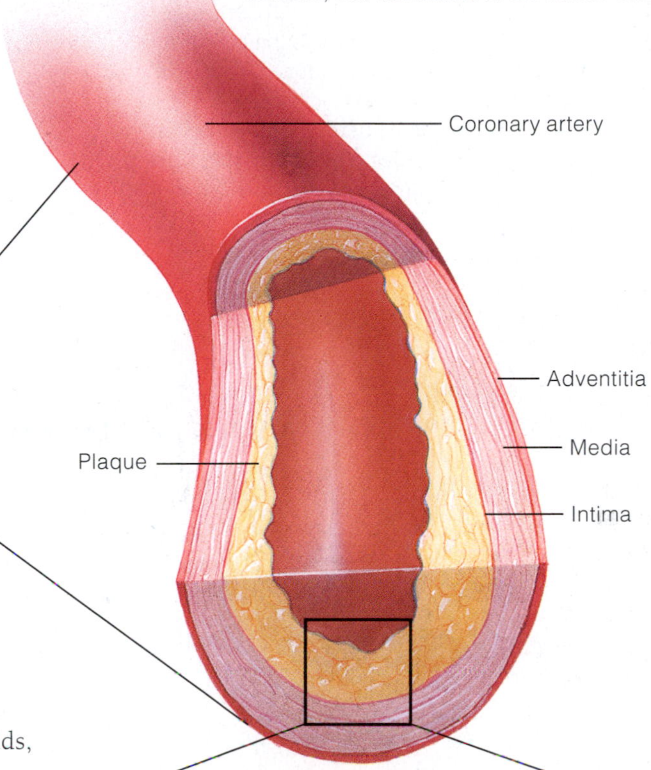
Coronary artery
Adventitia
Media
Plaque
Intima

Atherosclerosis

In atherosclerosis, lipids accumulate in the intimal layer of arteries. Fibroblasts in the area respond by producing collagen, and smooth muscle cells proliferate, together forming a complex lesion called plaque. Plaque consists mostly of cholesterol, triglycerides, phospholipids, collagen, and smooth muscle cells.

Plaque reduces the size of the lumen of the affected artery, impairing blood flow. In addition, plaque may ulcerate, causing a thrombus to form that may completely occlude the vessel.

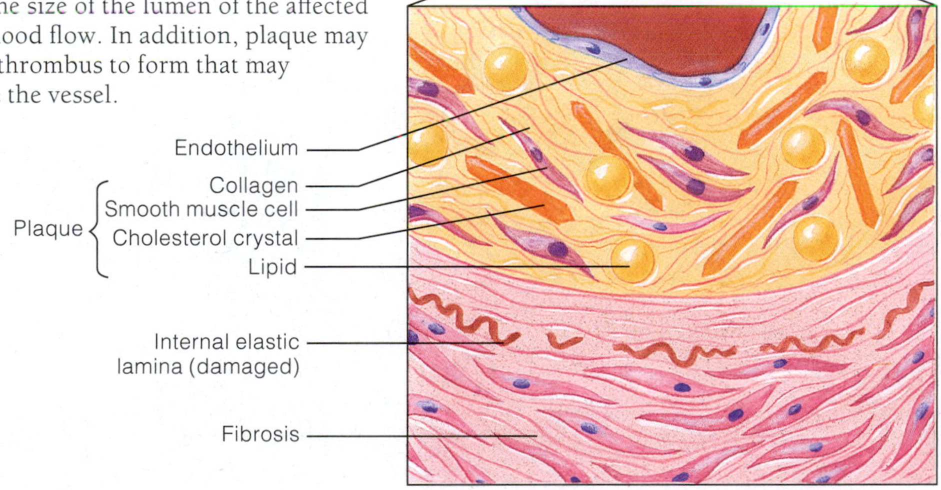
Endothelium
Plaque
Collagen
Smooth muscle cell
Cholesterol crystal
Lipid
Internal elastic
lamina (damaged)
Fibrosis

A

(continued)

Angina Pectoris

Angina is characterized by episodes of chest pain, usually precipitated by exercise and relieved by rest. When myocardial oxygen needs are greater than partially occluded vessels can supply, myocardial cells become ischemic and shift to anaerobic metabolism. Anaerobic metabolism produces lactic acid that stimulates nerve endings in the muscle, causing pain. The pain subsides when the oxygen supply again meets myocardial demand.

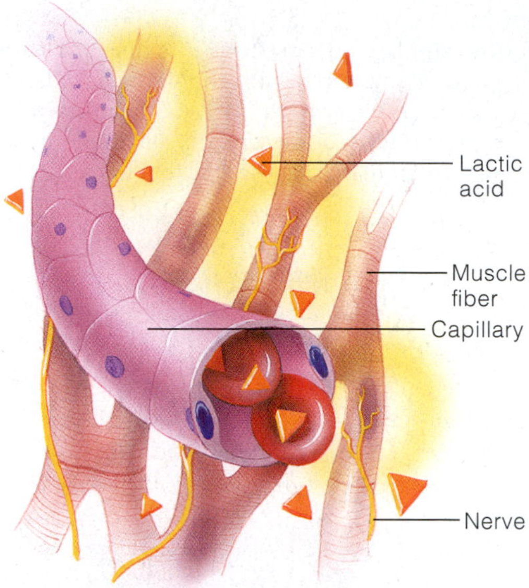
Lactic acid
Muscle fiber
Capillary
Nerve

Myocardial Infarction

Myocardial infarction occurs when complete obstruction of a coronary artery interrupts blood supply to an area of myocardium. Affected tissue becomes ischemic and eventually dies (infarcts) if the blood supply is not restored. The necrotic area is bordered by an area of injured or damaged tissue, which is in turn surrounded by an area of ischemic tissue. As myocardial cells die, they lyse and release various cardiac isoenzymes into the circulation. Elevated serum levels of creatinine kinase (CK) and cardiac-specific troponins are specific indicators of myocardial infarction.

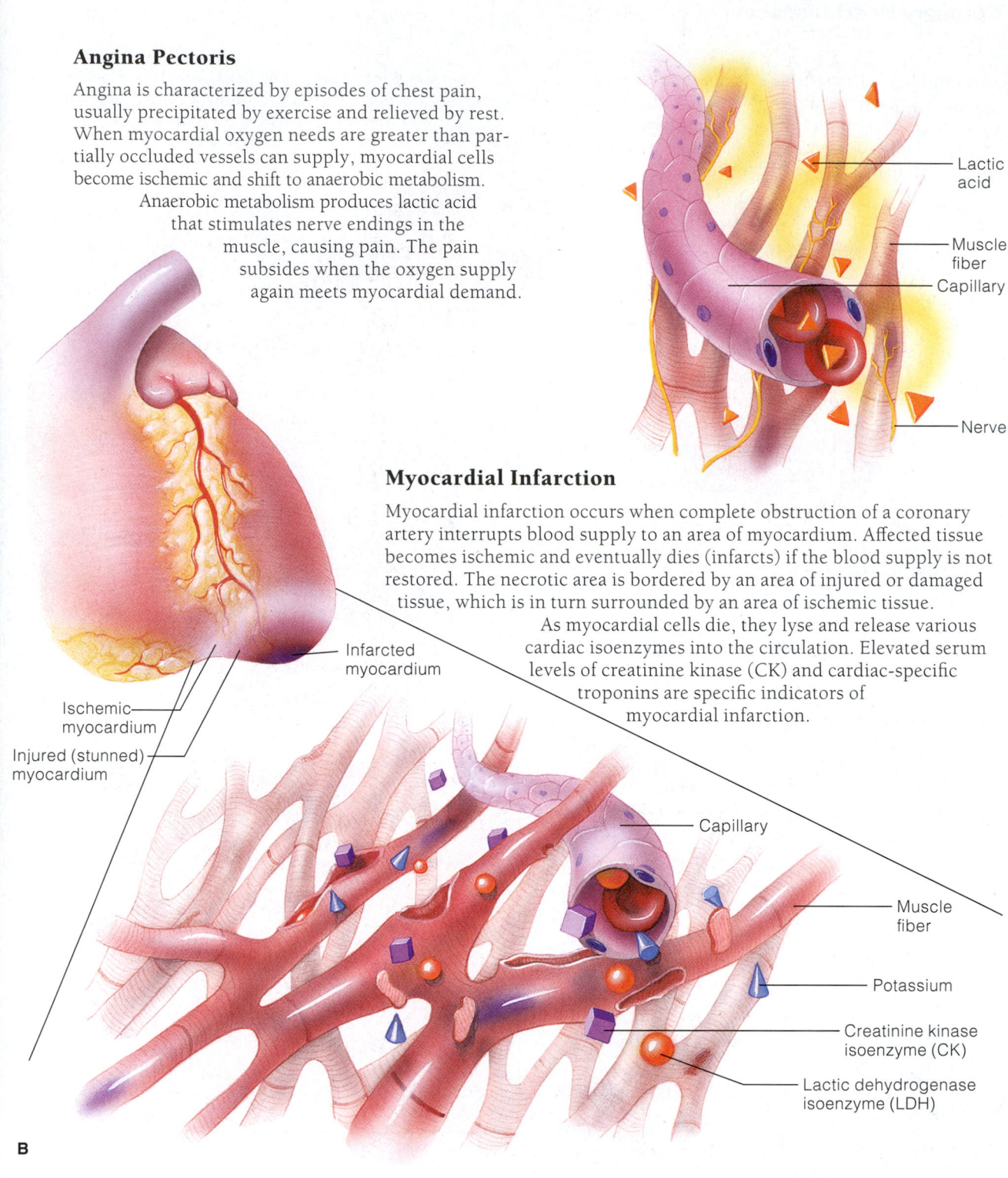

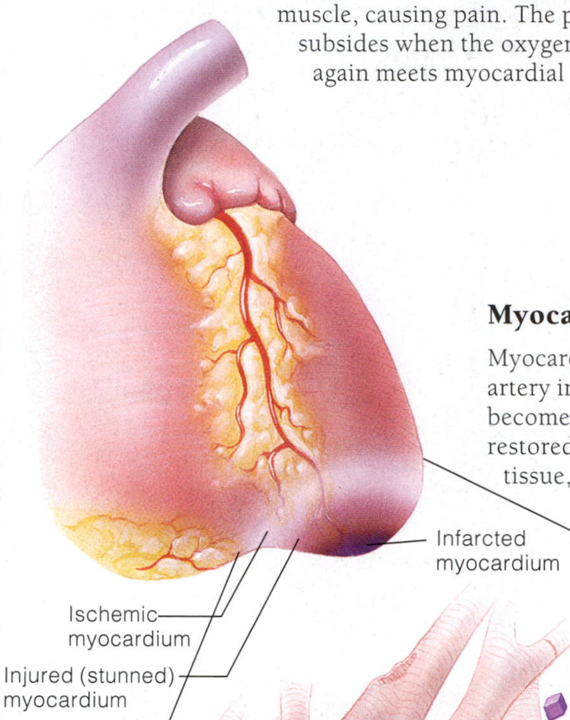
Infarcted myocardium
Ischemic myocardium
Injured (stunned) myocardium

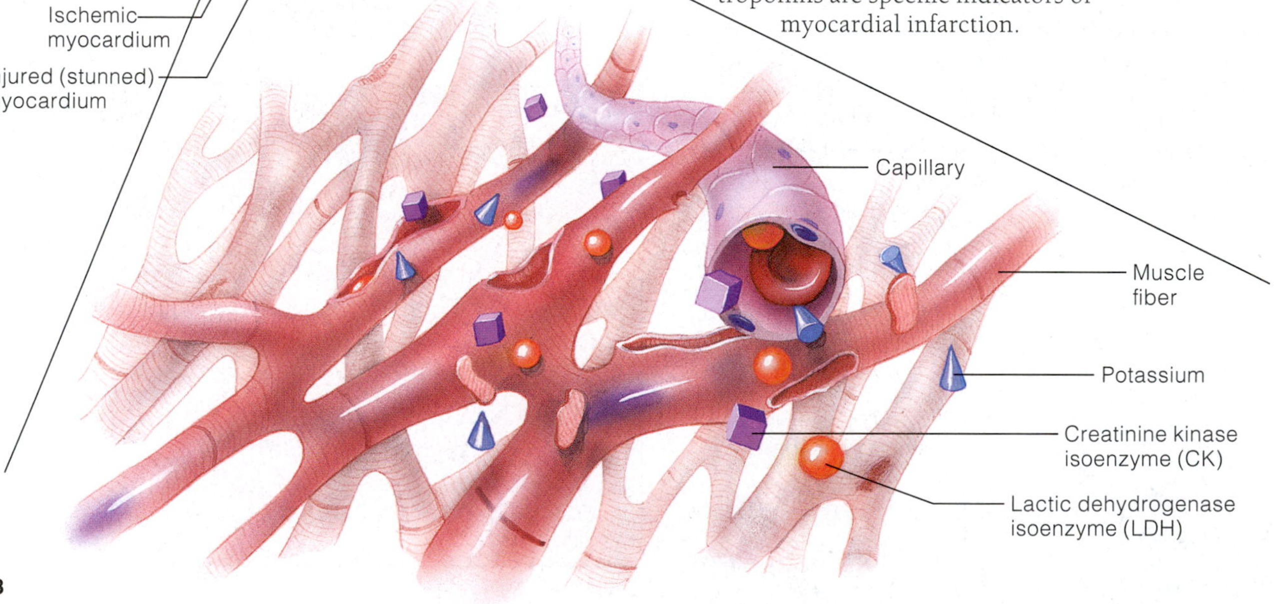
Capillary
Muscle fiber
Potassium
Creatinine kinase isoenzyme (CK)
Lactic dehydrogenase isoenzyme (LDH)

B

a yellowish fatty streak on the inner lining of the artery. Fibrous plaque develops as smooth muscle cells enlarge, collagen fibers proliferate, and blood lipids accumulate. The lesion protrudes into the arterial lumen and is fixed to the inner wall of the intima. It may invade the muscular media layer of the vessel as well. The developing plaque not only gradually occludes the vessel lumen but also impairs the vessel's ability to dilate in response to increased oxygen demands. Fibrous plaque lesions often develop at arterial bifurcations or curves or in areas of narrowing. As the plaque expands, it can produce severe stenosis or total occlusion of the artery.

The final stage of the process is the development of *atheromas*, complex lesions consisting of lipids, fibrous tissue, collagen, calcium, cellular debris, and capillaries. These calcified lesions can ulcerate or rupture, stimulating thrombosis. The vessel lumen may be rapidly occluded by the thrombus or it may embolize to occlude a distal vessel.

Plaque formation may be *eccentric*, located in a specific, asymmetric region of the vessel wall, or *concentric*, involving the entire vessel circumference. Manifestations of the process usually do not appear until about 75% of the arterial lumen has been occluded.

Atherosclerosis tends to develop where arteries *bifurcate* or branch. Certain vessels have a higher likelihood of being affected, including the coronary arteries (the left anterior descending artery in particular), the renal arteries, the bifurcation of the carotid arteries, and branching sections of peripheral arteries. In addition to obstructing or occluding blood flow, atherosclerosis weakens arterial walls and is a major cause of aneurysm in vessels such as the aorta and iliac arteries.

Myocardial Ischemia

Myocardial cells become ischemic when the oxygen supply is inadequate to meet metabolic demands. The critical factors in meeting the metabolic demands of cardiac cells are coronary perfusion and myocardial workload. Coronary perfusion can be affected by several different mechanisms:

- One or more vessels may be partially occluded by large, stable areas of plaque.
- Platelets can aggregate in narrowed vessels, forming a thrombus.
- Normal or already narrowed vessels may spasm.
- A drop in blood pressure may lead to inadequate flow through coronary vessels.
- Normal autoregulatory mechanisms that increase flow to working muscles may fail.

Workload is affected by the heart rate, myocardial contractility, preload (the amount of blood in the ventricles just prior to systole), and afterload (the peripheral pressure that must be overcome to move blood out of the heart into the circulation). The oxygen content of the blood and hematocrit are contributing factors to myocardial ischemia. **Box 30.1** lists factors that may lead to myocardial ischemia.

Myocardial cells have a limited supply of adenosine triphosphate (ATP). When myocardial workload increases or the supply of blood and oxygen falls, cellular ATP stores are quickly depleted, affecting contractility. Cellular metabolism switches from an efficient aerobic process to anaerobic metabolism. Lactic acid accumulates, and cells are damaged. If blood flow is restored within 20 minutes, aerobic metabolism and contractility are restored, and cellular repair begins. Continued ischemia results in cell necrosis and death (infarction).

Coronary heart disease is generally divided into two categories: Chronic ischemic heart disease and acute coronary syndromes. *Chronic ischemic heart disease* includes stable and vasospastic angina and silent myocardial ischemia. In women, fatigue is the most common presenting symptom of CHD. *Acute coronary syndromes* range from unstable angina to myocardial infarction. Acute coronary syndromes and myocardial infarction are the most common presenting symptoms of CHD in men. These disorders are discussed in the following sections of this chapter.

Incidence and Prevalence

Many risk factors for CHD can be controlled through lifestyle modification. In fact, with increased public awareness of risk factors related to CHD, mortality rates are declining by about 3.3% per year. Nevertheless, CHD remains a major public health problem. Heart disease is the leading cause of death for all U.S. ethnic groups except Asian American females (Benjamin et al., 2017). See the accompanying Focus on Cultural Diversity box. Nurses are in a prime position to encourage and support positive lifestyle changes by teaching and promoting healthy living practices. Individual choices can and do affect health.

BOX 30.1
Factors Contributing to Myocardial Ischemia

Coronary Perfusion	Myocardial Workload	Blood Oxygen Content
■ Atherosclerosis ■ Thrombosis ■ Vasospasm ■ Poor perfusion pressure	■ Rapid heart rate ■ Increased preload, afterload, or contractility ■ Increased metabolic demands (e.g., hyperthyroidism)	■ Reduced atmospheric oxygen pressure ■ Impaired gas exchange ■ Low red blood cells and hemoglobin content

Focus on Cultural Diversity
Heart Disease in the United States

- Caucasian American males have the highest prevalence of coronary heart disease (7.8%), followed by African American males (7.2%), African American females (7.0%), Hispanic males (6.7%), American Indians and Alaska Natives (6.0%), Hispanic females (5.9%), Caucasian American females (4.6%), and Asian American males and females (4.3%).
- Regionally, the rate of CHD is highest in the South and lowest in the West.

Source: Benjamin et al., 2017.

The highest incidence of CHD is in the Western world, mainly in Caucasian men age 45 and older (Benjamin et al., 2017). Both men and women are affected by coronary heart disease; in women, however, the onset is about 10 years later. After menopause, women's risk is equal to that of men.

Risk Factors

The causes of atherosclerosis are not known, but certain risk factors have been linked with the development of atherosclerotic plaques (NHLBI, 2017b). The Framingham Heart Study provided vital research into the relationship between risk factors and the development of heart disease (**Box 30.2**). Research into CHD is ongoing, looking at causative factors, manifestations, and protective measures for many populations.

Risk factors for CHD are frequently classified as *nonmodifiable*, or factors that cannot be changed, and *modifiable*, those factors that can be changed (**Table 30.1**).

Nonmodifiable Risk Factors

Age is a nonmodifiable risk factor. Over 50% of heart attack victims are age 65 or older; 80% of deaths due to MI occur in this age group. Gender and genetic factors are also nonmodifiable risk factors for CHD. Men are affected by CHD at an earlier age than women. A family history of CHD in a male first-degree relative younger than age 55 or a female first-degree relative younger than 65 years is identified as a risk factor for CHD (NHLBI, 2017a). Chromosome p921.3 has been associated with CHD. The region containing this chromosome also contains gene sequences for cyclin-dependent kinase inhibitors, which are implicated in the pathogenesis of atherosclerosis. See Chapter 29 for modifiable risk factors.

Interprofessional Care

Care of patients with coronary heart disease focuses on aggressive risk factor management to slow the atherosclerotic process and maintain myocardial perfusion. Until manifestations of chronic or acute ischemia are experienced, the diagnosis is often presumptive, based on history and the presence of risk factors.

Diagnosis

Laboratory testing assesses for risk factors such as an abnormal blood lipid profile (elevated triglyceride and LDL levels and decreased HDL levels) (Kee, 2014).

- ***Total serum cholesterol*** is elevated in hyperlipidemia. A *lipid profile* includes triglyceride, HDL, and LDL levels and enables calculation of the ratio of HDL to total cholesterol. The ratio should be at least 1:5, with 1:3 being the ideal ratio. Elevated lipid levels are associated with an increased risk of atherosclerosis. In patients with a strong family history of premature

BOX 30.2
The Framingham Heart Study

The Framingham Heart Study (FHS) is an ongoing, significant clinical research study that has provided data about cardiovascular disease for over 50 years. The study was initiated in 1948 with an original study group of 5209 participants in the town of Framingham, Massachusetts. Every 2 years, this original group is evaluated for cardiovascular events via their medical history, physical findings, and diagnostic testing. Children of the original group have also been studied as part of the Framingham Offspring Study. It was in reports of the FHS that the term *risk factor* first appeared (*www.framinghamheartstudy.org*).

Implications for Nursing

The data collected from both the FHS and the Framingham Offspring Study provide a rich database from which to develop evidence-based approaches for patients with heart disease. A major application of these research findings to practice is in primary preventive education, for example, through community cardiovascular health programs. As noted in the text, although research shows that increased public awareness of cardiovascular risk factors has lowered morbidity and mortality from heart disease, heart disease remains the number-one killer in the United States. Education about the effects of lifestyle on the cardiovascular system must begin in the early school years and be reinforced throughout the formative years. When healthy choices become habit, cardiac disease will be reduced.

A second application of these findings is in collaborative treatment. Nurses should keep up to date on the latest strategies for medical treatment so that they can provide accurate rationales to patients and formulate effective nursing treatment plans that complement medical management strategies. The result is better communication, a sense of collegiality and teamwork, and positive patient outcomes.

Moving Knowledge into Action

1. What kinds of strategies can be used in elementary school settings to teach cardiovascular health in a fun, informative manner?
2. Which healthcare providers should be included in a multidisciplinary effort to encourage patients to modify their lifestyles?
3. What changes do you need to make in your lifestyle to be a role model of heart-healthy living?

Table 30.1 Risk Factors for Coronary Heart Disease

Nonmodifiable	Modifiable	
	Pathophysiologic	**Lifestyle**
Age Men ≥ 45 years Women ≥ 55 years	Hyperlipidemia Elevated LDL cholesterol Elevated triglycerides Low HDL cholesterol	Cigarette smoking Obesity Physical inactivity Atherogenic diet
Gender	Hypertension	Women only: Use of oral contraceptives, hormone replacement therapy
Heredity	Diabetes mellitus	
Behavioral	Chronic stress Social isolation Anxiety and depression	
	Emerging risk factors: Elevated homocysteine levels Thrombogenic factors Inflammatory factors Impaired fasting glucose	

CHD or familial hypercholesterolemia, *lipoprotein Lp(a)* may also be measured. Elevated levels of Lp(a) may independently increase the risk of CHD. Other subsets of blood lipids may also be measured in selected patients. See the Diagnostic Tests table in Chapter 29 for nursing care related to lipid profile studies.

Diagnostic tests to identify subclinical (asymptomatic) CHD may be indicated when multiple risk factors are present.

- *C-reactive protein* is a serum protein associated with inflammatory processes. Recent evidence suggests that elevated blood levels of this protein may be predictive of CHD.
- *Ankle–brachial blood pressure index (ABI)* is an inexpensive, noninvasive test for peripheral vascular disease that may be predictive of CHD. Doppler is used to measure the systolic blood pressure in the brachial, posterior tibial, and dorsalis pedis arteries. An ABI of < 0.9 in either leg indicates the presence of peripheral arterial disease and a significant risk for CHD.
- *Exercise ECG testing* assesses the cardiac response to increased workload induced by exercise. The test is considered positive for CHD if myocardial ischemia is detected on the ECG (depression of the ST segment by > 3 mm; see Figure 30.1 later in the chapter), the patient develops chest pain, or the test is stopped due to excess fatigue, dysrhythmias, or other symptoms before the predicted maximal heart rate is achieved.
- *Electron beam computed tomography (EBCT)* creates a three-dimensional image of the heart and coronary arteries that can reveal coronary artery calcification and other abnormalities. A coronary artery calcium score can be calculated from this test, providing additional important information in the diagnosis of CHD. This noninvasive test requires no special preparation and can identify patients at risk for developing myocardial ischemia.
- *Myocardial perfusion imaging* (see the section on angina that follows) evaluates myocardial blood flow and perfusion, both at rest and during stress testing (exercise or mental stress).

These diagnostic tests are further explained in Chapter 29 and the later section on angina. Perfusion imaging studies are costly and are therefore not recommended for routine CHD risk assessment.

Risk Factor Management

Conservative management of CHD focuses on risk factor modification, including smoking, diet, exercise, and management of comorbidities.

Smoking. Smoking cessation reduces the risk for CHD within months after quitting and improves cardiovascular status. People who quit reduce their risk by 50%, regardless of how long they smoked before quitting. For women, the risk becomes equivalent to that of a nonsmoker within 3 to 5 years of smoking cessation. In addition, stopping smoking improves HDL levels, lowers LDL levels, and reduces blood viscosity. All smokers are advised to quit with health promotion activities focused on prevention.

Diet. The American Heart Association (AHA; 2017) Cholesterol Toolkit recommends reduced saturated fat and cholesterol intake with strategies to lower LDL levels (**Table 30.2**). Most fats are a mixture of saturated and unsaturated fatty acids. The highest proportions of saturated fat are found in whole-milk products, red meat, and coconut oil. Recommended proteins include nonfat dairy products, fish, and poultry. Solidified vegetable fats (e.g., margarine, shortening) contain trans fatty acids, which behave more like saturated fats. Soft margarines and vegetable oil spreads contain low levels of trans fatty acids and should be used instead of butter, stick margarine, and shortening. Monounsaturated fats—found in olive, canola, and peanut oils—actually lower LDL and cholesterol levels. Certain cold-water fish, such as tuna, salmon, and mackerel, contain

Table 30.2 Dietary Recommendations to Reduce Total Cholesterol, LDL Levels, and CHD Risk

Nutrient	Recommendation
Calories	Adjusted to attain/maintain desirable body weight
Total fat ■ Saturated fats ■ Polyunsaturated fat ■ Monounsaturated fat ■ Cholesterol	20–35% of total calories ■ < 10% of total calories ■ Up to 10% of total calories ■ Up to 20% of total calories ■ < 200 mg/day
Carbohydrate (primarily complex carbohydrates, such as whole grains, fruits, and vegetables)	45–65% of total calories
Dietary fiber	20–30 g/day
Protein	About 10–35% of total calories
Sodium	Less than 2300 mg/day and up to 1500 mg for those ages 51 and older or those who have hypertension, diabetes, or chronic kidney disease or are African American

Source: Compiled from U.S. Department of Agriculture and U.S. Department of Health and Human Services. (2015).

high levels of omega-3 (or Ω-3) fatty acids, which help raise HDL levels and decrease serum triglycerides, total serum cholesterol, and blood pressure.

In addition, increased intake of soluble fiber (found in oats, psyllium, pectin-rich fruits, and beans) and insoluble fiber (found in whole grains, vegetables, and fruits) is recommended. Folic acid and vitamins B_6 and B_{12} affect homocysteine metabolism, reducing serum levels. Leafy green vegetables (e.g., spinach and broccoli) and legumes (e.g., black-eyed peas, dried beans, and lentils) are rich sources of folate. Meat, fish, and poultry are rich in vitamins B_6 and B_{12}. Vitamin B_6 is also found in soy products; B_{12} is in fortified cereals. Increased intake of antioxidant nutrients (vitamin E in particular) and foods rich in antioxidants (fruits and vegetables) appears to increase HDL levels and has a protective effect on CHD.

In middle-aged and older adults, moderate alcohol intake may reduce the risk for CHD (AHA, 2017). Consumption of no more than two drinks per day for men or one drink per day for women is recommended. A drink is 5 ounces of wine, 12 ounces of beer, or 1.5 ounces of whiskey. People who do not drink alcohol, however, should not be encouraged to start consuming it as a heart-protective measure.

People who are overweight or obese are encouraged to lose weight through a combination of reduced calorie intake (maintaining a nutritionally sound diet) and increased exercise. High-protein, high-fat weight loss programs are not recommended for weight reduction.

Exercise. Regular physical exercise reduces the risk for CHD in several ways. It lowers VLDL, LDL, and triglyceride levels and raises HDL levels. Regular exercise reduces blood pressure and insulin resistance. Unless contraindicated, all patients are encouraged to participate in at least 30 minutes of moderate-intensity physical activity 5 to 6 days each week. To achieve weight loss and prevent weight gain, 60 to 90 minutes of moderate-intensity exercise daily is recommended.

Hypertension. Although hypertension often cannot be prevented or cured, it can be controlled. Hypertension control (maintaining a blood pressure lower than 130/80 mmHg) is vital to reduce atherosclerosis-promoting effects and to reduce the workload of the heart. Management strategies include reducing sodium intake, increasing calcium intake, regular exercise, stress management, and medications (Whelton et al., 2017). Hypertension management is discussed in Chapter 32.

Diabetes. Diabetes increases the risk of CHD by accelerating the atherosclerotic process. Weight loss (if appropriate), reduced fat intake, and exercise are particularly important for patients with diabetes. Because hyperglycemia apparently contributes to atherosclerosis, consistent blood glucose management is vital. See Chapter 20 for a detailed discussion about diabetes and blood glucose management.

Medications

Medication to lower total serum cholesterol and LDL levels and to raise HDL levels is an integral part of CHD management. Based on the patient's overall risk for CHD, drug therapy is used in conjunction with diet and other lifestyle changes (Nayor & Vasan, 2016).

Drugs used to treat hyperlipidemia act specifically by lowering LDL levels. The goal of treatment is to achieve an LDL level of > 130 mg/dL (AHA, 2017). Medications to treat hyperlipidemia are not inexpensive; the cost–benefit ratio needs to be considered because long-term treatment may be required. The four major classes of cholesterol-lowering drugs are statins, bile acid sequestrants, nicotinic acid, and fibrates (Shields, Fox, & Liebrecht, 2018). The nursing implications and patient teaching for these drug classes are outlined in **Medication Administration 30.A**.

The statins, including lovastatin (Mevacor), pravastatin (Pravachol), simvastatin (Zocor), and others, are first-line drugs for treating hyperlipidemia. They effectively lower LDL levels and may increase HDL levels. The statins can cause myopathy; all patients are instructed to report muscle pain and weakness or brown urine. Liver function tests are monitored during therapy because these drugs may increase liver enzyme levels.

The other cholesterol-lowering drugs, such as the bile acid sequestrants, nicotinic acid, and fibrates, are primarily used when combination therapy is required to lower serum cholesterol levels. They also may be used for selected patients, such as younger adults, women who wish to become pregnant, or to specifically lower triglyceride levels.

Medication Administration 30.A

Cholesterol-Lowering Drugs

STATINS

atorvastatin (Lipitor)

fluvastatin (Lescol)

lovastatin (Mevacor)

pravastatin (Pravachol)

rosuvastatin (Crestor)

simvastatin (Zocor)

Statins inhibit the enzyme HMG-CoA reductase in the liver, lowering LDL synthesis and serum levels. The statins are the first-line treatment for elevated LDL, used in conjunction with diet and lifestyle changes. Although their side effects are minimal, they may cause increased serum liver enzyme levels and myopathy. Rhabdomyolysis is a rare side effect resulting in the breakdown of muscle fibers.

Nursing Responsibilities

- Monitor serum cholesterol and liver enzyme levels before and during therapy (12 weeks and then at least yearly thereafter). Report elevated liver enzyme levels.
- Assess for muscle pain and tenderness. Monitor CPK level if present.
- If taking digoxin concurrently, monitor for and report digoxin toxicity.

Health Education for the Patient and Family

- Promptly report muscle pain, tenderness, or weakness; skin rash or hives or changes in skin color; abdominal pain or nausea and vomiting.
- Do not use these drugs if you are pregnant or plan to become pregnant.
- Inform your physician if you are taking any other medications concurrently.

BILE ACID SEQUESTRANTS

cholestyramine (Questran)

colestipol (Colestid)

colesevelam (Welchol)

Bile acid sequestrants lower LDL levels by binding bile acids in the intestine, reducing its reabsorption and cholesterol production in the liver. They are used in combination therapy regimens and for women who are considering pregnancy. Their primary disadvantages are inconvenience of administration due to bulk and gastrointestinal side effects such as constipation.

Nursing Responsibilities

- Mix cholestyramine and colestipol powders with 4 to 6 oz of water or juice; administer once or twice a day as ordered with meals.
- Store in a tightly closed container.

Health Education for the Patient and Family

- Promptly report constipation, severe gastric distress with nausea and vomiting, unexplained weight loss, black or bloody stools, or sudden back pain to your physician.
- Drinking ample amounts of fluids while taking these drugs reduces problems of constipation and bloating.
- Do not omit doses as this may affect the absorption of other drugs you are taking.

CHOLESTEROL ABSORPTION INHIBITORS

ezetimibe (Zetia)

Cholesterol absorption inhibitors block absorption in the small intestine. Their use is contraindicated with acute liver disease or hepatic insufficiency.

Nursing Responsibilities

- Can initially increase liver enzymes when used with statins; resolves with continued use.
- Can be taken without regard to meals.

NICOTINIC ACID

niacin (Nicobid, Nicolar, Niaspan, others)

Nicotinic acid in both prescription and nonprescription forms lowers total and LDL cholesterol and triglyceride levels. The crystalline form and Niaspan, a prescription extended-release tablet, also raise HDL levels. Because the doses required to achieve significant cholesterol-lowering effects are associated with multiple side effects, nicotinic acid is generally used in combination therapy, particularly with the statin drugs.

Nursing Responsibilities

- Give oral preparations with meals and accompanied by a cold beverage to minimize GI effects.
- Administer with caution to patients with active liver disease, peptic ulcer disease, gout, or type 2 diabetes.
- Monitor blood glucose, uric acid levels, and liver function tests during treatment.

Health Education for the Patient and Family

- Flushing of face, neck, and ears may occur within 2 hours following dose; these effects generally subside as treatment continues. Alcohol use during nicotinic acid therapy may worsen this effect.
- Report weakness or dizziness with changes in posture (lying to sitting; sitting to standing) to your physician. Change positions slowly to reduce the risk of injury.

FIBRIC ACID DERIVATIVES

gemfibrozil (Lopid)

fenofibrate (TriCor, Lipofen)

clofibrate (Atromid-S)

The fibrates are used to lower serum triglyceride levels; they have only a slight to modest effect on LDL levels. They affect lipid regulation by blocking triglyceride synthesis. They are used to treat very high triglyceride levels and may be used in combination with statins.

Nursing Responsibilities

- Monitor serum LDL and VLDL levels, electrolytes, glucose, liver enzymes, renal function tests, and CBC during therapy. Report abnormal values.
- Up to 2 months of treatment may be required to achieve a therapeutic effect; rebound, with decreasing benefit, may occur in the second or third month of treatment.

(continued)

Health Education for the Patient and Family

- Take with meals if the drug causes gastric distress.
- Promptly report flu-like symptoms (fatigue, muscle aching, soreness, or weakness) to your physician.
- Do not use this drug if you are pregnant or plan to become pregnant. Use reliable birth control measures while taking this drug.
- Contact your physician before stopping this drug and before taking any over-the-counter preparations.

Note: Drugs identified in blue are among the 200 most commonly prescribed medications in the United States.

Source: Adams, Holland, & Urban, 2017.

Patients at high risk for MI are often started on prophylactic low-dose aspirin therapy. The dose ranges from 80 to 325 mg/day. In women, the benefit of low-dose aspirin in reducing the risk for CHD is not clear prior to age 65. Aspirin is contraindicated for patients who have a history of aspirin sensitivity, bleeding disorders, or active peptic ulcer disease. Angiotensin-converting enzyme (ACE) inhibitors or angiotensin receptor blockers may also be prescribed for high-risk patients, including people with diabetes who have other CHD risk factors.

Nutrition

Two diet programs have been shown to have a beneficial effect on CHD. The Pritikin diet is basically vegetarian, high in complex carbohydrates and fiber, low in cholesterol, and extremely low in fat (< 10% of daily calories). Egg whites and limited amounts of nonfat dairy or soy products are allowed. In updates, the Pritikin diet also suggests awareness of caloric density. The Pritikin program requires 45 minutes of walking daily and recommends multivitamin supplements, including vitamins C and E and folate (Pritikin Longevity Center, 2017).

The Ornish diet is also vegetarian, although egg whites and a cup of nonfat milk or yogurt per day are allowed. No oil or fat is permitted, even for cooking. Two ounces of alcohol a day are permitted. The Ornish program also calls for stress reduction, emotional social support systems, daily stretching, and walking for 1 hour three times a week (Ornish Lifestyle Medicine, 2018).

Hypertension is a major, modifiable risk factor for CHD. When used with other lifestyle changes, the DASH (Dietary Approaches to Stop Hypertension) eating plan can help to prevent high blood pressure. The diet is heavy on grains (six to eight servings daily), vegetables (four to five servings daily), and fruits (four to five servings daily) and limits sodium (1500 to 2300 mg/day), fats, meats, and sweets (USDHHS, 2006). Refer to the U.S. Department of Health and Human Services website for a complete brochure.

Integrative Therapies

Diet and exercise programs that emphasize physical conditioning and a low-fat diet rich in antioxidants have been shown to be effective in managing CHD.

Supplements of vitamins C, E, B_6, B_{12}, and folic acid may be beneficial. Other potentially helpful complementary therapies include red wine or grape juice, foods containing bioflavonoids, green tea, nuts, and herbals and garlic (effective only for hypertension). Emphasize the need for patients to talk to their physician prior to taking any herbal preparations, as interactions with prescribed drugs are common. Behavioral therapies of benefit for patients with CHD include relaxation and stress management; guided imagery; treatment of depression; anger/hostility management; and meditation, tai chi, and yoga.

Nursing Care

Nurses are instrumental in educating adults about their risk for coronary heart disease, promoting participation in screening programs to identify that risk, and teaching all patients measures to reduce their risk for CHD.

Assessment

See the Course and Manifestations and Interprofessional Care sections for the assessment of the patient with coronary heart disease. Nursing assessment for CHD focuses on identifying risk factors:

- ***Health history:*** Current manifestations such as chest pain or heaviness, shortness of breath, weakness; current diet, exercise patterns, and medications; smoking history and pattern of alcohol intake; history of heart disease, hypertension, or diabetes; family history of CHD or other cardiac problems
- ***Physical assessment:*** Current weight and its appropriateness for height; body mass index; waist-to-hip ratio; blood pressure; strength and equality of peripheral pulses.

Priorities of Care

Collaborating with the interprofessional team to ensure adequate treatment of the underlying process while providing care that supports the physical and psychologic responses to the disorder is a priority.

Diagnoses, Outcomes, and Interventions

Maintain Appropriate Weight. Patients who are obese, have a waist-to-hip ratio > 0.8 (female) or 0.9 (male), or whose diet history or serum cholesterol levels indicate a need to reduce fat and cholesterol intake. See Chapters 21 and 22 for more information about assessing obesity.

Expected Outcome: Patient's weight will be within normal limits as a result of the application of therapeutic lifestyle changes.

The nurse will:

- Encourage assessment of food intake and eating patterns to help identify areas that can be improved. *Patients are often unaware of their fat and cholesterol intake, particularly when many meals are eaten away from home. Careful assessment increases awareness and allows the patient to make conscious changes.*

- Discuss American Heart Association and therapeutic lifestyle change dietary recommendations, emphasizing the role of diet in heart disease. Provide guidance regarding specific food choices with healthy alternatives. *Specific diet information and suggestions help the patient make better food choices.*
- Refer to clinical dietitian for diet planning and further teaching. Suggest cookbooks that offer low-fat recipes to encourage healthier eating, and provide American Heart Association and American Cancer Society recipe pamphlets and information on low-fat eating. *These resources provide tools for the patient to use as eating patterns change.*
- Encourage gradual but progressive dietary changes. *Drastic changes in eating patterns may cause frustration and discourage the patient from maintaining a healthy diet over the long term.*
- Discourage use of high-fat, low-carbohydrate, or other fad diets for weight loss. *These diets may adversely affect serum cholesterol and triglyceride levels and are often too drastic to maintain over the long term.*
- Encourage reasonable goals for weight loss (e.g., 1.0 to 1.5 lb per week and a 10% weight loss over 6 months). Provide information about weight loss programs and support groups such as Weight Watchers and Take Off Pounds Sensibly (TOPS). *Gradual but steady weight loss is more likely to be sustained. Recognized programs that emphasize healthy eating provide support and incentive for making lifetime dietary changes.*

Manage Risk Factors for CHD. Patients with risk factors for CHD may be unable to identify or independently manage their risk factors.

Expected Outcome: Patient will be independent in identifying and managing modifiable risk factors for CHD.

The nurse will:

- Discuss risk factors for CHD, stressing that changing or managing those factors that can be modified reduces the patient's overall risk for the disease. *Patients with significant nonmodifiable risk factors may be discouraged, reducing their ability to eliminate or control modifiable risk factors.*
- Discuss the immediate benefits of smoking cessation. Provide resource materials from the AHA, the American Lung Association, and the American Cancer Society. Refer to a structured smoking cessation program to increase the likelihood of success in quitting. *Long-time smokers may assume that the damage from smoking has already been done and quitting would not be worth the effort.*
- Help the patient identify specific sources of psychosocial and physical support for smoking cessation and dietary and lifestyle changes. *Support persons, groups, and aids such as nicotine patches help the patient achieve success and provide encouragement during difficult times (such as withdrawal symptoms).*
- Discuss the benefits of regular exercise for cardiovascular health and weight loss. Help identify favorite forms of exercise or physical activity. Encourage planning for 30 minutes of continuous aerobic activity (i.e., walking, running, bicycling, swimming) most days of the week. Encourage identification of an exercise buddy to help maintain motivation. *Engaging in preferred activities with a partner maintains motivation and increases the likelihood of maintaining an exercise program. Encourage continuation of the plan, even when days are missed.*
- Provide information and teaching about prescribed medications such as cholesterol-lowering drugs. Discuss the relationship between hypertension, diabetes, and CHD. *Teaching is important to promote understanding of and compliance with the prescribed drug regimen.*

Delegating Nursing Care Activities

As appropriate and allowed by the designated duties and responsibilities of unlicensed assistive personnel, the nurse may delegate nursing care activities such as measuring fluid intake and output, collecting vital signs (including orthostatic vital signs), encouraging oral or enteral fluid intake, and nonpharmacologic skin care.

Transitions of Care

Preventive information focuses on healthy lifestyle habits. See Chapter 29 for information on lifestyle modifications. Topics focus on increasing exercise and physical activity, smoking prevention/cessation, and healthy dietary choices. Be a model of healthy lifestyle habits, taking care of yourself, exercising, and eating right. In promoting healthy lifestyle habits, nurses can positively affect the incidence, morbidity, and mortality from CHD.

Strongly encourage all patients to avoid smoking in the first place and to stop all forms of tobacco use. Discuss the adverse effects of smoking and the benefits of quitting. Provide information about dietary recommendations to maintain a healthy weight and optimal cholesterol levels. Discuss the benefits and importance of regular exercise. Finally, encourage patients with cardiovascular risk factors to undergo regular screening for hypertension, diabetes, and abnormal blood lipids.

Encourage participation in some form of cardiac rehabilitation program. Formal programs provide comprehensive assessment of, interventions for, and teaching of patients with cardiac disease. Monitoring exercise and providing information about risk factors help patients identify ways to lower their risk for CHD.

Because patients themselves are primarily responsible for maintaining the lifestyle changes necessary to reduce the risk of CHD, provide teaching and support as outlined in the previous section. Assist the patient to make healthy choices and reinforce positive changes. Emphasize the importance of regular follow-up appointments to monitor progress.

The Patient with Angina Pectoris

Angina pectoris (angina) is chest pain resulting from reduced coronary blood flow, which causes a temporary imbalance between myocardial blood supply and demand (Sorenson et al., 2019). The imbalance may be due to coronary heart disease, atherosclerosis, or vessel constriction that impairs myocardial blood supply. Hypermetabolic conditions such as exercise, thyrotoxicosis, stimulant abuse (e.g., cocaine), hyperthyroidism, and emotional stress can increase myocardial oxygen demand, precipitating angina. Anemia, heart failure, ventricular hypertrophy, or pulmonary diseases may affect blood and oxygen supplies as well, causing angina.

Pathophysiology

The imbalance between myocardial blood supply and demand causes temporary and reversible myocardial ischemia. **Ischemia**, deficient blood flow to tissue, may be caused by partial obstruction of a coronary artery, coronary artery spasm, or a thrombus. Obstruction of a coronary artery deprives cells in the region of the heart normally supplied by that vessel of oxygen and nutrients needed for metabolic processes. Cellular processes are compromised as ATP stores are depleted. Reduced oxygen causes cells to switch from aerobic metabolism to anaerobic metabolism. Anaerobic metabolism causes lactic acid to build up in the cells. It also affects cell membrane permeability, releasing substances such as histamine, kinins, and specific enzymes that stimulate terminal nerve fibers in the cardiac muscle and send pain impulses to the central nervous system. The pain radiates to the upper body because the heart shares the same dermatome as this region. Return of adequate circulation provides the nutrients needed by cells and clears the waste products. More than 30 minutes of ischemia irreversibly damages myocardial cells (necrosis).

Three types of angina have been identified:

- ***Stable angina*** is the most common and predictable form of angina. It occurs with a predictable amount of activity or stress and is a common manifestation of CHD. Stable angina usually occurs when the work of the heart is increased by physical exertion, exposure to cold, or stress. Stable angina is relieved by rest and nitrates.
- ***Prinzmetal (variant) angina*** is atypical angina that occurs unpredictably (unrelated to activity) and often at night. It is caused by coronary artery spasm with or without an atherosclerotic lesion. The exact mechanism of coronary artery spasm is unknown. It may result from hyperactive sympathetic nervous system responses, altered calcium flow in smooth muscle, or reduced prostaglandins that promote vasodilation.
- ***Unstable angina*** occurs with increasing frequency, severity, and duration. Pain is unpredictable and occurs with decreasing levels of activity or stress and may occur at rest. Patients with unstable angina are at risk for myocardial infarction. Unstable angina is discussed further in the section on acute coronary syndromes.

Silent myocardial ischemia, or asymptomatic ischemia, is thought to be common in people with CHD. Silent ischemia may occur with either activity or with mental stress. Mental stress increases the heart rate and blood pressure, increasing myocardial oxygen demand (Sorenson et al., 2019). Like symptomatic angina, silent myocardial ischemia is associated with an increased chance of myocardial infarction and death.

Course and Manifestations

The cardinal manifestation of angina is chest pain. The pain is typically precipitated by an identifiable event, such as physical activity, strong emotion, stress, eating a heavy meal, or exposure to cold. The classic sequence of angina is activity–pain, rest–relief. The patient may describe the pain as a tight, squeezing, heavy pressure or a constricting sensation. It characteristically begins beneath the sternum and may radiate to the jaw, neck, shoulder, or arm. Less characteristically, the pain may be felt in the jaw, epigastric region, or back. Anginal pain usually occurs in a *crescendo–decrescendo* pattern (increasing to a peak, then gradually decreasing), typically lasting 2 to 5 minutes; it is generally relieved by rest. Additional manifestations of angina include dyspnea, pallor, tachycardia, and great anxiety and fear.

Women frequently present with atypical symptoms of angina, including fatigue, indigestion or nausea and vomiting, and upper back pain. The manifestations of angina include:

- ***Chest pain:*** Substernal or precordial (across the chest wall); may radiate to neck, arms, shoulders, or jaw
- ***Quality:*** Tight, squeezing, constricting, or heavy sensation; may also be described as burning, aching, choking, dull, or constant
- ***Associated manifestations:*** Dyspnea, pallor, tachycardia, anxiety, and fear
- ***Atypical manifestations:*** Indigestion, nausea and vomiting, upper back pain
- ***Precipitating factors:*** Exercise or activity, strong emotion, stress, cold, heavy meal
- ***Relieving factors:*** Rest, position change, nitroglycerin

The severity of angina can be graded by the degree to which it limits the patient's activities. Class I angina does not occur with ordinary physical activities. It is prompted by strenuous, rapid, or prolonged physical exertion. Class II angina may develop with rapid or prolonged walking or stair climbing, whereas Class III angina significantly limits ordinary physical activities. The patient with Class IV angina may have angina at rest, as well as with physical activity.

Interprofessional Care

The management of stable angina focuses on maintaining coronary blood flow and cardiac function. Stable angina can often be managed by medical therapy. Measures to restore coronary blood flow are discussed in the section on acute coronary syndrome. As for CHD, risk factor management is a vital component of care for the patient with angina (see the preceding section of this chapter).

Diagnosis

The diagnosis of angina is based on past medical history and family history, a comprehensive description of the chest pain, and physical assessment findings. Laboratory tests may confirm the presence of risk factors, such as an abnormal blood lipid profile and elevated blood glucose. Diagnostic tests provide information about overall cardiac function (Kee, 2014).

Common diagnostic tests to assess for coronary heart disease and angina include electrocardiography, stress testing, nuclear medicine studies, echocardiography (ultrasound), and coronary angiography.

Electrocardiography. A resting ECG may be normal, may show nonspecific changes in the ST segment and T wave, or may show evidence of previous myocardial infarction. Characteristic ECG changes are seen during anginal episodes. During periods of ischemia, the ST segment is depressed or downsloping, and the T wave may flatten or invert (**Figure 30.1** ■). These changes reverse when ischemia is relieved. For more details about the ECG, its waveforms, and its uses, see Chapter 29.

Stress Electrocardiography. *Stress electrocardiography* (exercise stress test) uses ECGs to monitor the cardiac response to an increased workload during progressive exercise. See the Diagnostic Tests table in Chapter 29 for more information about exercise stress tests.

Radionuclide Testing. *Radionuclide testing* is a safe, noninvasive technique to evaluate myocardial perfusion and left-ventricular function. The amount of radioisotope injected is very small; no special radiation precautions are required during or after the scan. Thallium-201 or a technetium-based radiocompound is injected intravenously, and the heart is scanned with a radiation detector. Ischemic or infarcted cells of the myocardium do not take up the substance normally, appearing as a "cold spot" on the scan. If the ischemia is transient, these spots gradually fill in, indicating the reversibility of the process. With severe ischemia or a myocardial infarction, these areas remain devoid of radioactivity.

Left-ventricular function can also be evaluated. Whereas the ejection fraction (portion of blood ejected from the left ventricle during systole) normally increases during exercise, it may actually decrease in coronary heart disease and stress-induced ischemia.

Radionuclide testing may be combined with pharmacologic stress testing for patients who are physically unable to exercise or to detect subclinical myocardial ischemia. A vasodilator is injected to induce the same ischemic changes that occur with exercise in the diseased heart. Coronary arteries unaffected by atherosclerosis dilate in response to the drugs, increasing blood flow to already well-perfused tissue. This reduces flow to ischemic muscle, called *myocardial steal syndrome*.

Echocardiography. *Echocardiography* is a noninvasive test that uses ultrasound to evaluate cardiac structure and function. It may be done at rest, during supine exercise, or immediately following upright exercise to evaluate movement of the myocardial wall and assess for possible ischemia or infarction.

Transesophageal echocardiography (TEE) uses ultrasound to identify abnormal blood flow patterns as well as cardiac structures. In TEE, the probe is on the tip of an endoscope inserted into the esophagus, positioning it close to the posterior heart (especially the left atrium and the aorta). It avoids interference by breasts, ribs, or lungs. See the Diagnostic Tests table in Chapter 29 for more information about these tests and the nursing implications.

Coronary Angiography. *Coronary angiography* is the gold standard for evaluating the coronary arteries. Guided by fluoroscopy, a catheter introduced into the femoral or brachial artery is threaded into the coronary artery. Dye is injected into each coronary opening, allowing visualization of the main coronary branches and any abnormalities, such as stenosis or obstruction. Narrowing of the vessel lumen by more than 50% is considered significant; most lesions that cause symptoms involve more than 70% narrowing. Vessel obstructions are noted on a coronary artery map that provides a guide for tracking disease progression and for elective treatment with angioplasty or cardiac surgery. During angiogram, the drug ergonovine maleate may be injected to induce coronary artery spasm and diagnose Prinzmetal angina. Nursing care of the patient undergoing a coronary angiogram is summarized in **Box 30.3** later in this chapter.

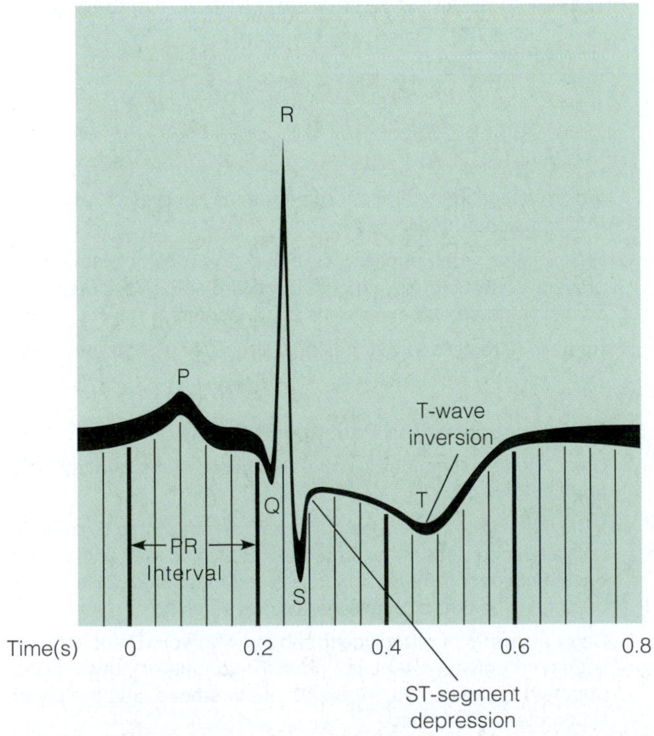
R
P
T-wave
inversion
Q
T
PR
Interval
S
Time(s)
0
0.2
0.4
0.6
0.8
ST-segment
depression

Figure 30.1 ■ ECG changes during an episode of angina. Note characteristic T-wave inversion and ST-segment depression of myocardial ischemia.

Medications

Drugs may be used for both acute and long-term relief of angina. The goal of drug treatment is to reduce oxygen demand and increase oxygen supply to the myocardium.

Three main classes of drugs are used to treat angina: Nitrates, beta-blockers, and calcium channel blockers.

Nitrates. Nitrates, including nitroglycerin and longer-acting nitrate preparations, are used to treat acute anginal attacks and prevent angina.

Sublingual nitroglycerin is the drug of choice to treat acute angina. It acts within 1 to 2 minutes, decreasing myocardial work and oxygen demand through venous and arterial dilation, which in turn reduce preload and afterload. It may also improve myocardial oxygen supply by dilating collateral blood vessels and reducing stenosis. Rapid-acting nitroglycerin is also available as a buccal spray in a metered system. For some patients, this may be easier to handle than small nitroglycerin tablets.

SAFETY ALERT: Sublingual nitroglycerin tablets and nitroglycerin spray are the only medications appropriate to treat an acute anginal attack. ■

Longer-acting nitroglycerin preparations (oral tablets, ointments, or transdermal patches) are used to prevent attacks of angina, not to treat an acute attack. The primary problem with long-term nitrate use is the development of *tolerance*, a decreasing effect from the same dose of medication. Tolerance can be limited by a dosing schedule that allows a nitrate-free period of at least 8 to 10 hours daily. This is usually scheduled at night, when angina is less likely to occur.

Headache is a common side effect of nitrates and may limit their usefulness. Nausea, dizziness, and hypotension are also common effects of therapy.

Beta-Blockers. Beta-blockers—including propranolol, metoprolol, nadolol, and atenolol—are considered first-line drugs to treat stable angina. They block the cardiac-stimulating effects of norepinephrine and epinephrine, preventing anginal attacks by reducing heart rate, myocardial contractility, and blood pressure, thus reducing myocardial oxygen demand. Beta-blockers may be used alone or with other medications to prevent angina.

Beta-blockers are contraindicated for patients with asthma or severe chronic obstructive pulmonary disease (COPD) (see Chapter 37) because they may cause severe bronchospasm. They are not used in patients with significant bradycardia or AV conduction blocks and are used cautiously in heart failure. Beta-blockers are not used to treat Prinzmetal angina because they may make it worse.

Calcium Channel Blockers. Calcium channel blockers reduce myocardial oxygen demand and increase myocardial blood and oxygen supply. These drugs, which include verapamil, diltiazem, and nifedipine, lower blood pressure, reduce myocardial contractility, and, in some cases, lower the heart rate, decreasing myocardial oxygen demand. They are also potent coronary vasodilators, effectively increasing oxygen supply. Like beta-blockers, calcium channel blockers act too slowly to effectively treat an acute attack of angina; they are used for long-term prophylaxis. Because they may actually increase ischemia and mortality in patients with heart failure or left-ventricular dysfunction, these drugs are usually not prescribed in the initial treatment of angina. They are used cautiously in patients with dysrhythmias, heart failure, or hypotension.

The nursing implications of antianginal medications are summarized in **Medication Administration 30.B.**

Aspirin. The patient with angina, particularly unstable angina, is at risk for myocardial infarction because of

Medication Administration 30.B

Antianginal Medications

ORGANIC NITRATES

amyl nitrite

isosorbide dinitrate (Isordil)

isosorbide mononitrate (ISMO)

nitroglycerin (Nitropaste, Nitro-Dur, Nitro-Bid, Nitrol, Transderm-Nitro, Nitrogard, Nitrodisc, Tridil)

Nitrates dilate both arterial and venous vessels, depending on the dose. Coronary artery vasodilation increases blood flow and myocardial oxygen supply. Venous dilation allows peripheral blood pooling, reducing venous return, preload, and cardiac work. Arterial dilation reduces vascular resistance and afterload, also reducing cardiac work. Sublingual nitroglycerin (NTG) tablets are used to treat and prevent acute anginal attacks (when taken prophylactically before activity). Nitrates are administered sublingually by buccal spray, intravenously for immediate effect, or orally or topically for sustained effect.

Nursing Responsibilities

- Dilute intravenous nitroglycerin before infusing; use only glass bottles for the mixture. Nitroglycerin adheres to PVC bags and tubing, affecting the amount of drug that is delivered. Use non-PVC infusion tubing.
- Wear gloves when applying nitroglycerin paste or ointment to prevent absorbing the drug through the skin. Measure dose carefully and spread evenly in a 2 × 3-inch area.
- Remove nitroglycerin patches or ointment at night to help prevent tolerance.

Health Education for the Patient and Family

- Use only the sublingual, buccal, and spray forms of nitrates to treat acute angina.
- If the first nitrate dose does not relieve angina within 5 minutes, take a second dose. After 5 more minutes, you may take a third dose if needed. If the pain is unrelieved or lasts for 20 minutes or longer, seek medical assistance immediately.
- Carry a supply of nitroglycerin tablets with you. Dissolve sublingual nitroglycerin tablets under the tongue or between the upper lip and gum. Do not eat, drink, or smoke until the tablet is completely dissolved.
- Keep sublingual tablets in their original amber glass bottle to protect them from heat, light, and moisture. Replace your supply every 6 months.

- You may experience a burning or tingling sensation under the tongue and develop a transient headache when you take the drug. These are expected; the headache will diminish over time.
- Use caution when standing from a sitting position; nitroglycerin may make you light-headed.
- Rotate ointment or transdermal patch application sites. Apply to a hairless area; spread ointment evenly without rubbing or massaging. Remove the patch or residual ointment at bedtime daily. Apply a fresh dose in the morning.
- If you are using a long-acting nitrate, keep a supply of immediate-acting nitrates to treat acute angina.

BETA-BLOCKERS

atenolol (Tenormin)
carvedilol (Coreg)
metoprolol (Lopressor, Toprol)
nadolol (Corgard)
propranolol (Inderal)

Beta-blockers decrease cardiac workload by blocking beta-receptors on the heart muscle, decreasing heart rate, contractility, myocardial oxygen consumption, and blood pressure. Beta-blockers also reduce *reflex tachycardia* (an increased heart rate in response to stimuli such as increased sympathetic nervous system [SNS] activity or vasodilation), which may develop with other antianginal drugs. Beta-blockers are frequently prescribed as antianginal and antihypertensive agents.

Nursing Responsibilities

- Document heart rate and blood pressure before administering the medication. Withhold drug if the heart rate is below 50 bpm or the blood pressure is below prescribed limits. Notify the physician.
- Assess for and report possible contraindications to therapy, including heart failure, bradycardia, AV block, asthma, or COPD.
- Concurrent use of beta-blockers and calcium channel blockers increases the risk for heart failure; notify the physician if these drugs are prescribed together.
- Do not abruptly discontinue these drugs after long-term therapy, as this can increase heart rate, contractility, and blood pressure and cause fatal dysrhythmia, myocardial infarction, or stroke.

Health Education for the Patient and Family

- Beta-blockers help prevent angina but will not relieve an acute attack. Keep a supply of fast-acting nitrates on hand for acute anginal attacks.
- Do not suddenly stop taking this medication. Discuss discontinuing this medication with your physician.
- Take your pulse daily. Do not take the drug, and contact your physician if your heart rate is below 50 bpm. Check your blood pressure frequently.
- Report a slow or irregular pulse, swelling or weight gain, or difficulty breathing to your physician.

CALCIUM CHANNEL BLOCKERS

amlodipine (Norvasc)
bepridil (Vascor)
diltiazem (Cardizem)
felodipine (Plendil)
isradipine (DynaCirc)
nicardipine (Cardene)
nifedipine (Adalat, Procardia)
nimodipine (Nimotop)
verapamil (Isoptin, Calan)

Calcium channel blockers are used to control angina, hypertension, and dysrhythmias. By blocking the entry of calcium into cells, these drugs reduce contractility, slow the heart rate and conduction, and cause vasodilation. Calcium channel blockers increase myocardial oxygen supply by dilating the coronary arteries; they decrease the workload of the heart by lowering vascular resistance and oxygen demand. Calcium channel blockers are often prescribed for patients with coronary artery spasm (Prinzmetal angina).

Nursing Responsibilities

- Do not mix verapamil in any solution containing sodium bicarbonate. Administer IV push verapamil over 2 to 3 minutes.
- Document blood pressure and heart rate before administering the drug. Withhold the drug if the heart rate is below 50 bpm. Notify the physician.
- Use caution when giving a calcium channel blocker with other cardiac depressants, such as beta-blockers. Concomitant administration with nitrates may cause excessive vasodilation.
- Manifestations of toxicity include nausea, generalized weakness, signs of decreased cardiac output, hypotension, bradycardia, and AV block. Report these findings immediately. Maintain intravenous access, and slowly administer intravenous calcium chloride. Do not infuse large volumes of fluid to treat hypotension as heart failure may result.

Health Education for the Patient and Family

- Take your pulse before taking the drug. If your heart rate drops below 50 bpm, do not take the drug and notify your physician.
- Keep a fresh supply of immediate-acting nitrate available to treat acute anginal attacks. Calcium channel blockers will not work fast enough to relieve an acute attack.

Note: Drugs identified in blue are among the 200 most commonly prescribed medications in the United States.

Source: Adams, et al., 2017.

significant narrowing of the coronary arteries. Low-dose aspirin (80 to 325 mg/day) is often prescribed to reduce the risk of platelet aggregation and thrombus formation.

Nursing Care

The focus of nursing care for patients with angina is similar to the collaborative care focus: To reduce myocardial oxygen demand and improve the oxygen supply. Angina is usually treated in community settings; the primary nursing focus is education.

Assessment

Focused assessment data for the patient with angina includes:

- *Health history:* Chest pain, including type, intensity, duration, frequency, aggravating factors and relief measures; associated symptoms; history of other cardiovascular disorders, peripheral vascular disease, or stroke; current medications and treatment; usual diet, exercise, and alcohol intake patterns; smoking history; use of other recreational drugs

- ***Physical assessment:*** Vital signs and heart sounds; strength and equality of peripheral pulses; skin color and temperature (central and peripheral); physical appearance during pain episode (e.g., shortness of breath, apparent anxiety, color, diaphoresis).

Priorities of Care

Collaborating with the interprofessional team to ensure adequate treatment of the cardiac perfusion limitations while providing care that supports circulatory support (including appropriate precautions) is a nursing priority. Teaching the patient and, as appropriate, caregivers strategies to identify early signs and symptoms of acute cardiac events and optimize safe home and work environments is another nursing priority. The nurse also focuses on promoting comfort and prevention of cardiac event recurrence.

Diagnoses, Outcomes, and Interventions

High-priority nursing care for the patient with angina includes managing ineffective cardiac tissue perfusion and managing the prescribed therapeutic regimen.

Promote Effective Cardiac Tissue Perfusion. Anginal pain results from impaired blood flow and oxygen supply to the myocardium. Nursing interventions can both prevent ischemia and shorten the duration of pain.

Expected Outcome: Patient will experience adequate cardiac perfusion as evidenced by freedom from chest pain related to angina and freedom from arrhythmias.

The nurse will:

- Keep prescribed nitroglycerin tablets at the patient's side so one can be taken at the onset of pain. *Anginal pain indicates myocardial ischemia. Nitroglycerin reduces cardiac workload and may improve myocardial blood flow, relieving ischemia and pain.*
- Start oxygen at 4 to 6 L/min per nasal cannula or as prescribed. *Supplemental oxygen reduces myocardial hypoxia.*
- Space activities to allow rest between them. *Activity increases cardiac workload and may precipitate angina. Spacing of activities allows the heart to recover.*
- Teach about prescribed medications to maintain myocardial perfusion and reduce cardiac workload. Emphasize that long-acting nitrates, beta-blockers, and calcium channel blockers are used to prevent anginal attacks, not to treat an acute attack. *It is important for the patient to understand the purpose and use of prescribed drugs to maintain optimal myocardial perfusion.*
- Instruct to take sublingual nitroglycerin before engaging in activities that precipitate angina (e.g., climbing stairs, sexual intercourse). *This prophylactic dose of nitroglycerin helps maintain cardiac perfusion when increased work is anticipated, preventing ischemia and chest pain.*
- Encourage to implement and maintain a progressive exercise program under the supervision of the primary care provider or a cardiac rehabilitation professional. *Exercise slows the atherosclerotic process and helps develop collateral circulation to the heart muscle.*
- Refer to a smoking cessation program as indicated. *Nicotine causes vasoconstriction and increases the heart rate, decreasing myocardial perfusion and increasing cardiac workload.*

Promote Adherence to Therapeutic Regimen. Denial may be strong in the patient with angina pectoris. Because many people think of the heart as the locus of life itself, problems such as angina remind people of their mortality, an uncomfortable fact. Denial may lead to forgetting to take prescribed medications or to attempting activities that will precipitate angina. Some patients, by contrast, may become afraid to engage in activities because of anticipated chest pain. Their inactivity may actually hasten the atherosclerotic process and inhibit collateral circulation development, worsening angina.

Expected Outcome: Patient will be knowledgeable about therapies used to manage angina as evidenced by verbalized understanding of the underlying pathophysiology of angina, correct medication plan, and early identification of the onset of anginal episodes.

The nurse will:

- Assess knowledge and understanding of angina. *Assessment allows tailoring of teaching and interventions to the needs of the patient.*
- Teach about angina and atherosclerosis as needed, building on current knowledge base. *This can help the patient understand that angina is a manageable disease and that pain can usually be controlled and the disease progress slowed.*
- Provide written and verbal instructions about prescribed medications and their use. *Written instructions reinforce teaching and are available to the patient for future reference.*
- Stress the importance of taking chest pains seriously while maintaining a positive attitude. *Although it is vital to recognize the significance of chest pain and deal with it appropriately, it is also important to maintain a positive outlook.*
- Refer patient to a cardiac rehabilitation program or other organized activities and support groups for patients with coronary artery disease. *Programs such as these help the patient develop risk factor management strategies, maintain a program of supervised activity, and gain coping skills.*

Delegating Nursing Care Activities

As appropriate and allowed by designated duties and responsibilities of assistive personnel, the nurse may delegate nursing care activities such as collecting vital signs (including orthostatic vital signs), measuring fluid intake and output, encouraging oral or enteral fluid intake, and skin care.

Transitions of Care

See Chapter 29 for discussion of health-promoting activities to prevent CHD. In addition to health promotion measures, emphasize the importance of active CHD risk factor management to slow progression of the disease. Encourage patients to stop smoking. Discuss the use of cholesterol-lowering drug therapy with patients who have hypercholesterolemia. Encourage regular aerobic exercise and a diet based on AHA or NCEP guidelines.

Many patients with stable angina manage their pain effectively, continuing to live active and productive lives. To promote effective management of this disorder, include the following topics in teaching for home care:

- Coronary heart disease and the processes that cause chest pain, including the relationship between the pain and reduced blood flow to the heart muscle.
- Use and effects (desired and adverse) of prescribed medications; importance of not discontinuing medications abruptly.
- Nitroglycerin use for acute angina: Always carry several tablets (not the entire supply); prophylactic use before activities that often cause chest pain; take tablet at first indication of pain rather than waiting to see if the pain develops; seek immediate medical assistance if three nitroglycerin tablets over 15 to 20 minutes do not relieve the pain. Instruct patient to not continue the series of nitroglycerin if dizziness or light-headedness develops but to seek immediate medical assistance.
- The importance of calling 911 or going to the emergency department immediately for unrelieved chest pain.
- Appropriate storage of nitroglycerin: This unstable compound needs to be stored in a cool, dry, dark place; no more than a 6-month supply should be kept on hand.

For the patient who has undergone cardiac surgery, also include:

- Respiratory care, activity, and pain management
- The importance of actively participating in rehabilitation
- Manifestations of infection or other potential complications and their management.

The Patient with Acute Coronary Syndrome

Acute coronary syndrome (ACS) is a condition of unstable cardiac ischemia. ACS includes unstable angina and acute myocardial ischemia with or without significant injury of myocardial tissue (Sorenson et al., 2019). Although the term ACS may, in some cases, be applied to acute myocardial infarction (myocardial tissue death), myocardial infarction is discussed separately in the next section of this chapter. An estimated 1.4 million Americans are admitted to the hospital annually with ACS, and it is the most common identified cause of sudden cardiac death (Benjamin et al., 2017).

Pathophysiology

ACS is a dynamic state in which coronary blood flow is acutely reduced, but not fully occluded. Myocardial cells are injured by the acute ischemia that results. Most people affected by ACS have significant stenosis of one or more coronary arteries.

ACS is precipitated by one or more of the following processes: (1) Rupture or erosion of atherosclerotic plaque with formation of a blood clot that does not fully occlude the vessel; (2) coronary artery spasm (e.g., Prinzmetal angina); (3) progressive vessel obstruction by atherosclerotic plaque or restenosis following a percutaneous revascularization (PCR) procedure; (4) inflammation of a coronary artery; or (5) increased myocardial oxygen demand and/or decreased supply (e.g., acute blood loss or anemia). Of these, ruptured or eroded plaque is the predominant pathophysiology underlying ACS. Plaque rupture is often triggered by hemodynamic factors such as increased heart rate, blood flow, and blood pressure in response to a surge of sympathetic nervous system activity. Increased SNS activity is also thought to contribute to the higher incidence of plaque rupture within the first hour of arising from bed in the morning.

When atherosclerotic plaque ruptures or erodes, the exposed lipid core of the plaque stimulates platelet aggregation and the extrinsic clotting pathway. Thrombin is generated and fibrin is deposited, forming a clot that severely impairs or obstructs blood flow to tissue distal to the area of plaque rupture. As a result, these cells become ischemic.

Injured myocardial cells contract less effectively, potentially reducing cardiac output if a large area of myocardium is affected. Lactic acid released from ischemic cells stimulates pain receptors, causing chest pain. Ischemia and injury affect electrical impulse conduction, producing inversion of the T wave and possibly elevation of the ST segment on the ECG.

Manifestations

The cardinal manifestation of ACS is chest pain, usually substernal or epigastric. The pain often radiates to the neck, left shoulder, and/or left arm. The pain may occur at rest and typically lasts longer than 10 to 20 minutes. In ACS, the chest pain is more severe and prolonged than that previously experienced by the patient. It may be a new onset of pain or may represent a pattern of increasing frequency and severity of anginal pain. Dyspnea, diaphoresis, pallor, and cool skin may be present. Tachycardia and hypotension may occur. The patient may be nauseated or feel light-headed. **Table 30.3** compares the features of stable angina, ACS, and acute myocardial infarction.

Interprofessional Care

The patient with ACS generally presents at the emergency department or physician's office with complaints of severe chest pain. The pain may be unrelieved by nitroglycerin or may be more severe and of longer duration than previous anginal episodes. The ECG is used in conjunction with blood levels of cardiac markers to differentiate between unstable angina and acute myocardial infarction. Patients with unstable angina are generally admitted to the acute care unit on bedrest with cardiac monitoring for 12 to 24 hours. Coronary revascularization procedures may be performed within 48 hours if significant CHD is identified.

Table 30.3 Comparing Stable Angina, Acute Coronary Syndrome, and Acute Myocardial Infarction

	Stable Angina	Acute Coronary Syndrome	Acute Myocardial Infarction
Pathophysiology	Myocardial ischemia occurs with increased workload (e.g., during exercise) due to stable atherosclerotic plaque narrowing coronary arteries.	Coronary artery spasm or partial occlusion by unstable plaque and thrombus formation occur, with increasing myocardial ischemia.	Obstruction of a coronary artery by a thrombus blocks blood supply to a portion of the myocardium, resulting in necrosis.
Chest pain	Stable and predictable, occurring with exertion or emotion Crescendo–decrescendo pattern May radiate to neck, shoulder, arms Usually lasts 5–10 min, relieved by rest	Occurs at rest; increasing frequency and severity Lasts 10 min or longer Radiates to neck, left shoulder, and arm Lasts longer than 10 min	Begins abruptly, unrelated to rest or exercise Severe, "crushing" Unrelieved by rest or nitroglycerin Radiates to arms, neck, jaw
Other manifestations	Indigestion, nausea Possible shortness of breath Anxiety	Epigastric pain Dyspnea Tachycardia, hypotension Cool, pale skin	Epigastric pain, nausea Dyspnea Pallor, diaphoresis Tachycardia or bradycardia, hyper- or hypotension
Diagnosis	ECG: T-wave inversion during anginal episodes Cardiac markers: Within normal range	ECG: ST-segment depression, T-wave inversion Cardiac markers: Within normal range or transient elevation	ECG: ST-segment elevation, possible Q wave Cardiac markers: Elevated

Diagnosis

The ECG and serum cardiac markers are the primary tests used to establish the diagnosis of ACS. Serum cardiac markers, proteins released from injured and necrotic heart muscle, can be measured (see the following section on acute myocardial infarction and **Table 30.4** for more information about serum cardiac markers).

- Cardiac muscle troponins, *cardiac-specific troponin T* (cT_nT) and *cardiac-specific troponin I* (cT_nI), are sensitive indicators of myocardial damage. Troponins may be elevated in ACS or may be within normal limits if chest pain is due to unstable angina.
- Creatine kinase (CK) and CK-MB (specific to myocardial muscle) levels are likely to be within normal limits or demonstrate transient elevation, returning to normal levels within 12 to 24 hours.

The ECG, particularly when done during the acute episode of chest pain, is a valuable diagnostic tool for ACS. ST-segment changes (elevation or depression) during chest pain that resolve when the pain abates usually indicate acute myocardial ischemia and severe underlying CHD.

Medications

Medications include drugs to reduce myocardial ischemia and those to reduce the risk for blood clotting. Fibrinolytic drugs (drugs that break down the fibrin in blood clots) may be given prior to or on admission to the emergency department. These drugs restore blood flow to ischemic cardiac muscle and can prevent permanent damage. (See the section on myocardial infarction and **Box 30.5** later in this chapter for more information about fibrinolytic drugs and their nursing implications.)

Nitrates and beta-blockers are used to restore blood flow to the ischemic myocardium and reduce the workload of the heart. Nitroglycerin is given by sublingual tablet or buccal spray. If chest pain is unrelieved after three doses 5 minutes apart, an intravenous nitroglycerin infusion is initiated. The infusion may be continued until the chest pain is relieved or for 12 to 24 hours. Topical or oral nitrates are then initiated. Beta-adrenergic blockers are initially given intravenously, followed by oral beta-blockers. Refer to Medication Administration 30.B for the nursing implications of these drugs.

Table 30.4 Cardiac Markers

Changes Occurring with MI						
Marker	**Normal Level**	**Primary Tissue Location**	**Significance of Elevation**	**Appears**	**Peaks**	**Duration**
CK (CPK)	Male: 12–80 units/L Female: 10–70 units/L	Cardiac muscle, skeletal muscle, brain	Injury to muscle cells	3–6 h	12–24 h	24–48 h
CK-MB	0–3% of total CK	Cardiac muscle	MI, cardiac ischemia, myocarditis, cardiac contusion, defibrillation	4–8 h	18–24 h	72 h
cT_nT	< 0.2 mcg/L	Cardiac muscle	Acute MI, unstable angina	2–4 h	24–36 h	10–14 days
cT_nI	< 3.1 mcg/L	Cardiac muscle	Acute MI, unstable angina	2–4 h	24–36 h	7–10 days

Aspirin, other antiplatelet drugs, and heparin are given to inhibit blood clotting and reduce the risk of thrombus formation. Aspirin and clopidogrel (Plavix) are given to patients with ACS who do not have an excessive bleeding risk. Aspirin and clopidogrel suppress platelet aggregation, interrupting the process of forming a stable blood clot. Both increase the risk of serious hemorrhage; for most patients, however, the benefit outweighs the risk. Intravenous antiplatelet drugs such as abciximab (ReoPro), eptifibatide (Integrilin), or tirofiban (Aggrastat) may be used when an invasive coronary revascularization procedure is anticipated in the immediate or near future. Nursing implications for the antiplatelet drugs are outlined in **Medication Administration 30.C.**

Revascularization Procedures

Several procedures may be used to restore blood flow and oxygen to ischemic tissue. Nonsurgical techniques include transluminal coronary angioplasty, laser angioplasty, coronary atherectomy, and intracoronary stents. Coronary artery bypass grafting (CABG) is a surgical procedure that may be used.

Percutaneous Coronary Revascularization. *Percutaneous coronary revascularization (PCR)* procedures are used to restore blood flow to the ischemic myocardium in patients

Medication Administration 30.C

Antiplatelet Drugs

ORAL ANTIPLATELET DRUGS

aspirin

clopidogrel (Plavix)

dipyridamole (Persantine)

prasugrel (Effient)

ticlopidine (Ticlid)

cilostazol (Pletal)

Antiplatelet drugs suppress platelet aggregation in arteries, preventing the development of an arterial thrombus. Aspirin, clopidogrel, and dipyridamole block different platelet activation pathways to inhibit platelet aggregation and clot formation. Ticlopidine alters the function of platelet membranes. The dose of aspirin given to achieve antiplatelet effects is low, typically 80 to 325 mg/day.

Nursing Responsibilities

- Inquire about a history of intracranial hemorrhage, upper gastrointestinal bleeding, peptic ulcer disease, or known bleeding tendency.
- Observe for and report increased bruising, petechiae, purpura, and apparent or occult bleeding (e.g., melena, hematemesis, hematuria, nosebleeds, bleeding from IV sites).
- Avoid needlesticks after administration.
- If a Foley catheter is ordered, insert prior to medication administration
- Only dipyridamole can be used concurrently with warfarin (Coumadin).

Health Education for the Patient and Family

- Take as directed. Take aspirin with food or milk; clopidogrel may be taken at any time of day.
- Do not use nonsteroidal anti-inflammatory drugs (NSAIDs) or other over-the-counter drugs that may contain aspirin or an NSAID unless prescribed by your physician.
- Check with your physician before taking any herbal remedies such as evening primrose oil, feverfew, garlic, ginkgo biloba, or grapeseed extract while taking these medications.
- Report unusual bruising or excessive bleeding.
- Inform all care providers (including dental professionals) of use of these drugs.

INTRAVENOUS ANTIPLATELET DRUGS

abciximab (ReoPro)

eptifibatide (Integrilin)

tirofiban (Aggrastat)

These intravenously administered antiplatelet drugs block the final common pathway of platelet activation and, thus, are more effective than oral antiplatelet drugs. However, the risk of bleeding is greater than with the orally administered antiplatelet drugs.

Nursing Responsibilities

- Determine history of bleeding disorders, intracranial hemorrhage, recent trauma, or surgery.
- Inquire about recent use of oral antiplatelet or anticoagulant drugs.
- Monitor CBC including hemoglobin, hematocrit, and platelet count; clotting studies, including PT, INR, PTT; vital signs; and ECG during therapy.
- Maintain a separate intravenous line for blood draws and administration of other drugs during infusion.
- Closely observe for and immediately report anaphylaxis or bleeding uncontrolled by pressure. Keep resuscitation equipment readily available.
- Maintain bedrest during infusion.

Health Education for the Patient and Family

- This drug is given to reduce the risk of clotting and myocardial infarction. It helps maintain blood flow through the affected vessel following angioplasty and stent placement.
- Immediately report any chest tightness, difficulty breathing, shortness of breath, or itching that develops during the infusion.
- Your risk of bleeding should return to normal within about 2 days following the infusion.
- Immediately report any unusual bruising or bleeding to your physician.

Note: Drugs identified in blue are among the 200 most commonly prescribed medications in the United States.

Source: Adams, et al., 2017.

with CHD. Approximately 600,000 PCR procedures are done annually in the United States (Patel et al., 2017). PCR is used to treat patients with the following:

- Moderately severe, chronic stable angina unrelieved by medical therapy
- Unstable angina
- Acute myocardial infarction
- Significant stenosis of the left anterior descending coronary artery
- Stenosis of a coronary artery bypass graft.

PCR procedures are similar to the procedure used for coronary angiography. A catheter introduced into the arterial circulation is guided into the opening of the narrowed coronary artery. A flexible guide wire is inserted through the catheter lumen into the affected vessel. The guide wire is then used to thread an angioplasty balloon, arterial stent, or other therapeutic device into the narrowed segment of the artery. The procedure is performed in the cardiac catheterization laboratory using local anesthesia. The hospital stay is short (1 to 2 days), minimizing costs.

In a *percutaneous transluminal coronary angioplasty (PTCA)*, a balloon-tipped catheter is threaded over the guide wire, with the balloon positioned across the area of narrowing (**Figure 30.2** ■). The balloon is inflated in a step-by-step fashion for about 30 seconds to 2 minutes to compress the plaque against the arterial wall, with the goal of reducing the vessel obstruction to less than 50% of the arterial lumen. PTCA is typically accompanied by placement of a stent. *Intracoronary stents* are metallic scaffolds used to maintain an open arterial lumen. Stents reduce the rate of restenosis following angioplasty by about one-third, and are now used in the majority of all PCR procedures. The stent is placed over a balloon catheter, guided into position, and expanded as the balloon is inflated. It then remains in the artery as a prop after the balloon is removed. Endothelial cells will completely line the inner wall of the stent to produce a smooth inner lining. Antiplatelet medications (aspirin and ticlopidine) are given following stent insertion to reduce the risk of thrombus formation at the site.

In contrast to stent procedures that enlarge the artery by displacing plaque, *atherectomy* procedures remove plaque from the identified lesion. The directional atherectomy catheter shaves the plaque off vessel walls using a rotary cutting head, retaining the fragments in its housing and removing them from the vessel. Rotational atherectomy catheters pulverize plaque into particles small enough to pass through the coronary microcirculation. Laser atherectomy devices use laser energy to remove plaque.

Complications following PCR procedures include hematoma at the catheter insertion site, pseudoaneurysm, embolism, hypersensitivity to contrast dye, dysrhythmias, bleeding, vessel perforation, restenosis, reocclusion of the treated vessel, or stroke. Nursing care of the patient undergoing PCR is outlined in **Box 30.3**.

Coronary Artery Bypass Grafting. Surgery for coronary heart disease involves using a section of a vein or an artery

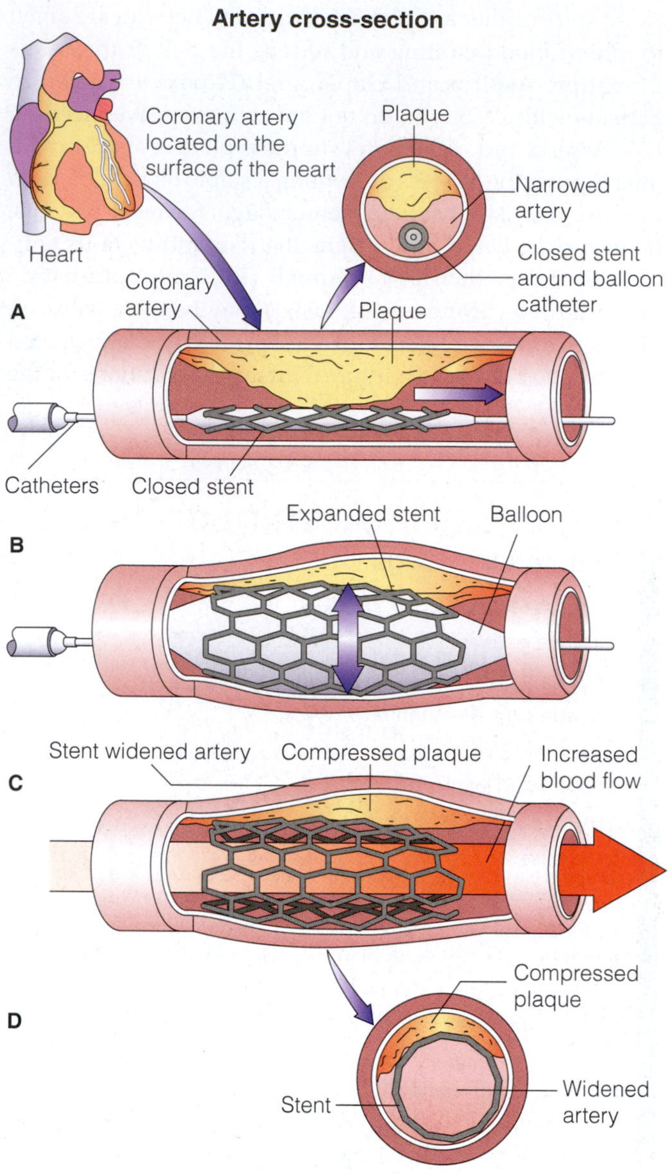
Artery cross-section
Coronary artery located on the surface of the heart
Plaque
Narrowed artery
Heart
Closed stent around balloon catheter
Coronary artery
Plaque
A
Catheters
Closed stent
Expanded stent
Balloon
B
Stent widened artery
Compressed plaque
Increased blood flow
C
D
Compressed plaque
Stent
Widened artery

Figure 30.2 ■ Percutaneous coronary revascularization. **A**, The balloon catheter with the stent is threaded into the affected coronary artery. **B** and **C**, The stent is positioned across the blockage and expanded. **D**, The balloon is deflated and removed, leaving the stent in place.

to create a connection (or bypass) between the aorta and the coronary artery beyond the obstruction (**Figure 30.3** ■). This then allows blood to perfuse the ischemic portion of the heart. The internal mammary artery in the chest and the saphenous vein from the leg are the vessels most commonly used for coronary artery bypass grafting (CABG).

Bypass grafts are safe and effective. Angina is totally relieved or significantly reduced in 90% of patients who undergo complete revascularization. Although anginal pain may recur within 3 years, it is rarely as severe as before surgery. CABG has a positive effect on mortality in many cases. It is recommended for patients who have multiple-vessel disease and impaired left-ventricular function or diabetes and for patients who have significant obstruction of the left main coronary artery (Perrin & MacLeod, 2018).

BOX 30.3
Nursing Care of the Patient Having PCR

BEFORE THE PROCEDURE

- Assess knowledge of the procedure and expectations of treatment. *This allows information to be tailored to the patient's needs and provides an opportunity to clarify misconceptions.*
- Describe the cardiac catheterization laboratory and the planned PCR procedure, including:
  - Preoperative preparation (refer to Chapter 4)
  - Planned anesthesia or sedation to be used
  - Drugs that may be given during the procedure, such as anticoagulants to reduce the risk of thrombus formation and intravenous nitroglycerin and a calcium channel blocker to dilate coronary arteries and prevent anginal pain
- Discuss possible sensations during the procedure, including flushing or warmth and a metallic taste in the mouth as the contrast dye is injected, and a feeling of pressure or chest pain during balloon inflation. *Advanced preparation for expected sensations reduces anxiety and improves outcomes.*
- Perform a comprehensive assessment, including hydration status (skin and mucous membrane moisture, turgor) and peripheral circulation (color, warmth, sensation, pulses, and capillary refill).

AFTER THE PROCEDURE

- Complete a head-to-toe assessment. Note any complaints of chest pain or evidence of decreased cardiac output or myocardial infarction. *Assessment provides a baseline for subsequent assessments and allows early identification of possible complications.*
- Monitor vital signs and cardiac rhythm continuously. Treat dysrhythmias as ordered. Obtain a 12-lead ECG if signs of ischemia develop, and notify physician. *Vital signs reflect cardiac output. Dysrhythmias may develop with reperfusion of the ischemic myocardium. ECG changes may indicate infarction or restenosis of the affected vessel.*
- Maintain intravenous nitroglycerin infusion. Administer anticoagulant and antiplatelet medications, nitrates, and calcium channel blockers as ordered. *These drugs decrease oxygen demand and increase oxygen supply by dilating the coronary arteries and systemic vasculature. They also reduce the risk of thrombus formation.*
- Monitor for and treat or report chest pain as indicated. *Chest pain may indicate ischemia and possible myocardial infarction.*
- Maintain bedrest as ordered with the head of the bed at 30 degrees or less. Prevent flexion of the leg on the affected side. Following sheath removal, follow protocol for pressure dressing or device or sandbag placement. *A large puncture wound occurs at the insertion site. Immobilization allows the wound to seal; a pressure dressing helps prevent bleeding.*
- Monitor distal pulses, color, movement, sensation, and temperature of the affected leg and insertion site every 15 minutes for the first hour, every 30 minutes for the next hour, every hour for the next 8 hours, and then every 4 hours. *A clot may form at the site, reducing perfusion of the affected leg. The site and dressing are monitored for excessive bleeding, hematoma formation, or pseudoaneurysm. Pseudoaneurysm occurs as a result of inadequate hemostasis after catheter removal.*
- Monitor intake and output, serum electrolytes, blood urea nitrogen (BUN), creatinine, complete blood count (CBC), partial thromboplastin time (PTT), and cardiac enzymes. Report abnormal results to the physician. *Contrast dye causes osmotic diuresis and may cause renal damage or a hypersensitivity reaction. Electrolyte imbalances increase the risk of dysrhythmias. Cardiac enzymes are monitored for indications of possible myocardial damage during the procedure. The PTT monitors the effectiveness of heparin therapy.*
- Monitor for bradycardia, light-headedness, hypotension, diaphoresis, and loss of consciousness during sheath removal. Keep atropine at bedside during sheath removal. *Bradycardia and signs of decreased cardiac output may occur during sheath removal because of a vasovagal reaction. Atropine decreases vagal tone and increases heart rate.*
- Monitor neurovascular status (level of consciousness, pupil size and reactivity, motor function). *A reduced level of consciousness may indicate development of stroke due to migration of clot particulates during PCR.*

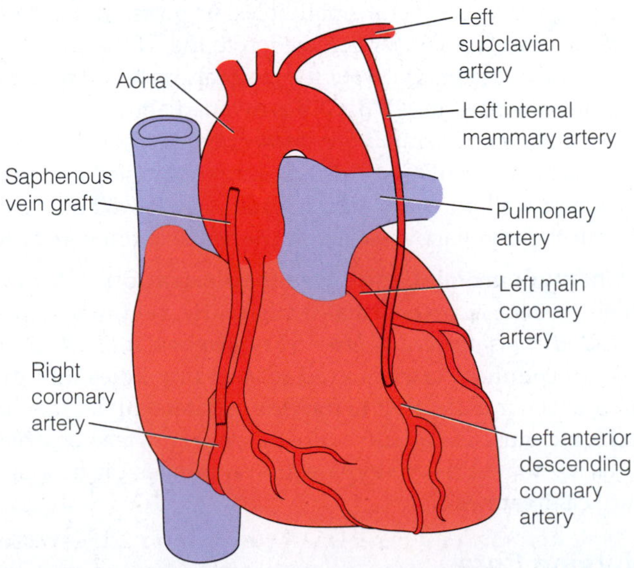
Left subclavian artery
Aorta
Left internal mammary artery
Saphenous vein graft
Pulmonary artery
Left main coronary artery
Right coronary artery
Left anterior descending coronary artery

Figure 30.3 ■ Coronary artery bypass grafting using the internal mammary artery and a saphenous vein graft.

A median sternotomy is commonly used to access the heart. The heart is usually stopped during surgery. The *cardiopulmonary bypass (CPB) pump* is used to maintain perfusion to the rest of the organs during open-heart surgery. Venous blood is removed from the body through a cannula placed in the right atrium or the superior and inferior venae cavae. Blood then circulates through the CPB pump, where it is oxygenated, its temperature is regulated, and it is filtered. Oxygenated blood is returned to the body through a cannula in the ascending aorta (**Figure 30.4** ■). Cardiopulmonary bypass enables surgeons to operate on a quiet heart and a relatively bloodless field. Hypothermia can be maintained to reduce the metabolic rate and decrease oxygen demand during surgery.

Newer techniques have been developed that allow surgeons to perform CABG without cardioplegia (stopping the heart) and CPB. Off-pump coronary artery bypass (OPCAB) allows use of a smaller incision for access. Although cardiopulmonary bypass is employed for the majority of coronary artery bypass procedures, OPCAB is a promising

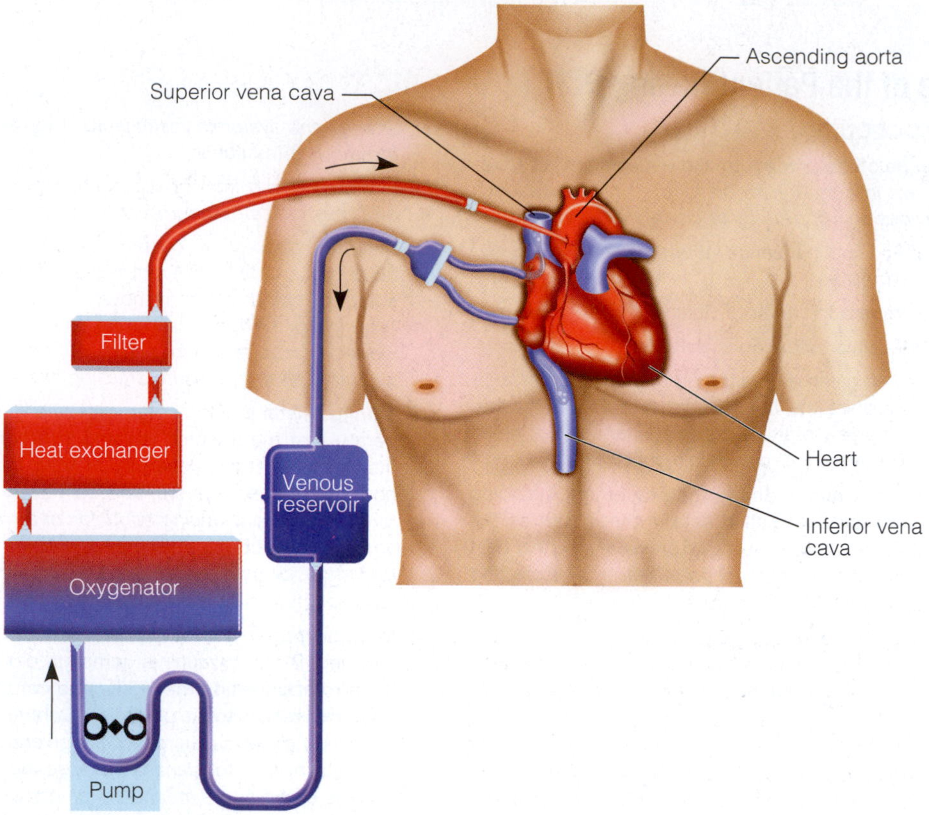
Superior vena cava
Ascending aorta
Filter
Heat exchanger
Venous reservoir
Oxygenator
Pump
Heart
Inferior vena cava

Figure 30.4 ■ A diagrammatic representation of cardiopulmonary bypass. A cannula in the superior and inferior venae cavae removes venous blood, which is then pumped through an oxygenator and heat exchanger. After filtering, oxygenated blood is returned to the ascending aorta.

alternative. Controlled studies demonstrate lower mortality and morbidity rates and faster recovery for patients undergoing OPCAB as compared to CABG with cardiopulmonary bypass.

When the saphenous vein is used, it is excised from its normal attachments in the leg, flushed with a cold heparinized saline solution, and then reversed so that its valves do not interfere with blood flow. When appropriate, a laparoscopic approach may be used to remove the vein. The vein is *anastomosed* (grafted) to the aorta and the coronary artery, distal to the occlusion (refer to Figure 30.3). This provides a bridge or conduit for blood flow past the obstruction. If the internal mammary artery (IMA) is used, its distal end is excised and anastomosed to the coronary artery distal to the obstruction. The IMA is often used to revascularize the left coronary artery because of the greater oxygen demand of the left ventricle.

Once grafting is completed, cardiopulmonary bypass is discontinued and the patient is rewarmed. Rewarming stimulates the heart to resume beating. Temporary pacing wires are sutured in place and passed through the chest wall in case temporary pacing is necessary. Chest tubes are placed in the pleural space and mediastinum to drain blood and reestablish negative pressure in the thoracic cavity. The sternum is closed using heavy wires and bone wax, the skin is closed with sutures or staples, and sterile dressings are applied over sternal and leg incisions.

Pre- and postoperative nursing care and teaching for the patient having a coronary artery bypass graft or other open-heart surgery are outlined in **Box 30.4**.

Minimally Invasive Coronary Artery Surgery. *Minimally invasive coronary artery surgery* is a potential future alternative to CABG. Two approaches may be used: *Port-access coronary artery bypass* uses several small holes, or ports, in the chest wall to access vessels for connection to the CPB pump and the surgical site; alternatively, the femoral artery and femoral vein may be used for CPB. CPB is avoided altogether using the *minimally invasive direct coronary artery bypass (MIDCAB)* approach. With MIDCAB, a small surgical incision and several chest wall ports are used to graft a chest wall artery to the affected coronary vessel while the heart continues to beat.

Transmyocardial Laser Revascularization. A new development in myocardial revascularization techniques is called *transmyocardial laser revascularization (TMLR)*. In this procedure, a laser is used to drill tiny holes into the myocardial muscle itself to provide collateral blood flow to ischemic muscle. Patients whose coronary artery obstructions are too diffuse to bypass are candidates for this new surgical treatment.

Nursing Care

Health promotion, assessment, nursing diagnoses, and interventions for the patient with ACS are similar to those

BOX 30.4
Nursing Care of the Patient Undergoing a Coronary Artery Bypass Graft

PREOPERATIVE CARE

- Provide routine preoperative care and teaching as outlined in Chapter 4.
- Verify presence of laboratory and diagnostic test results in the chart, including CBC, coagulation profile, urinalysis, chest x-ray, and coronary angiogram. *These baseline data are important for comparison of postoperative results and values.*
- Type and crossmatch four or more units of blood as ordered. *Blood is made available for use during and after surgery as needed.*
- Provide specific patient and family teaching related to the procedure and postoperative care. Include the following topics:
  - Cardiac recovery unit; sensory stimuli, personnel; noise and alarms; visiting policies
  - Tubes, drains, and general appearance
  - Monitoring equipment, including cardiac and hemodynamic monitoring systems
  - Respiratory support: Ventilator, endotracheal tube, suctioning; communication while intubated
  - Incisions and dressings
  - Pain management.

Preoperative teaching reduces anxiety and prepares the patient and family for the postoperative environment and expected sensations.

POSTOPERATIVE CARE

Provide routine postoperative care as outlined in Chapter 4. In addition to the care needs of all patients having major surgery, the cardiac surgery patient has specific care needs related to open-heart and thoracic surgery.

Monitor Cardiac Output

Cardiac output may be compromised postoperatively due to bleeding and fluid loss; depression of myocardial function by drugs, hypothermia, and surgical manipulation; dysrhythmias; increased vascular resistance; and a potential complication, *cardiac tamponade*, compression of the heart due to collected blood or fluid in the pericardium.

- Monitor vital signs, oxygen saturation, and hemodynamic parameters every 15 minutes. Note trends and report significant changes to the physician. *Initial hypothermia and bradycardia are expected; the heart rate should return to the normal range with rewarming. The blood pressure may fall during rewarming as vasodilation occurs. Hypotension and tachycardia, however, may indicate low cardiac output. Pulmonary artery pressure (PAP), pulmonary artery wedge pressure (PAWP), cardiac output, and oxygen saturation are monitored to evaluate fluid volume, cardiac function, and gas exchange.* Hemodynamic monitoring is further discussed in Chapter 31.
- Auscultate heart and breath sounds on admission and at least every 4 hours. *A ventricular gallop, or S_3, is an early sign of heart failure; an S_4 sound may indicate decreased ventricular compliance. Muffled heart sounds may be an early indication of cardiac tamponade. Adventitious breath sounds (wheezes, crackles, or rales) may be a manifestation of heart failure or respiratory compromise.*
- Assess skin color and temperature, peripheral pulses, and level of consciousness with vital signs. *Pale, mottled, or cyanotic coloring, cool and clammy skin, and diminished pulse amplitude are indicators of decreased cardiac output.*
- Continuously monitor and document cardiac rhythm. *Dysrhythmias are common and may interfere with cardiac filling and contractility, decreasing the cardiac output.*
- Measure intake and output hourly. Report urine output < 30 mL/h for 2 consecutive hours. *Intake and output measurements help evaluate fluid volume status. A fall in urine output may be an early indicator of decreased cardiac output.*
- Record chest tube output hourly. *Chest tube drainage > 70 mL/h or that is warm, red, and free flowing indicates hemorrhage and may necessitate a return to surgery. A sudden drop in chest tube output may indicate impending cardiac tamponade.*
- Monitor hemoglobin, hematocrit, and serum electrolytes. *A drop in hemoglobin and hematocrit may indicate hemorrhage that is not otherwise obvious. Electrolyte imbalances—potassium, calcium, and magnesium in particular—affect cardiac rhythm and contractility.*
- Administer intravenous fluids, fluid boluses, and blood transfusions as ordered. *Fluid and blood replacement helps ensure adequate blood volume and oxygen-carrying capacity.*
- Administer medications as ordered. *Medications ordered in the early postoperative period to maintain the cardiac output include inotropic drugs (e.g., dopamine, dobutamine) to increase the force of myocardial contractions; vasodilators (e.g., nitroprusside or nitroglycerin) to decrease vascular resistance and afterload; and antidysrhythmics to correct dysrhythmias that affect cardiac output.*
- Keep a temporary pacemaker at the bedside; initiate pacing as indicated. *Temporary pacing may be needed to maintain the cardiac output with bradydysrhythmias, such as high-level AV blocks.*

SAFETY ALERT: Assess for signs of cardiac tamponade: Increased heart rate, decreased BP, decreased urine output, increased central venous pressure, a sudden decrease in chest tube output, muffled/distant heart sounds, and diminished peripheral pulses. Notify physician immediately. Cardiac tamponade is a life-threatening complication that may develop postoperatively. Cardiac tamponade interferes with ventricular filling and contraction, decreasing cardiac output. Untreated, cardiac tamponade leads to cardiogenic shock and possible cardiac arrest. ■

Manage Rewarming

Hypothermia is maintained during cardiac surgery to reduce the metabolic rate and protect vital organs from ischemic damage. Although rewarming is instituted on completion of the surgery, the patient often remains hypothermic on admission to cardiac recovery. Gradual rewarming is necessary to prevent peripheral vasodilation and hypotension.

- Monitor core body temperature (e.g., tympanic membrane, pulmonary artery, bladder) for the first 8 hours following surgery. *Oral and rectal temperature measurements are not reliable indicators of core body temperature during this period.*
- Institute rewarming measures (e.g., warmed intravenous solutions or blood transfusion, warm blankets, warm inspired gases, radiant heat lamps) as needed to maintain a temperature above 36°C (96.8°F). Administer Thorazine, morphine, or diltiazem as ordered to relieve shivering. *Low body temperature may cause shivering, increasing oxygen demand and consumption. Hypothermia also increases the risk for hypoxia, metabolic acidosis, vasoconstriction and increased cardiac work, altered clotting, and dysrhythmias.*

Manage Acute Pain

Following a CABG, pain is experienced due to both the thoracic incision and removal of the saphenous vein from the leg. Dissection of the internal mammary artery (usually the left IMA) from the chest wall also causes chest pain on the affected side. Chest

(continued)

tube sites are also uncomfortable. The leg from which the saphenous vein graft was obtained may be more painful than the chest incision.

- Frequently assess for pain, including its location and character. Document its intensity using a standard pain scale. Assess for verbal and nonverbal indicators of pain. Validate pain cues with the patient. *Pain is subjective and differs among individuals. Incisional pain is expected; however, anginal pain may also develop. It is important to differentiate the type of pain.*

SAFETY ALERT: Promptly report anginal or cardiac pain. Cardiac pain may indicate a perioperative or postoperative myocardial infarction. ■

- Administer analgesics on a scheduled basis, by PCA, or by continuous infusion for the first 24 to 48 hours. *Research demonstrates that adequate pain management in the immediate postoperative period reduces complications from sympathetic stimulation and allows faster recovery. Pain causes muscle tension and vasoconstriction, impairing circulation and tissue perfusion, slowing wound healing, and increasing cardiac work.*
- Premedicate 30 minutes before activities or planned procedures. *Premedication and the subsequent reduction of pain improve patient participation and cooperation with care.*

Promote Adequate Gas Exchange

Atelectasis due to impaired ventilation and airway clearance is a common pulmonary complication of cardiac surgery. Gas exchange may also be affected by blood loss and decreased oxygen-carrying capacity following surgery. Phrenic nerve paralysis is a potential complication of cardiac surgery that may also contribute to impaired ventilation and gas exchange.

- Evaluate respiratory rate, depth, effort, symmetry of chest expansion, and breath sounds frequently. *Pain, anxiety, excess fluid volume, surgical injury, narcotics and anesthesia, and altered homeostasis can affect respiratory rate, depth, and effort postoperatively. Decreased chest expansion or asymmetrical movement may indicate impaired ventilation of one lung and needs further evaluation.*
- Note endotracheal tube (ETT) placement on chest x-ray. Mark tube position and secure in place. Insert an oral airway if an oral ETT is used. *The chest x-ray documents correct ETT placement above the bifurcation to the right and left mainstem bronchus. Marking its appropriate placement allows evaluation of potential tube movement. Secure the tube firmly in place to prevent slippage or inadvertent removal. An oral airway helps prevent obstruction of an oral ETT by biting.*
- Maintain ventilator settings as ordered. Monitor arterial blood gases (ABGs) as ordered. *Mechanical ventilation promotes optimal lung expansion and oxygenation postoperatively. ABGs are used to evaluate oxygenation and acid–base balance.*
- Suction as needed. *Suctioning is performed only as indicated to clear airway secretions.*
- Prepare for ventilator weaning and extubation, as appropriate. *The patient is removed from the ventilator and extubated as soon as possible to reduce complications associated with mechanical ventilation and intubation.*
- After extubation, teach use of the incentive spirometer, and encourage use every 2 hours. Encourage deep breathing; advise against vigorous coughing. Teach use of a cough pillow to splint chest incision and decrease pain. Frequently turn and encourage movement. Dangle on postoperative day 1. *Deep breathing, controlled coughing, and position changes improve ventilation and airway clearance and help prevent complications. Vigorous coughing may excessively increase intrathoracic pressure and cause sternal instability.*

Reduce Risk for Infection

Following an open-chest procedure, a sternal infection may develop that can progress to involve the mediastinum. Incisions for removal of the saphenous vein may also become infected. Patients with IMA grafts or who are diabetic, older, or malnourished are at high risk: Harvesting of IMA disrupts blood supply to the sternum, and these patients have impaired immune responses and healing.

- Assess sternal incision and leg wounds every shift. Document redness, warmth, swelling, and/or drainage from the site. Note wound approximation. *These assessments provide indicators of inflammation and healing.*
- Maintain a sterile dressing for the first 48 hours, and then leave the incision open to air. Use Steri-Strips as needed to maintain approximation of the wound edges. *The sterile dressing prevents early contamination of the wound, whereas exposing the incision after 48 hours promotes healing.*
- Report signs of wound infection: A swollen, reddened area that is hot and painful to the touch, drainage from the wound, impaired healing, or healed areas that reopen. *Evidence of infection or impaired healing requires further evaluation and treatment.*
- Culture wound drainage as indicated. *Identifying the infective organism facilitates the choosing of appropriate antibiotic therapy.*
- Collaborate with the dietitian to promote nutrition and fluid intake. *Good nutritional status is vital to healing and immune function.*

Promote Mental Clarity

Many factors affect neuropsychologic function after CABG, including the length of cardiopulmonary bypass, age, presurgery organic brain dysfunction, severity of illness, and decreased cardiac output. Sensory overload and deprivation, sleep disruption, and numerous drugs also affect thinking and mental clarity.

- Frequently reorient during initial recovery period. State that surgery is over and that the patient is in the recovery area. *Frequent reorientation provides emotional support and reality checks.*
- Explain all procedures before performing them. Speak in a clear, calm voice. Encourage questions, and give honest answers. *These measures provide information, decrease anxiety, and establish trust.*
- Secure all intravenous lines and invasive catheters/tubes (e.g., ETT, Foley catheter, nasogastric tube). *Disoriented patients may tug or pull at invasive equipment, disrupting them and increasing the risk of injury.*
- Note verbal responses to questions. Correct misconceptions immediately (e.g., "Mr. Snow, look at all the special equipment in this room. Does this room look like your bedroom at home?"). *Helping the patient recognize differences in the hospital environment offers a basis for continual reality checks.*
- Maintain a calendar and clock within the patient's view. *This provides current information regarding day, date, and time.*
- Involve family members in providing reorientation. Place familiar objects and photographs within view. Encourage family presence. *The family provides reassurance and contact with the familiar, assisting with orientation.*
- Promote patient participation in care and decision making as appropriate. *This allows the patient to maintain a degree of power and control and enables the patient to take an active role in recovery.*
- Report signs of hallucinations, delusions, depression, or agitation. *These may indicate progressive deterioration of mental status.*
- Administer sedatives cautiously. *Mild sedation may help prevent injury. Some sedatives may, however, have adverse effects, increasing confusion and disorientation.*
- Reevaluate neurologic status every shift. *These data allow evaluation of the effect of interventions.*

identified for patients with angina and with acute myocardial infarction. See the preceding and subsequent sections of this chapter for specific nursing care activities, as well as the Case Study & Nursing Care Plan that follows.

Case Study Nursing Care Plan

A Patient with Coronary Artery Bypass Surgery

Six weeks ago, John Clements, age 50, was discharged from the hospital after emergency triple bypass surgery. Despite having emergency surgery, his postoperative recovery was uneventful, and he was discharged 6 days after admission. He returns to the clinic for a postoperative stress test and to discuss his cardiac rehabilitation program. Anne Wagner, RN, CNS, a cardiac clinical nurse specialist and the program coordinator, meets Mr. Clements to obtain specific information regarding his medical status.

ASSESSMENT

Mr. Clements's medical history reveals significant CHD, an anterior wall myocardial infarction that led to his emergency triple bypass, and hyperlipidemia. Current medications include Cardizem, Isordil, Ecotrin, and Transderm Nitro 5. The ECG reveals sinus rhythm with some ST-segment and T-wave flattening. Resting heart rate 68 bpm, and blood pressure 136/84 mmHg.

Mr. Clements has a strong family history of CHD. He does not smoke, but does use alcohol occasionally in social situations. He enjoys "good Southern-style cooking" and watching television. Mr. Clements states his only regular exercise used to be an evening of dancing with his wife and friends about once a month, "But I get short of breath walking around the block now, so I guess I can't go dancing anymore!"

Mr. Clements owns his own contracting business and states that he typically works about 50 to 60 hours per week. He tells Ms. Wagner, "I don't know what this program is supposed to do for me. I have got to get back to work! You just can't sit around in my business—you have to make sure that the work is getting done on time, and you have to check on supplies and equipment and the like. But I feel like a weakling—I need to get my energy back!"

DIAGNOSES

- Intolerance to perform daily activities related to general weakness and fatigue
- Anxiety related to inability to work due to health crisis

EXPECTED OUTCOMES

- Patient will verbalize an understanding of the definition and components of his structured cardiac rehabilitation program.
- Patient will verbalize a desire to make lifestyle changes.
- Patient will identify resources available in the community to assist with lifestyle changes.
- Patient will participate in his activity program without suffering any complications.
- Patient will verbalize an increase in energy after 6 weeks on the program.
- Patient will accept the reality of the temporary change in his usual work responsibilities.

PLANNING AND IMPLEMENTATION

- Define the purpose and components of a cardiac rehabilitation program.
- Enroll in "heart health" classes, including cardiac anatomy, physiology, and coronary heart disease; exercise and activity prescriptions; lifestyle modifications, including diet counseling and stress management; emotional reactions to CAD; sexual activity; use of cardiac medications; and self-responsibility for health.
- Plan an exercise program based on stress test results, physical examination, and interview.
- Encourage to schedule rest periods before and after activity/exercise.
- Review signs and symptoms of overexertion.
- Provide information about community resources for emotional and educational support.
- Assist to identify strategies for dealing with concerns about his business role.

EVALUATION

Mr. Clements decides to "give the rehab program a try." Ms. Wagner and an exercise physiologist work with him to plan an individualized exercise/activity program. A registered dietitian provides dietary counseling. Ms. Wagner emphasizes stress management strategies. Mr. Clements is able to list manifestations of overexertion and states that he realizes the need for gradual activity progression.

After 6 weeks, Mr. Clements has reported a significant increase in energy and strength. "I am feeling much stronger, and have been sleeping better. Mary and I are taking evening walks around the neighborhood. My chest soreness is also gone." He has completed the 12-week cardiac rehabilitation program, and another stress test indicates that his cardiac function is adequate. Mr. Clements has joined the local Mended Hearts support group and states that he is now incorporating heart-healthy considerations into his daily routines.

(continued)

CLINICAL REASONING IN PATIENT CARE

1. Develop a personalized risk factor reduction plan for Mr. Clements.
2. How might denial affect Mr. Clements's ability to (a) accept the need for cardiac rehabilitation, (b) comply with the proposed lifestyle changes, and (c) make permanent adjustments to his daily life?
3. How does spousal support influence a patient's compliance with a structured cardiac rehabilitation program?
4. Mr. Clements tells you that since the surgery, his wife has been afraid that sexual activity will induce another heart attack. How would you respond to these concerns?

See Evaluating Your Response in Appendix B.

The Patient with Acute Myocardial Infarction

An **acute myocardial infarction (AMI)**, which is necrosis (death) of myocardial cells, is a life-threatening event. If circulation to the affected myocardium is not promptly restored, loss of functional myocardium affects the heart's ability to maintain an effective cardiac output. This may ultimately lead to cardiogenic shock and death (Sorenson et al., 2019).

Heart disease remains the leading cause of death in the United States. Of the major heart diseases, myocardial infarction (MI), or *heart attack*, and other forms of ischemic heart disease cause the majority of deaths. Annually, approximately 580,000 people in the United States experience their first MI; another 210,000 suffer an MI subsequent to the initial one. Approximately every 40 seconds, someone suffers a heart attack (Benjamin et al., 2017).

The majority of deaths from MI occur during the initial period after symptoms begin: Approximately 60% within the first hour and 40% prior to hospitalization. Heightening public awareness of the manifestations of MI, the importance of seeking immediate medical assistance, and training in cardiopulmonary resuscitation (CPR) techniques is vital to decrease deaths due to MI.

Myocardial infarction rarely occurs without preexisting coronary heart disease. Although no specific cause has been identified, the risk factors for MI are those for coronary heart disease: Age, gender, heredity, race, smoking, obesity, hyperlipidemia, hypertension, diabetes, sedentary lifestyle, diet, and others. See the previous section of this chapter on coronary heart disease for further discussion of these risk factors.

Pathophysiology

Atherosclerotic plaque may form stable or unstable lesions. *Stable* lesions progress by gradually occluding the vessel lumen, whereas *unstable* (or *complicated*) lesions are prone to rupture and thrombus formation. Stable lesions often cause angina; unstable lesions often lead to acute coronary syndromes or acute ischemic heart diseases. Acute coronary syndromes include unstable angina, myocardial infarction, and sudden cardiac death (Sorenson et al., 2019).

Myocardial infarction occurs when blood flow to a portion of cardiac muscle is completely blocked, resulting in prolonged tissue ischemia and irreversible cell damage. Coronary occlusion is usually caused by ulceration or rupture of a complicated atherosclerotic lesion. When an atherosclerotic lesion ruptures or ulcerates, substances are released that stimulate platelet aggregation, thrombin generation, and local vasomotor tone. As a result, the vessel constricts and a thrombus (clot) forms, occluding the vessel and interrupting blood flow to the myocardium distal to the obstruction.

Cellular injury occurs when the cells are denied adequate oxygen and nutrients. With prolonged ischemia lasting more than 20 to 45 minutes, irreversible hypoxemia causes cellular death and tissue necrosis. Oxygen, glycogen, and ATP stores of ischemic cells are rapidly depleted. Cellular metabolism shifts to an anaerobic process, producing hydrogen ions and lactic acid. Cellular acidosis increases cells' vulnerability to further damage with release of intracellular enzymes through the damaged cell membranes.

Cellular acidosis, electrolyte imbalances, and hormones released in response to cellular ischemia affect impulse conduction and myocardial contractility. Myocardial contractility decreases, increasing the risk for dysrhythmias and subsequently reducing stroke volume, cardiac output, blood pressure, and tissue perfusion.

Within 20 minutes of injury, the subendocardium, being most susceptible to changes in coronary blood flow, suffers the initial damage. If blood flow is restored at this point, the infarction is limited to subendocardial tissue (a *subendocardial* or *non-Q-wave infarction*). The damage progresses to the epicardium within 1 to 6 hours. When all layers of the myocardium are affected, it is known as a *transmural infarction*. A significant Q wave develops with a transmural infarction, so this also may be called a *Q-wave MI*. Complications such as heart failure are more frequently associated with Q-wave MIs; however, patients with non-Q-wave MIs frequently experience recurrent ischemia or subsequent MI within weeks or months of the event (Sorenson et al., 2019).

The necrotic, infarcted tissue is surrounded by regions of injured and ischemic tissues. Tissue in the ischemic area is potentially viable; restoration of blood flow minimizes the amount of tissue lost. The surrounding tissue also undergoes metabolic changes. It may be *stunned*, its contractility impaired for hours to days following reperfusion, or *hibernating*, a process that protects myocytes until perfusion is restored. *Myocardial remodeling* may occur, with cellular hypertrophy and loss of contractility in regions distant from the infarction. Rapid restoration of blood flow limits these changes.

When a larger artery is compromised, collateral vessels connecting smaller arteries in the coronary system dilate to maintain blood flow to the cardiac muscle. The degree of collateral circulation helps determine the extent of myocardial damage from ischemia. Acute occlusion of a coronary artery without any collateral flow results in massive tissue damage and possible death. Progressive narrowing of the larger coronary arteries allows collateral vessels to develop and enlarge, meeting the demand for blood flow. Good collateral circulation can limit the size of an MI.

MI usually affects the left ventricle because it is the major workhorse of the heart; its muscle mass is greater, as are its oxygen demands.

MIs are described by the damaged area of the heart. The coronary artery that is occluded determines the area of damage. Occlusion of the left anterior descending (LAD) artery affects blood flow to the anterior wall of the left ventricle (an anterior MI) and part of the interventricular septum. Occlusion of the left circumflex artery (LCA) causes a lateral MI. Right-ventricular, inferior, and posterior infarcts involve occlusions of the right coronary artery (RCA) and posterior descending artery (PDA). Occlusion of the left main coronary artery is the most devastating, causing ischemia of the entire left ventricle and a grave prognosis. Identifying the infarct site helps predict possible complications and determine appropriate therapy.

Cocaine-Induced MI

AMI may develop due to cocaine intoxication. Cocaine increases SNS activity by both increasing the release of catecholamines from central and peripheral stores and interfering with the reuptake of catecholamines. This increased catecholamine concentration stimulates the heart rate and increases its contractility, increases the automaticity of cardiac tissues and the risk of dysrhythmias, and causes vasoconstriction and hypertension. The patient with cocaine-induced MI may present with an altered level of consciousness, confusion and restlessness, seizure activity, tachycardia, hypotension, increased respiratory rate, and respiratory crackles.

Manifestations

Pain is a classic manifestation of MI. Chest pain due to MI is more severe than anginal pain. However, it is not the intensity of the chest pain that distinguishes MI from angina or acute coronary syndrome, but its duration and its continuous nature. The onset of pain is sudden and is usually not associated with activity. In fact, most MIs occur in the early morning. Patients with a history of angina may have more frequent anginal attacks in the days or weeks prior to an MI (unstable angina or ACS). Chest pain may be described as crushing and severe; as a pressure, heavy, or squeezing sensation; or as chest tightness or burning. The pain often begins in the center of the chest (*substernal*) and may radiate to the shoulders, neck, jaw, or arms. It lasts more than 15 to 20 minutes and is not relieved by rest or nitroglycerin.

Women and older adults often experience atypical chest pain, presenting with complaints of indigestion, heartburn, nausea, and vomiting. Women and older adults often present with atypical manifestations of MI but literature reports that many women report symptoms for weeks to months prior to the onset of acute MI (Blakemen & Bookman, 2016). However, heart disease is the number one cause of death in both groups, making early recognition and aggressive treatment vital. See Moving Evidence into Action.

Moving Evidence into Action

Warning Symptoms of Myocardial Infarction in Women

Clinical Issue

CHD is the leading killer of women in the United States. The risk of death and disability resulting from AMI is higher in women than in men. Part of the problem is the vague symptomatology and warning signs of AMI in women. Some researchers report that patients may experience symptoms months to weeks prior to the acute event (prodromal symptoms).

External Evidence

Blakeman and Booker (2016) conducted an integrative review of the literature to identify studies that described prodromal myocardial infarction symptoms in women. Their review included 12 studies (10 peer-reviewed articles and two doctoral dissertations). They found that prodromal MI symptoms were prevalent in almost all women. These symptoms included fatigue (most common); shortness of breath; chest, neck, and/or jaw pain; sleep disturbances; indigestion; and anxiety. The authors recommend that more study be done to further characterize the complex nature of these symptoms with the goal in using prodromal symptoms to recognize MI reliably in clinical practice.

Internal Evidence

As part of the evaluation of internal evidence, one must consider the clinical feasibility of evaluation of prodromal symptoms, the outcome of interest (early diagnosis of MI in women), current policies/procedures in place for MI diagnosis, and early intervention and identification of stakeholders that influence uptake of the proposed intervention. One question to ask: Is this problem (continued issues with diagnosis of MI in women) significant in the population of your care environment? Does the clinical environment support the use of the intervention? What about cost-benefit of the new intervention? In the use of monitoring women over time for prodromal symptoms, Blakeman and Booker (2016) noted that additional research is needed to characterize the complex symptomatology that may occur prior to the onset of a myocardial infarction.

Patient Considerations

When considering use of a new practice (like close assessment of symptoms in women at risk for MI), the nurse must consider the specific patient population where it will be used. Will patients and their families be amenable to such close assessment?

Putting the Pieces Together

Close monitoring of women at risk for MI for prodromal symptoms may be an answer to the problem of poor symptom identification in women. To effectively implement a plan, it is important to evaluate the external evidence and consider the internal implications and patient/family issues. With the implementation of new, more intensive monitoring of at-risk women, the outcome of early identification of MI in women is an important outcome to consider.

Reference

Blakeman, J. R., & Bookman, K. J. (2016). Prodromal myocardial infarction symptoms experienced by women. *Heart and Lung, 45*, 327–335.

Women are more likely than men to have a silent or unrecognized heart attack or to present in cardiac arrest or with cardiogenic shock. Women often experience epigastric pain and nausea, causing them to blame their discomfort on heartburn. Shortness of breath is common, as is fatigue and weakness of the shoulders and upper arms.

Older people often seek treatment for vague complaints of difficulty breathing, confusion, fainting, dizziness, abdominal pain, or cough. They often attribute their symptoms to a stroke. The prevalence of silent ischemia is greater in older adults.

Stress the importance of seeking medical help promptly for atypical manifestations of MI. Prompt diagnosis and intervention reduce the mortality and morbidity of MI in women and older adults, just as they do in men. Despite this fact, both women and older adults are more likely to delay seeking treatment and are less likely to be accurately diagnosed and aggressively treated for CHD. Younger women are a particularly important group to reach; their mortality rate when MI occurs is twice that of men.

Compensatory mechanisms cause many of the other symptoms of MI. SNS stimulation causes anxiety, tachycardia, and vasoconstriction, producing cool, clammy, mottled skin. Pain and blood chemistry changes stimulate the respiratory center, causing tachypnea. The patient often has a sense of impending doom and death. Tissue necrosis causes an inflammatory reaction that increases the white blood cell (WBC) count and elevates the temperature. Serum cardiac enzyme levels rise as enzymes are released from necrotic cardiac cells.

Other manifestations may vary, depending on the location and amount of infarcted tissue. Hypertension, hypotension, or signs of heart failure may develop. Vagal stimulation may cause nausea and vomiting, bradycardia, and hypotension. Hiccupping may develop due to diaphragmatic irritation. If a large vessel is occluded, the first sign of MI may be sudden death. Typical manifestations of MI include:

- Chest pain: Substernal or precordial (across the entire chest wall); may radiate to neck, jaw, shoulder(s), or left arm
- Tachycardia, tachypnea
- Dyspnea, shortness of breath
- Nausea and vomiting
- Anxiety, sense of impending doom
- Diaphoresis
- Cool, mottled skin; diminished peripheral pulses
- Hypotension or hypertension
- Palpitations, dysrhythmias
- Signs of left heart failure
- Decreased level of consciousness.

Complications

The risk of complications associated with MI is related to its size and location.

Dysrhythmias

Dysrhythmias, disturbances or irregularities of heart rhythm, are the most frequent complication of MI. Dysrhythmias are discussed in detail in the next section of this chapter.

Infarcted tissue is *arrhythmogenic*; that is, it alters the generation and conduction of electrical impulses in the heart, increasing the risk of dysrhythmias. Premature ventricular contractions (PVCs) are common following an MI, developing in more than 90% of patients with an AMI. Although not dangerous in themselves, they may be predictive of more dangerous dysrhythmias such as ventricular tachycardia or ventricular fibrillation. *Ventricular fibrillation (VF)* is a frequent cause of sudden cardiac death. The risk of VF is greatest in the first hour after MI, declining with time. Infarction around a conduction pathway will affect electrical conduction. *Atrioventricular (AV) block* may occur following anterior wall infarction. First-degree and Mobitz I (Wenckebach) blocks are most common, although complete heart block can occur. Bradydysrhythmias (abnormal slow rhythms) may develop when the inferior wall of the ventricle is affected.

Pump Failure

MI reduces myocardial contractility, ventricular wall motion, and compliance. Impaired contractility and filling may produce heart failure. The risk of heart failure is greatest when large portions of the left ventricle are infarcted. Severity of heart failure is dependent on the location and amount of myocardial damage. Anterior infarcts, affecting the left ventricle, result in more severe failure. Loss of 20 to 30% of the left-ventricular muscle mass may cause manifestations of left-sided heart failure, including dyspnea, fatigue, weakness, and respiratory crackles on auscultation. Inferior or right-ventricular MI may lead to right-sided heart failure with manifestations such as neck vein distention and peripheral edema. Hemodynamic monitoring is often initiated for patients with evidence of heart failure. Heart failure and its manifestations are discussed in greater depth in Chapter 31.

Cardiogenic Shock

Cardiogenic shock, impaired tissue perfusion due to pump failure, results when functioning myocardial muscle mass decreases by more than 40%. The heart is unable to pump enough blood to meet the needs of the body and maintain organ function. Low cardiac output due to cardiogenic shock also impairs perfusion of the coronary arteries and myocardium, further increasing tissue damage. Mortality from cardiogenic shock is greater than 70%, although this can be reduced by prompt intervention with revascularization procedures. Refer to Chapter 11 for a more extensive discussion of cardiogenic shock.

Infarct Extension

Approximately 10% of patients experience extension or reinfarction in the area of the original infarction during the first 10 to 14 days after an MI (Grass & Brener, 2014). Extension of the MI is characterized by increased myocardial necrosis from continued blood flow impairment and ongoing injury. Expansion of the MI is described as a permanent expansion of the infarcted area from thinning and dilation of the muscle. Infarct extension and expansion may cause manifestations such as continuing chest pain, hemodynamic compromise, and worsening heart failure.

Structural Defects

Necrotic muscle is replaced by scar tissue that is thinner than the ventricular muscle mass. This can lead to such complications as ventricular aneurysm, rupture of the interventricular septum or papillary muscle, and myocardial rupture. A *ventricular aneurysm* is an outpouching of the ventricular wall. It may develop when a large section of the ventricle is replaced by scar tissue. Because it does not contract during systole, stroke volume decreases. Blood may pool within the aneurysm, causing clots to form. Ischemia of the papillary muscle or chordae tendineae may cause structural damage, leading to papillary muscle dysfunction or rupture. Impaired AV valve function (usually the mitral valve) causes *regurgitation*, backflow of blood into the atria during systole. The interventricular septum may perforate or rupture due to ischemia and infarction. Myocardial rupture is a risk between days 4 and 7 after MI, when the injured tissue is soft and weak. This potential complication of MI is often fatal.

Pericarditis

Tissue necrosis prompts an inflammatory response. *Pericarditis*, inflammation of the pericardial tissue surrounding the heart, may complicate AMI, usually within 2 to 3 days. Pericarditis causes chest pain that may be aching or sharp and stabbing, aggravated by movement or deep breathing. A *pericardial friction rub* may be heard on auscultation of heart sounds.

Dressler syndrome, thought to be a hypersensitivity response to necrotic tissue or an autoimmune disorder, may develop days to weeks after AMI. It is a symptom complex characterized by fever, chest pain, and dyspnea. Dressler syndrome may spontaneously resolve or recur over several months, causing significant discomfort and distress.

Interprofessional Care

Immediate treatment goals for the MI patient are:

- Relieve chest pain.
- Reduce the extent of myocardial damage.
- Maintain cardiovascular stability.
- Decrease cardiac workload.
- Prevent complications.

Slowing the process of CHD and reducing the risk of future MI is a major long-term management goal for the patient.

Rapid assessment and early diagnosis are important in treating AMI. "Time is muscle" is a medical truism for the patient with AMI. The evolution of an AMI is dynamic: The quicker the artery is reopened (medically, surgically, or spontaneously), the more myocardium can be salvaged. Survival and long-term outcomes following AMI are improved by rapidly restoring blood flow to the "stunned" myocardium surrounding the infarcted tissue, reducing myocardial oxygen demand, and limiting the accumulation of toxic by-products of necrosis and reperfusion. The AHA recommends initiation of definitive treatment within 1 hour of entry into the healthcare system, as every minute of delay in treating patients with AMI affects the mortality risk during the first year.

The major problem interfering with timely reperfusion is delay in seeking medical care following the onset of symptoms. Many factors are cited as reasons for treatment delay, including advanced age, the perception of the seriousness of symptoms, denial, access to medical care, the availability of an emergency response system, and in-hospital delays. Immediate evaluation of the patient presenting with manifestations of myocardial infarction is essential to early diagnosis and treatment.

Diagnosis

Diagnostic testing is used to establish the diagnosis of AMI.

Serum cardiac markers are proteins released from necrotic heart muscle. The proteins most specific for diagnosis of MI are creatine kinase (CK; or creatine phosphokinase [CPK]) and cardiac-specific troponins (Table 30.4).

- ***Creatine kinase*** is an important enzyme for cellular function found principally in cardiac and skeletal muscle and the brain. CK levels rise rapidly with damage to these tissues, appearing in the serum 4 to 6 hours after AMI, peaking within 12 to 24 hours, and then declining during the next 48 to 72 hours. The CK level correlates with the size of the infarction; the greater the amount of infarcted tissue, the higher the serum CK level.
- ***CK-MB*** (also called *MB-bands*) is a subset of CK specific to cardiac muscle. This isoenzyme of CK is considered the most sensitive indicator of MI. Elevated CK alone is not specific for MI; elevated CK-MB greater than 5% is considered a positive indicator of MI. CK-MB levels do not normally rise with chest pain from angina or causes other than MI.
- ***Cardiac muscle troponins***, *cardiac-specific troponin T* (cT_nT), and *cardiac-specific troponin I* (cT_nI), are proteins released during myocardial infarction that are sensitive indicators of myocardial damage. These proteins are part of the actin-myosin unit in cardiac muscle and are normally not detectable in the blood. With necrosis of cardiac muscle, troponins are released and blood levels rise. The specificity of cT_nT and cT_nI to cardiac muscle necrosis makes these markers particularly useful when skeletal muscle trauma contributes to elevated CK levels (e.g., when CPR has been performed or traumatic injury occurred at the time of the MI). They are sensitive enough to detect very small infarctions that do not cause significant CK elevation. Both cT_nT and cT_nI remain in the blood for 10 to 14 days after an MI, making them useful for diagnosing MI when medical treatment is delayed.

Serum levels of cardiac markers are ordered on admission and for 3 succeeding days. Serial blood levels help establish the diagnosis and determine the extent of myocardial damage.

Other laboratory tests (Kee, 2014) may include:

- ***Myoglobin*** is one of the first cardiac markers to be detectable in the blood after an MI. It is released within a few hours of symptom onset. Its lack of specificity to cardiac muscle and rapid excretion (blood levels return to normal within 24 hours) limit its use (Perrin & MacLeod, 2017).
- ***Complete blood count (CBC)*** shows an elevated WBC count due to inflammation of the injured myocardium. The *erythrocyte sedimentation rate (ESR)* also rises because of inflammation.
- ***Arterial blood gases (ABGs)*** may be ordered to assess blood oxygen levels and acid–base balance.

Electrocardiography, echocardiography, and myocardial nuclear scans are the most common diagnostic tests performed when AMI is suspected. With the exception of the ECG, the timing of these tests depends on the patient's immediate condition. Hemodynamic monitoring may be initiated in the unstable patient following MI.

- ***Electrocardiography*** reflects changes in conduction due to myocardial ischemia and necrosis. Classic ECG changes seen in AMI include T-wave inversion, ST-segment elevation, and formation of a Q wave. Ischemic changes in the heart are seen as depression of the ST segment or inversion of the T wave (refer to Figure 30.2). With myocardial injury, elevation of the ST segment occurs (**Figure 30.5** ■). Significant Q-wave development indicates a transmural, or full-thickness, infarction. Myocardial damage can be localized using the 12-lead ECG. See Chapter 29 for more information about ECGs.
- ***Echocardiography*** is done to evaluate cardiac wall motion and left-ventricular function. Stunned and infarcted tissue does not contract as effectively (if at all) as healthy myocardium.
- ***Radionuclide imaging*** studies may be done to evaluate myocardial perfusion. These studies cannot differentiate between an acute MI and old scar tissue, but do help identify the specific area of myocardial ischemia and damage.
- ***Hemodynamic monitoring*** may be initiated when AMI significantly affects cardiac output and hemodynamic status. These invasive procedures are described in Chapter 31.

Medications

Aspirin, a platelet inhibitor, is now considered an essential part of AMI treatment. A 160- to 325-mg aspirin tablet is given by emergency personnel, with the instructions that it is to be chewed (for buccal absorption). This initial dose is followed by a daily oral dose of 160 to 325 mg of aspirin. Analgesics, fibrinolytic agents, and antidysrhythmic agents are among the principal classes of drugs used in treating AMI.

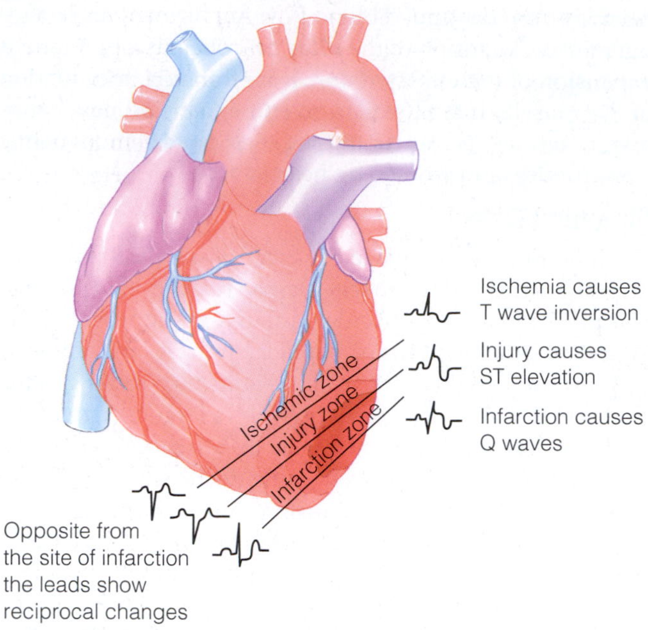
Ischemia causes
T wave inversion
Injury causes
ST elevation
Infarction causes
Q waves
Ischemic zone
Injury zone
Infarction zone
Opposite from
the site of infarction
the leads show
reciprocal changes

Figure 30.5 ■ ECG changes characteristic of MI.

Analgesia. Pain relief is vital in treating the patient with AMI. Pain stimulates the sympathetic nervous system, increasing the heart rate and blood pressure and, in turn, myocardial workload. Sublingual nitroglycerin may be given (up to three 0.4-mg doses at 5-minute intervals). Intravenous nitroglycerin may be continued for the first 24 to 48 hours to reduce myocardial work. In addition to pain relief, nitroglycerin decreases myocardial oxygen demand and may increase the supply of oxygen to the myocardium. Nitroglycerin is a peripheral and arterial vasodilator that reduces afterload. It dilates coronary arteries and collateral channels in the heart, increasing coronary blood flow to save myocardial tissue at risk. Nitrates may, however, cause reflex tachycardia or excessive hypotension, so close monitoring is necessary during administration. It is also important to ask the patient about use of sildenafil (Viagra) within the previous 24 hours before administering nitroglycerin, as the combination can precipitate a significant drop in blood pressure. See Medication Administration 30.B for the nursing implications of nitroglycerin and other drugs given to reduce myocardial workload following AMI.

Morphine sulfate is the drug of choice for pain unrelieved by nitroglycerin and for sedation. Following an initial intravenous dose of 4 to 8 mg, small doses (2 to 4 mg) may be repeated intravenously every 5 minutes until pain is relieved. It is important to assess frequently for pain relief and possible adverse effects of analgesia, such as excessive sedation. Pain unrelieved by expected or usual doses should be reported to the physician as it may indicate a complication such as extension of the infarct. Refer to Chapter 9 for more details about morphine administration. Antianxiety agents such as diazepam (Valium) may also be administered to promote rest.

Fibrinolytic Therapy Fibrinolytic agents, drugs that dissolve or break up blood clots, are first-line drugs used to treat acute MI when access to a cardiac catheterization lab for revascularization procedures is not immediately available. Fibrinolytic drugs activate the fibrinolytic system to *lyse* or destroy the clot, restoring blood flow to the obstructed artery. Early fibrinolytic administration (within the first 6 hours of MI onset) limits infarct size, reduces heart damage, and improves outcomes. Activation of the fibrinolytic system can cause multiple complications; approximately 0.5 to 5% of patients receiving fibrinolytic drugs experience serious bleeding complications. Not every patient is a candidate for fibrinolytic therapy; for example, it is contraindicated in patients with known bleeding disorders, history of cerebrovascular disease, uncontrolled hypertension, pregnancy, or recent trauma or surgery to the head or spine.

Several fibrinolytic agents are commonly used today. Among these, little difference in effectiveness has been demonstrated; there are, however, big differences in cost. Streptokinase, a biologic agent derived from group C *Streptococcus* organisms, is the least expensive of the drugs. Its primary drawback is the risk of a severe hypersensitivity reaction, including anaphylaxis. Streptokinase is administered by intravenous infusion. Anisoylated plasminogen-streptokinase activator complex (APSAC) is a related drug that can be administered by bolus over 2 to 5 minutes. It has many of the same effects as streptokinase, but is considerably more expensive. Tissue plasminogen activator (tPA), tenecteplase (TNK), and reteplase (rPA) are more effective in reestablishing myocardial perfusion, especially when the pain developed more than 3 hours previously. These drugs, however, are the most expensive. Nursing care of the patient receiving a fibrinolytic agent is outlined in Box 30.5.

Antidysrhythmics. Dysrhythmias are a common complication of AMI, particularly in the first 12 to 24 hours. Antidysrhythmic medications are used as needed to treat dysrhythmias. They may also be given prophylactically to prevent dysrhythmias. Ventricular dysrhythmias are treated with a Class I or Class III antidysrhythmic drug (see **Medication Administration 30.D**). Symptomatic bradycardia (bradycardia with associated hypotension and other signs of low cardiac output) is treated with

BOX 30.5
Nursing Care of the Patient Receiving Fibrinolytic Therapy

PREINFUSION CARE

- Obtain nursing history, and perform a physical assessment. *Information obtained from the history and physical exam helps determine whether fibrinolytic therapy is appropriate. The goal is to initiate fibrinolytic therapy within 30 minutes of arrival.*
- Evaluate for contraindications to fibrinolytic therapy: Recent surgery or trauma (including prolonged CPR), bleeding disorders or active bleeding, cerebrovascular accident, neurosurgery within the last 2 months, gastrointestinal ulcers, diabetic hemorrhagic retinopathy, and uncontrolled hypertension. *Fibrinolytic agents dissolve clots and therefore may precipitate intracranial, internal, or peripheral bleeding.*
- Inform the patient of the purpose of the therapy. Discuss the risk of bleeding and the need to keep the extremity immobile during and after the infusion. *Minimal movement of the extremity is necessary to prevent bleeding from the infusion site.*

DURING THE INFUSION

- Assess and record vital signs and the infusion site for hematoma or bleeding every 15 minutes for the first hour, every 30 minutes for the next 2 hours, and then hourly until the intravenous catheter is discontinued. Assess pulses, color, sensation, and temperature of both extremities with each vital sign check. *Vital signs and the site are frequently assessed to detect possible complications.*
- Remind the patient to keep the extremity still and straight. Do not elevate head of bed above 15 degrees. *Extremity immobilization helps prevent infusion site trauma and bleeding. Hypotension may develop; keeping the bed flat helps maintain cerebral perfusion.*
- Maintain continuous cardiac monitoring during the infusion. Keep antidysrhythmic drugs and the emergency cart readily available for treatment of significant dysrhythmias. *Ventricular dysrhythmias commonly occur with reperfusion of the ischemic myocardium.*

POSTINFUSION CARE

- Assess vital signs, distal pulses, and infusion site frequently as needed. *The patient remains at high risk for bleeding following fibrinolytic therapy.*
- Evaluate response to therapy: Normalization of ST segment, relief of chest pain, reperfusion dysrhythmias, and early peaking of the CK and CK-MB levels. *These are signs that the clot has been dissolved and the myocardium is being reperfused.*
- Maintain bedrest for 6 hours. Keep the head of the bed at or below 15 degrees. Reinforce the need to keep the extremity straight and immobile. Avoid any injections for 24 hours after catheter removal. *Precautions such as these are important to prevent bleeding.*
- Assess puncture sites for bleeding. On catheter removal hold direct pressure over the site for at least 30 minutes. Apply a pressure dressing to any venous or arterial sites as needed. Perform routine care in a gentle manner to avoid bruising or injury. *Fibrinolytic therapy disrupts normal coagulation. Peripheral bleeding may occur at puncture sites, and there may not be sufficient fibrin to form a clot. Direct or indirect pressure may be needed to control the bleeding.*
- Assess body fluids, including urine, vomitus, and feces, for evidence of bleeding; frequently assess for changes in level of consciousness and manifestations of increased intracranial pressure, which may indicate intracranial bleeding. Assess surgical sites for bleeding. Monitor hemoglobin and hematocrit levels, prothrombin time (PT), and partial thromboplastin time (PTT). *These provide additional means of assessing for bleeding.*
- Administer platelet-modifying drugs (e.g., aspirin, dipyridamole) as ordered. *Platelet inhibitors decrease platelet aggregation and adhesion and are used to prevent reocclusion of the artery.*
- Report manifestations of reocclusion, including changes in the ST segment, chest pain, or dysrhythmias. *Early recognition of reocclusion is vital to save myocardial tissue.*

intravenous atropine, 0.5 to 1 mg. Intravenous verapamil or the short-acting beta-blocker esmolol (Brevibloc) may be ordered to treat atrial fibrillation or other supraventricular tachydysrhythmias.

Other Medications. Beta-blockers such as propranolol (Inderal), atenolol (Tenormin), and metoprolol (Lopressor) reduce pain, limit infarct size, and decrease the incidence of serious ventricular dysrhythmias in AMI. These drugs decrease the heart rate, reducing cardiac work and myocardial oxygen demand. Initial doses are given intravenously. Oral beta-blocker therapy is continued to reduce the risk of reinfarction and death related to cardiovascular causes.

Angiotensin-converting enzyme (ACE) inhibitors also reduce mortality associated with AMI. These drugs reduce ventricular remodeling following an MI, reducing the risk for subsequent heart failure. They also may reduce the risk of reinfarction.

Anticoagulants and antiplatelet medications are often prescribed to maintain coronary artery patency following thrombolysis or a revascularization procedure. Abciximab (ReoPro) suppresses platelet aggregation and reduces the risk of reocclusion following angioplasty. It also improves vessel opening with fibrinolytic therapy, permitting lower doses of fibrinolytic drugs. Standard or low-molecular-weight heparin preparations are often given to patients with AMI. Heparin helps establish and maintain patency of the affected coronary artery. It is also used, along with long-term warfarin, to prevent systemic or pulmonary embolism in patients with significant left-ventricular impairment or atrial fibrillation following AMI. See Medication Administration 30.C for the nursing implications of antiplatelet drugs, and Chapter 34 for more information about anticoagulant therapy.

Patients with pump failure and hypotension may receive intravenous dopamine, a vasopressor. At low doses (< 5 mg/kg/min), it improves blood flow to the kidneys, preventing renal ischemia and possible acute renal failure (refer to Chapter 28). With increasing doses, dopamine increases myocardial contractility and causes vasoconstriction, improving blood pressure and cardiac output.

Antilipemic agents are used for the patient with hyperlipidemia. A stool softener such as docusate sodium is prescribed to maintain normal bowel function and reduce straining.

Treatments

The patient with a suspected or confirmed MI is monitored continuously. Care is provided in the intensive coronary care unit for the first 24 to 48 hours, after which time less intensive monitoring (e.g., telemetry) may be required. An intravenous line is established to allow rapid administration of emergency medications.

Bedrest is prescribed for the first 12 hours to reduce the cardiac workload. The bedside commode is generally allowed; studies have shown this to be less stressful than using a bedpan. If the patient's condition is stable, sitting in a chair at the bedside is permitted after 12 hours. Activities are gradually increased as tolerated. A quiet, calm environment with limited outside stimuli is preferred. Visitors are limited to promote rest. Oxygen is administered by nasal cannula at 2 to 5 L/min to improve oxygenation of the myocardium and other tissues.

A liquid diet may be prescribed for the first 4 to 12 hours to reduce gastric distention and myocardial workload. Following that, a low-fat, low-cholesterol, reduced-sodium diet is allowed. Sodium restrictions may be lifted after 2 to 3 days if no evidence of heart failure is present. Small, frequent feedings are often recommended. Drinks containing caffeine and very hot and cold foods may also be limited.

Revascularization Procedures

Many patients with AMI are treated with immediate or early percutaneous coronary revascularization (PCR) such as angioplasty and stent placement. PCR may follow fibrinolytic therapy or be used in place of fibrinolytic therapy to restore blood flow to ischemic myocardium. When compared with fibrinolytic therapy, prompt PCR reduces hospital mortality. In some cases, CABG surgery may be performed. The choice of procedure depends on the patient's age and immediate condition, the time elapsed from the onset of manifestations, and the extent of myocardial disease and damage. These procedures and related nursing care are covered in more depth in the preceding section on acute coronary syndrome.

Other Invasive Procedures

For patients with large MIs and evidence of pump failure, invasive devices may be used to temporarily take over the function of the heart, allowing the injured myocardium to heal. The intra-aortic balloon pump is widely used to augment cardiac output. Ventricular assist devices are indicated for patients requiring more or longer term artificial support than the intra-aortic balloon pump provides.

Intra-Aortic Balloon Pump. The *intra-aortic balloon pump (IABP)*, also called *intra-aortic balloon counterpulsation*, is a mechanical circulatory support device that may be used after cardiac surgery or to treat cardiogenic shock following AMI. The IABP temporarily supports cardiac function, allowing the heart to gradually recover by decreasing myocardial workload and oxygen demand and increasing perfusion of the coronary arteries.

A catheter with a 30- to 40-mL balloon is introduced into the aorta, usually via the femoral artery. The balloon catheter is connected to a console that regulates the inflation and deflation of the balloon. The IABP catheter inflates during diastole, increasing perfusion of the coronary and renal arteries, and deflates just prior to systole, decreasing afterload and cardiac workload (**Figure 30.6** ■). The inflation–deflation sequence is triggered by the ECG pattern. During the most acute period, the balloon inflates and deflates with each heart beat (1:1 ratio), providing maximal assistance to the heart. As the patient's condition improves, the IABP is weaned to inflate–deflate at varying intervals (e.g., 1:2, 1:4, 1:8). This provides a continually decreasing amount of support as the heart muscle recovers. When mechanical assistance is no longer required, the IABP catheter is removed.

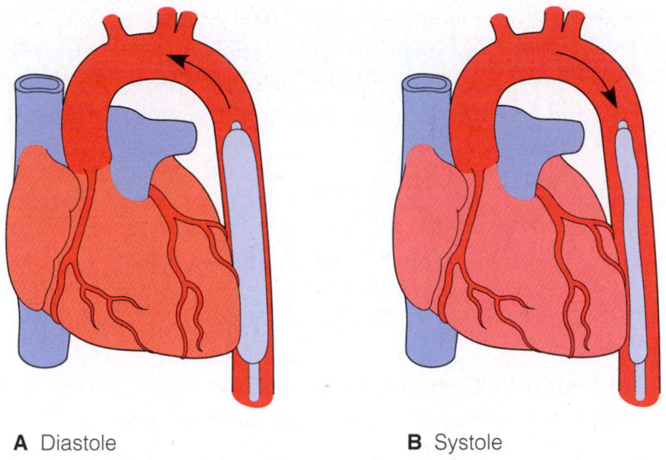
A Diastole
B Systole

Figure 30.6 ■ The intra-aortic balloon pump. **A**, When inflated during diastole, the balloon supports cerebral, renal, and coronary artery perfusion. **B**, The balloon deflates during systole, so cardiac output is unimpeded.

Ventricular Assist Devices. Use of *ventricular assist devices (VADs)* to aid the failing heart is becoming more common with advances in technology. Whereas the IABP can supplement cardiac output by approximately 10 to 15%, the VAD temporarily takes partial or complete control of cardiac function, depending on the type of device. VADs may be used as temporary or complete assist devices in AMI and cardiogenic shock when there is a chance for recovery of normal heart function after a period of cardiac rest. The device also may be used as a bridge to heart transplant. Nursing care for the patient with a VAD is supportive and includes assessing hemodynamic status and for complications associated with the device. Patients with VAD are at considerable risk for infection; strict aseptic technique is used with all invasive catheters and dressing changes. Pneumonia is also a risk due to immobility and ventilatory support. Mechanical failure of the VAD is a life-threatening event that requires immediate intervention (Perrin & MacLeod, 2018).

Cardiac Rehabilitation

Cardiac rehabilitation is a long-term program of medical evaluation, exercise, risk factor modification, education, and counseling designed to limit the physical and psychologic effects of cardiac illness and improve the patient's quality of life. Cardiac rehabilitation begins with admission for a cardiac event such as an AMI or a revascularization procedure. Phase 1 of the program is the inpatient phase. A thorough assessment of the patient's history, current status, risk factors, and motivation is obtained. During this phase, activity progresses from bedrest to independent performance of activities of daily living (ADLs) and ambulation within the facility. Both subjective and objective responses to increasing activity levels are evaluated. Excess fatigue, shortness of breath, chest pain, tachypnea, tachycardia, or cool, clammy skin indicates activity intolerance. Phase 2, immediate outpatient cardiac rehabilitation, begins within 3 weeks of the cardiac event. The goals for the outpatient program are to increase activity level, participation, and capacity; improve psychosocial status and treat anxiety or depression; and provide education and support for risk factor reduction. Continuation programs, phase 3 of cardiac rehabilitation, are directed at providing a transition to independent exercise and exercise maintenance. During this final phase, the patient may check in every 3 months for evaluation of risk factors, quality of life, and exercise habits.

Nursing Care

Nursing care of the patient with an acute myocardial infarction focuses on reducing cardiac work, identifying and treating complications in a timely manner, and preparing the patient for rehabilitation. See also the Case Study & Nursing Care Plan for a patient with an AMI.

Assessment

Nursing assessment for the patient with AMI must be both timely and ongoing. Assessment data related to AMI includes:

- *Health history:* Complaints of chest pain, including its location, intensity, character, radiation, and timing; associated symptoms such as nausea, heartburn, shortness of breath, and anxiety; treatment measures taken since onset of pain; past medical history, especially cardiac related; chronic diseases; current medications and any known allergies to medications; smoking history and use of recreational drugs and alcohol
- *Physical assessment:* General appearance including obvious signs of distress; vital signs; peripheral pulses; skin color, temperature, moisture; level of consciousness; heart and breath sounds; cardiac rhythm (on beside monitor); bowel sounds, abdominal tenderness.

Priorities of Care

Collaborating with the interprofessional team to ensure adequate treatment of the underlying process while providing care that supports the physical and psychologic responses to the acute cardiac event is a nursing priority.

Diagnoses, Outcomes, and Interventions

Priorities of nursing care include relieving chest pain, reducing cardiac work, and promoting oxygenation. Psychosocial support is especially important because an AMI can be devastating, bringing the patient face to face with his or her own mortality for the first time.

Manage Acute Pain. Chest pain occurs when the oxygen supply to the heart muscle does not meet the demand. Pain is caused by myocardial ischemia, infarction, and reperfusion of an ischemic area following fibrinolytic therapy or emergent PTCA. Pain stimulates the sympathetic nervous system, increasing cardiac work. Pain relief is a priority of care for the patient with AMI.

Expected Outcome: Patient's postevent pain will be controlled as evidenced by patient self-report of adequate pain management and reduction in pain-related behaviors.

The nurse will:

- Assess for verbal and nonverbal signs of pain. Document characteristics and the intensity of the pain, using a standard pain scale. Verify nonverbal indicators of pain with the patient. *Frequent, careful pain assessment allows early intervention to reduce the risk of further damage. Pain is a subjective experience; its expression may vary with location and intensity, previous experiences, and cultural and social background. Pain scales provide an objective tool for measuring pain and a way to assess pain relief or reduction.*

- Administer oxygen at 2 to 5 L/min per nasal cannula. *Supplemental oxygen increases oxygen supply to the myocardium, decreasing ischemia and pain.*
- Promote physical and psychologic rest. Provide information and emotional support. *Rest decreases cardiac workload and sympathetic nervous system stimulation, promoting comfort. Information and emotional support help decrease anxiety and provide psychologic rest.*
- Titrate intravenous nitroglycerin as ordered to relieve chest pain, maintaining a systolic blood pressure greater than 100 mmHg. *Nitroglycerin decreases chest pain by dilating peripheral vessels, reducing cardiac work, and dilating coronary vessels, including collateral channels, thus improving blood flow to ischemic tissue.*

SAFETY ALERT: Intravenous nitroglycerin causes peripheral vasodilation, which may lead to hypotension, reduced coronary blood flow, and tachycardia. Reduce the nitro flow rate and notify the physician if this occurs. ■

- Administer 2 to 4 mg morphine by intravenous push for chest pain as needed. *Morphine is an effective narcotic analgesic for chest pain. It decreases pain and anxiety, acts as a venodilator, and decreases the respiratory rate. The resulting reduction in preload and SNS stimulation reduces cardiac workload and oxygen consumption.*

Reassess for relief of chest pain. The goal of care is to achieve pain relief, not simply a reduction in pain to a manageable level.

Promote Effective Cardiac Tissue Perfusion. Cardiac muscle damage affects its compliance, contractility, and cardiac output. The extent of the effect on tissue perfusion depends on the location and amount of damage. Anterior wall infarcts have a greater effect on cardiac output than do right-ventricular infarcts. Infarcted muscle increases the risk for cardiac dysrhythmias, affecting the delivery of blood and oxygen to the tissues.

Expected Outcome: Patient will exhibit adequate cardiac perfusion as evidenced by freedom from chest pain related to angina and freedom from arrhythmias.

The nurse will:

- Assess and document vital signs. Report increases in heart rate and changes in rhythm, blood pressure, and respiratory rate. *Decreased cardiac output activates compensatory mechanisms that may cause tachycardia and vasoconstriction, increasing cardiac workload.*
- Assess for changes in level of consciousness (LOC); decreased urine output; moist, cool, pale, mottled, or cyanotic skin; dusky or cyanotic mucous membranes and nail beds; diminished/absent peripheral pulses; and delayed capillary refill. *These are manifestations of impaired tissue perfusion. A change in LOC is often the first manifestation of altered perfusion because brain tissue and cerebral function depend on a continuous supply of oxygen.*
- Auscultate heart and breath sounds. Note abnormal heart sounds (e.g., an S_3 or S_4 gallop or a murmur) or adventitious lung sounds. *Abnormal heart sounds or adventitious lung sounds may indicate impaired cardiac filling or output, increasing the risk for decreased tissue perfusion.*
- Monitor ECG rhythm continuously. *Dysrhythmias can further impair cardiac output and tissue perfusion.*
- Obtain a 12-lead ECG to assess complaints of chest pain. Report marked changes to the physician. Continued or unrelieved chest pain may indicate further myocardial ischemia and extension of the infarct; an ECG during episodes of chest pain provides a valuable diagnostic tool to assess myocardial perfusion.
- Monitor oxygen saturation levels. Administer oxygen as ordered. Obtain and assess ABGs as indicated. *Oxygen saturation is an indicator of gas exchange, tissue perfusion, and the effectiveness of oxygen administration. ABGs provide a more precise measurement of blood oxygen levels and allow assessment of acid–base balance.*
- Administer antidysrhythmic medications as needed. *Dysrhythmias affect tissue perfusion by altering cardiac output.*
- Obtain serial CK, isoenzyme, and troponin levels as ordered. *Levels of cardiac markers, CK isoenzymes in particular, correlate with the extent of myocardial damage.*
- Plan for invasive hemodynamic monitoring. *Hemodynamic monitoring facilitates AMI management and treatment evaluation by providing a means of assessing pressures in the systemic and pulmonary arteries, the relationship between oxygen supply and demand, cardiac output, and cardiac index.*

SAFETY ALERT: Continuously evaluate the response to interventions such as fibrinolytic therapy, drugs to improve cardiac output and tissue perfusion, and drugs to reduce cardiac work. Adverse effects of therapy may reduce the effectiveness of treatment. Bleeding due to fibrinolytic therapy may affect vascular volume and cardiac output; reperfusion dysrhythmias may affect cardiac output. Drugs used to improve cardiac output may increase cardiac workload, whereas those given to reduce cardiac workload may significantly affect contractility and cardiac output. ■

Promote Effective Coping. Coping mechanisms help an individual deal with a life-threatening event or with acute changes in health. However, certain coping mechanisms may be detrimental to restoring health, particularly if the patient relies on them for a prolonged period. Denial, for example, is a common coping mechanism among post-MI patients. In the initial stages, denial can reduce anxiety. Continued denial, however, can interfere with learning and compliance with treatment.

Expected Outcome: Patient will use effective coping behaviors as evidenced by decreased report of stress symptoms and verbalization and utilization of positive coping behaviors.

The nurse will:

- Establish an environment of caring and trust. Encourage the patient to express feelings. *Establishing a trusting nurse–patient relationship provides a safe environment for the patient to discuss feelings of helplessness, powerlessness, anxiety, and hopelessness. The nurse may then be able to provide additional resources to meet the patient's needs.*
- Accept denial as a coping mechanism, but do not reinforce it. *Denial may initially help by diminishing the psychologic threat to health, decreasing anxiety. However, its prolonged use can interfere with acceptance of reality and cooperation, possibly delaying treatment and hindering recovery.*
- Note aggressive behaviors, hostility, or anger. Document any failure to comply with treatments. *These signs can indicate anxiety and denial.*
- Help the patient identify positive coping skills used in the past (e.g., problem-solving skills, verbalization of feelings, asking for help, prayer). Reinforce use of positive coping behaviors. *Coping behaviors that have been successful in the past can help the patient deal with the current situation. These familiar methods can decrease feelings of powerlessness.*
- Provide opportunities for the patient to make decisions about the plan of care, as possible. *This promotes self-confidence and independence. Participating in care planning gives the patient a sense of control and the opportunity to use positive coping skills.*
- Provide privacy for the patient and significant other to share their questions and concerns. *Privacy provides an opportunity for the patient and partner to share their feelings and fears, offer support and encouragement to one another, relieve anxiety, and establish effective coping methods.*

Manage Fear. The fear of death and disability can be a paralyzing emotion that adversely affects the patient's recovery from AMI.

Expected Outcome: Patient will demonstrate reduced fear as evidenced by verbal and nonverbal indicators reflecting understanding by the patient and family of the current clinical condition.

The nurse will:

- Identify the patient's level of fear, noting verbal and nonverbal signs. *This information enables the nurse to plan appropriate interventions. Patients may not voice concerns; attention to nonverbal indicators is important. Controlling fear helps decrease SNS responses and catecholamine release that may increase feelings of fear and anxiety.*
- Acknowledge the patient's perception of the situation. Allow to verbalize concerns. *A sudden change in health status causes anxiety and fear of the unknown. Verbalizing these fears may help the patient cope with change and allow the healthcare team to provide information and correct misconceptions.*
- Encourage questions and provide consistent, factual answers. Repeat information as needed. *Accurate and consistent information can reduce fear. Honest explanations help strengthen the nurse–patient relationship and help the patient develop realistic expectations. Anxiety and fear decrease the ability to concentrate and retain information; therefore, information may need to be repeated.*
- Encourage self-care. Allow the patient to make decisions regarding the plan of care. *This promotes personal responsibility for health and allows some control over the situation. Patients' confidence increases as their dependence decreases.*
- Administer antianxiety medications as ordered. *These medications promote rest and relaxation and decrease feelings of anxiety, which may act as barriers to health restoration.*
- Teach nonpharmacologic methods of stress reduction (e.g., relaxation techniques, mental imagery, music therapy, breathing exercises, meditation, and massage). *Stress management techniques can help reduce tension and anxiety, provide a sense of control, and enhance coping skills.*

Delegating Nursing Care Activities

As appropriate and allowed by the designated duties and responsibilities of unlicensed assistive personnel, the nurse may delegate nursing care activities such as measuring fluid intake and output, collecting vital signs (including orthostatic vital signs), encouraging oral or enteral fluid intake, and nonpharmacologic skin care.

Transitions of Care

Preventative strategies focus on health promotion activities to prevent AMI. These strategies are outlined for CHD and angina in previous sections of this chapter and in Chapter 29. In addition, discuss risk factor management, use of prescribed medications, and cardiac rehabilitation to reduce the risk of complications or future infarctions.

Cardiac rehabilitation begins with admission to the healthcare facility and continues through the inpatient stay and after discharge into the rehabilitative period. The emphasis is on realistic application of information to maintain lifestyle changes.

Assessing readiness to learn is an important first step in preparing for home care. The patient in strong denial may not identify any relevance to the information being taught. Evaluate ability to learn, assessing physiologic and psychologic health, beliefs regarding personal responsibility for health, and expectations of the healthcare system. Also assess developmental level, ability to perform psychomotor skills, cognitive function, learning disabilities, existing knowledge base, and the influence of previous learning experiences. Provide written material to supplement teaching and encourage questions.

Include the following topics in teaching for home care:

- The normal anatomy and physiology of the heart, and the specific area of heart damage

- The process of CHD and implications of MI
- Purposes and side effects of prescribed medications.
- The importance of complying with the medical regimen and cardiac rehabilitation program and of keeping follow-up appointments
- Information about community resources, such as the local chapter of the AHA.

After discharge, follow up by telephone within 1 week and periodically thereafter during the recovery period. Provide telephone numbers of resource personnel who are available to respond to questions and concerns after discharge. While depressive symptoms can increase following AMI, research demonstrates that patients may report positive psychologic effects after AMI.

Because the patient who has had an MI is at high risk for sudden cardiac death, encourage family members to learn CPR and provide information about community resources for CPR training.

Case Study & Nursing Care Plan

A Patient with Acute Myocardial Infarction

Betty Williams, a 62-year-old psychologist, is admitted to the emergency department (ED) with complaints of severe substernal chest pain. Mrs. Williams states that the pain began after lunch, about 4 hours ago. She initially attributed the pain to indigestion. She described the pain, which now radiates to her jaw and left arm, as "really severe heartburn." It is accompanied by a "choking feeling," severe shortness of breath, and diaphoresis. The pain is unrelieved by rest, antacids, or three sublingual nitroglycerin tablets (0.4 mg).

Oxygen is started per nasal cannula at 5 L/min. Central and peripheral intravenous lines are inserted. A 12-lead ECG and the following lab work are obtained: Cardiac troponins, CK and CK isoenzymes, ABGs, CBC, and a chemistry panel. Morphine sulfate relieves Mrs. Williams's pain.

Mrs. Williams's medical history includes type 2 diabetes, angina, and hypertension. She has a 45-year history of cigarette smoking, averaging 1.5 to 2 packs per day. Family history reveals that Mrs. Williams's father died at age 42 of AMI, and her paternal grandfather died at age 65 of AMI. Mrs. Williams is taking the following medications: Tolbutamide (Orinase), hydrochlorothiazide, and isosorbide (Isordil).

Based on ECG changes and cardiac markers, an acute anterior MI is diagnosed. Mrs. Williams has no contraindications to fibrinolytic therapy and is deemed a good candidate. Intravenous alteplase (tPA, Activase) is given by bolus followed by intravenous infusions of alteplase and heparin. She is transferred to the coronary care unit (CCU).

ASSESSMENT

Dan Morales, RN, is Mrs. Williams's primary care nurse. Mrs. Williams is alert and oriented to person, place, and time. Vital signs are T 37.5°C (99.6°F), P 118 bpm, R 24/min with adequate depth, and BP 172/92 mmHg. Auscultation reveals an S_4 and fine crackles in the bases of both lungs. The ECG shows sinus tachycardia with occasional PVCs. Her skin is cool and slightly diaphoretic. Capillary refill is less than 3 seconds, and peripheral pulses are strong and equal. Her nail beds are pink.

A triple-lumen central line is in place. Nitroglycerin is infusing at 200 mcg/min in the distal lumen, the alteplase infusion is in the middle lumen, and a heparin infusion is in the proximal lumen. The peripheral intravenous line has a saline lock. Mrs. Williams states, "The pain is better since the nurse in the ED gave me a shot. But it has been coming and going. I would rate it a 4 right now, but it was terrible before. The doctor told me that this drug I'm getting will quickly open up the artery that is blocked. I hope it works! Do many people get this drug?"

DIAGNOSES

- Acute pain related to ischemic myocardial tissue
- Anxiety and fear related to change in health status
- Potential for changes in homeostasis related to the risk of bleeding secondary to fibrinolytic therapy
- Decreased cardiac function related to altered cardiac rate and rhythm

EXPECTED OUTCOMES

- Patient will rate chest pain as 2 or lower on a pain scale of 0 to 10.
- Patient will verbalize reduced anxiety and fear.
- Patient will demonstrate no signs of internal or external bleeding.
- Patient will maintain adequate cardiac output during and following reperfusion therapy.

PLANNING AND IMPLEMENTATION

The following interventions are planned and implemented during the immediate phase of Mrs. Williams's hospitalization:

- Instruct to report all chest pain. Monitor and evaluate pain using a scale of 0 to 10. Titrate intravenous nitroglycerin infusion for chest pain; stop infusion if systolic BP is below 100 mmHg. Administer 2 to 4 mg morphine intravenously for chest pain unrelieved by nitroglycerin infusion.
- Encourage verbalization of fears and concerns. Respond honestly, and correct misconceptions about the disease, therapeutic interventions, or prognosis.
- Assess knowledge of CHD. Explain the purpose of fibrinolytic therapy to dissolve the fresh clot and reperfuse the heart muscle, limiting heart damage.
- Explain the need for frequent monitoring of vital signs and potential bleeding.
- Assess for manifestations of internal or intracranial bleeding: Complaints of back or abdominal pain, headache, decreased level of consciousness, dizziness, bloody secretions or excretions, or pallor. Test all stools, urine, and vomitus for occult blood. Notify physician immediately of any abnormal findings.

- Monitor for signs of reperfusion: Decreased chest pain, return of ST segment to baseline, reperfusion dysrhythmias (e.g., PVCs, bradycardia, and heart block).
- Continuously monitor ECG for changes in cardiac rate, rhythm, and conduction. Assess vital signs.
- Treat dangerous dysrhythmias or other cardiac events per protocol. Notify the physician.
- Discuss continuing cardiac care and rehabilitation.

EVALUATION

The initial morphine dose reduces Mrs. Williams's chest pain from a rating of 8 to 4. The nitroglycerin infusion and fibrinolytic therapy further reduce her pain to 2. The nitroglycerin infusion is gradually discontinued after 24 hours. As her pain subsides, Mrs. Williams states that she feels "much better now that the pain is gone. I was afraid it would just get worse." She verbalizes an understanding of fibrinolytic therapy to limit myocardial damage. Bleeding problems are not noted. Reperfusion is indicated by relief of chest pain, return of the ST segment to baseline on the ECG, early peaking of CK levels, and increased frequency of PVCs but no significant dysrhythmias. Mrs. Williams remains in CCU for 36 hours and is transferred to the floor.

CLINICAL REASONING IN PATIENT CARE

1. How would the initial plan of care have changed if Mrs. Williams were not a candidate for fibrinolytic therapy?
2. Two days after her initial therapy, Mrs. Williams complains of palpitations. You notice frequent PVCs on the ECG monitor. What do you do?
3. What health promotion topics would you teach Mrs. Williams before discharge?
4. Mrs. Williams states, "I've been smoking for over 45 years, and I'm not going to stop now! Besides, it calms me down when I'm anxious." How would you respond to this statement?

See Evaluating Your Response in Appendix B.

30.2 Cardiac Rhythm Disorders

Heart muscle contracts in response to electrical stimulation. In the normal heart, electrical stimulation produces a synchronized, rhythmic heart muscle contraction that propels blood into the vascular system. Changes in cardiac rhythm affect this synchronized activity and the heart's ability to effectively pump blood to body tissues.

The Patient with a Cardiac Dysrhythmia

A *cardiac dysrhythmia* is a disturbance or irregularity in the electrical system of the heart. Cardiac dysrhythmias may be benign or have lethal consequences. Prompt recognition of a lethal dysrhythmia and quick action can save lives (Sorenson et al., 2019).

Dysrhythmias develop for many reasons. Not all are pathologic; some alterations in cardiac rhythm occur in response to events such as exercise or fear. For example, a rapid heart rate due to exercise, fever, or excitement is a normal response to the body's demand for oxygen or to stimulation of the SNS. Slow heart rates also may be normal. *Athletic heart syndrome*, which results from long-term training on the heart muscle, allows the heart to beat more slowly and forcefully while maintaining cardiac output and tissue perfusion. Many athletes have a heart rate of less than 60 bpm. Aging affects cardiac rhythm as well.

Regardless of cause, a dysrhythmia can significantly affect cardiac output, depending on heart muscle health. The patient's response to the dysrhythmia is key in determining the urgency and type of treatment needed. Treat the patient, not the monitor.

Physiology Review

The unique properties of cardiac cells allow effective heart function. Four properties are electrical; the fifth is the cardiac muscle's mechanical response to electrical stimulation.

- ***Automaticity*** is the ability of pacemaker cells to spontaneously initiate an electrical impulse (action potential). The sinoatrial (SA) node (also called the *sinus node*) is the dominant pacemaker, generating impulses at 60 to 100 times a minute. Myocardial muscle cells do not possess this ability.
- ***Excitability*** is the ability of myocardial cells to respond to stimuli generated by pacemaker cells.
- ***Conductivity*** is the ability to transmit an impulse from cell to cell. When one cell is stimulated, the impulse spreads rapidly throughout the heart muscle.
- ***Refractoriness*** is the inability of cardiac cells to respond to additional stimuli immediately following depolarization. In the absolute refractory period, depolarization will not occur in response to any stimulus. A stronger than normal stimulus is required to initiate depolarization during the relative refractory period. This is followed by the supernormal period, during which a mild stimulus will cause depolarization.
- ***Contractility*** is the ability of myocardial fibers to shorten in response to a stimulus. Heart muscle responds in an all-or-nothing manner: Stimulation of one muscle fiber causes the entire muscle mass to contract to its fullest extent as one unit.

Electrical activity of the heart is normally controlled by the cardiac conduction system (refer to Figure 29.7). The SA node, the primary pacemaker of the heart, usually generates impulses at a regular rate of 60 to 100 bpm. The impulse spreads through the atria, is briefly delayed at the AV node, and then spreads through conduction pathways of the ventricles and to ventricular muscle. The AV nodal delay allows the atria to contract, delivering an extra bolus of blood to the ventricles before they contract (the **atrial kick**). The AV node also controls the number of impulses that reach the ventricles, preventing extremely rapid heart rates.

Pathophysiology

Dysrhythmias arise through disruption of the very properties that stimulate and control the heartbeat: Automaticity, excitability, conductivity, and refractoriness.

Dysrhythmias due to altered impulse formation include changes in rate and rhythm and the development of ectopic beats. This category includes *tachydysrhythmias* (rapid heart rates), *bradydysrhythmias* (slow heart rates), and ectopic rhythms. These dysrhythmias result from a change in the automaticity of cardiac cells. The rate of impulse formation may abnormally increase or decrease. Aberrant (abnormal) impulses may originate outside normal conduction pathways, causing **ectopic beats**. Ectopic beats interrupt the normal conduction sequence and may not initiate a normal muscle contraction. Depending on the site and timing of abnormal impulses, they may have little effect on the patient or may pose a significant threat.

Ischemia, injury, and infarction of myocardial tissue affect its excitability and ability to conduct and respond to an electrical stimulus. Conduction abnormalities cause varying degrees of **heart block**, a block in the normal conduction pathways. Myocardial injury or infarction can obstruct or delay impulse conduction. Bundle branch blocks are common in acute myocardial infarction.

The *reentry phenomenon*, the occurrence of normal and slow conduction, is a major cause of tachydysrhythmias. A stimulus such as an ectopic beat triggers the reentry phenomenon. The impulse is delayed in one area of the heart (e.g., an area of ischemia or injury), but conducted normally through the rest. Muscle that has been depolarized by the normally conducted impulse is repolarized by the time the impulse traveling through the area of slow conduction reaches it, thus initiating another cycle of depolarization (Sorenson et al., 2019). The result is a dysrhythmia that propagates itself.

Several forms of reentry may occur. The impulse may travel through a set pathway to reenter repolarized tissue. Many atrial dysrhythmias follow this pattern, including atrial flutter. In functional reentry, local differences in the conduction of an impulse interrupt the normal wave of depolarization, sending it back on itself in a spiral pattern and setting up a permanent rotation. This type of pattern suppresses normal pacemaker activity and can lead to atrial fibrillation (Sorenson et al., 2019).

Cardiac rhythms are classified according to the site of impulse formation or the site and degree of conduction block. *Supraventricular rhythms* arise above the ventricles. These rhythms usually produce a QRS complex within the normal range. Sinus rhythms, atrial rhythms, and junctional (arising from the AV junction) rhythms are all supraventricular rhythms. *Ventricular rhythms* originate in the ventricles and may prove fatal if left untreated. *AV conduction blocks* result from a defect in impulse transmission from the atria to the ventricles. The major normal and abnormal cardiac rhythms are summarized in **Table 30.5**.

Table 30.5 Characteristics of Selected Cardiac Rhythms and Dysrhythmias

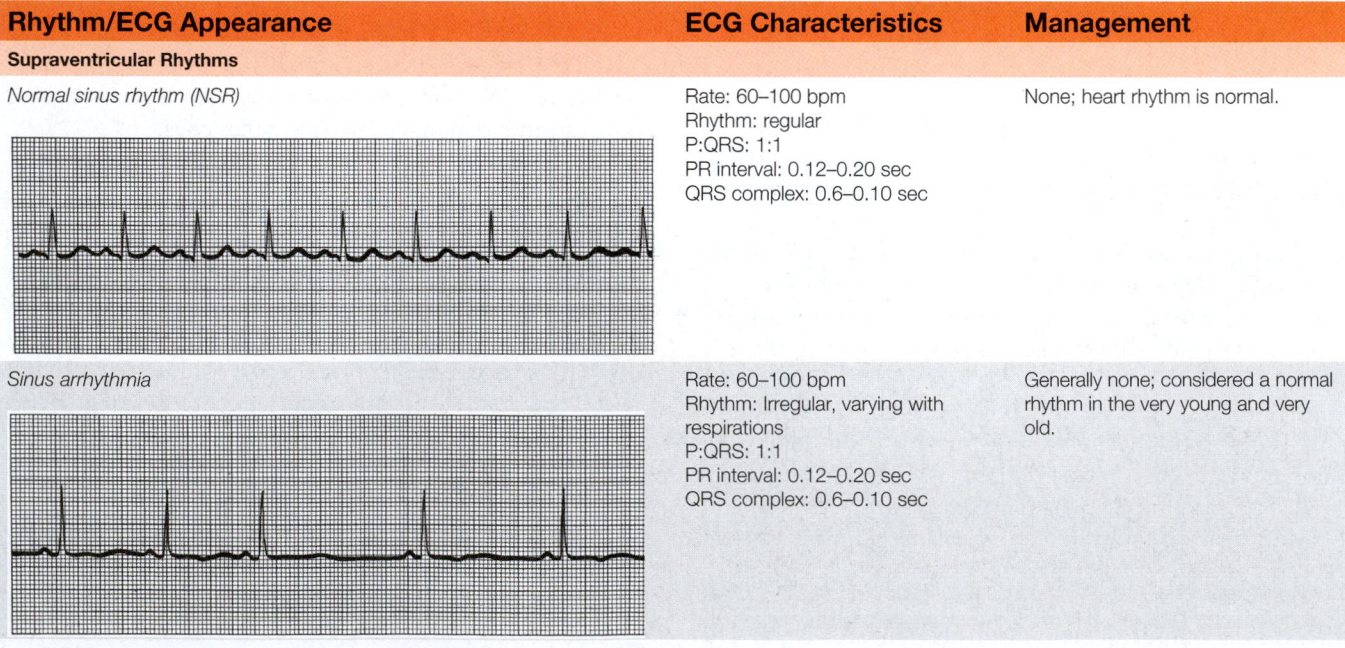

Rhythm/ECG Appearance	ECG Characteristics	Management
Supraventricular Rhythms		
Normal sinus rhythm (NSR) 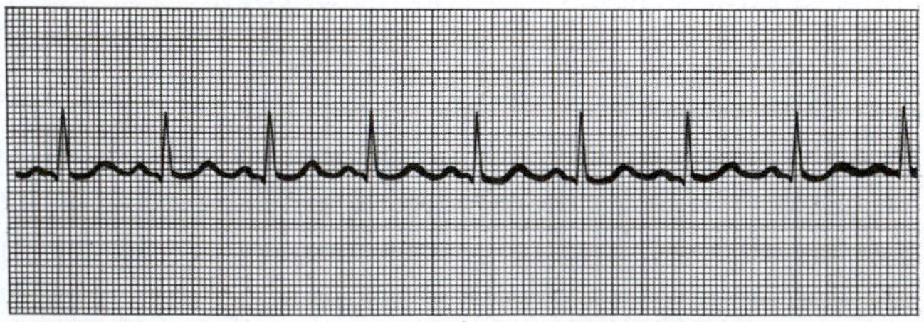	Rate: 60–100 bpm Rhythm: regular P:QRS: 1:1 PR interval: 0.12–0.20 sec QRS complex: 0.6–0.10 sec	None; heart rhythm is normal.
Sinus arrhythmia 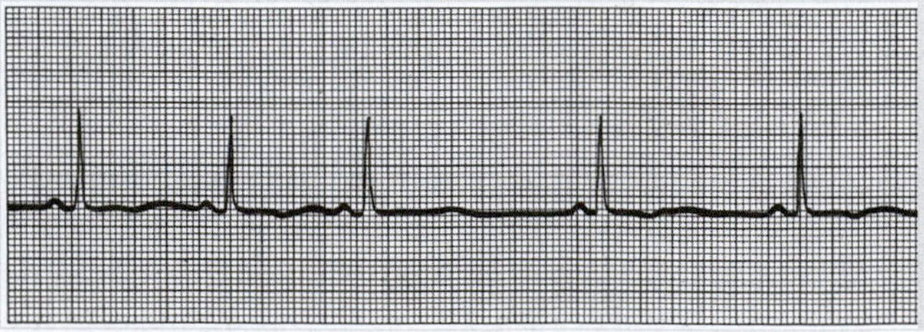	Rate: 60–100 bpm Rhythm: Irregular, varying with respirations P:QRS: 1:1 PR interval: 0.12–0.20 sec QRS complex: 0.6–0.10 sec	Generally none; considered a normal rhythm in the very young and very old.

Rhythm/ECG Appearance	ECG Characteristics	Management
Sinus tachycardia 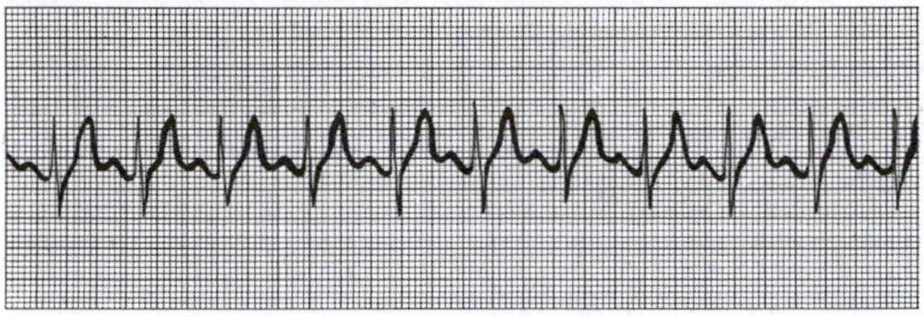	Rate: 101–150 bpm Rhythm: Regular P:QRS: 1:1 (With very fast rates, P wave may be hidden in preceding T wave.) PR interval: 0.12–0.20 sec QRS complex: 0.6–0.10 sec	Treated only if symptomatic or patient is at risk for myocardial damage. Treat underlying cause (e.g., hypovolemia, fever, pain). Beta-blockers or verapamil may be used.
Sinus bradycardia 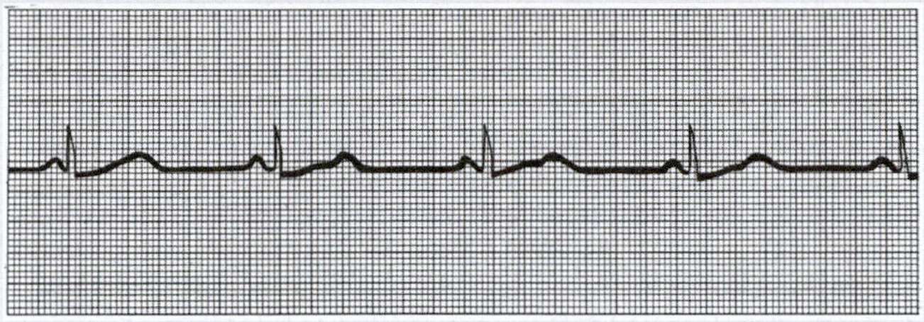	Rate: < 60 bpm Rhythm: regular P:QRS: 1:1 PR interval: 0.12–0.20 sec QRS complex: 0.6–0.10 sec	Treated only if symptomatic. Intravenous atropine or isoproterenol and/or pacemaker therapy may be used.
Premature atrial contractions (PACs) 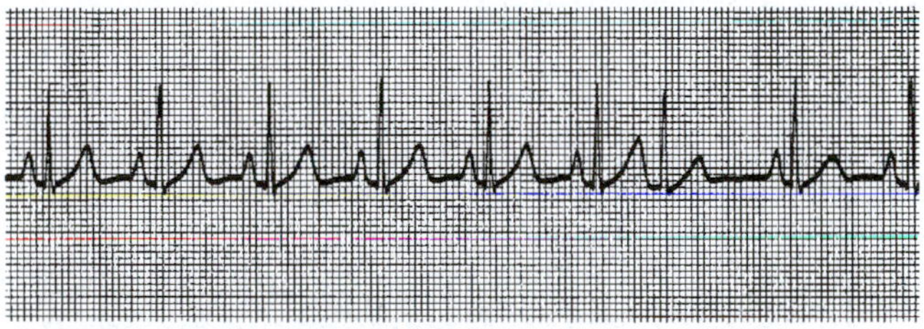	Rate: Variable Rhythm: Irregular, with normal rhythm interrupted by early beats arising in the atria P:QRS: 1:1 PR interval: 0.12–0.20 sec, but may be prolonged QRS complex: 0.6–0.10 sec	Usually require no treatment. Advise to reduce alcohol and caffeine intake, to reduce stress, and to stop smoking. Beta-blocker may be prescribed.
Paroxysmal supraventricular tachycardia (PSVT) 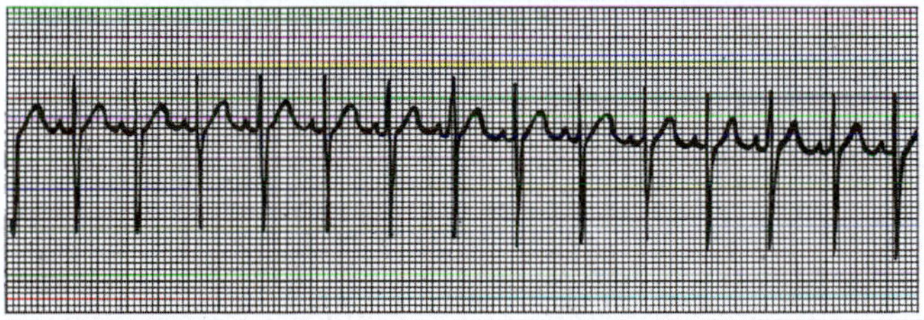	Rate: 100–280 bpm (usually 150–200 bpm) Rhythm: Regular P:QRS: P waves often not identifiable PR interval: Not measured QRS complex: 0.6–0.10 sec	Treat if symptomatic. Treatment may include vagal maneuvers (Valsalva, carotid sinus massage); oxygen therapy; adenosine or a beta-blocker; temporary pacing, or synchronized cardioversion.
Atrial flutter 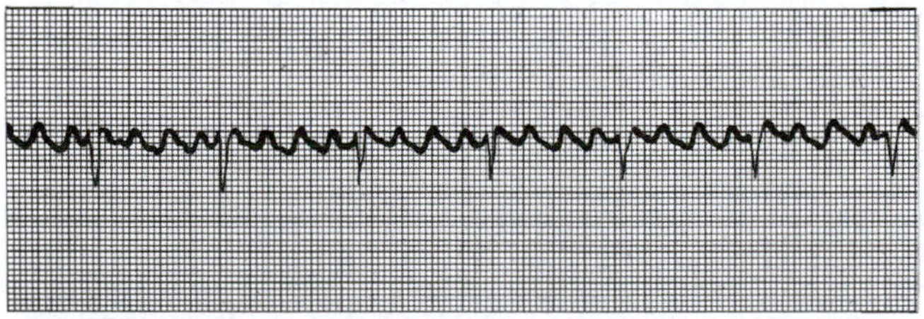	Rate: Atrial 240–360 bpm; ventricular rate depends on degree of AV block and usually is < 150 bpm Rhythm: Atrial regular; ventricular usually regular P:QRS: 2:1, 4:1, 6:1; may vary PR interval: Not measured QRS complex: 0.6–0.10 sec	Synchronized cardioversion; medications to slow ventricular response such as a beta-blocker or calcium channel blocker, followed by a Class I antidysrhythmic agent or amiodarone.
Atrial fibrillation 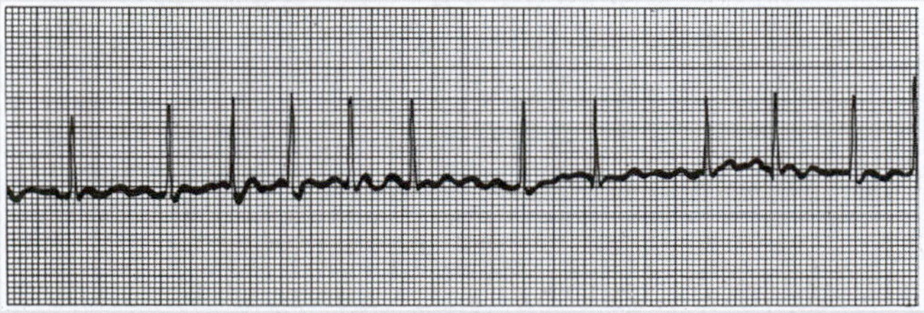	Rate: Atrial 300–600 bpm (too rapid to count); ventricular 100–180 bpm in untreated patients Rhythm: Irregularly irregular P:QRS: Variable PR interval: Not measured QRS complex: 0.06–0.10 sec	Synchronized cardioversion; medications to reduce ventricular response rate: Metoprolol, diltiazem, or digoxin; anticoagulant therapy to reduce risk of clot formation and stroke.

(continued)

Table 30.5 Characteristics of Selected Cardiac Rhythms and Dysrhythmias (*continued*)

Rhythm/ECG Appearance	ECG Characteristics	Management
Junctional escape rhythm 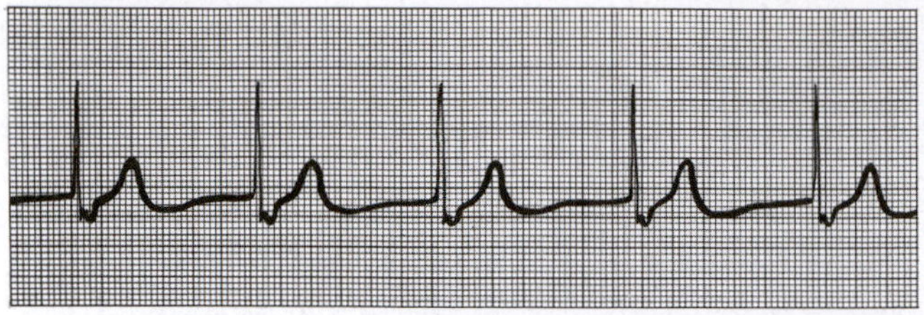	Rate: 40–60 bpm; junctional tachycardia 60–140 bpm Rhythm: Regular P:QRS: P waves may be absent, inverted, and immediately preceding or succeeding QRS complex or hidden in QRS complex. PR interval: < 0.10 sec QRS complex: 0.06–0.10 sec	Treat cause if symptomatic.
Ventricular Rhythms		
Premature ventricular contractions (PVCs) 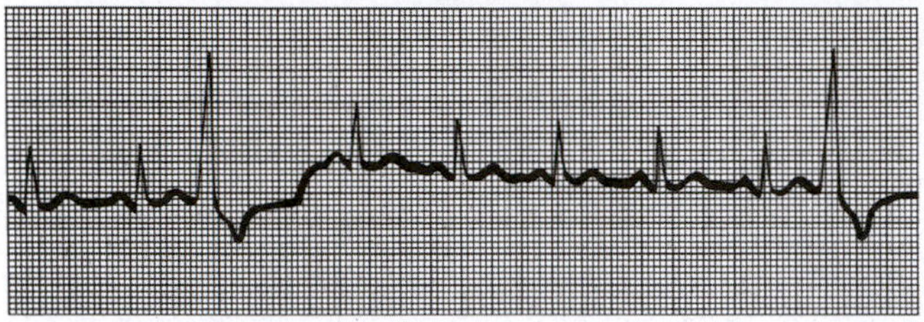	Rate: Variable Rhythm: Irregular, with PVC interrupting underlying rhythm and followed by a compensatory pause P:QRS: No P wave noted before PVC PR interval: Absent with PVC QRS complex: Wide (> 0.12 sec) and bizarre in appearance; differs from normal QRS complex	Treat if symptomatic or in presence of severe heart disease. Advise against stimulant use (caffeine, nicotine). Beta-blockers or Class I or III antidysrhythmic agents (see Medication Administration 30.D) may be used for patients with severe heart disease who are symptomatic.
Ventricular tachycardia (VT or V tach) 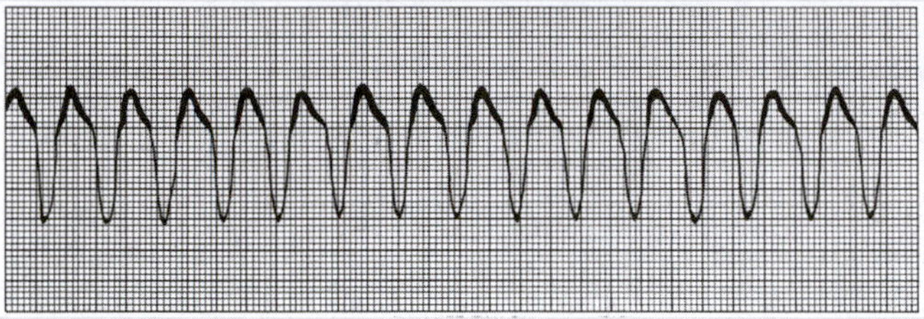	Rate: 100–250 bpm Rhythm: Regular P:QRS: P waves usually not identifiable PR interval: Not measured QRS complex: 0.12 sec or greater; bizarre shape	Treat if VT is sustained, symptomatic, or associated with organic heart disease. Treatment includes DC cardioversion or intravenous procainamide, lidocaine, or a Class III antidysrhythmic agent if hemodynamic instability is present. Surgical ablation or antitachycardia pacing with an implanted cardioverter/defibrillator (ICD) is used for repeated episodes.
Ventricular fibrillation (VF, V fib) 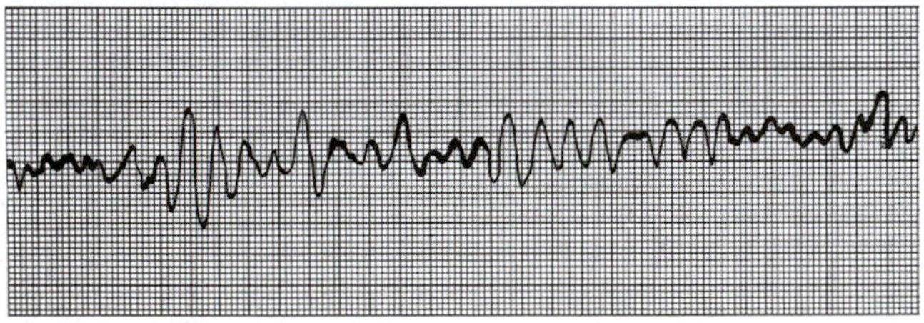	Rate: Too rapid to count Rhythm: Grossly irregular P:QRS: No identifiable P waves PR interval: None QRS: Bizarre, varying in shape and direction	Immediate defibrillation.
Atrioventricular Conduction Blocks		
First-degree AV block 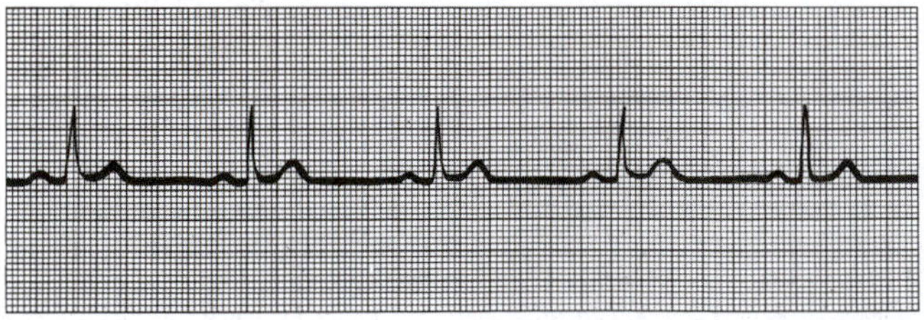	Rate: Usually 60–100 bpm Rhythm: Regular P:QRS: 1:1 PR interval: > 0.21 sec QRS complex: 0.06–0.10 sec	None required.

Rhythm/ECG Appearance	ECG Characteristics	Management
Second-degree AV block, type I (Mobitz I, Wenckebach) 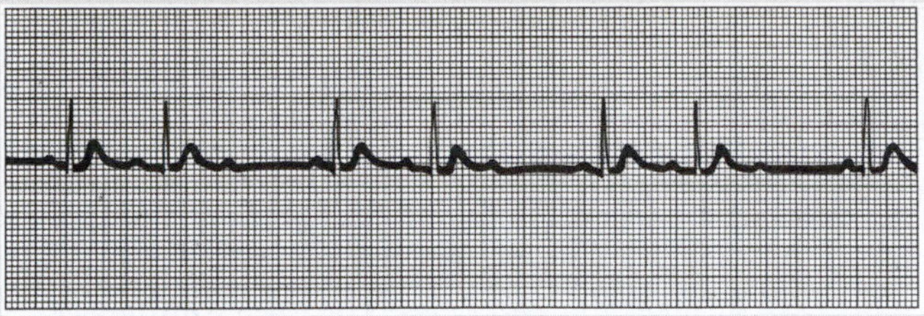	Rate: 60–100 bpm Rhythm: Atrial regular; ventricular irregular P:QRS: 1:1 until P wave blocked with no subsequent QRS complex PR interval: Progressively lengthens in a regular pattern QRS complex: 0.06–0.10 sec; sudden absence of QRS complex	Monitoring and observation; rarely progresses to a higher degree of block or requires treatment.
Second-degree AV block, type II (Mobitz II) 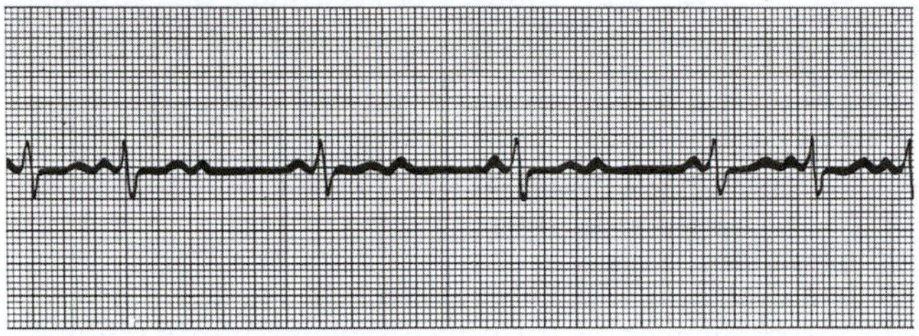	Rate: Atrial 60–100 bpm; ventricular < 60 bpm Rhythm: Atrial regular; ventricular irregular P:QRS: Typically 2:1, may vary PR interval: Constant PR interval for each conducted QRS complex QRS complex: 0.06–0.10 sec	Atropine or isoproterenol; pacemaker therapy.
Third-degree AV block (complete heart block) 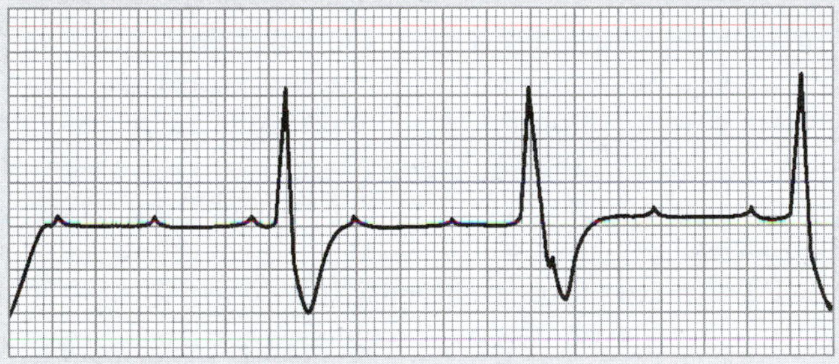	Rate: Atrial 60–100 bpm; ventricular 15–60 bpm Rhythm: Atrial regular; ventricular regular P:QRS: No relationship between P waves and QRS complexes; independent rhythms PR interval: Not measured QRS complex: 0.06–0.10 sec if junctional escape rhythm; > 0.12 sec if ventricular escape rhythm	Immediate pacemaker therapy.

Supraventricular Rhythms

Normal Sinus Rhythm. *Normal sinus rhythm (NSR)* is the normal heart rhythm, in which impulses originate in the SA node and travel through all normal conduction pathways without delay. All waveforms are of normal configuration, look alike, and have consistent (fixed) durations. The rate is between 60 and 100 bpm.

Sinus Node Dysrhythmias. *Sinus node dysrhythmias* may occur as a normal compensatory response (e.g., to exercise) or because of altered automaticity. In these rhythms, as in NSR, the initiating impulse is from the sinus node. They differ from NSR in rate or regularity of the rhythm. Sinus dysrhythmias include sinus arrhythmia, sinus tachycardia, and sinus bradycardia.

Sinus Arrhythmia. *Sinus arrhythmia* is a sinus rhythm in which the rate varies with respirations, causing an irregular rhythm. The rate increases during inspiration and decreases with expiration. Sinus arrhythmia is common in the very young and the very old. It can be caused by an increase in vagal tone, by digitalis toxicity, or by morphine administration.

Sinus Tachycardia. *Sinus tachycardia* has all of the characteristics of NSR, except that the rate is greater than 100 bpm. Tachycardia arises from enhanced automaticity in response to changes in the internal environment. SNS stimulation or blocked vagal (parasympathetic) activity increases the heart rate. Tachycardia is a normal response to any condition or event that increases the body's demand for oxygen and nutrients, such as exercise or hypoxia. In the patient on bed-rest, tachycardia is an ominous sign. Sinus tachycardia may be an early sign of cardiac dysfunction, such as heart failure. Tachycardia is detrimental in patients with cardiac disease because it increases cardiac workload and oxygen use.

Common causes of sinus tachycardia include exercise, excitement, anxiety, pain, fever, hypoxia, hypovolemia, anemia, hyperthyroidism, myocardial infarction, heart failure, cardiogenic shock, pulmonary embolism, caffeine intake, and certain drugs, such as atropine, epinephrine (Adrenalin), or isoproterenol (Isuprel).

Manifestations of sinus tachycardia include a rapid pulse rate. The patient may complain of feeling that the heart is racing, shortness of breath, and dizziness. In the presence of heart disease, sinus tachycardia may precipitate chest pain.

Sinus Bradycardia. *Sinus bradycardia* has all of the characteristics of NSR, but the rate is less than 60 bpm. Sinus bradycardia may result from increased vagal (parasympathetic) activity or from depressed automaticity due to injury or ischemia to the sinus node. Sinus bradycardia may be normal (e.g., in patients with athletic heart syndrome). The heart rate normally slows during sleep because the parasympathetic nervous system is dominant at this time. Other causes of sinus bradycardia include pain, increased intracranial pressure, sinus node disease, acute myocardial infarction (especially with inferior wall damage), hypothermia, acidosis, and certain drugs.

Sinus bradycardia may be asymptomatic; it is important to assess the patient before treating the rhythm. Manifestations of decreased cardiac output, such as decreased level of consciousness, syncope (faintness), or hypotension, indicate a need for intervention.

Sick Sinus Syndrome. *Sick sinus syndrome (SSS)* results from SA node disease or dysfunction that causes problems with impulse formation, transmission, and conduction. Sick sinus syndrome is often found in older adults. It may be caused by direct injury to sinus tissue, fibrosis of conduction fibers associated with aging, and such drugs as digitalis, beta-blockers, and calcium channel blockers.

ECG characteristics of SSS include sinus bradycardia, sinus arrhythmia, sinus pauses or arrest, and atrial tachydysrhythmias such as atrial fibrillation, atrial flutter, or atrial tachycardia. Bradycardia-tachycardia syndrome, characterized either by **paroxysmal** (abrupt onset and termination) atrial tachycardia followed by prolonged sinus pauses or alternating periods of bradycardia and tachycardia, also may indicate sinus node dysfunction.

Manifestations of sinus node dysfunction are often intermittent, related to a drop in cardiac output caused by the irregular rhythm. Fatigue, dizziness, light-headedness, and syncope are common. The heart rate may not increase in response to stressors such as exercise or fever.

Supraventricular Dysrhythmias

When an action potential originates in atrial tissue outside the sinus node, the resulting rhythm is classified as a *supraventricular rhythm*. In these dysrhythmias, an ectopic pacemaker takes over, or overrides, the SA node. They may occur when the SA node fails; an *escape rhythm* develops as a fail-safe mechanism to maintain the heart rate. The most common supraventricular dysrhythmias are premature atrial contractions, paroxysmal supraventricular tachycardia, atrial flutter, and atrial fibrillation. These rhythms may be paroxysmal; that is, they may occur in bursts with an abrupt beginning and end.

Premature Atrial Contractions. A *premature atrial contraction (PAC)* is an ectopic atrial beat that occurs earlier than the next expected sinus beat. PACs can arise anywhere in the atria. They are usually asymptomatic and benign, but they may initiate paroxysmal supraventricular tachycardia in susceptible individuals. PACs are common in older adults, often occurring without an obvious cause. Strong emotions, excessive alcohol intake, tobacco, and stimulants such as caffeine can precipitate PACs. They also may be associated with MI, heart failure and other cardiac disorders, hypoxemia, pulmonary embolism, digitalis toxicity, and electrolyte or acid–base imbalances. In patients with underlying heart disease, PACs may precede a more serious dysrhythmia.

The ECG tracing shows interruption of the underlying rhythm by a premature complex that looks similar to the underlying beats. The ectopic impulse of the PAC is usually conducted normally, leading to depolarization of cardiac muscle and a normal QRS complex. Because the impulse arises above the ventricles, it follows normal conduction pathways through the ventricles. The QRS complex is narrow or matches those of the underlying rhythm. The shape of the P wave of a PAC differs from normal P waves because its impulse arises outside the sinus node. A *noncompensatory pause* usually follows, as the PAC resets the SA node rhythm. Occasionally, the ectopic impulse may not be conducted through the heart, resulting in a lone P wave without a QRS or a nonconducted PAC.

PACs cause few manifestations. If frequent, they may cause palpitations or a fluttering sensation in the chest. Early beats may be noted on auscultating or palpating the pulse.

Paroxysmal Supraventricular Tachycardia. *Paroxysmal supraventricular tachycardia (PSVT)* is tachycardia of sudden onset and termination. PSVT is usually initiated by a reentry loop in or around the AV node; that is, an impulse reenters the same section of tissue over and over, causing repeated depolarizations.

PSVT occurs more frequently in women. Sympathetic nervous system stimulation and stressors such as fever, sepsis, and hyperthyroidism may precipitate PSVT. It also may be associated with heart diseases such as CHD, MI, rheumatic heart disease, myocarditis, or acute pericarditis. Abnormal conduction pathways associated with Wolff-Parkinson-White (WPW) or Lown-Ganong-Levine (LGL) may account for PSVT.

PSVT affects ventricular filling and cardiac output and decreases coronary artery perfusion. Its manifestations include complaints of palpitations and a racing heart, anxiety, dizziness, dyspnea, anginal pain, diaphoresis, extreme fatigue, and polyuria (urine output may reach up to 3 L in the first few hours after PSVT onset).

Atrial Flutter. *Atrial flutter* is a rapid and regular atrial rhythm thought to result from an intra-atrial reentry mechanism. Causes include sympathetic nervous system stimulation due to anxiety, caffeine and alcohol intake, thyrotoxicosis, CHD, or MI; pulmonary embolism; and abnormal conduction syndromes such as WPW or LGL syndromes. Older individuals with rheumatic heart disease and/or valvular disease are especially vulnerable.

Two types of atrial flutter have been identified. Type I atrial flutter has an atrial rate of 240 to 340 bpm. It develops due to a reentry mechanism in the right atrium. The mechanism leading to type II atrial flutter has not been identified. In this type of flutter, the atrial rate is faster, 350 to 350 bpm.

Patients with atrial flutter may complain of palpitations or a fluttering sensation in the chest or throat. If the ventricular rate is rapid, manifestations of decreased cardiac output—such as decreased level of consciousness, hypotension, decreased urinary output, and cool, clammy skin—may be noted. The atrial kick (additional ventricular filling with atrial contraction) is lost because of inadequate atrial filling.

ECG characteristics include what is commonly called a *sawtooth* or *picket fence* appearance of P waves, which are labeled flutter (F) waves. The atrial rate is rapid, often around 300 bpm. As a protective mechanism, many impulses are blocked at the AV node, and the ventricular rate is rarely greater than 150 to 170 bpm. Usually, atrial impulses are evenly conducted through the AV node, for example, two impulses to one QRS complex (2:1), four impulses to one QRS complex (4:1), or six impulses to one QRS complex (6:1). A constant conduction ratio results in a regular ventricular rhythm; the ventricular rhythm is irregular if the conduction ratio varies. The ventricular rate usually ranges from 150 to 170 bpm in 2:1 conduction and 60 to 75 bpm for lower conduction ratios. The T wave is usually hidden by overriding F waves; some F waves may be hidden in the QRS complex.

Atrial Fibrillation. *Atrial fibrillation* is a common dysrhythmia characterized by disorganized atrial activity without discrete atrial contractions. Multiple small reentry circuits develop in the atria. Atrial cells cannot repolarize in time to respond to the next stimulus (Sorenson et al., 2019). Extremely rapid atrial impulses bombard the AV node, resulting in an irregularly irregular ventricular response. Atrial fibrillation may occur suddenly and recur or it may persist as a chronic dysrhythmia. Atrial fibrillation is commonly associated with heart failure, rheumatic heart disease, CHD, hypertension, and hyperthyroidism.

Manifestations of atrial fibrillation relate to the rate of the ventricular response. With rapid response rates, manifestations of decreased cardiac output such as hypotension, shortness of breath, fatigue, and angina may develop. Patients with extensive heart disease may develop syncope or heart failure. Peripheral pulses are irregular and of variable amplitude (strength).

The specific ECG characteristics of atrial fibrillation include an irregularly irregular rhythm and the absence of identifiable P waves. The atrial rate is so rapid that it is not measurable. The ventricular rate varies.

Atrial fibrillation increases the risk for formation of thromboemboli. Organ infarction may occur as a result; the incidence of stroke is high.

Junctional Dysrhythmias

Rhythms that originate in AV nodal tissue are termed *junctional*. The AV junction includes the AV node and the bundle of His, which branches into the right and left bundle branches. An impulse arising from the AV junction may occur in response to failure of higher pacemakers, as in a *junctional escape rhythm*, or it may result from an abnormal mechanism, such as altered automaticity. An impulse arising from the AV junction may or may not be conducted back up to the atria. This conduction against the normal flow or pattern is called *retrograde conduction*. The resulting atrial wave, called a *P′ wave*, may be found before, during, or after the QRS complex, depending on the speed of conduction. The P′ wave is inverted in some ECG leads because the impulse moves from the AV node up to the atria instead of from the SA node down toward the AV node. In addition, the P′R interval is shorter than normal (< 0.12 second). The QRS complex is typically narrow.

A junctional rhythm may be due to drug toxicity (e.g., digitalis, beta-blockers, or calcium channel blockers), or other causes such as hypoxemia, hyperkalemia, increased vagal tone or damage to the AV node, MI, and heart failure. Loss of synchronized atrial contraction and the atrial kick may affect cardiac output, leading to manifestations of decreased cardiac output and impaired myocardial tissue perfusion. Heart failure may develop.

Premature junctional contractions (PJCs) occur before the next expected beat of the underlying rhythm. Isolated PJCs may occur in healthy people and are insignificant. *Junctional tachycardia* is a junctional rhythm with a rate greater than 60 bpm. It is caused by increased automaticity of AV nodal tissue. The ventricular rate is usually less than 140 bpm. Both rhythms are most commonly associated with digitalis toxicity, hypoxia, ischemia, or electrolyte imbalances.

Ventricular Dysrhythmias

Ventricular dysrhythmias originate in the ventricles. Because the ventricles pump blood into the pulmonary and systemic vasculature, any disruption of their rhythm affects cardiac output and tissue perfusion. A wide and bizarre QRS complex (> 0.12 second) is a characteristic feature of ventricular dysrhythmias. This occurs because ventricular ectopic impulses begin and travel outside normal conduction pathways. Other characteristics include no relationship of the QRS complex to a P wave, increased amplitude of the QRS complex, an abnormal ST segment, and a T wave deflected in the opposite direction from the QRS complex.

Premature Ventricular Contractions. *Premature ventricular contractions (PVCs)* are ectopic ventricular beats that occur before the next expected beat of the underlying rhythm. They usually do not reset the atrial rhythm and are followed by a full compensatory pause. PVCs often have no significance in people without heart disease. Frequent, recurrent, or multifocal PVCs may be associated with an increased risk for lethal dysrhythmias. PVCs result from either enhanced automaticity or a reentry phenomenon. They may be triggered by anxiety or stress; tobacco, alcohol, or caffeine use; hypoxia, acidosis, and electrolyte imbalances; sympathomimetic drugs; coronary heart disease, heart failure, or mechanical stimulation of the heart (e.g., the insertion of a cardiac catheter); or reperfusion after fibrinolytic therapy. The incidence and significance of PVCs is greatest after MI.

PVCs may be isolated or occur in a specific pattern. Two PVCs in a row are called a *couplet* or *paired* PVCs. Three consecutive PVCs (a *triplet* or *salvo*) is a short run of ventricular tachycardia. *Ventricular bigeminy* is characterized by a PVC following each normal beat; a PVC noted every third beat is called *ventricular trigeminy*. When the ventricular impulse arises from one ectopic site, all PVCs look the same (*monomorphic*) and are called *unifocal* PVCs. *Multifocal* PVCs arise from different ectopic sites and appear different from one another on the ECG (*polymorphic*).

The frequency and patterns of PVCs can be indicative of myocardial irritability and the risk for a lethal dysrhythmia. The following are considered warning signs in the patient with acute heart disease (e.g., an acute MI):

- PVCs that develop within the first 4 hours of an MI
- Frequent PVCs (six or more per minute)
- Couplets or triplets
- Multifocal PVCs
- R-on-T phenomenon (PVCs falling on the T wave).

In people without heart disease, isolated PVCs are usually insignificant and do not require treatment. Patients may complain of feeling their hearts skip a beat or of palpitations. In patients with preexisting heart disease, PVCs may indicate drug toxicity or an increased risk for lethal dysrhythmias and cardiac arrest. The risk is greatest following acute MI.

Ventricular Tachycardia. *Ventricular tachycardia (VT, V tach)* is a rapid ventricular rhythm defined as three or more consecutive PVCs. Ventricular tachycardia may occur in short bursts, or runs, or may persist for more than 30 seconds (sustained ventricular tachycardia). The rate is greater than 100 bpm, and the rhythm is usually regular. Reentry is the usual electrophysiologic mechanism responsible for VT. Myocardial ischemia and infarction are the most common predisposing factors for VT. It is also associated with cardiac structural disorders such as valvular disease, rheumatic heart disease, or cardiomyopathy. VT may occur in the absence of heart disease, with anorexia nervosa, metabolic disorders, and drug toxicity.

Nonsustained VT may occur paroxysmally and convert back to an effective rhythm spontaneously. The patient may experience a fluttering sensation in the chest or complain of palpitations and brief shortness of breath. Patients in sustained VT generally develop signs and symptoms of decreased cardiac output and hemodynamic instability, including severe hypotension, a weak or nonpalpable pulse, and loss of consciousness. Allowed to continue, VT can deteriorate into ventricular fibrillation. Sustained ventricular tachycardia is a medical emergency that requires immediate intervention, particularly in patients with cardiac disease.

Torsades de pointes is a type of ventricular tachycardia associated with *long QT syndrome*, a prolongation of the QT interval. Long QT syndrome may be genetic or acquired, occurring secondarily to electrolyte disruptions, MI, cocaine use, liquid protein diets, medications, or other conditions. In torsades de pointes, the QRS complexes vary in size, shape, and amplitude (**Figure 30.7** ■). Patients with torsades de pointes may have multiple bursts or episodes of VT or may develop ventricular fibrillation and sudden cardiac death (Sorenson et al., 2019; Perrin & MacLeod, 2018).

Ventricular Fibrillation. *Ventricular fibrillation (VF, V fib)* is extremely rapid, chaotic ventricular depolarization causing

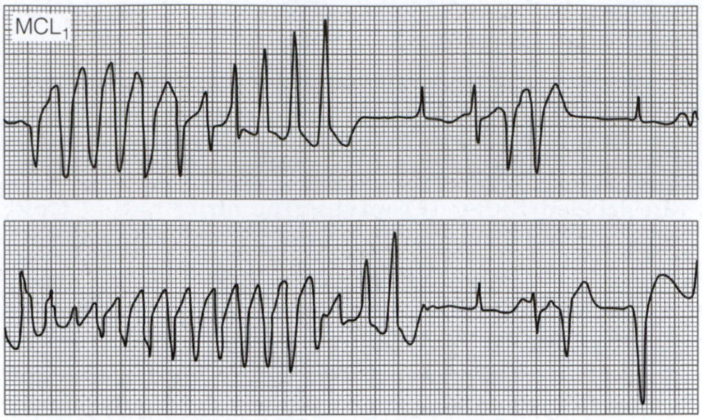
MCL$_1$

Figure 30.7 ■ Torsades de pointes. Note the wide and bizarre QRS complexes of varying size, shape (morphology), and amplitude.

the ventricles to quiver and cease contracting; there is no cardiac output. This is known as **cardiac arrest**; it is a medical emergency requiring immediate intervention with CPR. Death will follow the onset of VF within 4 minutes if the rhythm is not recognized and terminated and an effective perfusing rhythm reestablished.

VF is usually triggered by severe myocardial ischemia or infarction. It occurs without warning 50% of the time. It is the terminal event in many disease processes or traumatic conditions. VF may be precipitated by a single PVC or may follow VT. Other causes of VF include digitalis toxicity, reperfusion therapy, antidysrhythmic drugs, hypokalemia and hyperkalemia, hypothermia, metabolic acidosis, mechanical stimulation (as with the insertion of cardiac catheters or pacing wires), and electric shock.

Clinically, loss of ventricular contractions results in the absence of a palpable or audible pulse. The patient loses consciousness and stops breathing as perfusion ceases. The ECG shows grossly irregular, bizarre complexes with no discernible rate or rhythm.

Atrioventricular Conduction Blocks

Conduction defects that delay or block transmission of the sinus impulse through the AV node are called *atrioventricular (AV) conduction blocks.* Impaired conduction may result from tissue injury or disease, increased vagal (parasympathetic) tone, drug effects, or a congenital defect. AV conduction blocks vary in severity from benign to severe:

- ***First-degree AV block*** = delayed conduction through the AV node and a long PR interval
- ***Second-degree AV block*** = complete blockage of *some* impulses through the AV node; some P waves are not followed by a QRS complex
- ***Third-degree AV block*** = complete blockage of *all* impulses through the AV node; no relationship between P waves and QRS complexes.

First-Degree AV Block. *First-degree AV block* is a benign conduction delay that generally poses no threat, has no symptoms, and requires no treatment. Impulse conduction through the AV node is slowed, but all atrial impulses are conducted to the ventricles. It may result from injury or infarct of the AV node, other cardiac diseases, or drug effects. The ECG shows all characteristics of NSR; however, the PR interval is greater than 0.20 second.

Second-Degree AV Block. *Second-degree AV block* is characterized by failure to conduct one or more impulses from the atria to the ventricles. Two patterns of second-degree AV block are identified: Type I and type II.

- ***Second-Degree AV Block—Type I.*** *Type I second-degree AV block (Mobitz type I or Wenckebach phenomenon)* is characterized by a repeating pattern of increasing AV conduction delays until an impulse fails to conduct to the ventricles. On the ECG, PR intervals progressively lengthen until one QRS complex is not conducted, or dropped. The ventricular rate remains adequate to maintain cardiac output, and the patient is usually asymptomatic. Mobitz type I AV block is usually transient, associated with AMI or drug intoxication (e.g., digitalis, beta-blockers, or calcium channel blockers). It rarely progresses to complete heart block.
- ***Second-Degree AV Block—Type II.*** *Type II second-degree AV block (Mobitz type II)* involves intermittent failure of the AV node to conduct an impulse to the ventricles without preceding delays in conduction. The PR interval remains constant, but not all P waves are followed by QRS complexes (e.g., there may be two P waves for every QRS). Conduction through the His-Purkinje system is usually delayed as well, causing a widened QRS complex. Mobitz type II block is frequently associated with acute anterior wall MI and a high rate of mortality (Sorenson et al., 2019). Manifestations of Mobitz type II block depend on the ventricular rate. Pacemaker therapy may be required to maintain cardiac output.

Third-Degree AV Block. *Third-degree AV block (complete heart block)* occurs when atrial impulses are completely blocked at the AV node and fail to reach the ventricles. As a result, the atria and ventricles are controlled by different and independent pacemakers, with separate rates and rhythms. The ventricular impulse arises from either junctional fibers (with a rate of 40 to 60 bpm) or a ventricular pacemaker at a rate of less than 40 bpm. The width of the QRS complex depends on the location of the escape pacemaker. The QRS is wide and the rate is slow when the rhythm arises distal to the bundle of His.

Third-degree block is frequently associated with an inferior or anteroseptal myocardial infarction. Other causes include congenital conditions, acute or degenerative cardiac disease or damage, drug effects, and electrolyte imbalances. The slow escape rhythm significantly affects cardiac output, causing manifestations such as syncope (known as a *Stokes-Adams attack*), dizziness, fatigue, exercise intolerance, and heart failure. Third-degree AV block is life-threatening and requires immediate intervention to maintain adequate cardiac output.

AV Dissociation. Complete dissociation of atrial and ventricular rhythms can occur in conditions other than third-degree AV block. The two primary factors leading to AV dissociation are severe sinus bradycardia and a slower pacemaker (junctional or ventricular) that competes with or exceeds the normal sinus rhythm. AV dissociation may result from acute myocardial ischemia or infarction, cardiac surgery, or drug effects. The ECG shows separate and competing atrial (P waves) and ventricular (QRS complexes) rhythms.

Intraventricular Conduction Blocks

Once the impulse enters the ventricles, its conduction through the right and left bundle branches may be impaired (*bundle branch block*). As a result, the impulse is conducted more slowly than normal through the ventricles. On the ECG, the QRS complex is prolonged. Its appearance varies, depending on the affected bundle (right or left). Typically, no clinical manifestations are associated with bundle branch block unless it occurs in conjunction with an AV block.

Interprofessional Care

Cardiac dysrhythmias may be either benign or critical: Recognizing lethal dysrhythmias is a matter of life and death. Major goals of care include identifying the dysrhythmia, evaluating its effect on physical and psychosocial well-being, and treating underlying causes. This may involve correcting fluid and electrolyte or acid–base imbalances; treating hypoxia, pain, or anxiety; administering antidysrhythmic medications; or mechanical and surgical interventions.

Diagnosis

Diagnostic tests for dysrhythmias include the electrocardiogram, cardiac monitoring, and electrophysiology studies. Laboratory tests such as serum electrolytes, drug levels, and arterial blood gases may be done to help identify the cause of the dysrhythmia (Kee, 2014).

Electrocardiography. The 12-lead ECG may be required to accurately diagnose a dysrhythmia. It also provides information about underlying disease processes, such as MI or other cardiac disease. The ECG may also be used to monitor the effects of treatment. Refer to Chapter 29 for more information about the 12-lead ECG.

Cardiac Monitoring. Cardiac monitoring allows continuous observation of the cardiac rhythm. It is used in many different circumstances (**Box 30.6**). Different types of ECG monitoring are employed for different situations.

Continuous Cardiac Monitoring. Continuous monitoring of the cardiac rhythm is provided by bedside and central monitoring stations. Electrodes placed on the patient's chest attach to cables connected to a monitor. The heart rate and rhythm are displayed visually on a bedside monitor connected to a central monitoring station. The central station allows simultaneous monitoring of multiple patients within a nursing unit. Alarms on both bedside and central monitors warn of potential problems such as very rapid or very slow heart rates. Alarm limits are preset by the nurse for the individual patient.

BOX 30.6
Indications for Cardiac Monitoring

- Perioperative monitoring of heart rate and rhythm
- Detecting and identifying dysrhythmias
- Monitoring the effects of cardiac and noncardiac diseases on the heart
- Monitoring patients with potentially life-threatening conditions:
  - a. Major trauma (especially cardiac trauma)
  - b. Dissecting aneurysm
  - c. Acute myocardial infarction
  - d. Heart failure
  - e. Shock
  - f. Other emergency conditions
- Evaluating responses to procedures and interventions:
  - a. Drug therapies
  - b. Diagnostic procedures
  - c. Ablative techniques
  - d. Angioplasty or cardiac catheterization
  - e. Cardiac surgery
  - f. Pacemaker function
  - g. Automatic implantable cardioverter/defibrillator function

Telemetry may be used in acute care settings when the patient is ambulatory. Chest electrodes are connected to a portable transmitter worn around the neck or waist; the ECG is transmitted electronically to a central monitoring station for continuous monitoring.

Home Monitoring. Patients often complain of palpitations or other heart symptoms but are asymptomatic during evaluation in a hospital or community-based setting. Ambulatory or Holter monitoring may be used to identify intermittent dysrhythmias, to detect silent ischemia, to monitor the effects of treatment, and to assess pacemaker or automatic cardioverter/defibrillator function. Electrodes are applied and the leads attached to the portable telemetry monitor that records and stores all electrical activity. Patients are instructed to leave the electrode pads in place during monitoring and record any cardiac symptoms or events in a journal (such as chest pain, palpitations, syncope) and are told when to return to the clinic. After the prescribed period, usually 48 to 72 hours, the patient returns and the monitor is removed. Diary entries are compared to the recorded heart rhythms to identify the effects of dysrhythmias.

Electrophysiology Studies. Diagnostic cardiac *electrophysiology (EP) procedures* are used to identify dysrhythmias and their causes. EP studies are used to analyze components of the conduction system, identify sites of ectopic stimulation, and evaluate the effectiveness of treatment. EP procedures can be used for both diagnosis and as a therapeutic intervention.

In the electrophysiology laboratory, electrode catheters are guided by fluoroscopy into the heart through the femoral or brachial vein. The timing and sequence of electrical activation during normal and abnormal (aberrant) rhythms is observed and measured. Electrical stimulation may be used to induce dysrhythmias similar to the patient's clinical dysrhythmia. Following diagnosis, an EP procedure may be used to treat the dysrhythmia, for example, by overdrive pacing (stimulating the patient's heart rate to a rate faster than that of the tachydysrhythmia) to break the dysrhythmia's cycle or to perform ablative therapy to destroy the ectopic site. See the section on ablative techniques for further information.

Nursing care for the patient undergoing an EP procedure is similar to that for a coronary angiogram (refer to the Box 30.3). The procedure and expected sensations are explained. The patient remains awake during the procedure; antianxiety medications or sedatives are given to reduce apprehension. Intravenous heparin may be given during the procedure to reduce the risk of thromboembolism.

Complications of EP procedures are infrequent, but include fatal ventricular fibrillation, cardiac perforation, and major venous thrombosis. Careful post procedure monitoring is vital.

Medications

The goal of drug therapy is to suppress dysrhythmia formation. No drug has been found to be completely safe and effective. Antidysrhythmic drugs are primarily used for acute treatment of dysrhythmias, although they may also be used to manage chronic conditions. The overall goal of therapy is to maintain an effective cardiac output by stabilizing cardiac rhythm.

It is important to remember that virtually all antidysrhythmic drugs also have *prodysrhythmic* effects; that is, they can worsen existing dysrhythmias and precipitate new ones. Antidysrhythmic medications are used sparingly because of this tendency and because of studies that demonstrate higher mortality rates in patients receiving antidysrhythmic medications and the increasing safety and availability of interventional techniques.

Most antidysrhythmic drugs are classified by their effects on the cardiac action potential. Most are Class I drugs, or fast sodium channel blockers. By blocking sodium channels, these drugs slow impulse conduction in the atria and ventricles. This class is further divided into subclasses A, B, and C. Class II drugs are beta-blockers, which decrease SA node automaticity, AV conduction velocity, and myocardial contractility. Class III agents block potassium channels, delaying repolarization, and prolonging the relative refractory period. Class IV drugs are calcium channel blockers. Their effect is similar to that of beta-blockers. Adenosine and digoxin do not fit within the major classes. Both drugs reduce SA node automaticity and slow AV conduction. Ibutilide and magnesium also fall outside the major classes, but are used to treat dysrhythmias. **Medication Administration 30.D** outlines common antidysrhythmic drugs within each class and the nursing implications in caring for patients receiving these drugs.

Drugs that affect the autonomic nervous system may also be used to treat dysrhythmias. Sympathomimetics, such as epinephrine, stimulate the heart, increasing both heart rate and contractility. Anticholinergic agents such as atropine are used to decrease vagal tone and increase the heart rate. Magnesium

Medication Administration 30.D

Antidysrhythmic Drugs

CLASS I DRUGS: SODIUM CHANNEL BLOCKERS

Class IA

disopyramide (Norpace, Norpace CR)

procainamide (Pronestyl, Procan SR)

quinidine (Cardioquin, Quinidex, Quinaglute)

Class IA drugs decrease the flow of sodium into the cell and prolong the action potential. This decreases automaticity, slows the rate of impulse conduction, and prolongs refractiveness. They are used to treat both supraventricular and ventricular tachycardias.

Class IB

lidocaine (Xylocaine)

mexiletine (Mexitil)

phenytoin (Dilantin)

tocainide (Tonocard)

Class IB, or lidocaine-like, drugs decrease the refractory period but have little effect on automaticity. Drugs in this class are used primarily to treat ventricular dysrhythmias, including PVCs and ventricular tachycardia.

Class IC

flecainide (Tambocor)

propafenone (Rythmol)

Class IC drugs slow impulse conduction velocity but have little effect on refractoriness. They are used to reduce or eliminate tachydysrhythmias associated with reentry. Their significant prodysrhythmic effects limit their usefulness, but they may be used to treat supraventricular tachycardia.

CLASS II DRUGS: BETA-BLOCKERS

atenolol (Tenormin)

carvedilol (Coreg)

esmolol (Brevibloc)

metoprolol (Lopressor, Toprol)

nadolol (Corgard)

propranolol (Inderal)

Class II drugs are beta-blockers that decrease automaticity and conduction through the AV node. They also reduce the heart rate and myocardial contractility. They are used to treat supraventricular tachycardia and to slow the ventricular response rate to atrial fibrillation. These drugs may cause bronchospasm and are contraindicated for patients with asthma, chronic obstructive pulmonary disease (COPD), or other restrictive or obstructive lung diseases.

CLASS III DRUGS: POTASSIUM CHANNEL BLOCKERS

amiodarone (Cordarone)

bretylium (Bretylol)

dofetilide (Tikosyn)

ibutilide (Corvert)

sotalol (Betapace)

Class III drugs block potassium channels, prolonging repolarization and the refractory period. Drugs in this class are used primarily to treat ventricular tachycardia and ventricular fibrillation. Amiodarone may also be used for supraventricular tachycardias.

CLASS IV DRUGS: CALCIUM CHANNEL BLOCKERS

amlodipine (Norvasc)

diltiazem (Cardizem, Dilacor XR)

verapamil (Calan, Isoptin, Verelan)

Calcium channel blockers decrease automaticity and AV nodal conduction. They are used to manage supraventricular tachycardias. Like the beta-blockers, calcium channel blockers reduce myocardial contractility.

OTHER DRUGS

adenosine (Adenocard)

digoxin (Lanoxin)

Adenosine and digoxin decrease conduction through the AV node and are used to treat supraventricular tachycardias.

Nursing Responsibilities

- Obtain baseline data including vital signs, cardiac rhythm (including rate, PR and QT intervals, and QRS duration), and physical assessment (especially cardiac, neurologic, and respiratory status).
- Assess medication regimen to identify drugs that may interfere with antidysrhythmic therapy.
- Monitor ECG to evaluate the effectiveness of therapy and to assess for possible dysrhythmias precipitated by treatment.
- Immediately report manifestations of drug toxicity:
  a. Procainamide: Signs of heart failure; conduction delays or ventricular dysrhythmias; skin rash, myalgias or arthralgias, flu-like symptoms
  b. Disopyramide: Urinary retention, heart failure, eye pain
  c. Lidocaine: Changes in neurologic status, such as agitation, confusion, dizziness, nervousness
  d. Amiodarone: Pulmonary fibrosis (increasing dyspnea, cough, hepatic dysfunction—changes in liver function tests, jaundice); vision changes, photosensitivity
  e. Digoxin: Anorexia, nausea and vomiting; blurred or double vision; yellow-green halos; new-onset dysrhythmias.
- Use an infusion pump to administer intravenous infusions. Monitor the dose and assess its appropriateness (in mg/min or mcg/kg/min).

Health Education for the Patient and Family

- Take the drug exactly as prescribed. Do not skip or double doses. Check with your physician if a dose is missed.
- Take your pulse and record the rate daily before rising. Count the pulse for 1 full minute. Bring the record with you to each office or clinic visit.
- Report the following to the physician: Irregular pulse rate or rhythm, dizziness, eye pain, changes in vision, skin rashes or color changes, wheezing or other respiratory problems, changes in behavior.

Note: Drugs identified in blue are among the 200 most commonly prescribed medications in the United States.

Source: Adams, et al., 2017.

sulfate is an unclassified drug that has been shown to be safe and effective in treating ventricular tachycardias.

Countershock

Countershock is used to interrupt cardiac rhythms that compromise cardiac output and the patient's welfare. Delivery of a direct current charge depolarizes all cardiac cells at the same time. This simultaneous depolarization may stop a tachydysrhythmia and allow the sinus node to recover control of impulse formation. There are two types of countershock: Synchronized cardioversion and defibrillation.

Synchronized cardioversion. *Synchronized cardioversion* delivers direct electrical current synchronized with the patient's heart rhythm. Synchronization of the shock with the QRS complex prevents ventricular fibrillation by avoiding current delivery during the vulnerable period of repolarization. Cardioversion is usually done as an elective procedure to treat supraventricular tachycardia, atrial fibrillation, atrial flutter, or hemodynamically stable ventricular tachycardia.

The nurse assists with cardioversion by preparing the patient before the procedure; obtaining any laboratory tests ordered; obtaining and documenting ECG strips prior to, during, and after treatment; setting up the equipment; and monitoring the patient's response.

Patients in atrial fibrillation are at high risk for thromboembolism following cardioversion. Loss of atrial contractions with atrial fibrillation leads to blood pooling in the atria, increasing the risk of clot formation. When the atria begin to contract following successful cardioversion, clots may be dislodged, embolizing to the pulmonary or systemic circulation. If possible, anticoagulants are given for several weeks before cardioversion is attempted.

Defibrillation. Unlike carefully synchronized cardioversion, *defibrillation* is an emergency procedure that delivers direct current without regard to the cardiac cycle. Ventricular fibrillation is immediately treated as soon as the dysrhythmia is recognized. Early defibrillation has been shown to improve survival in patients experiencing VF.

Defibrillation can be delivered by external or internal paddles or pads. Conductive gel pads or paste is applied, and external paddles or pads are placed on the chest wall at the apex and base of the heart (**Figure 30.8 ■**). Internal paddles are applied directly on the heart, and may be used in surgery, the emergency department, or critical care. Internal defibrillation is done only by a physician; external defibrillation may be performed by any healthcare provider who has been trained in the procedure. Automatic external defibrillators (AEDs) are available on most hospital units to allow early defibrillation for cardiac arrest.

Pacemaker Therapy

A **pacemaker** is a pulse generator used to provide an electrical stimulus to the heart when the heart fails to generate or conduct its own at a rate that maintains the cardiac output. The pulse generator is connected to *leads* (insulated wires) passed intravenously into the heart or sutured directly to the epicardium. The leads sense the intrinsic electrical activity of the heart and provide an electrical stimulus to the heart when necessary (pacing).

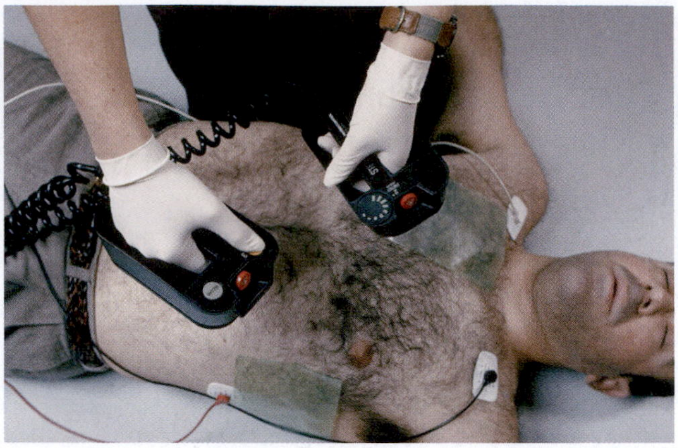

Figure 30.8 ■ Placement of paddles for defibrillation.

Pacemakers are used to treat both acute and chronic conduction defects such as third-degree AV block. They also may be used to treat bradydysrhythmias and tachydysrhythmias.

Temporary pacemakers use an external pulse generator (**Figure 30.9 ■**) attached to a lead threaded intravenously into the right ventricle, to temporary pacing wires implanted during cardiac surgery, or to external conductive pads placed on the chest wall for emergency pacing.

Permanent pacemakers use an internal pulse generator placed in a subcutaneous pocket in the subclavian space or abdominal wall. The generator connects to leads sewn directly onto the heart (*epicardial*) or passed transvenously into the heart (*endocardial*). Epicardial pacemakers (**Figure 30.10 ■**) require surgical exposure of the heart. Leads may be placed during cardiac surgery or using a small subxiphoid incision to expose the heart. Transvenous pacemaker leads are positioned in the right heart via the cephalic, subclavian,

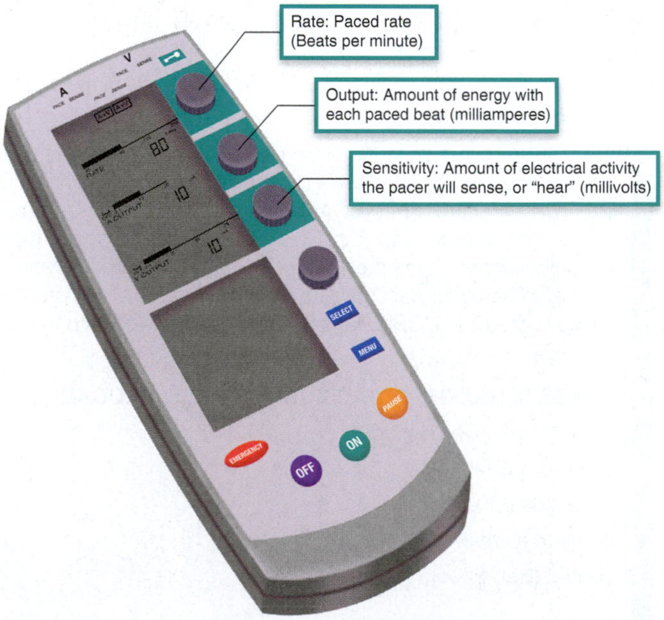
Rate: Paced rate
(Beats per minute)
Output: Amount of energy with
each paced beat (milliamperes)
Sensitivity: Amount of electrical activity
the pacer will sense, or "hear" (millivolts)
SELECT
MENU
PAUSE
ON
OFF
EMERGENCY

Figure 30.9 ■ Programmable settings on a temporary pacemaker.

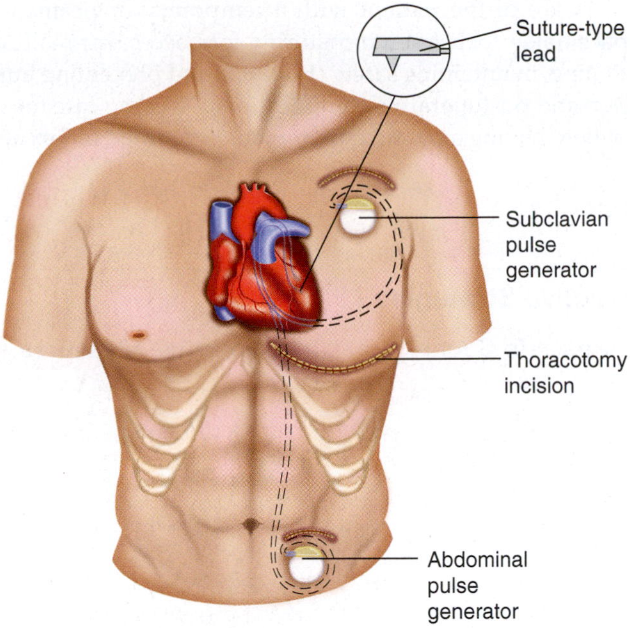
Suture-type lead
Subclavian pulse generator
Thoracotomy incision
Abdominal pulse generator

Figure 30.10 ■ A permanent epicardial pacemaker. The pulse generator may be placed in subcutaneous pockets in the subclavian or abdominal regions.

Table 30.6 Terms Used to Describe Pacemaker Functions

Term	Definition
Asynchronous pacing	Pacemaker delivers a pacing stimulus at a set rate regardless of intrinsic cardiac activity.
Base rate	Rate at which the pacemaker paces when no cardiac activity is sensed.
Capture	The ability of the pacing stimulus to generate a cardiac depolarization.
Demand pacing	Pacemaker delivers a pacing stimulus only when the intrinsic rate falls below the pacemaker's base rate.
Dual-chamber pacing	Allows both the atria and the ventricles to be paced; most frequently used permanent pacing mode.
Lead	An insulated wire that senses intrinsic cardiac activity and delivers a pacing stimulus as programmed.
Output	The electrical stimulus delivered by the pulse generator.
Pacing spike	A small vertical spike noted on the ECG with every pacemaker stimulus.
Sensing	The pacemaker's ability to identify and respond to intrinsic cardiac activity.
Single-chamber pacing	Pacing of only the atria or the ventricles, not both; most common temporary pacing mode used.

or jugular vein (**Figure 30.11** ■). Local anesthesia can be used for permanent pacer insertion.

Pacemakers are programmed to stimulate the atria or the ventricles (*single-chamber pacing*), or both (*dual-chamber pacing*). **Table 30.6** defines terms used to describe pacemaker modes and functions. The most commonly used pacemakers either (1) sense activity in and pace the ventricles only or (2) sense activity in and pace both the atria and the ventricles. Dual-chamber or *atrioventricular sequential pacing* stimulates both chambers of the heart in sequence. AV pacing imitates the normal sequence of atrial contraction followed by ventricular contraction, improving cardiac output.

Pacing is detected on the ECG strip by the presence of a pacing artifact (**Figure 30.12** ■). A sharp spike is noted before the P wave with atrial pacing and before the QRS

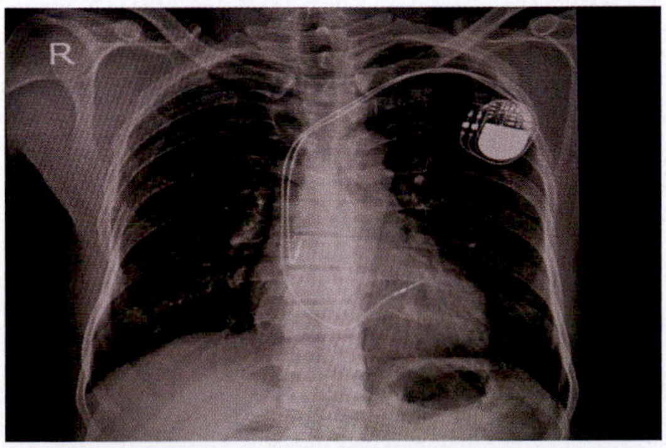
R

Figure 30.11 ■ A permanent transvenous (endocardial) pacemaker with the lead placed in the right ventricle via the subclavian vein.

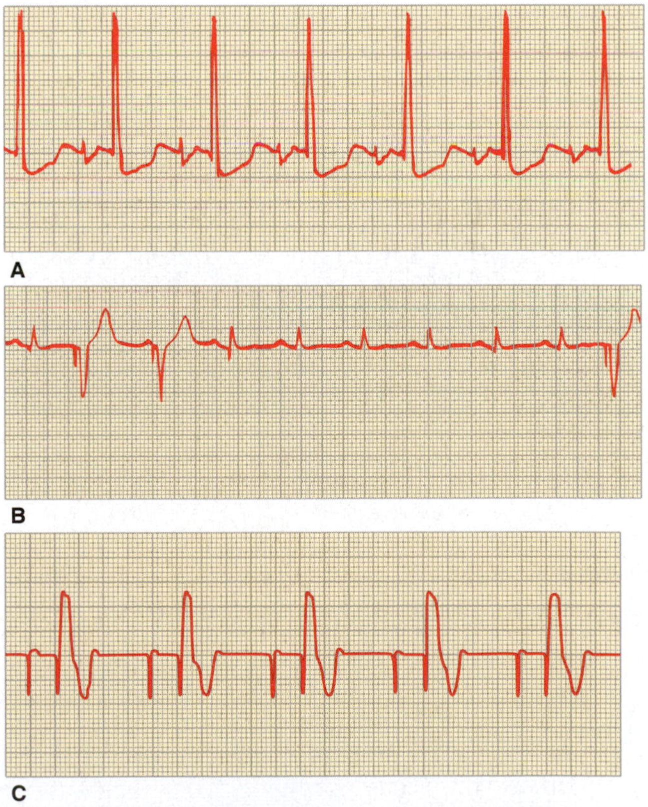
A
B
C

Figure 30.12 ■ Pacing artifacts. **A**, Atrial pacing and ventricular sensing. Note the pacer spike preceding the P wave. **B**, Ventricular demand pacing. Note the absence of pacer spikes when the patient's natural rhythm dominates. **C**, Atrioventricular pacing. Note the pacer spikes preceding both P waves and QRS complexes.

complex with ventricular pacing. Pacing spikes are seen before both the P wave and QRS complex in AV sequential pacing. Capture is noted if there is a contraction of the chamber immediately following the pacer spike. Problems in sensing, pacing, and capture are noted in **Table 30.7**.

Care of the patient with a temporary or permanent pacemaker focuses on monitoring for pacemaker malfunctioning, maintaining safety (**Box 30.7**) and preventing infection and postoperative complications. Nursing care for the patient having a pacemaker implant is outlined in **Box 30.8**.

Table 30.7 Potential Pacemaker Problems and Corrective Strategies

Problem	Possible Causes	Corrective Measures
Undersensing		
Device fails to detect existing cardiac depolarizations; therefore, it competes with the native rhythms. 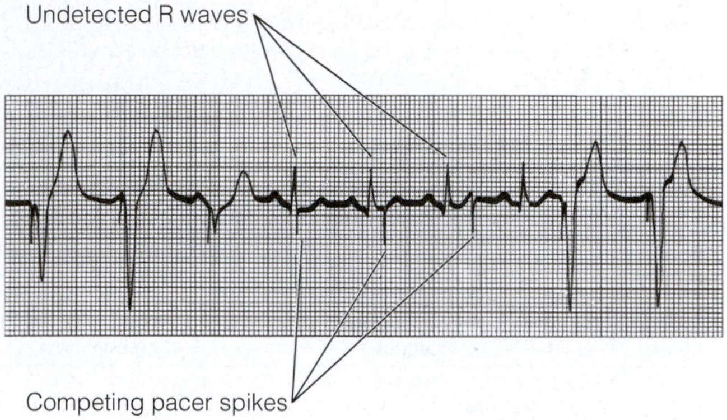 Undetected R waves Competing pacer spikes	Lead disconnected from pacer or from viable myocardium Sensitivity set too low Lead fracture Low battery	Check connection of lead to pacer. Increase sensitivity. Reposition or change lead. Change battery.
Oversensing		
Device detects noncardiac electrical events and interprets them as cardiac depolarizations; therefore, it is wrongly inhibited from pacing. 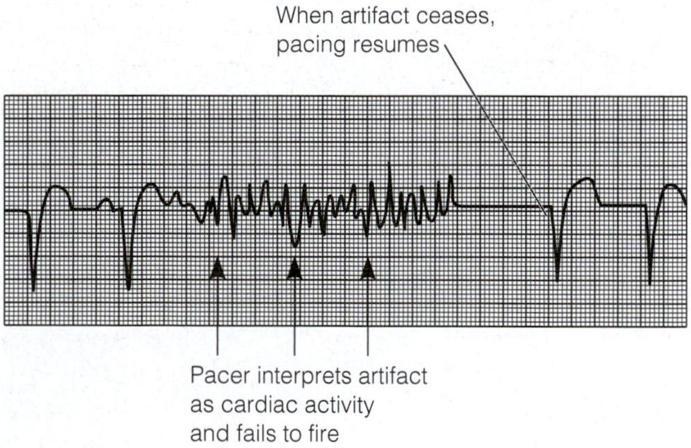 When artifact ceases, pacing resumes Pacer interprets artifact as cardiac activity and fails to fire	Sensitivity set too high Interference from electrical sources (ungrounded equipment, short circuits) is detected and misinterpreted by the device Lead disconnected from pacer or from viable myocardium	Decrease sensitivity (turn sensing control to a LARGER number). Remove all ungrounded electrical equipment or have it evaluated by hospital engineers. Check connection of lead to pacer.
Noncapture		
Device emits stimuli that fail to depolarize the myocardium. 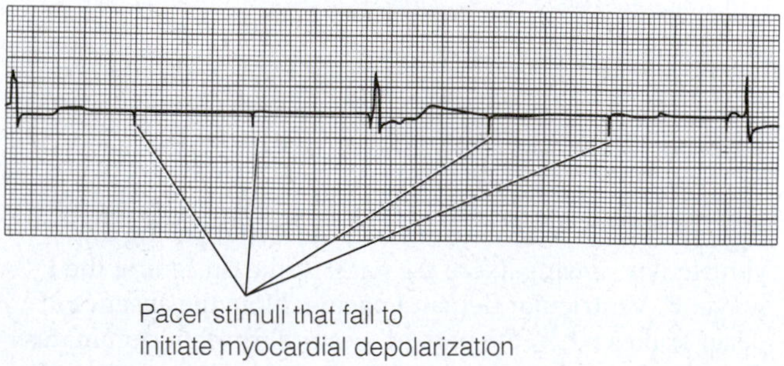 Pacer stimuli that fail to initiate myocardial depolarization	Output set too low in the noncaptured chamber Lead fracture High pacing threshold due to medication or metabolic changes Low battery	Increase output in the noncaptured chamber. Reposition or change lead. Alter medication regimen, correct metabolic changes. Change battery.

BOX 30.7
Safety Measures for Patients with a Temporary Pacemaker

- Ensure that all electrical equipment in use has a grounded plug; do not use adapters or extension cords.
- Encourage the use of battery-powered equipment (e.g., electric razor).
- Remove any damaged electrical equipment from the unit, including equipment
  a. that has been abused (e.g., has been dropped or in which liquid has been spilled).
  b. from which anyone has received a shock.
  c. that has frayed, worn, or otherwise damaged electrical cords or plugs.
  d. that has other evidence of impaired function, such as a hot smell during use or control knobs that are loose or do not consistently produce the expected response.
- Wear gloves when handling pacer electrodes or wires.
- Insulate pacemaker terminals and pacing wires with nonconductive, moisture-proof material (e.g., a rubber glove).
- Test the pacemaker battery prior to use.
- Keep a spare pacemaker, cable, batteries, and battery tester available at all times.
- Immediately report any apparent deviation from expected pacemaker function.

BOX 30.8
Nursing Care of the Patient Having a Permanent Pacemaker Implant

PREOPERATIVE CARE

- Provide routine preoperative care and teaching as outlined in Chapter 4.
- Assess knowledge and understanding of the procedure, clarifying and expanding on existing knowledge as needed. *Clarifying knowledge, providing information, and conveying emotional support reduce anxiety and fear and allow the patient to develop a realistic outlook regarding pacer therapy.*
- Place ECG monitor electrodes away from potential incision sites. *This helps preserve skin integrity.*
- Teach range-of-motion (ROM) exercises for the affected side. *ROM exercises of the affected arm and shoulder prevent stiffness and impaired function following pacemaker insertion.*

POSTOPERATIVE CARE

- Provide postoperative monitoring, analgesia, and care as outlined in Chapter 4.
- Obtain a chest x-ray as ordered. *A postoperative chest x-ray is used to identify lead location and detect possible complications, such as pneumothorax or pleural effusion.*
- Position for comfort. Minimize movement of the affected arm and shoulder during the initial postoperative period. *Restricting movement minimizes discomfort on the operative side and allows the leads to become anchored, reducing the risk of dislodging.*
- Assist with gentle ROM exercises at least three times daily, beginning 24 hours after pacemaker implantation. *ROM exercises help restore normal shoulder movement and prevent contractures on the affected side.*
- Monitor pacemaker function with cardiac monitoring or intermittent ECGs. Report pacemaker problems to the physician:
  a. Failure to pace. *This may indicate battery depletion, damage or dislodgement of pacer wires, or inappropriate sensing.*
  b. Failure to capture (the pacemaker stimulus is not followed by ventricular depolarization). *The electrical output of the pacemaker may not be adequate or the lead may be dislodged.*
  c. Improper sensing (the pacemaker is firing or not firing, regardless of the intrinsic rate). *This increases the risk for decreased cardiac output and dysrhythmias.*
  d. Runaway pacemaker (a pacemaker firing at a rapid rate). *This may be due to generator malfunction or problems with sensing.*
  e. Hiccups. *A lead positioned near the diaphragm can stimulate it, causing hiccups. Hiccups may occur in extremely thin patients or may indicate a medical emergency with perforation of the right ventricle by the pacing electrode tip.*
- Assess for dysrhythmias and treat as indicated. *Until the catheter is "seated" or adheres to the myocardium, its movement may cause myocardial irritability and dysrhythmias. Fibrotic tissue develops within 2 to 3 days.*
- Document the date of pacemaker insertion, the model and type, and settings. *This information is important for future reference.*
- Immediately report signs of potential complications, including myocardial perforation, cardiac tamponade, pneumothorax, hemothorax, emboli, skin breakdown, bleeding, infection, endocarditis, or poor wound healing (see Chapter 31 for more information about cardiac tamponade and endocarditis and Chapter 36 for pneumothorax and hemothorax). *Early identification of complications allows for aggressive intervention.*
- Provide a pacemaker identification card including the manufacturer's name, model number, mode of operation, rate parameters, and expected battery life. *This card provides a reference for the patient and future healthcare providers.*

HOME CARE

Provide appropriate teaching for the patient and family about the following:

- Placement of the pacemaker generator and leads in relation to the heart.
- How the pacemaker works and the rate at which it is set.
- Battery replacement. Most pacemaker batteries last 6 to 12 years. Replacement requires outpatient surgery to open the subcutaneous pocket and replace the battery.
- Notify healthcare provider of weakness, dizziness, or light-headedness.
- How to take and record the pulse rate. Instruct to assess pulse daily before arising and notify the physician if 5 or more bpm slower than the preset pacemaker rate.
- Incision care and signs of infection. Bruising may be present following surgery.

(continued)

- Signs of pacemaker malfunction to report, including dizziness, fainting, fatigue, weakness, chest pain, or palpitations.
- Activity restrictions as ordered. This is usually limited to contact sports (which may damage the generator) and avoiding heavy lifting for 2 months after surgery.
- Resume sexual activity as recommended by the physician. Avoid positions that cause pressure on the site.
- Avoid tight-fitting clothing over the pacemaker site to reduce irritation and avoid skin breakdown.
- Carry the pacemaker identification card at all times, and wear a medical alert bracelet or tag.
- Notify all care providers of the pacemaker.
- Do not hold or use certain electrical devices over the pacemaker site, including household appliances or tools, garage door openers, antitheft devices, or burglar alarms. Do not perform arc-welding. A pacemaker will set off airport security detectors; notify security officials of its presence.
- Maintain follow-up care with the physician as recommended.

Implantable Cardioverter/Defibrillator

Sudden cardiac death claims more than 300,000 lives per year in the United States. The *implantable cardioverter/defibrillator (ICD)* detects life-threatening changes in the cardiac rhythm and automatically delivers an electric shock to convert the dysrhythmia back into a normal rhythm. ICDs are used for sudden death survivors, patients with recurrent ventricular tachycardia, and patients with demonstrated risk factors for sudden death. ICDs can deliver a shock as needed, provide pacing on demand, and store ECG records of tachycardic episodes.

A pulse generator connected to lead electrodes for rhythm detection and current delivery is implanted in the left pectoral region. The lead is threaded transvenously to the apex of the right ventricle. The ICD is programmed to sense a change in heart rate or rhythm. When it detects a potentially lethal rhythm, it shocks the heart to convert the rhythm. The device can be programmed or reprogrammed at the bedside as necessary. The ICD may be tested prior to discharge.

Local or general anesthesia is used, and the patient may be discharged within 24 hours. The lithium-powered battery must be surgically replaced every 5 years. Complications and nursing care are similar to that for a patient having a permanent pacemaker implant (see Box 30.8).

The patient may briefly lose consciousness before the device discharges, typically regaining consciousness quickly after the episode. Some patients report significant discomfort with ICD discharge (like a blow to the chest). An individual in direct contact with the patient when the device discharges may experience a tingling sensation.

Cardiac Mapping and Catheter Ablation

Cardiac mapping and catheter ablation are used to locate and destroy an ectopic focus. These diagnostic and therapeutic measures use electrophysiology techniques and can be performed in the cardiac catheterization laboratory. *Cardiac mapping* is used to identify the site of earliest impulse formation in the atria or the ventricles. Intracardiac and extracardiac catheter electrodes and computer technology are used to pinpoint the ectopic site on a map of the heart. These same catheters can be used to deliver the ablative intervention.

Ablation destroys, removes, or isolates an ectopic focus. In most instances, radio-frequency energy produced by high-frequency alternating current is used to create heat as it passes through tissue. Catheter ablation is used to treat supraventricular tachycardias, atrial fibrillation and flutter, and, in some cases, paroxysmal ventricular tachycardia.

Anticoagulant therapy may be started after catheter ablation to reduce the risk of clot formation at the ablation site.

Other Therapies

In addition to medications and interventional techniques, other measures may be used to treat selected dysrhythmias. Vagal maneuvers that stimulate the parasympathetic nervous system may be used to slow the heart rate in supraventricular tachycardias. These maneuvers include *carotid sinus massage* and the *Valsalva maneuver*. Carotid sinus massage is performed only by a physician during continuous cardiac monitoring. Excessive slowing of the heart rate may result. The Valsalva maneuver, forced exhalation against a closed glottis (e.g., bearing down), increases intrathoracic pressure and vagal tone, slowing the pulse rate.

Nursing Care

Caring for the patient with cardiac dysrhythmias requires the ability to recognize, identify, and promptly treat the dysrhythmia. The urgency of intervention is determined by the effects of the dysrhythmia on the patient. Nursing care focuses on maintaining cardiac output, monitoring the response to therapy, and teaching. See the Case Study & Nursing Care Plan for a patient with supraventricular tachycardia.

Assessment

Assessment is vital before treating any suspected dysrhythmia. What appears to be ventricular tachycardia on the monitor may be the patient scratching or brushing his or her teeth. Apparent asystole on the monitor may be due to a loose electrode patch. Similarly, a heart rate of 52 bpm may not affect the overall cardiac output in some patients. Review Chapter 29 for complete assessment of the patient with a cardiac problem.

- *Health history:* Complaints of palpitations (ask for further definition of palpitations), fluttering sensations, or a sensation of the heart racing; episodes of dizziness, lightheadedness, or syncope (fainting); timing (duration, time of day); correlation with food or beverage intake, activity; presence of chest pain, shortness of breath, or other associated symptoms; history of heart or endocrine disease (such as hyperthyroidism); current medications
- *Physical assessment:* Level of consciousness (LOC); vital signs, including apical pulse for a full minute;

regularity and amplitude of peripheral pulses; color; presence of dyspnea, adventitious lung sounds; ECG rhythm analysis; oxygen saturation levels.

Priorities of Care

Collaborating with the interprofessional team to ensure adequate treatment of the cardiac perfusion limitations while providing care that supports circulation (including appropriate precautions) as well as teaching the patient and, as appropriate, caregivers strategies to identify early signs and symptoms of acute cardiac events and optimize safe home and work environments, should be considered priority nursing actions. The nurse also focuses on promoting comfort and prevention of cardiac event recurrence.

Diagnoses, Outcomes, and Interventions

The effect of the dysrhythmia on cardiac output is the priority of nursing care. Other potential nursing diagnoses related to dysrhythmias may include *Ineffective Tissue Perfusion*, *Activity Intolerance*, and *Fear* or *Anxiety*.

Monitor Cardiac Output. Dysrhythmias can affect cardiac output. Bradycardias decrease cardiac output if the stroke volume does not increase to compensate for the slow heart rate. Tachycardia reduces diastolic filling time, affecting stroke volume and coronary artery perfusion. Loss of the atrial kick in junctional rhythms, atrial fibrillation, and AV blocks also decreases ventricular filling and cardiac output. In ventricular fibrillation, loss of ventricular contractions causes cardiac arrest and no cardiac output.

Expected Outcome: Patient will demonstrate adequate cardiac output as evidenced by blood pressure and pulse rate and rhythm within normal limits.

SAFETY ALERT: Before treating any dysrhythmia, assess the patient, not just the monitor! Loose electrode pads, disconnected leads or cables, and muscle movement can simulate critical dysrhythmias. The patient's condition is the best indicator of the need for treatment. ■

The nurse will:

- Assess for decreased cardiac output: Decreased LOC; tachycardia; tachypnea; hypotension; low oxygen saturation; diaphoresis; low urine output; cool, clammy, mottled skin; pallor or cyanosis; and diminished peripheral pulses. *Initial signs of decreased cardiac output may be subtle, such as decreased LOC. Early recognition of the dysrhythmia's effect on cardiac output facilitates appropriate treatment and may prevent further adverse effects.*
- Monitor ECG; post ECG strip every shift and when rhythm changes occur. *Documenting cardiac rhythm provides a record of disease progression and treatment effectiveness.*

SAFETY ALERT: Assess vital signs, ECG, and oxygen saturation every 5 to 15 minutes during acute dysrhythmic episodes and during antidysrhythmic drug infusions. These data provide a record of cardiac output during the dysrhythmia. Antidysrhythmic drugs can adversely affect heart rate, rhythm, and blood pressure, further decreasing cardiac output. ■

- Assess for underlying causes of dysrhythmias, such as hypovolemia, hypoxia, anemia, electrolyte imbalance, vagal stimulation, or medications. *Sinus tachycardia often develops in response to tissue hypoxia. Vagal stimulation (such as the Valsalva maneuver) can precipitate bradycardia.*
- Assess serum electrolytes (especially potassium, calcium, and magnesium) and digitalis and antidysrhythmic drug levels as indicated. Report abnormal values. *Electrolyte imbalances affect cardiac depolarization and repolarization and may cause dysrhythmias. Toxic levels of digitalis and antidysrhythmic drugs can precipitate further dysrhythmias. Impaired renal or hepatic function increases the risk for toxicity, as does aging.*

Case Study & Nursing Care Plan

A Patient with Supraventricular Tachycardia

Elisa Vasquez, 53 years old, is admitted to the cardiac unit with complaints of palpitations, light-headedness, and shortness of breath. Her history reveals rheumatic fever at age 12 with subsequent rheumatic heart disease and mitral stenosis. An intravenous line is in place and she is receiving oxygen. Marcia Lewin, RN, is assigned to Ms. Vasquez.

ASSESSMENT	DIAGNOSIS	EXPECTED OUTCOMES
Ms. Lewin's assessment reveals that Ms. Vasquez is moderately anxious. Her ECG shows supraventricular tachycardia (SVT) with a rate of 154. Vital signs are T 37.1°C (98.8°F), R 26/min, BP 95/60 mmHg. Peripheral pulses weak but equal, mucous membranes pale pink, skin cool and dry. Fine crackles noted in both lung bases. A loud S_3 gallop and a diastolic murmur are noted. Ms. Vasquez is still complaining of palpitations and tells Ms. Lewin, "I feel so nervous and weak and dizzy." Ms. Vasquez's cardiologist orders 2.5 mg of verapamil to be given slowly via intravenous push and tells Ms. Lewin to prepare to assist with synchronized cardioversion if drug therapy does not control the ventricular rate.	■ Inadequate cardiac output related to inadequate ventricular filling associated with rapid tachycardia ■ Poor tissue perfusion related to decreased cardiac output ■ Anxiety related to unknown outcome of altered health state	■ Patient will maintain adequate cardiac output and tissue perfusion. ■ Patient will demonstrate a ventricular rate within normal limits and stable vital signs. ■ Patient will verbalize reduced anxiety. ■ Patient will verbalize an understanding of the rationale for the treatment measures to control the heart rate.

(continued)

PLANNING AND IMPLEMENTATION

- Provide oxygen per nasal cannula at 4 L/min.
- Continuously monitor ECG for rate, rhythm, and conduction. Assess vital signs and associated symptoms with changes in ECG. Report findings to physician.
- Explain the importance of rapidly reducing the heart rate. Explain the cardioversion procedure and encourage questions.
- Encourage verbalization of fears and concerns. Answer questions honestly, correcting misconceptions about the disease process, treatment, or prognosis.
- Administer intravenous diazepam as ordered before cardioversion.
- Document pretreatment vital signs, LOC, and peripheral pulses.
- Place emergency cart with drugs and airway management supplies in patient unit.
- Assist with cardioversion as indicated.
- Assess LOC, level of sedation, cardiovascular and respiratory status, and skin condition following cardioversion.
- Document procedure and postcardioversion rhythm and response to intervention.

EVALUATION

Intravenous verapamil lowers Ms. Vasquez's heart rate to 138 for a short time, after which it increases to 164 with BP of 82/64. Her cardiologist, Dr. Mullins, performs carotid sinus massage. The ventricular rate slows to 126 for 2 minutes, revealing atrial flutter waves, and then returns to a rate of 150. Dr. Mullins explains the treatment options, including synchronized cardioversion. Ms. Vasquez agrees to the procedure.

Ms. Vasquez is lightly sedated and synchronized cardioversion is performed. One countershock converts Ms. Vasquez to regular sinus rhythm at 96 bpm with BP 112/60.

Ms. Vasquez is sleepy from the sedation but recovers without incident. She states that she feels "much better," and her vital signs return to her normal levels. She remains in NSR with a rate of 86 to 92 beats per minute for the remainder of her hospital stay. Dr. Mullins places Ms. Vasquez on furosemide to treat manifestations of mild heart failure.

CLINICAL REASONING IN PATIENT CARE

1. What is the scientific basis for using carotid massage to treat supraventricular tachycardias? Was this an appropriate maneuver in the case of Ms. Vasquez?
2. What other treatment options might the physician have used to treat Ms. Vasquez's supraventricular tachycardia if she had been asymptomatic with stable vital signs?
3. Develop a teaching plan for Ms. Vasquez related to her prescription for furosemide.

See Evaluating Your Response in Appendix B.

- Be prepared to administer antidysrhythmic medications as indicated. Implement advanced cardiac life support (ACLS) protocols as needed. *Emergency drugs should be readily available, especially on units with high-risk patients. Refer to Table 30.5 and Medication Administration 30.D for drugs used to treat common dysrhythmias that may affect cardiac output.*
- If appropriate, instruct to perform the Valsalva maneuver (bear down as if straining or coughing) for supraventricular tachycardia or ventricular tachycardia without angina. *Vagal maneuvers stimulate the parasympathetic system and may terminate some dysrhythmias. The Valsalva maneuver is contraindicated if chest pain occurs with the dysrhythmia.*
- Prepare to assist with cardioversion. Prepare the patient per orders or hospital protocol. Explain the procedure to reduce anxiety. Have emergency equipment readily available. *Elective or emergency cardioversion is a treatment of choice for certain dysrhythmias.*

SAFETY ALERT: On recognizing ventricular fibrillation and cardiac arrest, begin emergency procedures. Call for help. Obtain defibrillator and immediately defibrillate. If the defibrillator will be brought by another healthcare provider, begin CPR. Initiate ACLS protocols and assist with resuscitation measures as directed. Cardiac output ceases with ventricular fibrillation. Immediate or early defibrillation has been shown to have the greatest impact on survival following cardiac arrest. ■

- After cardiac arrest, transfer to critical care. Perform and document head-to-toe assessment; obtain laboratory tests, 12-lead ECG, and chest x-ray as ordered; monitor and maintain oxygenation and intravenous infusions; and monitor vital signs and cardiac rhythm. *The period following resuscitation is critical, necessitating careful monitoring. Postarrest assessment allows comparison of the patient's condition with prearrest status and may identify CPR-related injuries. Correcting electrolyte disturbances, hypoxia, and acid–base imbalances is important to prevent further dysrhythmias and potential adverse effects on cardiac output. Intravenous access is crucial to maintain drug infusions. Hemodynamic monitoring may be instituted. The 12-lead ECG documents myocardial status, and the chest x-ray provides information about pulmonary status and possible thoracic injury due to CPR.*
- Notify the family of significant changes in the patient's condition or cardiac arrest, providing up-to-date information. Prepare family members prior to visits by explaining interventions (such as invasive tubes, a ventilator, or additional equipment) implemented since the last visit. *Concern for the family and significant others is*

part of holistic nursing. Researchers studying the needs of families have found that one of the most important needs was information about their loved one's condition. Patients and families need and appreciate honest communication and compassionate care. Preparing the family for critical changes in the patient's condition and plan of care helps them to cope with a situational crisis.

Transitions of Care

Prevention focuses on health promotion measures to prevent CHD also reduce the risk for dysrhythmias. In most cases, dysrhythmias develop as a result of ischemic or structural changes in the heart, rather than in isolation. Advise patients who are at risk or who complain of occasional palpitations or flutters in their chest to reduce their intake of caffeine and other SNS stimulants, such as excess chocolate.

Dysrhythmias have a significant physical and psychologic impact on the patient and all family members. Many of these patients and their families are under a great deal of stress from frequent hospitalizations, experimentation with therapies, frustration, and the fear of sudden cardiac death. A major teaching effort focuses on coping strategies and lifestyle changes, as well as specific management of prescribed therapies. Include the following topics as appropriate when teaching the patient and family for home care:

- Function, maintenance, precautions, and signs of malfunction or complications of any implanted device such as a pacemaker or ICD
- Monitoring pulse rate and rhythm
- Activity or dietary restrictions and any potential effects of the dysrhythmia or its treatment on lifestyle
- Medication management to reduce the risk of dysrhythmias, including the desired and potential adverse effects of antidysrhythmic drugs
- Specific instructions related to planned diagnostic tests or procedures
- The importance of follow-up visits with the cardiologist
- The importance of and where to obtain CPR training for the patient and family members.

In addition, discuss fears related to treatment or implanted devices, such as that of shocking a significant other during close contact or sexual activity. Explain that if a shock occurs, the partner may feel a slight buzz or tingling but should not be harmed. Refer to and encourage the patient and family to attend a peer support group for the specific condition.

Caring for the Older Adult with Cardiac Dysrhythmia

Aging affects the heart and the cardiac conduction system, increasing the incidence of dysrhythmias and conduction defects. Older adults may experience dysrhythmias even when no evidence of heart disease is found.

Older adults have a higher incidence than younger people of both ventricular and supraventricular dysrhythmias without detrimental effects. Ectopic beats, including short runs of ventricular tachycardia, occur more commonly during exercise in older adults. These dysrhythmias do not affect cardiac morbidity or mortality. Fibrosis of the bundle branches can lead to atrioventricular blocks; a prolonged PR interval is common in patients over the age of 65. Older adults also have a higher incidence of diseases that may affect heart rhythm. An older patient with hyperthyroidism, for example, may present with atrial fibrillation, syncope, and confusion instead of the usual manifestations of goiter, tremor, and exophthalmoses.

Assessing for Home Care

Assessment of older adults for problems related to cardiac dysrhythmias focuses on the effect of the dysrhythmia on functional health status:

- Ask about a history of cardiovascular disease and current medications.
- Inquire about symptoms such as episodes of dizziness, light-headedness, fainting, palpitations, chest pain, or shortness of breath.
- Ask about the relationship of symptoms such as palpitations to intake of certain foods and caffeine-containing beverages.
- Evaluate for other contributing factors such as smoking or alcohol intake.
- Inquire about a history of falls, particularly those occurring without apparent reason.

Teaching for Home Care

Teach measures to reduce the risk of cardiac dysrhythmias and the potential adverse consequences of dysrhythmias:

- Emphasize the importance of taking medications as prescribed. Discuss possible effects of over-the-counter medications on the heart.
- Encourage reducing or eliminating caffeine intake. Caffeine increases the risk of ectopic beats and rapid heart rates.
- Encourage participation in a smoking cessation program and reduce or eliminate alcohol intake if appropriate.
- Encourage engaging in regular exercise. Discuss the beneficial effects of exercise to maintain muscle mass, including cardiac muscle, and cardiovascular health.
- Instruct to contact primary care provider for evaluation of symptoms such as dizziness, fainting, frequent palpitations, shortness of breath, unexplained falls, or chest pain.

The Patient with Sudden Cardiac Death

Sudden cardiac death (SCD) is defined as unexpected death occurring within 1 hour of the onset of cardiovascular symptoms. It is usually caused by ventricular fibrillation and cardiac arrest (Sorenson et al., 2019). *Cardiac arrest* is the sudden collapse, loss of consciousness, and cessation of effective circulation that precedes biologic death. Worldwide, less than 5% of out-of-hospital cardiac arrest victims survive. In communities of North America that have organized lay rescuer and automated AED programs, the survival rate is significantly better, ranging from 49 to 67% when a witnessed arrest due to ventricular fibrillation occurs (Benjamin et al., 2017).

Arrhythmias related to CHD cause up to 81% of all sudden cardiac deaths in the United States (Benjamin et al., 2017). Other cardiac pathologies such as cardiomyopathy and valvular disorders may also lead to SCD. Noncardiac causes of sudden death include electrocution, pulmonary embolism, and rapid blood loss from a ruptured aortic aneurysm.

Ventricular fibrillation is the most common dysrhythmia associated with SCD, accounting for 65 to 80% of cardiac arrests (Benjamin et al., 2017). Sustained severe bradydysrhythmias, *asystole* or cardiac standstill, and pulseless electrical activity (organized cardiac electrical activity without a mechanical response) are responsible for most remaining SCDs. Selected cardiac and noncardiac causes of sudden cardiac death include:

CARDIAC CAUSES

- Coronary heart disease
- Reperfusion following ischemia
- Myocardial hypertrophy
- Cardiomyopathy
- Inflammatory myocardial disorders
- Valve disorders
- Primary electrical disorders
- Dissecting or ruptured aortic or ventricular aneurysm
- Cardiac drug toxicity

NONCARDIAC CAUSES

- Pulmonary embolism
- Cerebral hemorrhage
- Autonomic dysfunction
- Choking
- Electrical shock
- Electrolyte and acid–base imbalances

Risk factors for SCD are those associated with CHD. Advancing age and male gender are powerful risk factors. After age 65, the gap between male and female incidence of SCD narrows. Patients with dysrhythmias such as recurrent VT may have a higher risk of SCD. Women with AMI, however, are more likely to present with cardiac arrest and cardiogenic shock than with ventricular tachycardia.

Pathophysiology

Evidence of CHD with significant atherosclerosis and narrowing of two or more major coronary arteries is found in 75% of SCD victims. Although most have had a prior MI, only 20 to 30% have had a recent AMI. An acute change in cardiovascular status precedes cardiac arrest by up to 1 hour; however, often the onset is instantaneous or abrupt. Tachycardia develops, and the number of PVCs increases. This is followed by a run of VT that deteriorates into VF (Perrin & MacLeod, 2018).

Abnormalities of myocardial structure or function also contribute. Structural abnormalities include infarction, hypertrophy, myopathy, and electrical anomalies. Functional deviations are caused by such factors as ischemia followed by reperfusion, altered homeostasis, autonomic nervous system and hormone interactions, and toxic effects. The interactions of the two cause myocardial instability and may precipitate fatal dysrhythmias.

Manifestations

SCD may be preceded by typical manifestations of ACS or MI, including severe chest pain, dyspnea or orthopnea, and palpitations or light-headedness. The event itself is abrupt, with complete loss of consciousness and death within minutes. If VT precedes cardiac arrest, consciousness and mentation may be impaired prior to collapse and loss of consciousness.

Interprofessional Care

The goal of care is to restore cardiac output and tissue perfusion. Treatment measures are initiated as soon as clinical cardiac arrest is verified by the absence of respirations and carotid or femoral pulses. Basic and advanced cardiac life support measures must be instituted within 2 to 4 minutes of cardiac arrest to prevent permanent neurologic damage and ischemic injury to other organs.

Basic Life Support

Basic life support (BLS) begins with identification of the cardiac arrest and initiation of an emergency response.

Providers trained in the use of the *automated external defibrillator (AED)* should immediately defibrillate the patient in VF. Self-adhesive conductive pads attached to connecting cables are positioned on the chest (**Figure 30.13** ■). The AED analyzes the rhythm and advises the provider to charge the device if VF is detected. After warning all personnel to stand clear, the shock button is depressed to deliver a shock. Following the shock, CPR is immediately initiated. After approximately 2 minutes or five cycles of CPR, the rhythm is evaluated and circulation checked. The sequence of analysis, shock, and CPR is continued and ACLS protocols are initiated.

Cardiopulmonary resuscitation (CPR) is a mechanical attempt to maintain tissue perfusion using external cardiac compressions. All healthcare providers need to be proficient in CPR. The technique, as updated in 2015, should be performed according to American Heart Association or American Red Cross guidelines and hospital protocol (see **Box 30.9**). Research demonstrates clear benefit from sustained, effective chest compressions, yet compressions are often interrupted for ventilation, assessment of pulses, and other measures. Many patients are excessively ventilated and underperfused during CPR. In light of this finding, CPR now emphasizes chest compressions.

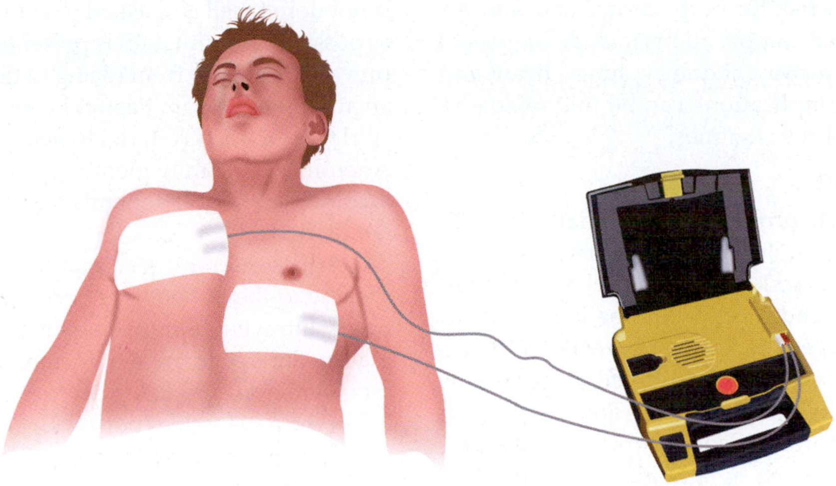

Figure 30.13 ■ Schematic of an automated external defibrillator attached to a patient.

BOX 30.9
Cardiopulmonary Resuscitation

1. Assess for responsiveness; shake the patient and shout.
2. Call for help. Dial 911 (if outside the healthcare facility) or initiate the institutional code or cardiac arrest procedure.
3. Initiate hard and fast cardiac compressions, pressing straight down to depress the sternum at least 2 inches, keeping the elbows locked and positioning the shoulders directly over the hands (Figure 1). Release pressure completely between compressions but do not lift the hands from the chest. The rate should be at least 100 to 120 compressions per minute (Figure 2).
4. After 30 compressions, open the airway using the head tilt–chin lift procedure by simultaneously pressing down on the forehead with one hand while lifting the chin upward with the other and deliver two ventilations (Figure 3).

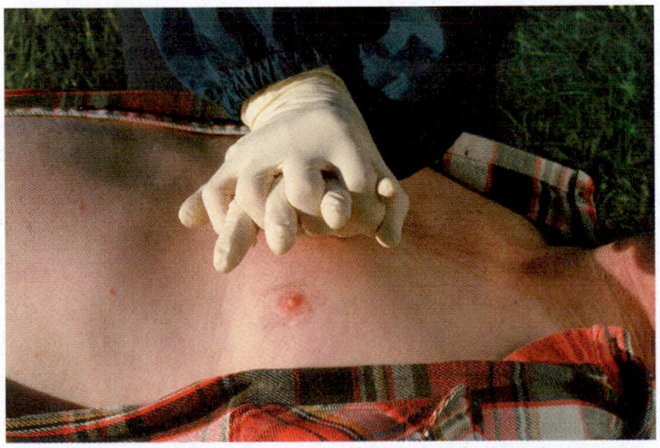

Figure 1. Placement of hands on the sternum between nipples.

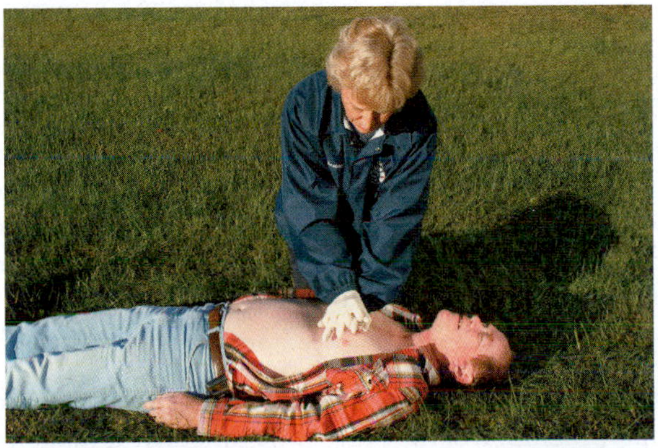

Figure 2. Arm, hand, and shoulder position for cardiac massage.

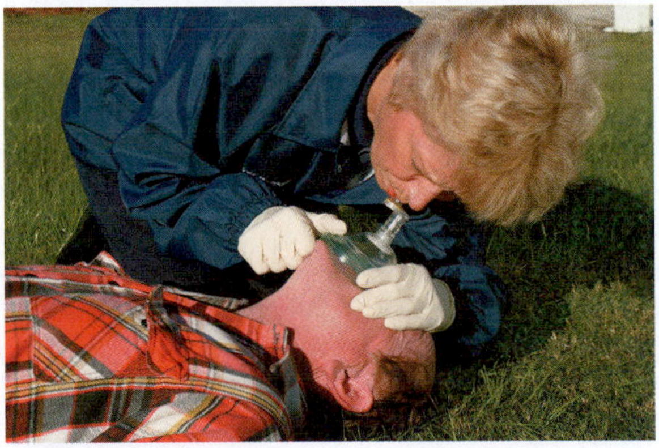

Figure 3. Head tilt–chin lift procedure and use of a bag-valve-mask unit.

5. Continue to compress the chest at a rate of at least 100 to 120 times per minute; continue CPR until help arrives.
6. When any rescuer witnesses an out-of-hospital arrest and an AED is immediately available on-site, the rescuer should start CPR with chest compressions and use the AED as soon as possible.

Source: American Heart Association, 2015.

CPR carries a high risk for both cardiac and noncardiac trauma. CPR-related complications include injuries to the skin, thorax, upper airway, abdomen, lungs, heart, and great vessels. These complications can be minimized by adhering to accepted CPR techniques.

Advanced Life Support

Advanced life support, provided by specially trained healthcare personnel, includes advanced airway support (insertion of a laryngeal mask airway [LMA], esophageal-tracheal Combitube, or endotracheal intubation) to maintain the airway and oxygenation, use of intravenous drugs following specific protocols, and additional interventions such as repeated defibrillation procedures and cardiac pacing. Epinephrine, vasopressin, sodium bicarbonate, and antidysrhythmic drugs such as amiodarone, lidocaine, procainamide, magnesium sulfate, and atropine may be used to attempt to restore and maintain an effective cardiac rhythm.

Postresuscitation Care

Patients who are resuscitated following a cardiac arrest that associated with ventricular fibrillation and acute MI have the best prognosis. The patient is transferred to a coronary care unit and MI treatment measures are instituted. Antidysrhythmic drugs may be continued for 24 to 48 hours to reduce the risk of subsequent episodes of VF.

Because the risk for recurrent cardiac arrest is significant in survivors, extensive diagnostic testing and interventions such as angioplasty or surgical revascularization of the myocardium, ablation, or an implantable cardioverter/defibrillator may be indicated.

Nursing Care

Nursing care of the patient experiencing SCD requires prompt recognition of the event and immediate initiation of BLS and ALS protocols. As noted before, fast and effective cardiac compressions and early defibrillation of unstable VT and VF are the most important keys to survival of cardiac arrest victims. Important concepts of emergency cardiac care are:

- Treat the patient, not the monitor. Recognize signs and symptoms of cardiac compromise early.
- Activate the emergency medical services system (i.e., call a code or call 911).
- Begin and continue basic cardiac life support principles throughout the resuscitation effort.
- Continually assess the effectiveness of emergency interventions.
- Defibrillate pulseless VT or VF as soon as possible.
- Initiate ALS protocols early.

The family is not forgotten during resuscitation. If family members are present, they are usually offered a private consultation room in which to await the outcome. If the family is not present, they are notified that their family member is not doing well and asked to come to the hospital as soon as possible. The situation is presented in a careful manner to prevent the family from racing to the hospital, precipitating an automobile crash. Pastoral care or the family's choice of spiritual support is offered to help during this difficult time. Attendance of family members during resuscitation efforts is controversial and depends on institutional protocols and family desires.

After successful resuscitation, the nurse provides care specific to the patient's underlying disease processes and needs. Intravenous infusions such as lidocaine or dopamine may be ordered to prevent further dysrhythmias and maintain hemodynamic stability.

If the patient does not survive the arrest, the nurse provides postmortem care and emotional and spiritual support to the family.

Nursing care to consider for the patient experiencing cardiac arrest includes:

- Promote effective cerebral tissue perfusion, which may be poor due to ineffective cardiac output
- Promote spontaneous ventilation, which may be inconsistent due to cardiac arrest
- Orient patient who may have disturbed thought processes related to compromised cerebral circulation
- Manage fear related to risk for future episodes of near sudden cardiac death.

The risk for a future episode of near SCD requires careful and effective teaching for home care prior to discharge. Discuss the following topics with the patient and family:

- Risk factor reduction for CHD
- Planned diagnostic studies to identify the cause of SCD, and possible interventions
- The risks and benefits of an ICD if appropriate
- The importance of carrying a card at all times listing all current medications and contact information for the patient's healthcare provider
- Early manifestations or warning signs of cardiac arrest
- The importance of CPR training and maintaining proficiency in performing CPR. (Provide referral to local CPR training providers or scheduled classes through the American Heart Association or American Red Cross.)

Nurses can impact death rates from cardiac arrest through community teaching as well. Survival rates from cardiac arrest related to SCD improve in communities in which a significant portion of the population is trained in CPR and early response by EMS agencies is stressed. Work with community groups and individuals can help create a population of people able to perform effective CPR.

CHAPTER HIGHLIGHTS

30.1 Disorders of Myocardial Perfusion

Describe the pathophysiology and manifestations of disorders of myocardial perfusion, and outline the interprofessional care and nursing care of patients with these disorders.

- Atherosclerosis is the primary underlying process in coronary heart disease, impaired perfusion of myocardial tissue.
- The risk factors for coronary heart disease are those for atherosclerosis: Age, gender, and genetic factors; hypertension, diabetes, abnormal blood lipids; cigarette smoking, obesity, physical inactivity, and diet; and emerging risk factors such as metabolic syndrome and homocysteine levels.
- Smoking cessation, exercise, diet modification, weight loss, medications to achieve desired blood lipid values, and effective hypertension and diabetes management are the primary treatment measures for coronary heart disease.
- Atherosclerosis of coronary vessels impairs the supply of blood, oxygen, and nutrients to the myocardium. Myocardial ischemia results in the manifestations of coronary heart disease, angina pectoris, acute coronary syndrome, and myocardial infarction.
- Stable angina develops with a predictable amount of activity or stress and typically follows an activity–pain, rest–relief pattern. Stable angina can often be managed effectively by medications and risk factor modification. The nursing focus is on education.
- Acute coronary syndrome or unstable angina is characterized by increasingly severe chest pain that occurs unpredictably. Acute coronary syndrome often requires aggressive interventions such as percutaneous coronary revascularization or coronary artery bypass surgery.
- Myocardial infarction, necrosis of myocardial tissue, results from complete blockage of a coronary artery, usually due to atherosclerotic plaque rupture and thrombus formation. Prompt restoration of blood flow through a revascularization procedure or administration of a fibrinolytic drug to dissolve the blood clot is necessary to preserve functional muscle tissue.
- The nursing focus for patients with acute coronary syndrome and myocardial infarction is on reducing myocardial work through measures such as pain relief and activity limitation, promoting blood flow and oxygenation through medication and oxygen administration and positioning, and early recognition and treatment of complications.

30.2 Cardiac Rhythm Disorders

Describe the pathophysiology and manifestations of cardiac dysrhythmias, and outline the interprofessional care and nursing care of patients with these disorders.

- Cardiac dysrhythmias may arise anywhere in conductive tissue of the myocardium. Dysrhythmias may be either benign or fatal, depending on their effect on cardiac output.
- Tachycardias increase the workload of the heart and may interfere with cardiac output if ventricular filling is impaired by the rapid rate.
- Bradycardias can affect cardiac output when the rate is too slow to meet the metabolic needs of the body.
- Atrial fibrillation is a common dysrhythmia that can lead to formation of blood clots within the heart and subsequent stroke if these clots lodge in cerebral blood vessels.
- Frequent ventricular dysrhythmias may indicate an increased risk for ventricular fibrillation and cardiac arrest.
- AV conduction blocks interfere with conduction of the sinus or atrial impulse through the AV node and to the ventricles.
- Although many antidysrhythmic medications are available, all increase the risk of dysrhythmia development, so they are used sparingly.
- The nurse's role in caring for patients with cardiac dysrhythmias focuses on prompt identification of the rhythm disruption, assessment of its effect on the patient, administration of medications and other treatment measures, and institution of life support procedures as indicated.

TEST YOURSELF NCLEX-RN® REVIEW

1. The nurse instructs a patient about modifiable risk factors for coronary artery disease. Which statements indicate that teaching has been effective? (Select all that apply.)
   A. "I should stop smoking to reduce my risk of heart disease."
   B. Restricting my activity reduces the onset of heart disease."
   C. "I should drink alcohol because this prevents heart disease."
   D. "There is not much that can be done to prevent heart disease."
   E. "Obesity is a risk factor that I can change to reduce the onset of heart disease."

2. A patient is prescribed lovastatin (Mevacor) for hyperlipidemia. What should the nurse instruct the patient about this medication? (Select all that apply.)
   A. Abstain from alcohol while taking this drug.
   B. Take the drug with meals to minimize gastric distress.
   C. Promptly report muscle pain or tenderness to the physician.
   D. Consume a diet that includes no more than 20% of calories from saturated fat.
   E. Expect periodic liver function tests while on this medication.
3. The nurse is caring for a patient with stable angina. Which assessment finding would be consistent with this medical diagnosis?
   A. Persistent ECG changes
   B. Increasing nocturnal pain
   C. Correlation between activity level and pain
   D. Evidence of impaired cardiac output such as weak peripheral pulses
4. The nurse is caring for a patient with acute coronary syndrome. The nurse prioritizes interventions to address which priority patient problem?
   A. Feelings of anxiety about the illness and future health
   B. Poor circulation to the extremities
   C. Need for education about personal health
   D. Poor perfusion of cardiac tissues
5. The nurse is caring for a patient recovering from a coronary angioplasty with stent placement. Which intervention is a priority for the patient at this time?
   A. Securing chest tubes to bedding
   B. Maintaining leg extension on the affected side
   C. Discontinuing intravenous lines when taking oral fluids
   D. Treating chest pain with intravenous morphine as needed
6. The nurse is planning care for a patient with acute myocardial infarction. What goals should the nurse use to guide this patient's care? (Select all that apply.)
   A. Relieve chest pain.
   B. Prevent complications.
   C. Increase blood viscosity.
   D. Decrease cardiac workload.
   E. Reduce myocardial damage.
7. A patient is a potential candidate for fibrinolytic therapy. The nurse understands that which findings may make that treatment contraindicated? (Select all that apply.)
   A. The patient is very anxious.
   B. The patient had gastric bypass surgery two months ago.
   C. The patient was in a motor vehicle crash last week.
   D. The patient's BMI falls in the obese category.
   E. The patient takes medication to control essential hypertension.
8. The nurse is reviewing laboratory results for a patient admitted with acute chest pain. Which laboratory value should cause the nurse the most concern?
   A. AST 65 units/L
   B. CK 320 units/L
   C. Hematocrit 35%
   D. APTT 35 seconds
9. The nurse recognizes that a patient has developed second-degree AV block, type II (Mobitz II). Which action should the nurse take at this time?
   A. Record the finding in the chart.
   B. Place the patient in Fowler position.
   C. Prepare for temporary pacemaker insertion.
   D. Administer a Class IB antidysrhythmic drug.
10. The nurse identifies that a patient has sinus bradycardia with a heart rate at 45 bpm. What should the nurse do first?
   A. Assess mental status and blood pressure.
   B. Prepare to administer intravenous atropine.
   C. Assess peripheral pulses on all four extremities.
   D. Determine if an apical-radial pulse deficit is present.

See Test Yourself answers in Appendix B.

REFERENCES

Adams, M. P., Holland, L. N., & Urban, C. (2017). *Pharmacology for nursing: A pathophysiologic approach* (5th ed.). Hoboken, NJ: Pearson Education.

American Heart Association (AHA). (2015). *Highlights of the 2015 American Heart Association Guidelines Update for CPR and ECC.* Retrieved from https://eccguidelines.heart.org/wp-content/uploads/2015/10/2015-AHA-Guidelines-Highlights-English.pdf.

American Heart Association (AHA). (2017). *Cholesterol toolkit.* Retrieved from www.ksw-gtg.com/aha-hcp-cholesterol/#/1/.

Benjamin, E. J., Blaha, M. J., Chiuve, S. E., Cushman, M., Das, S. R., Deo, R., . . . American Heart Association Statistics Committee and Stroke Statistics Subcommittee. (2017). Heart disease and stroke statistics—2017 update: A report from the American Heart Association. *Circulation, 135*(10), e146–e603.

Blakeman, J. R., & Bookman, K. J. (2016). Prodromal myocardial infarction symptoms experienced by women. *Heart and Lung, 45,* 327–335.

Grass, A. W., & Brener, S. J. (2014). *Complications of acute myocardial infarction.* Cleveland Clinic Center for Continuing Education. Retrieved from www.clevelandclinicmeded.com/medicalpubs/diseasemanagement/cardiology/complications-of-acute-myocardial-infarction/.

Kee, J. L. (2014). *Laboratory and diagnostic tests with nursing implications* (9th ed.). Boston, MA: Pearson.

National Heart, Lung, and Blood Institute (NHLBI), National Institutes of Health. (2017a). *High blood cholesterol. What you need to know.* Retrieved from https://www.nhlbi.nih.gov/health/resources/heart/heart-cholesterol-hbc-what-html.

National Heart, Lung, and Blood Institute (NHLBI), National Institutes of Health. (2017b). *What are the risk factors for heart disease?* Retrieved from https://www.nhlbi.nih.gov/health/educational/hearttruth/lower-risk/risk-factors.htm.

Nayor, M., & Vasan, R. S. (2016). Recent update to the US Cholesterol Treatment Guidelines: A comparison with international guidelines. *Circulation, 133,* 1795–1806.

Ornish Lifestyle Medicine. (2018). *Nutrition.* Retrieved from https://www.ornish.com/proven-program/nutrition/.

Patel, M. R., Calhoon, J. H., Dehmer, G. J., Grantham, J. A., Maddox, T. M., Maron, D. J., & Smith, P. K. (2017). ACC/AATS/AHA/ASE/ASNC/SCAI/SCCT/STS 2017 appropriate use criteria for coronary revascularization in patients with stable ischemic heart disease: A report of the American College of Cardiology Appropriate Use Criteria Task Force, American Association for Thoracic Surgery, American Heart Association, American Society of Echocardiography, American Society of Nuclear Cardiology, Society for Cardiovascular Angiography and Interventions, Society of Cardiovascular Computed Tomography, and Society of Thoracic Surgeons. *Journal of the American College of Cardiology 69,* 2212–2241.

Perrin, K. O., & MacLeod, C. E. (2018). *Understanding the essentials of critical care nursing* (3rd ed.) Hoboken, NJ: Pearson Education.

Pritikin Longevity Center. (2017). *Pritikin diet and eating plan.* Retrieved from https://www.pritikin.com/healthiest-diet/pritikin-eating-plan.

Shields, K. M., Fox, K. L., & Liebrecht, C. (2018). *Pearson Nurse's Drug Guide: 2018.* Boston, MA: Pearson.

Sorenson, M., Quinn, L., & Klein, D. (2019). *Pathophysiology: Concepts of human disease.* New York, NY: Pearson.

U.S. Department of Agriculture and U.S. Department of Health and Human Services. (2015). *Dietary guidelines for Americans, 2015–2020* (8th ed.). Washington, DC: U.S. Government Printing Office.

U.S. Department of Health and Human Services (USDHHS). (2006). *Your guide to lowering your blood pressure with DASH.* Retrieved from https://www.nhlbi.nih.gov/files/docs/public/heart/new_dash.pdf.

U.S. Department of Health and Human Services (USDHHS). (2018). *Healthy People 2020.* Retrieved from https://www.healthypeople.gov/2020/topics-objectives/topic/heart-disease-and-stroke.

Whelton, P. K., Carey, R. M., Aronow, W. S., Casey, D. E. Jr., Collins, K. J., Dennison Himmelfarb, C., . . . Wright, J. T. Jr. (2017). ACC/AHA/AAPA/ABC/ACPM/AGS/APhA/ASH/ASPC/NMA/PCNA guideline for the prevention, detection, evaluation, and management of high blood pressure in adults. *Hypertension.* [Epub ahead of print].

ADDITIONAL RESOURCES

Jellinger, P. S., Handelsman, Y., Rosenblit, P. D., Bloomgarden, Z. T., Fonseca, V. A., Garber, A. J., . . . Bush, M. A. (2017). American Association of Clinical Endocrinologists and American College of Endocrinology guidelines for management of dyslipidemia and prevention of cardiovascular disease. *Endocrine Practice, 23*(Suppl. 2), 1–87.

Lloyd-Jones, D. M., Morris, P. B., Ballantyne, C. M., Birtcher, K. K., Daly, D. D. Jr., DePalma, S, M., . . . Smith, S. C. Jr. (2017). 2017 focused update of the 2016 ACC Expert Consensus Decision Pathway on the role of non-statin therapies for LDL-cholesterol lowering in the management of atherosclerotic cardiovascular disease risk. *Journal of the American College of Cardiology, 70*(14), 1785–1822.

Stone, N. J., Robinson, J., Lichtenstein, A. H., Bairey Merz, C. N., Blum, C. B., Eckel, R. H., . . . Wilson, P. W. F. (2014). 2013 ACC/AHA guideline on the treatment of blood cholesterol to reduce atherosclerotic cardiovascular risk in adults: A report of the American College of Cardiology/American Heart Association Task Force on Practice Guidelines. *Circulation,* 63(25, Pt. B), 2889–2934.

Tracy, C. M., Epstein, A. E., Darbar, D., DiMarco, J. P., Dunbar, S. B., Estes, N. A. M., . . . Sweeney, M. O. (2012). 2012 ACCF/AHA/HRS focused update of the 2008 guidelines for device-based therapy of cardiac rhythm abnormalities: A report of the American College of Cardiology Foundation/American Heart Association Task Force on Practice Guidelines. *Circulation, 126*(14), 1784–1800.

U.S. Department of Health and Human Services (USDHHS). (2006). *Your guide to lowering your blood pressure with DASH.* Retrieved from https://www.nhlbi.nih.gov/files/docs/public/heart/new_dash.pdf.

Chapter 31

Nursing Care of Patients with Cardiac Disorders

Chapter Outline and Learning Outcomes

CLINICAL COMPETENCIES

- Apply knowledge of normal cardiac anatomy and physiology and assessment techniques in caring for patients with cardiac disorders.
- Assess the functional health status of patients with cardiac disorders, documenting and reporting deviations for expected findings.
- Based on patient assessment and knowledge of the disorder, determine priority nursing diagnoses.
- Plan, prioritize, and provide evidence-based, individualized care for patients with cardiac disorders.
- Safely and knowledgeably administer prescribed medications and treatments to patients with cardiac disorders.
- Actively participate in planning and coordinating interprofessional care for patients with cardiac disorders.
- Provide appropriate teaching and community-based care for patients with cardiac disorders and their families.
- Evaluate the effectiveness of nursing care, revising the plan of care as needed to promote, maintain, or restore the functional health status of patients with cardiac disorders.

KEY TERMS

aortic valve, 1088
cardiac tamponade, 1084
cardiomyopathy, 1097
endocarditis, 1077
heart failure, 1055
hemodynamics, 1061
heart failure with preserved ejection fraction (HFpEF), 1055
heart failure with reduced ejection fraction (HFrEF), 1055
mean arterial pressure (MAP), 1063
mitral valve, 1087
murmur, 1088
myocarditis, 1082
orthopnea, 1058
paroxysmal nocturnal dyspnea (PND), 1059
pericarditis, 1083
pulmonary edema, 1071
pulmonic valve, 1088
regurgitation, 1075
rheumatic fever, 1075
rheumatic heart disease (RHD), 1075
stenosis, 1075
tricuspid valve, 1087
valvular heart disease, 1087

Cardiac disorders affect the structure and/or function of the heart. These disorders interfere with the heart's primary purpose: To pump enough blood to meet the body's demand for oxygen and nutrients. Disruptions in cardiac function affect the functioning of other organs and tissues, potentially leading to organ system failure and death. Emergence of symptoms (fatigue, dyspnea, chest pain) is common with the progression of cardiac disorders. The New York Heart Association (NYHA) classification (American Heart Association [AHA], 2017a) is commonly used to describe the severity of exertional symptoms observed (see **Table 31.1**).

Heart failure is the most common cardiac disorder. Other cardiac disorders discussed in this chapter include structural cardiac disorders, such as valve disorders and cardiomyopathy, and inflammatory cardiac disorders, such

Table 31.1 New York Heart Association Classification

Class	Severity of Symptoms
I	No limitation in physical activity/asymptomatic
II	Symptoms with strenuous activity
III	Symptoms with mild activity
IV	Symptoms at rest

as endocarditis and pericarditis. Before continuing with this chapter, please review the heart's anatomy and physiology, nursing assessment, and diagnostic tests in Chapter 29.

31.1 Heart Failure

Heart failure is a complex syndrome resulting from cardiac disorders that impair the ventricles' ability to fill with and effectively pump blood. In heart failure, the heart is unable to pump enough blood to meet the metabolic demands of the body (Sorenson, Quinn, & Klein, 2019). It is the end result of many conditions. Frequently, it is a long-term effect of coronary heart disease and myocardial infarction (MI) when left-ventricular damage is extensive enough to impair cardiac output (refer to Chapter 29). Other diseases of the heart may also cause heart failure, including structural and inflammatory disorders. In a normal heart, failure can result from excessive demands placed on it. Heart failure may be acute or chronic.

The American Heart Association (2017a) classifies heart failure based on objective signs into stages A through D. Class C is further delineated into **heart failure with preserved ejection fraction (HFpEF)** and **heart failure with reduced ejection fraction (HFrEF)**. See **Table 31.2** for staging.

The Patient with Heart Failure

As mentioned, heart failure develops when the heart cannot effectively fill or contract with adequate strength to function as a pump to meet the needs of the body. As a result, cardiac output falls, leading to decreased tissue perfusion. The body initially adjusts to reduced cardiac output by activating inherent compensatory mechanisms to restore tissue perfusion. These normal mechanisms may result in vascular congestion—hence the commonly used term *congestive heart failure (CHF)*. As these mechanisms are exhausted, heart failure ensues, with increased morbidity and mortality.

Heart failure is a disorder of cardiac function. It is frequently due to *impaired myocardial contraction*, which may result from coronary heart disease and myocardial ischemia or infarct, or from a primary cardiac muscle disorder such as cardiomyopathy or myocarditis. Structural cardiac disorders, such as valve disorders or congenital heart defects, and hypertension can also lead to heart failure when the heart muscle is damaged by the long-standing *excessive workload* associated with these conditions. Other patients without a primary abnormality of myocardial function may present with manifestations of heart failure due to *acute excess demands* placed on the myocardium, such as volume overload, hyperthyroidism, and massive pulmonary embolus (see **Box 31.1**). Hypertension and coronary heart disease are the leading causes of heart failure in the United States. The high prevalence of hypertension in African Americans contributes significantly to their risk for and incidence of heart failure.

Incidence, Prevalence, and Risk Factors

More than 6.6 million people in the United States are currently living with heart failure; approximately 960,000 new cases of heart failure are diagnosed annually (Benjamin et al., 2017). Estimates predict an additional 3 million people will have heart failure by 2030. There is a rapid rise in heart failure prevalence after age 65. There is a gender differential for HF incidence. In males, HF incidence approximately doubles with each 10-year age increase from 65 to 85 years; however, the HF incidence rate triples for females between ages 65 to 74 and 75 to 84 years (Benjamin et al., 2017). At age 40, the lifetime risk of developing heart failure is 20 to 45% (Benjamin et al., 2017). There is a racial differential as well in the prevalence of HF as well. African Americans are disproportionately affected by HF (Sharma, Colvin-Adams, & Yancy, 2014). The estimated direct and indirect cost of heart failure in the United States in 2012 was $30.7 billion.

Ischemic heart disease (coronary heart disease) is the leading risk factor for heart failure. Up to 75% of individuals with heart failure have a history of hypertension.

The prognosis for a patient with heart failure depends on its underlying cause and how effectively precipitating factors can be treated. Most patients with heart failure die within 8 years of the diagnosis. The risk for sudden cardiac death is dramatically increased, occurring at a rate six to nine times that of the general population. In 2014, one in eight death certificates in the United States mentioned heart failure as the primary or a contributing cause of death (Benjamin et al., 2017).

Physiology Review

The mechanical pumping action of cardiac muscle propels the blood it receives to the pulmonary and systemic vascular systems for reoxygenation and delivery to the tissues. *Cardiac output (CO)* is the amount of blood pumped from the

Table 31.2 American Heart Association Heart Failure Stages

Stage	Substage	Defining Physiology, Characteristics
A		At high risk for HF but without structural heart disease or symptoms of HF
B		Structural heart disease but without signs or symptoms of HF
C	HFpEF HFrEF	Structural heart disease with prior or current symptoms of HF
D		Refractory HF

BOX 31.1

Selected Causes of Heart Failure

Impaired Myocardial Function	Increased Cardiac Workload	Acute Noncardiac Conditions
Coronary heart disease	Hypertension	Volume overload
Cardiomyopathies	Valve disorders	Hyperthyroidism
Rheumatic fever	Anemias	Fever, infection
Infective endocarditis	Congenital heart defects	Massive pulmonary embolus

ventricles in 1 minute. Cardiac output is used to assess cardiac performance, especially left-ventricular function. Effective cardiac output depends on adequate functional muscle mass and the ability of the ventricles to work together. Cardiac output is normally regulated by the oxygen needs of the body: As oxygen use increases, cardiac output increases to maintain cellular function. *Cardiac reserve* is the ability of the heart to increase CO to meet metabolic demand. Ventricular damage reduces the cardiac reserve.

Cardiac output is a product of heart rate and stroke volume. *Heart rate* affects cardiac output by controlling the number of ventricular contractions per minute. It is influenced by the autonomic nervous system, catecholamines, and thyroid hormones. Activation of a stress response (e.g., hypovolemia or fear) stimulates the sympathetic nervous system, increasing the heart rate and its contractility. Elevated heart rates increase cardiac output. Very rapid heart rates, however, shorten ventricular filling time (diastole), reducing stroke volume and cardiac output. On the other hand, a slow heart rate reduces cardiac output simply because of fewer cardiac cycles.

Stroke volume, the volume of blood ejected with each heartbeat, is determined by preload, afterload, and myocardial contractility. *Preload* is the volume of blood in the ventricles at end diastole (just prior to contraction). The blood in the ventricles exerts pressure on the ventricle walls, stretching muscle fibers. The greater the blood volume, the greater the force with which the ventricle contracts to expel the blood. *End-diastolic volume (EDV)* depends on the amount of blood returning to the ventricles (*venous return*), and the distensibility or stiffness of the ventricles (*compliance*). (See **Box 31.2**.)

Afterload is the force needed to eject blood into the circulation. This force must be great enough to overcome arterial pressures within the pulmonary and systemic vascular systems. The right ventricle must generate enough force to open the pulmonary valve and eject its blood into the pulmonary artery. The left ventricle ejects its blood into the systemic circulation by overcoming the arterial resistance behind the aortic valve. Increased systemic vascular resistance (e.g., hypertension) increases afterload, impairing stroke volume and increasing myocardial workload.

Contractility is the natural ability of cardiac muscle fibers to shorten during systole. Contractility is necessary to overcome arterial pressures and eject blood during systole. Impaired contractility affects cardiac output by reducing stroke volume. The *ejection fraction (EF)* is the percentage of blood in the ventricle that is ejected during systole. A normal ejection fraction is approximately 60%.

BOX 31.2

Explaining Physiologic Terms Using Practical Examples

The concepts of preload, the Frank-Starling mechanism, compliance, and afterload can be difficult to understand and to explain to patients. Use common analogies to make these concepts easier to understand:

- ***Preload:*** Think about a new rubber band. As you stretch the rubber band and then release it, it snaps back into shape with great force.
- ***Frank-Starling mechanism:*** When you repeatedly stretch that rubber band beyond a certain limit, it loses some elasticity and fails to return to its original shape and size.
- ***Compliance:*** Use a new rubber balloon to illustrate this concept. A new balloon is not very compliant—it takes a lot of work (force) to inflate it. As the balloon is repeatedly stretched, it becomes more compliant, expanding easily with less force.
- ***Afterload:*** When a hose is crimped or plugged, more force is required to eject a stream of water out its end.

Pathophysiology

When the heart begins to fail, mechanisms are activated to compensate for the impaired function and maintain the cardiac output. The primary compensatory mechanisms are (1) the Frank-Starling mechanism, (2) neuroendocrine responses including activation of the sympathetic nervous system (SNS) and the renin–angiotensin–aldosterone system (RAAS), and (3) ventricular hypertrophy. These mechanisms and their effects are summarized in **Table 31.3**.

Decreased cardiac output initially stimulates aortic baroreceptors, which in turn stimulate the SNS. SNS stimulation produces both cardiac and vascular responses through the release of norepinephrine. Norepinephrine increases heart rate and contractility by stimulating cardiac beta-receptors. Cardiac output improves as both heart rate and stroke volume increase. Norepinephrine also causes arterial and venous vasoconstriction, increasing venous return to the heart. Increased venous return increases ventricular filling and myocardial stretch, increasing the force

Table 31.3 Compensatory Mechanisms Activated in Heart Failure

Mechanism	Physiology	Effect on Body Systems	Complications
Frank-Starling mechanism	The greater the stretch of cardiac muscle fibers, the greater the force of contraction.	■ Increased contractile force leading to increased CO	■ Increased myocardial oxygen demand ■ Limited by overstretching
Neuroendocrine response	Decreased CO stimulates the sympathetic nervous system and catecholamine release.	■ Increased HR, BP, and contractility ■ Increased vascular resistance ■ Increased venous return	■ Tachycardia with decreased filling time and decreased CO ■ Increased vascular resistance ■ Increased myocardial workload and oxygen demand
	Decreased CO and decreased renal perfusion stimulate renin–angiotensin system.	■ Vasoconstriction and increased BP	■ Increased myocardial workload ■ Renal vasoconstriction and decreased renal perfusion
	Angiotensin stimulates aldosterone release from adrenal cortex.	■ Salt and water retention by the kidneys ■ Increased vascular volume	■ Increased preload and afterload ■ Pulmonary congestion
	ADH is released from posterior pituitary. Atrial natriuretic factor is released.	■ Water excretion inhibited ■ Increased sodium excretion ■ Diuresis	■ Fluid retention and increased preload and afterload
	Blood flow is redistributed to vital organs (heart and brain).	■ Decreased perfusion of other organ systems ■ Decreased perfusion of skin and muscles	■ Renal failure ■ Anaerobic metabolism and lactic acidosis
Ventricular hypertrophy	Increased cardiac workload causes myocardial muscle to hypertrophy and ventricles to dilate.	■ Increased contractile force to maintain CO	■ Increased myocardial oxygen demand ■ Cellular enlargement

of contraction (the Frank-Starling mechanism). Overstretching the muscle fibers past their physiologic limit results in an ineffective contraction.

Blood flow is redistributed to the brain and the heart to maintain perfusion of these vital organs. Decreased renal perfusion causes renin to be released from the kidneys. Activation of the RAAS produces additional vasoconstriction and stimulates the adrenal cortex to produce aldosterone and the posterior pituitary to release antidiuretic hormone (ADH). Aldosterone stimulates sodium reabsorption in renal tubules, promoting water retention. ADH acts on the distal tubule to inhibit water excretion and causes vasoconstriction. The effect of these hormones is significant vasoconstriction and salt and water retention, with a resulting increase in vascular volume. Increased ventricular filling increases the force of contraction, improving cardiac output. The increased vascular volume and venous return also increase atrial pressures, stimulating the release of an additional hormone, *atrial natriuretic factor (ANF)* or *atriopeptin.* ANF balances the effects of the other hormones to a certain extent, promoting sodium and water excretion and inhibiting the release of norepinephrine, renin, and ADH. This hormone is thought to be a natural preventative that delays severe cardiac decompensation.

Ventricular remodeling occurs as the heart chambers and myocardium adapt to fluid volume and pressure increases. The chambers dilate to accommodate excess fluid resulting from increased vascular volume and incomplete emptying. Initially, this additional stretch causes more effective contractions. *Ventricular hypertrophy* occurs as existing cardiac muscle cells enlarge, increasing their contractile elements (actin and myosin) and force of contraction.

Although these responses may help in the short-term regulation of cardiac output, it is now recognized that they hasten the deterioration of cardiac function. The onset of heart failure is heralded by *decompensation*, the loss of effective compensation. Heart failure progresses due to the very mechanisms that initially maintained circulatory stability.

The rapid heart rate shortens diastolic filling time, compromises coronary artery perfusion, and increases myocardial oxygen demand. Resulting ischemia further impairs cardiac output. Beta-receptors in the heart become less sensitive to continued SNS stimulation, decreasing heart rate and contractility. As the beta-receptors become less sensitive, norepinephrine stores in the cardiac muscle become depleted. In contrast, alpha-receptors on peripheral blood vessels become increasingly sensitive to persistent stimulation, promoting vasoconstriction and increasing afterload and cardiac workload.

Initially, ventricular hypertrophy and dilation increase cardiac output, but chronic distention causes the ventricular wall eventually to thin and degenerate. The purpose of hypertrophy is thus defeated. In addition, chronic overloading of the dilated ventricle eventually stretches the fibers beyond the optimal point for effective contraction. The ventricles continue to dilate to accommodate the excess fluid, but the heart loses the ability to contract forcefully. The heart muscle may eventually become so large that the coronary blood supply is inadequate, causing ischemia.

Chronic distention exhausts atrial stores of ANF. The effects of norepinephrine, renin, and ADH prevail, and the renin–angiotensin pathway is continually stimulated. This mechanism ultimately raises the hemodynamic stress on the heart by increasing both preload and afterload. As heart function deteriorates, less blood is delivered to the tissues and to the heart itself. Ischemia and necrosis of the myocardium further weaken the already failing heart, and the cycle repeats.

In normal hearts, the cardiac reserve allows the heart to adjust its output to meet metabolic needs of the body, increasing the cardiac output by up to five times the basal level during exercise. Patients with heart failure have minimal to no cardiac reserve. At rest, they may be unaffected; however, any stressor (e.g., exercise, illness) taxes their ability to meet the demand for oxygen and nutrients. Manifestations of activity intolerance when the person is at rest indicate a critical level of cardiac decompensation.

Classifications and Manifestations of Heart Failure

Heart failure is commonly classified in several different ways, depending on the underlying pathology. Classifications include:

- Systolic versus diastolic failure
- Left-sided versus right-sided failure
- Low-output versus high-output failure
- Acute versus chronic failure.

Systolic versus Diastolic Failure

Systolic failure occurs when the ventricle fails to contract adequately to eject a sufficient blood volume into the arterial system. Systolic function is affected by loss of myocardial cells due to ischemia and infarction, cardiomyopathy, or inflammation. The manifestations of systolic failure are those of decreased cardiac output: Weakness, fatigue, and decreased exercise tolerance.

Diastolic failure results when the heart cannot completely relax in diastole, disrupting normal filling. Passive diastolic filling decreases, increasing the importance of atrial contraction to preload. Diastolic dysfunction results from decreased ventricular compliance due to hypertrophic and cellular changes and impaired relaxation of the heart muscle. Its manifestations result from increased pressure and congestion behind the ventricle: Shortness of breath, tachypnea, and respiratory crackles if the left ventricle is affected; distended neck veins, liver enlargement, anorexia, and nausea if the right ventricle is affected. Many patients have components of both systolic and diastolic failure.

Left-Sided versus Right-Sided Failure

Depending on the pathophysiology involved, either the left or the right ventricle may be primarily affected. In chronic heart failure, however, both ventricles are typically impaired to some degree. Coronary heart disease and hypertension are common causes of *left-sided heart failure*, whereas *right-sided heart failure* is often caused by conditions that restrict blood flow to the lungs, such as acute or chronic pulmonary disease. Left-sided heart failure can also lead to right-sided failure as pressures in the pulmonary vascular system increase with congestion behind the failing left ventricle.

As left-ventricular function fails, cardiac output falls. Pressures in the left ventricle and atrium increase as the amount of blood remaining in the ventricle after systole increases. These increased pressures impair filling, causing congestion and increased pressures in the pulmonary vascular system. Increased pressures in this normally low-pressure system increase fluid movement from the blood vessels into interstitial tissues and the alveoli (**Figure 31.1** ■).

The manifestations of left-sided heart failure result from pulmonary congestion (*backward effects*) and decreased cardiac output (*forward effects*). Fatigue and activity intolerance are common early manifestations. Dizziness and syncope also may result from decreased cardiac output. Pulmonary congestion causes dyspnea, shortness of breath, and a cough. The patient may develop **orthopnea** (difficulty breathing while lying down), prompting use of two or three pillows or a recliner for sleeping. Cyanosis from impaired gas exchange may be noted. On auscultation of the lungs, inspiratory crackles (rales) and wheezes may be heard in lung bases. An S_3 gallop may be present, reflecting the heart's attempts to fill an already distended ventricle.

In right-sided heart failure, increased pressures in the pulmonary vasculature or right-ventricular muscle damage impair the right ventricle's ability to pump blood into the pulmonary circulation. The right ventricle and atrium become distended, and blood accumulates in the systemic venous system. Increased venous pressures cause abdominal organs to become congested and peripheral tissue edema to develop (**Figure 31.2** ■).

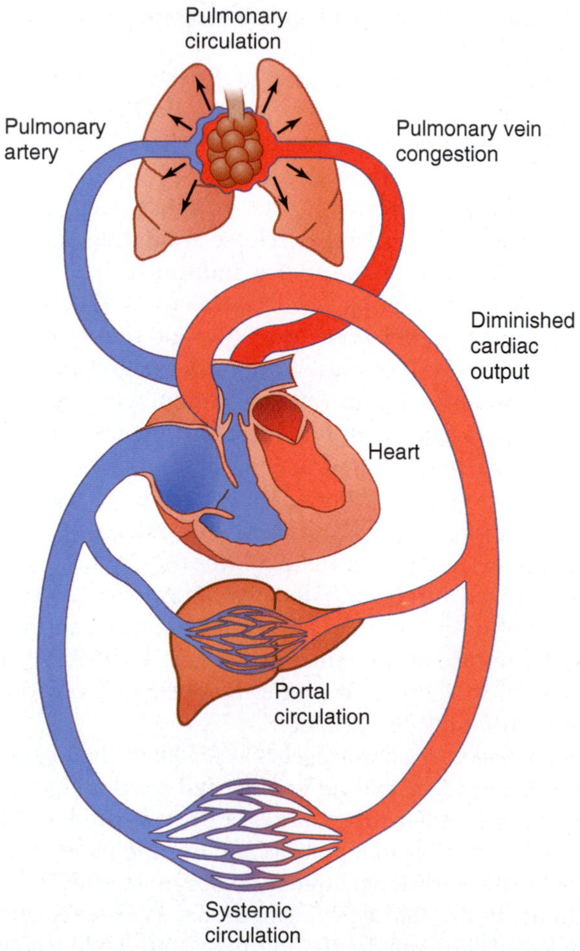
Pulmonary circulation
Pulmonary artery
Pulmonary vein congestion
Diminished cardiac output
Heart
Portal circulation
Systemic circulation

Figure 31.1 ■ The hemodynamic effects of left-sided heart failure.

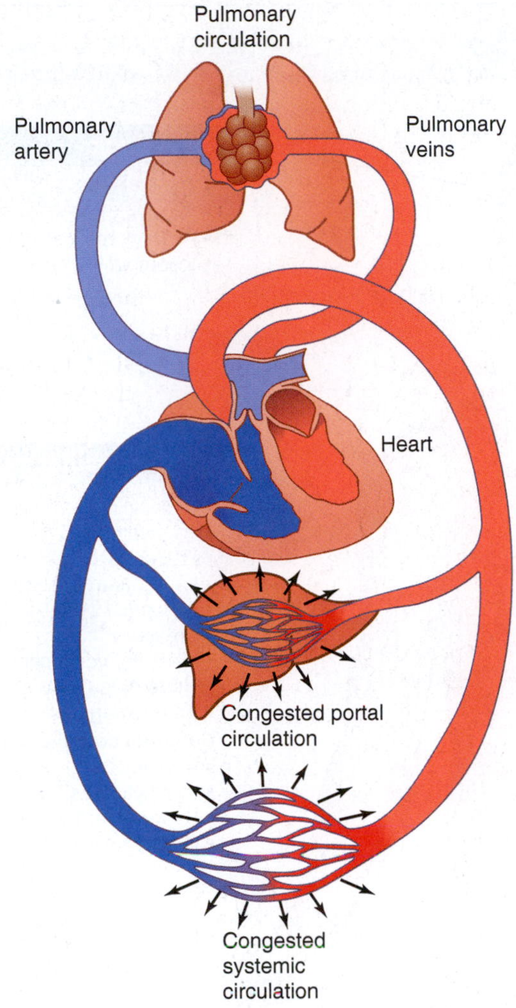
Pulmonary circulation
Pulmonary artery
Pulmonary veins
Heart
Congested portal circulation
Congested systemic circulation

Figure 31.2 ■ The hemodynamic effects of right-sided heart failure.

Dependent tissues tend to be affected because of the effects of gravity; edema develops in the feet and legs or, if the patient is bedridden, in the sacrum. Congestion of gastrointestinal tract vessels causes anorexia and nausea. Right upper quadrant pain may result from liver engorgement. Neck veins distend and become visible even when the patient is upright due to increased venous pressure.

Low-Output versus High-Output Failure

Patients with heart failure due to coronary heart disease, hypertension, cardiomyopathy, and other primary cardiac disorders develop *low-output failure* and manifestations such as those previously described. Patients in hypermetabolic states (e.g., hyperthyroidism, infection, anemia, or pregnancy) require increased cardiac output to maintain blood flow and oxygen to the tissues. If the increased blood flow cannot meet the oxygen demands of the tissues, compensatory mechanisms are activated to further increase cardiac output, which in turn further increases oxygen demand. Thus, even though cardiac output is high, the heart is unable to meet increased oxygen demands. This condition is known as *high-output failure*.

Acute versus Chronic Failure

Acute failure is the abrupt onset of a myocardial injury (such as a massive MI) resulting in suddenly decreased cardiac function and signs of decreased cardiac output. *Chronic failure* is a progressive deterioration of the heart muscle due to cardiomyopathies, valvular disease, or coronary heart disease (CHD).

Other Manifestations

In addition to the previous manifestations for the various classifications of heart failure, other signs and symptoms commonly are seen.

A fall in cardiac output activates mechanisms that cause increased salt and water retention. This causes weight gain and further increases pressures in the capillaries, resulting in edema. *Nocturia*, voiding more than one time at night, develops as edema fluid from dependent tissues is reabsorbed when the patient is supine. **Paroxysmal nocturnal dyspnea (PND)**, a frightening condition in which the patient awakens at night acutely short of breath, may also develop. PND occurs when edema fluid that has accumulated during the day is reabsorbed into the circulation at night, causing fluid overload and pulmonary congestion. Severe heart failure may cause dyspnea at rest as well as with activity, signifying little or no cardiac reserve. Both an S_3 and an S_4 gallop may be heard on auscultation.

See the Multisystem Effects of Heart Failure box on page 1062.

Complications

The compensatory mechanisms initiated in heart failure can lead to complications in other body systems. Congestive hepatomegaly and splenomegaly caused by engorgement of the portal venous system result in increased abdominal pressure, ascites, and gastrointestinal problems. With prolonged right-sided heart failure, liver function may be impaired. Myocardial distention can precipitate dysrhythmias, further impairing cardiac output. Pleural effusions and other pulmonary problems may develop. Major complications of severe heart failure are cardiogenic shock (described in Chapter 11) and acute pulmonary edema, a medical emergency described in the next section of this chapter.

Interprofessional Care

The main goals for care of heart failure are to slow its progression, reduce cardiac workload, improve cardiac function, and control fluid retention. Treatment strategies are based on the evolution and progression of heart failure (**Table 31.4**).

Diagnosis

Diagnosis of heart failure is based on the history, physical examination, and diagnostic findings.

- ***B-type natriuretic peptide (BNP)*** is a hormone released by the heart muscle in response to changes in blood volume. *N-terminal prohormone of brain natriuretic peptide (NT-proBNP)* is a rapid test (readable in 15 minutes) for

Multisystem Effects of
Heart Failure

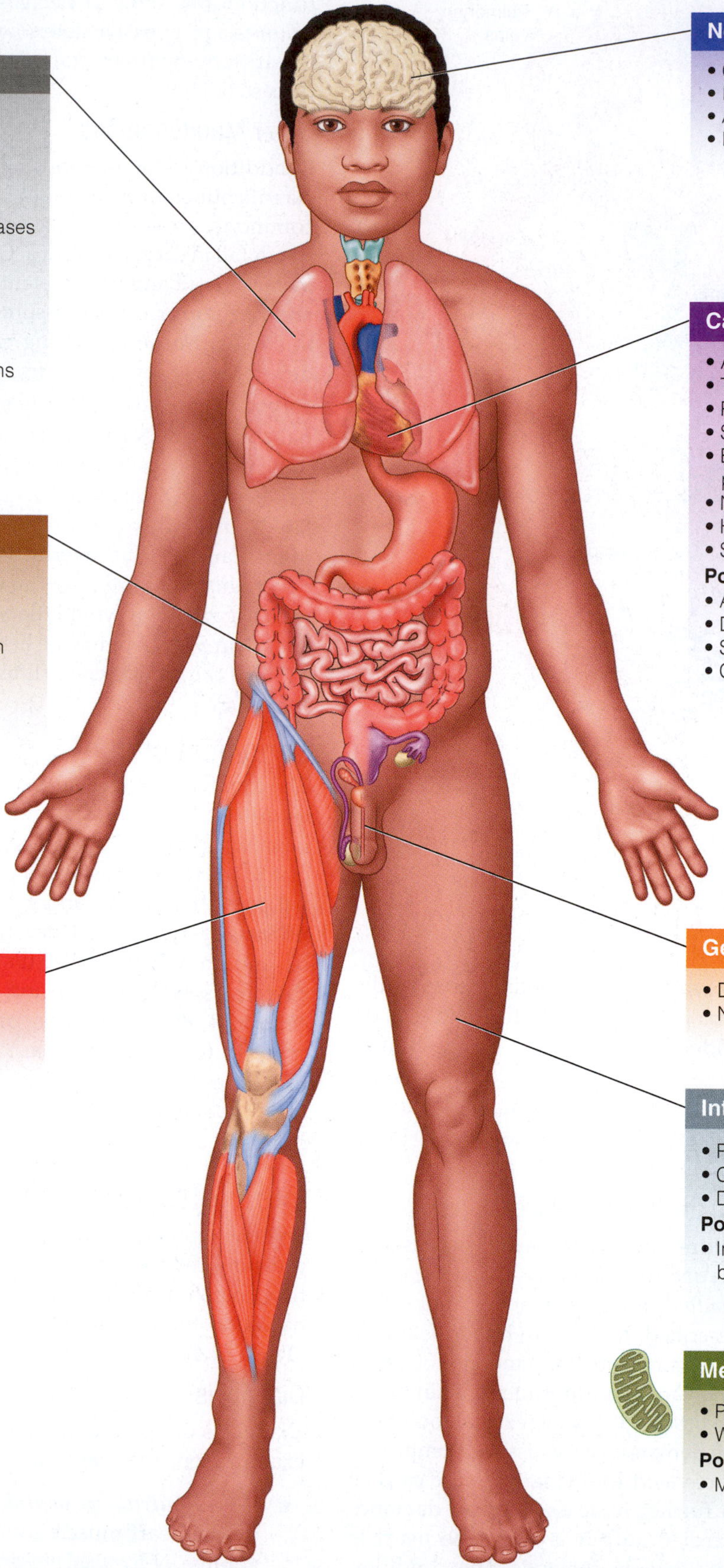

Respiratory
- Dyspnea on exertion
- Shortness of breath
- Tachypnea
- Orthopnea
- Dry cough
- Crackles (rales) in lung bases

Potential complications
- Pulmonary edema
- Pneumonia
- Cardiac asthma
- Pleural effusion
- Cheyne-Stokes respirations
- Respiratory acidosis

Neurologic
- Confusion
- Impaired memory
- Anxiety, restlessness
- Insomnia

Cardiovascular
- Activity intolerance
- Tachycardia
- Palpitations
- S_3, S_4 heart sounds
- Elevated central venous pressure
- Neck vein distention
- Hepatojugular reflux
- Splenomegaly

Potential complications
- Angina
- Dysrhythmias
- Sudden cardiac death
- Cardiogenic shock

Gastrointestinal
- Anorexia, nausea
- Abdominal distention
- Liver enlargement
- Right upper quadrant pain

Potential complications
- Malnutrition
- Ascites
- Liver dysfunction

Musculoskeletal
- Fatigue
- Weakness

Genitourinary
- Decreased urine output
- Nocturia

Integumentary
- Pallor or cyanosis
- Cool, clammy skin
- Diaphoresis

Potential complication
- Increased risk for tissue breakdown

Metabolic Processes
- Peripheral edema
- Weight gain

Potential complication
- Metabolic acidosis

Table 31.4 Recommended Treatment by Stages of Heart Failure

Stage	Recommended Treatment Measures
A High-risk for HF	Treat underlying risk factors (e.g., hypertension) including lipid disorders Angiotensin-converting enzyme (ACE) inhibitor or angiotensin-receptor blocker (ARB) therapy as appropriate Statins as appropriate Heart-healthy lifestyle (exercise; diet reducing salt, excess fats, and calories; tracking fluid intake) Smoking cessation, if indicated Discourage alcohol, illicit drug use Control blood glucose in patients with metabolic syndrome
B Structural heart changes without signs/symptoms of HF	As for stage A ACE inhibitor or ARB therapy as appropriate Beta-blocker therapy, if indicated In selected patients: Revascularization procedures, ICD
C Structural heart changes with signs/symptoms of HF	Stage C classified by preserved or reduced ejection fraction
C-HFpEF HF with preserved ejection fraction	Diuresis to relieve congestive symptoms Follow guidelines for management of comorbidities (e.g., HTN, AF, CAD, DM) Revascularization or valvular surgery when indicated
C-HFrEF HF with reduced ejection fraction	Diuretics for fluid retention ACE inhibitor or ARB therapy as appropriate Beta blockers as appropriate Aldosterone antagonists as appropriate In selected patients, other drugs may be used, including Hydralazine/isosorbide dinitrate, combined ACE inhibitor and ARB, Digoxin Other treatments in selected patients can include cardiac resynchronization therapy (biventricular pacing), implantable cardiac defibrillator, revascularization, or valvular surgery, when indicated
D	Chronic inotropes Temporary or permanent mechanical circulatory support Heart transplant Experimental surgery or drugs Palliative care and hospice ICD deactivation

BNP (Yancy et al., 2017). Blood levels of BNP increase in heart failure; however, it is important to remember that BNP levels may be elevated in women and in people over age 60 who do not have heart failure. These levels can also be lower in obese patients. Therefore, an elevated BNP cannot be used alone to diagnose heart failure.

- ***Serum electrolytes*** are measured to evaluate fluid and electrolyte status. Serum osmolality may be low due to fluid retention. Sodium, potassium, and chloride levels provide a baseline for evaluating the effects of treatment; serum calcium and magnesium are measured as well.
- ***Urinalysis, blood urea nitrogen (BUN)***, and ***serum creatinine*** are obtained to evaluate renal function.
- ***Liver function tests***, including ALT, AST, LDH, serum bilirubin, and total protein and albumin levels, are obtained to evaluate possible effects of heart failure on liver function.
- ***Thyroid function tests***, including TSH and TH levels, are obtained because both hyperthyroidism and hypothyroidism can be either a primary or a contributing cause of heart failure.
- ***Arterial blood gases (ABGs)*** are drawn for those with acute heart failure to evaluate gas exchange in the lungs and tissues.
- ***Chest x-ray*** may show pulmonary vascular congestion and cardiomegaly in heart failure.
- ***Electrocardiography*** is used to identify ECG changes associated with ventricular enlargement and to detect dysrhythmias, myocardial ischemia, or infarction.
- ***Echocardiography with Doppler flow studies*** are performed to evaluate left-ventricular function. Either *transthoracic echocardiography* or *transesophageal echocardiography* may be used.
- ***Radionuclide imaging*** is used to evaluate ventricular function and size.

Refer to Chapter 29 for more information and the nursing implications of these tests.

Hemodynamic Monitoring

Hemodynamics is the study of forces involved in blood circulation. Hemodynamic monitoring is used to assess cardiovascular function in patients who are critically ill or unstable. The main goals of invasive hemodynamic monitoring are to evaluate cardiac and circulatory function and the response to interventions.

Hemodynamic parameters include heart rate, arterial blood pressure, central venous or right atrial pressure, pulmonary pressures, and cardiac output. *Direct* hemodynamic parameters are obtained straight from the monitoring device (e.g., heart rate, arterial and venous pressures).

Indirect or *derived* measurements are calculated using the direct data (e.g., the cardiac index, mean arterial blood pressure, and stroke volume). Invasive hemodynamic monitoring is routinely used in critical care units.

Hemodynamic monitoring systems measure the pressure within a vessel and convert this signal into an electrical waveform that is amplified and displayed. The electrical signal may be graphically recorded on graph paper and displayed digitally on the monitor. System components include an invasive catheter threaded into an artery or vein connected to a transducer by stiff, high-pressure tubing. The pressure transducer translates pressures into an electrical signal that is relayed to the monitor. Additional components of the system include stopcocks and a continuous flush system with normal saline or heparinized saline and an infusion pressure bag to prevent clots from forming in the catheter. **Figure 31.3** ■ illustrates a pressure transducer and typical hemodynamic monitoring system.

Hemodynamic pressure monitoring may be used to measure peripheral arterial pressures, or central pressures, such as central venous pressure (CVP) or right atrial pressure (RAP) and pulmonary artery pressure (PAP). Although the information obtained from invasive monitoring is valuable, the procedure is not without risk. Pressure monitoring systems require calibration, leveling, and zeroing of the transducer to the level of the patient's left atrium. This is called the *phlebostatic axis*. Nursing care of the patient undergoing hemodynamic monitoring is outlined under acute nursing care later in the chapter. Potential complications of central pressure monitoring include:

- Bleeding
- Hematoma
- Pneumothorax
- Hemothorax
- Arterial puncture
- Dysrhythmias
- Venospasm
- Infection
- Air embolism
- Thromboembolism
- Brachial nerve injury
- Thoracic duct injury.

Intra-Arterial Pressure Monitoring. Intra-arterial pressure monitoring is commonly used in intensive and coronary care units. An indwelling arterial line, commonly called an *art line* or an *A line*, allows direct and continuous monitoring of systolic, diastolic, and mean arterial blood pressure and provides easy access for arterial blood sampling. Arterial lines are used to assess blood volume, monitor the effects of vasoactive drugs, and obtain frequent ABG determinations. Because the invasive catheter is inserted directly into the artery, it offers immediate access for blood gas measurements and blood testing.

The arterial blood pressure reflects the cardiac output and the resistance to blood flow created by the elastic arterial walls (*systemic vascular resistance [SVR]*). Cardiac output is determined by the blood volume and the ability of the ventricles to fill and effectively pump that blood. SVR is primarily determined by vessel diameter and distensibility (compliance). Factors such as SNS input, circulating hormones (e.g., epinephrine, norepinephrine, atrial natriuretic factor, and vasopressin), and the RAAS affect SVR.

The systolic blood pressure, normally about 120 mmHg in healthy adults, reflects the pressure generated during ventricular systole. During diastole, elastic arterial walls keep a

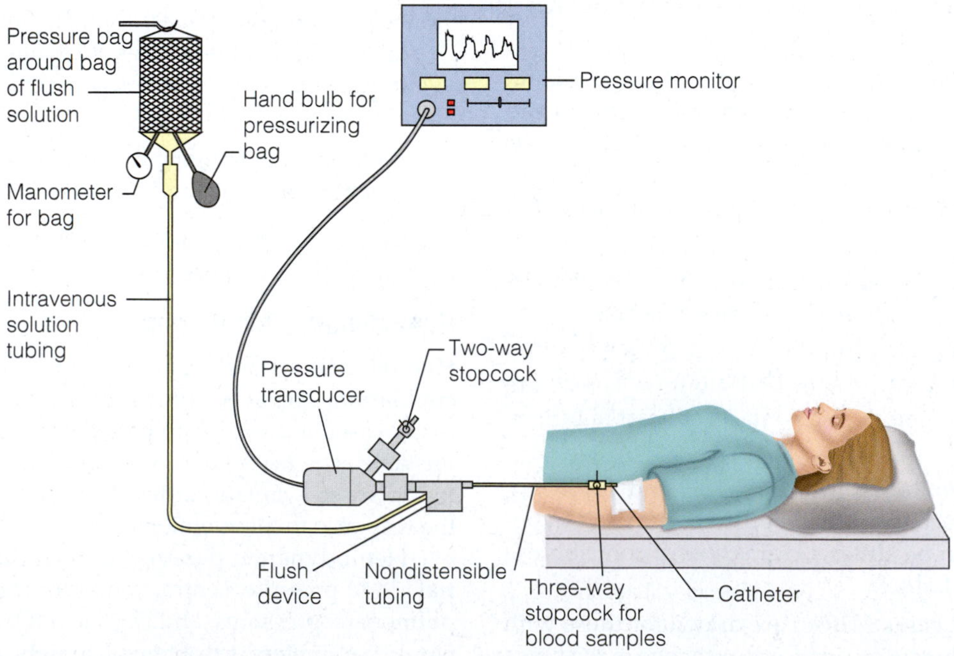
Pressure bag around bag of flush solution
Hand bulb for pressurizing bag
Pressure monitor
Manometer for bag
Intravenous solution tubing
Pressure transducer
Two-way stopcock
Flush device
Nondistensible tubing
Three-way stopcock for blood samples
Catheter

Figure 31.3 ■ A hemodynamic monitoring setup.

minimum pressure within the vessel (diastolic blood pressure) to maintain blood flow through the capillary beds. The average diastolic pressure in a healthy adult is 80 mmHg. The **mean arterial pressure (MAP)** is the average pressure in the arterial circulation throughout the cardiac cycle. It reflects the driving pressure, or perfusion pressure, an indicator of tissue perfusion. The formula MAP = CO × SVR is often used to show the relationships between factors determining the blood pressure. Mean arterial pressure can be calculated by adding one-third of the pulse pressure (PP) to the diastolic blood pressure (DBP): MAP = DBP + PP/3. For example, a blood pressure of 120/80 results in a mean arterial pressure of 93. Mean arterial pressures of 70 to 90 mmHg are desirable. Perfusion to vital organs is severely jeopardized at MAPs of 50 mmHg or less; MAPs > 05 mmHg may indicate hypertension or vasoconstriction.

Venous Pressure Monitoring. *Central venous pressure (CVP)* and *right atrial pressure (RAP)* are measures of blood volume and venous return. They also reflect right heart filling pressures. Pressures are elevated in right-sided heart failure. CVP and RAP are primarily used to monitor fluid volume status. To measure venous and atrial pressures, a catheter is inserted in the internal jugular or subclavian vein. The distal tip of the catheter is positioned in the superior vena cava just above or just inside the right atrium. CVP may be measured in either centimeters of water (cm H_2O) or in millimeters of mercury (mmHg). A water manometer is a clear tube with calibrated markings that is attached between a central catheter and an intravenous fluid bag. Pressure in the venous system causes fluid in the manometer to rise or fall. The CVP is recorded by noting the fluid level in the manometer. If the central line is connected to a pressure transducer, venous pressure is displayed digitally in millimeters of mercury.

The normal range for CVP is 2 to 8 cm H_2O or 2 to 6 mmHg, but CVP varies in individual patients. Hypovolemia and shock decrease the CVP; fluid overload, vasoconstriction, and cardiac tamponade increase CVP.

Pulmonary Artery Pressure Monitoring. The pulmonary artery (PA) catheter is a flow-directed, balloon-tipped catheter first used in the early 1970s. The PA catheter is often called a *Swan-Ganz catheter*, after the physicians who developed it. The PA catheter is used to evaluate left-ventricular and overall cardiac function. The PA catheter is inserted into a central vein, usually the internal jugular or subclavian vein, and threaded into the right atrium. A small balloon at the tip of the catheter allows the catheter to be drawn into the right ventricle and from there into the pulmonary artery (**Figure 31.4** ■). The inflated balloon carries the catheter forward until the balloon wedges in a small branch of pulmonary vasculature. Once in place, the balloon is deflated, and multiple lumens of the catheter allow measurement of pressures in the right atrium, pulmonary artery, and left ventricle. The normal PA pressure is around 25/10 mmHg; normal mean pulmonary artery pressure is about 15 mmHg (**Figure 31.5A** ■). Pulmonary artery pressure is increased in left-sided heart failure.

Inflation of the balloon effectively blocks pressure from behind the balloon and allows measurement of pressures generated by the left ventricle. This is known as *pulmonary capillary wedge pressure (PCWP, PWP)* and is used to assess left-ventricular function. The normal pulmonary capillary wedge pressure is 8 to 12 mmHg (**Figure 31.5B**). PCWP is increased in left-ventricular failure and pericardial tamponade and decreased in hypovolemia (Perrin & MacLeod, 2018).

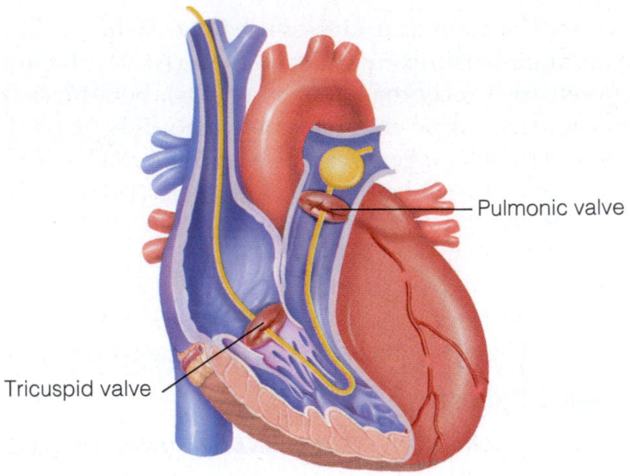
Pulmonic valve
Tricuspid valve

Figure 31.4 ■ Inflation of the balloon on the flow-directed catheter allows it to be carried through the pulmonic valve into the pulmonary artery.

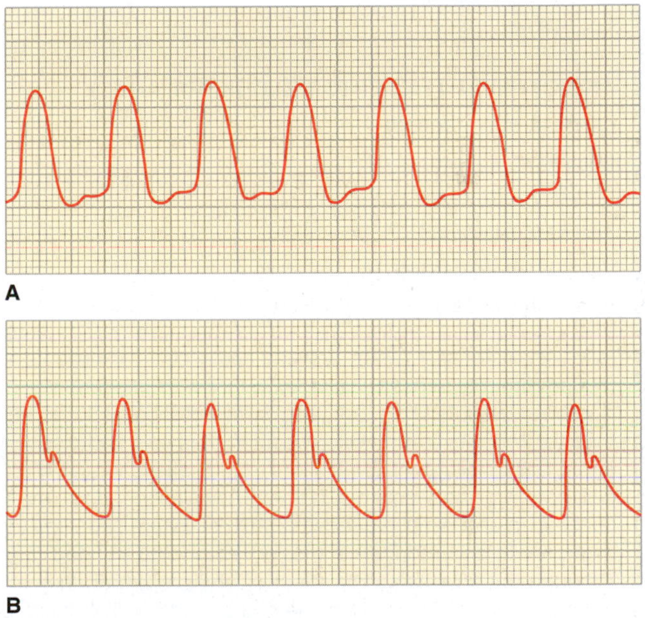
A
B

Figure 31.5 ■ Typical waveforms seen when measuring **A**, right-ventricular pressure, and **B**, pulmonary artery pressure.

Cardiac output can also be measured with the PA catheter using a technique called *thermodilution*. Cardiac output and the cardiac index are used to assess the heart's ability to meet the body's oxygen demands. Because body size affects overall cardiac output, the cardiac index is a more precise measure of heart function. The *cardiac index* is a calculation of cardiac output per square meter of body surface area. The normal cardiac index is 2.8 to 4.2 $L/min/m^2$.

Medications

Patients with heart failure often receive multiple medications to reduce cardiac workload and improve cardiac function. The main drug classes used to treat heart failure are the angiotensin-converting enzyme (ACE) inhibitors, angiotensin II receptor blockers (ARBs), beta-blockers, diuretics, inotropic medications (including digitalis, sympathomimetic agents, and phosphodiesterase inhibitors), direct vasodilators, and antidysrhythmic drugs. Combination drugs using neprilysin inhibitors and ARBs are also indicated in select HF patients (Yancy et al., 2016, 2017). Nursing implications for ACE inhibitors and ARBs, diuretics, inotropic medications, and neprilysin inhibitor/ARB combinations are found in **Medication Administration 31.A**.

Medication Administration 31.A

Heart Failure

ANGIOTENSIN-CONVERTING ENZYME (ACE) INHIBITORS

captopril (Capoten)

enalapril (Vasotec)

fosinopril (Monopril)

lisinopril (Prinivil, Zestril)

quinapril (Accupril)

ramipril (Altace)

ANGIOTENSIN II RECEPTOR BLOCKERS (ARBS)

candesartan (Atacand)

irbesartan (Avapro)

losartan (Cozaar)

nesiritide (Natrecor)

telmisartan (Micardis)

valsartan (Diovan)

ACE inhibitors and ARBs prevent acute coronary events and reduce mortality in heart failure. ACE inhibitors interfere with production of angiotensin II, resulting in vasodilation, reduced blood volume, and prevention of its effects in the heart and blood vessels. In heart failure, ACE inhibitors reduce afterload and improve cardiac output and renal blood flow. They also reduce pulmonary congestion and peripheral edema. ACE inhibitors suppress myocyte growth and reduce ventricular remodeling in heart failure. Although the pharmacologic effect of ARBs is similar, they block the action of angiotensin II at the receptor rather than interfering with its production.

Nursing Responsibilities

- Do not give these drugs to women in the second and third trimesters of pregnancy.
- Carefully monitor patients who are volume depleted or who have impaired renal function (assess BUN and creatinine).
- Use an infusion pump when administering ACE inhibitors intravenously.
- Monitor blood pressure closely for 2 hours following first dose and as indicated thereafter.
- Monitor serum potassium levels; ACE inhibitors can cause hyperkalemia (this is less of a concern with ARBs).
- Monitor white blood cell (WBC) count for potential neutropenia. Report to the physician.

Health Education for the Patient and Family

- Take the drug at the same time every day to ensure a stable blood level.
- Monitor your blood pressure and weight weekly. Report significant changes to your doctor.
- Avoid making sudden position changes; for example, rise from bed slowly. Lie down if you become dizzy or light-headed, particularly after the first dose.
- Report any signs of easy bruising and bleeding, sore throat or fever, edema, or skin rash. Immediately report swelling of the face, lips, or eyelids, and itching or breathing problems.
- A persistent, dry cough may develop if you are taking an ACE inhibitor. Contact your doctor if this becomes a problem.
- Take captopril or moexipril 1 hour before meals.

DIURETICS

acetazolamide (Diamox)

amiloride (Midamor)

bumetanide (Bumex)

chlorothiazide (Diuril)

ethacrynic acid (Edecrin)

furosemide (Lasix)

hydrochlorothiazide (HydroDIURIL)

metolazone (Zaroxolyn)

spironolactone (Aldactone)

torsemide (Demadex)

triamterene (Dyrenium)

Diuretics act on different portions of the kidney tubule to inhibit the reabsorption of sodium and water and promote their excretion. With the exception of the potassium-sparing diuretics—spironolactone, triamterene, and amiloride—diuretics also promote potassium excretion, increasing the risk of hypokalemia. Spironolactone, an aldosterone receptor blocker, reduces symptoms and slows the progression of heart failure. Aldosterone receptors in the heart and blood vessels promote myocardial remodeling and fibrosis, activate the sympathetic nervous system, and promote vascular fibrosis (which decreases compliance) and baroreceptor dysfunction.

Nursing Responsibilities

- Obtain baseline weight and vital signs.
- Monitor blood pressure, intake and output, weight, skin turgor, and edema as indicators of fluid volume status.
- Assess for volume depletion, particularly with loop diuretics (furosemide, ethacrynic acid, and bumetanide): Dizziness, orthostatic hypotension, tachycardia, and muscle cramping.
- Report abnormal serum electrolyte levels to the physician. Replace electrolytes as indicated.
- Do not administer potassium replacements to patients receiving a potassium-sparing diuretic.
- Evaluate renal function by assessing urine output, BUN, and serum creatinine.

- Administer intravenous furosemide slowly, no faster than 20 mg/min. Evaluate for signs of ototoxicity. Do not administer this drug or ethacrynic acid concurrently with aminoglycoside antibiotics (e.g., gentamicin), which are also ototoxic.

Health Education for the Patient and Family

- Drink at least six to eight glasses of water per day.
- Take your diuretic at times that will be the least disruptive to your lifestyle, usually in the morning and early afternoon if a second dose is ordered. Take with meals to decrease gastric upset.
- Monitor your blood pressure, pulse, and weight weekly. Report significant weight changes to your doctor.
- Report any of the following to your doctor: Severe abdominal pain, jaundice, dark urine, abnormal bleeding or bruising, flulike symptoms, signs of hypokalemia, hyponatremia, and dehydration (thirst, salt craving, dizziness, weakness, rapid pulse). See Chapter 10 for manifestations of electrolyte imbalances.
- Avoid sudden position changes. You may experience dizziness, light-headedness, or feelings of faintness.
- Unless you are taking a potassium-sparing diuretic, integrate foods rich in potassium into your diet. Limit sodium use.

POSITIVE INOTROPIC AGENTS

Digitalis Glycosides

digoxin (Lanoxin)

Digitalis improves myocardial contractility by interfering with ATPase in the myocardial cell membrane and increasing the amount of calcium available for contraction. The increased force of contraction causes the heart to empty more completely, increasing stroke volume and cardiac output. Improved cardiac output improves renal perfusion, decreasing renin secretion. This decreases preload and afterload, reducing cardiac workload. Digitalis also has electrophysiologic effects, slowing conduction through the AV node. This decreases the heart rate and reduces oxygen consumption.

Nursing Responsibilities

- Assess apical pulse before administering. Withhold digitalis and notify the physician if heart rate is below 60 bpm and/or manifestations of decreased cardiac output are noted. Record apical rate on medication record.
- Evaluate ECG for scooped (spoon-shaped) ST segment, AV block, bradycardia, and other dysrhythmias (especially premature ventricular contractions [PVCs] and atrial tachycardias).
- Report manifestations of digitalis toxicity: Anorexia, nausea and vomiting, abdominal pain, weakness, vision changes (diplopia, blurred vision, yellow-green or white halos seen around objects), and new-onset dysrhythmias.
- Assess potassium, magnesium, calcium, and serum digoxin levels before giving digitalis. Hypokalemia can precipitate toxicity even when the serum digitalis level is in the normal range.
- Monitor patients with renal insufficiency or renal failure and older adults carefully for digitalis toxicity.
- Prepare to administer digoxin immune fab (Digibind) for digoxin toxicity.

Health Education for the Patient and Family

- Take your pulse daily before taking your digoxin. Do not take the digoxin if your pulse is below 60 bpm or if you are weak, fatigued, light-headed, dizzy, short of breath, or having chest pain. Notify your physician immediately.
- Contact your doctor if you develop manifestations of digitalis toxicity: Palpitations, weakness, loss of appetite, nausea and vomiting, abdominal pain, blurred or colored vision, or double vision.
- Avoid using antacids and laxatives; they decrease digoxin absorption.
- Notify your physician immediately if you develop manifestations of potassium deficiency: Weakness, lethargy, thirst, depression, muscle cramps, or vomiting.
- Incorporate foods high in potassium into your diet: Fresh orange or tomato juice, bananas, raisins, dates, figs, prunes, apricots, spinach, cauliflower, and potatoes.

Sympathomimetic Agents

dopamine (Intropin)

dobutamine (Dobutrex)

Sympathomimetic agents stimulate the heart, improving the force of contraction. Dobutamine is preferred in managing heart failure because it does not increase the heart rate as much as dopamine, and it has a mild vasodilatory effect. These drugs are given by intravenous infusion and may be titrated to obtain their optimal effects.

Phosphodiesterase Inhibitors

inamrinone (Inocor)

milrinone (Primacor)

Phosphodiesterase inhibitors are used in treating acute heart failure to increase myocardial contractility and cause vasodilation. The net effects are an increase in cardiac output and a decrease in afterload.

Nursing Responsibilities

- Use an infusion pump to administer these agents. Monitor hemodynamic parameters carefully.
- Avoid discontinuing these drugs abruptly.
- Change solutions and tubing every 24 hours.
- Inamrinone is given as an intravenous bolus over 2 to 3 minutes, followed by an infusion of 5 to 10 mg/kg/min.
- Inamrinone may be infused full strength or diluted in normal saline or half-strength saline. Do not mix this drug with dextrose solutions. After dilution, inamrinone can be piggybacked into a line containing a dextrose solution.
- Monitor liver function and platelet counts; inamrinone may cause hepatotoxicity and thrombocytopenia.
- Do not confuse with amiodarone (Inocor).

Health Education for the Patient and Family

- Notify the nursing staff if you experience abdominal pain or notice a skin rash or bruising.

Combination Neprilysin Inhibitor/Angiotensin II Receptor Blocker

sacubitril/valsartan (Entresto)

This combination drug works on two pathways. The sacubitril converts to an active metabolite that inhibits the enzyme neprilysin, resulting in increased levels of natriuretic peptides. The valsartan works using the angiotension II receptor block pathway.

Nursing Responsibilities

- Monitor vital signs and blood pressure closely as hypotension risk increases with salt and/or fluid volume depletion.
- Monitor for angioedema.
- If currently on lithium, monitor for signs/symptoms of lithium toxicity.
- Monitor lab tests including liver and renal function and potassium, hemoglobin, and hematocrit.

(continued)

Health Education for the Patient and Family

- Seek medical care immediately if swelling of face, lips, tongue, or throat (angioedema).
- Change positions slowly.
- Avoid salt substitutes, nonprescribed potassium supplementation, or nonsteroidal anti-inflammatory drugs (NSAIDs). Consult with prescriber if use is planned.
- Women of childbearing age should use reliable contraception.
- Pregnancy and breastfeeding are contraindicated while taking this drug.

Note: Drugs identified in blue are among the 200 most commonly prescribed medications in the United States.

Source: Adams, Holland, & Urban, 2017.

ACE inhibitors, ARBs, and beta-blockers interfere with the neurohormonal mechanisms of sympathetic activation and the RAAS. ACE inhibitors interrupt the conversion of angiotensin I to angiotensin II by inhibiting the enzyme that mediates the conversion (angiotensin-converting enzyme). Angiotensin II causes intense vasoconstriction, increasing afterload and ventricular wall stress and increasing preload and ventricular dilation. It also stimulates aldosterone and ADH production, causing fluid retention. ACE inhibitors block this RAAS activity, decreasing cardiac work and increasing cardiac output. They reduce the progression and manifestations of heart failure, thus reducing the number and frequency of hospital admissions, decreasing mortality rates, and preventing cardiac complications. However, ACE inhibitors should be used with caution in African Americans due to increased risk for developing angioedema.

In contrast to ACE inhibitors, ARBs do not block the production of angiotensin II; instead, they block its action. The pharmacologic effect is similar, and they are also used in heart failure to slow its progression, reduce manifestations, and prevent cardiac complications.

Beta-blockers improve cardiac function in heart failure by inhibiting SNS activity. This prevents the long-term deleterious effects of sympathetic stimulation. Because beta-blockers reduce the force of myocardial contraction and may actually worsen symptoms, they are used in low doses. Beta-blockers are indicated for all classes of patients with heart failure. The combination of ACE inhibitors and beta-blockers improves patient outcomes. Beta-blockers are discussed further in Chapter 30.

Patients with symptomatic heart failure are often treated with diuretics as well. Diuretics relieve symptoms related to fluid retention. They may, however, cause significant electrolyte imbalances and rapid fluid loss. Patients with severe heart failure are often treated with a loop, or high-ceiling, diuretic such as furosemide (Lasix), bumetanide (Bumex), torsemide (Demadex), or ethacrynic acid (Edecrin). These drugs have a rapid onset of action, inhibiting chloride reabsorption in the ascending loop of Henle, which prompts sodium and water excretion. Their major drawback is their efficacy in promoting diuresis; loss of vascular volume can stimulate the SNS. Thiazide diuretics may be used for patients with less severe manifestations of heart failure. These agents promote fluid excretion by blocking sodium reabsorption in the terminal loop of Henle and the distal tubule.

Vasodilators relax smooth muscle in blood vessels, causing dilation. Arterial dilation reduces peripheral vascular resistance and afterload, reducing myocardial work. Venous dilation reduces venous return and preload. Pulmonary vascular relaxation reduces pulmonary capillary pressure, allowing reabsorption of fluid from interstitial tissues and the alveoli. Vasodilators include nitrates, hydralazine, and prazosin, an alpha-adrenergic blocker. See Chapter 32 for more information about vasodilators.

Nitrates produce both arterial and venous vasodilation. They may be given by nasal spray or by a sublingual, oral, or intravenous route. Sodium nitroprusside is a potent vasodilator that may be used to treat acute heart failure. It can cause excessive hypotension, so it is often given along with dopamine or dobutamine to maintain blood pressure. Isosorbide or nitroglycerin ointment may be used in long-term management of heart failure (refer to Chapter 30, page 995).

BiDil, a combination of two vasodilators, hydralazine and isosorbide, in fixed doses is an option for treatment of heart failure in African Americans. In African Americans with severe heart failure, BiDil improved symptoms and significantly reduced the number of hospitalizations and deaths attributed to heart failure (Ziaeian, Fonarow, & Heidenreich, 2017). The recommended dose is one to two tablets three times per day, although the dose may be as low as one-half tablet three times a day if side effects are intolerable.

Digitalis glycosides are used judiciously in symptomatic heart failure. Digitalis has a positive inotropic effect on the heart, increasing the strength of myocardial contraction by increasing the intracellular calcium concentrations. Digitalis also decreases SA node automaticity and slows conduction through the AV node, increasing ventricular filling time.

Digitalis has a narrow therapeutic index; in other words, therapeutic levels are very close to toxic levels. Early manifestations of digitalis toxicity include anorexia, nausea and vomiting, headache, altered vision, and confusion. A number of cardiac dysrhythmias are also associated with digitalis toxicity, including sinus arrest, supraventricular and ventricular tachycardias, and high levels of AV block. Low serum potassium levels increase the risk of digitalis toxicity, as do low magnesium and high calcium levels. Older adults are at particular risk for digitalis toxicity. The AHA's heart failure guidelines (Yancy et al., 2016, 2017) note that the risk of toxicity outweighs the benefits of this class of drug. Digitalis levels may be affected by a number of other drugs; check for potential interactions.

Dysrhythmias are common in patients with heart failure. Although PVCs may be frequent, they are often not associated with an increased risk of ventricular tachycardia and fibrillation. Because many antidysrhythmic medications depress left-ventricular function, PVCs are frequently left untreated in heart failure. Amiodarone is the drug of choice to treat nonsustained ventricular tachycardia, which is associated with a poor prognosis. (Refer to Chapter 30.)

Nutrition and Activity

A sodium-restricted diet is recommended to minimize sodium and water retention. Intake is generally limited to 1.5 to 2 g of sodium per day, a moderate restriction. Box 10.2 in Chapter 10 includes patient teaching regarding a sodium-restricted diet.

Exercise intolerance, decreased ability to participate in activities using large skeletal muscles due to fatigue or dyspnea, is a common early manifestation of heart failure. Activity may be restricted to bedrest during acute episodes of heart failure to reduce cardiac workload and allow the heart to compensate. Prolonged bedrest and continued activity limitations, however, are not recommended. A moderate, progressive activity program is prescribed to improve myocardial function. Exercise should be performed 3 to 5 days per week, and each session should include a 10- to 15-minute warm-up period, 20 to 30 minutes of exercise at the recommended intensity, and a cool-down period. Walking is encouraged on nontraining days. Cardiac rehabilitation service coverage for patients with chronic heart failure (defined as patients with left-ventricular ejection fraction of 35% or less and NYHA class II to IV symptoms despite being on optimal heart failure therapy for at least 6 weeks) has been covered by the Centers for Medicare and Medicaid Services (CMS) since 2013.

Other Treatments

In end-stage heart failure, devices to provide circulatory assistance or surgery may be required. Surgery may be used to treat the underlying cause of failure (e.g., replacement of diseased valves) or to improve quality of life. Valve replacement is discussed later in this chapter. Heart transplant is currently the only clearly effective surgical treatment for end-stage heart failure; its use is limited by the availability of donor hearts.

Circulatory Assistance. Devices such as the intra-aortic balloon pump or a left-ventricular assist device may be used when the patient is expected to recover or as a bridge to transplant (refer to Chapter 30). Newer devices that will allow longer-term support outside the hospital are in the developmental stages. These devices will serve either as a bridge to transplant or allow the myocardium to heal over an extended period of time.

Cardiac Transplantation. Heart transplantation is the treatment of choice for end-stage heart disease. Survival rates are good: 83% at 1 year and 76% at 3 years. More than 90% of patients return to normal, unrestricted functional abilities following transplantation. The most frequently used transplantation procedure leaves the posterior walls of the atria, the superior and inferior vena cavae, and the pulmonary veins of the recipient intact (**Figure 31.6** ■). The atrial walls of the donor heart are then anastomosed to the recipient's atria and the donor pulmonary artery and aorta are anastomosed to the recipient's vessels. Care is taken to avoid damaging the sinus node of the donor heart and to ensure integrity of the suture line to prevent postoperative bleeding. Donor organs are obtained from people with no evidence of cardiac trauma.

Nursing care of the patient having a heart transplantation is similar to care of any cardiac surgery patient (refer to Chapter 30). Bleeding is a major concern in the early postoperative period. Chest tube drainage is frequently monitored (initially every 15 minutes), as are the cardiac output, pulmonary artery pressures, and CVP. Cardiac tamponade (compression of the heart) can develop, presenting as either a sudden event or a gradual process. Chest tubes are gently milked (not stripped) as needed to maintain patency. Atrial dysrhythmias are relatively common following cardiac transplant. Temporary pacing wires are placed during surgery because surgical manipulation or postoperative swelling may disrupt the conduction system. Hypothermia is induced

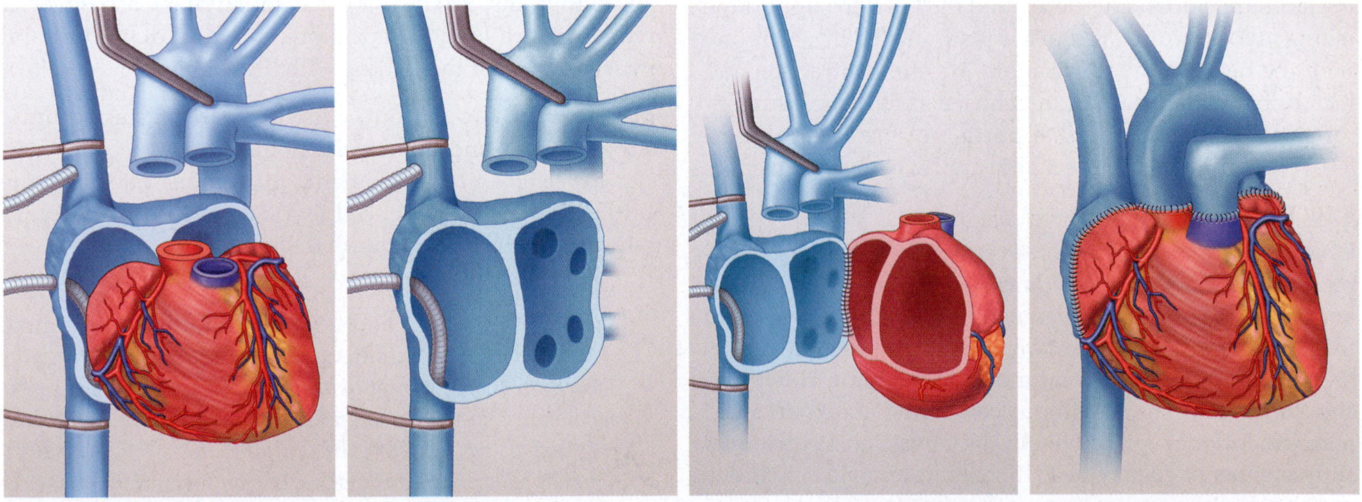
A
B
C
D

Figure 31.6 ■ Cardiac transplantation. **A**, The heart is removed, leaving the posterior walls of the atria intact. **B**, The donor heart is anastomosed to the atria, **C**, and the great vessels, **D**.

during surgery; postoperatively, the patient is gradually rewarmed over a 1- to 2-hour period. Prevention of rapid rewarming and shivering is important to maintain hemodynamic stability and reduce oxygen consumption. Cardiac function is impaired in up to 50% of transplanted hearts during the early postoperative period. Inotropic agents such as low-dose dopamine, dobutamine, or milrinone may be required to support cardiac function and circulation.

Infection and rejection are major postoperative concerns; these are the chief causes of mortality in patients with a transplantation. Rejection may develop immediately after transplantation (a rare occurrence), within weeks to months, or years after the transplantation. Acute rejection usually presents within weeks of the transplantation, developing when the transplanted organ is recognized by the immune system as foreign. Lymphocytes infiltrate the organ, and myocardial cell necrosis can be detected on biopsy. Acute rejection can often be treated using immunosuppressive drugs. These drugs are also given to prevent rejection of the transplanted organ, even when the tissue match is good (refer to Chapter 12). Although immunosuppressive medications help prevent organ rejection, they impair the patient's defenses against infection. Early postoperative infections are commonly bacterial or fungal (*candida*). Multiple invasive lines, prolonged ventilator support, and immunosuppressive therapy contribute to the transplant recipient's risk for infection. Aggressive nursing care directed at prevention of infection is vital: Limiting visitors with communicable diseases and practicing pulmonary hygiene measures, early ambulation, and strict aseptic technique.

The donor heart is denervated during the transplantation procedure. Lack of innervation by the autonomic nervous system affects the heart rate (usually between 90 and 110 bpm in transplanted hearts), its response to position changes, stress, exercise, and certain drugs.

Other Procedures. Other surgical procedures such as cardiomyoplasty and ventricular reduction surgery do not improve the prognosis or quality of life in patients with end-stage heart failure. *Cardiomyoplasty* involves wrapping the latissimus dorsi muscle around the heart to support the failing myocardium. The muscle is stimulated in synchrony with the heart, providing a more forceful contraction and increasing cardiac output. In ventricular reduction surgery (or *partial ventriculectomy*), a portion of the anteriolateral left-ventricular wall is resected to improve cardiac function.

Integrative Therapies

Evidence supports the use of several complementary therapies for heart failure. Hawthorn, a shrubby tree, contains natural cardiotonic ingredients in its blossoms, leaves, and fruit. It increases the force of myocardial contraction, dilates blood vessels, and has a natural ACE inhibitor. Hawthorn should never be used without consulting an experienced herb practitioner and advising the physician. Nutritional supplements of coenzyme Q10, magnesium, and thiamine may be used in conjunction with other treatments. Coenzyme Q10 improves mitochondria function and energy production. It can be lost with use of antilipemics.

Nursing Care

Assessment

See the Manifestations and Interprofessional Care sections for the assessment of the patient with heart failure.

Obtain both subjective and objective data when assessing the patient with heart failure.

- ***Health history:*** Complaints of increasing shortness of breath, dyspnea with exertion, decreasing activity tolerance, or paroxysmal nocturnal dyspnea; number of pillows used for sleeping; recent weight gain; presence of a cough; chest or abdominal pain; anorexia or nausea; history of cardiac disease, previous episodes of heart failure; other risk factors such as hypertension or diabetes; current medications; usual diet and activity and recent changes. Determine patient's NYHA class.
- ***Physical assessment:*** General appearance; ease of breathing, conversing, changing positions; apparent anxiety; vital signs including apical pulse; color of skin and mucous membranes; neck vein distention, peripheral pulses, capillary refill, presence and degree of edema; heart and breath sounds; abdominal contour, bowel sounds, tenderness; right upper abdominal tenderness, liver enlargement.

Priorities of Care

Collaborating with the interprofessional team to ensure adequate treatment of the underlying process while providing care that supports the physical and psychologic responses to the disorder is a priority of nursing care.

Diagnoses, Outcomes, and Interventions

Heart failure impacts quality of life, interfering with such daily activities as self-care and role performance. Reducing the oxygen demand of the heart is a major nursing care goal for the patient in acute heart failure. This includes providing rest and carrying out prescribed treatment measures to reduce cardiac workload, improve contractility, and manage symptoms. See also the accompanying Case Study & Nursing Care Plan for additional nursing diagnoses and interventions for the patient with heart failure.

Monitor Cardiac Output. As the heart fails as a pump, stroke volume and tissue perfusion decrease.

Expected Outcome: Patient will demonstrate adequate cardiac output as evidenced by blood pressure and pulse rate and rhythm within normal limits.

The nurse will:

- Monitor vital signs and oxygen saturation as indicated. *Decreased cardiac output stimulates the SNS to increase the heart rate in an attempt to restore CO. Tachycardia at rest is common. Diastolic blood pressure may initially be elevated because of vasoconstriction; in late stages, compensatory mechanisms fail, and BP falls. Oxygen saturation levels provide a measure of gas exchange and tissue perfusion.*
- Auscultate heart and breath sounds regularly. *S_1 and S_2 may be diminished if cardiac function is poor. A ventricular*

gallop (S_3) is an early sign of heart failure; atrial gallop (S_4) may also be present. Crackles are often heard in the lung bases; increasing crackles, dyspnea, and shortness of breath indicate worsening failure.

SAFETY ALERT: Report manifestations of decreased cardiac output and tissue perfusion: Changes in mentation; decreased urine output; cool, clammy skin; diminished pulses; pallor or cyanosis; or dysrhythmias. These are manifestations of decreased tissue perfusion to organ systems. ■

- Administer supplemental oxygen as needed. *This improves oxygenation of the blood, decreasing the effects of hypoxia and ischemia.*
- Administer prescribed medications as ordered. *Drugs are used to decrease the cardiac workload and increase the effectiveness of contractions.*
- Encourage rest, explaining the rationale. Elevate the head of the bed to reduce the work of breathing. Provide a bedside commode, and assist with ADLs. Instruct to avoid the Valsalva maneuver. *These measures reduce cardiac workload.*

Monitor Fluid Volume. As cardiac output falls, compensatory mechanisms cause salt and water retention, increasing blood volume. This increased fluid volume places additional stress on the already failing ventricles, making them work harder to move the fluid load.

Expected Outcome: Patient will maintain normal fluid volume as evidenced by weight loss and decreases in edema, jugular venous distention, and abdominal distention.

The nurse will:

- Assess respiratory status and auscultate lung sounds at least every 4 hours. Notify the physician of significant changes in condition. *Declining respiratory status indicates worsening left heart failure.*

SAFETY ALERT: Immediately notify the physician if the patient develops air hunger, an overwhelming sense of impending doom or panic, tachypnea, severe orthopnea, or a cough productive of large amounts of pink, frothy sputum. Acute pulmonary edema, a medical emergency, can develop rapidly, necessitating immediate intervention to preserve life. ■

- Monitor intake and output. Notify the physician if urine output is < 30 mL/h. Weigh daily. *Careful monitoring of fluid volume is important during treatment of heart failure. Diuretics may reduce circulating volume, producing hypovolemia despite persistent peripheral edema. A fall in urine output may indicate significantly reduced cardiac output and renal ischemia. Weight is an objective measure of fluid status: 1 L of fluid is equal to 2.2 lb of weight.*
- Record abdominal girth every shift. Note complaints of a loss of appetite, abdominal discomfort, or nausea. *Venous congestion can lead to ascites and may affect gastrointestinal function and nutritional status.*
- Monitor and record hemodynamic measurements. Report significant changes and negative trends. *Hemodynamic measurements provide a means of monitoring the patient's condition and response to treatment.*
- Restrict fluids as ordered. Allow choices of fluid type and timing of intake, scheduling most fluid intake during morning and afternoon hours. Offer ice chips and frequent mouth care; provide hard candies if allowed. *Providing choices increases the patient's sense of control. Ice chips, hard candies, and mouth care relieve dry mouth and thirst and promote comfort.*

Balance Activity and Rest. Patients with heart failure have little or no cardiac reserve to meet increased oxygen demands. As the disease progresses and cardiac function is further compromised, activity intolerance increases. The low cardiac output and inability to participate in activities may hinder self-care.

Expected Outcome: Patient will participate in physical activity as tolerated.

SAFETY ALERT: Monitor vital signs and cardiac rhythm during and after activities. Tachycardia, dysrhythmias, increasing dyspnea, changes in blood pressure, diaphoresis, pallor, complaints of chest pain, excessive fatigue, or palpitations indicate activity intolerance. Instruct to rest if manifestations are noted. The failing heart is unable to increase cardiac output to meet the increased oxygen demands associated with activity. Assessing response to activities helps evaluate cardiac function. Decreasing activity tolerance may signal deterioration of cardiac function, not overexertion. ■

The nurse will:

- Organize nursing care to allow rest periods. *Grouping activities together allows adequate time to rest and recharge.*
- Assist with ADLs as needed. Encourage independence within prescribed limits. *Assisting with ADLs helps ensure that care needs are met while reducing cardiac workload. Involving the patient promotes a sense of control and reduces helplessness.*
- Plan and implement progressive activities. Use passive and active ROM exercises as appropriate. Consult with physical therapist on activity plan. *Progressive activity slowly increases exercise capacity by strengthening and improving cardiac function without strain. Activity also helps prevent skeletal muscle atrophy. ROM exercises prevent complications of immobility in severely compromised patients.*
- Provide written and verbal information about activity after discharge. *Written information provides a reference for important information. Verbal information allows for clarification and validation of the material.*

Promote a Low-Sodium Diet. Diet is an important part of long-term management of heart failure to manage fluid retention.

Expected Outcome: Patient will comply with sodium restrictions prescribed as evidenced by reduction in fluid retention and edema.

The nurse will:

- Discuss the rationale for sodium restrictions. *Understanding fosters compliance with the prescribed diet.*
- Consult with dietitian to plan and teach a low-sodium and, if necessary for weight control, low-kilocalorie

diet. Provide a list of high-sodium, high-fat, high-cholesterol foods to avoid. Provide American Heart Association materials. *Dietary planning and teaching increase the patient's sense of control and participation in disease management. Food lists are useful memory aids.*

- Teach how to read food labels for nutritional information. Many processed foods contain hidden sodium, which can be identified by careful label reading. *Knowledge about hidden sodium can improve dietary selections.*
- Assist the patient to construct a 2-day meal plan choosing foods low in sodium. *This allows for learning assessment, clarification of misunderstandings, and reinforcement of teaching.*
- Encourage small, frequent meals rather than three heavy meals per day. *Small, frequent meals provide continuing energy resources and decrease the work required to digest a large meal.*

Delegating Nursing Care Activities

As appropriate and allowed by the designated duties and responsibilities of unlicensed assistive personnel, the nurse may delegate nursing care activities such as measuring fluid intake and output, collecting vital signs (including orthostatic vital signs), encouraging oral or enteral fluid intake, and ensuring nonpharmacologic skin care.

Transitions of Care

Preventive activities to reduce the risk for and incidence of heart failure are directed at the risk factors. Teach patients about coronary heart disease, the primary underlying cause of heart failure. Discuss CHD risk factors and ways to reduce those risk factors (see Chapter 30).

Hypertension is also a major cause of heart failure. Routinely screen patients for elevated blood pressure, and refer patients to a primary care provider as indicated. Discuss the importance of effectively managing hypertension to reduce the future risk for heart failure. Likewise, stress the relationship between effective diabetes management and reduced risk of heart failure.

Acute care of heart failure focuses on symptom management and hemodynamic monitoring. These both focus on fluid and electrolyte balance. For patients admitted for heart failure exacerbation, monitoring is a frequent interprofessional intervention. The nursing responsibilities for the patient undergoing hemodynamic monitoring include system management and patient supervision. With a newly placed central line, a chest x-ray should be obtained prior to IV fluid infusion to verify location of the catheter. Be sure to set alarm limits and turn the alarms on. Aseptic technique should be used with all central line interventions to prevent infection. Be sure to secure all connections and stopcocks to avoid disconnection and hemorrhage. Change intravenous solutions every 24 hours, site dressing every 48 hours, and tubing to the insertion site every 72 hours. Label solution, tubing, and dressing with date and time of change. Assess and document appearance of the insertion site at least every shift; observe for signs of infiltration, infection, or phlebitis. To ensure a continuous flow of flush solution through the pressure tubing and to prevent clot formation and catheter occlusion, maintain the pressure at 300 mmHg minimum at all times. Thoroughly flush stopcock ports after drawing blood samples from the pressure line to prevent catheter occlusion and bacterial colonization.

The nurse should calibrate and level the system at least once a shift using the right atrium as a constant reference level. Relevel the transducer after a change in patient position. Mark the right atrial position (at the fourth intercostal space, midaxillary line) on the chest wall, and use this as a reference point for all readings. All pressures should be measured between breaths to ensure that intrathoracic pressure does not influence the readings. Assess pulse and perfusion distal to the monitoring site. When assessing the patient's status, be sure to monitor pressure trends rather than individual readings for a better overall picture. When discontinuing the pressure line, apply manual pressure to the insertion site as soon as the catheter tip is out. Hold pressure for 5 to 15 minutes or until the bleeding stops, especially for arterial lines.

Heart failure is a chronic condition requiring active participation by the patient and family for effective management. In teaching for home care, include the following topics:

- The disease process and its effects on the patient's life
- Warning signals of cardiac decompensation that require treatment
- Desired and adverse effects of prescribed drugs; monitoring for effects; importance of compliance with drug regimen to prevent acute and long-term complications of heart failure
- Prescribed diet and sodium restriction; practical suggestions for reducing salt intake; recommend American Heart Association materials and recipes
- Exercise recommendations to strengthen the heart muscle and improve aerobic capacity (**Box 31.3**)
- The importance of keeping scheduled follow-up appointments to monitor disease progression and effects of therapy.

Provide referrals for home healthcare and household assistance (shopping, transportation, personal needs, and housekeeping) as indicated. Referrals to community agencies, such as local cardiac rehabilitation programs, heart support groups, or the AHA, can provide additional materials and psychosocial support. In older adults, heart failure may present with weakness and fatigue, somnolence, confusion, disorientation, or worsening dementia. Dependent edema and respiratory crackles may or may not indicate heart failure in older adults. Limited mobility or visual acuity may cause the older adult to rely on prepared foods that are high in sodium such as canned soups and frozen meals. Discuss normal daily activities and assess sleep and rest patterns. It is also important to assess the environment for safety and access to a pharmacy and medical care.

Unless a cardiac transplantation is performed, chronic heart failure is ultimately a terminal disease. The patient and family need honest discussions about the anticipated course of the disease and treatment options. It is important to discuss advance directives such as a living will

BOX 31.3
Home Activity Guidelines for the Patient with Heart Failure

- Perform as many activities as independently as you can.
- Space your meals and activities.
  a. Eat six small meals a day.
  b. Allow time during the day for periods of rest and relaxation.
- Engage in regular exercise such as walking five or more times a week.
  a. Start with a slow leisurely pace, walking as far as you can, up to 400 feet.
  b. Plan to walk twice a day at a comfortable, slow pace for the first couple of weeks at home, and then gradually increase the distance and pace.
- Perform all activities at a comfortable pace.
  a. If you get tired during any activity, stop what you are doing and rest for 15 minutes.
  b. Resume activity only if you feel up to it.
- Stop any activity that causes chest pain, shortness of breath, dizziness, faintness, excessive weakness, or sweating. Rest. Notify your physician if your activity tolerance changes and if symptoms continue after rest.
- Allow for longer warm-up and cool-down periods during exercise.
- Rest with feet elevated (e.g., in a recliner) when fatigued.
- Maintain adequate fluid intake.
- Prevent infection through pneumococcal and influenza immunizations.
- Avoid straining. Do not lift heavy objects. Eat a high-fiber diet and drink plenty of water to prevent constipation. Use laxatives or stool softeners, as approved by your physician, to avoid constipation and straining during bowel movements.

and medical power of attorney, differentiating potential acute events from which recovery would be anticipated (e.g., reversible exacerbation of heart failure, sudden cardiac arrest) from prolonged life support without reasonable expectation of functional recovery. Hospice services are available for patients with heart failure, and should be offered when appropriate. Severe dyspnea is common in the final stages of the disease. It may be managed with narcotic analgesics or with frequent intravenous diuretics and continuous infusion of a positive inotropic agent.

The Patient with Pulmonary Edema

Pulmonary edema is an abnormal accumulation of fluid in the interstitial tissue and alveoli of the lung. Both cardiac and noncardiac disorders can cause pulmonary edema. Cardiac causes include acute myocardial infarction, acute heart failure, and valvular disease. *Cardiogenic pulmonary edema*, the focus of this section, is a sign of severe cardiac decompensation. Noncardiac causes of pulmonary edema include primary pulmonary disorders, such as acute respiratory distress syndrome (ARDS), trauma, sepsis, drug overdose, or neurologic sequelae. Pulmonary edema due to ARDS is discussed in Chapter 37.

Pulmonary edema is a medical emergency: The patient is literally drowning in the fluid in the alveolar and interstitial pulmonary spaces. Its onset may be acute or gradual, progressing to severe respiratory distress. Immediate treatment is necessary.

Pathophysiology

In cardiogenic pulmonary edema, the contractility of the left ventricle is severely impaired. The ejection fraction falls as the ventricle is unable to eject the blood that enters it, causing a sharp rise in end-diastolic volume and pressure. Pulmonary hydrostatic pressures rise, ultimately exceeding the osmotic pressure of the blood. As a result, fluid leaking from the pulmonary capillaries congests interstitial tissues, decreasing lung compliance and interfering with gas exchange. As capillary and interstitial pressures increase further, the tight junctions of the alveolar walls are disrupted, and the fluid enters the alveoli, along with large red blood cells and protein molecules. Ventilation and gas exchange are severely disrupted, and hypoxia worsens.

Manifestations

The patient with acute pulmonary edema presents with classic multisystem manifestations including:

Respiratory

- Tachypnea
- Labored respirations
- Dyspnea
- Orthopnea
- Paroxysmal nocturnal dyspnea
- Cough productive of frothy, pink sputum
- Crackles, wheezes

Cardiovascular

- Tachycardia
- Hypotension
- Cyanosis
- Cool, clammy skin
- Hypoxemia
- Ventricular gallop

Neurologic

- Restlessness
- Anxiety
- Feeling of impending doom

Case Study & Nursing Care Plan

A Patient with Heart Failure

One year ago, Arthur Jackson, 67 years old, had a large anterior wall MI and underwent subsequent coronary artery bypass surgery. On discharge, he was started on a regimen of enalapril (Vasotec), digoxin, furosemide (Lasix), warfarin (Coumadin), and a potassium chloride supplement. He is now in the cardiac unit complaining of severe shortness of breath, hemoptysis, and poor appetite for 1 week. He is diagnosed with acute heart failure.

ASSESSMENT

Mr. Jackson refuses to settle in bed, preferring to sit in the bedside recliner in high-Fowler position. He states, "Lately, this is the only way I can breathe." Mr. Jackson states that he has not been able to work in his garden without getting short of breath. He complains of his shoes and belt being too tight.

When Mr. Jackson's nurse, Ms. Takashi, RN, obtains his nursing history, Mr. Jackson insists that he takes his medications regularly. He states that he normally works in his garden for light exercise. In his diet history, Mr. Jackson admits a fondness for bacon and Chinese food and sheepishly admits to snacking between meals "even though I need to lose weight."

Mr. Jackson's vital signs are BP 95/72 mmHg, HR 124 bpm and irregular, R 28/min and labored, and T 36.5°C (97.5°F). The cardiac monitor shows atrial fibrillation. An S_3 is noted on auscultation; the cardiac impulse is left of the midclavicular line. He has crackles and diminished breath sounds in the bases of both lungs. Significant jugular venous distention, 3+ pitting edema of feet and ankles, and abdominal distention are noted. Liver size is within normal limits by percussion. Skin is cool and diaphoretic. Chest x-ray shows cardiomegaly and pulmonary infiltrates.

DIAGNOSES

- Increased fluid volume due to impaired cardiac pump and salt and water retention
- Inability to tolerate daily activity related to impaired cardiac output
- Difficulty in managing diet due to lack of knowledge about diet restrictions

EXPECTED OUTCOMES

- Patient will demonstrate loss of excess fluid by weight loss and decreases in edema, jugular venous distention, and abdominal distention.
- Patient will demonstrate improved activity tolerance.
- Patient will verbalize understanding of diet restrictions.

PLANNING AND IMPLEMENTATION

- Take hourly vital signs and hemodynamic pressure measurements.
- Administer and monitor effects of prescribed diuretics and vasodilators.
- Weigh daily; strict intake and output.
- Enforce fluid restriction of 1500 mL/24 hours: 600 mL day shift, 600 mL evening shift, 300 mL at night.
- Auscultate heart and breath sounds every 4 hours and as indicated.
- Administer oxygen per nasal cannula at 2 L/min. Monitor oxygen saturation continuously. Notify physician if $< 94\%$.
- Place in high-Fowler or other position of comfort.
- Notify physician of significant changes in laboratory values.
- Teach about all medications and how to take and record pulse. Provide information about anticoagulant therapy and signs of bleeding.
- Design an activity plan with Mr. Jackson that incorporates preferred activities and scheduled rest periods.
- Instruct about sodium-restricted diet. Allow meal choices within allowed limits.
- Consult dietitian for planning and teaching Mr. and Mrs. Jackson about low-sodium diet.

EVALUATION

Mr. Jackson is discharged after 3 days in the cardiac unit. He has lost 8 pounds during his stay and states it is much easier to breathe and his shoes fit better. He is able to sleep in semi-Fowler position with only one pillow. His peripheral edema has resolved. Mr. and Mrs. Jackson met with the dietitian, who helped them develop a realistic eating plan to limit sodium, sugar, and fats. The dietitian also provided a list of high-sodium foods to avoid. Mr. Jackson is relieved to know that he can still enjoy Chinese food prepared without monosodium glutamate (MSG) or added salt. Ms. Takashi and the physical therapist designed a progressive activity plan with Mr. Jackson that he will continue at home. He remains in atrial fibrillation, a chronic condition. His knowledge of digoxin and Coumadin has been assessed and reinforced. Ms. Takashi confirms that he is able to accurately check his pulse and can list signs of digoxin toxicity and excessive bleeding.

CLINICAL REASONING IN PATIENT CARE

1. Mr. Jackson's medication regimen remains the same after discharge. What specific teaching does he need related to potential interactions of these drugs?
2. Mr. Jackson tells you, "Talk to my wife about my medications—she's Tarzan and I'm Jane now." How would you respond?
3. Design an exercise plan for Mr. Jackson to prevent deconditioning and conserve energy.
4. Mr. Jackson tells you, "Sometimes I forget whether I have taken my aspirin, so I'll take another just to be sure. After all, they are only baby aspirin. One or two extra a day shouldn't hurt, right?" What is your response?
5. Mr. Jackson is admitted to the neuro unit 6 months later with a cerebrovascular accident (CVA). What is the probable cause of his stroke?

See Evaluating Your Response in Appendix B.

Dyspnea, shortness of breath, and labored respirations are acute and severe, accompanied by orthopnea, the inability to breathe when lying down. Cyanosis is present, and the skin is cool, clammy, and diaphoretic. A productive cough with pink, frothy sputum develops due to fluid, RBCs, and plasma proteins in the alveoli and airways. Crackles are heard throughout the lung fields on auscultation. As the condition worsens, lung sounds become harsher. The patient often is restless and highly anxious, although severe hypoxia may cause confusion or lethargy.

As noted earlier, pulmonary edema is a medical emergency. Without rapid and effective intervention, severe tissue hypoxia and acidosis will lead to organ system failure and death.

Interprofessional Care

Immediate treatment for acute pulmonary edema focuses on restoring effective gas exchange and reducing fluid and pressure in the pulmonary vascular system. The patient is placed in an upright sitting position with the legs dangling to reduce venous return by trapping some excess fluid in the lower extremities. This position also facilitates breathing.

Diagnostic testing is limited to assessment of the acute situation. *Arterial blood gases (ABGs)* are drawn to assess gas exchange and acid–base balance. Oxygen tension (PaO_2) is usually low. Initially, carbon dioxide levels ($PaCO_2$) may also be reduced because of rapid respirations. As the condition progresses, the $PaCO_2$ rises and respiratory acidosis develops (see Chapter 10). *Oxygen saturation* levels are also continuously monitored. The *chest x-ray* shows pulmonary vascular congestion and alveolar edema. Provided the patient's condition allows, *hemodynamic monitoring* is instituted. In cardiogenic pulmonary edema, the pulmonary artery wedge pressure (PAWP) is elevated, usually over 25 mmHg. Cardiac output may be decreased.

Morphine is administered intravenously to relieve anxiety and improve the efficacy of breathing. It is also a vasodilator that reduces venous return and lowers left atrial pressure. Although morphine is very effective for patients with cardiogenic pulmonary edema, naloxone, its antidote, is kept readily available in case respiratory depression occurs.

Oxygen is administered using a positive pressure system that can achieve a 100% oxygen concentration. A continuous positive airway pressure (CPAP) mask system may be used or the patient may be intubated and mechanical ventilation employed (see Chapter 37). Positive pressure increases alveolar pressures and gas exchange while decreasing fluid diffusion into the alveoli.

Potent loop diuretics such as furosemide, ethacrynic acid, or bumetanide are administered intravenously to promote rapid diuresis. Furosemide is also a venous dilator, reducing venous return to the heart. Vasodilators such as intravenous nitroprusside are given to improve cardiac output by reducing afterload. Dopamine or dobutamine, and possibly digoxin, is administered to improve the myocardial contractility and cardiac output. Intravenous aminophylline may be used cautiously to reduce bronchospasm and decrease wheezing.

When the patient's condition has stabilized, further diagnostic tests may be done to determine the underlying cause of pulmonary edema, and specific treatment measures directed at the cause instituted.

Nursing Care

Nursing care of the patient with acute pulmonary edema focuses on relieving the pulmonary effects of the disorder. Interventions are directed toward improving oxygenation, reducing fluid volume, and providing emotional support.

Assessment

See the Manifestations and Interprofessional Care sections for the assessment of the patient with acute pulmonary edema.

The nurse is often instrumental in recognizing early manifestations of pulmonary edema and initiating treatment. As with many critical conditions, emergent care is directed toward the ABCs: Airway, breathing, and circulation.

Priorities of Care

Collaborating with the interprofessional team to ensure adequate treatment of the underlying process while providing care that supports the physical and psychologic responses to the disorder is a priority of nursing care.

Diagnoses, Outcomes, and Interventions

Promoting effective gas exchange and restoring an effective cardiac output are the priorities for nursing and interprofessional care of the patient with cardiogenic pulmonary edema. The experience of acute dyspnea and shortness of breath is terrifying for the patient; the nurse is instrumental in providing emotional support and reassurance.

Improve Gas Exchange. Accumulated fluid in the alveoli and airways interferes with ventilation of the lungs. As a result, alveolar oxygen levels fall and carbon dioxide levels may rise. Reduced alveolar oxygen decreases diffusion of the gas into pulmonary capillaries. In addition, pulmonary edema increases the distance over which gases must diffuse to cross the alveolar-capillary membrane, further reducing oxygen levels in the blood and oxygen delivery to the tissues.

Expected Outcome: Patient will experience improved ventilation and adequate oxygenation as evidenced by blood gas levels within normal limits for the individual patient.

The nurse will:

- Ensure airway patency. *A patent airway is absolutely vital for pulmonary function, including ventilation and gas exchange.*
- Assess the effectiveness of respiratory efforts and airway clearance. *Pulmonary edema increases the work of breathing. This increased effort can lead to fatigue and decreased respiratory effort.*
- Assess respiratory status frequently, including rate, effort, use of accessory muscles, sputum characteristics, lung sounds, and skin color. *The status of a patient in acute pulmonary edema can change rapidly for the better or worse.*
- Place in high-Fowler position with the legs dangling. *The upright position facilitates breathing and decreases venous return.*
- Administer oxygen as ordered by mask, CPAP mask, or ventilator. *Supplemental oxygen promotes gas exchange; positive pressure increases the pressure within the alveoli, airways, and thoracic cavity, decreasing venous return, pulmonary capillary pressure, and fluid leak into the alveoli.*
- Encourage patient to cough up secretions; provide nasotracheal suctioning, if necessary. *Coughing moves secretions from smaller airways into larger airways where they can be suctioned out, if necessary.*

SAFETY ALERT: Have emergency equipment readily available in case of respiratory arrest. Be prepared to assist with intubation and initiation of mechanical ventilation. Fatigue, impaired gas exchange, and respiratory acidosis can lead to respiratory and cardiac arrest. ■

Monitor Cardiac Output. Cardiogenic pulmonary edema is usually caused by either an acute decrease in myocardial contractility or increased workload that exceeds the ability of the left ventricle. The significant decrease in cardiac output increases pressure within the pulmonary vascular system and triggers compensatory mechanisms that increase the heart rate and blood volume. These compensatory mechanisms further increase the workload of the failing heart.

Expected Outcome: Patient will demonstrate adequate cardiac output as evidenced by blood pressure and pulse rate and rhythm within normal limits.

The nurse will:

- Monitor vital signs, hemodynamic status, and rhythm continuously. *Acute pulmonary edema is a critical condition, and cardiovascular status can change rapidly.*
- Assess heart sounds for possible S_3, S_4, or murmurs. *These abnormal heart sounds may be due to excess work or may indicate the cause of the acute pulmonary edema.*
- Initiate an intravenous line for medication administration. Administer morphine, diuretics, vasodilators, bronchodilators, and positive inotropic medications (e.g., digoxin) as ordered. *These drugs reduce cardiac work and improve contractility.*
- Insert an indwelling catheter as ordered; record output hourly. *Urine output of < 30 mL/h indicates impaired renal perfusion due to severely impaired cardiac output and a risk for renal failure or other complications.*
- Keep accurate intake and output records. Restrict fluids as ordered. *Fluids may be restricted to reduce vascular volume and cardiac workload.*

Manage Fear. Acute pulmonary edema is a very frightening experience for everyone (including the nurse).

Expected Outcome: Patient will demonstrate reduced fear as evidenced by verbal and nonverbal indicators that reflect understanding by the patient and family of the current clinical condition.

The nurse will:

- Provide emotional support for the patient and family members. *Fear and anxiety stimulate the sympathetic nervous system, which can lead to ineffective respiratory patterns and interfere with cooperation with care measures.*
- Explain all procedures and the reasons for the procedures to the patient and family members. Keep information brief and to the point. Use short sentences and a reassuring tone. *Anxiety and fear interfere with the ability to assimilate information; brief, factual information and reassurance reduce anxiety and fear.*
- Maintain close contact with the patient and family, providing reassurance that recovery from acute pulmonary edema is often as dramatic as its onset.
- Answer questions, and provide accurate information in a caring manner. *Knowledge reduces the anxiety and psychologic stress associated with this critical condition.*

Delegating Nursing Care Activities

As appropriate and allowed by the designated duties and responsibilities of unlicensed assistive personnel, the nurse may delegate nursing care activities such as measuring fluid intake and output, collecting vital signs (including orthostatic vital signs), encouraging oral or enteral fluid intake, and ensuring nonpharmacologic skin care.

Transitions of Care

Pulmonary embolism can be difficult to prevent if the patient has no history or known risk factors. Risk factors for pulmonary embolism can include history of deep vein thromboembolism (DVT), family history of clotting disorders, and obesity. Careful history taking can help identify a patient at risk for pulmonary embolism. If a positive history is noted, the risk should be discussed with the healthcare team to determine if any further intervention is indicated.

During the acute period, teaching is limited to immediate care measures. Once the acute episode of pulmonary edema has resolved, teach the patient and family about its underlying cause and prevention of future episodes. If pulmonary edema follows an acute myocardial infarction (AMI), include information related to CHD and the AMI, as well as information related to heart failure. Review the teaching and home care for patients with these disorders for further information.

Chronic management following pulmonary embolism focuses on anticoagulation therapy and patient instruction in risk factors to be avoided.

31.2 Inflammatory Heart Disorders

Any layer of cardiac tissue—the endocardium, myocardium, or pericardium—can become inflamed, thus damaging the heart valves, heart muscle, or pericardial lining. Manifestations of inflammatory heart disorders range from very mild to life-threatening. This section discusses the causes and management of rheumatic heart disease, endocarditis, myocarditis, and pericarditis.

The Patient with Rheumatic Fever and Rheumatic Heart Disease

Rheumatic fever is a systemic inflammatory disease caused by an abnormal immune response to pharyngeal infection by group A beta-hemolytic streptococci. Rheumatic fever is usually a self-limiting disorder, although it may become recurrent or chronic. Although the heart commonly is involved in the acute inflammatory process, only about 10% of people with rheumatic fever develop rheumatic heart disease. Rheumatic heart disease frequently damages the heart valves and is a major cause of the mitral and aortic valve disorders discussed in the next section of this chapter.

Incidence, Prevalence, and Risk Factors

In the United States and other industrialized nations, rheumatic fever and its sequelae are rare. The peak incidence of rheumatic fever is between ages 5 and 15 (Zuhlke et al., 2017); although it is rare after age 30, it may affect people of any age. About 3% of people with untreated group A streptococcal pharyngitis develop rheumatic fever. Rheumatic fever and rheumatic heart disease remain significant public health problems in many developing countries (Zuhlke et al., 2017).

Risk factors for streptococcal infections of the pharynx include environmental and economic factors such as crowded living conditions, malnutrition, immunodeficiency, and poor access to healthcare. Evidence also suggests an unknown genetic factor in susceptibility to rheumatic fever.

Pathophysiology

The pathophysiology of rheumatic fever is not yet totally understood. It is thought to result from an abnormal immune response to M proteins on group A beta-hemolytic streptococcal bacteria. These antigens can bind to cells in the heart, muscles, and brain. They also bind with receptors in synovial joints, provoking an autoimmune response. The resulting immune response to the bacteria also leads to inflammation in tissues containing these M proteins. Inflammatory lesions develop in connective tissues on the heart, joints, and skin. The antibodies may remain in the serum for up to 6 months following the initiating event. Refer to Chapters 11 and 12 for more information about the immune system and inflammatory response.

Carditis, inflammation of the heart, develops in about 50% of people with rheumatic fever. The inflammatory process usually involves all three layers of the heart—the pericardium, myocardium, and endocardium. *Aschoff bodies*, localized areas of tissue necrosis surrounded by immune cells, develop in cardiac tissues. Pericardial and myocardial inflammation tends to be mild and self-limiting. Endocardial inflammation, however, causes swelling and erythema of valve structures and small vegetative lesions on valve leaflets. As the inflammatory process resolves, fibrous scarring occurs, causing deformity.

Rheumatic heart disease (RHD) is a slowly progressive valvular deformity that may follow acute or repeated attacks of rheumatic fever. Valve leaflets become rigid and deformed; commissures (openings) fuse, and the chordae tendineae fibrose and shorten. This results in stenosis or regurgitation of the valve. In **stenosis**, a narrowed, fused valve obstructs forward blood flow. **Regurgitation** occurs when the valve fails to close properly (an *incompetent* valve), allowing blood to flow back through it. Valves on the left side of the heart are usually affected; the mitral valve is most frequently involved.

Manifestations

Manifestations of rheumatic fever typically follow the initial streptococcal infection by about 2 to 3 weeks. Fever and migratory joint pain are often initial manifestations. The knees, ankles, hips, and elbows are common sites of swelling and inflammation. *Erythema marginatum* is a temporary nonpruritic skin rash characterized by red lesions with clear borders and blanched centers usually found on the trunk and proximal extremities. Neurologic symptoms of rheumatic fever, although rare in adults, may range from irritability and an inability to concentrate to clumsiness and involuntary muscle spasms.

Manifestations of carditis include chest pain, tachycardia, a pericardial friction rub, or evidence of heart failure. On auscultation, an S_3, S_4, or a heart murmur may be heard. Cardiomegaly or pericardial effusion may develop. Other multisystemic manifestations of rheumatic fever include:

Cardiac

- Chest pain
- Friction rub
- Heart murmur

Musculoskeletal

- *Migratory polyarthritis*: Redness, heat, swelling, pain, and tenderness of more than one joint
- Usually affects large joints of extremities

Skin

- *Erythema marginatum*: Transitory pink, nonpruritic, macular lesions on trunk or inner aspect of upper arms or thighs
- *Subcutaneous nodules* over extensors of wrist, elbow, ankle, and knee joints

Neurologic

- *Sydenham's chorea*: Irritability; behavior changes; sudden, jerky, involuntary movements

Interprofessional Care

Management of the patient with rheumatic heart disease focuses on eradicating the streptococcal infection and managing the manifestations of the disease. Carditis and resulting heart failure are treated with measures to reduce the inflammatory process and manage the heart failure. Activities are limited, but bedrest is not generally ordered.

Diagnosis

In addition to the history and physical examination, a number of laboratory and diagnostic tests may be ordered for the patient with suspected rheumatic fever. **Table 31.5** identifies tests and values indicative of carditis associated with rheumatic fever.

- ***Complete blood count (CBC)*** and ***erythrocyte sedimentation rate (ESR)*** are indicators of the inflammatory process. The WBC count is elevated, and the number of red blood cells may be low due to the inflammatory inhibition of erythropoiesis. The ESR, a general indicator of inflammation, is elevated.
- ***C-reactive protein (CRP)*** is positive in an active inflammatory process.
- ***Antistreptolysin (ASO) titer*** is a test for streptococcal antibodies. It rises within 2 months of onset and is positive in most patients with rheumatic fever.
- ***Throat culture*** is positive for group A beta-hemolytic streptococcus in only 25 to 40% of patients with acute rheumatic fever.

Medications

As soon as rheumatic fever is diagnosed, antibiotics are started to eliminate the streptococcal infection. Penicillin is the antibiotic of choice to treat group A streptococci. Antibiotics are prescribed for at least 10 days. Erythromycin or clindamycin is used if the patient is allergic to penicillin. Prophylactic antibiotic therapy is continued for 5 to 10 years to prevent recurrences. Recurrences after 5 years or age 25 are rare. Penicillin G, 1.2 million units injected intramuscularly every 3 to 4 weeks, is the prophylaxis of choice. Oral penicillin, amoxicillin, sulfadiazine, or erythromycin may also be used.

Joint pain and fever are treated with salicylates (e.g., aspirin), ibuprofen, or another nonsteroidal anti-inflammatory drug (NSAID); corticosteroids may be used for severe pain due to inflammation or carditis. Refer to Chapter 9 for information about the use of these anti-inflammatory medications.

Nursing Care

Assessment

See the Manifestations and Interprofessional Care sections for the assessment of the patient with rheumatic fever/rheumatic heart disease. Assess patients at risk for rheumatic fever (prolonged, untreated, or recurrent pharyngitis) for possible manifestations.

- ***Health history:*** Complaints of recent sore throat with fever, difficulty swallowing, and general malaise; treatment measures; previous history of strep throat or rheumatic fever; history of heart murmur or other cardiac problems; current medications
- ***Physical assessment:*** Vital signs including temperature; skin color, presence of rash on trunk or proximal extremities; mental status; evidence of inflamed joints; heart and lung sounds.

Priorities of Care

Collaborating with the interprofessional team to ensure adequate treatment of the underlying process while providing care that supports the physical and psychologic responses to the disorder is a priority of nursing care.

Diagnoses, Outcomes, and Interventions

The nursing care focus for the patient with RHD is on providing supportive care and preventing complications. Teaching to prevent recurrence of rheumatic fever is extremely important. *Pain* and *Activity Intolerance* are priority nursing diagnoses for the patient with rheumatic fever and RHD.

Table 31.5 Diagnostic Tests for Rheumatic Heart Disease

Test	Values Characteristic of Rheumatic Heart Disease
White blood cell count (WBC)	$> 10,000/mm^3$
Red blood cell (RBC) count	< 4 million/mm^3
Erythrocyte sedimentation rate (ESR)	> 20 mm/h
C-reactive protein	Positive
Antistreptolysin (ASO) titer	> 250 International Units/mL
Throat culture	Usually positive for group A beta-hemolytic streptococci
Cardiac enzymes	Elevated in severe carditis
ECG changes	Prolonged PR interval
Chest x-ray	May show cardiac enlargement
Echocardiogram	May show valvular damage, enlarged chambers, decreased ventricular function, or pericardial effusion

Control Acute Pain. Joint and chest pain due to acute inflammation is common in rheumatic fever. Pain and inflammation may interfere with rest and healing.

Expected Outcome: Patient will achieve adequate pain control as evidenced by physical well-being.

The nurse will:

- Administer anti-inflammatory drugs as ordered. Promptly report manifestations of aspirin toxicity, including tinnitus, vomiting, and gastrointestinal bleeding. Give aspirin and other NSAIDs with food, milk, or antacids to minimize gastric irritation. *Joint pain and fever may be treated with anti-inflammatory agents such as aspirin and NSAIDs. Steroids may be prescribed for severe carditis.*
- Provide warm, moist compresses for local pain relief of acutely inflamed joints. *Moist heat helps relieve pain associated with inflamed joints by reducing inflammation.*
- Auscultate heart sounds as indicated (every shift or each home visit). Notify the physician if a pericardial friction rub or a new murmur develops. *A friction rub is produced as inflamed pericardial surfaces rub against each other. This also stimulates pain receptors and may increase discomfort.*

Promote Activity Tolerance. The patient with acute carditis or RHD may develop heart failure if the heart is unable to supply enough oxygen to meet the body's demand. Manifestations of fatigue, weakness, and dyspnea on exertion may result.

Expected Outcome: The patient will participate in physical activity as tolerated.

The nurse will:

- Explain the importance of activity limitations and reinforce teaching as needed. *Activities are limited during the acute phase of carditis to reduce the workload of the heart. Understanding the rationale improves cooperation with the limitations.*
- Encourage social and diversional activities such as visits with friends and family, reading, playing cards or board games, watching television, and listening to music or audio books. *Diversional activities provide a focus for the patient whose physical activities must be limited.*
- Encourage gradual increases in activity, monitoring for evidence of intolerance or heart failure. Consult a cardiac rehabilitation specialist to help design an activity progression schedule. *Gradual activity progression is encouraged as the patient's condition improves. Activity tolerance is monitored and activities modified as needed.*

Delegating Nursing Care Activities

As appropriate and allowed by the designated duties and responsibilities of unlicensed assistive personnel, the nurse may delegate nursing care activities such as measuring fluid intake and output, collecting vital signs (including orthostatic vital signs), encouraging oral or enteral fluid intake, and ensuring nonpharmacologic skin care.

Transitions of Care

Rheumatic fever is preventable. Good hand hygiene plays an important role. Prompt identification and treatment of streptococcal throat infections help decrease spread of the pathogen and the risk for rheumatic fever.

Characteristics of streptococcal sore throat include a red, fiery-looking throat, pain with swallowing, enlarged and tender cervical lymph nodes, fever range of 38.3° to 40.0°C (101° to 104°F), and headache. The nurse should emphasize the importance of finishing the complete course of medication to eradicate the pathogen.

Most patients with rheumatic fever and carditis do not require hospitalization. Teaching for home care focuses on both acute care and preventing recurrences and further tissue damage. Include the following topics:

- The importance of completing the full course of antibiotic therapy and continuing antibiotic prophylaxis as prescribed for the patient with chronic RHD; include the importance of antibiotic prophylaxis for invasive procedures (e.g., dental care, endoscopy, or surgery) to prevent bacterial endocarditis. Pamphlets on endocarditis prevention are helpful reminders and are available from the American Heart Association.
- Preventive dental care and good oral hygiene to maintain oral health and prevent gingival infections, which can lead to recurrence of the disease.
- Early recognition of streptococcal sore throat and appropriate treatment for both the patient and family members.
- Early manifestations of heart failure to report to the physician.
- Prescribed medications, including their dosage, route, intended and potential adverse effects, and manifestations to report to the physician.
- Dietary sodium restriction if ordered or recommended. A high-carbohydrate, high-protein diet may be recommended to facilitate healing and combat fatigue.

Refer for home health services or household assistance as indicated.

There are not indications for end-of-life care with rheumatic fever and rheumatic heart disease unless the valvular disease advances to significant valve dysfunction, in which case the end-of-life care would be the same as in heart failure.

The Patient with Infective Endocarditis

Endocarditis, inflammation of the endocardium, can involve any portion of the endothelial lining of the heart (AHA, 2017b). The valves are usually affected. Endocarditis is usually infectious in nature, characterized by colonization or invasion of the endocardium and heart valves by a pathogen.

Incidence and Risk Factors

Endocarditis is relatively uncommon, with an incidence of 1.5 to 6.2 cases per 100,000 people in developed countries. The greatest risk factor for endocarditis is previous heart damage.

Lesions develop on deformed valves, on valve prostheses, or in areas of tissue damage due to congenital deformities or ischemic disease. The left side of the heart, the mitral valve in particular, is usually affected. Intravenous drug use is also a significant risk factor. The right side of the heart is usually affected in these patients. Other risk factors include invasive catheters (e.g., a central venous catheter, hemodynamic monitoring, or an indwelling urinary catheter), dental procedures or poor dental health, and recent heart surgery.

Prosthetic valve endocarditis (PVE) may occur in patients with a mechanical or tissue valve replacement. This infection may develop in the early postoperative period (within 2 months after surgery) or later. Prosthetic valve endocarditis accounts for 10 to 20% of endocarditis cases. It usually affects males over the age of 60 and is more frequently associated with aortic valve prostheses than with mitral valve replacements. Early PVE is usually due to prosthetic valve contamination during surgery or perioperative bacteremia. Its course is often rapid, and mortality is high. Late-onset PVE more closely resembles subacute endocarditis.

Pathophysiology

Entry of pathogens into the bloodstream is required for infective endocarditis to develop. Bacteria may enter through oral lesions, during dental work or invasive procedures, such as intravenous catheter insertion, surgery, or urinary catheterization; during intravenous drug use; or as a result of infectious processes such as urinary tract or upper respiratory infection (Sorenson et al., 2019).

The initial lesion is a sterile platelet-fibrin vegetation formed on damaged endothelium (**Figure 31.7** ■). In acute infective endocarditis, these lesions develop on healthy valve structures, although the mechanism is unknown. In subacute endocarditis, they usually develop on already damaged valves or in endocardial tissue that has been damaged by abnormal pressures or blood flow within the heart.

Organisms that have invaded the blood colonize these vegetations. The vegetation enlarges as more platelets and fibrin are attracted to the site and cover the infecting organism. This covering "protects" the bacteria from quick removal by immune defenses such as phagocytosis by neutrophils, antibodies, and complement. Vegetations may be singular or multiple. They expand while loosely attached to edges of the valve. Friable vegetations can break or shear off, embolizing and traveling through the bloodstream to other organ systems. When they lodge in small vessels, they may cause hemorrhages, infarcts, or abscesses. Ultimately, the vegetations scar and deform the valves and cause turbulence of blood flowing through the heart. Heart valve function is affected, either obstructing forward blood flow or closing incompletely.

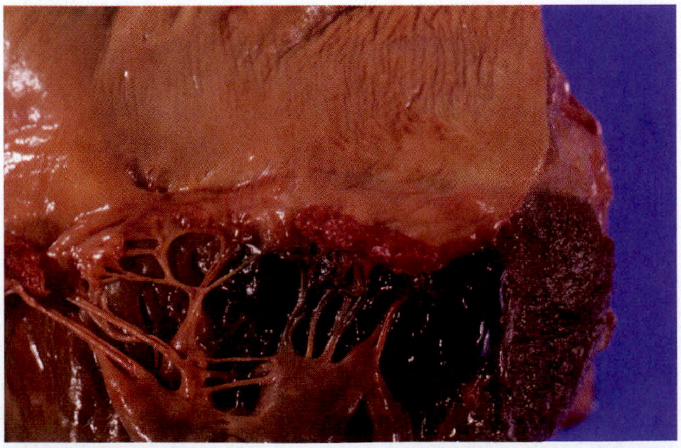

Figure 31.7 ■ A vegetative lesion of bacterial endocarditis.

Endocarditis is classified by its acuity and disease course (**Table 31.6**). *Acute infective endocarditis* has an abrupt onset and is a rapidly progressive, severe disease. Although almost any organism can cause infective endocarditis, virulent organisms such as *Staphylococcus aureus* cause a more abrupt onset and destructive course. *S. aureus* is commonly the infective organism in acute endocarditis. In contrast, *subacute infective endocarditis* has a more gradual onset, with predominant systemic manifestations. It is more likely to occur in patients with preexisting heart disease. *Streptococcus viridans*, enterococci, other gram-negative and gram-positive bacilli, yeasts, and fungi tend to cause the subacute forms of endocarditis (Sorenson et al., 2019).

Manifestations

The manifestations of infective endocarditis are often nonspecific and include:

- Chills and fever
- General malaise, fatigue
- Arthralgias
- Cough, dyspnea
- Heart murmur
- Anorexia, abdominal pain
- Petechiae, splinter hemorrhages
- Splenomegaly

A temperature above 39.4°C (101.5°F) and flulike symptoms develop, accompanied by cough, shortness of breath, and joint pain. The presentation of acute staphylococcal endocarditis is more severe, with a sudden onset, chills, and a high fever. Heart murmurs are heard in 90% of persons with infective endocarditis. An existing murmur may worsen, or a new murmur may develop.

Splenomegaly is common in chronic disease. Peripheral manifestations of infective endocarditis result from microemboli or circulating immune complexes. These manifestations include:

- ***Petechiae:*** Small, purplish-red hemorrhagic spots on the trunk, conjunctiva, and mucous membranes
- ***Splinter hemorrhage:*** Hemorrhagic streaks under the fingernails or toenails
- ***Osler nodes:*** Small, reddened, painful raised growths on finger and toe pads
- ***Janeway lesions:*** Small, nontender, purplish-red macular lesions on the palms of the hands and soles of the feet
- ***Roth spots:*** Small, whitish spots (cotton-wool spots) seen on the retina.

Table 31.6 Classifications of Infective Endocarditis

	Acute Infective Endocarditis	Subacute Infective Endocarditis
Onset	Sudden	Gradual
Usual organism	*Staphylococcus aureus*	*Streptococcus viridans*, enterococci, gram-negative and gram-positive bacilli, fungi, yeasts
Risk factors	Usually occurs in previously normal heart; intravenous drug use, infected intravenous sites	Usually occurs in damaged or deformed hearts; dental work, invasive procedures, and infections
Pathologic process	Rapid valve destruction	Valve destruction leading to regurgitation; embolization of friable vegetations
Presentation	Abrupt onset with spiking fever and chills; manifestations of heart failure	Gradual onset of febrile illness with cough, dyspnea, arthralgias, abdominal pain

Complications

Embolization of vegetative fragments may affect any organ system, particularly the lungs, brain, kidneys, and the skin and mucous membranes, with resulting organ infarction. Other common complications of infective endocarditis include heart failure, abscess, and aneurysms due to infiltration of the arterial wall by organisms. Without treatment, endocarditis is almost universally fatal; fortunately, antibiotic therapy is usually effective to treat this disease.

Interprofessional Care

Eradicating the infecting organism and minimizing valve damage and other adverse consequences of infective endocarditis are the priorities of care.

Diagnosis

There are no definitive tests for infective endocarditis, but diagnostic tests help establish the diagnosis.

- ***Blood cultures*** usually are positive for bacteria or other pathogens. Blood cultures are considered positive when a typical infecting organism is identified from two or more separate blood cultures (drawn from different sites and/or at different times, e.g., 12-hour intervals).
- ***Echocardiography*** (either transthoracic or transesophageal) to visualize vegetations can be diagnostic for infective endocarditis when combined with positive blood cultures. See Chapter 29 for more information about echocardiography.
- ***Serologic immune testing*** for circulating antigens to assess for typical infective organisms may be done.

Other diagnostic tests may include CBC, ESR, and serum creatinine levels; chest x-ray; and an electrocardiogram.

Medications

Preventing endocarditis in patients at high risk is important. Antibiotics are commonly prescribed for patients with preexisting valve damage or heart disease prior to high-risk procedures. In 2008, the AHA significantly altered the recommendations for endocarditis prophylaxis, reducing the groups of patients who require antibiotics prior to procedures (Nishimura et al., 2008) (see **Box 31.4**).

Antibiotic therapy effectively treats infective endocarditis in most cases. The goal of therapy is to eradicate the infecting organism from the blood and vegetative lesions in the heart. The fibrin covering that protects colonies of organisms from immune defenses also protects them from antibiotic therapy. Therefore, an extended course of multiple intravenous antibiotics is required.

Following blood cultures, antibiotic therapy is initiated with drugs known to be effective against the most common infecting organisms: Staphylococci, streptococci, and enterococci. The initial regimen may include nafcillin or oxacillin, penicillin or ampicillin, and gentamicin. Once the organism has been identified, therapy is tailored to that organism. Staphylococcal and enterococcal infections are treated with a combination of penicillin and gentamicin. If the patient is allergic to penicillin, ceftriaxone, cefazolin, or vancomycin may be used. Streptococcal infections are treated with nafcillin or oxacillin and gentamicin; cefazolin or vancomycin may be used if penicillin allergy is present. Intravenous drug therapy is continued for 2 to 8 weeks, depending on the infecting organism, the drugs used, and the results of repeat blood cultures. Refer to Chapter 12 for the nursing implications for antibiotic therapy.

The patient with prosthetic valve endocarditis requires extended treatment, usually 6 to 8 weeks. Combination therapy using vancomycin, rifampin, and gentamicin is used to treat these resistant infections.

Surgery

Some patients with infective endocarditis require the following from surgery:

- Replace severely damaged valves.
- Remove large vegetations at risk for embolization.
- Remove a valve that is a continuing source of infection that does not respond to antibiotic therapy.

The most common indication for surgery is valvular regurgitation that causes heart failure and does not respond to medical therapy. When the infection has not responded to antibiotic therapy within 7 to 10 days, the infected valve may be replaced to facilitate eradication of the organism. Patients with fungal endocarditis usually require surgical intervention. More information on valve replacement surgery is provided in the section on valve disorders.

Nursing Care

Assessment

See the Manifestations and Interprofessional Care sections for the assessment of the patient with endocarditis.

BOX 31.4

Updated Recommendations for Antibiotic Prophylaxis for Infective Endocarditis

Indications for Prophylaxis	Selected Procedures for which Prophylaxis Is Recommended	Suggested Antibiotics
■ Prosthetic valves ■ Previous episode(s) of infective endocarditis ■ Congenital heart disease ■ Unrepaired, cyanotic ■ Completely repaired up to 6 months postrepair ■ Repaired with residual defects ■ Cardiac transplant	■ Dental procedures in which bleeding is likely, including cleaning ■ Most surgeries ■ Bronchoscopy (only with incision of the respiratory tract mucosa) ■ Cystoscopy ■ Urinary catheterization when infection is present ■ Incision and drainage of infected tissue ■ Vaginal delivery if infection is present	■ Amoxicillin ■ Erythromycin ■ Ampicillin ■ Clindamycin ■ Vancomycin (recommended for MRSA) (*Note:* Choice of antibiotic depends on procedure.)

Note: Drugs identified in blue are among the 200 most commonly prescribed medications in the United States.

Assessment related to ineffective endocarditis includes identifying risk factors and manifestations of the disease.

- ***Health history:*** Complaints of persistent flulike symptoms, fatigue, shortness of breath, and activity intolerance; history of recent dental work or other invasive procedures; known heart murmur, valve or other heart disorder; recent intravenous drug use
- ***Physical assessment:*** Vital signs including temperature; apical pulse and heart sounds; rate and ease of respirations, lung sounds; skin color, temperature, and presence of petechiae or splinter hemorrhages.

Priorities of Care

Collaborating with the interprofessional team to ensure adequate treatment of the underlying process while providing care that supports the physical and psychologic responses to the disorder is a priority of nursing care.

Diagnoses, Outcomes, and Interventions

Nursing care focuses on managing the manifestations of endocarditis, administering antibiotics, and teaching the patient and family members about the disorder. In addition to the diagnoses identified next, nursing diagnoses and interventions for heart failure may also be appropriate for patients with infective endocarditis.

Monitor Body Temperature. Fever is common in patients with infective endocarditis. It may be acutely elevated and accompanied by chills, particularly with acute infective endocarditis. The inflammatory process initiates a cycle of events that affects the regulation of temperature and causes discomfort.

Expected Outcome: The patient's body temperature will be within normal limits as evidenced by measurements within normal range and skin warm and dry.

The nurse will:

- Record temperature every 2 to 4 hours. Report temperature above 39.4°C (101.5°F). Assess for complaints of discomfort. *Fever is usually low grade (below 39.4°C [101.5°F]) in infective endocarditis; higher temperatures may cause discomfort. The temperature usually returns to normal within 1 week after initiation of antibiotic therapy. Continued fever may indicate a need to modify the treatment regimen.*
- Obtain blood cultures as ordered, before initial antibiotic dose. *Initial blood cultures are obtained before antibiotic therapy is started to obtain adequate organisms to culture and identify. Follow-up cultures are used to assess the effectiveness of therapy.*
- Provide anti-inflammatory or antipyretic agents as prescribed. *Fever may be treated with anti-inflammatory or antipyretic agents such as aspirin, ibuprofen, or acetaminophen.*
- Administer antibiotics as ordered; obtain peak and trough drug levels as indicated. *Intravenous antibiotics are given to eradicate the pathogen. Peak and trough levels are used to evaluate the dose effectiveness in maintaining a therapeutic blood level.*

Promote Adequate Tissue Perfusion. Embolization of vegetative lesions can threaten tissue and organ perfusion. Vegetations from the left heart may lodge in arterioles or capillaries of the brain, kidneys, or peripheral tissues, causing infarction or abscess. A large embolism can cause manifestations of stroke or transient ischemic attack, renal failure, or tissue ischemia. Emboli from the right side of the heart become entrapped in pulmonary vasculature, causing manifestations of pulmonary embolism.

Expected Outcome: Patient's tissue perfusion will be adequate as evidenced by adequate arterial flow as seen by strong peripheral pulses and freedom from dyspnea.

The nurse will:

- Assess for, document, and report manifestations of decreased organ system perfusion:
  a. Neurologic: Changes in level of consciousness, numbness or tingling in extremities, hemiplegia, visual disturbances, or manifestations of stroke

b. Renal: Decreased urine output, hematuria, elevated BUN or creatinine
c. Pulmonary: Dyspnea, hemoptysis, shortness of breath, diminished breath sounds, restlessness, sudden chest or shoulder pain
d. Cardiovascular: Chest pain radiating to jaw or arms, tachycardia, anxiety, tachypnea, hypotension.

- All major organs and tissues, and the microcirculation, may be affected by emboli when vegetations break off due to turbulent blood flow. Emboli may cause manifestations of organ dysfunction. The most devastating effects of emboli are in the brain and the myocardium, with resulting infarctions. Intravenous drug users have a high risk of pulmonary emboli as a result of right-sided endocardial fragments.
- Assess and document skin color and temperature, quality of peripheral pulses, and capillary refill. *Peripheral emboli affect tissue perfusion, with a risk for tissue necrosis and possible extremity loss.*

Promote Effective Health Maintenance. The patient with endocarditis is often treated in the community. Teaching about disease management and prevention of possible recurrences of endocarditis is vital.

Expected Outcome: Patient will be knowledgeable about management of endocarditis as evidenced by patient being able to describe the components and rationale for the treatment plan.

The nurse will:

- Demonstrate intravenous catheter site care and intermittent antibiotic administration if the patient and family will manage therapy. Have the patient and/or significant other redemonstrate appropriate techniques. *Intermittent antibiotic infusions may be managed by the patient or family members or the patient may go to an outpatient facility to receive the infusions. Appropriate site care is necessary to reduce the risk of trauma and infection.*
- Explain the actions, doses, administration, and desired and adverse effects of prescribed drugs. Identify manifestations to be reported to the physician. Provide practical information about measures to reduce the risk of superinfection (e.g., consuming 8 oz of yogurt or buttermilk containing live bacterial cultures daily). *Careful compliance with prescribed drug therapy is vital to eradicate the infecting organism. Antibiotic therapy can, however, cause superinfections such as candidiasis due to elimination of normal body flora.*
- Teach about the function of heart valves and the effects of endocarditis on heart function. Include a simple definition of endocarditis, and explain the risk for its recurrence. *Information helps the patient and family understand endocarditis, its treatment, and its effects. Understanding increases compliance.*
- Describe the manifestations of heart failure to be reported to the physician. *Evidence of heart failure may necessitate modification of the treatment regimen or replacement of infected valves.*
- Stress the importance of notifying all care providers of valve disease, heart murmur, or valve replacement before undergoing invasive procedures. *Invasive procedures provide a portal of entry for bacteria. A history of valve disease increases the risk for the development or recurrence of endocarditis.*
- Encourage good dental hygiene and mouth care and regular dental checkups. Teach how to prevent bleeding from the gums and avoid developing mouth ulcers (e.g., gentle toothbrushing, ensuring that dentures fit properly, and avoiding toothpicks, dental floss, and high-flow water devices). *The oropharynx harbors streptococci, which are common causes of endocarditis. Bleeding gums offer an opportunity for bacteria to enter the bloodstream.*
- Encourage the patient to avoid people with upper respiratory infections. *Streptococci are normal pathogens in the upper respiratory tract; exposure to people with upper respiratory infections may increase the risk of infection.*
- If anticoagulant therapy is ordered, explain its actions, administration, and major side effects. Identify manifestations of bleeding to be promptly reported to the physician. *Patients with valve disease or a prosthetic valve following infective endocarditis may require continued anticoagulant therapy to prevent thrombi and emboli. Knowledge is vital for appropriate management of anticoagulant therapy and prevention of complications.*

Delegating Nursing Care Activities

As appropriate and allowed by designated duties and responsibilities of assistive personnel, the nurse may delegate nursing care activities such as measuring fluid intake and output, collecting vital signs (including orthostatic vital signs), encouraging oral or enteral fluid intake, and ensuring nonpharmacologic skin care.

Transitions of Care

Prevention of endocarditis is vital in susceptible people. Education is a key part of prevention. Use every opportunity to educate individuals and the public about the risks of intravenous drug use, including endocarditis. Discuss preventative measures with all patients with specific risk factors, such as a history of valve replacement, congenital heart defects, or cardiac transplantation (Nishimura et al., 2017).

Effective management of infective endocarditis starts with diagnosis. While many patients present with straightforward signs and symptoms such as persistent bacterial infection and valvular involvement, others may have more silent indicators. Echocardiography plays an important role in the diagnosis of infective endocarditis, providing visualization of valvular changes or the presence of vegetation. Depending on the severity of the clinical findings, surgical intervention to remove any vegetation may be indicated. Nursing management would follow nursing actions for cardiac surgery (see Chapter 30).

When preparing the patient with infective endocarditis for home care, provide teaching to promote adequate health maintenance as outlined previously. In addition, discuss the following topics:

- Although serious and frightening, infective endocarditis can usually be treated effectively with intravenous antibiotics.

- The importance of promptly reporting any unusual manifestation, such as a change in vision, sudden pain, or weakness, so that interventions to control complications can be promptly implemented.
- The rationale for all treatments and procedures.
- Preventing recurrences of infective endocarditis.
- The importance of maintaining contact with the physician for follow-up care and monitoring for long-term effects such as progressive valve damage and dysfunction.
- If appropriate, explain the risks associated with intravenous drug use.

Provide educational materials on infective endocarditis from the American Heart Association. Refer as appropriate to home health or home intravenous therapy services. Refer the patient and family members or significant others as appropriate to a drug or substance abuse treatment program or facility. Provide follow-up care to ensure compliance with the referral and treatment plan. There is not an indication for end-of-life care with infective endocarditis unless the valvular disease advances to significant valve dysfunction, in which case the care would be the same as that for patients with heart failure (Steiner, Cooper, & Kirkpatrick, 2017).

The Patient with Myocarditis

Myocarditis is inflammation of the heart muscle. It usually results from an infectious process, but also may occur as an immunologic response or due to the effects of radiation, toxins, or drugs (Sorenson et al., 2019). In the United States, myocarditis is usually viral, caused by coxsackievirus B. Approximately 10% of people with HIV disease develop myocarditis due to infiltration of the myocardium by the virus. Bacterial myocarditis, much less common, may be associated with endocarditis caused by *Staphylococcus aureus* or with diphtheria. Parasitic infections caused by *Trypanosoma cruzi* (Chagas disease) are common in Central and South America.

Incidence and Risk Factors

Myocarditis may occur at any age, and it is more common in men than in women. Factors that alter immune response (e.g., malnutrition, alcohol use, immunosuppressive drugs, exposure to radiation, stress, and advanced age) increase the risk for myocarditis. It is also a common complication of rheumatic fever and pericarditis.

Pathophysiology

In myocarditis, myocardial cells are damaged by an inflammatory process that causes local or diffuse swelling and damage. Infectious agents infiltrate interstitial tissues, forming abscesses. Autoimmune injury may occur when the immune system destroys not only the invading pathogen but also myocardial cells. The extent of damage to cardiac muscle ultimately determines the long-term outcome of the disease. Viral myocarditis is usually self-limited; it may progress, however, to become chronic, leading to dilated cardiomyopathy. Severe myocarditis may lead to heart failure.

Manifestations

The manifestations of myocarditis depend on the degree of myocardial damage. The patient may be asymptomatic. Nonspecific manifestations of inflammation such as fever, fatigue, general malaise, dyspnea, palpitations, arthralgias, and sore throat may be present. A nonspecific febrile illness or upper respiratory infection often precedes the onset of myocarditis symptoms. Abnormal heart sounds such as muffled S_1, an S_3, murmur, and pericardial friction rub may be heard. In some cases, manifestations of myocardial infarction, including chest pain, may occur.

Interprofessional Care

Myocarditis treatment focuses on resolving the inflammatory process to prevent further damage to the myocardium.

Diagnosis

Diagnostic studies may be ordered to help diagnose myocarditis.

- ***Electrocardiography*** may show transient ST segment and T-wave changes, as well as dysrhythmias and possible heart block.
- ***Cardiac markers***, such as the creatinine kinase, troponin T, and troponin I, may be elevated, indicating myocardial cell damage.
- ***Endomyocardial biopsy*** to examine myocardial cells is necessary to establish a definitive diagnosis; patchy cell necrosis and the inflammatory process can be identified.

Medications

If appropriate, antimicrobial therapy is used to eradicate the infecting organism. Antiviral therapy with interferon-α may be instituted. Immunosuppressive therapy with corticosteroids or other immunosuppressive agents (refer to Chapter 13) may be used to minimize the inflammatory response. Heart failure is treated as needed, using ACE inhibitors and drugs. Patients with myocarditis are often particularly sensitive to the effects of digitalis, so it is used with caution. Other medications used in treating myocarditis include antidysrhythmic agents to control dysrhythmias and anticoagulants to prevent emboli.

Bedrest and activity restrictions are ordered during the acute inflammatory process to reduce myocardial workload and prevent myocardial damage. Activities may be limited for as long as 6 months to a year.

Nursing Care

Nursing care is directed at decreasing myocardial workload and maintaining cardiac output. Both physical and emotional rest are indicated because anxiety increases myocardial oxygen demand. Hemodynamic parameters and the ECG are monitored closely, especially during the acute phase of the illness. Activity tolerance, urine output, and heart and breath sounds are frequently assessed for manifestations of heart failure. The following diagnoses for the patient with myocarditis may require nursing care:

- Poor activity and exercise tolerance related to impaired cardiac muscle function
- Reduced cardiac function related to myocardial inflammation
- Fatigue related to inflammation and impaired cardiac output
- Anxiety related to possible long-term effects of the disorder
- Fluid overload related to compensatory mechanisms for decreased cardiac output.

Transitions of Care

Prevention of myocarditis focuses on preventative actions to avoid infections. Myocarditis risk factors include viral, bacterial, and protozoal infections, exposure to radiation, and, in rare instances, autoimmune disorders.

Myocarditis develops acutely in most instances. Treatment focuses on the identification and removal of the causative agent. The clinical course follows that of a generalized inflammatory illness. Recovery may be spontaneous or heart failure may develop. Nursing care focuses on symptom management, careful cardiac assessment, and monitoring.

Include the following topics when preparing the patient with myocarditis for home care:

- Activity restrictions and other prescribed measures to reduce cardiac workload
- Early manifestations of heart failure to report to the physician
- The importance of following the prescribed treatment regimen
- Any recommended dietary modifications (such as a low-sodium diet for heart failure)
- Prescribed medications, their purpose, doses, and possible adverse effects
- The importance of adhering to the treatment plan and recommended follow-up appointments to reduce the risk of long-term consequences such as cardiomyopathy.

There are not indications for end-of life-care with myocarditis unless the process advances to heart failure, in which case the patient would be treated as described earlier for patients with heart failure.

The Patient with Pericarditis

The *pericardium* is the outermost layer of the heart. It is a two-layered membranous sac with a thin layer of serous fluid (normally no more than 30 to 50 mL) separating the layers. It protects and cushions the heart and the great vessels, provides a barrier to infectious processes in adjacent structures, prevents displacement of the myocardium and blood vessels, and prevents sudden distention of the heart.

Pericarditis is inflammation of the pericardium. Pericarditis may be a primary disorder or develop secondarily to another cardiac or systemic disorder. Some possible causes of pericarditis include:

Infectious

- Viruses
- Bacteria
- Tuberculosis
- Syphilis
- Parasites

Noninfectious

- Myocardial and pericardial injury
- Rheumatic fever
- Uremia
- Neoplasms
- Radiation
- Trauma or surgery
- Myxedema
- Autoimmune disorders
- Connective tissue diseases
- Prescription and nonprescription drugs
- Postcardiac injury.

Acute pericarditis is usually viral and affects men (usually under the age of 50) more frequently than women. Pericarditis affects 0.2 to 0.5% of hospitalized patients (Alwan et al., 2017) affecting many patients with end-stage renal disease and uremia (Black, 2018). Postmyocardial infarction pericarditis and postcardiotomy (following open-heart surgery) pericarditis are also common.

Pathophysiology

Pericardial tissue damage triggers an inflammatory response. Inflammatory mediators released from the injured tissue cause vasodilation, hyperemia, and edema. Capillary permeability increases, allowing plasma proteins, including fibrinogen, to escape into the pericardial space (Sorenson et al., 2019). White blood cells amass at the site of injury to destroy the causative agent. Exudate is formed, usually fibrinous or serofibrinous (a mixture of serous fluid and fibrinous exudate). In some cases, the exudate may contain red blood cells or, if infectious, purulent material. The inflammatory process may resolve without long-term effects, or scar tissue and adhesions may form between the pericardial layers.

Fibrosis and scarring of the pericardium may restrict cardiac function. Pericardial effusions may develop as serous or purulent exudate (depending on the causative agent) that collects in the pericardial sac. Pericardial effusion may be recurrent. Chronic inflammation causes the pericardium to become rigid.

Manifestations

Classic manifestations of acute pericarditis include chest pain, a pericardial friction rub, and fever. Chest pain, the most common symptom, has an abrupt onset. It is caused by inflammation of nerve fibers in the lower parietal pericardium and pleura covering the diaphragm. The pain is usually sharp, may be steady or intermittent, and may radiate to the back or neck. The pain can mimic myocardial ischemia; careful assessment is important to rule out myocardial infarction. Pericardial pain is aggravated by respiratory movements (i.e., deep inspiration and/or coughing), changes in body position, or swallowing. Sitting upright and leaning forward reduces the discomfort by moving the heart away from the diaphragmatic side of the lung pleura.

Although not always present, a *pericardial friction rub* is the characteristic sign of pericarditis. A pericardial friction rub is a leathery, grating sound produced by the inflamed pericardial layers rubbing against the chest wall or pleura. It is heard most clearly at the left lower sternal border with the patient sitting up or leaning forward. The rub is usually heard on expiration and may be constant or intermittent.

A low-grade fever (below 38.4°C [100°F]) often develops due to the inflammatory process. Dyspnea and tachycardia are common.

Complications

Pericardial effusion, cardiac tamponade, and constrictive pericarditis are possible complications of acute pericarditis.

Pericardial Effusion

A *pericardial effusion* is an abnormal collection of fluid between the pericardial layers that threatens normal cardiac function. The fluid may consist of pus, blood, serum, lymph, or a combination. The manifestations of a pericardial effusion depend on the rate at which the fluid collects. Although the pericardium normally contains about 30 to 50 mL of fluid, the sac can stretch to accommodate a gradual accumulation of fluid. Over time, the pericardial sac can accommodate up to 2 L of fluid without immediate adverse effects. Conversely, a rapid buildup of pericardial fluid (as little as 100 mL) does not allow the sac to stretch and can compress the heart, interfering with myocardial function. This compression of the heart is known as **cardiac tamponade**. Slowly developing pericardial effusion is often painless and has few manifestations. Heart sounds may be distant or muffled. The patient may have a cough or mild dyspnea.

Cardiac Tamponade

Cardiac tamponade is a medical emergency that must be aggressively treated to preserve life. Cardiac tamponade may result from pericardial effusion, trauma, cardiac rupture, or hemorrhage. Rapid collection of fluid in the pericardial sac interferes with ventricular filling and pumping, critically reducing cardiac output.

Classic manifestations of cardiac tamponade result from rising intracardiac pressures, decreased diastolic filling, and decreased cardiac output. A hallmark of cardiac tamponade is a paradoxical pulse, or *pulsus paradoxus*. A paradoxical pulse markedly decreases in amplitude during inspiration. Intrathoracic pressure normally drops during inspiration, enhancing venous return to the right heart. This draws more blood into the right side of the heart than the left, causing the interventricular septum to bulge slightly into the left ventricle. When ventricular filling is impaired by excess fluid in the pericardial sac, this bulging of the interventricular septum decreases cardiac output during inspiration (**Figure 31.8** ■). On palpation of the carotid or femoral artery, the pulse is diminished or absent during inspiration. A drop in systolic blood pressure of > 10 mmHg during inspiration also indicates pulsus paradoxus. Signs include muffled heart sounds, tachycardia, tachypnea, narrowed pulse pressure, and distended neck veins. Reduced urine output can be seen as well as cool, mottled skin. Late change would be decreased level of consciousness.

Chronic Constrictive Pericarditis

Chronic pericardial inflammation can lead to scar tissue formation between the pericardial layers. This scar tissue eventually contracts, restricting diastolic filling, and elevating venous pressure. Constrictive pericarditis may follow viral infection, radiation therapy, or heart surgery. Its manifestations include progressive dyspnea, fatigue, and weakness. Ascites is common; peripheral edema may develop. Neck veins are distended and may be particularly noticeable during inspiration (*Kussmaul sign*). This occurs because the right atrium is unable to dilate to accommodate increased venous return during inspiration. See **Figure 31.9** ■.

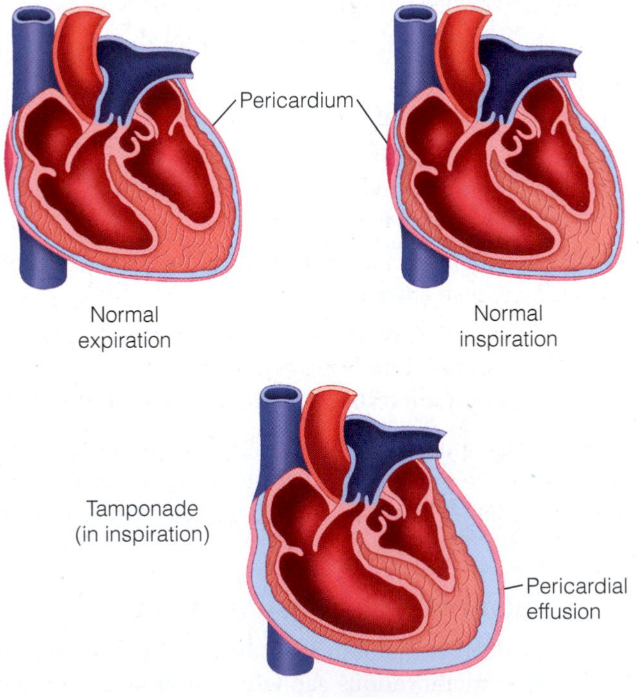
Pericardium
Normal expiration
Normal inspiration
Tamponade (in inspiration)
Pericardial effusion

Figure 31.8 ■ Cardiac tamponade. Note increased volume in the right ventricle during inspiration in both the normal heart and the heart affected by a pericardial effusion. In tamponade, fluid in the pericardial sac and the distended right ventricle restrict filling of the left ventricle and, consequently, cardiac output.

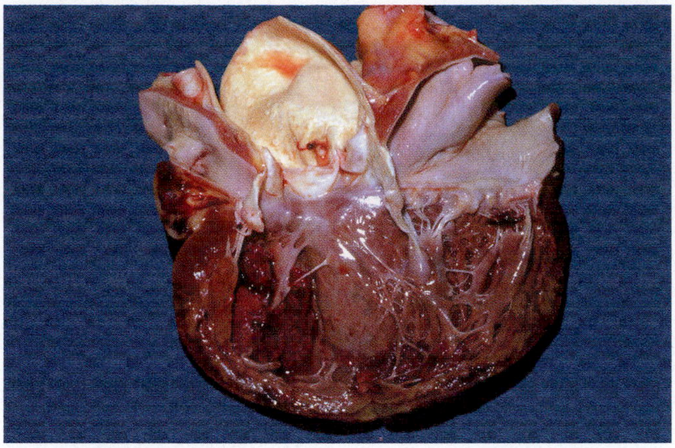

Figure 31.9 ■ Constrictive pericarditis.

Interprofessional Care

Care for the patient with pericarditis focuses on identifying its cause, if possible, reducing inflammation, relieving symptoms, and preventing complications. The patient is closely monitored for early manifestations of cardiac tamponade so that it can be treated promptly.

Diagnosis

There are no specific laboratory tests to diagnose pericarditis, but tests are often performed to differentiate pericarditis from myocardial infarction (Kee, 2014).

- *CBC* shows elevated WBCs and an ESR > 20 mm/h, indicating acute inflammation.
- *Cardiac enzymes* may be slightly elevated because the inflammatory process extends to involve the epicardial surface of the heart. Cardiac enzymes are typically much lower in pericarditis than in myocardial infarction.
- *Electrocardiography* shows typical changes associated with pericarditis, such as diffuse ST-segment elevation in all leads. This resolves more quickly than changes of AMI and is not associated with the QRS-complex and T-wave changes typically seen in MI. With a large pericardial effusion, the QRS amplitude may be decreased. Atrial dysrhythmias may occur in acute pericarditis.
- *Echocardiography* is used to assess heart motion, for pericardial effusion, and the extent of restriction.
- *Hemodynamic monitoring* may be used in acute pericarditis or pericardial effusion to assess pressures and cardiac output. Elevated pulmonary artery pressures and venous pressures occur with impaired filling due to pericardial effusion or constrictive pericarditis.
- *Chest x-ray* may show cardiac enlargement if a pericardial effusion is present.
- *Computed tomography (CT scan)* or *magnetic resonance imaging (MRI)* may be used to identify pericardial effusion or constrictive pericarditis.

Medications

Drug treatment for pericarditis addresses its manifestations. Aspirin and acetaminophen may be used to reduce fever. NSAIDs are used to reduce inflammation and promote comfort. In severe cases or with recurrent pericarditis, corticosteroids may be given to suppress the inflammatory response.

Pericardiocentesis

Pericardiocentesis may be done to remove fluid from the pericardial sac for diagnostic or therapeutic purposes (refer to Figure 29.18 in Chapter 29). The physician inserts a large (16- to 18-gauge) needle into the pericardial sac and withdraws excess fluid. The needle is attached to an ECG monitoring lead to help determine if the needle is touching the epicardial surface, which helps prevent piercing the myocardium. Pericardiocentesis may be an emergency procedure for the patient with cardiac tamponade.

Surgery

For recurrent pericarditis or recurrent pericardial effusion, a rectangular piece of the pericardium, or "window," may be excised to allow collected fluid to drain into the pleural space. Constrictive pericarditis may necessitate a partial or total *pericardiectomy*, removal of part or all of the pericardium, to relieve the ventricular compression and allow adequate filling.

Nursing Care

Assessment

See the Manifestations and Interprofessional Care sections for the assessment of the patient with pericarditis.

Assessment data to collect from the patient with suspected pericarditis includes:

- ***Health history:*** Complaints of acute substernal or precordial chest pain, effect of movement and breathing on discomfort, pain radiation, associated symptoms; recent AMI, heart surgery, or other cardiac disorder; current medications; chronic conditions such as renal failure or a connective tissue or autoimmune disorder
- ***Physical assessment:*** Vital signs including temperature, variation in systolic BP with respirations; strength of peripheral pulses, variations with respiratory movement; apical pulse, clarity, changes with respiratory movement, presence of a friction rub; neck vein distention; level of consciousness, skin color, and other indicators of cardiac output.

Priorities of Care

Collaborating with the interprofessional team to ensure adequate treatment of the underlying process while providing care that supports the physical and psychologic responses to the disorder is a priority of nursing care.

Diagnoses, Outcomes, and Interventions

Nursing care for the patient with pericarditis may occur in the acute or community setting. Closely observe for early manifestations of increasing effusion or cardiac tamponade. Priority nursing diagnoses relate to comfort, the risk for tamponade, and effects of the acute inflammatory process.

Manage Acute Pain. Inflamed pericardial layers rubbing against each other and the lung pleura stimulate phrenic nerve pain fibers in the lower portion of the parietal pericardium. Pain is usually acute and may be severe until inflammation resolves.

Expected Outcome: Patient will experience adequate pain control as evidenced by physical well-being.

The nurse will:

- Assess chest pain using a standard pain scale and noting the quality and radiation of the pain. Note nonverbal cues of pain (grimacing, guarding behaviors), and validate with the patient. *Careful assessment helps identify the cause of pain. The pain of pericarditis may radiate to the neck or back and is aggravated by movement, coughing, or deep breathing. A pain scale allows evaluation of the effectiveness of interventions.*
- Auscultate heart sounds every 4 hours. *Presence of a pericardial friction rub often correlates with the location and severity of the pain.*
- Administer NSAIDs on a regular basis as prescribed with food. Document effectiveness. *NSAIDs reduce fever, inflammation, and pericardial pain. They are most effective when administered around the clock on a consistent basis. Administering the medications with food helps decrease gastric distress.*
- Maintain a quiet, calm environment and position of comfort. Offer back rubs, heat/cold therapy, diversional activity, and emotional support. *Supportive interventions enhance the effects of the medication, may decrease pain perception, and convey a sense of caring.*

Promote Effective Breathing Pattern. Respiratory movement intensifies pericardial pain. In an effort to decrease pain, the patient often breathes shallowly, increasing the risk for pulmonary complications.

Expected Outcome: The patient will perform deep breathing using correct technique.

The nurse will:

- Document respiratory rate, effort, and breath sounds every 2 to 4 hours. Report adventitious or diminished breath sounds. *Shallow, guarded respirations may lead to increased respiratory rate and effort. Poor ventilation of peripheral alveoli may lead to congestion or atelectasis.*
- Encourage deep breathing and use of the incentive spirometer. Provide pain medication before respiratory therapy, as needed. *Deep breathing and an incentive spirometer promote alveolar ventilation and prevent atelectasis. Analgesia prior to respiratory treatments improves their effectiveness by decreasing guarding.*
- Administer oxygen as needed. *Supplementary oxygen promotes optimal gas exchange and tissue oxygenation.*
- Place in Fowler or high-Fowler position. Assist to a position of comfort. *Appropriate positioning reduces the work of breathing and decreases chest pain due to pericarditis.*

Reduce Risk for Decreased Cardiac Output. The acute inflammatory process of pericarditis can lead to significant pericardial effusion and cardiac tamponade. This potentially fatal complication can also occur with chronic pericardial effusion if the amount of fluid exceeds the ability of the pericardial sac to expand. Constrictive pericarditis increases the risk for decreased cardiac output because of restricted cardiac filling.

Expected Outcome: Patient will demonstrate adequate cardiac output as evidenced by blood pressure and pulse rate and rhythm within normal limits.

The nurse will:

- Document vital signs hourly during the acute inflammatory processes. *Frequent assessment allows early recognition of manifestations of decreased cardiac output, such as tachycardia, hypotension, or changes in pulse pressure.*

SAFETY ALERT: Assess heart sounds and peripheral pulses, and observe for neck vein distention and paradoxical pulse hourly. Promptly report distant, muffled heart sounds, new murmurs, or extra heart sounds, decreasing quality of peripheral pulses, and distended neck veins. Acute pericardial effusion interferes with normal cardiac filling and pumping, causing venous congestion and decreased cardiac output. As the amount of fluid increases in the pericardial sac, heart sounds are obscured. A drop in systolic blood pressure of >10 mmHg on inspiration signifies an abnormal response to changes in intrathoracic pressure. ■

- Report significant changes or trends in hemodynamic parameters and dysrhythmias. *Compression of the heart interferes with venous return, increasing CVP and right atrial pressures; dysrhythmias may also occur.*
- Promptly report other signs of decreased cardiac output: Decreased level of consciousness; decreased urine output; cold, clammy, mottled skin; delayed capillary refill; and weak peripheral pulses. *These signs of decreased organ and tissue perfusion indicate a significant drop in cardiac output.*
- Maintain at least one patent intravenous access site. *The patient in cardiac tamponade may require rapid intravenous fluid infusion to restore blood volume and administration of emergency drugs to support the circulation.*
- Prepare for emergency pericardiocentesis and/or surgery as necessary. Provide appropriate explanations and reassurance. Observe for adverse responses during pericardiocentesis. *Excess pericardial fluid must be rapidly evacuated to prevent further compromise of cardiac output and death. Emotional support and explanations reduce the patient's and family's anxiety and promote a caring atmosphere.*

Promote Activity Tolerance. In chronic constrictive pericarditis, pericardial adhesions and scarring restrict pericardial compliance, which in turn restricts heart filling and movement. Restricted filling and ineffective cardiac contraction decrease cardiac output. The heart cannot compensate for increased metabolic demands by increasing cardiac output, and cardiac reserve falls significantly.

Expected Outcome: Patient will participate in an activity program without suffering any complications.

The nurse will:

- Document vital signs, cardiac rhythm, skin color, and temperature before and after activity. Note any subjective complaints of fatigue, shortness of breath, chest pain, palpitations, or other symptoms with activity. *These parameters help determine the response to increased cardiac workload. Increased heart rate and respiratory rate and effort, decreased blood pressure, and dysrhythmias are indicators of activity intolerance. Pallor or cyanosis and cool, clammy, mottled skin are signs of decreased tissue perfusion. Complaints of weakness, shortness of breath, fatigue, dizziness, or palpitations are further evidence of activity intolerance.*
- Work with the patient and physical therapist to develop a realistic, progressive activity plan. Monitor response. Encourage independence, but provide assistance as needed. *Patient involvement in planning increases the likelihood of success, as well as the patient's self-esteem and sense of control. Promoting self-care provides additional control and independence and enhances self-image. Activity that significantly increases the heart rate (> 20 bpm over resting) should be stopped and reassessed for intensity.*
- Plan interventions and care activities to allow uninterrupted rest and sleep. *This supports healing and restoration of physical and emotional health.*

Delegating Nursing Care Activities

As appropriate and allowed by the designated duties and responsibilities of unlicensed assistive personnel, the nurse may delegate nursing care activities such as measuring fluid intake and output, collecting vital signs (including orthostatic vital signs), encouraging oral or enteral fluid intake, and ensuring nonpharmacologic skin care.

Transitions of Care

Although it may not yet be possible to identify many patients at risk for acute pericarditis or to prevent it, early identification and treatment of the disorder can reduce the risk of complications. Promptly report a pericardial friction rub or other manifestations of pericarditis in patients with recent AMI, cardiac surgery, or systemic diseases associated with a risk for pericarditis.

When caring for a patient with acute pericarditis, cardiac monitoring, symptom management, and interventions to promote function and reduce adverse effects are indicated. Oxygen therapy may be indicated for optimal perfusion and to avoid hypoxemia. Include the following topics when teaching the patient and family in preparation for home care:

- The importance of continuing anti-inflammatory medications as ordered. Advise to take NSAIDs with food, milk, or antacids to minimize gastric distress and to notify the physician if unable to tolerate the drug. Instruct to avoid aspirin or preparations containing aspirin while taking NSAIDs because it may interfere with activity.
- Prescribed medications, including dose, desired and possible adverse effects, and interactions with other drugs or food.
- Monitoring weight twice weekly because NSAIDs may cause fluid retention.
- Maintaining fluid intake of at least 2500 mL/day to minimize the risk of renal toxicity due to NSAID use.
- Measures to maintain activity restriction, if ordered. Activity will be gradually increased once the inflammatory process has resolved.
- Manifestations of recurrent pericarditis and the importance of reporting these manifestations promptly to the physician.

31.3 Disorders of Cardiac Structure

The Patient with Valvular Heart Disease

Proper heart valve function ensures one-way blood flow through the heart and vascular system. **Valvular heart disease** interferes with blood flow to and from the heart. Acquired valvular disorders can result from acute conditions, such as infective endocarditis, or from chronic conditions, such as rheumatic heart disease. Rheumatic heart disease is the most common cause of valvular disease (Sorenson et al., 2019) Acute myocardial infarction can also damage heart valves, causing tearing, ischemia, or damage to the papillary muscles that affects valve leaflet function. Congenital heart defects may affect the heart valves, often with no manifestations until adulthood. Aging affects heart structure and function and also increases the risk for valvular disease.

Physiology Review

The heart valves direct blood flow within and out of the heart. The valves are fibroelastic tissue supported by a ring of fibrous tissue (the annulus) that provides support.

The atrioventricular (AV) valves, the **mitral** (or *bicuspid*) **valve** on the left and the **tricuspid valve** on the right, separate the atria from the ventricles. These valves are normally fully open during diastole, allowing blood to flow freely from the atria into the ventricles. Rising pressure within the ventricles at the onset of systole (contraction) closes the AV valves, creating the S_1 heart sound ("lub"). The leaflets of the AV valves are connected to ventricular papillary muscles by fibrous *chordae tendineae*. The chordae tendineae prevent the valve leaflets from bulging back into the atria during systole.

The semilunar valves, the **aortic valve** and **pulmonic valve**, separate the ventricles from the great vessels. They open during systole, allowing blood to flow out of the heart with ventricular contraction. As the ventricle relaxes and intraventricular pressure falls at the beginning of diastole, the higher pressure within the great vessels (the aorta and pulmonary artery) closes these valves, creating the S_2 heart sound ("dub").

Pathophysiology

Valvular heart disease occurs as two major types of disorders: Stenosis and regurgitation (**Figure 31.10** ■). Stenosis occurs when valve leaflets fuse together and cannot fully open or close. The valve opening narrows and becomes rigid (Figure 31.10A). Scarring of the valves (from endocarditis or infarction) and calcium deposits can lead to stenosis. Stenotic valves impede the forward flow of blood, decreasing cardiac output because of impaired ventricular filling or ejection and stroke volume. Because stenotic valves also do not close completely, some backflow of blood occurs when the valve should be fully closed.

Regurgitant valves (called *insufficient* or *incompetent* valves) do not close completely (Figure 31.10B). This allows regurgitation, or backflow of blood, through the valve into the area it just left. Regurgitation can result from deformity or erosion of valve cusps caused by the vegetative lesions of bacterial endocarditis, by scarring or tearing from myocardial infarction, or by cardiac dilation. As the heart enlarges, the valve *annulus* (supporting ring of the valve) is stretched and the valve edges no longer meet to allow complete closure.

Valvular disease causes hemodynamic changes both in front of and behind the affected valve. Blood volume and pressures are reduced in front of the valve because flow is obstructed through a stenotic valve and backflow occurs through a regurgitant valve. By contrast, volumes and pressures characteristically increase behind the diseased valve. These hemodynamic changes may lead to pulmonary complications or heart failure. Higher pressures and compensatory changes to maintain cardiac output lead to remodeling and hypertrophy of the heart muscle.

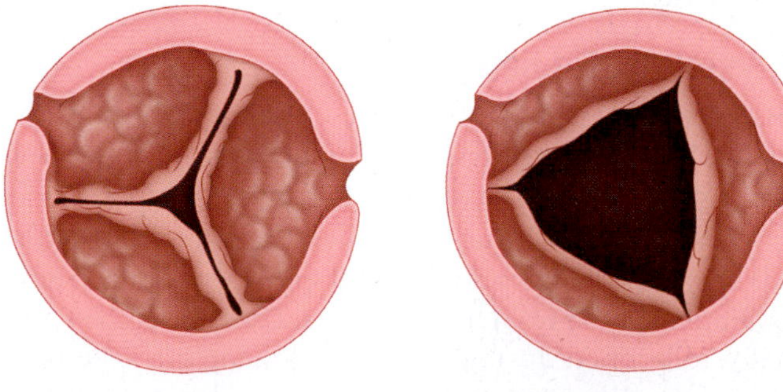
A Thickened and stenotic valve leaflets
B Retracted fibrosed valve openings

Figure 31.10 ■ Valvular heart disorders. **A**, Stenosis of a heart valve. **B**, An incompetent or regurgitant heart valve.

Stenosis increases the work of the chamber behind the affected valve as the heart attempts to move blood through the narrowed opening. Excess blood volume behind regurgitant valves causes dilation of the chamber. In mitral stenosis, for example, the left atrium hypertrophies to generate enough pressure to open and deliver its blood through the narrowed mitral valve. Not all of the blood is delivered before the valve closes, leaving blood to accumulate in the left atrium. This chamber dilates to accommodate the excess volume.

Eventually, cardiac output falls as compensatory mechanisms become less effective. The normal balance of oxygen supply and demand is upset, and the heart begins to fail. Increased muscle mass and size increase myocardial oxygen consumption. The size and workload of the heart exceed its blood supply, causing ischemia and chest pain. Eventually, necrosis occurs and functional muscle is lost. Contractile force, stroke volume, and cardiac output decrease. High pressures on the left side of the heart are reflected backward into the pulmonary system, causing pulmonary edema, pulmonary hypertension, and, eventually, right-ventricular failure.

Valvular disorders interfere with the smooth flow of blood through the heart. The flow becomes turbulent, causing a **murmur**, a characteristic manifestation of valvular disease. **Table 31.7** describes the murmurs associated with various types of valvular disorders.

Blood forced through the narrowed opening of a stenotic valve or regurgitated from a higher pressure chamber through an incompetent valve creates a jet stream effect (much like water spurting out of a partially occluded hose opening). The physical force of this jet stream damages the endocardium of the receiving chamber, increasing the risk for infective endocarditis.

The higher pressures on the left side of the heart subject its valves (the mitral and aortic valves) to more stress and damage than those on the right side of the heart (the tricuspid and pulmonic). Pulmonic valve disease is the least common of the valvular disorders.

Mitral Stenosis

Mitral stenosis narrows the mitral valve, obstructing blood flow from the left atrium into the left ventricle during diastole. It is usually caused by rheumatic heart disease or bacterial endocarditis; it rarely results from congenital defects. It affects females more frequently (66%) than males (Dima, 2018). Mitral stenosis is chronic and progressive.

In mitral valve stenosis, fibrous tissue replaces normal valve tissue, causing valve leaflets to stiffen and fuse. Resulting changes in blood flow through the valve lead to calcification of the valve leaflets. As calcium is deposited in and on the valve, the leaflets become more rigid and narrow the opening further. As the valve leaflets become less mobile, the chordae tendineae fuse, thicken, and shorten. Thromboemboli may form on the calcified leaflets.

The narrowed mitral opening impairs blood flow into the left ventricle, reducing end-diastolic volume and pressure and decreasing stroke volume. The narrowed opening

Table 31.7 Heart Murmur Timing and Characteristics

Murmur	Cardiac Cycle Timing	Auscultation Site	Configuration of Sound	Continuity
Mitral stenosis	Diastole	Apical	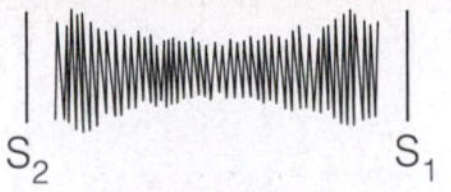 S_2 S_1	Rumble that increases in sound toward the end, continuous
Mitral regurgitation	Systole	Apex	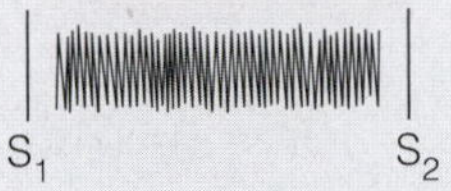 S_1 S_2	Holosystolic (occurs throughout systole), continuous
Aortic stenosis	Midsystolic	2nd intercostal space (ICS), right sternal border (RSB)	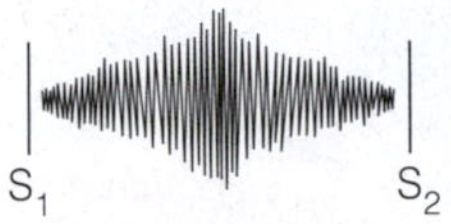 S_1 S_2	Crescendo–decrescendo, continuous
Aortic regurgitation	Diastole (early)	3rd ICS, left sternal border (LSB)	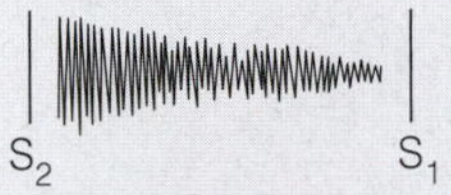 S_2 S_1	Decrescendo, continuous
Tricuspid stenosis	Diastole	Lower LSB	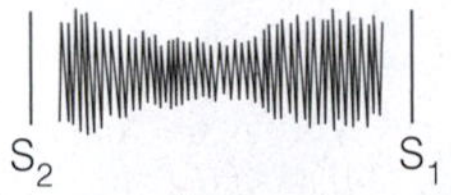 S_2 S_1	Rumble that increases in sound toward the end, continuous
Tricuspid regurgitation	Systole	4th ICS, LSB	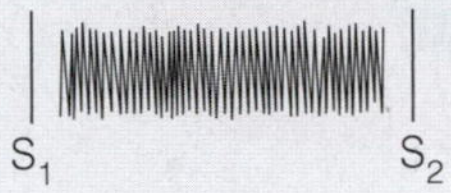 S_1 S_2	Holosystolic, continuous

also forces the left atrium to generate higher pressure to deliver blood to the left ventricle. This leads to left-atrial hypertrophy. The left atrium also dilates as obstructed blood flow increases its volume. As the resistance to blood flow increases, high atrial pressures are reflected back into the pulmonary vessels, increasing pulmonary pressures (**Figure 31.11** ■). Pulmonary hypertension increases the workload of the right ventricle, causing it to dilate and hypertrophy. Eventually, heart failure occurs.

Manifestations. Mitral stenosis may be asymptomatic or cause severe impairment. Its manifestations depend on cardiac output and pulmonary vascular pressures. Dyspnea on exertion (DOE) is typically the earliest manifestation. Others include cough, hemoptysis, frequent pulmonary infections such as bronchitis and pneumonia, paroxysmal nocturnal dyspnea, orthopnea, weakness, fatigue, and palpitations. As the stenosis worsens, manifestations of right heart failure, including jugular venous distention, hepatomegaly, ascites, and peripheral edema, develop. Crackles may be heard in the lung bases. In severe mitral stenosis, cyanosis of the face and extremities may be noted. Chest pain is rare but may occur.

On auscultation, a loud S_1, a split S_2, and a mitral opening snap may be heard. The opening snap reflects high left-atrial pressure. The murmur of mitral stenosis occurs during diastole and is typically a low-pitched, rumbling, crescendo–decrescendo sound. It is heard best with the bell of the stethoscope in the apical region. It may be accompanied by a palpable thrill (vibration).

Complications. Atrial dysrhythmias, particularly atrial fibrillation, are common due to chronic atrial distention. Thrombi may form and subsequently embolize to the brain, coronary arteries, kidneys, spleen, and extremities—potentially devastating complications.

Women with mitral stenosis may be asymptomatic until pregnancy. As the heart tries to compensate for increased circulating volume (30% more in pregnancy) by increasing cardiac output, left-atrial pressures rise, tachycardia reduces ventricular filling and stroke volume, and pulmonary pressures increase. Sudden pulmonary edema and heart failure may threaten the lives of the mother and fetus.

Mitral Regurgitation

Mitral regurgitation or *insufficiency* allows blood to flow back into the left atrium during systole because the valve does not close fully. Mitral valve prolapse, infective endocarditis, and rheumatic heart disease are common causes of mitral regurgitation (Gaasch, 2017). Degenerative calcification of the mitral annulus may cause mitral regurgitation in older women. Processes that dilate the mitral annulus or affect the supporting structures, papillary muscles, or the chordae tendineae may cause mitral regurgitation (e.g., left-ventricular hypertrophy and MI). Congenital defects may also cause mitral regurgitation.

In mitral regurgitation, blood flows into both the systemic circulation and back into the left atrium through the deformed valve during systole. This increases left-atrial volume (**Figure 31.12** ■). The left atrium dilates to accommodate its extra volume, pulling the posterior valve leaflet further away from the valve opening and worsening the defect. The left ventricle dilates to accommodate its increased preload and low cardiac output, further aggravating the problem.

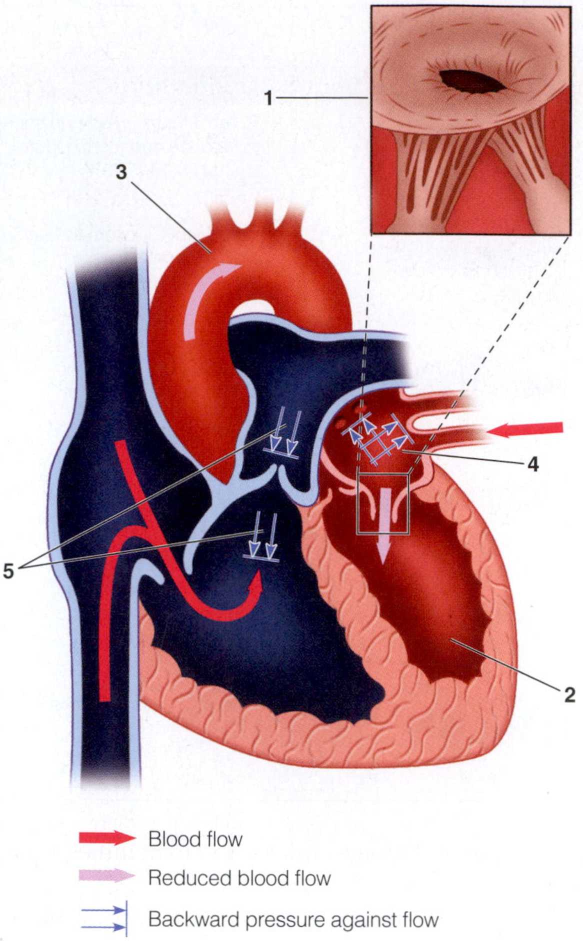
1
2
3
4
5
Blood flow
Reduced blood flow
Backward pressure against flow

Figure 31.11 ■ Mitral stenosis. Narrowing of the mitral valve orifice (1) reduces blood volume to left ventricle (2), which reduces cardiac output (3). Rising pressure in the left atrium (4) causes left-atrial hypertrophy and pulmonary congestion. Increased pressure in the pulmonary vessels (5) causes hypertrophy of the right ventricle and right atrium.

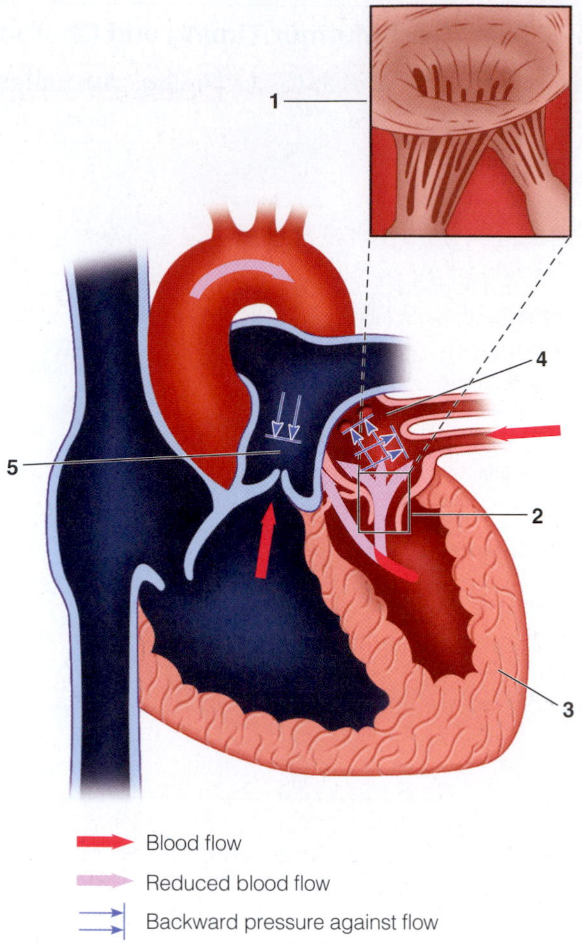
1
2
3
4
5
Blood flow
Reduced blood flow
Backward pressure against flow

Figure 31.12 ■ Mitral regurgitation. The mitral valve closes incompletely (1), allowing blood to regurgitate during systole from the left ventricle to the left atrium (2). Cardiac output falls; to compensate, the left ventricle hypertrophies (3). Rising left-atrial pressure (4) causes left-atrial hypertrophy and pulmonary congestion. Elevated pulmonary artery pressure (5) causes slight enlargement of the right ventricle.

Manifestations. Mitral regurgitation may be asymptomatic or cause symptoms such as fatigue, weakness, exertional dyspnea, and orthopnea. In severe or acute regurgitation, manifestations of left-sided heart failure develop, including pulmonary congestion and edema. High pulmonary pressures may lead to manifestations of right-sided heart failure.

The murmur of mitral regurgitation is usually loud, high pitched, rumbling, and holosystolic (occurring throughout systole). It is often accompanied by a palpable thrill and is heard most clearly at the cardiac apex. It may be characterized as a cooing or gull-like sound or as having a musical quality.

Mitral Valve Prolapse

Mitral valve prolapse (MVP) is a type of mitral insufficiency that occurs when one or both mitral valve cusps billow into the atrium during ventricular systole (Jelani, 2016). Its cause is often unclear. It also can result from acute or chronic rheumatic damage, ischemic heart disease, or other cardiac disorders. It commonly affects people with inherited connective tissue disorders such as Marfan syndrome

Genetic Considerations

Patients with Marfan Syndrome

Marfan syndrome is a genetic (autosomal dominant) connective tissue disorder that affects the skeleton, eyes, and cardiovascular system. Skeletal characteristics include a long, thin body, with long extremities and long, tapering fingers, sometimes called *arachnodactyly* (spider fingers). Joints are hyperextensible, and skeletal deformities such as kyphosis, scoliosis, pigeon chest, or pectus excavatum are common. The potentially life-threatening cardiovascular effects of Marfan syndrome include mitral valve prolapse, progressive dilation of the aortic valve ring, and weakness of arterial walls. People with Marfan syndrome may die young, between the ages of 30 and 40, often due to dissection and rupture of the aorta, but the majority survive into mid- to late adulthood (Genetics Home Reference, 2018).

(see the Genetic Considerations box). Mitral valve prolapse is usually benign, but about 0.01 to 0.02% of people with MVP have thickened mitral leaflets and a significant risk of morbidity and sudden death.

Excess collagen tissue in the valve leaflets and elongated chordae tendineae impair closure of the mitral valve, allowing the leaflets to billow into the left atrium during systole. Some ventricular blood volume regurgitates into the left atrium (**Figure 31.13** ■).

Manifestations and Complications. Mitral valve prolapse is usually asymptomatic. A midsystolic ejection click or murmur may be audible. A high-pitched late systolic murmur, sometimes described as a "whoop" or "honk," due to the regurgitation of blood through the valve, may develop in MVP. Atypical chest pain is the most common symptom of MVP. It may be left-sided or substernal and is frequently related to fatigue, not exertion. Tachydysrhythmias may develop with MVP, causing palpitations, lightheadedness, and syncope. Increased sympathetic nervous system tone may cause a sense of anxiety.

Mitral valve prolapse increases the risk for bacterial endocarditis. Progressive worsening of regurgitation can lead to heart failure. Thrombi may form on prolapsed valve leaflets; embolization may cause transient ischemic attacks (TIAs).

Aortic Stenosis

Aortic stenosis obstructs blood flow from the left ventricle into the aorta during systole. Aortic stenosis may be idiopathic or due to a congenital defect, rheumatic damage, or degenerative changes (Mayo Clinic, 2018). When rheumatic heart disease is the cause, mitral valve deformity is often also present. Rheumatic heart disease destroys aortic valve leaflets, with fibrosis and calcification causing rigidity and scarring. In the older adult, calcific aortic stenosis may result from degenerative changes associated with aging. Constant wear and tear on this valve can lead to fibrosis and calcification. Idiopathic calcific stenosis is generally mild and does not impair cardiac output.

As aortic stenosis progresses, the valve annulus decreases in size, increasing the work of the left ventricle to eject its volume through the narrowed opening into the aorta. To compensate, the ventricle hypertrophies to maintain an adequate stroke volume and cardiac output (**Figure 31.14** ■).

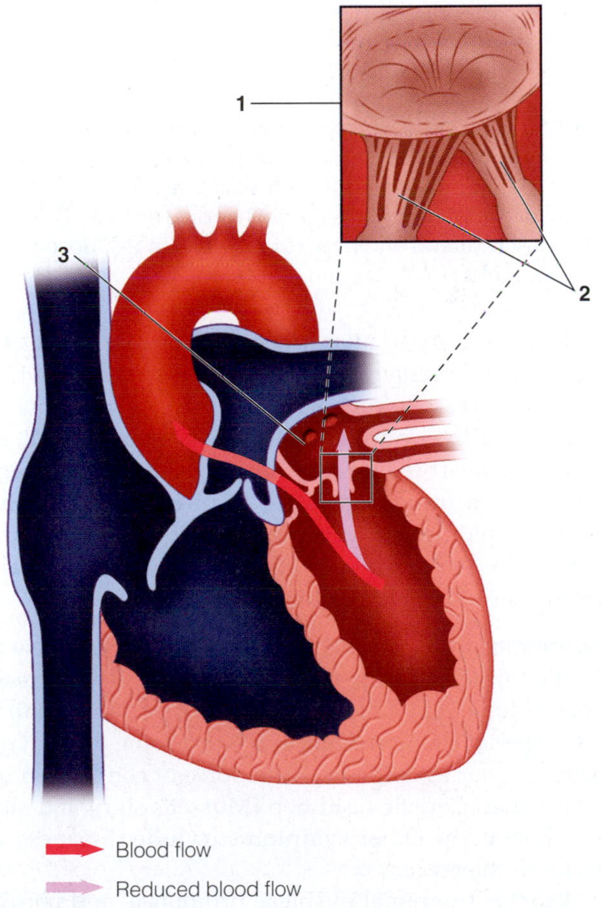
1
2
3
Blood flow
Reduced blood flow

Figure 31.13 ■ Mitral valve prolapse. Excess tissue in the valve leaflets (1) and elongated cordae tendineae (2) impair mitral valve closure during systole. Some ventricular blood regurgitates into the left atrium (3).

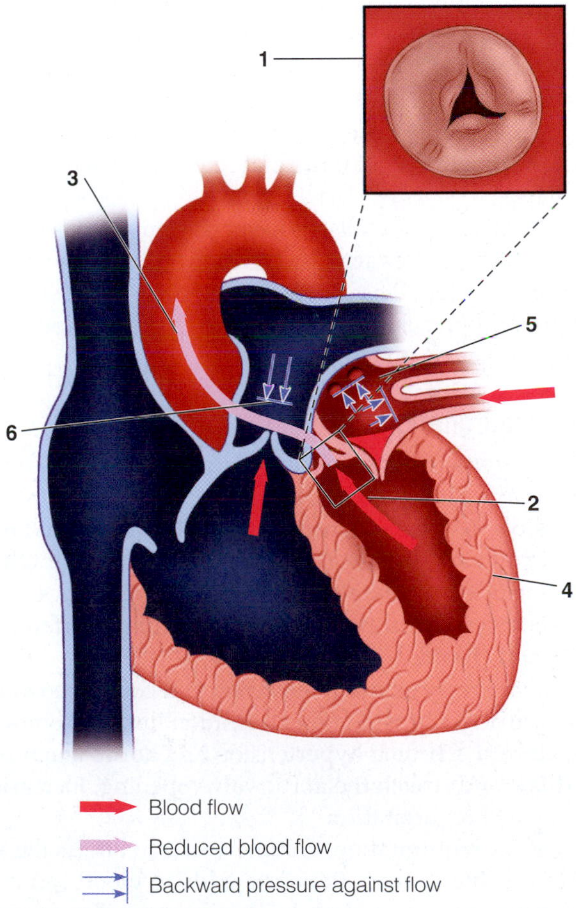
1
2
3
4
5
6
Blood flow
Reduced blood flow
Backward pressure against flow

Figure 31.14 ■ Aortic stenosis. The narrowed aortic valve orifice (1) decreases the left-ventricular ejection fraction during systole (2) and cardiac output (3). The left ventricle hypertrophies (4). Incomplete emptying of the left atrium (5) causes backward pressure through pulmonary veins and pulmonary hypertension. Elevated pulmonary artery pressure (6) causes right-ventricular strain.

Left-ventricular compliance also decreases. The additional workload increases myocardial oxygen consumption, which can precipitate myocardial ischemia. Coronary blood flow may also decrease in aortic stenosis. As left-ventricular end-diastolic pressure increases because of reduced stroke volume, left-atrial pressures increase. These pressures also affect the pulmonary vascular system; pulmonary vascular congestion and pulmonary edema may result.

Course and Manifestations. Aortic stenosis may be asymptomatic for many years. As the disease progresses and compensation fails, usually between ages 50 and 70, obstructed cardiac output causes manifestations of left-ventricular failure. Dyspnea on exertion, angina pectoris, and exertional syncope are classic manifestations of aortic stenosis. Pulse pressure, an indicator of stroke volume, narrows to 30 mmHg or less. Hemodynamic monitors show increased left-atrial pressure and pulmonary artery wedge pressure, as well as decreased stroke volume and cardiac output.

Aortic stenosis produces a harsh systolic murmur best heard in the second intercostal space to the right of the sternum. This crescendo–decrescendo murmur is produced by turbulence of blood entering the aorta through the stenotic valve. A palpable thrill is often felt. The murmur may radiate to the carotid arteries. Ventricular hypertrophy displaces the cardiac impulse to the left of the midclavicular line. As aortic stenosis progresses, S_3 and S_4 heart sounds may be heard, indicating heart failure and reduced left-ventricular compliance.

As cardiac output falls, tissue perfusion decreases. Late in the disease, pulmonary hypertension and right-ventricular failure develop. Untreated, symptomatic aortic stenosis has a poor prognosis; 10 to 20% of these patients experience sudden cardiac death.

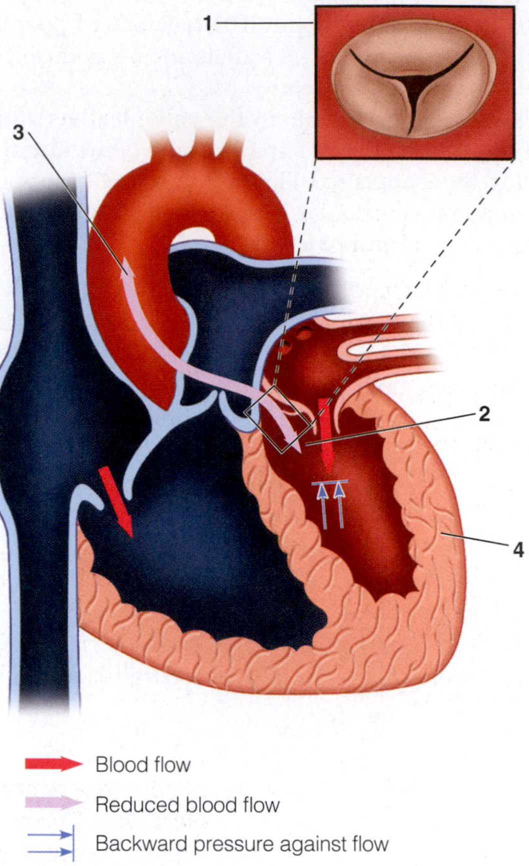
1
2
3
4
Blood flow
Reduced blood flow
Backward pressure against flow

Figure 31.15 ■ Aortic regurgitation. The cusps of the aortic valve widen and fail to close during diastole (1). Blood regurgitates from the aorta into the left ventricle (2), increasing left-ventricular volume and decreasing cardiac output (3). The left ventricle dilates and hypertrophies (4) in response to the increase in blood volume and workload.

Aortic Regurgitation

Aortic regurgitation, also called *aortic insufficiency*, allows blood to flow back into the left ventricle from the aorta during diastole. Most aortic regurgitation (67%) results from rheumatic heart disease (Nishimura et al., 2017). Other causes include congenital disorders, infective endocarditis, blunt chest trauma, aortic aneurysm, syphilis, Marfan syndrome, and chronic hypertension.

In aortic regurgitation, thickened and contracted valve cusps, scarring, fibrosis, and calcification impede complete valve closure. Chronic hypertension and aortic aneurysm may dilate and stretch the aortic valve opening, increasing the degree of regurgitation.

In aortic regurgitation, volume overload affects the left ventricle as blood from the aorta adds to blood received from the atrium during diastole. This increases diastolic left-ventricular pressure. Increased preload causes more forceful contractions and a high stroke volume (**Figure 31.15** ■). With time, muscle cells hypertrophy to compensate for increased cardiac workload and afterload; eventually this hypertrophy compromises cardiac output and increases regurgitation.

High left-ventricular pressures increase left atrial workload and pressure. This pressure is transmitted to the pulmonary vessels, causing pulmonary congestion. The workload of the right ventricle increases as a result, and right-sided heart failure may develop. Acute aortic regurgitation from traumatic injury or infective endocarditis causes a rapid decline in hemodynamic status from acute heart failure and pulmonary edema because compensatory mechanisms do not have time to develop.

Manifestations. Aortic regurgitation may be asymptomatic for many years, even when severe. The increased stroke volume may cause complaints of persistent palpitations, especially when recumbent. A throbbing pulse may be visible in arteries of the neck; the force of contraction may cause a characteristic head bob (Musset's sign) and shake the whole body. Other symptoms include dizziness and exercise intolerance.

Fatigue, exertional dyspnea, orthopnea, and paroxysmal nocturnal dyspnea are common in aortic regurgitation. Anginal pain may result from excessive cardiac workload and decreased coronary perfusion. Unlike CAD, angina often occurs at night and may not respond to conventional therapy.

The murmur of aortic regurgitation is heard during diastole as blood flows back into the left ventricle from the aorta. It is described as a blowing, high-pitched sound heard most clearly at the third left intercostal space. A palpable thrill and ventricular heave may be noted. An S_3 and S_4 may be heard as the heart fails and ventricular compliance diminishes. The apical impulse is displaced to the left.

High systolic and low diastolic pressures cause a widened pulse pressure. The arterial pressure waveform has a rapid upstroke and quickly collapsing downstroke, known as a *water-hammer pulse*. It is caused by the force of rapid and early delivery of the stroke volume into the aorta.

Tricuspid Valve Disorders

Tricuspid stenosis obstructs blood flow from the right atrium to the right ventricle. It usually results from rheumatic heart disease; mitral stenosis often occurs concurrently with tricuspid stenosis.

Fibrosed, retracted tricuspid valve cusps and fused leaflets narrow the valve orifice and prevent complete closure. Right-ventricular filling is impaired during diastole, and during systole, some blood regurgitates back into the right atrium. Pressure in the right atrium increases, and it enlarges in response to the increased pressure and workload. This increased right-atrial pressure is reflected backward into the systemic circulation. Right-ventricular stroke volume decreases, reducing the volume delivered to the pulmonary system and left heart. Stroke volume, cardiac output, and tissue perfusion fall.

Manifestations of tricuspid stenosis relate to systemic congestion and right-sided heart failure. They include increased central venous pressure, jugular venous distention, ascites, hepatomegaly, and peripheral edema. Low cardiac output causes fatigue and weakness. The low-pitched, rumbling diastolic murmur of tricuspid stenosis is most clearly heard in the fourth intercostal space at the left sternal border or over the xiphoid process.

Tricuspid regurgitation usually occurs secondarily to right-ventricular dilation. Stretching distorts the valve and its supporting structures, preventing complete valve closure. Left-ventricular failure is the usual cause of right-ventricular overload; pulmonary hypertension is another cause. The valve may be damaged by rheumatic heart disease, infective endocarditis, inferior MI, trauma, or other conditions.

Tricuspid regurgitation allows blood to flow back into the right atrium during systole, increasing right-atrial pressure. Increased right-atrial pressure causes manifestations of right-sided heart failure, including systemic venous congestion and low cardiac output. Atrial fibrillation due to atrial distention is common. The retrograde flow of blood over the deformed tricuspid valve causes a high-pitched, blowing systolic murmur heard over the tricuspid or xiphoid area.

Pulmonic Valve Disorders

Pulmonic stenosis obstructs blood flow from the right ventricle into the pulmonary system. It usually is a congenital disorder, although rheumatic heart disease or cancer may also cause pulmonic stenosis. The right ventricle hypertrophies to generate the pressure needed to pump blood into the pulmonary system. The right atrium also hypertrophies to overcome the high pressures generated in the right ventricle. Right-sided heart failure occurs when the ventricle can no longer generate adequate pressure to force blood past the narrowed valve opening.

Pulmonic stenosis is typically asymptomatic unless severe. Dyspnea on exertion and fatigue are early signs. As the condition progresses, right-sided heart failure develops, with peripheral edema, ascites, hepatomegaly, and increased venous pressures. Turbulent blood flow caused by the narrowed valve generates a harsh, systolic crescendo–decrescendo murmur heard in the pulmonic area, the second left intercostal space.

Pulmonic regurgitation is more common than pulmonary stenosis. It is a complication of pulmonary hypertension, which stretches and dilates the pulmonary orifice, causing incomplete valve closure. Infective endocarditis, pulmonary artery aneurysm, and syphilis may also cause pulmonic regurgitation.

Incomplete valve closure allows blood to flow back into the right ventricle during diastole, decreasing blood flow to the pulmonary circuit. The extra blood increases right-ventricular end-diastolic volume. When the ventricle can no longer compensate for the increased volume, right-sided heart failure develops. The murmur of pulmonic regurgitation is a high-pitched, decrescendo, blowing sound heard along the left sternal border during diastole.

Interprofessional Care

A heart murmur identified during routine physical examination often is the initial indication of valvular disease. If no symptoms are present, close observation for disease progression and prophylactic therapy to prevent infection of the diseased heart may be the only treatment.

Manifestations of heart failure are treated with diet and medications. When medical management is no longer effective, surgery is considered.

Diagnosis

The following diagnostic tests help to identify and diagnose valvular disease. See Chapter 30 for more information about these tests and related nursing care.

- *Echocardiography* is used routinely to diagnose valvular disease. Thickened valve leaflets, vegetations or growths on valve leaflets, myocardial function, and chamber size can be determined, and pressure gradients across valves and pulmonary artery pressures can be estimated. Either transthoracic or transesophageal echocardiography may be used.
- *Chest x-ray* can identify cardiac hypertrophy, chamber and great vessel enlargement, and dilation of the pulmonary vasculature. Calcification of the valve leaflets and annular openings may also be visible.
- *Electrocardiography* can demonstrate atrial and ventricular hypertrophy, conduction defects, and dysrhythmias associated with valvular disease.
- *Cardiac catheterization* may be used to assess contractility and to determine the pressure gradients across the

heart valves, in the heart chambers, and in the pulmonary system. It is used prevalvular surgery to assess CAD risk.

- *Exercise testing* should be used only with asymptomatic patients to assess for exercise-induced symptoms and abnormal blood pressure response. It is contraindicated for symptomatic aortic stenosis patients.

Medications

Heart failure resulting from valvular disease is treated with diuretics, ACE inhibitors, vasodilators, and possibly digitalis glycosides. Digitalis increases the force of myocardial contraction to maintain cardiac output. Diuretics, ACE inhibitors, and vasodilators reduce preload and afterload. (See Medication Administration 31.A.)

In patients with valvular disorders, atrial distention often causes atrial fibrillation. Digitalis or small doses of beta-blockers are given to slow the ventricular response (see Chapter 32 for information about atrial fibrillation and its treatment). Anticoagulant therapy is added to prevent clot and embolus formation, a common complication of atrial fibrillation as blood pools in the noncontracting atria. Anticoagulant therapy is also required following insertion of a mechanical heart valve. See Chapter 33 for information about anticoagulant therapy.

Valvular damage increases the risk for infective endocarditis as altered blood flow allows bacterial colonization. Antibiotics are prescribed prophylactically prior to any dental work, invasive procedures, or surgery to minimize the risk of bacteremia (bacteria in the blood) and subsequent endocarditis.

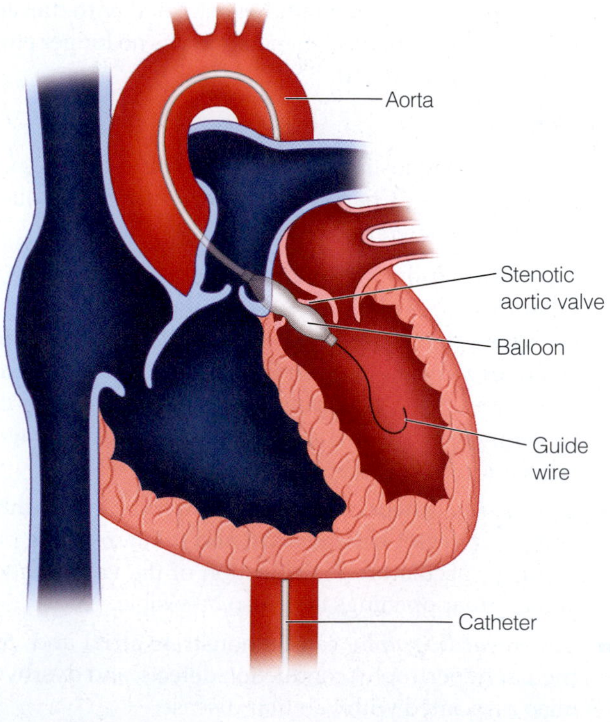
Aorta
Stenotic aortic valve
Balloon
Guide wire
Catheter

Figure 31.16 ■ Balloon valvotomy. The balloon catheter is guided into position straddling the stenosed valve. The balloon is then inflated to increase the size of the valve opening.

Percutaneous Balloon Valvotomy

A *percutaneous balloon valvotomy* is an invasive procedure performed in the cardiac catheterization laboratory. A balloon catheter similar to that used in coronary angioplasty procedures is inserted into the femoral vein or artery. Guided by fluoroscopy, the catheter is advanced into the heart and positioned with the balloon straddling the stenotic valve. The balloon is then inflated for approximately 90 seconds to divide the fused leaflets and enlarge the valve orifice (**Figure 31.16** ■). Balloon valvotomy is the treatment of choice for symptomatic mitral valve stenosis. It is used to treat children and young adults with aortic stenosis and may be indicated for older adults who are poor surgical risks and as a "bridge to surgery" when heart function is severely compromised. Nursing care of the patient with a balloon valvotomy is similar to that of the patient following coronary revascularization (refer to Chapter 30).

Surgery

Surgery to repair or replace the diseased valve may be done to restore valve function, alleviate symptoms, and prevent complications and death. Ideally, diseased valves are repaired or replaced before cardiopulmonary function is severely compromised. The diseased valve is repaired when possible because the risk for surgical mortality and complications is lower than with valve replacement.

Reconstructive Surgery. *Valvuloplasty* is a general term for reconstruction or repair of a heart valve. Methods include patching the perforated portion of the leaflet, resecting excess tissue, debriding vegetations or calcifications, and other techniques. Valvuloplasty may be used for stenotic or regurgitant mitral and tricuspid valves, mitral valve prolapse, and aortic stenosis. Common valvuloplasty procedures include:

- *Open commissurotomy*, surgical division of fused valve leaflets, is done to open stenotic valves. Fused commissures (junctions between valve leaflets or cusps) are incised, and calcium deposits are debrided as needed.
- *Annuloplasty* repairs a narrowed or an enlarged or dilated valve annulus, the supporting ring of the valve. A prosthetic ring may be used to resize the opening, or stitches and purse-string sutures may be used to reduce and gather excess tissue. Annuloplasty may be used for either stenotic or regurgitant valves.

Valve Replacement. Valve replacement is indicated when manifestations of valve dysfunction develop, preferably before left heart function is seriously impaired. In general, three factors determine the outcome of valve replacement surgery: (1) Heart function at the time of surgery, (2) intraoperative and postoperative care, and (3) characteristics and durability of the replacement valve.

Many different prosthetic heart valves are available, including mechanical and biologic tissue valves. Selection depends on the valve hemodynamics, resistance to clot formation, ease of insertion, anatomic suitability, and patient acceptance. The patient's age, underlying condition, and

Table 31.8 Advantages and Disadvantages of Prosthetic Heart Valves

Category	Types	Advantages	Disadvantages
Mechanical valves	Ball and cage Tilting disk	Long-term durability Good hemodynamics	Lifetime anticoagulation Audible click Risk of thromboembolism Infections are harder to treat
Biologic tissue valves	Porcine heterograft Bovine heterograft Human aortic homograft	Low incidence of thromboembolism No long-term anticoagulation Good hemodynamics Quiet Infections are easier to treat	Prone to deterioration Frequent replacement is required

contraindications to anticoagulation (such as a desire to become pregnant) are also considered in selecting the appropriate prosthesis. **Table 31.8** lists the advantages and disadvantages of biologic and mechanical valves.

Biologic tissue valves may be *heterografts*, excised from a pig or made of calf pericardium, or *homografts* from a human (obtained from a cadaver or during heart transplant). Biologic valves allow more normal blood flow and have a low risk of thrombus formation. As a result, long-term anticoagulation is rarely necessary. They are less durable, however, than mechanical valves. Up to 50% of biologic valves must be replaced by 15 years.

Mechanical prosthetic valves have the major advantage of long-term durability. These valves are frequently used when life expectancy exceeds 10 years. Their major disadvantage is the need for lifetime anticoagulation to prevent the development of clots on the valve.

Most mechanical valves have either a tilting disk or a ball-and-cage design. The tilting-disk valve designs are frequently used because they have a lower profile than the ball-and-cage types, allowing blood to flow through the valve with less obstruction (**Figure 31.17** ■). The St. Jude bileaflet design has good hemodynamics and low risk for clot formation. Both biologic and mechanical valves increase the risk of endocarditis, although its incidence is fairly low.

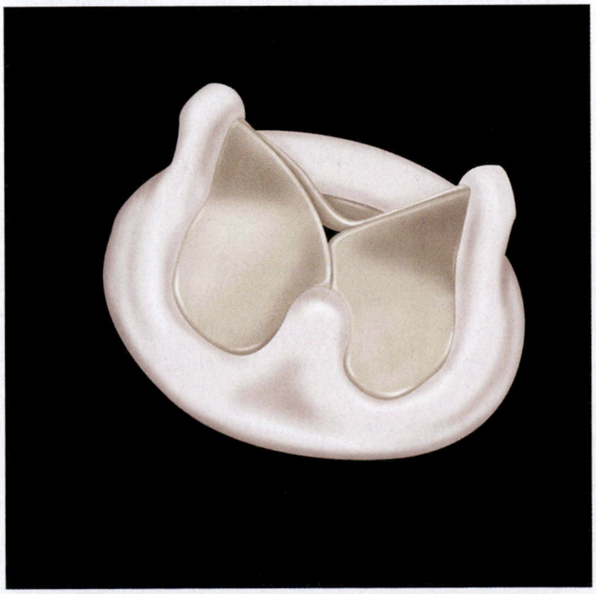

Figure 31.17 ■ Prosthetic heart valve, porcine valve.

Nursing Care

Assessment

See the Manifestations and Interprofessional Care sections for the assessment of the patient with valvular heart disease.

Assessment data related to valvular heart disease includes:

- *Health history:* Complaints of decreasing exercise tolerance, dyspnea on exertion, palpitations; history of frequent respiratory infections; previous history of rheumatic heart disease, endocarditis, or a heart murmur
- *Physical assessment:* Vital signs; skin color and temperature, evidence of clubbing or peripheral edema; neck vein distention; breath sounds; heart sounds and presence of S_3, S_4, or murmur; timing, grade, and characteristics of any murmur; palpate for cardiac heave and thrills; abdominal contour, liver, and spleen size.

Priorities of Care

Collaborating with the interprofessional team to ensure adequate treatment of the underlying process while providing care that supports the physical and psychologic responses to the disorder is a priority of nursing care.

Diagnoses, Outcomes, and Interventions

Nursing priorities include maintaining cardiac output, managing manifestations of the disorder, teaching about the disease process and its management, and preventing complications. Nursing care of the patient undergoing valve surgery is similar to that of the patient having other types of open-heart surgery (refer to Chapter 30), with increased attention to anticoagulation and preventing endocarditis.

Monitor Cardiac Output. Nearly all valve disorders affect ventricular filling and/or emptying, reducing cardiac output. Stenosis of the AV valves impairs ventricular filling and increases atrial pressures. Regurgitation of these valves reduces cardiac output as a portion of the blood in the ventricle regurgitates into the atria during systole. Stenosis of the semilunar valves obstructs ventricular outflow to the great vessels; regurgitation allows blood to flow back into the ventricles, creating higher filling pressures. When compensatory measures fail, heart failure develops.

Expected Outcome: Patient will demonstrate adequate cardiac output as evidenced by blood pressure and pulse rate and rhythm within normal limits.

The nurse will:

- Monitor vital signs and hemodynamic parameters, reporting changes from the baseline. *A fall in systolic blood pressure and tachycardia may indicate decreased cardiac output. Increasing pulmonary artery and pulmonary wedge pressures may also indicate decreased cardiac output, causing increased congestion and pressure in the pulmonary vascular system.*

SAFETY ALERT: Promptly report changes in level of consciousness; distended neck veins; dyspnea or respiratory crackles; urine output < 30 mL/h; cool, clammy, or cyanotic skin; diminished peripheral pulses; or slow capillary refill. These findings indicate decreased cardiac output and impaired tissue and organ perfusion. ■

- Monitor intake and output; weigh daily. Report weight gain of 1.4 to 2.3 kg (3 to 5 lb) within 24 hours. *Fluid retention is a compensatory mechanism that occurs when cardiac output decreases; 1 kg (2.2 lb) of weight equals 1 L of fluid.*
- Restrict fluids as ordered. *Fluid intake may be restricted to reduce cardiac workload and pressures within the heart and pulmonary circuit.*
- Monitor oxygen saturation continuously and ABGs as ordered. Report oxygen saturation $< 95\%$ (or as specified) and abnormal ABG results. *Oxygen saturation levels and ABGs allow assessment of oxygenation.*
- Elevate the head of the bed. Administer supplemental oxygen as ordered. *These measures improve alveolar ventilation and oxygenation.*
- Provide for physical, emotional, and mental rest. *Physical and psychologic rest decreases the cardiac workload.*
- Administer prescribed medications as ordered to reduce cardiac workload. *Diuretics, ACE inhibitors, and direct vasodilators may be prescribed to reduce fluid volume and afterload, reducing cardiac workload.*

Promote Activity Tolerance. Altered blood flow through the heart impairs delivery of oxygen and nutrients to the tissues. As the heart muscle fails and is unable to compensate for altered blood flow, tissue perfusion is further compromised. Dyspnea on exertion is often an early symptom of valvular disease.

Expected Outcome: Patient will participate in physical activity as tolerated.

The nurse will:

- Monitor vital signs before and during activities. *A change in heart rate of $>$ 20 bpm, a change of 20 mmHg or more in systolic BP, and complaints of dyspnea, shortness of breath, excessive fatigue, chest pain, diaphoresis, dizziness, or syncope may indicate activity intolerance.*
- Encourage self-care and gradually increasing activities as allowed and tolerated. Provide for rest periods, uninterrupted sleep, and adequate nutritional intake. *Gradual progression of activities avoids excessive cardiac stress. Encouraging self-care increases the patient's self-esteem and sense of power. Adequate rest and nutrition facilitate healing, decrease fatigue, and increase energy reserves.*
- Provide assistance as needed. Suggest use of a shower chair, sitting while brushing hair or teeth, and other energy-saving measures. *Reducing energy expenditure helps maintain a balance of oxygen supply and demand.*
- Consult with a cardiac rehabilitation specialist or physical therapist for in-bed exercises and an activity plan. *In-bed exercises may help improve strength.*
- Discuss ways to conserve energy at home. *Information provides practical ways to deal with activity limitations and empowers the patient to manage these limitations.*

Reduce Risk for Infection. Damaged and deformed valve leaflets and turbulent blood flow through the heart significantly increase the risk of infective endocarditis. Invasive diagnostic and monitoring lines (e.g., cardiac catheterization, hemodynamic monitoring) and disrupted skin with surgery also increase the risk of infection.

Expected Outcome: The patient will exhibit effective infection management as evidenced by skin integrity and body temperature within normal range.

The nurse will:

- Use aseptic technique for all invasive procedures. *Invasive procedures breach the body's protective mechanisms, potentially allowing bacteria to enter. Aseptic technique reduces this risk.*
- Record temperature every 4 hours; notify physician if temperature exceeds 38.5°C (100.5°F). *Fever may be an early indication of infection.*
- Assess wounds and catheter sites for redness, swelling, warmth, pain, or evidence of drainage. *These signs of inflammation may signal infection.*
- Administer antibiotics as ordered. Ensure completion of the full course. *Antibiotics are used to prevent and treat infection. Completion of the full course of therapy prevents drug-resistant organisms from multiplying.*
- Monitor WBC and differential. Notify physician of leukocytosis or leukopenia. *A high WBC and increased percentage of immature WBCs (bands) may indicate bacterial infection; a low WBC count may indicate an impaired immune response and increased susceptibility to infection.*

Prevent Bleeding. Anticoagulant therapy is commonly prescribed for patients with chronic atrial fibrillation, a history of emboli, and following valve replacement surgery. Although chronic anticoagulant therapy decreases the risk of clots and emboli, it increases the risk for bleeding and hemorrhage.

Expected Outcome: Patient will remain free of any evidence of new bleeding and take precautions to prevent bleeding.

SAFETY ALERT: Monitor the international normalized ratio (INR) or prothrombin time (PT or protime). Report an INR $>$ 3.5 or a PT $>$ 2.5 times the normal to the physician. An excessively high INR or PT indicates excessive anticoagulation and an increased risk for bleeding. ■

The nurse will:

- Test stools and vomitus for occult blood. *Bleeding due to excessive anticoagulation may not be apparent.*
- Instruct to avoid using aspirin or other NSAIDs. Encourage reading ingredient labels on over-the-counter drugs; many contain aspirin. *Aspirin and other NSAIDs interfere with clotting and may potentiate the effects of the anticoagulant therapy.*
- Advise using a soft-bristled toothbrush, electric razor, and gentle touch when cleaning fragile skin. *These measures decrease the risk of skin or gum trauma and bleeding.*

SAFETY ALERT: Monitor hemoglobin, hematocrit, and platelet count as ordered. Notify the physician of decreasing hemoglobin and hematocrit levels or if the platelet count falls below 50,000/mm^3. Low hemoglobin and hematocrit indicate blood loss. Platelet counts below 50,000/mm^3 significantly increase the risk of bleeding. ■

Delegating Nursing Care Activities

As appropriate and allowed by the designated duties and responsibilities of unlicensed assistive personnel, the nurse may delegate nursing care activities such as measuring fluid intake and output, collecting vital signs (including orthostatic vital signs), encouraging oral or enteral fluid intake, and ensuring nonpharmacologic skin care.

Transitions of Care

Preventing rheumatic heart disease is a key element in preventing heart valve disorders. Rheumatic heart disease is a consequence of rheumatic fever (see the previous section of this chapter), an immune process that may be a sequela to beta-hemolytic streptococcal infection of the pharynx (strep throat). Early treatment of strep throat prevents rheumatic fever. Teach individual patients, families, and communities about the importance of timely and effective treatment of strep throat. Emphasize the importance of completing the full prescription of antibiotics to prevent development of resistant bacteria. Prophylactic antibiotic therapy before invasive procedures to prevent infectious endocarditis is an important health promotion measure for patients with preexisting heart disease.

Careful evaluation of valvular disease is necessary to determine the best treatment. Physical examination, echocardiography, and other diagnostic tests are used to clarify the anatomic issues and to determine the type and severity of valvular disease. Surgical valve repair/replacement is commonly indicated in severe disease. Nursing care is the same as other cardiac surgery. See the accompanying Case Study & Nursing Care Plan for additional nursing care and teaching for a patient with mitral valve prolapse.

For most patients, valvular disease is a chronic condition. The patient has primary responsibility for managing the effects of the disorder. To prepare the patient and family for home care, discuss the following topics:

- Management of symptoms, including any necessary activity restrictions or lifestyle changes
- The importance of adequate rest to prevent fatigue
- Diet restrictions to reduce fluid retention and symptoms of heart failure
- Information about prescribed medications, including purpose, desired and possible adverse effects, scheduling, and possible interactions with other drugs
- The importance of keeping follow-up appointments to monitor the disease and its treatment
- Notifying all healthcare providers about valve disease or surgery to facilitate prescription of prophylactic antibiotics before invasive procedures or dental work
- Manifestations to immediately report to the healthcare provider: Increasing severity of symptoms, especially of worsening heart failure or pulmonary edema; signs of transient ischemic attacks or other embolic events; evidence of bleeding, such as joint pain, easy bruising, black and tarry stools, bleeding gums, or blood in the urine or sputum.

Provide referrals to community resources such as home maintenance services, home health services, and structured cardiac rehabilitation programs. Refer the patient and family (especially the primary food preparer) to a dietitian or nutritionist for teaching and assistance with menu planning. See the accompanying Case Study & Nursing Care Plan for additional nursing care and teaching for a patient with mitral valve prolapse.

Patients with severe valvular disease may advance to requiring end-of-life care if surgery or other interventions are not indicated. The goals of palliative care in the patient with severe valve disease would include:

- Promotion of quality of life
- Symptom management (dyspnea, fatigue, chest pain)
- Management of nonvalvular comorbidities
- Provision of psychosocial and spiritual support
- Communication regarding the prognosis and outcomes with the patient and family
- Prioritize care to meet patient values, goals, and preferences.

The Patient with Cardiomyopathy

Cardiomyopathies are disorders that affect the heart muscle itself. They are a diverse group of disorders that affect both systolic and diastolic functions. Cardiomyopathies may be either primary or secondary in origin. Primary cardiomyopathies are idiopathic; their cause is unknown. Secondary cardiomyopathies occur as a result of other processes, such as ischemia, infectious disease, exposure to toxins, connective tissue disorders, metabolic disorders, or nutritional deficiencies. In many cases, the cause of cardiomyopathy is unknown. Close to 24,000 deaths annually are directly attributed to cardiomyopathy. Mortality associated with cardiomyopathy is higher in older adults, men, and African Americans (Benjamin et al., 2017).

Case Study & Nursing Care Plan

A Patient with Mitral Valve Prolapse

Julie Snow, a 22-year-old college student, sees a nurse practitioner at the college health clinic for a physical examination after experiencing palpitations, fatigue, and a headache during midterm examinations. Ms. Snow tells Lakisha Johnson, FNP, "I'm scared that something is wrong with me."

During the past few months, Ms. Snow has had occasional palpitations that she describes as "feeling like my heart is doing flip-flops." Rarely, these palpitations have been accompanied by a sharp, stabbing pain in her chest that lasts only a few seconds. She initially attributed her symptoms to stress, but she is increasingly concerned because the "attacks" are becoming more frequent. Ms. Snow states that she has "always been healthy," does not smoke, uses alcohol socially, and exercises, albeit intermittently. Ms. Snow admits that she has been drinking a lot of coffee and cola and eating a lot of junk food lately.

ASSESSMENT

Ms. Johnson's assessment of Ms. Snow documents the following: Height 168 cm (66 in.), weight 63.6 kg (140 lb), T 37.4°C (99.3°F), BP 118/64 mmHg, P 82 bpm, and R 18/min. Slightly anxious but in no acute distress. Systolic click and soft crescendo murmur grade II/VI noted on auscultation. Apical impulse at 5th ICS left MCL. Lungs clear to auscultation. Review of remaining systems reveals no apparent abnormalities. An ECG shows sinus rhythm with occasional PACs. Based on the admission history, manifestations, and physical assessment, Ms. Johnson suspects mitral valve prolapse (MVP).

DIAGNOSES

- Anxiety related to fear of heart disease and implications for lifestyle
- Feeling powerless due to unpredictability of symptoms
- Potential for infection related to altered valve function

EXPECTED OUTCOMES

- Patient will verbalize an understanding of MVP and its management.
- Patient will discuss ways to decrease or relieve MVP symptoms.
- Patient will acknowledge the risk for endocarditis and identify precautions to prevent it.

PLANNING AND IMPLEMENTATION

- Consult with and refer to the cardiologist for continued monitoring and follow-up.
- Teach about MVP, including heart valve anatomy, physiology, and function, common manifestations of MVP, and treatment rationale.
- Discuss symptoms of progressive mitral regurgitation and the need to report these to the cardiologist.
- Discuss recommended follow-up care and its rationale.
- Allow to verbalize feelings and share concerns about MVP. Encourage to attend an MVP support group meeting.
- Discuss the prognosis for MVP, emphasizing that most patients live normal lives using diet and lifestyle management.
- Instruct to keep a weekly record of symptoms and their frequency for 1 month.
- Discuss lifestyle changes to manage symptoms: Aerobic exercise with warm-up and cool-down periods; maintaining adequate fluid intake, especially during hot weather or exercise; relaxation techniques (e.g., meditation, deep-breathing exercises, music therapy, yoga, guided imagery, heat therapy, or progressive muscle relaxation) to perform daily; avoiding caffeine and crash diets; forming healthy eating habits.
- Teach about infective endocarditis risk and prevention with prophylactic antibiotics. Encourage notifying dentist and other healthcare providers of MVP before dental or any other invasive procedures.

EVALUATION

After several educational sessions at the college health clinic, Ms. Snow verbalizes an understanding of MVP by explaining heart valve function, listing common manifestations of MVP, and describing indications of deteriorating heart function. She states she will report these manifestations to her cardiologist if they occur. She is given a booklet on MVP for additional reading. She verbalizes understanding of the risk of endocarditis, and states that she will notify her doctors of her MVP and the need for antibiotics before invasive procedures. Ms. Snow is attending a monthly MVP support group (led by a cardiology clinical nurse specialist) on campus and states, "I am so glad to know I'm not alone! It really helps to know that others are living well with MVP." Her weekly symptom log shows her symptoms are associated with late-night studying and drinking large amounts of coffee and cola. Ms. Snow has moderated her caffeine intake and increased her fluids, relieving her symptoms. In addition, Ms. Snow is taking a relaxation music therapy class. Ms. Snow states that she realizes that she has "the ability to control my life through the choices I make."

CLINICAL REASONING IN PATIENT CARE

1. Develop an action plan for Ms. Snow that outlines specific activities she can use to manage symptoms of MVP.
2. Why are patients with symptomatic MVP encouraged to include regular exercise in their health habits?
3. How does the support of family, friends, and other people with MVP assist MVP patients in managing their condition?
4. What manifestations would indicate a progressive worsening of Ms. Snow's mitral regurgitation?

See Evaluating Your Response in Appendix B.

Pathophysiology

The cardiomyopathies are categorized by their pathophysiology and presentation into three groups: Dilated, hypertrophic, and restrictive. **Table 31.9** compares the causes, pathophysiology, manifestations, and management of the cardiomyopathies.

Dilated Cardiomyopathy

Dilated cardiomyopathy is the most common type of cardiomyopathy, accounting for 85% of cases (Benjamin et al., 2017). Dilated cardiomyopathy is also a common cause of heart failure, accounting for about one in three cases. It is primarily a disease of middle age males; African American males have a higher risk than Caucasian American males.

The cause of dilated cardiomyopathy is unknown, although it appears to frequently result from toxins, metabolic conditions, or infection. Reversible dilated cardiomyopathy may develop due to alcohol and cocaine abuse, chemotherapeutic drug use, pregnancy, and systemic hypertension. Up to 20% of cases of dilated cardiomyopathy may be genetic in origin, most commonly transmitted in an autosomal dominant pattern, although autosomal recessive, X-linked, and mitochondrial patterns of inheritance are also seen (McMinn & Ross, 1995).

In dilated cardiomyopathy, heart chambers dilate and ventricular contraction is impaired. Both end-diastolic and end-systolic volumes increase, and the left-ventricular ejection fraction is substantially reduced, decreasing cardiac output. Left-ventricular dilation is prominent; left-ventricular hypertrophy is usually minimal. The right ventricle also may be enlarged. Extensive interstitial fibrosis (scarring) is evident; necrotic myocardial cells may also be seen.

Manifestations and Course. Manifestations of dilated cardiomyopathy develop gradually. Heart failure often presents years after the onset of dilation and pump failure. Both right- and left-sided failure occur, with dyspnea on exertion, orthopnea, paroxysmal nocturnal dyspnea, weakness, fatigue, peripheral edema, and ascites. Both S_3 and S_4 heart sounds are commonly heard, as well as an AV regurgitation murmur. Dysrhythmias are common, including supraventricular tachycardias, atrial fibrillation, and complex ventricular tachycardias. Untreated dysrhythmias can lead to sudden death. Mural thrombi (blood clots in

Table 31.9 Classifications of Cardiomyopathy

	Dilated	Hypertrophic	Restrictive
	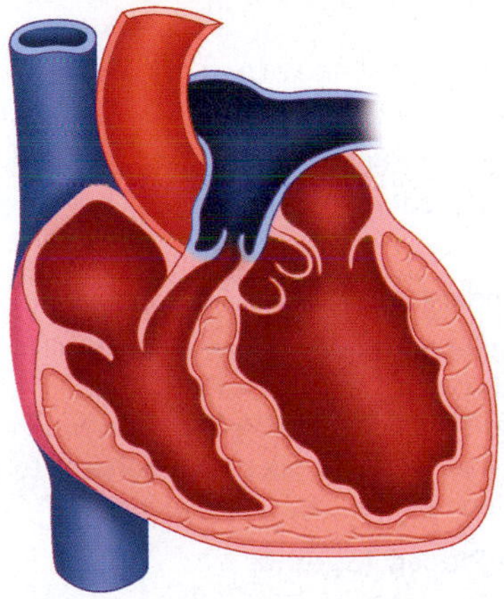	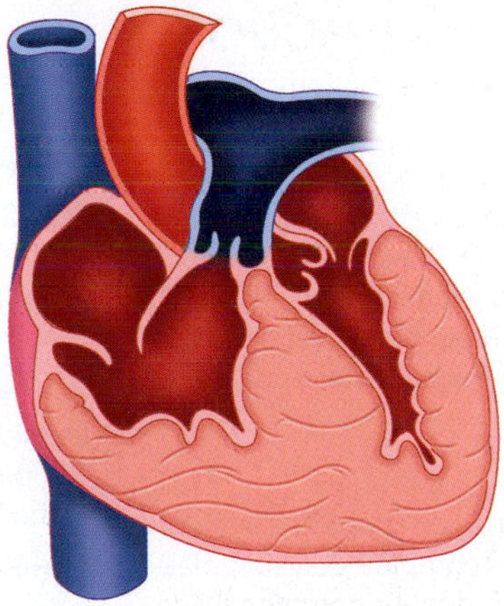	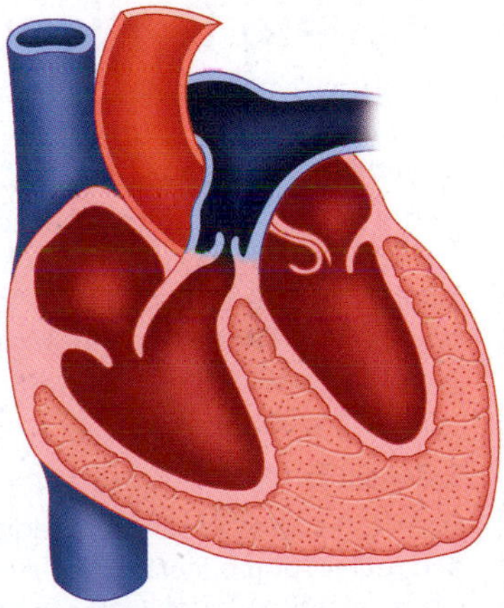
Causes	Usually idiopathic; may be secondary to chronic alcoholism or myocarditis	Hereditary; may be secondary to chronic hypertension	Usually secondary to amyloidosis, radiation, or myocardial fibrosis
Pathophysiology	Scarring and atrophy of myocardial cells Thickening of ventricular wall Dilation of heart chambers Impaired ventricular pumping Increased end-diastolic and end-systolic volumes Mural thrombi common	Hypertrophy of ventricular muscle mass Small left-ventricular volume Septal hypertrophy may obstruct left-ventricular outflow Left-atrial dilation	Excess rigidity of ventricular walls restricts filling Myocardial contractility remains relatively normal
Manifestations	Heart failure Cardiomegaly Dysrhythmias S_3 and S_4 gallop; murmur of mitral regurgitation	Dyspnea, anginal pain, syncope Left-ventricular hypertrophy Dysrhythmias Loud S_4 Sudden death	Dyspnea, fatigue Right-sided heart failure Mild to moderate cardiomegaly S_3 and S_4 heart sounds Mitral regurgitation murmur
Management	Management of heart failure ICD as needed Cardiac transplantation	Beta-blockers Calcium channel blockers Antidysrhythmic agents ICD, dual-chamber pacing Surgical excision of part of the ventricular septum	Management of heart failure Exercise restriction

the heart wall) may form in the left-ventricular apex and embolize to other parts of the body.

The prognosis of dilated cardiomyopathy is grim; most patients get progressively worse and 50% die within 5 years after the diagnosis; 75% die within 10 years (Benjamin et al., 2017).

Hypertrophic Cardiomyopathy

Hypertrophic cardiomyopathy is characterized by decreased compliance of the left ventricle and hypertrophy of the ventricular muscle mass. This impairs ventricular filling, leading to small end-diastolic volumes and low cardiac output. About half of all patients with hypertrophic cardiomyopathy have a family history of the disease (AHA, 2018). It is genetically transmitted in an autosomal dominant pattern.

The pattern of left-ventricular hypertrophy is unique in that the muscle may not hypertrophy equally. In a majority of patients, the interventricular septal mass, especially the upper portion, increases to a greater extent than the free wall of the ventricle. The enlarged upper septum narrows the passageway of blood into the aorta, impairing ventricular outflow. For this reason, this disorder is also known as *idiopathic hypertrophic subaortic stenosis (IHSS)* or *hypertrophic obstructive cardiomyopathy (HOCM)*.

Manifestations and Course. Hypertrophic cardiomyopathy may be asymptomatic for many years. Symptoms typically occur when increased oxygen demand causes increased ventricular contractility. They may develop suddenly during or after physical activity; in children and young adults, sudden cardiac death may be the first sign of the disorder. Hypertrophic cardiomyopathy is the probable or definite cause of death in 36% of young athletes who die suddenly (AHA, 2013). It is hypothesized that sudden cardiac death is due to ventricular dysrhythmias or hemodynamic factors. Predictors of sudden cardiac death in this population include age of less than 30 years, a family history of sudden death, syncopal episodes, severe ventricular hypertrophy, and ventricular tachycardia seen on ambulatory ECG monitoring. For a brief synopsis of a nursing research study regarding family presence during CPR and invasive procedures, see Moving Evidence into Action.

The usual manifestations of hypertrophic cardiomyopathy are dyspnea, angina, and syncope. Angina may result from ischemia due to overgrowth of the ventricular muscle, coronary artery abnormalities, or decreased coronary artery perfusion. Syncope may occur when the outflow tract obstruction severely decreases cardiac output and blood flow to the brain. Ventricular dysrhythmias are common;

Moving Evidence into Action

Decision Making in Heart Failure

Clinical Issue

Heart failure is a major disease process impacting function throughout the world. As HF is a chronic illness, ongoing decisions must be made related to treatments, pharmacologic options, and other, more invasive therapeutic options like surgery. How patients make decisions is an important concept for nurses to understand.

External Evidence

Hamel, Gaugler, Porta, and Hadidi (2018) conducted a systematic review of the literature to examine complex decision making to clarify key decision points and identify commonalities. Their review included 12 studies. Themes identified included "processing the decision," "timing and prognostication," and "considering the future." Some of the subthemes focused on when and how information was received, making the treatment decision, the role of the "future" in their decisions, and the influence of life and death decisions. Common themes were timing of discussions, the delivery of information, and considerations of the future.

Internal Evidence

As part of the evaluation of internal evidence, one must consider the patient's "real-time" response to the clinical decisions that must be made, the proposed treatment plan, and identification of stakeholders that influence the patient decision-making process. One question to ask: Are there patients with heart failure who are confronted with significant decisions regarding treatment planning within the population of your care environment? Does the clinical environment support the information related to patient decision making? How does providing more support for HF patients decision making in your environment impact costs?

Patient Considerations

When considering use of a new practice (like additional supportive decision making for patients with HF), the nurse must consider the specific patient population where it will be used. Will patients and their families be amenable to additional information related to their decision making?

Putting the Pieces Together

In the ideal world, the patient is a partner with the healthcare team, especially when making decisions related to the therapeutic plan when faced with a chronic illness like heart failure. Knowing the common themes that make up patient decision making can allow the healthcare team to support effective decision making by the patient and his or her family. To effectively implement a plan, it is important to evaluate the external evidence and consider the internal implications and patient/family issues. With the use of decision-making themes, more effective patient decisions can be supported. This will lead to increased patient participation in his or her therapeutic plan and patient satisfaction.

Reference

Hamel, A. V., Gaugler, J. E., Porta, C. M., & Hadidi, N. N. (2018). Complex decision-making in heart failure: A systematic review and thematic analysis. *Journal of Cardiovascular Nursing*, 33(3), 225–231.

atrial fibrillation may also develop. Other manifestations of hypertrophic cardiomyopathy include fatigue, dizziness, and palpitations. A harsh, crescendo–decrescendo systolic murmur of variable intensity heard best at the lower left sternal border and apex is characteristic in hypertrophic cardiomyopathy. An S_4 may also be noted on auscultation.

Restrictive Cardiomyopathy

The least common form of cardiomyopathy, *restrictive cardiomyopathy*, is characterized by rigid ventricular walls that impair diastolic filling. Causes of restrictive cardiomyopathy include myocardial fibrosis and infiltrative processes, such as amyloidosis. Fibrosis of the myocardium and endocardium causes excessive stiffness and rigidity of the ventricles. Decreased ventricular compliance impairs filling, with decreased ventricular size, elevated end-diastolic pressures, and decreased cardiac output. Contractility is unaffected, and the ejection fraction is normal.

Manifestations and Course. The manifestations of restrictive cardiomyopathy are those of heart failure and decreased tissue perfusion. Dyspnea on exertion and exercise intolerance are common. Jugular venous pressure is elevated, and the presence of S_3 and S_4 heart sounds is common. The prognosis for restrictive cardiomyopathy is poor. Most patients die within 3 years, and the systemic nature of the underlying disease process precludes effective treatment.

Interprofessional Care

With the exception of treating an underlying cause, little can be done to treat either dilated or restrictive cardiomyopathies. For these disorders, treatment focuses on managing heart failure and treating dysrhythmias. Refer to the section of this chapter on heart failure and Chapter 30 for specific treatment strategies. Treatment of hypertrophic cardiomyopathy focuses on reducing contractility and preventing sudden cardiac death. Strenuous physical exertion is restricted because it may precipitate dysrhythmias or sudden cardiac death. Dietary and sodium restrictions may help diminish the manifestations.

Diagnosis

Diagnosis begins with a history and physical assessment to rule out known causes of heart failure. Other tests may include:

- *Echocardiography* is done to assess chamber size and thickness, ventricular wall motion, valvular function, and systolic and diastolic function of the heart.
- *Electrocardiography* and *ambulatory ECG monitoring* demonstrate cardiac enlargement and detect dysrhythmias.
- *Chest x-ray* shows cardiomegaly, enlargement of the heart, and any pulmonary congestion or edema.
- *Hemodynamic studies* are used to assess cardiac output and pressures in the cardiac chambers and pulmonary vascular system.
- *Radionuclear scans* help identify changes in ventricular volume and mass, as well as perfusion deficits.
- *Cardiac catheterization* and *coronary angiography* may be done to evaluate coronary perfusion, the cardiac chambers, valves, and great vessels for function and structure, pressure relationships, and cardiac output.
- *Myocardial biopsy* uses the transvenous route to obtain myocardial tissue for biopsy. The cells are examined for infiltration, fibrosis, or inflammation.

Medications

The drug regimen used to treat heart failure is also used for dilated or restrictive cardiomyopathy. This includes ACE inhibitors, vasodilators, and digitalis (see the previous section of this chapter). Beta-blockers may also be used with caution in patients with dilated cardiomyopathy. Anticoagulants are given to reduce the risk of thrombus formation and embolization. Antidysrhythmic drugs are avoided if possible due to their tendency to precipitate further dysrhythmias.

Beta-blockers are the drugs of choice to reduce anginal symptoms and syncopal episodes associated with hypertrophic cardiomyopathy. The negative inotropic effects of beta-blockers and calcium channel blockers decrease the myocardial contractility, decreasing obstruction of the outflow tract. Beta-blockers also decrease heart rate and increase ventricular compliance, increasing diastolic filling time and cardiac output. Vasodilators, digitalis, nitrates, and diuretics are contraindicated. Amiodarone may be used to treat ventricular dysrhythmias.

Surgery

Without definitive treatment, patients with cardiomyopathy develop end-stage heart failure. Cardiac transplant is the definitive treatment for dilated cardiomyopathy. Ventricular assist devices may be used to support cardiac output until a donor heart is available. Transplantation is not a viable option for restrictive cardiomyopathy because transplantation does not eliminate the underlying process causing infiltration or fibrosis, and eventually the transplanted organ is affected as well. See the section on heart failure for more information about cardiac transplantation.

In severely symptomatic patients with obstructive hypertrophic cardiomyopathy, excess muscle may be surgically resected from the aortic valve outflow tract. The septum is incised, and tissue is removed. This procedure provides lasting improvement in about 75% of patients.

An implantable cardioverter–defibrillator (ICD) is often inserted to treat potentially lethal dysrhythmias, reducing the need for antidysrhythmic medications. A dual-chamber pacemaker may also be used to treat hypertrophic cardiomyopathy.

Nursing Care

Nursing assessment and care for patients with dilated and restrictive cardiomyopathy are similar to those provided to patients with heart failure. Teaching about the disease process and its management is vital. Some degree of activity restriction is often necessary; assist to conserve energy while encouraging self-care. Support coping skills and adaptation to required lifestyle changes. Provide information and support for decision making about cardiac transplantation if that is an option. Discuss the toxic and vasodilator effects of alcohol and encourage abstinence. See the Nursing Care section for heart failure earlier in this chapter for nursing diagnoses and suggested interventions.

The patient with hypertrophic cardiomyopathy requires care similar to that provided for myocardial ischemia; nitrates and other vasodilators, however, are avoided. If surgery is performed, nursing care is similar to that for any patient undergoing open-heart surgery or cardiac transplant. Discuss the genetic transmission of hypertrophic cardiomyopathy, and suggest screening of close relatives (parents and siblings).

Provide pre- and postoperative care and teaching as appropriate for patients undergoing invasive procedures or surgery for cardiomyopathy.

Nursing priorities that may be appropriate for patients with cardiomyopathy include:

- Monitoring cardiac function related to impaired left-ventricular filling, contractility, or outflow obstruction
- Reducing fatigue related to decreased cardiac output
- Promoting effective breathing related to heart failure
- Managing fear related to risk for sudden cardiac death
- Managing ADLs related to decreasing cardiac function and activity restrictions
- Supporting grieving patient and family related to poor prognosis.

Delegating Nursing Care Activities

As appropriate and allowed by the designated duties and responsibilities of unlicensed assistive personnel, the nurse may delegate nursing care activities such as measuring fluid intake and output, collecting vital signs (including orthostatic vital signs), encouraging oral or enteral fluid intake, and ensuring nonpharmacologic skin care.

Transitions of Care

While inherited forms of cardiomyopathy cannot be prevented, heart disease complications resulting in cardiomyopathy can be avoided by using heart-healthy lifestyle modifications. Management of hypertension, exercise, heart-healthy diet, and smoking cessation are important preventative measures.

The nursing management of acute cardiomyopathy focuses on symptom management and pharmacological interventions. Surgical interventions may be indicated. Cardiomyopathies are chronic, progressive disorders generally managed in home and community care settings unless surgery or a transplant is planned or end-stage heart failure develops. When teaching the patient and family for home care, include the following topics:

- Activity restrictions and dietary changes to reduce manifestations and prevent complications
- Prescribed drug regimen, its rationale, and intended and possible adverse effects
- The disease process, its expected ultimate outcome, and treatment options
- Cardiac transplantation, including the procedure, the need for lifetime immunosuppression to prevent transplant rejection, and the risks of postoperative infection and long-term immunosuppression
- Symptoms to report to the physician or for which immediate care is needed
- Cardiopulmonary resuscitation procedures and available training sites.

Refer the patient and family for home and social services and counseling as indicated. Provide information about community resources such as support groups or the American Heart Association.

Cardiomyopathy may progress to where end-of-life care is indicated. Palliative care may be needed if surgery or other interventions are not indicated. The goals of palliative care in the patient with cardiomyopathy would include the same goals as those of other patients with end-stage cardiac diseases (see sections on heart failure and valvular disease).

CHAPTER HIGHLIGHTS

31.1 Heart Failure

Describe the pathophysiology and manifestations of heart failure, and outline the interprofessional care and nursing care of patients with these disorders.

- Heart failure is the most common cardiac disorder, a condition in which the heart is unable to pump effectively to meet the body's need to provide blood and oxygen to the tissues.
- Heart failure is due to impaired myocardial contraction and is most commonly caused by coronary heart disease and myocardial ischemia or infarct.
- Heart failure can also occur due to long-standing excessive workload of the heart muscle such as in hypertension or valvular disorders.
- When the heart starts to fail, compensatory mechanisms are activated to help maintain tissue perfusion. Although these mechanisms, including increased contractile force, vasoconstriction, sodium and water retention, and remodeling of the heart, effectively maintain cardiac output in the short term, in the long term they hasten deterioration of heart function.
- Goals of heart failure management are to reduce the workload and improve its function. Medical

management includes medication use including ACE inhibitors, beta-blockers, diuretics, and vasodilators to reduce cardiac workload.

- Digitalis is no longer recommended as a first-line therapy due to the risk for digitalis toxicity outweighing the benefit due to the narrow therapeutic window.
- Nursing care of the patient with heart failure is primarily supportive and educative, providing the patient and family with the necessary knowledge and resources to manage this chronic condition.
- Cardiogenic pulmonary edema, a manifestation of severe cardiac decompensation, is a medical emergency, requiring immediate and effective treatment to preserve life. The nurse's role in managing pulmonary edema focuses on supporting respiratory and cardiac function through careful assessment and early intervention, administering prescribed medications, and providing reassurance to the patient and family.

31.2 Inflammatory Heart Disorders

Describe the pathophysiology and manifestations of inflammatory heart disorders, and outline the interprofessional care and nursing care of patients with these disorders.

- Inflammatory and infectious processes, such as rheumatic fever, endocarditis, myocarditis, and pericarditis, can affect any layer of the heart. While some, such as myocarditis and pericarditis, are typically mild and self-limiting, others can have long-term effects on cardiac structure and function.
- Processes such as rheumatic heart disease, endocarditis, and congenital conditions can affect the structure and function of the heart valves, resulting in either stenosis (narrowing) of the valve and restricted flow through it, or regurgitation, backflow of blood through a valve that does not fully close. The mitral and aortic valves are commonly affected due to the higher pressures and increased workload of the left side of the heart.

31.3 Disorders of Cardiac Structure

Describe the pathophysiology and manifestations of disorders of cardiac structure, and outline the interprofessional care and nursing care of patients with these disorders.

- Valve disorders may be mild, producing a heart murmur but no functional impairment for the patient, or severe, causing symptoms of heart failure even at rest. Repair or replacement of the valve may ultimately be required.
- Cardiomyopathies affect the heart muscle and its ability to stretch during filling and to contract effectively. Dilated cardiomyopathy, the most common type, is progressive, ultimately necessitating heart transplant. Hypertrophic cardiomyopathy affects both ventricular filling and outflow through the aortic valve. Surgical resection of excess tissue may relieve its manifestations.

TEST YOURSELF NCLEX-RN® REVIEW

1. A patient with heart failure has an ejection fraction of 25%. The nurse would prepare to care for a patient with which condition?
   - A. Ventricular function is severely impaired.
   - B. Cardiac output is greater than normal, which overtaxes the heart.
   - C. The amount of blood being ejected from the ventricles is within normal limits.
   - D. Twenty-five percent of the blood entering the ventricle remains in the ventricle after systole.
2. A patient admitted 24 hours previously with heart failure has lost 1 kg (2.2 lb) of weight, has a heart rate of 88, which was 105 on admission, and now has crackles only in the bases of the lungs. How should the nurse interpret these assessment findings?
   - A. More aggressive treatment is needed.
   - B. The patient's condition is unchanged from admission.
   - C. The treatment regimen is achieving the desired effect.
   - D. No further treatment is required at this time because the failure has resolved.
3. A patient is diagnosed with left-ventricular failure. Which findings are consistent with this diagnosis? (Select all that apply.)
   - A. Fatigue
   - B. Substernal chest pain during exercise
   - C. 5 cm jugular vein distention at 30 degrees
   - D. Bilateral inspiratory crackles to midscapulae
   - E. Complaints of shortness of breath with minimal exertion
4. The nurse is caring for a patient undergoing pulmonary artery pressure monitoring. What should the nurse include when caring for this patient? (Select all that apply.)
   - A. Maintain flush solution flow by gravity.
   - B. Calibrate and level the system every shift.
   - C. Secure the intravenous line to the bed linens.
   - D. Change tubing to the insertion site every 72 hours.
   - E. Measure pressure at the point of maximum inspiration.

5. A patient experiencing acute pulmonary edema is prescribed morphine sulfate 2 to 5 mg IV as needed for pain and dyspnea. What action should the nurse take with this prescribed medication?
   A. Administer the drug as ordered, monitoring respiratory status.
   B. Withhold the drug until the patient's respiratory status improves.
   C. Question the order because no time intervals have been specified.
   D. Administer the drug only when the patient complains of chest pain.
6. The nurse notes a grating heart sound when auscultating the apical pulse of a patient with pericarditis. What should the nurse do with this assessment data?
   A. Obtain an electrocardiogram.
   B. Initiate resuscitation measures.
   C. Immediately notify the physician.
   D. Note the finding in the patient's medical record.
7. The nurse is planning care for a patient with acute infective endocarditis. What would be an appropriate goal of nursing care for this patient?
   A. Resume usual activities within 1 week of treatment.
   B. Relate the benign and self-limiting nature of the disease.
   C. Consider cardiac transplantation as a viable treatment option.
   D. State the importance of continuing intravenous antibiotic therapy as ordered.
8. The nurse is assessing heart sounds of a patient scheduled for mitral valve replacement surgery secondary to mitral stenosis. Which sounds should the nurse expect to auscultate in this patient? (Select all that apply.)
   A. Loud S_1
   B. Muffled heart sounds
   C. S_3 and S_4 heart sounds
   D. Diastolic murmur heard at the apex
   E. A low pitched rumbling
9. A patient considering heart valve replacement asks if a biologic or mechanical valve is better to use. How should the nurse respond to the patient? (Select all that apply.)
   A. Biologic valves tend to be more durable than mechanical valves.
   B. The need to take drugs to prevent rejection of biologic tissue is a major consideration.
   C. Clotting is a risk with mechanical valves, necessitating anticoagulant drug therapy after insertion.
   D. Endocarditis is a risk following valve replacement that is more easily treated with mechanical valves.
   E. Good hemodynamics can be achieved with either type of valve.
10. The parents of a young athlete who collapsed and died due to hypertrophic cardiomyopathy ask how it is possible that their son had no symptoms of this disorder before experiencing sudden cardiac death. How should the nurse respond to the parents?
   A. "It is likely that your son had symptoms of the disorder before he died, but he may not have thought them important enough to tell someone about."
   B. "In this type of cardiomyopathy, the ventricle does not fill normally. During exercise, the heart may not be able to meet the body's needs for blood and oxygen."
   C. "Cardiomyopathy results in destruction and scarring of cardiac muscle cells. As a result, the ventricle may rupture during strenuous exercise, leading to sudden death."
   D. "Exercise causes the heart to contract more forcefully and can lead to changes in the heart's rhythm or the outflow of blood from the heart in people with hypertrophic cardiomyopathy."

See Test Yourself answers in Appendix B.

REFERENCES

Adams, M. P., Holland, L. N., & Urban, C. (2017). *Pharmacology for nursing: A pathophysiologic approach.* (5th ed.). Hoboken, NJ: Pearson Education.

Alwan, A., Tiruneh, F., Wessly, P., Khan, A., Iftikhar, H., Barned, S., & Larbi, D. (2017). Acute pericarditis: Descriptive study and etiology determination in a predominantly African American population. *Cureus, 9*(7), e1431.

American Heart Association (AHA). (2013). Heart disease and stroke statistics—2013 update. *Circulation, 127*(1), e6–e245. Retrieved from http://circ.ahajournals.org/content/127/1/e6.full.pdf+html?sid=4c0e1444-d592-434d-b2a0-d72abdb6a2ec.

American Heart Association (AHA). (2017a). *Classes of heart failure.* Retrieved from www.heart.org/HEARTORG/Conditions/HeartFailure/AboutHeartFailure/Classes-of-Heart-Failure_UCM_306328_Article.jsp#.WmThOq6nGUk.

American Heart Association (AHA). (2017b). *What is infective endocarditis?* Retrieved from www.heart.org/idc/groups/heart-public/@wcm/@hcm/documents/downloadable/ucm_300297.pdf.

American Heart Association (AHA). (2018). *Hypertrophic cardiomyopathy.* Retrieved from https://www.heart.org/idc/groups/heart-public/@wcm/@hcm/documents/downloadable/ucm_312225.pdf.

Benjamin, E. J., Blaha, M. J., Chiuve, S. E., Cushman, M., Das, S. R., Deo, R., . . . American Heart Association Statistics Committee and Stroke Statistics Subcommittee. (2017). Heart disease and stroke statistics—2017 update: A report from the American Heart Association. *Circulation, 135*(10), e146–e603.

Black, R. M. (2018). *Pericarditis in renal failure.* UpToDate. Retrieved from https://www.uptodate.com/contents/pericarditis-in-renal-failure.

Dima, C. (2018). *Mitral stenosis.* Medscape. Retrieved from https://emedicine.medscape.com/article/155724-overview#a6.

Gaasch, W. H. (2017). *Mitral regurgitation.* UpToDate. Retrieved from https://www.uptodate.com/contents/mitral-regurgitation-beyond-the-basics#H9.

Genetics Home Reference. (2018). *Marfan syndrome.* Retrieved from https://ghr.nlm.nih.gov/condition/marfan-syndrome.

Hamel, A. V., Gaugler, J. E., Porta, C. M., & Hadidi, N. N. (2018). Complex decision-making in heart failure: A systematic review and thematic analysis. *Journal of Cardiovascular Nursing* 33(3), 225–231.

Jelani, Q. (2016). *Mitral valve prolapse.* Medscape. Retrieved from https://emedicine.medscape.com/article/155494-overview.

Kee, J. L. (2014). *Laboratory and diagnostic tests with nursing implications* (9th ed.). Boston, MA: Pearson.

Mayo Clinic. (2018). *Aortic valve stenosis.* Retrieved from https://www.mayoclinic.org/diseases-conditions/aortic-stenosis/symptoms-causes/syc-20353139.

McMinn, T. R., & Ross, J. (1995). Hereditary dilated cardiomyopathy. *Clinical Cardiology, 18,* 7–15.

Nishimura, R. A., Otto, C. M., Bonow, R. O., Carabello, B. A., Erwin, J. P. III, Fleisher, L. A., . . . Thompson, A. (2017). 2017 AHA/ACC focused update of the 2014 AHA/ACC guideline for the management of patients with valvular heart disease: A report of the American College of Cardiology/American Heart Association Task Force on Clinical Practice Guidelines. *Circulation, 135*(25), e1159–e1195.

Perrin, K. O., & MacLeod, C. E. (2017). *Understanding the essentials of critical care nursing* (3rd ed.) Boston, MA: Pearson.

Sharma, A., Colvin-Adams, M., & Yancy, C. W. (2014). Heart failure in African Americans: Disparities can be overcome. *Cleveland Clinic Journal of Medicine, 81*(5), 301–311.

Sorenson, M., Quinn, L., & Klein, D. (2019). *Pathophysiology: Concepts of human disease.* Hoboken, NJ: Pearson Education.

Steiner, J. M., Cooper, S., & Kirkpatrick, J. N. (2017). Palliative care in end-stage valvular heart disease. *Heart, 103*(16), 1233–1237.

Yancy, C. W., Jessup, M., Bozkurt, B., Butler, J., Casey, D. E. Jr, Colvin, M. M., . . . Westlake, C. (2016). 2016 ACC/AHA/HFSA focused update on new pharmacological therapy for heart failure: An update of the 2013 ACCF/AHA guideline for the management of heart failure: A report of the American College of Cardiology Foundation/American Heart Association Task Force on Clinical Practice Guidelines and the Heart Failure Society of America. *Circulation, 134*, e282–e293.

Yancy, C. W., Jessup, M., Bozkurt, B., Butler, J., Casey, D. E. Jr, Colvin, M. M., . . . Westlake, C. (2017). 2017 ACC/AHA/HFSA focused update of the 2013 ACCF/AHA guideline for the management of heart failure: A report of the American College of Cardiology/American Heart Association Task Force on Clinical Practice Guidelines and the Heart Failure Society of America. *Circulation, 136*(6), e137–e161.

Ziaeian, B., Fonarow, G. C., & Heidenreich, P. A. (2017). Clinical effectiveness of hydralazine-isosorbide dinitrate in African-American patients with heart failure. *Journal of the American College of Cardiology, 5*(9), 632–639.

Zuhlke, L. J., Beaton, A., Engel, M. E., Hugo-Hamman, C. T., Karthikeyan, G., Katzenellenbogen, J. M., . . . Carapetis, J. (2017). Group A Streptococcus, acute rheumatic fever and rheumatic heart disease: Epidemiology and clinical considerations. *Current Treatment Options in Cardiovascular Medicine, 19*(2), 15.

ADDITIONAL RESOURCES

American Heart Association.
www.heart.org

Mended Hearts.
mendedhearts.org

National Coalition of Women with Heart Disease.
www.womenheart.org.

National Heart, Lung, and Blood Institute
www.nhlbi.nih.gov/health-topics.

Chapter 32

Nursing Care of Patients with Vascular and Lymphatic Disorders

Chapter Outline and Learning Outcomes

32.1 Disorders of Blood Pressure Regulation 1107

Describe the pathophysiology and manifestations of disorders of blood pressure, and outline the interprofessional care and nursing care of patients with these disorders.

32.2 Disorders of the Aorta and Its Branches 1122

Describe the pathophysiology and manifestations of disorders of the aorta and its branches, and outline the interprofessional care and nursing care of patients with these disorders.

32.3 Disorders of the Peripheral Arteries 1128

Describe the pathophysiology and manifestations of disorders of the peripheral arteries, and outline the interprofessional care and nursing care of patients with these disorders.

32.4 Disorders of Venous Circulation 1138

Describe the pathophysiology and manifestations of disorders of venous circulation, and outline the interprofessional care and nursing care of patients with these disorders.

32.5 Disorders of the Lymphatic System 1151

Describe the pathophysiology and manifestations of disorders of the lymphatic system, and outline the interprofessional care and nursing care of patients with these disorders.

CLINICAL COMPETENCIES

- Assess patients with peripheral vascular disorders, using data to select and prioritize appropriate nursing diagnoses and identify desired outcomes of care.
- Identify the effects of peripheral vascular disorders on the functional health status of assigned patients.
- Use research and an evidence-based plan to provide individualized care for patients with peripheral vascular disorders.
- Collaborate with the interprofessional care team in planning and providing care for patients with peripheral vascular disorders.
- Safely and knowledgably administer medications and prescribed treatments for patients with peripheral vascular disorders.
- Provide patient and family teaching to promote, maintain, and restore health in patients with common peripheral vascular disorders.

KEY TERMS

aneurysm, 1122
atherosclerosis, 1128
blood pressure (BP), 1107
chronic venous insufficiency, 1146
deep venous thrombosis (DVT), 1139
diastolic blood pressure, 1107
dissection, 1124
embolism, 1136
hypertension, 1107
intermittent claudication, 1124
lymphedema, 1152
mean arterial pressure (MAP), 1107
peripheral vascular disease (PVD), 1128
primary hypertension, 1108
pulse pressure, 1107
Raynaud disease/phenomenon, 1135
secondary hypertension, 1120
systolic blood pressure, 1107
thromboangiitis obliterans, 1132
thromboembolus, 1136
thrombus, 1136
varicose veins, 1148
vasoconstriction, 1128
vasodilation, 1128
venous thrombosis, 1139

The major processes that interfere with peripheral blood flow and movement of lymphatic fluid include constriction, obstruction, inflammation, and vasospasm. These conditions lead to disorders of blood pressure regulation, aortic structure, peripheral artery function, venous circulation, and lymphatic circulation.

A holistic approach is important when caring for patients with disorders of the peripheral vascular and lymphatic systems. The focus of care is on teaching long-term care measures, pain relief, improving peripheral blood and lymphatic circulation, preventing tissue damage, and promoting healing. The prescribed treatment may have emotional, social, and economic effects on the patient and family.

32.1 Disorders of Blood Pressure Regulation

Blood flows through the circulatory system from areas of higher pressure to areas of lower pressure. The amount of pressure in any portion of the vascular system is affected by a number of factors, including blood volume, vascular resistance, and cardiac output. The **blood pressure (BP)** is the tension or pressure exerted by blood against arterial walls. A certain amount of pressure within the system is necessary to maintain open vessels, capillary perfusion, and oxygenation of all body tissues. Excess pressure, however, has harmful effects, increasing the workload of the heart, altering the structure of the vessels, and affecting sensitive body tissues such as the kidneys, eyes, and central nervous system.

This section focuses on **hypertension**, or excess pressure in the arterial portion of systemic circulation. Excessively low blood pressure, *hypotension*, is discussed in Sections 11.3 and 11.4 of Chapter 11. Altered pulmonary vascular pressures are discussed in Chapter 37.

Physiology Review

Blood flow through the circulatory system requires *sufficient blood volume* to fill the blood vessels and *pressure differences* within the system that allow blood to move forward. The arterial, or supply side of circulation, has relatively high pressures created by the thick elastic walls of the arteries and arterioles. The venous, or return side of circulation, on the other hand, is a low-pressure system of thin-walled, distensible veins. Blood flows through the capillaries linking these two systems from the higher-pressure arterial side to the lower-pressure venous side.

The arterial blood pressure is created by the ejection of blood from the heart during systole (*cardiac output* or *CO*) and the tension, or resistance to blood flow, created by the elastic arterial walls (*systemic vascular resistance* or *SVR*). The blood pressure rises as the heart contracts during systole, ejecting its blood. This pressure wave, or the **systolic blood pressure**, is felt as the peripheral pulse and heard as the Korotkoff sounds during blood pressure measurement. In healthy adults, the average systolic pressure is < 120 mmHg. During diastole, or cardiac relaxation and filling, elastic arterial walls maintain a minimum pressure, the **diastolic blood pressure**, to maintain blood flow through the capillary beds. The average diastolic pressure in a healthy adult is < 80 mmHg. The difference between the systolic and diastolic pressure, normally about 40 mmHg, is known as the **pulse pressure**. The **mean arterial pressure (MAP)** is the average pressure in the arterial circulation throughout the cardiac cycle. It can be calculated using the formula [systolic BP + 2 (diastolic BP)] / 3.

Increased cardiac output (e.g., during exercise) or increased peripheral vascular resistance (e.g., vasoconstriction due to drug administration) cause the blood pressure to rise. Cardiac output is determined by the blood volume and the ability of the ventricles to fill and effectively pump that blood. A number of factors contribute to systemic vascular resistance, including vessel length, blood viscosity, and vessel diameter and distensibility (compliance). While vessel length and blood viscosity remain relatively constant, vessel diameter and compliance are subject to normal regulatory activities and disease.

The arterioles normally determine the SVR as their diameter changes in response to a variety of stimuli:

- ***Sympathetic nervous system (SNS)*** stimulation. Baroreceptors in the aortic arch and carotid sinus signal the SNS via the cardiovascular control center in the medulla when the MAP changes. A drop in MAP stimulates the SNS, increasing the heart rate and cardiac output, and constricting arterioles (except in skeletal muscle). As a result, BP rises. A rise in MAP has the opposite effect, decreasing the heart rate and cardiac output and causing arteriolar vasodilation.
- ***Circulating epinephrine*** and ***norepinephrine*** from the adrenal cortex (e.g., the fight-or-flight response) have the same effect as SNS stimulation.
- ***The renin–angiotensin–aldosterone system*** (RAAS) responds to renal perfusion. A drop in renal perfusion stimulates renin release. Renin converts angiotensinogen to angiotensin I, which is subsequently converted to angiotensin II in the lungs by angiotensin-converting enzyme (ACE). Angiotensin II is a potent vasoconstrictor. It also promotes sodium and water retention both directly and by stimulating the adrenal medulla to release aldosterone. Both SVR and CO increase, raising BP.
- ***Atrial natriuretic peptide*** is released from atrial cells in response to stretching by excess blood volume. It promotes vasodilation and sodium and water excretion, lowering BP.
- ***Adrenomedullin*** is a peptide synthesized and released by endothelial and smooth muscle cells in blood vessels. It is a potent vasodilator.
- ***Vasopressin*** or *antidiuretic hormone* (from the posterior pituitary gland) promotes water retention and vasoconstriction, raising BP.
- ***Local factors*** such as inflammatory mediators and various metabolites can promote vasodilation, affecting BP.

In addition to the preceding stimuli, the primary factor affecting vessel compliance is the extent of arteriosclerosis (hardening of the arteries) and atherosclerosis (plaque accumulation). **Figure 32.1** ■ summarizes the interrelationships of major factors regulating blood pressure.

The Patient with Primary Hypertension

Primary hypertension, also known as *essential hypertension*, is a persistently elevated systemic blood pressure. One in three, or 85.7 million, individuals in the United States have hypertension (Benjamin et al., 2017). More than 90% of these have primary hypertension, which has no identified cause.

Hypertension is defined as systolic blood pressure of 130 mmHg or higher or diastolic pressure of 80 to 89 mmHg, based on the average of three or more readings taken on separate occasions. **Table 32.1** identifies classifications of blood pressure for adults ages 18 and older as defined by the American Heart Association (2017a; Whelton et al., 2017).

Hypertension is an important public health issue: Although it rarely causes symptoms or noticeably limits the patient's functional health, hypertension is a major risk factor for coronary heart disease, heart failure, stroke, and renal failure. Hypertension and its consequences are not unique to the United States. The World Health Organization (2013) identifies blood pressure above optimal levels (a systolic BP > 115 mmHg) as responsible for 62% of cerebrovascular disease and 49% of ischemic heart disease worldwide.

The identification and treatment of hypertension in the United States has improved significantly in the past 25 years. It is estimated that about 34.5% of U.S. adults older than 20 years of age have hypertension. About 82% of adults with hypertension are aware that they have it. There is a gap between knowledge of diagnosis and adequate management; 75% of people with known hypertension are under current treatment, but only 53% of those have effective blood pressure control (Benjamin et al., 2017).

Pathophysiology

Primary hypertension is thought to develop from complex interactions among factors that regulate cardiac output and systemic vascular resistance. These interactions may include:

- Excess sympathetic nervous system with overstimulation of α- and β-adrenergic receptors, resulting in vasoconstriction and increased cardiac output.

Table 32.1 Classification of Blood Pressure for Adults

Category	Definition (mmHg)	Examples (mmHg)
Normal	< 120/80	112/75 119/79
Elevated	Systolic from 120 to 129 *and* diastolic < 80	125/72 129/79
Stage 1 hypertension	Systolic from 130 to 139 *or* diastolic from 80 to 89	130/79 129/80
Stage 2 hypertension	Systolic at least 140 *or* diastolic at least 90	135/90 140/85
Hypertensive crisis	Systolic over 180 *and/or* diastolic over 120	180/90 165/120

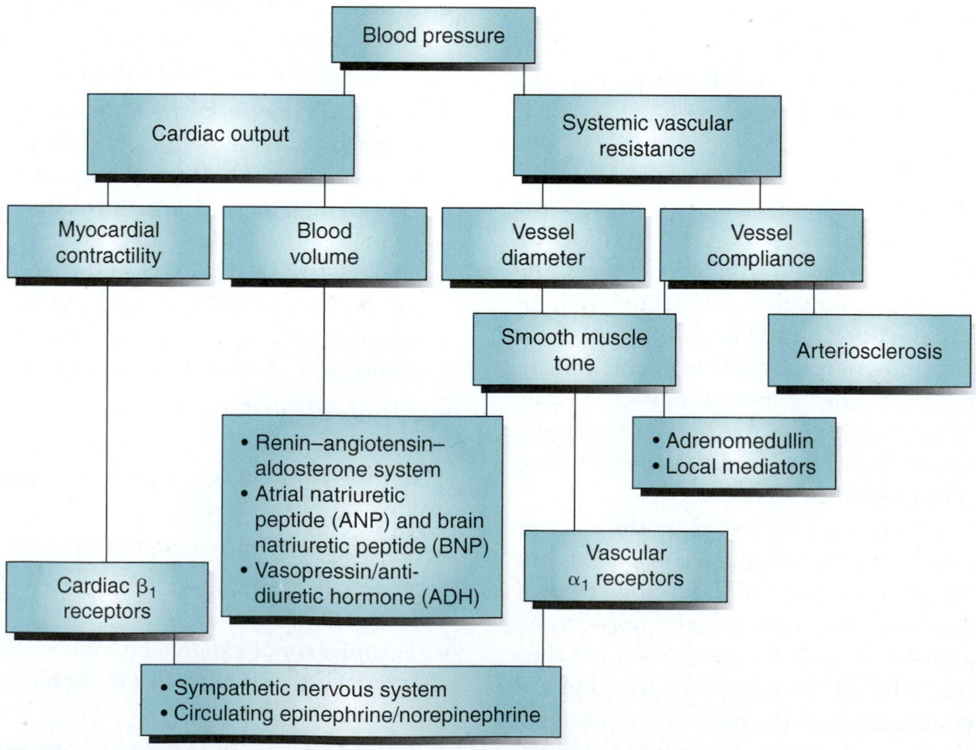

Blood pressure
Cardiac output
Systemic vascular resistance
Myocardial contractility
Blood volume
Vessel diameter
Vessel compliance
Smooth muscle tone
Arteriosclerosis
• Renin–angiotensin–aldosterone system
• Atrial natriuretic peptide (ANP) and brain natriuretic peptide (BNP)
• Vasopressin/anti-diuretic hormone (ADH)
• Adrenomedullin
• Local mediators
Cardiac β1 receptors
Vascular α1 receptors
• Sympathetic nervous system
• Circulating epinephrine/norepinephrine

Figure 32.1 ■ Factors affecting blood pressure.

- Altered function of the RAAS and its responsiveness to factors such as sodium intake and overall fluid volume. The RAAS affects vasomotor tone and salt and water excretion. Chronically high levels of angiotensin II lead to arteriolar remodeling, which permanently increases SVR. In approximately 20% of people with primary hypertension, renin levels are lower than normal. Increased sodium intake increases the blood pressure in these patients. Low plasma renin levels are more commonly seen in African Americans than in Whites. Another 15% of patients with hypertension have higher than normal plasma renin levels. For these patients, salt intake has less of an effect on blood pressure (Sorenson, Quinn, & Klein, 2019). Most people with hypertension have normal levels of renin activity.
- Other chemical mediators of vasomotor tone and blood volume such as atrial natriuretic peptide (factor) play a role by affecting vasomotor tone and sodium and water excretion. Vascular endothelium itself produces hormones (*endothelins*) that also affect vasomotor tone. Endothelin-1 is a potent vasoconstrictor (Sorenson et al., 2019).
- The interaction between insulin resistance, hyperinsulinemia, and endothelial function may be a primary cause of hypertension. Excess insulin has several effects that potentially contribute to hypertension: (1) Sodium retention by the kidneys, (2) increased sympathetic nervous system activity, (3) hypertrophy of vascular smooth muscle, and (4) changes in ion transport across cell membranes (Sorenson et al., 2019).

The result is sustained increases in blood volume and peripheral resistance. The cardiovascular system adapts to increased blood volume by increasing cardiac output. Autoregulatory mechanisms in the systemic arteries react to the increased volume, causing vasoconstriction. The increased systemic vascular resistance causes hypertension.

It appears unlikely that one single cause and pathologic process will be found to account for essential hypertension. Increasingly, evidence points to hypertension as a diverse group of pathophysiologic mechanisms resulting in the common manifestation of elevated blood pressure.

Incidence and Risk Factors

Hypertension primarily affects middle-age and older adults: More than 50% of people ages 60 to 74 and about 75% of those ages 75 and older are hypertensive (Benjamin et al., 2017). An age-related increase in the systolic blood pressure is the primary factor leading to the high incidence of hypertension in older adults. Unlike the diastolic blood pressure, which tends to rise until approximately age 50, then level off, the systolic blood pressure continues to rise with age. Hypertension increases the risk of stroke to about four times that of people with normal blood pressure and the risk for heart failure by two to three times that of people with normal blood pressure.

The prevalence of hypertension is significantly higher in Black populations than in White and Hispanic populations. Nearly 44% of Black adults are hypertensive, with Black women (46.3%) having a higher incidence than Black men (45%). Less than 34% of adult White and Hispanic people are affected. In Whites and Hispanics, more males than females are hypertensive; in Blacks, more women than men are affected (Benjamin et al., 2017).

A number of risk factors have been identified for primary hypertension (**Box 32.1**). Genetics plays a role, as do environmental factors.

- ***Family history.*** Studies show a genetic link in up to 40% of people with primary hypertension (Sorenson et al., 2019). Genes involved in the RAAS and others that affect vascular tone, salt and water transportation in the kidney, obesity, and insulin resistance are likely involved in the development of hypertension, although no consistent genetic linkages have been found.
- ***Age.*** The incidence of hypertension rises with increasing age. Aging affects baroreceptors involved in blood pressure regulation as well as arterial compliance. As the arteries become less compliant, pressure within the vessels increases. This is often most apparent as a gradual increase in the systolic pressure with aging.
- ***Race.*** Primary hypertension is more common and more severe in African Americans than in people of other ethnic backgrounds. It also tends to develop at an earlier age and is associated with more cardiovascular and renal damage. More African Americans with hypertension have low renin levels and altered renal excretion of sodium at normal blood pressure levels than people of other ethnic backgrounds (Sorenson et al., 2019).
- ***Mineral intake.*** High sodium intake is often associated with fluid retention. Hypertension related to sodium intake involves a number of different physiologic mechanisms, including the RAAS, nitric oxide, catecholamines, endothelin, and atrial natriuretic peptide. Low potassium, calcium, and magnesium intakes contribute to hypertension by unknown mechanisms. The ratio of sodium to potassium intake appears to play

BOX 32.1
Factors Contributing to Hypertension

MODIFIABLE FACTORS

- High sodium intake
- Low potassium, calcium, and magnesium intake
- Obesity
- Excess alcohol consumption
- Insulin resistance

NONMODIFIABLE FACTORS

- Genetic factors
- Family history
- Age
- Race

a role, possibly through the effects of increased potassium intake on sodium excretion. Potassium promotes vasodilation by reducing responses to catecholamines and angiotensin II. Calcium also has a vasodilator effect. Although magnesium has been shown to reduce blood pressure, its mechanism of action is unclear (Sorenson et al., 2019).

- ***Obesity.*** Central obesity (fat cell deposits in the abdomen), determined by an increased waist-to-hip ratio, has a stronger correlation with hypertension than body mass index or skinfold thickness. Although a clear correlation exists between obesity and hypertension, the relationship may be one common cause: Genetic factors appear to play a role in the common triad of obesity, hypertension, and insulin resistance.
- ***Insulin resistance.*** Insulin resistance with resulting hyperinsulinemia is linked with hypertension by its effects on the sympathetic nervous system, vascular smooth muscle, renal regulation of sodium and water, and changes in ion transport across cell membranes. Insulin resistance may be a genetic or an acquired trait. Although more commonly seen in obese individuals, insulin resistance has also been found in people of normal weight.
- ***Excess alcohol consumption.*** Regular consumption of three or more drinks a day increases the risk of hypertension. Decreasing or discontinuing alcohol consumption reduces blood pressure, particularly systolic readings. Lifestyle factors associated with excessive alcohol intake (obesity and lack of exercise) may contribute to hypertension as well.
- ***Stress.*** Physical and emotional stress cause transient elevations of blood pressure, but the role of stress in primary hypertension is less clear. Blood pressure normally fluctuates throughout the day, increasing with activity, discomfort, or emotional responses such as anger. Frequent or continued stress may cause vascular smooth muscle hypertrophy or affect central integrative pathways of the brain.

Manifestations

The early stages of primary hypertension are typically asymptomatic, marked only by elevated blood pressure. Blood pressure elevations are initially transient but eventually become permanent. When symptoms do appear, they are usually vague. Headache, usually in the back of the head and neck, may be present on awakening, subsiding during the day. Other symptoms result from target organ damage and may include nocturia, confusion, nausea and vomiting, and visual disturbances. Examination of the retina of the eye may reveal narrowed arterioles, hemorrhages, exudates, and *papilledema* (swelling of the optic nerve).

Complications

Sustained hypertension affects the cardiovascular, neurologic, and renal systems. The rate of atherosclerosis accelerates, increasing the risk for coronary heart disease and stroke. The workload of the left ventricle increases, leading to ventricular hypertrophy, which then increases the risk for coronary heart disease, dysrhythmias, and heart failure. The diastolic blood pressure is a significant cardiovascular risk factor until age 50; the systolic pressure then becomes the more important factor contributing to cardiovascular risk. Most deaths due to hypertension result from coronary heart disease and acute myocardial infarction or heart failure.

Accelerated atherosclerosis associated with hypertension increases the risk for cerebral infarction (stroke). Increased pressure in the cerebral vessels can lead to development of microaneurysms and an increased risk for cerebral hemorrhage. *Hypertensive encephalopathy* may develop. This syndrome is characterized by extremely high blood pressure, altered level of consciousness, increased intracranial pressure, papilledema, and seizures. Its etiology is unclear.

Hypertension can lead to nephrosclerosis and renal insufficiency. Proteinuria and microscopic hematuria develop, as well as signs of chronic renal failure. African Americans experience hypertensive kidney disease more frequently than Caucasian Americans (Sorenson et al., 2019).

Interprofessional Care

Hypertension management focuses on reducing blood pressure to < 140 mmHg systolic and 90 mmHg diastolic. The ultimate goal of hypertension management is to reduce cardiovascular and renal morbidity and mortality. The risk of cardiovascular complications (coronary heart disease, heart failure, stroke) decreases when the average blood pressure is < 120/80 mmHg; when the patient also has diabetes or renal disease, the treatment goal is a blood pressure < 120/80 mmHg. It is now recognized that most people with hypertension will require a combination of two or more drugs along with lifestyle changes to achieve recommended blood pressure levels (Whelton et al., 2017). Although there is no cure for hypertension, it can be controlled. **Figure 32.2** ■ shows the updated 2017 recommended algorithm for hypertension management.

Diagnosis

The patient is evaluated for the presence of identifiable causes of hypertension, cardiovascular risk factors, and the presence or absence of target organ damage (heart, brain, kidneys, peripheral vascular systems, and retina of the eye). Before treatment is started, the following diagnostic tests are performed:

- Electrocardiogram (ECG)
- Urinalysis
- Blood glucose
- Hematocrit
- Serum potassium, creatinine, and calcium
- Cholesterol and lipoprotein profile, including high-density lipoprotein (HDL), low-density lipoprotein (LDL), and triglycerides.

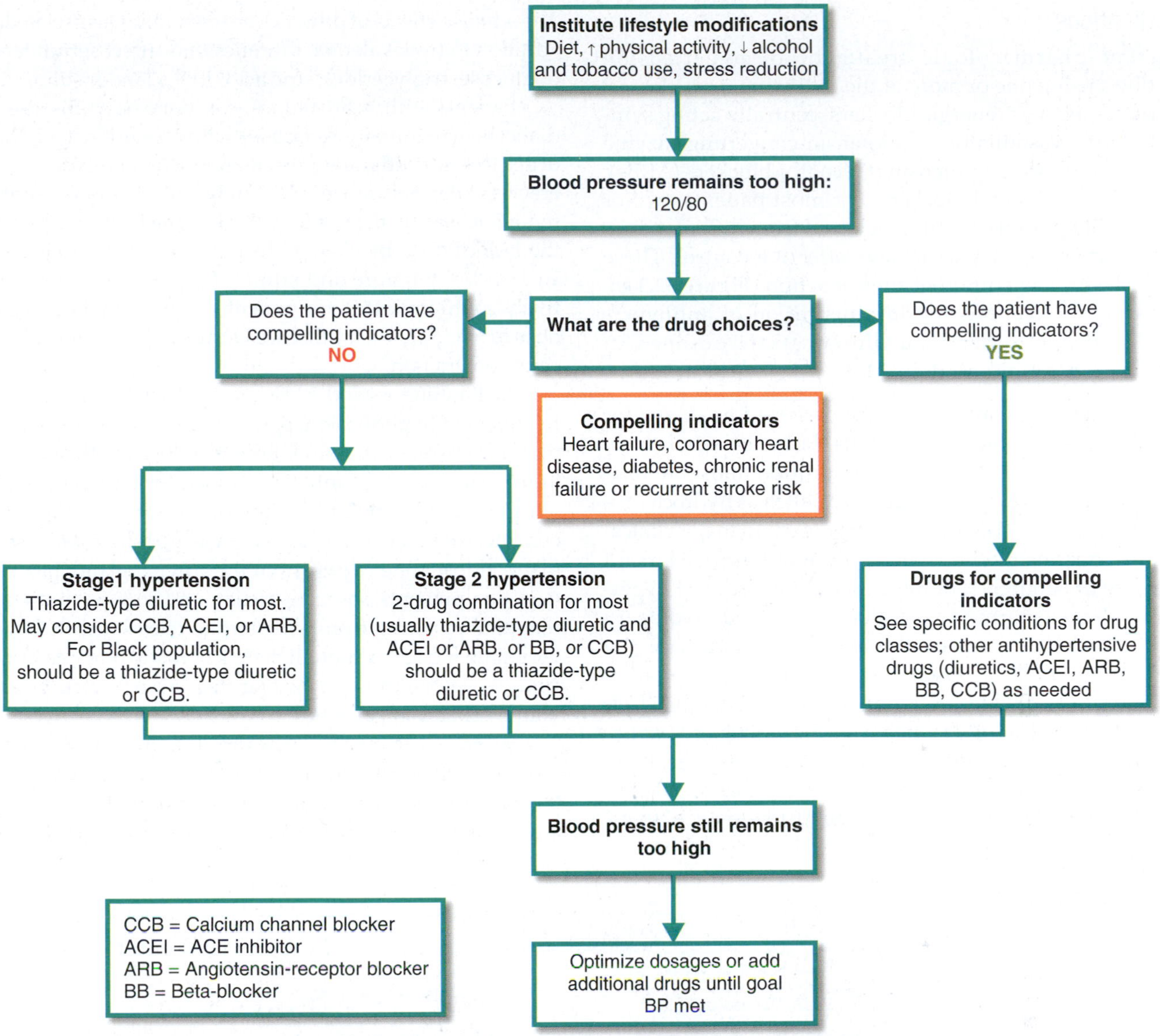
Institute lifestyle modifications
Diet, ↑ physical activity, ↓ alcohol and tobacco use, stress reduction
Blood pressure remains too high: 120/80
What are the drug choices?
Does the patient have compelling indicators? NO
Does the patient have compelling indicators? YES
Compelling indicators
Heart failure, coronary heart disease, diabetes, chronic renal failure or recurrent stroke risk
Stage1 hypertension
Thiazide-type diuretic for most. May consider CCB, ACEI, or ARB. For Black population, should be a thiazide-type diuretic or CCB.
Stage 2 hypertension
2-drug combination for most (usually thiazide-type diuretic and ACEI or ARB, or BB, or CCB) should be a thiazide-type diuretic or CCB.
Drugs for compelling indicators
See specific conditions for drug classes; other antihypertensive drugs (diuretics, ACEI, ARB, BB, CCB) as needed
Blood pressure still remains too high
Optimize dosages or add additional drugs until goal BP met
CCB = Calcium channel blocker
ACEI = ACE inhibitor
ARB = Angiotensin-receptor blocker
BB = Beta-blocker

Figure 32.2 ■ Algorithm for treating hypertension.

Additional tests that may be done include urinary albumin excretion, evaluation of the glomerular filtration rate (such as the creatinine clearance), and tests for emerging cardiovascular risk factors such as C-reactive protein and homocystine levels.

Lifestyle Modifications

Lifestyle modifications are recommended for all patients whose blood pressure falls within the elevated range (>120/>80 mmHg) and everyone with intermittent or sustained hypertension. These modifications include weight loss, dietary changes, restricted alcohol use and cigarette smoking, increased physical activity, and stress reduction.

Diet. Dietary approaches to managing hypertension focus on reducing sodium intake, maintaining adequate potassium and calcium intakes, and reducing total and saturated fat intake. A mild to moderate sodium restriction (no added salt) lowers blood pressure and potentiates the effect of antihypertensive drugs for most hypertensive patients. The DASH (Dietary Approaches to Stop Hypertension) diet has proven beneficial effects in lowering blood pressure. This diet focuses on whole foods rather than individual nutrients. It is rich in fruits and vegetables (up to 10 servings per day) and low in total and saturated fats. See Box 29.9 in Chapter 29 for more information.

Weight loss is recommended for patients who are obese. Loss of as little as 4.5 kg (10 lb) reduces blood pressure in many people. A balanced diet such as the DASH diet is recommended for weight loss.

Physical Activity. Regular exercise (such as walking, cycling, jogging, or swimming) reduces blood pressure and contributes to weight loss, stress reduction, and feelings of overall well-being. Previously sedentary patients are encouraged to engage in aerobic exercise for 30 to 45 minutes per day most days of the week (5 to 6 days). Isometric exercise (such as weight training) may not be appropriate because it can raise the systolic blood pressure.

Medications

Current pharmacologic treatment of hypertension involves using one or more of the following drug classes: Diuretics, beta-adrenergic blockers, centrally acting sympatholytics, vasodilators, angiotensin-converting enzyme (ACE) inhibitors, angiotensin II receptor blockers (ARBs), and calcium channel blockers. For most patients, two or more antihypertensive drugs selected from different drug classes are necessary to achieve effective control. These drug classes have different sites of action (**Figure 32.3** ■). Nursing implications for administration of antihypertensive drugs (other than diuretics) are outlined in **Medication Administration 32.A**.

Drug Classes. Diuretics are the preferred treatment for systolic hypertension in older adults. Diuretics are relatively safe and well-tolerated drugs; in addition, most are relatively inexpensive. Thiazide diuretics, such as hydrochlorothiazide (HydroDIURIL), are widely used. In major clinical studies, treatment with a single diuretic controlled blood pressure in about 50% of the patients and reduced hypertension-linked morbidity and mortality related to coronary heart disease. Diuretics control hypertension primarily by preventing tubular reabsorption of sodium, thus promoting sodium and water excretion and reducing blood volume. Thiazide diuretics reduce systemic vascular resistance through an unknown mechanism. Diuretics are particularly effective in Blacks and in patients who are obese, older, or who have increased plasma volume or low renin activity. The adverse effects of diuretics are generally dose related. In addition to hypokalemia, diuretics may affect serum levels of glucose, triglycerides, uric acid, LDLs, and insulin.

Patients with heart failure, coronary heart disease, or diabetes may initially be treated with a beta-blocker. These drugs lower blood pressure, apparently by reducing peripheral vascular resistance. They may reduce the amount of renin released by the kidneys by blocking $beta_1$ receptors in the kidney. Beta-blockers reduce the risk of complications such as heart failure and stroke. They are, however, relatively contraindicated for patients with asthma or chronic obstructive pulmonary disease because they promote bronchial constriction.

ACE inhibitors and ARBs are commonly used in initial treatment of hypertension, particularly for patients who are diabetic or who have heart failure, a history of MI, or chronic kidney disease. ACE inhibitors block formation of angiotensin II by inhibiting the action of angiotensin-converting enzyme. Angiotensin II is a potent vasoconstrictor that stimulates aldosterone release from the adrenal gland; blocking its action prevents vasoconstriction and sodium and water retention resulting from aldosterone release. ARBs have a very similar effect, although their action is to block angiotensin II receptors, thus preventing their vasoconstrictive and volume expansion effects.

Several drug classes work through their ability to promote vasodilation and reduce peripheral vascular resistance. Alpha-blockers such as prazosin and terazosin block stimulation of $alpha_1$-receptors on arterioles and veins,

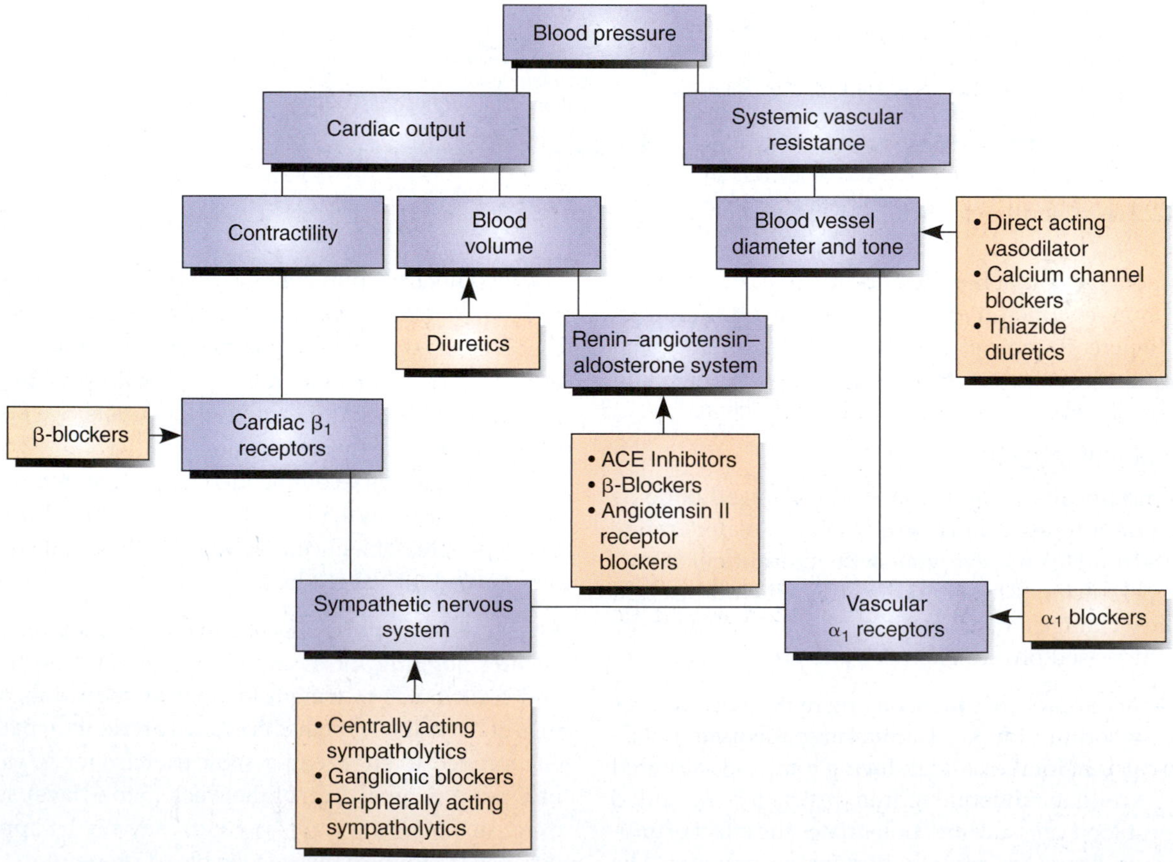

Blood pressure
Cardiac output
Systemic vascular resistance
Contractility
Blood volume
Blood vessel diameter and tone
• Direct acting vasodilator
• Calcium channel blockers
• Thiazide diuretics
Diuretics
Renin–angiotensin–aldosterone system
β-blockers
Cardiac β_1 receptors
• ACE Inhibitors
• β-Blockers
• Angiotensin II receptor blockers
Sympathetic nervous system
Vascular α_1 receptors
α_1 blockers
• Centrally acting sympatholytics
• Ganglionic blockers
• Peripherally acting sympatholytics

Figure 32.3 ■ Sites of antihypertensive drug action.

Medication Administration 32.A

Antihypertensive Drugs

PRIMARY AGENTS

Angiotensin-Converting Enzyme (ACE) Inhibitors

benazepril (Lotensin)	moexipril (Univasc)
captopril (Capoten)	perindopril (Aceon)
enalapril (Vasotec)	quinapril (Accupril)
fosinopril (Monopril)	ramipril (Altace)
lisinopril (Prinivil, Zestril)	trandolapril (Mavik)

Angiotensin II Receptor Blockers (ARBs)

azilsartan (Edarbi)	losartan (Cozaar)
candesartan (Atacand)	olmesartan (Benicar)
eprosartan (Teveten)	telmisartan (Micardis)
irbesartan (Avapro)	valsartan (Diovan)

The ACE inhibitors lower blood pressure by preventing conversion of angiotensin I to angiotensin II. This in turn prevents vasoconstriction and sodium and water retention. ARBs have the same effect, but they act by blocking the effect of angiotensin II on receptors. Both ACE inhibitors and ARBs are less effective in Black patients and are contraindicated in pregnancy (Adams, Holland, & Urban, 2017). Their primary adverse effects are persistent cough, first-dose hypotension, and hyperkalemia.

Nursing Responsibilities

- Assess blood pressure and WBC before giving the first dose. Monitor blood pressure for 2 hours after the first dose and regularly thereafter.
- Administer PO 1 hour before meals; tablets may be crushed.
- Report changes in WBCs or differential, hyperkalemia, or changes in BUN or serum creatinine to the primary care provider.
- Do not administer to patients with renal artery stenosis or who are pregnant.
- Immediately report and treat manifestations of angioedema (giant wheals and edema of the tongue, glottis, and pharynx). Initiate resuscitation measures as needed. Discontinue drug immediately and do not use in the future.

Health Education for the Patient and Family

- Report peripheral edema, signs of infection, or difficulty breathing to your primary care provider.
- Change position (lying to sitting and sitting to standing) slowly to prevent dizziness; sit down if dizziness or light-headedness develops.
- Do not take a potassium supplement or use a potassium-based salt substitute while taking this drug unless prescribed by your healthcare provider.
- Notify your healthcare provider if you become pregnant while taking this drug. Although it is safe early in pregnancy, taking the drug during the second and third trimesters may harm the fetus.

Calcium Channel Blockers

Dihydropyridines

amlodipine (Norvasc)	nicardipine (Cardene)
clevidipine (Cleviprex) (IV)	nifedipine (Procardia)
felodipine (Plendil)	nisoldipine (Sular)
isradipine (DynaCirc)	

Non-Dihydropyridines

diltiazem (Cardizem)	verapamil (Isoptin)

Calcium channel blockers inhibit the flow of calcium ions across the cell membrane of vascular tissue and cardiac cells. In doing so, they relax arterial smooth muscle, lowering peripheral resistance through vasodilation. Calcium channel blockers can cause reflex tachycardia, and some (e.g., verapamil and diltiazem) may impair cardiac function, worsening heart failure.

Nursing Responsibilities

- Assess blood pressure, apical pulse, and liver and renal function tests prior to giving these drugs.
- Calcium channel blockers may be given orally or intravenously.
- Do not administer verapamil or diltiazem to patients with severe hypotension, sinus, or atrioventricular blocks. Administer with caution to patients also taking digoxin or a beta-blocker.
- Periodically monitor blood pressure and apical pulse during therapy. Promptly report signs of bradycardia, AV block, or heart failure to the healthcare provider.

Health Education for the Patient and Family

- Take blood pressure and pulse daily as taught. Notify your healthcare provider if your pulse is < 60 bpm or your blood pressure is not within the specified range.
- This drug may cause constipation. Drink six to eight glasses of water each day, and increase fiber in diet.
- Report shortness of breath, weight gain, or swelling in feet or ankles to your primary care provider.

SECONDARY AGENTS

Alpha-Adrenergic Blockers

doxazosin (Cardura)	terazosin (Hytrin)
prazosin (Minipress)	

Alpha-adrenergic blocking agents block alpha-receptors in vascular smooth muscle, decreasing vasomotor tone and vasoconstriction. They also reduce serum levels of LDLs and very-low-density lipoproteins (VLDLs). However, vasodilation may cause orthostatic hypotension and reflex stimulation of the heart, resulting in tachycardia and palpitations. A beta-blocker may be ordered to minimize this effect.

Nursing Responsibilities

- Give the first dose at bedtime to minimize risk of fainting (called *first-dose syncope*). If the first dose is given in the daytime (or if the dose is increased), instruct to remain in bed for 3 to 4 hours.
- Assess blood pressure and apical pulse before each dose and as indicated thereafter.

Health Education for the Patient and Family

- There is a risk of fainting after taking the first dose of this drug. Take the drug at bedtime to reduce this risk, and do not drive or engage in other hazardous activities for 12 to 24 hours after the first dose.
- This drug may cause dizziness or light-headedness. Change positions slowly, and sit down if you become dizzy or light-headed.
- Notify your primary care provider if you develop nasal congestion or impotence while taking this drug.
- Notify your primary care provider before discontinuing this medication.

(*continued*)

Beta-Adrenergic Blocking Agents

acebutolol (Sectral)	nadolol (Corgard)
atenolol (Tenormin)	nebivolol (Bystolic)
betaxolol (Kerlone)	penbutolol (Levatol)
bisoprolol (Zebeta)	pindolol (Visken)
carteolol (Cartrol)	propranolol (Inderal)
esmolol (Brevibloc)	sotalol (Betapace)
metoprolol tartrate (Lopressor)	timolol (Blocadren)

Combined with an alpha-blocker:

carvedilol (Coreg)	labetalol (Normodyne)

Beta-adrenergic blockers are less commonly used as initial therapy to control hypertension (Adams et al., 2017). Beta-blockers reduce blood pressure by preventing beta-receptor stimulation in the heart, thereby decreasing heart rate and cardiac output. Beta-blockers also interfere with renin release by the kidneys, decreasing the effects of angiotensin and aldosterone. Potential adverse effects of beta-blockers include bronchospasm, fatigue, sleep disturbances, nightmares, bradycardia, heart block, worsening of heart failure, gastrointestinal disturbances, impotence, and increased triglyceride levels.

Nursing Responsibilities

- Before giving initial dose, assess for contraindications to beta-blockers such as asthma, chronic lung disease, bradycardia, or heart block.
- Assess blood pressure and apical pulse before giving dosage; notify primary care provider if vital signs are outside established parameters.
- Report adverse effects such as bradycardia, decreased cardiac output (fatigue, dyspnea with exertion, hypotension, decreased level of consciousness), heart failure, heart block, bronchoconstriction (wheezing, dyspnea), or altered blood glucose levels (in patients with diabetes).
- Carefully monitor responses of the older patient.

Health Education for the Patient and Family

- Monitor blood pressure and pulse daily as instructed.
- Change position (lying to sitting and sitting to standing) slowly to prevent dizziness and possible falls.
- Report effects such as fatigue, lethargy, and impotence to your healthcare provider.
- Notify your healthcare provider if you become short of breath or develop a cough or swelling of your extremities.
- If you have diabetes, check blood glucose levels more frequently because hypoglycemia may develop with few symptoms.
- Talk to your healthcare provider before taking any over-the-counter medications.
- Carry an adequate supply of the drug when traveling. Do not stop taking this drug without notifying your healthcare provider.

Centrally Acting Sympatholytics

clonidine (Catapres)	methyldopa (generic only)
guanfacine (Tenex)	reserpine (generic only)

The centrally acting sympatholytics stimulate the alpha$_2$-receptors in the CNS to suppress sympathetic outflow to the heart and blood vessels. A fall in cardiac output and vasodilation results, reducing blood pressure. Dry mouth and sedation are common adverse effects. Severe reflex hypertension may occur if abruptly discontinued. Clonidine is contraindicated during pregnancy; methyldopa is contraindicated for patients with active liver disease.

Nursing Responsibilities

- Assess for contraindications to therapy. Obtain baseline blood pressure, CBC, Coombs' test, and liver function studies.
- Administer oral doses at bedtime to minimize effects of sedation.
- Methyldopa may be given intravenously for hypertensive emergencies.
- Apply transdermal clonidine patch to dry, hairless area of intact skin on the chest or upper arm. Assess for rash, which indicates allergy, at area of application.
- Promptly report changes in laboratory values to the healthcare provider. Discontinue methyldopa if manifestations of liver dysfunction develop.

Health Education for the Patient and Family

- Relieve dry mouth by sipping water or chewing sugarless gum.
- Take with meals if gastric upset or nausea develops.
- Change position (lying to sitting and sitting to standing) slowly to prevent dizziness and possible falls.
- Do not suddenly discontinue medication or skip doses; this could cause serious hypertension.
- Report mental depression or decreased mental acuity to your healthcare provider.
- Side effects (such as dry mouth, nausea, and dizziness) tend to diminish over time.
- Do not drive a car if the medications cause drowsiness.

VASODILATORS

hydralazine (Apresoline)

Vasodilators reduce blood pressure by relaxing vascular smooth muscle (especially in the arterioles) and decreasing peripheral vascular resistance. These drugs are often prescribed in combination with a diuretic or beta-blocker because they can cause reflex tachycardia and fluid retention. Because these drugs can have significant toxic effects, they are not routinely used to manage chronic hypertension.

Nursing Responsibilities

- Hydralazine may be given orally or intravenously.
- Assess blood pressure and pulse before giving the drug and monitor during therapy as indicated. Report tachycardia or hypotension to the healthcare provider.
- Report peripheral edema and manifestations of volume overload and heart failure.
- Immediately report muffled heart sounds or paradoxical pulse as pericardial effusion and possible cardiac tamponade may develop during minoxidil therapy.
- Discontinue hydralazine and report manifestations of a systemic lupus erythematosus–like syndrome: Muscle or joint pain, fever, or symptoms of nephritis or pericarditis.

Health Education for the Patient and Family

- Change position (lying to sitting and sitting to standing) slowly to prevent dizziness and possible falls.
- Report muscle, joint aches, and fever to your healthcare provider.
- Headache, palpitations, and rapid pulse may develop but should abate in about 10 days.
- Do not discontinue the medication without talking to your healthcare provider.

Note: Drugs identified in blue are among the 200 most commonly prescribed medications in the United States.

Source: Adams, Holland, & Urban, 2017.

preventing vasoconstriction. Because of their ability to dilate both arterioles and veins, alpha-blockers can cause significant orthostatic hypotension, particularly following the initial dose.

Calcium channel blockers promote dilation of arterioles, the primary regulators of peripheral vascular resistance. These drugs can cause reflex tachycardia. Some calcium channel blockers, verapamil and diltiazem in particular, also suppress heart function, reducing stroke volume and cardiac output. Reflex tachycardia is minimal with these calcium channel blockers. Direct-acting vasodilators such as hydralazine and minoxidil directly affect the arterioles, reducing peripheral vascular resistance. These drugs have little effect on veins, so the risk of orthostatic hypotension is minimal. They are, however, associated with reflex tachycardia and fluid retention, so rarely are they administered as in single-drug treatment regimens.

Other factors considered in selecting drugs for treating hypertension include demographic characteristics of the patient, concurrent conditions, quality of life, cost, and possible interactions among prescribed drugs. In general, diuretics and calcium channel blockers are more effective for treating hypertension in Blacks than beta-blockers or ACE inhibitors. Beta-blockers are preferred to treat hypertension with concurrent coronary heart disease and angina, but are contraindicated for patients who have asthma or depression. Beta-blockers reduce exercise tolerance and may adversely affect lifestyle for some patients.

Drug Regimens. Treatment is usually initiated using a single antihypertensive drug at a low dose. Unless otherwise indicated, a diuretic is recommended as the initial drug of choice. The dose is slowly increased until optimal blood pressure control is achieved. If the drug does not effectively lower the blood pressure or has troubling side effects, a different drug from another class of antihypertensive medications is substituted. On the other hand, if the drug is tolerated well but has not lowered blood pressure to the desired level, a second drug from another class may be added to the treatment regimen.

Treatment of patients with stage 2 hypertension is generally more aggressive to minimize the risk of myocardial infarction (MI), heart failure, or stroke. When the blood pressure is > 180/120 mmHg (hypertensive crisis), immediate therapy, and possible hospitalization, is vital.

After a year of effective hypertension control, an effort may be made to reduce the dosage and number of drugs. This is known as *step-down therapy*. It is more successful in patients who have made lifestyle modifications. Careful blood pressure monitoring is necessary during and after step-down therapy because the blood pressure often rises again to hypertensive levels.

Integrative Therapies

Behavioral and mind–body therapies may be helpful for some patients in lowering blood pressure (see Moving Evidence into Action). The blood pressure increases in response to physiologic and psychologic stress and anxiety. Mind–body therapies such as yoga, tai chi, meditation, and guided imagery are designed to modify both physiologic and cognitive aspects of the stress response.

Nursing Care

Assessment

See the Manifestations and Interprofessional Care sections for the assessment of the patient with hypertension.

Moving Evidence into Action

Hypotensive Effect of Yoga Breathing Exercises

Clinical Issue

Standard therapies for hypertension include lifestyle changes and medications. The addition of a simple integrative therapy such as yoga breathing may have a positive benefit on blood pressure with minimal patient burden.

External Evidence

Brandani, Mizuno, Ciolac, and Monteiro (2017) conducted a systematic review of the impact of yoga breathing on blood pressure reduction. The review included 13 trials, assessing eight acute studies and five chronic studies of BP response to pranayama yoga breathing. They found significant BP reductions after yoga breathing in both short-term and long-term yoga studies. Limitations reported included low-quality studies, but the hypotensive effect of the yoga breathing was encouraging. Breathing with slower rhythms and nostril manipulation (left vs. right) had better results.

Internal Evidence

As part of the evaluation of internal evidence, one must consider the patient's interest in and willingness to use an integrative therapy. Additionally, the proposed intervention should also be considered in light of the healthcare team stakeholders that can influence patient willingness to use a new intervention.

Patient Considerations

When considering use of a new practice (like yoga breathing exercises), the nurse must consider the specific patient population where it will be used. Will patients and their families be amenable to the new intervention?

Putting the Pieces Together

Yoga is gentle for most patients. The use of yoga breathing would have minimal burden on the patient. A simple intervention such as this can be easily implemented with minimal cost and time. To effectively implement such a new intervention, it is important to evaluate the external evidence and consider the internal implications and patient/family issues. This simple intervention has the potential to improve blood pressure control.

Reference

Brandani, J. Z., Mizuno, J., Ciolac, E. G., & Monteiro, H. L. (2017). The hypotensive effect of Yoga's breathing exercises: A systematic review. *Complementary Therapy in Clinical Practice, 28*, 38–46. DOI: 10.1016/j.ctcp.2017.05.002

Focused assessment of the patient with hypertension includes:

- *Health history:* Complaints of morning headache, cervical pain; cardiovascular or central nervous system (CNS) manifestations; history of hypertension, renal disease, diabetes; family history of high blood pressure, heart failure, or kidney disease; current medications
- *Physical assessment:* Vital signs including blood pressure in both arms, apical and peripheral pulses; ophthalmologic exam of retinal fundus as appropriate
- *Laboratory data:* Serum electrolytes, glucose, and creatinine; cholesterol and lipoprotein profile; urinalysis.

Priorities of Care

Collaborating with the interprofessional team to ensure adequate treatment of the underlying process while providing care that supports the physical and psychologic responses to the disorder is a priority of nursing care.

Diagnoses, Outcomes, and Interventions

All patients with primary hypertension and their families need significant teaching to manage this chronic condition. Health maintenance is a high-priority problem. Depending on the stage of hypertension and concurrent illnesses, other appropriate nursing priorities may include promoting good nutrition, monitoring fluid volume, and ensuring adherence to the treatment regimen.

Promote a Healthy Lifestyle and Behaviors. An unhealthy lifestyle and behaviors can contribute to health problems such as hypertension. When hypertension has been identified, knowledge of the disease and its management is vital for the patient. Willingness to take responsibility for hypertension management is central to effective blood pressure control. Adopting healthy lifestyle changes enhances drug therapy; in some cases, the need for medications may be eliminated or reduced. Because hypertension is often an asymptomatic disease and many antihypertensive drugs have unpleasant side effects, it is vital that the patient understand the chronic progressive nature of the disease and its long-term consequences.

Expected Outcome: Patient will be knowledgeable about management of hypertension as evidenced by being able to describe the components and rationale for the treatment plan.

The nurse will:

- Assist with identifying current behaviors that contribute to hypertension. *The patient must first identify contributory behaviors before he or she can change them. Using knowledge of hypertension risk factors, the nurse can help identify behaviors and factors contributing to hypertension that can be changed. Including the family in this process is important to reduce potential sabotage of the patient's efforts to adopt healthier behaviors.*
- Assist in developing a realistic health maintenance plan. *Preparing a health maintenance plan for the patient does little to encourage personal responsibility for health. However, nurses can guide patients in developing realistic goals and expectations for the treatment plan and modifying risk factors such as smoking, exercise, diet, and stress.*
- Help the patient and family identify strengths and weaknesses in maintaining health. *Discussing areas of the health maintenance plan that are working well and those that present difficulties can help to identify necessary changes in the plan and additional strategies for implementing it.*

Monitor Adherence to Therapeutic Plan. Nonadherence, or failure to follow the identified treatment plan, is a continuing risk for any patient with a chronic disease. Recommended lifestyle changes such as diet, exercise, restricted alcohol intake, stress reduction, and smoking cessation are often difficult to maintain on a continuing basis. In addition, prescribed medications may have undesirable effects, whereas hypertension itself often has no symptoms or noticeable effects.

Expected Outcome: Patient will adhere to the treatment plan.

The nurse will:

- Inquire about reasons for nonadherence with the recommended treatment plan. Listen openly and without judging. *Nonthreatening discussion of factors contributing to nonadherence validates the patient's self-esteem and partnership in the treatment plan.*
- Assess factors contributing to nonadherence, such as adverse drug effects. Suggest measures to manage adverse effects or, if indicated, contact the primary care provider about possible alternative drugs. *Some adverse effects of antihypertensive drugs, such as gastric upset, light headedness, or nocturia, may be easily managed by changing the timing of the drug dose. Others, such as fatigue, decreased exercise tolerance, or impotence, may interfere with lifestyle and life roles to the extent that the patient finds them intolerable.*
- Evaluate knowledge of hypertension, its long-term effects, and treatment. Provide additional information and reinforce teaching as needed. *Knowledge increases the sense of control, which increases the likelihood of compliance with treatment.*
- Assist to develop realistic short-term goals for lifestyle changes. *Attempting to lose weight, exercise daily, stop smoking, and dramatically change the diet all at the same time may be overwhelming, leading to a sense of failure. Smaller, gradual changes are more easily incorporated into lifestyle and daily activities, improving compliance.*
- Work with the patient to develop mutual outcomes for the treatment plan. Discuss measures to improve compliance. The patient has absolute control over compliance with the treatment plan. *Demonstrating respect and involving the patient in decision making and planning can improve compliance.*
- Help the patient identify cues and develop reminders (e.g., written notes, a medication box filled weekly) to assist with maintaining a schedule for exercise

and medications. *Cues and other devices provide helpful reminders of activities and schedules until they are incorporated into habits.*

- Reassure the patient that relapse into old habits and behaviors is common. Encourage avoiding feelings of guilt associated with relapse, and use the circumstance to renew efforts to comply with treatment. *Guilt and feelings of failure can lead to further noncompliance unless the event is used to identify reasons for noncompliance and ways to prevent it from recurring in the future.*

Promote Balanced Nutrition. The relationship between obesity, excess alcohol intake, and hypertension is well documented. Hypertension is particularly associated with central obesity, identified by waist circumference greater than hip circumference. Although achieving weight loss is difficult and takes a commitment to changing eating and exercise habits, it is possible for most patients to achieve.

Expected Outcomes: If obese, patient will practice weight loss behaviors as evidenced by use of food diaries, selection of a healthy target weight, and following of a consistent exercise program.

The nurse will:

- Assess usual daily food intake, and discuss possible contributing factors to excess weight, such as sedentary lifestyle or using food as a reward or stress reliever. Inquire about diversional activities, exercise patterns, and previous weight reduction efforts (e.g., participation in weight reduction programs or using fad or crash diets). *Assessment data provides clues about contributing factors to obesity, the patient's knowledge base about the relationship between eating and exercise habits and weight, and safe weight loss strategies. This provides direction for further teaching and for developing a realistic weight reduction plan.*
- Mutually determine with the patient a realistic target weight (e.g., loss of 10% of current body weight over a 6-month period). Regularly monitor weight. Encourage a system of nonfood rewards for achieving small, incremental goals. *Setting weight loss goals helps formalize the process and provides motivation for continued progress. Developing realistic goals may be difficult; unrealistic goals, however, set the patient up for failure. Continuous incremental weight loss provides reassurance that it can be achieved and promotes permanent weight reduction.*
- Refer the patient to a dietitian for information about low-fat, low-calorie foods and eating plans. Focus on changing eating habits as opposed to "following a diet." *Focusing on changing eating habits promotes the sense that low-fat, low-calorie eating patterns should become a part of lifestyle rather than a short-term measure to be endured until the weight loss goal is achieved.*
- Recommend participating in an approved weight loss program such as Weight Watchers, Overeaters Anonymous, or Take Off Pounds Sensibly (TOPS). *Organized weight loss programs provide structure for a balanced weight reduction program, as well as mutual support from others trying to lose weight.*

Monitor Fluid Volume. Excess fluid volume often contributes to hypertension by increasing the cardiac output. A number of factors associated with hypertension can cause excess fluid volume, including sodium retention and disruption of the RAAS. In addition, some antihypertensive drugs, such as calcium channel blockers and vasodilators, can contribute to excess fluid in the interstitial spaces and peripheral edema.

Expected Outcome: Patient's fluid volume will be normal as evidenced by weight loss and decreases in edema, jugular venous distention, and abdominal distention.

The nurse will:

- Monitor blood pressure and other vital signs as indicated: Every 1 to 2 hours or more frequently during acute hypertensive states; or once a week or more frequently during initial treatment outside of the hospital setting. *Vital signs are an indicator of fluid balance and the effectiveness of treatment. An elevated blood pressure, pulse, and respiratory rate may indicate fluid retention, whereas orthostatic hypotension and tachycardia may indicate fluid volume deficit.*
- Monitor intake and output, and weigh daily (if in an acute or long-term care facility) or weekly (in the community). *Rapid weight changes (over days) more accurately reflect fluid balance than intake and output records. One liter of fluid weighs 1 kg (2.2 lb). Weight changes and intake and output records help monitor the effects of therapy.*
- Monitor for peripheral edema (sacral edema in the bedridden patient). *Drugs such as vasodilators can cause fluid accumulation in interstitial tissues, leading to peripheral or dependent edema. Adding a diuretic to the treatment plan may be necessary.*
- Refer to a dietitian for teaching about a restricted sodium diet. Discuss the relationship between sodium intake and fluid retention. Provide opportunities to choose low-sodium foods from simulated menus. Support efforts, and reassure that lifestyle changes such as consuming less sodium take time. *Knowledge provides the power to take control of sodium intake. Patience and perseverance are needed to succeed; positive reinforcement of efforts to change long-standing dietary patterns is important.*
- Monitor laboratory values, such as blood urea nitrogen (BUN), urine specific gravity, creatinine, electrolytes, and hematocrit and hemoglobin. Hypertension can alter renal perfusion and function, leading to fluid retention and altered laboratory values (Kee, 2014). *Changes in BUN and creatinine indicate impaired renal function, whereas changes in hematocrit and hemoglobin often reflect changes in fluid volume.*
- Discuss the importance of adhering to treatment plans such as dietary restrictions and medication schedules. *Understanding the rationale for treatment measures promotes the patient's sense of control and encourages compliance with the treatment regimen.*

Controlling high blood pressure is as important in the older adult as in younger adults. In the United States, the lifetime risk of hypertension is about 90% in men and women who live to age 80 to 85 (Benjamin et al., 2017). Systolic hypertension is common, as is an elevated pulse pressure (systolic BP minus diastolic BP), indicating decreased compliance of large arteries.

The Framingham Heart Study (2017) shows that cardiovascular deaths are two to five times more common in older adults with isolated systolic hypertension than in people with normal blood pressures. Stroke is more common in older adults with systolic hypertension. These findings appear to relate to changes in blood vessels associated with aging: Decreased compliance and decreased baroreceptor sensitivity. Decreased compliance impairs the ability of the vessels to expand and contract with varying amounts of blood, increasing peripheral vascular resistance and decreasing renal blood flow.

To obtain accurate blood pressure readings for older patients, slightly different procedures may be required. Palpation of the artery during cuff inflation is recommended to prevent inaccurate systolic readings due to an auscultatory gap, present in many older adults. The reflexes that maintain blood pressure during position changes diminish with age. Allow the older patient to sit upright or stand for 2 to 5 minutes before evaluating the blood pressure for true orthostatic readings.

Transitions of Care

Prevention of hypertension focuses teaching about the modifiable risk factors for hypertension. Advise all patients (as well as children and adolescents) to stop or never start smoking. Discuss the risks of obesity, excess alcohol intake, and a sedentary lifestyle with patients. Encourage all patients to eat a diet rich in fruits and vegetables and low in total and saturated fat. Discuss the potential benefits of following the DASH diet or a similar eating plan. Advise all patients to remain active and engage in aerobic exercise 5 or more days a week. Discuss the stress-reducing benefits of exercise.

Hypertensive crisis (BP > 180/> 120 mmHg) requires acute evaluation and treatment. With determination of the critical blood pressure, the evaluation for target organ damage (microvascular or macrovascular injuries) occurs next. If target organ damage is present, a hypertensive emergency is occurring, and ICU admission is required with treatment focused on BP reduction. Presence of life-threatening processes (aortic dissection, severe pre-eclampsia/eclampsia, or pheochromocytoma crisis) may result from rapid BP reduction (Whelton et al., 2017). Effective control of hypertension requires the patient to not only participate in the plan of care, but also to take an active role in managing the disease. Treatment is managed in community settings, with regular visits to a clinic or office to monitor blood pressure and effects of treatment measures. Include the following topics when teaching the patient and family about hypertension:

- ***Increase activity gradually.*** Develop a realistic exercise program that is enjoyable and fits into the patient's lifestyle. Identify an exercise buddy for additional motivation. Activity and exercise, through a gradual conditioning of muscles and blood vessels, lower blood pressure by reducing peripheral vascular resistance. As the heart becomes conditioned and pumps more efficiently, kidney perfusion improves and intravascular volume falls, further reducing blood pressure. Exercise reduces stress and contributes to weight loss and maintenance. Aerobic exercises, such as walking, jogging, swimming, and cycling, are appropriate; isometric activities (such as weight lifting) should be avoided without healthcare provider approval.
- ***Adopt healthy eating patterns.*** Follow a low-fat, low-cholesterol, moderate-sodium diet that is rich in fruits and vegetables and includes at least two servings of low-fat milk or milk products daily. Do not give up if you slip into old eating habits on occasion; use such occasions to identify ways to avoid future lapses.
- ***Stop smoking.*** Participate in organized smoking-cessation programs or use aids such as nicotine patches can help.
- ***Use alcohol in moderation if at all.*** Consume no more than 1.5 oz of hard liquor, 5 to 10 oz of wine, or 12 to 20 oz of beer per day.
- ***Use stress-reducing techniques*** such as meditation, relaxation, deep breathing, and exercise to manage stress. Anger and hostility intensify vasoconstriction; channeling these emotions into more positive responses such as using a change process to modify factors that provoke these emotions can reduce their harmful effects on blood pressure.
- ***Understand prescribed medications***, their intended effect, dose and timing, interactions, and possible adverse effects. Discuss effects that should be reported to the healthcare provider and those that can be managed by the patient or that will diminish over time.
- ***Know the importance of monitoring blood pressure*** and regular visits to the primary care provider or hypertension clinic to monitor treatment. During follow-up visits, assess the blood pressure and specific laboratory work (such as serum creatinine, BUN, and/or serum electrolytes) to evaluate the disease and the effects of antihypertensive medications.

Refer the patient to community blood pressure clinics and to home health services as needed for regular follow-up and reinforcement of teaching. Refer to a dietitian or to an organized weight loss program as indicated for further teaching and weight loss support. The accompanying Case Study & Nursing Care Plan provides additional information about community-based care for the patient with high blood pressure.

Offer blood pressure screening, and refer patients for follow-up as indicated (**Table 32.2**).

Table 32.2 Recommended Blood Pressure Follow-Up

Category	Blood Pressure (mmHg)	Recommended Follow-Up
Normal	< 120/80	Recheck in 1 year
Elevated	120–129/80	Recheck in 3 to 6 months
Stage 1 hypertension	130–139/80-89	Confirm within 1 month
Stage 2 hypertension	≥ 140/> 90	Evaluate within 1 month

Case Study & Nursing Care Plan

A Patient with Hypertension

Margaret Spezia is a married, 49-year-old woman with eight children whose ages range from 3 to 18 years. For the past 2 months, Mrs. Spezia has had frequent morning headaches and occasional dizziness and blurred vision. At her annual physical examination 1 month ago, her blood pressure was 168/104 and 156/94 mmHg. She was instructed to reduce her fat and cholesterol intake, to avoid using salt at the table, and to start walking for 30 to 45 minutes daily. Mrs. Spezia returns to the clinic for a follow-up.

ASSESSMENT

While escorting Mrs. Spezia to the exam room and obtaining her weight, blood pressure, and history, Lisa Christos, RN, notices that Mrs. Spezia seems restless and upset. Ms. Christos says, "You look upset about something. Is everything OK?" Mrs. Spezia responds, "Well, my head is throbbing, and I'm sort of dizzy. I think I'm just overdoing it and not getting enough rest. You know, raising eight children is a lot of work and expense. I just started working part time so we wouldn't get behind in our bills. I thought the extra money might relieve some of my stress, but I'm not so sure that's really happening. I'm not getting any better and I'm worried that I'll lose my job or become disabled and that my husband won't be able to manage the children by himself. I really need to go home, but first, I want to get rid of this awful headache. Would you please get me a couple of aspirin or something?"

Mrs. Spezia's history shows a steady weight gain during the past 18 years. She has no known family history of hypertension. Physical findings include height 160 cm (63 in.); weight 102 kg (225 lb); T 37.2°C (99°F); P 100 bpm and regular; R 16/min; BP 180/115 (lying), 170/110 (sitting), 165/105 mmHg (standing); average 10-point difference in readings between right and left arm (lower on left). Skin cool and dry, capillary refill 4 seconds right hand, 3 seconds left hand. Mrs. Spezia's total serum cholesterol is 245 mg/dL (normal < 200 mg/dL). All other blood and urine studies are within normal limits. Based on analysis of the data, Mrs. Spezia is started on enalapril 5 mg and hydrochlorothiazide 12.5 mg in a combination drug (Vaseretic) and placed on a low-fat, low-cholesterol, no-added-salt diet.

DIAGNOSES

- Fatigue due to effects of hypertension and stresses of daily life
- Obesity related to excessive food intake
- Inability to maintain a healthy lifestyle
- Insufficient understanding of effects of prescribed treatment

EXPECTED OUTCOMES

- Patient will reduce blood pressure readings to < 150 systolic and 90 diastolic by return visit next week.
- Patient will incorporate low-sodium and low-fat foods into her diet from a provided list.
- Patient will develop a plan for regular exercise.
- Patient will verbalize understanding of the effects of prescribed drug, dietary restrictions, exercise, and follow-up visits to help control hypertension.

PLANNING AND IMPLEMENTATION

- Teach to take own blood pressure daily and record it, bringing the record to scheduled clinic visits.
- Teach name, dose, action, and side effects of her antihypertensive medication.
- Instruct to walk for 15 minutes each day this week and to investigate swimming classes at the local pool.
- Discuss strategies for achieving a realistic weight loss goal.
- Refer patient to a dietary consultation for further teaching about fat and sodium restrictions.
- Discuss stress-reducing techniques, helping identify possible choices.

(continued)

EVALUATION

Mrs. Spezia returns to the clinic 1 week later. Her average blood pressure is now 138/80 mmHg. She has lost 1.5 lb and states that her oldest daughter has suggested that they join a weight reduction program together. Mrs. Spezia is walking for an average of 20 minutes at a local mall each day. She verbalizes an understanding of her medication and is taking it in the morning and before dinner each day. She met with the dietitian and discussed ways to reduce the sodium and fat in her diet. The dietitian provided a list of low-fat, low-sodium foods and recommended cookbooks to help Mrs. Spezia modify her cooking. Mrs. Spezia tells Ms. Christos, "I just can't believe how much better I feel already. My headaches are gone, I've actually lost some weight, and I feel motivated to keep going. If I had only known how much better I could feel! I don't expect I'll ever go back to my old habits again; it's just not worth it!"

CLINICAL REASONING IN PATIENT CARE

1. Identify the factors that contributed to Mrs. Spezia's hypertension. Which were modifiable and which were not?
2. What is the rationale for reducing sodium and fat in Mrs. Spezia's diet?
3. Suppose your hypertensive patient is homeless and has no source of income. How could you help ensure your patient would follow the treatment plan? What would you do if the patient did not follow it?
4. Discuss the role of stress in hypertension. What factors in Mrs. Spezia's life contribute to her stress level?

See Evaluating Your Response in Appendix B.

The Patient with Secondary Hypertension

Secondary hypertension is elevated blood pressure resulting from an identifiable underlying process. It accounts for only 5 to 10% of identified cases of hypertension. Kidney disease is the most common identifiable cause of high blood pressure in both adults and children (Sorenson et al., 2019). Other common identifiable causes of hypertension in adults include renovascular disease (reduced blood flow to the kidneys), disorders of the adrenal cortex, pheochromocytoma, coarctation of the aorta, and sleep apnea. The pathophysiology of selected causes of high blood pressure are summarized as follows:

- ***Kidney disease.*** Any disease that affects renal blood flow (e.g., renal artery stenosis) or renal function (e.g., glomerulonephritis, renal failure) can lead to hypertension. Disruption of the blood supply stimulates the RAAS, with resulting vasoconstriction and sodium and water retention. Altered kidney function affects the elimination of water and electrolytes, leading to hypertension.
- ***Coarctation of the aorta.*** Coarctation of the aorta is narrowing of the aorta, usually just distal to the subclavian arteries. Reduced renal and peripheral blood flow stimulates the RAAS and local vasoconstrictive responses, raising the blood pressure. A marked difference between pressures in the upper and lower extremities is common, with weak pulses and poor capillary refill in the lower extremities.
- ***Endocrine disorders.*** Adrenal gland disorders such as Cushing syndrome and primary aldosteronism can cause hypertension. A rare tumor of the adrenal medulla, *pheochromocytoma*, causes persistent or intermittent hypertension. Other endocrine disorders such as hyperthyroidism and pituitary disorders can also lead to hypertension.
- ***Neurologic disorders.*** Increased intracranial pressure causes an elevated blood pressure as the body attempts to maintain cerebral blood flow. Disorders that interfere with autonomic nervous system regulation (such as high spinal cord injury) may allow the sympathetic nervous system to predominate, increasing systemic vascular resistance and blood pressure.
- ***Drug use.*** Estrogen and oral contraceptive use may lead to hypertension, possibly by prompting sodium and water retention and affecting the RAAS. Stimulant drugs, such as cocaine and methamphetamines, increase systemic vascular resistance and cardiac output, resulting in hypertension.
- ***Pregnancy.*** Hypertension is the most common medical disorder among pregnant women. Hypertension may predate pregnancy or may occur as a direct response to the pregnancy. The mechanisms of hypertensive disorders of pregnancy are unclear, and they are a significant cause of maternal and fetal morbidity and mortality and require careful perinatal management.

The pattern of secondary hypertension varies, depending on its cause. Pheochromocytoma may cause attacks of hypertension that last for minutes to hours, accompanied by anxiety, palpitations, diaphoresis, pallor, and nausea and vomiting. Primary aldosteronism may cause hypertension, weakness, paresthesias, polyuria, and nocturia (see Chapter 19). Symptoms of kidney disease accompany hypertension when a renal disorder is the cause.

The following diagnostic tests may be ordered to differentiate primary from secondary hypertension.

- ***Renal function studies*** and *urinalysis* identify renal causes of hypertension. Elevated serum creatinine and BUN, reduced creatinine clearance, and hematuria, proteinuria, and casts often indicate kidney disease.
- ***Serum potassium*** is decreased in hyperaldosteronism.

- ***Blood chemistries***, including serum electrolytes, glucose, and lipid studies, are done to detect abnormalities indicative of endocrine or cardiovascular disease.
- ***Intravenous pyelography (IVP)***, *renal ultrasonography*, *renal arteriography*, and *computed tomography (CT)* or *magnetic resonance imaging (MRI)* may be done when secondary hypertension is suspected.

Interprofessional and nursing care for the patient with secondary hypertension is the same as that for primary hypertension, discussed in the previous section. In addition, the underlying process is treated. See chapters covering specific disorders for more information about treatment measures.

The Patient with Hypertensive Crisis

Some patients with hypertension may, for reasons not clearly understood, develop rapid, significant elevations in systolic and/or diastolic pressures. In a *hypertensive crisis* (also called *hypertensive emergency* or *malignant hypertension*) the systolic pressure is > 180 mmHg and the diastolic pressure is higher than 120 mmHg. Immediate treatment (within 1 hour) is vital to prevent cardiac, renal, and vascular damage and to reduce morbidity and mortality. Intense cerebral artery spasms help protect the brain from excess pressure; however, cerebral edema often develops. Prolonged severe hypertension damages walls of the arterioles and renal blood vessels and may lead to intravascular coagulation and acute renal failure.

Patients presenting with a hypertensive crisis may have manifestations such as:

- Rapid onset
- Blurred vision, papilledema (swelling of the optic nerve)
- Restlessness
- Systolic pressure > 180 mmHg
- Diastolic pressure > 120 mmHg
- Headache
- Confusion
- Motor and sensory deficits.

Most hypertensive emergencies occur when patients suddenly stop taking their medications or their hypertension is poorly controlled. Younger patients (30 to 50 years old), African American men, pregnant women with preeclampsia, and people with collagen and/or renal disease are also at higher risk for a hypertensive crisis (Sorenson et al., 2019).

The goal of care in hypertensive emergencies is to reduce the blood pressure by no more than 25% within minutes to 1 hour, then toward 160/100 within 2 to 6 hours. It is important to avoid rapid or excessive blood pressure decreases that may lead to renal, cerebral, or cardiac ischemia. Blood pressure is monitored frequently (every 5 to 30 minutes) during a hypertensive emergency (Whelton et al., 2017). The BUN, serum creatinine, calcium, and total protein levels are carefully monitored to help determine the prognosis for recovery. Drug treatment for malignant hypertension includes parenteral administration of a rapidly acting antihypertensive, such as the potent vasodilator sodium nitroprusside (Nipride). Other medications that may be used are outlined in **Table 32.3**. Management also focuses on treating any underlying or coexisting heart, kidney, and CNS disorders.

Nursing care for the patient with a hypertensive emergency focuses on continuous monitoring of blood pressure and titrating drugs (administered by intravenous bolus or infusion) as ordered to achieve desired blood pressure. Avoiding excessive or very rapid blood pressure reductions is as important as achieving the desired blood pressure

Table 32.3 Intravenous Drugs Used to Treat Hypertensive Emergencies

Class/Drug	Onset	Duration	Nursing Implications
Vasodilators			
Sodium nitroprusside (Nipride)	Seconds	1–2 min	■ Effective, easy to titrate. ■ May cause nausea and vomiting, muscle twitching, sweating. ■ Use with caution in increased intracranial pressure.
Nitroglycerin	2–5 min	5–10 min	■ Used when coronary ischemia accompanies hypertension. ■ May cause headache, vomiting. ■ Tolerance may develop with prolonged use.
Diazoxide (Hyperstat)	1–2 min	4–24 h	■ Avoided in patients with coronary artery disease. ■ Used with beta-blockers and diuretics. ■ Painful if it enters tissues.
Fenoldopam (Corlopam)	< 5 min	30 min	■ Use with caution in patients with glaucoma. ■ May cause tachycardia, headache, nausea, flushing. ■ Do not use concurrently with beta-blockers. ■ Monitor for heart failure, ischemic heart disease.
Hydralazine (Apresoline)	10–30 min	2–6 h	■ May be used for hypertension associated with eclampsia. ■ Avoided in patients with coronary heart disease. ■ May cause tachycardia, flushing, headache, vomiting, angina.
Calcium Channel Blockers			
Nicardipine (Cardene)	5–10 min	15–30 min; up to 4 h	■ Use with caution in coronary heart disease. ■ Avoid in patients with heart failure. ■ May cause tachycardia, headache, flushing, local phlebitis.

(continued)

Table 32.3 Intravenous Drugs Used to Treat Hypertensive Emergencies (*continued*)

Class/Drug	Onset	Duration	Nursing Implications
ACE Inhibitors			
Enalaprilat (Vasotec)	15–30 min	6–12 h	■ Monitor for hypotension. ■ Used in acute left heart failure. ■ Avoid in acute myocardial infarction.
Adrenergic Blockers			
Labetalol (Trandate)	5–10 min	3–6 h	■ Avoid in patients with acute heart failure and asthma. ■ May cause nausea and vomiting, dizziness. ■ Monitor for dyspnea, wheezing, heart block, orthostatic hypotension.
Esmolol (Brevibloc)	1–2 min	10–30 min	■ Avoided in patients with heart failure and asthma. ■ May cause nausea. ■ Monitor for hypotension, dyspnea, wheezing, heart failure, first-degree heart block.
Phentolamine (Regitine)	1–2 min	10–30 min	■ May cause tachycardia, flushing, headache.

readings. Reassure the patient and family of the rapid effect of prescribed drugs. Provide psychologic and emotional support as needed. Maintain an attitude of confidence that the treatment will achieve the desired effect. Following resolution of the hypertensive crisis, review causes of the crisis. Teach the patient and family measures to effectively manage hypertension and prevent future hypertensive emergencies.

32.2 Disorders of the Aorta and Its Branches

The aorta and its branches may be affected by occlusions, aneurysms, and inflammations. These disorders may be chronic or acute and life-threatening (e.g., a thoracic dissection). This section focuses on aneurysms of the aorta and its branches.

The Patient with an Aneurysm

An **aneurysm** is an abnormal dilation of a blood vessel, commonly at a site of a weakness or a tear in the vessel wall. Aneurysms commonly affect the aorta and peripheral arteries because of the high pressure in these vessels. An aneurysm may develop in the ventricular wall, usually affecting the left ventricle. Most arterial aneurysms are caused by arteriosclerosis or atherosclerosis; trauma may also lead to aneurysm formation.

Arterial aneurysms are most common in men over age 65 with a history of ever smoking (> 100 cigarettes in lifetime), most of whom are asymptomatic at the time of diagnosis. The incidence of aortic aneurysm is estimated to be 5.9 per 100,000 people per year (Benjamin et al., 2017). Aortic dissection affects about 5 to 30 per 1 million people each year. Hypertension is a major contributing factor in the development of some types of aortic aneurysms.

Pathophysiology

Aneurysms form due to weakness of the arterial wall (**Figure 32.4** ■). The major structural proteins of the aorta are collagen and elastin. Collagen provides tensile strength of the vessel, preventing excessive dilation. Elastin

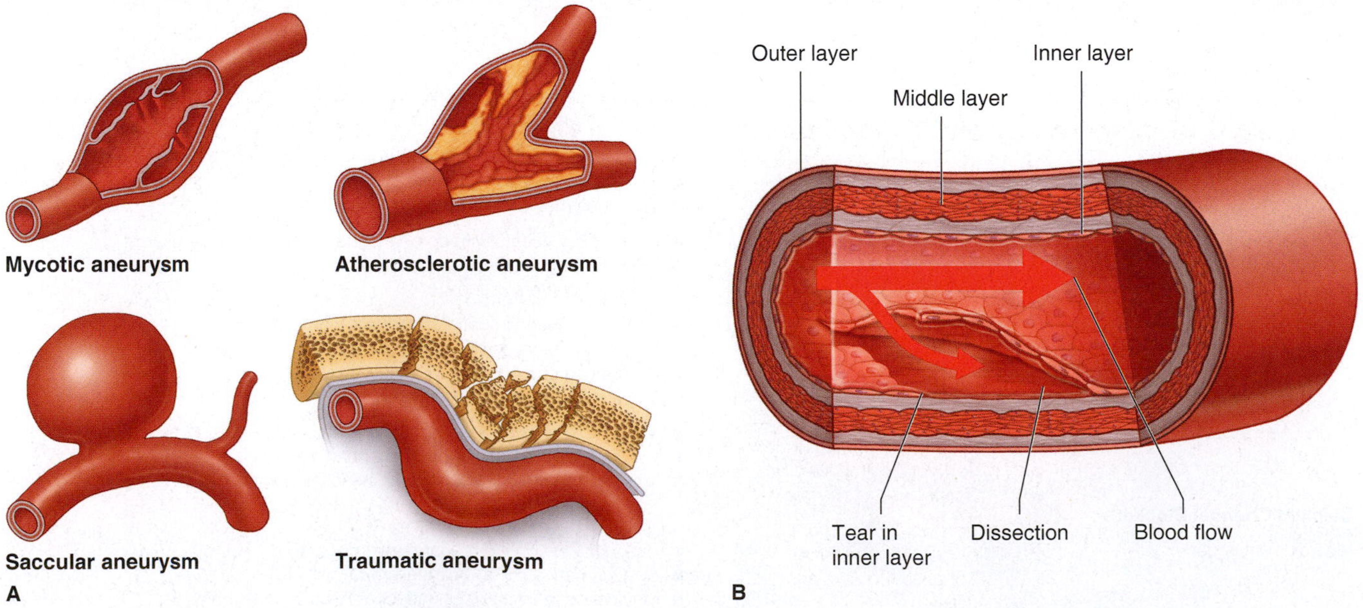
Mycotic aneurysm
Atherosclerotic aneurysm
Saccular aneurysm
Traumatic aneurysm
A
Outer layer
Middle layer
Inner layer
Tear in inner layer
Dissection
Blood flow
B

Figure 32.4 ■ Arterial abnormalities. **A**, Various types of aneurysms. **B**, Arterial dissection and clot formation.

allows vessel recoil, during which the vessel returns to its original size following systole. This recoil provides continued propulsion of the bolus of blood expelled from the ventricle. Elastin is a primary component of internal elastic lamina, which separates the intimal and medial layers of the aorta, and of the media, the smooth muscle layer of the aorta. Destruction of elastin can lead to abnormal dilation of the vessel; collagen destruction can allow the vessel to rupture (Sorenson et al., 2019).

True aneurysms are caused by the slow weakening of the arterial wall due to the long-term, eroding effects of atherosclerosis and hypertension. True aneurysms affect all three layers of the vessel wall, and most are fusiform and circumferential. Fusiform aneurysms are spindle shaped and taper at both ends. Circumferential aneurysms involve the entire diameter of the vessel. They generally grow slowly but progressively. Their length and diameter vary considerably among patients. A large fusiform aneurysm may affect most of the ascending aorta as well as a large portion of the abdominal aorta.

False aneurysms, also known as traumatic aneurysms, are caused by a traumatic break in the vessel wall rather than weakening of the vessel. They are often saccular, shaped like small outpouchings (sacs) on a portion of the vessel wall (see Figure 32.4A). A berry aneurysm is a type of saccular aneurysm. They are often small ($<$ 2 cm in diameter) and are caused by congenital weakness in the tunica media of the artery. Berry aneurysms are commonly found in the circle of Willis in the brain.

Dissecting aneurysms are unique, developing when a break or tear in the tunica intima and media allows blood to invade or *dissect* the layers of the vessel wall. The blood usually is contained by the adventitia, forming a saccular or longitudinal aneurysm (see Figure 32.4B).

Manifestations and Complications

Aneurysms affect different segments of the aorta and its branches. Their manifestations are generally due to pressure of the aneurysm on adjacent structures. **Table 32.4** summarizes the manifestations and complications of various types of aortic aneurysms.

Thoracic Aortic Aneurysms

Thoracic aortic aneurysms account for about 10% of aortic aneurysms, with an annual incidence of about 6 per 100,000 people (Saliba & Sia, 2015). They usually result from weakening of the aortic wall by arteriosclerosis and hypertension. Other causes include trauma, coarctation of the aorta, tertiary syphilis, fungal infections, and Marfan syndrome. The syphilis spirochete can invade and weaken aortic smooth muscle, causing an aneurysm to develop as long as 20 years after the primary infection. Marfan syndrome fragments elastic fibers of the aortic media, weakening the vessel wall. The Genetic Considerations box discusses genetic links associated with thoracic aortic aneurysms.

Thoracic aneurysms are frequently asymptomatic. When present, manifestations are caused by the effects of the aneurysm on blood flow (e.g., to the coronary arteries and great vessels of the head and upper body) and pressure

Genetic Considerations

Thoracic Aortic Aneurysms

About 20% of patients with aortic aneurysms have a family history of the disorder (Genetics Home Reference, 2018a). A condition known as *cystic medial necrosis* is prevalent in patients with Marfan syndrome and Ehlers-Danlos syndrome, inherited disorders involving connective tissues. In cystic medial necrosis, collagen and elastic fibers of the tunica media of the aorta degenerate. This loss of collagen and elastic tissues weakens the wall of the proximal aorta, leading to circumferential dilation of the ascending aorta and development of a fusiform aneurysm. In many other patients with thoracic aortic aneurysm (up to 20%), genetic syndromes affecting collagen and elastin are not recognized, but a strong family history of the disorder is present.

Table 32.4 Manifestations and Complications of Aortic Aneurysms

Type or Location	Manifestations	Complications
Thoracic	■ May be asymptomatic ■ Back, neck, or substernal pain ■ Dyspnea, stridor, or brassy cough if pressing on trachea ■ Hoarseness and dysphagia if pressing on esophagus or laryngeal nerve ■ Edema of the face and neck ■ Distended neck veins	■ Rupture and hemorrhage
Abdominal	■ Pulsating abdominal mass ■ Aortic calcification noted on x-ray ■ Mild to severe midabdominal or lumbar back pain ■ Cool, cyanotic extremities if iliac arteries are involved ■ Claudication (ischemic pain with exercise, relieved by rest)	■ Peripheral emboli to lower extremities ■ Rupture and hemorrhage
Aortic dissection	■ Abrupt, severe, ripping or tearing pain in area of aneurysm ■ Mild or marked hypertension early ■ Weak or absent pulses and blood pressure in upper extremities ■ Syncope	■ Hemorrhage ■ Renal failure ■ MI, heart failure, cardiac tamponade ■ Sepsis ■ Weakness or paralysis of lower extremities

placed by the distended aorta on surrounding structures. Consequently, manifestations vary by the location, size, and growth rate of the aneurysm. Substernal, neck, or back pain may occur. Pressure on the trachea, esophagus, laryngeal nerve, or superior vena cava may cause dyspnea, stridor, cough, difficult or painful swallowing, hoarseness, edema of the face and neck, and distended neck veins.

Aneurysms of the ascending aorta typically cause angina due to disruption of blood flow into the coronary arteries. Heart failure may develop as a result of disruption of the aortic valve and regurgitation of blood back into the left ventricle. Aneurysms of the aortic arch often cause dysphagia, dyspnea, hoarseness, confusion, and dizziness (due to disrupted cerebral blood flow). Thrombi that form within a thoracic aneurysm can embolize, causing a stroke, renal or mesenteric ischemia, or ischemia of the lower extremities. Aneurysms of the thoracic aorta tend to enlarge progressively and may rupture, causing death (AHA, 2017b).

Abdominal Aortic Aneurysms

Abdominal aortic aneurysms are associated with arteriosclerosis and hypertension. Increasing age and smoking are believed to contribute as well. Most abdominal aortic aneurysms are found in adults over age 65 (Benjamin et al., 2017). The vast majority (over 90%) develop below the renal arteries, usually where the abdominal aorta branches to form the iliac arteries (refer to Figure 32.4).

Most abdominal aneurysms are asymptomatic, but a pulsating mass in the mid and upper abdomen and a bruit over the mass are found on exam. When pain is present, it may be constant or intermittent, usually felt in the midabdominal region or lower back. Its intensity may range from mild discomfort to severe pain. Pain intensity often correlates with the size and severity of the aneurysm. Severe pain may indicate impending rupture.

Sluggish blood flow within the aneurysm may cause thrombi (blood clots) to form. These can become emboli (circulating clots), traveling to the lower extremities and occluding peripheral arteries. The aneurysm may rupture, with hemorrhage and hypovolemic shock. The risk of rupture increases as the size of the aneurysm increases; 20 to 40% of aneurysms > 5 cm in diameter rupture. After acute rupture, the mortality rate is greater than 50%, even when emergency surgery is performed (Sorenson et al., 2019).

Popliteal and Femoral Aneurysms

Most popliteal and femoral aneurysms are due to arteriosclerosis. They are often bilateral and usually affect men.

Popliteal aneurysms may be asymptomatic. Manifestations, if any, are due to decreased blood flow to the lower extremity and include **intermittent claudication** (cramping or pain in the leg muscles brought on by exercise and relieved by rest), rest pain, and numbness. A pulsating mass may be palpable in the popliteal fossa (behind the knee). Thrombosis and embolism are complications; gangrene may result, often necessitating amputation.

A *femoral aneurysm* is usually detected as a pulsating mass in the femoral area. The manifestations are similar to those of popliteal aneurysms, resulting from impaired blood flow. Femoral aneurysms may rupture.

Aortic Dissections

Dissection is a life-threatening emergency caused by a tear in the intima of the aorta with hemorrhage into the media. The hemorrhage dissects or splits the vessel wall, forming a blood-filled channel between its layers. Dissection can occur anywhere along the aorta. *Type A dissection* (*proximal dissection*) affects the ascending aorta; *type B dissection* (*distal dissection*) is limited to the descending aorta (refer to Figure 32.4B).

Hypertension is a major predisposing factor for aortic dissection, accounting for 70% of aortic dissections (Saliba & Sia, 2015). Cystic medial necrosis (see the Genetic Considerations box) is a major risk factor. Other risk factors include male gender, advancing age, pregnancy, congenital defects of the aortic valve, coarctation of the aorta, and inflammatory aortitis (Sorenson et al., 2019).

Dissection of the thoracic aortic walls progresses along the length of the vessel, moving both proximally and distally. As the aneurysm expands, pressure may prevent the aortic valve from closing or may occlude the branches of the aorta. Descending aortic dissection may extend into the renal, iliac, or femoral arteries.

The primary symptom of an aortic dissection is sudden, excruciating pain. The pain, often described as a ripping or tearing sensation, is usually over the area of dissection. Thoracic dissections cause chest or back pain. Other symptoms may include syncope, dyspnea, and weakness. The blood pressure may initially be increased, but rapidly falls and is often inaudible as the dissection occludes blood flow. Peripheral pulses are absent for the same reason.

Complications develop if major arteries are affected. Obstruction of the carotid artery causes neurologic symptoms such as weakness or paralysis. The myocardium, kidneys, or bowel may become ischemic or infarct if blood flow to the coronary arteries, renal arteries, or mesenteric artery is affected. Acute aortic regurgitation may develop with dissection of the ascending aorta. With treatment, the long-term prognosis is generally good, although the in-hospital mortality rate following surgery is 15 to 20% (Saliba & Sia, 2015).

Interprofessional Care

Most aneurysms are asymptomatic, detected through a routine physical examination. Treatment depends on the size of the aneurysm. Small, asymptomatic aneurysms may not be treated or are medically managed; large aneurysms (> 5 cm) at risk for rupture require surgery. In 2010 the American Heart Association updated the guidelines for management of thoracic aortic diseases (Hiratzka et al., 2010).

Diagnosis

Diagnostic studies done to establish the diagnosis and determine the size and location of the aneurysm may include:

- ***Chest x-ray*** to visualize thoracic aortic aneurysms.
- ***Abdominal ultrasonography*** to diagnose abdominal aortic aneurysms. One-time screening of men ages 65

to 75 who have ever smoked is recommended (U.S. Preventive Services Task Force, 2018).

- *Transesophageal echocardiography* to identify the specific location and extent of a thoracic aneurysm and to visualize a dissecting aneurysm.
- *Contrast-enhanced CT* or *MRI* allows precise measurements of aneurysm size.
- *Angiography* uses contrast solution injected into the aorta or involved vessel to visualize the precise size and location of the aneurysm.

Medications

Thoracic aortic aneurysms may be treated with long-term beta-blocker therapy and additional antihypertensive drugs as needed to control heart rate and blood pressure.

Patients with aortic dissection are initially treated with intravenous beta-blockers such as propranolol (Inderal), metoprolol (Lopressor), or esmolol (Brevibloc) to reduce the heart rate to about 60 bpm. Sodium nitroprusside (Nipride) infusion is started concurrently to reduce the systolic pressure to 120 mmHg or less. Calcium channel blockers (verapamil and diltiazem) also may be used. Direct vasodilators such as diazoxide (Hyperstat) and hydralazine (Apresoline) are avoided because they may actually worsen the dissection. Constant monitoring of vital signs, hemodynamic pressures (via Swan-Ganz catheter; refer to Chapter 30 for more information about hemodynamic pressure monitoring), and urine output are vital to ensure adequate perfusion of vital organs.

Following surgical correction of an aneurysm, anticoagulant therapy may be initiated. Heparin therapy is used initially, with conversion to oral anticoagulation prior to discharge. Many patients are maintained indefinitely on anticoagulant therapy; others may use lifelong, low-dose aspirin therapy to reduce the risk of clot formation.

Surgery

Operative repair of aortic aneurysms is indicated when the aneurysm is symptomatic or expanding rapidly. Thoracic aneurysms of > 6 cm in diameter are surgically repaired; asymptomatic abdominal aneurysms > 5 cm in diameter may be repaired, depending on the patient's operative risk factors (Perrin & MacLeod, 2017). Type A dissections are repaired as soon as feasible; type B dissections may be surgically repaired, depending on the extent of involvement and risk for rupture.

Endovascular aortic repairs (EVARs) are increasingly being used to treat abdominal and thoracic aortic aneurysms. The stent, which consists of a metal sheath covered with polyester fabric or a woven polyester tube, is usually placed percutaneously via the femoral artery. Fluoroscopy is used to guide its placement. Both straight and bifurcated grafts are available. Endovascular stent placement results in a shorter hospital stay and lower treatment cost. EVAR is associated with fewer pulmonary, renal, and cardiovascular complications than open surgical aneurysm repair (Cleveland Clinic, 2018). This option is generally preferred for patients who have a high surgical risk. The most common complication of endovascular aneurysm repair is persistent perfusion of the aneurysm (endoleak) caused by an ineffective seal at the proximal or distal end of the graft. Regular follow-up with abdominal CT scans is necessary to detect this complication, which can develop at any time postoperatively. Because stent grafts are handcrafted to fit the individual, repeated CT scans with contrast media are required preoperatively, increasing the risk for kidney damage and renal failure. On rare occasions, the graft may be malpositioned or may migrate from the desired location.

An open surgical procedure in which the aneurysm is excised and replaced with a synthetic fabric graft is the historical standard treatment for expanding abdominal aortic aneurysms (**Figure 32.5** ■). Although the aneurysm walls may be excised, they are usually left intact and used to cover the graft. Surgical repair of thoracic aneurysms is similar but more complex due to major vessels exiting at the aortic arch. Cardiopulmonary bypass is required if the ascending aorta is involved. The aortic valve also may be replaced during surgery.

SAFETY ALERT: Monitor for and report manifestations of graft leakage:

- Ecchymoses of the scrotum, perineum, or penis; a new or expanding hematoma
- Increased abdominal girth
- Weak or absent peripheral pulses; tachycardia; hypotension
- Decreased motor function or sensation in the extremities
- Fall in hemoglobin and hematocrit
- Increasing abdominal, pelvic, back, or groin pain
- Decreasing urinary output (< 30 mL/h)
- Decreasing CVP, pulmonary artery pressure, or pulmonary artery wedge pressure.

These manifestations may signal graft leakage and possible hemorrhage. Pain may be due to pressure from an expanding hematoma or bowel ischemia. Decreased renal perfusion causes the glomerular filtration rate and urine output to fall. ■

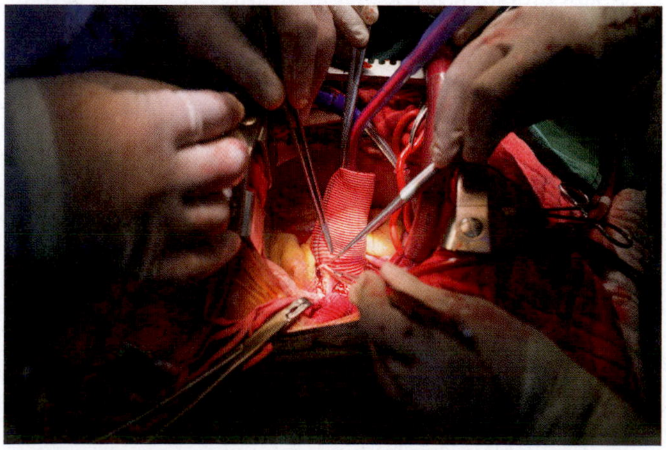

Figure 32.5 ■ Repair of an abdominal aortic aneurysm. The aorta is exposed and clamped between the renal and iliac arteries. Atherosclerotic plaque and thrombotic materials are removed. A synthetic graft is used to replace the aneurysm. The aneurysm walls are then sutured around the graft.

Nursing Care

Assessment

See the Manifestations and Interprofessional Care sections for the assessment of the patient with an aneurysm.

Focused assessment for the patient with a suspected aortic aneurysm includes:

- ***Health history:*** Complaints of chest, back, or abdominal pain; extremity weakness; shortness of breath, cough, difficult or painful swallowing, hoarseness; history of hypertension, coronary heart disease, heart failure, or peripheral vascular disease
- ***Physical assessment:*** Vital signs including blood pressure in upper and lower extremities; peripheral pulses; skin color and temperature; neck veins; abdominal exam including gentle palpation for masses and auscultation for bruits; neurologic exam including level of consciousness, sensation, and movement of extremities.

Priorities of Care

Collaborating with the interprofessional team to ensure adequate treatment of the underlying process while providing care that supports the physical and psychologic responses to the disorder is a priority of nursing care.

Diagnoses, Outcomes, and Interventions

Nursing care for patients with an aneurysm of the aorta or its branches focuses on monitoring and maintaining tissue perfusion, relieving pain, and reducing anxiety. Nursing care is usually acute, precipitated by a complication or surgical repair of the aneurysm.

Promote Effective Tissue Perfusion. Patients with aortic aneurysms are at risk for impaired tissue perfusion due to aneurysm rupture with resulting hemorrhage and lack of blood flow to tissues distal to the rupture. In addition, thrombi often form within the aneurysm and may become emboli, obstructing distal arterial blood flow.

Expected Outcome: Patient's tissue perfusion will be adequate as evidenced by adequate arterial flow (i.e., strong peripheral pulses).

SAFETY ALERT: Immediately report manifestations of impending rupture, expansion, or dissection of the aneurysm: Increased pain, discrepancy between upper and lower extremity blood pressures and peripheral pulses, increased mass size, change in LOC or motor or sensory function, and laboratory results. Rapid expansion may indicate increased risk for rupture, with resulting hemorrhage, shock, and possible death. Elective or planned surgery may rapidly become emergency surgery to prevent complications. ■

The nurse will:

- Implement interventions to reduce the risk of aneurysm rupture:
  a. Maintain bedrest with legs flat.
  b. Maintain a calm environment, implementing measures to reduce psychologic stress.
  c. Prevent straining during defecation and instruct to avoid holding the breath while moving.
  d. Administer beta-blockers and antihypertensives as prescribed.
- *Activity, stress, and the Valsalva maneuver increase blood pressure, increasing the risk of rupture. Elevating or crossing the legs restricts peripheral blood flow and increases pressure in the aorta or iliac arteries. Beta-blockers and antihypertensives are often ordered to reduce pressure in the dilated vessel.*
- Report manifestations of arterial thrombosis or embolism: Absent peripheral pulses; a pale or cyanotic, cool extremity; severe, diffuse abdominal pain with guarding; or increased groin, lumbar, or lower extremity pain. Sluggish blood flow within the aneurysm often causes thrombi to form. These thrombi can break loose, becoming emboli that can occlude peripheral arteries or arteries to the kidneys or mesentery. *Arterial occlusion may necessitate emergency surgery to restore blood flow and prevent tissue infarct or gangrene.*
- Continuously monitor cardiac rhythm. Report complaints of chest pain or changes in ECG tracing. Administer oxygen as indicated. *Aortic dissection and repair place the patient at significant risk for MI, a major cause of postoperative mortality and morbidity. Rapid identification and treatment of this complication can reduce the risk of death or the long-term adverse effects of MI.*
- Immediately report changes in mental status or symptoms of peripheral neurologic impairment (weakness, paresthesias, paralysis). The expanding aneurysm or dissection can affect carotid and cerebral blood flow or spinal cord perfusion, leading to neurologic symptoms. *Immediate restoration of blood flow is vital to prevent permanent neurologic deficits.*

Reduce Risk for Injury. Potent antihypertensive drugs are often given intravenously to reduce the pressure on an expanding or dissecting aneurysm. Continuous monitoring of infusions and hemodynamic parameters such as arterial pressure, pulmonary pressures, and cardiac output is vital to ensure that adequate tissue perfusion is maintained during infusions of these potent drugs.

Expected Outcome: Patient will experience effective risk control through use of close and careful drug monitoring.

The nurse will:

- Use an infusion control device for all drug infusions. *These devices prevent accidental or inadvertent changes in the rate of the infusion and dose of the drug.*
- Continuously monitor arterial pressure and hemodynamic parameters as indicated. Promptly report results outside the specified parameters to the healthcare provider. *Many of the drugs used are effective within minutes. Responses vary among individuals, particularly in the older adult, necessitating continuous monitoring.*
- Monitor urine output hourly. Report output < 30 mL/h. *The kidneys are very sensitive to reduced perfusion pressure; inadequate renal blood flow can lead to acute renal failure.*

Reduce Anxiety. Patients with aortic aneurysms are often highly anxious because of the urgent nature of the disorder. The nurse manages the anxiety levels of both the patient and family members to effectively address physiologic care needs. Stress reduction is necessary to help maintain the blood pressure within desired limits.

Expected Outcome: Patient's anxiety will be controlled as evidenced by verbalized decrease in subjective distress.

The nurse will:

- Explain all procedures and treatments, using simple and understandable terms. *Simplified explanations are necessary when anxiety levels interfere with learning and understanding.*
- Respond to all questions honestly, using a calm, empathetic, but matter-of-fact manner. *Honesty with the patient and family promotes trust and provides reassurance that the true nature of the situation is not being "hidden" from them.*
- Provide care in a calm, efficient manner. *Using a calm manner even during preparations for emergency surgery reassures the patient and family that although the situation is critical, the staff is prepared to handle things effectively.*
- Spend as much time as possible with the patient. Allow supportive family members to remain with the patient when possible. *The presence of a health professional and supportive family member reassures the patient that he or she is not alone in facing this crisis.*

Transitions of Care

Prevention of aortic aneurysms focuses on teaching about the risk factors for their development. A family history of aneurysm may increase the risks of developing an aneurysm, so careful physical assessment is indicated with this nonmodifiable risk factor. Modifiable risk factors include high blood pressure, high cholesterol, and smoking. Acute care focuses on the surgical correction of aortic aneurysms.

Preoperative Care

- As time permits, provide routine preoperative care and teaching, as outlined in Chapter 4. *Patients having vascular surgery have similar preoperative nursing care needs to other patients having major abdominal or thoracic surgery. If emergent surgery is required, time for preoperative care and teaching may be limited.*
- Implement measures to reduce fear and anxiety:
  a. Orient to the intensive care unit, if appropriate.
  b. Describe and explain the reason for all equipment and tubes, such as cardiac monitors, ventilators, nasogastric tubes, urinary catheters, intravenous lines and fluids, and intra-arterial lines.
  c. Explain what to expect following surgery (sights, sounds, frequency of taking vital signs, dressings, pain relief measures, communication strategies).
  d. Allow time for questions and expression of fears and concerns.

  These explanations provide a sense of control for the patient and family.
- Monitor for and implement care to reduce the risk of aneurysm rupture (see the following Diagnoses, Outcomes, and Interventions section). *Patients with a rapidly expanding or symptomatic aneurysm are at risk for rupture prior to surgical repair.*

Postoperative Care

- Provide routine postoperative care and specific measures as ordered by the healthcare provider. *Patients undergoing aneurysm repair require nursing care similar to that provided to all patients with major thoracic or abdominal surgery, in addition to specific measures related to vascular surgery.*
- Maintain fluid replacement and blood or volume expanders as ordered. Promptly report changes in vital signs, level of consciousness, and urine output. *Hypovolemic shock may develop due to blood loss during surgery, third spacing, inadequate fluid replacement, and/or hemorrhage if graft separation or leakage occurs.*
- Report manifestations of lower extremity embolism: Pain and numbness in lower extremities, decreasing pulses, and pale, cool, or cyanotic skin. *Pulses may be absent for 4 to 12 hours postoperatively due to vasospasm; however, absent pulses with pain, changes in sensation, and a pale, cool extremity are indicative of arterial occlusion.*
- Report manifestations of bowel ischemia or gangrene: Abdominal pain and distention, occult or fresh blood in stools, and diarrhea. *Bowel ischemia may result from an embolism or occur as a complication of surgery.*
- Report manifestations of impaired renal function: Urine output < 30 mL/h, fixed specific gravity, and increasing BUN and serum creatinine levels. *Hypovolemia or clamping of the aorta during surgery may impair renal perfusion, leading to acute renal failure.*
- Report manifestations of spinal cord ischemia: Lower extremity weakness or paraplegia. *Impaired spinal cord perfusion may lead to ischemia and impaired function.*

Topics to discuss when preparing patients and their families for home care or care in a community-based setting depend on the treatment plan. Discuss the following topics when surgical repair is not immediately planned and the aneurysm will be monitored:

- Measures to control hypertension, including lifestyle and prescribed drugs
- Benefits of smoking cessation
- Manifestations of increasing aneurysm size or complications to report to the healthcare provider.

Following surgery, discuss the following topics to prepare the patient and family for home care:

- Wound care and preventing infection; manifestations of impaired healing or infection to be reported
- Prescribed antihypertensive and anticoagulant medications and their expected and unintended effects
- The importance of adequate rest and nutrition for healing

- Measures to prevent constipation and straining at stool (such as increasing fluid and fiber in the diet)
- The importance of avoiding prolonged sitting, lifting heavy objects, engaging in strenuous exercise, and having sexual intercourse until approved by the healthcare provider (usually 6 to 12 weeks)
- Signs and symptoms of complications to report to the healthcare provider.

Provide referrals to a home health agency or community health service as necessary. Referrals are especially important for older adults and their caregivers, who may require additional assistance with complex care needs.

32.3 Disorders of the Peripheral Arteries

Disorders that impair peripheral arterial blood flow may be acute (e.g., arterial thrombosis) or chronic (e.g., peripheral arteriosclerosis). Chronic occlusive disorders may be due to structural defects of the arterial walls or spasm of affected arteries. Impaired peripheral arterial circulation limits the availability of oxygen and nutrients to the tissues and can have significant adverse effects. This section focuses on acute and chronic disorders affecting peripheral arteries. The nurse's role in caring for patients with peripheral arterial disorders focuses on maintaining tissue perfusion and educating the patient and family about the disorder and its management.

Physiology Review

Peripheral arteries are the part of the systemic circulation that delivers oxygen and nutrients to the skin and the extremities. Arterial walls have three layers: The *intima*, which includes the endothelium and a layer of connective tissue and the basement membrane; the *media*, composed of smooth muscle and elastic fibers; and the *adventitia*, a thin layer of connective tissue that contains collagen and elastic fibers. The smooth muscle of peripheral arteries controls blood flow as it contracts and relaxes. Contraction narrows the vessel lumen (**vasoconstriction**), whereas smooth muscle relaxation expands the vessel (**vasodilation**). Peripheral arteries become progressively smaller; arterioles are < 0.5 mm in diameter and are composed primarily of smooth muscle. The arterioles control blood flow through the capillary beds where gas, nutrient, and waste product exchange occurs. Capillary walls are very thin, consisting of a single layer of endothelial cells surrounded by a thin basement membrane.

Blood flows from an area of higher pressure to an area of lower pressure. *Resistance* opposes blood flow. Resistance is created by friction of the blood itself, although the primary determinants of vascular resistance are the diameter and length of the blood vessel. See the Physiology Review section under the Disorders of Blood Pressure Regulation section earlier in this chapter for more information about factors that determine vessel resistance.

The Patient with Peripheral Vascular Disease

Arteriosclerosis is the most common chronic arterial disorder, characterized by thickening, loss of elasticity, and calcification of arterial walls. **Atherosclerosis** is a form of arteriosclerosis in which deposits of fat and fibrin obstruct and harden the arteries (**Figure 32.6** ■). In the peripheral circulation, these pathologic changes impair the blood supply to peripheral tissues, particularly the lower extremities. This is known as **peripheral vascular disease (PVD)**.

Pathophysiology

The pathophysiology of atherosclerosis is detailed in Chapter 30. Atherosclerotic lesions involve both the intima and the media of the involved arteries. There are three types of PVD:

- Type 1 (10 to 15% of patients), involving the aorta and iliac arteries

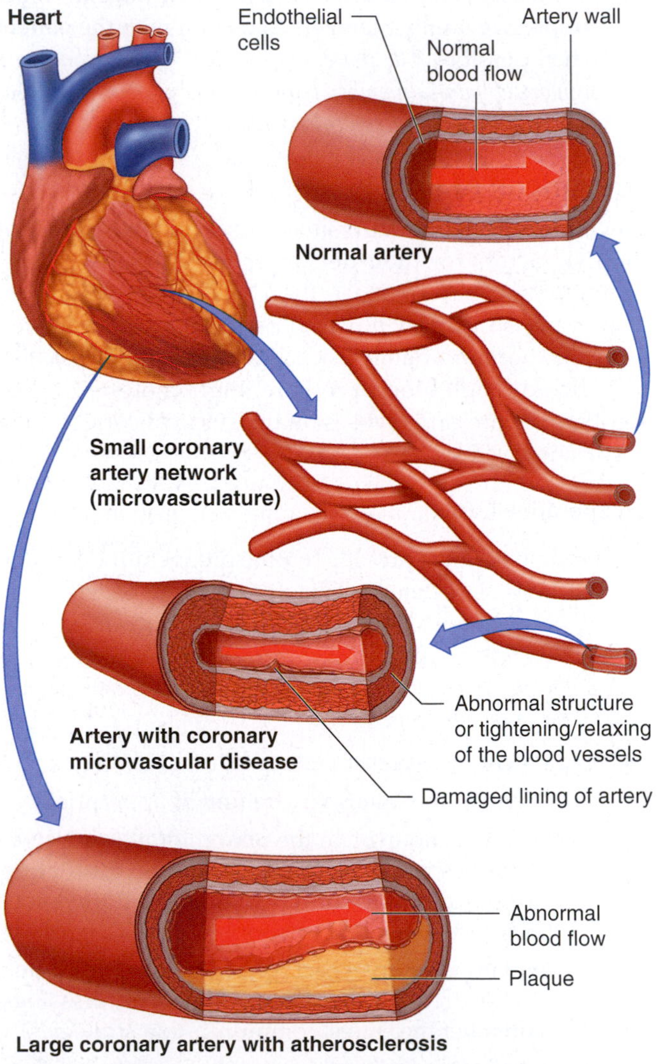

Heart
Endothelial cells
Artery wall
Normal blood flow
Normal artery
Small coronary artery network (microvasculature)
Abnormal structure or tightening/relaxing of the blood vessels
Artery with coronary microvascular disease
Damaged lining of artery
Abnormal blood flow
Plaque
Large coronary artery with atherosclerosis

Figure 32.6 ■ Atherosclerosis begins when endothelial cells are damaged. When LDL cholesterol reaches damaged endothelium, white blood cells attack the LDL and plaque begins to form.

- Type 2 (~25% of patients), involving the aorta and the common and external iliac arteries
- Type 3 (~60 to 70% of patients), in which the aorta and the iliac, femoral, popliteal, and tibial arteries are involved.

Arteriosclerosis in the abdominal aorta leads to the development of aneurysms as plaque erodes the vessel wall.

Plaque tends to form at arterial bifurcations. The vessel lumen is progressively obstructed, decreasing blood flow to the lower extremities. Tissue hypoxia or anoxia results. With gradual obstruction of the vessel, collateral circulation often develops. However, it is usually not adequate to supply tissue needs, especially when metabolic demand increases (e.g., during exercise). Manifestations typically develop only when the vessel is occluded by 60% or more.

Incidence and Risk Factors

PVD usually affects people in their 60s and 70s; men are more often affected than women. It is a common manifestation of atherosclerosis. Deaths attributed to peripheral arterial disease are about the same for Black and White males, but are higher among Black women than White women (Benjamin et al., 2017).

Risk factors for PVD are similar to those for atherosclerosis and coronary heart disease (refer to Chapter 30). Diabetes mellitus, hypercholesterolemia, hypertension, cigarette smoking, and high homocystine levels are risk factors for PVD (Sorenson et al., 2019).

Manifestations and Complications

Pain is the primary symptom of peripheral atherosclerosis. *Intermittent claudication*, a cramping or aching pain in the calves of the legs, the thighs, and the buttocks that occurs with a predictable level of activity, is characteristic of PVD. The pain is often accompanied by weakness and is relieved by rest.

Rest pain, in contrast, occurs during periods of inactivity. It is often described as a burning sensation in the lower legs. Rest pain increases when the legs are elevated and decreases when the legs are dependent (e.g., hanging over the side of the bed). The legs may feel cold or numb along with the pain. Sensation is diminished and the muscles may atrophy.

Peripheral pulses may be decreased or absent. A bruit may be heard over large affected arteries, such as the femoral artery and the abdominal aorta. The legs are pale when elevated, but often are dark red (*dependent rubor*) when dependent. The skin is often thin, shiny, and hairless, with discolored areas. Toenails may be thickened. Areas of skin breakdown and ulceration may be evident. Edema may develop with severe PVD. Manifestations of PVD include:

- Intermittent claudication
- Rest pain
- Paresthesias (numbness, decreased sensation)
- Diminished or absent peripheral pulses
- Pallor with extremity elevation, dependent rubor when dependent
- Thin, shiny, hairless skin; thickened toenails
- Areas of discoloration or skin breakdown.

Complications of peripheral atherosclerosis include gangrene and extremity amputation, rupture of abdominal aortic aneurysms, and possible infection and sepsis.

Interprofessional Care

Management of peripheral vascular disease focuses on slowing the atherosclerotic process and maintaining tissue perfusion.

Diagnosis

Although PVD can often be diagnosed by the history and physical examination, diagnostic tests may be ordered to evaluate its extent. Noninvasive studies are often sufficient.

- ***Segmental pressure measurements*** use sphygmomanometer cuffs and a Doppler device to compare blood pressures between the upper and lower extremities (normally similar) and within different segments of the affected extremity. In PVD, the BP may be lower in the legs than in the arms.
- ***Stress testing*** using a treadmill provides functional assessment of limitations. In PVD, pressure at the ankle may decline even further with exercise, confirming the diagnosis. Evaluation for coronary heart disease may be done simultaneously during exercise testing.
- ***Doppler ultrasound*** uses sound waves reflected off moving red blood cells within a vessel to evaluate blood flow. The impulses may be translated into an audible signal or a graphic waveform. With significant PVD, the waveform becomes progressively flatter as the transducer is moved distally along the affected vessel. Segmental pressures may be used to locate the site of obstruction.
- ***Duplex Doppler ultrasound*** combines the audible or graphic Doppler ultrasound with ultrasound imaging to identify arterial or venous abnormalities. Ultrasonic imaging provides views of the affected vessel while Doppler ultrasound evaluates blood flow. *Color-flow Doppler ultrasound (CDU)* provides color images of the vessel and blood flow.
- ***Transcutaneous oximetry*** evaluates oxygenation of tissues.
- ***Angiography*** or ***magnetic resonance angiography*** is done before revascularization procedures to locate and evaluate the extent of arterial obstruction. For angiography, a contrast medium is injected and vessels are visualized using fluoroscopy and x-rays. Magnetic resonance angiography does not require injection of a contrast medium and may replace angiography.

Medications

Drug treatment of peripheral atherosclerosis is less effective than with coronary heart disease. Medications to inhibit platelet aggregation, such as aspirin or clopidogrel (Plavix) are ordered to reduce the risk of arterial thrombosis. Cilostazol

(Pletal), a platelet inhibitor with vasodilator properties, improves claudication. Pentoxifylline (Trental) decreases blood viscosity and increases red blood cell flexibility, increasing blood flow to the microcirculation and tissues of the extremities. Parenteral vasodilator prostaglandins may be given on a long-term basis to decrease pain and facilitate healing in patients with severe limb ischemia (Adams et al., 2017).

Treatments

Smoking cessation is vital. Nicotine not only promotes atherosclerosis, but also causes vasospasm, further reducing blood flow to the extremities.

Meticulous foot care is vital to prevent ulceration and infection (**Box 32.2**). Elastic support hose, which reduce circulation to the skin, should not be used. Elevating the head of the bed on blocks may help relieve rest pain. Regular, progressively strenuous exercise, such as 30 to 45 minutes of walking daily, is important. The patient is taught to rest at the onset of claudication, resuming activity when the pain resolves.

BOX 32.2
Foot Care for the Patient with Peripheral Atherosclerosis

1. **Keep legs and feet clean, dry, and comfortable.**
   a. Wash legs and feet daily in warm water, using mild soap.
   b. Pat dry using a soft towel; be sure to dry between the toes.
   c. Apply moisturizing cream to prevent drying, but avoid lotion between toes.
   d. Use powder between the toes.
   e. Buy shoes in the afternoon (when feet are largest); never buy shoes that are uncomfortable. Be sure toes have adequate room.
   f. Wear a clean pair of cotton socks each day. Be sure sock seams are on the outside to reduce pressure.
2. **Prevent accidents and injuries to the feet.**
   a. Always wear shoes or slippers when getting out of bed.
   b. Walk on level ground and avoid crowds, if possible.
   c. Do not go barefoot.
   d. Inspect legs and feet daily; use a mirror to examine backs of legs and bottoms of feet.
   e. Have a professional foot care provider trim toenails and care for corns, calluses, ingrown toenails, or athlete's foot.
   f. Always check the temperature of the water before stepping into a tub.
   g. Do not get the legs or tops of the feet sunburned.
   h. Report leg or foot problems (increased pain, cuts, bruises, blistering, redness, or open areas) to your healthcare provider.
3. **Improve blood supply to the legs and feet.**
   a. Do not cross legs.
   b. Do not wear garters, girdles, or knee stockings.
   c. Do not swim or wade in cold water.

Other measures to slow the process of atherosclerosis, such as controlling diabetes and hypertension, lowering cholesterol levels, and weight loss, are also recommended (refer to Chapter 30).

Revascularization

Revascularization may be performed if symptoms are progressive, severe, or disabling. Other indications for surgery include symptoms that significantly interfere with activities of daily living, rest pain, and pregangrenous or gangrenous lesions. Either nonsurgical revascularization procedures or surgery may be performed.

Nonsurgical procedures include percutaneous transluminal angioplasty (PTA), stent placement, or atherectomy. Techniques may include balloon angioplasty to dilate the narrowed lumen, mechanical atherectomy to remove plaque, or laser or thermal angioplasty to vaporize the occluding material. In either case, a stent is typically placed at the time of PTA to maintain vessel patency. Iliac and femoral-popliteal PTA initially reestablish good blood flow and relieve symptoms in more than 80% of patients. Refer to Chapter 30 for more information about revascularization procedures.

Surgical options include endarterectomy to remove occlusive plaque from the artery and bypass grafts. Dacron or polytetrafluoroethylene (PTFE) is used as bypass grafts (Ambler & Twine, 2018). Both immediate and long-term graft patency is better with bypass grafting than with nonsurgical revascularization procedures, but the risk for operative complications such as myocardial infarction, stoke, infection, and peripheral embolization is higher. Nursing care for the patient having revascularization surgery is similar to that provided for patients having surgery of the aorta.

Integrative Therapies

Complementary therapies for peripheral vascular disease include interventions to improve circulation and to reduce stress. A number of complementary therapies may improve peripheral circulation, including aromatherapy with rosemary or vetiver; biofeedback; healing or therapeutic touch and massage; herbs such as ginkgo, garlic, cayenne, hawthorn, and bilberry; and exercise including yoga. Aromatherapy and yoga may reduce stress, as can breathing exercises, meditation, and counseling. In addition, complementary therapies to reduce atherosclerosis and lower cholesterol levels may slow the progress of PVD. Measures such as a very low-fat or vegetarian diet—including antioxidant nutrients or using vitamin C, vitamin E, or garlic supplements—may be useful.

Nursing Care

Assessment

See the Manifestations and Interprofessional Care sections for the assessment of the patient with peripheral vascular disease.

Focused assessment related to peripheral atherosclerosis includes:

- *Health history:* Complaints of pain, its relationship to exercise or rest, timing, associated symptoms, and relief measures; history of coronary heart disease, peripheral vascular disease, hyperlipidemia, hypertension, or diabetes; current medications; smoking history; usual diet and activity patterns

- ***Physical assessment:*** Vital signs; strength and equality of peripheral pulses of all extremities; capillary refill; skin color, temperature, hair distribution, presence of any discolorations or lesions; movement and sensation of lower extremities.

Priorities of Care

Collaborating with the interprofessional team to ensure adequate treatment of the underlying process while providing care that supports the physical and psychologic responses to the disorder is a priority of nursing care.

Diagnoses, Outcomes, and Interventions

Impaired tissue perfusion is an obvious problem in peripheral atherosclerosis. Acute and chronic pain may interfere with activities of daily living, and ambulation may be limited. The possibility of losing a lower extremity is frightening.

Promote Effective Perfusion of Peripheral Tissues. Impaired blood flow to the lower extremities affects gas, nutrient, and waste product exchange between the capillaries and cells. Oxygen and nutrient deprivation impairs cell function and tissue integrity, causing pain and impaired healing. Pain develops with exercise and when extremities are elevated.

Expected Outcome: Patient's tissue perfusion will be adequate as evidenced by adequate arterial flow (i.e., strong peripheral pulses).

The nurse will:

- Assess peripheral pulses, pain, color, temperature, and capillary refill every 4 hours and as needed. Use a Doppler device if pulses are not palpable. Mark pulse locations with an indelible marker. *Assessment data provide a baseline for evaluating the effectiveness of interventions and identifying changes in arterial blood flow.*
- Position with extremities dependent. *Gravity promotes arterial flow to the dependent extremity, increasing tissue perfusion and relieving pain.*
- Instruct to avoid smoking. If necessary, obtain an order for a nicotine patch or gum from the healthcare provider. Nicotine is a potent vasoconstrictor that further impairs arterial blood flow. Nicotine patches and gum contain less nicotine than cigarettes and can help reduce the stress of smoking cessation. *Smoking cessation is a vital component of care.*
- Discuss the benefits of regular exercise. *Exercise promotes development of collateral circulation to ischemic tissues and slows the process of atherosclerosis.*
- Use a foot cradle and lightweight blankets, socks, and slippers to keep extremities warm. Avoid electric heating pads or hot water bottles. *Keeping extremities warm conserves heat, prevents vasospasm, and promotes arterial flow. External heating devices are avoided to reduce the risk of burns in the patient with impaired sensation. The foot cradle protects tissues from compression by linens.*
- Encourage frequent position changes. Instruct to avoid crossing legs or using a pillow under the knees. *Position changes promote blood flow and reduce damage caused by pressure. Leg crossing and excessive flexion of the hip or knee joints can compress partially obstructed arteries and impair blood flow to distal tissues.*

Manage Pain. Impaired blood flow results in tissue ischemia. Metabolism shifts from an efficient aerobic process to an anaerobic process. Lactic acid and metabolic waste products accumulate in tissues, causing pain. Severe and cramping pain generally occurs with exercise early in the disease. Rest initially produces relief, similar to the process of angina (refer to Chapter 30). As the disease progresses, pain develops with less exercise and often occurs even at rest. Rest pain disrupts sleep, the sense of well-being, and has significant disruptive effects on life roles.

Expected Outcome: Patient's pain control will be adequate as evidenced by physical well-being.

The nurse will:

- Assess pain at least every 4 hours using a standard pain scale; assess more often as needed. *Pain is a subjective experience. Using a standard pain scale allows evaluation of treatment measures in relieving pain and restoring blood flow.*
- Keep extremities warm. *Cooling leads to vasoconstriction, increasing pain. Warming the extremities promotes vasodilation and improves arterial flow, reducing pain.*
- Teach pain relief and stress reduction techniques such as relaxation, meditation, and guided imagery. *Pain increases stress. The stress response leads to vasoconstriction, increasing pain. Stress reduction techniques, when combined with other measures to promote blood flow, can help reduce pain.*

Promote Skin Integrity. Patients with PVD are at risk for impaired skin integrity as a result of oxygen and nutrient deprivation. Chronic tissue ischemia leads to dry, scaly, and atrophied skin. Pruritus can lead to scratching; minor injuries may go unnoticed due to impaired sensation. Impaired tissue healing can lead to ulceration, infection, and potential gangrene.

Expected Outcome: Patient will demonstrate understanding of plan to heal skin and prevent reinjury.

The nurse will:

- Assess and document skin condition at least every 8 hours and with each home visit, more frequently as indicated. Tissue ischemia increases the risk for damage, even with minor trauma such as pressure from poorly fitting shoes or bed linens. *Frequent inspection and documentation of skin condition is vital to identify early indicators of impaired skin integrity and reduce the risk of complications such as infection.*
- Provide meticulous daily skin care, keeping the skin clean and dry. Apply a moisturizing cream to dry or

scaly areas. *Intact skin is the body's first defense against bacterial invasion. Ischemic tissues of the injured extremity provide an excellent medium for microorganism growth. Clean, dry, supple skin decreases the risk of breakdown.*

- Apply a bed cradle. *The bed cradle suspends bed linens over the legs, preventing them from placing pressure on extremities and injured tissues. Minimizing pressure on the tissues promotes capillary blood flow.*
- Provide an egg-crate mattress, flotation pad, sheepskin, or heel protectors. *Ischemic tissues may be damaged by minor trauma such as that created by the shearing forces of skin against bed linens.*

Promote Activity Tolerance. Pain and impaired perfusion of peripheral tissues may limit the patient's ability to engage in desired activities, even impairing self-care.

Expected Outcome: Patient will participate in activity program without suffering any complications.

The nurse will:

- Assist with care activities as needed. *Severe claudication or rest pain may limit activities. Muscle atrophy of affected extremities is common, leading to fatigue and weakness.*
- Unless contraindicated, encourage gradual increases in duration and intensity of exercise. Teach to rest with extremities dependent when claudication develops, resuming activity after pain has abated. *Gradual increases in the duration and intensity of exercise promote development of collateral circulation, improve exercise tolerance, provide a sense of well-being, and support self-esteem.*
- Provide diversional activities during periods of prescribed bedrest. Encourage relaxation techniques to reduce muscle tension. *Diversional activities help prevent boredom and stress associated with enforced rest. Relaxation techniques reduce vasoconstriction induced by stress, improving peripheral circulation.*
- Encourage frequent position changes and active range-of-motion exercises. Encourage self-care to the extent possible. *Position changes relieve pressure on tissues, improving capillary circulation and reducing tissue ischemia. Range-of-motion exercises help prevent muscle atrophy and joint contractures. Self-care supports self-esteem.*

Caring for Older Adults with PVD. With aging, blood vessels thicken and become less compliant. These changes reduce oxygen delivery to the tissues and impair carbon dioxide and waste product removal from the tissues. When normal effects of aging combine with an increased risk of atherosclerosis, the risk of peripheral vascular disease is high.

The older adult with peripheral vascular disease requires the same care and teaching as other patients. However, visual deficits and osteoarthritis may make foot care more difficult. Long-standing smoking habits are difficult to break. Mobility may be impaired by arthritis or the effects of neurologic disorders. The patient who lives alone may resist walking. Periodic visits by a community or home health nurse may be helpful, as may be encouraging the patient to join a support group for stopping smoking, changing eating habits, and taking part in regular physical activity

Transitions of Care

Discuss healthy lifestyle habits with community and religious groups, schoolchildren (grades K through 12), and through print media to reduce the incidence and slow the progression of atherosclerosis. Strongly encourage all patients to avoid smoking in the first place and to stop all forms of tobacco use. Discuss the adverse effects of smoking and the benefits of quitting. Provide information about dietary recommendations to maintain a healthy weight and optimal cholesterol levels. Discuss the benefits and importance of regular exercise. Regular daily exercise is a primary intervention for all types of peripheral arterial disease to promote development of collateral circulation and maintain tissue perfusion. Finally, encourage patients with cardiovascular risk factors to undergo regular screening for hypertension, diabetes, and hyperlipidemia.

Discuss the following topics when preparing the patient and family for home and community-based care.

- Smoking-cessation strategies and ways to avoid secondhand smoke
- Prescribed medications and anticoagulants, their purpose, doses, desired and adverse effects
- Signs of excess bleeding to report to the healthcare provider
- Skin surveillance and foot care (refer to Box 32.2)
- Recommended diet and exercise.

If revascularization or surgery has been performed, include the following topics as appropriate:

- Incision care
- Manifestations of complications (e.g., infection, graft leakage, or thrombosis) to be reported to the healthcare provider
- Activity limitations.

Provide referrals to home health services, physical or occupational therapy, and home maintenance assistance services as indicated. Consider resources such as Meals on Wheels for patients who are severely limited by their disease. PVD interferes with arterial blood flow to the lower extremities, increasing the risk for neuropathy and paresthesias, ulcers that do not heal, necrosis, gangrene, and amputation.

The Patient with Thromboangiitis Obliterans

Thromboangiitis obliterans (also called *Buerger disease*) is an occlusive vascular disease in which small and midsize peripheral arteries become inflamed and spastic, causing clots to form. This disease may affect either the upper or lower extremities; it often affects a leg or a foot. Its exact etiology is unknown, but there is evidence of significant T-cell activation, autoimmunity, and inflammation (Mayo Clinic, 2018).

Case Study & Nursing Care Plan

A Patient with Peripheral Vascular Disease

William Duffy, age 69, is retired. His wife convinces him to see his healthcare provider for increasing leg pain with walking and other exercise.

ASSESSMENT

Katie Kotson, RN, obtains Mr. Duffy's history before he sees his healthcare provider. He states that he can only walk about a block before the pain in his calves gets so bad that he has to stop and rest. As a result, he has been less and less active, spending most of his time the past few months watching sports on television. He denies rest pain. He was diagnosed with type 2 diabetes about 15 years ago, which he manages with daily glyburide (DiaBeta), an oral hypoglycemic. He has stable angina, for which he takes atenolol (Tenormin) and an occasional nitroglycerin tablet. His alcohol intake is moderate, averaging 1 to 2 beers per day, and he smokes about a pack of cigarettes per day. He states he tried to quit smoking after developing angina, but "after nearly 50 years of smoking, I think that's impossible!"

Physical exam findings include height 173 cm (68 in.), weight 107 kg (235 lb), BP 168/78 mmHg, P 66 bpm, R 16/min, T 36.5°C (97.6°F); upper extremities warm and pink, normal hair distribution, pulses strong and equal; lower extremities below knees cool and ruddy when dependent, pale to pink when elevated, skin shiny, scant hair; posterior tibial pulses weak bilaterally; weak pedal pulse on R, unable to palpate on L; 1+ to 2+ edema both feet and ankles.

The healthcare provider finds that Mr. Duffy's systolic blood pressure in his legs is an average of 28 mmHg lower than in his arms. He makes the diagnosis of peripheral atherosclerosis and schedules Mr. Duffy for an exercise stress test with ankle pressure measurements before and after exercise and a color-flow Doppler ultrasound. Mr. Duffy is to return in 3 weeks after these studies have been completed.

DIAGNOSES

- Inability to tolerate daily activity due to poor blood flow to lower extremities
- Difficulty maintaining a healthy lifestyle related to smoking and lack of information about disease management
- Risk for breaks in skin integrity related to ischemic tissues of legs and feet
- Risk for complications of peripheral extremities due to neurovascular complications

EXPECTED OUTCOMES

- Patient will walk for at least 15 minutes three to four times per day, gradually increasing his pace and duration of exercise.
- Patient will relate the benefits of smoking cessation.
- Patient will identify strategies to improve chances for success in stopping smoking.
- Patient will meet with dietitian before next visit to discuss dietary measures to promote weight loss and slow atherosclerosis.
- Patient will verbalize an understanding of appropriate foot care measures.
- Patient will identify measures to prevent inadvertent injury of feet and legs.

PLANNING AND IMPLEMENTATION

- Teach about peripheral atherosclerosis and its relationship to Mr. Duffy's symptoms.
- With Mr. and Mrs. Duffy, plan strategies to start and maintain a program of regular exercise.
- Instruct to warm up slowly and to stop exercise and rest for 3 minutes (or until pain is relieved) when claudication develops, then resume exercising.
- Discuss the effects of smoking on blood vessels.
- Help Mr. Duffy identify smoking-cessation strategies such as support groups, clinics, and nicotine patches.
- Schedule an appointment with the dietitian to develop a low-calorie, low-fat, and low-cholesterol American Diabetes Association (ADA) diet that includes preferred foods and considers usual eating patterns.
- Reinforce and supplement previous foot care teaching.
- Discuss effects of impaired circulation on sensation in feet and legs and measures to prevent injury.

EVALUATION

When Mr. Duffy returns to the office 3 weeks later, his diagnosis has been confirmed by the diagnostic studies. The healthcare provider decides to continue conservative therapy, now prescribing atorvastatin (Lipitor) to lower Mr. Duffy's serum cholesterol level and cilostazol (Pletal) to reduce the risk of thrombosis and improve symptoms of claudication. Mr. Duffy asks his healthcare provider for a prescription for nicotine patches, saying he is ready to quit smoking, but thinks he needs help to be successful. Mr. and Mrs. Duffy tell Miss Kotson that they are walking before every meal and really enjoying being outside more. They plan to walk in the local shopping mall in bad weather. Mrs. Duffy has bought an American Heart Association cookbook, and is carefully planning their meals. Both Mr. and Mrs. Duffy have lost 2.3 kg (5 lb) since the previous visit. Mr. Duffy's skin on his legs and feet remains intact, and he identifies the measures he is using to protect his lower extremities from injury.

CLINICAL REASONING IN PATIENT CARE

1. What additional lifestyle changes related to peripheral atherosclerosis might be appropriate to suggest to Mr. Duffy at this time? Why?
2. Explain the relationship between physical exercise and pain in the patient with peripheral atherosclerosis. Compare this relationship to that between exercise and angina.
3. Mr. Duffy uses a beta-blocker, atenolol, to prevent angina. Why is this drug not effective in preventing claudication?
4. Develop a nursing care plan for the diagnosis of difficulty in maintaining a healthy lifestyle.

See Evaluating Your Response in Appendix B.

Pathophysiology and Course

Inflammatory cells infiltrate the wall of small and midsize arteries in the feet and possibly the hands. This inflammatory process is accompanied by thrombus formation and vasospasms of arterial segments that impair blood flow. Adjacent veins and nerves may be affected. As the disease progresses, affected vessels become scarred and fibrotic.

The course of the disease is intermittent with dramatic exacerbations and marked remissions. The disease may remain dormant for periods of weeks, months, or years. As the disease progresses, collateral vessels are more extensively involved. Consequently, subsequent episodes are more intense and prolonged. Prolonged periods of tissue hypoxia increase the risk for tissue ulceration and gangrene.

Incidence and Risk Factors

Thromboangiitis obliterans primarily affects men under age 40 who smoke. Cigarette smoking is the single most significant cause of the disease. The disease is more prevalent in Asians and people of Eastern European descent. The incidence of HLA-B5 and 2A9 antigens is higher in people with thromboangiitis obliterans, suggesting a genetic link.

Manifestations and Complications

Pain in the affected extremities is the primary manifestation of thromboangiitis obliterans. Both claudication, cramping pain in the calves and feet or the forearms and hands, and rest pain in the fingers and toes may occur. Sensation is diminished. Eventually, the skin becomes thin and shiny and the nails are thickened and malformed. On examination, the involved digits and/or extremities are pale, cyanotic, or ruddy and cool or cold to touch. Distal pulses (e.g., the dorsalis pedis, posterior tibial, ulnar, or radial) are either difficult to locate or absent, even with a Doppler device.

Painful ulcers and gangrene may develop in the fingers and toes as a result of severely impaired blood flow. Amputation may be necessary to remove necrotic tissue.

Interprofessional Care

Thromboangiitis obliterans is usually diagnosed by the history and physical examination. Doppler studies may be used to locate and determine the extent of the disease. Angiography and magnetic resonance imaging may be used to evaluate the extent of the disease, but are usually unnecessary.

The one most important component in managing this disease is smoking cessation. While stopping smoking does not cure the disease, it may slow its extension to other vessels. With continued smoking, attacks become increasingly intense and last much longer, significantly increasing the risk for ulcerations and gangrene.

Additional conservative measures are used to prevent vasoconstriction, improve peripheral blood flow, and prevent complications of chronic ischemia. These measures include keeping extremities warm, managing stress, keeping affected extremities in a dependent position, preventing injury to affected tissues, and regular exercise. Walking for 20 or more minutes several times a day is recommended.

There are no specific drugs for thromboangiitis obliterans. A calcium channel blocker such as diltiazem (Cardizem) or verapamil (Isoptin), or pentoxifylline (Trental), which decreases blood viscosity and increases red blood cell flexibility to improve peripheral blood flow, may provide some symptom relief.

Surgical approaches for thromboangiitis obliterans include sympathectomy or arterial bypass graft. Sympathectomy interrupts sympathetic nervous system input to affected vessels, reducing vasoconstriction and spasm. Arterial bypass grafts may be useful when larger vessels are affected by the disease. Amputation of an affected digit or extremity may be necessary if gangrene develops. (See Chapter 39 for more information about amputation.) Only portions of digits or of limbs (e.g., below the knee) may be amputated, to preserve as much healthy tissue as possible.

The prognosis for thromboangiitis obliterans depends significantly on the patient's ability and willingness to stop smoking. With smoking cessation and good foot care, the prognosis for saving the extremities is good, even though no cure is available.

Nursing Care

Nursing assessment and care for patients with this disease is similar to that provided for patients with other arterial occlusive diseases. Refer to the Nursing Care section for peripheral atherosclerosis earlier in this chapter, as well as nursing care of the postsurgical patient (Chapter 4) and following amputation (Chapter 39).

Transitions of Care

Teaching the patient about health promotion activities to prevent thromboangiitis obliterans focuses on preventing smoking, especially in high-risk populations. Strongly encourage all patients to avoid smoking in the first place and to stop all forms of tobacco use. Discuss the adverse effects of smoking and the benefits of quitting.

Nursing care focuses on promoting arterial circulation and preventing prolonged tissue hypoxia. Because inflammatory, spastic episodes may be unpredictable, care focuses on smoking cessation and relieving acute manifestations. In addition, postsurgical care is necessary if surgery has been performed.

Discuss the following topics when preparing patients with thromboangiitis obliterans and their families for home or community-based care:

- Absolute necessity of smoking cessation
- Foot care
- Protecting affected extremities from injury
- Purpose, dose, desired and adverse effects, interactions, and any precautions associated with prescribed medications
- Signs and symptoms to report to the healthcare provider.

The Patient with Raynaud Disease

Pathophysiology

Raynaud disease and **Raynaud phenomenon** are characterized by episodes of intense vasospasm in the small arteries and arterioles of the fingers and sometimes the toes. Raynaud disease and phenomenon differ only in terms of cause. Raynaud disease has no identifiable cause; Raynaud phenomenon occurs secondarily to another disease (such as collagen vascular diseases like scleroderma and rheumatoid arthritis), other known causes of vasospasm, or long-term exposure to cold or machinery (Sorenson et al., 2019).

Raynaud disease primarily affects young women between the ages of 20 and 40. Genetic predisposition may play a role in its development, although the actual cause is unknown. **Table 32.5** compares thromboangiitis obliterans and Raynaud disease.

Manifestations

Raynaud disease and phenomenon are characterized by spasms of the small arteries in the digits. The arterial spasms limit arterial blood flow to the fingers and possibly the toes. Initial attacks may involve only the tips of one or two fingers; with disease progression, the entire finger and all fingers may be affected.

The manifestations of Raynaud occur intermittently when spasms develop. Raynaud disease has been called "the blue-white-red disease" because affected digits initially turn blue as blood flow is reduced due to vasospasm, then white as circulation is more severely limited, and finally very red as the fingers are warmed and the spasm resolves (**Figure 32.7** ■). Sensory changes may occur during attacks, including numbness, stiffness, decreased sensation, and aching pain.

The attacks tend to become more frequent and prolonged over time. With repeated attacks (and resultant decrease in oxygenation), the fingertips thicken and the nails become brittle. Ulceration and gangrene are serious complications that rarely occur.

Interprofessional Care

Raynaud disease and phenomenon are primarily diagnosed by the history and physical examination. There are no specific diagnostic tests for these disorders.

Vasodilators may be prescribed to provide symptomatic relief. Low doses of a sustained-release calcium

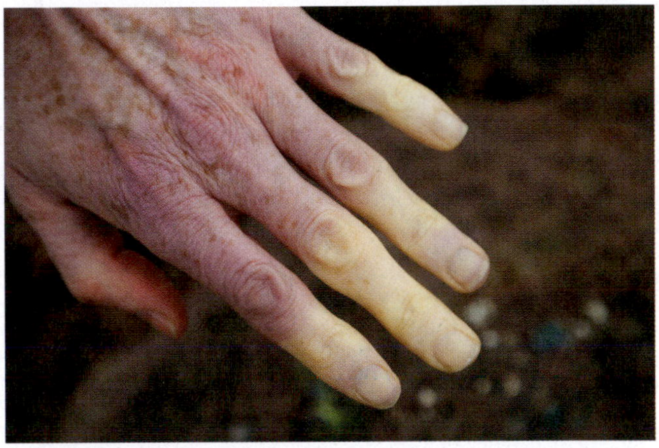

Figure 32.7 ■ Fingers of a patient with Raynaud phenomenon. Note the extreme pallor of the digits in response to exposure to cold.

Table 32.5 Comparison of Raynaud Disease and Thromboangiitis Obliterans

Topic	Raynaud Disease	Thromboangiitis Obliterans
Etiology	■ Unknown ■ Possible genetic predisposition	■ Cigarette smoking most probable single cause ■ Possible autoimmune response
Incidence/course of the disease	■ Onset commonly between 20 and 40 years of age ■ Usually affects young women ■ Becomes progressively worse over time	■ Occurs predominantly in men under 40 ■ More common in Asians and people of European heritage ■ Intermittent course with exacerbations and remissions ■ Increased severity and duration of attacks over time
Triggering stimuli	■ Emotional stress ■ Exposure to cold	■ Cigarette smoking
Assessment findings	■ Usually affects hands, sometimes toes ■ Pain becomes more severe and prolonged as disease progresses ■ "Blue-white-red" changes in color of hands with accompanying changes in skin temperature	■ Claudication and pain ■ Numbness or diminished sensation ■ Cool, pale, or cyanotic skin ■ Shiny, thin skin and white, malformed nails in affected extremities ■ Distal pulses difficult to find or absent ■ Trophic changes to nail beds ■ Ulceration and gangrene in later stages ■ Small, red, tender vascular cords in affected extremities
Management	■ Avoid unnecessary cold exposure ■ Emphasize smoking cessation ■ Medications such as calcium channel or alpha-adrenergic blockers as indicated ■ Teach stress management	■ Stop smoking (crucial) ■ Regular exercise ■ Protect extremities from cold injury ■ Teach stress management

channel blocker such as nifedipine (Procardia) or diltiazem (Cardizem) may be prescribed. The alpha-adrenergic blocker prazosin (Minipress) also may reduce the frequency and severity of attacks. Transdermal nitroglycerine (or longer-acting oral nitrates) helps some patients by decreasing the amount of time necessary for the hands to return to normal following an attack.

Conservative measures are a mainstay of treatment. Patients are instructed to keep their hands warm, wearing gloves when outside in cold weather and kitchen gloves when handling cold items (for instance, when preparing and serving cold foods and cleaning the refrigerator). Measures to avoid injury to the hands are taught. Sometimes attacks can be stopped by swinging the arms back and forth, increasing perfusion pressure in the small arteries by centrifugal force.

Smoking cessation is important. Stress reduction measures such as exercise, relaxation techniques, massage therapy, hobbies, aromatherapy, and counseling are taught or suggested. Additional lifestyle habits that contribute to vascular health are encouraged, such as reducing dietary fat, increasing activity level, and maintaining normal body weight.

Nursing Care

Nursing care for the patient with Raynaud disease is primarily educative and supportive. Protecting the hands and feet from exposure to cold and trauma is the major teaching topic. The diagnoses, outcomes, and interventions previously outlined for peripheral atherosclerosis are also appropriate for patients with Raynaud.

Transitions of Care

Raynaud prevention focuses on actions to avoid vascular constriction. Avoid cold weather and temperatures. Keep the body warm to avoid vasoconstriction of the skin. Nursing care to deal with the acute effects of Raynaud include warming of the affected body part and cessation of vasoconstricting agents such as nicotine.

Reassure patients with Raynaud disease that most people with the disorder experience only mild, infrequent episodes. Discuss the following topics in preparing the patient for managing the disorder:

- Dress warmly, keeping the trunk and hands warm.
- Avoid unnecessary exposure to cold.
- Stop smoking or do not start.
- Discuss the use, purpose, and desired and potential adverse effects of prescribed medications, if any.

The Patient with Acute Arterial Occlusion

A peripheral artery may be acutely occluded by development of a thrombus (blood clot) or by an embolism. Blood flow to tissues supplied by the artery is impaired, resulting in acute tissue ischemia and a risk for necrosis and gangrene.

Pathophysiology

Arterial Thrombosis

A **thrombus** is a blood clot that adheres to the vessel wall. Thrombi tend to develop in areas where intravascular factors stimulate coagulation (e.g., where a vessel lumen is partially obstructed and its wall is damaged and roughened by atherosclerosis). Other disorders, such as infection or inflammation of the vessel wall or pooling of blood (e.g., in an aneurysm), can also prompt coagulation and thrombus formation (Sorenson et al., 2019). A developing thrombus can occlude arterial blood flow through the vessel, leading to ischemia of tissues supplied by that artery. The extent of ischemia depends on the size of the affected artery and the degree of collateral circulation. In gradual processes of arterial occlusion such as atherosclerosis, collateral vessels often develop to compensate for impaired arterial flow. The extent of collateral circulation affects the degree of tissue ischemia distal to the thrombus.

Arterial Embolism

An **embolism** is sudden obstruction of a blood vessel by debris. A thrombus can break loose from the arterial wall to become a **thromboembolus**. Other substances can become emboli: Atherosclerotic plaque, masses of bacteria, cancer cells, amniotic fluid, bone marrow fat, and foreign objects such as air bubbles or broken intravenous catheters. Regardless of cause, an embolus eventually lodges in a vessel that is too small to allow it to pass.

Arterial emboli often originate in the left side of the heart. They are associated with myocardial infarction, valvular heart disease, left-sided heart failure, atrial fibrillation, or infectious heart diseases. Emboli from the left heart often enter the carotid arteries and become trapped in the cerebral circulation, causing neurologic deficits (see Chapter 42). Thromboemboli that develop in the aorta or peripheral arterial circulation tend to lodge in areas where the arterial lumen is narrowed by atherosclerotic plaque and at arterial bifurcations.

Manifestations

The manifestations of arterial thrombosis and embolism are those of tissue ischemia. Ischemic tissues are painful, pale, and cool or cold. Distal pulses are absent. Paresthesias (numbness and tingling) develop in the extremity. Cyanosis and mottling are common. Paralysis and muscle spasms may develop in the affected extremity. A line of demarcation between normal and ischemic tissue may be seen, particularly with embolism. Tissue below the line is cool or cold and pale, cyanotic, or mottled. Arterial occlusion can result in permanent vessel and limb damage. Complete arterial occlusion leads to tissue necrosis and gangrene unless blood flow is promptly restored.

Interprofessional Care

Acute arterial occlusions may require emergency treatment to preserve the limb if the obstructed vessel is large or collateral circulation is minimal. If the limb is not in jeopardy, more conservative management may be initiated.

Diagnosis

The diagnosis of acute arterial occlusion is often apparent by the signs and symptoms. *Arteriography* is used to confirm the diagnosis, locate the occlusion, and determine its extent.

Medications

Anticoagulation with intravenous heparin is initiated to prevent further clot propagation and recurrent embolism. Anticoagulation is continued with oral anticoagulants after discharge. See the section on venous thrombosis later in this chapter for more information about anticoagulant therapy (Adams et al., 2017).

Arterial thrombosis may be treated with intra-arterial thrombolytic therapy using streptokinase, urokinase, or tissue plasminogen activator (tPA) (refer to Chapter 30). Local intra-arterial injection of the thrombolytic drug allows use of lower doses and reduces the bleeding risk associated with thrombolytic drugs.

Surgery

Immediate *embolectomy* (within 4 to 6 hours) is the treatment of choice for acute arterial occlusion by an embolus to prevent tissue necrosis and gangrene. When the involved vessel is in an extremity, local anesthesia and a special balloon-tipped catheter known as a Fogarty catheter may be used for patients with high surgical risk. An embolus in the mesenteric circulation necessitates emergency laparotomy. The risk of complications and limb loss increases significantly if surgery is delayed by 12 or more hours. Potential major complications include compartment syndrome (Chapter 39), acute respiratory distress syndrome (Chapter 37), or acute renal failure (Chapter 28).

Arterial thrombosis may be treated surgically, although the required surgery may be more extensive due to the length of the vessel involved. *Thromboendarterectomy* is done to remove the thrombus and plaque in the artery. An arterial graft may be required. Nursing care for patients who have undergone embolectomy or thrombus removal is discussed in the nursing care section that follows.

Nursing Care

Assessment

See the Manifestations and Interprofessional Care sections for the assessment of the patient with acute arterial occlusion.

Nursing assessment for the patient with an acute arterial occlusion is highly focused due to the emergency nature of the problem.

- ***Health history:*** Complaints of pain, numbness, tingling, or weakness in the involved extremity; history of atherosclerotic vessel disease, heart disease, or recent invasive procedure (e.g., angiography, percutaneous revascularization procedure)
- ***Physical assessment:*** Vital signs; peripheral pulses in both extremities; color, temperature, sensation, and movement of involved extremity; skin condition; presence of a line of demarcation.

Priorities of Care

Collaborating with the interprofessional team to ensure adequate treatment of the underlying process while providing care that supports the physical and psychologic responses to the disorder is a priority of nursing care.

Diagnoses, Outcomes, and Interventions

Nursing care related to acute arterial occlusion focuses on protecting the affected extremity, managing anxiety, and reducing the risk of complications related to anticoagulant therapy.

Promote Effective Peripheral Tissue Perfusion. Protecting ischemic tissue from injury prior to surgery or medical thrombolysis is vital. Following surgery, there is a risk for thrombosis at the graft site or impaired perfusion due to edema of the surgical site.

Expected Outcome: Patient's tissue perfusion will be adequate as evidenced by adequate arterial flow (i.e., strong peripheral pulses).

The nurse will:

- Monitor extremity perfusion, comparing affected and unaffected extremities. Assess peripheral pulses (using the Doppler stethoscope as needed), skin temperature and color, capillary refill, movement, and sensation every 1 to 4 hours. Promptly report changes or complaints of increased or unrelieved pain. Propagation of a thrombus can further obstruct arterial flow, increasing tissue ischemia. Following surgery, arterial spasms may cause a cyanotic, pulseless extremity; normal color and pulses should return within 12 hours. *A thrombus may form at the surgical site or within a graft, causing tissue ischemia with pain and other manifestations of arterial occlusion. Further measures to restore circulation may be necessary.*
- Maintain intravenous fluids as ordered. *Adequate circulating blood volume is necessary to maintain cardiac output and tissue perfusion.*
- Protect the extremity, keeping it horizontal or lower than the heart. Use a cradle to keep bedclothes off the extremity and a sheepskin or foam pad to protect it from hard or abrasive surfaces. Do not apply heat or cold. *Keeping the extremity lower than the heart promotes collateral blood flow. Ischemic tissue is easily damaged by minimal trauma such as shearing by bed linens or heat or cold application.*
- Following surgery, avoid raising the knee, placing pillows under the knees, or sitting with 90-degree hip flexion. *These activities may impair blood flow through the affected vessel.*

Reduce Anxiety. Patients with an acute arterial occlusion are often very anxious. The rapid and intense nature of preoperative activities can be overwhelming, increasing anxiety about the disorder and its outcome. Manifestations of anxiety may include trembling, palpitations, restlessness, dry mouth, helplessness, inability to relax, irritability, forgetfulness, and lack of awareness of surroundings. Nursing measures focus on establishing trust and minimizing the effects of anxiety to decrease surgical risk and improve recovery.

Expected Outcome: Patient will be able to control anxiety as evidenced by verbalized decrease in subjective distress.

The nurse will:

- Spend as much time as possible with the patient. Provide opportunities to verbalize anxiety; offer reassurance and support. Support adaptive coping mechanisms. *The presence of a caring nurse provides a safe environment for expressing fears and anxieties. Coping mechanisms reduce the immediate perceived threat and increase the ability to deal with the situational crisis.*
- Perform required measures in an expedient but calm manner. *Calm, confident performance of treatment measures reassures the patient and family that appropriate care is being given to treat the problem at hand.*
- Assess anxiety level at least every 8 hours, and more often as needed. Intervene as indicated to reduce anxiety. *Assessment helps determine the intensity of anxiety and the patient's ability to control it and directs interventions to reduce it.*
- Decrease sensory stimuli as much as possible. *Reducing environmental stimuli provides the patient a degree of control over anxiety.*
- Speak slowly and clearly and avoid unnecessary interruptions when listening. Give concise directions, focusing on the present. Involve the patient in simple tasks and decisions to the extent possible. *High levels of anxiety interfere with learning. Keeping interactions focused on the present situation directs the patient's focus and provides reassurance that it is the most important focus of the nurse as well. Providing opportunities for self-care and decision making reinforces the patient's importance and power to control the situation.*

Reduce Risk for Injury and Bleeding. Thrombolytic and/or anticoagulant therapy used to dissolve existing clots and prevent further clot formation increases the risk for bleeding. Close monitoring of physical status and laboratory data is vital, as are measures to reduce the risk for injury and bleeding.

Expected Outcome: Patient will remain free of any evidence of new bleeding and take precautions to prevent bleeding.

The nurse will:

- Assess for and report manifestations of impaired clotting, including excessive incisional bleeding; prolonged oozing from injection sites; bleeding gums, nosebleed, or hematuria; petechiae, bruising, or purpura. *Anticoagulants and thrombolytics interfere with the clotting cascade and may cause abnormal bleeding.*
- Monitor activated partial thromboplastin time (aPTT) during heparin therapy and prothrombin time (PT) or International Normalized Ratio (INR) during oral anticoagulant therapy. Report values outside desired range. *The aPTT, PT, and INR are prolonged by anticoagulant therapy. Values higher than the desired range may indicate an increased risk for bleeding; values below the target may indicate inadequate anticoagulation.*
- Protect from injury: Use side rails or other measures as needed to prevent falls; avoid parenteral injections and other invasive procedures as much as possible; hold firm pressure over injection and intravenous sites for 5 minutes and over arterial punctures for 20 minutes; use a soft toothbrush or sponge for oral care; use an electric razor for shaving. *Minor trauma can lead to extensive bleeding, particularly in the patient who has received a thrombolytic drug.*

Transitions of Care

Education focusing on the risk factors for arterial occlusion are the same as those for other vascular beds and include the nonmodifiable factors of advanced age and male sex. Modifiable factors that are amenable to education include diabetes mellitus control, smoking cessation, blood pressure control, and lifestyle changes to control lipid levels. Acute care focuses on addressing impaired tissue perfusion. Surgical intervention is commonly required. When preparing the patient and family for home or community-based care related to an acute arterial occlusion, discuss the following topics as indicated:

- Care of the incision
- Manifestations of complications to be reported, including symptoms of infection or occlusion of the graft or artery
- Long-term anticoagulant therapy, including the reason, prescribed dose, follow-up laboratory testing and appointments, interactions with other drugs, and manifestations of excessive bleeding
- Any activity restrictions or dietary modifications
- Lifestyle modifications to slow atherosclerosis and control hypertension
- Measures to promote peripheral circulation and maintain tissue integrity (see the discussion of venous peripheral atherosclerosis that follows).

Refer for home care services (nursing care, physical therapy, housekeeping services) as indicated.

32.4 Disorders of Venous Circulation

The two primary categories of venous system disorders are occlusive disorders and those related to ineffective venous blood flow. Impaired venous blood flow can lead to stasis and clotting, as well as tissue changes associated with venous congestion.

Physiology Review

The venous system is a low-pressure system in comparison with the arterial circulation. Veins and venules are thin-walled, distensible vessels. Although they contain smooth muscle that allows them to contract or expand, the media (muscle layer) of veins is significantly thinner than that of arteries. The low pressures in the venous system allow it to serve as a reservoir for blood. Stimulation by the sympathetic nervous system causes veins to contract, helping maintain vascular volume. The low-pressure venous system relies on skeletal muscle contractions and pressure changes in the abdomen and thorax to facilitate blood return to the heart. Unlike arteries, veins of the extremities contain valves to prevent retrograde blood flow.

The Patient with Venous Thrombosis

Venous thrombosis (*thrombophlebitis*) is a condition in which a blood clot (thrombus) forms on the wall of a vein, accompanied by inflammation of the vein wall and some degree of obstructed venous blood flow.

Thrombi can form in either superficial or deep veins. **Deep venous thrombosis (DVT)** is a common complication of hospitalization, surgery, and immobilization. Obstetric and orthopedic procedures carry a higher risk for venous thrombosis; it may develop in more than 50% of patients having orthopedic surgery, particularly surgeries involving the hip or knee. Other significant risk factors for venous thrombosis include abdominal or thoracic surgery, certain cancers, trauma, pregnancy, and use of oral contraceptives or hormone replacement therapy. See **Box 32.3**.

Pathophysiology and Manifestations

Three pathologic factors, called *Virchow triad*, are associated with thrombophlebitis: (1) Stasis of blood, (2) vessel damage, and (3) increased blood coagulability. Vessel trauma stimulates the clotting cascade. Platelets aggregate at the site, particularly when venous stasis is present. Platelets and fibrin form the initial clot. Red blood cells are trapped in the fibrin meshwork, and the thrombus propagates (grows) in the direction of blood flow. The inflammatory response is triggered, causing tenderness, swelling, and erythema in the area of the thrombus. Initially the thrombus floats within the vein.

BOX 32.3
Factors Associated with Venous Thrombosis

- Immobilization: Myocardial infarction, heart failure, stroke, postoperative
- Surgery: Orthopedic, thoracic, abdominal, genitourinary
- Cancer: Pancreatic, lung, ovary, testes, urinary tract, breast, stomach
- Trauma: Fractures of the spine, pelvis, femur, tibia; spinal cord injury
- Pregnancy and delivery
- Hormone therapy: Oral contraceptives, hormone replacement therapy
- Coagulation disorders

Pieces of the thrombus may break loose and travel through the circulation as emboli. Fibroblasts eventually invade the thrombus, scarring the vein wall and destroying venous valves. Although patency of the vein may be restored, valve damage is permanent, affecting directional flow.

Manifestations of Deep Venous Thrombosis

The deep veins of the legs, primarily in the calf, and the pelvis provide the most hospitable environment for venous thrombosis. Approximately 80% of DVTs begin in the deep veins of the calf, often propagating into the popliteal and femoral veins (**Figure 32.8** ■). DVT is usually asymptomatic; in some patients, a pulmonary embolism may be the first indication.

When present, the manifestations of DVT are primarily due to the inflammatory process accompanying the thrombus. Calf pain, which may be described as tightness or a dull, aching pain in the affected extremity, particularly upon walking, is the most common symptom. Tenderness, swelling, warmth, and erythema may be noted along the course of involved veins. The affected extremity may be cyanotic and is often edematous. Rarely, a cord may be palpated over the affected vein. A positive Homans sign (pain in the calf when the foot is dorsiflexed) is an unreliable indicator of DVT. Manifestations of deep venous thrombosis include:

- Usually asymptomatic
- Dull, aching pain in affected extremity, especially when walking
- Possible tenderness, warmth, erythema along affected vein
- Cyanosis of affected extremity
- Edema of affected extremity

The major complications of DVT are chronic venous insufficiency and pulmonary embolism. Pulmonary embolism occurs when the clot fragments or breaks loose from the vein wall. As the clot travels, it moves through progressively larger veins and into the right side of the heart. From there it enters the pulmonary circulation, where it eventually occludes arterial flow to the lungs. The result is a mismatch between ventilation (air flow) and perfusion (blood flow) in a portion of the lungs. The effect on gas exchange depends on the size of the embolism and the vessel it occludes. See Chapter 37 for more information about pulmonary emboli.

Manifestations of Superficial Venous Thrombosis

Venous catheters and infusions are the primary risk factors for superficial venous thrombosis. Superficial venous thrombosis may develop in conjunction with thromboangiitis obliterans, varicose veins, or deep venous thrombosis. It may develop spontaneously in pregnant women or following delivery. In some cases, superficial venous thrombosis of the long saphenous vein is the earliest sign of an abdominal cancer such as pancreatic cancer.

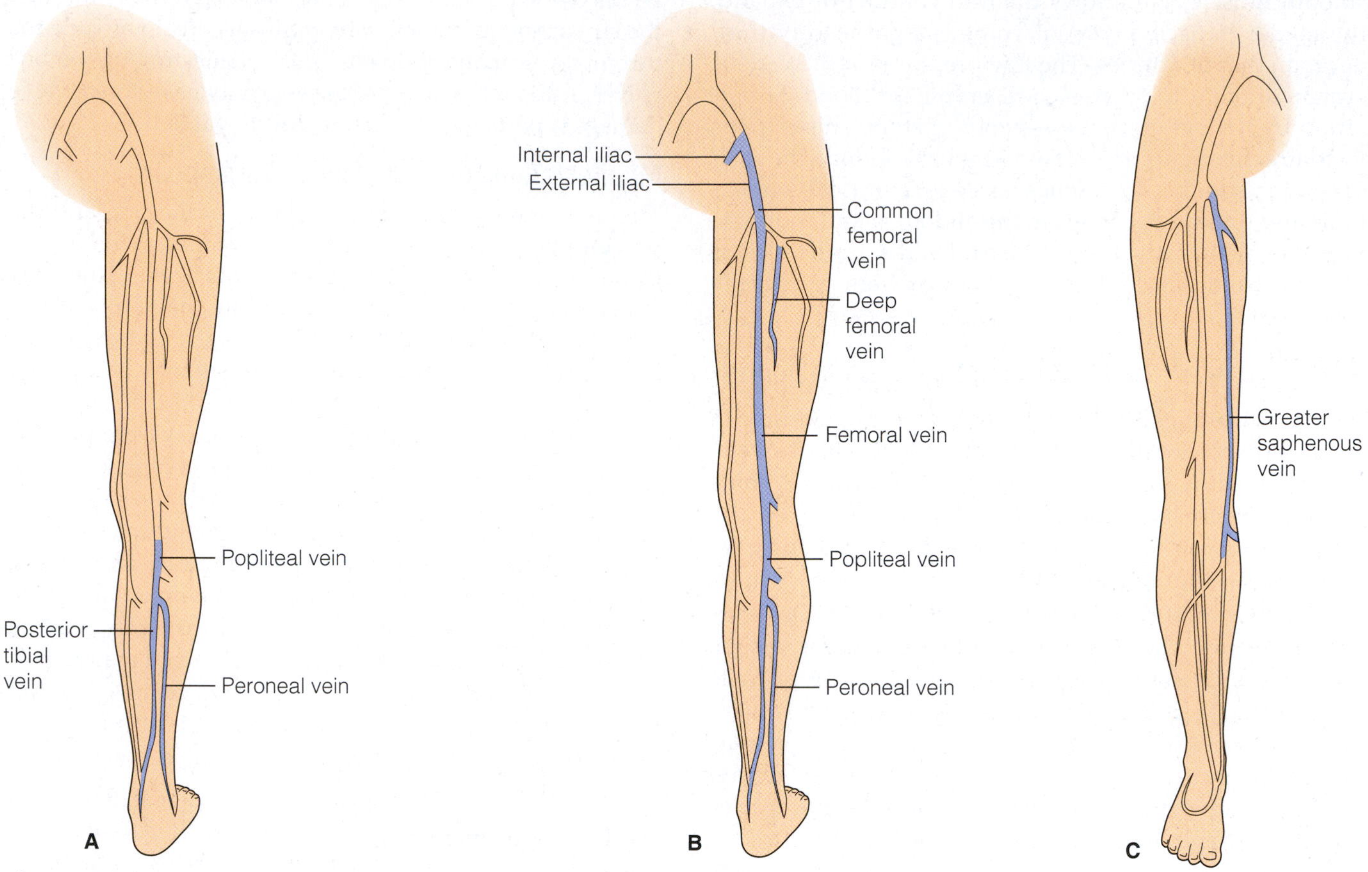
Popliteal vein
Posterior tibial vein
Peroneal vein
A
Internal iliac
External iliac
Common femoral vein
Deep femoral vein
Femoral vein
Popliteal vein
Peroneal vein
B
Greater saphenous vein
C

Figure 32.8 ■ Common locations of venous thrombosis. **A**, The most common sites of deep venous thrombosis. **B**, DVT extending from the calf to the iliac veins. **C**, Superficial venous thrombosis.

Superficial venous thrombosis is marked by pain and tenderness at the site of the thrombus. A reddened, warm, tender cord extending along the affected vein can be palpated. The area surrounding the vein may be swollen and red.

Interprofessional Care

It is important to differentiate venous thrombosis from other causes of extremity pain, such as cellulitis, muscle strain, contusion, and lymphedema. The history, physical examination, and diagnostic tests are used to establish the diagnosis. Treatment focuses on preventing further clotting or extension of the clot and addressing underlying causes.

Diagnosis

- ***Duplex venous ultrasonography*** is a noninvasive test used to visualize the vein and measure the velocity of blood flow in the veins. Although the clot often cannot be visualized directly, its presence can be inferred by an inability to compress the vein during the examination.
- ***Plethysmography*** is a noninvasive test that measures changes in blood flow through the veins. It is often used in conjunction with Doppler ultrasonography. Plethysmography is most valuable in diagnosing thromboses of larger or more superficial veins.
- ***MRI*** is another noninvasive means of detecting deep venous thrombosis. It is particularly useful when thrombosis of the vena cavae or pelvic veins is suspected.
- ***Ascending contrast venography*** uses an injected contrast medium to assess the location and extent of venous thrombosis. Although invasive, expensive, and uncomfortable, contrast venography is the most accurate diagnostic tool for venous thrombosis. It is used when the results of less invasive tests leave the diagnosis unclear.

Prophylaxis

Medications and other measures are used to prevent venous thrombosis when the risk is high. Low-molecular-weight heparins (see the following section) prevent DVT in patients who are undergoing general or orthopedic surgery, experiencing acute medical illness, or are on prolonged bedrest. Oral anticoagulation may be used as a prophylactic measure in patients with fractures or who are undergoing orthopedic surgery.

Elevating the foot of the bed with the knees slightly flexed promotes venous return. Early mobilization and leg exercises such as ankle flexion and extension assist venous flow by muscle compression. Intermittent pneumatic compression devices applied to the legs are effective to prevent

DVT. They are also used when anticoagulation is contraindicated due to the increased risk for bleeding. Elastic stockings are used to prevent venous thrombosis as well in patients at risk.

Medications

Anticoagulants to prevent clot propagation and enable the body's own lytic system to dissolve the clot are the mainstay of treatment for venous thrombosis. Thrombolytic drugs such as streptokinase or tissue plasminogen activator (tPA) may accelerate the process of clot lysis and prevent damage to venous valves. There is, however, no evidence that thrombolytic therapy is more effective in preventing pulmonary embolism in patients with existing DVT than anticoagulants. It also significantly increases the risk for bleeding and hemorrhage.

Nonsteroidal anti-inflammatory agents such as indomethacin (Indocin) or naproxen (Naprosyn) may be ordered to reduce inflammation in the veins and provide symptomatic relief, particularly for patients with superficial venous thrombosis.

Anticoagulants. Anticoagulants are given to prevent clot extension and reduce the risk of subsequent pulmonary embolism. Anticoagulation is initiated with unfractionated heparin or low-molecular-weight (LMW) heparin. Following an initial intravenous bolus of 7500 to 10,000 units of unfractionated heparin, a continuous heparin infusion of 1000 to 1500 International Units per hour is started. The dosage is calculated to maintain the activated partial thromboplastin time (aPTT) at approximately twice the control or normal value. An infusion pump is used to deliver the prescribed dosage. Frequent monitoring of the infusion is an important nursing responsibility. Subcutaneous heparin injections may be used as an alternate to intravenous infusion in some instances.

LMW heparins are increasingly used to prevent and treat venous thrombosis. They do not require the close laboratory monitoring of unfractionated heparins. LMW heparin is administered subcutaneously in fixed doses once or twice daily, allowing the option of outpatient treatment. LMW heparins have additional advantages, in that they are more effective and carry lower risks for bleeding and thrombocytopenia than conventional, unfractionated heparins.

Oral anticoagulation with warfarin may be initiated concurrently with heparin therapy. Overlapping heparin and warfarin therapy for 4 to 5 days is important because the full anticoagulant effect of warfarin is delayed, and it may actually promote clotting during the first few days of therapy. Warfarin doses are adjusted to maintain the INR at 2.0 to 3.0 (Shields, Fox, & Liebrecht, 2018).

Once this level is achieved, the heparin is discontinued and a maintenance dose of warfarin is prescribed to prevent recurrent thrombosis. Anticoagulation is generally continued for at least 3 months. When DVT is recurrent or risk factors such as altered coagulability or cancer are present, anticoagulant therapy may be prolonged. Regular follow-up is necessary to be sure prothrombin times (INR) remain within the desirable range for anticoagulation. See **Medication Administration 32.B** for the nursing implications for anticoagulant therapy.

Medication Administration 32.B

Anticoagulant Therapy

HEPARIN

Heparin interferes with the clotting cascade by inhibiting the effects of thrombin and preventing the conversion of fibrinogen to fibrin. This prevents the formation of a stable fibrin clot. At therapeutic levels, heparin prolongs the thrombin time, clotting time, and aPTT. When given intravenously, its effect is immediate. Given subcutaneously, its onset of action is within 1 hour (Adams et al., 2017; Shields et al., 2018). *Heparin-induced thrombocytopenia (HIT)* is a potential complication of therapy with unfractionated heparin. See Chapter 33 for more information about HIT and nursing responsibilities in monitoring for this dangerous potential complication.

Nursing Responsibilities

- Assess for history of unexplained or active bleeding. Assess laboratory results for abnormal clotting profile or evidence of active bleeding.
- Give a test dose as indicated to patients with a history of multiple allergies or a history of asthma.
- Administer by deep subcutaneous injection; abdominal sites are preferred. Avoid injecting within 2 inches of the umbilicus. Rotate sites. Do not aspirate prior to injecting or massage after the injection.
- Intravenous solutions may be diluted with dextrose, normal saline, or Ringer solution. Use an infusion pump.
- Keep protamine sulfate, a heparin antagonist, available to treat excessive bleeding.
- Monitor and report abnormal laboratory results and aPTT values outside the desired range.
- Promptly report evidence of bleeding such as hematemesis, hematuria, bleeding gums, or unexplained abdominal or back pain.

Health Education for the Patient and Family

- Report unusual bleeding or excessive menstrual flow.
- Use an electric razor and a soft-bristle toothbrush; prevent injury by clearing pathways, using a nightlight, and other measures.
- Do not consume alcohol.
- Avoid contact sports while on anticoagulant therapy.
- Do not consume large amounts of food rich in vitamin K (yellow and dark green vegetables).
- Do not use aspirin or NSAIDs while on heparin therapy unless advised to do so by your healthcare provider.
- Wear a medical alert tag and advise all healthcare providers (including dentists and podiatrists) of therapy.

LOW-MOLECULAR-WEIGHT HEPARINS

dalteparin (Fragmin)

enoxaparin (Lovenox)

(continued)

LMW heparins are the most bioavailable fraction of heparin. They provide a more precise and predictable anticoagulant effect than unfractionated heparins. Like unfractionated heparin, LMW heparin prevents conversion of prothrombin to thrombin, liberation of thromboplastin from platelets, and formation of a stable clot. LMW heparins cannot be used interchangeably with each other or with unfractionated heparin. Although the risk of heparin-induced thrombocytopenia is significantly lower with LMW heparin, patients who were previously treated with unfractionated heparin may develop HIT when treated with LMW heparin.

INJECTABLE ANTICOAGULANTS

antithrombin III (Thrombate III)
ardeparin (Normiflo)
argatroban (Acova)
bivalirudin (Angiomax)
desirudin (Iprivask)
fondaparinux (Arixtra)
tinzaparin (Innohep)

Nursing Responsibilities

- Assess for evidence of active bleeding, a history of bleeding disorders or thrombocytopenia, or sensitivity to heparin, sulfites, or pork products.
- Monitor for unusual or masked bleeding. PT and aPTT levels may be within normal levels even in the presence of hemorrhage.
- Administer by deep subcutaneous injection into abdominal wall, thigh, or buttocks. Rotate sites. Do not aspirate or massage.

Health Education for the Patient and Family

- Subcutaneous self-administration technique, timing of doses, and site rotation. Do not rub site after administering to minimize bruising.
- Do not take aspirin, NSAIDs, or other over-the-counter drugs unless recommended by your healthcare provider.
- Promptly report excessive bruising or bleeding, chest pain, difficulty breathing, itching, rash, or swelling to your healthcare provider.
- Keep follow-up appointments as scheduled.

ORAL ANTICOAGULANT

warfarin (Coumadin)

Warfarin interferes with synthesis of vitamin K–dependent clotting factors by the liver, leading to depletion of these factors. It has no effect on already circulating clotting factors or on existing clots. Warfarin inhibits extension of existing thrombi and the formation of new clots. Its action is cumulative and more prolonged than that of heparin.

Other Oral Anticoagulants

dabigatran (Pradaxa)
rivaroxaban (Xarelto)

Dabigatran is a direct thrombin inhibitor that helps to stop clots from forming by working directly on thrombin. Rivaroxaban acts as a selective factor X inhibitor, inactivating the cascade of coagulation. Neither requires monitoring like warfarin does; however, there is no reversal agent available for these drugs. Costs are also significantly higher for these drugs when compared to warfarin.

Nursing Responsibilities

- Assess laboratory results and history for evidence of abnormal bleeding.
- Multiple drugs affect the metabolism and protein binding of warfarin; note all medications and assess for interactions with warfarin.
- Do not give during pregnancy because warfarin may cause congenital malformations.
- Oral tablets may be crushed and given without regard to meals.
- Dilute intravenous warfarin with supplied diluent; administer within 4 hours by direct intravenous injection at a rate of 25 mg/min.
- Keep vitamin K available to reverse effects of warfarin in the event of excessive bleeding or hemorrhage.
- Monitor PT or INR; report values outside the desired range (warfarin only).

Health Education for the Patient and Family

- Do not take your prescribed dose and notify your healthcare provider immediately if bleeding occurs (hematemesis, bright red or black, tarry feces, hematuria, bleeding gums, excessive bruising, etc.). Report rash or manifestations of hepatitis (dark urine, malaise, yellow skin or sclera).
- Take your warfarin at the same time every day; do not change brands as their effects may differ.
- Menstrual bleeding may be slightly increased; contact your healthcare provider if it increases significantly. Use reliable birth control to prevent pregnancy while taking warfarin. Immediately contact your healthcare provider if you think you may be pregnant.
- Take precautions to prevent injury and bleeding: Use a soft-bristle toothbrush and electric razor, wear shoes, and use a nightlight. Avoid participating in contact sports.
- Do not smoke, use alcohol, or take any over-the-counter drugs unless specifically recommended by your healthcare provider. Notify all healthcare providers, including dentists and podiatrists, of therapy. Wear a medical alert tag.
- Obtain lab tests as scheduled and keep all scheduled follow-up appointments.

Note: Drugs identified in blue are among the 200 most commonly prescribed medications in the United States.

Source: Adams, et al., 2017.

Treatments

Treatment of venous thrombosis includes measures to relieve symptoms and reduce inflammation. With superficial venous thrombosis, applying warm, moist compresses over the affected vein, extremity rest, and anti-inflammatory agents usually provide relief of symptoms.

Bedrest may be ordered for DVT. The duration of bedrest is typically determined by the extent of leg edema. The legs are elevated 15 to 20 degrees, with the knees slightly flexed, above the level of the heart to promote venous return and discourage venous pooling. Elastic antiembolism stockings (TEDS) or pneumatic compression devices are frequently ordered to stimulate the muscle-pumping mechanism that promotes the return of blood to the heart. When permitted, walking is encouraged while avoiding prolonged standing or sitting. Crossing the legs is avoided, as are tight-fitting garments or stockings that bind.

Surgery

Venous thrombosis is usually effectively treated with conservative measures and anticoagulation. In some cases, however, surgery is required to remove the thrombus, prevent its extension into deep veins, or prevent the effects of embolization.

Venous thrombectomy is done when thrombi lodge in the femoral vein and their removal is necessary to prevent pulmonary embolism or gangrene. Successful thrombus removal rapidly improves venous circulation. The duration of this effect varies.

When venous thrombosis is recurrent and anticoagulant therapy is contraindicated, a filter may be inserted into the vena cava to capture emboli from the pelvis and lower extremities, preventing pulmonary embolism. Several different filters are available (**Figure 32.9** ■). The Greenfield filter is widely used for its ability to trap emboli within its apex while maintaining patency of the vena cava. The filter can be inserted under fluoroscopy with local anesthesia. Mortality and morbidity associated with the filter are very low.

Extensive thrombosis of the saphenous vein may necessitate ligation and division of the saphenous vein where it joins the femoral vein to prevent clot extension into the deep venous system. A vein affected by septic venous thrombosis is excised to control the infection. Antibiotic therapy is also initiated.

Nursing Care

Assessment

See the Manifestations and Interprofessional Care sections for the assessment of the patient with venous thrombosis.

Assess patients at risk for venous thrombosis for manifestations and risk factors.

- ***Health history:*** Ask about complaints of leg or calf pain, its duration and characteristics, and the effect of walking on the pain; history of venous thrombosis or other clotting disorders; current medications
- ***Physical assessment:*** Inspect affected extremity for redness, edema; palpate for tenderness, warmth, cordlike structures; body temperature

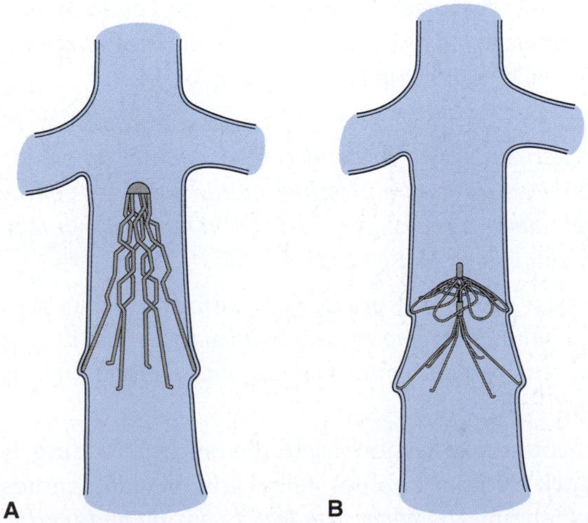
A
B

Figure 32.9 ■ Venal cava filters. **A**, Greenfield filter. **B**, Nitinol filter.

- ***Laboratory data:*** Tests include clotting studies (APTT, pro time, INR) (Kee, 2014).

See the accompanying Case Study & Nursing Care Plan for an example of an assessment of a patient with DVT.

Priorities of Care

Collaborating with the interprofessional team to ensure adequate treatment of the underlying process while providing care that supports the physical and psychologic responses to the disorder is a priority of nursing care.

Diagnoses, Outcomes, and Interventions

In addition to the preventative measures identified earlier, priority nursing diagnoses for the patient with venous thrombosis relate to pain, maintenance of tissue perfusion and integrity, and the potential adverse effects of prescribed treatments.

Manage Pain. The pain associated with venous thrombosis results from inflammation of the involved vein. It may be aggravated by use of the involved extremity. Associated edema and swelling may contribute to discomfort. Measures to reduce the inflammation often help relieve the pain.

Expected Outcome: Patient will exhibit adequate pain control as evidenced by physical well-being.

The nurse will:

- Regularly assess pain location, characteristics, and level using a standardized pain scale. Report increasing pain or changes in its location or characteristics. *Tissue substances released during the inflammatory process can stimulate pain receptors. In addition, localized swelling presses on pain-sensitive structures in the area of the inflammation, contributing to discomfort. As inflammation and swelling are reduced, pain should abate. Continued or increasing pain may indicate extension of the thrombosis. Sudden chest pain may indicate a pulmonary embolism, necessitating immediate intervention.*
- Measure calf and thigh diameter of the affected extremity on admission and daily thereafter. Report increases promptly. *The inflammatory process causes vasodilation and increases vessel permeability, causing edema of the affected extremity. Baseline and subsequent measurements provide a measure of treatment effectiveness.*
- Apply warm, moist heat to affected extremity at least four times daily, using warm, moist compresses or an aqua-K pad. *Moist heat penetrates tissues to a greater depth than dry heat. Warmth promotes vasodilation, allowing reabsorption of excess fluid into the circulation. Vasodilation also reduces resistance within the affected vessel, reducing pain. As edema subsides, pressure on surrounding tissues is relieved, thereby reducing pain.*
- Maintain bedrest as ordered. *Using leg muscles during walking exacerbates the inflammatory process and increases edema. This, in turn, increases venous compression and pain.*

Promote Effective Peripheral Tissue Perfusion. As thrombi develop, they occlude the lumen of the vein and obstruct blood flow. In addition, the accompanying inflammatory response may precipitate vessel spasms, further impairing arterial and venous blood flow and tissue perfusion. Impaired tissue perfusion, in turn, deprives tissues of nutrients and oxygen. As a result, distal tissues of the affected extremity are at risk for ulceration and infection.

Expected Outcome: Patient's tissue perfusion will be adequate as evidenced by adequate arterial flow (i.e., strong peripheral pulses).

The nurse will:

- Assess peripheral pulses, skin integrity, capillary refill times, and color of extremities at least every 8 hours. Report changes promptly. Assessment of both extremities allows comparison of the affected and unaffected limbs. *Weak or absent pulses, impaired capillary refill, or significant color changes in the affected extremity may indicate extension of the thrombus or a possible complication.*
- Assess the skin of the affected lower leg and foot at least every 8 hours and more often, as indicated. *Frequent assessment is important to rapidly detect early signs of tissue breakdown and implementation of measures to protect vulnerable tissues. Early intervention allows healing and restoration of tissue integrity; allowed to continue, the process can lead to necrosis and potential gangrene.*
- Elevate extremities at all times, keeping knees slightly flexed and legs above the level of the heart. *Elevation of the extremities promotes venous return and reduces peripheral edema. Knee flexion promotes muscle relaxation.*

SAFETY ALERT: Remove antiembolic stockings or pneumatic compression device for 30 to 60 minutes during daily hygiene. Antiembolic stockings (e.g., TED hose) and pneumatic compression devices exert pressure on the extremity and promote venous return. They can, however, impair perfusion of the dermis. Removing them periodically allows for assessment of the underlying tissue and restores perfusion of the dermis, reducing the risk for skin breakdown. Their use may be continued following discharge to reduce the risk of recurrent venous thrombosis. ■

- Use mild soaps, solutions, and lotions to clean the affected leg and foot daily. Pat dry after washing, and apply a non-alcohol-based lotion or moisturizing cream. *Daily hygiene with nondrying soaps and solutions removes potential pathogens from the skin surface and maintains skin integrity and the first line of defense against infection. Caustic or harsh soaps or solutions can dry and crack the skin. Dry, cracked skin permits bacteria and other microorganisms to enter and infect the tissue, potentially leading to ulceration and venous gangrene.*
- Use a weight-dispersion appliance such as an egg-crate mattress or sheepskin on the bed as needed. *Egg-crate mattresses and sheepskins distribute weight more evenly, preventing excess pressure on affected tissues.*
- Encourage frequent position changes at least every 2 hours while awake. *Frequent position changes reduce pressure on bony prominences and edematous tissue, reducing the risk of tissue breakdown.*

Reduce Risk for Bleeding. Anticoagulant therapy interferes with the body's normal clotting mechanisms, increasing the risk for bleeding and hemorrhage.

Expected Outcome: Patient will remain free of any evidence of new bleeding and take precautions to prevent bleeding.

The nurse will:

- Assess for and promptly report evidence of bleeding, such as petechiae; bruising; bleeding gums; obvious or occult blood in vomitus, stool, or urine; or unexplained back or abdominal pain. *Anticoagulants interfere with the ability to form a stable clot and prevent excessive bleeding. Even minor trauma such as toothbrushing or bumping into furniture can result in bleeding.*
- Monitor laboratory results, including the INR (prothrombin time), aPTT, hemoglobin, and hematocrit as indicated. Report values outside the normal or desired range. *Coagulation studies are used to monitor the effect of anticoagulant medications. Values within the desired range prevent further clot development while carrying a low risk for bleeding and hemorrhage. A fall in the hemoglobin and hematocrit levels may indicate undetected bleeding.*

Promote Mobility. Although prolonged bedrest is rarely required, when it is prescribed, it is associated with many problems including constipation, joint contractures, muscle atrophy, and boredom. Nursing care goals include maintaining joint range of motion, minimizing muscle atrophy, and reducing boredom.

Expected Outcome: Patient will demonstrate optimal independence in positioning, exercising, and performing functional activities in bed.

The nurse will:

- Encourage active range-of-motion (ROM) exercises at least every 8 hours. Provide passive ROM as needed. *ROM exercises maintain joint mobility and prevent contractures. Active ROM (performed by the patient) also helps prevent muscle atrophy and preserve function. While passive ROM exercises do not prevent muscle atrophy, they do maintain joint mobility.*
- Encourage frequent position changes, deep breathing, and coughing. *Prolonged immobility can lead to impaired airway clearance and respiratory complications, such as atelectasis or pneumonia. Turning, coughing, and deep breathing facilitate expulsion of secretions from the respiratory tract, airway clearance, and alveolar ventilation.*
- Encourage increased fluid and dietary fiber intake. *Constipation is a frequent complication of immobility due to decreased gastrointestinal motility and loss of abdominal muscle strength. Increasing fluid and fiber intake helps maintain soft, easily expelled stools.*
- Assist with and encourage ambulation as allowed. *Ambulation promotes venous blood flow, helps maintain muscle tone and joint mobility, and increases the sense of well-being.*
- Encourage diversional activities such as reading, handiwork or other hobbies, television or video games, and socializing. *Boredom may lead to dozing and inertia, with little physical movement or mental stimulation, increasing the risk for complications of immobility.*

Promote Effective Cardiopulmonary Tissue Perfusion. A thrombus that forms in the deep veins of the legs or pelvis may break loose or fragment, becoming an embolism. Emboli that originate in the venous system usually become trapped in the pulmonary circulation (pulmonary embolism). Gas exchange in the affected area is impaired as blood flow ceases or is reduced to an area of the lungs that is well ventilated (see Chapter 37).

Expected Outcome: Patient's tissue perfusion will be adequate as evidenced by adequate arterial flow (i.e., strong peripheral pulses) and freedom from dyspnea.

The nurse will:

- Frequently assess respiratory status, including rate, depth, ease, and oxygen saturation levels. *A mismatch of ventilation and perfusion can significantly affect gas exchange, leading to rapid, shallow respirations, dyspnea and air hunger, and a fall in oxygen saturation levels.*

SAFETY ALERT: Immediately report complaints of chest pain and shortness of breath, anxiety, or a sense of impending doom. The manifestations of pulmonary embolism are similar to those of myocardial infarction. Prompt intervention to restore pulmonary blood flow can reduce the risk of significant adverse effects. ■

- Initiate oxygen therapy, elevate the head of the bed, and reassure the patient who is experiencing manifestations of pulmonary embolism. *Oxygen therapy and elevating the head of the bed promote ventilation and gas exchange in those alveoli that are well perfused, helping maintain tissue oxygenation. Reassurance helps reduce anxiety and slow the respiratory rate, promoting greater respiratory depth and alveolar ventilation.*

Transitions of Care

Prevention of venous thrombosis is an important component of nursing care for all at-risk patients. Position patients to promote venous blood flow from the lower extremities, with the feet elevated and the knees slightly bent. Avoid placing pillows under the knees and positions in which the hips and knees are sharply flexed. Use a recliner chair or footstool when sitting. Ambulate patients as soon as possible, and maintain a regular schedule of ambulation throughout the day. Teach ankle flexion and extension exercises, and frequently remind patients to perform them. Apply elastic hose and pneumatic compression devices when appropriate. Instruct patients to avoid crossing legs when in bed or sitting. Inquire about possible prophylactic heparin or warfarin therapy for patients undergoing orthopedic surgery or other high-risk procedures. Frequently assess intravenous sites. Change the site and catheter as dictated by agency protocol and if evidence of local inflammation is noted.

Treatment measures for venous thrombosis may be initiated and carried out on an outpatient basis or continued for an extended period of time following hospital discharge.

Include the following topics when teaching for home care:

- Explanation of the disease process
- Treatment measures, including laboratory tests and their purposes, medications, and adverse effects that should be reported
- Appropriate methods of heat application
- Prescribed activity restrictions
- Measures to prevent future episodes of venous thrombosis
- The importance of follow-up visits and laboratory tests as scheduled.

Refer patients for community nursing services for continued assessment and reinforcement of teaching. Provide referrals for assistance with ADLs and home maintenance services as indicated. Consider referral for physical therapy, if needed.

Case Study & Nursing Care Plan

A Patient with Deep Venous Thrombosis

Mrs. Opal Hipps, age 75, lives alone with her dog, Chester, in her family home in the suburbs. She retired from her job as a postal clerk 10 years ago and now spends a lot of time reading and watching television. During the past week, she developed a vague aching pain in her right leg. She ignored the pain until last night when it developed into a much more severe pain in her right calf. She noticed that her right lower leg seemed larger than the left, and it was very tender to the touch. After seeing her healthcare provider and undergoing Doppler ultrasound studies, Mrs. Hipps is admitted to the hospital with the diagnosis of DVT in the right leg. She is placed on bedrest and intravenous heparin. Michael Cookson, RN, is assigned to admit and care for Mrs. Hipps.

ASSESSMENT	DIAGNOSES	EXPECTED OUTCOMES
Mr. Cookson notices that Mrs. Hipps was admitted 14 months ago for repair of a fractured femur. Mrs. Hipps says, "This business about a blood clot really has me worried." She also tells Mr. Cookson that she is worried about who will care for her dog while she is in the hospital. Physical findings include height 157 cm (62 in.), weight 68 kg (149 lb), T 37.3°C (99.2°F); vital signs within normal limits otherwise. Her left leg is warm and pink, with strong peripheral pulses and good capillary refill. Her right calf is dark red, very warm, and dry to the touch. It is tender to palpation. The right femoral and popliteal pulses are strong, but the pedal and posterior tibial pulses are difficult to locate. The right calf diameter is 1.27 cm (0.5 in.) larger than the left.	■ Pain related to inflammatory response in affected vein ■ Anxiety related to unexpected hospitalization and uncertainty about the seriousness of her illness ■ Poor peripheral perfusion related to decreased venous circulation in the right leg ■ Risk for breaks in skin integrity related to pooling of venous blood in the right leg	■ Patient will verbalize relief of right leg pain by day of discharge. ■ Patient will verbalize reduced anxiety by the second day of her hospitalization. ■ Patient will demonstrate reduced right leg diameter by 0.64 cm (0.25 in.) by the fifth day of hospitalization. ■ Patient will maintain intact skin on the right foot throughout the hospital stay.

(continued)

PLANNING AND IMPLEMENTATION

- Elevate legs, maintaining slight knee flexion, while in bed.
- Apply warm, moist compresses to right leg using a 2-hour-on, 2-hour-off schedule around the clock.
- Administer prescribed analgesics and evaluate effectiveness.
- Spend time with Mrs. Hipps to explain venous thrombosis and its treatment.
- Arrange for a friend or neighbor to care for Mrs. Hipps's dog.
- Apply antiembolism stockings as ordered; remove for 30 minutes every 8 hours.
- Monitor laboratory values to assess effect of anticoagulant therapy; report values outside desired range.
- Assist with progressive ambulation when allowed.
- Inspect legs and feet and record findings every 8 hours.

EVALUATION

Seven days after admission, the pain in Mrs. Hipps's right leg has subsided and the diameter of her right calf is equal to that of her left calf. Mrs. Hipps admits to Mr. Cookson that her fears really relate to a cousin who was hospitalized for a similar problem and had his leg amputated. After talking about her condition and the steps she can take to prevent its recurrence, she is much less anxious. Before discharge, Mr. Cookson reviews instructions for use of antiembolism stockings, daily walking, warfarin schedule, and scheduled follow-up appointment. Her neighbor, Kate, came to pick her up. As Mr. Cookson was helping Mrs. Hipps into the car, Kate handed her a small brown dog and said, "I took good care of Chester for you, but he's missed you." Mrs. Hipps smiled and assured Mr. Cookson that she would call the number he provided if she had any questions.

CLINICAL REASONING IN PATIENT CARE

1. Describe the pathophysiologic reasons for the pain in Mrs. Hipps's right leg.
2. How would you respond if Mrs. Hipps tells you she does not have the money to buy the prescribed anticoagulant when she goes home?
3. How would you change your teaching and discharge planning if Mrs. Hipps had difficulty caring for herself?
4. Design a plan of care for Mrs. Hipps for the diagnosis of poor peripheral perfusion.

See Evaluating Your Response in Appendix B.

The Patient with Chronic Venous Insufficiency

Chronic venous insufficiency is a disorder of inadequate venous return over a prolonged period. Deep venous thrombosis is the most frequent cause of chronic venous insufficiency. Other conditions, such as varicose veins or leg trauma, may contribute; in some instances, it develops without an identified precipitating cause (Sorenson et al., 2019).

Pathophysiology

Following DVT, large veins may remain occluded, increasing the pressure in other veins of the extremity. This increased pressure distends the veins, separating valve leaflets and impairing their ability to close (**Figure 32.10** ■). DVT also damages valve leaflets, causing them to thicken and contract. The result is impaired unidirectional blood flow and deep vein emptying (Sorenson et al., 2019).

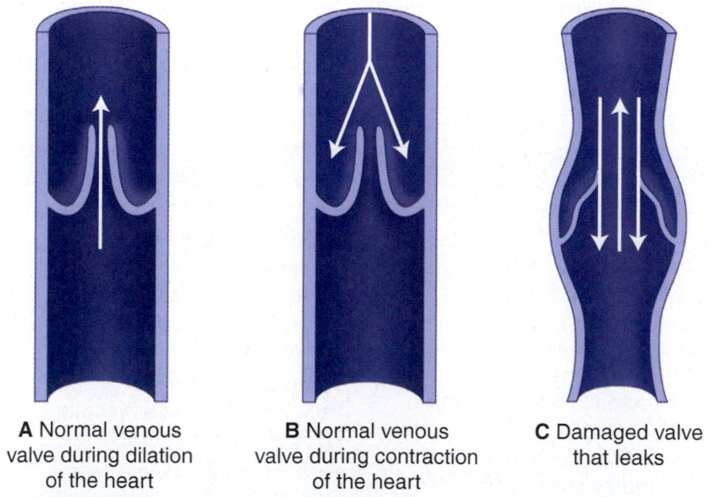
A Normal venous valve during dilation of the heart
B Normal venous valve during contraction of the heart
C Damaged valve that leaks

Figure 32.10 ■ Vein abnormalities. **A**, Normal venous valve during dilation of the heart. **B**, Normal venous valve during contraction of the heart. **C**, Damaged valve that leaks.

When venous valves are incompetent, the muscle-pumping action produced during activity cannot propel blood back to the heart. Venous blood collects and stagnates in the lower leg (*venous stasis*). Venous pressures in the calf and lower leg increase, particularly during ambulation. This increased pressure impairs arterial circulation to the lower extremities as well. The body's ability to provide sufficient oxygen and nutrients to the cells and remove metabolic waste products diminishes. Eventually, there is so little oxygen and nutrients that cells begin to die. The skin atrophies, and subcutaneous fat deposits necrose. Breakdown of red blood cells in the congested tissues causes brown skin pigmentation. Venous stasis ulcers develop. Congested tissues impair the body's ability to increase the supply of oxygen, nutrients, and metabolic energy to heal the ulcer. As a result, the condition worsens and, over time, the ulcers enlarge. The congested venous circulation also prevents the blood from mounting effective inflammatory and immune responses, significantly increasing the risk for infection in the ulcerated tissue (Sorenson et al., 2019).

Manifestations

Manifestations of chronic venous insufficiency include lower leg edema, itching, and discomfort of the affected extremity that increases with prolonged standing. The extremity is cyanotic. Recurrent stasis ulcers develop (**Figure 32.11** ■), usually forming just above the ankle, on the medial or anterior aspect of the leg. They heal poorly, forming scar tissue that breaks down easily. Tissue surrounding the ulcer is shiny, atrophic, and cyanotic, and there is a brownish pigmentation to the skin. Other skin changes may develop as well, such as eczema or stasis dermatitis. Necrosis and fibrosis of subcutaneous tissue cause the affected area of the leg to feel hard and somewhat leathery to the touch, but even the slightest trauma to the area can produce serious tissue breakdown. Symptoms of chronic venous insufficiency include:

- Lower extremity edema that worsens with standing
- Itching, dull leg discomfort or pain that increases with standing

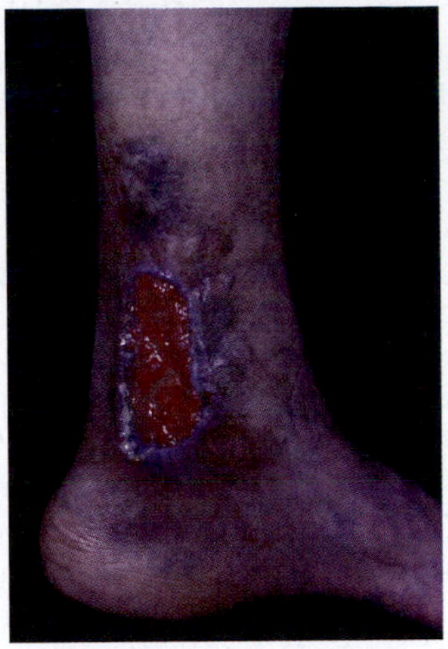

Figure 32.11 ■ Chronic venous insufficiency. Note the discoloration of the ankle and the stasis ulcer.

- Thin, shiny, atrophic skin
- Cyanosis and brown skin pigmentation of lower leg and foot
- Possible weeping dermatitis
- Thick, fibrous (hard) subcutaneous tissue
- Recurrent ulcerations of medial or anterior ankle.

Table 32.6 compares venous and arterial ulcers.

Interprofessional Care

Collaborative care for the patient with venous insufficiency focuses on relieving symptoms, promoting adequate circulation, and healing and preventing tissue damage.

The history and physical examination often establish the diagnosis of chronic venous insufficiency. Because a history of DVT is a major risk factor, careful evaluation of the past medical history and questioning of the patient are important. There are no specific diagnostic tests to confirm the diagnosis of chronic venous insufficiency.

Conservative management of venous insufficiency focuses on reducing edema and treating ulcerations. Prolonged standing or sitting is discouraged. Graduated

Table 32.6 Comparison of Arterial and Venous Leg Ulcers

Factor	Arterial Ulcers	Venous Ulcers
Location	Toes, feet, shin	Over medial or anterior ankle
Ulcer appearance	Deep, pale	Superficial, pink
Skin appearance	Normal to atrophic Pallor on elevation Rubor on dependency	Brown discoloration Stasis dermatitis Cyanosis on dependency
Skin temperature	Cool	Normal
Edema	Absent or mild	May be significant
Pain	Usually severe Intermittent claudication Rest pain	Usually mild Aching pain
Gangrene	May occur	Does not occur
Pulses	Decreased or absent	Normal

compression hosiery is ordered for daytime use, and frequent elevation of the legs and feet during the day is recommended. At night, the legs and feet should be elevated above the level of the heart by raising the foot of the mattress.

Treatment of associated stasis dermatitis varies, based on the duration of the condition. Wet compresses of boric acid, buffered aluminum acetate (Burrow solution), or isotonic saline solution are applied to acute weeping dermatitis four times a day for 1-hour periods. Following the compress, a topical corticosteroid (such as 0.5% hydrocortisone cream) is applied. Bedrest is prescribed during the acute period. Stasis dermatitis that is subsiding or chronic may be treated with a topical corticosteroid, zinc oxide ointment, or a topical broad-spectrum antifungal cream such as clotrimazole (Lotrimin) cream or miconazole (Monistat) cream.

Isotonic saline compresses or wet-to-dry dressings are applied to stasis ulcers to promote healing. A dilute topical antibiotic solution and an occlusive hydroactive or polyurethane foam may also be used. The ulcer may be treated by using a semirigid boot applied to the foot and lower leg. This device may be made of Unna's paste or Gauzetex bandage. Bony prominences must be well padded and the boot changed weekly. This device often allows ambulatory treatment.

A very large, chronic ulcer may require surgery. In this case, the incompetent veins are ligated, the ulcer is excised, and the area is covered with a skin graft (refer to Chapter 16).

Nursing Care

Nursing care for the patient with chronic venous insufficiency is primarily educative and supportive. See other sections of this chapter for specific nursing interventions related to many of these diagnoses. Patient teaching includes the following recommendations:

- Elevate the legs while resting and during sleep.
- Walk as much as possible, but avoid sitting or standing for long periods of time.
- When sitting, do not cross your legs or allow pressure on the back of the knees (such as sitting on the side of the bed).
- Do not wear anything that pinches your legs (such as knee-high hose, garters, or girdles).
- Wear elastic hose as prescribed. The elastic hose should be tighter over the feet than at the top of the leg. Be sure the tops of the elastic hose do not cut into your legs. Put on the hose after you have had your legs elevated.
- Keep the skin on your feet and legs clean, soft, and dry.
- Refer to the guidelines in Box 32.2 for care of the legs and feet.

Disorders of venous stasis are common after the fifth decade of life. Aging affects vessels and tissues, increasing the risk for venous insufficiency and varicose veins. In addition, mobility frequently declines with age, reducing the effect of the muscle pump in promoting venous return.

Regular exercise, walking in particular, is an important part of the treatment plan. Safety when walking is an important issue for older patients. Assess the patient's mobility and stability during ambulation. If appropriate, suggest using a walker and quad-cane as needed. Assist older patients holding jobs that require prolonged standing to identify strategies to minimize standing and incorporate periods of activity into their work.

Following surgery or during treatment for stasis ulcers, older patients may need additional assistance with home care and maintenance. Initiate referral to social services as needed to arrange for home nursing care, meals, assistance with ADLs, and home maintenance services as indicated. In some instances, temporary placement in an extended care facility is necessary until the patient and family can assume care.

The Patient with Varicose Veins

Varicose veins are irregular, tortuous veins with incompetent valves. Varicosities may develop in any veins, and may be called by other names, such as hemorrhoids in the rectum and varices in the esophagus. Varicosities usually affect the veins of the lower extremities; the long saphenous vein is often affected, and they also may develop in the short saphenous vein.

Pathophysiology

Varicose veins are classified as primary (with no involvement of deep veins) or secondary (caused by the obstruction of deep veins). In both cases, long-standing increased venous pressure stretches the vessel wall. This sustained stretching impairs the ability of the venous valves to close, causing them to become incompetent (Sorenson et al., 2019).

The erect position produces a twofold negative effect on the veins. When standing, the leg veins resemble vertical columns and must withstand the full force of venous blood pressure. Prolonged standing, the force of gravity, lack of leg exercise, and incompetent venous valves all weaken the muscle-pumping mechanism, reducing venous blood return to the heart. As standing continues, the amount of blood pooled in the veins increases, further stretching the vessel wall. The venous valves become increasingly incompetent.

Incidence and Risk Factors

Varicose veins affect about 15% of adults. They are more common in women over age 35 with an increased risk related to venous stasis during pregnancy. Aging is a risk factor, possibly related to decreased exercise and other factors that contribute to venous stasis. People in occupations that involve prolonged standing (such as beauticians, salespeople, and nurses) also have an increased incidence of varicose veins.

Most varicosities occur in the deep veins of the legs. Contributing causes include obesity, venous thrombosis, congenital arteriovenous malformations, or sustained pressure on abdominal veins (as in pregnancy and/or the presence of abdominal tumors). The effects of gravity, produced by long periods of standing, are a major causative factor.

Manifestations and Complications

Although varicose veins may be asymptomatic, most cause manifestations such as severe aching leg pain, leg fatigue, leg heaviness, itching, or feelings of heat in the legs. The degree of valvular incompetence does not seem to correlate well with the extent of symptoms. The menstrual cycle tends to worsen symptoms, suggesting a possible correlation with hormonal factors in women. Assessment reveals obvious dilated, tortuous veins beneath the skin of the upper and lower leg (**Figure 32.12** ■). If varicose veins are long-standing, the skin above the ankles may be thin and discolored, with a brown pigmentation. Symptoms of varicose veins include:

- Severe, aching pain in the leg
- Leg fatigue, heaviness
- Itching of the affected leg (stasis dermatitis)
- Feelings of warmth in the leg
- Visibly dilated veins
- Thin, discolored skin above the ankles
- Stasis ulcers.

Complications of varicose veins include venous insufficiency and stasis ulcers. Chronic stasis dermatitis may also develop. Superficial venous thrombosis may develop in varicose veins, especially during and after pregnancy, following surgery, and in patients on estrogen therapy (oral contraceptives or hormone replacement therapy).

Interprofessional Care

Varicose veins can usually be managed using conservative measures, although surgery may be required if symptoms are severe, when complications develop, or for cosmetic reasons.

Diagnosis

Although varicose veins are often diagnosed by the history and physical examination, diagnostic tests may be ordered.

- ***Doppler ultrasonography*** or ***duplex Doppler ultrasound*** may be performed to identify specific locations of incompetent valves. This test is particularly useful before surgery to identify valves that allow reflux of blood from the femoral, popliteal, or peripheral deep veins into the superficial veins.
- ***Trendelenburg test*** may be performed to determine the underlying cause of superficial venous insufficiency. The leg is elevated, then an elastic tourniquet is placed around the distal thigh. The varicosities are then observed as the patient stands. When valves of the deep veins are incompetent, the veins remain flat on standing; they rapidly distend when the superficial venous valves are the underlying cause.

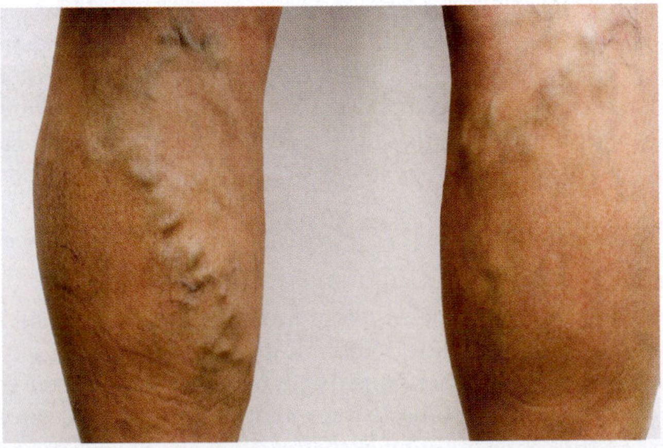

Figure 32.12 ■ A patient with varicose veins.

Treatments

Although there is no real cure, conservative measures are the core of treatment for most patients with uncomplicated varicose veins. These measures often relieve symptoms and prevent complications by improving venous circulation and relieving pressure on venous tissues. Properly fitted graduated compression stockings are commonly prescribed. They compress the veins, propelling blood back to the heart. Compression stockings augment the muscle pumping action of the legs. When worn during times of prolonged standing and in combination with frequent leg elevation, compression stockings often prevent progression of the condition and development of complications.

Regular, daily walking is also important. Prolonged sitting and standing are discouraged, although elevating the legs for specified periods during the day is beneficial. Leg elevation promotes venous return, prevents venous stasis, and decreases leg heaviness and fatigue.

Compression Sclerotherapy

In compression sclerotherapy, a sclerosing solution is injected into the varicose vein and a compression bandage is applied for a period of time. This obliterates the vein. Venous blood is rerouted through healthy vessels whose valves are not compromised. Compression sclerotherapy may be used to treat small, symptomatic varicosities. It may be the primary treatment, or it may be used in conjunction with varicose vein surgery. While compression sclerotherapy may be done for cosmetic reasons, complications such as phlebitis, tissue necrosis, or infection may occur and need to be considered prior to the procedures.

Surgery

Surgical treatment of varicose veins is generally reserved for patients who are very symptomatic, experience recurrent superficial venous thrombosis, and/or develop stasis ulcers. The objective of surgery is to remove the diseased veins. It may be considered for cosmetic reasons.

Surgery usually involves extensive ligation and stripping of the greater and lesser saphenous veins. The evening before surgery, the surgeon marks all incompetent superficial and perforating varicose veins with a permanent ink marker. Under either regional or general anesthesia, the greater saphenous vein is removed and the connected smaller tributaries that have not naturally clotted off are tied off. Multiple small incisions may be made over the varicosities, allowing removal of the affected segments of the vein. Incompetent tributaries that communicate with larger vessels are also ligated. For patients with less extensive disease or patients seeking cosmetic improvement, surgery may involve only the removal of the lesser saphenous vein through an incision in the popliteal fossa.

Postoperative care includes applying pressure bandages for a minimum of 6 weeks, elevating the extremities to minimize postoperative edema, and gradually increasing amounts of ambulation. Sitting and standing are prohibited during the initial recovery period and are gradually reintroduced as deemed appropriate by the surgeon.

Nursing Care

Assessment

See the Manifestations and Interprofessional Care sections for the assessment of the patient with varicose veins.

Focused assessment of the patient with varicose veins includes:

- ***Health history:*** Complaints of leg pain, aching, heaviness, or fatigue; ankle swelling; history of venous thrombosis
- ***Physical assessment:*** Visible, dilated, tortuous superficial veins in lower extremities.

Priorities of Care

Collaborating with the interprofessional team to ensure adequate treatment of the underlying process while providing care that supports the physical and psychologic responses to the disorder is a priority of nursing care.

Diagnoses, Outcomes, and Interventions

In planning and providing nursing care for patients with varicose veins, emphasis is placed on the importance of health teaching to manage the symptoms of varicose veins, particularly because there is no cure for the disease. Nursing care for patients who have undergone surgical treatment for varicose veins focuses on assessing and promoting wound healing and preventing infection. Nursing diagnoses may include those related to pain, impaired tissue perfusion and skin integrity, and a risk for impaired neurovascular function.

Manage Chronic Pain. Varicose veins can lead to pooling of venous blood in the lower extremities. Venous congestion can cause a dull ache or feeling of pressure in the legs, particularly after prolonged standing. As venous pressure rises, arterial circulation and delivery of oxygen and nutrients to tissues is impaired. Tissue ischemia contributes to the pain. The pain associated with varicose veins tends to be chronic, developing and progressing gradually over a long period of time.

Expected Outcome: Patient will exhibit adequate pain control as evidenced by physical well-being.

The nurse will:

- Assess pain, including its intensity, duration, and aggravating and relieving factors. *Pain assessment allows collaborative planning with the patient to identify appropriate interventions.*
- Inquire about current measures being used by the patient to manage pain and its effects. Ask about the effectiveness of current management strategies and the desire to change. *Chronic pain management ultimately falls to the patient. Strategies to address the pain must meet the patient's needs.*
- Suggest keeping a diary of pain intensity, timing, precipitating events, and effectiveness of relief measures. *Systematic tracking of pain is an important measure in improving its management.*
- Teach and reinforce nonpharmacologic pain management strategies such as progressive relaxation, imagery, deep breathing, distraction, and meditation. *The effectiveness of such strategies is well documented. Nonpharmacologic measures provide a variety of options for controlling pain while maintaining independence. These measures can also reduce reliance on analgesics.*
- Collaborate with the patient to establish a pain control plan. *Collaborative planning for pain management increases the patient's sense of control and reduces powerlessness. This, in turn, enhances the ability to cope with pain and its effects.*
- Regularly evaluate the effectiveness of planned interventions and pain management strategies. *Regular evaluation allows modification of the care plan as needed, as well as providing a measure of disease progression. Increasing or poorly controlled pain may necessitate additional collaborative interventions to manage the disorder.*

Promote Effective Peripheral Tissue Perfusion. Varicose veins and venous stasis impair delivery of nutrients and oxygen to peripheral tissues as elevated venous pressures interfere with blood flow through the capillary beds. Improving venous blood flow reduces venous pressures and promotes arterial flow to peripheral tissues.

Expected Outcome: Patient's tissue perfusion will be adequate as evidenced by adequate arterial flow (i.e., strong peripheral pulses).

The nurse will:

- Assess peripheral pulses, capillary refill, skin color and temperature, and extent of edema. *Assessment of arterial flow and tissue perfusion provides baseline and continuing data for evaluating the effectiveness of interventions.*
- Teach application and use of properly fitted elastic graduated compression stockings. *Elastic compression stockings compress the veins, promoting venous return from the lower extremities. During ambulation, the stockings enhance the blood-pumping action of the muscles. Because elastic stockings inhibit blood flow through small superficial vessels, they should be removed at least once each day for at least 30 minutes.*
- Instruct to maintain a program of regular exercise, such as walking for 20 to 30 minutes several times a day. When ambulation is restricted, active ROM exercises help maintain muscle tone, joint mobility, and venous return. *Exercise stimulates circulation and promotes blood flow through the vascular system.*

- Advise to elevate the legs for 15 to 20 minutes several times a day and to sleep with the legs elevated above the level of the heart. *Elevating the legs promotes venous return, reducing tissue congestion and improving arterial circulation. Improved venous return also increases cardiac output and renal perfusion, promoting elimination of excess fluid and decreasing peripheral edema.*

Reduce Risk for Skin Breakdown. Ineffective venous valve function impairs venous return and increases venous pressures. These increased pressures oppose arterial blood flow and the delivery of oxygen and nutrients to the cells. As a result, tissues are vulnerable to any additional insult and may break down.

Expected Outcome: Patient will demonstrate an understanding of plan to heal skin and prevent reinjury.

The nurse will:

- Assess lower extremity color, temperature, moisture, and for evidence of pressure or breakdown on admission and at each visit. *Initial and continuing assessment allows timely detection of early signs of skin and tissue breakdown. This, in turn, allows early institution of measures to prevent further tissue damage and promote healing.*
- Teach foot and skin care measures such as daily cleansing with nondrying soap, gentle drying, and lotions to prevent skin dryness and cracking. *Cleansing removes potentially harmful microorganisms and stimulates circulation. Care is taken to keep the skin moist and supple, promoting its function as the first line of defense against infection.*
- Discuss the importance of adequate nutrition and fluid intake. *Adequate nutrients are necessary to maintain tissue integrity and promote healing. A diet high in protein, carbohydrates, and vitamins and minerals promotes growth and maintenance of skin cells, provides energy, and helps prevent skin breakdown. Adequate hydration helps maintain the moisture and turgor of skin, reducing the risk of drying and breakdown.*

Reduce Risk for Neurologic Dysfunction. Severe varicose veins can lead to chronic venous insufficiency, impaired arterial circulation, and ultimately, disrupted sensation in the affected extremity. Impaired neurologic function increases the patient's risk for injury and infection of the extremity, as minor trauma may go unnoticed.

Expected Outcome: Patient will experience optimal peripheral neurovascular function as evidenced by freedom from pain, baseline peripheral sensation, and intact skin of the extremity.

The nurse will:

- Assess circulation, sensation, and movement of the lower extremities. *Disrupted circulation and venous congestion may interfere with sensory and motor function of the affected extremity. The potential for nerve and muscle involvement is especially high in patients with venous stasis ulcers.*
- Instruct to report signs of neurovascular dysfunction, such as numbness, coldness, pain, or tingling of an extremity. Early recognition of neurovascular dysfunction facilitates institution of interventions to prevent complications. Because the postoperative hospital stay following varicose vein surgery or venous stasis ulcer repair is brief, manifestations of neurovascular dysfunction may initially be detected by the patient. *Careful assessment and prompt reporting helps prevent potential complications such as skin breakdown, infection, and nerve damage.*
- Teach measures to protect the extremities from injury, such as always wearing shoes or firm slippers, wearing cotton socks to absorb moisture, and testing the temperature of bath water with a thermometer or the upper extremities before stepping in. *Sensation in the lower extremities may be affected by poor circulation, necessitating additional measures to protect the legs and feet from injury.*

Transitions of Care

Health promotion activities to reduce the incidence of varicose veins include teaching all patients, particularly young women, the benefits of regular exercise continued over the lifetime. Discuss the effect of prolonged sitting or standing on the legs, and encourage the patient whose occupation involves these activities to periodically get up and move or to sit with the legs elevated. Encourage all patients to maintain normal weight for their height.

Varicose vein acute care focuses on surgical preparation and post-operative care. Most patients with varicose veins provide self-care at home. Include the following topics when preparing the patient and family for home care:

- Leg elevation and exercise program
- Application and use of graduated elastic compression stockings
- Foot and leg care (refer to Box 32.2)
- Measures to avoid injury and skin breakdown
- Symptoms or potential complications to report to the healthcare provider.

32.5 Disorders of the Lymphatic System

The lymphatic system, which includes the lymphatic vessels and the lymph nodes, is a unique part of the circulatory system. The lymphatic system returns plasma and plasma proteins filtered out of the capillaries from interstitial tissues to the bloodstream. This fluid is called *lymph*. The lymphatic system consists of closed capillaries leading to larger lymphatic venules and lymphatic veins. These vessels contain smooth muscle and one-way valves that help move fluid toward the heart. Lymphatic vessels share the same sheath as arteries and veins; arterial pulsations and skeletal muscle contractions compress the lymphatic vessels to assist in maintaining lymph flow. As lymph moves through the lymphatic system, it is filtered through thousands of bean-shaped lymph nodes clustered along the vessels. Within these nodes, phagocytes remove foreign material from the lymph, preventing it from entering the bloodstream.

The Patient with Lymphadenopathy

Lymphadenopathy, enlarged lymph nodes, may be localized or generalized. Localized lymphadenopathy usually results from an inflammatory process (e.g., streptococcal pharyngitis or an infected wound). The node enlarges as lymphocytes and monocytes proliferate within the node to destroy infectious material. Palpable lymph nodes often develop in response to minor trauma or a localized infection. Generalized lymphadenopathy is usually associated with malignancy or disease. Malignant cells or other abnormal cells invade the node, causing it to enlarge.

Lymphangitis, inflammation of the lymph vessels draining an infected area of the body, is characterized by a red streak along the inflamed vessels, pain, heat, and swelling. Fever and chills may also be present. Local lymph nodes are swollen and tender.

Treatment for lymphadenopathy and lymphangitis focuses on identifying and treating the underlying condition. Elevating the body part and applying heat to inflamed lymphatic vessels help reduce swelling and promote blood flow to the affected area.

The Patient with Lymphedema

Pathophysiology and Risk Factors

Lymphedema may be a primary or a secondary disorder, resulting from inflammation, obstruction, or removal of lymphatic vessels. It is characterized by extremity edema due to accumulation of lymph. *Primary lymphedema* is uncommon, affecting about 1 in 10,000 people. It affects females more frequently than males and may be associated with a genetic disorder such as Turner syndrome (Genetics Home Reference, 2018b).

Secondary lymphedema is an acquired condition, resulting from damage, obstruction, or removal of lymphatic vessels. The most common worldwide cause of secondary lymphedema is *filariasis*, infestation of the lymphatic vessels by filaria, a nematode worm. Other important causes of secondary lymphedema include recurrent episodes of bacterial lymphangitis, obstruction of lymph vessels by tumors, and surgical or radiation treatment for breast cancer.

Manifestations

Obstruction of lymph drainage prevents fluid and protein molecules from interstitial tissues from returning to the circulation. The protein molecules increase the osmotic pressure in interstitial tissues, drawing in additional fluid that causes edema in the soft tissues. One or both extremities may be affected.

The edema begins distally, progressing up the limb to involve the entire extremity (**Figure 32.13** ■). Initial edema is soft and pitting; with chronic congestion, subcutaneous tissues become fibrotic, causing thick, rough skin and a woody texture of the limb (*brawny edema*). In contrast, the edema associated with venous disorders is softer, and the skin is often hyperpigmented with evidence of stasis dermatitis. Lymphedema is generally painless, although the limb may feel heavy.

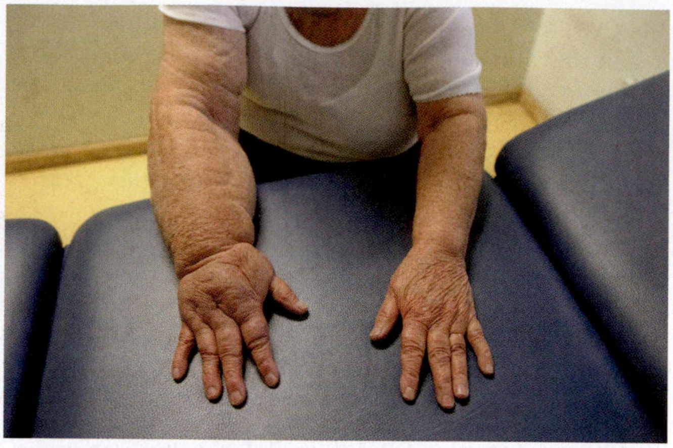

Figure 32.13 ■ A woman with lymphedema secondary to surgical treatment for breast cancer.

Interprofessional Care

Interprofessional care for the patient with lymphedema focuses on relieving edema and preventing or treating infection. The disorder may be difficult to treat effectively and can lead to progressive disability due to the weight and awkwardness of the affected extremity.

Diagnosis

Abdominal or pelvic ultrasound and CT scans are used to detect obstructing lesions. An MRI can show edema and identify lymph nodes and enlarged lymphatic vessels. More invasive procedures such as lymphangiography and radioactive isotope studies may occasionally be necessary to identify the lymphatic defect causing lymphedema.

- ***Lymphangiography*** uses injected contrast media to illustrate lymphatic vessels on x-rays. Organic dyes are used to identify a distal lymphatic vessel, and then a contrast medium is injected into the vessel for visualization of the lymphatic system of the limb. In primary lymphedema, lymph vessels are absent or hypoplastic (underdeveloped). In secondary lymphedema, lymph channels often are dilated; it may be possible to determine the level of obstruction.
- ***Lymphoscintigraphy*** involves injecting a radioactively tagged substance into distal subcutaneous tissues of the extremity, then mapping its flow through the lymphatic system. The pattern of lymph fluid distribution and transport is abnormal in patients with lymphedema.

Treatments

Meticulous skin and foot care is vital to prevent infection in the affected extremity. Shoes should always be worn to reduce the risk of injury. Careful cleansing and use of emollient lotions are recommended to prevent drying of the skin. Exercise is encouraged, as are frequent periods of leg elevation. The foot of the bed is raised by 15 to 20 degrees at night to promote lymph flow. Elastic graduated compression stockings may be ordered for use during the day. In some cases, an intermittent pneumatic compression device to reduce edema may be prescribed for home use.

Antibiotics are given to prevent and treat infection, which can be recurrent and difficult to eradicate. Diuretic therapy may be used intermittently, particularly when primary lymphedema is exacerbated by the menstrual cycle or seasonal variability.

Patients who do not respond to conservative treatment measures or who experience recurrent episodes of cellulitis and lymphangitis may require surgical treatment. Microvascular techniques may be used to create anastomoses between obstructed lymphatic vessels and adjacent veins, providing channels to redirect lymph into the venous system. Successful surgery may improve both extremity function and its cosmetic appearance.

Nursing Care

Nursing care for patients with lymphatic disorders focuses on reducing edema, preventing tissue damage related to the edema, and promoting effective coping with the effect of the disorder on body image and function.

Assessment

See the Manifestations and Interprofessional Care sections for the assessment of the patient with lymphatic disorders.

Priorities of Care

Collaborating with the interprofessional team to ensure adequate treatment of the underlying process while providing care that supports the physical and psychologic responses to the disorder is a priority of nursing care.

Diagnoses, Outcomes, and Interventions

Nursing care for the patient with lymphedema may include promoting skin integrity, monitoring fluid volume, and helping patients cope with the swelling of their body.

Promote Tissue Integrity. Obstructed lymphatic flow leads to fluid congestion of the interstitial spaces of subcutaneous tissue. The resulting edema compresses and damages tissues of the affected extremity. Subcutaneous tissues become fibrotic, reducing their protective functions of shock absorption and insulation. In addition, obstructed lymphatic flow reduces the effectiveness of lymph nodes in filtering and removing foreign material and pathogens from the body. This increases the risk for local tissue infection such as *cellulitis*, a diffuse bacterial infection of the skin. Cellulitis increases the risk for skin and tissue breakdown and, if not effectively treated, can lead to sepsis.

Expected Outcome: Patient will be able to describe measures to protect healthy tissue and prevent injury.

The nurse will:

- Frequently inspect the skin of the affected extremity, documenting the condition with each assessment. Promptly report areas of pallor, redness, or apparent inflammation. Breaks in the skin surface allow microbial invasion and increase the risk for infection. *Prompt identification and treatment of any lesions is vital to prevent further tissue breakdown and infection.*
- Apply well-fitting elastic graduated compression stockings or intermittent pneumatic pressure devices as ordered. *Elastic stockings and/or pneumatic pressure devices oppose the movement of fluid out of capillaries and improve its reabsorption into vascular spaces for transportation back to the heart.*
- Remove elastic stockings and intermittent pressure devices every 8 hours or at each home visit to inspect the underlying skin for evidence of redness, irritation, dryness, or breakdown. *Elastic graduated compression stockings, antiembolic stockings, and pneumatic compression devices compress small vessels nourishing the skin and subcutaneous tissue. Periodic removal not only allows inspection of the underlying skin, but also allows restoration of blood flow to these small vessels and the tissues.*
- Instruct to elevate the extremities while seated and during sleep. *Elevation of the extremities diminishes venous congestion, promotes venous return, facilitates arterial circulation and tissue perfusion, and helps reduce the accumulation of excess fluids in interstitial spaces of the affected extremity.*
- Use preventive skin care devices as indicated. Collected fluid in the affected extremity increases its weight and interferes with regular movement. The increased weight places greater pressure on surfaces of the limb that come in contact with furniture. *Protective devices such as egg-crate foam, sheepskin, pillows, or padding help prevent tissue compression, promoting circulation and reducing the risk of skin and tissue breakdown.*
- Keep skin clean and dry, especially in interdigital spaces. Teach skin and foot care to the patient and family. *Clean, dry skin provides the first line of defense against infection. Significant limb edema can interfere with reaching the distal extremity and cleaning interdigital spaces. The dark, moist spaces between the toes are an excellent environment for bacterial growth. Teaching fosters self-care and independence, as well as preparing the patient and family to manage this often chronic condition.*
- Discuss the importance of adhering to the therapeutic regimen. *Lymphedema is generally a chronic condition; effective management requires active patient participation in planning and implementing care to reduce edema and maintain tissue integrity.*

Monitor Fluid Volume. In lymphedema, obstruction, destruction, or congenital malformation of lymphatic vessels interferes with the normal circulation of lymphatic fluid. As a result, lymph collects in the subcutaneous tissues of the affected extremity, causing excess fluid volume of that extremity. Some patients may benefit from intermittent diuretic therapy and dietary sodium restriction.

Expected Outcome: Patient's fluid volume will be normal as evidenced by weight loss and decreases in edema, jugular venous distention, and abdominal distention.

The nurse will:

- Monitor intake and output and/or weight (daily or weekly). Use consistent scales, timing, and clothing for accurate weight measurements. *Intake and output records and short-term changes in weight reflect fluid balance.*

Measures of fluid balance permit evaluation of the effectiveness of interventions such as restricted sodium intake and diuretic therapy.

- Discuss the rationale for restricted sodium intake, if ordered. Teach ways to maintain the recommended sodium restriction, and assist to choose foods that are low in sodium. *Sodium causes retention of extracellular water; restricting dietary sodium may help prevent additional fluid accumulation in interstitial spaces.*
- During acute periods, assess the affected extremity daily for increased edema; measure girth of the extremity using consistent technique. *The size of the affected extremity provides a measure of the effectiveness of ordered interventions and progression of the disorder.*

Teach Coping Strategies. The disproportionate size of an extremity or extremities due to lymphedema can profoundly affect body image. During early stages of the disease, conservative measures may effectively reduce the edema and size of the affected limb. However, as the disease progresses, conservative measures may become less effective, leading to more permanent disfigurement. Mobility may be impaired, and the patient may develop an increasingly negative self-perception.

Expected Outcome: Patient will verbalize realistic expectations of lymphedema therapy impact on edema.

The nurse will:

- Encourage discussions about usual coping patterns and perception of self. *Knowledge of existing coping patterns and behaviors helps the nurse assess the patient's ability to cope with the current situation. This knowledge is then used to reinforce effective coping mechanisms and help develop more effective coping strategies. This exchange allows the patient to voice feelings related to actual or perceived changes in body image.*
- Accept the patient's perception of self and of the impact of the changes in appearance. *Nonjudgmental acceptance of the patient's view of self and of the effects of changes in appearance builds trust and promotes rapport. A trusting relationship promotes the patient's ability to take an active role in managing the disorder, participate in healthcare decisions, and adhere to the plan of care. Nonjudgmental listening also promotes mutual respect and demonstrates caring and compassion.*
- Encourage active participation in self-care. Assist with identifying alternative self-care strategies when the extent of edema interferes with performing some aspects of self-care such as trimming toenails or washing feet. *The patient may initially have difficulty viewing or touching the affected body part. Gentle encouragement and support from the nurse helps the patient assume self-care and accept the affected body part. Brainstorming to identify alternative care strategies promotes the patient's independence even when total self-care is not feasible.*

Transitions of Care

Lymphedema prevention focuses on protecting the skin from injury. Teach patients with interrupted lymphatic systems (which are common postoperatively) to avoid blood draws and to have their blood pressure measured on the unaffected extremity.

When preparing the patient with chronic lymphedema and family to manage the disorder, include the following teaching topics:

- Recommended program of exercise and elevation of the extremity
- Foot and skin care
- Use of elastic graduated compression stockings and/or intermittent pressure devices
- Importance of wearing elastic stockings during the majority of waking hours, removing them once during the daytime and while sleeping
- Measures to prevent infection in the affected extremity, such as wearing gloves while gardening
- Signs and symptoms to report to the healthcare provider (e.g., manifestations of tissue breakdown or infection, increasing edema, or evidence of compromised circulation)
- Use and precautions associated with any prescribed medications
- Sodium-restricted diet, if ordered.

Provide information about contacts for questions, and make referrals as needed. Evaluate the need for home health, home maintenance assistance, and other services such as physical or occupational therapy.

CHAPTER HIGHLIGHTS

32.1 Disorders of Blood Pressure Regulation

Describe the pathophysiology and manifestations of disorders of blood pressure regulation, and outline the interprofessional care and nursing care of patients with these disorders.

- Essential hypertension, blood pressure of 130/80 mmHg or higher with no clearly identified cause, rarely causes symptoms but is a major risk factor for coronary heart disease, heart failure, stroke, and renal insufficiency.
- Patients with prehypertension are advised to make lifestyle changes indicated for hypertension (weight loss, exercise, dietary changes, limited alcohol intake, and stress reduction), but generally are not treated with medications unless other risk factors such as diabetes or kidney disease are present.

- Systolic hypertension, an elevated systolic blood pressure without elevation of the diastolic pressure, is common in older adults and contributes to complications such as coronary heart disease and stroke.
- Medications to treat hypertension include diuretics, alpha- and beta-adrenergic blockers, ACE inhibitors and angiotensin II blockers, calcium channel blockers, and vasodilators. A combination of two or more drugs is often required for effective blood pressure control.

32.2 Disorders of the Aorta and Its Branches

Describe the pathophysiology and manifestations of disorders of the aorta and its branches, and outline the interprofessional care and nursing care of patients with these disorders.

- Aneurysms, abnormal dilation of a blood vessel, commonly affect the aorta and the iliac arteries, particularly in older men. A slowly expanding abdominal aortic aneurysm that does not produce symptoms or impair flow through the renal arteries may not be repaired, particularly in an older patient. Percutaneously inserted endovascular splints provide an alternative to surgery for abdominal aortic aneurysms.

32.3 Disorders of the Peripheral Arteries

Describe the pathophysiology and manifestations of disorders of the peripheral arteries, and outline the interprofessional care and nursing care of patients with these disorders.

- Peripheral vascular disease, obstruction or occlusion of peripheral arteries by atherosclerotic plaque, is common and a leading cause of disability and amputation.
- Smoking cessation and regular daily exercise are key components of treatment for peripheral vascular disorders such as atherosclerosis, thromboangiitis obliterans, and Raynaud disease.

32.4 Disorders of Venous Circulation

Describe the pathophysiology and manifestations of disorders of venous circulation, and outline the interprofessional care and nursing care of patients with these disorders.

- Venous thrombosis, particularly of the deep veins of the legs and pelvis, develops as a result of venous stasis, blood vessel damage, and increased coagulability of the blood. The developing clot may fragment or break loose, becoming an embolus that typically lodges in the pulmonary circulation (pulmonary embolus). Chronic venous insufficiency and venous stasis may develop as a result of deep venous thrombosis.
- Prophylactic anticoagulation and mobilization of the patient are the primary preventive measures for venous thrombosis. Monitoring coagulation studies and assessing for evidence of bleeding (overt or covert) are important nursing measures for the patient on anticoagulant therapy.

32.5 Disorders of the Lymphatic System

Describe the pathophysiology and manifestations of disorders of the lymphatic system, and outline the interprofessional care and nursing care of patients with these disorders.

- Lymphadenopathy (enlarged lymph nodes), lymphangitis (inflammation of the lymph vessels), and lymphedema are the most common disorders affecting the lymph system.

TEST YOURSELF NCLEX-RN® REVIEW

1. A patient whose blood pressure averages 180/106 mmHg on three different readings says to the nurse, "I don't understand how it could be so high—I feel just fine." What response should the nurse make to this patient?
   A. "This is probably just a false reading due to 'white coat syndrome.' Don't worry about it."
   B. "High blood pressure often has few or no symptoms; that's why it is called the 'silent killer.'"
   C. "It is unusual that you are not having some symptoms such as severe headaches and nosebleeds."
   D. "You probably should have your blood pressure rechecked in 3 months or so and then follow up with your primary care provider if it is still high."

2. The nurse instructs a patient about the DASH diet for blood pressure control. Which patient statement indicates that additional teaching is necessary?
   A. "It will be difficult to give up my pretzels as snacks."
   B. "I need to reduce my intake of saturated fats."
   C. "It will be a challenge to incorporate all those servings of fruits and vegetables into my diet."
   D. "As long as I follow the DASH diet, exercise is not as important."

3. A patient is prescribed valsartan (Diovan) for treatment of hypertension. What should the nurse include when teaching the patient about this medication? (Select all that apply.)
    A. Report a persistent disruptive cough to your healthcare provider.
    B. Use caution when rising from bed or a chair to prevent dizziness.
    C. Take the drug at bedtime to reduce the risk of falling due to light-headedness.
    D. Use a potassium-based salt substitute to prevent hypokalemia while taking this drug.
    E. You may stop taking this drug once your blood pressure is within the normal range for at least 2 months.
4. A patient is complaining of new-onset calf and foot pain. The nurse notes that the leg below the knee is cool and pale and that dorsalis pedis and posterior tibial pulses are absent. What should the nurse do first to help this patient?
    A. Notify the healthcare provider.
    B. Prepare to initiate heparin therapy.
    C. Position the leg flat, supported in anatomic position.
    D. Place a cradle over the leg to prevent pressure from bedding.
5. The nurse is caring for an 86-year-old patient with a newly diagnosed 5 cm abdominal aortic aneurysm. What information should the nurse use to plan care for this patient?
    A. Immediate surgery is indicated for type B aneurysms.
    B. The risk of surgical repair is lower than the risk that the aneurysm will rupture.
    C. Opening the abdomen for the surgical procedure greatly increases the risk of rupture.
    D. A percutaneously inserted endovascular stent may be considered because of the patient's age.
6. A patient is diagnosed with peripheral atherosclerosis. Which patient findings would the nurse attribute to that diagnosis? (Select all that apply.)
    A. Pallor of the legs and feet when dependent
    B. Impaired sensation in the affected extremity
    C. Increased hair growth on the affected extremity
    D. Higher blood pressure readings in the affected extremity
    E. Thickened toenails
7. The nurse is planning care for a patient being discharged with peripheral vascular disease. In which order should the nurse provide teaching to this patient?
    A. Foot and leg care
    B. Smoking cessation
    C. Weight loss strategies
    D. Regular daily exercise
    E. Daily inspection of feet and legs
8. The nurse provides discharge instructions to a patient with deep venous thrombosis. Which patient statement indicates that teaching has been effective?
    A. "I'll use a hard-backed, upright chair when sitting instead of my recliner."
    B. "I understand why I am not allowed to exercise for the next 6 weeks and will take it easy."
    C. "I'll get my blood drawn as scheduled and notify the doctor if I have any unusual bleeding or bruising."
    D. "I'll have my wife buy a low-cholesterol cookbook and we'll make an appointment with the dietitian to learn about a low-fat, low-cholesterol diet."
9. A patient with visible varicose veins wants to have surgery to remove them because of leg pain. What would be the most appropriate response for the nurse to make to this patient?
    A. "Surgery will have a good cosmetic effect, but will not relieve the discomfort associated with varicose veins."
    B. "All varicose veins should be surgically removed to restore adequate blood flow to your legs and prevent gangrene."
    C. "Often measures such as elevating your legs and elastic stockings can relieve the discomfort associated with varicose veins."
    D. "Surgery is never indicated unless the varicose veins are interfering with circulation. Have you tried cosmetic measures to cover them up?"
10. The nurse is caring for a patient with lymphedema. Which nursing interventions are indicated for this patient? (Select all that apply.)
    A. Elevate affected extremities at night.
    B. Reinforce the importance of taking prescribed diuretics.
    C. Assist to apply elastic compression stockings during the day.
    D. Carefully dry and apply emollient lotion to affected extremities after bathing.
    E. Reinforce bedrest until edema resolves.

See Test Yourself answers in Appendix B.

REFERENCES

Adams, M. P., Holland, L. N., & Urban, C. (2017). *Pharmacology for nursing: A pathophysiologic approach* (5th ed.). Hoboken, NJ: Pearson Education.

Ambler, G. K., & Twine, C. P. (2018). Graft type for femoropopliteal bypass surgery. *Cochrane Database of Systematic Reviews.* DOI: 10.1002/14651858.CD001487.pub3

American Heart Association (AHA). (2017a). *High blood pressure.* Retrieved from www.heart.org/HEARTORG/Conditions/HighBloodPressure/High-Blood-Pressure-or-Hypertension_UCM_002020_SubHomePage.jsp.

American Heart Association (AHA). (2017b). *Types of aneurysms.* Retrieved from www.heart.org/HEARTORG/Conditions/VascularHealth/AorticAneurysm/Types-of-Aneurysms_UCM_454436_Article.jsp#.WjXVNXlG33g.

Benjamin, E. J., Blaha, M. J., Chiuve, S. E., Cushman, M., Das, S. R., Deo, R., . . . American Heart Association Statistics Committee and Stroke Statistics Subcommittee. (2017). Heart disease and stroke statistics—2017 update: A report from the American Heart Association. *Circulation, 135*(10), e146–e603.

Brandani, J. Z., Mizuno, J., Ciolac, E. G., & Monteiro, H. L. (2017). The hypotensive effect of Yoga's breathing exercises: A systematic review. *Complementary Therapy in Clinical Practice, 28*, 38–46.

Cleveland Clinic. (2018). *Endovascular stent graft: Aortic aneurysm repair.* Retrieved from https://my.clevelandclinic.org/health/diseases/16964-endovascular-stent-graft-aortic-aneurysm-repair.

Framingham Heart Study. (2017). *Home page.* Retrieved from https://www.framinghamheartstudy.org.

Genetics Home Reference. (2018a). *Familial thoracic aortic aneurysm and dissection.* Retrieved from https://ghr.nlm.nih.gov/condition/familial-thoracic-aortic-aneurysm-and-dissection#statistics.

Genetics Home Reference. (2018b). *Turner syndrome.* Retrieved from https://ghr.nlm.nih.gov/condition/turner-syndrome#genes.

Hiratzka, L. F., Bakris, G. L., Beckman, J. A., Bersin, R. M., Carr, V. F., Casey, D. E. Jr., . . . Williams, D. M. (2010). 2010 ACCF/AHA/AATS/ACR/ASA/SCA/SCAI/SIR/STS/SVM Guidelines for the diagnosis and management of patients with thoracic aortic disease: A report of the American College of Cardiology Foundation/American Heart Association Task Force on Practice Guidelines, American Association for Thoracic Surgery, American College of Radiology, American Stroke Association, Society of Cardiovascular Anesthesiologists, Society for Cardiovascular Angiography and Interventions, Society of Interventional Radiology, Society of Thoracic Surgeons, and Society for Vascular Medicine. *Circulation, 121,* e266–e369.

Kee, J. L. (2014). *Laboratory and diagnostic tests with nursing implications* (9th ed.). Boston, MA: Pearson.

Mayo Clinic. (2018). *Buerger's disease.* Retrieved from https://www.mayoclinic.org/diseases-conditions/buergers-disease/symptoms-causes/syc-20350658.

Perrin, K. O., & MacLeod, C. E. (2017). *Understanding the essentials of critical care nursing* (3rd ed.). Boston, MA: Pearson.

Saliba, E., & Sia, Y. (2015). The ascending aortic aneurysm: When to intervene? *IJC Heart and Vasculature, 6,* 91–100.

Shields, K. M., Fox, K. L., & Liebrecht, C. (2018). *Pearson nurse's drug guide: 2018.* Boston, MA: Pearson.

Sorenson, M., Quinn, L., & Klein, D. (2019). *Pathophysiology: Concepts of human disease.* Hoboken, NJ: Pearson Education.

U.S. Preventive Services Task Force. (2018). *Abdominal aortic aneurysm screening.* Retrieved from https://www.uspreventiveservicestaskforce.org/Page/Document/UpdateSummaryFinal/abdominal-aortic-aneurysm-screening.

Whelton, P. K., Carey, R. M., Aronow, W. S., Casey, D. E. Jr., Collins, K. J., Dennison Himmelfarb, C., . . . Wright, J. T. Jr. (2017). ACC/AHA/AAPA/ABC/ACPM/AGS/APhA/ASH/ASPC/NMA/PCNA guideline for the prevention, detection, evaluation, and management of high blood pressure in adults. *Hypertension.* [Epub ahead of print].

World Health Organization. (2013).*Hypertension.* Retrieved from www.who.int/topics/hypertension/en/.

ADDITIONAL RESOURCES

American Heart Association

www.heart.org

National Heart, Lung, and Blood Institute

www.nhlbi.nih.gov/health-topics

Lymphedema Education and Research Network

lymphaticnetwork.org/living-with-lymphedema/lymphedema

Chapter 33

Nursing Care of Patients with Hematologic Disorders

Chapter Outline and Learning Outcomes

CLINICAL COMPETENCIES

- Assess the effects of hematologic disorders and prescribed treatments on patients' functional health status.
- Monitor and document continuing assessment data, including laboratory test results, subjective and objective information, and reporting data outside the normal or expected range.
- Based on knowledge of pathophysiology, prescribed treatment, and assessed data, identify and prioritize nursing diagnoses for patients with hematologic disorders.
- Use nursing research and evidence-based practice to identify and implement individualized nursing interventions for the patient with a hematologic disorder.
- Safely administer prescribed medications and treatments for patients with hematologic disorders.
- Collaborate with the interprofessional care team to plan and provide coordinated, effective care for patients with hematologic disorders.
- Provide appropriate teaching for patients with hematologic disorders, evaluating learning and the need for continued reinforcement of information.
- Use continuing assessment data to revise the plan of care as needed to restore, maintain, or promote functional health in the patient with a hematologic disorder.

KEY TERMS

anemia, 1159
aplastic anemia, 1167
bone marrow transplant (BMT), 1182
disseminated intravascular coagulation (DIC), 1207
hemolytic anemia, 1163
hemophilia, 1203
hemostasis, 1199
iron-deficiency anemia, 1160
leukemia, 1176
lymphoma, 1188
multiple myeloma, 1194
myelodysplastic syndrome (MDS), 1173
pernicious anemia, 1162
polycythemia, 1175
sickle cell crisis, 1163
sickle cell disease, 1163
stem cell transplant (SCT), 1182
thalassemia, 1164
thrombocytopenia, 1199

Disorders affecting the blood and blood-forming organs have effects that range from minor disruptions in daily activities to major life-threatening crises. Patients with hematologic disorders need holistic nursing care, including emotional support and care for problems involving major body systems. This chapter focuses on health changes resulting from changes in red cells, white cells, platelets, and clotting factors.

33.1 Red Blood Cell Disorders

Red blood cells (RBCs) transport oxygen to body tissues and help return carbon dioxide to the lungs for excretion. Alterations in the number, size, shape, or composition of RBCs affect their ability to carry out these functions effectively.

The Patient with Anemia

Anemia is an abnormally low number of circulating RBCs, low hemoglobin concentration, or both. A decrease in the number of circulating RBCs is the usual cause of anemia. This may result from acute or chronic blood loss, inadequate RBC production, or increased RBC destruction. Insufficient or defective hemoglobin within RBCs contributes to anemia. Depending on its severity, anemia may affect all major organ systems. Iron-deficiency anemia is the most common type of anemia. Risk for anemia increases with age. Persons older than 85 years are two to three times more likely to have anemia compared to other older adults.

Physiology Review

As blood flows through the pulmonary vascular system, oxygen diffuses from alveoli into capillary blood. The majority of the oxygen binds reversibly with the hemoglobin in RBCs; only about 3% of the oxygen remains in solution in the blood. When the blood reaches the capillaries serving body tissues, oxygen is released from the hemoglobin molecule and diffuses out of the capillary to reach the cells. The amount of oxygen that reaches the tissues depends on a number of factors, including:

- Available oxygen in the alveoli
- The diffusing surface and capacity of the lungs
- The number of RBCs and the amount and type of hemoglobin they contain
- The ability of the cardiovascular system to transport blood and oxygen to the tissues.

For more information about RBCs, hemoglobin, and their production and function, refer to Chapter 29.

Pathophysiology and Manifestations

A number of different pathologic mechanisms can lead to anemia (**Box 33.1**). Regardless of the cause, every type of anemia reduces the oxygen-carrying capacity of the blood due to a deficiency of RBCs or hemoglobin, leading to tissue hypoxia. The resulting manifestations depend on the severity of the anemia, how quickly it develops, and other factors such as age and health status.

When anemia develops gradually and the RBC reduction is moderate, successful compensatory mechanisms may result in few symptoms except when the oxygen needs of the body increase due to exercise or infection. Symptoms develop as RBCs and hemoglobin levels are further reduced. Pallor of the skin, mucous membranes, conjunctiva, and nail beds develops as a result of blood redistribution to vital organs and lack of hemoglobin (**Figure 33.1** ■). As tissue oxygenation decreases, the heart and respiratory rates rise in an attempt to increase cardiac output and tissue perfusion. Tissue hypoxia may cause angina, fatigue, dyspnea on exertion, and night cramps. It also stimulates erythropoietin release; increased erythropoietin activity stimulates

BOX 33.1
Pathophysiologic Mechanisms of Anemia

DECREASED RBC PRODUCTION

- Altered hemoglobin synthesis
  - a. Iron deficiency
  - b. Thalassemias
  - c. Chronic inflammation
- Altered DNA synthesis
  - a. Vitamin B_{12} or folic acid malabsorption or deficiency
- Bone marrow failure
  - a. Aplastic anemia (stem cell dysfunction)
  - b. Red cell aplasia
  - c. Myeloproliferative leukemias
  - d. Cancer metastasis, lymphoma
  - e. Chronic infection or inflammation, physical and emotional fatigue

INCREASED RBC LOSS OR DESTRUCTION

- Acute or chronic blood loss
  - a. Hemorrhage or trauma
  - b. Chronic gastrointestinal bleeding, menorrhagia
- Increased hemolysis
  - a. Hereditary cell membrane disorders
  - b. Defective hemoglobin—sickle cell disease or trait
  - c. Pyruvate kinase (PK) or glucose-6-phosphate dehydrogenase (G6PD) deficiency affecting glycolysis or cell oxidation
  - d. Immune mechanisms and disorders (e.g., blood reaction, hypersensitivity responses, autoimmune disorders)
  - e. Splenomegaly and hypersplenism
  - f. Infection
  - g. Erythrocyte trauma (e.g., due to cardiopulmonary bypass, hemolytic uremic syndrome)

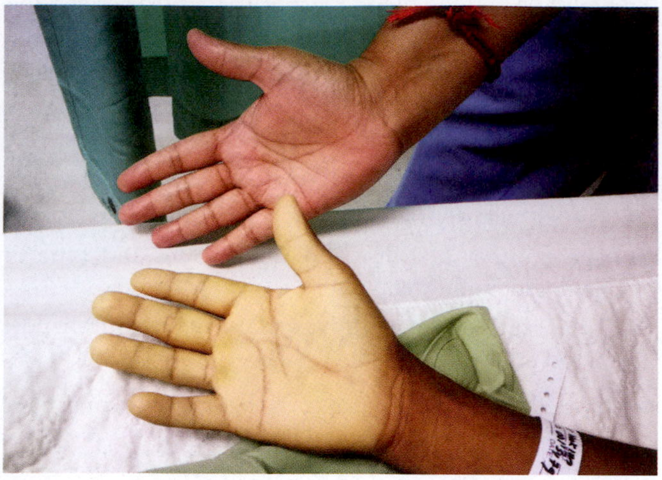

Figure 33.1 ■ The skin of the patient with anemia appears pale beside that of an individual with a normal hemoglobin and hematocrit.

RBC production in the bone marrow and may lead to bone pain. Cerebral hypoxia can lead to headache, dizziness, and dim vision. Heart failure may develop in severe anemia.

With rapid blood loss, blood volume is decreased as well as the oxygen-carrying capacity of the blood. Initial manifestations include tachycardia and tachypnea; the skin may be pale, cool, and clammy as peripheral vessels constrict to maintain blood flow to the heart and brain. With significant blood loss, signs of circulatory shock may occur, including hypotension, tachycardia, decreased level of consciousness, and oliguria. With chronic bleeding, fluid shifts from the interstitial spaces into the vessels, maintaining blood volume. Blood viscosity is reduced, which may result in a systolic heart murmur. See Multisystem Effects of Anemia.

Anemia is categorized by cause: Blood loss, nutritional, hemolytic, and bone marrow suppression (aplastic). Genetics also plays a role in some anemias. Discussions of the pathophysiology and specific manifestations of these types of anemias follow. Anemia is a significant problem in older adults. Unexplained anemia is found in 30 to 46% of older adults.

Blood Loss Anemia

When anemia results from acute or chronic bleeding, RBCs and other blood components (such as iron) are lost from the body. With acute blood loss, circulating volume decreases. As a result, the cardiac output falls. Compensatory mechanisms are activated to maintain the cardiac output: The heart rate increases, and peripheral blood vessels constrict. Vessels in the liver, a blood storage organ, also constrict, increasing circulating volume. Fluid shifts from the interstitial spaces into the vascular compartment to maintain blood volume, diluting the cellular components of the blood and reducing its viscosity. If hemorrhage continues, compensatory mechanisms become less effective, increasing the risk for shock and circulatory failure (refer to Chapter 11).

In acute blood loss, circulating RBCs are of normal size and shape (*normocytic*). Early in the hemorrhage, the RBC count, hemoglobin, and hematocrit may be normal; as fluid shifts from the interstitial space into the vascular space to maintain circulating volume, the RBC count, hemoglobin, and hematocrit fall. If sufficient iron is available, the number of circulating RBCs and hemoglobin levels return to normal within 3 to 4 weeks after the bleeding episode. Chronic blood loss, on the other hand, depletes iron stores as RBC production attempts to maintain the RBC supply. The resulting RBCs are *microcytic* (small) and *hypochromic* (pale).

Nutritional Anemias

A number of different nutrients are required for normal RBC development (erythropoiesis). Iron is a key nutrient necessary for hemoglobin synthesis. In addition, adequate supplies of protein (and its building blocks, amino acids), vitamins, and other minerals are required. The B vitamins, particularly B_{12} (cobalamin) and folate, have a key role in RBC development. Vitamins C and E are also necessary. Nutritional anemias result from nutrient deficits that affect RBC formation or hemoglobin synthesis. The nutrient deficit may be caused by inadequate diet, malabsorption of the nutrient, or an increased need for the nutrient. The most common types of nutritional anemias are iron-deficiency anemia, vitamin B_{12} anemia, and folic acid–deficiency anemia. Vitamin B_{12} and folic acid anemias are sometimes called *megaloblastic anemias* because enlarged nucleated RBCs called *megaloblasts* are seen in these anemias.

Iron-Deficiency Anemia. **Iron-deficiency anemia** is the most common type of anemia. It develops when the supply of iron is inadequate for optimal RBC formation. The body cannot synthesize hemoglobin without iron. Normally, the body efficiently recycles and stores iron, reusing much of the iron contained in RBCs that are removed from circulation due to age or damage. However, small amounts of iron are continually lost in the feces; therefore, adequate iron intake is necessary for normal hemoglobin synthesis and RBC production. Iron-deficiency anemia results in fewer numbers of RBCs, microcytic and hypochromic RBCs, and malformed RBCs (*poikilocytosis*) (**Figure 33.2** ■).

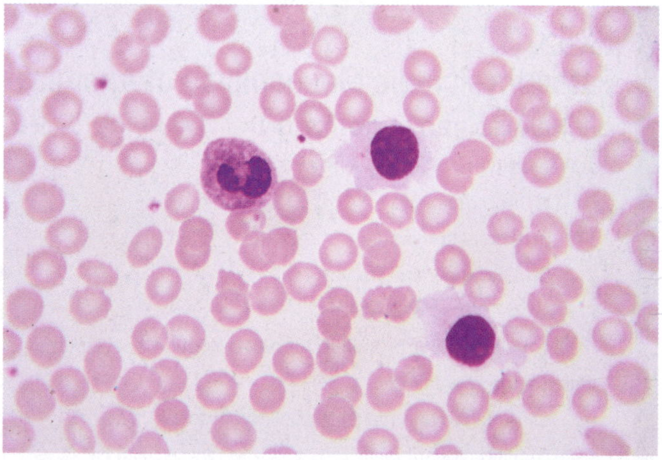

Figure 33.2 ■ A blood smear showing RBCs characteristically seen in iron-deficiency anemia. Note the pale color of the RBCs (hypochromic). Many of the cells are also smaller than normal (microcytic) and misshapen, reducing their oxygen-carrying capacity.

Multisystem Effects of
Anemia

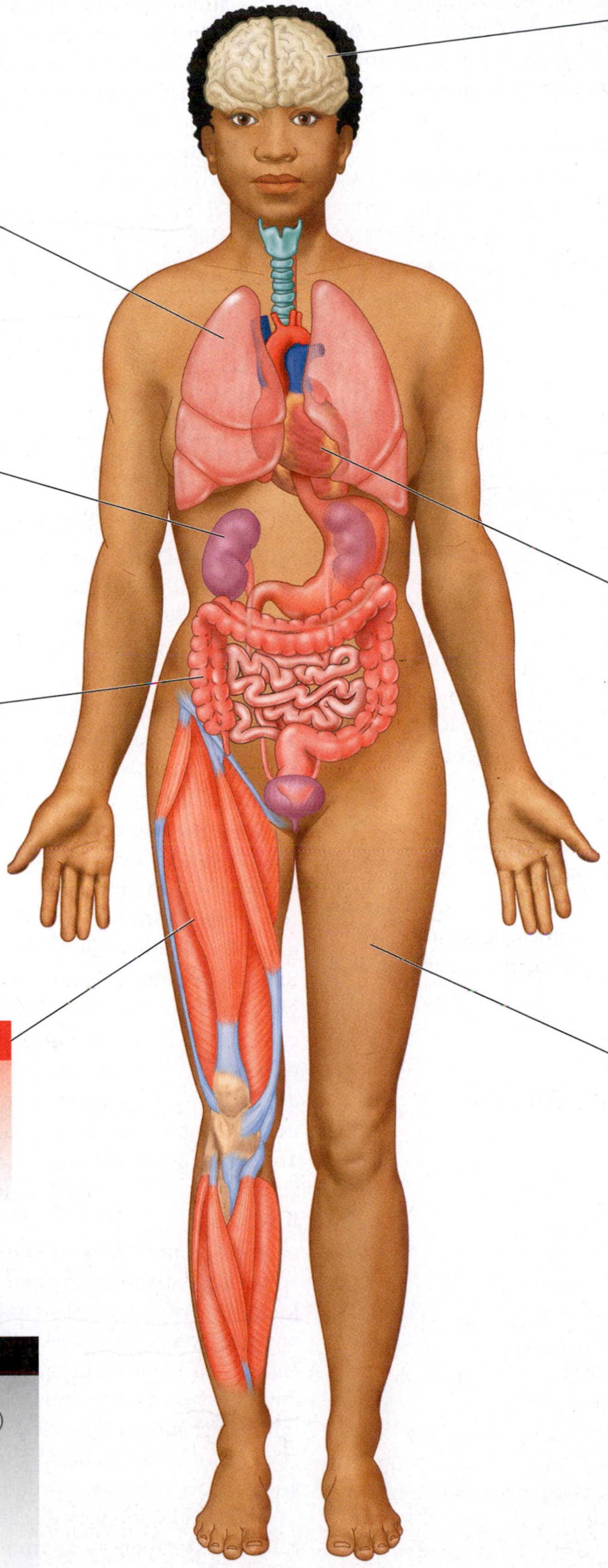

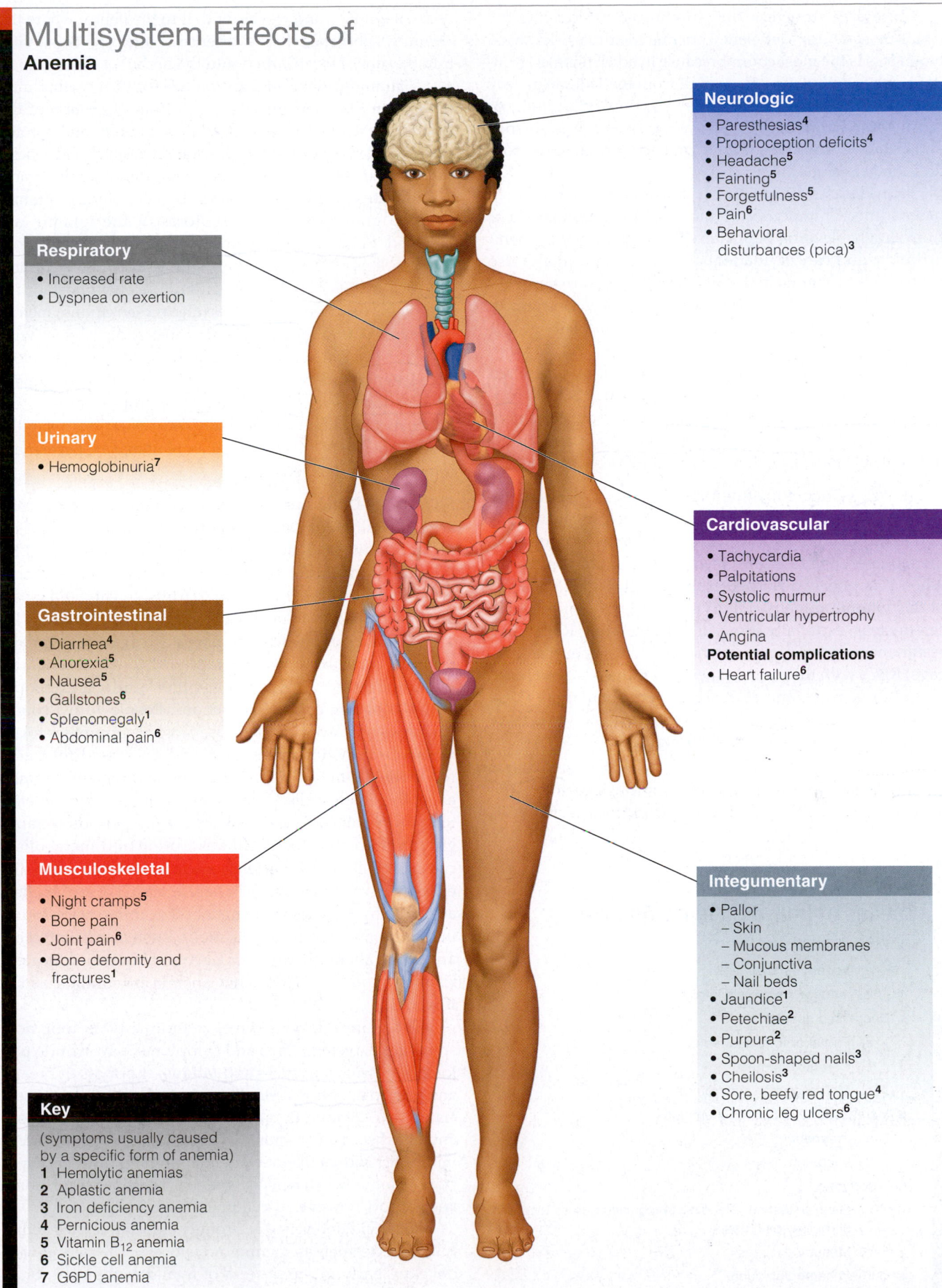

Neurologic
- Paresthesias[4]
- Proprioception deficits[4]
- Headache[5]
- Fainting[5]
- Forgetfulness[5]
- Pain[6]
- Behavioral disturbances (pica)[3]

Respiratory
- Increased rate
- Dyspnea on exertion

Urinary
- Hemoglobinuria[7]

Cardiovascular
- Tachycardia
- Palpitations
- Systolic murmur
- Ventricular hypertrophy
- Angina

Potential complications
- Heart failure[6]

Gastrointestinal
- Diarrhea[4]
- Anorexia[5]
- Nausea[5]
- Gallstones[6]
- Splenomegaly[1]
- Abdominal pain[6]

Musculoskeletal
- Night cramps[5]
- Bone pain
- Joint pain[6]
- Bone deformity and fractures[1]

Integumentary
- Pallor
  - Skin
  - Mucous membranes
  - Conjunctiva
  - Nail beds
- Jaundice[1]
- Petechiae[2]
- Purpura[2]
- Spoon-shaped nails[3]
- Cheilosis[3]
- Sore, beefy red tongue[4]
- Chronic leg ulcers[6]

Key
(symptoms usually caused by a specific form of anemia)

1 Hemolytic anemias
2 Aplastic anemia
3 Iron deficiency anemia
4 Pernicious anemia
5 Vitamin B_{12} anemia
6 Sickle cell anemia
7 G6PD anemia

Excessive iron loss due to chronic bleeding is the usual cause of iron-deficiency anemia in adults. Menstrual blood loss is the most common cause in adult females. Iron-deficiency anemia may also result from inadequate dietary iron intake (< 1 mg/day), malabsorption syndromes, or the increased iron requirements associated with pregnancy and lactation. **Box 33.2** summarizes common causes of iron-deficiency anemia.

Iron-deficiency anemia is particularly common in older adults. Chronic, occult (hidden) blood loss may occur from slowly bleeding peptic ulcers, GI inflammation, hemorrhoids, and cancer. Inadequate dietary iron intake also contributes to anemia in the older adult. Access to transportation may limit fresh food consumption, a factor contributing to poor iron intake among all adults, especially people with limited or fixed incomes.

In addition to the general manifestations of anemia described earlier, chronic iron deficiency may lead to brittle, spoon-shaped nails; cheilosis (cracks at the corners of the mouth); a smooth, sore tongue; and *pica* (a craving for unusual substances, such as clay or starch).

Vitamin B_{12}–Deficiency Anemia. Vitamin B_{12} is necessary for DNA synthesis and is found almost exclusively in foods derived from animals. Vitamin B_{12} deficiency occurs when inadequate vitamin B_{12} is consumed or, more commonly, when it is poorly absorbed from the GI tract. Deficiency of this vitamin impairs cell division and maturation of the cell nucleus, especially in rapidly proliferating RBCs. As a result, macrocytic (large), misshapen (oval rather than concave) RBCs with thin membranes are produced. Great numbers of these large, immature RBCs enter circulation. These cells are fragile, incapable of carrying adequate amounts of oxygen, and have a shortened lifespan.

Failure to absorb dietary vitamin B_{12} is called **pernicious anemia**. It develops due to a lack of intrinsic factor, a substance secreted by the gastric mucosa. Intrinsic factor binds with vitamin B_{12} and travels with it to the ileum, where the vitamin is absorbed. In the absence of intrinsic factor, vitamin B_{12} cannot be absorbed into the body.

Vitamin B_{12} deficiency may also result from other malabsorption disorders and dietary factors. Resection of the stomach or ileum, loss of pancreatic secretions, and chronic gastritis can affect vitamin B_{12} absorption. Dietary deficiencies of vitamin B_{12} are rare, usually occurring only among vegans.

Manifestations of vitamin B_{12}–deficiency anemia develop gradually as bodily stores of the vitamin are depleted. Pallor or slight jaundice and weakness develop. In pernicious anemia, a smooth, sore, beefy red tongue and diarrhea may occur. Because vitamin B_{12} is important for neurologic function, *paresthesias* (altered sensations, such as numbness or tingling) in the extremities and problems with *proprioception* (the sense of one's position in space) develop. These manifestations may progress to difficulty maintaining balance due to spinal cord damage. Central nervous system (CNS) manifestations of relatively short duration (6 months or less) are reversible with treatment but may be permanent if treatment is delayed.

Folic Acid–Deficiency Anemia. Like vitamin B_{12}, folic acid is required for DNA synthesis and normal maturation of RBCs. Folic acid–deficiency anemia is characterized by fragile, megaloblastic (large and immature) cells. Folic acid is found in green leafy vegetables, fruits, cereals, and meats and is absorbed from the intestines.

Folic acid–deficiency anemia due to inadequate intake is more common among people who are chronically undernourished. This includes older adults and people with alcoholism or drug addictions. People with alcoholism are especially at risk because alcohol suppresses folate metabolism, which forms folic acid. Increased folic acid requirements may also lead to anemia. Pregnant women are at the greatest risk. Infants and teenagers can develop temporary folic acid deficiencies during periods of rapid growth. Impaired folic acid absorption and metabolism can cause folic acid–deficiency anemia. Malabsorption disorders such as celiac sprue (a hereditary GI disorder characterized by an inability to metabolize amino acids found in gluten) and certain medications, such as methotrexate and some chemotherapeutic agents, may be implicated. Causes of folic acid–deficiency anemia are summarized in **Box 33.3**.

The manifestations develop gradually as folic acid stores are depleted. Signs and symptoms may include pallor, progressive weakness and fatigue, shortness of breath, and heart palpitations. Manifestations similar to those associated with vitamin B_{12} anemia, such as glossitis, cheilosis, and diarrhea, are common. No neurologic symptoms occur with folic acid–deficiency anemia, helping differentiate it from vitamin B_{12}–deficiency anemia. These two nutritional anemias do, however, sometimes coexist.

Folic acid deficiency is strongly associated with neural tube defects such as meningomyelocele. The neural tube develops early in the process of fetal development, often before pregnancy is recognized.

BOX 33.2
Causes of Iron-Deficiency Anemia

- Dietary deficiencies
  - a. Vegetarian diet
  - b. Inadequate protein intake
- Decreased absorption
  - a. Partial or total gastrectomy
  - b. Chronic diarrhea
  - c. Malabsorption syndromes
- Increased metabolic requirements
  - a. Pregnancy
  - b. Lactation
- Blood loss
  - a. Gastrointestinal bleeding (especially due to ulcers or chronic aspirin use)
  - b. Menstrual losses
- Chronic hemoglobinuria

BOX 33.3
Causes of Folic Acid–Deficiency Anemia

- Inadequate dietary intake

  At risk:
  a. Older adults
  b. People with alcoholism
  c. Patients receiving total parenteral nutrition
- Increased metabolic requirements

  At risk:
  a. Pregnant women
  b. Infants and teenagers
  c. Patients undergoing hemodialysis
  d. Patients with forms of hemolytic anemia
- Folic acid malabsorption and impaired metabolism
  a. Celiac sprue
  b. Chemotherapeutic agents, folate antagonists (methotrexate, pentamidine), or anticonvulsants
  c. Alcoholism

BOX 33.4
Causes of Hemolytic Anemia

INTRINSIC

- RBC cell membrane defects
- Hemoglobin structure defects (e.g., sickle cell disease, thalassemia)
- Inherited enzyme defects (e.g., G6PD deficiency)

EXTRINSIC

- Drugs, chemicals
- Toxins and venoms
- Bacterial and other infections
- Trauma, burns
- Mechanical damage (prosthetic heart valves)

Hemolytic Anemias

Hemolytic anemias are characterized by premature destruction (*lysis*) of RBCs. When RBCs break down, iron and other by-products of their destruction remain in the plasma. RBC lysis (hemolysis) may occur within the circulatory system or due to phagocytosis by WBCs such as circulating monocytes and macrophages in the spleen. In response to hemolysis, the hematopoietic activity of bone marrow increases, leading to increased reticulocytes (immature RBCs) in circulating blood. Most types of hemolytic anemia are characterized by normocytic and normochromic RBCs.

Hemolytic anemias have many different causes (**Box 33.4**). The cause may be *intrinsic*, arising from disorders within the RBC itself, or *extrinsic*, originating outside the RBC. Intrinsic disorders include cell membrane defects, defects in hemoglobin structure and function, and inherited enzyme deficiencies. See the accompanying Genetic Considerations box for more information about inherited intrinsic RBC disorders associated with hemolytic anemia. Extrinsic causes of hemolytic anemia include drugs, bacterial and other toxins, and trauma. This section discusses sickle cell disease, thalassemia, acquired hemolytic anemia, and glucose-6-phosphate dehydrogenase anemia.

Sickle Cell Disease. **Sickle cell disease** is a hereditary, chronic hemolytic anemia. It is characterized by episodes of *sickling*, during which RBCs become abnormally crescent shaped. The disorder is transmitted as an autosomal recessive genetic defect (**Figure 33.3** ■). This defect causes synthesis of an abnormal form of hemoglobin (HbS) within RBCs. Sickle cell disease can significantly shorten the lifespan, with most deaths occurring due to infection (Sorenson, Quinn, & Klein, 2019).

The disease is most common among people of African descent (refer to Genetics Consideration box). In the United States, 1 in 500 African Americans have sickle cell anemia (Genetics Home Reference, 2018d). They are at risk for **sickle cell crisis**, severe episodes of fever and intense pain that are the hallmark of this disorder.

The *HbS* gene changes the structure of the beta chain of the hemoglobin molecule. When hypoxemia develops and HbS is deoxygenated, it crystallizes into rodlike structures. Clusters of these rods form long chains that deform the erythrocyte into a crescent or sickle shape (**Figure 33.4** ■). The sickled cells tend to clump together and obstruct capillary blood flow, causing ischemia and possible infarction of surrounding tissue. See Pathophysiology Illustrated on page 1168.

When normal oxygen tension is restored, the sickled RBCs resume their normal shape; that is, they "unsickle." Repeated episodes of sickling and unsickling weaken RBC cell membranes. The weakened RBCs are hemolyzed and removed. Consequently, the normal lifespan of RBCs is greatly reduced in sickle cell disease, increasing the demand for RBC production. Conditions likely to trigger sickling include hypoxia, low environmental or body temperature, excessive exercise, anesthesia, dehydration, infections, or acidosis.

The acute and chronic manifestations of sickle cell disease arise from episodes of RBC sickling. Sickling causes general manifestations of hemolytic anemia, including pallor, fatigue, jaundice, and irritability. Extensive sickling can precipitate a crisis due to occluded circulation, impaired erythropoiesis, or sequestration of large amounts of blood in the liver or spleen (**Figure 33.5** ■).

A vasoocclusive or thrombotic crisis occurs when sickling develops in the microcirculation. Obstruction of blood flow triggers vasospasm that halts all blood flow in the vessel. Lack of blood flow leads to tissue ischemia and infarction. Vasoocclusive crises are painful and last an average of 4 to 6 days. Infarction of small vessels in the extremities causes painful swelling of the hands and feet; large joints may also be affected. Priapism (persistent, painful erection of the penis) may develop. Abdominal pain may signal infarction of abdominal organs and structures. Infarction

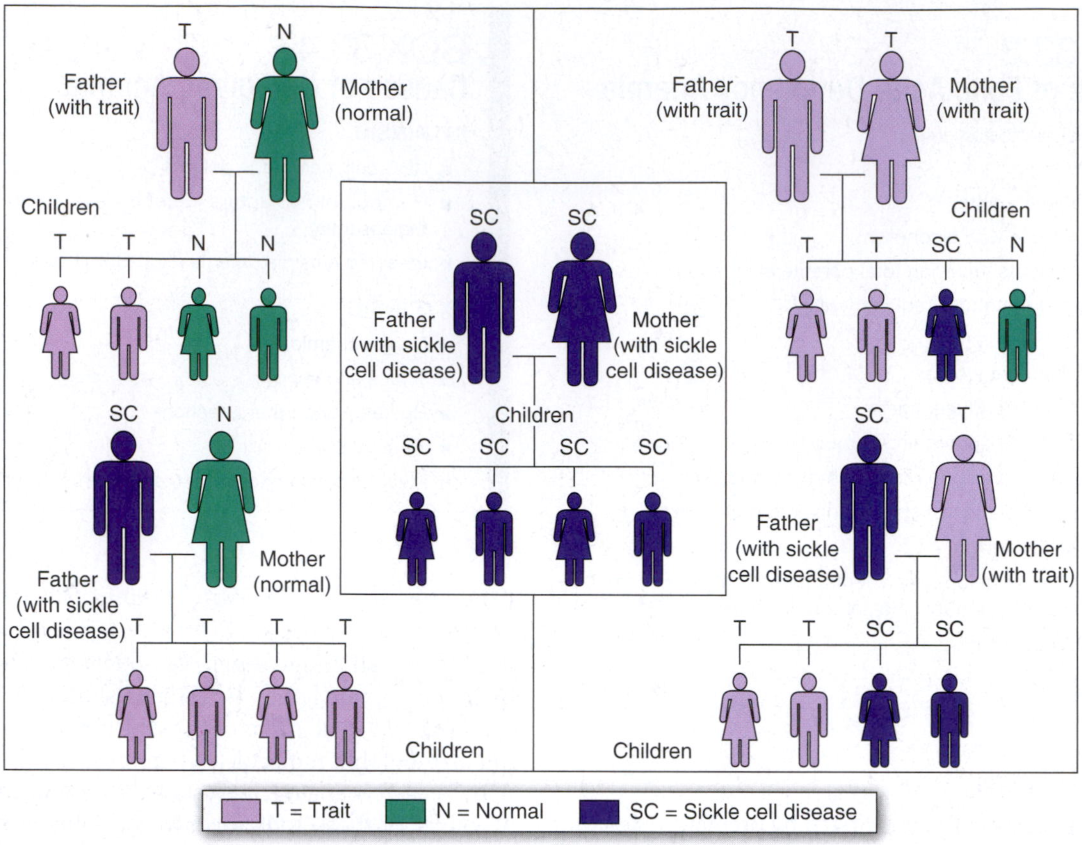
T
N
Father
(with trait)
Mother
(normal)
Children
T T N N
T
T
Father
(with trait)
Mother
(with trait)
Children
T T SC N
SC
SC
Father
(with sickle
cell disease)
Mother
(with sickle
cell disease)
Children
SC SC SC SC
SC
N
Father
(with sickle
cell disease)
Mother
(normal)
T T T T
Children
SC
T
Father
(with sickle
cell disease)
Mother
(with trait)
T T SC SC
Children
T = Trait
N = Normal
SC = Sickle cell disease

Figure 33.3 ■ Inheritance pattern for sickle cell disease.

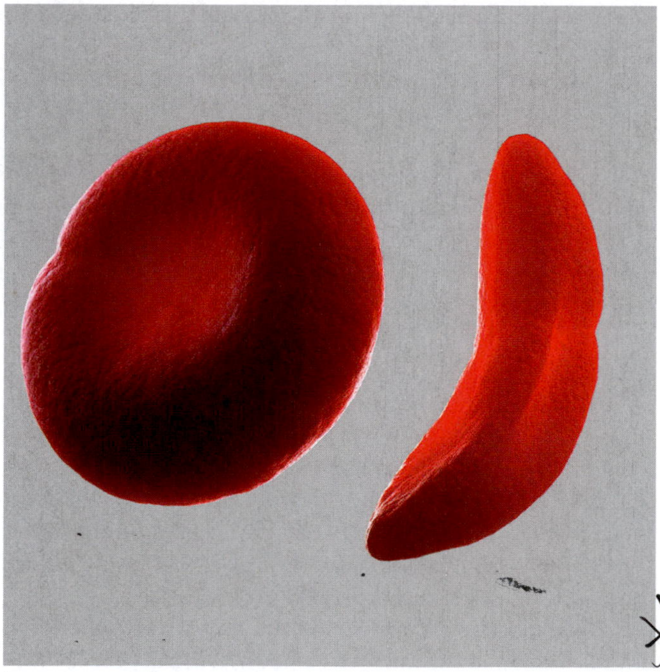

Figure 33.4 ■ Illustration of normal red blood cells and sickled cells.

may affect bone marrow or lead to aseptic necrosis of affected bones. Stroke may result from cerebral vessel occlusion (Sorenson et al., 2019). Skin ulcers may develop as a result of occluded vessels supplying the dermis. Repeated infarcts associated with sickling can affect the structure and function of nearly every organ system. People with sickle cell disease may develop an enlarged spleen and liver, renal insufficiency, gallstones, and other manifestations of organ dysfunction. *Acute chest syndrome*—a symptom complex that includes fever, chest pain, an increasing WBC count, and pulmonary infiltrates—may develop, as well as other pulmonary complications like pneumonia, pulmonary infarction, and pulmonary embolism.

The shortened RBC lifespan and compromised erythropoiesis can lead to profound *aplastic anemia* in sickle cell disease. *Sequestration crises* are marked by pooling of large amounts of blood in the liver and spleen. This sickle cell crisis only occurs in children, but is thought to be the cause of sickle cell disease–related deaths in early childhood (Sorenson et al., 2019).

Thalassemia. The **thalassemias** are inherited disorders of hemoglobin synthesis in which either the alpha or beta chains of the hemoglobin molecule are missing or defective. This leads to deficient hemoglobin production and fragile hypochromic, microcytic RBCs called *target cells* because of their distinctive bull's-eye appearance.

Thalassemia usually affects certain populations. People of Mediterranean descent (southern Italy and Greece) are more likely to have beta thalassemias (also called *Cooley anemia* or *Mediterranean anemia*). People of Asian ancestry, especially from Thailand, the Philippines, and China, more often have alpha thalassemia. Africans and African Americans may have both alpha and beta thalassemia. As with sickle cell disease, only one defective beta chain–forming

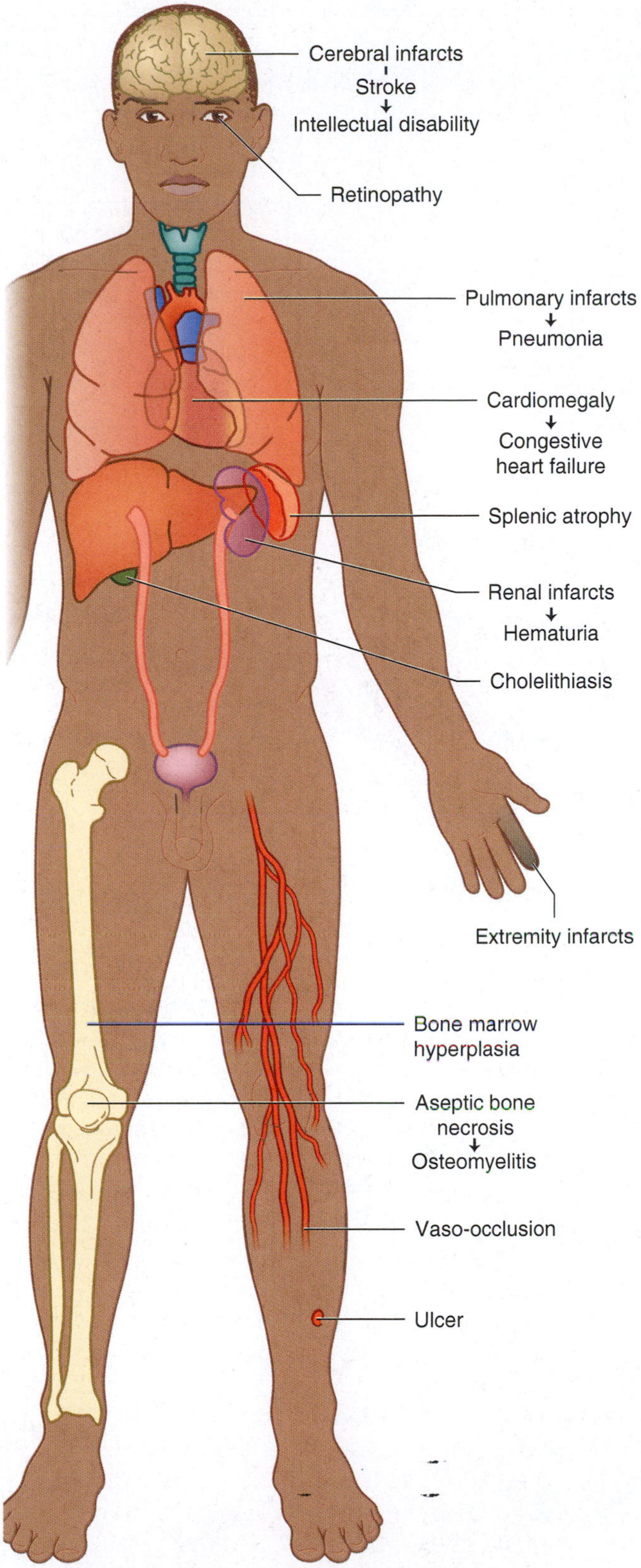

Cerebral infarcts
Stroke
Intellectual disability
Retinopathy
Pulmonary infarcts
Pneumonia
Cardiomegaly
Congestive heart failure
Splenic atrophy
Renal infarcts
Hematuria
Cholelithiasis
Extremity infarcts
Bone marrow hyperplasia
Aseptic bone necrosis
Osteomyelitis
Vaso-occlusion
Ulcer

Figure 33.5 ■ Manifestations and complications associated with sickle cell disease.

gene may be present (*beta thalassemia minor*), causing mild symptoms, or both may be defective (*beta thalassemia major*), leading to more severe symptoms. Children with thalassemia major rarely reach adulthood, although repeated blood transfusions may extend their lifespan (Sorenson et al., 2019). Four genes are responsible for alpha chain formation; one, two, three, or all four may be defective. In the latter case (*alpha-thalassemia major*), death is inevitable and usually occurs in utero. Genetic studies and counseling are recommended for people at risk for this illness.

People with thalassemia minor are often asymptomatic. When manifestations do occur, they include mild to moderate anemia, mild splenomegaly, bronze skin coloring, and bone marrow hyperplasia. The major form of the disease causes severe anemia, heart failure, and liver and spleen enlargement from increased red cell destruction. Fractures of the long bones, ribs, and vertebrae may result from bone marrow expansion and thinning due to increased hematopoiesis. Jaundice may develop due to hemolysis, as well as hepatomegaly and splenomegaly. Accumulation of iron in

Genetic Considerations

Inherited Hemolytic Anemias

Sickle Cell Disease

Mutations in the *HBB* gene cause sickle cell disease, which is inherited in an autosomal recessive pattern (Genetics Home Reference, 2018d).

- Sickle cell disease affects about 70,000 to 80,000 people in the United States.
- In African Americans, sickle cell disease occurs in 1 out of every 500 births.
- People from Central and South America, Cuba, Saudi Arabia, India, and Mediterranean countries such as Turkey, Greece, and Italy may also be at risk; sickle cell disease occurs in 1 of every 1000 to 1400 Hispanic American births.
- Sickle cell disease is a serious chronic and recurrent disease. The stress of the disease is compounded by the risk for its transmission to offspring. Recommend that all patients with sickle cell trait or disease obtain genetic counseling as part of their family planning process.

Alpha Thalassemia

Mutations in the *HBA1* or *HBA2* genes cause alpha thalassemia, which is inherited in a complex pattern depending on how many alleles the parents are missing (Genetics Home Reference, 2018a).

- Alpha thalassemia is fairly common, particularly in Southeast Asia. It also affects people from the Mediterranean countries, India, Africa, the Middle East, and Central Asia.

Beta Thalassemia

Mutations in the *HBB* gene cause beta thalassemia, which is inherited in an autosomal recessive pattern (Genetics Home Reference, 2018b).

- Beta-thalassemia is seen primarily in people of Mediterranean, Central and Southeast Asian, Middle Eastern, and North African origin.

G6PD Deficiency

Mutations of the *G6PD* gene cause G6PD deficiency, which is inherited in an X-linked recessive pattern. Therefore, it occurs almost entirely in males (Genetics Home Reference, 2018c).

- Approximately 1 out of 10 African American males are affected.
- An estimated 400 million people worldwide have G6PD deficiency, mostly those from certain areas of Africa, Asia, the Mediterranean countries, and the Middle East.

Pathophysiology Illustrated

Sickle Cell Disease

Hemoglobin S and Red Blood Cell Sickling

Sickle cell anemia is caused by an inherited autosomal recessive defect in Hb synthesis. Sickle cell hemoglobin (HbS) differs from normal hemoglobin only in the substitution of the amino acid valine for glutamine in both beta chains of the hemoglobin molecule.

When HbS is oxygenated, it has the same globular shape as normal hemoglobin. However, when HbS off-loads oxygen, it becomes insoluble in intracellular fluid and crystallizes into rodlike structures. Clusters of rods form polymers (long chains) that bend the erythrocyte into the characteristic crescent shape of the sickle cell.

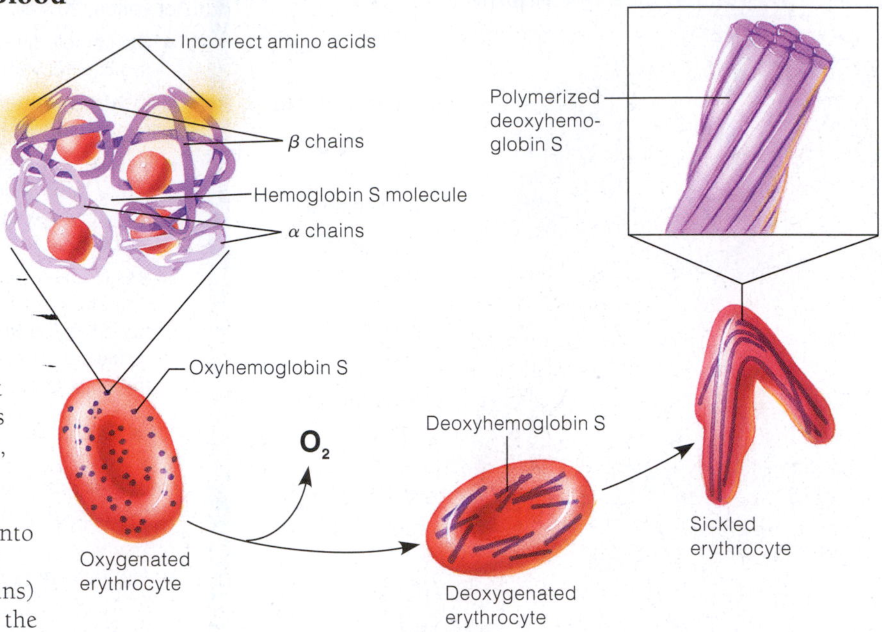
Incorrect amino acids
β chains
Hemoglobin S molecule
α chains
Polymerized deoxyhemoglobin S
Oxyhemoglobin S
O_2
Deoxyhemoglobin S
Oxygenated erythrocyte
Deoxygenated erythrocyte
Sickled erythrocyte

The Sickle Cell Disease Process

Sickle cell disease is characterized by episodes of acute painful crises. Sickling crises are triggered by conditions causing high tissue oxygen demands or that affect cellular pH. As the crisis begins, sickled erythrocytes adhere to capillary walls and to each other, obstructing blood flow and causing cellular hypoxia. The crisis accelerates as tissue hypoxia and acidic metabolic waste products cause further sickling and cell damage.

Sickle cell crises cause microinfarcts in joints and organs, and repeated crises slowly destroy organs and tissues. The spleen and kidneys are especially prone to sickling damage.

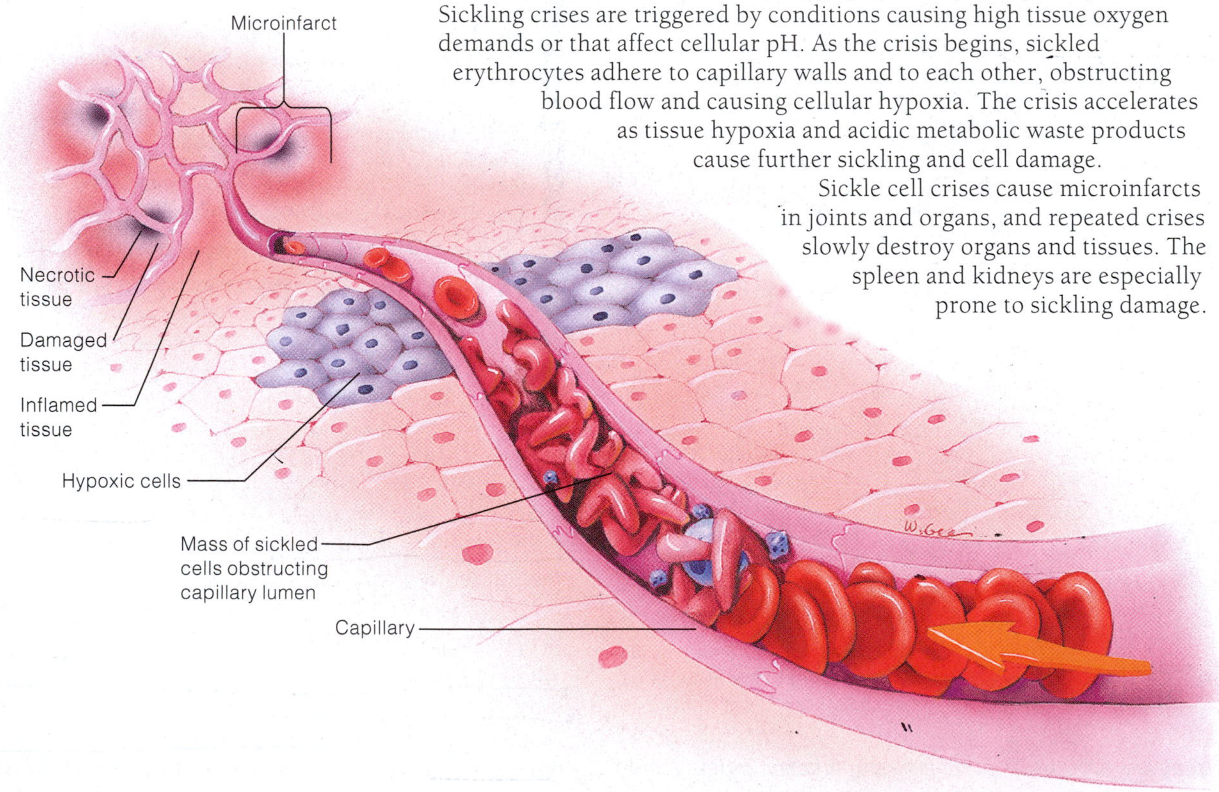
Microinfarct
Necrotic tissue
Damaged tissue
Inflamed tissue
Hypoxic cells
Mass of sickled cells obstructing capillary lumen
Capillary

the heart, liver, and pancreas following repeated transfusions for treatment may eventually cause failure of these organs.

Acquired Hemolytic Anemia. *Acquired hemolytic anemia* results from hemolysis due to factors outside of the RBC. Causes of acquired hemolytic anemias include:

- Mechanical trauma to RBCs produced by prosthetic heart valves, severe burns, hemodialysis, or radiation
- Autoimmune disorders
- Bacterial or protozoal infection
- Immune system–mediated responses, such as transfusion reactions
- Drugs, toxins, chemical agents, or venoms.

The manifestations of acquired hemolytic anemia depend on the extent of hemolysis and the body's ability to replace destroyed RBCs. The anemia itself is often mild to moderate as erythropoiesis increases to replace the destroyed RBCs. The spleen enlarges as it removes damaged or destroyed RBCs. If the breakdown of heme units exceeds the liver's ability to conjugate and excrete bilirubin, jaundice develops. When the condition is severe, bone marrow expands, and bones may be deformed or may develop pathologic fractures. The severity of generalized manifestations of anemia (tachycardia, pallor, etc.) depends on the degree of anemia and deficiency of tissue oxygenation.

Glucose-6-Phosphate Dehydrogenase Anemia. *Glucose-6-phosphate dehydrogenase (G6PD) anemia* is caused by a hereditary defect in RBC metabolism. It is relatively common in people of African and Mediterranean descent. The defective gene is located on the X chromosome and therefore affects more males than females. There are many variations of this genetic defect.

G6PD is an enzyme that catalyzes glycolysis, the process in which an RBC derives cellular energy. A defect in G6PD action causes direct oxidation of hemoglobin, damaging the RBC. Hemolysis usually occurs only when the affected person is exposed to stressors (e.g., drugs such as aspirin, sulfonamides, or vitamin K derivatives) that increase the metabolic demands on RBCs. The G6PD deficiency impairs the necessary compensatory increase in glucose metabolism and causes cellular damage. Damaged RBCs are destroyed over a period of 7 to 12 days.

When exposed to a stressor triggering G6PD anemia, symptoms develop within several days. These may include pallor, jaundice, hemoglobinuria (hemoglobin in the urine), and an elevated reticulocyte count. As new RBCs develop, counts return to normal.

Aplastic Anemia

In **aplastic anemia**, the bone marrow fails to produce all three types of blood cells, leading to *pancytopenia*. Normal bone marrow is replaced by fat. Fortunately, aplastic anemia is rare. *Fanconi anemia* is a rare aplastic anemia caused by defects of DNA repair. The underlying cause of about 50% of acquired aplastic anemia is unknown (*idiopathic aplastic anemia*). Other cases follow stem cell damage caused by exposure to radiation or certain chemical substances such as benzene, arsenic, nitrogen mustard, certain antibiotics (especially chloramphenicol), and chemotherapeutic drugs (Sorenson et al., 2019). Aplastic anemia may also occur with viral infections such as mononucleosis, hepatitis C, and HIV disease.

In aplastic anemia, the number of stem cells in the bone marrow is significantly reduced. The stem cell pool may be less than 1% of normal when the disease is recognized. Anemia develops as the bone marrow fails to replace RBCs that have reached the end of their lifespan. Remaining RBCs may be normochromic and normocytic or may be large with increased mean corpuscular volume.

Manifestations of aplastic anemia vary with the severity of the pancytopenia. Its onset is usually insidious but may also be sudden. Manifestations include fatigue, pallor, progressive weakness, exertional dyspnea, headache, and ultimately tachycardia and heart failure. Platelet deficiency leads to bleeding problems; bleeding gums, excessive bruising, and nosebleeds may be the initial symptoms. A deficiency of WBCs increases the risk of infection, causing manifestations such as sore throat and fever.

Interprofessional Care

Ensuring adequate tissue oxygenation is the priority of care in treating anemia. Specific therapy is determined by the underlying cause of the disorder. Usual treatments include medications, dietary modifications, blood replacement, or supportive interventions. **Table 33.1** outlines interprofessional care measures for selected types of anemia.

Diagnosis

When anemia is suspected, the following laboratory and diagnostic tests may be ordered:

- ***Complete blood count (CBC)*** is done to determine blood cell counts, hemoglobin, hematocrit, and RBC indices (refer to Table 33.1 for care details). The severity of the anemia, shape, volume, and iron content of the RBCs can help determine the cause of anemia.
- ***Iron level*** and ***total iron-binding capacity tests*** are performed to detect iron-deficiency anemia. A low serum iron concentration and elevated total iron-binding capacity are indicative of iron-deficiency anemia.
- ***Serum ferritin*** is low due to depletion of the total iron reserves available for hemoglobin synthesis. Ferritin is an iron-storage protein produced by the liver, spleen, and bone marrow. Ferritin mobilizes stored iron when metabolic needs are higher than dietary intake.
- ***Sickle cell test*** is a screening test to evaluate hemolytic anemia and detect HbS.
- ***Hemoglobin electrophoresis*** separates normal hemoglobin from abnormal forms. It is used to evaluate hemolytic anemia, diagnose thalassemia, and differentiate sickle cell trait from sickle cell disease.
- ***Schilling test*** measures vitamin B_{12} absorption before and after intrinsic factor administration to differentiate between pernicious anemia and intestinal malabsorption of the vitamin. A 24-hour urine sample is collected following administration of radioactive vitamin B_{12}.

Table 33.1 Interprofessional Care Focus for Major Anemias

Type of Anemia	Interprofessional Care
Iron-deficiency anemia	■ Increased dietary intake of iron-rich foods ■ Oral or parenteral iron supplements
Vitamin B_{12}–deficiency anemia	■ Increased dietary intake of foods containing vitamin B_{12} (e.g., meats, eggs, and dairy products) ■ Oral or parenteral vitamin B_{12} supplements ■ Parenteral vitamin B_{12} for deficiency due to malabsorption or lack of intrinsic factor
Folic acid–deficiency anemia	■ Increased dietary intake of foods rich in folic acid (folate) ■ Oral folic acid supplements ■ Folic acid supplements recommended for women who are pregnant or may become pregnant to prevent neural tube defects
Sickle cell disease	■ Treatment is primarily supportive ■ Hydroxyurea 10–30 mg/kg per day ■ Sickle cell crisis: a. Rest b. Oxygen therapy to maintain SaO_2 c. Narcotic analgesia d. Vigorous hydration e. Treatment of precipitating factors ■ Acute chest syndrome: a. Careful hydration; hemodynamic monitoring b. Oxygen therapy c. Transfusion ■ Folic acid supplements ■ Blood transfusions during surgery or pregnancy as necessary ■ Genetic counseling recommended
Thalassemia	■ Regular blood transfusions ■ Folic acid supplements ■ Possible splenectomy ■ Genetic counseling
Aplastic anemia	■ Withdrawal of the causative agent, if known ■ Blood transfusions ■ Bone marrow transplant as indicated

Lower-than-normal levels of the tagged B_{12} when intrinsic factor is given concurrently indicate malabsorption rather than pernicious anemia.

- *Bone marrow examination* is done to diagnose aplastic anemia. In aplastic anemia, normal marrow elements are significantly decreased as they are replaced by fat cells.
- *Quantitative assay of G6PD* may be performed to confirm a diagnosis of G6PD deficiency.

Medications

Medications used to treat anemia depend on its cause. Iron replacement therapy is ordered for iron-deficiency anemia. Supplemental iron may be given by mouth or parenterally. Intravenous administration of iron is becoming more common, particularly in patients with an acute deficiency and in anemia associated with chronic GI blood loss, chronic renal failure, and other chronic conditions that increase the need for blood cell production (e.g., cancers). The risk of anaphylaxis is a major concern when iron dextran is given intravenously. Other parenteral iron solutions, including intravenous sodium ferric gluconate (Ferrlecit) and iron sucrose (Venofer), carry a much lower risk of adverse and allergic reactions.

Parenteral vitamin B_{12} is given when malabsorption or lack of intrinsic factor leads to vitamin B_{12}–deficiency anemia. Folic acid is ordered for women of childbearing age, pregnant women, and patients with folic acid deficiency or sickle cell disease to meet the increased demands of the bone marrow. Hydroxyurea, a drug that promotes fetal hemoglobin production, may be prescribed for patients with sickle cell disease, particularly those with frequent crises or severe disease. Resulting increased levels of fetal hemoglobin interfere with the sickling process and reduce the incidence of painful crises. Nursing implications for patients receiving iron, vitamin B_{12}, and folic acid are found in **Medication Administration 33.A**.

Erythropoietin may be ordered for patients with low erythropoietin levels (e.g., patients with chronic renal failure) and people with anemia associated with other chronic diseases. Erythropoietin is given subcutaneously and may be given as often as three times a week in chronic renal failure. Because erythropoietin stimulates RBC production, adequate iron must be present. Patients receiving erythropoietin may require regular intravenous iron therapy as well (Adams, Holland, & Urban, 2018; Shields, Fox, & Liebrecht, 2018).

Immunosuppressive therapy with antithymocyte globulin (ATG), corticosteroids, and cyclosporine may be used to treat aplastic anemia. Androgens may stimulate blood cell production in some patients with aplastic anemia. See Chapter 12 for more information about immunosuppression.

Medication Administration 33.A

Drugs to Treat Anemia

IRON SOURCES

ferrous sulfate (Feosol, Fer-in-sol)

ferrous gluconate (Fergon, Ferralet, Fertinic)

iron dextran injection (Imferon)

iron polysaccharide

iron sucrose (Venofer)

sodium ferric gluconate (Ferrlecit)

Iron preparations are normally taken by mouth and are absorbed from the GI tract. They are given to treat anemias resulting from iron deficiency or blood loss. When absorbed, iron combines with transferrin. This complex is then transported to the bone marrow and incorporated into hemoglobin.

Nursing Responsibilities

- Prior to giving the drug, assess for use of drugs that might interact with iron (e.g., antacids, allopurinol, chloramphenicol, tetracyclines, vitamin E), GI bleeding, and manifestations of anemia.
- Administer iron preparations with orange juice to enhance absorption.
- If using an elixir, give it through a straw to prevent staining the teeth.
- Monitor for manifestations of iron toxicity: Nausea, diarrhea, or constipation; symptoms of anaphylactic shock (extreme cases).
- Monitor hemoglobin and reticulocyte counts.
- If the patient is also taking tetracyclines, schedule the dose of iron 2 hours before tetracycline (iron reduces the absorption of tetracycline).
- When administering IM or IV, monitor closely for anaphylaxis.

Health Education for the Patient and Family

- GI side effects may be reduced by taking iron with food (but not milk, which decreases absorption).
- Stools may be dark green or black; this is harmless.
- Increase fluids and fiber in diet to decrease constipation.

VITAMIN B_{12} SOURCES

cyanocobalamin (Kaybovite [oral], Anacobin [parenteral], Bedoz)

Cyanocobalamin is used to treat vitamin B_{12} deficiencies or malabsorption and pernicious anemia. It is rapidly absorbed when administered orally or by injection, and it is stored in the liver. Intrinsic factor is necessary for absorption from the GI tract.

Nursing Responsibilities

- Do not expose crystalline injection to light.
- Assess for other drugs that might interfere with the therapeutic response; chloramphenicol, cimetidine, colchicine, and timed-release potassium decrease its effectiveness.
- Do not mix cyanocobalamin in a syringe with other medications.
- Administer parenteral doses intramuscularly or deep subcutaneously to decrease local irritation.
- Monitor hemoglobin, RBC counts, reticulocyte counts, and potassium levels.

Health Education for the Patient and Family

- A burning sensation with injection is temporary.
- Avoid alcohol, which interferes with absorption.
- If used to treat pernicious anemia, the medication must be taken for life.

FOLIC ACID SOURCES

folic acid (Folvite, Novo-Folacid)

Synthetic folic acid is used to treat folic acid deficiency and megaloblastic or macrocytic anemia. It is absorbed from the GI tract and stored in the liver.

Nursing Responsibilities

- Prior to giving the medication, assess for use of drugs that alter its effect: Corticosteroids, methotrexate, oral contraceptives, phenytoin, sulfonamides.
- Do not mix folic acid with other medications in the same syringe.
- Monitor for possible hypersensitivity response of skin rash.

Health Education for the Patient and Family

- Large doses of folic acid may cause the urine to become darker yellow.
- Excess alcohol intake increases folic acid requirements.

Note: Medications identified in blue are among the 200 most frequently prescribed drugs in the United States.

Source: Adams, Holland, & Urban, 2017.

Nutrition

Dietary modifications are recommended for nutritional-deficiency anemias, such as iron-deficiency anemia, vitamin B_{12}–deficiency anemia, or folic acid–deficiency anemia. **Box 33.5** identifies good sources of dietary iron, folic acid, and vitamin B_{12}.

Blood Transfusion

Blood transfusions may be indicated to treat anemias resulting from major blood loss, such as from trauma or major surgery, and severe anemia regardless of cause. In acute hemorrhage, whole blood may be given to replace both blood cells and volume. A unit of packed RBCs may be given when anemia is severe and the patient demonstrates cardiovascular instability or compromise. Blood transfusions are discussed in-depth in Chapter 11.

Integrative Therapies

Complementary healthcare practitioners may recommend specific plant enzymes to treat nutritional anemias. Plant enzymes are believed to aid digestion of proteins, fats, and carbohydrates, facilitating absorption of their nutrients. Therapy is determined by the specific type of anemia. Plant enzymes should not be used alone to treat anemia, and it is important to check for possible interactions with prescribed medications before starting therapy.

BOX 33.5
Dietary Sources of Iron, Folic Acid, and Vitamin B_{12}

SOURCES OF IRON

Iron in the diet comes from two sources. *Heme iron* makes up about one-half of the iron from animal sources. *Nonheme iron* includes the remaining iron from animal sources and all the iron from plants, legumes, and nuts. Heme iron promotes absorption of nonheme iron from other foods when both forms are consumed at the same time. Absorption of nonheme iron is also enhanced by vitamin C and inhibited by tea and coffee.

Heme Iron

- Beef
- Chicken
- Egg yolk
- Clams, oysters
- Pork loin
- Turkey
- Veal

Nonheme Iron

- Bran flakes
- Brown rice
- Whole-grain breads
- Dried beans
- Dried fruits
- Leafy greens
- Oatmeal

SOURCES OF FOLIC ACID

- Green leafy vegetables
- Broccoli
- Organ meats
- Eggs
- Wheat germ
- Asparagus
- Liver
- Milk
- Yeast
- Kidney beans

SOURCES OF VITAMIN B_{12}

- Liver
- Fresh shrimp and oysters
- Eggs
- Milk
- Kidney
- Meats (muscle)
- Cheese

Nursing Care

For nursing care specific to the patient with a nutritional anemia, see the accompanying Case Study & Nursing Care Plan.

Assessment

See the Manifestations and Interprofessional Care sections for the assessment of the patient with anemia.

Assessment data to collect for patients with suspected anemia includes:

- ***Health history:*** Complaints of shortness of breath with activity, fatigue, weakness, dizziness or fainting, palpitations; history of previous anemia, bleeding episodes; menstrual history (if appropriate); medications; chronic diseases; usual diet and patterns of alcohol intake or cigarette smoking
- ***Physical assessment:*** General appearance, skin color; vital signs including temperature; heart and lung sounds; peripheral pulses, capillary refill; abdominal tenderness; obvious bleeding or bruising
- ***Laboratory data:*** CBC, hemoglobin and hematocrit; bone marrow studies; specialized tests (e.g., hemoglobin electrophoresis, Schilling test) (Kee, 2018).

Priorities of Care

Collaborating with the interprofessional team to ensure adequate treatment of the underlying process while providing care that supports the physical and psychologic responses to the disorder is a priority of nursing care.

Diagnoses, Outcomes, and Interventions

Anemia affects circulating oxygen levels and tissue oxygenation. Priority nursing care will be directed toward promoting activity, managing oral mucous membrane health, and helping patients to manage their activities of daily living (ADLs). With acute blood-loss anemia, reducing risk for insufficient cardiac output is also a priority. Patients with sickle cell disease have specific needs related to the effects of the disease on tissue perfusion; see the section on disseminated intravascular coagulation later in this chapter for nursing interventions appropriate to ineffective tissue perfusion, associated pain, and maintaining oxygenation.

Promote Activity Tolerance. Anemia causes weakness and shortness of breath on exertion. These symptoms are due to decreased circulating oxygen levels secondary to low hemoglobin levels. Weakness, fatigue, and/or vertigo may occur even during ADLs, including those associated with self-care, home life, job performance, and social roles.

Expected Outcome: Patient will participate in activity program without suffering any complications.

The nurse will:

- Help identify ways to conserve energy when performing necessary or desired activities. *Modifying the approach to a particular activity may reduce cardiorespiratory symptoms and activity-related fatigue. Alternative ways of performing tasks (e.g., sitting when performing hygiene care and kitchen tasks) may reduce oxygen demands. In some cases, assistance from others is necessary to conserve energy and reduce symptoms.*

- Help the patient and family establish priorities for tasks and activities. *Because family members may need to assume responsibility for additional tasks, the plan's success depends on mutually established goals.*
- Assist patient to develop a schedule of alternating activity and rest periods throughout the day. *Rest periods decrease oxygen needs, reducing strain on the heart and lungs and allowing restoration of homeostasis before further activities.*
- Encourage 8 to 10 hours of sleep at night. *Rest decreases oxygen demands and increases available energy for morning activities.*
- Monitor vital signs before and after activity. *Vital signs provide a measure of activity tolerance. Increased heart and respiratory rates or a change in blood pressure may indicate intolerance of the activity.*
- Discontinue activity if any of the following occurs:
  a. Complaints of chest pain, breathlessness, or vertigo
  b. Palpitations or tachycardia that does not return to normal within 4 minutes of resting
  c. Bradycardia
  d. Tachypnea or dyspnea
  e. Decreased systolic blood pressure.

  These changes may signify cardiac decompensation due to insufficient oxygenation. The intensity, duration, or frequency of the activity needs to be reduced.
- Instruct the patient not to smoke. *Smoking causes vasoconstriction and increases carbon monoxide levels in the blood, interfering with tissue oxygenation.*

Promote Oral Membrane Health. Glossitis and cheilosis may occur with nutritional deficiencies of iron, folate, and vitamin B_{12}. The tongue and lips become very red, and fissures or cracks may form at the corners of the mouth.

Expected Outcome: Patient will maintain intact, moist oral mucous membranes through use of measures to promote oral membrane health.

The nurse will:

- Monitor condition of lips and tongue daily. *Glossitis and cheilosis increase the risk for bleeding and infection and may require medical treatment. Pain and discomfort may interfere with oral intake, further worsening the nutritional deficiency.*
- Use a mouthwash of saline, saltwater, or half-strength peroxide and water to rinse the mouth every 2 to 4 hours. Avoid alcohol-based mouthwashes. *This cleanses and soothes oral mucous membranes. Alcohol-based mouthwashes further irritate and dry oral tissues.*
- Provide frequent oral hygiene (after each meal and at bedtime) with a soft-bristle toothbrush or sponge. *Removing food debris from painful fissures promotes comfort. A soft-bristle toothbrush reduces irritation or bleeding of oral mucosa. Keeping the oral cavity clean also reduces the risk of infection.*
- Apply a petroleum-based lubricating jelly or ointment to the lips after oral care. *Lubricating ointment helps to retain moisture, facilitate healing, and protect the lips from other drying agents.*
- Instruct patient to avoid hot, spicy, or acidic foods. *Such foods may further irritate and dry mucous membranes.*
- Encourage soft, cool, bland foods. *Foods that are soothing to the mucous membranes promote comfort and help maintain adequate food and fluid intake. Minimizing oral pain may also promote compliance with oral care routines.*
- Encourage eating four to six small meals daily with high protein and vitamin content. *Small, frequent meals may be better tolerated, increasing intake. Nutrient-rich meals promote healing of the mucous membranes.*

Reduce Risk for Decreased Cardiac Output. Cardiac output may be affected by acute bleeding and volume loss or by heart failure resulting from severe anemia. In addition, impaired tissue oxygenation leads to an increased respiratory rate and dyspnea.

Expected Outcome: Patient will demonstrate adequate cardiac output as evidenced by blood pressure and pulse rate being within normal parameters.

The nurse will:

- Monitor vital signs, breath sounds, and apical pulse. *Increased cardiac workload can affect the blood pressure, heart, and respiratory rates. Increased blood flow can lead to heart murmur or abnormal heart sounds such as S_3 or S_4. Tachypnea and dyspnea may affect the depth of respirations, alveolar ventilation, and blood and tissue oxygenation.*
- Assess for pallor, cyanosis, and dependent edema. *Blood is shunted to the vital organs, causing vasoconstriction of skin vessels. This, in addition to lower levels of hemoglobin, causes pallor. Cyanosis, especially of the lips and nail beds, indicates inadequate oxygenation of blood. Dependent edema occurs in response to right-ventricular failure.*

SAFETY ALERT: Report signs of decreased cardiac output to the healthcare provider. Severe anemia can lead to heart failure, necessitating additional treatment. ■

- Closely monitor for manifestations of anaphylaxis (urticaria, erythema or flushing, edema, wheezing, dyspnea, nausea and vomiting, anxiety) when administering parenteral iron preparations, particularly iron dextran. Immediately notify the healthcare provider, and prepare to administer prescribed drugs such as diphenhydramine (Benadryl) or epinephrine as ordered. Institute cardiopulmonary resuscitation measures as necessary. *Anaphylaxis, a systemic type I hypersensitivity (allergic) reaction, is a risk when administering parenteral iron preparations, iron dextran in particular. Anaphylaxis can lead to severe cardiopulmonary compromise, necessitating emergency measures to preserve life.*

Manage ADLs. Energy expenditures for ADLs may cause oxygen demands to exceed supply in the patient with severe anemia.

Expected Outcome: Patient will perform self-care activities to optimal potential.

The nurse will:

- Assist with ADLs, such as bathing, grooming, and eating, as needed. *Assistance decreases energy expenditures and tissue requirements for oxygen, reducing cardiac workload.*
- Discuss the importance of rest periods prior to such activities as dressing. *Rest reduces oxygen demand and cardiac workload. The person who is able to perform self-care in ADLs maintains independence, self-esteem, and morale.*

Transitions of Care

Nursing measures to prevent anemia focus on teaching good dietary habits to all patients, regardless of age. Stress the importance of consuming adequate amounts of iron, folate, and the B vitamins. Provide a list of dietary sources of these nutrients. Discuss alternate iron sources with vegetarian patients, and teach them that foods high in vitamin C enhance the absorption of iron from grains, legumes, and other sources. Emphasize the importance of adequate iron intake in women of childbearing age and older adults. Stress the increased need for these nutrients during pregnancy, and discuss strategies to ensure an adequate intake.

Nursing care of acute anemia focuses on treating and managing acute hemorrhage. The underlying cause of hemorrhage must be reversed or controlled. Blood replacement is commonly indicated.

With the exception of anemia resulting from acute hemorrhage, most patients with anemia are treated in the home and community setting. Include the following topics when preparing the patient and family for home care:

- Nutritional strategies to address deficiencies
- Prescribed medications, vitamins, or mineral supplements and their appropriate use, intended effect, possible adverse effects, and interactions with food or other medications
- Energy conservation strategies
- Other recommended treatment measures and follow-up
- If the anemia is genetically transmitted, such as sickle cell disease, include inheritance patterns of the disorder, symptoms of crisis, and manifestations to report to the healthcare provider.

Provide referrals for counseling to facilitate decisions about pregnancy as indicated. Also refer for nutritional assistance and teaching, home healthcare, or assistance with self-care and home maintenance activities as indicated. Older adults with nutritional anemias may benefit from community services such as senior meals or Meals on Wheels.

Anemia at the end of life is commonly secondary to another diagnosis such as cancer. Treatment to correct anemia is known to improve quality of life and reduce symptoms of fatigue and dyspnea.

Case Study & Nursing Care Plan

A Patient with Folic Acid–Deficiency Anemia

Sheri Matthews is a 76-year-old widow who lives alone. She tells Lisa Apana, RN, the nurse in her care provider's office, that she liked to cook when her husband was alive, but preparing an entire meal just for herself seems senseless. She relates that her typical day's menu includes coffee for breakfast; a bologna sandwich and coffee for lunch; and a hot dog or two, a few cookies, and a glass of milk for dinner.

ASSESSMENT	DIAGNOSES	EXPECTED OUTCOMES
Mrs. Matthews's nursing history includes a 9-kg (20-lb) weight loss since her husband died 8 months ago. She states that she sometimes has heart palpitations and always feels weak. Physical assessment: T 37.1°C (98.8°F), P 110 bpm, R 22/min, and BP 90/52 mmHg. Skin is warm, pale, and dry. Diagnostic tests indicate folic acid–deficiency anemia, and Mrs. Matthews is started on an oral folic acid supplement and instructed about foods containing folic acid.	■ Inability to tolerate activity related to weakness secondary to decreased tissue oxygenation ■ Decrease in nutrition related to lack of motivation to cook and understanding of nutritional needs, as manifested by weight loss of 9 kg and folic acid deficiency ■ Insufficient knowledge of information about a well-balanced diet and foods containing folic acid	■ Patient will verbalize the importance of taking folic acid supplements and eating a balanced diet. ■ Patient will gain at least 0.45 kg (1 lb) per week. ■ Patient will return to previous level of physical energy. ■ Patient will consume a balanced diet, including foods containing folic acid.

PLANNING AND IMPLEMENTATION

- Discuss foods required for a well-balanced diet, as well as dietary sources of folic acid.
- Develop a dietary plan with Mrs. Matthews that includes food preferences and foods that are easy and quick to prepare.
- Discuss the importance of taking the folic acid supplement. Advise to continue taking it even after she begins to feel better.
- Help Mrs. Matthews develop a schedule of activities that provides adequate rest and energy for cooking.

EVALUATION

Mrs. Matthews gained 0.45 kg (1 lb) during the first week of treatment. She has met with a nutritionist and has a better understanding of nutritional needs. She states that she can prepare hot meals when she schedules a rest period before and after lunch. Ms. Apana has provided written and verbal information about the folic acid supplement and diet. Mrs. Matthews verbalizes understanding, stating, "I will continue to take the folic acid until the doctor tells me to stop. I'm beginning to enjoy cooking again, now that I have a reason to cook!" Ms. Apana contacts the local senior services representative to determine if Mrs. Matthews is able to participate in the local Meals on Wheels program.

CLINICAL REASONING IN PATIENT CARE

1. What is the pathophysiologic basis for Mrs. Matthews's abnormal vital signs during her initial assessment?
2. Design a week's menu that includes foods high in folic acid.
3. Why was Mrs. Matthews placed on a folic acid supplement in addition to dietary modifications?
4. Why is the older adult at increased risk for developing folic acid–deficiency anemia? Consider physiologic, economic, and social factors.

See Evaluating Your Response in Appendix B.

The Patient with Myelodysplastic Syndrome

Myelodysplastic syndrome (MDS) is a group of blood disorders characterized by abnormal-appearing bone marrow and cytopenia (low numbers of circulating blood cells). MDS is not a single disease; at least five variations of the disorder have been identified. Anemia that does not respond to treatment (*refractory anemia*) is a characteristic of most forms of myelodysplasia.

Idiopathic MDS accounts for 70 to 80% of all cases. It primarily affects older adults; men have a slightly higher incidence of the disorder than women. Risk factors for secondary MDS include exposure to environmental toxins such as cigarette smoke, benzene and radiation, radiation therapy or chemotherapy for cancer treatment, and other anemias such as aplastic anemia or Fanconi anemia (American Cancer Society [ACS], 2018c).

Pathophysiology

MDS is a stem cell disorder in which stem cells fail to reproduce and differentiate into the various types of blood cells. The genetic components of stem cells (nuclear DNA and/or mitochondrial DNA) are altered. The bone marrow loses its ability to produce normal blood cells, instead producing abnormal (*dysplastic*) cells. With significant alterations, leukemia (proliferation of abnormal WBCs) may develop in people with MDS.

Manifestations

Anemia is the predominant early manifestation of MDS. The patient may develop symptoms of the anemia with increasing fatigue, weakness, dyspnea, and pallor. In many cases, the disorder is asymptomatic, identified when a routine blood count shows anemia. Splenomegaly may develop, leading to discomfort and a feeling of fullness in the left upper quadrant of the abdomen. Hepatomegaly may also develop, leading to right upper quadrant discomfort. Thrombocytopenia can lead to abnormal bleeding tendencies, and neutropenia increases the risk for infection (ACS, 2018c).

Interprofessional Care

Patients with MDS require long-term supportive care and therapy to maintain their quality of life. Stem cell transplant offers the only real hope for cure of MDS. See the Leukemia section later in this chapter for more information about stem cell transplant and associated nursing care.

Diagnosis

- **The** ***CBC*** reveals anemia. Although anemia may be the only abnormality of the blood count, the WBC count and the platelet count may also be low. Abnormalities of size and shape may be noted in all blood cells.
- ***Bone marrow*** often appears normal, although precursor cells may have an abnormal appearance. Increased numbers of myeloblasts (granulocyte precursor cells) may be present in the bone marrow.
- ***Serum erythropoietin, vitamin B12, serum iron, total iron-binding capacity, ferritin levels,*** and ***RBC folate levels*** are drawn to help guide supportive therapy.

Treatment

Management of MDS is based on the severity of the disease. Several classification systems are available, including the French-American-British (FAB) classification system, the International Prognostic Scoring System (IPSS), and the World Health Organization (WHO) classification system (ACS, 2018c). These systems are used to guide therapy for the patient with MDS.

All patients with MDS require monitoring, with regular healthcare provider visits and laboratory evaluations. Psychosocial support is provided to assist the patient and family dealing with a chronic, progressive, and ultimately fatal disease.

Patients with MDS may require frequent RBC transfusions to treat the predominant anemia. Each unit of packed

RBCs contains 250 to 300 mg of iron. The body is unable to excrete this excess iron, so it accumulates, leading to problems such as endocrine dysfunction, cirrhosis, pericarditis, and heart failure. *Iron chelation therapy* is used to remove excess iron from the body. Deferoxamine (Desferal) is administered by slow intravenous infusion or continuous subcutaneous infusion using an infusion pump to maintain a normal or negative iron balance. This drug is relatively safe, although local skin reactions such as rash and urticaria may develop. An oral form of the drug, deferasirox, is available, but not widely used.

Blood cell growth factors may be administered to stimulate stem cell development in MDS, although the response rate is low. Platelet transfusions are given when bleeding occurs due to low platelet levels. Antibiotic therapy is initiated for bacterial infections (ACS, 2018c). Chemotherapy regimens similar to those employed to treat leukemia may be used, but rarely are effective in treating MDS. Azacitidine (Vidaza), an antileukemic agent that acts on abnormal blood-forming cells in the bone marrow, may be more effective in treating MDS than standard chemotherapy regimens. As previously noted, stem cell transplant offers the only hope for cure. This high-risk therapy, however, is reserved for higher-risk patients. Factors such as age, functional ability, and other existing disease conditions help guide the decision to undergo stem cell transplant (ACS, 2018c).

Nursing Care

See the Manifestations and Interprofessional Care sections for the assessment of the patient with myelodysplastic syndrome.

Priorities of Care

Collaborating with the interprofessional team to ensure adequate treatment of the underlying process while providing care that supports the physical and psychologic responses to the disorder is a priority of nursing care.

Diagnoses, Outcomes, and Interventions

The inability to tolerate activity and the need for education about this disorder are the priorities of nursing care for the patient with MDS being managed in a community-based setting. Although neutropenia and thrombocytopenia may accompany the anemia of MDS, these problems are less common. See the section of this chapter on leukemia for additional potential nursing diagnoses and interventions for the patient with MDS.

Promote Activity Tolerance. The patient with MDS experiences fatigue, weakness, and shortness of breath on exertion related to the lack of RBCs and ineffective oxygen transport. These symptoms may affect the patient's ability to maintain self-care, home life, job performance, and social roles.

Expected Outcome: Patient will participate in activity program without suffering any complications.

The nurse will:

- Monitor vital signs, breath sounds, and apical pulse. *Increased cardiac workload due to anemia and impaired oxygen transport can affect the blood pressure, heart, and respiratory rates. Increased blood flow can lead to heart murmur or abnormal heart sounds such as S_3 or S_4. Accumulated iron can lead to pericarditis and a pericardial friction rub.*
- Help identify energy-conserving ways of performing necessary or desired activities. *Alternative ways of performing tasks (e.g., sitting while performing hygiene measures) may reduce oxygen demands and fatigue.*
- Help the patient and family establish priorities for tasks and activities. *Because family members may need to assume responsibility for additional tasks, the plan's success depends on mutually established goals.*
- Suggest planning recreational activities following a transfusion and adjusting activity level between transfusions to match energy and minimize fatigue. *The patient with MDS will have more energy and activity tolerance following a transfusion when RBC counts, hemoglobin, and hematocrit approach normal levels and oxygen transport is optimal.*
- Encourage 8 to 10 hours of sleep at night. *Rest decreases oxygen demands and increases available energy for morning activities.*
- Discontinue activity if any of the following occurs:
  a. Complaints of chest pain, breathlessness, or vertigo
  b. Palpitations or tachycardia that does not return to normal within 4 minutes of resting
  c. Bradycardia
  d. Tachypnea or dyspnea
  e. Decreased systolic blood pressure.

  These changes may signify cardiac decompensation due to insufficient oxygenation. The intensity, duration, or frequency of the activity needs to be reduced.
- Instruct the patient not to smoke. *Smoking causes vasoconstriction and increases carbon monoxide levels in the blood, interfering with tissue oxygenation.*

Teach Health Maintenance. MDS is a chronic, usually progressive disorder, requiring active management to maintain functional status and quality of life. Regular visits to the healthcare provider or clinic may be necessary. In addition, the patient or family members may need to learn to administer iron chelation therapy or chemotherapy drugs and measures to prevent complications (ACS, 2018c). The chronic nature of the disorder and the often advanced age of the patient and family caregivers may interfere with effective management of the disorder.

Expected Outcome: Patient will be knowledgeable about management of MDS as evidenced by being able to describe the components and rationale for the treatment plan.

The nurse will:

- Assess knowledge of disorder and the related treatments. *Assessment allows identification of knowledge gaps and provides a basis on which to provide additional information. Impaired disease management may be due to lack of knowledge or an inability to learn and perform psychomotor skills, for example, administration of parenteral drug therapy.*

- Provide information about the disorder, its effects, and prescribed medications and treatments. *Individualized instruction is more effective than general, possibly irrelevant information. The patient and caregivers need to be able to identify and manage possible adverse effects of drug therapy and to recognize potential complications to be reported to the healthcare provider.*
- Provide emotional support, expressing confidence in the patient's and caregivers' abilities to manage care. *Emotional support helps the patient and family caregivers incorporate the care regimen into their lifestyle.*
- Provide supervised learning and practice opportunities for administering parenteral medications, if ordered. *Successful practice sessions instill confidence in the ability to manage care and provide an opportunity for questions and exploring alternatives.*

Transitions of Care

There are no actions that can completely prevent MDS. As MDS is related to leukemia, smoking cessation may help to reduce the risk of leukemia and MDS. Chemotherapy and radiation therapy for cancer may play a role in MDS development, and research is ongoing to develop agents that reduce the risk for MDS development. Most patients diagnosed with MDS have no known preventable exposure to occupational and environmental radiation and chemicals.

Acute nursing care for MDS focuses on symptom management and reversal of blood cell loss. The use of growth factors can help return blood counts to more normal levels. Growth factors can focus on white blood cell production. Shortages of blood cells cause most of the symptoms in people with myelodysplastic syndromes, and growth factors can help the white blood cell counts to become more normal. Careful nursing care to avoid infections is imperative. The patient with myelodysplastic syndrome needs information about this chronic and ultimately fatal disease. Provide information about treatment options, including management of the infusion pump, if ordered. Discuss the timing of and options for stem cell transplant, and assist the patient to evaluate the potential benefits and risks of this treatment option.

End-of-life care for a patient with MDS focuses on symptom management, infection control, and comfort measures. As survival prognosis falls with increasing risk group assignment, MDS can be a fatal diagnosis. Prognosis based on the international risk groups ranges from 5 months to 12 years.

The Patient with Polycythemia

Polycythemia, or *erythrocytosis*, is an excess of RBCs characterized by a hematocrit higher than 55%. The two major types of polycythemia are primary and secondary. Primary polycythemia, where RBC production is increased, is uncommon. It mostly affects men of European Jewish ancestry between the ages of 40 and 70. Secondary polycythemia is the more common form, occurring when erythropoietin levels are elevated. It usually develops in response to chronic hypoxia such as in those who live at high altitude, smoke, or have chronic lung disease. A third type of polycythemia, relative polycythemia, results from a fluid volume deficit, not excess RBCs. It is corrected with rehydration.

Pathophysiology

Primary Polycythemia

Primary polycythemia, or *polycythemia vera (PV)*, is a neoplastic stem cell disorder characterized by overproduction of RBCs and, to a lesser extent, WBCs and platelets. It is classified as a myeloproliferative disorder. Its cause is unknown. In PV, colonies of endogenous erythroid stem cells develop. These colonies produce RBCs in the absence of erythropoietin, leading to excess RBC production.

Secondary Polycythemia

Secondary polycythemia, or *erythrocytosis*, is increased numbers of RBCs in response to excess erythropoietin secretion or prolonged hypoxia. Secondary polycythemia is the most common form of polycythemia.

Abnormally high erythropoietin levels can result from kidney disease or erythropoietin-secreting tumors (e.g., renal cell carcinoma). Chronic hypoxia that stimulates erythropoietin release is a more common cause of secondary polycythemia. People living at high altitudes, where the atmospheric oxygen pressure is lower, develop a degree of polycythemia, as do people with chronic heart or lung disease and smokers. Abnormal hemoglobin that forms tighter bonds with oxygen may also lead to secondary polycythemia.

Manifestations

Initially, PV is asymptomatic, and the diagnosis may be made during routine blood tests. Its manifestations are caused by increased blood volume and viscosity. Hypertension is common and may lead to complaints of headaches, dizziness, and vision and hearing disruptions. Venous stasis causes *plethora*, a ruddy, red color of the face, hands, feet, and mucous membranes. This is often accompanied by severe, painful itching of the fingers and toes. Retinal and cerebral vessels may be engorged. Hypermetabolism develops, causing weight loss and night sweats. Mental status may be altered, leading to drowsiness or delirium.

Thrombosis and hemorrhage are potential complications of PV. Thrombosis may cause transient ischemic attacks, angina, or manifestations of peripheral vascular disease. GI bleeding may occur, and portal hypertension may develop.

The manifestations of secondary polycythemia are similar to those of primary polycythemia. Splenomegaly, however, does not develop. Early symptoms are often overshadowed by the manifestations of the underlying disorder. Manifestations of polycythemia include:

- Hypertension
- Headache, tinnitus, blurred vision

- Plethora: Dark redness of the lips, feet, ears, fingernails, and mucous membranes
- Splenomegaly (polycythemia vera)
- Severe pruritus, extremity pain
- Weight loss, night sweats
- GI bleeding
- Intermittent claudication
- Symptoms from thrombosis within various organs.

Interprofessional Care

Diagnosis

In PV, serum erythropoietin levels are low. Bone marrow studies show hyperplasia of all hematopoietic elements. With secondary polycythemia, serum erythropoietin levels are usually high, and bone marrow studies show only red stem cell hyperplasia.

Treatments

For secondary polycythemia, treatment focuses on the underlying cause of the disorder. It is a physiologic response in people living at high altitudes, and unless the hematocrit is too high or oxygen saturation levels are low, no treatment is usually necessary. Smokers are urged to quit. Measures to raise oxygen saturation levels and reduce tissue hypoxia will often relieve the polycythemia. Patients with both primary and secondary polycythemia benefit from periodic phlebotomy (removing 300 to 500 mL of blood) to keep blood volume and viscosity within normal levels. For PV, chemotherapeutic agents such as hydroxyurea may be used to suppress marrow function but may increase the risk of developing leukemia (discussed later in this chapter). Pruritus may be relieved by antihistamines or may require more aggressive treatment with interferon-α or other treatments. One 325-mg aspirin tablet daily may be ordered to control thrombosis without increasing the risk of bleeding.

Nursing Care

Preventing polycythemia begins with educating children and adults about the dangers of smoking. Measures to reduce risk factors for cardiovascular disease may be beneficial.

This chronic condition is managed in community-based settings unless a complication develops. Teach the patient and family the importance of maintaining adequate hydration, increasing fluid intake during hot weather and when exercising. Discuss measures to prevent blood stasis: Elevating legs and feet when sitting, using support stockings, and continuing treatment measures. Instruct to report manifestations of thrombosis (leg or calf pain, chest pain, neurologic symptoms) or bleeding (black, tarry stools; vomiting blood or coffee-grounds emesis) immediately. Monitor the hematocrit and cell counts throughout treatment.

Clinical issues seen in patients with polycythemia include:

- Ambivalence regarding smoking cessation
- Discomfort related to effects of altered blood flow in distal extremities
- Potential poor tissue perfusion related to sluggish blood flow and increased risk for thrombosis.

33.2 White Blood Cell Disorders

Disorders of the white blood cells (WBCs) include the leukemias, malignant lymphomas (Hodgkin disease and non-Hodgkin lymphoma), multiple myeloma, neutropenia, and infectious mononucleosis. Review the physiology of WBCs and their function in Chapter 12.

The Patient with Leukemia

Leukemia (literally, "white blood") is a group of chronic malignant disorders of WBCs and WBC precursors. In leukemia, the usual ratio of red to white blood cells is reversed. Leukemias are characterized by replacement of bone marrow by malignant immature WBCs, abnormal immature circulating WBCs, and infiltration of these cells into the liver, spleen, and lymph nodes throughout the body.

Physiology Review

WBCs are the most diverse of the cellular components of the blood. They arise from three different precursor cells: Myeloblasts, which further differentiate into the granular leukocytes (granulocytes), neutrophils, eosinophils, and basophils; monoblasts, which mature into circulating monocytes, and ultimately into macrophages; and lymphoblasts, which become lymphocytes and mature in lymphoid tissue to B cells and T cells.

As a whole, the primary function of WBCs is to help maintain the body's immune defenses. Neutrophils, the most numerous WBCs in circulation, are active phagocytes, the first cells to arrive at injured tissue. Monocytes and macrophages are also phagocytic cells that dispose of foreign and waste material from tissues. Eosinophils and basophils are more specialized. Eosinophils are primarily involved in allergic responses and parasitic infections. Basophils are actively involved in the inflammatory response, releasing substances such as histamine and heparin into inflamed tissues. Lymphocytes, the smallest of the WBCs, are an integral part of the immune system. B cells are part of the humoral immune response, producing antibodies to specific antigens. T cells are part of the cell-mediated immune response. For more information about the inflammatory and immune responses, refer to Chapter 13. The normal WBC count and differential are presented in **Table 33.2**.

Pathophysiology

Leukemia begins with malignant transformation of a single stem cell. Leukemic cells proliferate slowly, but do not differentiate normally. They have a prolonged lifespan and accumulate in the bone marrow. As they accumulate, they compete with the proliferation of normal cells. Leukemic cells do not function as mature WBCs and are ineffective in the inflammatory and immune processes. Leukemic

Table 33.2 Normal White Blood Cell Count and Differential

Laboratory Test	Value
WBC count	5000–10,000/mm^3
Differential WBC count	
Neutrophils	60–70% or 3000–7000/mm^3
Eosinophils	1–3% or 50–400/mm^3
Basophils	0.3–0.5% or 25–200/mm^3
Lymphocytes	20–30% or 1000–4000/mm^3
Monocytes	3–8% or 100–600/mm^3

cells replace normal hematopoietic elements in the marrow. Because erythrocyte- and platelet-producing cells are crowded out, severe anemia, splenomegaly, and bleeding difficulties result.

Leukemic cells leave the bone marrow and travel through the circulatory system, infiltrating other body tissues such as the CNS, testes, skin, GI tract, and the lymph nodes, liver, and spleen. Death is usually due to internal hemorrhage and infections.

Incidence and Risk Factors

Although leukemia is often thought of as a childhood disease, it is diagnosed 10 times more often in adults than in children. Slightly more than half of diagnosed cases are acute leukemia and less than half are chronic leukemia. In 2017, the American Cancer Society (2017) estimated that 62,130 people were diagnosed with leukemia and 24,500 people died of leukemia.

Although the cause of most leukemias is unknown, certain risk factors have been identified. Men are affected more frequently than are women. People with certain genetic disorders such as Down syndrome have a higher incidence of leukemia. Environmental risk factors play a role as well. Risk factors for myeloid leukemia include cigarette smoking and exposure to chemicals such as benzene (present in cigarette smoke and gasoline). Exposure to ionizing radiation increases the risk for several types of leukemia. Patients who have undergone treatment for cancer have an increased risk. The human T-cell leukemia/lymphoma virus-1, a retrovirus, is known to cause certain leukemias and lymphomas (ACS, 2018a).

Manifestations

The general manifestations of leukemia (regardless of type) result from anemia, infection, and bleeding. These include pallor, fatigue, tachycardia, malaise, lethargy, and dyspnea on exertion. Infection may cause fever, night sweats, oral ulcerations, and frequent or recurrent respiratory, urinary, integumentary, or other infections. Increased bleeding due to thrombocytopenia leads to bruising, petechiae, bleeding gums, and bleeding within specific organs and tissues. See the Multisystem Effects of Leukemia box.

Other manifestations result from leukemic cell infiltration, increased metabolism, and increased leukocyte destruction. Infiltration of the liver, spleen, lymph nodes, and bone marrow causes pain and tissue swelling in the involved areas. Meningeal infiltration may cause manifestations of increased intracranial pressure, such as headache, altered level of consciousness, cranial nerve impairment, and nausea and vomiting. Infiltration of the kidneys may affect renal function, with decreased urine output and increased blood urea nitrogen and creatinine. Increased metabolism causes heat intolerance, weight loss, dyspnea on exertion, and tachycardia. Destruction of large numbers of WBCs releases substantial amounts of uric acid into the circulation; uric acid crystals may obstruct renal tubules, causing renal insufficiency.

Without treatment, leukemia is invariably fatal, usually due to complications of leukemic cell infiltration of bone marrow or vital organs. With treatment, prognosis varies. The overall 5-year survival rate is just over 50%. Survival rates differ by type of leukemia: People with acute myeloid leukemia have a 27% three-year survival rate, whereas the rate is 83% for people with chronic lymphocytic leukemia (ACS, 2018a; National Cancer Institute, 2017).

Classifications

Leukemias are classified by their acuity and by the predominant cell type involved. *Acute leukemias* are characterized by an acute onset, rapid disease progression, and immature or undifferentiated blast cells. *Chronic leukemias*, on the other hand, have a gradual onset, prolonged course, and abnormal mature-appearing cells. *Lymphocytic* (or *lymphoblastic*) *leukemias* involve immature lymphocytes and their precursor cells in the bone marrow. Lymphocytic leukemias infiltrate the spleen, lymph nodes, CNS, and other tissues. *Myeloid* (also called *myelogenous*, *myelocytic*, or *myeloblastic*) *leukemias* involve myeloid stem cells in the bone marrow, interfering with the maturation of all types of blood cells, including granulocytes, RBCs, and thrombocytes (Sorenson et al., 2019). Acute lymphoblastic leukemia is the most common type of leukemia in children. In adults, acute myeloid leukemia and chronic lymphocytic leukemia are the most common types (Sorenson et al., 2019). In summary, the general types of leukemia are as follows:

- Acute lymphocytic (lymphoblastic) leukemia (ALL)
- Chronic lymphocytic leukemia (CLL)
- Acute myeloid (myeloblastic) leukemia (AML)
- Chronic myeloid (myelogenous) leukemia (CML).

This general system of classifying leukemias does not differentiate subtypes of acute leukemias. The FAB system for classifying acute leukemias further differentiates acute leukemias by the predominant cell involved and the degree of cell differentiation (**Table 33.3**).

Acute Myeloid Leukemia

Acute myeloid leukemia (AML) is characterized by uncontrolled proliferation of myeloblasts (the precursors of granulocytes) and hyperplasia of the bone marrow and spleen

Multisystem Effects of
Leukemia

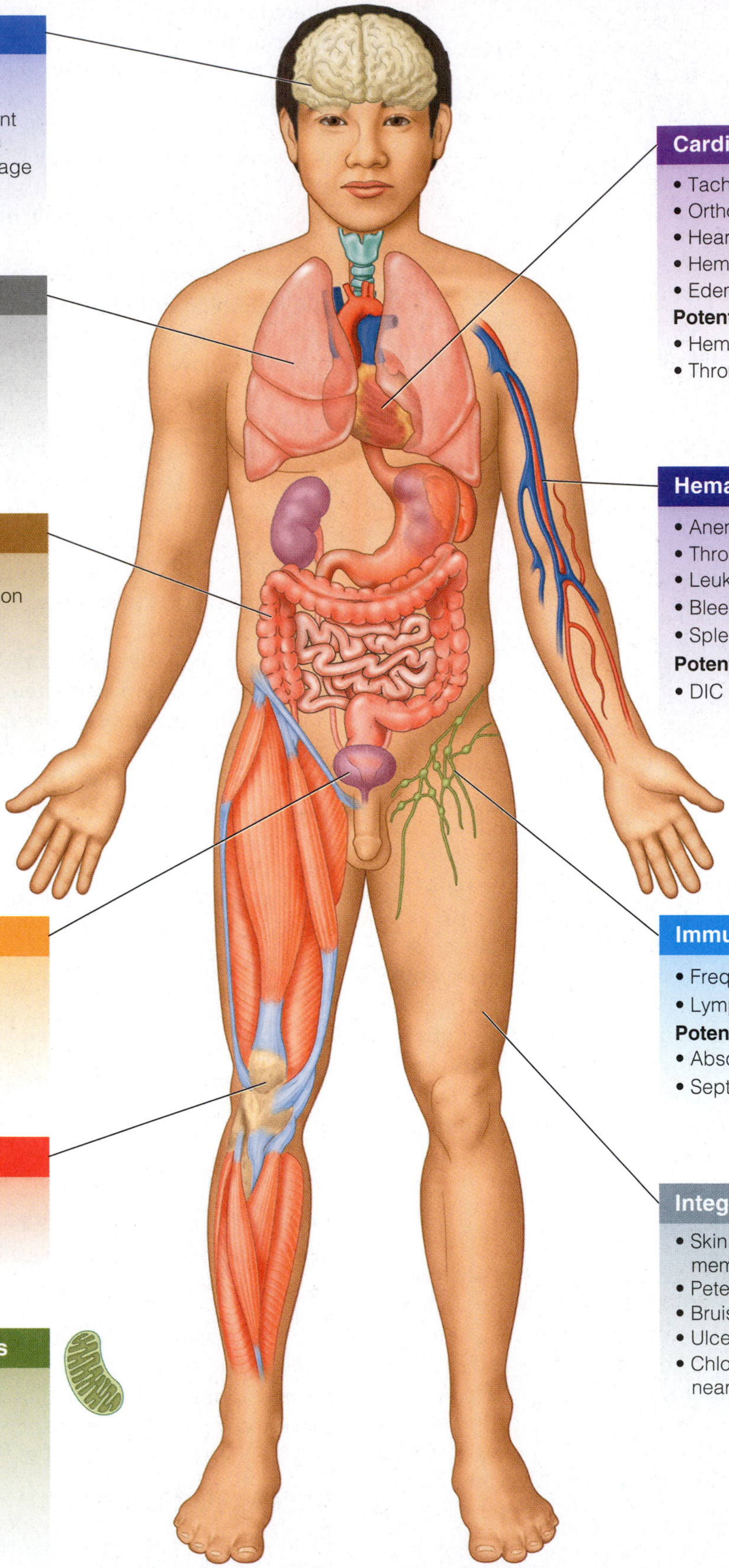

Neurologic
- Headache
- Altered LOC
- Cranial nerve impairment

Potential complications
- Subarachnoid hemorrhage
- Retinal hemorrhage
- Seizures, coma

Respiratory
- Dyspnea on exertion
- Pharyngitis, sore throat
- Frequent respiratory infections

Potential complication
- Pulmonary bleeding

Gastrointestinal
- Anorexia, nausea
- Oral ulcerations, infection
- Bleeding gums
- Gingival hyperplasia (gum overgrowth)
- Abdominal pain
- Hepatomegaly
- Occult GI bleeding

Urinary
- Urinary tract infection
- Hematuria

Potential complication
- Renal insufficiency or failure

Musculoskeletal
- Weakness
- Bone tenderness, pain
- Joint pain

Metabolic Processes
- Malaise, lethargy
- Heat intolerance
- Diaphoresis
- Chills, fever
- Night sweats
- Weight loss

Cardiovascular
- Tachycardia, palpitations
- Orthostatic hypotension
- Heart murmurs
- Hematomas
- Edema

Potential complications
- Hemorrhage
- Thrombophlebitis

Hematologic
- Anemia
- Thrombocytopenia
- Leukopenia
- Bleeding (epistaxis)
- Splenomegaly

Potential complication
- DIC

Immunologic
- Frequent or recurrent infections
- Lymphadenopathy

Potential complications
- Abscesses
- Septicemia

Integumentary
- Skin and mucous membrane pallor
- Petechiae
- Bruising, purpura
- Ulcerations
- Chloromas (skin infiltrations near bony prominences)

Table 33.3 FAB Classification of Acute Leukemia

Type	Class	Predominant Cells	Prognosis
Acute lymphocytic leukemia (ALL)	L_1	Immature lymphoblasts	> 90% remission rate in children
	L_2	Mature lymphoblasts	Relapse common after 2 or more years of remission
Acute myeloid leukemia (AML)	M_0	Undifferentiated cells	Poor
	M_1	Immature myeloblasts	Good; complete response in 65% or more
	M_2	Mature myeloblasts	Good for 2 or more years of remission
	M_3	Promyelocytes	Good in adults
	M_4	Myelocytes and monocytes	Poorest in adults
	M_5	Poorly or well-differentiated monocytes	Poor
	M_6	Predominant erythroblasts	Variable
	M_7	Megakaryocytes	Good in adults

(**Figure 33.6** ■). AML accounts for 80% of acute leukemia cases in adults. Treatment induces complete remission in 66% of patients, although only about 30 to 40% achieve cure or long-term remission (ACS, 2018a; Sorenson et al., 2019).

The manifestations of AML result from neutropenia and thrombocytopenia. Decreased neutrophils lead to recurrent severe infections, such as pneumonia, septicemia, abscesses, and mucous membrane ulceration. The manifestations of thrombocytopenia include petechiae, purpura, ecchymoses (bruising), epistaxis (nosebleeds), hematomas, hematuria, and GI bleeding. Bone infarctions or subperiosteal infiltrates of leukemic cells may cause bone pain. Anemia is a late manifestation, causing fatigue, headaches, pallor, and dyspnea on exertion. Death usually results from infection or hemorrhage.

Bone marrow aspiration shows a proliferation of immature WBCs. The CBC shows thrombocytopenia and normocytic, normochromic anemia.

Chronic Myeloid Leukemia

Chronic myeloid leukemia (CML) is characterized by abnormal proliferation of all bone marrow elements. This type of leukemia constitutes approximately 15% of adult leukemias. It affects men more frequently than women. The onset of CML is typically between ages 30 or 40 and 50, although it is seen in children and adolescents as well (Sorenson et al., 2019).

CML is usually associated with a chromosome abnormality called the *Philadelphia chromosome*, a balanced translocation of chromosome 22 to chromosome 9 (**Figure 33.7** ■). The fusion gene produced by this translocation, known as *bcr/abl*, is an *oncogene* capable of initiating a malignancy. Very large doses of ionizing radiation may also induce CML in some patients.

People with CML are often asymptomatic in the early stages and, in fact, are often diagnosed when a routine blood test reveals abnormal cell counts. Anemia causes weakness, fatigue, and dyspnea on exertion. The spleen is often enlarged, causing abdominal discomfort. Within 3 to 4 years, disease progresses to a more aggressive phase. Rapid cell proliferation and hypermetabolism cause fatigue, weight loss, sweating, and heat intolerance. The spleen enlarges, leading to a sensation of abdominal fullness and discomfort. Platelet function is affected in this stage, leading to bleeding

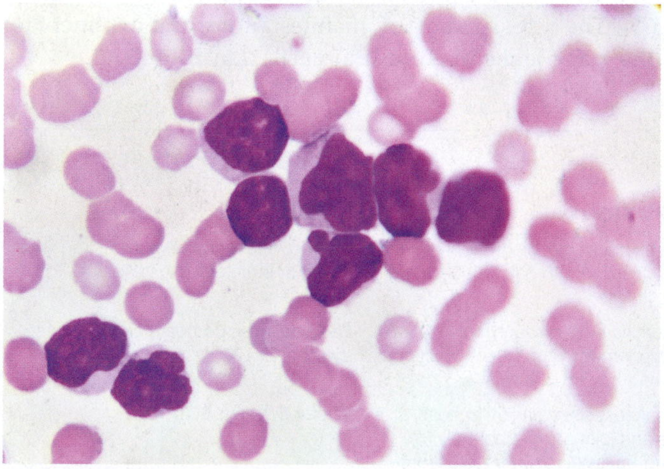

Figure 33.6 ■ A blood smear from the bone marrow of a patient with acute myeloid leukemia. Note the abnormally large number of myelocyte WBCs (stained purple) among the small RBCs.

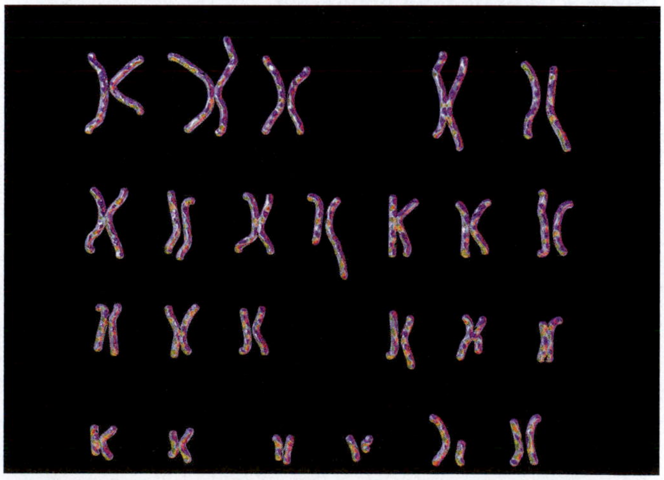

Figure 33.7 ■ The Philadelphia chromosome. Note the chromosomes of pairs 9 and 22. In each instance, the left-hand chromosome of the pair is normal, whereas an exchange of material between chromosomes has made the right-hand chromosome 9 larger and the right-hand chromosome 22 smaller. In stem cells within the bone marrow, the chromosome 22 defect leads to chronic myeloid leukemia.

and increased bruising. Finally, the disease evolves to acute leukemia, with blast cell proliferation. This stage, known as the *terminal blast crisis phase*, is characterized by significant constitutional manifestations, splenomegaly, and infiltration of leukemic cells into the skin, lymph nodes, bones, and CNS (Sorenson et al., 2019). Survival following the onset of this final stage averages only 2 to 4 months.

Acute Lymphocytic Leukemia

Acute lymphocytic leukemia (ALL) is the most common type of leukemia in children and young adults. In adults, ALL is rarely seen until late middle age, and then its incidence increases with aging. Genetic factors may play a role in its development, particularly the *bcr/abl* translocation also implicated in CML.

Most (80%) cases of ALL result from malignant transformation of B cells, with the remaining 20% arising from T cells (ACS, 2018a). The malignant cells resemble immature lymphocytes (*lymphoblasts*); however, they do not mature or function effectively to maintain immunity. These lymphoblasts accumulate in the bone marrow, lymph nodes, and spleen, as well as in circulating blood. Some types of lymphoma are thought to represent a later stage of the same disease.

The onset of ALL is usually rapid. Lymphoblasts proliferating in bone marrow and peripheral tissues crowd the growth of normal cells (**Figure 33.8** ■). Normal hematopoiesis is suppressed, leading to thrombocytopenia, leukopenia, and anemia. Manifestations of infections, bleeding, and anemia develop. Bone pain resulting from rapid generation of marrow elements, lymphadenopathy, and liver enlargement are also common. Infiltration of the CNS causes headaches, visual disturbances, vomiting, and seizures.

The CBC shows an elevated WBC count with increased lymphocytes on the differential. RBC and platelet counts are decreased. Bone marrow studies reveal a hypercellular marrow with growth of lymphoblasts. Combination chemotherapy produces complete remission in 80 to 90% of adults with ALL.

Chronic Lymphocytic Leukemia

Chronic lymphocytic leukemia (CLL) is characterized by proliferation and accumulation of small, abnormal, mature lymphocytes in the bone marrow, peripheral blood, and body tissues. The abnormal cells are usually B lymphocytes that

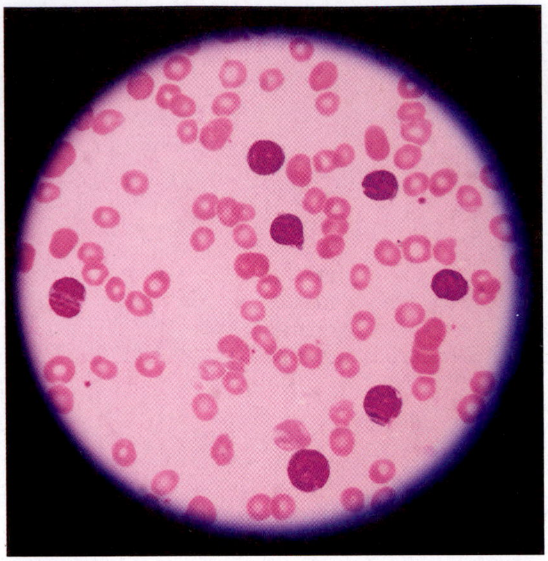

Figure 33.8 ■ A blood smear from the bone marrow of a patient with acute lymphocytic leukemia. Note the abnormally large number of lymphocytes (stained purple) crowding the bone marrow. As a result, normal production of RBCs, functional WBCs, and platelets is suppressed.

are unable to produce adequate antibodies to maintain normal immune function. Only about 5% of CLL involves T cells. CLL occurs more commonly in adults, especially in older adults (median age 65). CLL is the least common type of the major leukemias.

CLL has a slow onset and is often diagnosed during a routine physical examination. If symptoms are present, they usually include vague complaints of weakness or malaise. Possible clinical findings include anemia, infection, and enlarged lymph nodes, spleen, and liver. As in other leukemias, bone marrow hyperplasia is present. Erythrocyte and platelet counts are reduced. Leukocyte counts may either be elevated or reduced, but abnormal cells are always present. In CLL, years may elapse before treatment is required. Survival of this disease averages approximately 7 years.

The types, pathology, manifestations, and treatment for the major leukemias are summarized in **Table 33.4**.

Table 33.4 Major Types of Leukemia

Classification	Characteristics	Manifestations	Treatment
Acute lymphoblastic leukemia (ALL)	Primarily affects children and young adults; leukemic cells may infiltrate CNS	Recurrent infections; bleeding; pallor, bone pain, weight loss, sore throat, fatigue, night sweats, weakness	Chemotherapy; bone marrow transplant (BMT) or stem cell transplant (SCT)
Chronic lymphocytic leukemia (CLL)	Primarily affects older adults; insidious onset and slow, chronic course	Fatigue; exercise intolerance; lymphadenopathy and splenomegaly; recurrent infections, pallor, edema, thrombophlebitis	Often requires no treatment; chemotherapy; BMT
Acute myeloid leukemia (AML)	Common in older adults, may affect children and young adults. Strongly associated with toxins, genetic disorders, and treatment of other cancers	Fatigue, weakness, fever; anemia; headache; bone and joint pain; abnormal bleeding and bruising; recurrent infection; lymphadenopathy, splenomegaly, and hepatomegaly	Chemotherapy; SCT
Chronic myeloid leukemia (CML)	Primarily affects adults; early course slow and stable, progressing to aggressive phase in 3–4 years	Early: Weakness, fatigue, dyspnea on exertion; possible splenomegaly Later: Fever, weight loss, night sweats	Interferon-α; chemotherapy with imatinib mesylate (Gleevec), SCT

Table 33.5 Diagnostic Findings by Type of Leukemia

Test	AML	CML	ALL	CLL
RBC count	Low	Low	Low	Low
Hemoglobin	Low	Low	Low	Low
Hematocrit	Low	Low	Low	Low
Platelet count	Very low	High early, low late	Low	Low
WBC count	Varies	Increased	Varies	Increased
Myeloblasts	Present			
Neutrophils	Decreased	Increased	Decreased	
Lymphocytes		Normal		Normal
Monocytes		Normal/low		Increased
Blasts	Present	Present (crisis)	Present	
Bone marrow	Hypercellular		Hypercellular	
Myeloblasts	Present			
Lymphoblasts			Present	
Lymphocytes				Present

Interprofessional Care

Treatment for leukemia focuses on achieving remission or cure and relieving symptoms. The methods of treatment may include chemotherapy, radiation therapy, and bone marrow or stem cell transplantation. Cure is more often achieved in children with acute leukemia than in adults, although long-term remissions (disease-free periods with no signs or symptoms) can often be achieved.

Diagnosis

The following diagnostic tests are ordered when leukemia is suspected:

- *CBC* with differential is done to evaluate cell counts, hemoglobin and hematocrit levels, and the number, distribution, and morphology (size and shape) of WBCs.
- *Platelets* are measured to identify possible thrombocytopenia secondary to the leukemia and the risk of bleeding.
- *Bone marrow examination* provides information about cells within the marrow, the type of erythropoiesis, and the maturity of erythropoietic and leukopoietic cells.

Table 33.5 outlines the usual diagnostic test results in the various forms of leukemia.

Chemotherapy

Single agent or combination chemotherapy is the treatment of choice for most types of leukemia, with the goal of eradicating leukemic cells and producing remission. **Table 33.6** outlines typical chemotherapy regimens for different types of leukemia. Combination chemotherapy reduces drug resistance and toxicity and interrupts cell growth at various stages of the cell cycle, producing a complementary effect of the drugs used. Cancer treatment with chemotherapy is discussed in detail in Chapter 14.

Chemotherapy for leukemia is generally divided into the induction phase and postremission therapy. During induction, drug doses are high to eradicate leukemic cells from the bone marrow. These high doses also often damage stem cells and interfere with production of normal blood cells. Circulating mature blood cells are not affected because they are no longer dividing. The degree of bone marrow suppression is influenced by a number of factors, including age, nutritional status, concurrent chronic diseases such as impaired liver or renal function, the drug and drug dose, and prior treatment.

Colony-stimulating factors (CSFs), also called *hematopoietic growth factors*, are often administered to "rescue" the bone marrow following induction chemotherapy. CSFs are cytokines that regulate the growth and differentiation of blood cells. Factors that support neutrophil maturation, *granulocyte-macrophage CSF (GM-CSF)* and *granulocyte CSF*

Table 33.6 Chemotherapeutic Regimens Used to Treat Leukemia

Type of Leukemia	Chemotherapeutic Regimens
Acute myeloid leukemia	■ Cytarabine (Cytoxan; an alkylating agent), *with* daunorubicin (Cerubidine, an antitumor antibiotic) or idarubicin (Idamycin; an antitumor antibiotic) ■ All-*trans* retinoic acid (ATRA) added for patients with promyelocytic leukemia
Chronic myeloid leukemia	■ Imatinib mesylate (Gleevec), a *bcr/abl* tyrosine kinase (enzyme) inhibitor ■ Hydroxyurea (a DNA inhibitor) *or* homoharringtonine (HHT; a plant alkaloid) if imatinib not tolerated
Acute lymphocytic leukemia	■ Daunorubicin (Cerubidine; an antitumor antibiotic) *with* vincristine (Oncovin; a plant alkaloid) *with* prednisone with asparaginase (Elspar)
Chronic lymphocytic leukemia	■ Fludarabine (Fludara; an antimetabolite) *or* chlorambucil (Chloromycetin; an antitumor antibiotic) ■ Cyclophosphamide (Cytoxan; an alkylating agent), vincristine, and prednisone ■ Cyclophosphamide, doxorubicin (Adriamycin; an antitumor antibiotic), vincristine, and prednisone

(G-CSF), are commonly used. Bone pain is a common side effect of therapy with these agents. Patients may also experience fevers, chills, anorexia, muscle aches, and lethargy (Shields et al., 2018).

Once remission has been achieved, postremission chemotherapy is continued to eradicate any additional leukemic cells, prevent relapse, and prolong survival. A single chemotherapeutic agent, combination therapy, or bone marrow transplant may be used for postremission treatment.

Radiation Therapy

Radiation therapy damages cellular DNA. While the cell continues to function, it cannot divide and multiply. Cells that divide rapidly, such as bone marrow and cancer cells (radiosensitive cells), respond quickly to radiation therapy. Although normal cells are affected, they are better able to recover from the damage caused by the radiation than are cancer cells. The types of delivery, effects, and toxicities of radiation are discussed in greater detail in Chapter 14.

Bone Marrow Transplant

Bone marrow transplant (BMT) is the treatment of choice for some types of leukemia. BMT is often used in conjunction with or following chemotherapy or radiation. There are two major categories of BMT: In allogeneic BMT, the bone marrow of a healthy donor is infused into the patient with the illness; in autologous BMT, the patient is infused with his or her own bone marrow.

Allogeneic BMT. *Allogeneic BMT* uses bone marrow cells from a donor (often from a sibling with closely matched tissue antigens; closely matched unrelated donors may also be used). Prior to allogeneic BMT, high doses of chemotherapy and/or total body irradiation are used to destroy leukemic cells in the bone marrow. The donor's bone marrow is aspirated (**Figure 33.9 ■**) and infused through a central venous line into the recipient. Prior to BMT and reestablishment of bone marrow function, the patient is critically ill and at significant risk for infection and bleeding due to depletion of WBCs and platelets.

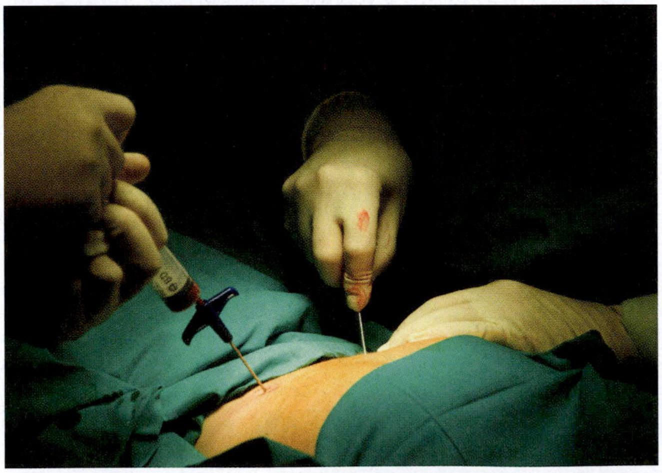

Figure 33.9 ■ Allogeneic bone marrow transplant. Bone marrow from the donor is aspirated, then filtered and infused into the recipient.

Autologous BMT. *Autologous BMT* uses the patient's own bone marrow to restore bone marrow function after chemotherapy or radiation. This procedure is often called *bone marrow rescue*. In autologous BMT, about 1 L of bone marrow is aspirated (usually from the iliac crests) during a period of disease remission. The bone marrow is then frozen and stored for use after treatment. If relapse occurs, lethal doses of chemotherapy or radiation are given to destroy the immune system and malignant cells and to prepare space in the bone marrow for new cells. The filtered bone marrow is then thawed and infused intravenously through a central line. The infused marrow cells slowly become a part of the patient's bone marrow, the neutrophil count increases, and normal hematopoiesis takes place.

As in allogeneic BMT, the patient is critically ill during the period of bone marrow destruction and immunosuppression. The patient is hospitalized in a private room for 6 to 8 weeks or more. Potential complications include malnutrition, infection, and bleeding.

Stem Cell Transplant

Allogeneic **stem cell transplant (SCT)** is an alternative to bone marrow transplant. SCT results in complete and sustained replacement of the recipient's blood cell lines (WBCs, RBCs, and platelets) with cells derived from the donor stem cells.

Donors must have tissue that is closely matched with that of the recipient. Prior to harvesting, hematopoietic growth factors, including G-CSF and GM-CSF, are administered to the donor for 4 to 5 days. This increases the concentration of stem cells in peripheral blood, allowing it to be used for the transplant instead of bone marrow. Peripheral blood is removed and white cells are separated from the plasma, then administered via a large central venous catheter. Large concentrations of stem cells are also present in umbilical cord blood. This may be stored and used in some cases.

The recipient undergoes similar treatment prior to SCT as for BMT. The risks for infection and other complications, as well as graft-versus-host disease, are similar.

Graft-versus-host Disease. Allogeneic BMT or SCT may precipitate *graft-versus-host disease (GVHD)*, which develops in up to 60% of all patients receiving an allogeneic BMT or SCT. In GVHD, immune cells of the donated bone marrow identify the recipient's body tissue as foreign. Consequently, T lymphocytes in the donated marrow attack the liver, skin, and GI tract, causing skin rashes progressing to desquamation (loss of skin), diarrhea, GI bleeding, and liver damage. *Acute GVHD* develops within days or weeks of the transplant and is usually marked by a pruritic, maculopapular rash that begins on the palms and soles of the feet and may extend over the entire body. Vaso-occlusive disease of the liver affects up to 25% of allogeneic bone marrow transplant recipients, with jaundice and elevated liver function tests (Sorenson et al., 2019). *Chronic GVHD* develops later, 100 or more days after the transplant, affecting 20 to 50% of patients who survive 6 months or more following allogeneic BMT or SCT. It may follow acute GVHD or develop in patients with no prior symptoms. GVHD is treated with antibiotics and steroids; immunosuppressant drugs such as thalidomide and immunotoxin (XomaZyme) may be used if necessary.

Biologic Therapy

Cytokines such as interferons and interleukins are biologic agents that may be used to treat some leukemias. These agents modify the body's response to cancer cells; in some cases, they are cytotoxic as well. Interferons are a complex group of messenger proteins normally produced in response to antigens such as viruses (refer to Chapter 12). They have multiple effects, including moderating immune function, and inhibiting abnormal cell proliferation and growth. Interferon-α may be used to treat some leukemias, particularly CML. Side effects commonly associated with interferon therapy include flulike symptoms, persistent fatigue and lethargy, weight loss, and muscle and joint pain.

Integrative Therapies

Although many complementary and alternative medicine therapies have been purported to treat cancer in general, at this time none have been shown to provide sustained benefit in treating leukemia. Clinical trials have demonstrated the efficacy of both coping skills training (relaxation and imagery) and hypnosis to significantly reduce the oral discomfort associated with leukemia and its treatment.

Nursing Care

For nursing care specific to the patient undergoing diagnostic testing for leukemia, see the accompanying Case Study & Nursing Care Plan.

Assessment

See the Manifestations and Interprofessional Care sections for the assessment of the patient with leukemia.

Focused assessment data related to leukemia includes:

- *Health history:* Complaints of fatigue, weakness, dyspnea on exertion, frequent infections, sore throat, night sweats, bleeding gums, or nosebleeds; recent weight loss; exposure to ionizing radiation (multiple x-rays, residence near a site of radiation or atomic testing) or chemicals (occupational); prior treatment for cancer; history of an immune disorder
- *Physical assessment:* Skin and mucous membranes for bruising, purpura, petechiae, ulcers or lesions; pallor; vital signs including orthostatic vitals; heart and lung sounds; abdominal examination; stool for occult blood
- *Laboratory data:* Blood count with differential; bone marrow studies.

Priorities of Care

Collaborating with the interprofessional team to ensure adequate treatment of the underlying process while providing care that supports the physical and psychologic responses to the disorder is a priority of nursing care.

Diagnoses, Outcomes, and Interventions

When caring for the patient with leukemia, the nurse considers the chronic and life-threatening nature of the disease as well as the effects of treatment. See the accompanying Moving Evidence into Action box. Priority nursing problems may include potential infection, poor nutrition, oral membrane issues, potential bleeding, and bereavement issues.

Moving Evidence into Action

Slow-Stroke Back Massage: Impact on Pain, Fatigue, and Sleep Problems in Patients with Leukemia

Clinical Issue

Patients with leukemia commonly experience fatigue, pain, and interrupted sleep. These symptoms impact their quality of life. Simple nursing interventions like massage therapy may show promise in ameliorating these symptoms.

External Evidence

Miladinia, Baraz, Shariati, and Malehi (2017) conducted a randomized controlled trial where 60 patients with leukemia were randomized to receive either slow-stroke massage therapy or usual care. The massage therapy was delivered for 10 minutes, three times per week, for 4 weeks. Numeric rating scales were used to measure perceptions of pain, fatigue, and disordered sleep, while sleep quality was measured using the Pittsburgh Sleep Quality Index. Results showed that the massage therapy intervention significantly reduced the progressive sleep disorder, pain, and fatigue and improved sleep quality over time.

Internal Evidence

As part of the evaluation of internal evidence, one must consider the patient's interest in and willingness to use massage therapy in addition to the rest of the therapeutic plan. Additionally, the proposed intervention should also be considered in light of the healthcare team stakeholders, which can influence patient willingness to use the new intervention.

Patient Considerations

When considering use of a new practice (like slow-stroke massage therapy), the nurse must consider the specific patient population where it will be used (in this case, patients with leukemia). Will patients and their families be amenable to the new intervention?

Putting the Pieces Together

Massage therapy is acceptable to most patients. The use of slow-stroke massage therapy would have minimal burden on the patient while being a positive experience. A simple

(continued)

intervention such as this can easily be implemented with minimal cost and time. To effectively implement such a new intervention, it is important to evaluate the external evidence and consider the internal implications and patient/family issues. This simple intervention has the potential to improve leukemia patient symptoms through a comforting activity.

Reference

Miladinia, M., Baraz, S., Shariati, A., & Malehi, A. S. (2017). Effects of slow-stroke back massage on symptom cluster in adult patients with acute leukemia: Supportive care in cancer nursing. *Cancer Nursing, 40*(1), 31–38.

Reduce Risk for Infection. Changes in WBC function impair the immune and inflammatory responses in leukemia, increasing the risk for infection. WBCs may be immature and ineffective or, in some cases, deficient. Chemotherapy or radiation therapy further depresses bone marrow function and increases the risk for infection.

Expected Outcome: Patient will describe measures to protect healthy tissue and prevent infection.

The nurse will:

- Promptly report manifestations of infection: Fever, chills, throat pain, cough, chest pain, burning on urination, purulent drainage, and itching and burning in vaginal or rectal areas. *Prompt reporting allows timely intervention to prevent overwhelming infection and sepsis.*
- Institute infection protection measures:
  a. Maintain protective isolation as indicated.
  b. Ensure meticulous hand hygiene among all people in contact with the patient.
  c. Assist as needed with appropriate hygiene measures.
  d. Restrict visitors with colds, flu, or infections.
  e. Provide oral hygiene after every meal.
  f. Avoid invasive procedures when possible, including injections, intravenous catheters, catheterizations, and rectal and vaginal procedures. When necessary, use strict aseptic technique for all invasive procedures and monitor carefully for infection.

  These precautions minimize exposure to bacterial, viral, and fungal pathogens. Infection is the major cause of death in patients with leukemia. Mucous membranes are especially susceptible to breakdown and infection as a result of tissue damage from chemotherapy or radiation.
- Monitor vital signs including temperature and oxygen saturation every 4 hours. Report temperature spikes with chilling, tachypnea, tachycardia, restlessness, change in PaO_2, and hypotension. *The inflammatory response may be impaired in leukemia, masking signs of infection until sepsis develops, indicated by manifestations such as those listed.*
- Monitor neutrophil levels (measured in cubic millimeters) for relative risk for infection:
  a. 2000 to 2500: No risk
  b. 1000 to 2000: Minimal risk
  c. 500 to 1000: Moderate risk
  d. Below 500: Severe risk.

  Neutrophils are the first line of defense against infection. As levels decrease, the risk for infection increases.
- Explain infection precautions and restrictions and their rationale; explain that these measures are usually temporary. *Patient and family understanding increases compliance and lowers the risk of infection.*

Promote Good Nutrition. The patient with leukemia may have difficulty meeting nutritional needs due to increased metabolism, fatigue, loss of appetite from radiation, nausea and vomiting from chemotherapy, or painful oral mucous membranes that make chewing and swallowing difficult and/or painful.

Expected Outcome: Patient will consume adequate nourishment to promote weight within normal range.

The nurse will:

- Weigh the patient regularly and evaluate weight loss over time to determine degree of malnutrition. A weight loss of 10 to 20% may indicate malnutrition. *A minimum intake of nutrients is necessary for health and tissue repair; cancer increases metabolic needs over this basal requirement. Weight loss occurs when metabolic requirements are not met. Both the disease process and its treatment can interfere with nutrient intake.*
- Address causative or contributing factors to inadequate food and fluid intake.
  a. Provide mouth care before and after meals; use a soft-bristle toothbrush or sponges as necessary.
  b. Provide liquids with different textures and tastes.
  c. Increase liquid intake with meals.
  d. Reduce intake of milk and milk products, which make mucus more tenacious.
  e. Assist to a sitting position for eating.
  f. Ensure that the environment is clean and odor free.
  g. Provide medications for pain or nausea 30 minutes before meals, if prescribed.
  h. Provide rest periods before meals.
  i. Offer small, frequent meals including low-fat, high-kilocalorie foods throughout the day.
  j. Provide commercial supplements, such as Ensure.
  k. Avoid painful or unpleasant procedures immediately before or after meals.
  l. Suggest measures to improve food tolerance, such as eating dry foods when arising, consuming salty foods if allowed, and avoiding very sweet, rich, or greasy foods.

Anorexia, nausea and vomiting, diarrhea, stomatitis, taste changes, and dysphagia often make eating difficult during cancer treatment when good nutrition is most important. Maintaining nutritional status decreases morbidity and mortality by preventing weight loss, improving the response to treatment, minimizing adverse effects, and improving quality of life. Small, frequent meals are often better tolerated, especially high-protein, high-kilocalorie foods.

Promote Oral Membrane Health. *Stomatitis,* inflammation and ulceration of the oral mucous membrane, is common in leukemia. Chemotherapy can further impair the integrity of constantly dividing oral tissues.

Expected Outcome: Patient will maintain intact, moist oral mucous membranes through use of measures to promote oral membrane health.

The nurse will:

- Inspect the buccal region, gums, sublingual area, and the throat daily for swelling or lesions. Ask about oral pain or burning. *Breakdown of the oral mucous membrane increases the risk of infection and bleeding, causes pain and discomfort with eating and swallowing, and may cause swelling that interferes with the airway.*
- Culture any oral lesions. *Herpes simplex virus and* Candida *(yeast) are more common in patients with neutropenia. Herpes lesions are usually red, raised, fluid-filled blisters;* Candida *causes a white coating and patches of white plaque.*
- Assist with mouth care and oral rinses with saline or a solution of hydrogen peroxide and water (1:1 or 1:3 hydrogen peroxide and water) every 2 to 4 hours. Apply petroleum jelly to the lips to prevent dryness and cracking. *These measures help prevent infection and increase comfort.*
- Encourage use of soft-bristle toothbrush or sponge to clean teeth and gums. *Toothbrushes with hard bristles may abrade inflamed mucosa, causing bleeding and increasing the risk of infection.*
- Administer medications as ordered to treat infection or relieve pain. *Topical antifungal agents such as nystatin may be prescribed to treat* Candida *infections. Topical anesthetics such as lidocaine may be prescribed to relieve comfort and facilitate good oral care.*
- Instruct patient to avoid alcohol-based mouthwashes, citrus fruit juices, spicy foods, very hot or very cold foods, alcohol, and crusty foods. Suggest bland, cool foods and cool liquids at least every 2 hours. *Avoiding mucosa-traumatizing foods and liquids increases comfort; bland, cool foods and liquids cause the least pain. Intake of adequate fluids is necessary to prevent dehydration.*

Reduce Risk of Bleeding. Bleeding is the second most common cause of leukemia deaths. As platelet counts decrease, the risk of bleeding increases (see the section later in this chapter on thrombocytopenia). Tumor lysis syndrome is also a risk in patients with leukemia who are undergoing their initial treatment with chemotherapy. Tumor lysis syndrome develops when a large number of malignant cells are destroyed by treatment with chemotherapy or radiation. The resultant by-products of cell lysis can overwhelm the body's ability to effectively eliminate them, leading to hyperkalemia, hyperphosphatemia with secondary hypocalcemia, and hyperuricemia.

Expected Outcome: Patient will remain free of any evidence of new bleeding and take precautions to prevent bleeding and to identify early onset of tumor lysis syndrome.

The nurse will:

- Assess vital signs every 4 hours for bleeding.
- Assess body systems every shift, including:
  a. Skin and mucous membranes for petechiae, ecchymoses, and purpura
  b. Gums, nasal membranes, and conjunctiva for bleeding
  c. Vomitus, stool, and urine for visible or occult blood
  d. Vaginal bleeding
  e. Prolonged bleeding from puncture sites
  f. Neurologic changes such as headache, visual changes, altered mentation, decreased level of consciousness, seizures
  g. Abdomen for complaints of epigastric pain, diminished bowel sounds, increasing abdominal girth, rigidity, or guarding.

  Early identification of bleeding helps prevent significant blood loss and potential shock. Internal hemorrhage may lead to tachycardia, hypotension, pallor, and diaphoresis. Bleeding into the lungs may cause dyspnea; bleeding into the abdomen causes increased girth, pain, and guarding. Intracranial bleeding affects mental status and level of consciousness.
- Avoid invasive procedures such as rectal temperatures and suppositories, vaginal douches, suppositories, tampons, urinary catheterization, and parenteral injections, if possible. Diagnostic procedures such as biopsy or lumbar puncture should not be done if the platelet count is $< 50{,}000$. *Invasive procedures can cause tissue trauma and bleeding. Procedures that use large-bore needles should be delayed until the platelet count is increased.*
- Apply pressure to injection sites for 3 to 5 minutes and to arterial punctures for 15 to 20 minutes. *Pressure prevents prolonged bleeding by prompting hemostasis and clot formation.*
- Instruct patient to avoid forcefully blowing or picking the nose, forceful coughing or sneezing, and straining to have a bowel movement. *These activities can damage mucous membranes, increasing the risk for bleeding.*
- Monitor and promptly report abnormal blood levels of electrolytes, uric acid, urea nitrogen, and creatinine or manifestations of tumor lysis syndrome. *Significant alterations in electrolyte levels can lead to complications such as cardiac dysrhythmias, muscle weakness or tetany, paresthesias, and mental status changes. Excess uric acid can compromise renal function and lead to metabolic acidosis and gout.*

- Maintain adequate hydration and administer prescribed medications such as allopurinol and diuretics as ordered. *Hydration is vital to maintain renal function and promote elimination of tumor lysis by-products. Allopurinol reduces the risk of uric acid crystallization in the kidneys and other tissues* (Shields et al., 2018).

Support the Grief Process. The diagnosis of cancer or another potentially life-threatening illness causes actual or perceived losses, such as loss of function, independence, normal appearance, friends, self-esteem, and self. Grieving is the emotional response to those losses. The adaptive process of mourning a loss and resolving grief is called grief work; grief work cannot begin until a loss is acknowledged. Refer to Chapter 5 for a detailed discussion of grief and loss.

Expected Outcome: Patient and family will discuss the meaning of losses (actual or perceived) to the patient and family's life.

The nurse will:

- Discuss roles of the patient and family and ways in which they have managed stressful situations in the past. Assess coping strategies and their effectiveness. Help identify sources of strength and support. Discuss changing roles resulting from a leukemia diagnosis and its effect on spiritual, social, and economic status and usual lifestyle. Evaluate cultural or ethnic factors that affect grief reactions. *Grieving is a normal response to a real or potential loss that begins at the time of diagnosis. The timing, duration, and intensity of grief and responses to grief may differ among family members. Share information on diagnosis, role change, and physical loss among all family members to build the foundation for mutual understanding and trust.*
- Use therapeutic communication skills to facilitate open discussion of losses and provide permission to grieve. *Encouraging discussion of the meaning of the loss helps decrease some of the anxiety associated with loss. This in turn allows the patient and family to examine the current situation and compare it with past situations with which they have coped successfully.*
- Provide information about agencies that may help in resolving grief, and make referrals as indicated. Consider self-help groups, cancer support groups, and bereavement groups. *Participating in support groups with others who are anticipating or experiencing a similar loss can decrease feelings of isolation.*

Transitions of Care

Prevention focused on health-promoting activities related to leukemia include teaching about leukemia risk factors, particularly those that can be controlled. Discuss the potential dangers of exposure to ionizing radiation and certain chemicals such as benzene. Encourage all patients to avoid smoking cigarettes. Discuss genetic counseling with patients at high risk for having a child with Down syndrome (over age 35).

Acute nursing care of the leukemia patient focuses on infection prevention, surveillance of body temperature, fluid and electrolyte balance and early symptoms of infection, initiation of neutropenia precautions (reverse isolation) and bleeding precautions, energy conservation, symptom management including pain control, and fatigue management. The nurse also promotes self-care and independence while providing assistance as needed with activities of daily living as indicated. Patient and family teaching for home care after treatment for leukemia focuses on encouraging self-care, providing information about the disease and the treatment, preventing infection and injury, and promoting nutrition. Teaching topics for each of these areas are as follows.

Encouraging Self-Care

- Hygiene measures and energy conservation during self-care activities
- Oral hygiene including using a soft-bristle toothbrush several times daily; avoid flossing
- Reporting lesions, bleeding, or signs of infection promptly
- Maintaining a balance of rest and activity

Providing Information about Leukemia and Treatment

- Bone marrow function, the pathophysiology of leukemia, and potential complications of leukemia
- Prognosis for the specific type of leukemia
- Treatment measures such as chemotherapy, radiation, bone marrow or stem cell transplant, their purpose and effects, where treatment is available, and potential adverse effects or risks
- Community, regional, and national resources for people with leukemia

Preventing Infection and Injury

- Hand hygiene and other measures to reduce exposure to pathogens such as avoiding people who are ill and avoiding crowds
- Avoiding foodborne illnesses by washing fruits and vegetables, proper food storage
- Dental hygiene measures
- Avoiding immunizations
- Manifestations to report: Fever, chills, burning on urination, foul-smelling urine, vaginal or rectal discharge, skin lesions
- Avoiding contact sports or strenuous exercise if platelet count is low
- Using an electric razor for shaving, avoiding rectal or vaginal suppositories, vaginal tampons, or enemas
- Increasing dietary fiber and using a bulk-forming laxative as needed to prevent straining
- Avoiding over-the-counter or prescription drugs that interfere with platelet function (see **Box 33.7** on page 1204)

Case Study & Nursing Care Plan

A Patient with Acute Myelocytic Leukemia

Catherine Cole is a 37-year-old secretary who lives with her husband, Ray, and teenage daughter, Amy, in an apartment in a large metropolitan area. About 2 months ago, Mrs. Cole began to tire easily and experience night sweats several times a week. She noted that she was pale, bruised easily, and was having heavier menstrual periods. Blood tests ordered by her healthcare provider are abnormal. She is admitted for a bone marrow biopsy.

ASSESSMENT

Mary Losapio, RN, obtains a nursing history and physical assessment for Mrs. Cole. Mrs. Cole tells her, "I'm so tired, and I have these bruises all over me. I'm so afraid of the results of the bone marrow examination. I don't know what we will do if I have cancer." Mrs. Cole clutches her husband's hand and then begins to cry. Physical assessment data include height 156 cm (64 in.), weight 48.1 kg (106 lb); vital signs T 37.8°C (100°F), P 102 bpm, R 22/min, BP 130/82 mmHg. Numerous petechiae scattered over trunk and arms; ecchymoses noted on lower right arm and right calf. Oral mucosa is red, with several small ulcerations in buccal areas.

Blood count shows reduced RBCs, hemoglobin, and hematocrit levels. The WBC is high, with myeloblasts seen on differential. The platelet count is very low. A tentative diagnosis of acute myelogenous leukemia is made.

DIAGNOSES

- Potential for infection related to altered WBC production and immune function
- Ineffectual defenses related to reduced platelet count and risk for bleeding
- Changes in oral mucosal membranes secondary to anemia and reduced platelets
- Fatigue related to anemia
- Anxiety related to fear of leukemia diagnosis

EXPECTED OUTCOMES

- Patient will remain free of infection.
- Patient will experience no significant bleeding.
- Patient will have intact oral mucous membranes.
- Patient will manage self-care activities despite fatigue.
- Patient will verbalize decreased anxiety.

PLANNING AND IMPLEMENTATION

- Place in a private room.
- Limit visitors to immediate family for the present.
- Instruct all staff, the family, and patient to carefully perform hand hygiene. Post a sign over the washbasin in the room as a reminder for handwashing.
- Record vital signs every 4 hours.
- Avoid invasive procedures unless absolutely necessary.
- Monitor for bleeding every 4 hours, including skin, oral mucosa, abdominal assessment, body fluids, and menstrual pad count.
- Instruct to perform oral hygiene every 2 to 4 hours, using a soft-bristle toothbrush.
- Ask the dietitian to work with Mrs. Cole to identify preferred foods. Instruct to avoid foods that may damage oral mucosa, such as very hot, very cold, or highly acidic or spicy foods.
- Provide for periods of rest alternating with activity.
- Teach about the bone marrow biopsy. Allow time for questions and to verbalize fears.
- Refer to the oncology nurse specialist for further teaching and support.

EVALUATION

The bone marrow biopsy confirms the diagnosis of acute myelogenous leukemia. Mrs. Cole is very upset, but calms as the healthcare provider and the oncology nurse discuss treatment plans and the possibility of remission. She decides to have outpatient chemotherapy. During her hospital stay, Mrs. Cole remained free of infection or further bleeding. She tells Ms. Losapio that her mouth feels better, although it is still painful. During routine assessment, Mrs. Cole remarks, "You know, I was so scared when I came here, but I think I am a little less so now. Sometimes not knowing what is wrong is worse than knowing."

CLINICAL REASONING IN PATIENT CARE

1. Describe how alterations in WBCs can increase a person's susceptibility to infection.
2. List sources of potential infection for the hospitalized patient.
3. What is the rationale for having the patient do her own oral and physical hygiene?
4. Outline a teaching plan for this patient and her family for home care to prevent infection.
5. Develop a care plan for Mrs. Cole for the diagnosis of potential for infection.

See Evaluating Your Response in Appendix B.

- The importance of reporting any bleeding (nosebleeds, rectal bleeding, vomiting blood, excessive menstrual periods, blood in the urine, bleeding gums, bruises, or collections of blood under the skin) or changes in behavior to the healthcare provider

Promoting Nutrition

- Eating several small, low-fat, high-calorie meals and drinking five to eight glasses of water daily
- Reporting continued weight loss, loss of appetite, or inability to eat for 24 hours
- Discussing dietary needs with the dietitian.

Assistance with physical care, finances, and transportation may be required following discharge. As needed, refer the patient and family to social services, support groups, home care services, and other agencies that can provide needed services (such as local chapters of the American Cancer Society, which can provide hospital beds and transportation for outpatient cancer treatment).

33.3 Lymphoid Tissue Disorders

The Patient with Malignant Lymphoma

Lymphomas are malignancies of lymphoid tissue. They are characterized by the proliferation of lymphocytes, histiocytes (resident monocytes or macrophages), and their precursors or derivatives. Lymphomas are closely related to lymphocytic leukemias. Some experts consider them to be different forms or stages of the same disease processes.

Pathophysiology

Although there are many types of malignant lymphoid cells, at this time lymphomas are commonly identified as Hodgkin disease or non-Hodgkin lymphoma.

Hodgkin Disease

Hodgkin disease is a lymphatic cancer, occurring most often in people between the ages of 15 and 35 or over age 50. It is somewhat more common in men than in women. Approximately 8260 new cases of Hodgkin disease were diagnosed in 2017 (ACS, 2017). The exact cause of Hodgkin disease is unknown, but both Epstein-Barr virus (EBV) infection and genetic factors appear to play a role in its development. Hodgkin disease is one of the most curable cancers. While as many as 60 to 90% of people with localized disease achieve cure with a normal lifespan, there may be an increased risk for a second cancer occurrence throughout life.

Hodgkin disease develops in a single lymph node or chain of nodes, spreading to adjoining nodes. Involved lymph nodes contain *Reed-Sternberg cells* (malignant cells) surrounded by host inflammatory cells. These malignant cells secrete inflammatory mediator substances, attracting inflammatory cells to the tumor site. They may invade almost any tissue in the body. The spleen is often involved; as the disease progresses, the liver, lungs, digestive tract, and CNS may be affected (Sorenson et al., 2019). Rapid proliferation of abnormal lymphocytes impairs the immune response, especially cell-mediated immune responses. Infections are common.

Hodgkin disease is classified as classic Hodgkin disease or as nodular lymphocyte-predominant Hodgkin disease. The classic form of the disease accounts for 95% of all cases; nodular lymphocyte-predominant Hodgkin is rare. Classic Hodgkin can be further divided into four subtypes by cells identified within the tumor, but the subtype does not affect the prognosis.

In both Hodgkin disease and non-Hodgkin lymphoma, the stage of the disease, the presence of systemic manifestations, and factors such as age help determine the prognosis. The prognosis is good when the disease is localized to one or two node regions. Factors such as anemia, thrombocytopenia, and older age reduce the likelihood of disease cure.

Non-Hodgkin Lymphoma

Non-Hodgkin lymphoma (NHL) is a diverse group of lymphoid tissue malignancies that do not contain Reed-Sternberg cells. Non-Hodgkin lymphomas tend to arise in peripheral lymph nodes and spread early to tissues throughout the body. Non-Hodgkin lymphoma is more common than Hodgkin disease, affecting an estimated 72,240 people in 2017 and causing about 20,140 deaths in 2017 (ACS, 2017). Older adults are more often affected, and it occurs more frequently in men than in women. Like Hodgkin disease, its cause is unknown, although both genetic and environmental factors (e.g., viral infections such as EBV, HTLV-1 and HTLV-2, and HIV) are thought to play a role.

As in most malignancies, non-Hodgkin lymphoma begins as a single transformed cell; it may arise from T cells, B cells, or tissue macrophages (histocytes). The primary types of non-Hodgkin lymphoma are identified in **Table 33.7**. Although non-Hodgkin lymphoma usually arises in a lymph node, it can originate in any lymphoid tissue. It tends to spread early and unpredictably to other lymphoid tissues and organs. Extranodal spread may involve the nasopharynx, GI tract, bone, CNS, thyroid, testes, and soft tissue.

The prognosis for non-Hodgkin lymphoma ranges from excellent to poor, depending on the identified cell type and grade of differentiation. Low-grade tumors (better differentiated) tend to be less aggressive and more curable. Higher-grade tumors are often disseminated at the time of diagnosis and have a poorer prognosis.

Incidence and Risk Factors

Malignant lymphomas are the seventh leading cause of cancer deaths in the United States. Approximately 80,500 new cases of lymphoma were diagnosed in 2017, and 21,210 deaths were attributed to the disease. The incidence of non-Hodgkin lymphoma has nearly doubled since 1970, but currently has stabilized, primarily due to a fall in its

Table 33.7 **Subtypes of Non-Hodgkin Lymphoma**

Subtype	Incidence	Course and Prognosis
B-Cell Lymphomas		
Diffuse large B-cell lymphomas	Most common adult type (40–50% of adult lymphomas) More common in males Incidence increases with age	Aggressive tumor 45–50% cure rate
Follicular lymphoma	Accounts for 40% of adult lymphomas, rare in children Incidence increases with age	Bone marrow frequently involved Course slow, indolent; 72% five-year survival
Extranodal marginal zone lymphoma (MALT lymphoma)	Accounts for about 5% of adult lymphomas, rare in children Incidence increases with age More common in Italy	Presents with tumors outside lymphatic system: GI tract, lung, thyroid, urinary tract, skin, CNS Slow, indolent course; 74% five-year survival
Mantle cell lymphoma	Accounts for 3–4% of adult lymphomas, rare in children Predominantly affects older men (74%)	Aggressive, difficult to cure 27% five-year survival
Burkitt lymphoma	Rare in adults (< 1% of lymphomas), more common in children (~30% NHL)	Rapidly progressive but responds well to therapy 45% five-year survival
T-Cell Lymphomas		
Precursor T-cell lymphoblastic leukemia/lymphoma	More common in children and young adults More common in males than in females	Can present either as ALL or lymphoma Aggressive disease; 26% five-year survival
Peripheral T-cell lymphoma	Most common T-cell lymphoma in adults	Often presents as disseminated disease 25% five-year survival
Mycosis fungoides/cutaneous T-cell lymphoma	Onset typically during mid-50s; more common in African Americans	Cutaneous lymphoma Slow course, progressing from patchy skin lesions to plaque to cutaneous tumors

incidence related to HIV infection and AIDS. The incidence of Hodgkin disease has significantly declined since 1990 (ACS, 2017).

While the cause of lymphoma is unknown, some risk factors have been identified. See the accompanying Genetic Considerations box for information about identified genetic links for lymphoma development. Immunosuppression due to drug therapy following organ transplant or to HIV disease increases the risk for non-Hodgkin lymphoma. Infectious agents such as human T-cell leukemia/lymphoma virus-1 (HTLV-1) and the Epstein-Barr virus (EBV) have also been identified as risk factors. Others may include occupational herbicide or chemical exposure.

Genetic Considerations

Focus on Lymphoma

Although specific genetic alterations have not been identified for all types of lymphoma, recurring genetic abnormalities associated with lymphomas point to a genetic link in disease development (ACS, 2018d). Three distinct genetic acquired abnormalities have been identified in non-Hodgkin lymphomas: Gross chromosomal changes such as translocations; rearrangements of specific genes; and altered expression of specific oncogenes (overexpression, underexpression, or mutation). Consistent genetic changes are associated with some lymphomas; in other cases, several genetic abnormalities may be seen. Hodgkin disease is unique from other lymphomas in that no specific genetic abnormalities have been identified. For more information about genetics and disease, refer to Chapter 8.

Manifestations

Hodgkin Disease

The most common symptom of Hodgkin disease is one or more painlessly enlarged lymph nodes, usually in the cervical or subclavicular region. Systemic manifestations such as persistent fever, night sweats, fatigue, and weight loss are associated with a poorer prognosis for the disease. Late symptoms such as malaise, pruritus, and anemia indicate spread of the disease (Sorenson et al., 2019). The spleen may be enlarged, and other organ systems such as the lungs and GI tract are occasionally involved.

Non-Hodgkin Lymphoma

The early manifestations of non-Hodgkin lymphoma are similar to those for Hodgkin disease. Painless lymphadenopathy may be localized or widespread (**Figure 33.10** ■). Systemic manifestations such as fever, night sweats, fatigue, and weight loss may be present, but are less common in non-Hodgkin lymphoma. Organ system involvement may cause symptoms such as abdominal pain and nausea and vomiting. Headaches, peripheral or cranial nerve symptoms, altered mental status, or seizures may signal CNS involvement.

The manifestations and clinical features of Hodgkin disease and non-Hodgkin lymphoma are compared in **Table 33.8**.

Interprofessional Care

Chemotherapy and radiation therapy, either alone or in combination, are the primary treatments for Hodgkin

Table 33.8 Features and Manifestations of Hodgkin Disease and Non-Hodgkin Lymphoma

Feature or Manifestation	Hodgkin Disease	Non-Hodgkin Lymphoma
Lymphadenopathy	Localized to a single node or chain, often cervical, subclavicular, or mediastinal	Multiple peripheral nodes, nodes of the mesentery often involved
Spread	Orderly and continuous	Diffuse and unpredictable
Extranodal involvement	Rare	Early and common
Bone marrow involvement	Uncommon	Common
Fever, night sweats, weight loss	Common	Uncommon until disease is extensive
Other manifestations	Fatigue, pruritus, splenomegaly; anemia, neutrophilia	Abdominal pain, nausea and vomiting; dyspnea, cough; CNS symptoms; lymphocytopenia

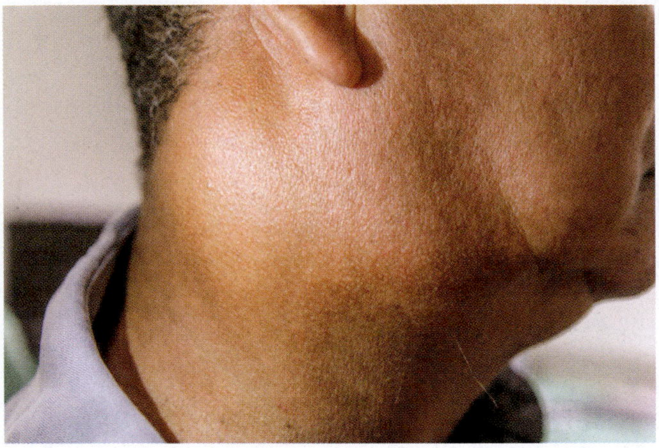

Figure 33.10 ■ Cervical lymphadenopathy in a patient with lymphoma of the neck.

disease and non-Hodgkin lymphoma. Use of monoclonal antibodies to target lymphoma cells, and bone marrow and peripheral stem cell transplants are under investigation for treating lymphomas as well. See the previous section on treatment of leukemia for more information about these transplants.

Diagnosis

The following diagnostic tests may be ordered for lymphomas:

- *CBC* results often show a mild normochromic, normocytic anemia in Hodgkin disease; other findings in Hodgkin disease may include leukocytosis with high neutrophil and eosinophil counts and an elevated sed rate. In non-Hodgkin lymphoma, the CBC typically remains normal until late in the disease, when pancytopenia may develop.
- An *erythrocyte sedimentation rate (ESR)* test is done to identify possible inflammatory causes of lymph node enlargement.
- *Chemistry studies of major organ function* (including liver function tests and renal function studies) are performed to identify possible organ involvement. *Serum LDH levels* and *protein electrophoresis* may also be done when Hodgkin disease is suspected.
- *Chest x-ray* is done to identify possible enlarged mediastinal lymph nodes and pulmonary involvement.
- *CT scans* of the chest, abdomen, and pelvis are performed to identify abnormal or enlarged nodes.
- *PET* or *gallium scans* may be performed in diagnosing the disease, as well as to evaluate the effectiveness of treatment.
- *Biopsy* of the largest, most central enlarged lymph node and of the bone marrow is done to establish the diagnosis for both Hodgkin disease and non-Hodgkin lymphoma. The presence of Reed-Sternberg cells confirms the diagnosis of Hodgkin disease.

Staging

Staging is used to determine the extent of the disease and appropriate treatment. The Ann Arbor Staging System is used to assess the extent and severity of lymphomas. The stages are:

Stage I: Involvement of a single lymph node region or lymphoid structure (e.g., spleen, thymus, lymphoid tonsillar tissue)

Stage II: Involvement of two or more lymph node regions on the same side of the diaphragm

Stage III: Involvement of lymph node regions or structures on both sides of the diaphragm:

III_1: Limited to upper abdomen (spleen, splenic, celiac, or portal nodes)

III_2: Involvement of lower abdominal nodes (para-aortic, iliac, or mesenteric)

Stage IV: Involvement of an extranodal site (not proximal or contiguous with an involved node) such as the liver, lung or pleura, bone or bone marrow, or skin.

The presence or absence of systemic symptoms is indicated by either an A (no systemic symptoms) or B (systemic symptoms of fever, night sweats, weight loss).

Chemotherapy

Combination chemotherapy is used to treat both Hodgkin disease and non-Hodgkin lymphoma. In both cases, chemotherapy is often followed by radiation therapy to involved lymph node regions. The choice of drug combination depends on the stage of the disease as well as the patient's age and general condition. Combination regimens used in the United States include CHOP (cyclophosphamide, doxorubicin, vincristine, and prednisone), ABVD (doxorubicin, bleomycin, vinblastine, and dacarbazine), MOPP (nitrogen mustard, vincristine, procarbazine, and prednisone), and ChlVPP (chlorambucil, vinblastine, procarbazine, and prednisone). These regimens may also be combined in alternating months to reduce the adverse effects and improve tumor cell kill. For more information about nursing care of the patient receiving combination chemotherapy, refer to Chapter 14.

Immunotherapy

Rituximab (Rituxan) is a monoclonal antibody used to destroy the CD20 antigen in B lymphocytes. This destruction results in cellular death of the lymphoma cell. It can be used alone or with cyclophosphamide, vincristine, and prednisone (CVP). The patient should be closely monitored for tumor lysis syndrome. It is recommended that patients be premedicated with diphenhydramine and acetaminophen. Rituximab should be used cautiously in patients with known cardiac disorders (Shields et al., 2018).

Radiation Therapy

Radiation therapy may be the primary treatment for early-stage Hodgkin disease, although early chemotherapy is becoming more common. In later stages and in non-Hodgkin lymphoma, it is usually combined with chemotherapy. Many lymphomas are highly responsive to radiation. The involved lymph node region is treated, with careful shielding to protect unaffected areas and minimize the extent of radiation burn and normal cell destruction (**Figure 33.11** ■). If the disease is advanced, total nodal irradiation may be done. Refer to Chapter 14 for nursing care of the patient receiving radiation therapy.

Stem Cell Transplant

Autologous peripheral blood stem cell transplant (PBSCT) is a treatment option for patients who experience remission of malignant lymphoma. Autologous PBSCT uses the patient's own stem cells to restore bone marrow function after chemotherapy or radiation. In autologous PBSCT, stem cells are obtained from peripheral blood following chemotherapy and treatment with colony-stimulating factors to promote development of normal blood cells. The blood containing these normal stem cells is then frozen and stored for use after treatment. If relapse occurs, lethal doses of chemotherapy or radiation are given to destroy the immune system and malignant cells. The blood is then thawed and infused intravenously through a peripheral line. The infused stem cells become a part of the patient's bone marrow and normal hematopoiesis takes place.

The patient is critically ill during the period of bone marrow destruction and immunosuppression. He or she is hospitalized in a private room for 6 to 8 weeks or more. See the accompanying Moving Evidence into Action box for discussion of the meaning of nurses' work related to BMT.

Complications of Treatment

Both chemotherapy and radiation therapy may have long-term effects. Permanent sterility is common, especially in older adults. Bone marrow depression can lead to immunosuppression, anemia, and bleeding. Secondary cancers and cardiac injury are the most serious late adverse effects of treatment. Chemotherapy regimens using MOPP or a related protocol carry a risk of acute leukemia. Cancers such as breast or lung cancer may develop 10 or more years after thoracic radiation. Thoracic radiation also increases the risk for coronary heart disease and hypothyroidism.

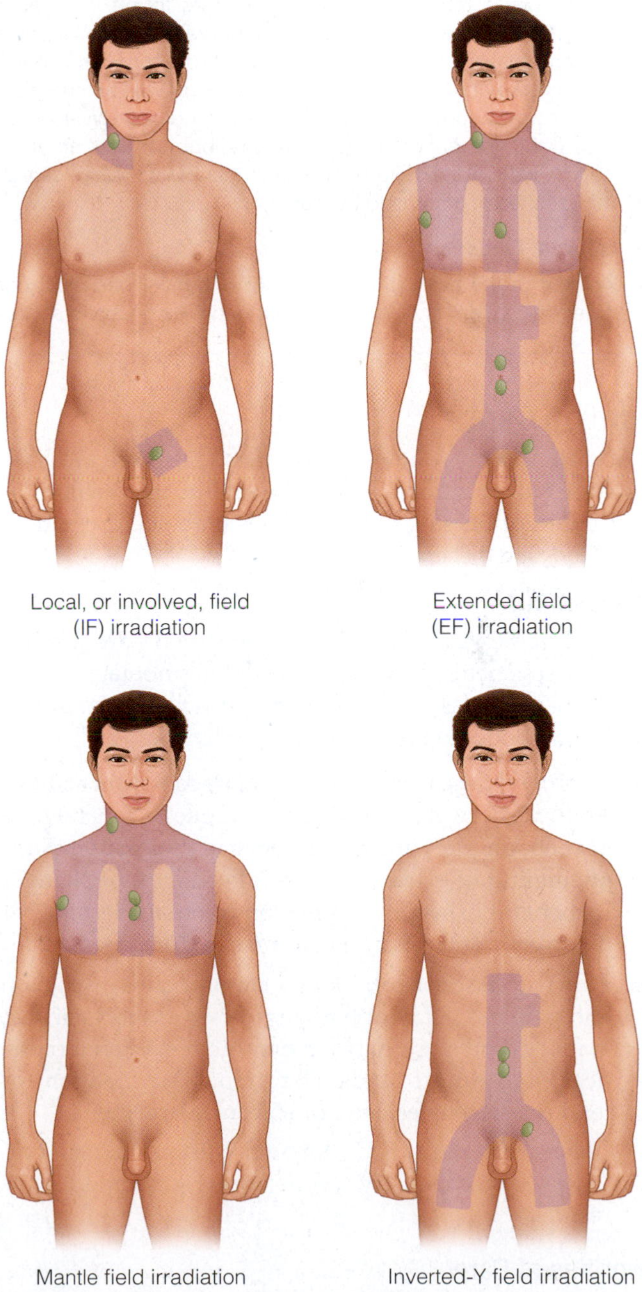
Local, or involved, field
(IF) irradiation
Extended field
(EF) irradiation
Mantle field irradiation
Inverted-Y field irradiation

Figure 33.11 ■ Patterns of radiation therapy used to treat lymphoma based on the location and extent of the disease.

Moving Evidence into Action
Caregiver Burden of Stem Cell Recipient Caregivers

Clinical Issue

Caring for someone undergoing a stem cell transplantation can be physically as well as emotionally taxing. As the patient is the center of focus, the burdens of the primary caregiver are often underrecognized.

External Evidence

Akgul and Ozdemir (2014) conducted a cross-sectional descriptive study of 55 stem-cell recipients and their primary caregivers. The study was conducted at three stem cell transplantation programs in Turkey. Caregiver burden was measured using the Zarit Burden Interview. The investigators found that patient symptoms of nausea and feeling undervalued were related to greater caregiver burden. Burden by score was also seen in caregivers with lower educational levels as well as caregivers with lower incomes. Also noted was higher caregiver burden when only the patient physical needs, but not their emotional needs, were addressed by the healthcare team. More caregiving resulted in increased burden.

Internal Evidence

As part of the evaluation of internal evidence, one must consider the patient and family interest and willingness to address caregiver issues. The healthcare team stakeholders can influence patient and family willingness to reveal concerns surrounding caregiving.

Patient Considerations

The nurse must consider the specific patient population where opening discussions around caregiving would be undertaken. Will stem cell recipients and their caregivers be amenable to such discussions?

Putting the Pieces Together

Stem cell transplantation is a situation fraught with not only physical but also emotional stress. Discussions and interventions to address caregiver burden of the primary caregiver of the stem cell recipient can improve not only the caregiver's experience, but also the support provided to the transplant recipient. To effectively implement such a discussion, it is important to evaluate the external evidence, consider the internal implications, and take into account patient/family issues.

Reference

Akgul, N., & Ozdemir, L. (2014). Caregiver burden among primary caregivers of patients undergoing peripheral blood stem cell transplantation: A cross sectional study. *European Journal of Oncology Nursing, 18*(4), 372–377.

Nursing Care

In addition to the following discussion, also see the Case Study & Nursing Care Plan at the end of this section for application of nursing care strategies for a specific patient with Hodgkin disease.

Assessment

See the Manifestations and Interprofessional Care sections for the assessment of the patient with lymphoma.

Focused assessment of the patient with Hodgkin disease or non-Hodgkin lymphoma includes:

- *Health history:* Complaints of enlarged lymph node(s), fever, night sweats, weight loss, fatigue or general malaise, abdominal pain, respiratory symptoms, numbness or tingling of extremities, visual changes, or changes in mentation; history of infectious mononucleosis, HIV disease, or other immunosuppressive disorders
- *Physical assessment:* Mental status exam; inspection and palpation of lymph nodes (cervical, subclavicular, axillary, and inguinal) for enlargement, tenderness; heart and lung sounds; abdominal examination for tenderness, masses, liver or spleen enlargement
- *Laboratory data:* CBC, hemoglobin and hematocrit, ESR; serum chemistry results; x-ray, scan, and biopsy results.

Priorities of Care

Collaborating with the interprofessional team to ensure adequate treatment of the underlying process while providing care that supports the physical and psychologic responses to the disorder is a priority of nursing care.

Diagnoses, Outcomes, and Interventions

Nursing care of the patient with malignant lymphoma involves both physical and emotional support during diagnosis and treatment. Common nursing care problems include impaired protection due to bone marrow suppression, fatigue, nausea, and altered body image. See the earlier Nursing Care section for leukemia for specific nursing interventions for reducing risk of bleeding.

Manage Fatigue. General malaise and fatigue may accompany malignant lymphoma and are side effects of chemotherapy. In addition, the physical and psychologic stress of dealing with a chronic, debilitating disease and its treatment may cause fatigue.

Expected Outcome: Patient will track patterns of fatigue and describe use of energy conservation techniques to offset fatigue.

The nurse will:

- Inquire about feelings of malaise (a vague feeling of body weakness or discomfort) and fatigue (a pervasive, drained feeling that cannot be eliminated). *Both malaise and fatigue are subjective experiences with physiologic, situational, and psychologic components.*
- Encourage verbalization of feelings about the impact of the disease and fatigue on lifestyle. *Discussion of feelings helps the patient clarify values and may assist in identifying priorities.*
- Encourage enjoyable but quiet activities, such as reading, listening to music, or hobbies. *Enjoyable activities help decrease feelings of fatigue. Quiet activities conserve energy while yielding a sense of accomplishment.*

- Encourage patient to establish priorities and include rest periods or naps when scheduling daily activities. *This provides a sense of control over activities and helps maintain self-esteem. Scheduled rest periods help restore energy and decrease fatigue.*
- Encourage delegation of some responsibilities to family members. *Delegation helps maintain the patient's involvement and role in family decisions and responsibilities, while conserving energy for those activities identified as high priority by the patient.*
- Identify and encourage the patient to use energy-saving equipment. *Performing tasks with less exertion and in less time helps conserve energy.*
- Encourage a diet high in carbohydrates and fluids. *A high-carbohydrate diet helps maintain muscle glycogen stores. A liberal fluid intake promotes excretion of metabolic by-products that may contribute to malaise and fatigue.*

Manage Nausea. The effects of malignant lymphoma and its treatment with chemotherapy and/or radiation therapy can contribute to nausea and interfere with nutritional status. Nausea, a sensation of abdominal fullness, and fear of vomiting often limit food intake. See the nursing care for promoting good nutrition in the earlier section on leukemia for additional interventions.

Expected Outcome: Patient will report relief from nausea and methods to decrease onset of nausea.

The nurse will:

- Assess precipitating factors for nausea and/or vomiting, the frequency of vomiting, and relief measures used by the patient. *Careful assessment allows development of interventions tailored to the patient's situation and needs.*

SAFETY ALERT: Provide ordered antiemetics before chemotherapy is started. Administering prescribed antiemetics before chemotherapy helps prevent nausea and the psychologic association of nausea with chemotherapy. ■

- Teach measures to prevent or relieve nausea and vomiting:
  a. Eat soda crackers and suck on hard candy.
  b. Eat soft, bland foods that are cold or at room temperature.
  c. Avoid unpleasant odors, and get fresh air.
  d. Eat prior to but not immediately before chemotherapy.
  e. Use distraction or progressive muscle relaxation when nauseated.
  f. If vomiting occurs, gradually resume oral intake with frequent sips of clear liquids or ice, progressing to bland foods.

  Crackers and hard candy often relieve queasiness, whereas hot, spicy, sweet, or strong-smelling foods may increase nausea. Alternative nausea relief measures may be effective.
- Provide small feedings of high-kilocalorie, high-protein foods, and fluids. *This increases nutritional intake.*
- Assist with oral care, general hygiene, and environmental control of temperature, appearance, and odors. *These measures enhance appetite.*
- Identify and provide preferred foods. *This promotes nutritional intake.*
- Assist patient to a sitting position during and immediately after meals. *The sitting position helps decrease early feelings of fullness.*

Manage Feelings About Changes to Appearance. The diagnosis of cancer is often devastating to the sense of trust in and the perception of one's body. Radiation and chemotherapy lead to changes in appearance and body function (e.g., hair loss, reduced libido, and infertility), further altering body image. Reactions to this diagnosis vary and may include refusal to look in a mirror, refusal to discuss the effects of the disease or treatment, unwillingness to participate in rehabilitation, inappropriate treatment decisions, increasing dependence on others or refusal to provide self-care, hostility, withdrawal, and signs of grieving.

Expected Outcome: Patient will verbalize realistic expectations of therapy impact on body appearance and function.

The nurse will:

- Assess perception of body image through subjective information such as:
  a. What the patient likes most and least about his or her body
  b. Preillness perception of people who are sick or have a disability
  c. Current understanding of health and limitations imposed by illness or treatment
  d. Feelings about the illness and its effect on perception of self and others.

  Body image is one's mental idea or picture of the body. It is based on past and present experiences and includes components of one's actual body and emotional responses to that body. Body image changes constantly. There is often a time lag between an actual body change and the changed body image; during this time, the diagnosis, teaching, and treatment may be rejected.
- Discuss the risk for and measures to cope with alopecia. Suggest wearing wigs, scarves, hats, or caps. Teach proper scalp care using baby shampoo or mild soap, a soft brush, sunscreen, and mineral oil to reduce itching. If eyelashes and eyebrows are lost, teach eye protection, such as wearing eyeglasses and caps with wide brims. *Chemotherapeutic agents attack rapidly dividing cells such as those responsible for hair growth. Hair loss usually begins 1 to 2 weeks after initiation of chemotherapy, with maximum loss 1 to 2 months later. Alopecia may range from thinning to total hair loss. Regrowth depends on the treatment schedule and doses; however, it usually begins 2 to 3 months after treatment ends. New hair may be softer, more curly, and slightly different in color. Teaching and emotional support help the patient anticipate hair loss, discuss its potential effect on body image, and learn self-care techniques.*

- Discuss available resources for financial assistance with purchase of wigs, including local American Cancer Society chapters and insurance plans. *A well-matched wig (or one the color the patient has always wished for!) can help maintain a positive body image.*

Promote Sexual Function. Sexual dysfunction may result from the malignancy and the effects of radiation and chemotherapy. Reproductive tissues are made of rapidly dividing cells, and cancer treatment may cause temporary or permanent sterility, changes in menstruation, and changes in libido.

Expected Outcome: Patient will identify underlying cause of sexual dysfunction and discuss alternative satisfying and acceptable sexual practices for self and partner.

The nurse will:

- Encourage discussion of actual or potential sexual dysfunction or sterility with the patient and significant other. *Patients may be reluctant to discuss this unintended effect of treatment unless encouraged.*
- Assess knowledge, provide information, and clarify misconceptions. Discuss realistic measures for coping (e.g., sperm banking prior to chemotherapy or radiation therapy). *Patients and their partners may be unclear about expected effects on sexuality, reproduction, and the permanency of these effects.*
- Refer for counseling as indicated. *Sexual counseling can help the patient and partner develop alternative strategies for expressing their sexuality.*

Reduce Risk for Injury to Skin. Malignant lymphomas may cause significant pruritus and drenching night sweats. As a result, skin integrity may be impaired. In addition, radiation therapy can cause superficial burns, which may also affect skin integrity.

Expected Outcome: Patient will demonstrate understanding of plan to heal skin and prevent reinjury.

The nurse will:

- Frequently assess skin, especially in areas undergoing radiation. Instruct to report any blistering. *Early identification of lesions allows timely treatment and can prevent further disruption of this important line of defense against infection.*
- Provide and teach measures to promote comfort and relieve itching: Use cool water and a mild soap to bathe; blot (rather than rub) dry skin; apply plain cornstarch or nonperfumed lotion or powder to the skin unless contraindicated; use lightweight blankets and clothing; maintain adequate humidity and a cool room temperature; wash bedding and clothes in mild detergent, and put them through a second rinse cycle. Also teach to avoid sunbathing and tanning beds and to protect the area from the sun. *Pruritus is aggravated by excessive warmth, excessive dryness, rough fabrics, fatigue, and stress. Lotions and some powders may be contraindicated during radiation therapy.*

Transitions of Care

Unfortunately, there are no known preventative measures for lymphoma. Risk may be reduced by avoiding known risk factors such as obesity or infections from HIV, Epstein-Barr virus, or *Helicobacter pylori*. Acute nursing care of the lymphoma patient focuses on infection prevention, surveillance of body temperature, fluid and electrolyte balance, early symptoms of infection, energy conservation, symptom management including pain control, and fatigue management. The nurse also promotes self-care and independence while providing assistance as needed with activities of daily living. When teaching the patient and family about home care, include the following topics in addition to those previously identified for specific nursing diagnoses:

- Information about the illness, planned treatment, and anticipated side effects of treatment
- Skin care and measures to relieve itching and protect areas of radiation
- Symptoms to report to the healthcare provider, including those of vertebral compression (decreased sensation or strength in lower extremities)
- Use of analgesics and alternative relief strategies for abdominal pain and peripheral neuropathies
- Respiratory care if mediastinal nodes are enlarged or lungs or pleurae are involved
- Planning ADLs to ensure adequate rest and exercise
- Measures to relieve nausea and maintain adequate nutrition.

Refer patients and family members to the local chapter of the American Cancer Society for information, assistance, and counseling. A list of state and local agencies that offer information about malignant lymphoma and financial assistance can be obtained from the Leukemia Society of America.

The Patient with Multiple Myeloma

Multiple myeloma is a malignancy in which plasma cells multiply uncontrollably and infiltrate the bone marrow, lymph nodes, spleen, and other tissues. *Plasma cells* are B-cell lymphocytes that develop to produce antibodies (immunoglobins).

Pathophysiology

Malignant plasma cells arise from one clone (*monoclonal*) of B cells that produces abnormally large amounts of a particular immunoglobin called the *M protein*. This abnormal protein interferes with normal antibody production and impairs the humoral immune response. It also increases blood viscosity and may damage kidney tubules. As myeloma cells proliferate, they replace the bone marrow and infiltrate the bone itself. Cortical bone is progressively destroyed by tumor growth and enzymes produced by myeloma cells. These enzymes facilitate bone destruction, its infiltration by tumor cells, development of new blood vessels to sustain the tumor, and growth of myeloma cells (Sorenson et al., 2019).

Case Study & Nursing Care Plan

A Patient with Hodgkin Disease

Albin Quito, age 28, is the nurse manager of a thoracic intensive care unit in a large teaching hospital. Lately he has been more tired than usual, often wakes up at night covered with sweat, and just does not feel well. He had thought that his symptoms were due to a viral illness and his busy work schedule. However, yesterday morning Mr. Quito noticed a large swollen area on the right side of his neck. He made an appointment with his primary healthcare provider who found a large cervical lymph node. A biopsy of the node and a CT scan of the chest were scheduled.

ASSESSMENT

David Herzog, the nurse in charge of the outpatient clinic, obtains a nursing history and assessment on Mr. Quito. His physical examination is essentially normal, with the exception of the enlarged node, which is not tender to palpation. When Mr. Quito is weighed, he tells Mr. Herzog that he has lost 3.2 kg (7 lb) in the past 2 months. In reviewing the results of the blood studies, Mr. Herzog notes mild anemia and an increased neutrophil count. The lymph node biopsy shows Reed-Sternberg cells. The clinic healthcare provider and Mr. Herzog tell Mr. Quito that the findings indicate stage I-B Hodgkin disease but that the prognosis is very good. The healthcare provider recommends a short course of combination chemotherapy followed by radiation therapy to involved sites.

DIAGNOSES

- Anxiety related to the diagnosis of Hodgkin disease and effects of treatment on job performance
- Potential for infection related to potential bone marrow depression due to chemotherapy
- Fatigue related to effects of cancer, chemotherapy, and radiation therapy

EXPECTED OUTCOMES

- Patient will verbalize reduced anxiety.
- Patient will remain free of infection.
- Patient will identify and use methods to preserve energy.

PLANNING AND IMPLEMENTATION

- Encourage to consider a leave of absence from work during course of treatment.
- Discuss joining a support group for people with cancer.
- Provide information about the illness, combination chemotherapy, and radiation therapy.
- Reinforce knowledge of actions to decrease the risk of infection.
- Discuss ways to decrease fatigue and maintain energy:
  a. Take a 1- to 2-hour nap once or twice a day.
  b. Avoid overexertion during weekends and time off.
  c. Maintain a well-balanced diet.

EVALUATION

When Mr. Quito returns the following week to begin chemotherapy, he brings his friend Nancy to meet Mr. Herzog and asks him to discuss his treatment with her. Mr. Quito says, "I am still really scared, but being able to talk about this with Nancy will help a lot." Mr. Quito has made arrangements to take a 4-month leave from work, with the understanding that his job will be held for him. He states that he will have some problems with money but is working them out. He also says he feels that taking a nap is silly but that he will rest to maintain his energy level. Mr. Quito and Nancy express confidence that he will be cured and say they plan to be active members of the cancer support group—even after recovery.

CLINICAL REASONING IN PATIENT CARE

1. Discuss the rationale for treating Hodgkin disease with chemotherapy and radiation.
2. Design a teaching plan to help Mr. Quito prevent infection while he is at home.
3. What effect does the diagnosis of cancer have on the developmental tasks of a young adult?
4. Develop a care plan for Mr. Quito for the nursing diagnosis of fatigue.

See Evaluating Your Response in Appendix B.

Affected bones (primarily the vertebrae, ribs, skull, pelvis, femur, clavicle, and scapula) are weakened and may break without trauma (pathologic fracture). With disease progression, malignant cells spread via the bloodstream to invade other organs (**Figure 33.12** ■).

Incidence and Risk Factors

The incidence of multiple myeloma is increasing slightly, with an estimated 30,280 cases diagnosed and 12,590 deaths due to the disease in 2017 (ACS, 2017). It affects African Americans nearly twice as often as Caucasian Americans, and men slightly more frequently than women. The incidence of multiple myeloma increases with age, rarely occurring before age 45; most cases are diagnosed in people over age 65 (ACS, 2018b). Its cause is unknown. Possible contributing factors include genetic alterations, radiation exposure, oncogenic virus, inflammatory stimuli, and chronic antigenic stimulation. The risk for developing multiple myeloma is higher in people of lower socioeconomic status. This increased risk may relate to environmental factors such as poor housing, occupational hazards, poor nutritional status, and other physical and psychosocial stressors such as exposure to infectious agents.

Manifestations

The disease develops slowly, and patients are sometimes diagnosed during evaluation for unrelated problems. Manifestations of multiple myeloma are due to its effects on the bone and the impaired immune response due to M protein production. Bone pain is the most common presenting symptom. With progression of the disease, the pain may increase in severity and become more localized. Rapid bone destruction releases calcium from the bone, leading to hypercalcemia and manifestations of neurologic dysfunction, such as lethargy, confusion, and weakness (**Figure 33.13** ■).

As functional antibody formation decreases and the humoral immune response is suppressed, recurrent infections develop. Cell-mediated immunity remains intact. *Bence Jones proteins* are found in the urine in multiple myeloma. These proteins are toxic to the renal tubules and may lead to renal failure with azotemia and uremia (refer to Chapter 28 for more information about renal failure).

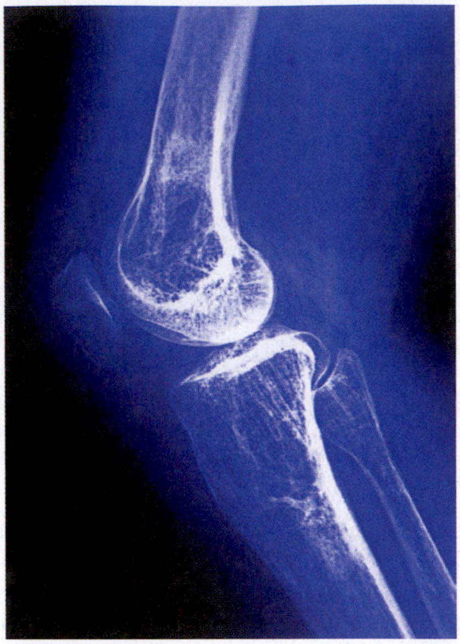

Figure 33.13 ■ X-ray of patient with multiple myeloma showing osteolytic lesions.

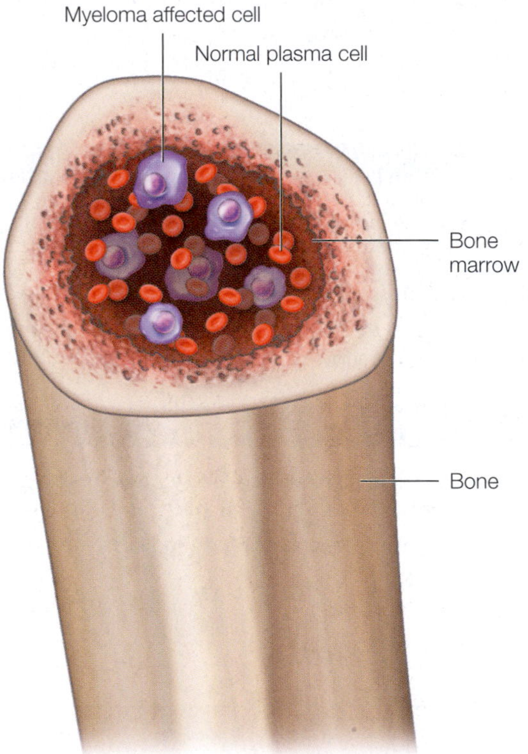
Myeloma affected cell
Normal plasma cell
Bone marrow
Bone

Figure 33.12 ■ An illustration of the progress of multiple myeloma. Abnormal plasma cells proliferate uncontrollably, gradually replacing bone marrow and infiltrating bone itself. As the disease progresses, these cells spread to other organs via the bloodstream.

Depending on the stage at diagnosis, median survival ranges from 29 to 62 months. The disease course is chronic, progressing more rapidly with each relapse after remission. The acute terminal stage of the disease is marked by pancytopenia and widespread organ infiltration by myeloma cells.

Interprofessional Care

Diagnosis and Staging

Diagnostic tests for multiple myeloma include:

- *X-rays* and other radiologic studies of the bone may reveal multiple punched-out lesions.
- *Bone marrow examination* shows an abnormal number of immature plasma cells.
- *CBC* shows moderate to severe anemia, and the *ESR* is usually elevated.
- *Protein electrophoresis* shows a spike of one type of antibody, usually IgG.
- *Serum calcium, creatinine, uric acid,* and *BUN levels* are often elevated.
- *Urinalysis* shows Bence Jones proteins in the urine.
- *Biopsy* of myeloma lesions confirms the diagnosis of multiple myeloma.

Staging of multiple myeloma is based on the hemoglobin and serum calcium levels, the amount of abnormal protein present, and the degree of bone involvement.

Treatment

There is no cure for multiple myeloma. In some patients, active observation is indicated, as the disease may continue with a slow, indolent (sluggish, not developing or progressing) course for many years. When indicated by disease stage or progression, standard treatment includes induction chemotherapy followed by stem cell transplant and maintenance chemotherapy to control progression of the disease. Supportive care is provided to reduce complications of the disease and their effects.

Combination chemotherapy with an alkylating agent (melphalan [Alkeran], cyclophosphamide [Cytoxan], or chlorambucil [Chloromycetin]) and prednisone administered for 4 to 7 days every 4 to 6 weeks is commonly used. Chemotherapy typically reduces bone pain, hypercalcemia, anemia, and the number of infections. Novel therapies that include immunomodulatory drugs lenalidomide (Revlimid) and thalidomide (Thalomid) and the proteasome inhibitor bortezomib (Velcade) contribute to improved survival rates and better response rates when compared to conventional chemotherapy. Localized radiation therapy may be used to treat painful bone lesions. High-dose chemotherapy followed by peripheral allogeneic stem cell transplant may be more effective in achieving cure, but is associated with a high mortality rate. When autologous SCT is used, G-CSF is administered prior to harvesting and preserving peripheral stem cells for collection, preservation, and transplant.

Supportive care may include treatment of hypercalcemia with hydration, possible bisphosphonate therapy to reduce bone loss (see Chapter 40), and calcium, vitamin D, and fluoride supplements to support bone structure. Plasma exchange therapy (plasmapheresis) to remove circulating M proteins is used as needed to treat acute renal failure. Infections are treated promptly when they develop.

Nursing Care

Assessment

See the Manifestations and Interprofessional Care sections for the assessment of the patient with multiple myeloma.

Focused assessment data for the patient with multiple myeloma includes:

- ***Health history:*** Complaints of back or bone pain, onset, duration, and intensity; complaints of weakness, fatigue, anorexia; history of frequent or recurrent infections; neurologic symptoms such as numbness and tingling or clumsiness
- ***Physical assessment:*** Level of consciousness and mental status; mobility, gait; localized tenderness or pain, bony crepitus with movement or palpation; movement and sensation in extremities.

Priorities of Care

Collaborating with the interprofessional team to ensure adequate treatment of the underlying process while providing care that supports the physical and psychologic responses to the disorder is a priority of nursing care.

Diagnoses, Outcomes, and Interventions

Nursing care of the patient with multiple myeloma focuses on problems of chronic pain, impaired mobility, and the risk for injury. Risk for infection is a major nursing care focus; see the previous section on leukemia for specific interventions to reduce this risk. Other nursing care needs are similar to those of patients with other cancers and chronic pain. Refer to Chapters 9 and 14 for additional specific nursing interventions for these problems.

Manage Chronic Pain. Patients with multiple myeloma typically experience chronic back pain and deep bone pain as myeloma cells saturate the bone marrow and invade the bone structure. Pathologic fractures are a common and reoccurring problem.

Expected Outcome: Patient will experience adequate pain control as evidenced by physical well-being.

The nurse will:

- Assess pain, including intensity (use a standard pain scale), onset, duration, precipitating factors, and effective relief measures. *Identifying the intensity, causes, and precipitating factors of pain helps determine and evaluate effective pain relief measures.*
- Determine position of greatest comfort, and assist as needed into this position. *The patient is best able to identify positions that minimize pain, but may need assistance with repositioning.*
- Support position with pillows. *Bony prominences may be painful due to infiltrates. Pillows can help relieve pressure on these prominences, thus reducing pain.*
- Provide uninterrupted rest periods. *Adequate rest facilitates pain relief and improves pain tolerance.*
- Teach adjunctive pain relief strategies such as relaxation or guided imagery. *A combination of pharmacologic and nonpharmacologic methods provides better management of chronic pain, especially bone pain.*
- Teach effective analgesic use, including the family in instruction. *Analgesics are most effective when taken before pain becomes severe. Patients and their families may be reluctant to use prescription analgesics on a regular basis.*
- Report unrelieved pain to the healthcare provider. *A different analgesic or addition of an adjunctive medication such as a nonsteroidal anti-inflammatory drug (NSAID) may be needed to effectively control pain.*

Promote Physical Mobility. Painful bony infiltrates and pathologic fractures may limit mobility. A brace or splint may be used to protect extremities or support the back. In addition, persistent weakness associated with the cancer and anemia may limit the patient's ability to participate in usual activities.

Expected Outcome: Patient will demonstrate optimal independence in positioning, exercising, and performing functional activities.

The nurse will:

- Assist to change position at least every 2 hours. *Assistance with repositioning is necessary due to weakness. Frequent repositioning improves comfort and reduces the risk for impaired skin and tissue integrity.*
- Provide a trapeze to assist in repositioning. *A trapeze provides better leverage, allowing the patient to assist with*

repositioning and providing a degree of independence. The ability to participate in self-care improves self-esteem.

SAFETY ALERT: Gently support extremities during repositioning. Weakened extremities due to infiltration of bone by myeloma cells and muscle atrophy from lack of use increase the risk for pathologic fractures. ■

Reduce Risk for Injury. The bone involvement of multiple myeloma places the patient at high risk for pathologic and traumatic fractures. Pathologic fractures can occur with simple activities such as turning or reaching for an item. The spine is usually affected; the ribs and bones of the extremities may also be at risk for fracture.

Expected Outcome: Patient will effectively control risk through use of close and careful positioning and activity monitoring.

The nurse will:

- Place needed items close at hand. *Straining to reach objects increases the risk of falling or sustaining other injury.*
- Provide safety measures to prevent falls from bed: Place the bed in a low position, use side rails as indicated, and place the call bell within reach. *Safety measures help prevent accidental injury. A secure environment minimizes risk and helps prevent falls.*
- Provide shoes with nonskid soles, a clear pathway, adequate lighting, and a level surface free of scatter rugs or other hazards when ambulating. Provide a walker as needed for support and security. *Weight-bearing exercise promotes bone repair. Safety measures, such as an unobstructed pathway and a firm walking surface, help prevent falls.*

Transitions of Care

There are no known preventative measures for multiple myeloma. No specific risk factors have been identified that can be managed.

The nursing care of the patient with multiple myeloma who is undergoing acute therapy focuses on managing the treatments (chemotherapy, radiation therapy, surgery, plasmapheresis therapy). Close surveillance of vital signs, fluid and electrolyte balance, and infection risk, as well as attention to symptom management, are priority goals for the nurse. When teaching patients and their families for home care, include the following topics:

- Strategies for home maintenance management
- Signs and symptoms of complications to be reported to the healthcare provider (e.g., symptoms of vertebral and extremity fractures)
- Manifestations of infection to report: Fever and chills; increased malaise, fatigue, or weakness; cough with or without sputum; sore throat; dysuria, nocturia, frequency, urgency, or malodorous urine.

Provide referrals for home health and home maintenance services, physical or occupational therapy, social services, and hospice care, as appropriate. End-of-life care for the patient with multiple myeloma focuses on symptom management and comfort measures. Family involvement is also essential. The nurse caring for the patient with multiple myeloma at the end of life also provides emotional support to the patient and family members.

The Patient with Neutropenia

Leukopenia is a decrease in the total circulating WBC count. Although any type of WBC may be affected, neutrophils, which make up the majority of WBCs, are affected most often. *Neutropenia* is a decrease in circulating neutrophils, usually < 1500 cells/µm. Neutropenia may be either congenital or acquired, developing secondarily to prolonged infection, hematologic disorders, starvation, or autoimmune disorders (such as rheumatoid arthritis). Chemotherapy and other drugs can suppress the bone marrow. Neutropenia develops in approximately half of patients undergoing chemotherapy to treat cancer. *Agranulocytosis* is severe neutropenia, with < 200 cells/µm. Numbers of other granulocytes are also reduced. It is usually a result of impaired leukocyte formation in the bone marrow or increased cell destruction in circulating blood. Agranulocytosis significantly increases the risk for infection. *Aplastic anemia* affects production of all blood cells, resulting in anemia, thrombocytopenia, and agranulocytosis.

Pathophysiology

Neutrophils are an integral component of the immune response. They are phagocytes, drawn to and activated by infection and inflammation to engulf and degrade invading microorganisms. Their lifespan in peripheral blood is short, less than 1 day. When *granulopoiesis* (the development and maturation of granulocytes) in the bone marrow is suppressed, the number of circulating neutrophils falls rapidly. As a result, the body's ability to defend itself against infection is significantly reduced.

Manifestations

The manifestations of neutropenia reflect the resulting impaired immunity and inflammatory response. Opportunistic bacterial, fungal, and protozoal infections develop, commonly affecting the respiratory tract and mucosa of the mouth, GI tract, and vagina. Malaise, chills, and fever with extreme weakness and fatigue are common manifestations.

Interprofessional Care

The diagnosis of neutropenia is made based on the patient's manifestations, risk factors, and the CBC. The total WBC is low, often $<1000/mm^3$.

Hematopoietic growth factors such as GM-CSF are administered to stimulate granulocyte maturation and differentiation. Infections are treated with antibiotic therapy. Protective isolation procedures may be initiated to prevent exposure to pathogens. When neutropenia is related to chemotherapy, cancer treatment often must be halted, at least temporarily, to allow the bone marrow to recover.

Nursing Care

The primary nursing care focus is early identification of neutropenia and protecting the patient from infection. The

WBC count is monitored on a regular basis and any decline reported to the healthcare provider. Protective isolation may be indicated, including restricting the number of visitors and people with apparent illness. See the entry on reducing risk for infection in the earlier section on leukemia for specific nursing interventions for the patient with neutropenia.

The Patient with Infectious Mononucleosis

Infectious mononucleosis is characterized by invasion of B cells in the oropharyngeal lymphoid tissues by the Epstein-Barr virus (EBV). This disease is usually benign and self-limiting. It often affects young adults between the ages of 15 and 30. Although many children are infected with EBV, symptomatic infectious mononucleosis is uncommon in early childhood. The virus is present in saliva, which appears to be the primary mode of transmission. As a result, infectious mononucleosis is sometimes called the "kissing disease."

EBV is also associated with some cancers, including Burkitt lymphoma and Hodgkin disease, B-cell lymphoma, and nasopharyngeal carcinoma.

Pathophysiology

When the virus enters the body, unaffected B cells produce antibodies against the virus, and T cells directly attack the virus. Infected B cells are destroyed as the virus replicates. The proliferation of B and T cells, as well as the removal of dead and damaged leukocytes, is responsible for the swelling of lymphoid tissues.

Manifestations

The incubation period for infectious mononucleosis is 4 to 8 weeks. Its onset is insidious, with headache, malaise, and fatigue. Fever, sore throat, and cervical lymphadenopathy (lymph node enlargement and pain) lasting 1 to 3 weeks are common. Symptom severity varies from person to person. Lymph node involvement may be generalized with some developing splenomegaly (enlarged spleen).

Interprofessional and Nursing Care

Laboratory findings include increased lymphocytes and monocytes, with about 20% of the cells atypical in form. Early in the infection, the WBC count is usually normal or low, but by the second week it increases and remains elevated for 4 to 8 weeks. Platelet counts are often low during the illness.

Recovery occurs in 2 to 3 weeks; however, debility and lethargy may last for up to 3 months. The treatment includes bedrest and analgesic agents to alleviate the symptoms. Nursing care is primarily educational to prevent further spread of the disease.

33.4 Platelet and Coagulation Disorders

Platelet and coagulation disorders affect **hemostasis**, control of bleeding. Hemostasis maintains a relatively steady state of blood volume, blood pressure, and blood flow through injured vessels. Bleeding disorders result from deficient platelets, disruption of the clotting cascade, or a combination of factors.

The Patient with Thrombocytopenia

Thrombocytopenia is a platelet count of < 100,000 per milliliter of blood. It can lead to abnormal bleeding. A continuing decline in circulating platelets to < 20,000/mL can lead to spontaneous bleeding and hemorrhage from minor trauma (**Figure 33.14** ■). Bleeding due to platelet deficiency usually occurs in small vessels, causing manifestations such as *petechiae* and *purpura*. The mucous membranes of the nose, mouth, GI tract, and vagina often bleed. Serious and potentially fatal bleeding occurs when the platelet count is < 10,000/mL.

Thrombocytopenia results from one of three mechanisms: Decreased production, increased sequestration in the spleen, or accelerated destruction. Primary thrombocytopenia that leads to increased platelet destruction is discussed next. Secondary thrombocytopenia may be caused by aplastic anemia, bone marrow malignancy, infection, radiation therapy, or drug therapy (**Box 33.6**). Heparin therapy is the most common drug-induced thrombocytopenia; it is included in the discussion that follows. Platelet sequestration is usually due to an enlarged spleen. Up to 90% of platelets may be removed from circulation with significant splenomegaly (Sorenson et al., 2019). Finally, thrombocytopenia may result from premature platelet destruction associated with disseminated intravascular coagulation (DIC).

Physiology Review

Effective control of bleeding requires a series of complex interactions between the damaged tissue and blood vessel, platelets, clotting factors, and processes to dissolve clots once bleeding has been controlled. Platelets are formed in the bone marrow under control of thrombopoietin, a protein produced by the liver, kidney, smooth muscle, and bone marrow. Platelets are attracted to the damaged vessel wall, where they aggregate and release mediators that activate

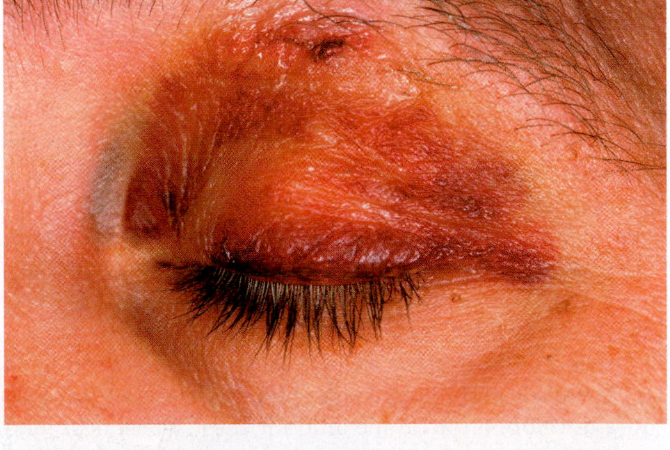

Figure 33.14 ■ Significant ecchymosis of the eyelid associated with minor trauma in a patient with thrombocytopenia.

BOX 33.6
Selected Causes of Secondary Thrombocytopenia

DISEASES

- Vitamin B_{12} anemia
- Folic acid anemia
- Aplastic anemia
- Leukemia
- Alcoholism
- DIC
- Infectious mononucleosis
- Viral infections
- HIV

DRUGS

- Thiazide diuretics
- Aspirin
- Ibuprofen
- Indomethacin
- Naproxen
- Sulfonamides
- Phenytoin
- Cimetidine
- Digoxin
- Furosemide
- Heparin
- Morphine

TREATMENTS

- Radiation therapy
- Chemotherapy
- Massive transfusion of stored blood

the clotting process. Refer to Chapter 29 for a more complete discussion about platelets, clotting, and hemostasis.

Pathophysiology and Manifestations

The two types of primary thrombocytopenia are immune thrombocytopenic purpura and thrombotic thrombocytopenic purpura.

Immune Thrombocytopenic Purpura

Immune thrombocytopenic purpura (ITP), also known as *idiopathic thrombocytopenic purpura*, is an autoimmune disorder in which platelet destruction is accelerated. In ITP, proteins on the platelet cell membrane stimulate autoantibody production, usually IgG antibodies. These autoantibodies adhere to the platelet membrane. Although the platelets function normally, the spleen reacts to them as being foreign and destroys the altered platelets after only 1 to 3 days of circulation.

The manifestations of ITP are due to bleeding from small vessels and mucous membranes. Petechiae and purpura develop, often on the anterior chest, arms, neck, and oral mucous membranes. Bruising may also be apparent. As bleeding progresses, epistaxis (nosebleed), hematuria, excess menstrual bleeding, and bleeding gums occur. Spontaneous intracranial bleeding is rare but does occur. Associated symptoms include weight loss, fever, and headache.

Acute ITP affects people of any age following a viral illness. Acute ITP typically lasts only 1 to 2 months, resolving without long-term consequences. In its chronic form, ITP typically affects adults between the ages of 20 and 50; women are affected more often than men. Its onset is insidious. Chronic (or adult) ITP often occurs in people with other immune-associated disorders such as systemic lupus erythematosus or HIV.

Thrombotic Thrombocytopenic Purpura

Thrombotic thrombocytopenic purpura (TTP) is a rare disorder in which thrombi occlude arterioles and capillaries of the microcirculation. Many organs are affected, including the heart, kidneys, and brain. The incidence of TTP is increasing (Sorenson et al., 2019). Its cause is unknown. Platelet aggregation is a key feature of the disorder. As RBCs circulate through partially occluded vessels, they fragment, leading to hemolytic anemia.

TTP may be acute, the more common and severe form, or chronic. Acute idiopathic TTP may be fatal within months if untreated. The manifestations of TTP include purpura and petechiae and neurologic symptoms such as headache, seizures, and altered consciousness.

Heparin-Induced Thrombocytopenia

Heparin-induced thrombocytopenia (HIT) develops as a result of an abnormal response to heparin therapy. Unfractionated heparin carries a greater potential to precipitate HIT; it can, however, develop in patients receiving low-molecular-weight heparin who have previously been treated with unfractionated heparin. Refer to Chapter 32 for further discussion of heparin therapy and the forms of heparin.

Heparin is a protein that occurs naturally in human tissues and inflammatory cells. It can react directly with platelets, causing them to agglutinate (clump) and be removed from circulation by phagocytosis. This form of HIT, called type I HIT, typically causes mild thrombocytopenia. The more severe form, type II HIT, results from an immune reaction to heparin. In type II HIT, heparin forms an immune complex with a platelet protein known as platelet factor 4 (PF4). This complex acts as a foreign antigen in some patients, stimulating antibody production. The antibody binds with the heparin–PF4 complex, and these antibody–heparin–PF4 complexes subsequently bind with circulating platelets, causing them to aggregate. As affected platelets aggregate, they are removed from circulation, leading to thrombocytopenia. In addition, small pieces of platelets can break loose, stimulating the clotting cascade and the development of thrombosis (clotting). The thrombocytopenia and the thrombosis can be reversed by prompt withdrawal of heparin therapy.

Despite thrombocytopenia, bleeding is usually a manifestation of HIT, probably because of the increased tendency to form clots. The patient may develop manifestations of an arterial thrombosis (severe pain, paresthesias, pallor and cool skin temperature, and pulselessness distal to the arterial occlusion) or of venous thrombosis (edema, redness, and warmth of the affected area). On rare occasions, an intravenous bolus of unfractionated heparin can precipitate an acute inflammatory response with manifestations that may mimic an acute pulmonary embolism—fever, chills, hypertension, tachycardia, dyspnea, chest pain, and cardiopulmonary arrest.

Interprofessional Care

The diagnosis of thrombocytopenia is based on history, manifestations, and diagnostic test results. Management focuses on treating or removing any causative factors and treating the platelet deficiency.

Diagnosis

The following diagnostic tests are used to identify thrombocytopenia:

- ***CBC with platelet count*** is done to evaluate blood cell counts, hemoglobin, and hematocrit.
- ***Antinuclear antibodies (ANA)*** are measured to assess for autoantibodies and identify possible contributing disorders such as systemic lupus erythematosus.
- ***Serologic studies*** for hepatitis viruses, cytomegalovirus (CMV), EBV, toxoplasma, and HIV may be done. Serologic testing may also be performed when HIT is suspected.
- ***Bone marrow examination*** evaluates for aplastic anemia and megakaryocyte production.

Medications

Oral glucocorticoids, such as prednisone, are prescribed to suppress the autoimmune response. Many patients who respond to glucocorticoid treatment relapse when the drug is withdrawn, however. Immunosuppressive drugs such as azathioprine, cyclophosphamide, and cyclosporine may be used.

Prompt withdrawal of heparin therapy is vital when HIT is the cause of thrombocytopenia. All sources of heparin are removed, including heparin used to flush intravenous or other catheters and heparin-coated catheters. A nonheparin anticoagulant such as lepirudin (Refludan) or argatroban may be substituted. Lepirudin is a thrombin inhibitor. It is a recombinant form of hirudin, originally isolated from the salivary glands of leeches. Its primary adverse effect is bleeding; as a protein, it can also stimulate antibody development, resulting in rare instances of anaphylaxis. Argatroban is a synthetic direct thrombin inhibitor with a short half-life. It clears quickly when the infusion is discontinued, an advantage if excessive bleeding develops or invasive procedures must be performed (Adams et al., 2018; Shields et al., 2018).

Treatments

Platelet transfusions may be required to treat acute bleeding due to thrombocytopenia. Platelets are prepared from fresh whole blood; one unit contains 30 to 60 mL of platelet concentrate. The expected increase in platelets after one unit is infused is 10,000/mL. *Plasmapheresis*, or *plasma exchange therapy*, is the primary treatment for acute thrombotic thrombocytopenic purpura. The patient's plasma is removed and replaced with fresh frozen plasma to remove autoantibodies, immune complexes, and toxins.

Surgery

A *splenectomy* (surgical removal of the spleen) is the treatment of choice if the patient with ITP relapses when glucocorticoids are discontinued. The spleen is the site of platelet destruction and antibody production. This surgery often cures the disorder, although relapse may occur years after splenectomy.

Nursing Care

Assessment

See the Manifestations and Interprofessional Care sections for the assessment of the patient with thrombocytopenia.

- ***Health history:*** Complaints of bruising with minor or no trauma, bleeding gums, nosebleed, heavy or prolonged menstrual periods; black, tarry, or bloody stools; hematemesis, headache, fever, or neurologic symptoms; recent weight loss; recent viral or other illness; current and recent medications; exposure to toxins; previous exposure to heparin
- ***Physical assessment:*** Skin and mucous membranes for color, temperature, petechiae, purpura, or bruises; vital signs; weight; mental status and level of consciousness; heart and breath sounds; abdominal exam; body fluids for occult blood
- ***Laboratory data:*** CBC, hemoglobin and hematocrit, platelet count; serologic and ANA test results; bone marrow examination results.

Priorities of Care

Collaborating with the interprofessional team to ensure adequate treatment of the underlying process while providing care that supports the physical and psychologic responses to the disorder is a priority of nursing care.

Diagnoses, Outcomes, and Interventions

Inadequate platelets impair hemostasis, placing the patient at risk for bleeding. Bleeding gums, an early sign of the disorder, affect oral mucous membrane integrity as well.

Reduce Risk of Bleeding. Bleeding is a serious complication associated with thrombocytopenia. As platelet counts (measured in cubic millimeters) decrease, the risk of bleeding increases: The risk is minimal with counts > 50,000 mm^3; moderate when the count is between 20,000 and 50,000 mm^3; and significant when the count falls below 20,000 mm^3.

Expected Outcome: Patient will remain free of any evidence of new bleeding and take precautions to prevent bleeding.

The nurse will:

- Monitor vital signs, heart, and breath sounds every 4 hours. Frequently assess for other manifestations of bleeding:
  a. Skin and mucous membranes for petechiae, ecchymoses, and hematoma formation
  b. Gums, nasal membranes, and conjunctiva for bleeding
  c. Overt or occult blood in emesis, urine, or stool

d. Vaginal bleeding
e. Prolonged bleeding from puncture sites
f. Neurologic changes: Headache, visual changes, altered mental status, decreasing level of consciousness, seizures
g. Abdominal: Epigastric pain, absence of bowel sounds, increasing abdominal girth, abdominal guarding or rigidity.

Early identification of bleeding is important to prevent serious blood loss and shock.

SAFETY ALERT: Avoid invasive procedures such as rectal temperatures, urinary catheterization, and parenteral injections to the extent possible. Diagnostic procedures such as biopsy or lumbar puncture should be avoided if the platelet count is $< 50{,}000$ mm^3. Invasive procedures can cause tissue trauma and bleeding. Procedures that use large-bore needles should be delayed until the platelet count is increased. ■

- Apply pressure to puncture sites for 3 to 5 minutes; apply pressure to arterial blood gas sites for 15 to 20 minutes. *Pressure promotes hemostasis and clot formation.*
- Instruct to avoid forcefully blowing the nose or picking crusts from the nose, straining to have a bowel movement, and forceful coughing or sneezing. *These activities increase the risk of external and internal bleeding.*

Promote Oral Membrane Health. Thrombocytopenia frequently leads to bleeding of the gums and oral mucosa. As a result, risk for infection and impaired nutrition increases.

Expected Outcome: Patient will maintain intact, moist oral mucous membranes through use of measures to promote oral membrane health.

The nurse will:

- Frequently assess the mouth for bleeding. Inquire about oral pain or tenderness. *Breakdown of oral mucous membranes increases the risk of infection and bleeding and causes discomfort with eating.*
- Encourage use of a soft-bristle toothbrush or sponge to clean teeth and gums. *Hard bristles may abrade oral mucosa, causing bleeding and increasing the risk of infection.*
- Instruct to rinse the mouth with saline every 2 to 4 hours. Apply petroleum jelly to lips as needed to prevent dryness and cracking. *Saline mouth rinses and petroleum jelly help maintain oral tissue integrity and promote cleansing and healing.*
- Instruct to avoid alcohol-based mouthwashes, very hot foods, alcohol, and crusty foods. Teach to drink cool liquids at least every 2 hours. *Avoiding foods and liquids that traumatize oral mucosa increases comfort; fluid intake prevents dehydration and helps maintain mucous membrane integrity.*

Transitions of Care

There are no risk factors that can be addressed to prevent the development of ITP. However, complications can be prevented.

Acute treatment of ITP focuses on increasing the platelet count to improve clotting and reducing risk of haemorrhage. Some patients experience a spontaneous remission. Others must learn to manage ITP as a chronic illness.

In the adult, ITP often is a chronic disorder that the patient and family must learn to manage. Secondary thrombocytopenia may be either acute or chronic. Discuss the following topics when preparing the patient and family for home care:

- Nature of the disorder, its usual course, and the treatment plan
- Use and desired and potential adverse effects of prescribed medications
- Risks and benefits of surgery or treatments such as plasma replacement therapy
- The importance of follow-up tests and visits for care
- Measures to reduce the risk of bleeding: Safety measures such as use of a soft-bristle toothbrush and electric razor, avoidance of contact sports and hazardous activities, and avoidance of medications that further interfere with platelet function (**Box 33.7**)

BOX 33.7
Medications That May Interfere with Platelet Function

OVER-THE-COUNTER MEDICATIONS

- Aspirin and salicylates, including:
  a. Alka-Seltzer
  b. Bufferin
  c. Doan's Pills
  d. Ecotrin
  e. Excedrin
  f. Midol
  g. Pepto-Bismol
  h. Vanquish
- NSAIDs such as:
  a. Advil
  b. Aleve
  c. Nuprin
  d. Pamprin IB

PRESCRIPTION MEDICATIONS

- Aspirin-containing analgesics
- Chemotherapy drugs
- Antibiotics such as penicillin
- Carbamazepine (Tegretol)
- Colchicine
- Dipyridamole (Persantine)
- Gold salts
- Heparin
- Quinine derivatives
- Sulfonamides
- Thiazide diuretics

Refer for home health or other community services (e.g., housekeeping, shopping) as indicated.

The Patient with Hemophilia

Hemophilia is a group of hereditary clotting factor disorders that lead to persistent and sometimes severe bleeding (see the accompanying Genetic Considerations box). Although often considered a disease of children, hemophilia may be diagnosed in adults. Deficiencies of three clotting factors, VIII, IX, and XI, account for 90 to 95% of the bleeding disorders collectively called *hemophilia* (Sorenson et al., 2019).

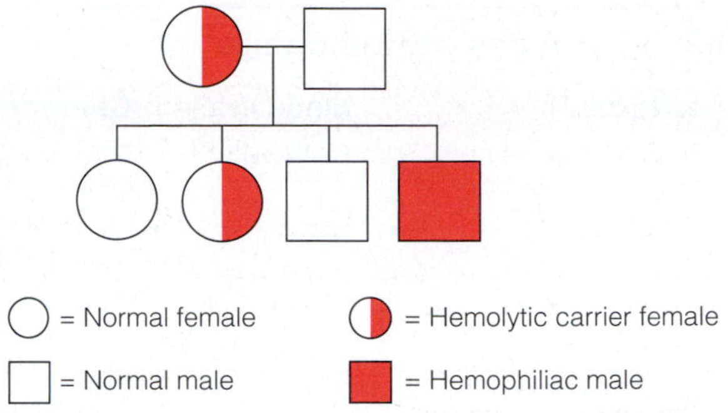
= Normal female
= Hemolytic carrier female
= Normal male
= Hemophiliac male

Figure 33.15 ■ The inheritance pattern of hemophilia A and B. Both are transmitted as X-linked recessive disorders. Females may be carriers, but only males develop these disorders.

Genetic Considerations

Focus on Hemophilia

The incidence and pattern of inheritance for the forms of hemophilia differ:

- Hemophilia A occurs in about 1 in 10,000 male births, transmitted on the X chromosome. Each male offspring has a 50% risk of inheriting the defective gene; each female offspring has a 50% risk of becoming a carrier.
- Hemophilia B occurs in about 1 in 100,000 male births, transmitted on the X chromosome.
- Von Willebrand disease affects about 1 in 100 to 500 people, usually inherited as an autosomal dominant trait: Offspring of an affected person have a 50% risk of inheriting the trait and the disorder.
- Factor XI deficiency is inherited as an autosomal recessive trait: Each offspring of a carrier and an unaffected individual has a 50% risk of inheriting the trait; each offspring of two carriers has a 50% risk of being a carrier and a 25% risk of having the disorder. This deficiency is common in Ashkenazi Jews.

Physiology Review

When tissue injury occurs, platelets collect at the site, adhering to the damaged vessel wall (the platelet plug). Activation of the clotting cascade, a sequential process of interactive reactions of clotting factors, is vital to form a stable clot. Clotting factors are plasma proteins primarily produced by the liver. A number of these factors require the presence of vitamin K for synthesis and activation. Once the clot has been formed and stabilized, it begins to retract, pulling together the edges of the damaged blood vessel to initiate the healing process.

Pathophysiology

Hemophilia A (or *classic hemophilia*) is the most common type of hemophilia, caused by deficiency or dysfunction of clotting factor VIII. It is transmitted as an X-linked recessive disorder from mothers to sons (**Figure 33.15** ■). The genetic defect of hemophilia A on the X chromosome may cause deficient Factor VIII production or a defective form of the protein. When the concentration of the clotting factor is 5 to 35% of normal, the disease is mild. Bleeding is infrequent and usually associated with trauma. Concentrations of 1 to 5% of normal result in moderate disease. Again, bleeding usually occurs secondarily to trauma. Severe hemophilia occurs when concentrations are less than 1% of normal. Bleeding is frequent, often occurring without trauma (Sorenson et al., 2019).

Hemophilia B (also called *Christmas disease*) accounts for about 15% of cases and is caused by a deficiency in Factor IX. Despite the difference in clotting factor deficits, hemophilia A and B are clinically identical.

Von Willebrand disease, often considered a type of hemophilia, is the most common hereditary bleeding disorder (Sorenson et al., 2019). It is caused by a deficit of or defective von Willebrand (vW) factor, a protein that mediates platelet adhesion. Reduced levels of Factor VIII are often also present because vW factor carries Factor VIII. This clotting disorder affects men and women equally. Bleeding associated with von Willebrand disease is rarely severe. It is often diagnosed when prolonged bleeding follows surgery or a dental extraction.

Factor XI deficiency (or *hemophilia C*) is usually a mild disorder, identified when postoperative bleeding is prolonged. A comparison of the types of hemophilia is found in **Table 33.9**.

People with hemophilia form a platelet plug at the site of bleeding, but the clotting factor deficit impairs formation of a stable fibrin clot. The effect of vW factor deficiency is somewhat different, in that platelet aggregation at the site of injury is impaired. In either case, prolonged or extensive bleeding may result. Often bleeding occurs in response to injury or as a result of surgery. However, a severe clotting factor deficit can lead to spontaneous bleeding into the joints (*hemarthrosis*), deep tissues, and CNS. Hemarthrosis often causes joint deformity and disability, usually of the elbows, hips, knees, and ankles.

Manifestations

The following are manifestations of hemophilia:

- Hemarthrosis
- Easy bruising and cutaneous hematoma formation with minor trauma (e.g., an injection)
- Bleeding from the gums and prolonged bleeding following minor injuries or cuts

Table 33.9 Types of Hemophilia

Type/Name	Deficiency	Characteristics	Treatment
Hemophilia A (classic hemophilia)	Factor VIII	Transmitted by females; occurs primarily in males; bleeding time normal; coagulation time prolonged	Factor VIII concentrate or cryoprecipitate
Hemophilia B	Factor IX	Transmitted by females; occurs primarily in males; bleeding time normal; coagulation time prolonged	Factor IX (Christmas disease concentrate)
Von Willebrand disease	vW Factor VIII	Occurs in both females and males; bleeding time and coagulation time are both prolonged	Cryoprecipitate and DDAVP
Factor XI deficiency	Factor XI	Occurs in both males and females; activated partial thromboplastin time (aPTT) is prolonged	Fresh frozen plasma

- GI bleeding, with hematemesis (vomiting blood), occult blood in the stools, gastric pain, or abdominal pain
- Spontaneous hematuria or epistaxis (nosebleed)
- Pain or paralysis due to the pressure of hematomas on nerves.

Intracranial hemorrhage is a potentially life-threatening manifestation of hemophilia.

Interprofessional Care

Treatment of hemophilia focuses on preventing and/or treating bleeding, primarily by replacing deficient clotting factors. Specific treatment depends on the severity of the disorder and the specific factor deficiency. Care may be complicated by hepatitis or HIV disease in people with hemophilia treated with clotting factor concentrates prepared from multiple units of donated blood. Today, routine testing of all blood, improved blood donor screening, and current methods of treating hemophilia have significantly reduced the risk for these bloodborne diseases.

Diagnosis

The following laboratory tests may be ordered:

- *Serum platelet levels* are measured and are usually normal.
- *Coagulation studies* such as aPTT, bleeding time, and prothrombin time are used to screen for hemophilia when abnormal bleeding occurs. The activated PTT is increased in all types of hemophilia. Prothrombin time is unaffected in these disorders but may be measured to rule out other disorders. Bleeding time is prolonged in von Willebrand's disease but normal in hemophilia A and B (Kee, 2014).
- *Factor assays* are performed; Factor VIII is decreased in hemophilia A and often in von Willebrand's disease, Factor IX is decreased in hemophilia B and Factor XI in hemophilia C.
- *Amniocentesis* or *chorionic villus sampling* is used to identify the genetic defect of hemophilia when there is a known family history of the disease.

Medications

Deficient clotting factors are replaced regularly, as a prophylactic measure before surgery and dental procedures and to control bleeding. Clotting factors may be given as fresh frozen plasma, cryoprecipitates, or concentrates. Factor levels are measured on a regular basis to determine whether the treatment is adequate. Clotting factors are often self-administered and may be taken on either a regular or intermittent schedule.

Fresh frozen plasma replaces all clotting factors (including both Factor VIII and Factor IX) except platelets. When the cause of bleeding is not yet determined, fresh frozen plasma may be administered intravenously until a definitive diagnosis is made.

Hemophilia A is usually treated with either heat-treated Factor VIII concentrate (heat treating reduces the risk of transmitting disease) or recombinant Factor VIII. Although recombinant Factor VIII, produced using recombinant DNA technology, eliminates the risk of viral disease transmission, its use is limited by cost. The dose of Factor VIII is determined by the severity of the deficit and the presence or prospect of active bleeding (e.g., planned surgery).

Desmopressin acetate (DDAVP, Stimate) may be given to people with mild hemophilia A or von Willebrand's disease prior to minor surgeries. This drug causes release of Factor VIII and will raise blood levels by two- or threefold for several hours, reducing the risk of bleeding and the need for clotting factor concentrate (Shields et al., 2018).

Factor IX concentrate (administered intravenously) is used to treat hemophilia B. Because Factor IX concentrates also contain a number of other proteins, there is risk of thrombosis with recurrent use. They are used judiciously, only when needed. Products produced by recombinant technology or that are monoclonally purified carry a lower risk of stimulating thrombus formation (Shields et al., 2018). Fresh frozen plasma replaces Factor XI and is used when necessary. It may be given daily until the risk for bleeding decreases.

Factor VIII concentrates contain functional vW factor, and may be used to treat von Willebrand's disease. Aspirin is avoided in all types of hemophilia.

Nursing Care

Although primary responsibility for care falls to the patient and family, nursing care presents challenges. For additional assessment and nursing care strategies, see the accompanying Case Study & Nursing Care Plan.

Assessment

Whereas severe hemophilia is usually diagnosed in childhood, milder cases may not be identified until surgery, invasive dental work, or a traumatic injury causes extensive or prolonged bleeding.

See the Manifestations and Interprofessional Care sections for the assessment of the patient with hemophilia.

Focused assessment related to hemophilia includes:

- ***Health history:*** Previous bleeding episodes with or without trauma; history of easy bruising, hematomas, epistaxis, bleeding gums, hematuria, vomiting blood, or joint pain; aspirin use; family history of hemophilia or bleeding disorders
- ***Physical assessment:*** Vital signs; bruising or bleeding of skin or mucous membranes; mental status; abdominal assessment; presence of joint deformity, decreased range of motion
- ***Laboratory data:*** CBC including hemoglobin, hematocrit, and platelet count; clotting factor assays; tests for occult blood (urine, stool, emesis); x-ray and scan results for evidence of bleeding.

Priorities of Care

Collaborating with the interprofessional team to ensure adequate treatment of the underlying process while providing care that supports the physical and psychologic responses to the disorder is a priority of nursing care.

Diagnoses, Outcomes, and Interventions

Impaired blood clotting, the need for continuing care and disease management, and the risk for genetic transmission of hemophilia are priority problems for the patient with hemophilia.

Reduce Risk of Bleeding. The inability to form stable clots and stem bleeding from injured blood vessels creates a significant risk for the patient with hemophilia. Nursing care measures focus on preventing injury and protecting the skin from damage.

Expected Outcome: Patient will remain free of any evidence of new bleeding and take precautions to prevent bleeding.

The nurse will:

- Monitor for signs of bleeding, including hematomas, ecchymoses, and purpura, as well as surface oozing or bleeding. Check emesis and stool for occult blood. *Bleeding may occur in cutaneous tissues as well as internal organs. Bleeding in the upper GI tract may not be readily apparent in the stool.*
- Notify the healthcare provider of any apparent bleeding. *Prompt intervention with administration of clotting factor concentrate decreases the risk of hemorrhage and subsequent hypovolemia.*
- Avoid intramuscular injections, rectal temperatures, and enemas. *These can pose a risk of tissue and vascular trauma, which can precipitate bleeding.*
- Use safety measures in personal care. For example, use an electric razor rather than a razor blade to shave. *Use of an electric razor minimizes the opportunity to develop superficial cuts that may result in bleeding.*
- If bleeding occurs, control blood loss using gentle pressure, ice, or a topical hemostatic agent, such as an absorbable gelatin sponge, microfibrillar collagen hemostat, or topical thrombin. *Direct pressure occludes bleeding vessels. Ice, a vasoconstrictor, may facilitate bleeding control, as do topical hemostatic agents.*
- Instruct to avoid activities that increase the risk of trauma, including contact sports, physical exertion associated with job performance, and to eliminate safety hazards in the home. *Depending on the severity of the clotting factor deficit, even minor trauma can lead to serious bleeding episodes. Safer activities such as noncontact sports (e.g., swimming, golf) and occupations that do not require physical labor may be substituted.*

Promote Health Maintenance. Hemophilia is a chronic disorder, requiring active management to prevent and control bleeding and complications. Frequent visits to the healthcare provider or clinic may be necessary. In addition, the patient may need to learn to self-administer clotting factors and measures to prevent complications. The lifelong nature of the disorder may interfere with compliance, especially during early adulthood.

Expected Outcome: Patient will be knowledgeable about management of hemophilia as evidenced by being able to describe the components and rationale for the treatment plan.

The nurse will:

- Assess knowledge of disorder and the related treatments. *Assessment allows identification of knowledge gaps and provides a basis on which to provide additional information. Impaired disease management may be due to lack of knowledge or a conscious decision not to follow the recommendations of the healthcare provider.*
- Provide information about the bleeding disorder and prescribed medications and treatments. *Individualized instruction is more effective than general, possibly irrelevant information.*
- Provide emotional support, expressing confidence in the patient's self-care abilities. *Emotional support helps the patient incorporate the care regimen into his or her lifestyle.*
- Provide supervised learning and practice opportunities for administering clotting factors and topical hemostatic agents. *Successful practice sessions instill confidence in the ability to manage care and provide an opportunity for questions and exploring alternatives.*

Transitions of Care

Encourage patients with a family history of hemophilia or bleeding disorders to seek genetic counseling during their family planning process. Although tests are available for the hemophilia gene, the technology to correct the disorder in utero does not yet exist. Refer to Chapter 8.

Acute management of a hemophilia crisis focuses on control of bleeding primarily by replacing deficient clotting factors. Close nursing assessment and surveillance is essential. Discuss the following topics when preparing the patient with a bleeding disorder and the family for home care:

- Recognizing the manifestations of internal bleeding: Pallor, weakness, restlessness, headache, disorientation, pain, swelling. These manifestations require emergency medical care and should be reported immediately.
- Applying cold packs and immobilizing the joint for 24 to 48 hours if hemarthrosis occurs.
- Using analgesics for pain; avoiding prescription and over-the-counter drugs containing aspirin.
- Ensuring a safe home environment (e.g., padding sharp edges of furniture, using transition lighting or a nightlight; avoiding scatter rugs; and wearing protective gloves when working in the house or yard).
- Using safe grooming practices such as electric razors.
- Wearing a medical alert bracelet in case of accident.
- Practicing good dental hygiene to decrease potential tooth decay and extractions. If dental procedures are necessary, discuss the need for prophylactic factor administration with the dentist and healthcare provider.
- Following safer-sex practices.
- Preparing and administering intravenous medications.

Refer the patient and family to a local hemophilia or bleeding disorders support group. Provide contact information for national organizations and information clearinghouses, such as the National Hemophilia Foundation.

Case Study & Nursing Care Plan

A Patient with Hemophilia

Jermiel Cruise is a 20-year-old student at a community college. He is admitted to the emergency department with a nosebleed that began when he fell during a touch football game. It has continued to bleed for over an hour.

ASSESSMENT	DIAGNOSES	EXPECTED OUTCOMES
Mr. Cruise states that he has hemophilia and realizes that playing contact sports "is probably a dumb thing to do." He adds that he has not had any recent bleeding episodes. An ice bag and manual pressure are applied in the emergency department. The healthcare provider orders Factor VIII concentrate to be administered. Physical assessment findings are T 36.2°C (97.2°F), BP 118/64 mmHg, P 78 BPM, R 18/min. Skin is pale but warm. Laboratory tests reveal a prolonged aPTT and a normal bleeding time and PT. Following treatment, Mr. Cruise's bleeding subsides.	■ Noncompliance with activity recommendations ■ Ineffectual defenses related to lack of clotting factor VIII	■ Patient will exhibit no further signs of bleeding. ■ Patient will maintain vital signs within his usual range. ■ Patient will maintain an open airway. ■ Patient will identify sports and recreation activities in which he can safely participate. ■ Patient will verbalize self-care measures to control bleeding.

PLANNING AND IMPLEMENTATION

- Monitor vital signs and for further signs of bleeding.
- Assess airway and auscultate breath sounds.
- Review emergency measures to help stop bleeding.
- Reiterate the importance of seeking prompt medical attention if bleeding should occur.
- Advise regarding the importance of wearing a medical alert bracelet identifying him as a hemophiliac.
- Discuss alternative noncontact sports and recreational activities.

EVALUATION

On discharge, Mr. Cruise has no further signs of bleeding, shock, or aspiration. He is able to verbalize methods to help stop local bleeding and the importance of seeking medical attention promptly when bleeding continues. Mr. Cruise agrees to stop at a local drugstore on the way home to order a medical alert bracelet. In addition, Mr. Cruise verbalizes an understanding of the importance of avoiding contact sports and has identified swimming and golf as alternative leisure activities that he might enjoy.

CLINICAL REASONING IN PATIENT CARE

1. What is the pathophysiologic basis for the bleeding that occurs in hemophilia A and B?
2. What was Mr. Cruise's priority nursing diagnosis? Why?
3. Why is family planning a special consideration with a patient who has hemophilia?
4. Outline a plan to teach the family of a patient diagnosed with hemophilia how to administer an intravenous infusion.
5. Develop a care plan for Mr. Cruise for the nursing diagnosis of noncompliance. Consider Mr. Cruise's age and developmental level in creating the plan.

See Evaluating Your Response in Appendix B.

The Patient with Disseminated Intravascular Coagulation

Disseminated intravascular coagulation (DIC) is a disruption of hemostasis characterized by widespread intravascular clotting and bleeding. It may be acute and life-threatening or relatively mild. DIC is a clinical syndrome that develops as a complication of a wide variety of other disorders (**Box 33.8**). Sepsis is the most common cause of DIC. Gram-negative and gram-positive bacteria as well as viruses, fungi, and protozoal infections may lead to DIC (Sorenson et al., 2019).

Pathophysiology

DIC is triggered by endothelial damage, release of tissue factors into the circulation, or inappropriate activation of the clotting cascade by an endotoxin. Both the intrinsic and the extrinsic clotting cascade may be activated, although the extrinsic cascade is usually the one activated. Extensive thrombin entering the systemic circulation overwhelms natural anticoagulants, leading to unrestricted clot formation (Sorenson et al., 2019). Clotting may be localized to an individual organ or widespread with deposition of small thrombi and emboli throughout the microvasculature. The widespread clotting consumes clotting factors (prothrombin, platelets, Factor V, and Factor VIII in particular) and activates fibrinolytic processes with anticoagulant production. As a result, hemorrhage occurs (**Figure 33.16** ■).

The sequence of DIC follows:

1. Endothelial damage, tissue factors, or toxins stimulate the clotting cascade.
2. Excess thrombin within the circulation overwhelms naturally occurring anticoagulants.

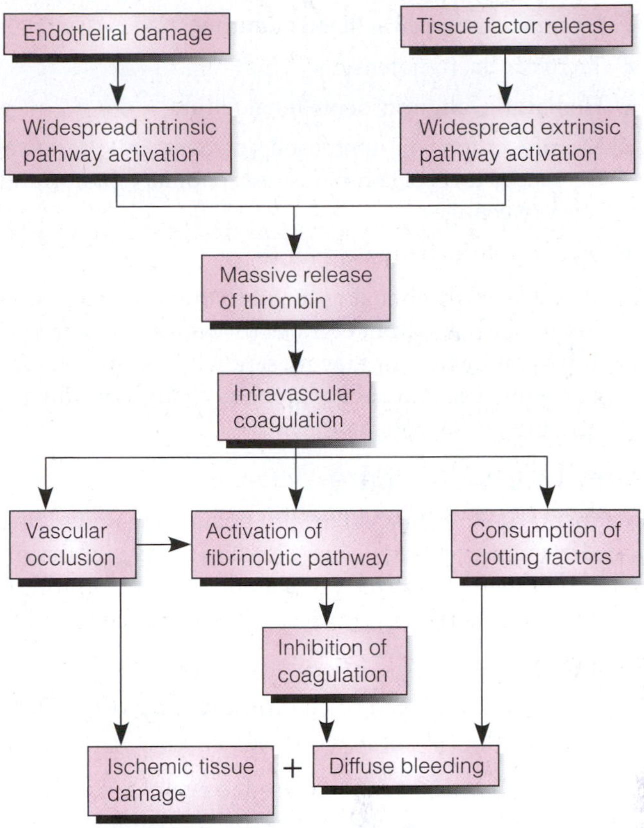
Endothelial damage
Tissue factor release
Widespread intrinsic pathway activation
Widespread extrinsic pathway activation
Massive release of thrombin
Intravascular coagulation
Vascular occlusion
Activation of fibrinolytic pathway
Consumption of clotting factors
Inhibition of coagulation
Ischemic tissue damage
+
Diffuse bleeding

Figure 33.16 ■ Disseminated intravascular coagulation. Endothelial cell injury or release of tissue factors activates the intrinsic or extrinsic clotting pathway (or both). As a result, numerous microthrombi form throughout the vasculature, causing ischemic tissue damage. Simultaneously, rapid consumption of clotting factors and activation of fibrinolytic mechanisms trigger widespread bleeding.

3. Widespread clotting occurs within the microvasculature.
4. Thrombi and emboli impair tissue perfusion, leading to ischemia, infarction, and necrosis.
5. Clotting factors and platelets are consumed faster than they can be replaced.
6. Clotting activates fibrinolytic processes that begin to break down clots.
7. Fibrin degradation products (FDPs; potent anticoagulants) are released, contributing to bleeding.
8. Clotting factors are depleted, the ability to form clots is lost, and hemorrhage occurs.

BOX 33.8
Conditions That May Precipitate Disseminated Intravascular Coagulation

TISSUE DAMAGE

- Trauma: Burns, gunshot wounds, frostbite, head injury
- Obstetric complications: Septic abortion, abruptio placentae, amniotic fluid embolus, retained dead fetus
- Neoplasms: Acute leukemia, adenocarcinomas
- Hemolysis
- Fat embolism

VESSEL DAMAGE

- Aortic aneurysm
- Acute glomerulonephritis
- Hemolytic uremic syndrome

INFECTIONS

- Bacterial infection or sepsis
- Viral or mycotic infections
- Parasitic or rickettsial infection

Manifestations

The manifestations of DIC result from both clotting and bleeding, although bleeding is more obvious, especially in acute DIC. Manifestations include:

- Frank hemorrhage from incisions
- Oozing of blood from punctures, intravenous catheter sites
- Purpura, petechiae, bruising
- Cyanosis of extremities
- GI bleeding or hemorrhage

- Dyspnea, tachypnea, bloody sputum
- Tachycardia, hypotension
- Hematuria, oliguria, acute renal failure
- Manifestations of increased intracranial pressure: Decreased level of consciousness, papillary, motor, and sensory changes
- Mental status changes

Bleeding ranges from oozing blood following an injection to frank hemorrhage from every body orifice. Chronic DIC may be asymptomatic or may present with peripheral cyanosis, thrombosis, and pregangrenous changes in the fingers and toes, nose, and genitalia.

Interprofessional Care

Treatment of DIC is directed toward treating the underlying disorder and preventing further bleeding or massive thrombosis. Treatment stabilizes the patient, reduces complications, and allows recovery to occur; it does not cure DIC.

Diagnosis

Diagnostic tests are used to confirm the diagnosis of DIC and evaluate the risk for hemorrhage:

- ***CBC*** and ***platelet count*** are used to evaluate the hemoglobin, hematocrit, and number of circulating platelets. *Schistocytes*, fragmented RBCs, may be noted due to cell trapping and damage within fibrin thrombi. The platelet count is decreased.
- ***Coagulation studies*** show prolonged prothrombin time (PT), partial thromboplastin time (PTT), and thrombin time and a low fibrinogen level due to depletion of clotting factors. The fibrinogen level helps predict bleeding in DIC: As it falls, the risk of bleeding increases.
- ***Fibrin degradation products (FDPs)*** or ***fibrin split products (FSPs)*** are increased due to the fibrinolysis that occurs with DIC.

Treatments

When bleeding is the major manifestation of DIC, fresh frozen plasma and platelet concentrates are given to restore clotting factors and platelets. Heparin, although controversial, may be administered. Heparin interferes with the clotting cascade and may prevent further clotting factor consumption due to uncontrolled thrombosis. It is used when bleeding is not controlled by plasma and platelets, as well as when the patient has manifestations of thrombotic problems such as acrocyanosis and possible gangrene. Long-term heparin therapy (administered by injection or continuous infusion using a portable pump) may be necessary for patients with chronic DIC.

Nursing Care

Assessment

Nurses can be instrumental in identifying early manifestations of DIC, facilitating timely intervention. See the Manifestations and Interprofessional Care sections for the assessment of the patient with myelodysplastic syndrome.

Focused nursing assessment for DIC includes:

- ***Health history:*** Recent abortion (spontaneous or therapeutic) or current pregnancy; presence of a known malignant tumor; history of abnormal bleeding episodes or a hematologic disorder
- ***Physical assessment:*** Bleeding from puncture wounds (e.g., injections), IV sites, incisions; hematuria, obvious or occult blood in emesis or stool, epistaxis, other abnormal bleeding; vital signs; heart and breath sounds; abdominal assessment including girth, contour, bowel sounds, tenderness or guarding to palpation; color, temperature, skin condition of hands, feet, and digits; petechiae or purpura of skin, mucous membranes
- ***Laboratory data:*** CBC with hemoglobin, hematocrit; platelet count; coagulation studies; evaluations of organ system function (e.g., liver and renal function tests); CT scans of the head and abdomen.

Priorities of Care

Collaborating with the interprofessional team to ensure adequate treatment of the underlying process while providing care that supports the physical and psychologic responses to the disorder is a priority of nursing care.

Diagnoses, Outcomes, and Interventions

Patients with acute DIC are often critically ill, with multiple nursing care needs. Priority nursing diagnoses discussed in this section focus on impaired tissue perfusion and gas exchange, pain, and fear (Perrin & MacLeod, 2017). Septic shock may precipitate DIC; hemorrhagic shock may occur as a complication of DIC. Refer to Chapter 11 for nursing diagnoses and interventions related to these problems.

Promote Effective Tissue Perfusion. Thrombi and emboli forming throughout the microcirculation affect the perfusion of multiple organs and tissues. Additionally, bleeding due to clotting factor consumption affects cardiac output and blood flow to these tissues.

Expected Outcome: Patient will achieve adequate tissue perfusion as evidenced by adequate arterial flow (i.e., strong peripheral pulses) and absence of symptoms of cardiac, pulmonary, and neurologic ischemia.

The nurse will:

- Assess extremity pulses, warmth, and capillary refill. Monitor level of consciousness (LOC) and mental status. *Monitoring central and peripheral tissue perfusion facilitates early treatment of impaired perfusion.*

SAFETY ALERT: Promptly report complaints of chest pain, changes in mental status, LOC, tissue perfusion, respirations, GI function, and urinary output. Chest pain or respiratory changes (tachypnea, dyspnea, orthopnea) may be due to angina, pulmonary embolism, or bleeding into lung tissue. Changes in mentation or LOC can indicate cerebral ischemia. A painful, pale, and cold extremity with no or diminished pulses indicates arterial occlusion. Prompt intervention is critical to save the extremity. Acute abdominal pain, decreased bowel sounds, and GI bleeding may indicate mesenteric occlusion, a surgical emergency. Decreased urine output may signify renal artery thrombosis; renal failure may develop. ■

- Carefully reposition at least every 2 hours. *Position changes facilitate circulation and tissue perfusion and provide an opportunity to assess for purpura, pallor, and bleeding.*
- Discourage crossing the legs, and do not elevate the knees on the bed or with a pillow. *These positions may impair arterial and venous flow to the lower legs and feet, increasing vascular stasis and the risk for thrombosis.*
- Minimize use of tape on the skin, using binders, nonadhesive dressings, and other devices as needed. *Preventing skin trauma reduces the risk for bleeding and potential infection.*

Promote Adequate Tissue Perfusion. Microclots in the pulmonary vasculature are likely to interfere with gas exchange in the patient with DIC.

Expected Outcome: Patient will achieve adequate tissue perfusion as evidenced by adequate arterial flow as evidenced by absence of symptoms of cardiac, pulmonary, and neurologic ischemia.

The nurse will:

- Monitor oxygen saturation continuously. Administer oxygen as ordered. *Oxygen saturation levels are a noninvasive means of assessing gas exchange. Supplemental oxygen promotes gas exchange and reduces cardiac work, relieving dyspnea.*

SAFETY ALERT: Monitor arterial blood gas results; report abnormal results to the healthcare provider. Low PaO_2 and rising $PaCO_2$ levels indicate impaired gas exchange and may signify the need for additional treatment. ■

- Place in Fowler or high-Fowler position as tolerated. *Elevating the head of the bed improves diaphragmatic excursion and alveolar ventilation.*
- Maintain bedrest. *Bedrest reduces oxygen demands and cardiac work.*
- Encourage deep breathing and effective coughing. *Increased respiratory depth and clearance of secretions from airways improve alveolar ventilation and oxygenation.*
- Cautious nasotracheal suctioning may be instituted if cough is ineffective or an endotracheal tube is in place. *Removal of secretions facilitates ventilation and oxygenation. However, care must be used to minimize suction-induced hypoxia and airway trauma.*
- Administer analgesics and antianxiety drugs as needed to control pain and anxiety. Provide reassurance and comfort measures. *Pain and anxiety increase the respiratory rate and decrease the depth of respirations, reducing effective ventilation and gas exchange.*

Manage Pain. Both the underlying cause of DIC and tissue ischemia from microvascular clots can cause pain. Identifying the etiology of pain is important to identify potential complications or harmful effects of DIC and to institute effective treatment.

Expected Outcome: Patient will exhibit adequate pain control as evidenced by physical well-being.

The nurse will:

- Use a standard pain scale chart to evaluate and monitor pain and analgesic effectiveness. *Monitoring pain and the response to medication facilitates development of an appropriate and effective treatment plan.*

SAFETY ALERT: Notify the healthcare provider promptly of new or a sudden increase in pain, especially when accompanied by changes in assessment findings. New or increased complaints of pain may signify increased circulatory impairment and ischemic changes in tissues such as the heart, bowel, or extremities. Circulation to a painful, pale or cyanotic, or cold extremity may be occluded by an arterial clot. Prompt intervention is necessary to save the extremity. Acute abdominal pain may signify mesenteric occlusion, a surgical emergency. Anginal pain may indicate occlusion of coronary arteries. ■

- Handle extremities gently. *Gentle handling reduces the risk of further injury to and pain in ischemic tissues.*
- Apply cool compresses to painful joints. *Application of cold decreases pain through the gate-control mechanism, inhibiting the dorsal horn of the spinal cord and reducing the sensation of pain.*

SAFETY ALERT: Continuously monitor effects of analgesics and mental and respiratory status. Analgesics may mask manifestations of neurologic impairment due to thromboembolism and may depress the respiratory center, further impairing gas exchange. Judicious analgesic administration with careful monitoring is vital to safely provide effective pain relief. ■

Manage Fear. The underlying serious illness and a complication such as DIC result in an uncertain prognosis, often accompanied by fear.

Expected Outcome: Patient will express fears about uncertain prognosis.

The nurse will:

- Encourage the patient and family to verbalize concerns. *This helps the patient and family identify their concerns and frame questions.*
- Answer questions truthfully. *Providing honest answers is vital to developing a therapeutic nurse–patient relationship. Accurate responses allow the patient and family to set priorities as they plan for an uncertain future.*
- Help the patient and family identify coping strategies to manage this significant situational stressor. *Implementing past effective coping methods may provide the skills to manage the current crisis.*
- Provide emotional support. *The presence of a caring nurse helps reduce the fear and anxiety associated with a crisis.*
- Maintain a calm environment. *A calm environment provides reassurance that the situation is in control, reduces anxiety, and promotes rest.*
- Respond promptly when the patient calls for help. *Prompt responses to expressed needs help develop a trusting relationship and a sense of security that assistance is readily available.*

- Teach relaxation techniques. *Relaxation techniques can reduce muscle tension and other signs of anxiety. Gaining control over physical responses can help the patient gain a sense of control over the situation.*

Transitions of Care

Prevention of DIC focuses on avoiding the risk factors for its development. The risk factors are primarily severe and complicated medical conditions. These include:

- Major trauma or burns
- Severe complicated obstetric conditions
- Solid tumors and hematologic malignancies
- Severe immune reactions

There is no specific treatment for DIC. The goal is to determine and treat the underlying cause of DIC. Although the immediate crisis of acute DIC is resolved prior to discharge, the patient may have some continuing effects of the disorder, such as impaired tissue integrity of distal extremities. Teach the patient and family about specific care needs, such as foot care or dressing changes. Provide instruction about any continuing medications and follow-up care.

Patients with chronic DIC may require continuing heparin therapy, using either intermittent subcutaneous injections or a portable infusion pump. Teach the patient and family members how to administer the injection or manage the infusion pump. Provide a referral to home healthcare or a home intravenous management service for assistance. Discuss the manifestations of excessive bleeding or recurrent clotting that need to be reported to the healthcare provider.

End-of-life care for the patient with DIC focuses on control of bleeding, symptom management, and comfort measures. Family involvement is also essential. The nurse caring for the patient with DIC at end of life also provides emotional support to the patient and family members.(*continued*)

CHAPTER HIGHLIGHTS

33.1 Red Blood Cell Disorders

Describe the pathophysiology and manifestations of red blood cell disorders, and outline the interprofessional care and nursing care of patients with these disorders.

- Anemia is the most common disorder of the red blood cells; nutritional deficiencies are the most common causes of anemia. Its manifestations relate to the function of RBCs and hemoglobin, transporting oxygen to the cells: Fatigue, increased respiratory and heart rates, shortness of breath with activity, and pallor.
- Genetically transmitted disorders such as sickle cell disease and thalassemia can cause significant anemia and associated problems in affected populations. These patients require teaching and episodic acute care for crises such as vaso-occlusive crisis in sickle cell disease.
- Nursing care related to anemia is primarily educational to prepare the patient for effective self-care, including diet, prescribed medications, and measures to prevent sickling episodes (for patients with sickle cell disease).

33.2 White Blood Cell Disorders

Describe the pathophysiology and manifestations of white blood cell disorders, and outline the interprofessional care and nursing care of patients with these disorders.

- Manifestations of the leukemias reflect the altered ability of abnormal WBCs to perform effective immune surveillance and crowding of the bone marrow and other organs by rapidly proliferating cells. Frequent sore throats, increased risk for infection, and manifestations of anemia and thrombocytopenia are seen, as well as an enlarged spleen and abdominal pain.
- Four major subgroups of leukemia are identified: Acute and chronic myeloid leukemias and acute and chronic lymphocytic (or lymphoblastic) leukemias. The primary population affected differs for each of these leukemias, as does their course.
- Genetic alterations and certain viruses are linked to the development of leukemia, as are exposure to chemotherapy drugs, environmental toxins, and ionizing radiation.
- Lymphocytic leukemias and lymphomas are closely related disorders.
- Nursing care for patients with leukemia and lymphoma focuses on reducing the risk for infection and bleeding, managing the effects of chemotherapy and radiation therapy, and, in some cases, caring for patients before and after bone marrow or stem cell transplant.
- The major risks associated with bone marrow and stem cell transplant are infection prior to and immediately following the transplant and graft-versus-host disease, a potentially fatal condition. A pruritic rash and desquamation of the palms and soles; abdominal pain, nausea, and diarrhea; and jaundice and elevated liver enzymes are common early manifestations of GVHD.

33.3 Lymphoid Tissue Disorders

Describe the pathophysiology and manifestations of lymphoid tissue disorders, and outline the interprofessional care and nursing care of patients with these disorders.

- The treatment of and nursing care for patients with lymphomas (including Hodgkin disease and non-Hodgkin lymphoma) is similar to that provided for patients with leukemia.
- Multiple myeloma is a malignancy of plasma cells, B lymphocytes that produce antibodies.
- Circulating M proteins and Bence Jones proteins in the urine are seen in multiple myeloma. The usual presenting manifestation is bone pain. Pathologic fractures and hypercalcemia are common complications of multiple myeloma as bone is destroyed.

33.4 Platelet and Coagulation Disorders

Describe the pathophysiology and manifestations of platelet and coagulation disorders, and outline the interprofessional care and nursing care of patients with these disorders.

- Bleeding and clotting disorders can result from either inadequate platelets (thrombocytopenia) or disruption of the clotting mechanisms (hemophilia, disseminated intravascular coagulation). Petechiae and purpura are common manifestations of bleeding/clotting disorders.
- Hemophilias are genetically transmitted disorders. Hemophilia A and B are transmitted on the X chromosome (sex-linked) from mother to son. Von Willebrand's disease, the most common bleeding disorder, is transmitted as an autosomal dominant disorder and affects men and women equally.
- Hemophilias are treated by replacement of the missing clotting factor and measures to prevent injury and bleeding.
- Disseminated intravascular coagulation is a disorder of widespread microvascular clotting. It is commonly precipitated by sepsis, but also may occur with conditions such as major trauma, malignancy, or as an obstetric emergency.
- In DIC, platelets and clotting factors are consumed by the abnormal clotting processes, leading to manifestations of bleeding, including frank hemorrhage, hematuria, oozing blood from parenteral and intravenous injection sites, and GI bleeding. Blood flow to organs and tissues is compromised by clot formation, leading to manifestations such as cyanosis of extremities, abdominal pain, renal failure, and changes in mental status and level of consciousness. Nursing care is supportive, focusing on administering prescribed treatments and monitoring and supporting cardiovascular, respiratory, and renal function.

TEST YOURSELF NCLEX-RN® REVIEW

1. The nurse is beginning an assessment of a patient with moderate anemia. Which manifestation should the nurse expect to assess in this patient?
   A. Pulse rate 140 bpm
   B. Hematocrit 45%
   C. WBC 14,000/µL
   D. Complaints of shortness of breath with exercise
2. The nurse is concerned that a patient recovering from gastric resection may develop nutritional-deficiency anemia related to malabsorption. For which manifestation should the nurse assess this patient? (Select all that apply.)
   A. Bone pain
   B. Steatorrhea
   C. Dark yellow or bronze skin color
   D. Numbness and tingling of extremities
   E. Sore, red tongue
3. The nurse is identifying potential patient problems for a patient receiving a bone marrow transplant for treatment of acute myelocytic leukemia. Which potential problems would be the immediate priority for this patient? (Select all that apply.)
   A. Anxiety regarding the nature of the diagnosis
   B. Increased risk for developing an infection
   C. Increased risk of bleeding
   D. Poor oxygenation
   E. Development of barriers to good nutrition
4. Which nursing interventions are priorities for a patient with acute myeloid leukemia? (Select all that apply.)
   A. Private room
   B. Soft, bland diet
   C. Rectal temperature q4h
   D. Oral hygiene after meals
   E. Airborne infection control precautions

5. A patient with non-Hodgkin lymphoma tells the nurse, "I might as well give up on dating. No woman will want me now." What is the most appropriate response for the nurse to make?
   A. "Lots of women find bald men attractive; besides, your hair may grow back soft and curly."
   B. "It sounds like you are concerned about the effects of this disease and the proposed treatment plan."
   C. "Don't worry. Malignant lymphomas are very treatable when caught in an early state of the disease."
   D. "Well, you may never be able to have children all right, but there are other ways to have a satisfying relationship with a woman."
6. A patient with lymphoma is prescribed the CHOP chemotherapy regimen. What should the nurse explain about the purpose of combining these medications as treatment for the disorder? (Select all that apply.)
   A. Targets different phases of the cell cycle
   B. Targets malignant cells in different organs
   C. Prevents the development of adverse effects
   D. Supports growth and development of normal cells
   E. Reduces drug resistance
7. A patient with multiple myeloma calls the home health nurse complaining of a new onset of severe back pain. What should the nurse respond to this patient?
   A. Suggest use of a back brace to reduce pain.
   B. Notify the healthcare provider of the onset of new pain.
   C. Reassure the patient that bone pain is expected with this disease.
   D. Inquire about the patient's use of NSAIDs and analgesics to manage pain.
8. During an assessment, the nurse observes reddish-purple spots and areas of purple bruising on a patient's arms and legs. Which laboratory result would be consistent with this assessment finding?
   A. INR 4.0
   B. Hematocrit 28%.
   C. WBC 4,500/mm^3
   D. Platelets 60 × 103/mm^3
9. A patient whose husband has hemophilia asks if her newborn baby girl could have the disease. What information should the nurse use when responding to this patient?
   A. Hemophilia is an autosomal dominant disorder; therefore, her daughter has a 50% chance of having the disorder.
   B. The most common forms of hemophilia are transmitted as sex-linked recessive disorders; her daughter is at risk for carrying the defective gene.
   C. Although hemophilia is genetically transmitted, its pattern of inheritance is unknown, and her daughter will need to be tested for the defective gene.
   D. Because hemophilia is a sex-linked recessive disorder carried on the Y chromosome, her daughter has no risk of having or carrying the disease.
10. The nurse is administering platelets to a patient with disseminated intravascular coagulation. What is the intended effect of this treatment?
   A. Replace depleted platelets.
   B. Restore tissue oxygenation.
   C. Promote intravascular clotting.
   D. Replace specific clotting factors.

See Test Yourself answers in Appendix B.

REFERENCES

Adams, M. P., Holland, L. N., & Urban, C. (2017). *Pharmacology for nursing: A pathophysiologic approach* (5th ed.). Hoboken, NJ: Pearson Education.

Akgul, N., & Ozdemir, L. (2014). Caregiver burden among primary caregivers of patients undergoing peripheral blood stem cell transplantation: A cross sectional study. *European Journal of Oncology Nursing, 18*(4), 372–377.

American Cancer Society (ACS). (2017). *Cancer facts and figures 2017*. Retrieved from https://www.cancer.org/content/dam/cancer-org/research/cancer-facts-and-statistics/annual-cancer-facts-and-figures/2017/cancer-facts-and-figures-2017.pdf.

American Cancer Society (ACS). (2018a). *Leukemia*. Retrieved from https://www.cancer.org/cancer/leukemia.html.

American Cancer Society (ACS). (2018b). *Multiple myeloma*. Retrieved from https://www.cancer.org/cancer/multiple-myeloma.html.

American Cancer Society. (2018c). *Myelodysplastic syndrome*. Retrieved from https://www.cancer.org/cancer/myelodysplastic-syndrome.html.

American Cancer Society (ACS). (2018d). *What causes non-Hodgkin lymphoma?* Retrieved from https://www.cancer.org/cancer/non-hodgkin-lymphoma/causes-risks-prevention/what-causes.html.

Genetics Home Reference. (2018a). *Alpha thalassemia.* Retrieved from https://ghr.nlm.nih.gov/condition/alpha-thalassemia#.

Genetics Home Reference. (2018b). *Beta thalassemia.* Retrieved from https://ghr.nlm.nih.gov/condition/beta-thalassemia.

Genetics Home Reference. (2018c). *Glucose-6-phosphate dehydrogenase deficiency.* Retrieved from https://ghr.nlm.nih.gov/condition/glucose-6-phosphate-dehydrogenase-deficiency#.

Genetics Home Reference. (2018d). *Sickle cell disease.* Retrieved from https://ghr.nlm.nih.gov/condition/sickle-cell-disease#.

Kee, J. L. (2018). *Laboratory and diagnostic tests with nursing implications* (10th ed.). Hoboken, NJ: Pearson Education.

Miladinia, M., Baraz, S., Shariati, A., & Malehi, A. S. (2017). Effects of slow-stroke back massage on symptom cluster in adult patients with acute leukemia: Supportive care in cancer nursing. *Cancer Nursing, 40*(1), 31–38.

National Cancer Institute. (2017). *Adult acute myeloid leukemia treatment* (PDQ®). Retrieved from https://www.cancer.gov/types/leukemia/hp/adult-aml-treatment-pdq.

Perrin, K. O., & MacLeod, C. E. (2018). *Understanding the essentials of critical care nursing* (3rd ed.). Hoboken, NJ: Pearson Education.

Shields, K. M., Fox, K. L., & Liebrecht, C. (2018). *Pearson nurse's drug guide: 2018.* Boston, MA: Pearson.

Sorenson, M., Quinn, L., & Klein, D. (2019). *Pathophysiology: Concepts of human disease.* Hoboken, NJ: Pearson Education.

ADDITIONAL RESOURCES

American Cancer Society

- Leukemia:
  - www.cancer.org/cancer/leukemia/index
- Non-Hodgkin lymphoma:
  - www.cancer.org/cancer/non-hodgkinlymphoma/index
- Hodgkin lymphoma:
  - www.cancer.org/cancer/hodgkindisease/index
- Multiple myeloma:
  - www.cancer.org/cancer/multiplemyeloma/index

Leukemia and Lymphoma Society

- www.lls.org

National Cancer Institute

- Leukemia:
  - www.cancer.gov/cancertopics/types/leukemia
- Non-Hodgkin lymphoma:
  - www.cancer.gov/cancertopics/types/non-hodgkin
- Hodgkin lymphoma:
  - www.cancer.gov/cancertopics/types/hodgkin
- Multiple myeloma:
  - www.cancer.gov/cancertopics/types/myeloma

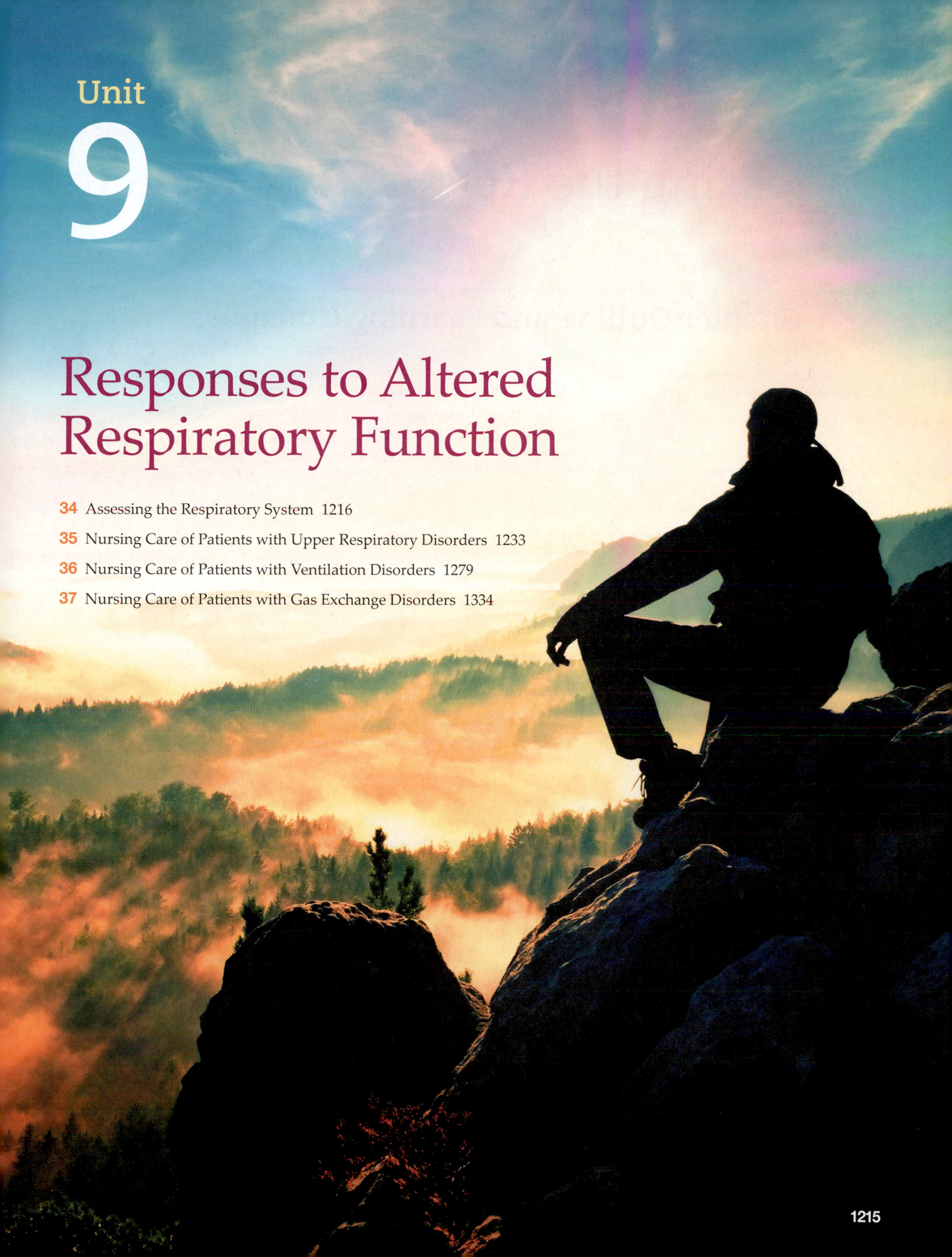

Unit

9

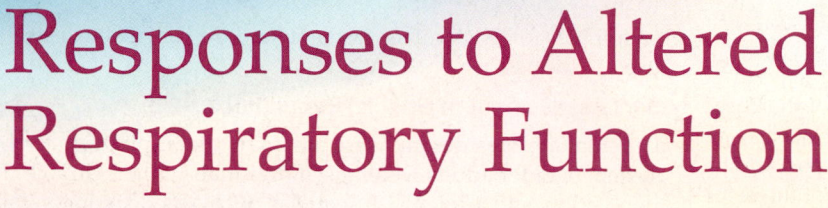

Responses to Altered Respiratory Function

Chapter 34

Assessing the Respiratory System

Chapter Outline and Learning Outcomes

34.1 Anatomy, Physiology, and Functions of the Respiratory System 1217

Describe the anatomy, physiology, and functions of the nose and sinuses, pharynx, larynx, trachea, lungs, pleura, bronchi and alveoli, and rib cage and intercostal muscles, and identify abnormal findings that may indicate impairment of the respiratory system.

34.2 Assessing Respiratory System Function 1223

Outline the components of the assessment of the respiratory system including topics for the health assessment interview, techniques for physical assessment, and the diagnostic tests used in the assessment.

34.3 Assessment of Special Populations 1229

Differentiate considerations for assessing the respiratory system of older adults, veterans, individuals in the LGBTQI population, and adults with sequelae of childhood/congenital conditions.

34.4 Health Promotion 1230

Summarize topics that nurses teach to promote healthy tissue integrity across the lifespan.

CLINICAL COMPETENCIES

- Complete a health history of the respiratory system, incorporating an appraisal of physiologic and psychosocial issues.
- Conduct and document a health history for patients having or at risk for alterations in the respiratory system.
- Conduct and document a physical assessment of respiratory structures and functions, demonstrating sensitivity and respect for the diversity of the human experience.
- Monitor the results of diagnostic tests and communicate abnormal findings within the interprofessional team.

KEY TERMS

apnea, 1224
atelectasis, 1224
bradypnea, 1224
crackles, 1226
friction rub, 1226
lung compliance, 1221
oxyhemoglobin, 1222
surfactant, 1222
tachypnea, 1224
tidal volume (TV), 1220
vital capacity (VC), 1220
wheezes, 1226

EQUIPMENT NEEDED

- Tongue blade
- Penlight
- Nasal speculum
- Metric ruler
- Marking pen
- Stethoscope with diaphragm

The respiratory system provides oxygen to cells and eliminates carbon dioxide, formed as a waste product of cellular metabolism. The events in this process, called *respiration*, are ventilation (the movement of air into and out of the lungs), perfusion (the flow of blood through the capillary system surrounding the lungs), and diffusion (the process of gas exchange between the blood and the alveoli of the lungs). The movement of respiratory muscles is controlled by the nervous system, and respiratory rate is adjusted to match body requirements during various activities. More than half of the population of the United States lives in an area impacted by unhealthy levels of air pollution (American Lung Association, 2018).

34.1 Anatomy, Physiology, and Functions of the Respiratory System

The respiratory system functions as a whole, but for discussion purposes is divided in this chapter into the upper respiratory system and the lower respiratory system.

The Upper Respiratory System

The upper respiratory system, composed of the conducting airways (nose and sinuses, pharynx, larynx, and trachea), serves as a passageway for air moving into the lungs and for carbon dioxide moving out to the external environment (**Figure 34.1** ■). As air moves through these structures, it is cleaned, filtered, humidified, and warmed.

Nose and Sinuses

The nose, the external opening of the respiratory system, is given structure by the nasal, frontal, and maxillary bones as well as plates of hyaline cartilage. The *nostrils* (also called the *external nares*) are two cavities within the nose, separated by the *nasal septum*. Nasal hairs filter the air as it enters the nares, and secreted mucus that contains lysozyme (an enzyme that destroys bacteria as they enter the nose) traps dust and bacteria. As mucus and debris accumulate, mucosal ciliated cells move it toward the pharynx, where it is swallowed. The mucosa is highly vascular, warming air that moves across its surface. The nasal cavity is surrounded by *paranasal sinuses* (**Figure 34.2** ■), located in the frontal, sphenoid, ethmoid, and maxillary bones. Sinuses lighten the skull, assist in speech, and produce mucus that drains into the nasal cavities to help trap debris. The mouth is an alternate airway, used if the nasal passages are plugged or a large intake of air is needed (for example, during strenuous exercise).

Pharynx

The *pharynx*, a funnel-shaped passageway about 13 cm (5 in.) long, extends from the base of the skull to the level of the C_6 vertebra. The pharynx serves as a passageway for both air and food. It is divided into three regions: The nasopharynx, the oropharynx, and the laryngopharynx.

The *nasopharynx* serves only as a passageway for air. Masses of lymphoid tissue (the tonsils and adenoids), located in the mucosa high in the posterior wall, trap and destroy infectious agents entering with the air. The eustachian tubes open into the nasopharynx, connecting it with the middle ear. The *oropharynx* lies behind the oral cavity and extends from the soft palate to the level of the hyoid bone. It serves as a passageway for both air and food. An upward rise of the soft palate prevents food from entering the nasopharynx during swallowing. The *laryngopharynx*, extending from the hyoid bone to the larynx, serves as a passageway for both food and air.

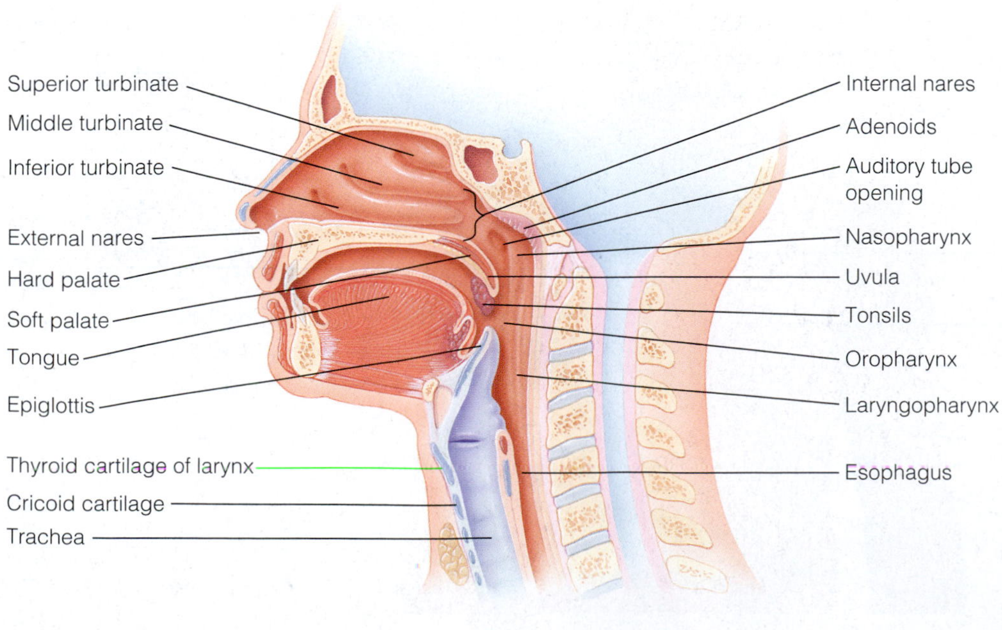

Superior turbinate
Middle turbinate
Inferior turbinate
External nares
Hard palate
Soft palate
Tongue
Epiglottis
Thyroid cartilage of larynx
Cricoid cartilage
Trachea
Internal nares
Adenoids
Auditory tube opening
Nasopharynx
Uvula
Tonsils
Oropharynx
Laryngopharynx
Esophagus

Figure 34.1 ■ The upper respiratory system.

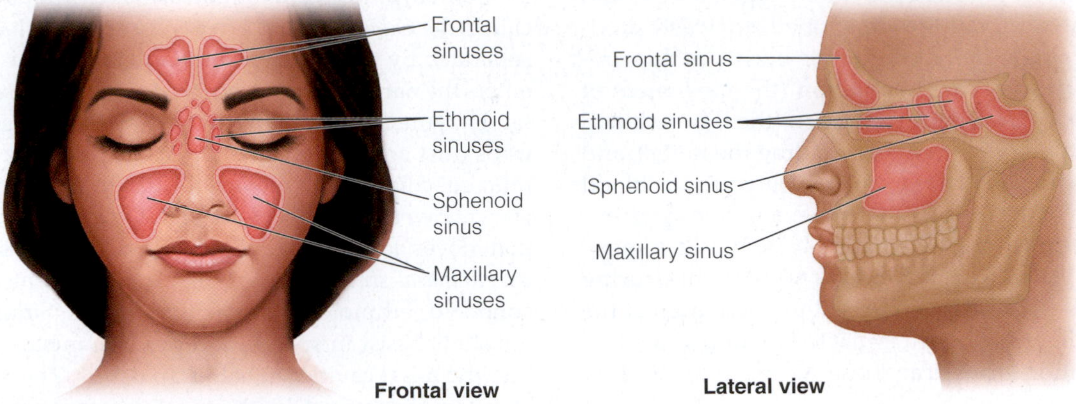
Frontal sinuses
Ethmoid sinuses
Sphenoid sinus
Maxillary sinuses
Frontal view
Frontal sinus
Ethmoid sinuses
Sphenoid sinus
Maxillary sinus
Lateral view

Figure 34.2 ■ Sinuses, frontal and lateral views.

Larynx

The *larynx* is about 5 cm (2 in.) long. It provides an airway, routes air and food into the proper passageway, and contains the vocal cords. As long as air is moving through the larynx, its inlet is open; however, the inlet closes during swallowing. The larynx is framed by the thyroid, the cricoid, and the epiglottis cartilages. The *thyroid cartilage* is formed by the fusion of two cartilages; the fusion point is visible as the Adam's apple. The *cricoid cartilage* lies below the thyroid cartilage. The *epiglottis* normally projects upward to the base of the tongue; however, during swallowing, the larynx moves upward and the epiglottis tips to cover the opening to the larynx. If anything other than air enters the larynx, a cough reflex expels the foreign substance before it can enter the lungs. This protective reflex does not work if the person is unconscious.

Trachea

The *trachea* begins at the inferior larynx and descends anteriorly to the esophagus to enter the mediastinum, where it divides to become the right and left primary bronchi of the lungs. The trachea is about 12 to 15 cm (4 to 5 in.) long and 2.5 cm (1 in.) in diameter. The mucosal lining of the trachea includes seromucous glands that produce thick mucus. Dust and debris in inspired air are trapped in this mucus, moved toward the throat by the cilia, and then either swallowed or coughed out through the mouth.

The Lower Respiratory System

The lower respiratory system includes the lungs, pleura, bronchi and alveoli, and the rib cage and intercostal muscles (**Figure 34.3** ■ and **Figure 34.4** ■).

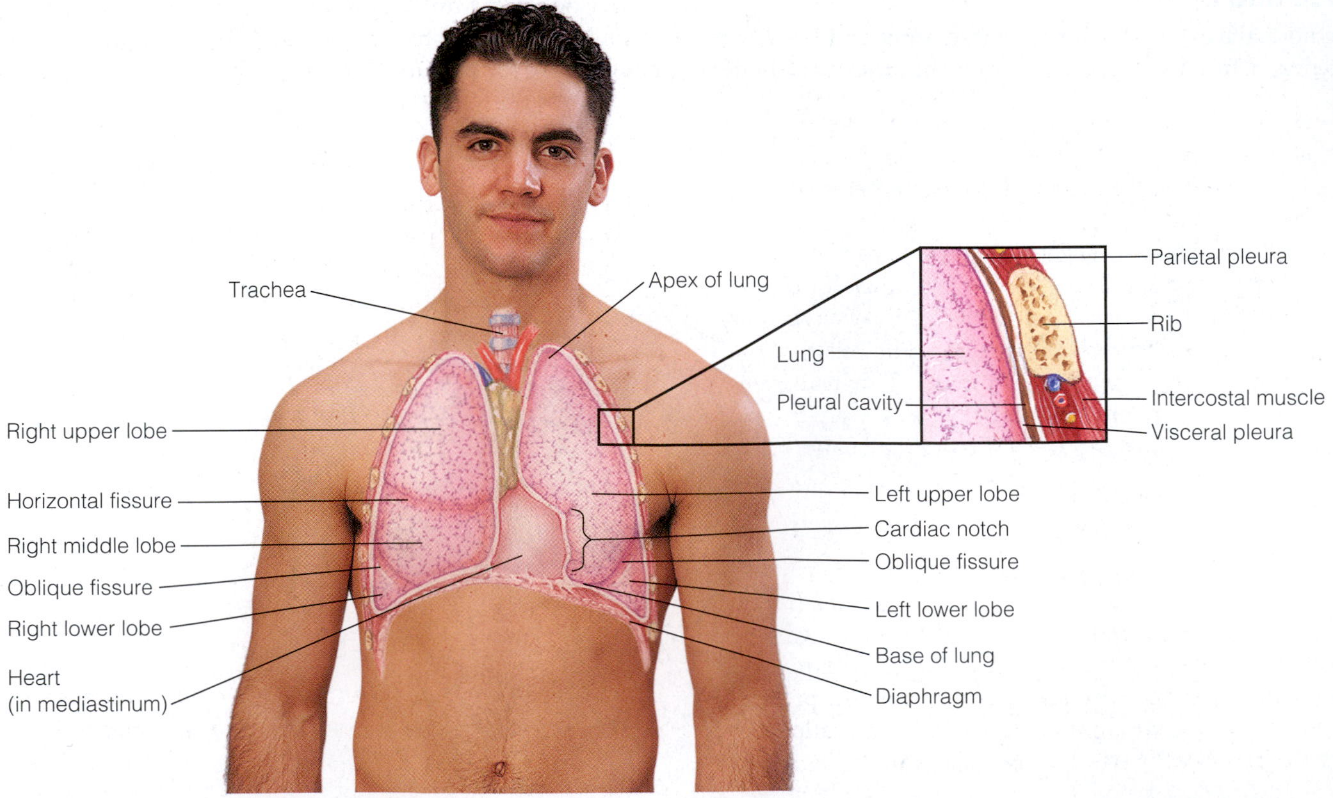
Trachea
Apex of lung
Right upper lobe
Horizontal fissure
Right middle lobe
Oblique fissure
Right lower lobe
Heart
(in mediastinum)
Lung
Pleural cavity
Parietal pleura
Rib
Intercostal muscle
Visceral pleura
Left upper lobe
Cardiac notch
Oblique fissure
Left lower lobe
Base of lung
Diaphragm

Figure 34.3 ■ The lower respiratory system, showing the location of the lungs, the mediastinum, and layers of visceral and parietal pleura.

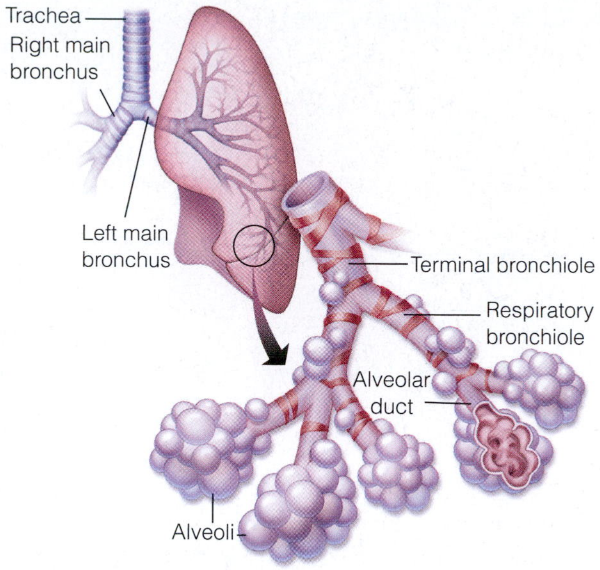
Trachea
Right main bronchus
Left main bronchus
Terminal bronchiole
Respiratory bronchiole
Alveolar duct
Alveoli

Figure 34.4 ■ Respiratory bronchi, bronchioles, alveolar ducts, and alveoli.

Lungs

The center of the thoracic cavity is filled by the *mediastinum*, which contains the heart, great blood vessels, bronchi, trachea, and esophagus. The mediastinum is flanked on either side by the lungs. Each lung is suspended in its own pleural cavity, with the anterior, lateral, and posterior lung surfaces lying close to the ribs. The *hilus*, on the mediastinal surface of each lung, is where blood vessels of the pulmonary and circulatory systems and the primary bronchus enter and exit the lungs. The apex of each lung lies just below the clavicle and the base of each lung rests on the diaphragm. The lungs are elastic connective tissue, called *stroma*, and are soft and spongy. The two lungs differ in size and shape. The left lung is smaller and has two lobes, whereas the right lung has three lobes.

The vascular system of the lungs consists of the *pulmonary arteries*, which deliver blood to the lungs for oxygenation, and the *pulmonary veins*, which deliver oxygenated blood to the heart. Within the lungs, the pulmonary arteries branch into a pulmonary capillary network that surrounds the alveoli. Lung tissue receives its blood supply from the bronchial arteries and drains by the bronchial and pulmonary veins.

Pleura

The *pleura* is a double-layered membrane that covers the lungs and the inside of the thoracic cavities (refer to Figure 34.3). The *parietal pleura* lines the thoracic wall and mediastinum. It is continuous with the *visceral pleura*, which covers the external lung surfaces. The pleura produces pleural fluid, a lubricating, serous fluid that allows the lungs to move easily over the thoracic wall during breathing. The structure of the pleura creates a slightly negative pressure in the pleural space (which is actually a potential rather than an actual space), necessary for lung function.

Bronchi and Alveoli

The trachea divides into right and left primary bronchi; the right primary bronchus is shorter, wider, and situated more vertically (making aspiration of foreign bodies into the right primary bronchus more likely). The point where the trachea divides is innervated with sensory neurons; coughing and bronchospasm may be induced by stimulation of these neurons through activities such as tracheal suctioning. The bronchi subdivide into smaller bronchi, and then into smaller bronchioles, ending in the terminal bronchioles, which are extremely small (refer to Figure 34.4). These branching passageways are collectively called the *bronchial tree*. From the terminal bronchioles, air moves into air sacs, which further branch into alveolar ducts that lead to alveolar sacs and then to the tiny alveoli. During inspiration, air enters the lungs through the primary bronchus and then moves through the increasingly smaller passageways of the lungs to the alveoli, where oxygen and carbon dioxide exchange occurs.

Alveoli cluster around the alveolar sacs, which open into a common chamber called the *atrium*. The adult lung has approximately 300 million alveoli, providing an enormous surface for gas exchange. The walls of alveoli are a single layer of squamous epithelial cells over a very thin basement membrane. The external surface of the alveoli is covered with pulmonary capillaries. The alveolar and capillary walls form the respiratory membrane. Gas exchange across the respiratory membrane occurs by simple diffusion. The alveolar walls also contain cells that secrete a surfactant-containing fluid, necessary for maintaining a moist surface and reducing the surface tension of the alveolar fluid to help prevent collapse of the lungs.

Rib Cage and Intercostal Muscles

The lungs are protected by the bones of the rib cage and the intercostal muscles. The 12 pairs of ribs articulate with the thoracic vertebrae (**Figure 34.5** ■). The sternum has three parts: The manubrium, the body, and the xiphoid process. The spaces between the ribs are called the *intercostal spaces*. Each intercostal space is named for the rib immediately above it (e.g., the space between the third and fourth ribs is designated as the third intercostal space). The intercostal muscles between the ribs, along with the diaphragm, are called the *inspiratory muscles*.

Factors Affecting Respiration

Many factors affect respiration. Those discussed here include changes in respiratory volume and capacity; air pressures; oxygen, carbon dioxide, and hydrogen ion concentrations in the blood; airway resistance, lung compliance, and elasticity; and alveolar surface tension.

Respiratory Volume and Capacity

Pulmonary function tests measure respiratory volumes and capacities and are described and illustrated in **Box 34.1**.

Air Pressures

Ventilation has two phases: *Inspiration*, during which air flows into the lungs; and *expiration*, during which gases

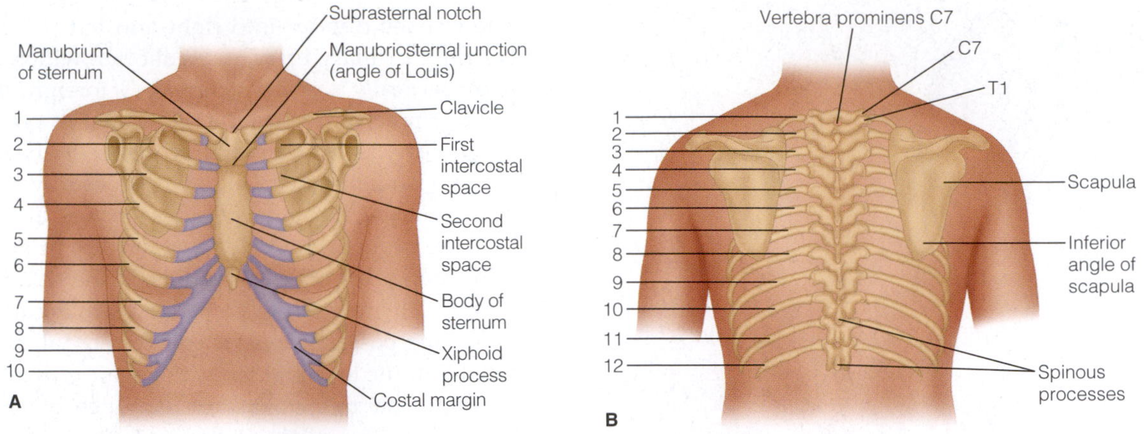
Suprasternal notch
Manubrium of sternum
Manubriosternal junction (angle of Louis)
Clavicle
First intercostal space
Second intercostal space
Body of sternum
Xiphoid process
Costal margin
1
2
3
4
5
6
7
8
9
10
A
Vertebra prominens C7
C7
T1
1
2
3
4
5
6
7
8
9
10
11
12
Scapula
Inferior angle of scapula
Spinous processes
B

Figure 34.5 ■ A, Anterior rib cage, showing intercostal spaces. B, Posterior rib cage.

BOX 34.1
Pulmonary Function Tests

Pulmonary function tests (PFTs) are performed in a pulmonary function laboratory. After preparing the patient, a nose clip is applied, and the patient breathes into a spirometer or body plethysmograph, a device for measuring and recording lung volume in liters versus time in seconds. The patient is instructed on how to breathe for specific tests; for example, to inhale as deeply as possible and then exhale to the maximal extent possible. Using measured lung volumes, respiratory capacities are calculated to assess pulmonary status. The specific values determined by PFT and illustrated in the accompanying figure include:

- ***Total lung capacity (TLC)*** is the total volume of the lungs at their maximum inflation. Four values are used to calculate TLC, with normal values for a healthy adult shown in parentheses:
  a. **Tidal volume (TV)**, the volume inhaled and exhaled with normal quiet breathing (500 mL)
  b. ***Inspiratory reserve volume (IRV)***, the maximum amount that can be inhaled over and above a normal inspiration (2000 to 3100 mL)
  c. ***Expiratory reserve volume (ERV)***, the maximum amount that can be exhaled following a normal exhalation (1000 mL)
  d. ***Residual volume (RV)***, the amount of air remaining in the lungs after maximal exhalation (1100 mL)
- **Vital capacity (VC)** is the total amount of air that can be exhaled after a maximal inspiration. It is calculated by adding together the IRV, TV, and ERV (4500 mL).
- ***Inspiratory capacity*** is the total amount of air that can be inhaled following a normal quiet exhalation. It is calculated by adding the TV and IRV.
- ***Functional residual capacity (FRC)*** is the volume of air left in the lungs after a normal exhalation. The ERV and RV are added to determine the FRC.
- ***Forced expiratory volume (FEV_1)*** is the amount of air that can be exhaled in 1 second.
- ***Forced vital capacity (FVC)*** is the amount of air that can be exhaled forcefully and rapidly after maximum air intake.
- ***Minute volume (MV)*** is the total amount or volume of air breathed in 1 minute.

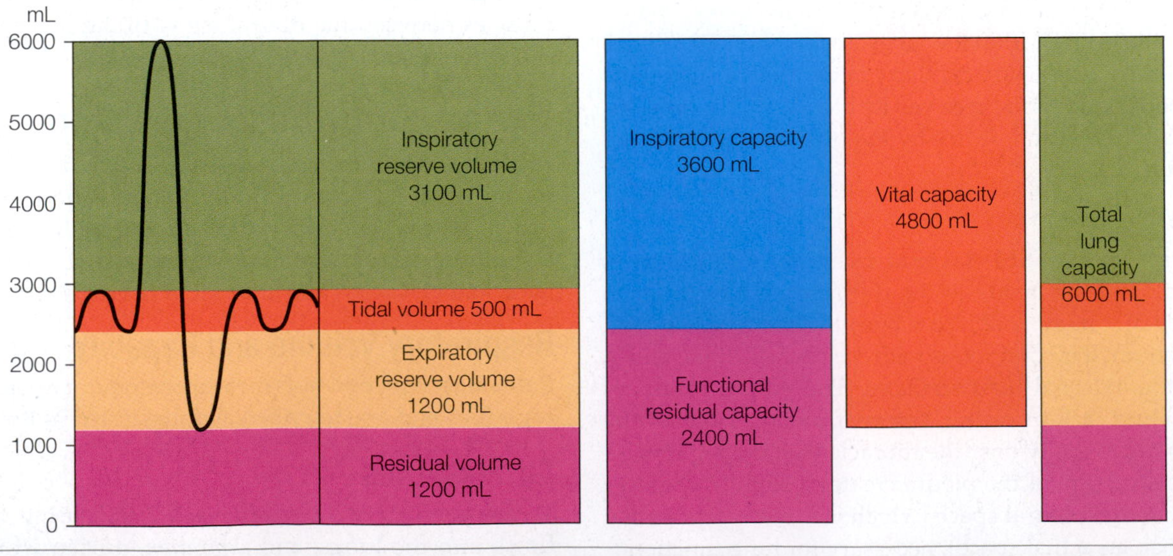
mL
6000
5000
4000
3000
2000
1000
0
Inspiratory reserve volume 3100 mL
Tidal volume 500 mL
Expiratory reserve volume 1200 mL
Residual volume 1200 mL
Inspiratory capacity 3600 mL
Functional residual capacity 2400 mL
Vital capacity 4800 mL
Total lung capacity 6000 mL

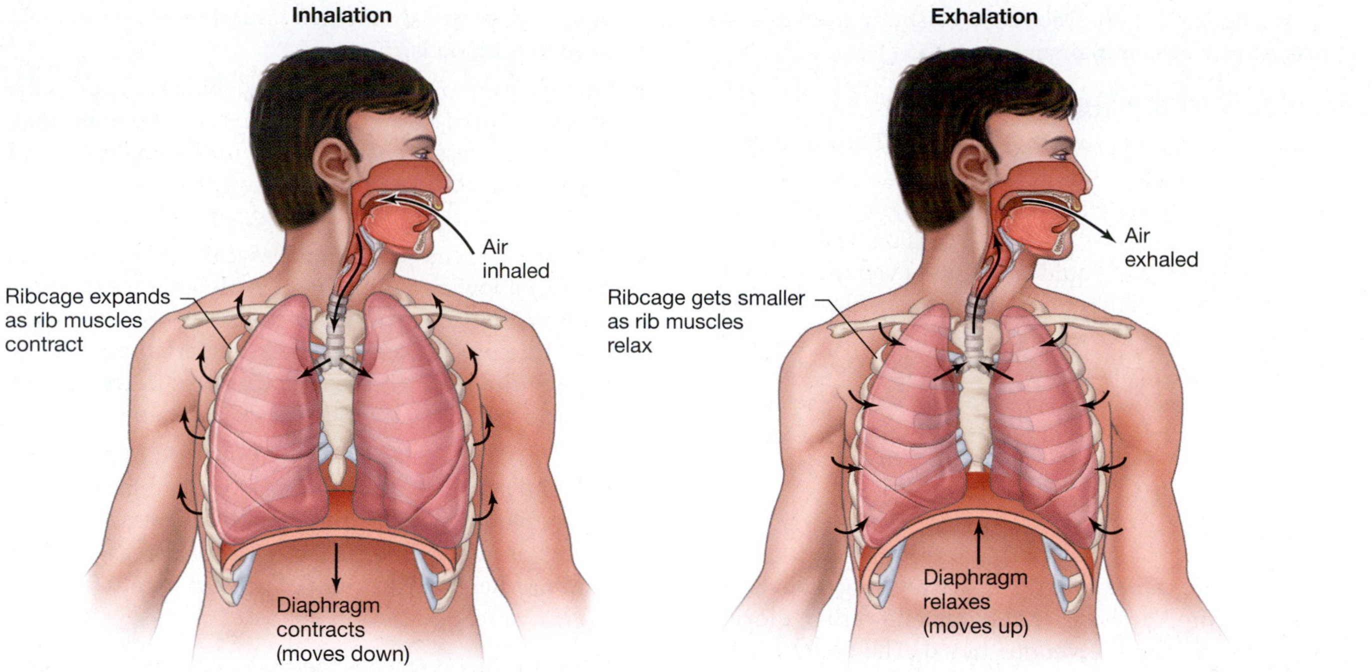
Inhalation
Air inhaled
Ribcage expands as rib muscles contract
Diaphragm contracts (moves down)
Exhalation
Air exhaled
Ribcage gets smaller as rib muscles relax
Diaphragm relaxes (moves up)

Figure 34.6 ■ Respiratory inspiration and expiration. Note the volume expansion of the thorax as the diaphragm flattens.

flow out of the lungs. The two phases make up a single breath and normally occur from 12 to 20 times each minute. A single inspiration lasts for about 1 to 1.5 seconds, whereas expiration lasts for about 2 to 3 seconds.

During inspiration, the diaphragm contracts and flattens to increase the vertical diameter of the thoracic cavity (**Figure 34.6** ■). The external intercostal muscles contract, elevating the rib cage and moving the sternum forward to expand the lateral and anteroposterior diameter of the thoracic cavity, decreasing intrapleural pressure. The lungs stretch and the intrapulmonary volume increases, decreasing intrapulmonary pressure slightly below atmospheric pressure. Air rushes into the lungs as a result of this pressure gradient until the intrapulmonary and atmospheric pressures equalize. In contrast, expiration is primarily a passive process that occurs as a result of the elasticity of the lungs (see Figure 34.6). The inspiratory muscles relax, the diaphragm rises, the ribs descend, and the lungs recoil. Both the thoracic and intrapulmonary pressures increase, compressing the alveoli.

Ventilation depends on volume changes within the thoracic cavity. A change in the volume of air in the thoracic cavity leads to a change in the air pressure within the cavity. Because gases always flow along their pressure gradients, a change in pressure results in gases flowing into or out of the lungs to equalize the pressure. The pressures normally present in the thoracic cavity are the intrapulmonary pressure and the intrapleural pressure. The *intrapulmonary pressure*, within the alveoli of the lungs, rises and falls constantly as a result of inhalation and exhalation. The *intrapleural pressure*, within the pleural space, also rises and falls with inhalation and exhalation, but it is always less than (or negative to) the intrapulmonary pressure. Intrapulmonary and intrapleural pressures are necessary not only to expand and contract the lungs, but also to prevent their collapse. The intrapulmonary pressure rises to a level greater than atmospheric pressure, and gases flow out of the lungs.

Oxygen, Carbon Dioxide, and Hydrogen Ion Concentrations

The rate and depth of respirations are controlled by respiratory centers in the medulla oblongata and pons of the brain and by chemoreceptors located in the medulla and in the carotid and aortic bodies. The centers and chemoreceptors respond to changes in the concentration of oxygen, carbon dioxide, and hydrogen ions in arterial blood. For example, when carbon dioxide concentration increases or the pH decreases, the respiratory rate increases. This process is further described in Chapter 10.

Airway Resistance, Lung Compliance, and Elasticity

Respiratory passageway resistance, lung compliance, and lung elasticity also affect respiration. *Respiratory passageway resistance* is created by the friction encountered as gases move along the respiratory passageways, by constriction of the passageways (especially the larger bronchioles), by accumulations of mucus or infectious material, and by tumors. As resistance increases, gas flow decreases. **Lung compliance** is the distensibility of the lungs. It depends on the elasticity of the lung tissue and the flexibility of the rib cage. Compliance is decreased by factors that decrease the elasticity of the lungs, block the respiratory passageways, or interfere with movement of the rib cage. Lung *elasticity* is essential for lung distention during inspiration and lung recoil during expiration. Decreased elasticity from disease such as emphysema impairs respiration.

Alveolar Surface Tension

A liquid film, primarily composed of water, covers the alveolar walls. At any gas–liquid boundary, the molecules of liquid are more strongly attracted to each other than to gas molecules. This produces a state of tension, called *surface tension*, that draws the liquid molecules even more closely together. The water content of the alveolar film compacts the alveoli and aids in the lungs' recoil during expiration. **Surfactant**, a lipoprotein produced by the alveolar cells, interferes with the adhesiveness of the water molecules, reducing surface tension and helping expand the lungs.

Oxygen and Carbon Dioxide Transport

The alveolar and capillary structures of the lungs allow oxygen to be restored to the arterial blood and carbon dioxide to be removed from the venous blood. The blood carries both oxygen and carbon dioxide as dissolved gases and in chemical combination with hemoglobin. In addition, carbon dioxide is changed to and transported as bicarbonate. When arterial blood gases are measured in the practice setting, they are given values that reflect the partial pressure of the gas in the alveoli (PO_2 = partial pressure of oxygen, PCO_2 = partial pressure of carbon dioxide). Arterial blood gases are used for clinical measurement as they reflect the gas exchange function of the alveoli (venous blood reflects the metabolic demands of the tissues). Normally, the PO_2 of arterial blood is greater than 80 mmHg and the PCO_2 of arterial blood ranges from 35 to 45 mmHg. The arterial blood gases reflect the partial pressure of the gas in the alveoli, increasing and decreasing as the alveolar pressure increases and decreases.

Oxygen Transport and Unloading

In the alveoli, oxygen moves to the pulmonary capillaries as a dissolved gas, moving down a concentration gradient. Oxygen is carried in the blood either dissolved or bound to hemoglobin. Because oxygen is relatively insoluble in solution, its ability to bind with hemoglobin is essential. Approximately 98 to 99% of oxygen is transported in the blood combined with hemoglobin as **oxyhemoglobin**; the remaining 1 to 2% is carried in the dissolved state.

Each hemoglobin molecule is made of four polypeptide chains, with each chain bound to an iron-containing heme group. The iron groups are the binding sites for oxygen; each hemoglobin molecule can form a loose and reversible bond with four molecules of oxygen. Oxygen binding is rapid and its affinity to hemoglobin is affected by temperature, blood pH, PO_2, PCO_2, and serum concentration of 2,3-DPG. These factors interact to ensure adequate delivery of oxygen to the cells.

- Under normal conditions, the hemoglobin in arterial blood is almost fully saturated at a PO_2 of 70 mmHg. As arterial blood flows through the capillaries, oxygen is unloaded, so that the oxygen saturation of hemoglobin in venous blood is 75%.
- The affinity of oxygen and hemoglobin decreases as the temperature of body tissues increases above normal. As a result, less oxygen binds with hemoglobin, and oxygen unloading increases. Conversely, as the body is chilled, oxygen unloading decreases.
- The oxygen–hemoglobin bond is weakened by increased hydrogen ion concentrations. As blood becomes more acidotic, oxygen unloading to the tissues increases. The same process occurs when the partial pressure of carbon dioxide increases because this decreases the Ph (acid–base balance is discussed in Chapter 10).
- The organic chemical 2,3-DPG is formed in red blood cells and increases the release of oxygen from hemoglobin by binding to it during times of increased metabolism (as when body temperature increases). This binding alters the structure of hemoglobin to facilitate oxygen unloading.

When the blood reaches the capillary level, it is critical that oxygen be able to dissociate from hemoglobin because only dissolved oxygen that is not bound to hemoglobin is able to pass through the capillary wall, diffuse through the cell membrane, and be available for use in cell metabolism. The relation between the oxygen carried in combination with hemoglobin and the PO_2 of the blood can be illustrated by an oxygen–hemoglobin dissociation curve, which demonstrates the release of oxygen from hemoglobin at the tissue capillaries (see **Figure 34.7** ■).

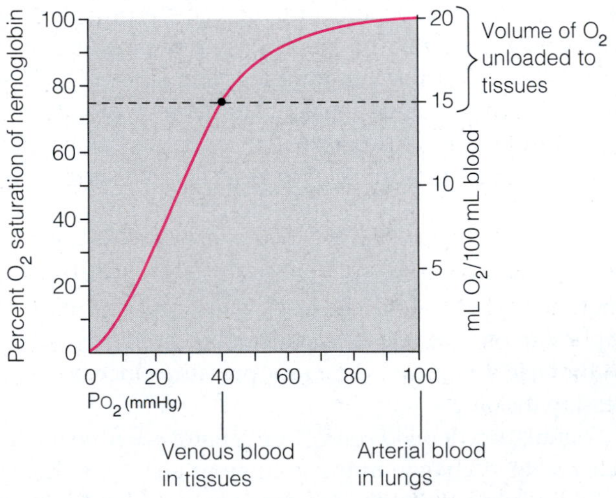
Percent O2 saturation of hemoglobin
100
80
60
40
20
0
0
20
40
60
80
100
PO2 (mmHg)
Venous blood in tissues
Arterial blood in lungs
20
15
10
5
mL O2/100 mL blood
Volume of O2 unloaded to tissues

Figure 34.7 ■ Oxygen–hemoglobin dissociation curve. The percent O_2 saturation of hemoglobin and total blood oxygen volume are shown for different oxygen partial pressures (PO_2). Arterial blood in the lungs is almost completely saturated. During one pass through the body, about 25% of hemoglobin-bound oxygen is unloaded to the tissues. Thus, venous blood is still about 75% saturated with oxygen. The steep portion of the curve shows that hemoglobin readily off-loads or on-loads oxygen at PO_2 levels below about 50 mmHg.

Carbon Dioxide Transport

Active cells produce about 200 mL of carbon dioxide each minute; this amount is exactly the same as that excreted by the lungs each minute. Excretion of carbon dioxide from the body requires transport by the blood from the cells to the lungs. Carbon dioxide is transported in three forms: As bicarbonate ions in the plasma (the largest amount is in this form), dissolved in plasma, and bound to hemoglobin.

The amount of carbon dioxide transported in the blood is strongly influenced by the oxygenation of the blood. When the PO_2 decreases, with a corresponding decrease in oxygen saturation, increased amounts of carbon dioxide can be carried in the blood. Carbon dioxide entering the systemic circulation from the cells causes more oxygen to dissociate from hemoglobin, in turn allowing more carbon dioxide to combine with hemoglobin and more bicarbonate ions to be generated. This situation is reversed in the pulmonary circulation, where the uptake of oxygen facilitates the release of carbon dioxide.

34.2 Assessing Respiratory Function

Function of the respiratory system is assessed by findings from a health assessment interview to collect subjective data, including consideration of genetic factors; a physical assessment to collect objective data; and diagnostic tests.

Health Assessment Interview

A health assessment interview to determine problems with respiratory structure and function may be conducted during a health screening, may focus on a chief complaint (such as shortness of breath), or may be part of a total health assessment. If the patient has a problem with respiratory function, analyze its onset, characteristics, course, severity, precipitating and relieving factors, and any associated symptoms, noting the timing and circumstances. For example, ask the patient:

- "Describe the problems you are having with your breathing. Is your breathing more difficult if you lie flat? Is it painful to breathe in or out?"
- "When did you first notice that your cough was becoming a problem? Do you cough up mucus? What color is the mucus?"
- "Have you had nosebleeds in the past?"

During the interview, carefully observe the patient for difficulty in breathing, pausing to breathe in the middle of a sentence, hoarseness, changes in voice quality, and cough. Ask about present health status, medical history, family health history, and risk factors for illness. To determine present health status, ask about pain in the nose, throat, or chest. Information about cough includes what type of cough (e.g., dry, constant, worse at night, painful), when it occurs, and how it is relieved. The patient should describe any sputum associated with the cough. Is the patient experiencing any dyspnea (difficult or labored breathing)? How is the dyspnea associated with activity levels and time of day? Is the patient having chest pain? How is this related to activity and time of day? Note the severity, type, and location of the pain. Explore problems with swallowing, smelling, or taste. Ask about nosebleeds and nasal or sinus stuffiness or pain and about current medication use, aerosols or inhalants, and oxygen use.

Document past medical history by asking questions about a history of allergies, asthma, bronchitis, emphysema, pneumonia, tuberculosis, or congestive heart failure. Other questions include a history of surgery or trauma to the respiratory structures and a history of other chronic illnesses such as cancer, kidney disease, and heart disease. If the patient has a health problem involving the respiratory system, ask about medications used to relieve nasal congestion, cough, dyspnea, or chest pain. Document a family history of allergies, tuberculosis, emphysema, and cancer.

Genetic Considerations

When conducting a health assessment interview and a physical assessment, the nurse should consider genetic influences on the health of the adult (National Institutes of Health, 2017). During the health assessment interview, ask about family members with health problems affecting respiratory function. In addition, ask about a family history of emphysema, asthma, cystic fibrosis, or lung cancer. During the physical assessment, assess for any manifestations that might indicate a genetic disorder. If data are found to indicate genetic risk factors or alterations, ask about genetic testing and refer for appropriate genetic counseling and evaluation. Examples of genetic disorders that affect the respiratory system follow.

- Deficiency of $alpha_1$-antitrypsin (a protein that protects the body from damage by its immune cells) is caused by a mutation of a gene located on chromosome 14. Deficiency of this protein leaves the lung susceptible to emphysema.
- Asthma, a disease that affects > 7% of the population, is an inheritable disease with a number of responsible genes (Centers for Disease Control and Prevention [CDC], 2017). (There are also other causes of asthma.)
- Cystic fibrosis is the most common fatal genetic disease in the United States today with a median predicted survival age of almost 40 years (Cystic Fibrosis Foundation, 2018). All gene defects result in defective transport of chloride and sodium by epithelial cells. As a result, the amount of sodium chloride is increased in body secretions. Thick mucus is produced that clogs the lungs, leads to infection, and blocks pancreatic enzymes from reaching the intestines to digest food.
- A familial history of lung cancer increases the risk of developing it, and small-cell lung cancer has a definite genetic component. In addition, researchers have found that patients with lung cancer who never smoked are more likely than smokers to have one of two genetic mutations linked to the disease (Kanwal, Ding, & Cao, 2017).

Chapter 8 provides further information about genetics in medical-surgical nursing.

The patient's personal lifestyle, environment, and occupation may provide clues to risk factors for actual or potential health problems. Question the patient about a history of smoking and/or exposure to environmental chemicals (including smog), dust, vapors, animals, coal dust, asbestos, fumes, or pollens. Other risk factors include a sedentary lifestyle and obesity. Ask the patient about use of alcohol and substances that are injected (such as heroin) or inhaled (such as cocaine or marijuana).

Physical Assessment

Physical assessment of the respiratory system may be performed either as part of a total assessment or alone for a patient with known or suspected problems (Shellenberger, Balakrishman, Avula, Ebel, & Shaik, 2017). The techniques used to assess the respiratory system are inspection, palpation, percussion, and auscultation. In addition, note the patient's level of consciousness, restlessness, and anxiety level, and assess the color of the lips and nail beds.

The room should be warm and well lighted. Ask the patient to remove all clothing above the waist; give women a gown to wear during the examination. Conduct the examination with the patient in the sitting position. Prior to the examination, collect all necessary equipment and explain the techniques to the patient to decrease anxiety.

Respiratory Assessments

Technique/Normal Findings	Abnormal Findings
Nasal Assessment **Inspect the nose for changes in size, shape, or color.** *The nose should be midline in the face, of the same color as the face, and the nares should be symmetric.*	■ The nose may be asymmetrical as a result of previous surgery or trauma. ■ The skin around the nostrils may be red and swollen in allergies or upper respiratory infections.
Inspect the nasal cavity. Use an otoscope with a broad, short speculum. Gently insert the speculum into each of the nares and assess the condition of the mucous membranes and the turbinates. *The septum should be midline with pink mucosa and without drainage.*	■ The septum may be deviated. ■ Perforation of the septum may occur with chronic cocaine abuse. ■ Red mucosa indicates infection. ■ Purulent drainage indicates nasal or sinus infection. ■ Watery nasal drainage, pale turbinates, and polyps on the turbinates may indicate allergies.
Assess ability to smell (cranial nerve I, olfactory). Ask the patient to breathe through one nostril while pressing the other one closed. Ask the patient to close his or her eyes. Place a substance with an aromatic odor under the patient's nose (use ground coffee or alcohol) and ask the patient to identify the odor. Test each nostril separately. *This test is usually done only if the patient has problems with the sense of smell, but the patient should be able to distinguish different odors.*	■ Changes in the ability to smell may be the result of damage to the olfactory nerve or to chronic inflammation of the nose. ■ Zinc deficiency may cause a loss of the sense of smell.
Sinus Assessment **Palpate the frontal and maxillary sinuses.** *The sinuses should not be tender to palpation.*	■ Frontal and maxillary sinuses are tender to palpation with allergies or sinus infections.
Thoracic Assessment **Assess respiratory rate.** *The normal respiratory rate is 12 to 20 breaths per minute.*	■ **Tachypnea** (rapid respiratory rate) is seen in **atelectasis** (collapse of lung tissue following obstruction of the bronchus or bronchioles), pneumonia, asthma, pleural effusion, pneumothorax, congestive heart failure, anxiety, and in response to pain. ■ Damage to the brainstem from a stroke or head injury may result in either tachypnea or **bradypnea** (low respiratory rate). ■ Bradypnea is seen with some circulatory disorders, lung disorders, and as a side effect of some medications. ■ **Apnea**, cessation of breathing lasting from a few seconds to a few minutes, may occur following a stroke or head trauma, as a side effect of some medications, or following airway obstruction.
Inspect the anteroposterior diameter of the chest. It should be less than the transverse diameter. *Normal ratio is 1:2.*	■ The anteroposterior diameter is equal to the transverse diameter in barrel chest, which typically occurs with emphysema.

Respiratory Assessments (*continued*)

Technique/Normal Findings	Abnormal Findings
Inspect for intercostal retraction or bulging. *There should be no retraction or bulging.*	■ Retraction of intercostal spaces may be seen in asthma. ■ Bulging of intercostal spaces may be seen in pneumothorax.
Inspect and palpate for chest expansion. Place your hands with the fingers spread apart palm down on the patient's posterolateral chest. Gently press the skin between your thumbs (**Figure 34.8 ■**). Ask the patient to breathe deeply. As the patient inhales, watch your hands for symmetry of movement. *Chest expansion should be bilaterally symmetric, with the examiner's hands moving 5 to 10 cm (2 to 4 in.) apart.*	■ Thoracic expansion is decreased on the affected side in atelectasis, pneumonia, pneumothorax, and pleural effusion. ■ Bilateral chest expansion is decreased in emphysema.
Gently palpate the location and position of the trachea. *The trachea should be midline.*	■ The trachea shifts to the unaffected side in pleural effusion and pneumothorax; it shifts to the affected side in atelectasis.
Percuss the lungs for dullness over shoulder apices and over anterior, posterior, and lateral intercostal spaces (**Figure 34.9 ■**). *The normal percussion tone over normal lung tissue is resonance.*	■ Dullness is heard in patients with atelectasis, lobar pneumonia, and pleural effusion. ■ Hyperresonance is heard in those with chronic asthma, emphysema, and pneumothorax.
Percuss the posterior chest for diaphragmatic excursion. Systematic percussion of the posterior chest from a level of lung resonance to the level of diaphragmatic dullness reveals diaphragmatic excursion, a measurement of the level of the diaphragm. First percuss downward over the posterior thorax while the patient exhales fully and holds the breath. Mark the spot at which the sound changes from resonant to dull. Then ask the patient to inhale and hold the breath while you percuss downward again to note the descent of the diaphragm. Again, mark the spot where the sound changes. Measure the difference. *Diaphragmatic excursion normally varies from about 3 to 5 cm (about 1 to 2 in.)* (**Figure 34.10 ■**).	■ Diaphragmatic excursion is decreased in emphysema, ascites, on the affected side in pleural effusion, and in pneumothorax. ■ A high level of dullness or a lack of excursion may indicate atelectasis or pleural effusion.

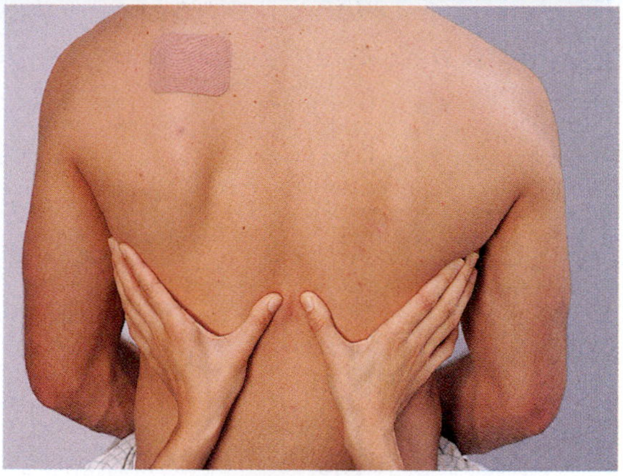

Figure 34.8 ■ Palpating for chest expansion.

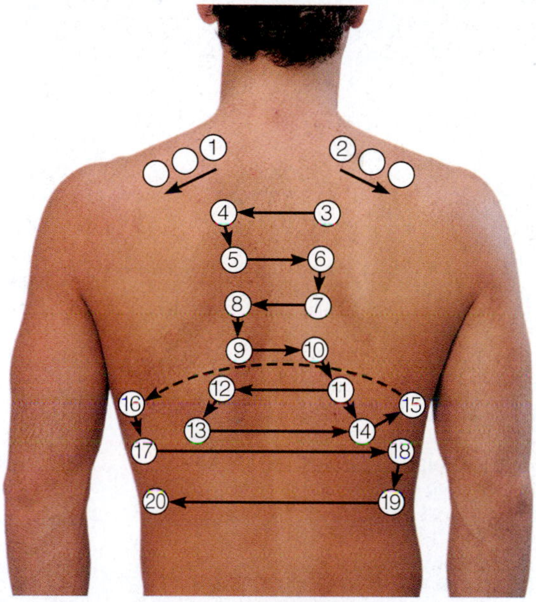
1
2
3
4
5
6
7
8
9
10
11
12
13
14
15
16
17
18
19
20

Figure 34.9 ■ Sequence for lung percussion.

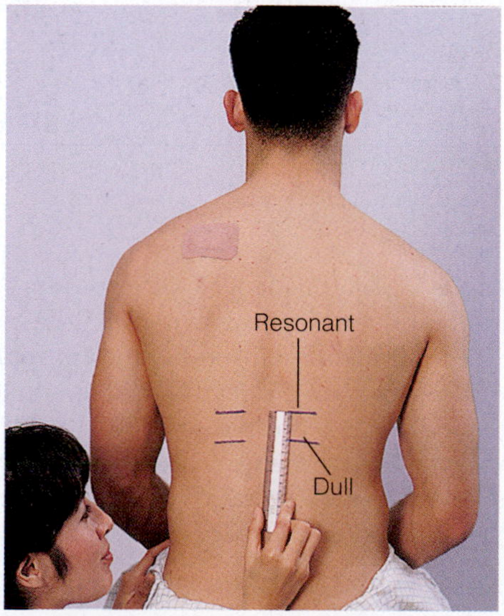
Resonant
Dull

Figure 34.10 ■ Measuring diaphragmatic excursion.

(*continued*)

Respiratory Assessments (*continued*)

Technique/Normal Findings	Abnormal Findings
Breath Sound Assessment Auscultate the lungs for breath sounds with the diaphragm of the stethoscope by having the patient take slow, deep breaths through the mouth. Listen over anterior, posterior, and lateral intercostal spaces (**Figure 34.11** ■). *The three different types of normal breath sounds are vesicular, bronchovesicular, and bronchial (***Table 34.1***).*	■ Bronchial breath sounds (expiration > inspiration) and bronchovesicular breath sounds (inspiration = expiration) are heard over lungs filled with fluid or solid tissue. ■ Breath sounds are decreased or diminished over atelectasis, emphysema, asthma, pleural effusion, and pneumothorax. ■ Breath sounds are increased over lobar pneumonia. ■ Breath sounds are absent over collapsed lung, surgical removal of lung, pleural effusion, and primary bronchus obstruction.
Auscultate for crackles, wheezes, and friction rubs. If crackles or wheezes are heard, ask the patient to cough and note if adventitious sound is cleared. *Normally, crackles, wheezes, and friction rubs are not present.*	■ **Crackles** (short, discrete, crackling or bubbling sounds) may be noted in pneumonia, bronchitis, and congestive heart failure. ■ **Wheezes** (continuous, musical sounds) may be heard in patients with bronchitis, emphysema, and asthma. ■ A **friction rub** is a loud, dry, creaking sound that indicates pleural inflammation.

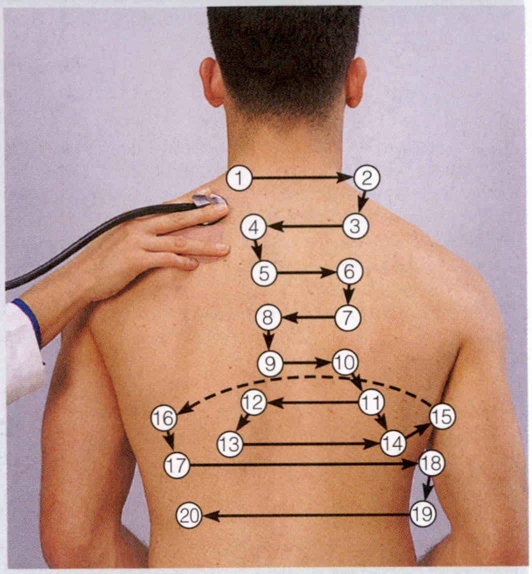
1
2
3
4
5
6
7
8
9
10
11
12
13
14
15
16
17
18
19
20
Figure 34.11 ■ Sequence for lung auscultation.

Table 34.1 Normal Breath Sounds

Type of Breath Sound	Characteristics
Vesicular	■ Soft, low-pitched, gentle sounds ■ Heard over all areas of the lungs except the major bronchi ■ Have a 3:1 ratio for inspiration and expiration, with inspiration lasting longer than expiration
Bronchovesicular	■ Medium pitch and intensity of sounds ■ Have a 1:1 ratio, with inspiration and expiration being equal in duration ■ Heard anteriorly over the primary bronchus on each side of the sternum and posteriorly between the scapulae
Bronchial	■ Loud, high-pitched sounds ■ Gap between inspiration and expiration ■ Have a 2:3 ratio for inspiration and expiration, with expiration longer than inspiration ■ Heard over the manubrium

Diagnosis

The results of diagnostic tests of respiratory function are used to support the diagnosis of a specific disease, to provide information to identify or modify the appropriate medications or therapy used to treat the disease, and to help nurses monitor the patient's responses to treatment and nursing care interventions. Diagnostic tests to assess the structures and functions of the respiratory system are described in the Diagnostic Tests feature. More information is included in the discussion of specific disorders in Chapters 35, 36, and 37.

Regardless of the type of diagnostic test, the nurse is responsible for explaining the procedure and any special preparation needed, assessing for medication use that may affect the outcome of the tests, supporting the patient during the examination as necessary, ensuring the consent form is signed (if necessary), documenting the procedures as appropriate, and monitoring the results of the tests.

Diagnostic Tests
of the Respiratory System

NAME OF TEST	PURPOSE AND DESCRIPTION	RELATED NURSING INTERVENTIONS
Arterial blood gases (ABGs)	This test of arterial blood is done to assess alterations in acid–base balance caused by a respiratory disorder, a metabolic disorder, or both. A pH of < 7.35 indicates acidosis and a pH of > 7.45 indicates alkalosis (see Chapter 10). To determine a respiratory cause, assess the $PaCO_2$: If pH is decreased and $PaCO_2$ is increased, respiratory acidosis is indicated. Normal values: pH: 7.35–7.45 $PaCO_2$: 35–45 mmHg PaO_2: 75–100 mmHg HCO_3: 22–26 mEq/L BE: ± 2 meq/L	Arterial blood is collected in a heparinized needle and syringe. Notify the person collecting the blood sample if the patient is taking anticoagulants or aspirin or has a clotting problem. The sample is placed on an ice-water bag and taken immediately to the lab. If patient is receiving oxygen, indicate the type, flow rate, administration device, and patient's temperature on lab slip. Apply pressure to puncture site for 5 minutes or longer, if needed (e.g., if taking anticoagulants or streptokinase). Do not collect blood from the same arm used for an IV infusion.
Biopsy of the lung	A biopsy of the lung is done to obtain tissue to differentiate benign from malignant tumors of the lungs. The biopsy may be done during a bronchoscopy or by surgical procedure.	Same as bronchoscopy or the same as a thoracotomy (incision through the chest wall) if a surgical biopsy is performed.
Bronchoscopy	A bronchoscopy is the direct visualization of the larynx, trachea, and bronchi through a bronchoscope to identify lesions, remove foreign bodies and secretions, obtain tissue for biopsy, and improve tracheobronchial drainage (**Figure 34.12** ■). The bronchoscope (in most cases, a fiberoptic scope) is passed through the nose or mouth and into the trachea. During the test, a catheter brush or biopsy forceps can be passed to obtain secretions or tissue for examination for cancer. The test is done in the hospital and may be done at the bedside, in a special procedure room, or in the surgical suite. 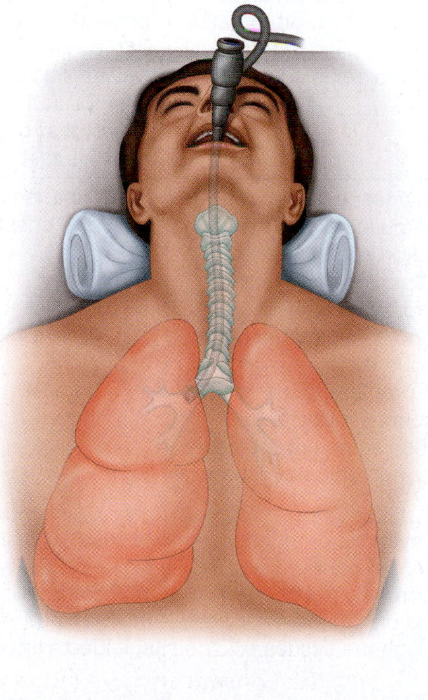 **Figure 34.12** ■ Fiberoptic bronchoscopy.	Assess for pregnancy and hypersensitivity to anesthetics, antibiotics, iodine, or contrast dyes; if any of these is present, notify the physician. Tell the patient not to eat or drink fluids for 8–12 h before the test. Remove dentures, contact lenses, and jewelry. Assess and record vital signs. Administer ordered premedications. After the procedure, assess for complications (laryngeal edema, bronchospasm, pneumothorax, cardiac dysrhythmias, and bleeding). Monitor for manifestations of respiratory difficulty (dyspnea, decreased breath sounds, decreased O_2 saturation), and hemoptysis (bloody sputum). Assess if the gag reflex is present before beginning food or fluids. Instruct the patient not to smoke for 6–8 h after the procedure because smoking may cause coughing and bleeding. Tell the patient it is normal to have some blood-tinged sputum, hoarseness, and/or a sore throat, but to notify the physician of any bleeding, pain, or respiratory difficulty.
Chest x-ray	Chest x-rays are used to identify abnormalities in chest structure and lung tissue, for diagnosis of diseases and injuries of the lungs, and to monitor treatment.	No special preparation is needed.

(continued)

Diagnostic Tests
of the Respiratory System (*continued*)

NAME OF TEST	PURPOSE AND DESCRIPTION	RELATED NURSING INTERVENTIONS
CT scan of the thorax	CT of the thorax may be performed when x-rays do not show some areas well, such as the pleura and mediastinum. It is also done to differentiate pathologic conditions (such as tumors, abscesses, and aortic aneurysms), to identify pleural effusion and enlarged lymph nodes, and to monitor treatment. Images are shown in cross-section.	If contrast dye is used, inform patient to not take oral food or fluids for 4 h before the test; if dye is not used, there are no food or fluid restrictions. Assess for allergies to iodine (e.g., to shellfish or previous procedures) and, if present, notify the physician. Medications such as diphenhydramine (Benadryl) and ranitidine (Zantac) may be given 1 h before the procedure. Assess medications: Oral hypoglycemic agents (including metformin) are contraindicated for use with iodinated contrast. Instruct the patient to increase oral fluid intake after the examination.
Magnetic resonance imaging (MRI) of the thorax	An MRI of the thorax is used to diagnose alterations in lung tissue that are more difficult to visualize by CT scan and to identify abnormal masses and fluid accumulation.	Inform patient of need to lie still during the examination. Assess for any metallic implants (such as pacemakers, clips on brain aneurysms, body piercing, tattoos, shrapnel). If present, notify imaging physician. Remove transdermal medication patches (both over-the-counter and prescribed) unless otherwise ordered. Replace the patch following the procedure. Tell the patient to inform the staff about the patch when making the appointment and when completing the admission information. Ask if patient is pregnant; if so, the test is not performed. Ask about claustrophobia; if it is a problem, request the patient to ask physician for a relaxing medication to take prior to the MRI.
Pulmonary angiography (angiogram)	This test, conducted in the hospital setting, is done to identify pulmonary emboli, tumors, aneurysms, vascular changes associated with emphysema, and pulmonary circulation. A catheter is inserted into the brachial or femoral artery, threaded into the pulmonary artery, and then dye is injected. ECG leads are applied to the chest for cardiac monitoring. Images of the lungs are taken.	Assess for hypersensitivity to iodine, seafood, or previous procedures using contrast dye. Take and record baseline vital signs. After the procedure, apply pressure to the injection site for 5–10 min (or until bleeding has stopped). Enforce bedrest for 12–24 h as ordered. Monitor vital signs, injection site, and peripheral pulses distal to the site after the test. Tell patient that coughing is a common occurrence after this test.
Pulmonary ventilation scan (V/Q scan)	This test is performed with two nuclear scans to measure breathing (ventilation) and circulation (perfusion) in all parts of the lungs. A ventilation scan is performed by scanning the lungs as the patient inhales radioactive gas. A perfusion scan is performed by injecting radioactive albumin into a vein and scanning the lungs. A decreased uptake of radioisotope during the perfusion scan indicates a blood flow problem, such as from a pulmonary embolus or pneumonitis. A decreased uptake of gas during the ventilation scan may indicate airway obstruction, pneumonia, or chronic pulmonary obstructive disease (COPD).	Tell the patient to remove all jewelry from the neck and chest.
Pulse oximetry	This noninvasive test is used to evaluate or monitor oxygen saturation of the blood. A device that uses infrared light is attached to an extremity (most commonly the finger, but can be used on the toe, earlobe, or nose) and light is passed through the tissues or reflected off bony structures. Normal value: 90–100%	Assess for factors that may alter findings, including faulty placement, movement, dark skin color, and acrylic nails. Light may affect the readings; the area of application should be shielded from external light sources.
Positron emission tomography (PET)	This relatively noninvasive test, when used to examine the lungs, is performed to identify lung nodules (cancers). The patient is given a radioactive substance and cross-sectional images are displayed on a computer.	Tell the patient that no alcohol, coffee, or tobacco is allowed for 24 h prior to the test. Encourage increased fluid intake posttest to help eliminate the radioactive material.

Diagnostic Tests
of the Respiratory System (*continued*)

NAME OF TEST	PURPOSE AND DESCRIPTION	RELATED NURSING INTERVENTIONS
Sputum studies: Culture and sensitivity	Culture and sensitivity of a single sputum specimen is done to diagnose bacterial infections, identify the most effective antibiotic, and evaluate treatment.	Instruct the patient to collect the specimen early in the morning. Explain that the sputum should come from deep in the lungs; take two or three deep breaths, and then cough the specimen into a sterile container. Sputum specimens may be obtained by a respiratory therapist or during bronchoscopy (described earlier) if the patient is unable to provide a specimen.
Acid-fast smear and culture	Sputum is examined for presence of acid-fast bacillus, specifically tuberculosis. A series of three early-morning sputum specimens is used.	
Cytology	Sputum is examined for presence of abnormal (malignant) cells. A single sputum specimen is collected in a special container of fixative solution.	
Thoracentesis	A thoracentesis is done to obtain a specimen of pleural fluid for diagnosis (and used as a procedure to remove pleural fluid or instill medication). A large-bore needle is inserted through the chest wall and into the pleural space. Following the procedure, a chest x-ray is taken to check for a pneumothorax.	Nursing care of the patient having a thoracentesis is provided in Chapter 36.

34.3 Assessment of Special Populations

Several changes associated with aging and disease affect respiratory function and airway clearance. The number of cilia decreases, and the cough weakens. Gag and cough reflexes diminish. The older adult is at greater risk for dehydration, leading to thick, viscous mucus that is difficult to expectorate. Immune function declines with age. These factors increase the risk of pulmonary infection and reduce the older adult's ability to respond effectively to infectious processes.

Other factors may also increase the risk for and severity of lower respiratory infections in the older adult: Immobility, smoking history, surgical procedures, use of multiple medications, malnutrition, and diseases such as COPD and heart disease.

Table 34.2 outlines age-related changes in the respiratory system and describes their significance.

The Veterans' Administration (VA) describes "presumption" of certain diagnoses related to military service. In Vietnam veterans who were exposed to agent Orange, presumption is described for respiratory cancers (lung, bronchus, larynx, trachea) in persons who have had symptoms appear within 1 year of exposure during active military duty. In atomic veterans (those exposed to ionizing radiation), presumption is described for bronchoalveolar carcinoma (VA, 2017). No differences have been noted for LGBTQI persons related to pulmonary disease and risk. All persons should be screened and treated based on physiologic findings.

Respiratory sequelae of congenital conditions primarily occur in four conditions: Restrictive lung disease, pulmonary hypertension, pulmonary hemorrhage, and plastic bronchitis (Lui et al., 2017; Sorenson, Quinn, & Klein, 2019). Up to 44% of adults with congenital heart disease have a pulmonary function test demonstrating a restrictive pulmonary pattern versus only 9% in the general population. Restrictive lung disease is seen most commonly in adults with a history of a Fontan procedure and tetralogy of Fallot repair (Lui et al., 2017). Pulmonary hypertension is believed to be related to the restrictive pattern. Pulmonary hemorrhage is more common in persons with a history of tetralogy of Fallot, pulmonary atresia, aortopulmonary collaterals or Eisenmenger syndrome (where up to 30% have hemoptysis) (Lui et al., 2017). Recurrent pneumonia has been shown to be a leading cause of death in adults with congenital heart

Table 34.2 Age-Related Changes in the Respiratory System

Age-Related Change	Significance
■ ↓ elastic recoil of lungs during expiration because of less elastic collagen and elastin ■ Calcification of the costal cartilage and weakening of the intercostal muscles ■ Loss of skeletal muscle strength in the thorax and diaphragm; flattening of the diaphragm ■ Alveoli are less elastic, more fibrotic, and have fewer functional capillaries ■ Cough is less effective ■ PO_2 reduces as much as 15% by age 80	The older adult often has an increased anterior–posterior chest diameter, with kyphosis and barrel chest. There is a reduction in vital capacity and an increase in residual volume, with decreased effectiveness in coughing up phlegm or sputum. All of these changes greatly increase the risk of respiratory infections (such as pneumonia), especially if the person becomes immobile. They also mean that respiratory infections are more difficult to treat.

disease (Lui et al., 2017). Plastic bronchitis is a lymphatic flow pathological process where lymph fluid collects in the airways, forming caulk-like plugs (called *casts*). These casts can block the airways, increasing breathing difficulty.

34.4 Health Promotion

Preventing lung disease focuses on avoidance of noxious inhalants, infection control, and healthy lifestyle choices. According to the Canadian Lung Association (2017), the following are general health-promoting recommendations:

- ***Stop smoking or never start.*** Smoking damages the lungs while increasing the risk for lung cancer and COPD. Teach patients that it is never too late to quit smoking and that multiple evidence-based methods have been shown to be effective. Encourage patients who do not smoke to avoid environments where smoking occurs. Simple strategies such as using smoke-free hotel rooms can promote lung health.
- ***Use good hand hygiene.*** Instruct patients that frequent handwashing with good technique (warm water, soap, friction for at least 15 seconds, rinse well) reduces most of the common shared bacteria.
- ***Use good cough technique.*** Teach patients that covering the mouth and nose with a tissue will help to stop the spread of germs. Coughing into a bent elbow is an option when no tissues are available. During peak flu and cold season, avoid crowds.
- ***Consider environmental changes to promote lung health.*** Encourage patients to maintain a clean house to reduce exposure to pet dander, dust, and mold. Indoor pollution (open wood-burning fires, overuse of aerosols) can cause lung damage. Teach patients to be aware of air pollution levels and limit exposure when particulate counts are high. Another teaching opportunity relates to radon, a naturally occurring radioactive gas. When present in the environment (home or work), it is the second leading cause of lung cancer when combined with smoking.
- ***Participate in healthy activity.*** Instruct the patient that 30 minutes of exercise each day will maintain oxygen transport efficiency.
- ***Get vaccinated.*** Teach patients that yearly influenza vaccinations are health-promoting behaviors, especially in those who are exposed to children, older adults, or persons who are sick. If the patient has a chronic lung disease, works in healthcare, or is over 65 years old, pneumonia vaccination is also recommended.

CHAPTER HIGHLIGHTS

34.1 Anatomy, Physiology, and Functions of the Respiratory System

Describe the anatomy, physiology, and functions of the nose and sinuses, pharynx, larynx, trachea, lungs, pleura, bronchi and alveoli, and rib cage and intercostal muscles, and identify abnormal findings that may indicate impairment of the respiratory system.

- Correct structure and function of the respiratory system is vital to ventilation, resulting in oxygenation of all body tissues.
- Normal anatomy, physiology, and functions of the upper and lower respiratory systems are the basis for assessment.

34.2 Assessing Respiratory System Function

Outline the components of the assessment of the respiratory system including topics for the health assessment interview, techniques for physical assessment, and the diagnostic tests used in the assessment.

- Manifestations of dysfunction, injury, and disorders affecting the respiratory system may be detected during a general health assessment as well as during a focused respiratory system assessment.
- Both general health and focused pulmonary system assessments can detect dysfunction, injury, and disorders.
- Assessment of the pulmonary system includes diagnostic tests, genetic considerations, a health interview, and a physical assessment.

34.3 Assessment of Special Populations

Differentiate considerations for assessing the respiratory system of older adults, veterans, individuals in the LGBTQI population, and adults with sequelae of childhood/congenital conditions.

- In older adults, physiological changes of the respiratory system lead to changes in pulmonary function that reduce efficiency. However, in the absence of chronic lung disease, these changes do not impact function.
- Respiratory sequelae of congenital conditions primarily occur in four conditions: Restrictive lung disease, pulmonary hypertension, pulmonary hemorrhage, and plastic bronchitis.

34.4 Health Promotion

Summarize topics that nurses teach to promote healthy tissue integrity across the lifespan.

- Preventing lung disease focuses on avoidance of noxious inhalants, infection control, and healthy lifestyle choices.

TEST YOURSELF NCLEX-RN® REVIEW

1. The nurse is assessing breath sounds. Where should the nurse place the diaphragm of the stethoscope to listen to the apex of the left lungs?
   A. In the mediastinum
   B. Just below the clavicle
   C. Within the parietal pleura
   D. Resting on the diaphragm
2. The nurse is concerned that a patient is at risk for developing lung cancer. What risk factor did the nurse most likely assess in this patient?
   A. Childhood obesity
   B. Family history of asthma
   C. Family history of lung cancer
   D. Frequent upper respiratory infections
3. Prior to providing care to a patient, the nurse reviews the previous day's vital sign assessments and notes that bronchovesicular breath sounds were documented. What should the nurse do next?
   A. Notify the physician.
   B. Measure and record vital signs as usual.
   C. Request a respiratory therapy treatment.
   D. Document the inability to hear breath sounds.
4. The nurse notes that a patient has an elevated body temperature. What processes are initiated between oxygen and hemoglobin as the temperature of body tissues increases? (Select all that apply.)
   A. Respiratory rate decreases.
   B. Lung compliance increases.
   C. Oxygen unloading is inhibited.
   D. Oxygen unloading is enhanced.
   E. 2,3 DGP is formed.
5. The nurse is teaching a patient about a thoracentesis. What should the nurse include in this teaching? (Select all that apply.)
   A. Fluid is removed from around the lung.
   B. A chest x-ray is done after the procedure.
   C. A needle is inserted through the chest wall.
   D. The procedure requires a thoracotomy.
   E. It is a specialized x-ray procedure.
6. The nurse is completing assessment of a patient's cough. Which questions should be included? (Select all that apply.)
   A. "When did you first notice your cough?"
   B. "Has anything you have tried made your cough go away?"
   C. "When do you have coughing episodes?"
   D. "Have you ever coughed before?"
   E. "Do you have pain in your chest when you cough?"
7. While auscultating a patient's breath sounds, the nurse notes continuous musical sounds. How should the nurse document this finding?
   A. Crackles
   B. Wheezes
   C. Murmurs
   D. Friction rub
8. While reviewing a patient's assessments, the nurse notes an absence of sounds in the right lower lung. Which information in the health history would explain this assessment finding?
   A. Admitted with pleural effusion
   B. History of tuberculosis
   C. Pneumonia 10 years ago
   D. Diagnosed with childhood asthma
9. The nurse is preparing to auscultate a patient's lung sounds. What direction should the nurse provide when making this assessment? (Select all that apply.)
   A. "Hold your breath."
   B. "Take slow, deep breaths."
   C. "Breathe through your nose."
   D. "Breathe through an opened mouth."
   E. "Repeat the number 99 several times."
10. While assessing a patient with a left pneumothorax, the nurse notes decreased diaphragmatic excursion on the left. What should the nurse do next?
    A. Document the assessment.
    B. Notify the physician immediately.
    C. Repeat the assessment several times.
    D. Tell the patient to hold his or her breath.

See Test Yourself answers in Appendix B.

BIBLIOGRAPHY

American Lung Association. (2018). *Homepage.* Retrieved from http://www.lung.org.

Canadian Lung Association. (2017). *Preventing lung disease.* Retrieved from https://www.lung.ca/lung-health/prevent-lung-disease.

Centers for Disease Control and Prevention. (CDC). (2017). *Most recent asthma data.* Retrieved from https://www.cdc.gov/asthma/most_recent_data.htm.

Cystic Fibrosis Foundation. (2018). *About cystic fibrosis.* Retrieved from https://www.cff.org/What-is-CF/About-Cystic-Fibrosis/.

Kanwal, M., Ding, X.-J., & Cao, Y. (2017). Familial risk for lung cancer. *Oncology Letters, 13*(2), 535–542.

Lui, G. K., Saidi, A., Bhatt, A. B., Burchill, L. J., Deen, J. F., Earing, M. G., . . . Yoo, S-J. (2017). Diagnosis and management of non-cardiac complications in adults with congenital heart disease: A scientific statement from the American Heart Association. *Circulation, 136.* [Epub ahead of print]

National Institutes of Health. (2017). *Genes and disease: Respiratory diseases.* Retrieved from www.ncbi.nlm.nih.gov/books/NBK22167.

Shellenberger, R. A., Balakrishnan, B., Avula, S., Ebel, A., & Shaik, S. (2017). Diagnostic value of the physical examination in patients with dyspnea. *Cleveland Clinical Journal of Medicine, 84*(12), 943–950.

Sorenson, M., Quinn, L., & Klein, D. (2019). *Pathophysiology: Concepts of human disease.* Hoboken, NJ: Pearson Education.

Veterans' Administration (VA). (2017). *Disability compensation: "Presumptive" disability benefits.* Retrieved from https://www.benefits.va.gov/BENEFITS/factsheets/serviceconnected/presumption.pdf.

ADDITIONAL RESOURCES

American Lung Association. (2018a). *Lung health and diseases.* Retrieved from www.lung.org/lung-health-and-diseases/.

American Lung Association. (2018b). *Our initiatives.* Retrieved from www.lung.org/our-initiatives/.

American Lung Association. (2018c). *Stop smoking.* Retrieved from www.lung.org/stop-smoking/

American Thoracic Society. (2017). *Patient resources: Fact sheets A to Z.* Retrieved from www.thoracic.org/patients/patient-resources/fact-sheets-az.php.

COPD Foundation. (2018). *Homepage.* Retrieved from https://www.copdfoundation.org.

Cystic Fibrosis Foundation. (2018). *Homepage.* Retrieved from https://www.cff.org/.

Lungs and You. (2018). *What is IPF?* Retrieved from https://www.lungsandyou.com/facts/what-is-ipf.

National Heart, Lung, and Blood Institute. (2018). *Health topics.* Retrieved from https://www.nhlbi.nih.gov.

Chapter 35

Nursing Care of Patients with Upper Respiratory Disorders

Chapter Outline and Learning Outcomes

35.1 Infectious and Inflammatory Disorders 1234

Describe the pathophysiology and manifestations of infectious and inflammatory upper respiratory disorders and outline the interprofessional care and nursing care of patients with these disorders.

35.2 Upper Respiratory Trauma or Obstruction 1254

Describe the pathophysiology and manifestations of disorders of upper respiratory trauma or obstruction and outline the interprofessional care and nursing care of patients with these disorders.

35.3 Upper Respiratory Tumors 1266

Describe the pathophysiology and manifestations of upper respiratory tumors and outline the interprofessional care and nursing care of patients with upper respiratory tumors.

CLINICAL COMPETENCIES

- Assess the functional health status of patients with upper respiratory disorders, using data to identify and prioritize holistic nursing care needs.
- Use nursing research and evidence-based practice to plan and implement nursing care for patients with upper respiratory disorders.
- Provide safe and effective nursing care for patients having surgery involving the upper respiratory system and/or with a tracheostomy.
- Safely administer medications and prescribed treatments for patients with disorders of the upper respiratory tract.
- Provide appropriate teaching for the patient and family affected by upper respiratory tract disorders.
- Evaluate the effectiveness of care, reassessing and modifying the plan of care as needed to achieve desired patient outcomes.

KEY TERMS

benign laryngeal tumors, 1267
coryza, 1234
epistaxis, 1254
influenza, 1239
laryngeal cancer, 1267
laryngeal obstruction, 1259
laryngeal trauma, 1259
laryngectomy, 1269
laryngitis, 1249
pertussis, 1252
pharyngitis, 1246
rhinitis, 1234
rhinoplasty, 1258
sinusitis, 1242
sleep apnea, 1263
tonsillitis, 1246

Upper respiratory disorders may affect the nose, paranasal sinuses, tonsils, adenoids, larynx, and pharynx, including nasopharynx and oropharynx. A patent (open and clear) upper airway is necessary for effective breathing. Upper respiratory disorders, such as the common cold, may be minor. However, acute and even life-threatening problems develop when upper airway patency is affected (e.g., by laryngeal edema). Upper respiratory disorders can affect breathing, communication, eating, swallowing, and body image. When breathing is compromised because of swelling, bleeding, or accumulation of secretions, fear and anxiety develop.

Nursing care focuses on maintaining the airway, managing pain and symptoms, promoting effective communication, and providing psychologic support for the patient and family.

35.1 Infectious and Inflammatory Disorders

Constant exposure of the upper respiratory tract to the environment makes it vulnerable to a variety of infectious and inflammatory conditions. Although most upper respiratory infections and inflammations are minor, complications may result. In the frail older adult, the risk of serious problems following an upper respiratory infection can be significant.

Rhinitis, inflammation of the nasal cavities, is the most common upper respiratory disorder. Rhinitis may be either acute or chronic. *Acute viral rhinitis*, or the common cold, is discussed next. Chronic rhinitis includes allergic, vasomotor, and atrophic rhinitis. *Allergic rhinitis*, or hay fever, results from a sensitivity reaction to allergens such as plant pollens. It tends to occur seasonally but can be perennial. The etiology of *vasomotor rhinitis* is unknown. Although its manifestations are similar to those of allergic rhinitis, it is not linked to allergens. *Atrophic rhinitis* is characterized by changes in the mucous membrane of the nasal cavities.

The Patient with a Viral Upper Respiratory Infection

Viral upper respiratory infections (URIs or the common cold) are the most common respiratory tract infections and are among the most common human diseases. URIs are highly contagious and are prevalent in schools and work environments. The incidence of acute URI peaks during September and late January, coinciding with the opening of schools, and again toward the end of April. Most adults experience two to four colds each year (Sorenson, Quinn, & Klein, 2019).

Pathophysiology

More than 200 strains of virus cause URIs, including rhinoviruses, adenoviruses, parainfluenza viruses, coronaviruses, and respiratory syncytial viruses. Occasionally, more than one virus may be present. Viruses causing acute URIs spread by aerosolized droplet nuclei during sneezing or coughing or by direct contact. The virus usually spreads when the hands and fingers pick it up from contaminated surfaces and carry it to the eyes and mucous membranes of the susceptible host. Infected patients are highly contagious, shedding virus for a few days prior to and after the appearance of symptoms. Although immunity is produced to the individual virus strain, the number of viruses causing URIs ensures that most people will experience colds throughout their lifetime.

Viscous mucus secretions in the upper respiratory tract trap invading organisms, preventing contamination of more vulnerable areas. Cells of the upper respiratory tract are infected when the virus attaches to receptors on the cell. Local immunologic defenses, such as secretory IgA antibodies in respiratory secretions, then attempt to inactivate the antigen, producing a local inflammatory response. The mucous membranes of the nasal passages swell and become hyperemic and engorged. Mucus-secreting glands become hyperactive. These responses to the virus produce the typical manifestations of viral URIs.

Manifestations

Acute viral upper respiratory infection often presents as the common cold. Nasal mucous membranes appear red (*erythematous*) and *boggy* (swollen). Swollen mucous membranes, local vasodilation, and secretions cause nasal congestion. Clear, watery secretions lead to **coryza** (nasal inflammation and profuse nasal discharge). Sneezing and coughing are common. Sore throat is common, and may be the initial symptom. Systemic manifestations of acute viral URIs infrequently include low-grade fever, headache, malaise, and muscle aches. Symptoms generally last for a few days up to 2 weeks.

Complications

Although acute viral URI is typically mild and self-limited, its effects on the immune defenses of the upper respiratory tract can increase the risk for more serious bacterial infections, such as sinusitis or otitis media.

Interprofessional Care

Because most acute viral URIs are self-limiting, self-care is appropriate and encouraged. Medical treatment is usually required only when complications such as sinusitis or otitis media develop.

Diagnosis

Diagnosis of acute viral URI is usually based on the history and physical examination. Diagnostic testing may be indicated if a complication such as bacterial infection is suspected. A white blood count (WBC) is generally not needed but may be ordered to assess for leukocytosis (an elevated WBC) if there are complications. Cultures of purulent discharge may also be obtained.

Treatment is symptomatic. Adequate rest, maintaining fluid intake, and avoiding chilling help relieve systemic symptoms such as fever, malaise, and muscle ache. Instruct patients to cover the mouth and nose with tissue when coughing or sneezing and to dispose of soiled tissues properly. Additionally, avoiding crowds helps prevent spread of the infection to others.

Medications

Medications may be recommended to shorten the duration of the illness and relieve symptoms. Mild decongestants or over-the-counter antihistamines may help relieve coryza and nasal congestion. Nasal sprays such as phenylephrine (Neo-Synephrine) rapidly relieve nasal congestion, but may lead to dependence and rebound congestion if used for more than a few days at a time. Warm saltwater gargles, throat lozenges, or mild analgesics may be used for sore throat. Although no specific antiviral therapy has been shown to be effective in shortening the duration of a URI, experimental vaccines to prevent acute viral URI are in developmental stages. For the nursing implications of decongestants and common antihistamines, see **Medication Administration 35.A.**

Integrative Therapies

Complementary therapies are appropriate for treating most acute viral URIs. Herbal remedies such as echinacea and garlic may have antiviral and antibiotic effects. Echinacea

Medication Administration 35.A

Decongestants and Antihistamines

NASAL AND ORAL DECONGESTANTS

naphazoline (Privine) nasal

oxymetazoline (Afrin 12 Hour, Neo-synephrine 12 hour, others) nasal and oral

phenylephrine (Afrin 4–6 hours, Neo-Synephrine 4–6 hours, others)

pseudoephedrine (Sudafed) oral

tetrahydrozoline (Tyzine) nasal

Decongestants promote vasoconstriction, reducing the inflammation and edema of nasal mucosa and relieving nasal congestion. They are very effective when applied topically (by nasal spray) because of their rapid onset of action. However, the duration of effect is short, followed by vasodilation and rebound congestion. Because of their rapid effect and short duration, these preparations are habit forming. Chronic use may lead to *rhinitis medicamentosa*, a rebound phenomenon of drug-induced nasal irritation and inflammation.

Nursing Responsibilities

- Assess for contraindications, such as hypertension or chronic heart disease. These drugs stimulate the sympathetic nervous system, increasing peripheral vascular resistance, blood pressure, and heart rate.
- Evaluate medication regimen for potential interactions such as antihypertensive medications and monoamine oxidase inhibitors (MAOIs).

Health Education for the Patient and Family

- Do not use more than the recommended dose.
- Check with the healthcare provider before taking decongestants if you are taking any prescription medications or are being treated for high blood pressure or heart disease.
- Use nasal sprays for no more than 3 to 5 days.
- Increase fluid intake to relieve mouth dryness.
- These drugs may cause nervousness, shakiness, or difficulty sleeping. Stop the drug if these effects occur.
- In some states, drugs containing pseudoephedrine may require a prescription or be kept behind the counter to reduce its use in preparing methamphetamine.

ANTIHISTAMINES (H_1-RECEPTOR ANTAGONISTS AND MAST CELL STABILIZERS)

brompheniramine (Dimetapp, others)

chlorpheniramine (Chlor-Trimeton, others)

clemastine (Tavist)

dexchlorpheniramine (Dexchlor, Poladex, Polaramine)

dimenhydrinate (Dramamine)

diphenhydramine (Benadryl, others)

Nonsedating

cetirizine (Zyrtec)

desloratadine (Clarinex)

fexofenadine (Allegra)

levocetirizine (Xyzal)

loratadine (Claritin)

Antihistamines are widely available with and without a prescription. They are frequently combined with decongestants in over-the-counter (OTC) cold and allergy preparations. Antihistamines relieve the systemic effects of histamine and dry respiratory secretions through an anticholinergic effect. Most antihistamines cause drowsiness; nonsedating forms are less likely to interfere with alertness. Diphenhydramine is used in numerous OTC sleep aids as well as in cold and allergy preparations.

Nursing Responsibilities

- Before administering or recommending these drugs, assess for possible contraindications, including:
  a. Acute asthma or lower respiratory disease that may be aggravated by drying of secretions
  b. Hypersensitivity to antihistamines
  c. Glaucoma (increased intraocular pressure)
  d. Impaired gastrointestinal motility or obstruction
  e. Prostatic hypertrophy or other urinary tract obstruction
  f. Heart disease.
- For patients who must remain alert while on antihistamine therapy, recommend nonsedating forms.

Health Education for the Patient and Family

- Do not drive or operate machinery while taking OTC or prescription forms of antihistamines known to be sedating.
- Stop the drug and notify your doctor immediately if you develop confusion, excessive sedation, chest tightness, wheezing, bleeding, or easy bruising while taking antihistamines.
- Do not use alcohol or other CNS depressants while taking antihistamines.
- Hard candy, gum, ice chips, and liquids help relieve mouth dryness caused by antihistamines.

Source: Data from Adams, Holland, & Urban, 2017.

is also thought to stimulate the immune system, improving the body's response to infection. Taken at the first sign of infection, echinacea may reduce the duration and symptoms, although clinical trials have shown no consistent benefit. The recommended dose of echinacea varies, depending on the part of the plant used in the preparation. It should not be used for longer than 2 weeks. It is contraindicated for use during pregnancy and lactation and in people who have an autoimmune disease such as rheumatoid arthritis (National Center for Complementary and Integrative Health [NCCIH], 2017).

Dietary supplements such as vitamin C and zinc are also promoted as measures to reduce the severity and duration of URI. Again, however, no consistent benefit is demonstrated in clinical trials (NCCIH, 2017). Although selected studies have shown a beneficial effect of zinc gluconate lozenges to reduce the duration of an induced URI, no such benefit was found when zinc was compared with placebo to treat naturally occurring URIs (NCCIH, 2017).

Aromatherapy with essential oils such as basil, cedarwood, eucalyptus, frankincense, lavender, marjoram, peppermint, or rosemary can reduce congestion and promote comfort and recovery. Teach patients that these essential oils are to be used only for inhalation, not for internal consumption. Acupuncture and acupressure may be effective in treating URIs in adults, particularly when combined with the use of Chinese herbs and when started early in the course of illness (Heo et al., 2016). Their beneficial effect is most likely related to stimulation of the immune response by acupuncture and acupressure.

Nursing Care

Assessment

Nursing assessment focuses on symptoms and history. Viral upper respiratory infections usually have a rapid onset and are time limited.

- ***Health history:*** Known exposure to virus; current symptoms, their onset and duration; presence of dyspnea, chest pain, productive cough, facial pain, or pressure in sinus areas; current medications, history of influenza vaccine; chronic diseases such as heart disease, COPD, or diabetes; smoking or alcohol abuse; institutionalized, communal living such as college dormitories; known medication allergies
- ***Physical assessment:*** General appearance; vital signs including temperature; skin color; lung sounds; abdominal exam; ear, nose, and throat examination
- ***Laboratory data:*** Throat and sputum cultures and chest x-ray unless suspect for evidence of bacterial infection or pneumonia.

Priorities of Care

Nursing care is supportive. The focus of nursing care for the adult with a viral URI is symptom management, surveillance for complications, teaching for self-care, and on identification of complications such as pneumonia, sinusitis, and prevention of viral spread.

Diagnoses, Interventions, and Outcomes

Although the symptoms of a viral URI can be distressing, most people provide self-care and do not contact a healthcare provider. Recommendations to rest in bed during the acute phase of the illness and limit activities until recovery are appropriate for viral URI.

Promote Effective Breathing. Due to the viral infection, the respiratory rate may increase and alter the depth of respirations, decreasing effective alveolar ventilation. Shallow respirations also increase the risk of *atelectasis*, lack of ventilation in an area of lung.

Expected Outcome: Patient will utilize techniques to promote adequate ventilation such as deep breathing and incentive spirometry.

The nurse will:

- Monitor respiratory rate and pattern. *Tachypnea and/or rapid, shallow respirations may impair effective alveolar ventilation and gas exchange.*
- Pace activities to provide for periods of rest. *Tachypnea increases the work of breathing, causing fatigue; fatigue, in turn, can further impair ventilation and reduce the effectiveness of coughing.*
- Elevate the head of the bed. *The upright position promotes drainage of nasal secretions, improves lung excursion, and reduces the work of breathing by lowering the diaphragm, which moves abdominal contents downward, creating less resistance to diaphragmatic excursion and slightly decreasing venous return.*

Promote Airway Clearance and Patency. Swelling and congestion of mucous membranes, extracellular fluid exudate, and impaired ciliary action due to cell damage increase the risk of impaired airway clearance in viral URI. The older adult is at particular risk because of normally reduced ciliary activity and increased lung compliance.

Expected Outcome: Patient will use techniques to promote airway clearance such as coughing and deep breathing.

The nurse will:

- Monitor the effectiveness of cough and ability to remove airway secretions. *Fatigue and general malaise may impair the ability to cough effectively and mobilize secretions.*
- Maintain adequate hydration. Assess mucous membranes and skin turgor for evidence of dehydration. *Fever, increased mucous membrane secretions, and decreased oral fluid intake may lead to dehydration and increased viscosity of secretions. Thick, viscous secretions are more difficult to expectorate.*
- Increase the humidity of inspired air with a bedside humidifier. *Increasing the water content of inhaled air helps loosen thick secretions and soothe mucous membranes.*
- Teach effective cough techniques. Administer analgesics as ordered. *The huff cough is effective to maintain open airways and spares energy (see Chapter 37 for patient teaching of this technique). Relieving muscle ache increases the ability to cough effectively.*

Assess Sleep Quality. Airway congestion, and persistent cough may interfere with the ability to rest, increasing fatigue and prolonging recovery.

Expected Outcome: Patient will verbalize techniques to reduce impact of upper respiratory symptoms on sleep patterns.

The nurse will:

- Assess sleep patterns using subjective and objective information. *The patient may appear to be sleeping but not achieving normal sleep patterns because of viral URI symptoms. Both subjective and objective data are important to accurately assess sleep.*

Reduce Risk for Infection. Infection control measures are recommended to prevent person-to-person transmission of viral URI control viral URI outbreaks in healthcare facilities.

Expected Outcome: Patient will describe measures to protect healthy tissue and prevent infection.

The nurse will:

- Use standard precautions and encourage all staff and visitors to wash hands frequently. *Hand hygiene is a primary infection control measure for infections transmitted via respiratory secretions.*
- Instruct patients and visitors to control respiratory secretions by using tissues and to maintain a distance of at least 3 feet from others when coughing or sneezing. Provide masks for patients and visitors who are coughing or sneezing. *Limiting the spread of aerosolized secretions by covering the nose and mouth and maintaining distance from other people can reduce the spread of the disease to vulnerable populations.*
- Use droplet precautions for patients with suspected or confirmed viral URI: Private room, masks for caregivers and visitors, and mask the patient when transporting within the facility. *These measures limit the spread of respiratory secretions.*

Delegating Nursing Care Activities

As appropriate and allowed by the designated duties and responsibilities of unlicensed assistive personnel, the nurse may delegate nursing care activities such as measuring vital signs, encouraging oral or enteral fluid intake, and providing skin care.

Transitions of Care

Patients can limit their incidence of acute viral URI by frequent handwashing and avoiding exposure to crowds. Maintaining good general health and participating in stress-reducing activities support the immune system and help prevent acute viral URIs. Teach the patient that becoming chilled or going out in the rain does not cause colds and that URIs are more likely to occur during periods of physical or psychologic stress.

The primary nursing role in caring for patients with acute viral URI is educational. Self-care is appropriate for most patients unless the problem is recurrent, or a complication occurs. Acute viral URI may interfere with work and recreational activities. Unless limited by symptoms, normal daily activities and roles can usually be maintained. Additional rest during the acute phase of illness is recommended. Additional fluid intake and a well-balanced diet help support the immune response, hastening recovery.

Include the following topics in teaching for home care:

- Use disposable tissues to cover the mouth and nose while coughing or sneezing to reduce airborne spread of the virus.
- Blow the nose with both nostrils open to prevent infected matter from being forced into the eustachian tubes.
- Wash hands frequently, especially after coughing or sneezing, to limit viral transmission.
- Use OTC preparations for symptomatic relief; understand precautions related to the sedating effects of antihistamines.
- Limit use of nasal decongestants to every 4 hours for only a few days at a time to prevent rebound effect.

The Patient with Respiratory Syncytial Virus (RSV)

Pathophysiology

Respiratory syncytial virus (RSV) is a common virus that is the primary cause of respiratory illnesses in young children and the majority of lower respiratory disease in infants. RSV is transmitted in much the same way as other URIs: Via contaminated hands or objects and by coarse droplets spread by coughing and sneezing. The incubation period is 4 to 6 days.

Risk Factors

Older children and adults are also commonly, and repeatedly, infected by RSV, but the disease is milder, usually presenting as a common cold. However, older adults and people who are immunocompromised may develop severe pneumonitis when exposed to RSV.

Manifestations

In adults, the manifestations of RSV are those of other common URIs, including rhinorrhea, sore throat, and cough. Headache, malaise, and low-grade fever may occur. In older adults, RSV may present as lower respiratory infection with fever or pneumonia (Sorenson et al., 2019).

Complications

While the illness also presents as URI in infants, it is more likely to progress to pneumonia, bronchiolitis, and tracheobronchiolitis in adults.

Interprofessional Care

Treatment for adults with upper respiratory RSV is symptomatic (see the section on URIs). When the lower respiratory tract is involved, hydration and other measures to mobilize respiratory secretions are important. Intubation and mechanical ventilation may be necessary if hypoxia develops.

Diagnosis

The diagnosis of RSV is based on history and clinical findings. A chest x-ray and WBC count may be done to rule out complications such as pneumonia. The WBC is commonly decreased in viral infections such as RSV; bacterial infections usually cause increased WBCs.

Medications

Aerosolized ribavirin (Virazole; an antiviral drug) may be prescribed for older adults and immunocompromised patients with RSV pneumonia.

Integrative Therapies

The National Center for Complementary and Integrative Health (2017) does not list any integrative therapies specific for RSV.

Nursing Care

Assessment

Nursing assessment focuses on symptoms and history.

- ***Health history:*** Known exposure to virus; current symptoms and their onset and duration; presence of dyspnea, chest pain, productive cough, facial pain, or pressure in sinus areas; current medications, history of influenza vaccine; chronic diseases such as heart disease, COPD, or diabetes; smoking or alcohol abuse; institutionalized, communal living such as college dormitories; known medication allergies
- ***Physical assessment:*** General appearance; vital signs including temperature; skin color; lung sounds; abdominal exam; ear, nose, and throat examination
- ***Laboratory data:*** Throat and sputum cultures and chest x-ray unless suspect for evidence of bacterial infection or pneumonia.

Priorities of Care

Nursing care is supportive. The focus of nursing care for the adult with URI manifestations of RSV is on teaching for self-care and on identification of complications such as pneumonia, sinusitis, and prevention of viral spread. When lower respiratory symptoms are present, nursing care is similar to that provided for patients with pneumonia (see Chapter 37).

Diagnoses, Interventions, and Outcomes

RSV signs and symptoms usually appear similar to those of a mild cold in adults. Most people provide self-care and may not contact a healthcare provider. Recommendations to rest in bed during the acute phase of the illness and limit activities until recovery are appropriate for RSV.

Promote Effective Breathing. Due to the viral infection, the respiratory rate may increase and alter the depth of respirations, decreasing effective alveolar ventilation. Shallow respirations also increase the risk of *atelectasis*, lack of ventilation in an area of the lungs.

Expected Outcome: Patient will utilize techniques to promote adequate ventilation such as deep breathing and incentive spirometry.

The nurse will:

- Monitor respiratory rate and pattern. *Tachypnea and/or rapid, shallow respirations may impair effective alveolar ventilation and gas exchange.*
- Pace activities to provide for periods of rest. *Tachypnea increases the work of breathing, causing fatigue; fatigue, in turn, can further impair ventilation and reduce the effectiveness of coughing.*
- Elevate the head of the bed. *The upright position promotes drainage of nasal secretions, improves lung excursion, and reduces the work of breathing by lowering the diaphragm, which moves abdominal contents downward, creating less resistance to diaphragmatic excursion and slightly decreasing venous return.*

Promote Airway Clearance and Patency. Swelling and congestion of mucous membranes, extracellular fluid exudate, and impaired ciliary action due to cell damage increase the risk of impaired airway clearance in viral URI. The older adult is at particular risk because of normally reduced ciliary activity and increased lung compliance.

Expected Outcome: Patient will use techniques to promote airway clearance such as coughing and deep breathing.

The nurse will:

- Monitor the effectiveness of cough and ability to remove airway secretions. *Fatigue and general malaise may impair the ability to cough effectively and mobilize secretions.*
- Maintain adequate hydration. Assess mucous membranes and skin turgor for evidence of dehydration. *Fever, increased mucous membrane secretions, and decreased oral fluid intake may lead to dehydration and increased viscosity of secretions. Thick, viscous secretions are more difficult to expectorate.*
- Increase the humidity of inspired air with a bedside humidifier. *Increasing the water content of inhaled air helps loosen thick secretions and soothe mucous membranes.*
- Teach effective cough techniques. Administer analgesics as ordered. *The huff cough is effective to maintain open airways and spares energy (see Chapter 37 for patient teaching of this technique). Relieving muscle ache increases the ability to cough effectively.*

Assess Sleep Quality. Airway congestion and persistent cough may interfere with the ability to rest, increasing fatigue and prolonging recovery.

Expected Outcome: Patient will verbalize techniques to reduce impact of upper respiratory symptoms on sleep patterns.

The nurse will:

- Assess sleep patterns using subjective and objective information. *The patient may appear to be sleeping but not achieving normal sleep patterns because of viral URI symptoms. Both subjective and objective data are important to assess sleep accurately.*

Reduce Risk for Infection. Infection control measures are recommended to prevent person-to-person transmission of viral URI and viral URI outbreaks in healthcare facilities.

Expected Outcome: Patient will describe measures to protect healthy tissue and prevent infection.

The nurse will:

- Use standard precautions and encourage all staff and visitors to wash hands frequently. *Hand hygiene is a primary infection control measure for infections transmitted via respiratory secretions.*
- Instruct patients and visitors to control respiratory secretions by using tissues and to maintain a distance of at least 3 feet from others when coughing or sneezing. Provide masks for patients and visitors who are coughing or sneezing. *Limiting the spread of aerosolized secretions by covering the nose and mouth and maintaining distance from other people can reduce the spread of the disease to vulnerable populations.*
- Use droplet precautions for patients with suspected or confirmed viral URI: Private room, masks for caregivers and visitors, and mask the patient when transporting within the facility. *These measures limit the spread of respiratory secretions.*

Delegating Nursing Care Activities

As appropriate and allowed by the designated duties and responsibilities of unlicensed assistive personnel, the nurse may delegate nursing care activities such as measuring vital signs, encouraging oral or enteral fluid intake, and providing skin care.

Transitions of Care

There is no vaccine for RSV. Preventive actions focus on good hand hygiene and frequent handwashing. RSV is common and most children have been exposed by the age of 2. Avoid others with colds and/or fevers.

The primary nursing role in caring for patients with RSV infection is educational. Self-care is appropriate for most patients unless the problem is recurrent or a complication occurs. RSV, as it presents like a mild cold, may interfere with work and recreational activities. Unless limited by symptoms, normal daily activities and roles can usually be maintained. Additional rest during the acute phase of illness is recommended. Additional fluid intake and a well-balanced diet help support the immune response, hastening recovery.

The Patient with Influenza

Influenza, or *flu*, is a highly contagious viral respiratory disease characterized by coryza, fever, cough, and systemic symptoms such as headache and malaise. Influenza usually occurs in epidemics or pandemics, although sporadic cases do occur. Localized outbreaks of influenza usually occur about every 1 to 3 years. Global epidemics (pandemics) are less frequent, developing every 10 to 15 years until the past two decades. In the last decade, an identified strain of avian (bird) influenza has raised concerns about a potential future pandemic. This strain of influenza virus has not yet demonstrated the ability to spread between humans; however, concerns are that it will mutate to allow person-to-person spread. See **Box 35.1** for more information about avian influenza.

Pathophysiology

Influenza virus is transmitted by airborne droplet and direct contact. Three major strains of the virus have been

BOX 35.1

Focus on Avian Influenza

Influenza viruses are common in nature, found in wild birds such as ducks and shore birds. Although these birds carry the virus, they usually are not harmed by it. Movement of the virus into domesticated flocks of ducks and chickens can not only devastate populations of these birds, but can also spread the virus to other domestic animals such as pigs.

Avian influenza is caused by a type A influenza virus identified as *H5N1*. Type A influenza viruses are subclassified by two proteins, hemagglutinin (HA) and neuraminidase (NA), found on the surface of the virus. HA allows the virus to attach to a cell and initiate an infection, whereas NA allows the virus to exit the host cell after replicating. Currently, there are only three known subtypes of influenza A circulating among humans: H1N1, H1N2, and H3N2. The H5N1 virus, which is particularly virulent and spread by migratory birds, raises fears of a potential human pandemic should it evolve to become transmissible from human to human.

Influenza viruses are very changeable, undergoing small, continuous changes as well as occasional large and abrupt changes. *Antigenic drift* is the term for small changes that occur continuously as a virus makes copies of itself. These changes help the virus elude the immune system and necessitate the production of new vaccines every year. Sudden, dramatic changes occur when two different strains of influenza virus (e.g., avian influenza and human influenza) infect the same cell and exchange genetic material. These changes, called *antigenic shift*, create a new subtype of the virus to which people have little or no immunity. Most reported cases of avian influenza A have occurred in previously healthy children and young adults, often with an underlying chronic illness.

Symptoms of avian influenza include typical flulike manifestations such as fever, cough, sore throat, and myalgias. In addition, affected people may develop eye infections, pneumonia, and respiratory distress, including acute respiratory distress syndrome (ARDS) (see Chapter 37 for more information about ARDS and its manifestations).

No vaccine to protect against the H5N1 virus has yet been developed for commercial use. The National Institute of Allergy and Infectious Diseases (NIAID; 2017b) continues research into influenza vaccine development. Some currently available antiviral medications may effectively treat avian influenza (World Health Organization, 2017).

A severe pandemic of H5N1 or avian influenza could disrupt all aspects of life, not only causing severe illness and death, but also overwhelming the healthcare system, impacting social services, and causing significant economic loss. Advance preparations such as those currently being undertaken by the World Health Organization and the United States and other countries can reduce the impact of a pandemic (Centers for Disease Control and Prevention [CDC], 2017c; NIAID, 2017b; World Health Organization, 2017).

identified: Influenza A virus, influenza B virus, and influenza C virus. Influenza A virus is responsible for most infections and the most severe outbreaks of influenza. This is primarily due to its ability to alter its surface antigens, bypassing previously developed immune defenses to the virus. New strains of influenza virus are named according to the strain, geographic origin, and year the strain was identified (e.g., A/Taiwan/89). Surface antigens of the specific virus may be used to further differentiate influenza A viruses. Outbreaks of influenza B virus are generally less extensive and less severe than those caused by influenza A virus. Illness associated with influenza C virus is mild and often goes unrecognized.

The incubation period for influenza is short, only 18 to 72 hours. The virus infects the respiratory epithelium. It rapidly replicates in infected cells and is released to infect neighboring cells. Inflammation leads to necrosis and shedding of serous and ciliated cells of the respiratory tract. This allows extracellular fluid to escape, producing rhinorrhea. With recovery, serous cells are replaced more rapidly than ciliated cells, leading to continued cough and coryza. Systemic manifestations of influenza are likely caused by release of inflammatory mediators such as tumor necrosis factor alpha, interleukin alpha, and interleukin 6 (Sorenson et al., 2019). The humoral and cell-mediated immune responses are activated by influenza infection and are supplemented by other local and systemic responses (such as interferons).

Risk Factors

Influenza attacks the respiratory system. Risk factors include age (highest risk in those under 5 or adults > 65 years), chronic illness (especially those with impaired immune or respiratory systems), pregnant and early postpartum women, residents of nursing homes or other long-term care facilities, and obese persons (BMI > 40).

Manifestations

Infection with influenza virus produces one of three syndromes: Uncomplicated nasopharyngeal inflammation, viral upper respiratory infection followed by bacterial infection, or viral pneumonia. The onset is rapid; profound malaise may develop in a matter of minutes.

Manifestations of influenza include abrupt onset of chills and fever, malaise, muscle aches, and headache. Respiratory manifestations include dry, nonproductive cough, sore throat, substernal burning, and coryza. Acute symptoms subside within 2 to 3 days, although fever may last as long as a week. The cough may be severe and productive. Along with fatigue and weakness, the cough can persist for days or several weeks.

Complications

Although influenza tends to be mild and self-limited in healthy adults, older adults and people with chronic heart or pulmonary disease have a high incidence of complications (such as pneumonia) and a higher risk for mortality related to the disease and its complications (CDC, 2017e; NIAID, 2017a).

The respiratory epithelial necrosis caused by influenza increases the risk for secondary bacterial infections. Sinusitis and otitis media are frequent complications of influenza. Tracheobronchitis, inflammation of the trachea and bronchi, may develop. Although tracheobronchitis is not a serious health risk, its manifestations may persist for up to 3 weeks.

Influenza is clearly linked to an increased risk for pneumonia, particularly in older adults. Changes in respiratory function associated with aging, including decreased effectiveness of cough and increased residual lung volume, pose little risk in the healthy older adult but greatly increase the risk for pneumonia associated with influenza. Primary influenza viral pneumonia, although uncommon, is a serious complication that may be fatal. It typically develops within 48 hours of the onset of influenza, often in patients with preexisting heart valve or pulmonary disease. Influenza pneumonia progresses rapidly and can cause hypoxemia and death within a few days. Secondary bacterial pneumonia is more likely to occur in older at-risk adults but also may affect otherwise healthy adults. It usually presents as a relapse of influenza, with a productive cough and evidence of pneumonia on the chest x-ray. See Chapter 37 for more information about pneumonia.

Other respiratory complications of influenza include exacerbation of chronic obstructive pulmonary disease (COPD), chronic bronchitis, or asthma. Sinusitis (discussed later in this chapter) may also may develop.

Reye syndrome is a rare but potentially fatal complication of influenza. Although it is more likely to affect children, it has also been identified in older adults. Most often associated with influenza B virus, Reye syndrome develops within 2 to 3 weeks after the onset of influenza. It has a 20% mortality rate (Weiner, 2015). Hepatic failure and encephalopathy develop rapidly in patients with Reye syndrome.

While uncommon, other potential complications of influenza include myositis (inflammation of skeletal muscles), myocarditis (inflammation of the heart muscle), and CNS disorders such as encephalitis and Guillain-Barré syndrome.

Interprofessional Care

Preventing community outbreaks and protecting vulnerable populations (e.g., older adults and people with chronic diseases) are the primary focus for interprofessional care related to influenza. Medical treatment of influenza focuses on establishing the diagnosis, providing symptomatic relief, and preventing complications.

Diagnosis

The diagnosis of influenza is based on history, clinical findings, and knowledge of an influenza outbreak in the community. A chest x-ray and WBC count may be done to rule out complications such as pneumonia. The WBC is commonly decreased in viral infections such as influenza; bacterial infections usually cause increased WBCs.

Medications

Yearly immunization with influenza vaccine is the single most important measure to prevent or minimize symptoms of influenza. Although the vaccine is readily available and inexpensive, only about 30% of at-risk patients are vaccinated each year (*Healthy People 2020*, 2018). Many may fear a reaction from the vaccine, although the vaccines are highly purified and reactions are rare. The rare person who experiences mild symptoms may have a low-grade fever, malaise, or myalgia for up to 24 hours after vaccination. Because the vaccine is produced in eggs, it should not be given to people who are allergic to egg protein. Serious adverse reactions to influenza vaccine are rare. Guillain-Barré syndrome, an acute neurologic disorder characterized by muscle weakness and distal sensory loss, has been associated with certain batches of vaccine.

Amantadine (Symmetrel) or rimantadine (Flumadine) may be used for prophylaxis in unvaccinated people who are exposed to the virus. If the drug is given before or within 48 hours of exposure, it inhibits viral shedding and prevents or decreases the symptoms of influenza. If possible, unvaccinated people should receive the vaccine along with the antiviral drug. The drug is continued for several weeks or for the duration of the influenza outbreak. Some strains of type A influenza virus have been found to be resistant to amantadine and rimantadine, potentially limiting their effectiveness in preventing or treating an influenza outbreak.

The antiviral drugs zanamivir (Relenza), oseltamivir (Tamiflu), and peramivir (Rapiva) also may be used to reduce the duration and severity of flu symptoms. Zanamivir is administered by inhalation; the other drugs are given orally. Because zanamivir can precipitate bronchospasm in patients with a history of asthma or chronic obstructive pulmonary disease (COPD), it is not recommended for use in these patients. All three drugs have reported effect on both influenza A and B (CDC, 2017e).

Over-the-counter analgesics such as aspirin, acetaminophen, or NSAIDs provide symptomatic relief of fever and muscle ache. Antitussives and mucolytics may decrease cough, promoting rest. Antibiotics are not indicated unless secondary bacterial infection occurs.

Integrative Therapies

While integrative therapies have reported use in viral upper respiratory infections, the National Center for Complementary and Integrative Health (2017) does not list any integrative therapies specific for influenza.

Nursing Care

Assessment

Unless there is a known outbreak of influenza in the community, it can be difficult to differentiate the manifestations of influenza from those of other URI.

See the Manifestations and Interprofessional Care sections for the assessment of the patient with influenza.

- ***Health history:*** Known exposure to virus; current symptoms and their onset and duration; presence of dyspnea, chest pain, productive cough, facial pain, or pressure in sinus areas; current medications, history of influenza vaccine; chronic diseases such as heart disease, COPD, or diabetes; smoking or alcohol abuse; institutionalized, communal living such as college dormitories; known medication allergies
- ***Physical assessment:*** General appearance; vital signs including temperature; skin color; lung sounds; abdominal exam; ear, nose, and throat examination
- ***Laboratory data:*** Influenza tests (nasal swabs, nasal aspirates), but usually not WBC, throat and sputum cultures, and chest x-ray unless suspect for evidence of bacterial infection or pneumonia.

Priorities of Care

Collaborating with the interprofessional team to ensure adequate treatment of the underlying process while providing care that supports the physical and psychologic responses to the disorder is a priority of nursing care.

Diagnoses, Outcomes, and Interventions

Although the symptoms of influenza are distressing, most people with the illness provide self-care and do not contact a healthcare provider. Recommendations to rest in bed during the acute phase of the illness and limit activities until recovery are appropriate for influenza.

Severe disease or complications of influenza may necessitate hospitalization for respiratory support and management. For these patients, nursing care focuses on maintaining breathing patterns, airway clearance, and adequate rest.

Promote Effective Breathing. Muscle aches, malaise, and elevated temperature may increase the respiratory rate and alter the depth of respirations, decreasing effective alveolar ventilation. Shallow respirations also increase the risk of *atelectasis*, lack of ventilation in an area of lung.

Expected Outcome: Patient will utilize techniques to promote adequate ventilation such as deep breathing and incentive spirometry.

The nurse will:

- Monitor respiratory rate and pattern. *Tachypnea and/or rapid, shallow respirations may impair effective alveolar ventilation and gas exchange.*
- Pace activities to provide for periods of rest. *Tachypnea increases the work of breathing, causing fatigue; fatigue, in turn, can further impair ventilation and reduce the effectiveness of coughing.*
- Elevate the head of the bed. *The upright position promotes drainage of nasal secretions, improves lung excursion, and reduces the work of breathing by lowering the diaphragm, which moves abdominal contents downward, creating less resistance to diaphragmatic excursion and slightly decreasing venous return.*

Promote Airway Clearance and Patency. Swelling and congestion of mucous membranes, extracellular fluid exudate, and impaired ciliary action due to cell damage increase the risk of impaired airway clearance in influenza. The older adult is at particular risk because of normally reduced ciliary activity and increased lung compliance.

Expected Outcome: Patient will use techniques to promote airway clearance such as coughing and deep breathing.

The nurse will:

- Monitor the effectiveness of cough and ability to remove airway secretions. *Fatigue and general malaise may impair the ability to cough effectively and mobilize secretions.*
- Maintain adequate hydration. Assess mucous membranes and skin turgor for evidence of dehydration. *Fever, increased mucous membrane secretions, and decreased oral fluid intake may lead to dehydration and increased viscosity of secretions. Thick, viscous secretions are more difficult to expectorate.*
- Increase the humidity of inspired air with a bedside humidifier. *Increasing the water content of inhaled air helps loosen thick secretions and soothe mucous membranes.*
- Teach effective cough techniques. Administer analgesics as ordered. *The huff cough is effective to maintain open airways and spares energy (see Chapter 37 for patient teaching of this technique). Relieving muscle ache increases the ability to cough effectively.*

Promote Sleep and Rest. Airway congestion, fever, malaise, muscle aches, and persistent cough may interfere with the ability to rest, increasing fatigue and prolonging recovery.

Expected Outcome: Patient will verbalize techniques to reduce impact of upper respiratory symptoms on sleep patterns.

The nurse will:

- Assess sleep patterns using subjective and objective information. *The patient may appear to be sleeping but not achieving normal sleep patterns because of influenza symptoms. Both subjective and objective data are important to accurately assess sleep.*
- Provide antipyretic and analgesic medications at or shortly before bedtime. *These drugs promote comfort by reducing fever and relieving muscle aches.*

Reduce Risk for Infection. Infection control measures are recommended to prevent person-to-person transmission of influenza and control influenza outbreaks in healthcare facilities.

Expected Outcome: Patient will describe measures to protect healthy tissue and prevent infection.

The nurse will:

- Use standard precautions and encourage all staff and visitors to wash hands frequently. *Hand hygiene is a primary infection control measure for infections transmitted via respiratory secretions.*
- Instruct patients and visitors to control respiratory secretions by using tissues and to maintain a distance of at least 3 feet from others when coughing or sneezing. Provide masks for patients and visitors who are coughing or sneezing. *Limiting the spread of aerosolized secretions by covering the nose and mouth and maintaining distance from other people can reduce the spread of the disease to vulnerable populations.*
- Use droplet precautions for patients with suspected or confirmed influenza: Private room, masks for caregivers and visitors, and mask the patient when transporting within the facility. *These measures limit the spread of respiratory secretions.*

Delegating Nursing Care Activities

As appropriate and allowed by the designated duties and responsibilities of unlicensed assistive personnel, the nurse may delegate nursing care/activities such as measuring vital signs, encouraging oral or enteral fluid intake, and providing skin care.

Transitions of Care

Preventing influenza by immunizing at-risk populations is an important aspect of care. Immunization with polyvalent (containing antigens of several viral strains) influenza virus vaccine is about 85% effective in preventing influenza infection for several months to a year (NIAID, 2017a). Annual immunization is recommended for all children (6 months to 18 years) and all adults who want it; at-risk patients, including people over the age of 50; residents of nursing homes; adults and children with chronic cardiopulmonary disorders (e.g., asthma) or chronic metabolic diseases such as diabetes; and healthcare workers who have frequent contact with high-risk patients. Additionally, family members of at-risk patients should be vaccinated to reduce the patient's risk of exposure. The vaccine is given in the fall, prior to the annual winter outbreak. Live attenuated vaccine, administered by internasal spray, is available for healthy people under age 50 (CDC, 2017e; Grohskopf et al., 2017).

Stress the importance of yearly influenza vaccination for everyone, unless contraindicated, especially patients in the high-risk groups and their families. Teach about spread of the disease, including not going to work or school if sick, and measures to reduce the risk of contracting influenza, such as handwashing, avoiding crowds, and avoiding people who are ill.

Encourage appropriate self-care for patients with influenza. Observe for complications that could lead to pneumonia or other acute respiratory process. Discuss the following topics related to home care:

- Increase rest during the acute, febrile phase of the illness.
- Increase fluid intake (to greater than normal level) even if anorexic.
- Use OTC medications at safe and effective dose and frequency for symptom relief.
- Employ hygiene measures such as using disposable tissues and frequent hand hygiene to reduce spread of the disease.
- Know manifestations of potential complications of influenza to report to the primary care provider.

The Patient with Sinusitis

Sinusitis is inflammation of the mucous membranes of one or more of the sinuses. Sinusitis is a common condition that usually follows an upper respiratory infection such as acute viral upper respiratory infection or influenza. Common causative organisms include viruses, streptococci, *S. pneumoniae*, *Haemophilus influenzae*, and staphylococci. The risk of sinusitis is higher when the immune system is suppressed by immunosuppressive drugs or HIV infection. Sinusitis is common and difficult to treat in people who have AIDS.

Pathophysiology

The sinuses (or *paranasal sinuses*) are air-filled cavities in the facial bones that open into the turbinates of the nasal cavity. They are lined with ciliated mucous membranes that help move fluid and microorganisms out of the sinuses into the nasal cavity. The sinuses are normally sterile. Air within the sinuses has a lower oxygen content than inspired air.

Sinusitis develops when nasal mucous membranes swell or when other disorders (such as polyps or tumors) obstruct sinus openings, impairing drainage. Mucus secretions collect in the sinus cavity, serving as a medium for viral or bacterial growth. The nasal and sinus mucous membranes are continuous; therefore, pathogens generally spread to the sinuses via the opening into the nasal turbinates. The inflammatory response provoked by pathogen invasion draws serum and leukocytes to the area to combat the infection, increasing swelling and pressure.

Any process that impairs drainage from the sinuses may precipitate sinusitis. Examples include nasal polyps, deviated septum, rhinitis, tooth abscess, and swimming or diving trauma. In hospitalized patients, sinusitis may develop following prolonged nasotracheal intubation. Usually more than one sinus is infected. The frontal and maxillary sinuses are usually involved in adults.

Sinusitis may be acute or chronic. Chronic sinusitis results when acute sinusitis is untreated, inadequately treated, or there are recurrent episodes or other factors that prevent sinus drainage. With continued infection, bacteria can become isolated, producing chronic inflammation. Over time, mucous membranes become thickened. Fungal infections may cause chronic infections, especially in immunosuppressed patients. Other factors that may contribute to chronic sinusitis are smoking, allergies, and habitual use of nasal sprays or inhalants.

Risk Factors

Risk factors for sinusitis are related to anatomy and other factors. Persons with nasal allergies and hay fever are at higher risk for sinusitis. An anatomical problem such as deviated septum, nasal polyps, or tumors also increase the risk for sinusitis. Persons with cystic fibrosis or immune-altering processes can also be at higher risk for sinusitis.

Manifestations

The patient with acute sinusitis often looks sick. Manifestations of sinusitis include pain and tenderness across the infected sinuses, headache, fever, and malaise. The pain usually increases with leaning forward. When the maxillary sinuses are involved, pain and pressure are felt over the cheek. The pain may be referred to the upper teeth. Frontal sinusitis causes pain and tenderness across the lower forehead. Infection of the ethmoid sinus produces retro-orbital pain and pain over the high lateral aspect of the nose. Sphenoid sinusitis, the rarest form, may cause pain in the occiput, vertex, or middle of the head. Symptoms often worsen for 3 to 4 hours after awakening and then become less severe in the afternoon and evening as secretions drain. The intensity and location of headache pain may change as sinuses drain. In acute sinusitis, the pain is usually constant and severe. In chronic sinusitis, the pain is described as dull and may be constant or intermittent.

Other symptoms include nasal congestion, purulent nasal discharge, and bad breath. The nasal mucous membrane is red and swollen. Purulent drainage may be noted at the opening to the middle turbinate. This may be the only sign of chronic sinusitis. Swallowed secretions from postnasal drip irritate and inflame the throat and may cause nausea or vomiting.

Complications

Complications develop when the infection spreads to surrounding structures (**Box 35.2**). These include periorbital abscess, or cellulitis, cavernous sinus thrombosis, meningitis, brain abscess, or sepsis. Eustachian tube edema may lead to temporary hearing loss.

Interprofessional Care

Treatment of sinusitis focuses on restoring drainage of obstructed sinuses, controlling infection, relieving pain, and preventing complications.

Diagnosis

The diagnosis of acute sinusitis can usually be made using the history and physical exam. Diagnostic studies such as CT scan or, less frequently, sinus x-rays are generally done only when sinusitis is persistent, chronic, or recurrent.

BOX 35.2
Potential Complications of Sinusitis

LOCAL COMPLICATIONS

- Orbital cellulitis
- Subperiosteal abscess
- Orbital abscess
- Cavernous sinus thrombosis
- Mucocele
- Osteomyelitis

INTRACRANIAL COMPLICATIONS

- Meningitis
- Epidural abscess
- Subdural abscess
- Brain abscess
- Venous sinus thrombosis

Refer to Chapter 34 for more information about diagnostic studies and their nursing implications.

- *Sinus x-rays* are used infrequently. Sinuses are normally translucent because they are filled with air; affected sinuses appear cloudy or opaque. A visible air-fluid level or thickening of the sinus mucosa may be seen in infected sinuses.
- *CT scan* is a more sensitive indicator of acute and chronic sinusitis and is often performed without preceding x-rays.
- *Magnetic resonance imaging (MRI)* may be ordered if malignancy of the sinus is suspected.

Medications

Antibiotic therapy directed at the usual organisms that cause sinusitis is typically prescribed if the symptoms have lasted for more than 7 days. Amoxicillin (possibly combined with clavulanate [Augmentin]), trimethoprim-sulfamethoxazole (Bactrim, Septra), cefuroxime (Ceftin), cefaclor (Ceclor), ciprofloxacin (Cipro), or clarithromycin (Biaxin) are commonly used antibiotics for sinusitis. Antibiotic therapy is continued for 10 to 14 days; occasionally a longer course is prescribed to prevent relapse. If the sinusitis does not respond to treatment with oral antibiotics, hospitalization and intravenous antibiotic therapy may be required. Refer to Chapter 12 for nursing care related to antibiotic therapy.

Topical steroids (such as fluticasone) and decongestants (in the form of nasal sprays) or oral decongestants such as pseudoephedrine or phenylephrine are also prescribed to reduce mucosal edema and promote sinus drainage. Antihistamines may decrease nasal congestion and facilitate sinus drainage, but they also tend to increase the viscosity of secretions and hinder drainage. For this reason, they may not be as effective as decongestants. Saline nose drops or sprays promote sinus drainage, as does inhalation of warm steam.

To administer topical drugs, the patient's head is kept in an upright position or leaned slightly forward.

Systemic mucolytic agents such as guaifenesin may be useful to liquefy secretions, promoting sinus drainage. Aerobic exercise also promotes mucous flow and may be recommended.

Surgery

Patients who do not respond to pharmacologic measures and who experience persistent facial pain, headache, or nasal congestion may require endoscopic sinus surgery. Detailed evaluation of the sinuses by CT scan is done prior to surgery. Under local or general anesthesia, a fiberoptic nasal endoscope is inserted to visualize the sinus opening. If obstruction is present, it can be removed, restoring patency and drainage. This surgery is most effective for local disease, for recurrent acute sinusitis, and for removing anatomic obstructions. Patients who have endoscopic sinus surgery usually do not require nasal packing postoperatively. Instead, frequent nasal cleaning and irrigation with normal saline are performed. The patient is instructed to sneeze with the mouth open and avoid blowing the nose, lifting, or straining for a week following surgery.

Antral irrigation can be done in the healthcare provider's office under local anesthesia. A 16-gauge needle is inserted under the inferior turbinate of the nose into the maxillary sinus on the affected side. Saline solution is instilled to irrigate the area and wash out the sinus of purulent exudate. The patient is seated with the head forward and mouth open to allow drainage of the solution through the nose and mouth. A culture of the exudate may be obtained to determine appropriate antibiotic therapy.

The *Caldwell-Luc procedure* may be necessary if endoscopic sinus surgery is unsuccessful. It is performed under local or general anesthesia. An incision is made under the upper lip into the maxillary sinus, and diseased mucous membrane and periosteum are removed. An opening between the maxillary sinus and lateral nasal wall, a "nasal antral window," is created to increase aeration of the sinus and promote drainage into the nasal cavity. The area is packed with gauze for 24 to 48 hours postoperatively. The gauze packing obstructs nasal breathing while it is in place. As the maxillary sinus heals, exposed bone is covered by mucosa. The upper lip and teeth may be numb for several months after the procedure because of nerve trauma. Chewing may be impaired on the affected side. Only liquids are given for the first 24 hours, followed by a soft diet. The patient is instructed to avoid wearing dentures and the Valsalva maneuver (no blowing the nose, coughing, or straining at stool) for about 2 weeks after the packing has been removed to prevent bleeding.

In *external sphenoethmoidectomy*, an incision along the side of the nose from the middle of the eyebrow is used to open and remove diseased tissue from the sphenoid or ethmoid sinuses (**Figure 35.1** ■). Nasal polyps may also be removed using this approach. Nasal packing is inserted, and an eye pressure patch is applied to decrease periorbital edema. Care is similar to that following the Caldwell-Luc procedure.

Integrative Therapies

Complementary therapies may help relieve symptoms of sinusitis and promote comfort. The use of high-volume, low-pressure nasal irrigation has expanded beyond postoperative management. A Cochrane review noted that there may be some benefit for low-pressure, high-volume

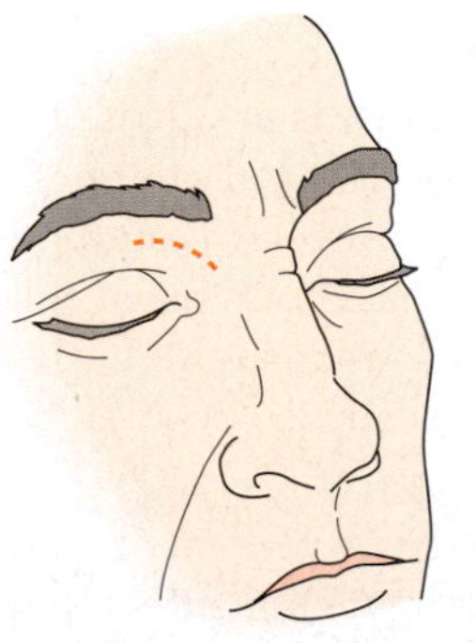

Figure 35.1 ■ Incision to access ethmoid and frontal sinuses. Resulting scar is nearly invisible in folds of the eye.

irrigation (Chong et al., 2016). Nasal irrigation systems such as neti pots are widely available over the counter. Aromatherapy using herbs such as basil, marjoram, or eucalyptus in a vaporizer or on a handkerchief; herbal teas made from goldenseal, yarrow, or coltsfoot; hot or cold compresses or steam inhalation; and acupressure may be employed.

Nursing Care

Assessment

See the Manifestations and Interprofessional Care sections for the assessment of the patient with sinusitis.

Focused assessment of the patient with suspected sinusitis includes:

- ***Health history:*** Complaints of frontal or periorbital headache, cheek, teeth, or ear pain; timing of pain and changes in intensity over course of the day; nasal discharge or postnasal drip; other symptoms like tenderness over the cheeks; previous sinus infections or trauma; current medications, known medication and environmental allergies (allergic rhinitis)
- ***Physical assessment:*** General appearance, vital signs including temperature; inspection of nasal and pharyngeal mucous membranes; percussion of sinuses for tenderness
- ***Laboratory data:*** CT of the sinuses, and infrequently sinus x-rays, WBC and differential, cultures of sinus drainage.

Priorities of Care

Collaborating with the interprofessional team to ensure adequate treatment of the underlying process while providing care that supports the physical and psychologic responses to the disorder is a priority of nursing care.

Diagnoses, Outcomes, and Interventions

The patient with sinusitis is often acutely uncomfortable. Obstructed and congested sinuses cause pain and pressure that increase with position changes and leaning forward. Treatment is usually community based, making education the key nursing role. When the patient is hospitalized for intravenous antibiotic therapy or sinus surgery, *Pain* and *Imbalanced Nutrition* are priority nursing diagnoses.

Manage Pain. Although sinus surgery is relatively minor, both the incision and postoperative swelling can cause discomfort. Nasal packing, if used, contributes to the discomfort.

Expected Outcome: Patient will experience adequate pain control as evidenced by physical well-being.

The nurse will:

- Assess pain using a standardized pain scale. Administer analgesics as ordered. *Relief of pain promotes a feeling of well-being and enhances recovery.*
- Apply ice packs to the nose. *Cold compresses reduce swelling, control bleeding, and provide local analgesia.*
- Elevate the head of the bed to Fowler or high-Fowler position for 24 to 48 hours after surgery. *Elevating the operative site minimizes tissue swelling and promotes comfort.*

Promote Balanced Nutrition. Postoperatively, the sense of smell, an appetite stimulus, is diminished by nasal packing. Mouth discomfort from the incision and numbness of the upper teeth may also impact appetite and eating.

Expected Outcome: Patient will consume adequate nourishment to promote weight within normal range.

The nurse will:

- Provide clear liquid diet progressing to soft foods as tolerated. High-calorie dietary supplements may be used. *A progressive diet is used to assess the ability to swallow without choking and allay fears. Foods high in calories and nutritional value provide for metabolic and healing requirements.*
- Monitor intake, output, and weight. *This information allows assessment of overall fluid balance and the adequacy of dietary intake.*
- Elevate the head of the bed during meals. *The upright position facilitates swallowing and minimizes risk of aspiration.*

Delegating Nursing Care Activities

As appropriate and allowed by the designated duties and responsibilities of unlicensed assistive personnel, the nurse may delegate nursing care/activities such as measuring vital signs, encouraging oral or enteral fluid intake, and providing skin care.

Transitions of Care

Measures to prevent sinusitis are those that promote nasal drainage: Encouraging increased fluid intake, judicious use of nasal decongestants as needed, and treating any obstructive process (e.g., with nasal steroid spray). Encourage patients with URI to blow their nose with both nares open. Advise patients that use of saline nasal sprays can help maintain patency of the opening to the sinuses, promoting drainage and reducing the risk of obstruction and infection.

Nursing care of the patient with sinusitis focuses on symptom management and close surveillance for complications.

- Use systemic or topical decongestants to promote sinus drainage.
- Maintain a liberal fluid intake to reduce the viscosity of mucous drainage.
- Use a humidifier or steam inhalation to promote sinus drainage.
- Sleep with the head of the bed elevated to a 45-degree angle and on the unaffected side to promote drainage of affected sinuses.
- Apply a warm, moist pack to the area of pain and tenderness to promote comfort.

Teaching for patients with recurrent sinusitis and their families focuses on following through with appropriate treatment and promoting comfort. Discuss the following topics when preparing for home care:

- Understand the importance of completing the entire course of prescribed antibiotics to achieve cure and prevent the development of antibiotic-resistant bacteria. Assist in developing a schedule that helps ensure all doses are taken.
- Use measures to prevent superinfections (such as vaginitis or oral thrush) during the prolonged course of treatment (e.g., consume 8 oz of yogurt containing live bacterial cultures daily while on antibiotics).
- Notify the healthcare provider if symptoms do not improve with treatment or if signs of a complication develop, such as increased pain and redness and swelling on the side of the nose or around the eyes.
- Understand postoperative instructions to prevent bleeding, such as avoiding blowing the nose for 7 to 10 days and avoiding strenuous activity such as heavy lifting for about 2 weeks.
- Use saline nasal sprays or nasal irrigation postoperatively to keep the nasal mucosa moist.

The Patient with Pharyngitis or Tonsillitis

Pharyngitis, acute inflammation of the pharynx, is one of the most commonly identified clinical problems. Although it is usually viral in origin, pharyngitis may also be caused by bacterial infection. *Group A beta-hemolytic streptococcus (GABHS)* (strep throat) is the most common cause of bacterial pharyngitis. Other bacteria that may cause pharyngitis include *Neisseria gonorrhoeae*, a gram-negative diplococcus that is sexually transmitted; *Mycoplasma*; and *Chlamydia trachomatis*. Pharyngitis may also be a result of postnasal drip from allergic rhinitis or as a result of gastroesophageal reflux into the throat.

Tonsillitis is acute inflammation of the palatine tonsils. Although it is sometimes viral in origin, tonsillitis is usually due to streptococcal infection. The incidence of streptococcal infections is greatest between late fall and spring, especially in cold climates. Viral tonsillitis may occur in epidemics in people living in crowded conditions, such as military recruits.

Pathophysiology

Pharyngitis and tonsillitis are contagious and spread by droplet nuclei. Incubation varies from a few hours to several days, depending on the organism. Viral infections are communicable for 2 to 3 days. Symptoms usually resolve within 3 to 10 days after onset.

Viral pharyngitis may be attributed to the same viruses causing the common cold: Rhinovirus, coronavirus, or parainfluenza virus. Pharyngitis caused by adenovirus, influenza virus, or Epstein-Barr virus (associated with infectious mononucleosis) may be particularly severe.

Risk Factors

Pharyngitis risk factors are primarily related to host factors. Prior colonization with group A Streptococcus (GAS) and exposure to someone who is colonized or immunocompromised are risk factors. Exposure risk factors include use of inhaled corticosteroids or ingestion of non-domestic meats.

Manifestations

Acute pharyngitis causes pain and fever. The pain may vary from a scratchy sore throat to one so painful that swallowing is difficult. Streptococcal pharyngitis is usually marked by an abrupt onset, with a fever of 38.3°C (101°F) or higher, severe sore throat with dysphagia, headache, malaise, and often arthralgias and myalgias and the absence of a cough. Anterior lymph nodes are often enlarged and tender. Exudate (pus) may be seen on the pharynx and tonsils (**Figure 35.2** ■). In contrast, the onset of viral pharyngitis is often gradual, with manifestations of low-grade fever, sore throat, mild hoarseness, headache, and rhinorrhea. The pharyngeal membranes appear mildly red with vascular congestion. Infectious mononucleosis, caused by the Epstein-Barr virus, often presents as acute pharyngitis, with visible patches of exudate on the pharynx or tonsils. The cervical lymph nodes are enlarged and tender as well.

In tonsillitis, the tonsils appear bright red and edematous. White exudate may be present on the tonsils; pressing on a tonsil may produce purulent drainage. The uvula may also be reddened and swollen. The tonsillar lymph nodes are usually tender and enlarged.

The patient with tonsillitis complains of a sore throat, difficulty swallowing, general malaise, fever, and otalgia (pain referred to the ear). Manifestations are often more severe in adolescents and adults than in children. Infection may extend via the eustachian tubes to cause acute otitis media. This may lead to further damage such as spontaneous rupture of the eardrums and mastoiditis. See Chapter 46 for more information about otitis media.

Complications

Although GABHS pharyngitis may be mild and indistinguishable from viral pharyngitis by its signs and symptoms, it can lead to significant complications such as abscess, scarlet fever, toxic shock syndrome, rheumatic fever, or acute

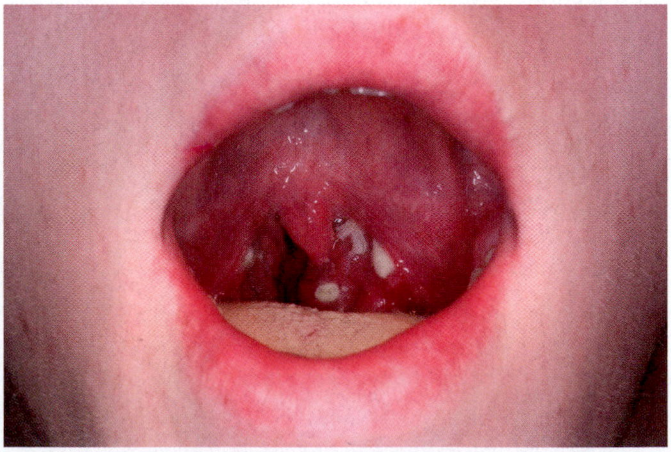

Figure 35.2 ■ The appearance of the oral pharynx and tonsils in acute pharyngitis and tonsillitis.

poststreptococcal glomerulonephritis. GABHS is treated with antibiotics to prevent these sequelae. *Peritonsillar abscess*, or *quinsy*, is a potential complication of tonsillitis. It usually results from GABHS infection extending from the tonsils to the surrounding tissue. The abscess causes pus formation behind the tonsil with marked swelling and asymmetric deviation of the uvula. The degree of swelling may make it difficult to swallow anything other than liquids. The patient may exhibit thickening of the voice, drooling, and a tonic contraction of the muscles of mastication, called *trismus*.

Rare but serious complications of GABHS pharyngitis and tonsillitis include acute glomerulonephritis and rheumatic fever, abnormal immune responses to the infection. Acute glomerulonephritis generally presents with sudden onset of hematuria, proteinuria, and, less commonly, hypertension and edema within 7 to 10 days after the acute infection. Rheumatic fever typically presents 3 to 5 weeks after acute infection with fever, painful or swollen joints, rash, and heart murmur. Other complications of bacterial infection include sinusitis, otitis media, mastoiditis, and cervical adenitis.

Interprofessional Care

Both viral and bacterial pharyngitis are usually self-limited diseases. However, because of the risk for serious complications associated with GABHS sore throat, an effort is usually made to identify this pathogen and treat only this pharyngitis with antibiotics.

Diagnosis

- ***Throat swab*** is obtained and examined for streptococcus antigen using the latex agglutination (LA) antigen test or enzyme immunoassay (ELISA) testing. These tests allow rapid identification of the antigen (in as little as 10 minutes for the LA test) but are not highly sensitive. When the test is positive, treatment for strep throat is initiated. If the test is negative, the swab is cultured to ensure that streptococcus organisms are not present. Throat cultures have a 90 to 95% specificity for GABHS. If the culture is initially negative, it will be held and reexamined after 24 hours (Khan, 2016).
- ***Complete blood count (CBC)*** may be done on severely ill patients or to rule out other causes of pharyngitis. The WBC count is usually normal or low in viral infections and elevated in bacterial infections.

Medications

Antipyretics and mild analgesics such as aspirin or acetaminophen provide symptomatic relief for throat pain and associated myalgias. Penicillin is the drug of choice for group A streptococci. Erythromycin, amoxicillin, or cefuroxime (Ceftin, Kefurox) may be used if the patient is allergic to penicillin. Antibiotic therapy is continued for at least 10 days. The patient is no longer contagious after 24 hours of antibiotic therapy.

Surgery

A peritonsillar abscess is drained by needle aspiration or by incision and drainage. The area is first sprayed with a topical anesthetic such as Cetacaine and then injected with a local anesthetic. The sitting position is preferred for the procedure because it enables expectoration of blood and pus. (See the Case Study & Nursing Care Plan for nursing care of the patient with a peritonsillar abscess.) Tonsillectomy is done either immediately or 6 weeks after incision and drainage of peritonsillar abscess.

Tonsillectomy (surgical removal of the tonsils) is indicated for recurrent or chronic infections that have not responded to antibiotic therapy, hypertrophy of the tonsils with risk of airway obstruction, peritonsillar abscess, repeated attacks of purulent otitis media, and tonsil malignancy. Adenoid tissue is usually removed at the same time. Bleeding is the most significant postoperative complication of tonsillectomy and may develop up to 2 weeks following the surgery.

Nursing Care

Because of the risk of significant complications associated with GABHS pharyngitis and tonsillitis, encourage all patients with symptoms that persist for several days or that include fever, lymphadenopathy, and myalgias to seek evaluation and treatment. Patients with tonsillitis who undergo surgical intervention require good perioperative nursing care and close observation for postoperative complications.

Assessment

See the Manifestations and Interprofessional Care sections for the assessment of the patient with pharyngitis and tonsillitis.

Focused assessment of the patient with suspected pharyngitis or tonsillitis includes:

- ***Health history:*** Complaints of sore throat, cheek, teeth, or ear pain; timing of pain and changes in intensity over course of the day; previous pharyngeal or tonsillar infections or trauma
- ***Physical assessment:*** General appearance; vital signs including temperature; inspection of pharyngeal mucous membranes.

Priorities of Care

Nursing care is supportive. The focus of nursing care for the adult with tonsillitis is on close surveillance for complications and teaching for self-care and prevention of causative organism spread. In the patient who undergoes surgery, perioperative care and close observation for postoperative complications are nursing priorities.

Diagnoses, Interventions, and Outcomes

Promote Airway Clearance and Patency. Whether the patient has severe pharyngitis or tonsillitis, local tissue edema may interfere with airway patency.

Expected Outcome: Patient will use techniques to promote airway clearance as indicated and tolerated in combination with maintenance of patent airway.

The nurse will:

- Apply cold packs to the neck or encourage oral intake of cold beverages/foods as ordered or indicated. *Cold application (whether external or internal) constricts local blood vessels and reduces edema development.*

Manage Acute Pain. Patients may experience acute pain due to postoperative swelling or infectious process edema.

Expected Outcome: Patient will have adequate pain management.

The nurse will:

- Assess patients for pain. For patients in the community, encourage pharmacological and nonpharmacological interventions as appropriate. *Adequate pain management promotes rest and healing.*
- Administer analgesics for postoperative patients as ordered. Encourage use of nonpharmacologic comfort measures. Reevaluate for effectiveness of the comfort intervention. *Pharmacological (pain medication) and nonpharmacological (application of cold compress [postoperative] or warm compress [pharyngitis]) impacts blood flow and improves comfort.*

Delegating Nursing Care Activities

As appropriate and allowed by the designated duties and responsibilities of unlicensed assistive personnel, the nurse may delegate nursing care/activities such as measuring vital signs, encouraging oral or enteral fluid intake, and providing skin care.

Transitions of Care

Patients can limit their incidence of pharyngitis and tonsillitis through good hygiene practices such as frequent handwashing and avoiding sharing utensils. Maintaining good general health and participating in stress-reducing activities support the immune system.

Following tonsillectomy, ensure a patent airway by placing the patient in semi-Fowler position with the head turned to the side to allow secretions to drain from the mouth and pharynx. Keep the airway in place until the gag and swallowing reflexes have returned. Apply an ice collar

Case Study & Nursing Care Plan

A Patient with a Peritonsillar Abscess

Monica Wunderman, age 27, was recently treated for tonsillitis caused by an infection by group A streptococcus. She presents to the emergency department (ED) 10 days later appearing acutely ill. She states that her throat is so sore that she has difficulty swallowing even liquids. Ms. Ironhorse, the ED nurse, completes an assessment of Ms. Wunderman.

ASSESSMENT	DIAGNOSIS	EXPECTED OUTCOMES
Findings include T 38.8°C (102°F). An acutely swollen and reddened area of the soft palate is noted in her mouth, half occluding the orifice from the mouth into the pharynx. Yellow exudate is present. CBC reveals an elevated WBC of 16,000/mm^3. A diagnosis of peritonsillar abscess is made. Needle aspiration of the abscess is performed.	■ Acute pain related to swelling ■ Potential for issues with airway clearance related to swelling of the oropharynx and pain ■ Decrease in fluid volume related to fever and decreased fluid intake	■ Patient will have minimal or no pain. ■ Patient will maintain a patent airway as demonstrated by normal respiratory rate and rhythm. ■ Patient will maintain optimal fluid intake as evidenced by consumption of fluids and semiliquid foods, moist mucous membranes, normal skin turgor, and normal temperature.

PLANNING AND IMPLEMENTATION

- Teach that ice-cold fluids may be easier to swallow than hot or room-temperature beverages and may provide a local analgesic effect.
- Advise to avoid citrus juices, hot or spicy foods, and rough-textured foods for 1 week.
- Teach pain management strategies such as applying an ice collar as desired and gargling with warm saline or mouthwash solution every 1 to 2 hours for the first 24 to 48 hours after aspiration of the abscess.
- Instruct to take medications (antibiotics) as prescribed.

EVALUATION

When Ms. Ironhorse contacts Ms. Wunderman by telephone 2 days after her visit to the ED, she reports complete relief of symptoms. She is afebrile, taking fluids without difficulty, and has had no difficulty breathing. She has not experienced any pain.

CLINICAL REASONING IN PATIENT CARE

1. Describe common symptoms of infectious or inflammatory diseases of the upper airway and discuss methods of symptom relief.
2. Describe common pharmacologic interventions for these disorders.
3. What themes of nursing diagnoses emerge for these patients?

See Evaluating Your Response in Appendix B.

to reduce swelling and pain. Notify the surgeon immediately if excessive bleeding or hemorrhage occurs. If there is no bleeding, allow water and cracked ice as desired. Warm saline mouthwashes are helpful in managing thick oral secretions following tonsillectomy. A liquid or semiliquid diet is recommended for several days.

For the patient who has had a peritonsillar abscess drainage or tonsillectomy, provide the following instructions:

- Postoperative mouth and throat care
- Avoiding use of aspirin for 2 weeks to reduce the risk of postoperative bleeding
- Manifestations of bleeding to report to the healthcare provider (delayed hemorrhage may occur for up to 1 week postsurgery).

Home care is appropriate for acute uncomplicated pharyngitis. Treatment focuses on adequate rest and relief of symptoms. A liquid or soft diet is useful when swallowing is difficult. Increased fluid intake is encouraged, especially when febrile. Warm saline gargles, moist inhalations, and application of an ice collar are soothing to the sore throat. Discuss the following topics when preparing the patient for home care:

- The importance of completing the full 10 days of antibiotic therapy, if prescribed
- Using warm saline gargles or throat lozenges for symptomatic relief
- Signs and symptoms of possible complications of GABHS streptococcal infection such as glomerulonephritis or rheumatic fever
- Monitoring temperature in the morning and evening until well to ensure that the infection has not spread to deeper tissues
- Proper use and disposal of tissues and frequent hand hygiene to prevent spreading the infection to others.

The Patient with a Laryngeal Infection

The *larynx*, located between the upper airways and the lungs, protects the lower respiratory tract from inhaled substances other than air and allows speech. The larynx includes the epiglottis, which covers the larynx during swallowing, and the glottis, or vocal cords. Either portion of the larynx may become inflamed.

Epiglottitis

Epiglottitis, inflammation of the epiglottis, is an uncommon disorder that presents as a medical emergency. *H. influenzae* infection is the most common cause of epiglottitis. Epiglottitis is a rapidly progressive cellulitis that begins between the base of the tongue and the epiglottis. The epiglottis itself becomes swollen and inflamed; swelling of adjacent tissues pushes the epiglottis posteriorly. This swelling and edema threaten the airway. Adults usually present with a 1- to 2-day history of sore throat, *odynophagia* (painful swallowing), dyspnea, and possibly drooling and stridor.

Use of a tongue blade to view the oropharynx is avoided; this may precipitate laryngospasm and airway obstruction. The epiglottis is visualized using a flexible fiberoptic laryngoscope to establish the diagnosis. The epiglottis appears red, swollen, and edematous. Nasotracheal intubation may be required to ensure airway patency. The patient is admitted to a critical care unit and intravenous antibiotic therapy is initiated. Ceftriaxone (Rocephin), cefuroxime (Ceftin), or ampicillin/sulbactam (Unasyn) may be prescribed. If allergic to penicillin, a combination of clindamycin (Cleocin) and either trimethoprim-sulfamethoxazole (TMP-SMZ) or ciprofloxacin (Cipro) may be used. Dexamethasone, a systemic corticosteroid, is also given to suppress the inflammatory response and rapidly reduce swelling of the epiglottis.

Nursing care for the patient with acute epiglottitis focuses on monitoring and maintaining airway patency. Monitor oxygen saturation continuously. Observe closely for signs of airway obstruction, including nasal flaring, restlessness, stridor, use of accessory muscles, and decreased oxygen saturation measurements. If the patient is not intubated, supplies for emergency intubation should be kept in the unit. Epiglottitis is frightening for both the patient and the nurse. Maintaining a calm, reassuring manner is an essential nursing role.

Laryngitis

Laryngitis, inflammation of the larynx, is a common disorder that may occur alone or in conjunction with other upper respiratory infections. It is commonly associated with viral URI such as influenza. It may also occur with bronchitis, pneumonia, other respiratory infections, or due to a tumor or polyp on the vocal cord. Excessive use of the voice, sudden changes in temperature or exposure to dust, irritating fumes, smoke, or other pollutants can also cause acute or chronic laryngitis. It is more common in the winter and in colder climates. Persistent laryngitis after URI resolution or removal of the irritant should be evaluated to rule out malignancy.

In laryngitis, the mucous membrane lining the larynx becomes inflamed; the vocal cords also may become edematous. The primary symptom of laryngitis is a change in the voice. Hoarseness or *aphonia*, complete loss of the voice, may occur. The throat is often sore and scratchy, and a dry, harsh cough may be present.

There is no specific treatment for viral laryngitis. Any identified precipitating factors such as overuse of the voice and exposure to irritants should be eliminated. Voice rest is advised, as is abstinence from tobacco and alcohol, which are chemical irritants. Treatment may also include inhaling steam or spraying the throat with antiseptic solutions. Identifying and eliminating irritants is helpful to prevent future attacks.

Impaired verbal communication is the priority nursing problem for patients with laryngitis. The meaning of messages is conveyed not only by the words used, but also by the tone and loudness of voice. Instruct to rest the voice as much as possible. Encourage speaking in short sentences or using alternate methods of communication, such as writing.

Resting the voice hastens recovery and decreases throat discomfort. Advise to use soothing throat lozenges, sprays, or other comfort measures such as gargling with a warm antiseptic solution. Help identify potential irritants, such as fumes, chemicals, or cold temperature, to prevent future bouts of laryngitis.

The Patient with Diphtheria

Diphtheria is an acute, contagious disease caused by *Corynebacterium diphtheriae*, a small aerobic pathogen. This disease, which primarily affects adults, is uncommon in the United States. Waning immunity due to lack of periodic booster immunizations is the primary risk factor for diphtheria in the United States.

The disease is spread through droplet nuclei and by contamination of articles such as eating utensils. Asymptomatic carriers can be a factor in spreading this infection. People who have recovered from diphtheria can harbor bacteria in their throats for up to 4 weeks. Diphtheria is easily spread in areas where sanitation is poor, living conditions are crowded, and access to healthcare is limited. Immunization is readily available, and infants and children are usually immunized against diphtheria, pertussis, and tetanus concurrently.

Pathophysiology

C. diphtheriae infects the mucous membranes of the respiratory tract and can invade skin lesions. The tonsils and pharynx are common sites of infection. Toxins released by the organism inflame mucosal surfaces of the pharynx. Exudate from inflamed tissues forms a thick, grayish, rubbery pseudomembrane over the posterior pharynx and sometimes into the trachea. This pseudomembrane adheres to inflamed, eroded surfaces and interferes with eating, drinking, and breathing. The airway may be obstructed, necessitating tracheostomy to maintain respirations. The toxins damage the heart and central nervous system (CNS) and may cause myocarditis and paralysis of cranial or peripheral nerves.

Risk Factors

Diphtheria risk factors include lack of or incomplete immunization against diphtheria and overcrowded or unsanitary environments. Persons who are immunocompromised are at greater risk. The nurse should teach the patient to maintain up-to-date immunization according to guidelines. According to the CDC (2017b), a diphtheria vaccination is recommended for all persons. The DTaP (diphtheria, tetanus, pertussis) vaccine is recommended for adults.

Manifestations

Patients with diphtheria develop fever, malaise, sore throat, and malodorous breath. In severe cases, the neck may be warm and swollen because of lymphadenopathy. Isolated patches of gray or white exudate grow and extend to form a gray membrane that becomes progressively thicker. Dislodging the membrane often causes bleeding. Symptoms of airway obstruction, such as stridor and cyanosis, can develop quickly.

Complications

Diphtheria can progress to life-threatening complications. Even with treatment about 10% of patients with diphtheria die from the disease. Without treatment, up to 50% of patients may die. Complications relate to progression of the infection and include airway occlusion, pulmonary infection that can progress to respiratory failure, myocarditis, or polyneuropathy that can progress to paralysis (CDC, 2017a).

Interprofessional Care

Interprofessional care goals for diphtheria are to prevent its transmission, treat the infection, neutralize toxins, and provide respiratory support.

Diagnosis

The diagnosis is confirmed by a throat culture. Gram-stain or immunofluorescent antibody stains may also be used.

Medications

Strict isolation procedures are instituted, and all contacts are screened and immunized. Booster shots are given to people who were immunized 5 or more years previously. Unimmunized contacts are treated with immunization and antibiotics.

Diphtheria antitoxin is given to neutralize free toxin and prevent further toxin production. It is delivered via IV over 1 hour or IM. Diphtheria antitoxin is produced in horses; a skin test for sensitivity to horse serum should precede immunization because about 1% of the population is sensitive to it (CDC, n.d.). Anaphylaxis is a risk during antitoxin therapy; epinephrine must be readily available. Antibiotics such as penicillin or erythromycin are administered to eliminate the organism.

Nursing Care

Assessment

See the Manifestations and Interprofessional Care sections for the assessment of the patient with diphtheria.

Focused assessment of the patient with suspected diphtheria includes:

- ***Health history:*** Complaints of weakness, sore throat, fever, difficulty swallowing due to swelling
- ***Physical assessment:*** General appearance, vital signs including temperature; inspection of nasal and pharyngeal mucous membranes; assessment of lymph glands of the neck
- ***Laboratory data:*** Sputum culture for diphtheria, WBC, and differential.

Priorities of Care

Patients with diphtheria require intensive nursing care. The patient is placed on bedrest and monitored closely for airway obstruction, cardiac manifestations, and CNS complications. Nutrition and fluid balance may be affected by difficulty swallowing. Upright positioning can promote fluid intake during the acute phase of the disease. Equipment for suction, emergency intubation, and tracheostomy are kept at the bedside.

Preventing further cases of diphtheria is a nursing responsibility. Symptomatic patients are isolated and treated until two negative throat cultures are obtained. Nasopharyngeal and throat cultures are also obtained from all close contacts. Asymptomatic disease carriers are confined to home until at least 3 days of antibiotic therapy have been completed. All contacts, including hospital personnel, receive tetanus and diphtheria toxoids (Td). Tetanus, diphtheria, and pertussis (Tdap) vaccine was licensed in 2005. It is the first vaccine for adolescents and adults that protects against pertussis as well as tetanus and diphtheria. It is given only once.

SAFETY ALERT: Diphtheria is a reportable disease. Immediately contact the local health department and the Centers for Disease Control and Prevention about all suspected and confirmed cases. ■

Diagnoses, Interventions, and Outcomes

Diphtheria is an acute and life-threatening illness. The disease first attacks the respiratory system and can progress to attacking the cardiac, renal, and nervous systems.

Promote Airway Clearance and Patency. When the patient has diphtheria, airway patency is of primary concern.

Expected Outcome: Patient will use techniques to promote airway clearance as indicated and tolerated in combination with maintenance of patent airway.

The nurse will:

- Monitor cough and the ability to move secretions. *Thickening of secretions may impair the ability to mobilize the secretions.*
- *Maintain adequate hydration. Assess mucous membranes and skin turgor for evidence of dehydration. Fever, increased mucus secretions, and decreased oral intake may lead to dehydration and increased viscosity of secretions. Thick, viscous secretions are more difficult to expectorate.*
- Increase the humidity of inspired air with a bedside humidifier. *Increasing the water content of inhaled air helps loosen thick secretions and soothe mucous membranes.*

Promote Effective Breathing. Due to the bacterial infection, the respiratory rate may increase and alter the depth of respirations, decreasing effective alveolar ventilation. Shallow respirations also increase the risk of *atelectasis*, lack of ventilation in an area of the lung.

Expected Outcome: Patient will utilize techniques to promote adequate ventilation such as deep breathing and incentive spirometry.

The nurse will:

- Monitor respiratory rate and pattern. *Tachypnea and/or rapid, shallow respirations may impair effective alveolar ventilation and gas exchange.*
- Pace activities to provide for periods of rest. *Tachypnea increases the work of breathing, causing fatigue; fatigue, in turn, can further impair ventilation and reduce the effectiveness of coughing.*
- Elevate the head of the bed. *The upright position improves lung excursion and reduces the work of breathing by lowering the diaphragm, which moves abdominal contents downward, creating less resistance to diaphragmatic excursion and slightly decreasing venous return.*

Assess Sleep Quality. Airway congestion and persistent cough may interfere with the ability to rest, increasing fatigue and prolonging recovery.

Expected Outcome: Patient will verbalize techniques to reduce impact of upper respiratory symptoms on sleep patterns.

The nurse will:

- Assess sleep patterns using subjective and objective information. *The patient may appear to be sleeping but not achieving normal sleep patterns because of viral URI symptoms. Both subjective and objective data are important to accurately assess sleep.*

Reduce Risk for Infection. Isolation is recommended to prevent person-to-person transmission of diphtheria.

Expected Outcome: Patient will describe measures to protect healthy tissue and prevent infection.

The nurse will:

- Use droplet isolation and encourage all staff and visitors to wash hands frequently. *Isolation procedures and good hand hygiene are primary infection control measures for infections like diphtheria transmitted via respiratory secretions.*
- Use droplet precautions for patients with suspected or confirmed diphtheria. These include providing a private room, masks for caregivers and visitors, and masking the patient when transporting within the facility. *These measures limit the spread of respiratory secretions.*

Delegating Nursing Care Activities

As appropriate and allowed by the designated duties and responsibilities of unlicensed assistive personnel, the nurse may delegate nursing care activities such as measuring vital signs, encouraging oral or enteral fluid intake, and providing skin care.

SAFETY ALERT: Adults should receive a diphtheria vaccine booster immunization every 10 years (usually given in combination with tetanus vaccine [Td]). However, the Tdap is administered only once and does not require booster injections (CDC, 2017d). ■

Transitions of Care

Diphtheria is best prevented by getting vaccinated. The nurse should teach the patient to get vaccinated and maintain up-to-date vaccinations.

The patient with diphtheria requires intensive nursing care and management. The patient must be placed in isolation until two negative throat cultures are found. The patient is placed on bedrest and monitored closely for airway obstruction, cardiac manifestations, and CNS complications. Nutrition and fluid balance may be affected by difficulty swallowing. Upright positioning can promote fluid intake during the acute phase of the disease. Equipment for suction, emergency intubation, and tracheostomy are kept at the bedside.

Diphtheria is an acute, life-threatening illness. The patient who recovers from the acute phase may require continued nursing care to regain function, strength, and endurance. Rehabilitation and recovery may occur in an inpatient or outpatient setting, depending on the individual. Without treatment, the underlying bacteria attaches to the airways and produces an endotoxin that destroys healthy tissue. The disease can progress beyond the respiratory system to the cardiac, renal, and nervous systems.

The Patient with Pertussis

Pertussis, or *whooping cough*, is a highly contagious acute upper respiratory infection caused by the bacterium *Bordetella pertussis*. Although it is thought to be a childhood disease that has been virtually eliminated by aggressive immunization of infants, pertussis still occurs in North America. Up to 45% of people affected by pertussis are adolescents and adults. Adults are thought to be an important reservoir for this disease (CDC, 2017d).

Pathophysiology

B. pertussis is a gram-negative rod that is spread by respiratory droplets. The bacteria attach to ciliated epithelial cells of the nasopharynx, multiplying and invading respiratory tissues. The damage and effects of pertussis are not due to the infection itself, but to toxins produced by the bacteria. These toxins damage the mucosa and paralyze the cilia. As a result, clearance of respiratory secretions is impaired, increasing the risk for pneumonia. The toxins also prompt an inflammatory response and inhibit immune defenses.

Although immunization does not appear to confer lifetime immunity, the disease tends to be milder in adolescents, adults, and people who have been immunized. These infected individuals can, however, transmit the disease to other susceptible people, including unimmunized or underimmunized infants (Sorenson et al., 2019).

Risk Factors

Pertussis occurs only in humans and is highly contagious. The two major risk factors are not being immunized and close contact with an infected person. Risk of developing pertussis without immunization is 80 to 100% with exposure (American Lung Association, 2018).

Manifestations

Classic pertussis follows a predictable pattern, with typical URI symptoms (coryza, sneezing, low-grade fever, and mild cough) beginning 7 to 10 days after exposure. After 1 to 2 weeks, the cough becomes more frequent, occurring in paroxysms or bursts of rapid coughs, often ending with an audible whoop caused by rapid inspiration. This whoop is less common in adolescents and adults, often delaying diagnosis. Vomiting commonly follows an episode of coughing. Coughing paroxysms vary in frequency from several per hour to 5 to 10 per day, interfering with eating and sleep. This stage of the disease, called the *paroxysmal stage*, commonly lasts about 6 weeks, after which coughing becomes less severe and gradually resolves over a period of up to 3 months.

In adolescents and adults, pertussis is suspected when an upper respiratory infection produces a cough that persists longer than 7 days, is accompanied by vomiting, and is worse at night.

Complications

Infants have the highest risk for complications of the disease, which may include pneumonia and neurologic complications. Neurologic complications are thought to result from hypoxia due to prolonged paroxysms of coughing. Complications in adolescents and adults may occur as a result of increased intrathoracic pressure during prolonged coughing spells. These may include pneumothorax, weight loss, inguinal hernia, rib fracture, and *cough syncope* (fainting due to hypoxia).

Interprofessional Care

Diagnosis

The diagnosis of pertussis is established by culture of nasopharyngeal secretions. However, nasopharyngeal secretions may remain positive for the organism for only about 3 weeks after the onset of symptoms, so blood tests for antibodies to the organism may be necessary to confirm the diagnosis. Lymphocytosis (elevated lymphocyte count) may be present.

Medications

Erythromycin is the antibiotic of choice to eradicate *B. pertussis* infection. TMP-SMZ may be used as an alternative to erythromycin. Respiratory isolation is instituted for 5 days after antibiotic therapy is started. Prophylactic erythromycin or TMP-SMZ is prescribed for all in the household and close contacts of the infected patient.

Hospitalization

Hospitalization is rarely required for adults, although children and infants with severe disease are often hospitalized to prevent complications such as the neurologic effects of hypoxia and malnutrition.

Nursing Care

Assessment

See the Manifestations and Interprofessional Care sections for the assessment of the patient with pertussis.

Focused assessment of the patient with suspected pertussis includes:

- ***Health history:*** Complaints of cough (initially intermittent, progresses to paroxysmal)
- ***Physical assessment:*** General appearance, vital signs including temperature; evaluation of cough
- ***Laboratory data:*** Nasopharyngeal culture for patients complaining of persistent cough, especially when the

cough is accompanied by vomiting or significantly worse at night, or if other members of the household or close contacts have a similar illness.

Priorities of Care

Nursing care is supportive. The focus of nursing care for the adult with pertussis is on close surveillance for complications and teaching for self-care and prevention of causative organism spread.

Diagnoses, Interventions, and Outcomes

Although the symptoms of pertussis can be distressing, some people provide self-care and do not contact a healthcare provider.

Promote Effective Breathing. Due to the presence of pertussis and the cardinal symptom of cough, the respiratory rate may increase and alter the depth of respirations, decreasing effective alveolar ventilation. Shallow respirations also increase the risk of *atelectasis*, lack of ventilation in an area of lung.

Expected Outcome: Patient will utilize techniques to promote adequate ventilation such as deep breathing and incentive spirometry.

The nurse will:

- Monitor respiratory rate and pattern. *Tachypnea and/or rapid, shallow respirations may impair effective alveolar ventilation and gas exchange.*
- Pace activities to provide for periods of rest. *Tachypnea increases the work of breathing, causing fatigue; fatigue, in turn, can further impair ventilation and reduce the effectiveness of coughing.*
- Elevate the head of the bed. *The upright position improves lung excursion and reduces the work of breathing by lowering the diaphragm, which moves abdominal contents downward, creating less resistance to diaphragmatic excursion and slightly decreasing venous return.*

Promote Airway Clearance and Patency. The increasing cough with thickening secretions increase the risk of impaired airway clearance in pertussis.

Expected Outcome: Patient will use techniques to promote airway clearance such as effective coughing and deep breathing.

The nurse will:

- Monitor the effectiveness of cough and ability to remove airway secretions. *Fatigue and general malaise may impair the ability to cough effectively and mobilize secretions.*
- Maintain adequate hydration. Assess mucous membranes and skin turgor for evidence of dehydration. *Fever, increased mucus secretions, and decreased oral fluid intake may lead to dehydration and increased viscosity of secretions. Thick, viscous secretions are more difficult to expectorate.*
- Increase the humidity of inspired air with a bedside humidifier. *Increasing the water content of inhaled air helps loosen thick secretions and soothe mucous membranes.*
- Teach effective cough techniques. Administer analgesics as ordered. *The huff cough is effective to maintain open airways and spares energy (see Chapter 37 for patient teaching of this technique). Relieving muscle ache increases the ability to cough effectively.*

Assess Sleep Quality. Airway congestion and persistent cough may interfere with the ability to rest, increasing fatigue and prolonging recovery.

Expected Outcome: Patient will verbalize techniques to reduce impact of upper respiratory symptoms on sleep patterns.

The nurse will:

- Assess sleep patterns using subjective and objective information. *The patient may appear to be sleeping but not achieving normal sleep patterns because of pertussis symptoms. Both subjective and objective data are important to accurately assess sleep.*

Reduce Risk for Infection. Infection control measures are recommended to prevent person-to-person transmission of pertussis.

Expected Outcome: Patient will describe measures to protect healthy tissue and prevent infection.

The nurse will:

- Use standard precautions and encourage all staff and visitors to wash hands frequently. *Hand hygiene is a primary infection control measure for infections transmitted via respiratory secretions.*
- Instruct patients and visitors to control respiratory secretions by using tissues and to maintain a distance of at least 3 feet from others when coughing or sneezing. Provide masks for patients and visitors who are coughing or sneezing. *Limiting the spread of aerosolized secretions by covering the nose and mouth and maintaining distance from other people can reduce the spread of the disease to vulnerable populations.*
- Use droplet precautions for patients with suspected or confirmed pertussis: Provide a private room, masks for caregivers and visitors, and mask the patient when transporting within the facility. *These measures limit the spread of respiratory secretions.*

Delegating Nursing Care Activities

As appropriate and allowed by the designated duties and responsibilities of unlicensed assistive personnel, the nurse may delegate nursing care/activities such as measuring vital signs, encouraging oral or enteral fluid intake, and providing skin care.

SAFETY ALERT: Pertussis is a reportable communicable disease. Report all probable and confirmed cases to the local health department and the Centers for Disease Control and Prevention. ■

Transitions of Care

Nurses are instrumental in promoting effective immunization of all infants and young children against pertussis. Active immunization with pertussis vaccine is the primary preventative strategy for pertussis. Acellular pertussis vaccines that are effective, but produce fewer adverse reactions than traditional whole-cell vaccines, are available and preferred for immunization.

Education is a key nursing role related to immunization because significant controversy currently exists about potential long-term adverse consequences of the vaccine. Recommend that all parents request acellular vaccine due to its lower risk of adverse effects.

Adult patients usually remain in the community for treatment. Teach respiratory isolation measures to be used until the disease is no longer communicable to others. Discuss ways to control respiratory secretions and the importance of disposing of tissues and secretions personally to prevent exposure of others. Stress the importance of prophylactic treatment for all household and close contacts. Discuss measures to maintain fluid and nutrient intake and use of a cough suppressant at night to promote rest. Encourage increased fluid intake to promote expectoration of respiratory secretions. Teach about the prescribed antibiotic, including its potential adverse effects and measures to reduce them, such as taking erythromycin with meals to prevent gastric upset.

Instruct the patient that the convalescent phase of pertussis is manifested with a reduction in paroxysmal coughing spells. The cough will continue to recede but occasional paroxysmal coughing spell can occur for many months after the onset of illness. Contact the local county health department for follow-up of contacts and compliance with prescribed treatment. Due to resurgence of pertussis among children, adults are recommended to obtain the Tdap vaccine to reduce risk of infection to children who have not been immunized or are underimmunized.

35.2 Upper Respiratory Trauma or Obstruction

Obstruction of the upper airway due to trauma (fracture of the nasal septum or the larynx), bleeding (e.g., epistaxis), or a tumor is frightening for the patient and may interfere with the ability to breathe.

The Patient with Epistaxis

The nose has a rich blood supply, receiving major arterial vessels from both the internal and external carotid artery systems. **Epistaxis**, a nosebleed, may be precipitated by a number of factors. Trauma (picking the nose or blunt trauma) can cause epistaxis, as can drying of nasal mucous membranes, infection, substance abuse (e.g., cocaine), arteriosclerosis, or hypertension. Epistaxis may also indicate a bleeding disorder related to acute leukemia, thrombocytopenia, aplastic anemia, or severe liver disease. Additionally, treatment with an anticoagulant or antiplatelet drug may cause a nosebleed. In adults, men have nosebleeds more frequently than women.

Pathophysiology

Ninety percent of all nosebleeds arise in the anterior nasal septum from Kiesselbach's area, a rich vascular plexus. Because of their location, these vessels are susceptible to trauma from nose picking, drying, and infection. Posterior epistaxis more often develops secondarily to systemic disorders such as blood dyscrasias, hypertension, or diabetes. In posterior epistaxis, bleeding is from the terminal branches of the sphenopalatine and internal maxillary arteries. Posterior epistaxis tends to be more severe and occurs more frequently in the older adult.

Risk Factors

Epistaxis has reported risk factors that include nasal perforation, nasal septum deviation, rhinitis, sinusitis, and upper respiratory tract infection. Significant risk factors for recurrent epistaxis include congestive heart failure, diabetes mellitus, hypertension, and a history of anemia.

Manifestations

Anterior nosebleeds usually produce obvious bleeding from the nares, as well as bleeding into the posterior nasal and oral pharynx. The bleeding from a posterior nosebleed may be less apparent, with most of the blood draining into the posterior nasopharynx and swallowed by the patient. Nausea and vomiting may occur due to swallowed blood.

Complications

Nosebleeds in and of themselves are usually self-limiting and do not usually cause complications. If the nosebleed is severe and treatment is not sought, the resulting hemorrhage can lead to anemia and, ultimately, to hypovolemic shock.

Interprofessional Care

The goal of treatment for epistaxis is to identify and control the source of bleeding.

Anterior bleeding can usually be managed by simple first-aid measures, such as applying pressure (pinching the nose toward the septum) for 5 to 10 minutes and applying ice packs to the nose and forehead to cause vasoconstriction. The patient is placed in a sitting position to decrease blood flow to the head and reduce venous pressure. Leaning forward reduces drainage of blood backward into the nasopharynx and decreases swallowing of blood. The patient is instructed to spit out the blood to help estimate the amount of bleeding and to prevent nausea and vomiting as a result of swallowed blood.

If applying pressure does not control the bleeding, medications, nasal packing, or surgery may be necessary.

Diagnosis

The diagnosis of epistaxis can be made using the history and physical exam.

Medications

Topical vasoconstrictors such as cocaine (0.5%), phenylephrine (Neo-Synephrine) (1:1000), or adrenaline (1:1000) may be used to control anterior bleeding. These medications may be applied by nasal spray or on a cotton swab held against the bleeding site. Chemical cauterization of the bleeding vessel may be done using agents such as silver nitrate or Gelfoam. A topical anesthetic such as tetracaine, lidocaine, or cocaine may be used prior to nasal packing. If posterior nasal packing is required, prophylactic antibiotic therapy is initiated to prevent sinusitis or possible toxic shock syndrome.

Nasal Packing

If bleeding cannot be controlled with pressure and local medications, a nasal tampon (a soft balloon filled with air) may be used to apply direct pressure to the bleeding vessel or the nasal cavity may be packed with 0.25-inch petroleum gauze. For an anterior pack, several feet of packing are placed carefully and systematically along the floor of the nasal cavity and then into the vault of the nose. Anterior nasal packs are usually left in place for 24 to 72 hours. If epistaxis is caused by a bleeding disorder, the packing may be left in place for 4 to 5 days while the disorder is treated.

Posterior nosebleeds are more difficult to control, requiring both anterior and posterior packing (**Figure 35.3** ■). Posterior packs are usually left in place for 2 to 5 days. A loose anterior nasal pack may also be inserted. Posterior nasal packing is very uncomfortable and can cause respiratory and cardiovascular complications. Hypoxemia is common; supplementary oxygen is administered. Endotracheal intubation may be necessary to maintain adequate ventilation and gas exchange. Narcotic analgesics are prescribed to manage the discomfort. Hypertension, dysrhythmias, and even acute myocardial infarction may occur in patients with severe cardiovascular disease. Toxic shock syndrome is another potential complication of posterior nasal packing. The pack may occlude the eustachian tube and sinus openings, resulting in ear discomfort, possible otitis media, or sinusitis. Oral and nasal dryness can be minimized by use of a high-humidity face tent. Nursing care of the patient with nasal packing is outlined in **Box 35.3**.

A Foley catheter or inflatable nasal balloons may be used as an alternative to posterior nasal packing for effective tamponade. The catheter or nasal balloon is inserted through the nose into the nasopharynx, inflated, and left in place for 2 to 3 days.

SAFETY ALERT: Assess the patient with nasal packing frequently for adequate oxygenation. Maintain supplemental oxygen as ordered. Cerebral hypoxia produces a sense of apprehension and fear. ■

Surgery

Chemical or surgical cautery procedures may be used to sclerose (shrink and tighten) involved vessels in the anterior aspect of the nose. The resulting scab must be left undisturbed until the mucosa has healed or further bleeding may occur.

Surgical procedures to control bleeding are often preferred to posterior nasal packing for posterior bleeding. The bleeding vessel may be cauterized using an endoscopic approach. In some cases, surgery is required to occlude the internal maxillary artery by ligation (tying off) or embolization. These procedures may be done under either conscious sedation and local anesthesia or general anesthesia. Facial paralysis, paresthesias, facial pain, and dental injury are potential complications.

Nursing Care

Assessment

See the Manifestations and Interprofessional Care sections for the assessment of the patient with nosebleed.

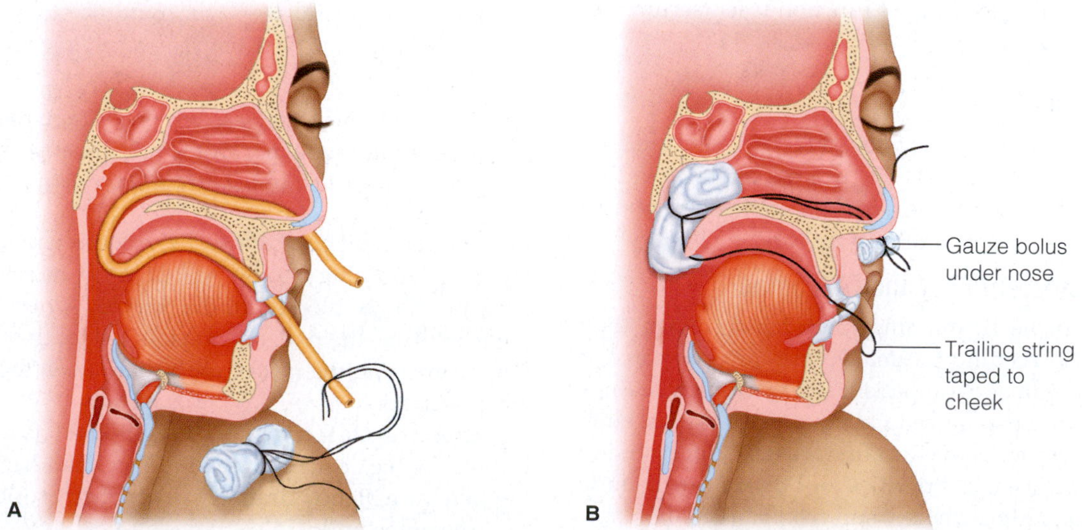
A
B
Gauze bolus under nose
Trailing string taped to cheek

Figure 35.3 ■ Posterior nasal packing. A, A rubber catheter is inserted through the nose and out the mouth and attached to the packing. B, The catheter is withdrawn through the nose to position the packing in the posterior nasopharynx. Ties exiting through the nose and mouth are used to stabilize the packing in position and remove it when it is no longer needed.

Box 35.3
Nursing Care of the Patient with Nasal Packing

For the patient who has nasal packing, the nurse will:

- Continuously monitor oxygen saturation. Administer supplementary oxygen as ordered. *Posterior nasal packing causes hypoxemia. Supplemental oxygen is given to maintain tissue oxygenation.*
- Frequently monitor vital signs and respiratory rate or pattern. *Posterior nasal packing increases the risk for respiratory and cardiovascular complications. Tachycardia and tachypnea may be early signs of cardiac or respiratory compromise.*
- Inspect the mouth and oropharynx. Notify the healthcare provider if the packing is seen in the oropharynx. *Misplacement of nasal packing can obstruct the upper airway.*
- Elevate the head of the bed. *Elevating the head of the bed facilitates ventilation.*
- Encourage deep, slow breathing through the mouth. Provide psychologic support, reassurance, and teaching. *Inability to breathe through the nose causes anxiety and fear.*
- Check for blood at the back of the throat and frequent swallowing. *Visible blood or frequent swallowing could indicate posterior bleeding.*
- Report hematemesis. *Bleeding from the posterior portion of the nose often drains down the nasopharynx and is swallowed. Hematemesis may indicate continued bleeding.*
- Apply cold compresses to nose. *An ice or cold compress decreases pain and promotes vasoconstriction, decreasing bleeding and swelling.*
- Provide for rest. *Rest reduces the metabolic demands and oxygen consumption.*
- Ensure adequate oral fluid intake. *Fluid intake helps maintain fluid balance and decreases dryness of oral mucous membranes because of mouth breathing.*
- Provide frequent oral hygiene. Use a bedside humidifier. *These measures reduce drying of oral mucous membranes and promote comfort.*

Nursing assessment of the patient with a nosebleed focuses on the immediate problem and possible underlying conditions.

- ***Health history:*** Duration of current bleed; any identified precipitating factors such as trauma; history of prior nosebleeds; current medications; chronic conditions such as hypertension, bleeding disorders, and so on
- ***Physical assessment:*** Estimated amount of bleeding; presence of blood in oropharynx; vital signs; evidence of facial or nasal trauma
- ***Laboratory data:*** Hemoglobin, hematocrit, platelets, and WBC as indicated; oxygen saturation; tests of organ function such as liver function tests (bilirubin, AST, ALT, LDH) or kidney function tests (serum creatinine, BUN).

Priorities of Care

Collaborate with the interprofessional team to ensure adequate treatment of the underlying process while providing care that supports the physical and psychologic responses to the disorder is a priority of nursing care.

Diagnoses, Interventions, and Outcomes

Nosebleeds can be frightening, particularly when they occur without preceding trauma. Nurses provide care for patients with epistaxis in outpatient and emergency settings and may care for hospitalized patients with nasal packing. Support, reassurance, and education are important nursing roles related to epistaxis. Priorities for nursing care include interventions to reduce anxiety and risk for aspiration.

Manage Anxiety. The amount of blood lost in a nosebleed can be frightening. The sensation of blood draining down the throat and the inability to breathe through the nose contribute to anxiety. Spontaneous epistaxis may lead to fear of a major health problem such as high blood pressure. This is not a life-threatening event. The nurse should model calmness for the patient and family.

Expected Outcome: Patient will be able to control anxiety as evidenced by verbalized decrease in subjective distress.

The nurse will:

- Maintain an attitude of calm reassurance. *By remaining calm and confident, the nurse reassures the patient that the nosebleed is not a life-threatening event.*
- Instruct the patient to pinch the nares together at the bridge of the nose. *Most nosebleeds are anterior in origin; direct pressure usually stops the bleeding. Having the patient place pressure on the nose provides a focus and helps restore a sense of control, reducing anxiety.*
- Encourage slow, deep breathing through the mouth. *Controlled mouth breathing maintains lung ventilation and reduces anxiety.*
- Provide a basin and tissues; encourage the patient to expectorate blood, not swallow it. *These measures give the patient greater control and reduce the fear of choking on blood.*

Reduce Risk for Aspiration. The combination of anxiety and blood draining into the nasopharynx increases the risk for aspiration of blood into the trachea. When nasal packing is in place, the patient is unable to breathe through the nose, increasing the risk of aspiration when food or fluids are consumed.

Expected Outcome: Patient will use vasoconstrictive techniques (i.e., cold compress to face) and head positioning to reduce bloody drainage down the nasopharynx.

The nurse will:

- Position upright with the head forward. Provide a basin for expectorating blood. *These measures minimize the amount of blood draining down the nasopharynx and swallowed, reducing the risk of aspiration and minimizing nausea from swallowed blood. Vomiting of swallowed blood increases the risk of aspiration.*

- Apply ice or a cold compress to the nose. *Cold causes vasoconstriction, reducing bleeding.*
- Position the patient with nasal packing with the head elevated and on the side when asleep. *This position reduces the risk of aspiration of oral secretions.*

Delegating Nursing Care Activities

As appropriate and allowed by the designated duties and responsibilities of unlicensed assistive personnel, the nurse may delegate nursing care/activities such as measuring vital signs, encouraging oral or enteral fluid intake, and providing skin care.

Transitions of Care

Following an episode of epistaxis, teaching for home care focuses on measures to prevent further bleeding. Include the following teaching topics:

- Avoid strenuous exercise for several days or weeks, depending on the severity of the nosebleed and its treatment.
- Do not blow the nose or engage in activities such as heavy lifting or bending that could increase pressure and dislodge the crust; sneeze with the mouth open to avoid increasing pressure in nasal vessels.
- For an anterior nosebleed, use petroleum jelly, a water-soluble lubricant, or bacitracin ointment to lubricate nasal mucosa and reduce the risk of spontaneous bleeding.
- Use a humidifier or vaporizer to minimize dryness of the mucous membranes.
- Do not forcefully blow the nose or pick the nose.
- For a spontaneous nosebleed, seek medical evaluation for any possible underlying problem, such as hypertension or a bleeding disorder.

The Patient with Nasal Trauma or Surgery

The nose is the most commonly broken bone of the face. A nasal fracture (broken nose) usually is caused by a sports injury or trauma related to violence or motor vehicle crashes. The nasal septum normally divides the nose into two equal parts. Deviation of the septum can result from nasal trauma. Soft tissue trauma commonly accompanies nasal fracture.

Pathophysiology

One or both sides of the nose may be broken. A *unilateral fracture* involves only one side of the nose. It causes little displacement or cosmetic deformity. It is usually not serious, but septal deviation and swelling can obstruct the airway. *Bilateral fractures* are more common, with depression or displacement of both nasal bones to one side. The nose appears flattened or deviated with an S or C configuration. *Complex fractures* may also involve the septum, ascending processes of the maxilla, and frontal bones of the face.

Soft tissue trauma commonly accompanies nasal fracture. Mucous membrane tears cause epistaxis. Soft tissue hematomas (black eyes) are also frequent. Swelling develops rapidly following the injury and may obscure the fracture. Boney crepitus may be felt on gentle palpation. Septal hematoma may develop, increasing the risk for infection.

Risk Factors

Nasal fracture risk factors are related to conditions that increase the risk for falls or facial trauma. These include increased age (balance issues), seizure disorders, alcohol or drug use/abuse, contact sports, reckless behaviors, and failure to wear a seat belt when travelling by car.

Manifestations

Manifestations of nasal fracture include epistaxis, deformity or displacement to one side, crepitus, periorbital edema and ecchymosis, and nasal bridge instability.

Complications

Potential complications of nasal fracture include septal hematoma and abscess formation, septal perforation or deviation, and cerebrospinal fluid (CSF) leakage. Septal hematoma can lead to complete and bilateral nasal obstruction. If undrained, hematoma increases the risk of staphylococcal abscess, which can lead to necrosis of septal cartilage and *saddle nose deformity*.

Septal deviation causes varying degrees of nasal obstruction. The septal cartilage bulges or deviates to one side, partially or totally obstructing the nares. Mild deviation is generally asymptomatic. Partial obstruction of airflow through one side may cause noisy breathing while awake and snoring during sleep. Major deviations can cause pain because of sinus obstruction or infection. They may also cause nosebleeds due to dryness of the nasal mucosa. Occasionally, the defect is severe enough to cause cosmetic deformity. Perforations are usually not serious and do not usually require repair unless obstruction or external deformity occurs.

Fractures of other facial bones may accompany a broken nose, particularly when facial trauma is severe. Fractures in the nasoethmoidal or frontal region can disrupt the dura, causing cerebrospinal fluid (CSF) leakage or rhinorrhea. CSF rhinorrhea is suspected when watery nasal drainage tests positive for glucose.

SAFETY ALERT: Test watery, clear fluid dripping from the ear or nose for glucose. CSF will test positive for glucose on a Dextrostrip. ■

Interprofessional Care

The major treatment goals for nasal fractures are to maintain a patent airway and prevent deformity. Respirations are closely monitored.

Diagnosis

Head and facial x-rays are done to identify the fracture and assess for other facial fractures. The intranasal cavity is examined using a nasal speculum to rule out septal hematoma. If a CSF leak is suspected, a CT scan is done. A radiopaque substance or fluorescein dye may be instilled into the intrathecal or lumbar subarachnoid space to identify the site of leakage.

Medications

Medications used in nasal fracture are usually related to the accompanying nosebleed. See medications under epistaxis.

Fracture Reduction

Ideally, the fracture is reduced early, before significant edema develops. Nasal fractures heal rapidly. Simple reduction may be done in the emergency department with local anesthesia. An external splint may be applied for 7 to 10 days to maintain proper alignment until healing occurs. The splint is padded to prevent skin breakdown. Ice may be gently applied to the face and nose to control edema and bleeding. Nasal packing may be used to control epistaxis.

Surgery

Complex nasal fractures, nasal septal deviation, or persistent CSF leakage may require surgical repair or realignment of nasal bones. Rhinoplasty with concurrent septoplasty is the most common procedure used to repair nasal fracture or a deviated nasal septum.

Rhinoplasty is surgical reconstruction of the nose. It is done to relieve airway obstruction and repair visible deformity of the nose following fracture. If edema is excessive after nasal fracture, surgery is delayed for 7 to 10 days to allow swelling to subside. Using an intranasal incision, the nasal skin is lifted, and the framework of the nose reshaped by removing, rearranging, or augmenting bone or cartilage. The skin is then repositioned over the reconstructed frame. Prosthetic implants may help reshape the nose. Either local or general anesthesia may be used; hospitalization is often unnecessary. Following surgery, nasal packing is left in place for up to 72 hours to minimize bleeding and provide tissue support. A temporary plastic splint molded to the shape of the nose is removed in 3 to 5 days. The splint protects the reshaped nose and helps to control swelling. Most swelling and bruising subside within 10 to 14 days; normal sensation returns within several months following surgery. Rhinoplasty generally has few complications.

Either a septoplasty or a submucous resection (SMR) may be done under local anesthesia to correct a deviated septum. *Septoplasty* involves incising one side of the septum, elevating the mucous membrane, and removing or straightening the deviated portion of septal cartilage. In a *submucous resection*, bone and cartilage are removed. In both procedures, packing is applied to both sides of the nose to prevent bleeding and to keep the septal mucosa in midline position.

Small defects in the cribriform plate, fovea ethmoidalis, or sphenoid sinus associated with persistent CSF leakage may require endoscopic repair. Either a tissue graft or fibrin glue may be used to repair the defect. The graft or glue is held in place with absorbable packing. Large defects may require craniotomy for repair.

SAFETY ALERT: Have suction equipment available. Airway patency is a priority; oropharyngeal suctioning may be necessary to remove secretions and maintain a clear airway. Suctioning of the nasopharynx is avoided to prevent additional tissue trauma. ■

Nursing Care

Assessment

See the Manifestations and Interprofessional Care sections for the assessment of the patient with nasal trauma.

Focused nursing assessment for the patient with a suspected nasal fracture includes:

- ***Health history:*** Nature and circumstances of the injury; pain; ability to breathe through the nose; complications from prior head injury
- ***Physical assessment:*** Evident trauma, swelling, ecchymosis, or deformity of the nose; vital signs, respiratory rate and ease; gentle palpation of nose and facial bones for crepitus; inspection of oropharynx for drainage; testing of nasal discharge for glucose.

Priorities of Care

Collaborate with the interprofessional team to ensure adequate treatment of the underlying process while providing care that supports the physical and psychologic responses to the disorder is a priority of nursing care.

Diagnoses, Outcomes, and Interventions

Nursing care for patients with nasal fracture focuses on controlling pain, bleeding, and swelling. Airway management is a priority. Most nasal fractures are managed on an outpatient basis, and education is a vital nursing function. See the accompanying Case Study & Nursing Care Plan for additional nursing diagnoses and interventions for the patient with nasal trauma.

Promote Airway Clearance and Patency. Immediately following nasal trauma and fracture, the airway is at risk for obstruction by bleeding and edema. Deformity resulting from inappropriate fracture position during healing can also impair nasal airway clearance. This is a consideration when inserting nasogastric tubes or suctioning patients with septal deviation.

Expected Outcome: Patient will use techniques to promote airway clearance such as coughing and deep breathing.

The nurse will:

- Monitor airway patency. *Edema and bleeding may obstruct the airway, causing signs of respiratory distress such as tachypnea, dyspnea, shortness of breath, tachycardia, and use of accessory muscles.*
- Monitor cough effectiveness and ability to clear airway secretions. *Pain, edema, and nasal bleeding may impair the ability to cough effectively.*
- Maintain adequate hydration. Assess mucous membranes and skin turgor for evidence of dehydration. *Decreased oral fluid intake may lead to dehydration and thick, viscous secretions that are more difficult to expectorate.*
- Assess patency of both nares before inserting a nasogastric tube or feeding tube. If airflow is obstructed through one side, insert the tube through the unobstructed nare. Carefully monitor respiratory status following tube insertion. *The nasogastric tube is inserted through the unobstructed nare to avoid mucosal trauma; however, a large gastric tube may interfere with nasal breathing, necessitating close monitoring.*

Reduce Risk for Infection. The patient with a nasal fracture is at increased risk for infection. The nasal mucosa is a natural barrier to infection, and trauma increases the risk for invasion by pathogens. Septal hematoma can lead to abscess formation and staphylococcal infection. A CSF leak indicates disruption of the dura, increasing the risk of ascending infection and meningitis.

Expected Outcome: Patient will describe measures to protect healthy tissue and prevent infection.

The nurse will:

- Avoid suctioning if possible. *Suctioning catheters could introduce microorganisms and cause additional trauma to tissues.*
- Monitor vital signs every 4 hours. *A rise in temperature may indicate infection.*
- Administer antibiotics as ordered. *Antibiotics may be prescribed to prevent abscess formation, and, if CSF leakage is present, to prevent meningitis.*

Delegating Nursing Care Activities

As appropriate and allowed by the designated duties and responsibilities of unlicensed assistive personnel, the nurse may delegate nursing care activities such as measuring vital signs, encouraging oral or enteral fluid intake, and providing skin care.

Transitions of Care

Teach all people, children and adolescents in particular, about the importance of wearing helmets and facial protectors when participating in high-risk sports such as football, hockey, and baseball. Promote the use of seat belts with a shoulder harness and airbags in vehicles to reduce the risk of facial injury in motor vehicle crashes.

Provide the following teaching when preparing the patient with a nasal fracture for home care:

- Elevate the head of the bed with blocks and apply ice or cold packs to the nose for 20 minutes four times a day to reduce swelling.
- Swelling usually subsides in several days; bruising may persist for several weeks.
- It is difficult to determine the final cosmetic outcome until swelling has subsided.
- If indicated by delayed fracture reduction or malformation, discuss rhinoplasty and its potential benefits.

If CSF leakage is present, also include the following instructions:

- Rest in bed with the head of the bed elevated to 30 to 45 degrees.
- Restrict fluid intake as ordered and take the prescribed diuretic to reduce intracranial pressure and CSF leakage.
- Distribute allowed fluids throughout the day.
- List name, purpose, effects, and precautions for any prescribed medication.
- Avoid straining, blowing the nose, sneezing, or vigorous coughing until allowed by the healthcare provider.
- Immediately report manifestations of infection, including stiff neck, headache, and fever to the healthcare provider.

Following rhinoplasty or septoplasty, provide the following instructions:

- Apply ice packs to the nose to relieve discomfort and reduce swelling.
- Elevate the head of the bed on blocks to decrease local edema.
- Do not blow the nose for 48 hours after the packing is removed to prevent bleeding.
- Vigorous coughing or straining at stool may cause bleeding and should be avoided.
- Clean teeth and mouth frequently and increase fluid intake to decrease oral dryness due to mouth breathing.
- Bruising around the eyes and nose will last for several days.

The Patient with Laryngeal Obstruction or Trauma

The larynx is the narrowest portion of the upper airway. As such, it is at risk for obstruction. Laryngeal obstruction is a life-threatening emergency. Blows to the neck or other traumatic injuries may damage the larynx, interfering with its patency and function.

Pathophysiology

In **laryngeal obstruction**, the larynx may be partially or fully obstructed by aspirated food or foreign objects, or by laryngospasm or edema due to inflammation, injury, anaphylaxis, or a tumor. Anything that occludes the larynx can obstruct the airway. The most common cause of obstruction in adults is ingested meat that lodges in the airway (the so-called *café coronary*).

Laryngeal trauma can occur in motor vehicle crashes or assaults (e.g., blows to the neck or attempted strangulation). The larynx may also be traumatized during endotracheal intubation or tracheotomy. Trauma may fracture thyroid and/or cricoid cartilage, resulting in loss of airway patency. Soft tissue injuries can cause swelling that further impairs the airway.

Risk Factors

Risk factors for food aspiration include ingesting large boluses of food and chewing them insufficiently, consuming excess alcohol, and wearing dentures. The only risk factor for laryngeal trauma is related to prolonged intubation or difficult intubation.

Manifestations

A foreign body in the larynx causes pain, laryngospasm, dyspnea, and inspiratory stridor. Aspirated foreign bodies may pass through the larynx into the trachea and lungs, causing pneumonitis.

Laryngospasm occurs due to repeated or traumatic intubation attempts, chemical irritation, or hypocalcemia. An

Case Study & Nursing Care Plan

A Patient with Nasal Trauma

Clifton Kavanaugh is a 36-year-old mailman who broke his nose when he was hit in the face by a baseball. He is admitted to the emergency department accompanied by a friend.

ASSESSMENT	DIAGNOSES	EXPECTED OUTCOMES
Mr. Kavanaugh presents with obvious deformity of the nose. It is swollen, bloody, and deviated to one side. The nose is bleeding slightly. Mr. Kavanaugh rates the pain as a 6 on a scale of 1 to 10. Vital signs are T 37°C (98.6°F) axillary, P 120 bpm and regular, R 22/min, and BP 132/70 mmHg. Mr. Kavanaugh is breathing through his mouth and holding an ice compress to his nose. Boney crepitus and edema are felt on palpation. There is no evidence of CSF leak from either nose or ears. X-ray confirms a nasal fracture.	■ Acute pain related to nasal fracture ■ Changes in breathing pattern related to obstruction (nasal swelling) ■ Anxiety related to pain ■ Concerns related to changes in appearance of face (e.g., swelling of nose, and patient statement of "I look like a raccoon")	■ Patient will verbalize relief of pain. ■ Patient will maintain a patent airway and normalize his breathing pattern. ■ Patient will demonstrate reduced anxiety. ■ Patient will express concerns about changes in facial appearance.

PLANNING AND IMPLEMENTATION

- Administer analgesics as ordered.
- Apply ice compress to nose.
- Inspect oropharynx for evidence of bleeding.
- Encourage deep, slow breathing through the mouth.
- Provide oral hygiene.
- Discuss concerns regarding injury.
- Assist with nasal splint application.

EVALUATION

Following treatment, Mr. Kavanaugh reports his pain has decreased to a level of 2 on a scale of 1 to 10. He appears more relaxed and is no longer grimacing. His respirations are easy at 18/min. The nasal splint is intact. Mr. Kavanaugh is able to look in a mirror and state with a laugh, "I look like a raccoon." He is admitted to the hospital for rhinoplasty.

CLINICAL REASONING IN PATIENT CARE

1. A patient in the emergency department with nasal trauma becomes extremely panicky because of blood draining down his throat. How would you intervene to reduce this patient's anxiety without using nasal suction? Why is it important to avoid suctioning the nasopharynx in the patient with nasal trauma?
2. Develop a plan of care for the patient with a leak of CSF from a nasal fracture.
3. Compare immediate versus delayed rhinoplasty for the patient with nasal fracture.

See Evaluating Your Response in Appendix B.

acute type I hypersensitivity response may cause anaphylaxis with release of inflammatory mediators, leading to angioedema of upper airways and severe laryngeal edema.

The most common manifestations of laryngeal obstruction are coughing, choking, gagging, obvious difficulty breathing with use of accessory muscles, and inspiratory stridor. As the airway is obstructed, signs of asphyxia become apparent. Respirations are labored and noisy with wheezing and stridor. Cyanosis may develop. Respiratory arrest and death may result without prompt treatment.

Manifestations of laryngeal trauma may include subcutaneous emphysema or crepitus, voice change, dysphagia and pain with swallowing, inspiratory stridor, hemoptysis, and cough.

Complications

Laryngeal trauma does not lead to complications but is an effect (complication) of prolonged endotracheal intubation. Prevention of this complication commonly leads to tracheostomy versus prolonged intubation in patients requiring long-term airway support and/or mechanical ventilation.

Interprofessional Care

Diagnosis and Treatment

Diagnosis is based on physical assessment. Poor or no air movement would trigger care. The treatment goal is to maintain an open airway. If airway obstruction is partial and the patient is able to cough and move air in and out of the lungs, radiologic and laryngoscopic examination may be done to locate the foreign body. An endotracheal tube may be inserted to maintain airflow through the larynx in spasm or an edematous larynx. For anaphylaxis, epinephrine may be administered to reduce laryngeal edema and relieve obstruction.

When airway obstruction due to a foreign body is complete, the Heimlich maneuver is performed immediately to clear the obstruction (**Figure 35.4** ■). For the conscious person, the rescuer wraps his or her arms around the victim from behind, places one fist between the umbilicus and xiphoid process, covers the fist with the other hand, and forcefully thrusts the hands upward. For the unconscious victim, the rescuer straddles the victim's thighs and delivers thrusts upward and inward on the upper abdomen. These moves are continued until the obstruction is relieved or more definitive care can be given. Endotracheal intubation may be attempted. If intubation is unsuccessful, an immediate cricothyrotomy or tracheotomy must be performed to open the airway.

CT scan is used to identify laryngeal fractures; however, emergency treatment may be required prior to diagnosis to ensure airway patency and preserve life. Soft tissue injuries may be managed conservatively with a bedside humidifier, intravenous fluids, antibiotics, and corticosteroids to reduce edema. More severe injuries require endotracheal intubation or immediate tracheostomy. Nursing care related to caring for the patient with a tracheostomy is presented later in this chapter. See Chapter 37 for more information about endotracheal intubation and nursing care for the intubated patient.

SAFETY ALERT: The priority of nursing care in laryngeal obstruction or trauma is restoring a patent airway to prevent cerebral anoxia and death. Laryngeal obstruction and trauma are medical emergencies requiring immediate intervention. ■

Nursing Care

Assessment

Closely monitor patients at risk for laryngeal obstruction (e.g., following neck trauma, newly extubated patients, and people receiving medications that carry a high risk of anaphylaxis, such as intravenous antibiotics or radiologic dyes) for manifestations of obstruction, including dyspnea, nasal flaring, tachypnea, anxiety, wheezing, and stridor.

Priorities of Care

Establishing a patent airway is the priority of care for the patient with a laryngeal obstruction. Suction the airway as needed; small aspirated foreign bodies might possibly be removed by suctioning. If obstruction is complete, initiate a cardiopulmonary arrest procedure and perform the Heimlich maneuver until the obstruction is relieved or the emergency response team arrives. Prepare to assist with emergency intubation or tracheotomy as needed. Provide emotional support, reassurance, and teaching for the patient and family to reduce anxiety.

Diagnoses, Interventions, and Outcomes

Nursing care for the patient with a laryngeal obstruction focuses on maintaining a patent airway and teaching about the disorder and strategies to prevent its recurrence. The risk for impaired verbal communication is significant. Dysphagia may interfere with swallowing and nutrition.

Promote Airway Clearance and Patency. Following treatment for laryngeal obstruction (vocal cord nodule, local tissue edema) may interfere with airway patency.

Expected Outcome: Patient will use techniques to promote airway clearance as indicated and tolerated in combination with maintenance of patent airway.

The nurse will:

- Apply cold packs to the neck as ordered or indicated. *Cold application constricts local blood vessels and reduces edema development.*
- Withhold food and fluids until the cough and gag reflexes have returned. *Local anesthesia used during treatment of laryngeal obstruction impairs the cough and gag reflexes, increasing the risk for aspiration.*

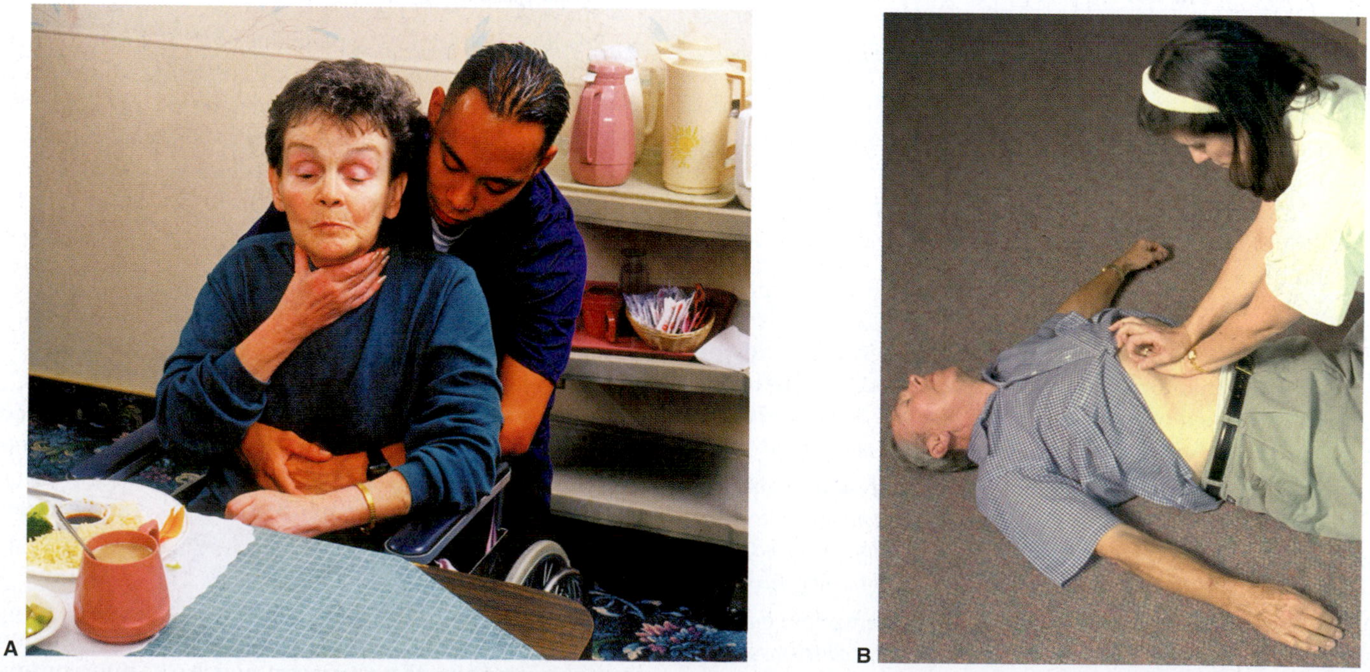
A
B

Figure 35.4 ■ Administering abdominal thrusts (the Heimlich maneuver) to **A**, a conscious victim, and **B**, an unconscious victim.

Promote Communication. Treatment of laryngeal obstruction may alter the quality of the voice or result in short-term restriction on speaking.

Expected Outcome: Patient will utilize alternative communication techniques.

The nurse will:

- Prior to treatment, if appropriate, assess for additional obstacles to communication. *Communication may be impaired by hearing loss, illiteracy, or weakness associated with the disease process, altering the ability to use alternative communication strategies.*
- Assess the importance of verbal communication to self-concept, occupation, and lifestyle. *Many factors influence adaptation to the loss of normal verbal communication. If the ability to speak is central to an occupation (e.g., school teacher, singer) or self-concept (e.g., a politician or attorney), adapting may be difficult.*
- Prior to surgery, introduce nonverbal communication strategies such as pencil and paper, white boards, or tablets. Encourage the patient to practice using each method and to choose the most acceptable one. *Having the patient determine a means of communication prior to surgery helps to alleviate anxiety and increases the sense of control.*
- Arrange consultation with a speech therapist about alternate forms of oral communication prior to surgery, if possible. *Determining a means of communicating on a continuing basis prior to surgery helps to relieve fear of inability to communicate.*
- Reinforce teaching about alternative communication strategies. *Anxiety or information overload may impair the ability to retain information; reinforcement facilitates learning.*
- Maintain a positive attitude about postoperative communication, but do not promote unrealistic expectations. *Not all patients are able to use all alternative methods of verbal communication. Some patients remain nonverbal.*

Reduce Risk for Choking. Disruption of laryngeal structures by the obstruction itself can impair the swallowing mechanism.

Expected Outcome: Patient will utilize modified food and fluid consistency to promote swallowing while using techniques to avoid choking.

The nurse will:

- Maintain intravenous fluids and enteral feedings or parenteral nutrition until adequate food and fluids can be ingested orally. *It is important to maintain nutritional and fluid balance until normal eating can be resumed.*
- Postoperatively, initiate oral intake with soft foods, not liquids. *Soft foods are easier than liquids to handle and swallow initially. As recovery progresses, thickened liquids can be swallowed, progressing to liquids, and, eventually, a normal diet.*
- Provide for privacy during initial attempts at eating. *Eating in the presence of others may cause embarrassment until confidence in eating is regained. Privacy also reduces distractions, allowing concentration on swallowing.*

Promote Balanced Nutrition. Laryngeal obstruction may cause dysphagia (difficulty swallowing) or odynophagia (painful swallowing). In either case, difficulty eating may ultimately impair nutrition. Enteral or parenteral feedings are usually needed initially to meet nutritional status.

Expected Outcome: Patient will consume adequate nourishment to promote weight within normal range.

The nurse will:

- Assess nutritional status using height and weight charts, reported weight loss, and anthropometric measurements such as skinfolds. *Thorough assessment of nutritional status is important in planning to meet current and anticipated calorie needs.*
- Monitor food and fluid intake and urinary output. *Pain or fatigue, rather than a sensation of fullness, may prompt the decision to stop eating, resulting in inadequate intake.*
- Evaluate current and preferred eating habits and foods, as well as understanding of nutrition. *This evaluation provides additional information about nutrition as well as a basis for future planning.*
- Weigh daily. *Daily weight is an accurate measure of both fluid balance and nutritional status.*
- Refer to a dietitian for further evaluation, planning, and education. *A professional can identify nutritional needs and help plan a diet that will meet them.*
- Refer to a swallowing therapist (specialized speech therapist) *for additional resources to improve nutritional intake.*
- Encourage experimentation with foods of different textures and temperatures. *Very cold foods or foods of a soft texture may be easier to swallow.*
- Encourage frequent, small meals rather than three large meals per day. *Frequent, small quantities of food improve overall intake when dysphagia, odynophagia, or fatigue interfere with nutrition.*
- Recommend liquid supplements such as Ensure when calorie needs are not being met. Provide information about where to obtain nutritional supplements. *Liquid dietary supplements provide balanced nutrition as well as additional calories and are an effective way of increasing intake. They are available without prescription in major supermarkets.*
- Provide mouth care before meals and supplemental feedings. *The treatment may cause altered taste in the mouth, which suppresses appetite.*

Delegating Nursing Care Activities

As appropriate and allowed by the designated duties and responsibilities of unlicensed assistive personnel, the nurse may delegate nursing care activities such as measuring vital signs, encouraging oral or enteral fluid intake, and providing skin care.

Transitions of Care

Health promotion and teaching for home care focus on preventing laryngeal obstruction and early intervention techniques. Everyone should be aware of the risk factors for adult aspiration. Caution patients who wear dentures to take small bites, chewing each bite carefully before swallowing. Discuss the relationship between excess alcohol intake and food aspiration.

Participate in promoting training of the general public in CPR and the Heimlich maneuver. The more people who are adequately trained in emergency procedures, the more likely it is that emergency procedures will be initiated in a timely manner. Patients with a known risk for anaphylaxis, such as people with a previous anaphylactic response and those allergic to bee venom, should wear a medical alert tag and carry a bee-sting kit to allow early intervention to prevent severe laryngeal edema and spasm.

The Patient with Obstructive Sleep Apnea

Sleep apnea, intermittent absence of airflow through the mouth and nose during sleep, is a serious and potentially life-threatening disorder. It affects at least 2% of middle-aged women and 4% of middle-aged men. Sleep apnea is a leading cause of excessive daytime sleepiness and may contribute to other problems such as poor work performance and motor vehicle crashes (Sorenson et al., 2019). Recent studies have linked sleep apnea with an increased risk for hypertension, ischemic heart disease, and exacerbation of heart failure (Sorenson et al., 2019).

Types of sleep apnea include obstructive and central. In *obstructive sleep apnea*, the more common type, the respiratory drive remains intact, but airflow ceases due to occlusion of the oropharyngeal airway. *Central sleep apnea* is a rare neurologic disorder that involves transient impairment of the neurologic drive to respiratory muscles.

Pathophysiology

During sleep, skeletal muscle tone decreases (except the diaphragm). The most significant decrease occurs during rapid eye movement (REM) sleep (Sorenson et al., 2019). Loss of normal pharyngeal muscle tone permits the pharynx to collapse during inspiration as pressure within the airways becomes negative in relation to atmospheric pressure. The tongue is also pulled against the posterior pharyngeal wall by gravity during sleep, causing further obstruction. Obesity or skeletal or soft tissue changes that decrease inspiratory tone, such as a relatively large tongue in a relatively small oropharynx, contribute to the problem. Airflow obstruction causes the oxygen saturation, Po_2, and pH to fall and the Pco_2 to rise. This progressive asphyxia causes brief arousal from sleep, which restores airway patency and airflow. Sleep can be severely fragmented because these episodes may occur hundreds of times each night.

Risk Factors

In addition to male gender, risk factors for obstructive sleep apnea include increasing age and obesity. Large neck circumference (> 43 cm [17 in.] in men and > 41 cm [16 in.] in women) is also a known risk factor for obstructive sleep apnea (Sorenson et al., 2019). Use of alcohol and other CNS depressants may contribute to sleep apnea.

Manifestations

Narrowed upper airways produce loud cyclic snoring during sleep, often years before obstructive sleep apnea occurs. The apneic periods can last 15 to 120 seconds during sleep. Other symptoms include grasping, choking, restlessness or thrashing during sleep. Excessive daytime sleepiness, headache, irritability, and restless sleep are also common manifestations. Later manifestations are personality changes, depression, intellectual impairment, impotence, and hypertension.

Complications

Recurrent episodes of apnea and arousal during sleep have secondary physiologic effects. Sleep fragmentation and loss of slow-wave sleep are thought to contribute to neurologic and behavior problems such as excessive daytime sleepiness, impaired intellect, memory loss, and personality changes. Recurrent nocturnal asphyxia and negative intrathoracic pressure due to airway obstruction increase the workload of the heart. People with coronary heart disease may develop myocardial ischemia and angina. Dysrhythmias, such as significant bradycardia and dangerous tachydysrhythmias, may develop. Left-ventricular function may be impaired and heart failure may occur. Systemic blood pressure remains high during sleep and may contribute to systemic hypertension that affects more than 50% of people with obstructive sleep apnea (Sorenson et al., 2019). Pulmonary hypertension may also develop. Sudden cardiac death is believed to be a potential fatal complication of obstructive sleep apnea.

Obstructive sleep apnea is a common condition in people who are morbidly obese. When these patients undergo gastric bypass surgery to treat their obesity, sleep apnea places them at significant risk for postoperative respiratory complications. Not only does the obesity interfere with chest movement and ventilation, it increases metabolic demands and carbon monoxide production. Anesthetic and analgesics used during surgery and in the postoperative period can lead to hypoxemia due to muscle relaxation and depression of the respiratory drive.

Interprofessional Care

The goal of care for obstructive sleep apnea is to restore airflow and prevent the adverse effects of the disorder. Sustained weight loss may cure obstructive sleep apnea.

Diagnosis

The diagnosis of obstructive sleep apnea is based on *polysomnography*, an overnight sleep study. Several variables are recorded during the study:

- Electroencephalogram and measurements of ocular activity and muscle tone
- Recordings of ventilatory activity and airflow
- Continuous arterial oxygen saturation readings
- Heart rate.

Transcutaneous arterial PCO_2 readings may also be monitored during the study. Because sleep studies are time consuming and expensive, overnight monitoring of oxygen saturation by pulse oximetry may be used to confirm the diagnosis of sleep apnea when symptoms indicate a high probability of the disorder. See Chapter 41 for more information about electroencephalography.

Treatments

Mild to moderate obstructive sleep apnea may be treated by losing weight, abstaining from alcohol, improving nasal patency, and avoiding the supine position for sleep. Although weight reduction often cures the disorder, maintaining optimal weight is difficult. Oral appliances designed to keep the mandible and tongue forward may also be prescribed.

Nasal continuous positive airway pressure (CPAP) is the treatment of choice for obstructive sleep apnea. Positive pressure generated by an air compressor and administered through a tight-fitting nasal mask (**Figure 35.5** ■) splints the pharyngeal airway, preventing collapse and obstruction. With proper training, this device is well tolerated by the patient. Nasal airways can become dry and irritated with CPAP, so an in-line humidifier or room humidifier is recommended. A newer device, the BiPAP ventilator, delivers higher pressures during inhalation and lower pressures during expiration, providing less resistance to exhaling.

Medications

Medications are not a usual or recommended treatment in obstructive sleep apnea.

Nutrition

In the patient with obstructive sleep apnea who is obese, weight loss may be recommended.

Surgery

Tonsillectomy and adenoidectomy may relieve upper airway obstruction in some patients. Excision of obstructive tissue from the soft palate, uvula, and posterior lateral pharyngeal wall may be accomplished by *uvulopalatopharyngoplasty* (*UPPP*). Response to surgical intervention varies based on a number of factors including severity and weight, with patients with milder cases of sleep apnea and weights < 125% of their ideal body weight more likely to experience benefits from surgery (Morgan, 2017). In severe cases, tracheostomy may also be performed to bypass the area of obstruction.

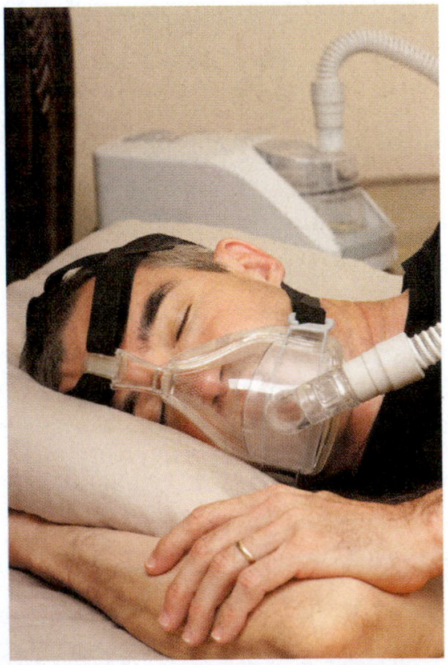

Figure 35.5 ■ A patient using a nasal mask and CPAP to treat sleep apnea.

Nursing Care

Assessment

Nursing assessment in OSA focuses on evaluation of sleep quality. Additionally, impact of poor sleep should be evaluated, such as daytime sleepiness, falling asleep during activities, safety, and interpersonal relationships.

- ***Health history:*** Sleep patterns and quality; daytime sleepiness; falling asleep during activities or inappropriate times; effect of sleep patterns and quality on partner
- ***Physical assessment:*** Weight and BMI; vital signs including temperature.

Priorities of Care

Nursing care is supportive. The focus of nursing care for the adult with obstructive sleep apnea is on teaching for self-care and use of medical devices in treatment of OSA.

Diagnoses, Interventions, and Outcomes

Obstructive sleep apnea is usually treated in the home. Nursing care focuses on teaching the patient and family about equipment use and strategies to decrease contributing factors such as obesity and alcohol intake.

Promote Sleep Quality. Obstructive sleep apnea may interfere with the ability to rest, increasing fatigue and prolonging recovery.

Expected Outcome: Patient will verbalize techniques to reduce impact of sleep apnea symptoms on sleep patterns.

The nurse will:

- Assess sleep patterns using subjective and objective information. *The patient may appear to be sleeping but not achieving normal sleep patterns because of symptoms of obstructive sleep apnea. Both subjective and objective data are important to accurately assess sleep.*

Promote Effective Breathing. Due to the viral infection, the respiratory rate may increase and alter the depth of respirations, decreasing effective alveolar ventilation. Shallow respirations also increase the risk of *atelectasis*, lack of ventilation in an area of lung.

Expected Outcome: Patient will utilize techniques to promote adequate ventilation such as deep breathing.

The nurse will:

- Monitor respiratory rate and pattern. *Tachypnea and/or rapid, shallow respirations may impair effective alveolar ventilation and gas exchange.*

- Elevate the head of the bed. *The upright position promotes drainage of nasal secretions, improves lung excursion, and reduces the work of breathing by lowering the diaphragm, which moves abdominal contents downward, creating less resistance to diaphragmatic excursion and slightly decreasing venous return.*

Promote Adequate Ventilation. Related to altered lung ventilation during obstructive episodes.

Expected Outcome: Patient will utilize techniques to promote adequate ventilation such as deep breathing.

The nurse will:

- Teach correct deep breathing techniques. *Tachypnea and/or rapid, shallow respirations may impair effective alveolar ventilation and gas exchange.*

Reduce Risk for Injury. Related to daytime somnolence and altered judgment.

Expected Outcome: Patient will display daytime alertness and sound judgment.

The nurse will:

- Monitor mental status. *Be especially observant of daytime somnolence and reduced judgment.*

Promote Sexual Function. Sleep apnea increases risk for impotence.

Expected Outcome: Patient will describe ways to use appropriate therapies to engage in sexual activity.

The nurse will:

- Establish rapport with patient and partner to promote discussion of feelings concerning changes in sexual functioning. *Nurse–patient rapport makes sensitive discussions more comfortable.*

Delegating Nursing Care Activities

As appropriate and allowed by the designated duties and responsibilities of unlicensed assistive personnel, the nurse may delegate nursing care activities such as measuring vital signs, encouraging oral or enteral fluid intake, and providing skin care.

Transitions of Care

There are no specific interventions that prevent sleep apnea. Maintaining normal body weight may help.

Effective sleep apnea management depends on the patient's willingness to participate in care. Provide teaching about the following topics:

- Relationship between obesity and sleep apnea
- Plans, resources, and referrals as needed for weight loss (e.g., programs such as Weight Watchers to provide additional support)
- Relationship of alcohol and sedatives to sleep apnea; referral to an alcohol treatment program or Alcoholics Anonymous as indicated
- How to use CPAP, if ordered
- The importance of using CPAP continuously at night
- Measures to reduce airway dryness, including supplemental humidity and an adequate fluid intake to maintain moist mucous membranes.

If a support group for people with sleep apnea syndrome is available in the local area, refer the patient and family to the group.

Moving Evidence into Action

Obstructive Sleep Apnea and Attention Impairment

Clinical Issue

In obstructive sleep apnea (OSA), continuous positive airway pressure (CPAP) is the standard therapy, but compliance with CPAP is low. OSA is known to impact not just sleep quality, but also quality of life, mood, and attention in persons with severe disease. It is unknown if these changes occur even in mild disease.

External Evidence

Luz and colleagues (2016) conducted a controlled study in which 39 mild OSA (apnea/hypopnea index 5–15) and 25 controls underwent a formal sleep study, as well as assessment of mood, sleep function, and a psychomotor vigilance test. The study showed that the mild OSA patients had increased sustained attention lapses compared with controls.

Internal Evidence

As part of the evaluation of internal evidence, the nurse needs to consider how the research findings impact the quality of the nurse–patient interaction.

Patient Considerations

When considering use of a new practice (such as modifications to healthcare education with OSA patients to address lapses in attention), the nurse must consider the specific patient population where it will be used (in this case, mild OSA patients). Will patients and their families be amenable to a new educational approach?

Putting the Pieces Together

Managing OSA can be complicated, resulting in low adherence with the treatment plan. For patients with reduced attention span, treatment failure can be expected. A simple change in educational approach could be easily implemented and potentially improve outcomes related to treatment compliance.

Reference

Luz, G. P., Guimarães, T. M., Weaver, T. E., Nery, L. E., Silva, L. O., Badke, L., . . . Bittencourt, L. (2016). Impaired sustained attention and lapses are present in patients with mild obstructive sleep apnea. *Sleep and Breathing, 20*(2), 681–687.

35.3 Upper Respiratory Tumors

Although tumors of the upper respiratory tract are relatively uncommon, they have the potential to impair the upper airways and interfere with breathing and ventilation of the lungs. Of the upper respiratory tract structures, the larynx is affected by abnormal growths most often.

The Patient with Nasal Polyps

Nasal polyps are benign grapelike growths of the mucous membrane lining the nose. These benign tumors can interfere with air movement through nasal passages or obstruct sinus openings, leading to sinusitis. They usually affect people who have chronic allergic rhinitis or asthma.

Pathophysiology

Chronic irritation and swelling of the mucous membranes from allergic rhinitis may cause slow polyp formation. Polyps form in areas of dependent mucous membrane, presenting as pale, edematous masses covered with mucous membrane. They are usually bilateral and have a stemlike base, making them fairly movable. Polyps can continue to enlarge, eventually becoming larger than a grape.

Risk Factors

Risk factors for nasal polyps include chronic inflammatory triggers such as nasal infections or allergies. Asthma is also a potential risk factor for nasal polyp development.

Manifestations

Polyps may be asymptomatic, although large polyps may cause nasal obstruction, rhinorrhea, and loss of sense of smell. Sinusitis may develop because sinus drainage is obstructed. The voice may have a nasal tone. Asthmatics who have nasal polyps may have an associated aspirin allergy of which they are not aware.

Complications

The presence of nasal polyps increases the likelihood of frequent or chronic sinus infections. They can also be an additive factor in sleep apnea.

Interprofessional Care

Diagnosis

Nasal polyps, while asymptomatic, are associated with chronic inflammation of the nasal and sinus lining. Emergent symptoms are related to sinusitis. Diagnosis is usually made with physical exam. Nasal endoscopy is the most common diagnostic test. CT scan can be used for polyps deeper in the sinus cavities and to evaluate the extent of the inflammation.

Medications

When polyps occur in conjunction with an acute upper respiratory infection, they may regress spontaneously with resolution of the infection. When symptomatic, polyps may be managed with topical corticosteroid nasal sprays or low-dose oral corticosteroids to shrink the edematous polyps and manage allergic symptoms. However, polyps continue to enlarge when corticosteroid therapy is discontinued.

Surgery

Surgery may be required to restore normal breathing. Surgical removal of polyps (*polypectomy*) is often done in the healthcare provider's office under local anesthesia. A wire snare is used to clip the polyps from their stemlike base. Nasal packing is inserted to control bleeding after removal. Alternatively, laser surgery may be used to remove polyps. Healing is more rapid following laser intervention, and the risk of bleeding is reduced. Because polyps tend to recur, repeated surgeries may be necessary.

Integrative Therapies

There are no evidence-based integrative therapies for nasal polyps.

Nursing Care

Assessment

See the Manifestations and Interprofessional Care sections for the assessment of the patient with nasal polyps.

Focused assessment of the patient with suspected nasal polyps includes:

- ***Health history:*** Complaints of sinusitis for more than 10 days; sensation of blockage of the nasal passage(s)
- ***Physical assessment:*** General appearance, vital signs including temperature; inspection of nasal and pharyngeal mucous membranes; percussion of sinuses for tenderness
- ***Laboratory data:*** CT of the sinuses, and infrequently sinus x-rays, WBC and differential, cultures of sinus drainage.

Priorities of Care

Collaborating with the interprofessional team to ensure adequate treatment of the underlying process while providing care that supports the physical and psychologic responses to the disorder is a priority of nursing care.

Diagnoses, Outcomes, and Interventions

The patient with nasal polyps may have some discomfort. Obstructed sinuses cause pain and pressure that increase with position changes and leaning forward. Treatment is usually community based, making education the key nursing role. When the patient is hospitalized for intravenous antibiotic therapy or sinus surgery, nurses must intervene to address pain and nutritional requirements.

Manage Pain. Although sinus surgery is relatively minor, both the incision and postoperative swelling can cause discomfort. Nasal packing, if used, contributes to the discomfort.

Expected Outcome: Patient will experience adequate pain control as evidenced by physical well-being.

The nurse will:

- Assess pain using a standardized pain scale. Administer analgesics as ordered. *Relief of pain promotes a feeling of well-being and enhances recovery.*

- Apply ice packs to the nose. *Cold compresses reduce swelling, control bleeding, and provide local analgesia.*
- Elevate the head of the bed to Fowler or high-Fowler position for 24 to 48 hours after surgery. *Elevating the operative site minimizes tissue swelling and promotes comfort.*

Promote Balanced Nutrition. Postoperatively, the sense of smell, an appetite stimulus, is diminished by nasal packing. Mouth discomfort from the incision and numbness of the upper teeth may also impact appetite and eating.

Expected Outcome: Patient will consume adequate nourishment to promote weight within normal range.

The nurse will:

- Provide clear liquid diet progressing to soft foods as tolerated. High-calorie dietary supplements may be used. *A progressive diet is used to assess the ability to swallow without choking and allay fears. Foods high in calories and nutritional value provide for metabolic and healing requirements.*
- Monitor intake, output, and weight. *This information allows assessment of overall fluid balance and the adequacy of dietary intake.*
- Elevate the head of the bed during meals. *The upright position facilitates swallowing and minimizes risk of aspiration.*

Delegating Nursing Care Activities

As appropriate and allowed by the designated duties and responsibilities of unlicensed assistive personnel, the nurse may delegate nursing care/activities such as measuring vital signs, encouraging oral or enteral fluid intake, and providing skin care.

Transitions of Care

Teaching about home care following polypectomy is the primary nursing responsibility for the patient with nasal polyps. Provide postoperative care instructions, and discuss measures to reduce the risk of bleeding.

- Apply ice or cold compresses to the nose to decrease swelling, promote comfort, and prevent bleeding.
- Avoid blowing the nose for 24 to 48 hours after nasal packing is removed.
- Avoid straining at stool, vigorous coughing, and strenuous exercise.

Discuss manifestations of possible bleeding, such as frequent swallowing or visible blood at the back of the throat. Swallowed blood may cause nausea and vomiting. Encourage the patient to rest for 2 to 3 days after surgery to reduce the risk of bleeding. Instruct to increase fluid intake and to clean mouth frequently to reduce oral dryness associated with mouth breathing while nasal packing is in place.

The Patient with a Laryngeal Tumor

Laryngeal tumors may be either benign or malignant. Benign tumors of the larynx include papillomas, nodules, and polyps. People who chronically shout, project, or vocalize in an abnormally high or low tone, abusing their voice, are at risk for developing benign laryngeal tumors. In adults, vocal cord nodules are often referred to as "singer's nodules"; cheerleaders and public speakers may also develop them. Voice abuse also contributes to the development of vocal cord polyps, as does cigarette smoking and chronic irritation from industrial pollutants.

Pathophysiology

Benign laryngeal tumors, or papillomas, are small, warty growths that are HPV viral in origin. Polyps and nodules may develop on the vocal cords of the larynx as a result of voice abuse (**Figure 35.6** ■). Nodules often occur as paired lesions on the free edges of the vocal cords.

Squamous cell carcinoma is the most common **laryngeal cancer**. Changes in the laryngeal mucosa occur over time as it is subjected to noxious irritants such as cigarette smoke. White, patchy, precancerous lesions known as *leukoplakia* appear. Red, velvety patches, called *erythroplakia*, are thought to represent a later stage of carcinoma development. The initial cancerous lesion, carcinoma in situ (CIS), is superficial. Malignant cells replace the lining layer, but do not invade into deeper tissues. Untreated, most CIS lesions develop into squamous cell cancer (National Cancer Institute [NCI], 2017b). Laryngeal cancer spreads by both direct invasion of surrounding tissues and by metastasis. It may metastasize to the lungs; however, metastases of other cancers to the larynx are rare.

Laryngeal cancer may develop in any of the three areas of the larynx: The glottis, supraglottis, or subglottis. Lesions of the true vocal cords or glottis account for nearly 60% of all laryngeal cancers (American Cancer Society [ACS], 2017b). Fortunately, these cancers tend to be well differentiated and slow growing. Metastasis occurs late in the course of the disease because of a limited lymphatic supply. The usual symptom of glottic cancer is hoarseness, or a change in the voice, because the tumor prevents complete closure of the vocal cords during speech.

Approximately 35% of laryngeal cancers develop in the supraglottic area, which includes the epiglottis, aryepiglottic

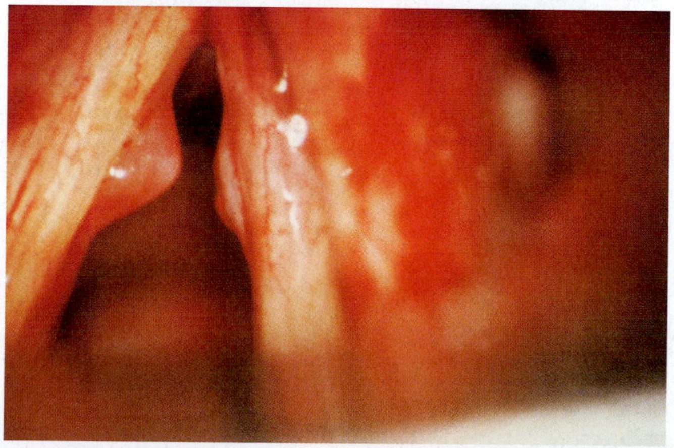

Figure 35.6 ■ Laryngoscopy showing a polyp on the right vocal cord.

folds, arytenoid muscles and cartilage, and false vocal cords (ACS, 2017b) (**Figure 35.7** ■). Lymphatic supply to this region of the larynx is rich; tumors often invade locally and metastasize early. Symptoms often do not develop until the tumor is relatively large, delaying diagnosis. Manifestations of supraglottic cancer include painful swallowing, sore throat, or a feeling of a lump in the throat. Later manifestations include dyspnea, foul breath, and pain that radiates to the ear (NCS, 2017b).

Subglottic tumors (below the vocal cords) are the least common, accounting for 5% of laryngeal tumors. They are often asymptomatic until the enlarging tumor obstructs the airway.

Risk Factors

Men are affected more than four times as often as women. Cancer of the larynx usually develops between ages 50 and 70. Tobacco use is the major risk factor for laryngeal cancer: The risk of developing laryngeal cancer is significantly greater in smokers (cigarette, pipe, or cigar) than in nonsmokers. Alcohol consumption is a significant cofactor in increasing the risk. When combined with smoking, the risk increases synergistically and significantly, perhaps as much as 100 times (NCI, 2017b). Other risk factors include poor nutrition, human papillomavirus (HPV) infection, exposure to asbestos and other occupational pollutants, and race (laryngeal cancer is more common in African Americans than among Caucasians, with African American men at greatest risk [NCI, 2014]).

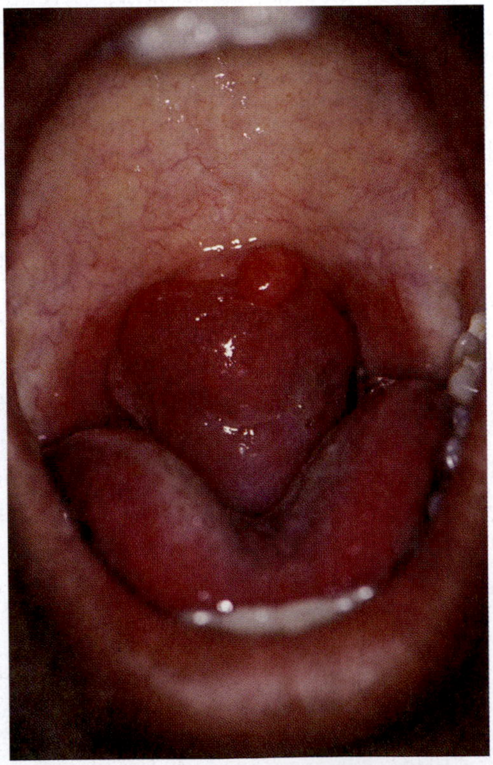

Figure 35.7 ■ Cancer of the larynx and epiglottis.

Manifestations

Manifestations of laryngeal cancer vary according to the site of the lesion, but may include hoarseness, change in the voice, painful swallowing, dyspnea, foul breath, a palpable lump in neck, and/or earache.

Complications

The primary complication of laryngeal cancer is airway obstruction. Disfigurement can be a complication/sequela of surgical intervention.

Interprofessional Care

Benign laryngeal tumors may resolve with correction of the underlying problem, such as voice training with a speech therapist or smoking cessation. Treatment of laryngeal malignancy varies with the extent of the cancer. Early diagnosis and treatment are important: The 5-year survival rate for those diagnosed while the tumor is still localized is approximately 77%, whereas the survival rate drops to 20% if the cancer metastasizes (American Cancer Society, 2017a; NCI, 2014).

Diagnosis

- ***Direct*** or ***indirect laryngoscopy*** is used for initial evaluation when laryngeal cancer is suspected. A fiberoptic laryngoscope is used for direct laryngoscopy; mirrors are used to visualize the larynx in indirect laryngoscopy.
- ***Biopsy*** is obtained from suspicious lesions to examine the cells. Biopsy is usually obtained under general anesthesia or conscious sedation. Tissue may be obtained via endoscopy or by fine-needle aspiration of the mass.
- ***Imaging studies*** such as CT scan, MRI, and chest x-ray are obtained to evaluate the size of the mass, possible extension into deeper tissues, involvement of lymph nodes, and possible metastasis to the lungs. A barium swallow may be done to evaluate the effects of the tumor on swallowing. A PET scan may also be done (possibly in conjunction with CT scan) to detect tumor metastasis.

Laryngeal cancer treatment is determined by *staging* the cancer. Information such as tumor size and location (T), number of involved lymph nodes (N), and presence or absence of metastases (M) is combined to assign a stage, designated by Roman numerals I to IV. **Table 35.1** outlines laryngeal cancer stages.

Treatments

An inhaled steroid spray may be used for vocal cord polyps.

Chemotherapy. Chemotherapy is used in combination with radiation therapy as the primary treatment for some laryngeal cancers. It is also used to treat distant metastasis and for palliation when the tumor is unresectable. The most commonly used chemotherapy drugs to treat laryngeal cancer are cisplatin (Platinol) and 5-fluorouracil (5-FU). Other drugs that may be used include methotrexate (Mexate), bleomycin sulfate (Blenoxane), and carboplatin (Paraplatin).

Table 35.1 Staging of Laryngeal Tumors

Stage	Description
Stage 0	■ Carcinoma *in situ* ■ No lymph node involvement or metastasis
Stage I	■ Tumor confined to site of origin with normal vocal cord mobility ■ No lymph node involvement or metastasis
Stage II	■ Tumor involves adjacent tissues ■ No lymph node involvement or metastasis
Stage III	■ Tumor confined to larynx with fixation of vocal cords; immediately surrounding supraglottic tissues may be involved ■ No lymph node involvement or a single positive node on the side of the tumor ■ No metastasis
Stage IV	■ Massive tumor that extends beyond boundaries of larynx to involve surrounding tissues ■ Single or multiple lymph nodes may be involved ■ Distant metastasis may be present

Source: Based on *AJCC Cancer Staging Manual, 7th Edition* (2010) published by Springer Science and Business Media LLC, www.springerlink.com; American Cancer Society. (2017). *Laryngeal cancer stages.* Retrieved from https://www.cancer.org/cancer/laryngeal-and-hypopharyngeal-cancer/detection-diagnosis-staging/staging.html.

A multiple-drug treatment regimen may be employed to maximize therapeutic effects. Refer to Chapter 14 for the nursing implications for chemotherapy.

Radiation Therapy. Radiation therapy is often the treatment of choice for early laryngeal cancer. Radiation disrupts the DNA of the cell, causing it to die. External radiation is commonly used; brachytherapy, implants of iridium seeds placed into hollow plastic needles that are inserted directly into or near the tumor site during surgery to deliver radiation, is less frequently used for laryngeal or hypopharyngeal cancer. Radiation therapy is extremely effective for treating glottic cancer, with cure rates equal to those achieved by surgery. Radiation therapy preserves the voice, although the tone or timber of the voice may be affected.

Radiation therapy may be used in combination with chemotherapy (*chemoradiotherapy*) to treat more advanced laryngeal cancers. Nearly two-thirds of patients with locally invasive cancers can avoid total laryngectomy when treated with combination radiation and chemotherapy. Survival rates are equal to those achieved with total laryngectomy (American Society of Clinical Oncologists, 2018).

Radiation therapy may also be used in conjunction with surgery to destroy any remaining cancerous cells or as a palliative treatment for advanced tumors. Refer to Chapter 14 for more information about radiation therapy and its nursing implications.

Surgery

In some cases, surgical excision of benign nodules or polyps is required. This is usually performed via laryngoscopy, using microforceps or a laser. A biopsy of the tumor is done to rule out malignancy.

The type of surgery used to treat laryngeal cancer is based on site, size, and invasiveness of the tumor into the larynx and surrounding tissues. The goals of surgery are to remove the malignancy, maintain airway patency, and achieve optimal cosmetic appearance.

Carcinoma in situ, vocal cord polyps, and early vocal cord cancers may be removed by laser during a laryngoscopy procedure. The cure rate for early tumors using this method is excellent. This surgery may be performed on an outpatient basis. The degree of trauma to the vocal cords varies, depending on the size of the lesion. The voice is preserved, but total voice rest with whispering only may be ordered for a week or more following surgery. In some cases, a temporary tracheostomy may be done at the time of surgery to ensure that swelling does not interfere with airway patency. Once the tracheostomy tube is removed and the opening is closed, the patient can eat, speak, and breathe normally.

Laryngectomy, removal of the larynx, may be necessary. A *partial laryngectomy* (hemilaryngectomy, vertical partial laryngectomy) may be used for tumors localized to a portion of the larynx with limited extension beyond the larynx. In a partial laryngectomy, 50% or more of the larynx is removed. The voice is generally well preserved, although it may be changed by the surgery. A tracheostomy tube may be inserted for early postoperative airway management. It is usually removed in 5 to 7 days as postoperative swelling subsides, and the stoma is allowed to close. Normal speaking, breathing, and swallowing are restored. If the epiglottis has been removed, careful monitoring for aspiration is necessary. Enteral tube feedings or parenteral nutrition may be required for several weeks after surgery. Swallowing techniques to prevent aspiration are taught.

A *total laryngectomy* is required for cancers that extend beyond the vocal cords. The entire larynx is removed, along with the epiglottis, thyroid cartilage, several tracheal rings, and the hyoid bone. Because the trachea and the esophagus are permanently separated by this surgery (**Figure 35.8** ■), there is no risk of aspiration during swallowing. Normal speech is lost, and a permanent tracheostomy is created in a total laryngectomy. The tracheostomy tube inserted during surgery may be left in place for several weeks and then removed, leaving a natural stoma, or it may be left in place permanently. See **Box 35.4** for nursing care of the patient having a total laryngectomy.

If cervical lymph nodes are involved but there is no evidence of distal metastasis, *radical* or *modified neck dissection*

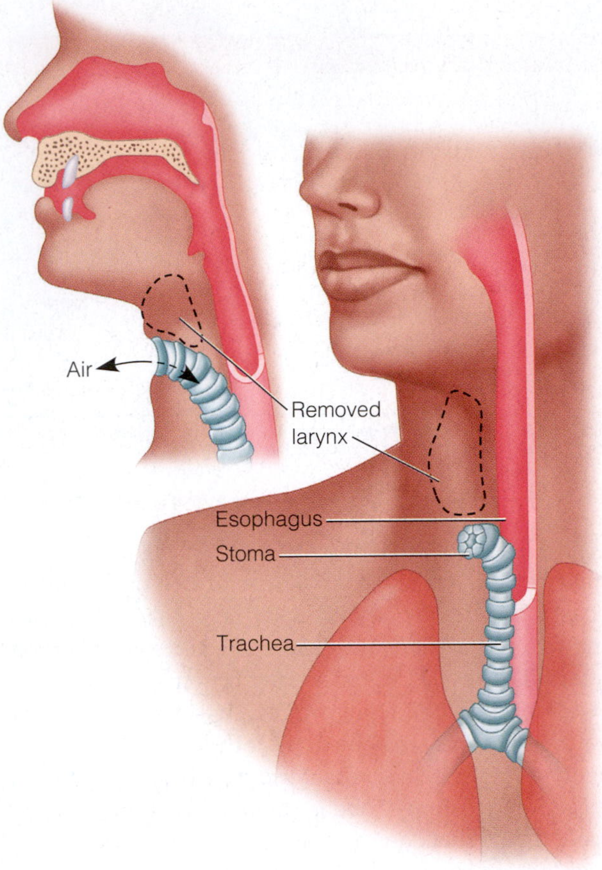
Air
Removed larynx
Esophagus
Stoma
Trachea

Figure 35.8 ■ Following a total laryngectomy, the patient has a permanent tracheostomy. No connection between the trachea and esophagus remains.

may be performed along with total laryngectomy. In a radical neck dissection, all soft tissue from the lower edge of the mandible down to the clavicle is removed, including cervical lymph nodes, the sternocleidomastoid muscle, internal jugular vein, cranial nerve XI (spinal accessory), and submaxillary salivary gland. Extensive tissue dissection can result in significant deformity. Skin grafts or flaps may be used to close the wound. Hemovac drains are placed in the wound to prevent hematoma and extensive edema formation. After surgery, the patient may have difficulty lifting and turning the head because of muscle loss. Resection of the spinal accessory nerve causes shoulder drop on the affected side. In a modified neck dissection, neck contents are removed, with the exception of the sternocleidomastoid muscle, internal jugular vein, and spinal accessory nerve.

A gastrostomy may also be performed to maintain nutrition in the patient with laryngeal or hypopharyngeal cancer. Refer to Chapter 23 for more information about caring for the patient with a gastrostomy tube.

SAFETY ALERT: During the immediate postoperative period, monitor closely for signs of airway obstruction, such as labored breathing or inspiratory stridor. The larynx is the narrowest portion of the upper airways. Tissue edema following surgery can further restrict the airway, interfering with lung ventilation and gas exchange. ■

Speech Rehabilitation

Various techniques may be used to restore speech after total laryngectomy. *Tracheoesophageal puncture (TEP)* is the usual method used to restore speech. A small fistula is created between the posterior tracheal wall and the anterior esophagus. A small, one-way shunt valve is fitted into the fistula (**Figure 35.9** ■). Occluding the tracheostomy stoma

Box 35.4
Nursing Care of the Patient Having a Total Laryngectomy

PREOPERATIVE CARE

- Assess knowledge and understanding of the diagnosis and proposed surgery. Clarify information and reinforce previous teaching as needed. *A clear understanding by the patient and family of the purpose, anticipated benefits, and consequences of total laryngectomy prior to surgery is vital to promote postoperative recovery.*
- Provide routine preoperative care and teaching, as explained in Chapter 4.
- Assess anxiety levels of the patient and family related to the diagnosis and proposed surgery. *High levels of anxiety interfere with learning and the ability to cooperate in care. Interventions to reduce anxiety may be required prior to teaching and providing preoperative instructions.*
- Without increasing fear, emphasize that total laryngectomy results in a loss of speech and that the patient will breathe through a permanent stoma in the neck. *Although patients and family members may verbalize an understanding of the loss of speech following surgery, they may believe that verbal communication will still be possible through the stoma.*
- Establish a means of communicating postoperatively, using pencil and paper, a tablet, white board, eye or hand signals, or other strategies. *Learning techniques for communicating preoperatively decreases the patient's and family's postoperative anxiety. Long-term speech rehabilitation measures, such as a tracheoesophageal puncture, are not appropriate for use in the immediate postoperative period.*
- Point out that surgery will affect the smell, taste, and eating in the initial postoperative period. Reassure that nutritional and fluid needs will be met with intravenous or enteral feedings until eating can be resumed. *The patient may not be prepared for the effect of surgery on taste and smell and, therefore, the enjoyment of food.*
- If possible and desired by the patient and family, arrange a visit by a postlaryngectomy patient who effectively uses an alternate form of verbal communication. *The patient and family may feel more comfortable expressing their fears and asking questions of someone who has gone through the same experience they are facing.*

POSTOPERATIVE CARE

- Provide routine postoperative nursing care and monitoring, as explained in Chapter 4.
- Frequently monitor airway patency and respiratory status, including respiratory rate and pattern, lung sounds, and oxygen

saturation. *Excessive or retained respiratory secretions can impair gas exchange, increase the work of breathing, and lead to complications such as pneumonia.*

- Encourage deep breathing and coughing. *Deep breathing helps ensure adequate ventilation of lower airways; coughing helps to move secretions out of airways.*
- Elevate the head of the bed. *The upright position promotes effective ventilation of the lungs and reduces edema and swelling of the neck.*
- Maintain humidification of inspired gases. *With a tracheostomy, humidification of inspired air in the upper airways is lost. Humidified air helps maintain moist mucous membranes and secretions, promoting secretion removal by coughing or suctioning.*
- Maintain an adequate fluid intake (intravenously, enterally, and orally when allowed). *Adequate hydration keeps secretions liquid and mucous membranes moist.*
- Suction via tracheostomy using sterile technique as needed. *Surgery, impaired nutrition, and the effects of radiation therapy may cause fatigue and a weak cough effort. Suctioning may be necessary to clear secretions and maintain airway patency.*
- Provide tracheostomy care as needed. *Periodic cleaning of the tracheostomy tube is necessary to remove accumulated secretions and maintain airway patency.*
- Teach to protect the stoma from particulate matter in the air with a gauze square or other stoma protector. *Permanent tracheostomy results in loss of the protective mechanisms of the upper airway that prevent foreign material from entering the lungs.*
- Instruct to support the head when moving in bed. *Additional head support reduces the strain on tissues in the operative area.*
- Place the call light within easy reach at all times; answer the call light promptly. *The patient who is unable to speak needs reassurance that help is within reach at all times.*
- Encourage family members to remain present when possible. *Supportive family presence helps reassure the patient that he or she will not be left alone or helpless.*
- Spend as much time as possible with the patient. When leaving the room, specify the time when you will return. *These measures help establish trust and relieve anxiety.*
- Arrange consultation with a speech therapist about alternate forms of oral communication prior to surgery if possible. *Determining a means of communicating on a continuing basis prior to surgery helps to relieve fear of inability to communicate and may guide the choice of a surgical procedure.*
- Reinforce teaching about alternative communication strategies. *Anxiety or information overload may impair the ability to retain information; reinforcement facilitates learning.*
- Maintain a positive attitude about postoperative communication, but do not promote unrealistic expectations. *Not all patients are able to use all alternative methods of verbal communication after the laryngectomy. Some patients remain nonverbal.*

with a finger forces exhaled air through the valve into the esophagus and hypopharynx, creating vibration and sound. The muscles of speech are used to form words. The one-way valve prevents aspiration from the esophagus into the trachea. An external tracheostoma valve may be used to avoid using the hand to occlude the stoma. This device covers the entire tracheal stoma and closes during exhalation, forcing air directly into the voice prosthesis. Not all postlaryngectomy patients are candidates for this device because its use requires motivation and manual dexterity.

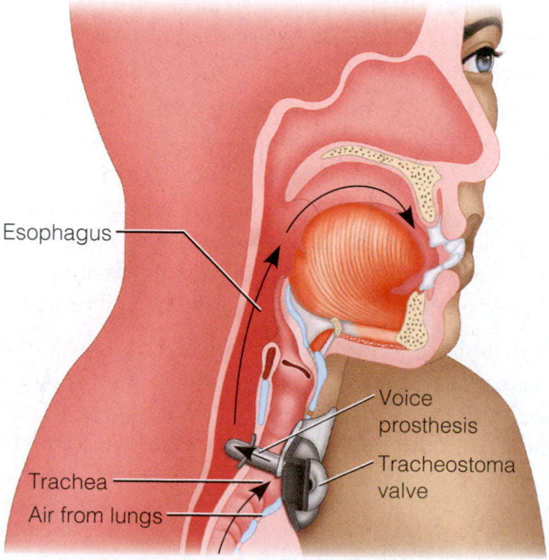
Esophagus
Voice prosthesis
Tracheostoma valve
Trachea
Air from lungs

Figure 35.9 ■ The tracheoesophageal prosthesis (TEP) allows diversion of air from the trachea through a one-way valve into the esophagus and oropharynx, producing speech when the tracheostomy stoma is occluded. The one-way valve prevents food from entering the trachea.

Esophageal speech uses swallowed air to create sound and form words as air is expelled in a controlled belch. The pharyngoesophageal segment vibrates with the belch, creating sound. Muscles of the mouth and tongue are used to control the sound and form words. This form of speech takes practice, and fluent speech may not be restored.

Several speech generators (electrolarynx) are available (**Figure 35.10** ■). One type is held to the neck and creates vibrations that are transmitted to the neck and into the mouth. The transmitted vibrations are formed into words using the normal muscles of speech. Another device delivers a tone into the mouth via a plastic tube inserted into the corner of the mouth. The lips, tongue, and mouth muscles are used to form the sound into words.

Nursing Care

Nurses can be instrumental in early identification and treatment of laryngeal disorders by emphasizing the need for patients with new chronic hoarseness to seek treatment.

Assessment

See the Manifestations and Interprofessional Care sections for the assessment of the patient with laryngeal cancer.

- ***Health history:*** Current symptoms, including voice change, difficulty swallowing, throat pain, weight loss; risk factors such as voice abuse (e.g., shouting), family history of cancer, occupational exposures (e.g., chemical inhalation); smoking, use of alcohol and amount
- ***Physical examination:*** Voice character; general appearance and apparent state of health, weight loss; swallowing ability; visible or palpable mass in neck.

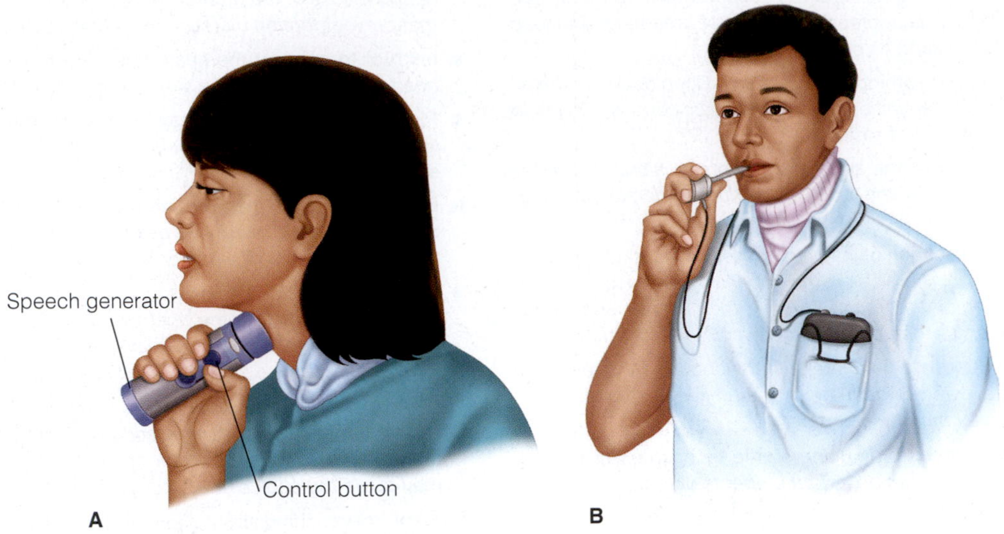
Speech generator
Control button
A
B

Figure 35.10 ■ Speech generators. **A**, The patient holds the vibrating tip of the speech generator against the throat, using the mouth to form words. **B**, A plastic handpiece of the generator is held in the corner of the mouth. The audible tone produced by the generator is formed into words.

Priorities of Care

Collaborating with the interprofessional team to ensure adequate treatment of the underlying process while providing care that supports the physical and psychologic responses to the disorder is a priority of nursing care.

Diagnoses, Interventions, and Outcomes

Nursing care for the patient with a benign tumor of the larynx focuses on maintaining a patent airway and teaching about the disorder and strategies to prevent its recurrence. The patient with laryngeal cancer has multiple nursing care needs. The risk for impaired verbal communication is significant. Dysphagia may interfere with swallowing and nutrition. Nutrition may also be impaired by radiation, chemotherapy, and surgery. Changes in body image may be due to weight loss due to increased metabolic demands of the malignancy. The diagnosis of cancer is frightening for most patients, no matter what the potential for cure is with treatment. See the Case Study & Nursing Care Plan that follows for additional nursing diagnoses and interventions.

Promote Airway Clearance and Patency. Following resection of a benign or malignant vocal cord nodule, local tissue edema may interfere with airway patency.

Expected Outcome: Patient will use techniques to promote airway clearance as indicated and tolerated in combination with maintenance of patent airway.

The nurse will:

- Apply cold packs to the neck as ordered or indicated. *Cold application constricts local blood vessels and reduces edema development.*
- Withhold food and fluids until the cough and gag reflexes have returned. *Local anesthesia used during removal of benign tumors and nodules impairs the cough and gag reflexes, increasing the risk for aspiration.*

Promote Communication. Treatment of laryngeal cancer often alters the quality of the voice, results in short-term restriction on speaking, or, in the case of total laryngectomy, causes loss of the voice. The patient ultimately determines treatment choices for laryngeal cancer; some choose to forgo laryngectomy to avoid voice loss when the chance for long-term success and cancer cure is minimal.

Expected Outcome: Patient will utilize alternative communication techniques.

The nurse will:

- Prior to surgery, assess for additional obstacles to communication. *Communication may be impaired by hearing loss, illiteracy, or weakness associated with the disease process, altering the ability to use alternative communication strategies.*
- Assess the importance of verbal communication to self-concept, occupation, and lifestyle. *Many factors influence adaptation to the loss of normal verbal communication. If the ability to speak is central to an occupation (e.g., school teacher, singer) or self-concept (e.g., politician, attorney), adapting to a total laryngectomy may be difficult. For these patients, laryngectomy may mean a loss of employment or career.*
- Prior to surgery, introduce nonverbal communication strategies such as pencil and paper, magic slate, white board, or tablet. Encourage the patient to practice using each method and to choose the most acceptable one. *Having the patient determine a means of communication prior to surgery helps to alleviate anxiety and increases the sense of control.*

SAFETY ALERT: After surgery, assess frequently. Place the call bell at hand. The presence of a caring nurse helps to decrease anxiety and promotes communication. Knowing that help is readily available enhances feelings of security and decreases anxiety. ■

Promote Swallowing. Disruption of laryngeal structures by the tumor itself or due to radiation or surgery can impair the swallowing mechanism. Additionally, even when a total laryngectomy has been performed and a connection between the oropharynx and trachea no longer exists, swallowing may cause fear of choking.

Expected Outcome: Patient will utilize modified food and fluid consistency to promote swallowing while using techniques to avoid choking.

- Maintain intravenous fluids and enteral feedings or parenteral nutrition until adequate food and fluids can be ingested orally. *It is important to maintain nutritional and fluid balance until normal eating can be resumed.*
- Postoperatively, initiate oral intake with soft foods, not liquids. *Soft foods are easier than liquids to handle and swallow initially. As recovery progresses, thickened liquids can be swallowed, progressing to liquids, and, eventually, a normal diet.*
- Following total laryngectomy, reassure that choking is not possible because there is no connection between the esophagus and trachea. *Patients often fear that swallowing will result in choking and they will be unable to cough effectively.*
- Instruct to initiate a swallow by placing a small amount of food on the back of the tongue, flex the head forward, and then think "swallow." *Swallowing is no longer an automatic function and needs to be relearned.*
- Provide for privacy during initial attempts at eating. *Eating in the presence of others may cause embarrassment until confidence in eating is regained. Privacy also reduces distractions, allowing concentration on swallowing.*

Promote Balanced Nutrition. Large laryngeal tumors often place pressure on the esophagus and may cause dysphagia (difficulty swallowing) or odynophagia (painful swallowing). In either case, difficulty eating may ultimately impair nutrition. Additionally, cancer often produces a hypermetabolic state, increasing calorie requirements. If surgery is performed, difficulty swallowing and a fear of aspiration in the early postoperative period also interfere with eating. Enteral or parenteral feedings are usually needed initially to meet nutritional status. After a total laryngectomy, the senses of taste and smell are disrupted. Although the sense of taste may be partially recovered, patients may complain that eating is no longer pleasurable.

Expected Outcome: Patient will consume adequate nourishment to promote weight within normal range.

The nurse will:

- Assess nutritional status using height and weight charts, reported weight loss, and anthropometric measurements such as skinfolds. *Thorough assessment of nutritional status is important in planning to meet current and anticipated calorie needs.*
- Monitor food and fluid intake and urinary output. *Pain or fatigue, rather than a sensation of fullness, may prompt the decision to stop eating, resulting in inadequate intake.*
- Evaluate current and preferred eating habits and foods, as well as understanding of nutrition. *This evaluation provides additional information about nutrition as well as a basis for future planning.*
- Weigh daily. *Daily weight is an accurate measure of both fluid balance and nutritional status.*
- Refer to a dietitian for further evaluation, planning, and education. *A professional can identify nutritional needs and help plan a diet that will meet them.*
- Refer to a swallowing therapist (specialized speech therapist) for additional resources to improve nutritional intake. *Initiating swallowing therapy early may help the patient relearn how to swallow more quickly, encouraging both confidence in the treatment plan and nutritional balance.*
- Reinforce swallowing instructions. *Reinforcement promotes learning.*
- Encourage experimentation with foods of different textures and temperatures. *Very cold foods or foods of a soft texture may be easier to swallow.*
- Encourage frequent, small meals rather than three large meals per day. *Frequent, small quantities of food improve overall intake when dysphagia, odynophagia, or fatigue interfere with nutrition.*
- Recommend liquid supplements such as Ensure when calorie needs are not being met. Provide information about where to obtain nutritional supplements. *Liquid dietary supplements provide balanced nutrition as well as additional calories and are an effective way of increasing intake. They are available without prescription in major supermarkets.*
- Provide mouth care before meals and supplemental feedings. Provide a topical anesthetic such as viscous lidocaine before eating for stomatitis or esophagitis related to radiation or chemotherapy. *The tumor or its treatment may cause bad breath or a foul taste in the mouth, which suppresses appetite. Inflamed mucosa may make eating uncomfortable. A topical anesthetic may relieve this discomfort and thus promote food intake.*
- Provide an antiemetic 30 minutes before eating as needed to relieve nausea. *Nausea interferes with food intake. An antiemetic can relieve nausea and make eating possible.*
- Suggest enteral (tube) feedings via nasogastric or gastrostomy tube if the patient is unable to consume enough food to maintain weight and nutritional status. *Both cancer and surgery increase calorie needs. Supplemental enteral feedings may be necessary to prevent catabolism and to promote healing and recovery.*
- Instruct to perform mouth rinses before initiating feeding postoperatively. *Rinsing helps clean the mouth and also practice in using tongue and cheek muscles to control fluid in the mouth.*

SAFETY ALERT: Following laryngectomy, place in semi-Fowler or Fowler position. Elevating the head of the bed facilitates swallowing of oral secretions and helps prevent regurgitation of tube feedings. ■

Promote Healthy Grief Responses. The patient with laryngeal cancer faces not only the diagnosis of cancer, which is often perceived as a death sentence, but also the prospect of mutilating surgery. If laryngectomy is necessary, the patient grieves the loss of both a body part and an important function, speech—a vital aspect of social interaction and interpersonal relationships and often necessary for one's career. It also enables people to express their needs when they cannot meet them alone. The loss of speech, therefore, is a major loss. In addition, the tracheal stoma changes the manner in which the patient breathes. If radical neck dissection is required, loss of neck musculature and function also alters body image and self-concept.

Expected Outcome: Patient and family will discuss the meaning of losses (anticipated or actual) to the patient and family's life.

The nurse will:

- Provide opportunities for expressing feelings of grief, anger, or fear about the diagnosis of cancer, the impending surgery, and the anticipated loss of speech. *The patient with laryngeal cancer needs the opportunity (and may need permission) to grieve anticipated losses. A cancer diagnosis may precipitate grieving for unfulfilled plans and expectations, even though a cure may be anticipated. Laryngectomy causes a major change in body image, with loss of a vital body part and creation of a stoma. The patient also grieves the loss of speech. This loss can have a significant impact on occupation and social interaction.*
- Provide a calm, supportive environment with adequate privacy and emotional support for the patient and family members as they work through the grieving process. *It is important for the patient and family to know that their feelings of loss are real and accepted by caregivers.*
- Help the patient and family discuss the potential impact of the loss on family structure and function. *Discussion helps family members understand each other's feelings and support one another.*
- Refer for psychologic or spiritual counseling, as appropriate. *Counseling and spiritual guidance can help the patient and family deal with the diagnosis and proposed treatment and help prevent a sense of defeat and hopelessness.*
- Help identify additional resources, such as coping strategies that have been successfully used in the past to deal with crises. *This exercise helps the patient and family identify strengths they can use to deal with the present situation.*

Delegating Nursing Care Activities

As appropriate and allowed by the designated duties and responsibilities of unlicensed assistive personnel, the nurse may delegate nursing care activities such as measuring vital signs, encouraging oral or enteral fluid intake, and providing skin care.

Transitions of Care

Health promotion activities to prevent laryngeal cancer focus on preventing smoking and chewing tobacco among children, adolescents, and young adults and promoting smoking cessation in people who do smoke. Activities to promote abstinence or moderate alcohol use are also beneficial in reducing a significant risk factor for laryngeal cancer.

Teaching for the patient with a benign laryngeal tumor emphasizes management of contributing factors. Stress the importance of not yelling or screaming. Refer patients, particularly singers, to a speech therapist for voice training. Emphasize the need to keep the voice within its normal range to reduce vocal cord stress. Encourage smoking cessation, particularly if the patient is also a singer. Discuss the relationship of industrial or occupational pollutants to laryngeal tumors and help explore ways of reducing pollutant exposure. Patient education that is covered in the acute setting includes:

- Clarification of treatment options, including risks and benefits.
- Importance of early intervention to reduce the risk of local spread and metastasis.
- If a total laryngectomy is proposed, options for communication after surgery, including the pros and cons of each:
  a. The tracheoesophageal puncture device requires some manual dexterity to manipulate.
  b. Only about 30% of patients are able to master esophageal speech.
  c. A trial of the speech generator prior to surgery may reduce frustration in learning to use it postoperatively.

Teaching the patient and family about laryngeal cancer, treatment options, and home care related to those treatments is an important nursing responsibility. Include the following topics when teaching:

- Care related to radiation therapy, including skin and mouth care and management of secretions. (Refer to Chapter 14 for more information about radiation therapy and its effects.)
- Strategies and resources for smoking cessation and alcohol abstinence.
- Ways to achieve and maintain optimal nutrition.
- Tracheostomy stoma care and preventing respiratory infection. Provide opportunities to practice and return demonstrated techniques. Clean technique (rather than sterile) is used; the tracheostomy tube may not be needed once the stoma is fully healed. Discuss these additional measures:
  a. Using a humidifier or vaporizer to add humidity to inspired air.
  b. Increasing fluid intake to maintain mucosal moisture and loosen secretions.
  c. Shielding the stoma with a stoma guard, such as a gauze square on a tie around the neck, to prevent particulate matter from entering the lower respiratory tract.
  d. Promptly removing secretions from skin surrounding the stoma to prevent irritation and skin breakdown.
  e. Water sports are contraindicated with a permanent tracheostomy; there is no restriction on other activities, although lifting may be more difficult because

of an inability to hold one's breath (the Valsalva maneuver).

f. Showering and bathing (without submerging the neck or head) are allowed; protect the stoma with a cupped hand or washcloth.

- Manifestations of potential complications of laryngectomy to be reported to the healthcare provider, including loss of hearing or facial expression due to auditory or facial nerve injury or shoulder drop due to damage to the spinal accessory nerve.

The patient and family need emotional and motivational support through this trying time. Refer to local support groups such as a laryngectomy club or lost cord club. If the patient and family are having difficulty adjusting to the diagnosis of cancer and the effects of treatment, provide referral to counseling

End-of-life care in the presence of laryngeal cancer focuses on symptom management, infection control, and comfort measures. Family involvement is also essential. The nurse caring for the head and neck cancer patient at end of life also provides emotional support to the patient and family members.

Case Study & Nursing Care Plan

A Patient with Total Laryngectomy

David Tom is a 61-year-old accountant who is divorced and has two adult children. He has smoked two packs of cigarettes daily since high school and usually has three or four cocktails each evening. After several months of a persistent sore throat and hoarseness, Mr. Tom was diagnosed with cancer of the larynx. He has been admitted to the surgical care unit from the ICU 2 days post–total laryngectomy.

ASSESSMENT

Mr. Tom's vital signs are stable: T 36.7°C (98°F) axillary, P 92 bpm and regular, R 18/min, and BP 146/84 mmHg. A tracheostomy tube is sutured in place, and he is receiving humidified oxygen at 28% per tracheostomy collar. Pulse oximetry is 94%. He is receiving continuous tube feeding per nasogastric feeding tube. Two Hemovac wound drains are present in the right neck area. A moderate amount of edema is noted in the right facial and submandibular area. Mr. Tom is ambulatory within the room.

DIAGNOSES

- Potential for ineffectual airway patency related to postoperative swelling
- Changes in breathing pattern related to pain, anxiety, and potentially from pain medications
- Changes in body image related to presence of tracheostomy stoma
- Compromised verbal communication related to total laryngectomy
- Pain related to surgical procedure
- Decrease in nutritional intake related to difficulty eating after surgery

EXPECTED OUTCOMES

- Patient will maintain clear airways and lung sounds.
- Patient will maintain oxygen saturation level > 92%.
- Patient will demonstrate interest in providing incision and stoma care.
- Patient will accept information about potential communication strategies.
- Patient will communicate effective pain management.
- Patient will maintain appropriate body weight, intake, and output.

PLANNING AND IMPLEMENTATION

- Assess respiratory status including rate, pattern, lung sounds, and cough effectiveness at least every 4 hours.
- Monitor quantity, color, and odor of secretions.
- Assess vital signs and pain at least every 4 hours. Administer analgesics as ordered.
- Schedule time to sit with Mr. Tom and discuss his concerns and feelings at least three times per day.
- Provide written information as requested.
- Monitor intake, output, and daily weight.
- Arrange dietary consultation to determine caloric requirements.

EVALUATION

Mr. Tom reports in writing that his pain is adequately controlled. His respiratory status is stable with clear breath sounds throughout and an oxygen saturation of 94%. He is afebrile. Mr. Tom is tolerating tube feedings well and expresses a desire to begin eating. The speech therapist has completed a swallowing evaluation, and the dietitian has visited and assisted in planning to begin oral feedings. Intake and output are stable, as is his weight. Mr. Tom has been receptive to receiving information about follow-up care and exploration of various modalities of speech.

CLINICAL REASONING IN PATIENT CARE

1. Compare and contrast advantages and disadvantages of various methods to allow speech following total laryngectomy.
2. Develop a plan of care for Mr. Tom for changes in body image related to presence of tracheostomy stoma.
3. Discuss nursing interventions to provide wound care for the patient with laryngectomy and radical neck dissection.
4. List strategies to optimize ventilation.

See Evaluating Your Response in Appendix B.

CHAPTER HIGHLIGHTS

35.1 Infectious or Inflammatory Disorders

Describe the pathophysiology and manifestations of infectious and inflammatory upper respiratory disorders, and outline the inter-professional care and nursing care of patients with these disorders.

- Upper respiratory infections (the common cold) are caused by a multitude of different viruses. Most are mild, self-limiting infections, appropriate for self-care; some viruses, however, such as RSV can cause serious lower respiratory illness in the very young or very old.
- Three different strains of influenza virus are identified; type A causes most outbreaks of influenza. Because this disease increases the risk of pneumonia in older adults, people with chronic diseases, and people who are immunocompromised, annual immunization is important for these populations and their caregivers.
- Influenza is differentiated from URI primarily by the presence of systemic manifestations, the duration and degree of fever, and the presence of persistent cough.
- Pharyngitis (sore throat) may be either viral or bacterial in origin; manifestations are similar. Patients with persistent or severe symptoms that include fever, enlarged lymph nodes, and myalgias should be evaluated to rule out GABHS pharyngitis, which can have significant complications such as rheumatic fever or poststreptococcal glomerulonephritis.
- The incidence of pertussis, a highly contagious reportable disease, is increasing due to waning immunity, decreased rates of childhood pertussis immunizations, and improved identification of the infection among adults. In adults, it is often recognized by prolonged and persistent coughing spells. Pertussis is treated in community settings with antibiotic therapy (usually erythromycin or TMP-SMZ).

35.2 Upper Respiratory Trauma or Obstruction

Describe the pathophysiology and manifestations of disorders of upper respiratory trauma or obstruction, and outline the interprofessional care and nursing care of patients with these disorders.

- Epistaxis (nosebleed) and nasal fracture are relatively common and pose a risk only when airway clearance is impaired. Emergency care for epistaxis includes pinching the nares or bridge of the nose, sitting upright leaning forward, and applying ice to the nose. When nasal packing is required to control bleeding, close monitoring of respiratory status (respiratory rate and effort, oxygen saturation) is critical.

35.3 Upper Respiratory Tumors

Describe the pathophysiology and manifestations of upper respiratory tumors, and outline the interprofessional care and nursing care of patients with upper respiratory tumors.

- Persistent voice hoarseness is the primary manifestation of laryngeal cancer. When identified and treated early, the rate of cure for laryngeal cancer is high. Some laryngeal tumors, however, have few manifestations until advanced. They may be treated by radiation therapy, chemotherapy, or surgery (laryngectomy and neck dissection).
- Following total laryngectomy, a permanent tracheostomy is created and the upper trachea and esophagus are separated, preventing aspiration when feedings are resumed. A tracheoesophageal puncture (TEP) may be created to allow verbal communication following total laryngectomy.

TEST YOURSELF NCLEX-RN® REVIEW

1. A patient with mild hypertension asks the nurse what can be done to relieve the symptoms of an acute URI. What should the nurse recommend to this patient?
   A. Ask his healthcare provider for an antibiotic prescription.
   B. Take 1000 mg of vitamin C and use zinc lozenges on a regular basis.
   C. Discuss the use of an over-the-counter nasal spray with the healthcare provider.
   D. Use an over-the-counter decongestant such as pseudoephedrine to relieve symptoms.

2. The community nurse is planning health promotion activities for a group of community-dwelling senior citizens. Which activity would most likely prevent influenza and pneumonia?
   A. Advising to avoid crowds
   B. Teaching effective hand hygiene
   C. Providing influenza vaccination clinics at the senior center
   D. Scheduling indoor exercise programs during winter months

3. The nurse is teaching a patient with bacterial sinusitis on care needed when at home. What should the nurse emphasize in this teaching? (Select all that apply.)
   A. Using a humidifier to promote sinus drainage
   B. Completing the antibiotic prescription as ordered
   C. Sleeping with the head of the bed elevated to 45 degrees
   D. Maintaining a liberal fluid intake to help liquefy secretions
   E. Applying cold packs to reduce swelling
4. The nurse is planning care for a patient with posterior nasal packing. Which nursing intervention is of the highest priority for this patient?
   A. Maintain oxygen therapy.
   B. Elevate the head of the bed.
   C. Provide frequent oral hygiene.
   D. Apply cold compresses to the nose.
5. A patient with facial trauma sustained in a motor vehicle crash complains of a "dripping" nose. The drainage appears like watery blood. What would be the most appropriate action for the nurse to take at this time?
   A. Provide a box of tissues.
   B. Suction the nasopharynx.
   C. Obtain a specimen for glucose testing.
   D. Reassure the patient that this is expected with a nasal fracture.
6. The nurse suspects that a patient is experiencing obstructive sleep apnea. What did the nurse most likely assess in this patient? (Select all that apply.)
   A. Loud cyclic snoring
   B. Elevated blood pressure
   C. Complaints of morning headache
   D. Complaints of daytime sleepiness
   E. Decreased oxygen saturation levels while awake
7. The nurse notes that a patient's voice is hoarse. What would be the most appropriate initial question for the nurse to ask the patient during the assessment?
   A. "Do you smoke?"
   B. "Do you have a sore throat?"
   C. "How long has your voice been hoarse?"
   D. "Would you like a prescription for throat lozenges?"
8. The nurse evaluates teaching provided to a patient with stage I laryngeal cancer. Which patient statement indicates teaching has been effective?
   A. "Thank goodness this type of cancer usually doesn't spread anywhere else."
   B. "I'm glad I don't have to worry about treating this cancer now because it was found so early."
   C. "I'm glad this was diagnosed early, when it can be treated with radiation so I won't lose my voice."
   D. "I hate to think about eventually losing the ability to speak, but I'd rather treat it aggressively than lose my life to cancer."
9. The nurse is caring for a patient recovering from a total laryngectomy and radical neck dissection. Place the interventions in the order in which the nurse should provide them to the patient.
   A. Frequently monitor airway patency.
   B. Suction via tracheostomy as needed.
   C. Instruct to support head when moving.
   D. Arrange consultation with speech therapist.
   E. Encourage to express feelings regarding loss of voice.
10. The nurse is teaching a patient about caring for a tracheostomy after discharge. What information should the nurse include? (Select all that apply.)
   A. Use sterile technique when changing dressings.
   B. Water sports are contraindicated.
   C. Recommend bathing rather than showering.
   D. Keep the area around the stoma clean and dry.
   E. Increase fluid intake.

See Test Yourself answers in Appendix B.

REFERENCES

Adams, M. P., Holland, L.N., & Urban, C. (2017). *Pharmacology for nursing: A pathophysiologic approach.* (5th ed.). Hoboken, NJ: Pearson Education.

American Cancer Society (ACS). (2017a). *Cancer facts and figures 2017.* Retrieved from https://www.cancer.org/content/dam/cancer-org/research/cancer-facts-and-statistics/annual-cancer-facts-and-figures/2017/cancer-facts-and-figures-2017.pdf.

American Cancer Society. (2017b). *Laryngeal and hypopharyngeal cancer.* Retrieved from www.cancer.org/cancer/laryngealandhypopharyngealcancer/index.

American Lung Association. (2018). *Pertussis symptoms, causes, and risk factors.* Retrieved from www.lung.org/lung-health-and-diseases/lung-disease-lookup/pertussis/pertussis-symptoms-causes.

American Society of Clinical Oncologists. (2018). *ASCO-SEP: Medical oncology self-evaluation program.* Alexandria, VA: Author.

Centers for Disease Control and Prevention (CDC). (2017a). *Diphtheria complications.*

Centers for Disease Control and Prevention (CDC). (2017b). *Diphtheria vaccination.* https://www.cdc.gov/vaccines/vpd/diphtheria/index.html.

Centers for Disease Control and Prevention (CDC). (2017c). *Influenza antiviral drug resistance.* Retrieved from www.cdc.gov/flu/about/qa/antiviralresistance.htm.

Centers for Disease Control and Prevention (CDC). (2017d). *Pertussis (whooping cough).* Retrieved from www.cdc.gov/pertussis/about/index.html.

Centers for Disease Control and Prevention (CDC). (2017e). *Seasonal flu.* Retrieved from www.cdc.gov/flu/.

Centers for Disease Control and Prevention. (n.d.). *Guide to skin testing for diphtheria antitoxin.* Retrieved from https://www.cdc.gov/diphtheria/downloads/skin-test-guide.pdf .

Chong, L., Head, K., Hopkins, C., Philpott, C., Glew, S., Scadding, G., . . . Schilder, A. G. M. (2016). Saline irrigation for chronic rhinosinusitis. *Cochrane Database of Systematic Reviews,* Issue 4. Article No.: CD011995. DOI: 10.1002/14651858.CD011995.pub2.

Grohskopf, L. A., Sokolow, L. Z., Broder, K. R., Olsen, S. J., Karron, R. A., Jernigan, D. B., & Bresee, J. S. (2017). Prevention and control of seasonal influenza with vaccines: Recommendations of the Advisory Committee on Immunization Practices — United States, 2017–18 influenza season. *Mortality and Morbidity Weekly Report Recommendations Report, 66*(RR-2), 1–20.

Healthy People 2020. (2018). Immunizations and Infectious diseases: IID 12.6. Retrieved from https://www.healthypeople.gov/2020/data-search/Search-the-Data#srch=influenza;topic-area=3527.

Heo, J.-S., Yang, S.-Y., Lim, S.-A., Lee, J.-M., Kang, J.-Y., Sun, S.-H., . . . Cho, J.-H. (2016). A manual acupuncture treatment attenuates common cold and its symptoms: A case series report from South Korea. *Journal of Traditional Chinese Medicine, 36*(6), 724–729.

Khan, Z. Z. (2016). *Group A streptococcal (GAS) infections workup.* Retrieved from https://emedicine.medscape.com/article/228936-workup.

Morgan, C. E. (2017). *Sleep-disordered breathing: Postsurgical prognosis.* Retrieved from https://emedicine.medscape.com/article/868770-overview#a9.

National Cancer Institute (NCI). (2014). *Cancer stat facts: Laryngeal cancer.* Retrieved from https://seer.cancer.gov/statfacts/html/laryn.html.

National Cancer Institute (NCI). (2017a). *Aromatherapy and essential oils.* Retrieved from https://www.cancer.gov/about-cancer/treatment/cam/hp/aromatherapy-pdq.

National Cancer Institute (NCI). (2017b). *Laryngeal cancer treatment: General information.* Retrieved from www.cancer.gov/cancertopics/pdq/treatment/laryngeal/healthprofessional/page2.

National Center for Complementary and Integrative Health (NCCIH). (2017). *5 tips: Natural products for the flu and colds: what does the science say?* Retrieved from http://nccam.nih.gov/health/tips/flucold.htm.

National Institute of Allergy and Infectious Diseases (NIAID). (2017a). *Influenza.* Retrieved from https://www.niaid.nih.gov/diseases-conditions/influenza.

National Institute of Allergy and Infectious Diseases (NIAID). (2017b). *Vaccine research center.* https://www.niaid.nih.gov/about/vrc.

Sorenson, M., Quinn, L., & Klein, D. (2019). *Pathophysiology: Concepts of human disease.* New York: Pearson.

Weiner, D. L. (2015). *Reye syndrome.* Retrieved from https://emedicine.medscape.com/article/803683-overview#a7.

World Health Organization (WHO). (2017). *Influenza (Avian and other zoonotic).* Retrieved from www.who.int/mediacentre/factsheets/avian_influenza/en/index.html.

ADDITIONAL RESOURCES

American Cancer Society. (2018). *Laryngeal and hypopharyngeal cancers.*

Retrieved from https://www.cancer.org/cancer/laryngeal-and-hypopharyngeal-cancer.html.

American Lung Association. (2018a). *Lung health and diseases.*

Retrieved from www.lung.org/lung-health-and-diseases/.

American Lung Association. (2018b). *Our initiatives.*

Retrieved from www.lung.org/our-initiatives/.

American Lung Association. (2018c). *Stop smoking.*

Retrieved from www.lung.org/stop-smoking/.

American Thoracic Society. (2017). *Patient resources: Fact sheets A to Z.*

Retrieved from www.thoracic.org/patients/patient-resources/fact-sheets-az.php.

National Heart, Lung, and Blood Institute. (2018). *Health topics.*

Retrieved from https://www.nhlbi.nih.gov.

Chapter 36

Nursing Care of Patients with Ventilation Disorders

Chapter Outline and Learning Outcomes

36.1 Infectious and Inflammatory Disorders 1280

Describe the pathophysiology and manifestations of infectious and inflammatory ventilation disorders, and outline the interprofessional care and nursing care of patients with these disorders.

36.2 Disorders of the Pleura 1307

Describe the pathophysiology and manifestations of disorders of the pleura, and outline the interprofessional care and nursing care of patients with these disorders.

36.3 Trauma of the Chest or Lung 1314

Describe the pathophysiology and manifestations of trauma of the chest or lung, and outline the interprofessional care and nursing care of patients with these injuries.

36.4 Lung Cancer 1321

Describe the pathophysiology and manifestations of lung cancer, and outline the interprofessional care and nursing care of patients with this disease.

CLINICAL COMPETENCIES

- Assess functional health status and the effects of lower respiratory and chest wall disorders on ventilation and gas exchange.
- Use assessment data and knowledge of the effects of the disorder and prescribed treatment to identify priority nursing diagnoses and plan care for patients with lower respiratory disorders.
- Use the nursing process and evidence-based nursing research to plan and implement individualized nursing care, including measures to promote ventilation and gas exchange for patients with lower respiratory disorders.
- Plan and provide appropriate teaching for health promotion among vulnerable populations and to prepare patients and families for continuity of care.
- Evaluate the effectiveness of nursing interventions and teaching, revising strategies and teaching plans as needed.
- Knowledgably and safely coordinate interprofessional care and administer prescribed medications and treatments for patients with lower respiratory disorders.

KEY TERMS

asphyxiation, 1318
bronchitis, 1280
cyanosis, 1280
dyspnea, 1280
empyema, 1283
flail chest, 1315
hemoptysis, 1280
hemothorax, 1314
hypoxemia, 1288
lung abscess, 1292
pleural effusion, 1307
pleuritis, 1307
pneumonia, 1281
pneumothorax, 1309
thoracentesis, 1308
tuberculosis (TB), 1293

Disorders affecting the lower respiratory system (below the larynx), pleural cavity, and chest wall can affect the ability to effectively move air into and out of the lungs (ventilation) and the exchange of oxygen and carbon dioxide across the alveolar-capillary membrane (respiration). The disorders discussed in this chapter—respiratory infections and inflammation, disorders and trauma of the chest wall and pleural cavity, and neoplasms of the lung—all affect the ability to maintain clear and patent airways and ventilate the lungs. Although these disorders can also affect gas exchange, nursing care for patients with these disorders generally focuses on maintaining airway patency and an effective breathing pattern.

The lower respiratory and chest wall disorders discussed in this chapter and in Chapter 37 (disorders of gas exchange) have both local and systemic effects. Local effects include cough, excess mucus production, shortness of breath or **dyspnea** (difficult or labored breathing), **hemoptysis** (bloody sputum), and chest pain. Systemic effects may include fever, anorexia and malaise, **cyanosis** (gray to blue or purple skin color caused by deoxygenated hemoglobin), and other manifestations of impaired gas exchange.

36.1 Infections and Inflammatory Disorders

Infections and inflammation of the lower respiratory system are common. The respiratory tree is constantly exposed to the environment as air moves into and out of the lower respiratory tract. In addition, the oropharynx is colonized by huge numbers of microorganisms that may be aspirated into the bronchial tree. Both anatomic and physiologic defenses help maintain the sterility of the lower respiratory tract. When these defenses are impaired, the risk for infection increases. For example, drugs, alcohol, or neuromuscular disease may suppress the cough reflex, and the influenza virus can leave the respiratory epithelium vulnerable to bacterial infection. Even in healthy people, microorganisms and other foreign material occasionally enter the bronchial tree and lung parenchyma.

The Patient with Acute Bronchitis

Bronchitis, inflammation of the bronchi, may be either an acute or a chronic condition. Acute bronchitis is relatively common in adults. The risk for acute bronchitis is increased by impaired immune defenses and cigarette smoking. In otherwise healthy adults, it typically follows a viral upper respiratory infection. Chronic bronchitis is a component of chronic obstructive pulmonary disease (COPD) and is discussed in Chapter 37.

Pathophysiology

Infectious bronchitis can be caused by either viruses or bacteria that damage the respiratory mucosa. In healthy adults, bacterial bronchitis generally only occurs as a complication of viral infection. Inhalation of toxic gases or chemicals can lead to inflammatory bronchitis.

The inflammatory response to infection or tissue damage from inhaled substances causes capillary dilation and edema of the mucosal lining of the bronchi. Inflammatory cells infiltrate the affected mucosa, leading to exudate formation and increased mucus production. Ciliated epithelium is damaged by the inflammatory response and ciliary function is impaired. The immune response of lymphocytes and tissue macrophages is inhibited by some viruses and mycobacteria, increasing the risk for bacterial infection. Mucosal irritation and increased mucus production initiate the cough reflex. The respiratory tract may become hyperirritable for an extended period of time, leading to paroxysms of coughing and bronchospasm.

Risk Factors

Risk factors for acute bronchitis include close exposure to someone with acute bronchitis, lack of current immunizations, and exposure to smoke, fumes, and pollution.

Manifestations

Acute bronchitis is typically heralded by a nonproductive cough that later becomes productive. The cough often occurs in paroxysms and may be aggravated by cold, dry, or dusty air. Chest pain, often substernal, is common. Other manifestations include moderate fever and general malaise.

Complications

Pneumonia is the primary complication of acute bronchitis. Recurrent bronchitis episodes are also seen in some patients.

Interprofessional Care

Diagnosis

The diagnosis of acute bronchitis is typically based on the history and clinical presentation. A chest x-ray may be ordered to rule out pneumonia because the presenting manifestations can be similar. Other diagnostic testing is rarely indicated. Treatment is symptomatic and includes rest, increased fluid intake, and the use of aspirin or acetaminophen to relieve fever and malaise.

Medications

While many healthcare providers prescribe a broad-spectrum antibiotic such as erythromycin or penicillin, only a small percentage of acute bacteria is found to be bacterial in origin. An expectorant cough medication is recommended for use during the day and a cough suppressant for night to facilitate rest.

Nursing Care

Assessment

See the Manifestations and Interprofessional Care sections for the assessment of the patient with acute bronchitis.

Focused assessment of the patient with acute bronchitis includes:

- *Health history:* Complaints of dyspnea, productive cough, previous bronchial infections
- *Physical assessment:* General appearance, vital signs including temperature; auscultation of lung sounds.

Priorities of Care

Nursing care is supportive. The focus of nursing care for the adult with acute bronchitis is on close surveillance for complications and teaching for self-care and prevention of causative organism spread.

Diagnoses, Interventions, and Outcomes

Promote Airway Clearance and Patency. When the patient has acute bronchitis, sputum production and local tissue edema may interfere with airway patency.

Expected Outcome: Patient will use techniques to promote airway clearance as indicated and tolerated in combination with maintenance of patent airway.

The nurse will:

- Teach effective cough technique to promote airway clearance.

Delegating Nursing Care Activities

As appropriate and allowed by the designated duties and responsibilities of unlicensed assistive personnel, the nurse may delegate nursing care activities such as measuring vital signs, encouraging oral or enteral fluid intake, and providing skin care.

Transitions of Care

Patients can limit their incidence of acute bronchitis by using good hygiene methods such as frequent handwashing. Maintaining good general health and participating in stress-reducing activities support the immune system.

Nursing care for patients with acute bronchitis is primarily educational, related to the following topics:

- Increase fluid intake to keep mucus thin and meet increased needs related to fever.
- Use over-the-counter analgesics and cough preparations containing guifanisen (thins secretions) and dextromethorphan (suppresses cough) for symptom relief.
- Be aware of the use and effects of any prescribed medications.
- Understand the importance of smoking cessation (as appropriate).

The Patient with Pneumonia

Inflammation of the lung parenchyma (the respiratory bronchioles and alveoli) is known as **pneumonia**. Despite significant advances in antibiotic therapy, pneumonia remains the eighth leading cause of death in the United States and the leading cause of death from infectious disease (American Lung Association, 2017; Centers for Disease Control and Prevention [CDC], 2017b). In 2014, there were 50,662 deaths in the United States attributed to pneumonia and influenza. Women have a higher death rate (16.2/100,000) than men (15.5/100,000) attributed to pneumonia and influenza. The differences in death rates attributed to influenza and pneumonia among different races and ethnicity are relatively small. Death rates are lowest in American Indian/Alaska Native populations at 8.0/100,00, Asian/Pacific Islanders at 9.3/100,000, Black populations at 11.8/100,000, and White populations at 17.3/100,000 (Kochanek, Murphy, Xu, & Tejada-Vera, 2016). Incidence and mortality are highest in older adults and people with debilitating diseases.

Pathophysiology

Pneumonia may be either infectious or noninfectious. Bacteria, viruses, fungi, protozoa, and other microbes can lead to infectious pneumonia. Other causes include aspiration of gastric contents and inhalation of toxic or irritating gases. Infectious pneumonias are often classified as community acquired, healthcare associated, or opportunistic. Different organisms are implicated in each of these classifications (**Box 36.1**). The most common causative organism for community-acquired pneumonia is *Streptococcus pneumoniae* (also called *pneumococcus*), a gram-positive bacterium. This organism causes about 36% of cases of community-acquired pneumonia and some 400,000 hospitalizations annually (CDC, 2015). *Mycoplasma pneumoniae, Chlamydia pneumoniae, Haemophilus influenzae*, and the influenza virus are also leading causes of community-acquired pneumonia. *Staphylococcus aureus* and gram-negative bacteria such as *Klebsiella pneumoniae, Pseudomonas aeruginosa*, and enteric bacilli, including *Escherichia coli*, are often implicated in healthcare-associated pneumonia. Organisms such as *Pneumocystis* generally cause infections only in immunocompromised people (opportunistic infections).

The lower respiratory tract is normally sterile. A number of defense mechanisms help maintain this sterile environment. Infectious particles trapped by the mucous membranes of the nose are removed by sneezing, whereas

BOX 36.1
Common Organisms Causing Pneumonia in Adults

COMMUNITY ACQUIRED

- *Streptococcus pneumoniae*
- *Mycoplasma pneumoniae*
- *Haemophilus influenzae*
- Influenza virus
- *Chlamydia pneumoniae*
- *Legionella pneumophila*

HEALTHCARE ASSOCIATED

- *Staphylococcus aureus*
- *Pseudomonas aeruginosa*
- *Klebsiella pneumoniae*
- *Escherichia coli*

OPPORTUNISTIC

- *Pneumocystis jiroveci*
- *Mycobacterium tuberculosis*
- Cytomegalovirus (CMV)
- Atypical mycobacteria
- Fungi

those deposited in the nasopharynx are usually swallowed or expectorated. Reflex closure of the epiglottis and the branching bronchial tree present anatomic barriers to entry of microorganisms and other possible contaminants. The cilia and mucus that line the respiratory tract and the cough reflex serve to trap and eliminate foreign matter that enters the lower respiratory tract. Organisms that make it past these barriers are usually rapidly phagocytized in the alveolus by resident macrophages, then attacked by the inflammatory and immune defenses of the body. Aging impairs these immune responses, increasing the risk for pneumonia.

The most common means of entry of pathogens into the lung is aspiration of oropharyngeal secretions containing microbes. Microorganisms may also be inhaled after having been released when an infected person coughs, sneezes, or talks. Contaminated aerosolized water may also be inhaled, an important means of spread for viral and some other types of pneumonia. Finally, bacteria may spread to the lungs through the bloodstream from infection elsewhere in the body. Host defenses must be overwhelmed either by the number of organisms or their *virulence* (disease-causing ability) in order for an infection to develop.

When the invading microorganisms colonize the alveoli, an inflammatory and immune response is initiated. The antigen–antibody response and endotoxins released by some organisms damage bronchial and alveolar mucous membranes, causing inflammation with vascular congestion and edema. Infectious debris and exudate can fill alveoli, interfering with ventilation and gas exchange (**Figure 36.1** ■). Pneumonia may develop in four distinct patterns: Lobar pneumonia, bronchopneumonia, interstitial pneumonia, and miliary pneumonia (**Table 36.1**).

Acute Bacterial Pneumonia

Of the bacterial pneumonias, the pathogenesis of pneumococcal (*Streptococcus pneumoniae*) pneumonia is best understood (**Figure 36.2** ■). These bacteria can reside in the upper

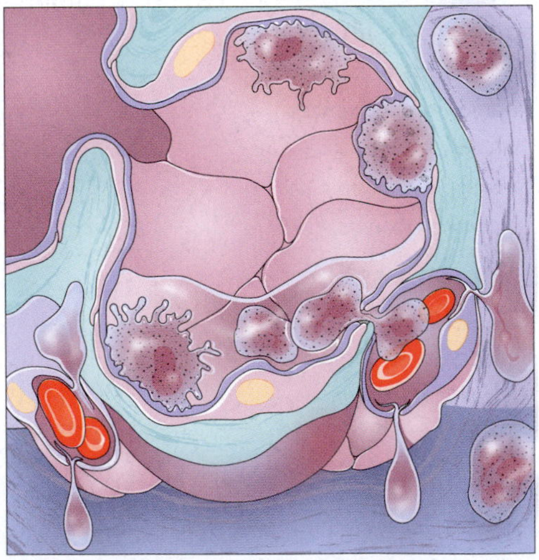

Figure 36.1 ■ In pneumonia, the inflammatory response causes fluid to accumulate in the alveoli and edema to form as alveolar capillaries dilate and allow fluid to leak into interstitial tissues.

Table 36.1 Patterns of Lung Involvement in Pneumonia

Pattern of Involvement	Description
Lobar pneumonia	Typically involves an entire lobe of a lung. Early in the process, when the immune response is minimal, bacteria spread throughout the affected lobe by rapid accumulation of edema fluid. As the immune and inflammatory responses develop, RBCs and neutrophils, damaged epithelial cells, and fibrin accumulate in the alveoli. Purulent exudate containing neutrophils and macrophages forms. As alveoli and respiratory bronchioles fill with exudate, blood cells, fibrin, and bacteria, *consolidation* (solidification) of lung tissue occurs. Finally, the process resolves as enzymes destroy the exudate and residual debris is reabsorbed, phagocytized, or coughed out.
Bronchopneumonia	Usually involves dependent portions of lung tissue, characterized by patchy consolidation. Exudate tends to remain primarily in the bronchi and bronchioles, with less edema and congestion of the alveoli than in lobar pneumonia.
Interstitial pneumonia	The inflammatory process primarily involves the interstitium: The alveolar walls and connective tissue supporting the bronchial tree. Involvement may be patchy or diffuse as lymphocytes, macrophages, and plasma cells infiltrate the alveolar septa. While alveoli typically do not contain significant exudates, protein-rich hyaline membranes may line the alveoli, interfering with gas exchange.
Miliary pneumonia	In miliary pneumonia, numerous discrete inflammatory lesions develop as a result of spread of the pathogen to the lungs via the bloodstream. Miliary pneumonia is primarily seen in people who are severely immunocompromised. As a result, the immune response is poor and damage to pleural tissue may be significant.

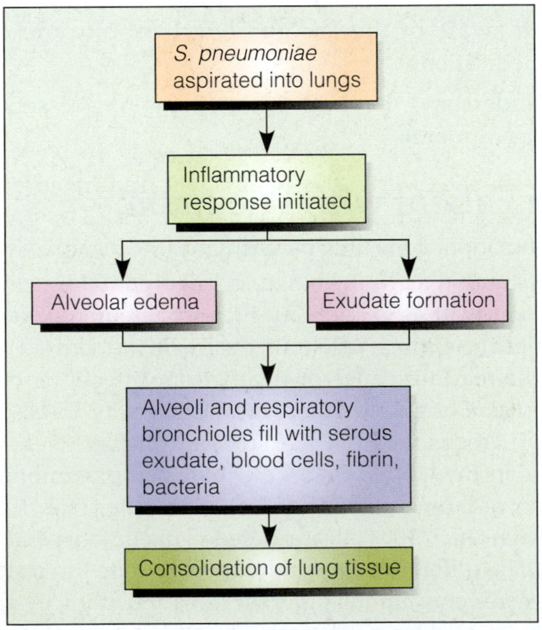
S. pneumoniae
aspirated into lungs
Inflammatory
response initiated
Alveolar edema
Exudate formation
Alveoli and respiratory
bronchioles fill with serous
exudate, blood cells, fibrin,
bacteria
Consolidation of lung tissue

Figure 36.2 ■ The pathogenesis of pneumococcal pneumonia.

respiratory tract of adults. They may be spread by direct person-to-person contact via droplets. In many cases, infection results from aspiration of resident bacteria. In the lower respiratory tract, the inflammatory response initiated by these organisms causes alveolar edema and the formation of exudate. As alveoli and respiratory bronchioles fill with serous exudate, blood cells, fibrin, and bacteria, *consolidation* (solidification) of lung tissue occurs. The lower lobes of the lungs are usually affected because of gravity. Consolidation of a large portion of an entire lung lobe is known as *lobar pneumonia*. This is the typical pattern for pneumococcal pneumonia. *Bronchopneumonia* is patchy consolidation involving several lobules. Other bacterial pneumonias often present with the patchy involvement of bronchopneumonia; pneumococcal pneumonia may also follow this pattern. The process resolves when macrophages dominate, digesting and removing inflammatory exudate from the infected lung.

Manifestations. The presentation of bacterial pneumonia is usually acute, with rapid onset of shaking chills (rigors), fever, and cough productive of rust-colored or purulent sputum. Chest aching or *pleuritic pain* (sharp, localized chest pain that increases with breathing and coughing) is common. Limited breath sounds and fine crackles or rales are heard over the affected area of lung. A pleural friction rub may be audible. If the involved area is large and gas exchange is impaired, dyspnea and cyanosis may be noted.

A more insidious onset with low-grade fever, cough, and scattered crackles is more typical of bronchopneumonia. Dyspnea is less commonly seen. The older adult or debilitated patient may have atypical manifestations of pneumonia, with little cough, scant sputum, and minimal evidence of respiratory distress. Fever, tachypnea, and altered mentation or agitation may be the primary presenting symptoms.

Complications. Pneumococcal pneumonia typically resolves uneventfully; normal lung structure is restored on completion of the process. Local extension of the infection to involve the pleura (*pleuritis*) is the most common complication. Pneumonias caused by *Staphylococcus aureus* and gram-negative bacteria often cause extensive parenchymal damage with necrosis, lung abscess, and empyema or pleural effusion. Progressive destruction of lung tissue and functional impairment is a possible consequence of *Klebsiella* pneumonia.

A *lung abscess* is a local area of necrosis and pus formation within the lung itself. Lung abscess is relatively uncommon. Manifestations develop slowly and include weight loss, malaise, night sweats, fever, and a productive cough. Sputum is foul smelling and tasting. Rupture of the abscess into a larger airway is heralded by production of copious amounts of purulent sputum.

Empyema is accumulation of purulent exudate in the pleural cavity, identified by chest x-ray or CT scan. Thoracentesis may be done or a chest tube inserted to remove purulent exudates. Bacteremia can spread the infection to other tissues, leading to meningitis, endocarditis or peritonitis, and increasing the risk of mortality.

Legionnaires' Disease

Legionnaires' disease is a form of bronchopneumonia caused by *Legionella pneumophila*, a gram-negative bacterium widely found in water, particularly warm standing water. Legionnaires' disease occurs sporadically and in outbreaks, such as that which occurred at an American Legion convention in 1976, when the disease was first recognized. Contaminated, water-cooled air-conditioning systems and other water sources have been implicated in its spread.

Smokers, older adults, and people with chronic diseases or impaired immune defenses are most susceptible to Legionnaires' disease. Symptoms develop gradually, beginning 2 to 10 days after exposure. Dry cough, dyspnea, general malaise, chills and fever, headache, confusion, anorexia and diarrhea, myalgias, and arthralgias are common manifestations. Consolidation of lung tissue is patchy or lobar. The overall mortality rate in Legionnaires' disease is reported to be between 5 and 10%, with rates among immunocompromised patients between 5 and 30% with appropriate care and treatment (World Health Organization, 2017a).

Primary Atypical Pneumonia

Pneumonia caused by *Mycoplasma pneumoniae* is generally classified as *primary atypical pneumonia* because its presentation and course differ significantly from those of other bacterial pneumonias. Mycoplasma infection often causes pharyngitis or bronchitis. When pneumonia develops, patchy inflammatory changes in the alveolar septum and interstitial tissue of the lung occur. Alveolar exudate and consolidation of lung tissue are not features of atypical pneumonia.

Young adults—college students and military recruits in particular—are the primary affected population. Primary atypical pneumonia is highly contagious. Its manifestations resemble those of viral pneumonia; systemic manifestations of fever, headache, myalgias, and arthralgias often dominate. The cough associated with atypical pneumonia is dry, hacking, and nonproductive. Because of the typically mild nature and predominant systemic manifestations, mycoplasmal and viral pneumonia are often referred to as *walking pneumonias*.

Viral Pneumonia

Up to 27% of hospitalized patients with pneumonia are found to have viral pneumonia (Jain, Self, Wunderink, & Fakhran, 2015). Influenza and adenovirus are the most common organisms; however, the incidence of cytomegalovirus (CMV) pneumonia is increasing in immunocompromised people. Other viruses such as herpes viruses and measles virus may also cause viral pneumonia. As in primary atypical pneumonia, lung involvement in viral pneumonia is limited to the alveolar septum and interstitial spaces.

Viral pneumonia is typically a mild disease that often affects older adults and people with chronic conditions. It usually occurs in community epidemics. Flulike symptoms of headache, fever, fatigue, malaise, and muscle aches are common, along with a dry cough.

Pneumocystis Pneumonia

People with acquired immunodeficiency syndrome (AIDS) and others with significant immunocompromise are at risk for developing an opportunistic pneumonia caused by *Pneumocystis jiroveci*, a common parasite found worldwide. Immunity to *Pneumocystis* is nearly universal, except in immunocompromised people. Opportunistic infection may develop in people treated with immunosuppressive or cytotoxic drugs for cancer or organ transplant and in people with genetic or acquired immunodeficiency. *Pneumocystis* pneumonia can be seen in up to 80% of patients with AIDS who do not receive prophylaxis (CDC, 1989).

Infection with *Pneumocystis* produces patchy involvement throughout the lungs, causing affected alveoli to thicken, become edematous, and fill with foamy, protein-rich fluid. Gas exchange is severely impaired as the disease progresses. *Pneumocystis pneumonia (PCP)* has an abrupt onset with fever, tachypnea and shortness of breath, and a dry, nonproductive cough. Respiratory distress can be significant, with intercostal retractions and cyanosis.

Table 36.2 compares the manifestations of infectious pneumonias.

Aspiration Pneumonia

Aspiration of gastric contents into the lungs results in a chemical and bacterial pneumonia known as *aspiration pneumonia*. Major risk factors for aspiration pneumonia include emergency surgery or obstetric procedures, depressed cough and gag reflexes, and impaired swallowing. Older surgical patients are at significant risk. Enteral nutrition by either nasogastric or gastric tube also increases the risk for aspiration pneumonia. Vomiting is not always apparent; silent regurgitation of gastric contents may occur when the level of consciousness is decreased. Measures to reduce the risk for aspiration pneumonia include minimizing the use of preoperative medications, promoting anesthetic elimination from the body, and preventing nausea and gastric distention.

The low pH of gastric contents causes a severe inflammatory response when aspirated into the respiratory tract. Pulmonary edema and respiratory failure may result. Common complications of aspiration pneumonia include abscesses, bronchiectasis (chronic dilation of the bronchi and bronchioles), and gangrene of pulmonary tissue.

Interprofessional Care

With early identification of the infecting organism, appropriate treatment, and support of respiratory function, most patients recover uneventfully. However, pneumonia remains a serious disease with significant mortality, especially in older adults and debilitated populations.

Diagnosis

Patient history, physical examination, and diagnostic testing are used to establish the diagnosis, determine the extent of lung involvement, and identify the causative organism.

- ***Chest x-ray*** is obtained to determine the extent and pattern of lung involvement. Fluid, infiltrates, consolidated lung tissue, and atelectasis (areas of alveolar collapse) appear as densities on the film. The *CT scan* provides a more detailed image of pulmonary tissue and may be used when the chest x-ray is not diagnostic.
- ***Sputum Gram stain*** rapidly identifies the infecting organisms as gram-positive or gram-negative bacteria. Antibiotic therapy can then be directed at the predominant type of organism until culture and sensitivity results are obtained.
- ***Sputum culture and sensitivity*** is ordered to identify the infecting organism and determine the most effective antibiotic therapy. When obtaining sputum for culture, it is important to obtain secretions from the lower respiratory tract, not the mouth and nasal passages.
- ***Complete blood count (CBC) with white blood cell (WBC) differential*** shows an elevated WBC (11,000/mm^3 or higher) with increased circulating immature leukocytes (a left shift) in response to the infectious process. WBC changes are minimal in viral and other pneumonias.
- ***Serology testing***, blood tests to detect antibodies to respiratory pathogens, may be used to identify the

Table 36.2 Manifestations of Infectious Pneumonias

Type	Onset	Respiratory Manifestations	Systemic Manifestations
Pneumococcal or lobar pneumonia	Abrupt	Cough productive of purulent or rust-colored sputum; pleuritic or aching chest pain; decreased breath sounds and crackles over affected area; possible dyspnea and cyanosis	Chills and fever
Bronchopneumonia	Gradual	Cough, scattered crackles; minimal dyspnea and respiratory distress	Low-grade fever
Legionnaires' disease	Gradual	Dry cough; dyspnea	Chills and fever; general malaise; headache; confusion; anorexia and diarrhea; myalgias and arthralgias
Primary atypical pneumonia	Gradual	Dry, hacking, nonproductive cough	Fever, headache, myalgias, and arthralgias dominate
Viral pneumonia	Sudden or gradual	Dry cough	Flulike symptoms
Pneumocystis pneumonia	Abrupt	Dry cough; tachypnea and shortness of breath; significant respiratory distress	Fever

infecting organism when blood and sputum cultures are negative.

- *Pulse oximetry*, a noninvasive method of measuring arterial oxygen saturation, is ordered to continuously monitor gas exchange. The Sao_2 is normally 95% or higher. An Sao_2 of < 95% may indicate impaired alveolar gas exchange.
- *Arterial blood gases (ABGs)* may be ordered to evaluate gas exchange. Respiratory secretions or pleuritic pain can interfere with alveolar ventilation. Alveolar inflammation can interfere with gas exchange across the alveolar-capillary membrane, especially if exudate or consolidation is present. An arterial oxygen tension (Po_2) of < 75 to 80 mmHg indicates impaired gas exchange or alveolar ventilation. See Chapters 10 and 34 for more information about gas transport, arterial blood gases, and normal or expected values.
- *Fiberoptic bronchoscopy* may be done to obtain a sputum specimen or remove secretions from the bronchial tree (refer to Figure 34.4 in Chapter 34). Nursing responsibilities related to bronchoscopy are summarized in the Diagnostic Tests table in Chapter 34.

Immunization

Vaccines offer some degree of protection against the most common bacterial and viral pneumonias. The CDC reports two versions of the pneumococcal vaccine: Pneumococcal conjugate vaccine 13 (PCV13, Prevnar) and pneumococcal polysaccharide vaccine (PPSV23, Pneumovax). The PCV13 protects against 13 types of pneumococcal bacteria, whereas the PPSV23 protects against 23 types of pneumococcal bacteria (CDC, 2017b).

PCV13 is the pneumonia vaccine used in children at 2, 4, 6, and 12 through 15 months. It can also be administered to adults who only need a single dose. PPSV23 is given to adults who need it and usually imparts lifetime immunity with a single dose. It is not effective in children less than 2 years of age. The PPSV23 is recommended for people who have a high risk of adverse outcome from bacterial pneumonias: People over age 65; those with chronic cardiac or respiratory conditions, diabetes mellitus, alcoholism, or other chronic diseases; and those who are immunocompromised. If an adult is receiving both the PCV13 and the PPSV23, the PCV13 should be administered first due to the immune response. The planned PPSV23 should then be administered 1 year later. In selected adults who received the PPSV23, two additional doses are recommended for people over age 65 who were immunized more than 5 years previously and before age 65, people with chronic renal failure or immunosuppressive conditions (e.g., malignancy), and people receiving chemotherapy with selected agents (CDC, 2017b).

Influenza vaccine is also recommended for high-risk populations. The predominant strain of influenza virus varies from year to year. A new vaccine formulation is prepared yearly, incorporating antigens of the influenza strains predicted to be the most prevalent for the upcoming flu season (typically the winter months). Vulnerable populations for whom yearly vaccine is recommended include those listed earlier as well as healthcare workers and residents of long-term care facilities. The vaccine contains egg protein and is not recommended for people who have a severe allergy to eggs or who have previously experienced a severe hypersensitivity response to the vaccine.

SAFETY ALERT: Inquire about allergic responses to eggs or previous influenza vaccinations prior to administering influenza vaccine. A significant hypersensitivity response may occur in patients who are allergic to egg protein. ■

Medications

Medications used to treat pneumonia may include antibiotics to eradicate the infection and bronchodilators to reduce bronchospasm and improve ventilation.

Initial antibiotic therapy is based on the results of sputum Gram stain and the pattern of lung involvement shown on the chest x-ray. Considerations such as the presence of cardiovascular disease or residence in a long-term care facility are also considered in the initial antibiotic choice. Typically, a broad-spectrum antibiotic such as a macrolide (e.g., clarithromycin, azithromycin, or erythromycin), a penicillin or a second- or third-generation cephalosporin, or a fluoroquinolone (e.g., ciprofloxacin) is ordered until the results of sputum culture and sensitivity tests are available. **Table 36.3** lists commonly prescribed antibiotics for

Table 36.3 Antibiotic Therapy for Selected Pneumonias

Causative Organism	Antibiotic of Choice	Alternative Antibiotics
Streptococcus pneumoniae	Penicillin G; amoxicillin	Erythromycin, *cephalosporins*, *doxycycline*, fluoroquinolones, clindamycin, vancomycin, *trimethoprim-sulfamethoxazole* (*TMP-SMZ*), linezolid
Haemophilus influenzae	Second- or third-generation cephalosporins, doxycycline, azithromycin, TMP-SMZ	Fluoroquinolones, *clarithromycin*
Staphylococcus aureus	Penicillinase-resistant penicillin (e.g., nafcillin); vancomycin for methicillin-resistant organisms	*Cephalosporins*, vancomycin, clindamycin; *ciprofloxacin*, fluoroquinolones, *TMP-SMZ*
Mycoplasma pneumoniae	Erythromycin, doxycycline	*Clarithromycin*, *azithromycin*, fluoroquinolones
Klebsiella pneumoniae	Third-generation cephalosporin (with aminoglycoside if severe); metronidazole	Aztreonam, imipenem-cilastatin, fluoroquinolones
Legionella pneumophila	Macrolide + rifampin; fluoroquinolones	*TMP-SMZ*, *doxycycline* + rifampin
Pneumocystis	TMP-SMZ, pentamidine + prednisone	Dapsone + *trimethoprim*, *clindamycin* + primaquine, trimetrexate + folinic acid
Chlamydia pneumoniae	Doxycycline	Macrolide, fluoroquinolones

Note: Drugs identified in blue are among the 200 most commonly prescribed medications in the United States.

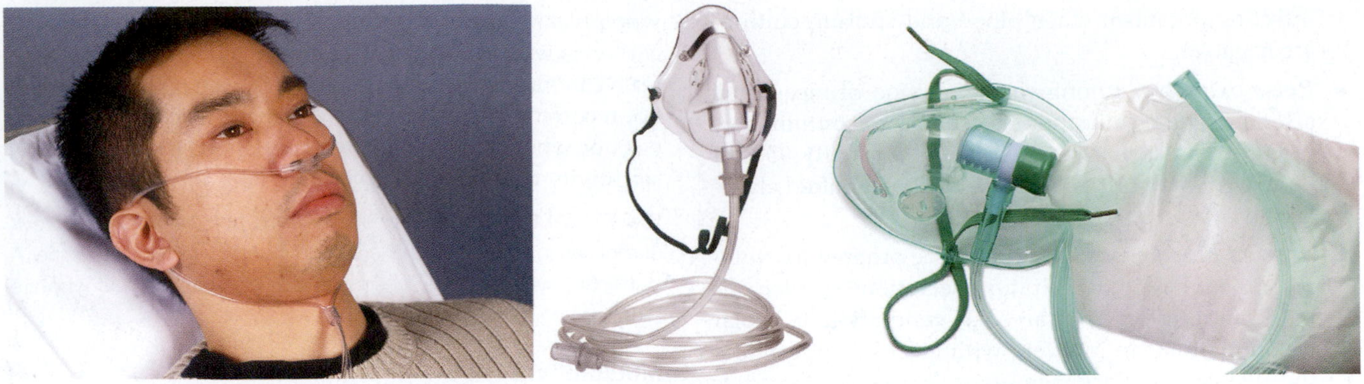

A Nasal cannula B Simple face mask C Nonrebreather mask

Figure 36.3 ■ Low-flow oxygen delivery devices. A, Nasal cannula. B, Simple face mask. C, Nonrebreather mask.

selected pneumonias; nursing implications for selected antibiotics are summarized in Medication Administration 12.A in Chapter 12, Nursing Care of Patients with Infections.

When an inflammatory response to the infection causes bronchospasm and constriction, bronchodilators may be ordered to improve ventilation and reduce hypoxia. Bronchodilators generally belong to one of two major groups: The sympathomimetic drugs, such as albuterol sulfate (Proventil) and metaproterenol (Alupent), or the methylxanthines, such as theophylline and aminophylline. Use of these drugs and related nursing implications are discussed in detail in the section on asthma.

An agent to break up mucus or reduce its viscosity may be prescribed. Acetylcysteine (Mucomyst), potassium iodide, and guaifenesin (a common ingredient in expectorant cough syrups) help to liquefy mucus, making it easier to expectorate. For many patients, however, increasing fluid intake is an effective means of liquefying mucus.

Treatments

When mucus secretions are thick and viscous, increasing fluid intake to 2500 to 3000 mL/day helps liquefy secretions, making them easier to cough up and expectorate. If the patient is unable to maintain an adequate oral intake, intravenous fluids and nutrition may be required.

Incentive spirometry may be used to promote deep breathing, coughing, and clearance of respiratory secretions. Endotracheal suctioning may be required if the cough is ineffective. This invasive technique is discussed in the section describing nursing care for the patient with acute respiratory failure in Chapter 37. On occasion, bronchoscopy is used to perform pulmonary toilet and remove secretions.

Oxygen Therapy. Oxygen therapy may be indicated for the patient who is tachypneic or hypoxemic.

Inflammation of the alveolar-capillary membrane interferes with diffusion of gases across the membrane. Diffusion is affected by several other factors, including the partial pressure of gases on each side of the membrane. Increasing the percentage of inspired oxygen above that of room air (21%) increases the partial pressure of oxygen in the alveoli and enhances its diffusion into the capillaries. Supplemental oxygen therefore improves oxygenation of the blood and tissues in patients with pneumonia.

Depending on the degree of hypoxia, oxygen may be administered by either a low-flow or high-flow system. Low-flow systems include the nasal cannula, simple face mask, partial rebreathing mask, and nonrebreathing mask (**Figure 36.3** ■). A nasal cannula can deliver 24 to 45% oxygen concentrations with flow rates of 2 to 6 L/min. The nasal cannula is comfortable and does not interfere with eating or talking. A simple face mask delivers 40 to 60% oxygen concentrations with flow rates of 5 to 8 L/min. Up to 100% oxygen can be delivered by the nonrebreather mask, the highest concentration possible without mechanical ventilation. When the amount of oxygen delivered must be precisely regulated, a high-flow system such as a Venturi mask is used (**Figure 36.4** ■). The Venturi mask regulates the ratio of oxygen to room air, allowing precise regulation of the oxygen percentage delivered, from 24 to 50%. High-flow oxygen can also be delivered via nasal cannula (Vapotherm). In these methods, oxygen and warmed normal saline are aerosolized. Flow at 15 L/min provides up to 90% FiO_2, whereas 10 L/min provides 65% FiO_2. Severe hypoxia may necessitate intubation and mechanical ventilation. Endotracheal intubation and methods of mechanical ventilation are discussed in Chapter 37.

Chest Physiotherapy. Chest physiotherapy, including percussion, vibration, and postural drainage, may be prescribed to reduce lung consolidation and prevent atelectasis. *Percussion* is performed by rhythmically striking or

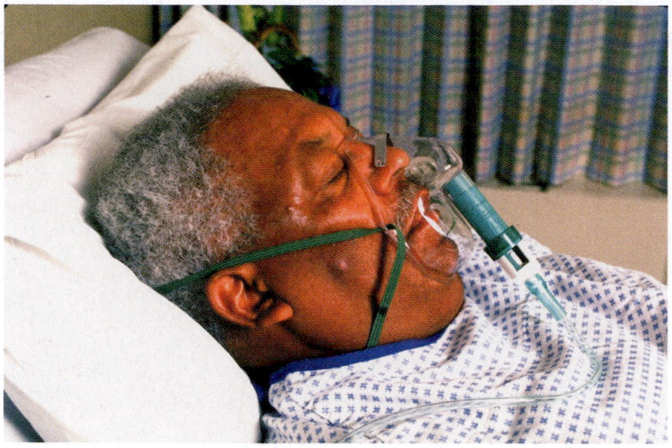

Figure 36.4 ■ Venturi mask, a high-flow oxygen delivery system.

clapping the chest wall with cupped hands, using rapid wrist flexion and extension. Cupping traps air between the palm and the patient's skin, setting up vibrations through the chest wall that loosen respiratory secretions. The trapped air also provides a cushion, preventing injury. When performed correctly, percussion produces a hollow, popping sound. Percussion may also be done using a mechanical percussion cup, vibration modes on certain hospital beds, or via a vest or chest wrap. The breasts, sternum, spinal column, and kidney regions are avoided during percussion.

Vibration facilitates secretion movement into larger airways. It is usually combined with percussion, although it may be used when percussion is contraindicated or poorly tolerated. Vibration is performed by repeatedly tensing the arm and hand muscles while maintaining firm but gentle pressure over the affected area with the flat of the hand.

Percussion and vibration are done in conjunction with *postural drainage*, which uses gravity to facilitate removal of secretions from a particular lung segment. The patient is positioned with the segment to be drained superior to or above the trachea or mainstem bronchus. Drainage of all lung segments requires a variety of positions (**Figure 36.5** ■); rarely do all segments require drainage. Bronchodilators or nebulizer (device that delivers medication via inhaled mist) treatments are administered as ordered prior to postural drainage. It is best to perform postural drainage before meals to avoid nausea and vomiting.

Integrative Therapies

Although complementary therapies do not replace conventional treatment for pneumonia, they often promote comfort and speed recovery. The herb echinacea is widely used to stimulate immune function and treat upper respiratory infections (URIs). Because viral URIs often precede pneumonia, it may be helpful in preventing pneumonia. Past research, however, shows mixed results for the effectiveness of echinacea in reducing the duration and severity of URI (National Center for Complementary and Integrative Health [NCCIH], 2015). Goldenseal, which is often sold in combination with echinacea, is used to treat bacterial, fungal, and protozoal infections of the mucous membranes of the respiratory tract.

Advise patients inquiring about the use of traditional Chinese medicine to reduce pneumonia symptoms to consult a qualified, trained practitioner first and determine if any of the products contain *ma huang* (a form of ephedra) or ephedra (University of Maryland Medical Center, 2016). Patients should avoid these products, which are banned in the United States, because ephedra use is linked to significant safety risks.

Nursing Care

Additional measures to screen for and detect pneumonia in older adults are appropriate. Frequent pulmonary assessment and aggressive interventions help prevent problems. Restoring and maintaining mobility improves ventilation and helps mobilize secretions. Promoting adequate fluid intake liquefies secretions, making them easier to expectorate.

Assessment

See the Manifestations and Interprofessional Care sections for the assessment of the patient with pneumonia.

Focused assessment of the patient with pneumonia includes:

- ***Health history:*** Current symptoms and their duration; presence of shortness of breath or difficulty breathing, chest pain and its relationship to breathing; cough, productive or nonproductive, color, consistency of sputum; other symptoms; recent upper respiratory or other acute illness; chronic diseases such as diabetes, chronic lung disease, or heart disease; current medications; medication allergies
- ***Physical assessment:*** Presentation, apparent distress, level of consciousness; vital signs including temperature; skin color, temperature; respiratory excursion, use of accessory muscles of respiration; lung sounds
- ***Laboratory data:*** WBC with differential, sputum Gram stain, culture and sensitivity, chest x-ray or CT scan.

Priorities of Care

Collaborate with the interprofessional team to ensure adequate treatment of the pneumonia infectious process while providing care that supports the physical and psychologic responses to the disorder throughout the acute and rehabilitative phases of care is a priority of nursing care.

Diagnoses, Interventions, and Outcomes

Patients with lower respiratory disorders such as pneumonia may have multiple nursing care needs, depending

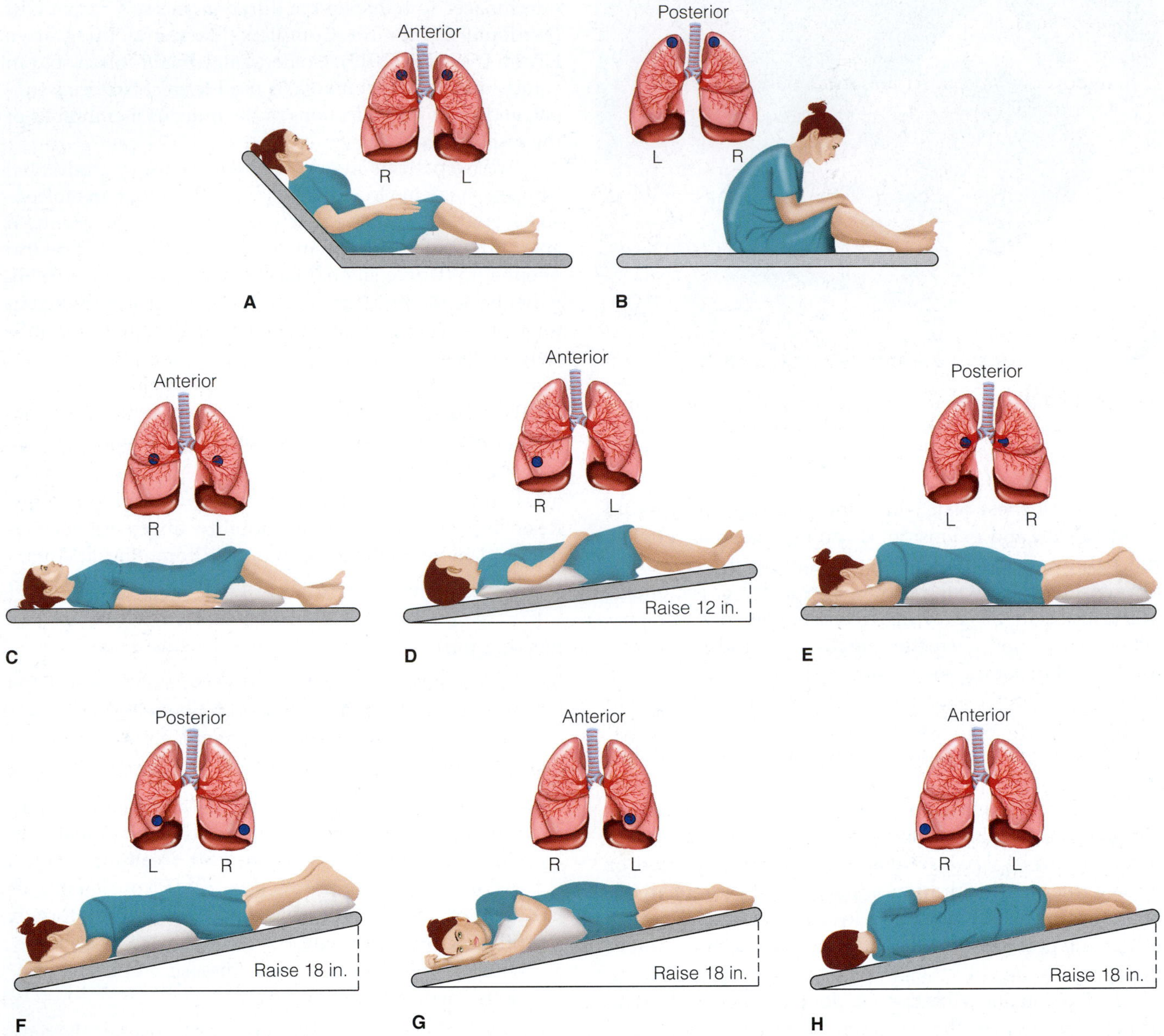
Anterior
R
L
A
Posterior
L
R
B
Anterior
R
L
C
Anterior
R
L
Raise 12 in.
D
Posterior
L
R
E
Posterior
L
R
Raise 18 in.
F
Anterior
R
L
Raise 18 in.
G
Anterior
R
L
Raise 18 in.
H

Figure 36.5 ■ Positions for postural drainage. A, Left and right anterior apical. B, Left and right posterior apical. C, Left and right anterior upper. D, Right middle lobe. E, Superior lower lobes. F, Left and right lower posterior. G, Left lower lateral. H, Right lower lateral.

on the severity of the illness. Alveolar ventilation and the process of alveolar respiration can be affected by inflammation and secretions. **Hypoxemia**, low levels of oxygen in the blood, and tissue hypoxia may result. Nursing care focuses on maintaining airway patency, supporting optimal respiratory function, and promoting rest to reduce metabolic and oxygen needs.

Promote Airway Clearance and Patency. The inflammatory response to infection causes tissue edema and exudate formation. In the lungs, the inflammatory response can narrow and potentially obstruct bronchial passages and alveoli. Assessment findings include adventitious breath sounds such as crackles (rales), rhonchi, and wheezes; dyspnea and tachypnea; coughing; and indicators of hypoxia such as cyanosis, reduced SaO_2 levels, anxiety, and apprehension.

Expected Outcome: Patient will use techniques to promote airway clearance such as coughing and deep breathing.

The nurse will:

- Assess respiratory status, including vital signs, breath sounds, SaO_2, and skin color at least every 4 hours. *Early identification of respiratory compromise allows intervention before tissue hypoxia is significant.*
- Assess cough and sputum (amount, color, consistency, and possible odor). *Assessment of the cough and nature*

of sputum produced allows evaluation of the effectiveness of respiratory clearance and the response to therapy.

- Monitor arterial blood gas results; report increasing hypoxemia and other abnormal results to the healthcare provider. *Blood gas changes may be an early indicator of impaired gas exchange due to airway narrowing or obstruction.*
- Place in Fowler or high-Fowler position. Encourage frequent position changes and ambulation as allowed. *The upright position promotes lung expansion; position changes and ambulation facilitate the movement of secretions.*
- Assist to cough, deep breathe, and use assistive devices. Provide endotracheal suctioning using aseptic technique as ordered. *Coughing, deep breathing, and suctioning help clear airways.*
- Provide a fluid intake of at least 2500 to 3000 mL/day. *A liberal fluid intake helps liquefy secretions, facilitating their clearance.*
- Work with the healthcare provider and respiratory therapist to provide pulmonary hygiene measures, such as incentive spirometry, postural drainage, percussion, and vibration. *These techniques help mobilize and clear secretions.*
- Administer prescribed medications as ordered, and monitor their effects. *If the infecting organism is resistant to the prescribed antibiotic, little improvement may be seen with treatment. Bronchodilators help maintain open airways but may have adverse effects such as anxiety and restlessness.*

Promote Effective Breathing. Pleural inflammation often accompanies pneumonia, causing sharp localized pain that increases with deep breathing, coughing, and movement, which can lead to rapid and shallow breathing. Distal airways and alveoli may not expand optimally with each breath, increasing the risk for atelectasis and decreasing gas exchange. Fatigue from the increased work of breathing is an additional problem in pneumonia. This, too, can lead to decreased lung inflation and an ineffective breathing pattern.

Expected Outcome: Patient will utilize techniques to promote adequate ventilation such as deep breathing and incentive spirometry.

The nurse will:

- Assess respiratory rate, depth, and lung sounds at least every 4 hours. *Tachypnea and diminished or adventitious breath sounds may be early indicators of respiratory compromise.*
- Provide for rest periods. *Rest reduces metabolic demands, fatigue, and the work of breathing, promoting a more effective breathing pattern.*
- Assess for pleuritic discomfort. Provide analgesics as ordered. *Adequate pain relief minimizes splinting and promotes adequate ventilation.*
- Provide reassurance during periods of respiratory distress. *Hypoxia and respiratory distress produce high levels of anxiety, which tends to further increase tachypnea and fatigue and decrease ventilation.*
- Administer oxygen as ordered. *Oxygen therapy increases the alveolar oxygen concentration and facilitates its diffusion across the alveolar-capillary membrane, reducing hypoxia and anxiety.*
- Teach slow abdominal breathing. *This breathing pattern promotes lung expansion.*
- Teach use of relaxation techniques, such as visualization and meditation. *These techniques help reduce anxiety and slow the breathing pattern.*

Reduce Energy Demands. Impaired airway clearance and gas exchange interfere with oxygen delivery to body cells and tissues. At the same time, the infectious process and the body's response to it increase metabolic demands on the cells. The net result of this imbalance between oxygen delivery and oxygen demand is a lack of physiologic energy to maintain normal daily activities.

Expected Outcome: Patient will participate in physical activity as tolerated.

The nurse will:

- Assess activity tolerance, noting any increase in pulse, respirations, dyspnea, diaphoresis, or cyanosis. *These assessment findings may indicate limited or impaired activity tolerance.*
- Assist with self-care activities, such as bathing. *Assistance with ADLs reduces energy demands.*
- Schedule activities, planning for rest periods. *Rest periods minimize fatigue and improve activity tolerance.*
- Provide assistive devices, such as an overhead trapeze. *These assistive devices facilitate movement and reduce energy demands.*
- Enlist the family's help to minimize stress and anxiety levels. *Stress and anxiety increase metabolic demands and can decrease activity tolerance.*
- Perform active or passive ROM exercises. *Exercises help maintain muscle tone and joint mobility and prevent contractures if bedrest is prolonged.*
- Provide emotional support and reassurance that strength and energy will return to normal when the infectious process has resolved and the balance of oxygen supply and demand is restored. *The patient may be concerned that activity intolerance will continue to be a problem after the acute infection is resolved.*

SAFETY ALERT: Activity intolerance may be an early sign of cardiorespiratory compromise, particularly in the older adult or patient with preexisting heart disease. New or worsening manifestations of activity intolerance should be reported to the healthcare provider. ■

Delegating Nursing Care Activities

As appropriate and allowed by the designated duties and responsibilities of unlicensed assistive personnel, the nurse may delegate nursing care activities such as measuring vital signs, encouraging oral or enteral fluid intake, and providing skin care.

Transitions of Care

Prevention is a key component in managing pneumonia. Identifying vulnerable populations and instituting preventative strategies are measures to reduce the mortality and morbidity associated with pneumonia. Health promotion activities focus on pneumonia prevention. Make patients in high-risk groups aware of the benefits of immunizations against influenza and pneumococcal pneumonia. A single dose of pneumococcus vaccine usually produces immunity to most strains of pneumococcal pneumonia, although repeat doses may be needed for older adults and people who are immunosuppressed. (Pneumococcal vaccine is contraindicated for people receiving immunosuppressive therapy.) Annual influenza vaccine helps prevent pneumonia because pneumonia often occurs as a sequela to influenza.

Patients require hospitalization for severe disease that compromises respiratory status. Manifestations of respiratory compromise include altered mental status, tachypnea, tachycardia, hypotension, hypo- or hyperthermia, and altered blood gases. Hospitalization may be necessary prior to respiratory compromise if risk factors such as advanced age and/or coexisting heart, kidney, or liver disease are present.

Most patients with pneumonia are treated in the community. Discuss the following topics when preparing the patient and family for home care:

- The importance of completing the prescribed medication regimen as ordered; potential drug side effects and their management, including manifestations that necessitate stopping the drug and notifying the healthcare provider
- Recommendations for limiting activities and increasing rest
- Maintaining adequate fluid intake to keep mucus thin for easier expectoration
- Ways to maintain adequate nutritional intake, such as small, frequent, well-balanced meals
- The importance of avoiding smoking or exposure to secondhand smoke to prevent further irritation of the lungs
- Manifestations to report to the healthcare provider, such as increasing shortness of breath, difficulty breathing, increased fever, fatigue, headache, sleepiness, or confusion
- The importance of keeping all follow-up appointments to ensure the pneumonia resolves.

Patients with respiratory compromise or who are older or debilitated may require home healthcare assistance to remain at home. Provide referrals for home health nursing and home maintenance services as indicated. Community services such as Meals on Wheels can provide support to reduce the energy demands of meal preparation.

The accompanying Case Study & Nursing Care Plan provides further nursing interventions for patients treated in the community.

The Patient with Severe Acute Respiratory Syndrome

Severe acute respiratory syndrome (SARS) is a lower respiratory illness of unknown etiology first described in people in Asia in February 2003. There have been no reported cases worldwide since 2004. Cases were identified in patients in North America, South America, Europe, and Asia before the 2003 outbreak was contained (CDC, 2017c). The primary population affected by SARS is previously healthy adults ages 25 to 70 years. In 2012, Middle East respiratory syndrome (MERS), a new SARS-like coronavirus, was identified (World Health Organization, 2017b). Genomic testing revealed the novel virus is closely related to the SARS virus. Vaccine development is under way (National Institute of Allergy and Infectious Diseases [NIAID], 2017).

Pathophysiology

A coronavirus not previously identified in humans is the infective agent responsible for SARS. This virus appears to spread primarily by contact with respiratory secretions. Other potential sources of the infection are through direct contact with an infected person or contaminated object and exposure of the eyes or mucous membranes to respiratory secretions (CDC, 2017c). Contact with contaminated water or sewage may transmit the disease, suggesting a fecal–oral transmission route as well.

The virus infects cells of the respiratory tract, leading to surface necrosis and sloughing of pneumocytes in the alveolar spaces and formation of hyaline membranes (a fibrin and protein film that interferes with gas exchange within the alveoli). The alveolar damage is accompanied by inflammation of interstitial pulmonary tissues with infiltration by lymphocytes and monocytes. The virus is also found in the blood, urine, and feces.

Manifestations

The incubation period for SARS generally has been 2 to 7 days, although in some people incubation has taken as long as 10 days. Fever higher than 38°C (100.4°F) is typically the initial manifestation of the disease. After 1 to 2 days, respiratory manifestations of SARS develop, including nonproductive cough, shortness of breath, dyspnea, and possible hypoxemia.

Complications

Respiratory symptoms may worsen, progressing to respiratory distress, during the second week of the illness. Acute respiratory distress syndrome (ARDS) or multiorgan dysfunction (refer to Chapter 11) may develop. The overall mortality rate for SARS is about 11%. The disease is less severe in children than in adults (CDC, 2017c).

Interprofessional Care

Prompt identification of SARS or related novel respiratory viruses, infection control measures, and reporting of the disease are vital to control these potentially fatal diseases. Healthcare providers and public health personnel should report cases of SARS or other nonpathogen-identified cases

Case Study & Nursing Care Plan

A Patient with Pneumonia

Mary O'Neal is a 35-year-old executive assistant and a part-time college student. On returning home from class one evening, she begins to feel chilled. She alternates between chills and sweats all night. Staying home from work, she remains in bed most of the next day. Her fever continues, and she develops a cough and dull aching chest pain. When the cough becomes productive of rust-colored sputum the following day, she seeks medical treatment from her family physician.

ASSESSMENT

Debby Kowalski, RN, the family practice clinic nurse, admits Mrs. O'Neal to the clinic and obtains the nursing assessment. Mrs. O'Neal denies any previous history of respiratory diseases "other than the usual colds, flu, and such." She also denies any history of smoking or medication allergies. She says her symptoms began abruptly with the onset of the chills. She describes her chest pain as a dull ache that was initially substernal but now is localized in her lower lateral right chest. The pain increases with deep breathing, coughing, and moving. Her cough is increasing in frequency and severity, and her sputum appears rusty brown. Her vital signs are BP 116/74 mmHg, P 104 bpm and regular, R 26/min, T 38.7°C (101.8°F). Skin is warm and flushed, with no evidence of cyanosis. Respirations shallow, unlabored; respiratory excursion equal. Diminished breath sounds in bases bilaterally, crackles noted in right posterior and lateral base. Faint pleural rub heard at right midaxillary line.

A STAT CBC shows a WBC of 18,900/mm^3; differential shows increased numbers of neutrophils and immature WBCs (bands). Ms. Kowalski has Mrs. O'Neal rinse with an antiseptic mouthwash and collect a sputum specimen for culture and Gram stain prior to seeing the healthcare provider.

The healthcare provider orders a chest x-ray after examining Mrs. O'Neal. Based on her history, examination, and the chest x-ray, he makes the diagnosis of acute bacterial pneumonia, probably pneumococcal. He prescribes oral penicillin V, 500 mg every 6 hours for 10 days. He asks Mrs. O'Neal to return for a follow-up appointment in 10 days and refers her back to Ms. Kowalski for appropriate teaching.

DIAGNOSIS

- Decreased ability to deeply breathe due to pleuritic chest pain
- Fever related to infection
- Insufficient knowledge related to diagnosis of pneumonia and its treatment

EXPECTED OUTCOMES

- Patient will maintain normal pulmonary function.
- Patient will describe measures to minimize elevations in body temperature.
- Patient will identify a schedule for taking her medication that will facilitate compliance with the regimen.
- Patient will describe manifestations that should be reported to the healthcare provider.

PLANNING AND IMPLEMENTATION

- Assess knowledge and understanding of pneumonia and its effects.
- Assist to develop a medication schedule that coordinates with normal daily routine.
- Teach about the following:
  a. Importance of avoiding use of a cough suppressant except at night to facilitate rest
  b. Ways to increase fluid intake to reduce fever and maintain thin mucus for easy expectoration
  c. Beneficial effects of rest, especially during the acute phase of her illness
  d. Safe use of aspirin and acetaminophen to reduce fever
  e. Importance of taking all prescribed medication doses as scheduled
  f. Common side effects of penicillin V and their management
  g. Early manifestations of penicillin allergy that necessitate stopping the medication and notifying the healthcare provider
  h. Signs of complications of pneumonia or worsening pneumonia to report.

EVALUATION

The sputum culture confirms *S. pneumoniae* as the cause of Mrs. O'Neal's pneumonia. When she returns for her follow-up appointment, she reports that she began to feel better after 2 days on the penicillin and returned to work the following Monday. Her examination reveals good breath sounds throughout with no adventitious sounds.

CLINICAL REASONING IN PATIENT CARE

1. Do any of the factors identified in the case study increase Mrs. O'Neal's risk for acute bacterial pneumonia?
2. Mrs. O'Neal's WBC differential showed increased neutrophil and band counts. Describe the reason for and effect of this change.
3. Even though Mrs. O'Neal has no history of medication allergies, anaphylactic shock remains a potential risk. Describe the sequence of events leading to anaphylactic shock, its initial symptoms, and immediate nursing interventions.
4. Had Mrs. O'Neal required hospitalization to treat her acute pneumonia, interruption of her usual activities and responsibilities could lead to anxiety. Develop a care plan for this situation.

See Evaluating Your Response in Appendix B.

to state and local health departments to determine if a novel virus may be the cause.

Infection Control

Because healthcare workers are at risk for developing SARS after caring for infected patients, infection control precautions should be immediately instituted if SARS is suspected. Standard precautions (see Appendix A) are implemented along with contact and airborne precautions. The CDC (2017c) recommends hand hygiene, gown, gloves, eye protection, and an N95 respirator to prevent transmission of SARS/novel coronavirus in healthcare settings.

When patients with SARS/novel coronavirus are managed in the community, they are advised to remain home for 10 days after the fever has resolved and until respiratory symptoms are absent or minimal. Members of the household are advised to wash hands frequently or use alcohol-based hand rubs. The patient is advised to cover the mouth and nose with tissue when coughing or sneezing and to wear a surgical mask during close contact with uninfected people. Sharing of utensils, towels, and bedding should be avoided. Routine cleaning (e.g., washing with soap and hot water) is adequate to disinfect objects and no special precautions are necessary for disposing of waste.

Treatments

Care of the patient with SARS/novel coronavirus is supportive. Oxygen may be administered to treat hypoxemia. Intubation and mechanical ventilation may be required if respiratory failure or acute respiratory distress syndrome (ARDS) develops.

The Patient with a Lung Abscess

A **lung abscess** is a localized area of lung destruction or necrosis and pus formation. The most common cause of lung abscess is aspiration and resulting pneumonia. Risk factors, therefore, are those for aspiration: Decreased level of consciousness due to anesthesia, injury or disease of the central nervous system (CNS), seizure, excessive sedation, or alcohol abuse; swallowing disorders; dental caries; and debilitation secondary to cancer or chronic disease. Lung abscess may also occur as a complication of some types of pneumonia, including those due to *Staphylococcus aureus*, *Klebsiella*, and *Legionella*.

Pathophysiology

A lung abscess forms after lung tissue becomes consolidated (i.e., after alveoli become filled with fluid, pus, and microorganisms). In up to 89% of patients, anaerobic organisms are identified. Consolidated tissue becomes necrotic. This necrotic process can spread to involve the entire bronchopulmonary segment and progress proximally until it ruptures into a bronchus. With rupture, the contents of the abscess empty into the bronchus, leaving a cavity filled with air and fluid, a process known as *cavitation*. If purulent material from the abscess is not expectorated, the infection may spread, leading to diffuse pneumonia or a syndrome similar to acute respiratory distress syndrome (discussed in Chapter 37).

Risk Factors

Risk for development of lung abscess is seen in those who abuse alcohol, in post-pneumonia patients, and in those who are immunocompromised (i.e., persons with cancer or HIV, organ transplant recipients, or persons with autoimmune disease).

Manifestations

Manifestations of lung abscess typically develop about 2 weeks after the precipitating event (aspiration, pneumonia, and so on). Onset may be either acute or insidious. Early symptoms are those of pneumonia: Productive cough, chills and fever, pleuritic chest pain, malaise, and anorexia. The temperature may be significantly elevated, 39.4°C (103°F) or higher. When the abscess ruptures, the patient may expectorate large amounts of foul-smelling, purulent, and possibly blood-streaked sputum. Breath sounds are diminished, and crackles may be noted in the region of the abscess. A dull percussion tone is also present.

Complications

Empyema (purulent exudate in the chest cavity) is the most common complication of a lung abscess. Lower-risk complications include hemoptysis and bronchoscopy-related aspiration.

Interprofessional Care

Diagnosis

The diagnosis of lung abscess is usually based on the history and presentation. The CBC may indicate leukocytosis. Sputum culture may not show the organism involved unless rupture occurs. Chest x-ray shows a thick-walled, solitary cavity with surrounding consolidation, although differentiating lung abscess from consolidation can be difficult until cavitation occurs.

Medications

Lung abscess is treated with antibiotic therapy, usually intravenous clindamycin (Cleocin), amoxicillin-clavulanate (Augmentin), or penicillin. Antibiotic therapy should be continued until the chest radiograph improves, usually at least 1 month.

Surgery

Postural drainage may be ordered to relieve obstruction and promote drainage. In some cases, bronchoscopy is used to drain the abscess. If the pleural space becomes involved, a chest tube (*tube thoracostomy*) may be used to drain the abscess. See the section on pneumothorax for further discussion of chest tubes.

Nursing Care

Assessment

See the Manifestations and Interprofessional Care sections for the assessment of the patient with a lung abscess.

Priorities of Care

Although most patients with lung abscess recover fully with appropriate antibiotic treatment, rupture and drainage of the abscess into a bronchus is a frightening experience. Nursing care needs of the patient relate primarily to maintaining a patent airway and adequate gas exchange.

Diagnoses, Interventions, and Outcomes

In addition to promoting airway clearance and patency and effective gas exchange, appropriate nursing interventions for the patient with a lung abscess will include:

- Administering antipyretics and other interventions to reduce hyperthermia related to the infectious process.
- Intervening to reduce anxiety by encouraging distraction and other nonpharmacologic techniques. If necessary, administer anxiolytics as ordered.
- Promoting patient comfort, sleep, and rest.

Patient and family teaching focuses on the importance of completing the prescribed antibiotic therapy. Most lung abscesses are successfully treated with antibiotics; however, treatment may last up to 1 month or more. Emphasize the importance of completing the entire course of therapy to eliminate the infecting organisms. Teach about the medication, including the name, dose, and desired and adverse effects. Stress the need to contact the healthcare provider if symptoms do not improve or if they become worse. Infection from lung abscess can spread not only to lung and pleural tissue but systemically, causing sepsis. If postural drainage is ordered, teach the patient and family how to perform this procedure. When procedures such as bronchoscopy or thoracostomy are performed to drain the abscess, provide preoperative teaching and instruction on postoperative care.

Delegating Nursing Care Activities

As appropriate and allowed by the designated duties and responsibilities of unlicensed assistive personnel, the nurse may delegate nursing care activities such as measuring vital signs, encouraging oral or enteral fluid intake, and providing skin care.

Transitions of Care

Nursing care for the patient focuses on education including appropriate pain control measures, oxygen therapy use and safety (if indicated), importance of rehydration (oral or IV fluids), and postural drainage techniques (if indicated). As most patients with a lung abscess are treated with antibiotics that resolve the underlying infection, patients should be reminded to complete the full course of antibiotics as prescribed. IV antibiotics may be prescribed for 2 to 3 weeks (involving home health care), followed by oral antibiotics for an additional 1 to 2 months. Teaching should also focus on any postoperative management, as indicated. Reassure the patient that the cure rate is more than 90% with antibiotic therapy.

The Patient with Tuberculosis

Tuberculosis (TB) is a chronic, recurrent infectious disease that usually affects the lungs, although any organ can be affected. Caused by *Mycobacterium tuberculosis*, TB is uncommon in the United States, especially among young adults of European descent.

M. tuberculosis is a relatively slow-growing, slender, rod-shaped, acid-fast organism with a waxy outer capsule, which increases its resistance to destruction. Although the lungs are usually infected, TB can involve other organs as well. It is transmitted by *droplet nuclei*, airborne droplets produced when an infected person coughs, sneezes, speaks, or sings. The tiny droplets can remain suspended in air for several hours. Infection may develop when a susceptible host breathes in air containing droplet nuclei and the contaminated particles elude the normal defenses of the upper respiratory tract to reach the alveoli.

Incidence and Prevalence

The incidence of TB fell steadily until the mid-1980s, thanks to improved sanitation, surveillance, and treatment of people with active disease. The late 1980s and early 1990s saw a resurgence of the disease, attributed primarily to the HIV/AIDS epidemic, the emergence of multiple-drug-resistant (MDR) strains of TB, and social factors such as immigration, poverty, homelessness, and drug abuse. Since the mid-1990s, TB rates have declined. In 2017 the CDC reported a 2.9% decrease from 2016 (CDC, 2017d). This decline can be attributed to TB-control programs that emphasize promptly identifying new cases and initiating and completing appropriate therapy.

Worldwide, TB continues to be a significant health problem, with an estimated 1.5 billion people (one-quarter of the world's population) infected by *M. tuberculosis*. An estimated 10.4 million cases of TB develop annually, with the majority (64%) occurring in the developing countries of Asia, Africa, the Middle East, and Latin America. TB accounts for an estimated 1.7 million deaths each year, with 40% of HIV deaths due to TB (World Health Organization, 2017c).

Today, TB in the United States primarily affects immigrants, those infected with HIV, and disadvantaged populations. See the Focus on Cultural Diversity box regarding the primary populations affected by TB. Poor urban areas—areas that are also affected by the epidemics of injection drug use, homelessness, malnutrition, and poor living conditions—are hit the hardest. Overcrowded institutions also contribute to the spread of TB; transmission in hospitals, homeless shelters, drug treatment centers, prisons, and residential facilities has been documented. People with altered immune function, including older adults and people with AIDS, are at particular risk for TB. Some strains of *M. tuberculosis* have become resistant to the first-line drugs used to treat the disease (isoniazid and rifampin), with the highest number of MDR TB cases at 18.7% in 2016 (CDC, 2017d, 2017e). In 2006, the WHO added the category of extensively drug-resistant TB (XDR TB) to describe the rare TB case that is resistant to the first-line TB drugs, as well as at least one of the second-line TB drugs (kanamycin, capreomycin, or amikacin) and at least one drug in the quinolone antibiotic subclass (CDC, 2017d, 2017e). Of MDR TB strains identified worldwide, 6.2% are XDR (WHO, 2017). Only one case of XDR TB was reported in the United States in 2016 (CDC, 2017d, 2017e).

Focus on Cultural Diversity

Tuberculosis

- The TB case rate for foreign-born U.S. residents is 14 times higher than that for people born in the United States (CDC, 2017d, 2017e).
- People from Asian and the Pacific Islands living in the United States have the highest case rates (18%) (CDC, 2017d, 2017e).

Pathophysiology

Tuberculosis is a systemic disease that manifests in specific ways across the organ systems. However, TB is most commonly thought of as a pulmonary disease. Extrapulmonary manifestations of TB are also discussed in this chapter.

Pulmonary Tuberculosis

Minute droplet nuclei containing one to three bacilli that elude upper airway defense systems to enter the lungs implant in an alveolus or respiratory bronchiole, usually in an upper lobe. As the bacteria multiply, they cause a local inflammatory response. The inflammatory response brings neutrophils and macrophages to the site. These phagocytic cells surround and engulf the bacilli, isolating them and preventing their spread. *M. tuberculosis* continues to slowly multiply; some mycobacteria enter the lymphatic system to stimulate a cellular-mediated immune response (refer to Chapter 13 to review immune responses). Neutrophils and macrophages isolate the bacteria but cannot destroy them. A granulomatous lesion called a *tubercle*, a sealed-off colony of bacilli, is formed. Within the tubercle, infected tissue dies, forming a cheeselike center, a process called *caseation necrosis*.

If the immune response is adequate, scar tissue develops around the tubercle, and the bacilli remain encapsulated. These lesions eventually calcify and are visible on x-ray. The patient, while infected by *M. tuberculosis*, does not develop TB disease. If the immune response is inadequate to contain the bacilli, the disease of TB can develop. Occasionally, the infection can progress, leading to extensive destruction of lung tissue. In *primary tuberculosis*, granulomatous tissue may erode into a bronchus or into a blood vessel, allowing the disease to spread throughout the lung or other organs. This severe form of TB is uncommon in adults (Sorenson, Quinn, & Klein, 2019).

A previously healed TB lesion may be reactivated. *Reactivation tuberculosis* occurs when the immune system is suppressed due to age, disease, or use of immunosuppressive drugs. The extent of lung disease can vary from small lesions to extensive cavitation of lung tissue. Tubercles rupture, spreading bacilli into the airways to form satellite lesions and produce tuberculosis pneumonia. Without treatment, massive lung involvement can lead to death, or a more chronic process of tubercle formation and cavitation may result. People with chronic disease continue to spread *M. tuberculosis* into the environment, potentially infecting others. The Pathophysiology Illustrated feature on pages 1297–1298 illustrates the pathogenesis of TB.

Patients with HIV disease are at high risk for developing active TB, due to primary infection or reactivation. HIV infection suppresses cellular immunity, which is vital to limiting the replication and spread of *M. tuberculosis*.

Extrapulmonary Tuberculosis

When primary disease or reactivation allows live bacilli to enter the bronchi, the disease may spread through the blood and lymph system to other organs. These distant disease metastases may produce an active lesion or they may become dormant and reactivate at a later time. Extrapulmonary TB is especially prevalent in people with HIV disease.

Miliary Tuberculosis. *Miliary tuberculosis* results from hematogenous spread (through the blood) of the bacilli throughout the body. Miliary tuberculosis causes chills and fever, weakness, malaise, and progressive dyspnea. Multiple lesions evenly distributed throughout the lungs are noted on x-ray. The sputum rarely contains organisms. The bone marrow is usually involved, causing anemia, thrombocytopenia, and leukocytosis. Without appropriate treatment, the prognosis is poor.

Genitourinary Tuberculosis. The kidney and genitourinary tract are common extrapulmonary sites for TB. The organism spreads to the kidney through the blood, initiating an inflammatory process similar to that which occurs in the lungs. Reactivation can occur years after the original infection. As the lesion then enlarges and caseates, a large portion of the renal parenchyma is destroyed. The infection can then spread to the rest of the urinary tract, including the ureters and bladder. Scarring and strictures commonly result. In men, the prostate, seminal vesicles, and epididymis may be involved. In women, TB may affect the fallopian tubes and ovaries.

Manifestations of genitourinary tuberculosis develop insidiously. Symptoms of a urinary tract infection, including malaise, dysuria, hematuria, and pyuria, develop. Flank pain may be present. Men may develop manifestations of epididymitis or prostatitis: Perineal, sacral, or scrotal pain and tenderness; difficulty voiding; and fever. Women may have manifestations of pelvic inflammatory disease, impaired fertility, or ectopic pregnancy.

Tuberculosis Meningitis. Tuberculosis meningitis results when TB spreads to the subarachnoid space. In the United States, this complication most often affects older adults, usually from reactivation of latent disease. Manifestations develop gradually, with listlessness, irritability, anorexia, and fever. Headache and behavior changes are common early symptoms in the older adult. As the disease progresses, the headache increases in intensity, vomiting develops, and the level of consciousness decreases. Convulsions and coma may follow. Without appropriate treatment, neurologic effects may become permanent.

Skeletal Tuberculosis. TB of the bones and joints is most likely to occur during childhood, when bone epiphyses are open and their blood supply is rich. The organisms spread via the blood to vertebrae, the ends of long bones, and joints.

Pathophysiology Illustrated
The Pathogenesis of Tuberculosis

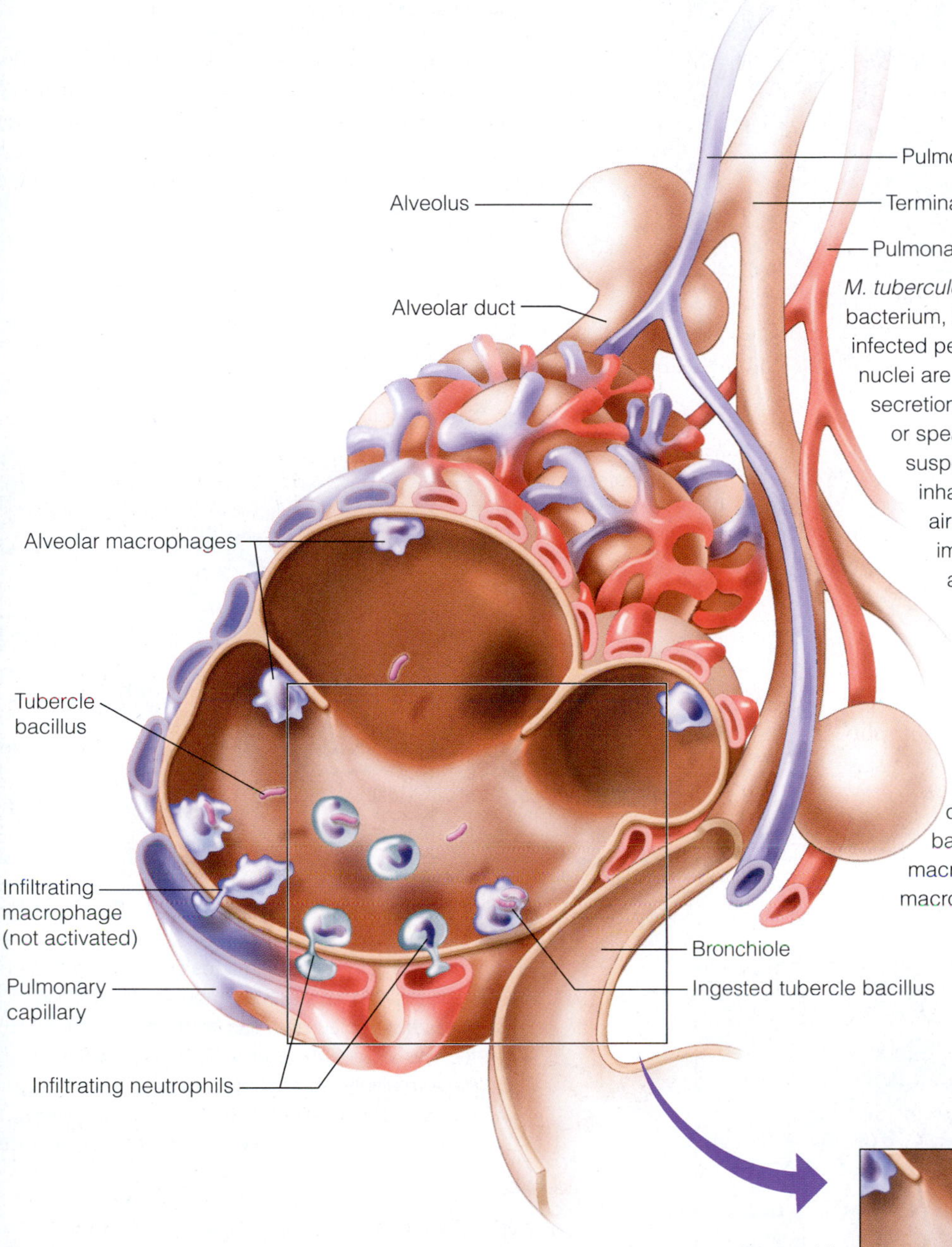

Pulmonary arteriole
Terminal bronchiole
Pulmonary venule
Alveolus
Alveolar duct
Alveolar macrophages
Tubercle bacillus
Infiltrating macrophage (not activated)
Pulmonary capillary
Infiltrating neutrophils
Bronchiole
Ingested tubercle bacillus

M. tuberculosis, a rod-shaped aerobic bacterium, is spread via droplet nuclei from an infected person to a susceptible host. Droplet nuclei are tiny droplets of respiratory secretions spread via coughing, sneezing, or speaking. When dried, they can remain suspended in air for several hours. Most inhaled bacilli are trapped in the upper airways; those reaching distal airways implant in the respiratory bronchioles and alveoli. Rarely, these tubercle bacilli multiply unchecked to cause primary tuberculosis. In most cases, activated alveolar macrophages ingest the bacilli. The bacilli may be destroyed; however, unique characteristics of the tuberculosis bacillus resist its destruction by the macrophage. The bacilli multiply within the macrophage, eventually killing the macrophage.

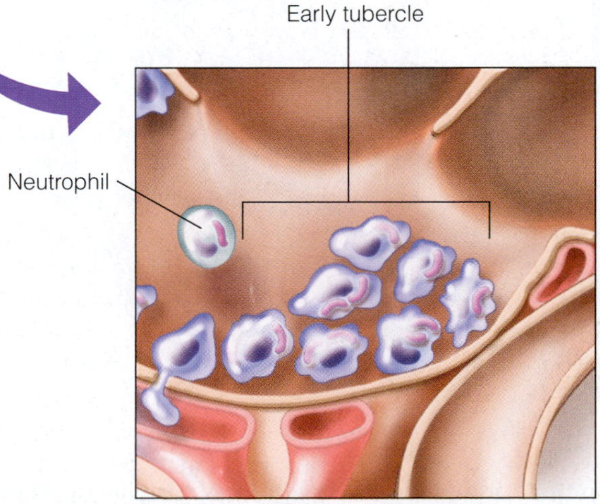

Early tubercle
Neutrophil

The dead macrophages lyse, releasing various chemotaxic factors into the bloodstream. Neutrophils and non-activated macrophages are attracted to the site. These phagocytic cells ingest the tubercle bacilli released from the lysed macrophages.

(continued)

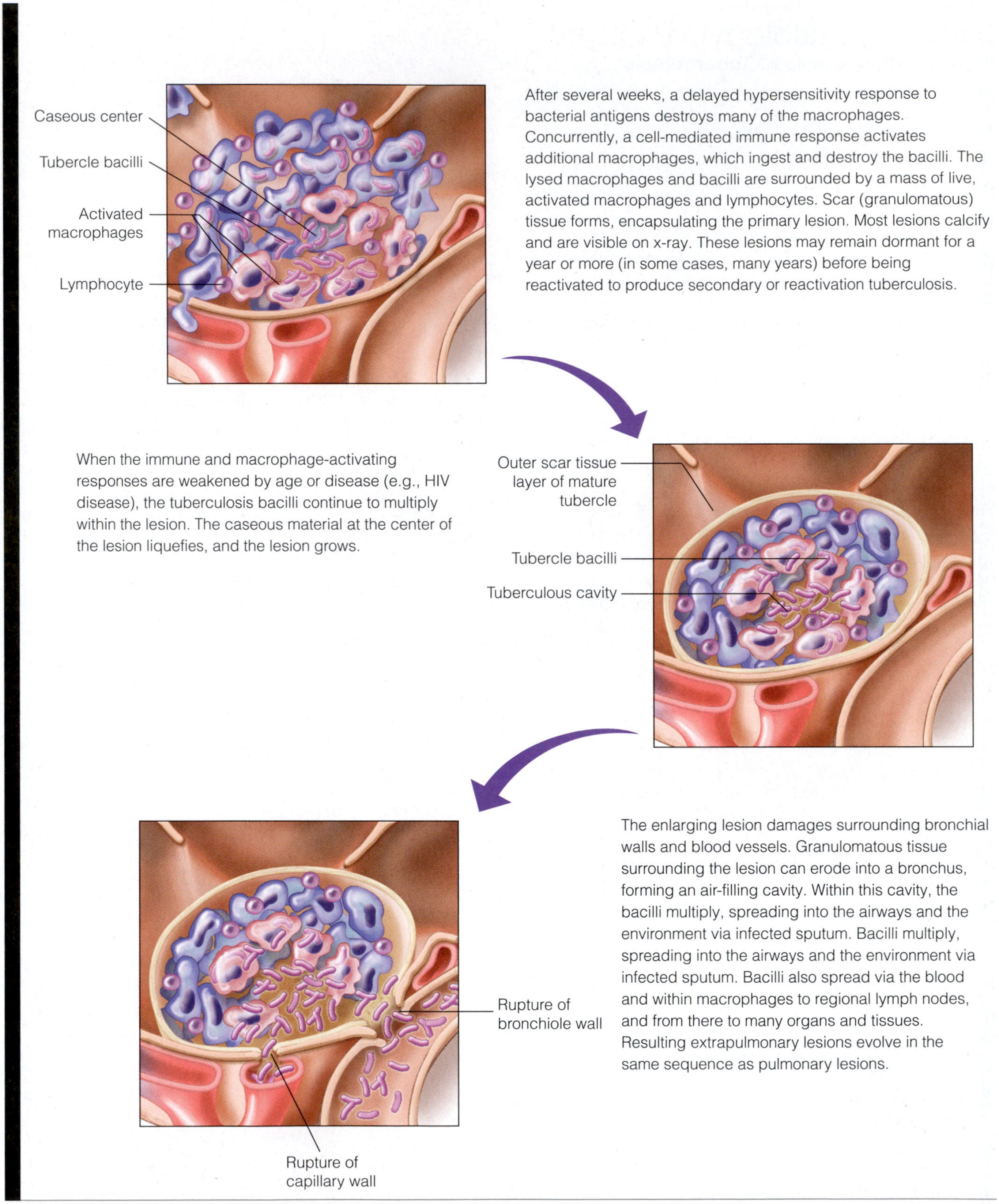
Caseous center
Tubercle bacilli
Activated macrophages
Lymphocyte
After several weeks, a delayed hypersensitivity response to bacterial antigens destroys many of the macrophages. Concurrently, a cell-mediated immune response activates additional macrophages, which ingest and destroy the bacilli. The lysed macrophages and bacilli are surrounded by a mass of live, activated macrophages and lymphocytes. Scar (granulomatous) tissue forms, encapsulating the primary lesion. Most lesions calcify and are visible on x-ray. These lesions may remain dormant for a year or more (in some cases, many years) before being reactivated to produce secondary or reactivation tuberculosis.
When the immune and macrophage-activating responses are weakened by age or disease (e.g., HIV disease), the tuberculosis bacilli continue to multiply within the lesion. The caseous material at the center of the lesion liquefies, and the lesion grows.
Outer scar tissue layer of mature tubercle
Tubercle bacilli
Tuberculous cavity
The enlarging lesion damages surrounding bronchial walls and blood vessels. Granulomatous tissue surrounding the lesion can erode into a bronchus, forming an air-filling cavity. Within this cavity, the bacilli multiply, spreading into the airways and the environment via infected sputum. Bacilli multiply, spreading into the airways and the environment via infected sputum. Bacilli also spread via the blood and within macrophages to regional lymph nodes, and from there to many organs and tissues. Resulting extrapulmonary lesions evolve in the same sequence as pulmonary lesions.
Rupture of bronchiole wall
Rupture of capillary wall

Immune and inflammatory processes isolate the bacilli, and the disease often becomes evident years or decades later.

Tuberculous spondylitis usually involves the thoracic vertebrae, eroding vertebral bodies and causing them to collapse. Significant kyphosis develops, and the spinal cord may be compressed. The large, weight-bearing joints (hips and knees) are most often affected by tuberculous arthritis, although other joints may be affected, particularly if they have been previously damaged. The involved joint is painful, warm, and tender.

Risk Factors

The risk for infection by *M. tuberculosis* is affected by characteristics of the infectious person, the extent of air contamination, duration of exposure, and susceptibility of the host. The number of microbes in the sputum, frequency and force of coughing, and behaviors such as covering the mouth when coughing affect the production of droplet nuclei. In a small, closed, or poorly ventilated space, droplet nuclei become more concentrated, increasing the risk of exposure. Prolonged contact, such as living in the same household, increases the risk. Less-than-optimal immune function—a problem for people in lower socioeconomic groups, injection drug users, the homeless, people with alcoholism, and people with HIV infection—increases the susceptibility of the host.

Manifestations

In pulmonary tuberculosis, the initial infection causes few symptoms and typically goes unnoticed until the tuberculin test becomes positive or calcified lesions are seen on chest x-ray. Manifestations of primary progressive or reactivation TB often develop insidiously and are initially nonspecific. Fatigue, weight loss, anorexia, low-grade afternoon fever, and night sweats are common. A dry cough develops, which later becomes productive of purulent and/or blood-tinged sputum. It is often at this stage that the patient seeks medical attention.

Complications

Tuberculosis empyema and bronchopleural fistula are the most serious complications of pulmonary TB. When a TB lesion ruptures, bacilli may contaminate the pleural space. Rupture also may allow air to enter the pleural space from the lung, causing pneumothorax.

Interprofessional Care

TB was a major public health concern earlier in this century, before the development of effective sanitation measures and drug treatment. Developing drug-resistant strains, susceptibility of people with HIV disease, and inadequate access to healthcare for high-risk populations contribute to the continuing significance of TB as a significant public health threat. Interprofessional care, therefore, focuses on:

- Early detection
- Accurate diagnosis
- Effective disease treatment
- Preventing TB spread to others.

Hospitalization is rarely required to treat TB. With appropriate treatment, patients become no longer infectious fairly rapidly. However, a patient with active TB may be admitted for a concurrent problem or a complication of the disease. Nurses and other healthcare workers are at risk for exposure if the disease has not yet been diagnosed. When a patient with TB is institutionalized, maintain respiratory isolation to minimize the risk of infection to other patients and to healthcare workers.

Failure to adhere to the prescribed treatment is a major problem in treating active TB: The patient can continue transmitting the disease to others, and drug-resistant strains of bacteria can develop when treatment is incomplete. TB must be reported to local and state public health departments; contacts are identified and examined. People who share living or work environments with the patient are tested and receive prophylactic treatment. Continuing contact with patients who have active TB is vital to ensure effective cure.

Screening

The tuberculin test is used to screen for TB infection. A cellular, or delayed hypersensitivity, response to *M. tuberculosis* develops within 3 to 10 weeks after the infection. Injecting a small amount of *purified protein derivative (PPD)* of tuberculin any time thereafter activates this response, attracting macrophages to the area and causing a pronounced local inflammatory response. The amount of induration surrounding the injection site is used to determine infection (see **Figure 36.6** ■). It is important to remember that a positive response indicates that infection and a cellular (T-cell) response have developed; however, it does not mean that active disease is present or that the patient is infectious to others.

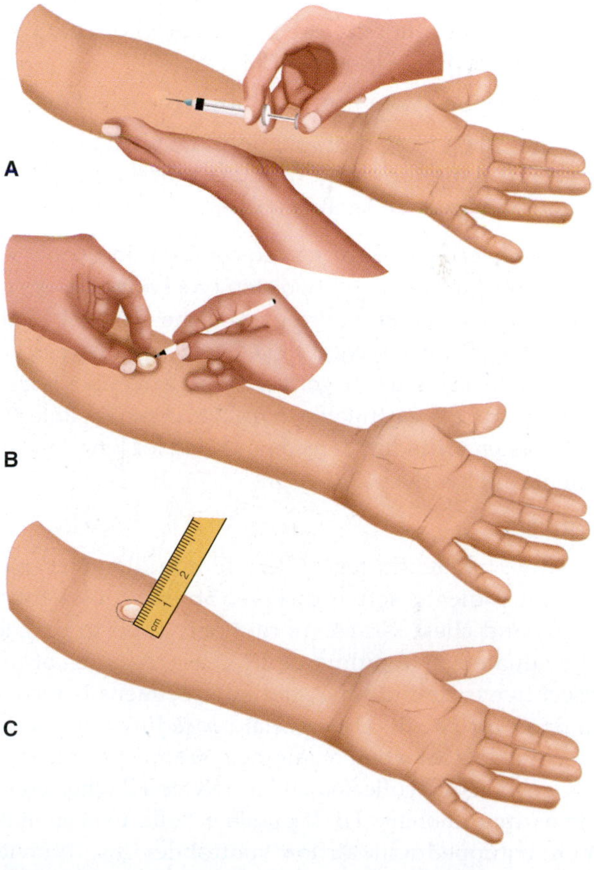
A
B
C

Figure 36.6 ■ A, Intradermal injection for tuberculin testing. B, The injection causes a local inflammatory response (wheal). C, Measurement of induration following tuberculin testing.

Two methods are currently available for tuberculin testing:

- ***Intradermal PPD (Mantoux) test:*** 0.1 mL of PPD (5 tuberculin units, or TU) is injected intradermally into the dorsal aspect of the forearm. This test is read within 48 to 72 hours, the peak reaction period, and recorded as the diameter of induration (raised area, not erythema) in millimeters. A response of 5 mm or greater after 48 hours is considered positive.
- ***Multiple-puncture (tine) test:*** A multiple-puncture device is used to introduce tuberculin into the skin. This test is less accurate than other testing methods. A vesicular reaction is considered positive; any other reaction must be confirmed using a Mantoux test.

Although it is impractical and unnecessary to screen the entire population, the CDC recommends screening people in the following risk groups:

- People with or at high risk for HIV infection
- Close contacts of people who have or are suspected of having infectious TB
- People with medical risk factors, such as silicosis, chronic malabsorption, end-stage renal failure, diabetes mellitus, immunosuppression, and hematologic and other malignancies
- People born in countries with a high prevalence of TB
- Infants and young children of adults who are at risk or who have been exposed to TB
- People with alcoholism and those who inject drugs
- Residents and staff of long-term residential facilities, such as long-term care facilities, correctional institutions, and mental health facilities.

False-negative responses are common in people who are immunosuppressed. A two-step procedure may be necessary to elicit a positive response. If the first test elicits a negative response, a second PPD test is given 1 week later. If the second test is also negative, the patient either is free of infection or is *anergic* (unable to react to common antigens). This two-step procedure is recommended for long-term care residents and workers.

Diagnosis

A positive tuberculin test (PPD > 5 mm diameter) alone does not indicate active disease. Sputum tests for the bacillus and chest x-rays are routinely used to diagnose and evaluate active pulmonary disease. A series of three consecutive early-morning sputum specimens is typically examined for bacilli. Use special procedures or personal protective devices when obtaining sputum specimens. Tissue specimens are collected and tested for TB when considering extrapulmonary TB. If possible, collect specimens in a room equipped with airflow control devices, ultraviolet light, or both. Alternatively, have the patient step outside to collect the specimen. Wear a mask capable of filtering droplet nuclei when collecting sputum specimens. Aerosol therapy, percussion, and postural drainage may help the patient produce sputum. Occasionally, tracheal suctioning, bronchoscopy, or gastric lavage may be necessary to obtain a specimen. See the Diagnostic Tests table in Chapter 34 for nursing care related to bronchoscopy.

- ***Sputum smear*** is microscopically examined for *acid-fast bacilli. M. tuberculosis* resists decolorizing chemicals after staining. This property is called *acid fast*. The acid-fast smear provides a rapid indicator of the tubercle bacillus.
- ***Sputum culture*** positive for *M. tuberculosis* provides the definitive diagnosis. However, *M. tuberculosis* is slow growing, requiring 4 to 8 weeks before it can be detected using traditional culture techniques. Automated radiometric culture systems (such as Bactec) allow detection of *M. tuberculosis* in several days.
- ***Sensitivity testing*** is performed, once the organism is detected, to identify appropriate drug therapy.
- ***Polymerase chain reaction (PCR)*** permits rapid detection of DNA from *M. tuberculosis*.
- ***Chest x-ray*** is ordered to diagnose and evaluate TB. Typical findings in pulmonary TB include dense lesions in the apical and posterior segments of the upper lobe and possible cavity formation.

Prior to initiating antituberculosis drug therapy, several additional diagnostic tests should be done to establish baseline data for monitoring potential adverse effects of the drugs:

- ***Liver function tests*** are obtained prior to treatment with isoniazid as this drug is hepatotoxic.
- ***Vision examination*** is done prior to treatment with ethambutol, a commonly used antituberculosis medication. Optic neuritis is a potential adverse effect of this drug. Periodic eye examinations are scheduled during the course of therapy.
- ***Audiometric testing*** is performed before streptomycin therapy is initiated. Ototoxicity is a significant adverse effect of streptomycin and other aminoglycoside antibiotics. Hearing is also evaluated periodically during the course of therapy to detect any hearing loss.

Medications

Chemotherapeutic medications are used both to prevent and treat TB infection. Goals of the pharmacologic treatment of TB are to do the following:

- Make the disease noncommunicable to others.
- Reduce symptoms of the disease.
- Effect a cure in the shortest possible time.

Prophylactic treatment is used to prevent active TB. Patients with a recent skin test conversion from negative to positive are often started on prophylactic therapy, especially when other risk factors are present. Prophylactic therapy is also used for people in close household contact with an individual whose sputum is positive for bacilli. Single-drug therapy is effective for prophylactic treatment, whereas treatment of active disease always involves two or more chemotherapeutic medications. For adults, INH at 300 mg per day for a period of 9 to 10 months is commonly used to prevent active TB.

When INH prophylaxis is contraindicated, bacillus Calmette-Guérin (BCG) vaccine may be prescribed. This vaccine is widely used in developing countries. BCG is made from an attenuated strain of *M. bovis*, a closely related bacillus that causes TB in cattle. In the United States, BCG vaccine is recommended only for infants, children, and healthcare workers with a negative tuberculin test who are repeatedly exposed to untreated or ineffectively treated people with active disease. After vaccination with BCG, a positive reaction to tuberculin testing is common. Periodic chest x-rays may be required for screening purposes.

The tuberculosis bacillus mutates readily to drug-resistant forms when only one anti-infective agent is used. Active disease is always treated with concurrent use of at least two antibacterial medications to which the organism is sensitive. The primary antituberculosis drugs can prevent development of resistance because all act by different mechanisms. However, the organism is protected within the tubercle, and 6 or more months of treatment is necessary to eradicate it.

Newly diagnosed TB is typically treated with an initial regimen of four oral antitubercular drugs, isoniazid (INH), rifampin, pyrazinamide, and ethambutol, daily (or several times per week on a decreasing schedule of frequency) for the first 2 months of treatment. This initial regimen is followed by at least 4 additional months of therapy with INH and rifampin, given daily, twice per week, or weekly. In the presence of HIV infection, treatment is continued for at least 9 months. The most common antituberculosis drugs are outlined in **Table 36.4**; their nursing implications are outlined in **Medication Administration 36.A**.

Nutrition

There is a known relationship between malnutrition and tuberculosis. Nutritional intervention in the presence of TB is based on a healthy diet with adequate protein intake. Assessment of fluid, electrolyte, vitamin, and mineral levels may be indicated in the malnourished TB patient. If deficiencies are found, nutritional supplementation and replacement are indicated.

Nursing Care

The primary preventative strategy used in the United States is treating people with latent TB infection demonstrated by a positive tuberculin test. A 9- to 10-month course of treatment with isoniazid reduces the risk of active TB by 90% or more. Isoniazid is also prescribed prophylactically for people with HIV infection who have been exposed to TB.

Assessment

See the Manifestations and Interprofessional Care sections for the assessment of the patient with tuberculosis.

Focused assessment for the patient with suspected TB includes:

- ***Health history:*** Complaints of fatigue, weight loss, night sweats, difficulty breathing, cough (productive or nonproductive), bloody sputum, or chest pain; known exposure to TB; most recent tuberculin test and results; living circumstances; alcohol and other recreational drug use
- ***Physical assessment:*** Vital signs including temperature; general appearance; respiratory rate and lung sounds
- ***Laboratory data:*** Tuberculin test results, presence of acid-fast bacilli in sputum, chest x-ray.

Priorities of Care

Collaborate with the interprofessional team to ensure adequate treatment and surveillance of tuberculosis while providing care that supports the physical and psychologic recovery from the infection is a priority of nursing care.

Diagnoses, Outcomes, and Interventions

Nursing care related to TB focuses primarily on infection control and compliance with prescribed treatment. See the accompanying Case Study & Nursing Care Plan on page 1306.

Table 36.4 Antituberculosis Medications

Drug and Dosage	Adverse Effects	Nursing Implications
Isoniazid (INH), oral: 300 mg daily or 900 mg one, two, or three times weekly	Peripheral neuropathy Hepatitis	Administer pyridoxine (vitamin B_6) concurrently. Monitor liver function studies (AST and ALT); avoid other hepatotoxins.
Rifampin (RMP), oral: 600 mg daily or two or three times weekly	Hepatitis Flulike syndrome; fever Colors body fluids—including sweat, urine, saliva, tears, and cerebrospinal fluid (CSF)—orange-red	As for INH. Do not miss or skip doses; flulike syndrome and fever occur when drug is resumed. Contact lenses may become discolored and should not be worn.
Pyrazinamide (PZA), oral: 1–2 g daily or 2–4 g twice weekly	Hyperuricemia Hepatotoxicity	Monitor uric acid levels. Monitor AST and ALT; avoid other hepatotoxins.
Ethambutol (EMB), oral: 800–1600 mg daily or 2–4 g twice weekly	Optic neuritis	Monitor red-green color discrimination and visual acuity.
Streptomycin (SM), intramuscular: 15 mg/kg, up to 1 g daily or 25–30 mg/kg twice weekly	Ototoxicity, vertigo Nephrotoxicity	Conduct periodic audiometric examinations. Monitor renal function studies, including BUN and serum creatinine.

Medication Administration 36.A

Antituberculosis Drugs

ISONIAZID (INH, LANIAZID, NYDRAZID)

Isoniazid is the drug of choice for TB prophylaxis and a first-line drug for treating active disease. It is effective against both intracellular and extracellular organisms. Isoniazid is used alone as a prophylactic medication and in combination with rifampin, ethambutol, or both. A fixed-dose combination form with 150 mg of INH and 300 mg of rifampin (Rifamate) is available as well.

Nursing Responsibilities

- Administer on an empty stomach 1 hour before or 2 hours after meals for maximum effect (if tolerated); may be given with meals to reduce gastrointestinal effects.
- Monitor for adverse effects:
  a. Numbness and tingling of the extremities (most likely to occur in patients who are malnourished, have diabetes, or abuse alcohol)
  b. Hepatotoxicity, as evidenced by abnormal liver function studies and scleral jaundice
  c. Hypersensitivity reactions, such as rash, drug fever, or evidence of anemia, bruising, bleeding, or infection related to agranulocytosis.
- Isoniazid interferes with the metabolism of diazepam (Valium), phenytoin (Dilantin), and carbamazepine. Doses of these drugs may need to be reduced to prevent toxicity.

Health Education for the Patient and Family

- Take the medication as prescribed for the entire treatment period to prevent incomplete eradication of the bacteria and development of resistant strains.
- Take the medication on an empty stomach. If nausea and vomiting occur, take with meals.
- If anorexia, nausea and vomiting, and jaundice (yellowing of the skin and the whites of the eyes) develop, notify your doctor immediately.
- Take pyridoxine as prescribed to prevent peripheral neuropathy.
- Avoid alcohol and other agents that may be harmful to the liver.
- Notify your doctor if you develop signs of an allergic reaction, such as rash, fever, easy bruising, bleeding gums, or fatigue.
- Use measures to prevent pregnancy while taking INH; this drug may be harmful to the developing fetus.

RIFAMPIN (RIFADIN, RIMACTANE)

Rifampin is commonly used in combination with INH and other antitubercular drugs. It is relatively low in toxicity, although it can cause hepatitis, a flulike immune response, and, rarely, renal failure. Rifampin stimulates the microsomal enzymes of the liver, increasing the rate of metabolism of many drugs and decreasing their effectiveness.

Nursing Responsibilities

- Administer on an empty stomach.
- Monitor CBC, liver function studies, and renal function studies for evidence of toxicity.
- Rifampin reduces the effect of oral contraceptives, quinidine, corticosteroids, warfarin, methadone, digoxin, and hypoglycemics. Monitor for the effectiveness of these drugs.

Health Education for the Patient and Family

- Rifampin causes body fluids, including sweat, urine, saliva, and tears, to turn red-orange. This is not harmful. Avoid wearing soft contact lenses, however, because they may be permanently stained.
- Aspirin may interfere with rifampin absorption and should not be taken concurrently.
- Fever, flulike symptoms, excessive fatigue, sore throat, or unusual bleeding may indicate an adverse reaction to the drug and should be reported to your doctor.

PYRAZINAMIDE (TEBRAZID)

Pyrazinamide is typically given with INH and rifampin for the first 2 months of TB treatment. Concurrent use of pyrazinamide allows a shorter course of therapy. As with many of the antitubercular agents, pyrazinamide is toxic to the liver. Its other principal adverse effect is hyperuricemia. Gout, however, rarely develops.

Nursing Responsibilities

- Administer with meals to reduce gastrointestinal side effects.
- Monitor liver function studies and serum uric acid levels. Notify the healthcare provider if changes are noted.

Health Education for the Patient and Family

- Notify your doctor if you develop loss of appetite, nausea and vomiting, jaundice, or symptoms of gout (a painful, red, hot, swollen joint, often the great toe or elbow).
- While taking this drug, avoid using alcohol or other substances that may be harmful to the liver.

ETHAMBUTOL (MYAMBUTOL)

Ethambutol is added to the initial treatment regimen or substituted for INH when an INH-resistant strain of TB is suspected. Ethambutol is a bacteriostatic drug that reduces the development of resistance to the bactericidal first-line agents. Its principal toxic effect is optic neuritis; fortunately, this is reversible. Early signs of optic neuritis include decreased visual acuity and loss of red-green discrimination. This drug may be safe for use in pregnancy.

Nursing Responsibilities

- Record a baseline visual examination prior to therapy. Schedule periodic eye exams during the course of treatment.
- Administer with meals to reduce gastrointestinal side effects.
- Monitor liver and renal function studies and neurologic status while taking this drug. Notify the healthcare provider of abnormal findings or significant changes.

Health Education for the Patient and Family

- Monitor vision daily by reading newspapers and looking at the same blue object (using usual corrective lenses, if appropriate). Notify your doctor if changes in vision or color perception occur.

STREPTOMYCIN

An aminoglycoside antibiotic, streptomycin is highly effective in treating most mycobacterial infections. Resistance may develop if it is used alone. Streptomycin has two primary drawbacks: (1) It must be administered parenterally because it is not absorbed in the gastrointestinal tract, and (2) it has toxic effects on the kidneys and ears.

Nursing Responsibilities

- Administer by deep intramuscular injection into a large muscle mass, rotating sites to minimize tissue trauma.

- Monitor urine output, weight, and renal function studies (including BUN and serum creatinine) to detect early signs of nephrotoxicity. Report significant changes to the healthcare provider.
- Maintain fluid intake at 2000 to 3000 mL/day to minimize the concentration of drug in the kidney tubules.
- Assess hearing and balance frequently. Have audiometric testing performed as indicated.

Health Education for the Patient and Family

- Maintain a daily fluid intake of at least 2.5 to 3 quarts.
- Weigh yourself on the same scale at least twice a week; report any significant weight gain to your doctor.
- Notify your doctor if hearing acuity decreases, ringing or buzzing sensations in the ear develop, or dizziness occurs.

If a drug-resistant strain is suspected, therapy is tailored to the resistance. In some cases, four or more anti-infective drugs may be used.

Antitubercular medications have many adverse and toxic effects. Close monitoring during therapy is necessary. Most have some degree of, or risk for, hepatotoxicity. For this reason, patients should avoid using alcohol and other drugs (such as acetaminophen) or chemicals that can damage the liver. Baseline liver and renal function studies are done prior to initiating therapy. Audiometric testing may also be done before treatment is started because several commonly used medications can affect hearing. Regular visits to a healthcare provider are necessary to evaluate regularly for adverse effects. Although none of these drugs have been proved to be teratogenic, potential adverse effects on the fetus are weighed against the benefit to the mother before they are prescribed during pregnancy.

Adherence to the prescribed regimen is also evaluated during follow-up visits. The urine can be examined for color changes characteristic of rifampin and tested for metabolites of INH. When adherence is a problem, medications are administered under direct supervision. Twice-weekly therapy is more cost effective in this instance, with a public health nurse watching the patient take and swallow the prescribed medication.

Repeat sputum specimens and chest x-rays are used to evaluate the effectiveness of therapy. In most cases, sputum cultures for *M. tuberculosis* are negative within 2 months of therapy; virtually all patients have negative sputum cultures within 3 months. If cultures remain positive at 3 months and beyond, treatment failure and drug resistance are suspected. In this case, cultures of the organism are tested for susceptibility to antitubercular agents, and two or three previously unused drugs are added to the treatment regimen.

With adherence to prescribed treatment, virtually all patients should have negative sputum cultures for *M. tuberculosis* within 3 months. The principal cause of treatment failure is noncompliance.

Provide Patient Teaching. Adequate knowledge and information are necessary to manage the disease and prevent its transmission to others. The patient needs to understand reasons for prolonged drug therapy and the importance of complying with treatment and follow-up. Antituberculosis drugs are relatively toxic. The patient needs to know how to minimize toxicity.

Expected Outcome: Patient will describe appropriate drug regimen and side effects for which they will monitor.

The nurse will:

- Assess knowledge about the disease process; identify misperceptions and emotional reactions. *Teaching based on previous learning enhances understanding and retention of information.*
- Assess ability and interest in learning, developmental level, and obstacles to learning. *Assessment allows presentation of information in a manner tailored to the learning needs and style of the patient, promoting learning.*
- Identify support systems, and include significant others in teaching. *A knowledgeable significant other provides reinforcement of learning, confirmation of understanding, and encouragement for the patient. Including significant others also reduces the risk of inadvertent sabotage of the treatment plan.*
- Establish a relationship of mutual trust with the patient and significant others. *An atmosphere of trust increases receptiveness to teaching and learning.*
- Develop mutually acceptable learning goals with the patient and significant other. *Working together to identify learning needs and establish goals increases the patient's "ownership" and interest in the process.*
- Select appropriate teaching strategies, using learning aids such as literature and visual materials that are appropriate for age, level of education, and intellect. *Teaching tailored to the patient is more effective and results in better learning.*
- Teach about TB and the prescribed treatment, including:
  a. Nature of the disease and its spread
  b. Purpose of treatment and follow-up procedures
  c. Measures to prevent spreading the disease to others
  d. Importance of maintaining good general health by eating a well-balanced, high-protein, high-carbohydrate diet; balancing exercise with rest; and avoiding crowds and people with upper respiratory infections
  e. Names, doses, purposes, and adverse effects of prescribed medications
  f. Importance of avoiding alcohol and other substances that may damage the liver while taking chemotherapeutic drugs
  g. Fluid intake needs of 2.5 to 3.0 quarts of fluid per day
  h. Manifestations to report to the healthcare provider: Chest pain, hemoptysis, difficulty breathing; anorexia, or nausea and vomiting; yellow tint to skin or sclera; sudden weight gain, swollen feet, ankles, legs, or hands; hearing loss, tinnitus, or vertigo; change in vision or difficulty discriminating colors.

  TB is a chronic disease requiring lengthy treatment with antitubercular medications. A good understanding of the disease and its treatment and potential adverse effects of therapy prepares the patient to manage care.

- Document teaching and level of understanding. Reinforce teaching and learning as needed. *Teaching is not complete until the patient can demonstrate learning of the information.*

Promote Adherence to the Treatment Plan. The populations at highest risk for developing active TB—the homeless and those who are in close contact with others who have TB—are also at high risk for being unable to manage its complex treatment regimen. Three or more costly medications that may have unpleasant or even dangerous side effects are prescribed. Frequent medical follow-up is required. Infectious diseases such as TB carry a stigma that may lead to denial of the disease or its seriousness. Patients with alcoholism and those who use IV drugs need to withdraw from their addiction to be successful in treating the disease. The patient with HIV infection faces a potentially fatal disease and costly treatment that may well override concerns about TB management.

Expected Outcome: Patient will comply with therapeutic regimen as evidenced by adherence to medication regimen and follow-up appointments.

The nurse will:

- Assess self-care abilities and support systems. *Assessment is used to help determine the patient's ability to follow the prescribed regimen.*
- Assess knowledge and understanding of the disease and its complications, treatment, and risks to others. Provide additional teaching and reinforcement as indicated. *Lack of understanding is a barrier to adherence with and management of the treatment regimen.*
- Work collaboratively to identify barriers or obstacles to managing the prescribed treatment. *Working collaboratively with the patient and other members of the healthcare team provides insight for overcoming identified barriers to effective treatment.*
- Assist the patient, significant others (if available), and healthcare team members to develop a plan for managing the prescribed regimen. *Including the patient in developing a plan to manage care increases the sense of control and ownership and helps ensure that personal, cultural, and lifestyle factors are considered. This increases the likelihood of adherence.*
- Provide verbal and written instructions that are clear and appropriate for level of literacy, language, knowledge, and understanding. *Clearly written directions provide support and reinforcement for the patient.*
- Provide active intervention for homeless people, including shelter placement or other housing and ongoing follow-up by easily accessed healthcare providers (clinics and public health workers in the neighborhood that do not present transportation or access problems, either real or perceived). *Simple referral will not ensure compliance, especially among disenfranchised populations. Active intervention is needed to help ensure treatment compliance.*
- Refer patients who are unlikely to adhere to the treatment regimen to the public health department for management and follow-up. *Because TB presents a significant public health risk, public health follow-up is essential. In some cases, it is necessary for nurses to administer medications, observing the patient swallow all pills.*

Reduce Risk for Infection. The spread of TB is a risk in any facility housing many people. It is especially high in residential care facilities for older patients and for people

Moving Evidence into Action

Testing for TB in Long-Term Care Facilities

Clinical Issue

Risk of tuberculosis (TB) is higher in communal living facilities such as long-term care facilities (LCFs). Understanding TB testing practices in these facilities is imperative to know the effectiveness of such testing.

External Evidence

Reddy and colleagues (2017) described the testing practices in three LCFs in the Boston, Massachusetts area. The study evaluated data on 291 LCF residents, finding that 63% were tested. Factors that impacted TB testing included a stay less than 90 days. The investigators found that 20% of the residents had latent TB but that testing was not always performed. This information provides evidence of a prevention opportunity. The importance of latent TB testing in LCFs needs to be promoted.

Internal Evidence

As part of the evaluation of internal evidence, one must consider the impact of the external evidence findings on how healthcare providers interact with this population.

Patient Considerations

When considering use of a new or promoting an existing practice (such as TB testing on residents of an LCF), the nurse must consider the specific patient population where it will be used (in this case, persons admitted to an LCF). Will patients and their families be amenable to the TB testing as a routine procedure?

Putting the Pieces Together

A TB outbreak in a communal living environment such as an LCF has the potential cause for significant morbidity in this population. The role of routine testing of TB in these residents is imperative to maintain a safe environment. The information from this study (showing that a less than 90-day stay was shown to be associated with reduced testing) is important information to consider when updating TB testing procedures in an LCF.

Reference

Reddy, D., Walker, J., White, L. F., Brandeis, G. H., Russell, M. L., Horsburgh, C. R., & Hochberg, N. S. (2017). Latent tuberculosis infection testing practices in long-term care facilities, Boston, Massachusetts. *Journal of the American Geriatrics Society, 65*(6), 1145–1151.

with AIDS. The increasing incidence of TB among homeless people and members of lower socioeconomic groups increases the risk in hospitals, emergency departments, and public and urgent care clinics. Respiratory precautions are necessary to prevent the spread of TB via microscopic airborne droplets to other patients and to healthcare workers.

Expected Outcome: Patient will describe measures to protect healthy tissue and prevent infection.

The nurse will:

- Place the patient in a private room with airflow control that prevents air within the room from circulating into the hallway or other rooms. A negative-flow room in which air is diluted by at least six fresh-air exchanges per hour is recommended. *A negative-flow room and multiple fresh-air exchanges dilute the concentration of droplet nuclei within the room and prevent their spread to adjacent areas.*
- Use standard precautions and TB isolation techniques as recommended by the CDC, including wearing masks and gowns when caring for patients who do not reliably cover the mouth when coughing. *These measures are important to prevent the spread of TB to others.*
- Discuss the reasons for and importance of respiratory isolation procedures during initial hospitalization. When treatment is provided as an outpatient, instruct to avoid crowds and close physical contact and maintain ventilation in living facilities, particularly during the first 3 weeks of treatment. *These measures help protect others during initial treatment, when sputum is still likely to contain significant numbers of bacilli.*
- Place a mask on the patient when transporting to other parts of the facility for diagnostic or treatment procedures. *Covering the patient's nose and mouth during transport minimizes air contamination and the risk to visitors and personnel.*
- Inform all personnel having contact with the patient of the diagnosis. *This allows personnel to take appropriate precautions.*
- Assist visitors to mask prior to entering the room. *Providing visitors with appropriate masks or respirators reduces their risk of infection.*
- Teach the patient how to limit transmitting the disease to others:

  a. Always cough and expectorate into tissues.

  b. Dispose of tissues properly, placing them in a closed bag.

  c. Wear a mask if you are sneezing or unable to control respiratory secretions.

  d. The disease is not spread by touching inanimate objects, so no special precautions are required for eating utensils, clothing, books, or other objects used.

  Teaching appropriate precautions helps prevent the spread of TB to others while allowing as much freedom from restraints as possible.

SAFETY ALERT: Use personal protective devices to reduce the risk of transmission during patient care. The Occupational Safety and Health Administration (OSHA) requires use of a HEPA-filtered respirator for protection against occupational exposure to TB. Surgical masks are ineffective to filter droplet nuclei, necessitating the use of protective devices capable of filtering bacteria and particles smaller than 1 micron. ■

- Teach how to collect sputum specimens. If necessary, have the patient step outside to collect a sputum specimen. *This minimizes the risk of exposure to healthcare personnel and provides for rapid dilution of any droplet nuclei produced and their exposure to ultraviolet light (which kills the bacteria).*
- Teach the importance of complying with prescribed treatment for the entire course of therapy. *Completion of the entire treatment regimen is important to reduce the risk of relapse and creation of drug-resistant organisms.*

The prevalence of active TB is significantly higher among older Caucasian adults in the United States than it is in young adults (CDC, 2017d, 2017e). Of cases among older adults, approximately 90% occur due to reactivation of the dormant bacteria. Older adults are at increased risk for reactivation TB due to age-related decreases in cell-mediated immunity. Chronic illnesses, poor nutrition, gastrectomy, alcoholism, or the long-term use of steroids and immunosuppressive agents may also reactivate dormant TB lesions.

Presenting symptoms of TB in the older adult are often vague, including coughing, weight loss, anorexia, or periodic fevers. These signs and symptoms should not be dismissed as a normal part of aging.

Residents of nursing homes are at increased risk for acquiring TB because of group living. Yearly tuberculin skin testing with purified protein derivative (PPD) is often required by state health departments. If the initial test is negative, a repeat PPD in 1 to 2 weeks is recommended. This improves sensitivity to the test so that silent cases of TB are not missed. A chest x-ray and sputum culture for acid-fast bacilli are obtained if the PPD is positive.

Successful treatment for TB includes taking at least two drugs for at least 6 to 9 months to totally eradicate the organism. Older adults usually do not develop drug-resistant forms of TB because they acquired the disease prior to emergence of drug-resistant strains.

Delegating Nursing Care Activities

As appropriate and allowed by the designated duties and responsibilities of unlicensed assistive personnel, the nurse may delegate nursing care activities such as measuring vital signs, encouraging oral or enteral fluid intake, and providing skin care.

Transitions of Care

TB today presents a greater threat to public health than it does to individuals. Nurses play a key role in maintaining public health. Education and TB screening are major nursing strategies to prevent TB. Public health teaching includes increasing awareness of TB as a reemerging threat. Teach patients

Case Study & Nursing Care Plan

A Patient with Tuberculosis

Harry Facée, age 53, arrives at a metropolitan public health clinic complaining of aching chest pain that has lasted for the past few days. He also says that his sputum is bloody. He is afraid he might have lung cancer, so he came in to see a healthcare provider.

ASSESSMENT

Raj Kamil, RN, the public health nurse at the clinic, obtains an admission history and physical examination of Mr. Facée. Mr. Kamil notes that Mr. Facée is a homeless person who has lived on the streets and in various shelters for the past "10 years or so." He usually prefers to sleep outdoors, taking refuge in shelters only during very cold or very wet weather. He has a small disability income, but usually scrounges for food or eats with other homeless people at soup kitchens. Mr. Facée states that he has had a cough for a long time that has become worse recently. It is now productive, especially in the mornings. He also admits that he has recently been waking up drenched with sweat in the middle of the night and is more tired than usual.

Although Mr. Facée's clothes are tattered, he is fairly clean. He answers questions appropriately and intelligently. Mr. Kamil does not detect any odor of alcohol on his breath. He is very thin, almost emaciated. Mr. Facée's vital signs are BP 152/86 mmHg, P 92 bpm, R 20/min, and T 37.8°C (100.2°F).

Suspecting tuberculosis, Mr. Kamil obtains a sputum specimen for Gram stain and culture, administers a tuberculin test, and sends Mr. Facée for a chest x-ray before he sees the clinic healthcare provider. Although the chest x-ray is inconclusive, the Gram stain is positive for acid-fast bacilli. The diagnosis of probable active pulmonary tuberculosis is made. The healthcare provider prescribes isoniazid, 300 mg orally; rifampin, 600 mg orally; and pyrazinamide, 1500 mg orally daily for 2 months, to be followed by twice-weekly isoniazid 900 mg orally and rifampin 600 mg orally. The healthcare provider also orders weekly sputum cultures for the first month.

DIAGNOSES

- Poor health maintenance related to homelessness
- Nonadherence to prescribed treatment, related to lack of understanding and resources
- Caloric intake less than needed, related to increased metabolic needs associated with infection
- Potential for peripheral neuropathy related to isoniazid therapy

EXPECTED OUTCOMES

- Patient will keep all follow-up appointments as scheduled.
- Patient will verbalize an understanding of his disease and its treatment.
- Patient will follow the prescribed plan of care.
- Patient will demonstrate measures to prevent spread of the organism to others.
- Patient will gain 0.5 to 1 kg (1 to 2 lb) of weight per week.
- Patient will promptly report symptoms of peripheral neuropathy, including numbness, tingling, or burning sensations.

PLANNING AND IMPLEMENTATION

- Teach about tuberculosis, and provide a patient education pamphlet about the disease.
- Instruct about the prescribed medications, potential adverse effects, and the importance of completing the entire prescribed regimen.
- Emphasize the importance of continued follow-up.
- Teach and demonstrate sputum and droplet control measures.
- Escort to the local incentive shelter program for directly observed medical therapy and meals.
- Identify verbally and in writing manifestations to report to the healthcare provider.

EVALUATION

Mr. Kamil successfully enrolls Mr. Facée in the local incentive shelter program. In this program, a healthcare worker administers Mr. Facée's medications daily, watching him swallow them. He is assigned a small individual room and can eat three daily meals at the shelter. He still prefers to sleep outside when the weather permits, but he complies with the requirement for supervised medication administration because he "likes the food there." Always a clean person, Mr. Facée is able to demonstrate appropriate sputum control measures and practices them faithfully. The sputum culture done after 2 months of treatment is negative for tubercle bacilli, and his chest x-ray indicates no disease progression.

CLINICAL REASONING IN PATIENT CARE

1. Many people who are homeless have schizophrenia or another mental illness. How would you adapt the care plan for a patient who is homeless with active tuberculosis who also has schizophrenia?
2. Mr. Kamil was fortunate in having access to an incentive shelter with healthcare workers to supervise medication compliance. Identify available resources in your area for patients who are homeless and infected with tuberculosis.
3. Develop a care plan for the nursing priority of ineffective airway clearance related to mucopurulent sputum and weak cough.

See Evaluating Your Response in Appendix B.

in all settings how to reduce the spread of TB by covering their mouths when coughing or sneezing and disposing of sputum appropriately. The benefit of screening programs to identify infected (though not necessarily infective) people also needs to be included in public health education.

The best TB prevention is early diagnosis of infections and appropriate treatment to achieve cure. BCG vaccine is recommended for infants born in countries where TB is prevalent, but is not widely used in the United States. It may be administered to healthcare workers in settings where the risk of infection with MDR strains of *M. tuberculosis* is high despite rigorous infection control measures.

Community-dwelling older adults are susceptible to TB as well as those in care facilities. The older adult with respiratory symptoms is often treated presumptively for pneumonia, without a sputum smear and Gram stain. Older adults living in the community may not have had a tuberculin test or chest x-ray for many years.

Assess risk factors for TB:

- General health and nutritional status, including intake of specific nutrients such as vitamin D (lack of vitamin D is associated with a higher risk of developing active TB)
- Presence of a chronic disease such as silicosis, diabetes, alcoholism, or HIV infection; past history of a gastrectomy
- Past history of a positive tuberculin test that now has converted to negative
- Medications such as corticosteroids or other immunosuppressive drugs.

Assess living and social situation:

- Natural light and ventilation in the home
- Access to clean water, cooking facilities, grocery stores, and other services
- Possible exposure to infected people, for example, sharing a household with someone with active TB, crowded living facilities, homelessness, frequent participation in senior activities, volunteer work in residential care facilities or other institutional settings
- Access to healthcare.

TB is typically treated in the community; hospitalization or institutionalization is rarely necessary or desirable. For the older adult being treated for active TB in the community, assess the following:

- Knowledge and understanding of the disease and the prescribed treatment regimen
- Mental status and ability to follow prescribed regimen and precautions to avoid exposing others to the disease
- Transportation and ability to access healthcare services on a regular basis
- Financial resources to complete treatment and follow-up care
- Need for home health or social services to ensure adequate treatment.

Most patients with TB are managed in community settings; few require institutionalization. The accompanying Case Study & Nursing Care Plan presents community-based nursing care for a patient with TB. In addition to the teaching topics and strategies identified earlier, discuss the following topics when preparing the patient and significant others for home care:

- Using disposable tissues to contain respiratory secretions, especially during the first 2 weeks of treatment when the disease may be transmitted to others
- Importance of screening close contacts for infection and possibly prophylactic treatment
- Effect, dose, and timing for all medications, and potential side effects and their management
- Importance of long-term therapy in eradicating the disease
- Principles of good nutrition, dietary guidelines for a patient with TB, and other measures to help maintain good health, such as balancing rest with exercise
- Signs and symptoms of complications to report to the healthcare provider.

Provide referrals as appropriate:

- Smoking cessation clinics or support groups
- Alcohol treatment facilities, Alcoholics Anonymous, other treatment programs or support groups
- Drug treatment facilities, Narcotics Anonymous, other outpatient or inpatient treatment programs or support groups
- Low-cost community clinics and incentive programs for people with TB
- Counseling, support groups, and other community resources that provide additional assistance and support.

The Patient with Inhalation Anthrax

Inhalation anthrax is a potential threat in the United States. This disease rarely affects humans in nature, even though both wild and domestic animals can be infected. However, *Bacillus anthracis*, the spore-forming rod responsible for causing anthrax, has been identified as an agent likely to be used as a biologic weapon. Anthrax spores can be aerosolized so they remain suspended in the air, allowing them to be inhaled into the lungs. Person-to-person transmission does not occur.

Inhalation anthrax causes initial flulike symptoms, including malaise, dry cough, and fever. This is followed by an abrupt onset of severe dyspnea, stridor, and cyanosis. Lymph nodes in the mediastinum and thorax become inflamed and enlarged. Septic shock and/or meningitis may develop. Untreated, death results from hemorrhagic thoracic lymphadenitis and hemorrhagic mediastinitis. Even with treatment, inhalation anthrax has a 45% mortality rate (CDC, 2017a).

Blood cultures and chest x-ray are used to diagnose inhalation anthrax. However, because death can quickly result from the disease, people who are known or suspected to have been exposed to anthrax spores are often treated prophylactically. Ciprofloxacin (Cipro) is used to both prevent and treat inhalation anthrax. Doxycycline (Vibramycin) is an alternative to ciprofloxacin. Although an anthrax vaccine exists, its use at this time is considered experimental (CDC, 2017a). See the section on bioterrorism in Chapter 7 for more information about anthrax and the section of this chapter on respiratory failure for nursing care measures for the patient with inhalation anthrax.

The Patient with a Fungal Infection

Fungal spores are endemic, present in the air everyone breathes. Normal respiratory defense mechanisms allow few of these spores to reach the lungs. If they reach the lungs, pulmonary macrophages and neutrophils efficiently remove them in most people. When they do cause infection, it is typically mild and self-limiting. Most fungi are opportunistic, able to cause infection only in people who are immunocompromised. For this reason, patients with AIDS, renal failure, leukemia, burns, or chronic diseases, as well as people receiving corticosteroids or immunosuppressants, are particularly susceptible to fungal diseases.

Many fungal lung diseases have a geographic distribution pattern. Histoplasmosis and blastomycosis are more common in the southeastern, mid-Atlantic, and central states. California, Arizona, and western Texas are the primary sites for coccidioidomycosis, also known as *San Joaquin Valley fever*.

The course and manifestations of fungal lung diseases resemble those of TB. Lung lesions are slow to develop, and symptoms are mild. The fungus can disseminate from the lung to other organs.

Pathophysiology

Histoplasmosis

Histoplasmosis, an infectious disease caused by *Histoplasma capsulatum*, is the most common fungal lung infection in the United States. The organism is found in the soil and is linked to exposure to bird droppings and bats. Infection occurs when the spores are inhaled and reach the alveoli. Most infections develop into *latent asymptomatic disease*, much like TB, or *primary acute histoplasmosis*, a mild, self-limiting influenza-like illness. Initial chest x-rays are nonspecific; later ones show areas of calcification. *Chronic progressive disease*, usually seen in older adults, is typically limited to the lungs but may involve any organ. Progressive lung changes and cavitation occur, with increasing dyspnea and eventual disabling pulmonary disease.

Regional lymph vessels spread the organism from the lungs to other parts of the body, much like the process that occurs in TB. In the healthy host, normal immune responses inactivate and remove the organism. In the immunocompromised host, however, macrophages remove the fungi but are unable to destroy them, resulting in *disseminated histoplasmosis*. This type of histoplasmosis is often fatal. Manifestations of fever, dyspnea, cough, weight loss, and muscle wasting are usual. Ulcerations of the mouth and oropharynx may be present, and the liver and spleen are enlarged.

Coccidioidomycosis

Coccidioidomycosis is an infectious disease caused by the fungus *Coccidioides immitis*. This mold grows in the soil of the arid Southwest, Mexico, and Central and South America. When inhaled, the fungus typically causes an acute, self-limiting pulmonary infection that is often asymptomatic and goes unrecognized. If manifestations do occur, they resemble those of influenza, with malaise, fever, body aches, and cough. Pleuritic pain, skin rash, and arthritis of the knees and ankles may also develop. Disseminated disease, which may affect the lymph nodes, meninges, spleen, liver, kidney, skin, and adrenal glands, is rare in immunocompetent people. When it does occur, the mortality rate is high. Meningitis is the usual cause of death.

Blastomycosis

The fungus *Blastomyces dermatitidis* causes the infectious disease *blastomycosis*. It occurs primarily in the south-central and Midwestern regions of the United States and in Canada. Men are affected more frequently than women. The lungs are the primary site for the disease, although it may spread to involve the skin, bones, genitourinary system, and, rarely, the CNS. Pulmonary symptoms include fever, dyspnea, pleuritic chest pain, and cough, which may become productive of bloody or purulent sputum. If untreated, the disseminated disease is slowly progressive and ultimately fatal.

Paracoccidioidomycosis

The fungus *Paracoccidioides brasiliensis* causes paracoccidioidomycosis. It is also known as *Brazilian blastomycosis* or *Lutz-Spendore-de Almeida disease*. As with blastomycosis, it often enters through the lungs but can spread to the lymph nodes and bone. It can occur in immunocompetent persons, often with onset in childhood. The pulmonary presentation includes lobar pneumonia or pleurisy that continues past the ninth day. Sulfa drugs and antifungals are used to eradicate the disease.

Aspergillosis

Aspergillus spores are common in the environment, but rarely cause disease except in persons who are immunocompromised. When they do cause infection, *Aspergillus* species invade blood vessels and produce hyphae that branch at acute angles, frequently causing venous or arterial thrombosis. In the lungs, aspergillosis can cause an acute, diffuse, self-limited pneumonitis. The manifestations of pulmonary *aspergillosis* include dyspnea, nonproductive cough, pleuritic chest pain, chills, and fever. If the organism invades a pulmonary blood vessel, hemoptysis or massive pulmonary hemorrhage can occur. In patients with underlying lung disease, balls of *Aspergillus* hyphae may form within cysts or cavities, usually in the upper lobes of the lung. Symptoms are often milder and more insidious in onset, with fever, weight loss, night sweats, and cough.

Interprofessional Care

Most fungal lung infections can be diagnosed by microscopic examination of a sputum specimen for the fungus. Blood cultures may be done, as well as cultures of cerebrospinal fluid, if indicated. Chest x-ray may show typical changes in lung tissue or widening of the mediastinum, depending on the infecting organism.

Acute pulmonary histoplasmosis and acute pulmonary coccidioidomycosis usually resolve without treatment, although antifungal drugs may be given to shorten the disease course. Oral itraconazole (Sporanox), a broad-spectrum antifungal agent, is commonly prescribed to treat histoplasmosis. Other fungal lung diseases and patients who are immunocompromised are often treated with intravenous amphotericin B. Surgery (lobectomy) may be indicated for patients with severe hemoptysis associated with aspergillosis.

Nursing Care

Patients with fungal lung infections have different nursing care needs, depending on the disease and their immune status. For most patients, nursing care focuses on education. People living in high-prevalence areas or who have specific risk factors such as exposure to bird droppings (for example, by cleaning chicken coops, pigeon lofts, or barns where birds roost), decomposed vegetation, rotting wood, or stored grain need to be aware of the risk, common symptoms, and measures to reduce the risk. Patients with latent histoplasmosis may need education to maintain good general health to prevent reactivation. Teach patients receiving antifungal drugs about the specific drug, its intended and adverse effects, the duration of therapy, and symptoms to report to the healthcare provider. Include teaching about any specific precautions such as drug or food interactions. Itraconazole interacts with many medications; verify the safety of concurrent usage with all other prescribed drugs. Its use is contraindicated during pregnancy and lactation; emphasize the importance of effective birth control and of notifying the healthcare provider immediately if pregnancy occurs. Amphotericin B is a toxic drug. Administer the initial intravenous dose slowly after premedicating with an antihistamine and antiemetic as ordered to manage its adverse effects. Monitor carefully during infusion and therapy for changes in vital signs, hydration, nutrition, weight, or urine output.

36.2 Disorders of the Pleura

The *pleura* is a thin membrane with two layers: The visceral pleura, which overlies the lung surface, and the parietal pleura, which lines the inner chest wall. Between the layers of pleura is a potential space, the *pleural cavity*, which contains a thin layer of serous fluid. As the thoracic cavity expands during inspiration, the pressure in this space becomes negative in relation to atmospheric and alveolar pressure. The expansible lung is drawn out, and air rushes into the alveoli. When the pleura is inflamed or affected by disease or injury, air or fluid can collect in the pleural cavity, restricting lung expansion, air movement, and ventilation.

The Patient with Pleuritis

Pleuritis (*pleurisy*), inflammation of the pleura, irritates sensory fibers of the parietal pleura, causing characteristic pain. Pleural inflammation usually occurs secondarily to another process, such as a viral respiratory illness, pneumonia, or rib injury.

The onset of pleuritis is typically abrupt. The pain is unilateral and well localized; it is usually sharp or stabbing in nature. Pain may be referred to the neck or the shoulder. Deep breathing, coughing, and movement aggravate the pain. Respirations are rapid and shallow, and chest wall movement is limited on the affected side. Breath sounds are diminished, and a pleural friction rub may be heard over the site.

The diagnosis of pleuritis is based on its manifestations. Chest x-ray and ECG may be ordered to rule out other causes of chest pain. Treatment for pleuritis is symptomatic. Analgesics and NSAIDs, indomethacin (Indocin) in particular, help relieve the pain. Codeine may be ordered, both to relieve pain and to suppress cough.

Nursing care for the patient with pleuritis is directed toward promoting comfort, including administration of NSAIDs and analgesics. Positioning and splinting the chest while coughing are also helpful. Although wrapping the chest with 6-inch-wide elastic bandages may help relieve pain, this may excessively restrict chest motion, increasing the risk of impaired airway clearance.

Teach the patient and family that pleuritis is generally self-limited and of short duration. Discuss symptoms to report to the healthcare provider: Increased fever, productive cough, difficulty breathing, or shortness of breath. Provide information about prescription and nonprescription NSAIDs and analgesics, including the drug ordered, how to use it, and its desired and possible adverse effects.

The Patient with a Pleural Effusion

The pleural space normally contains only about 10 to 20 mL of serous fluid. **Pleural effusion** is a collection of excess fluid in the pleural space. Pleural effusions result from either systemic or local disease. Systemic disorders that may lead to pleural effusion include heart failure, liver or renal disease, and connective tissue disorders, such as rheumatoid arthritis and systemic lupus erythematosus. Pneumonia, atelectasis, TB, lung cancer, and trauma are local conditions that may cause pleural effusion.

Pathophysiology

Excess pleural fluid may be either *transudate*, formed when capillary pressure is high or plasma proteins are low, or *exudate*, the result of increased capillary permeability. Heart failure is the most common precipitating factor in transudate formation, which may also accompany renal failure, nephrosis, liver failure, and malignancy. Exudate, a protein-rich fluid, is seen with inflammatory processes such as infections, systemic inflammation (e.g., rheumatoid arthritis or systemic lupus erythematosus), pulmonary infarction (leading to tissue necrosis and an inflammatory response), and malignancy (Sorenson et al., 2019). Other pleural fluid collections include *empyema*, pus in the pleural cavity; *hemothorax*, the presence of blood in the cavity; *hemorrhagic pleural effusion*, a mixture of blood and pleural fluid; and *chylothorax*, a collection of lymph in the pleural space. In adults, chylothorax may result from thoracic surgery or placement of a central catheter in one of the great veins (Sorenson et al., 2019).

Manifestations

A large pleural effusion compresses adjacent lung tissue. This causes the characteristic manifestation of dyspnea. Pain may develop, although with inflammatory processes pleuritic pain is often relieved by formation of an effusion because the fluid reduces friction between inflamed visceral and parietal pleura. Breath sounds are diminished or absent, and a dull percussion tone is heard over the affected area. Chest wall movement may be limited.

Complications

Complications of pleural effusion can lead to significant morbidity and to death. Some complications include lung scarring, pneumothorax (secondary to thoracentesis), empyema, or sepsis.

Interprofessional Care

Diagnosis

Chest x-ray often provides the first evidence of a pleural effusion. Because fluid typically collects in dependent regions, it is seen at the base of the affected lung on an upright chest x-ray and along the lateral wall when the patient is positioned on the affected side. CT scans and ultrasonography are also used to localize and differentiate pleural effusions.

Thoracentesis

If the cause of pleural effusion is not apparent, a thoracentesis may be done. **Thoracentesis** is an invasive procedure in which fluid (or occasionally air) is removed from the pleural space with a needle. Aspirated fluid is analyzed for appearance, cell counts, protein and glucose content, the presence of enzymes such as LDH and amylase, abnormal cells, and culture.

When pleural effusion is significant and interferes with respirations, thoracentesis is the treatment of choice to remove the fluid (**Figure 36.7 ■**). Thoracentesis may be performed at the bedside, in a procedure room, or in an outpatient setting. Local anesthesia is used, and the procedure requires less than 30 minutes to complete. Percussion, auscultation, radiography, or ultrasonography may be used to locate the effusion and needle insertion site. The amount of fluid removed is limited to 1200 to 1500 mL at one time to reduce the risk of cardiovascular collapse from rapid removal of too much fluid. Pneumothorax is a possible complication of thoracentesis if the visceral pleura is punctured or a closed-drainage system is not maintained during the procedure. Nursing care for the patient undergoing a thoracentesis is outlined in **Box 36.2**.

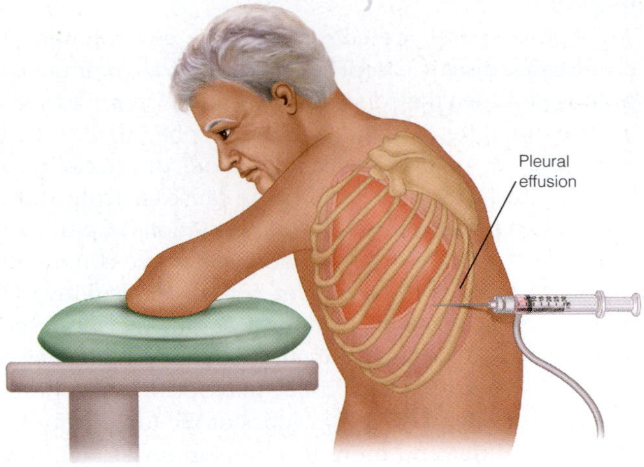
Pleural
effusion

Figure 36.7 ■ Thoracentesis. With the patient seated, a needle is inserted between the ribs into the pleural space to withdraw accumulated fluid.

Treatments

Because pleural effusion usually occurs secondary to another disease or disorder, medical management also focuses on treating the underlying condition to prevent further fluid accumulation. An empyema may require repeated drainage, as well as high doses of parenteral antibiotics. Occasionally, thoracotomy and surgical excision may be necessary. Recurrent pleural effusions, often due to cancer, may be prevented by instilling an irritant, such as doxycycline, bleomycin, or talc, into the pleural space to cause adhesion of the parietal and visceral pleura (*pleurodesis*). Water-seal chest tube drainage is often employed for hemothorax.

Nursing Care

Nursing care for the patient with a pleural effusion is directed toward supporting respiratory function and assisting with procedures to evacuate collected fluid. With a large pleural effusion and partial lung collapse, impaired gas exchange and activity intolerance are high-priority nursing problems. Risk for impaired gas exchange is also a priority problem during the initial period following thoracentesis.

Teaching for home care focuses on symptoms of recurrent effusion or complications following a thoracentesis to report to the healthcare provider: Increasing dyspnea or shortness of breath, cough, and hemoptysis. Pleuritic pain may be an early sign of effusion and should also be reported. Further teaching about an underlying condition

BOX 36.2
Nursing Care of the Patient Undergoing a Thoracentesis

PREPROCEDURE CARE

- Verify a signed informed consent for the procedure. *This invasive procedure requires informed consent.*
- Assess knowledge and understanding of the procedure and its purpose; provide additional information as needed. *An informed patient will be less apprehensive and more able to cooperate during the thoracentesis.*
- Fasting or sedation before the procedure is not required. *Only local anesthesia is used in this procedure, and the gag and cough reflexes remain intact.*
- Administer a cough suppressant, if indicated. *Movement and coughing during the procedure may cause inadvertent damage to the lung or pleura.*
- Obtain a thoracentesis tray; sterile gloves; injectable lidocaine, povidone-iodine, or chlorhexidine; dressing supplies; and an extra overbed table or Mayo stand. *These supplies are used by the healthcare provider performing the procedure.*
- Position the patient upright, leaning forward with arms and head supported on an anchored overbed table. *This position spreads the ribs, enlarging the intercostal space for needle insertion.*
- Inform the patient that although local anesthesia prevents pain as the needle is inserted, a sensation of pressure may be felt. *A pressure sensation occurs as the needle punctures the parietal pleura to enter the pleural space.*

POSTPROCEDURE CARE

- Monitor pulse, color, oxygen saturation, and other signs during thoracentesis. *These are indicators of physiologic tolerance of the procedure.*
- Apply a dressing over the puncture site, and position the patient on the unaffected side for 1 hour. *This allows the pleural puncture to heal.*
- Label obtained specimen with name, date, source, and diagnosis; send specimen to the laboratory for analysis. *Fluid obtained during thoracentesis may be examined for abnormal cells, bacteria, and other substances to determine the cause of the pleural effusion.*
- During the first several hours after thoracentesis, frequently assess and document vital signs; oxygen saturation; respiratory status, including respiratory excursion, lung sounds, cough, or hemoptysis; and puncture site for bleeding or crepitus. *Frequent assessment is important to detect possible complications of thoracentesis, such as pneumothorax.*
- Obtain a chest x-ray. *Chest x-ray is ordered to detect possible pneumothorax.*
- Normal activities can generally be resumed after 1 hour if no evidence of pneumothorax or other complication is present. *The puncture wound of thoracentesis heals rapidly.*

may also be necessary; for example, the patient with heart failure may need teaching about a salt-restricted diet.

Transitions of Care

There are no primary preventative measures for pleural effusion. Secondary prevention focuses on appropriate care for any processes listed as risk factors for a pleural effusion.

Acute nursing care is related to management of the patient undergoing a thoracentesis. See Box 36.2.

Teaching related to posthospital management after a pleural effusion is supportive and focuses on teaching related to comfort (use a pillow to splint the chest when coughing, rest as needed), prevention of complications such as atelectasis (coughing and deep breathing exercises, progressive return to activity as tolerated), and medication management as prescribed.

Malignant pleural effusion is a common complication seen in the palliative care setting. This is a distressing condition for the patient and family, resulting in symptoms such as dyspnea, a dry cough, chest heaviness, or pleuritic pain. Intervention is determined by severity of the condition as well as the care goals of the patient and family.

The Patient with Pneumothorax

Accumulation of air in the pleural space is called **pneumothorax**. Pneumothorax can occur spontaneously, without apparent cause, as a complication of preexisting lung disease, as a result of blunt or penetrating trauma to the chest, or from an iatrogenic cause (e.g., following thoracentesis).

Pathophysiology

Pressure in the pleural space is normally negative in relation to atmospheric pressure. This negative pressure is vital to the process of breathing. Contraction of the diaphragm and the intercostal muscles enlarges the thoracic space. Negative intrapleural pressure draws the lung outward, increasing its volume so air rushes in to fill the expanded lung space.

When either the visceral or parietal pleura is breached, air enters the pleural space, equalizing this pressure. Lung expansion is impaired, and the natural recoil tendency of the lung causes it to collapse to a greater or lesser extent, depending on the size and rapidity of air accumulation. **Table 36.5** illustrates the classifications of pneumothorax.

Spontaneous Pneumothorax

Spontaneous pneumothorax develops when an air-filled bleb, or blister, on the lung surface ruptures. Rupture allows air from the airways to enter the pleural space. Air accumulates until pressures are equalized or until collapse of the involved lung section seals the leak. Spontaneous pneumothorax may be either *primary* (*simple*) or *secondary* (*complicated*).

Primary pneumothorax affects previously healthy people, usually tall, slender men in their 20s and 30s (Daley, 2017). The cause of primary pneumothorax is unknown. Risk factors include smoking and familial factors. Air-filled blebs tend to form in the apices of the lungs. This is considered to be a benign condition, although recurrences are common. Certain activities, such as high-altitude flying and rapid decompression during scuba diving, also increase the risk of spontaneous pneumothorax.

Table 36.5 Types of Pneumothorax

Type	Pathophysiology	Manifestations
Spontaneous 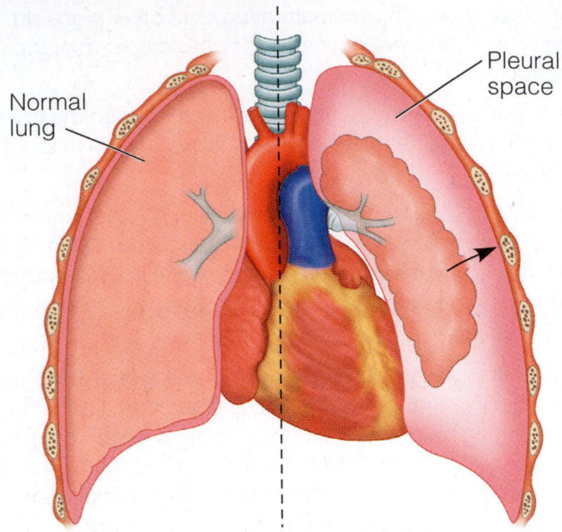Normal lung Pleural space	Rupture of a bleb on the lung surface allows air to enter pleural space from airways. ■ *Primary pneumothorax* affects previously healthy people. ■ *Secondary pneumothorax* affects people with preexisting lung disease (e.g., COPD).	■ Abrupt onset ■ Pleuritic chest pain ■ Dyspnea, shortness of breath ■ Tachypnea, tachycardia ■ Unequal lung excursion ■ Decreased breath sounds and hyperresonant percussion tone on affected side
Traumatic 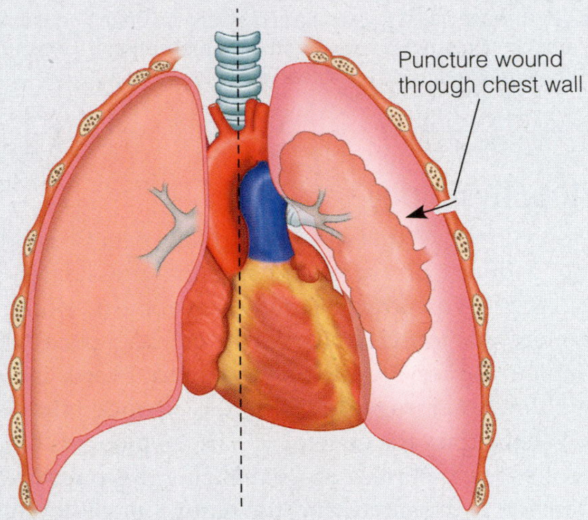Puncture wound through chest wall	Trauma to the chest wall or pleura disrupts the pleural membrane. ■ *Open* occurs with penetrating chest trauma that allows air from the environment to enter the pleural space. ■ *Closed* occurs with blunt trauma that allows air from the lung to enter the pleural space. ■ *Iatrogenic* involves laceration of visceral pleura during a procedure such as thoracentesis or central-line insertion.	■ Pain ■ Dyspnea ■ Tachypnea, tachycardia ■ Decreased respiratory excursion ■ Absent breath sounds in affected area ■ Air movement through an open wound
Tension 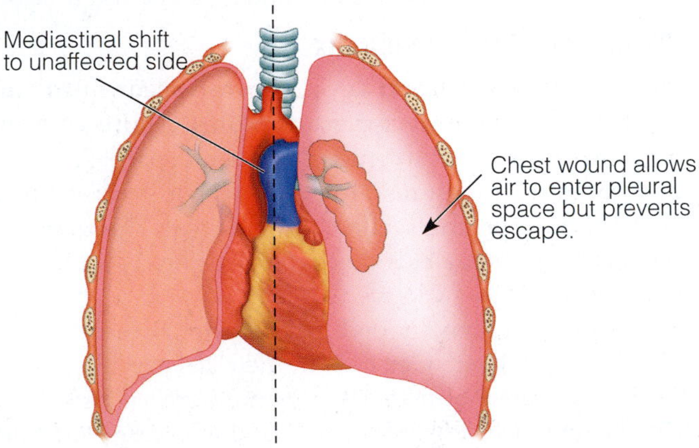Mediastinal shift to unaffected side Chest wound allows air to enter pleural space but prevents escape.	Air enters pleural space through chest wall or from airways but is unable to escape, resulting in rapid accumulation. Lung on affected side collapses. As intrapleural pressure increases, heart, great vessels, trachea, and esophagus shift toward the unaffected side.	■ Hypotension, shock ■ Distended neck veins ■ Severe dyspnea ■ Tachypnea, tachycardia ■ Decreased respiratory excursion ■ Absent breath sounds on affected side ■ Tracheal deviation toward unaffected side

Secondary pneumothorax, generally caused by overdistention and rupture of an alveolus, is more serious and potentially life-threatening. It develops in patients with underlying lung disease, usually COPD. Middle-aged and older adults are primarily affected. Secondary pneumothorax may also be associated with asthma, cystic fibrosis, pulmonary fibrosis, tuberculosis, acute respiratory distress syndrome (ARDS), and other lung diseases. Rarely, a form of secondary pneumothorax called *catamenial pneumothorax* can develop in affected women within 24 to 72 hours of the onset of menstrual flow (Daley, 2017).

Traumatic Pneumothorax

Blunt or penetrating trauma of the chest wall and pleura can cause pneumothorax. Blunt trauma, for example, due to a motor vehicle crash, fall, or during cardiopulmonary resuscitation (CPR), can lead to a *closed pneumothorax*. Fractured ribs penetrating the pleura are the leading cause of pneumothorax due to blunt trauma. Fracture of the trachea and a ruptured bronchus or esophagus may also result from blunt trauma, leading to closed pneumothorax.

Open pneumothorax (*sucking chest wound*) results from penetrating chest trauma such as a stab wound, gunshot wound, or impalement injury. With open pneumothorax, air moves freely between the pleural space and the atmosphere through the wound. Pressure on the affected side equalizes with the atmosphere, and the lung collapses rapidly. The result is significant hypoventilation.

Iatrogenic pneumothorax may result from puncture or laceration of the visceral pleura during central-line placement, thoracentesis, or lung biopsy. During bronchoscopy, bronchi or lung tissue can be disrupted. Alveoli can become overdistended and rupture during anesthesia, resuscitation procedures, or mechanical ventilation.

Tension Pneumothorax

Tension pneumothorax develops when injury to the chest wall or lungs allows air to enter the pleural space but prevents it from escaping. Pressure within the pleural space becomes positive in relation to atmospheric pressure as air rapidly accumulates with each breath. The lung on the affected side collapses, and pressure on the mediastinum shifts thoracic organs to the unaffected side of the chest, placing pressure on the opposite lung as well. Ventilation is severely compromised, and venous return to the heart is impaired. Tension pneumothorax is a medical emergency requiring immediate intervention to preserve respiration and cardiac output.

Risk Factors

Multiple lung conditions increase the risk for pneumothorax. These include COPD, cystic fibrosis, pulmonary tuberculosis, pneumonia, or asthma. In patients with COPD with bulla (air sac that enlarges like a bubble with very thin walls), risk for bulla rupture and resulting pneumothorax is increased.

Manifestations

The manifestations of spontaneous pneumothorax depend on the size of the pneumothorax, extent of lung collapse, and any underlying lung disease. Typically, pleuritic chest pain and shortness of breath begin abruptly, often while at rest. The respiratory and heart rates increase as gas exchange is affected. Chest wall movement may be asymmetrical, with less movement on the affected side than the unaffected side. The affected side is hyperresonant to percussion, and breath sounds may be diminished or absent. Hypoxemia may develop, although normal mechanisms that shunt blood flow to the unaffected lung often maintain normal oxygen saturation levels. Hypoxemia is more pronounced in secondary pneumothorax.

With traumatic pneumothorax, manifestations of pain and dyspnea may be masked or missed due to other injuries. Tachypnea and tachycardia may be attributed to the primary injury. Focused assessment for evidence of pneumothorax is vital. Chest wall movement on the affected side is diminished, and breath sounds are absent. If a penetrating wound is present, air may be heard and felt moving through it with respiratory efforts. Hemothorax frequently accompanies traumatic pneumothorax. The manifestations of iatrogenic pneumothorax are similar to those of spontaneous pneumothorax.

In tension pneumothorax, in addition to manifestations of pneumothorax, hypotension and distended neck veins are evident as venous return and cardiac output are affected. The trachea is displaced toward the unaffected side as a result of the mediastinal shift. Signs of shock may be present. Refer to Chapter 11 for the manifestations and treatment of shock.

Interprofessional Care

Treatment for pneumothorax depends on the severity of the problem. A small simple pneumothorax may require no treatment other than monitoring with serial x-rays. Air is absorbed from the pleural space, allowing most small pneumothoraces to resolve spontaneously. A large pneumothorax or significant symptoms usually requires treatment with *thoracostomy*, or the placement of chest tubes. Surgical intervention may be necessary to prevent recurrent spontaneous pneumothorax.

Diagnosis

Oxygen saturation measurements are obtained to evaluate the effect of pneumothorax on gas exchange. ABGs may be obtained to further assess gas exchange.

The chest x-ray is an effective diagnostic tool for pneumothorax. In tension pneumothorax, air is evident on the affected side, and mediastinal structures are shifted toward the opposite or unaffected side.

Treatments

Chest Tubes. The treatment of choice for significant pneumothorax is placement of a closed-chest catheter to allow the lung to reexpand. When a tube is placed in the pleural cavity to remove air or fluid, it must be sealed to prevent air from also entering the tube and, in essence, creating an open pneumothorax. Chest tubes are sealed with a Heimlich (one-way) valve (**Figure 36.8** ■) or connected

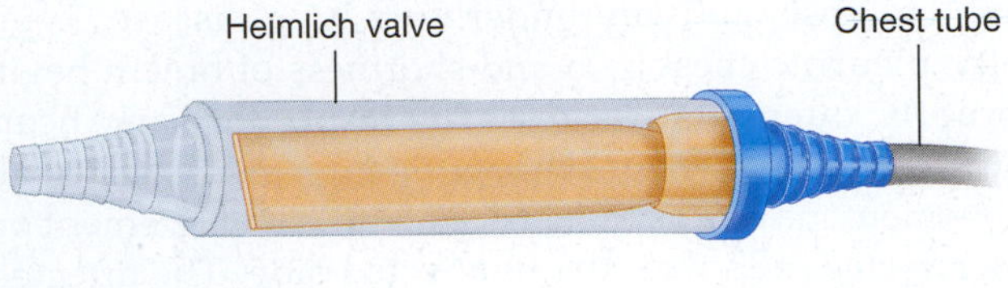

Heimlich valve
Chest tube

Figure 36.8 ■ The Heimlich one-way valve allows air to escape from the pleural space, helping reestablish negative pressure and allowing the lung to reexpand.

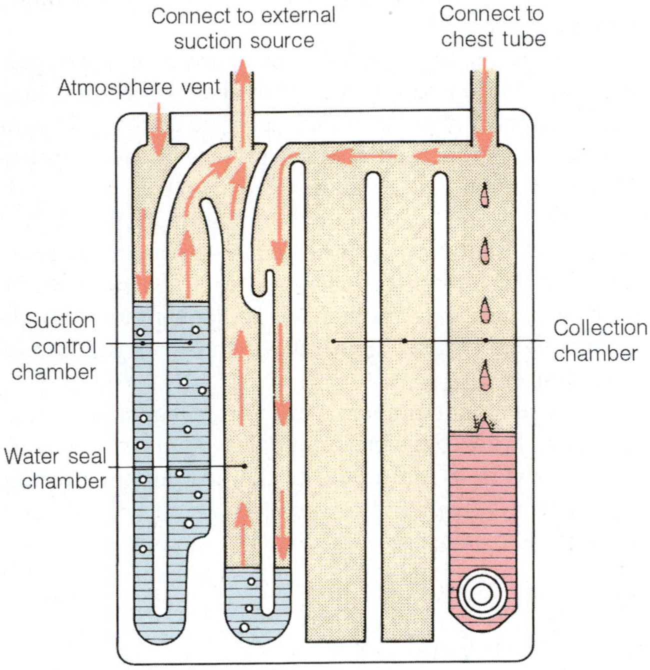

Connect to external suction source
Connect to chest tube
Atmosphere vent
Suction control chamber
Collection chamber
Water seal chamber

Figure 36.9 ■ A closed-chest drainage system.

to a closed-drainage system with a "water seal." The valve or water seal prevents air from entering the chest cavity during inspiration and allows air to escape during expiration. Applying a low level of suction to the system helps to reestablish negative pressure in the pleural space, allowing the lung to reexpand.

A number of closed-drainage chest tube systems are available. Most are self-contained disposable systems (**Figure 36.9** ■). Drainage from the chest tube is collected in the first collection chamber. This sealed chamber is connected to the water-seal chamber, which is in turn connected to the suction-control chamber. Nursing care of the patient with chest tubes is discussed in **Box 36.3**.

A large-bore needle or plastic intravenous catheter may be inserted through the chest wall as emergency treatment of a tension pneumothorax. This allows air to escape from the affected side, relieving pressure on mediastinal structures and the opposite lung.

SAFETY ALERT: Avoid placing tension on chest tubes during positioning, ambulation, and care activities. The chest tubes are minimally secured to the chest wall and can be dislodged if tension is placed on them. ■

BOX 36.3 Nursing Care of the Patient with Chest Tubes

PREPROCEDURE CARE

- Ensure a signed informed consent for chest tube insertion has been obtained. *This invasive procedure requires informed consent.*
- Provide additional information as indicated. Explain that local anesthesia will be used but that pressure may be felt as the trocar is inserted. Reassure the patient that breathing will be easier once the chest tube is in place and the lung reexpands. *The patient may be extremely dyspneic and anxious and may need reassurance that this invasive procedure will provide relief.*
- Gather all needed supplies, including thoracostomy tray, injectable lidocaine, sterile gloves, chest tube drainage system, sterile water, and a large sterile catheter-tipped syringe to use as a funnel for filling water-seal and suction chambers. *These supplies are used during the insertion procedure to establish a water-seal drainage system.*
- Position as indicated for the procedure. *Either an upright position (as for thoracentesis) or sidelying position may be used, depending on the site of the pneumothorax.*
- Assist with chest tube insertion as needed. The procedure may be performed in a procedure room, in the surgical suite, or at the bedside. *Although chest tube insertion is a relatively simple procedure, nursing assistance is necessary to support the patient and rapidly establish a closed-drainage system.*

POSTPROCEDURE CARE

- Assess respiratory status at least every 4 hours. *Frequent assessment is necessary to monitor respiratory status and the effect of a chest tube.*
- Maintain a closed system. Tape all connections, and secure the chest tube to the chest wall. *These measures are important to prevent inadvertent tube removal or disruption of the system integrity.*
- Keep the collection apparatus below the level of the chest. *Pleural fluid drains into the collection apparatus by gravity flow.*
- Check tubes frequently for kinks or loops. *These could interfere with drainage.*
- Check the water seal frequently. The water level should fluctuate with respiratory effort. If it does not, the system may not be patent or intact. Periodic air bubbles in the water-seal chamber are normal and indicate that trapped air is being removed from the chest. *Frequent assessment of the system is important to ensure appropriate functioning.*
- Measure drainage every 8 hours, marking the level on the drainage chamber. Report drainage that is cloudy, in excess of 70 mL per hour, or red, warm, and free flowing. *Red, free-flowing drainage indicates hemorrhage; cloudiness may indicate an infection.*
- Periodically assess water level in the suction control chamber, adding water as necessary. *Adequate water in the suction control chamber prevents excess suction from being placed on delicate pleural tissue.*
- Assist with frequent position changes and sitting and ambulation as allowed. *Chest tubes should not prevent performance of allowed activities. Care is needed to prevent inadvertent disconnection or removal of the tubes.*
- When the chest tube is removed, immediately apply a sterile occlusive petroleum jelly dressing. *An occlusive dressing prevents air from reentering the pleural space through the chest wound.*

Pleurodesis. Although controversial, *pleurodesis*, or creation of adhesions between the parietal and visceral pleura, may be used to prevent recurrent pneumothorax. This procedure involves instilling a chemical agent such as doxycycline into the pleural space. The subsequent inflammatory response creates scar tissue and adhesions between the pleural layers. This procedure reduces the recurrence rate to as low as 2% but can make subsequent surgery more difficult.

Surgery

The risk for recurrence of spontaneous pneumothorax increases with each attack. Patients at high risk for recurrent pneumothorax may have surgery to reduce the risk of future ruptures. A thoracotomy is done to excise or oversew blebs (usually at the apices of the lungs). The overlying pleura is then roughened or irritated to induce scarring and adhesion to the surface of the lung. In some cases, the parietal pleura may be partially excised. These procedures can be done using video-assisted thoracoscopic surgery (VATS), a minimally invasive surgical technique.

Nursing Care

Assessment

See the Manifestations and Interprofessional Care sections for the assessment of the patient with pneumothorax.

The patient with pneumothorax may be in acute respiratory distress, necessitating rapid and focused assessment.

- ***Health history:*** Current symptoms and their duration; precipitating factors or activities if known; previous episodes of pneumothorax; smoking history; chronic pulmonary diseases such as COPD
- ***Physical assessment:*** General appearance and degree of apparent respiratory distress; evidence of chest trauma; vital signs, oxygen saturation, skin color, level of consciousness; respiratory excursion, percussion tone, and breath sounds anterior and posterior chest; neck vein inspection, position of trachea; peripheral pulses
- ***Laboratory data:*** Chest x-ray, arterial blood gases.

Priorities of Care

Collaborate with the interprofessional team to ensure adequate treatment of the underlying etiology that led to the pneumothorax while providing care that promotes lung expansion and supports the physical and psychologic responses to the disorder.

Diagnoses, Interventions, and Outcomes

Maintaining or restoring adequate alveolar ventilation and gas exchange is of highest priority for the patient with a pneumothorax. Chest tubes may interfere with physical mobility, contributing to a high risk for injury.

Promote Effective Gas Exchange. Loss of negative pressure in the pleural cavity and the resulting collapse of lung tissue can cause poor chest expansion and loss of alveolar ventilation. As the pneumothorax is removed or reabsorbed, ventilation and gas exchange improve.

Expected Outcome: Improved ventilation and adequate oxygenation as evidenced by blood gas levels within normal limits for the individual patient.

The nurse will:

- Assess and document vital signs and respiratory status, including rate, depth, lung sounds, and oxygen saturation at least every 4 hours. *Frequent assessment is important to monitor the adequacy of respirations and lung expansion.*
- Evaluate chest wall movement, position of the trachea, and neck veins frequently. *Early identification of tension pneumothorax and appropriate interventions are vital to preserve cardiorespiratory function.*
- Place in Fowler or high-Fowler position. *This position facilitates lung expansion.*
- Administer oxygen as ordered. *Supplemental oxygen is given to improve oxygenation of the blood and tissues.*
- Provide emotional support, particularly in early stages and during chest tube insertion. *Dyspnea and hypoxemia can cause extreme anxiety and apprehension, impairing the ability to cooperate with procedures.*
- Assess chest tube, system function, and drainage at least every 2 hours. *The system must remain patent and intact to function effectively.*
- Provide for rest. *Adequate rest is important to conserve energy and reduce oxygen demand.*

Reduce Risk for Injury. Pain and the presence of chest tubes can reduce the perceived ability to ambulate and provide self-care. Moderate activity is encouraged unless respiratory function is significantly impaired. Caution is taken to maintain integrity of the chest tube system. If the tube is inadvertently pulled out or system integrity is disrupted, the pneumothorax may increase or infection may develop.

Expected Outcome: Patient will practice effective risk control through use of close and careful chest tube monitoring.

The nurse will:

- Secure a loop of drainage tubing to the sheet or gown. *Looping the drainage tubing prevents direct pressure on the chest tube itself.*
- When turning to the affected side, ensure that neither the chest tube nor drainage tubing is kinked or occluded under the patient. *This maintains patency of the system.*
- Teach the patient how to ambulate with the drainage system, keeping the system lower than the chest. In most cases, suction can be discontinued during ambulation. *Ambulation facilitates lung ventilation and expansion. Drainage systems are portable to allow ambulation while chest tubes are in place. Keeping the drainage system lower than the chest promotes drainage and prevents reflux.*

- Observe insertion site when changing chest tube dressings for redness, swelling, pain, or drainage. Report any signs of infection, including fever, to the healthcare provider. *Interruption of skin integrity by chest tube insertion increases the risk for infection.*
- Ensure all tubing connections are taped per hospital policy or provider preference. If a connection does come loose, reconnect it as soon as possible. *A closed, sealed system is vital to prevent air from entering the pleural space and an open pneumothorax.*

SAFETY ALERT: Seal the wound of an open pneumothorax or from inadvertent tube removal as soon as possible with a sterile occlusive dressing, such as gauze impregnated with petroleum jelly. If a sterile dressing is not available, other occlusive material such as foil or plastic wrap can be used. Tape the dressing on three sides only. An occlusive dressing taped on three sides prevents the development of a tension pneumothorax by inhibiting air from entering the wound during inhalation but allowing it to escape during exhalation. ■

Delegating Nursing Care Activities

As appropriate and allowed by the designated duties and responsibilities of unlicensed assistive personnel, the nurse may delegate nursing care activities such as measuring vital signs, encouraging oral or enteral fluid intake, and providing skin care.

Transitions of Care

Health promotion activities to prevent spontaneous and traumatic pneumothorax primarily involve health teaching. Initiate and participate in programs to prevent smoking among children and teenagers. Teach safe behaviors such as always wearing a seat beat in an automobile, driving safely, and using precautions to prevent falls when working or recreating in high places.

Following a pneumothorax, instruct the patient to gradually increase exercise and activity to previous levels. Stress the importance of follow-up care and monitoring. Discuss manifestations to report to the healthcare provider: Upper respiratory infections; fever, cough, or difficulty breathing; sudden, sharp chest pain; or redness, pain, swelling, tenderness, or drainage from the chest tube puncture wound.

Patients who have experienced spontaneous pneumothorax need education about their future risk. After a single episode of spontaneous pneumothorax, the risk of recurrence is 28 to 32% for primary pneumothorax and 43% for secondary pneumothorax (Daley, 2017). This risk increases with subsequent episodes. Stress the importance of quitting smoking to reduce the risk. Other activities that can precipitate recurrent episodes include mountain climbing or those involving exposure to high altitudes, flying in unpressurized aircraft, and scuba diving. The patient may be advised to avoid contact sports.

The Patient with Hemothorax

Hemothorax, or blood in the pleural space, usually occurs as a result of chest trauma, surgery, or diagnostic procedures. Hemothorax may develop in patients with chest trauma, usually due to laceration of the lung, an intercostal vessel, or the internal mammary artery. If a major thoracic vessel is disrupted, hemorrhage can be massive. Tumors, pulmonary infarction, and infections such as TB can also cause hemothorax. When blood collects in the pleural space, pressure on the affected lung impairs ventilation and gas exchange. With significant hemorrhage, a risk of shock exists.

Hemothorax causes symptoms similar to those of pneumothorax or pleural effusion. Lung sounds are diminished, and a dull percussion tone is noted over the collected blood, typically at the base of the lung. Chest x-ray is used to confirm the diagnosis of hemothorax.

Thoracentesis or thoracostomy with chest tube drainage is used to remove blood from the pleural space. With significant hemorrhage (e.g., due to trauma or surgery), the blood may be collected for subsequent autotransfusion. Blood for autotransfusion should be collected and reinfused within 4 hours. Strict aseptic technique is used when collecting the blood. It is collected through a gross particulate filter into a container primed with anticoagulant and reinfused when the container is full or when transfusion is necessary. Air is removed from the blood container prior to reinfusion and a filter used to eliminate debris, such as degenerating blood cells, fat particles, and fibrin.

Priority nursing care for the patient with hemothorax focuses on assessing and maintaining adequate respiratory function and cardiac output. The priority of care depends on the rate and extent of hemothorax. In a large, slow-developing hemothorax, ventilatory status may be affected significantly, making priorities for care those that support effective gas exchange and an effective breathing pattern (Perrin & MacLeod, 2012). When hemothorax develops rapidly and hemorrhage is significant, cardiac output and fluid volume become additional priorities for care.

When preparing the patient for home care following a hemothorax, discuss the importance of avoiding smoking and preventing respiratory infection. Include symptoms to report to the healthcare provider (cool, pale, clammy skin; low blood pressure; tachycardia). If trauma or infection caused the hemothorax, discuss measures to prevent future trauma and continuing treatment for the infection as indicated.

36.3 Trauma of the Chest or Lung

Chest injury is a contributing cause of death from trauma. It is commonly associated with motor vehicle crashes, violent crime, and falls. Chest injuries can range from mild, such as a simple rib fracture, to severe and fatal. Traumatic injury to the chest may involve both the chest wall and underlying thoracic structures, including the lungs, heart, great vessels, and esophagus. Chest and lung injury can result from several different mechanisms: Penetrating trauma, such as a stab or gunshot wound; blunt trauma, such as a fall, motor vehicle crash, vehicle–pedestrian impact, or crush injury; or inhalation injury, such as smoke inhalation or near-drowning.

Rapid and continuing assessment of the airway, breathing, and circulation (ABCs) is vital in chest or lung injuries. Chest trauma can disrupt any or all of these functions. Chest injuries that may be life-threatening include airway obstruction, tension pneumothorax, open pneumothorax, massive hemothorax, and flail chest with pulmonary contusion.

The Patient with a Thoracic Injury

Thoracic injuries may be minor and have little effect on respiratory status, for example, a simple rib fracture in a previously healthy patient. When pain or chest wall instability impair breathing or the underlying lung tissue is damaged, the risk is more significant. Motor vehicle crashes or falls are the usual causes of thoracic trauma.

Pathophysiology

Acceleration–deceleration injury and direct mechanisms of injury (e.g., crush injuries) are the most common mechanisms of thoracic injuries. Acceleration–deceleration injuries are caused by a rapid change in velocity as occurs in a motor vehicle crash or fall. The body stops suddenly, but the tissues and organs within the chest cavity continue to move forward until they impact the chest wall. Injuries sustained can be significant, depending on the velocity (speed) of the vehicle or body at the point of impact, the surface with which the body impacts, and individual characteristics (e.g., size and bone structure).

Rib Fracture

Simple rib fracture, usually involving a single rib, is the most common chest wall injury. Rib fracture is generally tolerated well and heals rapidly in a young, previously healthy person. In an older adult or person with preexisting lung disease, however, a fractured rib may lead to significant complications, such as pneumonia, atelectasis, and, potentially, respiratory failure. Displaced fractured ribs can penetrate the pleura, leading to pneumothorax and possible hemothorax. Fractures of certain ribs are more frequently associated with underlying tissue damage. Intrathoracic vessels may be damaged or torn with fractures of the first and second ribs. Fractures of the seventh through tenth ribs may cause liver or spleen injuries.

Flail Chest

Multiple rib fractures may impair chest wall stability and normal chest wall function. When two or more consecutive ribs are fractured in multiple places, a free-floating segment of the chest wall, or **flail chest**, results. Physiologic function of the chest wall is impaired as the flail segment sucks inward during inhalation and moves outward with exhalation. This is known as *paradoxic movement* (**Figure 36.10 ■**).

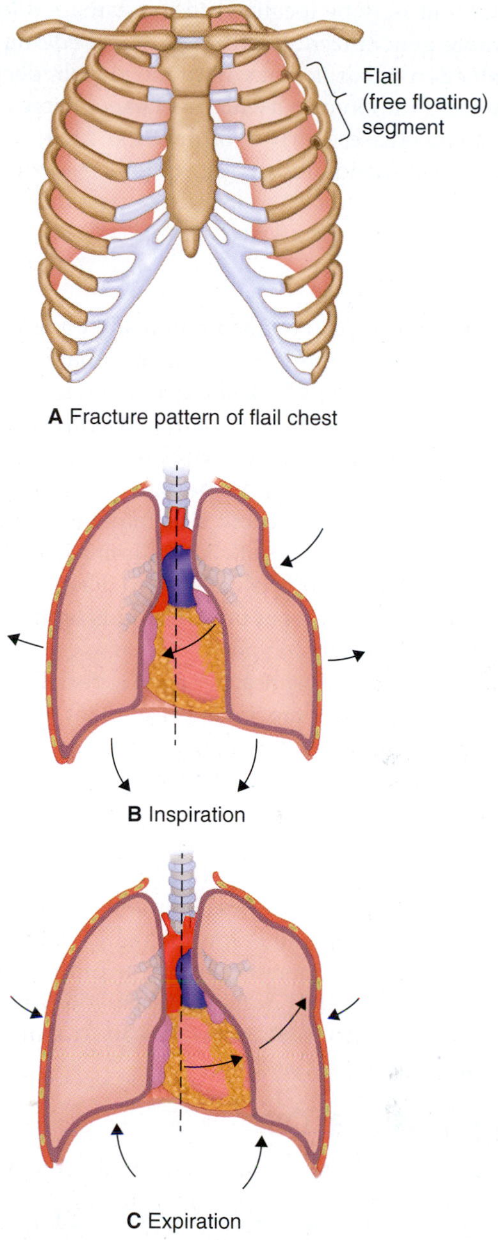
Flail
(free floating)
segment
A Fracture pattern of flail chest
B Inspiration
C Expiration

Figure 36.10 ■ Flail chest with paradoxical movement.

Flail chest can significantly affect ventilation and, consequently, gas exchange. Lung expansion is impaired and the work of breathing increases. Flail chest is frequently associated with underlying pulmonary contusion, which may lead to respiratory failure.

Pulmonary Contusion

Pulmonary contusion, or lung tissue injury, is frequently associated with flail chest and other blunt chest trauma. It may occur unilaterally or bilaterally. Pulmonary contusion often results from abrupt chest compression followed by sudden decompression, as can occur with a motor vehicle crash, significant fall, or crush injury. Alveoli and pulmonary arterioles rupture, causing intra-alveolar hemorrhage and interstitial and bronchial edema. The resulting inflammatory response increases capillary permeability, leading to edema that may be localized to the damaged lung tissue or more generalized. Inflammation and edema impair the production of surfactant within the alveoli, decreasing compliance. Pulmonary vascular resistance increases and blood flow decreases. Airway obstruction, atelectasis, and impaired gas diffusion result. Associated chest wall injury impairs the ability to clear secretions effectively, and the work of breathing is significantly increased.

Manifestations

Rib fracture causes pain on inspiration and coughing. This leads to voluntary splinting, with rapid, shallow respirations and inhibited cough. Bruising may be seen over the fracture, and crepitus may be palpated with respiratory movement. Breath sounds are diminished, especially in the bases, due to splinting. If pneumothorax develops, chest wall movement on the affected side may be reduced and breath sounds absent or significantly diminished. A hyperresonant percussion tone is usually noted. Hemothorax also causes diminished or absent breath sounds on the affected side, with a dull percussion note.

Flail chest causes dyspnea and pain, especially on inspiration. Paradoxic chest movement is evident with inspection. Chest expansion is unequal, and palpable crepitus is present. Breath sounds are diminished, and crackles may be heard on auscultation.

Manifestations of pulmonary contusion may not be apparent until 12 to 24 hours after the injury. Increasing shortness of breath, restlessness, apprehension, and chest pain are early signs. Copious sputum, which may be blood tinged, is present. Later manifestations include tachycardia, tachypnea, dyspnea, and cyanosis. Even with appropriate treatment, pulmonary contusion can lead to acute respiratory distress and potential death.

Interprofessional Care

Diagnosis

Chest x-ray is used to identify most chest wall injuries. Rib fractures are evident on x-ray. Pulmonary contusion may show as initial patchy opacifications progressing to diffuse opacification, or "white-out." Changes in oxygen saturation and arterial blood gases depend on the degree to which ventilation and gas exchange are affected by the injury.

Medications

Simple rib fractures typically heal uneventfully. Providing adequate analgesia to promote breathing, coughing, and movement is the primary intervention. With multiple rib fractures, an intercostal nerve block may be used to ensure adequate ventilation. Intercostal nerve blocks or continuous epidural analgesia may be employed to manage the pain associated with flail chest.

Treatments

Rib belts, binders, and taping to stabilize the rib cage are not recommended because they may interfere with ventilation and lead to atelectasis. Even with simple rib fracture, older patients and patients with preexisting lung disease require close monitoring to prevent and detect atelectasis, pneumonia, and other complications.

For a small flail chest, analgesia combined with supplemental oxygen therapy may be adequate. In some cases, internal or external fixation of the flail segment may be done.

The preferred treatment for flail chest is intubation and mechanical ventilation. Positive-pressure ventilation provides support and stabilization of the flail segment and improves ventilation and gas exchange. The work of breathing is decreased and healing improved.

Patients with pulmonary contusion are often critically ill, requiring intensive care management. Treatment is supportive, directed at maintaining adequate ventilation and alveolar gas exchange. Endotracheal intubation and mechanical ventilation are necessary in most cases. Repeated bronchoscopy may be done to remove secretions and cellular debris, preventing atelectasis. Although adequate hydration is necessary to prevent shock, overhydration can increase pulmonary edema. Pulmonary arterial pressure monitoring with a Swan-Ganz catheter and frequent arterial blood gas measurement is required for optimal fluid replacement and management of ventilatory support. Refer to Chapter 31 for more information about pulmonary artery pressure monitoring and Chapter 37 for nursing care of the patient who is intubated and ventilated.

Unilateral pulmonary contusion may present a unique management problem. Mechanical ventilation with positive end-expiratory pressure (PEEP) to maintain open alveoli and adequate gas exchange can damage the unaffected lung. Intubation with a double-lumen endotracheal tube that permits independent ventilation of each lung may be used.

Nursing Care

Assessment

See the Manifestations and Interprofessional Care sections for the assessment of the patient with a thoracic injury.

The nursing assessment of the patient with a thoracic injury may need to be rapid and focused.

- ***Health history:*** Pain, difficulty breathing; circumstances of the injury, including position in the motor vehicle, use of restraints, speed and type of impact; distance of a fall, surface and position on impact; history of chronic lung or heart disease; smoking history
- ***Physical assessment:*** Airway, breathing, circulation; level of consciousness; color, vital signs; respiratory rate, depth, ease; symmetry of chest movement; lung sounds and percussion tone; presence of bruising, crepitus, or paradoxical chest movement.

Priorities of Care

Collaborate with the interprofessional team to ensure adequate treatment of the underlying injury while providing care that supports the physical and psychologic responses to the injury, including pain management, is a priority of nursing care.

Diagnoses, Interventions, and Outcomes

Chest wall trauma can interfere with adequate chest expansion and alveolar ventilation. When a pulmonary contusion is also present, gas exchange is affected as well. Priorities for nursing management include controlling pain, ensuring adequate ventilation, and promoting gas exchange.

Manage Pain. With many thoracic injuries, pain interferes with lung expansion and coughing. Such pain can lead to complications such as pneumonia and atelectasis. Adequate pain management is a key component of medical and nursing management for these patients.

Expected Outcome: Patient will experience adequate pain control as evidenced by physical well-being.

The nurse will:

- Frequently assess pain, using a standard pain scale and objective data. *Increased respiratory rate, shallow respirations, diminished breath sounds, and reluctance to move and cough may indicate inadequate pain control in a thoracic injury.*
- Administer analgesics by patient-controlled analgesia or on a schedule to maintain pain control. *Analgesics are more effective when pain is not allowed to become intense.*
- Notify the healthcare provider if pain relief is inadequate or excess sedation and respiratory depression occur. *An intercostal nerve block may be done to reduce the need for narcotic analgesia. Assess for bleeding and adequate ventilation following a nerve block.*

SAFETY ALERT: Assess for possible respiratory depression due to narcotic analgesia. Respiratory depression can further compromise ventilation in the patient with thoracic injury. ■

Promote Airway Clearance and Patency. Aggressive respiratory hygiene may be necessary to maintain open airways and adequate ventilation.

Expected Outcome: Patient will use techniques to promote airway clearance such as coughing and deep breathing.

The nurse will:

- Assess lung sounds and respiratory rate, depth, and effort frequently. Encourage the patient to cough, use deep breathing techniques, and change position every 1 to 2 hours and use the incentive spirometer. *Frequent assessment and measures to maintain airway patency are vital to prevent complications in the patient with thoracic injury.*
- Teach the patient how to splint the affected area with a blanket or pillow when coughing. *Splinting reduces movement and discomfort of the affected area.*
- Suction airway as indicated. Work with respiratory therapy to maintain optimal mechanical ventilation. Secure the endotracheal tube to maintain appropriate position and lung ventilation. *Endotracheal tube security is particularly important when a double-lumen endotracheal tube is in place because malposition can occlude one main bronchus and prevent ventilation of the affected lung.*
- Elevate the head of the bed. *Elevating the head of the bed facilitates lung expansion and reduces the work of breathing.*

SAFETY ALERT: Promptly report to the healthcare provider signs of complications, such as diminished breath sounds, increasing crackles (rales) or rhonchi, dull or hyperresonant percussion tones, unequal chest movement, hemoptysis, chills or fever, or changes in vital signs. Prompt intervention for complications is vital to promote healing and recovery. ■

Promote Effective Gas Exchange. Impaired gas exchange is of particular concern in pulmonary contusion. Alveolar damage and pulmonary edema can significantly impair oxygenation of the blood and removal of carbon dioxide.

Expected Outcome: Patient will achieve improved ventilation and adequate oxygenation as evidenced by blood gas levels within normal limits for the individual patient.

The nurse will:

- Monitor vital signs, color, oxygen saturation, and arterial blood gases. Assess for manifestations such as anxiety or apprehension, restlessness, confusion or lethargy, or complaints of headache. *These assessment data alert the nurse and care providers to potential hypoxemia or hypercapnia due to impaired gas exchange.*
- Maintain oxygen therapy and mechanical ventilation, as ordered. Hyperoxygenate prior to suctioning. *Oxygen and mechanical ventilation support alveolar gas exchange. Hyperoxygenation prior to suctioning reduces the degree of hypoxemia that occurs during suctioning.*
- Monitor intake and output, weigh daily, and monitor central venous pressure and pulmonary artery pressure, as ordered. Maintain any ordered fluid restriction. *Fluid volume status is monitored to reduce the effects of pulmonary edema on lung tissues.*
- Maintain bedrest or activity restriction as ordered. Space activities to allow periods of uninterrupted rest. *Rest reduces the metabolic rate and oxygen consumption.*

Delegating Nursing Care Activities

As appropriate and allowed by the designated duties and responsibilities of unlicensed assistive personnel, the nurse may delegate nursing care activities such as measuring vital signs, encouraging oral or enteral fluid intake, and providing skin care.

Transitions of Care

Encourage the use of seat belts, shoulder harnesses, and supplemental restraint systems such as airbags to significantly reduce the incidence of thoracic injury associated with motor vehicle crashes. Discuss the importance of appropriate protective equipment and gear for people engaging in potentially hazardous activities such as contact sports, mountain climbing, and occupations such as roofing or house painting.

Simple rib fracture and minor chest wall injuries are often managed on an outpatient basis. Include the following topics when teaching for home care:

- Pain management and its importance in preventing respiratory complications
- Importance of coughing and deep breathing; how to splint the rib cage during coughing

- Reasons for not taping or wrapping the chest continuously
- Symptoms to report to the healthcare provider: Chills and fever, productive cough, purulent or bloody sputum, shortness of breath or difficulty breathing, and increasing chest pain
- Importance of avoiding respiratory irritants, such as cigarette smoke and occupational or environmental pollutants.

Significant pulmonary contusion can result in long-term respiratory insufficiency. Discuss activity modifications and occupational changes with the patient and family as indicated. Refer the patient to home care services such as respiratory therapy and home health, if needed.

The Patient with Inhalation Injury

The internal environment of the lungs normally is protected from noxious substances by respiratory defense mechanisms. If these defenses are breached, inhaled agents, such as gases, fumes, toxins, and water, can cause internal trauma to the lungs.

Pathophysiology

Smoke Inhalation

Pulmonary injury due to inhalation of hot air, toxic gases, or particulate matter is the leading cause of death in burn injury (Perrin & MacLeod, 2017). Smoke inhalation affects up to one-third of patients admitted to burn units. Smoke inhalation can significantly affect normal respiratory function through three different mechanisms:

- Thermal damage to the airways, leading to impaired ventilation
- Carbon monoxide or cyanide poisoning, resulting in tissue hypoxia
- Chemical damage to the lung from noxious gases, which can impair gas exchange.

Smoke inhalation is suspected whenever a burn occurs in a closed space; if there are burns to the face or upper torso or singed nasal hairs; if sputum contains ash-like material; and when manifestations such as dyspnea, wheezing, rales, or rhonchi develop.

The lower airways of the lungs are typically protected from thermal damage by cooling of the inhaled gases in the upper airway and laryngeal spasm. Upper airway obstruction due to tissue edema and laryngeal spasm can occur quickly, however, resulting in **asphyxiation**, or oxygen deprivation, without lung damage. Steam inhalation can cause thermal damage to tissues of the lower respiratory tract.

Inhalation of carbon monoxide or cyanide gas poses an immediate threat to life. Carbon monoxide is a colorless, odorless gas produced in a fire. It binds readily with hemoglobin. The affinity of carbon monoxide for hemoglobin is 200 to 250 times stronger than that of oxygen. Hemoglobin bound to carbon monoxide reduces the oxygen-carrying capacity of blood and oxygen delivery to cells of the body. Carbon monoxide poisoning is suspected if the burn occurred in a closed space, if there is evidence of inhalation injury, or if dyspnea develops.

Many other toxic chemicals may be present in smoke, especially in a house fire or industrial plant fire. Hydrogen cyanide can be lethal when inhaled. Inhalation of toxic chemicals causes bronchospasm and edema of the airways and alveoli. Acute respiratory distress syndrome may develop within 1 to 2 days. Sloughing of damaged mucosa leads to airway obstruction and atelectasis. Pneumonia is common following smoke inhalation.

Near-Drowning

Drowning is a leading preventable cause of accidental death in the United States. Approximately 3500 people die of drowning every year in the United States (CDC, 2017f). Alcohol ingestion is a factor in about 25% of adult drowning deaths. Other circumstances that may contribute to drowning and near-drowning include excessive fatigue, a sudden acute condition such as seizure or myocardial infarction, and head or spinal cord injury associated with diving.

Asphyxiation and aspiration are the primary problems associated with drowning and near-drowning. About 10% of victims do not aspirate water; instead, laryngeal spasm causes asphyxia. This is known as "dry drowning." In most cases, however, asphyxia and hypoxemia are the result of fluid aspiration. The effects of hypoxemia occur rapidly; loss of consciousness can occur within 3 to 5 minutes after total immersion. Circulatory impairment, brain injury, and brain death can occur within 5 to 10 minutes. Immersion in very cold water and the *dive reflex*, a protective mechanism that slows the heartbeat, constricts peripheral vessels, and shunts blood to the brain and heart, may prolong survival (CDC, 2017f).

Water aspiration can cause delayed death from near-drowning. Respiratory and systemic effects differ, depending on whether freshwater or saltwater has been aspirated. Freshwater is hypotonic; when aspirated, it is rapidly absorbed from the alveoli, leading to hypervolemia and hemodilution. Hemolysis occurs as blood cells are subjected to a hypotonic environment, and serum electrolytes are diluted. Electrolyte imbalances can cause cardiac dysrhythmias and death. Hemolysis can lead to acute tubular necrosis and acute renal failure. Aspiration of freshwater impairs pulmonary surfactant and damages the alveolar-capillary membrane. Respiratory failure can result.

Nearly the opposite effects occur with saltwater aspiration. As a hypertonic fluid, saltwater draws fluid into the alveoli, resulting in hypovolemia and hemoconcentration. Hemolysis is insignificant, and small elevations in serum sodium and chloride levels rarely cause life-threatening effects. With either type of near-drowning episode, inhaled microorganisms and debris can lead to pneumonia. The pathophysiologic changes associated with freshwater and saltwater near-drowning are illustrated in **Figure 36.11** ■.

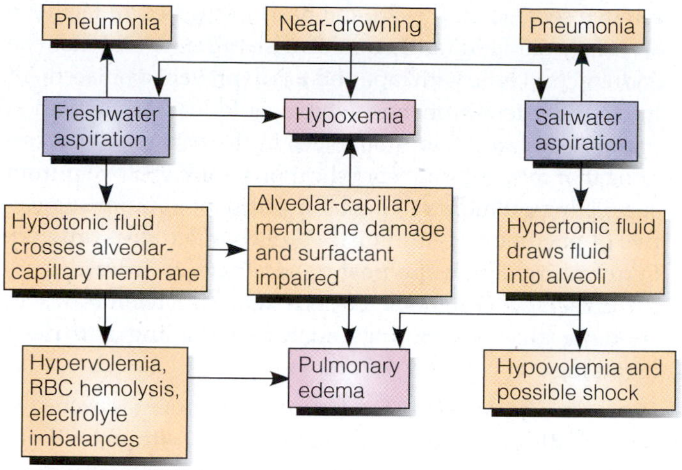
Pneumonia
Near-drowning
Pneumonia
Freshwater aspiration
Hypoxemia
Saltwater aspiration
Hypotonic fluid crosses alveolar-capillary membrane
Alveolar-capillary membrane damage and surfactant impaired
Hypertonic fluid draws fluid into alveoli
Hypervolemia, RBC hemolysis, electrolyte imbalances
Pulmonary edema
Hypovolemia and possible shock

Figure 36.11 ■ The pathogenesis of near-drowning, freshwater and saltwater.

The near-drowning victim who never loses consciousness or is conscious on admission to the emergency department has a good prognosis for recovery. The prognosis is less optimistic when neurologic damage has occurred.

Manifestations

Manifestations of smoke inhalation include dyspnea, wheezing, rales, and/or rhonchi.

The manifestations of carbon monoxide poisoning depend on the level of carboxyhemoglobin saturation. When hemoglobin is 10 to 20% saturated with carbon monoxide, symptoms include headache, dizziness, dyspnea, and nausea. A characteristic "cherry-red" skin color and mucous membranes may be seen. With increasing levels, confusion, visual disturbances, irritability, hallucinations, hypotension, seizures, and coma develop. Permanent neurologic deficit can occur in survivors of severe acute carbon monoxide poisoning.

Manifestations of near-drowning may include altered level of consciousness, restlessness, and apprehension. The patient may complain of headache or chest pain. Other signs include vomiting, possible cyanosis, apnea, tachypnea, and wheezing. If pulmonary edema is present, pink froth may be visible in the mouth and nose. Other manifestations include tachycardia, dysrhythmias, hypotension, shock, and cardiac arrest. Hypothermia may be present.

Interprofessional Care

After prevention, the second most important line of defense against death or permanent injury from inhalation injuries is removing the victim from the area of the fire or water and administering effective cardiopulmonary resuscitation. In many cases, immediate restoration of effective breathing and circulation is key to preserving life. Hypoxemia progresses rapidly until breathing is restored; reversal of tissue hypoxia depends on adequate circulation. In both smoke inhalation and near-drowning, intubation may be necessary to establish an airway. Oxygen is administered as soon as possible. Attempts to drain water from the lungs of the near-drowning victim waste time and are generally ineffective in restoring alveolar ventilation. External cardiac defibrillation may be necessary to reestablish an effective cardiac rhythm and circulation. When the victim is hypothermic, resuscitation measures are continued until the core body temperature reaches approximately 32°C (90°F). The basic rule in hypothermia is that the patient is not declared dead until the body has been rewarmed and signs of life remain absent.

Diagnosis

When inhalation injury is known or suspected, the following diagnostic tests may be done:

- ***ABGs*** are drawn to evaluate gas exchange and the degree of hypoxemia. Combined respiratory and metabolic acidosis may be apparent. With effective ventilation and supplemental oxygen, acidosis may reverse quickly. With carbon monoxide poisoning, arterial Po_2 may be normal, but oxyhemoglobin saturation is less than normal.
- ***Carboxyhemoglobin levels*** are drawn in suspected carbon monoxide poisoning. Normal levels are < 5% in nonsmokers and < 10% in smokers. Higher levels indicate carbon monoxide poisoning. Levels < 20% are considered mild poisoning; between 20 and 40% is moderate poisoning; and 40 to 60% is severe poisoning. Levels > 60% are generally fatal.
- ***Serum electrolytes*** and ***osmolality levels*** vary in near-drowning, depending on the type of water aspirated. In freshwater drowning, serum electrolyte levels and osmolality may be significantly reduced. With saltwater drowning, serum sodium and chloride may be somewhat high, and osmolality is increased because of hypovolemia.
- ***Chest x-ray*** is done, but may not show changes until 12 or more hours after the insult. Evidence of acute respiratory distress syndrome may be seen 24 to 48 hours after inhalation injury.
- ***Bronchoscopy*** may be ordered to inspect damaged lung tissue, particularly with smoke inhalation and possible thermal injury.

Treatments

Treatment of inhalation injury is generally supportive. Endotracheal intubation and mechanical ventilation are often required to maintain the airway and provide adequate alveolar ventilation and oxygenation. All patients with inhalation injury require supplemental oxygen, even when intubation and ventilation are not required. *Hyperbaric oxygen therapy*, the delivery of 100% oxygen at increased atmospheric pressure, may be used to treat carbon monoxide poisoning. This treatment carries some risks, such as oxygen toxicity and potential trauma to lung tissues, sinuses, and ears due to the increased pressures.

Other treatment measures may include bronchodilator therapy to manage bronchospasm. Bronchodilators can be administered by aerosol inhalation or intravenous infusion. Coughing and suctioning are important to remove secretions and debris. Chest physiotherapy with percussion and postural drainage may be performed.

Intravenous fluids may be ordered; if significant hemolysis has occurred, packed red blood cells may be given to improve the oxygen-carrying capacity of the blood. Fluid therapy is monitored carefully, using pulmonary artery or central venous pressures to reduce the risk of pulmonary edema.

With near-drowning victims, measures such as inducing hypothermia or barbiturate-induced coma and administering corticosteroids and osmotic diuretics may be employed to help prevent neurologic damage. Careful monitoring for complications such as pneumonia and acute respiratory distress syndrome is vital throughout the course of treatment. Respiratory status, vital signs, and other data are frequently assessed to identify complications and allow early intervention.

Nursing Care

Assessment

See the Manifestations and Interprofessional Care sections for the assessment of the patient with an inhalation injury.

Inhalation injuries may be medical emergencies, necessitating focused and timely nursing assessment.

- *Health history:* Circumstances of the injury, including duration of exposure to smoke or time under water, explosion or fire in a closed area, type and temperature of water immersed in; resuscitation measures used; allergies and current medical problems
- *Physical assessment:* Airway, breathing, circulation; level of consciousness; color, oxygen saturation level; vital signs; heart and lung sounds; urine output; evidence of burns or soot around nares or mouth
- *Laboratory data:* Carboxyhemoglobin levels, serum electrolytes, and osmolality; arterial blood gases; chest x-ray.

Priorities of Care

Collaborating with the interprofessional team to ensure adequate treatment of the underlying etiology in response to the inhalation injury while providing care that supports the physical and psychologic responses to the injury, including promoting salvage of optimal lung function, is a priority of nursing care.

Diagnoses, Interventions, and Outcomes

Nursing care priorities for the patient with an inhalation injury are determined by the type of injury or tissue damage. Airway clearance is a major concern in all inhalation injuries, as is impaired gas exchange. Tissue hypoxia can also be a significant problem.

Promote Airway Clearance and Patency. Nursing measures to maintain an adequate airway begin with careful and frequent assessment of respiratory status, including rate, depth, and effort, as well as breath sounds. Note amount, color, and consistency of sputum. Assist the patient to cough frequently, and suction the intubated patient as needed to remove secretions. Elevate the head of the bed to facilitate alveolar ventilation unless otherwise ordered. Stabilize the endotracheal tube with tape and ties to prevent displacement into a mainstem bronchus, which could lead to ventilation of only one lung. Report changes in the character of secretions that may indicate complications: Pink, frothy sputum suggesting pulmonary edema or purulent sputum suggestive of pneumonia. Administer bronchodilators as ordered. Perform percussion and postural drainage as ordered.

Expected Outcome: Patient will use techniques to promote airway clearance such as coughing and deep breathing.

Promote Effective Gas Exchange. Support gas exchange by administering supplemental oxygen, with or without mechanical ventilation. Frequently assess oxygen saturation, skin color, and mental status. Decreasing level of consciousness may be an early sign of hypoxemia. Monitor exhaled carbon dioxide, arterial blood gases, and pulmonary artery pressures as ordered and indicated. Report changes to the healthcare provider. Maintain oxygen flow rates as ordered. Provide frequent mouth care to reduce the discomfort of dry mucous membranes and prevent tissue breakdown. Work with respiratory therapy to maintain effective oxygen delivery with mechanical ventilation. Administer sedation as required. Maintain fluid restriction, if ordered.

Expected Outcome: Improved ventilation and adequate oxygenation as evidenced by blood gas levels within normal limits for the individual patient.

Promote Cerebral Tissue Perfusion. Impaired cerebral tissue perfusion is a priority problem, especially with near-drowning. Hypoxia and possible hypervolemia can lead to cerebral edema and increased intracranial pressure (IICP), further impairing blood flow. Monitor vital signs and neurologic status frequently. A change in level of consciousness or behavior is typically the earliest sign of IICP. Changes noted on an intracranial pressure monitor also provide early evidence of IICP. Increasing systolic blood pressure and pulse pressure and slowed heart rate are late signs. Other manifestations may include pupillary changes and decreasing muscle strength. Report changes promptly to the healthcare provider. Elevate the head of the bed and keep the head in neutral position to promote drainage from the cranial vault. Maintain effective ventilation and oxygenation; hypercapnia and hypoxemia increase cerebral edema. Administer sedation, osmotic diuretics, or corticosteroids as ordered to reduce cerebral edema. Maintain fluid restriction. Space activities and promote rest to reduce metabolic demands.

Expected Outcome: Patient will experience improved ventilation and adequate oxygenation as evidenced by blood gas levels within normal limits for the individual patient.

Delegating Nursing Care Activities

As appropriate and allowed by the designated duties and responsibilities of unlicensed assistive personnel, the nurse may delegate nursing care activities such as measuring vital signs, encouraging oral or enteral fluid intake, and providing skin care.

Transitions of Care

With inhalation injuries, the most effective treatment is prevention. A working smoke detector (with functioning batteries) could prevent the majority of deaths from smoke inhalation occurring in the home. The line "A smoke detector was found, but the batteries had been removed" is all too familiar in news reports of fire-related deaths.

To prevent drowning, life preservers and flotation vests or jackets should be worn on the body, not stored in the hold of the boat. These devices are designed to keep the head above water. Even accomplished swimmers should never enter the water alone in unguarded areas. Just as alcohol and driving do not mix, neither do alcohol and boating or other water sports.

Prevention of inhalation injuries is an important nursing responsibility. Teach everyone the value of a working smoke detector, especially in the sleeping areas of the house. Encourage families to develop an escape plan in case of fire and to use fire drills to rehearse getting out of the house. Smoldering cigarettes are a leading cause of house fires; help patients develop a plan to stop smoking. Teach people to drop and roll should clothing catch fire. (Flames and smoke rise, increasing the risk of respiratory injury when upright.)

Learning to swim safely is important to prevent drowning. Teach patients never to swim alone, when fatigued, or immediately following a meal. Remind patients that knowing how to swim will not prevent drowning in very cold water or in large bodies of water, such as lakes, rivers, or the ocean. Instruct to always wear flotation devices while boating, water-skiing, surfing, or wind-surfing. Wet suits help prevent hypothermia during activities in very cold water. Advise covering or fencing swimming pools, hot tubs, and ponds to prevent inadvertent entry and drowning.

A population well trained in effective, safe cardiopulmonary resuscitation (CPR) provides the best second line of defense against inhalation injury. Rapid restoration of breathing is essential to prevent hypoxia and brain damage. Encourage all people to be trained and regularly update CPR skills. Work with communities to increase the number of trained people. Refer patients to local chapters of the American Red Cross or American Heart Association for classes.

Teach patients who do not require hospitalization for inhalation injury about symptoms that may indicate a complication and should be reported to the healthcare provider: Increasing dyspnea, cough productive of purulent or pink frothy mucus, confusion, or other changes. Manifestations of respiratory damage may not be apparent for 24 to 48 hours following the injury.

Significant hypoxia due to near-drowning or carbon monoxide poisoning may cause permanent neurologic effects. Work with the family to develop communication techniques and identify remaining strengths. Help the family identify future care needs and means for meeting them, such as home health, personal care aides, or long-term care facilities. Provide social services and support group referrals.

36.4 Lung Cancer

The Patient with Lung Cancer

Lung cancer is the leading cause of cancer deaths in the United States, accounting for 25% of all cancer deaths. In 2017, about 155,870 people died from lung cancer in the United States; an estimated 222,500 new cases were diagnosed in that same year (American Cancer Society [ACS], 2017a). It is a major health problem with a grim prognosis: Most people with lung cancer die within 1 year of the initial diagnosis.

The incidence of lung cancer varies from state to state and among nations. It increases with age, occurring most commonly in patients over age 50. Family clusters of lung cancer suggest a genetic predisposition; however, exposure to tobacco smoke may be necessary for expression of the trait.

Pathophysiology

Lung cancer develops as damaged bronchial epithelial cells mutate over time to become neoplastic. The genetic abnormality commonly seen is on chromosome 3, with loss of genetic material. Alterations of tumor suppressor genes are also seen in some types of lung cancer. Lung cancer is the second most common cancer among men (after prostate cancer) and among women (after breast cancer). Lung cancer is the leading cause of cancer deaths (258%) in the United States, responsible for 84,5907,750 cancer deaths in men and 71,2803,590 cancer deaths in women (ACS, 2017a, 2017b).

The vast majority of primary lung lesions are *bronchogenic carcinoma*, tumors of the airway epithelium. These tumors are further differentiated by cell type: Small-cell carcinoma, adenocarcinoma, squamous cell carcinoma, and large-cell carcinoma. For clinical purposes, the latter three cell types are frequently classified together as non-small-cell carcinomas. *Small-cell carcinomas*, which account for approximately 15% of lung cancers, grow rapidly and spread early. These tumors have paraneoplastic properties; that is, they produce manifestations at sites that are not directly affected by the tumor. Small-cell lung carcinomas can synthesize bioactive products and hormones such as adrenocorticotropic hormones (ACTH), antidiuretic hormone (ADH), a parathormone-like hormone, and gastrin-releasing peptide. *Non-small-cell carcinoma* accounts for about 85% of lung cancers. Each cell type differs in its incidence, presentation, and manner of spread (ACS, 2017a, 2017b). **Table 36.6** outlines the incidence and unique characteristics of each cell type.

Bronchogenic cancer, regardless of cell type, tends to be aggressive, locally invasive, and have widespread metastatic lesions. Tumors begin as mucosal lesions that grow to form masses that obstruct the bronchi or invade adjacent lung tissue. All types frequently spread via the lymph system to nodes and other organs such as the brain, bones, and liver.

Risk Factors

Cigarette smoke, which contains 43 known chemical carcinogens and cancer promoters, is clearly the most significant cause of lung cancer (ACS, 2017b). More than 80% of lung cancer cases are related to smoking, and the disease is

Table 36.6 Comparison of Lung Cancer Cell Types

Cell Type	Prevalence	Presentation and Associated Manifestations	Spread
Small-cell (oat cell) carcinoma 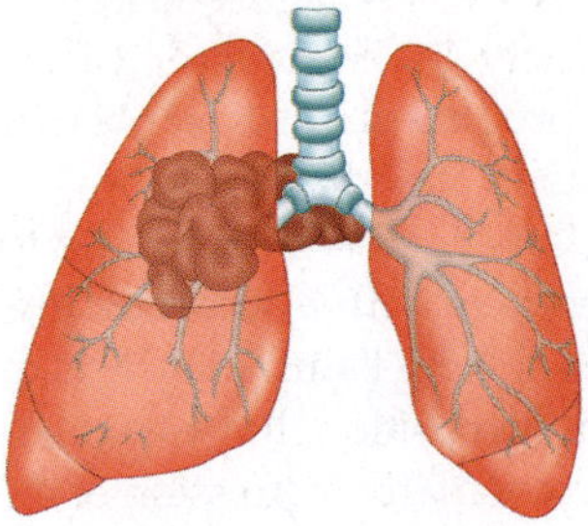	15% of all lung cancers	Central lesion with hilar mass common, early mediastinal involvement, no cavitation; SIADH, Cushing syndrome, thrombophlebitis	Aggressive tumor; > 40% of patients have distant metastasis at time of presentation
Adenocarcinoma 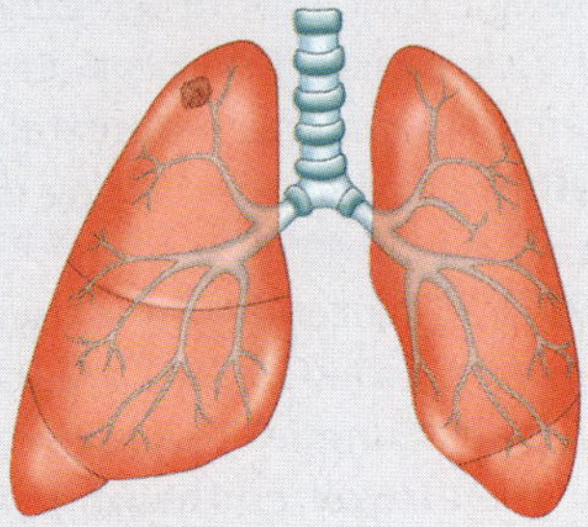	40% of all lung cancers	Peripheral mass involving bronchi; few local symptoms; hypertrophic pulmonary osteoarthropathy	Early metastasis to central nervous system, skeleton, and adrenal glands
Squamous cell carcinoma 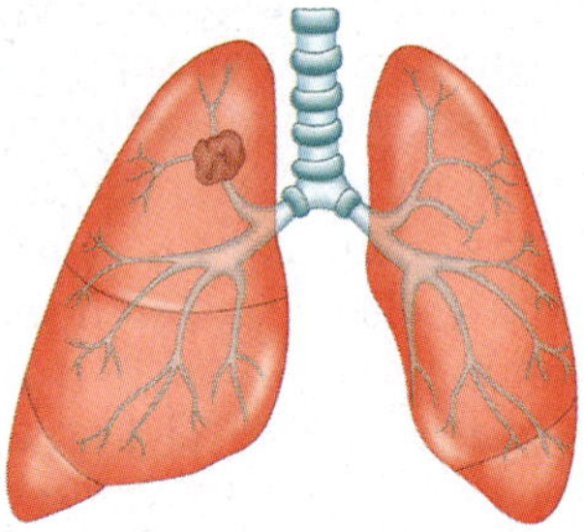	25–30% of all lung cancers	Central lesion located in large bronchi; patient presents with cough, dyspnea, atelectasis, and wheezing; hypercalcemia common	Spreads by local invasion
Large-cell carcinoma 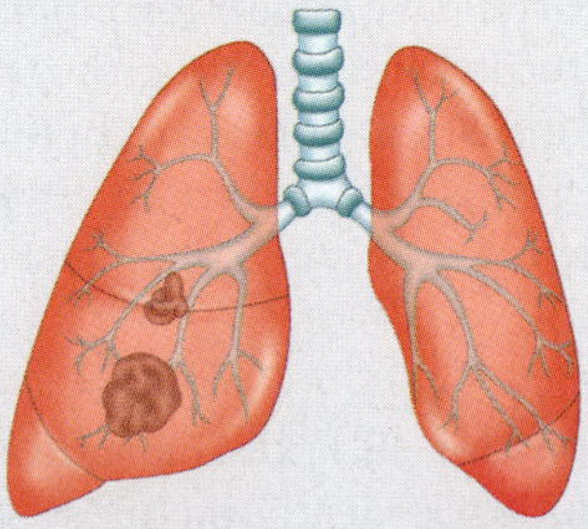	10–15% of all lung cancers	Usually peripheral lesion that is larger than that associated with adenocarcinoma and tends to cavitate; gynecomastia, thrombophlebitis	Early metastasis

23 times more common in male smokers than in male nonsmokers. There is a dose–response relationship between smoking and lung cancer; the more the person smokes and the longer the person smokes, the greater the risk. Even former smokers who have abstained for a number of years have a higher risk of developing lung cancer than nonsmokers. Exposure to ionizing radiation and inhaled irritants, asbestos in particular, is also recognized as a risk factor for lung cancer (Sorenson et al., 2019). Exposure to radon, a radioactive gas, also is identified as a lung cancer risk factor (ACS, 2017b). Radon forms as radium, an element present in the earth's crust, disintegrates. Radon tends to accumulate in closed spaces where air circulation is poor, such as caves, mines, and energy-efficient houses.

Manifestations

The manifestations of lung cancer are related to the location and spread of the tumor. Patients may present with symptoms related to the primary tumor, manifestations of metastatic disease, or with systemic symptoms. Initial symptoms are often attributed to smoking or chronic bronchitis. Chronic cough is common, as is hemoptysis. Wheezing and shortness of breath occur as a result of airway obstruction. Dull, aching chest pain occurs as the tumor spreads to the mediastinum; pleuritic pain occurs when the pleura is invaded. Hoarseness and/or dysphagia indicates pressure of the tumor on the trachea or esophagus.

Systemic and paraneoplastic manifestations of lung cancer include weight loss, anorexia, fatigue, and weakness; bone pain, tenderness, and swelling; clubbing of the fingers and toes; and various endocrine, neuromuscular, cardiovascular, and hematologic symptoms. See the Multisystem Effects of Lung Cancer on page 1326.

Confusion, impaired gait and balance, headache, and personality changes may indicate brain metastasis. Bone metastases cause bone pain, pathologic fractures, and possible spinal cord compression, as well as thrombocytopenia and anemia if bone marrow is invaded. When the liver is affected, symptoms of liver dysfunction and biliary obstruction—including jaundice, anorexia, and upper right quadrant pain—are evident.

Complications and Course

Superior vena cava syndrome, partial or complete obstruction of the superior vena cava, is a potential complication of lung cancer, particularly when the tumor involves the superior mediastinum or the mediastinal lymph nodes. Obstructed venous flow from the head and neck produces the symptoms of superior vena cava syndrome (edema of the neck and face, headache, dizziness, vision disturbances, and syncope) and may develop acutely or more gradually. Veins of the upper chest and neck are dilated; flushing occurs, followed by cyanosis. Cerebral edema may affect the level of consciousness; laryngeal edema may impair respirations.

Paraneoplastic syndromes commonly associated with lung cancer include syndrome of inappropriate ADH secretion (SIADH) with fluid retention, hyponatremia, edema, Cushing syndrome related to abnormal ACTH production, and hypercalcemia. Lung tumors may also produce procoagulation factors, increasing the risk for venous thrombosis, pulmonary embolism, and thrombotic endocarditis. In lung cancer, neuromuscular symptoms such as muscle weakness and wasting of the limbs may be the first indication of the disease (Sorenson et al., 2019).

At the time of diagnosis, cancer of the lung is typically well advanced, with distant metastasis present in 39% of patients and regional lymph node involvement in another 37%. The prognosis is generally poor: The overall 5-year survival rate is only 19% (ACS, 2017a, 2017b).

Interprofessional Care

Establishing an accurate diagnosis is the first step in treating lung cancer. Treatment decisions are based on the tumor location, type of cancer cell, staging of the tumor, and the patient's ability to tolerate treatment. Lung cancer is staged by the tumor size, location, degree of invasion of the primary tumor, and the presence of metastatic disease. Lung cancer staging is summarized in **Table 36.7**. Surgery is the treatment of choice for most forms of lung cancer.

Diagnosis

- ***Chest x-ray*** usually provides the first evidence of lung cancer. It is particularly reliable as a diagnostic tool when compared with a previous chest x-ray. In high-risk populations, the chest x-ray may be used as a screening tool for lung cancer.
- ***Sputum specimen*** is sent for *cytologic examination* to establish the diagnosis of lung cancer. The sputum sample is collected on arising in the morning. If malignant cells are found in the sputum, more expensive and invasive examinations may be unnecessary. However, a sputum sample negative for malignant cells does not rule out lung cancer; it may simply indicate that the tumor is not shedding cells into mucous secretions.
- ***Bronchoscopy*** is frequently done to visualize and obtain tissue for biopsy from the tumor. When a tumor mass or suspicious tissue is identified visually, a cable-activated instrument is used to obtain a biopsy specimen. If the tumor cannot be seen, the airways may be flushed with a saline solution (bronchial washing) to obtain cells for cytologic examination.
- ***CT scan*** is used to evaluate and localize tumors, particularly tumors in the lung parenchyma and pleura. It is also done prior to needle biopsy to localize the tumor. CT scanning can also detect distant tumor metastasis and evaluate tumor response to treatment.
- Cells or tissue for ***cytologic examination and biopsy*** may be obtained by aspirating fluid from a pleural effusion, percutaneous needle biopsy, and lymph node biopsy. These procedures may be done in an outpatient or a surgical setting.
- ***CBC, liver function studies,*** and ***serum electrolytes*** including calcium are obtained to evaluate for evidence of metastatic disease or paraneoplastic syndromes.
- ***Tuberculin test (PPD)*** is performed to rule out tuberculosis as the cause of symptoms and abnormalities seen on chest x-ray.

Multisystem Effects of
Lung Cancer

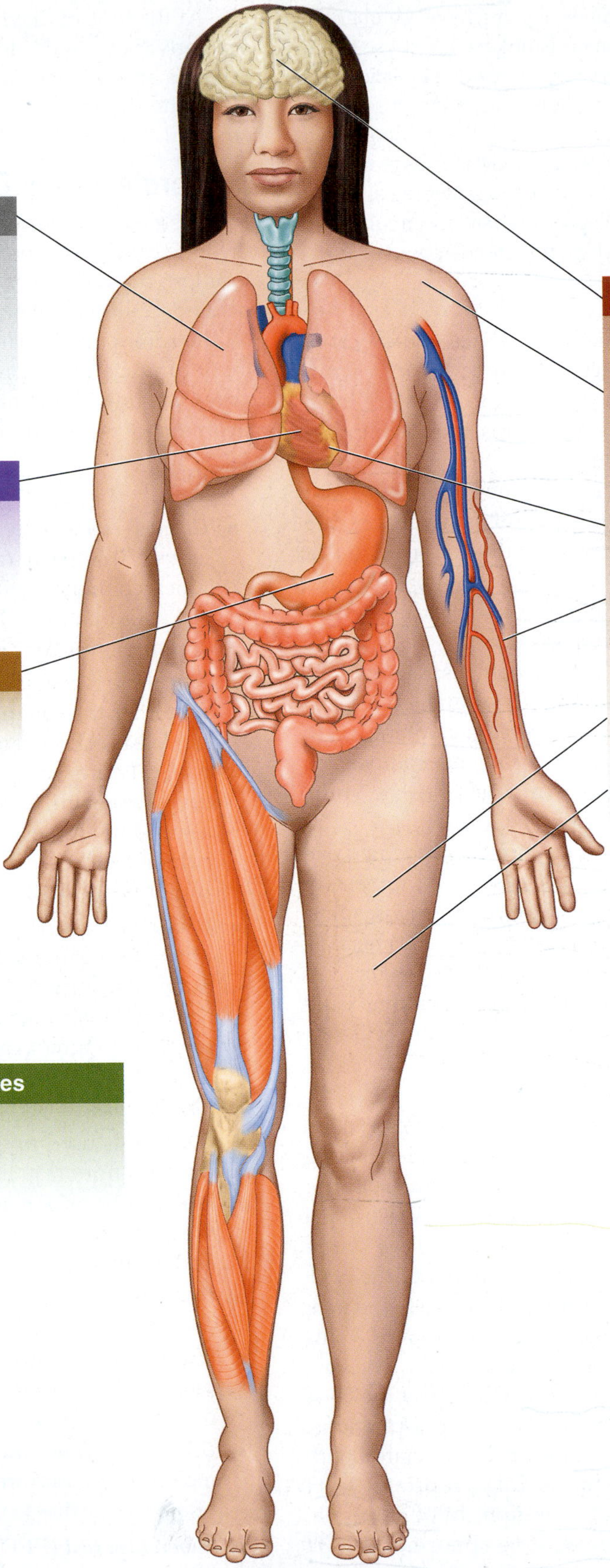

Respiratory
- Cough
- Hemoptysis
- Wheezing and dyspnea
- Chest pain, dull or pleuritic
- Hoarseness and dysphagia
- Pleural effusion

Cardiovascular
- Compression of the superior vena cava

Gastrointestinal
- Anorexia

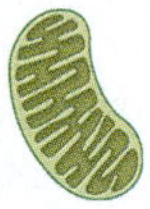

Metabolic processes
- Weight loss
- Fever

Paraneoplastic syndromes

Endocrine system
- Hypercalcemia
- Hyperphosphatemia
- Cushing syndrome
- Syndrome of inappropriate antidiuretic hormone (SIADH) with water retention and hyponatremia

Cardiovascular system
- Thrombophlebitis
- Endocarditis

Hematologic effects
- Anemia
- Disseminated intravascular coagulation (DIC)
- Eosinophillia

Connective tissue
- Osteoarthropathy with clubbing and periosteal inflammation

Neuromuscular effects
- Peripheral neuropathy
- Cerebellar degeneration
- Myasthenia-like muscle weakness

Table 36.7 Lung Cancer Staging

	Primary Tumor (T-Stage)	Regional Lymph Nodes (N)	Distant Metastasis (M)
	T_0—No evidence of primary tumor		
Stage 0	T_X—Malignant cells in bronchopulmonary secretions, but no tumor visualized		M_X—Presence of distant metastasis cannot be assessed
Stage I	T_1S—Carcinoma *in situ*	N_0—No regional lymph node metastasis	M_0—No distant metastasis
	T_1—Tumor that is 3 cm diameter or less, with no evidence of invasion		
Stage II	T_2—Tumor that is > 3 cm diameter, or invades visceral pleura, or has associated atelectasis or pneumonitis	N_1—Metastasis or direct extension to peribronchial or ipsilateral hilar nodes	
Stage III	T_3—Tumor with direct extension into an adjacent structure or any tumor with associated pleural effusion or atelectasis or pneumonitis of entire lung	N_2—Metastasis to ipsilateral mediastinal or subcarinal nodes	
Stage IV	T_4—Tumor that invades mediastinum or involves the heart, great vessels, trachea, esophagus, vertebral body, or carina; presence of malignant pleural effusion	N_3—Metastasis to contralateral mediastinal, scalene, or supraclavicular nodes	M_1—Distant metastasis present

Source: Based on Goldstraw, P., Crowley, J., Chanksky, K., Giroux, D. J., Groome, P. A., Rami-Porta, R., . . . Sobin, L. (2007). The IASLC Lung Cancer Staging Project: Proposals for the revision of the TMN stage groupings. The TNM classification of malignant tumors. *Journal of Thoracic Oncology, 2,* 706–714.

- *Pulmonary function tests (PFTs)* and *arterial blood gases* may be performed prior to the initiation of treatment if the patient has manifestations of respiratory insufficiency (e.g., dyspnea, activity intolerance, low oxygen saturation levels).

Medications

Combination chemotherapy (often combined with radiation therapy and/or surgery) is the treatment of choice for small-cell lung cancer because of its rapid growth, dissemination, and sensitivity to cytotoxic drugs. Used in combination, chemotherapeutic drugs allow tumor cells to be attacked at different parts of the cell cycle and in different ways, increasing the effectiveness of therapy. Five-year survival rates are 55% if treatment begins when the tumor is still localized within the lung; however, only 16% of lung cancers are diagnosed at this stage (American Lung Association, 2016). When a complete tumor response is achieved in the first few cycles of chemotherapy, the chances for long-term survival are much greater.

Combination chemotherapy is also used as an adjunct to surgery or radiation therapy for other types of lung cancer. It may be used to reduce the size of advanced local tumors prior to surgery, and to lengthen survival when distant metastases are present. Refer to Chapter 14 for further discussion of chemotherapy.

Bronchodilators may be prescribed to reduce airway obstruction. Analgesics and pain management strategies are vital when the cancer is advanced. Refer to Chapter 9 for more information about postoperative and cancer pain management.

Surgery

Surgery offers the only real chance for a cure in non-small-cell lung cancer. Unfortunately, most tumors are inoperable or only partially resectable at the time of diagnosis. The type of surgery performed depends on the location and size of the tumor, as well as the patient's pulmonary and general health. The goal of surgery is to remove all involved tissue while preserving as much functional lung as possible. **Table 36.8** outlines various surgical procedures used to treat lung cancer. Nursing care for the patient having lung surgery is outlined in **Box 36.4**.

Table 36.8 Types of Lung Surgery for Lung Cancer

Procedure	Description	Used For
Laser bronchoscopy	Bronchoscopy-guided laser used to resect tumor	Tumors localized in a main bronchus
Mediastinoscopy	Visualization of the mediastinum using an endoscope passed through a suprasternal incision	Evaluation and biopsy of a mediastinal tumor and lymph nodes
Thoracotomy	Incision into the chest wall	Access the lung and thoracic cavity for surgery
Wedge resection	Removal of a small section (wedge) of peripheral lung tissue	Small, peripheral lung tumors
Segmental resection	Removal of an individual bronchovascular segment of a lobe	Peripheral lung tumor with no evidence of extension to the chest wall or metastasis
Sleeve resection (bronchoplastic reconstruction)	Resection of a section of a major bronchus with reconstruction of remaining normal bronchus	Small lesion of a major bronchus
Lobectomy	Removal of a single lung lobe	Tumors confined to a single lobe
Pneumonectomy	Removal of an entire lung	Tumor widespread throughout the lung, involving the main bronchus, or fixed to the hilum

BOX 36.4
Nursing Care of the Patient Undergoing Lung Surgery

PREOPERATIVE CARE

- Provide routine preoperative nursing care, as outlined in Chapter 4.
- Note any history of smoking, respiratory and cardiac diseases, and other chronic conditions in the nursing history. *These factors may affect the response to surgery and the risk for postoperative complications.*
- Provide emotional and psychologic support for the patient and family. *In addition to facing surgery, the patient may be adjusting to a new diagnosis of cancer and the possibility that surgical intervention will only be partially successful.*
- Instruct the patient about postoperative procedures, including respiratory therapy, breathing exercises, and coughing techniques. Allow practice time. *Learning will be easier in the preoperative period, when pain and analgesia are not affecting mental function.*
- If the patient will return from surgery with an endotracheal tube and mechanical ventilation, establish a means of communication using alternative communication tools such as tablets. *Establishing a means of communication prior to surgery reduces postoperative anxiety at being unable to speak.*
- If the patient will return to the ICU, introduce the patient and family to the unit and any machines, such as ventilators and monitors, that will be used. *The knowledge that this is an expected part of surgical recovery reduces the patient's and family's postoperative anxiety.*

POSTOPERATIVE CARE

- Assess and provide routine postoperative care, as outlined in Chapter 4.
- Assess for adequate pain control, and provide analgesics as needed. *Incisional pain commonly causes altered breathing patterns in the patient who has undergone lung surgery.*
- Frequently assess respiratory status, including color, oxygen saturation, respiratory rate and depth, chest expansion, lung sounds, percussion tone, and arterial blood gases. *Maintaining adequate ventilation and gas exchange postoperatively is vital to reduce mortality and morbidity. Gas exchange may be impaired by complications of lung surgery, including pneumothorax, atelectasis, bronchospasm, pulmonary embolus, bronchopleural fistula, and acute respiratory distress syndrome.*
- Assist with effective coughing techniques, postural drainage, and incentive spirometry. Perform endotracheal suctioning as needed while intubated. *Surgical manipulation and anesthesia can increase mucus production, leading to airway obstruction. Aggressive pulmonary hygiene is important to prevent this complication.*
- Monitor and maintain effective mechanical ventilation. *This is vital to ensure adequate ventilation and gas exchange in the early postoperative period.*
- Maintain patent chest tubes and a closed-drainage system. Monitor chest tube output every hour initially, then every 2 to 4 or 8 hours as indicated. Notify the healthcare provider if chest tube output exceeds 70 mL per hour and/or is bright red, warm, and free flowing. *Maintaining a patent, intact chest drainage system is vital to reestablish negative pressure within the chest cavity and reexpansion of the lungs. Increased amounts of warm, free-flowing blood indicate intrathoracic hemorrhage that may necessitate surgical intervention.*
- Assess for signs of infection involving the incision or chest tube site(s). Use strict aseptic technique in caring for incisions and invasive monitoring devices. *The postoperative patient is at risk for incisional infections, empyema in the chest cavity, and pneumonia.*
- Assist with turning and to ambulate as soon as possible. *Early mobility is important to prevent possible complications, such as pneumonia or pulmonary embolus.*
- Assess and maintain nutritional status. Initiate enteral or parenteral nutrition early if intubation and mechanical ventilation will be required for an extended period. Provide frequent, small feedings once extubated. *Maintaining nutritional status promotes wound healing and prevents negative nitrogen balance. Frequent, small feedings reduce the fatigue associated with eating.*

Radiation Therapy

Radiation therapy is used alone or in combination with surgery or chemotherapy for lung cancer. The treatment goal may be either cure or symptom relief (palliative). Prior to surgery, radiation therapy is used to "debulk" tumors. When cancer has spread by direct extension to other thoracic structures and surgery is not feasible, radiation therapy may be the treatment of choice. It also may be used to relieve manifestations such as cough, hemoptysis, pain due to bone metastasis, and dyspnea from bronchial obstruction. Complications of lung cancer, such as superior vena cava syndrome, may be treated with radiation.

Radiation therapy may be delivered by external beam to the primary tumor site or by intraluminal radiation or brachytherapy. Radiation therapy and related nursing care are discussed further in Chapter 14. Specific nursing measures for the patient undergoing radiation therapy for lung cancer are outlined in **Box 36.5**.

Integrative Therapies

Research indicates that a significant number of patients diagnosed with lung cancer use complementary and alternative medicine (CAM). In a systematic review of CAM in lung cancer, between 10% and more than 60% of cancer patients use at least one form of CAM (National Institute of Integrative and Complementary Health, 2017). The CAM remedies used included herbal medicines, medicinal teas, homeopathy, animal extracts, aromatherapy (National Cancer Institute, 2018), and spiritual therapies. Although these therapies may be safe when used alone, the potential for interactions with conventional medical treatment must be considered. Inquire of patients about their use of complementary and alternative therapies, and inform members of the healthcare team when present.

Nursing Care

Assessment

See the Manifestations and Interprofessional Care sections for the assessment of the patient with lung cancer.

BOX 36.5
Nursing Care of the Patient Receiving Radiation Therapy for Lung Cancer

Although radiation therapy is well controlled and specifically directed toward the tumor cells, some normal cells are also damaged in the process of treatment. Nursing care and patient teaching help the patient cope with uncomfortable side effects associated with radiation therapy.

NURSING RESPONSIBILITIES

- Monitor for potential complications:
  a. Radiation pneumonitis—dyspnea on exertion, dry cough, fever
  b. Pericarditis—chest pain, pericardial friction rub; muffled heart sounds, paradoxical pulse, ECG abnormalities (Notify the healthcare provider if symptoms develop.)
  c. Esophagitis—pain, sore throat, difficulty swallowing.
- Encourage adequate fluid intake to liquefy respiratory secretions.
- Provide local analgesics and local anesthetics such as viscous lidocaine as ordered to relieve dysphagia and sore throat.
- Offer small, frequent meals of soft, cool foods and liquids to maintain nutritional status.

PATIENT AND FAMILY TEACHING

- If dyspnea or pneumonitis develop, teach positioning, pursed-lip techniques, and relaxation exercises to facilitate breathing.
- Reassure that pneumonitis is generally a self-limiting process and should resolve when the course of radiotherapy is completed.
- Teach the manifestations of pericarditis, which may develop during treatment or up to 1 year after its completion. Chest pain or pressure, rapid heartbeat, and fever may signal pericarditis; increasing fatigue, dyspnea, and light-headedness can indicate a chronic process with pericardial effusion and possible cardiac tamponade.
- Instruct to eliminate hot, spicy, or acidic foods from the diet if esophagitis is a problem. Alcohol and tobacco should also be avoided.
- Adequate rest and nutrition are important to alleviate the symptoms of radiation fatigue, which is common in patients receiving radiation therapy for lung cancer. The fatigue is generally temporary.

Nursing assessment related to lung cancer focuses on identifying risk factors for the disease, early manifestations of lung cancer, and respiratory function in the patient undergoing treatment.

- ***Health history:*** Current symptoms, including chronic cough, shortness of breath, blood-tinged sputum; systemic manifestations such as recent weight loss, fatigue, anorexia, bone pain; smoking history; occupational exposure to carcinogens; chronic diseases such as COPD
- ***Physical assessment:*** General appearance; skin color, evidence of clubbing; weight and height; vital signs; respiratory rate, depth, excursion; lung sounds to percussion and auscultation
- ***Laboratory tests:*** CBC and coagulation studies, serum electrolytes and osmolality, liver and renal function studies; chest x-ray and CT scan results; arterial blood gases and oxygen saturation levels.

Priorities of Care

Collaborate with the interprofessional team to ensure adequate treatment of the lung cancer while providing care that supports the physical and psychologic responses to the disease focusing on symptom management and treatment adherence is a priority of nursing care.

Diagnoses, Interventions, and Outcomes

The patient with lung cancer is facing invasive treatments with undesirable side effects, possibly surgery, and typically a poor prognosis for long-term survival. Nursing care needs are diverse, related to respiratory status, the cancer itself and possible metastases, and the treatment plan. Nursing care is directed toward promoting effective breathing and helping the patient return to normal activity levels. Pain and anticipatory grieving are also likely to be high-priority problems. See the accompanying Case Study & Nursing Care Plan on page 1332.

Promote Effective Breathing. Breathing pattern and ventilation may be affected by the tumor itself or by treatment of the tumor. Thoracic surgery increases the risk due to the incision and disruption of the muscles of respiration. Maintaining effective lung ventilation is particularly important postoperatively to reexpand remaining lung tissue and prevent surgical complications.

Expected Outcome: Patient will utilize techniques to promote adequate ventilation such as deep breathing and incentive spirometry.

The nurse will:

- Assess and document respiratory rate, depth, and lung sounds at least every 4 hours; evaluate more frequently in the immediate postoperative period or as indicated by condition. *Early detection of signs of respiratory compromise or adventitious lung sounds is vital for effective intervention.*
- Monitor oxygen saturation, exhaled carbon dioxide, and/or blood gas results, reporting changes from normal. *Changes in levels of blood oxygen or exhaled CO_2 may be early indications of respiratory compromise.*
- Frequently assess and document pain level (using a standard pain scale); provide analgesics as needed. *Pain and attempting to avoid chest movement to prevent additional pain can lead to rapid, shallow respirations and ineffective ventilation.*

- Elevate the head of the bed to 60 degrees. *Elevating the head of the bed reduces pressure on the diaphragm and permits optimal lung expansion.*
- Assist the patient to turn, cough, and deep breathe and use incentive spirometry. Help splint the chest with a pillow or blanket when coughing. *These measures promote airway clearance.*
- Suction airway as needed. *Suctioning may be required to remove secretions that the patient is unable to cough up and expectorate.*
- Provide chest physiotherapy with percussion and postural drainage as needed or ordered. *Percussion and postural drainage help maintain airway patency and effective respirations.*
- If mechanical ventilation is instituted, work with respiratory therapy and use analgesia or sedation as needed to synchronize respirations with the ventilator. *Coordination of the patient's respiratory effort with ventilator-delivered breaths is important for fully effective mechanical ventilation.*
- Provide reassurance and emotional support. *These measures help relieve anxiety and promote an effective breathing pattern.*

SAFETY ALERT: Maintain chest tube integrity and patency by ensuring uninterrupted gravity flow. Chest tubes help reestablish negative pressure in the thoracic cavity, allowing the lung to fully reexpand. ■

Promote Physical Activity as Tolerated. Both resectional lung surgery and inoperable lung cancer reduce the amount of functional lung tissue and surface area for gas diffusion. This can lead to activity intolerance if the oxygen supply is insufficient to meet the body's oxygen demand.

Expected Outcome: Patient will participate in physical activity as tolerated.

The nurse will:

- Assess and document physiologic responses to activity, including pulse, respiratory rate, dyspnea, and fatigue. *These assessments are good indicators of activity tolerance.*
- Plan rest periods between activities and procedures. *Rest periods reduce oxygen demands and fatigue.*
- Assist the postoperative patient to increase activities gradually. *Increasing activity levels gradually improves exercise tolerance.*
- Teach measures to conserve energy while performing ADLs, such as sitting while showering and dressing and wearing slip-on shoes. *These energy-conserving measures reduce oxygen demand and allow the patient to remain independent as long as possible.*
- Keep frequently used objects within easy reach. *This helps conserve energy.*
- Administer oxygen as prescribed. Teach the patient and family about home oxygen use, if appropriate. *Supplemental oxygen can help improve activity and exercise tolerance.*
- Encourage maintenance of physical activity to tolerance. *Maintaining activity levels to the degree possible improves physical and emotional well-being.*
- Allow family members to provide assistance as needed. *This helps the patient conserve energy and allows the family to retain a sense of usefulness.*

Manage Pain. Pain is a priority problem in both the postoperative period as well as in the terminal stages of cancer. Poorly managed pain prolongs recovery from surgery. In the terminal cancer patient, chronic and acute pain must be managed effectively to allow a peaceful death.

Expected Outcome: Patient will achieve adequate pain control as evidenced by physical well-being.

The nurse will:

- Assess and document pain using a standardized pain scale and objective data. *Pain is a subjective experience, best evaluated by the patient. Changes in vital signs, guarded movement, or unwillingness to move may indicate unreported pain.*
- Provide analgesics as needed to maintain comfort. *Postoperative recovery and restoration of function is facilitated by adequate pain management.*
- For cancer pain, maintain an around-the-clock medication schedule using narcotic, nonsteroidal anti-inflammatory drugs and other medications as ordered. *Addiction is not a concern in terminal cancer; providing adequate pain relief that does not allow "breakthrough" pain is important.*
- Provide or assist with comfort measures, such as massage, positioning, distraction, and relaxation techniques. *These techniques promote relaxation and enhance pain relief.*
- Assist the patient and family to plan and engage in activities that distract from pain such as reading, watching television, and engaging in social interactions. *Distraction helps the patient focus away from the pain.*
- Spend as much time with the patient as possible; allow family members to remain with the patient. *Physical presence of the nurse and family provides emotional support for the patient.*

Promote Healthy Grief Responses. Because lung cancer is often advanced when diagnosed, the patient faces the very real prospect of dying from the disease. Grieving for the anticipated loss of life is a normal response as the patient and family begin to adapt to the diagnosis. Nursing care goals are to promote expression of feelings and thoughts about the loss and to help the patient and family initiate grief work, make decisions, and use appropriate resources and coping mechanisms to deal with the loss.

Expected Outcome: Patient and family will discuss the meaning of losses (anticipated or actual) to the patient and family's life.

The nurse will:

- Spend time with the patient and family. *Time is necessary to develop a trusting, therapeutic relationship.*
- Answer questions honestly; do not deny the probable outcome of the disease. *Honesty reinforces reality and provides a sense of control over decisions to be made.*
- Encourage the patient and family to express their feelings, fears, and concerns. *Open expression of feelings helps to promote understanding and acceptance.*
- Assist with understanding the grieving process and acceptance of feelings as normal. *Feelings of guilt, anger, or depression may cause the patient to withdraw from others. Explanation of the grieving process enhances understanding and ability to cope.*
- Help identify strengths and coping measures that have been used effectively in the past. Provide positive reinforcement for effective coping behavior. *Past effective coping measures can help the patient and family deal with the present situation and regain a sense of control.*
- Help the patient and family make decisions regarding treatment and care. *This is also important to give them a sense of control.*
- Encourage use of other support systems, such as spiritual and social groups. Refer the patient and family to support groups, social support services, and hospice care, as indicated. Provide American Cancer Society literature and information as appropriate. *These support systems provide emotional support and help the patient and family cope with the diagnosis.*
- Discuss advance directives (the living will) and power of attorney for healthcare with the patient and family. *These documents give the patient and family a sense of control over medical care provided if the patient is no longer able to express his or her own wishes.*

Delegating Nursing Care Activities

As appropriate and allowed by the designated duties and responsibilities of unlicensed assistive personnel, the nurse may delegate nursing care activities such as measuring vital signs, encouraging oral or enteral fluid intake, and providing skin care.

Transitions of Care

Because lung cancer is typically advanced when diagnosed and the prognosis is generally poor, prevention of the disease must be a primary goal for all healthcare providers. With 80% of lung cancer related to cigarette smoking, reducing tobacco use can have a significant impact on the death rate from lung cancer—a far greater impact than advances in treatment.

The incidence of lung cancer is decreasing as the use of tobacco products declines. Teach people of all ages, particularly children and teenagers, about the link between cigarette smoking and lung cancer. Not smoking and avoiding exposure to secondhand smoke are the primary preventative measures for lung cancer. In addition, explain the risk of lung cancer to patients with occupational risk factors, exposure to asbestos products in particular.

A primary teaching need to prepare the patient and family affected by lung cancer for home care is information about the disease itself, expected prognosis, and planned treatment strategies. Provide honest information; do not promote false hope. Include the following additional topics in teaching for home care:

- Importance of quitting smoking, especially if surgery has been performed (The patient with lung cancer may have difficulty recognizing the need to stop smoking. Include information about the effects of nicotine and the tars in cigarette smoke on healing and already compromised lung tissue.)
- Planned treatments such as chemotherapy or radiation therapy, including expected effects and usual side effects of each
- Strategies to cope with noxious effects of radiation or chemotherapy
- Activities and exercises to improve strength and regain function for the postoperative patient
- The need to continue coughing and deep-breathing exercises at home
- Symptoms to report to the healthcare provider: Fever, increasing or continued shortness of breath, cough, increased or purulent sputum, redness, pain, swelling, or incisional drainage
- Use of prescribed medications, including desired and potential side effects and interactions with other drugs or foods
- Use of analgesics and other pain relief measures for postoperative or cancer pain
- Information about hospice services, home health, local cancer support groups for patients and caregivers, and American Cancer Society services.

Refer the patient and family for home health services including nursing care, assistance with ADLs, respiratory care, and respite care, as needed.

Case Study & Nursing Care Plan

A Patient with Lung Cancer

After coughing up bloody sputum one morning, James Mueller, a 68-year-old retired millworker, sees his healthcare provider. A chest x-ray shows a suspicious density in the central portion of his right lung. Mr. Mueller is admitted to the hospital the following Monday for diagnostic tests.

ASSESSMENT

Anita Sarros, RN, admits Mr. Mueller to the oncology unit and obtains a nursing history. Mr. Mueller is married and has three grown children. He worked in a local paper mill for 35 years before retiring at age 62. He describes himself as "pretty healthy," except for a chronic smoker's cough. He started smoking as a young man in the army. He has a 50 pack-year smoking history, having smoked a pack a day for 50 years, since age 18. Mr. Mueller says he briefly quit smoking following a small heart attack 3 years ago, but started again after 4 months. On further questioning, Mr. Mueller says his cough has been productive for the past few months, especially in the morning, and that he is shorter of breath than usual with activity.

Mr. Mueller's examination data includes BP 162/86 mmHg, P 78 bpm and regular, R 20/min, and T 36.9°C (98.4°F). Color good, skin warm and dry. Inspiratory and expiratory wheezes noted in right chest but good breath sounds throughout. No other abnormal findings are noted on examination. The healthcare provider orders early-morning sputum specimens times 3 days for cytologic examination and schedules a CT scan of the chest the morning after admission.

Mr. Mueller's CBC shows mild anemia, but remaining routine laboratory tests are essentially normal. Sputum cytology is positive for small-cell bronchogenic cancer. The CT scan shows a central mass approximately 4 cm in diameter with involved mediastinal and subclavicular lymph nodes. A small mass is also noted on the lumbar spine. After conferring with his healthcare provider and an oncologist, Mr. Mueller decides to undergo a trial course of chemotherapy.

DIAGNOSES

- Poor airway clearance related to tumor mass
- Inadequate nutrition related to effects of chemotherapy
- Limited knowledge about lung cancer and aids to smoking cessation

EXPECTED OUTCOMES

- Patient will maintain a patent airway.
- Patient will maintain current weight.
- Patient will participate in care.
- Patient will contact appropriate support groups.
- Patient will verbalize an understanding of the disease, its treatment, and prognosis.
- Patient will develop a plan to stop smoking.

PLANNING AND IMPLEMENTATION

- Teach coughing, deep breathing, and hydration measures to facilitate airway clearance.
- Discuss symptoms to report to the healthcare provider: Increased dyspnea or hemoptysis, severe stridor or wheezing, chest pain.
- Discuss measures to relieve nausea associated with chemotherapy, including premedication with a prescribed antiemetic.
- Have dietitian consult with Mr. and Mrs. Mueller to develop a diet plan for maintaining ideal weight.
- Discuss possible effects of lung cancer with Mr. and Mrs. Mueller.
- Encourage Mr. and Mrs. Mueller to call a family conference to discuss the disease with their children and grandchildren.
- Evaluate family members' knowledge and understanding of lung cancer, correcting misinformation and teaching as needed.
- Have an American Cancer Society volunteer contact the family.
- Refer to local cancer support group.
- Refer to home health department for follow-up and further teaching.
- Work with Mr. Mueller to develop a plan to stop smoking.
- Ask the healthcare provider for a prescription for nicotine patches or gum for Mr. Mueller.

Make Mr. Mueller aware of decisions that will need to be made regarding end-of-life issues. Encourage him to discuss his wishes with family if he is able.

EVALUATION

Mr. Mueller had his first chemotherapy treatment in the hospital and was discharged 4 days after admission. After 3 months of chemotherapy, his tumor shows little regression, and a liver scan reveals further metastasis. He and his wife decide to stop chemotherapy, a decision with which the children reluctantly agree. Mr. and Mrs. Mueller are referred to hospice services. With the help of hospice nurses and volunteers, Mr. Mueller is able to remain at home. His pain is managed initially with oral MS Contin, a sustained-release form of morphine sulfate, and later with an intravenous morphine infusion. Mr. Mueller dies at home with his family at his side 9 months after his diagnosis of lung cancer.

CLINICAL REASONING IN PATIENT CARE

1. The oncologist prescribed a chemotherapy regimen of cyclophosphamide, doxorubicin, and vincristine. Describe how each of these drugs works against cancer cells, and discuss the rationale for using this combination.
2. Develop a care plan to deal with the specific side effects for the treatment regimen given in question 1.
3. Mr. Mueller had small-cell (oat cell) cancer. How would his presentation and treatment differ if the diagnosis had been non-small-cell adenocarcinoma, stage $T_2N_2M_0$?

See Evaluating Your Response in Appendix B.

CHAPTER HIGHLIGHTS

36.1 Infectious and Inflammatory Disorders

Describe the pathophysiology and manifestations of infectious and inflammatory ventilation disorders, and outline the interprofessional care and nursing care of patients with these disorders.

- Pneumonia, inflammation of the respiratory bronchioles and alveoli, is usually bacterial in origin. Different organisms are commonly found in healthcare-associated pneumonia than in community-acquired pneumonia. Nursing care focuses on promoting airway clearance, supporting effective gas exchange, and promoting rest.
- Infection control measures, including standard, airborne, and contract precautions, are vital to prevent the spread of viral severe acute respiratory syndrome (SARS) or related novel respiratory viruses.
- Tuberculosis affects many people worldwide. In the United States, the primary affected populations are immigrants, people with compromised immunity, and people living in crowded or unsanitary conditions.
- The tuberculin test (PPD) detects a cellular immune response to *M. tuberculosis*, indicating infection, but not necessarily active disease.
- Effective tuberculosis treatment is a public health concern, requiring therapy and compliance monitoring, contact follow-up, and assessment for adverse treatment effects.
- Fungal lung infections tend to have a geographic pattern of distribution. People with compromised immune status are more likely to be affected. Their manifestations resemble those of pneumonia or tuberculosis.

36.2 Disorders of the Pleura

Describe the pathophysiology and manifestations of disorders of the pleura, and outline the interprofessional care and nursing care of patients with these disorders.

- Disorders of the pleura, such as pleural effusion and pneumothorax, can affect lung expansion, ventilation, and gas exchange when significant.
- Tension pneumothorax develops when air enters the pleural space but is unable to escape, collapsing the lung on the affected side and placing pressure on the unaffected lung and mediastinum. Ventilation, gas exchange, venous return, and cardiac output can be significantly affected.

36.3 Trauma of the Chest or Lung

Describe the pathophysiology and manifestations of trauma of the chest or lung, and outline the interprofessional care and nursing care of patients with these injuries.

- Trauma may affect the chest wall or the airways and alveoli. Flail chest and pulmonary contusion often occur concurrently; hemothorax also frequently develops with chest trauma. Chest trauma can endanger effective ventilation and gas exchange.

36.4 Lung Cancer

Describe the pathophysiology and manifestations of lung cancer, and outline the interprofessional care and nursing care of patients with this disease.

- Lung cancer, the leading cause of cancer deaths, typically is advanced when diagnosed. Surgery, radiation therapy, and chemotherapy are used to treat lung cancer, often in combination.
- Superior vena cava syndrome and paraneoplastic syndromes may complicate lung cancer.

TEST YOURSELF NCLEX-RN® REVIEW

1. The nurse is providing care to a patient newly admitted with bacterial pneumonia. Which action should the nurse perform first?
   A. Provide a meal for diet as tolerated.
   B. Obtain a sputum specimen for culture and sensitivity.
   C. Apply oxygen per nasal cannula at 5 L/min as prescribed.
   D. Insert an intravenous catheter and start the prescribed antibiotic.

2. The nurse notes that a patient with bacterial pneumonia has an overall gray skin tone with a bluish tinge around the lips. In which order should the nurse provide the listed interventions?
   A. Start oxygen.
   B. Assess breath sounds.
   C. Raise the head of the bed.
   D. Obtain oxygen saturation level
   E. Notify the healthcare provider.

3. The nurse evaluating an intradermal PPD tuberculin test notes large erythemic area surrounding the test site. What additional information indicates to the nurse that this is a positive result?
   A. The erythemic area is greater than 9 mm in size.
   B. The test was administered 24 hours ago.
   C. There is a 5 mm hardened area at the injection site.
   D. The patient resides in a long-term care facility.
4. The nurse is teaching a patient who is prescribed prophylactic daily isoniazid (INH) for conversion of a tuberculin test. What should the nurse include in this patient's teaching? (Select all that apply.)
   A. This drug turns the urine red-orange, which is harmless.
   B. Periodic eye examinations are required during treatment.
   C. Report numbness and tingling of extremities to the physician.
   D. Do not use aspirin while taking this drug because abnormal bleeding may occur.
   E. Expect to have liver function studies done periodically during treatment.
5. The nurse is evaluating teaching provided to a patient with lung cancer. Which patient statement indicates that teaching has been effective?
   A. "Having the 'big C' is very scary; I'm just glad it is one of the more curable forms of cancer."
   B. "Even though I can't undo the damage caused by cigarette smoking, I will try to quit preventing further damage to my lungs."
   C. "Well, since I'm going to die anyway, I may as well go home, put my affairs in order, and spend the rest of my time in the easy chair."
   D. "I understand that because the cancer has already spread I will be undergoing aggressive cancer treatment for the next several years to beat this thing."
6. The nurse caring for a patient following a lobectomy notes 100 mL of red drainage in the chest drainage container since checking it 30 minutes previously. What should the nurse do to help this patient? (Select all that apply.)
   A. Notify the surgeon.
   B. Empty the chest tube drainage system.
   C. Assess vital signs and level of consciousness.
   D. Apply pressure to the chest tube insertion site.
   E. Note the finding and reevaluate drainage in 30 minutes.
7. A patient is scheduled for a thoracentesis. What should the nurse do to assist the patient for this procedure? (Select all that apply.)
   A. Encourage to cough as the fluid is withdrawn.
   B. Coach to breathe deeply as the needle is inserted.
   C. Help to sit upright and lean forward during the procedure.
   D. Remind to remain on quiet bedrest for 4 hours following the procedure.
   E. Advise patient that a feeling of pressure will occur during insertion.
8. The nurse is providing discharge teaching to a patient with a fractured rib. What should the nurse instruct the patient to do?
   A. Use a small pillow to splint the area when coughing.
   B. Avoid using pain medications to prevent respiratory depression.
   C. Remain on bedrest for a week to allow the fracture to stabilize.
   D. Use elastic roller bandages like ACE wraps to stabilize the chest wall and promote comfort.
9. A victim of a house fire was transported to the emergency department for treatment of smoke inhalation. Which assessment finding should cause the nurse the greatest concern?
   A. Respiratory rate of 36
   B. Fine crackles in bilateral bases
   C. Ash-like material in the sputum
   D. Skin and mucous membranes pink
10. The nurse is planning care for a patient with a tension pneumothorax.
    The nurse should identify which interventions to achieve which goal as the highest priority for this patient?
    A. Manage acute pain
    B. Reduce risk for aspiration or other injury
    C. Promote effective gas exchange
    D. Prevent ineffective breathing pattern

See Test Yourself answers in Appendix B.

REFERENCES

American Cancer Society (ACS). (2017a). *Cancer facts and figures 2017*. Retrieved from https://www.cancer.org/content/dam/cancer-org/research/cancer-facts-and-statistics/annual-cancer-facts-and-figures/2017/cancer-facts-and-figures-2017.pdf.

American Cancer Society (ACS). (2017b). *Lung cancer*. Retrieved from https://www.cancer.org/cancer/lung-cancer.html.

American Lung Association. (2016). *Lung cancer fact sheet.* Retrieved from www.lung.org/lung-health-and-diseases/lung-disease-lookup/lung-cancer/resource-library/lung-cancer-fact-sheet.html.

American Lung Association. (2017). Pneumonia. *Lung Disease Data.* Retrieved from www.lung.org/lung-health-and-diseases/lung-disease-lookup/pneumonia/.

Centers for Disease Control and Prevention (CDC). (1989). *Guidelines for prophylaxis against Pneumocystis carinii pneumonia for persons infected with human immunodeficiency virus.* Retrieved from https://www.cdc.gov/mmwr/preview/mmwrhtml/00001409.htm.

Centers for Disease Control and Prevention (CDC). (2017a). *Anthrax.* Retrieved from https://www.cdc.gov/anthrax/index.html.

Centers for Disease Control and Prevention (CDC). (2017b). *Pneumonia.* Retrieved from https://www.cdc.gov/pneumonia/index.html.

Centers for Disease Control and Prevention (CDC). (2017c). *Severe acute respiratory syndrome (SARS).* Retrieved from https://www.cdc.gov/sars/about/fs-sars.html.

Centers for Disease Control and Prevention (CDC). (2017d). *Trends in tuberculosis, 2016* . Retrieved from https://www.cdc.gov/tb/publications/factsheets/statistics/tbtrends.htm.

Centers for Disease Control and Prevention (CDC). (2017e). *Tuberculosis data and statistics* Retrieved from https://www.cdc.gov/tb/statistics/default.htm.

Centers for Disease Control and Prevention (CDC). (2017f). *Unintentional drowning.* Retrieved from https://www.cdc.gov/homeandrecreationalsafety/water-safety/waterinjuries-factsheet.html.

Centers for Disease Control and Prevention. (2015). *Epidemiology and prevention of vaccine-preventable diseases* (13th ed.). (J. Hamborsky, A. Kroger, & S. Wolfe, Eds.). Washington, DC. Public Health Foundation. Retrieved from https://www.cdc.gov/vaccines/pubs/pinkbook/index.html.

Daley, B. J. (2017). *Pneumothorax: Epidemiology.* Retrieved from https://emedicine.medscape.com/article/424547-overview#a5.

Jain, S., Self, W. H., Wunderink, R. G., & Fakhran, S. (2015). Community-acquired pneumonias requiring hospitalization among US adults. *New England Journal of Medicine, 373,* 415–427.

Kochanek, K. D., Murphy, S. L., Xu, J. Q., & Tejada-Vera, B. (2016). Deaths: Final data for 2014. *National Vital Statistics Report, 65*(4). Hyattsville, MD: National Center for Health Statistics.

National Cancer Institute (NCI). (2018). *Aromatherapy and essential oils.* Retrieved from https://www.cancer.gov/about-cancer/treatment/cam/hp/aromatherapy-pdq.

National Center for Complementary and Integrative Health (NCCIH). (2017). *5 Tips: Natural products for the flu and colds: What does the science say?* Retrieved from https://nccih.nih.gov/health/tips/flucold.htm.

National Center for Complementary and Integrative Health (NCCIH). (2015). Three studies find echinacea ineffective against the common cold. Retrieved from https://nccih.nih.gov/research/results/spotlight/051805.htm.

National Institute of Allergy and Infectious Diseases (NIAID). (2017). *Vaccine research center.* https://www.niaid.nih.gov/about/vrc.

National Institute of Integrative and Complementary Health (NIICH). (2017). *Cancer prevention and treatment.* Retrieved from https://nccih.nih.gov/health/cancer.

Perrin, K. O., & MacLeod, C. E. (2017). *Understanding the essentials of critical care nursing* (3rd ed.) Boston: Pearson.

Shields, K. M., Fox, K. L., & Liebrecht, C. (2018). *Pearson nurse's drug guide: 2018.* Boston, MA: Pearson.

Sorenson, M., Quinn, L., & Klein, D. (2019). *Pathophysiology: Concepts of human disease.* New York: Pearson.

University of Maryland Medical Center. (2016). *Ephedra.* Retrieved from https://www.umm.edu/health/medical/altmed/herb/ephedra.

World Health Organization (WHO). (2017a). *Legionellosis.* Retrieved from www.who.int/mediacentre/factsheets/fs285/en/.

World Health Organization (WHO). (2017b). *Middle East respiratory syndrome coronavirus.* Retrieved from www.who.int/emergencies/mers-cov/en/.

World Health Organization (WHO). (2017c). *Tuberculosis.* Retrieved from www.who.int/mediacentre/factsheets/fs104/en/.

ADDITIONAL RESOURCES

American Lung Association. (2018a). *Lung health and diseases.* Retrieved from www.lung.org/lung-health-and-diseases/.

American Lung Association. (2018b). *Our initiatives.* Retrieved from www.lung.org/our-initiatives/.

American Thoracic Society. (2017). *Patient resources: Fact sheets A to Z.* Retrieved from www.thoracic.org/patients/patient-resources/fact-sheets-az.php.

National Heart, Lung, and Blood Institute. (2018). *Health topics.* Retrieved from https://www.nhlbi.nih.gov.

Chapter 37

Nursing Care of Patients with Gas Exchange Disorders

Chapter Outline and Learning Outcomes

37.1 Reactive Airway Disorders 1335

Describe the pathophysiology and manifestations of reactive airway disorders, and outline the interprofessional care and nursing care of patients with these disorders.

37.2 Interstitial Lung Disease 1361

Describe the pathophysiology and manifestations of interstitial lung disease, and outline the interprofessional care and nursing care of patients with this disorder.

37.3 Pulmonary Vascular Disorders 1364

Describe the pathophysiology and manifestations of pulmonary vascular disorders, and outline the interprofessional care and nursing care of patients with these disorders.

37.4 Respiratory Failure 1371

Describe the pathophysiology and manifestations of respiratory failure, and outline the interprofessional care and nursing care of patients with this condition.

CLINICAL COMPETENCIES

- Assess functional health status of patients with disorders affecting ventilation and gas exchange.
- Use assessed data and knowledge of the effects of a disorder and its prescribed treatment to identify priority nursing diagnoses and plan care for patients with disorders affecting ventilation and gas exchange.
- Use the nursing process and evidence-based nursing research to plan and implement individualized nursing care for patients, including measures to promote ventilation and gas exchange.
- Plan and provide appropriate teaching for health promotion among vulnerable populations and to prepare patients and families for continuity of care.
- Evaluate the effectiveness of nursing interventions and teaching, revising strategies and teaching plans as needed.
- Knowledgably and safely coordinate interprofessional care and administer prescribed medications and treatments for patients with disorders affecting ventilation and gas exchange.

KEY TERMS

acute respiratory distress syndrome (ARDS), 1381
asthma, 1335
atelectasis, 1360
bronchiectasis, 1361
chronic bronchitis, 1345
chronic obstructive pulmonary disease (COPD), 1345
cor pulmonale, 1370
cystic fibrosis (CF), 1356
emphysema, 1346
pulmonary embolism, 1364
pulmonary hypertension (PHTN), 1369
respiratory failure, 1371
sarcoidosis, 1363
status asthmaticus, 1337
terminal weaning, 1378
weaning, 1378

Normal function of the lower respiratory system depends on several organ systems: The central nervous system (CNS), which stimulates and controls breathing; chemoreceptors in the brain, aortic arch, and carotid bodies, which monitor the pH and oxygen content of blood; the heart and circulatory system, which provide for blood supply and gas exchange; the musculoskeletal system, which provides an intact thoracic cavity capable of expanding and contracting; and the lungs and bronchial tree, which allow air movement and gas exchange. Impaired function of any of these systems affects ventilation and respiration. As a result, tissues may become *hypoxic*, with inadequate oxygen to support metabolic activity.

Although some of the disorders discussed in this chapter can affect ventilation (air movement into and out of the airways and alveoli), all can have significant effects on gas exchange. The mechanisms by which they affect gas exchange differ:

- In reactive airway disease (asthma) and obstructive disorders, air trapping reduces the amount of oxygen available to drive gas exchange.
- Interstitial lung disorders affect the ability of the lungs to expand and the work of breathing, reducing alveolar oxygenation and gas exchange.
- Pulmonary vascular disorders affect blood flow to the lungs or a portion of the lungs, reducing gas exchange through their effects on perfusion of the lungs.
- Respiratory failure is the ultimate consequence of impaired gas exchange; the lungs cannot adequately oxygenate the blood or eliminate carbon dioxide.

With a few exceptions, the disorders discussed in this chapter are relatively common, chronic lung diseases (National Center for Health Statistics, 2016):

- Chronic obstructive pulmonary disease (COPD) is currently the third leading cause of death in the United States and worldwide.
- Since 2001, the death rate for chronic lower respiratory diseases has been higher for women, with women who smoke being 13 times as likely to die from COPD versus nonsmoking women.
- Whites have a higher death rate for chronic lower respiratory diseases than Blacks, Native Americans, or Hispanics. People of Asian heritage have the lowest death rate due to chronic lower respiratory diseases.
- Chronic lower respiratory diseases are the fourth leading cause of death for people ages 65 years and older and the sixth leading cause of death for adults 45 to 64 years old. They are not a leading cause of death for adults younger than age 45.

Disorders of other body systems, such as neurologic disorders (e.g., head injury, spinal cord trauma or disorders, amyotrophic lateral sclerosis [ALS], myasthenia gravis), can also affect gas exchange through their effects on the central or peripheral nervous systems. These disorders and their effects on the respiratory system are discussed in subsequent chapters of this text.

Aging affects pulmonary ventilation and gas exchange as well. The number of alveoli decrease, and emphysematous changes (senile emphysema) reduce the surface area for gas exchange. Alveoli become less elastic, causing increased air trapping and dead space. For most older adults who remain active, these changes have minimal effect on exercise tolerance and activities of daily living (ADLs). When combined with lung disease, however, age-related pulmonary changes increase the patient's risk for developing respiratory failure.

37.1 Reactive Airway Disorders

In reactive airway disorders, the airways narrow in response to a stimulus. Airway narrowing limits airflow both into and out of the alveoli. Limited airflow increases the work of breathing and the residual volume of the lungs as air is trapped distal to narrowed airways. Inspired air mixes with an abnormally large volume of residual air, effectively reducing the amount of oxygen available in the alveoli. Decreased alveolar ventilation further reduces oxygen available for exchange.

The Patient with Asthma

Asthma is a chronic inflammatory disorder of the airways characterized by recurrent episodes of wheezing, breathlessness, chest tightness, and coughing. Inflammation causes increased responsiveness of the airways to multiple stimuli. The widespread airflow obstruction that occurs during acute episodes usually reverses either spontaneously or with treatment. Although most episodes of asthma attacks are relatively brief, some patients with asthma may experience longer episodes with some degree of airway impairment daily. In rare cases, an acute episode of asthma is so severe that respiratory failure and death results.

In the United States, approximately 18.4 million adults had asthma in 2015. Asthma is a serious disease, causing about 3396 deaths in the United States in 2015 (Centers for Disease Control and Prevention [CDC], 2017a). Asthma is more common in children (13.1%) than in adults (10.9%) (CDC, 2017a). Across races, the mortality rate associated with asthma is higher in women than in men. The asthma mortality rate of Blacks is nearly three times that of Whites (Office of Minority Health, 2018). Deaths due to asthma are rare in children, but increase with age, particularly in middle and late adulthood and old age (CDC, 2017a).

Pathophysiology

Airways within the lungs contain crisscrossing strips of smooth muscle that control their diameter. This muscle is innervated by the autonomic nervous system. Parasympathetic (cholinergic) stimulation leads to *bronchoconstriction*, or narrowing of the airways. Sympathetic stimulation through $beta_2$-adrenergic receptors causes *bronchodilation*, or expansion of the airways. Slight bronchoconstriction normally dominates. However, when increased airflow is necessary (e.g., during exercise), the parasympathetic system is inhibited and stimulation of the sympathetic system causes bronchodilation. Inflammatory mediators (such as histamine) released during an antigen–antibody response act directly on bronchial smooth muscle to produce bronchoconstriction.

In asthma, the airways are in a persistent state of inflammation. During symptom-free periods, airway inflammation in asthma is subacute or quiet. Even during these periods, however, inflammatory cells such as eosinophils, neutrophils, and lymphocytes may be found in airway tissues and edema may be present. An acute inflammatory response, during which resident inflammatory cells interact with inflammatory mediators, cytokines, and additional infiltrating inflammatory cells, may be triggered by a variety of factors. Common triggers for an acute asthma attack include exposure to allergens, respiratory tract infection, exercise, inhaled irritants, and emotional upset.

Attack Triggers

Childhood asthma (which may continue into adulthood) is most often linked to inhalation of allergens such as pollen, animal dander, or household dust. Patients with allergic asthma often have a history of other allergies. Environmental pollutants, such as tobacco smoke and irritant gases (e.g., sulfur dioxide, nitrogen dioxide, and ozone), can provoke asthma. Exposure to secondhand smoke as a child is associated with a higher risk for and increased severity of asthma (CDC, 2017c). Agents found in the workplace, such as noxious fumes and gases, chemicals, and dusts, may cause occupational asthma.

Respiratory infections, viral in particular, are a common internal stimulus for an asthma attack. Exercise-induced asthma attacks are also common, affecting 40 to 90% of people with bronchial asthma (Sorenson, Quinn, & Klein, 2019). Loss of heat or water from the bronchial surface may contribute to exercise-induced asthma. Exercising in cold, dry air increases the risk of an asthma attack in susceptible people.

Emotional stress is a significant etiologic factor for attacks in patients with asthma. Common pharmacologic triggers include aspirin and other NSAIDs, beta-blockers, and sulfites (which are used as preservatives in wine, beer, fresh fruits, and salad).

Responses

When a trigger such as inhalation of an allergen or irritant occurs, an *acute* or *early response* develops in the hyperreactive airways predisposed to bronchospasm. Sensitized mast cells in the bronchial mucosa release inflammatory mediators such as histamine, prostaglandins, and leukotrienes. Resident and infiltrating inflammatory cells also produce inflammatory mediators such as cytokines, bradykinin, and growth factors. These mediators stimulate parasympathetic receptors and bronchial smooth muscle to produce bronchoconstriction. They also increase capillary permeability, which allows plasma to escape and leads to mucosal edema. Mucous production is stimulated; excess mucus collects in the narrowed airways.

The attack is prolonged by the *late-phase response*, which develops 4 to 12 hours after exposure to the trigger. Inflammatory cells such as basophils and eosinophils are activated, which damage airway epithelium, produce mucosal edema, impair mucociliary clearance, and produce or prolong bronchoconstriction. The degree of hyperreactivity depends on the extent of inflammation. Together, bronchoconstriction, edema and inflammation, and mucus secretion narrow the airway. Airway resistance increases, limiting airflow and increasing the work of breathing (**Figure 37.1** ■).

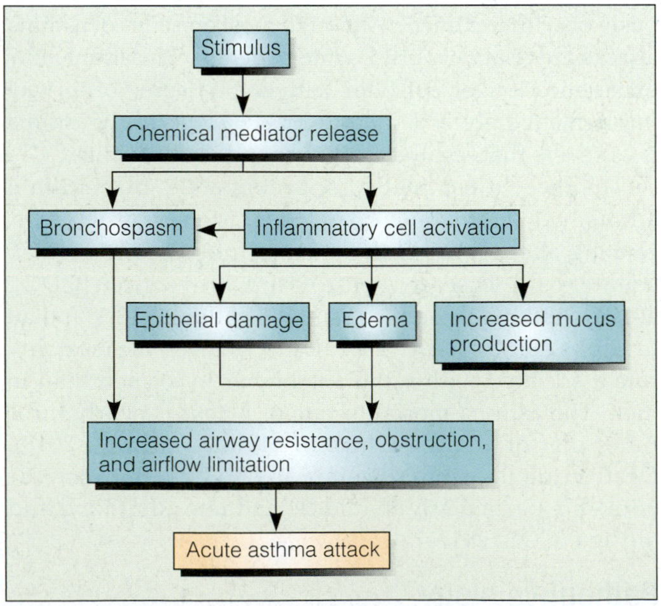

Stimulus
Chemical mediator release
Bronchospasm
Inflammatory cell activation
Epithelial damage
Edema
Increased mucus production
Increased airway resistance, obstruction, and airflow limitation
Acute asthma attack

Figure 37.1 ■ The pathogenesis of an acute episode of asthma.

Limited expiratory airflow traps air distal to the spastic, narrowed airways. Trapped air mixes with inspired air in the alveoli, reducing its oxygen tension and gas exchange across the alveolar-capillary membrane. Distended alveoli compress alveolar capillaries, reducing blood flow and further affecting gas exchange. As a result, hypoxemia develops. Hypoxemia and increased lung volume due to trapping stimulate the respiratory rate. Hyperventilation causes the $PaCO_2$ to fall, leading to respiratory alkalosis. (Refer to Chapter 10 for more information about acid–base imbalances.)

To summarize, in an acute asthma attack, inflammatory mediators are released from sensitized airways followed by activation of inflammatory cells. These events lead to bronchoconstriction, airway edema, and impaired mucociliary clearance. Airway narrowing limits airflow and increases the work of breathing; trapped air mixes with inhaled air, impairing gas exchange.

Risk Factors

A number of risk factors can be identified for asthma, although many patients develop the disease in the absence of known risk factors. Allergies play a strong role in childhood asthma, although less so in adults. There is a strong genetic component to the disease, although a specific pattern of inheritance has not been identified. Multiple regions on several chromosomes appear to contribute to asthma-related factors such as airway hyperreactivity and high IgE levels. Environmental factors, including air pollution and occupational exposure to industrial compounds, may contribute. Respiratory viruses such as rhinovirus and influenza can precipitate asthma attacks. Other contributory factors include exercise (particularly in cold air) and emotional stress.

Manifestations

An asthma attack is characterized by a subjective sensation of chest tightness, cough, dyspnea, wheezing, tachypnea, tachycardia, anxiety, and apprehension. The onset of symptoms may be either abrupt or insidious, and an attack may subside rapidly or persist for hours or days. A sense of chest constriction and nonproductive cough are common early manifestations of an attack. During an attack, tachycardia, tachypnea, and prolonged expiration are common. Diffuse wheezing is heard on auscultation. With more severe attacks, use of accessory muscles of respiration, intercostal retractions, loud wheezing, and distant breath sounds may be noted. Fatigue, anxiety, apprehension, and severe dyspnea that allows speaking only one or two words between breaths may occur with persistent severe episodes. The onset of respiratory failure is marked by inaudible breath sounds with reduced wheezing and an ineffective cough. Without careful assessment, this apparent relief of symptoms can be misinterpreted as an improvement.

The frequency of attacks and severity of symptoms vary greatly from person to person. Although some people have infrequent, mild episodes, others have nearly continuous manifestations of cough, dyspnea on exertion, and wheezing with periodic severe exacerbations (**Table 37.1**).

Complications

Status asthmaticus is severe, prolonged asthma that does not respond to routine treatment. Without aggressive therapy, status asthmaticus can lead to respiratory failure with hypoxemia, hypercapnia, and acidosis. Endotracheal intubation, mechanical ventilation, and aggressive drug treatment may be necessary to sustain life.

In addition to acute respiratory failure, other complications associated with acute asthma include dehydration, respiratory infection, atelectasis, pneumothorax, and cor pulmonale.

Asthma is one of the three most common causes of chronic cough (the other two being postnasal drip and gastroesophageal reflux disease [GERD]). Cough can be initiated by either upper airway irritants (e.g., postnasal drip or GERD) or by inflammation or constriction of the lower airways. Most commonly, cough associated with asthma is accompanied by classic asthma symptoms such as chest constriction, dyspnea, and wheezing. Patients with *cough-variant asthma*, however, have persistent cough without wheezing or dyspnea, often delaying diagnosis. These patients do have significant airway inflammation and demonstrate the pathophysiologic features of asthma.

Interprofessional Care

The diagnosis of asthma is based primarily on the history and manifestations. Treatment goals are twofold. Daily management focuses on controlling symptoms and preventing acute attacks. During an acute attack, therapy is directed toward restoring airway patency and alveolar ventilation.

Table 37.1 Classification of Asthma Severity

Classification	Symptom Frequency	Nighttime Symptoms
Mild intermittent	■ No more than twice a week ■ Brief attacks (hours to days) of varied intensity ■ Asymptomatic and normal peak expiratory flow (PEF) rate between attacks	No more than twice a month
Mild persistent	■ More than twice a week but less than once a day ■ Exacerbations may affect activity	More than twice a month
Moderate persistent	■ Daily symptoms ■ Daily short-acting bronchodilator use ■ Exacerbations affect activity ■ Exacerbations more than twice a week; may last for days	More than once a week
Severe persistent	■ Continual symptoms ■ Limited physical activity ■ Frequent exacerbations	Frequent

Source: National Heart, Lung, and Blood Institute, 2012.

Diagnosis

Diagnostic tests are used to determine the degree of airway involvement during and between acute episodes and identify causative factors such as allergens.

- ***Pulmonary function tests (PFTs)*** are used to evaluate the degree of airway obstruction. Pulmonary function testing done before and after use of an aerosolized bronchodilator helps determine the reversibility of airway obstruction. Airway reversibility is a cardinal sign seen on pulmonary function testing in asthma. The residual volume (RV) of the lungs may be increased and vital capacity decreased or normal even during periods of remission. The forced expiratory volume (FEV_1) and peak expiratory flow rate (PEFR), commonly referred to as *peak flow,* are the most valuable pulmonary function studies to evaluate the severity of an asthma attack and the effectiveness of treatment measures.
- ***Challenge*** or ***bronchial provocation testing*** uses an inhaled substance such as methacholine or histamine with PFTs to confirm the diagnosis of asthma by detecting airway hyperresponsiveness.
- ***Arterial blood gases (ABGs)*** are drawn during an acute attack in the hospital setting to evaluate oxygenation, carbon dioxide elimination, and acid–base status. ABGs initially show hypoxemia with a low PaO_2 and mild respiratory alkalosis with an elevated pH and low $PaCO_2$ due to tachypnea. Severe airflow obstruction causes significant hypoxemia and respiratory acidosis (pH < 7.35 and $PaCO_2 > 45$ mmHg), indicative of respiratory failure and the need for mechanical ventilation. Refer to Chapter 10 for more information about arterial blood gases and their interpretation.
- ***Skin testing*** may be done to identify specific allergens if an allergic trigger is suspected for asthma attacks. See Chapter 36 for more information about skin testing.
- ***Other testing*** may include blood sampling for serum immunoglobulin E for allergens and eosinophil count elevation. See Chapter 13 for information on IgE.

Disease Monitoring

Peak expiratory flow rate (PEFR) is used on a day-to-day basis to evaluate the severity of bronchial hyperresponsiveness. Small, inexpensive meters to measure PEFR are available. Readings taken at varying times of day over several weeks are used to establish the patient's personal best or normal PEFR. This value is then used to evaluate the severity of airway obstruction. Traffic signal colors are used for simplicity: *Green* (80 to 100% of personal best) indicates asthma that is under control; *yellow* (50 to 80%) is caution, indicating a need for further medication or treatment; and *red* (50% or less) signals an immediate need for a bronchodilator and medical treatment if the level does not immediately return to the yellow range (Sorenson et al., 2019).

Medications

Medications are used to prevent and control asthma symptoms, reduce the frequency and severity of exacerbations, and reverse airway obstruction. Drugs used for long-term control of asthma are taken daily to maintain control of the disease. The primary drugs in this group are anti-inflammatory agents, long-acting bronchodilators, and leukotriene modifiers. Quick-relief medications provide prompt relief of bronchoconstriction and airflow obstruction with associated wheezing, cough, and chest tightness. Short-acting adrenergic stimulants (rapid-acting bronchodilators), anticholinergic drugs, and methylxanthines fall into this category.

A stepwise approach for managing asthma is recommended (see **Table 37.2**). This approach is based on the severity of the disease (refer to Table 37.1). For all patients, a short-acting inhaled $beta_2$-agonist is recommended for quick relief of acute symptoms. Up to three treatments at 20-minute intervals or a single nebulizer treatment may be used as needed. Strategies for long-term control may need to be modified if a short-acting bronchodilator is needed more than twice a week (National Heart, Lung, and Blood Institute [NHLBI], 2012).

Many of the drugs used for continued asthma management and relief of an acute attack can be administered by a metered-dose inhaler (MDI), dry powder inhaler (DPI), or nebulizer. The advantages of administering medications locally by inhalation include rapid onset and reduced systemic effects of the drugs. In an MDI, a chemical propellant is used to deliver the medication when the canister is depressed. DPIs, in contrast, contain no propellant. Instead, the medication is released by inhaling rapidly through a mouthpiece. **Box 37.1** outlines patient teaching for use of an MDI or DPI.

Table 37.2 Stepwise Approach to Asthma Management for Adults

Step/Disease Severity	Preferred Treatment	Alternate or As-Needed Treatment
Step 1 Mild intermittent	No daily medication needed	Systemic corticosteroids for severe exacerbations
Step 2 Mild persistent	Low-dose inhaled corticosteroids	Cromolyn, leukotriene modifier, nedocromil, or sustained-release theophylline
Step 3 Moderate persistent	Low-to-moderate dose inhaled corticosteroids *and* long-acting inhaled $beta_2$-agonist	Increase inhaled corticosteroid dose *or* combine inhaled corticosteroid with leukotriene modifier or theophylline
Step 4 Severe persistent	High-dose inhaled corticosteroid *and* long-acting inhaled $beta_2$-agonist	Add systemic corticosteroid

Source: National Heart, Lung, and Blood Institute, 2012.

BOX 37.1
Patient Teaching: Using a Metered-Dose Inhaler, Dry Powder Inhaler, or Soft Mist Inhaler

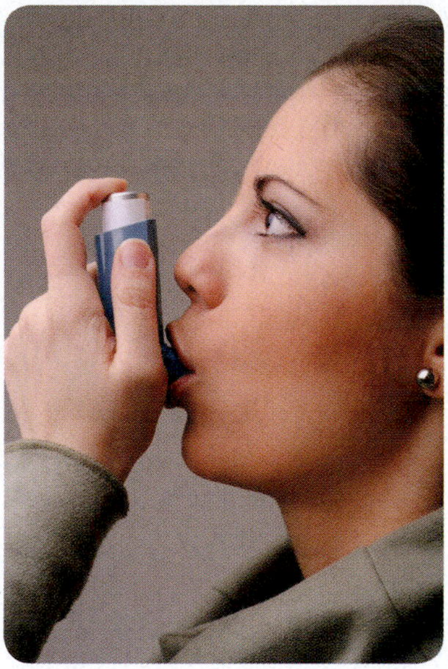

METERED-DOSE INHALER

- Firmly insert a charged MDI canister into the mouthpiece unit or spacer (if used).
- Remove mouthpiece cap. Shake canister vigorously for 3 to 5 seconds.
- Exhale slowly and completely.
- Holding the canister upside down, place the mouthpiece in the mouth, closing lips around it if a spacer is being used. When no spacer is used, hold the mouthpiece directly in front of the mouth.
- Press and hold the canister down while inhaling deeply and slowly for 3 to 5 seconds (see accompanying figure).
- Hold breath for 10 seconds, release pressure on the container, remove from mouth, and exhale. Wait 20 to 30 seconds before repeating the procedure for a second puff.
- Rinse the mouth after using the inhaler to minimize systemic absorption and drying of the mucous membranes.
- Rinse the inhaler mouthpiece and spacer after use; store in a clean location.

DRY POWDER INHALER

- Keep the inhaler and medication in a clean, dry location. Do not refrigerate or store in a humid place (e.g., the bathroom).
- Remove the cap and hold the inhaler upright. Inspect to be sure that the mechanism is clean and the mouthpiece is clear.
- If necessary, load the dose into the inhaler following the manufacturer's directions.
- Hold the inhaler level with the mouthpiece end facing down.
- Breathe slowly and completely. Tilt your head back slightly.
- Place the mouthpiece in your mouth with your teeth over the mouthpiece. Seal your lips around the mouthpiece. Do not block the inhaler with your tongue.
- Breathe in rapidly and deeply through your mouth over 2 to 3 seconds to activate the flow of medication.
- Remove the inhaler from your mouth and hold your breath for 10 seconds.
- Exhale slowly through pursed lips to allow the medication to enter distal airways. Never exhale into the inhaler mouthpiece to prevent clogging.
- Rinse your mouth or brush your teeth after using the inhaler to avoid a bad taste from the medication and to prevent a yeast infection (if a corticosteroid medication is being used).
- Store the inhaler in a clean, sealed plastic bag; do not wash the inhaler unless so directed by the manufacturer. The mouthpiece should be cleaned weekly using a dry cloth.

SOFT MIST INHALER

- Insert the metal cartridge into the plastic inhaler by pushing the narrow end of cartridge into inhaler.
- Prime the inhaler by turning the clear base in the direction of the arrows until a click is heard. Open the color cap and activate the device until a mist appears.
- Holding the device upright, turn the clear base until it clicks (primes the dose).
- Open the color cap.
- Breathe out and close your lips around the mouthpiece, pointing the inhaler to the back of your throat. Do not cover the air vents.
- Push the dose release button while taking in a slow, deep breath through your mouth. The mist is released over 8 seconds.
- Hold your breath for 10 seconds or as long as you can.
- Remove the inhaler and put the cap back on the mouthpiece.
- Rinse your mouth with water and then spit the water out. Do not swallow the water.

Bronchodilators. Most people with asthma need bronchodilator therapy to control their symptoms. Inhalation of nebulized medication is the preferred means of administration. The primary bronchodilators used include adrenergic stimulants, anticholinergic agents, and methylxanthines. These drugs are often administered in combination with an anti-inflammatory agent.

Adrenergic stimulants (beta$_2$-agonists) affect receptors on smooth muscle cells of the respiratory tract, causing smooth muscle relaxation and bronchodilation. Long-acting adrenergic stimulants such as inhaled salmeterol and oral sustained-release albuterol are used in conjunction with anti-inflammatory drugs to control symptoms, but are not appropriate to treat an acute episode of asthma. Inhaled short-acting beta-adrenergic agonists such as albuterol, bitolterol, pirbuterol, and terbutaline, administered by MDI, DPI, or soft mist inhaler, are the treatment of choice for quick relief. They act within minutes, but their duration is generally short, lasting only 4 to 6 hours. Tachycardia and muscle tremors, common side effects of adrenergic agonists, are minimal with inhalation therapy.

Anticholinergic medications prevent bronchoconstriction by blocking parasympathetic input to bronchial smooth muscle. Ipratropium bromide, an anticholinergic drug administered by MDI or handheld nebulizer, is useful when asthma symptoms are poorly controlled by adrenergic stimulants alone. Anticholinergic drugs act more slowly than adrenergic stimulants, requiring up to 60 to 90 minutes to achieve maximal effect.

Theophylline is a methylxanthine used as adjunctive treatment for asthma. It relaxes bronchial smooth muscle and may also inhibit the release of chemical mediators of the inflammatory response. Monitoring of serum theophylline levels is necessary because of wide individual variations in metabolism and elimination of the drug and its toxic effects. Serum levels of 10 to 20 μg/mL or lower are recommended. Theophylline may be used as a long-term bronchodilator, given once or twice daily. A related drug, aminophylline, may be administered intravenously to treat an acute, severe exacerbation of the disease.

Anti-Inflammatory Agents. Corticosteroids and two nonsteroidal anti-inflammatory agents, cromolyn sodium and nedocromil, are used to suppress airway inflammation and reduce asthma symptoms.

Corticosteroids block the late response to inhaled allergens and reduce bronchial hyperresponsiveness. The preferred route of administration is by MDI or DPI to minimize systemic absorption and reduce the adverse effects of prolonged steroid use (cushingoid effects). For a severe acute attack, corticosteroids may be given systemically to alleviate symptoms and induce remission.

Cromolyn sodium and nedocromil are used to prevent acute episodes of asthma. They reduce airway hyperreactivity and inhibit the release of mediator substances. These drugs are used for long-term control of asthma, not quick relief. They have a wide margin of safety and few side effects.

Leukotriene Modifiers. Leukotriene modifiers montelukast (Singulair), zafirlukast (Accolate), and zileuton (Zyflo Filmtab) are oral medications that reduce the inflammatory response in asthma. They appear to improve lung function, diminish symptoms, and reduce the need for short-acting bronchodilators. These drugs affect the metabolism and excretion of other medications such as warfarin and theophylline and may cause liver toxicity.

Nursing implications for medications used to treat asthma are outlined in **Medication Administration 37.A.**

Medication Administration 37.A

Asthma

ADRENERGIC STIMULANTS

albuterol (Proventil, Ventolin)
bitolterol (Tornalate)
epinephrine
isoetharine (Bronkosol, Bronkometer)
isoproterenol (Isuprel)
metaproterenol (Alupent, Metaprel)
pirbuterol (Maxair)
salmeterol (Serevent)
terbutaline (Brethaire, Brethine)

Combined Forms:

albuterol/ipratropium (Combivent)
salmeterol/fluticasone (Advair)

Adrenergic stimulants affect sympathetic receptors in the respiratory tract. Administered by MDIs or DPIs, these drugs are the treatment of choice for acute bronchial asthma. Nearly all of the drugs in this class (epinephrine and isoproterenol being the exceptions) selectively activate beta$_2$-receptors at the doses typically used to treat asthma. Beta$_2$-receptor activation results in smooth muscle relaxation and bronchodilation. Formoterol and salmeterol are highly selective to beta$_2$-receptors, resulting in fewer adverse effects. Formoterol and salmeterol have been shown to increase the risk of serious asthma exacerbations and death, however. The Food and Drug Administration recommends using these drugs only when the disease cannot be adequately controlled with other medications.

Oral forms of adrenergic agonists may be used for prophylaxis but are not effective in treating an acute attack because of their slow onset. When administered orally or parenterally, their effect on sympathetic nervous system receptors can produce undesirable side effects such as nervousness, irritability, tachycardia, and cardiac dysrhythmias.

Nursing Responsibilities

- Use with caution in patients with hypertension, cardiovascular disease, dysrhythmias, hyperthyroidism, or diabetes.
- When given to a patient who is hypoxemic and acidotic, these drugs may cause potentially dangerous cardiac stimulation.
- When given by MDI wait 1 to 2 minutes between puffs to allow airways to dilate, permitting the second dose to reach distal airways.
- Observe for desired effect of reduced dyspnea and wheezing. CNS stimulation (anxiety, irritability, and insomnia) and tremor are common side effects.

Health Education for the Patient and Family

- Use the prescribed inhaler or nebulizer as directed.
- If you are taking a bronchodilator along with another medication by inhalation, use the bronchodilator first to open airways and enhance the effectiveness of the second medication.
- Rinse the mouth after using inhalers to reduce systemic absorption of the medication.
- Keep a log to track your bronchodilator use. If the drug becomes less effective or if you need a higher dosage or more frequent doses than prescribed, contact your physician.
- Report palpitations, irregular pulse, and other side effects to your physician.

METHYLXANTHINES

aminophylline (Somophyllin)

theophylline (Bronkotabs, Quibron, Slo-Phyllin, Theolair, Theo-Dur, others)

The methylxanthines are CNS stimulants chemically related to caffeine. These drugs produce bronchodilation through relaxation of bronchial smooth muscle. As CNS stimulants, they produce adverse effects such as nervousness, insomnia, and tremors. When administered in large doses, convulsions may result.

Once the drugs of choice for preventing and treating asthma attacks, they are now used primarily to prevent nocturnal asthma in affected adult patients. Theophylline has a narrow margin of safety and high potential for toxicity. Because the metabolism and excretion of theophylline vary significantly from person to person—affected by such factors as age, smoking, genetics, and alcoholism and other chronic diseases—monitoring of serum levels is vital.

Nursing Responsibilities

- The therapeutic blood level for theophylline is 10 to 20 μg/mL.
- Monitor for manifestations of toxicity. Anorexia, nausea and vomiting, restlessness, insomnia, cardiac dysrhythmias, and seizures are early manifestations. Other manifestations include epigastric pain, hematemesis, diarrhea, headache, irritability, muscle twitching, palpitations, tachycardia, flushing, and circulatory failure.
- Administer with meals or a full glass of water or milk to minimize gastric irritation.
- Monitor the effect closely when administering concurrently with other medications such as barbiturates, anticonvulsants, thyroid hormone, beta-blockers, bronchodilators, and others.
- Aminophylline is incompatible with many other intravenous drugs. Use a separate line or flush the line with normal saline before and after administering any other preparation.

Health Education for the Patient and Family

- Oral methylxanthines are ineffective to treat an acute asthma attack; do not delay other treatment by using these drugs.
- Check with the physician before taking any over-the-counter (OTC) medications or other prescription drugs while on theophylline.
- Do not smoke while using this drug.
- Report adverse effects to the physician.

ANTICHOLINERGICS

atropine

ipratropium bromide (Atrovent)

tiotropium bromide (Spiriva)

Combined Form:

albuterol/ipratropium

Anticholinergics are potent bronchodilators, blocking muscarinic receptors of the parasympathetic nervous system. Activation of muscarinic receptors produces smooth muscle contraction and bronchoconstriction; blockade of these receptors facilitates smooth muscle relaxation and bronchodilation. Atropine is used infrequently because of its tendency to dry secretions of the mucous membranes and other side effects. Ipratropium and tiotropium bromide are available as inhalers and have fewer side effects than atropine.

Nursing Responsibilities

- Assess for possible contraindications to the drug, including hypersensitivity, glaucoma, prostatic hypertrophy, or bladder-neck obstruction.
- Assess for desired and/or adverse effects: Improving or worsening symptoms; nausea and vomiting, abdominal cramping, anxiety, dizziness; headache.
- Provide ice chips, fluids, or hard candy to relieve dry mouth.

Health Education for the Patient and Family

- To prevent overdose, take no more than the prescribed number of doses per day.
- If the drug becomes less effective over time, notify the physician; an adjustment in dosage may be needed.

CORTICOSTEROIDS

beclomethasone dipropionate (Vanceril, Beclovent)

dexamethasone sodium phosphate (Decadron Phosphate Respihaler)

flunisolide (AeroBid)

fluticasone propionate (Flovent)

triamcinolone acetonide (Azmacort)

Combined Form:

salmeterol/fluticasone (Advair)

The anti-inflammatory effect of corticosteroids helps both prevent and treat acute episodes. Corticosteroids are used to reduce the frequency and severity of asthma attacks and allow reduced dosages of other drugs. The beneficial effects of corticosteroids for asthma result from their ability to decrease the synthesis and release of inflammatory mediators (such as histamine and leukotrienes), reduce inflammatory cell activation and infiltration, and decrease airway edema. Corticosteroids also decrease mucous production in the airways and increase the number and receptivity of beta$_2$-receptors (Shields, Fox, & Liebrecht, 2018). The cushingoid side effects of corticosteroids, always a major concern with their use, are minimized when they are inhaled. It is a second-line drug, recommended for use only when asthma is inadequately controlled using other preparations.

Nursing Responsibilities

- Administer inhaler doses after bronchodilators to facilitate transit of the medication to distal airways.
- Assess for common side effects: Sore throat; hoarseness; and oropharyngeal or laryngeal ***Candida albicans*** infection.
- Administer antifungal medications or gargles as ordered.

Health Education for the Patient and Family

- Rinse the mouth after using the inhaler and maintain good oral hygiene to reduce the risk of fungal infections.
- These medications should not be used to alleviate the symptoms of an acute attack.
- Several weeks of continued therapy may be required before a beneficial effect is noticed.
- Notify the physician if you develop weight gain, fluid retention, muscle weakness, redistribution of fat, or mood changes.

MAST CELL STABILIZERS

cromolyn sodium (Intal, NasalCrom)

nedocromil (Tilade)

Cromolyn sodium and nedocromil inhibit inflammatory cells in the airway, blocking early and late responses to inhaled antigens. Both drugs also prevent bronchoconstriction in response to inhaling cold air. These drugs act primarily by stabilizing the cytoplasmic membrane of mast cells, preventing the cells from releasing inflammatory mediators such as histamine (Shields et al., 2018). These drugs are used only for preventing asthma attacks, not to treat an acute attack. They are administered by MDI and have a wide margin of safety. Patients using nedocromil may complain of an unpleasant taste.

(continued)

Nursing Responsibilities

- Evaluate for potential adverse effects of wheezing and bronchoconstriction.

Health Education for the Patient and Family

- Gargling or sipping water can decrease the throat irritation associated with nebulizer treatment.
- Use appropriate technique. Inhale deeply with head tipped back to open airways, hold breath, and then exhale. Repeat until all of the drug has been inhaled.
- These drugs are used only to prevent asthma attacks; they are not effective in treating an acute attack.
- Several weeks may be required before a beneficial effect is noted.

LEUKOTRIENE MODIFIERS

montelukast (Singulair)
zafirlukast (Accolate)
zileuton (Zyflo)

Leukotriene modifiers interfere with the inflammatory process in the airways by suppressing the effects of leukotrienes, a group of inflammatory mediators. Leukotrienes are powerful bronchoconstrictors and vasodilators; blocking their synthesis or their receptors improves airflow, decreases symptoms, and reduces the need for short-acting bronchodilators. They are used for maintenance therapy in adults and children over the age of 12 as an alternative to inhaled corticosteroid therapy. They are not used to treat an acute attack.

Nursing Responsibilities

- Administer at least 1 hour before or 2 hours after meals.
- These drugs inhibit some liver enzymes, affecting the metabolism of warfarin and possibly terfenadine and theophylline. Monitor prothrombin times and theophylline blood levels.
- Monitor liver enzymes because these drugs may be toxic to the liver.

Health Education for the Patient and Family

- Take the drugs as prescribed on an empty stomach.
- Notify the physician if a change in color of stools or urine is noted or if jaundice develops.

Note: Drugs identified in blue are among the 200 most commonly prescribed medications in the United States.

Source: Adams, et al., 2017

Integrative Therapies

A number of herbal preparations and other complementary therapies have historically been used in treating asthma. However, any complementary therapies should only be used in consultation with the primary provider or specialist. Dietary therapies, environmental considerations, and nutritional supplements are the complementary therapies used by asthma patients. Nutritional and dietary therapies may include elimination of certain foods or food additives (e.g., sulfite) from the diet, often in the absence of a documented food allergy or relationship between consumption and the onset of asthma symptoms. Although the evidence is inconsistent, increased intake of ascorbic acid (an antioxidant), zinc, and magnesium may help alleviate manifestations of asthma. People with mild asthma may benefit from addition of omega-3 polyunsaturated fatty acids to the diet, thereby experiencing less severe and fewer acute attacks.

Herbal preparations may include *Atropa belladonna* (the natural form of atropine) or ephedra (also called *ma huang*), an herb that contains ephedrine. These herbals have effects similar to those of drugs used to treat asthma and should not be used in combination with sympathetic stimulants or anticholinergic preparations. Because of the dangers associated with use of ephedra, sale of herbal products containing ephedra has been banned. Advise patients inquiring about the use of Chinese herbal remedies to treat asthma to inquire if any recommended product contains ma huang or ephedra and to avoid such products. Capsaicin may also relieve acute asthma symptoms. Other herbal preparations include quercetin and grape seed extract. Refer patients interested in using natural preparations to a qualified herbalist, and emphasize the importance of talking to a physician before using these preparations along with conventional treatment.

In addition to herbals, other complementary therapies such as biofeedback, yoga, breathing techniques, acupuncture, and massage have been found to alleviate or help control asthma symptoms.

Nursing Care

Nurses encounter patients with asthma both in the acute care setting during an acute exacerbation and as outpatients or in homes. The priority nursing care needs differ with each setting.

Assessment

See the Manifestations and Interprofessional Care sections for the assessment of the patient with acute asthma.

Assessment of the patient experiencing an acute asthma attack must be very focused and timely.

- *Health history:* Current symptoms, including chest tightness, shortness of breath, dyspnea; duration of current attack; measures used to relieve symptoms and their effect; identified precipitating factors for the attack; frequency of attacks; current medications; known allergies
- *Physical assessment:* Apparent level of distress; color; vital signs; respiratory rate and excursion, breath sounds throughout lung fields; apical pulse
- *Laboratory data:* Forced expiratory volume, peak expiratory flow rate; arterial blood gases.

Priorities of Care

Collaborate with the interprofessional team to ensure adequate treatment of the acute asthmatic process while providing care that supports the patient's optimal airway function and physical and psychologic responses to the disorder is a priority of nursing care.

Diagnoses, Outcomes, and Interventions

An acute asthma attack causes fear as breathing becomes increasingly difficult and hypoxemia develops. Anxiety in turn tends to increase the severity and manifestations of the attack. Priority nursing care needs during an acute attack focus on improving airway clearance and reducing fear and anxiety. Teaching about prevention of future attacks and home management must be postponed until adequate ventilation is restored.

Promote Airway Clearance and Patency. Bronchospasm and bronchoconstriction, increased mucus secretion, and airway edema narrow the airways and impair airflow during an acute attack of asthma. Both inspiratory and expiratory volume are affected, decreasing the oxygen available at the alveolus for the process of respiration. Narrowed air passages increase the work of breathing, increasing the metabolic rate and tissue demand for oxygen.

Expected Outcome: Patient will use techniques to promote airway clearance such as coughing and deep breathing.

The nurse will:

- Monitor skin color and temperature and level of consciousness. *Cyanosis, cool clammy skin, and changes in level of consciousness (agitation, lethargy, or confusion) indicate worsening hypoxia.*
- Assess arterial blood gas results and pulse oximetry readings; notify the healthcare provider of abnormal values or changes in status. *These values provide information about gas exchange and the adequacy of alveolar ventilation. A fall in oxygen saturation levels is an early indicator of impaired gas exchange.*
- Assess cough effort and sputum for color, consistency, and amount. *Ineffective cough may also signal impending respiratory failure.*
- Place in Fowler, high-Fowler, or orthopneic (with head and arms supported on the overbed table) position to facilitate breathing and lung expansion. *These positions reduce the work of breathing and increase lung expansion, especially of basilar areas.*
- Administer oxygen as ordered. If a mask is used, monitor closely for feelings of claustrophobia or suffocation. *Supplemental oxygen reduces hypoxemia. Although the mask is a very effective oxygen delivery system, it may increase anxiety.*
- Administer nebulizer treatments and provide humidification as ordered. *Nebulizer treatments are used to administer bronchodilators and other medications; humidity helps loosen secretions.*
- Initiate or assist with chest physiotherapy, including percussion and postural drainage. *Percussion and postural drainage facilitate the movement of secretions and airway clearance.*
- Increase fluid intake. *Increasing fluids helps keep secretions thin.*
- Provide endotracheal suctioning as needed. *Endotracheal suctioning may be necessary to remove secretions and improve ventilation if the patient is unable to clear secretions by coughing.*

SAFETY ALERT: Frequently assess respiratory status (at least every 1 to 2 hours): Respiratory rate and depth, chest movement or excursion, breath sounds, and peak expiratory flow rate. Respiratory status can change rapidly during an acute asthma attack and its treatment. A decreasing PEFR indicates worsening airflow restriction. Slowed, shallow respirations with significantly diminished breath sounds and decreased wheezing may indicate exhaustion and impending respiratory failure. Immediate intervention is necessary. ■

Promote Effective Breathing Pattern. The physiologic changes in lung ventilation that occur during an acute asthma attack impair both lung expansion and emptying. Anxiety caused by hypoxia and dyspnea compounds the problem by increasing the respiratory rate. Collaborative and nursing interventions can help restore a more normal breathing pattern and adequate lung ventilation.

Expected Outcome: Patient will demonstrate uncompromised ventilatory status as evidenced by absence of dyspnea, orthopnea, accessory muscle use, and adventitious lung sounds.

The nurse will:

- Frequently assess respiratory rate, pattern, and breath sounds. Note manifestations of ineffective breathing, including rapid rate, shallow respirations, nasal flaring, use of accessory muscles, intercostal retractions, and diminished or absent breath sounds. *Early identification of ineffective respirations allows timely initiation of interventions.*
- Monitor vital signs and laboratory results. *Tachypnea, tachycardia, an elevated blood pressure, and increasing hypoxemia and hypercapnia are signs of compromised respiratory status.*
- Assist with ADLs as needed. *This conserves energy and reduces fatigue.*
- Provide rest periods between scheduled activities and treatments. *Scheduled rest is important to prevent fatigue and reduce oxygen demands.*
- Teach and assist to use techniques to control breathing pattern:
  a. Pursed-lip breathing
  b. Abdominal breathing
  c. Relaxation techniques including visualization and meditation.

  Pursed-lip breathing helps keep airways open by maintaining positive pressure, and abdominal breathing improves lung expansion. Relaxation techniques reduce anxiety and its effect on the respiratory rate.
- Administer medications, including bronchodilators and anti-inflammatory drugs, as ordered. Monitor for desired and possible adverse effects. *Medications are used to improve airway status and facilitate breathing.*

Reduce Anxiety. Acute exacerbations of asthma can produce significant anxiety. Fear of being unable to breathe and feelings of suffocation associated with acute asthma are significant. Financial or other concerns may cause the patient to want to avoid hospitalization. Increasingly frequent and severe episodes may cause fear for the future. Hypoxia contributes to anxiety as well, stimulating the sympathetic nervous system and the fight-or-flight response.

Expected Outcome: Patient will be able to control anxiety as evidenced by verbalized decrease in subjective distress.

The nurse will:

- Assess level of anxiety. *Interventions for severe anxiety or panic differ from those for mild or moderate anxiety.*
- Assist to identify coping skills that have been successful in the past. *Successful coping helps the patient regain control of the situation, reducing anxiety.*
- Provide physical and emotional support. Remain with the patient during episodes of severe anxiety; schedule time every 1 to 2 hours to be with the mildly or moderately anxious patient, or more frequently if needed. Answer call lights promptly. *The severely anxious patient may fear being alone or believe that he or she will die if someone is not on hand. Knowing that the nurse is readily available and will return regardless if help is needed reduces anxiety.*
- Listen actively to concerns; do not deny or negate the fear of dying or of being unable to breathe. *Active listening promotes trust and helps the patient express concerns.*
- Provide clear, concise directions and explanations about procedures. Avoid presenting more information than the patient is able to assimilate. *Anxiety interferes with the ability to learn. Explanations may need to be repeated frequently.*
- Include the patient in care planning and decisions as appropriate, without making excessive demands. *Participating in decision making increases the patient's sense of control. Because high levels of anxiety interfere with the ability to make decisions, however, it is important to avoid placing demands on the patient that may further increase the level of anxiety.*
- Reduce excessive environmental stimuli, and maintain a calm demeanor. *This promotes rest.*
- Allow supportive family members to remain with the patient. *Significant others provide additional support and can help reduce anxiety.*
- Assist to use relaxation techniques, such as guided imagery, muscle relaxation, and meditation. *These techniques help restore psychologic balance and reduce sympathetic stimulation and responses.*

Promote Adherence to the Treatment Plan. Once acute asthma is under control and effective respirations have been reestablished, it is important to help the patient identify contributing factors to the attack and adhere to the therapeutic regimen. This helps the patient prevent future episodes.

Expected Outcome: Patient will comply with therapeutic regimen as evidenced by adherence to medication regimen and follow-up appointments.

The nurse will:

- Assess level of understanding about asthma and the prescribed treatment regimen. Provide additional information and teaching as indicated. *Assessment helps to identify and clarify misperceptions and difficulties with disease management.*
- Discuss the patient's perception of the illness and its effect on his or her lifestyle. *Open discussion can help identify conflicts between lifestyle and the treatment regimen.*
- Assist the patient and significant others to identify problems or difficulties integrating the treatment regimen into his or her lifestyle. *Asthma and its management may necessitate lifestyle modifications to prevent acute exacerbations. These modifications—such as eliminating cigarette smoking or pets from the household, removing carpets, or daily damp-dusting to remove dust mites—can significantly impact family members.*
- Assess knowledge and understanding of prescribed medications and use of OTC preparations. *This is important to determine misperceptions or possible misuse of medications.*
- Provide verbal and written instructions in the patient's primary language. *Written instructions reinforce teaching and allow future reference.*
- Refer to counseling, support groups, or self-help organizations. *Counseling, support groups, and self-help organizations can help the patient and family adapt to living with asthma and the treatment regimen.*

SAFETY ALERT: Assist to identify factors that contributed to the acute episode. Identifying contributing factors increases the patient's awareness of the disease and strategies to prevent future exacerbations. ■

Delegating Nursing Care Activities

As appropriate and allowed by the designated duties and responsibilities of unlicensed assistive personnel, the nurse may delegate nursing care activities such as measuring vital signs, encouraging oral or enteral fluid intake, and providing skin care.

Transitions of Care

Although specific measures to prevent asthma have not yet been identified, the link between parental smoking and childhood asthma is strong. Discuss this link with young people and families with children. Encourage all patients to not start smoking, and if they do smoke, to quit. Provide referrals to smoking-cessation clinics, help groups, or a care provider for nicotine patches as needed to facilitate quitting. Additional evidence suggests that early exposure to certain infectious diseases and to other children and limited use of antibiotics reduces the risk for developing asthma (NHLBI, 2012).

By avoiding allergens and environmental triggers, asthma attacks can often be prevented. Modifying the home environment by controlling dust, removing carpets, covering mattresses and pillows to reduce dust mite populations, and installing air filtering systems may be useful. Pets may need to be removed from the household. Eliminating all tobacco smoke in the home is vital. Wearing a mask that retains humidity and warm air while exercising in cold weather may help prevent attacks of exercise-induced asthma. Early treatment of respiratory infections is vital to prevent asthma exacerbations.

Asthma is a chronic disease that is best managed by the patient with assistance from medical personnel. Teaching for home care focuses on promoting the highest level of wellness and preventing and managing acute episodes and exacerbations of the disease. Topics to include in teaching are:

- Suggestions for lifestyle changes to avoid specific triggers for asthma attacks:
    a. Warm up slowly before exercising in cold weather; wear a special mask or scarf to retain air warmth and humidity while exercising.
    b. Substitute indoor exercises during cold, dry weather.
    c. Reduce the risk for respiratory infections (e.g., adequate rest, good nutrition, and stress management to maintain immune function, yearly influenza vaccines, and immunization against pneumococcal pneumonia).
    d. Use techniques to reduce or manage physical and psychologic stress.
- Using a PEFR meter to monitor airway status; how to manage the disease based on results.
- Using prescribed medications, including:
    a. Name, frequency, dose, and desired effect
    b. Potential adverse effects and their management, including effects to report to the physician
    c. Potential interactions with other drugs (including OTC herbal preparations) or foods
    d. If tolerance is a potential risk, how to identify it and steps to take.

Provide referrals to local or regional resources for further teaching and support as needed. Consider the need for home health services, home respiratory care services, and others as needed.

The Patient with Chronic Obstructive Pulmonary Disease

Patients with chronic airflow obstruction due to chronic bronchitis and/or emphysema are said to have **chronic obstructive pulmonary disease (COPD)**. In 2017, approximately 7 million Americans were affected by COPD (CDC, 2017b). It is more common among White people than Black people and affects men more frequently than women, although mortality rates are higher among women. It is the third leading cause of death in the United States (American Lung Association, 2017a). The incidence of COPD continues to rise in American Indian/Native Alaskans. In 2017, COPD and other chronic obstructive lung diseases accounted for 131,804 deaths (CDC, 2017b). In addition, COPD morbidity is significant. In people under age 65, COPD is second only to heart disease as a cause of disability, resulting in an estimated 250 million lost work hours each year.

Pathophysiology

COPD is characterized by slowly progressive obstruction of the airways. The disease is one of periodic exacerbations, often related to respiratory infection, with increased symptoms of dyspnea and sputum production. Unlike acute processes in which lung tissues recover, airways and lung parenchyma do not return to normal following an exacerbation; instead, they demonstrate progressive destructive changes.

Although one or the other may dominate, COPD typically includes components of both chronic bronchitis and emphysema, two distinctly different processes. Small airways disease, narrowing of small bronchioles, is also part of the COPD complex.

Through different mechanisms, these processes cause airways to narrow, resistance to airflow to increase, and expiration to become slow or difficult (**Figure 37.2** ■). The result is a mismatch between alveolar ventilation and blood flow or perfusion, leading to impaired gas exchange.

Chronic Bronchitis

Chronic bronchitis is a disorder of excessive bronchial mucus secretion. It is characterized by a productive cough lasting 3 or more months in 2 consecutive years (Sorenson et al., 2019). Cigarette smoke is the major factor implicated in the development of chronic bronchitis.

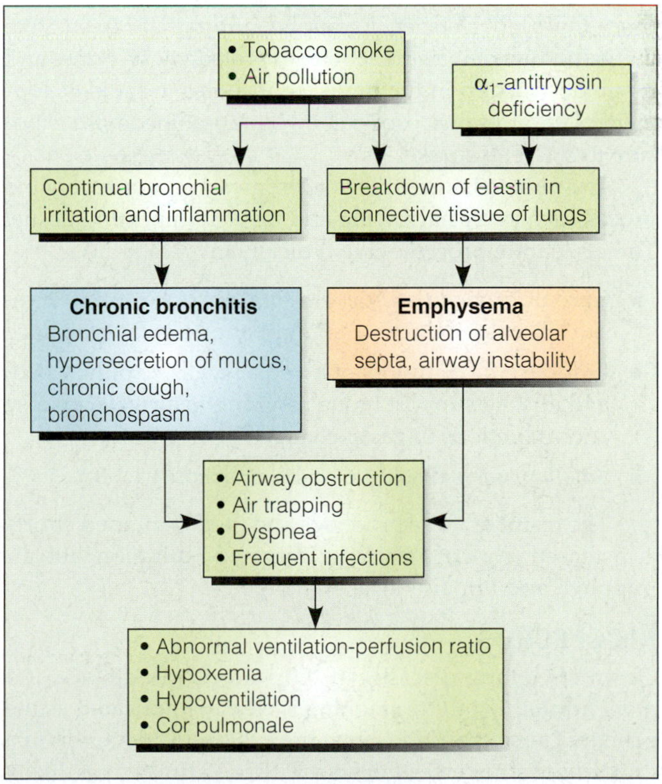

• Tobacco smoke
• Air pollution
α_1-antitrypsin deficiency
Continual bronchial irritation and inflammation
Breakdown of elastin in connective tissue of lungs
Chronic bronchitis
Bronchial edema, hypersecretion of mucus, chronic cough, bronchospasm
Emphysema
Destruction of alveolar septa, airway instability
• Airway obstruction
• Air trapping
• Dyspnea
• Frequent infections
• Abnormal ventilation-perfusion ratio
• Hypoxemia
• Hypoventilation
• Cor pulmonale

Figure 37.2 ■ The pathogenesis of chronic obstructive pulmonary disease.

Inhaled irritants lead to a chronic inflammatory process with vasodilation, congestion, and edema of the bronchial mucosa. Goblet cells increase in size and number, and mucous glands enlarge. Thick, tenacious mucus is produced in increased amounts. Changes in bronchial squamous cells impair the ability to clear mucus. Narrowed airways and excess secretions obstruct airflow; expiration is affected first, then inspiration. Because ciliary function is impaired, normal defense mechanisms are unable to clear the mucus and any inhaled pathogens. Recurrent infection is common in chronic bronchitis. An imbalance between ventilation and perfusion leads to hypoxemia, hypercapnia, and pulmonary hypertension. Pulmonary hypertension often leads to right-sided heart failure.

Emphysema

Emphysema is characterized by destruction of the walls of the alveoli, with resulting enlargement of abnormal air spaces. As in chronic bronchitis, cigarette smoking is strongly implicated as a causative factor in most cases of emphysema. Macrophages from the alveoli (air sacs) and CD-8 T lymphocytes increase and destroy lung tissue. Cytokines also play a role in the inflammation. Additionally, antiproteinases, which protect lung tissue, become inactivated, leading to reductions in lung repair. This results in alveolar wall destruction. Alveolar wall destruction causes alveoli and air spaces to enlarge, with loss of corresponding portions of the pulmonary capillary bed. As a result, the surface area for alveolar-capillary diffusion is reduced, affecting gas exchange. Elastic recoil is lost, reducing the volume of air that is passively expired. The loss of support tissue also affects airways, increasing the risk of expiratory collapse and further air trapping. Anatomically, either respiratory bronchioles or alveoli may be the primary tissue involved. Deficiency of alpha$_1$-antitrypsin, an enzyme that normally inhibits the activity of proteolytic enzymes and tissue destruction in the lungs, contributes to the development of emphysema, especially when combined with exposure to cigarette smoke.

To summarize, COPD is a progressive, nonreversible process of airway narrowing and loss of supporting tissue. Three separate processes are typically involved:

- Chronic bronchitis with persistent airway edema, excessive mucus production, and impaired airway clearance
- Emphysema with loss of alveolar walls, capillary bed, and airway support tissue resulting in airway collapse and reductions in gas exchange
- Small airways disease with bronchoconstriction.

The result of these processes and their combined effects is increased work of breathing, impaired expiration with air trapping, and impaired gas exchange.

Risk Factors

Obstructive lung disease typically affects middle-age and older adults. Cigarette smoking is clearly implicated as the primary cause of COPD. Even though COPD develops in a minority of smokers, smokers are 12 to 13 times more likely to die from COPD than nonsmokers. Cigarette smoke and the irritants it contains impair ciliary movement, inhibit the function of alveolar macrophages, and cause mucous-secreting glands to hypertrophy. Smoking also produces emphysema or airway destruction and constricts smooth muscle, increasing airway resistance. Other contributing factors include air pollution, occupational exposure to noxious dusts and gases, airway infection, and familial and genetic factors (see the Genetic Considerations box).

Manifestations

The clinical presentation of COPD varies from simple chronic bronchitis without disability to chronic respiratory failure and severe disability. **Box 37.2** outlines the classifications of COPD severity. Manifestations are typically absent or minor early in the disease. When the patient finally seeks care, productive cough, dyspnea, and exercise intolerance have often been present for as long as 10 years. The cough typically occurs in the mornings and is often attributed as *smoker's cough*. Initially, dyspnea occurs only on extreme exertion; as the disease progresses, activity tolerance spirals downward. Patients abandon activity to avoid dyspnea, leading to further deconditioning. This results in a patient so deconditioned

Genetic Considerations

Chronic Obstructive Pulmonary Disease

Severe alpha$_1$-antitrypsin (α_1AT or ATT) deficiency, present in about 1 to 2% of patients with COPD, is a proven risk factor for COPD. Normal α_1AT levels are associated with the common M allele. Two other alleles, the S allele and the Z allele, lead to reduced α_1AT levels. An estimated 25 million Americans carry a single gene associated with α_1AT deficiency and can pass that gene on to their offspring. People who inherit two Z alleles or one Z allele and one null allele have severe α_1AT deficiency. Approximately 1 in 2500 people in the United States inherit severe α_1AT deficiency. An estimated 100,000 people in the United States have emphysema related to α_1AT deficiency (Alpha 1 Foundation, 2017). Although studies suggest additional genetic factors in the development of COPD, at this time none have been proven.

BOX 37.2

Classification of COPD by Severity

Stage 0: At risk. Lung function normal, but chronic cough and sputum production are present

Stage 1: Mild COPD. Mild airflow limitation, usually with chronic cough and sputum production

Stage 2: Moderate COPD. Worsening airflow limitation, usually with progressing manifestations including dyspnea on exertion

Stage 3: Severe COPD. Further worsening of airflow limitation, increased shortness of breath, and repeated exacerbations impacting quality of life

Stage 4: Very severe COPD. Severe airflow limitation with significantly impaired quality of life and potentially life-threatening exacerbations.

Source: Adapted from Global Initiative for Chronic Obstructive Lung Disease (GOLD), 2017.

that dyspnea occurs with light activity or even at rest. The clinical features and manifestations of COPD are summarized in **Table 37.3**.

Manifestations of chronic bronchitis are a cough productive of copious amounts (at least ½ cup/day) of thick, tenacious sputum; cyanosis; and evidence of right-sided heart failure, including distended neck veins, edema, liver engorgement, and an enlarged heart. Adventitious sounds, including loud rhonchi and possible wheezes, are prominent on auscultation.

Emphysema is insidious in onset. Dyspnea is the initial symptom. Initially occurring only with exertion, dyspnea may progress to become severe even at rest. Cough is minimal or absent. Air trapping and hyperinflation increase the anteroposterior chest diameter, causing *barrel chest*. The patient is often thin, tachypneic, uses accessory muscles of respiration, and often assumes a position of sitting and leaning forward (**Figure 37.3** ■). The expiratory phase of the respiratory cycle is prolonged. On auscultation, breath sounds are diminished and the percussion tone is hyperresonant.

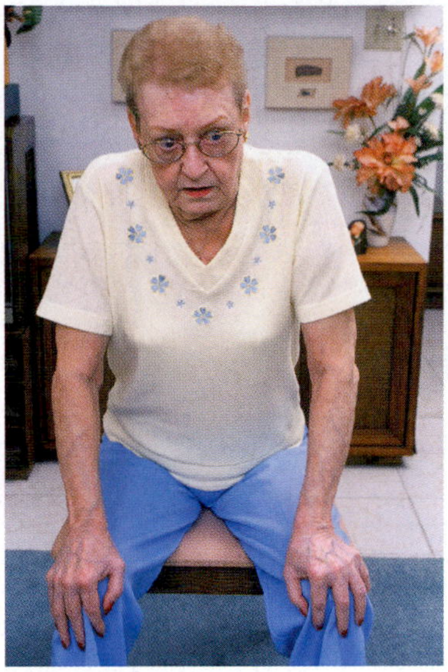

Figure 37.3 ■ Typical appearance of a patient with emphysema. Note the patient's anxious expression and assumption of the tripod position, leaning forward with the hands on the knees.

Interprofessional Care

Although COPD can be prevented in most people, it cannot be cured. Smoking abstinence is the only certain way to prevent COPD and to slow its progression. To a certain extent, airway obstruction can be reversed and disability minimized early in the disease. Treatment generally focuses on relieving symptoms, minimizing obstruction, and slowing disability.

Diagnosis

Diagnostic tests are used to help establish the diagnosis of COPD and identify the predominant component, emphysema or chronic bronchitis. These procedures are also used to assess respiratory status and monitor treatment effectiveness.

- ***Pulmonary function testing*** is performed to establish the diagnosis and evaluate the extent and progress of COPD (refer to Box 34.1). Results are based on calculated norms for each person by age, height, sex, and weight; note these as well as all current medications on the requisition. In COPD, the total lung capacity and residual volume are typically increased. The forced expiratory volume (FEV_1) and forced vital capacity (FVC) are decreased due to narrowed airways and resistance to airflow.
- ***Ventilation–perfusion scanning*** may be performed to determine the extent of ventilation–perfusion mismatch—that is, the extent to which lung tissue is ventilated but not perfused (dead space) or perfused but inadequately ventilated (physiologic shunting) (**Figure 37.4** ■). A radioisotope is injected or inhaled to illustrate areas of shunting and absent capillaries.

Table 37.3 Clinical Features and Manifestations of COPD

	Feature	Chronic Bronchitis	Emphysema
History	Onset	After age 35; recurrent respiratory infections	After age 50; insidious progressive dyspnea
	Smoking	Usual	Usual
	Cough	Persistent; productive of copious mucopurulent sputum	Absent or mild with scant clear sputum, if any
Physical examination	Appearance	Often obese; edematous and cyanotic; distended neck veins and other symptoms of right-sided heart failure	Usually thin and cachectic; barrel chest; prominent accessory muscles of respiration
	Chest	Adventitious sounds with wheezing and rhonchi; normal percussion note	Distant or diminished breath sounds; hyperresonant percussion note
Other features	Blood gases	Hypercapnia and hypoxemia; respiratory acidosis	Normal or mild hypoxemia; normal pH
	Pulmonary function studies	Normal or decreased total lung capacity; moderately increased residual volume	Increased total lung capacity; markedly increased residual volume
	Pulmonary hypertension	May be severe	Only when advanced

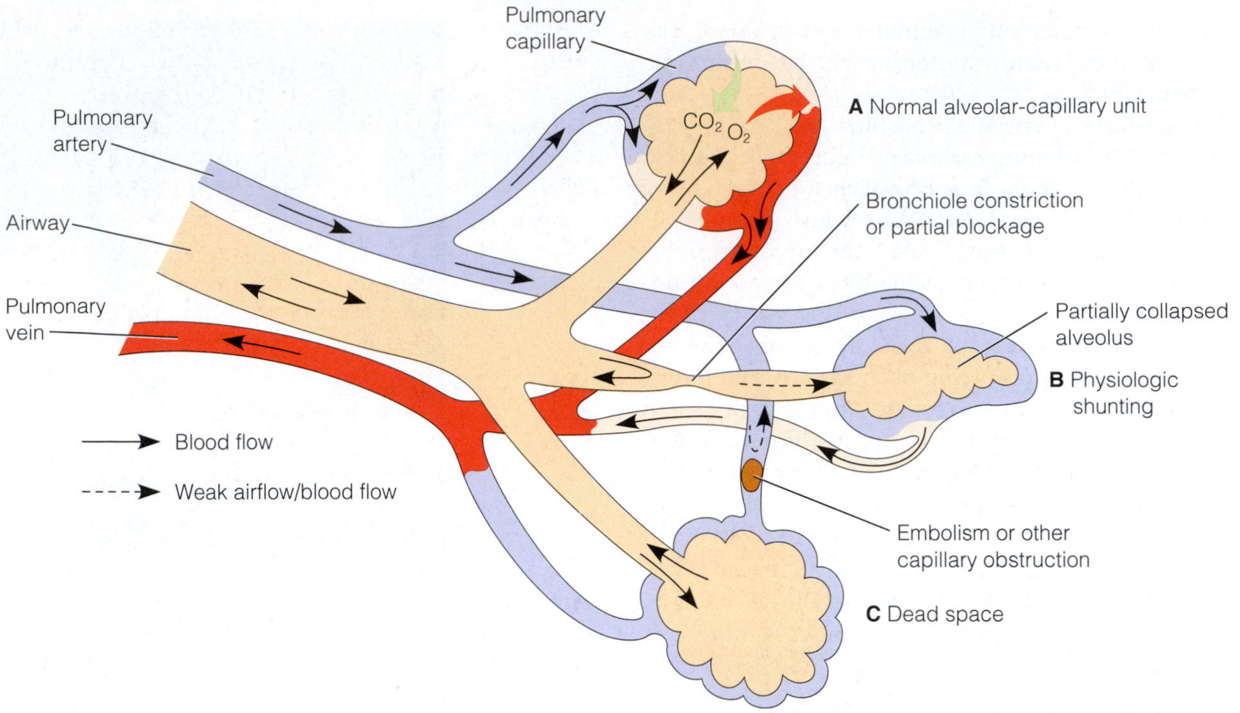
Pulmonary capillary
Pulmonary artery
Airway
Pulmonary vein
CO2 O2
A Normal alveolar-capillary unit
Bronchiole constriction or partial blockage
Partially collapsed alveolus
B Physiologic shunting
Blood flow
Weak airflow/blood flow
Embolism or other capillary obstruction
C Dead space

Figure 37.4 ■ Ventilation–perfusion relationships. **A**, Normal alveolar-capillary unit with an ideal match of ventilation and blood flow. Maximum gas exchange occurs between alveolus and blood. **B**, Physiologic shunting: A unit with adequate perfusion but inadequate ventilation. **C**, Dead space: A unit with adequate ventilation but inadequate perfusion. In the latter two cases, gas exchange is impaired.

- ***Serum alpha$_1$-antitrypsin levels*** may be drawn to screen for deficiency, particularly in patients with a family history of obstructive airway disease, those with an early onset, women, and nonsmokers. Normal adult serum alpha$_1$-antitrypsin levels range from 80 to 260 mg/dL. Fasting is not required prior to this test.
- ***Arterial blood gases (ABGs)*** are drawn to evaluate gas exchange, particularly during acute exacerbations of COPD. Patients with predominant emphysema often have mild hypoxemia and normal or low carbon dioxide tension. Respiratory alkalosis may be present due to an increased respiratory rate. Predominant chronic bronchitis and airway obstruction may cause marked hypoxemia and hypercapnia with respiratory acidosis. Oxygen saturation levels are low due to marked hypoxemia. Refer to Chapter 10, Box 10.8, for steps to interpret ABGs.
- ***Pulse oximetry*** is used to monitor oxygen saturation of the blood. Marked airway obstruction and hypoxemia often cause oxygen saturation levels < 95%. Pulse oximetry may be continuously monitored to assess the need for supplemental oxygen.
- ***Exhaled carbon dioxide*** **(*capnogram* or end-tidal carbon dioxide, ETCO$_2$)** may be measured in ventilated patients to evaluate alveolar ventilation. The normal ETCO$_2$ reading is 35 to 45 mmHg; it is elevated when ventilation is inadequate and decreased when pulmonary perfusion is impaired. ETCO$_2$ monitoring can reduce the frequency of ABG determinations.
- ***CBC with WBC differential*** often shows increased RBCs and hematocrit (erythrocytosis) as chronic hypoxia stimulates increased erythropoiesis to increase the oxygen-carrying capacity of the blood. *Polycythemia,* increased numbers of all blood cells, may be evident. Increased WBC count and a higher percentage of immature WBCs (bands) are often indicative of bacterial infection.
- ***Chest x-ray*** may show flattening of the diaphragm due to hyperinflation and evidence of pulmonary infection, if present.

Smoking Cessation

Smoking cessation can not only prevent COPD from developing, but can also improve lung function once the disease has been diagnosed. FEV$_1$ improves, and survival is prolonged, largely due to lower rates of lung cancer and heart disease. Sustained quitting is difficult; only 6% of smokers succeed in long-term abstinence from smoking. Use of nicotine patches or gum and an antidepressant such as bupropion (Wellbutrin, Zyban) or varenicline (Chantix) improve the chances of success (CDC, 2017d).

Medications

Immunization against pneumococcal pneumonia and a yearly influenza vaccine are recommended to reduce the risk of respiratory infections. A broad-spectrum antibiotic is prescribed if infection is suspected. Recent studies indicate that patients with purulent sputum and increased dyspnea will likely benefit from antibiotic therapy even if no other signs of infection are present. Prophylactic antibiotics may be ordered for patients who experience four or more disease exacerbations per year.

Bronchodilators improve airflow and reduce air trapping in COPD, resulting in improved dyspnea and exercise tolerance. Bronchodilators may be given by MDI, DPI, nebulizer, or orally. Oral administration may promote adherence, but is associated with much higher rates of adverse effects. A spacer or holding chamber may facilitate effective use of an MDI. Ipratropium bromide, an anticholinergic agent administered by MDI, is frequently prescribed. It has a longer duration of action than the short-acting beta$_2$-adrenergic stimulant bronchodilators and few side effects. Salmeterol, a longer-acting beta$_2$-agonist, may be used in combination therapy. Oral theophylline, a methylxanthine, is a weak bronchodilator and has a narrow therapeutic range, but is often prescribed for its other effects. Theophylline stimulates the respiratory drive, strengthens diaphragmatic contractions, and improves cardiac output. However, theophylline has a narrow therapeutic window, requiring careful monitoring. As a result, dyspnea, exercise tolerance, and quality of life improve for the patient with COPD. Bronchodilators are discussed in further detail in the section on asthma, and their nursing implications are outlined in Medication Administration 37.A earlier in this chapter.

Corticosteroid therapy may be used when asthma is a major component of COPD. It also improves symptoms and exercise tolerance, and may reduce the severity of exacerbations and the need for hospitalization. Oral corticosteroids, such as prednisone, are used initially. If a beneficial response occurs, the amount is reduced to the lowest effective dose. Every other day dosing or administration by inhaler is preferred to minimize steroid side effects, such as cushingoid effects and an increased risk for osteoporosis and vertebral fractures.

Alpha$_1$-antitrypsin (α_1AT) replacement therapy is available for patients with emphysema due to a genetic deficiency of the enzyme. Although expensive and inconvenient (α_1AT is administered weekly by intravenous infusion), it has been shown to reduce the rate of airflow decline and mortality.

Treatments

In addition to refraining from smoking, exposure to other airway irritants and allergens should be avoided. The patient should remain indoors during periods of significant air pollution to prevent exacerbations of the disease. Air filtering systems or air conditioning may be useful.

Pulmonary hygiene measures, including hydration, effective cough, percussion, and postural drainage, are used to improve clearance of airway secretions. Maintaining adequate systemic hydration is essential to keep secretions thin. Forceful coughing is often less effective than leaning forward and repeatedly "huffing," with relaxed breathing between huffs. Percussion and postural drainage may be necessary if the patient is unable to clear secretions by usual means. Cough suppressants and sedatives are generally avoided because they may cause retention of secretions.

While optimal medical management is helpful, it cannot reverse the pathologic changes of COPD. Pulmonary rehabilitation (PR) teaches patients how to manage their symptoms and attain their maximum level of functioning. PR includes exercise, education, and psychologic support. PR is most commonly delivered in the outpatient setting with exercise sessions of 30 to 90 minutes, three to five times per week. While PR does not change lung function, improvements in exercise and functional capacity and quality of life are seen. Both lower and upper extremity exercise should be used to promote activity tolerance during ADLs. See the accompanying Moving Evidence into Action box.

Breathing exercises are used to slow the respiratory rate and relieve accessory muscle fatigue. Pursed-lip breathing slows the respiratory rate and helps maintain open airways during exhalation by keeping positive pressure in the airways. Abdominal breathing relieves the work of accessory muscles of respiration.

Oxygen Therapy. Long-term oxygen therapy is used for severe and progressive hypoxemia. Oxygen therapy improves exercise tolerance, mental functioning, and quality of life in advanced COPD. It also reduces the rate of hospitalization and increases length of survival. Oxygen may be used intermittently, at night, or continuously. For severely hypoxemic patients, the greatest benefit is seen with continuous oxygen. Home oxygen may be supplied as liquid oxygen, compressed gas cylinders, or oxygen concentrators. Patients may be provided a combination of delivery systems to promote mobility outside of the home (i.e., oxygen concentrator and compressed gas).

An acute exacerbation of COPD may necessitate oxygenation and inspiratory positive-pressure assistance with a face mask or intubation and mechanical ventilation. The administration of oxygen without intubation and mechanical ventilation requires caution: Administering oxygen to patients with chronic elevated carbon dioxide levels in the blood can actually increase the $PaCO_2$, leading to increased somnolence and even respiratory failure. Close monitoring of level of consciousness and ABGs during oxygen therapy is vital (GOLD, 2017).

SAFETY ALERT: Hypercapnia (elevated $PaCO_2$ levels) is often chronic in patients with COPD (CO_2 retainers). In these patients, administering oxygen can actually increase the $PaCO_2$, leading to somnolence and acute respiratory failure. Although oxygen is the drug of choice for treating patients with COPD, close monitoring is necessary during oxygen therapy. ■

Surgery

When medical therapy is no longer effective, lung transplantation may be an option. Both single and bilateral transplants have been performed successfully, with a 1-year survival rate of 87.2% (Organ Procurement and Transplant

Moving Evidence into Action
Pulmonary Rehabilitation for COPD

Clinical Issue

Patients with COPD experience many challenges related to activity intolerance due to dyspnea. While pulmonary rehabilitation (PR) has been available for decades, less than 15% of patients are referred for PR. Advocating for PR with this patient group requires understanding the effectiveness of this intervention.

External Evidence

McCarthy and colleagues (2015) conducted a systematic review and meta-analysis of pulmonary rehabilitation to evaluate the impact on symptoms (dyspnea), activity performance (functional performance), and quality of life. The authors found that PR improves dyspnea and fatigue while also improving exercise capacity and health-related quality of life. The effects were noted to be moderately large and clinically significant. Pulmonary rehabilitation is an important component in the management of the COPD patient.

Internal Evidence

As part of the evaluation of internal evidence, one must consider the impact of the external evidence findings on how healthcare providers interact with this population.

Patient Considerations

When considering promoting an existing practice (such as pulmonary rehabilitation), the nurse must consider the specific patient population where it will be used (in this case, persons with COPD). Will patients and their families be amenable to enrolling in pulmonary rehabilitation? Will referral to PR become a routine procedure?

Putting the Pieces Together

The use of all evidence-based therapies in COPD will maximize patients' functioning and outlook on their chronic illness. Pulmonary rehabilitation, an outpatient program of exercise and education in a supportive setting, can positively impact patients with COPD. The systematic review and meta-analysis of randomized controlled trials is considered the highest level of evidence available and is supportive of this intervention. PR referral and encouragement of program participation should be the standard in caring for this population.

Reference

McCarthy, B., Casey, D., Devane, D., Murphy, K., Murphy, E., & Lacasse, Y. (2015). Pulmonary rehabilitation for chronic obstructive pulmonary disease. Cochrane Database *of Systematic Reviews*, Issue 2. DOI: 10.1002/14651858.CD003793.pub3.

Network, 2018). Lung reduction surgery is a surgical intervention for advanced diffuse emphysema and lung hyperinflation and is limited to selected patients. The procedure reduces the overall volume of the lung, reshapes it, and improves elastic recoil. As a result, pulmonary function and exercise tolerance improve and dyspnea is reduced. Refer to Box 36.4 in Chapter 36 for nursing care of the patient undergoing lung surgery. Special nursing care considerations related to lung or heart–lung transplant are summarized in **Box 37.3**.

Integrative Therapies

Complementary therapies may be useful to help manage symptoms of COPD. Dietary measures such as minimizing intake of dairy products and salt may help reduce mucus production and keep mucus more liquefied. Be sure to recommend measures to replace the protein and calcium in dairy products to help maintain nutritional balance.

Herbal teas made with peppermint and yarrow, coltsfoot, or comfrey may act as expectorants to help relieve chest congestion. Licorice root, which may be taken in several forms, also has expectorant and anti-inflammatory effects that may be beneficial. Licorice root can, however, cause toxicity when used for extended periods of time. Refer patients to a qualified herbalist for treatment.

Acupuncture may help the patient with smoking cessation and has also been used to treat asthma and other respiratory conditions. Hypnotherapy and guided imagery are used to assist with smoking cessation. These techniques can also help the patient control anxiety and breathing patterns. Refer patients to a trained professional. Nurses, physicians, psychologists, counselors, social workers, and others can take professional training in hypnotherapy and guided imagery.

Nursing Care

Assessment

See the Manifestations and Interprofessional Care sections for the assessment of the patient with COPD.

Focused assessment for the patient with chronic obstructive pulmonary disease includes:

- *Health history:* Current symptoms, including cough, sputum production, shortness of breath or dyspnea, activity tolerance; frequency of respiratory infections and most recent episode; previous diagnosis of emphysema, chronic bronchitis, or asthma; current medications; smoking history (in pack-years—packs per day times number of years smoked), history of exposure to secondhand smoke, occupational or other pollutants
- *Physical assessment:* General appearance, weight for height, mental status; vital signs including temperature; skin color and temperature; anteroposterior-to-lateral chest diameter ratio, use of accessory muscles, nasal flaring or pursed-lip breathing; respiratory excursion and diaphragmatic excursion; percussion tone; breath sounds throughout; neck veins, apical pulse and heart sounds, peripheral pulses, edema

BOX 37.3
Nursing Considerations Related to Lung Transplant

Although immediate postoperative care for patients undergoing lung or heart–lung transplant is provided by specially trained interprofessional teams in transplant centers, increased survival following transplant means that these patients are increasingly seen in community-based settings, nontransplant hospitals, and on general nursing care units. An understanding of common post-transplant complications and the care needs of the post-transplant patient facilitates appropriate nursing care.

COMMON POST-TRANSPLANT COMPLICATIONS

In the early post-transplant period, the most common complications relate to the surgical procedure itself or to rejection of the transplanted organ(s).

Rejection. Acute organ rejection can occur at any time following the transplant. An acute change in FEV_1 and FVC on home spirometry is often the first indication of acute rejection. Other manifestations of rejection include fever, shortness of breath, and an elevated WBC. Because these manifestations are similar to those of infection, the patient is instructed to return to the transplant clinic or center for a transbronchial biopsy. Acute rejection is treated with increased corticosteroids and adjustment of the immunosuppressive regimen (see Chapter 13). Chronic rejection is less amenable to therapy, ultimately necessitating retransplant.

Infection. Prevention of infection is vital in lung transplant patients. The patient is encouraged to reduce his or her risk of infection by avoiding contact with people who have an infectious disease (e.g., URI, shingles, diseases of childhood). Prophylactic trimethoprim-sulfamethoxazole (TMP-SMZ) is administered weekly to prevent *Pneumocystis* pneumonia (see Chapter 36).

Bacterial endocarditis prophylaxis is also provided as needed (see Chapter 31). The post-transplant patient may not have typical manifestations of infection due to immunosuppression. Any vague symptoms with or without fever or leukocytosis are investigated. Recurrent viral infections such as CMV have been associated with chronic rejection, so are aggressively treated with antiviral therapy. Treatment of other infections is targeted to the infectious organism.

NURSING CONSIDERATIONS FOR THE POST-TRANSPLANT PATIENT

Reverse isolation procedures are not necessary unless the neutrophil count is very low (< $500/mm^3$). Use good hand hygiene and standard precautions at all times and aseptic technique for dressing changes, IV starts and site care, and other invasive procedures (such as urinary catheterization). Do not allow caregivers or visitors with URI to have contact with the patient; a mask may be provided for short visits if contact is unavoidable. Skin surveillance and care are vital following transplant. Intact skin reduces the risk of infection; however, corticosteroid therapy increases the risk for skin tears and breakdown.

The effect of all medications on immunosuppressive therapy and the transplanted organ(s) should be carefully investigated prior to administration. Some antibiotics and other drugs can affect blood levels of immunosuppressants.

Particular attention must be paid to pulmonary hygiene. Denervation of the transplanted lung eliminates the usual cough stimuli. Regularly scheduled coughing and deep breathing, and the use of vibration, percussion, and postural drainage, are important to prevent accumulation of secretions.

- *Laboratory data:* Forced vital capacity (FVC) and forced expiratory volume in 1 second (FEV_1), ABGs, and hematocrit.

Priorities of Care

Collaborate with the interprofessional team to ensure adequate treatment of the underlying process while providing care that supports the physical and psychologic responses to the disorder is a priority of nursing care.

Diagnoses, Interventions, and Outcomes

Patients with chronic obstructive pulmonary disease, whether hospitalized or in the community, have multiple nursing care needs. Because of the obstructive nature of the disease, airway clearance is a high priority. Nutritional deficit is common, particularly when emphysema is predominant. Because this chronic disease affects all functional health patterns, psychosocial issues are also of concern in planning nursing care. In addition to the nursing diagnoses presented here, see the Case Study & Nursing Care Plan that follows.

Promote Airway Clearance and Patency. Both chronic bronchitis and emphysema affect the ability to maintain open airways. In chronic bronchitis, copious amounts of thick, tenacious mucus are produced. Ciliary action is impaired, making it difficult to clear mucus from the airways. The loss of supporting tissue caused by emphysema increases the risk for airway collapse. In both cases, air is trapped distally, and less oxygen is available to the alveoli for diffusion. Normal respiratory defense mechanisms are impaired, and mucous-plugged airways provide an ideal environment for bacterial growth. Respiratory infection further impairs airway clearance and is often the cause of an acute exacerbation.

Expected Outcome: Patient will demonstrate movement of air into and out of the lungs.

The nurse will:

- Assess respiratory status every 1 to 2 hours or as indicated. Assess rate and pattern; cough and secretions (color, amount, consistency, and odor); and breath sounds, both normal and adventitious. *Frequent assessment is vital to monitor current status and response to treatment. Adventitious sounds should decrease with effective intervention. Diminished or absent breath sounds may indicate increasing airway obstruction and possible atelectasis.*
- Promptly report changes in oxygen saturation, skin color, or mental status. *A drop in oxygen saturation*

levels, increasing cyanosis, or altered level of consciousness indicates hypoxemia, possibly related to airway obstruction.

- Monitor ABG results. *Increasing hypoxemia, hypercapnia, and respiratory acidosis may indicate increasing airway obstruction.*
- Weigh daily, monitor intake and output, and assess mucous membranes and skin turgor. *Dehydration causes respiratory secretions to become thicker, more tenacious, and difficult to expectorate; fluid overload can further compromise respiratory status.*
- Encourage a fluid intake of at least 2000 to 2500 mL per day unless contraindicated. *Adequate fluid intake helps keep mucous secretions thin.*
- Place in Fowler, high-Fowler, or orthopneic position; encourage movement and activity to tolerance. *Upright positions improve ventilation and reduce the work of breathing. Activity helps mobilize secretions and prevent them from pooling.*
- Assist with coughing and deep breathing at least every 2 hours while awake. Position seated upright, leaning forward during coughing. *The upright position promotes chest expansion, increasing the effectiveness of coughing and reducing the work involved.*
- Provide tissues and a paper bag to dispose of expectorated sputum. *This important infection control measure reduces the spread of respiratory organisms to other people.*
- Refer to a respiratory therapist, and assist with or perform percussion and postural drainage as needed. *Percussion helps loosen secretions in airways; postural drainage facilitates movement of these secretions out of the respiratory tract.*
- Provide endotracheal, oral, or nasopharyngeal suctioning as necessary. *Suctioning may be necessary to clear secretions and may stimulate a cough.*
- Provide rest periods between treatments and procedures. *The patient with COPD fatigues easily; adequate rest is important to conserve energy and reduce fatigue.*
- Administer expectorant and bronchodilator medications as ordered. Correlate timing with respiratory treatments. *Using expectorants and bronchodilators prior to coughing, percussion, and postural drainage increases their effectiveness in clearing airways.*
- Provide supplemental oxygen as ordered. *Supplemental oxygen helps maintain adequate blood and tissue oxygenation.*

SAFETY ALERT: Prepare for intubation and mechanical ventilation if respiratory status deteriorates (increasing hypoxemia and hypercapnia, decreased level of consciousness, cyanosis, or worsening airway obstruction). Respiratory failure is a possible complication of an acute exacerbation of COPD and requires immediate intervention to preserve life. ■

Promote Balanced Nutrition. With advanced COPD, minimal activity, including eating, can cause fatigue and dyspnea. The patient may be unable to consume a full meal without resting. At the same time, the increased work of breathing (8 to 10 times that of normal) increases metabolic demands, and more calories are required. The patient may appear cachectic (thin and wasted). Poor nutritional status further impairs immune function and increases the risk of a complicating infection.

Expected Outcome: Patient will consume adequate nourishment to promote weight within normal range.

The nurse will:

- Assess nutritional status, including diet history, weight for height (use reference tables of desired weights), and anthropometric (skinfold) measurements. *It is important to differentiate nutritional status from body type rather than assume a nutritional impairment.*
- Observe and document food intake, including types, amounts, and caloric intake. *This information can provide direction for supplementation, if needed.*
- Monitor laboratory values, including serum albumin, prealbumin, and electrolyte levels. *These values provide information about the adequacy of nutritional intake, including protein.*
- Consult with a dietitian to plan meals and nutritional supplements that meet caloric needs. *More concentrated sources of high-energy foods may be required to maintain caloric intake without excess fatigue. A diet high in proteins and fats without excess carbohydrates is recommended to minimize carbon dioxide production during metabolism (carbohydrates are metabolized to form CO_2 and water).*
- Provide frequent, small feedings with between-meal supplements. *Frequent, small meals help maintain intake and reduce fatigue associated with eating.*
- Place seated or in high-Fowler position for meals. *An upright position promotes lung expansion and reduces dyspnea.*
- Assist to choose preferred foods from the menu; encourage family members to bring food from home if allowed. *Providing preferred foods encourages eating.*
- Keep snacks at the bedside. *Snacks provide additional caloric intake.*
- Provide mouth care prior to meals. *This helps enhance the appetite.*
- If unable to maintain oral intake, consult with the physician about enteral or parenteral feedings. *Maintenance of caloric and nutrient intake is vital to prevent catabolism.*

Promote Healthy Family Coping. Chronic illness affects the entire family structure. Roles and relationships change; additional demands are placed on the family. Family members may become overprotective of the patient. Conversely, family members may blame the patient for causing the illness or have distorted perceptions about it, even denying its existence. In the most severe cases, they may refuse to assist or participate in care. The patient may develop an attitude of helplessness or dependence or may demonstrate anger, hostility, or aggression.

Expected Outcome: Patient will identify three healthy coping behaviors that family members can employ to facilitate a shift toward improved family functioning.

The nurse will:

- Assess interactions between patient and family. *Assessment helps identify desired and potential destructive behaviors.*
- Assess the effect of the illness on the family. *Assessment of family interactions, roles, and relationships assists in planning appropriate interventions.*
- Help the patient and family identify strengths for coping with the situation. *Identifying personal and family strengths helps the family regain a sense of control.*
- Provide information and teaching about COPD. *Education helps the family gain an understanding of the patient's condition and needs.*
- Encourage expression of feelings. Avoid judging feelings expressed or family members as "good" or "bad," "right" or "wrong." *It is important for the nurse to remain objective to maintain the therapeutic relationship.*
- Help family members recognize behaviors and attitudes that may hinder effective treatment, such as continuing to smoke in the house. *Family members may be unaware of the effect of their behavior on the patient's ability to change habits and cope with a disabling disease.*
- Encourage family members to participate in care. *This helps develop skills for use at home.*
- Initiate a "care conference" involving the patient, family, and healthcare team members from a variety of disciplines. *A wide range of perspectives and areas of expertise aids in problem solving and facilitates communication.*
- If dysfunctional family relationships interfere with measures to enhance coping, advocate for the patient, reaffirming his or her right to make decisions. *Dysfunctional family relationships are not likely to change simply because of illness. The nurse can better meet the patient's needs by accepting his or her limitations in dealing with family members.*
- Refer the patient and family to support groups and pulmonary rehabilitation programs, as available. *Support groups and structured rehabilitation programs enhance coping abilities.*
- Arrange a social services consultation. *This can help the patient and family identify care and support service needs.*
- Refer community agencies or services such as home health, homemaker services, or Meals on Wheels as appropriate. *Agencies or community services can provide additional support beyond the family's means or capability.*

Encourage Smoking Cessation. Smoking is more than a habit; it is an addiction. The patient who must quit is facing a significant loss, not only of nicotine but also of a lifestyle. Although the patient may fully comprehend the consequences of continuing to smoke, the decision to give up a part of his or her life is not easy. This fear may be expressed in such concerns as "I'll gain weight" or "What will I do with my hands?" In addition to providing practical information, a plan, and assistance with nicotine withdrawal, the nurse must support the patient's decision-making process to comply with an order to stop smoking.

Expected Outcome: Patient will express an interest in smoking cessation.

The nurse will:

- Assess knowledge and understanding of the choices involved and possible consequences of each. *The decision to quit smoking ultimately belongs to the patient. He or she needs a full understanding of the consequences of quitting or continuing to smoke.*
- Acknowledge concerns, values, and beliefs; listen nonjudgmentally. *The nurse needs to avoid imposing his or her values and beliefs about smoking on the patient.*
- Spend time with the patient, encouraging expression of feelings. *This demonstrates acceptance of the patient and his or her right to make the decision.*
- Help plan a course of action for quitting smoking and adapt it as necessary. *When the patient develops the plan, he or she has more ownership in it and interest in making it work.*
- Demonstrate respect for decisions and the right to choose. *Respect supports self-esteem and the ability to cope.*
- Provide referral to a counselor or other professional as needed. *Counselors or other people trained to assist with smoking cessation can help with decision making.*

Delegating Nursing Care Activities

As appropriate and allowed by the designated duties and responsibilities of unlicensed assistive personnel, the nurse may delegate nursing care activities such as measuring vital signs, encouraging oral or enteral fluid intake, and providing skin care.

Transitions of Care

Avoiding smoking is the best preventative measure for chronic obstructive pulmonary disease. Even in patients with COPD, smoking cessation improves lung function and increases survival. Educate all patients, including preschool and school-age children, about the risks of smoking (see **Box 37.4**).

Case Study & Nursing Care Plan

A Patient with COPD

Helen Mercurio, known as "Happy" to all her friends, is an 83-year-old widow who lives with her two adult sons. During the past 15 years, Mrs. Mercurio has become increasingly short of breath while gardening and walking, two of her favorite activities. She has also developed a chronic cough that is particularly bad in the mornings. Ten years ago, her family physician told her that she had emphysema. She is admitted to the hospital with possible pneumonia and acute exacerbation of COPD.

ASSESSMENT

Jeff Harris, RN, admits Mrs. Mercurio to the medical unit. In the nursing history, Mr. Harris notes that she denies ever smoking, but says that her husband and two sons have been smokers "for practically their whole lives." She says she lived an active life before developing lung disease, but now her breathing and cough have progressed so that she now must rest after just a few minutes of housework or other activity. Her cough is productive of moderate to large amounts of sputum, particularly in the mornings. She developed increasing shortness of breath and sputum 2 days ago; this morning, she could not complete her morning activities without resting, so she contacted her physician.

On physical examination, Mr. Harris notes the following: Skin is very warm and dry, color dusky. Pauses frequently while speaking to breathe. Respiratory rate 36/min, fairly shallow; coughs frequently, producing large amounts of thick, tenacious green sputum. Other vital signs: P 115 bpm and irregular, BP 186/60 mmHg, T 39°C (102.4°F). Appears very thin; weight 43.6 kg (96 lb), height 160 cm (63 in.). Anteroposterior-to-lateral chest diameter ratio approximately 1:1, indicating barrel chest; moderate kyphosis noted. Chest hyperresonant to percussion. Auscultation reveals distant breath sounds with scattered wheezes and rhonchi throughout lung fields. Chest x-ray shows flattening of diaphragm, slight cardiac enlargement, prominent vascular and bronchial markings, and patchy infiltrates. Initial laboratory work reveals moderate erythrocytosis, leukocytosis, and low serum albumin. Arterial blood gas results: pH 7.19; PaO_2 54 mmHg; $PaCO_2$ 59 mmHg; HCO_3^- 30 mg/dL, and O_2 saturation 88%. Admitting orders include sputum specimen for culture; intravenous penicillin G, 2 million units every 4 hours; tiotropium bromide (Spiriva) two puffs once a day; bedrest with bathroom privileges; oxygen per nasal cannula at 2 L continuously; and regular diet.

DIAGNOSES

- Difficulty with airway clearness related to pneumonia and COPD
- Decreased gas exchange related to acute and chronic lung disease
- Potential for respiratory failure related to respiratory muscle fatigue and loss of hypoxemic respiratory drive
- Inadequate nutrition related to increase metabolism due to increased work of breathing

EXPECTED OUTCOMES

- Patient will expectorate secretions effectively.
- Patient will return to level of pulmonary function prior to acute exacerbation.
- Patient will demonstrate improved arterial blood gas and oxygen saturation values.
- Patient will maintain spontaneous respirations without excess fatigue.
- Patient will demonstrate adequate nutritional intake to meet body needs.

PLANNING AND IMPLEMENTATION

- Assess respiratory status and level of consciousness every 1 to 2 hours until stable, then at least every 4 hours.
- Closely monitor response to oxygen therapy, including skin color, oxygen saturation, sputum consistency, and respiratory drive.
- Increase fluid intake to at least 2500 mL/day and provide bedside humidifier.
- Elevate head of bed to at least 30 degrees at all times.
- Teach huff coughing technique.
- Administer medications as ordered. Provide mouth care after inhaler.
- Contact respiratory therapy for percussion and postural drainage following inhaler treatments.
- Provide for uninterrupted rest periods following treatments and procedures.
- Promote adequate nutritional intake using high-protein, small, frequent meals.
- Meet with Mrs. Mercurio and her sons to develop a postdischarge care plan including referral to pulmonary rehabilitation following home health care.
- Refer to home health department for nursing follow-up.
- Refer to social services for possible assistance with home maintenance.

EVALUATION

After the first day in the hospital, Mrs. Mercurio's condition begins to improve slowly. On discharge 6 days later, she is able to provide self-care with less fatigue and dyspnea. She is using oxygen at night only, admitting that it is just for security. Although a few scattered wheezes and rhonchi are still present in her lungs, Mrs. Mercurio's sputum is thinner, white, and easily expectorated. She will continue taking oral penicillin V for an additional 10 days at home. She will also continue using the Spiriva inhaler as prescribed at home. Although Mrs. Mercurio's sons admit they will probably never be able to quit smoking, they have agreed to smoke only in the garage or outside. Her sons will also promote a nutritionally balanced diet of small, frequent meals. A home health nurse will initially evaluate Mrs. Mercurio's progress three times weekly. Arrangements have been made for a housekeeper to come twice a week for cleaning and laundry. Mrs. Mercurio is glad to be returning home and grateful for the arrangements that have been made.

CLINICAL REASONING IN PATIENT CARE

1. Mrs. Mercurio has never been a smoker but had long-term exposure to secondhand smoke. How does secondhand smoke contribute to lung diseases in adults and children?
2. Mrs. Mercurio's nursing care plan included the nursing diagnosis of potential for respiratory failure related to respiratory muscle fatigue and loss of hypoxemic respiratory drive. Identify the normal physiologic events that stimulate breathing, and describe how these differ for the patient with chronic hypoxemia and hypercapnia.
3. The patient with an acute exacerbation of COPD is at risk for respiratory failure. What changes in Mrs. Mercurio's assessment findings could indicate this complication?
4. Develop a nursing care plan for Mrs. Mercurio for her difficulty with conducting preferred activities due to respiratory condition.

See Evaluating Your Response in Appendix B.

BOX 37.4
Cigarette Smoking and Tobacco Use

The use of tobacco reaches back to early civilizations, when it was used in religious ceremonies and as an offering of friendship. At one time, tobacco was thought to have medicinal qualities effective against all common diseases. Widespread use of tobacco among the male population of the industrialized world began during World War I.

Tobacco is now recognized as the leading cause of preventable illness in the world. Diseases directly related to tobacco use are responsible for the deaths of approximately 480,000 Americans every year, and smoking is implicated in the etiology of a number of wide-ranging conditions from cardiovascular diseases to respiratory diseases to diabetes and obesity (U.S. Department of Health and Human Services, 2014). In spite of this knowledge, aggressive marketing of the product continues, and its worldwide use is increasing, especially in underdeveloped countries.

The link between tobacco use and lung cancer was reported as early as 1912. In 1987, lung cancer became the leading cause of cancer-related death in the United States among both men and women (Parker, Tong, Bolden, & Wingo, 1997).

Cigarette smoke contains over 4800 chemicals (69 of which are known to cause cancer), including nicotine (CDC, 2017d). Nicotine is a highly addictive psychoactive substance that is relatively cheap and readily available. It produces euphoria, which acts as a positive reinforcer for continued use. In North American society, tobacco is more acceptable than many other dependency-producing drugs.

Tar is the particulate matter in cigarette smoke that is responsible for most of its carcinogenic and pathologic effects on the lungs. Smoke also paralyzes the cilia, reducing their ability to remove tars from contact with the respiratory epithelium. The risk for cancer and other lung diseases is dose related, affected by the age at which smoking began, the number of cigarettes smoked per day, and the number of years smoked. Smoking cessation reduces the risks associated with tobacco use. For some, such as the risk of coronary heart disease, quitting smoking yields rapid benefits. For others, the degree of risk reduction is less immediate, but still significant.

Nurses need to do more than simply advise patients to quit smoking and talk about the risks of smoking. Nurses can take an active role in smoking cessation. Identify smoking habits, smoking-related illnesses, and previous efforts to quit. Work with the patient to identify barriers and obstacles to quitting. Educate about the addictive nature of nicotine, and explain the manifestations of nicotine withdrawal (anxiety, irritability, headache, and disturbed sleep). Develop a plan with the patient that specifies a target date to quit and includes ways to deal with obstacles to quitting, withdrawal symptoms, and the temptation to resume smoking. Offer self-help material at an appropriate reading level. Refer to a counselor, physician, self-help group, or smoking-cessation clinic. If a relapse occurs, accept it as a normal part of rehabilitation from any addictive substance. Continue to provide support and encouragement, helping the patient avoid further relapses.

Nurses can be especially effective in primary prevention of cigarette smoking and the diseases associated with it. Just as tobacco companies direct advertising at women and teens, nurses can target these populations and younger children for programs to prevent smoking. In addition, nurses need to become active in reducing minors' access to tobacco products, especially cigarettes and chewing tobacco (often the first product used by teens).

As with any chronic disease, the patient and family will have primary responsibility for disease management. Teaching is vital to promote optimal health and slow disease progression. Teaching for home care focuses on effective coughing and breathing techniques (**Box 37.5**), preventing exacerbations, and managing prescribed therapies.

In addition, include the following topics when teaching for home care:

- Maintaining adequate fluid intake, at least 2.0 to 2.5 quarts of fluid daily

(*continued*)

- Avoiding respiratory irritants, including cigarette smoke, both primary and secondary, other smoke sources, dust, aerosol sprays, air pollution, and very cold, dry air
- Preventing exposure to infection, especially upper respiratory infections
- Importance of pneumococcal vaccine and annual influenza immunization
- Prescribed exercise program, maintaining ADLs, and balancing rest and exercise
- Maintaining nutrient intake (e.g., eating small, frequent meals and using nutritional supplements to provide adequate calories)
- Ways of reducing sodium intake, if prescribed
- Identifying early signs of an infection or exacerbation and the importance of seeking medical attention for fever, increased sputum production, purulent (green or yellow) sputum, upper respiratory infection, increased shortness of breath or difficulty breathing, decreased activity tolerance or appetite, increased need for oxygen
- Prescribed medications, including purpose, proper use, and expected effects
- Avoiding use of OTC medications unless approved by the physician
- Other prescribed therapies, such as use of home oxygen, percussion, postural drainage, and nebulizer treatments
- Use, cleaning, and maintenance of any required special equipment
- Importance of wearing an identification band and carrying a list of medications at all times in case of an emergency.

Provide referrals to home care services such as home health, assistance with ADLs as needed, home maintenance services, respiratory therapy and home oxygen services, and other agencies such as Meals on Wheels and senior services as indicated.

BOX 37.5
Patient Teaching: Effective Coughing and Breathing Techniques

Pursed-lip and diaphragmatic breathing techniques help minimize air trapping and fatigue.

PURSED-LIP BREATHING

Pursed-lip breathing helps maintain open airways by maintaining positive pressures longer during exhalation. Teach the patient to do the following:

1. Inhale through the nose with the mouth closed.
2. Exhale slowly through pursed lips, as though whistling or blowing out a candle, making exhalation twice as long as inhalation.

DIAPHRAGMATIC BREATHING

Diaphragmatic or abdominal breathing helps conserve energy by using the larger and more efficient muscles of respiration. Teach the patient to do the following:

1. Place one hand on the abdomen, the other on the chest.
2. Inhale, concentrating on pushing the abdominal hand outward while the chest hand remains still.
3. Exhale slowly, while the abdominal hand moves inward and the chest hand remains still.

Repeat these exercises as often as necessary until the techniques become incorporated into normal breathing.

CONTROLLED COUGHING

Several different coughing techniques may be useful. For controlled cough technique, teach the patient to do the following:

1. Following prescribed bronchodilator treatment, inhale deeply and hold breath briefly.
2. Cough twice, the first time to loosen mucus, the second to expel secretions.
3. Inhale by sniffing to prevent mucus from moving back into deep airways.
4. Rest. Avoid prolonged coughing to prevent fatigue and hypoxemia.

HUFF COUGHING

For huff coughing, teach the patient to do the following:

1. Inhale deeply while leaning forward.
2. Exhale sharply with a "huff" sound, to help keep airways open while mobilizing secretions.

The Patient with Cystic Fibrosis

Cystic fibrosis (CF) is an autosomal recessive disorder that affects epithelial cells of the respiratory, gastrointestinal, and reproductive tracts and leads to abnormal exocrine gland secretions. Although it can affect many organ systems, CF is particularly damaging to the lungs, leading to COPD in childhood and early adulthood. Respiratory manifestations of CF are the usual cause of morbidity and death from this disease. The gastrointestinal tract is also affected significantly; exocrine pancreatic insufficiency is characteristic of CF. Abnormally high sweat electrolytes also occur in CF.

CF is the most common lethal genetic disease in Caucasian Americans, affecting about 1 in 2500 to 3500 live births. It is less common in African Americans (1 in 17,000) and rare in Asian Americans (1 in 100,000). About 5% of Caucasians in the United States carry the CF trait. Although the manifestations of CF usually develop in childhood, about 7% of patients with CF are diagnosed as adults. Adults now make up more than 45% of the CF population in the United States, with the median survival rate at 41 years. Children born in 2018 and later with CF can expect to survive into their 50s and beyond (Cystic Fibrosis Foundation [CFF], 2017).

Pathophysiology

The CFTR protein is involved in membrane transport of chloride and sodium in cells lining the ducts of exocrine glands (sweat glands, pancreas, liver, and reproductive systems). The genetic abnormality of CF leads to a lack or abnormality of this protein, with resulting abnormal electrolyte transport across epithelial cell membranes. Defective chloride transport causes more water and sodium reabsorption than normal. Secretions in affected organs become thick and viscous, obstructing glands and ducts. This obstruction causes dilation of secretory glands and damage to exocrine tissue. The hallmark pathophysiologic effects of CF include:

Genetic Considerations
Cystic Fibrosis

The gene responsible for cystic fibrosis is at a single locus on the long arm of chromosome 7. This gene codes for a protein known as the *cystic fibrosis transmembrane conductance regulator (CFTR)*. More than 1000 mutations of this gene have been identified. The most common mutation, identified as ΔF508, accounts for about 66% cases of cystic fibrosis. Cystic fibrosis is an autosomal recessive disorder: It is not transmitted as a sex-linked trait, and the normal gene is dominant. People with one abnormal gene do not have the disorder, but they can transmit the abnormal gene to their offspring. When a child inherits an abnormal gene from both parents, the disorder manifests. Genetic screening of family members of a patient with CF can detect 70 to 75% of carriers of the CF gene. Screening for the CF gene is not recommended for the general population.

- Excess mucus production in the respiratory tract with impaired ability to clear secretions and progressive COPD
- Pancreatic enzyme deficiency and impaired digestion
- Abnormal elevation of sodium and chloride concentrations in sweat.

In the lungs, viscous mucus plugs small airways and impairs mucociliary clearance, leading to atelectasis, infection, bronchiectasis, and dilation of distal airways. Lower respiratory infections with *Staphylococcus aureus* and *Pseudomonas* are common (Sorenson et al., 2019). Acute and chronic damage to lung parenchyma causes tissue loss and extensive scarring and fibrosis. The upper lobes are involved to a greater extent than the lower lobes. Severe airway obstruction and chronic hypoxemia lead to pulmonary hypertension, right-ventricular hypertrophy, and eventual cor pulmonale. Death usually results from a combination of cardiovascular changes and respiratory failure.

Pancreatic insufficiency is a frequent component of CF. It can range from slight pancreatic dysfunction to complete absence of function due to obstruction of pancreatic ducts with thick mucus and degenerative and fibrotic changes. Pancreatic insufficiency and impaired enzyme secretion lead to impaired digestion and absorption of proteins, carbohydrates, and fats.

Complications

About 8% of patients with CF develop diabetes mellitus (Sorenson, Quinn & Klein, 2018). Liver failure is another potential complication of the disease. Because the genetic defect also affects cells of the reproductive tract, males with CF are usually sterile. Although females may have difficulty conceiving, pregnancies are usually carried to term.

Manifestations

Manifestations of CF in a young adult include a history of chronic lung disease. Recurrent pneumonia, exercise intolerance, and chronic cough are typical. Other pulmonary manifestations include *clubbing* of the fingers and toes (**Figure 37.5 ■**), increased anteroposterior chest diameter (barrel chest), hyperresonant percussion tone, and basilar crackles on auscultation. Distended neck veins, ascites, and peripheral edema accompany right-sided heart failure. Abdominal pain and *steatorrhea* (excess fat in the stools, causing frequent, bulky, foul-smelling stool) commonly result from associated pancreatic insufficiency. Growth and development are often retarded, resulting in small stature. See Multisystem Effects of Cystic Fibrosis.

Interprofessional Care

The treatment plan for cystic fibrosis is multidisciplinary, with the goals of preventing or treating respiratory complications and maintaining adequate nutrition. Psychosocial care is vital, as is genetic and occupational counseling.

Diagnosis

Although evidence of lung disease and pancreatic insufficiency suggest CF, analysis of Cl^- concentration in sweat is used to confirm the diagnosis. In CF, the Cl^-concentration is greater than 70 mEq/L. Pilocarpine (a parasympathomimetic agent) and a small electric current are used to increase sweat production on the forearm. Absorbent paper or gauze is used to collect the sweat for analysis.

ABGs and oxygen saturation levels show hypoxemia. Pulmonary function studies reveal reduced airflow, reduced forced vital capacity, and reduced total lung capacity. Alveolar-capillary diffusion is also typically reduced.

Medications

Immunization against respiratory infections is vital to promote optimal health. Yearly influenza vaccine is recommended, along with measles and pertussis boosters as needed.

Bronchodilator inhalers may be used to control airway constriction. Acute pulmonary infections are treated with appropriate antibiotic therapy as determined by sputum culture and sensitivity tests. A prolonged treatment course or multiple antibiotics may be required to eradicate pulmonary infections. Antibiotics may be administered by several routes, including inhalation, to achieve the desired concentration in large airways. Dornase alfa, recombinant human DNase, breaks down the excess DNA in the sputum of patients with

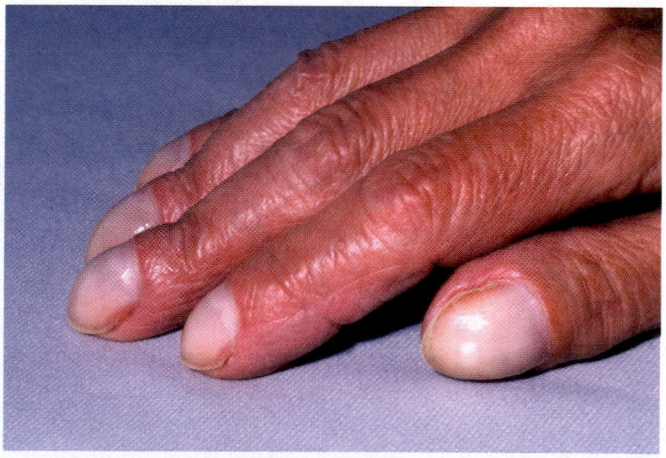

Figure 37.5 ■ Clubbing of fingers caused by chronic hypoxemia.

Multitsystem Effects of
Cystic Fibrosis

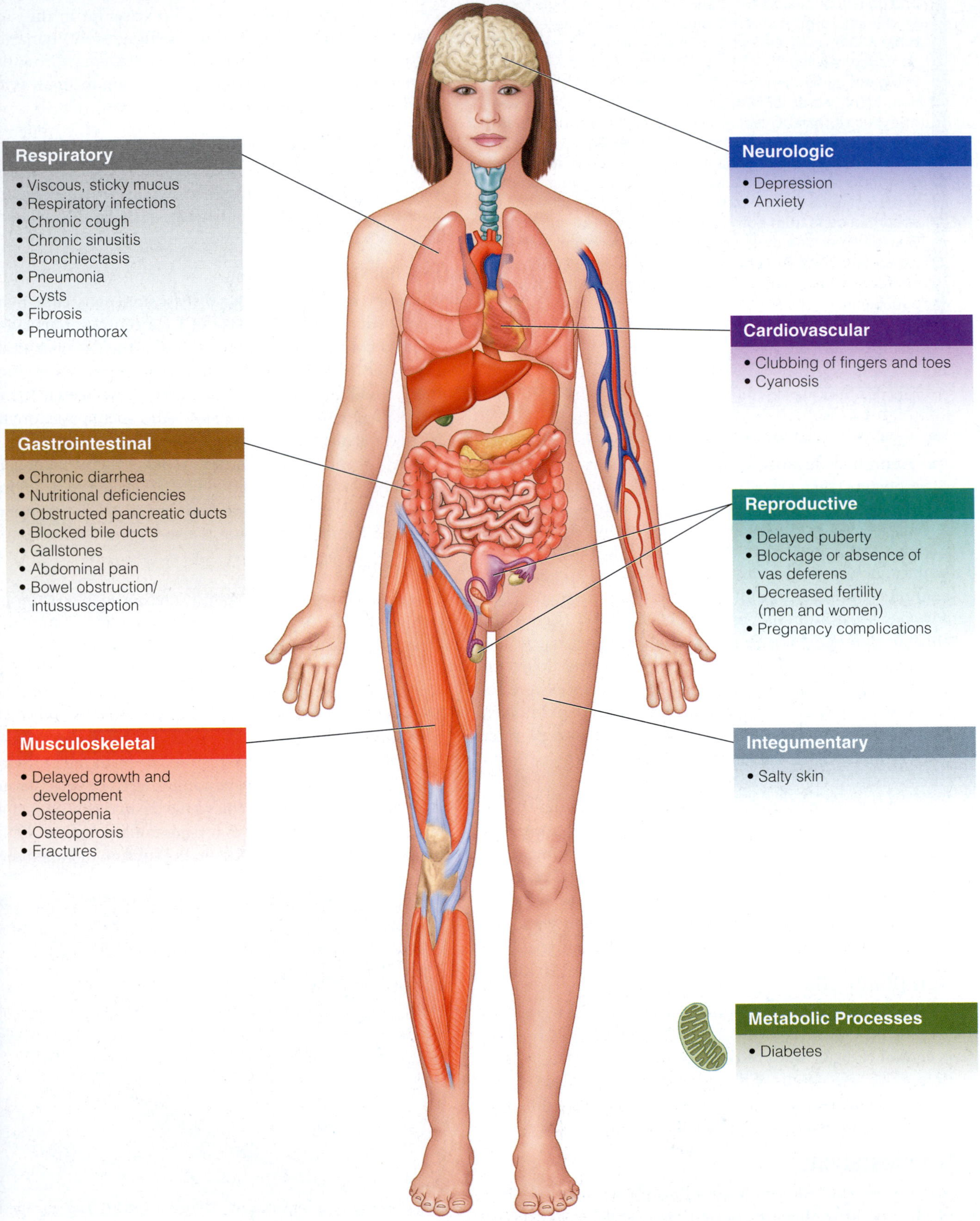

Respiratory
• Viscous, sticky mucus
• Respiratory infections
• Chronic cough
• Chronic sinusitis
• Bronchiectasis
• Pneumonia
• Cysts
• Fibrosis
• Pneumothorax
Neurologic
• Depression
• Anxiety
Cardiovascular
• Clubbing of fingers and toes
• Cyanosis
Gastrointestinal
• Chronic diarrhea
• Nutritional deficiencies
• Obstructed pancreatic ducts
• Blocked bile ducts
• Gallstones
• Abdominal pain
• Bowel obstruction/ intussusception
Reproductive
• Delayed puberty
• Blockage or absence of vas deferens
• Decreased fertility (men and women)
• Pregnancy complications
Musculoskeletal
• Delayed growth and development
• Osteopenia
• Osteoporosis
• Fractures
Integumentary
• Salty skin
Metabolic Processes
• Diabetes

CF, decreasing its viscosity and making it easier to clear. Dornase alfa, administered by aerosol, reduces the frequency of hospitalizations and the need for antibiotics for some patients.

Nutrition

In CF, good nutrition is a key component of disease management. Research has supported that good nutritional management improves survival. Nutritional interventions focus on adequate energy intake secondary to malabsorption and chronic pulmonary bacterial colonization increasing inflammation. Due to the underlying pathophysiological process involving the exocrine glands (including the pancreas), pancreatic enzyme replacement therapy is needed by a majority of CF patients. Nutritional complications include liver disease and diabetes. Additionally, fat-soluble vitamin deficiencies (especially A, E, and K) are a common problem. In patients with liver involvement, vitamin D deficiency is seen.

Treatments

Chest physiotherapy with percussion and postural drainage is used to promote airway clearance. Newer airway clearance techniques include the use of the huff cough technique with specified breathing cycles or patterns. In one technique, a valved mask or mouthpiece is used to maintain positive expiratory pressure (PEP) for approximately 20 breaths, followed by three to five huff coughs. This cycle is repeated for a total of 20 minutes. The autogenic drainage technique, a form of biofeedback, involves controlled breathing at specific lung volumes and patterns to facilitate the movement of mucus into larger airways, where it can be cleared with the huff cough. Oscillating positive expiratory pressure uses a flutter valve device, which looks like a fat pipe and contains a steel ball within an inner cone. The weight of the ball provides intermittent PEP, which vibrates airway walls to loosen secretions (CFF, 2017).

Oxygen therapy may be required for hypoxemia. A liberal fluid intake helps reduce the viscosity of mucus secretions. A diet high in protein, fat, and calories may be necessary to maintain weight. Vitamins and minerals are supplemented to counteract excess losses in the sweat and stools. Enteral or parenteral nutrition may be required during acute exacerbations of the disease.

Surgery

Lung transplantation currently offers the only definitive treatment for CF, but it is not considered a cure—the patient trades CF for the lifelong management of transplanted organs. Lung transplantation lengthens lifespan and improves quality of life. In CF, double lung transplant is indicated. Single-lung transplant is contraindicated due to the chronic infection in the lungs. Because the donor lungs do not have the CF gene, they do not develop the pathophysiologic changes of CF. Although the other defects characteristic of CF remain, these can be managed with pharmacologic therapy.

Nursing Care

Nursing care for the patient with cystic fibrosis is much the same as that for any chronic obstructive lung disease. The genetic component of the disease and the patient's age are important considerations. Adults with CF are just entering their productive years and face a lifespan that is likely to be shortened significantly. Women who do conceive face the prospect of transmitting the defective gene to their offspring.

Assessment

Focused assessment for the patient with cystic fibrosis includes:

- *Health history:* Current symptoms, including cough, sputum production, shortness of breath or dyspnea, activity tolerance; frequency of respiratory infections and most recent episode; previous diagnosis of cystic fibrosis; current medications
- *Physical assessment:* General appearance, weight for height, mental status; vital signs including temperature; skin color and temperature; anteroposterior-to-lateral chest diameter ratio, use of accessory muscles, nasal flaring or pursed-lip breathing; respiratory excursion and diaphragmatic excursion; percussion tone; breath sounds throughout; neck veins, apical pulse and heart sounds, peripheral pulses, edema
- *Laboratory data:* Forced vital capacity (FVC) and forced expiratory volume in 1 second (FEV_1), ABGs, hematocrit (as indicated), genetic testing for the specific genetic mutation.

Priorities of Care

Promoting airway clearance is the priority of nursing care.

Diagnoses, Interventions, and Outcomes

In addition to risk for impairment of the airway, patients with CF and their families may experience anticipatory grieving. Promoting healthy grief responses not only helps patients and their families cope with the diagnosis, it also helps them better manage the illness and adhere to the therapeutic regimen.

Promote Airway Clearance and Patency. Bronchial hygiene measures, including vibration, percussion, and postural drainage, are the mainstay of treatment for patients with CF.

Expected Outcome: Patient will use techniques to promote airway clearance such as coughing, deep breathing, and mechanical clearance techniques including chest physical therapy.

The nurse will:

- Assess respiratory status, including vital signs, breath sounds, SaO_2, and skin color at least every 4 hours. *Early identification of respiratory compromise allows intervention before tissue hypoxia is significant.*
- Assess cough and sputum (amount, color, consistency, and possible odor). *Assessment of the cough and nature of sputum produced allows evaluation of the effectiveness of respiratory clearance and the response to therapy.*
- Monitor arterial blood gas results; report increasing hypoxemia and other abnormal results to the physician. *Blood gas changes may be an early indicator of impaired gas exchange due to airway obstruction.*
- Place in Fowler or high-Fowler position. Encourage frequent position changes and ambulation as allowed. *The upright position promotes lung expansion; position changes and ambulation facilitate the movement of secretions.*

- Assist to cough, deep breathe, and use assistive devices. Provide endotracheal suctioning using aseptic technique as ordered. *Coughing, deep breathing, and suctioning help clear airways.*
- Provide a fluid intake of at least 2500 to 3000 mL/day. *A liberal fluid intake helps liquefy secretions, facilitating their clearance.*
- Work with the healthcare provider and respiratory therapist to provide pulmonary hygiene measures, such as postural drainage, percussion, and vibration. *These techniques help mobilize and clear secretions.*
- Administer prescribed medications as ordered, and monitor their effects. *If the infecting organism is resistant to the prescribed antibiotic, little improvement may be seen with treatment. Bronchodilators help maintain open airways but may have adverse effects such as anxiety and restlessness.*

Promote Healthy Grief Responses. The patient with CF and family members face the knowledge that lifespan may be short: The median survival rate is 41 years (CFF, 2017).

Expected Outcome: Patient and family will discuss the meaning of losses (actual or perceived) to the patient and family's life.

The nurse will:

- Spend time with the patient and family. *Time is necessary to develop a trusting therapeutic relationship.*
- Answer questions honestly; do not deny the probable outcome of the disease. *Honesty reinforces reality and provides a sense of control over decisions to be made.*
- Encourage the patient and family to express their feelings, fears, and concerns. *Open expression of feelings helps to promote understanding and acceptance.*
- Assist with understanding the grieving process and acceptance of feelings as normal. *Feelings of guilt, anger, or depression may cause the patient to withdraw from others. Explanation of the grieving process enhances understanding and ability to cope.*
- Help the patient and family make decisions regarding treatment and care. *This is also important to give them a sense of control.*
- Encourage use of other support systems, such as spiritual and social groups. Refer the patient and family to support groups, social support services, and hospice care as indicated. *These support systems provide emotional support and help the patient and family cope with the diagnosis while developing healthy coping skills.*
- Discuss advance directives (the living will) and power of attorney for healthcare with the patient and family. *These documents give the patient and family a sense of control over medical care provided if the patient is no longer able to express his or her own wishes.*

Delegating Nursing Care Activities

As appropriate and allowed by the designated duties and responsibilities of unlicensed assistive personnel, the nurse may delegate nursing care activities such as measuring vital signs, encouraging oral or enteral fluid intake, and providing skin care.

Transitions of Care

Education of the patient and family affected by cystic fibrosis is essential to maintaining optimal health. The adult whose disease was diagnosed in infancy or childhood has grown up with the disease and often has a much greater knowledge level than many caregivers. However, when the initial diagnosis is made, regardless of the patient's age the teaching needs are significant. Include the following topics when teaching for home care:

- Respiratory care techniques, including percussion, postural drainage, and controlled cough techniques
- Specific breathing and coughing exercises and procedures
- The importance of avoiding respiratory irritants, such as cigarette smoke, air pollution, and occupational dusts and gases
- Measures to prevent respiratory infection, such as maintaining immunizations and optimal general health and avoiding exposure to large crowds and infected people.

Refer the patient and/or family to a dietitian for planning and teaching to maintain adequate nutrition and minimize gastrointestinal symptoms. Referral to community agencies and support groups is also helpful.

Discuss the genetic transmission of cystic fibrosis and refer for counseling and possible genetic testing. Help the patient and family sort through the impact of the disease on future pregnancies and generations. Remember that the possibility of CF may present an ethical dilemma regarding future pregnancies. Provide support as needed.

The Patient with Atelectasis

Atelectasis is not a disease but a condition associated with many respiratory disorders. It is a state of partial or total lung collapse and airlessness. It may be acute or chronic. The most common cause of atelectasis is obstruction of the bronchus ventilating a segment of lung tissue. The affected segment may be small or an entire lobe. Other causes include compression of the lung by pneumothorax, pleural effusion, or tumor or loss of pulmonary surfactant and inability to maintain open alveoli.

The manifestations of atelectasis depend on its size. Diminished breath sounds over the affected area may be the only sign of a small atelectasis. If a large lung segment is affected, manifestations may include tachycardia, tachypnea, dyspnea, cyanosis, and other signs of hypoxemia. Chest expansion may be reduced and breath sounds absent on the affected side. Fever and other manifestations of infection may be present.

Chest x-ray shows an area of airless lung. CT scan may help determine the cause of atelectasis.

The primary therapy for atelectasis is prevention. High-risk patients—such as those with COPD, smokers undergoing surgery, and people on prolonged bedrest or mechanical ventilation—should have vigorous chest physiotherapy to maintain open airways. Frequently assess respiratory status, including rate, breath sounds, and spirometry readings for early detection and treatment.

When atelectasis develops, treatment focuses on the underlying cause. Vigorous coughing and chest therapy may relieve obstruction by a mucus plug. Bronchoscopy may be necessary to remove the obstruction. Antibiotic therapy is ordered to treat infectious causes.

Nursing care to prevent and treat atelectasis is directed toward airway clearance. Position the patient with atelectasis on the unaffected side to promote gravity drainage of affected segment. Encourage frequent position changes, ambulation, coughing, and deep breathing. Unless contraindicated, encourage fluids to help liquefy secretions. Teach the patient at high risk for developing atelectasis about pulmonary care measures, fluid intake, and preventing pulmonary infections.

The Patient with Bronchiectasis

Bronchiectasis is characterized by permanent abnormal dilation of one or more large bronchi and destruction of bronchial walls. Infection is often present. The destructive process of bronchiectasis is initiated by inflammation, usually due to recurrent airway infection. About half of all cases of bronchiectasis are related to cystic fibrosis. Other causes include infections, such as severe pneumonia, tuberculosis, or fungal infections; lung abscess; exposure to toxic gases; abnormal lung or immunologic defenses; and localized airway obstruction due to a foreign body or tumor. Inflammation and airway obstruction are common to all these processes. Bronchial walls become weakened and dilated as a result, leading to pooling of secretions and further infection and inflammation.

A chronic cough productive of large amounts of mucopurulent sputum is characteristic. Other manifestations of bronchiectasis include hemoptysis, recurrent pneumonia, wheezing and shortness of breath, malnutrition, right-sided heart failure, and cor pulmonale.

Collaborative care for bronchiectasis focuses on maintaining optimal pulmonary function and preventing progression of the disorder. The diagnosis is typically based on the history and physical examination. Chest x-ray and CT scan may be ordered to help confirm the diagnosis and determine the extent of lung damage.

Antibiotics are prescribed at the first indication of infection and may also be used prophylactically. Inhaled bronchodilators may be ordered. Chest physiotherapy is a vital component of continuing care for bronchiectasis. Percussion and postural drainage help mobilize secretions. Oxygen may be prescribed. Bronchoscopy may be used to clear retained secretions or obstruction or to evaluate hemoptysis. If lung destruction is localized and unresponsive to conservative management, surgical lung resection may be necessary.

Nursing care of the patient with bronchiectasis is similar to that for patients with other obstructive lung diseases. Airway clearance is a primary problem, as is ineffective breathing pattern. Nurses should also assess and be prepared to plan interventions to address impairment of gas exchange, nutrition deficits, and self-care deficits.

37.2 Interstitial Lung Disease

There are more than 130 pulmonary disorders that are considered interstitial lung diseases (ILDs). These damage the interstitial or connective tissue of the lung. Occupational lung diseases, sarcoidosis, and rheumatologic diseases such as scleroderma or systemic lupus erythematosus can result in ILD. Toxic drugs and radiation also cause interstitial damage. **Table 37.4** identifies common causes of interstitial lung disorders.

These disorders may be acute or insidious. Their rate of progression varies from person to person, as does the degree of disability they produce.

The Patient with an Occupational Lung Disease

Occupational lung diseases are a diverse group of disorders directly related to inhalation of noxious substances in the work environment. In the United States, occupational illnesses and injuries account for more than $67 and $183 billion, respectively, in direct and indirect costs per year (National Center for Health Statistics, 2016).

There are two major classifications of occupational lung diseases:

- ***Pneumoconioses***, chronic fibrotic lung diseases caused by inhalation of inorganic dusts and particulate matter. These include silicosis, coal worker's pneumoconiosis, and asbestosis.
- ***Hypersensitivity pneumonitis***, allergic pulmonary diseases caused by exposure to inhaled organic dusts. These include farmer's lung, hot tub lung, and pigeon-breeder's lung.

Pathophysiology

Lung tissue contains elastin and collagen fibers. Elastin fibers are easily stretched, facilitating lung expansion. Collagen fibers, in contrast, resist stretching. This increases the work of breathing. Both elastin and collagen affect lung

Table 37.4 Selected Causes of Interstitial Lung Disorders

Cause	Examples
Inorganic dusts	Silica (silicosis), asbestos (asbestosis), coal (coal worker's pneumoconiosis), talc (talcosis)
Organic dusts	Cotton (byssinosis), sugar cane (bagassosis), moldy hay (farmer's lung)
Drugs	Antineoplastic agents, antibiotics, gold salts, phenytoin
Radiation	External radiation or inhaled radioactive materials
Infections	Widespread TB or fungal infections, viral or *Pneumocystis jiroveci* pneumonia
Poisons and noxious gases	Paraquat, nitrogen dioxide, chlorine, ammonia, sulfur dioxide
Systemic diseases	Uremia, pulmonary edema
Unknown causes	Sarcoidosis, idiopathic pulmonary fibrosis, connective tissue disorders

compliance, or the ease with which the lungs are inflated. Other factors affecting compliance include the water content of lung tissue and surface tension (Sorenson et al., 2019).

When a noxious substance is inhaled, the response to that substance depends on the following:

- The size of particulates
- Its nature (organic or inorganic)
- Where it deposits in the respiratory tract
- The susceptibility of the individual.

Relatively large particles, larger than 6 microns, are too big to reach lower airways and are often deposited in the nose. Smaller particles can be carried with inspired air into the alveoli. Normal lung defenses, including alveolar macrophages, lymph channels, and the mucociliary escalator, attempt to remove particulate matter from the alveoli. Cigarette smoking, alcohol ingestion, or hypersensitivity reactions can impair these defenses.

The inhaled substance damages alveolar epithelium, leading to an inflammatory process of the alveoli and interstitial tissue of the lung. The inflammatory response produces further damage, and abnormal fibrotic (scar) tissue replaces the elastin fibers of normal lung tissue. As a result, the lungs become stiff and noncompliant. Lung volumes decrease, the work of breathing increases, and alveolar-capillary diffusion is impaired, leading to hypoxemia.

Asbestosis

Inhalation of asbestos fibers is a common cause of occupational lung disease. *Asbestosis* is a diffuse interstitial fibrotic disease involving the terminal airways, alveoli, and pleurae. Exposure to asbestos fibers occurs during mining, milling, manufacturing, and application of asbestos products. Although symptoms may not become apparent until 20 years after exposure, they tend to progress, even when further exposure has been halted. Asbestosis is also associated with an increased risk of bronchogenic carcinoma, especially in cigarette smokers. *Mesothelioma*, a rare cancer of the pleural membrane, is also associated with asbestos exposure. The period between asbestos exposure and tumor development in mesothelioma is long, ranging from 20 to 30 years. People exposed to asbestos prior to imposition of strict environmental controls may only now be developing manifestations of this disease.

Silicosis

Inhalation of silica dust by hard-rock miners, foundry workers, sandblasters, pottery makers, and granite cutters can lead to *silicosis*, a nodular pulmonary fibrosis. Approximately 2 million workers in the United States are at risk for exposure to silica (American Lung Association, 2018b). Although generally associated with long-term exposure to silica, it can develop in as little as 10 months of intense exposure. In silicosis, macrophages are destroyed as they engulf silica particles, releasing substances that damage lung tissue and lead to fibrosis and scarring.

Coal Worker's Pneumoconiosis

Ingestion of coal dust by alveolar macrophages causes "coal macules" to form, leading to *coal worker's pneumoconiosis*, or *black lung disease*. This occupational lung disease affects between 5 and 12% of all miners, with a higher incidence in the eastern United States than in the West (National Institute for Occupational Safety and Health, 2016). Coal macules appear on chest x-ray as diffuse, small opacities primarily affecting the upper lungs (American Lung Association, 2017b).

Hypersensitivity Pneumonitis

Workers exposed to organic dusts and gases may develop *hypersensitivity pneumonitis*, an allergic pulmonary disease affecting the airways and alveoli. Byssinosis (resulting from cotton dust exposure), bagassosis (due to exposure to moldy sugar cane fiber), farmer's lung, and pigeon-breeder's lung are examples of hypersensitivity pneumonitis.

Manifestations

The manifestations of asbestosis include exertional dyspnea, exercise intolerance, and inspiratory crackles. Diffuse, small, irregular, or linear opacities appear on chest x-ray, primarily in the lower lobes. As the disease progresses, respiratory failure and marked hypoxemia may develop.

Simple silicosis is asymptomatic with no demonstrable respiratory impairment. In contrast, complicated silicosis is characterized by large conglomerate densities in the upper lungs. These patients may be severely dyspneic and have a productive cough. Pulmonary function testing shows both restrictive and obstructive changes. Increasing size of conglomerate masses can lead to severe disability, cor pulmonale, and death.

Simple coal worker's pneumoconiosis (CWP) is generally asymptomatic. Progressive massive fibrosis, a complication of CWP that destroys the pulmonary vascular bed and airways of the upper lungs, was almost eradicated in the 1990s due to protections instituted under the Coal Mine and Health Safety Act. However, there is evidence of a resurgence of progressive massive fibrosis in eastern Kentucky, with implications for other areas of the country (Blackley, Crum, Halldin, Storey, & Laney, 2016). This progressive form of the disease causes symptoms similar to those of complicated silicosis.

In hypersensitivity pneumonitis, either acute or subacute illness can occur. Acute illness occurs 4 to 8 hours after exposure and is heralded by sudden onset of malaise, chills and fever, dyspnea, cough, and nausea. The subacute syndrome is characterized by an insidious onset of chronic cough, progressive dyspnea, anorexia, and weight loss. Diffuse fibrosis occurs after repeated exposure to the organic material, leading to respiratory insufficiency.

Interprofessional Care

Chest x-ray, pulmonary function studies, bronchoscopy, and possibly lung biopsy are used to establish the diagnosis of pneumoconioses. Characteristic patterns are seen for each disorder on x-ray. Pulmonary function testing shows restrictive impairment of lung ventilation, with reduced vital capacity and reduced total lung capacity. The diffusing capacity of the lungs is also decreased. Blood gas analysis reveals hypoxemia, especially with exercise. Bronchoscopy may be performed to obtain tissue for biopsy.

Specialized lung scans may be used to determine the extent of fibrosis.

Eliminating further exposure to the offending agent is an important part of disease management. There is no specific therapy. Anti-inflammatory drugs, such as corticosteroids, may reduce the inflammatory response and slow the progression of the disease. Preventing exposure to other damaging substances such as cigarette smoke and pollution is vital. Pneumococcal vaccine and annual influenza immunizations are recommended to reduce the risk of lower respiratory infections. Other care is supportive, similar to that for COPD.

Nursing Care

Assessment

See the Manifestations and Interprofessional Care sections for the assessment of the patient with occupational lung diseases.

Priorities of Care

Collaborate with the interprofessional team to ensure adequate treatment of the underlying process while providing care that supports the physical and psychologic responses to the disorder is a priority of nursing care.

Diagnoses, Interventions, and Outcomes

Nursing care for patients with occupational lung diseases is similar to that for patients with COPD. Activity intolerance is a high-priority problem for many patients. Severe dyspnea can significantly interfere with ADLs. Nursing measures to reduce energy expenditures and provide for rest are essential. Caregiver role strain, either actual or potential, must be considered when the patient with severe disability is being cared for at home.

Both patient and family coping may be compromised. Many of these diseases develop after 20 to 30 years of exposure to the hazardous material. Patients who entered the industry following high school may develop evidence of disease in their 40s and face the possibility of changing their occupation or developing significant disability. The resulting role strain affects all members of the family.

In addition to family coping, nursing interventions to promote effective breathing, healthy grief responses, and self-esteem may be appropriate for the patient with an occupational lung disease.

Delegating Nursing Care Activities

As appropriate and allowed by the designated duties and responsibilities of unlicensed assistive personnel, the nurse may delegate nursing care activities such as measuring vital signs, encouraging oral or enteral fluid intake, and providing skin care.

Transitions of Care

Prevention is a key strategy for all occupational lung diseases. Containing dust and wearing personal protective devices that limit the amount of inhaled particles are essential for people who work in industries with known risks.

Teaching about the dangers of occupational lung diseases and ways to reduce their risk needs to begin early, before the disease develops. Nurses in industrial and public health settings can begin by recognizing potential dangers and teaching workers about measures to reduce dust in their work area and the use of personal protective devices such as masks. Nurses working with affected families have an excellent opportunity to begin educating children about the risks associated with the occupation.

The affected patient and family need teaching in preparation for home care, including:

- Prevention of further lung damage (e.g., avoiding cigarette smoke and heavy air pollution)
- Recommendations for pneumococcal and annual influenza immunizations; yearly tuberculin testing for patients with silicosis
- Pulmonary hygiene measures, such as liberal fluid intake, coughing, and deep-breathing exercises
- Use and care of oxygen therapy equipment, if required
- Use and effects of any prescribed or recommended OTC medications.

In addition to teaching related to disease prevention and management, patients and their families may need information on how to access programs and other resources offered through agencies such as the Office of Safety and Health Administration (OSHA) and the Social Security Administration. For example, the federal government has established specific clinics and benefits for coal workers, as well as a surveillance program to track trends in the health of coal miners. Information on these resources is available at the website of the Coal Workers' Health Surveillance Program (https://www.cdc.gov/niosh/topics/cwhsp/default.html).

The Patient with Sarcoidosis

Sarcoidosis is a chronic, multisystem disease characterized by an exaggerated cellular immune response in involved tissues. This abnormal immune response leads to granuloma formation in the lungs, lymph nodes, liver, eyes, skin, and other organs. Its cause is unknown. Sarcoidosis primarily affects adults over the age of 20. In the United States, the incidence is highest in African Americans. Women are affected at a slightly higher rate than men (ALA, 2018a).

In sarcoidosis, multiple granulomas form; these lesions may resolve spontaneously or proceed to fibrosis. The lungs are affected in about 90% of patients with sarcoidosis. Mortality rates range from 1 to 8%, depending on factors such as care settings, age, ethnicity, gender, and severity of the disease. Sarcoidosis has a relatively high rate of serious disability from ocular, respiratory, or other organ damage. Risk factors for greater severity and new organ involvement include lower socioeconomic status. African American populations also tend to experience greater severity (Gerke, 2014). Pulmonary hemorrhage and cardiac and respiratory failure from pulmonary fibrosis are the leading causes of death from sarcoidosis.

The manifestations of sarcoidosis vary, depending on the organ system affected. It may be asymptomatic, diagnosed by characteristic findings on routine chest x-ray. Symptoms may be insidious, with anorexia, fatigue, weight loss, fever, dyspnea, arthralgias, and myalgias. Skin lesions, uveitis, lymphadenopathy, hepatomegaly, or other manifestations may also develop.

Leukopenia, eosinophilia, and an elevated erythrocyte sedimentation rate (ESR) are typically noted in sarcoidosis. The chest x-ray helps to determine the extent of pulmonary involvement. Biopsy of a granulomatous lesion may be required to confirm the diagnosis. Pulmonary function tests reveal decreased compliance and impaired diffusing capacity.

Sarcoidosis often resolves spontaneously, therefore treatment is indicated only when symptoms are severe or disabling. Corticosteroid therapy is prescribed to suppress the inflammatory process when indicated. Relapse frequently occurs when corticosteroids are discontinued. Other anti-inflammatory or immune-modifier medications may also be used, including chloroquine, indomethacin, azathioprine, and methotrexate.

Nursing care for patients with sarcoidosis is directed by involved organ systems and related manifestations. Respiratory care is supportive and includes avoiding respiratory irritants and maintaining adequate ventilation. Refer for smoking-cessation assistance as needed.

Teach patients with limited symptoms about the disease and symptoms to report to a healthcare provider, including shortness of breath, tearing and eye inflammation, chest pain or irregular pulse, skin lesions, and swollen and painful joints. If corticosteroid therapy is prescribed, teach the importance of taking the drug as prescribed and not stopping it abruptly. Include information about managing the side effects of corticosteroids by limiting sodium and increasing potassium in the diet, taking the medication with food or milk to minimize gastric irritation, and identifying early signs of infection.

37.3 Pulmonary Vascular Disorders

The cardiovascular and respiratory systems are closely interrelated. As blood flows through the capillary network of the pulmonary vascular system, oxygen diffuses into it and carbon dioxide diffuses out. An effective match of alveolar ventilation and capillary perfusion is essential to maintain this process and, ultimately, tissue oxygenation and function of all organ systems. Both vascular and alveolar changes can alter gas exchange. Arteriosclerotic changes in pulmonary vasculature reduce blood flow to the alveolus. Nearly all lower respiratory system disorders can potentially affect ventilation. Many also have a secondary effect on lung perfusion because breakdown or fibrosis of alveolar walls destroys the capillary network as well. This section focuses on primary disorders of the pulmonary vascular system.

The Patient with a Pulmonary Embolism

A **pulmonary embolism** (or *thromboembolism*) is obstruction of blood flow in part of the pulmonary vascular system by an embolus. Thromboemboli, or blood clots, that develop in the venous system (deep venous thrombosis [DVT]) or right side of the heart are the most frequent cause of pulmonary embolism. Other sources of emboli include tumors that have invaded venous circulation, fat or bone marrow entering the circulation due to fracture or other trauma, amniotic fluid released into the circulation during childbirth, and intravenous injection of air or other foreign substances.

Pulmonary embolism causes an estimated 60,000 deaths annually, occurring in more than 600,000 patients per year. Although many substances can become emboli, thrombus arising from the deep veins of the legs is the leading cause of pulmonary embolism. *Deep venous thrombosis (DVT)* develops in approximately 5 million people per year in the United States (CDC, 2017e).

Pulmonary embolism (PE) is a medical emergency. Sudden death occurs in 25% of PE onset. Up to 30% of patients die within the first month following onset (CDC, 2018). In many cases, DVT has not been recognized or treated; often embolization also goes undetected. Prevention is the most effective treatment strategy for pulmonary embolism.

Pathophysiology

The right heart receives deoxygenated blood from the systemic venous circulation. The entire output of the right ventricle enters the pulmonary circulation via the pulmonary artery. This artery branches into successively smaller arteries, arterioles, and capillaries of the pulmonary vascular system. Each alveolus of the lungs is surrounded by a meshwork of capillaries. Oxygen and carbon dioxide readily diffuse across the alveolar-capillary membrane, driven by a concentration gradient. The partial pressure of oxygen in the alveolus is greater than in the capillary, therefore it diffuses into the blood. Carbon dioxide diffuses from the capillaries into the alveoli, driven by the higher pressure of dissolved carbon dioxide in venous blood.

A match between blood flow through the pulmonary vascular system (perfusion) and lung ventilation is necessary for effective *respiration* (gas exchange) (refer to Figure 37.4). Local factors regulate ventilation and perfusion to maintain this match. A low alveolar PaO_2 constricts alveolar capillaries, directing blood flow to better ventilated areas of the lung. High alveolar $PaCO_2$ levels cause local bronchodilation, increasing airflow and eliminating excess carbon dioxide.

Thrombi affecting only the deep veins of the calf rarely embolize to the pulmonary circulation. However, thrombi often propagate proximally to the popliteal and ileofemoral veins. From there, they may break loose to become an embolus. As vessels of the venous system become progressively larger, the embolus moves freely until it enters the pulmonary arterial system with its progressively smaller vessels leading to the pulmonary capillary beds (**Figure 37.6** ■).

The impact of a pulmonary embolus depends on the extent to which pulmonary blood flow is obstructed, the size of the embolus, its nature, and secondary effects of the obstruction. The effects can range widely:

- Occlusion of a large pulmonary artery with sudden death. Gas exchange is significantly reduced or prevented, and cardiac output falls dramatically as blood

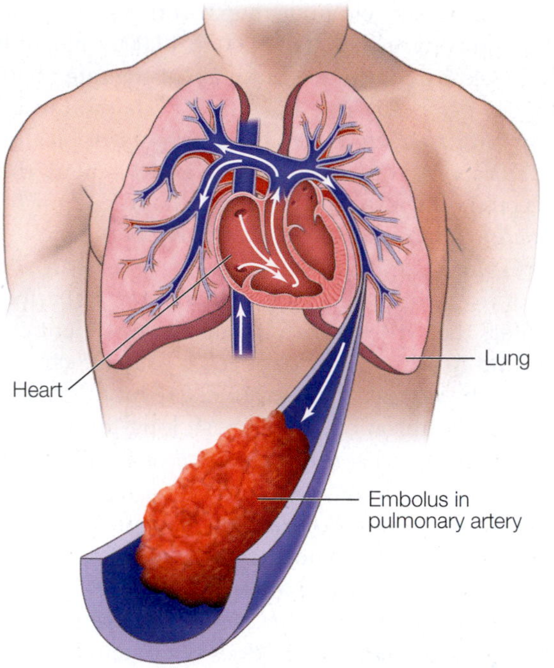
Heart
Lung
Embolus in pulmonary artery

Figure 37.6 ■ A thromboembolism lodged in a pulmonary vessel.

fails to move through the pulmonary vascular system and return to the left heart.

- Lung tissue infarction due to occlusion of a significant portion of pulmonary blood flow. Fewer than 10% of pulmonary emboli result in pulmonary infarction.
- Obstruction of a small segment of the pulmonary circulation with no permanent lung injury.
- Chronic or recurrent small emboli, which may be multiple.

Obstruction of pulmonary blood flow by an embolus affects both perfusion and ventilation. Neurohumoral reflexes triggered by obstruction cause vasoconstriction, increasing pulmonary vascular resistance. In severe cases, this can lead to pulmonary hypertension and right-ventricular heart failure. Systemically, hypotension and a drop in cardiac output may develop. Bronchoconstriction occurs in the affected area of lung. Dead space (areas of the lung that are ventilated but not perfused) increases. Alveolar surfactant decreases, increasing the risk for atelectasis.

If infarction does not occur, the fibrinolytic system (refer to Chapter 30) ultimately dissolves the clot, and pulmonary function returns to normal. Infarcted tissue becomes scarred and fibrotic.

Fat emboli are the most common nonthrombotic pulmonary emboli. A fat embolism usually occurs after fracture of long bone (typically the femur) releases bone marrow fat into the circulation. Adipose tissue or liver trauma may also lead to fat emboli.

Risk Factors

The risk factors for pulmonary embolus are those for DVT: Stasis of venous blood flow, vessel wall damage, and altered blood coagulation. Prolonged immobility; trauma, including hip and femur fractures; surgery (orthopedic, pelvic, and gynecologic surgery in particular); myocardial infarction and heart failure; obesity; and advanced age are risk factors for DVT. Women who use oral contraceptives or estrogen therapy are at risk, as are women during pregnancy and childbirth. See Chapter 32, Section 32.4, for more information about DVT.

Manifestations

The manifestations of pulmonary embolism depend on its size and location. Small emboli may be asymptomatic. Manifestations usually develop abruptly, over a period of minutes. The most common symptoms are dyspnea, shortness of breath, and pleuritic chest pain. Anxiety, a sense of impending doom, and cough are also common. Diaphoresis and hemoptysis may develop. Massive pulmonary embolus can cause syncope and cyanosis. On examination, tachycardia and tachypnea are noted. Crackles may be heard on auscultation of the chest, and a cardiac gallop (S_3 and possibly S_4) may be noted. A low-grade fever may develop. It is difficult to differentiate pulmonary embolism from myocardial infarction or pneumonia by manifestations.

Less common manifestations of pulmonary embolism are diaphoresis, hemoptysis, syncope, cyanosis, and S_3 and/or S_4 gallop. Characteristic manifestations of fat emboli include sudden onset of cardiopulmonary and neurologic symptoms: Dyspnea, tachypnea, tachycardia, confusion, delirium, and decreased level of consciousness. Petechiae often develop on the chest and arms.

Interprofessional Care

Because deep venous thrombosis may not be identified until pulmonary embolism occurs, prevention is the primary goal in treating pulmonary embolism. Prophylactic anticoagulation can be used to prevent the development of DVT. Early ambulation of medical and surgical patients is an effective means of preventing venous stasis and reducing the incidence of pulmonary embolism. External pneumatic compression of the legs is also effective for patients undergoing neurosurgery, urologic surgery, or major surgery of the hip or knee, or when anticoagulant therapy is contraindicated. Other preventative measures include elevating the legs and active and passive leg exercises.

When pulmonary embolism occurs, treatment is supportive. Oxygen therapy is initiated, and analgesics may be ordered to relieve severe pleuritic pain and anxiety. Pulmonary artery and wedge pressures may be monitored with a balloon (Swan-Ganz) catheter. Although cardiac outputs may also be assessed, this is rarely done in this population. Cardiac rhythm is monitored to detect dysrhythmias.

Diagnosis

The studies performed to identify DVT differ from those used to diagnose a pulmonary embolism. Refer to Chapter 32 for diagnostic studies for venous thrombosis.

- *Plasma D-dimer levels* are highly specific to the presence of a thrombus. D-dimer is a fragment of fibrin formed during lysis of a blood clot; elevated blood levels indicate thrombus formation and lysis (e.g., DVT and pulmonary embolism).

- ***Chest CT with contrast*** is the principal test used to diagnose pulmonary embolism. Chest CT effectively shows large, central PE; newer-generation scanners can also detect peripheral emboli.
- ***Lung scans***, including perfusion and ventilation scans, may be used. In a perfusion lung scan, radiotagged albumin is injected intravenously and distributed in the lungs by the pulmonary blood flow. The lungs are then scanned for distribution of the isotope. An area of lung in which the isotope is undetectable is suggestive of occluded blood flow and pulmonary embolism. For a ventilation scan, a radiotagged gas is inhaled and the lungs are scanned for gas distribution. Combined perfusion and ventilation scans allow identification of areas of the lungs that are ventilated but not perfused, a characteristic of pulmonary embolism.
- ***Pulmonary angiography*** is the definitive test for pulmonary embolism when other, less invasive tests are inconclusive. It is possible to detect very small emboli with angiography. A contrast medium injected into the pulmonary arteries illustrates the pulmonary vascular system on x-ray.
- ***Chest x-ray*** often shows pulmonary infiltration and occasionally pleural effusion.
- ***Electrocardiogram (ECG)*** is ordered to rule out acute myocardial infarction as the cause of symptoms. ECG findings commonly associated with pulmonary embolism include tachycardia and nonspecific T-wave changes.
- ***ABGs*** usually show hypoxemia (PaO_2 < 80 mmHg), and often respiratory alkalosis (pH > 7.45, $PaCO_2$ < 38 mmHg) due to tachypnea and hyperventilation.
- ***Exhaled carbon dioxide ($ETCO_2$)*** may be measured to evaluate alveolar perfusion. The normal $ETCO_2$ reading is 35 to 45 mmHg; it is decreased when pulmonary perfusion is impaired.
- ***Coagulation studies*** are ordered to monitor the response to therapy. The *activated partial thromboplastin time* (*aPTT* or *PTT*) is used to assess the intrinsic clotting pathway and the response to heparin therapy. Desired levels with anticoagulant therapy are 1.5 to 2 times the control value. The risk of recurrent thromboembolism is high at lower levels; the risk of bleeding increases at higher levels. The *International Normalized Ratio (INR)* is used to assess the extrinsic clotting system and oral anticoagulation with warfarin (Coumadin). The goal of anticoagulant therapy is to achieve a therapeutic range of 2.0 to 3.0.

Medications

Anticoagulant therapy is the standard treatment to prevent pulmonary emboli. It is often instituted in high-risk patients who have no evidence of pulmonary embolism, to prevent possible devastating effects (Adams, Holland, & Urban, 2017). In the patient with DVT or a pulmonary embolus, anticoagulants are administered to prevent further clotting and embolization. Refer to Chapter 32, Medication Administration 32.B, for the nursing implications for anticoagulant therapy.

For pulmonary embolus, heparin therapy is initiated with an intravenous bolus of 5000 to 10,000 units of heparin, followed by continuous infusion at the rate of 1000 to 1500 units per hour. The aPTT or PTT is monitored frequently until stabilized. Heparin therapy is typically continued for about 5 days or until oral anticoagulant therapy has become fully effective. Refer to Chapter 32 for further information on low-molecular-weight heparin.

Oral anticoagulant therapy with warfarin sodium (Coumadin) is initiated at the same time as heparin. Warfarin alters the synthesis of vitamin K–dependent clotting factors and requires 5 to 7 days to be fully effective. Anticoagulant therapy is continued for 2 to 3 months when few risk factors for thromboemboli exist; long-term therapy is used when chronic disorders that increase the risk of thromboemboli are present.

Bleeding is a risk associated with anticoagulant therapy. Although major hemorrhage is uncommon, it occurs in approximately 5% of patients receiving intravenous heparin. Cardiac, hepatic, and renal disease increase the risk of significant bleeding, as does age over 60 years. Protamine, a protein that combines with heparin to inactivate it, is used to stop its anticoagulant effect if major bleeding occurs. Vitamin K is given to treat bleeding associated with Coumadin therapy.

Thrombolytic therapy may be used to treat massive pulmonary embolus and hypotension. Streptokinase, urokinase, or tissue plasminogen activator (tPA) is used to *lyse* (disintegrate) the embolus, restore pulmonary blood flow, and reduce pulmonary artery and right heart pressures. Although thrombolytic therapy may not reduce mortality associated with pulmonary embolus, it may reduce the incidence of pulmonary hypertension, which develops 3 to 5 years after an embolism. Thrombolysis significantly increases the risk of bleeding, particularly cerebral bleeding. Contraindications to thrombolysis include intracranial disease, recent stroke, active bleeding or a bleeding disorder, pregnancy, severe hypertension, and recent surgery or trauma. Because of the increased risk of hemorrhage, invasive procedures are avoided after thrombolysis. Refer to Chapter 30 for further discussion of thrombolytic therapy and its nursing implications.

Surgery

When anticoagulant therapy fails to prevent recurrent emboli, an umbrella-like filter may be inserted into the inferior vena cava to trap large emboli while allowing continued blood flow (refer to Figure 32.11A). The filter is usually inserted percutaneously, via either the femoral or jugular vein.

Nursing Care

Assessment

See the Manifestations and Interprofessional Care sections for the assessment of the patient with a pulmonary embolism.

Because pulmonary embolus can be a medical emergency, assessment may be very focused. In other instances, when emboli are small and not life-threatening, a more extensive nursing assessment may be done.

- ***Health history:*** Chest pain, shortness of breath, other symptoms, including onset, severity, precipitating factors; history of recent surgery, venous thrombosis, or other risk factors such as childbirth or malignancy; current medications
- ***Physical assessment:*** Level of consciousness, presence of respirations and pulse; color, skin temperature, and moisture; vital signs including apical pulse and temperature; breath sounds and heart sounds; oxygen saturation level; neck vein distention, peripheral edema
- ***Laboratory data:*** Plasma D-dimer levels, coagulation studies; chest x-ray and other imaging studies; oxygen saturation and ABGs; ECG.

Priorities of Care

Collaborate with the interprofessional team to ensure adequate treatment of the underlying process while providing care that supports the physical and psychologic responses to the disorder is a priority of nursing care.

Diagnoses, Interventions, and Outcomes

A large pulmonary embolus can cause a significant mismatch between pulmonary ventilation and circulation. Impaired gas exchange is a priority problem and focus for interventions. Cardiac output may be significantly affected by obstructed pulmonary blood flow. Thrombolytic and anticoagulant therapy affect the clotting process, increasing the risk for bleeding. Anxiety accompanies pulmonary embolism almost universally.

Promote Effective Gas Exchange. Pulmonary embolism results in areas of the lung that are ventilated but not perfused; they receive no capillary blood flow. If the embolus is large and a major segment of the lung is not perfused, gas exchange is significantly affected. Nursing interventions are directed toward compensating for impaired gas exchange.

Expected Outcome: Patient's tissue perfusion will be effective as indicated by adequate arterial flow as evidenced by absence of symptoms of cardiac, pulmonary, and neurologic ischemia.

The nurse will:

- Frequently assess respiratory status, including rate, depth, effort, lung sounds, and oxygen saturation. *Impaired ventilation will further compromise gas exchange and worsen hypoxemia. Oxygen saturation can be monitored continuously and noninvasively to evaluate gas exchange.*
- Monitor and record level of consciousness, mental status, and skin color. *Hypoxemia often causes confusion and agitation; hypercapnia may reduce level of consciousness. Cyanosis indicates significant hypoxemia.*
- Place in Fowler or high-Fowler position, with the lower extremities dependent. *This position facilitates maximal lung expansion and reduces venous return to the right side of the heart, lowering pressures in the pulmonary vascular system.*
- Monitor arterial blood gas results, reporting abnormal findings as indicated. *ABGs are used to assess gas exchange and tissue oxygenation. An arterial line may be inserted for monitoring arterial pressure and arterial blood sampling.*
- Maintain bedrest. *Bedrest reduces metabolic demands and tissue needs for oxygen.*

SAFETY ALERT: Start oxygen per nasal cannula or mask. Obtain an order from the healthcare provider if one has not been written. Supplemental oxygen increases alveolar and arterial oxygenation. Oxygen is a drug that requires a prescription. It may, however, be initiated by the nurse in an emergency to prevent tissue hypoxia. ■

Promote Adequate Cardiac Output. The impact of a large pulmonary embolus on hemodynamic status can be significant. Pressures in the pulmonary vascular system and right heart increase; blood return to the left heart and cardiac output may significantly decrease. Nursing interventions focus on preserving an adequate blood pressure and organ function until cardiopulmonary status stabilizes. A central line for hemodynamic monitoring may be instituted (refer to Chapter 30 for nursing care related to hemodynamic monitoring).

Expected Outcome: Patient will demonstrate adequate cardiac output as evidenced by blood pressure and pulse rate within normal parameters for the patient.

The nurse will:

- Auscultate heart sounds every 2 to 4 hours, reporting any abnormalities. *Sounds such as an S_3 or S_4 gallop may indicate cardiac compromise.*
- Record intake and output hourly. *Decreased urinary output is often an early indicator of decreased cardiac output. Maintaining renal perfusion is vital to preserve renal function and prevent acute renal failure.*
- Assess skin color and temperature. *These assessments monitor tissue perfusion.*
- Monitor cardiac rhythm. *A drop in cardiac output and other hemodynamic alterations resulting from pulmonary embolism can precipitate dysrhythmias. Dysrhythmias, in turn, can further impair cardiac output.*
- Administer vasopressors and other medications as ordered. Carefully monitor the response to prescribed medications. *Drugs may be prescribed to maintain adequate arterial pressure and tissue perfusion. Potent drugs such as vasopressors require careful monitoring for desired and adverse effects.*
- Monitor pulmonary artery pressures, neck vein distention, and peripheral edema. Report findings as indicated. *Right-sided heart failure is a potential complication of pulmonary embolism because of increased pulmonary artery pressures.*
- Maintain intravenous and arterial access sites as well as central lines. *The patient may be in unstable and critical condition, potentially needing immediate interventions to maintain life.*

- Provide frequent skin care. *Impaired tissue perfusion and oxygenation increase the risk of skin and tissue breakdown.*
- Instruct to report chest pain or other symptoms. *Decreased cardiac output and an increased workload due to pulmonary hypertension may cause anginal pain.*

SAFETY ALERT: Assess and record vital signs and cardiopulmonary status every 15 to 30 minutes initially, then every 2 to 4 hours as condition stabilizes. Frequent assessment facilitates timely interventions to maintain cardiovascular status and preserve organ function. ■

Reduce Risk for Bleeding and Hemorrhage. Thrombolytics and anticoagulant therapy impair normal clotting mechanisms, increasing the risk for bleeding and hemorrhage. This risk is particularly acute during the first 24 to 48 hours following thrombolytic drug administration.

Expected Outcome: Patient will remain free of any evidence of new bleeding and take precautions to prevent bleeding.

The nurse will:

- Assess frequently for overt and covert signs of bleeding: Bleeding gums; hematuria; obvious or occult blood in stool or vomitus; incisional bleeding, bleeding or bruising of injection sites or with minor trauma; joint pain or immobility; abdominal or flank pain. *Careful monitoring is necessary to identify early signs of abnormal bleeding and prevent potential hemorrhage.*
- Report coagulation study results outside the desired range for anticoagulant therapy. *Levels below the target range may indicate an increased risk for further clot development and pulmonary emboli; levels above the target range indicate an increased risk for bleeding.*
- Keep protamine sulfate available for heparin therapy and vitamin K available for warfarin (Coumadin) therapy. *Bleeding or hemorrhage due to excess anticoagulant may require antidote administration to rapidly reverse anticoagulant effects.*
- Assess medication regimen for possible drug interactions that could potentiate or inhibit anticoagulant effects. *Drug interactions can increase the risk for hemorrhage or further embolus formation.*
- Avoid invasive procedures, injections, and venous punctures when possible, particularly during and following thrombolytic therapy. *Invasive procedures increase the risk of tissue trauma and bleeding.*
- Maintain firm pressure on injection and venipuncture sites. Maintain pressure for 30 minutes following arterial puncture. *Firm pressure reduces the risk for bleeding into the tissues.*
- Maintain adequate fluid intake. Administer stool softeners as ordered. *These measures help prevent constipation and straining, which may precipitate bleeding of hemorrhoids.*

SAFETY ALERT: Promptly report changes in neurologic status. Although cerebral bleeding is not evident externally, changes in level of consciousness and other neurologic signs suggest it and should be reported immediately. ■

Reduce Anxiety. Pulmonary embolism is a physiologic and psychologic threat to safety and integrity. It is a major physiologic stressor, eliciting a strong neuroendocrine stress response. The feeling of suffocation and inability to catch one's breath that accompanies a pulmonary embolus is also a strong psychologic stressor. Fear, anxiety, and apprehension are common responses.

Expected Outcome: Patient will be able to manage anxiety as evidenced by verbalized decrease in subjective distress.

The nurse will:

- Assess anxiety level. *Appropriate interventions are determined by the level of anxiety.*
- Provide reassurance and emotional support, listening to fears. Do not negate the fear of dying, but reassure that treatment usually restores effective respiratory function. *The fear of death is very real and must not be discounted; however, it is important to provide reassurance to alleviate excess anxiety.*
- Remain with the patient as much as possible. *The presence of a caring nurse helps reduce fear.*
- Explain procedures and treatments using short, simple sentences. *Providing clearly understood, simple instructions reduces fear of the unknown.*
- Reduce environmental stimuli, and use a calm, reassuring manner. *These measures help reduce anxiety (for both the nurse and the patient).*
- Allow supportive family members to remain with the patient as much as possible. *Calm, supportive family members provide further reassurance.*
- Administer morphine sulfate as ordered. *Morphine is given to reduce pain and anxiety.*

SAFETY ALERT: Use an infusion device to administer heparin, which helps prevent administration of excess medication. ■

Delegating Nursing Care Activities

As appropriate and allowed by the designated duties and responsibilities of unlicensed assistive personnel, the nurse may delegate nursing care activities such as measuring vital signs, encouraging oral or enteral fluid intake, and providing skin care.

Transitions of Care

Nurses are key in preventing pulmonary embolism. Encouraging patients to ambulate after surgery or illness, applying compression stockings or pneumatic compression devices, teaching and encouraging leg exercises, discouraging the use of pillows under the knees—all these measures help prevent DVT and subsequent pulmonary emboli.

Teach patients to reduce the risks associated with long periods of immobility, stopping every 1 to 2 hours during long automobile trips for a brief stretch and walk, getting up every hour or so and doing leg exercises while seated during long flights, and avoiding crossing the legs to prevent venous stasis and pooling. Regular exercise such as walking also reduces the risk of DVT. Instruct patients who stand for long periods to use well-fitted elastic stockings, being careful to avoid hose that bind around the knee or thigh.

Discuss the following topics when preparing the patient with pulmonary embolism and family members for home care:

- Use of prescribed anticoagulant, including drug interactions, scheduled laboratory testing, and manifestations of bleeding to report to the primary care provider
- Using a soft-bristle toothbrush and electric razor to reduce the risk of bleeding
- Avoiding aspirin (unless prescribed) and other over-the-counter medications (including herbal supplements) without approval by the physician
- Importance of wearing a medical alert tag for anticoagulant use
- Health promotion measures to reduce the risk of recurrent pulmonary embolism
- Symptoms of recurrent pulmonary embolism, such as sudden chest pain, shortness of breath, and possibly bloody sputum.

The Patient with Pulmonary Hypertension

The pulmonary vascular system is normally a high-flow, low-pressure, low-resistance system that can accommodate large increases in blood flow when necessary (e.g., during exercise). The normal mean arterial pressure in the pulmonary system is 12 to 15 mmHg (25 to 28 systolic/8 diastolic). **Pulmonary hypertension (PHTN)** is abnormal elevation of the pulmonary arterial pressure. An estimated 500 to 1000 new cases of primary pulmonary hypertension are diagnosed annually, primarily in women between age 20 and 40 (American Heart Association, 2017).

Pathophysiology

Pulmonary hypertension can develop as a primary disorder, but it can also occur secondarily to another condition. In both instances, changes in the pulmonary artery lead to abnormal growth and remodeling of pulmonary vessels. Smooth muscle cells and fibroblasts proliferate, leading to abnormal vasoconstriction and fibrosis of pulmonary vessels. Once initiated, pulmonary vascular changes are progressive and irreversible. Vasoconstrictive substances such as endothelin 1 and thromboxane A2 are produced in excess, while the production of vasodilating substances such as nitric oxide is reduced. This further contributes to vasoconstriction and increased pulmonary artery pressures. Thromboxane A2 also stimulates platelet aggregation, promoting clot formation in pulmonary vessels. The development of plexiform lesions is also a hallmark of PHTN. Inflammation may contribute to progression of the disease. Vasoconstriction and increased pressures in the pulmonary system increase the workload of the right ventricle, ultimately leading to right-ventricular failure.

World Health Organization PHTN Groups

The World Health Organization has established categories of pulmonary hypertension, which emphasize treatment of the underlying disease and can be used to better inform efforts such as morbidity and mortality rates, resource allocation, and health information for patients (Ferreira, n.d.). The categories are listed in **Box 37.6**.

Primary Pulmonary Hypertension

Primary pulmonary hypertension is an uncommon disorder without an identified cause. It occurs in both familial and sporadic patterns. In the 50% of persons with the familial form, the bone morphogenetic protein receptor (*BMPR2*), a gene transmitted in an autosomal dominant pattern, affects the walls of pulmonary arteries, leading to abnormal vessel growth and remodeling. This gene is located at chromosomal region 2q32. Presence of the mutation carries a 10 to 20% risk of developing pulmonary arterial hypertension (PAH) over the lifetime. Primary pulmonary hypertension affects primarily women in their 30s and 40s.

Secondary Pulmonary Hypertension

Secondary pulmonary hypertension is more common than primary. HIV infection and collagen diseases such as

BOX 37.6
WHO Categories of Pulmonary Hypertension

GROUP 1 PULMONARY ARTERIAL HYPERTENSION (PAH)
- No known cause (Primary)
- Inherited
- Drugs or toxins causes
- Connective tissue disease
- HIV infection
- Liver disease
- Congenital heart disease
- Sickle cell disease
- Schistosomiasis
- Conditions of the veins and small blood vessels of the lungs

GROUP 2 PULMONARY HYPERTENSION
- Left heart disease (mitral valve disease, high blood pressure)

GROUP 3 PULMONARY HYPERTENSION
- Related to lung problems (COPD, ILD, sleep apnea)

GROUP 4 PULMONARY HYPERTENSION
- Blood clots in the lungs
- General clotting disorders

GROUP 5 PULMONARY HYPERTENSION (SECONDARY TO:)
- Polycythemia vera, essential thrombocytopenia
- Sarcoidosis and vasculitis
- Metabolic disorders (thyroid, glycogen storage disease)
- Kidney disease, pulmonary artery compression

scleroderma and lupus may lead to secondary pulmonary hypertension. However, its usual cause is reduced size of the pulmonary vascular bed, which may be due to vasoconstriction or widespread vessel destruction or obstruction. Hypoxemia is a potent pulmonary vasoconstrictor and a common initiating factor in pulmonary hypertension. Chronic lung diseases, sleep apnea, and hypoventilation due to obesity or neuromuscular disease can lead to hypoxemia. Alveolar wall destruction associated with emphysema leads to loss of pulmonary capillaries. Large or multiple pulmonary emboli may cause significant vessel obstruction. Other factors such as left-ventricular failure or mitral stenosis can also lead to elevated pulmonary pressures. Once initiated, pulmonary hypertension becomes self-sustaining, as pulmonary vessels undergo changes that further narrow the pulmonary bed.

Manifestations

The manifestations of pulmonary hypertension are progressive dyspnea, fatigue, angina, and syncope with exertion. In secondary pulmonary hypertension, the signs and symptoms are often masked by those of the underlying disease. Dull, retrosternal chest pain may occur in addition to the manifestations of the primary disease. Primary pulmonary hypertension is a progressive disorder that generally causes a steady decline to death within 3 to 4 years.

Complications

Cor pulmonale is a condition of right-ventricular hypertrophy and failure resulting from long-standing pulmonary hypertension. Chronic obstructive pulmonary disease is the most common cause of cor pulmonale.

The manifestations of cor pulmonale are those of the underlying pulmonary disorder and right-sided heart failure. Chronic productive cough, progressive dyspnea, and wheezing are common. With right-sided heart failure, peripheral edema and distended neck veins are seen. Skin is warm, moist, and both ruddy and cyanotic because of increased numbers of RBCs and hypoxemia.

Interprofessional Care

Diagnosis

The CBC commonly shows *polycythemia*, increased numbers of red blood cells. ABGs and oxygen saturation measurements reveal hypoxemia. The chest x-ray shows right heart enlargement and dilation of central pulmonary arteries. Typical ECG changes are those of right-ventricular hypertrophy. An echocardiogram may be done to identify cardiac changes occurring either as a cause or result of pulmonary hypertension. Doppler ultrasonography is a noninvasive means of estimating pulmonary artery pressure, but cardiac catheterization may be required for definitive diagnosis. Refer to Chapter 30 for nursing care of the patient having a percutaneous coronary revascularization procedure.

Treatment for pulmonary hypertension focuses on slowing the course of the disease, preventing thrombus formation, and reducing pulmonary vasoconstriction. Oxygen is administered to reduce hypoxemia and improve activity tolerance. If polycythemia is present, phlebotomy is performed to reduce the viscosity of the blood.

Medications

The calcium channel blockers nifedipine (Procardia) or diltiazem (Cardizem) may be given to reduce pulmonary vascular resistance and improve cardiac output. Short-acting direct vasodilators such as intravenous epoprostenol (Flolan) or treprostinil (Remodulin), or oral bosentan (Tracleer), may be used for patients who do not respond to calcium channel blockers. An oral anticoagulant (warfarin [Coumadin]) is given to prevent clotting.

Surgery

Bilateral lung or heart–lung transplant is the most effective long-term treatment for primary pulmonary hypertension. When cor pulmonale is present, salt and water restrictions as well as diuretic therapy are added to the previously mentioned regimen to manage the right-sided heart failure.

Nursing Care

Nursing care for the patient with pulmonary hypertension or cor pulmonale is largely supportive. The focus is toward the underlying lung disease. Impaired gas exchange due to contraction of the pulmonary vascular system is a significant problem that causes many secondary problems, such as activity intolerance, anxiety, and fatigue. Nursing interventions for impaired gas exchange are directed toward maintaining adequate alveolar ventilation, oxygenation, and perfusion. The following measures may be included:

- Monitoring breath sounds, respiratory rate, skin color, and use of accessory muscles
- Positioning for optimal lung expansion
- Coughing, deep breathing, and chest physiotherapy
- Administering prescribed vasodilators.

It is important to assess fatigue and dyspnea with activities and to plan frequent rest periods. Assist with self-care as needed to conserve energy.

With primary pulmonary hypertension, patients and family members may experience anticipatory grieving and hopelessness. When cor pulmonale is present, nurses must monitor for impaired cardiac output and excess fluid volume. In addition, nurses should assess individual coping and help patients identify coping mechanisms that have helped them in the past.

Transitions of Care

Most care for these chronic conditions is provided in the home and community settings. Teaching is directed both at the underlying lung disease, if present, and the resulting hypertensive process. Refer to the section on COPD for teaching related to this disease, the most frequent underlying cause of cor pulmonale.

In addition, provide teaching about the following topics for the patient and family:

- Disease process, its management, and the prognosis
- Manifestations or changes in condition to report to the primary care or specialty provider, such as a change in

activity tolerance, increased edema, and signs of respiratory infection or exacerbation

- Importance of planned rest periods between activities and measures to conserve energy, such as using a shower chair
- Importance of not smoking due to its irritant and vasoconstrictive effects
- Prescribed medications, including their use and effects.

37.4 Respiratory Failure

Many of the conditions discussed in this chapter and in Chapter 36, from pneumonia to acute respiratory distress syndrome (ARDS), can lead to respiratory failure. In **respiratory failure**, the lungs are unable to oxygenate the blood and remove carbon dioxide adequately to meet the body's needs, even at rest.

The Patient with Acute Respiratory Failure

Respiratory failure is not a disease but a consequence of severe respiratory dysfunction. It is often defined by arterial blood gas values. An arterial oxygen level (PaO_2) of lesser than 50 to 60 mmHg and an arterial carbon dioxide level ($PaCO_2$) of greater than 50 mmHg are generally accepted as indicators of respiratory failure. However, patients with advanced COPD may be alert and functional with blood gas values that would indicate respiratory failure in someone whose respiratory function was previously normal. In patients with COPD, respiratory failure is indicated by an acute drop in blood oxygen levels along with increased carbon dioxide levels.

Respiratory failure can result from inadequate alveolar ventilation (hypoventilation), impaired gas exchange, or a significant ventilation–perfusion mismatch. COPD is the most common cause of respiratory failure. Other lung diseases, chest injury, inhalation trauma, neuromuscular disorders, and cardiac conditions can also lead to respiratory failure. Selected causes of acute respiratory failure are identified in **Table 37.5**.

Pathophysiology

Respiratory failure may be characterized by primary hypoxemia or a combination of hypoxemia and hypercapnia (**Figure 37.7** ■). In hypoxemic respiratory failure, PaO_2 is significantly reduced, whereas $PaCO_2$ remains normal or is low due to stimulation of the respiratory center and tachypnea. Impaired diffusion across the alveolar-capillary membrane and a ventilation–perfusion mismatch can cause a drop in arterial oxygen levels that is more rapid than the rise in carbon dioxide. Metabolic acidosis results from tissue hypoxia. The increased work of breathing can eventually lead to respiratory muscle fatigue and hypoventilation.

Hypoventilation, or reduced movement of air into and out of the lung, causes carbon dioxide retention. With significant hypoventilation, the carbon dioxide level in the blood rises rapidly, leading to respiratory acidosis. Hypoxemia develops more slowly and responds readily to administration of oxygen unless gas exchange is also impaired.

In summary, hypoxemia without a corresponding rise in carbon dioxide levels indicates a failure of oxygenation; hypoxemia with hypercapnia is the result of lung hypoventilation.

Manifestations

The manifestations of respiratory failure are caused by hypoxemia and hypercapnia, as well as the underlying disease process. Hypoxemia causes dyspnea and neurologic symptoms such as restlessness, apprehension, impaired

Table 37.5 Selected Causes of Respiratory Failure

Types of Dysfunction	Examples
Impaired Ventilation	
Airway obstruction	■ Laryngospasm ■ Foreign body aspiration ■ Airway edema
Respiratory disease	■ Asthma ■ COPD
Neurologic causes	■ Spinal cord injury ■ Poliomyelitis ■ Guillain-Barré syndrome ■ Drug overdose ■ Stroke
Chest wall injury	■ Flail chest ■ Pneumothorax
Impaired Diffusion	
Alveolar disorders	■ Pneumonia ■ Pneumonitis ■ COPD
Pulmonary edema	■ Heart failure ■ Acute respiratory distress syndrome ■ Near-drowning
Ventilation–perfusion mismatch	■ Pulmonary embolism

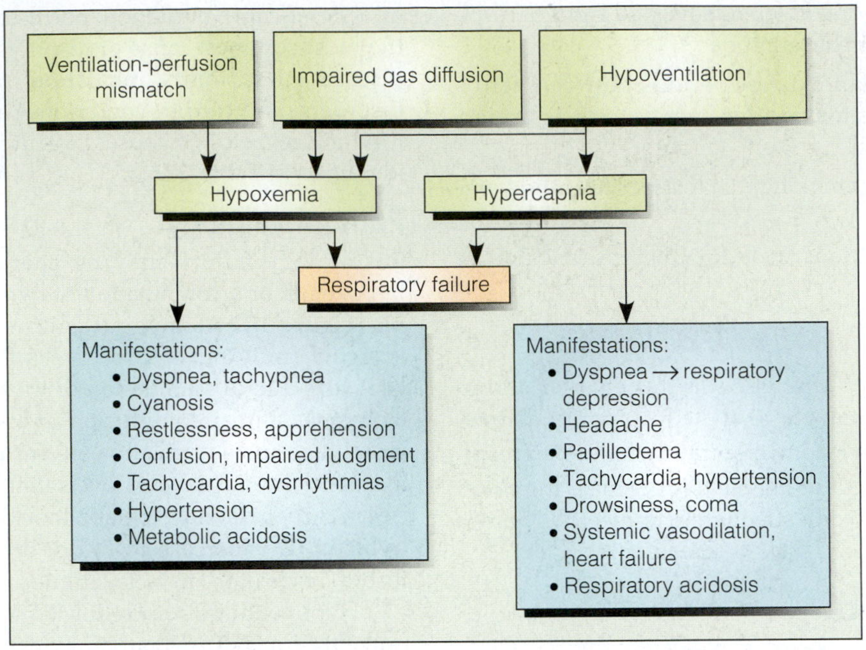
Ventilation-perfusion mismatch
Impaired gas diffusion
Hypoventilation
Hypoxemia
Hypercapnia
Respiratory failure
Manifestations:
• Dyspnea, tachypnea
• Cyanosis
• Restlessness, apprehension
• Confusion, impaired judgment
• Tachycardia, dysrhythmias
• Hypertension
• Metabolic acidosis
Manifestations:
• Dyspnea ⟶ respiratory depression
• Headache
• Papilledema
• Tachycardia, hypertension
• Drowsiness, coma
• Systemic vasodilation, heart failure
• Respiratory acidosis

Figure 37.7 ■ Causes and manifestations of respiratory failure.

judgment, and motor impairment. Tachycardia and hypertension develop as the cardiac output increases in an effort to bring more oxygen to the tissues. Cyanosis is present. As hypoxemia progresses, dysrhythmias, hypotension, and decreased cardiac output may develop.

Increased carbon dioxide levels depress CNS function and cause vasodilation. Dyspnea and headache are early signs. Other manifestations include peripheral and conjunctival vasodilation, papilledema, neuromuscular irritability, and decreased level of consciousness. As hypercapnia worsens, the respiratory center may be depressed, reducing dyspnea and slowing respirations. Increased carbon dioxide and hydrogen ion concentrations no longer stimulate the respiratory center; hypoxemia provides the primary active breathing stimulus. Administering oxygen without ventilatory support may further reduce the drive to breathe, leading to respiratory arrest.

The prognosis for acute respiratory failure varies, depending on the underlying disease process. Respiratory failure resulting from uncomplicated drug overdose generally resolves quickly without long-term effects. The course may be prolonged and the outcome less favorable when respiratory failure results from underlying lung disease.

Interprofessional Care

Treatment of respiratory failure focuses on correcting the underlying cause or disease, supporting ventilation, and correcting hypoxemia and hypercapnia. Care related to disorders that can precipitate respiratory failure is discussed in the sections specific to each disorder.

Diagnosis

Exhaled carbon dioxide and arterial blood gases are used to diagnose and monitor treatment of respiratory failure.

- ***Exhaled carbon dioxide ($ETCO_2$)*** is used to evaluate alveolar ventilation. The normal $ETCO_2$ is 35 to 45 mmHg; it is elevated when ventilation is inadequate and decreased when pulmonary perfusion is impaired.
- ***ABGs*** are also used to evaluate alveolar ventilation and gas exchange. With hypoxemic respiratory failure, the $PaCO_2$ may be normal, 35 to 45 mmHg, or even low due to tachypnea. A pH of < 7.35 and low bicarbonate levels indicate metabolic acidosis, typical of hypoxemic respiratory failure.

In respiratory failure due to hypoventilation, the $PaCO_2$ is elevated, usually greater than 50 mmHg. The pH is low due to respiratory acidosis. Acidosis develops rapidly in hypoxemia and hypercapnia because of increased acid production (metabolic) and decreased acid elimination (respiratory).

Medications

Drugs used in treating respiratory failure depend on the underlying cause of the failure and the need for intubation and mechanical ventilation.

Beta-adrenergic (sympathomimetic) or anticholinergic medications may be administered by inhalation to promote bronchodilation. If mechanical ventilation is required, the drugs may be given by nebulizer attached to the ventilator. Methylxanthine bronchodilators (theophylline derivatives) may be given intravenously. See Medication Administration 37.A and the asthma section earlier in this chapter for more information about bronchodilators and their nursing implications. Corticosteroids, administered by inhalation or intravenously, may be ordered to reduce airway edema. Antibiotics are given to treat any underlying infection.

Sedation and analgesia are often required during mechanical ventilation to decrease pain and anxiety. Benzodiazepines such as diazepam (Valium), lorazepam (Ativan), or midazolam (Versed) may be used for sedation and to inhibit the respiratory drive. Intravenous morphine or fentanyl provides analgesia and also inhibits the respiratory drive, allowing more effective mechanical ventilation. Occasionally, the patient's respiratory drive competes with the ventilator despite sedation, decreasing its effectiveness and increasing the work of breathing. A neuromuscular blocking agent in combination with sedation may be necessary to induce paralysis and suppress the ability to breathe. Nursing implications of neuromuscular blockers are described **Medication Administration 37.B.**

Oxygen Therapy

Oxygen is administered to reverse hypoxemia in acute respiratory failure. In general, the goal is to achieve an oxygen saturation of 90% or greater without oxygen toxicity. A PaO_2 of about 60 mmHg is usually adequate to meet the oxygen needs of body tissues. Higher levels do not significantly increase oxygen saturation and may lead to hypoventilation in patients with chronic hypercapnia. As little as 1 to 3 L of oxygen per nasal cannula or 28% oxygen per Venturi mask may correct hypoxemia in advanced COPD. Oxygen concentrations of 40 to 60% may be required when diffusion is impaired (e.g., in pneumonia or acute respiratory distress syndrome). High concentrations are used only for short periods to avoid oxygen toxicity. Both the oxygen concentration and duration of therapy contribute to oxygen toxicity. Continued high oxygen concentrations impair the synthesis of surfactant, reducing lung compliance (ease of inflation). Acute respiratory distress syndrome or absorption atelectasis may develop.

When respiratory failure is caused by hypoventilation or usual oxygen delivery systems do not correct hypoxemia, a tight-fitting mask to maintain *continuous positive airway pressure (CPAP)* may be used. CPAP increases lung volume, opening previously closed alveoli, improving ventilation of underventilated alveoli, and improving ventilation–perfusion relationships.

Airway Management

If the upper airway is obstructed or positive-pressure mechanical ventilation is necessary to correct hypoxemia and hypercapnia, an endotracheal tube that extends from the mouth or nose into the trachea is inserted (**Figure 37.8** ■). To maintain positive-pressure ventilation, the tube is cuffed with an air-filled or foam sac just above the end of the tube. When the cuff is inflated, it obstructs the upper airway, preventing air from escaping back into the nose or mouth. Excess pressure of the cuff can cause tissue ischemia and necrosis of the trachea. To minimize this risk, high-volume, low-pressure ("floppy") cuffs are used. Tubes with low-pressure cuffs may be left in place for 3 to 4 weeks.

A tracheostomy may be performed if long-term ventilatory support is required. Although a tracheostomy is more comfortable and easier to secure in place, complications such as cuff necrosis and increased risk of infection are associated with tracheostomy as well as endotracheal intubation. **Table 37.6** compares the advantages, disadvantages, and possible complications of the various types of endotracheal tubes and a tracheostomy.

Medication Administration 37.B

Neuromuscular Blockers

NONDEPOLARIZING NEUROMUSCULAR BLOCKERS

atracurium besylate (Tracrium)
cisatracurium (Nimbex)
pancuronium bromide (Pavulon)
rocuronium (Zemuron)

Nondepolarizing neuromuscular blockers competitively block the action of acetylcholine (ACh) at skeletal muscle receptors, preventing muscle depolarization and contraction. Complete muscle paralysis is achieved within minutes. Facial muscles are affected first, followed by muscles of the limbs, neck, and trunk. The muscles of respiration (the diaphragm and intercostal muscles) are the least sensitive to the effects of neuromuscular blockers and are paralyzed last. When the drug is discontinued or an antagonist is given, respiratory function is recovered first, as the muscle groups recover in reverse order.

Nursing Responsibilities

- Prior to administering, assess endotracheal tube placement and ensure effective mechanical ventilator function. The risk of hypoxemia and organ damage is significant if respiratory muscles are paralyzed without adequate ventilatory support in place.
- Administer the drug by slow intravenous injection and/or intravenous infusion as prescribed.
- Keep an acetylcholinesterase (AChE) inhibitor such as neostigmine (Prostigmin) available at the bedside to rapidly reverse neuromuscular effects, if needed.
- Administer morphine sulfate, diazepam (Valium), or other antianxiety agent or sedative as ordered. Neuromuscular blockers provide no sedation or pain relief; muscle paralysis produces extreme anxiety.
- Instill artificial tears every 2 to 4 hours.
- Suction oral cavity as needed to remove saliva.
- ***Never*** turn off ventilator alarms when administering neuromuscular blockers. Should the tubing become disconnected or unplugged or the patient is unable to breathe independently, call for help.
- Treat the patient as though awake and alert. Although unable to respond, mental function is unaffected.

Health Education for the Patient and Family

- Reassure that the ability to move and communicate will return when the drug is discontinued.
- Teach the family about the effects of the drug and the reason for its use. Explain that the patient can hear and understand what is going on.

Source: Adams, et al., 2017.

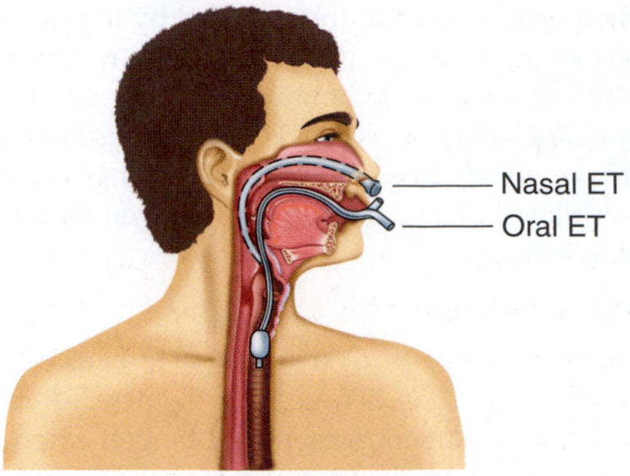
Nasal ET
Oral ET

Figure 37.8 ■ Illustration of nasal and oral endotracheal tubes.

When the patient is able to maintain effective respirations and ventilatory support is no longer required, the endotracheal tube is removed (*extubation*). Gag, cough, and swallow reflexes must be intact to prevent aspiration. After oxygenation and suctioning, the cuff is deflated and the tube removed. Humidified oxygen is provided immediately following removal. Close observation for respiratory distress is vital following extubation. Inspiratory stridor within the first 24 hours indicates laryngeal edema, which may necessitate reintubation. Sore throat and a hoarse voice are common after extubation. Oral intake is reinitiated slowly, with careful assessment of swallowing.

Mechanical Ventilation

Mechanical ventilation is indicated when alveolar ventilation is inadequate to maintain blood oxygen and carbon dioxide levels. Specific indications for mechanical ventilation include:

- Apnea or acute ventilatory failure
- Hypoxemia unresponsive to oxygen therapy alone
- Increased work of breathing with progressive patient fatigue.

The most common indicator for ventilation support is actual or potential respiratory muscle fatigue. Drug overdose, neural disorders, chest wall injury, and airway problems such as severe asthma or COPD can lead to acute ventilatory failure. Disorders that affect alveolar-capillary diffusion, such as pulmonary contusion, pneumonia, and ARDS, may necessitate mechanical ventilation to attain adequate oxygenation. Positive-pressure ventilation increases lung volume, helps redistribute fluid from the alveolar to the interstitial space, and helps reduce the oxygen demand caused by increased work of breathing.

Types of Ventilators. Two broad general classifications of mechanical ventilators are available. Negative-pressure ventilators create negative (subatmospheric) pressure externally to draw the chest outward and air into the lungs, mimicking spontaneous breathing. The iron lung, cuirass ventilator, and PulmoWrap are examples of negative-pressure ventilators. Patients with neuromuscular disorders (e.g., postpolio syndrome, amyotrophic lateral sclerosis) that interfere with the ability to maintain adequate ventilation are the primary users of negative-pressure ventilators. They may also be used by patients who require ventilator support during sleep.

Positive-pressure ventilators are more commonly used than negative-pressure ventilators, especially in treating acute respiratory failure (**Figure 37.9** ■). These ventilators push air into the lungs, rather than drawing it in like negative-pressure ventilators. Either invasive ventilation using an endotracheal tube or tracheostomy or noninvasive positive-pressure ventilation may be used. Increasingly, noninvasive techniques, which use a nasal or face mask, nasal plugs, or an oral mouthpiece, are used.

Several variables are used to trigger, cycle, and limit airflow with positive-pressure ventilators. The *trigger* prompts the ventilator to deliver a breath. The patient's inspiratory effort triggers *ventilator-assisted breaths. Ventilator-controlled breaths* are usually triggered by a preset time interval (e.g., a breath is delivered every 5 seconds for a rate of 12 breaths per minute). The ventilator *cycle*, or duration of inspiration,

Table 37.6 A Comparison of Endotracheal Tubes and Tracheostomy

	Advantages	Disadvantages	Potential Complications
Oral endotracheal tube	■ More easily inserted ■ Larger tube can be used, facilitating work of breathing, suctioning	■ More difficult to secure ■ Can be obstructed by biting ■ Communication and mouth care more difficult ■ Increased risk of lower respiratory infection	■ Obstruction or displacement ■ Pressure necrosis of lip ■ Tracheoesophageal fistula
Nasal endotracheal tube	■ More easily secured and stabilized ■ Well tolerated by patient ■ Facilitates communication and oral hygiene	■ Necessitates smaller tube, which may impede removal of secretions ■ Increased risk of lower respiratory infection	■ Obstruction or displacement ■ Pressure necrosis of nares ■ Obstruction of sinus drainage, possible sinusitis ■ Tracheoesophageal fistula
Tracheostomy	■ Easily secured and stabilized ■ Enables swallowing, speech, and oral hygiene ■ Avoids upper airway complications	■ Requires surgical incision ■ Increased risk of lower respiratory infection	■ Hemorrhage due to incision or vessel erosion by tube ■ Wound infection ■ Subcutaneous emphysema ■ Tracheoesophageal fistula ■ Tracheal infarction and stenosis

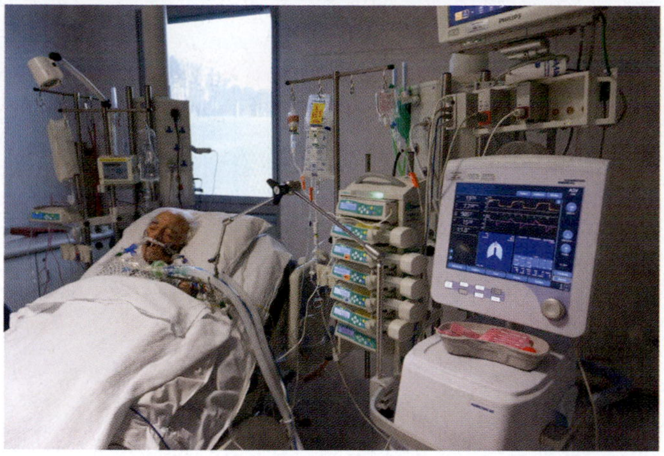

Figure 37.9 ■ A patient on a positive-pressure ventilator in an ICU.

can be limited by volume, pressure, flow, or time. *Volume-cycled ventilators* deliver air until a preset volume is delivered. *Pressure-cycled ventilators* cycle off when a preset pressure is achieved within the airways. *Flow-cycled ventilators* are cycled by a preset inspiratory flow rate, and *time-cycled ventilators* deliver air for a set time interval. Airflow delivered by the ventilator can also be limited by factors such as airway pressure (e.g., a volume-cycled ventilator can be set to immediately stop inspiratory flow if airway pressure exceeds a preset value).

Modes of Ventilation. A number of different *modes* or patterns of ventilation may be used with positive-pressure ventilators. The mode determines whether a breath is initiated by the patient or the ventilator and the pattern of airway support provided by the ventilator. Continuous positive airway pressure, bilevel airway pressure support, assist-control mode ventilation, synchronized intermittent mandatory ventilation, positive end-expiratory pressure, pressure support ventilation, and pressure-control ventilation are common modes and adjuncts of ventilation in use today (**Table 37.7**).

- ***Noninvasive ventilation (NIV)*** provides ventilator support using a tight-fitting face mask, thus avoiding intubation. Its primary use is to support patients with obstructive sleep apnea, neuromuscular disease, or impending respiratory failure (e.g., advanced COPD). NIV can also be used for patients in respiratory failure who refuse intubation. The degree of success varies, primarily limited by patient intolerance due to the physical and psychologic discomfort of wearing a mask when dyspneic. NIV tends to be more successful in patients without significant underlying lung disease (e.g., respiratory failure related to neuromuscular disease).
- ***Continuous positive airway pressure (CPAP)*** applies positive pressure to the airways of a spontaneously breathing patient. CPAP may be used with either endotracheal intubation or a tight-fitting face mask. All breathing is spontaneous (patient triggered) and pressure controlled. CPAP is used to help maintain open airways and alveoli, decreasing the work of breathing. *BiPAP* provides inspiratory positive airway pressure as well as airway support during expiration. BiPAP ventilation is primarily used at night with a tight-fitting mask (nasal, facial, or oral). Bilevel ventilation is a ventilator mode with high PEEP and low PEEP. Three modes of ventilation can be used with BiPAP: Spontaneous breathing (S); timed mode (T), in which pressure-supported breaths are delivered at a predetermined rate; and spontaneous/timed (S/T), in which the ventilator switches to timed mode if spontaneous breathing falls below a preset rate.
- ***Assist-control mode ventilation* (*ACMV* or *AC*)** is frequently used to initiate mechanical ventilation and when the patient is at risk for respiratory arrest (e.g., overdose or head injury). Assisted breaths are triggered by inspiratory effort; however, if the respiratory rate falls below a preset number (e.g., 14 per minute), ventilator-controlled breaths are delivered. All breaths, assisted and controlled, are delivered at a specific tidal volume or pressure and inspiratory flow rate.
- ***Synchronized intermittent mandatory ventilation (SIMV)*** allows the patient to breathe spontaneously, without ventilator assistance, between delivered ventilator breaths. Mandatory or ventilator-controlled breaths are delivered at a preset rate, volume, and/or pressure, coordinated with the patient's inspiratory efforts. This mode of ventilation is used to support ventilation, to exercise respiratory muscles between ventilator-assisted breaths, and during the weaning process.
- ***Positive end-expiratory pressure (PEEP)*** requires intubation and can be applied to any of the previously described ventilator modes. With PEEP, a positive pressure is maintained in the airways during exhalation and between breaths. Keeping alveoli open between breaths improves ventilation–perfusion relationships and diffusion across the alveolar-capillary membrane. This reduces hypoxemia and allows use of lower percentages of inspired oxygen. PEEP is particularly useful for treating ARDS.
- ***Pressure support ventilation (PSV)*** delivers ventilator-assisted breaths when the patient initiates an inspiratory effort. The cycle is flow limited; inspiration is terminated when inspiratory airflow falls below a preset rate. This mode decreases the work of breathing. It can be used in combination with SIMV when the respiratory drive is depressed. Ventilatory support can be gradually withdrawn during weaning.
- ***Pressure-control ventilation (PCV),*** in contrast, controls pressure within the airways to reduce the risk of airway trauma (e.g., following thoracic surgery). Ventilation is time triggered and time cycled, but pressure is limited. The ventilator maintains a preset airway pressure throughout inspiration. Because all breaths are controlled by the ventilator, heavy sedation may be

Table 37.7 Modes of Positive-Pressure Ventilator Operation

Mode	Description	Pattern
Spontaneous breathing	Patient has full control of rate, tidal volume, pressures.	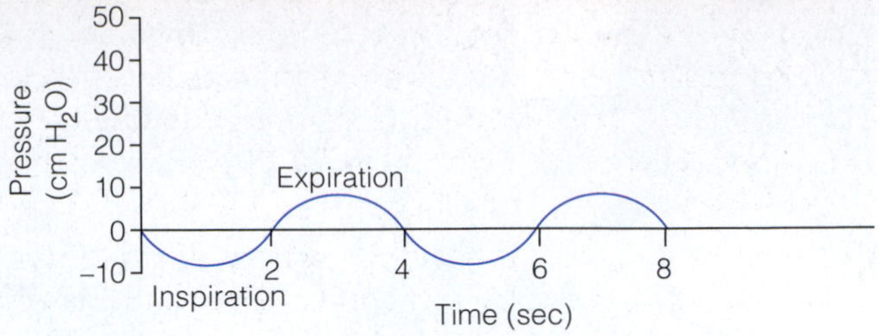Pressure (cm H_2O) 50 40 30 20 10 0 −10 Expiration Inspiration 2 4 6 8 Time (sec)
Assist-control mode ventilation (ACMV)	Patient can trigger ventilator to deliver breaths at preset volume or pressure and inspiratory flow rate; breaths will be delivered at preset rate if patient does not initiate.	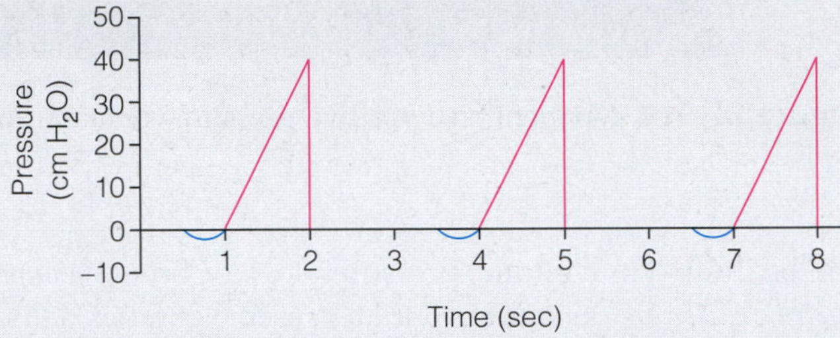Pressure (cm H_2O) 50 40 30 20 10 0 −10 1 2 3 4 5 6 7 8 Time (sec)
Synchronized intermittent mandatory ventilation (SIMV)	Mandatory breaths delivered by ventilator are synchronized with patient's inspiratory effort.	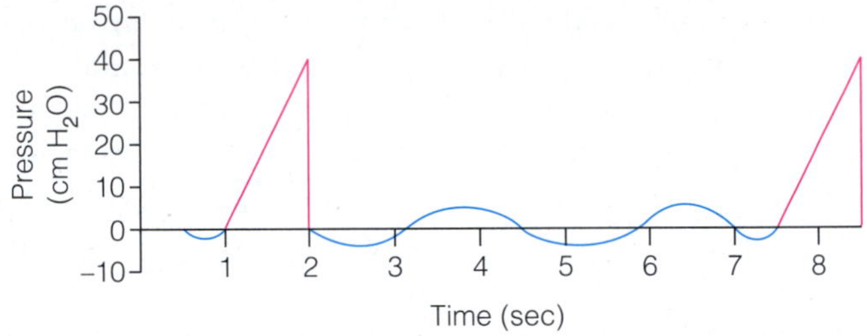Pressure (cm H_2O) 50 40 30 20 10 0 −10 1 2 3 4 5 6 7 8 Time (sec)
Continuous positive airway pressure (CPAP)	Positive pressure is maintained in airways; all breaths are spontaneous.	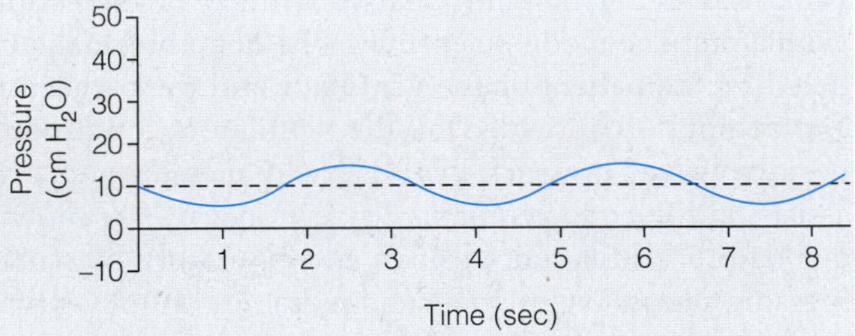Pressure (cm H_2O) 50 40 30 20 10 0 −10 1 2 3 4 5 6 7 8 Time (sec)
Positive end-expiratory pressure (PEEP)	Used in conjunction with other ventilator modes; positive airway pressure is maintained throughout respiratory cycle.	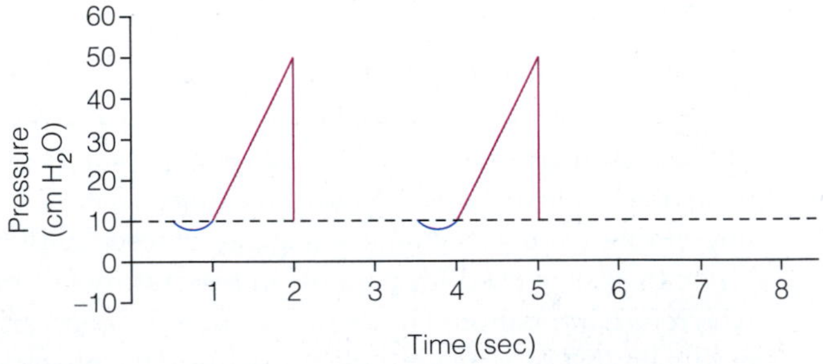Pressure (cm H_2O) 60 50 40 30 20 10 0 −10 1 2 3 4 5 6 7 8 Time (sec)
Pressure support ventilation (PSV)	Pressurized inspiratory flow supports the patient's inspiratory effort, decreasing the work of breathing.	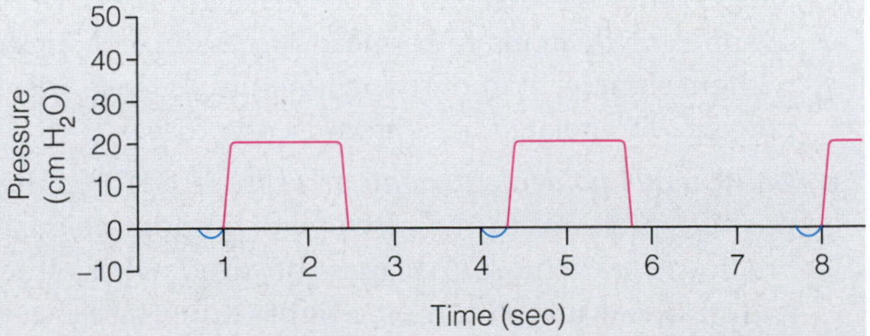Pressure (cm H_2O) 50 40 30 20 10 0 −10 1 2 3 4 5 6 7 8 Time (sec)

required to prevent competition between inspiratory effort and ventilator control.

- ***Independent lung ventilation*** provides separate ventilation for each lung. Indications include unilateral lung disease. It can be used after lung transplantation to address pulmonary pressure differences between the native lung and allograft. It requires a double-lumen endotracheal tube and two ventilators. Patients may require heavy sedation.
- ***High-frequency ventilation*** provides small gas volumes delivered at a rapid rate. It is indicated in patients who are hemodynamically unstable and intolerant of conventional MV. Use requires sedation and possibly pharmacologic paralysis (Perrin & MacLeod, 2012).

Ventilator Settings. In addition to choosing the mode of ventilation, other parameters are set to meet individual patient needs when positive-pressure ventilation is used (**Table 37.8**).

For most adult patients, the rate is initially set between 12 and 15 breaths per minute. With ACMV or SIMV, the patient's respiratory rate is often higher than the ventilator setting due to spontaneous breathing. Exhaled carbon dioxide ($ETCO_2$) or the $PaCO_2$ may be used to determine the rate. A $PaCO_2$ lesser than 35 mmHg indicates hyperventilation and respiratory alkalosis; the set rate is reduced. A $PaCO_2$ greater than 45 mmHg or an $ETCO_2$ greater than 45 mmHg indicates hypoventilation and a need to increase the rate.

The tidal volume setting controls the amount of gas delivered with each ventilator breath. The normal adult tidal volume at rest is about 7 mL/kg of body weight, or 400 to 550 mL. The tidal volume delivered by mechanical ventilation is slightly higher (500 to 750 mL) to compensate for tubing dead space. Higher tidal volumes can cause lung tissue trauma.

The percentage of oxygen delivered with ventilator breaths is adjusted to maintain the oxygen saturation and PaO_2 within acceptable ranges. Because prolonged delivery of high oxygen concentrations increases the risk of oxygen toxicity and pulmonary fibrosis, the FIO_2 is set at the lowest possible level for adequate tissue oxygenation. For most patients, the goal is to maintain an oxygen saturation greater than 90%. Lower oxygen saturation levels may be appropriate for patients with long-standing COPD.

Complications. Although endotracheal intubation and mechanical ventilation can be lifesaving in respiratory failure, they are not without risk. Improper endotracheal tube placement or advancement of the tube into a mainstem bronchus can result in ventilation of one lung only. The inflated lung becomes overdistended and traumatized, and the uninflated lung develops atelectasis. In noninvasive ventilation, associated complications include gastric dilation, aspiration, facial skin necrosis, drying of the eyes and mucous membranes, stress, and claustrophobia.

- ***Ventilator-associated pneumonia.*** Infection is a significant risk associated with intubation and mechanical ventilation. Normal upper respiratory tract defense mechanisms are bypassed, with loss of air humidification and trapping of pathogens. Oral secretions and gastric contents can enter the respiratory tree through the open epiglottis. Frequent, meticulous oral hygiene is vital in preventing ventilator-associated pneumonia. Often the cough reflex is inhibited or impaired by the underlying disease process and the continued presence of the endotracheal tube. Even when strict asepsis is used for suctioning and other respiratory procedures, the lower airways are contaminated within 24 hours of intubation. Secretions often become thick and tenacious, increasing the risk of atelectasis.
- ***Barotrauma*** (also called *volutrauma*) is lung injury due to alveolar overdistention. Both the volume of delivered gas and the pressures under which it is delivered can contribute to barotraumas. As a result, overdistended alveoli rupture, allowing air to escape into the pulmonary interstitial spaces and the mediastinum, pleural space, and other tissues. Subcutaneous emphysema, pneumothorax, and pneumomediastinum are possible results of barotrauma. *Subcutaneous emphysema,* or air in the subcutaneous tissue, causes tissue swelling of the chest, neck, and face. A "crackling" or air-bubble-popping sensation is felt on palpation of subcutaneous emphysema. Swelling may be massive. Once the cause is corrected, the air is gradually reabsorbed over weeks.
- ***Pneumothorax*** is identified by signs of unequal chest expansion, a sudden loss or significant decrease in breath sounds on the affected side, and a hyperresonant percussion tone. Rapid chest tube insertion is necessary to prevent tension pneumothorax and cardiovascular compromise.

Table 37.8 Ventilator Settings

Parameter	Description
Rate (*f*)	Number of ventilator-delivered breaths per minute; usually 12 to 15 in adults using ACMV, may be lower in SIMV
Tidal volume (V_t)	Amount of gas delivered with each ventilator breath; usually 8 to 10 mL/kg of body weight
Oxygen concentration (FIO_2)	Percentage of oxygen delivered with ventilator breaths; can be set between 21 (room air) and 100%
I:E ratio	Duration of inspiration to expiration; usually 1:2 to 1:1.5
Flow rate	Speed at which air is delivered
Sensitivity	Effort required by patient to initiate a ventilator-assisted breath
Pressure limit	Maximal pressure within airways that will terminate a ventilator breath

- *Pneumomediastinum* is the presence of air in the mediastinum, the space between the lungs that contains the heart, great vessels, trachea, and esophagus. Air in the mediastinal space can interfere with the function of all these organs and lead to such complications as pneumopericardium (air in the pericardial sac). Pneumomediastinum may have few manifestations, but the chest x-ray shows widening of the mediastinal space.
- ***Cardiovascular effects.*** Positive-pressure ventilation increases intrathoracic pressure, which can interfere with venous return to the heart and ventricular filling. As a result, cardiac output falls. Use of PEEP increases the effects of mechanical ventilation on cardiac output. The decreased cardiac output can affect liver and kidney function secondarily.
- ***Gastrointestinal complications*** are commonly associated with prolonged mechanical ventilation. Stress ulcers (erosive gastritis) may develop, leading to painless gastrointestinal hemorrhage. Histamine H_2-receptor blockers or sucralfate are often used to prevent stress ulcers. Air leaks around the endotracheal tube can cause gastric distention; a nasogastric tube is often inserted to prevent vomiting. Sedation and other medications used during mechanical ventilation can slow intestinal motility, leading to constipation.

Nutrition and Fluids. Attention must also be paid to fluid and electrolyte status and adequate nutrition. Mechanical ventilation promotes sodium and water retention due to its effects on cardiac output. Renal perfusion is decreased, stimulating the renin–angiotensin–aldosterone system to retain sodium and water. A Swan-Ganz catheter is often inserted to monitor pulmonary artery pressures and cardiac output. An arterial line allows repeated blood gas analysis and continuous arterial pressure monitoring. Serum electrolytes are drawn frequently, and intake, output, and daily weight are carefully monitored.

Enteral or parenteral nutrition is provided during mechanical ventilation because the endotracheal tube prohibits eating. A nasogastric, gastrostomy, or jejunostomy feeding tube is placed for enteral nutrition. A jejunostomy tube may be used to reduce the risk of regurgitation and aspiration.

Weaning. The process of removing ventilator support and reestablishing spontaneous, independent respirations is called **weaning**. Weaning begins only after the underlying process causing respiratory failure has been corrected or stabilized. The process and time required for weaning depend on factors such as preexisting lung condition, duration of mechanical ventilation, and the patient's general condition, both physical and psychologic. In all cases, the vital signs, respiratory rate, extent of dyspnea, blood gases, and clinical status are used to evaluate weaning and its progress.

Following a brief period of mechanical ventilation, T-piece or CPAP may be used for weaning. In T-piece weaning, the ventilator is removed for brief periods during which oxygen is delivered using a T-piece (**Figure 37.10** ■). The duration of periods off the ventilator is gradually increased until the patient can maintain adequate independent respirations for several hours. Vital signs, oxygen saturation, $ETCO_2$, and PaO_2 are carefully monitored during the process. The patient is placed back on the ventilator at previous settings if signs of respiratory distress develop. When mechanical ventilation is no longer needed, the endotracheal tube is removed. CPAP weaning follows a similar process, with trials of spontaneous breathing supported by the ventilator in CPAP mode.

SIMV and PSV are used for weaning when the duration of mechanical ventilation has been longer and reconditioning of respiratory muscles is needed. When SIMV is used, the number of mandatory ventilator-assisted breaths is gradually decreased as ABGs, $ETCO_2$, and the respiratory rate are monitored. When the patient is able to tolerate SIMV at 4 breaths per minute without rest periods of greater ventilatory support, CPAP or T-piece weaning is attempted prior to extubation.

Weaning is the primary use for PSV. Initially, PSV is set slightly below the peak inspiratory pressures required during volume-cycled ventilation. Pressure support levels are gradually decreased, often in a cyclic pattern of periods of minimal support alternating with higher support to recondition respiratory muscles. When the PSV level is just enough to overcome endotracheal tube resistance, support is discontinued and the patient is extubated.

When an illness is terminal or irreversible with a poor prognosis, terminal weaning may be requested by the patient or family. **Terminal weaning** is the gradual withdrawal of mechanical ventilation when survival without assisted ventilation is not expected. Unlike weaning when recovery is expected, which usually occurs in an intensive care unit (ICU), the patient is moved to a quiet medical-surgical or hospice room or even home prior to initiating terminal weaning. Family members are encouraged to remain with the patient throughout the process. If possible, decisions about sedation and analgesia prior to and during weaning are made with the patient, as are decisions about hydration and nutritional support following weaning. Ventilator support is withdrawn using the same modes described earlier (SIMV, PSV). Analgesia and sedation are given to promote comfort during weaning.

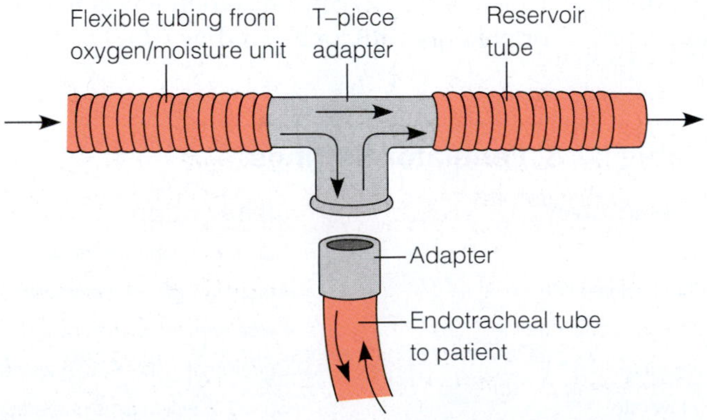
Flexible tubing from oxygen/moisture unit
T–piece adapter
Reservoir tube
Adapter
Endotracheal tube to patient

Figure 37.10 ■ A T-piece, or "blow-by" unit, for weaning from mechanical ventilation.

Nursing Care

Assessment

See the Manifestations and Interprofessional Care sections for the assessment of the patient with respiratory failure.

Focused assessment data related to respiratory failure includes:

- ***Health history:*** Current manifestations, their duration, and identified precipitating factors (may need to be obtained from family members if mental status is affected); history of previous episodes; chronic diseases such as COPD, occupational lung disease; current medications
- ***Physical assessment:*** Level of consciousness, mental status; vital signs; color and oxygen saturation; respiratory assessment including rate and depth, use of accessory muscles, respiratory excursion, auscultation; cardiovascular assessment including heart rate and sounds, neck vein distention, peripheral pulses, evidence of clubbing
- ***Laboratory data:*** ABGs, chest x-ray, pulmonary artery pressure and wedge pressure readings, cardiac output.

SAFETY ALERT: Frequently assess respiratory rate, chest movement, lung sounds, oxygen saturation, $ETCO_2$, and ABGs. Intubation and mechanical ventilation do not ensure adequate oxygenation and ventilation. Displacement of the endotracheal tube or obstruction by respiratory secretions impairs ventilation. ■

Priorities of Care

Collaborate with the interprofessional team to ensure adequate treatment of the underlying process while providing care that supports the physical and psychologic responses to the disorder is a priority of nursing care.

Diagnoses, Interventions, and Outcomes

Patients in respiratory failure are often unstable and critically ill. They require both intensive medical care and intensive nursing care. Priority nursing needs relate to maintaining ventilation and a patent airway. Perhaps less obvious, but no less critical, nursing care needs relate to preventing injury and managing anxiety.

Promote Adequate Ventilation. In acute respiratory failure, fatigue from the work of breathing may impair the ability to maintain adequate ventilation. This is a concern both prior to initiation of mechanical ventilation and during the weaning process.

Expected Outcome: Patient will maintain arterial blood gases within safe parameters while effectively maintaining airway and secretion mobilization.

The nurse will:

- Assess and document respiratory rate, vital signs, and oxygen saturation every 15 to 30 minutes. *Close monitoring is vital to detect early signs of increasing respiratory distress and inability to sustain adequate breathing.*
- Promptly report worsening arterial blood gases and oxygen saturation levels. *Close assessment of these values allows timely intervention as needed.*
- Administer oxygen as ordered, monitoring response. Observe closely for respiratory depression, especially in the patient with COPD. *Oxygen administration reduces the hypoxemic respiratory drive. Chronically high* $PaCO_2$ *levels depress the respiratory center; hypoxemia may provide the only respiratory drive.*
- Place in Fowler or high-Fowler position. *Sitting positions decrease pressure on the diaphragm and chest, improving lung ventilation and decreasing the work of breathing.*
- Minimize activities and energy expenditures by assisting with ADLs, spacing procedures and activities, and allowing uninterrupted rest periods. *Rest is vital to reduce oxygen and energy demands.*
- Avoid sedatives and respiratory depressant drugs unless mechanically ventilated. *These medications can further depress the respiratory drive, worsening respiratory failure.*
- Prepare for endotracheal intubation and mechanical ventilation:
  a. Obtain an intubation tray with a selection of sterile endotracheal tubes and a laryngoscope with a variety of adult blades.
  b. Check laryngoscope lamp; replace battery pack or bulb as needed.
  c. Set up for endotracheal suction, bringing continuous suction head, container, tubing, sterile catheter and glove kits, and sterile normal saline to the bedside.
  d. Notify respiratory therapy to set up the ventilator.
  e. Notify radiology that a portable chest x-ray will be needed on completion of intubation to verify correct placement of the endotracheal tube.

  Intubation and mechanical ventilation may be required to maintain ventilation and gas exchange.
- Explain the procedure and its purpose to the patient and family, providing reassurance that this is a temporary measure to reduce the work of breathing and allow rest. Alert that talking is not possible while the endotracheal tube is in place, and establish a means of communication. *Thorough explanation is important to relieve anxiety.*

SAFETY ALERT: Promptly report signs of respiratory distress, including tachypnea, tachycardia, nasal flaring, use of accessory muscles, intercostal retractions, cyanosis, increasing restlessness, anxiety, or decreased level of consciousness. These may be early manifestations of respiratory failure and inability to maintain ventilatory effort. ■

Promote Airway Clearance and Patency. Ineffective airway clearance may either cause respiratory failure or occur as a result of interventions. Impaired ventilation frequently leads to acute respiratory failure, particularly in patients with COPD or asthma. Chest trauma can also impair airway patency as a result of pulmonary contusion and ineffective cough. Although intubation and mechanical ventilation can be lifesaving measures, they also increase the risk of respiratory infection and ineffective secretion management.

Expected Outcome: Patient will use techniques to promote airway clearance such as coughing and deep breathing when able. Patient's airway clearance will be maintained by the nurse during mechanical ventilation via suctioning as needed.

The nurse will:

- Suction as needed to maintain a patent airway. Indicators for suctioning include crackles and rhonchi on auscultation, frequent coughing or setting off the high-pressure alarm, and increasing restlessness or anxiety. *Although patients with a tracheostomy can usually cough up secretions, the length and diameter of endotracheal tubes make this extremely difficult. Even with humidification, secretions often become thick and tenacious, further inhibiting their removal.*
- Obtain sputum for culture if it appears purulent or is odorous. *Culture is necessary to identify pathogens and guide antibiotic therapy.*
- Perform percussion, vibration, and postural drainage as ordered. *These techniques help loosen secretions and move them into larger airways for removal by coughing or suctioning.*
- Firmly secure endotracheal or tracheostomy tube. Provide adequate slack on ventilator tubing to prevent tension on the tube when turning, positioning, or transferring to chair or stretcher. If necessary, loosely restrain hands. *These measures are important to ensure proper airway placement and prevent its inadvertent removal.*
- Assess fluid balance and maintain adequate hydration. *Adequate hydration helps liquefy secretions.*

SAFETY ALERT: Evaluate endotracheal tube cuff pressure by measurement (should have no more than 20 to 25 mmHg of pressure) or by auscultating the suprasternal notch for a hissing sound at the end of inspiration. The minimum effective cuff pressure to maintain alveolar ventilation is used to reduce the risk of tracheal ischemia and necrosis. ■

Reduce Risk for Injury. Many factors increase the risk for injury in acute respiratory failure. Hypoxemia and hypercapnia affect the level of consciousness and may impair mental status. Endotracheal intubation and mechanical ventilation carry risks of tracheal damage and trauma to the lungs. Neuromuscular blockade, if used, presents a significant risk for injury because the patient is unable to breathe spontaneously, communicate, and move.

Expected Outcome: Patient will demonstrate understanding of plan to promote safe environment related to therapeutic needs (endotracheal tube, medications) as appropriate for patient condition.

The nurse will:

- Assess frequently, noting the following:
  a. Neurologic: Level of consciousness, orientation, and awareness
  b. Tissue integrity: Condition of mucosa of mouth and nose, skin, and extremities
  c. Respiratory: Lung sounds, chest excursion, and ventilator pressures
  d. Cardiovascular: Vital signs, skin color, capillary refill, and peripheral pulses
  e. Gastrointestinal: Bowel sounds; test gastric secretions and feces for occult blood
  f. Genitourinary: Urine output, daily weight

  Complications associated with respiratory failure and mechanical ventilation can affect many body systems. Frequent assessment allows early detection and intervention.
- Report condition changes such as increasing air leak around the cuff and decreased breath sounds or chest movement. *These may be manifestations of a complication of intubation and ventilation, such as tracheal necrosis, displacement of the endotracheal tube into the right mainstem bronchus, pneumothorax, or atelectasis.*
- Turn and reposition frequently, taking care to stabilize endotracheal tube during movement. *Repositioning helps maintain tissue perfusion and prevent skin and tissue breakdown.*
- Keep skin and linens clean, dry, and wrinkle free. Protect pressure areas with padding, egg crate, or heal and elbow protectors. *The patient may not be able to perceive and report pain or move voluntarily to reduce pressure, necessitating excellent skin care and potential specialty bed use.*
- Perform passive ROM exercises every 4 to 8 hours. *These exercises maintain joint flexibility and help prevent contractures associated with long-term immobility.*
- Keep side rails up and use soft restraints as needed. *These safety measures are important to prevent falls, inadvertent disconnection of the ventilator, or dislodging of the endotracheal tube.*
- Administer histamine H_2-blockers and sucralfate as ordered. *Stress gastritis and possible gastrointestinal hemorrhage are common, preventable complications of mechanical ventilation.*

SAFETY ALERT: Do not bypass or turn off any ventilator alarms. The intubated patient is unable to communicate verbally and cannot call for help. If neuromuscular blockers are used, the patient is also unable to breathe without ventilator support. ■

Reduce Anxiety. Critical illness creates anxiety for any patient. In acute respiratory failure, this anxiety is compounded by the presence of an endotracheal tube or tracheostomy, mechanical ventilator, numerous monitors and equipment, and, potentially, neuromuscular blockade and paralysis of voluntary muscles. Fear of continued dependence on the mechanical ventilator and inability to return to a normal life may compound this anxiety.

Expected Outcome: Patient will control anxiety as evidenced by verbalized decrease in subjective distress.

The nurse will:

- Frequently monitor anxiety level. *High levels of anxiety increase oxygen use and often interfere with the ability to work with the respirator. This can increase hypoxemia and further increase anxiety; intervention is necessary to break this cycle.*

- Remain with the patient as much as possible. *The frequent and continuing presence of a caregiver provides reassurance that help is readily available.*
- Explain all monitors, procedures, unusual sounds, and machinery. *Understanding of the environment and various sounds and alarms reduces anxiety.*
- Provide a simple means of communication, such as a tablet or other communication-assistive device. If neuromuscular blockade is used, use methods such as looking to the right for "yes" and left for "no." Reassure that endotracheal tube removal restores the ability to speak. *The inability to speak and call out for help is frightening for the patient. Providing an alternate means of communication helps reduce anxiety.*
- Encourage frequent family visits, especially if the time of visitations is being limited. Encourage family participation in care. *Family visits help reduce anxiety and feelings of abandonment. Allowing family members to participate in care helps reduce their anxiety as well.*
- Explain to the family that the patient can hear and understand. Emphasize the importance of talking to the patient, not over or about the patient. *The family may not understand that the patient may be mentally alert although unable to respond. Talking to the patient about everyday things reduces the patient's sense of isolation and fear.*
- Provide distraction with radio or television, if allowed. *Distraction helps reduce the focus on machines and unusual sounds of monitors and alarms.*
- Attend to physical needs promptly and completely. *This provides reassurance that needs will be met even though the patient is unable to ask for assistance.*
- Reassure that intubation and mechanical ventilation are temporary measures to allow the lungs to rest and heal. Reinforce that the patient will be able to breathe independently again. *The patient may fear continued dependence on mechanical ventilation.*

SAFETY ALERT: Provide sedation and antianxiety medications as needed, especially when neuromuscular blockade is used. Although neuromuscular blockade paralyzes voluntary muscles, the level of consciousness is unimpaired. ■

Delegating Nursing Care Activities

As appropriate and allowed by the designated duties and responsibilities of unlicensed assistive personnel, the nurse may delegate nursing care activities such as measuring vital signs, encouraging oral or enteral fluid intake, and providing skin care.

Transitions of Care

Education is a primary strategy to prevent respiratory failure. Teach all patients and the public about the risks of smoking, water safety, the value of a working smoke detector, and measures to prevent smoke inhalation during a fire. Discuss the importance of pneumococcal vaccine and annual influenza immunizations for people who are at high risk, including those over age 65 and people with chronic diseases. Teach patients with spinal cord injury or neuromuscular disease to use effective breathing and coughing techniques to maintain airway patency. Work with patients addicted to narcotic drugs to attain and maintain drug-free status. Teach patients with COPD about measures to reduce their risk of respiratory infection and symptoms to report to the physician.

Prior to hospital discharge, teach the patient and family about the following topics:

- Factors that precipitated respiratory failure and measures to prevent it in the future (e.g., the impact of respiratory irritants on compromised lungs)
- Measures to prevent future episodes such as remaining indoors with an air filter or air conditioning when pollution levels are high, obtaining influenza and pneumonia immunizations, and avoiding exposure to cigarette smoke
- Effective coughing and pulmonary hygiene measures such as percussion, vibration, and postural drainage.

Acute respiratory failure resulting from an acute insult such as pneumonia or near-drowning often resolves with few long-term sequelae. When respiratory failure results from an underlying disease such as COPD, the prognosis is less optimistic. Patients with end-stage COPD may have repeated episodes of respiratory failure, with a gradual loss of respiratory function and reserve. These patients may choose terminal weaning rather than a future of increasing disability. Discuss what to expect during the terminal weaning process with the patient and family. Discuss use of sedation prior to and during the weaning process. Explain that medications are used to reduce respiratory distress and dyspnea during weaning. Assure the patient and family that nursing support is continuously available during the weaning process and that family and other supporters such as clergy are allowed to remain with the patient.

The Patient with Acute Respiratory Distress Syndrome

Acute respiratory distress syndrome (ARDS) is characterized by noncardiac pulmonary edema and progressive refractory hypoxemia. First identified in 1967, ARDS has been known by various names, such as shock lung and adult hyaline membrane disease. It is widely recognized as a severe form of acute respiratory failure. Approximately 190,000 Americans experience ARDS each year, with most of them recovering near-normal lung function within 6 months. Despite this, the mortality rate associated with ARDS is about 40% and is often due to multiple organ system dysfunction related to ineffective tissue oxygenation (NHLBI, 2012).

Although the exact cause of ARDS is unclear, it is known that ARDS does not occur as a primary process but may follow a number of diverse conditions producing direct or indirect lung injury (**Table 37.9**). Patients who develop ARDS as a complication of an acute lung injury or condition are more likely to fully recover than patients with chronic conditions (NHLBI, 2012).

Table 37.9 Conditions Associated with the Development of ARDS

Condition	Examples
Shock	Hemorrhagic shock, septic shock
Inhalation injuries	Aspiration of gastric contents, smoke and toxic gases, near-drowning, oxygen toxicity
Infections	Gram-negative sepsis, viral pneumonias, *Pneumocystis jiroveci* pneumonia, miliary tuberculosis
Drug overdose	Heroin, methadone, propoxyphene, aspirin
Trauma	Burns, head injury, lung contusion, fat emboli
Other	Disseminated intravascular coagulation (DIC), pancreatitis, uremia, amniotic fluid and air emboli, multiple transfusions, open heart surgery with cardiopulmonary bypass

Pathophysiology

The underlying pathology in ARDS is acute lung injury resulting from an unregulated systemic inflammatory response to acute injury or inflammation. Inflammatory cellular responses such as tumor necrosis factor (TNF), leukotrienes, macrophage inhibitory factor along with platelet sequestration and activation, as well as biochemical mediators, damage the alveolar-capillary membrane. This damage develops rapidly, often within 90 minutes of the systemic inflammatory response and within 24 hours of the initial insult (**Figure 37.11** ■). Damaged capillary membranes allow plasma and blood cells to escape into the interstitial space. Increased interstitial pressure and damage to the alveolar membrane allow fluid to enter the alveoli. Within the alveolus, the fluid dilutes and inactivates surfactant. Surfactant-producing cells are damaged by the inflammatory process, leading to a deficit of surfactant, increased alveolar surface tension, and alveolar collapse with atelectasis. The lungs become less compliant, and gas exchange is impaired. As the syndrome progresses, hyaline membranes form, further reducing gas exchange and compliance. Finally, fibrotic changes occur in the lungs. Intra-alveolar septa thicken, and alveolar surface area for gas exchange is reduced. Hypoxemia becomes refractory or resistant to improvement with supplemental oxygen, and the $PaCO_2$ rises as diffusion is further impaired. The Pathophysiology Illustrated feature shows the pathophysiology of ARDS.

As ARDS progresses, tissue hypoxia becomes significant and metabolic acidosis develops. Carbon dioxide exchange is impaired as well as oxygen exchange, leading to combined respiratory and metabolic acidosis. Sepsis and multiple organ system dysfunction of the kidneys, liver, gastrointestinal tract, CNS, and cardiovascular system are the leading causes of death in ARDS. If the process is halted before this occurs, the long-term prognosis for recovery is good.

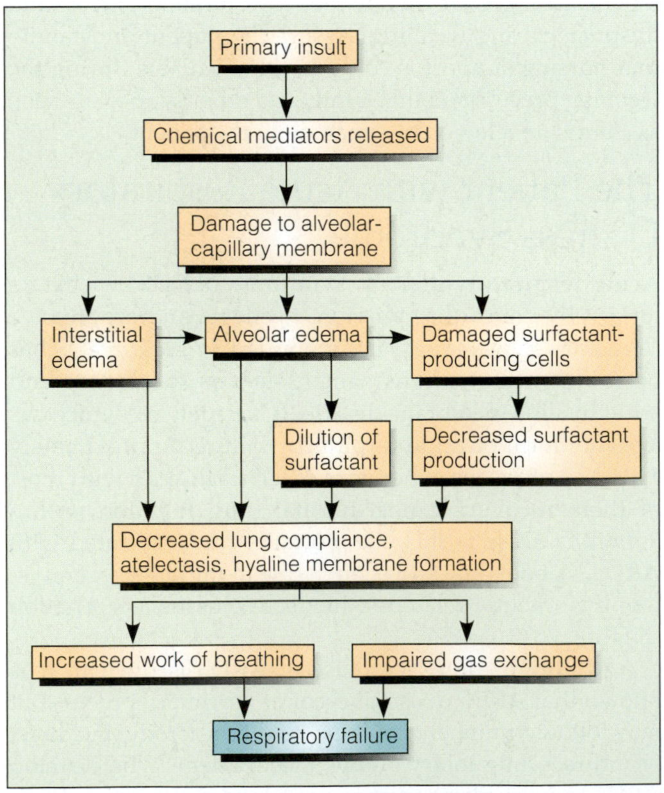

Primary insult
Chemical mediators released
Damage to alveolar-capillary membrane
Interstitial edema
Alveolar edema
Damaged surfactant-producing cells
Dilution of surfactant
Decreased surfactant production
Decreased lung compliance, atelectasis, hyaline membrane formation
Increased work of breathing
Impaired gas exchange
Respiratory failure

Figure 37.11 ■ The pathogenesis of ARDS.

Manifestations

Initial manifestations of ARDS typically develop 24 to 48 hours after the initial insult. Dyspnea, tachypnea, and anxiety are early manifestations. Progressive respiratory distress develops with increasing respiratory rate, intercostal retractions, and use of accessory muscles of respiration. Cyanosis develops that may not improve with oxygen administration. Breath sounds are initially clear, but crackles (rales) and rhonchi develop later. As respiratory failure progresses, mental status changes such as agitation, confusion, and lethargy occur.

Interprofessional Care

ARDS management is directed toward identifying and treating its underlying cause and providing aggressive respiratory support.

Diagnosis

Refractory hypoxemia (hypoxemia that does not improve with oxygen administration) is the hallmark of ARDS.

- ***ABGs*** initially show hypoxemia with a PaO_2 of < 60 mmHg and respiratory alkalosis due to tachypnea.
- ***Chest x-ray*** changes may not be evident for as long as 24 hours after the onset of ARDS. Diffuse infiltrates are seen initially, progressing to a "white-out" pattern. Chest *CT scan* provides a better illustration of the pattern of alveolar consolidation and atelectasis in ARDS.
- ***Pulmonary function testing*** shows decreased lung compliance with reduced vital capacity, minute volume, and functional vital capacity.
- ***Pulmonary artery pressure monitoring*** shows normal pressures in ARDS, helping distinguish ARDS from cardiogenic pulmonary edema.

Pathophysiology Illustrated
Acute Respiratory Distress Syndrome

Acute respiratory distress syndrome (ARDS) is a severe form of acute respiratory failure that occurs in response to pulmonary or systemic insults. ARDS is characterized by noncardiogenic pulmonary edema caused by inflammatory damage to alveolar and capillary walls. Many disorders may precipitate ARDS, although sepsis is the most common.

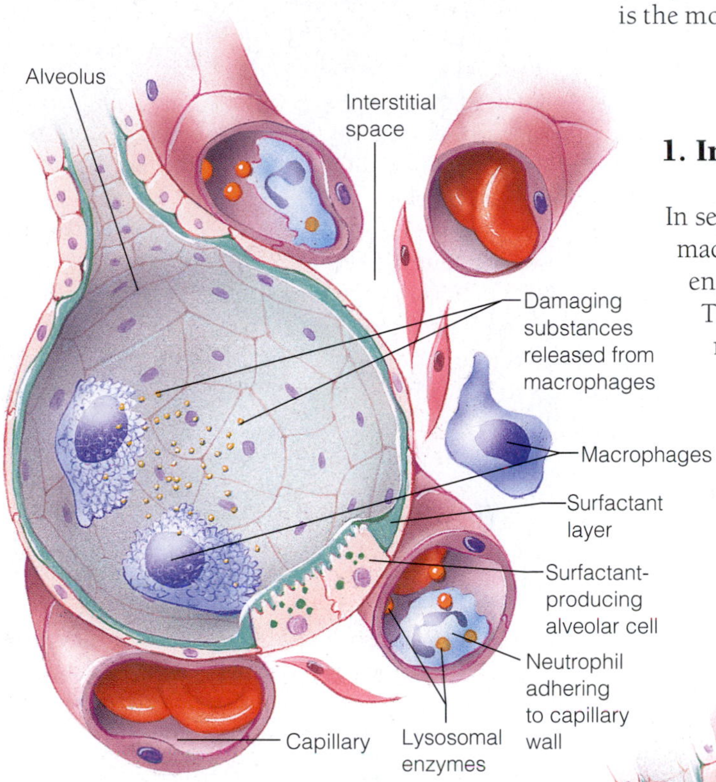
Alveolus
Interstitial space
Damaging substances released from macrophages
Macrophages
Surfactant layer
Surfactant-producing alveolar cell
Neutrophil adhering to capillary wall
Capillary
Lysosomal enzymes

1. Initiation of ARDS

In sepsis-induced ARDS, bacterial toxins cause macrophages and neutrophils to adhere to endothelial surfaces of the alveoli and capillaries. The macrophages release oxidants, inflammatory mediators, enzymes, and peptides that damage the capillary and alveolar walls. In response, neutrophils release lysosomal enzymes causing further damage.

2. Onset of Pulmonary Edema

The damaged capillary and alveolar walls become more permeable, allowing plasma, proteins, and erythrocytes to enter the interstitial space. As interstitial edema increases, pressure in the interstitial space rises and fluid leaks into alveoli. Plasma proteins accumulating in the interstitial space lower the osmotic gradient between the capillary and interstitial compartment. As a result, the balance is disrupted between the osmotic force that pulls fluid from the interstitial space into the capillaries and the normal hydrostatic pressure that pushes fluid out of the capillaries. This imbalance causes even more fluid to enter alveoli.

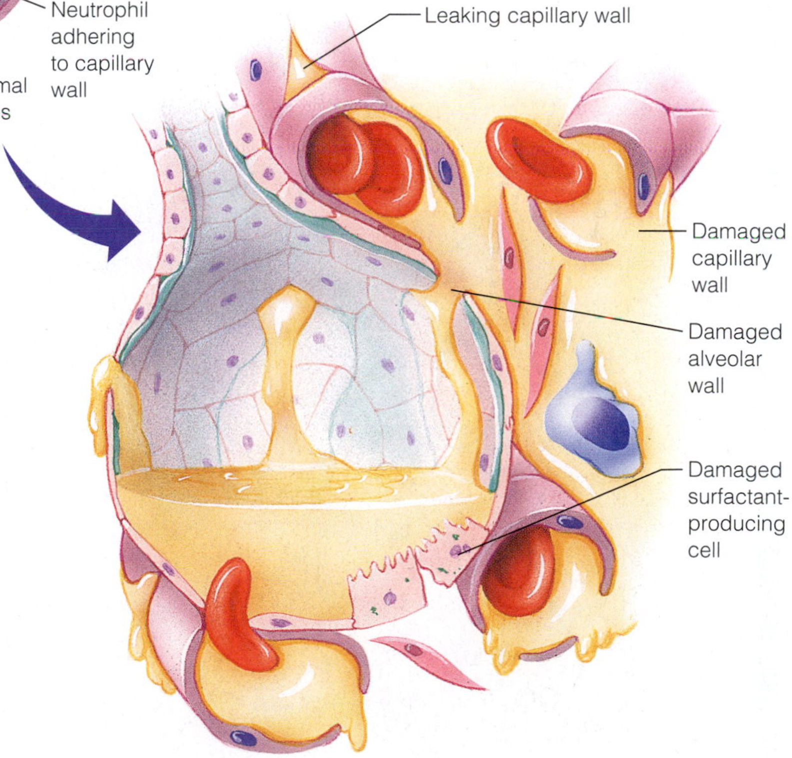
Leaking capillary wall
Damaged capillary wall
Damaged alveolar wall
Damaged surfactant-producing cell

(*continued*)

4. End-Stage ARDS

Fibrin and cell debris from necrotic cells combine to form hyaline membranes, which line the interior of the alveoli and further reduce alveolar compliance and gas exchange. Because carbon dioxide cannot diffuse across hyaline membranes, $PaCO_2$ levels now begin to rise while PaO_2 levels continue to fall. Rising $PaCO_2$ levels can lead to respiratory acidosis. Without respiratory support, respiratory failure will develop.
Even with aggressive treatment, almost 50% of clients with ARDS die.

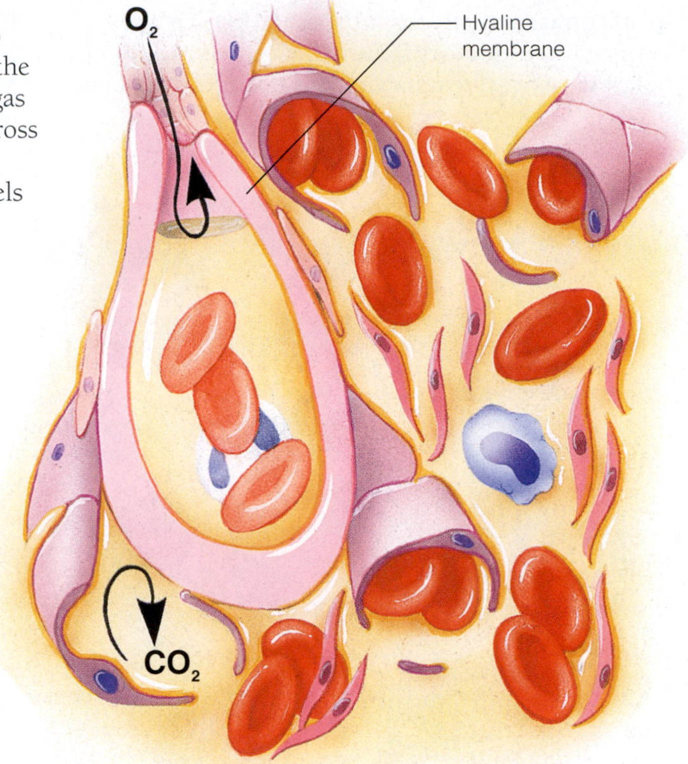
O2
Hyaline membrane
CO2

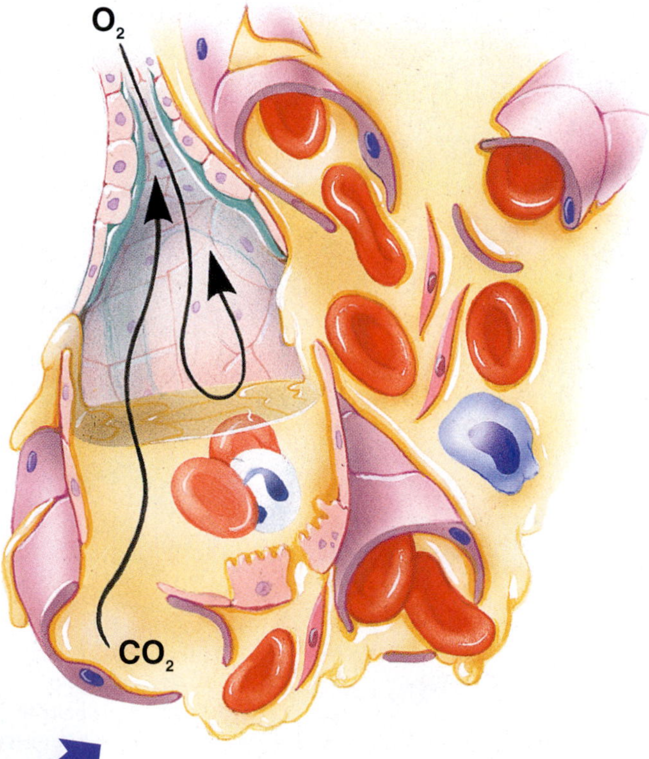
O2
CO2

3. Alveolar Collapse

Protein-rich fluid accumulates in the alveoli, inactivating surfactant and damaging type II alveolar cells that produce surfactant. (Surfactant is important in maintaining alveolar compliance—the ability of tissue to stretch or distend.) As active surfactant is lost, the alveoli stiffen and collapse, leading to atelectasis, which increases breathing effort.

Decreased alveolar compliance, atelectasis, and fluid-filled alveoli interfere with gas exchange across the alveolar-capillary membrane. Blood oxygen (PaO_2) levels fall. Because carbon dioxide diffuses more readily than oxygen, however, blood carbon dioxide ($PaCO_2$) levels also fall initially as tachypnea causes more CO_2 to be expired.

In addition to the hallmark refractory hypoxemia, healthcare providers may use the Berlin definition, which includes:

- Onset: < 7 days from the predisposing clinical insult
- Imaging: Bilateral opacities on chest x-ray or CT that is not fully explained by effusion, atelectasis, or nodules
- Noncardiac pulmonary edema: Respiratory failure without a cardiac problem or fluid overload
- Oxygen requirements: PaO_2/FiO_2 ratio with ≥5 cm H_2O positive end-expiratory pressure

  Mild ARDS: 201–300

  Moderate ARDS: 101–200

  Severe ARDS: < 100
- Any predisposing conditions? If none, an echocardiogram may be ordered to rule out cardiac problem.

Medications

Although there is no definitive drug therapy for ARDS, a number of medications may be used. Inhaled nitric oxide reduces intrapulmonary shunting and improves oxygenation by dilating blood vessels in better-ventilated areas of the lungs. Surfactant therapy may be prescribed. Surfactant is a complex mixture of phospholipids, neutral lipids, and proteins that forms a thin layer atop a thin layer of water on the inner surface of the alveolus, reducing the surface tension within the alveoli. Surface tension tends to pull the walls of the alveoli together, increasing the likelihood of collapse during exhalation. Surfactant, by reducing surface tension, helps maintain open alveoli, decreasing the work of breathing, improving compliance and gas exchange, and preventing atelectasis.

Interventions to block the inflammatory response are under investigation, such as using nonsteroidal anti-inflammatory agents and corticosteroids. Corticosteroids may be used late in the course of ARDS to improve oxygenation and lung mechanics when fibrotic changes occur.

Mechanical Ventilation

The mainstay of ARDS management is endotracheal intubation and mechanical ventilation. With ARDS, it is rarely possible to maintain adequate tissue oxygenation with oxygen therapy alone.

With mechanical ventilation, the FIO_2 is set at the lowest possible level to maintain a PaO_2 higher than 60 mmHg and oxygen saturation of approximately 90%. When the PaO_2 cannot be maintained with lesser than 50% inspired oxygen, there is a risk that oxygen toxicity will accentuate ARDS. Often it is necessary to use PEEP during mechanical ventilation settings to maintain blood and tissue oxygenation. Maintaining open airways and alveoli enhances gas diffusion and reduces ventilation–perfusion mismatch. PEEP decreases cardiac output and increases the risk of barotrauma, necessitating close monitoring. Either assist-control or SIMV may be used along with PEEP or CPAP in treating ARDS.

It is important to remember that mechanical ventilation does not cure ARDS; it simply supports respiratory function while the underlying problem is being identified and treated.

Treatments

The use of low-dose corticosteroids remains controversial in the treatment of ARDS. However, in a meta-analysis of research studies, low-dose corticosteroids were associated with improved mortality and morbidity without increased risk for adverse reactions (Lamontagne et al., 2010).

Atelectasis occurs frequently in dependent lung regions in ARDS. Prone positioning in conjunction with mechanical ventilation reduces the pressure of surrounding tissue on dependent regions and improves oxygenation.

Other management strategies include careful fluid replacement, attention to nutrition, treatment of any infection, and correction of the underlying condition. A Swan-Ganz line is sometimes placed to monitor pulmonary artery pressures and cardiac output. Fluid replacement is carefully tailored to these measurements to avoid fluid imbalances, which may worsen hypoxia and ARDS. Enteral or parenteral feeding is necessary to maintain nutritional status and prevent tissue catabolism. Infections are treated with intravenous antibiotic therapy tailored to the causative organism. Low-molecular-weight heparin may be ordered to prevent thrombophlebitis and possible pulmonary embolus or disseminated intravascular coagulation, a possible complication of ARDS.

Nursing Care

The nursing care needs of the patient with ARDS are very similar to those of any patient with acute respiratory failure. See the Manifestations and Interprofessional Care sections for the assessment of the patient with ARDS.

Diagnoses, Interventions, and Outcomes

Maintaining adequate ventilation and respirations are of highest priority, along with preventing injury and managing anxiety. See the section on acute respiratory failure for nursing care related to these diagnoses. Additional high-priority nursing care concerns for the patient with ARDS are related to the effects of PEEP on cardiac output and potential problems of weaning ventilatory support. See the Case Study & Nursing Care Plan that follows for additional nursing interventions for the patient with ARDS.

Promote Adequate Cardiac Output. With positive-pressure ventilation, increased intrathoracic pressure decreases cardiac output. When PEEP is applied, intrathoracic pressure increases further; this can significantly decrease venous return, ventricular filling, stroke volume, and cardiac output. Manifestations of decreased cardiac output include hypotension and compensatory tachycardia as the heart attempts to maintain cardiac output despite decreased stroke volume. In the patient who is already hypoxic because of ARDS, this drop in cardiac output can increase tissue damage. Urine output falls, and dysrhythmias may develop.

Expected Outcome: Patient will demonstrate adequate cardiac output as evidenced by blood pressure and pulse rate within normal parameters for the patient.

The nurse will:

- Monitor and record vital signs, including apical pulse, at least every 2 hours, and more frequently immediately following initiation of mechanical ventilation or addition of PEEP. *Frequent assessment is vital to detect early signs of decreased cardiac output.*

- Record urine output hourly. *Because a significant portion of the cardiac output goes directly to the kidneys, a fall in urine output to < 30 mL/h is often the first sign of decreased cardiac output.*
- Assess level of consciousness at least every 4 hours. *Altered level of consciousness, confusion, and restlessness are early signs of cerebral hypoxia due to decreased cardiac output.*
- Monitor pulmonary artery pressures, central venous pressure, and cardiac output readings every 1 to 4 hours. *Changes in these measurements may indicate worsening cardiac status.*
- Assess heart and lung sounds frequently. *Increasing crackles or abnormal heart sounds may indicate heart failure.*
- Weigh daily at the same time. *Accurate daily weights are the best indicator of fluid volume status.*
- Frequently provide good skin care, keeping skin clean and dry and protecting pressure points. *Tissue hypoxia increases the risk of skin breakdown, which in turn increases the risk of infection and sepsis.*
- Maintain intravenous fluids as ordered. *Intravenous fluids are given to maintain vascular volume and prevent dehydration.*
- Administer analgesics, sedatives, and neuromuscular blockers as needed. *These medications may be prescribed to decrease cardiac workload.*

SAFETY ALERT: Frequently assess respiratory status following weaning and extubation. Keep an intubation kit readily available following extubation; be prepared for emergency reintubation. Laryngeal spasm or laryngeal edema may develop following extubation, necessitating reintubation to maintain respirations. ■

Reduce Risk for Dysfunctional Ventilatory Weaning Response. The patient with dysfunctional ventilatory weaning response has difficulty adjusting to reduced mechanical ventilator support, prolonging the weaning process. Airway congestion, inadequate rest or nutrition, pain, anxiety, and an unsupportive environment are factors that can contribute to difficulty weaning. With ARDS, the pathologic processes of the disease and its effects on gas exchange may be responsible for a prolonged or ineffective weaning process.

Expected Outcome: Patient will maintain arterial blood gases within safe parameters while effectively maintaining airway and secretion mobilization.

Assessment findings indicative of dysfunctional weaning include:

- Dyspnea, apprehension, or agitation
- Decreasing oxygen saturation level
- Cyanosis or pallor, diaphoresis
- Increased blood pressure, pulse, and respiratory rate
- Diminished or adventitious breath sounds, use of accessory muscles
- Decreased level of consciousness
- Deteriorating arterial blood gas values
- Shallow, gasping breaths or paradoxic abdominal breathing.

Nursing interventions for dysfunctional weaning include:

- Assess vital signs every 15 to 30 minutes following changes in ventilator settings and during T-piece trials. *Vital signs, heart and respiratory rates in particular, can provide early signs of hypoxemia and poor tolerance of the weaning process.*
- Place in Fowler or high-Fowler position. *Fowler position facilitates lung expansion and reduces the work of breathing.*
- Fully explain all weaning procedures, along with expected changes in breathing. *Adequate explanations help reduce anxiety and improve the ability to cooperate.*
- Remain with the patient during initial periods following changes of ventilator settings or T-piece trials. *This provides reassurance and allows close monitoring of the response.*
- Limit procedures and activities during weaning periods. *Reducing energy expenditures and cardiac work facilitates the weaning process.*
- Provide diversion, such as television or radio. *Diversion helps distract the focus from breathing.*
- Begin weaning procedures in the morning, when the patient is well rested and alert; weaning may be discontinued overnight to provide rest. *The work of breathing increases during the weaning process; adequate rest is important.*
- When SIMV is used for weaning, decrease the SIMV rate by increments of two breaths per minute. *Slow reduction of ventilator support allows respiratory muscle reconditioning and gradual resumption of the work of breathing.*
- Avoid administering drugs that may depress respirations during the weaning process (except as ordered at night to facilitate rest when ventilator support is provided). *Sedatives or analgesics that depress respirations can impair the weaning process.*
- Keep oxygen at the bedside following weaning and extubation. *Supplemental oxygen may be necessary to maintain adequate blood and tissue oxygenation.*
- Provide pulmonary hygiene with percussion and postural drainage. *Maintaining patent airways and adequate alveolar ventilation is vital during the weaning process.*

SAFETY ALERT: Frequently monitor oxygen saturation, $ETCO_2$, and ABGs following changes in ventilator settings. These values are used to assess the adequacy of ventilation and gas exchange during the weaning process. ■

Delegating Nursing Care Activities

As appropriate and allowed by the designated duties and responsibilities of unlicensed assistive personnel, the nurse may delegate nursing care activities such as measuring vital signs, encouraging oral or enteral fluid intake, and providing skin care.

Case Study & Nursing Care Plan

A Patient with ARDS

Peggy Adamson is a 36-year-old single woman admitted to the hospital following a near-drowning in a local lake. On admission to the emergency department, Ms. Adamson is alert and oriented, having been rescued and resuscitated within 2 minutes of the accident. Rescuers report that she seemed to have aspirated "a lot" of water as she was water-skiing when the accident occurred. She is admitted to the intensive care unit for observation. Oxygen is started per nasal cannula at 6 L/min, intravenous fluids are administered to correct electrolyte imbalances, and 40 mg of furosemide (Lasix) is given intravenously for hypervolemia.

ASSESSMENT

Nadia Mucha cares for Ms. Adamson the evening of the day after her admission. Throughout her stay, Ms. Adamson has remained alert and oriented with stable vital signs. Her respiratory rate has been 20 to 24/min, with scattered crackles, oxygen saturations of around 94%, and a PaO_2 of 75 to 80 mmHg on 6 L/min of oxygen. Her pulse has been 96 to 100 bpm and regular. On her initial assessment, Ms. Mucha notes that Ms. Adamson seems apprehensive and anxious.

Although her blood pressure is 116/74 mmHg, unchanged from previous levels, her heart rate is up to 106 bpm and respiratory rate is 28/min. Her lungs have scattered crackles but good breath sounds throughout, unchanged from previous assessments. Ms. Adamson's oxygen saturation has dropped to 84%, so Ms. Mucha orders ABGs and increases the oxygen to 8 L/min. ABG results show PaO_2 65 mmHg, respiratory alkalosis pH 7.48, and $PaCO_2$ 32 mmHg.

Ms. Mucha orders a portable chest x-ray and notifies the attending physician of the ABG results and the change in Ms. Adamson's status. The physician orders a nonrebreather mask at 8 L/min and repeat ABGs in 1 hour. The chest x-ray reveals scattered infiltrates and a normal heart size.

Ms. Adamson's oxygen saturation continues to fall, and subsequent blood gases show a PaO_2 of 55 mmHg. The attending physician diagnoses probable ARDS and orders nasotracheal intubation and mechanical ventilation.

DIAGNOSES

- Decreased gas exchange related to near drowning
- Anxiety related to hypoxemia
- Potential for decreased cardiac output related to positive pressure ventilation
- Risk for injury related to endotracheal intubation

EXPECTED OUTCOMES

- Patient will breathe effectively with the mechanical ventilator.
- Patient will demonstrate improved oxygen saturation, $ETCO_2$, and ABG values.
- Patient will express fears related to intubation and mechanical ventilation.
- Patient will demonstrate reduced anxiety levels (relaxed facial expression, ability to rest).
- Patient will maintain adequate cardiac output and tissue perfusion.
- Patient will tolerate endotracheal intubation and mechanical ventilation without evidence of infection or barotrauma.

PLANNING AND IMPLEMENTATION

- Obtain all necessary supplies and notify respiratory therapy and radiology in preparation for intubation and mechanical ventilation.
- Explain the purpose and procedure of intubation.
- Provide an opportunity to express fears related to intubation and mechanical ventilation; answer questions and provide reassurance.
- Discuss communication strategies while intubated; obtain a magic slate.
- Administer analgesics and/or sedatives as ordered.
- Monitor oxygen saturation and $ETCO_2$ levels every 30 to 60 minutes initially after instituting mechanical ventilation; report changes to the physician.
- Obtain ABGs as ordered or indicated; monitor and report results.
- Suction via endotracheal tube as needed to maintain clear airways.
- Allow periods of uninterrupted rest.
- Monitor vital signs every 1 to 2 hours.
- Assess skin color, capillary refill, and the presence of edema every 4 hours.
- Monitor urine output hourly; report output of < 30 mL/h.
- Assess lung sounds and chest excursion every 1 to 2 hours.

EVALUATION

Ms. Adamson is intubated and placed on a volume-cycled ventilator at 50% FIO_2 and a tidal volume of 700 mL in the assist-control mode at 16 breaths per minute. She has difficulty working with the ventilator initially, so a fentanyl drip is ordered to reduce her anxiety. Ms. Adamson's oxygen saturation, $ETCO_2$, and ABG results do not begin to improve until 5 mmHg of PEEP is added to ventilator settings. After 3 days of mechanical ventilation with PEEP and aggressive fluid and diuretic therapy, Ms. Adamson begins to improve. She is placed on SIMV, and over the course of another 3 days she is gradually weaned off the ventilator to a face mask with CPAP. She eventually recovers fully, with minimal apparent long-term effects.

(continued)

CLINICAL REASONING IN PATIENT CARE

1. Endotracheal intubation and mechanical ventilation were effective in supporting Ms. Adamson's respiratory status as she recovered from ARDS. Discuss a possible sequence of events had it not been possible to wean her from the ventilator.
2. How might the presentation and management of an acute episode of respiratory failure due to ARDS differ from respiratory failure related to COPD?
3. What measures can nurses take to prevent the development of ARDS?
4. Develop a nursing care plan for Ms. Adamson for her feeling of helplessness related to endotracheal intubation and mechanical ventilation.

See Evaluating Your Response in Appendix B.

Transitions of Care

When preparing the patient who has recovered from ARDS and the family for home care, discuss the following topics:

- ARDS did not result from something they did or did not do, but developed as a consequence of serious illness. Provide factual information about ARDS.
- Maximal respiratory function following ARDS is usually achieved within 6 months; respiratory function may remain significantly impaired. This may necessitate changes in occupation, lifestyle, and family roles.
- Avoiding smoking and exposure to secondhand smoke and environmental pollutants is vital to prevent further lung damage.
- Obtain immunization for pneumococcal pneumonia and annual influenza immunizations to prevent further episodes of serious respiratory disease.

Provide referrals to home health and respiratory care services as indicated, as well as for occupational therapy and counseling as needed.

CHAPTER HIGHLIGHTS

37.1 Reactive Airway Disorders

Describe the pathophysiology and manifestations of reactive airway disorders, and outline the interprofessional care and nursing care of patients with these disorders.

- Obstructive disorders of the lower respiratory system, including asthma, COPD, and cystic fibrosis, impair airflow into and out of the lungs, often affecting the outflow of air to a greater extent than inflow. As a result, air trapping in the alveoli increases the residual volume of the lungs and reduces functional residual capacity. Alveolar ventilation is reduced as well. The net result is less available oxygen in the alveoli and impaired gas exchange.
- In many instances, acute episodes of asthma can be avoided through the use of inhaled steroids to reduce airway inflammation, inhaled long-acting bronchodilators, and frequent self-monitoring of expiratory flow rate. Nursing care focuses on teaching for self-management and providing care during acute episodes of airway constriction.
- Chronic obstructive pulmonary disease (COPD) is a long-term process of progressive lung dysfunction. COPD involves two different disease processes: Chronic bronchitis, characterized by airway edema and excessive mucous production, and emphysema, characterized by destruction of supporting tissue with enlargement of respiratory bronchioles and alveolar spaces and loss of surface area for gas exchange.
- Smoking and exposure to tobacco smoke is the single greatest risk factor for COPD. A small percentage of cases result from an inherited deficiency of alpha$_1$-antitripsin, an enzyme that inhibits lung tissue destruction. Although smoking cessation does not reverse COPD, it does slow the progress of the disease.
- Cystic fibrosis, inherited as an autosomal recessive disorder, causes thick, viscous secretions in affected organs, primarily the lungs, pancreas, sweat glands, and reproductive tract. In the lungs, small airway clearance is impaired, leading to atelectasis, bronchiectasis, infection, and dilation of distal airways with air trapping and impaired gas exchange. Chest physiotherapy and early treatment of respiratory infections are key components of disease management. Ultimately, lung or heart–lung transplant may be required.

37.2 Interstitial Lung Disease

Describe the pathophysiology and manifestations of interstitial lung disease, and outline the interprofessional care and nursing care of patients with this disorder.

- Occupational lung diseases, such as pneumoconiosis and hypersensitivity pneumonitis, damage interstitial tissues of the lungs, leading to fibrosis and scarring that cause the lungs to become stiff and noncompliant. Lung volumes decrease, the work of breathing increases, and gas diffusion is impaired. Most occupational lung diseases are progressive and irreversible. Interprofessional care is similar to that provided for patients with COPD.

37.3 Pulmonary Vascular Disorders

Describe the pathophysiology and manifestations of pulmonary vascular disorders, and outline the interprofessional care and nursing care of patients with these disorders.

- Pulmonary vascular disorders affect blood flow through the pulmonary vascular system and gas exchange. Pulmonary embolism, obstruction of pulmonary blood flow, is a potentially critical condition usually resulting from deep venous thrombosis. Sudden onset of chest pain and dyspnea with changes in hemodynamic status are possible manifestations of pulmonary embolism. Prevention through early ambulation, lower extremity exercises, and sequential compression devices is the most effective treatment for pulmonary embolism.
- In primary and secondary forms of pulmonary hypertension, constriction of pulmonary vessels and remodeling of the pulmonary vascular bed increase pressure in the pulmonary system and right heart, ultimately leading to right-sided heart failure (cor pulmonale). Treatment focuses on slowing disease progression through oxygen therapy, administration of vasodilators and anticoagulants, and supporting patient function.

37.4 Respiratory Failure

Describe the pathophysiology and manifestations of respiratory failure, and outline the interprofessional care and nursing care of patients with this condition.

- Hypoventilation, impaired gas exchange, and significant ventilation–perfusion mismatch (e.g., pulmonary embolism) can lead to respiratory failure. Hypoventilation leads to hypoxemia and hypercapnia, whereas in impaired gas exchange or ventilation–perfusion mismatch, hypoxemia dominates.
- The manifestations of respiratory failure relate directly to the effects of hypoxemia and hypercapnia.
- Respiratory support is often required, using positive-pressure ventilators. Variables of mechanical ventilation include the mode or cycle of ventilation, the flow rate and amount, pressures delivered, and the oxygen concentration. Either invasive or noninvasive techniques may be used.
- Complications of mechanical ventilation include lung and mucous membrane trauma and infection, reduced cardiac output, gastric dilation, impaired communication, and stress.
- ARDS is noncardiac pulmonary edema caused by a diffuse inflammatory response with increased pulmonary capillary permeability leading to interstitial and alveolar edema and impaired gas exchange. As the process continues, lung compliance decreases, increasing the work of breathing, and atelectasis and consolidation of lung tissue develop. Respiratory failure with refractory hypoxemia results.
- Mechanical ventilation and measures to support physiologic function are the primary treatments for ARDS. The mortality rate, however, remains high at about 40%.

TEST YOURSELF NCLEX-RN® REVIEW

1. The nurse identifies these problems for a patient with an acute asthma attack. Which problem is of the highest priority?
   A. The patient is anxious because breathing is difficult.
   B. Because the patient is anxious, respirations are irregular.
   C. Patient has impaired airflow due to bronchoconstriction and abundance of thick mucus.
   D. Patient is unaware of personal asthma triggers and of how to use medications.
2. The nurse caring for a patient with asthma notices that the patient's respirations have slowed and coughing has stopped. Breath sounds are diminished throughout his lung fields and absent in the bases. Which action should the nurse take?
   A. Obtain a chest x-ray.
   B. Ask family members to leave.
   C. Notify the healthcare provider.
   D. Allow the patient to rest undisturbed.
3. The nurse is instructing a patient with asthma on the use of a metered-dose inhaler (MDI) for medication administration. What should the nurse teach the patient about the medications being provided through this device? (Select all that apply.)
   A. Shake the canister vigorously for 3 to 5 seconds before use.
   B. Take quick, shallow breaths in rapid succession while holding the canister down.
   C. Rinse the mouth after using the inhaler to reduce systemic absorption of the drug.
   D. Use the inhaler containing the anti-inflammatory drug first, then the bronchodilator.
   E. Wait one full minute before repeating the procedure for a second puff of medication.

4. The nurse is assessing a patient with chronic obstructive airway disease. Which finding would be expected when conducting the physical examination of this patient? (Select all that apply.)
   A. Mental confusion and lethargy
   B. Oxygen saturation readings of 85% or less
   C. 3+ pitting edema of ankles and lower legs
   D. AP chest diameter equal to or greater than lateral chest diameter
   E. Use of accessory muscles of respiration
5. The nurse is determining goals of care for a patient with chronic obstructive pulmonary disease. Which would be an appropriate goal for this patient?
   A. Will maintain SaO_2 of 90% or higher.
   B. Will verbalize self-care measures to regain lost lung function.
   C. Arterial blood gases will be within normal limits by discharge.
   D. Will identify strategies to help reduce number of cigarettes smoked per day.
6. The nurse is planning care for a patient with chronic obstructive pulmonary disease. Which information should the nurse consider when determining if the patient should have supplemental oxygen?
   A. Oxygen is used only at night for patients with COPD.
   B. Because oxygen is flammable, the patient should not smoke when using oxygen.
   C. The patient needs to be closely monitored for signs of respiratory depression.
   D. Oxygen is never used for patients with COPD because they may become dependent on it.
7. The home care nurse is providing direction to a home care aide who is scheduled to care for a patient with cystic fibrosis. Which information should the nurse instruct the aide to report immediately? (Select all that apply.)
   A. Fever
   B. Bulky, fatty stools
   C. Difficulty clearing mucous secretions
   D. Increasing shortness of breath and fatigue
   E. Thick, tenacious, milky, and white sputum
8. A patient in skeletal traction suddenly develops right-sided chest pain and shortness of breath. What should the nurse do? (Select all that apply.)
   A. Check for Homans sign.
   B. Start oxygen per nasal cannula.
   C. Place in the high-Fowler position.
   D. Administer the prescribed analgesic.
   E. Auscultate heart sounds every 2 to 4 hours.
9. The nurse caring for a patient with COPD is concerned that the patient is developing respiratory failure. What did the nurse assess as an early sign of possible respiratory failure?
   A. Deep coma
   B. Decreased urine output
   C. Restlessness and tachypnea
   D. Hypotension and tachycardia
10. The nurse is caring for a patient undergoing mechanical ventilation for acute respiratory failure. Which measure should the nurse use to help maintain effective alveolar ventilation?
    A. Keep the patient in the supine position.
    B. Maintain ordered oxygen concentration.
    C. Increase the tidal volume on the ventilator.
    D. Perform endotracheal suctioning as indicated.

See Test Yourself answers in Appendix B.

REFERENCES

Adams, M., Holland, N., & Urban, C. (2017). *Pharmacology for nurses: A pathophysiologic approach.* Boston, MA: Pearson.

Alpha 1 Foundation. (2017). *Home page.* Retrieved from https://www.alpha1.org.

American Heart Association. (2017). *Pulmonary hypertension: High blood pressure in the heart to lung system. What is pulmonary hypertension?* Retrieved from www.heart.org/HEARTORG/Conditions/HighBloodPressure/GettheFactsAboutHighBloodPressure/Pulmonary-Hypertension---High-Blood-Pressure-in-the-Heart-to-Lung-System_UCM_301792_Article.jsp.

American Lung Association (ALA). (2017a). *Chronic obstructive pulmonary disease (COPD).* Retrieved from www.lung.org/lung-health-and-diseases/lung-disease-lookup/copd/.

American Lung Association (ALA). (2017b). *Pneumoconiosis.* Retrieved from www.lung.org/lung-health-and-diseases/lung-disease-lookup/pneumoconiosis/.

American Lung Association. (2018a). *Learn about sarcoidosis.* Retrieved from www.lung.org/lung-health-and-diseases/lung-disease-lookup/sarcoidosis/learn-about-sarcoidosis.html.

American Lung Association. (2018b). *Learn about silicosis.* Retrieved from www.lung.org/lung-health-and-diseases/lung-disease-lookup/silicosis/learn-about-silicosis.html.

Blackley, D. J., Crum, J. B., Halldin, C. N., Storey, E., & Laney, A. S. (2016). Resurgence of progressive massive fibrosis in coal miners — Eastern Kentucky, 2016. *Morbidity and Mortality Weekly Report, 65*(49), 1385–1389.

Retrieved from https://www.cdc.gov/mmwr/volumes/65/wr/mm6549a1.htm.

Centers for Disease Control and Prevention (CDC). (2017a). *Asthma fast facts*. Retrieved from https://www.cdc.gov/asthma/pdfs/asthma_fast_facts_statistics.pdf.

Centers for Disease Control and Prevention (CDC). (2017b). *Chronic obstructive pulmonary disease (COPD)*. Retrieved from https://www.cdc.gov/copd/index.html.

Centers for Disease Control. (2017c). *Health effects of secondhand smoke*. Retrieved from https://www.cdc.gov/tobacco/data_statistics/fact_sheets/secondhand_smoke/health_effects/index.htm.

Centers for Disease Control and Prevention (CDC). (2017d). *Smoking cessation*. Retrieved from https://www.cdc.gov/tobacco/data_statistics/fact_sheets/cessation/quitting/index.htm.

Centers for Disease Control and Prevention (CDC). (2017e). *Venous thromboembolism (blood clots)*. Retrieved from https://www.cdc.gov/ncbddd/dvt/data.html.

Centers for Disease Control and Prevention (CDC). (2018). *Venous thromboembolism: data and statistics*. Retrieved from https://www.cdc.gov/ncbddd/dvt/data.html.

Cystic Fibrosis Foundation. (2017). *Home page*. Retrieved from https://www.cff.org/.

Ferreira, L. M. (n.d.) Pulmonary hypertension WHO classification. *Pulmonary Hypertension News*. Retrieved from https://pulmonaryhypertensionnews.com/pulmonary-hypertension-who-classification/.

Gerke, A. K. (2014). Morbidity and mortality in sarcoidosis. *Current Opinion in Pulmonary Medicine, 20*(5), 472–478.

Global Initiative for Obstructive Lung Disease (GOLD). (2017). *Global strategy for the diagnosis, management and prevention of chronic obstructive pulmonary disease*. Retrieved from www.goldcopd.org.

Lamontagne, F., Briel, M., Guyatt, G. H., Cook, D. J., Bhatnagar, N., & Meade, M. (2010). Corticosteroid therapy for acute lung injury, acute respiratory distress syndrome, and severe pneumonia: A meta-analysis of randomized controlled trials. *Journal of Critical Care, 25*(3), 420–435.

McCarthy, B., Casey, D., Devane, D., Murphy, K., Murphy, E., & Lacasse, Y. (2015). Pulmonary rehabilitation for chronic obstructive pulmonary disease. *Cochrane Database of Systematic Reviews*, Issue 2. DOI: 10.1002/14651858.CD003793.pub3.

National Center for Health Statistics. (2016). *Health, United States, 2016 with chartbook*. Retrieved from https://www.cdc.gov/nchs/data/hus/hus16.pdf.

National Heart, Lung, and Blood Institute. (2012). *Asthma care quick reference*. Retrieved from https://www.nhlbi.nih.gov/files/docs/guidelines/asthma_qrg.pdf.

National Heart, Lung, and Blood Institute (NHLBI). (2017). *ARDS*. Retrieved from http://www.nhlbi.nih.gov/health/health-topics/topics/ards.

National Institute for Occupational Safety and Health. (2016). *Coal Workers' Health Surveillance Program: CWHSP frequently asked questions*. Retrieved from https://www.cdc.gov/niosh/topics/cwhsp/faq.html.

Office of Minority Health. (2018). Asthma and African Americans. Retrieved from https://minorityhealth.hhs.gov/omh/browse.aspx?lvl=4&lvlid=15.

Organ Procurement and Transplant Network. (2018). Lung Kaplan-Meier graft survival rates for transplants performed: 2008–2015. Retrieved from https://optn.transplant.hrsa.gov/data/view-data-reports/national-data/#.

Parker, S. L., Tong, T., Bolden, S., & Wingo, P. A. (1997). Cancer statistics, 1997. *CA: A Cancer Journal for Clinicians, 47*(1), 5–27.

Perrin, K. O., & MacLeod, C. E. (2017). *Understanding the essentials of critical care nursing* (3rd ed.). Boston, MA: Pearson.

Shields, K. M., Fox, K. L., & Liebrecht, C. (2018). *Pearson nurse's drug guide: 2018*. Boston, MA: Pearson.

Sorenson, M., Quinn, L., & Klein, D. (2019). *Pathophysiology: Concepts of human disease*. New York: Pearson.

U.S. Department of Health and Human Services. (2014). *The health consequences of smoking–50 years of progress: A report of the Surgeon General*. Retrieved from https://www.surgeongeneral.gov/library/reports/50-years-of-progress/full-report.pdf.

ADDITIONAL RESOURCES

American Lung Association. (2018a). *Lung health and diseases*. Retrieved from www.lung.org/lung-health-and-diseases/

American Lung Association. (2018b). *Our initiatives*. Retrieved from www.lung.org/our-initiatives/

American Lung Association. (2018c). *Stop smoking*. Retrieved from www.lung.org/stop-smoking/

American Thoracic Society. (2017). *Patient resources: Fact sheets A to Z*.
Retrieved from www.thoracic.org/patients/patient-resources/fact-sheets-az.php

COPD Foundation. (2018). *Homepage*.
Retrieved from https://www.copdfoundation.org

Cystic Fibrosis Foundation. (2018). *Homepage*.
Retrieved from https://www.cff.org/

Lungs and You. (2018). *What is IPF?*
Retrieved from https://www.lungsandyou.com/facts/what-is-ipf

National Heart, Lung, and Blood Institute. (2018). *Health topics*.
Retrieved from https://www.nhlbi.nih.gov

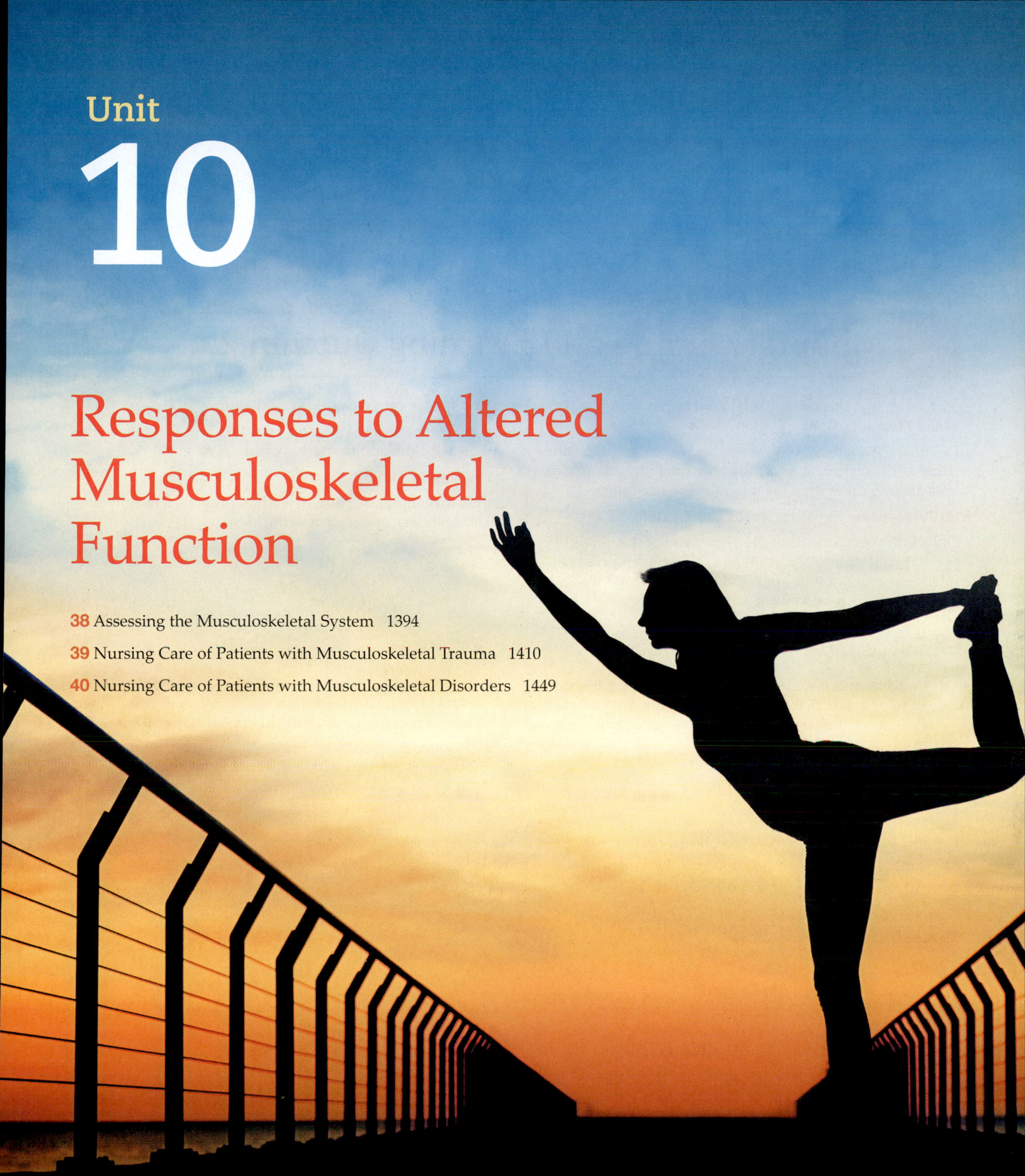

Unit

10

Responses to Altered Musculoskeletal Function

Chapter 38

Assessing the Musculoskeletal System

Chapter Outline and Learning Outcomes

CLINICAL COMPETENCIES

- Conduct and document a health history for patients who have or are at risk for alterations in the musculoskeletal system, eliciting patient values, preferences, and expressed needs as part of the interview.
- Conduct and document a physical assessment of musculoskeletal structures and functions, demonstrating sensitivity and respect for the diversity of human experience.
- Monitor the results of diagnostic tests and communicate abnormal findings within the interprofessional team.

KEY TERMS

bursitis, 1402
crepitation, 1401
hematopoiesis, 1395
kyphosis, 1401
lordosis, 1401
ossification, 1397
osteoblast, 1395
osteoclast, 1395
scoliosis, 1401
synovitis, 1403
tendonitis, 1402

EQUIPMENT NEEDED

- Tape measure
- Goniometer

The tissues and structures of the musculoskeletal system perform many functions, including support, protection, and movement. The musculoskeletal system has two subsystems: The bones and joints of the skeleton and the skeletal muscles. These subsystems work together to allow the body to perform both gross, simple movements such as closing a door, and fine, complex movements such as repairing a watch. Alterations in the structure and/or function of the musculoskeletal system affect and are affected by the integrity of the neurologic system; disorders of both of the systems place the patient at risk for functional alterations, including activity, self-care, and self-concept.

38.1 Anatomy, Physiology, and Functions of the Musculoskeletal System

The musculoskeletal system is composed of bones of the skeletal system, cartilage (a connective tissue), ligaments, tendons, and skeletal muscles and joints. The bones serve as the framework for the body and for the attachment of muscles, tendons, and ligaments. Innervated by the nervous system, contraction and relaxation of muscles permit movement at joints.

Bones

The human skeleton is made up of 206 bones (**Figure 38.1** ■). Bones of the skeletal system are divided into the axial skeleton (the skull, thorax, and vertebrae) and the appendicular skeleton (shoulder, arms, pelvic girdle, and legs).

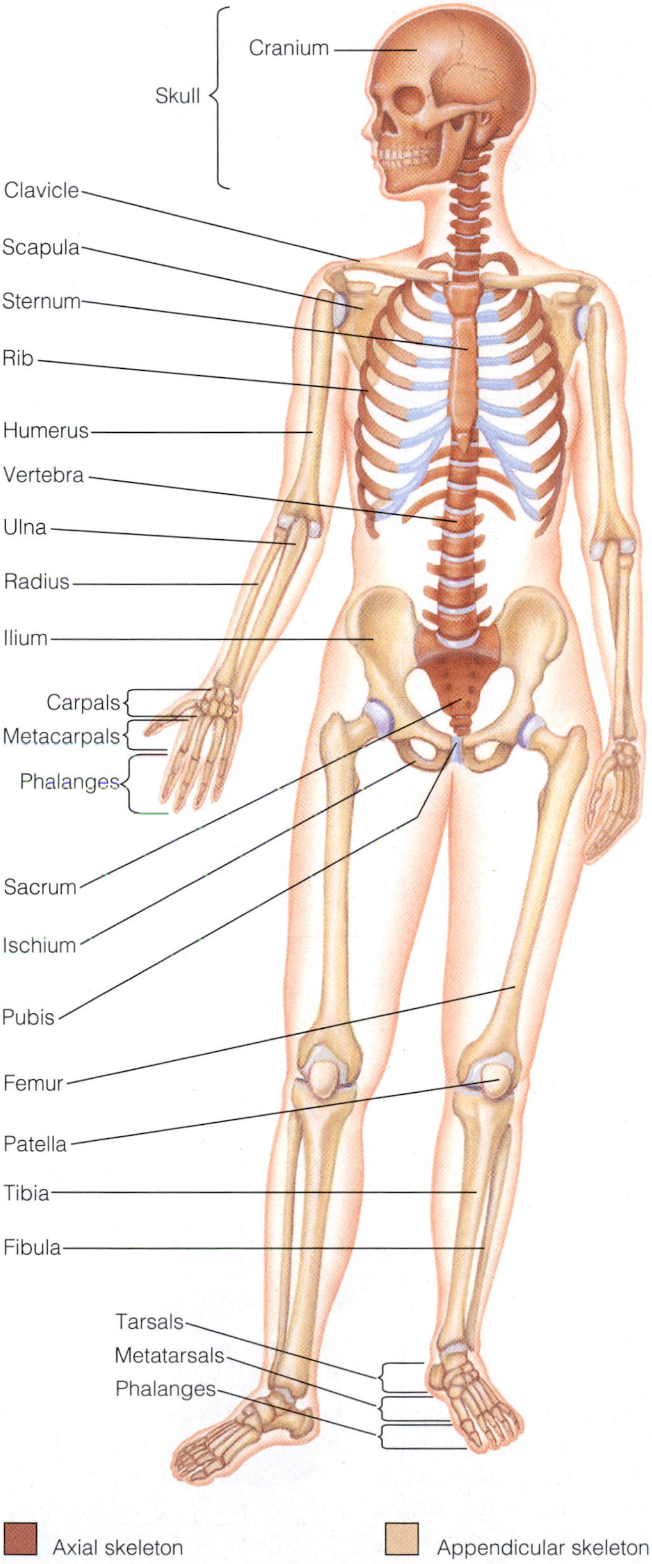
Skull
Cranium
Clavicle
Scapula
Sternum
Rib
Humerus
Vertebra
Ulna
Radius
Ilium
Carpals
Metacarpals
Phalanges
Sacrum
Ischium
Pubis
Femur
Patella
Tibia
Fibula
Tarsals
Metatarsals
Phalanges
Axial skeleton
Appendicular skeleton

Figure 38.1 ■ Bones of the human skeleton.

Bones form the body's structure and provide support for soft tissues. They protect vital organs from injury and serve to move body parts by providing points of attachment for muscles. Bones also store minerals and serve as a site for **hematopoiesis** (blood cell formation).

Bone Structure

Bone cells include **osteoblasts** (cells that form bone), osteocytes (cells that maintain bone matrix), **osteoclasts** (cells that resorb bone), and osteoprogenitor cells (the source of all bone cells except osteoclasts). Bone matrix is the extracellular element of bone tissue; it consists of collagen fibers, minerals (primarily calcium and phosphate), proteins, carbohydrates, and ground substance. *Ground substance* is a gelatinous material that facilitates diffusion of nutrients, wastes, and gases between the blood vessels and bone tissue. Bones are covered with *periosteum*, a double-layered connective tissue. The outer layer of the periosteum contains blood vessels and nerves; the inner layer is anchored to the bone.

Bones consist of a rigid connective tissue called *osseous tissue*, of which there are two types: Laminar bone (strong, mature bone found in the adult skeleton) and woven bone (which provides a temporary framework for support and is found in the developing fetus, as part of healing fractures, and in areas surrounding tumors and infections of bones). There are two types of mature bones: Compact and spongy bone. *Compact bone* forms the outer shell of a bone, whereas spongy bone is found in the interior of bones. *Spongy bone* is composed of lattice-like structures (trabeculae), lined with osteogenic cells and filled with red or yellow bone marrow (Sorenson, Quinn, & Klein, 2019).

The basic structural unit of laminar bone is the *Haversian system* (also called an *osteon*). The Haversian system consists of a central canal, called the *Haversian canal*; concentric layers of bone matrix, called lamellae; spaces between the lamellae, called *lacunae*; osteocytes within the lacunae; and small channels, called *canaliculi* (**Figure 38.2** ■). The spongy sections of long bones and flat bones contain tissue for hematopoiesis. In the adult, these sections, called *red marrow cavities*, are present in the spongy center of flat bones (especially the sternum) and in only two long bones: The humerus and the head of the femur.

Bone Shapes

Bones are classified by shape (**Figure 38.3** ■):

- ***Long bones*** have a midportion, or shaft, called a diaphysis and two broad ends, called *epiphyses* (**Figure 38.4** ■). The diaphysis is compact bone and contains the marrow cavity, which is lined with endosteum. Long bones include the bones of the arms, legs, fingers, and toes.
- ***Short bones***, also called *cuboid bones*, include the bones of the wrist and ankle.
- ***Flat bones*** are thin and flat, and most are curved. Flat bones include most bones of the skull, the sternum, and the ribs.

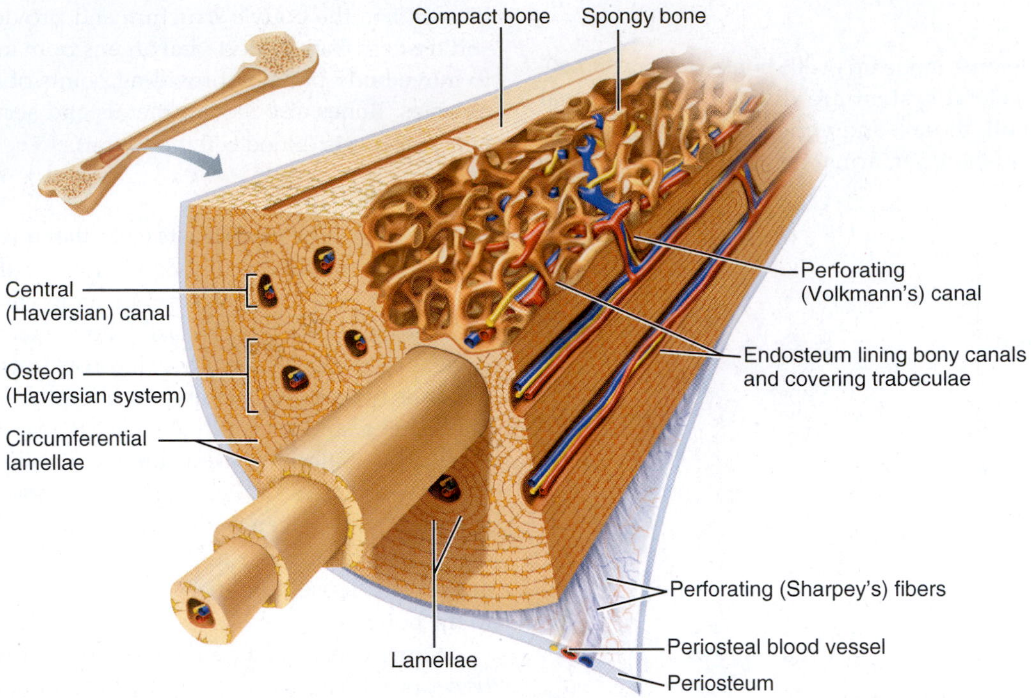
Compact bone
Spongy bone
Central (Haversian) canal
Osteon (Haversian system)
Circumferential lamellae
Perforating (Volkmann's) canal
Endosteum lining bony canals and covering trabeculae
Perforating (Sharpey's) fibers
Periosteal blood vessel
Periosteum
Lamellae

Figure 38.2 ■ The structure of compact bone and the Haversian system.

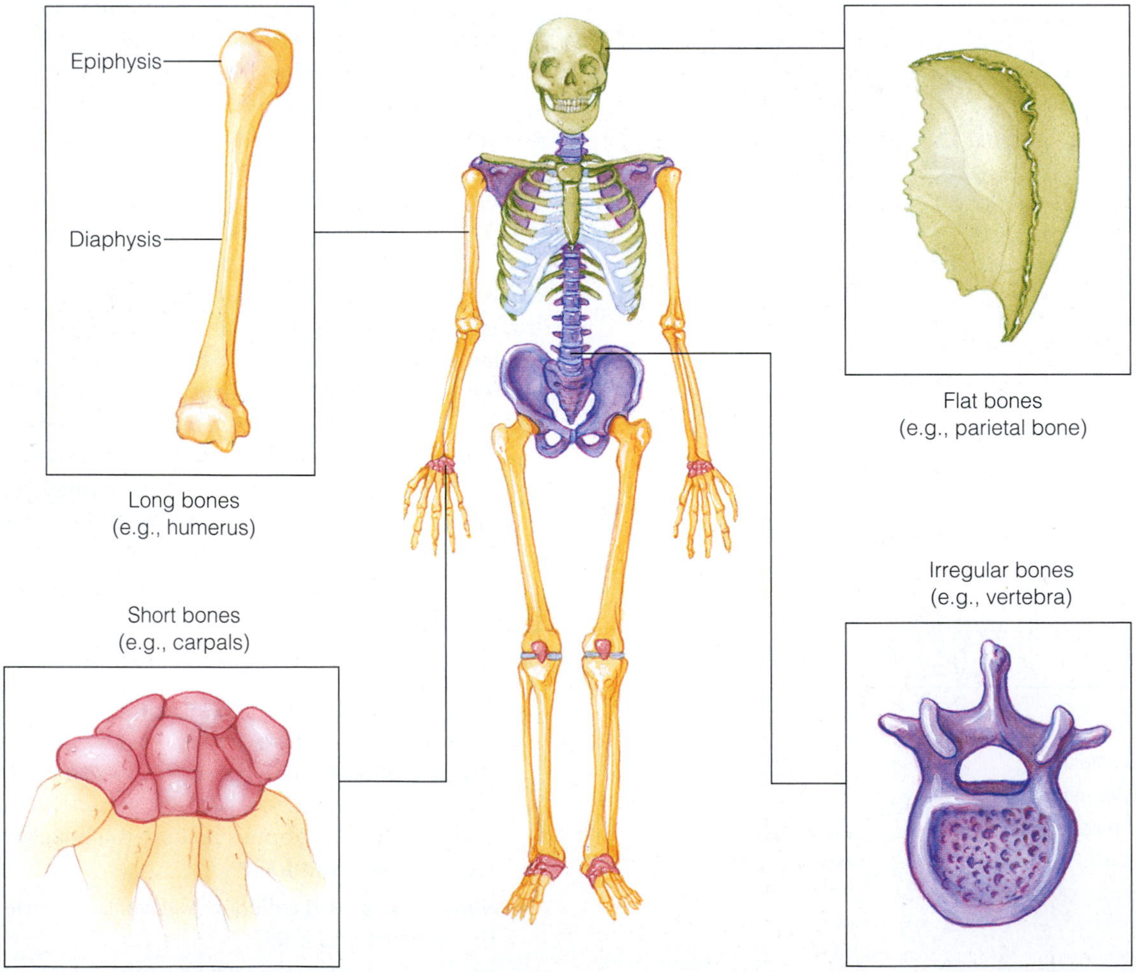
Epiphysis
Diaphysis
Long bones (e.g., humerus)
Flat bones (e.g., parietal bone)
Short bones (e.g., carpals)
Irregular bones (e.g., vertebra)

Figure 38.3 ■ Classification of bones according to shape.

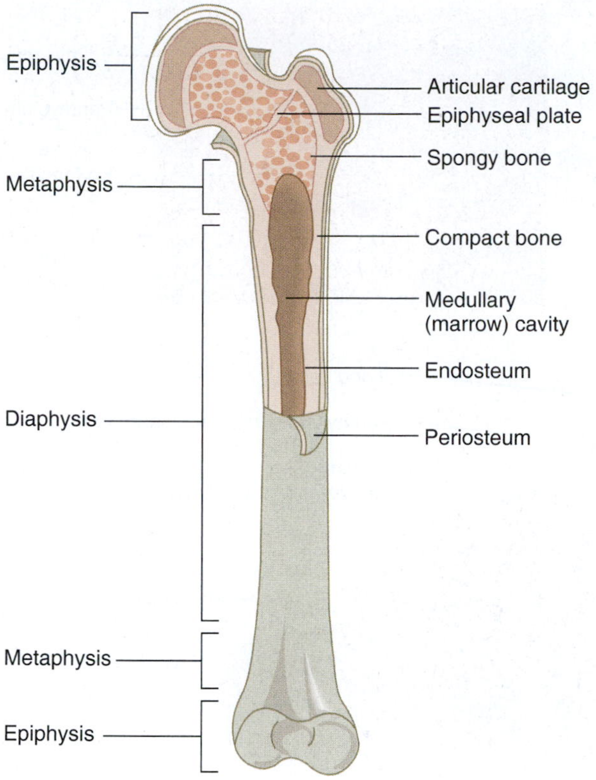
Epiphysis
Articular cartilage
Epiphyseal plate
Spongy bone
Metaphysis
Compact bone
Medullary (marrow) cavity
Endosteum
Diaphysis
Periosteum
Metaphysis
Epiphysis

Figure 38.4 ■ Parts of a long bone.

- ***Irregular bones*** are of various shapes and sizes. Irregular bones include the vertebrae, the scapulae, and the bones of the pelvic girdle.

Bone Remodeling in Adults

Although the bones of adults do not normally increase in length and size, constant remodeling of bones, as well as repair of damaged bone tissue, occurs throughout life. In the bone remodeling process, bone resorption and bone deposit occur at all periosteal and endosteal surfaces. Hormones and forces that put stress on the bones regulate this process, which involves a combined action of the osteocytes, osteoclasts, and osteoblasts. Bones that are in use, and are therefore subjected to stress, increase their osteoblastic activity to increase **ossification** (the development of bone). Bones that are inactive undergo increased osteoclast activity and bone resorption.

The hormonal stimulus for bone remodeling is controlled by a negative feedback mechanism that regulates blood calcium levels. This stimulus involves the interaction of parathyroid hormone (PTH) from the parathyroid glands and calcitonin from the thyroid gland. When blood levels of calcium decrease, PTH is released. PTH then stimulates osteoclast activity and bone resorption so that calcium is released from the bone matrix. As a result, blood levels of calcium rise, and the stimulus for PTH release ends. Rising blood calcium levels stimulate the secretion of calcitonin, inhibit bone resorption, and cause the deposit of calcium salts in the bone matrix. Thus, bones are necessary to regulate blood calcium levels. Calcium ions are necessary for the transmission of nerve impulses, the release of neurotransmitters, muscle contraction, blood clotting, glandular secretion, and cell division. Bone remodeling is also regulated by the response of bones to gravitational pull and to mechanical stress from the pull of muscles. Bones that undergo increased stress are heavier and larger.

Cartilage

Cartilage is a firm, flexible connective tissue. There are three types of cartilage: Elastic cartilage (found in the ear), hyaline cartilage (the cartilage that joins the ribs to the sternum and vertebrae, many cartilages of the respiratory tract, the articular cartilages, and the epiphyseal plates), and fibrocartilage (found in the intervertebral disks, the symphysis pubis, and the areas where tendons connect to bones).

Muscles

The three types of muscle tissue in the body are skeletal muscle, smooth muscle, and cardiac muscle (**Table 38.1**). This discussion focuses on skeletal muscle, the only type of muscle that allows musculoskeletal function. Skeletal muscles attach to and cover the bones of the skeleton. Skeletal muscles promote body movement, help maintain posture, and produce body heat. They may be moved by conscious, voluntary control or by reflex activity. The body has approximately 600 skeletal muscles.

Skeletal muscles are thick bundles of parallel multinucleated contractile cells called *fibers* (**Figure 38.5** ■). Each single muscle fiber is itself a bundle of smaller structures called *myofibrils*. Myofibrils are strands of smaller repeating units called *sarcomeres*, which consist of thick filaments of myosin and thin filaments of actin, proteins that contribute to muscle contraction. Skeletal muscle cells have typical functional properties:

- ***Excitability:*** The ability to receive and respond to a stimulus. The stimulus is usually a neurotransmitter released by a neuron, and the response is the generation and transmission of an action potential along the plasma membrane of the muscle cell.
- ***Contractibility:*** The ability to respond to a stimulus by forcibly shortening

Table 38.1 Types of Body Muscle

Type	Description	Examples
Skeletal	Striated, voluntary muscle (can consciously move)	Biceps, triceps, deltoid, gluteus maximus
Smooth	Nonstriated, involuntary muscle (cannot consciously move)	Muscles in the walls of the bladder, stomach, and bronchi
Cardiac	Striated, involuntary muscle	Heart muscle

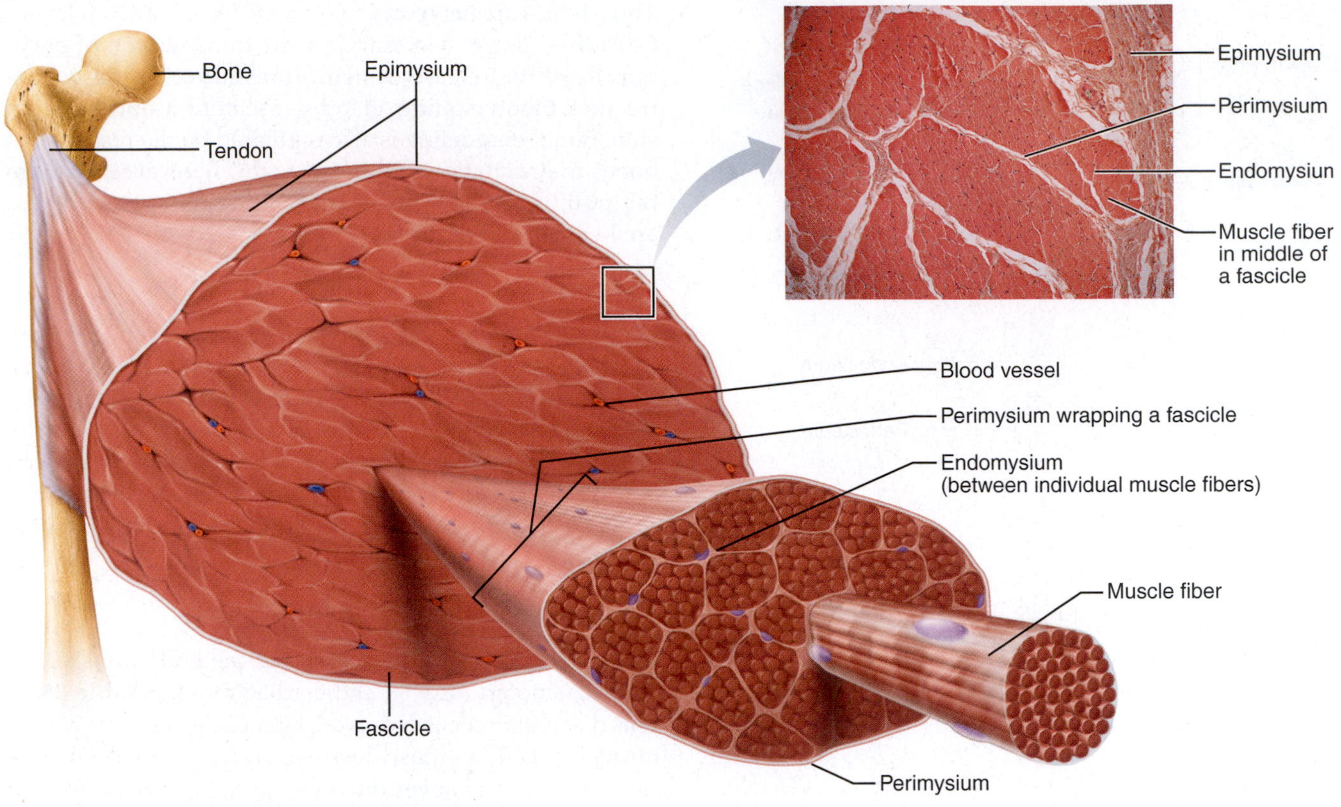
Bone
Epimysium
Tendon
Epimysium
Perimysium
Endomysiun
Muscle fiber in middle of a fascicle
Blood vessel
Perimysium wrapping a fascicle
Endomysium (between individual muscle fibers)
Muscle fiber
Fascicle
Perimysium

Figure 38.5 ■ Structure of skeletal muscle.

- ***Extensibility:*** The ability to respond to a stimulus by extending and relaxing
- ***Elasticity:*** The ability to resume its resting length after it has shortened or lengthened.

Skeletal muscle movement is triggered when motor neurons release acetylcholine, a neurotransmitter that crosses the neuromuscular junction and alters the permeability of the muscle fiber. Sodium ions enter the fiber, producing an action potential that causes muscle contraction. The more fibers that contract, the stronger the contraction of the entire muscle.

Prolonged strenuous activity causes continuous nerve impulses and eventually results in a buildup of lactic acid and reduced energy in the muscle, or muscle fatigue. However, continuous nerve impulses are also responsible for maintaining muscle tone. Regular exercise increases the size and strength of muscles, while lack of use results in muscle atrophy.

Joints

Joints, or articulations, are regions where two or more bones meet. Joints hold the bones of the skeleton together while allowing the body to move. Joints may be classified by function as *synarthroses*, immovable joints; *amphiarthroses*, slightly movable joints; or *diarthroses*, freely movable joints. Joints are also classified by structure as fibrous, cartilaginous, or synovial. **Table 38.2** describes each of these types. Fibrous joints permit little or no movement because the articulating bones are joined either by short connective tissue fibers that bind the bones together or by short cords of fibrous tissue called *ligaments* that permit slight give but no true movement. Some cartilaginous joints, such as the sternocostal joints of the rib cage, are composed of hyaline cartilage growths that fuse together the articulating bone ends. These joints are immobile. In other cartilaginous joints, such as the intervertebral disks, the hyaline cartilage fuses to an intervening plate of flexible fibrocartilage. This structural feature accounts for the flexibility of the vertebral column.

Bones in synovial joints are enclosed by a cavity that is filled with synovial fluid, a filtrate of blood plasma (**Figure 38.6** ■). Synovial joints are freely movable, allowing many kinds of movements, as listed and described in

Table 38.2 Structural Classification of Joints

Type	Description	Examples
Fibrous	Bones united or connected by collagen fibers	Skull sutures Ligament connecting distal tibia and fibula Connection between a tooth and its socket
Cartilaginous	Bones united or connected by cartilage	Vertebral joints Joint between first rib and manubrium of sternum Joint of the symphysis pubis
Synovial	Bones separated by a cavity containing synovial fluid	Joints of the extremities Shoulder joints Hip joints

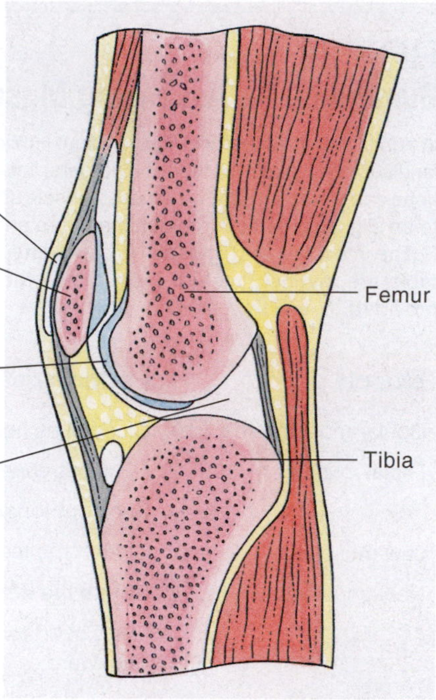
Bursa
Patella
Articular cartilage
Synovial cavity with synovial fluid
Femur
Tibia

Figure 38.6 ■ Structure of a synovial joint (knee).

Table 38.3. Synovial fluid fills the free spaces of the joint capsule, enhancing the smooth movement of the articulating bones. *Bursae* are small sacs of synovial fluid that cushion and protect bony areas that are at high risk for friction, such as the knee and the shoulder. *Tendon sheaths* are a form of bursae, but they are wrapped around tendons in high-friction areas.

Ligaments and Tendons

The fibrous capsules that surround synovial joints are supported by ligaments, dense bands of connective tissue that connect bones to bones. Ligaments limit or enhance movement, provide joint stability, and enhance joint strength.

Tendons are fibrous connective tissue bands that connect muscles to the periosteum of bones and enable the bones to move when skeletal muscles contract. When muscles contract, increased pressure causes the tendon to pull, push, or rotate the bone to which it is connected.

Table 38.3 Movements Allowed by Synovial Joints

Movement	Description
Abduction	Move limb away from body midline
Adduction	Move limb toward body midline
Extension	Straighten limbs at joint
Flexion	Bend limbs at joint
Dorsiflexion	Bend ankle to bring top of foot toward shin
Plantar flexion	Straighten ankle to point toes down
Pronation	Turn forearm to place palm down
Supination	Turn forearm to place palm up
Eversion	Turn out
Inversion	Turn in
Circumduction	Move in circle
Internal rotation	Move inward on a central axis
External rotation	Move outward on a central axis
Protraction	Move forward and parallel to ground
Retraction	Move backward and parallel to ground

38.2 Assessing the Musculoskeletal System

Structures and functions of the musculoskeletal system are assessed by findings from diagnostic tests, a health assessment interview to collect subjective data, and a physical assessment to collect objective data.

Health Assessment Interview

A health assessment interview to determine problems with musculoskeletal structure and/or function may be conducted during a health screening, may focus on a chief complaint (such as joint pain), or may be part of a complete health assessment (Bickley, 2016). Health problems affecting the neurologic system may manifest as problems with musculoskeletal function and an assessment of both systems may be necessary. If the patient has problems with musculoskeletal structure or function, analyze its onset, characteristics, course, severity, precipitating and relieving factors, and any associated symptoms, noting the timing and circumstances. For example, ask the patient:

- "Describe the pain. Can you point to its location? Does the pain increase with movement? Have you noticed any redness or swelling?"
- "Did you injure your ankle before you began to experience difficulty walking?"
- "Is your pain worse in the morning, or does it get worse throughout the day?"

The primary manifestations of altered musculoskeletal function are pain and limited mobility. Specific descriptors of the pain, its location, and its nature are important. Other significant information includes fever, fatigue, changes in weight, rash, and/or swelling. Collect information about the patient's lifestyle, including type of employment, ability to carry out activities of daily living (ADLs), self-care, exercise or participation in sports, use of alcohol or drugs, and nutrition. Explore past injuries and measures to self-treat pain (such as over-the-counter medications, prescribed medications, application of heat or cold, splinting, wrapping, or rest).

Physical Assessment

Physical assessment of the musculoskeletal system may be performed either as part of a total assessment or as a focused assessment for a patient with known or suspected problems. The techniques used to assess the musculoskeletal system are inspection, palpation, and measurement of muscle mass and joint range of motion (ROM). The patient should be comfortably dressed in clothing so that the movement of all joints is seen clearly. The patient may be standing, sitting, or lying down; the sequence of the examination should be such that the patient is not required to make frequent position changes. An assessment of the older adult, the patient in pain, or the patient who is weak may take extra time. Normal age-related findings for the older adult are summarized in the Assessment of Special Populations section.

Prior to the examination, collect all equipment and explain the techniques to decrease the patient's anxiety. The sequence for a musculoskeletal examination follows.

1. Begin the examination with an assessment of gait and posture. Inspect for overall appearance, posture, and position. Observe the patient's ability to rise from a chair, how the patient walks and pivots/turns, sits, and/or moves about in bed.
2. Proceeding in a cephalocaudal direction:
   a. Inspect and palpate the bones for any obvious deformity or changes in size or shape. Palpation will also elicit tenderness or pain.
   b. Inspect the extremities for symmetry, having equal length and muscle mass. If a difference is noted, measure extremity length and circumference, comparing limbs bilaterally.
   c. Inspect and palpate joints for swelling, pain, redness, or warmth. Palpate large joints for crepitus as the patient moves the joint through ROM. For the patient with an upright posture, a relaxed, coordinated gait, and no specific complaints of joint pain, stiffness, or swelling, ROM may be assessed on selected joints only.
   d. Providing resistance by gently pushing in the opposite direction, assess and document muscle strength on a scale of 0 to 5 (**Table 38.4**). **Box 38.1** provides guidelines for testing the strength of various muscle groups.

BOX 38.1
Guidelines for Assessing Muscle Strength

In adults, muscles are bilaterally strong. However, neuromuscular diseases, disuse, metabolic disorders, inflammation, or infections can cause muscle weakness. Muscle strength is expected to be slightly greater in the dominant arm and leg.

The muscles and muscle groups listed in the following table are routinely tested. Instructions for patients are also provided.

Muscle	Patient Instructions
Ocular muscles and lids	Close eyes tightly.
Facial muscles	Blow out cheeks.
	Stick out tongue.
Jaw muscles	Clench the teeth.
Neck muscles	Rotate the head side to side.
	Bend head forward and backward.
Shoulder muscles	Shrug shoulders.
Deltoid muscles	Hold arms up out to the side (abduction).
Biceps muscle	Bend the arm at the elbow.
Triceps muscle	Straighten the arm.
Wrist muscles	Bend hand forward and backward.
Finger muscles	Shake hands.
	Make a fist.
	Spread fingers.
Hip muscles	Raise straight leg while supine.
Gluteal and leg muscles	Alternately cross legs while sitting.
Quadriceps muscle	Straighten leg (extend the knee).
Ankle and foot muscles	Bend foot up and down.

Diagnosis

The results of diagnostic tests of musculoskeletal structure and function are used to support the diagnosis of a specific injury or disease, to provide information to identify or modify treatment of the disease, and to help the interprofessional team monitor the patient's responses to treatment and interventions. Diagnostic tests to assess the structures and functions of the musculoskeletal system are described in the Diagnostic Tests feature on page 1405. Many of these tests are invasive or require use of a contrast agent; hence, signed consent is required prior to the procedure.

Regardless of the type of diagnostic test, the nurse is responsible for explaining the procedure and any special preparation needed, assessing for medication use that may affect the outcome of the tests, supporting the patient during the examination as necessary, documenting the procedures as appropriate, ensuring the consent form is signed (if required), and monitoring the results of the tests (Kee, 2018). The nurse is also responsible for postprocedure care and patient teaching for self-care at home.

Table 38.4 Muscle Grading Scale

Grading Scale	Assessment Description
0	No muscle contraction
1	Can feel contraction of muscle but there is no movement of limb
2	Passive ROM
3	Full ROM against gravity
4	Full ROM against some resistance
5	Full ROM against full resistance

Musculoskeletal Assessments

Technique/Normal Findings	Abnormal Findings
Gait and Body Posture Assessment	
Inspect posture and gait. *Posture should be upright; gait should be smooth and steady.*	■ Joint stiffness, pain, deformities, and muscle weakness can cause changes in gait and posture.
Inspect the spine. Ask the patient to stand and bend back slowly as far as possible, bend slowly to the right and then to the left as far as possible, turn slowly to the right and left, and bend forward slowly and try to touch fingers to toes. *When viewed from the back, the cervical and lumbar spine are concave, the thoracic spine is convex, and the spine is straight; the hips and shoulders are level.*	■ With herniated lumbar disks and some types of arthritis, the lumbar curve flattens and spinal mobility is decreased. ■ An increased lumbar curve, called **lordosis**, may be seen in obesity or pregnancy. ■ A lateral, S-shaped curvature of the spine is called **scoliosis**. Functional scoliosis is usually a compensatory response to painful paravertebral muscles, herniated disks, or discrepancy in leg length. It disappears with forward flexion. Structural scoliosis is often congenital and tends to become apparent during adolescence. It is accentuated with bending forward. ■ **Kyphosis** is an exaggerated thoracic curvature of the spine associated with disorders such as osteoporosis and Paget disease.
Joint Assessment	
Inspect the joints for deformity, swelling, and redness. *There should be no visible deformity, swelling, or redness of joints.* Palpate the joints for tenderness, warmth, crepitation, consistency, and muscle mass. *Joints should be nontender and consistent bilaterally and without visible or palpable excess warmth, crepitation, or enlargement.*	■ Diseases of the joints may be manifested by signs of inflammation or such deformities as tissue loss, tissue overgrowth, or contractures; irreversible shortening of muscles and tendons may occur. ■ Edema in a joint and surrounding tissue may cause swelling; the joint may feel spongy to palpation. ■ Excess fluid in the synovial space may cause obvious bulging. ■ Redness, swelling, and pain are evidence of inflammation or infection in the joint. ■ Inflammation and injury cause joint pain. ■ Inflammatory arthritis, bursitis, tendonitis, and osteomyelitis (infection of a bone) result in painful, hot joints. ■ **Crepitation** (a grating sound and sensation) is present in a joint when the articulating surfaces have lost their cartilage, such as in arthritis.
Range-of-Motion Assessment	
Assess joint ROM by asking the patient to perform movements specific to each joint. *All bilateral joints should move through full range of motion.* *Temporomandibular joint:* "Open your mouth wide, and then close your mouth." (As the patient opens and closes the mouth, palpate the temporomandibular joints with your index and middle fingers, as shown in **Figure 38.7** ■.)	■ Clicking or popping noises, decreased ROM, pain, and swelling may indicate temporomandibular joint syndrome or, in rare cases, osteoarthritis.

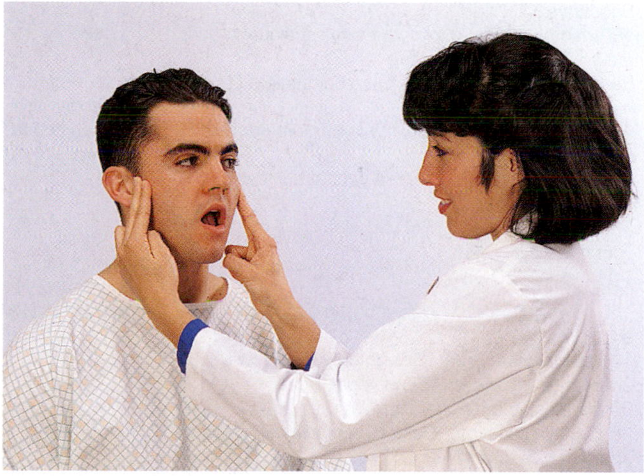

Figure 38.7 ■ Palpating the temporomandibular joints.

Technique/Normal Findings	Abnormal Findings
Cervical spine: 45-degree flexion: "Touch your chin to your chest." 55-degree extension: "Look at the ceiling." 38-degree lateral flexion: "Try to touch your right ear to your right shoulder." Repeat with the left side. 70-degree rotation: "Try to touch your chin to each shoulder."	■ Neck pain and limited extension with lateral flexion are seen with herniated cervical disks and in cervical spondylosis. ■ An immobile neck with head and neck thrust forward is seen with ankylosing spondylitis.

(continued)

Technique/Normal Findings	Abnormal Findings
Lumbar spine: 75- to 90-degree flexion: "Touch your toes with your fingers" (**Figure 38.8A** ■). 30-degree extension: "Bend backward slowly." 35-degree lateral flexion: "Bend right and left" (**Figure 38.8B** ■). 30-degree rotation: "Twist your shoulders right and left" (**Figure 38.8C** ■).	■ Decreased movement or pain with movement may indicate an abnormal spinal curvature, arthritis, herniated disk, or spasm of paravertebral muscles.

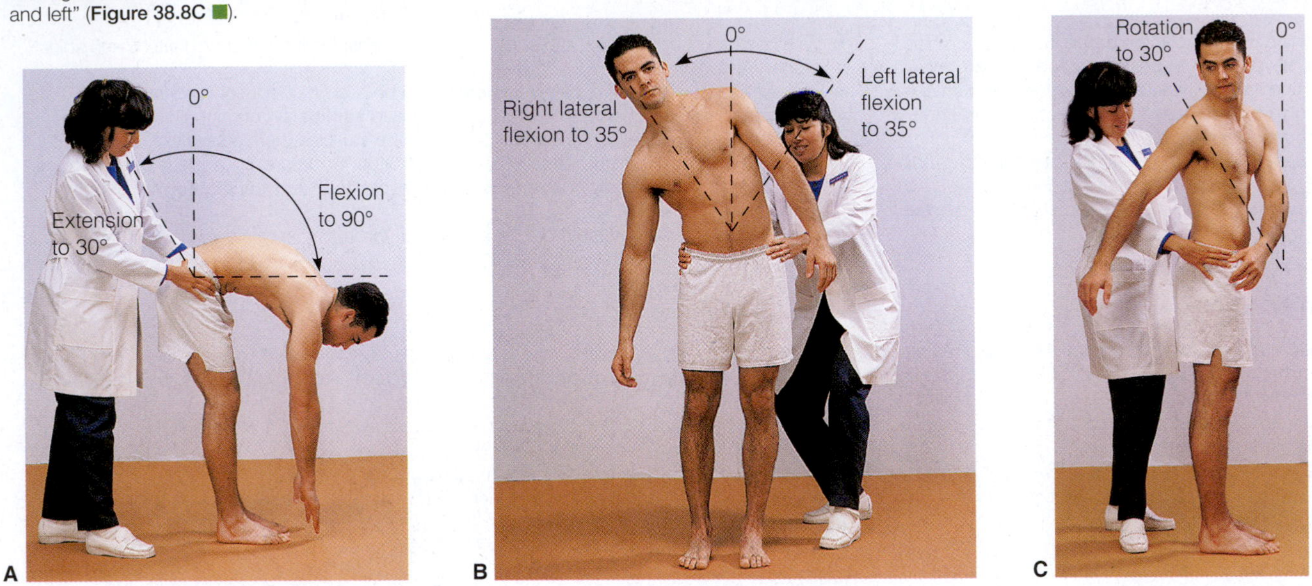
0°
Extension to 30°
Flexion to 90°
A
Right lateral flexion to 35°
0°
Left lateral flexion to 35°
B
Rotation to 30°
0°
C

Figure 38.8 ■ **A,** Forward flexion of spine. **B,** Lateral flexion of spine. **C,** Rotation of spine.

Technique/Normal Findings	Abnormal Findings
Shoulders: 180-degree flexion: "Hold your arms straight up and out." 50-degree hyperextension: "Put your straight arm behind your back." 90-degree internal rotation: "Put your forearm behind your lower back." 180-degree abduction: "Raise your straight arm up and out to your side." 50-degree adduction: "Put your straight arm across your chest."	■ Pain and tenderness over the biceps tendon occurs with **tendonitis** (inflammation of a tendon). ■ In a rotator cuff injury, the arm cannot be abducted fully and the movement causes pain and tenderness. ■ Pain and limited abduction is also seen with **bursitis** (inflammation of a bursa) and calcium deposits in this area.
Elbows: 160-degree flexion: "Touch your hands to your shoulders." 180-degree extension: "Straighten your elbows." 90-degree supination: "Bend your elbows 90 degrees, and turn hands palm up." 90-degree pronation: "Bend your elbows 90 degrees, and turn fists down."	■ Swollen, tender, inflamed elbows occur in gouty arthritis and rheumatoid arthritis. ■ Pain and tenderness at the lateral epicondyle occur in tennis elbow.
Wrists: 90-degree flexion: "Bend wrist down." 70-degree extension: "Bend wrist up." 55-degree ulnar deviation: "Bend wrist toward little finger." 20-degree radial deviation: "Bend wrist toward thumb."	■ Bilateral chronic tenderness and swelling in the wrist is seen in arthritis.
Fingers: Flexion: "Make a fist." Extension: "Open your hand." Abduction: "Spread your fingers." Adduction: "Close your fingers."	■ Flexion and extension of fingers are decreased in arthritis. ■ Heberden nodes and Bouchard nodes are hard, nontender nodules on the dorsolateral parts of the distal and proximal interphalangeal joints, respectively. They are common in osteoarthritis. ■ Stiff, painful, swollen finger joints are seen in acute rheumatoid arthritis. ■ Boutonnière and swan-neck deformities are seen in chronic rheumatoid arthritis. ■ Swollen finger joints with a white chalky discharge may be seen in chronic gout. ■ Dupuytren contracture, inability to extend the fourth and/or fifth fingers, may be seen in some older adults.

Technique/Normal Findings	Abnormal Findings
Hips (patient is lying down): 120-degree flexion: "Bring bent knee up to your chest." 30-degree hyperextension: "Lie on the abdomen, and lift up one leg at a time." 45-degree abduction: "Hold your leg straight, and move it out to the side." 38-degree internal rotation: "Bend your knee, and swing it toward your other leg." 45-degree external rotation: "Bend your knee, and swing it out to the side."	■ Movement of the hip is limited and/or painful in arthritis.

SAFETY ALERT: Unless approved by the physician, do not have the patient who has a hip prosthesis perform these movements due to the risk of prosthesis dislocation. ■

Technique/Normal Findings	Abnormal Findings
Knees: 130-degree flexion: "Do a deep knee bend." 180-degree extension: "Sit down and hold your legs straight out in front of you."	■ Swelling over the suprapatellar pouch is seen with inflammation and fluid in the articular capsule of the knee. **Synovitis** is inflammation of the synovial membrane lining the articular capsule of a joint. It is common with knee trauma. ■ Swelling over the patella is seen in bursitis.
Ankles: 20-degree dorsiflexion: "Point your foot to the ceiling." 45-degree plantar flexion: "Point your foot to the floor." 30-degree inversion: "Walk on the outside of your feet." 20-degree eversion: "Walk on the inside of your feet."	■ Contractures of the Achilles tendon may occur in patients with rheumatoid arthritis or following prolonged bedrest.
Toes: 90-degree flexion: "Walk on your toes."	■ The great toe is excessively abducted in hallux valgus (bunion). ■ The joint of the great toe is swollen, inflamed, and painful in acute gouty arthritis. ■ There is hyperextension of the metatarsophalangeal joint and flexion of the proximal interphalangeal joint with hammer toes.

Special Assessments

The following special techniques may be used to assess for suspected abnormalities.

Perform Phalen test. Ask the patient to hold the wrist in acute flexion for 60 seconds (**Figure 38.9** ■).
There should be no tingling, numbness, or pain.

■ Numbness and burning in the fingers during Phalen test may indicate carpal tunnel syndrome.

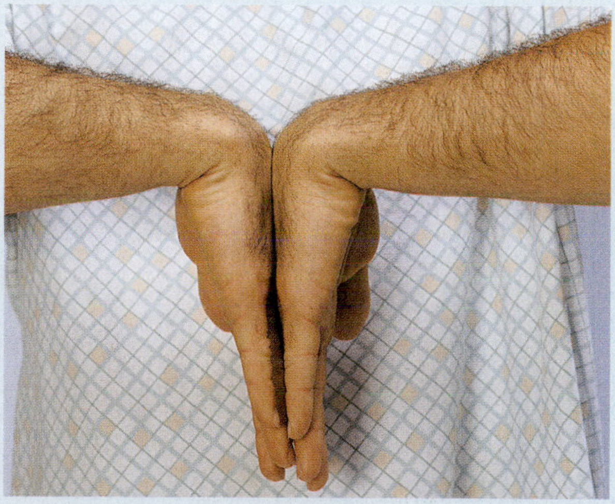

Figure 38.9 ■ Phalen test.

Check for small amounts of fluid on the knee by assessing the bulge sign. Milk upward on the medial side of the knee, and then tap the lateral side of the patella (**Figure 38.10** ■).
No fluid bulge should appear on the medial side of the knee.

■ A fluid bulge indicates increased fluid in the knee joint rather than soft tissue swelling.

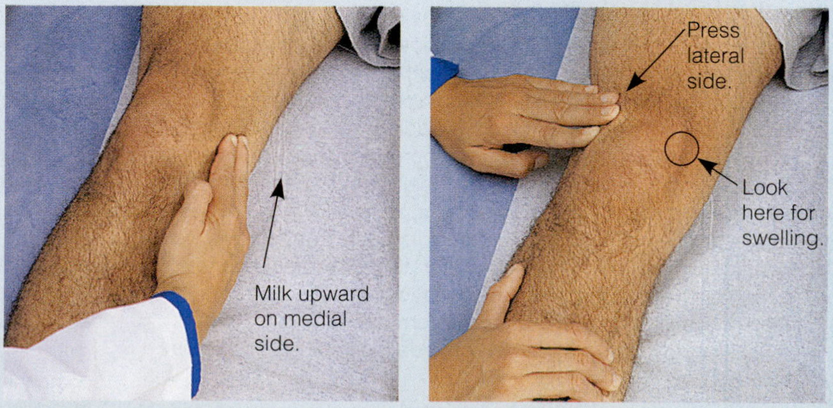
Milk upward on medial side.
Press lateral side.
Look here for swelling.

Figure 38.10 ■ Assessing the bulge sign.

(continued)

Technique/Normal Findings	Abnormal Findings
Assess for ballottement, a maneuver to detect large amounts of fluid in the knee. Apply downward pressure on the knee with one hand while pushing the patella backward against the femur with the other hand (**Figure 38.11** ■). *There should be little or no movement of the patella. The patella should rest firmly over the femur.*	■ Increased fluid will cause a clicking sensation as the patella displaces the fluid and hits the femur.
Perform McMurray test. With the patient reclining, flex the hip and knee 90 degrees or until the patient experiences pain. Palpating the medial and lateral aspects of the knee, externally rotate the foot and extend the knee; repeat the maneuver, internally rotating the foot and extending the knee (**Figure 38.12** ■). *There should be no pain or clicking.*	■ Pain, locking (inability to fully extend the knee), or a popping sound may indicate an injury to a meniscus, a disk of cartilaginous tissue in the knee.
Perform the Thomas test. Ask the patient to lie down and extend one leg while bringing the knee of the opposite leg to the chest. *The extended leg should not rise off the table.*	■ A hip flexion contracture will cause the extended leg to rise off the table.

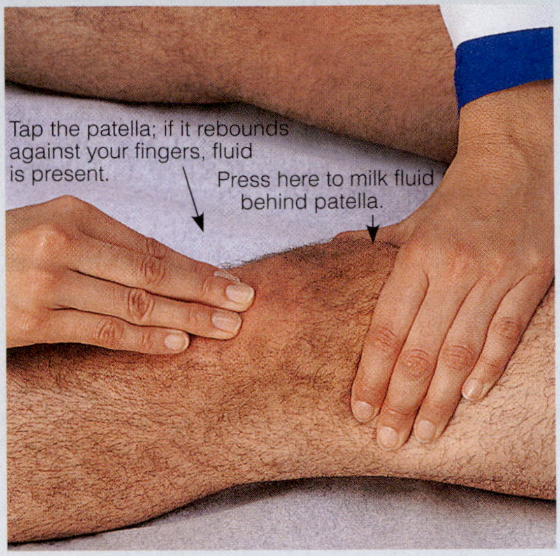
Tap the patella; if it rebounds against your fingers, fluid is present.
Press here to milk fluid behind patella.

Figure 38.11 ■ Assessing ballottement.

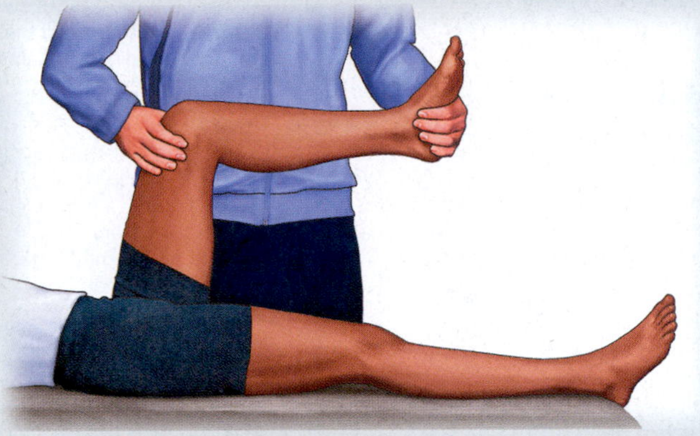

Figure 38.12 ■ McMurray test.

Genetic Considerations

When conducting a health assessment interview and a physical assessment, the nurse needs to consider genetic influences on the health of the adult. During the health assessment interview, ask about family members with health problems affecting musculoskeletal structure or function. In addition, ask about a family history of arthritis, abnormally long bones, children with muscular dystrophy, and anyone with amyotrophic lateral sclerosis (ALS). During the physical assessment, assess for any manifestations that might indicate a genetic disorder. If data are found to indicate genetic risk factors or alterations, ask about genetic testing and refer for appropriate genetic counseling and evaluation (Genetic and Rare Diseases Information Center, 2018).

Examples of musculoskeletal disorders with a genetic basis include:

- Myotonic dystrophy is an inherited disorder in which the muscles become weak, have a decreased ability to relax, and eventually waste away. Other manifestations are mental deficiency, hair loss, and cataracts. Although rare, the disease does increase in severity with each successive generation.
- Marfan syndrome, an autosomal dominant disorder of connective tissue, affects the bones, lungs, eyes, heart, and blood vessels. It is characterized by abnormally long extremities, hyperextensible joints, and a variety of spinal, skeletal, and other deformities. It is believed to have affected Abraham Lincoln. The aspect of the disease that is most life-threatening is the effect on the cardiovascular system (Sorenson et al., 2019).
- Duchenne muscular dystrophy, an X-linked disorder, affects primarily males. It is one of the most common muscular dystrophies and is characterized by rapid muscle degeneration early in life.
- Other musculoskeletal diseases believed to have a genetic component include rheumatoid arthritis, osteoarthritis, gout, muscular dystrophy, ankylosing spondylitis, lupus erythematosus, and scleroderma.

Diagnostic Tests
of the Musculoskeletal System

NAME OF TEST	PURPOSE AND DESCRIPTION	RELATED NURSING INTERVENTIONS
Arthrocentesis	This procedure is done to obtain synovial fluid from a joint for diagnosis (such as infections) or to remove excess fluid. A needle is inserted through the joint capsule and fluid is aspirated.	After the procedure, apply a compression dressing and tell the patient to report any bleeding, leakage of fluid, or excessive pain to the healthcare provider.
Arthroscopy	An endoscopic examination of the interior surfaces of a joint, arthroscopy is used to perform surgery and diagnose diseases of the patella, meniscus, and synovial and extrasynovial membranes. In addition, fluid may be drained from the joint and tissue removed for biopsy. A fiberoptic endoscope is inserted into the joint, either with local anesthesia or general anesthesia. An arthrography (x-ray examination of the joint) is performed prior to an arthroscopy.	Instruct the patient about orders for fasting and use of current medications prior to the procedure. Following the procedure, assess for bleeding and swelling, apply ice to the area if prescribed, and instruct patient to avoid excessive use of the joint for 2 to 3 days.
Blood chemistry	See **Table 38.5**.	No special preparation is needed.

Table 38.5 Blood Tests with Purposes Specific to the Musculoskeletal System

Name of Test	Purpose	Normal Value
Alkaline phosphatase (ALP)	To identify bone diseases. Increased in bone cancer, Paget disease, healing fractures, rheumatoid arthritis, osteoporosis.	42–136 units/L ALP^1: 20–130 units/L ALP^2: 20–120 units/L (increases slightly with aging)
Calcium (Ca)	To monitor calcium levels and detect calcium imbalances. Decreased with inadequate calcium and vitamin D intake and malabsorption from the gastrointestinal tract. Increased in bone cancer and multiple fractures.	4.5–5.5 mEq/L or 9–11 mg/dL (serum)
Creatine kinase (CK), creatinine phosphokinase (CPK)	To diagnose muscle trauma or disease. Increased in muscular dystrophy and traumatic injuries (specifically, CPK-MM isoenzyme).	Male: 50–170 units/L Female: 25–140 units/L CPK-MM: 94–100%
Human leukocyte antigen (HLA)	To diagnose diseases such as juvenile RA or ankylosing spondylitis.	No normal value
Phosphorus (P), phosphate (PO_4)	To assess phosphorous levels. Increased with bone tumors and healing fractures.	1.7–2.6 mEq/L or 2.5–4.5 mg/Dl
Rheumatoid factor (RF)	To diagnose rheumatoid arthritis (RA) (positive for RA at > 1:80). Also increased in lupus erythematosus and scleroderma.	< 1:20 titer
Uric acid	To diagnose and monitor the treatment of gout. Panic level considered >12 mg/dL.	Male: 3.5–8.0 mg/dL Female: 2.8–6.8 mg/dL

NAME OF TEST	PURPOSE AND DESCRIPTION	RELATED NURSING INTERVENTIONS
Bone mineral density (BMD), bone absorptiometry **Dual-energy x-ray absorptiometry (DEXA)** **Quantitative ultrasonography (QUS)**	These examinations are done to evaluate bone density, diagnose osteoporosis, and determine risk for osteoporosis-related fracture. DEXA of the hip and lumbar spine can calculate the size and thickness of bone. QUS, which does not expose the patient to ionizing radiation, evaluates density of the calcaneus (heel bone). Osteoporosis is diagnosed if the bone mass is more than 2.5 standard deviations below peak bone mass. Normal value: 1 standard deviation below peak bone mass	Instruct patient to remove all metal objects from the area to be scanned (such as jewelry, belt buckles, zippers).

NAME OF TEST	PURPOSE AND DESCRIPTION	RELATED NURSING INTERVENTIONS
Bone scan	During a bone scan, the concentration of an injected radioisotope in bone is determined using a scintillation (gamma) camera detector. Uptake is increased in osteomyelitis, osteoporosis, cancers of the bone, and in some fractures. Uptake is decreased in avascular necrosis.	No special preparation is needed, although the patient should be well hydrated. Advise the patient to drink three glasses of water during the waiting period (after the isotope is injected and before the scan is obtained). Instruct the patient to remove metal objects, jewelry, and keys prior to the scan.
Computed tomography (CT) scan—long bones and joints, spine	A CT of long bones and joints provides a three-dimensional picture used to evaluate musculoskeletal trauma (fractures) and bony abnormalities (such as tumors). A CT of the spine can identify tumors, cysts, vascular malformations, and herniated intervertebral disks.	If contrast dye is used, assess for allergy to iodine, seafood, or radiologic contrast (many contain iodine). Assess medications; noniodated contrast media may be necessary for patients taking oral hypoglycemic agents. Have spine x-rays available. If scheduling myelogram and spine CT, patient should have myelogram first. After the test, if contrast dye was used, monitor for delayed allergic reaction (rash, itching, headache, vomiting) and instruct patient to increase fluid intake.
Electromyogram (EMG)	An EMG measures the electrical activity of skeletal muscles at rest and during contraction; this information is useful in diagnosing neuromuscular diseases. Needle electrodes are inserted into affected skeletal muscles, allowing electrical activity to be heard, viewed on an oscilloscope, and recorded on graph paper. Normally, there is no electrical activity at rest.	Tell the patient not to drink fluids containing caffeine or to smoke for 3 hours before the test and not to take medications such as muscle relaxants, anticholinergics, or cholinergics as ordered by the physician. If serum enzymes such as SGOT, CPK, or LDH are ordered, the specimen should be drawn before the EMG or 5 to 10 days after the EMG.
Magnetic resonance imaging (MRI)	An MRI of bony structures is used in diagnosis and evaluation of avascular necrosis, osteomyelitis, tumors, disk abnormalities, and tears in ligament or cartilage. It uses radio waves and magnetic fields; gadolinium may be injected to increase visualization of bony or muscular structures.	Inform patient of need to lie still during the examination. Assess for tattoos and any metallic implants (such as pacemakers, clips on brain aneurysms, body piercings, shrapnel). If present, notify imaging healthcare provider. Ask if patient is pregnant; if so, the test is not performed. Ask about claustrophobia; if a problem, instruct patient to ask for a relaxing medication to take prior to the MRI.
Musculoskeletal ultrasound (US)	Musculoskeletal ultrasound provides images of muscles, tendons, ligaments, joints, and soft tissue. It is used to help diagnose muscle and tendon tears; bleeding into muscle, soft tissue, or joints; tumors; and joint abnormalities.	This noninvasive test requires no special preparation, although the patient may be asked to remove jewelry in the area to be examined.
Skeletal x-ray	X-rays are done to identify and evaluate bone density and structure.	Ask women if they are pregnant; x-rays should be avoided during the first trimester. No special preparation is needed for skeletal x-rays.

38.3 Assessment of Special Populations

Key age-related musculoskeletal system changes and their significance are outlined in **Table 38.6**.

Patient assessments should include evaluation of military service and information regarding any interface with the Veteran's Administration (Veteran's Administration, 2017a). The nurse should be aware that the Veteran's Administration provides specialized programs and rehabilitation for veterans who have experienced an amputation. Starting in 2007, the VA established the Amputation System of Care (ASoC) designed to reduce variance and increase access to state-of-the-art rehabilitation techniques and prosthetic technology (Veteran's Administration, 2017b).

38.4 Health Promotion

Trauma prevention can save lives. Trauma is the leading cause of death among adults under age 45 (National Center for Health Statistics, 2016). Young adults face a high risk of sustaining trauma. They need to be taught the importance of safety equipment—such as automobile seat belts, helmets for bicycle and motorized vehicle riders, football pads, proper footwear, protective eyewear, and hard hats—in preventing or decreasing the severity of injury from trauma. Older adults should have regular screenings for osteoporosis (with a bone density test), activity levels,

Table 38.6 Age-Related Changes in the Musculoskeletal System

Age-Related Change	Significance
Bones and Joints	
■ Decreased bone mass and minerals. ■ Decreased calcium reabsorption, a slow resorption of the interior of long bones, and slower production of new bone on the outside surface of bones. ■ Thinning of intervertebral disks, erosion of vertebrae, and kyphosis often develop. ■ Cartilage on bone surfaces in joints deteriorates and bone spurs may occur. ■ Synovial fluid becomes less viscous.	Decreased bone mass and decreased calcium absorption contribute to bones that are often thinner and weaker, with an increased risk of fractures with trauma. As the spinal column shortens, height decreases. Changes in spine can shift center of gravity, increasing the risk for falls. Loss of joint cartilage and formation of bone spurs make movement more painful and may even limit mobility.
Muscles, Ligaments, and Tendons	
■ Muscle fibers atrophy and fibrous tissue slowly replaces muscle tissue. ■ Decreased muscle mass and strength. ■ Ligaments and tendons lose elasticity resulting in loss of joint range of motion (Tabloski, 2014).	Regular exercise is very important in decreasing the loss of muscle mass and strength associated with aging.

cognitive and affective disorders, vision impairments, and assessment for risk for falls. Older adults can reduce their risk of falling by increasing lower body strength and balance through regular physical activity and by asking their healthcare provider or pharmacist to review their medications. Educational programs about workplace and farm safety, including information about ergonomic principles, can also help prevent musculoskeletal injuries.

Exercising regularly and avoiding obesity are important factors in maintaining good bone health in all adults. An adequate intake of calcium is essential to ensure proper growth, development, and maintenance of strong bones throughout life. It is important that women ensure good bone health prior to menopause because the loss of estrogen during and after menopause decreases calcium use and increases the risk of osteoporosis. Strong bones are formed by calcium intake and weight-bearing exercise, both of which are equally important in the postmenopausal woman.

CHAPTER HIGHLIGHTS

38.1 Anatomy, Physiology, and Functions of the Musculoskeletal System

Describe the anatomy, physiology, and functions of the musculoskeletal system, and identify abnormal findings that may indicate impairments of the musculoskeletal system.

- Intact structure and function of the musculoskeletal system is vital to the ability to independently perform usual activities of daily living and other activities.

38.2 Assessing the Musculoskeletal System

Outline the components of the assessment of the musculoskeletal system, including topics for the health assessment interview, techniques for physical assessment, and the diagnostic tests used in the assessment.

- Manifestations of dysfunction, injuries, and disorders affecting the musculoskeletal system may be detected during a general health assessment as well as during focused and functional musculoskeletal assessments.
- Musculoskeletal disorders are diagnosed primarily using a targeted medical history, physical assessment, and functional assessments of the musculoskeletal system. Diagnostic tests help to identify and diagnose musculoskeletal injuries and disorders.

38.3 Assessment of Special Populations

Differentiate considerations for assessing the musculoskeletal systems of older adults and veterans.

- There are many musculoskeletal impacts found in the older adult patient. Changes related to aging and chronic illness are the most common changes.
- All patients should be assessed for military service. If the patient had served, determination of VA involvement in care helps to maintain coordination of care.

38.4 Health Promotion

Summarize topics that nurses can teach to promote a healthy musculoskeletal system across the lifespan.

- Musculoskeletal health promotion focuses on two overarching topics: Trauma prevention (especially with young adults) and the importance of regular exercise and maintenance of normal body weight.

TEST YOURSELF NCLEX-RN® REVIEW

1. The nurse is caring for a patient with an epiphyseal fracture. What bone classification should the nurse keep in mind when planning this patient's care?
   A. Flat
   B. Long
   C. Short
   D. Irregular
2. During an assessment the nurse asks the patient to move an extremity away from the body midline. The nurse would document the patient's ability to make which movement?
   A. Flexion
   B. Extension
   C. Abduction
   D. Adduction
3. A patient with gout asks, "Why is my blood being examined for uric acid?" What should the nurse respond to this patient?
   A. "We are testing to see why you have that big bruise on your hip."
   B. "A uric acid test is done to diagnose rheumatoid arthritis."
   C. "It will help us determine if you have inherited a familial muscle disease."
   D. "A uric acid test is done to see if your gout medication is effective."
4. The nurse is assessing the musculoskeletal status of a 70-year-old patient. What findings should the nurse consider as expected age-related changes in this body system? (Select all that apply.)
   A. The patient's upper arm and thigh circumference has decreased.
   B. The patient says, "I don't think I am as strong in my muscles as I was a few years ago."
   C. There is significant edema in the patient's ankles, hips, and knees.
   D. The patient has difficulty raising arms up above the head.
   E. There has been a loss of 1/2 inch in height from previous assessment one year ago.
5. A patient is scheduled for an electromyogram. What should the nurse instruct the patient to do in preparation for this diagnostic test? (Select all that apply.)
   A. Do not smoke for 3 hours before the test.
   B. Avoid taking muscle relaxants before the test.
   C. Avoid taking oral hypoglycemic agents before the test.
   D. Alert the healthcare provider about an allergy to shellfish.
   E. Avoid fluids containing caffeine for 3 hours before the test.
6. The nurse is assessing muscle strength. What should the nurse ask the patient to do to assess jaw muscle strength? (Select all that apply.)
   A. "Clench your teeth."
   B. "Stick out your tongue."
   C. "Close your eyes tightly."
   D. "Bend your head forward."
   E. "Blow out your cheeks."
7. The nurse hears a grating sound while assessing range of motion of a patient's hip. How should the nurse document this finding?
   A. Crackles
   B. Arthritis
   C. Synovitis
   D. Crepitation
8. While assessing for ballottement, a nurse notes that the patella rebounds against the fingers. What does this finding indicate?
   A. Fluid in the knee joint
   B. Deformity of the elbow
   C. Crepitus in the hip joint
   D. Infection of the metatarsals
9. During the physical assessment of a young adult, the nurse notes a lateral, S-shaped curve of the spine. What should the nurse suspect is occurring with this patient?
   A. Lordosis
   B. Scoliosis
   C. Kyphosis
   D. Musculosis
10. The nurse is preparing to assess a patient's musculoskeletal system. What should the nurse keep in mind as being the most common manifestations of musculoskeletal disorders? (Select all that apply.)
    A. Pain
    B. Cyanosis
    C. Decreased pulses
    D. Exaggerated reflexes
    E. Limited mobility

See Test Yourself answers in Appendix B.

REFERENCES

Bickley, L. (2016). *Bates' guide to physical examination and history taking* (12th ed.). Philadelphia, PA: Lippincott Williams & Wilkins.

Genetic and Rare Diseases Information Center (GARD). (2018). *Musculoskeletal diseases.* Retrieved from https://rarediseases.info.nih.gov/diseases/diseases-by-category/15/musculoskeletal-diseases.

Kee, J. L. (2018). *Laboratory and diagnostic tests with nursing implications* (10th ed.). Hoboken, NJ: Pearson Education.

National Center for Health Statistics. (2016). *Health, United States, 2016 with chartbook.* Retrieved from https://www.cdc.gov/nchs/data/hus/hus16.pdf.

Sorenson, M., Quinn, L., & Klein, D. (2019). *Pathophysiology: Concepts of human disease.* Hoboken, NJ: Pearson Education.

Veterans' Administration (VA). (2017a). *Disability compensation: "Presumptive" disability benefits.* Retrieved from https://www.benefits.va.gov/BENEFITS/factsheets/serviceconnected/presumption.pdf.

Veterans' Administration (VA). (2017b). *Rehabilitation and prosthetic services.* Retrieved from https://www.prosthetics.va.gov.

ADDITIONAL RESOURCES

American College of Sports Medicine
https://www.acsm.org/

Arthritis Foundation
https://www.arthritis.org/

National Institute of Arthritis, Musculoskeletal and Skin Diseases
https://www.niams.nih.gov/

National Institute for Occupational Health and Safety, Musculoskeletal Health Program
https://www.cdc.gov/niosh/programs/msd/default.html

Chapter 39

Nursing Care of Patients with Musculoskeletal Trauma

Chapter Outline and Learning Outcomes

39.1 Traumatic Injuries of the Muscles, Ligaments, and Tendons 1411

Describe the pathophysiology and manifestations of traumatic injuries of the muscles, ligaments, and tendons, and outline the interprofessional care and nursing care of patients with these injuries.

39.2 Traumatic Injuries of Bones 1417

Describe the pathophysiology and manifestations of traumatic injuries of bones, and outline the interprofessional care and nursing care of patients with these injuries.

CLINICAL COMPETENCIES

- Assess health status of patients with musculoskeletal injuries, including the patient's perception of the injury, its impact on lifestyle, and expectations for care.
- Use current evidence and evidence-based guidelines to plan, coordinate, and implement care for patients who have experienced musculoskeletal trauma.
- Determine priority nursing problems, based on assessed data, to plan and implement individualized nursing interventions and teaching for patients with musculoskeletal injuries.
- Provide skilled care for patients with a cast, fixation device, traction, or amputation, maintaining patient and caregiver safety at all times.
- Coordinate and integrate interprofessional care into care of patients with musculoskeletal trauma.
- Communicate and document care for patients with traumatic injuries of the musculoskeletal system using electronic medical records and other communication methods as appropriate.

KEY TERMS

amputation, 1439
compartment syndrome, 1436
contracture, 1441
contusion, 1411
dislocation, 1413
fat embolism syndrome (FES), 1436
flail chest, 1423
fracture, 1417
phantom limb pain, 1441
sprain, 1411
strain, 1411
subluxation, 1413

Musculoskeletal trauma refers to injuries to muscle, bone, and soft tissue that result from excessive external force. With trauma, the external force transmits more kinetic energy than the tissue can absorb, and injury results. The severity of the injury depends not only on the amount of force but also on the location of the impact because different parts of the body can withstand different amounts of force. A wide variety of external forces can cause trauma, and the force involved can vary in severity (e.g., a step off the curb, a fall, being tackled in a football game, and a motor vehicle crash).

Traumatic musculoskeletal injuries include blunt tissue trauma, damage to tendons and ligaments, and fractures of bones. Various forces that cause musculoskeletal trauma are typical for a specific environment, activity, or age group. Regardless of the cause, the injury may require rehabilitation and temporary or permanent changes in lifestyle. Occupational musculoskeletal disorders accounted for 286,350 healthcare visits in the United States in 2015 (Bureau of Labor Statistics [BLS], 2017). Nine percent of these resulted in at least one day absent from work. Nursing assistants accounted for 43% of these cases and RNs accounted for 20% (BLS, 2017).

Musculoskeletal trauma can result in mild to severe injuries, from a minor soft tissue injury, to a fracture, to a complete amputation. In addition, trauma to one part of the musculoskeletal system often produces dysfunction in adjacent structures. For example, a fracture of the femur prevents the adjacent muscles from abducting and adducting.

Nursing care helps minimize the effects of musculoskeletal trauma, prevents complications, and hastens restoration of function. This chapter discusses injuries to the muscles, ligaments, and tendons, including contusions, strains, and sprains; joint trauma; repetitive use injuries; fractures; and amputations.

39.1 Traumatic Injuries of the Muscles, Ligaments, and Tendons

The Patient with a Contusion, Strain, or Sprain

Contusions, strains, and sprains are among the most commonly reported musculoskeletal injuries. They account for about 50% of work-related injuries, with lower back injuries being the most commonly reported occupational injury (BLS, 2016). However, many sprains and strains are not work related and are often not reported. The lower back and cervical region of the spine are the most common sites for muscle strains, and the ankle is the most commonly sprained joint, usually caused by forced inversion of the foot (Feger et al., 2017). In the United States, sprains and strains account for over 41% of all sports and recreation-related injuries (Sheu, Chen, & Hedegaard, 2016).

Pathophysiology

A **contusion**, the least serious form of musculoskeletal injury, is bleeding into soft tissue that results from a blunt force, such as a kick or striking a body part against a hard object. The skin remains intact, but small blood vessels rupture and bleed into soft tissues. A contusion with a large amount of bleeding is referred to as a *hematoma*.

A **strain** is a stretching injury to a muscle or a muscle–tendon unit caused by mechanical overloading. A muscle that is forced to extend past its elasticity will develop microscopic tears. Lifting heavy objects without bending the knees or a sudden acceleration–deceleration, as in a motor vehicle crash, can cause strains. Common sites for a muscle strain are the lower back and the hamstring muscle in the back of the thigh. A **sprain** is a stretch and/or tear of one or more ligaments surrounding a joint. Forces going in opposite directions cause the ligament to overstretch and/or tear. The ligaments may be partially or completely torn. Grades of sprain severity are presented in **Table 39.1**.

Table 39.1 Grades of Sprain Severity

Grade	Description	Manifestations
Grade 1 (mild)	Overstretching or minimal tear of ligaments with no joint instability	■ Mild pain, edema, tenderness ■ Little or no bruising ■ Minimal or no loss of joint function or ability to bear weight
Grade 2 (moderate)	Partial tear of the ligament	■ Moderate pain, bruising, and edema ■ Mild to moderate joint instability, functional disability ■ Weight bearing difficult
Grade 3 (severe)	Complete tear or rupture of the ligament	■ Severe pain, edema, and bruising ■ Significant functional loss and joint instability ■ Inability to bear weight

Risk Factors

Falls are the number one risk factor for contusions, sprains, and strains. Mechanisms of falls vary with age. In adolescents and young adults, participation in athletic events most commonly leads to falls. In middle age, fall injuries can be related to participation in sports or be work related. For sports-related falls, improper physical conditioning, a growing musculoskeletal system, contact sports (wrestling, football, soccer, etc.), and running and jumping sports (basketball, volleyball, etc.) are notable risk factors (Agarwal & Mann, 2016; Nguyen, Sheehan, Davis, & Gill, 2017). Additionally, females are more likely to be seen in emergency departments for lateral ankle sprains (Shah, Thomas, Noone, Blanchette, & Wikstrom, 2016). In the very young and in older adults, balance issues and tripping are common etiologies of falls.

Manifestations

The manifestations of a contusion include edema and discoloration of the skin. The blood in the soft tissue initially results in a purple and blue color commonly referred to as a *bruise*. As the blood begins to reabsorb, the area involved becomes brown and then yellow until it disappears.

The manifestations of a strain include pain, limited motion, muscle spasms, edema, and possible muscle weakness. Severe strains that partially or completely tear the muscle or tendon can be disabling with significant bleeding, edema, and bruising around the muscle.

Manifestations of sprains include loss of the functional ability of the joint, a feeling of a pop or tear, discoloration, pain, and rapid edema. Motion increases the joint pain. The intensity of the manifestations depends on the severity of the sprain.

Interprofessional Care

Diagnosis

Physical exam alone can lead to a diagnosis. However, when soft tissue trauma occurs, musculoskeletal ultrasound or x-rays and magnetic resonance imaging (MRI) may be done to determine the extent of tissue damage and rule out fracture.

Medications

Nonsteroidal anti-inflammatory drugs (NSAIDs) are used to reduce pain, edema, and inflammation associated with the injury. Alternately, acetaminophen may provide comparable pain relief (Shawen, Dworak, & Anderson, 2016).

Treatment

The goal of the initial stage of treating soft tissue trauma is to reduce edema and pain. Patients should follow a regimen of **PRICE** for the first 24 to 48 hours (see **Table 39.2**).

Protection

Rest

Ice

Compression

Elevation.

Early weight bearing as tolerated has been shown to hasten healing in the lower extremities (McGovern & Martin, 2016).

Ankle sprains may be immobilized with a cast or splint, with no limitations on weight bearing. A knee injury often requires a knee immobilizer. If an upper extremity is injured, a sling is provided. Physical therapy may be recommended for rehabilitation. Time required for healing depends on the severity of the injury; for example, a mild ankle sprain may require up to 3 to 6 weeks of rehabilitation, whereas a severe sprain may require up to 8 to 12 months to return to full activities (National Institute of Arthritis and Musculoskeletal and Skin Diseases, 2015).

Surgery

Surgery to repair the torn ligament, muscle, or tendon may be required for severe sprains or strains.

Nursing Care

The nursing care of each patient is individualized. For example, a strain or sprain may not be as devastating to an attorney as it is to a professional athlete; therefore, the nurse should determine what the injury means to the particular patient.

Assessment

Nursing assessment centers on the injured area and the patient's reaction to the injury. Immediately postinjury, the nurse should assess for head injury and level of consciousness. Once the patient is stable, a focused assessment is performed including skin, neurovascular (if an extremity is involved), musculoskeletal in the area of injury, pain, and psychosocial.

Priorities of Care

Nursing care priorities for the patient with a sprain or strain focus on reduction of inflammation, immobilization of the joint, associated acute pain, impaired physical mobility, and the risks for impaired tissue perfusion and neurovascular compromise.

Diagnoses, Outcomes, and Interventions

Patient care priorities focus on providing information about self-care to decrease pain and return physical mobility to preinjury levels.

Manage Acute Pain. The pain results from soft tissue trauma is primarily due to the injury to the muscle or ligament and secondarily to bleeding and edema at the injury site.

Expected Outcome: Patient will verbalize pharmacologic and nonpharmacologic measures to manage pain within acceptable levels.

The nurse will:

- Teach the patient to use PRICE (protection, rest, ice, compression, elevation) therapy to care for the injury. *The interventions included in PRICE therapy prevent further injury and allow the injured muscle, ligament, or tendon to heal (rest), cause vasoconstriction and reduce pain (ice), decrease edema formation and pain (compression), and promote venous return to decrease edema and pain (elevation).*
- Teach effective use of prescription and over-the-counter (OTC) analgesics and NSAIDs to manage pain. *An understanding of effective analgesic and NSAID use allows the patient to maintain comfort and activity within recommended limits.*

Promote Physical Mobility. Pain causes the patient to avoid using or bearing weight with the injured extremity, therefore limiting their mobility.

Expected Outcome: Patient will regain preinjury level of mobility.

The nurse will:

- Teach the reason why early ambulation and weight bearing, as ordered, are important. *Patient may be reluctant to move due to pain, therefore teaching the complications*

Table 39.2 PRICE Therapy for Musculoskeletal Injuries

Action	Patient and Family Education
Protection	■ Immobilization with splinting above and below the injured area, including the joints, as needed, protects the area from further injury
Rest	■ Decrease regular daily living activities and exercise as needed. ■ Limit weight bearing on the injured extremity for 48 hours for severe injuries. ■ If you use a cane or crutch to avoid weight bearing, use it on the uninjured side so you can lean away from and relieve weight on the injured leg.
Ice	■ To avoid cold injury or frostbite, apply an ice pack to the injured area for no more than 20 minutes at a time, four to eight times a day. ■ An ice bag, cold pack, plastic bag filled with crushed ice and wrapped in a towel, or a bag of frozen peas may be used.
Compression	■ Loosen the compression bandage if you experience numbness, tingling, or edema distal to the injury, or if the distal extremity becomes cool or cyanotic (bluish-gray).
Elevation	■ Keep the injured extremity elevated on a pillow above heart level to help reduce edema and pain.

of immobility can add motivation to his or her participation in activities.

- Teach the correct use of crutches, walkers, canes, or slings if prescribed. *Use of the correct technique increases safety and encourages use of these devices.*
- Teach signs and symptoms of healing and complications and when to report these to the care provider. *Patient needs to be aware of the signs and symptoms of complications in order to prevent further compromise.*
- Encourage follow-up care. *Severe sprains may require further evaluation to determine if physical therapy or surgical intervention is indicated.*

Delegating Nursing Care Activities

Unlicensed assistive personnel (UAP) may be assigned the task of ice application and elevation of an extremity with specific parameters for the length of time the ice should be applied. They may also assist with mobility of the patient once the nurse or physical therapist has taught the patient to use any assistive devices.

Transitions of Care

In the general population, physical conditioning, good lighting, and being careful will help prevent falls and thus these injuries. Athletes can help prevent contusions, strains, and sprains through appropriate physical conditioning and proper training in the sport and the position played. Bracing has been shown to be effective in preventing recurrent ankle sprains (Janssen, van Mechelen, & Verhagen, 2014). The National Athletic Trainer's Association (Kaminski et al., 2013) holds the position that the best prevention is a multi-intervention prevention program for 3 months prior to activity focusing on balance and neuromuscular control.

The Patient with Joint Trauma

The synovial joints of the upper and lower extremities can be subjected to injury from trauma as a result of recreational activities or accidents. Hip joint trauma is covered extensively in Chapter 40.

Pathophysiology

Joint trauma affects the joint structure itself and/or the soft tissues supporting the joint: Muscles, ligaments, and tendons. These injuries can be made worse if there is an underlying issue, such as osteoarthritis or rheumatoid arthritis. Additionally, systemic disease processes can have an influence on the joint structures, making the joints more vulnerable to serious issues. These systemic processes include osteoporosis, diabetes mellitus, and some autoimmune diseases, such as systemic lupus erythematous.

Rotator Cuff Injuries

The shoulder joint is particularly vulnerable to injuries due to its wide range of motion, complexity, and exposed position. Most shoulder issues result from rotator cuff injuries. The rotator cuff is the group of muscles that control shoulder movement. The four muscles that make up the rotator cuff all have their insertion point in the humeral head. Rotator cuff disorders include tendinitis, bursitis, and partial and complete muscle tears. These injuries can be acute or may result from repetitive use injury or degenerative changes of the involved tissues.

Knee Injuries

The knee is vulnerable to ligament tears, meniscal injury, and patellar dislocation. These injuries are frequently associated with sports activities that lead to falls or abnormal twisting of the knee joint. The medial collateral ligament (MCL) is the most commonly injured knee ligament; anterior cruciate ligament (ACL) tears are also common sports injuries (Luke & Ma, 2017). The menisci, two C-shaped plates of cartilage within each knee joint, act as shock absorbers. A tear of the medial meniscus is a common knee injury. The patella, or knee cap, can become partially or completely dislocated or be fractured.

Joint Dislocation

A **dislocation** is an injury in which the ends of bones are displaced out of their normal position and joint articulation is lost. Dislocations usually follow trauma such as a fall or blow. They commonly occur during contact sports such as football or from falls resulting from activities such as skiing. Pathologic dislocations result from disease of the joint, including infection, rheumatoid arthritis, paralysis, neuromuscular diseases, and tumors.

Although dislocations may occur in any joint, they occur most frequently in the shoulder, acromioclavicular joints, and the patella. A **subluxation** is a partial dislocation in which the bones of the joint remain in partial contact.

Risk Factors

Risk factors for joint injury include participation in athletic events and joint overuse. Additionally, females of childbearing age have an increased risk of anterior cruciate ligament (ACL) injury due to laxity in the ligaments, which is influenced by the hormone levels associated with the menstrual cycle (Bell et al., 2014).

These injuries can be made worse if there is an underlying issue, such as osteoarthritis or rheumatoid arthritis. Additionally, systemic disease processes can have an influence on the joint structures, making the joints more vulnerable to serious issues. These systemic processes include osteoporosis, diabetes mellitus, and some autoimmune diseases, such as systemic lupus erythematous.

Manifestations

Manifestations of rotator cuff damage include shoulder pain, which may be worse at night or when lying on the involved shoulder and is most often felt in the deltoid (Buti, 2013). Range of motion, internal rotation and adduction in particular, increases discomfort and is often limited.

The patient with a knee injury often relates a history of an acute injury, with immediate pain, a tearing or popping sensation, or the knee "giving out." Edema of the affected joint may develop immediately or over several hours after the injury. With meniscus injuries the patient may complain of pain with ambulation, a locking sensation of the joint (with large tears), and edema (Davis & Saulog-Wendel, 2013).

Joint dislocation causes pain, deformity, and limited motion of the affected joint.

Complications

Pain is the most common complication of untreated conditions. A frozen (immovable) shoulder and functional limitations are complications of an untreated rotator cuff injury (Buti, 2013). Mobility difficulties can result with delayed treatment of knee injuries. Nerve impingement is a potential complication with joint dislocation or subluxation, as well as functional limitations.

Interprofessional Care

Care of the patient with a joint injury focuses on relieving pain, managing or correcting the resulting disorder, and preventing complications.

Diagnosis

The history and physical are often sufficient to identify joint trauma. Specific examination maneuvers may be performed. X-rays of the affected joint are obtained; an MRI may also be performed.

Treatment

The treatment is dictated by the type of injury. A dislocation is usually *reduced* (bone ends realigned) using manual traction. Dislocations of the shoulder joint are most often being managed with closed reduction and a limited period of post reduction immobilization. A dislocated hip requires immediate reduction to prevent necrosis of the femoral head and injury to the sciatic and femoral nerves. After reduction, the patient is placed on bedrest for several days and then the patient is fitted with a brace to lend strength to the hip muscles so that ambulation may be resumed. Physical therapy will be prescribed for hip muscle strengthening. If a hip dislocation is accompanied by a fracture, the patient will undergo surgery to increase mobility, decrease complications, and rapidly stabilize the joint.

Treatment for rotator cuff injuries is usually conservative, including joint rest, NSAIDs, moist heat, and, for persistent problems, physical therapy. Some patients require surgery to repair a torn rotator cuff.

Joint protection, rest with compression, ice, elevation, and restricted weight bearing are initially prescribed for knee injuries. Physical therapy is ordered during rehabilitation. Patients with recurrent pain, edema, or injuries may require surgery to repair the joint damage.

Surgery

If closed reduction fails, surgery may be necessary to realign the joint and prevent complications such as neurovascular injury. The goal of this surgery is to repair the tendon(s) and reattach it to the bone to reestablish as much joint mobility as possible. Ligament repairs, meniscal tear repairs, and patella tendon repairs (for dislocation) are the surgical intervention employed for knee issues.

Nursing Care

Nursing care of the patient with joint trauma is individualized to the cause of injury and the age of the patient.

Assessment

- *Health history:* Ask about history of trauma, including circumstances of injury if known; pain, including location, character, timing, and activities or movements that aggravate or relieve it; history of prior musculoskeletal injuries; chronic illnesses; medications
- *Physical assessment:* Compare the position, color, size, and temperature of the affected joint to the corresponding unaffected joint. Palpate for pulses, tenderness, crepitus, temperature, and edema. Ask the patient if he or she experiences any altered sensation, which may indicate nerve impingement or damage. Instruct the patient or assist to move the joint through its normal range of motion, stopping and noting where pain is experienced. Do not move the affected joint beyond that point. When a joint dislocation is suspected, assess color, temperature, pulses, movement, and sensation of the limb distal to the affected joint.

Priorities of Care

Relieving pain, preventing complications, and teaching for self-care and rehabilitation are priorities of care for the patient with joint trauma. Teach about the specific joint injury or disorder and its causes and treatments. Joint injuries often tend to be recurring for patients actively participating in sports and vigorous physical activities. Prolonged immobilization (for several weeks after the injury) and aggressive rehabilitation following the initial injury can reduce the risk of recurrent problems. The following topics should be addressed:

- Importance of complying with the prescribed length of immobilization
- Skin care and ways to prevent skin-to-skin contact, particularly in the axillary area
- Referrals to physical and occupational therapy as needed
- Prescribed rehabilitation exercises to strengthen muscles and other supportive structures in the affected joint, decreasing the risk of future trauma
- Alternatives to activities that precipitate recurrent trauma.

Diagnoses, Outcomes, and Interventions

Reduce Risk for Peripheral Neurovascular Dysfunction. The patient with a dislocation, in particular, requires frequent assessments to ensure that neurovascular compromise does not develop; however, all joint trauma cases should have routine neurovascular assessments.

Expected Outcome: Patient's circulation, movement, and sensation distal to injury will remain intact.

The nurse will:

- Monitor neurovascular status by assessing the **five P's**:

  Pain
  Pulses
  Pallor
  Paralysis
  Paresthesia.

- Teach patient the signs and symptoms of neurovascular compromise. *Neurovascular compromise is indicated by increased pain, decreased or absent pulses, pale skin with decreased capillary refill, inability to move a body part or extremity, and changes in sensation (such as "pins and needles" sensations or loss of sense of sharp/dull touch).*
- Maintain immobilization as ordered after reduction. *Immobilization prevents the joint from dislocating again.*
- Maintain proper application of immobilization devices (immobilizers, slings, casts, etc.) and teach the patient the proper application of the device. *Improperly placed immobilization devices can cause undue pressure over blood vessels and nerves, which can lead to neurovascular compromise.*
- Encourage patient to begin mobilization as soon as indicated to prevent complications. *Complications of deep venous thrombosis can occur, even in the healthiest patient, when mobility is drastically limited.*

Manage Acute Pain. The pain resulting from joint trauma may be acute, especially at the moment of injury, or chronic, such as pain from rotator cuff damage, which may be worse at night or when lying on the involved shoulder.

Expected Outcome: Patient will use pharmacologic and nonpharmacologic strategies to manage pain and maintain comfort.

The nurse will:

- Encourage use of an appropriate splint or joint immobilizer. *Splinting maintains joint alignment and reduces pain and inflammation.*
- Teach safe application of ice or heat to the affected joint as indicated. *Ice causes vasoconstriction and numbs the tender area; heat decreases edema by increasing venous return. Inappropriately applied, both ice and heat can damage tissues.*
- Instruct about using NSAIDs, as ordered. *Taken on a regular basis (not as needed for pain), NSAIDs decrease edema and inflammation, reducing pain.*
- Teach use of assistive devices such as a sling, crutches, or cane to reduce stress on the affected joint or minimize weight bearing. *When used appropriately, assistive devices help minimize use of and stress on the affected joint, promoting joint rest and healing. When used inappropriately, these assistive devices can increase the risk of further injury or damage.*

Promote Mobility and Self-Care. Encouraging mobility and self-care will reduce immobility complications and promote circulation, speeding recovery.

Expected Outcome: Patient will regain preinjury level of mobility.

The nurse will:

- Encourage patients to be as independent as possible in their mobility and self-care. *Encouraging independence will help the patient and hasten healing.*
- Refer to physical therapy for appropriate exercises. *The physical therapist can teach exercises to strengthen supportive joint tissues and maintain or restore joint mobility.*
- Refer to occupational therapy for assistance with performing activities of daily living (ADLs). *Occupational therapy can help the patient learn new ways to perform tasks to prevent recurring symptoms.*

Delegating Nursing Care Activities

UAP can assist with mobilization and proper application of immobilization devices (after RN or PT/OT has first properly fitted the device), as well as encourage independence with mobility and ADLs.

Transitions of Care

In addition to good physical conditioning, using caution during physical activity and avoiding situations where these types of injuries occur are the best means of prevention. Rotator cuff injuries could arise from repetitive movements, therefore exploring a different means of performing the same activity may be called for to prevent further damage. (See the next section for a further discussion of repetitive use injuries.)

Preventing the condition from becoming a chronic issue consists of good initial and follow-up care after the injury. Taking precautions to avoid the circumstances that led to the injury in the first place is another way to prevent a recurring injury.

If there is a significant impact on mobility or ADLs then home care may include referrals to outpatient or home physical and occupational therapy.

The Patient with a Repetitive Use Injury

Repeatedly twisting and turning the wrist, pronating and supinating the forearm, kneeling, or raising arms over the head can result in repetitive use injuries. Patients with repetitive use injuries often appear puzzled as they relate a history of manifestations that have worsened over time. They deny abrupt trauma and often worry about the ability to return to work. Repetitive use injuries are common; they account for 2.2% of all workplace injuries (BLS, 2016).

Pathophysiology

Common repetitive use injuries include carpal tunnel syndrome, bursitis, and tendonitis.

Carpal Tunnel Syndrome

The carpal tunnel is a compartment through which flexor tendons and the median nerve pass from the elbow to the hand. The syndrome develops from narrowing of the tunnel and irritation of the median nerve. The narrowing can be to multiple issues, but all result in a narrowing of the carpal tunnel and compression of the median nerve. Inflammation and edema of the synovial lining of the tendon sheaths are some causes, An anatomically narrow carpal tunnel, noninflammatory fibrosis of the synovial lining of the tendon sheaths, or a mass lesion are other causes of the narrowed carpal tunnel (Kothari, 2018).

Bursitis

Bursitis is an inflammation of a bursa, an enclosed sac found between muscles, tendons, and bony prominences. The bursae that commonly become inflamed are in the shoulder, hip, knee, and elbow. Constant friction between the bursa and the musculoskeletal tissue around it causes irritation, edema, and inflammation. Occasionally, bursitis may be caused by an infection.

Tendonitis

Tendonitis is inflammation of the tendon at its point of origin. Common sites for tendonitis include the patella (jumper's knee), elbow (epicondylitis), and shoulder (impingement syndrome). Epicondylitis is also referred to as *tennis elbow* or *golfer's elbow*. This disorder typically results from chronic repetitive wrist extension and pronation or supination.

Risk Factors

Carpal tunnel syndrome risk factors include obesity, pregnancy, diabetes, rheumatoid arthritis, hypothyroidism, connective tissue disorders, genetic predisposition, workplace factors, and being female. Additionally preexisting median mononeuropathy and aromatase inhibitor use have been found to be risk factors (Kothari, 2018).

Bursitis risk factors include aging, occupations or hobbies that have repetitive motion or place pressure on a specific bursae, and some chronic conditions, including rheumatoid arthritis, gout, and diabetes (Mayo Clinic, 2018a). Like bursitis, age and repetitive motion occupations and hobbies contribute to tendonitis occurrences (Mayo Clinic, 2018b).

Manifestations

Patients with carpal tunnel syndrome typically complain of numbness and tingling of the thumb, index finger, and lateral ventral surface of the middle finger. They may also complain of pain in this area that interferes with sleep and is alleviated by shaking or massaging the hand and fingers. The affected hand may become weak and the patient may be unable to hold utensils or perform activities that require precision.

Manifestations of bursitis develop as the bursa becomes engorged. The area around the sac is tender, and extension and flexion of the joint near the bursa produce pain. The inflamed bursa is hot, red, and edematous, which may indicate an infection. The patient guards the joint to decrease pain and may point to the area of the bursa when identifying joint tenderness.

Manifestations of tendonitis include point tenderness, pain with flexion and extension of the joint or against resistance, and a history of repetitive use.

Complications

Ongoing pain and reduced mobility in the joint accompany untreated conditions. With untreated impingement syndrome the anterior shoulder may become unstable, especially if the underlying cause is not identified and remedied (Buti, 2013). With epicondylitis, flexion contractions may develop if left untreated (Perz, 2013).

Interprofessional Care

Medical management of repetitive use disorders focuses on relieving pain and increasing mobility. Once the diagnosis is made, treatment can range from conservative measures such as rest, medications, and physical therapy to aggressive measures such as surgery.

Diagnosis

Carpal tunnel syndrome is diagnosed by the patient's history and physical examination. The history may reveal an occupation that involves areas such as computer work, jackhammer operation, mechanical work, or gymnastics. History of a radial bone fracture or rheumatoid arthritis also increases the risk of carpal tunnel syndrome. Tests specific for carpal tunnel include the Phalen test. Ultrasound or MRI, electromyography (EMG), and nerve conduction studies may be done to confirm the diagnosis. Bursitis and tendonitis are diagnosed by history and physical examination. Movements such as shaking hands may reproduce the pain of epicondylitis. If septic bursitis is suspected, the fluid may be aspirated and sent for cultures.

Medications

The patient with a repetitive use injury usually receives NSAIDs. Narcotics may be administered for acute flare-ups and severe pain. For the patient who has tendonitis or carpal tunnel syndrome, corticosteroids may be injected into the joint. For septic bursitis, appropriate anti-infectives will be prescribed. Corticosteroids should not be utilized if septic bursitis is suspected (Perz, 2013).

Treatments

Initial treatment for repetitive use injuries is conservative, followed, if necessary, by surgery.

Conservative Management. The first steps in the care of all repetitive use injuries are to immobilize and rest the involved joint. The joint may be splinted, and ice may be applied (as described in Table 39.2) in the first 24 to 48 hours to decrease pain and inflammation. Ice application may be followed by heat application every 4 hours to relieve pain. Physical and occupational therapy may be prescribed to strengthen the supporting joint structures (Buti, 2013).

Additionally, working with an expert in ergonomics can help to prevent the conditions that produce the injuries. In a study of radiologists, Thompson (2014) found that implementing ergonomic training using ergonomic equipment (computer mouse) and using adjustable chairs and tables significantly reduced pain levels.

Surgery. Surgery is usually reserved for the patient who does not obtain relief with conservative treatment. Surgery for carpal tunnel syndrome includes resection of the carpal ligament to enlarge the tunnel. In tendonitis and bursitis, calcified deposits may be removed from the area surrounding the tendon or bursa. With shoulder impingement, surgical repair will depend on the specific joint involved. These surgeries can range from arthroscopic subacromial decompression to open rotator cuff repair (Buti, 2013).

Integrative Therapies

Wolfe (2015) describes the use of a specific type of acupuncture, acumoxa therapy, to help alleviate the symptoms of repetitive use injuries in those with moderate to mild cases of the injury.

Nursing Care

The nursing care of a patient with a repetitive use injury focuses on relieving pain, teaching about the disease process and treatment, improving physical mobility, and improving performance of ADLs.

Assessment

- *Health history:* Ask about history of trauma, including circumstances of injury if known or if there has been a history of repetitive movements. If the patient cannot state anything, ask about their job and what it entails. Assess for pain, including location, character, timing, and activities or movements that aggravate or relieve it; range of motion to the joints above and below the area of concern; history of prior musculoskeletal injuries; chronic illnesses; and medications. Patients may report pain when lying or standing in certain positions.
- *Physical assessment:* Compare the position, color, size, and temperature of the affected extremity to the corresponding unaffected extremity. Palpate for pulses, tenderness, crepitus, temperature, and edema. Ask the patient if he or she is experiencing any altered sensation, which may indicate nerve impingement or damage. Assess strength in the affected extremity, comparing bilaterally. Instruct the patient or assist to move the joint through its normal range of motion, stopping and noting where pain is experienced. Do not move the affected joint beyond that point. Note the position in which the pain and other symptoms occur. In the joints, palpate for crepitus, edema, or pain with palpation.

SAFETY ALERT: Do not move the affected joint beyond the point of pain. ■

Diagnoses, Outcomes, and Interventions

Manage Acute Pain. Edema and nerve inflammation cause pain in the patient with a repetitive use injury.

Expected Outcome: Patient will report improved comfort and rest.

The nurse will:

- Ask the patient to rate the pain on a scale of 0 to 10 (with 10 being the most severe pain) before and after any intervention. *This facilitates objective assessment of the effectiveness of the chosen pain relief strategy.*
- Encourage the use of immobilizers, as prescribed and for the amount of time prescribed. *Splinting maintains joint alignment and prevents pain due to movement of inflamed tissues.*
- Teach the patient to apply ice and/or heat, as prescribed. *Ice causes vasoconstriction and decreases the pooling of blood in the inflamed area. Ice may also numb the tender area. Heat decreases edema by increasing venous return.*
- Encourage use of NSAIDs, as prescribed. *NSAIDs decrease edema by inhibiting prostaglandins and interrupting the inflammatory process.*

Promote Mobility and Self-Care. Joint pain and edema can limit range of motion of the affected joint.

Expected Outcome: Patient will regain previous level of mobility without pain.

The nurse will:

- Suggest interventions to manage pain: Immobilization, ice/heat, and pain medications, as prescribed. *If the joint is pain free, the patient will be more likely to take an active role in therapy.*
- Encourage patients to be as independent as possible in their mobility and self-care. *Encouraging independence will help the patient and hasten healing.*
- Refer to physical therapy for appropriate exercises. *The physical therapist can teach exercises to strengthen supportive joint tissues and maintain or restore joint mobility.*
- Refer to occupational therapy for assistance with performing ADLs. *Occupational therapy can help the patient learn new ways to perform tasks to prevent recurring symptoms.*

Delegating Nursing Care Activities

UAP can assist with mobilization and proper application of immobilization devices (after RN or PT/OT has first properly fit the device), as well as encourage independence with mobility and ADLs.

Transitions of Care

Teach patients ways to avoid unnecessary exposure to the activities that increase risk of redeveloping the injury. Suggest evaluation of the patient's work environment by an environmental risk manager or ergonomic specialist who can prescribe measures to reduce the risk of repetitive use injuries. Wrist supports or an ergonomic keyboard may be useful for the patient who uses a computer extensively. Appropriate desk and chair height are also important in maintaining the correct anatomic position while working. These interventions work in both initial prevention and prevention of further or repeat injuries.

39.2 Traumatic Injuries of Bones

The Patient with a Fracture

A **fracture** is any break in the continuity of a bone. Fractures vary in severity according to the location and the type of fracture. Although fractures occur in all age groups, they are more common in people who have sustained trauma and in older patients.

Pathophysiology

A fracture occurs when the bone is subjected to more kinetic energy than it can absorb. Fractures may result from a direct blow, a crushing force (compression), a sudden twisting motion (torsion), a severe muscle contraction, or disease that has weakened the bone (called a *stress* or *pathologic fracture*). Two basic mechanisms produce fractures: Direct force and indirect force. With direct force, the kinetic energy is applied at or near the site of the fracture. The bone cannot withstand the force. With indirect force, the kinetic energy is transmitted from the point of impact to a site where the bone is weaker. The fracture occurs at the weaker point.

Fractures in adults are classified as shown in **Figure 39.1** ■.

- If the skin is intact, the fracture is considered a *closed (simple) fracture*. If the skin integrity is interrupted, the fracture is considered an *open (compound) fracture*. An open fracture allows bacteria to enter the injured area and increases the risk of complications.
- *Complete* fractures involve the entire width of the bone whereas *incomplete* fractures involve only a part of the width of the bone.
- The fracture line may be *oblique* (at an angle to the bone) or *spiral* (curves around the bone). An *avulsed* fracture occurs when the fracture pulls bone and other tissues away from the point of attachment. Fractures may also be described as *comminuted* (the bone breaks in many pieces; *compressed* (the bone is crushed), *impacted* (the broken bone ends are forced into each other), or *depressed* (the broken bone is forced inward).
- A *stable* (nondisplaced) fracture is one in which the bones maintain their anatomic alignment. An *unstable* (displaced) fracture occurs when the bones move out of correct anatomic alignment. If a fracture is displaced, immediate interventions are required to prevent further damage to soft tissue, muscle, and bone.

Fractures may also be classified by the affected portion of the bone, such as proximal, midshaft, or distal. The point of reference may also be specific, such as intra-articular or diaphyseal.

Risk Factors

Trauma from various causes result in fractures in adolescents and young adults. Falls are the most common cause of injury in people aged 65 and older, with fractures of the vertebrae, distal radius, and hip common (Sorenson, Quinn, & Klein, 2019). Osteoporosis is a great contributor to fractures in older adults. The nonprofit organization American Bone Health (2016) lists the following as risk factors for fractures: Smoking, alcohol abuse, chronic steroid use, diabetes mellitus, a history of low-impact fractures, and a family history of hip fractures. It states that 50% of women and 25% of men over the age of 50 will sustain at least one fracture in their lifetime.

Fracture Healing

Fracture healing progresses over four phases: Hematoma formation, fibrocartilaginous callus formation, bony callus formation, and remodeling. (See Pathophysiology Illustrated on page 1420.) When a bone fractures, bleeding and tissue damage at the site of the fracture initiate an inflammatory response. A hematoma forms between the fractured bone ends and around the bone surfaces. The fractured bone surfaces and fragments are deprived of oxygen and nutrients, leading to localized cellular necrosis, which heightens the inflammatory response and release of inflammatory mediators. These chemicals in turn cause vasodilation and edema. Fibroblasts, lymphocytes, and macrophages migrate to the fracture site, and fibroblasts within the hematoma form a fibrin meshwork. Lymphocytes and macrophages wall off the area, localizing and containing the inflammation.

Within 48 hours, fibroblasts and new capillaries growing into the fracture form granulation tissue that gradually replaces the hematoma. Phagocytes remove cell debris. Osteoblasts (bone-forming cells) migrate to the fracture site, where they build a web of collagen fibers from both sides of the fractured bone. Chondroblasts lay down patches of cartilage as a base for bone growth. This fibrocartilaginous callus connects bone fragments, splinting the fracture and maintaining bone alignment. However, it cannot yet support weight bearing.

The third stage of fracture healing, bony callus formation, begins 3 to 4 weeks after the injury and continues for 2 to 3 months. Osteoblasts continue to form collagen fibers and bone matrix, which are gradually mineralized with calcium and mineral salts. Osteoclasts migrate to the repair site to remove damaged and excess bone in the callus. Fibrocartilaginous callus is gradually replaced with cancellous bone. This process progresses from the outer surface of the bone toward the fracture site.

In the final phase of healing, remodeling, excess callus is removed and new bone is laid down along the fracture line. As the bone heals and is subjected to the mechanical stress of everyday use, osteoblasts and osteoclasts remodel the repair site along the lines of force. Cancellous bone is replaced by compact bone, and the remodeled area closely resembles the original, unbroken bone.

The age, physical condition of the patient, and the type of fracture influence healing. Other factors, both local and systemic, also influence bone healing either positively or negatively (**Box 39.1**). Healing time varies with the individual. An uncomplicated fracture of the arm or foot can heal in 6 to 8 weeks. A fractured vertebra will take at least 12 weeks to heal. Healing of a fractured hip may take from 12 to 16 weeks.

Etiology and Manifestations

Causes and manifestations are described for the following fractures: Skull, face, spine, clavicle, humerus, elbow, radius/ulna, wrist/hand, ribs, pelvis, hip, femur, tibia/fibula, and ankle/foot.

Closed

- Bone breaks but skin remains intact.
- Also called a simple fracture.

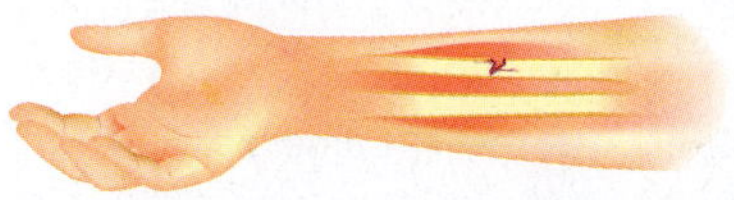

Open

- Bone breaks and protrudes through the skin; increased risk of osteomyelitis,
- Also called a compound fracture.

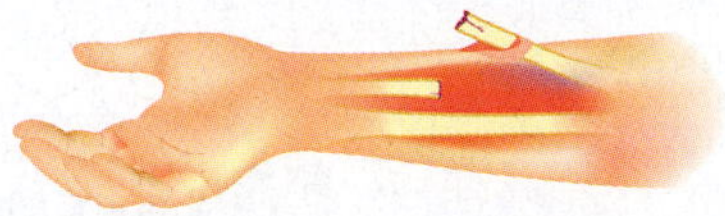

Complete

- Fracture involves the entire width of the bone.

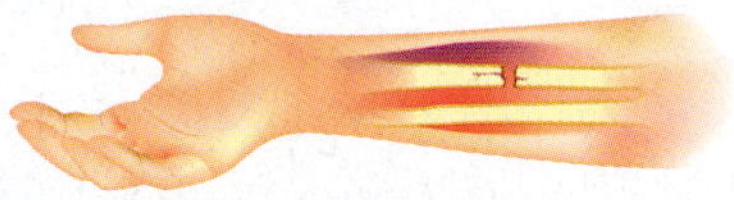

Greenstick

- Bone fragments are still partially joined.
- Also called an incomplete fracture.
- Occurs commonly in children.

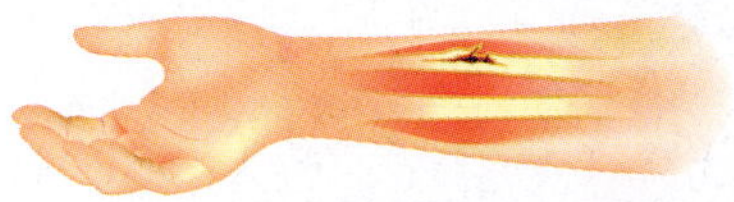

Comminuted

- Bone fragments into many pieces.
- Common in individuals with brittle bones, such as patients with osteogenesis imperfecta.

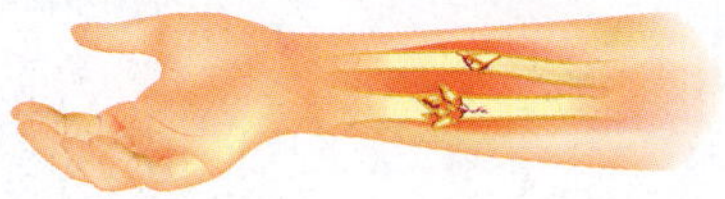

Impacted

- The two ends of the bone are forced together.
- Also called a buckle fracture.
- Often seen with children's arm and hip fractures.

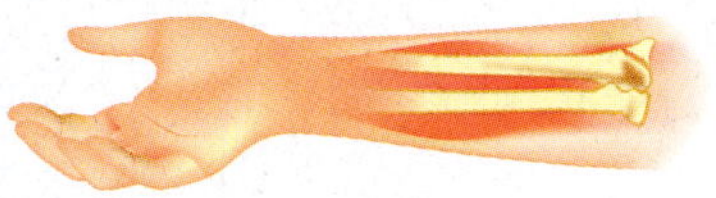

Oblique

- Fracture occurs diagonal to the bone's axis.

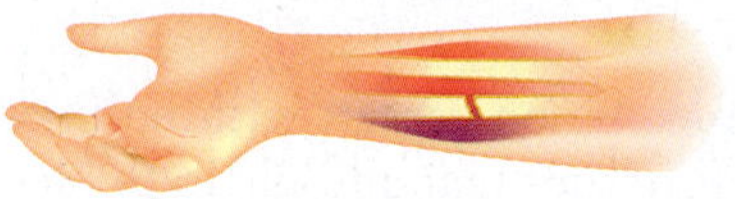

Transverse

- Fracture occurs at a right angle to the bone's axis.

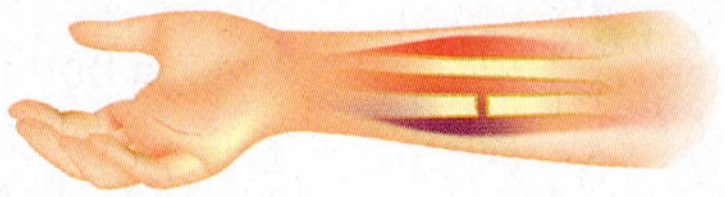

Linear

- Fracture occurs parallel to the bone's axis.

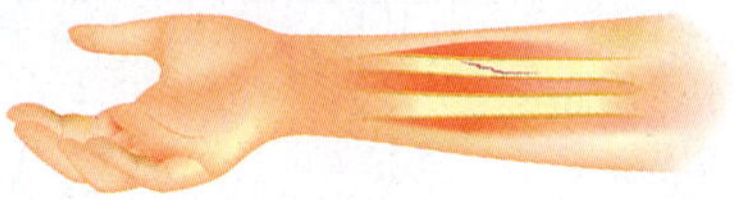

Displaced

- Broken ends of bones move out of correct anatomical alignment.
- Also called an unstable fracture.
- Requires immediate attention to prevent further damage.

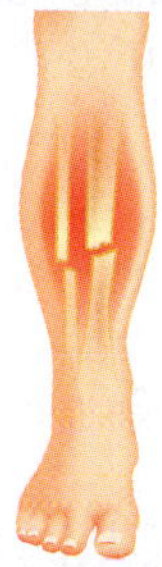

Nondisplaced

- Broken ends of bones remain aligned.
- Also called a stable fracture.

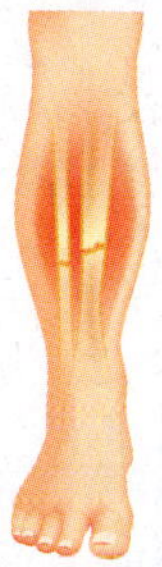

Avulsion

- A fragment of bone is separated from the rest of the bone.
- May also involve displacement of surrounding tissues.

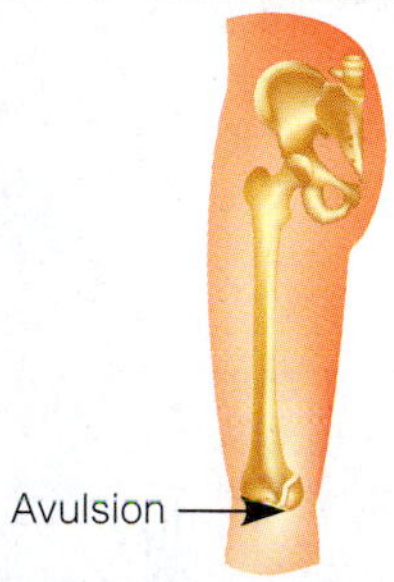
Avulsion

Stress

- Caused by small repetitive forces on the bone.
- Often caused by participation in sports or exercise.

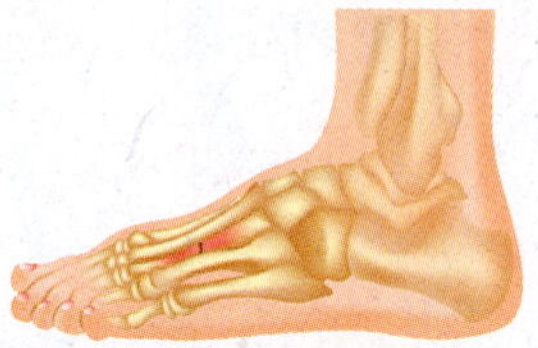

Spiral

- Fracture spirals around the bone.
- Occurs as the result of a twisting force, often during sports.
- Occurs commonly in children.

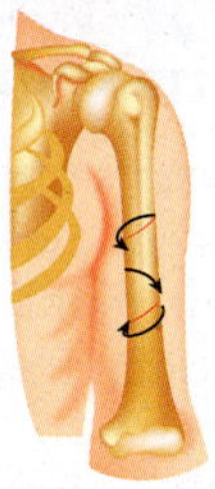

Depression

- Bone is forced inward.
- Occurs commonly in skull fractures.

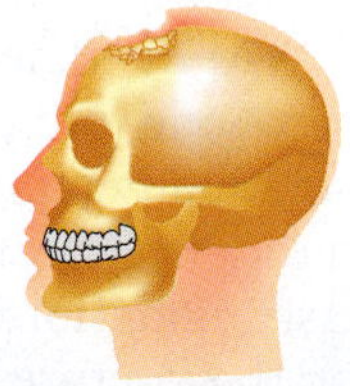

Pathologic

- Caused by a disease that weakens the bone such as osteoporosis, bone cancer, and osteogenesis imperfecta.

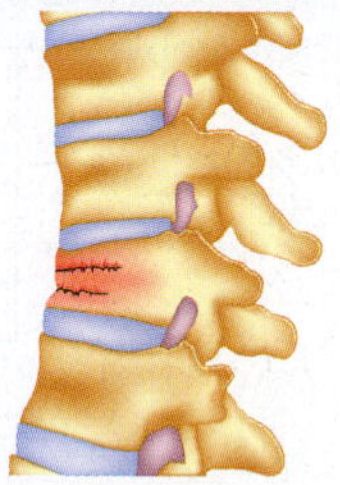

Compression

- Bone is crushed; occurs most commonly in vertebrae.
- Common in patients with osteoporosis.

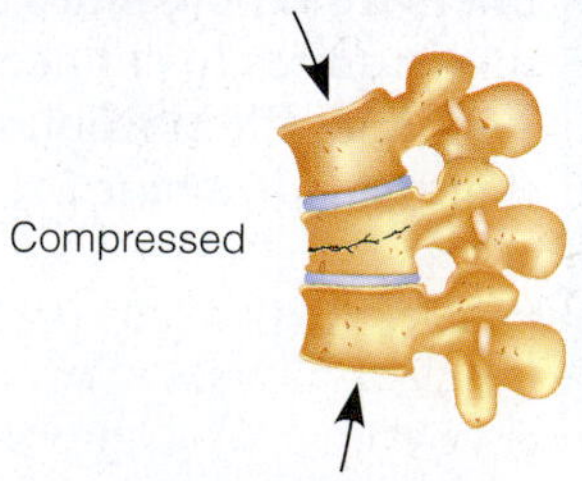
Compressed

Figure 39.1 ■ Common fractures in adults.

Pathophysiology Illustrated
Bone Healing

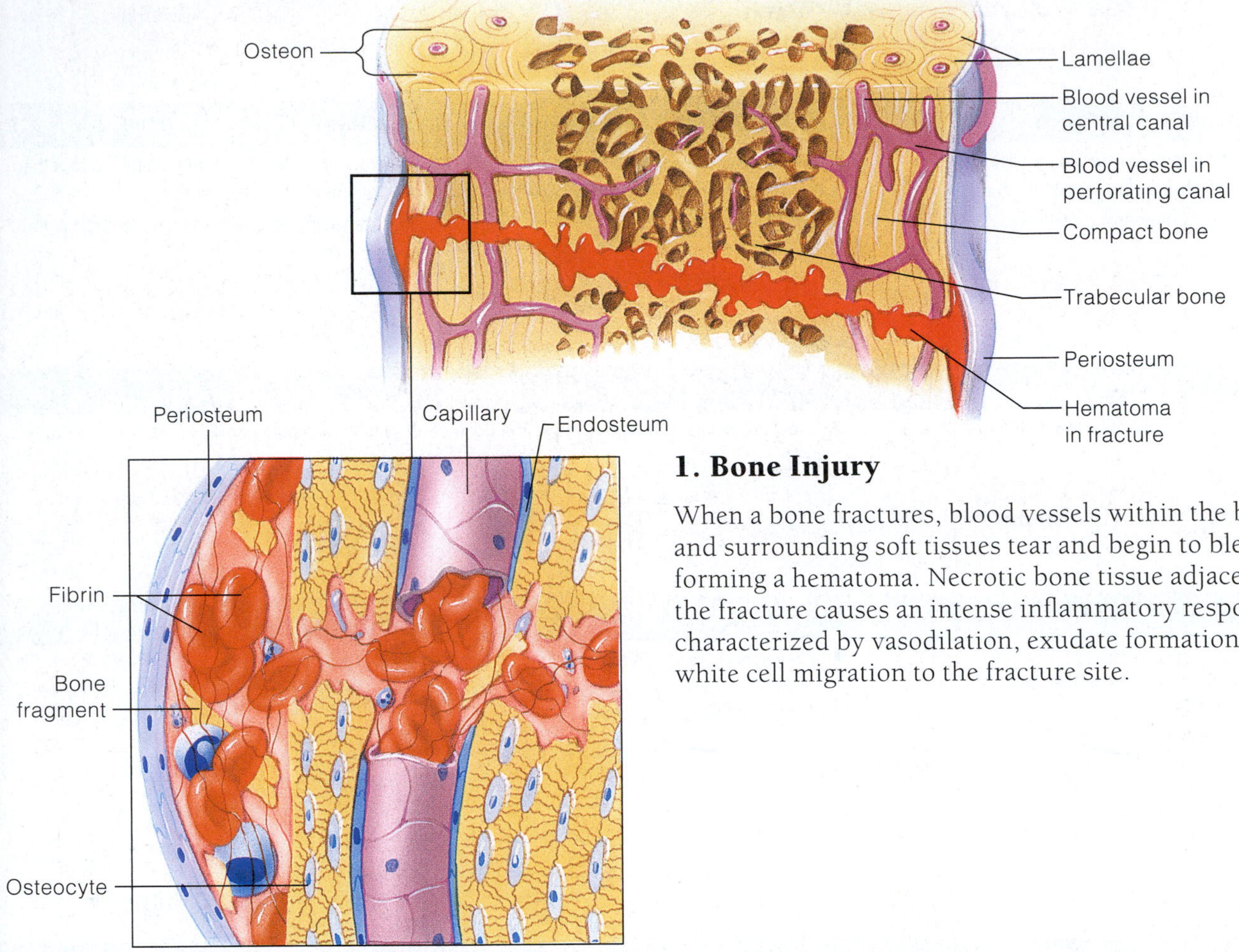
Osteon
Lamellae
Blood vessel in central canal
Blood vessel in perforating canal
Compact bone
Trabecular bone
Periosteum
Hematoma in fracture
Periosteum
Capillary
Endosteum
Fibrin
Bone fragment
Osteocyte

1. Bone Injury

When a bone fractures, blood vessels within the bone and surrounding soft tissues tear and begin to bleed, forming a hematoma. Necrotic bone tissue adjacent to the fracture causes an intense inflammatory response characterized by vasodilation, exudate formation, and white cell migration to the fracture site.

2. Fibrocartilaginous Callus Formation

Clotting factors within the hematoma form a fibrin meshwork. Within 48 hours, fibroblasts and new capillaries growing into the fracture form granulation tissue that gradually replaces the hematoma. Phagocytes begin to remove cell debris.

Osteoblasts, bone-forming cells, proliferate and migrate into the fracture site, forming a fibrocartilaginous callus. The osteoblasts build a web of collagen fibers from both sides of the fracture site that eventually unites to connect bone fragments, thus splinting the bone. Chondroblasts lay down patches of cartilage that provide a base for bone growth.

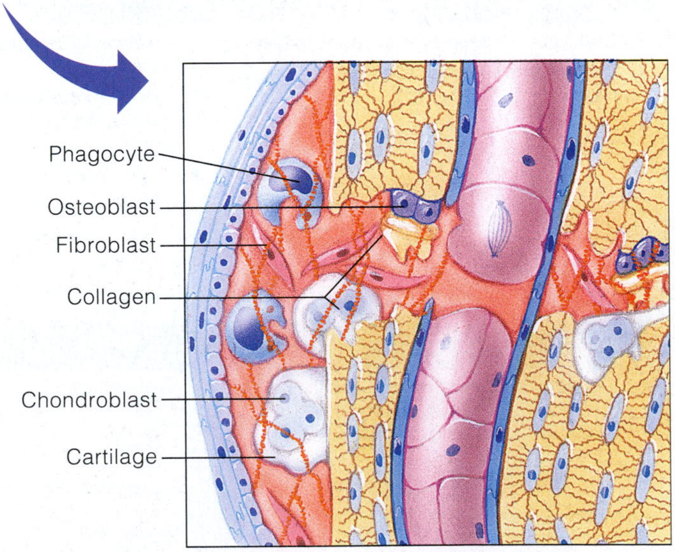
Phagocyte
Osteoblast
Fibroblast
Collagen
Chondroblast
Cartilage

Pathophysiology Illustrated

Bone Healing

4. Bone Remodeling

Osteoblasts continue to form new woven bone, which is in turn organized into the lamellar structures of compact bone. Osteoclasts resorb excess callus as it is replaced by mature bone.

As the bone heals and is subjected to the mechanical stress of everyday use, osteoblasts and osteoclasts respond by remodeling the repair site along the lines of force. This ensures that the repaired section of bone eventually resembles the structure of the uninjured part.

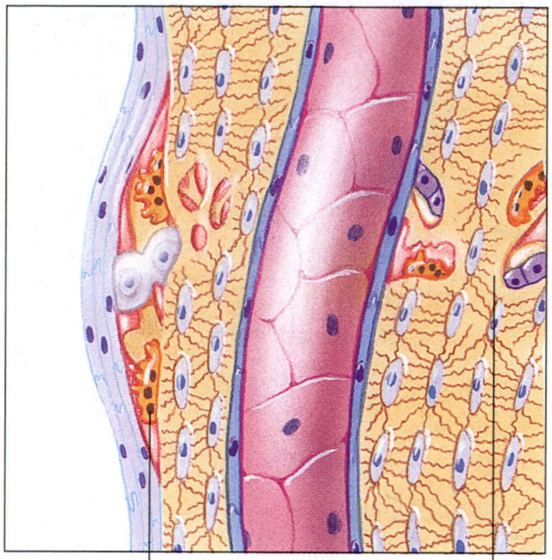
Osteoclast
New compact bone

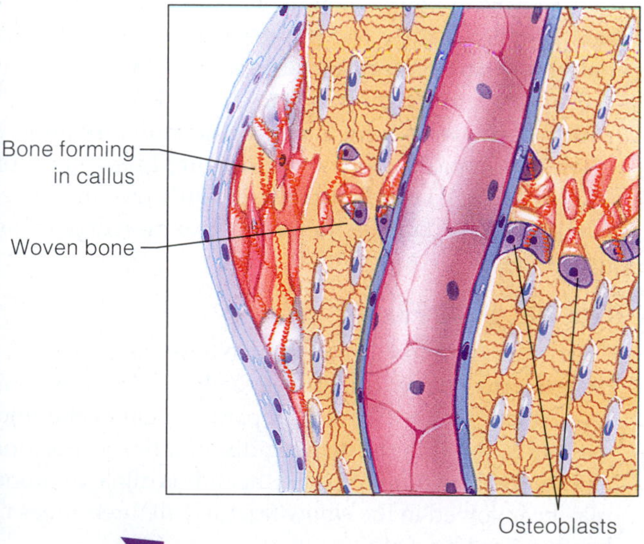
Bone forming in callus
Woven bone
Osteoblasts

3. Bony Callus Formation

Osteoblasts continue to proliferate and synthesize collagen fibers and bone matrix, which are gradually mineralized with calcium and mineral salts to form a spongy mass of woven bone. The trabeculae of woven bone bridge the fracture. Osteoclasts migrate to the repair site and begin removing excess bone in the callus. Bony callus formation usually continues for 2 to 3 months.

BOX 39.1
Factors Influencing Bone Healing

POSITIVE FACTORS

Local

- Immobilization
- Timely correction of displacement
- Application of ice
- Electrical stimulation

Systemic

- Adequate amounts of growth hormone, vitamin D, and calcium
- Adequate blood supply
- Absence of infection or diseases
- Younger age
- Moderate activity level prior to injury

NEGATIVE FACTORS

Local

- Delay in correction of displacement
- Open fracture (increases risk of infection)
- Presence of foreign body at fracture site

Systemic

- Immunocompromised status
- Decreased circulation (as in diabetes or peripheral vascular disease)
- Malnutrition
- Osteoporosis
- Advanced age

Fracture of the Skull

A skull fracture may result from either a fall or a direct blow. The patient must be assessed for neurologic changes and any loss of consciousness must be documented. A complete neurologic assessment is conducted. Level of consciousness (LOC) and orientation to person, place, and time; pupillary reaction to light; movement and strength of all extremities; and complaints of nausea and vomiting are noted. A displaced skull fracture, which is referred to as *depressed*, may press on the brain and cause neurologic damage.

Fracture of the Face

Fracture of the facial bones may result from a direct blow. The patient presents with hematomas, pain, edema, and bony deformity. Nondisplaced fractures are monitored to ensure the airway is not compromised. The patient is observed for any neurologic deficits. Severely displaced or multiple facial fractures are treated with ORIF with wires or plates.

Fracture of the Spine

The spine can be injured in many ways, including sports injuries, falls, and motor vehicle crashes. Cervical and lumbar fractures occur most commonly, but the thoracic and sacral spine can also be fractured. The most severe complication of spine fracture is injury to the spinal cord. A displaced or unstable fracture of the vertebrae may apply pressure on the spinal cord. This pressure on the spinal cord may result in ischemia and permanent paralysis.

Fracture of the Clavicle

A fracture of the clavicle commonly results from a direct blow or a fall. The most common location is midclavicular. An individual with a midclavicular fracture typically assumes a protective slumping position to immobilize the arm and prevent shoulder movement. A less common fracture occurs along the distal third of the clavicle. This type of fracture may be associated with ligament damage. Injuries to the clavicle may be associated with skull or cervical fractures. Displaced clavicular fractures may damage subclavian vessels, leading to hemorrhage, or the lung, with resulting pneumothorax. Injury to the brachial plexus may result in numbness and decreased movement of the arm on the affected side. Malunion of a clavicular fracture can result in asymmetry of the shoulders.

Fracture of the Humerus

The severity of humerus fractures and appropriate treatment is determined by the location of the fracture, the presence of displacement, and the presence of neurovascular compromise. Treatment focuses on immobilizing the fractured bone in normal anatomic position. Common complications of humeral fracture include nerve and ligament damage, frozen or stiff joints, and malunion. Early interventions may prevent permanent damage.

Fractures of the proximal humerus are common in older adults. A simple nondisplaced fracture of the proximal humerus (near the humeral head) with a normal neurovascular assessment can be safely treated with immobilization. A more complicated displaced fracture of the proximal humerus with bone fragmentation requires surgical intervention. The risk for impaired range of motion (ROM) of the shoulder increases with fracture severity and soft tissue damage. Rehabilitative measures focus on increasing ROM.

Fracture of the Elbow

The most common location of an elbow fracture is the distal humerus. Elbow fractures usually result from a fall or direct blow to the elbow. The patient guards the injured extremity, holding the arm rigidly in a flexed position or an extended position. Because the radius, ulna, or humerus may be involved in the elbow fracture, all three bones must be visualized by x-ray.

Complications of an elbow fracture include nerve or artery damage and *hemarthrosis*, a collection of blood in the elbow joint. The most serious complication of an elbow fracture is Volkmann contracture, which results from arterial occlusion and muscle ischemia. The patient complains of forearm pain, impaired sensation, and loss of motor function. Rapid interventions are aimed at relieving pressure on the brachial artery and nerve and preventing muscle atrophy.

Fracture of the Radius and/or Ulna

Fractures of the radius and ulna may result from either indirect injury, such as twisting or pulling on the arm, or direct injury, such as that resulting from a fall. The usual treatment of radius fractures depends on the location. The proximal radial head may be fractured from a fall on an outstretched hand. Blood commonly collects in the elbow joint and must be aspirated. If the fracture is nondisplaced, a sling is applied.

When both bones are broken, the fracture is usually displaced. The patient complains of pain and cannot supinate the hand (turn the palm up).

Complications after a radius and/or ulnar fracture include compartment syndrome, delayed healing, and decreased wrist and finger movement. After surgery, the patient also has an increased risk of infection.

Fractures in the Wrist and/or Hand

Wrist fractures often result from a fall onto an outstretched hand or onto the back of the hand. A common type of wrist fracture is *Colles fracture*, in which the distal radius fractures after a fall onto an outstretched hand. The patient with a wrist fracture presents with a bony deformity, pain, numbness, weakness, and decreased ROM of the fingers. The capillary refill and sensation of the hand must be assessed.

The hand is composed of many bones. Most commonly, the metacarpals and phalanges are involved in a hand fracture. The injuring mechanism varies from striking an object with a closed fist to closing a hand in a door. The patient presents with complaints of pain, edema, and decreased ROM.

Comparative x-rays of both the injured and uninjured wrist and hand may be obtained to identify the fracture. Complications of wrist and hand fractures are compartment syndrome, nerve damage, ligament damage, and delayed union. A wrist fracture is commonly treated with closed reduction, cast application, and elevation of the injured extremity. A hand fracture is splinted and elevated.

Fracture of the Ribs

Rib fractures commonly result from blunt chest trauma. The location of the fracture and involvement of underlying organs determine the severity of the injury. Fractures of the first through third ribs may damage the subclavian artery or vein. Fractures of the lower ribs may cause spleen and liver injuries.

The patient typically presents with a history of recent chest trauma and complaints of pain along the lateral portion of the rib. Palpation of the rib reveals a bony deformity and increases pain. Deep inspiration also increases pain. The skin over the fracture site may be ecchymotic (bruised).

Flail chest results from the fracture of two or more adjacent ribs in two or more places and the formation of a free-floating segment that moves in the opposite direction of the rib cage. The bony instability impairs respirations. The flail segment is surgically stabilized and respirations are supported.

Potential complications of rib fractures include pulmonary contusion, pneumothorax, and/or hemothorax. The fractured rib may pierce the lung and injure it. The lower ribs may pierce the liver or spleen, resulting in intra-abdominal bleeding. Pneumonia may also develop from ineffective clearing of respiratory secretions.

Fracture of the Pelvis

Pelvic fractures are often caused by trauma, such as a fall or an automobile crash. Pelvic fracture may result from a fall from a standing position in the older adult. Hemorrhage with significant blood loss and damage to organs contained within the pelvis (e.g., the bladder, urethra, reproductive organs, and bowel) are significant risks associated with pelvic fracture. Trauma to extrapelvic organs such as the kidneys is common.

The patient with a pelvic fracture presents with pain in the back or hip area. A single fracture in the pelvis is treated conservatively with analgesia and activity limitation. In more severe fractures, internal or external fixation may be used (Xianping et al., 2017). Logrolling increases patient comfort.

Fracture of the Hip

A hip fracture refers to a fracture of the femur at the head, neck, or trochanteric regions (**Figure 39.2** ■). Hip fractures are classified as intracapsular or extracapsular. *Intracapsular fractures* involve the head or neck of the femur; *extracapsular fractures* involve the trochanteric region. The majority of hip fractures involve the neck or trochanteric regions. The femoral head and neck lie within the joint capsule and are not covered in periosteum; thus, they do not have a large blood supply. Fractures at this location usually fragment, further decreasing blood supply and increasing the risk of nonunion and avascular necrosis. The trochanteric region is covered in periosteum and therefore has more blood supply than the head or neck.

Hip fractures result from falls and are the most common injury in the older population, requiring hospitalization of more than 258,000 older adults each year in the United States. They result in serious health problems and increase the risk of dying in people age 65 and older. The annual number of hip fractures has remained relatively stable in recent years, even declining among some age groups (Centers for Disease Control and Prevention, [CDC], 2016a, 2016b). Factors contributing to falls include problems with gait and balance, neurologic and musculoskeletal impairments, dementia, psychoactive medications, and visual impairments. Modifiable risk factors, identified through research, include lower body weakness, problems with walking and balance, and taking four or more medications or any psychoactive medications. See Moving Evidence into Action for evidence-based fall prevention for older adults.

Hip fractures are common in older adults as a result of decreases in bone mass and the increased tendency to fall.

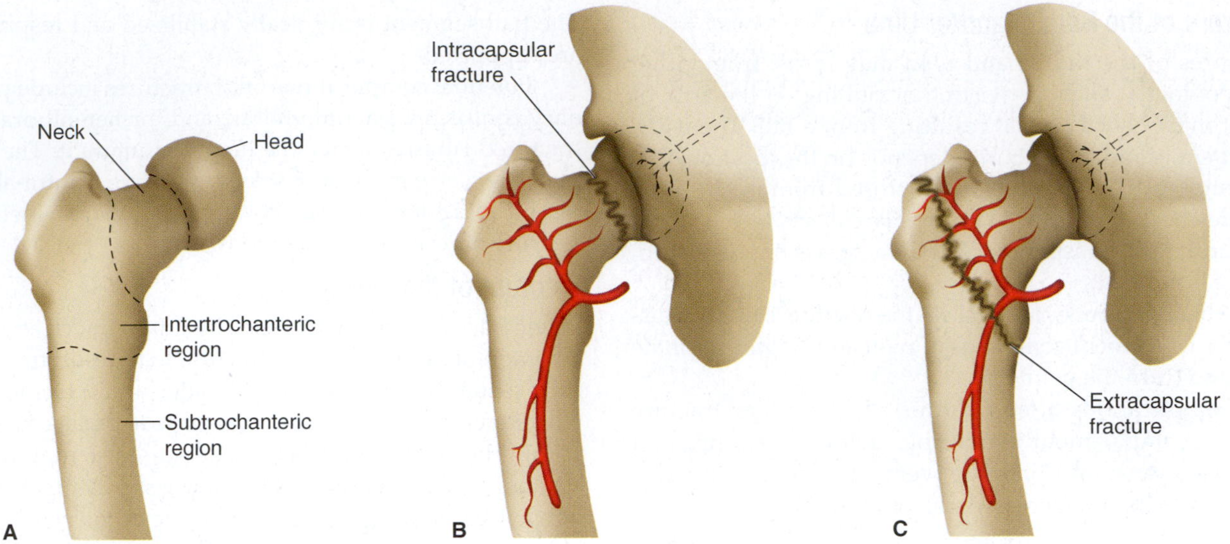
Neck
Head
Intertrochanteric region
Subtrochanteric region
A
Intracapsular fracture
B
Extracapsular fracture
C

Figure 39.2 ■ Hip fractures. **A**, The head of the femur, the neck of the femur, and the trochanteric regions of the femur. **B**, Femoral neck fractures are common. Fractures of the femoral neck and head, located within the hip capsule, are classified as intracapsular fractures. **C**, Intertrochanteric fractures, classified as extracapsular fractures, occur in the intertrochanteric region between the greater and lesser trochanters. Note how both femoral neck fractures and intertrochanteric fractures disrupt the blood supply to the bone.

Moving Evidence into Action

Falls Prevention

Clinical Issue

Evidence-based clinical guidelines exist for fall prevention and are considered a standard of nursing care. This emphasis arose from the Institute of Medicine describing hospital-acquired life-threatening conditions. Hospital falls occur between 2.7 and 7 per 1000 hospital days. In response, the Centers for Medicare and Medicaid Services implemented non-reimbursement for hospital-acquired conditions including hospital falls and trauma.

External Evidence

The Hartford Institute for Geriatric Nursing has identified falls as a geriatric syndrome with identifiable risk factors and precipitating causes. Assessment for fall risk includes intrinsic factors such as age (particularly over 75 years); chronic conditions (e.g., dementia, arthritis, Parkinson disease, diabetes, or depression); use of an assistive device; impaired vision, gait, or balance; urge urinary incontinence; and use of high-risk medications. Regular assessment of the patient care environment for factors such as spills, lighting, grab bars, and equipment repair is recommended. Care planning to prevent falls is individualized to identify risks and involves an integrated, multidisciplinary team (Gray-Micelli & Quigley, 2012).

Internal Evidence

As part of the evaluation of internal evidence, one must consider the patient's "real-time" response to the clinical decisions that must be made, the proposed falls prevention plan, and identification of stakeholders who influence the patient decision-making process. One question to ask: Are there patients at risk for falling within the population of your care environment? Does the clinical environment support a systematic falls prevention program? How does using a falls prevention program in your environment impact costs?

Patient Considerations

When considering use of a new practice (like a falls prevention program), the nurse must consider the specific patient population where it will be used. Will patients and their families be amenable to the assessment and interventions to help prevent falls?

Putting the Pieces Together

In the ideal world, patient falls would never occur, but they do. Based on the evidence, intrinsic and extrinsic factors have identified the patient at higher risk for falling. Using this information to systematically assess patients as well as implementing safe environment practices and appropriate assistive devices, falls can be prevented. To effectively implement a plan, it is important to evaluate the external evidence and consider the internal implications and patient/family issues. With the use of an evidence-based falls prevention program, unnecessary and injurious falls can be prevented.

Reference

Gray-Micelli, D., & Quigley, P. A. (2012). *Nursing standard of practice protocol: Falls prevention.* New York: The Hartford Institute for Geriatric Nursing. Retrieved from https://consultgeri.org/geriatric-topics/falls.

Whether the femur breaks spontaneously and causes the fall or whether the fall causes the fracture is not always clear; regardless of the cause of the fracture, rapid interventions are required to prevent bone necrosis. Assessment findings commonly associated with a hip fracture are pain, inability to walk, and shortening and external rotation of the affected lower extremity. Rarely, the fracture dislocates posteriorly; if that occurs, the extremity may internally rotate. However, some patients with a hip fracture have only vague pain in the buttocks, knees, thighs, groin, or back, and their ability to walk is unaffected. If the fracture is not visible on x-ray, a bone scan or MRI may be done to confirm the presence of the fracture.

Fracture of the Femoral Shaft

A large amount of force—such as from motor vehicle crashes, falls, or acts of violence—is required to fracture the shaft of the femur. Patients with femoral shaft fractures often have associated multiple traumas. Pathologic fractures may also occur in the femoral shaft (Rothrock, 2011). A fracture of the femoral shaft is manifested by an edematous, deformed, painful thigh. The patient is unable to move the hip or knee. Initial assessment focuses on the circulation and sensation present in the affected extremity. Pedal pulses and capillary refill in the affected extremity are compared to the unaffected extremity. Complications of a femoral shaft fracture include hypovolemia due to blood loss (which may be as great as 1.0 to 1.5 L), fat embolism, dislocation of the hip or knee, muscle atrophy, and ligament damage.

Fracture of the Tibia and/or Fibula

Fractures of the lower extremities often result from automobile or motorcycle crashes or sports injuries. The patient presents with edema, pain, bony deformity, and a hematoma at the level of injury.

Circulation and sensation are assessed to rule out common complications of the fracture, including damage to the peroneal nerve or tibial artery, compartment syndrome, hemarthroses, and ligament damage. An inability to point the toe upward on the affected side may indicate peroneal nerve damage. Absence of the dorsalis pedis pulse on the affected side may indicate tibial artery damage. Potential manifestations of compartment syndrome include pain on passive movement and paresthesias. An edematous knee may indicate a collection of blood in the knee joint. Ligament damage may be present if the patient cannot move the knee and/or ankle.

Fracture of the Ankle and/or Foot

The patient with an ankle fracture presents with pain, limited ROM, hematoma, edema, and difficulty ambulating. Nondisplaced ankle fractures are often treated by closed reduction and casting. Multiple or displaced fractures are treated by surgical intervention and splinting.

The patient with a foot fracture presents with similar symptoms; however, ROM of the ankle is not usually affected. Most foot fractures are nondisplaced and treated with closed reduction and casting. More severe displaced foot fractures may require surgery and the placement of wires to maintain reduction of the fracture.

Interprofessional Care

A fracture requires treatment to stabilize the fractured bone(s), maintain bone alignment, prevent complications, and restore function. The diagnosis of a fracture is primarily based on physical examination and x-rays.

Emergency Care

Emergency care of the patient with a fracture includes immobilizing the fracture, maintaining tissue perfusion, and preventing infection. In the case of serious trauma, the cervical spine is immobilized and normal body alignment is maintained. Once the patient is in a secure location, he or she is assessed for instability or deformity of the bone. If any deformity or instability is detected, the extremity is immobilized. The joints above and below the deformity are immobilized. Open wounds are covered with sterile dressings, and bleeding is controlled with a pressure dressing. The extremities are assessed for the presence and equality of pulses, movement, and sensation.

The fracture is splinted to maintain normal anatomic alignment and prevent the fracture from dislocating. Splinting relieves pain and prevents further damage to the arteries, nerves, and bones. Pulses, movement, and sensation are reevaluated after splinting.

Diagnosis

Diagnosis of a fracture usually is confirmed by radiographic tests. X-rays and bone scans are used to identify fractures (**Figure 39.3** ■). Blood chemistry studies, complete blood count (CBC), and coagulation studies may be used to assess blood loss, renal function, muscle breakdown, and the risk of excessive bleeding or clotting.

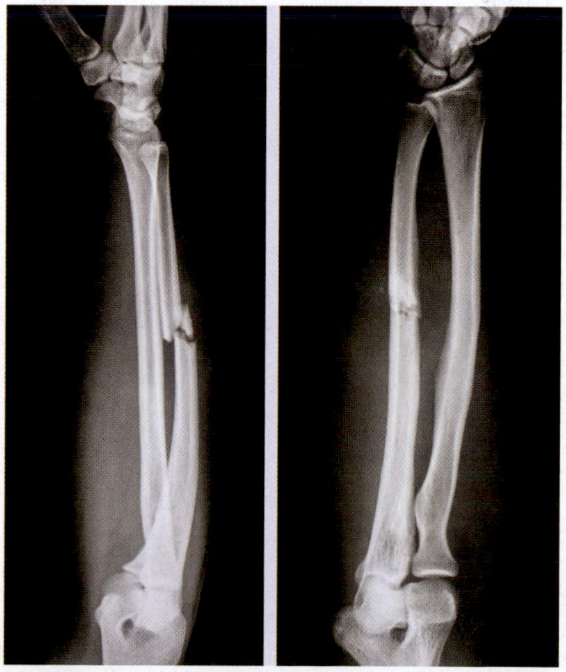

Figure 39.3 ■ X-ray of an oblique fracture of the femur.

BOX 39.2
Pain Management for the Patient with a Fracture

The patient who has had musculoskeletal trauma experiences pain from many different causes:

- Disruption of the continuity of the bone
- Damage to ligaments and tendons
- Inflammation and edema of tissues around the trauma site
- Muscle spasms
- Tissue ischemia from edema inside a cast, splint, or the muscle fascia sheath
- Hematoma formation
- Pressure over bony prominences from casts or splints.

The pain associated with the fracture and surrounding tissue damage is often severe and may be described as sharp, aching, or burning. Carefully assess any complaint of pain, including the location, character, and duration of pain. Nursing interventions for acute pain due to fracture include:

1. Administer prescribed analgesics, including NSAIDs and opioid analgesics. For serious fractures or following orthopedic surgery, patient-controlled analgesia (PCA) or epidural analgesia may be used. Administer NSAIDs and analgesics at regular intervals, around-the-clock, for the first 24 to 48 hours, then instruct the patient to request or take the medication before the pain is severe. Reassure the patient that addiction does not result from taking medications to relieve fracture or surgical pain. Most patients require only oral analgesics by the third or fourth day after orthopedic surgery.
2. Assist the patient to frequently change positions to relieve pressure and use pillows to provide support.
3. Elevate the involved extremity, and apply cold (if prescribed) to help decrease edema.
4. Monitor and drain accumulated fluids in any drainage devices to ensure patency, reduce edema, and decrease the possibility of hematoma formation.
5. Encourage the patient to wiggle fingers or toes on an extremity in a cast or traction to improve venous return and decrease edema.
6. Teach the patient adjunctive pain management techniques, such as relaxation and guided imagery.
7. Notify the physician of severe or unrelieved pain, which may indicate a serious complication such as compartment syndrome or neurovascular impairment.

Medications

Most patients with a fracture initially require analgesia to relieve pain. In the case of multiple fractures or fractures of large bones, opioids are administered initially. NSAIDs are prescribed to decrease inflammation and supplement analgesia. Pain management for the patient with a fracture is described in **Box 39.2**.

Antibiotics are typically administered prophylactically, particularly to patients with open or complex fractures. Anticoagulants may be prescribed to prevent DVT, particularly if surgery or prolonged immobilization is necessary. Stool softeners may be given to decrease the risk of constipation secondary to narcotics and immobility. Patients who have sustained trauma are often placed on antiulcer medications or antacids to reduce the risk of gastrointestinal bleeding.

Nutrition

Promotion of a high-protein diet with adequate calcium and vitamin D will assist in the healing of the tissues and bones. Also, ensure that the patient stays hydrated, which also assists in healing, prevents constipation, and decreases the risk of blood clots.

Treatment

Before the fractured bone is stabilized for healing, the fracture is *reduced* or restored to its normal alignment. In *closed reduction*, the bone is repositioned using external manipulation. Local or regional anesthesia or conscious sedation is usually given before closed reduction. The fracture is then immobilized with a splint, cast, or traction. An x-ray may be done to verify proper position, and pulses, movement, and sensation are assessed distal to the fracture. An *open reduction* is done in surgery. The bone is exposed and realigned; plates, wires, nails, and/or screws may be used to maintain its position.

Traction. Muscle spasms usually accompany fractures and may pull bones out of alignment. Traction applies a pulling force to return or maintain the fractured bones in normal anatomic position (**Figure 39.4** ■). All traction needs a counter weight. Often the patient's own body is the counter weight. Suspended weights may also be used. Types of traction are:

- ***Manual traction*** is applied by physically pulling on the extremity. Manual traction is often used to reduce a fracture or dislocation (Figure 39.4A).
- ***Skin traction (straight traction)*** is used to control muscle spasms and to immobilize a part of the body during transport or before surgery, with traction exerting its grabbing and pulling force on the patient's skin (Figure 39.4B). Skin traction is noninvasive and is relatively comfortable for the patient. The most common type of skin traction is Buck's traction, used to immobilize the leg before surgery to repair a hip or proximal femur fracture. Buck's traction uses traction tape or a foam boot applied to the lower leg attached to a free-hanging weight to immobilize the leg.
- ***Balanced suspension traction*** involves more than one force of pull to raise and support the injured extremity off the bed and maintain its alignment (Figure 39.4C). Balanced suspension traction increases bed mobility while maintaining bone position. It also makes it easier to change linens and perform back care.
- ***Skeletal traction*** involves inserting pins into the bone to apply the pulling force directly (Figure 39.4D). Local,

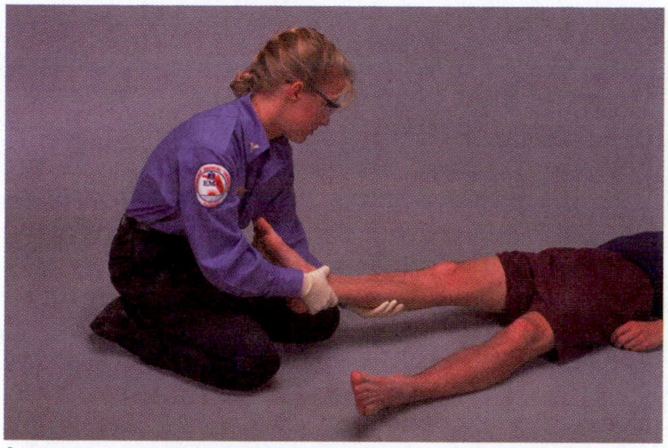

A

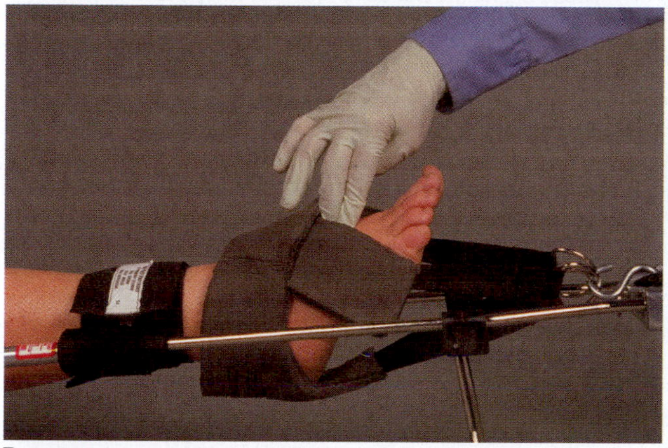

B

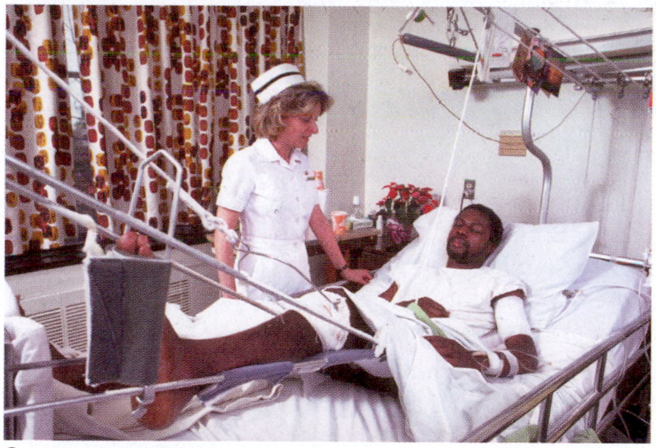

C

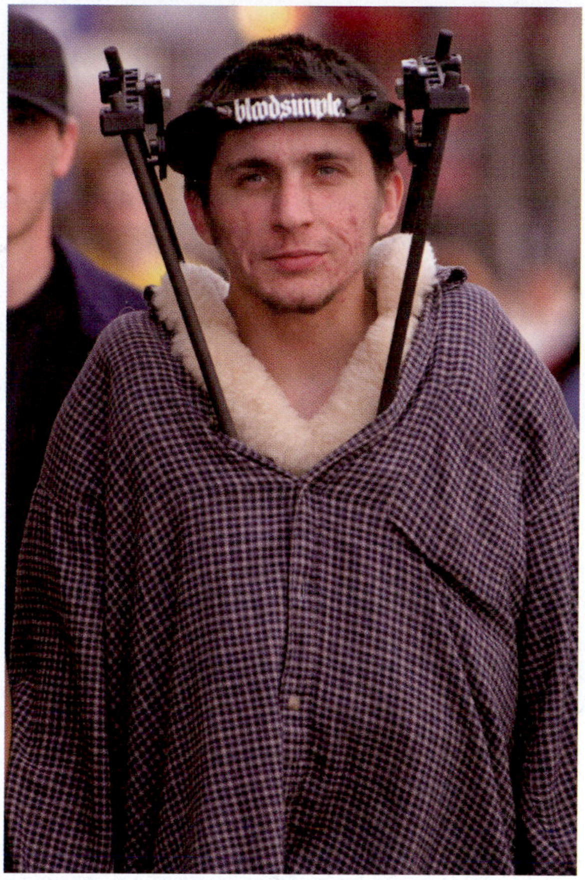

D

Figure 39.4 ■ Traction is the application of a pulling force to restore or maintain bone alignment for fracture healing. **A**, Manual traction is applied to restore or maintain alignment during emergency treatment of a fracture. **B**, Skin traction (also called straight traction), such as is shown here, is often used to temporarily maintain alignment. **C**, Balanced suspension traction is commonly used for fractures of the femur. **D**, Skeletal traction, in which the pulling force is applied directly to the bone, may be used to treat fractures of the spine and other bones.

spinal, or general anesthetic is provided during pin placement. One or more pulling forces may be applied with skeletal traction. Skeletal traction allows more weight to be used to maintain the proper anatomic alignment. The risk of infection is greater, however, and it may cause more discomfort. The weights used for skeletal traction are not removed by the nurse. Nursing interventions for patients in traction are described in **Box 39.3**.

Casts. A *cast* is a rigid device applied to immobilize the injured bones and promote healing. The cast immobilizes the joint above and the joint below the fractured bone so that the bone will not move during healing. A fracture is first reduced manually and a cast is then applied. Casts are applied on patients who have relatively stable fractures.

The cast, which may be composed of plaster or fiberglass, is applied over a thin cushion of padding and molded to the normal contour of the body (**Figure 39.5** ■). The cast must be allowed to dry before any pressure is applied to it; simply palpating a wet cast with the fingertips will leave dents that may cause pressure ulcers. A plaster cast may require up to 48 hours to dry, whereas a fiberglass cast dries within an hour. The type of cast applied is determined by

BOX 39.3
Nursing Interventions for Patients in Traction

- Maintain the pulling force and direction of the traction.
    a. In most instances, the patient's weight provides countertraction.
    b. Center the patient on the bed; maintain body alignment with the direction of pull.
    c. Do not wedge the patient's foot or place it flush with the footboard of the bed.
    d. Ensure that weights hang freely and do not touch the floor.
    e. Ensure that nothing is lying on or obstructing the ropes.
    f. Do not allow the knots at the end of the rope to come into contact with the pulley.
- Perform neurovascular assessments frequently.
- Assess for common complications of immobility, including pressure ulcer formation, renal calculi, deep venous thrombosis, pneumonia, paralytic ileus, and loss of appetite.
- If a problem is detected, assist in repositioning. Stabilize the fracture site during repositioning.
- Teach the patient and family about the type and purpose of the traction.
- For skin traction:
    a. Frequently assess skin, bony prominences, and pressure points for evidence of pressure, shearing, or pending breakdown.
    b. Protect pressure sites with padding and protective dressings, as indicated.
    c. Remove weights only if intermittent traction has been ordered to alleviate muscle spasm.
- For skeletal traction:
    a. Never remove the weights.
    b. Frequently assess pin insertion sites and provide pin site care per policy.
    c. Report signs of infection at the pin sites, such as redness, drainage, and increased tenderness.

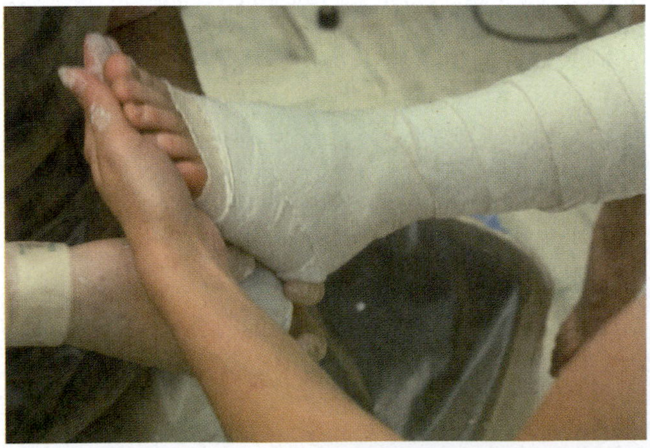

Figure 39.5 ■ Padding to protect the skin is applied under the cast.

BOX 39.4
Nursing Care of the Patient with a Cast

Nursing Interventions

- Perform frequent neurovascular assessments.
- Inspect the cast for drainage and palpate for "hot spots" that may indicate the presence of underlying infection.
- Promptly report increased or severe pain, changes in neurovascular status, or a hot spot or drainage on the cast.
- If crutches are used, arrange for physical therapist to teach correct crutch walking.

Health Education for the Patient and Family

- The cast dries from the inside out; do not use a blow dryer to speed drying; do not cover the cast while it is drying.
- A sensation of warmth during drying is normal.
- Do not put anything into the cast.
- Keep the cast clean and dry; use plastic wrap as needed to protect it.
- If the cast is made of fiberglass, dry it with a blow dryer on the cool setting if it becomes wet.
- Notify your doctor immediately if you develop increased pain, coolness, changes in color, increased edema, and/or loss of sensation.
- Use a blow dryer on the cool setting to relieve itching by blowing cool air into the cast.
- A sling may be used to distribute the weight of the cast evenly around the neck. Do not roll the sling; this can impair circulation to the neck.
- When the cast is removed, an oscillating cast saw will be used. It is noisy and you will feel its vibration, but a guard prevents it from penetrating past the depth of the cast, so it will not cut the skin.

the location of the fracture (**Figure 39.6** ■). Nursing care of the patient with a cast is discussed in **Box 39.4**. During follow-up appointments, the physician may x-ray the bone to assess alignment and healing and possibly remove the cast for skin assessment.

Electrical Bone Stimulation. Electrical bone stimulation is the application of an electrical current at the fracture

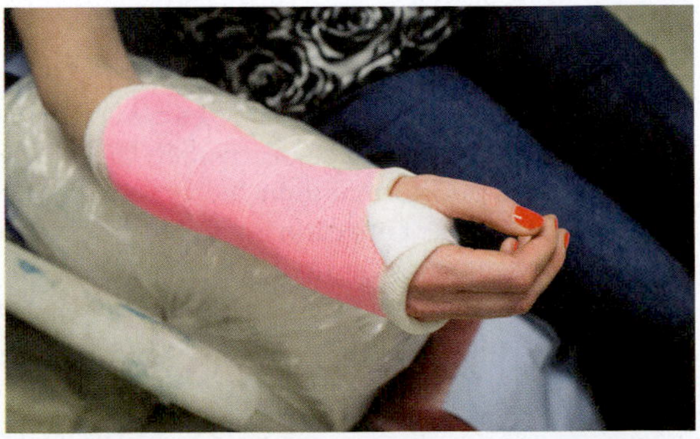

Figure 39.6 ■ A short arm cast that also immobilizes the thumb is used to stabilize a wrist fracture.

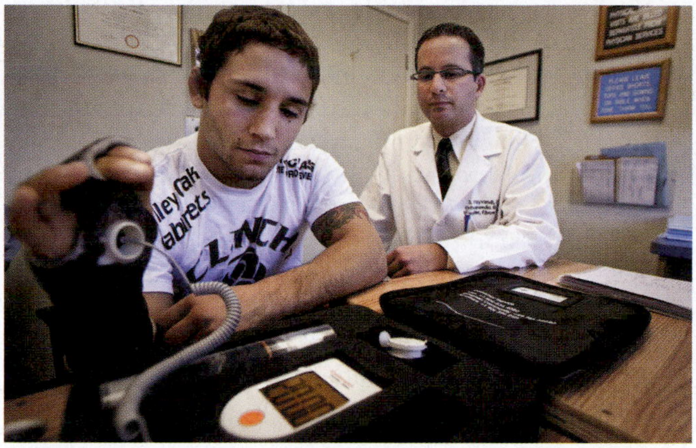

Figure 39.7 ■ External electrical bone growth stimulator.

site. It is a painless method of treating fractures that are not healing appropriately. The electrical stress increases the migration of osteoblasts and osteoclasts to the fracture site. Mineral deposition increases, promoting bone healing. Electrical bone stimulation can be accomplished invasively or noninvasively (**Figure 39.7** ■). In invasive stimulation, the surgeon inserts a cathode and a lead wire at the fracture site. The lead wire is attached to an internal or external generator, which delivers electricity to the cathode 24 hours a day. In noninvasive inductive stimulation, a treatment coil encircles the cast or skin directly over the fracture site. The coil is attached to an external generator that runs on batteries. The electricity goes through the skin to the fracture site. The time period for external stimulation can vary from 3 to 10 hours per day. The patient may be taught to self-administer noninvasive electrical stimulation. Electrical bone stimulation is contraindicated in the presence of infection and for upper extremities if the patient has a pacemaker.

Surgery. Surgery is indicated for a fracture that requires direct visualization and repair, a fracture with common long-term complications, or a fracture that is severely comminuted and threatens vascular supply.

The simplest type of surgery is application of an external fixator device. An external fixator consists of a frame connected to pins that are inserted perpendicular to the long axis of the bone (**Figure 39.8** ■). The number of pins inserted varies with the type and site of the fracture; in general, the same number of pins is inserted above and below the fracture line. The pins require care similar to that provided for skeletal traction pins. The patient is monitored for infection, and frequent neurovascular assessment is performed. The fixator increases independence while maintaining immobilization.

Internal fixation can be accomplished through a surgical procedure called an *open reduction and internal fixation (ORIF)* or through closed reduction followed by percutaneous intramedullary (IM) fixation. In ORIF, the fracture is reduced (placed in correct anatomic alignment) and nails, screws, plates, or pins are inserted to hold the bones in place

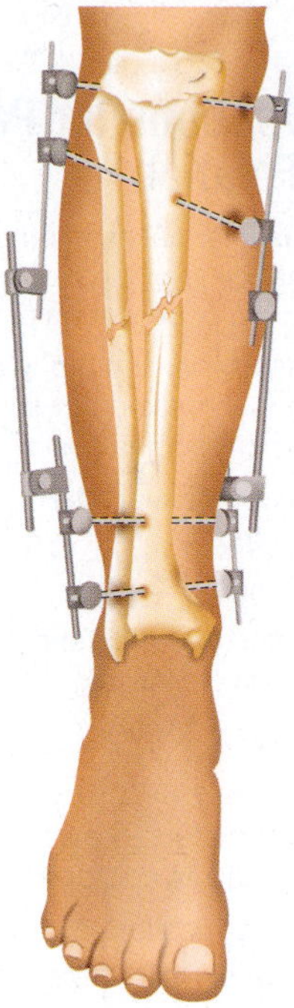

Figure 39.8 ■ In external fixation, pins are placed through the bone above and below the fracture site to immobilize the bone. External fixation rods hold the pins in place.

(**Figure 39.9** ■). Open fractures of the extremities are most commonly repaired in this way. Hip fractures in older patients are frequently repaired with ORIF to prevent complications and to allow early rehabilitation. Interventions for postoperative nursing care are presented in **Box 39.5**. In percutaneous IM fixation, the intramedullary nail or rod is inserted into the marrow cavity and across the fracture site through a small incision. Because of the small incision required, scarring and the risk for significant blood loss and infection are lower with this procedure. IM fixation allows for early return to ADLs with limited weight bearing and use of the extremity, promotes bone healing, and minimizes muscle wasting and loss of range of motion (ROM). In a study of pelvic fraction

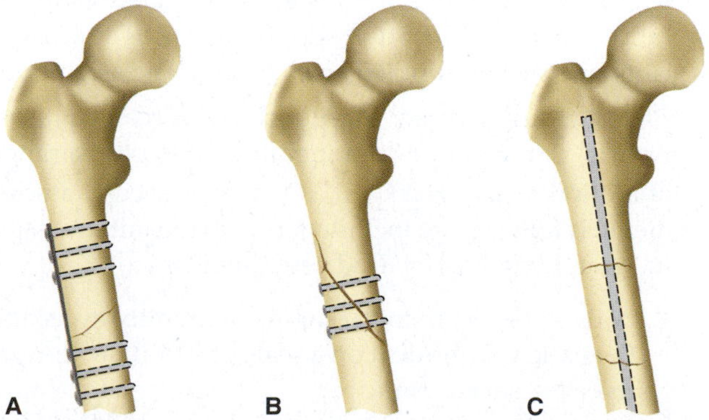
A
B
C

Figure 39.9 ■ Internal fixation hardware is entirely within the body. **A**, Fixation of a short oblique fracture using a plate and screws above and below the fracture. **B**, Fixation of a long oblique fracture using screws through the fracture site. **C**, Fixation of a segmental fracture using a medullary nail.

BOX 39.5
Nursing Interventions for Patients with Internal Fixation

- Perform neurovascular assessments frequently, promptly reporting any change in pulses, color, temperature, capillary refill, movement, or sensation of the affected extremity
- Frequently assess type, location, and severity of pain. Report pain that is increasing in severity, unexpected, or unrelieved by prescribed analgesia.
- Administer medications, such as analgesics and antibiotics, per physician's orders.
- Assess the following:
  a. Amount, color, and odor of drainage on dressing and in wound drain device (e.g., Hemovac, Jackson-Pratt)
  b. Bowel sounds
  c. Lung sounds.
- Maintain position of affected part or extremity as ordered, using positioning aids as appropriate.
- Encourage early mobilization, coughing, and deep breathing, as appropriate, to help prevent complications.
- Arrange for physical and occupational therapy, as ordered.
- Collaborate with physical therapists to promote allowed activity.

fixation, Ma et al. (2017) concluded that internal fixation resulted in less blood loss, shorter operating room times, and better postoperative recovery than external fixation.

Nursing Care

In planning and implementing nursing care for the patient with fractures, the nurse should consider the patient's physical and psychologic responses to the traumatic experience, as well as teaching needs to promote self-care.

Assessment

Collect the following data through the health history and physical examination:

- ***Health history:*** Age, history of traumatic event, history of prior musculoskeletal injuries, chronic illnesses, medications (ask the older adult specifically about anticoagulants and calcium supplements), tobacco and alcohol use
- ***Physical assessment:*** Pain with movement, pulses, edema, skin color and temperature, deformity, range of motion, touch. The **five Ps** of neurovascular assessment, as follows, are included in both the initial assessment and ongoing focused assessments:

  1. **Pain.** Assess pain in the injured extremity by asking the patient to grade it on a scale of 0 to 10, with 10 as the most severe pain.
  2. **Pulses.** Assess distal pulses beginning with the unaffected extremity. Compare the quality of pulses in the affected extremity to those of the unaffected extremity.
  3. **Pallor.** Observe for pallor and skin color in the injured extremity. Paleness and coolness may indicate arterial compromise, whereas warmth and a bluish tinge may indicate venous blood pooling. Assess capillary refill, comparing the affected and unaffected extremities.
  4. **Paralysis/paresis.** Assess ability to move body parts distal to the fracture site. Inability to move indicates paralysis. Loss of muscle strength (weakness) when moving is paresis. A finding of limited ROM may lead to early recognition of problems such as nerve damage and paralysis.
  5. **Paresthesia.** Ask the patient to identify any changes in sensation such as burning, numbness, prickly feeling, or stinging. Assess sensation distal to the injury, including ability to discriminate sharp and dull touch and two-point discrimination.

Priorities of Care

Nursing care priorities for the patient with a fracture focus on associated acute pain, impaired physical mobility, and the risks for impaired tissue perfusion and neurovascular compromise.

Diagnoses, Outcomes, and Interventions

Nursing care for patients with fractures ranges from teaching for home care following treatment in the emergency or urgent care department to providing interventions to maintain health and decrease the risk of complications in patients with complex or multiple fractures. Teaching is also necessary for caregivers of a patient who is discharged home or to a long-term care or rehabilitation facility following a fracture. See the accompanying Case Study & Nursing Care Plan for a patient with hip fracture on page 1435.

Manage Acute Pain. Pain is caused by impaired bone integrity and soft tissue damage and is compounded by muscle spasms and edema.

Expected Outcome: Patient will report pain within acceptable range on a standardized pain scale.

The nurse will:

- Monitor vital signs. *Some analgesics decrease respiratory effort and blood pressure.*
- Ask the patient to rate the pain on a scale of 0 to 10 (with 10 as the most severe pain) before and after any intervention. *This facilitates objective assessment of the effectiveness of the chosen pain relief strategy. Pain that increases in intensity or remains unrelieved with analgesics can indicate compartment syndrome.*
- For the patient with a hip fracture, apply Buck's traction per healthcare provider's orders. Keep the traction weights hanging freely. *Buck's traction immobilizes the fracture and decreases pain and additional trauma.*
- Move the patient gently and slowly. Support a fractured extremity above and below the fracture when moving. *Gentle moving and support of the injured extremity help prevent the development of severe muscle spasms.*
- Elevate the injured extremity above the level of the heart. *Elevating the extremity promotes venous return and decreases edema, which decreases pain.*
- Encourage distraction or other adjunctive methods of pain relief, such as deep breathing and relaxation.

Distraction, deep breathing, and relaxation help decrease the focus on the pain and may lessen the intensity of pain.

- Administer NSAIDs and pain medications as prescribed. For home care, explain the importance of taking pain medications before the pain becomes severe. *Analgesics alleviate pain by stimulating opiate receptor sites. NSAIDs mediate inflammation and provide an analgesic effect.*

Reduce Risk for Impaired Peripheral Neurovascular Function. In the patient with a fracture, compartment syndrome or deep venous thrombosis can impair circulation and, in turn, tissue perfusion. Furthermore, peripheral nerves may be damaged as a result of the initial trauma, during movement of the affected extremity, or as a consequence of compartment syndrome.

Expected Outcome: Peripheral circulation and neurologic function will remain within expected parameters.

The nurse will:

- Support the injured extremity above and below the fracture site when moving the patient. *Supporting the injured extremity above and below the fracture site helps prevent displacement of bony fragments and decreases the risk of further nerve damage.*
- Assess the five Ps every 1 to 2 hours immediately postinjury until stable then per protocol. Report abnormal findings immediately. *Unrelenting pain, pallor, paresthesias, and paresis are strong indicators of compartment syndrome.*
- Assess nail beds for capillary refill. If nails are too thick or discolored, assess the skin around the nail. *Delayed capillary refill may indicate decreased tissue perfusion.*
- Monitor the extremity for edema and hematoma. *Excessive edema and hematoma formation can compromise circulation.*
- Assess for deep, throbbing, unrelenting pain. *Pain that is not relieved by analgesics may indicate neurovascular compromise.*
- Assess the ability to differentiate between sharp and dull touch and the presence of paresthesias and paralysis every 1 to 2 hours immediately postinjury until stable then per protocol. *Paresthesias develop as a result of pressure on nerves and may indicate compartment syndrome. Paralysis is a late sign of nerve entrapment and requires that the physician be notified immediately.*
- Monitor the tightness of the cast. *Edema can cause the cast to become tight; a tight-fitting cast may lead to compartment syndrome or paralysis. Two finger breadths should fit around the edge of the cast. If unable to fit two fingers around the edge of the cast, notify the care provider as soon as possible. Refer to Box 39.4.*
- If the cast is tight, be prepared to assist the physician with bivalving (**Figure 39.10** ■). *Bivalving, the process of splitting a cast down both sides, alleviates pressure on an injured extremity.*
- If compartment syndrome is suspected, assist the healthcare provider in measuring compartment pressure. *Compartment pressure that rises to within 10 to 30 mmHg of diastolic pressure indicates compartment syndrome and circulatory compromise* (Stracciolini & Hammerberg, 2018).

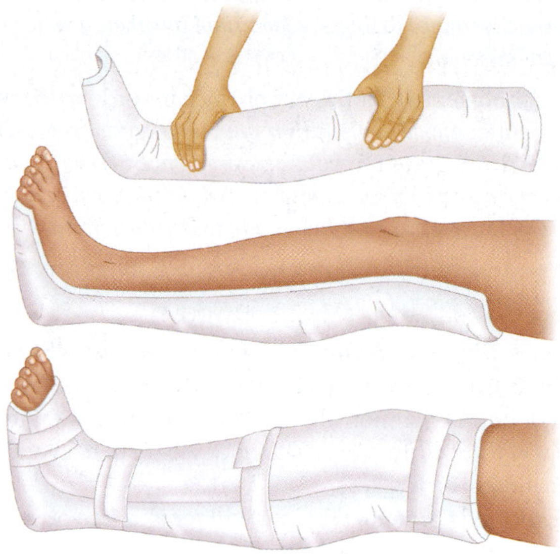

Figure 39.10 ■ Bivalving is the process of splitting a cast down both sides to alleviate pressure on or allow visualization of an extremity.

- Unless contraindicated, elevate the injured extremity above the level of the heart. *Elevating the extremity increases venous return and decreases edema. It may be contraindicated, however, if compartment syndrome develops because elevation may further reduce arterial flow to the extremity.*
- Administer anticoagulant per physician's order. *Prophylactic anticoagulation decreases the risk of clot formation.*

SAFETY ALERT: Pulses may remain strong while capillary circulation within the affected extremity is severely impaired in compartment syndrome. ■

Reduce Risk for Infection. An open fracture carries significant risk for wound contamination and subsequent infection. Wound healing in orthopedic patients is affected by the cause of the wound as well as the therapies used to repair musculoskeletal structures. It is important to understand normal wound healing processes, characteristics of musculoskeletal wounds, contamination, and drainage, and potential complications to plan for and implement appropriate interventions.

Expected Outcome: Patient will remain free of infection until healing is complete.

The nurse will:

- For patients with skeletal pins, follow established guidelines for skeletal pin site care. *Pins or wires attached to traction, casts, or external fixators stabilize a segment of bone so optimal healing can occur.*
- Monitor vital signs and lab reports of WBCs. *Increases in pulse rate, respiratory rate, temperature, and WBCs may indicate infection.*
- Use sterile technique for dressing changes. *Aseptic technique is necessary to avoid introducing organisms into the operative site.*

- Assess the wound for size, color, and the presence of any drainage. *Redness, edema, and purulent drainage indicate infection.*
- Administer antibiotics per physician's orders. *Prophylactic antibiotic administration inhibits bacterial reproduction and thereby helps prevent skin flora from entering the wound. In the case of "dirty wounds," such as those occurring from vehicular crashes, antibiotics are routinely administered.*
- Promote nutritional intake. *Adequate nutrition assists in preventing infection.*

Promote Physical Mobility. The patient who has experienced a fracture requires immobilization of the fractured bone(s). Immobilization alters normal gait and mobility. The patient will need to use assistive devices such as crutches, canes, slings, or walkers.

Expected Outcome: Patient will remain free of injury or adverse effects of reduced mobility.

The nurse will:

- Teach or assist patient with ROM exercises of the unaffected limbs. *ROM exercises help prevent muscle atrophy and maintain strength and joint function. Flexion and extension exercises prevent the development of foot drop, wrist drop, or frozen joints.*
- Teach isometric exercises, and encourage the patient to perform them every 4 hours. *Isometric exercises help prevent muscle atrophy and force synovial fluid and nutrients into the cartilage.*
- Encourage ambulation when able; provide assistance as necessary. *Ambulation maintains and improves circulation, helps prevent muscle atrophy, and helps maintain bowel function.*
- Turn the patient on bedrest every 2 hours. If the patient is in traction, teach the patient to shift his or her weight every hour. *Turning and shifting weight increase circulation and help prevent skin breakdown.*

SAFETY ALERT: Teach and observe the patient's use of assistive devices (such as canes, crutches, walkers, and slings) in conjunction with the physical therapist. Proper use of devices is necessary for safe ambulation and helps prevent the loss of joint function secondary to complications and falls. ■

A summary of the treatment of, complications of, and nursing interventions for specific fractures is found in **Table 39.3**.

Table 39.3 Treatment, Complications, and Nursing Interventions of Specific Fractures

Treatment	Complications	Specific Nursing Interventions
Skull		
Nondisplaced: Monitor level of consciousness and protect area from further pressure ***Displaced/depressed:*** Surgical repair displacement with plates and screws, especially if causing traumatic brain injury	■ *Displaced/depressed:* Often associated with traumatic brain injury ■ *Basilar skull fractures:* May lead to cerebral spinal fluid (CSF) leaks from the ears or nose, exposing the spine to potential infection	■ A complete neurologic assessment: Level of consciousness (LOC) and orientation to person, place, time, and situation; pupillary reaction to light; movement and strength of all extremities; and complaints of nausea and vomiting ■ Elevate head of bed at least 30 degrees ■ Assess for potential CSF leaks ■ Monitor for pain and treat accordingly ■ Apply ice/cold packs to bruised area, as tolerated
Face		
Severely displaced or multiple facial fractures: Open reduction and internal fixation (ORIF) with wires or plates and screws	■ Airway compromise related to edema from trauma ■ Older adults are more likely to have associated injuries (e.g., brain, chest, spine) than younger adults (Toivari, Suominen, Lindqvist, & Thoren, 2016) ■ *Orbital fractures:* Severe edema may impact vision	■ Maintain patent airway ■ Monitor respiratory effort ■ Assist patient with airway clearance with oral and tracheal suctioning as needed ■ Elevate head of bed at least 30 degrees ■ Monitor for pain and treat accordingly ■ Apply ice/cold packs to bruised areas, as tolerated ■ Support patient's body image and provide reassurance as needed
Spine		
Nondisplaced cervical spinal fracture: Cervical collar or halo immobilizing brace (refer to Figure 39.4) ***Displaced cervical fracture:*** Reduced by manual or skeletal traction followed by the application of a brace and/or surgical stabilization of the bones with wires, plates, and screws ***Nondisplaced thoracic and lumbar fractures:*** Generally treated with thoracolumbar braces ***Displaced thoracic and lumbar fractures:*** Treated with surgical stabilization with wires, plates, and screws	■ *Spinal cord injury:* Displaced or unstable fracture of the vertebrae may apply pressure on or puncture the spinal cord, which may result in temporary or permanent paralysis	■ Assess and monitor for neurologic dysfunction distal to the site of injury ■ Monitor for complications of immobility (e.g., pressure injuries, DVT) ■ Monitor bowel and bladder habits ■ Assess pain and treat accordingly ■ Initiate bowel and bladder training as indicated ■ Encourage participation in self-care ■ Seek occupational and physical therapy consults ■ Support patient's psychosocial wellness ■ Seek counseling with social services or clergy as appropriate ■ Teach about use and care of any immobilization devices prescribed ■ Seek consult for rehabilitation facility to assist with transition to home

Treatment	Complications	Specific Nursing Interventions
Clavicle		
Nondisplaced: Cervical strap (immobilization and pain control) ***Displaced:*** Surgical fixation with plates and screws and then cervical strap for support	■ Displaced clavicular fractures may damage subclavian vessels or the lung ■ Injury to the brachial plexus may result in numbness and decreased movement of the arm on the affected side ■ Malunion of a clavicular fracture can result in asymmetry of the shoulders	■ Assess pain and treat accordingly ■ For patients with untreated displaced fractures, monitor for signs of complications: Low blood pressure, pale skin, other signs of hemorrhage, respiratory effort, and reduced lung sounds
Humerus		
Nondisplaced: Immobilization with sling and swath or hanging arm cast ***Displaced proximal humerus fracture:*** ORIF, or if not a surgical candidate, patient may be placed in skeletal traction to maintain alignment after manual reduction; this type of traction places the injured arm in an upright position over the patient's head and traction is applied to the distal portion of the humerus	■ Nerve and ligament damage ■ Frozen or stiff joints and malunion ■ Risk for impaired ROM of the shoulder increases with fracture severity and soft tissue damage ■ Rehabilitative measures focus on increasing ROM ■ Early interventions may prevent permanent damage	■ Assess neurovascular status in affected extremity, more frequently immediately postinjury or surgery, moving to every 4 to 8 hours after 24 hours ■ Assess pain and treat accordingly ■ Encourage exercises: a. *Finger exercises:* Move each finger of the affected arm through complete range of motion b. *Pendulum shoulder exercises:* Dangle the affected arm at the side, and move it forward and backward about 30 degrees in each direction, once released to do so by surgeon ■ Seek occupational therapy consult ■ Instruct the patient and family in cast care and sling application, neurovascular assessments, exercises, prescribed pain medications, and manifestations of complications and when to report these
Elbow, Radius, Ulna, Wrist, and Hand		
Elbow ***Nondisplaced:*** Posterior splint and sling for several weeks ***Displaced fracture:*** ORIF with wires or plates and screws	■ Most common is decreased ROM due to applied limited mobility of the joint (Perz, 2013) ■ Nerve or artery damage ■ Hemarthrosis, a collection of blood in the elbow joint ■ *Myositis ossificans:* Heterotropic bone growth causing capsular tightness and decreased ROM (Perz, 2013)	■ Assess pain and treat accordingly ■ Assess neurovascular status ■ Maintain immobilization ■ Teach use and care of sling, splint, and/or cast ■ Encourage use of unaffected areas (fingers, wrist, or elbow) to prevent muscle stiffness and wasting ■ Seek occupational therapy consult if patient's dominant extremity is affected ■ Instruct the patient regarding: a. Neurovascular assessments b. Maintaining immobilization c. Importance of elevation of the extremity, as ordered d. When to call the care provider about changes in sensation or an increase in pain
Radius/Ulna ***Nondisplaced:*** Splint and sling initially. After swelling has stopped, a cast will be placed ***Displaced:*** ORIF with posterior splint	■ Compartment syndrome ■ Delayed healing ■ Decreased wrist ROM ■ Contractures	
Wrist/Hand ***Nondisplaced:*** Casting with or without sling ***Displaced:*** If unable to achieved appropriate alignment with manual reduction of the fracture, ORIF will be performed with casting/splinting for support	■ Compartment syndrome ■ Nerve damage ■ Ligament damage ■ Delayed or nonunion	
Ribs		
Nondisplaced: Supportive splinting and monitor ***Displaced:*** Surgical repair, ORIF ***Flail rib:*** Two or more adjacent ribs in two or more places and the formation of a free-floating segment that moves in the opposite direction of the rib cage; segment is surgically stabilized with plates	■ Pulmonary contusion ■ Pneumothorax and/or hemothorax ■ Subclavian artery or vein damage (first through third rib fractures) ■ Spleen and liver damage (lower rib fractures) ■ Pneumonia or atelectasis due to ineffective clearing of respiratory secretions	■ Monitor respiratory effort and depth ■ Assess pain and treat accordingly ■ Teach patient about splinting and importance of deep breathing with or without the use of an incentive spirometer ■ Teach to return to the emergency department if shortness of breath develops and call care provider should signs of pneumonia develop (fever, cough, difficulty breathing)

(continued)

Table 39.3 (*Continued*)

Treatment	Complications	Specific Nursing Interventions
Pelvis		
Nondisplaced/stable: Bedrest, progressing to ambulation with limited weight bearing; skeletal traction or pelvic sling traction (Kahn-Kastell, 2013) ***Displaced/unstable:*** ORIF; in immediate posttrauma period or if unstable and patient has other conditions from the trauma that need to be stabilized prior to surgery, an external fixator may be applied to stabilize the pelvis	■ Hypovolemic shock secondary to hemorrhage ■ Nerve damage ■ Thromboembolism ■ Malunion/nonunion (Kahn-Kastell, 2013) ■ Complications of immobility	■ Assess pain and treat accordingly ■ Monitor for signs of hypovolemic shock ■ Monitor urine for blood (indicating bladder injury) ■ Logrolling and maintaining pelvic alignment increases patient comfort ■ Assess and monitor for neurologic dysfunction distal to the site of injury ■ Monitor for complications of immobility (e.g., pressure injuries, DVT) ■ Monitor bowel and bladder habits ■ Seek occupational and physical therapy consults ■ Seek consult for rehabilitation facility to assist with transition to home
Hip, Femur, Tibia, Fibula, Ankle, and Foot		
Hip ***Initial:*** Prior to surgery, placement in Buck skin traction ***Conservative:*** Nonsurgical treatment may be used for a patient who is nonambulatory prefracture, has a poor prognosis to return to functional level of mobility, or is not able to medically undergo surgery Surgical treatment depends on the exact location of the fracture: ***Intracapsular or femoral neck:*** Threaded pins, compression hip screws, femoral head replacement, primary THA, or hemiarthroplasty ***Intertrochanteric:*** ORIF with nails, pins, and compression hip screws ***Subtrochanteric:*** ORIF with intramedullary nails, sliding nail plate, or fixed plate (Kahn-Kastell, 2013) (**Figure 39.11** ■)	■ Neurovascular compromise ■ Complications of immobility ■ Postoperative infection ■ Hip dislocation (with THA) ■ DVT	■ Assess pain and treat accordingly ■ Assess neurovascular status ■ Maintain skin integrity ■ Tibia/fibula and foot/ankle injuries may be elevated and ice applied ■ Preoperative: Routine preoperative teaching ■ Postoperative: Prevent infection and administer postoperative antibiotics, as ordered; encourage postoperative respiratory and leg exercises; routine postoperative discharge teaching ■ Seek physical therapy consult and reinforce instruction of exercises, mobility parameters, and use of mobility assistive devices ■ Seek occupational therapy for assistance with ADLs and reinforce instruction and use of assistive devices ■ Teach patient signs and symptoms of the potential complications and when to report these to the care provider ■ Teach use and care of splints, casts, and/or other immobilization devices

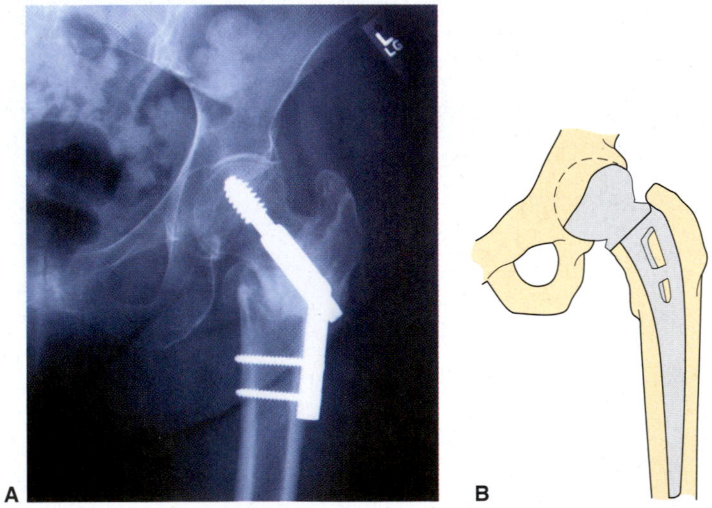
A
B

Figure 39.11 ■ Surgical fixation of hip fractures. **A**, A surgical nail or screw used to stabilize an intertrochanteric fracture. **B**, Use of a hip prosthesis (artificial hip) to replace a damaged femoral head.

Treatment	Complications	Specific Nursing Interventions
Femur ***Initial nondisplaced and displaced:*** Skeletal traction for reduction and immobilization of the fracture until stable, followed by surgical fixation with an intramedullary rod	■ Hypovolemia due to blood loss (may be as great as 1.0 to 1.5 L) ■ Fat embolism ■ DVT ■ Compartment syndrome (rare)	

Treatment	Complications	Specific Nursing Interventions
Tibia/Fibula ***Nondisplaced:*** Casting or immobilization brace/boot with no touch-down weight bearing for 10 days to 2 weeks; after 3 to 4 weeks, the cast is replaced with a functional/walking brace/boot that provides continued support and protection ***Displaced:*** External fixation or ORIF using an intermedullary rod; following surgery, a cast or immobilization brace may be applied; weight bearing begins according to the physician's orders **Ankle** ***Nondisplaced:*** Closed reduction and casting ***Displaced or multiple fractures:*** ORIF with plates, screws or nails, and splinting/casting or external fixation **Foot** ***Nondisplaced:*** Most foot fractures are nondisplaced and treated with closed reduction and casting ***Displaced:*** May require surgery and the placement of wires to maintain reduction of the fracture	■ Damage to the peroneal nerve or tibial artery ■ Compartment syndrome ■ Hemarthroses ■ Ligament damage	

Delegating Nursing Care Activities

Once patients have learned to use assistive devices, UAP may help with mobilization and assist the patient with ADLs. They will also assist with emptying and recording drainage, application, and removal of antithromboembolism stockings and use of SCDs.

Case Study & Nursing Care Plan

A Patient with a Hip Fracture

Stella Carbolito is a 74-year-old woman with a history of osteoporosis. She lives alone in a two-story row home. She is retired and takes pride in making all her own food from scratch. While walking to the market one day, Mrs. Carbolito falls and fractures her left hip. She is transported by ambulance to the nearest emergency department.

ASSESSMENT	DIAGNOSES	EXPECTED OUTCOMES
During the initial assessment, abnormal findings are that Mrs. Carbolito's left leg is shorter than her right leg and is externally rotated. Distal pulses are present and bilaterally strong; both legs are warm. Mrs. Carbolito complains of severe pain but denies any numbness or burning. She is able to wiggle the toes on her left leg and has full movement of her right leg. Initial vital signs are T 36.6°C (98.0°F), P 100 bpm, R 18/min, BP 120/58 mmHg. Diagnostic tests include CBC, blood chemistry, and x-ray studies of the left hip and pelvis. The CBC reveals a hemoglobin of 11.0 g/dL and a WBC count within normal limits. Blood chemistry findings are within normal limits. The x-ray reveals a fracture of the left femoral neck. Mrs. Carbolito is admitted to the hospital with an order for 10 lb of straight (Buck) leg traction. An open reduction and internal fixation (ORIF) is planned for the following day.	■ Acute pain related to fractured left femoral neck and muscle spasms ■ Decreased mobility related to bed rest and fractured left femoral head ■ Potential for peripheral nerve damage related to unstable bones and swelling	■ Patient will verbalize a decrease in pain. ■ Patient will verbalize the purpose of traction and surgery. ■ Patient will maintain normal neurovascular status. ■ Patient will demonstrate postoperative exercises.

PLANNING AND IMPLEMENTATION

- Assess pain on a scale of 0 to 10 before and after implementing measures to reduce pain.
- Administer analgesics per the physician's order.
- Perform neurovascular assessment every 2 to 4 hours, and document findings.
- Apply straight leg traction per physician's order.
- Teach the purpose of traction and surgery.
- Teach the purpose of and the procedure for performing isometric and flexion/extension exercises.

(Continued)

EVALUATION

On the day after surgery, Mrs. Carbolito is out of bed and in a chair. She verbalizes a decrease in pain. There have been no abnormal neurovascular assessments. She is able to independently perform isometric and flexion/extension exercises in both lower extremities. Discharge planning includes referrals for home care. A home health nurse will visit, and the social worker at the hospital has ordered a trapeze for her bed, an elevated toilet seat, an elevated cushion for her chair, and a walker.

CLINICAL REASONING IN PATIENT CARE

1. What factors placed Mrs. Carbolito at risk for a hip fracture?
2. Mrs. Carbolito says, "I don't understand why they had to put that heavy thing on my leg before I went to surgery to get my hip fixed." What would you tell her? What preoperative factors might have decreased teaching effectiveness?
3. Describe how each of the following, if manifested by Mrs. Carbolito, would increase her risk for postoperative complications: Urinary incontinence, weight more than 20% under normal for her height, chronic constipation. What nursing diagnoses and interventions would you include in her plan of care to decrease the risk?

See Evaluating Your Response in Appendix B.

Complications

Complications of musculoskeletal trauma include compartment syndrome, fat embolism, deep venous thrombosis, infection, delayed or nonunion, or *complex regional pain syndrome*.

Compartment Syndrome

Muscles, nerves, and blood vessels of the extremities are enclosed by a fibrous membrane or fascia. The fascia, which is nonexpansile, supports these tissues. **Compartment syndrome** occurs when increased pressure within this confined space constricts the structures within it, compromising circulation and tissue function. Acute compartment syndrome may result from hemorrhage and edema within the compartment following a fracture, crush injury, or surgery. External compression of the limb by a cast or dressing that constricts the limb can also lead to compartment syndrome.

Compression of nerves within the compartment causes severe pain, paresthesias (burning, tingling, or loss of sensation), and diminished reflexes. Entrapment of the blood vessels limits tissue perfusion, beginning a cycle of events that may result in the loss of the limb. Inadequate oxygen supply causes cellular acidosis, which intensifies as cellular energy requirements are met through anaerobic metabolism. The capillaries inside the compartment dilate in an attempt to increase the supply of blood and oxygen. Additional blood and oxygen are not available, and plasma proteins leak out into the interstitial tissues. The interstitial tissue then pulls fluid in to balance the protein load. As a result, edema within the compartment increases. The edema causes further compression of the vascular network, and the cycle continues. Uninterrupted, this cycle threatens the patient's limb and increases the risk of sepsis. Acute kidney injury is also a risk if pressure is unrelieved because the breakdown of muscle cells releases myoglobin, a protein toxic to the kidney tubules.

Compartment syndrome usually develops within the first 48 hours of injury, when edema is at its peak. It is important to note that because major arteries are outside muscle compartments, arterial pulses often remain normal, even when pressure within the compartment significantly impairs tissue perfusion. Necrosis of affected muscle can develop within 4 to 8 hours, necessitating timely identification and treatment of the syndrome (Sorenson et al., 2019).

Early manifestations of compartment syndrome include pain and normal or decreased peripheral pulses. Later manifestations include cyanosis; tingling; loss of sensation (paresthesias); weakness (paresis); and severe pain, especially when the extremity is passively flexed.

If compartment syndrome develops, interventions to alleviate pressure are implemented. Restrictive dressings are removed or a tight-fitting cast is split. *Fasciotomy*, surgical incision of the muscle fascia to relieve pressure within the compartment, may be necessary. After a fasciotomy, the incision is left open, leading to a potential infection risk.

Volkmann contracture, an uncommon complication of elbow or forearm fractures, can result from unresolved compartment syndrome. Arterial blood flow decreases, leading to ischemia, degeneration, and contracture of forearm muscles. The severity of Volkmann contracture varies from mild, limited to wrist flexors, to severe, affecting both flexor and extensor muscles of the forearm.

Fat Embolism Syndrome

Fat emboli are commonly released from adipose tissue or bone marrow after long bone fractures. In most cases, these are benign and asymptomatic (Kosova, Bergmark, & Piazza, 2015). **Fat embolism syndrome (FES)** is a rare complication characterized by neurologic dysfunction, pulmonary insufficiency, and a petechial rash on the chest, axilla, and upper arms (Sorenson et al., 2019). Long bone fractures and other major trauma are the principal risk factors for fat emboli; hip replacement surgery also poses a risk for FES.

According to the mechanical theory of FES development, increased interstitial pressure at the site of the injury causes fat droplets from damaged adipose tissue and bone marrow to enter the circulation. These fat globules then lodge in small vessels, causing local ischemia and inflammation, with release of inflammatory mediators and vasoactive chemicals. The biochemical theory states that fat globules are released from tissue in response to stress-related catecholamines. Embolized fat is then broken down into free fatty acids, which cause pulmonary tissue inflammation and acute lung injury (Kosova et al., 2015).

Manifestations, the result of vascular occlusion and injury and the inflammatory response, usually develop within 12 to 72 hours after injury. Respiratory manifestations of dyspnea, tachypnea, and hypoxemia are often the first indicators of FES. Pulmonary edema, impaired surfactant production, and atelectasis can result in significant respiratory insufficiency and manifestations of acute respiratory distress syndrome. Neurologic symptoms, including restlessness, acute confusion, and altered level of consciousness, follow (Kosova et al., 2015). Fat droplets activate the clotting cascade, causing thrombocytopenia. Petechiae appearing on the skin, soft palate, and conjunctiva are thought to result from either microvascular clotting or the accompanying thrombocytopenia.

Early immobilization of long bone fractures reduces the risk of FES. Surgical stabilization further reduces the risk. Prompt identification and treatment of the syndrome are necessary to maintain adequate pulmonary function. In severe cases, the patient may require intubation and mechanical ventilation to prevent hypoxemia. Fluid balance is closely monitored. Prophylactic corticosteroids in patients with long bone fractures have been shown to decrease the incidence of FES, including inhaled corticosteroids (Sen, Prakash, Tripathy, Argarwal, & Sen, 2017). Corticosteriods may also be administered to decrease the inflammatory response in the lung, stabilize lipid membranes, and reduce bronchospasm (Sorenson et al., 2019).

Deep Venous Thrombosis

Deep venous thrombosis (DVT) is a condition in which a blood clot forms along the intimal lining of a large vein, accompanied by inflammation of the vein wall. Risk factors for DVT are (1) venous stasis, or decreased blood flow; (2) injury to blood vessel walls; and (3) altered blood coagulation (**Table 39.4**). Trauma to the vein stimulates the clotting cascade. Platelets aggregate (clump together) at the site, forming the thrombus. Fibrin, white blood cells (WBCs), and red blood cells (RBCs) begin to cling to the thrombus, and the inflammatory response is initiated. The tail of the clot or the entire thrombus may dislodge and become an embolus, ultimately lodging in the pulmonary circulation (pulmonary embolism). Pulmonary embolism is a leading cause of death in patients who have had hip fracture surgery (Sorenson et al., 2019). If the thrombus remains in the vein, venous insufficiency may result from scarring and valve damage.

Although DVT is often asymptomatic, it may cause edema, pain, tenderness, or cramping of the affected extremity. Doppler ultrasonography is commonly used to identify DVT. In some cases, MRI or a venogram may be required for diagnosis.

The best treatment for DVT is prevention. Early immobilization of the fracture and early ambulation of the patient are imperative. Prophylactic anticoagulation is beneficial. Antiembolism stockings and sequential compression devices (SCDs) increase venous return and prevent venous stasis. See Chapter 32 for more information about preventing venous thromboembolism.

Table 39.4 Risk Factors for Deep Venous Thrombosis

Risk Factor	Implications for Fractures
Decreased blood flow	Muscle contractions facilitating venous flow may be impaired by immobility or stabilization of the fracture (e.g., with a cast or fixation device).
Injury to blood vessel wall	May occur as a direct result of trauma or from surgical manipulation.
Altered blood coagulation	The body's attempt to maintain homeostasis leads to increased production of platelets and clotting factors.

Infection

Infection is more likely to occur in an open fracture than a closed fracture, but any complication that decreases blood supply increases the risk of infection. Infection may result from contamination at the time of injury or during surgery. *Pseudomonas*, *Staphylococcus*, or *Clostridium* organisms may invade the wound or bone. *Clostridium* infection is particularly serious because it may lead to severe gas gangrene and cellulitis, but any infection may delay healing and result in osteomyelitis, infection within the bone that can lead to tissue death and necrosis.

Delayed Union and Nonunion

Delayed healing can affect any fracture, but it most commonly affects the long bones: The humerus, femur, or tibia. *Delayed union* is the prolonged healing of bones beyond the usual time period. Both injury-related factors (the type and location of fracture and accompanying soft tissue injury) and systemic factors (age, general health, immune status, chronic diseases, and smoking) can affect healing, Delayed union is diagnosed by means of serial x-ray studies. It is important to note that x-ray findings may lag 1 to 2 weeks behind the healing process; for example, a patient may be completely healed by week 13, but this fact may not be apparent on the x-ray until week 14.

Delayed union may lead to nonunion, which can cause persistent pain and movement at the fracture site. Nonunion may require surgical interventions, such as internal fixation and bone grafting. If infection is present, the bones are surgically debrided. Electrical or ultrasonic stimulation of the fracture site may be effective to promote healing. Biologic agents such as growth hormone or parathyroid hormone may be given to stimulate bone growth.

Complex Regional Pain Syndrome

Complex regional pain syndrome (CRPS) may occur after musculoskeletal or nerve trauma. It is characterized by pain that is disproportionate to the injury in the affected limb, as well as sensory, temperature, motor, and skin changes of the extremity, in addition to edema and diaphoresis (Lo, Cavazos, & Burnett, 2017). Female gender and older age are risk factors for CRPS. The pain of CRPS is severe, diffuse, and burning. Initially the affected extremity appears inflamed and edematous, later becoming cool and pale. Muscle wasting, skin and nail changes, and bone abnormalities can develop. In CRPS, it appears that pain receptors in the affected extremity become sensitized to catecholamines, neurotransmitters associated with sympathetic nervous system activity. Its cause is unclear; it may be related to central or peripheral nervous system damage, an inflammatory process, disrupted healing, or an autoimmune process. Diagnosis is made by the patient's history and physical examination. X-rays may demonstrate spotty osteoporosis, and bone scans may reveal increased uptake of radionuclide. Treatment requires an interprofessional team approach, including physical therapy with pharmacologic treatment of the neuropathic pain and inflammation (short term) (Lo et al., 2017). Nerve blocks may be required for patients who do not respond to other treatments.

Transitions of Care

Preventing fractures is particularly important in older adults. Educate patients and their families on the importance of exercise, home safety, medication reviews, and vision checks:

- Begin a regular exercise program; lack of exercise leads to weakness and an increased chance of falling. Exercises that improve balance and coordination (such as yoga or tai chi) are the most helpful.
- Make your home safer:
  a. Remove any items in your pathway, including from stairs, to avoid tripping.
  b. Remove small throw rugs or use double-sided tape to keep rugs from slipping.
  c. Place frequently used items within easy reach to avoid use of a step stool.
  d. Install grab bars next to your toilet and in the tub or shower.
  e. Use nonslip mats in the bathtub and on shower floors.
  f. Improve lighting, using lamp shades or frosted bulbs to reduce glare. Install nightlights in hallways and bathroom.
  g. Install handrails and lights in all staircases.
  h. Wear shoes that give good support and have thin, nonslip soles. Avoid wearing slippers and athletic shoes with deep treads.
- Ask your healthcare provider to review your medications, including prescriptions and over-the-counter medications. Some medications or a combination of medications may cause dizziness or drowsiness, leading to falls.
- Have your vision checked by an eye doctor. Your glasses may no longer have the correct prescription, or you may have developed an eye condition such as cataracts or glaucoma that limits your vision.

For the patient who is recovering from a fracture, patient and family teaching focuses on individualized needs. Discharge teaching will focus on self-care, pain management, prevention of complications, and what and when to report any changes or concerns to the care provider based on the patient's injury and comorbid conditions. Written and verbal teaching is necessary. Return demonstration of appropriate care and use of devices is needed to prevent complications, such as skin irritation with immobilization devices or injury from improper use of crutches.

In particular, address the following topics for home care of the patient who has fractured a hip:

- Encourage independence in ADLs:
  a. Explain that the patient should sit only on high chairs to prevent excess flexion of the hip; an elevated toilet seat can be added to a regular toilet seat.
  b. Encourage the patient and family to equip the shower with a hand rail to aid stability and prevent falls.
  c. If a walker is needed, teach the patient its proper use. Do not carry the walker, but lift it, advance it, and then take two steps, or use a rolling walker.
  d. If a cane is needed, instruct the patient to use it on the affected side.
- Stress the importance of well-balanced meals, and explain all prescribed medications.

Patients who have experienced a fracture or who have had orthopedic surgery often have a cast and may require an extended period of limited activities. Address the following topics for home care:

- Cast care (see Box 39.4)
- Follow the physician's order for weight bearing
- Physical therapy can evaluate the home environment for safety and suggest modifications as needed. Physical therapists also teach crutch walking, limited weight bearing, transferring, and other activities.
- Home care agency nurses can teach wound care and provide ongoing monitoring of wound healing
- Local medical equipment and supply sources rent or sell durable equipment such as crutches, walkers, wheelchairs, overhead trapeze units, shower chairs, elevated toilet seats, grab bars, and bedside commodes. Slings or braces may be purchased through medical equipment dealers. Often the hospital social service department can assist with these arrangements.
- Local pharmacies are good resources for dressing supplies such as antiseptic solutions or ointments, dressings, and tape
- Fitness equipment suppliers may be able to provide rehabilitation equipment such as hand or ankle weights for strengthening exercises.

Fractures, or complications from them, can be fatal. When caring for a patient with a fracture at the end of life, the extent of fracture treatment is dependent on overall condition and tolerance for procedures. Commonly at end of life, fractures may be treated using conservative means, focusing on correct bone placement, immobilization, pain management, and reduction of neurovascular compromise.

The Patient with an Amputation

An **amputation** is the partial or total removal of an extremity or body part. Amputation may be the result of a traumatic event or a chronic condition such as peripheral vascular disease or diabetes mellitus. It is estimated that 2 million people with amputations live in the United States, and that 185,000 new amputations occur each year (Amputee Coalition, 2017). Most of these are due to peripheral vascular disease or diabetes. Trauma is the second leading cause of amputations. People age 65 and older with diabetes are more likely to have an amputation than younger diabetics (Amputee Coalition of America, n.d.). As of June 2015, a total of 1,645 soldiers have suffered a major limb amputation in the Middle East wars (Fischer, 2015). However, no service-related amputations were reported in 2016 (Montgomery, 2017).

The loss of all or part of an extremity has a significant physical and psychosocial effect on the patient and family. Adaptation may take a long time and require much effort. Interprofessional healthcare is always important, but is especially necessary to meet the patient's physical, socioeconomic, spiritual, cultural, and emotional needs after an unexpected or planned amputation.

Pathophysiology

Amputations result from or are necessitated by interruption in blood flow, either acute or chronic. In acute trauma situations, the limb is partially or completely severed, and tissue death ensues. However, replantation of fingers, small body parts, and entire limbs has been successful. In chronic disease processes, circulation is impaired, venous pooling begins, proteins leak into the interstitium, and edema develops. Edema increases the risk of injury and further decreases circulation. Stasis ulcers develop and readily become infected because impaired healing and altered immune processes allow bacteria to proliferate. The presence of progressive infection further compromises circulation and ultimately leads to gangrene, which requires amputation.

Levels of Amputation

The level of amputation is determined by local and systemic factors. Local factors include ischemia and gangrene; systemic factors include cardiovascular status, renal function, and severity of diabetes mellitus. The goals are to alleviate symptoms, to maintain healthy tissue, and to increase functional outcome. When possible, the joints are preserved because they allow greater function of the extremity. **Figure 39.12** ■ illustrates common sites of amputation.

Terms used to refer to amputations are defined in **Table 39.5**.

Amputation Site Healing

For the prosthesis to fit well, the amputation site must heal properly. To promote healing, a compression dressing is

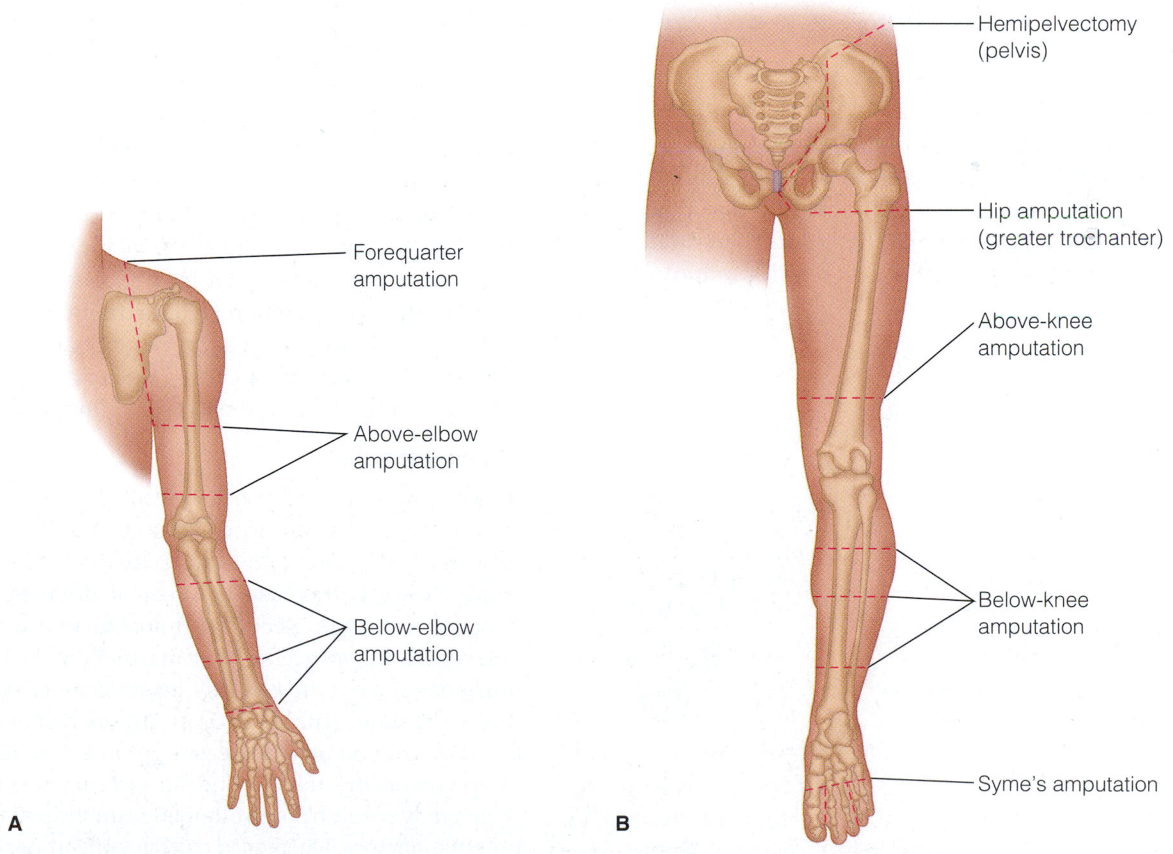
Forequarter amputation
Above-elbow amputation
Below-elbow amputation
A
Hemipelvectomy (pelvis)
Hip amputation (greater trochanter)
Above-knee amputation
Below-knee amputation
Syme's amputation
B

Figure 39.12 ■ Common sites of amputation. **A**, The upper extremities. **B**, The lower extremities. The surgeon determines the level of amputation based on blood supply and tissue condition.

Table 39.5 Amputation Terms

Term	Meaning
Arm	Amputation of a portion of the arm, either above or below the elbow
Disarticulation	Amputation through a joint
Forequarter	Removal of the entire arm and disarticulation of the shoulder
Closed (flap)	Amputation in which a flap of skin is formed to cover the end of the wound
Open (guillotine)	Perpendicular cutting of the extremity in which the wound is left open; used when infection is present
Leg	Amputation below the knee (BK)
Thigh	Amputation above the knee (AK)
Finger or toe	Amputation of one or all of the fingers or toes
Syme	Modified disarticulation of the ankle
Foot	Amputation of part of the foot and toes

applied to prevent infection and minimize edema. A soft compression dressing is applied when frequent wound checks are necessary. When this type of dressing is used, a splint is sometimes applied to help mold the extremity to fit the prosthesis. After the wound is dressed, the patient is encouraged to toughen the stump skin by pushing it into first soft and then harder surfaces. The stump is wrapped in an elastic bandage to allow a conical shape to form and to prevent edema. The bandage is applied from the distal to the proximal extremity (**Figure 39.13** ■). A commercial "stump shrinker" sheath may be used as well.

Risk Factors and Causes

Peripheral vascular disease (PVD) is the major cause of amputation of the lower extremities. Common risk factors for the development of PVD include hypertension, diabetes, smoking, and hyperlipidemia. Peripheral neuropathy also places the person with diabetes at risk for amputation. In peripheral neuropathy, loss of sensation frequently leads to unrecognized injury and infection. Untreated infection may lead to gangrene and the need for amputation.

The incidence of traumatic amputations is highest among young men. Most amputations in this group result from motor vehicle crashes or accidents involving machinery at work. Combat-related trauma also accounts for a significant number of traumatic amputations in young adults. Other traumatic events that may necessitate an amputation are frostbite, burns, or electrocution.

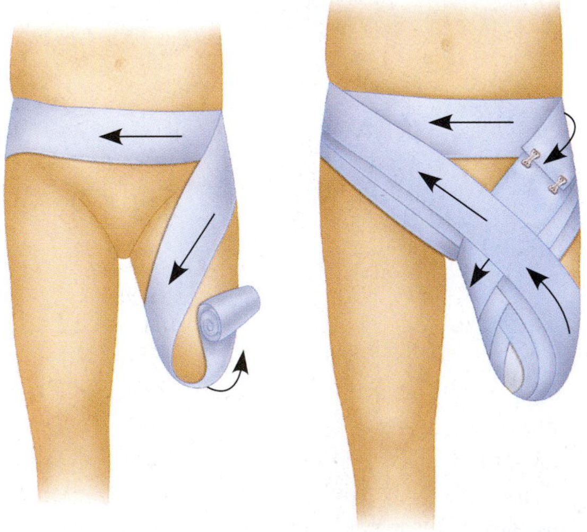

Figure 39.13 ■ Stump dressings increase venous return, decrease edema, and help shape the stump for a prosthesis. With an above-knee amputation, a figure-eight bandage is started by bringing the bandage down over the stump and back up around the hips.

Manifestations

In a typical situation, the patient presents to the trauma center with an injury that may be life threatening; significant loss of blood and tissue may have already occurred, and shock may develop. The completely amputated portion may be intact and brought to the hospital on ice for potential replantation. The wound may be a clean cut, as in a guillotine amputation, or the tissue may be severely damaged, mangled and completely or partially separated from the area. The condition of the site will depend on the mechanism of injury.

Complications

Complications that may occur after an amputation include infection, delayed healing, chronic stump pain and phantom pain, and contractures.

Infection

Generally, the patient who experiences a traumatic amputation has a greater risk of infection than the person who has a planned amputation due to the environmental conditions where the amputation occurred. However, even planned amputations carry a risk of infection. The patient who is older, has diabetes mellitus, or suffers peripheral neurovascular compromise is at a particularly high risk for infection. Infection may present itself locally or systemically. Local manifestations of infection include drainage, odor, redness, and increased discomfort at the suture line. Systemic manifestations include fever, an increased heart rate, a decrease in blood pressure, chills, and positive wound or blood cultures.

Delayed Healing

If infection is present or if the circulation remains compromised, delayed healing (occurring at a slower rate than expected) will result. In older patients, other preexisting conditions can increase the risk of delayed healing. In patients of any age, electrolyte imbalances can contribute to delayed healing processes, as can a diet that lacks the proper nutrients to meet the body's increased metabolic demands during healing. Smoking compromises healing by causing vasoconstriction and decreasing blood flow to the stump. Deep venous thrombosis and compromised venous return, which may result from prolonged immobilization, are other potential factors. Decreased cardiac output decreases blood flow and thus also delays healing.

Chronic Stump Pain and Phantom Limb Pain

Chronic stump pain is the result of neuroma formation, causing severe burning pain. Interventions to relieve this pain include medications, nerve blocks, transcutaneous electrical nerve stimulation (TENS), and surgical stump reconstruction. **Phantom limb pain** is not the same as phantom limb sensation. A majority of amputees experience phantom limb sensation (sensations such as tingling, numbness, cramping, or itching in the phantom foot or hand) early in the postoperative period. It is often self-limited, but may last for decades in some patients. When phantom limb sensation is painful, it is referred to as *phantom limb pain*. Phantom limb pain more frequently affects people who had pain in the amputated limb prior to its removal than those who did not. Several theories for phantom limb pain have been developed. These include regeneration of severed peripheral nerves and abnormal impulses generated by spinal cord neurons that no longer receive normal sensory input from the body (Sorenson et al., 2019). Treatments include pain management, TENS, mirror therapy, and a variety of surgical procedures. Mirror therapy uses visualization of the intact extremity to allow the patient to "see" the movement of the amputated extremity by watching the intact extremity in a mirror. The management of phantom limb pain is difficult for both patients and healthcare professionals. Patients with phantom limb pain often benefit from referral to a pain clinic for a comprehensive pain management program.

Contractures

A **contracture** is an abnormal flexion and fixation of a joint caused by muscle atrophy and shortening. Contracture of the joint above the amputation is a common complication. The patient needs to be taught to extend the joint and to perform muscle-strengthening exercises. The patient with an above-the-knee amputation should not sit for prolonged periods of time; prolonged sitting can lead to hip contracture. He or she should not elevate the stump for prolonged periods of time after the first 48 hours. Additionally, the patient should lie prone for periods throughout the day. The patient with a below-the-knee amputation may place the end of their stump on a pillow in order to keep the knee extended. Placing it on a pillow with the knee bent encourages the development of knee and hip contractures and should be avoided. A knee immobilizer may be used to help maintain joint extension. The same principles apply to the upper extremities. All joints should receive either active or passive ROM exercises every 4 to 6 hours. A trapeze frame should be added to the bed to encourage the patient to change position every 2 hours. The patient who has an upper extremity amputation should exercise both shoulders. Postural exercises can help prevent the patient from hunching over secondary to the loss of weight on the affected side.

Interprofessional Care

Interprofessional care is essential for the patient who has sustained an amputation. Physical therapy and occupational retraining are necessary, and the patient may also benefit from the presence of clergy or a social work or psychology consult. The entire healthcare team must view both the positive and the negative effects of amputation; that is, they must see amputation as a means to increase the patient's independence and to relieve symptoms. The patient should be able to become familiar with the members of the healthcare team and their roles; this allows the patient greater control over his or her care and rehabilitation and promotes independence.

Diagnosis

In nonemergent situations, preoperatively, the patient has routine laboratory and diagnostic tests. Preoperative tests, including Doppler flowmetry, segmental blood pressure determination, transcutaneous partial pressure oxygen readings, and angiography, are performed to assess the circulation present in the limb at different levels and to determine the level of viable tissue. Postoperative tests include CBC to monitor for hemorrhage, WBC count to monitor for infection, blood chemistries to evaluate electrolytes and fluid balance, and a vascular Doppler ultrasonography, if a DVT is suspected.

Medications

Medications are used to manage pain, to prevent or treat infection, prevent deep venous thrombosis, and, as needed, to maintain cardiac output and tissue perfusion. Postoperatively, the patient resumes any routinely prescribed medications. A gastric acid–reducing medication (H_2 antagonist or proton pump inhibitor) may also be ordered to decrease the risk of peptic ulcer formation. Stool softeners may be administered to prevent constipation from immobility or opioids.

Surgery

For traumatic amputations in which the amputated portion of the limb or digit is available and the ends of the amputation are relatively intact, replantation surgery can be considered. Other items taken into consideration when deciding if replantation is possible are the types of fractures present at the site, if there is multilevel involvement, if there is damage to the vascular endothelium, and if there is debris in the wound. Severe damage to the vascular endothelium, as well as the amount of debris in the wound, may lead to poor outcomes and therefore amputation may be the best choice for the patient (Nicholson & Platt, 2014).

Surgical amputations may be open (*guillotine*) or closed (*flap*). Open amputations are most often performed when infection is present or it is highly suspected that the wound may become infected. The wound is not closed but remains open to drain. When infection is no longer present or the risk of infection has passed, surgery is performed to close the wound. In closed amputations, the wound is closed with a flap of skin that is sutured in place over the stump.

Prosthetics

The type of prosthesis selected for the patient with an amputation depends on the level of the amputation as well as the patient's occupation and lifestyle. Each prosthesis is based on a detailed prosthetic prescription and is custom-made for the patient. Most are made of plastic and foam materials. Many factors influence the patient's use of the prosthesis, including the status of the remaining limb, cognitive status, cardiovascular status, preoperative activity level, and motivation to use the prosthesis.

Patients with a lower extremity amputation are often fitted with early walking aids. Pneumatic devices that fit over the stump are used in the immediate postoperative period to allow early ambulation, decrease postoperative edema, and improve morale. Patients may begin weight bearing as soon as 2 weeks after surgery. Patients with upper extremity amputations may be fitted for a prosthesis immediately after surgery. Rehabilitation of the patient with an amputation is a team effort, involving the patient, nurse, physician, physical therapist, occupational therapist, social worker, prosthetist, and vocational counselor.

Nursing Care

Assessment

Collect the following data through the health history and physical examination. Further focused assessments are described in the following nursing interventions sections.

- ***Health history:*** Mechanism of injury, current and past health problems, pain, occupation, ability to perform ADLs preinjury or presurgery, changes in sensation in the feet, cultural and/or religious guidelines for handling the amputated part
- ***Physical assessment:*** Bilateral neurovascular status of the extremities, bilateral capillary refill time, skin over the lower extremities (discoloration, edema, ulcerations, hair, gangrene) or a thorough wound assessment.

Priorities of Care

Effective pain management is an immediate priority of care for the patient undergoing amputation. Monitoring for and preventing complications are also high-priority nursing activities. Although a focus toward rehabilitation begins prior to surgery, rehabilitation is the primary focus of nursing and interprofessional care following amputation.

Diagnoses, Planning, and Interventions

The goals of nursing care for an individual with an amputation are to relieve pain, promote healing, prevent complications, support the patient and family during the process of grieving and adaptation to alterations in body image, and restore mobility. Care is individualized, and the circumstances that led to the amputation (e.g., traumatic injury or disease) must also be addressed. See the accompanying Case Study & Nursing Care Plan on page 1444.

Manage Acute Pain. Pain from the surgical procedure and/or injury can be compounded by muscle spasms, edema, and phantom limb pain.

Expected Outcome: Patient will report pain at an acceptable level using a standardized pain scale.

The nurse will:

- Ask the patient to rate the pain on a scale of 0 to 10 (with 10 as the most severe pain) before and after any intervention. *This facilitates objective assessment of the effectiveness of the chosen pain relief strategy. Pain that increases in intensity or remains unrelieved with analgesics can indicate compartment syndrome.*
- Splint and support the injured area. *Splinting prevents additional injury by immobilizing the stump and decreasing edema while molding the stump for a good prosthetic fit.*
- Unless contraindicated, elevate the stump on a pillow for the first 24 to 48 hours after surgery. *Elevating the stump promotes venous return and decreases edema, which will decrease pain.*
- Move and turn the patient gently and slowly, supporting the limb as the patient moves. *Gentle moving, turning, and limb support prevents the development of severe muscle spasms.*
- Administer pain medications as prescribed. A PCA pump may be ordered by the physician. *Analgesics alleviate pain by binding to opiate receptor sites blocking the pain sensation. PCA pumps increase patient control and allow early relief of pain before it intensifies.*
- Encourage deep breathing and relaxation exercises. *These techniques increase the effectiveness of analgesics and modify the pain experience.*
- Reposition patient every 2 hours; turn from side to side and onto abdomen. *Repositioning alleviates pressure from one area and distributes it throughout the body and helps prevent cramping of muscles.*

Reduce Risk of Infection. The patient who has an amputation is at risk for wound infection. Early recognition of infection can lead to early treatment and prevent wound dehiscence.

Expected Outcome: Patient's wound will heal without evidence of infection.

The nurse will:

- Assess the wound for redness, drainage, temperature, edema, and suture line approximation. *Redness is normal in the immediate postoperative period; if it persists, however, it can indicate infection. A hot area that is palpated over the incision or increased drainage may also indicate infection.*
- Take the patient's temperature every 4 to 8 hours. *Increased body temperature may indicate infection.*
- Monitor WBC count. *The WBC count rises in the presence of infection.*
- Use aseptic technique to change the wound dressing. *Aseptic technique prevents the contamination of the wound with bacteria.*
- Administer antibiotics, as ordered. *Antibiotics inhibit bacterial cell replication and help prevent or eradicate infection.*
- Teach the patient stump-wrapping techniques. *Correctly wrapping the stump from the distal to proximal extremity increases venous return and prevents pooling of fluid, thereby reducing the chance of infection.*

Reduce Risk of Impaired Skin Integrity. Stump care is essential, not only in the postoperative healing period, but also throughout life with a prosthesis. A variety of skin problems may be caused by a prosthesis, including epidermoid cysts, abrasions, blisters, and hair follicle infections. The patient must be taught stump care prior to discharge.

Expected Outcome: Patient's skin will remain intact without evidence of adverse effects of prosthesis.

The nurse will:

- Each day, preferably at night, wash the stump with soap and warm water and dry thoroughly. Inspect the stump for redness, irritation, or abrasions. *It is essential to maintain intact skin to ensure successful use of the prosthesis.*
- Massage the end of the stump, beginning 3 weeks after surgery. *Massage helps desensitize the remaining part of the limb and prevents scar tissue formation. If the skin adheres to the underlying tissue, it will tear when stressed by wearing a prosthesis.*
- Expose any open areas of skin on the remaining part of the limb for 1 hour four times a day. *Air exposure promotes healing.*
- Change stump socks and elastic wraps each day. Wash these in mild soap and water, and allow to completely dry before using again. *Stump socks and elastic wraps must be kept clean and dry to prevent skin breakdown.*

Reduce Risk for Psychosocial Issues. The patient who has lost an extremity is at risk for complicated grieving. Denial of the need for surgery and the inability to discuss feelings compound this risk.

Expected Outcome: Patient will verbalize grief and the meaning of the loss.

The nurse will:

- Encourage verbalization of feelings, using open-ended questions. *Asking open-ended questions allows the patient to discuss feelings and communicates willingness to listen.*
- Actively listen and maintain eye contact. *Active listening and eye contact communicate respect for what the patient is expressing.*
- Reflect on the patient's feelings. *Reflection statements such as "You seem angry" allow the patient to recognize feelings and perhaps develop a plan for resolution.*
- Allow the patient to have unlimited visiting hours, if possible. *Unlimited visiting hours allow increased social support.*
- If desired by the patient, provide spiritual support by encouraging activities such as visits from a spiritual leader, prayer, and meditation. *These activities often provide support during the grieving process.*

Promote Healthy Body Image. Although amputation is a reconstructive surgery, the patient's body image may still be disturbed. Risk for body image disturbance is higher in young trauma patients, in whom body image is a particularly important component of self-image.

Expected Outcome: Patient will demonstrate acceptance of appearance and resume self-care activities.

The nurse will:

- Encourage verbalization of feelings. *This allows the patient to communicate concerns and fears and lets the patient know the nurse is willing to listen.*
- Allow the patient to wear clothing from home. *Familiar clothing provides emotional comfort and helps the patient retain a sense of his or her own identity.*
- Encourage the patient to look at the stump. *Looking at and touching the stump helps the patient face his or her fear of the unknown and move from denial to acceptance.*
- Encourage the patient to care for the stump. *Active participation in care increases self-esteem and independence.*
- Offer to have a fellow amputee visit the patient. *A support person who has experienced the same change gives the patient the hope that he or she can regain independence.*
- Encourage active participation in rehabilitation. *Active participation in rehabilitation increases independence and mobility.*

Promote Physical Mobility. If time allows, the patient should begin strengthening muscles preoperatively. If the amputation is the result of an emergency, exercises begin within 24 to 48 hours of surgery. The return of independent mobility boosts self-esteem and promotes adaptation to amputation.

Expected Outcome: Patient will participate in prescribed activities, demonstrating correct use of assistive devices.

The nurse will:

- Perform ROM exercises on all joints, active and passive. *ROM exercises help prevent the development of joint contractures that limit mobility.*
- Maintain postoperative stump shrinkage devices. These may be elastic bandages, shrinker socks, an elastic stockinette, or a rigid plaster cast. *Postoperative dressings decrease edema and shape the stump for prosthetic wear.*
- Turn and reposition the patient every 2 hours. *The patient with a lower extremity amputation should lie prone every 4 hours. Repositioning increases blood flow to muscles, forces synovial fluid into joints, and helps prevent contractures.*
- Reinforce teaching by the physical therapist in crutch walking or the use of assistive devices. *These devices increase mobility by balancing the patient and facilitating ambulation.*
- Encourage active participation in physical therapy. *Physical therapy will fatigue the patient in the early stage of healing. Encouragement may increase the patient's participation in the physical therapy regimen and thereby increase activity tolerance.*

Delegating Nursing Care Activities

Mobility and daily care activities may be delegated to UAP once the patient has been taught by physical or occupational therapy and nursing.

Transitions of Care

Health promotion activities focus on preventing the progression of chronic diseases such as PVD and diabetes mellitus and on safety. Patients with PVD from any cause need education about foot care and early recognition of decreased circulation. Education within both urban and rural populations should provide knowledge about working safely with lawn care equipment as well as farm and occupational machinery.

In addition, it is important for the public to know what to do if a traumatic amputation occurs in the home,

Case Study & Nursing Care Plan

A Patient with a Below-the-Knee Amputation

John Rocke is a 45-year-old divorced man with a history of type 1 diabetes mellitus and poor control of blood glucose levels. Mr. Rocke is unemployed and lives alone. Mr. Rocke failed to seek prompt medical attention for a foot infection; as a result, a left below-the-knee amputation was necessary.

Mr. Rocke is in his second postoperative day and his vital signs are stable. The stump is splinted and has a soft dressing. The wound is approximating well without signs of infection. He has not performed ROM exercises or turning since his surgery, complaining of severe pain. When the nurse goes into the room, he yells, "Get out! I don't want anyone to see me like this." No one has visited him since his hospitalization. He is tolerating an 1800-kcal diabetic diet and is using a urinal independently. He has an order for morphine, 10 mg IM every 3 to 4 hours prn for pain, and cefazolin (Ancef), 1 g IV every 8 hours. He is on blood glucose and carbohydrate coverage with insulin glargine subcutaneously after meals in addition to his routine lantus injections.

ASSESSMENT	DIAGNOSES	EXPECTED OUTCOMES
Jane Simmons, RN, is now assigned to his care. She notes that Mr. Rocke will not let anyone enter the room to give him medication or assess his vital signs.	■ Disturbed image of self related to amputation of left lower leg ■ Anger and grief related to amputation ■ Acute pain related to amputation ■ Nonadherence to therapeutic regimen	■ Patient will verbalize his feelings about the amputation. ■ Patient will allow the staff to monitor his vital signs and administer medications. ■ Patient will be allowed to control his pain with a PCA pump. ■ Patient will verbalize a decrease in pain. ■ Patient will verbalize the importance of turning. ■ Patient will turn every 2 hours.

PLANNING AND IMPLEMENTATION

- Encourage verbalization of feelings.
- Actively listen to the patient.
- Offer to arrange a visit with a fellow amputee.
- Ask the physician if the patient can be placed on a PCA pump or work with patient to see what pain relief measures or medication schedule he feels would be beneficial.
- Teach the patient the importance of turning every 2 hours to prevent contractures.
- Encourage turning and lying prone.
- Teach the importance of antibiotics in preventing and treating infection.

EVALUATION

One week after his surgery, Mr. Rocke is actively participating in his care. He has apologized for his behavior and has explained to Ms. Simmons that he was angry about the loss of his leg. He states, "I thought I knew what to expect but I didn't."

CLINICAL REASONING IN PATIENT CARE

1. How would you respond when Mr. Rocke yells at you to leave?
2. What do you believe is the highest priority of nursing care for Mr. Rocke at this time?
3. What members of the interprofessional healthcare team should the nurse ensure are involved in Mr. Rocke's care at this time?
4. Once Mr. Rocke is ready to assist with his stump care, how would you proceed? Would you give him full responsibility for care and dressings, or would you gradually increase his participation? Why?
5. What factors in Mr. Rocke's home environment and medical history may make self-care more difficult? Do you expect Mr. Rocke to follow up on care after his discharge? Why or why not?
6. Mr. Rocke states, "Why should I exercise this leg—it was already cut off!?" How would you respond? What is the purpose of exercising the stump?

See Evaluating Your Response in Appendix B.

community, or workplace. Preserving life is the first priority: First ensure that the patient can breathe; administer CPR as necessary, and control bleeding with direct pressure. The following guidelines may help preserve the amputated part until it can be surgically reattached:

- Keep the person in a supine position with the legs elevated
- Apply firm pressure to the bleeding area, using a towel or article of clothing
- Wrap the amputated part in a clean cloth. If possible, soak the cloth in saline (such as contact lens solution)
- Put the amputated part in a plastic bag and put the bag on ice. Do not let the amputated part come into direct contact with the ice or water.
- Send the amputated part to the emergency department with the injured person, and be sure the emergency personnel know what it is.

Amputation of a limb has significant long-term consequences for the patient. Patient and family teaching includes stump care, prosthesis fitting and care, medications, assistive devices, exercises, rehabilitation, counseling, support services, and follow-up appointments. The patient will grieve the loss of a body part and must adjust to a new self-image. The patient's ability to perform normal daily living activities and to maintain his or her usual family and social roles may be significantly affected, at least initially. Depending on the patient's occupation, job performance may be affected, necessitating a change of career.

The nurse may be responsible for involving multiple members of the healthcare team in the patient's care and rehabilitation and coordinating their activities. Following an amputation, the patient may need the services of any or all of the following:

- Social services to help with rehabilitative and financial arrangements
- Physical therapists to teach ambulation techniques and to provide deep heat or massage
- Occupational therapists to assist the patient in developing adaptive techniques to deal with the loss of a limb
- Prosthetists to develop a prosthesis for the missing limb that will meet the patient's needs for ADLs and other activities
- Home health services for nursing care such as assessments and wound care
- Support group services to assist in adapting to the body image change and effects of amputation on ADLs.

Preparing the amputee for home care includes a careful assessment of the patient, the family, available support services, and the home for possible barriers to the patient's safety and independence.

Assess the patient's acceptance of the amputation and knowledge base about care needs, any activity restrictions or special needs, and resources for home care. Discuss home management—who is responsible for household activities such as cleaning and cooking. Inquire about arrangements that have been made for home care activities and ADLs. Evaluate the patient's use of prescription and nonprescription medications, paying particular attention to possible interactions and drugs that may affect the patient's balance, mental alertness, or appetite. Ask about social habits—such as cigarette smoking, alcohol use, or other drug use—that may affect healing or the patient's ability to provide self-care.

Assess the patient's home environment for possible safety hazards or barriers to ambulation, such as:

- Scatter rugs
- Stairs between living areas of the house
- Presence of grab bars to facilitate toileting and bathing
- Access to clean water and other needs for wound care.

The new amputee needs a great deal of teaching to learn to adapt to loss of a limb, whether it is an upper or lower extremity that has been lost. Because the patient must be ready to learn before teaching can be effective, use therapeutic communication techniques to encourage the patient to verbalize feelings about the amputation and its effects. Use active listening and teach the patient ways to reduce anxiety and deal with feelings of helplessness and loss. Encourage the patient to participate in care of the stump to build self-esteem and reinforce teaching. Include the following in teaching for home care:

- Teach the patient to wrap the stump appropriately in preparation for fitting the prosthesis
- Discuss positioning of the stump. Contractures are a particular problem for patients with an above-knee amputation and can interfere with the ability to effectively use a prosthesis.
- Teach the patient how to perform stump exercises to maintain joint mobility and muscle tone of the affected limb
- Encourage the patient to resume physical activities as soon as possible. This improves the patient's health and well-being, as well as the patient's self-esteem.
- Discuss household modifications to promote independence, such as grab bars in the bathroom, faucets with single-handle controls for water flow and temperature, and handheld shower heads and shower chairs for bathing.

Holistic nursing care is especially important for the older patient with an amputation. The normal aging process decreases renal and liver function; hence, medications have longer half-lives. Altered circulation prolongs wound healing, and slowing of reflexes and alterations in gait may disrupt balance. A walker may be more appropriate than crutches because older patients have less strength in the upper extremities. Safety issues, such as decreasing the risk for recurrent falls, must be addressed. The nurse should also assess the patient's need for in-home assistance and make appropriate referrals to visiting nurses and home health aides.

In addition, suggest the following resources:

- The Amputee Coalition of America
- Amputee Resource Foundation of America.

CHAPTER HIGHLIGHTS

39.1 Traumatic Injuries of the Muscles, Ligaments, and Tendons

Describe the pathophysiology and manifestations of traumatic injuries of the muscles, ligaments, and tendons, and outline the interprofessional care and nursing care of patients with these injuries.

- Musculoskeletal injuries, including strains, sprains, fractures, and joint injuries, are common, often associated with recreational activities or trauma. Nursing care includes assessing the circumstances and impact of the injury as well as neurovascular status distal to the injury and teaching prescribed treatment and rehabilitation.

- Immediate treatment for contusions, strains, and sprains includes PRICE (protection, rest, ice, compression, elevation) therapy.
- Joint trauma may damage soft tissue, cartilage, or even result in joint dislocation. Monitor neurovascular status, assessing the affected extremity for increased pain, decreased or absent pulses, pale skin, inability to move the extremity, and changes in sensation.
- Repetitive use injuries, especially common in the workplace, include carpal tunnel syndrome, bursitis, and tendonitis.

39.2 Traumatic Injuries of Bones

Describe the pathophysiology and manifestations of traumatic injuries of bones, and outline the interprofessional care and nursing care of patients with these injuries.

- Fractures are usually uncomplicated, but place the patient at risk for both acute and long-term complications and may necessitate surgery or other invasive procedures for healing. Nurses must promptly recognize complications and initiate appropriate care.
- Fractures are closed or simple (skin is intact) or open or compound (skin integrity is interrupted); open fractures are at risk for infection. Other fracture descriptors include oblique or spiral, avulsed, comminuted, compressed, impacted, or depressed.
- Fractures heal through four phases: Hematoma, fibrocartilaginous callus, bony callus, and remodeling. Healing is influenced by the age and physical condition of the patient and by the type of fracture.
- Fracture complications include compartment syndrome, fat embolism syndrome, deep venous thrombosis, infection, delayed union and nonunion, and complex regional pain syndrome.
- Fractures are treated with surgery—both internal and external fixation, traction, and/or casts/splints to stabilize the fractured bone, maintain bone alignment and immobilization, prevent complications, and restore function.
- Fractures of the hip, most often sustained by older adult women, are usually the result of a fall. Hip fractures present a serious health problem for people age 65 and older, potentially impacting the patient's independence and even shortening the lifespan.
- Nursing care for the patient with a fracture focuses on interventions for acute pain, risk for impaired peripheral neurovascular function, risk for infection, and impaired physical mobility.
- Amputation, the partial or total removal of an extremity, has significant physical and psychosocial effects on the patient and on the family. In addition to providing care and support for the patient and family, the nurse is actively involved in coordinating the interprofessional team for optimal patient care and rehabilitation.
- The most common cause for amputation of a lower extremity is peripheral vascular disease. Trauma is the most common cause for upper extremity amputation.
- Complications that may follow an amputation include infection, delayed healing, chronic stump pain, phantom pain, and contractures. Stump care is necessary to prevent complications and to prepare the stump for a prosthesis.
- Nursing care for the patient with an amputation is focused on a return to functional health, with interventions to meet needs for acute pain, impaired skin integrity, grieving, disturbed body image, and impaired physical mobility.

TEST YOURSELF NCLEX-RN® REVIEW

1. The nurse is teaching a patient self-care approaches for a sprained ankle. For which reason should the nurse emphasize the use of ice after this type of injury?
   A. Increases white blood cells.
   B. Lowers the blood pressure and pulse.
   C. Promotes venous return.
   D. Constricts local blood vessels.
2. A patient with a compound, open fracture of the femur is scheduled for immediate surgery. Which patient problem does the nurse prioritize when planning care for the immediate postoperative period?
   A. The patient is unstable and may fall.
   B. There is a high risk of infection
   C. It will require more than one nurse to help the patient transfer.
   D. The patient may be fearful of another injury.
3. The nurse is concerned after performing a neurovascular assessment on an older patient with a lower arm cast. Which finding caused the nurse to become concerned?
   A. Pale, cold fingers
   B. Slightly edematous fingers
   C. Warm, pink skin above the cast
   D. Pain rating of 2 on a 0-to-10 scale
4. The nurse is preparing instructional materials for a patient recovering from a fractured leg. The nurse should teach the patient to take in adequate amounts of which mineral essential to bone healing?
   A. Sodium
   B. Calcium
   C. Potassium
   D. Magnesium

5. Documentation from the previous shift reveals that a patient in a long leg cast had a decreased pedal pulse. The patient was medicated for a report of pain rated at an 8 on the scale of 1 to 10. Which additional findings, occurring on this shift, should the nurse immediately report to the healthcare provider? (Select all that apply.)
   A. Fever
   B. Weakness
   C. Cyanotic foot
   D. Tingling in the foot
   E. Severe pain with passive flexion
6. The nurse is caring for a patient with a deep venous thrombosis of the left lower extremity. What additional body system should the nurse carefully monitor in this patient?
   A. Renal
   B. Digestive
   C. Respiratory
   D. Hematologic
7. A patient has been diagnosed with complex regional pain syndrome (CRPS). The nurse reviews the medical record for which factors that increase risk for this syndrome? (Select all that apply.)
   A. Female gender
   B. History of cardiac disease
   C. Older age
   D. Injury to upper rather than lower extremity
   E. Fair skin and auburn hair
8. The nurse is caring for a patient recovering from a below-the-knee amputation. What should be included in this patient's plan of care for the first 48 hours? (Select all that apply.)
   A. Elevate the stump.
   B. Keep the knee extended.
   C. Apply a knee immobilizer.
   D. Out of bed in bedside chair as much as possible.
   E. Provide passive ROM exercises every 4 hours.
9. The week following a below-the-knee amputation, the patient complains of toes cramping in the amputated foot. What strategies can the nurse use to help alleviate this discomfort? (Select all that apply.)
   A. TENS unit therapy
   B. Increased vitamin D in the diet
   C. Mirror therapy
   D. Fluid restriction
   E. Tightening of stump dressing
10. The nurse is preparing an educational session for employees of a manufacturing plant regarding emergency care of amputated digits. What should the nurse include when teaching about this type of injury?
   A. Immediately transport the person to the hospital.
   B. Place the amputated digit in a storage bag filled with warm water.
   C. Wrap the amputated digit in a towel, place in a plastic bag, and lay it on ice.
   D. Place the digit in a plastic bag and tape the bag to the patient's extremity.

See Test Yourself answers in Appendix B.

REFERENCES

Agarwal, S., & Mann, E. (2016). Knee injuries in wrestlers: A prospective study from the Indian subcontinent. *Asian Journal of Sports Medicine, 7*(4), 1–6.

American Bone Health. (2016). *Fracture risk factors.* Retrieved from https://americanbonehealth.org/what-you-should-know/fracture-risk-factors/.

Amputee Coalition. (2017). *Limb loss statistics.* Retrieved from www.amputee-coalition.org/resources/limb-loss-statistics/.

Amputee Coalition of America. (n.d.). *People with amputation speak out.* Retrieved from www.amputee-coalition.org/wp-content/uploads/2014/11/lsp_people-speak-out_120115-113243.pdf.

Bell, D. R., Blackburn, J. T., Hackney, A. C., Marshall, S. W., Beutler, A. I., & Padua, D. A. (2014). Jump-landing biomechanics and knee-laxity change across the menstrual cycle in women with anterior cruciate ligament reconstruction. *Journal of Athletic Training, 49*(2), 154–162.

Bureau of Labor Statistics (BLS). (2016). *Nonfatal occupational injuries and illnesses requiring days away from work, 2015.* Retrieved from https://www.bls.gov/news.release/pdf/osh2.pdf.

Bureau of Labor Statistics (BLS). (2017). *Frequently asked questions.* Retrieved from https://www.bls.gov/iif/oshfaq1.htm#q15.

Buti, R. L. (2013). The shoulder. In L. Schoenly (Ed.), *Core curriculum for orthopaedic nursing* (7th ed.). Chicago: National Association of Orthopaedic Nursing.

Centers for Disease Control and Prevention (CDC). (2016a). *Falls among older adults: An overview.* Retrieved from www.cdc.gov/HomeandRecreationalSafety/Falls/adultfalls.html.

Centers for Disease Control and Prevention (CDC). (2016b). *Hip fractures among older adults.* Retrieved from www.cdc.gov/HomeandRecreationalSafety/Falls/adulthipfx.html.

Davis, J. & Saulog-Wendel, P. (2013). The knee. In L. Schoenly (Ed.), *Core curriculum for orthopaedic nursing* (7th ed.). Chicago: National Association of Orthopaedic Nursing.

Feger, M. A., Glaviano, N. R., Hart, J. M., Saliba, S. A., Park, J. S., Hertel, J., & Donovan, L. (2017). Current trends in the management of lateral ankle sprain in the United States. *Clinical Journal of Sport Medicine, 27*(2), 145–152.

Fischer, H. (2015). U.S. military casualty statistics: Operation New Dawn, Operation Iraqi Freedom, and Operation Enduring Freedom. *CRS Report for Congress.* Congressional Research Service, No. 7-5700. Retrieved from www.fas.org/sgp/crs/natsec/RS22452.pdf.

Gray-Micelli, D., & Quigley, P. A. (2012). *Nursing standard of practice protocol: Falls prevention.* New York: The Hartford Institute for Geriatric Nursing. Retrieved from https://consultgeri.org/geriatric-topics/falls.

Janssen, K. W., van Mechelen, W., & Verhagen, E. M. (2014). Bracing superior to neuromuscular training for the prevention of self-reported recurrent ankle sprains: A three-arm randomised controlled trial. *British Journal of Sports Medicine, 48*(16), 1235–1239.

Kaminski, T. W., Hertel, J., Amendola, N., Docherty, C. L., Dolan, M. G., Hopkins, J. Y. Nussbaum, E., . . . Richie, D. (2013). National Athletic Trainers' Association position statement: Conservative management and prevention of ankle sprains in athletes. *Journal of Athletic Training, 48*(4), 528–545.

Kosova, E., Bergmark, B., & Piazza, G. (2015). Fat embolism syndrome. *Circulation,* 131:317-320.

Kothari, M. J. (2018). *Carpel tunnel syndrome: Treatment and prognosis.* Retrieved from www.uptodate.com/contents/carpal-tunnel-syndrome-treatment-and-prognosis.

Lo, J. C., Cavazos, J., & Burnett, C. (2017). Management of complex regional pain syndrome. *Baylor University Medical Center Proceedings, 30*(3): 286-288.

Luke, A., & Ma, C. B. (2017). Sports medicine and outpatient orthopedics. In S. J. McPhee & M. W. Rabow (Eds.), *Current medical diagnosis and treatment* 2017. New York, NY: McGraw-Hill.

Ma, X., Zheng, X., Zhao, W., Lu, Z., Xu, L., Liu, Y., & Liu, Z. (2017). Internal versus external fixation for the treatment of pelvic fractures: A comparative study. Clinical and Investigative Medicine, 40(3): E102. Retrieved from https://www.ncbi.nlm.nih.gov/pubmed/28653611.

Mayo Clinic. (2018a, August). *Diseases and conditions: Bursitis: Risk factors.* Retrieved from www.mayoclinic.org/diseases-conditions/bursitis/basics/risk-factors/con-20015102.

Mayo Clinic. (2018b, November). *Diseases and conditions: Tendinitis: Risk factors.* Retrieved from www.mayoclinic.org/diseases-conditions/tendinitis/basics/risk-factors/con-20020309.

McGovern, R. P., & Martin, R. L. (2016). Managing ankle ligament sprains and tears: Current opinion. *Open Access Journal of Sports Medicine, 7,* 33–42. Retrieved from https://www.ncbi.nlm.nih.gov/pmc/articles/PMC4780668/pdf/oajsm-7-033.pdf.

Montgomery, N. (2017, March 16). 2016 marks first year without combat amputation since Afghan, Iraq wars began. *Stars and Stripes.* Retrieved from https://www.stripes.com/2016-marks-first-year-without-combat-amputation-since-afghan-iraq-wars-began-1.459288.

National Institute of Arthritis and Musculoskeletal and Skin Diseases. (NIAMS). (2015). *Sprains and strains treatment.* Retrieved from https://www.niams.nih.gov/health-topics/sprains-and-strains#tab-treatment.

Nguyen, J. C., Sheehan, S. E., Davis, K. W., & Gill, K. G. (2014). Sports and the growing musculoskeletal system: Sports imaging series. *British Journal of Sports Medicine, 48*(6), 1235–1239.

Nicholson, S., & Platt, A. (2014). Management of traumatic digital amputations. *British Journal of Hospital Medicine, 75*(4), C50–C54.

Perz, R. A. (2013). The elbow. In L. Schoenly (Ed.), *Core curriculum for orthopaedic nursing* (7th ed., pp. 509–526). Chicago: National Association of Orthopaedic Nursing.

Sen, R. K., Prakash, S., Tripathy, S. K., Argarwal, A., & Sen, I. M. (2017). Inhalational ciclesonide found beneficial in prevention of fat embolism syndrome and improvement of hypoxia in isolated skeletal trauma victims. *European Journal of Trauma and Emergency Surgery,* 43(3), 313–318.

Shah, S., Thomas, A. C., Noone, J. M., Blanchette, C. M., & Wikstrom, E. A. (2016). Incidence and cost of ankle sprains in United States emergency departments. *Sports Health, 8*(6), 547–552.

Shawen, S. B., Dworak, T., & Anderson, R. B. (2016). Return to play following ankle sprain and lateral ligament reconstruction. *Clinics in Sports Medicine, 35*(4), 697–709.

Sheu, Y., Chen, L., & Hedegaard, H. (2016, November 18). Sports- and recreation-related injury episodes in the United States, 2011–2014. *National Health Statistics Reports, 99.* Retrieved from https://www.cdc.gov/nchs/data/nhsr/nhsr099.pdf.

Sorenson, M., Quinn, L., & Klein, D. (2019). *Pathophysiology: Concepts of human disease.* Hoboken, NJ: Pearson Education.

Stracciolini, A., & Hammerberg, E. M. (2018). Acute compartment syndrome of the extremities. *UpToDate.* Retrieved from https://www.uptodate.com/contents/acute-compartment-syndrome-of-the-extremities.

Thompson, A. C. (2014). Factors associated with repetitive strain, and strategies to reduce injury among breast-imaging radiologists. *Journal of the American College of Radiology 11*(11) 1074–1079.

Toivari, M. M., Suominen, A. L., Lindqvist, C., & Thoren, H. (2016). Among patients with facial fractures, geriatric patients have an increased risk for associated injuries. *Journal of Oral and Maxillofacial Surgery, 74*(7), 1403–1409.

Wolfe, H. L. (2015). Managing repetitive strain injuries with channel-based Acumoxa therapy. *California Journal of Oriental Medicine, 26*(1), 3–7.

Xianping, M., Xudong, Z., Wei, Z., Zifeng, L., Lei, X., Yi, L., & Zhongcai, L. (2017). Interval versus external fixation for the treatment of pelvic fractures: A comparative study. *Clinical and Investigative Medicine, 40*(3), E102–E110.

Chapter 40

Nursing Care of Patients with Musculoskeletal Disorders

Chapter Outline and Learning Outcomes

40.1 Metabolic Musculoskeletal Disorders 1450

Describe the pathophysiology and manifestations of metabolic musculoskeletal disorders, and outline the interprofessional care and nursing care of patients with these disorders.

40.2 Degenerative Musculoskeletal Disorders 1465

Describe the pathophysiology and manifestations of degenerative musculoskeletal disorders, and outline the interprofessional care and nursing care of patients with these disorders.

40.3 Autoimmune and Inflammatory Musculoskeletal Disorders 1475

Describe the pathophysiology and manifestations of autoimmune and inflammatory musculoskeletal disorders, and outline the interprofessional care and nursing care of patients with these disorders.

40.4 Infectious Musculoskeletal Disorders 1497

Describe the pathophysiology and manifestations of infectious musculoskeletal disorders, and outline the interprofessional care and nursing care of patients with these disorders.

40.5 Neoplastic Musculoskeletal Disorders 1501

Describe the pathophysiology and manifestations of neoplastic musculoskeletal disorders, and outline the interprofessional care and nursing care of patients with these disorders.

40.6 Other Musculoskeletal Disorders 1504

Describe the pathophysiology and manifestations of other musculoskeletal disorders, including low back pain, fibromyalgia, spinal deformity, and common foot disorders, and outline the interprofessional care and nursing care of patients with these disorders.

CLINICAL COMPETENCIES

- Assess functional status of patients with musculoskeletal disorders, eliciting patient values, preferences, and expressed needs.
- Use research and evidence-based practice guidelines to plan, provide, and manage safe and effective individualized care for patients with musculoskeletal disorders.
- Determine priority nursing diagnoses, based on assessed data, to select and implement patient-centered nursing interventions for patients with musculoskeletal disorders.
- Monitor patient responses to interprofessional and nursing interventions, recognizing, documenting, and reporting adverse or unanticipated responses.
- Demonstrate effective use of strategies to reduce the risk of harm to patients with musculoskeletal disorders.
- Integrate and coordinate interprofessional care into care of patients with musculoskeletal disorders.
- Use quality measures to identify gaps between local and best practices when caring for patients with musculoskeletal disorders.
- Use the electronic medical record to plan care, document care provided, and revise plan of care as appropriate.

KEY TERMS

arthroplasty, 1468
arthroscopy, 1468
fibromyalgia, 1507
gout, 1460
kyphosis, 1508
osteoarthritis (OA), 1466
osteomyelitis, 1497
osteoporosis, 1450
rheumatoid arthritis (RA), 1475
scoliosis, 1508
systemic lupus erythematosus (SLE), 1487

Musculoskeletal diseases affect more than half of all adults in the United States. Trauma, back pain, and arthritis are the three most common reasons for seeking health care (United States Bone and Joint Initiative, 2018). Musculoskeletal disorders are one of the major reasons medical care is sought. Throughout a person's lifetime at least one visit to a primary care provider or emergency department will be for some type of musculoskeletal problem, traumatic or acquired. In this chapter, metabolic, degenerative, autoimmune and inflammatory, infectious, neoplastic, and other musculoskeletal diseases are reviewed and nursing care is explored.

40.1 Metabolic Musculoskeletal Disorders

Metabolic bone disorders disrupt the bone remodeling process, which normally involves a sequence of bone reabsorption and formation. Cancellous (spongy) bone has a significantly higher turnover rate than cortical (compact) bone. Adults constantly replace existing bone through resorption of old bone by osteoclasts and formation of new bone by osteoblasts. Ideally, the amount of new bone formed is equal to the amount of bone resorbed. Metabolic bone disorders may result from a variety of factors, including aging, calcium and phosphate imbalances, genetics, and changes in hormone levels. Gout, also a metabolic joint disorder, results from altered uric acid metabolism and elimination.

The Patient with Osteoporosis

Osteoporosis, literally defined as "porous bones," is a metabolic bone disorder characterized by loss of bone mass, increased bone fragility, and an increased risk of fractures. The reduced bone mass is caused by an imbalance of the processes that influence bone growth and maintenance. Although osteoporosis may result from an endocrine disorder or malignancy, it is most often associated with aging.

The National Osteoporosis Foundation (NOF; 2014) has found that osteoporosis is a health threat for an estimated 54 million Americans; 10.2 million people have osteoporosis and 43.4 million have low bone mass, increasing their risk for the disease. Although osteoporosis can occur at any age and in both men and women, 80% of those with osteoporosis are women. One in two women and one in four men over age 50 will have an osteoporosis-related fracture in his or her remaining lifetime.

Pathophysiology

Although the exact pathophysiology of osteoporosis is unclear, it is known to involve an imbalance of the activity of osteoblasts and osteoclasts. Bone formation occurs more rapidly than does resorption until adulthood, when peak bone mass is reached. After peak bone mass is achieved at about age 30, resorption exceeds formation and slightly more bone is lost than is gained. Cortical bone loss for women can be between 30 and 40% and between 15 and 20% for men (Bethel, Carbone, Lohr, & Machua, 2017). This loss is accelerated if the diet is deficient in vitamin D and calcium. In women, bone loss further increases after menopause (with loss of estrogen), then slows, but does not stop, at about age 60. While testosterone levels in men decline with aging, this is a more gradual process and associated bone loss occurs more slowly.

The rate of bone loss varies both among individuals and at different skeletal sites. The spine, which is 66 to 75% cancellous bone, may show significant osteoporotic changes before bones such as the forearm or wrist, which are predominantly cortical bone. *Postmenopausal osteoporosis* particularly affects bones such as vertebral bodies. Accelerated bone loss at one site magnifies the imbalance of bone resorption and formation. Cortical bone becomes more porous with increased remodeling activity. When coupled with changes to microarchitecture, this reduces the biomechanical strength of bones and increases the risk for fracture (Curtis, Moon, Dennison, Harvey, & Cooper, 2016). *Senile osteoporosis*, associated with aging, tends to affect cortical bone (Mayo Clinic, 2016).

Risk Factors

The risk of developing osteoporosis depends on how much bone mass is achieved between ages 25 and 35, and how much is lost later. Certain diseases, lifestyle habits, and ethnic backgrounds increase the risk of developing osteoporosis. Different variables affect one's risk of osteoporosis—some can be modified and others cannot.

Nonmodifiable Risk Factors

Both men and women are susceptible to osteoporosis as they age because the activity of osteoblasts and osteoclasts diminishes. Women have a significantly higher risk for manifestations and complications of osteoporosis because their peak bone mass is 10 to 15% less than that of men. In addition, age-related bone loss begins earlier and proceeds more rapidly in women, beginning in their 30s and accelerating before menopause. Estrogen in women and testosterone in men appear to help prevent bone loss; decreasing levels of these hormones associated with aging contribute to bone loss. Age-related bone loss in men occurs 15 to 20 years later than in women and at a slower rate. Individuals who are thin and/or have a small frame are considered at higher risk for osteoporosis.

A family history of osteoporosis is a risk factor for the disorder, as well as a history of fracture in a first-degree relative. Caucasian Americans and Asians are at a higher risk for osteoporosis than African Americans. The highest percentage of cases occurs in Caucasian and Asian women ages 50 and older, with 20% estimated to have osteoporosis and more than half estimated to have low bone mass. Ten percent of Latinas age 50 and older are affected, with half of all Latinas estimated to have low bone mass (NOF, 2017d). African American women over the age of 50 have a lower incidence, with an estimated 5% having osteoporosis and 35% low bone mass (NOF, 2017d). Caucasian men are more likely to develop osteoporosis than men of other ethnic backgrounds (National Institute of Arthritis and Musculoskeletal and Skin Diseases [NIAMS], 2015).

Patients who have an endocrine disorder such as hyperthyroidism, hyperparathyroidism, Cushing syndrome, or diabetes mellitus are at high risk for osteoporosis. These disorders affect the metabolism, in turn affecting nutritional status and bone mineralization. Malabsorption disorders such as celiac disease, pancreatic disorders, and inflammatory bowel disease affect calcium absorption and increase the risk for osteoporosis.

Modifiable Risk Factors

Modifiable risk factors include behaviors that place an individual at risk for developing osteoporosis, as well as physical changes such as menopause whose contribution to osteoporosis can be modified by preventive strategies. Calcium deficiency is an important modifiable risk factor contributing to osteoporosis. Calcium is an essential mineral in the process of bone formation and other significant body functions. When dietary intake of calcium is insufficient, the body compensates by removing calcium from the skeleton, weakening bone tissue. Acidosis, which may result from a high-protein diet, contributes to osteoporosis in two ways. Calcium is withdrawn from the bone as the kidneys attempt to buffer the excess acid. Acidosis may directly stimulate osteoclast function. A high intake of diet soda containing significant phosphate can also deplete calcium stores.

In women, estrogen levels affect osteoporosis risk. Estrogen promotes the activity of osteoblasts, increasing new bone formation, and inhibits osteoclast activity. In addition, estrogen enhances calcium absorption and stimulates the thyroid gland to secrete calcitonin, a hormone that suppresses osteoclast activity and increases osteoblast activity. With menopause and decreasing estrogen levels, bone loss accelerates in women. Premature osteoporosis is increasing in female athletes, who have a greater incidence of eating disorders and amenorrhea. Poor nutrition and intense physical training can result in a deficient production of estrogen. Decreased estrogen, combined with a lack of calcium and vitamin D, results in a loss of bone density (Sorenson, Quinn, & Klein, 2019). In men, low testosterone levels increase the risk for osteoporosis.

Both cigarette smoking and excess alcohol intake (more than three drinks per day) are risk factors for osteoporosis. Smoking decreases the blood supply to bones. Nicotine slows the production of osteoblasts and impairs the absorption of calcium, contributing to decreased bone density. Alcohol has a direct toxic effect on osteoblast activity, suppressing bone formation during periods of alcohol intoxication. In addition, heavy alcohol use may be associated with nutritional deficiencies that contribute to osteoporosis. Moderate alcohol consumption in postmenopausal women may increase bone mineral content, possibly by increasing levels of estrogen and calcitonin.

Sedentary lifestyle is another modifiable risk factor that can cause osteoporosis. Weight-bearing exercise, such as walking, influences bone metabolism in several ways. The stress of this type of exercise increases blood flow to bones, which brings growth-producing nutrients to the cells. Walking increases osteoblast growth and activity.

Anyone who takes a glucocorticoid medication (prednisone or dexamethasone, for example) for more than 3 months is at risk for glucocorticoid-induced osteoporosis. These medications, often prescribed to manage rheumatic diseases, can directly affect bone cells, slowing the rate of bone formation. They also interfere with how the body uses calcium and affect levels of sex hormones, leading to bone loss. The American College of Rheumatology (2017a) recommends counseling about calcium and vitamin D supplements for all patients starting glucocorticoid treatment. Other medications known to increase the risk for osteoporosis and fracture include anticonvulsants, immunosuppressants, and some other drugs.

The word **ACCESS** can be used to remember the primary risk factors for osteoporosis:

Alcohol
Corticosteroid
Calcium low
Estrogen low
Smoking
Sedentary lifestyle.

Manifestations

The most common manifestations of osteoporosis are loss of height, progressive curvature of the spine, low back pain, and fractures of the forearm, spine, or hip. Osteoporosis is often called the "silent disease" because bone loss occurs without symptoms.

The loss of height occurs as vertebral bodies collapse. Acute episodes are generally painful, with radiation of the pain around the flank into the abdomen. Vertebral collapse can occur with little or no stress; minimal movements such as bending, lifting, or jumping may precipitate the pain. In some patients, vertebral collapse may occur slowly, accompanied by little discomfort. Along with loss of height, characteristic dorsal kyphosis and cervical lordosis develop, accounting for the "dowager's hump" often associated with aging. The abdomen tends to protrude and knees and hips flex as the body attempts to maintain its center of gravity (**Figure 40.1** ■).

Complications

Fractures are the most common complication of osteoporosis, with the disease being responsible for an estimated 2 million fractures each year (NOF, 2017b). There may be no obvious manifestations of osteoporosis until fractures occur. Some fractures are spontaneous; others may result from everyday activities.

Interprofessional Care

Care of the patient with osteoporosis focuses on early identification of risk, stopping or slowing the process, alleviating symptoms, and preventing complications. Proper nutrition and exercise are important components of treatment. The U.S. Preventive Services Task Force (2011) recommends osteoporosis screening for all women ages 65 years and older; Caucasian women with an increased fracture risk

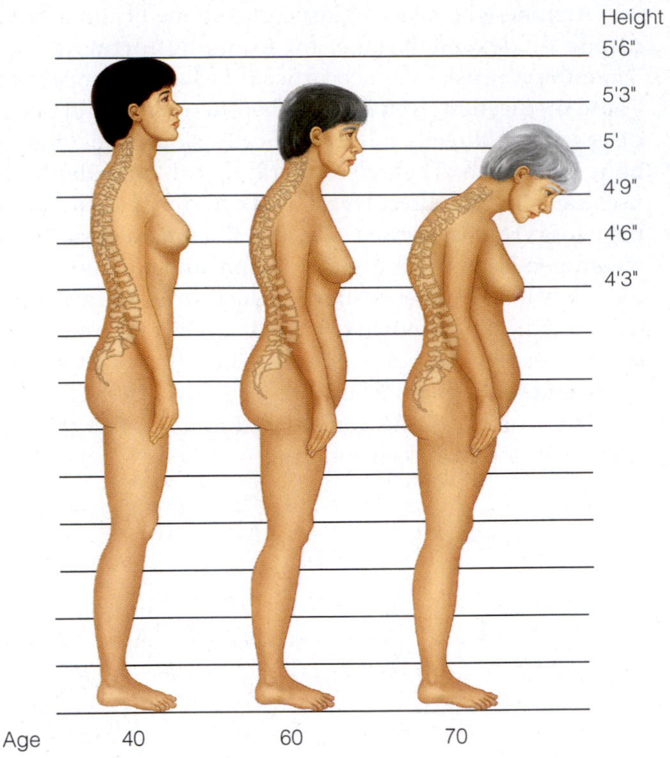
Height
5'6"
5'3"
5'
4'9"
4'6"
4'3"
Age
40
60
70

Figure 40.1 ■ Spinal changes caused by osteoporosis. As the condition progresses, height can be reduced by as much as 18 cm (7 in.).

benefit from earlier screening. A further study by the U.S. Preventive Services Task Force (Viswanathan et al., 2017) was not able to identify the best screening tool for osteoporosis. However, the FRAX (Fracture Risk Assessment) tool, which uses clinical data such as age, body mass index (BMI), parental fracture history, and tobacco and alcohol use, is commonly used to assess fracture risk. The task force found insufficient evidence to recommend screening for men who have not had previous fractures or known causes of osteoporosis.

Diagnosis

Bone mineral density (BMD) tests are used to estimate skeletal mass or density in patients at risk for osteoporosis. Dual-energy x-ray absorptiometry (DEXA) measures bone density in the lumbar spine or hip. Current diagnostic and treatment recommendations rely on DEXA measurements. Quantitative ultrasonography, which transmits painless sound waves through the heel of the foot to measure bone density, is a less expensive screening test that may be used. CT scanning of the spine, hip, forearm, or tibia may also be used to evaluate fracture risk. It is costlier, however, and exposes the patient to more radiation. Laboratory tests such as a complete blood count (CBC), serum and urine calcium, and liver and renal function studies may be done to rule out other causes of bone loss. The serum 25(OH) D test measures total body vitamin D levels and may be ordered for patients at risk for deficiencies, for example, older adults with minimal sun exposure. Biochemical markers of bone turnover, including serum bone-specific alkaline phosphatase, osteocalcin, and others, may be used to monitor treatment response; however, evidence is inconclusive regarding measurement of actual patient response to treatment and adherence to the medication regimen (Ensrud & Crandall, 2017). A comparison of laboratory tests for metabolic bone diseases is outlined in **Table 40.1**.

Medications

Bisphosphonates are the current drugs of choice for preventing and treating osteoporosis. Bisphosphonates are potent inhibitors of bone resorption that preserve bone mass and increase bone density in the hip and vertebrae. Alendronate, risedronate, and oral ibandronate are approved for preventing and treating postmenopausal osteoporosis. Alendronate and risedronate may also be prescribed for men and to prevent or treat glucocorticoid-induced osteoporosis. The nursing implications of bisphosphonates are found in **Medication Administration 40.A**. Adverse effects such as heartburn, difficulty swallowing, and gastric upset may limit long-term adherence to bisphosphonate therapy. The American Society for Bone and Mineral Research recommends reassessment of risk factors after 5 years on a bisphosphonate orally and 3 years intravenously (Adler et al., 2016). Denosumab (Prolia) is a monoclonal antibody for treating postmenopausal osteoporosis in women. This drug has a different mechanism of action, blocking the formation of osteoclasts, the cells that break down bone. It is

Table 40.1 Differential Features of Osteoporosis, Osteomalacia, and Paget Disease

Differentiating Features	Osteoporosis	Osteomalacia	Paget Disease
Pathophysiology	Bone resorption outpaces bone formation	Inadequate mineralization of bone matrix	Excessive osteoclastic activity and formation of poor-quality bone
Calcium level (serum)	Normal	Low or normal	Normal or elevated (especially in immobilized patients)
Phosphate level (serum)	Normal	Low or normal	Normal
Parathyroid hormone level (serum)	Normal	High or normal	Normal
Alkaline phosphatase level (serum)	Normal	Elevated	Increased; not a reliable test for patients who have liver disease or are pregnant
Hydroxyproline (urine)	Not applicable	Not applicable	Increased
Radiographic findings	Osteopenia, fractures	Decreased bone density, radiolucent bands known as Looser's zones, or pseudofractures	"Punched-out" appearance of bone, increase in bone thickness, linear fractures, mosaic pattern of bone matrix

Medication Administration 40.A

The Patient with Osteoporosis

BISPHOSPHONATES

alendronate (Fosamax)
etidronate (Didronel)
ibandronate (Boniva)
pamidronate (Aredia)
risedronate (Actonel)
tiludronate (Skelid)
zoledronic acid (Reclast, Zometa)

The bisphosphonates inhibit bone resorption by inhibiting osteoclast activity, increasing the mineral density of bones, and reducing the incidence of fractures. They are used both in the prevention and treatment of osteoporosis. When used for Paget disease, bisphosphonates slow the accelerated bone turnover associated with this disease.

Nursing Responsibilities

- Administer oral forms with 6 to 8 ounces of water 30 minutes before food or other medications. Other liquids decrease absorption.
- Do not crush, break, or chew tablets.
- Do not give foods high in calcium, vitamins with mineral supplements, or antacids within 2 hours of administering oral bisphosphonates.
- Instruct the patient to avoid lying down for 30 to 60 minutes after taking the drug to minimize irritation to the esophagus.
- Assess renal function studies before initiating therapy; alendronate is not recommended for use in patients with renal insufficiency.
- Dilute the prescribed dose of intravenous preparations and administer by slow intravenous injection or infusion as recommended. Do not add to calcium-containing solutions such as Ringer or lactated Ringer solutions.
- Monitor the IV site for signs of thrombophlebitis.
- Assess the patient for signs of electrolyte imbalance or other adverse responses such as a drug fever.

Health Education for the Patient and Family

- Take the medication as directed with clear water only. Consuming other beverages or food within 30 minutes of taking the drug may interfere with its absorption and effectiveness.
- Do not lie down until after you have eaten because the drug can irritate the esophagus.
- Report symptoms such as new or worsening heartburn, difficult or painful swallowing, or jaw pain to your primary care provider.
- Fever with or without chills and flulike symptoms may occur while receiving intravenous bisphosphonates; this will subside without treatment.
- Report any abnormal symptoms such as tingling around the mouth or numbness and tingling of the fingers or toes, which may indicate an imbalance of electrolytes in the blood.
- Take calcium and vitamin D supplements as instructed by your primary care provider.
- Response to these medications is gradual and continues for months after the drug is stopped.

CALCITONIN

calcitonin (Fortical, Miacalcin)

In postmenopausal osteoporosis (and treatment of Paget disease), calcitonin prevents further bone loss and increases bone mass if the patient consumes adequate amounts of calcium and vitamin D. Calcitonin may be used in combination therapy with a bisphosphonate or for patients who cannot use bisphosphonates.

Nursing Responsibilities

- Calcitonin is protein in nature; both the parenteral and nasal spray forms may cause an anaphylactic-type allergic response. Observe the patient for 20 minutes after administration; have appropriate emergency equipment and drugs available to treat anaphylaxis.
- Alternate nostrils daily when administering calcitonin nasal spray. Assess nasal mucosa daily for irritation.
- Review medical history for conditions that contraindicate use of calcitonin products: hypersensitivity to calcitonin–salmon and lactation (calcitonin is secreted in breast milk and may inhibit lactation).
- Observe for side effects: Nausea and vomiting, anorexia, mild transient flushing of the palms of the hands and the soles of the feet, and urinary frequency.
- Teach the patient the proper technique for handling and injecting the drug at home.

Health Education for the Patient and Family

- Take the medication in the evening to minimize side effects.
- Warm nasal spray to room temperature before using.
- Rhinitis (runny nose) is the most common side effect with calcitonin nasal spray. Other possible side effects include sores, itching, or other nasal symptoms. Report nosebleeds to your primary care provider.
- Nausea and vomiting may occur during initial stages of therapy; they disappear as treatment continues.
- While taking the medication, be sure to consume adequate amounts of calcium and vitamin D.

Note: Drugs identified in blue are among the 200 most commonly prescribed medications in the United States.

Source: Data from Adams, Holland, & Urban, 2017.

administered by subcutaneous injection every 6 months. Its long-term safety is not yet known; however, estrogen replacement therapy is not currently recommended as a treatment of osteoporosis (Bethel et al., 2017).

Raloxifene (Evista) and tamoxifen (Nolvadex, Tamofen) are selective estrogen receptor modulators (SERMs) that prevent bone loss by mimicking estrogen's beneficial effects on bone density in postmenopausal women. SERMs do not have the risks of estrogen and have the added benefit of reducing the risk for invasive breast cancer. Hot flashes are a common side effect. These drugs should not be taken by women with a history of blood clots (Bethel et al., 2017).

Calcitonin (Fortical, Miacalcin) is a hormone that increases bone formation and decreases bone resorption. Calcitonin increases spinal bone density and reduces the risk of compression fractures; it may reduce the risk of hip fracture

Table 40.2 Recommended Adult Intake of Calcium and Vitamin D

Ages	Elemental Calcium (mg)	Vitamin D (units)
19–50 years	1000	400 – 800
51–70 years	1000	800 – 1,000
Over 70 years	1200	800 – 1,000

Source: Data from NOF, 2015.

as well. Calcitonin is usually prescribed as a nasal spray, although it is also available in parenteral form. Because calcitonin is a protein, it can precipitate anaphylactic-type allergic responses. Teriparatide (Forteo) is a synthetic parathyroid hormone, administered subcutaneously to stimulate new bone formation and mass. It is used to decrease the risk of bone fracture from osteoporosis in postmenopausal women and in men with high risk for fracture (Bethel et al., 2017). Use of teriparatide and denosumab in combination has been found to be more effective in increasing bone mineral density than when taken alone (Cosman, 2014).

Nutrition

An adequate intake of calcium and vitamin D beginning in childhood is critical to prevent and treat osteoporosis. By ages 18 to 25, 85 to 90% of adult bone mass is present (NOF, 2017d). See **Table 40.2** for recommended calcium and vitamin D intakes for adults. Food sources of calcium include dairy products (milk, yogurt, and cheese), as well as foods fortified with calcium.

For patients of all ages, stress the importance of maintaining a daily calcium intake that meets National Osteoporosis Foundation (NOF) recommendations (refer to Table 40.2). This is particularly important for adolescent girls and young adult women who may avoid eating many high-calcium foods such as dairy products because of concerns about weight. Optimal calcium intake before ages 30 to 35 probably increases peak bone mass. Emphasize that low-fat (or nonfat) dairy products also contain calcium, although some fat in the product may enhance calcium absorption.

Milk and milk products are the best sources of calcium. The lactose in milk facilitates calcium absorption as well. Other food sources of calcium include sardines, clams, oysters, and salmon, as well as dark green, leafy vegetables such as broccoli, collard greens, bok choy, and spinach. For patients who avoid dairy products because of lactose intolerance or a vegetarian diet, suggest alternate sources.

Calcium supplements are available in many forms. Most supplements (including Tums) provide calcium carbonate in the range of 200 to 600 mg per tablet. Recommend limiting doses to no more than 500 mg of calcium as the amount absorbed declines at higher doses (Rosen, 2017). A combination of calcium with vitamin D is recommended, particularly for older adults who may have a vitamin D deficiency that impairs their ability to absorb and use calcium.

Surgery

There are no specific surgeries for osteoporosis. Any surgeries in patients with osteoporosis would be related to the complications of the disease, such as fracture repair.

Integrative Therapies

Exercise, such as yoga and tai chi, have been found to be effective in preventing osteoporosis and maintaining bone mineral density in postmenopausal women (Kogan, Cheng, Rao, DeMocker, & Koroma Nelson, 2017).

Nursing Care

Osteoporosis is both preventable and treatable; therefore, nursing care focuses primarily on planning and implementing interventions to prevent the disease, its manifestations, and the resulting injuries. An important aspect of preventing osteoporosis is educating patients under age 35. See Case Study & Nursing Care Plan for a patient with osteoporosis.

Assessment

Collect the following data through the health history and physical examination:

- ***Health history:*** Age, risk factors, history of fractures, smoking history, alcohol intake, medications, usual diet, menstrual history including menopause, usual exercise/activity level, low back pain
- ***Physical assessment:*** Height, spinal curves; FRAX assessment (**Box 40.1**).

Priorities of Care

Although the immediate nursing focus for the patient with osteoporosis may change, depending on the setting and patient's condition, maintaining safety and preventing fractures are priorities of care.

Diagnoses, Outcomes, and Interventions

Nursing care of patients who have osteoporosis focuses on teaching about the disease process, helping maintain physical mobility and nutrition, and solving problems associated with pain and injury.

Promote Self-Health Management. At multiple points in the patient's lifetime, nurses can provide vital information that will help patients use self-care strategies to reduce their risk of developing osteoporosis.

BOX 40.1 Using FRAX to Assess Fracture Risk

FRAX (Fracture Risk Assessment) is a computer-based algorithm used to assess the probability of osteoporosis-related fracture in people age 40 and older. It is readily available online and uses easily obtained clinical data, including:

- Age and gender
- Height and weight (to calculate BMI)
- Current smoking and alcohol consumption
- Previous personal or parental fracture
- Other risk factors (e.g., use of glucocorticoids, rheumatoid arthritis, diabetes)
- BMD, if known.

Although the FRAX tool has limitations (Kanis et al., 2017), it can be used by nurses and other health professionals to help the patient and interprofessional team make informed decisions regarding BMD testing and osteoporosis treatment.

Expected Outcome: Patient will verbalize dietary, activity, and lifestyle measures to maintain bone health and prevent fracture.

The nurse will:

- Assess the patient's health habits, including diet, exercise, smoking, and alcohol use. *The risk of developing osteoporosis in later life is affected by such things as diet, regular participation in weight-bearing exercise, and personal habits such as smoking and alcohol consumption* (Cosman et al., 2014).
- Teach women and men of all ages the importance of maintaining an adequate calcium intake. Provide a list of calcium-rich foods, and discuss the use of calcium supplements with patients who do not consume adequate dietary calcium. *Calcium needs vary during the course of a lifetime; however, many patients never consume adequate amounts of calcium. This affects their peak bone mass and the rate of bone loss with aging. Calcium in foods is more completely absorbed than that supplied by calcium supplements.*
- Discuss the importance of maintaining a regular schedule of exercise, weight-bearing or other forms, either through an exercise program or regular physical activity. *Weight-bearing exercise promotes osteoblast activity, helping maintain bone strength and integrity. All forms of exercise promote bone health.*
- Refer patients to smoking-cessation programs and alcohol treatment programs as appropriate. *Smoking interferes with estrogen's protective effects on bones, promoting bone loss. Excess alcohol intake affects the nutritional status of the patient, increasing the risk of calcium and vitamin D deficiency.*
- Refer patients with significant risk factors for osteoporosis or fracture to primary care providers or clinics for bone density evaluation. *Early identification and treatment of osteoporotic changes in bones can reduce the risk and possible long-term consequences of falls and fractures.*

Reduce Risk for Injury. Falls that would result in little or no injury in the healthy adult may cause fractures in the patient with osteoporosis. Even normal movements such as twisting, bending, lifting, or rising from bed can precipitate a vertebral fracture.

Expected Outcome: Patient will remain free of osteoporosis-related fracture.

The nurse will:

- Implement safety precautions as necessary for the patient who is hospitalized or in a long-term care facility. Maintain the bed in low position; use side rails if indicated to prevent the patient from getting up alone; provide nighttime lighting to toilet facilities. *Most falls are preventable, particularly in hospitals and long-term care facilities.*
- Avoid using restraints (if hospitalized or a resident in a long-term care facility) if at all possible. *Restraints may actually increase the patient's risk of falling and increase the risk of injury associated with a fall.*

SAFETY ALERT: Patients may fracture osteoporotic bones when pulling against restraints. ■

- Teach patients who are able to participate in weight-bearing exercises/activity to perform exercises at least three times a week for a sustained period of 30 to 40 minutes. The mechanical force of weight-bearing exercises promotes bone growth. *Bones weaken and demineralize without exercise. Walking is an easy, low-impact form of exercise. Swimming (including walking on the bottom of the pool) does not provide the needed weight-bearing activity.*
- Encourage older adults to use assistive devices to maintain independence in ADLs. *Walking sticks, canes, and other assistive devices encourage patient independence and support activities that promote bone growth.*
- Teach older patients about safety and fall precautions. *An assessment of the patient's home for safety and fall risks may reduce the risk of fractures and, in turn, the cost of hospitalization and potential disability and/or death.*

Promote Good Nutrition. Most Americans do not maintain their recommended daily intake of calcium. Patients must therefore be made aware of the relationship between an adequate calcium intake and maintaining strong bones.

Expected Outcome: Patient will consume recommended amounts of calcium, vitamin D, and other nutrients daily.

The nurse will:

- Teach adolescents, pregnant or lactating women, and adults through age 50 to eat foods high in calcium and to maintain a daily calcium intake of 1000 mg. *The NOF recommends a daily calcium intake of 1000 mg per day for all adults until age 70 years (see Table 40.2).*
- Encourage adults over age 70 to maintain a calcium intake of 1200 mg daily, either through diet or a calcium supplement. *Calcium needs for older adults are higher than for young adults.*
- Teach patients taking calcium supplements the importance of taking the medication at the proper time and the side effects that may occur. *Free hydrochloric acid is needed for calcium absorption. Calcium carbonate supplements (e.g., Tums) should be taken with food to allow adequate absorption. Calcium citrate supplements should be taken with meals to prevent gastrointestinal (GI) distress.*

SAFETY ALERT: Calcium supplements should be taken in divided doses (two to three times daily) for improved absorption. ■

Relieve Acute Pain. Advanced stages of osteoporosis can result in pain and limit mobility. Acute pain usually results from a complicating fracture, especially a compression fracture of the vertebrae.

Expected Outcome: Patient will report pain within an acceptable range.

The nurse will:

- Suggest anti-inflammatory pain medications for treatment of both acute and chronic phases of pain. Patients should be instructed in the amount and frequency as noted on the manufacturer's labels. *Continuous administration of ibuprofen or other nonsteroidal anti-inflammatory drugs (NSAIDs) can be useful to provide relief from pain, but patients must be cautioned not to exceed dosage recommendations due to potential for kidney damage.*

- Suggest the application of heat to relieve pain. *A heating pad may offer temporary pain relief. To avoid the "rebound effect," the heat should be removed every 20 to 30 minutes.*

SAFETY ALERT: Gastrointestinal bleeding is a risk for patients taking NSAIDs. Teach patients to watch for bright red bleeding from the stomach (in vomitus) or dark black bowel movements. Avoid use in patients with a history of stomach ulcers or bleeding tendencies. ■

Delegating Nursing Care Activities

Nursing care activities such as assisting with ambulation and daily living activities and ensuring safety for the patient with osteoporosis may be delegated to assistive personnel as allowed within their designated duties and responsibilities.

Transitions of Care

Health promotion activities to prevent or slow osteoporosis focus on calcium intake, exercise, and health-related behaviors. Behaviors that help prevent osteoporosis include not smoking, avoiding excessive alcohol intake, and limiting caffeine intake to two or three cups of coffee each day.

Teach patients the importance of physical activity and weight-bearing exercises in preventing and slowing bone loss and reducing fall risk (Kemmler, Kohl, & von Stengel, 2017). Suggest that patients participate in regular exercise such as walking, stair climbing, or tai chi for at least

Case Study & Nursing Care Plan

A Patient with Osteoporosis

Nancy Bauer is a 53-year-old woman who has smoked one pack of cigarettes a day for 30 years and drinks one to two glasses of wine with dinner each evening. She does not routinely exercise. Mrs. Bauer has had symptoms of menopause for 8 years, including hot flashes in the early years and mood swings of late. She has never been on hormone replacement therapy.

Mrs. Bauer is currently seeking medical advice for continuous low back pain. The pain is not relieved with an over-the-counter (OTC) analgesic, and she frequently wakes up during the night because of the pain. She is diagnosed with osteoporosis.

ASSESSMENT	DIAGNOSES	EXPECTED OUTCOMES
The nurse practitioner notes that Mrs. Bauer's vital signs are within normal limits. She has full range of motion (ROM) of all extremities and is able to stand and bend over, but she reports discomfort when returning to the upright position. Mrs. Bauer has a slightly pronounced "hump" on her upper back and is 1 inch shorter than her stated height on admission. Her current height is 65 inches; weight is 145 pounds. Her muscle strength is symmetric and strong.	■ Acute pain of the lower spine related to vertebral compression ■ Need for education related to osteoporosis to prevent further damage ■ Potential for injury due to effects of change in bone structure secondary to osteoporosis	■ Patient will verbalize a decrease in back pain. ■ Patient will be able to describe ways to treat her osteoporosis and prevent further complications. ■ Patient will verbalize how stopping smoking can help prevent further progression of osteoporosis. ■ Patient will seek consultation for supplements and medications to prevent further bone loss. ■ Patient will design a program of physical activity to prevent complications of osteoporosis. ■ Patient will verbalize safety precautions to prevent fractures due to falls.

PLANNING AND IMPLEMENTATION

- Teach back-strengthening exercises.
- Refer to an osteoporosis support group, if available.
- Provide realistic, yet optimistic, feedback about loss of height and bone integrity and the potential outcomes of treatment.
- Assess current knowledge base, and correct misconceptions regarding treatment of osteoporosis.
- Instruct on dietary and calcium supplements that help prevent effects of osteoporosis.
- Discuss physical exercises that help prevent complications due to osteoporosis.
- Review safety and fall precautions and provide literature regarding how to create a safe home environment.

EVALUATION

On her return visit 6 months later, Mrs. Bauer reports that she feels much better. She is no longer irritable and does not experience mood swings because she has been taking her prescribed hormone replacements for 6 months. She is eating products rich in calcium and taking a daily supplement of calcium with vitamin D. Mrs. Bauer has reduced her wine intake to one glass in the evening and now drinks decaffeinated coffee and tea. She also states that since she stopped smoking, she has been walking 30 to 45 minutes every day.

CLINICAL REASONING IN PATIENT CARE

1. Locate the FRAX WHO Fracture Risk Assessment Tool online. Using the data provided, determine Mrs. Bauer's 10-year risk for experiencing a fracture.
2. Do you need additional data to complete this assessment? If so, what additional subjective and objective data will you obtain?
3. How will you explain the results of this calculation to Mrs. Bauer?
4. What is the rationale for stopping smoking and limiting caffeine and alcohol intake in the treatment of osteoporosis?
5. What foods would you encourage for patients at high risk for osteoporosis whose serum cholesterol and LDL/HDL ratios indicate a high risk for cardiovascular disease?
6. What physical activities would you consider beneficial in helping to prevent the effects of osteoporosis in the female patient who is wheelchair-bound or has limited mobility?

See Evaluating Your Response in Appendix B.

20 minutes five or more times a week. Inform patients that swimming and pool aerobic exercises are not as beneficial for maintaining bone density because of the lack of weight-bearing activity.

The patient who has osteoporosis needs education on safety and fall prevention. In addition to home safety, outdoor safety is important, too. Patients should be taught to use assistive devices for added stability, to wear rubber-soled shoes for traction, to walk on the grass when sidewalks are slippery, and to sprinkle salt or cat litter on icy sidewalks in the winter. Address the following topics when discussing home care:

- Resources for medical supplies and assistive devices
- Diet, exercise, and medications
- Pain management
- Maintaining good posture to help prevent stress on the spine
- Helpful resources:
  a. National Osteoporosis Foundation
  b. Osteoporosis and Related Bone Diseases National Resource Center (NIH)
  c. National Women's Health Resource Center
  d. Older Women's League
  e. American College of Rheumatology.

The Patient with Paget Disease of Bone

Paget disease of bone, also called *osteitis deformans*, is a progressive metabolic skeletal disorder that results from localized excessive metabolic activity in bone, with excessive bone resorption followed by excessive bone formation (NOF, 2017a). This chronic remodeling results in the affected bones being larger and softer, causing bone pain, arthritis, obvious skeletal deformities, and fractures. The disorder can affect any bone or bones; however, the femur, tibia, pelvis, vertebrae, and skull are most commonly involved. It is the second most common bone disease in the United States.

Both genetic and environmental factors appear to play a role in the development of Paget disease. A reported 15 to 25% of patients report a family history of Paget disease. Viral particles have been found in osteoclasts of people with Paget disease, suggesting that viral infection plays a role in its development (NOF, 2017b; Sorenson et al., 2019).

Pathophysiology

In Paget disease, the number, size, and activity of osteoclasts increase significantly, resulting in excessive osteoclastic bone resorption and hyperemia in affected segments of bone. This initial phase of hyperactive bone resorption is followed by very active bone formation. In this phase, normal laminar bone is replaced by haphazard or disorganized bone. This bone is not as structurally sound as normal bone and can bow and fracture more easily. During this phase, normal bone marrow may be replaced by fibrous connective tissue. When the excessive bone cell activity decreases in the third or "burned-out" phase of the disease, the newly formed bone becomes hard and brittle. This brittleness may lead to fractures. Multiple areas of the skeleton may be affected by Paget disease, often in different phases at various sites.

Risk Factors

Paget disease occurs slightly more in men than in women, affecting from 1.5 to 8% of the population over the age of 40, depending on age and location (NOF, 2017b). It is more common in people of European and Greek descent and less common in people from Scandinavia and Asia (NOF, 2017b). There appears to be a genetic link in some Paget disease cases (Cundy, 2017).

Manifestations

Most patients with Paget disease are asymptomatic for years, and the disease is often discovered when typical changes are seen on an incidental x-ray (**Figure 40.2** ■). Manifestations are often vague and depend on the specific area involved. The most common manifestation is localized pain of the long bones of the lower extremities; joints; spine; pelvis; and/or cranium (i.e., headache with skull involvement). The pain is described as a mild to moderate deep ache that is worse at rest, especially at night (Cundy, 2017). The pain is often relieved by moving. The pain is usually due to metabolic

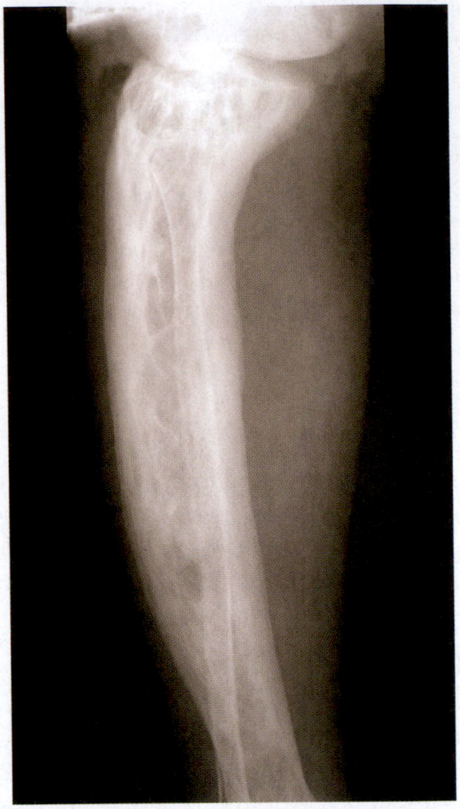

Figure 40.2 ■ An x-ray of a leg bone affected by Paget disease. Note how the bone is misshapen, curved, and has a "punched-out" appearance.

bone activity, secondary degenerative osteoarthritis, fractures, or nerve impingement. Because of the increase in blood flow to pagetic bone, flushing and warmth of the overlying skin may be apparent. Other manifestations presenting as musculoskeletal effects include deformity (enlargement of skull, bowing of lower extremities, and deformity of elbows and knees); abnormal gait; increased head size; pathologic fractures (upper femur, pelvis); compression fractures; collapse of the vertebrae, resulting in kyphosis and loss of height; and muscle weakness. Metabolic manifestations of Paget disease include symptoms of hypercalcemia in immobilized patients; hypercalciuria and renal calculi; and increased skin temperature over affected bone.

Complications

Pathologic fractures resulting from loss of bone structure are a serious complication of Paget's disease. Involvement of the skull and vertebrae may cause neurologic complications such as cranial nerve palsies, headache, paresis, and hearing loss. Heart failure in patients with preexisting cardiac disease may develop secondary to increased metabolic demand and is a serious complication of Paget disease (NOF, 2017b; Sorenson et al., 2019). Sarcomas, an uncommon complication, may develop.

Interprofessional Care

Care of the patient with Paget disease focuses on relieving pain, suppressing active disease, and preventing or minimizing the effects of complications. Pharmacologic therapy is commonly used to treat Paget disease.

Diagnosis

Many of the diagnostic tests that are useful for the diagnosis of osteoporosis are equally useful for patients with Paget disease (refer to Table 40.1). These include x-rays and bone scintigraphy (scan) to illustrate localized areas of demineralization in the early stages, seen as "punched-out" areas showing a coarse, irregular appearance to the bone (refer to Figure 40.2). In the later phase, x-rays show enlargement of the bones, tiny cracks in the long bones, and/or bowing of the weight-bearing bones. Computed tomography (CT) scans and magnetic resonance imaging (MRI) help identify possible causes of pain, including degenerative problems, spinal stenosis, or nerve root impingement. A bone scan may be performed to determine the full extent of the disease (Cundy, 2017).

Laboratory tests used in diagnosis include a serum alkaline phosphatase, which can increase dramatically in active disease; the normal level (30 to 115 International Units/L) may be elevated to over 3000 International Units/L when the disease is active.

Medications

Bisphosphonates such as alendronate (Fosamax), pamidronate (Aredia), and tiludronate (Skelid) are the primary treatments used for Paget disease. These drugs inhibit bone resorption, possibly by attaching to the surface of the calcium/phosphate phase of bone and inhibiting osteoclast activity. They are safe and are usually well tolerated by the patient. Bone pain is relieved, and the incidence of pathologic fractures is reduced. Cardiac and vascular manifestations of the disease also improve. Alendronate and several other bisphosphonates are available for oral administration. Oral preparations are poorly absorbed from the GI tract and may cause gastric or esophageal irritation. They should be given with a full glass of water on an empty stomach, at least 30 minutes before other medications or food. Pamidronate is given as an intravenous infusion in D_5W or normal saline. It is given for 3 successive days, generally promoting a rapid response with reduced urinary excretion of hydroxyproline and pyridinium and a fall in alkaline phosphatase. Intravenous pamidronate may cause flulike symptoms, but these are generally brief. Intravenous zoledronic acid (Zometa) is also approved for treating Paget disease; one 5-mg infusion of this drug produces a prolonged response (1 to 2 years) in most patients (Charles, 2016). Calcium and vitamin D supplements are also prescribed for patients receiving bisphosphonates. After bisphosphonate treatment, patients often experience remission of symptoms for a year or more. See Medication Administration 40.A for nursing implications for bisphosphonates.

Patients who cannot tolerate bisphosphonate drugs may be treated with calcitonin. Calcitonin inhibits osteoclastic resorption of bone. Calcitonin is available in both parenteral and nasal spray forms. The parenteral form of calcitonin is used in treating Paget disease (NOF, 2017c). (Refer to Medication Administration 40.A for nursing implications.)

Treatments to suppress Paget disease activity (bisphosphonates or calcitonin) are generally effective to relieve pain associated with the disease. Pain due to complications such as bone deformity, arthritis, or neurologic complications may be treated with an analgesic such as acetaminophen or with NSAIDs.

Nutrition

There has been no link found between nutrition and Paget disease. The National Osteoporosis Foundation (NOF, 2017c) suggests maintaining adequate levels of calcium and vitamin D, as recommended by health care professionals

Surgery

Surgical interventions may be necessary for patients with Paget disease, such as repairing a complete fracture through pagetic bone, realigning a knee through tibial osteotomy to decrease pain, or replacing a hip and/or knee for osteoarthritis. Excessive operative bleeding is a risk in Paget disease due to increased vascularity of affected bone. Pretreatment with a potent bisphosphonate reduces disease activity prior to surgery and decreases the risk of excessive operative blood loss (NOF, 2017d).

Nursing Care

Assessment

Because Paget disease often goes unrecognized until it is advanced, it is important for nurses to recognize its manifestations and seek additional information from the patient when those manifestations are present. Therefore, assessment will focus on the patient's complaints, including a complete pain assessment, assessment of range of motion, a nutrition assessment, and a review of medications. The nurse will also assess the patient's home routines and level of activity prior to and after the symptoms started to manifest. This will help to determine the extent of disability and potential need for rehabilitation services to assist the patient to return to their desired level of activity.

Priorities of Care

The nursing interventions for the patient with Paget disease focus on pain control, prevention of injury or fractures, and education regarding the disease process and prescribed therapies.

Diagnoses, Outcomes, and Interventions

Because Paget disease often goes unrecognized until it is advanced, it is important for nurses to recognize its manifestations and seek additional information from the patient when those manifestations are present.

Manage Chronic Pain. The most common manifestation of Paget disease is bone pain. This is usually the manifestation that prompts the patient to seek healthcare.

Expected Outcome: Patient will verbalize an understanding of the relationship of pain to disease activity.

The nurse will:

- Assess the location and extent of the pain to determine the bone areas involved. *Bone pain in Paget disease may be poorly localized and described as "aching and deep."*
- Explain the relationship between pain and disease activity and the importance of overall disease management to improve comfort. *Pain associated with Paget disease is often relieved by treatment to suppress disease activity.*
- Teach the patient to take NSAIDs on a regular basis, as prescribed. Acetaminophen may be taken as needed for pain. *Pain is most noticeable at night or when the patient is resting. The pain can become evident when it is aggravated by pressure and weight bearing.*
- Ensure correct placement of prescribed brace or corset. The patient may be required to wear a light brace or corset to relieve back pain and provide support when assuming an upright position. *The patient may need instruction in the correct application of the device and in the evaluation of pressure areas that may result from wearing the device.*

Promote Physical Mobility. Patients with Paget disease need to maintain or improve mobility so that they can perform necessary self-care activities and prevent complications of immobility.

Expected Outcome: Patient will be able to maintain activities and mobility without experiencing complications such as fracture.

The nurse will:

- Provide an assistive device for use when ambulating. *During the active phase of Paget disease, the patient is prone to fractures. Bone deformities, activity intolerance, fear of falling, and pain are all factors that may make the patient more prone to falls. An assistive device can provide both physical and psychologic support during ambulation, permit the patient to ambulate further, and provide a device for resting during ambulation.*
- Teach good body mechanics. *The patient with bone deformities should avoid activities that require lifting and twisting. In the patient with Paget disease, activities as seemingly simple as lifting a heavy box may result in a fracture.*
- Reinforce information about exercise protocols and activity regimens. *Exercise and activity protocols should be planned carefully to prevent injury and to minimize fatigue.*

Delegating Nursing Care Activities

Nursing care that can be delegated to an unlicensed assistive person include assistance with the application of support devices, mobility, and activities of daily living.

Transitions of Care

There is no known prevention for Paget disease, as the exact cause is unknown. A diagnosis of Paget disease can be frightening for the patient and family. It is important that they understand that this is a treatable disease and that many manifestations of the disease will be relieved with treatment. Inform the patient that remissions of the disease often last for a year or more after effective treatment. The Paget Foundation should be suggested as a resource. Discuss the following topics:

- The importance of following the prescribed treatment regimen and keeping scheduled follow-up appointments
- Because it may take several weeks to notice a response to treatment, the importance of continuing therapy during this time and after a response is obtained
- If bisphosphonates such as alendronate or pamidronate are ordered, the importance of taking supplemental calcium to prevent low blood calcium levels
- The importance of remaining active
- Safety in the home and outdoor environment to prevent falls
- The need to report to the primary care provider any sudden pain or disability, even if no trauma has occurred, because pathologic fractures are possible.

Because there is no cure for Paget disease, long-term care and follow-up are essential to managing the disease symptoms and preventing complications. Education regarding the importance of seeing the healthcare provider on a regular basis, taking medications as prescribed, and obtaining laboratory tests, as prescribed, to periodically monitor the effectiveness of the medications are important to emphasize. Referral to support groups, such as the Paget Foundation, will connect patients and family members with other people dealing with this issue as well.

The Patient with Gout

Gout is a metabolic disorder characterized by an episodic acute inflammatory arthritis triggered by crystallization of urate within the joints. It develops in response to an excess of uric acid in the body, resulting in high levels of uric acid in the blood (hyperuricemia) and deposition of urate crystals in synovial fluid and other tissues (Ragab, Elshahaly, & Bardin, 2017). Deposits in the synovial fluids cause acute inflammation of the joint (*gouty arthritis*). Acute gouty arthritis typically has an abrupt onset, usually at night, and often involves the first metatarsophalangeal joint (great toe). The initial acute attack is usually followed by a period of months or years without manifestations. As the disease progresses, urates are deposited in various other connective tissues. Urate deposits in subcutaneous tissues cause the formation of small white nodules called *tophi*. Deposits of crystals in the kidneys can form urate kidney stones and result in kidney failure.

Gout affects an estimated 8 million Americans, the majority of whom are men (American College of Rheumatology, 2017b). Gout occurs in 1 to 4% of the population (Ragab et al., 2017).

Pathophysiology

Uric acid is the breakdown product of purine metabolism. Normally, a balance exists between its production and excretion, with approximately two-thirds of the amount produced each day excreted by the kidneys and the rest in the feces. The serum uric acid level is normally maintained between 3.5 and 8.0 mg/dL in men and 2.8 and 6.8 mg/dL in women. At levels greater than 8.0 mg/dL, the serum is saturated with urate, the ionized form of uric acid. As the concentration increases, plasma becomes supersaturated, creating a risk for formation of monosodium urate crystals. Hyperuricemia results from either an underexcretion of uric acid by the kidneys or an overproduction of uric acid. In hyperuricemia, increased urate levels are present in other extracellular fluids, including synovial fluid, as well as in plasma. Synovial fluid, however, is a poor solvent for urate than plasma, increasing the risk for urate crystal formation.

Monosodium urate crystals may form in the synovial fluid or in the synovial membrane, cartilage, or other joint connective tissues. Crystals tend to form in peripheral tissues of the body, where lower temperatures reduce the solubility of the uric acid. They may also form in connective tissue and the kidneys. These crystals stimulate and continue the inflammatory process, during which neutrophils respond by ingesting the crystals. The neutrophils release their phagolysosomes, causing tissue damage, which perpetuates the inflammation. Ultimately, the inflammatory process destroys joint cartilage and underlying bone.

Risk Factors

A number of risk factors for gout have been identified. Of these, male gender and aging cannot be modified; the others can be. The role of diet as a risk factor for gout appears to relate primarily to its contribution to chronic diseases such as obesity, metabolic syndrome, and type 2 diabetes (Ragab et al., 2017). Consumption of a diet rich in meat and seafood is associated with a higher risk of developing gout. Although alcohol intake, especially beer, has long been known to increase the risk for hyperuricemia and gout, recent studies have shown that consumption of soft drinks sweetened with sugar or fructose (corn syrup) also increases the risk for gout in men (Ragab et al., 2017). Chronic kidney disease and use of certain medications, such as diuretics and aspirin, are also considered risk factors for gout.

Manifestations

The manifestations of gout range from asymptomatic hyperuricemia to repeated episodes of acute gouty arthritis, and advanced gout with chronic arthritis and the development of tophi.

Early gout is characterized by asymptomatic hyperuricemia, with serum levels averaging 9 to 10 mg/dL. Most people with hyperuricemia do not progress to further stages of the disease.

An acute gouty arthritis attack, usually affecting a single joint, occurs unexpectedly, often beginning at night. An attack may be triggered by trauma, alcohol ingestion, dietary excess, or a stressor such as surgery. The affected joint becomes erythematous, hot, edematous, and extremely painful and tender. Approximately 50% of initial attacks of acute gouty arthritis occur in the metatarsophalangeal joint of the great toe. Other sites for acute attacks include the instep of the foot, ankles, heels, knees, wrists, fingers, and elbows. The pain, often intense, peaks within several hours and may be accompanied by fever, chills, malaise, and an elevated white blood cell (WBC) count and sedimentation rate. The skin over the joint becomes warm and dusky red (**Figure 40.3 ■**).

Acute attacks of gouty arthritis last from several hours to up to 10 days and typically subside spontaneously. Approximately 60% of people experience a recurrent attack within 1 year. Successive attacks tend to last longer, occur with increasing frequency, involve more than one joint, and resolve less completely than the initial attack.

When hyperuricemia is not treated, an advanced gout state, the urate pool expands and urate crystal deposits (tophi) develop in cartilage, synovial membranes, tendons, and soft tissues. They are seen most often in the helix of the ear, in tissues surrounding joints and bursae (especially around the elbows and knees), along tendons of the fingers or ankles, and on ulnar surfaces of the forearms. The skin over tophi may ulcerate, exuding chalky material containing inflammatory cells and urate crystals. Tophi can also develop in the tissues of the heart and spinal epidura. Although tophi themselves are not painful, they may restrict joint movement and cause pain and deformities of the affected joints. Tophi may also compress nerves and erode and drain through the skin. Patients will complain of joint stiffness and limited ROM, with deformity of the joints evident.

Complications

Kidney disease may occur in patients with untreated gout, particularly when hypertension is also present. Urate crystals are deposited in interstitial tissue of the kidneys. Uric acid crystals also form in the collecting tubules, renal pelvis, and ureter, forming stones. The stones can range in size from a grain of sand to a massive structure filling the spaces of the kidney. Uric acid stones can potentially obstruct urine flow and lead to acute kidney injury. Advanced gout and

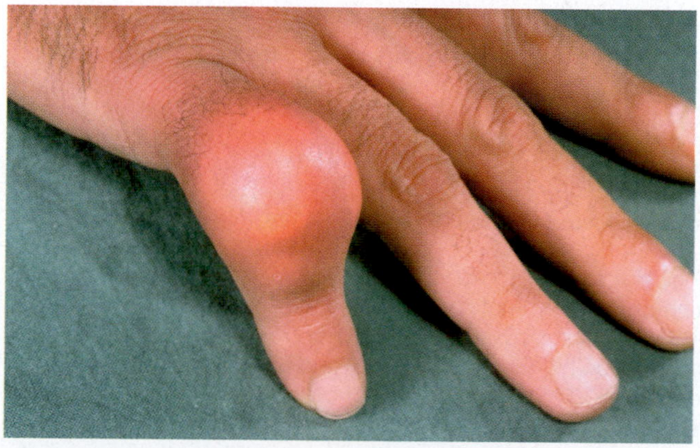

Figure 40.3 ■ Acute gouty arthritis affecting the distal interphalangeal joint of a man.

hyperuricemia has also been shown to be associated with heart failure (Bardin & Richette, 2017).

Interprofessional Care

The classic presentation of acute gouty arthritis is so distinctive that the diagnosis can often be based on the patient's history and physical examination. Treatment is directed toward terminating an acute attack, preventing recurrent attacks, and reversing or preventing complications resulting from crystal deposition in tissues and formation of uric acid kidney stones. Lifestyle changes such as weight loss, exercise to achieve physical fitness, smoking cessation, reduced intake of foods rich in purines or containing high-fructose corn syrup, and limited alcohol intake are important to reduce serum uric acid levels. Because of the association between hyperuricemia, hypertension, and metabolic syndrome, patients with asymptomatic hyperuricemia and gout should undergo cardiovascular risk factor screening.

Diagnosis

Diagnostic testing is performed to establish an accurate diagnosis and direct long-term therapy. The serum uric acid level is nearly always elevated (usually above 8.5 mg/dL) in patients with gout but may actually be low or within the normal range during an acute attack (Becker, 2018a). The WBC count shows significant elevation, reaching levels as high as 20,000/mm^3 during an acute attack. Erythrocyte sedimentation rate (ESR or sed rate) is elevated during an acute attack from the acute inflammatory process that accompanies deposits of urate crystals in a joint. Serum creatinine is obtained to evaluate kidney function. In addition, a 24-hour urine specimen is analyzed to determine uric acid production and excretion, and analysis of fluid aspirated from the acutely inflamed joint or material aspirated from a tophus shows typical needle-shaped urate crystals, providing the definitive diagnosis of gout.

Medications

Medications are used to terminate an acute attack, prevent further attacks, and reduce serum uric acid levels to prevent long-term sequelae of the disease. It is important to treat the acute attack of gouty arthritis before initiating treatment to reduce serum uric acid levels because an abrupt decrease in serum uric acid may lead to further acute manifestations. Pharmacologic therapy is a mainstay of treatment in achieving these goals.

Acute Attack. Treatment for an acute gouty arthritis attack may be initiated with a nonsteroidal anti-inflammatory drug, oral glucocorticoids, or colchicine (Becker, 2018d). NSAIDs are the treatment of choice for most patients experiencing an acute attack of gout. Indomethacin (Indocin) or naproxen (Naprosyn, Anaprox) are the most frequently used NSAIDs for acute attacks (Becker, 2018d). Although extremely effective, NSAIDs are contraindicated for patients with active peptic ulcer disease, impaired renal function, or a history of hypersensitivity reactions to the drugs. As with other anti-inflammatory drugs, patients should be aware of possible risks and follow recommended doses carefully.

Colchicine may be used to terminate an acute attack. Joint pain begins to diminish within 12 hours of the initiation of treatment and disappears within 2 days. Colchicine apparently acts by interrupting the cycle of urate crystal deposition and inflammation in an acute attack of gout. It has no anti-inflammatory effect in other forms of arthritis, and its use is limited to gout. The use of colchicine is limited by significant side effects. When administered orally, many patients develop abdominal cramping, diarrhea, or nausea and vomiting. It is contraindicated for patients who have significant gastrointestinal (GI), renal, hepatic, or cardiac disease.

Corticosteroids may be prescribed for the patient with acute gouty arthritis. The intra-articular route may be used for monoarticular arthritis to avoid the multiple systemic effects of steroid therapy. When multiple joints are involved, corticosteroids may be administered either orally or parenterally.

Prophylactic Therapy. In addition to dietary and lifestyle modifications, pharmacologic therapy to lower uric acid levels is recommended for patients with gout. Allopurinol (Zyloprim) is the drug of choice for lowering serum urate levels (Becker, 2018c). Febuxostat (Uloric) is another drug that can be used to lower uric acid levels. These drugs are xanthine oxidase inhibitors that lower plasma uric acid levels and facilitate the mobilization of tophi. Because of their effectiveness in lowering serum uric acid levels, initiation of therapy may trigger an attack of acute gout.

Pegloticase (Krystexxa), an enzyme that prompts the conversion of uric acid to a metabolite excreted by the kidneys, is a relatively new antigout medication. This drug is used in patients who do not respond well to other urate-lowering medications; it is administered by intravenous infusion and carries a risk for anaphylaxis (Becker, 2018c).

The nursing implications for medications used to treat gout are included in **Medication Administration 40.B**.

Nutrition

Dietary purines contribute only slightly to uric acid levels in the body, and no specific diet may be recommended.

Medication Administration 40.B

The Patient with Gout

XANTHINE OXIDASE INHIBITORS

allopurinol (Alloprin, Zyloprim, Others)

febuxostat (Uloric)

Xanthine oxidase inhibitors act on purine metabolism, reducing the production of uric acid and decreasing serum and urinary concentrations of uric acid. They are used for patients with manifestations of primary or secondary gout, including acute attacks, tophi, joint destruction, urinary stones, and nephropathy.

Nursing Responsibilities

- Monitor intake and output.
- Monitor for desired effect of decreased serum uric acid levels and for adverse effects such as nausea, diarrhea, and rash.
- Assess renal and liver function tests prior to the initiation of and during treatment. Report signs of impaired renal or liver function to the physician.
- Administer with meals to minimize gastric distress.
- Monitor CBC periodically because allopurinol therapy may cause bone marrow depression.
- Allopurinol interacts with multiple drugs; check for potential interaction before administering any other medications.
- Discontinue allopurinol and notify the physician immediately if the patient develops a rash or fever. These symptoms may indicate potentially life-threatening drug toxicity.

Health Education for the Patient and Family

- Stop taking the drug and report any skin rash, painful urination, blood in the urine, eye irritation, or swelling of the lips or mouth to the physician immediately.
- Take the medication after meals to minimize gastric distress.
- Drink 3 to 4 quarts of fluid daily to maintain a urinary output greater than 2 L/day.
- Acute gouty attacks may occur during the initial stages of therapy; continue therapy prescribed for attacks (such as colchicine or an NSAID) to minimize acute episodes.
- Do not take a double dose of medication if you miss a dose.

ANTIGOUT MEDICATION

Colchicine

Colchicine is used to treat acute gouty arthritis and prevent recurrent episodes of the disease. Colchicine does not alter serum uric acid levels, but appears to interrupt the cycle of urate crystal deposition and inflammatory response. It is given once or twice daily by mouth. Colchicine is also available as a fixed-dose combination with a uricosuric agent, probenecid (Benemid).

Nursing Responsibilities

- Assess for possible contraindications to colchicine therapy, including serious GI, renal, hepatic, or cardiac disease.
- Administer oral colchicine on an empty stomach to facilitate absorption.
- Evaluate for adverse effects, including abdominal cramping, nausea and vomiting, and diarrhea, and report promptly because these side effects may necessitate discontinuation of the drug.

Health Education for the Patient and Family

- Drink 3 to 4 quarts of liquid per day.
- Report adverse responses, including GI problems, fatigue, bleeding, easy bruising, or recurrent infections, to the physician.
- Do not drink alcohol.

URICOSURIC DRUGS

probenecid (Benemid)

sulfinpyrazone (Anturane)

Probenecid is a uricosuric drug that inhibits the tubular reabsorption of urate, promoting the excretion of uric acid and decreasing serum uric acid levels. Sulfinpyrazone is a uricosuric drug that potentiates the renal excretion of uric acid, reducing serum uric acid levels. These drugs are used to prevent recurrent attacks of acute gouty arthritis and treat chronic gout.

Nursing Responsibilities

- Assess for prior hypersensitivity responses to the drug.
- Administer after meals or with milk to minimize gastric distress.

- Do not administer these drugs during or within the 2 to 3 weeks following an attack of acute gouty arthritis.
- Increase fluid intake to at least 3 L/day to prevent the formation of uric acid kidney calculi.
- Do not administer aspirin or products containing aspirin to patients receiving these drugs because salicylates interfere with the action of the drug.
- These drugs interact with multiple other medications; check for interactions before administering any drug to a patient taking one of these drugs.
- Monitor for and report possible adverse or toxic effects, including headache, dizziness, nausea and vomiting, bone marrow depression, hypersensitivity responses, and impaired kidney or liver function.
- Assess for contraindications to therapy with sulfinpyrazone, including active peptic ulcer disease, a history of hypersensitivity to phenylbutazone or other pyrazoles, or blood dyscrasias.

Health Education for the Patient and Family

- Do not take aspirin or products containing aspirin while taking this drug. Use acetaminophen for relief of mild pain.
- Drink at least 3 quarts of fluids per day to minimize the risk of kidney stone formation.
- Take the drug with or after meals to minimize gastric distress, and report epigastric pain, nausea, or black stools to the physician promptly.

Note: Drugs identified in blue are among the 200 most commonly prescribed medications in the United States.

Source: Data from Adams et al., 2017.

Current evidence-based recommendations are that patients with gout limit their intake of purine-rich foods such as high amounts of meats and seafood, as well as drinks sweetened with high-fructose corn syrup (Becker, 2018b). Intake of low-fat or nonfat dairy products and vegetables is encouraged. Purine-rich vegetables like spinach, asparagus, cauliflower, and mushrooms should be avoided. The patient who is obese is advised to lose weight, but fasting is contraindicated for patients with gout. Alcohol intake should be limited and avoided altogether during an acute gouty arthritis attack. A liberal fluid intake to maintain a daily urinary output of 2000 mL or more is recommended to increase urate excretion and reduce the risk of urinary stone formation.

Treatment

Treatment for gout, in addition to medications, include dietary management and rest. During an acute attack of gouty arthritis, rest of the involved joint(s) is prescribed. The affected joint may be elevated and ice packs applied for comfort.

Nursing Care

Patients with gout provide self-care at home. Teaching focuses on self-management of pain and altered mobility.

Assessment

Reviewing the patient's medical record and history will give the nurse the information needed to assist in developing a care plan appropriate for the patient. Assessing the patient's knowledge of the issue as well as physical assessment for manifestations will add data to develop the care plan.

Priorities of Care

Pain is a primary focus for nursing interventions in the patient experiencing an acute attack of gout. The patient's mobility is also impaired during an acute attack, both because of pain and prescribed activity limitations

Diagnoses, Outcomes, and Interventions

Pain is a primary focus for nursing interventions in the patient experiencing an acute attack of gout. The patient's mobility is also impaired during an acute attack, both because of pain and prescribed activity limitations.

Relieve Acute Pain. The pain associated with an attack of acute gouty arthritis is intense and accompanied by intense tenderness of the affected joint. Measures to alleviate the pain are vital in the initial period until anti-inflammatory medications become effective and the acute inflammatory response is relieved. The following are important in teaching about pain relief.

Expected Outcome: Patient will verbalize measures to effectively manage the pain of acute gouty arthritis.

The nurse will:

- Position the affected joint for comfort. Elevate the joint or extremity (usually the foot) on a pillow, maintaining alignment. A cold pack or ice may be applied intermittently to the affected joint(s), protecting the skin from cold injury. *Elevation and normal body alignment facilitate blood return from the affected joint, alleviating some of the edema. Ice is identified as an appropriate adjunctive measure to reduce pain and inflammation associated with acute gouty arthritis.*
- Protect the affected joint from pressure, placing a foot cradle on the bed to keep bed covers off the foot or wearing a protective shoe that keeps pressure off the joint. *A foot cradle keeps bed linens from applying pressure on the affected joint.*
- Take anti-inflammatory and antigout medications as prescribed. In the initial period, colchicine may be given several times a day. *These medications reduce the acute inflammatory response, gradually relieving discomfort. Taking the medications around the clock is important to attain and maintain a therapeutic blood level.*
- Take analgesics as prescribed. Avoid aspirin. *Supplemental analgesia may be necessary in the acute period until the inflammatory response is mediated. Aspirin interferes with the action of some anti-inflammatory drugs* (Adams et al., 2017).
- Maintain joint rest. *It is important to immobilize the affected joint and promote rest to prevent exacerbation of joint inflammation.*

Transitions of Care

If this is a recurrent issue, assist the patient to identify potential triggers for the flare-up of the tissue and include teaching to help minimize the triggers.

Discuss the following topics with the patient:

- Inform the patient that initial attacks cause no permanent damage but that recurrent attacks can lead to permanent damage and joint destruction. Discuss other potential effects of continued hyperuricemia, including tophaceous deposits in subcutaneous and other connective tissues. Discuss the potential for kidney damage and kidney stones.
- Stress the need to continue the medication until the physician discontinues it, even though the patient is free of manifestations of gout. Tell the patient to avoid, if possible, drugs that increase uric acid blood levels: Hydrochlorothiazide (HydroDIURIL), cyclosporine (Neoral, Sandimmune), furosemide (Lasix), and high doses of aspirin. Patients who need to reduce their risk of heart attack may safely take one baby aspirin each day.
- The importance of a high intake of fluids each day and avoiding the use of alcohol.

The Patient with Osteomalacia

Osteomalacia, often referred to as adult rickets, is a metabolic bone disorder characterized by inadequate or delayed mineralization of bone matrix in mature bone, resulting in softening of bones. Bone mineralization requires adequate calcium and phosphate ions in extracellular fluid. When either of these ions is insufficient, the bone matrix is not mineralized and cannot sustain weight bearing. Marked deformities of weight-bearing bone and pathologic fractures occur. Vitamin D deficiency is the most common cause of osteomalacia.

Osteomalacia has been rare in the United States because many foods are fortified with vitamin D, but its incidence is increasing among older adults and people who have limited sun exposure in the Americas, Europe, and parts of the Middle East (Creo, Thacher, Pettifor, Strand, & Fischer, 2016).

Pathophysiology

The two main causes of osteomalacia are (1) insufficient calcium absorption in the intestine due to a lack of calcium intake or vitamin D deficiency or resistance and (2) decreased phosphate absorption or increased losses of phosphate through the urine. In its natural form, vitamin D is obtained from certain foods and ultraviolet radiation of the sun. Vitamin D maintains adequate serum levels of calcium and phosphate for normal mineralization of the bone. Vitamin D deficiency or resistance to its action disrupts the normal mineralization of the bone, causing it to soften.

Impaired bone mineralization causes abnormalities in both cancellous and compact bone. The osteoid (the soft, noncalcified part of the matrix) continues to be produced but is not mineralized. This abnormal buildup of demineralized bone leads to gross deformities of the long bones, spine, pelvis, and skull because the bone is soft and unable to bear the weight and stress of body movement.

The causes of osteomalacia are summarized in **Box 40.2**.

BOX 40.2
Causes of Osteomalacia

VITAMIN D DEFICIENCY

- Inadequate dietary intake
- Lack of sun exposure
- Malabsorption: Gastric bypass, small-bowel disorders, gallbladder disease, chronic pancreatic insufficiency, treatment with orlistat (Alli, Xenical) or cholestyramine (LoCHOLEST, Questran)
- Drug effects: Isoniazid, rifampin, anticonvulsants

PHOSPHATE DEPLETION

- Inadequate intake
- Impaired absorption due to chronic antacid use
- Impaired renal tubular reabsorption due to either acquired or genetic disorders

SYSTEMIC ACIDOSIS

- Renal tubular acidosis
- Ureterosigmoidostomy
- Fanconi syndrome

BONE MINERALIZATION INHIBITORS

- Hypophosphatasia
- Sodium fluoride or disodium etidronate (Didronel)
- Aluminum intoxication

CHRONIC KIDNEY DISEASE

CALCIUM MALABSORPTION

Risk Factors

The major risk factors for vitamin D deficiency are a diet low in vitamin D, inadequate sun exposure, impaired intestinal absorption of fats (vitamin D is a fat-soluble vitamin), liver or kidney disorders that interfere with the metabolism of vitamin D to its active forms, and certain drugs. Aging plays a role; the body's ability to synthesize vitamin D in response to sun exposure declines with aging (Tabloski, 2014).

Hypophosphatemia can result from insufficient dietary intake, excessive losses through the urine or stool, or a shift into the cells. Alcohol abuse is the most common cause of hypophosphatemia because of related dietary deficiencies, vomiting, antacid use, and increased renal excretion of phosphate. Ingesting large amounts of nonabsorbable antacids increases phosphate losses in the stool. Several acquired and genetic disorders cause increased losses of phosphate in the urine.

Older adults, as a group, are at high risk for osteomalacia because of dietary deficiencies, age-related intestinal malabsorption, less effective vitamin D synthesis, and possible physical mobility limitations that restrict their exposure to sunlight.

Manifestations

Muscle fatigue and weakness, manifestations of vitamin D deficiency, may be noted before overt manifestations of osteomalacia are seen. This may be as simple as having difficulty changing from a lying to a sitting position and a sitting to a standing position. The manifestations of osteomalacia include bone pain and tenderness, which may be vague and generalized at first, then become more intense with activity as the disease progresses. This pain occurs most frequently in the pelvis, long bones of the extremities, spine, and ribs. A waddling gait may be due to pain and muscle weakness. Fractures occur as the disease progresses. Dorsal kyphosis may occur in severe cases. In contrast to osteoporosis, osteomalacia is not associated with a significant occurrence of hip fractures. Instead, pathologic fractures occur in the commonly weakened areas (e.g., distal radius and proximal femur).

Interprofessional Care

Osteomalacia may be difficult to differentiate from osteoporosis because the manifestations are very similar; however, once the specific cause is determined, appropriate therapy will correct the disorder.

Diagnosis

A history of inadequate dietary intake, chronic kidney disease, or some malabsorption states may suggest osteomalacia. Refer to Table 40.1, which compares the diagnostic findings of osteomalacia with those of osteoporosis and Paget disease. X-rays demonstrate the effects of generalized bone demineralization: Cancellous bone loss, cyst formation, compression fractures, bowing and bending deformities of the long bones, and osteoid deposits, particularly in the vertebral bodies and pelvis.

Laboratory tests include serum calcium, parathyroid hormone, phosphate, vitamin D (25-hydroxy $[OH]D_3$ or $1.25[OH]_2D_3$), and alkaline phosphatase levels. Calcium may be normal or low, depending on the cause of the disease. Calcium levels may be reduced when calcium absorption is impaired or in severe vitamin D deficiency. Secondary hypoparathyroidism may shift calcium from the bone into extracellular fluid, maintaining a normal serum calcium level. Parathyroid hormone is frequently elevated as a compensatory response to hypocalcemia in renal failure or vitamin D deficiency. Alkaline phosphatase is usually elevated.

Nutrition

Therapeutic management of osteomalacia usually involves administration of calcium and vitamin D supplements (800 International Units daily). Patients in whom metabolic activation of vitamin D is impaired may require a metabolite of the vitamin that does not require activation, such as ergocalciferol (D_2). Phosphate supplements may be indicated. Radiologic evidence of healing is often apparent within weeks of initiating therapy.

Nursing Care

Managing the patient with osteomalacia includes assessing the patient's current dietary intake of vitamin D, calcium, and phosphorus and exposure to ultraviolet light. It also includes managing patient responses to bone pain and tenderness, fractures, and muscle weakness.

Diagnoses, Outcomes, and Interventions

Provide Patient Teaching. A knowledge deficit regarding the causes and prevention of osteomalacia is the primary concern for the nurse to address.

Expected Outcome: The patient will be able to express adequate knowledge to manage or prevent osteomalacia and its complications.

The nurse will:

- Teach that the causes and the consequences of osteomalacia are important, not only for the patient with osteomalacia, but also for people at risk for developing the disease. *When milk and other dairy products began to be fortified with vitamin D, the incidence of childhood rickets decreased dramatically. Now many patients are unaware of the importance of vitamin D, calcium, and phosphorus to bone health.*
- Teach older adults about the importance of maintaining an adequate intake of milk and other dairy products that are not only rich in calcium and phosphorus, but are also fortified with vitamin D. Few other food sources provide enough vitamin D to meet recommended levels. Cod liver oil may be used as a supplement because it contains significant amounts of vitamin D. *Supplements are not recommended, however, for patients who get adequate vitamin D through dietary sources and sun exposure because this fat-soluble vitamin may become toxic at very high levels. Instruct patients who are taking supplements to report to their primary care provider symptoms such as anorexia, nausea and vomiting, frequent urination, muscle weakness, and constipation that may be indicative of hypervitaminosis D.*
- Teach the patient with osteomalacia about safety measures to prevent falls. Discuss the importance of eliminating scatter rugs and clutter from living areas to prevent tripping. Teach the patient to place a nightlight in hallways and in the bathroom to prevent falls associated with nighttime toileting. Suggest installing grab bars in the shower and tub and next to the toilet for safety. *Prevention is the best way to prevent associated fractures with osteomalacia.*
- Teach patients with bone pain and muscle weakness to use assistive devices such as walkers, canes, or crutches when ambulating. Provide referrals to physical therapy for teaching patients how to safely use these devices. *The use of assistive devices will increase stability, thus reducing the risk for falls.*
- Encourage patients to participate in a supervised exercise program such as water aerobics or tai chi to improve muscle strength and balance. *Exercise increases muscle strength and balance, reducing the risk for falls.*

40.2 Degenerative Disorders

Degenerative musculoskeletal disorders, osteoarthritis in particular, are among the most common causes of pain and disability in adults and older adults. Muscular dystrophy, a degenerative muscle disorder, affects significantly fewer people but can have devastating effects.

The Patient with Osteoarthritis

Osteoarthritis (OA) (also called *degenerative joint disease*) is the most commonly occurring of all forms of arthritis and a leading cause of pain and disability in older adults (Centers for Disease Control and Prevention [CDC], 2018b). This disease is characterized by progressive loss of joint cartilage, synovitis (inflammation of the synovium lining the joint), joint pain, stiffness, and loss of joint motion. OA may be idiopathic or secondary, although it may be difficult to differentiate between primary and secondary OA.

OA affects nearly 54.4 million Americans; it is uncommon in adults under age 40 and prevalent in older adults (CDC, 2017). Women are more often affected by OA than men (Barbour, Helmick, Boring, & Brady, 2017). The joints most affected are in the hand, neck, lower back, hip, and knee. Men are more likely than women to have hip OA, whereas postmenopausal women more often have hand OA.

Pathophysiology

The cartilage that lines joints provides a smooth surface, so that the bones of the joint glide over one another without friction, and it distributes the load from one bone to the next, dissipating the mechanical stress that occurs with joint loading. This cartilage normally contains more than 70% water. More than 90% of its dry weight is collagen, which provides strength, and proteoglycans, which provide elasticity and stiffness to compression. Chondrocytes, cartilage cells, nest in this meshwork of collagen and proteoglycans. Chondrocytes regularly break down worn joint cartilage and synthesize the components to replace it. Normal articular cartilage exudes some of its water with compression, providing lubrication for joint surfaces. This water is reabsorbed during relaxation of the joint.

In OA, proteoglycans and collagen are lost from the cartilage as a result of enzymatic degradation. The water content of the cartilage increases as the collagen matrix is destroyed. With the loss of proteoglycans and collagen fibers, the cartilage becomes yellow or brownish gray and loses its tensile strength. Surface ulcerations occur, and fissures develop in deeper layers of the cartilage. Eventually, large areas of articular cartilage are lost, and underlying bone is exposed. The bone thickens in exposed areas, reducing its ability to absorb energy in joint loading. Cysts can develop in the bone as synovial fluid leaks through damaged cartilage. Cartilage-coated *osteophytes* (bony outgrowths) change the anatomy of the joint. As these spurs or projections enlarge, small pieces may break off, leading to mild synovitis (inflammation of the synovial membrane).

Risk Factors

Increasing age is the primary risk factor for OA. Its incidence and prevalence increase significantly with age. Joint cartilage thins with aging and is less able to respond to joint loading than cartilage in younger adults. Genetics can also play a role: A strong genetic linkage has been identified for OA of the hand and the knee (Kalunian, 2017).

Excessive weight contributes to the development of OA, especially in the hip and knee. Increasing body weight significantly increases the load placed on the knees during walking. An increased risk for OA of the hands suggests there also may be a metabolic risk factor associated with obesity. Inactivity is another risk factor. Moderate recreational exercise has been shown to both decrease the chance of developing OA and the progression of manifestations when OA is present. Repetitive joint use, however, also increases the risk for OA. People involved in occupations that require regular bending of the knee or hips or carrying heavy loads have increased risk for hip, knee, or spine OA. Textile mill workers have a higher rate of OA involving the interphalangeal joints. People involved in strenuous, repetitive exercise (such as participating in sports) have an increased risk of developing OA, particularly of the hip or knee.

Manifestations

The onset of OA is usually gradual and insidious and slowly progressive. Pain and stiffness in one or more joints (usually weight bearing) are the first manifestations of OA. The pain is localized to the affected joints and may be described as a deep ache. It is typically associated with use or motion of the joint and relieved by rest, although it may become persistent as the disease progresses. Pain at night may be accompanied by paresthesias (numbness, tingling). Pain may be referred to other parts of the body; for example, OA of the lumbosacral spine may cause severe pain along the path of the sciatic nerve. Following periods of immobility, such as sleeping all night or after a long automobile ride, involved joints may stiffen. Usually only a few minutes of activity are necessary to relieve the stiffness. Range of motion (ROM) of the joint decreases as the disease progresses and grating or crepitus may be noted during movement. Bony overgrowth may cause joint enlargement (**Figure 40.4** ■), and flexion contractures may occur because of joint instability. In OA, enlarged joints are characteristically bony-hard and cool on palpation. Manifestations specific to affected joints are outlined in **Table 40.3**.

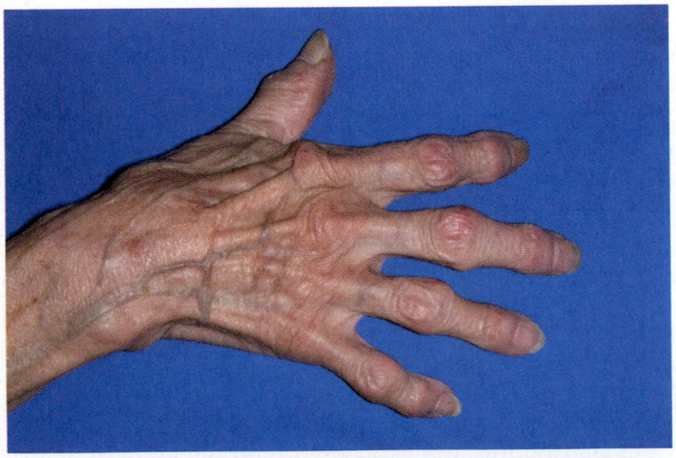

Figure 40.4 ■ Typical interphalangeal joint changes associated with osteoarthritis.

Table 40.3 Manifestations of Osteoarthritis by Affected Joint

Affected Site	Manifestations
Interphalangeal joints	■ *Heberden nodes*—bony enlargements of distal interphalangeal (DIP) joints ■ *Bouchard nodes*—bony enlargement of proximal interphalangeal (PIP) joints
First carpometacarpal	■ Edema, tenderness at base of thumb ■ Crepitus with movement ■ "Squared" appearance of joint
Spine	■ Localized pain and stiffness ■ Muscle spasm ■ Limited range of motion ■ Nerve root compression with radicular pain and motor weakness
Hips	■ Pain referred to inguinal area, buttock, thigh, or knee ■ Loss of internal rotation ■ Limited extension, adduction, and flexion
Knees	■ Pain and bony enlargement ■ Effusions ■ Crepitus ■ Instability (buckling) and deformity with advanced disease ■ Flexion contracture may develop

The presentation of OA in older patients is similar to that in younger adults. However, in this population, the risk of debilitation because of OA is greater, and the disease may progress faster. In addition, pain, stiffness, and limited ROM increase the risk of falls and fractures in the older adult.

Complications

Complications associated with osteoarthritis include pain, stiffness, limited mobility, and destruction of the articulation surfaces of the joint. These issues often lead to the necessity of surgical intervention.

Interprofessional Care

The primary treatment goals for the patient with osteoarthritis are to (1) control discomfort, (2) improve or maintain joint function and mobility, and (3) reduce or prevent physical disability.

Diagnosis

The diagnosis of OA is generally based on the patient's history, physical examination, and x-rays of affected joints. Characteristic changes of OA are visible in x-ray studies of affected joints. Initially, irregular joint space narrowing is seen. Progressive changes include increased density of subchondral (under cartilage) bone, osteophyte formation at the joint periphery, and the formation of cysts in the bone. In some cases, MRI may be done to determine the extent of joint damage. Examination of synovial fluid from involved joints can help rule out other types of arthritis (e.g., inflammatory arthritis, gout).

Medications

When the pain of OA cannot be managed by conservative treatment (see the following section) it often can be managed through the use of mild analgesics such as OTC NSAIDs (ibuprofen). NSAIDs such as ibuprofen (Motrin) or naproxen (Aleve) are prescribed to relieve the pain and stiffness associated with OA of the hip or knee. Treatment guidelines recommend that NSAIDs be given together with a proton-pump inhibitor to reduce the risk for gastrointestinal bleeding (Deveza, 2017). Acetaminophen (Tylenol) has been found to not have a lot of benefit for osteoarthritis patients (Machado et al., 2015). A selective COX-2 inhibitor (celecoxib or Celebrex) may be ordered for patients with a history of GI bleeding or who do not tolerate other NSAIDs. The following section on rheumatoid arthritis provides more information about these drugs.

Strong evidence also supports the use of topical NSAIDs (e.g., diclofenac topical gel [Pennsaid]) and capsaicin (Capzasin, Zostrix) for relief of OA pain, particularly for people age 75 and older (Deveza, 2017). These drugs have the advantage of minimizing systemic adverse effects. The patient should be taught to keep the medications away from the eyes, nose, mouth, or any open skin and not to bandage or apply heat to the treated area. The products should be used no more than three or four times a day and discontinued immediately if severe irritation occurs. Up to 2 weeks of regular use may be necessary for full effect.

Potent anti-inflammatory medications, such as systemic corticosteroids, are seldom prescribed for patients with OA, although intra-articular corticosteroid injections may be used. With intra-articular injections, a long-acting corticosteroid medication, often mixed with a local anesthetic such as lidocaine, is injected directly into the joint space of the affected joints. However, there is little evidence to support the use of corticosteroid injections (Juni et al., 2015). Intra-articular hyaluronic acid (HA) is an option for patients with OA of the knee joint. HA is a component of synovial fluid; it also appears to have anti-inflammatory effects. It is given in a series of three or five weekly intra-articular injections and may be effective for as long as 6 months following completion of the series. A recent review of the research studies performed using HA have shown only small clinical benefits for patients receiving these injections (Deveza, 2017).

Prescription analgesics such as tramadol or an opioid analgesic may be necessary for patients with advanced OA and moderate to severe pain. See Chapter 9 for a more detailed discussion about acute and chronic pain management.

Treatment

Conservative measures, including regular exercise and weight loss as indicated, are primary components of the treatment plan for OA. These may include any or all of the following:

- ROM exercises, muscle-strengthening exercises, aerobic exercises; walking, quadriceps-strengthening exercises, yoga, tai chi, and water-based exercises are recommended
- Heat and ice
- A balance between exercise and rest

- Use of a cane, crutches, or a walker as needed
- Weight loss, if indicated.

Surgery

Surgical procedures can provide dramatic results for patients with significant chronic pain and loss of joint function. Although elective surgical procedures are frequently avoided in the older adult, even they can benefit significantly if they do not have a chronic medical condition that contraindicates surgery.

Arthroscopy. **Arthroscopy** is a surgical procedure in which an arthroscope is inserted into a joint to diagnose the type of arthritis or to perform debridement by smoothing rough cartilage and flushing out the joint to remove debris. Although arthroscopic debridement and lavage of involved joints have been used, arthroscopy has not proven effective in the treatment of knee OA (Mandl & Martin, 2017). It may be useful to remove large pieces of debris or repair torn cartilage or to introduce autologous chondrocyte grafts for patients with localized articular surface damage (Mandl & Martin, 2017).

Osteotomy. An *osteotomy*, an incision into or transection of the bone, may be performed to realign an affected joint, particularly when significant bony overgrowth or osteophyte formation has occurred. This procedure may also be used to shift the joint load toward areas of less severely damaged cartilage. Although osteotomy does not halt the progress of OA, it may have a beneficial effect on joint function and pain, delaying the need for a joint replacement by several years.

Joint Arthroplasty. A joint **arthroplasty** is the reconstruction or replacement of a joint. Arthroplasty is usually indicated when the patient has severely restricted joint mobility and pain at rest. Pain from the osteoarthritis (OA) is virtually eliminated, and the function of the joint is generally improved. Arthroplasty may involve partial joint replacement (hemiarthroplasty) or, for most patients with OA, both surfaces of the affected joint are replaced with prosthetic parts in a procedure known as a *total joint replacement*. Joints that may be replaced include the hip, knee, shoulder, elbow, ankle, wrist, and joints of the fingers and toes.

In a total joint replacement, some or all of the synovium, cartilage, ligaments, and bone on both sides of the joint are removed. A metallic (cobalt and chromium alloy or titanium) prosthesis is inserted to replace one joint surface (generally the load-end or distal portion of a weight-bearing joint). The other joint surface is replaced with a corresponding metallic prosthesis; however, these are usually lined polyethylene (a type of plastic) to allow smooth movement of the joint.

Prosthetic joints may be either cemented or uncemented. Uncemented prosthetics are made with a porous outer coating on the components that are inserted so they fit tightly into existing bone. The implant is secured by new bone growth into the prosthesis, a process that requires approximately 3 months. Although a longer period of limited weight bearing is necessary until the prosthesis is fixed in place by the bony growth, the implant appears to have a longer useful lifespan than cemented prostheses. In a cemented joint replacement, a pliable polymer that hardens to hold the prosthesis in place is used to secure the prosthesis to existing bone. Cemented joint replacements are more commonly used in older adults and in those who have osteoporosis.

- ***Total hip replacement*** involves replacing the articular surfaces of the acetabulum and femoral head. The entire head of the femur and part of the femoral neck are removed and replaced with a prosthesis (**Figure 40.5** ■). The acetabulum is remodeled and an appropriately shaped prosthesis of high-molecular-weight polyethylene is inserted. The success rate for total hip replacement is reported to be greater than 90%. Approximately 310,000 total hip replacements are done each year in the United States; most are for treatment of OA (Wolford, Palso, & Bercovitz, 2015). Most hip replacements last 10 to 15 years, after which a second joint replacement, a revision, can be performed. Potential problems associated with a total hip replacement include venous thromboembolic events, dislocation within the prosthesis, loosening of joint components from surrounding bone, and infection. Minimally invasive total hip arthroplasty may shorten healing time, reduce blood loss, and has a lower risk of associated complications; however, evidence has been mixed for these claims (Erens & Crowley, 2017). Minimally invasive surgical techniques use the same size of prosthetic components but consist of smaller incisions with smaller instruments through which the components are inserted.
- ***Total knee replacement*** is performed if the patient has intractable pain and x-ray films show evidence of arthritis of the knee. An estimated 693,400 knee replacements were performed in the United States in 2010 (Williams, Wolford & Bercovitz, 2015). Several prosthetic devices

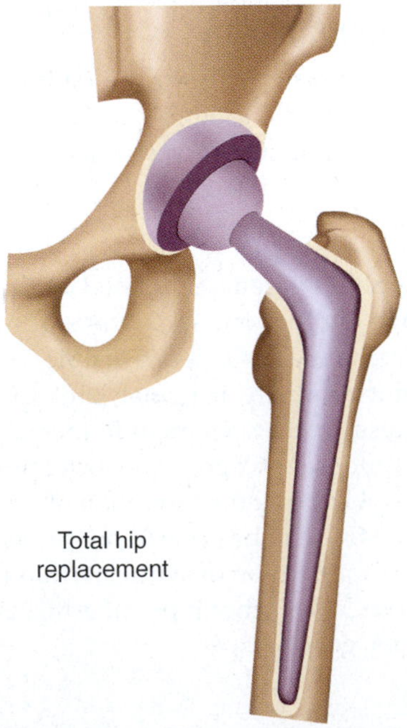
Total hip
replacement

Figure 40.5 ■ Total hip prosthesis.

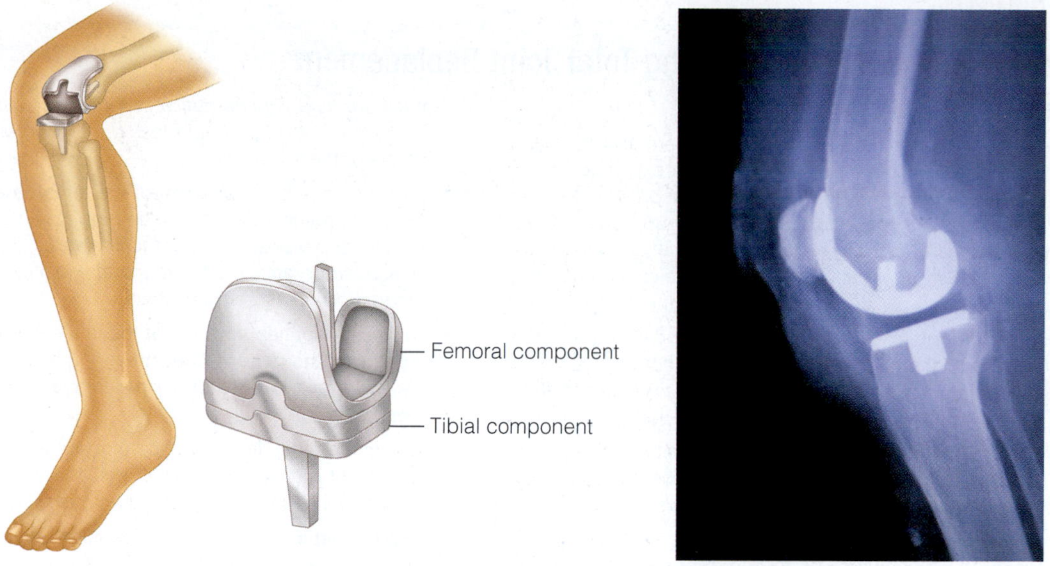
Femoral component
Tibial component

Figure 40.6 ■ One type of total knee implant.

involving removal of varying amounts of bone are available for knee joint replacement (**Figure 40.6** ■). The femoral side of the joint is replaced with a metallic surface, and the tibial side with polyethylene. More than 80% of patients obtain significant or total relief of pain with a total knee replacement. They must, however, engage in a vigorous program of rehabilitation to achieve the best results. Joint failure is more common with knee replacement than with a total hip replacement. Loosened joint components, often on the tibial side, are the most common cause of failure. The possible complications following a total knee replacement are the same as for a total hip replacement.

- ***Total shoulder replacement*** is indicated for unremitting pain and marked limitation of ROM because of arthritic involvement of both the humeral and glenoid joint surfaces of the shoulder. Following surgery, the joint is immobilized in a sling or abduction splint for 2 to 3 weeks following arthroplasty. Dislocation, loosening of the prosthesis, and infection are potential problems associated with total shoulder replacement.
- ***Total elbow replacement*** involves replacement of the humeral and ulnar surfaces of the elbow joint with a metal and polyethylene prosthesis. Pain and disabling stiffness of the joint are indications for an elbow arthroplasty. Complications, including dislocation, fracture, tricep weakness, loosening, and infection, occur frequently.

Infection is the major complication associated with total joint replacement. Not only does infection interfere with healing and prolong recovery, but it may also necessitate removal of the prosthesis and may lead to loss of joint function. Other potential complications include circulatory impairment to the affected limb, thromboembolism, nerve damage, and dislocation of the joint.

Nursing care for the patient undergoing total joint replacement is outlined in **Box 40.3**.

Physical Therapy and Rehabilitation

Recovery from all types of joint replacement requires postoperative physical therapy, focusing on building strength and regaining joint flexibility. Rehabilitation begins in the hospital, most often the day following surgery, and may be continued during home care. Recovery from a hip replacement is 80% complete in 4 weeks and 100% complete in 6 months. Recovery from a knee replacement is 80% complete in 4 weeks and 100% complete after 1 year. During rehabilitation, the patient must follow a regimen of exercise, rest, and medication.

Integrative Therapies

The following complementary therapies are examples of those that may be used by people with OA to relieve pain and stiffness. These same therapies are used by people with rheumatoid arthritis.

- Biomagnetic therapy
- Acupuncture; studies have demonstrated a beneficial effect of acupuncture for relieving pain and promoting mobility in patients with OA (Barrows, 2013)
- Eliminating nightshade foods such as potatoes, tomatoes, peppers, eggplant, and tobacco
- Taking nutritional supplements, such as glucosamine, chondroitin, boron, zinc, copper, selenium, manganese, flavonoids, and/or SAM-e. The evidence supporting use of glucosamine with or without chondroitin shows these agents are often helpful to reduce pain associated with hip and knee osteoarthritis. There is limited evidence that glucosamine and/or chondroitin slow the progression of OA (Barrows, 2013).
- Herbal therapy
- Massage therapy

BOX 40.3
Nursing Care of the Patient Having Total Joint Replacement

PREOPERATIVE CARE

- Assess the patient's knowledge and understanding of the planned operative procedure. Provide further explanations and clarification as needed. *It is important for the patient to have a clear and realistic understanding of the surgical procedure and expected results. Knowledge decreases anxiety and increases the patient's ability to assist with postoperative care procedures.*
- Obtain a health history and physical assessment, including ROM of the affected joints. *This information not only allows nurses to tailor care to the needs of the individual but also serves as a baseline for comparison of postoperative assessment data.*
- Explain necessary postoperative activity restrictions. Teach how to use the overhead trapeze for changing positions. *The patient who learns and practices moving techniques before surgery can use them more effectively in the postoperative period.*
- Provide or reinforce teaching of postoperative exercises specific to the joint on which surgery is to be performed. *Exercises are prescribed postoperatively to (1) strengthen muscles providing joint stability and support, (2) prevent muscle atrophy and joint contractures, and (3) prevent venous stasis and possible thromboembolism.*
- Teach respiratory hygiene procedures such as the use of incentive spirometry, coughing, and deep breathing. *Adequate respiratory hygiene is imperative for all patients undergoing joint replacement to prevent respiratory complications associated with immobility and the effects of anesthesia. In addition, many patients undergoing total joint replacement are elderly and may have reduced mucociliary clearance.*
- Discuss postoperative pain control, including use of patient-controlled analgesia (PCA) or epidural infusion as appropriate. *It is important for the patient to understand the purpose and use of postoperative pain control measures to allow early mobility and reduce complications associated with immobility.*
- Teach or provide prescribed preoperative skin preparation such as shower, shampoo, and skin scrub with antibacterial solution. *These measures help reduce transient bacteria that may be introduced into the surgical site.*
- Administer intravenous antibiotic as ordered. *Antibiotic therapy is initiated before or during surgery and continued postoperatively to further reduce the risk of infection.*

POSTOPERATIVE CARE

- Monitor vital signs, including temperature and level of consciousness, every 4 hours or more frequently as indicated. Report significant changes or unanticipated findings to the physician. *These routine assessments provide information about the patient's cardiovascular status and can give early indications of complications such as excessive bleeding, fluid volume deficit, and infection.*
- Perform neurovascular checks (color, temperature, pulses and capillary refill, movement, and sensation) on the affected limb hourly for the first 12 to 24 hours, then every 2 to 4 hours. Report abnormal findings to the physician immediately. *Surgery can disrupt the blood supply to or innervation of the affected extremity. If so, rapid intervention is important to preserve the function of the extremity.*
- Monitor incisional bleeding by emptying and recording suction drainage every 4 hours and assessing the dressing frequently. *Significant blood loss can occur with a total joint replacement, particularly a total hip replacement.*
- Reinforce the dressing as needed. *The dressing is usually changed 24 to 48 hours after surgery but may need reinforcement if excess bleeding occurs.*
- Maintain intravenous infusion and accurate intake and output records during the initial postoperative period. *The patient is at risk for fluid volume deficit in the initial postoperative period because of blood and fluid loss during surgery, as well as the effects of the anesthetic.*
- Maintain prescribed position of the affected extremity using a sling, abduction splint, brace, immobilizer, or other prescribed device. *Proper positioning of the affected extremity is vital in the initial postoperative period so that the joint prosthesis does not become dislocated or displaced.*
- Remind the patient to use the incentive spirometer, to cough, and to breathe deeply at least every 2 hours. *These measures are important to prevent respiratory complications such as pneumonia.*
- Assess the patient's level of comfort frequently. Maintain PCA, epidural infusion, or other prescribed analgesia to promote comfort. *Adequate pain management promotes healing and mobility.*
- Help the patient get out of bed as soon as allowed. Teach and reinforce the use of techniques to prevent weight bearing on the affected extremity, such as the overhead trapeze, pivot turning, and toe touch. *Early mobility prevents complications such as pneumonia and thromboembolism, but appropriate techniques must be used to prevent injury to the operative site.*
- Initiate physical therapy and exercises as prescribed for the specific joint replaced, such as quadriceps setting, leg raising, and passive and active ROM exercises. *These exercises help prevent muscle atrophy and thromboembolism and strengthen the muscles of the affected extremity so that it can support the prosthetic joint.*
- Use sequential compression devices or antiembolism stockings as prescribed. *These help prevent thromboembolism and pulmonary embolus for the patient who must remain immobile following surgery.*
- For the patient with a total hip replacement, prevent hip flexion of greater than 90 degrees or adduction of the affected leg. Provide a seat riser for the toilet or commode. *These measures prevent dislocation of the joint.*
- Assess the patient with a total hip replacement for signs of prosthesis dislocation, including pain in the affected hip or shortening and internal rotation of the affected leg.
- For the patient with a total knee replacement, use a continuous passive range-of-motion (CPM) device or ROM exercises as prescribed. *Dislocation is not a problem with a knee replacement, and more emphasis is placed on ROM exercises in the early postoperative period.*
- Maintain fluid intake and encourage a high-fiber diet. Administer stool softeners or rectal suppositories as needed. *Immobility and analgesia contribute to the potential problem of constipation; these measures help maintain regular fecal elimination.*
- Encourage consumption of a well-balanced diet with adequate protein. *Adequate nutrition promotes tissue healing.*
- Teach or reinforce postdischarge exercises and activity restrictions. Emphasize the importance of scheduled follow-up physician visits. *Patients are discharged from the acute care facility before healing is complete. Exercises are prescribed and activities are resumed gradually to protect the integrity of the joint replacement and prevent contractures.*
- For those patients needing additional direct care after discharge, arrange placement in a long-term care or rehabilitation facility. *Activity restrictions may preclude discharge to home for some patients.*
- Make referrals as needed to home health agencies and physical therapy. *Patients often require home healthcare for both nursing care needs and continued physical therapy following discharge from acute or long-term care.*

- Osteopathic manipulation
- Vitamin therapy
- Yoga.

Nursing Care

OA is a chronic process for which there is no cure. The focus of nursing care for the patient with OA is providing comfort, helping maintain mobility and ADLs, teaching, and assisting with adaptations to maintain life roles. See the Case Study & Nursing Care Plan for a patient with OA.

Assessment

Collect the following data through the health history and physical examination:

- ***Health history:*** Family history of OA; occupation; recreational activities; joint pain, stiffness; ability to carry out daily living activities
- ***Physical assessment:*** Height/weight; gait; joints: symmetry, size, shape, color, appearance, temperature, pain, crepitus, ROM, Heberden nodes, Bouchard nodes, muscle strength.

Priorities of Care

Nursing care priorities for the patient with OA vary with the circumstances of the patient's interaction with the healthcare system. Maintaining circulation and tissue perfusion is of highest priority for the patient admitted with acute gastrointestinal bleeding related to chronic aspirin or NSAID use, whereas promoting comfort and mobility are priorities for the patient for whom osteoarthritis is either the primary or a secondary health issue.

Diagnoses, Outcomes, and Interventions

Nursing interventions for patients with OA are directed toward managing chronic pain, facilitating physical mobility, and improving ability to provide self-care.

Manage Chronic Pain. Pain is a primary manifestation of OA. As joint tissues degenerate and changes in joint structure occur, the amount of discomfort generally increases. The pain associated with OA increases with activity and tends to be relieved with rest. Nonpharmacologic comfort measures are appropriate, with mild analgesics used to supplement these as needed.

Expected Outcome: Patient will report pain within an acceptable level.

The nurse will:

- Monitor the level of pain, including intensity, location, quality, and aggravating and relieving factors. *Accurate assessment of pain provides a basis for evaluation of the effect of interventions.*
- Teach patients to take prescribed analgesic or anti-inflammatory medication as directed. *Analgesics reduce the perception of pain and may decrease muscle spasm as well. Anti-inflammatory medication may be ordered to decrease local inflammatory response in affected joints. Regularly scheduled doses of an analgesic or NSAID may be prescribed to prevent severe pain, muscle spasm, or inflammation.*
- Encourage rest of painful joints. *The pain of OA is often relieved by joint rest.*
- Suggest applying heat to painful joints using the shower, a tub or sitz bath, warm packs, hot wax baths, heated gloves, or diathermy, which uses high-frequency electrical currents to generate heat. *Heat application reduces pain and disability and improves quality of life in patients with osteoarthritis.*
- Emphasize the importance of proper posture and good body mechanics for walking, sitting, lifting, and moving. *Good body mechanics and posture reduce stress on affected joints.*
- Encourage the overweight patient to reduce weight. *Excess weight places abnormal stress on joints, particularly the knees.*
- Encourage the use of nonpharmacologic pain relief measures such as progressive relaxation, meditation, visualization, and distraction. *These adjunctive pain relief measures can reduce the patient's reliance on analgesics and increase comfort.*

Promote Physical Mobility. As intra-articular cartilage degenerates and joint structures are altered, the patient with OA experiences pain, stiffness, and decreased ROM in affected joints. When the spine, large weight-bearing joints of the hips and knees, or the ankles and feet are affected, physical mobility can be significantly reduced.

Expected Outcome: Patient will maintain physical mobility and ability to perform desired and daily living activities.

The nurse will:

- Assess the ROM of affected joints. *Assessing joint mobility is important as a basis for planning appropriate interventions.*
- Perform a functional mobility assessment, evaluating gait, ability to sit and rise from a sitting position, ability to step into and out of the tub or shower, and negotiation of stairs. *The functional assessment provides vital data about the patient's ability to maintain ADLs.*
- Teach active and passive ROM exercises as well as isometric, progressive resistance, and low-impact aerobic exercises. *Active ROM exercises help maintain muscle tone and mobility of affected joints and prevent contractures. Isometric and progressive resistance exercises improve muscle tone and strength; aerobic exercise improves endurance and cardiovascular fitness.*
- Collaborate with physical and/or occupational therapists to recommend braces or mobility aids as appropriate. *Use of braces to support unstable joints or mobility aids such as a cane reduce the pressure on and risk of injury to joints affected by OA.*

Promote Self-Care. Just as OA of the lower extremities can reduce the patient's mobility, OA of the upper extremities (the wrist, hand, and finger joints in particular) can significantly interfere with performance of ADLs such as cooking and brushing the hair. When the lower extremities are affected, bathing and toileting can be difficult.

Expected Outcome: The patient will identify strategies to enhance self-care.

The nurse will:

- Perform a functional assessment of the upper and lower extremities. For upper extremities, assess the ability to touch the back of the head and to hold and use small items such as eating utensils. *The functional assessment provides important data about the patient's ability to provide self-care.*
- Assess the home setting to determine the need for assistive devices such as handrails, grab bars, walk-in shower stall, or shower chair and handheld showerhead. *Many assistive devices are relatively easy and inexpensive to obtain and can significantly improve the patient's independence.*
- Assist in obtaining other assistive devices such as long-handled shoehorns, zipper grabbers, long-handled tongs or grippers for retrieving items from the floor, jar openers, and special eating utensils. Collaborate with occupational therapy as needed. *These devices can prolong independence in performing ADLs. Occupational therapy has the knowledge to add to these devices as appropriate.*

Delegating Nursing Care Activities

As appropriate and allowed by the designated duties and responsibilities of unlicensed assistive personnel, the nurse may delegate nursing care activities such as assisting with ambulation, hygiene, and ADLs for the patient with osteoarthritis. With appropriate training and supervision, assistive personnel may assist with heat and cold application to affected joints as ordered.

Transitions of Care

Although OA cannot be prevented, maintaining a normal weight and having a program of regular, moderate exercise will reduce risk factors. Moderate exercise is protective; however, sports-related injuries have been shown to

Case Study & Nursing Care Plan

A Patient with Osteoarthritis

Robert Cerulli, a 72-year-old retired fisherman, seeks medical attention for pain in his right hip that has become severe during the past year. Significant degenerative changes in both hip joints are noted on x-ray films. The physician recommends a total replacement of the right hip. Mr. Cerulli has preoperative teaching and tests the afternoon prior to his surgery, scheduled for 0800 the following morning.

ASSESSMENT	DIAGNOSES	EXPECTED OUTCOMES
Christie Phlaugh, RN, completes an admission health history and examination. She notes that Mr. Cerulli has mild Parkinson disease and is taking carbidopa/levodopa (Sinemet 25-100) four times a day to control his symptoms. No other chronic medical conditions have been reported. Mr. Cerulli says he has been essentially healthy his entire life. He has no known allergies to medications, has never smoked, and consumes only small amounts of alcohol. On examination, Ms. Phlaugh notes that he is alert and oriented. His vital signs are BP 116/64 mmHg, P 68 bpm and regular, R 18/min, T 36.3°C (97.4°F) PO. Peripheral pulses are 2+ and equal in the upper extremities, and 1+ but equal in the lower extremities. His feet are cool to touch but have immediate capillary refill. He has full ROM of his shoulders, elbows, and wrists. The ROM of both hips is significantly restricted. Hip flexion beyond 90 degrees prompts pain on both sides. Both flexion and extension of the knees are limited slightly. Mr. Cerulli walks with a limp, favoring his right hip, and has a shuffling gait. Preoperative laboratory studies including CBC, coagulation studies, chemistry panel, and urinalysis show a serum creatinine of 1.7 mg/dL and BUN of 30 mg/dL, with no other abnormal values noted. Cefazolin (Ancef) 500 mg is to be administered intravenously at 0600 prior to surgery, and Mr. Cerulli is to shower and shampoo with antibacterial soap at bedtime. The physical therapist meets with Mr. Cerulli to evaluate his mobility and begin teaching him about postoperative weight-bearing restrictions.	■ Acute pain related to surgical incision ■ Potential for infection related to surgical incision ■ Potential for peripheral neurovascular complicates related to vascular disruption and edema ■ Limited physical mobility related to decreased muscle strength secondary to Parkinson disorder and surgical repair of the hip	■ Patient will maintain an adequate level of comfort postoperatively as demonstrated by verbal reports of pain at 2 or lower on a standard pain scale of 0 to 10. ■ Patient will remain free of infection. ■ Patient will maintain circulation, sensation, and movement within the patient's own normal limits. ■ Patient will remain free of injury postoperatively. ■ Patient will verbalize feeling of increased strength and ability to move.

PLANNING AND IMPLEMENTATION

- Instruct in the use of PCA and monitor its effectiveness with pain assessments.
- Assess pain and sedation level at least hourly during first 24 to 48 hours postoperatively and as needed thereafter.
- Assess the surgical site frequently; report signs of excess bleeding or inflammation.
- Monitor temperature every 4 hours.
- Encourage the use of an incentive spirometer hourly for first 24 hours, then at least every 2 hours while awake.
- Maintain sequential compression device while in bed and/or antiembolic stockings, as ordered. Remove stockings daily for 1 hour.
- Maintain abduction of the right hip with pillows.
- Assess pulses, color, movement, and sensation of right foot hourly for the first 4 hours, then every 2 hours for 4 hours, then every 4 hours.
- Assist out of bed three times a day after the first 24 hours.
- Collaborate with physical therapy to increase ambulation, with appropriate assistive devices.

EVALUATION

Mr. Cerulli returns to the orthopedic unit from the postanesthesia care unit. He becomes confused and disoriented during the first 36 hours after surgery, but his orientation and thought processes gradually clear. His family has stayed with him, and he has not experienced injury or other adverse consequences from his confusion. Otherwise, Mr. Cerulli has had an uneventful postoperative recovery. Four days after surgery, he is transferred to an extended care rehabilitation facility for further therapy until he is able to ambulate with weight bearing, as tolerated, on his affected leg. He returns home 3 weeks after surgery, able to use a walker for ambulation. Arrangements are made for an overbed trapeze, elevated toilet seat, and shower chair in his home. A home health nurse and physical therapist visit Mr. and Mrs. Cerulli twice weekly for a month following his discharge. During this time, he gradually resumes full weight bearing. Mr. Cerulli expresses pleasure with the relief of his hip pain and says he has no fear of having his left hip replaced in the future.

CLINICAL REASONING IN PATIENT CARE

1. Patients rarely enter the healthcare system with a single diagnosis; Mr. Cerulli has Parkinson disease in addition to his osteoarthritis. Should Ms. Phlaugh develop nursing diagnoses and plan interventions related to this diagnosis and its current treatment?
2. What postoperative assessment findings should be anticipated related to Mr. Cerulli's diagnosis of Parkinson disease?
3. Does Parkinson disease or its management increase Mr. Cerulli's risk for intra- or postoperative complications? If so, what complications could be anticipated?
4. Mr. Cerulli's preoperative laboratory work showed a modest elevation in his serum creatinine and BUN. What do these studies indicate? How might these changes affect nursing responsibilities related to medication administration for Mr. Cerulli?
5. Mr. Cerulli became confused postoperatively. What factors in his history might have alerted the nurses to this possibility? How might anesthesia and postoperative analgesics have contributed to his confusion?
6. Develop a care plan for Mr. Cerulli to address his postoperative confusion.

See Evaluating Your Response in Appendix B.

increase the risk for OA. Advise patients that protective devices such as a knee brace can reduce this risk, particularly when a joint is unstable due to previous damage (e.g., ligament tears).

Because of the chronicity of OA, patients and their families need appropriate teaching to manage the disease and its consequences effectively. Much of the teaching focus is on preservation of joint function and mobility. Discuss the following topics:

- Safeguard against hazards to safe mobility, such as scatter rugs. Encourage installation of safety devices such as handrails and grab bars.
- Understand the disease process and its chronic degenerative nature.
- Learn exercise techniques, including ROM, isometric, postural, stretching, and strengthening, to maintain healthy cartilage, preserve ROM, and develop supportive muscles and tendons. A walking program is beneficial for patients with OA of the knee. Older adults may be more willing to exercise as part of a group or organized activity.
- Do not overuse or stress affected joints with heavy lifting, excessive stair climbing or bending, or other repetitive actions.
- Sit in a straight chair without slumping, avoid soft chairs or recliners, and sleep on a firm mattress or use a bed board.
- Use pain relief measures including prescribed or OTC analgesic medications and nonpharmacologic pain relief measures such as heat, rest, massage, relaxation, and meditation.

For the patient who has had a total joint replacement, discuss:

- Use and weight bearing of the affected limb
- Appropriate environmental modifications, such as an overhead trapeze for getting out of bed, elevated toilet seats, and types of chairs to use and avoid when sitting

- Prescribed exercises
- Use of assistive devices for ambulation, such as crutches or a walker
- Possible complications, including signs of infection or dislocation, and the need to notify the physician promptly if these occur.

Make referrals to home care, physical or occupational therapy, or other community agencies as indicated, and suggest the following resources:

- National Institute of Arthritis and Musculoskeletal and Skin Diseases
- Arthritis Foundation
- American College of Rheumatology
- Moss Rehab Resource Net.

The Patient with Muscular Dystrophy

Muscular dystrophy (MD) is a group of inherited muscle diseases that cause progressive muscle degeneration and wasting. The differences in the types of MD relate to the genetic pattern of transmission, the age at onset, the gender affected, the muscles involved, and the rate at which the disease progresses. These factors are summarized in **Table 40.4**. In most cases of MD, there is a positive family history.

Pathophysiology

Although the underlying genetic defect and cellular pathology differ among the muscular dystrophies, all are primary diseases characterized by progressive necrosis of muscle tissue. Fat and connective tissue replace muscle fibers, increasing size of the muscle while causing progressive weakness. Muscle weakness has an insidious onset but is relentlessly progressive. DMD, the best understood of the muscular dystrophies, results from mutation of the gene that codes for dystrophin, a protein necessary for stability of the sarcolemma. Instability leads to membrane tears, muscle necrosis, and a continuous process of repair, regeneration, and muscle fibrosis. Ultimately, there is almost complete loss of muscle fibers (Mayo Clinic, 2018).

Risk Factors

The most common form of MD, *Duchenne muscular dystrophy (DMD)*, is inherited as a recessive single-gene defect on the X chromosome (a sex-linked recessive disorder) and is transmitted from the mother to male children. This disorder predominantly affects males and occurs in 1 of 3500 live male births. Although rare, spontaneous mutation may cause the disorder in girls (Mayo Clinic, 2018). It can be recognized as early as the 12th week of pregnancy by DNA analysis of a chorionic villi sample. DNA analysis can also be used to identify female relatives who may carry the defective gene.

Manifestations and Complications

Manifestations of DMD appear in early childhood, with progressive muscle weakness ultimately leading to death from respiratory and cardiac muscle involvement by the late teens or early adulthood. Other types of MD have an onset at any age, and a slow progression with a normal lifespan.

All forms of MD exhibit manifestations of muscle weakness. The specific muscles involved depend on the type of MD. As the disease progresses, the person develops difficulty with ambulation and eventually becomes wheelchair-bound and finally bed-bound. Cardiac abnormalities, endocrine abnormalities, and mental retardation may also occur. The complications associated with the MD are related to the progression of the disease (see Table 40.4).

Interprofessional Care

Because there is no cure or specific treatment for MD, care focuses on preserving and promoting mobility. An interprofessional approach involving many members of the healthcare team is necessary to meet the physical and psychologic needs of these patients and their families. Diagnosis and classification of the muscular dystrophies are most

Table 40.4 Types of Muscular Dystrophy

Type	Sex and Age at Onset	Clinical Manifestations	Progression
Duchenne	Males Ages 3–5	■ Weakness of pelvic and shoulder girdles ■ Waddling gait ■ Toe walking ■ Lordosis ■ Cardiac abnormalities ■ Low IQ in 50% of cases	Rapid; patient usually confined to wheelchair by age 15; death occurs by age 20
Myotonic	Males and females Any age	■ Weakness and atrophy of facial muscles ■ Muscle weakness of distal extremities ■ Cardiac abnormalities ■ Endocrine abnormalities ■ Mental retardation (common)	Slow; death usually occurs in early 50s
Becker	Males Ages 5–20	■ Weakness of pelvic and shoulder girdles ■ Cardiac involvement, possible heart failure	Slow; patient usually confined to wheelchair at 25 years after onset; life span into 30s to 50s
Facioscapulohumeral	Males and females Ages 10–20	■ Weakness of face and shoulder girdles ■ Eventual involvement of abdominal, feet, and pelvic muscles	Slow; normal lifespan
Limb-girdle	Males and females Ages 15–40	■ Weakness of shoulder and pelvic girdles	Extremely variable; usually slow

often based on the manifestations and the pattern of muscle involvement. Biochemical examination, muscle biopsy, and electromyography confirm the diagnosis.

Diagnosis

Tests include measuring creatine kinase (CK-MM, the isoenzyme found in skeletal muscle), which is elevated in the patient with suspected MD; performing a muscle biopsy to identify fibrous connective tissue and fatty deposits that displace functional muscle fibers; and conducting an electromyogram (EMG), which will show a decrease in amplitude in MD. Genetic testing may be done to identify the specific defect. Muscle biopsy may be performed to establish the diagnosis.

Medications

There are no specific medications used to treat MD. However, a successful phase 1 clinical trial has been completed, using the drug omigapil (Callisto), to combat the muscle "floppiness" that occurs in children 5 to 16 years old with congenital MD (National Institutes for Health, 2018). Omigapil has been shown to be safe in use in patients with Parkinson and amyotrophic lateral sclerosis (AML). Omigapil was shown to regenerate muscle in mice (Olanow et al., 2006). This muscle regeneration is the aim of the clinical trial in hopes of increasing muscular strength and mobility in patients with congenital MD.

Nursing Care

Nursing care for a patient with MD focuses on promoting independence and mobility and providing psychologic support for both the patient and family. A holistic approach is essential in planning and implementing care.

Diagnoses, Outcomes, and Interventions

Promote Balance of Independence and Acceptance. The progressive muscle weakness that is associated with MD impairs the patient's ability to perform self-care.

Expected Outcome: Patient will accept assistance or total care from caregivers as needed.

The nurse will:

- Provide patients and family with supportive care during the progress of the disease. *The goal of treatment is to prolong each functional stage and delay or prevent deformity. When transition from ambulation to a wheelchair occurs, there may be feelings of depression and grief.*
- Promote realistic tasks for patients to avoid patient frustration. When the patient struggles with tasks beyond their functional level, frustration develops. *All forms of MD result in progressive muscle weakness. Management of the disease is directed toward keeping the patient as functional as possible while preventing any deformities.*
- Collaborate with physical and occupational therapy. *Collaboration with PT and OT can allow additional modes and methods of promoting self-care.*

Transitions of Care

Teaching the patient with MD focuses on maintaining function and independence and preventing deformities. Teach prescribed exercises such as stretching and counterposturing exercises. For the patient with braces, discuss skin care and ways to prevent irritation under the brace. Because the patient may have weakness involving muscles of respiration, teach the patient how to prevent respiratory infections, such as avoiding crowds during flu season and being immunized against pneumococcal pneumonia and influenza. Provide information about support services and organizations such as the Muscular Dystrophy Association.

40.3 Autoimmune and Inflammatory Musculoskeletal Disorders

Autoimmune and inflammatory disorders of the musculoskeletal system are characterized by diffuse inflammatory lesions and degenerative changes in connective tissues. The disorders have similar clinical features and may affect many of the same structures and organs.

The Patient with Rheumatoid Arthritis

Rheumatoid arthritis (RA) is a chronic systemic autoimmune disease that causes inflammation of connective tissue, primarily in the joints. Its course and severity are variable, and the range of manifestations is broad. Manifestations of RA may be minimal, with mild inflammation of only a few joints and little structural damage, or relentlessly progressive, with multiple inflamed joints and marked deformity. Most patients exhibit a pattern of symmetric involvement of multiple peripheral joints and periods of remission and exacerbation.

RA is less common than osteoarthritis. An estimated 27 million adults in the United States are affected by OA, whereas about 1.3 million Americans and as much as 1% worldwide have RA (Rheumatoid Arthritis Support Network, 2016). RA affects two to three times as many women as men. It is important to establish an accurate diagnosis because the management of these disorders differs significantly.

The cause of RA is unknown. Genetic factors have been found to play a role in its development, likely in combination with environmental factors. The role of estrogens in the immune response may account for the significantly higher incidence of RA among women when compared to men (Gabriel & Crowson, 2018). It is speculated that an infectious agent, such as mycoplasma, Epstein-Barr virus, or another virus, may play a role in initiating the abnormal immune responses present in RA. Several studies have found that cigarette smoking increases the risk for developing RA.

The course of RA is variable and fluctuating. Remissions are most likely to occur in the first year of the disease. Some people with RA have a single episode that resolves within 2 to 5 years after its onset, whereas others may have fluctuating disease activity. In the most severe disease course, RA was seen as progressive and unremitting before the introduction of disease-modifying antirheumatic drugs (DMARDs), which has increased the long-term functional outlook for patients (Venables & Maini, 2017). Life expectancy is shortened in people with RA, with cardiovascular disease, infection, renal impairment, and lymphoproliferative disorders being the leading causes of death (Venables & Maini, 2017).

Pathophysiology

It is believed that exposure to an unidentified antigen (e.g., a virus) causes an aberrant immune response in a genetically susceptible host. As a result, normal antibodies (immunoglobulins) become autoantibodies and attack host tissues. These transformed antibodies, usually present in people with RA, include *rheumatoid factors (RFs)* and *anti-CP antibodies*. The self-produced antibodies bind with their target antigens in blood, collagen, cartilage, and other proteins and tissues, forming immune complexes. Complement is activated by the immune complexes, prompting an inflammatory response in synovial and other involved tissues.

Leukocytes from the circulation are attracted to the synovial membrane of involved joints, where neutrophils and macrophages ingest the immune complexes and release enzymes that degrade synovial tissue and articular cartilage. Activation of B and T lymphocytes results in increased production of rheumatoid factors, anti-CP antibodies, and enzymes that increase and continue the inflammatory process.

The inflammatory and immune processes damage the synovial membrane. It swells from infiltration of the leukocytes and thickens as cells proliferate and abnormally enlarge. Prostaglandins promote vasodilation, and synovial cells and tissue become hyperactive. New blood vessels grow to support synovial hyperplasia, forming a vascular granulation tissue called *pannus*.

The joint damage that occurs in RA is the result of at least three processes:

- Inflammatory pannus spreads to cover joint cartilage and produces enzymes such as collagenase and other proteases that promote tissue damage (**Figure 40.7** ■)
- Cytokines, especially interleukin-1 (IL-1) and tumor necrosis factor alpha (TNF-α), activate chondrocytes to attack joint cartilage

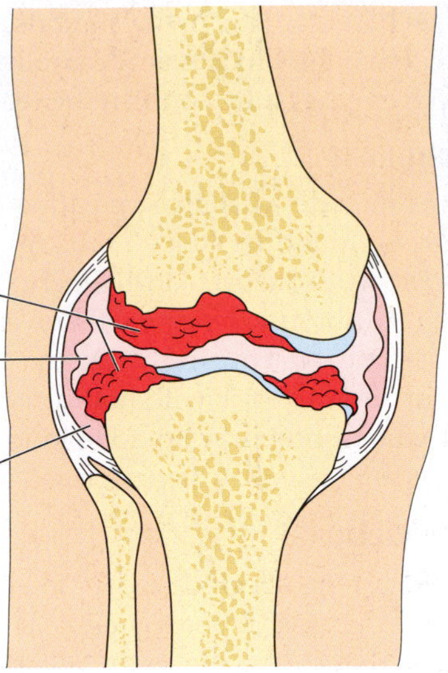
Pannus with areas of eroded cartilage and bone
Increased joint fluid
Inflamed synovium

Figure 40.7 ■ Joint inflammation and destruction in rheumatoid arthritis. Note synovial inflammation with pannus formation and the erosion of cartilage and underlying bone.

- These cytokines, along with IL-6, also activate osteoclasts, leading to resorption and demineralization of underlying bone.

Circulating immune complexes and the cytokines IL-1, TNF-α, and IL-6 account for the systemic features of RA as well, including malaise, fatigue, and vasculitis.

Risk Factors

Risk factors for the development of RA include genetic links, cigarette smoking, viral or bacterial triggers, and occupational exposure to silica and asbestos (Gabriel & Crowson, 2018).

Manifestations

Clinical features distinguishing RA from OA are listed in **Table 40.5** and manifestations of RA are shown in the Multisystem of Effects Rheumatoid Arthritis feature.

Table 40.5 Comparison of the Manifestations of Rheumatoid Arthritis and Osteoarthritis

Feature	Rheumatoid Arthritis	Osteoarthritis
Onset	■ Usually insidious, may be abrupt	■ Insidious
Course	■ Generally progressive ■ Characterized by remissions and exacerbations	■ Slowly progressive
Pain and stiffness	■ Predominant on arising, lasting >1 h ■ Also occurs after prolonged inactivity	■ Pain with activity ■ Stiffness following periods of immobility generally relieved within minutes
Affected joints	■ Appear red, hot, swollen; "boggy" and tender to palpation; decreased ROM, weakness ■ Multiple joints affected in symmetric pattern; PIP, MCP, wrists, knees, ankles, and toes often involved	■ Affected joints may appear swollen; cool and bony-hard on palpation; decreased ROM ■ One or several joints affected including hips, knees, lumbar and cervical spine, PIP and DIP, and first MTP joint
Systemic manifestations	■ Fatigue, weakness ■ Anorexia, weight loss ■ Fever ■ Rheumatoid nodules ■ Anemia	■ Fatigue

Multisystem Effects of Rheumatoid Arthritis

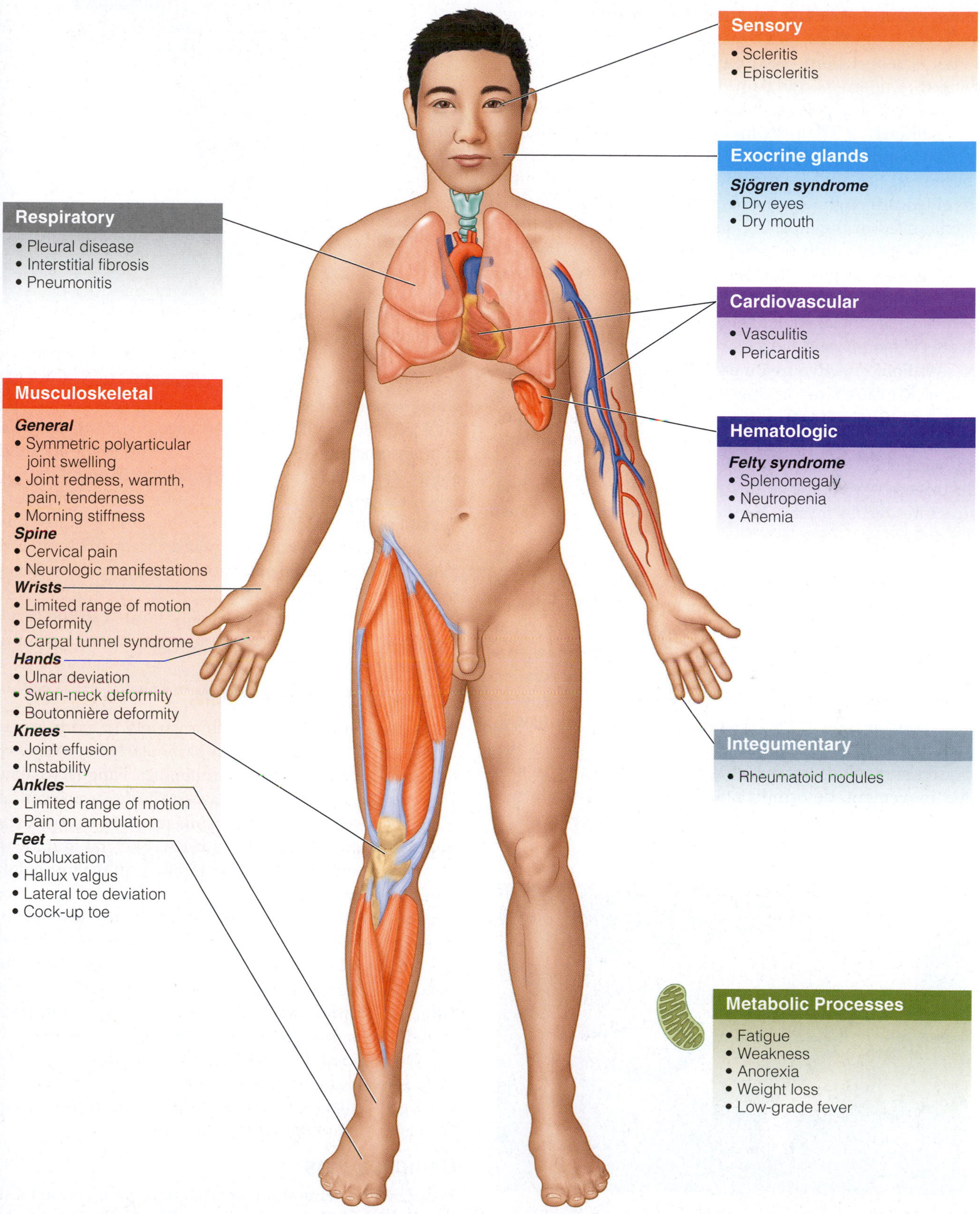
Sensory
• Scleritis
• Episcleritis
Exocrine glands
Sjögren syndrome
• Dry eyes
• Dry mouth
Respiratory
• Pleural disease
• Interstitial fibrosis
• Pneumonitis
Cardiovascular
• Vasculitis
• Pericarditis
Musculoskeletal
General
• Symmetric polyarticular joint swelling
• Joint redness, warmth, pain, tenderness
• Morning stiffness
Spine
• Cervical pain
• Neurologic manifestations
Wrists
• Limited range of motion
• Deformity
• Carpal tunnel syndrome
Hands
• Ulnar deviation
• Swan-neck deformity
• Boutonnière deformity
Knees
• Joint effusion
• Instability
Ankles
• Limited range of motion
• Pain on ambulation
Feet
• Subluxation
• Hallux valgus
• Lateral toe deviation
• Cock-up toe
Hematologic
Felty syndrome
• Splenomegaly
• Neutropenia
• Anemia
Integumentary
• Rheumatoid nodules
Metabolic Processes
• Fatigue
• Weakness
• Anorexia
• Weight loss
• Low-grade fever

Joint Manifestations

The onset of RA is typically insidious, although it may be acute, precipitated by a stressor such as infection, surgery, or trauma. Joint manifestations are often preceded by systemic manifestations of inflammation, including fatigue, anorexia, weight loss, and nonspecific aching and stiffness. Patients report joint swelling with associated stiffness, warmth, tenderness, and pain. The pattern of joint involvement is typically polyarticular (involving multiple joints) and symmetric. The proximal interphalangeal (PIP) and metacarpophalangeal (MCP) joints of the fingers, the wrists, the knees, the ankles, and the toes are most frequently involved, although RA can affect any joint. Stiffness is most pronounced in the morning, lasting more than 1 hour. It may also occur with prolonged rest during the day and may be more severe following strenuous activity. Swollen, inflamed joints feel "boggy" or sponge-like on palpation because of synovial edema (**Figure 40.8** ■). ROM is limited in affected joints, and muscular weakness may be evident.

Without effective treatment, the persistent inflammation of RA causes deformities of the joint and supporting structures (ligaments, tendons, and muscles). As the joint is destroyed, ligaments, tendons, and the joint capsule are weakened or destroyed. Joint cartilage and bone are destroyed. Weakening or destruction of these supporting structures results in lack of opposition to muscle pull, causing deformity.

Characteristic changes in the hands and fingers include ulnar deviation of the fingers and subluxation at the MCP joints. *Swan-neck deformity* is characterized by hyperextension of the PIP joint with compensatory flexion of the distal interphalangeal (DIP) joints (**Figure 40.9** ■). A flexion deformity of the PIP joints with extension of the DIP joint is called a *boutonnière deformity*. The ability to form a pinch is limited by hyperextension of the interphalangeal joint and flexion of the MCP joint of the thumb.

Wrist involvement is nearly universal, leading to limited movement, deformity, and carpal tunnel syndrome. Inflammation of the elbows often causes flexion contracture.

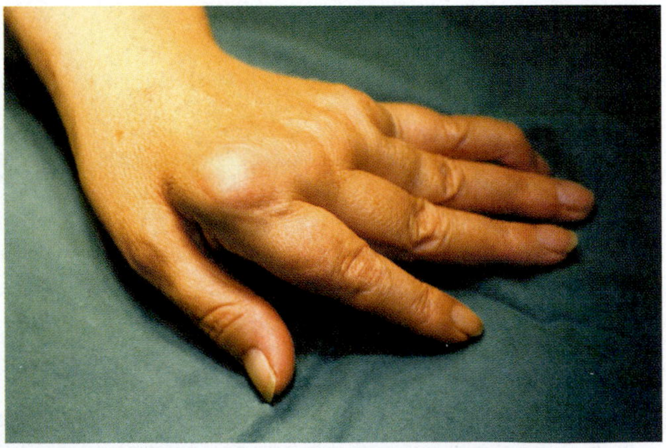

Figure 40.8 ■ Edema and inflammation of the second and third PIP joints of the hand in a patient with rheumatoid arthritis.

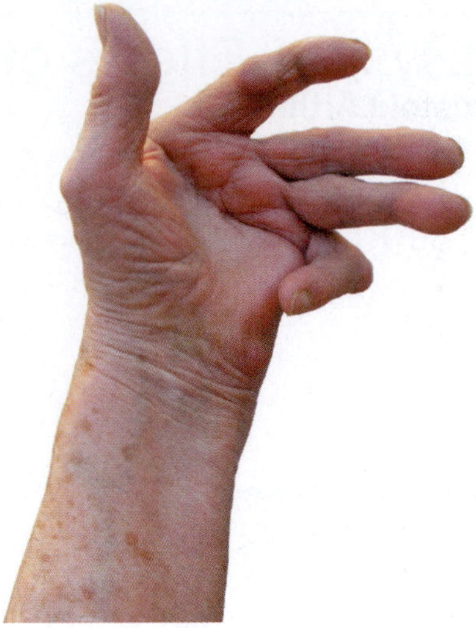

Figure 40.9 ■ Typical hand deformities associated with rheumatoid arthritis.

The knees are frequently affected in RA, with visible edema often obliterating normal contours. Instability of the knee joint along with quadriceps atrophy, contractures, and valgus (knock-knee) deformities can lead to significant disability. Ambulation may be limited by pain and deformities when the ankles and feet are involved. Typical deformities of the feet and toes include subluxation, hallux valgus (deviation of the great toe toward the other digits of the foot), lateral deviation of the toes, and interphalangeal joint hyperextension (cock-up toes).

Spinal involvement is usually limited to the cervical vertebrae. Neck pain is common, and neurologic complications can occur.

Extra-Articular Manifestations

RA is a systemic disease with a variety of extra-articular manifestations. These are seen particularly in patients with high levels of circulating autoantibodies. Fatigue, weakness, anorexia, weight loss, and low-grade fever are common when the disease is active. Anemia resistant to iron therapy frequently affects patients with RA. Skeletal muscle atrophy is common, usually most apparent in the musculature around affected joints.

Rheumatoid nodules may develop, usually in subcutaneous tissue in areas subject to pressure: On the forearm, olecranon bursa, over the MCP joints, and on the toes. Rheumatoid nodules are granulomatous lesions that are firm and either movable or fixed. They may also be found in viscera, including the heart, lungs, intestinal tract, and dura.

Other possible extra-articular manifestations of RA include pleural effusion, vasculitis, pericarditis, and splenomegaly (enlargement of the spleen). See the Multisystem Effects of Rheumatoid Arthritis feature.

Complications

People with rheumatoid arthritis have an increased risk of developing cardiovascular disease (CVD). The increased risk of developing CVD seems to be correlated with the activity and length of time the RA has been present (Venables &

BOX 40.4
Classification Criteria for Rheumatoid Arthritis

- ***Joint involvement:*** Number of large and small joints involved
- ***Serology testing:*** Presence of RF and/or anti-CP antibody
- ***Markers of acute inflammation:*** Abnormal levels of C-reactive protein (CRP) or erythrocyte sedimentation rate (ESR)
- ***Duration of symptoms:*** 6 weeks or longer.

Maini, 2017). Although not necessarily linked to the RA, patients with RA tend to develop infections, renal disease, and lymphoproliferative disorders (leukemia or lymphoma) more frequently than those without RA. This may be due to the immunosuppressant drugs used to control the inflammation associated with RA (Venables & Maini, 2017).

Interprofessional Care

The diagnosis of RA is based on the patient's history, physical assessment, and diagnostic tests. Classification criteria developed by the American College of Rheumatology (Aletaha et al., 2010) are used to help identify patients during early onset of the disease (**Box 40.4**). These criteria are applied to patients who present with synovitis involving at least one joint that is not better explained by another disease.

Once the diagnosis of RA has been established, the goals of therapy are to prevent joint damage and disability and to improve well-being and ability to function. No cure currently exists for RA; however, current treatment regimens can often significantly limit joint damage and preserve function. A multidisciplinary approach is used, with a balance of rest, exercise, physical therapy, and suppression of the inflammatory processes.

Diagnosis

Diagnostic tests are used to help establish the diagnosis of RA. Testing is also used to rule out other forms of arthritis and connective tissue disorders.

Laboratory tests are used to measure levels of autoantibodies, C-reactive protein levels, and the ESR, which is typically elevated. The anti-CPA blood test, which detects antibodies to cyclic citrullinated peptide (CP), provides a more specific marker for RA. Anti-CPA and rheumatoid factor may be present in only about 50% of patients with early disease, however. A CBC is done to identify anemia.

Synovial fluid examination will demonstrate changes associated with inflammation, including increased turbidity (cloudiness), decreased viscosity, and increased protein and WBC levels. X-rays of affected joints are the most specific test for diagnosis of RA. Early in the disease, few changes may be evident other than soft tissue edema and joint effusions. As the disease progresses, joint space narrowing and erosions are seen.

Medications

Several different drug classifications are used in the pharmacologic management of patients with RA based on the Guideline for the Treatment of Rheumatoid Arthritis from the American College of Rheumatologists (Singh et al., 2015).

- NSAIDs and mild analgesics are used to help manage manifestations of the disease early in the diagnosis and for flare-ups. Although these drugs may relieve symptoms of RA, they appear to have little effect on disease progression.
- Low-dose oral corticosteroids are used to rapidly reduce pain and inflammation. Corticosteroids may also slow the development and progression of bone erosions associated with RA. These drugs may be used early in the disease, before disease-modifying antirheumatic drugs have achieved full effect, and for acute disease flare-ups. Intra-articular corticosteroids may be used to provide temporary relief in patients with one or a limited number of affected joints during acute flare-ups to avoid systemic corticosteroid use.
- A diverse group of drugs classified as disease-modifying antirheumatic drugs (DMARDs) is employed to slow or prevent the progression of joint damage. These drugs, which include synthetic (or nonbiologic) DMARDs such as methotrexate, sulfasalazine, and antimalarial agents, and biologic DMARDs such as anti-TNF-α, abatacept, and rituximab, appear to alter the course of the disease, reducing its destruction of joints. These drugs should be introduced early after the diagnosis of RA because much of the joint damage associated with RA occurs early in the disease process.

Nonsteroidal Anti-Inflammatory Drugs. A number of NSAIDs are available for use in the management of RA. All NSAIDs act by inhibiting prostaglandin synthesis. Although the efficacy of all NSAIDs, including aspirin, is equivalent, patient responses are individual. Several trials of different NSAIDs may be necessary to find the most effective drug.

Gastric irritation, ulceration, and bleeding are the most common toxic effects of NSAIDs. They can also affect the lower intestinal tract, leading to perforation or aggravation of inflammatory bowel disorders. All NSAIDs can also be toxic to the kidneys. With the exception of the COX-2 inhibitor celecoxib, most NSAIDs also inhibit platelet function, increasing the risk for bleeding. Aspirin is the only drug in this group that has been found to lower the risk of cardiovascular disease; all others actually increase cardiovascular risk.

NSAIDs commonly prescribed for patients with RA are listed in **Table 40.6**.

Corticosteroids. Systemic corticosteroids can dramatically relieve the symptoms of RA and appear to slow the progression of joint destruction. The long-term use of corticosteroids is associated with multiple side effects, such as poor wound healing, increased risk of infection, osteoporosis, and GI bleeding. Severe rebound manifestations can occur when these medications are discontinued. For these reasons, the use of systemic corticosteroids is limited to acute disease flare-ups, or, when necessary, low daily dosages.

Table 40.6 Selected Nonsteroidal Anti-Inflammatory Drugs Used in Rheumatoid Arthritis

Drug	Average Dose	Comments and Precautions
aspirin	600–900 mg four to six times daily	Least expensive NSAID; associated with risk of GI ulceration, bleeding, and possible hemorrhage; may cause hepatotoxicity
etodolac (Lodine)	200–400 mg q6h	Expensive; may have less GI toxicity
ibuprofen (Motrin, Advil, others)	300 mg four times/day; 400–800 mg three or four times/day	Available in prescription and OTC forms; less gastric distress reported than with aspirin or indomethacin; discontinue if visual disturbances develop
indomethacin (Indocin)	25–50 mg two to four times/day	A potent NSAID used for moderate to severe RA and acute episodes of chronic disease; higher incidence of adverse GI effects and CNS effects such as headache, dizziness, and depression
meloxicam (Mobic)	7.5–15 mg/day	Daily dosing and rare adverse effects are advantages
nabumetone (Relafen)	1000–2000 mg/day	Most common adverse effects include diarrhea and abdominal pain
naproxen (Aleve, Anaprox, Naprosyn)	250–500 mg twice a day	Available in prescription and OTC preparations
piroxicam (Feldene)	10–20 mg/day in a single or divided dose	Expensive; GI side effects dyspepsia, nausea and vomiting, and discomfort may occur more frequently than with other NSAIDs
sulindac (Clinoril)	150–200 mg twice a day	May be safer for use than other NSAIDs in patients with chronic renal disease and for patients with Stevens-Johnson syndrome

Note: Drugs identified in blue are among the 200 most commonly prescribed medications in the United States.
Source: Data from Adams et al., 2017.

Disease-Modifying Antirheumatic Drugs. Disease-modifying antirheumatic drugs (DMARDs) are the treatment of choice for RA with the goal of achieving remission or significantly lower disease activity (Singh et al., 2015). DMARDs are a diverse group of medications including drugs that modify immune and inflammatory responses (**Table 40.7**). They share characteristics that make them useful in the treatment of RA. DMARDs may be used individually (monotherapy) or in combination. Although beneficial effects are not apparent for several weeks or months following the initiation of therapy, they can produce not only clinical improvement but also evidence of decreased disease activity. Because the desired effects of DMARDs are delayed, NSAIDs are often continued during initial therapy. All of these drugs are fairly toxic, and close monitoring is necessary during the course of therapy. Treatment for active infections such as hepatitis B or C or known latent tuberculosis infection should be started prior to initiation of DMARD therapies (Singh et al., 2015).

Nonbiologic DMARDs. Commonly used nonbiologic DMARDs include methotrexate, sulfasalazine, leflunomide (Arava), and hydroxychloroquine.

Methotrexate is the DMARD of choice, used in both monotherapy and in combination with other DMARDs (Seo, 2017). A weekly dose can produce a beneficial effect in as few as 2 to 4 weeks. Gastric irritation and stomatitis are the most frequent side effects associated with methotrexate, but side effects may be better controlled if folic acid is taken at the same time. Alcoholism, diabetes, obesity, advanced age, and renal disease increase the risk of toxic effects (hepatotoxicity, bone marrow suppression, interstitial pneumonitis).

Sulfasalazine, a drug regularly prescribed for chronic inflammatory bowel disease, may also be prescribed for RA. Adverse effects such as neutropenia and thrombocytopenia are relatively common with sulfasalazine, necessitating frequent CBCs to monitor its effects. Leflunomide reversibly inhibits an enzyme involved in the autoimmune process. Because this drug is teratogenic, it is contraindicated for premenopausal women and for men who desire children. Hydroxychloroquine (Plaquenil) is an antimalarial agent sometimes employed in the treatment of RA. Three to 6 months of therapy is required to achieve the desired response, and many patients do not experience significant benefit. Although hydroxychloroquine has a relatively low toxicity, it can cause pigmentary retinitis and vision loss. Patients receiving this drug require a thorough vision examination every 6 months.

Drugs such as penicillamine or gold salts, used in the past to treat RA, are rarely prescribed. Although these agents may be effective for some patients, toxic reactions are common and can be severe, including bone marrow suppression, proteinuria, and nephrosis.

Biologic Dmards. Biologic DMARDs may be used alone, but often are prescribed in combination with methotrexate to reduce disease activity and induce remission (Moreland & Cannella, 2016; Singh et al., 2015). These drugs act by inhibiting components of the immune or inflammatory response, such as TNF-α or IL-1. They control the manifestations of RA in most patients, slow the progression of joint damage, and reduce disability. Biologic DMARDs increase the risk for infection and have been associated with an increased risk for reactivation tuberculosis. Patients are screened for tuberculosis prior to treatment.

Several biologic DMARDs act by inhibiting tumor necrosis factor, thus interrupting the inflammatory cascade of RA. Etanercept (Enbrel) inhibits the binding of tumor necrosis factor to receptor sites. Infliximab (Remicade) is a

Table 40.7 Disease-Modifying Antirheumatic Drugs Used to Treat Rheumatoid Arthritis

Class/Medications	Usual Dose	Adverse Effects	Comments/Nursing Responsibilities
Nonbiologic DMARDs			
hydroxychloroquine (Plaquenil)	200–600 mg/day with meals	■ CNS reactions including irritability, nightmares, psychoses, seizures ■ Retinopathy ■ Alopecia, pruritus, Stevens-Johnson syndrome ■ Blood dyscrasias ■ GI disturbances	■ Should not be used during pregnancy. ■ Regular ophthalmologic examinations are required. ■ Assess for rash. ■ Assess for suicidal tendencies. ■ Administer with milk or food to minimize GI distress.
leflunomide (Arava)	100 mg for 3 days, then 10–20 mg daily	■ Diarrhea ■ Nausea ■ Rash ■ Alopecia ■ Liver toxicity ■ Weight loss ■ Interstitial lung disease	■ Contraindicated for patients with liver impairment. ■ Instruct to use reliable contraception. ■ Instruct to stop taking the drug and promptly report infection. ■ Monitor respiratory status.
methotrexate	7.5–15 mg orally once per week	■ Stomatitis, gastric distress ■ Blood dyscrasias ■ Liver toxicity ■ Interstitial pneumonitis, pulmonary fibrosis ■ Nephropathy	■ Maintain high fluid intake. ■ Inspect mouth daily; report ulcerations, necrotic areas, bleeding, or discomfort. ■ Monitor liver and kidney function tests, CBC, chest x-rays, reporting abnormal or unexpected results. ■ Instruct to avoid alcohol and exposure to sunlight or ultraviolet light. ■ Instruct to practice effective contraception during treatment. ■ Instruct to report immediately any signs or symptoms of infection, low back or side pain, easy bruising, blood in stool or urine.
sulfasalazine (Azulfidine)	2 g/day in divided doses with meals	■ Anorexia, nausea and vomiting, diarrhea ■ Infertility ■ Headache ■ Rash ■ Blood dyscrasias ■ Stevens-Johnson syndrome ■ Fever	■ Maintain high fluid intake. ■ May cause yellow-orange skin or urine discoloration. ■ Monitor CBC and liver function tests every 3 months ■ Assess for rash.
Biologic DMARDs			
abatacept (Orencia)	500–1000 mg per IV infusion every 2 weeks for additional two doses, then every month; Available subcutaneously; initial dose may be IV as above, then 125 mg within one day, then weekly after that or subcutaneous 125 mg every week without initial IV dose	■ Headache ■ Nausea ■ Upper respiratory tract infection	■ Screen for tuberculosis prior to initiating treatment. ■ Stop infusion and notify physician if hypotension, urticaria, or dyspnea develops. ■ Instruct to promptly report signs of allergic response or infection. ■ Advise to avoid live-virus vaccines while taking abatacept and for 3 months after discontinuing the drug. ■ SC: Administer at room temperature in front of thigh (preferred site); do not rub the injection site.
anakinra (Kineret)	100 mg/day subcutaneously	■ Bacterial infections (URI, sinusitis) ■ Injection-site reactions (erythema, inflammation, pain)	■ Monitor for and report manifestations of infection. ■ Monitor blood counts and renal function studies. ■ Assess for injection-site reactions.
rituximab (Rituxan)	1000 mg per IV infusion on days 1 and 15	■ Infusion reactions: Fever, chills, pruritus, urticaria, flushing, dyspnea ■ Hypotension	■ Monitor BP and ECG during infusion; promptly report hypersensitivity responses. ■ Instruct to use effective contraception during and for 12 months after treatment.
tocilizumab (Actemra)	4 mg/kg per IV infusion every 4 weeks 162 mg every 2 weeks subcutaneously (<100 kg) 162 mg every week (>100 kg)	■ Serious infections including opportunistic infections ■ Elevated ALT and AST levels ■ Headache ■ Nasopharyngitis ■ Hypertension ■ Upper respiratory infections	■ Monitor for allergic responses during and immediately following infusion. ■ Monitor for and report manifestations of infection. ■ Monitor CBC and liver function studies.
Tumor necrosis factor inhibitors: ■ adalimumab (Humira) ■ etanercept (Enbrel) ■ infliximab (Remicade) ■ certolizumab (Cimzia, Pegol) ■ golimumab (Simponi)	 40 mg subcutaneously every other week 50 mg subcutaneously weekly 3 mg/kg IV infusion weeks 0, 2, 6, then every 8 wks 400 mg subcutaneously weeks 0, 2, 4; then 400 mg every 4 weeks 50 mg subcutaneously monthly	■ Injection-site reactions ■ Increased risk for infection ■ Possible flulike symptoms (headache, malaise) ■ Headache ■ Rash	■ Obtain tuberculin test results before treatment is started. ■ Instruct to promptly report signs of infection. ■ Stop infusion of infliximab and promptly notify physician if signs of anaphylaxis develop.

Note: Drugs identified in blue are among the 200 most commonly prescribed medications in the United States.

Source: Adams et al., 2017.

biologic response modifier and TNF-α receptor antagonist. Given by intravenous infusion, the drug is administered to reduce infiltration of inflammatory cells and TNF-α production. Adalimumab (Humira), given by subcutaneous injection, binds with TNF receptor sites.

Abatacept (Orencia) and rituximab (Rituxan) are generally reserved for patients with high levels of disease activity. Abatacept acts by interfering with the formation of T cells, whereas rituximab is a monoclonal antibody that depletes B cells. Tocilizumab (Actemra) and Anakinra (Kineret) work by inhibiting IL-1 and IL-6 receptors. Like other biologic DMARDs, these drugs are given parenterally, most by intravenous infusion.

Nutrition

For most patients with RA, an ordinary, well-balanced diet is recommended. Some patients may benefit from fish oils, when added to three DMARDs, to help achieve remission of symptoms with the DMARDs alone (Proudman et al., 2015). Active RA may cause anorexia. Continuing to encourage adequate nutrition and hydration can help to prevent malnutrition and dehydration.

Treatment

The primary objectives in treating RA are to prevent joint damage and disability, reduce pain and inflammation, and minimize side effects of treatment.

Rest and Exercise. A balanced program of rest and exercise is an important component in the management of patients with RA. Physical and occupational therapists can design and monitor individualized activity and rest programs.

Regular rest periods during the day may be beneficial to reduce manifestations of the disease. Additionally, splinting of inflamed joints reduces unwanted motion and provides local joint rest. A variety of orthotic devices are available to reduce joint strain and help maintain function.

A balanced program of physical therapy and exercise is critical to maintain muscle strength and joint mobility. Dynamic strength training (e.g., isometric exercises, use of resistance bands) is used to improve muscle strength without increasing joint stress. Low-impact aerobic exercises, such as swimming and walking, have been shown to benefit patients with RA without adversely affecting joint inflammation or prompting acute episodes.

Heat and Cold. Heat and cold are used for their analgesic and muscle-relaxing effects. Moist heat is generally the most effective and can be provided by a tub bath or shower. Joint pain is relieved in some patients through the application of cold.

Assistive Devices and Splints. Occupational therapists can work with patient with RA to suggest and develop assistive devices, such as a cane, walker, or raised toilet seat, which are useful for patients with significant hip or knee arthritis. Splints provide joint rest and prevent contractures and can be custom-made for the patient. Night splints for the hands and/or wrists should maintain the extremity in a position of maximum function. The best "splint" for the hip is lying prone for several hours a day on a firm bed. In general, splints should be applied for the shortest period needed, should be made of lightweight materials, and should be easily removed to perform ROM exercises once or twice a day.

Surgery

Surgical intervention may be employed for the patient with RA when medical management has failed to prevent joint damage. Arthrodesis (joint fusion) may be used to stabilize joints such as cervical vertebrae, wrists, and ankles. Arthroplasty, or total joint replacement, may be necessary in cases of gross deformity and joint destruction. Total joint replacement and nursing care of patients undergoing this surgery are discussed in the preceding section on OA.

Nursing Care

Patients with chronic, progressive, systemic disorders such as RA have multiple nursing care needs involving many functional health patterns. Physical manifestations of the disease often result in acute and chronic pain, fatigue, impaired mobility, and difficulty performing routine tasks. Treatments to reduce disease activity or prompt remission can have significant side effects and often increase the patient's risk of infection. The disease also has many psychosocial effects. The patient has an incurable chronic disease and may be facing a lifetime of therapy. Pain and fatigue can interfere with the patient's ability to perform expected roles, such as home maintenance or job responsibilities. Even though the patient's hands may appear swollen or deformed, other people may not understand the systemic nature of the disease or realize the difference between RA and OA. See the Case Study & Nursing Care Plan for a patient with RA.

Assessment

Collect the following focused data through the health history and physical examination:

- *Health history:* Pain; duration of morning stiffness; fatigue; joint inflammation: number, location, duration, onset, effect on function; fever; sleep patterns; current RA treatment; past illnesses (including tuberculosis or hepatitis) or surgery; ability to carry out ADLs and self-care activities
- *Physical assessment:* Height/weight; gait; joints: symmetry, size, shape, color, appearance, temperature, range of motion, pain; skin: nodules, purpura; respiratory: cough, crackles; cardiovascular: pericardial friction rub, apical impulse, S_3.

Priorities of Care

Nursing care priorities for the patient with RA will vary depending on the circumstances of the nurse–patient interaction. The newly diagnosed patient who is just starting treatment to reduce disease activity with the goal of achieving remission has very different care needs than the patient experiencing a treatment complication such as infection or gastrointestinal bleeding or the patient who has undergone a total joint arthroplasty.

Diagnoses, Outcomes, and Interventions

Many nursing diagnoses may be appropriate for the patient with RA. This section focuses on those related to its predominant manifestations and their effect on the patient's life.

Promote Self-Health Management. Patients newly diagnosed with RA need to become actively involved in managing their disease. To do so, the patient needs to understand his or her condition, the prescribed therapeutic regimen and treatment goals, and how to manage both treatment and manifestations of RA. Disease manifestations such as fatigue, pain, and weakness and medication effects such as increased risk for infection can interfere with the patient's ability to maintain health. Psychosocial issues such as denial, poor coping, lack of financial and other resources, and inadequate support can also be significant for the patient with RA.

Expected Outcome: Patient will demonstrate willingness and the ability to effectively manage prescribed therapeutic regimen.

The nurse will:

- Assess the patient's understanding of RA, its manifestations and effects, and the anticipated course of the disease. Reinforce and clarify information as needed, providing written material at the patient's level. *Newly diagnosed patients need understandable information that is readily available to develop an understanding of their disease and its treatment and their role in managing RA.*
- Initiate an interprofessional care conference with the patient and family. *Patients and families need opportunities to discuss management strategies and their concerns and perceptions to develop a better understanding of interprofessional team member roles and services.*
- Encourage the patient and family members to discuss the effect of the disease on their lives. *Open discussion helps identify the need for practical skills to manage pain, fatigue, and physical limitations of the disease, as well as psychosocial and emotional challenges associated with RA and its treatment.*
- Refer the patient and family to community and social service agencies and local support groups. *These groups and agencies are valuable resources for the patient and family.*

Manage Chronic Pain. Pain is a constant feature of RA when the disease is active. Some patients say the pain in joints and surrounding tissue is like a deep, constant toothache. Pain can significantly affect the patient's ability to provide self-care and maintain daily activities. It also contributes to the patient's fatigue.

Expected Outcome: Patient will report minimal joint pain 2 or lower as measured on a standard pain scale of 0 to 10.

The nurse will:

- Monitor the level of pain and duration of morning stiffness. *Pain and morning stiffness are indicators of disease activity* (Venables & Maini, 2017). *Increased pain may necessitate changes in the therapeutic treatment plan.*
- Teach the use of heat and cold applications to provide pain relief. The patient may apply heat by showering or taking tub baths or by using local applications such as warm compresses or paraffin dips. During periods of acute inflammation, cold packs may relieve pain more effectively. *Both heat and cold have analgesic effects and can help relieve associated muscle spasms.*
- Teach about the use of prescribed anti-inflammatory medications and the relationship of pain and disease activity. *Anti-inflammatory agents reduce chemical mediators of inflammation and edema, relieving pain. Increasing pain (level, duration, number of painful joints) is an indicator of increased disease activity and may necessitate a change in the therapeutic regimen.*

Reduce Fatigue. The pain and chronic inflammatory processes associated with RA lead to fatigue. Other factors such as disrupted sleep, anemia, and muscle weakness contribute as well.

Expected Outcome: Patient will demonstrate reduced fatigue with increased ability and desire to participate in daily activities.

The nurse will:

- Encourage a balance of periods of activity with periods of rest. *Both joint and whole-body rest are important; regular activity is important to maintain muscle strength and reduce fatigue* (Schur, Maini, & Gibofsky, 2016).
- Help patient to prioritize activities, performing the most important ones early in the day. *Assigning priorities helps the patient avoid performing relatively unimportant activities at the expense of more meaningful and important ones.*
- Encourage dynamic (aerobic) physical activity in addition to prescribed ROM exercises. *Aerobic exercise promotes a sense of well-being and restful sleep patterns.*
- Refer to counseling or support groups. *Counseling and support groups can help the patient develop effective coping strategies and deal with depression and hopelessness.*

Facilitate Role Changes. RA can interfere with the patient's ability to pursue a career and fill other life roles, such as parent, spouse, or homemaker. As the patient's role changes, so must the roles of other family members. This can contribute to changes in family processes, increased stress, and further difficulty coping with the effects of RA.

Expected Outcome: Patient will acknowledge impact of disease on roles and relationships and express willingness to use available resources.

The nurse will:

- Discuss the effects of the disease on the patient's career and other life roles. Encourage the patient to identify changes brought on by the disease. *Discussion helps the patient to accept the changes and begin to identify strategies for coping with them.*
- Encourage the patient and family to discuss their feelings about role changes and grieve lost roles or abilities. *Verbalization allows family members to validate and accept*

feelings about losses and changes, thus helping them to move into new roles.

- Listen actively to concerns expressed by the patient and family members; acknowledge the validity of concerns about the disease, prescribed treatment, and the prognosis. *Demonstrating acceptance of these feelings and concerns promotes trust and validates their reality.*
- Help the patient and family identify strengths they can use to cope with role changes. *Identifying strengths helps the patient and family to consider role changes that maintain self-esteem and dignity.*
- Encourage the patient to make decisions and assume personal responsibility for disease management. *Patients who assume a personal and active role in managing their disease maintain a greater sense of self-control and self-esteem.*

Delegating Nursing Care Activities

As appropriate and allowed within the designated duties and responsibilities of unlicensed assistive personnel, the nurse may delegate nursing care activities such as assisting with daily living activities and ROM exercises and application of splints for the patient with rheumatoid arthritis.

Transitions of Care

There is no way to prevent RA. With vigilant adherence to medication and exercise routines, the patient with RA can

Case Study & Nursing Care Plan

A Patient with Rheumatoid Arthritis

Janice James is a 40-year-old high school science teacher who began noticing vague joint pain, fatigue, poor appetite, and general malaise about 3 months ago. Her symptoms have continued, and she reports feeling very stiff in the mornings, often taking until 10:00 or 11:00 a.m. to begin to feel normal. She initially attributed aching pain in her hands and wrists to the quilting she loves to do in the evenings but made an appointment with her family physician when she noticed that her knuckles and finger joints were not just achy but also swollen and hot. Noting that Mrs. James has a significantly elevated ESR, the physician refers her to the rheumatology clinic for further evaluation. Following examination and laboratory and radiologic testing, the rheumatologist establishes a diagnosis of rheumatoid arthritis and initiates an interprofessional team conference to plan its management.

ASSESSMENT	DIAGNOSES	EXPECTED OUTCOMES
Cathy Greenstein, RN, completes an assessment of Mrs. James. She notes that Mrs. James appears fatigued and ill and states that she feels unable to keep up with all her responsibilities as a teacher and a parent due to her fatigue. Mrs. James's past medical history reveals only the usual childhood diseases and three uncomplicated pregnancies. Physical assessment findings include BP 124/78 mmHg, P 82 bpm and regular, R 18/min, T 37.8°C (100.2°F) oral. Hands: Edema of the proximal interphalangeal (PIP) and metacarpophalangeal (MCP) joints of both hands; second and third PIP and second MCP joints on right hand are red, shiny, hot, spongy, and tender to palpation; able to extend fingers to 180 degrees but cannot make a complete fist with either hand, with flexion limited to less than 90 degrees; grip strength is weak bilaterally; wrist ROM is limited in all directions. Knees have edema, and flexion is slightly limited; positive bulge sign in the right knee. Diagnostic findings are an ESR of 52 mm/h, elevated CRP, and positive for rheumatoid factor and anti-CCP antibodies. Few changes other than soft tissue edema are evident on hand and wrist x-rays.	▪ Chronic pain related to joint inflammation ▪ Limited activity related to the effects of inflammation ▪ Inability to perform activities of daily living related to fatigue and pain ▪ Need for education related to diagnosis and therapeutic regimen	▪ Patient will verbalize effective pain management strategies: a. Use of assistive devices to minimize joint stress with ADLs b. A plan to reduce responsibilities for home maintenance c. An understanding of appropriate use of prescribed NSAID to relieve pain and reduce inflammation. ▪ Patient will demonstrate understanding of the prescribed therapeutic regimen and its importance for both short- and long-term benefit.

PLANNING AND IMPLEMENTATION

- Teach techniques for relieving pain and morning stiffness, including:
  a. Schedule NSAIDs at equal intervals throughout the day.
  b. Take morning NSAID dose with milk and crackers approximately 30 minutes before rising.
  c. Perform ROM exercises in shower or bathtub.
  d. Apply local heat with paraffin dip or compress; use cold packs as needed.
  e. Teach techniques to minimize joint stress while performing ADLs.
- Provide Arthritis Foundation literature and information.
- Discuss ways to delegate household tasks to other family members.
- Explore ways to incorporate 30-minute rest breaks into work schedule.
- Provide information about the disease process and its manifestations, prescribed medications with desired and adverse effects, and the importance of balancing rest and activity.

EVALUATION

The initial treatment regimen of NSAIDs, methotrexate, rest, exercise, and physical therapy succeeded in reducing Mrs. James's disease activity. However, complete remission has not been achieved. She has had difficulty scheduling rest periods at work and has had to struggle to delegate household tasks. "I don't look sick to the kids, and they seem to think housecleaning is a terrible imposition on their time. It's often easier to just do it myself than to fight about it. Besides, that way it gets done right." Mrs. James has faithfully followed the prescribed medication regimen and exercise routines, and she has kept her scheduled appointments and maintained contact with the treatment team.

CLINICAL REASONING IN PATIENT CARE

1. Review the diagnostic criteria for rheumatoid arthritis. What laboratory and radiologic tests are used to help establish the diagnosis of RA?
2. Are these tests specific for RA or might abnormal results occur with other diseases or in other circumstances?
3. Do these tests require any specific patient preparation or teaching? If so, what teaching does Mrs. James require?
4. Mrs. James is 40 years old. Would your nursing interventions differ if she were 72 years old? If so, how?
5. Rheumatoid arthritis is a chronic illness. What are the physical, emotional, and economic implications of a chronic illness that results in chronic pain and deformity?
6. Develop a nursing care plan for Mrs. James to address her inability to perform ADLs

See Evaluating Your Response in Appendix B.

prevent the sequelae of the disease and remain as mobile as possible for as long as possible.

RA is typically a chronic, progressive disease. As with most diseases of this nature, involvement of the patient and family in its management is vital. Education is an important nursing role in caring for patients with RA and their families, improving quality of life and motivation to adhere to the prescribed therapeutic regimen. Address the following topics for home care of the patient and for family members:

- Disease process and treatments, including rest and exercise
- Medications, including their desired effects and anticipated onset of action, common adverse effects, and precautions specific to each medication
- Management of stiffness and pain
- Energy conservation
- Use of assistive devices to maintain independence, including self-care aids such as handheld showers, long-handled brushes and shoehorns, and eating utensils with oversized or special handles
- How to apply splints and take care of skin
- Home and equipment modifications, such as a raised toilet seat, grab bars in the bathroom, a bath chair, or adapted counter heights for patients in a wheelchair
- Physical therapy, occupational therapy, home health and homemaker services
- Helpful resources:

    a. National Institute of Arthritis and Musculoskeletal and Skin Diseases
    b. American College of Rheumatology Research and Education Foundation
    c. Arthritis Foundation
    d. The Arthritis Society
    e. American Physical Therapy Foundation
    f. American Chronic Pain Association.

The Patient with Ankylosing Spondylitis

Ankylosing spondylitis (AS), also known as *axial spondyloarthritis*, is a chronic inflammatory arthritis that primarily affects the axial skeleton, leading to pain and progressive stiffening and fusion of the spine. The typical age of onset is between 17 and 35, with an estimated 2.7 million adults affected in the United States (Spondylitis Association of America, 2018a). The incidence is greater in men than in women, and men have more severe disease. AS is difficult to diagnose in the early stages but may be a major cause of persistent back pain in young adults.

The cause of ankylosing spondylitis is unknown. As with the other forms of arthritis primarily affecting the spine, there is a strong genetic component. Approximately 90% of people with ankylosing spondylitis have the HLA-B27 antigen; about 8% of the general population has this antigen (Spondylitis Association of America, 2018a). Being related to someone who has AS and being male are risk factors for AS (Yu & van Tubergen, 2017). Although a specific trigger for AS has not been identified, evidence suggests that enteric bacteria may play a role in its development. Patients with AS may be prone to microlesions in the intestines, which allow the bacteria into the systemic circulation. These bacteria then settled in the spine, leading to inflammation and the symptoms that accompany the AS (Yu & van Tubergen, 2018).

Pathophysiology

The inflammation of ankylosing spondylitis initially affects sites where ligaments attach to the bone (entheses). Early inflammatory changes are often first noted in the sacroiliac joints. The joints of the spine are also affected. Bone destruction can occur following the inflammation. As the bone begins to attempt to repair itself the bony growth occurs in the cartilaginous joints and gradual calcification and ossification that leads to ankylosis, or joint consolidation and immobility, often referred to as a "bamboo spine" (Yu & van Tubergen, 2018). Other organ systems may be affected as well, including the eyes, lungs, heart, and kidneys.

Manifestations and Complications

The onset of ankylosing spondylitis is usually gradual and insidious. Patients may have persistent or intermittent bouts of low back pain. The pain is worse at night, followed by morning stiffness that is relieved by activity. Pain may radiate to the buttocks, hips, or down the legs. As the disease progresses, back motion becomes limited, the lumbar curve is lost, and the thoracic curvature is accentuated. In severe cases, the entire spine becomes fused, preventing any motion. Patients with ankylosing spondylitis may experience peripheral arthritis, primarily affecting the hip, shoulders, and knee joints. Systemic manifestations include anorexia, weight loss, fever, and fatigue. Many patients develop uveitis (inflammation of the iris and the middle, vascular layer of the eye). Extra-articular manifestations of the disease may also include inflammatory bowel disease, psoriasis, and, uncommonly, pulmonary or cardiac dysfunction (Yu & van Tubergen, 2017).

For most patients with ankylosing spondylitis, the disease is intermittent with mild to moderate acute episodes. These patients have a good prognosis with little risk of severe disability.

In patients with AS, complications that may occur are osteopenia, which is the most common, vertebral fractures, neurologic changes secondary to changes in the spinal structure, and, on rare occasions, renal compromise (Yu & van Tubergen, 2017).

Interprofessional Care

Diagnosis

Diagnostic testing shows an elevated ESR and CRP during periods of active disease and typically a positive HLA-B27 antigen. The diagnosis of ankylosing spondylitis is usually confirmed with x-ray examination of the sacroiliac joints and spine. The sacroiliac joint becomes blurred and gradually obliterated. As the disease progresses, vertebrae become squared and disk spaces narrow. MRI allows earlier identification of active sacroiliitis and may be used for diagnosis.

Medications

NSAIDs relieve pain and stiffness and allow the patient to perform necessary ADLs and exercises. Patients who fail to respond to treatment with NSAIDs may be treated with a biologic DMARD that targets TNF-α. These drugs, including infliximab (Remicade), etanercept (Enbrel), and adalimumab (Humira) or golimumab (Simponi), significantly reduce disease activity and improve manifestations and function for patients with AS (Yu, 2016a). Refer to Table 40.7 for nursing implications of these drugs.

Treatment

As with other forms of arthritis, the management of ankylosing spondylitis is multidimensional. The goals of therapy include relieving symptoms, maintaining function, prevention complications, and minimizing systemic symptoms (Yu, 2016a). Physical therapy and daily exercises are important to maintain posture and joint ROM.

Surgery

Severe hip joint involvement may necessitate total hip arthroplasty. Spinal deformities may require stabilization to reduce pressure of the spinal column (Yu, 2016a).

Nursing Care

Diagnoses, Outcomes, and Interventions

The primary nursing role in ankylosing spondylitis is to provide supportive care and education. Most interactions are on an outpatient basis and teaching and evaluation should occur with each encounter to assess the patient's adherence to the therapeutic regimen.

Teach Therapeutic Regimen. *Expected Outcome:* Patient will verbalize understanding of and willingness to employ measures to manage ankylosing spondylitis.

The nurse will:

- Promote mobility by teaching the patient to take NSAIDs at regular intervals throughout the day with food, milk, or antacid. *Mobility prevents complications and promotes healthy self-esteem. Taking NSAIDs regularly helps to alleviate discomfort that can prevent mobility and can lessen the progression of skeletal changes* (Yu, 2016a). *Taking NSAIDs with food, milk or antacids helps to prevent stomach irritation that may occur with these medications.*
- Suggest that the patient perform exercises in the shower. *Warm, moist heat promotes mobility.*
- Stress the importance of following the prescribed physical therapy and exercise program to maintain mobility. *Often patients find it difficult to maintain a therapeutic exercise program due to limitations. Having the knowledge of why this is so important may help them to continue the routine.*
- If the patient is receiving a DMARD, provide information about possible adverse effects and when to contact the healthcare provider. *Due to the immunosuppressant nature of these medications, patients should be aware of the possible signs of infection that are different from the typical signs.*
- Educate the patient that proper positioning and posture are important. Suggest that when sleeping, a board be placed under the mattress to provide firmness, and the person should sleep in the supine position using either no pillow or only one small pillow. *These interventions are helpful to prevent abnormal spinal curvature.*
- Promote self-care activities including maintenance of proper weight, quitting smoking, and muscle-strengthening exercises. *These activities promote bone and muscle strength and prevent complications of AS.*
- Suggest occupational counseling if pain and deformity are severe enough to cause work-related problems.

Occupational counselors can assist in finding work that is less strenuous and/or suggest training for other occupations that would be more appropriate for the patient if pain and deformity are an issue.

The Patient with Reactive Arthritis

Pathophysiology

Reactive arthritis (ReA) (Reiter syndrome) is an acute, nonpurulent inflammatory arthritis that is believed to be a response to an exposure or infection with certain types of bacteria, including *Chlamydia* or *Salmonella, Shigella, Yersinia*, or *Campylobacter* (Spondylitis Association of America, 2018b). Like ankylosing spondylitis, this type of arthritis often affects people who have an inherited HLA-B27 antigen.

Manifestations and Complications

Manifestations of ReA typically occur 2 to 4 weeks after the infection and subside in 3 to 12 months. The condition has a tendency to recur. Nonbacterial urethritis may be the initial manifestation of ReA in men. In women, urethritis and cervicitis may be asymptomatic. Fatigue, malaise, fever, and weight loss are common. Conjunctivitis and acute inflammatory arthritis follow. The arthritis is usually asymmetric, affecting weight-bearing joints of the lower extremities, such as the knees, ankles, metatarsal, and toe joints. The wrists and fingers may also be involved. Tendinitis, fasciitis, and back pain are common. Mouth ulcers, inflammation of the glans penis, and skin lesions may occur. The heart and aorta may also be affected.

Reactive arthritis is typically self-limited, although it can be recurrent or progressive. About 15 to 20% of people with ReA develop chronic arthritis or spondylitis (Spondylitis Association of America, 2018b).

Interprofessional Care

Diagnosis

The diagnosis of reactive arthritis is based on the patient's history and presenting symptoms. No test is specific for the disorder. Urethral or cervical cultures are obtained to rule out gonococcal infection.

Medications

When *Chlamydia* is suspected, the patient may be treated with erythromycin or a 6-month course of rifampin plus azithromycin or doxycycline. Reactive arthritis is treated symptomatically, usually with NSAIDs. Patients with persistent ReA may respond to treatment intra-articularly or systemic glucocorticoids (Yu, 2016b). If the symptoms are still not controlled, treat with a DMARD such as sulfasalazine or an immunosuppressive agent such as azathioprine (Imuran) or methotrexate. In severe chronic ReA, a biologic TNF inhibitor such as adalimumab (Humira) or etanercept (Embrel) may be used (Yu, 2016b).

Nursing Care

Patients with reactive arthritis are usually seen in primary care settings such as a clinic or physician's office, making the nursing role primarily one of education. Teach the patient about the association of the arthritis with the precipitating infection (if identified). Stress the importance of treating the infection effectively if it is still present. Use this opportunity to provide information about sexually transmitted infections and protective measures to prevent their transmission. Discuss the usual self-limited nature of reactive arthritis, the appropriate use of prescribed NSAID preparations, and symptomatic relief measures such as application of heat and rest.

The Patient with Systemic Lupus Erythematosus

Systemic lupus erythematosus (SLE) is a chronic inflammatory autoimmune disease that affects almost all body systems, including the musculoskeletal system. The manifestations of SLE are widely variable and are thought to result from cell and tissue damage caused by deposition of antigen–antibody complexes in connective tissues. SLE can range from a mild, episodic disorder to a rapidly fatal disease process. The CDC (2018c) lists the number of definite or probable SLE cases at between 161,000 and 322,000. Although the exact etiology of SLE is unknown, genetic, environmental, and hormonal factors play a role in its development. Twin studies and a familial pattern of the disease point to a genetic component, as does an increased incidence of other connective tissue diseases in relatives of people with SLE. Certain human leukocyte antigen (HLA) genes are seen more frequently in people with SLE. Environmental factors such as viruses (e.g., Epstein-Barr virus), occupational exposure to silica dust, ultraviolet light, and cigarette smoking may play a role in activation of the pathologic mechanisms of the disease. In addition, an imbalance of sex hormones may contribute to the development of SLE. Women who use estrogen-containing oral contraceptives or hormone replacement have a higher risk of developing SLE (Schur & Hahn, 2017).

Pathophysiology

The pathophysiology of SLE involves the production of a large variety of autoantibodies against normal body components such as nucleic acids, erythrocytes, coagulation proteins, lymphocytes, and platelets. Autoantibody production results from hyperreactivity of B cells (humoral response) because of disordered T-cell function (cellular immune response). The most characteristic autoantibodies in SLE are produced in response to nucleic acids, including DNA, histones, ribonucleoproteins, and other components of the cell nucleus.

SLE autoantibodies bind with their target tissue to form immune complexes, which are then deposited in the connective tissue of blood vessels, lymphatic vessels, and other tissues. The deposits trigger an inflammatory response with release of chemotaxins, cytokines, vasoactive peptides, and destructive enzymes, which results in local tissue damage. The kidneys are a frequent site of complex deposition and damage; other tissues affected include the musculoskeletal system, brain, heart, spleen, lung, GI tract, skin, and peritoneum. The autoantibodies produced and their target tissue determine the manifestations of SLE.

Risk Factors

SLE usually affects women of childbearing age but it can occur at any age, affect either gender, and is found in all ethnic groups. In the United States, African Americans, Hispanics/Latinos, American Indians/Native Alaskans, and Asians are affected more than Caucasians (CDC, 2018c).

A number of drugs can cause a syndrome that mimics lupus in patients with no other risk factors for the disease. Procainamide (e.g., Procan-SR, Pronestyl) and hydralazine (Apresoline, Hydralyn) are the most common drugs implicated, along with isoniazid (INH).

Manifestations

SLE can affect the majority of systems in the body. The course of SLE is mild in most patients, with periods of remission and exacerbation. Typical early manifestations of SLE mimic those of rheumatoid arthritis, including systemic manifestations of unexplained fever, anorexia, extreme fatigue, and weight loss, and musculoskeletal manifestations of multiple arthralgias and symmetric polyarthritis. Joint symptoms affect more than 90% of patients with SLE (Gladman, 2018). Although synovitis may be present, the arthritis associated with SLE is rarely deforming.

Most people affected by SLE have skin manifestations at some point during their disease. In fact, SLE was originally described as a skin disorder and named for the characteristic red butterfly rash across the cheeks and bridge of the nose (**Figure 40.10** ■). Many patients with SLE are photosensitive; a diffuse maculopapular rash on skin exposed to the sun is common. Other cutaneous manifestations include discoid lesions (raised, scaly, circular lesions with an erythematous rim), hives, erythematous fingertip lesions, and splinter hemorrhages. Alopecia is common in patients with SLE, although the hair usually grows back. Painless mucous membrane ulcerations may occur on the lips or in the mouth or nose. Other common manifestations of SLE include vascular symptoms of pale, cyanotic fingers or toes; edema in legs and around eyes; ulcers in the mouth; and enlarged lymph nodes.

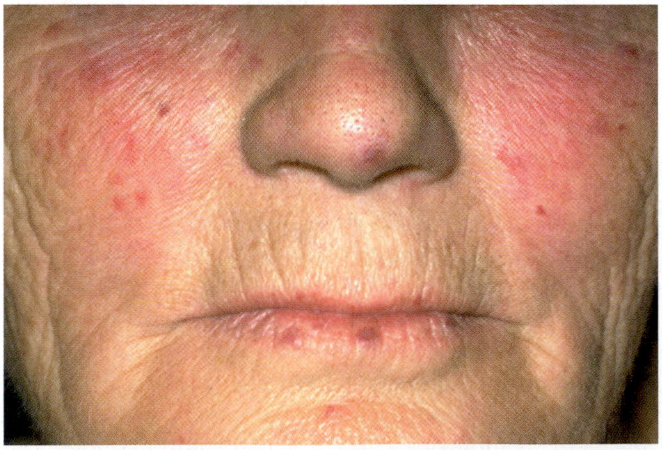

Figure 40.10 ■ The butterfly rash of systemic lupus erythematosus.

The other body systems that can be affected include the renal, gastrointestinal, pulmonary, cardiac, neuropsychiatric, and hematologic systems, as well as the eyes. Approximately 50% of people with SLE experience renal manifestations of the disease, including proteinuria, cellular casts, and nephrotic syndrome. Up to 10% develop renal failure because of the disease.

Hematologic abnormalities such as anemia, leukopenia, and thrombocytopenia are common with SLE. Up to 40% of patients with SLE develop pericarditis. Myocarditis is less common but may develop. Vascular disorders such as vasculitis and Raynaud phenomenon often occur. Patients with SLE have an increased risk for acute thrombotic events such as transient ischemic attack (TIA), stroke, and myocardial infarction. Pleuritis, pleural effusions, and lupus pneumonitis are common pulmonary manifestations of SLE.

Nervous system effects of the disease are common, including cognitive dysfunction with a decline in intellect, memory loss, and disorientation. Other possible neurologic manifestations include headache, psychosis, and seizures. Ocular manifestations of SLE include conjunctivitis, photophobia, and transient blindness due to retinal vasculitis.

GI manifestations of SLE, such as anorexia, nausea, abdominal pain, and diarrhea, may affect up to 45% of patients with the disease. The liver may be enlarged, and liver function tests may yield abnormal results.

Renal and CNS manifestations of SLE rarely occur with drug-induced lupus, but arthritic and other systemic symptoms are common. Manifestations of drug-induced lupus usually resolve when the medication is discontinued. See Multisystem Effects of Systemic Lupus Erythematosus.

Complications

A common complication of SLE is osteoporosis (Gladman, 2018). Serious infections are another complication due to the immunocompromised state of the patient with SLE.

Interprofessional Care

As with RA, effective management of SLE requires teamwork, with active participation by both the patient and members of the healthcare team. Although there is no cure for SLE, the 10-year survival rate is approximately 90% among patients with this disease, which was once considered fatal in most cases.

Because of the diversity of organ system involvement and manifestations of SLE, diagnosis can be difficult. No one specific test is available to confirm the presence of this disease in all people suspected of having it. Instead, the diagnosis is based on the patient's history and physical assessment, as well as laboratory studies.

Multisystem Effects of
Systemic Lupus Erythematosus

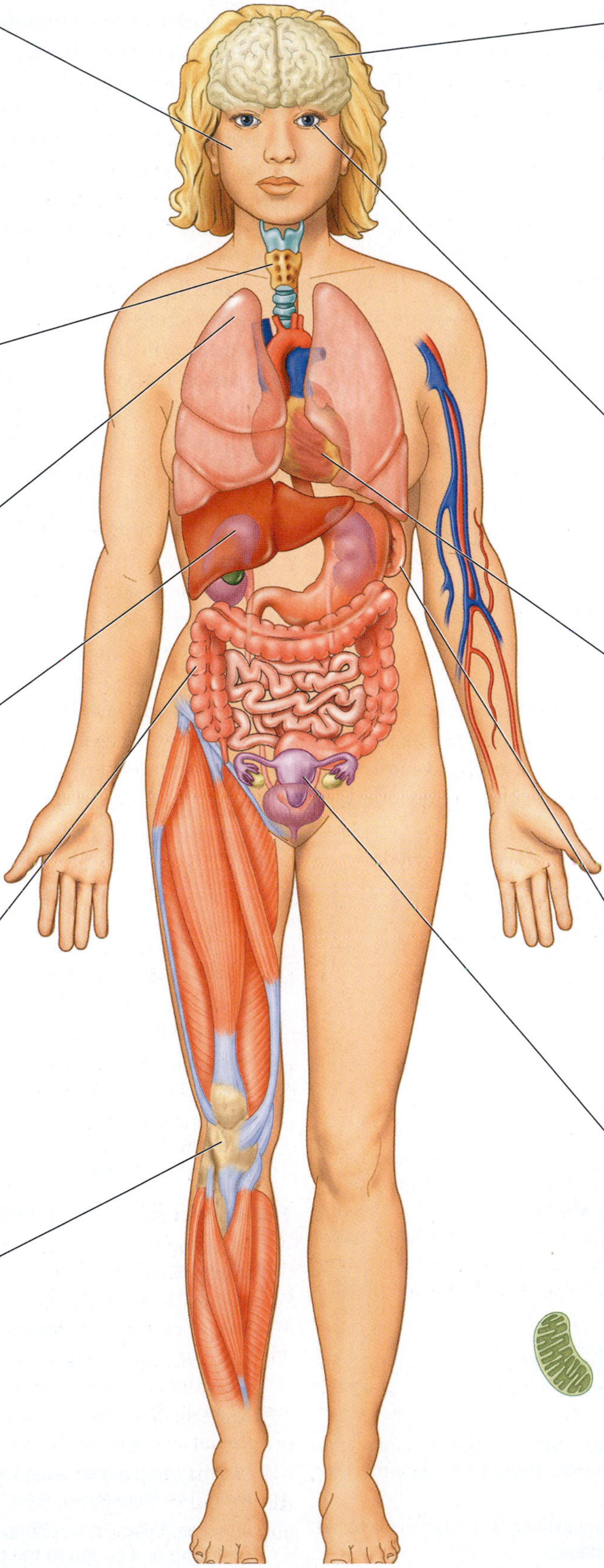

Integumentary
- Butterfly rash on face
- Photosensitivity
- Maculopapular rash on exposed body surfaces
- Discoid lesions
- Erythematous fingertip lesions
- Splinter hemorrhages
- Alopecia
- Ulcers (lip, mouth, nose)

Endocrine
- Thyroid abnormalities
- Hyperparathyroidism
- Glucose intolerance

Respiratory
- Pleurisy
- Pleural effusion
- Pneumonitis
- Interstitial fibrosis

Urinary
- Proteinuria
- Cellular casts

Potential complications
- Nephrotic syndrome
- Renal failure

Gastrointestinal
- Anorexia
- Nausea
- Abdominal pain
- Diarrhea
- Hepatomegaly

Musculoskeletal
- Arthralgias
- Symmetric polyarthritis
- Joint swelling and effusion
- Morning stiffness

Neurologic
- Neuropathies (peripheral and central)
- Seizures
- Depression
- Psychosis

Potential complications
- Stroke
- Organic brain syndrome
  - Intellectual impairment
  - Memory loss
  - Personality changes
  - Disorientation

Sensory
- Conjunctivitis
- Photophobia
- Retinal vasculitis with transient blindness
- Cotton-wool spots on retina

Cardiovascular
- Pericarditis
- Myocarditis
- Endocarditis
- Vasculitis
- Venous or arterial thrombosis

Hematologic
- Anemia
- Leukopenia
- Thrombocytopenia
- Splenomegaly

Reproductive
- Pregnancy-induced hypertension edema, and proteinuria
- Fetal loss

Metabolic Processes
- Low-grade fever
- Malaise
- Weight loss

Diagnosis

The multiple autoantibodies produced in SLE cause a number of abnormalities in laboratory tests.

- ***Antinuclear antibody (ANA) testing*** is positive in more than 98% of patients with SLE
- ***Anti-DNA antibody testing*** is a more specific indicator of SLE because these antibodies are rarely found in any other disorder
- ***ESR*** is typically elevated, occasionally to greater than 100 mm/h
- ***Serum complement levels*** are usually decreased as complement is consumed or "used up" by the development of antigen–antibody complexes
- ***CBC*** abnormalities include moderate to severe anemia, leukopenia, and lymphocytopenia, and possible thrombocytopenia
- ***Urinalysis*** shows mild proteinuria, hematuria, and blood cell casts during exacerbations of the disease when the kidneys are involved. Renal function tests including *serum creatinine*, *blood urea nitrogen (BUN)*, and *eGFR* may also be obtained to evaluate the extent of renal disease.
- ***Kidney biopsy*** may be performed to assess the severity of renal lesions and guide therapy.

Medications

The patient with mild or remittent SLE may need little or no therapy other than supportive care. Arthralgias, arthritis, fever, and fatigue can often be managed with acetaminophen, aspirin, or NSAIDs. Aspirin is particularly beneficial for patients with SLE because its antiplatelet effects help prevent thrombosis. It may, however, cause liver toxicity and hepatitis. NSAIDs are used with caution because they may increase the risk of renal dysfunction or myocardial infarction.

Skin and arthritic manifestations of SLE may be treated with antimalarial drugs such as hydroxychloroquine (Plaquenil). Hydroxychloroquine has also been shown to be effective in reducing the frequency of acute episodes of SLE in people with mild or inactive disease. Retinal toxicity and possibly irreversible blindness are the primary concerns with this drug. For this reason, the patient taking hydroxychloroquine undergoes an ophthalmologic exam frequently (every 6 months, or as indicated) (Wallace, 2017).

Patients with severe and life-threatening manifestations of SLE (such as nephritis, hemolytic anemia, myocarditis, pericarditis, or CNS lupus) require corticosteroid therapy in high doses. Intravenous methylprednisolone is utilized, 0.5 to 1 g/day for 3 days in acutely ill patients or 1 to 2 mg/kg/day in less acutely ill patients (Wallace, 2017). The dosage is tapered as rapidly as the patient's disease allows, although lowering the dosage may precipitate an acute episode. Some patients with SLE require long-term corticosteroid therapy to manage symptoms and prevent major organ damage. These patients are at increased risk for corticosteroid side effects, such as cushingoid effects, weight gain, hypertension, infection, accelerated osteoporosis, and hypokalemia.

Immunosuppressive agents such as cyclophosphamide (Cytoxan), mycophenolate (CellCept), azathioprine (Imuran), or rituximab (Rituxan) may be used, alone or in combination with corticosteroids, to treat patients with active SLE or lupus nephritis (see **Medication**

Medication Administration 40.C

Immunosuppressive Agents for SLE

CYTOTOXIC AGENTS

azathioprine (Imuran)
cyclophosphamide (Cytoxan)
cyclosporine (Sandimmune)
mycophenolate mofetil (CellCept)

Certain cytotoxic or antineoplastic drugs are effective as immunosuppressive agents. They act by decreasing the proliferation of cells within the immune system and are widely used to prevent rejection following a tissue or organ transplant. They are usually administered concurrently with corticosteroid therapy, allowing lower doses of both preparations and resulting in fewer side effects.

Nursing Responsibilities

- Monitor blood count, with particular attention to the WBC and platelet counts. Notify the physician if WBCs fall below 4000 or platelets below 75,000.
- Monitor renal and liver function studies including creatinine, BUN, eGFR, and liver enzyme levels. Report any abnormal levels to the physician.
- Oral preparations should be administered with food to minimize GI effects. Antacids may be ordered.
- Increase fluids to maintain good hydration and urinary output.
- Monitor intake and output.
- Monitor for signs of abnormal bleeding: Bleeding gums, bruising, petechiae, joint pain, hematuria, and black or tarry stools.
- Use meticulous hand hygiene and other appropriate measures to protect the patient from infection. Assess for signs of infection.
- Pulmonary fibrosis is a potential adverse effect of cyclophosphamide. Therefore, monitor the results of pulmonary function studies and be alert to clinical signs of dyspnea or cough.

Health Education for the Patient and Family

- Avoid large crowds and situations where you might be exposed to infections.
- Report signs of infection such as chills, fever, sore throat, fatigue, or malaise to the physician.
- Use contraceptive measures to prevent pregnancy while you are taking these drugs because they cause birth defects.
- Avoid the use of aspirin or ibuprofen while taking these drugs. Report any signs of bleeding to the physician.
- You may stop menstruating while you are taking cyclophosphamide. The menses will resume after the drug is discontinued.
- If you are taking cyclophosphamide, be sure to report difficulty breathing or a cough to the physician.

Source: Adams, et al., 2017.

Administration 40.C). When these agents are used in combination, lower, less toxic doses of each drug can be used. The patient receiving immunosuppressive agents is at increased risk for infection, malignancy, bone marrow depression, and toxic effects specific to the drug prescribed. Studies involving use of biologic therapies targeted at T or B lymphocytes are ongoing.

Nutrition

There is no specific nutritional treatment for SLE, however, the majority of patients have low serum vitamin D levels (Wallace, 2017). Sun exposure, the key way to help the body naturally produce vitamin D (25-hydoxyvitamin D), can exacerbate a flare-up of SLE, therefore patients are encouraged to avoid sun exposure. These levels should be monitored occasionally, and patients should be encouraged to seek a dietary consult for ways to increase vitamin D intake. Of note, during an acute exacerbation or in the presence of a fever, metabolism in increased and caloric intake may need to be increased.

Treatment

Because exposure to ultraviolet light can trigger a disease flare-up, the patient with SLE should be cautioned to avoid sun exposure. Patients should use sunscreens with a sun protection factor (SPF) rating of 15 or higher when outside. Topical corticosteroids may be used to treat skin lesions. Some physicians recommend avoiding the use of oral contraceptives because estrogen can trigger an acute episode.

Patients with lupus nephritis who progress to develop end-stage renal disease are treated with dialysis (hemodialysis or peritoneal dialysis) and kidney transplantation.

SAFETY ALERT: The warning signs of an SLE flare-up include:

- Increased fatigue
- Pain, abdominal discomfort
- Rash
- Headache
- Fever
- Dizziness ■

Nursing Care

Priorities of Care

Nursing care for the patient with mild SLE may be limited to teaching about the disease and strategies to maintain remission or low disease activity. The patient with severe disease, however, has many diverse nursing needs, which vary according to the organ systems involved. Because of the close link between RA and SLE, many of the nursing diagnoses and interventions identified for the patient with arthritis may be appropriate for the patient with lupus. The nursing care needs of the patient with lupus nephritis or end-stage renal disease are outlined in Chapter 28. This section focuses on the needs of the patient related to the dermatologic manifestations of lupus, an increased risk for infection, and health maintenance. The nursing care of patients with RA symptoms were discussed earlier in this chapter.

Diagnoses, Outcomes, and Interventions

The priority nursing interventions for the patient with SLE are focused on problems with impaired skin integrity, risk for infection, and health maintenance.

Promote Skin Integrity. Skin lesions are a common manifestation of SLE. A rash or discoid lesion interrupts the integrity of the skin, which is the first line of protection against infection, increasing the patient's already high risk of infection. These lesions, which usually appear on exposed parts of the skin, can also be disfiguring and cause the patient emotional distress.

Expected Outcome: Patient will verbalize understanding of and willingness to employ measures to reduce risk for epidermal manifestations of SLE.

The nurse will:

- Assess knowledge of SLE and its possible effects on the skin. *Assessment allows the nurse to base teaching and information on the patient's existing knowledge, improving learning and retention.*
- Discuss the relationship between sun exposure and disease activity, both dermatologic and systemic. *It is important for the patient to understand that sun exposure may not only cause dermatologic manifestations but also trigger an acute episode.*
- Suggest the following strategies to limit sun exposure:
  a. Avoid being out of doors during hours of greatest sun intensity (10:00 a.m. to 3:00 p.m.).
  b. Use sunscreen with an SPF of 15 or higher when sun exposure cannot be avoided. Apply it 30 minutes before going out into the sun.
  c. Reapply sunscreen after swimming, exercising, or bathing.
  d. Wear loose clothing with long sleeves and wide-brimmed hats when out of doors.

  These strategies can help the patient maintain a normal lifestyle while helping to prevent acute episodes.
- Keep skin clean and dry; apply therapeutic creams or ointments to lesions as prescribed. *These measures promote healing and reduce the risk for infection.*

Reduce Risk for Infection. Ineffective protection can be a problem for the patient with SLE, who is at increased risk for infection and multiple organ system problems because of the disease. In addition, treatment with corticosteroids or immunosuppressive agents further impairs immune responses and the ability to fight infection. The following interventions are for the patient who is hospitalized.

Expected Outcome: Patient will remain free of infection.

The nurse will:

- Wash hands before and after providing direct care. *Hand hygiene removes transient organisms from the skin, reducing the risk of transmission to the patient.*
- Use strict aseptic technique in caring for intravenous lines and indwelling urinary catheters or performing

any wound care. *Aseptic technique offers protection against external and resident host microorganisms.*

- Assess patient frequently for infection. Monitor temperature and vital signs every 4 hours. Assess for signs of cellulitis, including tenderness, redness, edema, and warmth. Report signs of infection to the physician promptly. *Therapy can suppress usual responses, such as elevated temperature and inflammation. The fever of infection may be mistaken for the fever commonly associated with lupus. The patient receiving immunosuppressive therapy for the disease has an even higher risk for infection.*
- Monitor laboratory values, including CBC and tests of organ function; report changes to the physician. *An elevation in the WBC count with a shift to the left (increased numbers of immature leukocytes in the blood) may be an early indication of infection. Changes in liver function studies, renal function studies, myocardial enzymes, or other laboratory values may indicate organ system involvement.*
- Initiate reverse or protective isolation procedures as indicated by the patient's immune status. *These procedures provide further protection from infection for the severely immunocompromised patient.*
- Ensure an adequate nutrient intake, offering supplementary feedings as indicated or maintaining parenteral nutrition, if necessary. *Adequate nutrition is important for healing and immune system function.*
- Teach the patient the importance of good hand hygiene after using the bathroom and before eating. *Hand hygiene reduces the risk of infection with endogenous organisms.*
- Monitor for potential adverse effects of medications including thrombocytopenia and possible bleeding, fluid retention with edema and possible hypertension, loss of bone density, osteoporosis, and possible pathologic fractures, renal or hepatic toxicity, and cardiac effects, particularly in the patient with fluid retention and hypervolemia. *Medications used to treat SLE have many potential adverse effects that can impair normal protective and homeostatic mechanisms.*

Promote Self-Health Management. As with other chronic diseases, much of the responsibility for maintaining optimal health rests with the patient. Disease manifestations such as fatigue, arthralgias, arthritis, and increased risk for infection can interfere with the patient's ability to maintain health. Psychosocial issues can also be a significant factor in health maintenance for the patient with lupus. These issues may include denial of the significance of the disease, poor coping, lack of financial and other resources, and an inadequate support system.

Expected Outcome: Patient will demonstrate an understanding of and ability to manage prescribed therapeutic regimen.

The nurse will:

- Assess the ability to maintain optimal health, identifying physical and psychosocial factors that may affect health maintenance. *Before intervening to improve the patient's health maintenance, the nurse must identify and understand factors affecting it.*
- Provide care and teaching in a nonjudgmental manner. *To intervene effectively, the nurse must accept the patient and family as they are.*
- Encourage the patient and family members to discuss the effect of the disease on their lives. *Open discussion helps the patient and the nurse identify barriers to health maintenance and begin exploring alternative strategies.*
- Initiate an interprofessional care conference with the patient and family. *In this care conference, a number of perspectives can be expressed, improving the planning of strategies for health maintenance activities.*
- Refer the patient and family to counseling as needed. *Counseling may help the patient and family develop the necessary coping skills to accept and deal with the disease.*
- Refer the patient and family to community and social service agencies and local support groups. *These groups and agencies are valuable resources for the patient and family.*

Transitions of Care

Teaching is a critical factor in preparing patients with SLE to manage their chronic disease. Address the following topics:

- The disease and its potential effects. Promote an optimistic outlook, stressing that the majority of patients do not require long-term corticosteroid therapy and that the disease may improve over time.
- The importance of skin care.
- The importance of avoiding exposure to infection.
- The need to follow the prescribed treatment plan, including rest and exercise, medications, and follow-up appointments. Discuss manifestations of an acute episode (often called a *flare-up* or *flare*) and stress the importance of contacting the physician promptly if any of these manifestations occur.
- The importance of wearing a medical alert tag identifying the condition and therapy such as corticosteroids or immunosuppressives.
- Family planning with the patient and spouse. The use of oral contraceptives may be contraindicated for the patient; if appropriate, provide information about alternative means of birth control. Pregnancy is not contraindicated for most women with lupus. However, the pregnant patient requires close monitoring because acute episodes sometimes accompany pregnancy.
- The need for preventive healthcare for both men and women with SLE. Women should have gynecologic and breast examinations and men should have prostate examinations each year. Both men and women should have regular screenings for cholesterol and blood pressure. Annual influenza vaccinations are important, as is pneumococcal vaccination for older patients. If patients are taking corticosteroids or antimalarial medications, annual eye examinations should be conducted to screen for and treat any eye problems.

- Helpful resources:
    a. National Institute of Arthritis and Musculoskeletal and Skin Diseases
    b. Lupus Foundation of America.

The Patient with Systemic Sclerosis (Scleroderma)

Systemic sclerosis, also known as *scleroderma* (hardening of the skin), is a chronic disease characterized by deposition of excess collagen tissue in the skin and internal organs. The cause of systemic sclerosis is unknown, but genetic, immune, and environmental factors are thought to play a role. Although this uncommon disease is distributed worldwide, a higher incidence is noted in miners exposed to silica and in people exposed to certain chemicals such as polyvinyl chloride, epoxy resins, and aromatic hydrocarbons.

Systemic sclerosis affects from 4 to 489 cases per million people in the United States. The U.S. and Australia have higher occurrence rates than in Japan or Europe (Varga, 2017a).

Pathophysiology

Early systemic sclerosis is characterized by functional and structural abnormalities of the small arteries and arterioles that lead to progressive vessel obstruction, increased permeability, and fibrosis. Blood flow to surrounding tissues and organs is reduced; inflammatory changes may be noted in affected tissues prior to the development of fibrosis. Autoimmunity and vascular damage are believed to lead to fibrosis in systemic sclerosis. This process is characterized by progressive replacement of normal tissue with dense connective tissue (Denton, 2017b). Abnormal proliferation of fibrous connective tissue occurs in the skin, blood vessels, lungs, GI tract, and other organs. Nearly all patients with systemic sclerosis develop Raynaud phenomenon, a vascular disorder characterized by reversible arterial vasospasm.

Scleroderma may be either limited, with limited visceral organ involvement, or diffuse, with both skin and visceral organ involvement. Limited cutaneous systemic sclerosis (lcSSc) affects the fingers, distal extremities, and face. Involvement of visceral organs tends to be slow and insidious, and the long-term prognosis is better than that for patients with diffuse sclerosis, with a 75% 10-year survival rate (Denton, 2017b). In diffuse cutaneous systemic sclerosis (dcSSc), skin involvement is progressive, beginning at the distal extremities and progressing to involve the face and trunk. These patients tend to develop pulmonary fibrosis and renal involvement early in the disease. This disease is usually progressive; complete remission is rare. Infections and diseases of the cardiovascular, renal, pulmonary, and CNS are the most common causes of death in people with systemic sclerosis.

Risk Factors

Development of systemic sclerosis has been shown in those patients who have the genetic predisposition to the development after an exposure to viruses or certain environment toxins or drugs (Varga, 2017b).

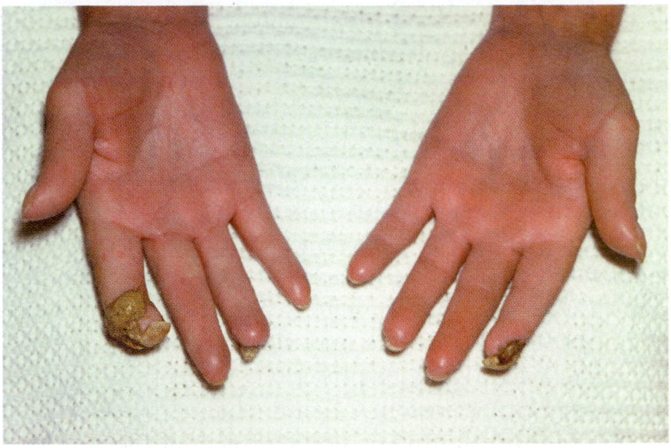

Figure 40.11 ■ Patient with scleroderma and Raynaud phenomenon.

Manifestations

The initial manifestations of systemic sclerosis are usually noted in the skin, which thickens markedly. Diffuse, nonpitting edema is also noted. As the disease progresses, the skin begins to atrophy, becoming taut, shiny, and hyperpigmented (**Figure 40.11** ■). Facial skin tightening leads to loss of skin lines and a pursed-lip appearance. Skin tightness may limit mobility, particularly of the face and hands. Other skin manifestations include *telangiectasias* (flat, red areas caused by dilation of small blood vessels, usually noted on the face, hands, and in the mouth) and calcium deposits, usually noted around joints.

Arthralgias and Raynaud phenomenon are common early manifestations of systemic sclerosis. Raynaud phenomenon (intermittent attacks of small artery vasospasm) is characterized by pallor of the fingers followed by cyanosis, and then reactive hyperemia with redness. Attacks are usually triggered by cold temperatures.

Complications

The patient with visceral organ involvement may have varied symptoms. Dysphagia is common because the motility of the esophagus is affected. Pulmonary involvement can lead to exertional dyspnea due to impaired gas exchange and right-sided heart failure due to pulmonary hypertension. Involvement of the heart may cause manifestations of pericarditis and dysrhythmias. Diarrhea or constipation, abdominal cramping, and malabsorption can occur when the GI tract is affected. Renal effects can lead to proteinuria, hematuria, hypertension, and renal failure (Varga, 2017a).

Interprofessional Care

The manifestations of systemic sclerosis often allow diagnosis with little or no testing. No cure is currently available; treatment is symptomatic and supportive.

Diagnosis

No single diagnostic test is specific for systemic sclerosis, although a titer of 1:40 or higher for antinuclear antibody (ANA) is the most sensitive for diagnosis. Other laboratory studies that are done include an ESR, which is typically elevated from the chronic inflammatory process, and a CBC, which will demonstrate anemia. A skin biopsy may be done to confirm the diagnosis.

Medications

Medications to treat systemic sclerosis are chosen based on the organ manifestations presented by each patient. Immunosuppressive agents and corticosteroids are of limited benefit but may be used to slow or prevent pulmonary fibrosis and in life-threatening disease. Cyclophosphamide (Cytoxan) or methotrexate may slow disease progression. Sildenafil (Viagra) may be prescribed to treat symptomatic pulmonary hypertension. Calcium channel blockers such as nifedipine (Procardia) or alpha-adrenergic blockers such as prazosin (Minipress) may be prescribed for patients with Raynaud phenomenon (Denton, 2017a). When manifestations of esophagitis accompany systemic sclerosis, H_2-receptor blockers such as cimetidine (Tagamet) or ranitidine (Zantac), antacids, or proton pump inhibitors, such as omeprazole (Prilosec), which blocks all gastric secretion, may be ordered. Tetracycline or another broad-spectrum antibiotic may be prescribed to suppress intestinal flora and relieve symptoms of malabsorption. Patients with kidney disease are usually treated with angiotensin-converting enzyme (ACE) inhibitors such as captopril (Capoten) to control hypertension and preserve renal function. End-stage kidney disease is managed with dialysis and transplantation (Denton, 2017a).

Therapies

Physical therapy is an important part of the management of systemic sclerosis to maintain mobility of affected tissues, the hands and face. Because the mouth opening, if involved, becomes increasingly smaller as the disease progresses, stretching and strengthening of facial muscles can be vital to maintaining oral food intake. Therefore, speech therapy should be consulted to assist with these exercises.

Nursing Care

Nursing care needs of patients with systemic sclerosis are individualized to the effects and manifestations of the disease. Skin manifestations are present to some degree in nearly all patients with systemic sclerosis. Nursing care related to the skin focuses on maintaining skin integrity and flexibility. Measures to maintain supple skin are important because elasticity cannot be regained once it is lost. Apply moisturizers to prevent dryness and cracking. Protect the skin where it is stretched taut over joints or bony prominences. Perform ROM exercises to help prevent joint contractures due to increasingly tight skin.

Difficulty swallowing and recurrent esophagitis may interfere with the patient's nutritional status. Provide frequent, small meals. Consult with a dietitian, a speech therapist, and the patient to determine which foods are easy to swallow. Keep the patient in a sitting or Fowler position after meals and elevate the head of the bed at night to minimize esophageal reflux.

The dermatologic and systemic effects of the disease may have significant psychologic effects on the patient, leading to feelings of helplessness and hopelessness and self-esteem disturbance. Establish an atmosphere of trust with the patient. Listen actively and acknowledge concerns about the disease and its effects on the patient's life and appearance. Encourage the patient to share these concerns with family members and significant others. Provide referral to social services or counseling as appropriate.

The patient with predominant pulmonary disease has nursing care needs similar to those of other patients with restrictive respiratory disorders. If the patient with systemic sclerosis has impaired renal function, nursing care is similar to that for patients with chronic kidney disease.

Transitions of Care

Teach the patient with systemic sclerosis about the disease and introduce measures to help manage its effects. Stress the importance of good skin care and physical therapy exercises to maintain mobility, particularly of the hands and face. Discuss the need to avoid chilling (local and whole body) to prevent episodes of Raynaud phenomenon. Teach the role of proper dress in the winter: Loose, warm clothing, gloves, and warm stockings. If needed, stress the need to stop smoking because of the vasoconstrictive effect of nicotine and the respiratory effects of the disease. Provide the patient with information about manifestations of disease progression and organ involvement. Teach the patient to report new or worsening symptoms to the physician. In addition, suggest the following resources:

- National Institute of Arthritis and Musculoskeletal and Skin Diseases
- Scleroderma Foundation
- Scleroderma Research Foundation
- International Scleroderma Network.

The Patient with Sjögren Syndrome

Sjögren syndrome is a chronic, progressive autoimmune disorder that causes inflammation and dysfunction of exocrine glands throughout the body. Although it can occur as a primary disorder, Sjögren syndrome is often associated with other rheumatic disease, including rheumatoid arthritis, SLE, primary biliary cirrhosis, systemic sclerosis, Hashimoto thyroiditis, and interstitial pulmonary fibrosis.

Pathophysiology

In this disease, exocrine glands in many areas of the body are destroyed by infiltration of lymphocytes and deposits of immune complexes. The salivary and lacrimal glands are particularly affected, leading to the characteristic manifestations of *xerophthalmia* (dry eyes) and *xerostomia* (dry mouth).

Risk Factors

Sjögren syndrome primarily affects women, with a ratio of women to men at 9:1. The highest incidence is between the ages of 40 and 60 years (Patel & Shanane, 2014).

Manifestations and Complications

Patients often experience dry, gritty-feeling eyes and may develop corneal ulcerations. Mucosal dryness affects taste, smell, chewing, and swallowing and leads to increased dental caries. Parotid gland enlargement is common. Excess dryness can also affect the nose, throat, larynx, bronchi, vagina, and skin. Systemic effects of Sjögren syndrome include arthritis, dysphagia, pancreatitis, pleuritis, neurologic manifestations including migraine, and vasculitis.

Nephritis may occur, but renal failure rarely results. Patients with Sjögren syndrome have a greatly increased risk of developing malignant lymphoma.

Interprofessional Care

Diagnosis

The diagnosis of Sjögren syndrome is often based on the patient's history and clinical presentation. A Schirmer test, which measures the quantity of tears secreted in a 5-minute period in response to irritation; ocular staining; and slit-lamp examination of the eye may be performed. A definitive diagnosis can be made by biopsy of a salivary gland for evidence of lymphoid foci.

Treatment

Treatment is supportive. Artificial tears are used to decrease eye irritation and dryness. The patient can keep the mouth moist by drinking fluids, using a saliva substitute, and chewing sugarless gum. Medications that increase mouth dryness, such as atropine and decongestants, should be avoided.

Nursing Care

Nurses caring for patients with Sjögren syndrome need to teach measures to protect the patient's eyes and oral mucosa. Instill artificial tears as needed. Encourage the patient to sip fluids throughout the day. Provide frequent oral hygiene, particularly before and after meals. Ensure that the patient has sufficient fluids to drink during meals because fluids help with chewing and swallowing.

The Patient with Inflammatory Myopathy

The inflammatory myopathies include polymyositis and dermatomyositis. *Polymyositis (PM)* is a systemic connective tissue disorder characterized by inflammation of connective tissue and muscle fibers leading to muscle weakness and atrophy. When muscle fiber inflammation is accompanied by skin lesions secondary to capillary damage, the disease is known as *dermatomyositis (DM)* (Greenberg, 2018).

Pathophysiology and Risk Factors

The immune mechanism causing the inflammatory response is not clear, but autoantibodies can be identified in most people with the disease. The activation of complement is thought to contribute to the inflammatory process. Inflammation leads to muscle fiber necrosis and degeneration.

Inflammatory myopathies are rare, affecting people of all ages and ethnic groups. Women are about twice as likely to be affected as men (Femia, 2017).

Manifestations

Initial manifestations of PM and DM include muscle tenderness and weakness, rash, arthralgias, fatigue, fever, and weight loss. Skeletal muscle weakness is the predominant manifestation. Its onset may be either insidious or abrupt. Muscle weakness tends to progress over weeks to months. Muscles of the shoulder and pelvic girdles are particularly affected, making it difficult for the patient to get out of chairs, climb stairs, and reach overhead. Weakness of neck flexor muscles may make it difficult to raise the head from a pillow. Affected muscles may also be tender and painful. A characteristic dusky red rash may be present on the face and upper trunk. Other manifestations include Raynaud phenomenon, dysphagia, dyspnea, and cough (due to interstitial pneumonitis).

Skin manifestations will occur with DM but not PM. The skin manifestations include Gottron papules (erythematous papules over the dorsal aspects of the fingers), Gottron sign (erythematous macules, patches or papules on sites other than the hands), erythematous skin irritation on the upper eyelids, facial erythema, and multiple other forms of skin changes (Miller & Vleugels, 2017).

Complications

Interstitial lung disease, malignancy—most often adenocarcinoma, esophageal disease, and myocarditis—are all complications that can occur with both PM and DM (Miller & Vleugels, 2017).

Interprofessional Care

Diagnosis

There is no specific test to diagnose inflammatory myopathy. Autoantibodies may be identified in blood serum. Serum levels of muscle enzymes are elevated, particularly creatine kinase (CK) and aldolase levels. Biopsy of involved muscle shows patchy muscle fiber necrosis and the presence of inflammatory cells.

Medications

A combination of rest and corticosteroid therapy is prescribed to reduce the inflammatory response. Long-term corticosteroid therapy may be necessary to manage the disease. Immunosuppressive agents such as methotrexate, cyclophosphamide, and azathioprine may be used in combination with corticosteroids to induce remission (Miller, 2018).

Nursing Care

The nursing role in caring for the patient with an inflammatory myopathy is supportive. Measures to promote comfort are important. Muscle weakness may interfere with the patient's ability to provide self-care and manage health and home. The patient may have difficulty with speech because of pharyngeal muscle weakness. Provide alternate means of communication as needed and use patience in listening. Observe closely while the patient eats because aspiration is a potential problem. Modify the patient's diet as needed to maintain nutrition and safety. A speech therapy consult may be necessary.

Transitions of Care

Education of the patient and family is an important component of care. Emphasize the need to balance periods of rest and activity. Discuss skin care to prevent dryness and infection. Teach the patient about prescribed medications and their short- and long-term side effects. Provide information about safety measures while eating. Encourage family members to become trained in performance of the Heimlich maneuver and CPR. Discuss signs of respiratory infection and other possible complications of inflammatory myopathy, including renal failure and malignancy.

The Patient with Lyme Disease

Lyme disease is an inflammatory disorder caused by the spirochete *Borrelia burgdorferi*, which is transmitted primarily by ticks. It is the most commonly reported tickborne illness in the United States. Geographically, Lyme disease is more prevalent in the areas where ticks are found. The majority are found in the Northeast and Middle Atlantic states, the upper Midwest, and still present, but much less so, in Northern California and the Pacific Northwest regions of the United States (Beard, 2016). It has also been reported throughout Europe, Asia, and Australia. Ticks that act as vectors for Lyme disease, primarily *Ixodes dammini*, *I. pacificus*, and *I. scapularis* in the United States, are usually carried by mice or deer, although other animals may be infected. The most frequent time of onset is the summer months. Lyme disease occurs most often in children and adults living in rural areas (Beard, 2016). Fortunately, all stages of Lyme disease can be cured by antibiotics, but some people with late neurologic or arthritic involvement may not improve.

Pathophysiology

B. burgdorferi enters the skin at the site of the tick bite. After an incubation period of up to 30 days, it migrates outward in the skin, forming a characteristic lesion called *erythema migrans*. It may also spread via lymph or blood to other skin sites, nodes, or organs. The inflammatory joint changes associated with Lyme disease closely resemble those of rheumatoid arthritis (vascular congestion, tissue infiltration by inflammatory cells, possible pannus formation, and erosion of cartilage and bone).

Manifestations

Manifestations are often seen in the skin, musculoskeletal system, and CNS. Lyme disease begins with flulike manifestations and a skin rash, followed weeks or months later by neurologic symptoms, including facial nerve palsy and meningitis, and months to years later by arthritis. This progression is highly individualized.

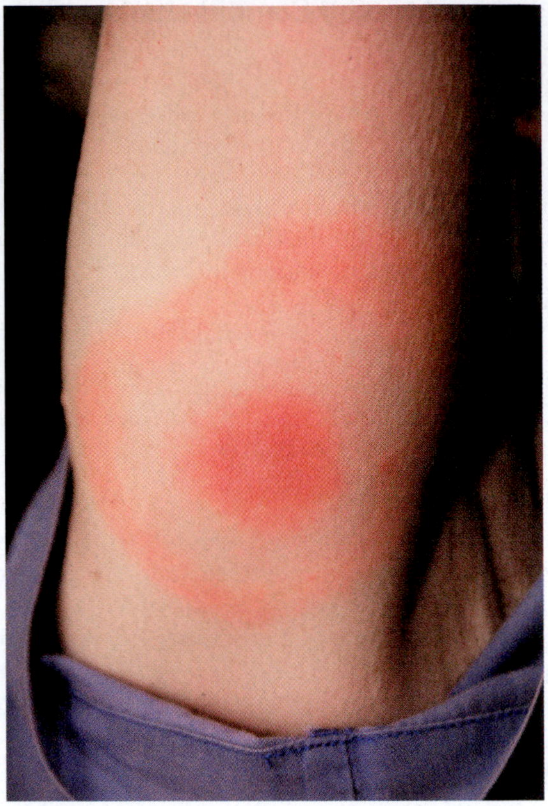

Figure 40.12 ■ The characteristic erythema migrans (bull's-eye) lesion of Lyme disease on a patient's arm.

Erythema migrans is the initial manifestation of Lyme disease (**Figure 40.12** ■). This flat or slightly raised red lesion at the site of the tick bite expands over several days (up to a diameter of 20 cm [8 in.]), with the central area clearing as it expands (Hu, 2016). Systemic symptoms such as fatigue, malaise, fever, chills, and myalgias often accompany the initial lesion. As the disease spreads, secondary skin lesions develop, as do migratory musculoskeletal symptoms, including arthralgias, myalgias, and tendinitis. Persistent fatigue is common during this stage of the disease. Headache and stiff neck are characteristic neurologic manifestations.

Complications

With untreated infection, complications can develop months to years after the initial infection. Chronic recurrent arthritis, primarily affecting large joints (especially the knee), is common. Permanent disability may result. Other effects that may be seen weeks to months after the initial infection include meningitis, encephalitis, and neuropathies, as well as cardiac complications including myocarditis and heart block.

Interprofessional Care

Diagnosis

Both manifestations and laboratory studies are used to establish the diagnosis of Lyme disease. For early disseminated disease and late Lyme disease, positive IgM and IgG antibodies of *B. burgdorferi* can be detected (Hu, 2016).

Medications

The early diagnosis and proper antibiotic treatment of Lyme disease are important to preventing the complications of infection. A number of antibiotics may be used to treat Lyme disease, including doxycycline (Doxy-Caps, Vibramycin), amoxicillin (Amoxil), cefuroxime axetil (Ceftin), or erythromycin (Hu, 2017). Therapy may be continued for up to 21 days to ensure eradication of the organism from affected tissues. In addition to antibiotic treatment, aspirin or an NSAID may be prescribed for relief of arthritic symptoms. The affected joint may be splinted to rest the joint. When the knee is involved, weight bearing may be restricted and the use of crutches indicated.

Nursing Care

Nursing care focuses on prevention of the disease. Many people do not protect themselves from tick bites. This protection is becoming increasingly important with a higher incidence of Lyme disease, due in part to an overpopulation of deer and the encroachment of the suburbs on once rural areas. Simple measures that can help prevent tick bites are:

- Avoid tick-infested areas, especially in spring and summer, such as woods and rural areas with brush and tall weeds.
- Cover exposed skin with long-sleeved shirts and tuck pants into socks. Wearing high rubber boots may provide additional protection.
- Use insect repellents that contain DEET on clothing and exposed skin and apply permethrin to clothing prior to exposure.
- Inspect skin, especially in areas of tight-fitting clothing, after exposure.
- Remove attached ticks with fine-tipped tweezers. Grasp the tick firmly as close to the skin as possible and pull the tick's body up and away from the skin. If the tick's head remains in the skin, it will not cause Lyme disease (the bacteria are in the tick's midgut). Most cases occur when the tick has been feeding for at least 24 hours. Clean the area with an antiseptic.

40.4 Infectious Musculoskeletal Disorders

The Patient with Osteomyelitis

Osteomyelitis is an infection of the bone. Osteomyelitis may occur as an acute, subacute, or chronic process. It occurs because of a penetrating wound, bacteremia (hematogenous osteomyelitis), invasion from a contiguous locus of infection, or direct contamination related to surgery or trauma (Lalani, 2017). Foreign material, such as prosthetic joint implants and devices used to stabilize fractures, can be sites in which osteomyelitis originates. Hemodialysis and injection drug use are also risk factors for osteomyelitis.

Pathophysiology

The cause of osteomyelitis is usually bacterial; however, fungi, parasites, and viruses can also cause bone infection. *Staphylococcus aureus* is the most common infecting organism (Sopirala, 2017). Other organisms include *Escherichia coli*, *Pseudomonas*, *Serratia*, *Salmonella*, and *M. tuberculosis*.

After entry, bacteria lodge and multiply in the bone, resulting in the inflammatory and immune system response. Phagocytes attempt to contain the infection, releasing enzymes in the process that destroy bone tissue. Pus forms, followed by edema and vascular congestion. The Haversian canals in the medullary cavity of the bone allow the infection to travel to other segments of the bone. If the infection reaches the outer margin of the bone, it raises the periosteum of the bone, spreading along the surface (**Figure 40.13** ■). Lifting of the periosteum from the cortex disrupts the blood vessels that enter the bone. Pressure increases, further compromising the vascular supply and leading to ischemia and eventual necrosis of the bone. Blood and antibiotics cannot reach the bone tissue once the pressure compromises the vascular and arteriolar systems. In addition, bacteria adhere to damaged bone, coating the underlying bony matrix, including fibrinogen, collagen, and other substances, with a protective film that further impedes host defenses (Sopirala, 2017).

Hematogenous Osteomyelitis

Hematogenous infections are caused by pathogens that are carried in the blood from sites of infection elsewhere in the

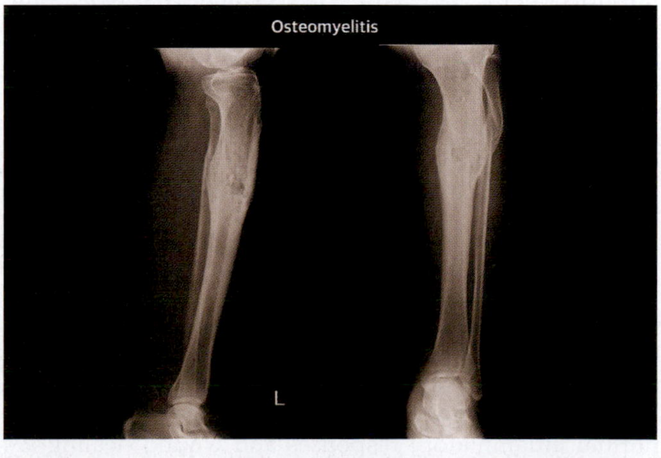
Osteomyelitis
L

Figure 40.13 ■ X-ray of patient with osteomyelitis.

body. This type of osteomyelitis occurs more in children than in adults (Lalani, 2017). Three circumstances must be present for hematogenous osteomyelitis to occur: Local or systemic immunocompromise, the number of pathogens present, and the virulence of the pathogen (Sopirala, 2017). Hematogenous osteomyelitis primarily affects older adults, people with sickle cell disease, and intravenous drug users (immunocompromised). The spine is the usual site of infection in adults. Pathogens enter the well-perfused vertebral bodies of adults via the spinal arteries (number). From there, the infection spreads into the disk space. The lumbar spine is involved more frequently than the thoracic or cervical spine. Urinary tract infections, soft tissue infection, endocarditis, and infected intravenous sites are sources of pathogens (virulence).

Patients with acute hematogenous osteomyelitis experience an acute onset of pain, tenderness, and fever. Soft tissue edema over the affected bone may be noted. The course of vertebral osteomyelitis in intravenous drug users is often subacute, with vague, dull pain in the affected region and a normal or low-grade fever. The pain intensifies over 2 to 3 months and is accompanied by tenderness, muscle spasm, and limited ROM.

Osteomyelitis from a Contiguous Infection

Infections caused by an extension of infection from adjacent soft tissues fall into this category of osteomyelitis. The infection is a result of, or complication of, direct penetrating wounds, joint replacements, decubitus ulcers, and neurosurgery. This is the most common cause of osteomyelitis in adults.

Risk Factors

Osteomyelitis can occur at any age, but adults over age 50 are more commonly affected. The older adult is at risk for osteomyelitis for several reasons. Immune function tends to decline with age; the older adult is also more likely to have a chronic disease process such as diabetes mellitus that affects immune function. Circulatory status in older adults is often compromised by atherosclerotic processes, impairing blood flow to the bone. Older adults have a higher risk of pressure ulcers because of circulatory, skin, sensation, and mobility changes associated with aging. Pressure ulcers that cannot be staged and treated because of eschar formation pose a particular risk. In addition, the older adult may not demonstrate the typical signs of infection and inflammation, which allows an infectious process to become well established before it is detected.

People with diabetes and peripheral vascular disease are at risk for developing osteomyelitis involving the feet and lower extremities (Lalani, 2017). Diabetic neuropathy exposes the foot and lower extremities to trauma and pressure ulcers. The patient may be unaware of the infection as it spreads into the bone. When tissue perfusion is poor, normal inflammatory responses and wound healing are impaired. The infection is often diagnosed when the patient seeks treatment for a nonhealing sore, swollen toe, or acute cellulitis.

Manifestations

Manifestations of osteomyelitis vary according to the age of the patient, the cause and site of involvement, and whether the infection is acute, subacute, or chronic. If the infection occurs near a joint, osteomyelitis can appear to be septic arthritis (see below) and must be ruled out as the cause to ensure proper management (Lalani, 2017).

Acute osteomyelitis symptoms develop gradually over several days. Dull pain in the affected area gradually increases in intensity. Tenderness, warmth, erythema, and edema may be present (Lalani, 2017). Fever and rigors may also be present. Subacute symptoms include mild pain that develops over several weeks, with a low-grade fever but with minimal other symptoms (Lalani, 2017).

Chronic osteomyelitis symptoms are sometimes related to a sinus tract that develops. These manifestations include pain, erythema, and edema. The symptoms can be associated with other medical conditions, ulcers, soft tissue trauma, prosthetic material, or vascular insufficiency, with nonhealing areas, making it difficult to diagnose (Lalani, 2017).

Complications

Osteomyelitis can be considered a complication itself, related to issues discussed above. However, if left untreated, osteomyelitis can become chronic, leading to development of sinus tracts, which can cause osteolysis and lead to pathologic fractures (Lalani, 2017). Sepsis may occur as well. Cancers, such as squamous cell carcinoma and others, have been known to develop with chronic osteomyelitis (Lalani, 2017).

Interprofessional Care

Care of the patient with osteomyelitis focuses on relieving pain, eliminating the infection, and preventing or minimizing complications. Early diagnosis is important to prevent bone necrosis by early administration of the appropriate antibiotic. A thorough history and physical examination are important to identify risk factors and possible causes of the infection.

Diagnosis

The diagnosis of osteomyelitis is based on standard x-rays, bone scans, MRI, blood tests, and biopsy. An MRI, CT scan, and bone scan may be conducted to identify abscesses, sinus tracts, and bone changes. An ultrasound can detect subperiosteal fluid collections, abscesses, and periosteal thickening and elevation associated with osteomyelitis. During an acute infection, ESR and WBC are elevated. Blood and tissue cultures (from affected bone or soft tissue) are obtained to identify the infecting organism and direct antibiotic therapy.

Medications

Antibiotic therapy is mandatory to prevent acute osteomyelitis from progressing to the chronic phase. Parenteral antibiotic therapy begins as soon as cultures (blood and/or wound) are obtained. A penicillinase-resistant semisynthetic penicillin (e.g., nafcillin, oxacillin) or a cephalosporin such as cefazolin (Ancef) or ceftriaxone (Rocephin) may be given until the culture and sensitivity results are known. These antibiotics are used initially because many cases of osteomyelitis are caused by *S. aureus*. When the detailed sensitivity report is obtained from the cultures, more definitive antibiotics are prescribed.

For the patient with acute or chronic osteomyelitis, antibiotics are continued for 4 to 6 weeks. Intravenous antibiotic administration (preferred method) or oral therapy is common. The type of antibiotic is dependent on culture results and any allergies the patient may have. Home IV therapy can be arranged to avoid costly hospital stays.

Surgery

Surgical debridement may be performed early in the course of the infection to remove necrotic tissue and identify the infecting organism. Debridement is the primary treatment for the patient with chronic osteomyelitis. The periosteum is excised, and the cortex is drilled to release the pressure from accumulated pus. During this procedure, cultures may be obtained and sent to the laboratory for analysis. The wound holes are irrigated, and the wound is then closed. The cavity may be kept clean by inserting drainage tubes that are connected to an irrigation and suction system.

A musculocutaneous (myocutaneous) flap is another approach used for the treatment of the dead space caused by extensive debridement of the infected site. The procedure involves moving or rotating a muscle and the section of skin fed by the arteries from that muscle into the cavity created by the surgery. A skin graft is performed later.

Adjuvant Therapies

Hyperbaric oxygen (HBO) therapy and negative-pressure wound therapy (NPWT) (WoundVac) have been used as adjuvant therapies for patients with chronic osteomyelitis. Due to the often poor blood flow through the bone, HBO seems to be assistive in promoting healing in these chronic wounds (Lalani, 2017). NPWT can speed up the wound healing process in open, slow-healing wounds (Gestring, 2017).

Nursing Care

The patient with acute osteomyelitis, no matter the etiology, will be required to be on long-term antibiotics. This lifestyle change, although temporary, can disrupt the patient's role and be stressful on the patient's significant other and family. Supportive nursing care is key to assist the patient to cope with all the changes that are occurring in his or her life.

The patient with chronic osteomyelitis faces frequent and lengthy hospitalizations and/or treatment modalities. The prognosis is uncertain, and functional deficits and amputation are a constant concern. The ongoing expenses, loss of financial support, and role changes within the family are also patient concerns.

Assessment

No matter the type of osteomyelitis, acute or chronic, there are focused assessments that the nurse needs to perform to determine the best way to assist the patient with his or her current and anticipated needs. Focused assessments to perform include vital signs, wound and skin assessment, peripheral neurovascular assessment, and psychosocial assessment. General assessments of the other body systems will alert the nurse to any potential complications or side effects from medications.

Priorities of Care

Care priorities focus on assisting the patient to eradicate the infection using the prescribed medications, wound care, and activity restrictions, as needed. Additionally, focusing on the prevention of further infection, especially once home, will aid in the recovery process and prevent complications.

Diagnoses, Outcomes, and Interventions

Nursing diagnoses associated with acute osteomyelitis focus on preventing the transmission of infection and problems due to immobility. Providing comfort and patient teaching are also very important.

Promote Tissue Integrity. The patient who has undergone surgical debridement of infected bone has an increased risk for an additional infection due to disruption of the skin barrier. Aggressive antibiotic therapy also disrupts the patient's usual body flora, an important factor in preventing pathogenic organisms from establishing infection. Infection is a hypermetabolic state that increases the patient's kilocalorie needs.

Expected Outcome: Patient will experience no adverse consequences of surgical or antibiotic therapy.

The nurse will:

- Maintain strict hand hygiene practices and teach the patient and family about hand hygiene. *Meticulous hand hygiene helps prevent the spread of infection by minimizing the entry of organisms into susceptible patients.*
- Administer antimicrobial therapy at specified time intervals. *Optimal blood levels of antibiotic therapy are mandatory in patients with infectious processes.*
- Monitor site of infection, surgical wound, and systemic manifestations for evidence of desired therapeutic effect (reduced inflammation, evidence of healing, improved overall physical status). Promptly report deviations from expected course, as well as manifestations of superinfection or complications of therapy. *Monitoring patient responses to therapy is an important nursing responsibility in acute care settings, extended care or rehabilitation facilities, and in the patient's home.*
- Maintain the patient's optimal dietary kilocalorie and protein intake. *High kilocalorie and protein intake provide the patient with sufficient nutritional support for the body's needs during the stressful event of the inflammatory process.*

Promote Physical Mobility. Pain, infection, inflammation, and the use of immobilizers can all impair the mobility of the patient with osteomyelitis.

Expected Outcome: Patient will experience no adverse effects of required immobilization.

The nurse will:

- Maintain the affected limb in functional position when immobilized. *The patient may hesitate to move the involved extremity because of continuous pain; therefore, the extremity must be maintained in functional position to avoid flexion contracture.*

- Maintain rest and avoid subjecting the affected extremity to weight-bearing activities. *The involved extremity must be immobilized to avoid pathologic fractures caused by stress on the weakened bone.*
- Ensure active or passive ROM exercises every 4 hours. *Flexion contracture occurs when the patient remains immobile or when there is only minimal joint movement. Consult a physical therapist for a plan of exercises to avoid contracture.*

Relieve Acute Pain. The patient with osteomyelitis experiences pain due to edema.

Expected Outcome: Patient will verbalize an acceptable level of comfort.

The nurse will:

- Use a splint or immobilizer when the patient experiences acute pain from edema. *Splinting or immobilizing the involved extremity provides support and reduces pain caused by movement.*
- Ask the healthcare provider to order scheduled administration of narcotic and nonnarcotic analgesics on a 24-hour basis rather than as needed. *The use of 24-hour administration allows blood levels of pain-relieving medications to remain constant.*
- Use nonpharmacologic strategies (e.g., distraction, relaxation techniques) for adjunctive pain management. *Pain of the muscles and joints may be controlled through nonpharmacologic interventions. Warm moist packs, warm baths, or heating pads to the involved extremity provide comfort due to vasodilation.*
- Avoid excessive manipulation of the involved area; handle the area gently. Carefully assess the patient for guarding, limping, or unwillingness to move the affected part. Communicate to other healthcare professionals the patient's preferences for assistive devices and means of manipulating the involved area. *Gentle handling and minimal manipulation help reduce pain.*

Transitions of Care

Although patients may be hospitalized for acute treatment and surgery, most care is provided at home. Home health services can provide intravenous medications, if prescribed. Discuss the following topics for home care:

- The importance of careful hand hygiene, especially after toileting and dressing changes.
- The importance of taking all antibiotics as prescribed. Include information about helping prevent the yeast infections (of the mouth or vagina) and diarrhea often associated with prolonged antibiotic therapy by eating 8 oz of live-culture yogurt each day.
- The need to take pain medications on a regular basis to prevent pain from becoming severe. Provide information about how to deal with side effects, such as constipation, by increasing fluid and fiber intake.
- How to perform wound care and sources for needed equipment and supplies.
- Rest or limited weight bearing for the affected extremity or body part. Teach how to avoid complications associated with prolonged immobilization, such as frequently shifting position, keeping skin and linens clean and dry, and doing active ROM exercises for unaffected joints.
- The importance of maintaining good nutrition. An adequate supply of kilocalories, protein, and other nutrients is necessary for immune function and healing. Suggest frequent, small meals and using nutritional supplements such as Ensure to help maintain nutritional intake.

The Patient with Septic Arthritis

Pathophysiology

Septic arthritis can develop if a joint space is invaded by a pathogen. The most common bacteria implicated in septic arthritis include gonococci and *S. aureus*. Methicillin-resistant *S. aureus* (MRSA) and Gram-positive streptococci infections are increasingly seen. Infections by Gram-negative bacteria such as *E. coli* and *Pseudomonas* more commonly affect people who inject recreational drugs, are immunocompromised, or have been involved in a trauma (Goldenberg & Sexton, 2017).

Infection of the joint leads to inflammation with resulting synovitis and joint effusion. Abscesses may form in synovial tissues or bone underlying joint cartilage. If not treated promptly and effectively, septic arthritis can lead to destruction of the affected joint. A single joint, often the knee, is usually affected. Septic arthritis may also affect hip, fingers, or elbow (Goldenberg & Sexton, 2017).

Risk Factors

The primary risk factors for septic arthritis are persistent bacteremia (bacteria in the blood) (e.g., due to use of injectable drugs, endocarditis), previous joint damage (e.g., due to trauma or rheumatoid arthritis), impaired immunity (e.g., diabetes, renal failure, alcoholism), and loss of skin integrity. Previous intra-articular corticosteroid injections, arthroscopic surgery, and total joint replacements that allow potential direct contamination of the joint are additional risk factors (Goldenberg & Sexton, 2017).

Manifestations and Complications

The onset of septic arthritis is typically abrupt, marked by pain and stiffness of the infected joint. The joint appears red and swollen and is hot and tender to the touch. Effusion (increased fluid within the joint space) is usually present. Systemic manifestations of infection, such as chills and fever, often accompany local manifestations, although these may be muted if the patient is immunocompromised or taking anti-inflammatory medications.

Destruction of the joint or severe joint dysfunction, leading to the need for amputation, arthrodesis, or joint replacement, is the major complication of septic arthritis (Goldenberg & Sexton, 2017). Additionally, mortality associated with septic arthritis often occurs in the presence of comorbid conditions that leave patients immunocompromised (Goldenberg & Sexton, 2017).

Interprofessional Care

Diagnosis

Septic arthritis is a medical emergency requiring prompt treatment to preserve joint function. When it is suspected, fluid from the affected joint is aspirated and sent for Gram stain and culture. Cultures are also obtained from all likely sources of the infection, including blood, sputum, or wounds. The synovial fluid culture is always positive in nongonococcal septic arthritis, but is often negative for bacteria in early gonococcal arthritis. Infected synovial fluid is usually cloudy, with a high WBC count and a low glucose level. Joint x-ray films are often normal in the initial stages, but soon show demineralization, bony erosions, and joint space narrowing.

Medications

Treatment with a broad-spectrum parenteral antibiotic is initiated before the results of culture are obtained. The medication may be changed or adjusted once the organism has been identified. Antibiotic therapy is continued for at least 2 weeks after inflammatory manifestations have abated. This is followed by 2 weeks of oral antibiotic therapy (Goldenberg & Sexton, 2017).

Surgery

The infected joint is treated with drainage of infected pus and debris, rest, and systemic antibiotics. Needle aspiration of the infected joint may be effective to remove infected synovial fluid, although in some cases arthroscopy or arthrotomy are necessary. Repeated joint aspirations may be necessary.

Joint rest with no weight bearing is prescribed, but immobilization of the joint is not generally required. Physical therapy is implemented during the recovery period to ensure maintenance of optimal joint function.

Nursing Care

Septic arthritis can be frightening to the patient who experiences a sudden onset of joint pain and edema and is faced with the possibility of rapid functional loss of movement. Nursing care is both supportive and educative. Patients may be hospitalized for initial treatment with intravenous antibiotics. It is important to monitor the patient's response to therapy, including systemic manifestations such as fever. Position the affected joint appropriately, using pillows to elevate it as needed. Warm compresses may be ordered for comfort. Active ROM exercises preserve joint mobility and should be initiated as soon as the healthcare provider allows.

Transitions of Care

The patient with septic arthritis needs information about the disorder, its etiology, and its treatment. Teach the patient how organisms may gain entry into the joint space. Discuss the role that the use of injected drugs and sexually transmitted infections play in septic arthritis and means to prevent infection as appropriate (e.g., using clean "works," practicing safer sex). Refer the patient to a drug treatment program, if necessary. Emphasize the importance of complying with all aspects of the treatment plan to prevent joint destruction and disability. A social services consult may be necessary to assist with transition to home and continuing antibiotic therapy, if ordered.

40.5 Neoplastic Musculoskeletal Disorders

Bone tumors may be either primary or metastatic. Like other tumors, bone tumors can be either benign or malignant. Virtually every malignant tumor can metastasize to bone. However, the most common metastatic bone tumors originate from primary tumors of the prostate, breast, kidney, thyroid, and lung. The focus for discussion in this section is care of the patient with a primary bone tumor.

The Patient with a Bone Tumor

Benign bone tumors, which are far more common than malignant bone tumors, tend to grow slowly and do not often destroy surrounding tissues. Primary malignant tumors of the bone, known as sarcomas, are rare, accounting for less than 0.2% of all adult cancers (American Cancer Society [ACS], 2018a). Malignant tumors grow rapidly and metastasize.

Primary bone tumors arise from bone tissue itself, that is, cartilage (chondrogenic), bone (osteogenic), collagen (collagenic), and bone marrow cells (myelogenic). The tissue type, neoplasm classification, sites, and incidence of the most common primary bone tumors are summarized in **Table 40.8**.

Pathophysiology

The etiology of bone tumors is unknown, but there is a connection between increased bone activity and the development of primary bone tumors. Bone tumors frequently occur when primary bone growth is at its peak in adolescence or is overstimulated during disease, such as Paget disease.

Primary tumors cause *osteolysis*, which weakens the bone, resulting in bone fractures. Normal bone adjacent to the tumor responds to tumor pressure by altering its normal pattern of remodeling. The bone's surface becomes altered, and the contours enlarge in the area of the tumor growth.

Malignant bone tumors invade and destroy adjacent bone tissue by producing substances that promote bone resorption or by interfering with a bone's blood supply. Benign bone tumors, unlike malignant ones, have a symmetric, controlled growth pattern. As they grow, they push against neighboring bone tissue. This weakens the bone's structure until it becomes unable to withstand the stress of ordinary use, frequently resulting in pathologic fracture.

Table 40.8 Common Primary Bone Tumors

Tumor	Tissue Origin	Site	Population Affected
Benign Bone Tumors			
Osteochondroma	Cartilage	■ On bone surface near growth plate ■ Long bones	■ Most common benign tumor ■ Children and adolescents
Enchondroma	Cartilage	■ Medullary bone ■ Hands, feet ■ Humerus ■ Femur	■ Adolescents and young adults
Osteoid osteoma	Bone	■ Long bones ■ May also affect hands, fingers, or spine	■ Children to young adults ■ 3:1 males to females
Malignant Bone Tumors			
Osteosarcoma	Bone	■ Long bones around the knee (distal femur, proximal tibia) ■ Other long bones (proximal humerus)	■ Most common malignant bone tumor after multiple myeloma, 45% of bone sarcomas ■ Adolescents and young adults ■ Males more frequently than females
Ewing sarcoma	Bone	■ Shaft of long bones ■ Flat bones	■ Adolescents and young adults
Chondrosarcoma	Cartilage	■ Flat bones (pelvis, scapula) ■ Diaphysis (shaft) of long bones	■ Adults and older adults ■ Accounts for 20–25% of sarcomas
Multiple myeloma	Bone marrow (plasma cells)		■ Most common malignant bone tumor; considered a hematologic cancer

Source: Data from ACS, 2018c.

Risk Factors

There are some genetic disorders that cause some gene mutations and increase the likelihood of a person developing some type of bone tumor. Paget disease is considered a precancerous condition, in which approximately 1% of those with the disease develop bone cancer. Exposure to radiation (e.g., cancer radiation therapy) and bone marrow transplant are known to increase the risk for developing bone cancer, as are certain rare genetic disorders (ACS, 2018b).

Manifestations

The three main manifestations of bone tumors are pain, a mass, and impaired function. Bone pain usually develops over several months, is constant or intermittent, and may be worse at night (Wang, Gebhardt, & Rainusso, 2017). The mass is described as edema or a lump on the bone that is firm, slightly tender, and may be felt through the skin. The mass may interfere with normal movement and/or cause the bone to break. The manifestations of bone tumors are often associated with a history of a fall or blow to the extremity that brings the mass to the patient's attention. The injury, rather than the growth itself, usually causes the patient to seek medical attention. Manifestations of bone tumors by site are outlined in **Table 40.9**.

Interprofessional Care

Treatment and care of the patient with a bone tumor focuses on prompt diagnosis, removal of the tumor, prevention of complications, and patient education.

Table 40.9 Manifestations of Bone Tumors by Site

Site	Manifestations
Bony Sarcomas	
Upper or lower extremity and pelvis	■ Worsening deep bony pain ■ Pain at night or during rest that may radiate and become severe ■ Muscular weakness or atrophy
Metaphysis of distal femur, proximal tibia, proximal humerus, and pelvis	■ Soft tissue mass extending from bone with erythematous or warm skin over tissue mass ■ Change in ability to perform ADLs ■ Fever
Soft Tissue Sarcomas	
Upper or lower extremity and pelvis	■ Enlarging firm mass with irregular borders, which causes pain in surrounding soft tissue structures
Thigh; shoulder and pelvis	■ Erythema or warmth and venous dilation over skin ■ Muscular weakness and atrophy with limited range of motion, change in ability to perform ADLs, and change in gait ■ Paresthesias with neurologic involvement and distal edema ■ Palpable local lymph nodes
Pelvis	■ Altered bowel and bladder habits or pain with intercourse

Diagnosis

The diagnosis of bone tumors is critical to the survival of the patient and possible preservation of the affected limb.

Radiologic studies include x-rays, CT scans, and MRI. X-rays show the location of the tumors and the extent of bone involvement. Benign tumors are characterized by sharp margins that are clearly separate from the surrounding normal bone. Malignant bone destruction has a characteristic "moth-eaten" pattern in which the growth has a less-defined margin that cannot be separated from the normal bone. CT scan and MRI are useful in evaluating the extent of tumor invasion into bone, soft tissues, and neurovascular structures. Percutaneous needle biopsy or needle biopsy at the time of surgery is used to determine the exact type of bone tumor.

Laboratory tests include an alkaline phosphatase (elevated with malignant bone tumor) and a calcium level (increased with massive bone destruction).

Treatment

As with other malignant tumors, bone tumors are treated with chemotherapy, radiation therapy, and surgery.

Chemotherapy. Chemotherapeutic agents are administered to shrink the malignant tumor before surgery, to control recurrence of tumor growth after surgery, or to treat metastasis of the tumor. Chemotherapeutic agents used to treat bone tumors are listed in **Box 40.5**. See Chapter 14 for further discussion of chemotherapy and its nursing implications.

Radiation Therapy. Radiation therapy may be used in combination with chemotherapy for tumors sensitive to its effects. Most primary malignant bone tumors in adults are resistant to radiation, so its role is generally adjunctive (Janeway & Maki, 2018). Radiation therapy is frequently applied to metastatic bone carcinomas as a method of pain control. It is also used to eliminate bony tumors or to eliminate any remaining tumor after a surgical procedure.

Surgery. Surgery is the primary treatment for osteosarcoma. The goal of surgery for the treatment of primary bone tumors is to eliminate the tumor completely. Tumors are removed either by excising the tumor itself or by amputating the affected limb. Wide excision of the tumor involves removing the tumor along with a small margin of normal tissue surrounding the tumor. In limb-sparing (or limb-salvage) surgery, cadaver allografts or metal prostheses are used to replace missing bone, avoiding amputation (Honicek, 2016).

> **BOX 40.5**
> **Chemotherapeutic Agents Used for Bone Tumors**
>
> **ALKYLATING AGENTS**
> Carboplatin
> Cyclophosphamide
> Ifosfamide
>
> **ANTIBIOTICS**
> Bleomycin
> Dactinomycin
> Doxorubicin
>
> **ANTIMETABOLITES**
> Methotrexate
>
> **MITOSIS INHIBITORS**
> Etoposide
>
> **PLANT ALKALOIDS**
> Vincristine
>
> **SYNTHETIC AGENTS**
> Cisplatin
>
> *Source:* Data from Janeway & Maki, 2018.

Nursing Care

Nursing care for the patient with a bone tumor requires innovative interventions from the time of diagnosis through the rehabilitation phase. In the acute phase, problems associated with pain, lack of knowledge, immobility, coping, and anxiety are foremost. If the patient develops complications from treatment or if a malignancy metastasizes, problems related to health management, home maintenance, self-concept, and prevention of further complications take priority.

Diagnoses, Outcomes, and Interventions

The patient with a bone tumor requires nursing care to address many health problems, including prevention of injury, relief of pain, assistance with mobility, and teaching about the disease process and treatment.

Reduce Risk for Injury. In the patient with a bone tumor, changes in bone tissue can cause pathologic fractures.

Expected Outcome: Patient will remain free of injury related to effects of bone tumor or treatment.

The nurse will:

- Teach patient how to avoid falls or injury to the tumor site, such as by using assistive devices when walking and ensuring the home environment is safe (e.g., remove throw rugs and use nightlights). *Pathologic fractures may occur at the tumor site because bone destruction can weaken the area.*
- Provide referral to physical or occupational therapy for fitting of and teaching about assistive devices for ambulating, such as a cane, crutches, or a walker. *Assistive devices can reduce the risk of falling when the patient has significant weakness of an extremity or when balance has been affected by treatment of the disease.*

Manage Acute and Chronic Pain. In the patient with a bone tumor, pain may be related to direct invasion of the tumor or to pathologic fractures. Patients may experience both acute and chronic pain.

Expected Outcome: Patient will be able to verbalize strategies to effectively manage pain.

The nurse will:

- Develop strategies for controlling both acute pain (from surgery, fracture, or inflammation) and chronic pain (from progression of the disease). *Analgesics combined with nonpharmacologic methods of pain control provide optimum relief of pain. Chronic pain, when mild in nature, is best managed with NSAIDs or aspirin. Moderate pain is best managed with a combination of narcotic analgesics and NSAIDs. Severe pain is best relieved with long-acting or sustained-relief narcotic analgesics.*

- Provide assistive devices (e.g., canes, walkers, crutches) when the patient ambulates. *Assistive devices lessen the pain by supporting weight bearing during ambulation.*

Promote Physical Mobility. Pain, muscle wasting, or surgical procedures can impair the physical mobility of the patient with a bone tumor.

Expected Outcome: Patient will participate in exercises and rehabilitation activities to regain physical mobility.

The nurse will:

- Begin muscle-strengthening and active and passive ROM exercises immediately after surgery. A continuous passive motion (CPM) machine may be used after surgical procedures to either upper or lower extremities. *Muscle-strengthening exercises must be encouraged as soon as possible to prevent muscle wasting and shorten the rehabilitation period.*
- Encourage exercises that help strengthen the triceps muscles. *The triceps are the major muscles in the arms and must be strengthened to assist in use of crutches or other assistive devices.*
- For the patient who has undergone an amputation of a lower extremity, encourage quadriceps and gluteal setting exercises and leg raises. *These exercises will benefit the patient when the rehabilitation period begins.*

Transitions of Care

The patient with a primary bone tumor needs information about the disease, its potential consequences, and treatment options. Present information in a matter-of-fact manner, taking time to listen to and address the patient's and family's concerns. Discuss expected effects and potential side effects of surgery, chemotherapy, and radiation therapy. Provide information about how to minimize side effects. Teach the post-surgical patient about wound care, demonstrating dressing changes and stump care (if amputation has occurred). Provide the patient with a list of local resources for obtaining supplies. Discuss activity and weight-bearing restrictions. Refer the patient to physical therapy for teaching about ambulation and appropriate muscle-group strengthening exercises. Ensure that the patient who has experienced an amputation is working with or has a referral to a prosthetic specialist.

For the patient with metastatic disease, discuss palliative care and hospice services and support groups for patients with cancer. Consultation of social services and chaplain services are usually indicated at this time.

40.6 Other Musculoskeletal Disorders

Other musculoskeletal disorders include low back pain (LBP), fibromyalgia, and disorders affecting the back and feet. Herniated intervertebral disk, a common back disorder, is discussed in Chapter 43.

The Patient with Low Back Pain

A systematic review by Hoy et al. (2014) found that "LBP causes more global disability than any other condition" (p. 968). Acute or chronic low back pain involves the lumbar, lumbosacral, or sacroiliac areas of the back. In most cases, low back pain is nonspecific, without an identifiable anatomic explanation (Wheeler, Wipf, Staiger, Deyo, & Jarvik, 2018). Back pain is a major health issue and frequent reason for physician visits in the United States, with an annual cost exceeding $100 billion. Back pain is the leading cause of disability among adults under age 45 years (Wheeler et al., 2018). Low back pain caused by degenerative disk disease and herniated vertebral disks is discussed in Chapter 43.

Pathophysiology

The pathophysiology of back pain varies with its many associated factors (**Box 40.6**). In general, the five causes and types of back pain are:

1. Local pain is caused by compression or irritation of sensory nerves. Fractures, strains, and sprains are common causes of local pain.

BOX 40.6
Factors Associated with Back Pain

MECHANICAL INJURY OR TRAUMA

- Muscle strain or spasm
- Compression fracture
- Lumbar disk disease

DEGENERATIVE DISORDERS

- Spondylosis
- Spinal stenosis
- Osteoarthritis

SYSTEMIC DISORDERS

- Osteomyelitis
- Osteoporosis or osteomalacia
- Neoplasms, primary or metastatic

REFERRED PAIN

- Gastrointestinal disorders
- Genitourinary disorders
- Gynecologic disorders
- Abdominal aortic aneurysm
- Hip pathology

OTHER

- Fibromyalgia
- Psychiatric syndromes
- Chronic anxiety
- Depression

2. Referred pain may originate from abdominal or pelvic viscera. This type of pain is generally not affected by posture or movement.
3. Pain of spinal origin, that is, pain associated with pathology of the spine such as disk disease or arthritis, may be referred to other structures such as the buttocks, groin, or legs.
4. Radicular back pain is sharp, radiating from the back to the leg along a nerve root. This pain may be aggravated by movements such as coughing, sneezing, or sitting.
5. Muscle spasm pain is associated with many spine disorders, although its origin may be unclear. This type of back pain is dull and may be accompanied by abnormal posture and taut spinal muscles.

Although an injury may account for initiation of the pain, factors such as deconditioning, psychologic issues, other chronic illnesses, genetics, and culture may be responsible for symptoms that extend past the normal healing time for damaged tissues.

Risk Factors

Risk factors as outlined by Wheeler et al. (2018) include smoking, obesity, age, female gender, physically strenuous work, sedentary work, psychologically strenuous work, low educational attainment, job dissatisfaction, somatization disorder, anxiety, and depression.

Manifestations

Patients with low back pain report pain ranging from mild discomfort lasting a few hours to chronic debilitating pain. Acute low back pain is defined by a symptom duration of 6 weeks or less, subacute as having lasted 7 to 12 weeks, and chronic low back pain by a duration of more than 12 weeks (Chou, 2017). Acute pain is usually thought to be injury related; however, most patients with acute low back pain are unable to identify a specific event associated with its onset.

Back pain may be localized, near the affected part of the back, or more generalized. Back pain may be referred to the buttocks, groin, or thighs. Radicular pain is generally sharp, radiating to a leg along a nerve pathway, and aggravated by coughing, sneezing, or contracting the abdominal muscles (e.g., to lift a heavy object). Muscle spasm pain may be accompanied by abnormal posture and tense muscles along the spine.

Complications

When back pain is nonspecific as to etiology, it usually resolves within 4 weeks. Chronic back pain is the complication of nonspecific back pain. Unless the pain has an identifiable origin, the complications are minimal.

Interprofessional Care

Care of the patient with low back pain focuses on evaluating the cause of the pain (when identifiable), relieving pain, correcting the condition, if possible, preventing complications, and educating the patient. A multimodal approach is often the best choice in meeting these goals.

Diagnosis

The choice of diagnostic tests for the patient with low back pain depends on the suspected diagnoses, clinical findings, and history. Current guidelines for care recommend that radiography, CT scans, and MRI be used only with clinical signs of a potentially serious underlying condition. Diagnostic testing may be considered if pain and other manifestations continue to limit the patient after 4 to 6 weeks of conservative treatment (Wheeler et al., 2018).

Medications

The medications of choice for low back pain are nonprescription NSAIDs, ibuprofen (Motrin), and naproxen (Aleve). NSAIDs block prostaglandin production and reduce inflammation, thus relieving the pain. Acetaminophen has not been shown to be effective in pain relief for acute low back pain (Chou et al., 2017). Muscle relaxants, prescribed medications, such as cyclobenzaprine (Flexeril), methocarbamol (Robaxin), or carisoprodol (Soma), may be used and have shown some benefit over placebo, but the studies looking at combining NSAIDs and muscle relaxants have shown mixed efficacy (Chou et al., 2017). Opioids have not been shown to provide any significant relieve over placebo medications (Chou et al., 2017).

Treatment

The majority of patients with acute low back pain need only a short-term treatment regimen or conservative treatment. Limited rest, with early resumption of normal physical activity and education, is often the primary method of treatment. There is no evidence that activity is harmful or aggravating to the source of pain. In fact, activity promotes bone and muscle strength and may increase endorphin levels. Therefore, active rehabilitation helps to restore function and reduce pain.

Pain may be relieved by application of heat to the back. Exercise programs are helpful provided that the patient begins gradually and increases activity over time as the recovery process continues. Physical therapy procedures include diathermy (deep heat therapy), ultrasonography, hydrotherapy, and transcutaneous electrical nerve stimulation (TENS) units. These therapies reduce the muscle spasms and pain temporarily. They are frequently used in combination with exercise to provide early mobilization for the patient.

Integrative Therapies

Complementary and alternative medicine strategies for low back pain include chiropractic, acupuncture, and massage. Evidence supports the use of spinal manipulation (chiropractic) for treating acute low back pain, finding its effectiveness to be equivalent to conservative medical management (Chou et al., 2017).

Nursing Care

Nursing care of the patient with low back pain focuses on educating the patient. Most patients have very little understanding of the anatomy of the spine, the reasons for the pain, the choices for treatment, and the importance of self-management. Therefore, education is an essential aspect of treating low back pain.

Assessment

Collect the following data through the health history and physical examination:

- ***Health history:*** Location, type (description), intensity, duration, aggravating and relieving factors; identifiable precipitating event, if known; previous episodes; current general health; ability to carry out ADLs and self-care activities; use of prescription, nonprescription, or recreational drugs or alcohol
- ***Physical assessment:*** Appearance; posture and gait; height and weight; tenderness; lumbar spine ROM; lower extremity movement and sensation.

Priorities of Care

Educating the patient to become an active collaborator in treating his or her back pain is a priority for nurses and the whole interprofessional team.

Diagnoses, Outcomes, and Interventions

Teach Self-Health Management. The patient with low back pain requires information regarding treatment, rehabilitation, and preventing injury.

Expected Outcome: Patient will become an active partner in managing back pain.

The nurse will:

- Teach appropriate comfort measures, such as use of nonprescription analgesics or NSAIDs. Ensure the patient has a clear understanding of the appropriate use of muscle relaxants or opioid analgesics, if prescribed, or the rationale for not using these drugs to treat acute back pain. *Patients who have a clear understanding of appropriate treatment of their back pain and who participate in the plan of care have greater satisfaction with their treatment outcomes.*
- Discuss use of nonprescription analgesics and NSAIDs for low back pain. Instruct the patient to initially take analgesics or NSAIDs on a routine schedule. *Mild analgesics or NSAIDs may help the patient remain active, preventing muscle deconditioning that can occur with prolonged rest. Maintaining a constant blood level of NSAIDs or analgesics reduces inflammation and provides continuous pain relief.*
- Encourage patients to stay active and continue daily living activities as allowed by symptoms. *There is little scientific evidence to show that bedrest is beneficial, but there is ample evidence about the adverse effects of bedrest. Staying in bed for more than 1 to 2 days can actually increase pain and cause joint stiffness and muscle weakness.*
- Instruct patient about appropriate use of heat to relieve back pain. Teach about the "rebound phenomenon" of prolonged heat or ice therapy. *Applying heat longer than 30 minutes causes a reverse effect known as the rebound phenomenon. Heat produces maximum vasodilation in 20 to 30 minutes. Continuation of the application beyond 30 to 45 minutes causes tissue congestion and the blood vessels constrict. Although cold (e.g., an ice pack or massage with ice) may be used, evidence for its effectiveness in relieving back pain is lacking.*
- Teach the use of appropriate body mechanics in lifting and reaching. The patient should be instructed to plan the lift, keep the object being lifted close to the body, and avoid twisting when lifting. Encourage the patient to obtain help when lifting. *An item is considered excessively heavy if it equals 35% of the lifter's body weight.*
- Instruct the patient to modify the workplace or environment to minimize stress to the lower back. *Lumbar supports in chairs, adjustment of chair or table height, and rubber floor mats help prevent back strain or injury.*
- Encourage patients who are obese to lose weight. *The trunk of the body must carry excess weight when the patient is obese. People who are obese are farther away from the objects they lift because of their greater abdominal girth. They may also have more difficulty squatting to lift. The greater the distance between an object and the patient's center of gravity, the higher the risk for straining the lower back.*
- Discuss the use of integrative therapies in treating acute low back pain. *Spinal manipulation (chiropractic) has been shown to be equally effective to conventional medicine for treating low back pain.*

Transitions of Care

Recommendations for preventing back pain from the National Institute of Neurological Disorders and Stroke (NINDS; 2014) include:

- Always stretch before exercise or other strenuous physical activity.
- Don't slouch when standing or sitting. The lower back can support a person's weight most easily when the curvature is reduced. When standing, keep your weight balanced on your feet.
- At home or at work, make sure work surfaces are at a comfortable height.
- Sit in a chair with good lumbar support and proper position and height for the task. Keep shoulders back. Switch sitting positions often and periodically walk around the office or gently stretch muscles to relieve tension. A pillow or rolled-up towel placed behind the small of the back can provide some lumbar support. During prolonged periods of sitting, elevate feet on a low stool or a stack of books.
- Wear comfortable, low-heeled shoes.
- Sleeping on one's side with the knees drawn up in a fetal position can help open up the joints in the spine and relieve pressure by reducing the curvature of the spine. Always sleep on a firm surface.
- Don't try to lift objects that are too heavy. Lift from the knees, pull the stomach muscles in, and keep the head

down and in line with a straight back. When lifting, keep objects close to the body. Do not twist when lifting.

- Maintain proper nutrition and diet to reduce and prevent excessive weight gain, especially weight around the waistline that taxes lower back muscles. A diet with sufficient daily intake of calcium, phosphorus, and vitamin D helps to promote new bone growth.
- Quit smoking. Smoking reduces blood flow to the lower spine, which can contribute to spinal disk degeneration. Smoking also increases the risk of osteoporosis and impedes healing. Coughing due to heavy smoking may also cause back pain.

In industrial and work settings, nurses should be alert for situations that increase the risk of back pain and injury. Office workers should have chairs with appropriate seat height and length and back support. Modifications of work space or machinery may be necessary for industrial workers to avoid excess stresses on back muscles. Finally, it is important to remember that back pain is a leading cause of lost work time for nurses themselves. Remind coworkers to use good body mechanics and to seek help when lifting or moving patients.

Back pain is a common problem in the United States and other industrialized countries. Nurses can have an effect on this significant problem by teaching health practices to prevent back injury to patients of all ages. Teach patients how to safely lift, bend, and turn when engaging in physical activity. Stress the importance of using large muscle groups of the legs to lift rather than bending and lifting with the smaller muscles of the back. Teach other aspects of good body mechanics, including posture, sleeping on a firm mattress, and sitting in chairs that provide good support. Discuss the positive effect of maintaining optimal body weight and good physical fitness.

The Patient with Fibromyalgia

Fibromyalgia is a common rheumatic syndrome characterized by chronic widespread musculoskeletal pain, stiffness, and tenderness. Fibromyalgia is estimated to affect 2% of the U.S. population (CDC, 2018a). It is found in most countries, among most ethnic groups, and across socioeconomic classes. Women are affected more frequently than men. Fibromyalgia can develop at any age and is the most common cause of generalized, musculoskeletal pain in women age 20 to 55 (Goldenberg, 2017a). The cause is unknown, but a combination of genetic and environmental factors is thought to contribute.

Pathophysiology

The pathogenesis of fibromyalgia appears to be complex, involving several levels of the central nervous system as well as the autonomic and somatic peripheral nervous systems and the endocrine system. A genetic predisposition, disordered central pain processing, with abnormal CSF levels of neurotransmitters (substance P, serotonin, and norepinephrine) and abnormal hypothalamic–pituitary–adrenal (HPA) axis responses, is increasingly shown to be central to fibromyalgia (Goldenberg, 2017c). As a result, patients with fibromyalgia perceive pain at a lower level of stimulation than people who are unaffected by the disorder.

Manifestations

A gradual onset of chronic muscle pain is typical, although the onset may be sudden. The pain may be localized or involve the entire body and may be exacerbated by disrupted sleep, exercise, or stress (Goldenberg, 2017a). The neck, spine, shoulders, and hips are often affected. Pain is produced by palpating localized "tender points" (**Figure 40.14** ■). Local tightness or muscle spasm may also occur. Systemic manifestations of fibromyalgia include fatigue, sleep disruptions, headaches, morning stiffness, painful menstrual periods, and problems with thinking and memory (called *fibro fog*) (Goldenberg, 2017a). Pain and fatigue may be aggravated by exertion.

Complications

Although there are no real complications associated with the pathophysiology of fibromyalgia, there are still complications that occur in patients' lives. The chronic nature of the disease can be psychologically difficult. An increased risk of suicide has been found in patients with fibromyalgia in older demographic and retrospective studies (Dreyer, Kendall, Danneskiold-Samsoe, Bartels, & Bliddal, 2010; Ratcliffe, Enns, Belik, & Sareen, 2008).

Another nonphysiologic complication has to do with a patient's work life. Whereas most patients with fibromyalgia report that they can still work, there are 10 to 30% who report they are unable to work due to the chronic pain and fatigue (Goldenberg, 2017b).

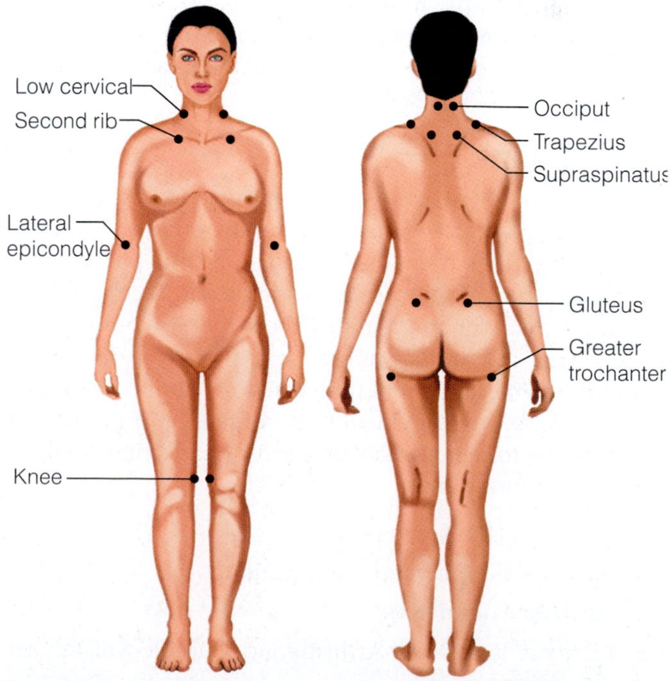
Low cervical
Second rib
Lateral epicondyle
Knee
Occiput
Trapezius
Supraspinatus
Gluteus
Greater trochanter

Figure 40.14 ■ Location of "tender points" in fibromyalgia.

Interprofessional Care

Diagnosis

The diagnosis of fibromyalgia is based on the history and physical assessment. The American College of Rheumatology criteria used for diagnosis are a history of widespread pain and symptoms of fatigue, waking unrefreshed, and cognitive symptoms (such as thinking or remembering difficulties) that have been present for at least 3 months (Goldenberg, 2017a). There are no laboratory or diagnostic tests for the disorder.

Medications

Tricyclic antidepressants (e.g., amitriptyline) have been shown to promote better sleep and relieve manifestations of fibromyalgia. Only three medications are approved by the U.S. Food and Drug Administration for treating fibromyalgia. Two of these drugs, duloxetine (Cymbalta) and milnacipran (Savella), are mixed reuptake inhibitors that increase both serotonin and norepinephrine levels. The third approved drug, pregabalin (Lyrica), was developed to treat neuropathic pain. Lower dosages of all these medications are usually initiated and then slowly increased until symptom relief is achieved or the maximum dosage is reached (Goldenberg, 2017b).

Integrative Therapies

Acknowledgment of the patient's symptoms and the chronic but treatable nature of this disease is important. Treatment focuses on improving function and quality of life rather than on eliminating pain. Integrative therapies may include a program of structured low-impact aerobic exercise for conditioning, as well as stretching exercises. Heated pool treatments with or without exercise have been shown to be beneficial. Other treatments such as cognitive-behavioral therapy, hypnotherapy, biofeedback, tai chi, yoga, meditation, qigong, and acupuncture have all been found to show positive results (Lauche, Cramer, Häuser, Dobos, & Langhorst, 2015).

Nursing Care

Nursing care for patients with fibromyalgia is supportive and educational, provided in community settings. Acknowledgment of the patient's symptoms and the chronic but treatable nature of this disease is important. Teach patients about the disorder and reassure them that its course is not progressive, and it does not cause crippling or deformity. Provide verbal and written instructions about the use of heat, exercise, stress-reduction techniques, and prescribed medications to relieve manifestations. In addition, suggest the following resources:

- Fibromyalgia Network
- National Fibromyalgia Association
- Arthritis Foundation
- National Institute of Arthritis and Musculoskeletal and Skin Diseases.

The Patient with Spinal Deformity

Scoliosis and kyphosis are the two most common deformities of the spinal column. **Scoliosis** is a lateral curvature of the spine. **Kyphosis** is excessive angulation of the normal posterior curve of the thoracic spine (**Figure 40.15** ■).

An estimated 600,000 people in the United States are affected by scoliosis. It is usually diagnosed in adolescence. Although the incidence is equal between genders, females are eight times more likely to require treatment for significant curvature (National Scoliosis Foundation, n.d.). Idiopathic scoliosis is the most common form of the disorder, accounting for approximately 85% of cases. Congenital and neuromuscular disorders such as cerebral palsy, poliomyelitis, and MD account for the rest (National Scoliosis Foundation, n.d.).

Pathophysiology

Scoliosis

Scoliosis is classified as *postural* when the small curve corrects with bending, and *structural* when the curve does not correct with bending. Most patients requiring treatment have structural scoliosis, a curve caused by a fixed deformity.

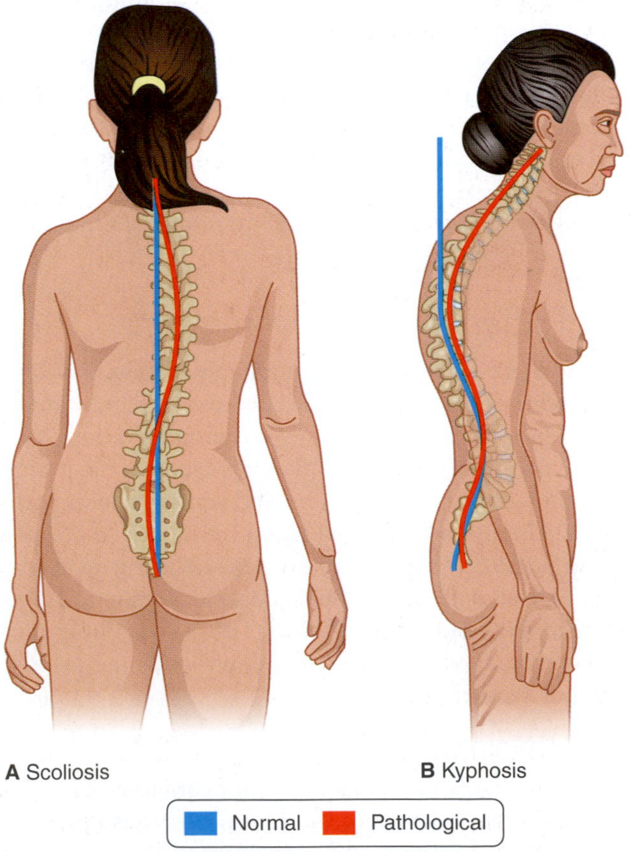

A Scoliosis
B Kyphosis
Normal
Pathological

Figure 40.15 ■ Common deformities of the spinal column: **A**, Scoliosis is a lateral curvature of the spine. **B**, Kyphosis is an exaggerated posterior curvature of the thoracic spine.

The lateral curve that occurs in scoliosis is usually evident in the thoracic, lumbar, or thoracolumbar regions of the spine. A right thoracic curve is the most common. The vertebral bodies in these spinal regions can be rotated as well as curved to one side or the other. Curves greater than 40 degrees are considered severe and require treatment.

As scoliosis emerges in adolescence, the soft tissues (muscles and ligaments) shorten on the concave side of the curvature. Over time, progressive deformities of the vertebral column and ribs develop, causing one-sided compression of the vertebral bodies. The degree of compression and twisting varies according to the location of each vertebra within the curved portion of the spine.

Kyphosis

Like scoliosis, kyphosis is classified as postural or structural. Postural kyphosis is caused by a slumping posture. Structural kyphosis may result from congenital malformations or pediatric disorders such as rickets or poliomyelitis. However, kyphosis may also occur during adulthood because of vertebral tuberculosis and Paget disease or metabolic disorders such as osteoporosis and osteomalacia. The condition can also result from the surgical removal or radiation of intervertebral disks for the treatment of spinal cord tumors or cysts. Kyphosis can be seen in people of all ages, when there are other structural spine issues present, but is most common in older adults.

Risk Factors

There seems to be a genetic predisposition for scoliosis, but there are no other identifiable risk factors (Sherl, 2018). Risk factors for kyphosis are centered on the strength and structure of the vertebrae. Vertebral fractures, low bone density, short vertebral height, degenerative disk disease, poor posture, muscle weakness, loss of elastic tissue in intervertebral ligaments, and genetic or metabolic conditions have all been found to be risk factors for developing kyphosis (Kado, 2017).

Manifestations

Scoliosis is usually first noted by the deformity it causes, such as one shoulder that is higher than the other, a prominent hip, or a projecting scapula. The manifestations of scoliosis include asymmetry of the shoulders, scapulae, and waist creases; prominence of the thoracic ribs or paravertebral muscles on forward bend; and lateral curvature and vertebral rotation on posteroanterior x-ray. Pain is present in severe cases, usually in the lumbar region. Pain may also be caused by pressure on the ribs or the crest of the ilium. Shortness of breath may result from diminished chest expansion, and GI disturbances (anorexia, nausea) may occur because of crowding of the abdominal organs.

The manifestations of kyphosis include moderate back pain, posterior rounding at the thoracic level as viewed from the side (*hunchback*), and a kyphotic curve of over 45 degrees on x-ray.

Complications

Pain, impaired mobility, and respiratory problems may occur in cases of severe curvature of scoliosis. The same complications occur in patients with kyphosis. Additionally, patients with kyphosis are at an increased risk of falls, fractures, and GI issues (Kado, 2017).

Interprofessional Care

Diagnosis of scoliosis and kyphosis is important to prevent severe spinal deformity and back pain in the adult. The patient stands with the arms relaxed and hanging freely at the sides while the examiner evaluates him or her from both the back and the front for symmetry of the shoulders, scapulae, waist creases, and the length of the arms. The patient then bends forward, and the examiner observes for prominence of the thoracic ribs or vertebral muscles. The patient is then viewed from the side while the screener looks for increased thoracic rounding or lumbar swayback.

Diagnosis

Upright posteroanterior and lateral x-rays are used to confirm the diagnosis of curvature of the spine. For the patient with scoliosis, the degree of curvature is measured by determining the amount of lateral deviation to the left or right. For the patient with kyphosis, anteroposterior and lateral views typically reveal wedging of the vertebrae.

Treatment

Scoliosis and kyphosis may be treated conservatively or with surgery.

Braces can be used to prevent progression of scoliosis and kyphosis in younger patients whose skeletons have not yet matured. Bracing is the treatment of choice for adolescents with curves of 25 to 40 degrees. Bracing can also be effective in improving muscle strength in patients with kyphosis (Kado, 2017). Conservative treatment for adults with scoliosis and kyphosis may include weight reduction, active and passive exercises, and the use of braces for support.

Surgery

The decision to surgically correct spinal deformities depends on factors such as the degree of curvature and the patient's overall physical, emotional, and neurologic status. Even with surgery, it is not possible to correct the abnormal curvature completely. The surgical procedure involves attaching metal reinforcing rods to the vertebrae and is usually performed using an anterior approach, although more severe curvature may require both an anterior and a posterior approach. The types of straightening devices most frequently use bilateral rods with wire hooks or screws that stabilize the spine and correct the deformity.

Nursing Care

Nursing interventions for patients with scoliosis or kyphosis focus on minimizing the risk for injury and neurologic impairment and educating the patient and family about the condition. See the section on herniated disk in Chapter 43 for nursing care of the patient undergoing back surgery.

Assess the environment for safety hazards. Some braces do not allow the patient to flex or hyperextend the spinal column. The older adult with kyphosis or a fixed curvature may also have limited spinal movement and difficulty seeing environmental hazards. Advise the patient to use handrails on stairways and take precautions when walking on slippery surfaces or areas with throw rugs.

Teach the patient for whom a brace is prescribed how to apply the brace and ways to reduce skin irritation beneath the brace: Wearing a smooth cotton t-shirt or cotton tube under the brace at all times, changing undergarments at least once daily, and washing them with a mild soap. Undergarments should be changed more frequently in warmer weather. Advise the patient to avoid lotion and body powders; they may irritate the skin. Suggest loosening the brace during meals and for the first 30 minutes after each meal to promote comfort and allow adequate nutritional intake.

Transitions of Care

Patients with structural scoliosis or kyphosis need reassurance that the condition was not caused by poor posture. If a brace is prescribed to relieve pain and other symptoms associated with the disorder, provide verbal and written instructions for wearing the brace, such as the number of hours per day it is to be worn and activity restrictions to follow when wearing or not wearing the brace. Teach the patient how to protect and care for skin under the brace.

Surgical patients need postoperative teaching regarding site care and activities. Patients who have spinal surgery are often allowed to ambulate soon after surgery but sitting may be restricted because of the stresses it places on the spine. Instruct the patient to notify the physician if numbness, tingling, pain, or weakness of an extremity develops after surgery.

Discuss the importance of not smoking and of avoiding respiratory infections for patients with scoliosis or kyphosis that restricts respiratory excursion. Encourage these patients to obtain pneumococcal pneumonia and influenza immunizations.

The Patient with a Common Foot Disorder

Foot disorders often cause pain or difficulty in walking. These disorders may be congenital; related to a systemic disorder; caused by wearing poorly fitting, confining, or high-heeled shoes; or due to physical stress on the foot. These disorders are more prevalent among women. Common foot disorders are summarized in **Table 40.10**.

Interprofessional Care

Diagnosis

Care of the patient with a foot disorder focuses on relieving pain, correcting any structural deformity, and preventing reoccurrence. In most cases, foot disorders are diagnosed by the patient's history and by inspection. X-rays of the affected foot are taken if the need for surgery arises.

Medications

Analgesics may be prescribed to relieve pain and inflammation. In severe cases, corticosteroid drugs may be injected into the affected joints or surrounding tissue to relieve acute inflammation.

Surgery

Surgery is reserved for patients with intractable toe deformities or pain. Hallux valgus is treated with bunionectomy; ligaments are lengthened or shortened as needed, and pins are drilled into place so the toe remains in position. Similarly, the correction of hammertoe also involves straightening the affected toe and inserting pins to retain the correction. A cast may be applied over the foot following surgery to correct toe deformities. Surgery for Morton neuroma causes loss of sensation to a portion of the foot because removing the neuroma involves cutting out a portion of the plantar nerve.

Integrative Therapies

Conservative treatment usually involves the use of corrective shoes or orthotic devices that support the arch or cushion and stretch the affected joints. For Morton neuroma, metatarsal pads are used to spread the patient's toes and decompress the affected nerve. Exercises that stretch the plantar fascia and calf muscles are beneficial in plantar fasciitis.

Nursing Care

Pain relief, prevention of infection, and patient education are important priorities for the nursing care of patients with foot disorders.

Instruct patients to wear appropriate or corrective footwear to assist in the conservative treatment of foot problems. Pain related to foot problems can result from footwear that does not provide proper toe room; in addition, heels higher than 1 inch can cause constant flexion and hyperextension problems. In some instances, the patient must purchase special shoes or orthotics to ensure correct fit and relief of symptoms.

Suggest purchasing protective pads to wear over painful bunions, calluses/corns, and the ball of the foot. Instruct to remove pads and inspect the skin every other day. Patients who have difficulty reaching or observing the involved foot should ask another person to do the inspection for them. It is especially important to emphasize the need for inspection to patients who have

Table 40.10 Common Foot Disorders

Disorder	Description/Pathophysiology	Manifestations
Hallux valgus (bunion)	Enlargement and lateral displacement of the first metatarsal (great toe) (**Figure 40.16** ■) with gradual loss of stabilizing action of the great toe	■ Lateral deviation of the great toe with MTP joint enlargement ■ Joint pain ■ Calluses ■ Limited joint ROM, possible crepitus

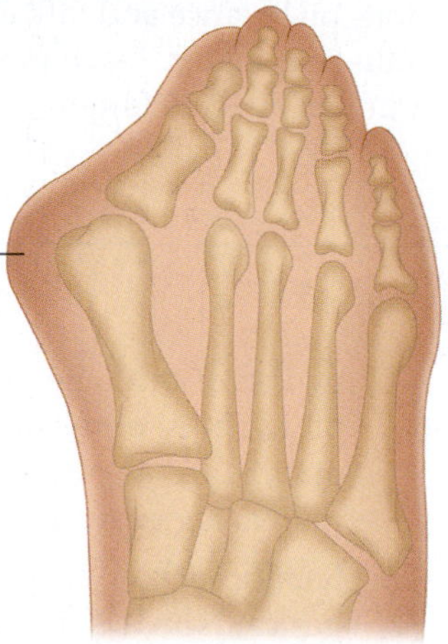
Bunion

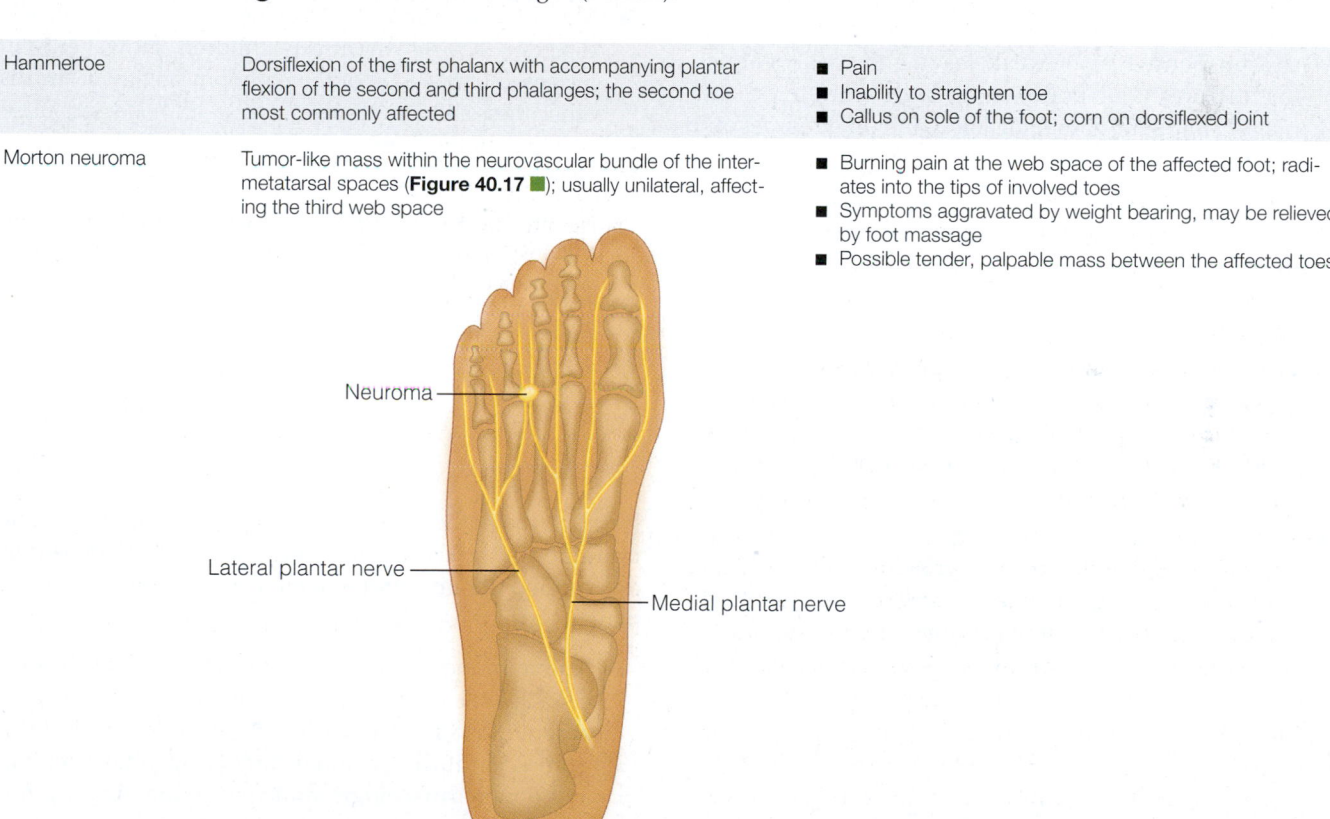

Figure 40.16 ■ Hallux valgus (bunion).

Disorder	Description/Pathophysiology	Manifestations
Hammertoe	Dorsiflexion of the first phalanx with accompanying plantar flexion of the second and third phalanges; the second toe most commonly affected	■ Pain ■ Inability to straighten toe ■ Callus on sole of the foot; corn on dorsiflexed joint
Morton neuroma	Tumor-like mass within the neurovascular bundle of the intermetatarsal spaces (**Figure 40.17** ■); usually unilateral, affecting the third web space	■ Burning pain at the web space of the affected foot; radiates into the tips of involved toes ■ Symptoms aggravated by weight bearing, may be relieved by foot massage ■ Possible tender, palpable mass between the affected toes

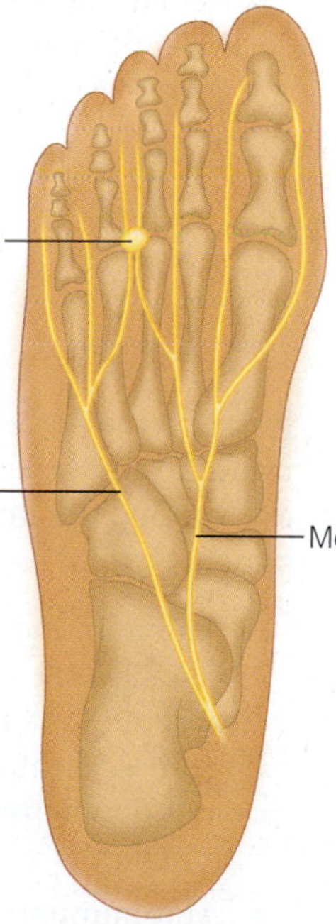
Neuroma
Lateral plantar nerve
Medial plantar nerve

Figure 40.17 ■ Morton neuroma.

Disorder	Description/Pathophysiology	Manifestations
Plantar fasciitis	Inflammation of the plantar fascia (connects the heel bone to the toes and creates the arch of the foot)	■ Severe foot pain with first steps on arising in the morning or after a period of inactivity ■ Aggravated by walking barefoot, climbing stairs

experienced loss of sensation of the feet due to such disorders as diabetes and chronic peripheral vascular disease.

Teach patients who have undergone surgery proper care and cleaning of exposed pins implanted during the surgical procedure. Instruct how to keep pins and casts dry while bathing or ambulating in inclement weather; for example, wearing a plastic bag over the cast or pins when bathing or walking in rain or snow.

For patients in all age groups, teach the importance of well-fitting footwear. Discuss the long-term effects of wearing high-heeled shoes with constricting toes with women. Suggest alternatives for stylish footwear and encourage patients to wear supportive and nonrestrictive footwear at all times. Discuss the possible effects of bunions on balance and talk about safety measures to prevent falls and injury. Teach patients techniques to relieve pressure on affected joints.

CHAPTER HIGHLIGHTS

40.1 Metabolic Musculoskeletal Disorders

Describe the pathophysiology and manifestations of metabolic musculoskeletal disorders, and outline the interprofessional care and nursing care of patients with these disorders.

- Metabolic bone and joint disorders arise from disrupted processes or impaired elimination of wastes. As a result, bones may be weak, leaving the patient at risk for fractures. Metabolic wastes such as urate crystals may accumulate, damaging joints and other tissues and causing acute pain.
- Metabolic bone disorders, including osteoporosis, Page disease, and osteomalacia, begin in the bone remodeling process. Aging, calcium and phosphate imbalances, genetics, and changes in hormone levels contribute to these disorders.
- Osteoporosis is a major health problem in the United States, with fractures being the most common complication. Health promotion activities to prevent osteoporosis include a calcium-rich diet, weight-bearing exercise, and a healthy lifestyle.
- Gout is characterized by hyperuricemia and urate crystal formation in the joint synovium. Attacks of the disease typically begin with an acutely painful inflammation of the first joint of the great toe, although other joints such as the knee or elbow may be affected.

40.2 Degenerative Musculoskeletal Disorders

Describe the pathophysiology and manifestations of degenerative musculoskeletal disorders, and outline the interprofessional care and nursing care of patients with these disorders.

- Degenerative disorders of the joints and muscles can lead to impaired mobility and chronic pain. These problems may in turn cause disability, especially in the performance of daily living activities.
- Osteoarthritis (OA) is the most commonly occurring of all forms of arthritis and a leading cause of pain and disability in older adults. The disease is characterized by loss of cartilage in articulating joints and hypertrophy of bone at the articular margins. Pain and inflammation are most often managed conservatively with mild analgesics and NSAIDs.
- Significant pain and disability not controlled with analgesics, NSAIDs, exercise, and physical therapy may necessitate total joint replacement.
- Muscular dystrophy is a degenerative musculoskeletal disorder that mostly affects children. However, with increased knowledge of the pathophysiology of the disorder, these children are living into adulthood and nurses will encounter them in both inpatient and outpatient settings.
- Knowledge of the disease processes and potential complications will assist the nurse in caring for the patient with this disorder in their history.

40.3 Autoimmune and Inflammatory Musculoskeletal Disorders

Describe the pathophysiology and manifestations of autoimmune and inflammatory musculoskeletal disorders, and outline the interprofessional care and nursing care of patients with these disorders.

- Autoimmune and inflammatory disorders of the musculoskeletal system are systemic in nature and often chronic, potentially leading to significant disability. Care is multidimensional, involving pharmacologic and nonpharmacologic strategies to maintain optimal function.
- Autoimmune and inflammatory musculoskeletal disorders include rheumatoid arthritis (RA), ankylosing spondylitis (AS), reactive arthritis (ReA), systemic lupus erythematosus (SLE), inflammatory myopathy, and Lyme disease.
- Although the cause of RA is unknown, it is believed to involve a combination of genetic and environmental factors. RA is a systemic disease, affecting one or many joints and also causing fatigue, weakness, anorexia, weight loss, and fever. The primary objectives of

treatment and care are to reduce pain and inflammation, preserve function, and prevent deformity.

- Connective tissue is the most abundant and widely distributed body tissue. It connects body parts and provides support; forms bones, cartilage, and the walls of blood vessels; and attaches muscles to bones. Disorders that affect connective tissue have diverse manifestations, and patients need interprofessional team support for effective disease management.
- Systemic lupus erythematosus (SLE) is a chronic inflammatory connective tissue disease, affecting almost all body systems, including the musculoskeletal system. Skin lesions are a common manifestation, exhibited by a characteristic rash on the face. The patient with SLE is at increased risk for infection.
- Systemic sclerosis is a chronic disease characterized by the formation of excess connective tissue and diffuse fibrosis of the skin and internal organs. It may be either localized or generalized.
- Lyme disease is caused by the spirochete *Borrelia burgdorferi*, carried and transmitted primarily by ticks. The disease can be treated effectively with antibiotics.

40.4 Infectious Musculoskeletal Disorders

Describe the pathophysiology and manifestations of infectious musculoskeletal disorders, and outline the interprofessional care and nursing care of patients with these disorders.

- Infectious disorders of bone and joints are caused by a pathogen and are often difficult to treat. Effective treatment is vital, however, to prevent chronic pain, deformity, and disability. The nurse coordinates, provides, and monitors treatment measures and responses in acute care and the home and provides patient, family, and caregiver education.
- Osteomyelitis and septic arthritis are infectious musculoskeletal disorders. Osteomyelitis may be the result of a bloodborne pathogen, a contiguous infection, or a complication of vascular insufficiency. Septic arthritis is a medical emergency requiring immediate treatment to preserve joint function.

40.5 Neoplastic Musculoskeletal Disorders

Describe the pathophysiology and manifestations of neoplastic musculoskeletal disorders, and outline the interprofessional care and nursing care of patients with these disorders.

- Bone tumors may be benign or malignant, primary or metastatic. The primary manifestations of a bone tumor are pain, a mass, and impaired function. Nursing care is directed toward teaching to prevent injury and interventions to relieve pain.
- Musculoskeletal disorders characterized by chronic pain and discomfort can have significant physical and psychosocial effects on the patient. The nursing role in caring for these patients focuses on providing support and educating the patient about his or her condition so the patient can be an active partner in managing the condition.

40.6 Other Musculoskeletal Disorders

Describe the pathophysiology and manifestations of other musculoskeletal disorders, including low back pain, fibromyalgia, spinal deformity, and common foot disorders, and outline the interprofessional care and nursing care of patients with these disorders.

- Low back pain is among the most common problems causing adults to seek medical care. Unless risk factors or manifestations indicating a secondary origin (e.g., a tumor or infection) are present, this condition is appropriate for conservative management with mild analgesics, NSAIDs, or chiropractic. Patients are encouraged to stay active, avoiding only strenuous lifting or activity.
- Fibromyalgia is characterized by chronic widespread musculoskeletal pain and tenderness that has a significant negative impact on physical and psychosocial functioning. A combination of physical conditioning, cognitive-behavioral strategies, and pharmacologic treatment is commonly employed to treat fibromyalgia.
- Structural musculoskeletal disorders include scoliosis, kyphosis, hallux valgus, hammertoe, and Morton neuroma. Plantar fasciitis is a common cause of foot pain in adults.

TEST YOURSELF NCLEX-RN® REVIEW

1. A patient with osteoporosis is prescribed the bisphosphonate alendronate (Fosamax). What should the nurse include when teaching the patient about this medication? (Select all that apply.)
   A. Take the medication as directed with clear water only.
   B. Avoid lying down for 30 to 60 minutes after taking the drug.
   C. Consume no food or fluids for 30 minutes after taking the drug.
   D. Take calcium and vitamin D supplements as instructed by your healthcare provider.
   E. For ease in swallowing, you may chew the tablet thoroughly.

2. The nurse is preparing teaching for a patient with mild osteoarthritis of the knees. Which medication treatments should the nurse include in these instructions? (Select all that apply.)
   A. Opioids
   B. NSAIDs
   C. Hormones
   D. Antibiotics
   E. Hyaluronic acid
3. The nurse is reviewing laboratory values for a patient with an acute attack of gout. Which laboratory value should the nurse expect to be increased? (Select all that apply.)
   A. WBC
   B. Creatinine
   C. Hematocrit
   D. Alkaline phosphatase
   E. Sed rate
4. The nurse is preparing a teaching session for community members on osteoporosis and osteomalacia. What should the nurse include as a potential complication for both health problems?
   A. Infection
   B. Fractures
   C. Blood clots
   D. Contractures
5. During an assessment the nurse determines that a patient with knee pain is at risk for osteoarthritis. What did the nurse assess in this patient?
   A. Having a history of falls
   B. Eating a diet high in calcium
   C. Walking 30 minutes each day
   D. Being overweight by 30 pounds
6. The nurse is planning postoperative care for a patient who had a knee replacement. What interventions will the nurse include? (Select all that apply.)
   A. Maintain knee immobilizer to prevent joint dislocation.
   B. Use sequential compression devices.
   C. Keep the patient on bedrest for the first 24 hours after surgery.
   D. Encourage a high fiber diet
   E. Initially maintain non-weight-bearing on the affected extremity.
7. The nurse is determining the type of arthritis a patient is experiencing. Which assessment finding would be present if the patient has rheumatoid arthritis?
   A. Stiffness is relieved by activity.
   B. Health history includes weight loss and fever.
   C. Abnormal joint findings are limited to the hands.
   D. Heberden nodes are located on the finger joints.
8. The nurse identifies that a patient with systemic lupus erythematosus has ineffective protection. Which intervention is priority when caring for this patient?
   A. Monitor laboratory findings.
   B. Provide appropriate skin care.
   C. Practice careful hand hygiene.
   D. Administer prescribed medications.
9. The community nurse is preparing a presentation on Lyme disease for community members. What should the nurse explain about the spread of the organism for this disease?
   A. The bite of an infected mosquito
   B. Brief contact with an infected tick
   C. An infected tick embedded for over 24 hours
   D. Primarily by droplets from infected people
10. A patient has just been diagnosed with septic arthritis. The nurse would question which medical order for this patient?
   A. Sputum culture
   B. Ambulate three time daily
   C. Prepare for arthrotomy
   D. Broad spectrum antibiotic

See Test Yourself answers in Appendix B.

REFERENCES

Adams, M. P., Holland, L. N., & Urban, C. (2017). *Pharmacology for nursing: A pathophysiologic approach* (5th ed.). Hoboken, NJ: Pearson Education.

Adler, R. A., El-Hajj Fuleihan, G., Bauer, D. C., Camacho, P. M., Clarke, B. L., Clines, G. A., . . . Sellmeyer, D. E. (2016), Managing osteoporosis in patients on long-term bisphosphonate treatment: Report of a task force of the American Society for Bone and Mineral Research. *Journal of Bone Mineral and Research*, *31*, 16–35.

Aletaha, D., Neogi, T., Silman, A. J., Funovits, J., Felson, D. T., Bingham III, C. O., . . . Hawker, G. (2010). 2010 Rheumatoid Arthritis Classification Criteria: An American College of Rheumatology/European League Against Rheumatism collaborative initiative. *Arthritis and Rheumatism*, *62*(9), 2569–2581.

American Cancer Society (ACS). (2018a). *Key statistics for osteosarcoma.* Retrieved from https://www.cancer.org/cancer/osteosarcoma/about/key-statistics.html.

American Cancer Society (ACS) (2018b). *Risk factors for bone cancer.* Retrieved from https://www.cancer.org/cancer/bone-cancer/causes-risks-prevention/risk-factors.html.

American Cancer Society (ACS) (2018c). *What is bone cancer?* Retrieved from https://www.cancer.org/cancer/bone-cancer/about/what-is-bone-cancer.html.w

American College of Rheumatology. (2017a). *Glucocorticoid-induced osteoporosis.* Retrieved from https://www.rheumatology.org/I-Am-A/Patient-Caregiver/Diseases-Conditions/Glucocorticoid-induced-Osteoperosis.

American College of Rheumatology. (2017b). *Prevalence statistics.* Retrieved from https://www.rheumatology.org/Learning-Center/Statistics/Prevalence-Statistics.

Barbour, K. E., Helmick, C. G., Boring, M. A., & Brady, T. J. (2017). Vital signs: Prevalence of doctor-diagnosed arthritis and arthritis-attributable activity limitation—United States, 2013–2015. *Morbidity and Mortality Weekly Report*, *66*(9), 246–253.

Bardin, T., & Richette, P. (2017). Impact of comorbidities on gout and hyperuricaemia: An update on prevalence and treatment options. *BMC Medicine*, *15*(123).

Barrows, K. (2013). Complementary and alternative medicine. In M. Papadakis & S. McPhee (Eds.), *Current medical diagnosis and treatment 2013.* New York, NY: McGraw-Hill. Retrieved from http://www.accessmedicine.com

Beard, C. B. (2016). Epidemiology of Lyme disease. UpToDate.com. Retrieved from https://www.uptodate.com/contents/epidemiology-of-lyme-disease?search=Epidemiology%20of%20Lyme%20disease&source=search_result&selectedTitle=1~150&usage_type=default&display_rank=1.

Becker, M. A. (2018a). Clinical manifestations and diagnosis of gout. *UpToDate.com.* Retrieved from https://www.uptodate.com/contents/clinical-manifestations-and-diagnosis-of-gout?search=gout%20diagnosis&source=search_result&selectedTitle=1~150&usage_type=default&display_rank=1.

Becker, M. A. (2018b). Lifestyle modification and other strategies to reduce the risk of gout flares and progression of gout. *UpToDate.com.* Retrieved from https://www.uptodate.com/contents/lifestyle-modification-and-other-strategies-to-reduce-the-risk-of-gout-flares-and-progression-of-gout?search=Lifestyle%20modification%20and%20other%20strategies%20to%20reduce%20the%20risk%20of%20gout%20flares%20and%20progression%20of%20gout&source=search_result&selectedTitle=1~150&usage_type=default&display_rank=1.

Becker, M. A. (2018c). Pharmacologic urate-lowering therapy and treatment of tophi in patients with gout. UpToDate.com. Retrieved from https://www.uptodate.com/contents/pharmacologic-urate-lowering-therapy-and-treatment-of-tophi-in-patients-with-gout?search=Pharmacologic%20urate-lowering%20therapy%20and%20treatment%20of%20tophi%20in%20patients%20with%20gout&source=search_result&selectedTitle=1~150&usage_type=default&display_rank=1.

Becker, M. A. (2018d). Treatment of gout flares. UpToDate.com. Retrieved from https://www.uptodate.com/contents/treatment-of-gout-flares?search=Treatment%20of%20gout%20flares&source=search_result&selectedTitle=1~150&usage_type=default&display_rank=1.

Bethel, M., Carbone, L. D., Lohr, K. M., & Machua, W. (2017). *Osteoporosis.* Retrieved from https://emedicine.medscape.com/article/330598-overview#a3.

Centers for Disease Control and Prevention (CDC). (2017). *Arthritis: National statistics.* Retrieved from https://www.cdc.gov/arthritis/data_statistics/national-statistics.html.

Centers for Disease Control and Prevention (CDC). (2018a). *Fibromyalgia.* Retrieved from https://www.cdc.gov/arthritis/basics/fibromyalgia.htm.

Centers for Disease Control and Prevention (CDC). (2018b). *Osteoarthritis.* Retrieved from www.cdc.gov/arthritis/basics/osteoarthritis.htm.

Centers for Disease Control and Prevention (CDC). (2018c). *Systemic lupus erythematosus.* Retrieved from https://www.cdc.gov/lupus/facts/detailed.html.

Charles, J. F. (2016). Treatment of Paget disease of bone. UpToDate.com. Retrieved from https://www.uptodate.com/contents/treatment-of-paget-disease-of-bone?search=Treatment%20of%20Paget%20disease%20of%20bone&source=search_result&selectedTitle=1~36&usage_type=default&display_rank=1.

Chou, R. (2017). Subacute and chronic pain: Non-pharmacologic and pharmacologic treatment. UpToDate.com. Retrieved from https://www.uptodate.com/contents/subacute-and-chronic-low-back-pain-nonpharmacologic-and-pharmacologic-treatment?search=Subacute%20and%20chronic%20low%20back%20pain:%20Nonpharmacologic%20and%20pharmacologic%20treatment&source=search_result&selectedTitle=1~150&usage_type=default&display_rank=1.

Chou, R., Deyo, R., Friedly, J., Skelly, A., Weimer, M., Fu, R., . . . Grusing, S. (2017). Systemic pharmacologic therapies for low back pain: A systematic review for an American College of Physicians clinical practice guideline. *Annals of Internal Medicine*, *166*(7), 480–492.

Cosman, F., deBeur, S. J., LeBoff, M. S., Lewiecki, E. M., Tanner, B., Randall, S., & Lindsay, R. (2014). Clinician's guide to prevention and treatment of osteoporosis. *Osteoporosis International*, *25*(10), 2359–2381.

Creo, A. L., Thacher, T. D., Pettifor, J. M., Strand, M. A., & Fischer, P. R. (2016). Nutritional rickets around the world: An update. *Paediatrics and International Child Health*, *37*(2), 84–98.

Cundy, T. (2017). Paget's disease of bone. *Metabolism*, *80*, 5–14.

Curtis, E. M., Moon, R. J., Dennison, E. M., Harvey, N. C., & Cooper, C. (2016). Recent advances in the pathogenesis and treatment of osteoporosis. *Clinical Medicine, 16*(4), 360–364.

Denton, C. P. (2017a). Overview of the treatment and prognosis of systemic sclerosis (scleroderma) in adults. UpToDate.com. Retrieved from https://www.uptodate.com/contents/overview-of-the-treatment-and-prognosis-of-systemic-sclerosis-scleroderma-in-adults?search=Overview%20of%20the%20treatment%20and%20prognosis%20of%20systemic%20sclerosis%20(scleroderma)%20in%20adults&source=search_result&selectedTitle=1~150&usage_type=default&display_rank=1.

Denton, C. P. (2017b). Pathogenesis of systemic sclerosis (scleroderma). UpToDate.com. Retrieved from https://www.uptodate.com/contents/pathogenesis-of-systemic-sclerosis-scleroderma?search=Pathogenesis%20of%20systemic%20sclerosis%20(scleroderma)&source=search_result&selectedTitle=1~150&usage_type=default&display_rank=1.

Deveza, L. A. (2017). Overview of the management of osteoarthritis. UpToDate.com. Retrieved from https://www.uptodate.com/contents/overview-of-the-management-of-osteoarthritis?search=Overview%20of%20the%20management%20of%20osteoarthritis&source=search_result&selectedTitle=1~150&usage_type=default&display_rank=1.

Dreyer, L., Kendall, S., Danneskiold-Samsøe, B., Bartels, E. M., & Bliddal, H. (2010). Mortality in a cohort of Danish patients with fibromyalgia: Increased frequency of suicide. *Arthritis and Rheumatology, 62*(10), 3101–3108.

Ensrud, K. E., & Crandall, C. J. (2017). Osteoporosis. *Annals of Internal Medicine, 167*(3), ITC17–ITC32.

Erens, G. A., & Crowley, M. (2017). Total hip arthroplasty. UpToDate.com. Retrieved from https://www.uptodate.com/contents/total-hip-arthroplasty

Femia, A. (2017). Dermatomyositis. *Medscape.* Retrieved from https://emedicine.medscape.com/article/332783-overview#a6.

Gabriel, S. E., & Crowson, C. S. (2018). Epidemiology of, risk factors for, and possible causes of rheumatoid arthritis. UpToDate.com. https://www.uptodate.com/contents/epidemiology-of-risk-factors-for-and-possible-causes-of-rheumatoid-arthritis?search=risk%20factors%20for%20rheumatoid%20arthritis&source=search_result&selectedTitle=1~150&usage_type=default&display_rank=1.

Gestring, M. (2017). Negative pressure wound therapy. UpToDate.com. Retrieved from https://www.uptodate.com/contents/negative-pressure-wound-therapy?search=Negative%20pressure%20wound%20therapy&source=search_result&selectedTitle=1~46&usage_type=default&display_rank=1.

Gladman, D. D. (2018). Overview of the clinical manifestations of systemic lupus erythematosus in adults. UpToDate.com. Retrieved from https://www.uptodate.com/contents/overview-of-the-clinical-manifestations-of-systemic-lupus-erythematosus-in-adults?search=Overview%20of%20the%20clinical%20manifestations%20of%20systemic%20lupus%20erythematosus%20in%20adults&source=search_result&selectedTitle=1~150&usage_type=default&display_rank=1.

Goldenberg, D. L. (2017a). Clinical manifestations and diagnosis of fibromyalgia in adults. UpToDate.com. Retrieved from https://www.uptodate.com/contents/clinical-manifestations-and-diagnosis-of-fibromyalgia in-adults?search=Clinical%20manifestations%20and%20diagnosis%20of%20fibromyalgia%20in%20adults&source=search_result&selectedTitle=1~140&usage_type=default&display_rank=1.

Goldenberg, D. L. (2017b). Initial treatment of fibromyalgia in adults. UpToDate.com. Retrieved from https://www.uptodate.com/contents/initial-treatment-of-fibromyalgia-in-adults?search=Initial%20treatment%20of%20fibromyalgia%20in%20adults&source=search_result&selectedTitle=1~150&usage_type=default&display_rank=1.

Goldenberg, D. L. (2017c). Pathogenesis of fibromyalgia. UpToDate.com. Retrieved from https://www.uptodate.com/contents/pathogenesis-of-fibromyalgia?search=Pathogenesis%20of%20fibromyalgia&source=search_result&selectedTitle=1~140&usage_type=default&display_rank=1.

Goldenberg, D. L., & Sexton, D. J. (2017). Septic arthritis in adults. UpToDate.com. Retrieved from https://www.uptodate.com/contents/septic-arthritis-in-adults?search=septic%20arthritis%20in%20adults&source=search_result&selectedTitle=1~150&usage_type=default&display_rank=1.

Greenberg, S. A. (2018). Pathogenesis of inflammatory myopathies. UpToDate.com. Retrieved from https://www.uptodate.com/contents/pathogenesis-of-inflammatory-myopathies?search=Pathogenesis%20of%20inflammatory%20myopathies&source=search_result&selectedTitle=1~150&usage_type=default&display_rank=1.

Honicek, F. J. (2016). Bone sarcomas: Preoperative evaluation, histologic classification, and principles of surgical management. UpToDate.com. Retrieved from https://www.uptodate.com/contents/search?search=Bone%20sarcomas:%20Preoperative%20evaluation,%20histologic%20classification,%20and%20principles%20of%20surgical%20management&sp=0-&searchType=PLAIN_TEXT&source=USER_INPUT&searchControl=TOP_PULLDOWN&searchOffset=1&autoComplete=false&language=en&max=10&index=&autoCompleteTerm=.

Hoy, D., March, L., Brooks, P., Blyth, F., Woolf, A., Bain, C., . . . Buchbinder, R. (2014). The global burden of low back pain: estimates from the Global Burden of Disease 2010 study. *Annals of the Rheumatic Diseases, 73*(6), 968–974.

Hu, L. (2016). Clinical manifestations of Lyme disease in adults. UpToDate.com. Retrieved from https://www.uptodate.com/contents/clinical-manifestations-of-lyme-disease-in-adults?search=Clinical%20manifestations%20of%20Lyme%20disease%20in%20adults&source=search_result&selectedTitle=1~150&usage_type=default&display_rank=1.

Hu, L. (2017). Treatment of Lyme disease. UpToDate.com. Retrieved from https://www.uptodate.com/contents/treatment-of-lyme-disease?search=Treatment%20of%20Lyme%20disease&source=search_result&selectedTitle=1~150&usage_type=default&display_rank=1.

Janeway, K. A., & Maki, R. (2018). Chemotherapy and radiation therapy in the management of osteosarcoma. UpToDate.com. Retrieved from https://www.uptodate.com/contents/chemotherapy-and-radiation-therapy-in-the-management-of-osteosarcoma?search=Chemotherapy%20and%20radiation%20therapy%20in%20the%20management%20of%20osteosarcoma&source=search_result&selectedTitle=1~150&usage_type=default&display_rank=1.

Juni, P., Hari, R., Rutjes, A. W., Fischer, R., Silletta, M. G., Reichenbach, S., & da Costa, B. R. (2015). Intra-articular corticosteroid for knee osteoarthritis. *Cochrane Database Systematic Review, 10*, CD005328.

Kado, D. (2017). Overview of hyperkyphosis in older persons. UpToDate.com. Retrieved from https://www.uptodate.com/contents/overview-of-hyperkyphosis-in-older-persons?search=Overview%20of%20hyperkyphosis%20in%20older%20persons&source=search_result&selectedTitle=1~150&usage_type=default&display_rank=1.

Kalunian, K. C. (2017). Risk factors for and possible causes of osteoarthritis. UpToDate.com. Retrieved from https://www.uptodate.com/contents/risk-factors-for-and-possible-causes-of-osteoarthritis?search=Risk%20factors%20for%20and%20possible%20causes%20of%20osteoarthritis&source=search_result&selectedTitle=1~150&usage_type=default&display_rank=1#H4497799.

Kanis, J. A., Harvey, N. C., Johansson, H., Oden, A., Leslie, W. D., & McCloskey, E. V. (2017). FRAX update. *Journal of Clinical Densitometry*, 20(3), 360–367.

Kemmler, W., Kohl, M., & von Stengel, S. (2017). Long-term effects of exercise in postmenopausal women: 16-year results of the Erlangen Fitness and Osteoporosis Prevention Study (EFOPS). *Menopause, 24*(1), 45–51.

Kogan, M., Cheng, S., Rao, S., DeMocker, S., & Koroma Nelson, M. (2017). Integrative medicine for geriatric and palliative care. *Medical Clinics of North America, 101*(5), 1005–1029.

Lalani, T. (2017). Overview of osteomyelitis in adults. UpToDate.com. Retrieved from https://www.uptodate.com/contents/overview-of-osteomyelitis-in-adults?search=Overview%20of%20osteomyelitis%20in%20adults&source=search_result&selectedTitle=1~150&usage_type=default&display_rank=1.

Lauche, R., Cramer, H., Häuser, W., Dobos, G., & Langhorst, J. (2015). A systematic overview of reviews for complementary and alternative therapies in the treatment of the fibromyalgia syndrome. *Evidence-Based Complementary and Alternative Medicine, 2015*, 610615.

Machado, G. C., Maher, C. G., Ferreira, P. H., Pinheiro, M. B., Lin, C. W., Day, R. O., . . . Ferreira, M. L. (2015). Efficacy and safety of paracetamol for spinal pain and osteoarthritis: Systematic review and meta-analysis of randomised placebo controlled trials. *British Medical Journal, 350*, h1225.

Mandl, L. A., & Martin, G. M. (2017). Overview of surgical therapy of knee and hip osteoarthritis. UpToDate.com. Retrieved from https://www.uptodate.com/contents/overview-of-surgical-therapy-of-knee-and-hip-osteoarthritis?search=Overview%20of%20surgical%20therapy%20of%20knee%20and%20hip%20osteoarthritis&source=search_result&selectedTitle=1~150&usage_type=default&display_rank=1.

Mayo Clinic. (2016). *Osteoporosis*. Retrieved from https://www.mayoclinic.org/diseases-conditions/osteoporosis/symptoms-causes/syc-20351968.

Mayo Clinic. (2018). *Muscular dystrophy*. Retrieved from https://www.mayoclinic.org/diseases-conditions/muscular-dystrophy/symptoms-causes/syc-20375388.

Miller, M. L. (2018). Initial treatment of dermatomyositis and polymyositis in adults. UpToDate.com. Retrieved from https://www.uptodate.com/contents/initial-treatment-of-dermatomyositis-and-polymyositis-in-adults?search=Initial%20treatment%20of%20dermatomyositis%20and%20polymyositis%20in%20adultsadults&source=search_result&selectedTitle=1~150&usage_type=default&display_rank=1.

Miller, M. L., & Vleugels, R. A. (2017). Clinical manifestations of dermatomyositis and polymyositis in adults. UpToDate.com. Retrieved from https://www.uptodate.com/contents/clinical-manifestations-of-dermatomyositis-and-polymyositis-in-adults?search=Tools%20%20Clinical%20manifestations%20of%20dermatomyositis%20and%20polymyositis%20in%20adults&source=search_result&selectedTitle=1~150&usage_type=default&display_rank=1.

Moreland, L. W., & Cannella, A. (2016). General principles of management of rheumatoid arthritis in adults. UpToDate.com. Retrieved from https://www.uptodate.com/contents/general-principles-of-management-of-rheumatoid-arthritis-in-adults?search=General%20principles%20of%20management%20of%20rheumatoid%20arthritis%20in%20adults&source=search_result&selectedTitle=1~150&usage_type=default&display_rank=1.

National Institute of Arthritis and Musculoskeletal and Skin Diseases (NIAMS). (2015). *Osteoporosis in men.*

Retrieved from https://www.niams.nih.gov/Health_Info/Bone/Osteoporosis/men.asp.

National Institutes for Health (NIH). (2018). Congenital muscular dystrophy ascending multiple dose cohort study analyzing pharmacokinetics at three dose levels in children and adolescents with assessment of safety and tolerability of omigapil (CALLISTO). ClinicalTrials.gov. Retrieved from https://clinicaltrials.gov/ct2/show/NCT01805024?term=OMIGAPIL&rank=1.

National Institute of Neurological Disorders and Stroke (NINDS). (2014). *Low back pain fact sheet.* Retrieved from https://www.ninds.nih.gov/Disorders/Patient-Caregiver-Education/Fact-Sheets/Low-Back-Pain-Fact-Sheet#3102_8.

National Osteoporosis Foundation (NOF). (2014). *NOF releases updated data detailing the prevalence of osteoporosis and low bone mass in the U.S.* Retrieved from https://www.nof.org/2014/06/02/54-million-americans-affected-by-osteoporosis-and-low-bone-mass/.

National Osteoporosis Foundation (NOF). (2015). *NOF statement on calcium and vitamin D.* Retrieved from https://www.nof.org/2015/08/03/nof-statement-on-calcium-and-vitamin-d/.

National Osteoporosis Foundation (NOF). (2017a). *Frequently asked questions about Paget's disease.* Retrieved from https://www.nof.org/pagets/pagets-frequently-asked-questions/.

National Osteoporosis Foundation (NOF). (2017b). *Symptoms, risk factors and complications.* Retrieved from https://www.nof.org/pagets-symptoms/.

National Osteoporosis Foundation (NOF). (2017c). *Treatment options.* Retrieved from https://www.nof.org/pagets/pagets-treatment-options/

National Osteoporosis Foundation (NOF). (2017d). *What women need to know.* Retrieved from https://www.nof.org/preventing-fractures/general-facts/what-women-need-to-know/.

National Scoliosis Foundation. (n.d.). *Information and support.* Retrieved from www.scoliosis.org/info.php.

Olanow, C. W., Schapira, A. H., LeWitt, P. A., Kieburtz, K., Sauer, D., Olivieri, G., . . . Hubble, J. (2006). TCH346 as a neuroprotective drug in Parkinson's disease: A double-blind, randomised, controlled trial. *Lancet Neurology, 5*(12), 1013–1020.

Patel, R., & Shahane, A. (2014). The epidemiology of Sjogren's syndrome. *Clinical Epidemiology, 6,* 247–255.

Proudman, S. M., James, M. J., Spargo, L. D., Metcalf, R. G., Sullivan, T. R., Rischmueller, M., . . . Cleland, L. G. (2015). Fish oil in recent onset rheumatoid arthritis: A randomised, double-blind controlled trial within algorithm-based drug use. *Annals of the Rheumatic Diseases, 74*(1), 89–95.

Ragab, G., Elshahaly, M., & Bardin, T. (2017). Gout: An old disease in new perspective—A review. *Journal of Advanced Research, 8*(5), 495–511.

Ratcliffe, G. E., Enns, M. W., Belik, S. L., & Sareen, J. (2008). Chronic pain conditions and suicidal ideation and suicide attempts: An epidemiologic perspective. *Clinical Journal of Pain, 24*(3), 204–210.

Rheumatoid Arthritis Support Network. (2016). *Rheumatoid arthritis: Fast facts.* Retrieved from https://www.rheumatoidarthritis.org/ra/facts-and-statistics/.

Rosen, H. H. (2017). Patient education: Calcium and vitamin D for bone health (Beyond the Basics). UpToDate.com. Retrieved from https://www.uptodate.com/contents/prevention-of-osteoporosis?search=Prevention%20of%20osteoporosis&source=search_result&selectedTitle=1~150&usage_type=default&display_rank=1.

Schur, P. H., & Hahn, B. H. (2017). Epidemiology and pathogenesis of systemic lupus erythematosus. UpToDate.com. Retrieved from https://www.uptodate.com/contents/epidemiology-and-pathogenesis-of-systemic-lupus-erythematosus?search=Epidemiology%20and%20pathogenesis%20of%20systemic%20lupus%20erythematosus&source=search_result&selectedTitle=1~150&usage_type=default&display_rank=1.

Schur, P. H., Maini, R. N., & Gibofsky, A. (2016). Nonpharmacologic therapies and preventive measures for patients with rheumatoid arthritis. UpToDate.com. Retrieved from https://www.uptodate.com/contents/nonpharmacologic-therapies-and-preventive-measures-for-patients-with-rheumatoid-arthritis?search=Nonpharmacologic%20therapies%20and%20preventive%20measures%20for%20patients%20with%20rheumatoid%20arthritis&source=search_result&selectedTitle=1~150&usage_type=default&display_rank=1.

Seo, P. (2017). Overview of immunosuppressive and conventional (non-biologic) disease-modifying drugs in the rheumatic diseases. UpToDate.com. Retrieved from https://www.uptodate.com/contents/overview-of-immunosuppressive-and-conventional-non-biologic-disease-modifying-drugs-in-the-rheumatic-diseases?search=Overview%20of%20immunosuppressive%20and%20conventional%20(non-biologic)%20disease-modifying%20drugs%20in%20the%20rheumatic%20diseases&source=search_result&selectedTitle=1~150&usage_type=default&display_rank=1.

Sherl, S. A. (2018). Adolescent idiopathic scoliosis: Clinical features, evaluation, and diagnosis. UpToDate.com. Retrieved from https://www.uptodate.com/contents/adolescent-idiopathic-scoliosis-clinical-features-evaluation-and-diagnosis?search=Adolescent%20idiopathic%20scoliosis:%20Clinical%20features,%20evaluation,%20and%20diagnosis&source=search_result&selectedTitle=1~10&usage_type=default&display_rank=1.

Singh, J., Saag, K., Bridges, S. L., Akl, E. A., Bannuru, R. R., Sullivan, M. C., . . . McAlindon, T. (2015). 2015 American College of Rheumatology guidelines for the treatment of rheumatoid arthritis. *Arthritis Care and Research, 68*(1), 1–26.

Sopirala, M. M. (2017). Pathogenesis of osteomyelitis. UpToDate.com. Retrieved from https://www.uptodate.com/contents/pathogenesis-of-osteomyelitis?search=Pathogenesis%20of%20osteomyelitis&source=search_result&selectedTitle=1~150&usage_type=default&display_rank=1.

Sorenson, M., Quinn, L., & Klein, D. (2019). *Pathophysiology: Concepts of human disease.* Hoboken, NJ: Pearson Education.

Spondylitis Association of America. (2018a). *Ankylosing spondylitis.* Retrieved from www.spondylitis.org/about/as.aspx.

Spondylitis Association of America. (2018b). *Reactive arthritis.* Retrieved from www.spondylitis.org/about/reative.aspx.

Tabloski, P. (2014). *Gerontological nursing* (3rd ed.). Upper Saddle River, NJ: Pearson.

United States Bone and Joint Initiative. (2018). *The burden of musculoskeletal diseases in the United States: Musculoskeletal diseases* (4th ed.). Retrieved from www.boneandjointburden.org.

U.S. Preventive Services Task Force. (2011). Screening for osteoporosis: U.S. Preventive Services Task Force recommendation statement. *Annals of Internal Medicine, 154*(5), 356–364.

Varga, J. (2017a). Overview of the clinical manifestations of systemic sclerosis (scleroderma) in adults. UpToDate.com. Retrieved from https://www.uptodate.com/contents/overview-of-the-clinical-manifestations-of-systemic-sclerosis-scleroderma-in-adults

Varga, J. (2017b). Risk factors for and possible causes of systemic sclerosis (scleroderma). UpToDate.com. Retrieved from https://www.uptodate.com/contents/risk-factors-for-and-possible-causes-of-systemic-sclerosis-scleroderma?search=Risk%20factors%20for%20and%20possible%20causes%20of%20systemic%20sclerosis%20(scleroderma&source=search_result&selectedTitle=1~150&usage_type=default&display_rank=1.

Venables, P. J. W., & Maini, R. N. (2017). Disease outcome and functional capacity in rheumatoid arthritis. UpToDate.com. Retrieved from https://www.uptodate.com/contents/disease-outcome-and-functional-capacity-in-rheumatoid-arthritis?search=Disease%20outcome%20and%20functional%20capacity%20in%20rheumatoid%20arthritis&source=search_result&selectedTitle=1~150&usage_type=default&display_rank=1.

Viswanathan, M., Reddy, S. Berkman, N., Cullen, K., Middleton, J. C., Nicholson, W. K., & Kahwati, L. C. (2017). Screening to prevent osteoporotic fractures: An evidence review for the U.S. Preventive Services Task Force. Rockville, MD: Agency for Healthcare Research and Quality, U.S. Department of Health and Human Services. Retrieved from https://www.uspreventiveservicestaskforce.org/Page/Document/draft-evidence-review/osteoporosis-screening1.

Wallace, D. J. (2017). Antimalarial drugs in the treatment of rheumatic disease. UpToDate.com. Retrieved from https://www.uptodate.com/contents/antimalarial-drugs-in-the-treatment-of-rheumatic-disease?search=Antimalarial%20drugs%20in%20the%20treatment%20of%20rheumatic%20disease&source=search_result&selectedTitle=1~150&usage_type=default&display_rank=1.

Wang, L. L., Gebhardt, M. C., & Rainusso, N. (2017). Osteosarcoma: Epidemiology, pathogenesis, clinical presentation, diagnosis, and histology. UpToDate.com. Retrieved from https://www.uptodate.com/contents/osteosarcoma-epidemiology-pathogenesis-clinical-presentation-diagnosis-and-histology?search=Osteosarcoma:%20Epidemiology,%20pathogenesis,%20clinical%20presentation,%20diagnosis,%20and%20histology&source=search_result&selectedTitle=1~82&usage_type=default&display_rank=1.

Wheeler, S. G., Wipf, J. E., Staiger, T. O., Deyo, R. A., & Jarvik, J. G. (2018). Evaluation of low back pain in adults. UpToDate.com. Retrieved from https://www.uptodate.com/contents/evaluation-of-low-back-pain-in-adults?search=Evaluation%20of%20low%20back%20pain%20in%20adults&source=search_result&selectedTitle=1~150&usage_type=default&display_rank=1.

Williams, S. N., Wolford, M. L., & Bercovitz, A. (2015). Hospitalization for total knee replacement among inpatients aged 45 and over: United States, 2000–2010. *NCHS Data Brief, 210.* Retrieved from https://www.cdc.gov/nchs/data/databriefs/db210.pdf.

Wolford, M. L., Palso, K., & Bercovitz, A. (2015). Hospitalization for hip knee replacement among inpatients aged 45 and over: United States, 2000–2010. *NCHS Data Brief, 186.* Retrieved from https://www.cdc.gov/nchs/data/databriefs/db186.pdf.

Yu, D. T. (2016a). Assessment and treatment of ankylosing spondylitis in adults. UpToDate.com. Retrieved from https://www.uptodate.com/contents/assessment-and-treatment-of-ankylosing-spondylitis-in-adults?search=Assessment20and%20treatment%20of%20ankylosing%20spondylitis%20in%20adults&source=search_result&selectedTitle=1~150&usage_type=default&display_rank=1.

Yu, D. T. (2016b). Reactive arthritis. UpToDate.com. Retrieved from https://www.uptodate.com/contents/reactive-arthritis?search=reactive%20arthritis&source=search_result&selectedTitle=1~118&usage_type=default&display_rank=1.

Yu, D. T., & van Tubergen, A. (2017). Clinical manifestations of axial spondyloarthritis (ankylosing spondylitis and nonradiographic axial spondyloarthritis) in adults. UpToDate.com. Retrieved from https://www.uptodate.com/contents/clinical

-manifestations-of-axial-spondyloarthritis-ankylosing-spondylitis-and-nonradiographic-axial-spondyloarthritis-in-adults?search=Clinical%20manifestations%20of%20axial%20spondyloarthritis%20(ankylosing%20spondylitis%20and%20nonradiographic%20axial%20spondyloarthritis)%20in%20adults&source=search_result&selectedTitle=1~148&usage_type=default&display_rank=1.

Yu, D. T., & van Tubergen, A. (2018). Pathogenesis of spondyloarthritis. UpToDate.com. Retrieved from https://www.uptodate.com/contents/pathogenesis-of-spondyloarthritis?search=Pathogenesis%20of%20spondyloarthritis&source=search_result&selectedTitle=1~150&usage_type=default&display_rank=1.

ADDITIONAL RESOURCES

Arthritis Foundation
www.arthritis.org

National Institute of Health Osteoporosis and Related Bone Diseases National Resource Center
https://www.niams.nih.gov/Health_Info/Bone/

National Osteoporosis Foundation
https://www.nof.org/patients/patient-support/nof-support-groups/

Unit

11

Responses to Altered Neurologic Function

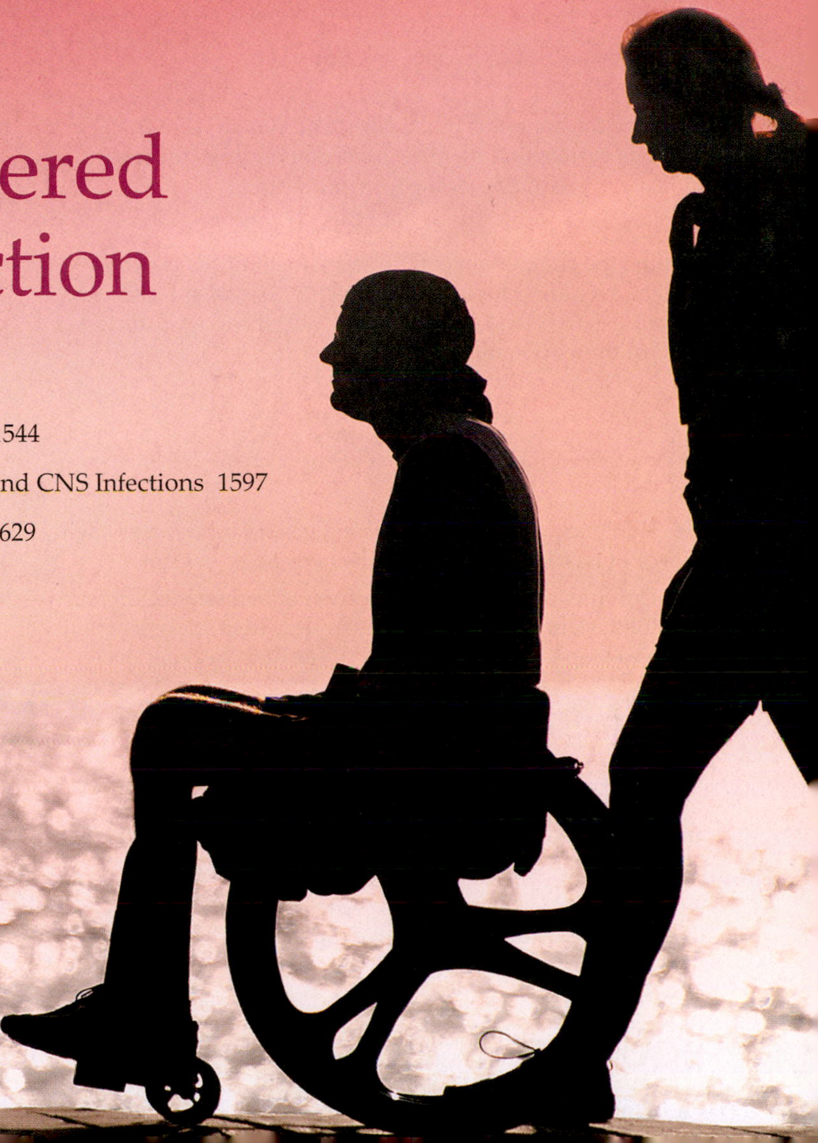

Chapter 41

Assessing the Nervous System

Chapter Outline and Learning Outcomes

41.1 Anatomy, Physiology, and Functions of the Nervous System 1523

Describe the anatomy, physiology, and functions of the nervous system and identify abnormal findings that may indicate impairments of the nervous system.

41.2 Assessing Neurologic Function 1531

Outline the components of the assessment of the nervous system, including topics for the health assessment interview, techniques for physical assessment, and the diagnostic tests used in the assessment.

41.3 Assessment of Special Populations 1541

Differentiate considerations for assessing the nervous systems of older adults and veterans.

41.4 Health Promotion 1541

Summarize topics that nurses teach to promote healthy tissue integrity across the lifespan.

CLINICAL COMPETENCIES

- Conduct and document a health history for patients having or at risk for alterations in the neurologic system.
- Conduct and document a physical assessment of neurologic structures and functions demonstrating sensitivity and respect for the diversity of the human experience.
- Monitor the results of diagnostic tests and communicate abnormal findings within the interprofessional team.
- Perform specific neurologic assessments for patients with suspected meningeal irritation and for patients who are disoriented or comatose.

KEY TERMS

anosmia, 1534
aphasia, 1533
ataxia, 1536
decerebrate posturing, 1538
decorticate posturing, 1538
diaphoresis, 1529
dysarthria, 1533
dysphagia, 1535
dysphonia, 1533
fasciculations, 1535
flaccidity, 1536
kinesthesia, 1535
nystagmus, 1534
ptosis, 1534
spasticity, 1536
tremors, 1536

EQUIPMENT NEEDED

- Cotton balls
- Safety pin
- Tongue depressor
- Tuning fork
- Reflex hammer
- Pencil and paper
- Penlight
- Printed materials
- Substances to test the senses of smell and taste

The nervous system regulates and integrates all body functions, muscle movements, senses, mental abilities, and emotions. It collects information from the internal and external environments as sensory input, processes and interprets the input, and initiates and coordinates responses that are manifested as motor or sensory output. Alterations in structure and/or function of the nervous system have the potential to affect a wide variety of human functions, such as activity and exercise, comfort, cardiovascular and respiratory function, elimination, and sexuality. Changes in appearance and abilities for self-care further increase the risk for alterations in self-concept and relationships.

Worldwide, neurological disorders are a prevalent cause of disability and death. The most common neurological disorders are headache and Alzheimer disease (Global Burden of Disease Study, 2017).

41.1 Anatomy, Physiology, and Functions of the Nervous System

The nervous system is divided into two regions: The *central nervous system (CNS)*, which consists of the brain and spinal cord, and the *peripheral nervous system (PNS)*, which consists of the cranial nerves, the spinal nerves, and the autonomic nervous system.

Neurons, Action Potentials, and Neurotransmitters

The highly integrated CNS and PNS consist of just two types of cells: Neurons, which receive impulses and send them on to other cells, and neuroglia, which protect and nourish the neurons. This section focuses on the neurons.

Neurons

Each neuron consists of a dendrite, a cell body, and an axon (**Figure 41.1** ■). The *dendrite* is a short projection from the cell body that conducts impulses toward the cell body. *Cell bodies*, most of which are located within the CNS, are clustered in ganglia or nuclei. The cell bodies and dendrites comprise what is often called the *gray matter of the CNS*. The *axon*, a long process, conducts impulses away from the cell body. Many axons are covered with a *myelin sheath*, a white lipid substance. It is interrupted at intervals in unmyelinated areas called *nodes of Ranvier*, which allow movement of ions between the axon and the extracellular fluid. The myelin sheath serves to increase the speed of nerve impulse conduction in axons and is essential for the survival of larger nerve processes. Myelinated nerve fibers comprise the white matter of the brain and spinal cord.

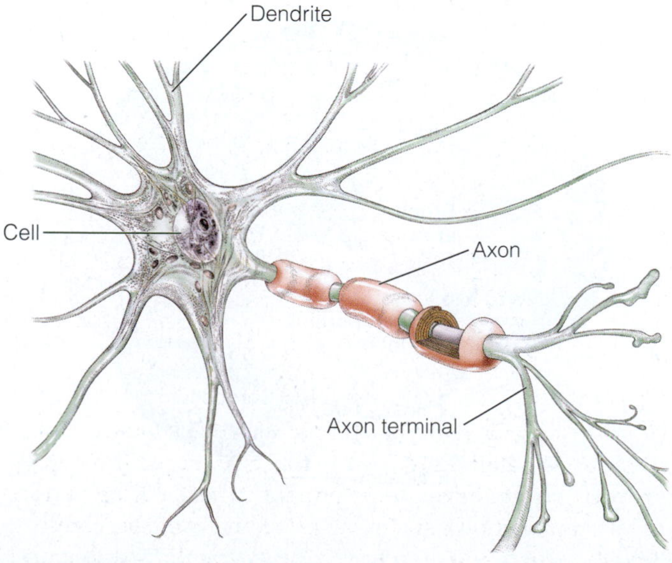
Dendrite
Cell
Axon
Axon terminal

Figure 41.1 ■ A typical neuron.

Action Potentials

Action potentials are impulses (movements of electrical charge along an axon membrane) that allow neurons to communicate with other neurons and body cells. They are initiated by stimuli and propagated by the rapid movement of charged ions through the cell membrane. When a neuron reaches a certain level of stimulation, an electrical impulse is generated and conducted along the length of its axon. The movement of impulses to and from the CNS is made possible by afferent and efferent neurons. Afferent, or sensory, neurons have receptors in skin, muscles, and other organs and relay impulses to the CNS. Efferent, or motor, neurons transmit impulses from the CNS to cause some type of action.

Nerve impulses occur when a stimulus reaches a point great enough to generate a change in electrical charge across the cell membrane of a neuron. A neuron that is not involved in impulse conduction is in a resting, or polarized, state, in which the number of positive ions in the fluid outside of the cell membrane is greater than in the fluid within the cell. The chief regulators of membrane potential are sodium and potassium: Sodium is the major positive ion in the extracellular fluid, and potassium is the major positive ion in the intracellular fluid. In response to an electrical stimulus, the cell membrane becomes permeable to sodium, which moves into the cell. This changes the polarity of the cell membrane, and the neuron is said to depolarize. This event stimulates an action potential (a nerve impulse) to travel down the axon. When the charges and ions return to their original resting state, the neuron is repolarized.

The events in an action potential are:

1. Initially, sodium permeability increases. As the membrane is depolarized, sodium channels open and sodium rushes into the cell to a point of depolarization (the inside of the cell becomes less negative in comparison to the outside of the cell).
2. This is followed by a decrease in sodium permeability, lasting only about 1 millisecond. The sodium gates close and the sodium influx stops.
3. The final event is an increase in potassium permeability. The potassium gates open, potassium rushes out of the cell, and the cell interior becomes progressively less positive. The membrane potential moves back to its resting state and is repolarized.

The action potential is generated only at the point of the stimulus; once generated, it is propagated along the entire length of the axon regardless of whether the stimulus continues. Conduction of the impulse is rapid in myelinated fibers, with the action potential "jumping" from one node of Ranvier to the next. The conduction of the impulse is slower in unmyelinated fibers.

Neurotransmitters

Neurotransmitters are the chemical messengers of the nervous system. When the action potential reaches the end of the axon at the presynaptic terminal, a neurotransmitter is released and travels across the synaptic cleft to bind with receptors in the postsynaptic neuron dendrite or cell body. The neurotransmitter may either be inhibitory or excitatory. The excitatory neurotransmitter is almost always *acetylcholine (ACh)*, which is rapidly degraded by the enzyme acetylcholinesterase. Nerves that transmit impulses through the release of ACh are called *cholinergic*. Receptors that bind ACh are found in the viscera, skeletal muscle cells, and the adrenal medulla (where they stimulate the release of epinephrine). The effect of ACh binding may be either to stimulate or to inhibit a response.

Norepinephrine (NE), which may be either excitatory or inhibitory, is another major neurotransmitter. Nerves that transmit impulses through the release of NE are called *adrenergic*. Receptors that bind NE are found in the heart, lungs, kidneys, blood vessels, and all target organs stimulated by the sympathetic division except the heart. Adrenergic receptors are further divided into alpha and beta types. Alpha-adrenergic receptors help control such varied functions as arterial vasoconstriction and pupil dilation. Beta-adrenergic fibers may be either beta$_1$- or beta$_2$-receptors. *Beta$_1$-receptors* are found in the heart, where they regulate the rate and force of contraction. *Beta$_2$-receptors* are found in receptor cells of the lungs, arteries, liver, and uterus; they help regulate bronchial diameter, arterial diameter, and glycogenesis. Generally, binding of NE to alpha-receptors stimulates a response, whereas binding to beta-receptors inhibits a response.

Other neurotransmitters include *gamma aminobutyric acid (GABA)*, which inhibits CNS function; *dopamine*, which may be inhibitory or excitatory and helps control fine movement and emotions; and *serotonin*, which is usually inhibitory and controls sleep, hunger, and behavior and also affects consciousness.

The Central Nervous System

The *central nervous system* consists of the brain and spinal cord, highly evolved clusters of neurons that act to accept, interconnect, interpret, and generate a response to nerve impulses originating throughout the body.

The Brain

The *brain* is the control center of the nervous system and also generates thoughts, emotions, and speech. The brain has four major regions: The cerebrum, the diencephalon, the brainstem, and the cerebellum (**Figure 41.2** ■). The general functions of these regions are summarized in **Table 41.1**.

The two hemispheres of the cerebrum account for almost 60% of brain weight. The surface of the cerebrum is folded into elevated ridges of tissue called *gyri*, which are separated by shallow grooves (sulci) and deep grooves (fissures). The longitudinal fissure separates the hemispheres, and the transverse fissure separates the cerebrum from the cerebellum. In addition, each cerebral hemisphere is divided into frontal, parietal, temporal, and occipital lobes (**Figure 41.3** ■).

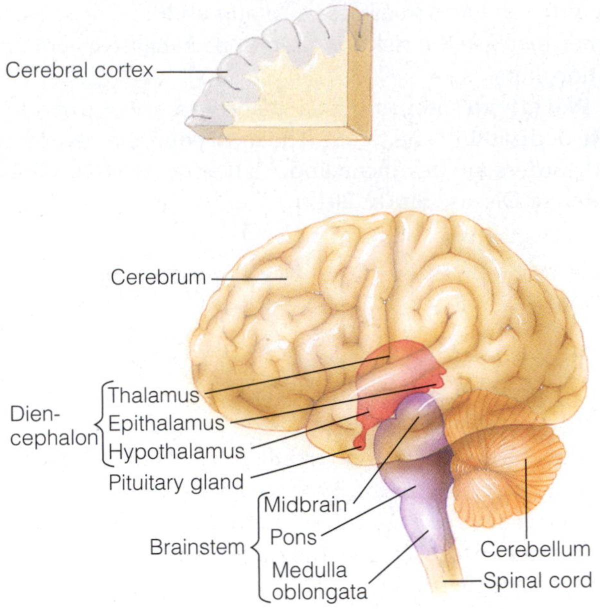
Cerebral cortex
Cerebrum
Dien-
cephalon
Thalamus
Epithalamus
Hypothalamus
Pituitary gland
Brainstem
Midbrain
Pons
Medulla
oblongata
Cerebellum
Spinal cord

Figure 41.2 ■ The four major regions of the brain.

Table 41.1 General Functions of the Four Regions of the Brain

Region	Functions
Cerebrum	■ Interprets sensory input ■ Controls skeletal muscle activity ■ Processes intellect and emotions ■ Contains skills memory
Diencephalon	■ Conducts sensory and motor impulses ■ Regulates autonomic nervous system ■ Regulates and produces hormones ■ Mediates emotional responses
Brainstem	■ Serves as conduction pathway ■ Serves as site of decussation of tracts ■ Contains respiratory nuclei ■ Helps regulate skeletal muscles
Cerebellum	■ Processes information ■ Provides information necessary for balance, posture, and coordinated muscle movement

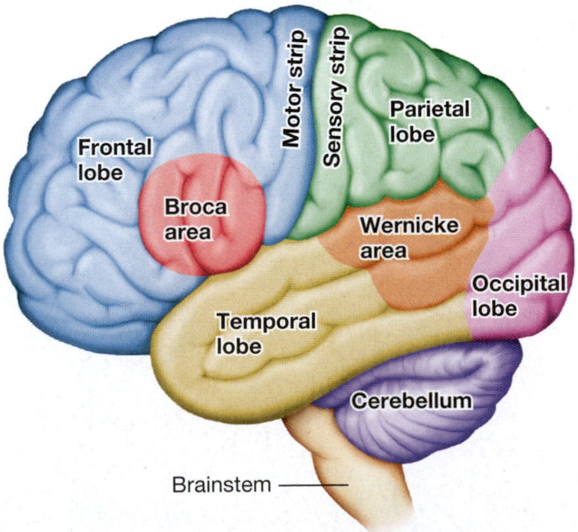
Motor strip
Sensory strip
Parietal lobe
Frontal lobe
Broca area
Wernicke area
Occipital lobe
Temporal lobe
Cerebellum
Brainstem

Figure 41.3 ■ Lobes of the cerebrum and functional areas of the cerebral cortex.

The cerebral hemispheres are connected by a thick band of nerve fibers called the *corpus callosum*, which allows communication between the two hemispheres. Each hemisphere receives sensory and motor impulses from the opposite side of the body. Most people have a more highly developed left hemisphere, which is responsible for the control of language. The right hemisphere has greater control over nonverbal perceptual functions.

The *cerebral cortex* is the outer surface of the cerebrum. It consists of neuron cell bodies, unmyelinated fibers, neuroglia, and blood vessels. The functions of the different lobes of the cerebrum and the specific areas of the cerebral cortex are listed in **Table 41.2**.

The *diencephalon* is embedded in the cerebrum superior to the brainstem. It consists of the thalamus, hypothalamus, and epithalamus. The *thalamus* begins to process sensory impulses before they ascend to the cerebral cortex. It serves as a sorting, processing, and relay station for input into the cortical region. The *hypothalamus*, located inferior to the thalamus, regulates temperature, water metabolism, appetite, emotional expressions, part of the sleep–wake cycle, and thirst. The *epithalamus* forms the dorsal part of the diencephalon and includes the pineal body, which is part of the endocrine system that affects growth and development.

Brainstem

The *brainstem* consists of the midbrain, pons, and medulla oblongata. The *midbrain* is a center for auditory and visual reflexes and functions as a nerve pathway between the cerebral hemispheres and lower brain. The *pons* is located just below the midbrain. It consists mostly of fiber tracts, but it also contains nuclei that control respiration. The *medulla oblongata*, located at the base of the brainstem, is continuous with the superior portion of the spinal cord. Nuclei of the medulla oblongata play an important role in controlling cardiac rate, blood pressure, respiration, and swallowing.

The cerebellum is connected to the midbrain, pons, and medulla. Its functions include coordinating skeletal muscle activity, maintaining balance, and controlling fine movements.

Table 41.2 Functions of Lobes of the Cerebrum and Areas of the Cerebral Cortex

Area	Functions
Parietal lobe (somatosensory area of cerebral cortex)	Promotes recognition of pain, cold, and light touch. The left side receives input from the right side of the body, and vice versa.
Occipital lobe	Receives and interprets visual stimuli.
Temporal lobe	Receives and interprets olfactory and auditory stimuli.
Frontal lobe	Controls movements of voluntary muscles.
Primary motor area	Facilitates voluntary movement of skeletal muscles.
Speech area	Promotes understanding of spoken and written words.
Motor speech area (Broca area)	Promotes vocalization of words.

Ventricles

The brain contains four *ventricles*, which are chambers filled with cerebrospinal fluid (CSF). They are linked by ducts that allow the CSF to circulate. One lateral ventricle is located within each hemisphere. These communicate with the third ventricle through the foramen of Monro. The third ventricle communicates with the fourth ventricle through the cerebral aqueduct that runs through the midbrain. The cerebral aqueduct is continuous with the central canal of the spinal cord.

Cerebrospinal Fluid

Cerebrospinal fluid, a clear and colorless liquid, is formed by the choroid plexus, which is made up of groups of specialized capillaries located in the brain ventricles. Derived from blood plasma, CSF consists of 99% water and contains protein, sodium, chloride, potassium, bicarbonate, and glucose (**Table 41.3** outlines normal laboratory values for CSF). The usual amount of CSF ranges from 80 to 200 mL and is replaced several times each day. CSF is normally produced and absorbed in equal amounts. CSF circulates from the lateral ventricles of the cerebral hemispheres into the third ventricle, through the midbrain, and into the fourth ventricle. Some CSF flows down the center of the spinal cord as the rest of it circulates into the subarachnoid space and returns to the blood through the arachnoid villi. CSF forms a cushion for the brain tissue, protects the brain and spinal cord from trauma, helps provide nourishment for the brain, and removes waste products of cerebrospinal cellular metabolism.

Meninges

The brain and spinal cord are covered and protected by three connective tissue membranes called *meninges*. The meninges form divisions within the skull, enclose venous sinuses, and contain CSF. The meninges have three layers (**Figure 41.4** ■). The outermost double layer, the *dura mater*, is attached to the inner surface of the skull. The middle layer is the *arachnoid mater*, which encloses the entire CNS and forms the subarachnoid space that contains CSF. The innermost layer, the *pia mater*, clings to the brain, spinal cord, and segmental nerves and is filled with small blood vessels.

Table 41.3 Normal Laboratory Values for Cerebrospinal Fluid

Component	Normal Value
Appearance	Clear and colorless
Ph	7.35
Specific gravity	1.007
WBCs	0–8 mm^3
Protein	40 mg/dL
Glucose	40–70 mg/dL
Chloride	118–132 mmol/L
Pressure	70–180 mmH_2O

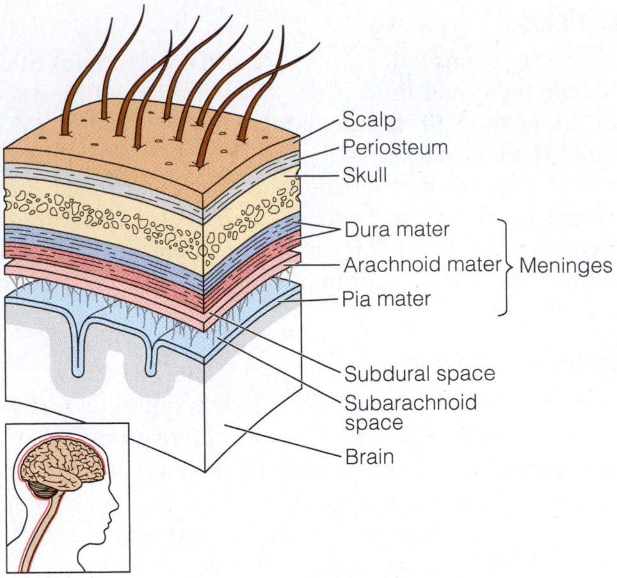
Scalp
Periosteum
Skull
Dura mater
Arachnoid mater
Pia mater
Meninges
Subdural space
Subarachnoid space
Brain

Figure 41.4 ■ Anatomy of the meninges.

Cerebral Circulation and the Blood–Brain Barrier

The brain receives about 750 mL of blood each minute and uses 20% of the body's total oxygen uptake. The large amount of oxygen is necessary for metabolism of glucose, which is the brain's sole source of energy. Blood flow to the brain is mostly controlled by autoregulatory or local mechanisms that respond to the brain's metabolic needs. *Autoregulation* is the ability of the brain to maintain constant cerebral blood flow despite changes in systemic blood pressure. At least three metabolic factors affect cerebral blood flow: Carbon dioxide, hydrogen ion, and oxygen concentrations. Of these, increased carbon dioxide is the major stimulus for vasodilation with resultant increased cerebral blood flow.

The anterior part of the brain is supplied with blood by the two internal carotid arteries, and the posterior part of the brain is supplied with blood by the vertebral arteries. The internal carotid artery branches into further arteries: The ophthalmic, posterior communicating, anterior choroidal, anterior cerebral, and middle cerebral. The brainstem and cerebellum receive their blood supply from the basilar artery. These major arteries are connected by small anterior and posterior communicating arteries, which form a circle of connected blood vessels called the *circle of Willis* (**Figure 41.5** ■). This circle serves as a protective device, providing alternative routes for brain tissues to receive their blood supply.

The capillaries in the brain have low permeability because the cells that compose their walls join at very tight junctions and are surrounded by a basement membrane and by the processes of astrocytes in the brain. This blood–brain barrier allows lipids, glucose, some amino acids, water, carbon dioxide, and oxygen to pass through it, thus maintaining a controlled environment. Substances such as urea, creatinine, proteins, some toxins, and most antibiotics cannot pass this barrier and enter brain tissue. However, injury to or infection of the brain may cause increased permeability of the blood–brain barrier, altering concentrations of proteins, water, and electrolytes.

The Limbic System and the Reticular Formation

The limbic system and the reticular formation are functional brain systems. These systems, made of networks of neurons, communicate across areas of the brain.

The *limbic system* consists of structures that form a ring of tissue in the medial side of each hemisphere, surrounding the upper portion of the brainstem and corpus callosum. The limbic system integrates and modulates input to make up the affective part of the brain, providing emotional and behavioral responses to environmental stimuli.

The *reticular formation* is located through the central core of the medulla oblongata, pons, and midbrain. This system has widespread connections throughout the brain

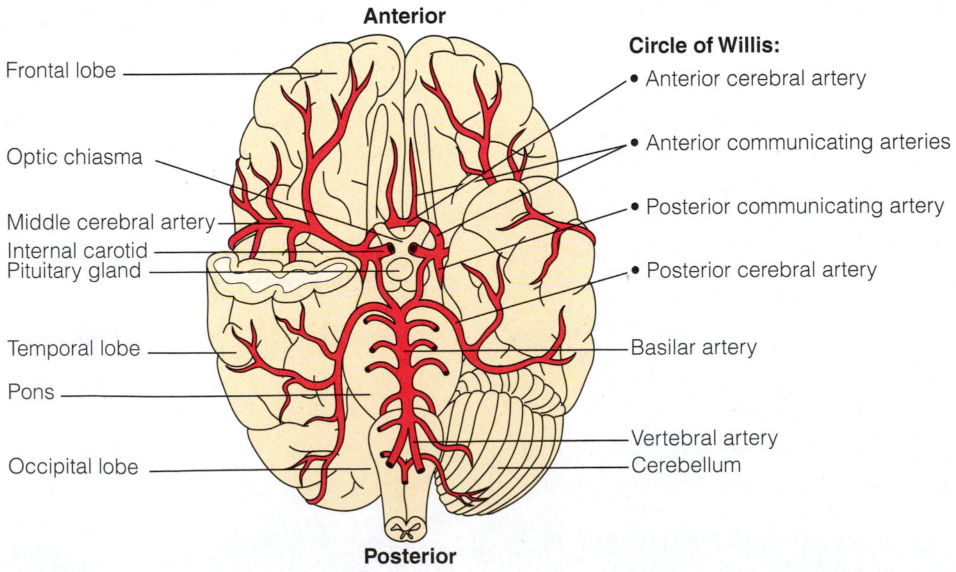
Anterior
Frontal lobe
Optic chiasma
Middle cerebral artery
Internal carotid
Pituitary gland
Temporal lobe
Pons
Occipital lobe
Circle of Willis:
• Anterior cerebral artery
• Anterior communicating arteries
• Posterior communicating artery
• Posterior cerebral artery
Basilar artery
Vertebral artery
Cerebellum
Posterior

Figure 41.5 ■ Major arteries serving the brain and the circle of Willis.

and relays sensory input from all body systems to all levels of the brain. The reticular formation includes the *reticular activating system (RAS)*. The RAS is a stimulating system for the cerebral cortex, keeping it alert and responsive to incoming sensory stimuli while filtering out repetitive or unwanted stimuli. The sleep center inhibits activity of the RAS, and drugs and alcohol may depress it. Other parts of the reticular formation include motor nuclei that help maintain muscle tone and coordinated movements through interconnections with spinal nerves, and the vasomotor and cardiovascular regulatory centers, which are part of autonomic regulation of the cardiovascular system.

The Spinal Cord

The *spinal cord*, protected by the vertebrae, the meninges, and CSF, extends from the medulla to the level of the first lumbar vertebra (**Figure 41.6** ■). It serves as a center for conducting messages to and from the brain and as a reflex center. The spinal cord is about 42 cm (17 in.) long and 1.8 cm (0.75 in.) thick. The gray matter of the cord is on the inside, and the white matter is on the outside (the reverse of the arrangement in the brain).

The spinal cord is surrounded by 33 vertebrae: Eight cervical, 12 thoracic, five lumbar, five sacral, and four fused vertebrae that form the coccyx. Each vertebra consists of a body and a vertebral arch formed by projections from the body. This arch encloses a space called the *vertebral foramen*. The vertebral foramina of all the vertebrae form the vertebral canal through which the spinal cord passes. Intervertebral foramina are spaces between the vertebrae through which spinal nerve roots pass as they exit the vertebral column. Intervertebral disks are located between each of the movable vertebrae. Each disk is made of a thick capsule surrounding a gelatinous core called the *nucleus pulposus*. Ligaments that provide mobility and protection surround the vertebral column.

Functions of the Spinal Cord and Spinal Roots

Messages to and from the brain are conducted via pathways called either *ascending* (sensory) or *descending* (motor) (**Figure 41.7** ■). The major ascending tracts are the *lateral* and *anterior spinothalamic tracts*, which carry sensations for pain, temperature, and crude touch; and the *posterior tracts*, which carry sensations for fine touch,

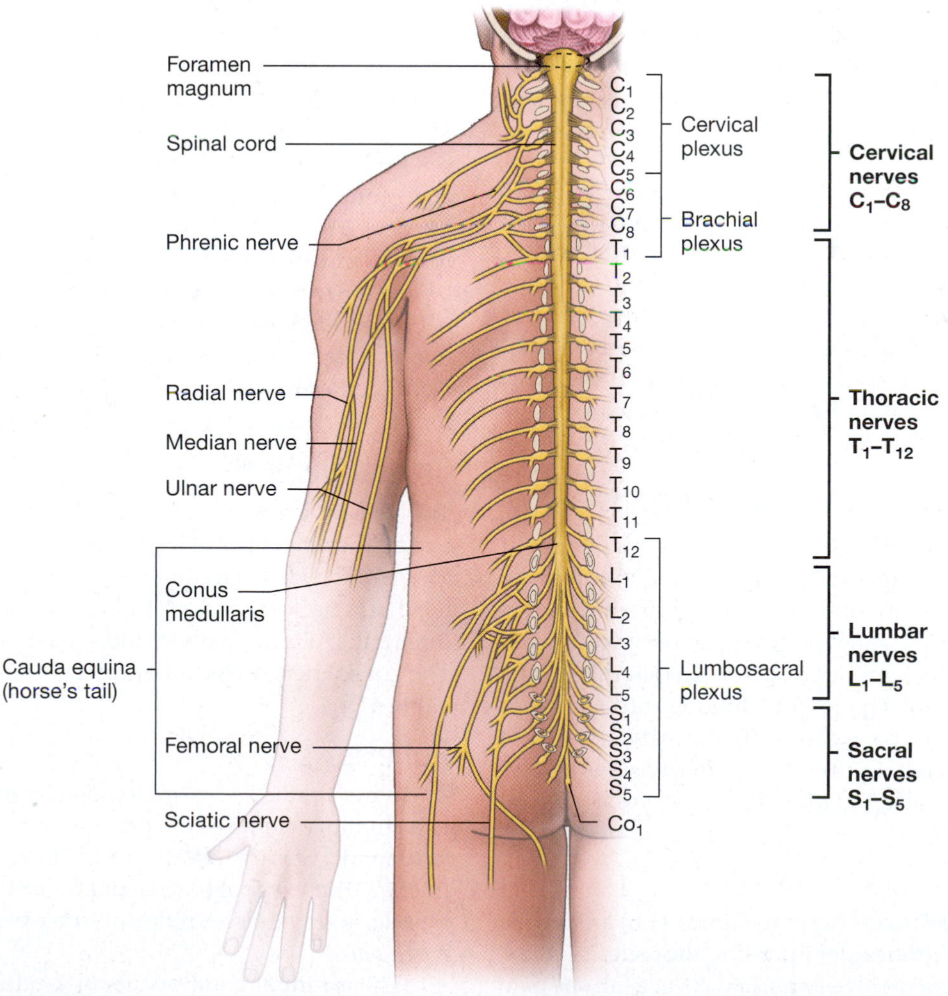

Foramen magnum
Spinal cord
Phrenic nerve
Radial nerve
Median nerve
Ulnar nerve
Conus medullaris
Cauda equina (horse's tail)
Femoral nerve
Sciatic nerve
C_1
C_2
C_3
C_4
C_5
C_6
C_7
C_8
T_1
T_2
T_3
T_4
T_5
T_6
T_7
T_8
T_9
T_{10}
T_{11}
T_{12}
L_1
L_2
L_3
L_4
L_5
S_1
S_2
S_3
S_4
S_5
Co_1
Cervical plexus
Brachial plexus
Lumbosacral plexus
Cervical nerves C_1–C_8
Thoracic nerves T_1–T_{12}
Lumbar nerves L_1–L_5
Sacral nerves S_1–S_5

Figure 41.6 ■ Distribution of spinal nerves.

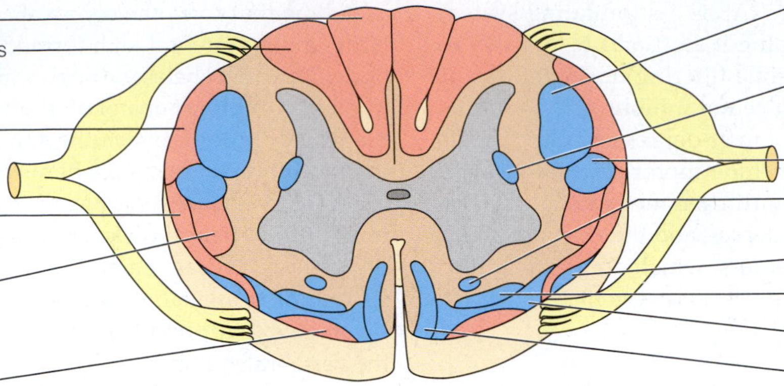
Ascending (sensory) tracts
Fasciculus gracilis
Fasciculus cuneatus
Posterior spinocerebellar tract
Anterior spinocerebellar tract
Lateral spinothalamic tract
Anterior spinothalamic tract
Descending (motor) tracts
Lateral corticospinal tract
Lateral reticulospinal tract
Rubrospinal tract
Anterior reticulospinal tract
Olivospinal tract
Tectospinal tract
Vestibulospinal tract
Anterior corticospinal tract

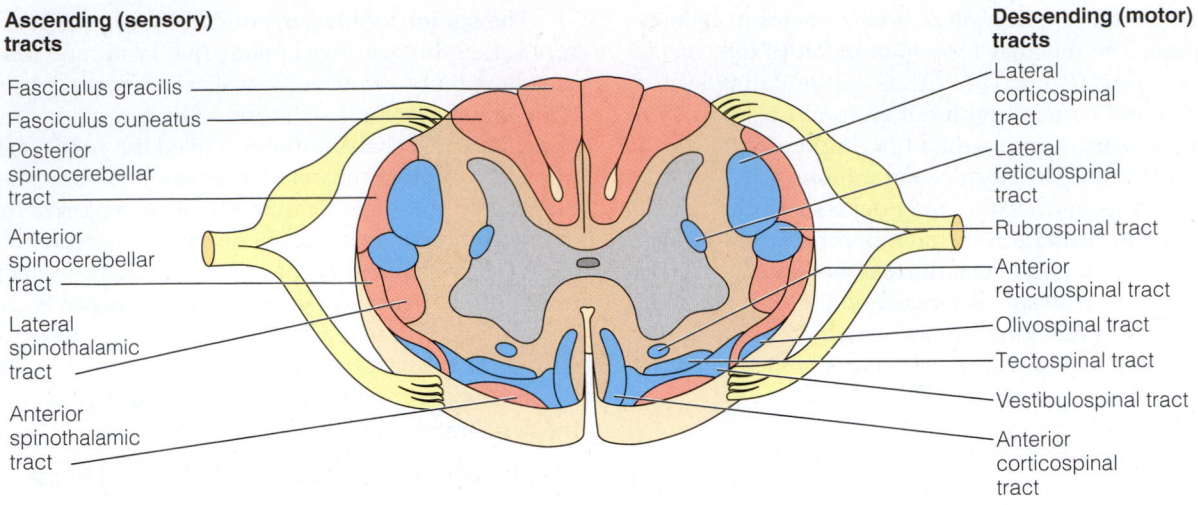

Figure 41.7 ■ Ascending and descending tracts of the spinal cord.

position, and vibration. The *pyramidal tracts* are descending tracts consisting of fibers that originate in the motor cortex of the brain and travel to the brainstem and then down the spinal cord. They mediate voluntary purposeful movements and stimulate certain muscular actions while inhibiting others. They carry fibers that inhibit muscle tone. The *extrapyramidal tracts* include the pathways between the cerebral cortex, basal ganglia, brainstem, and spinal cord outside the pyramidal tract. They maintain muscle tone and gross body movements.

Upper and Lower Motor Neurons

Upper motor neurons carry impulses from the cerebral cortex to the anterior gray column of the spinal cord. Damage to upper motor neurons results in increased muscle tone, decreased muscle strength, decreased coordination, and hyperactive reflexes. *Lower motor neurons* begin in the anterior gray column of the spinal cord and end in the muscle. Damage to lower motor neurons results in decreased muscle tone, muscle atrophy, fasciculations, and loss of reflexes.

The Peripheral Nervous System

The *peripheral nervous system* links the CNS with the rest of the body. It is responsible for receiving and transmitting information from and about the external environment. The PNS consists of nerves, ganglia (groups of nerve cells), and sensory receptors located outside—or peripheral to—the brain and spinal cord. The PNS is divided into a sensory (afferent) division and a motor (efferent) division. Most nerves of the PNS contain fibers for both divisions and all are classified regionally as either spinal nerves or cranial nerves.

Spinal Nerves

The 31 pairs of *spinal nerves* (refer to Figure 41.6) are named by their location: Cervical, eight pairs; thoracic, 12 pairs; lumbar, five pairs; sacral, five pairs; and coccygeal, one pair. Spinal nerves exit the vertebral column through intervertebral foramina to travel to the body regions they serve. The spinal cord does not reach the end of the vertebral column; as a result, the lumbar and sacral nerve roots travel inferiorly through the vertebral canal for some distance before exiting the vertebral column through their associated intervertebral foramina. This collection of descending nerve roots is called the *cauda equina*.

Each spinal nerve contains both sensory and motor fibers. The sensory fibers are located in the dorsal root, and their cell bodies are located within the dorsal root ganglion. The motor fibers are located in the ventral root, and their cell bodies are located within the spinal cord. The dorsal and ventral roots merge outside the vertebral canal just past the dorsal root ganglion, forming a spinal nerve. Each spinal nerve further divides into branches called *rami*. An area of skin innervated by cutaneous branches of a single spinal nerve is called a *dermatome*. The dorsal roots of the spinal nerves carry sensations from these specific dermatomes. Dermatomes provide anatomic landmarks that are useful for locating neurologic lesions (**Figure 41.8** ■).

Cranial Nerves

Twelve pairs of *cranial nerves (CNs)* originate in the forebrain and brainstem (**Figure 41.9** ■). The vagus nerve extends into the ventral body cavity, but the other 11 pairs innervate only head and neck regions. Although most are mixed nerves, three pairs (olfactory, optic, and acoustic) are solely sensory. The cranial nerves and their related functions are listed in **Table 41.4**.

Reflexes

A *reflex* is a rapid, involuntary, predictable motor response to a stimulus. Reflexes are categorized as either somatic or autonomic. *Somatic reflexes* result in skeletal muscle contraction. *Autonomic reflexes* activate cardiac muscle, smooth muscle, and glands. A reflex occurs over a pathway called a *reflex arc*.

The essential components of a reflex arc are a receptor, a sensory neuron to carry afferent impulses to the CNS, an integration center in the spinal cord or brain, a motor

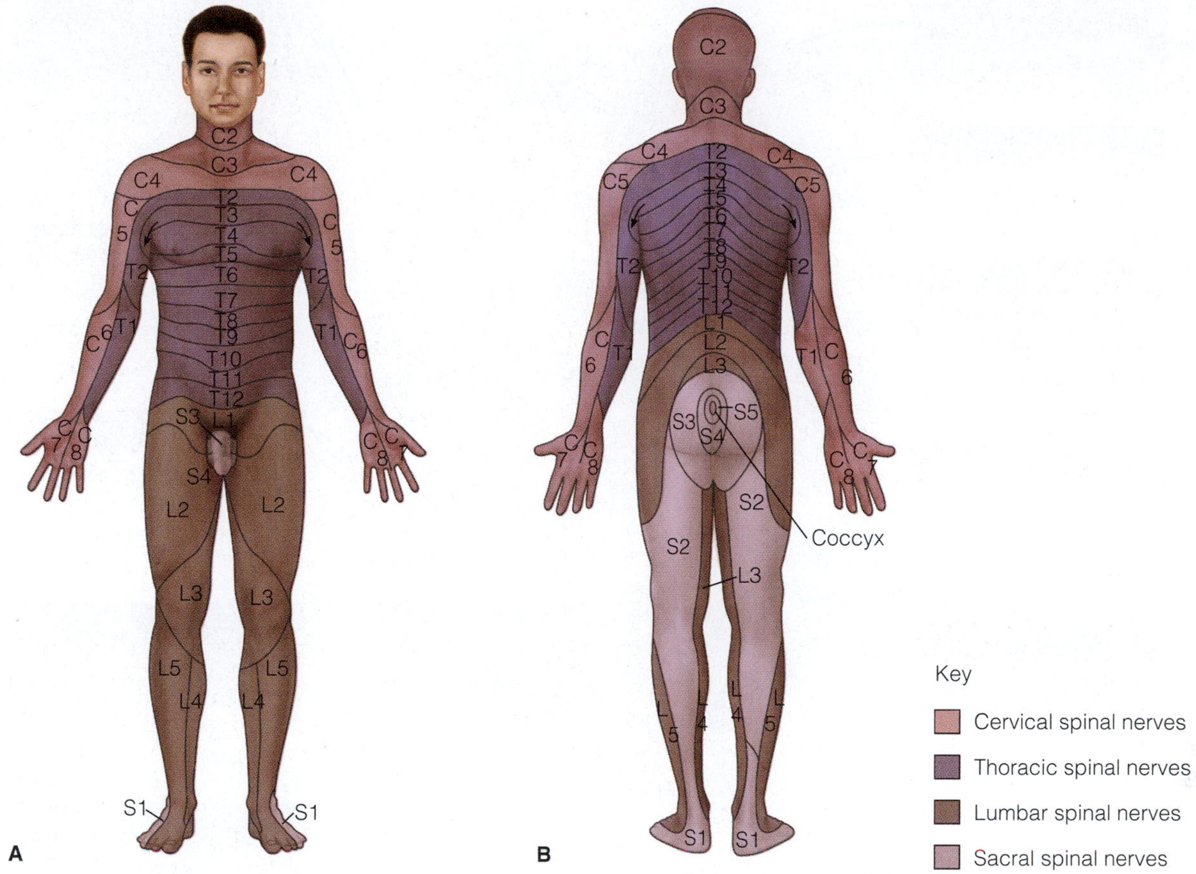
A
B
Coccyx
Key
Cervical spinal nerves
Thoracic spinal nerves
Lumbar spinal nerves
Sacral spinal nerves

Figure 41.8 ■ **A**, Anterior, and **B**, posterior dermatomes of the body.

neuron to carry efferent impulses, and an effector (the tissue that responds by contracting or secreting) (**Figure 41.10** ■).

Somatic reflexes mediated by the spinal cord are called *spinal reflexes*. Many spinal reflexes occur without impulses traveling to and from the brain, with the cord serving as the integration center. *Deep tendon reflexes (DTRs)* occur in response to muscle contraction and cause muscle relaxation and lengthening. DTRs depend on intact sensory and motor nerve roots, functional synapses in the spinal cord, a functional neuromuscular junction, and a competent muscle. Thus, an abnormal DTR could indicate a variety of health problems, including a lesion of a spinal nerve. *Flexor*, or *withdrawal*, *reflexes* are caused by actual or perceived painful stimuli and result in withdrawal of the part of the body that is threatened. Superficial responses result from gentle stimulation of the skin. These responses depend on functional upper motor pathways and an intact reflex arc.

The Autonomic Nervous System

The *autonomic nervous system (ANS)* is a division of the PNS that regulates the internal environment of the body. It is also called the *general visceral motor system* because it consists of motor neurons that innervate the body's viscera. Whereas skeletal muscle activity and reflexes are regulated by a division of the PNS called the *somatic nervous system*, the ANS regulates the activity of cardiac muscle, smooth muscle, and glands. The ANS is primarily controlled by the reticular formation in the brainstem. Stimulation of centers in the medulla initiates reflexes that regulate cardiac rate, blood vessel diameter, and gastrointestinal function.

The ANS has sympathetic and parasympathetic divisions. Although fibers from both divisions affect the same structures, the actions of the two divisions are opposite in effect, and they serve to counterbalance each other. The major neurotransmitters for impulse transmission in the ANS are norepinephrine and acetylcholine.

Sympathetic Division

Norepinephrine is the primary neurotransmitter of the sympathetic division. The *sympathetic division* of the ANS prepares the body to handle situations that are perceived as harmful or stressful and to participate in strenuous activity. Cell bodies for this division arise in the lateral horns of the spinal cord in the area from T_1 through L_2. The fibers separate after leaving the cord and form a chain of ganglia that extends from the neck to the pelvis. Long fibers then extend to the organs that are supplied by the sympathetic division. Stimulation of the sympathetic division can exert the following effects on target organs or tissues:

- Dilated pupils
- Inhibited secretions
- **Diaphoresis** (copious production of sweat)
- Increased rate and force of heartbeat

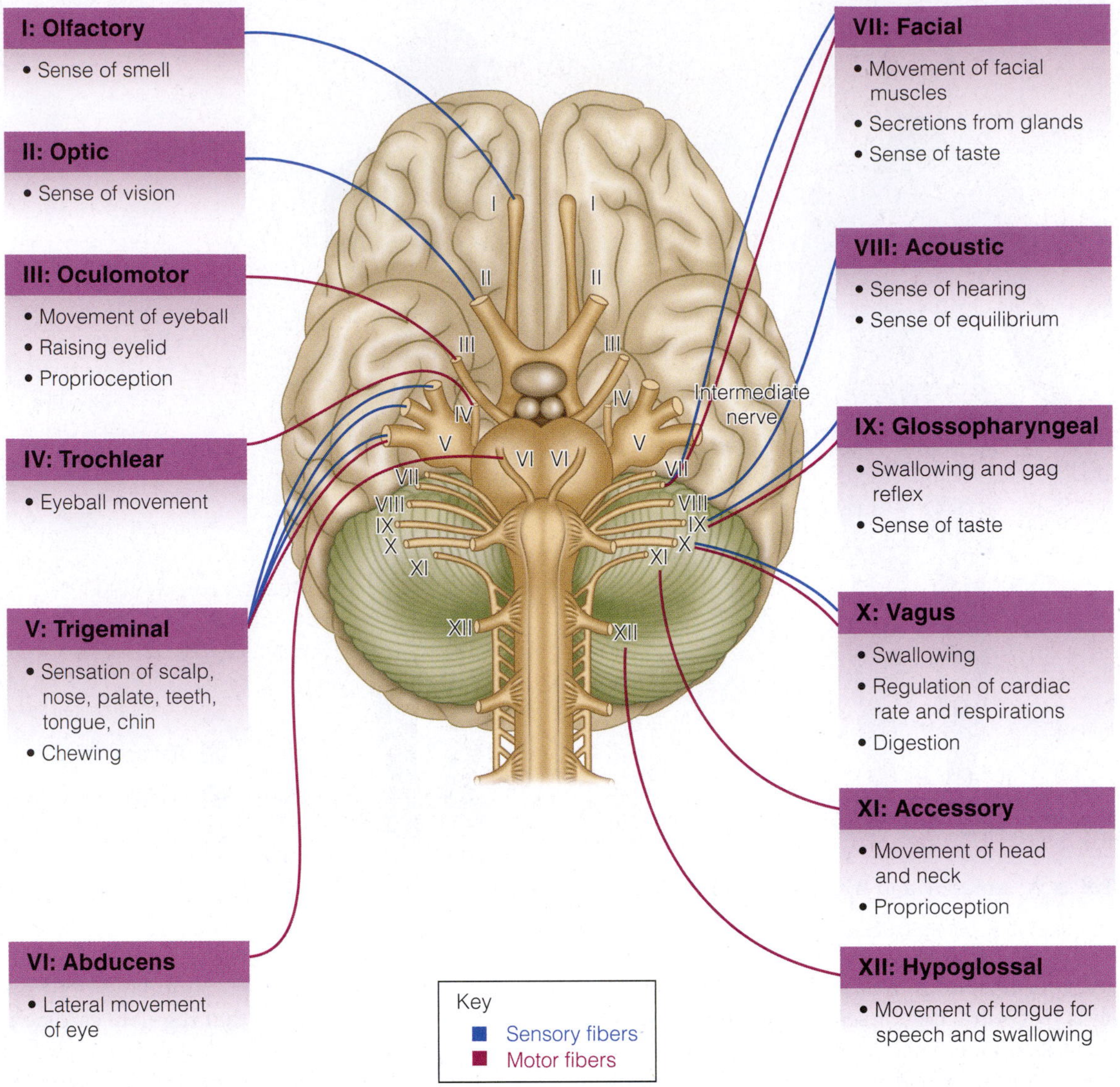
I: Olfactory
• Sense of smell
II: Optic
• Sense of vision
III: Oculomotor
• Movement of eyeball
• Raising eyelid
• Proprioception
IV: Trochlear
• Eyeball movement
V: Trigeminal
• Sensation of scalp, nose, palate, teeth, tongue, chin
• Chewing
VI: Abducens
• Lateral movement of eye
VII: Facial
• Movement of facial muscles
• Secretions from glands
• Sense of taste
VIII: Acoustic
• Sense of hearing
• Sense of equilibrium
IX: Glossopharyngeal
• Swallowing and gag reflex
• Sense of taste
X: Vagus
• Swallowing
• Regulation of cardiac rate and respirations
• Digestion
XI: Accessory
• Movement of head and neck
• Proprioception
XII: Hypoglossal
• Movement of tongue for speech and swallowing
Intermediate nerve
Key
Sensory fibers
Motor fibers

Figure 41.9 ■ Cranial nerves.

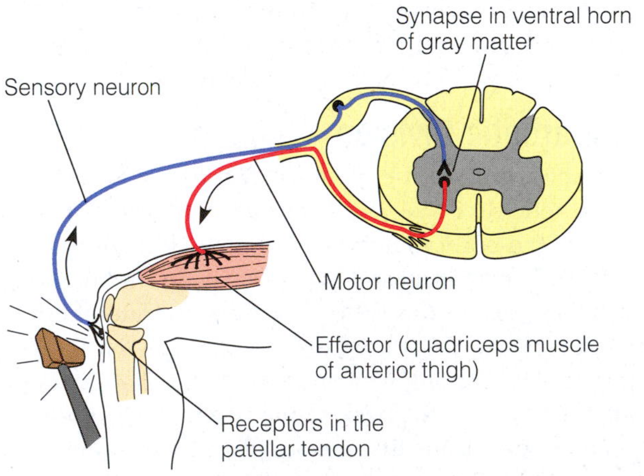
Synapse in ventral horn of gray matter
Sensory neuron
Motor neuron
Effector (quadriceps muscle of anterior thigh)
Receptors in the patellar tendon

Figure 41.10 ■ A typical reflex arc of a spinal nerve. In the two-neuron reflex arc, the stimulus is transferred from the sensory neuron directly to the motor neuron at the point of synapse in the spinal cord.

- Vasodilation of the coronary arteries
- Dilation of the bronchioles
- Decreased digestion
- Increased release of glucose by the liver
- Decreased urine output
- Vasoconstriction of arteries
- Vasoconstriction of abdominal and skin blood vessels
- Increased blood clotting
- Increased metabolic rate
- Increased mental alertness.

Parasympathetic Division

Acetylcholine is the primary neurotransmitter of the parasympathetic division. The *parasympathetic division* of the ANS operates during nonstressful situations. Cell bodies for this division are located in the brainstem (for the cranial nerves)

Table 41.4 Cranial Nerves

Name	Function
I Olfactory	■ Sense of smell
II Optic	■ Vision
III Oculomotor	■ Eyeball movement ■ Raising of upper eyelid ■ Constriction of pupil ■ Proprioception
IV Trochlear	■ Eyeball movement
V Trigeminal	■ Sensation of the upper scalp, upper eyelid, nose, nasal cavity, cornea, and lacrimal gland ■ Sensation of the palate, upper teeth, cheek, top lip, lower eyelid, and scalp ■ Sensation of the tongue, lower teeth, chin, and temporal scalp ■ Chewing
VI Abducens	■ Lateral movement of the eyeball
VII Facial	■ Movement of facial muscles ■ Secretions of lacrimal, nasal, submandibular, and sublingual glands ■ Sensation of taste
VIII Acoustic	■ Sense of equilibrium ■ Sense of hearing
IX Glossopharyngeal	■ Swallowing ■ Gag reflex ■ Secretions of parotid salivary gland ■ Sense of taste ■ Touch, pressure, and pain from pharynx and posterior tongue ■ Pressure from carotid arteries ■ Receptors to regulate blood pressure
X Vagus	■ Swallowing ■ Regulation of cardiac rate ■ Regulation of respirations ■ Digestion ■ Sensation from thoracic and abdominal organs ■ Proprioception ■ Sense of taste
XI Accessory	■ Movement of head and neck ■ Proprioception
XII Hypoglossal	■ Movement of tongue for speech and swallowing

and in the lateral gray matter of S_2 through S_4. Other than the fibers supplying cranial nerves III, VII, IX, and X, the fibers are carried by the vagus nerve to body tissues, thoracic organs, and visceral organs. Stimulation of the parasympathetic division of the ANS produces the following effects:

- Constriction of pupils
- Stimulation of glandular secretions
- Decreased heart rate
- Vasoconstriction of coronary arteries
- Constriction of the bronchioles
- Increased peristalsis and secretion of gastrointestinal fluid.

41.2 Assessing Neurologic Function

Structures and functions of the neurologic system are assessed by findings from a health assessment interview to collect subjective data, a physical assessment to collect objective data, and diagnostic tests.

Health Assessment Interview

A health assessment to determine problems with neurologic structure and/or function may be conducted during a health screening, may focus on a chief complaint (such as headaches), or may be part of a total health assessment. Health problems affecting the neurologic system may manifest as problems with musculoskeletal function and an assessment of both systems may be necessary. If the patient's level of consciousness is altered, the nurse may need to rely on family members for information (Bickley, 2016).

If the patient has problems with neurologic structure or function, analyze its onset, characteristics, course, severity, precipitating and relieving factors, and any associated symptoms, noting the time and circumstances. For example, ask the patient:

- "Describe the location and intensity of the pain you have experienced in your left leg. Is it made worse by coughing, sneezing, or walking?"
- "When did you first notice that you were having numbness in your fingers?"
- "What kind of difficulty do you have when you try to walk?"

Questions about present health status include information about numbness, tingling sensations, tremors, problems with coordination or balance, or loss of movement in any part of the body. Ask the patient about difficulty with speaking, seeing, hearing, tasting, or detecting odors. In addition, elicit information about memory, feeling state (such as anxiety or depression), recent changes in sleep patterns, ability to perform self-care and activities of daily living, sexual activity, and weight. If the patient is taking prescribed medications, over-the-counter medications, or herbal supplements, ask about the type and purpose, as well as the frequency and duration of use.

Ask about any past history of seizures, fainting, dizziness, headaches, and any trauma, tumors, or surgery of the brain, spinal cord, or nerves. Discuss illnesses that may cause neurologic manifestations, including cardiac disease, stroke, pernicious anemia, sinus infections, liver disease, and/or renal failure. Also ask the patient about family history of neurologic health problems, diabetes mellitus, hypertension, seizures, or mental health problems.

Question the patient about occupational hazards, such as exposure to toxic chemicals or materials, use of protective headgear, and the amount of time spent performing repetitive

Genetic Considerations

When conducting a health assessment interview and a physical assessment, it is important to consider genetic influences on the health of the adult. Several neurologic diseases that directly affect the nervous system have a genetic component, some are due to mutation of a single gene, and others have a more complex method of inheritance (Genetic and Rare Diseases Information Center, 2017). During the health assessment interview, ask about family members with health problems affecting neurologic structure or function. In addition, ask about a family history of problems with muscular coordination, Parkinson disease, narcolepsy, tremor, seizures, Alzheimer disease, multiple sclerosis, or amyotrophic lateral sclerosis. During the physical assessment, assess for any manifestations that might indicate a genetic disorder. If data are found to indicate genetic risk factors or alterations, ask about genetic testing and refer for appropriate genetic counseling and evaluation. Chapter 8 provides further information about genetics in medical-surgical nursing.

Examples of neurologic disorders with a genetic component include:

- ***Parkinson disease (PD)*** is a neurodegenerative disease manifested by tremor, muscular stiffness, and difficulty with balance and walking. One risk factor for PD is a positive family history of the disease.
- ***Multiple sclerosis (MS)*** is not directly inherited, but genetic factors may influence a predisposition to MS within families as well as the severity and course of the disease.
- ***Narcolepsy***, a sleep disorder, has a familial connection.
- ***Huntington disease (HD)*** is an inherited degenerative disorder that results in degeneration of neurons in certain areas of the brain. A child of a parent with HD has a 50–50 chance of inheriting the gene for the disease.
- ***Friedreich ataxia*** is a rare inherited disease that causes a progressive loss of voluntary muscle coordination and enlargement of the heart.
- ***Essential tremor***, as a primary disorder, affects as many as 3 to 4 million people. In more than half of cases, essential tremor is inherited as an autosomal dominant trait, meaning that children of an individual with the disease have a 50% chance of also developing the disorder.
- ***Epilepsy*** is one of the most common neurologic diseases, characterized by abnormal cell firing in the brain that causes recurring seizures. A genetic predisposition is found in many cases.
- ***Charcot-Marie-Tooth syndrome*** is the most common inherited peripheral neuropathy in the world, characterized by a slowly progressive degeneration of the muscles of the foot, lower leg, hand, and forearm.
- ***Alzheimer disease (AD)*** is a leading cause of death in adults, increasing in incidence with age and more common in women. AD tends to run in families, with mutations in four genes believed to be responsible for the disease.
- ***Amyotrophic lateral sclerosis (ALS)*** is a neurologic disease that causes progressive degeneration of motor neurons in the brain and spinal cord, resulting in paralysis and death. Chromosome abnormalities have been linked to familial ALS.
- ***Tay-Sachs disease*** is most often considered a disease of children, but there is a chronic adult form that causes neuron dysfunction and psychosis.

motions (e.g., data entry and assembly). Ask questions about self-care to assess the patient's diet and use of tobacco, drugs, or alcohol, and ask whether the patient wears a helmet when riding a bike or motorcycle or participating in contact sports or if seat belts are used when driving a motor vehicle.

Physical Assessment

Physical assessment begins when the nurse first meets the patient and makes an overall evaluation of the patient's mental and physical status (Bickley, 2016). The mental status examination is conducted with both the nurse and the patient seated. The rest of the neurologic examination may be performed with the patient either sitting or standing. A thorough neurologic examination is discussed here, but in most instances, the nurse will conduct a focused assessment specific to the patient's health status.

The neurologic system is assessed through inspection, palpation, and percussion (with a reflex hammer). When conducting the mental status and cognitive portions of the examination, be aware that fatigue or illness may alter findings. Provide rest periods for the patient as needed. When interpreting findings, consider the patient's age, educational background, and cultural orientation.

The assessment should take place in a private, comfortable setting. Ask the patient to remove outer clothing, shoes, and stockings. Provide a gown for the patient to wear. It is important to explain that the neurologic examination is lengthy and may consist of questions and requests that seem strange to the patient. Explain the rationale for each part of the examination.

A brief version of this physical assessment, often referred to as a *neuro check*, may be performed in a shorter time period when a patient requires frequent ongoing assessments of neurologic status (**Box 41.1**).

Another simple assessment commonly used by first responders is the **AVPU** scale, which stands for:

Alert: Is the patient fully alert (not necessarily oriented)?

Verbal: Does the patient make some kind of response when verbally addressed?

Pain: Does the patient respond to painful stimuli?

Unresponsive: Is the patient nonresponsive to verbal or painful stimuli?

BOX 41.1
Abbreviated Neurologic Assessment (Neuro Check)

1. Assess level of consciousness (response to auditory and/or tactile stimulus).
2. Obtain vital signs (BP, P, R).
3. Check pupillary response to light.
4. Assess strength of hand grip and movement of extremities bilaterally.
5. Determine ability to sense touch/pain in extremities.

Neurologic Assessments

Technique/Normal Findings	Abnormal Findings
MENTAL STATUS ASSESSMENT	
Assess appearance, including dress, hygiene, grooming, gait, and posture. *The patient should be appropriately dressed and clean, with normal gait and posture.* Assess behavior, including actions and affect, content and quality of speech, and level of consciousness (LOC). Use the Glasgow Coma Scale (**Table 41.5**) to document findings. *A score of 15 on the Glasgow Coma Scale indicates the patient is alert and oriented.*	■ Unilateral neglect (inattention to one side of body) may occur with some strokes. Poor hygiene and grooming may be seen in patients with dementing disorders. ■ Abnormal gait and posture may be seen in transient ischemic attacks (TIAs), strokes, and Parkinson disease. ■ Emotional swings or changes in personality may be observed in patients who have had a stroke. ■ The face appears masklike (very little expressive movement of facial muscles) in patients with Parkinson disease. ■ Apathy is seen in dementing disorders. ■ **Aphasia** (defective or absent language function) may occur in TIAs and strokes. Aphasias are seen with damage to the left cerebral cortex. Aphasias are more often seen with strokes of the left hemisphere than the right hemisphere. ■ **Dysphonia** (change in the tone of the voice) is common in strokes. Dysphonia is seen with paralysis of the vocal cords (cranial nerve X). ■ **Dysarthria** (difficulty speaking) is seen with lesions of upper and lower motor neurons, the cerebellum, and the extrapyramidal tract. ■ Damage to the brainstem and/or cerebral cortex may alter LOC. ■ Drowsiness and decreased LOC may be associated with brain trauma, infection, TIA, stroke, and brain tumor. ■ Level of consciousness, ranging from confusion to coma, is usually altered with a stroke.

Table 41.5 Glasgow Coma Scale

Assessment	Response	Score
Eyes Open	Spontaneously	4
Record *C* if eyes are closed by swelling.	To sound	3
	To pressure	2
	No response	1
	Not testable	NT
Verbal Response	Oriented	5
Record *T* if an endotracheal or tracheostomy tube is in place.	Confused	4
	Single words	3
	Sounds (moans/groans)	2
	No response	1
	Not testable	NT
Best Motor Response	Obeys commands	6
Record best upper arm response.	Localizes pain	5
	Flexion-withdrawal	4
	Abnormal flexion	3
	Abnormal extension	2
	No response	1
	Not testable	NT
Total Score:		

Note: *A higher score indicates a higher level of functioning.

Source: Adapted from Glasgow Coma Scale, 2014.

(*continued*)

Neurologic Assessments (*continued*)

Technique/Normal Findings	Abnormal Findings
Assess cognitive function. Note orientation to time, place, and person. Note attention span and recent and remote memory. Ask the patient to: 1. Repeat five to seven numbers. 2. Recall three items after 5 min. 3. Recall his or her address, breakfast, or birthday. Assess thought processes (both content and perceptions) by noting responses to questions. Note ability to understand what is said and to express thoughts. Note ability to make logical and safe judgments. *The patient should be oriented to time, place, and person; demonstrate attention and ability to remember recent and past events; respond appropriately to questions; and be able to make judgments.*	■ Disorientation to time and place may occur in patients with stroke of the right cerebral hemisphere. ■ Memory deficits are often seen in patients with a stroke. ■ Perceptual deficits may be seen in stroke. These same deficits may occur following brain trauma and in dementing disorders. ■ Impaired cognition is often noted with stroke, cerebral trauma, and brain tumor.
CRANIAL NERVE ASSESSMENTS	
Test CN I (olfactory). Note patient's ability to smell scents (e.g., soap, coffee) with each nostril. This test is usually done only if a problem with the ability to smell is reported. *Sense of smell should be equal in both nostrils.*	■ **Anosmia** (an inability to smell) may be seen with lesions of the frontal lobe and may also occur with impaired blood flow to the middle cerebral artery.
Test CN II (optic). Assess vision in each eye with Snellen chart (see Chapter 45 for guidelines). *Based on previous ability to see and use of visual aids, patient should be able to see with both eyes.*	■ Blindness in one eye may be seen with stroke or with TIA. Impaired vision or blindness in one side of both eyes (homonymous hemianopia) is associated with stroke. ■ Impaired vision may be seen with stroke and brain tumor. ■ Blindness or double vision may be noted with stroke and TIA. ■ Diplopia (double vision) may occur in multiple sclerosis.
Test CNs III, IV, and VI (oculomotor, trochlear, and abducens). Assess extraocular movements by asking the patient to follow your finger as you write an *H* in the air (see Chapter 45). Assess **PERRL**, **P**upils **E**qually **R**ound **R**eactive to **L**ight, by covering one eye at a time and shining a bright light directly into the uncovered eye (use a penlight or an ophthalmoscope). See Chapter 45 for detailed assessment guidelines. *Extraocular movements should be present bilaterally, and pupils should be equally round and reactive to light.*	■ **Nystagmus** (involuntary eye movement) may be seen with stroke. ■ Constricted pupils are associated with impaired blood flow from a stroke or medication/drug use.
Assess for ptosis (drooping eyelids). *Eyelids should not droop.* Test CN V (trigeminal). Assess ability to feel light, dull, and sharp sensations on the face. With the patient's eyes closed, check whether sensation is the same on both sides of the face. Stroke the cheek with a wisp of cotton for light touch, with a closed safety pin for dull touch, and with a tongue depressor for sharp touch. If the sharp point of a safety pin is used to assess sharp touch, be sure to avoid scratching the surface of the skin, and discard the pin after it is used. Assess the corneal reflex by touching the corneal surface with a wisp of cotton. The reflex may be absent or decreased in patients who wear contact lenses. *Ability to feel light, dull, and sharp sensations should be intact. Normally the patient blinks.*	■ Ptosis (also called *Horner syndrome*) occurs with strokes, myasthenia gravis, and palsy of CN III. ■ Changes in facial sensations are noted with impaired blood flow to the carotid artery. ■ Decreased sensations to the face and cornea on the same side of the body, as well as numbness of the lip and mouth, occur with stroke. ■ Loss of facial sensation or contraction of the masseter and temporal muscles is seen with lesions of CN V. ■ Severe facial pain is seen with trigeminal neuralgia (tic douloureux). ■ The corneal reflex may be impaired with lesions of CN V or VII.

Technique/Normal Findings	Abnormal Findings
Test CN VII (facial). Assess ability to taste sweet, sour, and salt on the anterior two-thirds of the tongue by asking the patient to stick out the tongue and applying a salty, sweet, or sour substance. Assess ability to frown, show teeth, blow out cheeks, raise eyebrows, smile, and close eyes tightly. *Patient should be able to taste sweet, sour, and salt substances. Should be able to frown, show teeth, blow out cheeks, raise eyebrows, smile, and close eyes tightly. Muscle movement should be equal bilaterally.*	■ Loss of ability to taste may occur with brain tumors or with nerve impairment. ■ Asymmetry or decreased movement of facial muscles is noted with lesions of the upper and lower motor neurons. ■ Paralysis of the lower motor neurons from injury to CN VII results in the inability to close eyes, a flat nasolabial fold, paralysis of lower face, and inability to wrinkle forehead. ■ Paralysis of the upper motor neurons from a stroke results in weakness of eyelids and paralysis of lower face. ■ Pain, paralysis, and sagging of facial muscles are seen on the affected side in Bell's palsy.
Test CN VIII (acoustic). Assess ability to hear the ticking of a watch and whispered and spoken words (see Chapter 45). *Patient should be able to hear with both ears.*	■ Decreased hearing or deafness may occur with strokes and/or tumors of CN VIII.
Test CN IX and X (glossopharyngeal and vagus). If gag reflex is intact, observe patient swallowing a small drink of water. Observe for a symmetrical rise of the soft palate and uvula as the patient says "ah." Assess gag reflex by touching back of patient's throat with tongue depressor. *Patient should have intact gag reflex.* Assess ability to taste salty, sweet, and sour substances on the posterior third of the tongue (see previous description). *Patient should be able to swallow without difficulty, have symmetrical rise of the soft palate, and taste appropriately.*	■ **Dysphagia** (difficulty swallowing) is common with impaired blood flow to the brain. ■ Unilateral loss of the gag reflex occurs with lesions of CN IX and X.
Test CN XI (spinal accessory). Assess the patient's ability to shrug the shoulders and turn head against resistance: Ask the patient to turn the head to one side against the resistance of your hand; ask the patient to shrug the shoulders while you exert downward pressure. Observe symmetry, strength, and size of muscles. *Patient should be able to shrug shoulders and turn head against resistance.*	■ Muscle weakness is noted with lower motor neuron disease. Contralateral hemiparesis is seen with stroke.
Test CN XII (hypoglossal). Assess the patient's ability to stick out the tongue and move the tongue from side to side against resistance of a tongue depressor. *Patient should be able to stick out tongue and move it from side to side against resistance.*	■ Atrophy and **fasciculations** (twitches) of the tongue are seen in lower motor neuron disease. The tongue may deviate toward involved side of body.
SENSORY FUNCTION ASSESSMENTS	
Assess ability to feel touch. Touch both sides of various parts of the body (the chest, abdomen, arms, and legs) with one or more of the following: ■ Cotton wisp ■ Sharp object ■ Dull object Vibrating tuning fork placed on bony prominences. *Patient can differentiate between soft and sharp and can feel vibrations appropriately.* Assess sense of position (**kinesthesia**). Move the patient's finger or big toe up or down. Ask the patient to describe the movement. *Patient can accurately describe position of finger or toe when moved up or down.*	■ Decreased sensation of pain occurs with injury to the spinothalamic tract. ■ Decreased vibratory sensations are seen with injuries to the posterior column tract. ■ Transient numbness of face, arm, or hand is seen with TIA. ■ Sensory loss on one side of the body is seen with lesions of higher pathways to the spinal cord. ■ Bilateral sensory loss is seen in polyneuropathy (a disease in which multiple peripheral nerves are affected, such as Guillain-Barré syndrome or diabetes mellitus). Sensations are impaired with stroke, brain tumor, and spinal cord trauma or compression. ■ Lesions of the posterior column of the spinal cord may affect sense of position.

(*continued*)

Neurologic Assessments (*continued*)

Technique/Normal Findings	Abnormal Findings
Assess ability to discriminate fine touch. Ask the patient to identify the following: 1. Object in hand, such as a coin or key (tests stereognosis) 2. Number written on hand (tests graphesthesia) (**Figure 41.11** ■) 3. Two points of simultaneous pinpricks on the hand (tests two-point discrimination) (**Figure 41.12** ■) 4. Where he or she is being touched (tests localization) 5. How many sensations are felt when touched simultaneously on both sides of the body (tests extinction). *Patient can identify and discriminate fine touch.*	■ Inability to discriminate fine touch (stereognosis, graphesthesia, two points, point localization, and extinction) may occur with injury to the posterior columns or sensory cortex.

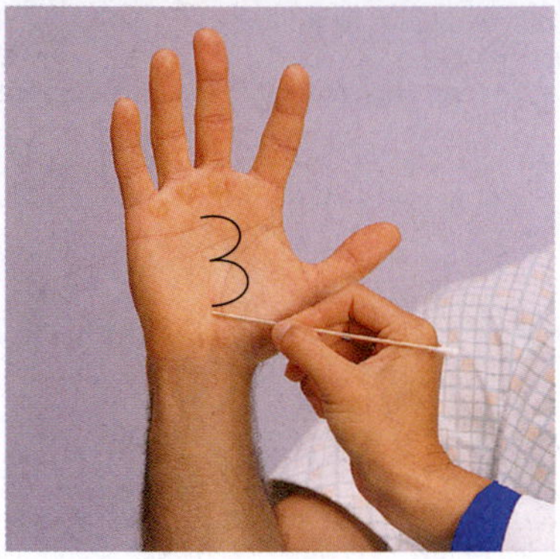

Figure 41.11 ■ Testing graphesthesia.

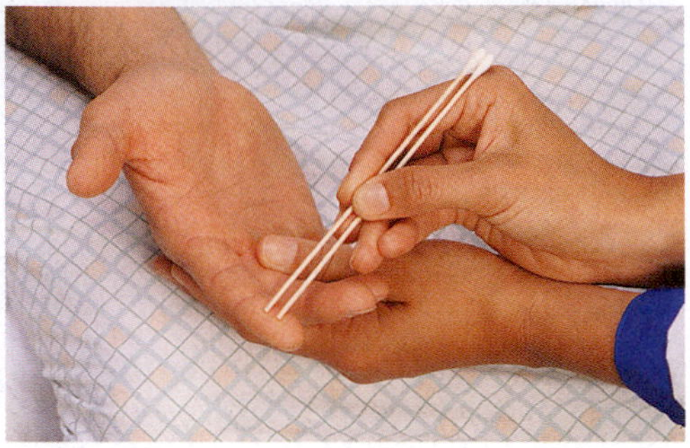

Figure 41.12 ■ Testing two-point discrimination.

Technique/Normal Findings	Abnormal Findings
MOTOR FUNCTION ASSESSMENTS	
Assess bilateral symmetry and size of muscles. Assess for **tremors** (rhythmic movements) and fasciculations (irregular movements). Observe movements as patient is at rest (not making a purposeful movement) and with activity (making a purposeful movement, such as reaching for a glass of water). *Muscles are bilaterally symmetrical and of equal size. Tremors or fasciculations are not present.*	■ Atrophy of muscles is seen with disease of the lower motor neurons. ■ Tremors that occur with activity are seen in multiple sclerosis and diseases of the cerebellar system. ■ Tremors that occur at rest and disappear with movement are common in Parkinson's disease. ■ Fasciculations occur in disease or trauma to the lower motor neurons, as a side effect of medications, in fever, in sodium deficiency, and in uremia.
Assess muscle tone. *Muscle tone is appropriate.*	■ Muscle tone is decreased (**flaccidity**) in disease or trauma of the lower motor neurons and early stroke. ■ Muscle tone is increased (**spasticity**) in disease of the corticospinal motor tract. ■ Muscles are rigid in disease of the extrapyramidal motor tract. ■ Muscles move in small, regular jerky movements (cogwheel rigidity) in Parkinson disease.
Assess bilateral muscle strength and movement. Ask the patient to: 1. Squeeze your hands. 2. Push feet against the resistance of your hands. 3. Raise both legs off the bed. *See* Chapter 38 *for a scale to grade muscle strength. Muscle strength and movement are bilaterally equal and strong.*	■ Weakness of the arms, legs, or hands is often seen with TIA. ■ Hemiplegia (paralysis of one-half of the body vertically) is noted with stroke. ■ Flaccid paralysis is noted with stroke. ■ Paralysis or decreased movement is seen in multiple sclerosis and myasthenia gravis. ■ There is total loss of motor function below the level of injury in complete spinal cord transection and in injuries to the anterior portion of the spinal cord. ■ Spasticity of muscles may occur as a result of incomplete spinal cord injuries.
CEREBELLAR FUNCTION ASSESSMENTS	
Assess the gait. Ask the patient to walk normally, then in a heel-to-toe fashion, then on toes, and finally on heels. *Patient has appropriate gait and can walk heel-to-toe, on toes, and on heels.* Perform Romberg test: Ask the patient to stand with the feet together and eyes closed. (Stand close to patient to prevent falling.) *There should be minimal swaying for up to 20 seconds.*	■ **Ataxia** is a lack of coordination and a clumsiness of movements, with staggering, wide-based, and unbalanced gait. Ataxia is often seen with stroke and cerebellar tumor. Swaying and falling are seen in cerebellar ataxia. Inability to walk on toes, then heels, may indicate disease of the upper motor neurons. ■ Spastic hemiparesis is often associated with stroke or upper motor neuron disease. The patient walks with one leg stiffly dragging while the other leg circles out and forward. One arm is held flexed and close to the side. ■ Steppage gait is noted with disease of the lower motor neurons. The patient drags or lifts the foot high, then slaps the foot onto the floor. The patient cannot walk on the heels. ■ Sensory ataxia may be associated with polyneuropathy or damage to the posterior columns. The patient walks on the heels before bringing down the toes and the feet are held wide apart. Gait worsens with the eyes closed. ■ Parkinsonian gait is often seen in Parkinson disease. The patient stoops over while walking and shuffles the feet. The arms are held close to the side. ■ A positive Romberg test may be seen in cerebellar ataxia.

Technique/Normal Findings	Abnormal Findings
Assess coordination. Observe ability to pat knees, alternating front and back of hands and increasing speed. Observe ability to touch each finger of one hand to the thumb. Observe ability to touch the nose, then one of the fingers, then the nose again. Observe ability to run each heel down each shin, while in a supine position (**Figure 41.13** ■). *Patient demonstrates coordinated movements.*	■ Ataxic movements are apparent in cerebellar disease.

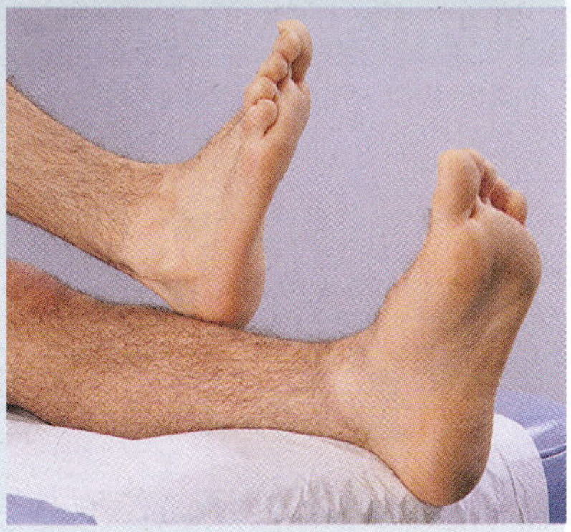

Figure 41.13 ■ Heel-to-shin test.

Reflex Assessments

A reflex hammer is used to strike the tendon of various reflex sites. To test deep tendon reflexes, ask the patient to lock the fingers of both hands together and then pull; this encourages relaxation and promotes reflexes of lower extremities. Superficial reflexes are assessed by lightly stroking the area with the end of a tongue depressor. Criteria often used to record reflexes are listed in the right-hand column.

0 = absent or no response
1 = hypoactive; weaker than normal (+)
2 = normal (++)
3 = stronger than normal (+++)
4 = hyperactive, sustained clonus (++++)
A score of 2 is considered normal.

Technique/Normal Findings	Abnormal Findings
Assess the patellar, biceps, brachioradialis, triceps, and Achilles deep tendon reflexes (Figure 41.14 ■). *Average responses are normal (neither hyperactive or no response).*	■ Hyperactive reflexes are present with lesions of upper motor neurons. ■ Decreased reflexes are present with lower motor neuron involvement.

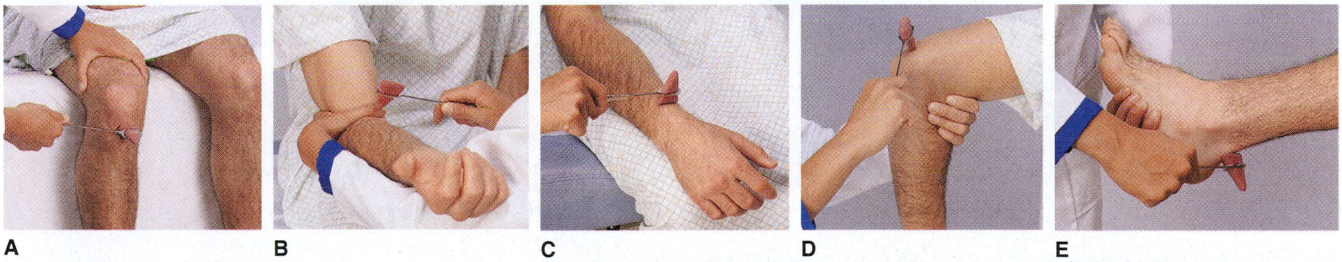
A
B
C
D
E

Figure 41.14 ■ Deep-tendon reflexes. **A**, Using reinforcement technique to test the patellar reflex. **B**, Biceps reflex. **C**, Brachioradialis reflex. **D**, Triceps reflex. **E**, Achilles reflex.

Technique/Normal Findings	Abnormal Findings
Assess for clonus by dorsiflexing the patient's foot. *No rhythmic oscillations are observed between dorsiflexion and plantar flexion.*	■ *Clonus*, a hyperactive, rhythmic dorsiflexion and plantar flexion, is noted with upper motor neuron disease.
Assess the superficial abdominal and cremasteric reflexes. **Abdominal reflex: Lightly stroke the abdomen with a tongue depressor from the side to the midline.** *Normally the side of the abdomen being stroked will contract toward the umbilicus* (**Figure 41.15** ■). Cremasteric reflex: Lightly stroke the inner thigh of the male patient with a tongue depressor. *Normally, the testicle on the side being stroked will rise.*	■ Superficial reflexes may be absent with disease of the lower and upper motor neurons.

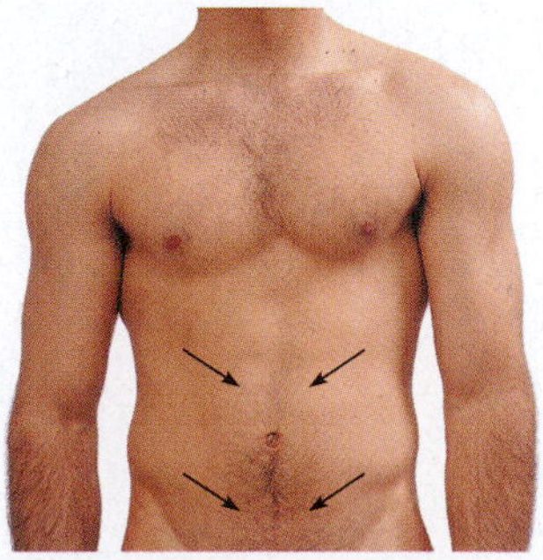

Figure 41.15 ■ Location of superficial abdominal reflexes.

(*continued*)

Reflex Assessments (*continued*)

Technique/Normal Findings	Abnormal Findings
Assess the Babinski (plantar response) reflex (Figure 41.16 ■). *Normally, the toes curl inward.*	■ Dorsiflexion of the big toe and fanning of the other toes is seen with upper motor neuron disease of the pyramidal tract.

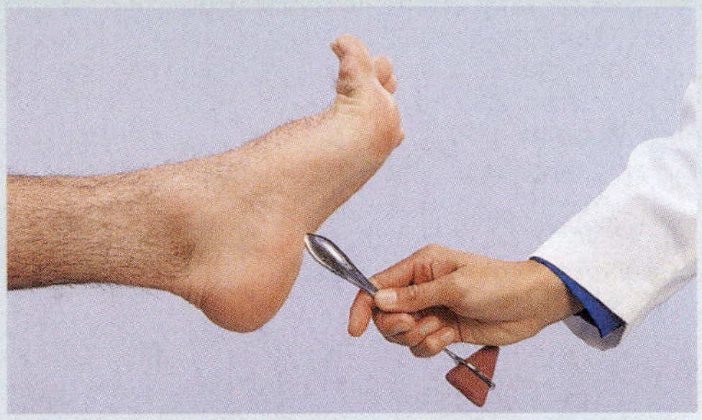

Figure 41.16 ■ Assessing the Babinski reflex.

Special Neurologic Assessments

Technique/Normal Findings	Abnormal Findings
Assess for Brudzinski sign. With the patient supine, flex the head to the chest (Figure 41.17 ■). *There should be no pain, resistance, or flexion of the hips or knees.*	■ Pain, resistance, and flexion of hips and knees occur with meningeal irritation. ■ Excessive pain and/or resistance occurs with meningeal irritation.
Assess for Kernig sign. With the patient supine, flex the knees and hips, then straighten the knee (Figure 41.18 ■). *There should be no pain or resistance.*	■ Resistance and pain may occur in a patient with multiple sclerosis.

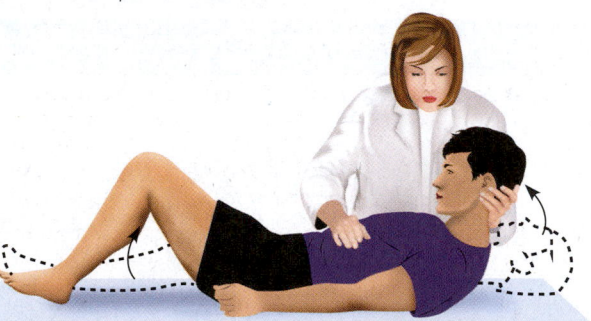

Figure 41.17 ■ Assessing the Brudzinski sign.

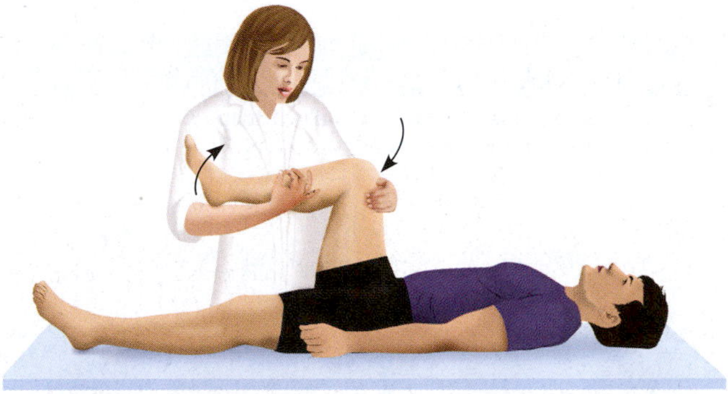

Figure 41.18 ■ Assessing the Kernig sign.

Technique/Normal Findings	Abnormal Findings
Assess for abnormal postures in patients who are unconscious (Figure 41.19 ■). *There should be no abnormal posturing.*	Observe for **decorticate posturing**, in which the upper arms are close to the sides; the elbows, wrists, and fingers are flexed; the legs are extended with internal rotation; and the feet are plantar flexed (**Figure 41.19A**). ■ Decorticate posturing occurs with lesions of the corticospinal tracts. Observe for **decerebrate posturing**, in which the neck is extended, with the jaw clenched; the arms are pronated, extended, and close to the sides; the legs are extended straight out; and the feet are plantar flexed (**Figure 41.19B**). ■ Decerebrate posturing occurs with lesions of the midbrain, pons, or diencephalon.

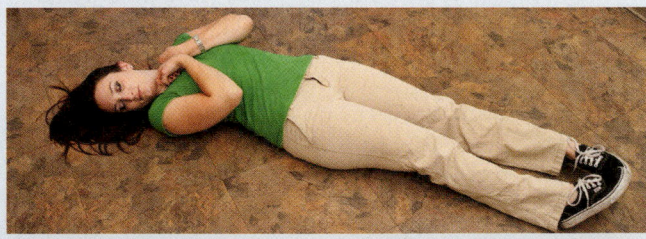

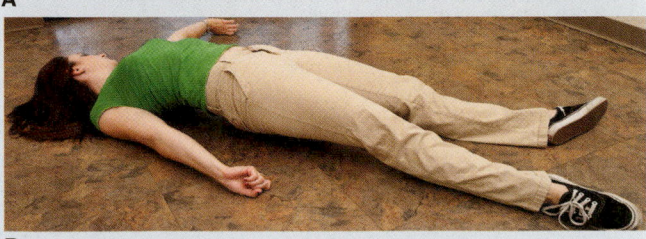

Figure 41.19 ■ **A**, Decorticate posturing. **B**, Decerebrate posturing.

Diagnostic Tests

The results of diagnostic tests of neurologic structure and function are used to support the diagnosis of a specific injury or disease, to provide information to identify or modify the appropriate medications or therapy used to treat the disease, and to help nurses monitor the patient's responses to treatment and nursing care interventions. Diagnostic tests to assess the structures and functions of the neurologic system are described in the table below. More information is included in the discussion of specific injuries or diseases in Chapters 42, 43, and 44.

Regardless of the type of diagnostic test, the nurse is responsible for explaining the procedure and any special preparation needed, assessing for medication use that may affect the outcome of the tests, ensuring the consent form is signed (if necessary), supporting the patient during the examination as necessary, documenting the procedures as appropriate, and monitoring the results of the tests. The nurse is also responsible for postprocedure care and patient teaching for self-care at home.

Diagnostic Tests of the Neurologic System

NAME OF TEST	PURPOSE AND DESCRIPTION	RELATED NURSING INTERVENTIONS
Carotid duplex study **Transcranial Doppler study**	A carotid duplex study evaluates the velocity of blood flow through the carotid arteries and identifies occlusive disease. Sound waves produced by the blood flow are used to produce an image. A transcranial Doppler study follows the same procedure, but is used to evaluate intracranial blood vessels.	No special preparation is needed.
Cerebral angiogram	A cerebral angiogram is the definitive diagnostic procedure for aneurysms, arteriovenous malformations, blood vessel patency and stenosis, thrombosis, vasospasm, aneurysm, and space-occupying lesions (such as tumors or hematomas). It may be performed either as part of a surgical procedure or with local anesthesia. In radiology, a contrast medium is injected and films are taken at various time intervals.	Tell the patient not to eat or drink fluids 8 hours prior to the procedure. Assess for history of allergy to iodine, seafood, or previous contrast dye; if present, notify physician. After the procedure, vital signs are monitored, and fluids are forced to clear the contrast medium. Bedrest is maintained for 12–24 h. Monitor for manifestations of a transient ischemic attack (weakness or numbness in an extremity, confusion, slurred speech) and delayed allergic reaction to the contrast dye (itching, rash, tachycardia, dyspnea, hypotension).
Computed tomography (CT) scan—brain, spine	A CT scan of the brain is used to identify intracerebral hemorrhage, tumors, cysts, aneurysms, edema, ischemia, atrophy, and tissue necrosis. It may also be used to evaluate a shift in intracranial contents and differentiate type of stroke. CT scans of the spine are primarily done to assess bony abnormalities. The tests involve computer-assisted x-rays of several levels of cross-sections of the body part being examined; they may be done with or without contrast.	If a contrast dye is used, tell the patient to not eat or drink liquids for 8 hours prior to the test, or if the test is in the afternoon to not eat or drink fluids after a liquid breakfast. Assess medications; if an iodinated contrast is used, oral hypoglycemic agents are contraindicated. Ask the patient to remove hairpins, clips, jewelry, and dentures if contrast dye is used. Explain to the patient that when a brain scan is done, the head is positioned in a cradle and a strap is applied snugly around the head during the test (the test lasts from 5 to 10 min). After a scan with contrast, monitor for and report signs of a delayed allergic reaction, such as rash, itching, headache, or vomiting.
Electroencephalogram (EEG) **Magnetoencephalogram (MEG)**	An EEG is used to measure the electrical activity of the brain to diagnose brain disease and brain death. Electrodes are applied to the scalp with skin clips and a graphic picture is obtained (similar to an ECG of the heart). An MEG detects magnetic fields generated by activity of neurons and can identify the area of the brain affected by a stroke, brain disorders or trauma, or seizures.	Assess medications and tell the patient not to take prescribed medications or liquids that may stimulate or depress brain waves as ordered (usually for 24–48 h) before the test. These include anticonvulsants, tranquilizers, depressants, and caffeine-containing foods and beverages (e.g., coffee, tea, colas, alcohol, and chocolate). Instruct the patient to wash his or her hair the night before the procedure, but to not use oil or hairspray on the hair. After the test, acetone may be used to remove the paste from the patient's head.
Electromyogram (EMG)	An EMG measures the electrical activity of skeletal muscles at rest and during contraction and so is useful in diagnosing neuromuscular diseases. Needle electrodes are inserted into skeletal muscle (as on the legs) and electrical activity can be heard, viewed on an oscilloscope, and recorded on graph paper. Normally, there is no electrical activity at rest.	Tell patient not to drink fluids containing caffeine or to smoke for 3 h before the test. Assess medications: If approved by healthcare provider, patient should not take medications such as muscle relaxants, anticholinergics, and cholinergics. If serum enzymes are ordered (such as SGOT, CPK, or LDH), the specimen should be drawn before an EMG or 5–10 days after the test.

(continued)

NAME OF TEST	PURPOSE AND DESCRIPTION	RELATED NURSING INTERVENTIONS
Evoked potentials	This test measures nerve conduction along pathways to evaluate the evoked potential of muscle contractions. It is used to diagnose and evaluate neuromuscular diseases and identify nerve damage. Transcutaneous or percutaneous electrodes are applied to the skin and provide recordings.	No special preparation is needed.
Lumbar puncture (LP)	An LP is used to measure CSF pressure and to obtain a sample of CSF to use in diagnosis of multiple sclerosis or increased intracranial pressure from meningitis, subarachnoid hemorrhage, brain tumor, brain abscess, encephalitis, and viral infections. A needle is inserted in L_3–L_4 or L_4–L_5 and fluid is aspirated.	Ask the patient to void. Assess and document vital signs. Collect sterile lumbar puncture tray, an antiseptic solution, a local anesthetic, sterile gloves, and tape. Label the test tubes 1, 2, and 3. Place the patient on his or her side in the fetal position with back bowed, head flexed on the chest, and the knees drawn up to the abdomen. Assist the healthcare provider with the procedure. Following the LP, assess and document vital signs at specified intervals. Monitor for changes in neurologic status (fever, hypertension, irritability, lower extremity numbness or tingling, nonreactive pupils). Administer ordered analgesic for headache. Instruct the patient to lie flat in bed in the prone or supine position for 4–8 h. Monitor the puncture site for leakage of cerebrospinal fluid or hematoma formation. Encourage increased intake of fluids (up to 3000 mL in 24 h).
Magnetic resonance imaging (MRI) **Functional MRI** **Magnetic resonance angiography (MRA)** **Magnetic resonance spectroscopy (MRS)**	An MRI is done to identify and monitor conditions of the brain and spinal cord, including stroke, tumors, trauma, seizures, and multiple sclerosis. It uses magnetic energy to provide images, and a gadolinium contrast media may be used to enhance visualization. An MRI is more sensitive than a CT scan to the subtle vascular changes seen in Alzheimer disease. A functional MRI is done to evaluate metabolic or blood flow responses of the brain to specific tasks, such as activity and rest. An MRA can provide information about the blood vessels of the brain and identify vascular lesions. It uses the signals from blood vessels to reconstruct only those vessels with blood flow. An MRS uses a scanner to confirm the presence of Alzheimer disease, determine the extent of head injury from trauma or stroke, and identify the causes of coma.	Assess for any metallic implants (such as clips on brain aneurysms, pacemaker, body piercings, tattoos, and shrapnel). If present, notify physician. Remove transdermal medication patches (both OTC and prescribed) unless otherwise ordered. Replace the patch following the procedure. Tell the patient to inform the staff about the patch when making the appointment and when completing the admission information. Ask if patient is pregnant; if so, the test is not performed. Ask about claustrophobia; if a problem exists, request patient to ask the referring physician for a relaxing medication prior to the MRI. If the patient is very claustrophobic, obese, or confused, an open MRI may be used.
Myelogram	A myelogram is used to identify lesions of the spinal cord, such as tumors or a herniated intervertebral disk. A lumbar puncture is done, a contrast medium is injected into the subarachnoid space, and x-rays are taken.	Instruct the patient to drink additional fluids the day before the test and then to stop all food and fluids for 4 h prior to the test. Assess medications; antipsychotics, antidepressants, and anticoagulants may be withheld for several days before the procedure, depending on physician orders. Tell the patient not to smoke the day before the test. Assess for history of allergy to iodine, seafood, or previous contrast dye; if present, notify physician. Ask the patient to void immediately before the test. After the procedure, position the patient in a supine position with the head slightly elevated for several hours. Encourage oral fluid intake. Monitor for and notify the physician of a fever, excessive nausea and vomiting, a severe headache, or a stiff neck. Take and record vital signs as specified. Monitor lumbar insertion site for CSF leakage or hematoma. Monitor neurologic status and ensure patient voids within 8 h. Encourage increased oral fluids. Administer prescribed analgesic for headache.
Positron emission tomography (PET) **Single-photon emission computed tomography (SPECT)**	When used to study the brain, a PET can assess normal brain function and cerebral blood flow and volume; it can differentiate different types of dementia; and it can identify stages of brain tumors. A substance containing a radionuclide is given by gas or by injection and cross sections of tissue are detected and displayed by computer. A SPECT is similar to a PET, but uses different substances. It can be used to diagnose stroke, brain tumor, and seizure disorders.	Tell the patient not to drink coffee or alcohol or smoke for 24 h before the test. Assess glucose levels pretest. Post-test, encourage oral fluids to facilitate excretion of the radioactive substance.
X-rays of skull and spine	Standard x-rays of the skull and spine are done to identify fractures, displacement of vertebrae, spinal curves, and tissue displacement (as by tumors).	No special preparation is needed.

41.3 Assessment of Special Populations

Key age-related neurologic system changes and their significance are outlined in **Table 41.6**.

For years, epilepsy was believed to be a disease that only affected children. However, 300,000 senior citizens have an epilepsy diagnosis (Epilepsy Foundation, 2018). Having a seizure disorder at this age increases the risk of falls and fractures and threatens independence. These data have important implications for nursing assessments and care.

- The most common cause of epilepsy in older adults is arteriosclerosis of the cerebrovascular system and stroke.
- The most common type of seizure in older adults is a complex partial seizure.
- Older adults tend to have longer postseizure manifestations than do younger adults.

Epilepsy that begins in older adults is often easier to control with antiepileptic drugs (AEDs) than that in younger people. However, some AEDs decrease the effect of statins used to treat elevated cholesterol levels.

Many older adults experience mild problems with memory, but do not have Alzheimer disease. Careful evaluation of the older adult is done in order to avoid misdiagnosing dementia in these cases.

Parkinson disease is a common disorder in older adults, who are already at greater risk for falls resulting from orthostatic hypotension, osteoporosis, poor vision, and other problems that cause disorientation and confusion, such as AD.

Older adults are particularly susceptible to psychologic disturbances. For this reason, an environment of reduced stimulation as well as other pharmacologic and nonpharmacologic measures may be necessary. A priority is to protect the older adult from injury and maintain safety and supervision at all times if signs of psychologic dysfunction are present.

Older adults are especially susceptible to heat stroke and psychologic side effects, including confusion, depression, delusions, and hallucinations. Anticholinergics should be tapered slowly when discontinued to avoid enhancing parkinsonian symptoms.

Patient assessments should include evaluation of military service and information regarding any interface with the Veteran's Administration (VA). The nurse should be aware that the VA provides specialized programs and rehabilitation for veterans who have experienced a neurological injury such as traumatic brain injury. The Epilepsy Foundation (2018) provides information about caring for veterans with epilepsy. The VA has established the Polytrauma System of Care (PSC). This integrated network of specialized rehabilitation programs provides care and rehabilitation for polytrauma and traumatic brain injuries (Veterans' Administration, 2018).

41.4 Health Promotion

Nervous system health promotion is based on injury prevention and healthy behavior maintenance. Neurologic injuries due to trauma can be prevented with correct use of safety equipment such as helmets when bicycling or riding a motorcycle and using vehicular safety and seat belts.

Older adults and their caregivers should consider screenings for neurological disorders or memory changes if symptoms appear. For everyone, general health promotion such as physical activity, healthy diet, and sufficient sleep positively impact neurological function.

Table 41.6 Age-Related Changes in the Neurologic System

Age-Related Change	Significance
■ ↓ number of brain cells, cerebral blood flow, and metabolism ■ Slower nerve conduction velocity	Delayed response to multiple stimuli and slower reflexes; may need additional time to process and respond to verbal stimuli.
■ Slower retrieval of information from long-term memory	There is some age-related forgetfulness, which can be improved by using memory aids such as making lists.
■ Slower response to changes in balance	May contribute to increased risk for falls.
■ May exhibit less readiness to learn and depend on prior experiences to solve problems. ■ Is more easily distracted and has a decrease in the ability to maintain attention.	Learning new skills or knowledge is improved when they are related to previously learned information and when limits are set on times for learning (e.g., no more than 30 minutes at one time).

CHAPTER HIGHLIGHTS

41.1 Anatomy, Physiology, and Functions of the Nervous System

Describe the anatomy, physiology, and functions of the nervous system and identify abnormal findings that may indicate impairments of the nervous system.

- Correct structure and function of the nervous system are vital to enervate, regulate, and integrate all of the body's functions.

41.2 Assessing Neurologic Function

Outline the components of the assessment of the nervous system, including topics for the health assessment interview, techniques for physical assessment, and the diagnostic tests used in the assessment.

- Manifestations of dysfunction, injury, and disorders affecting the nervous system may be detected during a general health assessment as well as during a focused nervous system assessment.

41.3 Assessment of Special Populations

Differentiate considerations for assessing the nervous systems of older adults and veterans.

- Several age-related changes are noted for the neurological system. Neurological diseases such as AD and PD and other disorders are more prevalent in the older adult.
- All patients should be assessed for military service. If the patient had served, determination of VA involvement in care helps to maintain coordination of care.

41.4 Health Promotion

Summarize topics that nurses teach to promote healthy tissue integrity across the lifespan.

- Neurological health promotion focuses on two overarching topics: Trauma prevention and healthy behaviors (regular exercise, good nutrition, adequate sleep).

TEST YOURSELF NCLEX-RN® REVIEW

1. A patient has a systemic illness but demonstrates no signs of neurologic involvement. Which physiologic mechanism should the nurse recall that protects the brain from harmful substances?
   A. Blood–brain barrier
   B. Structure of neurons
   C. Large oxygen demand
   D. Circulation of cerebrospinal fluid
2. The nurse is assessing a patient with damage to the lower motor neurons. Which findings should the nurse expect to assess in this patient? (Select all that apply.)
   A. Loss of reflexes
   B. Increased muscle tone
   C. Decreased coordination
   D. Fasciculations
   E. Muscle atrophy
3. The nurse is preparing a teaching session on the neurologic system for a group of nursing students. What should the nurse include about the purpose and function of cerebrospinal fluid? (Select all that apply.)
   A. Cushions the brain
   B. Helps nourish the brain
   C. Prevents glucose from entering brain cells
   D. Protects the brain and spinal cord from trauma
   E. Removes waste products of cellular metabolism
4. A patient's assessment reveals lack of movement of the left eye. The nurse will conduct additional assessment of which cranial nerves that control this movement? (Select all that apply.)
   A. Olfactory
   B. Optic
   C. Oculomotor
   D. Trochlear
   E. Trigeminal
5. A patient reports narrowly missing having an automobile crash when merging onto the freeway. Which division of the autonomic nervous system should the nurse recall as causing body responses to stress?
   A. Adrenergic
   B. Cholinergic
   C. Sympathetic
   D. Parasympathetic
6. The nurse is preparing to assess a patient's neurologic system. The nurse will prepare to use which assessment techniques in this assessment? (Select all that apply.)
   A. Palpation
   B. Percussion
   C. Inspection
   D. Auscultation
   E. History review

7. The nurse is assessing a patient's cranial nerve function. What equipment should the nurse use to assess function of cranial nerve V, the trigeminal nerve?
   A. Cotton ball and safety pin
   B. Measuring tape and pencil
   C. Scents such as coffee and vanilla
   D. Stethoscope with bell and diaphragm
8. The nurse assesses decreased corneal reflex in a newly admitted patient. This reflex may normally be decreased due to which history?
   A. Over age 50
   B. Wears contact lenses
   C. Takes diuretic medications
   D. Wears dentures
9. The nurse is planning to assess a patient's gag reflex. What equipment should the nurse use to test this reflex?
   A. Safety pin
   B. Cotton ball
   C. Stethoscope
   D. Tongue depressor
10. The nurse is documenting that a patient is demonstrating decorticate posturing. What does this statement indicate about the patient's physical posture? (Select all that apply.)
   A. Arms extended
   B. Fingers flexed
   C. Feet plantar flexed
   D. Legs internally rotated
   E. Wrists extended

See Test Yourself answers in Appendix B.

REFERENCES

Bickley, L. (2016). *Bates' guide to physical examination and history taking* (12th ed.). Philadelphia, PA: Lippincott Williams & *Wilkins*.

Epilepsy Foundation. (2018). *Special populations*. Retrieved from https://www.epilepsy.com/learn/special-populations.

Genetic and Rare Diseases Information Center (GARD). (2017). *Nervous system diseases*. Retrieved from https://rarediseases.info.nih.gov/diseases/diseases-by-category/17/nervous-system-diseases.

Glasgow Coma Scale. (2014). *The Glasgow structured approach to assessment of the Glasgow Coma Scale*. Retrieved from www.glasgowcomascale.org.

Global Burden of Disease Study. (2017). Global, regional, and national burden of neurological disorders during 1999–2015: A systematic analysis for the Global Burden of Disease Study 2015. *Lancet Neurology, 16*(11), 877–897. Retrieved from https://www.thelancet.com/journals/laneur/article/PIIS1474-4422(17)30299-5/fulltext.

Veterans' Administration (VA). (2018). *Polytrauma/TBI system of care*. Retrieved from https://www.polytrauma.va.gov.

ADDITIONAL RESOURCES

Epilepsy Foundation
www.epilepsy.com

Glasgow Coma Scale
www.glasgowcomascale.org

Chapter 42

Nursing Care of Patients with Intracranial Disorders

Chapter Outline and Learning Outcomes

CLINICAL COMPETENCIES

- Assess the functional status of patients with intracranial disorders and monitor, document, and report abnormal manifestations.
- Use assessed data, individual and cultural patient values and variations, expressed patient needs and preferences, clinical expertise, and evidence to determine priority nursing diagnoses and select and implement individualized nursing interventions for patients with intracranial disorders.
- Administer medications used to treat intracranial disorders knowledgeably and safely.
- Provide appropriate interventions to patients having intracranial pressure monitoring, tonic–clonic seizures, and intracranial surgery.
- Effectively communicate with and function within the interprofessional team to plan and provide care for patients with intracranial disorders.
- Use evidence-based practice to provide care for patients undergoing awake craniotomy.
- Provide appropriate teaching to facilitate safety and to provide information and support necessary for long-term care of patients with intracranial disorders.
- Revise plan of care as needed to provide effective interventions to promote, maintain, or restore functional health status to patients with intracranial disorders.

KEY TERMS

The patient with an intracranial disorder presents a unique nursing challenge. Problems the patient experiences in the acute stage of the disorder are often a prelude to long-term problems requiring ongoing management. These long-term problems range from alterations in the body's basic functions to dysfunctions in the complex processes of the human mind. Systemic problems may accompany or develop secondary to an intracranial disorder. Intracranial disorders may affect both the patient's quality of life and that of the patient's family.

The manifestations of altered cerebral function discussed in this chapter occur as a result of illness or injury. Assessing the patterns of these manifestations helps determine the extent of the cerebral dysfunction and improvement or deterioration of cerebral function. Except in the case of direct damage to the brainstem and reticular activating system (RAS), brain function deterioration usually follows a predictable progression, that is, a pattern in which higher levels of function are impaired initially, progressing to impairment of more primitive functions. Altered level of consciousness (LOC) and behavior changes are early manifestations of the deterioration of the function of the cerebral hemispheres. Structures in the midbrain and brainstem are affected sequentially, with characteristic changes in LOC; patterns of respiration, pupillary, and oculomotor responses; and motor function. Manifestations of progressive deterioration of cerebral function are outlined in **Table 42.1**.

42.1 Altered Level of Consciousness

Consciousness is a condition in which the individual is aware of self and environment and is able to respond appropriately to stimuli. Full consciousness requires both normal arousal and full cognition. Arousal, or alertness, depends on the RAS, a diffuse system of neurons in the thalamus and upper brainstem. *Cognition* is a complex process involving all mental activities controlled by the cerebral hemispheres, including thought processes, memory, perception, problem solving, and emotion. These two components of consciousness depend on the normal physiologic functions of and connections between the arousal mechanisms of the reticular formation and the cognitive functions of the cerebral hemispheres. Because arousal and cognition are independent components of consciousness, each can act separately on stimuli. For example, the RAS reacts to the discomfort caused by a full bladder by waking the person in the middle of the night. Once awake, however, the frontal cortex alerts the person that the bladder is full and prompts the person to go to the bathroom and empty it.

Conditions that affect either the RAS or the function of the cerebral hemispheres can interfere with the normal LOC. Terms commonly used to describe altered LOC are listed and defined in **Table 42.2**. A patient may pass from

Table 42.1 Manifestations of Progressive Deterioration of Brain Function

Level of Consciousness	Pupillary Response	Oculomotor Responses	Motor Responses	Breathing
Alert; oriented to time, place, and person	Brisk and equal; pupils regular	Eyes move as head turns Caloric testing (ear irrigation) produces nystagmus	Purposeful movement; responds to commands	Regular pattern with normal rate and depth
Responds to verbal stimuli; decreased concentration; agitation, confusion, lethargy; disoriented	Small and reactive	Roving eye movements; doll's eyes positive, with gaze fixed straight ahead; eye deviation away from cold caloric stimulus and toward warm stimulus	Purposeful movement in response to pain stimulus	Yawning, sighing respirations
Requires continuous stimulation to rouse			Decorticate posturing with upper extremity flexion	Cheyne-Stokes respirations with crescendo–decrescendo pattern in rate and depth followed by period of apnea
Reflexive positioning to pain stimulus	Pupils fixed (nonreactive) in midposition	Caloric testing produces nystagmus	Decerebrate posturing with adduction and rigid extension of upper and lower extremities	Central neurogenic hyperventilation with rapid, regular, and deep respirations; apneustic breathing with prolonged inspiration and pauses at full inspiration and following expiration
No response to stimuli	Pupils fixed in midposition	No spontaneous eye movement or nystagmus	Extension of upper extremities with flexion of lower extremities; flaccidity (lack of muscle tone)	Cluster or ataxic breathing with irregular pattern and depth of respirations; gasping respirations or apnea

Table 42.2 Terms Used to Describe Level of Consciousness

Term	Characteristics of the Patient
Full consciousness	Alert; oriented to time, place, and person; comprehends spoken and written words
Confusion	Unable to think rapidly and clearly; easily bewildered, with poor memory and short attention span; misinterprets stimuli; judgment is impaired
Disorientation	Not aware of or not oriented to time, place, or person
Obtundation	Lethargic, somnolent; responsive to verbal or tactile stimuli but quickly drifts back to sleep
Stupor	Generally unresponsive; may be briefly aroused by vigorous, repeated, or painful stimuli; may shrink away from or grab at the source of stimuli
Semicomatose	Does not move spontaneously; unresponsive to stimuli, although vigorous or painful stimuli may result in stirring, moaning, or withdrawal from the stimuli, without actual arousal
Coma	Unarousable; will not stir or moan in response to any stimulus; may exhibit nonpurposeful response (slight movement) of area stimulated but makes no attempt to withdraw
Deep coma	Completely unarousable and unresponsive to any kind of stimulus, including pain; absence of brainstem reflexes; corneal, papillary, and pharyngeal reflexes; and tendon and plantar reflexes

full consciousness to coma within hours or experience a slow diminishment of consciousness that does not become evident for weeks or months. The nurse can help provide effective care for a patient with an altered LOC by looking beyond the diagnostic labels of consciousness and accurately assessing the patient's behavior and response to stimuli.

To help remember the major causes of altered consciousness, use the following mnemonics:

AEIOU or **TIPSS**

Alcohol	**T**umor
Epilepsy	**I**njury
Insulin	**P**sychiatric
Opium	**S**troke
Uremia	**S**epsis

The Patient with Altered Level of Consciousness

Pathophysiology

An individual's level of consciousness can be altered by processes that affect the arousal functions of the brainstem, the cognitive functions of the cerebral hemispheres, or both.

Arousal and Cognition

The physiologic seat of consciousness, the reticular formation, is a mass of nerve cells and fibers that make up the core of the brainstem, extending from the medulla to the midbrain. The axons of reticular neurons are exceptionally long and branch outward to cells in the hypothalamus, thalamus, cerebellum, and spinal cord. A system of reticular neurons within the RAS passes steady streams of impulses through thalamic relays in order to stimulate the cerebral cortex into wakefulness. The body's sensory tracts interact with RAS neurons; this interrelationship helps control the strength of the rousing effect on the cerebrum.

Damage to the RAS impairs an individual's ability to maintain wakefulness and arousal. Stroke is the most common cause of RAS destruction. Other causes include demyelinating diseases such as multiple sclerosis, tumors, abscesses, and head injury. Function of the RAS may be suppressed by compression of the brainstem with edema and ischemia. Pressure and compression of the brainstem may be due to tumors, edema, increased intracranial pressure (IICP), hematomas or hemorrhage, or aneurysm. Although it is possible to assess LOC or arousal in the patient with RAS damage, an impairment in arousal may make it impossible to assess cognitive function.

The function of the cerebral hemispheres depends on continuous blood flow with unimpeded supplies of oxygen and glucose. Processes that disrupt this flow of blood and nutrients may cause widespread damage, impairing arousal and cognition. Bilateral hemispheric lesions (such as global ischemia) and metabolic disorders (such as hypoglycemia) are the most common causes of altered LOC related to cerebral dysfunction of the hemispheres. Localized masses, such as a hematoma or cerebral edema, that displace normal structures and cause direct or indirect pressure on the opposite hemisphere or brainstem can also affect LOC. The patient who has widespread damage to the cerebral hemispheres but an intact RAS has sleep–wake cycles and may rouse in response to stimuli; the patient cannot be said to be alert, however, because cognition is impaired.

Any systemic condition that affects the delivery of blood, oxygen, and glucose to the brain or alters cell membranes may also alter LOC. If cerebral blood flow is impaired or the patient becomes hypoxic or hypoglycemic, cerebral metabolism is impaired and level of consciousness declines rapidly. Severe hypoxia quickly leads to ischemia. Ischemia may be focal (for example, following a stroke) or global (as from cardiac arrest or hypovolemic shock). Patients at particular risk include those with poorly controlled diabetes and those with cardiac or respiratory failure. Other metabolic alterations that can affect LOC include fluid and electrolyte imbalances, such as hyponatremia or hyperosmolality, and acid–base alterations, such as hypercapnia (an elevated arterial carbon dioxide level) (refer to Chapter 10). Accumulated waste products and toxins from liver or renal failure can affect neuronal and neurotransmitter function, altering

LOC. Drugs that depress the central nervous system (e.g., alcohol, analgesics, anesthetics) suppress metabolic and membrane activities in the RAS and cerebral hemispheres, thereby affecting LOC. Glutamate, the main excitatory neurotransmitter in the brain, may accumulate during prolonged ischemia, resulting in acute glutamate toxicity and cell death.

Seizure activity, with abnormal electrical discharges from a local area of the brain or from the entire brain, commonly affects LOC. It appears that the spontaneous, disordered discharge of activity that occurs during a seizure exhausts energy metabolites or produces locally toxic molecules, altering LOC for a time after the seizure. Consciousness returns when the metabolic balance of the neurons is restored. (Seizures are discussed later in this chapter.)

As impairment of brain function progresses, higher-intensity stimuli are required to elicit a response from the patient. Initially, the patient may rouse to verbal stimuli and respond appropriately to questions, remaining oriented to time, place, and person. With deterioration of neurologic function, the patient becomes more difficult to rouse and may become agitated and confused when awakened. Orientation to time is lost initially, followed by orientation to place and then to person. Continuous stimulation or vigorous shaking is required to maintain wakefulness as LOC decreases. Eventually, the patient does not respond, even with deep painful stimuli.

Patterns of Respiration

Progressive impairment of neural function also causes predictable changes in respiratory patterns as respiratory centers are affected. In normal respirations, a rhythmic pattern is maintained by neural centers in the pons and medulla that respond to changes in arterial levels of oxygen (PaO_2) and carbon dioxide ($PaCO_2$). When there is damage to the RAS or cerebral hemispheres, neural control of these centers is lost, and lower brainstem centers regulate breathing patterns by responding only to changes in $PaCO_2$, resulting in irregular respiratory patterns. The initial manifestations of deteriorating brain function are yawning and sighing. As outlined earlier in Table 42.1, progressive deterioration in brain function is accompanied by decreasing LOC and changes in breathing patterns. The types of respirations, by area of cerebral damage, are:

- *Diencephalon:* Cheyne-Stokes respirations (alternating periods of deep, rapid breathing followed by periods of apnea)
- *Midbrain:* Neurogenic hyperventilation (may exceed 40 breaths per minute), the result of uninhibited stimulation of the respiratory centers
- *Pons:* Apneustic respirations, characterized by sighing on midinspiration or prolonged inhalation and exhalation; results from excessive stimulation of the respiratory centers
- *Medulla:* Ataxic/apneic respirations (totally uncoordinated and irregular), probably as a result of the loss of responsiveness to CO_2.

Pupillary and Oculomotor Responses

The areas of the brainstem that control arousal are adjacent to areas that control the pupils. A predictable progression of pupillary and oculomotor responses occurs as level of consciousness deteriorates toward coma (refer to Table 42.1). If the lesion or process affecting neurologic function is localized, effects may initially be seen in the ipsilateral pupil (the pupil on the same side as the lesion). With generalized or systemic processes, pupils are affected equally. If the pupils are small and equally reactive, metabolic processes affecting LOC may be present. With compression of cranial nerve III at the midbrain, the pupils may become oval or eccentric (off center). As the level of functional impairment progresses, the pupils become fixed (unresponsive to light) and dilated. The sudden appearance of fixed and dilated pupils may be described in an informal medical term as *blown pupils*.

In deteriorating LOC and coma, spontaneous eye movement is lost and reflexive ocular movements are altered. Normally, both eyes move simultaneously in the same direction; injury to the cranial nerve nuclei in the midbrain and pons can impair normal movement. Doll's-eye movements are reflexive movements of the eyes in the opposite direction of head rotation; they are an indicator of brainstem function (**Figure 42.1** ■). As a result of the oculocephalic

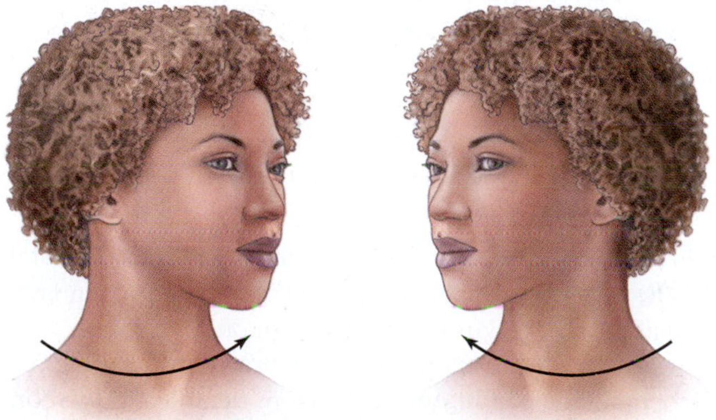

Positive doll's eyes response

As head is turned to the side, the eyes are still facing forward.

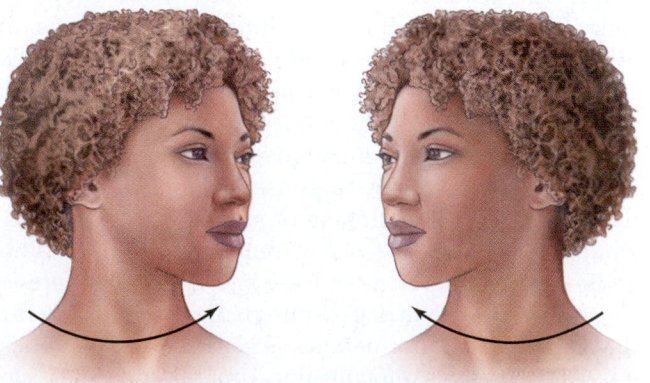

Negative doll's eyes response

As the head turns to the side, the eyes deviate in the opposite direction of the head turning.

Figure 42.1 ■ Doll's-eye movements characteristic of altered level of consciousness.

reflex, the eyes move upward with passive flexion of the neck and downward with passive neck extension. As brainstem function deteriorates, this reflex is lost. The eyes fail to turn together and, eventually, remain fixed in the midposition as the head is turned.

Motor Responses

The level of brain dysfunction and the side of the brain affected may be assessed by motor responses. These responses are the most accurate identifier of changes in mental status. In altered LOC, motor responses to stimuli range from an appropriate response to a command (e.g., "squeeze my hand") to flaccidity (refer to Table 42.1). Initially, the patient may be able to move purposefully away from a noxious stimulus, for example, to brush the examiner's hand away from the face. As function declines, movements become more generalized (withdrawal, grimacing) and less purposeful. Reflexive motor responses may occur, including decorticate posturing with flexion of the upper extremities accompanied by extension of the lower extremities. With further decline, decerebrate posturing is seen, with adduction and rigid extension of the upper and lower extremities. Without intervention, the patient eventually becomes flaccid, with little or no motor response to stimuli.

Coma States and Brain Death

Possible outcomes of altered LOC and coma include full recovery with no long-term residual effects, recovery with residual damage (such as learning deficits, emotional difficulties, or impaired judgment), or more severe consequences such as persistent vegetative state (cerebral death), locked-in syndrome, and brain death.

Persistent Vegetative State. **Persistent vegetative state (PVS)** is a permanent condition of complete unawareness of self and the environment and loss of all cognitive functions. Usually the result of severe brain trauma or global ischemia, this condition results from death of the cerebral hemispheres with continued function of the brainstem and cerebellum. While the homeostatic regulatory functions of the brain continue, the ability to respond meaningfully to the environment is lost. The patient has sleep–wake cycles and retains the ability to chew, swallow, and cough but cannot interact with the environment. When awake, the eyes may wander back and forth across the room, but they cannot track an object or person. In a minimally conscious state, the patient is aware of the environment and can follow simple commands, manipulate objects, gesture or verbalize to indicate yes/no responses, and make meaningful movements (such as blinking or smiling) in response to a stimulus. The diagnosis of PVS requires that the condition be present at 1 month after acute brain injury and present for at least 1 month in degenerative/metabolic disorders or developmental malformations (Sorenson, Quinn, & Klein, 2019). PVS presents difficult ethical, moral, and legal issues.

Locked-In Syndrome. **Locked-in syndrome** is distinctly different from persistent vegetative state in that the patient is alert and fully aware of the environment and has intact cognitive abilities, but is unable to communicate through speech or movement because of blocked efferent pathways from the brain. Motor paralysis affects all voluntary muscles, although the upper cranial nerves (I through IV) may remain intact, allowing the patient to communicate through eye movements and blinking. In essence, the patient is locked inside a paralyzed body while remaining fully conscious of self and environment. Infarction or hemorrhage of the pons that disrupts outgoing nerve tracts but spares the RAS is the usual cause of locked-in syndrome. This condition may also result when the corticospinal tracts between the midbrain and pons are interrupted. Disorders of the lower motor neurons or muscles, such as poliomyelitis, myasthenia gravis, or amyotrophic lateral sclerosis, may also paralyze motor responses, leading to locked-in syndrome.

Brain Death. **Brain death** is the cessation and irreversibility of all brain functions, including the brainstem. Although the exact criteria for establishing brain death may vary somewhat from state to state, it is generally agreed that brain death has occurred when there is no evidence of cerebral or brainstem function for an extended period (usually 6 to 24 hours) in a patient who has a normal body temperature and is not affected by a depressant drug or alcohol poisoning. Generally recognized criteria are:

- Unresponsive coma with absent motor and reflex movements
- No spontaneous respiration (apnea)
- Pupils fixed (unresponsive to light) and dilated
- Absent ocular responses to head turning and caloric stimulation (Caloric stimulation is performed by irrigating the ear with ice-cold water to test the oculovestibular reflex, a reflex controlled by the brainstem. Normally, the cold causes the eyes to first move toward the irrigated side, followed by a return to midline.)
- Flat electroencephalogram (EEG) and no cerebral blood circulation present on angiography (if performed)
- Persistence of these manifestations for 30 minutes to 1 hour and for 6 hours after onset of coma and apnea.

Apnea in the comatose patient is determined by the apnea test. The ventilator is removed while maintaining oxygenation by tracheal cannula and allowing the PCO_2 to increase to 60 mmHg or higher. This level of carbon dioxide is high enough to stimulate respiration if the brainstem is functional. The EEG may be used to establish the absence of brain activity when brain death is suspected. A flat EEG over a period of 6 to 12 hours in a patient who is not hypothermic or under the influence of drugs that depress the central nervous system (CNS) is generally accepted as an indicator of brain death.

Prognosis

The prognosis for patients with altered LOC and coma varies according to the underlying cause and pathologic process. Age and general medical condition also play a role in determining outcome. Young adults may fully recover following deep coma from, for example, head injury or drug overdose. Recovery of consciousness within 2 weeks is associated with a favorable outcome. In general, the prognosis is poor for patients who lack pupillary reaction or reflex eye movements 6 hours after the onset of coma.

Interprofessional Care

Management of the patient with an altered LOC or coma must begin immediately. The focus of management is to identify the underlying cause, preserve function, and prevent deterioration, if possible. Airway and breathing must be maintained during the initial acute stage until the diagnosis and prognosis can be established. Intravenous fluids are used to support circulation and to correct fluid, electrolyte, and acid–base imbalances. Treatment protocols to reduce IICP or control seizure activity (discussed later in this chapter) may be initiated. Changes in LOC associated with craniocerebral trauma often require immediate surgical intervention.

Diagnosis

Although the patient's history and physical examination findings often indicate the cause of alterations in LOC, several diagnostic tests may be useful in establishing the diagnosis. The tests used to evaluate possible metabolic, toxic, or drug-induced disorders include both radiologic and laboratory tests.

CT and MRI scanning are done to detect neurologic damage due to hemorrhage, tumor, cyst, edema, myocardial infarction, or brain atrophy. These tests may also identify displacement of brain structures by large or expanding lesions. Radioisotope brain scan is performed to identify abnormal lesions in the brain and evaluate cerebral blood flow. Cerebral angiography allows radiographic visualization of the cerebral vascular system. This exam can identify lesions such as aneurysms, occluded vessels, or tumors, and may also be used to determine cessation of cerebral blood flow and brain death. Transcranial Doppler studies are used to assess cerebral blood flow. Lumbar puncture with cerebrospinal fluid (CSF) analysis is performed when infection and possible meningitis are suspected as a cause of altered LOC. EEG is used to evaluate the electrical activity of the brain.

Laboratory tests are used to identify and monitor altered LOC. These may include any or all of the following (Kee, 2018):

- ***Blood glucose*** is measured immediately when coma is of unknown origin and hypoglycemia is suspected or possible. When the blood glucose falls to less than 40 to 50 mg/dL, cerebral function declines rapidly.
- ***Serum electrolytes***—sodium, potassium, bicarbonate, chloride, and calcium in particular—are measured to assess for metabolic disturbances and guide intravenous therapy. Hyponatremia, in which serum sodium levels are below 115 mEq/L (normal level: 135 to 145 mEq/L), is associated with coma and convulsions, especially if it develops rapidly.
- ***Serum osmolality*** is evaluated. Both hyperosmolar and hypo-osmolar states may be associated with coma. Hyperosmolality (above 320 mOsm/kg H_2O) causes cellular dehydration of brain tissue as fluid is drawn into the vascular system by osmosis. Hypo-osmolality (less than 250 mOsm/kg H_2O), by contrast, leads to cerebral edema and swelling, impairing consciousness.
- ***Arterial blood gases (ABGs)*** are drawn to evaluate arterial oxygen and carbon dioxide levels as well as acid–base balance. Hypoxemia is a frequent cause of altered LOC; increased levels of carbon dioxide are also toxic to the brain and can induce coma, particularly when the onset of hypercapnia is acute.
- ***Liver function tests,*** including bilirubin, AST, ALT, LDH, serum albumin, and serum ammonia levels, are determined to evaluate hepatic function. High ammonia levels seen in hepatic failure interfere with cerebral metabolism and neurotransmitters, affecting LOC.
- ***Toxicology screening*** of blood and urine is done to determine if altered LOC is the result of acute drug or alcohol toxicity. Serum alcohol levels are measured and the blood is assessed for the presence of substances such as barbiturates, carbon monoxide, or lead.

Medications

Medications are used to support homeostasis and normal function for the patient with altered LOC, as well as to treat specific underlying disorders. An intravenous catheter is inserted, and fluid balance is maintained using isotonic or slightly hypertonic solutions, such as normal saline or lactated Ringer solution. The patient's response to fluid administration is monitored carefully for evidence of increased cerebral edema.

If hypoglycemia is present, 50% glucose is administered intravenously to rapidly restore cerebral metabolism. Conversely, insulin is administered to the patient with hyperglycemia to reduce the blood glucose level and thus the serum osmolality. With narcotic overdose, naloxone is administered. Naloxone is a narcotic antagonist that competes for narcotic receptor sites, effectively blocking the depressant effect of the narcotic. Thiamine may be administered with glucose, particularly if the patient is malnourished or known to abuse alcohol, to prevent exacerbation of Wernicke's encephalopathy, a hemorrhagic encephalopathy due to thiamine deficiency that is associated with chronic alcoholism.

Any underlying fluid and electrolyte imbalance is corrected by administering medications or appropriate electrolytes. For the patient who is hyponatremic and has a low serum osmolality, furosemide (Lasix) or an osmotic diuretic such as mannitol may be administered to promote water excretion. Appropriate antibiotics are administered intravenously to the patient with suspected or confirmed meningitis.

Nutrition

In patients with long-term alterations in consciousness, such as PVS or locked-in syndrome, measures to maintain nutritional status are initiated. Enteral feedings with a gastrostomy tube are preferred if the patient is unable to take enough food by mouth without aspirating. In some cases, total parenteral nutrition (TPN) may be used.

Surgery

Although surgery is not indicated for most patients with altered LOC, it may be necessary if the cause of coma is an intracerebral tumor, hemorrhage, or hematoma. When there is a risk of IICP, the patient is monitored continuously. Intracranial monitoring is discussed in the following section.

Other Treatments

Support of the airway and respirations is vital in the patient with an altered LOC. The patient who is drowsy but rousable may need little more than an oral pharyngeal airway. With more severe alterations in consciousness, the patient may need endotracheal intubation to maintain airway patency, particularly if the cough and gag reflexes are absent. Mechanical ventilation is indicated when hypoventilation or apnea is present. Unless a do-not-resuscitate (DNR) order is in effect, mechanical ventilation should be initiated even if it has not been established that the disorder is reversible; without ventilatory support, cerebral anoxia develops rapidly, and brain death may ensue. ABGs are monitored frequently to determine the adequacy of ventilation. Cautious hyperventilation may be used to reduce $PaCO_2$ and promote cerebral vasoconstriction to reduce cerebral edema.

Nursing Care

Nursing care of the patient with an altered LOC is planned and implemented for a variety of responses of both the patient and the family of the patient.

Assessment

See the Manifestations and Interprofessional Care sections for the assessment of the patient with altered LOC.

Priorities of Care

Collaborating with the interprofessional team to ensure adequate treatment of the underlying process while providing care that supports the physical and psychologic responses to the disorder is a priority of nursing care.

Diagnoses, Outcomes, and Interventions

Diagnoses, outcomes, and interventions discussed in this section are directed toward the unconscious patient and focus on problems with airway maintenance, skin integrity, contractures, and nutrition.

Maintain Adequate Airway Clearance. Ineffective airway clearance related to loss of the cough reflex and the inability to expectorate is a major problem for the unconscious patient. The cough reflex may be absent or impaired when conditions that produce coma depress the function of the medullary centers.

Expected Outcome: Adequate airway clearance will be maintained by the nurse through safety measures and appropriate suctioning.

The nurse will:

- Assess ability to clear secretions. Monitor breath sounds, rate and depth of respirations, dyspnea, pulse oximeter, and the presence of cyanosis. *The patient's ability to clear secretions serves as the initial assessment base for developing further interventions.*
- In unconscious patients or those without an intact cough reflex, maintain an open airway by periodic suctioning, limiting the time of suctioning to 10 seconds (Perrin & MacLeod, 2018). Periodic suctioning may be necessary to clear the airway of mucus, blood, or other drainage. *Suctioning for more than 10 seconds in the patient with IICP may cause hypercapnia, which in turn vasodilates cerebral vessels, increases cerebral blood volume, and increases ICP.*
- Turn from side to side every 2 hours, and maintain a side-lying position with the head of the bed elevated approximately 30 degrees. Do not position the unconscious patient on the back. *Turning the patient from side to side facilitates respirations, prevents the tongue from obstructing the airway, and helps prevent pooling of secretions in one area of the lungs (thus decreasing the risk of pneumonia).*
- Monitor the results of arterial blood gas analysis and pulse oximetry. Maintain records of trends. *ABGs and pulse oximetry directly measure the oxygen content of blood and are good indicators of the lungs' ability to oxygenate the blood.*

SAFETY ALERT: If the patient has a basilar skull fracture or CSF draining from the ears or nose, never suction nasally. ■

Reduce Risk for Aspiration. The unconscious patient with a depressed or absent gag and swallowing reflex is at high risk for aspiration. Drainage, mucus, or blood may obstruct the airway and interfere with oxygenation. Pooling of aspiration secretions in the lungs also increases the risk of pneumonia.

Expected Outcome: Patent airway and clear lung sounds will be maintained.

The nurse will:

- Assess swallowing and gag reflexes every shift as appropriate to the patient's level of consciousness. *Deepening levels of unconsciousness may cause a loss of the swallow and gag reflexes.*
- Monitor for and report manifestations of aspiration: Crackles and wheezes, dullness to percussion over an area of the lungs, dyspnea, tachypnea, and cyanosis. *Early recognition facilitates prompt intervention.*
- Provide interventions to prevent aspiration: Maintain NPO status, position on the side, and provide suctioning as needed. *The side-lying position allows secretions to drain from the mouth rather than into the pharynx. Oral hygiene and suctioning remove secretions that might otherwise be aspirated.*

SAFETY ALERT: Never give unconscious patients oral food and fluids because of the risk of aspiration. ■

Reduce Risk for Impaired Skin Integrity. On average, healthy people change positions during sleep every 11 minutes; the unconscious patient often cannot maintain the movement needed to prevent pressure on the skin, especially over bony prominences. As a result, the skin and subcutaneous tissues may become ischemic and prone to develop pressure ulcers. Perspiration and incontinence of urine and stool may exacerbate the problem. Nursing interventions are directed to maintaining the integrity not only of the skin, but also of the lips and mucous membranes. Nursing care to prevent pressure ulcer development is discussed in Chapter 16.

Expected Outcome: Patient will experience effective wound healing and infection management as evidenced by skin integrity and body temperature within normal range.

Promote Physical Mobility. Patients who are unconscious are unable to maintain normal musculoskeletal movement and are at high risk for contractures related to decreased movement. Because the flexor and adductor muscles are stronger than the extensors and abductors, flexor and adductor contractures develop quickly without preventive measures. Passive range-of-motion (ROM) exercises must be performed routinely to maintain muscle tone and function, to prevent additional disability, and to help restore impaired motor function.

Expected Outcome: Patient's joint range of motion will be maintained with progression to transfers and ambulation as LOC alteration resolves.

The nurse will:

- Maintain extremities in functional positions by providing proper support devices. Remove support devices every 4 hours for skin care and passive ROM exercises. Provide pillows for the axillary region; rolled washcloths may be placed in elevated hands; use splints to prevent plantar flexion (foot drop). *Pillows in the axillary region help prevent adduction of the shoulder. Rolled washcloths help decrease edema and flexion contracture of the fingers. Splints are useful in preventing plantar flexion.*
- Collaborate with a physical therapist to develop and implement passive ROM exercises (unless contraindicated, e.g., for the patient with IICP) at least four times a day. *ROM exercises help prevent contractures by stretching muscles and tendons and maintaining joint mobility.*

Promote Adequate Nutritional Intake. The unconscious patient is at risk for an alteration in nutrition related to a reduced or complete inability to eat. This is especially true for the patient who is unconscious as the result of an infection or trauma, both of which increase metabolic requirements.

Expected Outcome: Patient's nutritional intake will be adequate to meet physiologic processes as evidenced by oral or enteral intake of high-protein, high-nutrient diet.

The nurse will:

- Monitor nutritional status through daily weights (on bed scales) and laboratory data. For accuracy, weigh the patient at the same time each day, wearing the same clothing, and using the same scales. *Changes in laboratory data with decreased nutrition include a decrease in the levels of serum prealbumin and serum transferrin.*
- Assess the need for alternative methods of nutritional support (tube feeding or total parenteral nutrition) through collaboration with dietitian. *Patients unable to take oral food require parenteral nutrition or liquid feedings through a nasogastric, gastrostomy, or jejunostomy tube. Protein, calorie, zinc, and vitamin C needs increase during wound healing.*

Delegating Nursing Care Activities

As appropriate and allowed by the designated duties and responsibilities of unlicensed assistive personnel, the nurse may delegate nursing care activities such as measuring vital signs (including orthostatic vital signs), encouraging oral or enteral fluid intake, and providing skin care.

Transitions of Care

Prevention of altered level of consciousness is dependent on the underlying and/or precipitating etiology leading to the changes.

Reinforce information provided by the physician, and encourage the family to talk to the patient as though he or she were able to understand. Explain that this communication may initially seem awkward, but in time it will feel appropriate. The presence of many tubes (e.g., intravenous line, urinary catheter, ventilator) may be overwhelming to the family. They may not perceive the seriousness of the situation if a thorough explanation is not given. Include family members in the patient's care as much as they wish to be involved.

Allow significant others to stay with the patient when possible. Reinforce the need for family members to care for themselves by encouraging adequate meals and rest. Offer to contact support services such as friends, neighbors, and social services that the hospital may provide. Ask family members to leave a telephone number where they can be reached, and assure them that they will be called if any significant changes occur. Encourage family members to call if they have questions or concerns.

Family members of a patient with an altered level of consciousness are often very anxious. It is difficult for the family to deal with the patient's uncertain prognosis. They may experience various conflicting emotions, such as guilt and anger.

42.2 Increased Intracranial Pressure

In the adult, the rigid cranial cavity created by the skull is normally filled to capacity with three essentially noncompressible elements: The brain (80%), cerebrospinal fluid (8%), and blood (12%). A state of dynamic equilibrium exists: If the volume of any of the three components increases, the volume of the others must decrease to maintain normal pressures within the cranial cavity. This is known as the Monro-Kellie hypothesis. The normal intracranial pressure is 5 to 10 mmHg (measured intracranially with a pressure transducer while the patient is lying with the head elevated 30 degrees) or 60 to 180 cm H_2O (measured with a water manometer while the patient is lying in a lateral recumbent position).

Increased intracranial pressure (IICP), also labeled *intracranial hypertension*, is sustained elevated pressure (greater than 10 mmHg) within the cranial cavity. Sustained IICP can result in significant tissue ischemia and damage to delicate neural tissue. Cerebral edema is the most frequent cause of sustained increases in ICP. Other causes include head trauma, tumors, abscesses, stroke, inflammation, and hemorrhage.

The Patient with Increased Intracranial Pressure

Pathophysiology

Cerebral blood flow and perfusion are important concepts for understanding the development and effects of IICP. Whereas blood and CSF contribute an equal percentage to normal intracranial volume, vascular factors account for twice the amount of increase in ICP that CSF does. The brain requires a constant supply of oxygen and glucose to meet its metabolic demands; 15 to 20% of the resting cardiac output goes to the brain to meet its metabolic needs. Interruption of the cerebral blood flow leads to ischemia and disruption of the cerebral metabolism.

Pressure and chemical autoregulation are compensatory mechanisms in which cerebral arterioles change diameter to maintain cerebral blood flow when ICP increases. In pressure autoregulation, stretch receptors within small blood vessels of the brain cause smooth muscle of the arterioles to contract. Increased arterial pressure stimulates these receptors, leading to vasoconstriction; when arterial pressure is low, stimulation of these receptors decreases, causing relaxation and vasodilation. Chemical, or metabolic, autoregulation works in much the same way as pressure autoregulation. In this case, the stimulus is a buildup of metabolic by-products of cell metabolism, including lactic acid, pyruvic acid, carbonic acid, and carbon dioxide. Carbon dioxide and increased hydrogen ion concentration are potent cerebral vasodilators that may act locally or systemically to increase cerebral blood flow. Conversely, a fall in $PaCO_2$ causes cerebral vasoconstriction. Arterial oxygen tension (PaO_2) also affects cerebral blood flow, although it is a less powerful mechanism than that exerted by carbon dioxide and hydrogen ions.

IICP may result from an increase in intracranial contents from a space-occupying lesion, hydrocephalus, cerebral edema, excess cerebrospinal fluid, or intracranial hemorrhage. Displacement of some CSF to the spinal subarachnoid space and increased CSF absorption are early compensatory mechanisms. The low-pressure venous system is also compressed, and cerebral arteries constrict to reduce blood flow. The brain tissue's ability to accommodate change is relatively restricted. The relationship between the volume of the intracranial components and intracranial pressure is known as *compliance*. When the capacity to compensate for IICP is exceeded, increased intracranial pressure (hypertension) develops. Intracranial hypertension is a sustained state of IICP and is potentially life-threatening.

Autoregulatory mechanisms have a limited ability to maintain cerebral blood flow. When autoregulation fails, cerebrovascular tone is reduced and cerebral blood flow becomes dependent on changes in blood pressure. Autoregulation may be lost either locally or globally because of several factors, including IICP, local or diffuse cerebral tissue ischemia or inflammation, prolonged hypotension, and hypercapnia or hypoxia.

Cerebral Edema

Cerebral edema is an increase in the volume of brain tissue due to abnormal accumulation of fluid. Cerebral edema is associated with IICP; it may occur as a local process in the area of a tumor or injury, or it may affect the entire brain. Two types of cerebral edema are vasogenic edema and cytotoxic edema. Both types may occur at the same time (Sorenson et al., 2019):

- *Vasogenic edema*, an extracellular edema of the white matter, results from an increase in the capillary permeability of cerebral vessels. Localized cerebral edema occurs around brain tumors and globally around cerebral trauma and meningitis.
- *Cytotoxic edema* is an increase in fluid in neurons, glia, and endothelial cells as a result of failure of the sodium-potassium pump with accumulation of water and sodium in the cells. Diffuse brain swelling results. Both white and gray matter can be involved. Cytotoxic edema is associated with an event causing anoxia or hypoxia, such as a cardiac arrest. It may also occur with hypo-osmolar conditions such as hyponatremia or the syndrome of inappropriate secretion of antidiuretic hormone (SIADH).

Hydrocephalus

Hydrocephalus in adults refers to a syndrome in which abnormal overproduction, circulation, or reabsorption of CSF occurs. It is classified as either noncommunicating or communicating hydrocephalus. *Noncommunicating hydrocephalus* occurs when CSF drainage from the ventricular system is obstructed. It may develop when a mass or tumor, inflammation or hemorrhage, or congenital malformation obstructs the ventricular system. *Communicating hydrocephalus* is a condition in which CSF is not effectively reabsorbed through the arachnoid villi. It may occur secondarily to subarachnoid hemorrhage or scarring from infection. In normal-pressure hydrocephalus, seen most often in adults age 60 or older, ventricular enlargement causes cerebral tissue compression but the CSF pressure on lumbar puncture is normal. This condition may follow cerebral trauma or surgery or the cause may not be known.

Brain Herniation

If IICP is not treated, cerebral tissue is displaced toward a more compliant area. This can result in brain herniation, the displacement of brain tissue from its normal compartment under dural folds of the falx cerebri or through the tentorial notch or incisura of the tentorium cerebelli (Sorenson et al., 2019). Herniation of the cerebellum through the tentorium exerts pressure on the brainstem, with subsequent herniation through the foramen magnum. This is a lethal complication of IICP because it puts pressure on the vital centers of the medulla.

Brain herniation syndromes are generally categorized as supratentorial or infratentorial, depending on their location above or below the tentorium cerebelli (**Figure 42.2** ■). Supratentorial herniation syndromes include cingulate herniation, central or transtentorial herniation, uncal or lateral transtentorial herniation, and infratentorial herniation.

- *Cingulate herniation* (**Figure 42.2A**) occurs when the cingulate gyrus is displaced under the falx cerebri. Local blood supply and cerebral tissue are compressed, resulting in ischemia and further increases in intracranial pressure.
- *Central* or *transtentorial herniation* is the downward displacement of brain structures, including the cerebral hemispheres, basal ganglia, diencephalon, and midbrain through the tentorial incisura (**Figure 42.2B**). The patient's neurologic signs may deteriorate rapidly, with decreased LOC progressing to coma, Cheyne-Stokes respirations progressing to central neurogenic hyperventilation, and pupils progressing from small and reactive to midsize and fixed. The patient may demonstrate abnormal motor responses with unilateral decorticate posturing.
- *Uncal* or *lateral transtentorial herniation* occurs when a lateral mass displaces cerebral tissue centrally, forcing the medial aspect of the temporal lobe under the edge of the tentorial incisura (**Figure 42.2C**). The oculomotor nerve (cranial nerve III) often becomes trapped between the uncus and the tentorium, causing ipsilateral pupillary dilation. Other manifestations include alterations in LOC, motor deficits (which may occur on the same side as the herniation because of compression of the cerebral peduncle on the opposite side), decreased sensation, respiratory changes, abnormal positioning, and eventual respiratory arrest.
- *Infratentorial herniation* results from increased pressure within the infratentorial compartment. Herniation may occur either upward, with structures displaced through the tentorial incisura, or downward, with displacement through the foramen magnum (**Figure 42.2D**). Downward displacement compresses the medulla, including its centers for controlling vital functions. Manifestations associated with medullary compression include coma, altered respiratory patterns, fixed pupils, and decorticate or decerebrate posturing. Respiratory or cardiac arrest may occur.

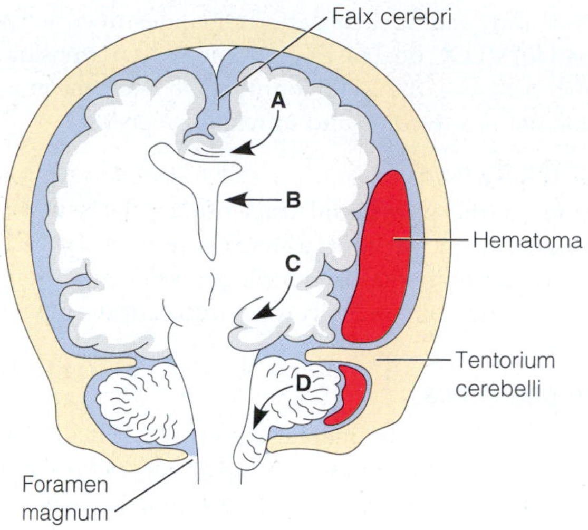
Falx cerebri
A
B
C
D
Hematoma
Tentorium cerebelli
Foramen magnum

Figure 42.2 ■ Forms of brain herniation due to IICP. **A**, Cingulate herniation occurs when the cingulate gyrus is compressed under the falx cerebri. **B**, Central herniation occurs when a centrally located lesion compresses central and midbrain structures. **C**, Lateral herniation occurs when a lesion at the side of the brain compresses the uncus or hippocampal gyrus. **D**, Infratentorial herniation occurs when the cerebellar tonsils are forced downward, compressing the medulla and top of the spinal cord.

Manifestations

With loss of autoregulation, intracranial pressure continues to rise and cerebral perfusion falls. Cerebral tissue becomes hypoxic, and manifestations of cellular ischemia appear. The manifestations of IICP include:

- Decreasing level of consciousness: Early there is confusion, restlessness, lethargy, disorientation that progresses first to time, then to place and person. Higher levels of function (mental processing) are affected first; as pressure increases, midbrain and deeper, more primitive functions are affected. Late in the process there is coma without response even to painful stimuli.
- Pupillary dysfunction, sluggish response to light progresses to dilated and fixed pupils. Vision becomes blurred and diplopia (double vision) is common. There may be an inability to move the eyes upward and drooping (ptosis) of the eyelids.
- Papilledema (edema of the optic disc)
- Abnormal motor responses, including weakness of the contralateral (opposite) side (hemiparesis) early; followed by hemiplegia, decorticate or decerebrate posturing
- Increase in mean arterial pressure, with a significant increase in systolic blood pressure and pulse pressure
- Decreased pulse rate
- Dramatic increase in body temperature
- Altered respirations
- Headache, worse on rising to an upright position and when changing positions
- Nausea with projectile vomiting.

Level of Consciousness

Because the neurons of the cerebral cortex are most sensitive to oxygen deficit, changes in cortical function are the most sensitive indicator of neurologic change (Sorenson et al., 2019). Behavior and personality changes occur; the patient may become irritable and agitated. Memory and judgment are impaired, and speech pattern changes may be noted. The patient's LOC decreases. As cerebral hypertension and hypoxia progress, the LOC continues to decrease in a predictable pattern to coma and unresponsiveness.

Motor Responses

Pressure on the pyramidal tract often causes weakness (hemiparesis) on the contralateral side early in IICP. As ICP continues to increase, hemiplegia and abnormal motor responses, such as decorticate or decerebrate posturing, develop.

Vision and Pupils

Altered vision is an early manifestation of IICP; it is caused by pressure on the visual pathways and cranial nerves. Blurred vision, decreased visual acuity, and diplopia are common. Pupillary and oculomotor responses are affected as well. Because the cause of IICP is often localized at first, pupillary changes, including gradual dilation and sluggish response to light, may initially be limited to the ipsilateral side.

Vital Signs

Ischemia of the vasomotor center in the brainstem triggers the CNS ischemic response, a late sign of IICP. Neuronal ischemia in the vasomotor center causes a marked increase in the mean arterial pressure (MAP), with a significant increase in systolic blood pressure and increased pulse pressure. The increased MAP causes reflexive slowing of the cardiac rate. This trio of manifestations (rising systolic blood pressure, widening pulse pressure, bradycardia) is known as Cushing's response and represents a compensatory response to try to maintain cerebral perfusion pressure. The loss of compensatory mechanisms and brainstem function is a late sign indicated by hypertension, bradycardia, and respiratory abnormalities and is called *Cushing's triad* (Perrin & MacLeod, 2017; Sorenson et al., 2019). Although the temperature is usually normal in early stages, as ICP continues to increase, hypothalamic function is impaired and the temperature may rise dramatically.

Other Manifestations

Additional manifestations of IICP include headache, particularly on rising, that worsens with position changes. Headache is more common with slowly developing IICP and occurs because of pressure on pain-sensitive structures, such as the middle meningeal arteries, the venous sinuses, and the dura at the base of the skull. Papilledema (edema and swelling of the optic disc) may be noted on funduscopic examination. Vomiting, often projectile and occurring without warning, may develop.

Interprofessional Care

Management of the patient with IICP is directed toward identifying and treating the underlying cause of the disorder and controlling ICP to prevent herniation syndrome. IICP is a medical emergency, and there is little time to complete lengthy diagnostic tests. The diagnosis must be made on the basis of observation and neurologic assessment; even subtle changes may be clinically significant.

Diagnosis

Diagnostic tests focus on identifying the presence of IICP and its underlying cause. A CT scan or MRI is generally the initial test used to identify the possible causes of IICP (such as space-occupying lesions or hydrocephalus) and to evaluate therapeutic options. In general, a lumbar puncture is not performed when IICP is suspected because the sudden release of the pressure in the skull may cause cerebral herniation.

In addition to the diagnostic tests listed in the previous section for altered LOC, the following specific tests are usually ordered and their results closely monitored:

- *Serum osmolality* is an indicator of hydration status in the patient with IICP. The test measures the number of dissolved particles (electrolytes, urea, glucose) in the serum. The normal range for the adult is 280 to 300 mOsm/kg H_2O. In addition to the restriction of fluids in the patient with IICP, serum osmolality is maintained at a slightly elevated level (325 mOsm/kg H_2O) to draw excess intracellular fluid into the vascular system.
- *ABGs* are monitored frequently to assess pH and levels of oxygen and carbon dioxide. Hydrogen ions and carbon dioxide are both potent vasodilators; hypoxemia also causes vasodilation, although to a lesser degree.

Medications

Medications play an important role in the management of IICP. These medications with nursing implications are described in **Medication Administration 42.A**.

In addition, sedation and paralysis are used as chemical restraints to control restlessness and agitation because these movements increase blood pressure, ICP, and cerebral metabolism. Paralysis with neuromuscular blockage is most often accomplished with pancuronium. Patients must be closely monitored during treatment for residual muscle weakness and signs of respiratory distress.

Surgery

Patients with IICP may undergo various intracranial surgical techniques to treat the underlying cause (see the discussion in the later section on brain tumors). In addition, infarcted or necrotic tissue may be resected to reduce brain mass. A drainage catheter or shunt may be inserted laterally via a burr hole into a ventricle to drain excess cerebrospinal fluid and reduce hydrocephalus. The removal of even a small amount of CSF may dramatically reduce IICP and restore cerebral perfusion pressure.

ICP Monitoring

Critical to preserving brain function and preventing secondary brain damage from IICP are careful assessments and monitoring with ICP monitors, measuring cerebral blood flow and cerebral perfusion pressure, and measuring oxygen levels of brain tissue. Intracranial pressure monitors facilitate continual assessment of ICP and the effects of medical therapy and nursing interventions. In addition, cerebral perfusion pressure (the difference between MAP and ICP) can be readily calculated, allowing more precise

Medication Administration 42.A

Increased Intracranial Pressure

OSMOTIC DIURETICS

glucose

mannitol (Osmitrol)

urea

Osmotic diuretics (hyperosmotic agents) draw fluid out of brain cells by increasing the osmolality of the blood. The effects of these drugs vary with the type of injury. Mannitol therapy is often initiated if the patient's ICP has exceeded 15 to 20 mmHg for at least 10 minutes. Both IV bolus and continuous infusion techniques are used. Repeated use of mannitol can lead to continual elevations in serum osmolality, with attendant risk of seizures and a serious fluid and electrolyte imbalance. Urea is seldom administered IV because a severe local reaction may result if leakage occurs at the injection site. Mannitol and urea are used cautiously if renal disease is present.

Nursing Responsibilities

- Monitor vital signs, urinary output, central venous pressure (CVP), and pulmonary artery pressures (PAP) before and every hour throughout administration.
- Assess for manifestations of dehydration.
- Assess for muscle weakness, numbness, tingling, paresthesia, confusion, and excessive thirst.
- Assess for pulmonary edema while administering the medication.
- Monitor neurologic status and intracranial pressure readings.
- Monitor renal function and serum electrolytes throughout therapy.
- Do not administer the medication if crystals are present in the solution. Administer with an inline filter. Observe infusion site frequently for infiltration.
- Do not administer mannitol solution with blood.

LOOP DIURETICS

ethacrynic acid (Edecrin)

furosemide (Lasix)

Loop diuretics such as furosemide and ethacrynic acid inhibit sodium and chloride reabsorption at the ascending loop of Henle. They cause a reduction in the rate of CSF production, thus reducing ICP.

Nursing Responsibilities

- Monitor vital signs and electrolyte values closely.
- Assess fluid status throughout therapy.
- Monitor blood pressure and pulse before and during administration.
- Monitor renal laboratory studies closely.
- Use infusion pump to ensure accurate dosage.

INTRAVENOUS FLUIDS

Keeping the patient moderately dehydrated to maintain serum osmolality can be effective in reducing cerebral edema. When giving IV fluids, closely monitor the osmolality of the solutions; if patients with IICP are given hypo-osmolar solutions, increased cerebral edema can occur. Preferred solutions include 0.45 to 0.9% sodium chloride solutions.

Nursing Responsibilities

- Monitor fluid status closely.
- Monitor neurologic status closely.
- Avoid administering solutions that become hypo-osmolar, such as 5% dextrose in water.

OTHER PHARMACOLOGIC INTERVENTIONS FOR ICP

- Antipyretics, such as acetaminophen, are used in conjunction with a hypothermia blanket to reduce hyperthermia, thereby decreasing the high cerebral metabolism that contributes to IICP.
- Antiulcer drugs, such as histamine H_2 antagonists (e.g., ranitidine [Zantac]) or sucralfate (Carafate), are used in patients with ICP to decrease the development of stress ulcers.
- Antihypertensive agents, such as beta-adrenergic blocking agents, may be used if the mean arterial pressure is high.
- Vasopressors may be used if the mean arterial pressure is low.
- Anticonvulsants may be given to prevent or treat seizures.

Because the patient with IICP often has an altered level of consciousness, patient and family teaching are not discussed in this feature.

Note: Drugs identified in blue are among the 200 most commonly prescribed medications in the United States.

Source: Adams, et al., 2017.

manipulation of therapeutic measures to maintain cerebral perfusion and thereby prevent ischemia. The criteria for ICP monitoring depends on the patient, but in general, patients who are comatose and have a Glasgow Coma Scale score of 8 or less should be monitored. (The Glasgow Coma Scale is provided in Table 41.5 in Chapter 41.)

Basic monitoring systems include an epidural probe, subarachnoid bolt or screw, and intraventricular catheter (**Figure 42.3** ■). Intraventricular fluid-filled catheters are placed in the anterior horn of the lateral ventricle (most often in the right side). Ventricular catheters can both drain CSF and measure ICP. The ICP value is measured deep in the brain and is considered the most reflective of the whole brain pressure. Subarachnoid devices are placed in the subarachnoid space. A fiberoptic transducer-tipped catheter can be placed in the epidural, subdural, or parenchymal space, with ICP values considered very accurate. Once the intracranial sensor is implanted, it is connected to a transducer that converts the impulses to a signal that the recording device can translate into an oscilloscope tracing, digital value, or graphic recording.

Transcranial blood flow is monitored with transcranial Doppler (TCD) studies to measure the velocity of blood flow in the cerebral vessels. Cerebral perfusion pressure (CPP) is the pressure it takes for the heart to provide the brain with blood, calculated by subtracting the ICP from mean arterial pressure (normal CPP is 70 to 95 mmHg). Brain oxygenation monitoring may be conducted by using

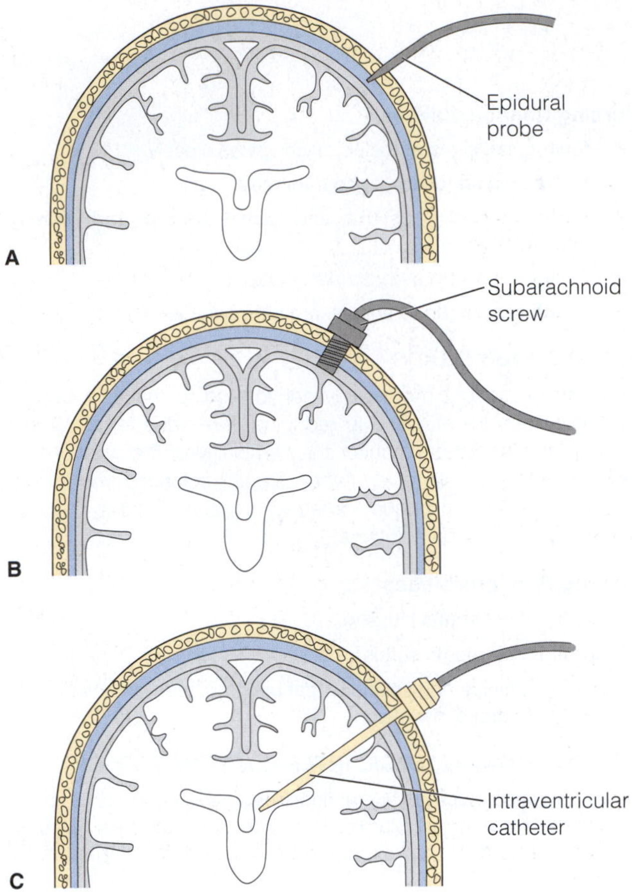
Epidural
probe
A
Subarachnoid
screw
B
Intraventricular
catheter
C

Figure 42.3 ■ Types of intracranial pressure monitoring. **A**, Epidural probe. **B**, Subarachnoid screw. **C**, Intraventricular catheter.

a jugular bulb oxygen saturation (SjO_2) monitor connected to a small fiberoptic catheter inserted into the jugular vein (normal SjO_2 is 50 to 75%). Another device used to monitor brain tissue oxygenation is the LICOX system, which includes information about oxygen status and temperature status within the brain tissue itself. In addition, cerebral microdialysis catheters can provide information about the nature of the cerebral interstitial fluid.

Mechanical Ventilation

Patients with ICP often require intubation and are placed on a ventilator for respiratory management. Mechanical ventilation may be used to maintain partial pressure of oxygen and carbon dioxide, thus preventing hypoxemia and hypercapnia, both of which can increase intracranial pressure. It is important to maintain adequate oxygenation with a partial pressure of arterial oxygen at about 100 mmHg and a partial pressure of arterial carbon dioxide of about 35 mmHg. The patient with IICP and signs of impending herniation may be carefully hyperventilated to cause cerebral vasoconstriction; however, this also increases cerebral ischemia.

Nursing Care

The nursing care of patients with IICP involves identifying those at risk and managing factors known to increase intracranial pressure. A major focus is protecting the patient from sudden increases in ICP or a decrease in cerebral blood flow.

Assessment

See the Manifestations and Interprofessional Care sections for the assessment of the patient with IICP.

Priorities of Care

Collaborating with the interprofessional team to ensure adequate treatment of the underlying process while providing care that supports the physical and psychologic responses to the disorder is a priority of nursing care.

Diagnoses, Outcomes, and Interventions

Nursing interventions include monitoring neurologic status, maintaining airway patency, ensuring adequate ventilation, positioning and moving, instituting seizure precautions (described later in this chapter), and monitoring fluids and electrolytes. Additionally, both patient and family need emotional support during this period.

Maintain Normal ICP. A number of disorders may lead to IICP, including cerebral edema, hydrocephalus, tumors, hematoma and hemorrhage, herniation syndromes, trauma, and changes in carbon dioxide concentrations. IICP alters cerebral perfusion and oxygenation of brain cells. The patient with IICP requires intensive care and often needs ventilator assistance.

Expected Outcome: Patient's ICP will be maintained within normal range as evidenced by motor/sensory functions, papillary size and reaction, and behaviors.

The nurse will:

- Assess for and report manifestations of IICP every 15 minutes to 1 hour and as necessary. Assessment areas include LOC, behavior, motor/sensory functions, pupillary size and reaction to light, and vital signs, including temperature. Look for trends because vital signs alone do not correlate well with early deterioration. *Assessment of neurologic status establishes the patient's clinical condition and provides a baseline for measuring changes. Sudden changes in neurologic signs often indicate deterioration. An elevated temperature with increased oxygen consumption further increases intracranial pressure. Pupillary responses mirror the status of the midbrain and pons. Pressure on the brainstem may compromise the function of cranial nerves IX and X and protective mechanisms, such as the gag and cough reflexes.*
- For the patient on a ventilator: Maintain patency of the airway; preoxygenate with 100% oxygen before suctioning; limit suctioning to 10 seconds; suction gently. *Preoxygenation helps maintain oxygen levels during suctioning. Suctioning stimulates the cough reflex and Valsalva maneuver. Correct suctioning minimizes the risk of hypoxemia.*
- Monitor ABGs. *ABGs provide a reliable indicator of oxygen and carbon dioxide levels. If oxygen concentration is low, oxygen may be given or increased.*
- Elevate head of the bed to 30 degrees or keep flat, as prescribed; maintain the alignment of the head and

neck to avoid hyperextension or exaggerated neck flexion; avoid prone position. *Keeping the head of the bed elevated facilitates venous drainage from the cerebrum. Obstruction of jugular veins can impede venous drainage from the brain.*

- Teach the patient at risk for or experiencing IICP (and able to follow instructions) to avoid coughing, blowing the nose, straining to have a bowel movement, pushing against the bed rails, or performing isometric (muscle contracting) exercises. *These actions increase ICP.*
- Monitor bladder distention and bowel constipation. Administer stool softeners and use the Credé technique (applying pressure to the suprapubic region with the fingers of one or both hands) to empty the bladder (if ordered). If the Credé technique is not effective, discuss with the physician urinary catheterization if the bladder remains distended. *Constipation and bladder distention increase intrathoracic or intra-abdominal pressure and place the patient at risk for impaired venous drainage from the brain.*
- If alert, assist in moving up in bed. Do not ask to push with heels or arms or push against a footboard. Avoid a footboard and restraints. *Moving up in bed requires pushing. Helping the patient move prevents initiation of the Valsalva maneuver, which increases intracranial pressure.*
- Plan nursing care so that activities are not clustered together; avoid turning the patient, getting the patient on the bedpan, or suctioning within the same time period. Schedule nursing care to provide rest periods between procedures. *Multiple procedures, including certain nursing care activities, can increase ICP. Constant stimulation tends to increase ICP. Individualized nursing care ensures optimal spacing of activities and rest.*
- Provide a quiet environment, limiting noxious stimuli. Avoid jarring the bed. Try to limit situations that cause emotional upset; maintain a calm, reassuring manner; caution family members to refrain from unpleasant conversations or conversations that may be emotionally stimulating to the patient. *Noxious stimuli and emotional upsets cause an elevation in ICP.*
- Maintain fluid limitations, if prescribed. *Restricting fluids helps decrease cerebral edema by reducing total body water.*

SAFETY ALERT: Often, the earliest manifestations of a change in intracranial pressure are alterations in the level of consciousness and respirations. ■

Reduce Risk for Infection. Although any patient with an open head wound is at risk for infection, the interventions discussed here are for the patient with an intracranial monitoring device. Most clinical units have written protocols for managing these systems. The following nursing actions serve only as a general guide.

Expected Outcome: Infection management and control will be maintained as evidenced by freedom from symptoms of infection, maintenance of white blood cell count and differential, and vital signs within normal limits.

The nurse will:

- Keep dressings over the catheter dry, and change dressings on a prescribed basis (usually every 24 to 48 hours). *Wet dressings are conducive to bacterial growth.*
- Monitor the insertion site for leaking CSF, drainage, or infection. Monitor for manifestations of infection, including changes in vital signs, chills, increased WBC counts, and positive cultures of drainage. *Close monitoring helps detect the earliest signs of infection and helps prevent major complications. Fever is usually considered the key assessment. However, fever in a patient with a neurologic disorder may be due to damage to the hypothalamus. Headache, generalized muscle aches, shivering, and chills may also be seen in the patient with infection.*
- Use strict aseptic technique when in contact with the device. Check drainage system for loose connections. *The use of aseptic technique and monitoring drainage systems for loose connections help prevent nosocomial infections. Most nosocomial infections are transmitted by healthcare workers who fail to wash their hands properly, to change gloves between patients, or to follow aseptic technique protocols. Invasive procedures provide an excellent opportunity for microbes to enter the body.*

Delegating Nursing Care Activities

As appropriate and allowed by the designated duties and responsibilities of unlicensed assistive personnel, the nurse may delegate nursing care activities such as measuring vital signs (including orthostatic vital signs) and providing skin care.

Transitions of Care

The underlying etiology of increased intracranial pressure is multifactorial. Preventive strategies focus on these etiologies.

Encourage the family to talk to the patient, but maintain a quiet environment with a minimum of stimuli. Inform family members that upsetting the patient may increase intracranial pressure and that they should avoid discussions that may distress the patient.

For patients unable to make decisions about treatment and to sign informed consent, the family must carry out these functions.

42.3 Seizures

A **seizure** is abnormal electrical discharge in the brain (Epilepsy Foundation, 2018b). This abnormal neuronal activity, which may involve all or part of the brain, disturbs skeletal motor function, sensation, autonomic function of the viscera, behavior, and/or consciousness. Although many of the disorders discussed in this chapter may cause seizures, this section focuses on **epilepsy** (seizure disorder), a chronic disorder of abnormal, recurring, excessive, and self-terminating electrical discharge from neurons. All people with epilepsy have seizures, but not all people who have a seizure have epilepsy. Only after an individual has two or more seizures is the diagnosis of epilepsy made (Epilepsy Foundation, 2018a).

Epilepsy is characterized by recurring seizures accompanied by some type of change in behavior. The time period between seizures may range from minutes to years.

Seizures and epilepsy are estimated to affect more than 3.4 million people of all ages, races, and ethnic backgrounds in the United States (Epilepsy Foundation, 2018a). There is a strong genetic component. Although people of any age may be affected, the prevalence and incidence of epilepsy increases in older adults (Sorenson et al., 2019).

Pathophysiology

Seizures occur when there is an excessive imbalance in excitation and inhibition in either focal areas of the cerebral cortex (causing focal seizures) or over the entire cerebral cortex (causing generalized seizures). Either a focal or a generalized increase in the excitability of neurons may result from energy failure of neurons, producing either transient depolarization or lack of local inhibition. Seizures may also result from alterations in membrane potentials that increase the risk of hypersensitive neurons responding abnormally to changes in the cellular environment.

All people have a seizure threshold; when this threshold is exceeded, a seizure may occur. In some people, the seizure threshold may be abnormally low, increasing their risk for seizure activity; in other people pathologic processes may alter the seizure threshold. The hypersensitive neurons that initiate seizure activity are called the *epileptogenic focus*. The epileptogenic focus generates a large number of discharges that are either enhanced or minimized, depending on the active neurotransmitter present on the postsynaptic membrane. Secondary epileptogenic foci may be induced in the same hemisphere through synapses or may spread to involve the opposite hemisphere through connecting pathways (Sorenson et al., 2019).

People who have epilepsy often experience triggers that provoke a seizure. Triggers may be individualized, such as specific music or odors and flashing lights. General triggers include fatigue, hypoglycemia, fever, alcohol consumption, constipation, hyperventilation, and menstruation.

Risk Factors

Although some precipitating factors for seizures are known (such as birth defects, trauma, brain tumors, IICP, metabolic disorders, Alzheimer's disease, and cardiovascular diseases), the cause is unknown in 70% of all cases (Sorenson et al., 2019). Isolated seizure episodes may occur in otherwise healthy people for a variety of reasons, including fever, infection, metabolic or endocrine disorder (such as hypoglycemia), or exposure to toxins.

Manifestations

Although seizures may be categorized in several different ways, the classification developed by the International League Against Epilepsy is the most useful clinically (Scheffer et al., 2017). It categorizes seizures as seizure types, epilepsy types, and epilepsy syndrome.

Seizure Types

The seizure type classes include: Focal, generalized, or unknown.

Focal Seizures. *Focal seizures* involve the activation of only a restricted part of one cerebral hemisphere. Manifestations may include alterations in motor function, sensory signs, or autonomic or psychic symptoms. Typically, the motor portion of the cortex is affected, causing recurrent muscle contractions of the face or a contralateral part of the body, such as a finger or hand. This motor activity may stay confined to one area or spread sequentially to adjacent parts, a phenomenon known as a *Jacksonian march* or *Jacksonian seizure*. Manifestations can also include the sensory portion of the brain, resulting in abnormal sensations or hallucinations. Disruptions in the function of the autonomic nervous system, with resulting tachycardia, flushing, hypotension, and hypertension, or psychic manifestations, such as a sense of déjà vu (a feeling that "this has happened before") or inappropriate fear or anger, may also be experienced. Focal seizures may be preceded by an **aura**, a warning sign of an impending seizure, such as an unusual smell, a sense of déjà vu, or a sudden intense emotion.

Generalized Seizures. *Generalized seizures* involve both hemispheres of the brain as well as deeper brain structures, such as the thalamus, basal ganglia, and upper brainstem. Consciousness is always impaired with generalized seizures. Absence and tonic–clonic seizures are the common forms of generalized seizure activity.

In an *absence seizure*, a sudden brief cessation of all motor activity accompanied by a blank stare and unresponsiveness can occur. Absence seizures are more common in children but also occur in adults. The seizure typically lasts only 5 to 10 seconds, although some may last for 30 seconds or more. Movements such as eyelid fluttering or automatisms such as lip smacking may occur during an absence seizure. Seizure activity may vary from occasional episodes to several hundred per day.

Tonic–clonic seizures (formerly called *grand mal*) are the most common type of seizure activity in adults. This type of seizure activity follows a typical pattern. A warning aura may precede generalized seizure activity. The aura may be a vague sense of uneasiness or an abnormal gustatory, visual, auditory, or visceral sensation (such as a metallic taste in the mouth, a smell of burning rubber, or seeing a bright light). Often, however, the seizure occurs without warning.

The seizure begins with a sudden loss of consciousness and sharp tonic muscle contractions (the tonic phase of the seizure). With the muscle contraction, air is forced out of the lungs, and the patient may cry out. Postural control is lost, and the patient falls to the floor in the opisthotonic posture (**Figure 42.4** ■). Muscles are rigid, with the arms and legs extended and the jaw clenched (**Figure 42.4A**). Urinary incontinence is common; bowel incontinence may also occur. Breathing ceases and cyanosis develops during the tonic phase of a seizure. The pupils are fixed and dilated. The tonic phase lasts an average of 15 seconds, although it may persist for up to a minute.

The clonic phase, which follows the tonic phase, is characterized by alternating contraction and relaxation of the muscles in all the extremities along with hyperventilation (**Figure 42.4B**). The eyes roll back, and the patient froths at the mouth. The clonic phase varies in duration and subsides

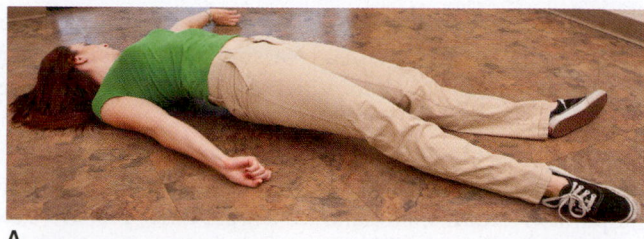

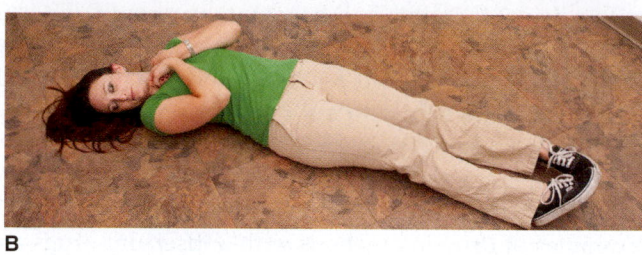
A
B

Figure 42.4 ■ Tonic–clonic seizures in grand mal seizures. **A**, Tonic phase. **B**, Clonic phase.

gradually. The entire tonic–clonic portion of the seizure generally lasts no more than 60 to 90 seconds.

Following the clonic phase of seizure activity, the person remains unconscious and unresponsive to stimuli. This period is known as the postictal period or phase. The person is relaxed and breathes quietly; he or she regains consciousness gradually and may be confused and disoriented on waking. Headache, muscle aches, and fatigue often follow the seizure, and the person may sleep for several hours. Amnesia of the seizure is usual; the person also may not recall events just prior to the seizure activity.

Because of the lack of warning with tonic–clonic seizures, head injury, fractures, burns, or motor vehicle crashes may occur secondarily to seizure activity.

Unknown Onset. Seizures when the onset is not determined.

Epilepsy Types

Epilepsy types require an existing epilepsy diagnosis. This usually requires that the patient has experienced more than one seizure.

Focal Epilepsy. This type of epilepsy includes unifocal and multifocal seizures. These also include single hemisphere seizures. There can be a range of seizure types, including focal aware, focal impaired awareness, focal motor, focal nonmotor, and bilateral tonic–clonic.

Generalized Epilepsy. This type of epilepsy has generalized spike-wave activity on EEG. There can be a range of seizure types, including absence, myoclonic, atonic, tonic, and tonic–clonic.

Combined Generalized and Focal Epilepsy. This new classification as of 2017 is for patients who have experienced both focal and generalized seizures. Dravet syndrome and Lennox-Gastaut syndrome are examples of combined generalized and focal epilepsy.

Unknown Epilepsy Type. This classification is used when a patient has a diagnosis of epilepsy but it cannot be determined by epilepsy type.

Epilepsy Syndrome

Epilepsy syndrome is the third level of classification, referring to a cluster of features including seizure type, EEG, and imaging features. The level of classification provides a guide for the many well-recognized syndromes (such as Dravet syndrome), although the ILAE has not approved any current syndromes.

Terms No Longer Used in Epilepsy Classification

The following terms are no longer used by the ILAE classification:

- Simple partial seizures
- Complex partial seizures
- Partial seizures
- Psychic seizures
- Dyscognitive seizures
- Secondarily generalized tonic–clonic seizures.

Status Epilepticus

Status epilepticus can develop during seizure activity. In this case, the seizure activity becomes continuous, with only very short periods of calm between intense and persistent seizures. The repetitive seizures may be of any type, although they are usually generalized tonic–clonic (Sorenson et al., 2019). Repeated seizures have a cumulative effect, producing muscular contractions that can interfere with respirations. Hypoxia, acidosis, hypoglycemia, hyperthermia, and exhaustion may occur if the convulsive activity is not halted.

Status epilepticus requires immediate intervention to preserve life. Establishing and maintaining the airway is a priority. A solution of 50% dextrose is administered IV to prevent hypoglycemia. Diazepam (Valium) or lorazepam (Ativan) is given intravenously, and the dose repeated in 10 minutes if necessary to stop seizure activity. Phenytoin (Dilantin) is administered IV for longer-term control of seizures. Phenobarbital may also be administered to patients in status epilepticus.

The Patient with Seizures

Interprofessional Care

Initial treatment focuses on controlling the seizure; the long-term goal is to determine the cause and prevent future seizures. Interprofessional care includes diagnostic testing, medications, and, in some cases, surgery.

Diagnosis

Diagnostic testing is performed to confirm the diagnosis and to determine any treatable causes and precipitating factors. Radiologic examinations include an MRI or CT scan to determine abnormalities in the brain and a skull x-ray to identify any bony abnormalities. An electroencephalogram (EEG) helps localize any brain lesions and confirm the diagnosis. A lumbar puncture may be performed to assess spinal fluid for CNS infections (increased WBCs) or tumors (increased protein levels). Blood studies are used to assess blood count, electrolytes, blood urea, and blood glucose.

Medications

Antiseizure drugs do not cure seizures or epilepsy, but they can reduce or control most seizure activity. More than 20 drugs are available for use in the treatment of epilepsy. Antiseizure drugs generally act in one of three ways: By potentiating gamma-aminobutyric acid (GABA), suppressing sodium influx, or suppressing calcium influx. These drugs suppress neuronal activity enough to prevent seizures.

The goals of medications for epilepsy are to protect the patient from harm and to reduce or prevent seizure activity without impairing cognitive function or producing undesirable side effects. Ideally, the lowest possible dose of a single medication that will control the patient's seizures is prescribed; however, several medications must be tried before the most effective is identified, and a combination of drugs may be needed to manage the patient's seizures. Therapy is individualized, based on the type of seizure activity and the patient's response to the medication. In most patients with seizures of a single type, satisfactory control can be established with a single antiseizure drug. Drugs that may be used with adults having either partial or mixed seizures include gabapentin (Neurontin), lamotrigine (Lamictal), oxcarbazepine (Trileptal), and topiramate (Topamax) (Adams, Holland, & Urban, 2017; Shields, Fox, & Liebrecht, 2018). Antiseizure drugs have been associated with suicidal thoughts and behavior; as a result, the U.S. Food and Drug Administration has issued a list of the warning signs. Nurses should assess for these manifestations and instruct the family to call the healthcare provider to report any unusual changes in the patient's mood or behavior. Examples of and nursing implications for antiseizure drugs are described in **Medication Administration 42.B**. Examples of drug interactions with antiseizure drugs are listed in **Box 42.1**.

Medication Administration 42.B

Seizures

ANTISEIZURE DRUGS

Potentiate GABA Action (Barbiturates, Benzodiazepines, and Other Drugs)

clonazepam (Klonopin)
diazepam (Valium)
gabapentin (Neurontin)
lorazepam (Ativan)
phenobarbital (Luminol)
pregabalin (Lyrica)
primidone (Mysoline)
topiramate (Topramax)

Suppress Sodium Influx (Hydantoins and Related Drugs)

carbamazepine (Tegretol)
fosphenytoin (Cerebrex)
lamotrigine (Lamictal)
levetiracetam (Keppra)
phenytoin (Dilantin)
valproic acid (Depakene)
zonisamide (Zonegran)

Suppress Calcium Influx

ethosuximide (Zarontin)
methsuximide (Celontin)

Antiseizure drugs are used to control chronic seizures and involuntary muscle spasms or movements characteristic of certain neurologic diseases. These drugs act in the motor cortex of the brain to reduce the spread of electrical discharges from the rapidly firing epileptic foci in this area. These agents control seizures without impairing the normal functions of the CNS. Drugs effective against one type of seizure may not be effective against another; anticonvulsant therapy must be individualized.

Nursing Responsibilities

- Monitor blood pressure, pulse, and respirations.
- Note evidence of CNS side effects, such as blurred vision, dimmed vision, slurred speech, nystagmus, or confusion. Gingival hyperplasia may be noted in patients taking phenytoin.
- Recognize that if patients are to be on prolonged therapy, they may need a diet rich in vitamin D.
- Monitor the serum calcium level as ordered; phenytoin can contribute to demineralization of bone.
- When administering anticonvulsants intravenously, monitor closely for respiratory depression and cardiovascular collapse.
- Administer gabapentin 2 hours after antacids.
- Administer tiagabine HCl with food.

Health Education for the Patient and Family

- Take the exact dosage prescribed. Do not increase, decrease, or discontinue the dosage without obtaining the primary care provider's approval; doing so may lead to convulsions.
- Avoid hazardous tasks until the drug has been regulated. Antiseizures may at first decrease mental alertness and cause drowsiness, headache, dizziness, and uncoordination of muscles. These effects are usually dose related and may disappear with a change of dosage or continued therapy. See **Box 42.1** for drug interactions with antiseizures
- If you are taking phenytoin (Dilantin), maintain good oral hygiene. Use a soft-bristled toothbrush, massage the gums, and floss daily.
- It is very important to obtain liver function studies regularly as ordered by the primary care provider. This will help detect early signs of hepatitis and other liver problems. Report for all scheduled laboratory studies, including complete blood count, kidney and liver function studies, and drug levels.
- Carry identification indicating the type of seizures for which you are being treated.
- Do not take gabapentin 1 hour before or less than 2 hours after an antacid.
- If you are taking lamotrigine and develop a rash, tell your healthcare provider.
- Take tiagabine HCl (Gabitril) with food.

Note: Drugs identified in blue are among the 200 most commonly prescribed medications in the United States.

Source: Adams, et al., 2017.

BOX 42.1
Drug Interactions with Antiseizure Drugs

- *Valproic acid (Depakene) and phenobarbital.* Blood levels of phenobarbital may rise significantly when valproic acid is added to the patient's medication regimen.
- *Phenobarbital and digoxin.* This combination may increase the metabolism of digoxin, resulting in decreased digoxin levels.
- *Phenobarbital and sodium warfarin (Coumadin).* Phenobarbital may decrease the absorption of sodium warfarin from the gastrointestinal tract and decrease the drug's anticoagulant response.
- *Disulfiram (Antabuse) and phenobarbital.* This combination may inhibit the metabolism of the antiseizure drug and increase the incidence of side effects associated with them.
- *Carbamazepine and oral contraceptives.* Carbamazepine decreases the effectiveness of oral contraceptives.
- *Other drugs.* Other drugs reported to interact with antiseizure drugs include aspirin, certain antibiotics, isoniazid, acetazolamide (Diamox), antacids, folic acid, and narcotics.

If the patient has been seizure free for at least 3 years, withdrawal of medications may be considered, with the dose of one drug at a time reduced over weeks or months. There is no way to predict which patients can remain seizure free without medication, but if seizures reoccur, the same medications usually provide good control.

Surgery

Resective surgery, with removal of the epileptogenic focus, is an option for patients whose seizures are not well controlled with antiseizure drugs. Candidates for this type of surgery include those who are unresponsive to medical management, who have a unilateral focus, and who have impaired quality of life from seizures. The goal of surgery is to reduce the patient's uncontrollable seizures. General postoperative care for the patient with intracranial surgery follows the nursing management guidelines outlined later in the chapter. Another surgical option is the Responsive Neurostimulator System, which uses electrodes implanted in the brain that are stimulated by low-level electrical current to suppress a seizure.

Vagal Nerve Stimulation Therapy

This therapy is designed to send regular, small pulses of electrical energy to the brain via the vagus nerve. A flat, round battery (about the size of a silver dollar) is implanted in the chest wall, and electrodes are threaded under the skin and wound around the vagus nerve in the neck. The battery is programmed to deliver a small amount of electrical energy every few seconds. The therapy does not stop the seizures, but rather reduces the number and improves the patient's quality of life.

Integrative Therapies

A ketogenic diet is a diet high in fat and low in carbohydrates and protein. This diet may have a beneficial impact on select patients with seizures (Adams et al., 2017). Cannabidiol (CBD), a component of marijuana, has been reported to reduce seizures in some children (National Center for Complementary and Integrative Medicine [NCCIM], 2018b).

Nursing Care

Nursing care is described for patients with a seizure disorder, but the care of the person during a seizure is the same regardless of the cause. See the Case Study & Nursing Care Plan for a patient with seizures on page 1563.

Assessment

See the Manifestations and Interprofessional Care sections for the assessment of the patient with seizures.

Collect the following data through the health history and physical examination:

- ***Health history:*** Past seizures; age when the first seizure occurred, most recent seizure; factors precipitating a seizure, any warning signs (aura); prophylactic anticonvulsant therapy; and specific concerns the patient may have about the seizures
- ***Physical assessment:*** Important data used in determining an accurate diagnosis describes manifestations obtained from nursing assessments before, during, and after a seizure. (**Table 42.3** lists nursing assessments before, during, and after a seizure, with rationale.)

Priorities of Care

Collaborating with the interprofessional team to ensure adequate treatment of the underlying process while providing care that supports the physical and psychologic responses to the disorder is a priority of nursing care.

Diagnoses, Outcomes, and Interventions

Nursing care of patients with seizures focuses on providing care during and immediately after the seizure and on patient/family teaching. The patient with seizures has a wide variety of responses to actual or potential changes in health status; interventions discussed in this section focus on facilitating physical and psychologic comfort and safety.

Maintain Adequate Airway Clearance. During a seizure, the tongue may fall back and obstruct the airway, the gag reflex may be depressed, and secretions may pool at the back of the throat. These may put the patient at risk for an obstructed airway. Most seizures occur in the home or community; therefore, teach these interventions to the patient's family:

Expected Outcome: Adequate airway clearance will be maintained through the use of protective interventions to maintain patent airway.

The nurse will:

- Provide interventions to maintain a patent airway:
  - a. Loosen clothing around the neck.
  - b. Turn on the side.
  - c. Do not force anything into the mouth.
  - d. If prescribed and available, administer oxygen by mask.

Although it was at one time believed that it was necessary to place a padded tongue blade in the patient's mouth during a

Table 42.3 Nursing Assessments Before, During, and After a Seizure

Assessment	Rationale
What was the patient's level of consciousness? If consciousness was lost, at what point?	Indicates area of brain involved and type of seizure.
What was the patient doing just before the attack?	May suggest precipitating factors.
In what part of the body did the seizure start?	May indicate the site of seizure activity in the brain tissue; for example, if jerking movements were first observed in the right hand, the seizure focus may be in the left motor cortex.
Was there an epileptic cry?	Usually indicates the tonic stage of a generalized tonic–clonic seizure.
Were any automatisms such as eyelid fluttering, chewing, lip smacking, or swallowing observed?	Often seen in complex, partial, and absence seizures.
How long did movements last? Did the location or character change (tonic to clonic)? Did movements involve both sides of the body or just one?	Indicates areas in which focal activity originated.
Did the head and/or eyes turn to one side and, if so, which side?	Helps localize the focus of the seizure. During the seizure, the head and eyes will typically turn away from the side of the epileptogenic focus.
Were there changes in pupillary reactions?	Indicates involvement of the autonomic nervous system.
If the patient fell, was the head hit?	Skull x-ray studies may be needed to rule out subdural hematoma or fracture.
Was there foaming or frothing from the mouth?	Usually indicates a tonic–clonic seizure.
Was there urinary or bowel incontinence?	Usually indicates a tonic–clonic seizure.

seizure, this is no longer recommended; an improperly placed tongue blade can obstruct the airway. Turning the patient on the side allows secretions to drain from the mouth.

- Teach family members or significant others how to care for the patient during a seizure to prevent airway obstruction. *Family members are often the only people present to provide this emergency intervention.*

Relieve Anxiety. The patient with a seizure disorder is understandably anxious about the future, with questions about ability to go to school or work, have a family, and drive a car. Feelings of embarrassment about having a seizure in public and rejection by others are common and also increase the patient's anxiety.

Expected Outcome: Patient will be able to control anxiety as evidenced by verbalized decrease in subjective distress.

The nurse will:

- Provide support by explaining that concerns are normal. *It is important to be sensitive to the effect of seizures on the patient's self-concept and body image; alterations in these areas not only increase anxiety but also cause withdrawal from socialization with others. Demonstrating acceptance of the patient's concerns allows further discussion.*
- Help identify safe leisure activities. *Worrying about being hurt if a seizure occurs may cause withdrawal from social activities that are pleasurable.*
- Provide information about sources and support groups. *Sharing information with other people with similar health problems allows for a more realistic viewpoint; accurate information can clear up misconceptions that cause anxiety.*
- Provide accurate information about hiring practices and legal limitations on driving or operating heavy or dangerous machinery. *Accurate information decreases anxiety about the unknown. The Americans with Disabilities Act prohibits discrimination; however, there are legal limitations on driving until the person is proven free of seizures.*

Provide Special Instructions for Women. Women with epilepsy require specific knowledge related to their menstrual cycle, contraception, and childbearing.

Expected Outcome: Patient will explain how to incorporate new health regimen into lifestyle.

The nurse will:

- Encourage discussion with the woman's healthcare provider about the increased probability of seizures at the time of menses. *Medications to prevent seizures may require dosage adjustments, and avoidance of other triggers is important.*
- Discuss the effects of antiseizure drugs. *These drugs decrease the effectiveness of oral contraceptives (decreased effectiveness is indicated by breakthrough bleeding); other forms of birth control (such as intrauterine devices) may be necessary. In addition, some antiseizures can cause birth defects if pregnancy does occur.*

Transitions of Care

Health promotion activities for the patient with seizures focus on teaching to reduce the incidence of seizure activity and to promote safety. Stress the following:

- Stress the importance of follow-up care, of keeping medical appointments, and of continuing to take antiepileptics as prescribed even when no seizures are experienced.
- Review any state and local laws that apply to people with seizure disorders. Driving a motor vehicle is usually prohibited for 6 months to 2 years after a seizure episode. Usually, a driver's license can be reinstated or obtained after a seizure-free period and a letter from the healthcare provider.

Case Study & Nursing Care Plan

A Patient with a Seizure Disorder

Janet Carlson is a 19-year-old college student who lives with her parents and one younger sister. Although Janet had seizures while she was in grade school, they have been controlled with medication. However, she had a tonic–clonic seizure yesterday and immediately made an appointment with her family physician. She is currently taking phenytoin (Dilantin) 300 mg/day as a maintenance medication to prevent seizures.

ASSESSMENT

Evita Farias, RN, completes a health history for Ms. Carlson. During the history, she tells Ms. Farias that she has been under stress because of difficulties in completing her course requirements this semester. She has not been sleeping as many hours per night, and sometimes she forgets to take her medication. Janet's serum phenytoin level is 8 mg/mL. Therapeutic level is 10 to 20 mg/mL.

DIAGNOSES

- Injury related to recurrence of generalized tonic–clonic seizure activity and low serum phenytoin levels
- Need for education about activities that may trigger seizure occurrence, the effect of stress on seizures, and medication information

EXPECTED OUTCOMES

- Patient will verbalize precipitating and triggering factors related to the onset of seizures.
- Patient will verbalize the relationship between emotional and physical stress and seizures.
- Patient will verbalize the importance of taking antiseizure medication.

PLANNING AND IMPLEMENTATION

- Teach patient and her family the following:
  - Current information about seizures
  - Care during and after a seizure
  - Medication protocols
  - Factors and activities that can trigger seizures
  - The importance of follow-up care.
- Refer patient and her family to a local epilepsy support group.
- Recommend that she purchase and wear a medical alert bracelet.

EVALUATION

Ms. Carlson is instructed to continue taking Dilantin 300 mg/day. She states the importance of nutrition, rest, and measures to reduce stress. She also discusses the importance of maintaining the proper blood levels of her medication, stating that too little or too much of the medication could cause problems. Ms. Carlson recognizes that the seizures had recurred during a busy time in school during which she had forgotten to take her medication. She is now wearing a medical alert bracelet. Ms. Farias provides the Carlsons with the telephone number of the Epilepsy Foundation of America.

CLINICAL REASONING IN PATIENT CARE

1. If you were Ms. Carlson's nurse, would your teaching differ if she were living alone? If so, how?
2. Ms. Carlson tells you that although she knows she should not drive a car, she often drives her friend to work. How would you approach this problem?
3. Ms. Carlson states, "It's embarrassing to wear a medical alert bracelet." How would you respond, and what recommendation(s) would you make?

See Evaluating Your Response in Appendix B.

- Know drug interactions with other prescribed drugs, over-the-counter (OTC) drugs, street drugs, and alcohol.
- Teach family members first aid for a seizure: Cushion the head, loosen anything tight around the neck, turn on the side, do not hold down.
- Teach family members to call for medical assistance if the seizures last for more than 5 minutes, recovery is slow, a second seizure occurs, there is difficulty breathing after recovery, or if there are signs of injury (such as bleeding from the mouth).

Teaching follows a systematic assessment of the needs of both the patient and family. Include family members so that they can learn seizure management, including the care and observations necessary before and during a seizure. Stress the importance of safety and keeping the airway patent during a seizure.

Help both the patient and family adjust to a diagnosis of epilepsy. Address the following topics:

- The importance of wearing a medical alert band or carrying a medical alert card at all times
- Avoiding alcoholic beverages and limiting coffee intake
- Taking showers versus tub baths, because of safety issues during a generalized seizure
- Factors that may trigger a seizure, and paying attention to an aura if one occurs
- Helpful resources, including the American Epilepsy Society and the Epilepsy Foundation.

42.4 Stroke

A **stroke** (cerebral vascular accident [CVA] or brain attack) is an emergency condition in which neurologic deficits result from a sudden decrease in blood flow to a localized area of the brain. Strokes may be ischemic (when blood supply to a part of the brain is suddenly interrupted by a thrombus, embolus, or blood vessel stenosis) or hemorrhagic (when a blood vessel ruptures, spilling blood into spaces surrounding neurons). The neurologic deficits caused by ischemia and the resultant necrosis of cells in the brain vary according to the area of the brain involved, the size of the affected area, and the length of time blood flow is decreased or stopped. A major loss of blood supply to the brain can cause severe disability or death. When the duration of decreased blood flow is short and the anatomic area involved is small, the person may not be aware that damage has been done.

On average, someone in the United States has a stroke every 40 seconds and dies of a stroke every 3 minutes and 45 seconds. Stroke is the fifth leading cause of death and the leading cause of adult disability in North America, where 795,000 people suffer a stroke each year. Of those, 160,000 die and many patients who survive are left with some type of functional impairment (American Heart Association [AHA], 2018). The risk doubles for every decade after age 55, and two-thirds of all strokes occur in people over the age of 65. As the population of baby boomers reaches and exceeds this age, stroke will be even more significant to healthcare providers.

Pathophysiology

The brain, which makes up only 2% of total body weight, receives approximately 20% of the cardiac output each minute (about 750 mL) and accounts for 20% of the body's oxygen consumption. Cerebral blood flow, especially in the deep cerebral vessels, is largely self-regulated by the brain to meet metabolic needs. This self-regulation (also called *autoregulation*) allows the brain to maintain a constant blood flow despite changes in systemic blood pressure. However, autoregulation is not effective when systemic blood pressure falls below 50 mmHg or rises above 160 mmHg. In the latter case, the increased systemic pressure causes an increase in cerebral blood flow with resultant overdistention of cerebral vessels. Cerebral blood flow also increases in response to increased carbon dioxide concentrations, increased hydrogen ion concentrations, and decreased oxygen concentrations.

When blood flow to and oxygenation of cerebral neurons are decreased or interrupted from a stroke, pathophysiologic changes at the cellular level take place in 4 to 5 minutes. Each minute during a stroke, 2 million brain cells die. The changes that take place are the result of a chain of chemical reactions called the *ischemic cascade* (Sorenson et al., 2019). This process occurs in three stages: Primary cell death, secondary cell death, and inflammation and immune response.

Primary cell death begins as blood supply is cut off to a part of the brain, resulting in ischemia in the core area of involved brain tissue. Anoxia and lack of nutrients to the cells affect the mitochondria of the cells, essentially depriving the cells of their energy source. As the mitochondria break down, they release oxygen-free radicals (such as glutamate) into the cytoplasm, destroying other intercellular structures. Cell membrane channels open, allowing calcium, sodium, and potassium to enter the cells. At the same time, the affected cells release excitatory amino acids into the intracellular spaces. Homeostasis is lost and water enters the cell (called *cytoxic edema*) to the point that the cells burst and quickly become infarcted and necrotic. This process begins in 4 to 5 minutes and may last as long as 2 to 3 hours.

Secondary cell death ensues from exposure to excessive amounts of glutamate, nitric oxide, free radicals, and excitatory amino acids released from necrotic cells. These cells, surrounding the area of initial damage, have only enough blood supply to remain alive for a few hours. If blood supply is restored to these cells within 2 to 3 hours, some cells can live and become functional. The area of living cells in and around the area of dead and necrotic cells is called the *penumbra*.

As secondary cell death is taking place, the body's immune system does further damage through an inflammatory reaction mediated by the vascular system. The initial damage attracts leukocytes to the damaged area; these white cells penetrate the endothelial wall, move through the blood–brain barrier, and invade the substance of the brain, causing further injury and cell death. Monocytes and macrophages release inflammatory chemicals (cytokines, interleukins, and tissue necrosis factor) at the site of injury to inhibit the release of natural tissue plasminogen activator and inactivate anticlotting factors. These effects make it more difficult for the body to dissolve a clot.

A stroke is characterized by a gradual or rapid onset of neurologic deficits due to compromised cerebral blood flow. The neurologic deficits that occur as a result of a stroke can often be used to identify its location. Because the motor pathways cross at the junction of the medulla and spinal cord (decussation), strokes lead to loss or impairment of sensorimotor functions on the side of the body *opposite* the side of the brain that is damaged. This effect, known as a **contralateral deficit**, means that a stroke in the right hemisphere of the brain is manifested by deficits in the left side of the body (and vice versa).

Ischemic Stroke

Ischemic strokes account for 87% of all strokes (Centers for Disease Control and Prevention [CDC], 2018b). The blockage may result from a blood clot (either as a thrombus or an emboli) or from stenosis of a vessel resulting from a buildup of plaque. Plaque may cause stenosis in large blood vessels or small blood vessels. Large vessel blockage usually is the result of thrombi. Small vessel strokes are small to very small infarcts in the deep, noncortical areas of the brain or the brainstem. Cardiogenic embolic strokes are caused by a blood clot (most commonly from atrial fibrillation) moving through cerebral blood vessels until the vessel is too small to allow further movement.

Transient Ischemic Attack. A **transient ischemic attack (TIA)**, sometimes called a *mini-stroke*, is a brief period of localized cerebral ischemia that causes neurologic deficits lasting for less than 24 hours (CDC, 2018b). TIAs are often warning signals of an ischemic thrombotic stroke. One or many TIAs may precede a stroke, with the time between the TIA and a stroke ranging from hours to months. The etiology of TIA includes inflammatory artery disorders, sickle cell disease, atherosclerotic changes in carotid and cerebral arteries, thrombosis, and emboli. Neurologic manifestations of a TIA vary according to the location and size of the cerebral vessel involved and have a sudden onset. Commonly occurring deficits include contralateral numbness or weakness of the leg, hand, forearm, and corner of the mouth; aphasia; and visual disturbances such as blurring. The patient may also experience a visual disturbance called *amaurosis fugax* (a fleeting blindness of one eye, described as a shade coming down over vision in the affected eye).

Large Vessel (Thrombotic) Stroke. A thrombotic stroke is caused by occlusion of a large cerebral vessel by a thrombus (blood clot). Thrombotic strokes most often occur in older people who are resting or sleeping. The blood pressure is lower during sleep, so there is less pressure to push the blood through an already narrowed arterial lumen, and ischemia may result (CDC, 2018b).

Thrombi tend to form in large arteries that bifurcate and have narrowed lumens as a result of deposits of atherosclerotic plaque. The plaque involves the intima of the arteries, causing the internal elastic lamina to become thin and frayed with exposure of underlying connective tissue. This structural change causes platelets to adhere to the rough surface and release the enzyme adenosine diphosphate. This enzyme initiates the clotting sequence, and a thrombus forms. A thrombus may remain in place and continue to enlarge, completely occluding the lumen of the vessel, or a part of it may break off and become an embolus. These strokes commonly affect a single cerebral artery supplying the cerebral cortex, causing aphasia, neglect syndrome, and/or visual field defects.

Small Vessel Stroke (Lacunar Infarct). Thrombotic strokes affecting the smaller cerebral vessels are called *lacunar (small vessel) strokes* because the infarcted areas slough off, leaving a small cavity or "lake" in the brain tissue. They occur in the deeper parts of the brain or the brainstem from occlusion of small branches of large cerebral arteries, most often the middle cerebral and posterior cerebral arteries. Manifestations include motor hemiplegia, sensory hemiplegia, and dysarthria.

Cardiogenic Embolic Stroke. A cardiogenic embolic stroke results when a blood clot from atrial fibrillation, ventricular thrombi, myocardial infarction, congestive heart disease, or atherosclerotic plaque (and other sources) enters the circulatory system and becomes lodged in a cerebral vessel too narrow to permit further movement. The blood vessel is then occluded. The most frequent sites of cerebral emboli are at bifurcations of vessels, particularly those of the middle cerebral artery.

Hemorrhagic Stroke

A hemorrhagic stroke, or intracranial hemorrhage, occurs when a cerebral blood vessel ruptures. There are two types of hemorrhagic strokes: Intracerebral hemorrhage and subarachnoid hemorrhage. An intracerebral hemorrhage often occurs in older adults with sustained increase in systolic–diastolic blood pressure. A subarachnoid hemorrhage is commonly seen in younger people. Intracranial hemorrhage usually occurs suddenly, often when the affected person is engaged in some activity. Although hypertension is the most common cause, a variety of factors may contribute to a hemorrhagic stroke, including rupture of a brittle plaque-encrusted artery wall, ruptured intracranial aneurysms, trauma, erosion of blood vessels by tumors, arteriovenous malformations, anticoagulant therapy, and blood disorders. Of all forms of stroke, this form is most often fatal. (Hemorrhagic strokes that result from ruptured cerebral aneurysm or an arteriovenous malformation are discussed in the next sections of the chapter.)

As a result of rupture of the blood vessel, blood enters the brain tissue, the cerebral ventricles, or the subarachnoid space, compressing adjacent tissues and causing blood vessel spasm and cerebral edema. Blood in the ventricles or subarachnoid space irritates the meninges and brain tissue, causing an inflammatory reaction and impairing absorption and circulation of CSF. The onset of manifestations from a hemorrhagic stroke is rapid. Manifestations depend on the location of the hemorrhage, but may include vomiting, headache, seizures, hemiplegia, and loss of consciousness. Pressure on brain tissue from IICP may cause coma and death.

Risk Factors

Certain diseases, lifestyle habits, and ethnic backgrounds increase the risk of a stroke. Risk factors include hypertension, sickle cell disease, atrial fibrillation, diabetes mellitus, hyperlipidemia, sleep apnea, smoking, and substance and alcohol abuse. Other risk factors include a previous stroke or TIA, family history of stroke, obesity, a sedentary lifestyle, and recent viral and bacterial infections. Risk factors specific to women are oral contraceptive use, pregnancy, childbirth, menopause, migraine headaches with aura, autoimmune disorders (such as diabetes and lupus), hormone replacement therapy, and clotting disorders. African Americans have about a one-third higher risk of having a stroke as do Caucasian Americans. Hispanics have a higher incidence of ischemic stroke at an earlier age and also have a higher incidence of intracerebral hemorrhage and subarachnoid hemorrhage (National Institute of Neurological Disorders and Stroke [NINDS], 2018a).

Risk factors are classified as unmodifiable (age, gender, race, and heredity) and modifiable (all disease and lifestyle risks). **Box 42.2** describes the risk factors for stroke in women.

Modifiable risk factors can be altered by prevention. The NINDS (2018a) recommends the following preventive

BOX 42.2
Risk Factors for Stroke in Women

Some risk factors for stroke apply only to women, most specifically pregnancy, childbirth, and menopause. These risks are the result of fluctuations in hormones that occur at different stages of life. However, other risks are also more common for women, and information should be collected during a health history. For accurate assessment, ask the following questions, depending on the woman's age:

- How many pregnancies have you had?
- Have you had a miscarriage? If so, how many?
- How many births have you had? When was your last delivery?
- When was your last menstrual period?
- Do you take any type of hormone replacement therapy?
- Do you take birth control pills?
- Do you have migraine headaches? If so, do you have an aura?
- Have you ever been diagnosed with diabetes or lupus?
- Have you ever been diagnosed with a clotting disorder? Have you ever had a clot in your leg?

measures for the most important treatable conditions that increase the risk of stroke:

- Hypertension: ***Treat it***. Eat a balanced diet, maintain a healthy weight, and exercise to reduce blood pressure.
- Cigarette smoking: ***Quit it***. Medical help is available.
- Heart disease: ***Manage it***. Healthcare providers can treat heart disease and prescribe medications to help prevent the formation of clots. For those over the age of 50, discuss aspirin therapy with your provider.
- Diabetes: ***Control it***. Treatment can delay complications that increase the risk of stroke.
- TIAs: ***Seek help***. TIAs should never be ignored and can be treated.

Early detection of stroke is critical to reducing extent of injury, complication, and morbidity. The American Stroke Association developed the mnemonic for stroke detection **Act FAST**:

Face: Ask the person to smile. Does one side of the face droop?

Arm: Ask the person to raise both arms. Does one arm drift downward?

Speech: Ask the person to repeat a simple sentence. Does the speech sound slurred or strange?

Time: If you observe any of these symptoms, it is time to call 9-1-1 or get to the nearest stroke center or hospital (National Stroke Association, 2018b).

Manifestations

Manifestations of a stroke vary according to the cerebral artery involved and the area of the brain affected. Women with stroke are more likely to report nontraditional manifestations (especially disorientation, confusion, or loss of consciousness) than men. Manifestations are always sudden in onset, focal, and usually one-sided. The various deficits associated with involvement of a specific cerebral artery are collectively referred to as stroke syndromes, although the deficits often overlap (American Stroke Association, 2018a). See **Table 42.4**.

Complications

Typical complications include sensory-perceptual deficits, cognitive and behavioral changes, communication disorders, motor deficits, and elimination disorders. These may be transient or permanent, depending on the degree of ischemia and necrosis as well as time of treatment. As a result of the neurologic deficits, the patient with a stroke has complications that involve many different body systems (**Table 42.5**). The disabilities resulting from a stroke often cause serious alterations in functional health status.

Sensory-Perceptual Deficits

A stroke may involve pathologic changes in neurologic pathways that alter the ability to integrate, interpret, and attend to sensory data. The patient may experience deficits in vision, hearing, equilibrium, taste, and sense of smell. The ability to perceive vibration, pain, warmth, cold, and pressure may be impaired, as may proprioception (the body's sense of its position). The loss of these

Table 42.4 Manifestations of a Stroke by Involved Cerebral Vessel

Vessel	Manifestations
Internal carotid artery	■ Contralateral paralysis of the arm, leg, and face ■ Contralateral sensory deficits of the arm, leg, and face ■ If the dominant hemisphere is involved: Aphasia ■ If the nondominant hemisphere is involved: Apraxia, agnosia, unilateral neglect ■ Homonymous hemianopia (see **Figure 42.5**)
Middle cerebral artery	■ Drowsiness, stupor, coma ■ Contralateral hemiplegia of the arm and face ■ Contralateral sensory deficits of the arm and face ■ Global aphasia (if dominant hemisphere involved) ■ Homonymous hemianopia
Anterior cerebral artery	■ Contralateral weakness or paralysis of the foot and leg ■ Contralateral sensory loss of the toes, foot, and leg ■ Loss of ability to make decisions or act voluntarily ■ Urinary incontinence
Vertebral artery	■ Pain in face, nose, or eye ■ Numbness and weakness of the face on involved side ■ Problems with gait ■ Dysphagia

Table 42.5 Manifestations and Complications of Stroke by Body System

Body System	Manifestations and Complications
Integument	■ Pressure injuries
Neurologic	■ Hyperthermia ■ Neglect syndrome ■ Seizures ■ Agnosia ■ Communication deficits: Expressive aphasia, receptive aphasia, global aphasia, agraphia ■ Visual deficits: Homonymous hemianopia, diplopia, decreased acuity ■ Cognitive changes: Memory loss, short attention span, distractibility, poor judgment, poor problem solving, disorientation ■ Behavioral changes: Emotional lability, loss of social inhibitions, fear, hostility, anger, depression ■ IICP ■ Alterations in consciousness ■ Sensory loss to touch, pain, heat, cold, pressure
Respiratory	■ Respiratory center damage ■ Airway obstruction ■ Decreased ability to cough
Gastrointestinal	■ Dysphagia ■ Constipation, stool impaction
Genitourinary	■ Incontinence, frequency, urgency ■ Urinary retention ■ Renal calculi
Musculoskeletal	■ Hemiplegia ■ Contractures ■ Bony ankylosis ■ Disuse atrophy ■ Dysarthria

sensory abilities increases the risk for injury. Deficits may include:

- **Hemianopia:** The loss of half of the visual field of one or both eyes; when the same half is missing in each eye, the condition is called *homonymous hemianopia* (refer to Figure 42.5).
- **Agnosia:** The inability to recognize one or more subjects that were previously familiar; agnosia may be visual, tactile, or auditory.
- **Apraxia:** The inability to carry out some motor pattern (e.g., drawing a figure, getting dressed) even when strength and coordination are adequate.

Another form of sensory-perceptual deficit is **neglect syndrome** (or *unilateral neglect*), in which the patient has a disorder of attention. In this syndrome, the person cannot integrate and use perceptions from the affected side of the body or from the environment on the affected side, and ignores that part. In severe cases, the patient may even deny the paralysis. This deficit is more common following a stroke of the right hemisphere where damage to the parietal lobe (a center for mediation of directed attention) results in perceptual deficits.

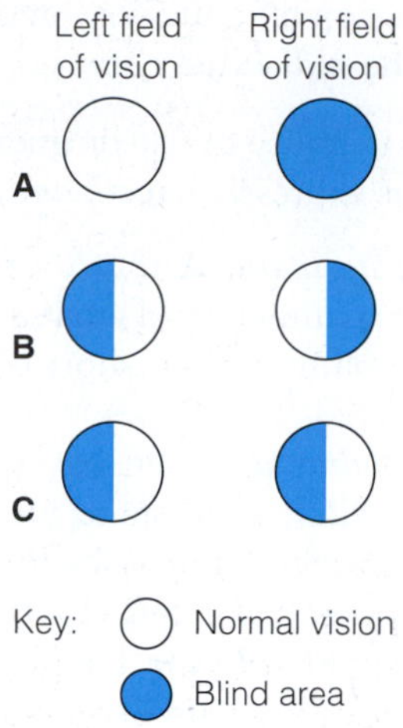
Left field of vision
Right field of vision
A
B
C
Key:
Normal vision
Blind area

Figure 42.5 ■ Abnormal visual fields. **A**, Normal left field of vision with loss of vision in right field. **B**, Loss of vision in temporal half of both fields (bitemporal hemianopia). **C**, Loss of vision in nasal field of right eye and temporal field of left eye (homonymous hemianopia).

Pain and discomfort may accompany a stroke, with the patient experiencing acute pain, numbness, or strange sensations. Although not common, damage to the thalamus may cause central stroke pain or central pain syndrome (CPS). The pain in this syndrome includes hot and cold, burning, tingling, and sharp stabbing pain, most often in the extremities. It is worsened by movement and temperature changes. The painful sensations are not relieved by pain medications, nor are there any specific treatments.

Cognitive and Behavioral Changes

A change in consciousness, ranging from mild confusion to coma, is a common manifestation of a stroke. It may result from tissue damage following ischemia or hemorrhage involving either the carotid or vertebral arteries. Altered consciousness may also be the result of cerebral edema or IICP.

Behavioral changes include emotional lability (in which the patient may laugh or cry inappropriately), loss of self-control (manifested by behavior such as swearing or refusing to wear clothing), and decreased tolerance for stress (resulting in anger or depression). Intellectual changes may include memory loss, decreased attention span, poor judgment, and an inability to think abstractly.

Communication Disorders

Communication is a complex process, involving motor functions, speech, language, memory, reasoning, and emotions. Communication disorders are usually the result of a stroke affecting the dominant hemisphere. The left hemisphere is dominant in about 95% of right-handed people and 70% of left-handed people (Sorenson et al., 2019). Many different impairments may occur, and most are partial. Disorders of communication affect both speech (the mechanical act of articulating language through the spoken word) and language (the vocal or written formulation of ideas to communicate thoughts and feelings). Language involves oral and written expression and auditory and reading comprehension. Among these disorders are:

- **Aphasia:** The inability to use or understand language; aphasia may be expressive, receptive, or mixed (global).
  - ***Expressive aphasia:*** A motor speech problem in which one can understand what is being said but can respond verbally only in short phrases; also called *Broca aphasia*.
  - ***Receptive aphasia:*** A sensory speech problem in which one cannot understand the spoken (and often written) word. Speech may be fluent but with inappropriate content; also called *Wernicke aphasia*.
  - ***Mixed or global aphasia:*** Language dysfunction in both understanding and expression.
- ***Dysarthria:*** Any disturbance in muscular control of speech.

Motor Deficits

Body movement results from a complex interaction between the brain, spinal cord, and peripheral nerves. The motor areas of the cerebral cortex, the basal ganglia, and the cerebellum initiate voluntary movement by sending messages to the spinal cord, which then transmits the messages to the peripheral nerves. A stroke may interrupt the CNS component of this relay system and produce effects in the contralateral side ranging from mild weakness to severe limitation of any kind of movement.

Depending on the area of the brain involved, strokes may cause weakness, paralysis, and/or spasticity. The deficits include:

- **Hemiplegia:** Paralysis of the left or right half of the body (**Figure 42.6** ■).
- **Hemiparesis:** Weakness of the left or right half of the body.
- ***Flaccidity:*** Absence of muscle tone (hypotonia).
- ***Spasticity:*** Increased muscle tone (hypertonia), usually with some degree of weakness. The flexor muscles are usually more strongly affected in the upper extremities, and the extensor muscles are more strongly affected in the lower extremities.

When the corticospinal tract is involved, the affected arm and leg almost always are initially flaccid and then become spastic within 6 to 8 weeks. Spasticity often causes characteristic body positioning: Adduction of the shoulder, pronation of the forearm, flexion of the fingers, and extension of the hip and knee. There is often foot drop, outward rotation of the leg, and dependent edema in the involved extremities.

The motor deficits may result in altered mobility, further impairing body function. The complications of immobility involve multiple body systems and include orthostatic hypotension, increased thrombus formation, decreased cardiac output, impaired respiratory function, osteoporosis, formation of renal calculi, contractures, and decubitus ulcer formation.

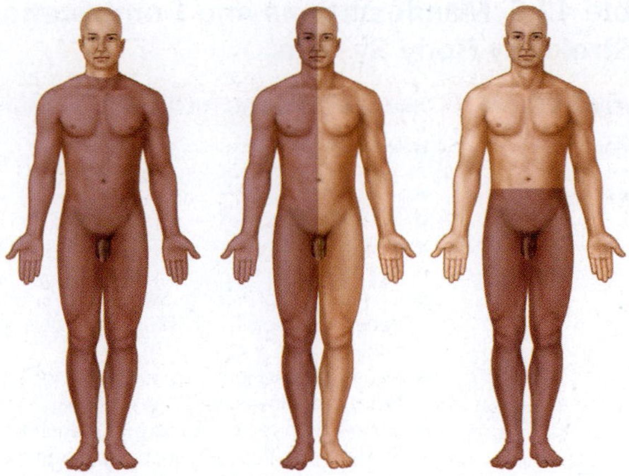

A Quadriplegia
B Hemiplegia
C Paraplegia

Figure 42.6 ■ Types of paralysis. **A**, Quadriplegia is complete or partial paralysis of the upper extremities and complete paralysis of the lower part of the body. **B**, Hemiplegia is paralysis of one-half of the body when it is divided along the median sagittal plane. **C**, Paraplegia is paralysis of the lower part of the body.

Elimination Disorders

Disorders of bladder and bowel elimination are common. A stroke may cause partial loss of the sensations that trigger bladder elimination, resulting in urinary frequency, urgency, or incontinence. Control of urination may be altered as a result of cognitive deficits. Changes in bowel elimination are common, resulting from changes in LOC, immobility, and dehydration.

The Patient with a Stroke

Interprofessional Care

The type of treatment a patient with a stroke receives depends on the stage of the disease. In general, there are three treatment stages: Stroke prevention, acute care immediately after a stroke, and rehabilitation after a stroke. The patient with an acute stroke may receive medical and/or surgical treatment. The focus in the acute care phase is on diagnosing the type and cause of the stroke, supporting cerebral circulation, and controlling or preventing further deficits. The goals of stroke care are to minimize brain injury and maximize patient recovery. The focus of acute care has shifted from the nearest hospital to certified stroke centers (if possible) where patients with a stroke can be provided appropriate care from entrance to the emergency department to discharge following rehabilitation.

Diagnosis

Diagnosis begins with a complete history and careful physical assessment, including a thorough neurologic examination. The time of the onset of stroke manifestations is a critical part of assessment. The National Institutes of Health (NIH; 2003) Stroke Scale is the seminal clinical evaluation tool widely used to assess neurologic outcome and degree of recovery. Part of the scale is illustrated in **Table 42.6**. The

Table 42.6 NIH Stroke Scale: Assessment of Level of Consciousness

Instructions	Scale Definition	Score*
1a. Level of Consciousness		
The investigator must choose a response, even if a full evaluation is prevented by such obstacles as an endotracheal tube, language barrier, orotracheal trauma/bandages. A 3 is scored only if the patient makes no movement (other than reflexive posturing) in response to noxious stimulation.	0 = Alert, keenly responsive 1 = Not alert, but arousable by minor stimulation to obey, answer, or respond 2 = Not alert, requires repeated stimulation to attend, or is obtunded and requires strong or painful stimulation to make movements (not stereotyped) 3 = Responds only with reflex motor or autonomic effects or totally unresponsive, flaccid, movements are dysreflexic	______
1b. LOC Questions		
The patient is asked the month and his or her age. The answer must be correct. There is no partial credit for being close. Aphasic and stuporous patients who do not comprehend the questions will score 2. Patients unable to speak because of endotracheal intubation, orotracheal trauma, severe dysarthria from any cause, language barrier, or any other problem not secondary to aphasia are given a 1. It is important that only the initial answer be graded and that the examiner not help the patient with verbal or nonverbal cues.	0 = Answers both questions correctly 1 = Answers one question correctly 2 = Answers neither question correctly	______
1c. LOC Commands		
The patient is asked to open and close the eyes and then to grip and release the nonparetic hand. Substitute another one-step command if the hands cannot be used. Credit is given if an unequivocal attempt is made but not completed due to weakness. If the patient does not respond to command, the task should be demonstrated to him or her (pantomime) and score the results (i.e., follows none, one, or two commands). Patients with trauma, amputation, or other physical impediments should be given suitable one-step commands. Only the first attempt is scored.	0 = Performs both tasks correctly 1 = Performs one task correctly 2 = Performs neither task correctly	______

*A lower score indicates better function.
Adapted from *https://stroke.nih.gov/documents/NIH_Stroke_Scale.pdf*.

tool measures LOC, vision, facial paralysis, motor abilities, ataxia, sensation, language, and attention. The entire scale may be accessed at the website for the National Institute of Neurological Disorders and Stroke.

Imaging tests are used to identify an increased risk for a stroke or to identify pathophysiologic changes after a stroke has occurred. Computed tomography (CT) is the first imaging technique used to demonstrate the presence of hemorrhage, tumors, aneurysm, ischemia, edema, and tissue necrosis. A CT scan can also demonstrate a shift in intracranial contents and is useful in distinguishing the type of stroke (e.g., a hemorrhagic stroke results in an increase in density). Cerebral infarctions are usually visible with a CT scan 6 to 8 hours after a stroke; hemorrhage is visible immediately. Other imaging tests that may be used for diagnosis include a cerebral arteriogram, a transcranial ultrasound Doppler, an MRI, an MRA, a PET, and a SPECT. A perfusion- and diffusion-weighted imaging (DWI) test can be used to identify cerebral ischemia immediately after onset of the stroke and also identify areas of possibly reversible damage (the penumbra). In addition to imaging tests, a blood test has recently been approved to screen for recurrent stroke risk. The PLAC test scans the blood for high levels of lipoprotein-associated phospholipase A2 (Lp-Pla2), found to be more common in people who have had strokes.

A lumbar puncture may be performed to obtain CSF for examination if there is no danger of IICP. An ischemic stroke may elevate CSF pressure; after a hemorrhagic stroke blood may be seen in the CSF.

Medications

Medications are administered to prevent a stroke in patients with TIAs or a previous stroke and to treat the patient during the acute phase of a stroke. Treatment for IICP was discussed in a previous section of the chapter.

Prevention. Antiplatelet agents are often used to treat patients with TIAs or who have had a previous stroke. Platelets are concentrated in high blood flow arteries, where they adhere to endothelial tissue damaged by atherosclerosis and occlude the vessel. The drugs used to prevent clot formation and blood vessel occlusion include aspirin, clopidogrel (Plavix), dipyridamole (Persantine), and ticlopidine (Ticlid). Daily low-dose aspirin reduces TIA occurrence and stroke risk by interfering with platelet aggregation. Ticlopidine (Ticlid) is a platelet-aggregation inhibitor that has shown reduction in thrombotic stroke risk.

Acute Stroke. Medications are used to treat the patient during the acute phase of an ischemic stroke to prevent further thrombosis formation, increase cerebral blood flow, and protect cerebral neurons. The type of medication used varies according to the type of stroke.

Fibrinolytic therapy, using a tissue plasminogen activator such as recombinant tissue-type plasminogen activator alteplase (tPA), sometimes given concurrently with an anticoagulant, is used to treat ischemic stroke. The drug converts plasminogen to plasmin, resulting in fibrinolysis of the clot. To be effective, it must be given IV within 3 hours of the onset of manifestations, after confirming (with a CT scan) that the patient has not had a hemorrhagic stroke. However, a European study found that tPA administered between 3 and 4.5 hours after the onset of manifestations significantly improved clinical outcomes, although it also increased the risk of intracranial hemorrhage. Antithrombotic drugs, which inhibit the platelet phase of clot formation, have been used as a preventive measure for patients at risk for ischemic stroke. Both aspirin and dipyridamole have been used for this purpose. These drugs are sometimes also used in combination with other drugs during acute treatment. Antiplatelet agents are contraindicated in patients with a hemorrhagic stroke.

Anticoagulant drug therapy (refer to Chapter 30) may be ordered for an ischemic stroke. The most commonly used anticoagulants are warfarin (Coumadin), heparin, and enoxaparin (Lovenox). Anticoagulants do not dissolve an existing clot but rather prevent further extension of the clot and formation of new clots. Sodium heparin may be given subcutaneously or by continuous IV drip, or warfarin sodium (Coumadin) may be given orally. It is recommended that the use of antifactor Xa be used to monitor blood coagulation (Adams et al., 2017).

Management of hypertension is controversial but if the patient is eligible for fibrinolytic therapy, blood pressure control is essential to decrease the risk of bleeding. If the blood pressure is sustained at systolic levels >185 mmHg or diastolic levels >110 mmHg, the patient cannot be treated with IV tPA.

SAFETY ALERT: Anticoagulants are never administered to a patient with a hemorrhagic stroke. ■

Nutrition

While there are no specific dietary recommendations to help prevent a stroke, a healthy diet includes a wide variety of fruits and vegetables and lean protein and avoids overuse of saturated fats and concentrated sugar.

Surgery

Surgery may be performed to prevent the occurrence of a stroke, to restore blood flow when a stroke has already occurred, or to repair vascular damage or malformations. In people who have had TIAs or are in danger of having another stroke, a carotid endarterectomy at the carotid artery bifurcation may be performed to remove atherosclerotic plaque (**Figure 42.7** ■). Nursing care for the patient in the initial postoperative period following a carotid endarterectomy is described in **Box 42.3**.

When an occluded or stenotic vessel is not directly accessible, an extracranial–intracranial bypass may be performed through bypass of the internal carotid, middle cerebral, or vertebral arteries. The procedure reestablishes blood flow to the affected area of the brain. A carotid angioplasty with stenting is an option for treating cerebral stenosis. During the procedure an angioplasty balloon catheter is inserted through an artery in the patient's arm or leg. Under

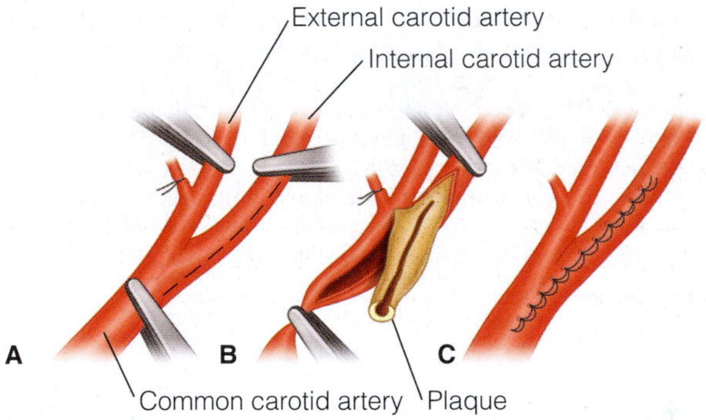
External carotid artery
Internal carotid artery
A
B
C
Common carotid artery
Plaque

Figure 42.7 ■ Carotid endarterectomy. **A**, The occluded area is clamped off and an incision is made in the artery. **B**, Plaque is removed from the inner layer of the artery. **C**, To restore blood flow through the artery, the artery is sutured or a graft is completed.

BOX 42.3
Nursing Care of the Patient Having a Carotid Endarterectomy

POSTOPERATIVE CARE

- Position on the unoperated side and either maintain a flat position or elevate the head of the bed 30 degrees as prescribed. Maintain head and neck alignment and avoid rotating, flexing, or hyperextending head. *Pressure on the wound is undesirable. Elevating the head decreases edema in the operative site. Maintaining head and neck alignment prevents additional tension or pressure on the operative side.*
- Support the head when changing position. Teach to support the head with the hands when able to move about. *Supporting the head helps prevent stress on the operative site (which may cause bleeding and hematoma formation); it also helps reduce stress on the suture line.*
- Assess respirations and oxygen saturation.
  a. *Hemorrhage.* Assess the dressing and the area under the neck and shoulders for drainage. Assess for increased pulse and decreased blood pressure. *The most common cause of respiratory problems is pressure on the trachea from a hematoma formation.*
  b. *Respiratory distress.* Assess respiratory rate, rhythm, depth, and effort. Observe for restlessness. Keep a tracheostomy tray at the bedside. *Respiratory distress may result from edema and hematoma formation, which may compress the trachea.*
  c. *Cranial nerve impairment.* Observe and record any facial drooping, tongue deviation, hoarseness, dysphagia, or loss of facial sensation. *Cranial nerves may be stretched during surgery, leading to temporary deficits in cranial nerve function.*
  d. *Hypertension or hypotension.* Take and record blood pressure at least hourly. Report any changes immediately and implement orders for medications to treat hypertension or hypotension. *About one-half of all patients having a carotid endarterectomy develop unstable blood pressure related to surgical denervation of the carotid sinus. Uncontrolled hypertension may precipitate a stroke. The most common problem is hypotension, possibly related to stimulation of the carotid body baroreceptors, which are exposed during surgery. Hypotension may result in myocardial ischemia.*

fluoroscopy, the catheter is advanced to the area of carotid artery stenosis and a small filter is inserted to catch any clots or pieces of debris that might break loose. The balloon is then inflated to widen the artery, followed by insertion of a permanent stent in the area of the angioplasty.

Other treatments include suctioning the clot out of the artery or threading a wire through the clot and pulling it out. A noninvasive method of improving recovery from a stroke, called *noninvasive transcranial direct current stimulation (TDCS)*, has been shown to improve motor outcomes and is under study.

Rehabilitation

Various types of interprofessional therapy are necessary for poststroke rehabilitation. These are most often provided in a setting dedicated to rehabilitation. Patients are frequently transferred to these settings for poststroke care for several weeks before being discharged to home. Listed next are the types and goals of therapies used.

- ***Physical therapy*** may help prevent contractures and improve muscle strength and coordination. Physical therapists teach exercises to enable the patient to relearn how to walk, sit, lie down, and change from one type of movement to another.
- ***Occupational therapy*** provides assistive devices and a plan for regaining lost motor skills that greatly improve quality of life after a stroke. These skills include eating, drinking, bathing, cooking, reading, writing, and toileting.
- ***Speech and language therapy*** is provided to help the patient improve swallowing as well as how to relearn language and communication skills.

Nursing Care

Even though many people who have a stroke have full recovery, a substantial number are left with disabilities that affect their physical, emotional, interpersonal, and family status. The required nursing care is often complex and multidimensional, requiring consideration of continuity of care for patients in acute care settings, long-term care settings, rehabilitation centers, and the home.

Nurses caring for patients who have had a stroke require knowledge and skill to meet patient and family needs during both the acute and the rehabilitative phases of care. The patient may have multiple losses: Loss of mobility, ability to provide self-care, communications, concept of self, and interpersonal or intimate relationships with others. Holistic, individualized nursing care is essential in all settings and focuses on promoting the achievement of maximum potential and quality of life.

The patient's family is often faced with many changes. The young to middle-age adult with a family member who has had a stroke may be faced with economic difficulties and social isolation. The middle-age adult family member may become the caretaker for an older parent. An older adult may not be able to care for a spouse and may have to accept long-term care placement. In addition, the older adult who has no family may have to struggle alone to regain the ability to function independently. Although not all of these problems are amenable to nursing solutions, the nurse is most often the healthcare provider who assesses and identifies the needs of each individual and provides information and referrals to patients and families to help meet those needs.

Because a stroke has the potential to cause many different health problems, a wide variety of nursing diagnoses may be appropriate. It is important to remember that each person will be affected differently, depending on the degree of ischemia and the area of the brain involved. Nursing diagnoses discussed in this section focus on problems with cerebral tissue perfusion (specific to nursing care during the acute phase), physical mobility, self-care, communication, sensory-perceptual deficits, bowel and urine elimination, and swallowing (specific to prevention of complications and rehabilitation). In addition, many of the diagnoses, outcomes, and interventions provided for the patient with alterations in consciousness, IICP, and seizures may be appropriate. See the Case Study & Nursing Care Plan for a patient with a stroke on page 1575.

Assessment

See the Manifestations and Interprofessional Care sections for the assessment of the patient with stroke.

The following data are collected through the health history and physical examination. Further focused assessments are described with nursing interventions. If the patient is a woman, she has risks for stroke that are different than those of a man and should be asked questions specific to her gender (see Box 42.2).

- ***Health history:*** Risk factors, previous stroke, drug use (prescribed, OTC, and street drugs), smoking history, when manifestations began, severity of manifestations, presence of incontinence, family support system, advance directives or medical power of attorney
- ***Physical assessment:*** Stroke scale, level of consciousness, vital signs, motor strength, coordination, communication, cranial nerves, sensory function, skin integrity, mobility status.

Priorities of Care

Collaborating with the interprofessional team to ensure adequate treatment of the underlying process while providing care that supports the physical and psychologic responses to the disorder is a priority of nursing care.

Diagnoses, Outcomes, and Interventions

Depending on the severity of the stroke, the patient may be admitted to the intensive care unit. Regardless of the hospital setting, the nurse provides interventions to maintain functional status and prevent complications.

Maintain Adequate Cerebral Perfusion. The initial assessment and care of the patient admitted for intensive care focuses on identifying changes that may indicate altered cerebral perfusion. The patient's airway, breathing, circulation, and neurologic status are monitored and interventions are provided to maintain cerebral perfusion.

Expected Outcome: Patient will demonstrate appropriate orientation to person, place, time and situation as indicated. Patient's cerebral perfusion will be adequate as evidenced by motor/sensory functions, pupillary size and reaction, and behaviors.

The nurse will:

- Monitor respiratory status, oxygen saturation, and airway patency. Auscultate pulmonary sounds and monitor respiratory rate and results of studies of arterial blood gases.
- Suction as necessary, using care to suction no longer than 10 seconds at any one time, using sterile technique.
- Administer oxygen as prescribed.

  The patient may be unconscious and breathing may be impaired. Suctioning removes secretions that obstruct air flow, but also decreases O_2, increases CO_2, and partially obstructs the airway. Suctioning for longer than 10 seconds at a time may increase intracranial pressure (Perrin & MacLeod, 2018). *Respiratory complications develop rapidly, as manifested by crackles and wheezes, rapid respirations, and respiratory acidosis. The administration of oxygen decreases the risk for hypoxia and hypercapnia, which can increase cerebral ischemia and intracranial pressure.*
- Position the patient on the side. *Side positioning allows secretions to drain out of the mouth, helping to prevent aspiration.*

SAFETY ALERT: When lying on the affected side, patients may be restless because they do not have normal sensation and may feel as if they are going to fall. ■

- Monitor mental status and LOC: Restlessness, drowsiness, lethargy, inability to follow commands, unresponsiveness. *Changes in mental status and LOC are often initial manifestations of IICP.*
- Assess for pain, headache, decreased muscle strength, sluggish pupillary reflexes, absent gag or swallowing reflexes, hemiplegia, Babinski's sign, and decerebrate or decorticate posturing. *Frequent monitoring of neurologic status is necessary to detect changes. Alterations in mental status, LOC, movement, strength, and reflexes indicate IICP, the major cause of death in the acute phase of a stroke.*
- Continuously monitor cardiac status, observing for dysrhythmias. *A stroke may cause cardiac dysrhythmias, including bradycardia, PVCs, tachycardia, and AV block. Characteristic ECG changes include a shortened PR interval, peaked T waves, and a depressed ST segment.*
- Monitor body temperature and maintain temperature at less than 37°C (98.6°F) at all times during acute care. *In a large meta-analysis, fever was consistently found to be associated with worse outcomes in patients with stroke.*
- Maintain accurate intake and output records. Measure urinary output via a Foley catheter. *A stroke may damage the pituitary gland, resulting in diabetes insipidus and the possibility of dehydration from greatly increased urinary output. If a Foley catheter is inserted, follow strict guidelines to prevent infection and for securing the catheter.*
- Monitor for diabetes insipidus and dehydration. *Diabetes insipidus is indicated by a large output of dilute urine; dehydration is indicated by scanty amounts of dark, concentrated urine. Clarification of the difference in symptoms promotes appropriate intervention delivery.*
- Monitor for seizures. Pad the side rails, and administer prescribed antiseizure drugs. *Seizures may be the result of cerebral tissue damage or IICP. Padded side rails prevent injury if a seizure occurs. Antiseizure drugs prevent or treat seizures.*

Promote Physical Mobility. The goals of care for patients with impaired mobility are to maintain and improve functional abilities (by maintaining normal function and alignment, preventing edema of extremities, and reducing spasticity) and to prevent complications.

Expected Outcome: Patient's joint range of motion will be maintained with progression to transfers and ambulation as tolerated and appropriate for condition.

The nurse will:

- Encourage active ROM exercises for unaffected extremities and perform passive ROM exercises for affected extremities every 4 hours during day and evening shifts and once during the night shift. Support the joint during passive ROM exercises. *Active ROM exercises maintain or improve muscle strength and endurance and help to maintain cardiopulmonary function. Passive ROM exercises do not strengthen muscles but do help maintain joint flexibility.*
- Turn every 2 hours around the clock, following a posted schedule for side-to-side and supine-to-prone position changes (verify prone positioning with the physician). Maintain body alignment and support extremities in proper position with pillows. *Turning on a regular basis, accompanied by proper positioning, maintains joint function, alleviates pressure on bony prominences that can lead to skin breakdown, decreases dependent edema in hands and feet, and lessens the risk of complications resulting from immobility.*
- Monitor the lower extremities each shift for manifestations of thrombophlebitis. Assess for increased warmth and redness in calves; measure the circumference of the calves and thighs. Provide care for sequential compression stockings (per agency protocol), if prescribed. *Patients on bedrest (especially those with loss of muscle strength and tone) are particularly prone to the development of deep venous thrombosis. Promptly report manifestations of thrombophlebitis.*
- Collaborate with the physical therapist as the patient gains mobility, using consistent techniques to move the patient from the bed to the wheelchair and to help the patient ambulate. *The use of consistent techniques facilitates rehabilitation.*

SAFETY ALERT: Both active and passive exercises increase venous return, decreasing the risk of thrombophlebitis. ■

Promote Self-Care. The patient who has had a stroke may be unable to perform self-care (bathing, dressing, feeding, and/or toileting) as a result of impaired mobility or mental confusion. It is important for patients to perform as much of their own physical care and grooming as possible to promote functional ability, increase independence, decrease feelings of powerlessness, and improve self-esteem. Before establishing a plan to increase self-care, determine which hand was dominant before the stroke. If the patient's dominant side is affected, self-care will be more difficult.

Expected Outcome: Patient will be able to complete self-care activities to optimal potential.

The nurse will:

- Screen for executive cognitive dysfunction (abstract thought, actions planned and taken toward a goal, adaptation to the unexpected). *Executive cognitive dysfunction can more reliably predict loss of autonomy than memory impairment can. This assessment is essential to helping a patient remain as safe and independent as possible.*
- Encourage use of the unaffected arm to bathe, brush teeth, comb hair, dress, and eat. *Use of the unaffected arm promotes functional ability and independence.*
- Teach the patient to put on clothing by first dressing the affected extremities and then dressing the unaffected extremities. *This technique facilitates self-dressing with minimal assistance.*
- Collaborate with the occupational therapist in scheduling times for training for upper extremity functioning necessary for activities of daily living (ADLs). Encourage the use of assistive devices (if required) for eating, physical hygiene, and dressing. *Following a regular schedule in daily routines promotes learning. The use of assistive devices promotes independence and decreases feelings of powerlessness. Optimal grooming facilitates positive self-concept.*

Assist with Communication. The patient who loses communication abilities requires intensive speech therapy and emotional support. It is important to determine the specific nature of the impairment when planning interventions and helping family members understand specific problems. Although the speech therapist is usually most involved with speech rehabilitation, nurses must plan interventions to meet communication needs during all phases of care.

Expected Outcome: Patient will be able to use alternative methods of communication effectively.

The nurse will:

- Approach and treat the patient as an adult.
- Do not assume that the patient who does not respond verbally cannot hear. Do not use a raised voice when addressing the patient.
- Allow adequate time for the patient to respond.
- Face the patient and speak slowly.
- When you do not understand the patient's speech, be honest and say so.
- Use short, simple statements and questions. *Accepting the patient and providing dignity and respect enhances the nurse–patient relationship. Allowing adequate response time and using short verbal statements or questions while facing the patient motivates the patient to communicate and decreases frustration.*
- Accept frustration and anger as a normal reaction to the loss of function. *Anger represents the patient's frustration at the inability to control the loss of function.*
- Try alternate methods of communication, including writing tablets, flash cards, and computerized talking boards. *Patients unable to communicate verbally may use other methods effectively.*

Promote Normal Urinary and Bowel Elimination. Both urinary and bowel elimination may be altered because of neurologic deficits, impaired mobility, cognitive impairment, communication deficits, or preexisting problems (especially if the patient is an older adult). Other causes include changes in food and fluid intake and side effects of medications. Urinary incontinence or retention and constipation, fecal incontinence, and fecal impaction are the usual manifestations.

Expected Outcome: Patient will be able to perceive and recognize cues for toileting and independently conduct toileting activities to their optimal function.

The nurse will:

- Assess for urinary frequency, urgency, incontinence, nocturia, and voiding in small amounts. In addition, assess the patient's ability to respond to the need to void, the ability to use the call light, and the ability to use toileting equipment. Use established guidelines to assess and manage patients with urinary incontinence. *Assessment needed for early detection of bladder dysfunction.*
- Assess for a distended bladder. *Voiding small amounts of urine frequently may be a manifestation of a bladder dysfunction.*
- Encourage bladder training by having patient void on schedule, such as every 2 hours, rather than in response to the urge to void.
- Teach Kegel exercises. To perform Kegel exercises, the patient contracts the perineal muscles as though stopping urination, holds the contraction for 5 seconds, and then releases.
- Use positive reinforcement (verbal praise) for successful management of urinary elimination. *Voiding every 2 hours or on schedule promotes bladder tone and urine storage. Kegel exercises increase pubococcygeal muscle tone and bladder control, decreasing incontinence. Positive reinforcement can be a useful part of the teaching program.*
- Discuss prestroke bowel habits, as well as the pattern of bowel elimination since the stroke.
- If the patient is able to swallow without difficulty, encourage fluids (up to 2000 mL/day) and a high-fiber diet.
- Increase physical activity as tolerated.
- Assist in using the toilet facilities at the same time each day (based on usual patterns of bowel elimination), ensuring privacy and having the patient sit in an upright position if at all possible.

- Administer prescribed stool softeners if the patient is following a bowel elimination routine or is not drinking sufficient fluids.

  Increased fluids, fiber, and activity stimulate intestinal motility. Establishing a regular daily time for bowel movements in the upright position and in privacy promotes normal bowel elimination. Stool softeners help prevent the formation of hard stool that is more difficult to expel.

Prevent Aspiration and Ensure Adequate Nutrition. A stroke may impair the ability to swallow. Weakness or lack of coordination of the tongue, attention deficits, and deficits involving the swallowing reflex all play a role. Dysphagia (difficulty swallowing) may result in choking, drooling, aspiration, or regurgitation. Nursing care focuses on maintaining safety by preventing aspiration and on ensuring adequate nutrition.

Expected Outcome: Patient will remain free from aspiration as evidenced by clear lung sounds and temperature within normal range.

The nurse will:

- Monitor results of swallowing studies (often conducted by a physical therapist) prior to providing oral food and fluids.
- When eating, do the following to avoid aspiration and ensure safety:
  a. Put in upright sitting position with neck slightly flexed.
  b. Order puréed or soft food. Liquids should be of the same consistency as honey.
  c. Feed or teach patient to eat by putting food behind the front teeth on the unaffected side of the mouth and tilting the head slightly backward. Teach to swallow one bite at a time.
  d. Assess for coughing with eating or drinking.
  e. Have suction equipment available at the bedside in case of choking or aspiration.

  Sitting upright with the head and neck first slightly flexed and then tilted back helps the patient swallow. The patient can usually swallow puréed or soft foods more easily than liquid or solid foods. Using the unaffected side of the mouth helps prevent food from collecting in the mouth and makes swallowing safer; in addition, food is less likely to fall out of the mouth.
- Monitor lung sounds. *Coarse lung sounds heard in the right upper and/or lower lobes may indicate aspiration because the right bronchus is the first division of the bronchi and where the majority of aspirations occur.*
- Minimize distractions and, if necessary, give step-by-step instructions for eating. *Distractions increase the risk of aspiration. Complex activities are easier to perform when broken down into small steps.*

SAFETY ALERT: After eating, check the mouth for "pocketing" of food, especially in the affected cheek. ■

Delegating Nursing Care Activities

As appropriate and allowed by the designated duties and responsibilities of unlicensed assistive personnel, the nurse may delegate nursing care activities such as measuring vital signs (including orthostatic vital signs), encouraging oral or enteral fluid intake, and providing skin care.

Transitions of Care

Health promotion activities focus on stroke prevention, especially for those people with known risk factors. More lives are saved by preventing strokes than by treating them. It is important to discuss, as appropriate, the importance of stopping smoking and drug use with patients of all ages. Maintaining a normal weight through diet and exercise can help reduce obesity, which increases the risk of hypertension and type 2 diabetes mellitus (both in turn increase the risk of a stroke). Cholesterol levels should be screened regularly to monitor for hyperlipidemia. Regular healthcare to monitor for and treat cardiovascular disorders and to detect and treat infections such as infective endocarditis is important.

It is also important to increase public awareness of the signs of a TIA or stroke and of the need to call 911 or to seek care immediately if warning signs or symptoms occur. There are several public awareness campaigns that are useful. The symptoms listed next are those publicized by NINDS (2018a). The American Stroke Association provides clues to recognizing a stroke (remember the Act FAST mnemonic). In addition, The Stroke Collaborative (2015) describes five warning signs of stroke as follows:

1. ***Weakness:*** Sudden loss of strength or sudden numbness in the face, arm, or leg, even if temporary
2. ***Trouble speaking:*** Sudden difficulty speaking or understanding or sudden confusion, even if temporary
3. ***Vision problems:*** Sudden trouble with vision, even if temporary
4. ***Headache:*** Sudden severe and unusual headache
5. ***Dizziness:*** Sudden loss of balance, especially with any of the above signs.

Throughout the rehabilitation process, it is important not only to encourage self-care as much as possible but also to involve family members in the plan of care. Stress that ADLs may take twice as long as they did before the stroke. Emphasize that physical function may continue to improve for up to 3 months, and speech may continue to improve for even longer. Address the following topics in preparing the patient and family for continuity of care:

- Physical care, medications, physical therapy, occupational therapy, speech therapy
- Home environment conducive to using equipment (such as a wheelchair or walker) and equipment modifications (e.g., a raised toilet seat, grab bars in the bathroom, a bath chair, a vise lid opener, a long-handled shoehorn)
- Home health services

- Community resources, such as Meals on Wheels, senior centers, older adult care, large-print telephone dials, stroke clubs, and an emergency alerting system; financial assistance may be available within the community for housekeeping and personal care assistance
- Helpful organizational resources include the American Heart Association, the National Stroke Association, Stroke Clubs International, and the National Institute of Neurological Disorders and Stroke.

Case Study & Nursing Care Plan

A Patient with a Stroke

Orville Boren is a 63-year-old African American who had a stroke due to a right cerebral thrombosis 1 week ago. He is a history instructor at the local community college. His hobbies are wood carving and gardening. Mr. Boren is also an active member of his church. For the past 2 years, Mr. Boren has been taking medication for hypertension, but his wife Emily reports that he often forgets to take it and that his blood pressure was high at his last physical examination. Mrs. Boren tells the staff that she has never had to worry about her husband's health before and that she wants to learn everything she can to care for him at home. However, she says that her husband was always the one to make the decisions and pay the bills. Mrs. Boren adds that all the children, grandchildren, neighbors, and family pastor want to see Mr. Boren back at home as soon as possible.

ASSESSMENT

Carol Merck, RN, the nurse assigned to Mr. Boren, completes a health history and physical assessment, with Mrs. Boren providing information for the history. Mrs. Boren reports that her husband did have several spells of dizziness and blurred vision the week before his stroke, but they lasted only a few minutes and he believed them to be due to "old age and working out in the sun." On the morning of admission, Mr. Boren woke up and could not move his left arm or leg; he also could not speak sensibly. Mrs. Boren called 911, and an ambulance took her husband to the hospital.

Physical assessment findings include the following: Mr. Boren is drowsy but responds to verbal stimuli. Although he does not respond verbally, he can nod his head to indicate "yes" when asked questions. Flaccid paralysis is present in his left arm and left leg, with no response noted to touch in those extremities (he is left-handed). Visual fields are decreased in a pattern consistent with homonymous hemianopia. A CT scan, negative on admission, is repeated on the day after admission and confirms the medical diagnosis of a right-brain stroke due to a thrombus of the middle cerebral artery.

Mr. Boren's medical treatment includes heparin sodium administered by continuous intravenous drip, with clotting studies to be performed every 4 hours and the dose adjusted accordingly.

DIAGNOSES

- Inability to feed self, related to loss of the ability to use the left hand and arm
- Risk for immobility related to neurologic deficits causing left hemiplegia
- Risk for skin damage related to inability to change position
- Visual disturbance related to changes in visual fields
- Inability to talk related to cerebral injury

EXPECTED OUTCOMES

- Patient will learn to use his right hand to feed himself.
- Patient will participate in exercises necessary to maintain muscle strength and tone.
- Patient will maintain skin integrity.
- Patient will indicate understanding that visual fields may improve in a few weeks.
- Patient will practice and implement speech therapy activities while at the same time using alternative methods of communication.

PLANNING AND IMPLEMENTATION

- Arrange mealtimes so that he is sitting up by the window in a clean and private environment.
- Provide adaptive devices (silverware with thick handles and nonslip plates).
- Encourage Mrs. Boren to visit at mealtimes, to assist with meals, and to periodically bring a favorite food from home.
- Provide passive ROM exercises for his left arm and leg; schedule active ROM exercises for his right extremities as well as quadriceps and gluteal sets every 4 hours during waking hours.
- Keep his skin clean and dry at all times.
- Establish and maintain a regular schedule for turning when he is in bed.
- Place objects (e.g., call bell, tissues) on unaffected side and approach him from that side.
- Support attempts to communicate verbally; when he is not understood, he prefers to use a large marker and tablet.

(*continued*)

EVALUATION

Mr. Boren is discharged to his home with home health visits ordered for physical therapy, occupational therapy, speech therapy, and skilled nursing care. During the first 2 months after discharge, Martha Grimes, RN, the home health nurse, visits Mr. and Mrs. Boren at home. At the end of 2 months, Mr. Boren is using his right hand to feed himself. He has regained partial use of his left arm and leg and is using a walker to move around the house and yard; he is even able to work in his flower garden. His skin has remained intact, and his vision is back to normal. He is slowly relearning speech; this has been the most difficult change for him to accept. Once he writes on his tablet, "I think God has forgotten me."

CLINICAL REASONING IN PATIENT CARE

1. Hypertension is sometimes referred to as "the silent killer." Provide justifications for this statement.
2. The functional changes Mr. Boren has experienced may make a return to teaching difficult. What other uses of his knowledge and abilities might you suggest?
3. If after you had completed passive ROM on Mr. Boren's left arm, he wrote, "I just ignore that part of my body—it doesn't work anyway." What would be your reply?

See Evaluating Your Response in Appendix B.

42.5 Intracranial Vascular Disorders

The Patient with an Intracranial Aneurysm

An *intracranial aneurysm* is a saccular outpouching of a cerebral artery that occurs at the site of a weakness in the vessel wall. It is believed to be the result of a congenital defect in a cerebral vessel wall. A ruptured cerebral aneurysm is the most common cause of a hemorrhagic stroke. Seen most often in adults over age 50, a ruptured intracranial aneurysm often results in death or severe disability in those who survive (Sorenson et al., 2019).

Pathophysiology

Intracranial aneurysms tend to occur at the bifurcations in the circle of Willis. Intracranial aneurysms often enlarge over time, making the vessel wall thin and increasing the probability of rupture. There are several types, but most are small saccular aneurysms called *berry aneurysms* (because of their small, berry-like projections). Rupture of these aneurysms results in bleeding into the subarachnoid space (causing a subarachnoid hemorrhage).

Risk Factors

Risk factors for intracranial aneurysms include inherited and lifestyle risk factors. Inherited factors can include connective tissue disorders that can weaken arterial walls, polycystic kidney disease, arteriovenous malformations and a family history of aneurysms. Lifestyle risk factors include hypertension and cigarette smoking and/or drug abuse (NINDS, 2018c).

Manifestations

The manifestations of a ruptured intracranial aneurysm (and subsequent subarachnoid hemorrhage) include a sudden, explosive headache and neck pain; nausea and vomiting; a stiff neck and photophobia (due to meningeal irritation); cranial nerve deficits; and stroke syndrome. Hypertension and cardiac dysrhythmias may occur from the massive release of catecholamines triggered by the subarachnoid hemorrhage. Fibrin and platelets seal off the bleeding point, but the escaped blood forms a clot that irritates the brain tissue. The resulting inflammatory response causes cerebral edema, and both the edema and the hemorrhage increase intracranial pressure. The pituitary gland is in proximity to the circle of Willis and is often affected secondary to edema and irritation, with resulting diabetes insipidus and hyponatremia (NINDS, 2018c).

Complications

The major complications of a ruptured intracranial aneurysm are rebleeding and vasospasm. Hypothalamic dysfunction, hydrocephalus, and seizures are also potential complications. The greatest risk for rebleeding is within the first 2 weeks after the initial rupture, although it may occur at any time following the initial occurrence. Approximately 70% of patients who have rebleeding will die (NINDS, 2018c). Cerebral vasospasm is a common but dangerous complication that is associated with a large number of deaths and disability. A cerebral vasospasm narrows the lumen of one or more cerebral vessels, causing ischemia and infarction of brain tissue supplied by the affected vessels. It occurs in blood vessels surrounded by thick blood clots and is thought to be the result of the release of ET-1, a potent vasoconstrictor of cerebral arteries (Hickey, 2013). The manifestations vary according to the degree of spasm and the area of brain affected. Regional alterations may cause focal deficits (such as hemiplegia), whereas global alterations cause loss of consciousness.

Interprofessional Care

The care of the patient with a ruptured intracranial aneurysm includes determining the location of the aneurysm, treating the manifestations of the hemorrhage, and preventing rebleeding and vasospasm. Interventions using radiology, angiography, and a variety of procedures may be used to prevent aneurysm rupture or to stop the bleeding. Surgery is usually the treatment of choice to repair the bleeding artery.

Diagnosis

The diagnostic tests conducted to identify the site and extent of a ruptured intracranial aneurysm, as well as rebleeding, are a CT scan, a spiral computed tomography angiogram (CTA), and bilateral carotid and vertebral cerebral angiograms. A CT is used to initially detect the hemorrhage, and a CTA can rapidly identify the arterial anatomy. Angiograms provide visualization of all four major cerebral vessels and their branches, providing early diagnosis and treatment. A lumbar puncture will reveal blood-tinged spinal fluid.

Medications

Calcium channel blockers, such as nimodipine (Nimotop), are used to improve neurologic deficits due to vasospasm following subarachnoid hemorrhage from ruptured intracranial aneurysms. Administered orally or by feeding tube (never IV), it has been found to enhance collateral blood flow and improve outcomes (Adams et al., 2017).

Other medications that may be prescribed include anticonvulsants, such as phenytoin (Dilantin), to prevent seizures if the patient has IICP; analgesics for headache; antacids and H_2-receptor antagonists (such as ranitidine [Xanax]) to prevent gastric irritation; and stool softeners to prevent constipation and straining with a bowel movement (which increases intracranial pressure and blood pressure and may cause rebleeding).

Treatment

Treatments for an intracranial aneurysm are performed either to prevent rupture or to isolate the vessel to prevent further bleeding. Patients with good neurologic status may have surgery soon after the rupture. In patients with significant neurologic deficits, surgery may be delayed until they are more stable and less at risk for vasospasm; however, the trend is toward surgery as soon as possible.

Several different types of procedures are used to repair a ruptured intracranial aneurysm or to prevent the rupture of an existing large aneurysm. The neck of the aneurysm may be clipped with a metal clip to prevent entry of blood into the aneurysm. Endovascular techniques that may be used include balloon embolization and platinum coil electrothrombosis.

Nursing Care

Nursing care is planned and implemented for the patient with a ruptured intracranial aneurysm to prevent rebleeding as well as to meet needs resulting from neurologic deficits. Appropriate diagnoses, outcomes, and interventions are described earlier in the chapter in the discussion of nursing care for the patient with a stroke. The priority interventions in the acute care stage of a ruptured intracranial aneurysm focus on treating ineffective cerebral tissue perfusion.

Transitions of Care

Preventive measures for intracranial aneurysms focus on healthy lifestyle choices. Maintaining a normal blood pressure, getting regular exercise, eating a healthy diet, and stopping smoking will all help prevent an aneurysm.

Immediate medical treatment is imperative with the development of an intracranial aneurysm. Treatment focuses on reversal of the underlying cause of vessel rupture to reduce neurological impacts of the injury.

The Patient with an Arteriovenous Malformation

An *arteriovenous (AV) malformation* is a congenital intracranial lesion, formed by a tangled collection of dilated arteries and veins that allows blood to flow directly from the arterial into the venous system, bypassing the normal capillary network. Most AV malformations (90%) are located in the cerebral hemispheres; the remainder are found in the cerebellum and brainstem. Rupture of vessels in AV malformations account for 2% of all strokes (NINDS, 2017).

Pathophysiology

AV malformations, believed to arise from failure of development of the capillary network in the embryo, displace rather than encompass normal brain tissue. AV malformations range in size from very small to very large. The pathophysiologic effects of an AV malformation are the result of the shunting of blood from the arterial to the venous system and of altered perfusion of cerebral tissue near the malformation. The shunting of arterial blood directly into the venous system within the malformation transfers the higher arterial pressure directly into the lower-pressure venous system. This increased pressure is likely to cause spontaneous bleeding or progressive expansion and rupture of a blood vessel. Altered cerebral perfusion results when blood flow through a large, high-flow malformation is diverted from the normal cerebral circulation, causing tissue ischemia of the area surrounding the malformation. This is sometimes called a *vascular steal phenomenon*.

Risk Factors

Patients with this condition develop manifestations before 40 years of age; it affects men and women equally (NINDS, 2017).

Manifestations

The manifestations are the result of spontaneous bleeding from the lesion into the subarachnoid space or brain tissue. Large malformations are usually initially manifested by seizure activity. In contrast, the manifestations of a small malformation are more often due to a hemorrhage that causes neurologic deficits. In both instances, the patient may have recurrent headaches that do not respond to treatment.

Interprofessional Care

AV malformations are diagnosed with the same diagnostic tests used to diagnose an intracranial aneurysm. Treatment is by surgical excision, vascular occlusion, and radiosurgery. When the malformation is excised or obstructed, blood flow is no longer shunted, and cerebral perfusion improves.

Nursing Care

Nursing care depends on the condition of the malformation. If hemorrhage has not occurred, teach the patient to avoid activities that raise blood pressure or could cause injury. The patient is usually given medications to control blood pressure and prevent seizures. If the malformation ruptures and causes an intracranial hemorrhage, nursing care is the same as that provided to a patient who has had a stroke.

42.6 Traumatic Brain Injury

Traumatic brain injury (TBI) refers to any injury of the scalp, skull (cranium or facial bones), or brain. TBI is a leading cause of death and disability in the United States. Each year, 2.8 million people suffer a TBI; of those, 282,000 are hospitalized and survive and 50,000 will die (Bob Woodruff Foundation, 2018). The Centers for Disease Control and Prevention (2018a) define TBI as "caused by a bump, blow, or jolt to the head or a penetrating head injury that disrupts the normal function of the brain." A TBI may be classified as a penetrating (or open) head injury (when an object pierces the skull and enters the brain) or a closed head injury (the head suddenly and violently hits an object but the object does not break through the skull). Damage to the brain may be focal (confined to one area) or diffuse (involving more than one area of the brain).

TBI may cause problems with cognition, movement, sensation, and emotions. Even mild brain injuries, if repeated over an extended period of time, can result in cumulative neurologic and cognitive deficits. TBI is a major public health problem, especially among males ages 15 to 24. Blasts are the leading cause of TBI among military personnel in war zones; veterans' advocates believe 150,000 to 300,000 Iraq veterans have suffered TBI (CDC, 2018a).

According to NINDS (2018d), more than 50% of all TBIs in adults under the age of 75 are the result of crashes involving cars, motorcycles, bicycles, and pedestrians. TBIs in adults over the age of 75 are the result of falls. People ages 75 and older have the highest rates of TBI-related hospitalizations and death (NINDS, 2018d).

Other causes of TBI include violence and sports injuries. At least half of all TBIs involve alcohol or other drug use. The cause often determines the outcome; 91% of TBI from firearms (two-thirds of which may involve suicides) result in death, while 11% of TBIs from falls result in death.

Specific damage following craniocerebral injuries is related to the mechanism of the injury (how it occurs), the nature of the injury (type), and the location of the injury (where it occurs).

Head injuries may occur through several mechanisms:

- *Contact phenomena injury* is sustained when the head is struck by a moving object, such as a swinging bat. It includes local effects such as scalp lacerations and/or skull fractures and intracerebral contusions, lacerations, hematoma, and hemorrhage.
- *Acceleration–deceleration injury* (linear injury) occurs when the head hits an object and the brain rebounds within the skull (**Figure 42.8** ■). The brain is injured at the point of impact (the *coup*) and on the opposite side of the impact (the *contrecoup*). Strain on cerebral tissue produces injury by compression, tension, or shearing. This type of injury is responsible for acute subdural hematoma and diffuse axonal injury.
- *Rotational injury* occurs when the brain rotates within the skull and hits bony buttresses in the cranial vault; these injuries are more severe than those from linear injuries.

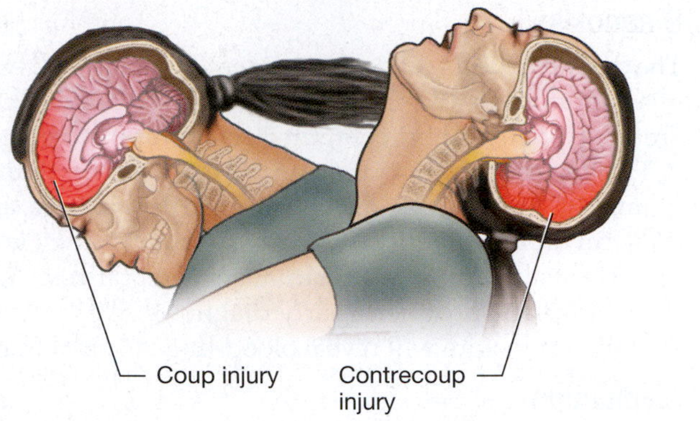
Coup injury
Contrecoup injury

Figure 42.8 ■ Coup–contrecoup head injury. Following the initial injury (coup), the brain rebounds within the skull and sustains additional Much better art! Thanks, Laura! injury (contrecoup) in the opposite part of the brain.

Types of craniocerebral trauma include injuries to the skull, injuries to the brain (including concussion and contusion), and intracranial hematomas and hemorrhage. Brain injury can result either from the direct effects of the trauma on brain tissue or from secondary responses to trauma, such as cerebral edema, hematoma, or IICP.

Focal or Diffuse Traumatic Brain Injury

The brain is protected from injury by enclosure in the bones of the skull and the cushioning effects of cerebrospinal fluid. Metabolic stability is maintained by a variety of mechanisms, including the blood–brain barrier and autoregulation of blood supply. However, damage to the brain can occur from the direct effects of trauma as well as from injury from ischemia, cerebral edema, IICP, hypoxia, and infection. These mechanisms of injury are often interrelated.

Pathophysiology

Brain injury results from both primary and secondary mechanisms. Primary injury results from the impact. A blow to the head, even with no break in the skull, can cause serious and diffuse brain injury. Injury to axons disrupts oligodendroglia, and direct mechanical disruption is caused by debris and leakage.

Secondary injury is the progression of the initial injury resulting from events that affect perfusion and oxygenation of brain cells. The theories of cause and mechanisms of secondary injury are summarized here. They include the effects of hypoxia, ischemia, and inflammation. Hypoxia interferes with the delivery of oxygen; ischemia interferes with the delivery of oxygen and glucose and with the removal of metabolic wastes. The consequences of cerebral ischemia include increased cellular permeability to sodium (cytotoxic edema) and release of free fatty acids and lactic acidosis. The release of excitatory amino acids (such as glutamate and aspartate) causes an influx of calcium with changes in electrophysiology. The inflammatory process begins immediately, resulting in the release of cytokines. It is unknown if these cytokines are protective or injurious, but it is known that inflammatory mediators such as tumor necrosis factor increase with TBI and are associated with cerebral edema, disruption of the blood–brain barrier, and death of neurons (Sorenson et al., 2019).

Acute brain injury affects all body systems as well as the central nervous system. Systemic effects of acute brain injury are listed in **Table 42.7**.

Focal Brain Injuries

Focal brain injuries are specific brain lesions confined to one area of the brain. They include contusions and hemorrhage/hematomas. The force of an impact produces contusions from direct contact with the inside of the skull that in turn may cause epidural hemorrhage and subdural and intracerebral hematomas. The mechanisms of injury are damage to the brain at the point of the impact and the rebound effect. The damaged area is surrounded by edema, contributing to IICP. Infarction and necrosis, multiple hemorrhages, and edema are found within the contused areas.

Intracranial hemorrhage can result directly from the trauma or from the shearing forces on cerebral arteries and veins that occur with acceleration–deceleration. Depending on the site and rate of bleeding, manifestations may appear immediately or may not become evident for hours or even weeks. Intracranial hemorrhages and the hematomas they cause place pressure on surrounding structures, causing manifestations of an expanding focal lesion. They also cause IICP, leading to altered levels of consciousness and potential herniation syndromes. Intracranial hematomas are classified by their location as epidural, subdural, or intracerebral. **Table 42.8** compares the frequency, locations, common sites, precipitating factors, and manifestations of intracranial hematomas; **Figure 42.9** ■ illustrates their locations.

Contusion. A cerebral contusion is a bruise of the surface of the brain, typically accompanied by small, diffuse venous hemorrhages. Both white and gray matter may have a bruised, discolored appearance. Contusions (and other focal brain injuries) occur when the brain strikes the inner skull, often with a coup (point of impact) lesion and a contrecoup lesion on the opposite side of the brain. Contusions occur most frequently near bony prominences of the skull. Cerebral edema can follow contusion, resulting in IICP. Contusions; small, diffuse venous hemorrhages; and brain swelling are at their peak 12 to 24 hours after injury.

Manifestations of the contusion depend on the size and location of the brain injury. An initial loss of consciousness occurs; LOC may remain altered, and behavior changes such as combativeness may persist for an extended period. Full consciousness may be regained extremely slowly, and residual deficits may persist; in some patients, full LOC never really returns. Focal effects of the contusion may cause loss of reflexes, hemiparesis (muscular weakness of one-half of the body), or abnormal posturing. Manifestations of IICP may occur if cerebral edema develops. Regaining full LOC may take an extended period of time and residual deficits may persist.

Epidural Hematoma. An **epidural hematoma** (also called an *extradural hematoma*) develops in the potential space between the dura and the skull, which normally adhere to one another. As the blood collects, the expanding hematoma pulls the dura away from the skull. Epidural hematomas affect young to middle-age adults more frequently than older adults because the dura becomes more tightly attached to the skull with aging.

Table 42.7 Systemic Effects of Acute Brain Injury

Cause	Effect
Stimulation of the sympathetic nervous system (SNS), which stimulates the adrenal cortex and medulla to increase glucocorticoid and mineralocorticoid levels	■ Increased metabolism of carbohydrates, fats, and proteins ■ Retention of sodium and water
Stimulation of the SNS, increasing the serum catecholamine levels	■ Hypertension ■ EEG changes ■ Dysrhythmias (bradycardia, sinus tachycardia)
Altered release of antidiuretic hormone (ADH) from the posterior pituitary	■ Retention of water or diuresis and diabetes insipidus
Neurogenic pulmonary dysfunction	■ Abnormal respiratory patterns ■ Reduced residual capacity with retention of CO_2, vasodilation, and increased ICP ■ Pulmonary edema
Stress response to trauma	■ Hyperglycemia
Increased platelet, plasma fibrinogen, and thromboplastin levels	■ Decreased clotting and prothrombin times ■ Vascular occlusion ■ Disseminated intravascular coagulation ■ Anemia
Immunosuppression	■ Infection
Decreased gastric motility and increased gastric acidity	■ Gastritis ■ Gastric ulcers

Table 42.8 Comparison of Intracranial Hematomas

Location/Common Site	Precipitating Factors	Manifestations
Epidural Hematoma (2–6% of all types of head injuries)		
Located in the space between the skull and the dura mater Common site: The temporal bone (over the middle meningeal artery)	Skull fractures Contusion	■ Momentary loss of consciousness followed by a lucid period lasting from a few hours to 1–2 days ■ Rapid deterioration in level of consciousness (drowsiness to confusion to coma) ■ Seizures ■ Headache ■ Hemiparesis (may be ipsilateral or contralateral) ■ Fixed dilated ipsilateral pupil ■ Rise in blood pressure with decreases in pulse and respirations indicates a rapidly increasing hematoma
Subdural Hematoma (approximately 29% of all types of head injuries)		
Located in the space below the dural surface (between the dura and arachnoid and pia mater layers of meninges) Common site: May occur any place in cranium	Closed head injury Acceleration–deceleration injury Cerebral atrophy (seen in older adults) Chronic alcoholism Use of anticoagulants Contusion	Acute: ■ Headache ■ Drowsiness ■ Agitation ■ Slowed thinking ■ Confusion Subacute: ■ Same as those of acute subdural hematoma but develop more slowly Chronic: ■ Manifestations may not appear until weeks to months after injury ■ Confusion, slowed thinking, drowsiness
Intracerebral Hematoma (14–15% of all types of head injuries)		
Located directly in the brain tissue Common site: Frontal or temporal region	Gunshot wounds Depressed bone fractures Stab injury Long history of systemic hypertension Contusions	■ Headache ■ Deteriorating consciousness to deep coma ■ Hemiplegia on contralateral side ■ Dilated pupil on the side of the clot

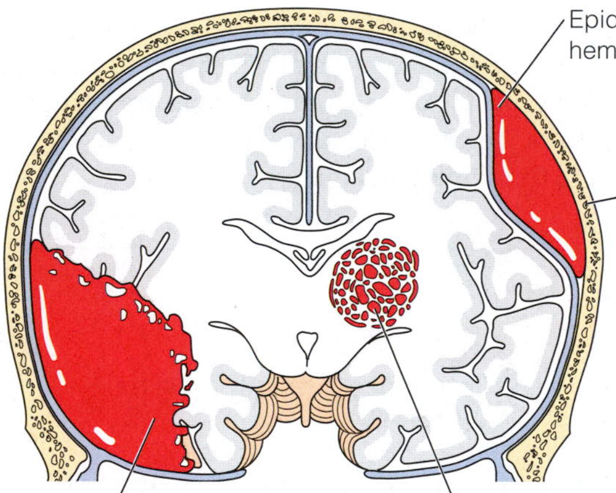
Epidural hematoma
Skull
Subdural hematoma
Intracerebral hematoma

Figure 42.9 ■ Three types of hematomas: epidural hematoma, subdural hematoma, and intracerebral hematoma.

Epidural hematomas usually result from a skull fracture that tears an artery, often the middle meningeal artery. Because epidural hematomas are arterial in origin, they tend to develop rapidly. The patient may lose consciousness with the initial injury and then have a brief lucid period before the LOC rapidly declines from drowsiness to coma as the hematoma expands, compressing brain tissue. Other manifestations include headache; vomiting; a fixed, dilated pupil on the same side (ipsilateral) as the hematoma; contralateral (opposite-side) hemiparesis or hemiplegia; and possible seizures. Because epidural hematomas usually develop rapidly, timely intervention is vital to prevent significant increases in ICP and herniation.

Subdural Hematoma. **Subdural hematomas**, in which a localized mass of blood collects between the dura mater and the arachnoid mater, are more common than epidural hematomas. Acute subdural hematomas are usually located at the top of the head and develop within 48 hours of the initial head injury. Although a lucid period may occur, the patient commonly develops drowsiness, confusion, and enlargement of the ipsilateral pupil within minutes or hours of the injury. If responsive, the patient may complain of a unilateral headache. Hemiparesis and respiratory pattern changes may occur.

Chronic subdural hematomas develop over weeks or months. The chronic type is seen most often in older adults and people who have some brain atrophy with subsequent enlarged epidural space. Chronic subdural hematomas are often associated with relatively minor trauma such as a fall or may occur spontaneously in the older adult or in patients with bleeding disorders. Manifestations of the hematoma develop slowly and may be mistaken for the onset of dementia in the older adult. Slowed thinking, confusion, drowsiness, and lethargy are common early manifestations. Other manifestations include headache, dilation and sluggishness of the ipsilateral pupil, and possible seizures.

Intracerebral Hematoma. Intracerebral hematomas may be single or multiple and are associated with contusions. They may occur in any location but are usually found in the frontal or temporal lobes. They may result from closed head trauma, particularly contusion or shearing of small blood vessels deep within the hemispheres. Intracerebral hematomas can also accompany other types of head trauma such as lacerations. Older adults are particularly vulnerable to intracerebral hemorrhage because cerebral blood vessels are more fragile and easily torn. The manifestations of intracerebral hematoma vary according to the location of the hematoma. Headache may develop, along with decreasing LOC, hemiplegia, and dilation of the ipsilateral pupil. The expanding clot increases intracranial pressure, and herniation may occur.

Diffuse Cerebral Injury

A diffuse cerebral injury (concussion and diffuse axonal injury) affects the entire brain and is caused by a shaking motion, with twisting movement (rotational injury) as the primary mechanism of injury. Shearing stresses on brain tissue cause axonal damage from shearing, tearing, or stretching of nerve fibers. The most serious axonal injuries are located farthest from the brainstem, with the frontal and temporal axonal tracts being most vulnerable to injury. Physical deficits include spastic paralysis, peripheral nerve injury, swallowing disorders, visual and hearing impairments, and taste and smell disorders. Damage to axons decreases the speed of information processing and responding and disrupts attention, resulting in serious cognitive and affective impairments. Cognitive deficits that may result include disorientation and confusion, short attention span, problems with memory and learning, perceptual problems, and poor judgment. Possible behavioral deficits include agitation, impulsivity, depression, and social withdrawal.

Initially, the damage involves tearing of axons, blood vessels, and brain tissue (visible only by electron microscope). The number of damaged axons progressively increases, with pathology involving the nuclei and axons. The damaged axons, which resemble sausage links, regress into round balls called *retraction balls* (visible with light microscopy). After several weeks, the retraction balls are replaced by clusters of microglia. In the final phase, astrocytosis (equivalent to scarring) occurs at the site of axonal damage, accompanied by demyelination of long axon tracts.

Mild Concussion. The word ***concussion*** means "violent shaking." A concussion involves temporary axonal disturbances. It is defined as a momentary interruption of brain function. A concussion is associated with an immediate, brief loss of consciousness on impact. Altered consciousness may last only seconds or persist for several hours. Amnesia for events immediately preceding (antegrade amnesia) and following (retrograde amnesia) the injury is common.

Classic Cerebral Concussion. A classic cerebral concussion involves diffuse cerebral disconnection from the brainstem RAS. An immediate loss of consciousness occurs, lasting less than 6 hours. Both retrograde and antegrade amnesia occur, and cerebral contusions may be present. In a severe concussion, a brief seizure and respiratory arrest may occur; transient pallor, bradycardia, and hypotension may accompany loss of consciousness. Patients may develop postconcussion syndrome with persistent headache, dizziness, irritability, insomnia, impaired memory and concentration, and learning problems. Postconcussion syndrome may last for several weeks or, rarely, up to a year.

Diffuse Axonal Injury. *Diffuse axonal injury (DAI)* is a brain injury in which a high-speed acceleration–deceleration injury, typically associated with motor vehicle crashes, causes widespread disruption of axons in the white matter. Focal lesions may be found in the corpus callosum, midbrain, and brainstem. An immediate loss of consciousness occurs. DAI accounts for approximately 50% of primary brain injuries and accounts for 35% of deaths from all TBIs (CDC, 2018a).

DAIs may range from mild to severe. In mild DAI, coma lasts 6 to 24 hours, and cognitive, psychologic, and sensorimotor deficits may persist. In moderate DAI, injury and impairment is spread throughout the cerebral cortex and diencephalon. There is axonal tearing, coma lasting more than 24 hours, and often incomplete recovery. In severe DAI, axonal injury occurs in both cerebral hemispheres, the diencephalon, and the brainstem. Immediate autonomic dysfunction occurs, and IICP is manifested. Profound cognitive and sensorimotor deficits occur, involving movement, verbal and written communication, ability to learn and reason, and ability to modulate behavior.

Manifestations

Manifestations of concussion include:

- Immediate loss of consciousness (lasting usually no longer than 5 minutes)
- Amnesia for events surrounding injury
- Headache
- Drowsiness, confusion, dizziness
- Visual disturbances (diplopia, blurred vision)
- Possible brief seizure activity with transient apnea, bradycardia, pallor, and hypotension.

Manifestations of postconcussion syndrome include persistent headache, dizziness, irritability, insomnia, impaired memory and concentration, and learning problems.

Interprofessional Care

The patient with a brain injury may receive medical and/or surgical treatment. Although patients with a mild concussion may be assessed and sent home for recovery, most people who have a TBI require intensive care at a trauma center. Evidence-based guidelines for medical care have been established by the Brain Trauma Foundation in the document *Guidelines for the Management of Severe Traumatic Brain Injury* (Carney et al., 2016) and are updated periodically. A summary of the immediate care of the patient with a TBI follows:

- ***Concussion:*** Following a concussion, the patient may be observed for 1 to 2 hours in the emergency department (ED), and then discharged home with instructions for further observation to detect manifestations of secondary injury. If the loss of consciousness extended more than 2 minutes, the patient may be admitted to the hospital for observation.

- *Acute TBI:* Recognition and management of acute TBI with transport to an ED is essential to patient outcomes. Morbidity and mortality increase with hypotension (systolic pressure < 90 mmHg) and hypoxia (PaO_2 < 60 mmHg), so fluids are given to support a mean systolic arterial blood pressure at more than 90 mmHg. The fluid of choice for IV fluids is hypertonic saline because it reduces IICP. Assessment of the patient's airway, breathing, and circulation (ABCs), with management of dysfunction, is necessary to decrease the secondary effects of the brain injury. An intracranial pressure monitor probe may be inserted to assess ICP and monitor therapy to reduce cerebral edema and maintain cerebral perfusion. Osmotic diuretics such as mannitol may also be administered to reduce cerebral edema. Adequate oxygenation is vital to maintain cerebral metabolism; carbon dioxide is a potent vasodilator, and increased levels may contribute to cerebral edema and IICP.

On admission to the ICU from the ED, the patient may be placed on a special bed and connected to various monitoring devices. Invasive lines are inserted, including a central venous pressure (CVP) catheter, arterial line, pulmonary catheter, ventriculostomy, ICP monitor, and perhaps a retrograde jugular catheter. In most instances, an endotracheal tube is inserted and connected to a mechanical ventilator, cardiac monitoring is initiated, bilateral sequential pressure boots are applied, pulse oximetry is started, and a rectal temperature probe is inserted. Laboratory values are monitored for changes to ensure early detection of cerebral hypoxia and impending ischemia to prevent secondary brain injury.

Diagnosis

Diagnostic testing may be done to monitor hemodynamic status and detect conditions that may contribute to cerebral edema. Radiologic examinations include skull x-rays (to identify skull fractures and assess penetrating objects) and CT scan or MRI to detect contusions and lacerations associated with diffuse axonal injury. ABGs are analyzed, with particular attention to oxygen and carbon dioxide levels.

Managing IICP

IICP is managed to reestablish equilibrium of the intracranial contents and prevent secondary brain damage. Treatments include airway management, hyperventilation (used if signs of herniation appear), fluid resuscitation, positioning, temperature regulation, and medications. Medications other than those previously discussed include a category of drugs called *neuroprotectants*. These drugs are used to treat or alter some of the pathologic pathways that occur in ischemia and must be administered within a short time of the injury to be effective. Classifications of the drugs include lipid peroxidase inhibitors, free radical scavengers, receptor antagonists, calcium channel blockers, and gangliosides.

Surgery

Small subdural hematomas can frequently be reabsorbed and may be treated conservatively with close observation and supportive care. However, the treatment of choice for epidural hematomas and large acute subdural hematomas is surgical evacuation of the clot. This can often be performed through burr holes made into the skull (**Figure 42.10** ■). In an epidural hematoma, the bleeding vessel can also be ligated during this procedure, preventing further bleeding. Rebleeding may occur following evacuation of an acute subdural hematoma in older adults and patients with chronic alcoholism. A craniotomy is necessary to evacuate chronic subdural hematomas because the hematoma tends to solidify, making it difficult or impossible to remove through burr holes. Surgery is less successful in treating intracerebral hematomas because of widespread tissue damage. Supportive care to manage intracranial pressure and prevent complications is provided.

Nursing Care

In addition to the nursing care discussed in this section, see the Case Study & Nursing Care Plan for a patient with a subdural hematoma on page 1584.

Assessment

See the Manifestations and Interprofessional Care sections for the assessment of the patient with subdural hematoma.

Collect the following data through the health history and physical examination:

- *Health history:* A history of the injury is helpful in understanding the nature of the craniocerebral trauma; knowledge about loss of consciousness assists the nurse in planning care; however, most patients with severe

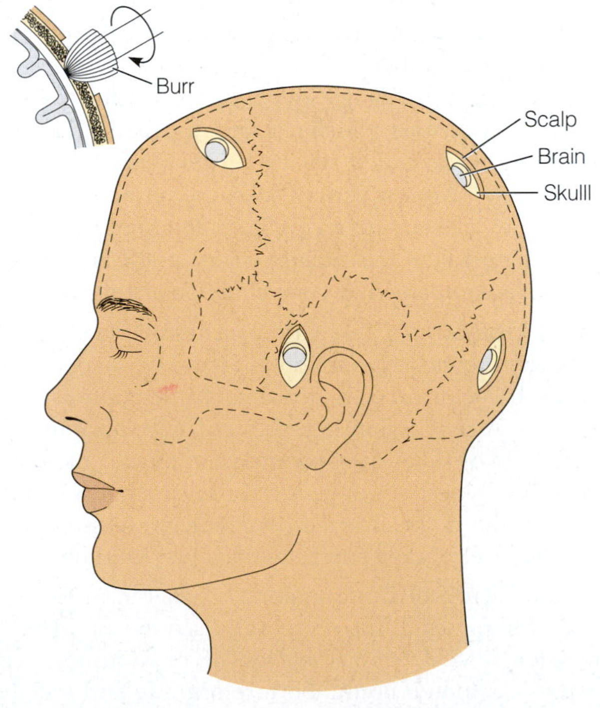
Burr
Scalp
Brain
Skulll

Figure 42.10 ■ Possible location of Burr holes.

TBI will not be able to communicate (either from the injury itself or from intubation)

- *Physical assessment:* Neurologic assessment, including pupils, LOC, Glasgow Coma Scale (a finding of 3 to 8 denotes severe TBI as defined by the Brain Trauma Foundation), brainstem reflexes (cornea, cough, gag, extraocular movements), spontaneous movement; response to pain; vital signs; skull and face (deformity, lacerations, bruising, bleeding); movement of extremities, other injuries.

Priorities of Care

Collaborating with the interprofessional team to ensure adequate treatment of the underlying process while providing care that supports the physical and psychologic responses to the disorder is a priority of nursing care.

Diagnoses, Outcomes, and Interventions

Nursing care of the patient in the acute care phase initially focuses on maintaining an effective airway and breathing pattern. Nursing care is also directed toward continuous assessment and monitoring of neurologic function as well as other body systems. This close monitoring provides early recognition and treatment of problems and complications and initiation of aggressive forms of therapy that may be needed.

Many nursing diagnoses associated with traumatic brain injury correspond with those outlined previously for the patient with altered LOC, IICP, and seizures. Specific nursing diagnoses discussed in this section focus on problems with intracranial adaptive capacity, airway clearance, and breathing patterns.

SAFETY ALERT: Overhydration from rapid infusion of IV fluids may cause or further increase IICP. ■

Monitor Intracranial Pressure. The patient with a traumatic brain injury has or is at high risk for IICP. Because the mechanisms that normally compensate for changes in intracranial pressure are compromised, intracranial pressure increases in disproportion to a variety of stimuli. (See the discussion earlier in the chapter for other diagnoses, outcomes, and interventions for the patient with IICP.)

Expected Outcome: Patient will experience fewer than five episodes of disproportionate increases in intracranial pressure in 24 hours.

The nurse will:

- Monitor for manifestations of IICP, including eye opening response, motor response, and verbal response. *These responses evaluate the ability to integrate commands with conscious and involuntary movement.*
- Monitor for changes in vital signs: Bradycardia or tachycardia, varying breathing patterns, hypertension, and/or widening pulse pressure. Vital signs vary depending on the site of impairment. *Cushing triad (bradycardia, increased systolic blood pressure, and increased pulse pressure) indicates brainstem ischemia leading to cerebral herniation.*
- Monitor for vomiting, headache, lethargy, restlessness, purposeless movements, and changes in mentation. *These manifestations may be early indicators of intracranial pressure changes.*
- Monitor temperature and initiate hypothermia treatment as prescribed. *Impaired hypothalamic function can interfere with temperature regulation. Hyperthermia may increase ICP.*
- Monitor fluid status: Regularly compare intake and output (a urinary catheter is inserted to assess renal perfusion), review serum osmolality, and use an infusion pump to administer IV fluids (if prescribed). *Osmotic diuretics, if used to treat cerebral edema, may cause hypotension and decreased cardiac output.*

Maintain Adequate Airway Clearance. The primary objective in the care of any trauma patient is maintaining a patent airway to prevent hypoxia. However, in the initial acute care phase, the risk of cervical vertebral fractures and spinal cord injury may complicate the process of establishing a patent airway. In addition, other multisystem injuries may complicate the interpretation of vital signs. In general, all unconscious people with a head injury should be intubated with an endotracheal tube to prevent aspiration. Patients with head trauma may also require a tracheostomy to provide an airway and be placed on a ventilator.

Expected Outcome: Adequate airway clearance will be maintained by use of protective interventions to maintain airway patency and suctioning as indicated.

The nurse will:

- Monitor neurologic manifestations on a regular schedule. *Changes in neurologic manifestations may indicate IICP, with the risk of further depression of the respiratory system and respiratory arrest.*
- Maintain head and neck in neutral alignment, immobilized until injury is determined. *Head rotation and neck flexion are associated with IICP, decreased jugular venous outflow, and localized changes in cerebral blood flow. Immobilization prevents spinal cord injury in suspected or actual fractures of the cervical spine; spinal cord injury at this level would further impair respiratory function.*
- Clear the nose and mouth of mucus and blood. *This helps maintain patency of the upper airway.*
- Suction the airway as needed, limiting suctioning time to no more than 10 seconds at one time. Do not suction the nasal passages until a dural tear has been ruled out. *Suctioning is usually necessary to maintain a patent airway.*

Promote Effective Breathing Pattern. The patient with a traumatic brain injury and hematoma is at high risk for ineffective breathing pattern related to IICP. If ICP increases dramatically, tentorial herniation may occur, leading to sudden respiratory arrest.

Expected Outcome: Patient will experience nursing interventions to promote adequate ventilation such as deep breathing and slowing respirations. The patient will accept nursing interventions to promote effective breathing.

The nurse will:

- Monitor the respiratory pattern for rate, depth, and rhythm every 2 hours or as needed if the patient is not on a ventilator. Assess breath sounds, presence of cyanosis, restlessness, and use of accessory respiratory muscles. Monitor pulse oximetry and blood gas levels. *Head injuries may cause alterations in respirations. An increased respiratory rate may indicate hypoxia. A decrease in respiratory rate may be the result of depression of the medullary respiratory center.*
- Monitor ICP readings. Continuous measurement of ICP is used to diagnose and monitor IICP. *As ICP increases, herniation may occur, leading to respiratory arrest and death.*
- If the patient is not intubated, prepare for oxygen administration and/or tracheal intubation if respiratory distress occurs. *Supplying oxygen prevents hypoxia until a hematoma can be evacuated, relieving pressure on the respiratory center.*
- Prepare for cranial surgery if deteriorating respiratory pattern and neurologic changes are noted. *Surgical intervention usually consists of placing several burr holes in the skull or performing a craniotomy to remove the hematoma. (Intracranial surgery is discussed later in the chapter.) However, the cerebral edema and IICP may cause death even if surgery is performed.*

SAFETY ALERT: In general, an initial increase in intracranial pressure causes respirations to slow; as the pressure continues to increase, respirations become rapid. ■

Case Study & Nursing Care Plan

A Patient with a Subdural Hematoma

Wong Lee is a 50-year-old tug boat mechanic who is married and has three sons. Although Mr. Lee has been through rehabilitation twice for alcoholism, he has not been able to quit drinking. His physician has explained the physical consequences and the possible interaction between alcohol and the anticoagulant Mr. Lee is taking for chronic atrial fibrillation. While attending a family reunion, during which he eats a large meal and drinks several beers, Mr. Lee joins a game of softball. Mrs. Lee is concerned that Mr. Lee has consumed too much alcohol to play ball in the heat, but Mr. Lee is adamant and states that he wants to pitch. During the end of the second inning, the batter hits a ball that strikes Mr. Lee in the head. Mr. Lee stumbles and drops to the ground, holding his head. He does not lose consciousness and gets up on his own. His sons and wife try to persuade him to go to the hospital, but Mr. Lee insists he feels fine.

Two weeks later, after an evening of consuming several mixed drinks, Mr. Lee develops a headache. He attributes the headache to a hangover, but instead of improving the next day, the headache becomes steadily worse. He becomes confused and disoriented. His wife, concerned that his drinking is increasing again, calls the physician, who admits Mr. Lee to the detoxification center at the local hospital. A CT scan is performed. The diagnosis of a subdural hematoma is made, and Mr. Lee is transferred to the neurosurgical unit.

ASSESSMENT	DIAGNOSES	EXPECTED OUTCOMES
When Saundra Knight, the nurse on the neurosurgical unit, enters the room, she notices that Mr. Lee is sitting in bed, laughing and giddy. As she begins to talk to Mr. Lee, he states, "Don't ask me anything—I can't think. My headache is getting worse." Over the next few hours, the giddiness subsides, and Mr. Lee becomes drowsy. Ms. Knight reports a Glasgow Coma Scale score of 11. An ICP monitor is inserted and reveals IICP. Mr. Lee is scheduled to have burr holes and hematoma evacuation that afternoon.	■ Poor ventilation related to pressure on respiratory center by intracranial hematoma ■ Inadequate cerebral perfusion related to IICP secondary to cerebral edema	■ Patient will maintain a respiratory rate and rhythm within normal limits. ■ Patient will maintain adequate cerebral perfusion, as evidenced by stable vital signs, stable neurologic status, and no decrease in level of consciousness.

PLANNING AND IMPLEMENTATION

- Perform neurologic assessment every 2 hours or as needed.
- Monitor vital signs every 2 hours or as needed.
- Explain to the family the procedure for intracranial surgery.

EVALUATION

The first day postoperatively, Mr. Lee begins breathing on his own without ventilatory support. His respiratory rate and rhythm are within normal limits, with no signs of abnormal breath sounds. The ICP monitor readings are appropriate, and Mr. Lee shows significant improvement in level of consciousness, with a Glasgow Coma Scale score of 15. Mr. Lee continues to improve and is discharged to home 5 days after surgery.

CLINICAL REASONING IN PATIENT CARE

1. Describe the similarities and differences between Mr. Lee's disorder and the manifestations of other types of intracranial hematomas.
2. Mr. Lee kept trying to pull out his ICP line. You know he should not be restrained because pulling against restraints increases restlessness and increases intracranial pressure. What would you do?
3. Write a care plan for Mr. Lee to address his acute confusion.

See Evaluating Your Response in Appendix B.

Delegating Nursing Care Activities

As appropriate and allowed by the designated duties and responsibilities of unlicensed assistive personnel, the nurse may delegate nursing care activities such as measuring vital signs (including orthostatic vital signs) and providing skin care.

Transitions of Care

The best way to treat any injury is to prevent it from happening. Public education must continue to stress the importance of safe driving, the dangers of driving under the influence of alcohol or drugs, and the necessity of wearing seat belts and cycle helmets. Legislation has mandated such motor vehicle changes as seat belts, child safety seats, air bags, use of headsets with cell phones, and prohibition of texting while driving. Other behaviors that can reduce the morbidity and mortality associated with TBI are following gun safety rules, promoting farm safety, and teaching older adults about safety (such as preventing falls) in the home.

Inform the patient and family that a postconcussion syndrome sometimes occurs. If the patient experiences persistent headaches and dizziness, is uncharacteristically emotional, seems overly tired, or has difficulty paying attention or remembering, the healthcare provider should be notified. Explain that these manifestations may persist for some time. Rehabilitation may help the patient compensate for memory impairment and attention deficits.

Patients who survive an acute brain injury will require long-term physical care and rehabilitation. Although recovery is highly individualized, many patients who regain consciousness require lifelong care; others remain in a coma or vegetative state. The family members often expect the patient to recover fully after the coma subsides, and they need information about the real possibility of residual deficits in self-care, emotional responses, cognition, communication, and movement. Topics that should be addressed for home care include:

- The need to encourage self-care and independence as much as possible
- Information to enhance recovery (CDC, 2017):
  a. Get lots of rest. Don't rush back to work or school.
  b. Avoid anything that could cause another blow or jolt to the head.
  c. Consult with physician about when it will be safe to drive a car, ride a bike, or use heavy equipment (reaction time is often slower after a TBI).
  d. Take only prescribed drugs and don't drink alcohol.
  e. Write things down if you are having problems remembering.
  f. If the injury was severe, therapy may be needed to learn lost skills, such as speaking, walking, or reading.
- Safety issues
- Equipment needs, such as a wheelchair and hospital bed
- Vocational counseling and services
- Referral to community resources and support groups
- Helpful resources:
  a. National Head Injury Foundation
  b. Brain Injury Association of America
  c. Brain Trauma Foundation
  d. International Center for Individuals with Disabilities.

42.7 Brain Tumors

Brain tumors are growths of abnormal cells in brain tissue, meninges, the pituitary gland, or blood vessels. Brain tumors may be benign or malignant, primary or secondary (metastatic), and intracerebral or extracerebral. Regardless of type or location, brain tumors are potentially lethal because they grow within a closed cranial vault and displace or impinge on CNS structures. Chapter 14 provides information about cancer in adults.

It is estimated that 25,000 new cases of primary malignant brain tumors are diagnosed annually in the United States and approximately 16,000 people die each year (American Brain Tumor Association [ABTA], 2018b; American Cancer Society [ACS], 2018b).

The cause of many brain tumors is largely unknown. The brain itself is relatively protected from cancer-causing chemicals that are inhaled or eaten, including cigarette smoke. DNA mutations may affect oncogenes (speed up cell division) or tumor suppressor genes (slow cell division or cause cell death) so that the risk for or actual abnormal cell growth occurs. These mutations may be genetic or may occur as cells continually divide, die, and are replaced. Research is ongoing in this area (ABTA, 2018a).

The Patient with a Brain Tumor

Pathophysiology

Brain tumors may be classified as benign or malignant, based on the tissue type and characteristics of the cells. The use of the term *benign* may be misleading. A tumor that is benign by histologic examination but is surgically inaccessible may continue to grow and expand, increasing intracranial pressure and causing neurologic deficits, herniation, and finally death. In discussions of brain tumors, the term *malignant* is used to describe the lack of cell differentiation and the invasive nature of the tumor.

Brain tumors may also be classified as primary or metastatic, depending on their origin (**Table 42.9**). Primary tumors of CNS tissue arise from the cells and structures that are found within the brain, for example, neurons and neuroglia. The primary intracranial tumors that originate in the skull cavity but not from brain tissue itself arise from the supporting structures, including the meninges, pituitary gland, and pineal gland. Primary brain tumors are the most common type of brain tumor and rarely metastasize outside the CNS. Metastatic brain tumors originate from structures outside the brain, such as the lungs (most common origination), breasts, and prostate gland.

Table 42.9 Classification of Primary Brain Tumors

Tumor Name	Characteristics
Primary Tumors	
Glioma	
Astrocytoma	■ Most common glioma (30% of all brain tumors; 80% of all malignant brain tumors)
Glioblastoma multiforme	■ Most malignant form
Ependymoma	■ Fast growing
Oligodendroglioma	■ Tumor that develops from lining of ventricles
Astroblastoma	■ Rare, slow growing ■ May be encapsulated, benign
Extracerebral Tumors	
Medulloblastoma	■ Rare (1% of all brain tumors) ■ Fast growing and malignant ■ Found in cerebellum
Meningioma	■ Most common primary brain tumor (34%) ■ Slow growing ■ Develops in meninges (especially dura) ■ Firm and encapsulated
Acoustic neuroma (neurofibromatosis)	■ About 9% of all brain tumors ■ Slow growing ■ Benign ■ Originates from Schwann cells of cranial nerve XIII ■ May also affect cranial nerves V, VII, IX, and X ■ Genetic origin due to autosomal-dominant Mendelian trait ■ Firm, encapsulated lesions attached to nerve
Congenital (Developmental) Tumors	
Hemangioblastoma	■ Vascular tumor ■ Slow growing
Craniopharyngioma	■ Solid or cystic tumor ■ Compresses pituitary gland ■ Presses on the third ventricle and may cause blockage of CSF
Pituitary Adenomas	
Chromophobic	■ About 13% of all brain tumors ■ Account for most pituitary tumors ■ Nonsecreting tumor ■ Slow growing
Eosinophilic	■ Secreting tumors that produce growth hormone
Basophilic	■ Secreting tumors that produce adrenocorticotropic hormone ■ Fast growing

Focal disturbances from both primary and metastatic tumors take place when there is compression of brain tissue, tumor infiltration, or direct invasion of brain parenchyma with destruction of neural tissue, altered blood flow, and brain edema. Vasogenic edema occurs as the tumor grows and compresses adjacent tissue. Increased capillary permeability allows plasma to seep into the extracellular space and between the layers of the myelin sheath, altering electrical potential and impairing cell activity. Venous obstruction and edema due to breakdown of the blood–brain barrier by substances released by the tumor cells increase intracranial volume and intracranial pressure.

Manifestations

Manifestations can develop as a result of the growth of the tumor, while others are related to the location of the lesion. Some of the more common manifestations include changes in cognition or consciousness, a headache that is usually worse in the morning, seizures, and vomiting. Compression of brain tissue and the invasion of the brain tumor into the cerebral tissue may lead to changes typically seen with cerebral edema and IICP (described earlier in the chapter). Cerebral blood supply may diminish as the tumor compresses blood vessels. Shifts in brain tissue can occur, leading to brain herniation syndromes and, if untreated, death. **Table 42.10** outlines the manifestations of brain tumors by location.

Interprofessional Care

Treatment for a brain tumor may involve chemotherapy, radiation therapy, surgery, or any combination of these, as discussed in Chapter 14. Several variables are considered when selecting the appropriate treatment modality: The size and location of the tumor, the type of tumor, related symptoms (such as neurologic deficits), and the patient's overall condition.

Diagnosis

A thorough history and physical examination are conducted, with abnormal findings from an examination of the fundus of the eye, visual fields, neurologic assessment, and EEG used to identify a possible tumor. An MRI with gadolinium enhancement, the test of choice, can locate the tumor and define its size, shape, extent to which normal anatomy is distorted, and the degree of any associated cerebral edema. Arteriograms may show stretching or displacement of cerebral vessels by the tumor, as well as the presence of tumor vascularity. Endocrine studies are conducted if a pituitary tumor is suspected (Kee, 2014). (Refer to Chapters 18 and 41 for further information about diagnostic tests of the endocrine and neurologic systems.)

Chemotherapy

The use of chemotherapy to treat brain tumors has been limited by the blood–brain barrier. Various methods are

Table 42.10 Manifestations of Brain Tumors by Location

Lobe	Manifestations
Frontal lobe tumors	■ Inappropriate behavior ■ Recent memory loss ■ Personality changes ■ Headache ■ Inability to concentrate ■ Expressive aphasia ■ Impaired judgment ■ Motor dysfunctions
Parietal lobe tumors	■ Sensory deficits: Paresthesia, loss of two-point discrimination, visual field deficits
Temporal lobe tumors	■ Psychomotor seizures
Occipital lobe tumors	■ Visual disturbances
Cerebellum tumors	■ Disturbances in coordination and equilibrium
Pituitary tumors	■ Endocrine dysfunction ■ Visual deficits ■ Headache

used to overcome the barrier. An intraventricular method of medication administration uses an Ommaya reservoir that is surgically implanted into a lateral ventricle of the brain (**Figure 42.11** ■). Convection-enhanced delivery (CED) is the continuous injection of chemotherapy (as a fluid) directly to the tumor site through a catheter with positive pressure (in this case, the blood–brain barrier keeps the chemotherapy inside the brain). Biodegradable anhydrous wafers, which are impregnated with a chemotherapeutic drug, may be implanted into the tumor at the time of surgery as another option.

An oral chemotherapeutic medication, temozolomide (Temodar), is used for palliative therapy for glioblastoma. Research is ongoing to develop agents that will specifically target the genetic features and molecular profiles of a tumor (Adams et al., 2018).

Surgery

Surgery is the preferred treatment of primary tumors. The goal is to remove the tumor, if possible, reduce the size of the tumor, or provide symptom relief (palliation). The type of procedure, the surgical approach, and the timing of surgery (emergency vs. planned procedure) influence the overall nursing management of the patient having intracranial surgery.

Some of the more common intracranial neurosurgical procedures follow.

- *Burr hole:* A hole made in the skull with a special drill. The hole may facilitate the evacuation of an extracerebral clot or a series of holes may be made in preparation for craniotomy (refer to Figure 42.10).
- *Craniotomy:* A surgical opening into the cranial cavity (**Figure 42.12** ■). A series of burr holes is made and the bone between the holes is cut with a special saw called a *craniotome*. The tumor is excised, and the bone flap is returned to the opening. A craniotomy may also be performed to repair defects associated with traumatic head injuries or to repair a cerebral aneurysm.
- *Craniectomy:* An excision of a portion of the skull and complete removal of the bone flap. This procedure may be done to provide decompression after cerebral edema. Pressure on the brain structures is reduced by providing space for expansion.
- *Cranioplasty:* Plastic repair to the skull in which synthetic material is inserted to replace the cranial bone that was removed. This procedure may be performed after a large craniectomy. The plastic repair restores the contour and integrity of the cranium.

Radiation Therapy

Radiation therapy may be administered alone or as adjunctive therapy with surgery. Radiation is often the treatment of choice for surgically inaccessible tumors; it may also be used to decrease the size of a tumor prior to surgery. Tumors that were not completely excised by surgery may also be treated with radiation.

Specialty Procedures

Technologic advances—including the development of special instruments, the use of stereotaxic techniques for localizing a specific target, and the use of the laser beam—have greatly advanced neurosurgical practice. Microsurgery involves an operating microscope with microinstruments and supportive illumination equipment. Using stereotaxic techniques to precisely locate a specific target point allows for location of discrete areas of the brain that control specific functions and exact locations of deep brain lesions. The use of a laser beam for excision of a tumor results in less damage

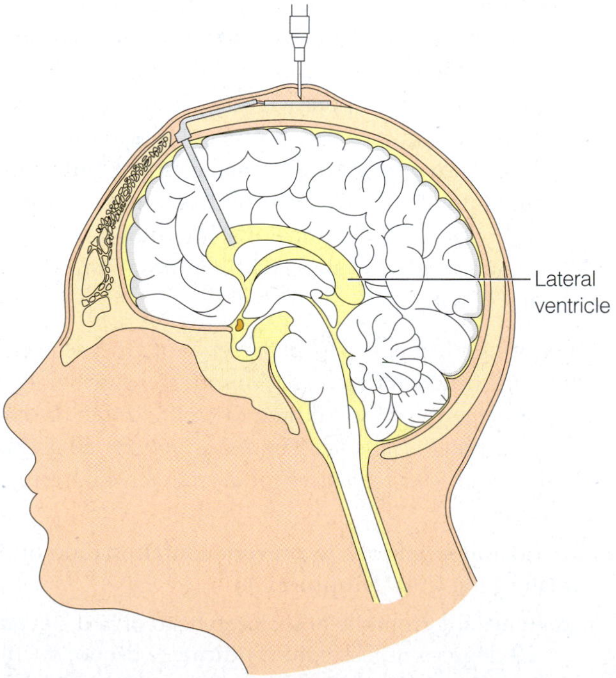
Lateral
ventricle

Figure 42.11 ■ Ommaya reservoir for medication administration.

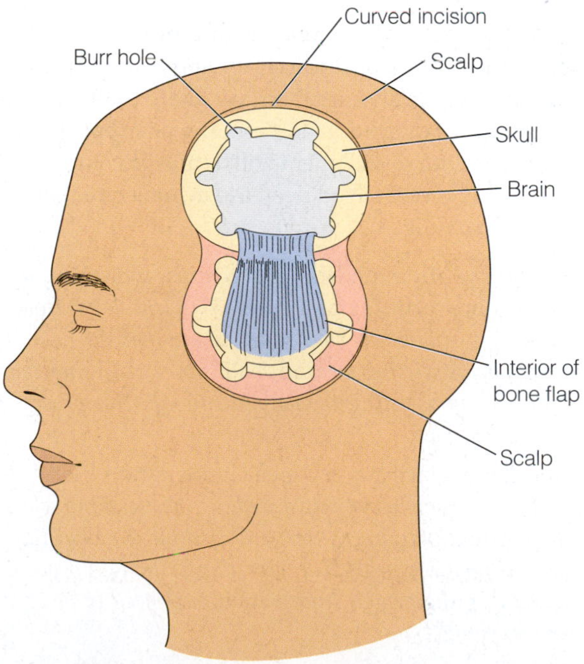
Curved incision
Burr hole
Scalp
Skull
Brain
Interior of
bone flap
Scalp

Figure 42.12 ■ In a craniotomy, a portion of the skull and overlying scalp is removed to allow access to the brain.

to surrounding tissue and less postoperative swelling. The gamma knife, which is not actually a knife but a heavily shielded helmet, is capable of destroying deep and otherwise inaccessible lesions in a single treatment session (ACS, 2018a). Research is being conducted on other methods of treating brain tumors, including hyperthermia and duplicating the immune response.

Nursing Care

The nursing care of the patient with a brain tumor includes support during the diagnostic period and specific management as directed by the selected treatment. The foundation for care is data from the health history and physical assessment, which includes identifying neurologic deficits. Many of the alterations in health commonly experienced by the patient with a brain tumor have been discussed throughout this chapter, including altered level of consciousness, IICP, and seizures. The patient will require intensive care in the immediate postoperative period. In addition to the nursing care described in this section, see the Case Study & Nursing Care Plan for a patient with a brain tumor on page 1591.

Assessment

See the Manifestations and Interprofessional Care sections for the assessment of the patient with a brain tumor.

Priorities of Care

Collaborating with the interprofessional team to ensure adequate treatment of the underlying process while providing care that supports the physical and psychologic responses to the disorder is a priority of nursing care.

Diagnoses, Outcomes, and Interventions

This section of the chapter focuses on nursing interventions for the patient who has intracranial surgery. The nursing diagnoses discussed are anxiety, risk for infection, ineffective protection, acute pain, and low self-esteem.

Relieve Anxiety. The diagnosis of a brain tumor brings anxiety and feelings of uncertainty about the future. Both the patient and family members are likely to be apprehensive and require education and emotional support.

Expected Outcome: Patient will be able to control anxiety as evidenced by verbalized decrease in subjective distress.

The nurse will:

- Explain routine medical procedures, including bloodwork and radiologic studies. *Baseline laboratory and radiologic studies are needed to ensure that the patient has no other preexisting medical condition. Explaining the procedures and assisting the patient through this process help decrease anxiety.*
- Reinforce, clarify, and repeat information. *Both patient and family may have limited understanding of the scheduled diagnostic tests, procedures, and treatment modalities. The patient may be confused or have altered thought processes as a result of the tumor. Information may need to be repeated or reexplained.*
- Encourage patient and family to verbalize feelings, questions, and fears. Provide realistic information appropriate to their level of understanding. *Verbalization helps reduce anxiety and fear.*
- Review patient and family strengths and effective coping skills. *Personal strengths, support systems, and coping skills can aid in the development of appropriate strategies to reduce anxiety.*
- Arrange for a member of the clergy to visit, if desired. *Faith in a higher being is often a strong source of strength and support.*
- Provide preoperative teaching, including the following information:
  a. Type of anesthesia and surgery
  b. Time surgery will begin and expected length of procedure and recovery room stay
  c. Where the patient will be taken after surgery (CCU, ICU) (if possible, show the patient and family the CCU or ICU and introduce them to the nurse who will be in charge of care after the surgery)
  d. Where family can wait during and following surgery
  e. Appearance of the patient after surgery, which may include swollen, bruised eyelids and other facial features; a large dressing covering the head; a partially or fully shaved head; and a tracheostomy or endotracheal tube
  f. Behavior of the patient after surgery, which will differ depending on the site of surgery, although cognitive and behavioral changes are common

  Information about what to expect reduces anxiety.
- Allow time for patient and family to be together. *Patients and families need quiet time together to support each other and prepare emotionally for surgery.*

Reduce Risk for Infection. The patient who has had intracranial surgery is at risk for infection from multiple invasive lines, the scalp wound, and the risk of introduction of bacteria into the operative area. The nurse provides interventions to monitor for and prevent infection.

Expected Outcome: Infection management and control will be maintained as evidenced by freedom from symptoms of infection, maintenance of white blood cell count and differential, and vital signs within normal limits.

The nurse will:

- Monitor for leakage of CSF: Presence of glucose in clear drainage from ears, nose, or wound; constant swallowing; statements of "something dripping down the back of my throat." *These manifestations indicate an opening in the dura, which provides an avenue for an ascending infection.*
- Provide interventions to prevent contamination of the area leaking CSF, if appropriate:
  a. If leaking from the nose: Keep head of bed elevated 20 degrees unless contraindicated; do not suction nasally; do not clean nose; tell patient not to put finger in nose; do not insert packing.

Moving Evidence into Action

Cognitive Dysfunction in Patients with Metastases of the Brain

Clinical Issue

Cognitive impairments in patients with brain tumors raise challenges for the patient, their caregivers and the treatment team. The use of personalized coping strategies may help caregivers when delivered as part of the patient's care.

External Evidence

Saria and colleagues (2017) described coping and resilience in 56 caregivers of patients with brain tumors. The caregivers reported that memory impairment occurred more frequently than depressive symptoms or disruptive behavior. The caregivers reported that acceptance was the most commonly used coping strategy. In conclusion, the authors reported that an individualized approach promotes positive coping in caregivers of patients with brain metastatic tumors.

Internal Evidence

As part of the evaluation of internal evidence, one must consider the impact of the external evidence findings on how healthcare providers interact with this population.

Patient Considerations

When considering use of a new or promoting an existing practice (like personalizing teaching and counseling about coping strategies), the nurse must consider the specific patient population where it will be used (in this case, the caregivers of patients with metastatic brain tumors). Will patients and their caregivers be amenable to more personalized coping strategy instruction?

Pulling the Pieces Together

Caregivers dealing with a diagnosis of metastatic brain cancer is challenging enough. Add to that emerging symptoms like cognitive decline, depression, or disruptive behaviors makes caregiving even more challenging. Coping strategies are important skills for the nurse to promote with caregivers of seriously ill patients. The information from this study (supporting personalized coping skills teaching) is important information to consider when attempting to meet the needs of caregivers of this population.

Reference

Saria, M. G., Courchesne, N., Evangelista, L., Carter, J., MacManus, D. A., Gorman, M. K., . . . Maliski, S. (2017). Cognitive dysfunction in patients with brain metastases: Influences on caregiver resilience and coping. *Supportive Care in Cancer, 25*, 2247–1256.

b. If leaking from the ear: Position patient on side of leakage unless contraindicated; do not clean ear; tell patient not to put finger in ear; do not insert packing.

c. Place a sterile dressing over the area of drainage and change as soon as it becomes damp.

Leakage of CSF indicates a break in the dura and increases the risk of an ascending infection. Surgery may be necessary to repair the break; however, the leak usually heals spontaneously in about 1 week.

- Monitor for and report manifestations of infection:
  - a. Take and record temperature on a regular basis.
  - b. Assess IV insertion sites for redness, swelling, drainage, and pain.
  - c. Assess scalp wound for redness, swelling, bulging, drainage, and pain.
  - d. Assess for manifestations of meningitis: Fever and chills, increasing headache, neck stiffness, positive Kernig's or Brudzinski sign, photophobia.
  - e. Monitor laboratory reports for increased WBC count.

Intact skin is the first line of defense against infection. Any break in the skin increases the risk of infection. Intracranial surgery increases the risk of meningitis, with infectious agents ascending into the brain.

- Implement interventions to prevent infection:
  - a. Use strict aseptic technique when changing dressings and when caring for wound drains and ICP monitor lines.
  - b. Keep the patient's hands away from drains and dressings; use mitten restraints, if necessary.
  - c. Administer prescribed antibiotics.

Sterile technique decreases the risk of introducing infection into a wound. Antibiotics are usually prescribed prophylactically to prevent infection.

Reduce Risk of IICP and Bleeding. The patient who has intracranial surgery does not have normal human defenses against changes in intracranial pressure and is also at risk from cerebral edema, IICP (with seizures), and a shift of intracerebral contents. In addition, the surgery may cause cerebral bleeding or hematoma formation. Assessments and interventions for IICP and seizures were described earlier in the chapter.

Expected Outcome: Patient will remain free of any evidence of new increased intracranial pressure or bleeding.

If a shunt has been inserted, the following applies:

- ***For internal shunts:*** Avoid pressure on the shunt, reservoir, or tubing. Pump the shunt only if prescribed.
- ***For external shunts:*** Avoid kinks in tubing, and maintain the drainage collecting device and patient's head at the prescribed levels.

Relieve Acute Pain. The patient who has intracranial surgery has a headache as a result of either compression or displacement of brain tissue or from IICP.

Expected Outcome: Patient will achieve adequate pain control as evidenced by rest and sleep behaviors and reduced pain-related behaviors.

The nurse will:

- Assess the location, duration, and intensity of the pain, using a scale of 0 (no pain) to 10 (worst pain) in the patient who can communicate verbally. *The patient is the best source of information about pain.*
- Implement interventions to reduce the pain:
  a. Raise the head of the bed slightly.
  b. Reduce noise and bright lights in the room.
  c. If allowed, loosen head dressing.
  d. Administer narcotic analgesics with caution.

  Nonpharmacologic measures and medications may be used to reduce IICP and headache.

SAFETY ALERT: Narcotic analgesics mask changes in eye signs and depress respirations. ■

Promote Acceptance and Independence. The patient who has intracranial surgery has many alterations that affect self-esteem and body image. Physical changes include a loss of hair on the scalp, swelling and bruising in the eyelids and face, and perhaps an indentation in the skull. The patient must depend on others to meet basic needs. There are often long-term neurologic deficits, affecting areas such as speech, vision, and motor abilities, which require changes in roles and relationships.

Expected Outcome: Patient will demonstrate that self-perceptions are accurate given their physical capabilities.

The nurse will:

- Assess for verbal and nonverbal manifestations of negative self-esteem: Denial of changes, preoccupation with changes, refusal to look in the mirror, withdrawal from family and friends, expressions of grief and loss. *Low self-esteem can be initiated by stressful situations and changes in body image.*
- Provide interventions to improve self-concept:
  a. Limit negative self-assessment.
  b. Help focus on positive areas of life.
  c. Help identify sources of support and strength.
  d. Help identify and use helpful coping methods.
  e. Encourage significant others to visit.
  f. Encourage independence in self-care.

  Self-esteem is derived from one's own perceptions of competence and from the responses of others. When one's self-concept and self-ideal are congruent, self-esteem is enhanced.

Transitions of Care

The effect of the possible outcomes following the surgery often produces fear in both patient and family, interfering with their ability to retain information. The patient may have cognitive or neurologic deficits that interfere with learning. Family members must be assessed for their ability to cope with the stress of the surgery. Information may have to be repeated several times.

Patients and their families who have experienced intracranial surgery require emotional support. The process of recovery is often extended and may involve adaptation to changes in body image and management of any motor or sensory deficits. If family members are willing, they may begin to assist with ADLs while the patient is in the hospital, such as assisting with personal hygiene and meals. Patients should also be encouraged to take an active role in their own care. Discharge planning includes a discussion of the following topics: Medication information; wound care; the use of wigs, turbans, hats, or colorful scarves; and the importance of follow-up visits. In addition, emphasize the importance of reporting manifestations such as stiff neck, increasing headache, elevated temperature, new motor or sensory deficits, vision changes, or seizures.

Provide information about the overall treatment plan, management of deficits and/or disabilities, and future needs. Specific teaching topics are:

- Safety measures for motor deficits, sensory deficits, lack of coordination, seizures, and cognitive deficits
- Comfort measures for nausea and vomiting and pain
- Measures for communication, if aphasia is present
- Measures to improve vision, if visual deficits are present
- How to buy wigs and hairpieces
- Referrals to support groups and community resources
- Helpful resources:
  a. American Cancer Society
  b. American Brain Tumor Association
  c. National Brain Tumor Foundation
  d. Brain Tumor Society.

42.8 Headache

Headache, one of the most frequent manifestations of a health problem, is pain within the cranial vault. Headaches may occur as a result of benign or pathologic conditions, intracranial or extracranial conditions, diseases of other body systems, stress, musculoskeletal tension, or a combination of these factors. Most tension headaches are mild, transient, and relieved by a mild analgesic. However, some headaches are chronic, intense, and recurrent. Manifestations of headache vary according to the cause, type, and precipitating symptoms.

Pathophysiology

The bones of the skull and the brain tissue lack pain-sensitive nerve fibers, but selected structures within and surrounding the cranial vault are sensitive to pain. There are many different types of headaches, and headaches may be primary or secondary to many other illnesses and injuries. This discussion focuses on migraine headache and cluster headache.

Migraine Headache

Migraine headache is a recurring primary headache, often initiated by a triggering event and usually accompanied by a neurologic dysfunction. It affects about 20 million people

Case Study & Nursing Care Plan

A Patient with a Brain Tumor

Claire Lange is a 42-year-old television announcer. During one night's broadcast, she confuses several major news items so badly that her coanchor tries to correct her. Ms. Lange responds angrily that she does not need any help and then rises and storms off the set. As she leaves the camera area, she limps noticeably and appears to drag her left leg. The show's producer asks her what is wrong; she screams that nothing is wrong—she simply has another headache. He follows her to her dressing room and inquires about her headaches. She tells him that they come and go but have been getting worse lately. He then asks her if she has injured her left leg; she responds that the leg was weak because she was tired. As the producer leaves the dressing room, Ms. Lange begins to shake and collapses on the floor. The producer recognizes that she is having a seizure and calls for an ambulance.

Ms. Lange is admitted to the neurology floor of the local hospital for evaluation. A CT scan, MRI, and EEG are completed and identify an intracranial mass. A biopsy of the mass is positive for malignant cells. A glioma in the frontal lobe is identified, and surgery is scheduled for that week.

ASSESSMENT

When Clara Rosetti, RN, enters Ms. Lange's room, she sees Ms. Lange looking at her shoulder-length hair in the mirror. Ms. Lange tells Ms. Rosetti that she has never in her life worn her hair any shorter, and "Now you're going to cut it all off!" She paces the room and makes the statement, "I guess the hair isn't really important if I survive this situation." She also says that she has a headache.

DIAGNOSES

- Headache related to tumor and increase in intracranial pressure
- Anxiety related to upcoming hair loss, cranial incision, and unknown future following surgery

EXPECTED OUTCOMES

- Patient will verbalize the causes of pain.
- Patient will verbalize an understanding of the changes in body appearance that are associated with the scheduled intracranial surgery (e.g., shaving of the head prior to surgery, cranial incision, facial swelling postoperatively).
- Patient will identify measures that will help minimize the effect of the hair loss.
- Patient will verbalize a reduction in anxiety.

PLANNING AND IMPLEMENTATION

- Assess level of discomfort using a rating scale of 0 to 10.
- Provide a quiet, nonstimulating environment.
- Position the patient for comfort, keeping the head of the bed elevated to promote venous drainage.
- Assess level of consciousness for potential increases in ICP.
- Encourage patient to verbalize feelings about the surgery.
- Suggest measures that may help minimize the hair loss, such as the use of turbans, scarves, hats, and wigs.
- Suggest relaxation techniques to decrease anxiety.

EVALUATION

By the time of surgery, Ms. Lange has recognized the relationship between the brain tumor and the headache. She states that lying in a flat position and coughing increase the headache. The head of the bed is kept at a 30- to 42-degree angle. Daily activities are spaced to provide periods of rest. Ms. Lange demonstrates no significant changes in level of consciousness. She has talked about the effect of the loss of her hair and television responsibilities. Ms. Lange has learned that the hair preparation would be done in surgery and that the hair would be saved for her. She states she has already consulted her hair stylist and that "scarves and turbans are on the way."

CLINICAL REASONING IN PATIENT CARE

1. Outline interventions to decrease intracranial pressure both before and after surgery.
2. When making your initial assessments on the morning of surgery, you find that Ms. Lange has a decreased pulse and increased blood pressure. She tells you her headache is worse and suddenly vomits. What do you do now?
3. Ms. Lange asks you to be sure that she has absolutely no visitors after surgery because she knows how ugly she will look. How would you respond?
4. Design a plan of care for Ms. Lange to address her feelings of acute anxiety and lack of control over her circumstances.

See Evaluating Your Response in Appendix B.

in the United States and is more common in women than in men. The headaches have a familial association and are thought to be inherited as an autosomal-dominant trait. Migraine headaches may occur daily or as infrequently as once a year.

The two most common types of migraine headaches are migraine without an aura (occurring in about 85% of cases) and classic migraine with aura (Sorenson et al., 2019). In a migraine with aura, some type of sensory manifestation (such as visual disturbances) occurs prior to the manifestations. The manifestations, except for the aura, are the same for both types. The exact causes of migraine are not fully understood, but there is a relationship between serotonin and migraine headaches. It is thought that cerebral blood vessels narrow and reduce blood flow, followed by vasodilation, swelling, and pain.

A variety of factors are believed to trigger the onset of a migraine headache. Rapid changes in blood glucose levels, stress, emotional excitement, fatigue, alcohol intake, stimuli such as bright lights, and food high in tyramine or other vasoactive substances (e.g., aged cheese, nuts, chocolate, and alcoholic beverages) have been associated with migraine attacks. Hypertension and fever may make the disorder worse. The menstrual cycle is a trigger for many women.

In a migraine headache, the pain is unilateral and throbbing, but can become bilateral as the headache continues. Physical activity or even moving the head can intensify pain. Chills, nausea and vomiting, fatigue, and sensitivity to light, sound, or odor are often present. Other manifestations may include blurred vision, anorexia, hunger, diarrhea, abdominal cramping, facial pallor, sweating, and stiffness or tenderness of the neck. The headache lasts 4 to 72 hours and then gradually subsides. The patient may be acutely ill and is often extremely irritable. The sensory organs often become hypersensitive, and the patient withdraws from sound and light. The scalp is tender. After the headache, the headache area is sensitive to touch and a deep aching is present. The patient is exhausted.

Cluster Headache

A *cluster headache* is an extremely severe, unilateral, burning pain located behind or around the eyes; it is predominantly experienced by men between 20 and 40 years of age. The headaches occur in groups or "clusters" of one to eight each day for several weeks or months, followed by remission lasting months to years (NINDS, 2018c). The physiologic mechanism underlying cluster headaches is not well understood, but involves a vascular disorder, a disturbance of serotonergic mechanisms, a sympathetic defect, or dysregulation of the hypothalamus. The headaches often occur in the spring and fall and then disappear for an extended period. Triggers for cluster headaches are individualized and include alcohol intake, certain foods, smoking, high altitude, and sleep cycle disturbances.

Although the headache may occur at any time, it typically begins 2 to 3 hours after falling asleep, awakens the person, and then lasts from 15 minutes to 3 hours. Intense unilateral pain around or behind one eye is accompanied by rhinorrhea, lacrimation, flushing, sweating, facial edema, and possible miosis or ptosis on the affected side. The same side of the head is involved in each cluster of attacks.

The Patient with a Headache

Interprofessional Care

Therapeutic management of migraine and cluster headache includes a combination of patient teaching, medications, and measures to control contributing factors.

Diagnosis

Diagnosis and treatment are based on history, identifying triggering or precipitating events, and the type of headache. A thorough history and physical examination are integral parts of the assessment. Neurodiagnostic testing may be done to rule out a structural disease process. Testing may include a brain scan, MRI, x-ray studies of the skull and cervical spine, EEG, or lumbar puncture for CSF if inflammation is suspected. Serum metabolic screens and hypersensitivity testing may also be performed if systemic problems are suspected.

Medications

The management of migraine and cluster headaches includes administering medications to prevent pain (prophylactic therapy) as well as drugs to stop (or abort) a headache in progress. The patient with frequent migraine headaches is a candidate for prophylactic therapy. When the manifestations of migraine are recognized early, medications may be used to abort or limit the severity and duration of the headache. Drug categories used to treat migraine headaches, followed by examples, include beta-blockers (*propranolol* [Inderal]), tricyclic antidepressants (*amitriptyline* [Endep]), ergot alkaloids (methysergide [Sansert]), selective serotonin reuptake inhibitors (SSRIs) (*paroxetine* [Paxil]), and calcium channel antagonists (*verapamil* [Calan]).

Sumatriptan (Imitrex) is available in oral, nasal spray, or subcutaneous injection forms. It binds with serotonin$_1$ receptors and is rapidly effective. Zolmitriptan (Zomig), a serotonin 5-HT$_1$-receptor agonist, is administered orally or by nasal spray and is effective in the treatment of acute headache. Once a migraine is in progress, a narcotic analgesic such as codeine may be required. Antiemetics may be prescribed to control nausea and vomiting.

(*Note:* Drugs identified in *italics* are among the 200 most commonly prescribed medications in the United States.)

Many of the same medications used to treat migraine headaches are used to treat cluster headaches. Medications such as ergotamine tartrate may be given in suppository form at bedtime to prevent headache during the episodic attacks. Patients may find that inhaling 100% oxygen at 7 L/min for 15 minutes at the onset of an attack relieves their headache. Preventive treatment includes calcium channel blockers, lithium carbonate, topiramate, and baclofen. Intranasal lidocaine may be effective. Deep-brain surgical neurostimulation is an experimental approach that is having some success in eliminating cluster headaches (Adams et al., 2017).

Integrative Therapies

Multiple complementary and integrative therapies have been described to effectively treat headaches. Evidence supports use of acupuncture generally for headaches. Biofeedback has been shown to be effective for tension headaches. Equivocal findings continue for massage, relaxation techniques, or spinal manipulation, so these should be used with caution. Herbs that have been reported effective for migraine headaches include butterbur while feverfew, magnesium, and riboflavin have been reported as effective. Additionally, coenzyme Q10 is reported as possibly effective (NCCIH, 2018a).

Nursing Care

The primary response of the patient requiring nursing interventions is teaching for self-care at home. Provide suggestions for strategies to control the pain (see **Box 42.4**). In addition, suggest the patient keep a diary of duration, onset, location, relation to menstruation or food intake, and precipitating triggers. Referrals for methods of stress reduction may be necessary for patients with long-term or migraine headaches.

BOX 42.4
Suggestions to Decrease Incidence of Migraine Headaches

- Wake up at the same time every morning.
- Eat your meals and exercise on a regular schedule.
- No smoking or caffeine after 3:00 p.m.
- No artificial sweeteners or MSG.
- Reduce or eliminate red wine, cheese, alcohol, chocolate, and caffeine.
- Practice relaxation techniques, such as yoga, meditation, or biofeedback.

CHAPTER HIGHLIGHTS

42.1 Altered Level of Consciousness

Describe the pathophysiology and manifestations of altered level of consciousness, and outline the interprofessional care and nursing care of patients with this condition.

- Altered level of consciousness (LOC) is a common response to intracranial disorders and is an early manifestation of deterioration of the function of the cerebral hemispheres. The alteration in cerebral function occurs in a sequential pattern, with characteristic changes in LOC, respiratory patterns, pupillary and oculomotor responses, and motor function.
- Coma states include persistent vegetative state and locked-in syndrome.

42.2 Increased Intracranial Pressure

Describe the pathophysiology and manifestations of increased intracranial pressure, and outline the interprofessional care and nursing care of patients with this condition.

- Increased intracranial pressure (IICP) is a sustained elevated pressure (greater than 10 mmHg) within the cranial cavity. IICP may result from cerebral edema, hydrocephalus, head trauma, tumors, abscesses, inflammation, hemorrhage, or stroke.
- The manifestations of IICP include a decreasing LOC, abnormal motor weakness and responses, altered vision, altered vital signs, headache, papilledema, and projectile vomiting. If untreated, IICP causes a displacement (herniation) of cerebral tissue and herniation of the cerebellum through the tentorium, followed by herniation of the brainstem through the foramen magnum. This is a lethal complication of IICP because it puts pressure on the vital centers in the medulla. IICP is primarily managed with osmotic diuretics and monitored with continuous intracranial pressure monitors.

42.3 Seizures

Describe the pathophysiology and manifestations of seizures, and outline the interprofessional care and nursing care of patients with seizures.

- A seizure is a single event of abnormal electrical discharge.
- Epilepsy is a chronic seizure disorder of abnormal, recurring, excessive, and self-terminating electrical discharges from neurons.
- Seizures are categorized into those that affect only a part of the brain (partial seizures) and those that affect all of the brain (generalized). The most common type of seizure in adults is a tonic–clonic generalized seizure.

42.4 Stroke

Describe the pathophysiology and manifestations of stroke, and outline the interprofessional care and nursing care of patients with stroke.

- A stroke is a condition in which neurologic deficits result from a sudden decrease in blood flow to a localized area of the brain. Strokes may be ischemic or hemorrhagic. Ischemic strokes result from a blockage of a cerebral artery by formation of a blood clot or by a clot or foreign substance lodging in a blood vessel; they include transient ischemic attacks, thrombotic strokes, or embolic strokes. Hemorrhagic strokes occur when a cerebral blood vessel ruptures. Depending on the size and location of cerebral tissue damage, strokes may cause cognitive and behavior changes, sensory-perceptual deficits, language disorders, and motor deficits. Treatment of an ischemic stroke with fibrinolytic therapy within 3 hours of the onset of manifestations may reverse damage to cerebral neurons. Nursing care is directed toward both prevention of a stroke through community-based educational programs and interventions to promote recovery and decrease complications.

42.5 Intracranial Vascular Disorders

Describe the pathophysiology and manifestations of intracranial vascular disorders, and outline the interprofessional care and nursing care of patients with these disorders.

- Intracerebral hemorrhage may follow rupture of an intracranial aneurysm or arteriovenous malformation. Intracranial aneurysms occur at the site of a weakness in a cerebral blood vessel. AV malformations are a tangled collection of dilated arteries and veins.
- An epidural hematoma develops in the potential space between the dura and the skull. A subdural hematoma collects between the dura mater and the arachnoid mater. Diffuse brain injuries include contusions, concussions, and diffuse axonal injury. Patients with an acute TBI must have immediate transport and treatment in an ED, followed by care in an ICU. They will require long-term physical care and rehabilitation.
- Arteriovenous malformations are a tangled collection of dilated arteries and veins, increasing the risk for rupture.

42.6 Traumatic Brain Injury

Describe the pathophysiology and manifestations of traumatic brain injuries, and outline the interprofessional care and nursing care of patients with this condition.

- Traumatic brain injury (TBI) refers to any injury of the scalp, skull, or brain and is a leading cause of death and disability.
- Traumatic brain injuries can include focal or diffuse brain injury. An acute brain injury affects all body systems and carries the risk of secondary injury to the brain from hypoxia and ischemia.

42.7 Brain Tumors

Describe the pathophysiology and manifestations of brain tumors, and outline the interprofessional care and nursing care of patients with brain tumors.

- Brain tumors are growths within the cranium, including on or in brain tissue, the meninges, the pituitary gland, or blood vessels.
- Brain tumors may be benign or malignant, primary or metastatic, and intracerebral or extracerebral.
- Regardless of the type or location, brain tumors are potentially lethal because they displace or impinge on CNS structures within a closed bony system.

42.8 Headache

Describe the pathophysiology and manifestations of headaches, and outline the interprofessional care and nursing care of patients with headaches.

- Headaches, a common type of intracranial pain, are categorized as tension, migraine, and cluster.
- A classic migraine is characterized by an aura; a common migraine does not have an aura.

TEST YOURSELF NCLEX-RN® REVIEW

1. The nurse is assessing the breathing pattern of a patient with a head injury who has a change in level of consciousness. Which pathophysiologic event causes an irregular respiratory pattern as level of consciousness decreases?
   A. Pressure on the meninges
   B. Reflexive motor responses
   C. Loss of the oculocephalic reflex
   D. Lower brainstem responses to changes in $PaCO_2$
2. The nurse assesses a depressed gag reflex in an unconscious patient. The nurse's priority interventions will relate to which patient problem?
   A. Increased risk of aspiration
   B. Ineffectiveness of breathing pattern
   C. Risk for increased intracranial pressure
   D. Risk for poor nutrition
3. The nurse is caring for a patient with a closed head injury. The nurse evaluates that the prescribed hyperosmotic agents are having their intended effects when which assessment is made? (Select all that apply.)
   A. Body temperature decreases
   B. Patient is seizure-free
   C. Stools for occult blood are negative
   D. Urine output increases
   E. Intracranial pressure decreases
4. The nurse is monitoring the neurologic status of a patient in a coma. Which command should the nurse use to accurately identify changes in mental status?
   A. "Squeeze my hand."
   B. "Tell me your name."
   C. "Are you having trouble breathing?"
   D. "Look at this light when I shine it in your eyes."

5. Laboratory tests are being prescribed for a patient with altered level of consciousness. Which tests should the nurse expect to be prescribed for this patient? (Select all that apply.)
   A. Blood glucose
   B. Urine for WBCs
   C. Serum electrolytes
   D. Liver function tests
   E. Blood and urine toxicology
6. The nurse is caring for a patient with altered level of consciousness. On which laboratory value should the nurse focus as the most accurate indicator of hydration status in the patient?
   A. CBC
   B. Urinalysis
   C. Blood culture
   D. Serum osmolality
7. The nurse is concerned that a patient is experiencing a transient ischemic attack. What did the nurse most likely assess in this patient? (Select all that apply.)
   A. Sudden severe pain over the left eye
   B. Visual disturbance of one or both eyes
   C. Loss of sensation and reflexes in both legs
   D. Complete paralysis of the right arm and leg
   E. Numbness and tingling in the corner of the mouth
8. The nurse is instructing a patient on ways to prevent a stroke. What should the nurse emphasize as being the greatest risks for a stroke? (Select all that apply.)
   A. Diabetes
   B. History of head trauma
   C. Heart disease
   D. Hypertension
   E. Hyperlipidemia
9. The nurse is providing care for a patient who has had an acute ischemic stroke of a left cerebral vessel. The medical record includes information that the patient has contralateral deficits. What does this information suggest to the nurse?
   A. Both sides of the body are involved.
   B. Deficits will be present below the level of the stroke.
   C. The patient will have neurologic deficits on the left side of the body.
   D. The patient will have neurologic deficits on the right side of the body.
10. A patient has had a carotid endarterectomy. The nurse plans which care for this patient? (Select all that apply.)
   A. Position on the operative side.
   B. Support the head during position changes.
   C. Keep the head of bed elevated at least 45 degrees.
   D. Maintain head and neck alignment.
   E. Keep a tracheostomy tray at the bedside.

See Test Yourself answers in Appendix B.

REFERENCES

Adams, M., Holland, N., & Urban, C. (2017). *Pharmacology for nurses: A pathophysiological approach* (5th ed.). Boston, MA: Pearson.

American Brain Tumor Association (ABTA). (2018a). *Brain tumor information.* Retrieved from www.abta.org/brain-tumor-information/.

American Brain Tumor Association (ABTA). (2018b). *Brain tumor statistics.* Retrieved from www.abta.org/about-us/news/brain-tumor-statistics/.

American Cancer Society (ACS). (2018a). *Brain and spinal cord tumors in adults.* Retrieved from https://www.cancer.org/cancer/brain-spinal-cord-tumors-adults.html.

American Cancer Society (ACS). (2018b). *Cancer facts and figures 2018.* Retrieved from https://www.cancer.org/content/dam/cancer-org/research/cancer-facts-and-statistics/annual-cancer-facts-and-figures/2018/cancer-facts-and-figures-2018.pdf.

American Heart Association. (2018). *Heart disease and stroke statistics at-a-glance.* Retrieved from www.heart.org/idc/groups/ahamah-public/@wcm/@sop/@smd/documents/downloadable/ucm_498848.pdf?utm_campaign=sciencenews17-18&utm_source=science-news&utm_medium=heart&utm_content=phd01-31-18.

American Stroke Association. (2018a). *Effects of strokes.* Retrieved from www.strokeassociation.org/STROKEORG/AboutStroke/EffectsofStroke/Effects-of-Stroke_UCM_308534_SubHomePage.jsp.

American Stroke Association. (2018b). *Warning signs and symptoms of stroke.* Retrieved from www.strokeassociation.org/STROKEORG/WarningSigns/Stroke-Warning-Signs-and-Symptoms_UCM_308528_SubHomePage.jsp.

Bob Woodruff Foundation. (2018). *Get the stats on traumatic brain injury in the United States.* Retrieved from https://www.brainline.org/article/get-stats-traumatic-brain-injury-united-states.

Carney, N., Totten, A. M., O'Reilly, C., Ullman, J. S., Hawryluk, G. W. J., & Bell, M. J. (2016). *Guidelines for the management of severe traumatic brain injury* (4th ed.). Retrieved from https://braintrauma.org/uploads/03/12/Guidelines_for_Management_of_Severe_TBI_4th_Edition.pdf.

Centers for Disease Control and Prevention. (2017). *Recovery from concussion.* Retrieved from https://www.cdc.gov/headsup/basics/concussion_recovery.html.

Centers for Disease Control and Prevention. (2018a). *Traumatic brain injury and concussions.* Retrieved from https://www.cdc.gov/traumaticbraininjury/index.html

Centers for Disease Control and Prevention. (2018b). *Types of stroke.* Retrieved from https://www.cdc.gov/stroke/types_of_stroke.htm.

Epilepsy Foundation. (2018a). *About epilepsy: The basics.* Retrieved from https://www.epilepsy.com/learn/about-epilepsy-basics.

Epilepsy Foundation. (2018b). *Types of seizures.* Retrieved from https://www.epilepsy.com/learn/types-seizures.

Hickey, J. V. (2013). *The clinical practice of neurological and neurosurgical nursing* (7th ed.). Philadelphia, PA: Lippincott Williams & Wilkins.

Kee, J. L. (2018). *Laboratory and diagnostic tests with nursing implications* (10th ed.). Hoboken, NJ: Pearson Education.

National Center for Complementary and Integrative Health (NCCIH). (2018a). *Headaches.* Retrieved from https://nccih.nih.gov/health/pain/headaches.htm.

National Center for Complementary and Integrative Health (NCCIH). (2018b). *In the News: Component of marijuana reduces seizures in some children with epilepsy.* Retrieved from https://nccih.nih.gov/news/cannabidiol.

National Institute of Neurological Disorders and Stroke (NINDS). (2017). *Arteriovenous malformations and other vascular lesions of the brain.* Retrieved from https://www.ninds.nih.gov/Disorders/Patient-Caregiver-Education/Fact-Sheets/Arteriovenous-Malformation-Fact-Sheet.

National Institute of Neurological Disorders and Stroke (NINDS). (2018a). *Brain basics: Preventing Stroke.* Retrieved from https://www.ninds.nih.gov/Disorders/Patient-Caregiver-Education/Preventing-Stroke.

National Institute of Neurological Disorders and Stroke (NINDS). (2018b). *Cerebral aneurysms.* Retrieved from https://www.ninds.nih.gov/Disorders/Patient-Caregiver-Education/Fact-Sheets/Cerebral-Aneurysms-Fact-Sheet.

National Institute of Neurological Disorders and Stroke (NINDS). (2018c). *Headache information page.* Retrieved from https://www.ninds.nih.gov/Disorders/All-Disorders/Headache-Information-Page.

National Institute of Neurological Disorders and Stroke (NINDS). (2018d). *Traumatic brain injury.* Retrieved from https://www.ninds.nih.gov/Disorders/All-Disorders/Traumatic-Brain-Injury-Information-Page.

National Institutes of Health (NIH). (2003). *NIH Stroke Scale.* Retrieved from www.ninds.nih.gov/doctors/NIH_Stroke_Scale.pdf.

Perrin, K. O., & MacLeod, C. E. (2018). *Understanding the essentials of critical care nursing* (3rd ed.). Upper Saddle River, NJ: Pearson Prentice Hall.

Saria, M. G., Courchesne, N., Evangelista, L., Carter, J., MacManus, D. A., Gorman, M. K., . . . Maliski, S. (2017). Cognitive dysfunction in patients with brain metastases: Influences on caregiver resilience and coping. *Supportive Care in Cancer, 25*, 2247–1256.

Scheffer, I. E., Berkovic, S., Capovilla, G., Connolly, M. B., French, J., Guilhoto, L., . . . Zuberi, S. M. (2017). International League Against Epilepsy [ILAE]: LAE classification of the epilepsies: Position paper of the ILAE Commission for Classification and Terminology. *Epilepsia, 58*(4), 512–521. Retrieved from https://onlinelibrary.wiley.com/doi/epdf/10.1111/epi.13709.

Shields, K. M., Fox, K. L., & Liebrecht, C. (2018). *Pearson nurse's drug guide.* Boston, MA: Pearson.

Sorenson, M., Quinn, L., & Klein, D. (2019). *Pathophysiology: Concepts of human disease.* Hoboken, NJ: Pearson Education.

The Stroke Collaborative. (2015). *Give me five.* Retrieved from www.strokeassociation.org/STROKEORG/StrokeConnectionMagazine/ReadSCNow/SCM-JulyAugust-2008_UCM_310442_Article.jsp#.WvYtu8kh1PY.

ADDITIONAL RESOURCES

American Brain Tumor Association (ABTA)
www.abta.org

American Stroke Association
www.strokeassociation.org/STROKEORG/

Epilepsy Foundation
www.epilepsy.com

National Institute of Neurological Disorders and Stroke (NINDS)
www.ninds.nih.gov/Disorders/All-Disorders/Traumatic-Brain-Injury-Information-Page

Chapter 43

Nursing Care of Patients with Spinal Cord Disorders and CNS Infections

Chapter Outline and Learning Outcomes

43.1 Spinal Cord Disorders 1598

Describe the pathophysiology and manifestations of spinal cord injuries, and outline the interprofessional care and nursing care of patients with these disorders.

43.2 Infectious Disorders of the Central Nervous System 1617

Describe the pathophysiology and manifestations of central nervous system infections, and outline the interprofessional care and nursing care of patients with these disorders.

CLINICAL COMPETENCIES

- Assess and monitor the functional health status of patients with spinal cord disorders and CNS infections, communicating findings to appropriate interprofessional team members.
- Demonstrate effective use of individualized and patient-centered strategies as well as evidence-based practice to prioritize care and implement interventions for patients with spinal cord disorders and CNS infections.
- Adapt individual and cultural values and variations as well as expressed needs and preferences into the plan of care for patients with spinal cord disorders and CNS infections.
- Administer oral and injectable medications used to treat spinal cord disorders and CNS infections knowledgeably and safely.
- Provide appropriate and safe care to patients having a halo fixation and a posterior laminectomy.
- Effectively communicate with and function within the interprofessional team to plan and provide care.
- Utilize assessed data, patient values, and evidence to provide teaching to facilitate self-catheterization, self-care of a ruptured intervertebral disk, and community-based self-care of disabilities resulting from spinal cord disorders and CNS infections.
- Use evidence-based research to prevent ventilator-associated pneumonia in patients in the neurologic ICU.
- Revise plan of care as needed to provide effective interventions to promote, maintain, or restore functional health status to patients with spinal cord disorders and CNS infections.
- Document care in the electronic medical record and use information management tools to monitor outcomes of care.
- Provide appropriate patient and family education for prevention of injury and infection.
- Participate in studies and projects to improve the quality and safety of care for patients with spinal cord disorders and CNS infections.

KEY TERMS

autonomic dysreflexia, 1601
botulism, 1624
cauda equine syndrome, 1611
Creutzfeldt-Jakob disease (CJD), 1623
diskectomy, 1612
encephalitis, 1618
herniation, 1611
meningitis, 1617
neurogenic shock, 1600
paraplegia, 1599
paresthesia, 1611
postpolio syndrome (PPS), 1624
rabies, 1624
radiculopathy, 1611
ruptured intervertebral disk, 1611
sciatica, 1611
spinal cord injury (SCI), 1598
spinal cord tumors, 1615
spinal shock, 1600
tetanus, 1622
tetraplegia (quadriplegia), 1599
ventilator-associated pneumonia (VAP), 1606

The health problems discussed in this chapter result from disorders of the spinal cord and infections of the central nervous system (CNS). Patients with these disorders experience a wide variety of neurologic deficits that affect functional health patterns. They often also require treatment and care for both acute and long-term health problems.

Nursing care for patients with these disorders is tailored to meet the needs of the patient and is individualized by the patient's responses to alterations in structure and function. The disabilities and long-term effects from spinal cord disorders, spinal cord injuries, and CNS infections have the potential to cause feelings of loss and grief for the patient and their families.

43.1 Spinal Cord Disorders

The Patient with a Spinal Cord Injury

Nursing care of patients with a spinal cord injury takes place from acute care through ongoing rehabilitation in a variety of settings. Although priorities may change depending on the patient and setting, care focuses on maximizing functional health status to preserve quality of life. The nurse provides evidence-based care and collaborates with other members of the interprofessional team in meeting this goal.

Approximately 17,500 people suffer a spinal cord injury each year (National Spinal Cord Injury Statistical Center [NSCISC], 2017). A **spinal cord injury (SCI)** involves damage to the neural elements of the spinal cord. Because the spinal cord contains the tracts that connect sensory afferent neurons and lower motor neurons with centers in the brain, both sensory and motor functions are often involved. The major causes of SCI are contusion, compression, laceration, transection, hemorrhage, damage to blood vessels that supply the spinal cord, and damage to blood vessels in the spinal cord, resulting in ischemia and possible necrosis (Mataliotakis & Tsirikos, 2016; Sorenson, Quinn, & Klein, 2019).

Fractures to vertebrae and tears to ligaments can damage the cord and spinal nerves and make the spinal column unstable. Injury to blood vessels supplying the cord can cause ischemia, leading to permanent damage. This discussion focuses on traumatic injuries, but the information is also applicable to congenital deformities, primary or metastatic tumors, ischemia and infarction, and bone disease with pathologic fractures of the vertebrae.

Pathophysiology

The spinal cord provides a two-way pathway for the conduction of impulses and information to and from the brain and the body. It also serves as a major reflex center; through its attached spinal nerves, it is involved in the sensory and motor innervation of the entire body below the head. The spinal cord consists of an outer region of white matter and an inner region of gray matter. The gray matter comprises the central canal of the cord, including the posterior (dorsal) horns, the anterior (ventral) horns, and the lateral horns. It is divided into a sensory half (dorsal) and a motor half (ventral) and innervates somatic and visceral regions of the body. The white matter consists of tracts or pathways that convey information. The ascending (sensory) pathways carry information about proprioception, fine touch, discrimination, pain, temperature, deep pressure, and touch. The descending (motor) pathways carry information about movement.

Spinal cord injuries involve damage to the vertebrae and supporting ligaments as well as the spinal cord itself. Damage to vertebrae and ligaments may in turn damage the spinal cord. The pathophysiology of SCI involves primary (initial trauma or injury to structures surrounding the spinal cord or the spinal cord itself) and secondary injury (damage to vasculature or cells that occur as a result of the primary injury). When primary spinal cord injury occurs, the irreversible neurologic injury leads to microscopic hemorrhages in the gray matter of the cord and edema of the white matter of the cord that can lead to necrosis of neural tissue. Neuronal injury causes loss of reflexes below the level of injury. The hemorrhages extend, eventually involving the entire gray matter. Microcirculation to the cord is impaired by edema and hemorrhage, causing ischemia.

When ischemia is prolonged, necrosis of both gray and white matter begins within a few hours, and within 24 hours the function of nerves passing through the injured area is lost. Although circulation returns to the white matter of the cord in about 24 hours, decreased circulation in the gray matter continues (Sorenson et al., 2019). Because edema extends the level of injury for two cord segments above and below the affected level, the extent of injury cannot be determined for up to 1 week.

Tissue repair occurs over a period of 3 to 4 weeks. Phagocytes enter the area in 36 to 48 hours after the initial injury. Neurons degenerate and are removed by microphages in the first 10 days after the injury. Red blood cells (RBCs) disintegrate, and the hemorrhages are reabsorbed. Eventually the area of injury is replaced by acellular collagenous tissue, and the meninges thicken (Sorenson et al., 2019).

Forces Resulting in Spinal Cord Injury

SCIs are the result of the application of excessive force to the spinal column. The most common causes of abnormal spinal column movements are acceleration and deceleration (forces that are applied to the body, for example, in automobile crashes and falls). *Acceleration* occurs when an external force is applied (the head and neck are suddenly sent into motion, such as in a rear-end motor vehicle accident leading to hyperextension). *Deceleration* occurs in a head-on collision (the external force causes an abrupt stop in movement causing hyperflexion of the neck). The alteration of the spinal cord and soft tissues caused by these abnormal movements is called *deformation*. The following forces and movements (**Figure 43.1** ■) may cause a variety of spinal cord injuries, with the extent of injury depending on the amount and direction of motion and the rate of application of force:

- ***Hyperflexion***, or forcible forward bending, may compress vertebral bodies and disrupt ligaments and intervertebral disks.

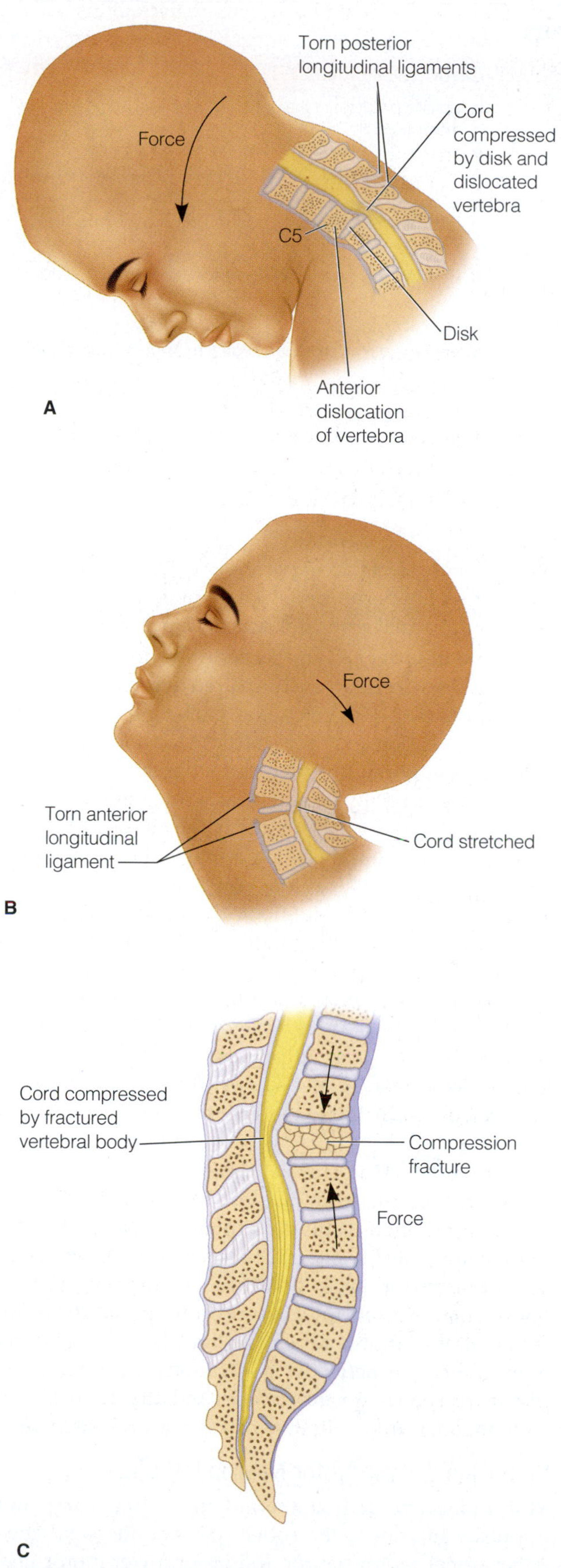
Torn posterior longitudinal ligaments
Force
Cord compressed by disk and dislocated vertebra
C5
Disk
Anterior dislocation of vertebra
A
Force
Torn anterior longitudinal ligament
Cord stretched
B
Cord compressed by fractured vertebral body
Compression fracture
Force
C

Figure 43.1 ■ Spinal cord injury mechanisms. **A**, Hyperflexion. **B**, Hyperextension. **C**, Axial loading, a form of compression.

- ***Hyperextension***, or forcible backward bending, often disrupts ligaments and causes vertebral fractures.
- ***Axial loading***, a form of compression, is the application of vertical force to the spinal column (e.g., by falling and landing on the feet or buttocks, or by diving into shallow water).
- ***Excessive rotation***, in which the head is excessively turned, may tear ligaments, fracture articular surfaces, and cause compression fractures.

The spinal cord may be penetrated by bullets and other foreign objects (e.g., knife wounds, shrapnel from explosions). Penetrating injuries may cause vertebral fractures or blood vessel damage, tear ligaments and muscles, or cut through part or all of the spinal cord. Complete severing of the cord is rare.

Sites of Pathology

The injury is identified by vertebral level. For example, a C_6 spinal cord injury is at the sixth cervical vertebra. The most frequent sites of injury of the cord are at the first, second, and fourth to seventh cervical vertebrae (C_1, C_2, C_4 to C_7) and the 10th thoracic to second lumbar vertebrae (T_{10} to L_2) (Sorenson et al., 2019). These areas are more prone to injury due to the increased capacity for movement. In addition, the cord fills most of the vertebral canal in the cervical and lumbar regions and thus is more easily injured. Damage to vertebrae and ligaments causes the spinal column to become unstable, increasing the possibility of compression or stretching of the cord with any further movement.

Classification of Spinal Cord Injuries

SCIs are further classified according to the amount of cord involvement. **Tetraplegia** (or *quadriplegia*) occurs with damage to the neural structures in the cervical area of the cord, resulting in loss or impairment of motor and/or sensory function in the arms, trunk, legs, and pelvic organs. **Paraplegia** occurs with damage to the neural structures in the thoracic, lumbar, or sacral area of the cord, resulting in loss or impairment of motor and/or sensory function in the trunk, legs, and pelvic organs. Function of the arms is spared; the other losses depend on the level of injury. Complete SCIs involve complete interruption of the motor and sensory neural pathways. This results in a total loss of motor and sensory function below the level of the injury, although complete does not necessarily mean the spinal cord has been severed. An incomplete SCI is a partial interruption of the motor and sensory pathways, with variable loss of function below the level of injury. Incomplete SCIs are further classified into syndromes, as outlined in **Table 43.1**. Both complete and incomplete injuries can occur in paraplegia and tetraplegia. Alterations in function that occur as the result of spinal cord injury vary depending on the amount of tissue damage and level of injury.

Risk Factors

The majority (81%) of SCIs occur in young males, and the majority of injuries are caused by motor vehicle crashes (38.4%). The second most common cause is falls (30.5%),

Table 43.1 Incomplete Spinal Cord Injury Syndromes

Type	Cause	Location	Deficits
Central cord syndrome	Cord transection Hyperextension	Cervical	■ Spastic paralysis of the upper extremities; decrease of fine motor control ■ Variable paralysis of the lower extremities ■ Variable effects on the bowel, the bladder, and sexual function
Anterior syndrome	Damage to the anterior spinal artery Infarction of the anterior spinal artery	Anterior two-thirds of the cord	■ Paralysis below the level of injury ■ Loss of temperature and pain sensation below the level of injury
Posterior syndrome (rare)	Vertebral dislocation Herniated disk Compression	Nerve roots	■ Loss of deep touch, proprioception, and vibration sense
Brown-Séquard syndrome	Penetrating trauma	Hemisection of the anterior and posterior cord	■ Paralysis below the level of injury on the ipsilateral (same) side of the body ■ Contralateral loss of temperature and pain sensation below the level of injury ■ Ipsilateral loss of proprioception below the level of injury
Horner syndrome	Incomplete cord transection	Cervical sympathetic nerves	■ Ipsilateral ptosis of the eyelid, constricted pupil, and facial anhidrosis (inability to perspire)

followed by acts of violence (most commonly gunshot wounds) and sports and recreational activities (NSCISC, 2017). Most SCIs are preventable and education is an important tool in this prevention. Education should include use of protective equipment (helmets, seat belts) as well as environmental changes (removing throw rugs, other obstacles from floors). In general, young males (age 16 to 30) have been considered at higher risk for SCIs than other patient populations. However, the older population is also at a high risk of SCI, due to the risk of falls (related to disease processes and medications) as well as degenerative spine diseases.

Manifestations

The spinal cord, vertebrae, intervertebral disks, spinal nerves, ligaments, and surrounding soft tissue structures are in such close anatomic proximity that any condition or injury affecting one structure may affect any one or all surrounding structures. Pneumonia and septicemia are the most common causes of death in those who survive SCIs (NSCISC, 2017) and are an important consideration for nursing interventions and prevention.

Injuries of the spinal cord have the potential to affect movement, perception, sensation, sexual function, and elimination. Manifestations and complications of SCI by body system are listed in **Table 43.2**.

Spinal shock is the response of the cord itself to injury. It involves temporary loss of reflex function (*areflexia*) below the level of injury at the cervical and upper thoracic spinal cord. As a result of the injury, sympathetic function is interrupted and parasympathetic function is unopposed. This condition is characterized by flaccid paralysis, deep tendon reflexes, and loss of all sensations below the level of injury. There is loss of urinary bladder tone, intestinal peristalsis, perspiration, and vasomotor tone. Additionally, the autonomic dysfunction results in hypotension and bradycardia (Mataliotakis & Tsirikos, 2016).

Spinal shock can begin immediately after injury to the spinal cord and may last for a few weeks. Return of function includes bladder tone, hyperreflexia, and sacral reflexes. The initial phase of flaccid paralysis is then followed by various states of hyperreflexia (Mataliotakis & Tsirikos, 2016).

An individual with a cervical or upper thoracic SCI may also have **neurogenic shock**, resulting in cardiovascular changes. As a result of the impaired sympathetic nervous system, vascular beds below the level of injury dilate, leading to hypotension and bradycardia (Mataliotakis & Tsirikos, 2016). It is important to note that a patient with traumatic SCI could potentially be suffering from extreme blood loss as well, depending on the nature of the injuries. Neurogenic shock presents similarly to hemorrhagic shock, with the key difference being the heart rate; neurogenic shock causes *bradycardia* and hemorrhagic shock leads to *tachycardia*.

It is difficult initially to differentiate spinal shock from neurogenic shock. Spinal shock will manifest the signs and symptoms related to the flaccidity of muscles and the loss of reflexes (Winter, Pattani, & Temple, 2017). Recovery from spinal shock is a gradual process, usually lasting from 4 to 6 weeks. Weakness and sensory loss lasting longer than 6 weeks are likely due to the injury.

Complications

The complications of an SCI involve many different body systems and often result in permanent disability and loss of functional health status. The complications include but are not limited to upper and lower motor neuron deficits, paraplegia and tetraplegia, and autonomic dysreflexia. Other complications, depending on the level and severity of the injury, are ineffective respirations; altered skin integrity; increased risk of thrombosis; and alterations in bowel elimination, urinary elimination, and sexual patterns.

Upper and Lower Motor Neuron Deficits

Motor neurons are functional units that carry motor impulses. Injuries to the spinal cord are often classified as either upper motor neuron lesions or lower motor neuron lesions. The upper motor neurons (located in the cerebral cortex, brainstem, and corticospinal and corticobulbar tracts) are responsible for voluntary movement. When these

Table 43.2 Manifestations and Complications of Spinal Cord Injury by Body System

Body System	Manifestations	Complications
Integumentary	■ Pressure injury	■ Infections ■ Septicemia
Neurologic	■ Pain ■ Areflexia ■ Hypotonia ■ Psychiatric complications	■ Suicidal ideation ■ Depression ■ Low self-esteem ■ Loss of bladder control
Cardiovascular	■ Spinal shock ■ Paroxysmal hypertension ■ Cardiac dysrhythmias ■ Decreased venous return ■ Coronary artery disease	■ Deep vein thrombosis ■ Bradycardia ■ Orthostatic hypotension
Respiratory	■ Limited chest expansion ■ Decreased cough reflex ■ Decreased vital capacity ■ Pulmonary embolism	■ Pneumonia ■ Atelectasis
Gastrointestinal	■ Stress ulcers ■ Paralytic ileus ■ Stool impaction ■ Stool incontinence	■ Autonomic dysreflexia ■ Chronic constipation
Genitourinary	■ Urinary retention ■ Urinary incontinence ■ Neurogenic bladder ■ Impotence ■ Testicular atrophy ■ Inability to ejaculate ■ Decreased vaginal lubrication	■ Infections ■ Autonomic dysreflexia ■ Skin breakdown ■ Difficulty conceiving children
Musculoskeletal	■ Joint contractures ■ Osteoporosis ■ Muscle spasms ■ Muscle atrophy ■ Pathologic fractures ■ Paraplegia ■ Tetraplegia	■ Pain ■ Overuse injuries ■ Inability to reposition self

motor pathways are interrupted, the patient experiences spastic paralysis and hyperreflexia and may be unable to carry out skilled movement.

Lower motor neurons (located in the anterior horn of the spinal cord, the motor nuclei of the brainstem, and the axons that reach the motor end plate of skeletal muscles) are responsible for innervation and contraction of skeletal muscles. Interruption of lower motor neurons results in muscle flaccidity and extensive muscle atrophy, with loss of both voluntary and involuntary movement. If only some of the motor neurons supplying a muscle are affected, the patient experiences partial paralysis; if all motor neurons to a muscle are affected, the patient experiences complete paralysis and hyporeflexia.

Paraplegia and Tetraplegia

Two common neurologic deficits resulting from an SCI are paraplegia and tetraplegia, described earlier and illustrated in the previous chapter (refer to Figure 42.6).

Autonomic Dysreflexia

Autonomic dysreflexia (also called *autonomic hyperreflexia*) is an exaggerated sympathetic response that occurs in patients with SCIs at or above the T_6 level (Matthews & Lee, 2016). This response is generally seen only after recovery from spinal shock and occurs due to a lack of control of the autonomic nervous system by higher centers. Mass reflex stimulation of the sympathetic nerves below the level of the injured cord area occurs, which therefore increases blood pressure. The body then attempts to compensate for this increased blood pressure by triggering the parasympathetic nervous system. This causes bradycardia and vasodilation above the level of the injury. Untreated autonomic dysreflexia is potentially fatal.

Autonomic dysreflexia is triggered by stimuli that would normally cause abdominal discomfort, by stimulation of pain receptors, and by visceral contractions. Causes include a full bladder (the most common cause) resulting from a blocked urinary catheter, fecal impaction, bladder infections or stones, sexual intercourse, intrauterine contractions, pressure ulcers or ingrown toenails, dressing changes, and surgical procedures. Evidence of this syndrome may not occur right after injury, however, symptoms typically occur within the first year if the patient will experience this complication (Abrams & Wakasa, 2014). It is important that nurses and families are skilled at recognizing the signs and symptoms of autonomic dysreflexia. Symptoms include pounding headache, bradycardia, flushing, blurred vision, nausea, diaphoresis above the lesion, and hypertension (with readings as high as 240/120 mmHg). Autonomic dysreflexia is a neurologic emergency and requires immediate treatment.

Interprofessional Care

The patient with an acute SCI requires emergency assessment, immobilization, and possibly medications and surgery. The patient is first assessed and stabilized at the accident scene, transported for treatment to an emergency department (ED), and then admitted to an intensive care unit. Management requires an interprofessional team for this complex multisystem injury.

Emergency Care

The danger of death from SCI is greatest when there is damage to or transection of the upper cervical region. When the injury is at the C_1 to C_4 level, respiratory paralysis is common, and the patient who survives requires ventilator assistance to breathe. Injuries below C_4 may increase the risk of respiratory failure if edema ascends the cord. It is of critical importance not to complicate the initial injury by allowing the fractured vertebrae to damage the cord further during transport to the hospital. Although at one time injuries to the high cervical cord were almost always fatal, advances in trauma care have greatly improved the survival rate.

All people who have sustained trauma to the head or spine, or who are unconscious, should be treated as though they have a spinal cord injury. Prehospital management includes rapid assessment of the ABCs (airway, breathing, circulation), immobilizing and stabilizing the head and neck, removing the individual from the site of injury, stabilizing other life-threatening injuries, and rapidly transporting the individual by ambulance or helicopter to the appropriate facility (a trauma center, if available). Guidelines for emergency care are as follows:

- Do not flex, extend, or rotate the neck.
- Immobilize the neck, using rolled towels or blankets, or apply a cervical collar before moving the patient onto a backboard.
- Secure the head by placing a belt or tape across the forehead and securing it to the stretcher.
- Secure patient to the backboard.
- Maintain the patient in the supine position.
- Transfer directly from the stretcher with backboard still in place to the type of bed that will be used in the hospital.

Assessment findings at the scene of the accident or in the ED vary according to the level of injury. The assessment findings common to the level of injury are outlined in **Box 43.1**. Manifestations of spinal shock are also assessed.

The patient in the ED with a suspected or identified SCI is also treated for respiratory problems, bladder distention, and cardiovascular alterations (Hansebout & Kachur, 2014). Respiratory distress in the patient with a cervical-level injury is treated with intubation and mechanical ventilation. Oxygen is administered to the patient with a thoracic-level injury. To prevent overdistention of an atonic bladder, an indwelling catheter is inserted and connected to gravity drainage. Cardiovascular status is assessed continuously using telemetry as well as invasive monitoring devices, such as a pulmonary artery catheter and/or arterial line.

BOX 43.1

Assessment Findings in Acute SCI

CERVICAL INJURY

- Paralysis or weakness of extremities
- Respiratory distress manifested by changes in ABG studies, cyanosis, flaring of the nostrils, use of accessory muscles of respiration, and restlessness
- Bradycardia and hypotension
- Decreased peristalsis

THORACIC AND LUMBAR INJURY

- Paralysis or weakness of extremities

Steroid protocols may be instituted using methylprednisolone (Solu-Medrol) if the drug can be given within 8 hours of injury. Evidence does not show significant improvement with use of corticosteroids and in fact may lead to increased complications. At this time, the use of corticosteroids is no longer part of the guidelines in initial treatment of SCI, however, it may still be prescribed (Hansebout & Kachur, 2014).

Diagnosis

Diagnostic tests are ordered to identify the level and extent of injury and to detect any complications. The tests include x-rays of the spine, CT or magnetic resonance imaging (MRI) of the spine, and somatosensory-evoked potential studies to locate the level of spinal cord injury by stimulating peripheral nerves and measuring response times. Arterial blood gases (ABG) are measured to establish a baseline or to identify problems due to respiratory insufficiency. A trauma screen (blood type and cross-match, blood alcohol level, urine drug screen, and pregnancy test for women up to age 45) is conducted in the ED.

Fluid Management

Crystalloids such as D_5 45NS or Ringer lactate solution are often administered. Potassium and multivitamins may be added to the IV fluids. If the patient becomes hypotensive in the early stage of treatment, IV fluids are administered to increase blood pressure. Fluid administration should be closely monitored, as too many fluids could lead to additional cord swelling (Hansebout & Kachur, 2014). Close monitoring of fluid intake and urine output are essential.

Medications

Pharmacologic treatment of the patient with SCI is primarily symptomatic. Medications focus on decreasing edema from the injury, treating hypotension and bradycardia, relieving pain, treating spasticity, preventing immobility complications, and maintaining bowel function.

- Corticosteroids may be used to decrease or control inflammation and edema of the cord.
- Vasopressors are used in the immediate acute care phase to treat bradycardia or hypotension due to spinal and neurogenic shock. Examples of these drugs are dopamine (Intropin) to treat hypotension in neurogenic shock and

dobutamine (Dobutrex) to support cardiac function. Atropine should be available at the bedside to treat bradycardia.

- Antispasmodics such as baclofen (Lioresal), diazepam (Valium), and dantrolene (Dantrium) may be used to treat spasticity in patients with spinal cord injury.
- Antiemetics may be administered to prevent vomiting.
- Analgesics such as nonsteroidal anti-inflammatory drugs (NSAIDs) and narcotics are administered to reduce pain.
- Proton pump inhibitors, such as esomeprazole (Nexium), omeprazole (Prilosec), or pantoprazole (Protonix), are often administered to prevent stress-related gastric ulcers, a common complication in SCI. (*Note:* Drugs identified in blue are among the 200 most commonly prescribed medications in the United States.)
- Unless contraindicated, anticoagulants including enoxaparin (Lovenox) may be given to prevent thrombophlebitis.
- Stool softeners such as docusate (Colace) may be administered as part of a bowel training program (Abrams & Wakasa, 2014).

Nutrition

A regular diet should be started for patients with spinal cord injury within a couple of days of injury (Hansbout & Kachur, 2014). For patients that are unable to ingest foods and liquids orally an enteral feeding tube or parenteral nutrition may need to be started. Patients should be encouraged to eat a high-fiber diet and consume plenty of liquids to aid in gastric motility.

Treatments

The treatments used in the management of an SCI include surgery, stabilization, and immobilization.

Surgery. Early surgical treatment may be necessary if there is evidence of compression of the spinal cord by bone fragments or a hematoma. Surgery may also be done to stabilize and support the spine. However, many patients are treated with stabilization devices and do not require surgery. Surgeries that may be performed include a decompression laminectomy, a spinal fusion, and insertion of metal rods. Surgeries of the spine are discussed later in the chapter.

Stabilization and Immobilization. As a result of one or more dislocations or fractures of the cervical vertebrae, the patient with an SCI may be immobilized in some type of traction or external fixation device to stabilize the vertebral column and prevent further damage to the cord (**Figure 43.2** ■). Traction may also be used to stabilize the spinal column for patients who are not yet in a condition to have surgery or who have severe bleeding and edema of the injured cord. The physician applies the traction or fixation device; the nurse is responsible for assessments and interventions following the application.

Although used less frequently today, various devices provide cervical traction. For example, Gardner-Wells tongs may be used (**Figure 43.3** ■). In this type of traction, the physician applies pins to the skull, approximately 1 cm above each ear, and weights are attached to the device.

The halo external fixation device is often used to provide stabilization if there is no significant involvement of the ligaments (**Figure 43.4** ■). It is most often used to provide stability for fractures of the cervical and high thoracic vertebrae without cord damage. This device allows greater mobility, self-care, and participation in rehabilitation programs. The device is secured with four pins inserted into

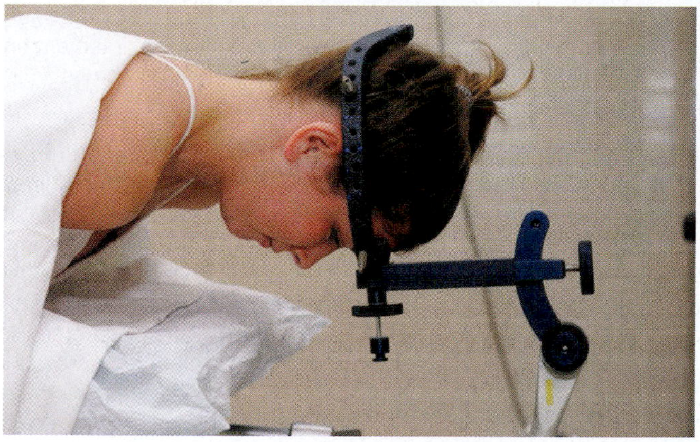

Figure 43.2 ■ Traction device.

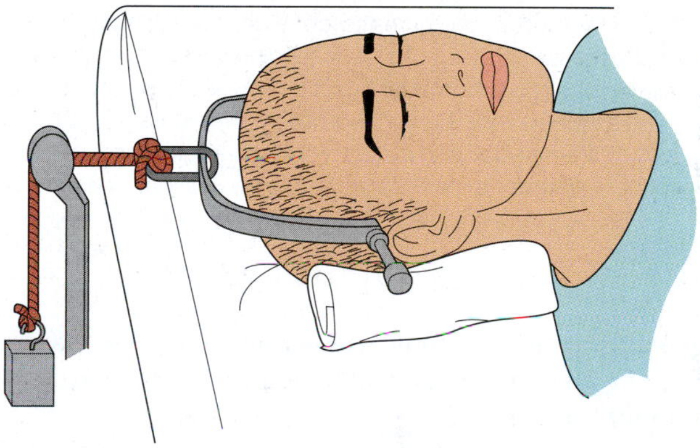

Figure 43.3 ■ Cervical traction may be applied by several methods, including Gardner-Wells tongs.

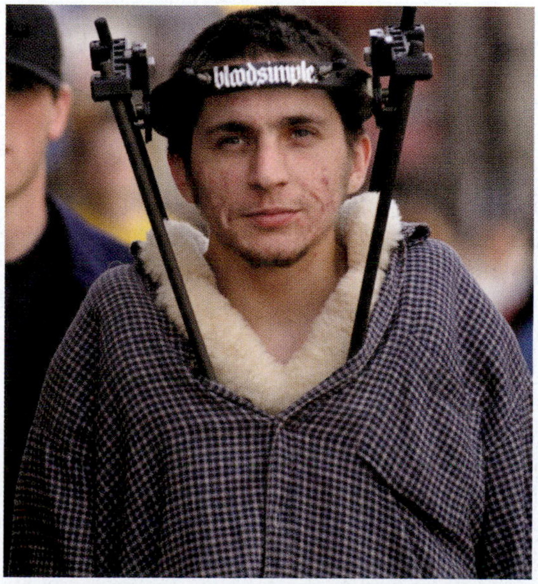
bloodsimple

Figure 43.4 ■ The halo external fixation device.

Moving Evidence into Action

Preventing Respiratory Complications in Patients with SCI

Clinical Issue

In patients with SCI, deep vein thrombosis (DVT) can be a very serious complication, especially in the acute stages after injury. Understanding the manifestations and efficacy of interventions for DVT prophylaxis can help improve patient outcomes.

External Evidence

The Consortium for Spinal Cord Medicine (Consortium for Spinal Cord Medicine, 2016) created several different clinical practice guidelines for SCIs in order to help ensure the best outcomes for patients. The guideline for DVT prophylaxis reviews the best practices for prevention based on a systematic review of the literature. Starting prophylactic treatment for DVT within the first 2 weeks of injury provided the greatest outcomes for patients. Based on the findings from the systematic review, it is recommended that pneumatic compression devices be applied as soon as possible to the lower extremities and low-molecular-weight heparin be used. Other interventions have been tested, however, they were not as effective.

Internal Evidence

It is important for the nurse to consider the institution's policies regarding use of pneumatic devices to prevent DVT. Prior to administering any medications, review the risks and potential complications as well as the prescribed order. The nurse should work as part of the interdisciplinary team, including pharmacists and prescribers, in order to provide individualized patient-centered care.

Patient Considerations

Prior to implementation of these recommendations, the nurse should assess the patient for any contraindications for DVT prophylaxis. If the patient has a break in the lower extremities or a known clot, then the use of pneumatic compression devices is contraindicated. Use of anticoagulants could put the patient at risk for bleeding. Lab values and patient assessments including vital signs should be reviewed regularly and any abnormalities reported to the prescriber immediately.

Putting the Pieces Together

Due to venous stasis, which is often related to both blood pressure and heart rate as well as the flaccidity of the muscles, SCI patients are at very high risk for developing DVT. The nurse must be aware of ways in which to prevent DVT in order to prevent serious complications such as pulmonary emboli, myocardial infarction, or even stroke. If appropriate interventions have not been ordered for the patient, the nurse must work with the interdisciplinary team and advocate for the appropriate evidence-based interventions.

Reference

Consortium for Spinal Cord Medicine. (2016). Prevention of venous thromboembolism in individuals with spinal cord injury: Clinical practice guidelines for health care providers, 3rd ed. *Topics in Spinal Cord Injury Rehabilitation, 22*(3), 209–240.

the skull, two in the frontal bone and two in the occipital bone. The halo ring is then attached to a rigid plastic vest lined with sheepskin.

Research to Improve SCI Management

An SCI is costly in terms of human life, human function, and healthcare costs. For the patient with a high cervical injury, improving the ability of even one spinal segment to function may make an enormous difference in quality of life. Research is currently being conducted on neurons of the spinal cord, stimulators to improve muscle function, and equipment to aid activities of daily living (ADLs) (National Institute of Neurologic Disorders and Stroke [NINDS], 2013).

Scientists are focusing on methods of advancing our knowledge of spinal cord repair, including protecting surviving neurons from further damage, replacing damaged neurons, stimulating the regrowth of axons and correctly targeting their connections, and retraining neural circuits to restore body functions.

Clinical research to improve rehabilitation is ongoing. A functional electrical stimulation (FES) system uses electrical stimulators to encourage functional walking and gripping. The stimulators must be implanted and the computer interface system is still limited. Devices implanted in the brain might be used to send a signal to a computer that in turn signals a robotic arm to move. New technologies include improved, lighter-weight wheelchairs; some can climb stairs and lift an individual to eye level. Voice-activated software can be used for many self-care activities, including banking, using a smartphone, and reading or listening to music (NINDS, 2017).

Nursing Care

The patient with an SCI has complex needs during both the acute phase and the rehabilitative phase that involve a multidisciplinary approach to care. Patients are typically younger and will therefore require consideration of the lifelong effects on themselves and their families. The nurse coordinates and plans patient care, implementing interventions that are individualized. The focus of the plan is to prevent the secondary complications of immobility and altered body functions, to promote self-care, and to educate the patient and family. See the Case Study & Nursing Care Plan for a patient with an SCI on page 1611.

Assessment

The following data are collected through the health history and physical examination (refer to Chapter 41). Further focused assessments are described with nursing interventions in the next section.

- *Health history:* Time, location, and type of event causing injury; location, duration, quality, and intensity of pain; dyspnea; sensation; paresthesia
- *Physical assessment:* Vital signs, motor strength, movement, spinal reflexes, bowel sounds, bladder distention, urinary output, level of consciousness.

Priorities of Care

Nursing care priorities for the patient with SCI evolve over time. Interventions to preserve life and prevent or manage complications have priority during the initial period following the injury. As the acuity of the injury resolves, the focus moves to restoring functional capabilities to the greatest extent possible and prevention of secondary complications.

Diagnoses, Outcomes, and Interventions

Because an SCI has many possible effects, many nursing diagnoses may be appropriate. Nursing diagnoses discussed in this section focus on problems with physical mobility, respirations, dysreflexia, bowel and bladder elimination, sexual dysfunction, and self-esteem.

Promote Physical Mobility. After the initial period of spinal shock and areflexia, the patient regains spinal reflex activity and muscle tone that is not under the control of higher centers. Patients with injuries above the level of T_{12} experience involuntary spastic movements of skeletal muscles. These muscle spasms may lead to pain and contractures (Abrams & Wakasa, 2017). Spasms may impair the ability to carry out ADLs, however, by increasing the tone, there may actually be some benefit with standing and transfers (Abrams & Wakasa, 2017). If present, paraplegia or tetraplegia increases the potential for impaired skin integrity, thrombophlebitis, and contractures.

The goals of care for patients with impaired mobility related to a spinal cord injury are to reduce the effects of spasticity and to prevent complications involving the skin, the cardiovascular system, and joint function.

Expected Outcome: Patient will demonstrate minimal spasticity and optimal motor functioning.

The nurse will:

- Perform passive ROM exercises for all extremities at least twice a day. Identify stimuli that cause spastic movements and either avoid the stimuli (such as certain exercises) or teach the patient to expect the movements. Use braces as appropriate to prevent contractures. *ROM exercises help prevent contractures and stretch spastic muscles, promoting rehabilitation.*
- Maintain skin integrity by turning every 2 hours, assessing pressure points at least once each shift, and using a special bed, if indicated. In addition, the nurse should ensure that skin remains dry. The patient may be placed on a regular or special bed, such as a kinetic bed. *Immobility compresses soft tissues and promotes the development of decubitus ulcers. The lack of sensory warning mechanisms and of voluntary motor control of skin dermatomes further increases the risk for altered skin integrity. Special beds allow movement or turning while keeping the spinal column in alignment.*
- Assess the lower extremities each shift for manifestations of DVT. Observe for redness, swelling, and increased heat; measure thigh and calf circumference daily. If antiembolic stockings or sequential compression devices are ordered, remove each shift and assess for skin impairment and provide skin care. *Patients with neurologic deficits are at high risk for DVT as a result of immobility, vasomotor dysfunction, and decreased venous return with venous stasis, especially during the first 2 weeks after injury (Hansebout & Kachur, 2014). Thigh-high graduated compression stockings and/or sequential compression boots help prevent pooling of blood in the lower extremities and increase venous return, lessening the risk for venous stasis and thrombus formation. Nurses must ensure the stockings are properly sized and used.*

Promote Oxygenation. Injuries at the level of C_3 to C_5 affect the diaphragm and the phrenic nerve. An injury at level T_1 through T_7 impairs phrenic nerve innervation of the intercostal muscles, and at T_6 to T_{12}, the abdominal muscles are denervated, compromising exhalation and overall respiratory function. Patients will have an ineffective cough due to abdominal muscle paralysis, thereby increasing the risk of pneumonia. Patients with cord injuries at C_3 or above have paralysis of the respiratory muscles and cannot breathe without a ventilator (Berlowitz, Wadsworth, & Ross, 2016) (see the Moving Knowledge into Action box for related nursing care). Goals of care are to maintain a patent airway, promote oxygenation, and prevent respiratory complications.

Expected Outcome: Patient will demonstrate effective respiratory pattern and adequate gas exchange.

The nurse will:

- Monitor vital capacity and respiratory effectiveness, assessing for tachycardia, restlessness, cyanosis, pallor, low PaO_2, high $PaCO_2$, and vital capacity less than 1 L. *Patients with cervical cord injuries frequently require ventilatory support; injuries at other levels may reduce deep breathing, vital capacity, and effective coughing.*
- Monitor for signs of ascending edema of the spinal cord, including difficulty swallowing or coughing, respiratory stridor, use of accessory muscles of respiration, bradycardia, and increasing motor and sensory loss. Report these manifestations immediately. *Hemorrhage and edema can further impair respiratory function. Patients with injuries above C_7 may need a tracheostomy in addition to mechanical ventilation.*

SAFETY ALERT: Changes in ABGs and vital capacity signal respiratory insufficiency. ■

Monitor Breathing Pattern. In patients with SCI injury at higher levels, assisted ventilation and a tracheostomy are often necessary; when the injury is at lower levels, the patient's ability to take a deep breath and cough is also diminished. The goals of nursing interventions are to maintain normal respiratory rate (12 to 20 breaths per minute), maintain a patent airway and effective breathing patterns, and prevent pulmonary complications such as atelectasis and pneumonia.

Expected Outcome: Patient will demonstrate effective respiratory patterns and an absence of infectious and mechanical complications.

The nurse will:

- Assess respiratory rate, rhythm, and depth every 4 hours (or more frequently if needed). Auscultate breath sounds as a part of a respiratory assessment.

Injury to the cervical or thoracic cord can decrease respiratory function and increase the risk for respiratory problems.

- Monitor results of oxygen saturation with pulse oximetry and arterial blood gas (ABG) studies. *ABG studies provide information about gas exchange; decreasing pH, oxygen, and oxygen saturation levels and increasing carbon dioxide levels signal respiratory acidosis.*
- Administer supplemental oxygen as prescribed. *Oxygen saturation must be maintained with supplemental oxygen to prevent hypoxemia and secondary SCI.*
- Assist the patient to turn, cough, and deep-breathe at least every 2 hours. *Paralysis of intercostal or abdominal muscles decreases the ability to expectorate secretions by coughing; retained secretions increase the risk for pneumonia. The inability to breathe deeply may result in atelectasis.*

Prevent Autonomic Dysreflexia. Autonomic dysreflexia is an emergency that requires immediate assessment and intervention to prevent complications of extremely high blood pressure (loss of consciousness, seizure, intracranial hemorrhage and even death) (Tyler, 2015).

Expected Outcome: The patient will not develop autonomic dysreflexia.

The nurse will:

- Elevate the head of the patient's bed and remove compression stockings or boots. *These measures create a position that induces orthostatic hypotension, thereby causing pooling of blood in the lower extremities and decreased venous return, thus decreasing blood pressure.*
- Assess blood pressure every 2 to 3 minutes while at the same time assessing for stimuli that initiated the response (such as a full bladder, impacted stool, or skin pressure). *The most serious danger in dysreflexia is elevated blood pressure (an increase of more than 20 to 30 mmHG greater than the patients baseline)* (Tyler, 2015), *which could precipitate a stroke, myocardial infarction, dysrhythmias, or seizures. If the patient has a Foley catheter, ensure that there are no kinks in the tubing. If there is no Foley catheter, drain the bladder with a straight catheter. If manifestations persist, assess for a fecal impaction.*
- Administer prescribed medications. If blood pressure remains dangerously elevated, the physician may prescribe intravenous administration of nitroprusside (Nitropress). Other medications that may be used include nifedipine (Procardia), hydralazine (Apresoline), or labetalol (Normodyne). *Nitroprusside is an antihypertensive drug used in emergency situations to lower blood pressure in adults with dangerously high readings. Nifedipine and hydralazine are vasodilators that are administered to decrease the elevated blood pressure. Labetalol is a beta-blocker that results in vasodilation and thereby lowers BP.*

SAFETY ALERT: It is important to closely monitor for hypotension following administration of these medications, especially if the stimulus for dysreflexia has been removed. If labetalol is ordered, the heart rate must be at least 60 for safe administration of the medication. ■

Promote Normal Urinary and Bowel Elimination. Depending on the level of the injury, the patient with an SCI may have alterations in bowel and bladder function. Patients with injuries to the cord at or above the S_2 to S_4 levels will have a neurogenic bladder, with deficits in control of micturition. Voluntary and involuntary bowel control are

Moving Evidence into Action

Reducing Incidence of Ventilator-Associated Pneumonia

Clinical Issue

Ventilator-associated pneumonia (VAP) is a preventable secondary complication from intubation and mechanical support. Mechanically ventilated patients are at increased risk of VAP from factors such as a decreased level of consciousness; dry, open mouth; and aspiration of secretions. While all of these are risk factors for VAP, aspiration of secretions containing pathogens is likely the biggest risk factor (Zuckerman, 2016).

External Evidence

A comprehensive literature review was conducted to examine the use of chlorhexadine solution for oral care to prevent VAP (Zuckerman, 2016). Results demonstrated that the use of chlorhexadine as part of a VAP bundle, resulted in a significant reduction in the VAP rate in mechanically ventilated patients (Zuckerman, 2016).

Internal Evidence

It is important to note that the use of chlorhexadine is just one piece to be added to the VAP bundle to prevent VAP. The VAP bundle should be reviewed for specific interventions at individual institutions, however, in general, the bundle will include raising the head of bed greater than 30 degrees, peptic ulcer prophylaxis, deep vein thrombosis prophylaxis, periods of rest from sedation, and reduction in sedatives if warranted (Zuckerman, 2016).

Patient Consideration

Always review individual patient allergies and other contraindications prior to using a treatment such as chlorhexadine. The patient should be weaned from mechanical ventilation as soon as possible in order to help prevent infection.

Putting the Pieces Together

For a patient to be diagnosed with VAP, they must be on a mechanical ventilator for at least 48 hours. Nurses should ensure compliance with the institution's VAP bundle and consider the addition of chlorhexidine mouthwash in order to prevent this serious hospital-acquired infection.

Reference

Zuckerman, L. M. (2016). Oral chlorhexidine use to prevent ventilator-associated pneumonia in adults: Review of current literature. *Dimensions of Critical Care Nursing, 35*(1), 25–36.

affected in the patient with a lower motor neuron injury. Bowel and bladder retraining are possible, but if not then assisted elimination is necessary. Although an indwelling catheter may be used in the acute phase of care, the goal is to reestablish a catheter-free state where intermittent self-catheterization is possible, as this helps to decrease the risk of infection (Abrams & Wakasa, 2014). Goals of care are to restore effective elimination patterns.

Expected Outcome: Patient will demonstrate normal bladder and bowel patterns.

The nurse will:

- Monitor for manifestations of a full bladder. *Overdistention stretches the bladder and can lead to backflow of urine into the ureters and kidney. Stasis of urine in an incompletely emptied bladder increases the risk for infection.*
- Monitor for bowel sounds, bowel patterns, and stool consistency. *Good bowel function is imperative for effective elimination and to prevent complications.*
- Teach self-catheterization to patients who will be able to carry out the procedure alone or with minimal assistance (**Box 43.2**). *Straight catheterization at regular intervals is part of bladder training because periodic distention and relaxation of bladder muscles promote reflex bladder activity. In addition, self-care fosters independence.*
- Monitor residual urine throughout the bladder retraining program. *A residual urine amount of less than 80 mL after a triggered voiding is considered satisfactory.*
- Monitor for elimination of frequent, small, liquid, foul-smelling stools. *Injuries to sacral cord elements or higher often result in loss of defecation reflex. Even if peristalsis is present, the ability to have a bowel movement is impaired by loss of this reflex. Fecal impactions are an ongoing problem and are manifested by this type of bowel elimination.*
- Institute a bowel retraining program as follows:
  a. Assess patterns of bowel elimination to establish the best times for an individualized program.
  b. Maintain high-fluid, high-fiber diet.
  c. Use stool softeners as prescribed; rectal suppositories and enemas may be used 30 minutes after meals to stimulate stronger peristalsis and facilitate evacuation.
  d. Maintain upright position if at all possible and ensure privacy.
  e. If patient is unable to evacuate, digital stimulation or manual removal on a regular basis may be the most effective long-term management.

A bowel retraining program to regulate the bowel through reflex activity may be instituted in patients with upper motor neuron injuries. The patient with a lower motor neuron injury loses defecation reflex, and bowel retraining is more difficult.

SAFETY ALERT: A distended bladder can be palpated over the lower abdomen above the symphysis pubis. Voiding frequently in small amounts may signal a neurogenic bladder. ■

BOX 43.2
Patient Teaching of Self-Catheterization

Self-catheterization on an intermittent basis (usually a part of self-care at home) is a clean rather than a sterile procedure. The hands should be washed before and after the procedure, and the urinary meatus should be gently cleansed with soap and water.

FEMALE SELF-CATHETERIZATION

- Attempt to void. If urine is not of sufficient quantity (at least 100 mL) or if you cannot void at all, do self-catheterization. *A large amount of residual urine means that more frequent catheterizations (every 4 to 6 hours) are necessary.*
- While sitting on the wheelchair or the commode, locate urethra. Visualize urethra by looking in a mirror or palpate urethra with fingertip. *Visualization or palpation of the meatus is necessary for accurate catheter insertion.*
- Lubricate meatus with a water-soluble lubricant. *Lubrication facilitates insertion of catheter and reduces trauma to tissues.*
- Take a deep breath and insert the catheter tip 5 to 7.5 cm (2 to 3 in.) or until urine flows. *The catheter enters the bladder more easily when the sphincter is relaxed. The deep breath relaxes the sphincter. The female urethra is 3.8 to 6.4 cm (1.5 to 2.5 in.) long.*
- Hold catheter securely and allow urine to drain until flow stops. *Withdrawing and reinserting catheter increases risk of infection.*
- Withdraw catheter and wash with soap and water. Store catheter in a clean airtight container. *The catheter can be reused until it is too soft or too hard to be directed into and through the urinary meatus. Clean technique (not sterile) is sufficient for home self-catheterization.*

MALE SELF-CATHETERIZATION

- Attempt to void. If urine is not of sufficient quantity (e.g., less than 100 mL) or if you cannot void at all, do self-catheterization. *A large amount of residual urine means that more frequent catheterizations (every 4 to 6 hours) are necessary.*
- Sit either on the commode or in wheelchair. Hold penis with slight upward tension and extend it to its full length. *Extending the penis straightens the urethra.*
- Lubricate the catheter from tip to about 15 cm (6 in.) downward. *Lubrication is crucial to male catheterization because of length of urethra.*
- Take a deep breath and insert catheter 15 to 18 cm (6 to 7 in.) or until urine flows. *The catheter enters the bladder more easily when the sphincter is relaxed. The deep breath relaxes the sphincter. The male urethra is about 15 cm (6 in.) long.*
- Hold catheter securely and allow urine to drain until flow has stopped. *Withdrawing and reinserting catheter increase risk of infection.*
- Withdraw catheter and wash with soap and water. Store catheter in a clean and airtight container. *The catheter can be reused until it is too soft or too hard to be directed into and through the urethra. Clean technique (not sterile) is used for home self-catheterization.*

Promote Optimal Sexual Function. Sexual intercourse is often still possible for the SCI patient. In men, the general rule is that the higher the level of injury, the greater the potential to have reflexogenic erections, although ejaculation or orgasm may not occur. Fertility is diminished due to a lack of temperature control of the testes. Ejaculation can be stimulated so that the patient's sperm can inseminate his partner so that fatherhood is a possibility. Men who have sacral-level injuries do not have reflexogenic erections but may have psychogenic erections and are more likely to remain fertile.

Women with SCI generally do not have sensation during sexual intercourse, but pregnancy is possible. There is an increased risk of autonomic dysreflexia in pregnant females with SCI, particularly during labor and delivery. Birth control options should be discussed on an ongoing basis.

A patient with an SCI may be deeply concerned about sexual dysfunctions, and these concerns may lead to lowered self-esteem, altered self-image, and/or changes in feelings about being an attractive and desirable person. The nurse must assess concerns and provide a climate that is receptive to discussion about sexuality. Examples of objectives for sexual counseling for the SCI patient are that the patient will understand how the injury has altered sexual functioning, will be aware of alternative ways of achieving sexual pleasure, and will have a positive self-concept and body image.

Patients with SCIs will be assessed in terms of their physical limitations and educated regarding the potential for sexual functioning and fertility.

Expected Outcome: Patient will experience optimal sexual functioning with minimal complications related to sexual interactions.

The nurse will:

- Include data about sexuality when obtaining the nursing history and database. *Sexuality is a private matter for most people, and the patient may not discuss it unless the nurse introduces the topic.*
- Provide accurate information about the effect of the SCI on sexual function. *Accurate information gives the patient a realistic picture of how the injury will affect sexuality.*
- Initiate a discussion with the patient and partner of alternative means of gaining sexual satisfaction; these include the use of vibrators and oral–genital and manual stimulation. *Alternatives to intercourse can meet sexual needs and help maintain the relationship with a significant other.*
- Refer for sexual counseling, if appropriate, or to local support groups where questions can be answered by others with similar experiences. *Knowing that others have had similar experiences can decrease social isolation and provide a means of learning alternative methods of sexual functioning.*

Promote Optimal Self-Esteem. An SCI is the result of sudden trauma. Within moments, a formerly independent, fully functioning individual is suddenly unable to move and faces enormous adjustments in social, economic, and personal roles and relationships. Body image, self-esteem, and role performance are affected by the damage. Patients often demonstrate behaviors that may be difficult for the nurse to handle, including depression, denial, and anger, immediately after the injury. In addition to these responses, the young adult patient may act out by making sexually overt statements.

The goals of care for the SCI patient and family include acceptance of changes in biopsychosocial functioning while optimizing the patient's ability for self-care and independence.

Expected Outcome: Patient will demonstrate optimal self-esteem.

The nurse will:

- Encourage talking about all aspects of physical function and care. *Talking provides a safe outlet for fears and frustrations and increases self-awareness. Acceptance of self facilitates rehabilitation.*
- Encourage self-care and independent decision making. *Participating in self-care can promote positive coping; making decisions decreases feelings of powerlessness.*
- Help identify strategies to increase independence in desired roles; include both short- and long-term goals. Discuss assistive devices (such as hand-operated automobiles). *Identifying strategies to increase independence fosters a positive self-concept and motivates the patient to achieve rehabilitation goals.*
- Include family members and important others in discussions. *The realization that others do care and will continue to provide support is important in fostering positive self-regard.*
- Refer the patient and family to support groups or for psychologic counseling. *Adjustment to change is more likely when the patient and family seek peer and professional assistance.*

Delegating Nursing Care Activities

As appropriate and allowed by the designated duties and responsibilities of unlicensed assistive personnel, the nurse may delegate nursing care activities such as measuring vital signs (including orthostatic vital signs), encouraging oral or enteral fluid intake, and providing skin care.

Transitions of Care

Health promotion for SCI primarily involves preventing injuries. Nurses can provide valuable information in the community and in the workplace to prevent SCI. Programs that focus on wearing seat belts and using approved infant seats and child booster chairs in automobiles can do much to help decrease the number of SCIs each year. Educational programs that promote workplace safety and farm safety should include information about how to prevent falls and how to use heavy equipment safely.

In the acute phase of treatment, it is most important to ensure hemodynamic stability of the patient. These

Case Study & Nursing Care Plan

A Patient with an SCI

Jim Valdez, a 19-year-old college sophomore, is admitted to the hospital by ambulance following an automobile crash. His family (father, mother, and sister) lives 100 miles away and cannot visit often, although they are very concerned. On admission to the hospital, a computed tomography (CT) scan of the spine shows a fracture and partial laceration of the cord at the C_7 level. Mr. Valdez is in halo traction. One night, he tells the nurse, "I wish I had just died when I got hurt. I don't think I can stand to live like this."

ASSESSMENT

When Mr. Valdez is admitted to the intensive care unit, he has flaccid paralysis involving all extremities. He has no sensation below the clavicle or in portions of his arms and legs. His bladder is distended and bowel sounds are absent. Other assessment findings include BP 90/56 mmHg, P 50 bpm, T 36.1°C (97°F), arterial blood gases pH 7.4, PaO_2 96, $PaCO_2$ 37, SaO_2 96%. Oxygen per nasal cannula is given at 2 L/min, and halo traction is applied. A Foley catheter is inserted into his bladder, and a nasogastric tube is inserted and attached to low-pressure continuous suction.

After 3 days, Mr. Valdez is moved from the intensive care unit to the neurosurgical unit for continuing care and planning for transfer to a rehabilitation hospital in his hometown. His vital signs have stabilized and are normal for his age; respirations and oxygenation are normal. Other neurologic assessments remain the same.

DIAGNOSES

- Lack of mobility related to paralysis of lower and upper extremities
- Fecal incontinence related to lack of voluntary sphincter control
- Anger and grief related to denial of loss

EXPECTED OUTCOMES

- Patient will be actively involved in exercise programs.
- Patient will have a soft, formed stool every second or third day.
- Patient will verbally express his grief to parents and staff.

PLANNING AND IMPLEMENTATION

- Conduct passive exercises on all extremities four times a day.
- Provide progressive mobilization by initially raising the head of the bed 90 degrees (repeat two to three times during the first day of movement); if blood pressure remains normal, dangle for 5 minutes before transferring him to a chair.
- His usual time for a bowel movement is after breakfast; schedule retraining program for that time.
- Encourage a diet high in fiber and fluids. Likes whole-wheat bread, orange juice, and cola; does not like water.
- Promote grief work by providing time to express feelings. Explain to the family that his denial and anger are part of the grieving process.
- Determine food likes and dislikes and order preferred foods from the menu. Encourage his friends to bring in his favorite foods periodically.
- Take and record weight every third day, using the bed scales.

EVALUATION

By the time Mr. Valdez is transferred to the rehabilitation hospital he is looking forward to learning how to use special equipment and getting his own motorized wheelchair. He is able to sit up in a chair without dizziness or hypotension. The use of ordered stool softeners combined with a high-fiber diet and fluid intake of 2000 to 3000 mL per day has maintained bowel elimination. Mr. Valdez and his parents have spent 3 hours talking about their feelings related to the accident and the future. Although the discussion is emotionally difficult, all three say they now feel much better. Mr. Valdez still has episodes of angry outbursts and tears, but he is more optimistic about what can be done and believes he can finish college. He selects foods from the menu each day and eats most of his meals, but he especially enjoys the times his friends bring in pizza or hamburgers.

CLINICAL REASONING IN PATIENT CARE

1. Considering Mr. Valdez's age and developmental level, do you think his emotional responses to his injury are appropriate?
2. Issues of sexuality are obviously important for the patient with a spinal cord injury. How would you approach Mr. Valdez about this topic?
3. What would be your response if Mr. Valdez allows only male nurses to provide care?
4. Outline a teaching program to help Mr. Valdez meet long-term urinary elimination needs.

See Evaluating Your Response in Appendix B.

treatments include maintaining immobilization of the neck and spinal column, care of life-threatening injuries (bleeding, pneumothorax), securing an airway, maintaining adequate ventilation, and stabilization of vital signs. Prevention of secondary injury is a main goal in the acute phase of spinal cord injury. Hypoxia and hypotension can greatly increase the incidence of secondary injury (Ropper, Neal, & Theodore, 2015). Maintaining perfusion to the spinal cord and preventing additional swelling or compression on the cord can prevent extension of injury. Once stabilized, the patient may need to be prepped for surgical decompression.

Throughout the hospital stay, nursing care should include prevention of pressure ulcers, deep vein thrombosis, and urinary tract infections. Monitoring of airway, breathing, and circulation and signs and symptoms of spinal shock and neurogenic shock are important throughout the stay.

Rehabilitation of the patient with an SCI is an ongoing process that moves from intensive care through intermediate care to rehabilitation and then community-based and home care. Nursing interventions are necessary at all points in the process to prevent the complications of altered physical mobility and body functions and to teach the patient and family measures that promote independence in self-care.

Discharge planning should be addressed even in the initial plan of care while the patient is in the critical care setting. Advance planning ensures continuity of care when the patient leaves the hospital setting.

The following should be included in teaching the patient and family about care at home:

- Self-care activities (ADLs, exercises, bowel and bladder programs, skin care)
- Mobility (use of assistive devices: Wheelchair, crutches, special automobiles)
- Preparation of the home environment: If the patient is in a wheelchair, will steps, stairs, doors, or carpeted floors present physical barriers? If a special bed is necessary, have arrangements been made to provide it?
- Psychologic support
- Independent activities
- Community resources, such as emergency alerting systems through a local hospital or agency, support groups, career centers for job retraining, counseling
- Coping skills for patient and caregiver
- Referral to a home health agency and physical therapist for the patient who is returning home
- Helpful resources:

  a. American Spine Injury Association
  b. National Spinal Cord Injury Association
  c. American Paralysis Association
  d. Christopher and Dana Reeve Paralysis Foundation
  e. Paralyzed Veterans of America.

The Patient with a Herniated Intervertebral Disk

A *herniated intervertebral disk* (also called a *ruptured disk, herniated nucleus pulposus*, or *slipped disk*) is a rupture of cartilage surrounding the intervertebral disk with protrusion of the nucleus pulposus (**Figure 43.5 ■**). This complication is seen more commonly in men than in women and is most often seen in patients between the ages of 30 and 50 (Sorenson, et al., 2019).

Pathophysiology

The intervertebral disks, located between the vertebral bodies, are made of an inner nucleus pulposus and an outer collar (the annulus fibrosus). The disks allow the spine to

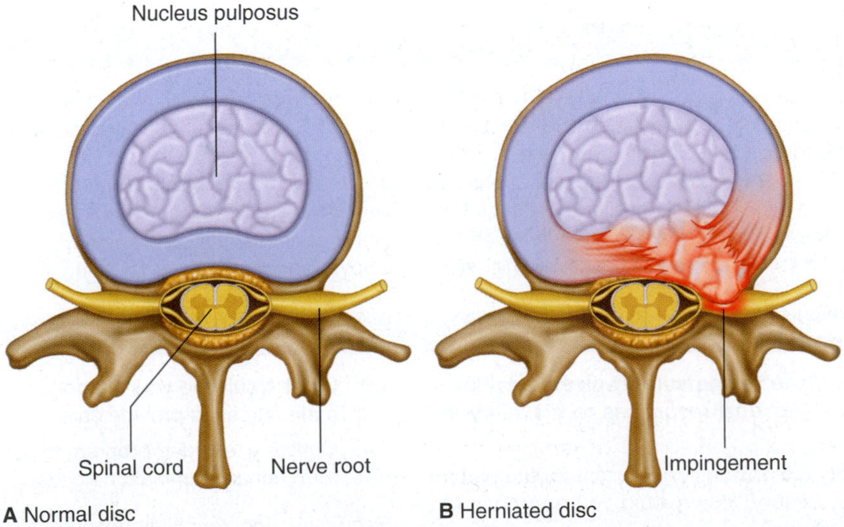
Nucleus pulposus
Spinal cord
Nerve root
A Normal disc
Impingement
B Herniated disc

Figure 43.5 ■ A, Normal intervertebral disc. **B**, A herniated intervertebral disk. The herniated nucleus pulposus is applying pressure against the nerve root.

absorb compression by acting as shock absorbers. A herniated intervertebral disk occurs when the nucleus pulposus protrudes through a weakened or torn annulus fibrosus of an intervertebral disk (refer to Figure 43.5). This protrusion may occur anywhere along the vertebral column, with the majority of herniated disks occurring in the lumbar region (L_4 or L_5 to S_1). Cervical **herniation** is most often seen in older patients and often involves C_6 to C_7 (Sorenson et al., 2019). Herniation of thoracic disks is uncommon.

A herniated intervertebral disk may result from trauma, degenerative disorders of the spine, or aging. The protrusion may occur spontaneously or as a result of trauma, such as lifting heavy objects while in the flexed position or falling on the buttocks or back. It may result from degenerative diseases, such as osteoarthritis, and aging. Aging causes degeneration in the annulus fibrosus and the posterior longitudinal ligaments, and the vertebrae and disks are less able to respond to movement and are more easily injured.

Rupture of the disk most often allows herniation of the nucleus pulposus in a posterolateral direction, with compression of the associated nerve root. The resulting pressure on adjacent spinal nerves causes characteristic manifestations, which vary with the location and the amount of protruding disk material. Occasionally the herniation is central rather than posterolateral, with pressure on the spinal cord.

The herniation may be abrupt or gradual. Lifting incorrectly or suddenly twisting the spine can cause rupture with immediate intense pain and muscle spasms. Gradual herniation is the result of degenerative changes, osteoarthritis, or ankylosis spondylitis. Patients with a gradual herniation have a slow onset of pain and neurologic deficits. Both motor and sensory manifestations occur and are localized to the area of the body innervated by the nerve root. The manifestations may be described as **radiculopathy** (a condition in which one or more nerves, especially nerve roots, do not function normally) and/or **paresthesia** (an abnormal sensation of the skin, such as numbness, burning, or pricking).

Risk Factors

A herniated disk may be due to normal wear and tear of the vertebrae as in cases of degenerative disk disease. However, it can also be related to trauma. Risk factors include repeated lifting (as may be common with certain occupations) as well as weight-bearing sports (Sorenson et al., 2019).

Manifestations

Manifestations of a herniated intervertebral disk are based on the location and the extent of the herniation. These manifestations can be categorized as lumbar disk or cervical disk.

Lumbar Disk Manifestations

The classic manifestation of a ruptured lumbar disk is recurrent episodes of pain in the lower back. The pain typically radiates across the buttock and down the posterior leg. **Sciatica** is a term used to describe lumbar back pain that radiates down the posterior leg to the ankle and is increased by sneezing or coughing (the result of pressure on nerve roots L_4, L_5, S_1, S_2, or S_3, which give rise to the sciatic nerve). The patient feels pain when lifting one leg while dorsiflexing the foot of that leg. Sciatica pain varies in intensity, ranging from mildly uncomfortable to excruciating. It is aggravated by a variety of positions and activities, including sitting, straining, coughing, sneezing, climbing stairs, walking, and riding in a car. Prolonged sitting and climbing of stairs are especially painful.

Additional manifestations that the patient may experience with herniation in the lumbar region include paresthesia, muscle spasms, weakness, motor deficits, and sensory deficits as well as some changes in reflexes.

Cervical Disk Manifestations

A majority of cervical herniations are the result of degeneration; other causes include trauma and physical exertion (Robinson & Kothari, 2016). Cervical disks that herniate laterally cause radicular pain in the shoulder, neck, and arm and paresthesias along the dermatome of the compressed nerve root. Other manifestations of lateral cervical herniation include muscle spasms and stiff neck and decreased or absent arm reflexes. Central cervical herniations result in a dull, intermittent pain; however, the patient may also experience lower extremity weakness, unsteady gait, muscle spasms, urinary elimination problems, altered sexual function, and hyperactive lower extremity reflexes. A cervical herniation due to acute trauma may be manifested by immediate weakness of the extremity or, if severe, by paralysis. Any suspected herniation that is not related to degeneration and has significant neurologic involvement should be evaluated with radiologic testing (Robinson & Kothari, 2016).

Complications

Many disk herniations are self-limiting and symptoms typically resolve within 6 weeks without intervention (Robinson & Kothari, 2016). **Cauda equina syndrome** is a complication that can occur with complete nerve root compression. Symptoms include bowel and bladder incontinence along with paralysis of the lower extremities. This is considered a medical emergency and will require immediate surgical intervention to decompress the herniation.

Interprofessional Care

Considerations for the patient with a **ruptured intervertebral disk** include identifying the location of herniation and determining whether conservative treatment or surgery is indicated. Diagnostic tests may also be performed to differentiate a herniated disk from other causes of acute back pain.

Diagnosis

Diagnostic tests are ordered to differentiate the cause of back pain; for example, back and leg pain is also caused by spinal tumors, degenerative processes, or abdominal diseases. Assessing pain is an important part of diagnosis. The tests (refer to Chapter 41) include x-rays and CT scans of the lumbosacral or cervical area to identify skeletal deformities and narrowing of the disk spaces. Electromyography (EMG), which measures electrical activity of skeletal muscles at rest and during voluntary contraction, may be conducted to identify specific muscles affected by the pressure of the herniation on the nerve roots. A myelogram with contrast medium is performed to rule out tumors and illustrate areas of herniation, although it does not provide the detail found with CT or MRI.

Muscle strength and reflexes are tested, with the straight leg test being an important diagnostic test. In order to conduct this, the patient is placed in the supine position while the leg is passively raised. This movement places traction on the nerve root, which increases the pain if the nerve root is inflamed.

Medications

The patient with a ruptured intervertebral disk is treated with medications to relieve pain and reduce swelling and muscle spasms. Pain is usually managed with NSAIDs. Muscle spasms are treated with muscle relaxants.

Treatments

A ruptured intervertebral disk may be treated conservatively or with surgery.

Conservative Treatment. A ruptured intervertebral disk is usually managed conservatively unless the patient is experiencing severe neurologic deficits. The goals of treatment are pain relief and healing of the involved disk by fibrosis. Conservative treatment is usually prescribed for 2 to 6 weeks. If the patient continues to have pain after that time, surgery may be considered. The treatment regimen depends on the severity of the manifestations. Decreasing activity level with bedrest is no longer recommended; in many cases, the patient is advised to continue with normal activities while taking prescribed medications for pain, inflammation, and muscle spasms.

Surgery. Surgery is indicated for patients with unrelenting pain, those who fail to respond to conservative management, or those with serious neurologic deficits (Levin, Hsu, & Armon, 2017). Several surgical interventions are used to treat a ruptured intervertebral disk. The type of surgery chosen depends on the location of the disk and the stability of the spinal column:

- ***Laminectomy***, the type of surgery most often performed, is the removal of a part of the vertebral lamina (bony arch on dorsal surface). The surgery is done to relieve pressure on the nerves. It is often combined with removal of the protruding nucleus pulposus (nucleotomy). Nursing care for the patient having a laminectomy is discussed in **Box 43.3**. A **diskectomy** is the removal of the nucleus pulposus of an intervertebral disk. Diskectomy may be performed alone or in conjunction with a laminectomy (Levin et al., 2017).
- ***Spinal fusion*** is the insertion of a wedge-shaped piece of bone or bone chips (which can be harvested from the patient or from cadaver bone) between the vertebrae to stabilize them. Although not appropriate for all patients requiring a spinal fusion, this does facilitate a short hospital stay and convalescence.
- ***Foraminotomy*** is a surgical procedure to enlarge the space (passageway or neuroforamen) where a spinal nerve exits the spinal canal. The bone or tissue obstructing the passageway is removed. The posterior approach is taken for lumbar surgery while cervical disk surgery can be approached posteriorly or anteriorly (Nguyen et al., 2017).
- ***Microdiskectomy***, in which microsurgical techniques are used, is performed through a very small incision. This type of surgery decreases the possibility of trauma to surrounding structures during surgery and allows early postoperative mobility and a short hospital stay.

Nursing Care

Nursing care for the patient with a ruptured intervertebral disk may be provided through information in community and work settings, during conservative treatment, and during pre- and postoperative treatment. The pain of the ruptured disk is often discouraging and debilitating and may affect the patient's ability to work.

Assessment

The following data are collected through the health history and physical examination (refer to Chapter 41):

- ***Health history:*** Type of employment, risk factors, pain (location, duration, intensity)
- ***Physical assessment:*** Muscle strength and coordination, sensation, reflexes.

Priorities of Care

The goals of care are to maximize comfort, provide effective pain management techniques, promote correct body alignment, and prevent further injury.

Diagnoses, Outcomes, and Interventions

Nursing care for patients with a herniated intervertebral disk focuses largely on pain management, both during conservative management and after surgery.

Relieve Acute Pain. Patients with a ruptured intervertebral disk experience acute back and leg pain. Acute pain may be related to preoperative muscle spasms or nerve root compression. After surgery, the patient may have pain at the site of the incision and in the surgical area.

Expected Outcome: Patient will be free of acute leg and back pain.

The nurse will:

- Assess the degree of pain on a scale of 0 to 10, with 10 being greatest pain, and identify contributing and relieving factors. *Pain is a subjective experience requiring a thorough nursing assessment prior to any interventions.*
- Use a firm mattress or place a board under the mattress. *A firm bed supports the spinal column and muscles.*
- Teach the patient to avoid turning or twisting the spinal column and to assume positions that decrease stress on the vertebral column (e.g., when in the supine position,

BOX 43.3
Nursing Care of the Patient Having a Posterior Laminectomy

PREOPERATIVE TEACHING

- Demonstrate and ask for a return demonstration of logrolling; patient should avoid bending or twisting the spine. *To ensure healing, the spinal column must remain in alignment when turning and moving.*
- Explain the importance of taking pain medications regularly and of asking for them before the pain is severe. Inform the patient that pain may not improve for several days or weeks after surgery. *Pain is easier to control if medications are taken before the pain is severe. Pain may be prolonged in the post-op laminectomy patient because edema due to surgery irritates and compresses the nerve roots.*
- Demonstrate the use of a fracture bedpan and ask the patient to practice its use. *The patient usually must remain flat in bed for a period of time following surgery. A fracture bedpan is more comfortable for patients who must lie flat.*
- Demonstrate and ask for a return demonstration of deep breathing, use of the incentive spirometer, and leg exercises. *These measures prevent respiratory and circulatory complications.*

POSTOPERATIVE CARE

- Maintain a position that minimizes stress on the surgical wound. Depending on the physician's orders, the patient may need to lay flat for a period of time. Be sure to instruct the patient not to bend or twist the spine and maintain the position of the cervical collar as appropriate. *Positioning should minimize stress on the surgical wound and suture line. A cervical collar provides stability and prevents flexing or twisting of the neck for patient's status post cervical laminectomy.*
- Turn every 2 hours, using the logrolling technique. Teach the patient not to use the side rails to change position. Maintain proper body alignment in all positions. *The patient's body is turned as a single unit (usually with a turning sheet) to avoid movement of the operative area. Pulling on the side rails puts stress on the operative area and may also cause misalignment of the vertebral column.*
- Monitor for signs of nerve root compression.
  a. Cervical laminectomy: Assess hand grips, arm strength, ability to move the fingers, and ability to detect touch.
  b. Lumbar laminectomy: Assess leg strength, ability to wiggle the toes, and ability to detect touch.
  c. Compare bilateral findings. Report muscle weakness or sensory impairment to the physician immediately. *Loss of motor and sensory function may indicate nerve root compression.*
- Assess for hematoma formation as manifested by severe incisional pain unrelieved by analgesics and a decrease in motor function. Report these findings immediately. *A hematoma may form at the surgical site. If untreated, it may cause irreversible neurologic deficits including paraplegia and bowel/bladder dysfunctions (Eisen, 2015).*
- Assess for leakage of cerebrospinal fluid (CSF). Assess the dressing for increased moisture. Check the sheets for wet area when the patient is lying supine; check for clear liquid running down the back when the patient is sitting or standing. Gently palpate edges of wound to detect a bulge. Leakage can also be assessed for the presence of glucose, which is a positive indicator of CSF. If leakage is noted, the patient should lie flat in bed and findings should be immediately reported. *Although uncommon, leakage of CSF greatly increases the risk for infection of the wound and of the meninges.*
- Assess for nerve root injury. Assess the ability to dorsiflex the foot (lumbar laminectomy) and the grip strength (cervical laminectomy). Assess the patient who has had a cervical laminectomy for hoarseness. Report hoarseness and further assess ability to swallow. *Nerve root compression may cause permanent damage, resulting in foot drop (in lumbar laminectomy patients) and hand weakness (in cervical laminectomy patients). Damage to the laryngeal nerve (in anterior approach) may cause permanent hoarseness. Impaired ability to swallow puts the patient at risk for aspiration.*
- Assess for urinary retention. The patient should void within 8 hours after surgery. If the physician allows, let males stand to void. Compare intake and output for each 8-hour period. Use a bladder scanner to identify urinary retention or residual urine. *All patients who have received a general anesthetic are at risk for urinary retention. The patient who has had a lumbar laminectomy may have even more difficulty voiding as a result of stimulation of sympathetic nerves during surgery.*
- Assess for pain using a scale from 0 (no pain) to 10 (severe pain). Administer prescribed analgesics on a regular basis, or teach patient to use patient-controlled analgesia (PCA) pump, if prescribed. Discuss concerns about pain that is unrelieved by surgery. *Compression of the nerve root over time results in edema and inflammation. Because of surgery-induced edema, the patient is likely to experience either the same pain or perhaps more severe pain in the period immediately after surgery. This pain usually persists for several weeks after surgery. In addition, many patients who have had a lumbar laminectomy have muscle spasms in the lower back, abdomen, and thighs for the first few days after surgery.*
- Assess for infection by taking and recording vital signs at least every 4 hours; report increased body temperature. Assess the wound and dressing for signs of infection including erythema, purulent drainage, and pain. Use sterile technique to change dressings. *The surgical patient is always at risk for infection; the patient with a laminectomy is also at risk for arachnoiditis. This inflammation of the arachnoid layer of the spinal meninges results from contamination during surgery and may cause painful adhesions.*
- Encourage deep breathing and the use of incentive spirometry every 2 hours; coughing may be discouraged. *Anesthesia and immobility depress respiratory function. Coughing may be discouraged because it can disrupt healing tissues, especially in patients having a cervical laminectomy.*
- Increase mobility as prescribed. (The time frame for ambulation is prescribed by the physician; the routine here is representative.) Patients often sit on the side of the bed and dangle their legs the evening after surgery or the first day thereafter. Most patients ambulate the first postoperative day. To help the patient out of bed, first elevate the head of the bed. Then bring the patient's legs over the side of the bed at the same time that the upper body moves into the upright position. Patients should only ambulate without assistance if there is no dizziness or weakness. *Early ambulation increases respiratory and circulatory function and decreases the risk of thrombophlebitis of the lower extremities. The vertebral column should remain in alignment while the patient sits and stands. Safety must be a priority during the postoperative period.*

flex the hips slightly). A small pillow may be placed under the knees (for patients with a herniated lumbar disk) or under the neck (for patients with a herniated cervical disk). *Correct body positions can decrease intradisk pressure.*

- Provide analgesic medications around the clock. *Intense pain can increase muscle spasms, making it crucial to maintain therapeutic levels of analgesics in the bloodstream.*

Manage Chronic Pain. The patient with a ruptured intervertebral disk often has pain for an extended period of time. Despite conservative treatment or previous surgery, pain may be ongoing or intermittent. If previous surgery has not relieved the pain, the patient may be depressed or angry. Caring for a patient with chronic pain can be frustrating, and the patient is often regarded as difficult.

Expected Outcome: Patient's pain will be managed effectively with optimal pain relief.

The nurse will:

- Treat the patient's reports of pain with respect. *The patient is the person experiencing the pain and is thus the expert about it.*
- Not refer to the patient as being addicted to pain medication. *All types of analgesics may be used legitimately to manage pain.*
- Monitor patient carefully for any changes in condition. *Significant changes in the patient's condition may go unrecognized when pain is present for a prolonged period of time.*
- Maintain written plans of care for pain management that are individualized and ensure continuity of care. *When the patient makes several visits (for instance, to an ED or a pain clinic), medical records provide a past history of effective pain management.*
- Teach alternative methods of pain management. Assess and consider the patient's coping style when recommending methods. *Patients who have a passive coping style are more likely to manage pain by depending on others, taking medications, and resting. Patients with an active coping style are more likely to manage pain by learning self-management methods and staying active.*
- Develop effective methods of improving rest and sleep. Problems with rest and sleep make pain management more difficult. *Sleeping poorly at night contributes to decreased motivation, confused thinking, depression, and muscle aches.*
- Refer patient to a physical therapist for an exercise program, if appropriate. *The patient needs to know exactly what exercises to do, how many repetitions are recommended, for how long, and how often. The patient should not exercise to the point of causing increased pain.*
- Assess need for referrals (and make them, if necessary) for the patient who is depressed or anxious. *Anxiety and depression are often linked to long-term chronic pain, making pain management more difficult. Suggesting that referrals help with the frustration (rather than depression) may make a significant difference in the effectiveness of pain management strategies.*

SAFETY ALERT: Although the patient may develop tolerance to a narcotic analgesic, tolerance does not imply addiction. Pain is unique for each patient and must be assessed objectively. Using the pain scale and administering medications and treatments to reduce pain is essential in those with chronic pain. ■

Promote Normal Bowel Elimination. The patient with a ruptured intervertebral disk often has problems with constipation because of reduced mobility and use of pain medications. Nursing interventions to alleviate and prevent constipation are important because straining to have a bowel movement can increase intradisk pressure, thus increasing pain. The goal of care is to prevent constipation and restore normal bowel elimination patterns.

Expected Outcome: Patient's bowel elimination patterns will be within normal limits.

The nurse will:

- Assess the patient's usual bowel routine, including diet, fluid intake, and the use of laxatives or enemas. *Effective interventions are based on individualized needs.*
- Encourage a fluid intake of 2500 to 3000 mL/day unless contraindicated by the presence of renal or cardiac disease. *Adequate fluid intake facilitates the passage of feces.*
- Increase fiber and bulk in the diet. If the patient is unable to tolerate increased fiber, consult with the physician about the use of stool softeners or bulk-forming agents. *Bulk and fiber promote regularity by retaining water in the large intestine.*

SAFETY ALERT: Individuals who use laxatives or enemas for long periods of time may be dependent on them to have a bowel movement. Accurate assessments of patterns and management techniques is essential to avoid bowel dysfunction. ■

Delegating Nursing Care Activities

As appropriate and allowed by the designated duties and responsibilities of unlicensed assistive personnel, the nurse may delegate nursing care activities such as measuring fluid intake and output, collecting vital signs (including orthostatic vital signs), encouraging oral or enteral fluid intake, positioning the patient, and providing skin care.

Transitions of Care

Most patients with a herniated disk will be treated conservatively and will not require invasive treatments. Pain management is the priority during the acute phase. Patients should take analgesics as prescribed and continue with their daily routines as much as possible. The nurse should help guide the patient in techniques that will help with pain management (see **Box 43.4**).

It is the nurse's responsibility to teach the patient and family about chronic pain control, including specific interventions to alleviate pain. The nurse's role may be that of advocate and creative problem solver (see Box 43.4). The following topics should be addressed:

- Often the goal is to control pain so that the patient can perform normal ADLs, rather than to reach a pain-free state.

BOX 43.4
Teaching the Patient with a Ruptured Intervertebral Disk

- Sleep on a firm mattress; use a bed board, if necessary.
- When lying in the supine position, flex the knees to approximately a 45-degree angle with a small pillow and use a small pillow under the head.
- Avoid any activities that flex the spine, such as bending or lifting, and do not twist the back.
- Follow a diet to maintain body weight or to lose weight, if needed.
- Follow the prescribed exercise program; for example, do the following:
    a. Lie flat on your back on the floor. Tighten your abdominal and buttock muscles and tilt your pelvis forward so that your lower back is flat on the floor (this is called a *pelvic tilt*). Hold the position for 3 seconds and repeat for the prescribed number of times.
    b. Lying on the back on a firm surface, press the feet to the floor, tighten the abdominal muscles, and lift the upper half of the body off the floor. Hold the position for 3 seconds, and repeat as prescribed.
    c. Lying on your back on a firm surface, bring your knees up to the chest. Put your hands around your knees and raise the buttocks off the floor. Repeat as prescribed.
    d. Sit upright on the floor or a firm surface. Keep one leg straight and bend the other knee. Reach for the toes of the straightened leg. Switch legs. Repeat as prescribed.
    e. Stand upright. Squat down, flexing the hips and knees. Straighten your back. Stand upright by straightening the knees. Repeat as prescribed.
- Wear flat-heeled shoes that provide good support.
- Use proper lifting techniques. For instance, squat and use your thigh muscles to lift an object from the floor, and spread your feet to get a wide base of support when you lift while you are standing.

- Nonpharmacologic methods of pain management include relaxation techniques, guided imagery, distraction, hypnosis, and music. Joining a support group may be an effective intervention in coping with and managing pain.
- Patients may be referred to a physical therapist for education about body mechanics and back-strengthening exercises. Nurses should have the patient demonstrate the exercises to reinforce teaching.

The Patient with a Spinal Cord Tumor

Spinal cord tumors may be benign or malignant, primary or metastatic. Tumors of the spinal cord are seen equally in men and in women, most often occur between the ages of 20 and 60 years, and are rare in older adults.

Tumors of the spinal cord are classified as either primary or secondary (metastatic). Primary tumors are rare and have an unknown cause. They may arise at any level of the spinal column, with the majority being thoracic. Most spinal cord tumors are metastatic. Metastatic tumors occur in approximately 20% of all patients with cancer (Schiff, 2016) and are most commonly the result of malignancies of the lung, breast, and prostate (Welch, Schiff, & Gerszten, 2017).

Spinal cord tumors may also be classified by anatomic location as either intramedullary or extramedullary tumors. Intramedullary tumors arise from within the neural tissues of the spinal cord; those that occur most frequently are ependymomas and gliomas. Extramedullary tumors, the most common type, arise from tissues outside the spinal cord, with commonly occurring tumors including neurofibromas, meningiomas, sarcomas, chordomas, and vascular tumors. Extramedullary tumors are further categorized as intradural (arising from the nerve roots or meninges within the subarachnoid space) or extradural (arising from epidural tissue or the vertebrae outside the dura). Extradural tumors are the most common location for metastatic cancer. Both primary and metastatic intradural tumors can involve the cerebrospinal fluid, a condition called *leptomeningeal disease (LMD)*.

Pathophysiology

Depending on their anatomic location, spinal cord tumors lead to pathologic changes as a result of compression, invasion, or ischemia secondary to arterial or venous obstruction. Extramedullary tumors (whether benign or malignant) alter normal function through compression of the spinal cord, with destruction of white matter and eventual filling of the space around the spinal cord. Cord compression is a serious complication, with symptoms ranging from weakness, minor sensory disturbance and autonomic changes to severe pain and irreversible paralysis (Schiff, 2016). Compression of the cord interferes with normal blood flow and membrane potentials, altering afferent and efferent motor, sensory, and reflex impulses. Compression causes edema, which can ascend the cord and cause further neurologic deficits. Intramedullary tumors both compress and invade the cord, resulting in cord enlargement and distortion of the white matter.

The vertebral column is the most common site in the bony skeleton for cancer metastasis. Metastatic tumors can involve the vertebrae, grow through the vertebral foramina, or directly affect the dura, spinal fluid, or spinal cord. The lesion, as it grows, causes epidural compression of the cord or spinal nerves.

Risk Factors

Primary spinal tumors are rare; genetics or exposure to carcinogens may play a part in the formation of these tumors (American Association of Neurological Surgeons, 2017b). Patients that have previously been diagnosed with breast, prostate, or lung cancer are at risk for extramedullary spinal tumors.

Manifestations

The manifestations of a spinal cord tumor depend on the anatomic location, level of occurrence, type of tumor, and spinal nerves involved (see **Table 43.3**). General manifestations of a spinal cord tumor include pain, motor and sensory deficits, changes in bowel and/or bladder elimination, and changes in sexual function.

Pain is often the first manifestation of a spinal cord tumor. It is caused by compression of the spinal cord, tension on the spinal nerves, or tumor attachment to the proximal dura (the covering of the spinal cord). The pain may be either localized or radicular. Localized pain is felt when pressure is applied over the spinous process of the involved area and often accompanies metastatic vertebral tumors. Radicular pain is sensed along the path of a nerve as a result of compression, irritation, or tension of a nerve root and is often made worse by any activity that causes intraspinal pressure, such as sneezing or coughing.

Motor manifestations resulting from a spinal cord tumor include paresis and paralysis below the level of the tumor, spasticity, and hyperactive reflexes. The Babinski reflex may be positive. These deficits are the result of involvement of the corticospinal tracts.

Many different sensory manifestations may occur, depending on the location and level of the tumor. Lateral tumor growth and compression affect the lateral spinothalamic tracts, causing pain, numbness, tingling, and coldness. If the tumor involves the posterior columns, the senses of vibration and proprioception of body parts are affected.

Bladder and bowel elimination and sexual function are often affected. Bowel elimination deficits include constipation that may progress to paralytic ileus. Initial bladder elimination deficits include frequency, urgency, and difficulty voiding and may progress to urinary retention and a neurogenic bladder. The male patient may be impotent.

Syringomyelia is a complication of spinal cord tumors involving formation of a fluid-filled cystic cavity in the central intramedullary gray matter, causing pain, motor weakness, and spasticity.

Complications

One of the common complications for patients with spinal cord tumor is spinal cord compression, which can lead to infarction and paralysis. Immediate recognition and intervention is important to prevent permanent damage.

Interprofessional Care

The medical management of the patient with a spinal cord tumor focuses first on diagnosis. Treatment depends on the type of tumor, its location, and the patient's condition. Prognosis and quality of life are related to the patient's prediagnosis health status, rapid diagnosis, and type of tumor (American Association of Neurological Surgeons, 2017b; Schiff, 2016).

Diagnosis

The patient with a spinal cord tumor undergoes many of the same diagnostic tests as does the patient with a ruptured intervertebral disk, including x-rays, CT scans, MRI, and myelogram (refer to Chapter 41). MRI is the go-to for primary diagnosis, as this test is noninvasive and allows the practitioner to visualize the entire area of the spine (Schiff, 2016).

Medications

The patient with a spinal cord tumor is prescribed medications (typically opioid analgesics) to control pain and edema. Severe pain can result from a metastatic tumor and may necessitate insertion of an epidural catheter for narcotic analgesia. Steroids such as dexamethasone (Decadron) are administered to control cord edema.

Immobilization

Spinal stability must be determined before treatments can be planned, particularly because some treatments have the potential to destabilize the spine (radiotherapy, laminectomy). The biomechanics, anatomy, and flexibility of the

Table 43.3 Manifestations of Spinal Cord Tumors

Location	Manifestations
Cervical cord tumors	■ Ipsilateral arm motor involvement, followed by ipsilateral and contralateral leg involvement, followed by contralateral arm involvement ■ Paresis of the arms and legs ■ Stiffness of the neck ■ Paraplegia ■ Pain in the shoulders and arms ■ Hyperactive reflexes
Thoracic cord tumors	■ Paresis and spasticity of one leg, followed by paresis and spasticity of the other leg ■ Pain in the back and chest ■ Positive Babinski reflex ■ Bowel and bladder dysfunction ■ Sexual dysfunction
Lumbosacral cord tumors	■ Paresis and spasticity of one leg, followed by paresis and spasticity of the other leg ■ Pain in the lower back, radiating to the legs and perineal area ■ Loss of sensation in the legs ■ Bowel and bladder dysfunction ■ Sexual dysfunction ■ Decreased or absent ankle and knee reflexes

spine are assessed to determine if the spine is unstable. A patient with an unstable spine may suffer from significant pain. External spinal support such as bracing has not been shown to help with the pain related to an unstable spine; surgery with internal fixation would be required (Schiff, Brown, & Shaffrey, 2017).

Surgery

Intramedullary and intradural tumors are surgically excised when possible by performing a laminectomy. Advances in microsurgical techniques and laser surgery have increased the possibility that tumors can be removed. Metastatic tumors that cause cord compression require surgical decompression and/or partial removal to preserve motor, bowel, or bladder function.

Other Treatments

Stereotactic Radiosurgery. Stereotactic radiosurgery may be an alternative to surgery for some patients. This process provides a painless, noninvasive treatment that delivers high doses of precisely targeted radiation to destroy tumors while minimizing damage to healthy tissue. This procedure is sometimes referred to by its trade name of *Cyberknife* or *Gammaknife*.

Radiation Therapy. Radiation therapy is used to treat metastatic spinal cord tumors for several different reasons. It may be used on an emergency basis to treat the patient with rapidly progressing neurologic deficits. It may be used to reduce pain, and it may be used following surgical excision of as much tumor mass as possible.

Radiation of the spinal cord may cause radiation-induced myelopathy to develop. This complication of radiation exposure occurs over time, with manifestations of *Brown-Séquard syndrome* (weakness or paralysis on one side of the body and loss of sensation on the opposite side) developing greater than 6 months after therapy (Oh, 2017). The manifestations may progress to paraplegia, sensory loss, and loss of bowel and bladder control (Oh, 2017).

Nursing Care

Nursing care for the patient with a spinal cord tumor is individualized to the type of tumor and the type of treatment. The patient with a benign tumor that is removed by surgery has different healthcare needs than the patient with a metastatic tumor, even though they may have similar neurologic deficits. The patient with a spinal cord tumor (regardless of type) requires nursing care to monitor for neurologic changes, to provide pain management, and to manage motor and sensory deficits in order to preserve quality of life.

Assessment

The assessments and nursing interventions and delegation of care for the patient with a spinal cord tumor are much the same as those described for the patient with an SCI or the patient undergoing surgery for a ruptured intervertebral disk. The nurse should ensure regular and thorough neurological assessments every 2 hours and report changes immediately (Kaplow & Iyere, 2016).

Transitions of Care

Patients diagnosed with a primary spinal tumor will be treated based on the stage of the tumor. Patient teaching regarding the spinal cord tumor as well as signs and symptoms of neurologic changes are important.

Following surgical treatment, the patient may be transferred to a rehabilitation center or be discharged to home for the recovery period. Referrals for home care, occupational therapy, and physical therapy can restore functional abilities. Family members and caregivers must be taught how to position and transfer the patient from bed to chair. Teaching must also include methods for providing physical care, managing any devices (such as an indwelling catheter), and preventing or treating constipation as well as signs and symptoms to report to the provider (Kaplow & Iyere, 2016).

The goal of treatment in metastatic tumors is more palliative and is geared to alleviate pain symptoms as well as regain functioning in order to enhance quality of life (Ciftdemir, Kaya, Selcuk et al., 2016).

43.2 Infectious Disorders of the Central Nervous System

The Patient with a CNS Infection

The CNS—including the brain, spinal cord, meninges, neural tissues, and blood vessels—may be directly affected by bacteria, viruses, fungi, protozoans, and rickettsiae. In general, organisms enter the brain in two ways: By bacteria that cross the blood–brain barrier due to infections of nearby structures (such as sinusitis, otitis media, or pneumonia) or by direct invasion through, for example, a skull fracture or bullet hole. The incidence of pathogenic CNS infections increases in the presence of HIV and AIDS because of the risk of opportunistic infections such as toxoplasmosis, cryptococcus, tuberculosis, herpes simplex virus (HSV), or cytomegalovirus (CMV).

Pathophysiology

When pathogens enter the CNS and the meninges, an infectious inflammatory process results. As edema occurs, intracranial pressure (ICP) increases. The pathogenic invasion and increased ICP (IICP) may result in brain damage and life-threatening complications.

Meningitis

Meningitis is a pyogenic (purulent) infection that involves the pia mater, the arachnoid, and the subarachnoid space, including the cerebrospinal fluid. The infection spreads rapidly throughout the CNS because of the circulation of CSF around the brain and spinal cord. Meningitis may be acute or chronic and bacterial, viral, fungal, or parasitic in origin.

The causative organism must overcome nonspecific and specific host defense mechanisms to invade and replicate in the CSF. These defenses include the skin barrier, the blood–brain barrier, the nonspecific inflammatory response, and the immune response. The organisms that initiate the host response in meningitis initially colonize and invade the nasopharyngeal mucosa. Organisms invade the vascular system and then penetrate the CNS if the blood–brain barrier is damaged by surgery, the inflammatory response, or cerebral edema.

Infection of the CSF and meninges causes an inflammatory response in the pia mater, arachnoid space, and CSF. Because the meninges and subarachnoid space are continuous around the brain, spinal cord, and optic nerves, the infection and inflammatory response are always cerebrospinal, involving both the brain and spinal cord. Increased capillary permeability causes leakage of fluids into the interstitial spaces while purulent exudate infiltrates cranial nerve sheaths and blocks the choroid plexus and subarachnoid villi. IICP causes decreased cerebral perfusion and a loss of cerebral autoregulation.

Bacterial Meningitis. According to the Centers for Disease Control and Prevention (CDC, 2017a), the most common causative organisms of bacterial meningitis include *Neisseria meningitidis*, group B streptococcus, *Streptococcus pneumoniae*, *Haemophilus influenzae*, and *Listeria monocytogenes*. The incidence of meningitis from *H. influenzae* has been greatly reduced because of vaccination against the organism.

Epidemics of meningococcal meningitis occur in populations who live in close contact, such as military recruits and students living in college dormitories. Infants less than 1 year old and adolescents and young adults have the greatest occurrence of meningococcal meningitis in the United States (CDC, 2017b), vaccinations are available to prevent meningococcal meningitis.

Pathogen entry into the CNS initiates the inflammatory response in the meninges, CSF, and ventricles. Meningeal vessels become engorged and permeability increases. Phagocytic white blood cells (WBCs) migrate into the subarachnoid space, forming a purulent exudate that thickens and clouds the CSF and impairs its flow. Rapid exudate formation causes further inflammation and edema of meningeal cells with resulting IICP.

Viral Meningitis. Acute viral meningitis, also called *aseptic meningitis*, is less severe than bacterial meningitis. Numerous viruses, such as HSV, herpes zoster, Epstein-Barr virus, or West Nile virus, can cause viral meningitis. Although the inflammatory response is also provoked, this disease is typically benign, short lived, and with an uneventful recovery.

Encephalitis

Encephalitis is a generalized infection of the parenchyma of the brain or spinal cord. It is typically caused by a virus but can also be caused by bacteria, fungi, and other organisms. See **Table 43.4** for a list of common causes.

Viral Encephalitis. Viruses depend on living tissue for reproduction and become highly destructive when invading brain tissue. They gain access to the CNS via the bloodstream or via a preexisting case of meningitis. An inflammatory response extends over the cerebral cortex, white matter, and meninges. Degeneration of neurons occurs along with local necrotizing hemorrhage. Generalized hemorrhage, edema, and progressive degeneration of nerve cell bodies occur. Unlike meningitis, there is no exudate formation. Certain viruses show a propensity for specific areas of the brain (e.g., HSV involves frontal and temporal lobes).

Arbovirus Encephalitis. The arboviruses are arthropod-borne (mosquito and tick) agents that infect humans. They include many different types, including western equine encephalitis, St. Louis encephalitis, and West Nile encephalitis. The most common arboviral encephalitis in the United States is West Nile encephalitis (Gluckman, 2017), which has become endemic in the United States.

The arthropod-borne agents cause widespread degeneration of nerve cells, resulting in edema, necrosis, and possible hemorrhage. IICP may develop.

Table 43.4 Causes of Encephalitis

Cause	Comments
Arboviruses	Transmitted most often by bites from mosquitoes. Bites from mosquitoes occur in middle to late summer. Most common types are St. Louis, eastern and western equine encephalitis, and West Nile encephalitis. May destroy major parts of lobe or hemisphere. Mortality rates associated with arboviruses are higher than those associated with enteroviruses.
Enteroviruses, such as echovirus, coxsackievirus, poliovirus, paramyxovirus (the virus that causes mumps), and varicella-zoster (the virus that causes chickenpox)	Infection occurs more frequently in summer (except infection by the mumps virus, which occurs more frequently in early winter). A degree of protection can be provided by immunization against measles, mumps, and poliomyelitis. Mortality rates are lower than those associated with herpes simplex type 1 virus.
Herpes simplex type 1 virus	Can occur any time of year and throughout the world. Has an affinity for frontal and temporal lobes. Prognosis is grave but not hopeless; mortality rate can be as high as 20 to 30% (Klein, 2017).
Amebic meningoencephalitis due to infection by *Naegleria* and *Acanthamoeba* protozoa	Both protozoa are found in warm freshwater and enter nasal mucosa of people swimming in ponds or lakes. May also be found in soil and decaying vegetation. Incidence of infection is increasing in North America.
Exogenous poisoning	May occur after ingestion of lead or arsenic or inhalation of carbon monoxide.

Brain Abscess

A brain abscess is an infection with a collection of purulent material within the brain tissue. The causes of a brain abscess include open trauma and neurosurgery; infections of the mastoid, middle ear, nasal cavity, or nasal sinuses; metastatic spread from distant foci (such as heart, lungs, skin, abscessed teeth, and dirty needles); and arising from other associated areas of infection. Immunocompromise increases the risk for abscesses. The most common pathogens causing an abscess are streptococci and staphylococci. Yeast, fungi, and parasites may also cause brain abscesses.

A brain abscess results from the presence of microorganisms in the brain tissue. If the abscess is encapsulated, it may enlarge and behave as a space-occupying lesion within the cranium. This predisposes the patient to a systemic inflammatory process and to the serious consequences of IICP. Occasionally, the abscess does not become encapsulated but spreads through brain tissue to the subarachnoid space and ventricular system.

Risk Factors

Risk factors for meningitis include otitis media, mastoiditis, sinusitis, neurosurgery, systemic sepsis, immunocompromise, diabetes, intravenous drug use, basal skull fractures, or crowded living conditions. Age is the biggest risk factor for encephalitis, older adults and young children have the highest incidence; patients that are immunocompromised are also at risk for infection.

Patients that are immunocompromised or those that use intravenous drugs are at highest risk for brain abscesses.

Manifestations

Bacterial meningitis typically presents with fever and chills, severe headache, and nausea and vomiting. The older adult may not have a high fever, but may instead exhibit confusion. Meningeal irritation causes nuchal rigidity (stiff neck), a positive Brudzinski sign (neck flexion that causes hip and knee flexion; see **Figure 43.6** ■), and a positive Kernig sign (inability to extend knee while hip is flexed at a 90-degree angle). Photophobia and possibly diplopia are present.

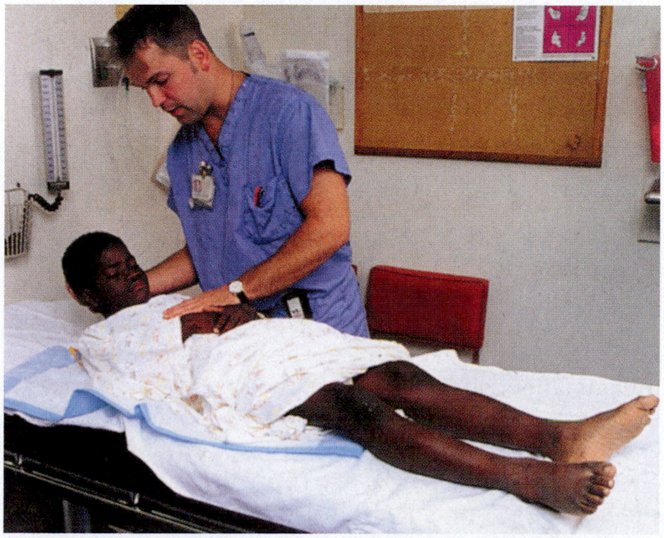

Figure 43.6 ■ Positive Brudzinski sign.

In meningococcal meningitis, skin hemorrhages and ecchymosis occur related to the vasculitis caused by the rapidly replicating pathogens. IICP may be present and cause decreased LOC, seizures, changes in vital signs and respiratory pattern, and papilledema.

The manifestations of viral meningitis, although similar to bacterial meningitis, are milder. The patient may have mild flulike symptoms that progress to an intense headache and malaise, fever, nausea and vomiting, and lethargy. Photophobia and drowsiness can occur but the patient typically remains oriented. Neck stiffness, positive Brudzinski sign, and positive Kernig sign are usually present, as these are signs of inflammation in the meninges (Pentima, 2016).

Manifestations of viral encephalitis vary depending on the organism and area of the brain affected and are similar to those of meningitis. These include fever, headache, seizures, stiff neck, and altered LOC. The patient may be disoriented, agitated, restless, lethargic, or drowsy. Disease progression can lead to coma.

Manifestations of arbovirus encephalitis include fever, malaise, sore throat, nausea and vomiting, stiff neck, tremors, paralysis, exaggerated deep tendon reflexes, seizures, and altered LOC.

With brain abscess, patients initially exhibit general symptoms of infection, such as chills, fever, malaise, and anorexia. Because a brain abscess generally forms after infection, the patient may think that he is having an exacerbation of that initial infection and may experience seizures, altered LOC, and manifestations of IICP. As the abscess enlarges, symptoms will reflect its location in the brain. For example, a frontal lobe abscess may cause contralateral hemiparesis, expressive aphasia, focal seizures, and frontal headache.

Complications

In bacterial meningitis, the arachnoid layer may have fibrotic changes and formation of scar tissue from the infection. Adhesions and effusions can develop, interfering with the normal circulation of CSF. Complications of bacterial meningitis include cranial nerve damage and hydrocephalus that affects cranial nerve VIII (auditory nerve), causing deafness.

The manifestations of encephalitis vary from meningitis in relation to the neurologic deficits that are seen in the patient. The patient may experience symptoms of decreased level of consciousness (LOC), confusion, or even slurred speech. Depending on the amount of cerebral swelling the patient experiences, the neurologic deficits may become irreversible or even lead to death (Gluckman, 2017).

Serious complications for brain abscesses include seizures and hydrocephaly (swelling), which can lead to neurologic deficits. Patient outcomes for brain abscesses have greatly improved; approximately 70% of patients recover with little residual neurological effects (Brouwer, 2014).

Interprofessional Care

Both meningitis and encephalitis can be fatal if they are not promptly diagnosed and treated. Even with treatment, CNS damage can cause serious neurologic deficits. Bacterial meningitis is a medical emergency and must be treated with appropriate antibiotics and supportive interventions. The treatments for viral meningitis and encephalitis are primarily symptomatic. Brain abscesses are treated with antibiotics; if this is not effective, the abscess may need to be decompressed through aspiration (Brouwer, 2014).

Diagnosis

The diagnosis of bacterial or viral meningitis is based on manifestations and diagnostic test results. Gram stain and culture of the CSF are used to determine if a bacterial infection is present and to identify the specific infectious agent. Polymerase chain reaction (PCR) techniques may be used to detect viral DNA or RNA in spinal fluid. CT scan will show an area of increased contrast surrounding a low-density core with brain abscess.

Lumbar puncture with examination of the CSF is utilized to diagnose bacterial meningitis. Data that indicate bacterial meningitis include turbid, cloudy CSF; markedly increased WBC counts and protein content; and a decreased glucose content. Opening pressures on the lumbar puncture are elevated. In contrast, encephalitis displays a normal CSF analysis. The patient with a brain abscess will have a markedly elevated pressure with elevated protein content and elevated WBC count. (Because a lumbar puncture in the presence of a space-occupying lesion can result in brain herniation and death, a CT scan is performed first if neurologic findings support such a lesion.)

Medications

Immediate intravenous administration of a broad-spectrum antibiotic that crosses the blood–brain barrier into the subarachnoid space is instituted in cases of bacterial meningitis. Once culture reports identify the causative organism, drug therapy with a high dose of one or more specific intravenous antibiotics is continued for 2 weeks. Vancomycin as well as a cephalosporin (such as cefotaxime or ceftriaxone) antibiotic are currently the preferred treatment regimen (Tunkel, 2017). As antibiotic-resistant organisms continue to be identified, it can be expected that this antibiotic regimen will be adjusted based on the sensitivity of bacteria present in the CSF. Steroids such as dexamethasone (Decadron) are often given with the antibiotics to suppress inflammation. Fungal meningitis is treated with antifungal agents, such as amphotericin-B (Amphotec) and voriconazole (Vfend).

Treatment for encephalitis consists of administering specific medications and preventing complications. Viral encephalitis is treated with intravenous *acyclovir* (Zovirax).

Antibiotic therapy is the primary treatment for brain abscess and should be started immediately. A combination of broad-spectrum antibiotics is used if the infecting organism is unknown. Antipyretic and analgesic medications may provide symptomatic relief; however, analgesics that have a depressant effect on the CNS (such as opiates) are avoided to prevent masking of early manifestations of deteriorating LOC. The patient may initially require antiemetics to control nausea and vomiting. Fluid and electrolyte status is maintained through intravenous fluid replacement until the patient is able to resume oral intake.

Surgery

Surgical drainage of an encapsulated abscess may be necessary. The decision to perform surgery is based on the patient's general condition, the stage of abscess development, and the site of the abscess.

Nursing Care

CNS infections are serious illnesses, with potentially life-threatening effects and complications. Nursing assessments and interventions are critical in identifying changes in the patient's neurologic status and preventing complications from IICP. In addition to the nursing care described in this section, see the Case Study & Nursing Care Plan for a patient with bacterial meningitis on page 1622.

Assessment

Collect the following data through the health history and physical examination (refer to Chapter 41). Further focused assessments are described in the following interventions section.

- *Health history:* Risk factors (place of residence, exposure to someone with meningitis or encephalitis, concurrent infections, other illnesses, travel), when manifestations began, severity of manifestations, current nausea, headache and stiff neck, seizures
- *Physical assessment:* Glasgow Coma Scale, LOC, vital signs, motor function, pupillary check, cranial nerves, neck ROM, Brudzinski sign, Kernig sign, skin (rash, petechiae, purpura), muscle movement and strength, speech.

Priorities of Care

The goals of care for the patient with a CNS infection are an absence of infection, normal neurologic functioning, and normal vital signs.

Diagnoses, Outcomes, and Interventions

In planning and implementing nursing care for the patient with a CNS infection, the prognosis may depend on the supportive care given. The patient is often very ill, and the combination of fever, dehydration, and IICP may predispose him or her to seizures. Airway obstruction, respiratory arrest, or cardiac dysrhythmias may occur. Nursing diagnoses and interventions for the patient with an altered LOC, IICP, and seizures are also appropriate for the patient with a CNS infection. Nursing interventions in this section focus on inability to defend against disease insults and risk for fluid volume deficit.

Reduce Risk of Infection. Patients with CNS infections are less able to protect themselves against insults from both internal and external sources. The effects of the infection, inflammation, and resulting pathophysiologic processes may include pain, fever, altered LOC, seizures, IICP, and cranial nerve dysfunction. In addition, pathophysiologic effects on the brain may lead to permanent neurologic deficits, such as loss of motor function or dementia.

Expected Outcome: Patient will be adequately protected against infection.

The nurse will:

- Monitor neurologic status on a regular basis. *Many complications are evidenced by changes in neurologic manifestations.*
- Monitor vital signs, including temperature, on a regular basis. *The patient often has a high temperature throughout the illness, ranging from 38° to 40.5°C (101° to 105°F).*
- Monitor levels of consciousness. Assess levels of orientation, memory, attention span, and response to stimuli. *Early in the infection, the patient often has problems with memory and orientation. There may be problems with following commands, restlessness, irritability, and combativeness. As the illness progresses, the LOC decreases to lethargy and finally into deep coma.*
- Monitor for manifestations of seizure activity, and institute seizure precautions:
  a. Monitor twitching of hands or face and tonic–clonic movements.
  b. Have oral airway and suction equipment readily available.
  c. Pad side rails, maintain bed in low position, and keep side rails up. *Irritation of the cerebral cortex secondary to meningeal inflammation may cause seizures. Careful monitoring and seizure precautions are necessary to prevent injury.*
- Monitor for manifestations of cranial nerve damage; monitor extraocular movements, facial movement, dizziness, ability to hear, double vision, drooping upper eyelids (ptosis), and pupillary changes. *Cranial nerve dysfunction may result from inflammation or vascular changes in the brain.*
- Monitor for manifestations of IICP: Decreased pulse, increased blood pressure, widening pulse pressure, respiratory changes, and vomiting. *IICP results from infectious or inflammatory exudate, cerebral edema, and hydrocephalus.*
- Administer prescribed medications and fluids. *Antibiotics are prescribed to eradicate the bacteria. Mannitol may be prescribed to reduce IICP. IV fluids are administered to replace fluids lost through vomiting and diaphoresis.*

SAFETY ALERT: Hyperthermia may result from IICP, while an increased temperature can also increase ICP. The presence of any fever must be recognized promptly and treated effectively to prevent further increases in ICP. ■

Maintain Hydration. The patient is at risk for fluid volume deficit related to increased metabolic rate and diaphoresis. The goals of care are to provide hydration and maintain adequate intake and output.

Expected Outcome: Patient will be adequately hydrated.

The nurse will:

- Monitor for presence, or worsening, of fluid volume deficit.
  a. Measure and compare intake and output every 2 to 4 hours.
  b. Monitor daily body weights.
  c. Monitor skin turgor and condition of mucous membranes and tongue.
  d. Monitor urine amount, color, and odor.
  e. Monitor BUN:creatinine ratio.

  The elastic property of the skin depends partially on interstitial fluid volume. If the patient has a fluid volume deficit, skin flattens more slowly after a pinch is released. Mucous membranes and tongue are dry, urine output is decreased, urine is dark in color and concentrated with a strong odor, urine specific gravity is greater than 1.020, and BUN will rise out of proportion to serum creatinine.
- When administering fluids, either orally or parenterally, consider concurrent illnesses. *Patients with IICP or renal failure require complex management. Refer to Chapter 10 for a further discussion of fluid volume deficit.*

SAFETY ALERT: A weight loss of 0.5 kg (1 lb) represents a fluid loss of approximately 500 mL. Close monitoring of intake and output is essential for prompt recognition of fluid deficits. Renal function can be permanently impaired in states of dehydration. ■

Delegating Nursing Care Activities

A patient suffering from an infection in the CNS will need to have vital signs and intake and output closely monitored. As appropriate, the nurse can delegate these tasks to the unlicensed assistive personnel. In addition, as disease processes progress, the patient may have difficulty repositioning on his or her own and may require assistance for turns every 2 hours.

Transitions of Care

As with many other intracranial injuries and disorders, educational activities to promote health by preventing meningitis and encephalitis are important nursing interventions. The following information to reduce risk should be provided:

- Vaccinations for meningococcal meningitis are recommended by the CDC (Centers for Disease Control and Prevention, 2017c) for teens, with a booster shot at the age of 16. The CDC also recommends the vaccine for those traveling to an underdeveloped country where meningococcal disease is common (i.e., parts of Africa), those who are immunocompromised, or those with possible exposure to the infection.
- Adults over the age of 65 should receive the pneumococcal vaccine.
- Wash hands with soap and water before and after contact with an individual who may be infected with meningitis or encephalitis and after using the bathroom.
- Do not share food, drinking glasses, eating utensils, tissues, towels, lipstick, or cigarettes.
- Control mosquitos with repellants, insecticides, and protective clothing. Community programs conduct spraying to destroy the insect larvae and eliminate breeding places, such as pools of stagnant water.
- Prompt diagnosis and treatment are crucial for infections of the head, neck, and respiratory system as well as for signs and symptoms of meningitis.

Case Study & Nursing Care Plan

A Patient with Bacterial Meningitis

Monty Cook is a 22-year-old musician who plays in a local rock band. He is unmarried and lives with his parents. He is known by everyone in the community as a quiet, low-key, easygoing person and an excellent guitar player. During a performance 2 days ago, he had difficulty playing his guitar, complaining of bright stage lights blazing in his eyes. When he tried to keep his head down to prevent the lights from hurting his eyes, he noticed his neck was very stiff. After the performance, one of the newest members of the band remarked that it certainly was not their best performance. Monty responded angrily that maybe the new members of the group needed more practice. Then he stomped out and went home to bed.

He wakes at 4:00 a.m. with a severe headache, sweating, chills, and a temperature of 38.9°C (102°F). He is unable to bend his neck without severe pain. His mother is alarmed at his agitation and irritability and rushes him to the ED. A lumbar puncture performed in the ED reveals turbid, cloudy fluid; Mr. Cook also has a markedly increased WBC count, increased protein, and a decreased glucose content. Bacterial meningitis is diagnosed and Mr. Cook is admitted.

ASSESSMENT	DIAGNOSES	EXPECTED OUTCOMES
When the nurse, Agatha Aldi, enters the patient's room, Mr. Cook is thrashing in the bed and talking incoherently. On assessment, the nurse notes dry mucous membranes, cracked lips, and small petechiae over the upper torso and abdomen. Mr. Cook's temperature is now 40°C (104°F) and a positive Kernig sign is present. Intravenous broad-spectrum antibiotics are prescribed and initiated. After 2 hours nurse Aldi notes that Mr. Cook's LOC has decreased significantly.	■ Fever related to infection and abnormal temperature regulation by hypothalamus ■ Restlessness and agitation related to intracranial infection	■ Patient's body temperature will decrease. ■ Patient will become less restless and agitated.

PLANNING AND IMPLEMENTATION

- Monitor vital signs every 2 hours.
- Provide sponge baths if temperature continues to rise.
- Provide a quiet, nonstimulating environment with the shades drawn.
- Provide oral care every 4 hours.
- Measure and compare intake and output every 2 hours.
- Perform neurologic assessments every 2 to 4 hours.
- Monitor for and report seizure activity and decreasing LOC.
- Keep bed in low position with side rails elevated.
- Administer prescribed intravenous antibiotics.

EVALUATION

After 4 days of antibiotic therapy, Mr. Cook's temperature has returned to near normal. Ms. Aldi notes that he has begun opening his eyes and visually tracking her as she moves about the room. Mr. Cook responds to a request to squeeze Ms. Aldi's fingers and after several hours asks her what has happened. On day 5, Mr. Cook states that he feels better and his headache is gone. He asks for sips of juice and begins urinating regularly. Seven days after admission, Mr. Cook is discharged and is able to go home with his mother. He has some weakness in his legs, but otherwise has no evidence of neurologic deficits.

CLINICAL REASONING IN PATIENT CARE

1. What strategies should the nurse use to decrease the environmental stimuli for Mr. Cook, and what is the rationale for doing so?
2. If you were caring for Mr. Cook in the initial phase of the illness and he became combative, what would you do?
3. Develop a plan of care to address Mr. Cook's acute pain. Consider the effect of narcotics on respiratory function in designing the plan.

See Evaluating Your Response in Appendix B.

The Patient with Tetanus

Tetanus, or lockjaw, is a disorder caused by the neurotoxin *Clostridium tetani*. This anaerobic bacillus lives in the soil, and spores enter the body through open wounds contaminated with dirt, street dust, or feces (animal or human).

Pathophysiology

When the spores of *C. tetani* enter a wound, they germinate and produce a toxin called *tetanospasmin*. Incubation occurs over an average of 7 to 10 days (Mayo Clinic, 2017). Toxins are then absorbed by the peripheral nerves and carried to the spinal cord, where they block the action of inhibitory enzymes at spinal synapses. This impairs transmission of neuromuscular impulses and even minor stimuli will cause uncontrolled muscle spasms.

Risk Factors

Incidence is highest among people who have never been immunized and adults that have maintained immunity with the 10-year booster shot.

Manifestations

Manifestations begin with pain at the infection site followed by neck and jaw stiffness and dysphagia. Profuse perspiration, increased salivation, and drooling can occur followed by hyperreflexia and spasms of the jaw muscles (trismus) or facial muscles. Rigidity and painful spasms of the abdomen, neck, and back then follow. Generalized tonic seizures may result from minor stimuli and the patient assumes a typical opisthotonic position during the seizures, characterized by retraction of the head, arching of the back, and extension of the feet. Breathing may be impaired by spasms of the glottis and respiratory muscles. Throughout these changes, the patient retains normal mental status.

Complications

The complications of tetanus include laryngospasms, fractures, hypertension, pneumonia, and death (CDC, 2017e). Cardiac and respiratory failure are late, life-threatening complications. Fatal outcomes are more likely in older adults (CDC, 2014).

Interprofessional Care

There are no specific diagnostic tests for tetanus; diagnosis is based on manifestations. Tetanus is completely preventable by active immunization. Immunization for children includes tetanus toxoid, administered as part of the diphtheria–tetanus–pertussis (DTaP) immunization series. In adults that have not received previous tetanus vaccination, immunization is obtained by administering tetanus toxoid (Td) in two doses 4 to 6 weeks apart, with a third dose in 6 to 12 months. All individuals should have a booster dose every 10 years throughout life or at the time of a major injury if the last booster dose was given more than 5 years prior to the injury (CDC, 2017e).

If a wound is contaminated or if the individual's immunization status is uncertain, passive immunization with tetanus immune globulin is administered. Active immunization with tetanus toxoid is begun at the same time. The wound is carefully and thoroughly cleaned and debrided, and antibiotics are administered only if there are signs or symptoms of infection in the wound, not as prophylaxis for tetanus.

The patient with tetanus requires intensive care in an area of minimal stimulation. Muscle spasms and seizures are controlled by diazepam (Valium) or another benzodiazepine, often combined with a sedative. Anticoagulants may be prescribed to prevent venous thrombosis. In severe cases, seizures and spasms are controlled with paralysis by a neuromuscular blocking agent, and airway obstruction is managed by mechanical ventilation.

Nursing Care

Nursing care for the patient with tetanus is intensive and focuses on assessments and interventions to promote safety, prevent injury, maintain nutrition, and maintain pulmonary and cardiovascular function. The patient usually requires in-hospital care for several weeks. The nursing care plan commonly includes:

- Place in a quiet, darkened room to decrease stimuli that cause muscle spasms and seizures.
- Provide only necessary physical care, and do so during periods of maximal sedation to decrease tactile stimulation that causes muscle spasms.
- Maintain oxygenation through mechanical ventilator and frequent suctioning of secretions.
- Maintain intravenous access for the administration of fluids and medications.
- Administer prescribed antibiotics, anticonvulsants, and sedatives. In the case of cardiovascular complications, administer prescribed beta-adrenergic blocking agents such as propranolol (Inderal).
- Provide adequate nutrition through prescribed nutritional support, such as total parenteral nutrition.
- Monitor respiratory and cardiovascular status and provide immediate interventions for respiratory or cardiovascular failure.
- Monitor fluid and electrolyte status. Ensure adequate fluid intake to maintain hydration and urinary output.
- Monitor urinary output, which should be maintained at 1.5 to 2 L/day.
- Monitor for the hazards of immobility, including constipation, pneumonia, deep venous thrombosis, and pressure ulcers.

Transitions of Care

Tetanus is a preventable disorder, and nurses have a major role in promoting immunizations for all children and for educating adults about the need for booster doses. The older population is at risk if there is no history of immunization or a lapsed immunization. Community health fairs and programs targeting senior citizen groups can address this issue.

Wound care must be taught and must include the use of soap and water. All foreign material should be carefully flushed or removed from a wound and medical care sought for wounds that are more extensive or contaminated.

The Patient with Creutzfeldt-Jakob Disease

Classic **Creutzfeldt-Jakob disease (CJD)** (*spongiform encephalopathy*) is a rapidly progressive, degenerative, neurologic disease that causes brain degeneration without inflammation. The disease is not transmissible and is always fatal. The causative agent is believed to be an abnormal form of a cellular glycoprotein known as a *prion protein*. Transmission of the agent is by direct contamination with infected neural tissue, such as during eye and brain surgery.

A different form of the disease, called *new-variant CJD (vCJD)*, is a rare, degenerative, fatal brain disorder, but differs from the classic form of CJD. New-variant CJD, referred to as "mad-cow disease," is believed to result from consumption of cattle products contaminated with bovine spongiform encephalopathy (BSE) and affects primarily young adults. Because the illness is fatal and is associated with infected cattle, severe restrictions have been placed on the importation of cattle, sheep, and goats as well as related animal products from countries in which BSE occurs.

Disease symptoms progress rapidly and include myoclonus, dementia, and behavior changes. There is no known cure for this disease; fatalities generally occur within 6 to 12 months of onset of symptoms (Brown & Lee, 2017).

Nursing care focuses on maximizing comfort, preventing injury, preventing transmission, and providing support.

The Patient with Postpolio Syndrome

Postpolio syndrome (PPS) is a complication of a previous infection by the poliomyelitis virus. Polio was an epidemic in the 1940s and 1950s, but has largely been eradicated through immunization with oral live trivalent virus vaccine. According to the CDC (Centers for Disease Control and Prevention, 2016), it is estimated that 25 to 40% of the people in the United States who had contracted the disease experience postpolio syndrome. Those individuals previously affected with the polio virus have struggled for years to rehabilitate themselves and lead productive lives but as they approach retirement age, they are again experiencing manifestations that may be physically and psychologically incapacitating. Symptoms of such a recurrence include weakness in both previously affected and unaffected muscles. The manifestations include progressive muscle weakness, fatigue, and pain, leading to muscle atrophy and scoliosis.

The cause of postpolio syndrome is not known. The new weakness of muscles is believed to be due to degeneration of individual nerve terminals in the motor units that remain after the initial illness. Gradually, nerve terminals malfunction and permanent weakness occurs.

Postpolio syndrome is diagnosed by a previous history of polio and manifestations that persist for at least 1 year. Diagnostic studies of nerve conduction, muscle strength, and pulmonary function determine current physical status. Treatment addresses the manifestations and often involves physical therapy and pulmonary rehabilitation programs.

The patient with postpolio syndrome faces the challenge of unexpected physical changes. Patients are often anxious about how others will react or what the future holds. Respiratory dysfunction may result in the need for oxygen. Muscle weakness and decreased pulmonary function may make walking difficult, if not impossible. ADLs, independent self-care, and careers are threatened.

Many former polio patients have not fully recovered psychologically and may respond to a recurrence of manifestations with denial and disbelief. Older patients may not know they had polio as children. Nurses are responsible for assessing and identifying the manifestations of the disease, and it is essential to question middle-age and older adults about a past history of polio when conducting the health history. The nurse individualizes teaching to meet the physical and psychosocial needs of the patient and family by providing candid explanations. Patients are taught how to prevent fatigue, promote optimal respiratory function, meet self-care needs, modify ADLs, and maintain safety. Follow-up care with nurses, physicians, physical therapists, respiratory therapists, and counselors is indicated. Referral to a support group can make a positive difference in the coping strategies of the patient and family.

The Patient with Rabies

Rabies is a viral infection of the CNS most often transmitted through the bite of an infected rabid animal (CDC, 2017d). If bitten by an animal that is suspected of having rabies, patients should receive postexposure treatment; if untreated, rabies is fatal.

The manifestations occur in stages. During the initial, or prodromal, stage, the site of the wound is painful and exhibits various paresthesias. General manifestations of infection (such as headache, loss of appetite, and sore throat) may appear. Patients may have increased sensitivity to light and sounds, and the skin is especially sensitive to changes in temperature. The prodromal stage is followed by an excitement stage where periods of agitation alternate with periods of quiet. Attempts to drink cause painful laryngospasms that prevent the individual from drinking fluids (a phenomenon called *hydrophobia*). Large amounts of thick, tenacious mucus are present. The patient experiences convulsions, muscle spasms, and periods of apnea. Untreated cases lead to death within about 7 days and are typically due to respiratory failure.

Nursing care for patients with rabies is provided in an intensive care unit, with the patient in a quiet, darkened room to decrease stimulation. Interventions are required to maintain the airway, maintain oxygenation, and control seizures. Universal precautions are vigilantly maintained as the rabies virus is present in the patient's saliva. If an open wound of a healthcare provider is contaminated with infected saliva, the provider must receive postexposure immunizations.

Patient and family teaching focuses on the importance of immunizing pets, providing proper care of wounds, and seeking immediate medical attention for animal bites. Because the untreated disease is almost always fatal, the best intervention is prevention.

The Patient with Botulism

Botulism is food poisoning caused by ingestion of food contaminated with a toxin produced by the bacillus *Clostridium botulinum*. This anaerobic spore-forming bacillus is found in the soil. Infection occurs from eating improperly canned or cooked foods, especially home-canned vegetables and fruits, smoked meats, and vacuum-packed fish. Untreated cases can lead to death.

The toxins liberated by *C. botulinum* are absorbed by the gastrointestinal tract and bound to nerve tissues, blocking the release of acetylcholine from nerve endings and causing respiratory paralysis due to skeletal muscle paralysis.

Manifestations for botulism appear 12 to 36 hours after ingestion of contaminated food and begin with visual disturbances including diplopia; loss of accommodation; fixed, dilated pupils; and possible ptosis. Gastrointestinal manifestations include nausea and vomiting, diarrhea, dysphagia, and dry mouth. Impaired laryngeal muscle tone leads to dystonia. Paralysis of all muscle groups leads to respiratory paralysis and death.

Patients diagnosed with botulism are treated in an intensive care environment with close monitoring of respiratory function. Many patients will need mechanical ventilator support.

CHAPTER HIGHLIGHTS

43.1 Spinal Cord Disorders

Describe the pathophysiology and manifestations of spinal cord injuries, and outline the interprofessional and nursing care of patients with these disorders.

- Spinal cord injuries are typically related to trauma, with the major risk factors being age (young adults), gender (male), and alcohol or drug abuse. The causes of SCIs include direct trauma, fractures, torn ligaments, circulatory impairment, contusions, lacerations, or transections of the cord. Complete or incomplete SCIs are determined by the degree of interruption in motor and sensory pathways. Movement, perception, sensation, sexual function, and elimination are potentially affected by these injuries.
- Complications of SCIs include spinal shock, which is the temporary loss of all reflexes (areflexia) below the level of injury. Manifestations of spinal shock include bradycardia, hypotension, and flaccid paralysis. Autonomic dysreflexia (AD) is an exaggerated sympathetic response when SCI injuries are at or above T_6. AD is triggered by noxious stimuli and results in severe and life-threatening hypertension.
- Community education and use of protective equipment (such as car seats, seat belts, and bicycle helments) are essential for prevention of SCI.
- Rehabilitation of the SCI patient is an ongoing process from intensive care to home care. Nursing interventions are necessary in all settings to promote independence in self-care.
- A herniated intervertebral disk is a rupture of the cartilage surrounding the intervertebral disk with protrusion of the nucleus pulposus. The major manifestation of lumbar disks is lower back and sciatic pain on the affected side.
- Spinal cord tumors may be benign or malignant, primary or metastatic. Depending on tumor size and location, pathologic changes in function can result from compression, invasion, or ischemia.

43.2 Infectious Disorders of the Central Nervous System

Describe the pathophysiology and manifestations of central nervous system infections, and outline the interprofessional and nursing care of patients with these disorders.

- CNS infections are caused by bacteria, bacterial toxins, viruses, fungi, protozoans, and rickettsiae. Organisms enter the CNS through the bloodstream or by direct invasion. The major CNS infections are meningitis and encephalitis. Treatments include broad-spectrum antibiotics or antifungal agents. Community-based health education can provide important preventive information.

TEST YOURSELF NCLEX-RN® REVIEW

1. A patient is admitted to the ED with a cervical SCI following an automobile crash. What should the nurse explain to the family as the reason for the patient being placed on mechanical ventilation?
   A. The accident injured the patient's lungs.
   B. The nerves that control lung function have been injured.
   C. The patient is unable to breathe because of being unconscious.
   D. The ventilator is temporary to ensure the patient receives adequate oxygen until recovery.
2. The nurse is planning care for a patient with an acute SCI. According to best practices, which medications should the nurse prepare during this patient's initial care? (Select all that apply.)
   A. Analgesics
   B. Antibiotics
   C. Vasopressors
   D. Antihistamines
   E. Corticosteroids
3. A patient with a thoracic spinal cord injury is experiencing spinal shock. How should the nurse explain this pathophysiologic process to the patient? (Select all that apply.)
   A. There is damage to the lower motor neurons.
   B. There is an exaggerated sympathetic response.
   C. There is a loss of control of cardiovascular mechanisms.
   D. There is a temporary loss of reflex function below the level of injury.
   E. There is loss of sensation below the level of the injury that may be temporary.
4. A patient is demonstrating manifestations of autonomic dysreflexia. What will the nurse most likely assess as the reason for this health problem?
   A. Diarrhea
   B. Distended bladder
   C. Elevated blood pressure
   D. Respiratory wheezes and stridor

5. An industrial nurse is conducting a class for manufacturing plant employees on methods to prevent back pain. What should the nurse include in this teaching? (Select all that apply.)
   A. Use large leg muscles to push when lifting.
   B. Bend from the waist to lift articles from the floor.
   C. Spread the feet apart to broaden the base of support.
   D. Avoid squatting while lifting.
   E. Always twist to the side while lifting.
6. A nurse is assessing a patient recovering from a posterior cervical laminectomy for manifestations of spinal cord compression. How should this assessment be conducted? (Select all that apply.)
   A. Ask the patient to wiggle his or her toes.
   B. Ask the patient to grip the nurse's hands.
   C. Use a stethoscope to auscultate heart sounds.
   D. Use a reflex hammer to assess Babinski's reflex.
   E. Assess the patient's ability to detect touch on hands.
7. A patient with a lumbar spinal cord tumor reports sudden onset of numbness in one leg. Which intervention is the nurse's priority?
   A. Ask the patient to rate the amount of numbness on a scale similar to the pain scale.
   B. Reposition the patient and recheck in 15 minutes.
   C. Discuss this report with the health care provider.
   D. Check the patient's indwelling catheter for kinking.
8. A patient with meningitis is drowsy and confused. What should the nurse explain to the patient's family as being the cause for these mental status changes?
   A. Decreased intracranial pressure
   B. Bleeding in the central nervous system
   C. Elevated serum white blood cell count
   D. Sluggish flow of cerebrospinal fluid
9. A nurse is planning a seminar for city public health workers on ways to reduce the onset of West Nile encephalitis in the community. On which topic should the nurse focus in this seminar?
   A. Garbage pickup
   B. Sanitation services
   C. Mosquito spraying
   D. Washing fruits and vegetables
10. A patient with a spinal cord injury is prescribed pantoprazole (Protonix). The nurse will explain which rationale for this administration?
   A. Prevents stress-related gastric ulcers.
   B. Encourages healing of gastric nerves.
   C. Promotes digestion of enteral feedings.
   D. Supports healthy bacteria in the gastrointestinal tract.

See Test Yourself answers in Appendix B.

REFERENCES

Abrams, G. M., & Wakasa, M. (2014). *Chronic complications of spinal cord injury and disease.* Retrieved from https://www.uptodate-com.proxy.lib.ohio-state.edu/contents/chronic-complications-of-spinal-cord-injury-and-disease?source=search_result&search=autonomic%20dysreflexia&selectedTitle=1~28.

American Association of Neurological Surgeons. (2017a). *Herniated disc.* Retrieved from www.aans.org/Patients/Neurosurgical-Conditions-and-Treatments/Herniated-Disc.

American Association of Neurological Surgeons. (2017b). *Spinal tumors.* Retrieved from www.aans.org/Patients/Neurosurgical-Conditions-and-Treatments/Spinal-Tumors.

Berlowitz, D. J., Wadsworth, B., & Ross, J. (2016). Respiratory problems and management in people with spinal cord injury. *Breathe, 12*(4), 328–340.

Brouwer, M. C. (2014). Brain abscess. *New England Journal of Medicine, 371*(5), 447–456.

Brown, H. G., & Lee, J. M. (2017). *Cruetzfeldt-Jakob disease.* Retrieved from https://www.uptodate-com.proxy.lib.ohio-state.edu/contents/creutzfeldt-jakob-disease?source=search_result&search=creutzfeldt%20jakob%20disease&selectedTitle=1~77#H29.

Centers for Disease Control and Prevention (CDC). (2014). *Manual for the surveillance of vaccine-preventable diseases.* Retrieved from https://www.cdc.gov/vaccines/pubs/surv-manual/chpt16-tetanus.html.

Centers for Disease Control and Prevention (CDC). (2016). *Polio: For healthcare professionals.* Retrieved from https://www.cdc.gov/polio/us/hcp.html.

Centers for Disease Control and Prevention (CDC). (2017a). *Bacterial meningitis.* Retrieved from https://www.cdc.gov/meningitis/bacterial.html.

Centers for Disease Control and Prevention (CDC). (2017b). *Meningococcal disease: Technical and clinical information.* Retrieved from https://www.cdc.gov/meningococcal/clinical-info.html.

Centers for Disease Control and Prevention (CDC). (2017c). *Meningococcal vaccination.* Retrieved from https://www.cdc.gov/vaccines/vpd/mening/index.html.

Centers for Disease Control and Prevention (CDC). (2017d). *Rabies.* Retrieved from https://www.cdc.gov/rabies/index.html.

Centers for Disease Control and Prevention (CDC). (2017e). *Tetanus: For clinicians.* Retrieved from https://www.cdc.gov/tetanus/clinicians.html#symptoms.

Ciftdemir, M., Kaya, M., Selcuk, E., Yalniz, E. (2016). Tumors of the spine. *World Journal of Orthopedics, 7*(2), 109–116.

Consortium for Spinal Cord Medicine. (2016). Prevention of venous thromboembolism in individuals with spinal cord injury: Clinical practice guidelines for health care providers, 3rd ed. *Topics in Spinal Cord Injury Rehabilitation, 22*(3), 209–240.

Eisen, A. (2015). *Anatomy and localization of spinal cord disorders.* Retrieved from https://www.uptodate-com.proxy.lib.ohio-state.edu/contents/anatomy-and-localization-of-spinal-cord-disorders?source=search_result&search=spinal%20cord%20injury&selectedTitle=6~150.

Gluckman, S. J. (2017). *Viral encephalitis in adults.* Retrieved from https://www.uptodate-com.proxy.lib.ohio-state.edu/contents/viral-encephalitis-in-adults?source=search_result&search=encephalitis&selectedTitle=1~150.

Hansebout, R. R., & Kachur, E. (2014). *Acute traumatic spinal cord injury.* Retrieved from https://www.uptodate-com.proxy.lib.ohio-state.edu/contents/acute-traumatic-spinal-cord-injury/print?source=search_result&search=tetraplegia&selectedTitle=3~137.

Kaplow, R., & Iyere, K. (2016). Understanding spinal cord compression. *Nursing, 46*(9), 44–51.

Klein, R. S. (2017). *Herpes simplex virus type 1 encephalitis.* Retrieved from https://www-uptodate-com.proxy.lib.ohio-state.edu/contents/herpes-simplex-virus-type-1-encephalitis?source=see_link.

Levin, K., Hsu, P. S., & Armon, C. (2017). *Acute lumbosacral radiculopathy: Treatment and prognosis.* Retrieved from https://www.uptodate-com.proxy.lib.ohio-state.edu/contents/acute-lumbosacral-radiculopathy-treatment-and-prognosis?source=search_result&search=herniated%20disc%20treatment&selectedTitle=1~95.

Mataliotakis, G., & Tsirikos, A. (2016). Spinal cord trauma: Pathophysiology classification of spinal cord injury syndromes, treatment principles and controversies. *Orthopaedics and Trauma, 30*(5), 440–449.

Matthews, L., & Lee, L. A. (2016). *Anesthesia for adults with acute spinal cord injury.* Retrieved from https://www.uptodate-com.proxy.lib.ohio-state.edu/contents/anesthesia-for-adults-with-acute-spinal-cordinjury/print?source=search_result&search=spinal%20shock&selectedTitle=3~32.

Mayo Clinic. (2017). *Tetanus.* Retrieved from https://www.mayoclinic.org/diseases-conditions/tetanus/symptoms-causes/syc-20351625

National Institute of Neurological Disorders and Stroke (NINDS). (2017). *Spinal cord injury: Hope through research.* Retrieved from https://www.ninds.nih.gov/Disorders/Patient-Caregiver-Education/Hope-Through-Research/Spinal-Cord-Injury-Hope-Through-Research.

National Spinal Cord Injury Statistical Center (NSCISC). (2017). *Spinal cord injury facts and figures at a glance.* Retrieved from https://www.nscisc.uab.edu/Public/Facts%20and%20Figures%20-%202017.pdf.

Nguyen, J., Chu, B., Kuo, C. C., Leasure, J. M., Ames, C., & Kondrashov, D. (2017). Changes in foraminal area with anterior decompression versus keyhole foraminotomy in the cervical spine: A biomechanical investigation. *Journal of Neurosurgery: Spine, 27*(6), 620–626.

Oh, K. (2017). *Complications of spinal cord irradiation.* Retrieved from https://www.uptodate-com.proxy.lib.ohio-state.edu/contents/complications-of-spinal-cord-irradiation?source=see_link.

Pentima, C. D. (2016). *Viral meningitis: Clinical features and diagnosis in children.* Retrieved from https://www.uptodate-com.proxy.lib.ohio-state.edu/contents/viral-meningitis-clinical-features-and-diagnosis-in-children?source=search_result&search=viral%20meningitis&selectedTitle=3~150.

Ropper, A. E., Neal, M. T., & Theodore, N. (2015). Acute management of traumatic cervical spinal cord injury. *Practical Neurology, 15,* 266–272.

Robinson, J., & Kothari, M. J. (2016). *Clinical features and diagnosis of cervical radiculopathy.* Retrieved from https://www.uptodate-com.proxy.lib.ohio-state.edu/contents/clinical-features-and-diagnosis-of-cervical-radiculopathy?source=search_result&search=cervical%20herniated%20disc&selectedTitle=2~23.

Schiff, D. (2016). *Clinical features and diagnosis of neoplastic epidural spinal cord compression, including cauda equine syndrome.* Retrieved from https://www.uptodate-com.proxy.lib.ohio-state.edu/contents/clinical-features-and-diagnosis-of-neoplastic-epidural-spinal-cord-compression-including-cauda-equina-syndrome?source=see_link.

Schiff, D., Brown, P., & Shaffrey, M. E. (2017). *Treatment and prognosis of neoplastic epidural spinal cord compression, including cauda equine syndrome.* Retrieved from https://www.uptodate-com.proxy.lib.ohio-state.edu/contents/treatment-and-prognosis-of-neoplastic-epidural-spinal-cord-compression-including-cauda-equina-syndrome?source=search_result&search=spinal%20cord%20tumor&selectedTitle=7~114.

Sorenson, M., Quinn, L., & Klein, D. (2019). *Pathophysiology: Concepts of human disease.* Hoboken, NJ: Pearson Education.

Tunkel, A. R. (2017). *Treatment of bacterial meningitis caused by specific pathogens in adults.* Retrieved from https://www.uptodate-com.proxy.lib.ohio-state.edu/contents/treatment-of-bacterial-meningitis-caused-by-specific-pathogens-in-adults?source=see_link.

Tyler, C. L. (2015). Intraoperative cardiac emergencies. *Critical Care Nursing Clinics of North America, 27*(1), 17–31.

Welch, W. C., Schiff, D., & Gerszten, P. C. (2017). *Spinal cord tumors.* Retrieved from https://www.uptodate-com.proxy.lib.ohio-state.edu/contents/spinal-cord-tumors?source=search_result&search=spinal%20cord%20tumor&selectedTitle=1~114.

Winter, B., Pattani, H., & Temple, E. (2017). Spinal cord injury. *Anaesthesia and Intensive Care Medicine, 18*(8): 404–409.

Zuckerman, L. M. (2016). Oral chlorhexidine use to prevent ventilator-associated pneumonia in adults: Review of current literature. *Dimensions of Critical Care Nursing, 35*(1), 25–36.

ADDITIONAL RESOURCES

American Spinal Cord Injury Association (ASIA)
asia-spinalinjury.org

Christopher & Dana Reeve Foundation
www.christopherreeve.org

Paralyzed Veterans of America
www.pva.org

Chapter 44

Nursing Care of Patients with Neurologic Disorders

Chapter Outline and Learning Outcomes

CLINICAL COMPETENCIES

- Assess and monitor functional status of patients with neurologic disorders, and communicate findings to appropriate interprofessional team members.
- Demonstrate effective use of individualized and patient-centered strategies as well as evidence-based research to prioritize care and design nursing interventions that are specific to the needs of aging patients with multiple sclerosis.
- Incorporate assessments, patient needs and preferences (including individual and cultural values), clinical expertise, and evidence-based practice into the formation of priorities and interventions for patients with neurologic disorders.
- Safely and accurately administer oral and injectable medications used to treat Alzheimer disease, multiple sclerosis, Parkinson disease, and myasthenia gravis.
- Effectively communicate with and function within the interprofessional team to plan and provide care for patients with neurologic disorders.
- Provide appropriate and effective teaching to facilitate safety, communication, and community-based self-care for patients with acute and chronic healthcare needs that result from neurologic disorders.
- Revise plan of care as needed to provide effective interventions to promote, maintain, or restore functional health status to patients with neurologic disorders.
- Document care in the electronic medical record and use information management tools to monitor outcomes of care.
- Participate in studies and projects to improve the quality and safety of care for patients with neurologic disorders.

KEY TERMS

Alzheimer disease (AD), 1630
amyotrophic lateral sclerosis (ALS), 1655
basal ganglia, 1645
Bell palsy, 1665
chorea, 1655
dementia, 1630
dopaminergic, 1647
Guillain-Barré syndrome (GBS), 1661
Huntington disease (HD), 1655
multiple sclerosis (MS), 1638
myasthenia gravis (MG), 1657
myelin sheaths, 1638
neuralgia, 1663
neurotransmitters, 1647
Parkinson disease (PD), 1645
trigeminal neuralgia (TN), 1663

This chapter discusses degenerative neurologic disorders, peripheral nervous system disorders, and cranial nerve disorders. For many of the disorders, care is based on similar nursing diagnoses. To avoid repeating those diagnoses and interventions for each disorder, they have been divided among the nursing care discussions as appropriate.

44.1 Degenerative Neurologic Disorders

Degenerative neurologic disorders affect the central nervous system (CNS) and the peripheral nerves. By progressively disrupting cognitive processes or motor functions, disorders such as Alzheimer disease, Parkinson disease, and multiple sclerosis strike at the core of an individual's sense of personal autonomy and well-being and can be psychologically and emotionally devastating to family members and caregivers.

Ongoing medical research into degenerative neurologic disorders offers an increasing measure of hope to patients and their families. The discovery of genetic or biochemical markers associated with some of these disorders is leading to the development of effective screening and diagnostic methods. In addition, new drugs may halt the progression of the disorders in some patients, transforming them into manageable conditions. The chapter begins with a discussion of dementia, which is not a specific disease but rather a collection of manifestations that are caused by a variety of disorders that affect the brain.

Dementia

Dementia (meaning "deprived of mind") is cognitive decline caused by any disorder that permanently damages areas of the brain necessary for memory and learning. The hallmark of dementia is impairment of both short- and long-term memory, with resultant deficits in critical reasoning and judgment, communication, and/or changes in behavior (Alzheimer's Association, 2017f; Larson, 2017). Impairments of cognitive function are usually accompanied by deterioration in emotional control, social behavior, and motivation. People with dementia may have agitation, delusions, and hallucinations. All forms of dementia result from death of neurons and/or the loss of communication among the cells. Although the exact cause is not always known, there is clearly a genetic component in the development of some types of dementia. It is important to remember that although the incidence of dementia increases with age, it is not a normal component of aging.

To be diagnosed with dementia, the following criteria must be met (National Institute on Aging, 2017a):

- Two or more deficits in the following cognitive abilities:
  a. Memory loss
  b. Ability to generate coherent speech or understand spoken or written language
  c. Ability to recognize or identify objects, assuming intact sensory function
  d. Ability to focus and pay attention
  e. Ability to reason and problem-solve
- The decline in cognitive abilities must be severe enough to interfere with daily life.

Although exact numbers are difficult to determine, it is estimated that in the United States 8.8% of all people 65 years or older have dementia, and of those 60 to 80% have Alzheimer disease (Alzheimer's Association, 2017f; Healthy People 2020, 2017). Many different diseases and conditions may cause dementia, including Alzheimer disease, vascular dementia, Parkinson disease, normal-pressure hydrocephalus, Creutzfeldt-Jakob disease, metabolic disorders, medications, poisoning, chronic traumatic encephalopathy (CTE), and anoxia. Even though the actual cause of all dementias may not be known, factors that increase the risk of developing one or more kinds of dementia have been identified. These include aging, a family history of dementia, smoking and alcohol use, atherosclerosis, high cholesterol, elevated plasma homocysteine levels, diabetes mellitus, and Down syndrome.

The Patient with Alzheimer Disease

Alzheimer disease (AD) is the most common form of dementia, with an estimated 5.5 million people living with this disease (Alzheimer's Association, 2017a). AD is characterized by progressive, irreversible deterioration of general intellectual functioning. AD most commonly occurs in individuals over the age of 65 (Alzheimer's Association, 2017a). It affects almost twice as many women as men, but this is believed to be the result of women living relatively longer than men (Keene, Montine, & Kuller, 2017). AD is currently the sixth leading cause of death in the United States (Alzheimer's Association, 2017a). People with AD die an average of 4 to 8 years after diagnosis, but the disease duration can be as long as 20 years (Alzheimer's Association, 2017a).

Memory loss is usually the first sign of Alzheimer disease. Memory deficits are initially subtle and family members and friends may not suspect a problem until the disease progresses and manifestations become more noticeable. It is important to involve family members in the process of diagnosing AD or other forms of dementia; it is often a family member expressing concerns regarding cognitive symptoms that helps inform a diagnosis (Wolk & Dickerson, 2017). Progression of the disease varies, but the course is one of deteriorating cognition and judgment with eventual physical decline and total inability to perform activities of daily living (ADLs). With the loss of the ability to perform even the most basic ADLs, the burden of meeting the patient's needs shifts to the caregiver.

Pathophysiology

Characteristic findings in the brains of patients with AD are loss of nerve cells and the presence of neuritic plaques, neurofibrillary tangles, and amyloid angiopathy (**Figure 44.1** ■). Several theories are proposed for the cause of AD. The theories include the amyloid hypothesis (AD is the result of an

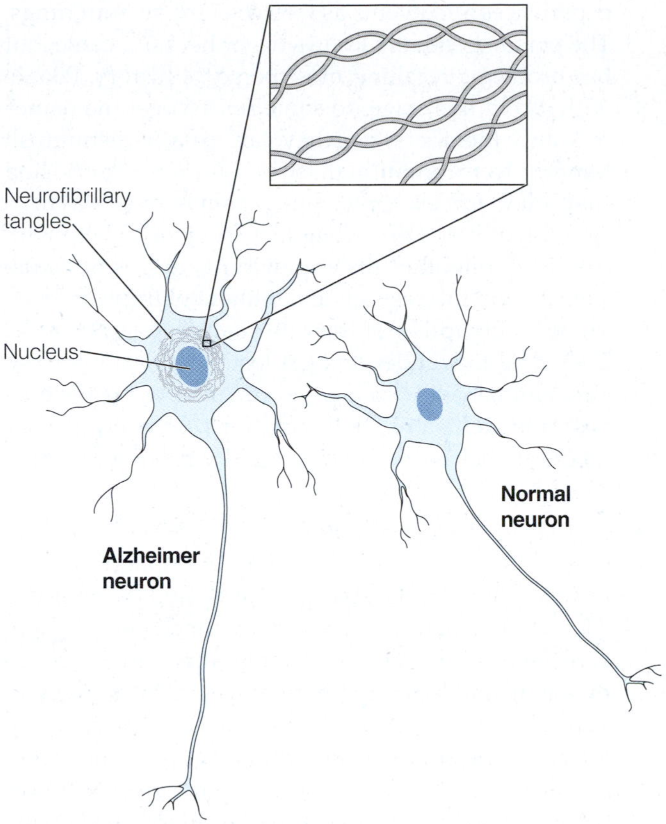
Neurofibrillary tangles
Nucleus
Normal neuron
Alzheimer neuron

Figure 44.1 ■ Neuron with neurofibrillary tangles seen in Alzheimer disease.

accumulation of beta-amyloid in plaques), the tau hypothesis (AD is the result of tau protein dysfunction), and the vascular hypothesis (many AD patients also have vascular dementia, the result of cardiovascular and cerebrovascular disease causing endothelial damage). Making diagnosis more difficult is that some people have these same pathophysiologic changes, but do not develop AD.

Neuritic plaques are groups of nerve cells (and especially the terminal axons) that degenerate and clump around an amyloid core as plaques, found in the spaces between the neurons of the brain. These plaques, which develop first in areas used for memory and cognition, disrupt transmission of nerve impulses. The plaques consist primarily of insoluble deposits of beta-amyloid, a protein fragment from a larger protein called amyloid precursor protein, mixed with other neurons and nonnerve cells.

Neurofibrillary tangles, found in the cytoplasm of abnormal neurons, are composed of fibrous proteins wound around each other in a helical way. The fibrous proteins contain the protein tau. Tau normally holds together the microtubules, which guide nutrients and molecules to the end of the axon. Because tau no longer maintains the transport system, communication is lost between neurons. Death of neurons may follow, contributing to the development of dementia.

Blood flow to the affected areas of the brain is decreased. The brain atrophies, and corresponding enlargement of ventricles and sulci is evident (**Figure 44.2** ■). As AD progresses, more areas of the brain are affected. Neuronal

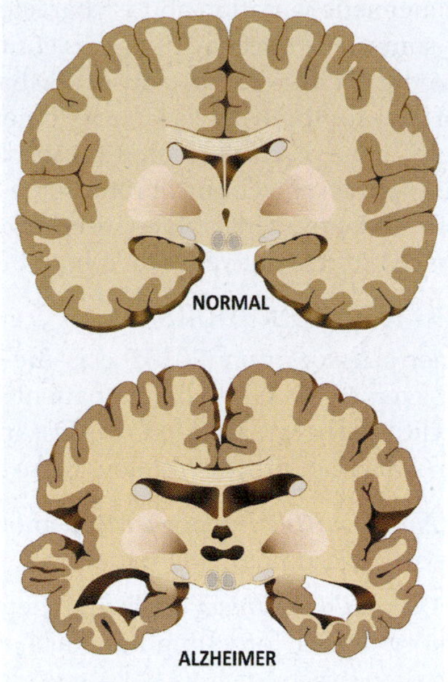
NORMAL
ALZHEIMER

Figure 44.2 ■ Changes in neuroanatomy associated with Alzheimer disease. Note areas of cortical atrophy, narrowing of the gyri, enlargement of sulci, and ventricular dilation.

and neurotransmitter losses (such as acetylcholine, a neurotransmitter associated with memory) are correlated with the number of neuritic plaques and the severity of AD. Researchers are currently working on ways to use both beta-amyloid and tau proteins as diagnostic indicators for AD, in order to help with earlier diagnosis of the disease (Alzheimer's Association, 2017a).

AD is characterized by atrophy of the cortical area of the brain and loss of neurons, especially in the hippocampus and temporal lobes. With significant atrophy and loss of brain tissue, the ventricles enlarge (a form of hydrocephalus). Several structural and chemical changes in the brain occur with AD, especially in the hippocampus and the frontal and temporal lobes of the cerebral cortex. As AD destroys neurons in the hippocampus and related structures, short-term memory fails and the ability to perform easy and familiar tasks declines. The effect of AD on neurons in the cerebral cortex is loss of language skills and judgment. Emotional outbursts and behavior changes (such as wandering and agitation) begin to occur and become more frequent as the disease progresses. Eventually, other areas of the brain are affected; all affected areas begin to atrophy, and the person becomes unresponsive.

Risk Factors

Although the exact cause is unknown, it appears that AD develops from the interaction of multiple factors. Age is the major risk factor, but other risk factors include head trauma, inflammatory factors, and oxidative stress. Other risk factors to evaluate include low educational level, lack of mental stimulation, migraines, and heavy smoking and alcohol consumption. People who develop AD under age 65 are said to have early-onset AD; those who develop AD after age 65 have late-onset AD. A small percentage of AD is caused by a genetic variation and is characterized by an early onset—sometimes affecting people as young as age 30. Research into the genetics of early-onset AD has identified mutations of at least three genes: The *APP* gene on chromosome 21, *PSI* gene on chromosome 14, and *PS2* gene on chromosome 1. The *ApoE* gene on chromosome 19 increases the risk for the development of late-onset AD and lowers the age of onset, but it is not yet known how this occurs.

Stages and Manifestations

The Alzheimer's Association (2017c) classifies Alzheimer disease into seven stages based on the patient's manifestations and abilities. The progression of AD varies for each individual and may not precisely follow these stages.

- *Stage 1: No Cognitive Impairment:* Memory problems are not experienced nor evident to others.
- *Stage 2: Very Mild Decline:* People find themselves having memory lapses, forgetting familiar names, or losing everyday objects such as keys and glasses. These memory problems are not evident to others nor are they detectable during a medical examination.
- *Stage 3: Mild Cognitive Decline:* Early-stage AD may be diagnosed in some, but not all, people with AD in this stage. Family and friends begin to notice problems and the deficits may be measured or detected during a medical examination. Common problems include trouble finding words or names, decreased ability to remember names when introduced to new people, retaining little information when reading a passage, decreased ability to plan or organize, losing or misplacing valuable objects, and having performance issues in social and work settings that are noticeable to others.
- *Stage 4: Moderate Cognitive Decline:* A careful medical interview will identify deficiencies in knowledge of recent events, impaired ability to perform challenging mental arithmetic (such as counting backward from 100 by 7s), decreased capacity to perform complex tasks (such as buying groceries or paying bills), and a reduced memory for personal history. The person often appears subdued and withdrawn, especially in social or mentally challenging situations.
- *State 5: Moderately Severe Cognitive Decline:* In this stage major deficits in memory and a decline in cognitive function emerge. Some assistance with ADLs becomes essential, but the person can usually eat and use the toilet. People with AD in this stage do usually retain knowledge about themselves and know their name and the names of family members. Problems include inability to recall current address or telephone number; confusion about where they are as well as the date, day of the week, or season; and trouble with less challenging mental arithmetic (such as counting backward by 4s from 40).
- *Stage 6: Severe Cognitive Decline:* This stage is characterized by worsening memory, emergence of personality changes, and the need for extensive help with ADLs. There is loss of most awareness of recent experiences and events as well as of the surroundings. The person generally knows his or her own name, but has problems recalling most personal history. People with AD in this stage do sometimes forget the names of family members, but they can usually distinguish familiar from unfamiliar faces. Without supervision they may, for example, put pajamas over daytime clothing or shoes on wrong feet. They need help with details of toileting (flushing, wiping, disposing of tissue) and are increasingly incontinent of urine or feces. There is disruption of their normal sleep–wake cycle. They tend to wander and get lost. Significant personality and behavior changes occur, such as suspiciousness and delusions, hallucinations, or compulsive/repetitive behavior (such as hand wringing or tissue shredding).
- *Stage 7: Very Severe Cognitive Decline:* This is the final stage. The person loses the ability to respond to his or her environment, the ability to speak, and the ability to control movement. Some words or phrases may be spoken, but they are not recognizable. Total care is needed for eating and toileting (there is general incontinence). The ability to walk without assistance is lost first, followed by the ability to sit without support, the ability to smile, and the ability to hold up the head. Reflexes become abnormal, muscles grow rigid, and swallowing is impaired. There are many possible causes of death as the person with AD reaches the final stage. The affected person is at increased risk for aspiration pneumonia from impaired swallowing. Loss of neurons impairs sensations such as hunger or thirst, leading to complications of malnutrition or dehydration. Infections can result in sepsis.

Interprofessional Care

There is no cure for AD, and the main objective of care is to provide an environment that matches the patient's functional abilities. Nurses, physicians, physical therapists, and social workers collaborate with the patient's family to provide the least restrictive environment in which the patient can safely function.

Diagnosis

There is no specific diagnostic test for AD. The only definitive method of diagnosis is postmortem examination of brain tissue. As a result, AD is diagnosed by ruling out causes for the patient's manifestations. An extensive workup is especially important because the dementia may be due to a reversible or treatable condition. For example, an older patient's misuse of medications can lead to overdosing and resulting confusion. Other conditions that may be considered are depression, infection, hypothyroidism, dehydration, heart disease, stroke, and chronic obstructive respiratory disease. Mental status is assessed with quick tests, the most common of which is the Folstein Mini Mental State Examination (measures orientation, registration, attention, calculation, recall, and language) (Tsoi, Chan, Hirai, et al., 2015). Another simple test that is often used is the mini-cog, which consists of a memory test and a clock drawing test (Alzheimer's Association, 2017e). The mini-cog is a quick test to administer and can help show the need for further assessment.

A diagnosis of AD requires the documented presence of dementia established by clinical examination and the results of a mental status test and absence of systemic or brain disorders that could cause deficits in memory and cognition (National Institute on Aging, 2017b).

Medications

No drugs have demonstrated effectiveness in halting the AD process but those medications listed in **Medication Administration 44.A** are considered to slow the progression of cognitive decline. Other medications are prescribed for manifestations such as sleep disturbances and agitation. In general, patients should see an improvement in cognition and ADLs within 3 months of starting pharmacologic treatment (Glynn-Servedio & Seys Ranola, 2017).

Depression often accompanies AD and is treated with the appropriate medication. Antihistamines and tricyclic antidepressants that have high anticholinergic activity are usually avoided because they can increase AD manifestations. Occasionally, patients with AD require atypical antipsychotic medications such as risperidone (Risperdal) to manage severe agitation, delusions, or aggression. When antipsychotic drugs are prescribed, considerations need to be taken for the risk of extrapyramidal symptoms; for this reason, use of traditional antipsychotic medications are limited (Adams, Holland, & Urban, 2017).

Nutrition

Since there is no cure for AD, prevention is key. There are several risk factors for AD that are associated with diet, including obesity, diabetes mellitus, and high cholesterol (Bane & Cole, 2015). The Mediterranean diet has been shown to have neuroprotective benefits likely associated with the high intake of fresh fruits and vegetables as well as omega 3 fatty acids (Bane & Cole, 2015).

Integrative Therapies

Integrative therapies have been used in treating the manifestations of AD and include:

- Huperzine A, a traditional Chinese medicine, which acts as an acetylcholinesterase inhibitor
- Coenzyme Q10, an antioxidant that naturally occurs in the body
- Supplements, such as zinc, ginkgo biloba, B vitamins, and vitamin E
- Therapies involving acupuncture, exercise, massage, art, music, sound, dance, and pet therapy.

Medication Administration 44.A

The Patient with Alzheimer Disease

ACETYLCHOLINESTERASE INHIBITORS (AChEIs)

donepezil hydrochloride (Aricept)

In the early stages of AD, the pathologic changes in neurons result in a deficiency of acetylcholine (a key neurotransmitter involved in cognitive functioning). Cholinesterase inhibitors slow the breakdown of acetylcholine release by the remaining intact neurons. The drugs are used to improve memory in mild to moderate AD dementia. In this group, donepezil is considered first-line therapy because of its once-daily dosing, narrower adverse effect profile, and efficacy.

NMDA RECEPTOR ANTAGONIST (N-METHYL-D-ASPARTATE)

memantine hydrochloride (Namenda)

rivastigmine tartrate (Exelon)

Namenda binds to NMDA receptor-operated cation channels, slowing death of neurons. It temporarily delays more severe AD manifestations.

Nursing Responsibilities

- Monitor for nausea and vomiting, anorexia, and diarrhea.
- Monitor for bradycardia if AChEIs are being administered with beta-blockers, digoxin, or antiarrhythmic drugs.
- Administer donepezil hydrochloride at bedtime.
- Administer rivastigmine tartrate (both capsules and liquid) with food. Liquid form may be administered undiluted or mixed with water, juice, or soda. Stir to completely dissolve. The rivastigmine patch is applied once every 24 hours at the same time of day, using the upper chest, upper or lower back, or upper arm, ensure site is rotated application site daily.
- Monitor for jaundice, increased bilirubin levels, and other signs of liver involvement, such as rising serum aminotransferase (AST, ALT) levels. Dosage adjustment or drug discontinuation may be required.
- Observe for GI bleeding and gastric pain.
- Monitor for cholinergic-related problems: Bladder outlet obstruction, seizures, and slowed cardiac rate.
- Assist with ambulation because dizziness is a common side effect.
- Monitor glycemic control in patients with diabetes.
- Assess for improvement in AD symptoms, especially in reasoning, memory, and ADLs.

Health Education for the Patient and Family

- Notify the physician promptly if jaundice, seizures, slowed heart rate, GI bleeding, or difficulty urinating occurs.
- Follow directions for times and instructions for administration of specific medication.
- Follow healthcare provider's recommendation for periodic EEGs, blood tests, and urine tests.
- Medications do not cure AD and eventually become ineffective as the disease progresses.

Note: Drugs identified in blue are among the 200 most commonly prescribed medications in the United States.

Source: Adams, et al., 2017.

Nursing Care

Patients with AD often require intensive, supportive nursing interventions directed at the physical and psychosocial responses to illness. Equally important, the nurse can facilitate the long-term support of these patients by providing teaching and referrals to follow-up care in the community. See the Case Study & Nursing Care Plan for a patient with AD on page 1639.

Assessment

Collect the following data through the health history and physical examination (refer to Chapter 41). Further focused assessments are described with nursing interventions that follow.

- ***Health history:*** Family member/caregiver support, living arrangements, ability to carry out ADLs, changes in self-care, drug use, work history (e.g., exposure to metals), previous history of depression, multiple strokes, brain injury or brain infection, family history of dementia, sleep pattern, changes in cognition and memory, ability to communicate, changes in behavior
- ***Physical assessment:*** Height/weight, orientation, abstract reasoning, mental status.

Priorities of Care

The goals of care for a patient with an impaired memory are to maintain a safe environment and to optimize that environment to the patient's functional level.

Falls Prevention. Patients with AD are at high risk for falls due to decreased cognition and polypharmacy as well as inability to complete ADLs. Patients and families should be educated on ways to decrease falls in the home. The Centers for Disease Control and Prevention (2017) recommends the following modifications be made in the home:

- Trip hazards are eliminated (including removal of throw rugs)
- Place items within easy reach (avoid using stool or ladder)
- Install grab bars and hand rails in shower/tub, next to toilets, and along staircases
- Provide for adequate lighting, especially at stairs
- Wear shoes that fit with nonskid soles.

Memory Loss. Techniques to help with the memory loss should be included in teaching for both the patient and the caregiver. Techniques for communicating with patients with AD are outlined in **Box 44.1**.

- Suggest complementary therapies, such as meditation, massage, or exercise. *These activities can help reduce stress; stress can aggravate memory loss.*
- Suggest using a calendar, keeping lists of reminders, or asking someone else to remind of appointments and events. *Written or verbal reminders are helpful if memory is impaired.*

BOX 44.1
Communicating with the Patient with Alzheimer Disease

- Face the patient, make eye contact, and talk directly to him or her; call the patient by name.
- When first approaching the patient, identify yourself.
- Use respectful phrases and language, do not talk down to the patient or use childlike phrases.
- Avoid outside distractions.
- Use simple sentences and words with few syllables.
- Speak in a calm, low voice.
- Ask one question at a time. Use questions that require only a yes or no response.
- Keep nonverbal communication relaxed and parallel to the verbal communication.
- Avoid giving the impression of being in a hurry; try to have a relaxed approach.
- Observe for anxiety—wringing hands, pacing, darting eye movements—and alter your approach to decrease anxiety.
- Avoid arguing with patients; do not insist on orienting patient to reality; the patient's point of reference may not be based in reality.
- Give plenty of time for the patient with AD to process what you are trying to say; do not expect patients to perform skills beyond their abilities.
- Repeat explanations in simple terms.

General Safety Considerations. It is important for caregivers to evaluate the patient's home environment to protect the patient from hazards that may post a safety risk. These considerations were adapted from the Alzheimer's Association (2017b).

- Secure items that may be mistakenly ingested, such as cleaning preparations and house plants. Keep medications locked up to avoid overdose.
- Modify potentially unsafe areas, such as unenclosed porches.
- Provide double lock systems to outside doors and doors to rooms that are off-limits.
- Protect from fire hazards; for example, make matches and cigarettes inaccessible.
- Modify the controls on the oven and stove.
- Adjust the water heater to a safe temperature.
- Keep a list of emergency phone numbers accessible.
- Ensure that the family member with a cognitive impairment has no access to dangerous objects in the home such as knives and guns.

SAFETY ALERT: Risk for falls and medication errors are both factors in the care of patients with AD. Any change in the physical environment or placement of household belongings or increased stimulation can contribute to an increased risk for falls and to the possibility of medication errors. Patients with AD frequently require supervision with physical tasks, ambulation, and medication administration, particularly in an unfamiliar environment. ■

Diagnoses, Outcomes, and Interventions

During the early stage of AD, nursing care focuses on helping the patient make minor adaptations to his or her environment. As the patient becomes progressively unable to manage self-care tasks, more adaptations are required. Equally important, the caregiver needs much support—both physical and psychosocial—as the patient becomes increasingly dependent.

Reduce Risk for Harm. Due to progressive changes in the AD patient's ability for self-care and safety, caregivers and nurses must take on increasing responsibility to protect AD patients in their environment.

Expected Outcome: Patient with impaired memory will be in a safe environment where the risk for harm is eliminated.

The nurse will:

- Recommend using a medication box labeled with days and times. *A medication box is a good way to remember to take medications.*
- Provide information to the healthcare staff about the individual's memory problems if treatment or professional care of the individual with AD is necessary. *Families provide much of the care and support of older adults living with dementia. Family caregivers are an important source of information and should be regarded as an integral part of the healthcare team.*
- Provide continuity in nursing staff. *This not only promotes consistency of care for the patient but also allows the nurse to determine more accurately changes in the patient's condition.*
- Repeat explanations simply and as needed to decrease anxiety. *Loss of short-term memory leads to loss of a point of reference; eventually, AD patients think they are experiencing everything for the first time.*

SAFETY ALERT: It may be necessary to teach the caregiver how to refill the medication box or to stress the importance of spot checking if the patient fills it. ■

Relieve Anxiety. Managing the AD patient's behaviors associated with anxiety, restlessness, and confusion is a major challenge confronting nurses and caregivers. Frequently, patients are relatively calm in the morning hours, only to experience increasing periods of agitation in the afternoon and evening hours. The AD patient may wake from the night's sleep with confusion, fearfulness, or panic attacks.

Expected Outcome: Patient's anxiety will be minimized/controlled so as to ensure patient safety and manageability, as well as patient comfort.

The nurse will:

- Monitor for early behaviors of fatigue and agitation. *Early assessment of problems results in prompt intervention to promote rest or to remove the patient from the situation causing anxiety.*
- Remove from situations that are causing increased anxiety, such as noisy activities involving large groups. *High-stimulus situations may increase anxious feelings and agitation.*
- Keep daily routine as consistent as possible. *Providing a structured day enhances feelings of familiarity and decreases stress.*
- Schedule rest periods or quiet times throughout the day. *Fatigue contributes to anxiety and lowers the ability to tolerate stress.*
- Provide quiet activities, such as listening to favorite music, in the afternoon or early evening. *Quiet activities may help decrease sundowning.*
- If confusion and agitation persist or escalate, assess for physical causes such as decreased oxygenation, infections, fatigue, constipation, and electrolyte imbalance. *Physical factors can increase agitation in patients with AD.*
- Use therapeutic touch or gentle hand massage. *These activities induce relaxation and have a calming effect.*

Instill Hope. As the patient and family recognize the effect of AD on their lives, they may feel a sense of hopelessness. They may not have the coping skills to deal effectively with the diagnosis and anticipated problems. The increasingly degenerative, irreversible nature of the disorder tends to diminish hope; only the ability to adapt to the many problems can restore it.

Expected Outcome: Signs and symptoms of hopelessness will be minimized by use of coping skills and family/community resources.

The nurse will:

- Assess the patient's and family's response to the diagnosis and understanding of AD; encourage expression of feelings. *Understanding the patient's and family's perspective enables the nurse to dispel myths about AD.*
- Provide realistic information about the disorder; provide information at the patient's and family's level of understanding. *Patient and family may need to have separate sessions. Factual information provides a foundation for decision making.*
- Avoid criticizing or judging expressed feelings. *An environment accepting of the expression of real feelings promotes both further expression of feelings and willingness to discuss other issues.*
- Support positive family bonds and enhance communication among family members; promote mutual positive regard. *Strong family relationships can provide direction for living and convey a willingness to share the burden.*
- Encourage the patient to make as many decisions as possible. *Self-determination enhances a feeling of control over a situation and may give a sense of hope.*
- Encourage the patient and family to seek spiritual guidance that previously inspired hope. *The patient's church is a legitimate support system. Faith and belief in a higher power can inspire hope beyond present circumstances.*

Reduce Caregiver Stress. Most caregivers of patients with AD are spouses or other family members. Because AD is a chronic and debilitating disorder, caregivers may feel overwhelmed by their responsibilities. The caregiving spouse faces not only the responsibility for the patient's multiple physical demands but also economic and psychosocial stressors. The patient may have to cease driving, and the loss of independence represented by this loss of the ability to drive may trigger anxiety and anger. Fear of the future, loss of income, loss of companionship and a mate—combined with fatigue—make the caregiver vulnerable. Caregivers may become physically and mentally exhausted and socially isolated because of the overwhelming responsibilities of providing total care to the incapacitated family member. Although most families prefer to keep the person with AD at home as long as possible, most people with the disease eventually need more assistance than family members can provide and must move to a facility for professional care.

Expected Outcome: Caregivers will manage stress of role by acknowledging and accessing resources that reduce responsibilities and minimize stress/exhaustion/demands.

The nurse will:

- Teach the caregivers self-care techniques, such as taking rest periods and avoiding fatigue. *Fatigue adds to stress and potentially leads to poor decision making.*
- Have the caregivers list and regularly take part in physical activities they enjoy, such as walking or swimming. *Regular physical exercise decreases stress.*
- Refer the caregivers to local AD support groups. Suggest books pertinent to the subject. *Providing explicit suggestions for locating support systems and providing specific information promote coping.*
- Refer the caregivers to Meals on Wheels, home health, respite care, and other community services. *Community agencies can relieve some of the daily care burdens, thus providing time for other activities. Programs that support caregivers have been shown to delay nursing home placement.*
- Ensure that the family knows that hospice care is available during the end stages of AD. *Hospice services can support the family during this difficult time.*

Delegating Nursing Care

As appropriate and allowed by the designated duties and responsibilities of unlicensed assistive personnel, the nurse may delegate nursing care activities such as close monitoring of environment for safe conditions (e.g., avoiding scatter rugs, moving furniture, and providing lighting so that patient can ambulate safely).

Transitions of Care

Health promotion for the patient with AD focuses on maintaining functional abilities and safety. If the patient will be cared for at home, address safety considerations as well as the caregivers' abilities to meet the patient's basic needs, such as maintaining hygiene and other ADLs. Adapt nursing interventions and teaching to the patient's stage of AD. Nurses promote caregiver health; information about caregiver support systems and respite care should be provided.

The public needs to be aware of the warning signs of AD and seek medical care when they are observed. The 10 warning signs of AD are memory loss, difficulty with problem solving, challenges in performing familiar tasks, disorientation to time and place, vision problems, problems with language, poor or decreased judgment, misplacing things, changes in mood and personality, and avoiding social settings (Alzheimer's Association, 2017d). Although there is no proven way to prevent AD, recommendations have been made to delay the onset of manifestations. These include staying active mentally, physically, and socially. Activities such as walking each day, reading the newspaper, visiting the library, or writing a letter are important in maintaining cognitive ability in old age. Other recommendations are generally beneficial for health, including eating a healthy diet (with an emphasis on fruits, vegetables, and fiber), controlling cardiovascular and diabetes mellitus risk factors (weight, smoking, blood pressure, and cholesterol), and avoiding head injuries (by wearing seat belts and helmets and avoiding falls).

Family caregiving takes an enormous toll on mental, physical, emotional, and financial resources. Family members see a former fully functioning and independent loved one become progressively more impaired and dependent on others for total care. The patient with AD drains time and energy, leading to high rates of stress, depression, symptoms of "burnout," and frequent illnesses in the caregiver. The stress of caregiving can even have a negative effect on the care provided to a loved one (Krishnan, York, Bakus, et al, 2017). Teaching self-care, coping and providing resources for caregivers is an important nursing intervention that can help alleviate some of the symptoms of burnout.

Teaching for patients and families centers initially on explaining the disorder and exploring available support systems. Anticipate the need to reexplain the disorder and its consequences because patients and families may be in shock or denial during the initial period of the disease. In addition to explaining the anticipated changes with AD, suggest practical solutions to identified problems. It is important to evaluate both the patient and caregivers; interventions must be appropriate for the family's situation and resources. Maintaining the least restrictive environment that promotes safety for the patient is a major goal of teaching. Using memory cues, such as labeling drawers to indicate specific types of clothing and labeling rooms, can help orient the patient and foster independence. Consistency in the environment and daily routine is an essential part of care. Emphasizing realistic expectations means adjusting care and communication techniques to the patient's level of ability.

Address the following topics for home care of the patient and for the caregiver:

- Support groups and peer counseling are helpful in handling caregiver stress.
- An individual with AD who is confused or agitated is not comfortable and is usually frightened.

- Plan care that matches the person's level of coping, using a consistent routine.
- Provide regular rest periods to decrease the patient's stress and fatigue (these do not increase nighttime wandering).
- Plan care for the caregiver. Periodic adult daycare or respite care during the initial stages, with plans for increasing assistance to meet the patient's daily needs as the disease progresses, may be sufficient. Referrals to the appropriate agency for long-term care, including skilled nursing facilities, may be indicated. Family members may need help adjusting to the idea of extended care but may be relieved to relinquish the physical care needs.
- Suggest the following resources: Alzheimer's Association, Alzheimer's Disease and Related Disorders Association, Alzheimer's Disease Education and Referral Center, and the National Institute of Neurological Disorders and Stroke.

A patient can suffer with AD for many years before it leads to their death. Early recognition of AD can not only help preserve some cognitive functioning for a period of time, but it can also help patients to participate in end-of-life decisions and planning. Toward the end of the disease process, it becomes difficult or impossible for the patient to communicate and it is important for family to have an understanding of the patient's wishes. Nearing the end of the disease process, referrals to palliative or hospice care may be appropriate.

Case Study & Nursing Care Plan

A Patient with Alzheimer Disease

Arthur and Ruth Joste, both age 73, have been married for 47 years; he is a retired history teacher, she has been a homemaker. They have four children; two live in the same town, and two live out of state. Arthur has noticed that he is having problems remembering friends' names and phone numbers; his wife has been asking him if he is driving in the correct direction when they go shopping.

Mrs. Joste has severe osteoarthritis and is unable to lift heavy objects; she is only able to perform light housekeeping tasks. For about 18 months, Mrs. Joste has been aware of her husband's progressive cognitive decline, including forgetting current news from last night's newspaper, miscalculating checkbook balances, neglecting his hygiene needs, and confusing their children's and grandchildren's names. The Jostes are referred to a neurologist for evaluation.

ASSESSMENT	DIAGNOSES	EXPECTED OUTCOMES
Martha Spital, RN, assesses Mr. Joste at the neurologist's office. She notes that he is unable to recall his home address without prompting, to name the correct date (although he does know the day of the week), to subtract serial 7s more than twice, and to recall two of three objects. He is alert to his surroundings. Mrs. Joste states that the problems seem to be getting worse with time. Mr. Joste seems easily agitated, and his wife reports that his sleep habits are "jumbled"; he has long periods of wakefulness in the nighttime hours. Following a thorough evaluation and diagnostic testing to rule out other possible disorders, the neurologist tells the couple that Mr. Joste has probable dementia of the Alzheimer type. Both have feared this diagnosis; they want to know how they can be sure that Mr. Joste has this disease and what they can do to prevent further decline. Both are obviously saddened, and they verbalize their feelings of being overwhelmed. The Jostes intend to remain in their home "for as long as we can."	■ Confusion related to deterioration of brain function and dementia ■ Inability to perform self-care related to forgetfulness and declining physical abilities ■ Increased risk of injury related to decreased orientation ■ Sleep deficit related to time disorientation ■ Caregiver (wife) stress related to need to care for self and husband	■ Patient will remain free of injury. ■ Patient will navigate home environment with modifications as needed. ■ Patient will participate in grooming and hygiene activities with prompting and supervision. ■ Patient will obtain a minimum of 7 uninterrupted hours of sleep a night. ■ Mrs. Joste will participate in a minimum of two out-of-home activities a week.

PLANNING AND IMPLEMENTATION

The home health nurse, Erick Montane, RN, makes a home visit to evaluate the environment, assess available support, and determine needs. He meets two of the Jostes' children, Dawn and Jay, who live in the same community and are willing to participate as much as possible in providing care and modifying the home.

Mr. Montane discusses the importance of establishing and maintaining a consistent daily routine. He emphasizes the importance of matching activities to Mr. Joste's mental abilities to avoid frustration and increased agitation. Mr. Montane recommends labeling drawers with their contents, such as Mr. Joste's sock drawer. Labeling rooms may eventually be necessary.

Because his inability to comprehend and process information distresses and agitates Mr. Joste, Mr. Montane teaches the family to modify their communications to fit Mr. Joste's cognitive ability, such as using simple, direct statements and directions. Mr. Montane recommends that family members keep background noise to a minimum because this may be a source of confusion.

After assessing the home, Mr. Montane makes the following recommendations about safety:

- Remove throw rugs from hallways, and tack down any remaining carpets. Ensure that stairs are carpeted to protect Mr. Joste from injury.

(continued)

- Secure the kitchen, bathroom, and workshop cabinets as well as the controls on the oven and stove.
- Modify the doors so that operating the locks requires a two-step system of unlocking, such as with a deadbolt and a key.
- Provide extra lighting in dark areas, especially a nightlight in the hallway and bathroom.

Mr. Montane explains that Mrs. Joste will need assistance with housekeeping as Mr. Joste continues to decline. Mr. Montane provides referrals to community services, including Meals on Wheels, which can supply a daily meal. He also suggests that the Jostes obtain the services of a home health aide to provide daily hygiene care. Most of the remaining home maintenance needs can be met with the children's help.

Mr. and Mrs. Joste and the two children attend the weekly local support group meetings for Alzheimer disease and related disorders for approximately 3 months; thereafter, Mrs. Joste attends with her daughter.

EVALUATION

Six months after the initial home visit and family planning session, Mr. Joste's assessment is as follows:

- Has not had a fall, burn, or other injury.
- Has periods of confusion when outside his home, but 90% of the time is oriented to place when at home.
- Has attended several support group meetings until 3 months ago. Currently, his wife attends weekly, and a daughter occasionally accompanies her. She has continued to participate in their church and maintains contact with a few friends. She is finding it harder to leave her husband unattended for even a few minutes.
- Is able to clean and dress himself with prompting; he is not able to choose his own clothing. If hygiene articles are "set up" (e.g., if the toothpaste is placed on the toothbrush), he remembers to perform the hygiene activity. The children have been replacing buttons and zippers with Velcro closures on his clothing.
- Sleeps an average of 6 hours a night with a 30-minute nap in the afternoon; this pattern is consistent with his previous sleep pattern.
- Has seemed to be more easily agitated for the past month. He wanders from room to room, apparently looking for something. These behaviors are worse in the evening and on cloudy days. Mrs. Joste sadly acknowledges her progressive inability to care for her husband.

CLINICAL REASONING IN PATIENT CARE

1. Develop a tool to teach safety needs for the patient with Alzheimer disease and his family.
2. List five interventions to decrease agitation in older adults with cognitive impairment; give three additional examples of activities suited to an older adult with AD who has osteoarthritis.
3. You are caring for a patient in stage 5 Alzheimer disease. She is 165 cm (65 in.) tall and weighs 59.9 kg (132 lb); she has lost 1.4 kg (3 lb) within the past month. The patient has difficulty focusing on eating and is easily agitated. Describe your plan for ensuring that she has adequate nutrition. (Consult current literature to help devise an evidence-based plan.)

See Evaluating Your Response in Appendix B.

The Patient with Multiple Sclerosis

Multiple sclerosis (MS) is a chronic demyelinating disease of the CNS (brain, optic nerves, and spinal cord). The disease ranges from relatively mild to totally disabling. The manifestations of MS vary according to the area of the nervous system affected. The initial onset may be followed by a total remission, making diagnosis difficult. In many patients, MS is characterized by periods of exacerbation, when manifestations are highly pronounced, followed by periods of remission, when manifestations are not obvious. The end result is progression of the disease with increasing loss of function.

The onset of MS is usually between 20 and 40 years of age, but the disease has been diagnosed in children and elderly patients (Faguy, 2016). MS is the most prevalent CNS demyelinating disorder and is a leading cause of neurologic disability in young adults. Women are affected by MS up to three times more often than men and it is more prevalent in colder northern latitudes (Faguy, 2016). The risk of developing MS is seven-fold greater when MS is also present in a first-degree relative, although it is not considered a hereditary disease.

Pathophysiology

MS is believed to occur as a result of an autoimmune response occurring more frequently in a genetically susceptible individual. The target antigen has not been identified, but is suggested to be an immune response to a protein in the CNS. As with other demyelinating disorders, MS is characterized by inflammation and selective destruction of CNS myelin (Faguy, 2016).

Myelin sheaths are fatty, segmented wrappings that normally protect and insulate nerve fibers and increase the speed of transmission of nerve impulses. In multiple sclerosis, these myelin sheaths of the white matter of the spinal cord, brain, and optic nerve are destroyed in patches, called *plaques*, along the axon (see Pathophysiology Illustrated on pages 1640–1641). The demyelination of nerve fibers slows and distorts the conduction of nerve impulses and sometimes results in the total absence or distortion of impulse transmission. The neurons affected by MS are located in the spinal cord, brainstem, cerebral and cerebellar areas, and the optic nerve.

Plaques typically are scattered through the white matter of the CNS, although they may extend into adjacent gray matter. Early manifestations are the result of inflammatory edema in and around the plaque and partial demyelination. These manifestations typically disappear within weeks after the initial episode. With progression of the disease, the demyelination and plaque formation result in scarring of glia (gliosis) and degeneration of axons. MS develops in two stages. In the first stage small inflammatory lesions develop sequentially. During the second stage these lesions extend and consolidate as gliosis and demyelination occurs. It is unknown whether the inflammatory process is directed against the myelin or against oligodendrocytes that produce myelin. Evidence suggests that remyelination occurs in the CNS if the disease process is stopped before the oligodendrocytes are destroyed (Multiple Sclerosis Association of America [MSAA], 2017a).

There are four possible courses of MS: Relapsing-remitting (characterized by periodic remission and exacerbation of manifestations), primary progressive (almost continuous neurologic deterioration from onset of manifestations), secondary progressive (gradual deterioration with or without relapses), and progressive-relapsing (gradual progression of neurologic deterioration with superimposed relapses). Most individuals with MS present with the relapsing-remitting type.

Risk Factors

Several risk factors have been associated with MS, including genetics, geographic location, diagnosis of other autoimmune disorders (type 1 diabetes), low levels of vitamin D, obesity, smoking, and high salt intake (Faguy, 2016; MSAA, 2017b).

Manifestations

The manifestations of MS vary according to the areas destroyed by demyelination and the affected body system (see Multisystem Effects of Multiple Sclerosis on page 1642). The most common manifestations include (Newsome et al., 2017):

- Fatigue
- Pain
- Visual deficits, with visual blurring, diplopia, decreased central visual acuity, area of diminished vision in the visual fields, nystagmus
- Cognitive dysfunctions involving concentration, short-term memory, word finding, and planning
- Mood alterations are most often manifested as depression and anxiety
- Weakness and/or numbness in one or both extremities (most often the legs)
- Upper motor neuron involvement is manifested by stiffness, slowness, and weakness (spastic paresis)
- Bladder dysfunctions include urgency, hesitancy, and incontinence
- Bowel dysfunction is most often seen as constipation
- Sexual dysfunction.

In many patients, the initial manifestation involves paresthesia, visual deficits, urinary incontinence, and compromised gait (Sorenson, Quinn, & Klein, 2019). Fatigue is one of the most disabling manifestations and affects almost all patients with MS.

The manifestations (individualized to each patient) typically last for several days or weeks and then completely or partially resolve. After a period of relatively normal function, manifestations reappear.

Complications

Increased risk of falls is of great concern for patients diagnosed with MS. These patients tend to have an impaired gait related to pain, weakness, spasticity, and other manifestations, which put them at high risk for falls and injury (Newsome et al., 2017). Patient teaching and symptom management are important interventions to prevent fall-related injuries.

Interprofessional Care

Management of the patient with MS varies according to the severity of the manifestations. The focus is on retaining the optimal level of functioning possible, given the degree of disability. Rehabilitation—physical, occupational/vocational, and psychosocial—is a cornerstone of an interprofessional approach to treatment. During exacerbations, the focus of interventions shifts to controlling manifestations and quickly returning to remission. Recent guidelines for the treatment of MS show the importance of interprofessional care and communication, ensuring that all team members have a good understanding of the disease process, treatment goals, and plan of care (Newsome et al., 2016).

Diagnosis

Previously, an MS diagnosis was only based on the patient having two or more exacerbations followed by remission in addition to diagnostic testing. However, waiting for the patient to have two exacerbations can delay diagnosis, and early intervention is imperative to delay worsening of the disease (Luzzio, 2017). New guidelines have been identified to include use of magnetic resonance imaging (MRI) to identify lesions in addition to clinical history (Luzzio, 2017). Diagnostic tests (refer to Chapter 41) vary with the presenting complaints. MRI with findings of lesions is the most definitive test available; however, it is only one of several laboratory and diagnostic tests that may be performed when establishing the diagnosis. Cerebrospinal fluid (CSF) analysis reveals an increased number of T lymphocytes that are reactive with antigens, indicating the presence of an immune response. The majority of patients with MS have elevated levels of immunoglobulin G (IgG) in the CSF. A CT scan of the brain may reveal atrophy and white-matter lesions.

Medications

Medications slow the progression of MS and decrease the number of attacks (see **Medication Administration 44.B**). Medications are used for a variety of reasons, including treatment of manifestations, to modify the course of the disease, or to interrupt the progression of the disease.

The medications used during an exacerbation are aimed at decreasing inflammation to inhibit manifestations and induce remission. A combination of adrenal corticosteroid hormone (ACTH) and glucocorticoids are

Pathophysiology Illustrated
Multiple Sclerosis

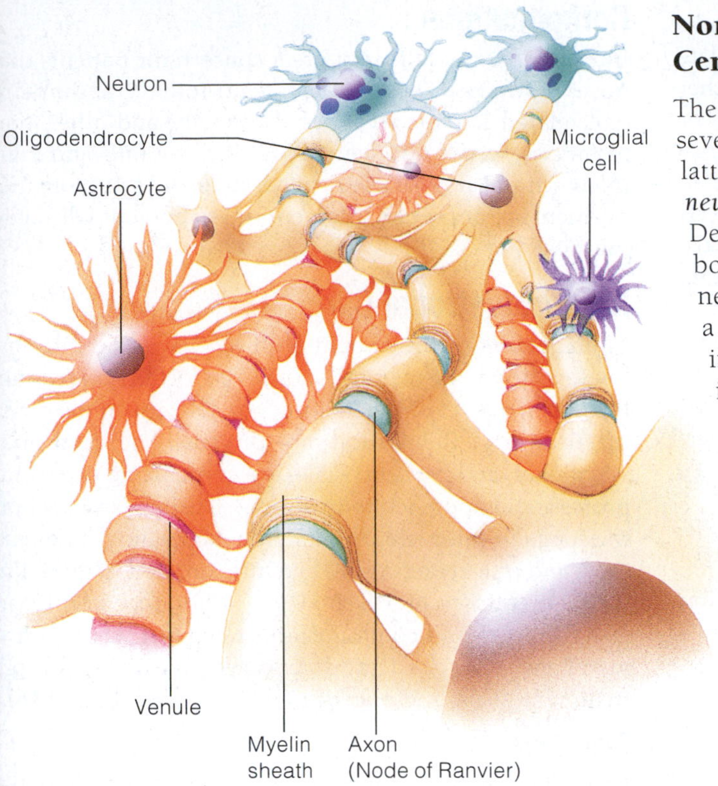
Neuron
Oligodendrocyte
Astrocyte
Microglial cell
Venule
Myelin sheath
Axon (Node of Ranvier)

Normal Anatomy of the Central Nervous System

The central nervous system (CNS) is composed of several cell types arranged in a dense, interconnected lattice. The basic functional cell of the CNS is the *neuron*, which transmits electrochemical impulses. Dendrites, thin projections extending from the neuron body, receive impulses that are passed down the neuronal axon for transmission to other cells. Myelin, a lipid-protein substance, surrounds the axons, insulating them and speeding nerve impulse transmission.

Neurons are surrounded by a network of cells:

- *Astrocytes* support neurons and connnect them to surrounding capillaries and venules.
- *Microglia* are motile phagocytic cells.
- *Oligodendrocytes* wrap concentric layers of myelin around nearby axons.

Acute Attack

Multiple sclerosis (MS) is a demyelinating disease in which axonal myelin in the central nervous system is eroded, destroyed, and replaced by scar tissue.

An autoimmune process apparently triggered by genetic and environmental factors is believed to cause inflammation of venules in the CNS. This disrupts the blood–brain barrier, allowing lymphocytes to enter CNS tissue. These lymphocytes proliferate and produce IgG, an antibody that attacks and damages myelin and causes the release of inflammatory chemicals and edema. As the inflammation subsides, the myelin regenerates and manifestations of the disease subside.

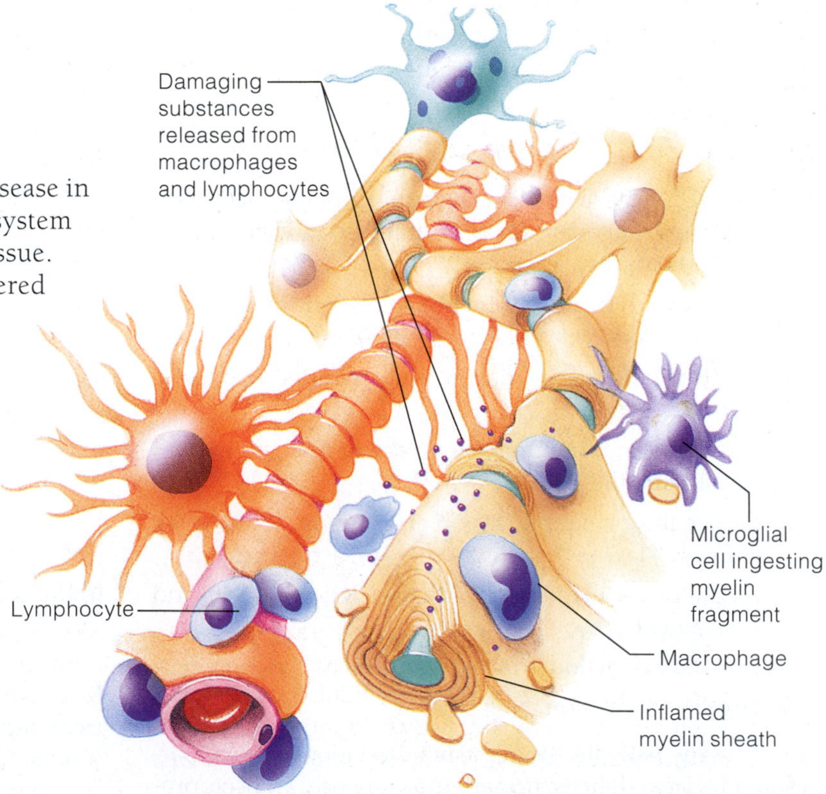
Damaging substances released from macrophages and lymphocytes
Microglial cell ingesting myelin fragment
Lymphocyte
Macrophage
Inflamed myelin sheath

Chronic Lesion

After repeated inflammatory attacks, myelin is irreparably damaged. Segments of axons become totally demyelinated and may degenerate. Astrocytes proliferate in damaged regions of the CNS (a process called *gliosis*), forming plaques. The plaques are scattered throughout the CNS, appearing as gray or pinkish lesions. The relapsing-remitting character of MS and the scattered areas of damage within the CNS account for the variable nature of MS manifestations.

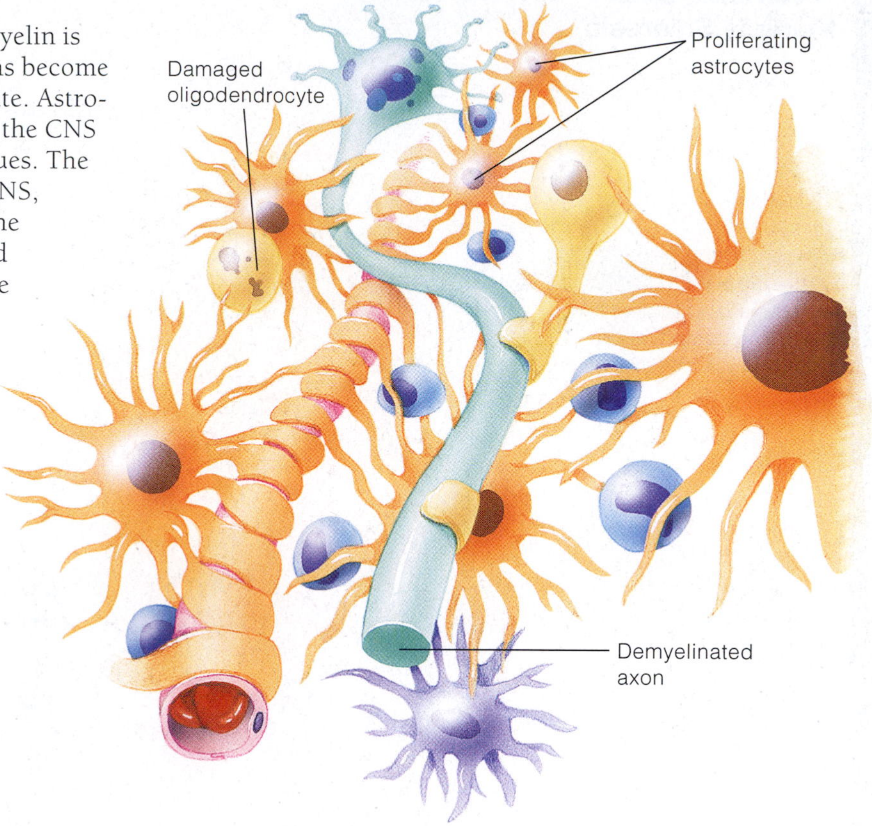
Damaged oligodendrocyte
Proliferating astrocytes
Demyelinated axon

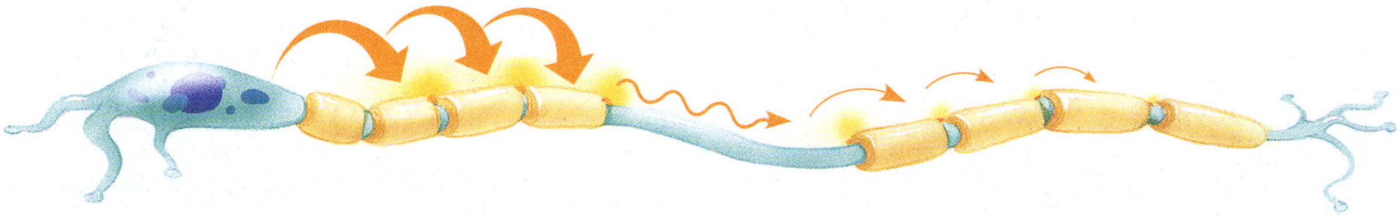

Abnormal Nerve Impulse Transmission

In an undamaged neuron, nerve impulses travel down the axon by "leaping" from one node of Ranvier to the next, thus greatly increasing the speed of impulse transmission. When nerve impulses travel down an axon damaged by MS, they are significantly slowed and weakened as they pass across the surface of demyelinated areas. Impulses may be blocked entirely when axons degenerate. The weakening or interruption of the transmission of nerve impulses and plaque formation within the CNS cause the manifestations of MS, including extremity weakness, paresthesias, visual disturbances, bladder dysfunction, and vertigo.

often used to decrease inflammation and suppress the immune system. Immunosuppressive agents, including alemtuzumab (Lemtrada) and mitoxantrone (Novantrone), are also used. Interferon and glatiramer acetate are used to reduce exacerbations in patients with relapsing-remitting MS. Interferon alpha, beta, and gamma (Avonex, Rebif, Betaseron) enhance immune function, while glatiramer acetate (Copaxone) stimulates parts of the myelin basic protein to reduce the relapse rate of MS. Both drugs are given by injection and are usually well tolerated. An oral medication given once daily, called fingolimod (Gilenya), is now available. It works to trap immune cells in lymph nodes. The first dose is monitored due to the risk of bradycardia, and other side effects include diarrhea, cough, and headache. Medication therapies should be chosen based on the progression of the disease, adverse effects, patient compliance (willingness to inject medications), and clinician experience (Faguy, 2016).

Medications may be used to treat the specific manifestations of MS. Anticholinergics are administered for bladder spasticity; cholinergics are given for bladder flaccidity. Fatigue may be treated with amantadine (Symmetrel).

Multisystem Effects of
Multiple Sclerosis

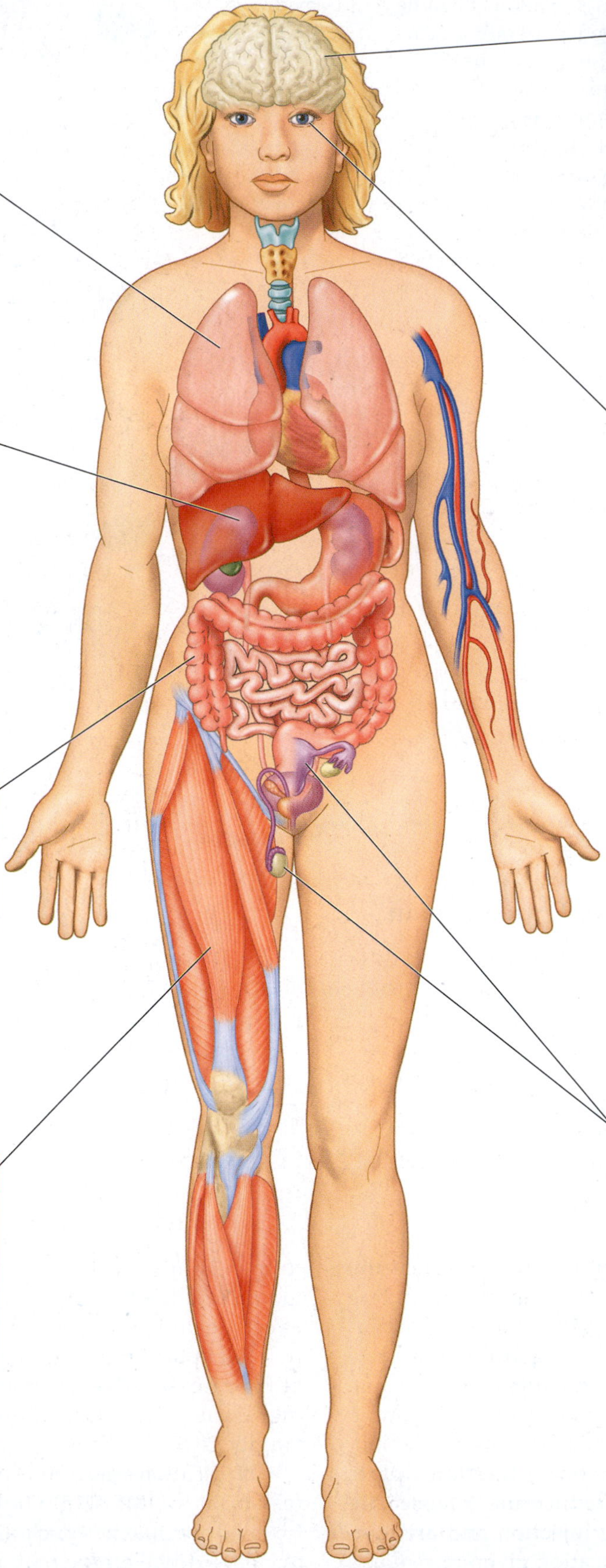

Neurologic

- Emotional lability (euphoria or depression)
- Forgetfulness
- Apathy
- Scanning speech
- Impaired judgment
- Irritability

Potential complications

- Convulsive seizures
- Dementia

Respiratory

- Diminished cough reflex

Potential complication

- Respiratory infections

Urinary

- Hesitancy
- Frequency
- Retention
- Reflex bladder emptying

Potential complications

- Recurring UTIs
- Incontinence

Sensory

Visual

- Blurred vision
- Diplopia
- Nystagmus
- Visual field defects (blind spots)
- Eye pain

Auditory

- Vertigo
- Nausea

Tactile (especially hands or legs)

- Numbness
- Paresthesias (tingling, burning sensation)
- Diminished sense of temperature
- Pain with spasms
- Loss of proprioception

Potential complication

Visual

- Blindness

Gastrointestinal

Oral/esophageal

- Difficulty chewing
- Dysphagia

Upper/lower GI

- ↓ or absent sphincter control
- Bowel incontinence
- Constipation

Musculoskeletal

- Fatigue
- Limb weakness
- Ataxic movements (shaky, irregular, uncoordinated)
- Intention tremors
- Spasticity
- Muscular atrophy
- Dragging of foot and foot drop
- Dysarthria with slurred speech

Reproductive

- Impotence (male)
- Loss of genital sensation
- Painfully heightened sensation (female)
- Vaginal dryness

Medication Administration 44.B

The Patient with Multiple Sclerosis

IMMUNOMODULATORS

glatiramer acetate

interferon beta-1a

interferon beta-1b

Administered to patients with relapsing-remitting MS to prolong the time of onset to disability. Their use is based on the assumption that MS is an immunologically mediated disease. Interferon beta-1b produces a decrease in the MS lesions in some patients. Anxiety, confusion, and depression with suicidal tendencies have also been reported. Adverse reactions include liver toxicity, anxiety, pain at the injection site, and generalized flulike manifestations (Adams et al., 2017).

Nursing Responsibilities

- Assess baseline parameters to evaluate drug side effects: Psychologic profile, liver function tests, and CBC with differential.
- Monitor CBC and liver function tests as prescribed.
- Assess injection site and report ulceration promptly (pain and redness are common reactions).
- Evaluate patient's baseline neurologic, sensory, and motor function. Monitor changes in condition and function.
- Report if patient is pregnant or breastfeeding.

Health Education for the Patient and Family

- These drugs may cause depression and thoughts of suicide; report these feelings immediately to the physician.
- Rotate injection sites; avoid areas that show skin reactions.
- Seek follow-up care to monitor neurologic changes, CBC, and liver function.
- Avoid individuals who are sick.
- Flulike symptoms may occur within hours to days of an injection.

ADRENOCORTICOSTEROID THERAPY

dexamethasone (Decadron)

methylprednisolone (Medrol, Solu-Medrol)

prednisone (Deltasone, Meticorten, Orasone)

Adrenocorticosteroids are used to treat exacerbations of MS. The drugs are given to suppress the immune system, implicated in the etiology of MS. If the drug is used long term, the usual steroid precautions are indicated, such as tapering of doses on discontinuation, monitoring for glucose intolerance, osteoporosis, and cataract formation. Use with caution in pregnant and lactating women.

MUSCLE RELAXANTS

baclofen (Lioresal)

dantrolene (Dantrium)

Muscle relaxants are given to patients with MS to relieve muscle spasms. Most muscle relaxants act by suppressing CNS reflexes that regulate muscle activity. Baclofen (Lioresal) is the first-line muscle relaxant used for MS (Luzzio, 2017). Caution should be used with baclofen therapy. Sudden withdrawal may cause seizures and paranoid ideation and should be discontinued over a slow taper. In contrast, dantrolene (Dantrium) is not a centrally acting muscle relaxant; rather, it acts directly on skeletal muscles. Use of muscle relaxants is contraindicated in patients with hepatitis or cirrhosis.

Nursing Responsibilities

- Evaluate baseline muscle strength and spasticity, range of motion (ROM), and dexterity.
- Maintain safety or fall precautions; dizziness and drowsiness are common side effects.
- Monitor liver function tests (enzymes and bilirubin) for signs of hepatotoxicity.

Health Education for the Patient and Family

- These drugs may cause sedative effects. Take appropriate safety measures (e.g., avoid driving).
- Avoid CNS depressants (antihistamines, alcohol); they can increase the sedative effects of the medication.
- If you are taking baclofen, do not suddenly stop the medication.
- Increase fiber and fluids in the diet to prevent constipation.
- Change positions slowly to minimize dizziness and other effects of orthostatic hypotension.

IMMUNOSUPPRESSANTS

azathioprine (Imuran)

methotrexate (Rasuvo)

Immunosuppressants are given to patients with MS because of the autoimmune component of the disease. Because these medications suppress the immune system, they put the patient at risk for opportunistic infections. Patients should be aware of this increased risk and avoid persons that are acutely ill.

Nursing Responsibilities

- Monitor baseline parameters: CBC with platelet count and differential, urinalysis, liver function tests, hepatitis profile.
- Assess for anemia: Fatigue, lethargy, pallor
- Watch for bleeding.
- Protect against and observe for subtle signs of infection.

Health Education for the Patient and Family

- Report infection, bleeding, and anemia immediately.
- Drink at least 2 L of fluid a day, and observe urine for blood.
- Report jaundice immediately.
- Check oral cavity daily for changes or ulcers.
- Avoid becoming pregnant while taking these drugs.
- Obtain follow-up care, including frequent blood tests.

Nutrition

Patients with MS may be overweight because of their inability to ambulate. Ideally, the patient should maintain a weight as close as possible to that recommended for the patient's height and body type; maintaining a healthy weight will help aid mobility.

As MS progresses, the patient's ability to prepare food and eat may be compromised. Changes in muscle tone, tremor, weakness, and ataxia all contribute to nutritional problems. Dysphagia is a common problem. The diet is adapted to accommodate changes in the patient's ability to chew and swallow, and collaboration with a dietitian will be important.

Rehabilitation

Physical and rehabilitative therapies are tailored to the patient's level of functioning. The long-term goal is to enable the patient to retain as much independence as possible, thereby enhancing the quality of life. One major intervention is to maintain and increase existing muscle strength. Many of the symptoms that are seen in MS can be helped with exercise and physical therapy, including spasticity, fatigue, and pain.

Spasticity is managed with stretching exercises, gait training, and braces, splints, or other assistive devices. To maintain balance, the patient is encouraged to widen the base of support by standing with the feet slightly apart. Walkers and canes may be weighted to provide support and balance for the ataxic patient.

An interprofessional approach to rehabilitation will provide supportive services: Speech therapy for problems with phonation, occupational therapy to maintain strength in the upper extremities and carry out ADLs, and occupational counseling. Referrals to an urologist are indicated for problems with urinary incontinence, urinary tract infections, retention, and impotence.

Surgery

Surgery may be indicated for patients who experience severe spasticity and deformity. However, physical therapy can prevent most severe problems. Surgical procedures that may be seen in MS patients include tendon release procedures (to help with range of motion) or placement of an intrathecal Baclofen pump (for spasticity) (Luzzio, 2017).

Nursing Care

Because the disease most often affects young adults, the psychosocial and economic effects can be devastating. People with MS have to make adjustments to body-image changes while simultaneously adapting to altered relationships and decreased earnings usually encountered with the disease. A once-healthy spouse may become wheelchair bound; an individual once independent may eventually become dependent for even the most basic ADLs. The unpredictable course of MS is a challenge for long-term planning. See the Case Study & Nursing Care Plan for the patient with MS on page 1646.

Assessment

Collect the following data through the health history and physical examination (see Chapter 41):

- *Health history:* History of childhood viral illnesses, geographic residence as a child, exposure to physical or emotional stressors (pregnancy/delivery, extremes of heat), medications, symptom onset, severity of manifestations
- *Physical assessment:* Affect, mood, speech, eye movements, gait, tremors, vision and hearing, reflexes, muscle strength and movement, sensation.

Priorities of Care

Interprofessional collaboration is extremely important for the care of the patient with MS (Newsome et al., 2016). Patients will need to interact with a variety of healthcare professionals and it is important that everyone is working toward the same goal. Patient education is an important nursing priority as compliance to treatment regimens is instrumental in preventing exacerbations.

Diagnoses, Outcomes, and Interventions

Interventions for the patient with MS vary with the acuity of exacerbations and the presenting problems. Many diagnoses relate to the inability to perform ADLs. Others reflect problems with musculoskeletal changes or altered nerve conduction.

Prevent Fatigue. Fatigue is experienced by almost all patients with MS. Fatigue in the patient with MS may be both primary and secondary. Primary fatigue is caused by the disease itself; secondary fatigue is the result of some of the pathophysiologic consequences of the disease. It is experienced both mentally and physically. Fatigue affects every aspect of the MS patient's life: The ability to remain independent and perform self-care, sexual function, mobility, airway clearance, and ultimately self-concept and coping. Fatigue will increase the MS patient's risk for falls. It is important to remember that the fatigue from chronic illnesses such as MS is very different from being tired and that rest and sleep may not result in improvement.

A great deal of teaching is needed to help the patient and family understand fatigue and how to adapt. Patients and families need assistance managing fatigue in a society in which energy is highly valued.

Expected Outcomes: The patient will be free of fatigue as evidenced by ability to complete self-care activities and other ADLs. The patient will be able to optimize independence and self-care by demonstrating ADL abilities, taking frequent rest periods, and maintaining adequate nutrition.

The nurse will:

- Assess degree of fatigue and identify contributing factors. The Fatigue Impact Scale may be used to assess the effect of fatigue on ADLs. *Fatigue is a subjective experience that needs to be evaluated thoroughly before planning can begin.*
- Arrange daily activities and ADLs to include rest periods, with regular rest periods between activities and preserving energy by eliminating unnecessary tasks or using an assistive device to perform tasks (Baixinho et al., 2016). *Rest is essential to manage feelings of fatigue; periods of relaxation may help replenish energy reserves.*
- Ask the patient to consider which activities are really necessary and to set priorities. *Prioritizing activities promotes independence and self-control.*

- Suggest performing tasks in the morning hours. *People usually have greater energy reserves in the morning hours and diminished reserves in the afternoon.*
- Advise to avoid temperature extremes, such as hot showers or exposure to cold. *Maintaining a relatively constant body temperature may avoid exacerbation of the disorder. Heat can delay impulse transmission across demyelinated nerves, which contributes to fatigue.*
- Provide interventions to relieve pain (a fairly common manifestation of MS). *Pain can increase fatigue; fatigue can increase the experience of pain. Greater than half of patients with MS will experience pain (Newsome et al., 2017).*
- Refer to the appropriate professionals to manage fatigue: Stress management groups, support groups, occupational or physical therapist, as indicated. *Support groups and therapy can facilitate self-management and improve coping.*

Encourage Self-Care. Patients with MS may need assistance with bathing, toileting, dressing, grooming, and feeding. The help needed can range from minimal guidance to total dependence. The patient's ability to perform self-care activities is the gauge by which family members and caregivers need to adjust assistance. Self-care encompasses both the decisions about care and the provision of care; most patients are capable of making decisions even after physical limitations prevent physical self-care. The need to maintain self-determination cannot be overemphasized and must be incorporated into each intervention. As the patient with MS ages, there may be even more need for teaching to provide self-care.

Delegating Nursing Care Activities

As appropriate and allowed by the designated duties and responsibilities of unlicensed assistive personnel, the nurse may delegate nursing care activities such as measuring fluid intake and output, collecting vital signs (including orthostatic vital signs), encouraging oral or enteral intake, positioning the patient, and providing skin care.

Transitions of Care

Following an overview of the disorder, the patient needs to understand how to prevent fatigue and exacerbations. Teach the patient to avoid stress, extremes of cold and heat, high humidity, physical overexertion, and infections because these may trigger a relapse of manifestations. Because approximately 30% of women in the postpartum period tend to relapse (Fugay, 2016), counseling about this risk is indicated. However, pregnancy itself seems to be protective against relapse. Also, address preventive measures to avoid risk of respiratory and urinary tract infections.

The inconsistent and erratic nature of MS can make teaching for self-care difficult. Initial teaching focuses on a realistic explanation of MS. Referral to a support group early in the course of the disease is indicated. Social support can make a positive difference in a patient's and family's ability to cope with MS. Address the following topics in preparing the patient for home care:

- Various treatment options and their side effects
- Ongoing care from nurses, counselors, and physical, occupational, and speech therapists, as well as the physician and community health nurse
- Helpful resources: National MS Society, Multiple Sclerosis Association of America, and the National Institute of Neurological Disorders and Stroke (NINDS).

Symptomatic treatment should be focused first on symptoms that pose an increased risk to the patient such as skin breakdown and falls (Newsome et al., 2017). Then, the priority should shift to symptom management that most affects quality of life and patient preferences. It is important to have open dialogue with the patient to understand how the symptoms are affecting them and what they see as the priority.

Patients with MS will require ongoing follow-up with their healthcare provider to evaluate effectiveness and adverse effects of medications and evaluation of lesions through MRI.

The Patient with Parkinson Disease

Parkinson disease (PD) is a progressive, degenerative neurologic disorder of **basal ganglia** function characterized by tremor (shaking), muscle rigidity, bradykinesia (slowness of movement), and postural instability (DeMaagd & Philip, 2015a). People with PD are faced with multiple problems involving independence in ADLs, emotional well-being, financial security, and relationships with others. Prognosis is poor, owing to the progressive degeneration that ultimately affects multiple physiologic systems and their function. Psychosocial effects are equally devastating, and the family needs more support as the patient's debilitation increases. The progression of PD is patient dependent and can eventually lead to total disability, leaving the patient wheelchair or bed bound (Oliver & Veronese, 2017).

PD is one of the most common neurologic disorders, affecting more than 1 million people in North America and more than 10 million people worldwide (Parkinson's Foundation, 2017b). It is estimated that approximately 60,000 new cases are identified each year in the United States (Parkinson's Foundation, 2017b).

The disorder usually develops later in life, but has been noted in adults under age 40 (DeMaagd & Philip, 2015a). Men are affected more often than women. There is a genetic link, with about 10 to 15% of PD patients having a family history of the disease (Parkinson's Foundation, 2017a). The cause of PD is still unknown, but is believed to be the result of environmental and genetic factors (Hauser, 2017).

Case Study & Nursing Care Plan

A Patient with Multiple Sclerosis

George McMurphy, a 45-year-old from northern Minnesota, was diagnosed with MS approximately 5 years ago. He states that he probably had mild symptoms as long ago as 10 years. He works as a manager for a large grocery store chain near his home. He lives at home with his wife and two children, ages 12 and 15. Recently, Mr. McMurphy has had increasing problems with urinary incontinence, lack of energy, weakness, extreme fatigue, and altered mobility from spasticity in his leg muscles. He has a fever, chest congestion, and a cough productive of green sputum. He is admitted to the hospital for evaluation and treatment of pneumonia and exacerbation of his MS.

ASSESSMENT

Denise Miller, RN, primary care nurse, is assigned to care for Mr. McMurphy. His major complaint is the inability to "bring up all this sputum; I feel rotten from being so congested. I hate not being able to get to work and for my wife having to tend to my personal needs." Vital signs are BP 134/84 mmHg, P 94 bpm, R 30/min, T 38.8°C (102°F). Mr. McMurphy is admitted for an acute exacerbation of the disorder, probably triggered by pneumonia. He will be treated with ACTH and intravenous antibiotics during this admission.

Mr. McMurphy is discharged 3 days following admission. He states that he feels stronger; on discharge, he has no problem clearing his airway. Although he continues to pace his activities to avoid fatigue, his muscle strength and "tiredness" have improved. He is able to complete ADLs unassisted.

Pulmonary function has returned to normal prehospitalization levels: ABGs and pulse oximetry are within normal limits. Both Mr. McMurphy and his wife have listed several ways to modify their daily routine to allow more rest and decreased stress. Follow-up visits to his primary care physician have been arranged, and the couple has been provided with information about the local MS support group.

DIAGNOSES

- Blocked airway related to lung infection and thick mucus
- Lack of mobility related to fatigue and spasticity
- Inability to perform ADLs related to muscle weakness

EXPECTED OUTCOMES

- Patient will be able to clear airway, with clear lungs on auscultation and pulse oximetry readings above 95%.
- Patient will be able to ambulate using assistive devices, if needed, and to take frequent rest periods during episodes of mobility.
- Patient will be able to perform self-care activities such as bathing, dressing, and feeding oneself without becoming overly fatigued and tired.
- Patient will be able to verbalize methods to adapt daily routine to patient's level of tolerance.

PLANNING AND IMPLEMENTATION

- Initiate pulmonary hygiene measures (e.g., incentive spirometry, turning, deep breathing and coughing, breathing exercises, and postural drainage) at least every 2 hours. Assess lung sounds, oxygen saturation, and ability to clear airway.
- Teach the importance of maintaining an oral fluid intake of at least 2000 mL/day to prevent tenacious sputum and urinary tract infections. Teach signs and symptoms of urinary and respiratory infections.
- Encourage participation in decision making about care.
- Assist with ADLs only as needed, based on level of fatigue and muscle weakness.
- Plan self-care activities so that they are performed during periods of peak level of energy; intersperse rest periods throughout the day.
- Refer to an MS support group.
- Refer to physical and occupational therapists for counseling regarding control of spasticity and possible splinting of spastic muscles.
- Consult a urologist for assessment of bladder incontinence; teach intermittent catheterization. Alternatively, the use of an external condom catheter may be indicated.

CLINICAL REASONING IN PATIENT CARE

1. Describe approaches the nurse could take to ensure that Mr. McMurphy does not exceed his activity tolerance.
2. Develop a teaching plan for Mr. McMurphy to help prevent future respiratory infections.
3. Develop a care plan for Mr. McMurphy to address his potential for injury related to fatigue, muscle weakness, and spasticity.

See Evaluating Your Response in Appendix B.

Parkinson-like manifestations, called *secondary parkinsonism*, may result from other disorders such as stroke, brain trauma, encephalitis, brain tumors, toxins, and drugs. Drug-induced parkinsonism, which is usually reversible, may occur in people taking neuroleptics, antiemetics, antihypertensives, and illegal designer drugs containing MPTP, a toxic chemical. Carbon monoxide or cyanide poisoning can also cause secondary parkinsonism. This discussion focuses on primary Parkinson disease.

Pathophysiology

Coordinated, voluntary body movement is achieved through the actions of **neurotransmitters** in the basal ganglia of the brain. Some neurotransmitters facilitate the transmission of excitatory nerve impulses, while other neurotransmitters inhibit their transmission. Together, this system allows control of movement. A disturbed balance between excitatory and inhibitory neurotransmitters causes disorders of voluntary motor function, such as PD.

In PD, neurons in the cerebral cortex atrophy and are lost, the **dopaminergic** nigrostriatal (pigmented) pathway degenerates, and the number of specific dopamine receptors in the basal ganglia decreases. These pathologic processes cause a decrease in the production of dopamine (a neurotransmitter that helps regulate nerve impulses involved in motor function) from the substantia nigra. The usual balance of dopamine (an inhibitory neurotransmitter) and acetylcholine (an excitatory neurotransmitter) in the brain is disrupted, and dopamine no longer inhibits acetylcholine. The failure to inhibit acetylcholine is the underlying basis for the manifestations of the disorder. In PD, 50 to 80% of the neurotransmitter dopamine may have been depleted before symptoms occur (DeMaagd & Philip, 2015a).

Throughout the progression of PD, Lewy bodies form in the brain, which cause lesions or plaques to form. It is thought that the Lewy bodies gradually spread throughout the nervous system, leading to increasing motor and nonmotor manifestations (Williams-Gray & Worth, 2016).

Manifestations

Parkinson disease begins with subtle nonmotor manifestations, which can be present for years before motor symptoms are realized (Williams-Gray & Worth, 2016). These early manifestations may include sleep disturbance, depression, and loss of sense of smell (Kalia & Lang, 2015). There are four common motor symptoms experienced by PD patients, including a resting tremor, rigidity, bradykinesia, and postural instability (DeMaagd & Philip, 2015a). See also Multisystem Effects of Parkinson Disease.

Tremor

Tremor at rest is usually the most visible manifestation, affecting the hands and feet, head, neck, face, lips and tongue, or jaw. The characteristic tremor is rhythmic, alternating flexion and contraction, and is initially unilateral. The tremor disappears with movement and sleep. As the disorder progresses, the tremor becomes bilateral. Patients have progressive impairment in performing skills that require dexterity and fine muscle control, such as writing and eating.

Rigidity and Bradykinesia

Manifestations related to motor and postural effects include rigidity, bradykinesia, and uncoordinated movements. Rigidity (resulting from involuntary contraction of all skeletal muscles) makes both active and passive movement difficult. It is manifested as increased resistance to passive ROM. Although the extremity moves, it does so in a jerky motion, called *cogwheel rigidity*. The first manifestation of rigidity may be muscle cramps in the toes or hands, but most often the patient describes stiffness, heaviness, or aching in muscles. Rigidity, which may result in flexion contractures, begins on one side of the body and progresses to become bilateral.

Bradykinesia, experienced as difficulty in starting, continuing, or coordinating movements, is the most common and crippling manifestation. All striated muscles are affected, including those that involve walking, turning, chewing, swallowing, and speaking. Slowed or delayed movements affect the eyes, mouth, and voice, causing a masklike face and softened or muffled voice. Disorders of swallowing result in problems with eating and with drooling. Patients have a staring gaze with minimal change in expression (**Figure 44.3** ■). Patients describe a sense of being frozen in place as voluntary movement is lost, and they stand, sit, or lie in one position without movement for long periods of time.

Abnormal Posture

The loss of normal postural reflexes results in postural abnormalities, including disorders of postural fixation, equilibrium, and righting. Involuntary flexion of the head

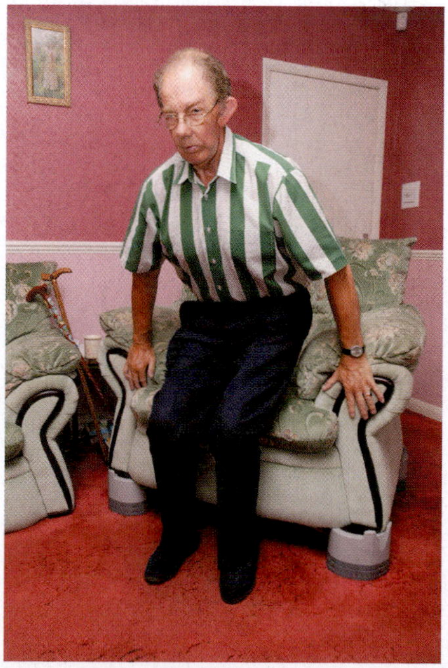

Figure 44.3 ■ Patients with Parkinson disease lack facial expression or animation.

Multisystem Effects of
Parkinson Disease

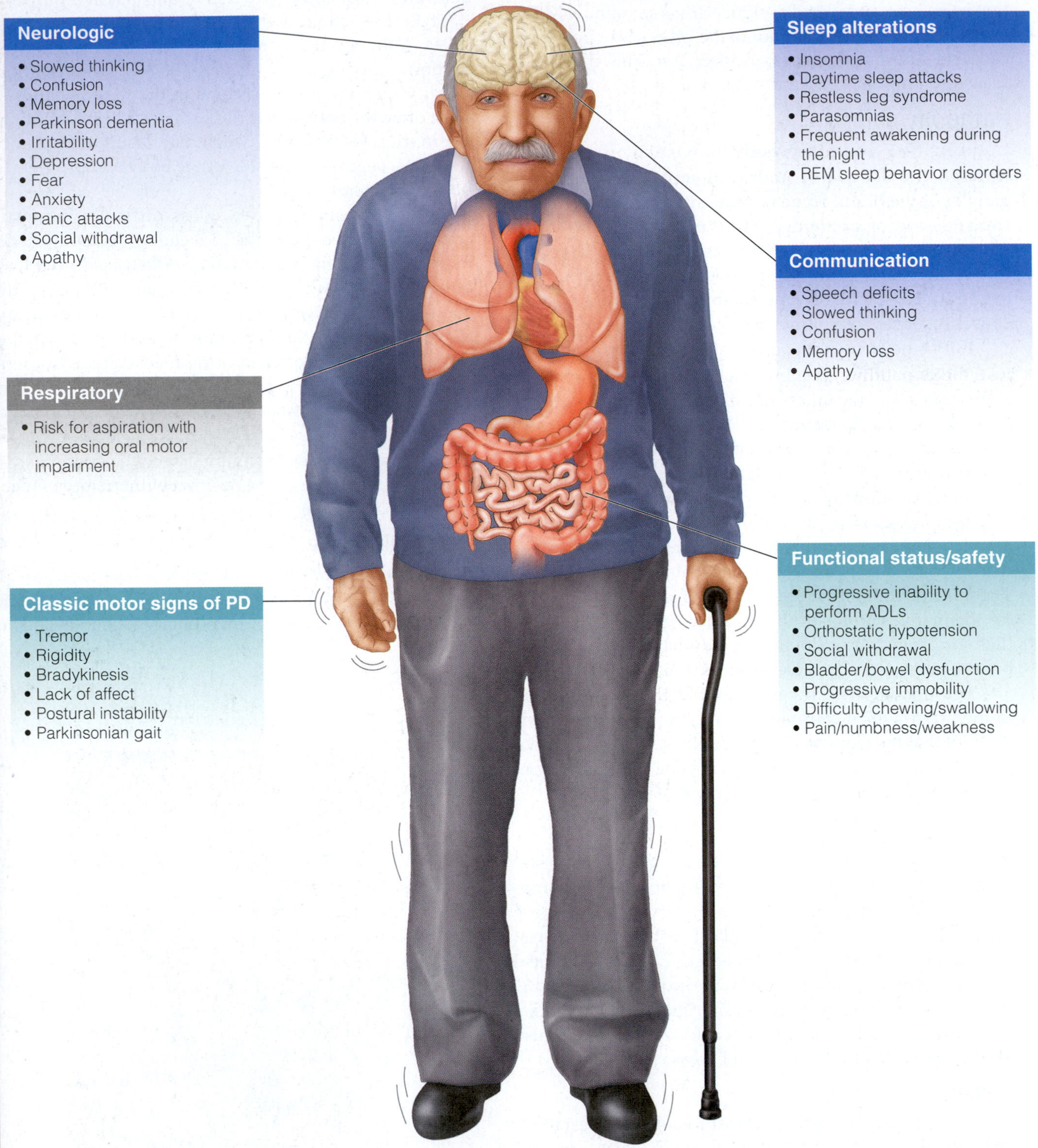
Neurologic
• Slowed thinking
• Confusion
• Memory loss
• Parkinson dementia
• Irritability
• Depression
• Fear
• Anxiety
• Panic attacks
• Social withdrawal
• Apathy
Sleep alterations
• Insomnia
• Daytime sleep attacks
• Restless leg syndrome
• Parasomnias
• Frequent awakening during the night
• REM sleep behavior disorders
Communication
• Speech deficits
• Slowed thinking
• Confusion
• Memory loss
• Apathy
Respiratory
• Risk for aspiration with increasing oral motor impairment
Functional status/safety
• Progressive inability to perform ADLs
• Orthostatic hypotension
• Social withdrawal
• Bladder/bowel dysfunction
• Progressive immobility
• Difficulty chewing/swallowing
• Pain/numbness/weakness
Classic motor signs of PD
• Tremor
• Rigidity
• Bradykinesis
• Lack of affect
• Postural instability
• Parkinsonian gait

and shoulders means the person with PD cannot maintain an upright position of the trunk when sitting or standing. This problem of postural fixation results in the characteristic stooped, leaning-forward position. Disorders of equilibrium follow loss of postural fixation with an inability to make adjustments when leaning or falling, increasing the risk of injury from falls (forward or backward). The patient takes short, shuffling steps to try to maintain an upright position when walking.

Autonomic and Neuroendocrine Effects

Many manifestations result from the loss of functions controlled by the autonomic nervous system. Elimination problems include constipation and urinary hesitation or frequency. Patients may experience problems related to orthostatic hypotension, including dizziness with position change. Eczematous skin changes and seborrhea are related to the increase in sweat gland activity secondary to increased sebotrophic hormone production.

Mood and Cognition

Both depression and dementia are pathologies associated with PD. Dementia occurs later in the disease process and is often associated with increased Lewy body formation (Sorenson et al., 2019). The patient has manifestations similar to the person with Alzheimer disease, including confusion, disorientation, memory loss, distractibility, and changes in abstraction and judgment.

Sleep Disturbances

Patients with PD commonly have sleep disturbances, although they may experience decreased manifestations during sleep in the early stages. The ability to fall and stay asleep is affected by acetylcholine. Muscle rigidity may compromise sleep because of the inability to change position. This lack of muscle movement causes the patient to awaken and consciously shift positions.

Interrelated Effects

Some of the manifestations that patients with PD experience have multiple contributing factors. For example, constipation is common because of decreased peristalsis. However, decreased peristalsis is not the only cause: Immobility, tremors (resulting in being unable to drink from a glass easily), and dietary changes from dysphagia all contribute to the problem of constipation.

Complications

The following complications are associated with Parkinson disease:

- Paranoia and hallucinations, which may accompany dementia
- Impaired communication due to changes in speech, handwriting, and expressiveness
- Falls from balance, posture, and motor changes as well as from postural hypotension
- Infections, such as pneumonia
- Malnutrition related to dysphagia and inability to prepare meals
- Altered sleep patterns due to loss of dopamine, Levodopa side effects (nightmares, dreams) or side effects of anticholinergics (hyperreflexia, muscle twitching), and depression
- Skin breakdown and pressure ulcers associated with urinary incontinence, malnutrition, and sweat reflex changes
- Depression and social isolation.

Interprofessional Care

At present there is no cure for PD, but medications bring dramatic improvement in manifestations. Diagnosis is based primarily on a thorough history and physical examination and is made based on having two of the three cardinal manifestations: Tremor at rest, bradykinesia, and rigidity. Interventions vary with the clinical stage of the disorder and include medication, surgery, and rehabilitation to retain the optimal level of functioning possible. An interprofessional approach is essential for these patients. Speech and swallowing problems can be addressed by a speech therapist, while a physical therapist helps the patient maintain independence and therefore increased quality of life. The pharmacy should be directly involved in the teaching related to medications, as should any community organizations that may enhance the patient's ability to remain independent. The team should work together to help improve the patient's quality of life, which should include both pharmacologic and alternative therapies (Cascaes da Silva et al., 2016; DeMaagd & Philip, 2015b). Evidence-based practice guidelines for the management of PD are available and should be utilized as appropriate.

Diagnosis

No diagnostic test differentiates Parkinson disease from other neurologic disorders; it is important to rule out other potential causes of symptoms in order to make an accurate diagnosis (Hauser, 2017).

Medications

The goal of drug therapy is to control manifestations to the greatest extent possible. Generally, medications vary with the stage of the disease; however, response is individualized and guides the selection of medications. Types of drugs used include monoamine oxidase B (MAO-B) inhibitors, dopaminergics, dopamine agonists, catelchol-o-methyltransferase inhibitors (COMT), and anticholinergics. Information about these drugs is presented in **Medication Administration 44.C**. It is important for patients and family members to know that each person must be individually evaluated, and if medications for PD become ineffective, others may be prescribed.

Other medications may be used to treat problems related to Parkinson disease, including antidepressants and laxatives or stool softeners.

Medication Administration 44.C

The Patient with Parkinson Disease

DOPAMINE PRECURSORS

carbidopa

levodopa

levodopa-carbidopa (Parcopa, Sinemet)

These drugs have their major effect on the akinesia of Parkinson disease, improving mobility while decreasing muscle rigidity and tremor. Levodopa is a metabolic precursor of dopamine, but unlike dopamine, it can cross the blood–brain barrier. Levodopa is converted to dopamine in the brain by decarboxylase, a catalytic enzyme, and stimulates dopamine receptors to balance the dopamine/acetylcholine concentrations. Carbidopa prevents decarboxylase from converting levodopa to dopamine in the peripheral tissues; therefore, carbidopa is frequently given in combination with levodopa. Amantadine is actually an antiviral drug that is often used in the early stages of PD to treat dyskinesia and also elevates mood.

Levodopa is avoided in patients with narrow-angle glaucoma, renal impairment, hepatic insufficiency, or melanoma. The "on–off" phenomenon occurs after the patient takes levodopa for several years; this phenomenon is characterized by unexpected dyskinesias (abnormal movements) and lack of symptom control.

Common side effects are nausea and vomiting; darkening of urine and sweat; dyskinesias, especially in the first few months of therapy; orthostatic hypotension; and psychologic reactions, such as hallucinations and vivid dreams.

Nursing Responsibilities

- Establish the patient's baseline functional abilities in performing ADLs and administering medication; assess motor control and coordination.
- To avoid adverse reactions, assess the patient's overall health status before initiating therapy.
- Monitor medications known to cause adverse drug interactions: Anticholinergics, pyridoxine, and antipsychotic agents alter the effectiveness of levodopa; MAO-B inhibitors can cause severe hypertension because of their vasoconstrictive effects.

Health Education for the Patient and Family

- Levodopa may not take effect for several weeks to months.
- Do not alter dosages of medications; taking more of a medication can cause severe side effects.
- Do not abruptly stop this medication as it could cause severe withdrawal symptoms that can mimic neuroleptic malignant syndrome (Adams et al., 2017).
- Divide protein intake into equal amounts for the day's meals. Avoid foods high in pyridoxine, such as pork, beef, ham, avocado, beans, and oatmeal.
- Levodopa may cause urine to darken, but this is harmless.
- To prevent side effects: Change position slowly to avoid a drop in blood pressure; prevent constipation by increasing fluid intake and exercising regularly.
- Notify practitioner if you begin to have difficulty making voluntary movements or if cardiac or psychologic symptoms develop.
- Watch for the "on–off" phenomenon, in which periods of symptom control alternate with periods when the drug fails to control symptoms.

MONOAMINE OXIDASE B INHIBITORS (MAO-B INHIBITORS)

rasagiline (Azilect)

selegiline (Eldepryl, Zelapar)

MAO-B inhibitors work by inhibiting the enzyme system that would otherwise break down and destroy dopamine as well as stimulating the dopamine receptors (Adams et al., 2017). Serious adverse effects include hallucinations, hepatotoxicity, and seizures. Based on adverse effects the dosages of these medications may need to be adjusted. Because it is highly selective for the MAO-A enzyme, selegiline does not have antidepressant.

Nursing Responsibilities

- Establish baseline functional abilities: Motor control and movements, position changes, and mental status.
- Monitor problems with insomnia.
- Assess for orthostatic hypotension; look for unsteadiness with position change and complaints of dizziness.
- Assess for hypertension, which can occur with higher-than-usual doses.

Health Education for the Patient and Family

- It is very important to take the medication as directed.
- Notify the practitioner if insomnia occurs.
- Report signs of dizziness when changing positions or standing, changes in ability to move, or psychologic changes.
- Change positions slowly, especially when moving from a sitting to a standing position.
- Keep follow-up appointments for evaluation of the medication's effectiveness.

DOPAMINE AGONISTS

bromocriptine (Parlodel)

pramipexole (Mirapex)

Dopamine agonists act by mimicking the role of dopamine in the brain. They can be used alone or in combination with levodopa therapy: When dopamine agonists are given with levodopa, they increase the therapeutic effects of levodopa and reduce fluctuations in motor symptoms. Adverse reactions are similar to those of levodopa: Nausea, orthostatic hypotension, and psychologic disturbances are common. Nursing responsibilities and patient and family teaching information are similar to those that apply to the dopaminergics; however, family members should know that these drugs may cause compulsive behavior.

CATECHOL-*O*-METHYLTRANSFERASE INHIBITORS

entacapone (Comtan)

tolcapone (Tasmar)

COMT inhibitors inhibit catechol-*O*-methyltransferase (COMT), which is responsible for metabolizing dopamine. The concurrent administration of a COMT inhibitor with levodopa increases the amount of levodopa available to the brain to control Parkinson disease.

Nursing Responsibilities

- Monitor liver function test results and manifestations of liver impairment (dark urine, jaundice).
- Administer with food.
- If given concurrently with warfarin, monitor PT and INR.

Health Education for the Patient and Family

- Avoid using alcohol and sedatives.
- Rise slowly from a sitting or lying position to avoid falling.
- Nausea is common at the beginning of therapy.
- Report increased loss of muscle control, yellow skin or eyes, dark urine, hallucinations, and severe diarrhea.

ANTICHOLINERGICS

benzotropine (Cogentin)

trihexyphenidyl (Artane)

Anticholinergics are effective in Parkinson disease because they block the excitatory action of the neurotransmitter acetylcholine. They are frequently used during the early stages of the disease. They may be given in combination with carbidopa-levodopa therapy. These medications ease drooling, tremors, and rigidity; however, side effects are common and may include blurred vision, dry mouth, constipation, and tachycardia.

Nursing Responsibilities

- Perform baseline assessment for presence of glaucoma, cardiac dysfunction, and prostatic hypertrophy.
- Note other medications, including OTC medications that have anticholinergic effects, such as antihistamines and tricyclic antidepressants.
- Monitor for side effects, especially changes in vision, urinary elimination, gastric emptying, and mentation.

Health Education for the Patient and Family

- Inform your practitioner if you begin taking any new medications or notice any new symptoms.
- Avoid overexposure to heat; take precautions to avoid heat stroke: Drink fluids, keep cool, avoid strenuous activity on hot days.
- Practice home safety to prevent falls.
- Avoid taking OTC antihistamines or sleeping aids; these have anticholinergic activity.
- Have the eyes examined annually to check for glaucoma; wear dark glasses if photophobia develops.

Moving Evidence into Action

Improving Motor Symptoms in Patients with Parkinson Disease

Clinical Issue

Parkinson disease causes progressive disabilities, which lead to the patient's inability to perform activities of daily living (ADLs) as well as a decreased quality of life. Improving motor function to help increase quality of life is one goal of medication treatment in PD. Unfortunately, after patients have been on their medications for several years, they are not as effective and can lead to increased "off-time," meaning the period when the medications wear off and are not as effective.

External Evidence

In a medication review, multiple studies were analyzed regarding the efficacy of carbidopa/levodopa extended release (ER) (Greig & McKeage, 2016). There is evidence to show carbidopa/levodopa ER medication helps to decrease the amount of off-time in PD patients without increasing dyskinesia by maintaining a steady release of the drug (Greig & McKeage, 2016).

Internal Evidence

Patients should be assessed for their compliance with medications and their ability to adequately prepare and self-administer the medications. Adverse effects of this medication are similar to immediate release carbidopa/levidopa (Greig & McKeage, 2016). The nurse should assess the patient for adverse effects including postural hypotension prior to administration.

Patient Consideration

Cost and availability of the medication should be evaluated. Patient teaching should be completed regarding potential adverse effects, dosing, and administration schedule. The nurse should work as part of the interdisciplinary team including the pharmacists and prescribers in order to provide individualized patient-centered care.

Putting the Pieces Together

Medication "off-time" can make the completion of ADLs difficult, which can lead to patient dissatisfaction. The nurse should be aware of interventions that can help improve motor symptoms. If appropriate interventions have not been ordered for the patient, the nurse must work with the interdisciplinary team and advocate for the appropriate evidence-based interventions.

Reference

Greig, S. L., & McKeage, K. (2015). Carbidopa/levodopa ER capsules (Rytary, Numient): A review in Parkinson's disease. *CNS Drugs, 30,* 79–90.

Nutrition

Patients should be encouraged to drink plenty of fluids and they should be monitored for signs of weight loss. High-protein diets should be avoided as this can interfere with the efficacy of some of the medications (DeMaagd & Philip, 2015a).

Surgery

Surgical treatment of PD may be used for patients who have had the disease for a long time and are no longer able to control manifestations with medications. The most commonly used procedure is deep brain stimulation (DBS). Treatment by DBS is used for carefully selected patients with advanced tremors. Contraindications for DBS include psychiatric issues and dementia (DeMaggd & Philip, 2015b).

In the surgery, an implanted pacemaker-like neurostimulator (about the size of a stopwatch) is implanted into the subthalamus area (a small structure deep in the subcortical area) of the brain. A lead wire is then connected to an implanted pulse generator (similar to an advanced cardiac pacemaker) (Pahwa, 2014). The electrical impulses from the generator stimulate the targeted area of the brain to interfere with and block the brain's electrical signals that cause the manifestations of PD. Although most people with PD will need to continue medications after having DBS, many are able to reduce the dosage as well as side effects (such as dyskinesias from long-term levodopa use). Following surgery, the patient is closely monitored for neurologic complications (such as weakness, confusion, decreasing LOC, seizures, or dysrhythmias), intracranial infections, and technology malfunction. Intracranial disorders are discussed in Chapter 42.

Research for the treatment and potential cure of PD is ongoing and currently include gene therapy, cell replacement therapy and vaccine therapy. Time will tell the success or failure of these treatments (William-Gray & Worth, 2016).

Integrative Therapies

Exercise is beneficial in helping increase strength and decrease the incidence of falls in PD patients (Cascaes da Silva, 2016; DeMaggd & Philip, 2015a). All therapies should be aimed at improving patient mobility and increasing quality of life.

Nursing Care

The chronic and eventually debilitating nature of PD poses many challenges to patients, families, and healthcare professionals. Dependence due to declining physical and mental abilities is of major concern. In the early stages, most patients are able to remain at home, with the family assisting with or providing many of the patient's ADL needs. As the disease progresses and the burden of care increases, the patient and family may prefer placement in a long-term care facility. See the Case Study & Nursing Care Plan for the patient with PD on page 1654.

Assessment

Collect the following data through the health history and physical examination (refer to Chapter 41). Further focused assessments are described with nursing interventions.

- ***Health history:*** Brain trauma, stroke, infection, exposure to heavy metals or carbon monoxide, medication and drug use, incontinence, constipation, weight loss, sweating, sleep problems, muscle pain, mood
- ***Physical assessment:*** Affect; appearance; speech; scalp, eyelashes, and skin; drooling; tremor; coordination; posture; gait; muscle rigidity; mental status.

Diagnoses, Outcomes, and Interventions

Patients with PD have complex and, ultimately, multisystem needs. Deficits in mobility and self-care are common. Psychosocial needs may include problems related to changes in body perception, coping, and feelings of powerlessness. This section focuses on the nursing diagnoses related to physical mobility, verbal communication, nutrition, and sleep patterns.

Promote Physical Mobility. Patients with PD have impaired mobility for several reasons, including tremors, gait pattern disturbances, and alterations in body positioning, such as forward bending of the trunk. Poor self-esteem may contribute to the patient's lack of motivation and willingness to be mobile.

Expected Outcome: Patient's deficits in mobility and self-care will be eliminated or minimized as evidenced by the patient being able to perform ADLs independently or with minimal assistance.

The nurse will:

- Suggest referral to a physical therapist to develop an individualized exercise program. *A program specific to the patient supplies motivation and also helps the patient maintain muscle tone, flexibility, and mobility.*
- Request the physical therapist teach caregivers how to do ROM exercises at least twice a day, emphasizing the trunk, neck, arms, hips, and legs. *Maintaining joint mobility promotes better function and strength, improving gait pattern. Consistent ROM exercises can prevent contractures.*
- Ask caregivers to ambulate the patient at least four times a day, if possible. *Exercise fosters independence and self-esteem.*
- Recommend assistive devices, such as lift chairs, canes, splints, or braces, as indicated. *Adaptive equipment improves balance, protects joints, and promotes proper anatomic positioning.*
- Promote mobility and safety by instructing the patient to:
  a. Slightly elevate the back legs of chairs and raise the toilet seat to help rise from a sitting position to a standing position.
  b. Wear shoes with Velcro closures.
  c. Remove potential hazards, such as unanchored throw rugs.
  d. Install handrails and nonskid surfaces in bathtubs and showers.
  e. Ensure adequate lighting throughout the home and in outside areas, especially in areas where transfers are common.

  Safety measures prevent potential complications that may result from falls or other accidents and promote self-esteem and quality of life through self-care. Individuals who have fallen, often have a fear of falling and will decrease activity to prevent a future occurrence; patient education on factors that lead to falls can help with overall understanding and future fall prevention (Lamont, 2017).

Promote Verbal Communication. Diminished vocal amplitude and loss of muscular control can impair the patient's ability to speak. Both caregivers and family members must remember to give patients enough time for self-expression; an unhurried approach is recommended. Seek input from family members when determining alternative methods of communicating with the patient.

Expected Outcome: The patient will use effective communication techniques.

The nurse will:

- Assess current communication abilities in speech, hearing, and writing. *Communication involves both sending and receiving messages.*
- Develop methods of communication appropriate to coordination abilities, such as a magic slate, flash cards with common phrases, and pointing to objects.

Individualizing a method of communication decreases anxiety and isolation.

- Suggest referral to a speech pathologist to develop oral exercises and interventions that will facilitate speaking. *The muscles of speech and swallowing are affected by the Parkinson disease process.*
- Remind patient to speak more loudly, if possible. *A low, monotonous voice is characteristic of the patient with Parkinson disease.*

Promote Adequate Nutrition. Tremors, altered gait, and impaired chewing and swallowing can cause nutritional problems in the patient with PD. As the disorder progresses, interventions for ensuring optimal nutrition need to be adapted to the patient's functional abilities. Assess the patient's swallow reflex before starting any feeding program.

Expected Outcome: The patient will maintain adequate nutrition by use of appropriate and safe individualized interventions.

The nurse will:

- Assess nutritional status and self-feeding abilities; suggest referral to an occupational or speech therapist, if needed. *An initial assessment of abilities ensures that interventions are personalized to the patient's current functional abilities.*
- Teach caregivers how to prepare foods of proper consistency as determined by swallowing function. *The patient may aspirate food that is too liquid.*
- Weigh weekly. *Early recognition of weight loss allows for intervention.*
- Teach eating methods to decrease tremors, such as holding a piece of bread in the hand that is not holding an eating utensil. *Nonintention tremor may be reduced through purposeful activity.*
- Encourage diet that is high in bulk and fluids. *Several anti-Parkinson medications and inactivity can cause constipation.*

Manage Sleep Pattern. Rigidity and weakness can cause patients with Parkinson disease to lose the ability to move and change positions during sleep. The resulting discomfort causes periods of wakefulness. Medications to treat Parkinson disease contribute to sleep pattern disturbance; for example, levodopa can cause vivid dreams. Nurses can help accurately assess the sleep pattern disturbance and can plan interventions to improve or increase sleep time.

- Assess sleep pattern and existing conditions that may affect sleep, such as depression or pain. *Patients experiencing anxiety, depression, and dementia have a difficult time falling asleep and may wake up more often at night.*
- Explain the disease process and the effects of decreased dopamine on the sleep–wake cycle. *Depending on the dosage, levodopa causes less REM sleep and deep sleep.*
- Review the patient's medication. *Levodopa can cause vivid dreams. Other medications (diuretics and hypnotics) may also interfere with sleep.*
- Teach how to modify lifestyle activities that affect sleep and mobility (refer also to BOX 3.1, Good Sleep Hygiene, in Chapter 3):
    a. Institute a routine of activities with limited rest periods during the day; avoid napping close to bedtime. Avoid strenuous exercise in the evening. *Daytime sleeping may contribute to a decrease in nighttime sleeping. Vigorous exercise just before bedtime may act as a stimulant.*
    b. Incorporate diet modifications, such as limiting caffeine and alcohol intake. *Caffeine is a stimulant, and alcohol may cause early-morning awakenings, increased daytime sleepiness, and nightmares.*
    c. Adapt the environment to aid in sleep (e.g., darken the room and decrease noise). *Reducing environmental stimuli decreases external sleep disturbances.*

SAFETY ALERT: Remember to assess pain status; lack of adequate pain control may interfere with sleep as well as with mobility/balance. ■

Delegating Nursing Care Activities

As appropriate and allowed by the designated duties and responsibilities of unlicensed assistive personnel, the nurse may delegate nursing care activities such as monitoring diet intake and output to determine diet restrictions (limiting alcohol/caffeine, promoting milk at bedtime). Other activities to be delegated are promoting patient exercise during the day and restricting it at night and creating an optimal environment for sleep (darkened and quiet room).

Transitions of Care

Teaching preventive measures is extremely important when caring for patients who have symptoms of Parkinson disease. Preventing malnutrition, falls and other environmental accidents, constipation, skin breakdown from incontinence or immobility, and joint contracture requires teaching and reinforcement.

In addition to incorporating information about safety needs, teach ways to prevent orthostatic hypotension when the patient changes positions; some patients may benefit from wearing individually fitted compression hose. Address safety considerations for proper administration of medications.

It is important for both the patient and the family to maintain independence and self-care as long as possible. To maintain function and quality of life, the following topics should be addressed:

- Realistic expectations
- Equipment suppliers
- Home environment conducive to using equipment
- Referrals to speech therapist, occupational therapist, physical therapist, and dietitian
- Gait training and exercises for improving ambulation, speech, swallowing, and self-care
- Increased fluid intake of 3000 mL/day and increased fiber in every meal

- Stool softeners or laxatives as needed for bowel elimination
- Swallowing during eating and taking medications (Have suction equipment available and know the Heimlich maneuver if choking occurs.)
- Foods that can be easily swallowed (such as pureed or soft) and have six small meals a day, if possible
- Helpful resources:
  a. American Parkinson's Disease Association
  b. National Parkinson Foundation, Inc.
  c. Parkinson's Disease Foundation
  d. National Institute of Neurological Disorders and Stroke.

Case Study & Nursing Care Plan

A Patient with Parkinson Disease

Stanley Ralph, age 78, was diagnosed with PD at age 64. His wife died 5 years ago and he has no other living family. Mr. Ralph worked for more than 40 years as a mechanic in a large factory. He is a resident of a long-term care facility. During a clinic visit for a review of his medications, the following assessment was made.

ASSESSMENT

While the nurse practitioner, José Martenaz, is conducting the assessment on Mr. Ralph, he makes the following assessments. Mr. Ralph has had a history of PD for 14 years, The physical assessment demonstrates oily and damp skin, lack of face expressions, tremors in both hands and feet, and slurred speech that is also slow in tempo. Mr. Ralph's gait is slow and shuffling. José reviews the medical record and notes that Mr. Ralph has lost 4.5 kg (10 lb) in the past 3 months. There has not been a change in Mr. Ralph's medication of levodopa with carbidopa. Finally when asked, Mr. Ralph stated his major problems are "eating, bowels, and walking."

DIAGNOSES

- Constipation related to lack of exercise, decreased food intake, and effects of medications
- Difficulty speaking related to lip tremors, slow/slurred speech, and facial muscle involvement of PD
- Inadequate nutrition related to difficulty swallowing and chewing
- Limited mobility related to rigidity and bradykinesia

EXPECTED OUTCOMES

- Patient will have a soft stool at least every other day.
- Patient will practice exercises provided by physical therapist twice a day.
- Patient will increase number of calories, fluids, and fiber in diet provided at long-term care facility.
- Patient will improve joint mobility and ability to ambulate.

PLANNING AND IMPLEMENTATION

- Discuss problems with bowel elimination with staff at long-term care facility; suggest increasing fluids to 3000 mL/day and also increasing fiber in the diet with oatmeal for breakfast, and more fruits and vegetables at meals.
- Encourage exercises provided by speech therapist to improve speech and swallowing. If these are not effective, make a referral for another evaluation.
- Discuss diet plan with dietitian at the long-term care facility, including consistency of foods and number of calories. Suggest dietitian be a part of swallowing evaluation conducted by the speech therapist.
- Refer for physical therapy and occupational therapy for a program to improve gait and joint mobility and to decrease risk of falling.

EVALUATION

In a return visit 3 months later, Mr. Ralph reports that "my bowels are working better." He has gained 3.2 kg (7 lb), and the staff report that this is related to multiple factors, including practicing his swallowing exercises, getting more exercise that stimulated his appetite, and changing his diet to six small meals a day of soft or pureed foods. The staff is offering him liquids at meals and snack times, and he usually drinks all they give him. His speech is not much improved. His posture and gait are somewhat better, and he is doing the exercises provided by the physical therapist and occupational therapist. Mr. Ralph's functional abilities have improved so much that the staff is considering training sessions specific to care of residents with PD.

CLINICAL REASONING IN PATIENT CARE

1. Although Mr. Ralph did not mention it, the staff reports that he is frustrated by not being able to dress himself. What suggestions could you make to facilitate his independence?
2. Mr. Ralph spends most of his time alone, although he enjoys the company of the other residents. List assessments and interventions to increase his diversional activity.
3. The loss of his wife and the debilitating effects of his disease increase Mr. Ralph's risk for experiencing complicated grief. What might you suggest the long-term staff do to reduce this risk? Are there other resources that might assist him with this problem?

See Evaluating Your Response in Appendix B.

The Patient with Huntington Disease

Huntington disease (HD) is a progressive, degenerative, inherited neurologic disease characterized by increasing dementia and **chorea** (jerky, rapid, involuntary movements). It is an autosomal-dominant inherited disease that is generally fatal within 15 to 20 years of diagnosis (Dayalu & Albin, 2015). There is no cure for the disease; treatment is focused on symptom management.

Because the patient is usually asymptomatic until age 30 to 40, he or she may already have passed the gene to the next generation. The psychologic effect is devastating to patients and their families. The family not only experiences guilt from passing the disease from one generation to the next, but is also faced with the overwhelming long-term care needs of those affected. It is common for several family members to have the disease.

Early manifestations of personality change include severe depression, memory loss with decreased ability to concentrate, emotional lability, and impulsiveness. The patient experiences frequent mood swings ranging from uncontrollable periods of anger to apathy. Eventually, signs of dementia, including disorientation, confusion, and lack of sense of time, become evident and interfere with self-care.

Initially, movement problems are described as fidgeting or restlessness, followed by progressive worsening of abnormal movements. Choreiform movements, which begin in the face and arms and then involve the entire body, are manifested by facial grimaces, tongue protrusion, jerky movement of the distal arms or legs, and a rhythmic, lurching gait that almost resembles a dance. (The term *chorea* comes from *choreia*, a Greek word meaning "dance.") Gait changes cause uncoordinated movements and contribute to frequent falls.

The manifestations slowly progress after initial manifestations appear. Prognosis is poor, with inevitable debilitation and total dependence. Death usually results from aspiration pneumonia or another infectious process.

Initially, much of the nursing care focuses on teaching about the disease, psychologic support, and genetic counseling. As manifestations become more severe, nursing considerations center on problems related not only to immobility and altered nutrition, but also to the increasing self-care deficits.

The Patient with Amyotrophic Lateral Sclerosis

Amyotrophic lateral sclerosis (ALS), or *Lou Gehrig's disease* (named for a famous baseball player who died of the disease), is a rapidly progressive and fatal degenerative neurologic disease characterized by weakness and wasting of muscles under voluntary control, without any accompanying sensory changes. For most patients cognitive functioning remains intact, however, dementia may be seen in some patients (Bellomo & Cichminski, 2015).

ALS is a rare disorder that affects approximately 20,000 to 30,000 individuals in the United States (Bellomo & Cichminski, 2015). In up to 90 to 95% of cases, the disease occurs at random without clearly associated risk factors. About 5 to 10% of all cases are inherited in what is termed *familial ALS*. Most of the health problems a patient with ALS encounters are related to swallowing and managing secretions, communication, and dysfunction of the muscles used in respiration. The average survival after onset of ALS manifestations is 3 to 5 years, with most deaths caused from respiratory failure (Bellomo & Cichminski, 2015).

Pathophysiology

ALS causes degeneration of upper and lower motor neurons and eventual death of the motor neuron. Once death of the neuron occurs, the patient is no longer able to voluntarily control muscle movement (Bellomo & Cichminski, 2015). Scarring or sclerosis also occurs on the lateral corticospinal tract (Sorenson et al., 2019).

Manifestations

The initial manifestations relate to dysfunction of upper motor neurons, lower motor neurons, or both. Dysfunction of UMNs results in spastic, weak muscles with increased deep tendon reflexes. Dysfunction of LMNs results in muscle flaccidity, paresis (weakness), paralysis, and atrophy.

Muscle twitches or weakness in an extremity and slurred speech are common early manifestations. The weakness may initially affect only one muscle group. Manifestations vary according to the particular muscle group involved; fasciculations (twitching) of involved muscles are common in the early stage of the disorder. With the loss of muscle innervation, the muscles atrophy, and paralysis results. Muscle mass decreases, and patients complain of progressive fatigue.

Increasing brainstem involvement causes progressive atrophy of the tongue and facial muscles with eventual dysphagia and dysarthria. Emotional lability and loss of control occur. Muscle weakness and atrophy eventually mean that as the disease progresses, the patient is unable to stand, walk, or use the hands or arms and requires ventilatory support to breathe.

Interprofessional Care

Because many treatable disorders may cause manifestations similar to those that appear in the initial stage of ALS, a thorough evaluation is required. Once ALS is diagnosed, the primary goal is to support the patient and family in meeting physical and psychosocial needs, particularly as the disease progresses. There is no cure for ALS.

Medical and nursing care for patients with ALS is primarily supportive. Referral for home health management is indicated. Occupational, physical, speech, and respiratory therapy are major supportive and rehabilitative treatments. As the disorder progresses and swallowing becomes ineffective, a gastrostomy tube may be necessary to provide adequate nutritional intake. Ventilatory assistance should be discussed with patients before the need occurs.

Medications

Riluzole (Rilutek), an antiglutamate, is the first medication developed to treat ALS. It inhibits the presynaptic release of glutamic acid in the CNS and protects neurons against the excitotoxicity of glutamic acid.

In 2014, the "ice bucket challenge" became a popular way to bring awareness to ALS and, ultimately, millions of dollars in donations. According to the ALS Association (2017), these donations helped with approval of a new medication, Radicava, to help treat ALS. This medication is used to help slow down degeneration of motor function (ALS, 2017).

Nursing Care

Nursing care focuses on current health problems and on anticipating future difficulties. As with other disorders causing incapacitation and dependence, individualized nursing goals and interventions relate to decreasing complications, especially those associated with loss of muscular function and immobility; promoting independence to the extent possible; initiating referrals, particularly to a support group for both patient and family; and providing physical and psychosocial support as indicated.

Of special consideration is planning for the patient's eventual inability to communicate. Because the patient's eye muscles and movements remain intact, signals can be prearranged before the loss of speech.

Diagnoses, Interventions, and Outcomes

Two priorities of care that are frequently needed for patients with ALS are promoting physical mobility and promoting effective breathing

Promote Physical Mobility. Patients with ALS are at risk for developing problems associated with bedrest, not only because they cannot move and reposition themselves, but also because they frequently have altered nutritional and hydration status. Nursing interventions focus on preventing skin breakdown and infections, such as urinary tract infections.

Expected Outcome: In patients with ALS, independence in physical mobility will be maintained or improved by demonstration of physical movement, exercise, and performance of daily activities that are consistent with patient's abilities.

The nurse will:

- Assess current condition for baseline parameters, particularly skin over bony prominences, lung sounds, and vital signs. *Understanding patient's current condition allows accurate future assessment and realistic planning.*
- Assess skin, provide skin care, and obtain an alternating-pressure mattress. *Pressure points are at risk for breakdown; early detection is crucial to instituting appropriate care.*
- Institute active ROM exercises as the patient is able. Perform passive ROM exercises every 2 hours, when the patient is turned. *Contractures can develop within a week because extensor muscles are weaker than flexor muscles.*
- Maintain positive nitrogen balance and hydration status. Monitor prealbumin levels, hemoglobin and hematocrit levels, and urine specific gravity. *Adequate protein is required to maintain osmotic pressure and prevent edema; positive nitrogen balance promotes optimal body functioning.*

SAFETY ALERT: Urinary tract infection (UTI) is indicated by cloudy, foul-smelling urine, pain on urination, fever, and general malaise. Nursing priorities are early detection of such symptoms in order to prevent urosepsis. ■

Promote Effective Breathing. As the muscle weakness of ALS continues, patients become less able to breathe. The respiratory muscles are affected, and patients eventually may require ventilatory assistance. The nurse initiates measures to support the existing respiratory effort.

Expected Outcome: Patient's ineffective breathing patterns will be eliminated by demonstration of coughing, deep breathing, and expectoration of any secretions, as well as evidence of normal respiratory rate, lungs that are clear to auscultation, well-perfused skin and mucous membranes (pink), and normal range of pulse oximetry.

The nurse will:

- Obtain a baseline assessment of breathing pattern, air movement, and oxygen saturation. *Assessments indicating the patient's current condition provide data to plan individualized interventions.*
- Turn at least every 2 hours. *Movement enhances the ability to move pulmonary secretions and prevents stasis.*
- Elevate the head of the bed at least 30 degrees, suction as indicated, and provide oxygen. *This supports ventilation and enhances lung expansion as the patient's condition changes.*
- Monitor temperature and lung sounds routinely; obtain sputum culture as indicated. *Early detection of a possible infectious process leads to prompt treatment.*

Transitions of Care

Initial teaching centers on explaining the disease process, expected course, and prognosis. Referral to a social worker to determine home care needs and financial assistance is helpful. Counseling and referrals to a home health agency, dietitian, and physical, speech, and occupational therapists can help the family meet the patient's changing needs and abilities. The realistic anticipation of needs cannot be overemphasized.

As the patient becomes more debilitated, family members or other care providers focus on preventing complications. For example, family members need to know how to suction the patient and perform the Heimlich maneuver to prevent aspiration. Teaching the family how to prevent problems related to immobility is a primary consideration for the nurse. Another focus of teaching is basic care needs, such as care required to meet elimination needs. Teach families methods to establish a bowel routine, considerations related to a urinary catheter, and the need to promptly report manifestations of an infection.

Moving Evidence into Action
Respiratory Failure in Patients with ALS

Clinical Issue

Mortality in ALS is generally due to respiratory failure related to diaphragm weakness. Some patients will choose to be placed on mechanical ventilation as a means of life support. However, only around 5 to 10% of all ALS patients will choose permanent mechanical ventilation (Bellomo & Cichminski, 2015). Other methods of assisting patients with ventilation have been evaluated, including the use of diaphragm pacing.

External Evidence

Diaphragm pacing is a technique used to help stimulate the muscle contraction of the diaphragm to aid in respiration (Onders, Elmo, Kaplan et al., 2014). A pilot study was conducted on 16 patients with ALS to assess the therapeutic effects of diaphragm pacing (Onders et al., 2014). This study showed diaphragm pacing helped prolong life by a few months when tracheostomy ventilation was not used as treatment. The FDA has cleared diaphragm pacing for use in ALS patients as an intervention with few adverse effects and likely benefit (Onders et al., 2014). As this was a pilot study, further evaluation of the diaphragm pacing is needed to show efficacy in ALS patients.

Internal Evidence

ALS is generally fatal within 3 to 5 years. Diaphragm pacing helps to prolong life without tracheostomy ventilation; however, this is not a cure. It is important for the nurse to talk with the patient and their families and understand their goals of treatment.

Putting the Pieces Together

There is evidence to suggest that diaphragm pacing can be beneficial for ALS patients. The nurse should work with the patient and their families to educate them on diaphragm pacing and let them know the risks and potential benefits. The nurse should collaborate with the interdisciplinary team to advocate for their patients' treatment goals.

Reference

Onders, R. P., Elmo, M. J., Kaplan, C., Katirji, B., & Schilz, R. (2014). Final analysis of the pilot trial of diaphragm pacing in amyotrophic lateral sclerosis with long-term follow-up: Diaphragm pacing positively affects diaphragm respiration. *American Journal of Surgery, 207,* 393–397.

44.2 Peripheral Nervous System Disorders

Many etiologic agents are responsible for peripheral nervous system (PNS) disorders. Autoimmune disorders, viruses, environmental toxins such as heavy metals, and nutritional deficiencies can affect the PNS.

The Patient with Myasthenia Gravis

Myasthenia gravis (MG) is a chronic autoimmune neuromuscular disorder characterized by fatigue and severe weakness of skeletal muscles. Patients experience periods of remission and exacerbation, and mild forms of the disorder exist. Weakness may remain limited to a few muscle groups, especially the ocular muscles, or may become generalized with all muscles eventually becoming weakened. MG is another rare neurological disease with approximately 36,000 to 60,000 patients suffering with MG in the United States (Howard, 2015).

Pathophysiology

MG is an autoimmune disorder that affects the neurotransmitter acetylcholine. Acetylcholine helps to stimulate muscle contraction. In MG, antibodies destroy or block neuromuscular junction receptor sites. Even though there is enough acetylcholine in the body, acetylcholine is not able to attach to receptor sites and stimulate muscle contraction. The result is a decrease in the muscle's ability to contract. A comparison of a normal neuromuscular junction and one affected by MG is shown in **Figure 44.4** ■.

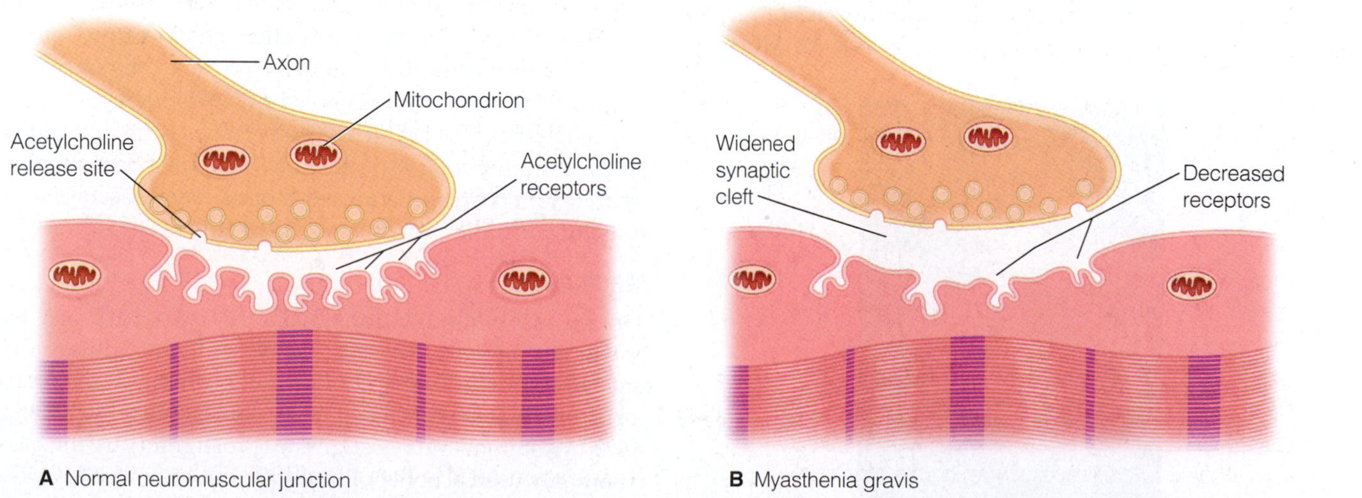
Axon
Mitochondrion
Acetylcholine release site
Acetylcholine receptors
Widened synaptic cleft
Decreased receptors
A Normal neuromuscular junction
B Myasthenia gravis

Figure 44.4 ■ **A**, A normal neuromuscular junction and **B**, one showing the changes seen in myasthenia gravis. These changes interfere with the transmission of nerve impulses to the muscle.

In most patients with MG, the thymus gland, which is usually inactive after puberty, continues to produce antibodies because of hyperplasia of the gland or because of tumors. It is believed that the thymus is a source of an autoantigen that triggers an autoimmune response in MG. The exact mechanism and reason for the thymus gland's antibody production are unknown. MG is sometimes associated with thyrotoxicosis (hyperthyroidism), rheumatoid arthritis, and lupus erythematosus. The disorder is often diagnosed when a patient seeks treatment for a coincidental infection that exacerbates manifestations. Exacerbations may also occur before the menstrual period and during or soon after pregnancy.

Manifestations

The manifestations of MG correspond to the muscles involved. Initially, the eye muscles are affected and the patient experiences either diplopia (unilateral or bilateral double vision) or ptosis (drooping of the eyelid) (**Figure 44.5** ■). Next, the facial, speech, and mastication muscles become weak, and patients may have periods of dysarthria (speech disorder) and dysphagia (difficulty swallowing). Fatigue is evident even when the patient tries to eat a meal; the chewing muscles tire, and the patient is forced to stop eating momentarily. A smile becomes a snarl or grimace, and the voice is weak with a muffled nasal quality. Problems performing fine motor movements of the hands, such as writing, appear early in the disease.

As the disease progresses, the muscles of the neck and extremities are affected. When the muscles of the neck become affected, the head juts forward. Deep tendon reflexes are usually normal, however, even in weak muscles. Fatigue and weakness are exacerbated with stress, fever, overexertion, and exposure to heat and are relieved by rest. Manifestations vary on a daily basis.

Complications

Complications are directly related to the degree of muscle weakness and the specific muscles involved. For example, when the pharyngeal and palatal muscles are affected, the patient cannot manage swallowing and may aspirate food or fluids. The patient is at increased risk for pneumonia because weakness of the diaphragm and muscles of respiration compromises gas exchange. Patients with MG can develop life-threatening emergencies, including myasthenic crisis and cholinergic crisis. Ventilation and oxygenation take priority when the patient is in crisis (Goldenberg, 2016).

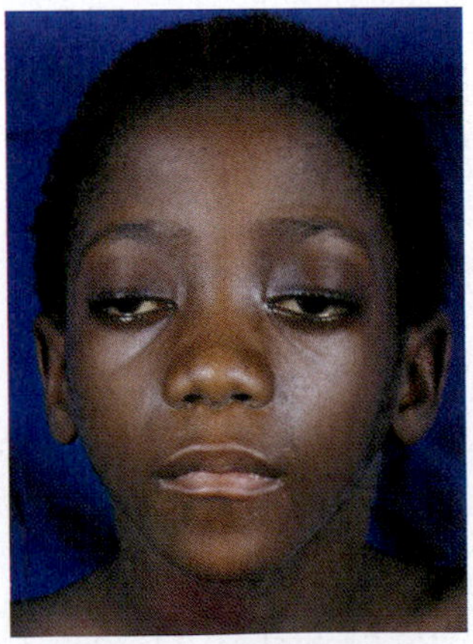

Figure 44.5 ■ In myasthenia gravis, the patient experiences unilateral weakness of the facial muscles.

Myasthenic Crisis

Myasthenic crisis is a sudden exacerbation of motor weakness, putting the patient at risk of respiratory failure and aspiration. Myasthenic crisis is most often due to undermedication, missed doses of medication, or a developing infection. Manifestations of myasthenic crisis include tachycardia, tachypnea, severe respiratory distress, dysphagia, restlessness, impaired speech, and anxiety.

Cholinergic Crisis

Cholinergic crisis is the result of overdosage with the anticholinesterase (cholinergic) medications used to treat MG. Gastrointestinal manifestations, severe muscle weakness, vertigo, and respiratory distress are signs of cholinergic crisis. Both types of crises are emergency, life-threatening situations; patients frequently require ventilatory assistance. As both myasthenic crisis and cholinergic crisis present similarly, it can be difficult to differentiate between the two (Goldenberg, 2016).

Interprofessional Care

Care of the patient with MG focuses on providing appropriate treatment, preventing complications, and supporting the patient and family in meeting physical and psychosocial needs, especially as the disease progresses.

Diagnosis

Diagnostic tests are conducted following a thorough history and physical examination, with special attention to the facial, oculomotor, laryngeal, and respiratory muscles. Diagnostic tests include the anticholinesterase (Tensilon) test, nerve stimulation studies, and an analysis of antiacetylcholine receptor antibodies.

In the Tensilon test, the patient is injected with edrophonium chloride (Tensilon), a short-acting anticholinesterase. Patients with MG show a significant improvement in muscle strength that lasts approximately 5 minutes. This test is also used to differentiate myasthenic crisis (caused by insufficient medication, so the patient shows improvement with the drug) from cholinergic crisis (caused by overmedication, so the patient does not show improvement).

Single-fiber electromyography can detect delayed or failed neuromuscular transmission in muscle fibers supplied by a single nerve fiber. Serum assay of circulating acetylcholine receptor antibodies, if increased, is strongly diagnostic of MG.

Medications

The primary medications used to treat MG are the anticholinesterases. These drugs act at the neuromuscular junction and allow acetylcholine to concentrate at the receptor sites, thus promoting muscle contraction. Pyridostigmine (Mestinon) and neostigmine (Prostigmin) are the most commonly used acetylcholinesterase inhibitors for MG. The patient's decrease in manifestations guides dosage.

Immunosuppression with glucocorticoids, typically prednisone, is another pharmacologic therapy aimed at improving muscle strength. Patients must be aware of the need to stay on the drug at the prescribed dose to determine the least amount required for efficacy. If patients do not respond to prednisone alone, it may be combined with other immunosuppressive agents, such as cyclosporine or azathioprine (Imuran). Medications used to treat MG are discussed in **Medication Administration 44.D**.

Surgery

Thymectomy is often recommended for patients younger than age 60. The two surgical approaches used are the transcervical approach, which is considered less invasive, and the transsternal approach. The latter approach allows a more extensive removal of the gland; however, it also poses more potential complications because it involves splitting the sternum.

Preoperatively, patients may be tapered from steroid therapy. Usually, pyridostigmine is administered to prevent muscular manifestations during the perioperative period. Postoperative nursing care focuses on preventing complications and controlling pain. Remission may take several years to achieve. Refer to Chapter 36 for care of the patient having a thoracotomy and chest tubes. A tracheostomy may be required when the diaphragm or intercostal muscles are involved.

Plasmapheresis

Plasma exchange in MG is used as a temporary solution to worsening symptoms (Howard, 2015). The goal of therapy is to remove the antiacetylcholine receptor antibodies, thus improving severe muscle weakness, fatigue, and other manifestations. The procedure is frequently performed when respiratory muscle involvement is evident. See **Figure 44.6** ■ and **Box 44.2** for nursing care of the patient undergoing plasmapheresis.

Nursing Care

Because avoiding fatigue is a major part of teaching, it is important to incorporate interventions to enhance rest and conserve energy. For example, suggest sitting while preparing meals and while performing hygiene and grooming. Anticipating problems, such as impaired communication, and developing alternative solutions can be helpful in promoting independence.

Diagnoses, Interventions, and Outcomes

Nursing care of patients with MG focuses not only on present problems but also on anticipated needs. Preventing myasthenic and cholinergic crises and providing psychologic support to patients and families are two important aspects of care. Individualized care depends on the specific therapy instituted.

Maintain Effective Airway Clearance. The underlying causes of ineffective airway clearance for the person with MG include poor cough mechanism, decreased rib cage expansion, diminished diaphragm movement, and decreased expiratory effort. The following interventions require particular attention if the patient undergoes a thymectomy.

Medication Administration 44.D

The Patient with Myasthenia Gravis

ANTICHOLINESTERASES/CHOLINESTERASE INHIBITORS

neostigmine (Prostigmin)

pyridostigmine (Mestinon, Regonol)

Cholinesterase inhibitors are used in MG to enhance the effects of acetylcholine at the remaining skeletal muscle receptors. Cholinesterase inhibitors do not cure or change the underlying pathophysiologic processes, but they can provide effective, lifelong improvement of symptoms. Because the cholinesterase inhibitors are nonselective, the neuromuscular, muscarinic, and ganglionic junctions are each affected.

Adjusting the dose to obtain maximum benefit with minimal side effects is a major consideration when administering cholinesterase inhibitors. Initially, small doses are given followed by incremental increases until optimal muscle strength is obtained. The dose may need to be adjusted when activities result in symptoms of undermedication, such as increased ptosis. Severe undermedication results in myasthenic crisis.

Cholinesterase inhibitors should not be administered to patients experiencing obstruction of the intestinal or urinary tract. Caution is advised when administering these drugs to patients with asthma, hyperthyroidism, bradycardia, or peptic ulcer disease. Cholinesterase inhibitors can cross the placenta; reproductive counseling is indicated.

Nursing Responsibilities

- Obtain a baseline assessment of muscle strength and abilities, concentrating on swallowing and ptosis.
- Administer the medication parenterally if the patient has dysphagia. Check the dose of the medication carefully when changing from oral to parenteral routes.
- Evaluate the effectiveness of the medication and document the response, for example, time when fatigue occurs.
- Promptly recognize and respond to manifestations of excessive stimulation of muscarinic receptors: Excess salivation, urinary urgency, bradycardia, gastrointestinal hypermotility, diaphoresis. Atropine can be administered to combat these manifestations. Respiratory depression and failure can occur.

Health Education for the Patient and Family

- Balancing symptom control with dosage is crucial; record time of dose and response in a journal. Note the time of day when fatigued and any adverse effects, such as excess salivation, sweating, slow heartbeat, and diarrhea.
- Take the medication about 30 minutes prior to meals to enhance swallowing and chewing.
- Report manifestations of myasthenic crisis immediately: Severe muscle weakness, fast heartbeat, restlessness, difficulty breathing, increasing difficulty swallowing or speaking.
- Report slow heartbeat, increased salivation or sweating, and/or decreased blood pressure immediately.
- Review possible causes of myasthenic crisis: Physical or emotional stress, infection, or reduction in dosage.
- Wear or carry medical alert identification.

Expected Outcome: Ineffective airway clearance will be minimized as evidenced by patient's ability to expectorate secretions, maintain clear lungs, and demonstrate normal pulse oximetry and oxygenation patterns on assessment.

The nurse will:

- Assist with turning, deep breathing, and coughing at least every 2 hours. Teach proper coughing techniques; use an incentive spirometer every 2 hours while the patient is awake. *Position changes promote lung expansion; coughing helps clear secretions from the tracheobronchial tree.*
- Place in a semi-Fowler position. *This position expands the lungs and alleviates pressure from the diaphragm, especially important if the patient is obese.*
- Maintain hydration status and monitor for dehydration; use a humidifier as needed. If needed, teach family how to perform percussion, postural drainage, and suction. *Interventions to liquefy secretions, such as ensuring a daily fluid intake of up to 2500 mL (perhaps via feeding tube or parenteral route), help the patient mobilize and expectorate sputum.*

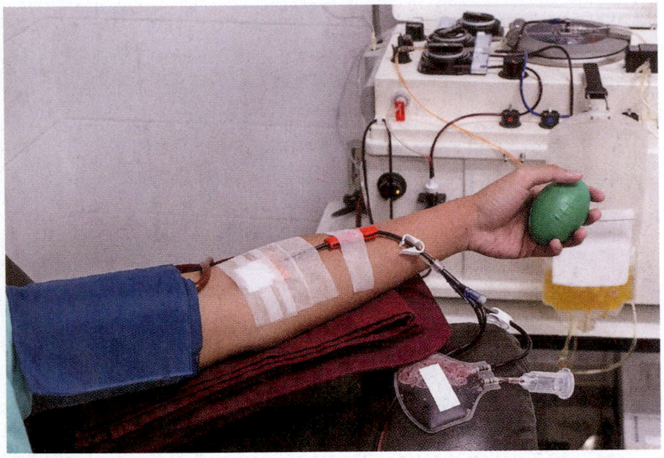

Figure 44.6 ■ Plasmapheresis is a procedure used to separate the blood's cellular components from plasma. About 50 mL/min is withdrawn to the centrifuge in the plasmapheresis machine. The plasma is replaced with donor plasma or colloids and returned to the patient.

BOX 44.2
Patient and Family Teaching: Myasthenia Gravis

- Schedule periods of rest and avoid stress; conserve energy when possible.
- Avoid cigarette smoke, alcohol, and beverages with quinine (e.g., tonic water).
- Take medications as prescribed. If manifestations change, consult the physician; the dose may need to be adjusted.
- Avoid extremes of temperature; an environment that is too hot or too cold may cause an exacerbation of MG.
- Avoid people with upper respiratory infections; infections can result in an exacerbation and extreme weakness.

Reduce Risk of Aspiration. Patients with MG have weakness of the laryngeal and pharyngeal muscles involved with swallowing. Alterations in swallowing place the patient at risk for poor nutrition as well as for possible aspiration. Family members need to be included in teaching, particularly the person who prepares and assists with meals.

Expected Outcome: Risk for aspiration related to impaired swallowing will be prevented by sitting the patient in high-Fowler position if able to maintain oral intake and by avoiding thin liquids that increase that risk.

The nurse will:

- Assess the ability to safely manage various consistencies of foods; consult with a speech therapist for evaluation. *Dysphagic patients are at risk for aspiration; matching food consistency to the patient's ability to swallow enhances safety.*
- Plan meals to promote medication effectiveness. *Pyridostigmine should be given 30 minutes before the meal to provide optimal muscle strength for swallowing and chewing.*
- Have the patient eat slowly, using small bites of food. Schedule meals during periods when the patient is adequately rested; develop a daily schedule incorporating rest periods. *Fatigue may add to dysphagia, putting the patient at greater risk for aspiration.*
- If necessary, give cues while eating, such as "Chew your food thoroughly; swallow." *Keeping patient focused may enhance swallowing.*
- Teach caregivers the Heimlich maneuver and how to suction. *Knowing specific measures to take in case of aspiration decreases both the patient's and family's anxiety and promotes confidence in managing potential problems.*
- Monitor lung sounds, the rate and character of respirations, and pulse oximetry readings at least every 4 hours or as indicated by patient's condition. *Frequent assessments are critical to early identification of ineffective respirations and oxygenation of tissues.*

Delegating Nursing Care Activities

As appropriate and allowed by the designated duties and responsibilities of unlicensed assistive personnel, the nurse may delegate nursing care activities such as mobilizing, positioning, and turning the patient as well as encouraging coughing and deep breathing. Delegation can include encouraging fluids and monitoring intake and output, as well as feeding patient and monitoring consistency of liquids if taking orally (e.g., thickening of liquids).

Transitions of Care

Teaching the patient and family with MG focuses on prevention and recognition of crisis situations, understanding the disorder, and methods for coping with both physical and psychosocial problems. Setting realistic goals with the patient and family provides opportunities for self-assessment and promotes active participation in rehabilitation. Address the following topics:

- The importance of maintaining consistency in medication dosage and management

- Realistic expectations
- Methods to avoid fatigue and undue stress; specific measures for avoiding upper respiratory infections and exposure to extreme heat or cold
- Birth control measures or referral for counseling (Pregnancy can exacerbate manifestations; also, medications used to control MG, such as neostigmine bromide [Prostigmin], cross the placenta.)
- Referral to support groups
- Helpful resources such as the Myasthenia Gravis Foundation of America, Inc.

The Patient with Guillain-Barré Syndrome

Guillain-Barré syndrome (GBS) is a rare and acute autoimmune disease. It has a similar morbidity across all age ranges, affecting less than 2 people per 100,000 every year (Van den Berg et al., 2014). GBS is an acute inflammatory demyelinating disorder of the PNS characterized by an acute onset of motor paralysis (usually ascending). The cause is unknown, but precipitating events include acute infection, surgery, viral immunizations, and other viral illnesses. In approximately half of cases, *Campylobacter jejuni* is identified as the cause of the preceding infection (Van den Berg et al., 2014). The majority of patients recover within two years of disease onset; many patients will see residual effects of the disease, including weakness and fatigue (Sorenson et al., 2019; Van den Berg et al., 2014).

The disease is characterized by progressive ascending flaccid paralysis, accompanied by paresthesias and numbness. About 25% of patients have respiratory involvement to the point that ventilatory assistance is required (Van den Berg et al., 2014). GBS is often a medical emergency.

Pathophysiology

The primary pathophysiologic process in GBS is the destruction of myelin sheaths covering the axons of peripheral nerves. The demyelination is thought to be the result of both a humoral- and cell-mediated immunologic response. Myelin insulates the neuron and facilitates conduction of impulses. The loss of myelin results in poor conduction of nerve impulses, causing sudden muscle weakness and loss of reflex response. In the worst cases, complete paralysis occurs. Other manifestations occur when nerve conduction to various muscles is interrupted. The stages of Guillain-Barré syndrome and their usual manifestations are presented in **Table 44.1**.

Interprofessional Care

Care of the patient with GBS requires an interprofessional approach. From the initial progressive phase through rehabilitation, many members of the healthcare team are involved. An accurate and rapid diagnosis is needed to ensure prompt supportive treatment, particularly if there is respiratory involvement combined with widespread paralysis.

Diagnosis

GBS is diagnosed after a thorough history and clinical examination, differentiating from several disorders, among them influenza, heavy metal poisoning, Lyme disease, and cranial hemorrhage. Diagnosis is made based on manifestations, history of a recent viral infection, elevated CSF protein levels, and EMG studies reflecting decreased nerve conduction. Although there is no specific test to diagnose this syndrome, several findings support and confirm the diagnosis. Physical exam will reveal progressive weakness in legs and arms as well as decreased deep tendon reflexes in the affected limbs (Van den Berg et al., 2014).

Medications

During the progressive phase of GBS, patients will often be prescribed IVIG, which is an immune globulin that helps suppress the antibodies that are attacking the myelin sheaths. Morphine is commonly administered to control muscle pain. Anticoagulation therapy is usually instituted to prevent thromboembolic complications, such as deep venous thrombosis and pulmonary embolism, which are associated with prolonged bedrest. If hypotension is a problem, vasopressors are prescribed.

Nutrition and Fluids

Nutritional support for the patient who is immobilized for prolonged periods of time is crucial. Maintaining positive nitrogen balance, ensuring sufficient fluid intake and electrolyte balance, and ensuring recommended caloric intake are goals of therapy. When swallowing problems occur,

Table 44.1 Stages and Manifestations of Guillain-Barré Syndrome

Stage	Manifestations
I: Progressive stage	■ Characterized by severe and rapid weakness, especially in the lower extremities; loss of muscle strength progressing to quadriplegia and respiratory failure; decreasing deep tendon reflexes; decreasing vital capacity; paresthesias, numbness; pain, especially nocturnal; facial muscle involvement (inability to wrinkle forehead or change expressions) ■ Symptoms generally peak within four weeks of onset (Van den Berg et al., 2014) ■ Involvement of the autonomic nervous system manifested by bradycardia, sweating, fluctuating blood pressure
II: Stabilizing/plateau stage	■ This stage can last anywhere from 2 days to 6 months (Van den Berg et al., 2014) ■ Marks the end of changes in condition; characterized by a "leveling-off" of symptoms ■ Generally, the labile autonomic functions stabilize
III: Recovery stage	■ May take from several months to 2 years ■ Marked by improvement in symptoms ■ Generally, muscle strength and function return in descending order

total parenteral nutrition may be indicated if feeding via a nasogastric or gastrostomy tube is ineffective.

Plasmapheresis

Plasma exchange has been beneficial, particularly when performed early in the syndrome's development. Antibodies are removed, and immunosuppressive agents are administered concurrently. Patients typically have three to four exchanges during an 8- to 10-day period.

Physical and Occupational Therapy

Long-term physical and occupational therapy are crucial to recovery. Patients with Guillain-Barré syndrome usually require prolonged rehabilitation care, which begins during the acute phase and focuses on preventing complications and limiting the effects of immobility. The severe muscle atrophy and loss of muscle tone require that patients relearn many functions and skills, such as walking. Compromise in respiratory function may delay physical rehabilitation; patients need positive reinforcement when they make even small gains in their progress. Continued attention to pain control is essential because paresthesia and pain can interfere with physical therapy.

Nursing Care

Many of the nursing interventions for patients with this syndrome involve monitoring neurologic function, preventing problems of immobility, ensuring adequate hydration and nutrition, and promoting respiratory function. Anticipating needs of both the patient and family is an important aspect of care. For example, developing an alternative method of communication before it is necessary may decrease anxiety.

Assessment

Assessment for the patient with GBS is similar to other neurologic disorders. The initial stage of GBS can be a medical emergency and the priority needs to be with maintaining the patient's airway. Assessing oxygenation, vital signs, and work of breathing are important aspects of the assessment. As GBS is a progressive neurologic disease, the nurse should regularly assess patient strength and movement of extremities. Changes in assessment should be reported immediately. Pain is a symptom that the majority of patients with GBS experience (Van den Berg et al., 2014). It is important that the nurse regularly assess the patient's pain and provide appropriate pharmacologic and nonpharmacologic treatments to provide comfort.

Priorities of Care

Nursing care focuses on preventing complications that may be fatal by following a rigorous predetermined schedule for turning and respiratory care (e.g., coughing, deep breathing, suctioning), by using strict aseptic technique, and by providing continuous psychosocial support.

Diagnoses, Interventions, and Outcomes

Anxiety and powerlessness are major nursing considerations. The patient is almost always admitted to the ICU for care, and is mentally alert but suddenly mute, ventilator dependent, and immobile. Refer to previous nursing care sections in this chapter for interventions related to anxiety, imbalanced nutrition, impaired swallowing, impaired verbal communication, and ineffective airway clearance. This section focuses on pain and impaired skin integrity.

Control Acute Pain. Pain experienced with Guillain-Barré syndrome varies. Frequently, there is a "stocking–glove" pattern, with pain in the hands, feet, and legs. Pain and tenderness in muscles can be severe; interventions are individualized to meet patient needs. The intense pain combined with altered sensations leads to anxiety; nursing interventions can make a difference in breaking the cycle of increasing pain that leads to increased anxiety and in turn causes more pain.

Expected Outcome: Patient's acute pain related to muscle atrophy will be controlled as evidenced by assessments of pain of 1 to 3 on a 0-to-10 pain scale, minimal grimacing, and optimal movement and comfort expressed by the patient.

The nurse will:

- Listen to the description of pain; determine presence of triggers or a pattern. *Acknowledging the patient's perception of pain is a basis for treatment; listening establishes trust.*
- Use a pain scale for determining extent of pain. *Consistent measurement is essential to evaluate degree of pain and effectiveness of intervention.*
- Use complementary therapies to help manage pain:
  a. Application of heat/cold
  b. Guided imagery
  c. Relaxation techniques
  d. Massage

  Presenting options for managing pain gives the patient control over the situation and helps reduce anxiety. Noninvasive interventions may augment the therapeutic benefit of medications.
- Provide analgesics as indicated; administer on a regular schedule rather than waiting until pain becomes severe. *Anticipating and managing pain before it becomes severe decreases anxiety and averts the cycle of increased anxiety, leading to increased pain.*
- Monitor for side effects of analgesics, particularly respiratory depression; assess respirations and lung sounds. Perform routine pulmonary care measures and monitor for aspiration. *Patients with Guillain-Barré syndrome have weakened thoracic muscles; frequent respiratory monitoring is indicated.*

Promote Good Skin Integrity. During the acute and plateau stages of Guillain-Barré syndrome, patients are at risk for problems related to immobility and malnutrition. Impaired skin integrity is one such problem. Preventing areas of skin breakdown is important. Prophylactic interventions will help ensure that ingested protein and calories are used to maintain ideal body weight and other body functions rather than to heal an avoidable problem. Implicit in interventions is maintenance of adequate nutrition.

Expected Outcome: Patient's risk for impaired skin integrity will be eliminated or minimized as evidenced by absence of skin breakdown.

The nurse will:

- Inspect bony prominences and provide skin care at least every 2 hours. Reposition the patient and clean, dry, and lubricate the skin as needed. *These activities stimulate circulation and ensure an even distribution of body weight; baseline observations allow discovery of early signs of altered integrity.*
- Pad bony prominences, such as sacral area, heels, and elbows. *This decreases shearing tears on these pressure points.*
- Use an alternating-pressure mattress or water bed. *Relieving pressure stimulates circulation and promotes oxygenation of tissues.*
- Monitor for incontinence and provide thorough skin care following each episode of incontinence. *Urine is caustic to the skin, and the moisture promotes skin breakdown.*

Transitions of Care

In general, there is no way to prevent GBS. It can reoccur in patients that have had an episode of GBS in the past. Although a very rare occurrence, GBS can be triggered by vaccination administration. It is important to assess the patient for previous history of GBS prior to administering vaccinations.

Patients and family members are frequently stunned by the rapid deterioration of function and fear that the paralysis will be permanent. Regularly reinforce teaching because the patient's high anxiety level may interfere with listening and understanding. When possible, include the patient and family in decision making; seek their input when planning a daily schedule of care that incorporates various therapies.

Teaching the rationales for preventive measures reinforces the patient's and family's understanding and may promote compliance during the lengthy rehabilitation. For example, because of autonomic nerve involvement, patients need to be monitored for cardiac dysrhythmias and taught to avoid changing position suddenly to prevent orthostatic hypotension.

Referrals to appropriate therapists are a component of anticipating needs; speech, nutritional, occupational, and physical therapists are an integral part of rehabilitation. Another focus of care is teaching both the patient and family; incorporate explanations for interventions aimed at promoting self-care. For further information, refer the patient and family to the Guillain-Barré Syndrome Foundation, International.

44.3 Cranial Nerve Disorders

Disorders of the cranial nerves may be caused by intracranial trauma or by pathologic processes. The pairs of cranial nerves, described in Chapter 41, are numbered in the order in which they arise in the brain and are named according to their anatomic characteristic or primary function. The most common cranial nerve disorders are those affecting the trigeminal (cranial nerve V) and the facial (cranial nerve VII) nerves. These disorders, discussed in the following sections, result primarily in pain or loss of sensory or motor function.

The Patient with Trigeminal Neuralgia

Neuralgia is characterized by severe, brief, repetitive attacks of stabbing pain, occurring along the distribution of a spinal or cranial nerve. The pain usually follows stimulation of the cutaneous region supplied by that nerve. **Trigeminal neuralgia (TN)**, also called *tic douloureux*, is a chronic disease of the trigeminal cranial nerve (V) that causes unilateral excruciating facial pain. The trigeminal nerve has three divisions: Ophthalmic, maxillary, and mandibular (**Figure 44.7** ■). The maxillary and mandibular divisions are affected in almost all cases of this disorder.

TN is more common in women than in men, occurring most often in middle or late adult life.

Pathophysiology

The actual cause of TN is unclear, but it is generally accepted that TN follows vascular compression and demyelination of the trigeminal nerve (Singh, 2016). Contributing factors include trauma, dental or jaw infections, flulike illnesses, aneurysm, tumor, and MS.

Stimulating specific areas of the face, called trigger zones, may initiate the onset of pain. These trigger zones are small areas on the cheek, lip, gum, or forehead that are

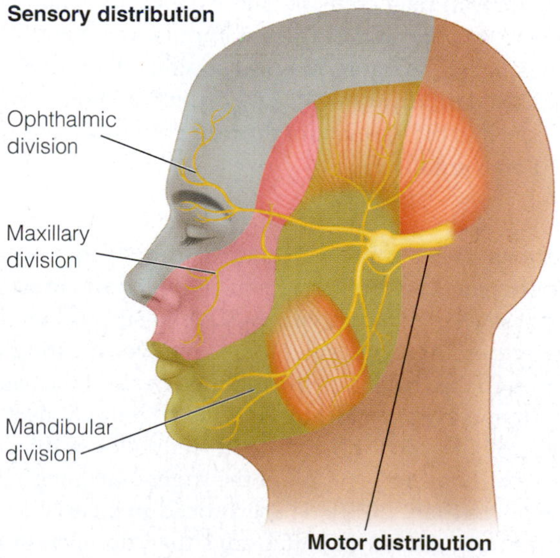
Sensory distribution
Ophthalmic division
Maxillary division
Mandibular division
Motor distribution

Figure 44.7 ■ Sensory and motor distribution of the trigeminal nerve. The three sensory divisions are ophthalmic, maxillary, and mandibular.

sensitive to even minimal stimuli. The pain episodes are initiated by many factors, including light touch, eating, swallowing, talking, sneezing, shaving, chewing gum, brushing the teeth, or washing the face. Other factors that may trigger a pain episode include changes in temperature and exposure to wind. In an attempt to control the pain, patients may refuse to wash, shave, eat, or talk.

Manifestations

Trigeminal neuralgia is characterized by brief (lasting a few seconds to a few minutes), repetitive episodes of sudden severe facial pain. The pain may occur as often as hundreds of times a day to as infrequently as a few times a year. The pain is experienced over the surface of the skin. It most often begins near one side of the mouth and rises toward the ear, eye, or nostril on the same side of the face.

The episodes of pain may recur for several weeks or months. The disease then spontaneously goes into remission, and the patient is free of pain for periods lasting from days to years. As the patient grows older, the remissions tend to become shorter, and a dull ache may be present between episodes of acute pain.

Interprofessional Care

Diagnosis

There are no specific diagnostic tests for TN. The disorder is diagnosed by the characteristic location and type of pain. The disorder is treated by pharmacologic or surgical interventions.

Medications

The drug most useful in controlling the pain is the tricyclic anticonvulsant carbamazepine (Tegretol). If carbamazepine is ineffective, other medications such as the anticonvulsant gabapentin (Neurontin) or the skeletal muscle relaxant baclofen (Lioresal) may be used. These drugs are administered to decrease paroxysmal afferent impulses and stop the pain. Drugs in this category may cause side effects of dizziness, nausea, and drowsiness. Liver function, bone marrow function, and blood levels of the medications should be monitored on a regular basis.

Surgery

If medications do not control the pain, surgical procedures may be performed, including various types of rhizotomy, the surgical severing of a nerve root. Closed surgical interventions by percutaneous rhizotomy involve inserting a needle through the cheek into the foramen ovale at the base of the brain and partially destroying the trigeminal nerve with glycerol (an alcohol), by radiofrequency-induced heat, or by balloon compression of the trigeminal ganglion (Bajwa, Ho, & Khan, 2017). These procedures carry less risk and result in shorter hospital stays than do open procedures, but there is a possibility of recurrence of pain. Following surgery, the patient may have some facial numbness, but there is usually no residual paralysis. The patient will have some loss of facial sensation (e.g., to temperature, pain, and/or touch) and is at risk for loss of the corneal reflex.

Nursing Care

Priorities of Care

Nursing care for the patient with TN involves teaching self-management at home after medical or surgical intervention. Primary patient concerns are managing pain, maintaining nutrition, and preventing injury.

Diagnoses, Outcomes, and Interventions

Interventions for managing pain and improving nutritional intake are addressed here; teaching to prevent injury following surgery is discussed under patient and family teaching.

Control Acute Pain. The patient with TN has excruciating pain and often avoids ADLs and socializing with others in an attempt to prevent the onset of pain. Pain management is fully discussed in Chapter 9. Nursing interventions for pain in patients with this disorder focus on strategies for self-management.

Expected Outcome: Patient's acute pain will be controlled at a tolerable level as evidenced by objective and subjective pain assessment (use of pain scale, lack of grimacing, verbal assessment of pain, interaction with others, and vital signs).

The nurse will:

- Identify factors that trigger an attack, and discuss strategies to avoid these precipitating factors. *Most patients can clearly identify trigger zones and triggering factors. Identification is the first step in pain control.*
- Determine usual response to pain. *Sensitivity and reaction to pain are influenced by previous experiences with pain and by age, gender, emotional factors, and cultural background.*
- Assess factors that affect the ability to influence pain tolerance, including the knowledge and cause of the pain, the meaning of the pain, the ability to control the pain, cultural background, and support systems. *Pain tolerance, which is the duration and intensity of pain an individual is willing to endure, differs greatly among individuals and may also vary within particular patients in different situations.*
- Monitor the effects of the medication prescribed for the neuralgia. *If the prescribed medication does not provide relief, other medications or methods of treatment may be used to control the pain.*

Promote Balanced Diet. Patients often refuse to eat during periods of pain attacks, fearing that the movements of chewing may precipitate the pain. In addition, the chronic nature of the illness often causes depression, which may depress the appetite.

Expected Outcome: Patient's risk for altered nutrition will be eliminated/minimized by patient's consumption of a healthy and well-balanced diet and weight stability.

The nurse will:

- Monitor dietary intake and weight at each visit, and ask the patient to keep a weekly weight record. *Ongoing assessments are necessary for early detection of nutritional deficiencies.*

- Discuss the temperature and consistency of foods eaten, and suggest referral to a dietitian, if necessary. *Hot or cold foods may trigger an attack; soft, warm, or cool foods are less likely to act as triggers.*
- Suggest chewing on the unaffected side of the mouth. *Chewing on the unaffected side is less likely to trigger an attack of pain and so facilitates food intake.*
- If unable to tolerate oral food, tube feedings may be necessary. *Adequate kilocalories and nutrients for metabolic processes are essential.*

Delegating Nursing Care Activities

As appropriate and allowed by the designated duties and responsibilities of unlicensed assistive personnel, the nurse may delegate nursing care activities such as prompt reporting of any change in patient's behavior (e.g., complaints of pain to assistive personnel, restlessness, changes in vital signs); maintenance of a quiet, dark, relaxed environment; monitoring intake and daily weights; and reporting a reduced intake and/or anorexia.

Transitions of Care

As the disease progresses, attacks may occur more frequently and become more severe (Singh, 2016). Some sensory loss will be noted on assessment. Treatment generally begins with one medication and may be increased as needed to two or three medications before surgery becomes inevitable (Singh, 2016). Depression is a serious complication of this disease, as patients experience significant pain; they often choose to limit certain activities to prevent triggering an attack. The nurse should be aware of the signs and symptoms of depression and discuss findings with the interdisciplinary team. The patient with TN who is receiving medical treatment and providing self-care at home requires teaching about the disease process, the medication(s) being taken, and ways to reduce the incidence of attacks of pain. For example, if the home setting is drafty and attacks of pain are triggered by cold air blowing across the face, it may be necessary to encourage the patient to put weather stripping around windows and doors. See **Box 44.3** for patient teaching to prevent injury to affected areas.

BOX 44.3
Teaching for Home Care of Trigeminal Neuralgia

EYE CARE

- Do not rub the eyes; use artificial tears four times a day if the eyes are dry or irritated.
- Wear an eye patch at night.
- Wear protective sunglasses or goggles when outside, when working in dusty areas, when mowing the lawn, and when using any type of spray material (e.g., hairspray, cleaning materials, paint, insecticides).
- Remember to blink frequently.
- Check your eyes for redness or swelling each day.
- Schedule regular eye examinations.

FACE AND MOUTH CARE

- Chew on the unaffected side of the mouth.
- Avoid eating hot foods or drinking hot liquids.
- After every meal, brush your teeth and inspect the inside of your mouth for food that may collect between the gums and cheek.
- Have regular dental examinations; you will not be able to feel pain associated with gum infection or tooth decay.
- Use an electric razor to shave the face.
- Protect your face from very cold or windy conditions.

The Patient with Bell Palsy

Bell palsy, also called *facial paralysis*, is a disorder of the seventh cranial (facial) nerve, characterized by unilateral weakness of the facial muscles. This disorder can occur at any age but is seen most often in adults between the ages of 20 and 40 (Taylor, 2017). The incidence is equal in men and women. More than 70% of patients recover completely within a few weeks to a few months (Phan, Panizza, & Wallwork, 2016). It may occur as a distinct classic disease or may accompany other diseases such as Guillain-Barré syndrome, tumor, Lyme disease, or stroke.

Pathophysiology

The cause of the classic disorder is believed to be the herpes simplex virus type 1 and herpes zoster virus, which lead to nerve inflammation.

Manifestations

The onset of Bell palsy is usually sudden and almost always involves one side of the face. Pain behind the ear or along the jaw may precede the paralysis. The patient initially notices numbness or stiffness of one side of the face that distorts the appearance. As the disease progresses, the distortion becomes more obvious, and the face appears asymmetric. The facial paralysis causes the entire side of the face to droop, and the patient cannot wrinkle the forehead, close the eye, or pucker the lips on the affected side. When the patient attempts to smile, the lower facial muscles are pulled to the opposite side of the face. Some patients have only mild manifestations, whereas others have complete facial paralysis (**Figure 44.8** ■). Patients often believe they have had a stroke.

Interprofessional Care

There are no definitive laboratory or diagnostic tests for Bell's palsy; diagnosis is made by excluding other causes. Treatment includes medications and physical therapy. Steroid treatment should be initiated within 72 hours of diagnosis (Phan et al., 2016). Studies have shown that antiviral drugs such as acyclovir combined with steroid treatment may be effective by limiting damage to the nerve. Physical therapy to stimulate the facial nerve and help maintain muscle tone may help prevent permanent contractures before recovery takes place. Moist heat applied to the affected side of the face may decrease pain.

Nursing Care

Priorities of Care

- Use artificial tears four times a day to lubricate the eye; wear an eye patch or tape the eye shut at night. Wear sunglasses or goggles when outside, when working in dusty conditions, and when using any type of spray.
- Massage combined with warm, moist heat is often effective in relieving the pain.
- A soft diet that does not require chewing and six small meals a day are helpful. Chew slowly on the unaffected side and avoid hot foods. Clean the mouth and carefully inspect the area between the gums and cheek for food after each meal.
- As function returns, practice wrinkling the forehead, closing the eyes, blowing air out of the puckered mouth, and whistling for 5 minutes three or four times a day.

Transitions of Care

There are several risk factors for Bell palsy, including pregnancy, obesity, hypertension, diabetes, and upper respiratory illness (Phan et al., 2016). Teaching patients how to maintain a healthy diet and incorporate exercise into daily routines in order to prevent some of these risk factors may be helpful. Although patients provide self-care at home, the nurse plays a key role in teaching the patient and family about Bell palsy and how to prevent injury and maintain nutrition. The patient is often anxious about his or her appearance and may require counseling if any deficits in facial expression become permanent.

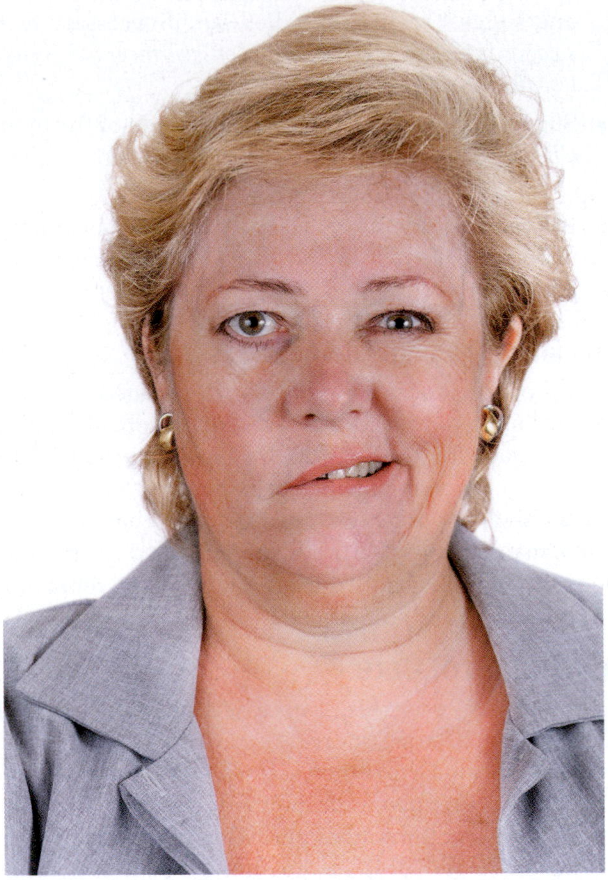

Figure 44.8 ■ The patient with Bell palsy shows the typical drooping of one side of the face.

CHAPTER HIGHLIGHTS

44.1 Degenerative Neurologic Disorders

Describe the pathophysiology and manifestations of degenerative neurologic disorders, and outline the interprofessional care and nursing care of patients with these disorders.

- Dementia involves impairment in short- and long-term memory; impairment in language, motor activity, recognition, and/or abstract thinking; and a clinical course characterized by gradual onset and continuing cognitive decline.
- Alzheimer disease (AD) is progressive and relentless and is characterized by cognitive and functional decline. The disease is characterized by atrophy of brain tissue, loss of neurons, neurofibrillary tangles, and amyloid plaques. There are no effective treatments for preventing AD, although pharmacologic and nonpharmacologic therapies may slow its course. Education of caregivers addresses burdens and expectations and provides instruction regarding community resources. The goal is to maximize the environment to the patient's functional abilities and safety needs.
- Multiple sclerosis (MS) is an autoimmune, demyelinating disease of the central nervous system. MS is multifactorial, with genetic and environmental factors linked to its incidence. Exposure to UVB light and exposure to the Epstein-Barr virus have both been implicated as environmental factors that interact with genes to lead to the onset of MS. The loss of myelin leads to axon dysfunction, which slows and distorts nerve impulses. Medications are used to slow the progression of the disease, decrease the number of exacerbations, and treat manifestations.
- Parkinson disease (PD) is a progressive degenerative neurologic disease characterized by tremor, muscle rigidity, and bradykinesia. The loss of voluntary motor control is the result of pathologic processes resulting in a decrease of dopamine (an inhibitory neurotransmitter) so that it can no longer inhibit acetylcholine (an excitatory neurotransmitter). Medications to treat

manifestations include MAO inhibitors, dopaminergics, dopamine agonists, and anticholinergics.

- Huntington disease (chorea) is a progressive, degenerative inherited neurologic disease characterized by increasing dementia and chorea.
- Amyotrophic lateral sclerosis (ALS) is a rapidly progressive and fatal degenerative motor neuron disease characterized by weakness and wasting of voluntary control muscles, but without sensory or cognitive changes. The patient eventually loses the ability to communicate and breathe.

44.2 Peripheral Nervous System Disorders

Describe the pathophysiology and manifestations peripheral nervous system disorders, and outline the interprofessional care and nursing care of patients with these disorders.

- Myasthenia gravis (MG) is a chronic autoimmune PNS disorder characterized by fatigue and severe skeletal muscle weakness. It results from a decreased number of acetylcholine receptors at the neuromuscular junction, so muscles are unable to contract. Life-threatening emergencies include myasthenic crisis (sudden increase in motor weakness) and cholinergic crisis (from an overdose of the anticholinesterase medications used to treat MG).
- Guillain-Barré syndrome (GBS) is an acute inflammatory demyelinating disease of the PNS characterized by an acute onset of flaccid motor paralysis that begins in the lower extremities and ascends to involve the upper extremities, torso, and cranial nerves. Paralysis of intercostal and diaphragmatic muscles often necessitates ventilatory assistance. The progressive phase lasts up to 4 weeks, followed by recovery, which takes from 6 months to 2 years.

44.3 Cranial Nerve Disorders

Describe the pathophysiology and manifestations of cranial nerve disorders, and outline the interprofessional care and nursing care of patients with these disorders.

- Cranial nerve disorders include trigeminal neuralgia (TN) and Bell palsy. TN is a chronic disorder of cranial nerve V and causes severe facial pain. Bell palsy is an acute disorder of cranial nerve VII, characterized by unilateral paralysis of the facial muscles.

TEST YOURSELF NCLEX-RN® REVIEW

1. The nurse is reviewing a patient's manifestations to determine if dementia is present. What information will help the nurse with this determination? (Select all that apply.)
   A. Dementia causes impaired short- and long-term memory.
   B. Dementia is an acute disorder, resulting from an injury to the brain.
   C. Dementia is the primary manifestation of Guillain-Barré syndrome.
   D. Dementia describes the cognitive and behavioral manifestations of Alzheimer disease.
   E. Dementia is a general term used to describe manifestations of damage or death of neurons.
2. A patient is concerned about developing Alzheimer disease with aging. What manifestation should the nurse instruct as usually being the first indication of the disease?
   A. Inability to perform basic ADLs
   B. Mild and subtle memory deficits
   C. Inability to communicate verbally
   D. Wandering and changes in sleep patterns at night
3. The nurse is identifying interventions appropriate for a patient with multiple sclerosis. These interventions should focus on which patient goal that occurs in all patients with MS, regardless of type or severity?
   A. Preventing fatigue
   B. Relieving pain
   C. Reducing risk of aspiration
   D. Improving gas exchange
4. The nurse is preparing medication teaching for a patient with multiple sclerosis. Which medications should be included in this teaching? (Select all that apply.)
   A. Antibiotics
   B. Antihistamines
   C. Immunomodulators
   D. Dopamine precursors
   E. Adrenocorticosteroids
5. The nurse is teaching a young adult patient with multiple sclerosis about the disease process. What information should the nurse include during this teaching? (Select all that apply.)
   A. Onset is usually between 20 and 40.
   B. The disease is treatable, but not curable.
   C. It is important to avoid extremes of heat and cold.
   D. Few drugs are available for the treatment of MS.
   E. Alternating relapses and remissions are a common disease pattern.

6. The nurse is preparing to talk with the family of a patient newly diagnosed with Parkinson disease. How should the nurse explain the cause of this disorder?
   A. Genetic defect
   B. Effects of a neurotoxin
   C. Autoimmune responses to a viral infection
   D. Failure of dopamine to inhibit acetylcholine
7. The nurse is preparing instructions for the caregiver of a patient with Parkinson disease regarding care that will be needed at home. What information should the nurse provide to the caregiver? (Select all that apply.)
   A. Ways to prevent falls
   B. Interventions to maintain nutrition
   C. The need to avoid daily baths and showers
   D. Ways to prevent an overdose of medications
   E. How to prevent constipation
8. The nurse is preparing medication teaching for a patient with amyotrophic lateral sclerosis. On which drug classification should the nurse focus when providing these instructions?
   A. Antiglutamate
   B. Anticholinergic
   C. Dopamine agonist
   D. Anti-inflammatory
9. The nurse is preparing a teaching plan for a patient with Bell palsy. What information should the nurse include?
   A. "One side of your face will not move normally."
   B. "The disease affects your muscles so you can't walk."
   C. "You will experience severe facial pain during attacks."
   D. "Be sure to boil all home-canned foods before eating them."
10. The nurse is preparing teaching for the family of a patient with myasthenia gravis. The nurse would teach the family to immediately report which manifestations that indicate possible myasthenic crisis? (Select all that apply.)
    A. Severe muscle tetany
    B. Fast heartbeat
    C. Increased difficulty speaking
    D. Incontinence of urine
    E. Depressed affect

See Test Yourself answers in Appendix B.

REFERENCES

Adams, M. P., Holland, L. N. & Urban, C. Q. (2017). *Pharmacology for nurses: A pathophysiologic approach* (5th ed.). Boston, MA: Pearson.

Alzheimer's Association. (2017f). *What is dementia?* Retrieved from https://www.alz.org/what-is-dementia.asp.

Alzheimer's Association. (2017a). 2017 Alzheimer's disease facts and figures. *Alzheimer's and Dementia, 13,* 325–373.

Alzheimer's Association. (2017b). *Home safety and Alzheimer's.* Retrieved from https://www.alz.org/care/alzheimers-dementia-home-safety.asp.

Alzheimer's Association. (2017c). *Seven stages of Alzheimer's.* Retrieved from https://m.alz.org/stages-of-alzheimers.asp?sp=true.

Alzheimer's Association (2017d). *10 warning signs of Alzheimer's.* Retrieved from https://m.alz.org/10-warning-signs.asp.

Alzheimer's Association. (2017e). *Tests for diagnosis.* Retrieved from https://m.alz.org/tests-for-diagnosis.asp#mental.

Amyotrophic Lateral Sclerosis (ALS) Association. (2017). *Every drop adds up.* Retrieved from http://www.alsa.org/fight-als/ice-bucket-challenge.html.

Bajwa, Z. H., Ho, C. C., & Khan, S. A. (2017). *Trigeminal neuralgia.* Retrieved from https://www-uptodate-com.proxy.lib.ohio-state.edu/contents/trigeminal-neuralgia?source=search_result&search=rhizotomy&selectedTitle=1~7.

Baixinho, C. L., Mertens, J., Duarte, A. F., Teixeira, F. M., Quental, I. A., & Silva Martens, S. (2016). Nursing interventions promoting functionality among adults with multiple sclerosis: Integrative review. *Journal of Nursing, 10*(2), 838–847.

Bane, T. J., & Cole, C. (2015). Prevention of Alzheimer disease: The roles of nutrition and primary care. *The Nurse Practitioner, 40*(5), 30–35.

Bellomo, T. L., & Cichminski, L. (2015). Amyotrophic lateral sclerosis: What nurses need to know. *Nursing, 45*(10), 46-51.

Cascaes da Silva, F., da Rosa Iop, R., Domingos dos Santos, P., Aguiar Bezerra de Melo, L. M., Barbosa Gutierres Filho, P. J., & da Silva, R. (2016). Effects of physical-exercise-based rehabilitation programs on the quality of life of patients with Parkinson's disease: A systematic review of randomized controlled trials. *Journal of Aging and Physical Activity, 24*(3), 484–496.

Centers for Disease Control and Prevention. (2017). *What you can do to prevent falls.* Retrieved from https://www-cdc-gov.proxy.lib.ohio-state.edu/steadi/pdf/What_You_Can_Do_brochure-a.pdf.

Dayalu, P., & Albin, R. L (2015). Huntington disease pathogenesis and treatment. *Neurologic Clinics, 33*(1), 101–114.

DeMaagd, G., & Philip, A. (2015a). Parkinson's disease and its management part 1: Disease entity, risk factors, pathophysiology, clinical presentation and diagnosis. *P & T, 40*(8), 504–510.

DeMaagd, G., & Philip, A. (2015b). Parkinson's disease and its management part 3: Nondopaminergic and nonpharmacological treatment options. *P & T, 40*(10), 668–679.

Faguy, K. (2016). Multiple sclerosis: An update. *Radiologic Technology, 87*(5), 529–553.

Glynn-Servedio, B. E., & Seys Ranola, T. (2017). AChE inhibitors and NMDA receptor antagonists in advanced Alzheimer's disease. *The Consultant Pharmacist, 32*(9), 511–518.

Goldenberg, W. D. (2016). *Emergent management of myasthenia gravis.* Retrieved from https://emedicine.medscape.com/article/793136-overview?pa=liMFlhmkxBIvT5rnPLkEY9pgt3Kq9UHMJfOMAmHaEbZzIElgmSJi8dDUJGCMOG8ecFrqow%2Bf2%2F37XuRaZT6JAA%3D%3D#a1.

Greig, S. L., & McKeage, K. (2015). Carbidopa/levodopa ER capsules (Rytary, Numient): A review in Parkinson's disease. *CNS Drugs, 30,* 79–90.

Hauser, R. A. (2017). *Parkinson disease.* Retrieved from https://emedicine.medscape.com/article/1831191-overview?pa=MODRhV878fjKlQxu4fR%2FST6PFMmvmLUHcWcBN%2BcUeMFKxppjG8S6trm4FyMII41dLCEJNCrbkqLWYvqLrhntWA%3D%3D#a1.

Healthy People 2020. (2017). *Dementias including Alzheimer's disease.* Retrieved from https://www.healthypeople.gov/2020/topics-objectives/topic/dementias-including-alzheimers-disease.

Howard, J. F. (2015). *Clinical overview of MG.* Retrieved from www.myasthenia.org/HealthProfessionals/ClinicalOverviewofMG.aspx.

Kalia, L. V., & Lang, A. E. (2015). Parkinson's disease. *Lancet, 386*(9996), 896–912.

Krishnan, S., York, M. K., Bakus, D., & Heyn, P. C. (2017). Coping with caregiver burnout when caring for a person with neurodegenerative disease: A guide for caregivers. *Archives of Physical Medicine & Rehabilitation, 98*(4), 805–807.

Keene, C. D., Montine, T. J., & Kuller, L. H. (2017). *Epidemiology, pathology, and pathogenesis of Alzheimer disease.* Retrieved from https://www-uptodate-com.proxy.lib.ohio-state.edu/contents/epidemiology-pathology-and-pathogenesis-of-alzheimer-disease?source=search_result&search=alzheimers&selectedTitle=2~150.

Lamont, R. M. (2017). Falls in people with Parkinson's disease: A prospective comparison of community and home-based falls. *Gait & Posture, 55,* 62–67.

Larson, E. B. (2017). *Evaluation of cognitive impairment and dementia.* Retrieved from https://www-uptodate-com.proxy.lib.ohio-state.edu/contents/evaluation-of-cognitive-impairment-and-dementia?source=search_result&search=dementia&selectedTitle=1~150.

Luzzio, C. (2017). *Multiple sclerosis.* Retrieved from https://emedicine.medscape.com/article/1146199-overview.

Multiple Sclerosis Association of America (MSAA). (2017a). *The immune system and multiple sclerosis.* Retrieved from https://mymsaa.org/ms-information/overview/immune-system/.

Multiple Sclerosis Association of America (MSAA). (2017b). *Who gets multiple sclerosis.* Retrieved from https://mymsaa.org/ms-information/overview/who-gets-ms/.

National Institute on Aging. (2017a). *Basics of Alzheimer's disease and dementia: What is dementia?* Retrieved from https://www.nia.nih.gov/health/what-dementia.

National Institute on Aging. (2017b). *Symptoms and diagnosis of Alzheimer's disease: How is Alzheimer's disease diagnosed?* Retrieved from https://www.nia.nih.gov/health/how-alzheimers-disease-diagnosed.

Newsome, S. D., Aliotta, P. J., Bainbridge, J., Bennett, S. E., Cutter, G., Fenton, K., . . . Jones, D. E. (2016). A framework of care in multiple sclerosis, part 1. *International Journal of MS Care, 18*(6), 314–323.

Newsome, S. D., Aliotta, P. J., Bainbridge, J., Bennett, S. E., Cutter, G., Fenton, K., . . . Jones, D. E. (2017). A framework of care in multiple sclerosis, part 2: Symptomatic care and beyond. *International Journal of MS Care, 19*(1), 42–56.

Oliver, D., & Veronese, S. (2017). *Palliative approach to Parkinson disease and parkinsonian disorders.* Retrieved from https://www-uptodate-com.proxy.lib.ohio-state.edu/contents/palliative-approach-to-parkinson-disease-and-parkinsonian-disorders?source=search_result&search=parkinsons&selectedTitle=4~150.

Onders, R. P., Elmo, M. J., Kaplan, C., Katirji, B., & Schilz, R. (2014). Final analysis of the pilot trial of diaphragm pacing in amyotrophic lateral sclerosis with long-term follow-up: Diaphragm pacing positively affects diaphragm respiration. *American Journal of Surgery, 207,* 393–397.

Pahwa, R. (2014). *Deep brain stimulation for Parkinson's disease.* Retrieved from https://emedicine.medscape.com/article/1965354-overview#a4.

Parkinson's Foundation. (2017a). *Understanding Parkinson's: Genetic factors.* Retrieved from www.parkinson.org/Understanding-Parkinsons/Causes-and-Statistics/Genetic-Factors.

Parkinson's Foundation. (2017b). *Understanding Parkinson's: Statistics.* Retrieved from www.parkinson.org/Understanding-Parkinsons/Causes-and-Statistics/Statistics.

Phan, N, T., Panizza, B., & Wallwork, B. (2016). A general practice approach to Bell's palsy. *Australian Family Physician, 45*(11), 794–797.

Singh, M. K. (2016). *Trigeminal neuralgia.* Retrieved from https://emedicine.medscape.com/article/1145144-overview#a1.

Sorenson, M., Quinn, L., & Klein, D. (2019). *Pathophysiology: Concepts of human disease.* Hoboken, NJ: Pearson Education.

Taylor, D. C. (2017). *Bell palsy.* Retrieved from https://emedicine.medscape.com/article/1146903-overview#a7.

Tsoi, K. K., Chan, J. Y., Hirai, H. W., Wong, S. Y., & Kwok, T. C. (2015). Cognitive tests to detect dementia a systematic review and meta-analysis. *JAMA Internal Medicine, 175*(9), 1450–1458.

Van den Berg, B., Walgaard, C., Drenthen, J., Fokke, C., Jacobs, B. C., & Van Doorn, P. A. (2014). Guillain-Barre syndrome: Pathogenesis, diagnosis, treatment and prognosis. *Nature Reviews Neurology, 10*, 469–482.

Williams-Gray, C. H., & Worth, P. F. (2016). Parkinson's disease. *Medicine, 44*(9), 542–546.

Wolk, D. A., & Dickerson, B. C. (2017). *Clinical features and diagnosis of Alzheimer disease.* Retrieved from https://www.uptodate-com.proxy.lib.ohio-state.edu/contents/clinical-features-and-diagnosis-of-alzheimer-disease?source=search_result&search=alzheimers&selectedTitle=1~150.

ADDITIONAL RESOURCES

ALS Association
alsa.org

Alzheimer's Foundation of America
alzfdn.org/

American Parkinson Disease Association
www.apdaparkinson.org

Huntington's Disease Society of America
www.hdsa.org

Les Turner ALS Foundation
lesturnerals.org

Michael J. Fox Foundation for Parkinson's Research
www.michaeljfox.org

Multiple Sclerosis Association of America
www.msassociation.org

Multiple Sclerosis Foundation
msfocus.org

National Parkinson Foundation
parkinson.org

Unit

12

Responses to Altered Sensory Function

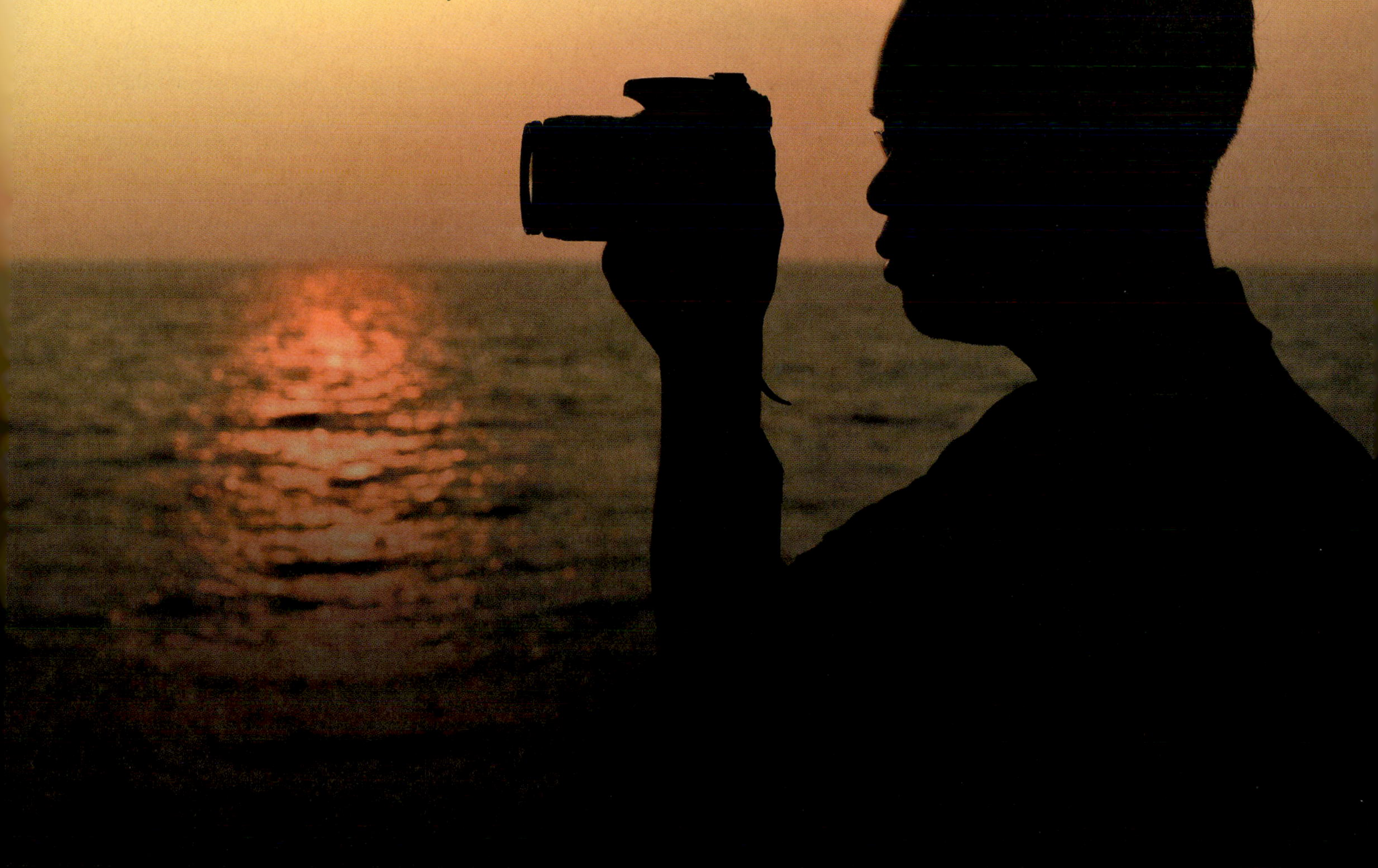

Chapter 45

Assessing the Eye and Ear

Chapter Outline and Learning Outcomes

45.1 Anatomy, Physiology, and Functions of the Eyes 1673

Describe the anatomy, physiology, and functions of the eye, and identify abnormal findings that may indicate visual impairment.

45.2 Assessing the Eyes 1676

Outline the components of the assessment of the eye and vision, including topics for the health assessment interview, techniques for physical assessment, and the diagnostic tests used in the assessment.

45.3 Anatomy, Physiology, and Functions of the Ears 1682

Describe the anatomy, physiology, and functions of the ear, and identify abnormal findings that may indicate hearing impairment.

45.4 Assessing the Ears 1684

Outline the components of the assessment of the ear and hearing, including topics for the health assessment interview, techniques for physical assessment, and the diagnostic tests used in the assessment.

45.5 Assessment of Special Populations 1688

Differentiate considerations for assessing vision and hearing of older adults, veterans, and adults with sequelae of childhood/congenital conditions.

45.6 Health Promotion 1689

Summarize topics that nurses teach to promote healthy vision and hearing across the lifespan.

CLINICAL COMPETENCIES

- Conduct and document a health history for patients having or at risk for alterations in the structure or functions of the eye and ear, eliciting patient preferences, values, and expressed needs.
- Safely and effectively assess the structure and functions of the eye and ear, documenting and reporting, as appropriate, unexpected findings.
- Provide appropriate teaching for patients undergoing diagnostic tests of the eyes, ears, vision, or hearing.
- Monitor the results of diagnostic tests and report abnormal findings.

KEY TERMS

accommodation, 1676
cerumen, 1682
convergence, 1676
corneal reflex, 1673
hyperopia, 1678
myopia, 1678
nystagmus, 1678
presbycusis, 1689
presbyopia, 1678
ptosis, 1679
pupillary light reflex, 1673
refraction, 1676

EQUIPMENT NEEDED

- Visual acuity charts
- Opaque eye cover
- Pen
- Penlight
- Cotton-tipped applicator
- Ophthalmoscope
- Otoscope
- Tuning fork

The eyes and ears provide pathways for visual and auditory stimuli to reach the brain. In addition, specialized structures within the ear help maintain position sense and equilibrium. Deficits in vision and hearing may limit self-care, mobility, safety, independence, communication, and relationships with others.

45.1 Anatomy, Physiology, and Functions of the Eyes

The eyes are complex structures containing 70% of the sensory receptors of the body. Each eye is a sphere measuring about 2.5 cm (1 in.) in diameter, surrounded and protected by a bony orbit and cushions of fat. The primary functions of the eyes are to encode the patterns of light from the environment through photoreceptors and to carry the coded information from the eyes to the brain. The brain gives meaning to the coded information, allowing us to make sense of what we see (Sorenson, Quinn, & Klein, 2019).

Accessory Structures of the Eye

Although the accessory structures of the eye are outside the eyeball, they are vital to its protection. These include the eyebrows, eyelids, eyelashes, conjunctiva, lacrimal apparatus, and extrinsic eye muscles (**Figure 45.1** ■).

The *eyebrows* shade the eyes. The *eyelashes*, short hairs that project from the top and bottom borders of the eyelids, protect the eye from foreign bodies, regulate the entry of light into the eye, and distribute tears by blinking. An unexpected touch to the eyelashes initiates the blinking reflex, which protects the eyes from foreign objects. The *conjunctiva* is a thin, transparent mucous membrane that lines the inner surfaces of the eyelids and also folds over the anterior surface of the eyeball, lubricating the eyes. The *palpebral conjunctiva* lines the upper and lower eyelids, whereas the *bulbar conjunctiva* loosely covers the anterior sclera (the white part of the eye). The *lacrimal apparatus* is composed of the lacrimal gland, the puncta, the lacrimal sac, and the nasolacrimal duct. Together, these structures secrete, distribute, and drain tears to cleanse and moisten the eye's surface.

The six extrinsic eye muscles control movement of the eye, allowing it to follow a moving object and move precisely. The muscles also help maintain the shape of the eyeball. The cranial nerves control the extrinsic muscles (**Figure 45.2** ■).

The Eye

The eye receives and transmits visual stimuli to the brain for interpretation. The wall of the eyeball is composed of three layers: The fibrous, vascular, and inner layers. The inner layer of the eye contains photoreceptors (visual receptors). The cavity of the eye is filled with fluids called *humors*. This cavity is divided into anterior and posterior cavities by the lens, the focusing apparatus of the eye (**Figure 45.3** ■).

Sclera and Cornea

The white *sclera*, the outer fibrous layer of the eyeball, protects and gives shape to the eyeball. The sclera gives way to the cornea over the iris and pupil. The *cornea* is transparent, avascular, and sensitive to touch. It forms a window that allows light to enter the eye and is a part of its focusing apparatus. When the cornea is touched, the eyelids blink (the **corneal reflex**) and tears are secreted.

Iris

The *iris*, part of the vascular layer of the eye, is a disc of muscle surrounding the pupil and lying between the cornea and the lens. The iris gives the eye its color and regulates light entry by controlling the size of the pupil. The *pupil* is the dark center of the eye through which light enters. The pupil constricts when bright light enters the eye and when it is used for near vision; it dilates when light conditions are dim and when the eye is used for far vision. In response to intense light, the pupil constricts rapidly in the **pupillary light reflex**.

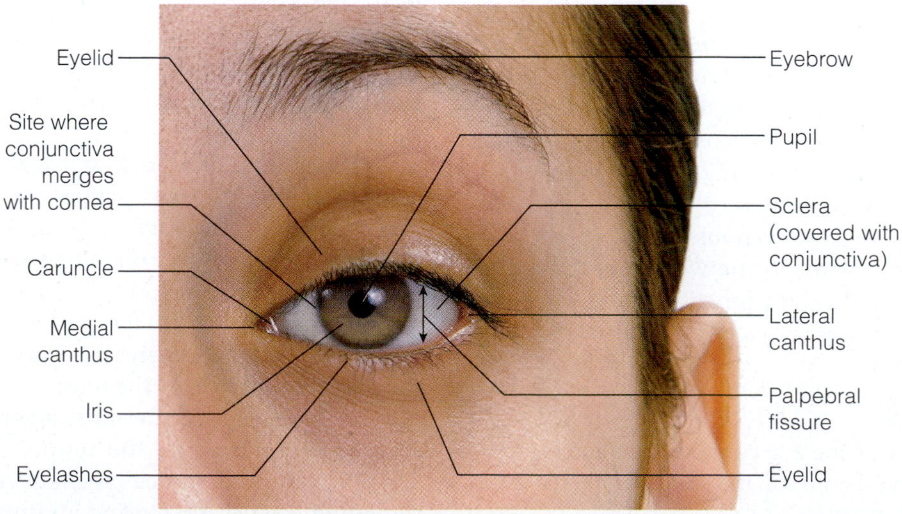
Eyelid
Site where conjunctiva merges with cornea
Caruncle
Medial canthus
Iris
Eyelashes
Eyebrow
Pupil
Sclera (covered with conjunctiva)
Lateral canthus
Palpebral fissure
Eyelid

Figure 45.1 ■ Accessory and external structures of the eye.

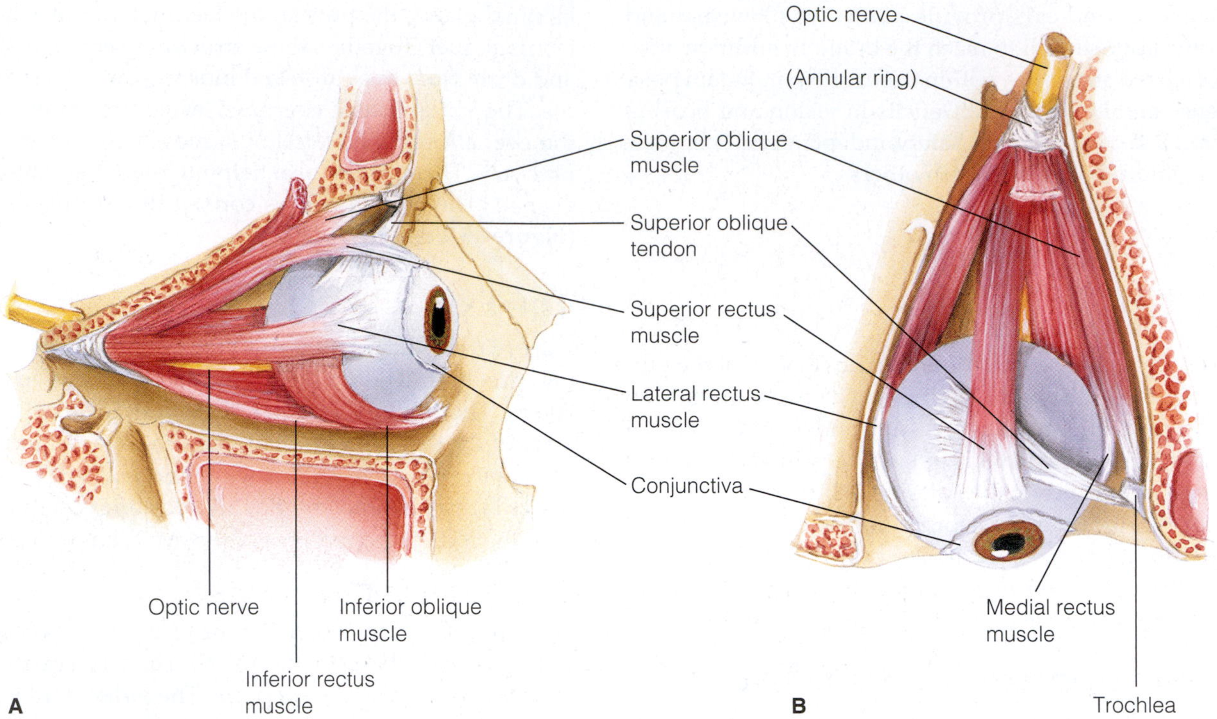
Superior oblique muscle
Superior oblique tendon
Superior rectus muscle
Lateral rectus muscle
Conjunctiva
Optic nerve
Inferior oblique muscle
Inferior rectus muscle
A
Optic nerve
(Annular ring)
Medial rectus muscle
Trochlea
B

C

Name	Controlling cranial nerve	Action
Lateral rectus	VI (abducens)	Moves eye laterally
Medial rectus	III (oculomotor)	Moves eye medially
Superior rectus	III (oculomotor)	Elevates eye or rolls it superiorly
Inferior rectus	III (oculomotor)	Depresses eye or rolls it inferiorly
Inferior oblique	III (oculomotor)	Elevates eye and turns it laterally
Superior oblique	IV (trochlear)	Depresses eye and turns it laterally

Figure 45.2 ■ Extraocular muscles. **A**, Lateral view of the right eye. **B**, Superior view of the right eye. **C**, Innervation of the extraocular muscles by the cranial nerves.

Aqueous Fluid

The anterior cavity is filled with *aqueous humor*, a clear fluid that circulates through the anterior chamber (the space between the cornea and the iris) and the posterior chamber (the space between the iris and the lens). Aqueous humor is constantly formed by the ciliary body (refer to Figure 45.3) and drained to maintain a relatively constant intraocular pressure. The fluid drains into venous blood via the *scleral venous sinus* (canal of Schlemm), a network of channels that circles the eye in the angle at the junction of the sclera and the cornea. Aqueous humor provides nutrients and oxygen to the cornea and the lens.

Internal Chamber

The internal chamber of the eye contains the lens, the posterior cavity and vitreous humor, the ciliary body, the uvea, and the retina.

The *lens* is a biconvex, avascular, transparent structure located directly behind the pupil. It can change shape to focus and refract light onto the retina. The *posterior cavity* lies behind the lens. It is filled with a clear gelatinous substance, the *vitreous humor*, which supports the posterior surface of the lens, maintains the position of the retina, and transmits light.

The vascular layer, also called the *uvea*, is the middle layer of the eyeball. This pigmented layer has three components: The iris, ciliary body, and choroid. The *ciliary body* encircles the lens and, along with the iris, regulates the amount of light reaching the retina by controlling the shape of the lens. Most of the uvea is made up of the *choroid*, which includes an extensive capillary network that delivers oxygen and nutrients to the retina.

The *retina* is the innermost layer of the eye. The pigmented outer layer of the retina, next to the choroid, absorbs light and serves biochemical functions such as removing wastes and storing vitamin A. The transparent inner neural layer is made up of millions of light receptors in structures called *rods* and *cones*. Rods enable vision

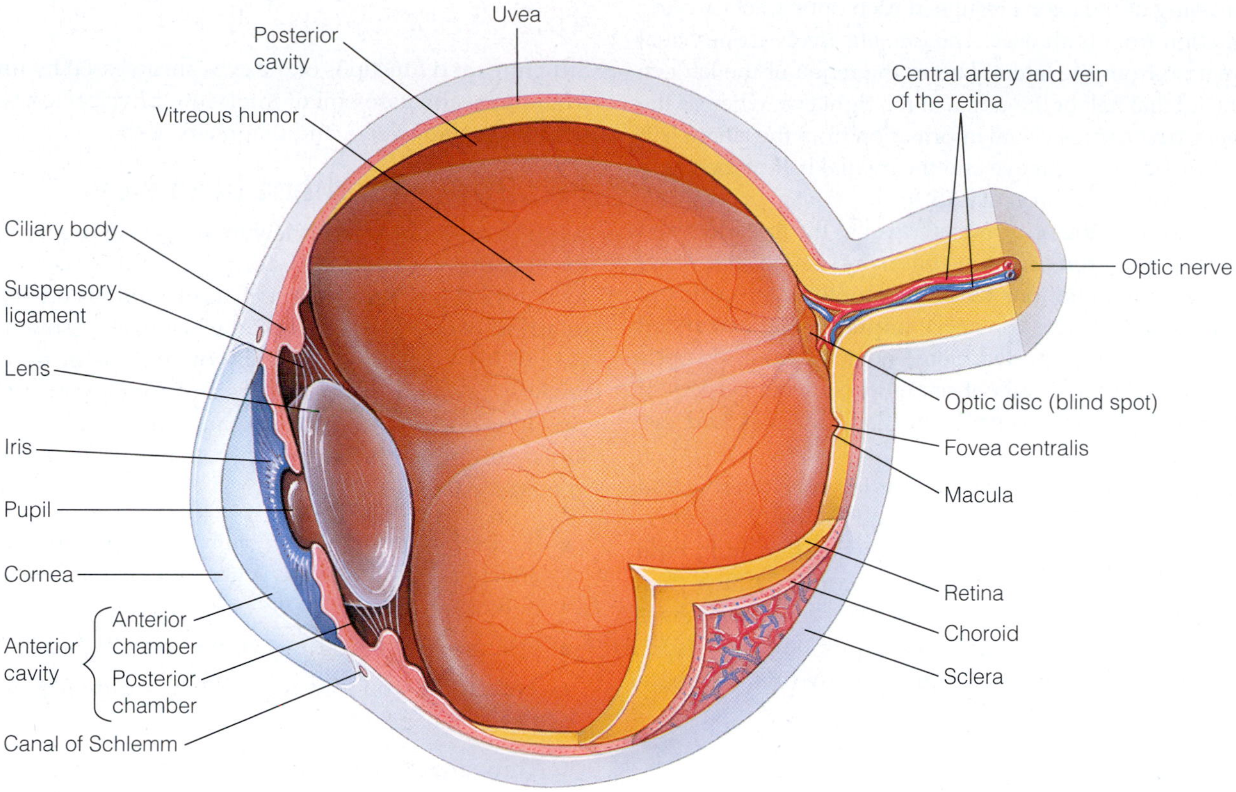
Uvea
Posterior cavity
Central artery and vein of the retina
Vitreous humor
Ciliary body
Optic nerve
Suspensory ligament
Lens
Optic disc (blind spot)
Iris
Fovea centralis
Pupil
Macula
Cornea
Retina
Anterior chamber
Choroid
Anterior cavity
Posterior chamber
Sclera
Canal of Schlemm

Figure 45.3 ■ Internal structures of the eye.

in dim light as well as peripheral vision. Cones enable vision in bright light and the perception of color. The *optic disc*, a cream-colored round or oval area within the retina, is the point at which the optic nerve enters the eye. The slight depression in the center of the optic disc is called the *physiologic cup*. The *macula*, located laterally to the optic disc, primarily contains cones. The *fovea centralis*, a slight depression in the center of the macula that contains only cones, is the area of sharpest and most detailed color vision.

The Visual Pathway

Signals produced when photoreceptors are stimulated by light are transmitted to bipolar cells and then to ganglion cells. The optic nerves are cranial nerves formed of the axons of ganglion cells. The two optic nerves meet at the *optic chiasma*, just anterior to the pituitary gland in the brain. At the optic chiasma, axons from the medial half of each retina cross to the opposite side to form pairs of axons from each eye. These pairs continue as the left and right optic tracts (**Figure 45.4** ■).

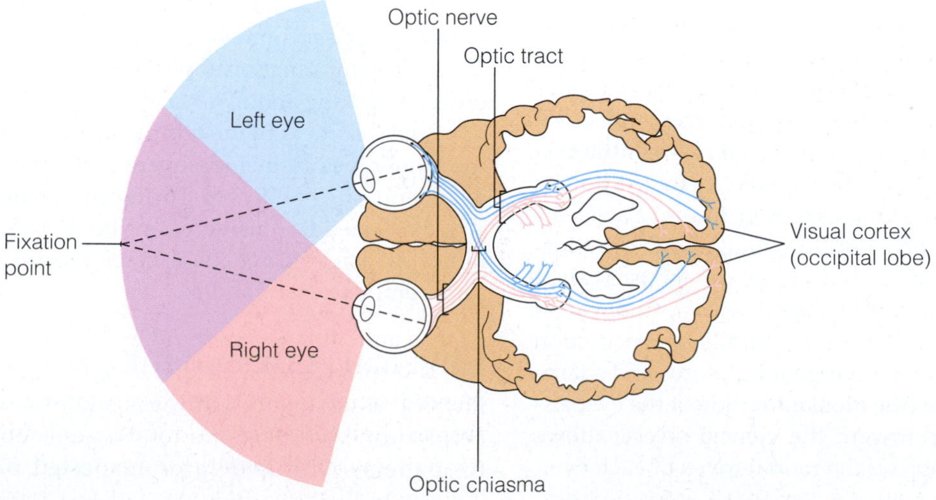
Optic nerve
Optic tract
Left eye
Fixation point
Visual cortex (occipital lobe)
Right eye
Optic chiasma

Figure 45.4 ■ The visual fields of the eye and the visual pathways to the brain.

The crossing of the axons results in each optic tract carrying information from both eyes. The *left optic tract* carries visual information from the lateral half of the retina of the left eye and the medial half of the retina of the right eye, whereas the *right optic tract* carries visual information from the lateral half of the retina of the right eye and the medial half of the retina of the left eye (Sorenson et al., 2019).

The axons in the optic tracts travel to the thalamus and synapse with neurons, forming pathways called *optic radiations*. The optic radiations terminate in the visual cortex of the *occipital lobe*, where the nerve impulses that originated in the retina are interpreted. Some neurons from the optic tracts send signals to subconscious processing centers of the midbrain, which control pupillary reflexes and eye movement.

The visual fields of each eye overlap considerably and each eye sees a slightly different view. Because of this overlap and the crossing of the axons, information from both eyes reaches each side of the visual cortex, which then fuses the information into one image. This fusion of images accounts for the ability to perceive depth; however, depth perception depends on visual input from two eyes that both focus well.

Refraction

Refraction is the bending of light rays as they pass from one medium to another medium of different density. As light rays pass through the eye, they are refracted at several points: As they enter the cornea, as they leave the cornea and enter the aqueous humor, as they enter the lens, and as they leave the lens and enter the vitreous humor. At the lens, the light is bent so that it converges at a single point on the retina. This focusing of the image is called **accommodation**. Because the lens is convex, the image projected onto the retina (the real image) is upside down and reversed from left to right. This real image is coded as electric signals that are sent to the brain. The brain decodes the image so that the person perceives it as it occurs in space.

The eyes are best adapted to see distant objects. When both eyes fix on the same distant image, the ciliary muscle is relaxed and the lens is flattened. For people with emmetropic (normal) vision, the distance from the viewed object at which the eyes require no accommodation is 6 m (20 ft). This point is called the *far point of vision*. To focus for near vision, the ciliary muscles contract, the pupils constrict, and the eyeballs converge. Ciliary muscle contraction reduces the tension on the lens capsule so that it bulges outward (becomes rounder). This change in shape achieves a shorter focal length, focusing close images on the retina. The closest point at which an individual can focus is called the *near point of vision*; in young adults with normal vision this is usually 20 to 25 cm (8 to 10 in.). Pupillary constriction helps eliminate most of the divergent light rays and sharpens focus. **Convergence** (the medial rotation of the eyeballs so that each is directed toward the viewed object) allows the focusing of the image on the retinal fovea of each eye.

45.2 Assessing the Eyes

Structures and functions of the eyes are assessed by findings from the health assessment interview, physical assessment of the eyes and vision, and diagnostic tests.

Health Assessment Interview

A health assessment interview to determine problems with the eyes may be conducted during a health screening, may focus on a chief complaint (such as blurred vision or an eye infection), or may be part of a total health assessment. If the patient has a health problem involving one or both eyes, analyze its onset, characteristics and course, severity, precipitating and relieving factors, and any associated symptoms, noting the timing and circumstances. For example, you may ask the patient:

- "Describe the type of eye pain you experience. Does it affect one or both eyes? When did it begin? How long does it last?"
- "Have you noticed rings around streetlights at night?"
- "When did you first notice having difficulty reading the newspaper?"

Throughout the interview, be alert to nonverbal behaviors (such as squinting or abnormal eye movements) that suggest problems with eye function. Explore problems such as watery, dry, or irritated eyes or changes in vision. Assess the patient's use of corrective eyewear and care of eyeglasses or contact lenses. If the patient uses eye medications, ask about the type and purpose as well as the frequency and duration of use. When taking the history, inquire about eye trauma, surgery, or infections, as well as the date and results of the last eye examination. In addition, ask about a history of diabetes, hypertension, thyroid disorders, glaucoma, cataracts, and eye infections. Include questions about a family history of nearsightedness or farsightedness, cancer of the retina, color blindness, and any other eye or vision disorders.

Collect information about environmental or work exposure to irritating chemicals, participation in sports or hobbies that pose the risk of eye injury, and the use of protective eyewear during dangerous activities, such as sawing wood or using a grass trimmer.

Collect information about possible inherited vision disorders by asking about visual disorders of family members or visual disorders in the family history. For example, does the family history include open-angle glaucoma? Macular degeneration? Follow up during the physical assessment (see the Genetics Considerations box). If the family history indicates increased genetic risk, refer to an ophthalmologist for a complete examination.

Physical Assessment

Physical assessment of the eyes and of visual acuity may be performed as part of a total assessment or separately for patients with known or suspected problems of the

Genetic Considerations

Eye Diseases with a Genetic Component

When conducting a health assessment interview and a physical assessment, it is important for the nurse to consider genetic influences on the health of an adult (National Center for Biotechnology Information, 2016). Several diseases of the eyes have a genetic component. During the health assessment interview, ask about a family history of glaucoma or blindness. Examples of eye disorders include:

- *Glaucoma* is a term used for a group of diseases that damage the optic nerve and cause blindness. Increased intraocular pressure (IOP) is commonly associated with glaucoma. Primary, open-angle glaucoma is hereditary and is influenced by mutations across multiple genes. The genetic impact on other types of glaucoma is less clear. (Glaucoma Research Foundation, 2018). If the patient has family members with glaucoma, they are at higher risk of developing the condition. Glaucoma is the leading cause of blindness in African Americans (Glaucoma Research Foundation, 2017).
- Leber hereditary optic neuropathy, which causes gradual painless loss of central vision, usually affects young men (Genetics Home Reference, 2018b).
- Retinitis pigmentosa may be transmitted in an autosomal recessive, dominant, or X-linked pattern, resulting in progressive night blindness, with loss of visual acuity and peripheral vision (Genetics Home Reference, 2018e).

eyes. The eyes and vision are primarily assessed through inspection of external structures and assessment of visual fields and visual acuity, extraocular muscle function, and internal structures. Palpation (e.g., of a blocked lacrimal duct) may be used if a problem is identified. Prior to the examination, explain the techniques to the patient to decrease anxiety. The patient may sit or stand during the assessment.

Visual acuity is assessed with an eye chart such as the Snellen chart or the E chart for distance vision and the Rosenbaum chart for near vision. The Snellen chart contains rows of letters in various sizes, with numbers at the end of each row to indicate the visual acuity of a patient who can read the row at a distance of 20 ft (6 m). (The E chart is used for the patient who is unable to read or does not read English.) The top number at the end of the row is always 20, representing the distance between the patient and the chart. The bottom number is the distance (in feet) at which an individual with normal vision can read the line. An individual with normal vision can read the row marked 20/20. To conduct the assessment, position the person 20 ft from the chart in a well-lit area. Ask the patient to cover one eye with an opaque cover (**Figure 45.5** ■). Then ask the patient to read the smallest row discernible. Measure visual acuity in the other eye in the same way, and then assess visual acuity with the patient using both eyes. The patient who wears corrective lenses may be tested with and without the lenses.

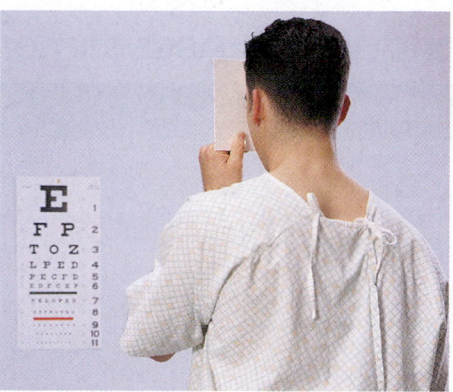
E
F P
T O Z

Figure 45.5 ■ Testing distant vision using the Snellen eye chart.

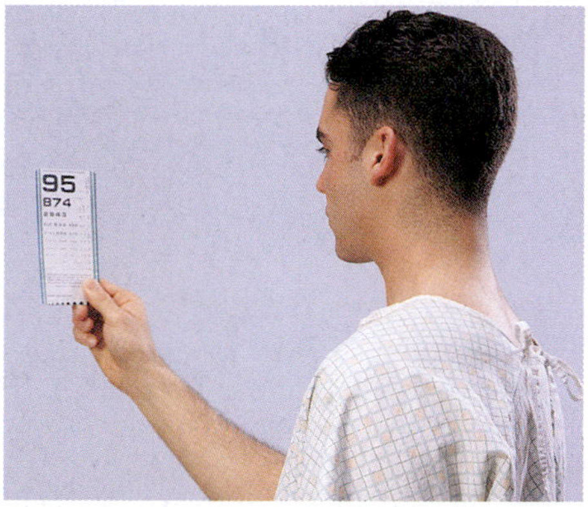
95
874

Figure 45.6 ■ Testing near vision using the Rosenbaum eye chart.

The Rosenbaum chart is held at a distance of 30 to 36 cm (12 to 14 in.) from the eyes, with visual acuity measured in the same manner as with the Snellen chart (**Figure 45.6** ■). A gross estimate of near vision may also be assessed by asking the person to read from a magazine or newspaper.

Diagnosis

Diagnostic tests to assess the structure and functions of the eyes are used to support the diagnosis of a specific injury, disease, or vision problem; to provide information to guide treatment; and to monitor the patient's responses to treatment and interventions. These tests are most often conducted in a healthcare provider's office. Diagnostic tests of the eyes are described in the Diagnostic Tests table on page 1682 (Kee, 2017).

Regardless of the type of diagnostic test, the nurse is responsible for explaining the procedure and any special preparation, for assessing any medication use that might affect the test outcome, for supporting the patient during the examination as necessary, for ensuring the consent form is signed (if required), and for monitoring the results of the tests. The nurse is also responsible for postprocedure care and patient teaching for self-care at home.

Eye and Vision Assessments

Technique/Normal Findings	Abnormal Findings
Vision Assessment	
Assess distant vision, using the Snellen or E chart. *When standing 20 ft from the chart, the patient can read the smallest line of letters with or without corrective lenses (recorded as 20/20).*	■ Changes in distant vision are often the result of **myopia** (nearsightedness). For example, a reading of 20/100 indicates impaired distance vision. An individual has to stand 20 ft from the chart to read a line that an individual with normal vision could read 100 ft from the chart.
Assess near vision, using a Rosenbaum chart or a card with newsprint held 12–14 in. from the patient's eyes. *Normal near visual acuity is 14/14 with or without corrective lenses.*	■ Changes in near vision, especially in patients over age 45, can indicate **presbyopia**, impaired near vision resulting from a loss of elasticity of the lens related to aging. In younger patients, this condition is referred to as **hyperopia** (farsightedness).
Visual Fields Assessment Assess visual fields using the confrontation test to evaluate peripheral vision (**Figure 45.7** ■). The visual fields of the examiner (which must be normal for this assessment) are used as the standard. Sit directly opposite the patient at a distance of 18–24 in. and instruct the patient to look directly at you. Ask the patient to cover one eye while you cover your own eye opposite to the patient (e.g., the patient's right eye and examiner's left eye). Move the penlight from the periphery toward the center from right to left, above and below, and from the middle of each of these directions. *Both you and the patient should see the penlight enter the field of vision at the same time if the examiner has normal peripheral vision.*	■ Narrowing of visual fields may occur with aging or may indicate an eye disorder such as glaucoma or retinal detachment or a neurologic disorder.

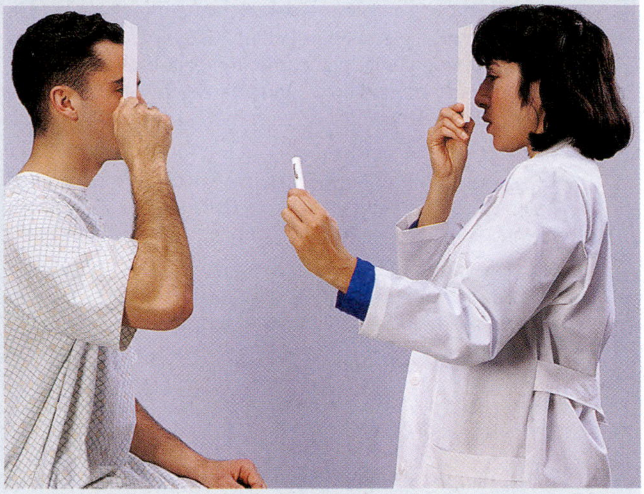

Figure 45.7 ■ Visual field testing.

Technique/Normal Findings	Abnormal Findings
Eye Movement Assessment	
Assess the cardinal fields of gaze to evaluate extraocular eye movements. Ask the patient to follow a pen while keeping the head stationary. Move the pen through the six fields one at a time, returning to the central starting point before proceeding to the next field (**Figure 45.8** ■). *The eyes should move through each field without involuntary movements.* The cover test is used to evaluate alignment of the eyes. To conduct the test, hold a pen or your finger about 1 ft from the eyes and ask the person to focus on that object. Cover one of the patient's eyes and note any movement in the uncovered eye; as you remove the cover, assess for movement in the eye that was just uncovered. Repeat the procedure with the other eye. *The gaze should remain steady and fixed with covering and uncovering of the eye.*	■ Failure of one or both eyes to follow the object in any given direction may indicate extraocular muscle weakness or cranial nerve dysfunction. ■ An involuntary rhythmic movement of the eyes, **nystagmus**, is associated with neurologic disorders and the use of some medications. ■ Movement of an eye with the cover test indicates weakness of eye muscles.

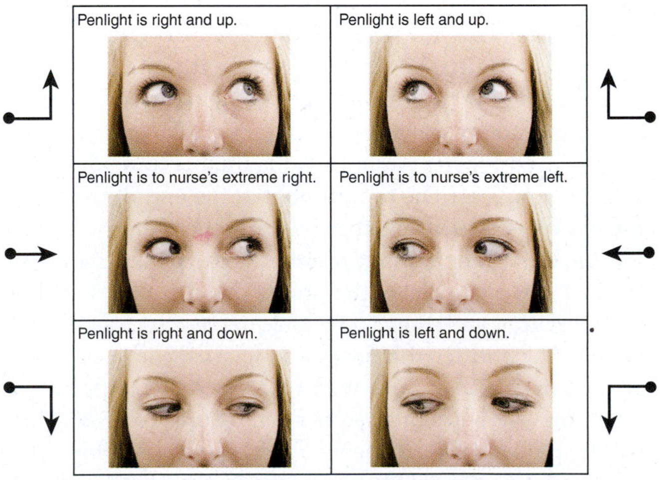
Penlight is right and up.
Penlight is left and up.
Penlight is to nurse's extreme right.
Penlight is to nurse's extreme left.
Penlight is right and down.
Penlight is left and down.

Figure 45.8 ■ The six cardinal fields of gaze.

Technique/Normal Findings	Abnormal Findings
Assess the corneal light reflex. Direct a light source onto the bridge of the nose from 12 to 15 in. away. *Observe for symmetric reflection of the light from each eye.*	■ Reflections of the light from different sites on the eyes reveal extraocular muscle weakness.
Assess convergence. Ask the patient to follow an object as you move it toward the patient's eyes. *Normally, both eyes converge toward the center.*	■ Failure of the eyes to converge equally on an approaching object may indicate a neuromuscular disorder or extraocular muscle weakness.
Pupillary Assessment	
Observe pupil size, shape, and equality. *Pupils should be round and of equal size, 3–5 mm.*	■ Pupils that are unequal in size may indicate previous eye surgery or a serious neurologic problem, such as increased intracranial pressure.
Assess direct and consensual pupil response. Ask the patient to look straight ahead. Shine a light obliquely into one eye at a time. Observe for constriction of the pupil in the illuminated eye. Test both eyes. To test consensual pupil response, again shine a light obliquely into one eye at a time as the patient looks straight ahead. Observe constriction of the pupil in the opposite eye. *The normal direct and consensual pupillary response is prompt constriction.*	■ Failure of the pupils to respond to light may indicate degeneration of the retina or destruction of the optic nerve. ■ A patient who has one dilated and unresponsive pupil may have paralysis of the oculomotor nerve. ■ Some eye medications may cause unequal dilation, constriction, or inequality of pupil size. Morphine and narcotic drugs may cause small pupils with poor responses to light, and anticholinergic drugs such as atropine may cause dilated, poorly responsive pupils.
Test for accommodation. Hold an object at a distance of a few feet from the patient. The pupils should dilate. Ask the patient to follow the object as you bring it to within a few inches of his or her nose. *The pupils should constrict and converge as they change focus to follow the object.*	■ Failure of accommodation along with lack of pupil response to light may signal a neurologic problem. ■ Lack of response to light with appropriate response to accommodation is often seen in patients with diabetes.
External Eye Assessment	
Inspect the eyelids. *Eyelids should be the color of the patient's facial skin, without redness, discharge, or drooping. The lids should just cover the upper and lower borders of the iris.*	■ Unusual redness or discharge may indicate inflammation due to trauma, allergies, or infection. ■ Drooping of one eyelid, called **ptosis**, may be the result of a stroke, indicate a neuromuscular disorder, or be congenital (**Figure 45.9** ■). ■ Unusual widening of the lids may be due to exophthalmos (protrusion of the eyeball). Exophthalmos is often associated with hyperthyroid conditions. ■ An acute localized inflammation of a hair follicle is known as a hordeolum (sty) and is generally caused by staphylococcal organisms. ■ A chalazion is an infection or retention cyst of the meibomian glands.

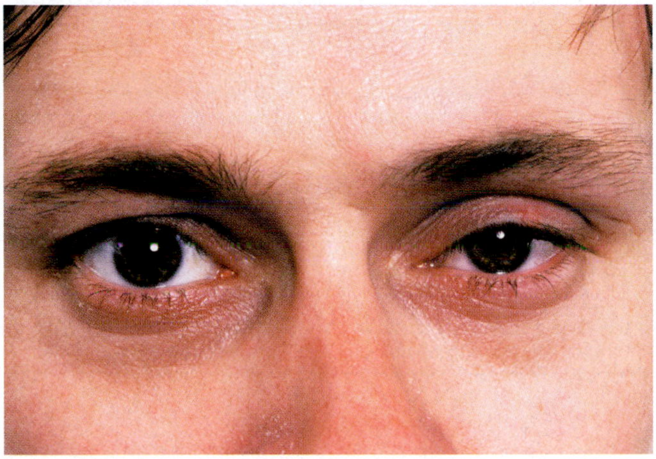

Figure 45.9 ■ Ptosis.

Technique/Normal Findings	Abnormal Findings
Inspect the puncta. *The puncta should be free of redness or discharge.*	■ Unusual redness or discharge from the puncta may indicate an inflammation due to trauma, infection, or allergies.
Inspect the bulbar and palpebral conjunctiva. *The conjunctiva should be clear, moist, and smooth. The upper and lower palpebral conjunctiva should be clear, without redness or swelling.*	■ Increased erythema or the presence of exudate may indicate acute conjunctivitis. ■ Conjunctival pallor may indicate anemia. ■ A fold in the conjunctiva, called a pterygium, may be seen as a clouded area that extends over the cornea. This is an abnormal growth of the bulbar conjunctiva, usually seen on the nasal side of the cornea. It may interfere with vision if it covers the pupil.
Inspect the sclera. *The sclera is white in people of European descent; people with darker skin normally have yellow sclera.*	■ Unusual redness may indicate an inflammatory state as a result of trauma, allergies, or infection. ■ Yellow discoloration of the sclera in patients with fair skin may be seen in conditions involving the liver, such as hepatitis. ■ Bright red areas in the sclera are often subconjunctival hemorrhages and may indicate trauma or bleeding disorders. They may also occur spontaneously.
Inspect the cornea. *The cornea is normally transparent.*	■ Dullness, opacities, or irregularities of the cornea may be abnormal. ■ Corneal arcus is a thin, grayish-white arc seen toward the edge of the cornea. It is normal in older adults.

(continued)

Eye and Vision Assessments (*continued*)

Technique/Normal Findings	Abnormal Findings
Assess corneal sensitivity. Lightly touch a wisp of cotton to the patient's cornea. *This action should cause a corneal reflex (blinking of the eye).*	■ Failure of the corneal reflex may indicate a neurologic disorder.
Inspect the iris. *The iris is normally round, flat, and evenly colored.*	■ Lack of clarity of the iris may indicate a cloudiness of the cornea. ■ Constriction of the pupil accompanied by pain and circumcorneal redness indicates acute iritis.
Palpate over the lacrimal glands, puncta, and nasolacrimal duct. (Wear gloves if you see any drainage.) *There should be no tenderness, drainage, or excessive tearing.*	■ Tenderness over any of these areas or drainage from the puncta may indicate an infectious process. ■ Excessive tearing may indicate a blockage of the nasolacrimal duct.
Internal Eye Assessment	
Assess internal structures of the eye using the ophthalmoscope, an instrument that allows visualization of the lens, the vitreous humor, and the retina. **Box 45.1** provides guidelines for using an ophthalmoscope.	
Inspect for the red reflex. *The red reflex should be clearly visible.*	■ Absence of a red reflex often indicates improper position of the ophthalmoscope, but also may indicate total opacity of the pupil by a cataract or a hemorrhage into the vitreous humor.
Inspect the lens and vitreous body. *The lens should be clear.*	■ A cataract is an opacity of the lens, often seen as a dark shadow on ophthalmoscopic examination. It may be a result of aging, trauma, diabetes, or a congenital defect.
Inspect the retina. *There should be no visible hemorrhages, exudate, or white patches.*	■ Areas of hemorrhage, exudate, and white patches may be a result of diabetes or long-standing hypertension.
Inspect the optic disc. *The optic disc should be round to oval in shape with clear, well-defined borders.*	■ Loss of definition of the optic disc, as well as an increase in the size of the physiologic cup, is seen in papilledema from increased intracranial pressure.
Inspect the blood vessels of the retina. *The retinal blood vessels should be distinct.*	■ Glaucoma may cause displacement of blood vessels from the center of the optic disc due to increased intraocular pressure. ■ Hypertension may cause a narrowing of the vein where an arteriole crosses over. ■ Engorged veins may occur with diabetes, atherosclerosis, and blood disorders.
Inspect the retinal background. *The retina should be a consistent red-orange color, becoming lighter around the optic disc.*	■ Variations in color or a pale color overall may indicate disease.
Inspect the macula. *The macula should be visible on the temporal side of the optic disc.*	■ Absence of the *fovea centralis is common in older patients. It* may indicate macular degeneration, a cause of loss of central vision.

BOX 45.1
Guidelines for Using an Ophthalmoscope

The ophthalmoscope has a head and a handle.

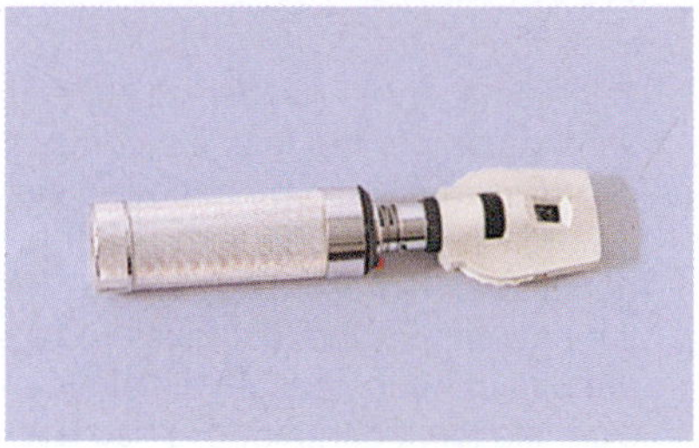

An ophthalmoscope.

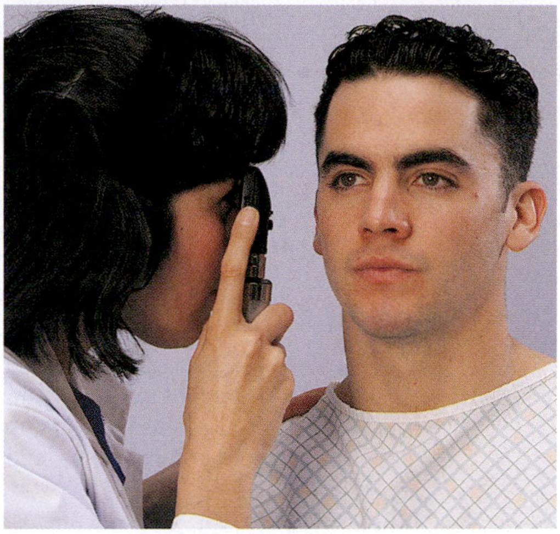

Technique for holding an ophthalmoscope.

The head contains a focus wheel (also called a *lens selector dial*) located on the side, lenses of varying magnification, and an opening through which the eye structures are visualized. The focus wheel adjusts the lens refraction, which is measured in diopters. The diopter measurements range from 0 to +40 when the lens is rotated clockwise, and from 0 to –25 when the lens is rotated counterclockwise. By moving the focus wheel, the examiner can focus light rays to visualize the retina. The handle usually contains batteries that can be recharged. *Note:* Assessing the internal eye with the ophthalmoscope is a skill that takes practice.

Before the examination, explain the procedure to the patient. Assemble the ophthalmoscope. Wash your hands and wear disposable gloves if the patient has any drainage from the eyes. Darken the room (to allow the pupils of the patient to dilate) and ask the patient to look straight ahead, focusing on a fixed point such as an object on the wall. Hold the ophthalmoscope in one hand, resting the index finger on the focus wheel.

1. Turn on the ophthalmoscope light, and set the focus wheel to 0 diopters. Hold the ophthalmoscope in your right hand with your index finger on the focus wheel. Standing in front of the patient, position yourself at a 15-degree angle to the patient's line of vision.
2. Hold the opening of the ophthalmoscope up to your right eye and direct the light toward the patient's right eye from a distance of about 12 in.
3. As the beam of light falls on the patient's pupil, observe for the red reflex, which appears as a sharply outlined orange glow from within the pupil. This glow is the reflection of the light from the retina.
4. Move closer to the patient, turning the focus wheel clockwise toward the positive numbers as needed to maintain clear focus.
5. Examine the lens and the vitreous body, both of which should be clear.
6. Gradually rotate the focus wheel counterclockwise toward the negative numbers as needed, focusing on a structure of the retina (such as the disc or a blood vessel). Turn the focus wheel until the image is clear. Examine the structures of the retina as follows:
   a. *Optic disc:* Assess for size, shape, color, distinct margins, and the physiologic cup. The disc is round to slightly oval and about 1.5–2 mm in diameter. It has a yellow to pink color that is lighter than the retina itself. The margins should be sharp and clear. The physiologic cup is a small depression that occupies about one-third of the optic disc, lying temporal to the center of the disc.

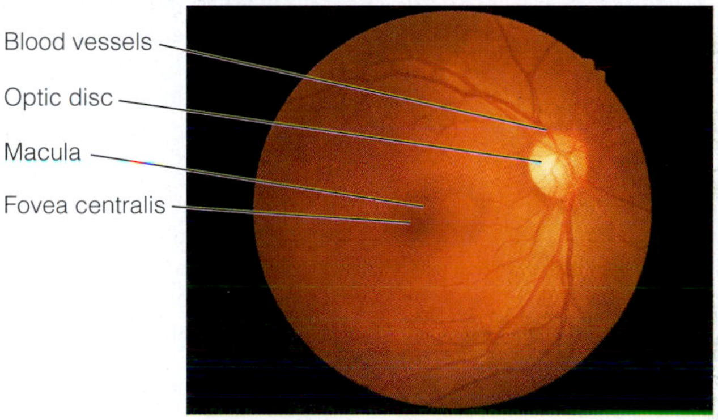
Blood vessels
Optic disc
Macula
Fovea centralis

The optic disc as seen through an ophthalmoscope.
Source: Don Wong/Science Source/Photo Researchers, Inc.

   b. *Vessels of the retina:* Assess for color, arteriolar light reflex, ratio of arterioles to veins, and arteriovenous crossings. The arterioles are red, brighter than the veins, and about one-fourth smaller. The arterioles normally have a narrow light reflex from the center of each vessel; veins do not have this light reflex. The ratio of arterioles to veins is usually 2:3 or 4:5. The vessels normally cross and become smaller toward the periphery.
   c. *Retinal background:* Assess color and changes in color. The retina is normally reddish-orange and regular in color.
   d. *Macula:* Assess size and color. To assess the macula, ask the patient to look directly into the ophthalmoscope light. The macula is temporal to the optic disc, appears slightly darker than the retina, and has no visible vessels. The fovea centralis may be seen as a bright spot of light. Because looking directly into the light causes some discomfort, conduct this portion of the examination last. The macula is often difficult to visualize.
7. Using the same technique, examine the left eye.

Diagnostic Tests of the Eye

NAME OF TEST	PURPOSE AND DESCRIPTION	RELATED NURSING INTERVENTIONS
Computed tomography (CT) scan and magnetic resonance imaging (MRI) of the eye	Imaging techniques used to identify foreign objects or tumors within the eye, orbit, or optic nerve. The head is positioned in a cradle and a wide strap is applied around the head to keep it immobilized during the test. MRI is contraindicated if a metallic foreign body is suspected.	Tell the patient to remove all hairpins, clips, and earrings before the test. If a contrast dye is used, dentures must also be removed. Assess for allergies to iodine (e.g., to shellfish or previous procedures) and, if present, notify the physician. Inform the patient that the test takes 5–10 min. Instruct the patient to increase oral fluid intake after the examination if contrast dye has been used.
Fluorescein angiography	Fluorescein solution is injected IV to evaluate blood vessels in the eye in conditions such as diabetes, macular degeneration, or retinal vessel occlusion.	Informed consent is required for this test. Note current medications and notify the physician if the patient is pregnant. Inform the patient that a hot flush and transient nausea may be experienced when the dye is injected. Monitor for anaphylactic hypersensitivity responses that may occur. Fluorescent yellow-colored urine and a yellow skin color may be noted for 1–2 days after the procedure; these are not harmful.
Refraction, retinoscopy, refractometry	These tests are used to measure refractive error. Either a handheld retinoscope or an instrument with multiple lenses is used; with the latter method the patient chooses lenses that provide best vision.	No special preparation is needed; tell the patient that pupils will be dilated with medication and may be enlarged for several hours.
Tonometry	This test is used to diagnose increased intraocular pressure in glaucoma. A handheld tonometer or computerized device may be used. The cornea is anesthetized prior to being touched with the device. Normal value: 10–22 mmHg.	No special preparation is needed. Instruct the patient not to rub the eyes.
Ultrasonography	Ultrasonography may be used to assess retinal tumors or detachments and vitreous hemorrhage or to locate foreign bodies.	This noninvasive test is painless and requires no special patient preparation.

45.3 Anatomy, Physiology, and Functions of the Ears

As a sensory organ, the ears have two primary functions: Hearing and maintaining equilibrium. Anatomically, each ear is divided into three areas: The external ear, the middle ear, and the inner ear (**Figure 45.10** ■). All three are involved in hearing, but only the inner ear is involved in equilibrium (Sorenson et al., 2019).

The External Ear

The *external ear* consists of the auricle (or pinna), the external auditory canal, and the tympanic membrane. The *auricles* contain sebaceous and sweat glands and sometimes hair. Each auricle has a rim (the helix) and a lobe. The auricle serves to direct sound waves into the ear. The *external auditory canal*, which is about 2.5 cm (1 in.) long, extends from the auricle to the tympanic membrane. The canal is lined with skin that contains hair, sebaceous glands, and ceruminous glands. The external auditory canal serves as a resonator for the range of sound waves typical of human speech and increases the pressure that sound waves in this frequency range place on the tympanic membrane. The canal's ceruminous glands secrete a yellow to brown waxy substance called **cerumen**. Cerumen traps foreign bodies; it also has bacteriostatic properties, protecting the tympanic membrane and the middle ear from infections.

The *tympanic membrane* lies between the external ear and the middle ear. It is a thin, semitransparent, fibrous structure covered with skin on the external side and mucosa on the inner side. The membrane vibrates as sound waves strike it; these vibrations are transferred as sound waves to the middle ear.

The Middle Ear

The *middle ear* is an air-filled cavity in the temporal bone. The middle ear contains the three auditory ossicles: The malleus, the incus, and the stapes. These bones extend across the middle ear to the tympanic membrane. The medial side of the middle ear is a bony wall containing two membrane-covered openings: The oval window and the round window. The posterior wall of the middle ear

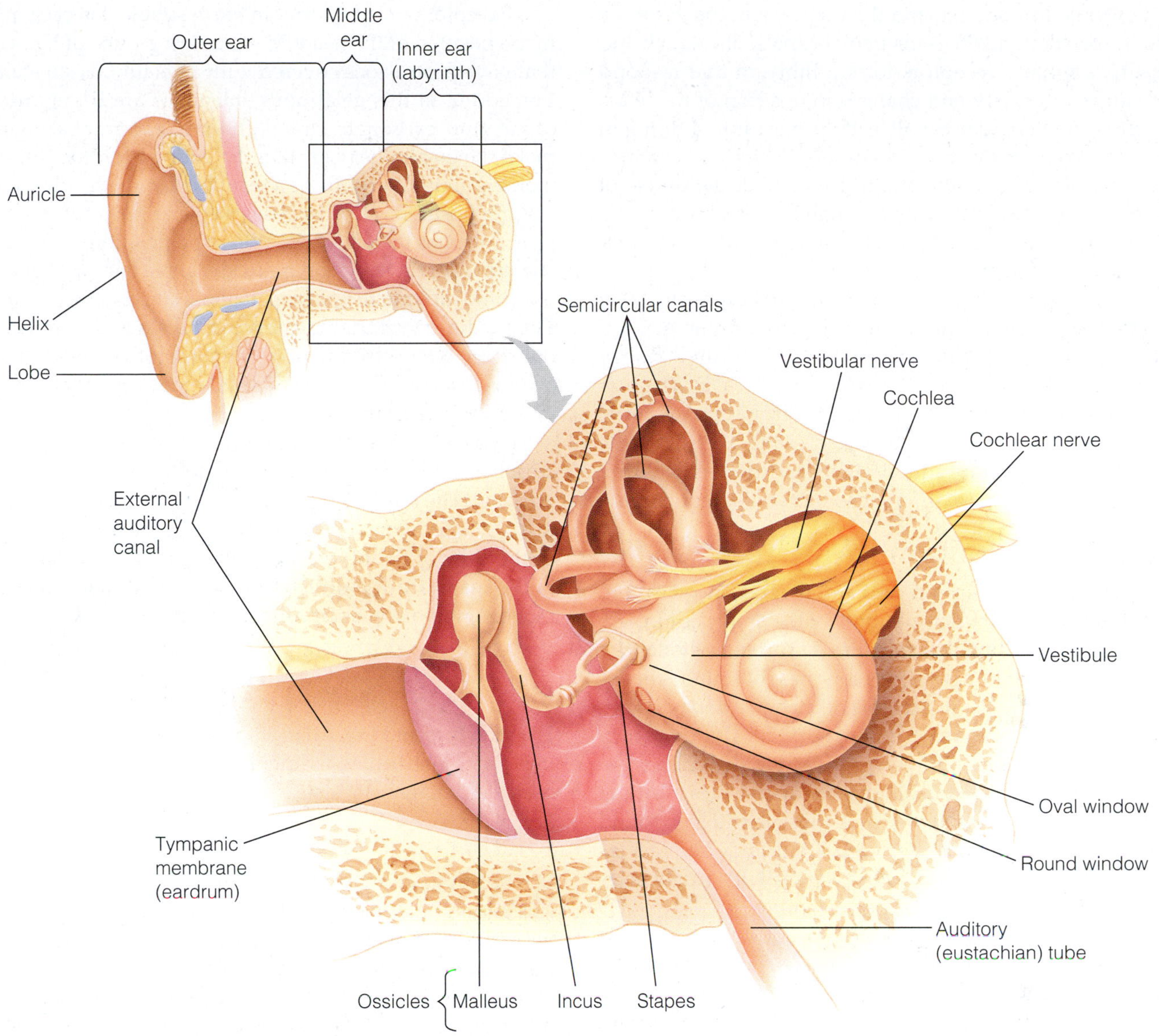
Outer ear
Middle ear
Inner ear (labyrinth)
Auricle
Helix
Lobe
External auditory canal
Semicircular canals
Vestibular nerve
Cochlea
Cochlear nerve
Vestibule
Oval window
Round window
Auditory (eustachian) tube
Tympanic membrane (eardrum)
Ossicles
Malleus
Incus
Stapes

Figure 45.10 ■ Structures of the external ear, middle ear, and inner ear.

contains the *mastoid antrum*, which communicates with the mastoid sinuses. The mastoid sinuses help the middle ear adjust to changes in pressure. The middle ear also opens into the auditory tube (also called the *pharyngotympanic* or *Eustachian tube*), which connects with the nasopharynx. The *auditory tube* helps to equalize the air pressure in the middle ear by opening briefly in response to differences between middle ear pressure and atmospheric pressure. The mucous membrane lining the middle ear is continuous with the mucous membranes lining the pharynx.

The *malleus* attaches to the tympanic membrane and articulates with the *incus*, which in turn articulates with the *stapes*. The stapes fits into the oval window. When the tympanic membrane vibrates, the vibrations are conducted across the middle ear to the oval window by the ossicles. The vibrations set in motion the fluids of the inner ear, which in turn stimulate the hearing receptors. Two small muscles attached to the ossicles contract reflexively in response to sudden loud noises, decreasing the vibrations and protecting the inner ear.

The Inner Ear

The *inner ear*, also called the *labyrinth*, is a maze of bony chambers (the bony labyrinth) located deep within the temporal bone, just behind the eye socket. The *membranous labyrinth*, a delicate network of interconnected fluid-filled tubes, lies within this maze. *Perilymph*, a fluid similar to cerebrospinal fluid, flows between the bony and the membranous labyrinth. Within the chambers of the membranous labyrinth is a fluid called *endolymph*. These fluids conduct sound vibrations and respond to changes in body position and movement.

The bony labyrinth has three regions: The vestibule, the semicircular canals, and the cochlea. The *vestibule* is the central portion of the inner ear, one side of which is a bony wall containing the oval window. Two sacs within the vestibule (the saccule and the utricle) join the vestibule with the cochlea and the semicircular canals. The *saccule* and the *utricle* contain receptors for equilibrium that respond to changes in gravity and changes in position of the head. The three semicircular canals each project into a different plane (anterior, posterior, and lateral). Each canal contains a semicircular duct that communicates with the utricle of the vestibule. Each duct has an enlarged area at one end containing an equilibrium receptor that responds to angular movements of the head.

The *cochlea* is a tiny bony chamber that houses the *organ of Corti*, the receptor organ for hearing. The organ of Corti is a series of sensory hair cells, arranged in a single row of inner hair cells and three rows of outer hair cells. The hair cells are innervated by sensory fibers from cranial nerve VIII. The organ of Corti is supported in the cochlea by the flexible basilar membrane, which has fibers of varying lengths that respond to different sound wave frequencies.

Sound Conduction

Hearing is the perception and interpretation of sound. Sound is produced when the molecules of a medium are compressed, resulting in a pressure disturbance evidenced as a sound wave. The intensity or loudness of sound is determined by the amplitude (height) of the sound wave, with greater amplitudes causing louder sounds. The frequency of the sound wave in vibrations per second determines the pitch or tone of the sound, with higher frequencies resulting in higher sounds. The human ear is most sensitive to sound waves with frequencies between 1000 and 4000 cycles per second, but can detect sound waves with frequencies between 20 and 20,000 cycles per second.

Sound waves enter the external auditory canal and cause the tympanic membrane to vibrate at the same frequency. The ossicles not only transmit the motion of the tympanic membrane to the oval window but also amplify the energy of the sound wave. As the stapes moves against the oval window, the perilymph in the vestibule is set in motion. The increased pressure of the perilymph is transmitted to fibers of the basilar membrane and then to the organ of Corti. The up-and-down movements of the fibers of the basilar membrane pull the hair cells in the organ of Corti, which in turn generates action potentials that are transmitted to cranial nerve VIII and then to the brain for interpretation.

Several brainstem auditory nuclei transmit impulses to the cerebral cortex. Fibers from each ear cross, with each auditory cortex receiving impulses from both ears. Auditory processing is so finely tuned that a wide variety of sounds of different pitch and loudness can be heard at any one time. In addition, the source of the sound can be localized.

Equilibrium

The inner ear also provides information about the position of the head. This information is used to coordinate body movements so that equilibrium and balance are maintained (Sorenson et al., 2019). The types of equilibrium are static balance (affected by changes in the position of the head) and dynamic balance (affected by the movement of the head).

Receptors called *maculae* in the vestibule detect changes in the position of the head. Maculae are groups of hair cells that have protrusions covered with a gelatinous substance. Embedded in this gelatinous substance are tiny particles of calcium carbonate called *otoliths* (ear stones), which make the gelatin heavier than the endolymph that fills the membranous labyrinth. As a result, when the head is in the upright position, gravity causes the gelatinous substance to bear down on the hair cells. When the position of the head changes, the force on the hair cells also changes, bending them and altering the pattern of stimulation of the neurons. Thus, a different pattern of nerve impulses is transmitted to the brain, where stimulation of the motor centers initiates actions that coordinate various body movements according to the position of the head.

The receptor for dynamic equilibrium is in the crista, a crest in the membrane lining the ampulla of each semicircular canal. The cristae are stimulated by rotatory head movement (acceleration and deceleration) as a result of changes in the flow of endolymph and of movement of hair cells in the maculae. The direction of endolymph and hair cell movement is always opposite to the motion of the body.

45.4 Assessing the Ears

The structure and functions of the ears are assessed by findings from a health assessment interview, physical assessment, and diagnostic tests.

Health Assessment Interview

The health history to collect subjective data about the ears and hearing may be part of a health screening, may focus on a chief complaint (such as hearing problems or pain in the ear), or may be part of a total health assessment. If the patient has a problem involving one or both ears, analyze its onset, characteristics and course, severity, precipitating and relieving factors, and any associated symptoms, noting the timing and circumstances. For example, you may ask the following questions:

- "Have you noticed any difficulty hearing high-pitched sounds, low-pitched sounds, or both?"
- "When did you first notice the ringing in your ears? Is it constant or intermittent?"
- "Is your workplace very noisy? If so, do you wear protective ear equipment at work?"
- "Do you or have you listened to music with headphones or earbuds?"
- "Do you attend loud concerts or other types of entertainment?"

Throughout the examination, be alert to nonverbal behaviors (such as inappropriate answers, requests to repeat statements, or tilting the head toward you) that suggest problems with ear function. Explore changes in hearing, ringing in the ears (tinnitus), ear pain, drainage from the ears, or the use of hearing aids. When taking the history, ask about trauma, surgery, or infections of the ear as well

Genetic Considerations

Hearing Impairments with a Genetic Component

When conducting a health assessment interview and a physical assessment, it is important for the nurse to consider genetic influences on the health of an adult. Several diseases of the ears and types of hearing impairment have a genetic component. During the health assessment interview, ask about a family history of presbycusis, congenital hearing impairment, hearing impairment associated with another disorder such as vision loss or a kidney or thyroid disorder, or tumors of the auditory nerve.

During the physical assessment, assess for any manifestations that might indicate a genetic syndrome such as symptoms of thyroid, kidney, or vision disorders. If data are found to indicate genetic risk factors or alterations, ask about genetic testing and refer for appropriate genetic counseling and evaluation.

Examples of ear disorders include:

- Hereditary hearing impairment (HHI) is believed to account for more than 50% of childhood hearing loss and can also manifest later in life. Most HHI follows an autosomal recessive inheritance pattern (Shearer, Hildebrand, & Smith, 2017).
- Heredity is increasingly recognized as a contributor to presbycusis (hearing loss associated with aging) (Genetics Home Reference, 2018a).
- Pendred syndrome is an inherited disorder that accounts for as much as 10% of hereditary deafness. The deafness is usually accompanied by a thyroid goiter (Genetics Home Reference, 2018d).
- Neurofibromatosis type 2, a rare inherited disorder, is characterized by the development of acoustic neuromas (benign tumors of the auditory nerve) and malignant central nervous system tumors (Genetics Home Reference, 2018c).

as the date of the last ear examination. In addition, ask the patient about a medical history of infectious diseases, such as meningitis or mumps, as well as the use of medications that may affect hearing. Because ear problems tend to run in families, ask about a family history of hearing loss, ear problems, or diseases that could result in such problems (see the Genetic Considerations box). If the patient has a hearing aid, ascertain the type and assess measures for its care.

Physical Assessment

Physical assessment of the ears and hearing may be performed as part of a total health assessment or separately for patients with known or suspected problems with the ears. The ears and hearing are assessed primarily through inspection of external structures, the auditory canal, and the tympanic membrane. Hearing acuity is assessed by the whisper test and using a tuning fork.

The patient should be sitting, and the examiner's head should be level with the head of the patient. Prior to the assessment, collect all necessary equipment and explain the techniques to the patient to decrease anxiety. The auditory canal and tympanic membrane are inspected with an otoscope. Guidelines for use of the otoscope are listed in **Box 45.2**.

BOX 45.2

Guidelines for Using an Otoscope

The otoscope is used to inspect the auditory canal and the tympanic membrane. The handle contains batteries for the light; specula of varied sizes are used to direct the light.

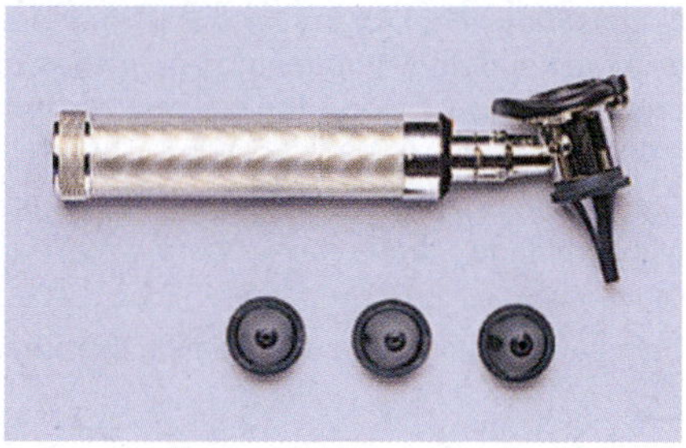

An otoscope.

Before the examination, explain the procedure to the patient. Assemble the otoscope, using the largest speculum that will fit into the patient's auditory canal without discomfort. Wash your hands; wear disposable gloves if the patient has any drainage from the ears. Turn on the otoscope light. Ask the patient to tip the head slightly toward the shoulder opposite the ear being examined. When the patient is in this position, the auditory canal is aligned with the speculum.

1. Hold the handle of the otoscope in your dominant hand. If the patient is restless, hold the otoscope handle upward, resting the hand against the patient's head.
2. For adult patients, grasp the superior portion of the auricle and pull up, out, and back to straighten the auditory canal.

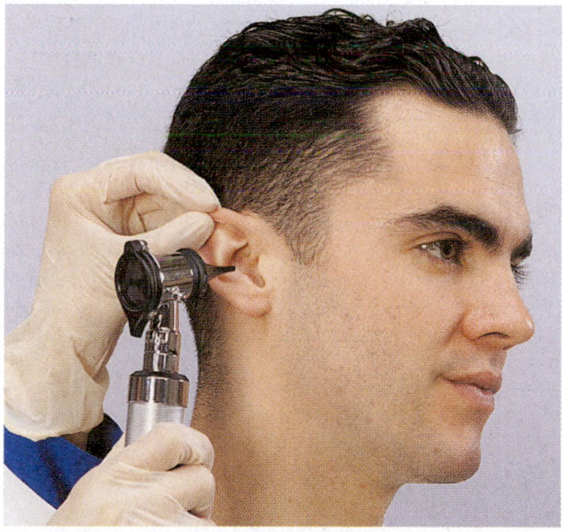

Technique for using an otoscope.

3. Insert the speculum into the ear. While gently advancing the speculum, inspect the walls of the auditory canal for color, obstructions, hair growth, and cerumen. Old cerumen is very dark and may obstruct visualization of part or all of the tympanic membrane.
4. Adjusting auditory canal alignment and otoscope position as needed, inspect the tympanic membrane. A normal membrane is translucent, allowing a portion of the malleus to be seen as a shadow behind the membrane. A cone-shaped light reflection should be visible.
5. Note the color and surface of the membrane. The normal tympanic membrane is pearly gray, shiny, and

(*continued*)

semitransparent. The surface should be continuous, intact, and either flat or concave.

6. Identify the landmarks on the tympanic membrane:
   a. The cone of light, located in the anteroinferior quadrant (5 o'clock position on the right side; 7 o'clock on the left)
   b. The malleus, pars tensa, annulus, pars flaccida, and malleolar folds.
7. Assess movement of the tympanic membrane. If the auditory tube is patent, the membrane moves in and out when air is injected or when the patient performs the Valsalva maneuver.
8. Gently withdraw the speculum. If the speculum is soiled with drainage or cerumen, use a clean speculum for the other ear.
9. Using the same technique, examine the other ear.

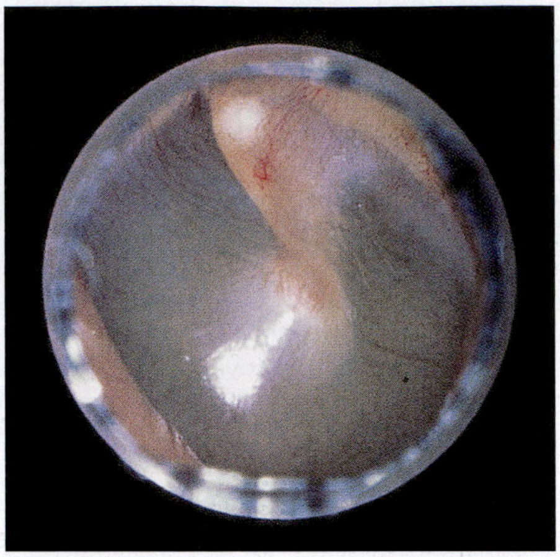

The tympanic membrane as it appears through the otoscope.

Ear and Hearing Assessments

Technique/Normal Findings	Abnormal Findings
Hearing Assessment	
Perform the whisper test. Ask the patient to occlude one ear with a finger. Standing behind and 1–2 ft away from the patient, whisper numbers and ask the patient to repeat them. Repeat the procedure, having the patient occlude the other ear. Note whether you need to raise your voice or to stand closer to make the patient hear you. *The patient with no hearing loss will accurately repeat whispered numbers or a phrase.*	■ Inability to repeat what is said may indicate a hearing loss.
Assess auditory acuity using a tuning fork. A tuning fork with a frequency of 512 Hz is preferred for auditory evaluation. Hold the tuning fork at the base and make it vibrate by stroking, squeezing, or lightly tapping the prongs on the heel of the opposite hand. The following tests are performed to evaluate conductive versus perceptive hearing loss.	
Perform the Weber test. Place the base of a vibrating tuning fork on the midline vertex of the patient's head (**Figure 45.11** ■). Ask whether the patient hears the sound equally in both ears or better in one than the other. *Sound is normally heard equally in both ears.*	■ Sound heard in, or lateralized to, one ear indicates either a conductive loss in that ear or a sensorineural loss in the other ear. The sound will be louder on the impaired side with a conductive hearing loss. The sound will be softer on the impaired side with a sensorineural hearing loss. Conductive losses may be due to a buildup of cerumen, an infection such as otitis media, or perforation of the eardrum.
Perform the Rinne test. Place the base of a vibrating tuning fork on the patient's mastoid bone. Ask the patient to indicate when the sound is no longer heard. When the patient does so, quickly reposition the tuning fork in front of the patient's ear close to the ear canal. Ask whether the patient can hear the sound. If the patient says yes, ask the patient to indicate when the sound is no longer heard. Repeat over the opposite mastoid bone (**Figure 45.12** ■). *The patient will normally hear the sound twice as long by air conduction (AC) as by bone conduction (BC), recorded as AC > BC (air conduction greater than bone conduction).*	■ With conductive hearing loss, bone conduction is equal to or greater than air conduction in the affected ear.

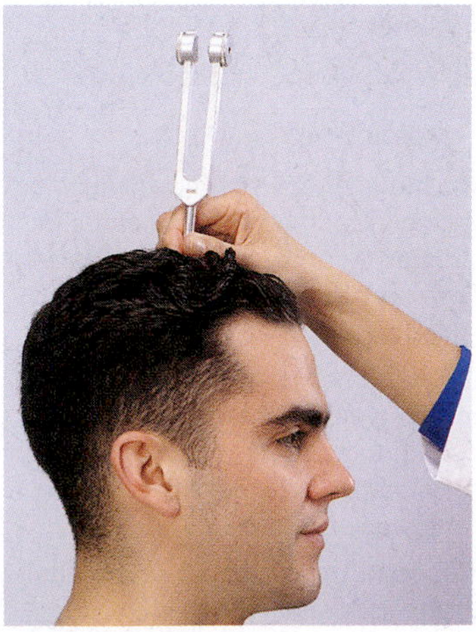

Figure 45.11 ■ Performing the Weber test.

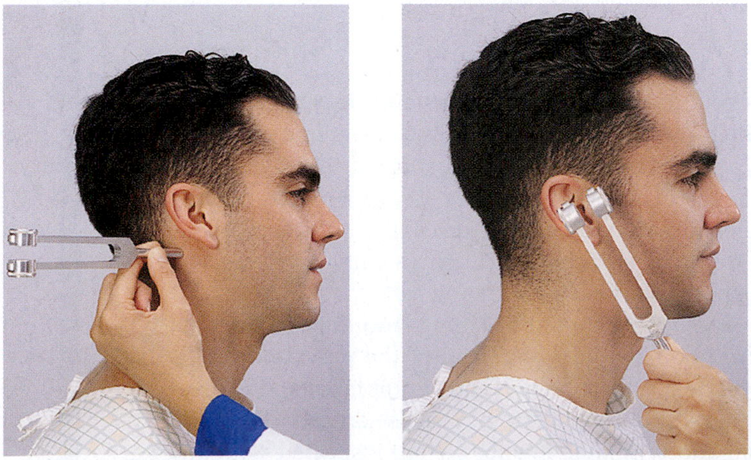

Figure 45.12 ■ Performing the Rinne test for conductive hearing loss.

Technique/Normal Findings	Abnormal Findings
Ear Assessment	
Inspect the external ears for symmetry, proportion, color, and integrity. *External ears are normally equal in size, of a color that matches the patient's face, and without redness or lesions.*	■ Unusual redness or drainage may indicate an inflammatory response to infection or trauma. ■ Scales or skin lesions around the rim of the auricle may indicate skin cancer. ■ Small, raised lesions on the rim of the ear are known as tophi and may indicate gout.
Palpate the auricles and over each mastoid process. *There should be no pain or swelling on palpation.*	■ Tenderness, swelling, or nodules may indicate inflammation of the external auditory canal or mastoiditis.
Inspect the external auditory canal with the otoscope. *Canal walls should be pink and smooth without lesions. Cerumen is normally present in small, odorless amounts. People with darker skin tend to have darker cerumen.*	■ Unusual redness, lesions, or purulent drainage may indicate an infection. ■ Cerumen varies in color and texture, but hardened, dry, or foul-smelling cerumen may indicate an infection or impacted cerumen.
Inspect the tympanic membrane. *The tympanic membrane should be pearly gray, shiny, and translucent without bulging or retraction.*	■ White, opaque areas on the tympanic membrane are often scars from previous perforations (**Figure 45.13 ■**). ■ Inconsistent texture and color may be due to scarring from previous perforations caused by infection, allergies, or trauma. ■ Bulging membranes are indicated by a loss of bony landmarks and a distorted light reflex. Such bulges may be the result of otitis media or auditory tube dysfunction. ■ Retracted tympanic membranes are indicated by accentuated bony landmarks and a distorted light reflex. Such retraction is often due to an obstructed auditory tube.

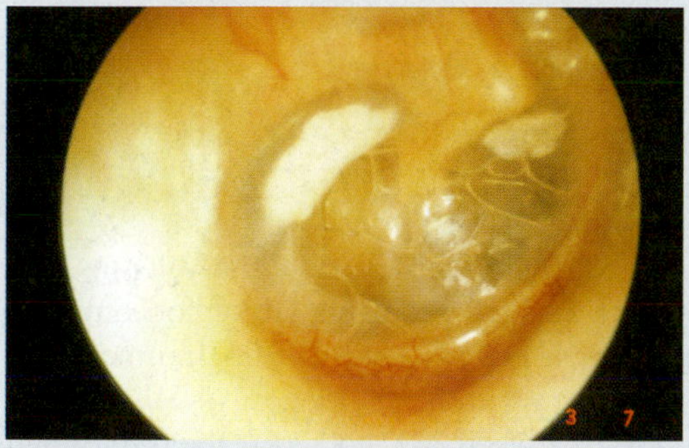

Figure 45.13 ■ Scarring of the tympanic membrane.

Technique/Normal Findings	Abnormal Findings
Tympanometry may be performed to evaluate the response of the tympanic membrane to changes in air pressure and middle ear function. The results are plotted on a tympanogram. Insert the device into the ear canal. Tell the patient he or she will hear a loud tone as the measurements are taken, and instruct not to speak, move, swallow, or jump when the sound is heard. Repeat for the other ear. *The graphic results indicate normal tympanic membrane movement.*	■ Abnormal findings may include little or no tympanic membrane movement, indicative of fluid in the middle ear, or negative pressure in the middle ear, indicative of auditory tube dysfunction.

Diagnosis

The results of diagnostic tests are used to support the diagnosis of a specific injury, disease, or hearing problem; to provide information to identify or modify appropriate medications or assistive devices used to treat the disease or problem; and to help monitor the patient's responses to treatment and nursing care interventions. Diagnostic tests of the ear, especially for hearing, are most often conducted in a healthcare provider's office. Diagnostic tests to assess the structure and functions of the ears are described in the Diagnostic Tests table.

Diagnostic Tests for Ear Disorders

NAME OF TEST	PURPOSE AND DESCRIPTION	RELATED NURSING INTERVENTIONS
Audiometry	Audiometry is used to evaluate and diagnose conductive and sensorineural hearing loss. Patient sits in soundproof room and responds when sounds are heard. Speech audiometry tests word recognition and word discrimination.	No special preparation is needed.

(*continued*)

Diagnostic Tests for Ear Disorders (*continued*)

NAME OF TEST	PURPOSE AND DESCRIPTION	RELATED NURSING INTERVENTIONS
Auditory brainstem response (ABR) and auditory evoked potential (AEP)	The ABR and AEP tests measure the electrical activity of the auditory pathway from inner ear to brain to identify the site of sensorineural hearing loss or to diagnose brainstem pathology, stroke, and acoustic neuroma.	No special preparation is needed.
Electronystagmography (ENG) or videonystagmography (VNG)	This test is used to detect eye movements (nystagmus) in response to changes in head position or stimulation of balance sensors in the inner ear using warm and cool water or air. It may be used to evaluate vertigo or help diagnose Ménière's disease.	Instruct the patient to avoid consuming caffeine or alcohol for 24 h prior to the test. Food intake may be restricted for 6 h prior to testing to prevent vomiting.
Vestibular evoked myogenic potentials (VEMP)	This test is used to diagnose inner ear disorders such as Ménière's disease or vertigo by detecting neck and eye muscle contractions in response to the stimulus of sound.	No special preparation is needed.

Regardless of the type of diagnostic test, the nurse is responsible for explaining the procedure and any special preparation needed, for assessing for any medication use that might affect the outcome of the tests, for supporting the patient during the examination as necessary, for ensuring the consent form is signed (if necessary), for documenting the procedures as appropriate, and for monitoring the results of the tests.

45.5 Assessment of Special Populations

Key age-related changes in the eyes and ears and their significance are outlined in **Table 45.1**.

According to reports from the Veterans Administration, both eye and ear problems are of concern in persons who served in the military. Up to 245,000 traumatic eye injuries and penetrating wounds resulting in visual disorders have been reported. Between 2000 and 2010, the Department of Defense reports that 186,555 people with eye injuries sought care in medical military facilities (VisionAware, 2017). A study by Wells and colleagues (2015) reported that 7.5% of military participants had new-onset hearing loss. This study also noted that combat experience was associated with a 64% increased risk for hearing loss. This evidence supports the importance of careful history taking by the nurse that should include questions related to military service and any health outcomes related to the service (Veterans' Administration [VA], 2017a, 2017b).

Table 45.1 Age-Related Changes in the Eyes and Ears

Age-Related Change	Significance
The Eyes	
Accessory Structures	
■ Decreased musculature of eyelids ■ Atrophy of lacrimal glands ■ Loss of orbital fat ■ Raised, soft yellow plaques called *xanthelasma* on lids	Eyes appear sunken; upper and lower lids may droop. Decreased tear production leads to dry eyes, with itching and burning. Xanthelasma have cosmetic significance only.
The Cornea	
■ Lipid deposits around the periphery of the cornea ■ ↓ corneal sensitivity	A partial or complete white circle may form around the cornea (arcus senilis). Decreased sensitivity increases the risk of eye injury.
The Pupil	
■ ↓ pupil size and responsiveness to light	Increased light is needed to see clearly and for depth perception. Slowed pupillary reaction causes difficulty adapting to light changes (e.g., moving from a light environment into a dark one or from dark to light).
The Lens	
■ Lens loses elasticity, with reduced ability to change shape and focus light. ■ Lens becomes thicker and loses clarity, increasingly opaque.	Presbyopia, difficulty accommodating for near vision, develops. Light rays scatter, causing glare; color discrimination decreases. Ability to adapt to the dark declines.

Age-Related Change	Significance
The Posterior Cavity	
■ Vitreous humor shrinks and pulls away from the retina.	Vision is less acute and contains vitreous floaters; risk of retinal detachment increases.
The Retina and Visual Pathways	
■ Visual fields narrow. ■ Photoreceptor cells atrophy and are lost. ■ Light scatter in the retina increases. ■ Retinal blood vessels thin and sclerose. ■ Transmission and interpretation of stimuli slow.	Peripheral vision is decreased and color perception is impaired, particularly of blue-green tones. Increased risk of falls as a result of changes in depth perception and adaptation to changes in light. Vision progressively declines with age.
The Ears	
The Inner Ear	
■ Loss of hair cells, ↓ blood supply, less flexible basilar membrane, degeneration of spiral ganglion cells, and ↓ production of endolymph result in progressive hearing loss with age (**presbycusis**). ■ High-frequency sounds are lost; middle- and low-frequency sounds may also be lost or decreased. ■ Vestibular structures degenerate; organ of Corti and cochlea atrophy.	Older adults may require hearing aids to hear well. With loss of high-frequency sounds, speech may be distorted, contributing to a risk for communication problems. Degeneration and atrophy of inner ear structures concerned with balance and equilibrium increase the risk for falls.
The Middle Ear	
■ Muscles and ligaments weaken and stiffen, decreasing the acoustic reflex.	Sounds made from one's own body and speech are louder and may further interfere with hearing, speech, and communications.
The External Ear	
■ Cerumen is dryer and harder and tends to accumulate in the ear canal. ■ Decreased apocrine gland activity in ear canal contributes to cerumen accumulation, as well as dryness and itching.	Accumulated cerumen may impair hearing. The lining of the ear canal is more easily irritated or damaged, increasing the risk of external ear infection.

45.6 Health Promotion

Health promotion of the eye and ear focuses on regular examinations. An eye exam should be conducted at least every 2 years until the age of 60, then yearly after that by an optometrist or ophthalmologist (American Academy of Opthalmology, 2015). Ear examination should be conducted yearly with the physical examination. If any symptoms related to the ear (reduced hearing, ringing in the ears) are noted, this should trigger referral to an ear or hearing specialist (Bickley, 2016).

CHAPTER HIGHLIGHTS

45.1 Anatomy, Physiology, and Functions of the Eyes

Describe the anatomy, physiology, and functions of the eye, and identify abnormal findings that may indicate visual impairment.

- Abnormalities in the structure or function of the eyes and their accessory structures can threaten or impair vision and the patient's safety, independence, and social interactions.

45.2 Assessing the Eyes

Outline the components of the assessment of the eye and vision, including topics for the health assessment interview, techniques for physical assessment, and the diagnostic tests used in the assessment.

- Careful examination of the eyes are an important part of the comprehensive assessment.
- Careful history taking is imperative to evaluate for hereditary eye conditions.

45.3 Anatomy, Physiology, and Functions of the Ears

Describe the anatomy, physiology, and functions of the ear, and identify abnormal findings that may indicate hearing impairment.

- For hearing to occur, sound waves must travel from the external auditory meatus, through the ear canal, to vibrate the tympanic membrane and bony structures of the middle ear, which in turn activate the receptors of the cochlea.

45.4 Assessing the Ears

Outline the components of the assessment of the ear and hearing, including topics for the health assessment interview, techniques for physical assessment, and the diagnostic tests used in the assessment.

- Careful examination of the ears are an important part of the comprehensive assessment.
- Careful history taking related to personal and environmental exposure to loud sounds provides information for the primary risk factors for hearing loss.

45.5 Assessment of Special Populations

Differentiate considerations for assessing vision and hearing of older adults, veterans, and adults with sequelae of childhood/congenital conditions.

- Changes of normal gaining lead to changes in both the eyes and ears. Environmental exposures can also trigger changes (cataracts, hearing loss).
- Veterans have a higher risk for traumatic eye injury and hearing injury while deployed.

45.6 Health Promotion

Summarize topics that nurses teach to promote healthy vision and hearing across the lifespan.

- Regular examinations are the most important health-promoting practice for eye and ear health.

TEST YOURSELF NCLEX-RN® REVIEW

1. During an eye assessment, a nurse touches the part of the eye covering the iris and pupil. Which patient response should the nurse expect?
   A. Dilated pupil
   B. Excess tearing
   C. Blinking of eyelids
   D. Bilateral nystagmus
2. The nurse is conducting a health history with an older patient. Which statement would indicate that the patient is experiencing presbyopia?
   A. "I think I have a lot of earwax in my ears."
   B. "My arms just don't seem long enough to read."
   C. "I can't seem to remember anything these days."
   D. "I am having so much trouble hearing music."
3. The nurse is planning to assess a patient's sound conduction. What equipment should the nurse use to make this assessment?
   A. Penlight
   B. Otoscope
   C. Tuning fork
   D. Ophthalmoscope
4. The nurse is preparing to assess a patient's eyes for accommodation. Which findings should the nurse expect when conducting this assessment? (Select all that apply.)
   A. Rhythmical blinking occurs.
   B. Eyes move in six different directions.
   C. Pupils dilate when focused on a distant object.
   D. Pupils constrict when focused on a near object.
   E. Eyes move in the direction that the head is turned.
5. A patient is scheduled to have eye refraction completed. What should the nurse say to the patient before this test is done? (Select all that apply.)
   A. "Are you allergic to seafood?"
   B. "You will be blindfolded during the test."
   C. "Your pupils will be dilated for several hours."
   D. "This test is uncomfortable, but it doesn't take long."
   E. "There is nothing special you should do before coming for this test."
6. The nurse is concerned that an older patient is experiencing age-related changes in the inner ear. What did the nurse most likely assess in this patient? (Select all that apply.)
   A. Loss of balance when walking
   B. Loss of ability to hear high-frequency sounds
   C. Self-speech sounds louder to the patient
   D. Decreased middle- and low-frequency sounds
   E. Impacted cerumen and itchy external ear canal
7. The nurse is preparing to assess a patient using the Snellen chart. What is the nurse planning to assess in this patient?
   A. Near vision
   B. Visual fields
   C. Convergence
   D. Distant vision
8. The nurse wants to make a rough estimate of a patient's ability to hear. Which assessment should the nurse use to make this estimation?
   A. Rinne test
   B. Weber test
   C. Audiometry
   D. Whisper test
9. After an assessment the nurse determines that an older patient is experiencing an age-related change to the lens of the eyes. What did the nurse assess in this patient?
   A. Complaints of glare
   B. Slow reaction to light
   C. Dry, itchy, and burning eyes
   D. Difficulty with far vision
10. The nurse is preparing to assess a patient's visual fields. Which criterion should be present to accurately assess the patient's visual fields? (Select all that apply.)
    A. Patient must be able to follow directions.
    B. Examiner must not wear glasses.
    C. Patient must wear corrective lenses.
    D. Examiner must have normal visual fields.
    E. Patient must have no less than 20/30 vision.

See Test Yourself answers in Appendix B.

REFERENCES

American Academy of Opthalmology. (2015). *Frequency of ocular exams-2015.* Retrieved from https://www.aao.org/clinical-statement/frequency-of-ocular-examinations.

Bickley, L. (2016). *Bates' guide to physical examination and history taking* (12th ed.). Philadelphia, PA: Lippincott Williams & Wilkins.

Genetics Home Reference. (2018a). *Age-related hearing loss.* Retrieved from https://ghr.nlm.nih.gov/condition/age-related-hearing-loss.

Genetics Home Reference. (2018b). *Leber hereditary optic neuropathy.* Retrieved from https://ghr.nlm.nih.gov/condition/leber-hereditary-optic-neuropathy.

Genetics Home Reference. (2018c). *Neurofibromatosis type 2.* Retrieved from https://ghr.nlm.nih.gov/condition/neurofibromatosis-type-2.

Genetics Home Reference. (2018d). *Pendred syndrome.* Retrieved from https://ghr.nlm.nih.gov/condition/pendred-syndrome.

Genetics Home Reference. (2018e). *Retinitis pigmentosa.* Retrieved from https://ghr.nlm.nih.gov/condition/retinitis-pigmentosa.

Glaucoma Research Foundation. (2017). *Glaucoma facts and stats.* Retrieved from https://www.glaucoma.org/glaucoma/glaucoma-facts-and-stats.php.

Glaucoma Research Foundation. (2018). *The genetics of glaucoma.* Retrieved from https://www.glaucoma.org/glaucoma/the-genetics-of-glaucoma-what-is-new.php.

Kee, J. L. (2018). *Laboratory and diagnostic tests with nursing implications* (10th ed.). Hoboken, NJ: Pearson Education.

National Center for Biotechnology Information. (2016). *Genes and disease: Diseases of the eye.* Retrieved from www.ncbi.nlm.nih.gov/books/NBK22174.

Shearer, A. E., Hildebrand, M. S., & Smith, R. J. H. (2017). *Hereditary hearing loss and deafness overview.* Retrieved from https://www.ncbi.nlm.nih.gov/books/NBK1434/.

Sorenson, M., Quinn, L., & Klein, D. (2019). *Pathophysiology: Concepts of human disease.* Hoboken, NJ: Pearson Education.

Veterans' Administration (VA). (2017a). *Center for the Prevention and Treatment of Vision Loss.* Retrieved from https://www.vision.research.va.gov/index.asp.

Veterans' Administration (VA). (2017b). *Disability Compensation: "Presumptive" disability benefits.* Retrieved from https://www.benefits.va.gov/BENEFITS/factsheets/serviceconnected/presumption.pdf.

VisionAware. (2017). *Statistics on vision loss and the military and policy implications.* Retrieved from www.visionaware.org/info/everyday-living/essential-skills/information-for-veterans-coping-with-vision-loss/statistics-on-vision-loss-and-the-military/1235.

Wells, T. S., Seelig, A. D., Ryan, M. A. K., Jones, J. M., Hooper, T. I., Jacobson, I. G., & Boyko, E. J. (2015). Hearing loss associated with U.S. military deployment. *Noise Health, 17*(74), 34–42.

ADDITIONAL RESOURCES

American Academy of Audiology
www.audiology.org

Genetics Home Reference
https://ghr.nlm.nih.gov

National Eye Institute (NEI)
https://www.nei.nih.gov

National Eye Institute
www.nei.nih.gov/eyedata

National Institute on Deafness and Other Communication Disorders
https://www.nidcd.nih.gov

Chapter 46

Nursing Care of Patients with Eye and Ear Disorders

Chapter Outline and Learning Outcomes

CLINICAL COMPETENCIES

- Assess vision, hearing, functional health, and safety of patients with eye and ear disorders.
- Using assessed data and current evidence-based practice guidelines, determine priority nursing diagnoses and interventions for patients with eye and ear disorders.
- Communicate, collaborate, and coordinate with the interprofessional team to provide safe, effective care for patients with eye and ear disorders.
- Considering patient preferences, values, and expressed needs, plan and implement appropriate and individualized evidence-based nursing interventions and teaching for the patient with an eye or ear disorder.
- Safely and effectively administer eye and ear medications and prescribed treatments.
- Critically evaluate the healthcare environment for threats to the safety of patients with eye and ear disorders.
- Evaluate the effectiveness of care provided for patients with eye and ear disorders, sharing data and revising practices and individual plans of care as indicated.

KEY TERMS

age-related macular degeneration (AMD), 1714
astigmatism, 1697
cataract, 1705
conjunctivitis, 1694
diabetic retinopathy, 1715
enucleation, 1719
glaucoma, 1707
hyperopia, 1697
hyphema, 1703
Ménière disease, 1727
myopia, 1697
myringotomy, 1724
nystagmus, 1727
otitis media, 1722
presbycusis, 1731
tinnitus, 1731
vertigo, 1723

Vision and hearing provide the primary means of input for much of what we know about the world. The ability to receive and organize information orients us to our surroundings. These senses allow us to communicate, gain access to information, and derive pleasure from the sights and sounds of the world around us.

This chapter discusses conditions affecting vision and hearing as the result of eye and ear disorders. Nursing care focuses on patients with vision and hearing deficits that can result from the disorders presented.

46.1 Eye Disorders

Visual impairment exists on a continuum from blindness to decreased visual acuity that can be corrected with refractive lenses to normal or near normal. *Visual impairment* is defined as 20/40 vision in the better eye, even with corrective lenses. The legal definition of *blindness* is visual acuity no better than 20/200 in the better eye with optimal correction or a visual field of lesser than 20 degrees in diameter (compared to the normal of 180 degrees) (National Federation of the Blind, 2017). Total blindness usually indicates that the patient has no light perception at all. In practical terms, an individual with a visual deficit sufficient to need assistive devices or aid from other people for normal activities of daily living is considered blind.

Nearly 10 million Americans are blind or have some visual impairment (National Federation of the Blind, 2017). More than 1.2 million Americans are legally blind. In the United States, blindness is more prevalent among White populations than it is among Black and Hispanic populations (National Eye Institute, 2017a; National Federation of the Blind, 2017). In the United States, cataracts, age-related macular degeneration, glaucoma, and diabetic retinopathy remain significant causes of blindness in adults.

Although blindness can often be prevented or cured, it remains a significant problem worldwide because of lack of access to care, fear of surgery or treatment, poor sanitation and nutrition, and ignorance of need. Worldwide, between 30 and 40 million people have visual impairment significant enough to be considered blind.

Any portion of the eye and its protective structures may be affected by an acute or chronic condition. Although many eye disorders are minor and have little or no effect on vision, others can and often do result in vision impairment. Disorders and diseases of the outer, visible portion of the eye often cause discomfort and may have cosmetic effects. With appropriate treatment, vision impairment can often be prevented or reversed. Disorders of the cornea present the greatest risk to vision in this group. The patient who has had eye surgery or minor trauma may have either temporary or permanent visual impairment. Disorders affecting the internal structures or the function of the eye are more likely to have adverse effects on vision. These disorders are more likely to affect adults over the age of 40, and older adults in particular. The prevalence of impaired vision and blindness increases significantly after age 75. Other common conditions affecting the vision of middle and older adults, in order of prevalence in 2016 were cataracts, 24,409,978; diabetic retinopathy, 7,685,237; glaucoma, 2,719,379; and macular degeneration, 2,069,403 (National Eye Institute, 2017c).

Although disorders that commonly affect vision often cannot be prevented or cured, some can be controlled and vision corrected to normal or near normal. In addition to the real threat a disorder poses to vision, the patient may experience anxiety related to a perceived threat. **Box 46.1** outlines the major causes of significantly impaired vision and nursing care for the patient who is blind. These principles of nursing care may apply to patients with many of the disorders discussed in this chapter.

The Patient with Conjunctivitis

The *conjunctiva*—the thin, transparent membrane that covers the anterior surface of the eye and lines the inner surfaces of the eyelids—is vulnerable to inflammation and infection because of its constant exposure to the environment.

BOX 46.1
Nursing Care of the Patient Who Is Blind

People who are blind need to cope not only with the loss of a major sense but often also with societal attitudes that make them feel inferior, helpless, and inadequate. The idea of losing the ability to see is uniformly feared, leaving sighted people often unable to understand the magnitude and impact of the loss in those who have experienced it. Because of this fear and confusion, sighted people are unsure of what people who are blind expect from them.

The adjustment of the individual who is born blind and raised to become an independent member of society differs from that of the individual who has been sighted and becomes blind. The individual who has been blind from birth has developed numerous adaptive strategies that the newly blind individual has yet to learn.

Although adaptation may be easier for the patient who experiences a gradual loss of vision than for someone with an abrupt loss, both must grieve the lost sense. The patient who becomes blind needs to grieve the lost body function as well as the loss of mobility, self-sufficiency, perhaps economic security, and, to a certain extent, contact with reality as it has been perceived. The patient's self-concept and self-esteem are threatened. Anger, denial, remorse, and self-pity are not uncommon in the initial period following loss of sight. Interpersonal relationships and roles are affected. Communication patterns change with the loss of the ability to perceive many nonverbal cues. Expressions of sexuality may be impaired.

Acceptance of the change from sighted to blind is characterized by releasing the hope that vision will be regained. Self-esteem increases as the patient attempts and masters activities of self-sufficiency such as completing activities of daily living (ADLs), cooking, and becoming mobile outside the known home environment.

Health professionals often confuse the role of someone who is blind with the role of a patient, seeing the individual as helpless, dependent, and lacking in personal identity and control. Although nurses need to take blindness into account in planning care and maintaining patient safety, it is vital to give the patient who is blind the same respect and decision-making power that all patients deserve. Nurses who have dealt with their own emotions and responses to vision loss are better prepared to help the patient adapt.

Nurses can foster independence in the hospitalized patient with a significant vision deficit by doing the following:

- ***Orient to the environment verbally and physically:*** Describe the room using a central point such as the bed. Lead the patient around the room, identifying chairs, sink, bathroom, and other landmarks. Be sure that objects such as chairs, personal items,

(*continued*)

and clothing remain in the same place unless moved by the patient. Leave doors either fully open or closed as the patient wishes, but, to preserve safety, do not leave doors partially open. Keep the room and hallways free of clutter.

- ***Use verbal communication freely:*** Describe activities going on around the patient. Introduce yourself as you enter the room and let the patient know when you are leaving.
- ***Provide other sensory stimuli*** such as radio and television as desired by the patient.
- ***Orient to food trays by using the face of a clock*** to describe the position of food items on the plate and tray (unless the patient has always been blind and cannot visualize a clock face).
- ***Allow the patient to hold your arm as you walk slightly ahead*** when assisting with ambulation. Do not hold the patient's arm. Verbally describe the environment, such as "There will be two steps up 5 feet ahead."
- ***Do not hesitate to ask what assistance the patient desires.***

For the patient with a new loss of sight, refer to available services. Counseling can help the patient cope with and eventually adapt to the loss of sight. People who are blind can receive mobility training, assistance with relearning self-care activities, education in the use of Braille to communicate, and vocational and other forms of rehabilitation. Local, state, and national agencies such as the American Foundation for the Blind, National Braille Association, and National Federation for the Blind coordinate services for the blind. Many assistive devices are available, including guide or pilot dogs, large print books, audio books, speech recognition software, and low-vision aids.

Conjunctivitis, inflammation of the conjunctiva, is the most common eye disease. Its usual cause is a bacterial or viral infection. These infections can be transmitted to the eye by direct contact (e.g., hands, tissues, towels). Allergens, chemical irritants, and exposure to radiant energy such as ultraviolet light from the sun or tanning devices can also lead to this common condition. Its severity can range from mild irritation with redness and tearing to conjunctival edema, hemorrhage, or a severe necrotizing process with tissue destruction.

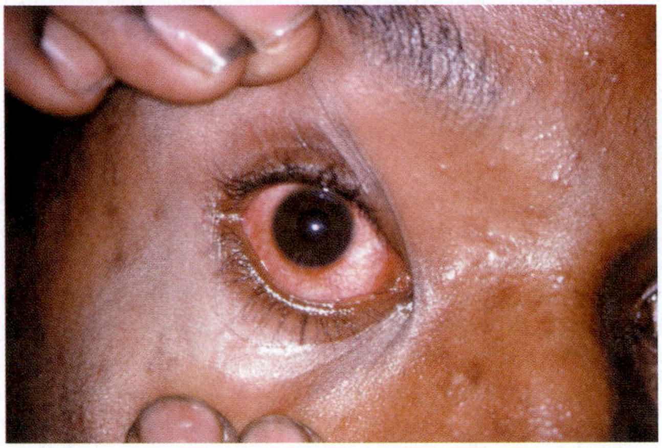

Figure 46.1 ■ The appearance of an eye with conjunctivitis.

Pathophysiology

Acute Conjunctivitis

Infectious conjunctivitis may be bacterial, viral, or fungal in origin. Bacterial conjunctivitis, also known as *pink eye*, is highly contagious, and is often caused by *Staphylococcus* or *Haemophilus* (Sorenson et al., 2019). Adenovirus infection is the leading cause of conjunctivitis in adults. Systemic infections that may affect the eyes include herpes simplex and other viral infections. Contact with genital secretions infected with *Gonococcus* can cause gonococcal conjunctivitis, a medical emergency that can lead to corneal perforation.

Trachoma

Trachoma, a chronic conjunctivitis caused by *Chlamydia trachomatis*, is a significant preventable cause of blindness worldwide. Trachoma is endemic in northern and sub-Saharan Africa, the Middle East, and parts of Asia. Although the prevalence is lower than in endemic regions, trachoma is also found in parts of Australia, the South Pacific, and South America. Trachoma is contagious, transmitted primarily by close personal contact (eye-to-eye, hand-to-eye) or by fomites such as towels, handkerchiefs, and flies (National Eye Institute, 2017e).

Manifestations

Redness and itching of the affected eye are common manifestations of acute conjunctivitis (**Figure 46.1** ■). The patient may also complain of a scratchy, burning, or gritty sensation. Pain is not common; however, photophobia (sensitivity to light) may occur. Tearing and discharge accompany the inflammatory process. The discharge may be watery, purulent, or mucoid, depending on the cause of conjunctivitis. The patient may have associated manifestations such as pharyngitis, fever, malaise, and swollen preauricular lymph nodes.

Early manifestations of trachoma include redness, eyelid edema, tearing, and photophobia. Small conjunctival follicles develop on the upper lids. The inflammation also causes superficial corneal vascularization and infiltration with granulation tissue. Scarring of the conjunctival lining of the lid causes entropion (inversion of the lid margin) (**Figure 46.2** ■). The lashes then abrade the cornea, eventually causing ulceration and scarring. The scarred cornea is opaque, resulting in loss of vision.

Interprofessional Care

Management of the patient with conjunctivitis focuses on establishing an accurate diagnosis and prompt treatment.

Diagnosis

Accurate diagnosis of conjunctivitis is especially important because other potentially vision-threatening conditions, such as acute uveitis or acute angle-closure glaucoma, can also cause a red eye (**Table 46.1**). Diagnostic procedures may include:

- ***Culture and sensitivity*** of exudates to determine presence of an infection and identify the infecting organism
- ***Fluorescein stain*** with slit-lamp examination to identify possible corneal ulcerations or abrasions, which appear green with staining
- ***Conjunctival scrapings*** are examined microscopically or cultured to identify the organisms.

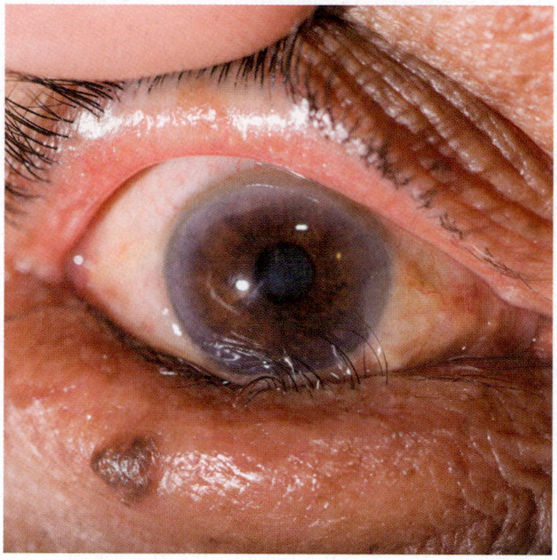

Figure 46.2 ■ Entropion.

Additional laboratory testing such as blood counts or antibody titers may be used to identify underlying infectious or autoimmune processes.

Medications

Conjunctivitis is treated with antibiotic, antiviral, or anti-inflammatory drugs as appropriate. Topical anti-infectives applied as either eyedrops or ointment may include erythromycin, gentamicin, penicillin, bacitracin, sulfacetamide sodium, amphotericin B, or idoxuridine. For severe infections or cellulitis, anti-infectives may be administered by subconjunctival injection or systemic intravenous infusion. Antihistamines are used to minimize symptoms of conjunctivitis when an allergic response underlies the inflammatory process.

Integrative Therapies

Frequent eye irrigations may be ordered to remove the copious purulent discharge associated with conjunctivitis. Soaking the lids with warm saline compresses prior to cleansing promotes comfort and facilitates the removal of crusts and exudate in conjunctivitis.

Nursing Care

The nursing role in treating conjunctivitis is primarily one of education to prevent the disorder and to prevent its spread when it does occur.

Assessment

- ***Health history:*** Presence of redness, discomfort, tearing, photophobia, and drainage; symptom onset; care measures; use of contact lenses; exposure to "pink eye" or recent travel; allergies; previous history of conjunctivitis; presence of any chronic diseases
- ***Physical assessment:*** Visual acuity; inspection of eyelids, conjunctiva, sclera, and cornea; vital signs including temperature.

Priorities of Care

Nursing care priorities for the patient with conjunctivitis focus on preventing the infection from spreading to others and preventing complications.

Diagnoses, Interventions, and Outcomes

Reduce Risk for Infection. Acute conjunctivitis is highly contagious. Although most patients experience no more than discomfort from the disease, the infection carries a risk for scarring and damage to the delicate cornea of the eye. Preventing the spread of this infection is a vital nursing role.

Expected Outcome: Patient will verbalize an understanding of and willingness to follow measures to prevent infection spread to others.

The nurse will:

- Teach patient to wash hands thoroughly before instilling eye medications. Instruct to avoid touching or rubbing the eyes. Advise to use a new, clean cotton-tipped swab or cotton ball for cleaning each eye. *Hand hygiene is the single most important measure to prevent transmission of infection to the eye. Touching or rubbing the eyes increases the risk of infection and corneal trauma. Using a new swab or cotton ball prevents cross-contamination between eyes.*
- Teach patient to instill prescribed eyedrops or ointment as ordered (see **Box 46.2**). *Prescribed medications reduce inflammation and eliminate infection.*
- Discuss the importance of avoiding contact lens use until the infectious process has cleared and of completing the prescribed treatment. *Use of contact lenses in the inflamed eyes can lead to further damage and impair healing.*

Table 46.1 Possible Causes of Acute Red Eye

	Acute Conjunctivitis	Corneal Trauma or Infection	Acute Uveitis	Acute Angle-Closure Glaucoma
Incidence	Very common	Common	Common	Rare
Pain	Mild	Moderate to severe	Moderate	Severe
Vision	Normal	Blurred	Blurred	Markedly blurred
Discharge	May be copious	Watery, may be purulent	None	None
Conjunctival erythema	Diffuse	Primarily around cornea	Primarily around cornea	Primarily around cornea
Cornea	Clear	Depends on cause	Usually clear	Cloudy
Pupils	Normal size, response to light	Normal size, response to light	Small, minimal response to light	Moderately dilated, fixed

BOX 46.2
Patient Teaching for Instilling Eyedrops and Eye Ointments

To ensure safe, effective delivery of eye medication, patient teaching should include:

- Wash hands with soap and water. Rinse and dry hands.
- Read directions to determine whether drops need to be gently shaken.
- Check applicator/dropper tip for cracks or chips.
- Avoid touching the applicator tip to your eye or hands. It must be kept clean.
- Tilt your head back slightly, and pull down the lower eyelid with your index finger to form a pocket.
- Hold the applicator with the other hand, tip facing down, as close to the eye as possible without touching it.
- Use the other fingers on that hand as a brace against your face to stabilize your hand.
- Look up and gently squeeze medication into the lower eyelid pocket. Instill the prescribed amount of medication.
- Tip your head slightly down and close your eyes for 2–3 minutes. Try not to squint or blink.
- Apply gentle pressure to the lacrimal duct.
- Wipe any excess medication from your face with a tissue.
- Replace and tighten the applicator lid.
- To remove any medication, wash your hands.

Reduce Risk for Impaired Vision. Conjunctivitis can potentially disrupt the integrity or clarity of the cornea. Because of its vital role in focusing light on the retina, corneal damage can impair visual acuity.

Expected Outcome: Patient's infectious process will resolve without adverse effects such as scarring or injury related to impaired vision.

The nurse will:

- Assess vision with and without corrective lenses. *Assessment provides a baseline to evaluate possible changes in vision resulting from the infection.*
- Instruct patient to avoid activities requiring high visual acuity until the infection has cleared. *The inflammatory process, edema of the conjunctiva, and local antibiotic applications can decrease visual acuity and cloud vision.*
- Instruct patient to use dark sunglasses with appropriate UV protection when out of doors, even on cloudy days. *Photophobia, a common manifestation of conjunctivitis, causes eye pain with increased light intensity.*

Delegating Nursing Care Activities

Because of the importance of maintaining asepsis when caring for the eyes of a patient with conjunctivitis, it is appropriate for the nurse to retain direct responsibility for care activities such as cleansing the lids and instilling eye medications.

Transitions of Care

Education is a vital strategy for preventing conjunctivitis. Teach all patients about proper eye care, including the importance of not sharing towels, makeup, or contact lenses and avoiding rubbing or scratching the eyes. Instruct to avoid using old eye makeup, which can cause eye infections. Teach contact lens users appropriate care (**Box 46.3**). Emphasize the need to follow cleaning instructions precisely to avoid bacterial contamination of lenses. If the eyes become red, irritated, or develop discharge, instruct the patient to avoid wearing contact lenses until the inflammatory process has cleared.

Patients with conjunctivitis are typically managed in the community, reinforcing the need for effective teaching for home care. Emphasize to the family ways to prevent transmission of infection. If the patient is unable to administer eye medications, involve the family in teaching. Include the following topics:

- Safety and medical asepsis when cleansing the eye
- Instillation of prescribed eyedrops and ointments
- Comfort measures such as reducing lighting intensity and wearing sunglasses
- Avoidance of activities such as excessive reading while eye is inflamed.

The Patient with a Corneal Disorder

The clear cornea allows light rays to enter the eye and transmits images onto the retina. It helps to focus light on the retina and protects the internal eye structures. The cornea can be affected by a variety of disorders, including infection and trauma. Although the cornea heals quickly after minor injuries or abrasions, injury to its deeper layers can delay healing or result in scarring.

Currently, 42.5% of persons age 12 to 54 in the United States are diagnosed with myopia. In contrast, 9.9% of the U.S. population age 40 and older are farsighted (hyperopia). Keratitis is the most serious potential complication of contact lens use. Scarring that occurs as a result of keratitis is a leading cause of blindness worldwide (National Eye Institute, 2017c).

Pathophysiology

The cornea has three major layers: The outermost epithelium, which consists of five or six layers of cells that are constantly being renewed; the stroma, which makes up 90% of corneal tissue; and the single-cell thickness endothelium adjacent to the aqueous humor of the anterior chamber. The cornea is avascular tissue; the central cornea is dependent on atmospheric oxygen to meet its metabolic needs. Because there is no blood supply, immune defenses have

BOX 46.3
Contact Lens Care

- Wash hands thoroughly before handling contact lenses.
- Keep storage case clean.
- Remove lenses before sleep, cleaning and storing as recommended by manufacturer.
- Use cleaning and wetting solutions recommended by an eye care professional or lens manufacturer. Do not use water or homemade solutions for wetting or cleaning lenses.
- If eye redness, tearing, vision loss, or pain occurs, remove lenses and contact an eye care professional as soon as possible.
- Do not share contact lenses or allow another person to "try on" lenses.

difficulty fending off infections of the cornea (Sorenson et al., 2019).

Light enters the eye through the normally clear cornea. As light passes through the curved cornea, it is bent or *refracted* onto the lens, which then focuses the light on sensory cells of the retina. A change in the curvature of the cornea or in its clarity affects the ability of the eye to clearly focus; as a result, vision is distorted or blurred. Refractive errors such as **myopia** (nearsightedness), **hyperopia** (farsightedness), and **astigmatism** (an irregularly shaped cornea or lens that prevents light from focusing properly on the retina) are common. Corneal scarring and ulceration are two major causes of blindness worldwide. **Table 46.2** summarizes major disorders of the cornea.

Interprofessional Care

Management of the patient with a corneal disorder focuses on establishing an accurate diagnosis and prompt treatment to reduce the risk of permanent vision deficit. The history and physical assessment are key in diagnosing these disorders.

Although many eye disorders can be treated in the community, the patient with a severe corneal infection or ulcer may require hospitalization. Corneal ulcers are medical emergencies, requiring prompt referral to an ophthalmologist for treatment. Pressure dressings may be applied to both eyes for comfort and to reduce the risk of perforation and loss of eye contents.

Diagnosis

Visual acuity is tested on all patients presenting with refractory or corneal disorders. The following tests may be ordered to identify the cause and extent of eye infections or inflammations:

Table 46.2 Major Disorders of the Cornea

Disorder	Pathophysiology	Manifestations
Refractive Errors		
Myopia	Excessive curvature of the cornea or elongation of the eyeball causes the image to focus in front of the retina instead of on it.	Objects in close range are seen clearly and those at a distance are blurred.
Hyperopia	Flattening of the cornea or an eyeball that is too short causes the image to focus behind the retina.	Objects at a distance are seen more clearly than those that are close.
Astigmatism	Irregular or abnormal curvature of the cornea causes light rays to focus on more than one area of the retina.	Both near and distance vision are distorted.
Keratitis		
	Inflammation of the cornea. In *nonulcerative keratitis*, all layers of corneal epithelium are affected, but remain intact. *Ulcerative keratitis*, a possible consequence of bacterial conjunctivitis, affects the epithelium and stroma of the cornea, leading to tissue destruction and ulceration.	■ Tearing, decreased visual acuity ■ Discomfort ranging from a gritty sensation in the eye to severe pain ■ *Blepharospasm* (spasm of the eyelid and inability to open the eye) ■ Presence of discharge, especially if the conjunctiva is also inflamed ■ Corneal ulceration may be visible on direct examination
Corneal Ulcer		
	Local necrosis of the cornea, with destruction of epithelium and/or stroma. Scarring and opacity of the cornea may result. Ulcers may be superficial or deep, penetrating underlying layers and leading to infection of deeper eye structures or extrusion of eye contents. Causes include infection (bacterial conjunctivitis, trachoma, gonorrhea, herpes simplex, or herpes zoster), exposure trauma, or the misuse of contact lenses. Immunosuppression is a risk factor for infection-related corneal ulcer.	■ Decreased visual acuity ■ Conjunctival redness ■ Eye pain, foreign body sensation ■ Photophobia, tearing ■ Partial or total vision loss ■ Ulceration visible on fluorescein staining and direct examination
Corneal Dystrophies		
	Accumulation of cloudy material in part or parts of the cornea. Usually inherited disorders that progress gradually and affect both eyes. *Keratoconus*, the most common corneal dystrophy, involves progressive thinning and outward bulging of the center of the cornea, affecting its shape and ability to focus light on the lens of the eye.	■ Decreased visual acuity ■ Corneal swelling and possible scarring

- *Fluorescein stain* with slit-lamp examination allows visualization of any corneal ulcerations or abrasions, which appear green with staining
- *Conjunctival or ulcer scrapings* are examined microscopically or cultured to identify the organisms.

Additional laboratory testing such as blood counts or antibody titers may be used to identify any underlying infectious or autoimmune processes.

Medication

Infectious processes are treated with antibiotic or antiviral therapy as appropriate. Topical anti-infectives applied as eyedrops or ointment may include erythromycin, gentamicin, penicillin, bacitracin, sulfacetamide sodium, amphotericin B, or idoxuridine. For severe infections, central ulcers, or cellulitis, anti-infectives may be administered by subconjunctival injection and/or systemic intravenous infusion. Corticosteroids may be prescribed for keratitis related to systemic inflammatory disorders or trauma; however, it is important to avoid their use with local infections to avoid suppressing the immune and inflammatory responses.

Corrective Lenses

Corrective lenses, either in the form of eyeglasses or contact lenses, are generally prescribed to restore visual acuity for patients with refractive errors such as myopia, hyperopia, and astigmatism. Specially fitted contact lenses to reduce vision distortion are ordered for patients with keratoconus. Because contact lenses are a risk factor for corneal infection and ulcers, teaching appropriate care is vital (refer to Box 46.3).

Surgery

Laser Eye Surgery. Laser eye surgery is commonly performed to correct refractive errors such as myopia, hyperopia, and astigmatism. In these surgeries, a laser is used to permanently change the shape of the cornea. In most cases, the need to use corrective lenses is reduced or eliminated. Several surgical procedures are available:

- Laser *in situ* keratomileusis (LASIK)
- Photorefractive keratectomy (PRK)
- Laser epithelial keratomileusis (LASEK)
- Laser thermokeratoplasty (LTK).

These procedures reshape the cornea using laser technology to remove a thin layer of epithelial cells or to shrink and reshape the cornea. Candidates for laser vision-correction surgery should be in good health and must have adequate corneal thickness such that perforation is not a risk.

Following surgery, patients may experience a temporary loss of contrast sharpness (images do not appear as crisp as with corrective lenses), over- or undercorrection of visual acuity, dry eyes, or temporarily decreased night vision with halos, glare, and starbursts. Diffuse lamellar keratitis (DLK) is a rare complication of surgery that, while treatable, can lead to vision impairment if not identified and treated early.

Phototherapeutic keratectomy (PTK) provides an alternative to corneal transplant in treating corneal dystrophies, scars, and some infections. In this procedure, diseased corneal tissue is vaporized and surface irregularities are corrected with little trauma to surrounding tissue. Healing occurs rapidly.

Corneal Transplant. Once the cornea has become scarred and opaque, no treatment can restore its clarity. The first successful corneal transplant (or *keratoplasty*), replacement of diseased cornea by healthy corneal tissue from a donor, was performed in 1906. Current corneal transplant procedures have a success rate of approximately 90% (National Eye Institute, 2017b).

Corneas are harvested from the cadavers of uninfected adults who were under the age of 65 and who died as a result of acute trauma or illness. After harvesting, the cornea can be stored in a tissue-culture medium for up to 4 weeks before being used as a graft. Corneal transplantation is usually an elective surgery, although emergency transplantation may be required for perforation of the cornea.

Corneal transplant may be either lamellar or penetrating. In a lamellar keratoplasty, the superficial layer of cornea is removed and replaced with a graft. The anterior chamber remains intact. In a penetrating keratoplasty, a button or full thickness of cornea is removed and replaced by donor tissue (**Figure 46.3 ■**). The graft is then sutured in place using suture finer than human hair and a continuous or interrupted stitch. Because the cornea is avascular, these sutures remain in place for up to a year to ensure healing.

Most corneal transplants do not require hospitalization. The eye is patched for 24 hours following surgery. Narcotic analgesia may be required initially because the cornea is extremely sensitive. Corticosteroid eyedrops are ordered to reduce the inflammatory response and prevent edema of the graft. Antibiotic drops may be prescribed to prevent infection.

The risk of transplant rejection is low. Because the cornea is avascular, there is little exposure of the transplanted corneal tissue to the host's immune defenses (Sorenson, Quinn & Klein, 2019). Research suggests that matching of blood type (not tissue type, as is required for major organ transplants) between the donor and the transplant recipient

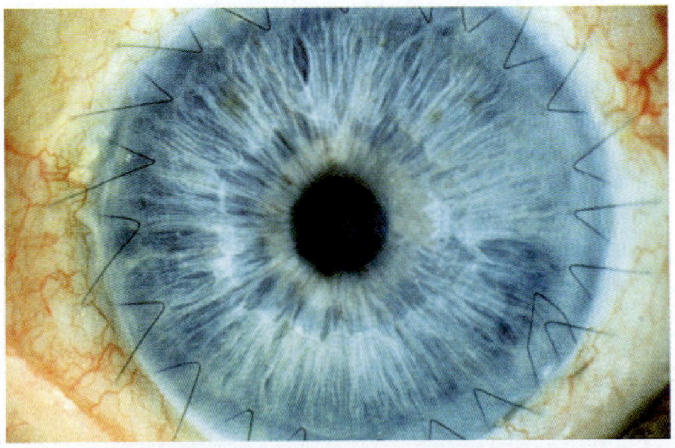

Figure 46.3 ■ Corneal transplant. The diseased cornea is removed and a corneal graft is sutured in place using material finer than a human hair.

may reduce the risk of transplant rejection (National Eye Institute, 2017b). When rejection does occur, it occurs within 3 weeks of the transplant, beginning with inflammation at the edge of the grafted tissue and spreading to involve the entire graft. In many cases, rejection can be successfully treated using corticosteroid therapy, preserving the graft.

See **Box 46.4** for nursing care of the patient having eye surgery.

Nursing Care

The nursing role in caring for patients with corneal disorders may involve direct care, but more often focuses on prevention and education. Nurses working in clinics and outpatient surgical settings care for patients undergoing corneal transplant and surgeries to correct refractive errors.

BOX 46.4
Nursing Care of the Patient Having Eye Surgery

PREOPERATIVE CARE

- Provide routine preoperative care as ordered.
- Assess visual acuity of the nonoperative eye prior to surgery. *The patient with limited vision in the nonoperative eye may need additional attention and ADL assistance postoperatively to ensure safety.*
- Assess the patient's support systems and the possible effect of impaired vision on lifestyle and ability to perform ADLs in the postoperative period. *Safety measures such as installing handrails and removing throw rugs from the home can help promote mobility and safety, especially if the patient has limited vision in the unaffected eye.*
- Teach measures to prevent eye injury postoperatively: Avoid vomiting, straining at stool, coughing, sneezing, lifting more than 5 lb, and bending over at the waist. *These activities temporarily increase intraocular pressure and may lead to postoperative complications.*
- Remove all eye makeup and contact lenses or glasses prior to surgery. Store corrective lenses in a safe place, and make them readily available to the patient on return from surgery. *Maintaining visual acuity in the unaffected eye helps reduce fear and maintain safety.*
- Administer preoperative medications and eyedrops or ointments as prescribed. *Mydriatic (pupil-dilating) or cycloplegic (ciliary-paralytic) drops and drops to lower intraocular pressure may be prescribed preoperatively.*

POSTOPERATIVE CARE

- Provide routine postoperative care as ordered.
- Assess eye dressing for bleeding or drainage following surgery. *Bleeding or drainage may indicate a surgical complication.*
- Maintain the eye patch or shield in place. *The eye patch or shield helps prevent inadvertent injury to the operative site.*
- Place in semi-Fowler or Fowler position on the unaffected side. *Elevating the head of the bed and lying on the unaffected side reduce intraocular pressure in the affected eye.*
- Remind the patient to avoid coughing, sneezing, or straining as needed. *These activities increase intraocular pressure.*
- Assess and medicate as necessary for complaints of pain, aching, or a scratchy sensation in the affected eye. Immediately report complaints of sudden, sharp eye pain to the physician. *An abrupt increase in or onset of eye pain may indicate hemorrhage or other ocular emergency requiring immediate intervention to preserve sight.*
- Assess for potential complications:
  a. Pain in or drainage from the affected eye
  b. Hemorrhage with blood in the anterior chamber of the eye
  c. Flashes of light, floaters, or the sensation of a curtain being drawn over the eye (indicators of retinal detachment)
  d. Cloudy appearance to the cornea (corneal edema).

  Evidence of complications or unusual complaints should be reported to the healthcare provider at once. Early intervention is often necessary to preserve sight.
- Approach the patient on the unaffected side. *This approach facilitates eye contact and communication.*
- Place personal articles and the call light within easy reach. *These measures prevent stretching and straining by the patient.*
- Administer antibiotic, anti-inflammatory, and other systemic and topical eye medications as prescribed. *Medications are prescribed to prevent infection or inflammation of the operative site, maintain pupil constriction, and control intraocular pressure.*
- Administer antiemetic medication as needed. *It is important to prevent vomiting to maintain normal intraocular pressures.*

Health Education for the Patient and Family

- Teach the patient and family about home care:
  a. How to instill eyedrops
  b. The name, dosage, schedule, duration, purpose, and side effects of medications
  c. How and when to use the eye patch and eye shield
  d. The importance of avoiding scratching, rubbing, touching, or squeezing the affected eye
  e. Measures to avoid constipation and straining
  f. Activity limitations, if ordered
  g. Symptoms to report, including eye pain or pressure, redness or cloudiness, drainage, decreased vision, floaters or flashes of light, or halos around bright objects
  h. The need to wear sunglasses with side shields when outdoors to reduce photophobia.
- Remind the patient that vision may not stabilize for several weeks following eye surgery. New corrective lenses, if necessary, are not prescribed until vision has stabilized. *Patients may be alarmed that vision seems worse after surgery than before and need reassurance that visual acuity usually improves with time and healing of the affected eye.*
- Emphasize the importance of keeping recommended follow-up appointments. Provide referral to a community home health agency for assistance with home care after discharge as needed.

Assessment

Collect the following data through the health history and physical examination. Additional focused assessments are described in Chapter 45 and with the interventions that follow.

- ***Health history:*** Risk factors; presence of redness, discomfort, tearing, photophobia, edema, and drainage; symptom onset; presence of pain, effect on vision
- ***Physical assessment:*** Visual acuity; inspection of external eye, including conjunctiva, sclera, and cornea; extraocular movements.

Priorities of Care

Corneal disorders often affect visual acuity and can cause acute pain. The priority nursing focus is on preventing complications and promoting healing and comfort, and preventing injury.

Diagnoses, Interventions, and Outcomes

Reduce Risk for Impaired Vision. Disorders affecting the cornea may disrupt its integrity or clarity. Because the cornea plays a vital role in focusing light on the retina, corneal damage can affect vision, impairing visual acuity and even causing legal blindness.

Expected Outcome: Patient's visual acuity will be preserved or restored to previous level.

The nurse will:

- Assess vision with and without corrective lenses. *Assessment provides a baseline to evaluate possible vision changes resulting from the disorder or treatment.*
- Instruct about thorough hand hygiene before inserting or removing contact lenses or instilling any eye medications. Teach to avoid touching or rubbing the eyes. Instruct to use a new, clean cotton-tipped swab or cotton ball for cleaning each eye. *Hand hygiene is the single most important measure to prevent transmission of infection to the eye. Touching or rubbing the eyes increases the risk of infection and corneal trauma. Using a new swab or cotton ball prevents cross-contamination between eyes.*
- Emphasize the importance of proper care of contact lenses specific to the type of lens used. *Patients who wear hard contact lenses must remove them daily because the central cornea needs exposure to atmospheric oxygen. Although soft and extended-wear lenses allow the cornea to "breathe," improper cleaning carries a major risk for infection.*
- Teach the importance of using eye protection when engaging in potentially dangerous activities. *Trauma increases the risk of infection and scarring of the cornea.*
- If corneal perforation is suspected, place the patient in the supine position, close the eye, and cover it with a dry, sterile dressing. Notify the physician immediately. *Corneal perforation may occur without warning in patients with corneal ulcers. It places the patient at risk for loss of eye contents. Emergency measures are taken to reduce intraocular pressure and maintain eye integrity to preserve vision.*

SAFETY ALERT: Suspect corneal perforation with complaints of sudden, severe eye pain and photophobia. ■

Manage Acute Pain. The cornea of the eye is extremely sensitive; therefore, corneal disorders frequently cause significant pain. Pain, in turn, increases the stress response and interferes with rest, potentially impairing healing.

Expected Outcome: Patient will demonstrate pain relief through verbal expressions of comfort and nonverbal expressions such as relaxed body posture and ability to rest and focus.

The nurse will:

- Assess pain, using verbal and nonverbal cues. *Pain is a subjective experience and can be evaluated only by the patient's response and in terms of its effect on the patient.*
- Administer prescribed analgesia routinely in the first 12 to 24 hours after corneal surgery. *Routine administration of analgesics prevents pain from reaching a level of severity at which it becomes difficult to relieve.*
- Patch both eyes if necessary. *Patching both eyes reduces eye movement and irritation of the affected eye.*
- Teach to apply warm compresses to reduce inflammation and pain. *The use of warm compresses for 15 minutes, three to four times a day, promotes comfort for patients with keratitis or corneal injury.*
- Instruct to use dark sunglasses with appropriate UV protection when out of doors, even on cloudy days. *True photophobia, often associated with corneal disorders, causes eye pain with increased light intensity.*
- Teach to instill prescribed eyedrops as ordered. *Prescribed medications may reduce inflammation and eliminate infection, reducing discomfort.*

Reduce Risk for Injury. The patient who has undergone corneal transplantation has an increased risk for injury for several reasons. The eye on which surgery was performed is patched for 24 hours after surgery, changing depth perception and increasing the risk for falls. Increased intraocular pressure or trauma to the eye may damage the graft, resulting in graft rejection.

Expected Outcome: The patient will participate in safe postoperative management.

The nurse will:

- Instruct to call for help before getting up or ambulating after surgery. Ensure access to the call light. *It may take time for the patient to adjust to changes in depth perception caused by the eye patch. Assistance helps prevent falls that may not only injure the patient but also traumatize the operative site.*
- Administer prescribed antiemetics and stool softeners postoperatively. *Vomiting and straining at stool increase intraocular pressure, potentially damaging suture lines.*
- Teach how to apply an eye shield at night after the eye patch is removed. *An eye shield may be recommended at night to prevent inadvertent rubbing or trauma to the eye during sleep.*
- Instruct not to rub or scratch the eye. *Rubbing or scratching may disrupt suture lines or damage the grafted tissue.*

- Reinforce the importance of using eye protection during hazardous activities. *Following a corneal transplant, the patient has the same risk of eye injury as other people who perform hazardous activities.*

Delegating Nursing Care Activities

For the visually impaired patient, the unlicensed assistive personnel may help set up meal trays using the clock description (i.e., the drink is at 10 o'clock, the meat is on the plate from 2 o'clock to 6 o'clock, etc.), assist with bathing by setting up bath supplies per patient wishes, and assist with ambulation if the patient requires assistance.

Transitions of Care

Education is a vital strategy for preventing many corneal disorders. Teach all patients about proper eye care, including the importance of not sharing towels and makeup, avoiding rubbing or scratching the eyes, and preventing trauma and infection. Teach contact lens users appropriate care and cleaning techniques. Stress the importance of periodic removal of lenses, even extended-wear lenses. In general, lenses should be removed at night, even though manufacturers may claim it is safe to wear them while sleeping. Emphasize the need to follow cleaning instructions precisely to avoid bacterial contamination of lenses and possible corneal infection. If the patient experiences a corneal abrasion or keratitis, instruct to avoid wearing contact lenses until the cornea has healed completely.

Following treatment, teach patients to manage their condition at home. Emphasize to the family ways to prevent transmission of infection. If the patient is unable to administer eye medications or to perform other eye care techniques, involve the family in the teaching session. The following topics should be included:

- Safety and medical asepsis when cleansing the eye
- Instillation of prescribed eyedrops and ointments
- Application of an eye patch and where to obtain supplies
- Avoidance of activities such as excessive reading while eye is inflamed
- Follow-up appointments after corneal transplant surgery
- Signs of graft rejection
- Avoidance of activities that increase intraocular pressure such as straining, coughing, sneezing, bending over, lifting heavy objects
- Helpful resource: National Eye Institute and Lighthouse International.

The Patient with a Disorder Affecting the Eyelids

The eyelids and eyelashes are constantly exposed to the environment, as they protect the eye from damage. When these structures are inflamed, deformed, or their function is impaired, it affects both appearance and their protective functions.

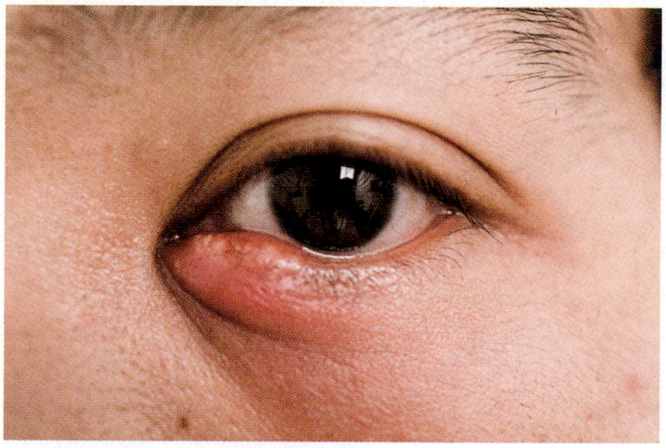

Figure 46.4 ■ Hordeolum.

Pathophysiology

The most common disorder affecting the eyelids is *marginal blepharitis*, an inflammation of the glands and lash follicles on the margins of the eyelids. This inflammatory disorder can be caused by a staphylococcal infection or it may be seborrheic in origin; commonly, both types are present. Seborrheic blepharitis is usually associated with seborrhea (dandruff) of the scalp or eyebrows.

Infection of one or more of the sebaceous glands of the eyelid may cause a hordeolum (sty) (Sorenson et al., 2019). *Hordeolum* is a staphylococcal abscess that may occur on either the external or internal margin of the lid (**Figure 46.4** ■).

Chronic inflammation of a meibomian gland may lead to formation of a *chalazion*, a granulomatous cyst or nodule of the lid (**Figure 46.5** ■). Chalazion may also follow a hordeolum that was inadequately treated. A lid lesion that ulcerates or does not heal may indicate basal or squamous cell carcinoma and should be further investigated.

Entropion, inversion of the lid margin (refer to Figure 46.2), may be associated with the normal aging process (senile entropion) or result from an infectious process such as trachoma. Entropion can lead to corneal irritation and, potentially, scarring as the lashes rub on the conjunctiva and cornea during blinking and sleep. *Ectropion*, or eversion of the lid margin, occurs primarily as an effect of aging (**Figure 46.6** ■). Other conditions may also lead to ectropion, including facial nerve paralysis or palsy (Bell palsy), scarring, or infection. With ectropion, the eye

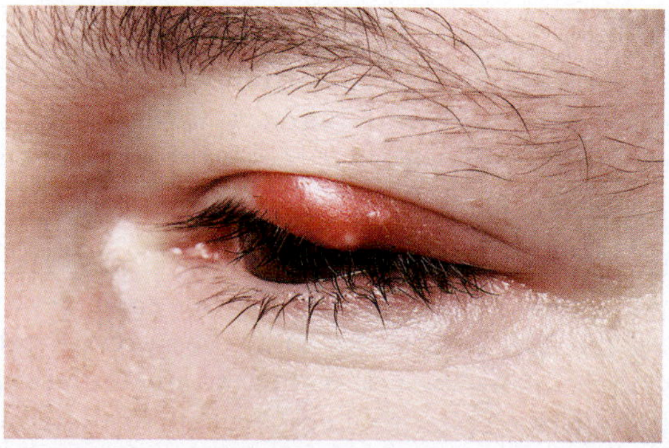

Figure 46.5 ■ Chalazion.

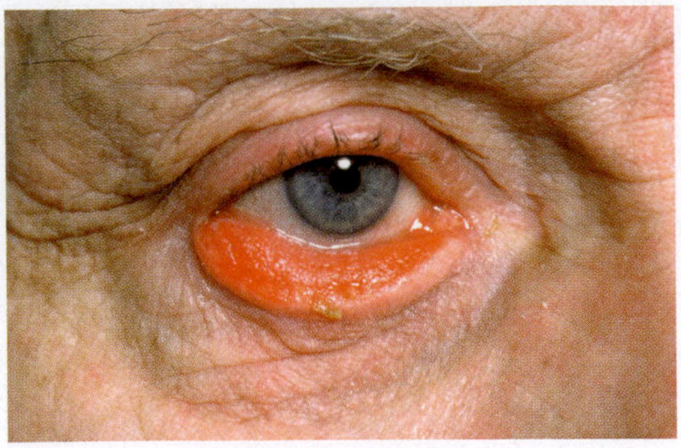

Figure 46.6 ■ Ectropion.

does not close effectively, increasing the risk for drying and damage to conjunctival membrane and the cornea. Both entropion and ectropion have cosmetic effects as well, altering the appearance of the eye and face.

Manifestations

Irritation, burning, and itching of eyelid margins are common manifestations of blepharitis. The eye appears red rimmed with mucous discharge, and there is crusting or scaling of lid margins. Lid margins may ulcerate, resulting in a loss of eyelashes.

An external hordeolum is characterized initially by acute pain at the lid margin and redness. A small tender raised area is visible. The patient may also experience photophobia, tearing, and the sensation of a foreign body in the affected eye. Internal hordeola are seen on the conjunctival side of the lid and may have more severe manifestations.

Chalazions present as a hard swelling on the lid, and surrounding conjunctival tissue is reddened. Unlike a hordeolum, a chalazion is painless. It may slowly increase in size and eventually require removal, but most resolve within several months.

Interprofessional Care

Diagnosis

Disorders affecting the eyelids are typically managed in the community. Diagnosis is usually made through the history and physical examination. Diagnostic tests are rarely required except to identify corneal or conjunctival damage resulting from the condition.

Medications

Topical antibiotics (eyedrops or ointments) may be prescribed for the patient with hordeolum and to treat infection resulting from irritation of the eye by a deformed lid.

Treatment

Careful cleansing of the lid margins using a "no-tears" baby shampoo is often recommended for marginal blepharitis. Soaking the lids with warm saline compresses prior to cleansing facilitates the removal of the crusts and exudate that result from blepharitis. Local heat applications may be used to treat hordeolum or chalazion; excision and drainage may be required if this is not effective. In entropion or ectropion, surgery may be performed to correct the defect, reduce the risk of damage to the eye, and improve cosmetic appearance.

Nursing Care

The nursing role focuses on education and comfort measures. Teach patients about appropriate eye care, including avoiding rubbing or scratching the eyes. Discuss the importance of not using old eye makeup, which can cause lid infections. Instruct to wash hands well before cleansing the eyelids or instilling any eye medications. Instruct to use a new, clean cotton-tipped swab or cotton ball for cleaning each eye. Teach to instill prescribed eyedrops and apply ointments as ordered. If the patient is unable to administer eye medications, involve the family in teaching. Teach to apply warm compresses to reduce inflammation and discomfort.

The Patient with Eye Trauma

More than 2 million eye injuries occur each year (American Academy of Ophthalmology, 2017). Many eye injuries are minor, but without timely and appropriate intervention, even a minor injury can threaten vision. For this reason, all eye injuries should be considered medical emergencies requiring immediate evaluation and intervention.

Pathophysiology

Any part of the eye, especially the exposed parts, may be affected by trauma. Foreign bodies, abrasions, and lacerations are the most common types of eye injury. Traumatic injury may also be due to a burn, penetrating object, or blunt force.

Corneal Abrasion

Corneal abrasion is disruption of the superficial epithelium of the cornea. Objects commonly causing corneal abrasion include contact lenses, eyelashes, small foreign bodies such as dust and dirt, and fingernails. Drying of the eye surface and chemical irritants may also result in a corneal abrasion.

When the stroma is damaged by a deep abrasion or laceration, there is an increased risk of infection, slowed healing, and scar formation.

Burns

The outer surface of the eye may be subjected to burns caused by heat, radiation, or explosion, but chemical burns are the most common. Either acid or alkaline substances may burn the eye. Ammonia, products that contain lye (such as oven and drain cleaners), and acids from car batteries or other sources are often implicated in eye injuries. Burns caused by alkaline substances are particularly serious because tiny particles of the chemical may remain in the conjunctival sac, causing progressive damage. Acid causes rapid damage to the eye, but generally causes less serious burns than alkaline substances.

Explosions and flash burn injuries pose the greatest risk for thermal burns of the eye. Ultraviolet rays can also cause corneal damage ranging in severity from mild to extensive. Depending on the source of the ultraviolet light, these burns may be known by various names such as snowblindness, arc welder's burn, or flash burn.

Penetrating Trauma

Perforation of the eye occurs from a variety of causes. Metal flakes or other particles produced by high-speed drilling or grinding, glass shards, or other substances may penetrate the eye. Gunshots (including BBs), arrows, and knives can penetrate the eye. In a penetrating injury, the layers of the eye spontaneously reapproximate after entry of a sharp-pointed object or small missile into the globe. These injuries may not be readily apparent with inspection of the eye. In a perforating injury, the layers of the eye do not spontaneously reapproximate, resulting in rupture of the globe and potential loss of ocular contents.

Penetrating injuries may be hidden because of tissue swelling or missed when the patient has other significant injuries that command attention. When the eyelid is lacerated or has a puncture wound, inspection of the underlying eye tissue for possible damage is vital.

Blunt Trauma

Sports injuries are a common cause of blunt trauma to the eye: It may be struck with a ball (baseball, tennis, racquetball, and handball are frequently implicated) or injured in contact sports such as basketball, football, boxing, or wrestling. Motor vehicle crashes, falls, and physical assault are examples of other causes of blunt eye trauma.

Blunt trauma may lead to a minor eye injury such as lid ecchymosis (black eye) or subconjunctival hemorrhage, caused by rupture of a blood vessel in the conjunctiva (**Figure 46.7** ■).

Hyphema, bleeding into the anterior chamber of the eye, is a potential result of blunt eye trauma. When the highly vascular uveal tract of the eye is disrupted by blunt force, hemorrhage may result, filling the anterior chamber.

An orbital blowout fracture is another potential result of blunt eye trauma. Although any part of the eye orbit may be fractured, the ethmoid bone on the orbital floor is the most likely site. Orbital contents, including fat, muscles, and the eye itself, may herniate through the fracture into the underlying maxillary sinus.

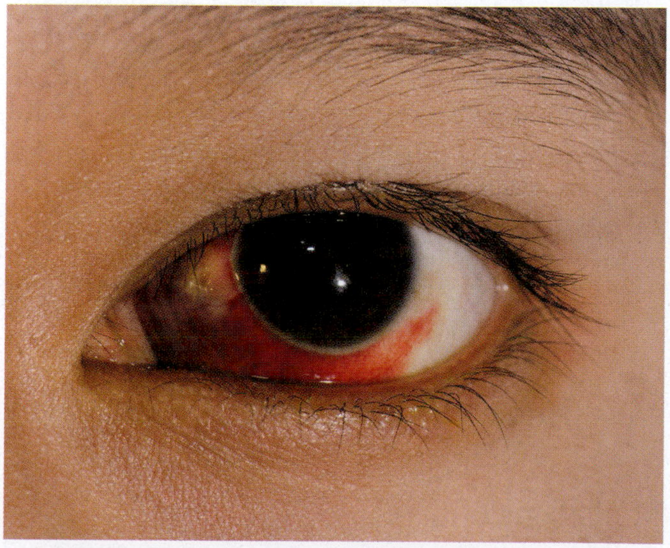

Figure 46.7 ■ Subconjunctival hemorrhage.

Manifestations

Superficial abrasions of the cornea are extremely painful but generally heal rapidly without complication or scarring. Photophobia and tearing are commonly present.

In patients with burns, in addition to giving a history of face and eye contact with a caustic substance or other burning agent, the patients often complain of eye pain and decreased vision. Eyelids are often swollen. Burns may also affect the face or lids. The appearance of the eye may vary, depending on the type of burn. The conjunctiva is reddened and edematous; sloughing may be seen, particularly with chemical burns. The cornea often appears cloudy or hazy, and ulcerations may be evident.

Eye perforations cause pain, partial or complete loss of vision, and possibly bleeding or extrusion of eye contents.

With lid ecchymosis and subconjunctival hemorrhage, a well-defined bright area of erythema appears under the conjunctiva. No pain or discomfort is associated with the hemorrhage and no treatment is necessary. The blood typically reabsorbs within 2 to 3 weeks. Patients with hyphema complain of eye pain, decreased visual acuity, and seeing a reddish tint. Blood is visible in the anterior chamber.

Patients with orbital blowout fractures complain of diplopia (double vision), pain with upward movement of the affected eye, and decreased sensation on the affected cheek. The eye appears sunken (enophthalmos) and has limited movement on examination.

Interprofessional Care

Diagnosis

When trauma to the eye is known or suspected, a thorough examination is conducted to determine the type and extent of the injury. Unless immediate treatment is indicated, as with a chemical burn, vision is evaluated initially. If the patient normally wears corrective lenses, vision assessment is performed while glasses are worn. Eye movement is evaluated unless a penetrating object is present, and the lid and eye are inspected for lacerations. Inspection is performed using strong light and magnification with a headband loupe or slit lamp. Topical anesthesia may be used prior to inspection if eye pain and photophobia make eye opening difficult. Fluorescein staining can help identify foreign bodies and abrasions. Any conjunctival or anterior chamber hemorrhage is noted, as is the presence or absence of the red reflex. Ophthalmoscopic examination is used to detect hemorrhage or trauma to the interior chamber.

Facial x-rays and CT scans are used to identify orbital fractures or foreign bodies within the globe. Ultrasonography may be employed to detect a detached retina or vitreous hemorrhage.

Treatment

Foreign bodies are removed using irrigation, a sterile cotton-tipped applicator, or a sterile needle or other instrument. Antibiotic ointment—erythromycin or sulfacetamide sodium—is applied after their removal. In patients with corneal abrasions and large foreign bodies in the eye, an

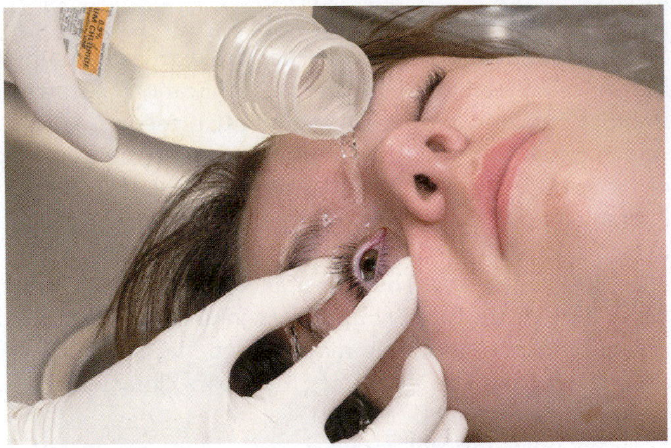

Figure 46.8 ■ A nurse uses sterile normal saline to flush the eye of a patient with a suspected chemical burn.

eye patch is applied firmly after the antibiotic application to keep the eye closed for approximately 24 hours.

The immediate priority of care for patients with chemical burns is flushing the affected eye with copious amounts of fluid (**Figure 46.8** ■). Physiologic (normal) saline is preferred; however, water may be used if saline is not available. A special contact lens irrigating unit (Morgan lens) or a bottle of irrigant with intravenous tubing held to flush all eye surfaces may be useful. The eyelid is everted to identify and remove material from the conjunctival sac. A topical anesthetic, such as tetracaine drops, helps relieve pain, making inspection and irrigation easier. During irrigation, fluid is directed from the inner canthus of the eye to the outer or lateral canthus. Tipping the patient's head slightly to the affected side prevents contamination of the unaffected eye. Irrigation is continued until the pH of the eye is normal (in the range of 7.2 to 7.4). Following irrigation, a topical antibiotic ointment such as gentamicin ophthalmic is applied.

Penetrating wounds of the eye generally require surgical intervention by an ophthalmic surgeon. Immediate care focuses on relieving pain and protecting the eye from further injury. To prevent loss of intraocular contents, do not place pressure on the eye itself, but gently cover with sterile gauze or an eye pad. If a foreign body is embedded in or sticking out of the eye, no attempt is made to remove it. The object should be immobilized and the eye protected with a metal eye shield until an ophthalmologist can see the patient. A paper cup or other protective device may be used if the object is too large to use an eye shield. Patching the unaffected eye as well decreases ocular movement. Pain is managed using narcotic analgesics such as morphine. The patient may also require sedation (e.g., diazepam) and antiemetic medications to prevent vomiting. Antibiotics such as intravenous cefazolin (Ancef) or gentamicin (Garamycin) are prescribed to prevent infection.

Interventions for the patient with blunt trauma to the eye include placing the patient on bed rest in semi-Fowler position and protecting the eye from further injury with an eye shield. The unaffected eye is also patched to minimize eye movement. A carbonic anhydrase inhibitor such as acetazolamide (Diamox) or dichlorphenamide (Daranide) may be prescribed to reduce intraocular pressure.

Nursing Care

The nursing role involves educating people about the prevention of eye injuries and providing direct care to patients with eye injuries.

Priorities of Care

Ocular injuries require immediate interventions simultaneously with assessment and accurate history collection. The time, type, and extent of injury and the circumstances under which it occurred are determined. In addition, ask about preexisting vision problems.

Diagnoses, Interventions, and Outcomes

Reduce Risk of Vision Loss. All types of eye trauma pose the risk of violating the integrity of the eye and, hence, threatening vision. The goals of nursing care, therefore, are preserving vision and the integrity of the eye and preventing further damage.

Expected Outcome: Patient's injured ocular tissue will heal without complications and previous visual acuity will be restored.

The nurse will:

- Assess vision in each eye and both eyes, with and without corrective lenses, on entry into the emergency department or primary care setting. *An initial assessment provides valuable information about the effect of the injury on the patient's vision and a baseline for future comparisons.*
- Inspect eye(s) carefully for evidence of foreign bodies, burns, penetrating injury, or blunt trauma. Note if lacerations, burns, or other trauma are evident in tissues surrounding the eye. *Eye trauma may be hidden by other injuries and, as a result, remain untreated.*
- If a burn or foreign body is present, anesthetic drops may be instilled and the eye irrigated either before or after the physician evaluates the patient. *Blepharism and eye pain may impair assessment of the injured eye. Irrigation to remove the chemical is of higher priority than assessment of the eye.*
- Loose foreign bodies may be removed using a moist, sterile, cotton-tipped applicator. *Prompt removal of foreign bodies may prevent corneal abrasion.*
- For a severe or penetrating injury, promote rest and stabilize the injured eye by applying an eye pad or gauze dressing loosely over both the affected and unaffected eye. Stabilize any penetrating object, if possible. *These measures reduce eye movement and can help preserve the patient's vision.*
- Following treatment, apply eyedrops or ointment as prescribed and apply an eye pad or shield if ordered. *An eye pad is applied to the affected eye to reduce pain and photophobia and to promote healing.*

Transitions of Care

Teaching related to eye injuries focuses on prevention and first-aid measures. Teaching individuals and groups how to prevent eye injuries is an important nursing role, especially for people involved in hazardous occupations and activities. Teach employees and participants in high-risk sports or activities how and when to use eye protection devices. Stress the importance of using seat belts and air bags to prevent eye injury in automobile crashes. Instruct patients to immediately flush the eye with copious amounts of water if a chemical splash occurs. Loose, visible foreign bodies can be removed using a clean, moistened cotton-tipped swab. If an abrasion, penetrating, or blunt injury is suspected, the eye should be covered loosely with sterile gauze and medical attention sought immediately. Instruct patients not to remove objects that penetrate the eye.

Following an injury, discuss the following topics with the patient and family:

- Prescribed medications and possible adverse effects
- Strategies to prevent further trauma
- Application of an eye pad or shield
- Avoidance of activities that increase intraocular pressure
- Importance of activity restrictions.

The Patient with Uveitis

The middle vascular layer of the eye, including the choroid, the ciliary body, and the iris, is known as the uvea and uveal tract. *Uveitis* is inflammation of all or part of this vascular layer. *Iritis*, inflammation of the iris only, occurs more commonly than uveitis.

Uveitis is usually a disease limited to the eye; it may be idiopathic or caused by an autoimmune process, infection, parasitic disease, or trauma. Many cases can be linked to a systemic disease, often an arthritic or autoimmune disorder such as ankylosing spondylitis, Reiter's syndrome, rheumatoid arthritis, or sarcoidosis (see Chapter 40). Uveitis has also been linked with tuberculosis and syphilis. Manifestations of uveitis include pupillary constriction and erythema around the limbus. The patient may complain of severe eye pain and photophobia, as well as blurred vision.

Immunosuppressive therapy may be used to suppress the inflammatory response in patients with severe uveitis. Atropine may also be prescribed for associated inflammation of the iris. The patient may require analgesics such as acetaminophen and/or codeine for pain management. Nursing care is supportive, focusing on promotion of comfort and teaching about the disorder and its management.

The Patient with Cataracts

A **cataract** is an opacification (clouding) of the lens of the eye. This opacification can significantly interfere with light transmission to the retina and the ability to perceive images clearly.

Cataracts are a common and significant cause of visual deficits, affecting more than 22 million people over age 40 in the United States. By age 80, over half of the population is affected (National Eye Institute, 2017c). In many cases, however, cataracts do not significantly impair vision. Cataracts affect slightly more women than men, and more Whites than people of other ethnicities. More than 3 million cataract removal surgeries are performed annually in the United States. (National Eye Institute, 2017e). To remember risk factors for cataracts, use the mnemonic **CATARACt**:

Congenital

Aging

Toxicity (steroids, etc.)

Accidents

Radiation (sunlight)

Altered metabolism (diabetes mellitus)

Cigarette smoking

Pathophysiology

The majority of cataracts are senile cataracts, formed as a result of the aging process (Sorenson et al., 2019). As the lens ages, its fibers and proteins change and degenerate. The proteins clump, clouding the lens and reducing light transmission to the retina. This process generally begins at the periphery of the lens, gradually spreading to involve the central portion. As the cataract continues to develop, the entire lens may become opaque. When only a portion of the lens is affected, the cataract is called *immature*. A *mature* cataract is opacity of the entire lens. In addition to clouding, the lens may discolor over time, affecting the ability to accurately discriminate colors.

Risk Factors

Age is the greatest single risk factor for cataracts. Genetics may contribute to the risk, although the link is unclear. Environmental and lifestyle factors play a role: Long-term exposure to sunlight (ultraviolet B [UVB] rays) contributes; cigarette smoking and heavy alcohol consumption are associated with earlier cataract development. Although senile cataracts are by far the most common, cataracts may also be congenital or acquired in origin. Eye trauma, including injury to the lens capsule by a foreign body, blunt trauma, or exposure to heat or radiation, can precipitate cataract formation. Diabetes mellitus is associated with earlier development of cataracts, especially when the blood glucose level is not carefully controlled at or near normal levels. Certain drugs such as systemic or inhaled corticosteroids, chlorpromazine (Thorazine), and busulfan (Myleran) also prompt the formation of cataracts.

Manifestations

Cataracts tend to occur bilaterally unless related to eye trauma. Fortunately, they tend to develop at different rates, and one cataract generally matures more rapidly than the other. Because a cataract interferes with light transmission through the lens, visual acuity decreases, affecting both close and distance vision (**Figure 46.9** ■). Light rays are scattered as they pass through the lens, causing complaints of glare. Glare affects the ability to adjust between light and dark environments. Color discrimination is impaired, particularly in the blue-to-purple range. When the cataract is

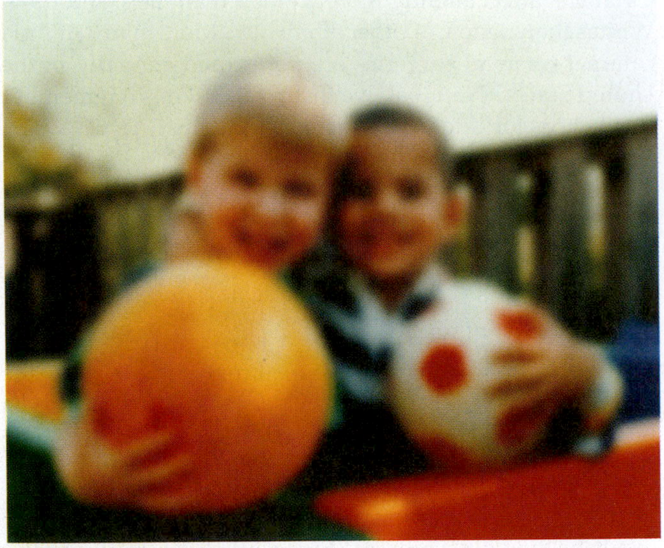

Figure 46.9 ■ A scene as viewed by a patient with cataracts.

mature, the pupil may appear cloudy gray or white rather than black.

Interprofessional Care

Diagnosis

The diagnosis of a cataract is made based on the history and eye examination. Ophthalmoscopic examination confirms the diagnosis by identifying the location and extent of a cataract. As the cataract matures, ophthalmoscopy reveals a dark area instead of the red reflex.

Surgery

Surgical removal is the only treatment used at this time for cataracts; no medical treatment is available to prevent or treat them. If the patient presents with bilateral cataracts, surgery is generally performed on one eye at a time. If an intraocular lens (an artificial lens to replace the diseased lens of the eye) is to be implanted during surgery, the corneal curvature and anteroposterior diameter of the eye are measured prior to surgery to determine the lens power needed for the intraocular lens implant.

Surgical removal of the cataract and lens is indicated when the cataract has developed to the point that vision and performance of ADLs are affected. A mature cataract may also be removed when it causes a secondary condition such as glaucoma or uveitis.

Cataract surgery is usually done on an outpatient basis, using local anesthesia. If general anesthesia is required, the patient may be hospitalized overnight. Extracapsular extraction, in which the anterior capsule, nucleus, and cortex of the lens are removed, leaving the posterior capsule intact, is the procedure of choice (**Figure 46.10** ■). Using an operating microscope, the surgeon makes a small incision at the edge of the clear cornea and extracts the lens via emulsification and aspiration. In this technique, ultrasound vibrations are used to break the lens material into fragments (phacoemulsification), which are then suctioned out of the eye. The remaining posterior capsule supports the lens implant and protects the retina.

After removal of the lens, a silicone or acrylic resin intraocular lens is implanted to replace the light-focusing functions of the diseased lens. This implant rapidly restores binocular vision and depth perception. Following extracapsular lens removal, the intraocular lens (IOL) is positioned in the posterior capsule behind the iris (refer to Figure 46.10). Currently available intraocular lenses allow for correction of refractive disorders of distance vision or astigmatism, often allowing the patient to no longer rely on corrective lenses for visual acuity. Bifocal and multifocal IOLs are also available (National Eye Institute, 2017e).

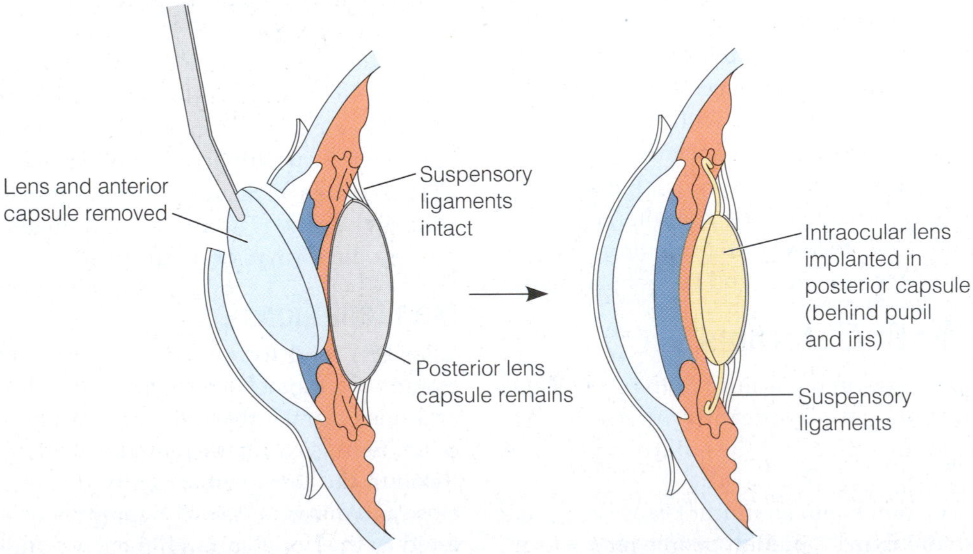
Lens and anterior capsule removed
Suspensory ligaments intact
Posterior lens capsule remains
Intraocular lens implanted in posterior capsule (behind pupil and iris)
Suspensory ligaments

Figure 46.10 ■ Extracapsular cataract extraction with removal of the lens and anterior capsule, leaving the posterior capsule intact. The intraocular lens is implanted within the posterior capsule.

These specialized lenses are not always appropriate, however. The patient with a preexisting refractive error may continue to require corrective lenses and often needs a prescriptive change after surgery.

Complications of cataract surgery are unusual and occur in lesser than 1% of the surgeries. Loss of vitreous humor, corneal edema, increased intraocular pressure, hemorrhage, inflammation or infection, retinal detachment, and displacement of the implanted lens are potential complications. Months or years after cataract removal, opacification of the remaining posterior capsule may develop. Vision can be restored using laser capsulotomy (creating an opening for light to pass through the opacified capsule) or surgical incision into the posterior capsule to allow light to reach the retina (National Eye Institute, 2017e).

Nursing Care

Assessment

- *Health history:* Effect of vision changes on lifestyle and activities (e.g., ability to read, watch television, participate in work and recreational activities); history of smoking, diabetes, use of prescription drugs associated with increased risk of cataract or cataract surgery
- *Physical assessment:* General health; visual acuity (using corrective lenses and Snellen chart) in each eye; presence of red reflex.

Priorities of Care

The patient with cataracts often has few physical care nursing needs. Patient advocacy, psychologic and emotional support, and teaching/learning needs are typically of higher priority for these patients. Review nursing care of the patient having eye surgery as outlined in Box 46.4.

Diagnoses, Interventions, and Outcomes

Promote Knowledge and Reduce Anxiety. With the initial diagnosis of cataract, the nurse often becomes an important information resource for the patient.

Expected Outcome: Patient will be able to relate the risks and potential benefits of cataract surgery to current lifestyle and roles.

The nurse will:

- Explain the nonemergent nature of the condition and help the patient determine the extent to which the cataract is affecting daily life. *This helps the patient decide when to proceed with surgery. Providing information about cataracts and their surgical removal also assists with decision making.*
- Attend to verbalized concerns about surgery and its outcome. Address questions factually and completely. *Fear of blindness is second only to fear of cancer for many patients. Careful listening, teaching, and a caring, understanding attitude can help the patient deal with this fear prior to surgery.*

Promote Self-Care Following Cataract Surgery. Minimal care is needed following cataract surgery.

Expected Outcome: Patient will achieve effective self-care postoperatively.

The nurse will:

- Assess for factors that may interfere with the patient's ability to provide self-care postoperatively. *A chronic condition such as arthritis that may affect the ability to administer eyedrops may indicate the need to include a family member in teaching.*
- Assess for other care needs that may be impacted by vision changes in the early postoperative period. *Other care needs, such as insulin injections, may suggest the need for home health or nursing care postoperatively.*

Transitions of Care

Advise all patients about the importance of protecting the eyes from UVB rays by wearing eye protection during activities such as welding and sunglasses with UVB protection when out of doors. Discuss the link between heavy smoking and cataract development. Provide anti–tobacco use education for young people and resources to stop smoking for people who do smoke.

With the initial diagnosis, teaching focuses on the disorder, indications for surgery, and vision restoration following cataract removal. Teaching adaptive strategies to deal with effects of the cataract on vision and depth perception are also useful. When surgery is scheduled, provide pre- and postoperative teaching, including a significant other in teaching sessions. Reinforce the following information with written instructions:

- Initial limitations such as avoiding lifting, strenuous activity, sleeping on operative side, or getting water in the eye
- Importance of not rubbing or scratching the eye
- Prescribed medications and side effects
- Importance of follow-up appointments
- Manifestations of postoperative complications such as eye pain, decreased visual acuity or other change in vision, headache, nausea, or itching and redness of the affected eye
- Instillation of eyedrops and application of eye shield (for nighttime use)
- Anticipated vision changes as appropriate.

The Patient with Glaucoma

Glaucoma is a condition characterized by optic neuropathy with gradual loss of peripheral vision and, usually, increased intraocular pressure of the eye. Glaucoma is a silent thief of vision. The patient typically experiences no manifestations other than narrowing of the visual field, which occurs so gradually that it often goes unnoticed until late in the disease process.

Glaucoma affects about 3 million people over the age of 40 in the United States; it remains undetected in approximately 50% of these cases. Glaucoma is a leading cause of blindness worldwide and the leading cause of blindness among African Americans. Age and race are the primary identified risk factors; it is more common in Blacks and Hispanics than in Whites (Glaucoma Research Foundation, 2017, 2018).

Pathophysiology

Aqueous humor, a thick fluid, occupies both the anterior and posterior chambers of the eye. The normal intraocular pressure of approximately 10 to 20 mmHg is maintained by a balance between the production of aqueous humor in the ciliary body, its flow through the pupil from the posterior to the anterior chamber of the eye, and its outflow or absorption through the trabecular meshwork and scleral venous sinus (canal of Schlemm) (refer to Figure 45.3 in the previous chapter). When this balance is disrupted, usually because of a decrease in the outflow or absorption of aqueous humor, the intraocular pressure increases (Sorenson et al., 2019). Although the exact relationship is unclear, it appears that increased intraocular pressure injures the optic nerve, either by compressing it or by impairing blood flow to the nerve. Axons in the periphery of the optic disc are damaged first. As optic fibers are destroyed, the rim of the optic disc shrinks and the normal depression in its center (the *optic cup*) becomes larger and deeper (called optic "cupping"). These changes to the optic disc are visible before visual field changes can be detected. As the disease progresses, there is a painless, progressive narrowing of the visual field (**Figure 46.11** ■) and eventual blindness. Vision loss is often significant before the patient seeks treatment and glaucoma is diagnosed.

Primary glaucoma in adults has two major forms: Open-angle glaucoma and angle-closure glaucoma. Both terms refer to the angle formed at the point where the iris meets the cornea in the eye's anterior chamber (**Figure 46.12** ■). Forms of primary glaucoma are compared in **Table 46.3**.

Open-Angle Glaucoma

Open-angle glaucoma, often called *chronic simple glaucoma*, is the most common form in adults, accounting for approximately 90% of all glaucoma. Its cause is unknown; it is thought to have a hereditary component, but no clear inheritance pattern can be identified. Open-angle glaucoma occurs more frequently and at an earlier age in African Americans than in Caucasians.

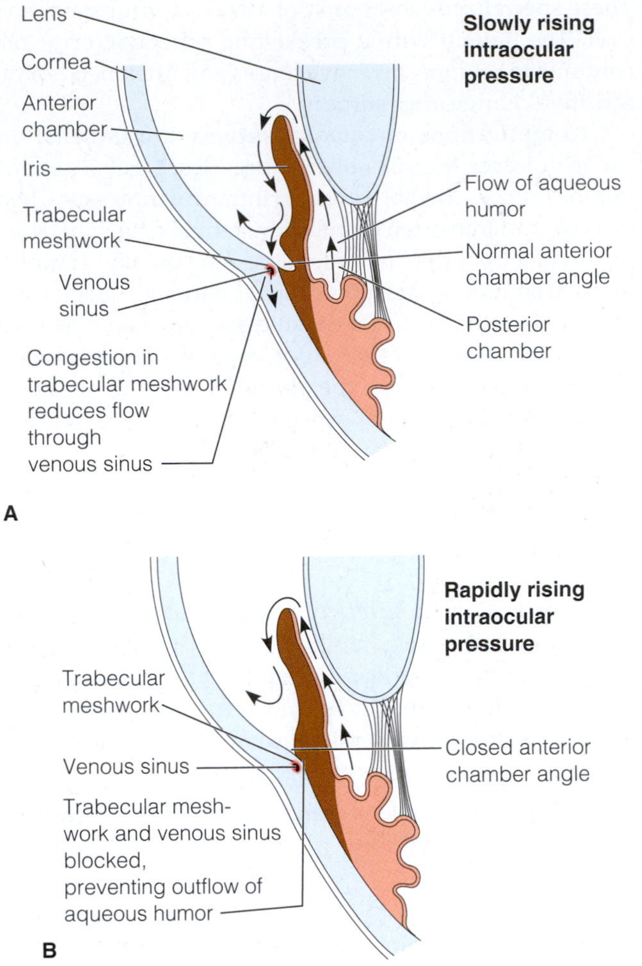
Lens
Cornea
Anterior chamber
Iris
Trabecular meshwork
Venous sinus
Congestion in trabecular meshwork reduces flow through venous sinus
Slowly rising intraocular pressure
Flow of aqueous humor
Normal anterior chamber angle
Posterior chamber
A
Rapidly rising intraocular pressure
Trabecular meshwork
Venous sinus
Trabecular meshwork and venous sinus blocked, preventing outflow of aqueous humor
Closed anterior chamber angle
B

Figure 46.12 ■ Forms of primary adult glaucoma. **A**, In chronic open-angle glaucoma, the anterior chamber angle remains open, but drainage of aqueous humor through the scleral venous sinus is impaired. **B**, In acute angle-closure glaucoma, the angle of the iris and anterior chamber narrows, obstructing the outflow of aqueous humor.

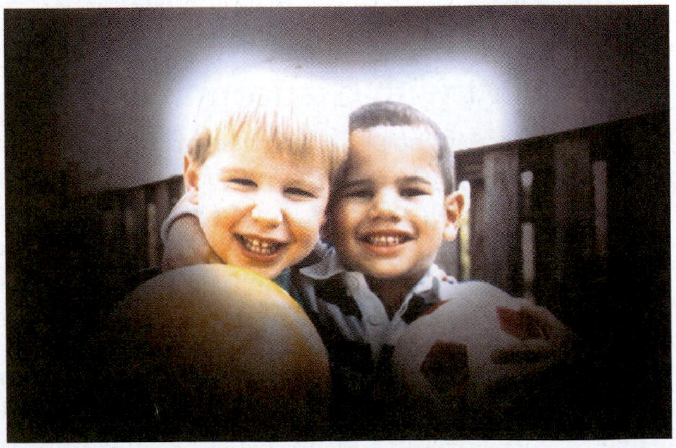

Figure 46.11 ■ Narrowing of visual fields typical of untreated glaucoma.

In open-angle glaucoma, the anterior chamber angle between the iris and cornea is normal (Figure 46.12A), hence the term *open angle*. However, the flow of aqueous humor through the trabecular meshwork and into the scleral venous sinus is relatively obstructed; the cause of this obstruction is unknown. Restricted outflow leads to an increased amount of fluid in the eye and increased intraocular pressure. Open-angle glaucoma tends to be a chronic, gradually progressive disease. The trabecular meshwork increasingly inhibits the outflow of aqueous humor, and the intraocular pressure gradually increases. The result is neuronal ischemia and optic nerve degeneration, leading to gradual loss of vision.

Open-angle glaucoma typically affects both eyes, although the pressures and progression may not be symmetric.

Table 46.3 A Comparison of Open-Angle and Angle-Closure Glaucoma

	Open-Angle Glaucoma	Angle-Closure Glaucoma
Incidence	■ Common ■ Accounts for 90% of all cases of glaucoma	■ Uncommon
Risk factors	■ Over age 40 ■ Genetic link ■ African American ancestry	■ Narrow anterior chamber angle ■ Aging ■ Asian or Inuit ancestry
Pathophysiology	■ Impaired aqueous outflow through the scleral venous sinus ■ Damage to axons of retinal ganglion cells with optic nerve atrophy ■ Gradual, consistent increase in intraocular pressure ■ Usually bilateral	■ Pupil dilation or lens accommodation causes already narrowed angle to close, blocking aqueous outflow ■ Rapid rise in intraocular pressure ■ Usually unilateral
Manifestations	■ No initial manifestations ■ Frequent lens changes in glasses ■ Impaired dark adaptation ■ Halos around lights ■ Gradual reduction of visual fields with preservation of central vision until late in the disease ■ Mild to severe increased intraocular pressure	■ Abrupt onset of eye pain, headache ■ Decreased visual acuity ■ Nausea and vomiting ■ Reddened conjunctiva ■ Cloudy cornea ■ Fixed pupil ■ Rapid, significant increase in intraocular pressure
Management	■ Topical medications such as beta-blockers, adrenergics, prostaglandin analogs ■ Carbonic anhydrase inhibitors ■ Laser trabeculoplasty, trabeculectomy	■ Topical miotics or beta-blockers ■ Systemic osmotic agents, carbonic anhydrase inhibitors ■ Laser iridotomy or peripheral iridectomy

Angle-Closure Glaucoma

Acute angle-closure (also called *narrow-angle* or *closed-angle*) *glaucoma* is the other, less common form of primary glaucoma in adults. It usually affects people with a shallow anterior chamber caused by an inherited defect (Sorenson et al., 2019). Approximately 1% of people over the age of 35 have narrowed anterior chamber angles; the incidence is higher in older adults and in people of Asian or Inuit (Alaska Native) ancestry (Glaucoma Research Foundation, 2018).

Narrowing of the anterior chamber angle (refer to Figure 46.12A for an illustration of the normal anterior chamber angle) occurs because of corneal flattening or bulging of the iris into the anterior chamber. When the lens thickens during accommodation or the iris thickens during pupil dilation, this angle can close completely. Closure of the angle blocks the outflow of aqueous humor through the trabecular meshwork and scleral venous sinus, and the intraocular pressure rises abruptly (Figure 46.12B). This abrupt increase in intraocular pressure damages the neurons of the retina and the optic nerve, leading to a rapid and permanent loss of vision if not treated promptly.

Episodes of angle-closure glaucoma are typically unilateral. However, a history of angle-closure glaucoma of one eye increases the risk that it will occur in the other eye.

Because of the effect of pupil dilation on aqueous outflow in angle-closure glaucoma, episodes often occur in association with darkness, emotional upset, or other factors that cause the pupil to dilate. Patients may have intermittent episodes lasting several hours before having a more typical prolonged attack of angle-closure glaucoma. For patients with a history of the condition, it is vital to avoid medications such as atropine and other anticholinergics, which have a mydriatic or pupil-dilating effect.

Risk Factors

Glaucoma is usually a primary condition without an identified cause. Primary glaucoma is most common in adults over the age of 60, but may be a congenital condition in infants and children (Glaucoma Research Foundation, 2018). Secondary glaucoma can develop as a result of infection or inflammation of the eye, cataract, tumor, hemorrhage, or eye trauma.

Manifestations

Open-angle glaucoma is painless, with gradual loss of visual fields. This loss of peripheral vision generally occurs so gradually that the patient is often unaware of it and only when it is detected through a comprehensive vision examination is it found. Intraocular pressure usually, but not always, is elevated (Glaucoma Research Foundation, 2017).

Symptoms such as severe eye and face pain, general malaise, nausea and vomiting, seeing colored halos around lights, and an abrupt decrease in visual acuity are associated with acute episodes of angle-closure glaucoma. The conjunctiva of the affected eye may be reddened and the cornea clouded with corneal edema. The pupil may be fixed (nonreactive to light) at midpoint. Some patients may experience periodic mild attacks, usually in the evening, with eye discomfort, impaired vision, and colored rings around lights.

Interprofessional Care

Although glaucoma cannot be predicted, prevented, or cured, in most cases it can be controlled and vision preserved if diagnosed early. Because the most prevalent type of glaucoma, open-angle glaucoma, has few symptoms, routine eye examinations are recommended for early detection. Optic disc examination, measurement of intraocular pressure, and visual field testing are used for diagnosis and monitoring of treatment effectiveness.

Diagnosis

The following diagnostic studies are used to detect and evaluate for the presence, severity, type, and effects of glaucoma (Kee, 2017):

- *Tonometry* indirectly measures intraocular pressure (**Figure 46.13** ■). Contact or noncontact tonometry may be used. Routine tonometry screening is recommended for all people over the age of 60. A single elevated pressure reading does not warrant a diagnosis of glaucoma; variations in intraocular pressure occur throughout the day.
- *Fundoscopy* (visual inspection of the optic fundus using an ophthalmoscope) identifies pallor and an increase in the size and depth of the optic cup on the optic disc. These changes are significant for diagnosing glaucoma.
- *Gonioscopy* uses a gonioscope to measure the depth of the anterior chamber. This test differentiates open-angle from angle-closure glaucoma.
- *Visual field testing* identifies the degree of central visual field narrowing and peripheral vision loss. The patient with glaucoma may retain 20/20 central vision even though there is severe peripheral vision loss.

Medications

Although medications cannot cure glaucoma, many patients with open-angle glaucoma can control intraocular pressure and preserve vision indefinitely with medications. Medications are used alone or in combination with the timing and dosage individually determined by pressure measurements. The primary drugs used to treat glaucoma are topical beta-adrenergic blocking agents, adrenergics (mydriatics), prostaglandin analogs, or carbonic anhydrase inhibitors. An oral carbonic anhydrase inhibitor may also be used.

Prostaglandin analogs such as latanoprost (Xalatan) are generally the drugs of choice for treating chronic glaucoma because they can be administered daily and have a low adverse effect rate. These drugs increase aqueous outflow. Although they have fewer systemic effects, these drugs may cause conjunctival hyperemia and permanent changes in the color of the iris and eyebrows.

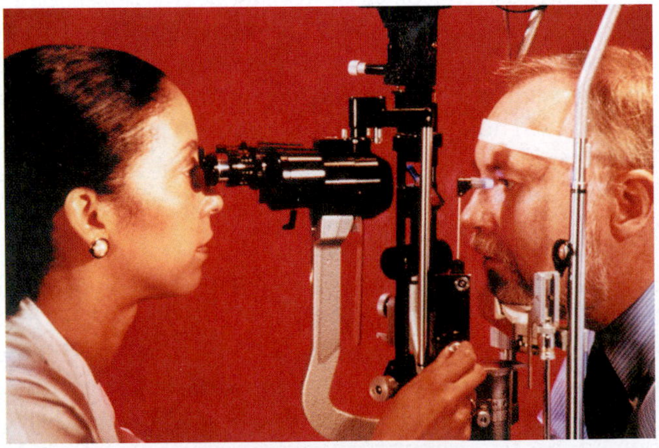

Figure 46.13 ■ An eye professional uses a tonometer to indirectly measure the intraocular pressure of a patient's eye.

Topical beta-adrenergic blocking agents decrease the production of aqueous humor in the ciliary body. Beta-adrenergic blockers can be used once or twice a day, depending on the drug and dosage form. When administering beta-blockers or teaching about their use, it is important to remember that ophthalmic preparations can produce systemic effects, including bronchospasm, bradycardia, and heart failure.

The adrenergic agonist brimonidine may be prescribed along with a beta-blocker or if beta-blockers are contraindicated (e.g., in a patient with heart failure, asthma, or chronic obstructive pulmonary disease [COPD]). Another adrenergic agonist, apraclonidine, may be prescribed when other drugs do not sufficiently reduce intraocular pressure, but adverse effects make it inappropriate for long-term use (Adams, Holland, & Urban, 2017).

Dorzolamide (Trusopt), a carbonic anhydrase inhibitor, decreases the production of aqueous humor and reduces intraocular pressure. It is used with other drugs to control pressures and in patients for whom beta-blockers are contraindicated because of heart failure or reactive airway disease (asthma). Acetazolamide (Diamox), a systemic carbonic anhydrase inhibitor, also may be used for some patients.

Nursing implications for the medications used to control chronic glaucoma are outlined in **Medication Administration 46.A.**

In acute angle-closure glaucoma, diuretics may be administered intravenously to achieve a rapid decrease in intraocular pressure prior to surgical intervention. Both the carbonic anhydrase inhibitor acetazolamide and osmotic diuretics, such as mannitol, are used. Fast-acting miotic drops, such as pilocarpine, are also administered to constrict the pupil and draw the iris away from the angle and from the scleral venous sinus. Prostaglandin analogs, beta-blockers, and adrenergic agents may also be given by topical application.

Surgery

Surgical intervention is indicated for patients with acute angle-closure glaucoma and for patients with chronic open-angle glaucoma that is not effectively controlled by medication.

Surgical management of chronic open-angle glaucoma involves improving the drainage of aqueous humor from the anterior chamber of the eye. Trabeculoplasty and trabeculectomy filtration surgery are the most commonly used procedures.

In a *laser trabeculoplasty*, an argon laser is aimed through a gonioscope to create multiple laser burns spaced evenly around the trabecular meshwork. As the burns heal, the scars they create cause tension, stretching and opening the meshwork. This noninvasive technique is the treatment of choice because it requires no incision and can be performed as an outpatient procedure.

Trabeculectomy is a type of filtration surgery in which a permanent fistula is created to drain aqueous humor from the anterior chamber of the eye. A portion of trabecular meshwork

Medication Administration 46.A

The Patient with Glaucoma

Adrenergic Agonists (Mydriatics)

apraclonidine

brimonidine (Alphagan)

Adrenergic agonists dilate the pupil, reduce the production of aqueous humor, and increase its absorption, effectively reducing intraocular pressure in open-angle glaucoma.

Nursing Responsibilities

- Assess for contraindications and adverse reactions to adrenergic agonists, including acute angle-closure glaucoma, hypertension, cardiac dysrhythmias, and coronary heart disease.
- Assess for central nervous system side effects of anxiety, nervousness, and muscle tremors. If these side effects are severe, notify the healthcare provider.
- Assess for a hypersensitivity reaction, including itching, lid edema, and discharge from the eyes. Notify the healthcare provider if you notice these signs.

Health Education for the Patient and Family

- Report any change in visual acuity or eye pain. (Eye pain may indicate an attack of angle-closure glaucoma and must be reported to the healthcare provider immediately.)
- Avoid over-the-counter (OTC) sinus and cold medications containing pseudoephedrine and phenylephrine. They may accentuate the side effects of this drug.

Beta-Adrenergic Blockers

betaxolol (Betoptic)

carteolol (Cartrol, Ocupress)

levobunolol (Betagan)

metipranolol (OptiPranolol)

timolol (Timoptic)

Selected beta-adrenergic blockers reduce intraocular pressure by decreasing the production of aqueous humor. Because beta-blockers do not affect pupil size and lens accommodation, they do not have the adverse effects on visual acuity that adrenergic agonists do. Their systemic effects, however, may limit their usefulness for certain patients.

Nursing Responsibilities

- Assess for allergies or contraindications to beta-blocker therapy, including asthma, COPD, heart block, and heart failure.
- Maintain pressure over the lacrimal sac after administration to prevent systemic absorption.
- Assess for side effects such as bradycardia, hypotension, and depression.

Health Education for the Patient and Family

- After instilling the eyedrops, put pressure on the lacrimal sac, at the corner of the eye near the bridge of the nose, to keep the drug from entering your system.
- Your vision may be blurred during the initial period of therapy, but it will improve as you continue to use the drug.
- Report adverse effects, including worsening vision, difficulty breathing, reduced exercise tolerance, and sweating or flushing, to the healthcare provider.

Carbonic Anhydrase Inhibitors

acetazolamide (Diamox)

brinzolamide (Azopt)

dorzolamide (Trusopt)

The carbonic anhydrase inhibitors lower intraocular pressure and are used primarily as adjunctive therapy. Dorzolamide and brinzolamide are administered as eyedrops, whereas acetazolamide may be given PO, IM, or IV.

Nursing Responsibilities

- Assess for allergies or other contraindications to the use of carbonic anhydrase inhibitors, including known allergy to sulfa or severe renal or hepatic disease.
- Monitor for increased drug interactions of amphetamines, procainamide, quinidine, tricyclic antidepressants, and ephedrine and pseudoephedrine.
- Assess daily weight, intake and output, serum electrolytes, and vital signs in patients taking oral or parenteral carbonic anhydrase inhibitors.
- Administer PO in the morning to prevent sleep disruption because of the diuretic effect.
- If used with another topical ophthalmic, administer 10 minutes apart.

Health Education for the Patient and Family

- For oral medications, maintain a fluid intake of 2 to 3 L/day and rise slowly from lying or sitting positions because you may feel dizzy when you first stand (orthostatic hypotension).
- For topical medications, notify the healthcare provider if you have prolonged eye irritation.

Prostaglandin Analogs

bimatoprost (Lumigan)

latanoprost (Xalatan)

travoprost (Travatan)

The prostaglandin analog drugs relax the ciliary muscle, improving the outflow of aqueous humor and reducing intraocular pressure. These drugs have the advantage of requiring only a single daily dose. They do, however, have some adverse effects such as blurred vision and stinging and, when used long term, cause permanent darkening of the iris of the eye and eyebrows, increased growth of eyelashes, and conjunctival hyperemia (redness).

Nursing Responsibilities

- Assess and note eye color and presence of inflammation, exudates, or pain.
- Note vital signs and most recent liver function test results because these may be altered by the drug.

Health Education for the Patient and Family

- Use once daily at bedtime as directed. This drug may blur vision; use at bedtime minimizes associated safety risks.
- Remove contact lenses before administering this drug.
- Minor eye discomfort, including burning and tearing, may occur with this drug. Notify your healthcare provider if adverse effects are severe or intolerable.
- This drug may cause darkening of your iris, the skin around the eyes, and the eyebrows, as well as increased growth of the eyelashes. These color changes are permanent but will not progress if the drug is discontinued by your doctor.

Note: Drugs identified in blue are among the 200 most commonly prescribed medications in the United States.

Source: Data from Adams et al., 2017.

is removed, and a flap of sclera is left unsutured to create a channel or fistula between the anterior chamber and the subconjunctival space. Aqueous humor is able to drain into the space under the conjunctiva, where it can be absorbed into the systemic circulation. A trabeculectomy is usually performed under general anesthesia and requires hospitalization.

If these procedures are not fully effective, either photocoagulation using an argon laser (heat) or cyclocryotherapy using a probe to freeze tissue may be employed to destroy portions of the ciliary body. This tissue destruction reduces the production of aqueous humor, subsequently reducing intraocular pressure. Another surgical procedure involves insertion of a glaucoma drainage device that regulates the outflow of aqueous humor.

Surgical procedures used in the treatment of acute angle-closure glaucoma include gonioplasty, laser iridotomy, and peripheral iridectomy. Because of the high risk for a future attack of angle-closure glaucoma in the unaffected eye, these procedures are often performed prophylactically.

In *gonioplasty*, the healing and scarring of microscopic lesions created at the periphery of the iris draw the iris away from the cornea, widening the anterior chamber. This widening of the chamber increases the angle and opens drainage channels for aqueous humor.

Laser iridotomy is a noninvasive procedure using a laser to create multiple small perforations in the iris of the eye. These perforations allow aqueous humor to drain from the posterior chamber to the anterior chamber and out through the trabecular meshwork and the scleral venous sinus. During an *iridectomy*, a small segment of the iris is removed to facilitate the flow of aqueous humor between the posterior and anterior chambers and to open the anterior chamber angle.

Nursing Care

When planning and providing nursing care for the patient with glaucoma, both the specific form of the disease and its actual or potential effects on the patient's vision, lifestyle, safety, and psychosocial well-being must be considered. In the hospitalized patient, glaucoma is typically a concurrent diagnosis rather than the primary reason for seeking care, unless the diagnosis is acute angle-closure glaucoma. For additional nursing activities for the patient with glaucoma, see the accompanying Case Study & Nursing Care Plan.

Assessment

Collect the following data through a health history and physical examination.

- ***Health history:*** Family history; presence of altered vision, halos, and excessive tearing; sudden, severe eye pain; use of corrective lenses; most recent eye examination
- ***Physical assessment:*** Distant and near vision, peripheral fields, retina for optic nerve cupping.

Priorities of Nursing Care

Teaching for effective management of this chronic disease and preventing vision loss is the nursing care priority for the patient newly diagnosed with glaucoma. When vision loss has occurred, the visual deficit and reducing the risk for injury are priority nursing care focuses.

Diagnoses, Interventions, and Outcomes

Nursing care planning focuses on problems associated with the temporary or permanent visual impairment, the resultant increased risk for injury, and the psychosocial problems of anxiety and coping.

Provide Orientation to Environment. Whether glaucoma, and its resulting impaired vision, is the patient's primary problem or a preexisting condition in a patient with another disorder, it must be a primary consideration in nursing care planning.

Expected Outcome: Patient will adapt to functioning in healthcare environment without experiencing injury or adverse effects related to impaired vision.

The nurse will:

- Address by name and identify yourself with each interaction. Orient to time, place, person, and situation as indicated. State the purpose of your visit. *The patient with impaired vision must rely on input from the other senses. A lack of visual cues increases the importance of verbal ones. For example, the patient with impaired vision cannot see the nurse checking an intravenous infusion and needs a verbal explanation of who is in the room and why. When the patient's normal daily routine is disrupted by illness or hospitalization, additional sensory input such as a radio, television, and explanations of the routine and activities are useful to maintain the patient's orientation.*
- Provide any visual aids that are routinely used. Keep them close, making sure that the patient knows where they are and can reach them easily. *Easy access encourages the patient to use these items and enhances the ability to provide self-care.*
- Orient to the environment. Explain the location of the call bell, personal items, and the furniture in the room. *Patients with visual impairments are usually very capable of providing self-care in a known environment.*
- Provide other tools or items that can help compensate for diminished vision:
  a. Bright, nonglare lighting
  b. Books, magazines, and instructions in large print
  c. Audio books
  d. Telephones with oversize pushbuttons
  e. A clock with numbers and hands that can be felt.
- Assist with meals by doing the following:
  a. Reading menu selections and marking choices
  b. Describing the position of foods on a meal tray according to the clock system
  c. Placing the utensils in a readily accessible position
  d. Removing lids from containers, buttering bread, and cutting meat, as needed
  e. If the visual impairment is new or temporary, the patient may need continued assistance during the meal.

Providing assistance during eating is important to maintain the patient's nutritional status. The patient may be ashamed of needing help or embarrassed to request it and may respond by not eating or by claiming not to be hungry.

- Assist with mobility and ambulation as needed:
  a. Have the patient hold your arm or elbow, and walk slightly ahead as a guide. Do not hold the patient's arm or elbow.
  b. Describe the surroundings and progress as you proceed. Warn in advance of potential hazards, turns, and steps.
  c. Teach to feel the chair, bed, or commode with the hands and the back of the legs before sitting.

These measures help ensure the patient's safety while providing for mobility and helping prevent complications associated with immobility.

- If the vision loss is unilateral and recent, provide instructions related to unilateral vision loss and change in depth perception:
  a. Caution about the loss of depth perception and teach safety precautions, such as reaching slowly for objects and using visual cues as to distance, especially when driving.
  b. Teach to scan, turning the head fully toward the affected side to identify potential hazards and looking up and down to compensate for the loss of depth perception.

The patient with a unilateral vision loss is often unaware of its effect on peripheral vision and depth perception.

Reduce Risk for Injury. Whether the patient is experiencing a sudden loss of vision due to acute angle-closure glaucoma or significant visual impairment due to inadequately managed chronic glaucoma, both are at an increased risk for injury. Patients who have had surgical interventions for glaucoma are at even greater risk.

Expected Outcome: Patient will remain free of injury while in healthcare environment.

The nurse will:

- Assess ability to perform ADLs. *Patients may be reluctant to request assistance, believing that they should be able to perform these familiar tasks. Careful assessment and provision of needed assistance help prevent injury and maintain the patient's self-esteem.*
- Notify all personnel to avoid changing the arrangement of the patient's room. *The patient with impaired vision is at high risk for falling when in an unfamiliar environment. It is important to maintain a safe, familiar room when the patient is hospitalized.*
- Discuss possible adaptations in the home to help the patient remain as independent as possible and prevent falls or other injuries. *Often minor changes in the home environment, such as removing scatter rugs and small items of furniture, allow the patient to navigate safely in this already familiar environment.*

SAFETY ALERT: Keep traffic areas free of clutter to reduce the risk for injury in patients with impaired vision. ■

Reduce Anxiety. The actual or potential loss of sight threatens the patient's self-concept, role functioning, patterns of interaction, and, potentially, environment. The patient with impaired vision who functions well in a familiar environment will feel anxious in the unfamiliar setting of a hospital or care facility.

Expected Outcome: Patient will report and demonstrate reduced levels of anxiety.

The nurse will:

- Assess for verbal and nonverbal indications of level of anxiety and for normal coping mechanisms. Repeated expressions of concern or denial that the vision change will affect the patient's life indicate anxiety. Nonverbal indicators include tension, difficulty concentrating or thinking, restlessness, poor eye contact, and changes in vocalization (rapid speech, voice quivering). Physical indicators include tachycardia, dilated pupils, cool and clammy skin, and tremors. *The patient may not recognize this feeling as anxiety. Identifying and acknowledging the anxiety state can help the patient recognize and deal with it.*
- Encourage to verbalize fears, anger, and feelings of anxiety. *Verbalizing helps externalize the anxiety and allows fears to be addressed.*
- Discuss perception of the eye condition and its effects on lifestyle and roles. *Discussion provides an opportunity to correct misperceptions and introduce alternative activities and assistive devices for patients with visual impairments.*
- Introduce yourself when entering the room, explain all procedures fully before and as they are being performed, and use touch to convey proximity and caring. *The patient with impaired vision must rely on the other senses to make up for the loss of sight. Because the patient cannot see what you are doing, complete explanations of even simple tasks such as refilling a water glass help to relieve anxiety.*
- Identify coping strategies that have been useful in the past and adapt these strategies to the present situation. *Previously successful coping strategies may be employed to increase the patient's sense of control.*

Delegating Nursing Care Activities

For the visually impaired patient, the unlicensed assistive personnel may help set up meal trays using the clock description (i.e., the drink is at 10 o'clock, the meat is on the plate from 2 o'clock to 6 o'clock, etc.), assist with bathing by setting up bath supplies per patient wishes, and assist with ambulation if the patient requires assistance.

Transitions of Care

Although glaucoma cannot be prevented, its severity and potentially deleterious permanent effects can be limited with early visual screening. The nurse assumes an important role in educating the public about risk factors for glaucoma such as increased age and the higher incidence in African Americans and Asians. All people over the age of 40 are encouraged to receive an eye examination every 2 to 4 years, including tonometry screening. Those with a predominant family history should be evaluated more frequently, every 1 to 2 years. After the age of 65, yearly ophthalmologic examinations are recommended.

Patients with glaucoma require teaching about lifetime strategies for managing the disease at home. Poor adherence to prescribed therapy is a significant problem in many patients with chronic glaucoma (Glaucoma Research Foundation, 2017). They need to understand the importance of lifelong therapy to control the disease and prevent blindness. If a permanent visual impairment has resulted, the patient needs information on achieving the maximum possible independence while maintaining safety. The following topics should be discussed with the patient and family:

- Prescribed medications, including proper storage and how to instill eyedrops
- Importance of not taking certain prescription and OTC medications without consulting a physician
- The need for periodic eye examinations with intraocular pressure measurement
- Risks, warning signs, and management of acute angle-closure glaucoma
- Possible surgical options
- Community resources, such as Visually Impaired Society, local library, and transportation services
- Helpful resources: National Glaucoma Foundation, Young and Under Pressure Glaucoma Foundation, Glaucoma Research Foundation, and Prevention of Blindness Society.

The Patient with Age-Related Macular Degeneration

Age-related macular degeneration (AMD) is a leading cause of legal blindness and impaired vision in older adults (National Eye Institute, 2017a). Age-related macular degeneration rarely affects people under the age of 50 and the incidence and prevalence increase rapidly with age (National Eye Institute, 2017a).

Pathophysiology

The macula is the area of the retina that provides sharp central vision, receiving light from the center of the visual field. Two forms of age-related macular degeneration are identified, a nonexudative (dry) form and an exudative (wet) form. Although both are progressive disorders, their manifestations and management differ (Sorenson et al., 2019).

Nonexudative, or dry, *macular degeneration* is the more common form of AMD. It is a gradual process that begins with accumulation of deposits called *drusen* beneath the pigment epithelium of the retina. Over time, these deposits enlarge and become more numerous. The pigment epithelium detaches in small areas and becomes atrophic, interfering with sensory function of the macula. Vision loss is typically not significant, and the disorder progresses slowly. There is, however, a risk that the disorder will progress to an exudative stage of the disease.

Exudative macular degeneration is characterized by the formation of new, weak blood vessels in the potential space between the choroid (vascular layer of the eye) and the retina (neurosensory layer). These new vessels are prone to leak, elevating the retina from the choroid and distorting vision. Although exudative macular degeneration is typically a gradual process, bleeding can lead to acute vision loss in some cases. With significant or repeated bleeding episodes, scar tissue forms, and central vision is permanently lost (National Eye Institute, 2017a).

Risk Factors

Although the exact cause of AMD is unknown, factors associated with it include aging, smoking, race, and genetic factors. Caucasian Americans have a significantly higher risk of developing AMD than all people of other racial backgrounds or ethnicities. Recent evidence suggests that inflammation plays a role in the development of AMD, as does the interaction of certain genes with the immune system (National Eye Institute, 2017a). Evidence suggests that the risk for developing AMD may be reduced by consumption of omega-3 fatty acids in fish and vegetables high in lutein and zeaxanthin (carotenoids found in vegetables such as spinach, kale, and broccoli).

Manifestations

When the macula is damaged, central vision becomes blurred and distorted, but peripheral vision remains intact. Distortion of vision in one eye is a common initial manifestation; straight lines appear wavy or distorted. With the loss of central vision, activities that require close central vision, such as reading and sewing, are particularly affected (**Figure 46.14** ■).

Interprofessional Care

Diagnosis

AMD is diagnosed through vision and retinal examination. The Amsler grid (**Figure 46.15** ■) can be used to identify

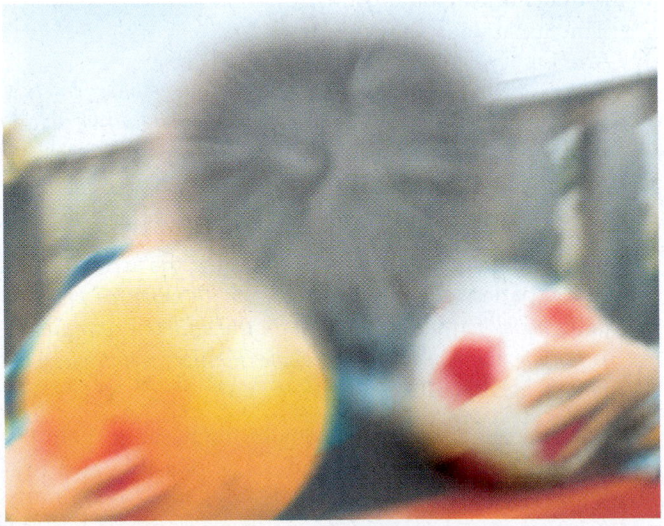

Figure 46.14 ■ Loss of central vision with advanced age-related macular degeneration.

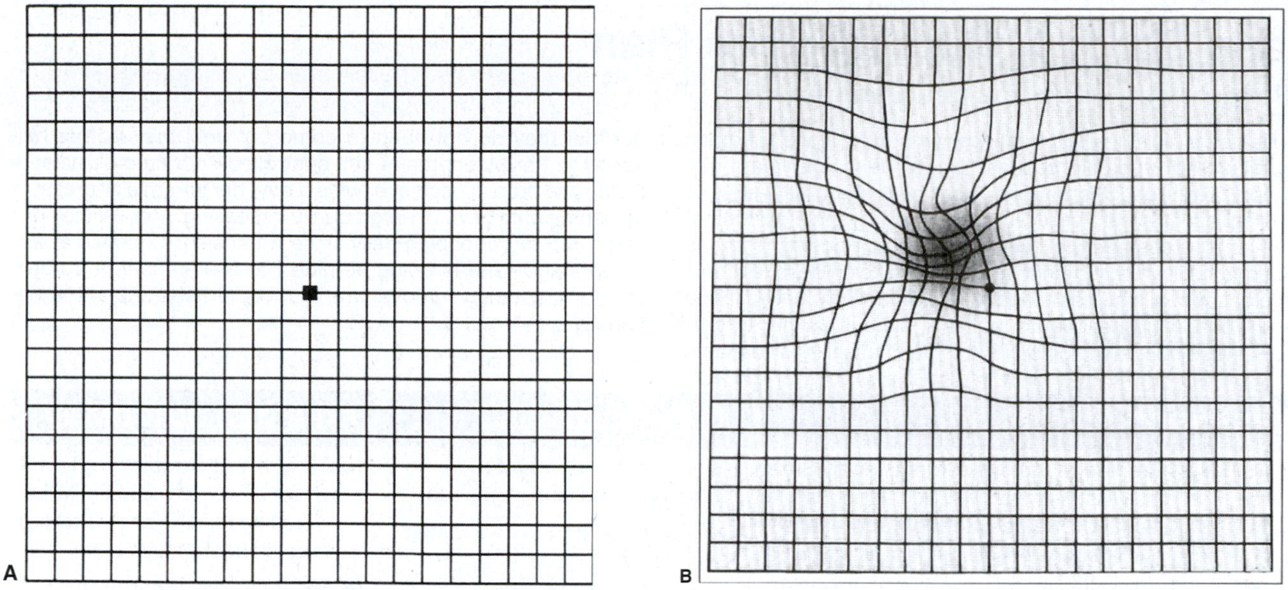
A
B

Figure 46.15 ■ **A**, Amsler grid. **B**, Amsler grid as it might appear to someone with age-related macular degeneration.

distortion of central vision caused by AMD. If treatment for wet AMD is planned, a *fluorescein angiogram* may be done. Pictures are taken as the dye passes through the blood vessels of the retina, allowing detection of leaks.

Medications

Two drugs that inhibit the growth of new blood vessels, bevacizumab (Avastin) and ranibizumab (Lucentis), have been shown to improve vision and prevent vision loss in patients with advanced AMD. The drug may be administered monthly or on an as-needed basis (National Eye Institute, 2017a).

Nutrition

In its early or intermediate stages, the progress of dry AMD can be slowed through the use of vitamins C and E, beta-carotene (vitamin A), and zinc (National Eye Institute, 2017a).

Treatment

Wet AMD may also be treated with laser surgery or photodynamic therapy. Although these treatments do not cure the disease, they may slow the rate of vision loss. In laser surgery, fragile blood vessels are destroyed, preventing bleeding. There is a risk, however, of damage to surrounding healthy tissue, some vision loss, and continued growth of new vessels. In photodynamic therapy, verteporfin, a drug that tends to adhere to the surface of new blood vessels, is injected systemically. Light is then shined into the affected eye, activating the drug and destroying new blood vessels. This treatment is relatively fast and painless, but does require avoidance of exposure to direct sunlight or bright indoor light for 5 days following treatment (National Eye Institute, 2017a).

Nursing Care

Nurses should be alert for patients demonstrating new and rapid-onset manifestations of macular degeneration and promptly refer these patients for ophthalmologic evaluation. Early intervention may preserve a greater degree of vision and slow the progress of the disease. For patients with slowly progressive manifestations, the nursing focus is on helping the patient and family members adapt to the gradual decline in vision by recommending visual aids and other coping strategies. Large-print books and magazines, the use of a magnifying glass, and high-intensity lighting can help the patient to cope with the reduced vision of macular degeneration. Patient education materials should be in a large-print format.

The Patient with Diabetic Retinopathy

Diabetic retinopathy is a vascular disorder affecting the capillaries of the retina. The capillaries become sclerotic and lose their ability to transport sufficient oxygen and nutrients to the retina. In the United States, more than 4.1 million people have diabetic retinopathy, and it is the leading cause of new blindness in people ages 20 to 74 (National Eye Institute, 2017d). Hispanic individuals are disproportionately affected by diabetic retinopathy (8% of adults), whereas approximately 5.1% of White adults and 5.4% of Black adults in the United States have diabetic retinopathy (National Eye Institute, 2017e).

Pathophysiology

Diabetic retinopathy has two stages: *Nonproliferative* or background retinopathy and *proliferative* retinopathy (Sorenson et al., 2019). Nonproliferative retinopathy is typically the initial form seen, usually about 10 years after diabetes is diagnosed. The venous capillaries of the eye dilate and develop microaneurysms that may then leak, causing retinal edema, or they may rupture, causing small hemorrhages into the retina. On ophthalmoscopic examination, yellow exudates, cotton-wool patches indicative of

Case Study & Nursing Care Plan

A Patient with Glaucoma and Cataracts

Lila Rainey is an 80-year-old widow who lives alone. She has worn glasses for nearsightedness since she was a young girl, and now wears bifocals to correct her near vision as well. She was diagnosed 4 years ago with chronic open-angle glaucoma, for which she uses timolol (Timoptic) 0.5%. Recently she has noticed difficulty reading and watching television despite a new lens prescription. She has stopped driving at night because the glare of oncoming headlights makes it difficult for her to see. Mrs. Rainey's ophthalmologist has told her that she has cataracts but that they do not need to come out until they bother her. Although her glaucoma is still controlled with timolol maleate 0.5%, one drop in each eye twice a day, her intraocular pressure measurements have been gradually increasing. Mrs. Rainey has taken 325 mg of aspirin daily since a transient ischemic attack 8 years ago. She is being admitted to the outpatient surgery unit for a cataract removal and intraocular lens implant in her right eye.

ASSESSMENT

Mrs. Rainey is admitted to the eye surgery unit by Susan Schafer, RN. In her assessment, Ms. Schafer finds Mrs. Rainey to be alert and oriented, though apprehensive about her upcoming surgery. Assessment findings include BP 134/72 mmHg, P 86 bpm, R 18/min. Mrs. Rainey's physical assessment is essentially normal. Her pupils are round and equal and react briskly to light and accommodation. Her conjunctivae are pink; sclera and corneas are clear. Using the ophthalmoscope, Ms. Schafer notes that the red reflex in Mrs. Rainey's right eye is diminished. Ophthalmic examination shows visual acuity of 20/150 OD (right eye) and 20/50 OS (left eye) with corrective lenses. Ms. Schafer reviews the operative procedure with Mrs. Rainey, answering her questions and telling her what to expect after surgery. Following preoperative protocols, Mrs. Rainey is prepared and transported to surgery.

DIAGNOSES

- Impaired vision related to myopia and lens extraction
- Anxiety related to anticipated surgery
- Decreased knowledge related to postoperative care

EXPECTED OUTCOMES

- Patient will regain sufficient visual acuity to maintain ADLs, including reading and watching television for enjoyment.
- Patient will demonstrate a reduced level of anxiety.
- Patient will demonstrate the procedure for instilling eyedrops postoperatively.
- Patient will demonstrate knowledge of the home care she will require after surgery, signs of complications, and actions to take if complications occur.

PLANNING AND IMPLEMENTATION

- Provide a safe environment, placing the call light and personal care items within easy reach.
- Encourage Mrs. Rainey to express her fears about surgery and its potential effect on vision.
- Explain all procedures related to surgery and recovery.
- Instruct her to avoid rubbing the eye, shutting the eyelids tightly, lifting, or straining to have a bowel movement. Teach her to wear glasses during the day and an eye shield at night to prevent injury to the surgical site.
- Provide verbal and written instructions about postoperative care, including a schedule of follow-up examinations, potential complications, and actions to take in response.

EVALUATION

Mrs. Rainey is discharged the morning after her surgery. She is visibly relieved when the eye patch is removed because her vision in the operated eye is better than before surgery, even without her glasses. She is able to relate the recommended activity restrictions. Mrs. Rainey administers her own eyedrops before discharge and relates an understanding of the prescribed postoperative care and safety precautions. Mrs. Rainey's daughter plans to visit her mother two to three times a week until Mrs. Rainey is able to resume all her previous activities. Mrs. Rainey says that she won't "be so scared when I need my other eye done." She understands the chronic nature of her glaucoma and says that her vision is too important for her to neglect her timolol drops and routine eye exams.

CLINICAL REASONING IN PATIENT CARE

1. Why did it become more difficult to control Mrs. Rainey's intraocular pressure as her cataract matured?
2. Identify medications that are commonly prescribed following cataract surgery. What are the risks of interactions between these medications and Mrs. Rainey's timolol drops?
3. Develop a care plan for decreased knowledge related to self-care and activities of daily living.

See Evaluating Your Response in Appendix B.

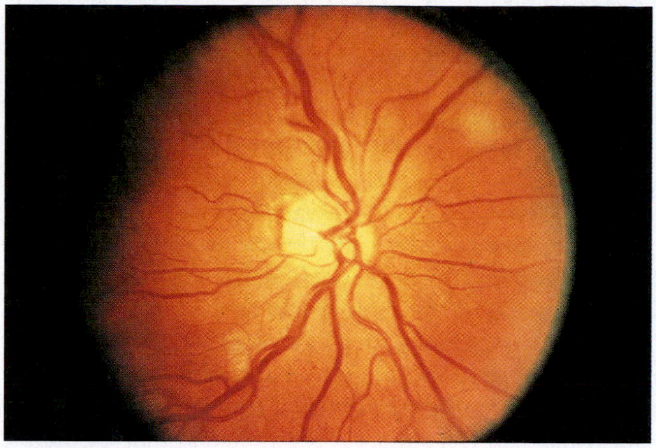

Figure 46.16 ■ Appearance of the ocular fundus in diabetic retinopathy.

retinal ischemia, and red-dot hemorrhages are observed (**Figure 46.16** ■). When the peripheral retina is involved, the patient may experience few symptoms other than light glare. Edema of the macula or a large hemorrhage may cause vision loss.

Diabetic retinopathy may progress to the proliferative form. This disease is marked by large areas of retinal ischemia and the formation of new blood vessels (neovascularization) spreading over the inner surface of the retina and into the vitreous body. These vessels are fine and fragile, making them permeable and easily ruptured. Blood and blood protein leakage contribute to retinal edema, and hemorrhage into the vitreous body may occur. The vessels gradually become fibrous and firmly attached to the vitreous body, increasing the risk of retinal detachment.

Risk Factors

The risk of developing diabetic retinopathy is related to the duration of the diabetes and the degree of glycemic control. Hypertension is also a risk factor (National Eye Institute, 2017d). Retinopathy is seen in both type 1 and type 2 diabetes. Nursing care of the patient with diabetes is discussed in Chapter 20.

Interprofessional Care

Diagnosis

Patients with diabetes should be examined yearly by an ophthalmologist. The development of any new visual manifestations is an additional indication for prompt ophthalmologic examination and possibly retinal angiography.

Treatment

Laser photocoagulation is used to treat both the nonproliferative and proliferative forms of diabetic retinopathy. Leaking microaneurysms are sealed and proliferating vessels destroyed, reducing the risk of hemorrhage, retinal edema, and retinal detachment. This treatment also slows the progress of aneurysms and new vessel formation; however, it does not cure the disorder. Injections of the drug ranibizumab (Lucentis) into the eye in combination with laser treatment improve outcomes for patients with diabetic macular edema (fluid accumulation on the retina) (National Eye Institute, 2017d).

Nursing Care

Diagnoses, Interventions, and Outcomes

As with many other eye disorders, the nursing care focus for diabetic retinopathy is primarily educational. The patient who is newly diagnosed with diabetes needs to understand the importance of regular eye examinations beginning approximately 5 years after the onset of type 1 diabetes and at the time of diagnosis of type 2 diabetes. Changes of diabetic retinopathy may already be present when type 2 diabetes is diagnosed.

Delegating Nursing Care Activities

As appropriate and allowed by the designated duties and responsibilities of unlicensed assistive personnel, the nurse may delegate nursing care activities such as measuring vital signs, encouraging oral or enteral fluid intake, and providing skin care. For the visually impaired patient, the unlicensed assistive personnel may help set up meal trays using the clock description, assist with bathing by setting up bath supplies per patient wishes, and assist with ambulation if the patient requires assistance.

Transitions of Care

Strict control of blood glucose levels and blood pressure are important preventative measures and may slow the progression of retinopathy as well. Although conclusive research is lacking, patients with advanced diabetic retinopathy may be advised to avoid physical activity associated with the Valsalva maneuver (e.g., weight training).

Teach the patient to report promptly any new visual manifestation, including blurred vision; black spots (floaters), cobwebs, or flashing lights in the visual field; or a sudden loss of vision in one or both eyes. Emphasize to the patient that careful blood glucose control may help prevent diabetic retinopathy from developing; it may also slow its progress. The patient's blood pressure should also be maintained within normal limits to prevent further damage to retinal vessels. Although diabetic retinopathy cannot be halted or cured, its progress can be slowed with aggressive management. Much of the burden for this management falls on the patient, increasing the importance of good teaching.

The Patient with a Retinal Detachment

The retina contains the photoreceptors of the eye, which allow the perception of light and initial processing of images and stimuli for transmission to the optic center of the brain. Disruption of this neural layer of the eye by trauma or disease interferes with light perception and image transmission, potentially resulting in blindness.

Both primary eye conditions and systemic diseases can affect the retina and interfere with vision. Retinal tears or detachments can occur either spontaneously or as a result of trauma.

Pathophysiology

Separation of the retina or sensory portion of the eye from the choroid, the pigmented vascular layer, is known as a *retinal detachment*. Although retinal detachment may be precipitated by trauma, it usually occurs spontaneously. The vitreous humor normally adheres to the retina at the optic disc, the macula, and the periphery of the eye.

The retina may actually tear and fold back on itself or it may remain intact but no longer adhere to the choroid. A break or tear in the retina allows fluid from the vitreous cavity to enter the defect. This, along with fluid that escapes from choroid vessels, the pull of gravity, and traction exerted by the vitreous humor, separates the retina from the choroid. The detached area may rapidly increase in size, increasing loss of vision. Unless contact between the retina and choroid is reestablished, the neurons of the retina become ischemic and die, causing permanent vision loss. For this reason, retinal detachment is a true medical emergency, requiring prompt ophthalmologic referral and treatment.

Risk Factors

With aging, the vitreous humor shrinks and may pull the retina away from the choroid. Aging therefore is a common risk factor, as are myopia and aphakia, absence of the lens (e.g., following lens removal for cataracts).

Manifestations

When the retina detaches, the patient may experience floaters, or irregular dark lines or spots, as well as flashes of light in the visual field. Often the patient describes the sensation of having a curtain or veil drawn across the visual field from the top, side, or bottom, much like a curtain being drawn over a window. The area of the visual field affected is directly related to the area of detachment. For example, because light rays cross as they pass through the lens, a retinal tear in the superior portion of the eye results in a deficit in the lower part of the visual field. The patient feels no pain, and the eye appears normal to visual inspection. Other common manifestations of retinal detachment include blurred vision and progressive deterioration of vision. If the macula is involved, there is a loss of central vision.

Interprofessional Care

Diagnosis

Retinal detachment is a medical emergency; prompt treatment is necessary to preserve vision. The manifestations and examination of the ocular fundus by ophthalmoscopy establish the diagnosis of retinal detachment. Early diagnosis and intervention are vital. If the condition is left untreated, the detached portion will become necrotic because of lost contact with the vascular supply of the choroid. The result is permanent blindness in that portion of the eye. If an ophthalmologist is not readily available, the patient's head is positioned so that gravity pulls the detached portion of the retina into closer contact with the choroid.

Treatment

Interventions are directed toward bringing the retina and choroid back into contact and reestablishing the blood and nutrient supply to the retina. Either cryotherapy, using a supercooled probe, or laser photocoagulation may be used to seal retinal holes and to create an area of inflammation and adhesion to "weld" the layers together.

A surgical procedure called *scleral buckling* may also be used. In this procedure, an indentation or fold is created in the sclera, bringing the choroid into contact with the retina. Contact is maintained with a local implant on the sclera or an encircling strap or "buckle." An inert gas may also be injected into the vitreous cavity, a procedure called *pneumatic retinopexy*. The patient is positioned so that the bubble pushes the detached portion of the retina into contact with the choroid. Silicone oil may also be injected into the eye to reestablish contact between the retina and choroid.

With a retinal tear, it may be necessary to use surgical instruments to manipulate the detached section of retina into place. Air or a liquid is then injected into the vitreous to maintain retinal contact with the choroid or laser therapy is used to create a bond.

Nursing Care

The nursing focus for the patient with a detached retina is on early identification and treatment. Retinal detachment can be successfully treated on an outpatient basis, often in an ophthalmologist's office. For these patients, the nursing focus is on education.

Priorities of Care

Because early intervention is vital to preserve the patient's sight, nurses must recognize early manifestations of retinal detachment and intervene appropriately to obtain definitive treatment for the patient.

Diagnoses, Interventions, and Outcomes

Promote Effective Retinal Tissue Perfusion. Restoring contact between the retina and choroid is a priority of nursing and medical care for the patient with retinal detachment. Vitreous humor may leak through a retinal tear and fluid exudate may collect behind the tear, causing further detachment. If the macula is detached, central vision is lost, and the prognosis for full vision restoration is poorer.

Expected Outcome: Patient's visual acuity and field will be restored to previous level.

The nurse will:

- Assess for other manifestations of eye disease. *Retinal detachment is painless and has no outward manifestations. The patient with a red eye or cloudy cornea may be experiencing acute angle-closure glaucoma rather than retinal detachment.*
- Notify physician and the ophthalmologist immediately. *Immediate medical intervention is required in patients with retinal detachment to preserve vision.*
- Position so the area of detachment is inferior. For instance, for a superior temporal retinal detachment of the right eye (with corresponding vision loss in the

inferior medial visual field of that eye), place supine with the head turned to the right. *Correct positioning allows the contents of the posterior portion of the eye to place pressure on the detached area, bringing the retina in closer contact with the choroid.*

SAFETY ALERT: Carefully assess anyone who complains of a sudden rapid loss of vision because this often signals a medical emergency. ■

Reduce Anxiety. Retinal detachment causes a rapid decline in vision in the affected eye, often occurring spontaneously and without pain. Unless previous episodes have occurred, the patient usually does not know what is causing the problem. Anxiety and fear of complete vision loss are common, expected reactions.

Expected Outcome: Patient will report and demonstrate reduced levels of anxiety.

The nurse will:

- Maintain a calm, confident attitude while carrying out priority interventions. *Administering care in a calm although urgent manner helps reassure the patient that the problem is treatable and that appropriate measures are being taken.*
- Reassure that most retinal detachments are successfully treated, usually on an outpatient basis. *Reassurance can help allay the patient's fear of permanent vision loss.*
- For spontaneous detachments, assure the patient that he or she did not cause the detachment to occur. *The patient may believe that the detachment is related to a specific activity and feel guilty for somehow causing this loss of vision.*
- Explain all procedures fully, including the reason for positioning. *Explanations facilitate understanding and help relieve anxiety in unfamiliar settings.*
- Allow supportive family members or friends to remain with the patient as much as possible. *Additional support helps lower the patient's anxiety level.*

Transitions of Care

Teaching for the patient undergoing treatment for retinal detachment is similar to that for patients experiencing other types of eye surgery (see Box 46.4). If the retina remains detached, provide instructions about the change in peripheral vision or other visual fields and changes in depth perception.

Discuss the following topics with the patient and family to prepare for home care:

- Limitations on positioning the head before or following repair
- Activity restrictions such as no bending or straining at stool
- Use of eye shield
- Early manifestations and the importance of seeking immediate treatment
- Follow-up treatment with the ophthalmologist.

The Patient with Retinitis Pigmentosa

Retinitis pigmentosa is a hereditary degenerative disease characterized by retinal atrophy and loss of retinal function progressing from the periphery to the central region of the retina. It is inherited as an autosomal dominant, autosomal recessive, or X-linked trait and may be associated with other genetic defects.

In retinitis pigmentosa, the genetic defect appears to cause production of an unstable form of rhodopsin, the receptor protein of rod cells in the retina. Rod cells degenerate, initially at the periphery of the retina. The areas of degeneration and cell death slowly expand, causing vision to narrow. Central vision is finally lost as well.

The initial manifestation of retinitis pigmentosa, difficulty with night vision, is often noted during childhood. As the disease progresses, there is slow loss of visual fields, photophobia, and disrupted color vision. The progression to tunnel vision and blindness is gradual; the patient may be totally blind by age 40.

Currently, there is no effective treatment for retinitis pigmentosa. Research into the role that defective rhodopsin plays in the disease holds future promise for the development of therapy that may at least slow its progress.

Patients with retinitis pigmentosa may benefit from low-vision aids, much like those for the patient with macular degeneration. Additionally, information about the disease and its progress is vital so the patient can plan for the eventual total loss of sight. Patients with retinitis pigmentosa should be referred for genetic counseling prior to starting a family to determine the risk of transmitting the disease to their children.

The Patient with an Enucleation

Occasionally surgical removal of an eye is necessary because of trauma, infection, glaucoma, intractable pain, or malignancy. This procedure is known as **enucleation**.

Enucleation is performed under local or general anesthesia. After the globe is removed, the conjunctiva and eye muscles are sutured to a round implant inserted into the orbit to maintain its shape. A pressure dressing is left in place for 24 to 46 hours. The patient is permitted out of bed on the day of surgery. Hemorrhage and infection are the most commonly seen complications.

Postoperative nursing care includes teaching, psychologic support, and observation for potential complications. The patient may be instructed to apply warm compresses and instill antibiotic ointment or drops postoperatively. If irrigation of the eye socket is ordered, have the patient lean over a sink or basin, if possible, or position on the affected side with a clean emesis basin to hold the irrigant as it flows out of the socket. Gently hold the lids open and irrigate the socket using a bulb syringe and clean warm water.

Within 1 week, a temporary prosthesis called a *conformer* is fitted into the empty socket. The permanent prosthesis is individually designed to closely resemble the patient's other eye. The prosthesis can be fitted 1 to

2 months after surgery. Often it is difficult to discern which eye is functional and which is the prosthesis.

46.2 Ear Disorders

For an individual to hear, sound waves must enter the external auditory meatus and travel through the ear canal to vibrate the tympanic membrane and bony structures of the middle ear, which in turn activate the receptors of the cochlea. Trauma or disease involving any portion of this pathway can affect hearing or cause symptoms such as tinnitus, the perception of sound such as ringing, buzzing, or roaring in the ears.

Disorders of the external ear, including the auricle, auditory meatus, and ear canal, can affect the conduction of sound waves and hearing. Obstruction of the external auditory canal or damage to the tympanic membrane, which separates the outer from the middle ear, may lead to conductive hearing loss. Infection or inflammation, trauma, and obstruction of the ear canal with cerumen (wax) or a foreign body are the most common conditions affecting the external ear.

Disorders of the middle ear may be either acute or chronic. Unless these disorders are treated promptly and effectively, damage and scarring of middle ear structures can result in a permanent conductive hearing loss. Infectious or inflammatory disorders such as otitis media and mastoiditis are the most common conditions affecting the middle ear. Otosclerosis, a genetic condition, may also affect the structures of the middle ear.

The Patient with Otitis Externa

Otitis externa is inflammation of the ear canal. Commonly known as *swimmer's ear*, it is most prevalent in people who spend significant time in the water and those who live in warm, humid climates. Competitive athletes, including swimmers, divers, and surfers, are particularly prone to otitis externa. Wearing a hearing aid or ear plugs, which hold moisture in the ear canal, is an additional risk factor. Although *Pseudomonas aeruginosa* or other bacterial infection is the most common cause, external otitis may also be due to fungal infection, mechanical trauma (such as cleaning the ear with a toothpick), or a local hypersensitivity reaction.

Pathophysiology

Disruption of the normal environment within the external auditory canal typically precedes the inflammatory process (Sorenson et al., 2019). Retained moisture, cleaning, or drying of the ear canal removes the protective layer of cerumen, an acidic, water-repellent substance with antimicrobial properties. Its removal leaves the skin of the ear canal vulnerable to invasion and infection. For surfers, the presence of *exostoses*, bony growths in the ear canals resulting from prolonged exposure to cold, predisposes to impaction and retained moisture within the canal.

Manifestations

The patient with otitis externa often complains of a feeling of fullness in the ear. Ear pain is typically present and may be severe. The pain of otitis externa can be differentiated from that associated with otitis media by manipulation of the auricle. In external otitis, this maneuver increases the pain, whereas the patient with otitis media experiences no change in pain perception. Odorless watery or purulent drainage may be present. The ear canal appears inflamed and edematous on examination.

Complications

Cellulitis of the surrounding tissue is a possible complication of external otitis. Instruct the patient to report to the primary care provider any increase in pain, swelling, or redness of surrounding tissues; fever; or other manifestations of infection such as malaise or increased fatigue.

Interprofessional Care

Medications

A topical antibiotic is often prescribed for the treatment of otitis externa. A topical corticosteroid may be ordered in combination with the antibiotic to provide immediate relief of the pain, swelling, and itching. Polymyxin B-neomycin-hydrocortisone (Cortisporin Otic) is a typical combination preparation used to treat external otitis; these antibiotics are effective against *Pseudomonas*. It is important to identify known sensitivity to any of the drugs in this preparation prior to initiating therapy. Patients who are sensitive to neomycin may develop dermatitis, in which case the drug must be stopped. Other preparations such as 1% tolnaftate solution (Tinactin) may be prescribed for a fungal infection of the ear canal.

Treatment

Management of the patient with an external ear disorder focuses on restoring the normal balance of the external ear canal and teaching the patient how to prevent future problems.

For otitis externa, the following steps are recommended in treatment:

- Thorough cleansing of the ear canal, particularly if drainage or debris is present
- Treatment of the infection with local antibiotics; if cellulitis is present, systemic antibiotics may be necessary
- Medication to relieve the pain and itching
- Teaching to prevent future episodes of swimmer's ear.

Nursing Care

External otitis can cause severe pain and discomfort. Although the disorder is rarely serious enough to require hospitalization, the nurse teaches the patient about the disorder, comfort measures, and prevention of future episodes.

Diagnoses, Interventions, and Outcomes

Provide Teaching to Restore Tissue Integrity. External otitis may result from attempts to clean the ear canal with a toothpick, cotton-tipped applicator, or other implement that damages the skin, allowing an infectious organism to invade the tissue. Even if the canal is not damaged by attempts to clean it, the cleaning process often interrupts normal mechanisms, causing cerumen and debris to collect in the canal. This collected debris, in turn, tends to trap water within the canal, causing maceration of the skin.

Expected Outcome: Integrity of tissues in the patient's external ear canal will be restored.

The nurse will:

- Inform patient that ear canals rarely need cleansing beyond washing of the external meatus with soap and water. Teach patients of all ages not to clean ear canals with any implement. *"Cleaning" increases the risk of tissue damage and impairs the normal mechanism that clears the canal of accumulated cerumen and debris.*
- Teach patient (and, if necessary, a family member) how to instill prescribed eardrops (see **Box 46.5**).
- Teach patient to avoid getting water in the affected ear until it is fully healed. Cotton balls may be used while showering to prevent water from entering the ear canal. The patient should refrain from water sports and activities for 7 to 10 days or until approved by the primary care provider. *Retained moisture in the ear canal can further impair skin integrity, increasing inflammation.*

Transitions of Care

The patient is ultimately responsible for carrying out the prescribed treatment regimen in external otitis and for implementing measures to prevent future episodes. Teaching is vital. Provide verbal and written instructions on use of the prescribed medications. Teach the patient care measures to prevent recurrent episodes, which is especially important for swimmers, divers, and surfers. Teach the patient to:

- Keep the ear canal as dry as possible while in the water:
  a. Use silicone earplugs, which can keep water out of the ear without reducing hearing significantly.
  b. Wear a tight-fitting swim cap or wet suit hood, especially in cold ocean water. These protect the ear from the cold and from sand and other water debris.
- Dry the ear canal immediately after swimming or showering. Allow water to drain by tilting the head and pulling the earlobe in various directions to straighten the ear canal. Dry the outer ear with a towel, then use a hair dryer on the lowest setting several inches from the ear to dry the canal.
- Not insert cotton swabs or other objects into the ear canal. This removes the protective layer of cerumen and may damage the canal, increasing the risk of infection. In addition, if debris such as sand is present, the swab may actually push debris farther into the canal, forming an impacted mass.
- Consult their primary care provider about using a drying agent in the ear canal after swimming. Commercial alcohol-based eardrops or a 1:1 mixture of white vinegar and rubbing alcohol is effective in drying the canal and restoring its normal acidic environment.
- If it is necessary to remove impacted debris from the ear canal, irrigate the ear with warm tap water. A bulb syringe available over the counter or a 20-mL syringe attached to a short Teflon intravenous catheter (with the needle removed) is effective. With the head tilted toward the affected side, direct a stream of warm water toward the upper wall of the ear canal, allowing the water to run out into a bowl or sink. Repeated instillations may be necessary to break up and flush out impacted wax and debris.
- Follow manufacturer's directions for cleaning and disinfecting pools and hot tubs. Use pool test strips to check pools and hot tubs for adequate disinfectant and pH levels before entering.

BOX 46.5
Patient Teaching for Instilling Eardrops

- Wash hands.
- Warm the medication briefly by holding the container in the hand or placing it in a pocket for approximately 5 minutes before instilling the drops. *Warming the medication promotes comfort.*
- Lie on the unaffected side; if sitting, tilt the head toward the unaffected side. *This position allows gravity to assist in moving the medication to the inner portion of the ear canal.*
- Partially fill the ear dropper with medication.
- Using the nondominant hand, straighten the ear canal by pulling the pinna of the ear up and back. *Straightening helps the medication travel along the length of the canal.*
- Administer the prescribed number of drops into the ear canal. *It is important that the full amount of prescribed medication be administered to penetrate the length of the canal and achieve full effectiveness.*
- Remain in the sidelying position for approximately 5 minutes after the instillation of drops. *This position allows the medication to penetrate into deeper portions of the canal and prevents it from running out when the head is moved upright.*
- Loosely place a small piece of cotton in the auditory meatus for 15 to 20 minutes. *The cotton helps keep the medication in the canal.*

The Patient with Impacted Cerumen or a Foreign Body

The external auditory canal can be obstructed by cerumen or foreign bodies. The curved shape and narrow lumen of the canal make it particularly vulnerable to obstruction.

Pathophysiology

As cerumen dries, it moves down and out of the ear canal. In some individuals it tends to accumulate, narrowing the canal. A variety of objects become foreign bodies in the ear canal. In adults, implements used to clean the ear canal may break and become lodged. Insects also may enter the ear canal and be unable to exit.

Risk Factors

Aging is a risk factor for impaction because less cerumen is produced and it is harder and drier. The accumulation of cerumen is often aggravated by attempting to remove it using cotton-tipped swabs or hairpins, which pack it more deeply into the ear canal.

Manifestations

When the ear canal becomes occluded with either cerumen or a foreign body, the patient experiences a conductive hearing loss in the affected ear. Manifestations include a sensation of fullness, along with tinnitus and coughing due to stimulation of the vagal nerve. The foreign body or impacted cerumen may be visualized on otoscopy. Impacted cerumen appears as a yellow, brown, or black mass in the canal.

Interprofessional Care

Treatment

Treatment focuses on clearing the canal. If there is no evidence of tympanic membrane perforation, irrigation of the canal is often the initial therapy.

Impacted wax, objects, or insects may require physical removal using an ear curet, forceps, or right-angle hook inserted via an otoscope and ear speculum. When an organic foreign body such as a bean or an insect is suspected, water should not be instilled into the ear canal because it may cause the object to swell, making its removal more difficult. Smooth, round objects present the biggest challenge to remove from the ear canal. Suction applied using a piece of soft intravenous tubing may be effective.

Medications

Mineral oil or topical lidocaine drops are used to immobilize or kill insects prior to their removal from the ear.

Nursing Care

Nurses are often involved in identifying and relieving obstructions of the ear canal, especially in outpatient and community settings. Any patient with evidence of a new conductive hearing loss or complaints of discomfort and fullness in one ear should be evaluated for possible obstruction. Inability to visualize the tympanic membrane or observation of a dark, shiny mass obstructing the canal may indicate a need for an irrigation or other procedure to clear the canal. It is important to determine that the tympanic membrane is intact before irrigating; assessment by a physician or advanced practitioner may be necessary if a ruptured membrane is suspected.

Transitions of Care

Because obstruction of the ear canal with cerumen or a foreign body is generally preventable, teaching is a key component of nursing care. Patients need to know appropriate care measures for the external ear. Although the ear canal rarely needs cleaning, the patient prone to cerumen impaction needs teaching about the use of mineral oil or commercial products to soften wax and of irrigation to remove it. All patients should understand the importance of not inserting anything smaller than a finger wrapped with a washcloth into the ear canal to avoid trauma to the canal or eardrum. Stress the risk of impacting cerumen against the tympanic membrane when using cotton-tipped swabs to clean the ear canal. Additionally, the swab may break and lodge in the canal. If eardrops have been prescribed, teach the patient and a family member how to instill them (see Box 46.5).

The Patient with Otitis Media

Otitis media, inflammation or infection of the middle ear, primarily affects infants and young children but may also occur in adults. The tympanic membrane, which separates the middle ear from the external auditory canal, protects the middle ear from the external environment. The auditory (eustachian) tube connects the middle ear with the nasopharynx to help equalize the pressure in the middle ear with the atmospheric pressure. Unfortunately, this connecting tube also provides a route by which infectious organisms enter the middle ear from the nose and throat, causing otitis media, the most common disease of the middle ear.

Pathophysiology

There are two primary forms of otitis media: Serous and acute. Both forms are associated with upper respiratory infection and auditory tube dysfunction (Sorenson et al., 2019). The auditory tube is narrow and flat, normally opening only during yawning and swallowing. Allergies or upper respiratory tract infections can cause edema of the tube lining, impairing its function. Air within the middle ear is trapped and gradually absorbed, creating negative pressure in this space.

Serous Otitis Media

Serous otitis media (also called *otitis media with effusion*) occurs when the auditory tube is obstructed for a prolonged time, impairing air pressure equalization in the middle ear. Air within the middle ear space is gradually absorbed; the tube obstruction prevents more air from entering the middle ear. The resulting negative pressure in the middle ear causes sterile serous fluid to move from the capillaries into the space, forming a sterile effusion of the middle ear.

Acute Otitis Media

The auditory tube also provides a route for the entry of pathogens into the normally sterile middle ear, resulting in acute otitis media. Acute otitis media typically follows an upper respiratory infection. Edema of the auditory tube impairs drainage of the middle ear, causing mucus and serous fluid to accumulate. This fluid is an excellent environment for the growth of bacteria, which may enter from the oronasopharynx via the auditory tube. Although a viral upper respiratory infection may predispose the patient to a middle ear infection, the bacteria *Streptococcus pneumoniae*, *Haemophilus influenzae*, and *Streptococcus pyogenes* account for most cases of otitis media in adults. Invasion and colonization of the middle ear by bacteria and the resultant migration of white blood cells cause pus formation.

Risk Factors

Upper respiratory infection or allergies such as hay fever predispose the patient to serous otitis media. In addition, patients with narrowed or edematous auditory tubes may also be subject to barotrauma. In these patients, the middle ear cannot adapt to rapid changes in barometric pressure such as those that occur during air travel or underwater diving. Barotrauma tends to occur during descent in an airplane because negative pressure within the middle ear causes the auditory tube to collapse and lock. Underwater diving places even greater stress on the auditory tube and middle ear.

Manifestations

Typical manifestations of serous otitis media include decreased hearing in the affected ear and complaints of "snapping" or "popping" in the ear. On examination, the tympanic membrane demonstrates decreased mobility and may appear retracted or bulging. Fluid or air bubbles are often visible behind the drum (**Figure 46.17** ■). Pressure differences such as those occurring with flying or underwater diving may cause acute pain, hemorrhage into the middle ear, rupture of the tympanic membrane, or even rupture of the round window with sensory hearing loss and severe **vertigo** (a sensation of whirling or rotation). *Hemotympanum*, bleeding into or behind the tympanic membrane, may be observed on otoscopic examination.

The patient with acute otitis media experiences mild to severe pain in the affected ear. The patient's temperature is often elevated. Diminished hearing, dizziness, vertigo, and tinnitus are common associated complaints. Pus within the mastoid air cells often causes mastoid tenderness in acute otitis media. On otoscopic examination, the tympanic membrane appears red and inflamed or dull and bulging (**Figure 46.18** ■). Decreased movement of the membrane is demonstrated by tympanometry or air insufflation. Spontaneous rupture of the tympanic membrane releases a purulent discharge.

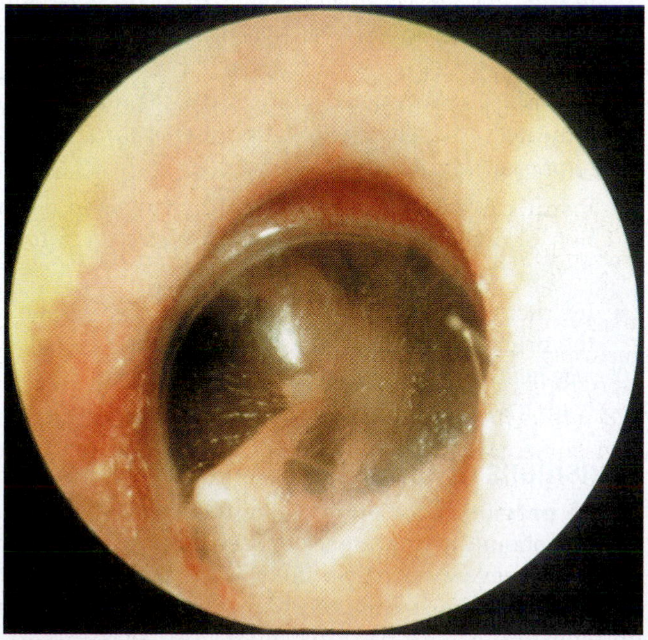

Figure 46.17 ■ The appearance of the tympanic membrane in serous otitis media.

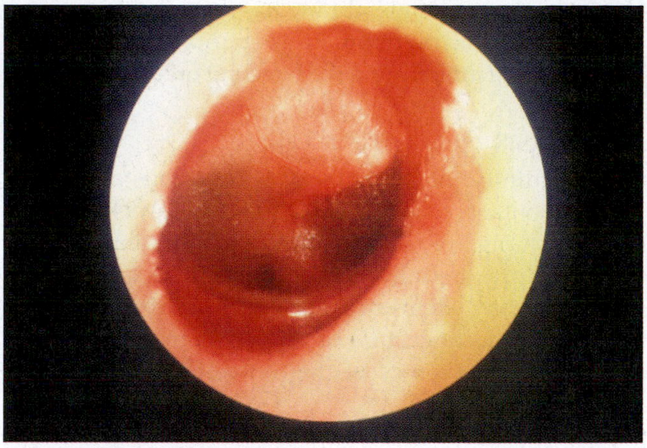

Figure 46.18 ■ A red, bulging tympanic membrane indicative of acute otitis media.

Manifestations such as persistent fever, nausea and vomiting, irritability, lethargy, or persistent headache may indicate a complication such as meningitis and should be reported immediately to the care provider.

Complications

Accumulated pus can increase middle ear pressure sufficiently to rupture the tympanic membrane. The bacterial infection may also migrate internally, causing mastoiditis, brain abscess, or bacterial meningitis. A more common complication of otitis media is a persistent conductive hearing loss, which typically resolves when the middle ear effusion clears.

Interprofessional Care

The diagnosis of otitis media is usually based on the history and physical examination. The tympanic membrane can be visualized and its mobility evaluated using a pneumatic otoscope that allows a puff of air to be instilled into the ear canal. Generally, the tympanic membrane moves slightly when air is instilled or the patient performs the Valsalva maneuver. Less movement is seen in patients with auditory tube dysfunction and acute otitis media with effusion.

Diagnosis

- ***Impedance audiometry***, also known as *tympanometry*, is an accurate diagnostic test for otitis media with effusion. A continuous tone is delivered to the tympanic membrane by an audiometer with a sealed probe tip. Compliance of the tympanic membrane and middle ear is measured by recording energy reflected from the membrane surface. With middle ear effusion, compliance is reduced.
- ***Complete blood count (CBC)*** may be done to assess for an elevated WBC count and increased numbers of immature cells indicative of acute bacterial infection.

- If the tympanic membrane has ruptured or a tympanocentesis or myringotomy is performed, drainage is cultured to determine the infecting organism.

Medications

When auditory tube dysfunction and serous otitis media do not spontaneously resolve within 2 to 4 weeks or if they lead to hearing loss, a short course of an anti-inflammatory drug (e.g., oral prednisone for 7 days) may be prescribed to reduce mucosal edema of the tube and improve its patency. Although a decongestant or antihistamine may be used, there is little evidence of their effectiveness in treating serous otitis media.

The patient with auditory tube dysfunction may be taught to autoinflate the middle ear by performing the Valsalva maneuver or by forcefully exhaling against closed nostrils. Additionally, the patient is advised to avoid air travel and underwater diving.

Acute otitis media is usually treated with antibiotic therapy, especially amoxicillin, cefdinir (Omnicef), cefuroxime, or azithromycin, for 5 to 10 days. This course of treatment is long enough to ensure eradication of the infective organism, yet short enough to reduce the incidence of bacterial resistance. Analgesics, antipyretics, antihistamines, and local application of heat may provide symptomatic relief.

Surgery

Myringotomy (an incision of the tympanic membrane) or tympanocentesis may be performed to relieve excess pressure in the middle ear and prevent spontaneous rupture of the eardrum. To perform a tympanocentesis, the healthcare provider inserts a 20-gauge spinal needle through the inferior portion of the tympanic membrane, allowing aspiration of fluid and pus from the middle ear to relieve pressure and, if necessary, obtain a specimen for culture. Myringotomy may be performed to relieve severe pain or when complications of acute otitis media, such as mastoiditis, are present. As soon as the pressure is released, pain subsides and hearing improves.

Patients who do not respond to antibiotic therapy may require myringotomy with insertion of ventilation (tympanostomy) tubes. Small tubes are inserted into the inferior portion of the tympanic membrane, providing for ventilation and drainage of the middle ear during healing. The tube is eventually extruded from the ear, and the tympanic membrane heals. While the tube is in place, it is important to avoid getting any water in the ear canal because it may then enter the middle ear space.

Nursing Care

Patients with otitis media are commonly treated in outpatient and community settings. The nursing role is primarily one of support and education.

Assessment

Collect assessment data through a health history and physical examination:

- ***Health history:*** Recent upper respiratory infection; presence, intensity, and nature of pain in affected ear; sense of fullness or pressure in the ear; change in hearing; snapping or popping sensation in the affected ear; presence of vertigo
- ***Physical assessment:*** Temperature; hearing test; inspect tympanic membrane.

Priorities of Care

Patient teaching is a nursing care priority for the patient with otitis media. Just as it is important for the patient to understand the importance of seeking care for acute symptoms, it is also important to understand that antibiotic therapy is not always indicated and the risks of inappropriate antibiotic use.

Diagnoses, Interventions, and Outcomes

Pain can be a significant problem for patients with otitis media, as can the risk of damage to delicate tissues of the middle ear by the infectious and inflammatory processes.

Manage Acute Pain. Tissue edema, effusion of the middle ear, and the inflammatory response can affect the pain-sensitive tissues of the middle ear in otitis media, causing acute discomfort. This discomfort is increased by pressure changes, such as those that occur during air travel or underwater diving.

Expected Outcome: Patient will report an understanding of measures to relieve pain and promote comfort.

The nurse will:

- Assess pain for severity, quality, and location. *A thorough assessment is important to determine the source of the pain. The pain of otitis media, unlike that of external otitis, is not aggravated by movement of the external ear.*
- Encourage the use of mild analgesics such as aspirin or acetaminophen every 4 hours as needed to relieve pain and fever. *These nonprescription medications are effective in reducing the perception of pain. Aspirin also has anti-inflammatory properties that may help relieve the inflammation of the ear.*
- Advise to apply heat to the affected side unless contraindicated. *Heat dilates blood vessels, promoting the reabsorption of fluid and reducing swelling.*
- Instruct to avoid air travel, rapid changes in elevation, or diving. *A rapid change in barometric pressure can increase the patient's pain significantly.*
- Instruct to report promptly an abrupt relief of pain to the primary care provider. *Pain that subsides abruptly may indicate spontaneous perforation of the tympanic membrane with relief of pressure within the middle ear.*

Transitions of Care

Health promotion for otitis media focuses on educating patients about the importance of seeking medical care for prolonged, severe ear pain with or without drainage combined with an upper respiratory tract infection. Untreated or repeated attacks of otitis media can progress to a chronic form of otitis media, acute mastoiditis, or eardrum perforation.

The patient who has otitis media needs teaching about the disorder, its causes and prevention, and any specific treatment recommended or prescribed. Discuss the following topics with the patient and family:

- Antibiotic therapy and its indications, use, and potential side effects
- Importance of completing all ordered doses
- Follow-up examinations in 2 to 4 weeks
- Avoidance of swimming, diving, or submerging the head while bathing if ventilation tubes are in place.

If surgical intervention is necessary, teach the patient and family members about the surgery and postoperative care. Provide instruction about any special postoperative precautions, such as avoiding water in the ear canals or avoiding sudden changes in air pressure.

The Patient with Acute Mastoiditis

The mastoid process is a portion of the temporal bone of the skull lying adjacent to the middle ear. It is full of air cavities called *mastoid air cells* or *mastoid sinuses*. The infection of acute otitis media generally extends into the mastoid air cells; effective treatment of acute otitis media eliminates the infection from the mastoid cells as well. When treatment is ineffective, pus remains in the mastoid air cells, and acute *mastoiditis*, bacterial infection of the mastoid process, may develop.

Pathophysiology

In acute mastoiditis, pressure created by pus in mastoid air cells destroys the bony septa between the cells, forming large spaces. Portions of the mastoid process are eroded. With chronic infection, an abscess may form or bony sclerosis of the mastoid may result. Acute mastoiditis increases the risk of meningitis because only a very thin bony plate separates mastoid air cells from the brain.

Manifestations

Manifestations of acute mastoiditis usually develop approximately 2 to 3 weeks after an episode of acute otitis media and include recurrent earache and hearing loss on the affected side. The pain is persistent and throbbing; tenderness is present over the mastoid process (behind the ear). It may also be red and inflamed. Swelling of the process can cause the auricle of the ear to protrude more than normal. Fever may be accompanied by tinnitus and headache. Profuse drainage from the affected ear may be noted.

Interprofessional Care

Acute mastoiditis is treated aggressively with intravenous antibiotic therapy tailored to the infecting organism. Antibiotics are continued for at least 14 days. Infections that do not respond to medical therapy or that pose a high risk of spreading to the brain may necessitate *mastoidectomy*—surgical removal of the infected mastoid air cells, bone, and pus—and inspection of the underlying dura for possible abscess.

Nursing Care

Following surgical intervention, carefully assess the wound and drainage for evidence of infection or other complications. The patient's hearing may be temporarily or permanently affected, depending on the extent of the surgery. If the patient has impaired hearing in the unaffected ear as well, develop a means of communication with the patient prior to surgery. If the hearing is preserved in the unaffected ear, position the patient with that ear toward the door. Speak slowly and clearly; do not shout or speak unusually loudly. Be sure that family and staff know about the patient's hearing loss and use appropriate communication techniques. Assist the patient with ambulation initially because dizziness and vertigo are common following surgery. Nursing care of the patient having ear surgery is discussed in **Box 46.6**.

BOX 46.6
Nursing Care of the Patient Having Ear Surgery

PREOPERATIVE CARE

- Provide preoperative care as ordered or per standard protocol.
- Assess hearing or verify documentation of preoperative hearing assessment. *These data are important in evaluating the results of the surgical procedure.*
- Establish a means of communication to be used after surgery. *Hearing may be impaired after surgery.*
- Explain that blowing of the nose, coughing, and sneezing are restricted postoperatively to prevent pressure changes in the middle ear and potential disruption of the surgical site. Keeping the mouth open during a cough or sneeze minimizes pressure changes in the middle ear. *Providing teaching and the opportunity to practice before surgery promotes cooperation in the postoperative period.*

POSTOPERATIVE CARE

- Assess for bleeding or drainage from the affected ear. *Infection and hemorrhage are possible complications.*
- Administer antiemetics as ordered to prevent vomiting. *Vomiting may increase the pressure in the middle ear, disrupting the surgical site.*
- Elevate the head of bed and position the patient on the unaffected side. *This position minimizes the pressure in the middle ear.*
- Assess for vertigo or dizziness, especially with ambulation or movement in bed. Avoid unnecessary movements such as turning. Take measures to ensure safety during ambulation. *Surgery on the ear may disrupt equilibrium, increasing the risk of falling.*
- Assess hearing postoperatively. Stand on the unaffected side to communicate and use other measures such as written messages as needed for effective communication with the patient with impaired hearing. Reassure the patient that decreased hearing acuity immediately after surgery is expected. *Hearing improvement, if an expected result of the ear surgery, typically does not occur until earplugs are removed and edema and drainage at the operative site have resolved. If no reconstruction*

(continued)

of the middle ear is done or the cochlea is involved, permanent hearing loss in the affected ear may be an expected result.

- Remind to avoid coughing, sneezing, or blowing the nose. *These increase pressure in the middle ear.*

Health Education for the Patient and Family

- Provide instructions for home care:
  a. To prevent contamination of the ear canal, avoid showers, shampooing, and immersing the head until the healthcare provider says you can do so.
  b. Keep the outer earplug clean and dry, changing it as needed. Do not remove inner ear dressing until instructed to do so by the healthcare provider.
  c. Avoid blowing the nose; if you need to cough or sneeze, keep the mouth open.
  d. Do not swim or dive without healthcare provider approval. Check with your doctor regarding air travel.
  e. Meclizine hydrochloride (Antivert) or other antiemetic/antihistamine medication may be necessary for up to 1 month following surgery.
  f. Fever, bleeding, increased drainage, increased dizziness, or decreased hearing after discharge may indicate a complication. Notify the healthcare provider if any of these occur.

The Patient with Chronic Otitis Media

Chronic otitis media involves permanent perforation of the tympanic membrane, with or without recurrent pus formation. Changes in the mucosa and bony structures (ossicles) of the middle ear often accompany chronic otitis media. It is usually the result of recurrent acute otitis media and auditory tube dysfunction, but may also result from trauma or other diseases.

Marginal perforations, which usually occur in the posterior-superior portion of the tympanic membrane, are associated with more complications than central perforations. With marginal perforations, squamous epithelium may migrate from the ear canal into the middle ear, where it begins to desquamate and accumulate, forming a *cholesteatoma* (a cyst or mass filled with epithelial cell debris). Its incidence is highest in children and young adults. The desquamating epithelium continues to accumulate and remains infected, producing collagenases (enzymes) that destroy adjacent bone. The inflammatory process impairs the blood supply to the stapes, causing its destruction and conductive hearing loss. Cholesteatomas are benign and slow-growing tumors, which can enlarge to fill the entire middle ear. Untreated, the cholesteatoma can progressively destroy the ossicles and erode into the inner ear, causing profound hearing loss.

Systemic antibiotics are prescribed for exacerbations of purulent otitis media. Tympanic membrane perforation is repaired with a tympanoplasty to restore sound conduction and the integrity of the middle ear. A cholesteatoma may require delicate surgery for its removal. If at all possible, radical mastoidectomy with removal of the tympanic membrane, ossicles, and tumor is avoided.

As with other complications of acute otitis media, a priority of nursing care is prevention of chronic otitis media and cholesteatoma. Patients with chronic otitis media need to understand various treatment options and their risks and benefits, as well as the long-term risk of not treating a perforated tympanic membrane. They are also taught how to instill eardrops, to clean the external auditory meatus, and to not irrigate the ear when the tympanic membrane is perforated or if they think it might be.

If surgical treatment of chronic otitis media will affect the patient's hearing, include this information in preoperative teaching. Teach the patient and family how to use alternative means of communication if this will be necessary postoperatively. When an assistive device is ordered, teach the patient and a family member about its use (National Institute on Deafness and Other Communication Disorders [NIDCD], 2017a).

The Patient with Otosclerosis

Otosclerosis is a common cause of conductive hearing loss. Abnormal bone formation in the osseous labyrinth of the temporal bone causes the footplate of the stapes to become fixed or immobile in the oval window. The result is a conductive hearing loss.

Otosclerosis is a hereditary disorder with an autosomal dominant pattern of inheritance (Shearer, Hildebrand, & Smith, 2017). It occurs most commonly in Caucasian populations and in females. The progressive hearing loss typically begins in adolescence or early adulthood and seems to be accelerated by pregnancy. Although both ears are affected, the rate of hearing loss is asymmetric. Because bone conduction of sound is retained, the patient may be able to use the telephone but have difficulty conversing in person. Tinnitus may also be associated with otosclerosis.

On examination, a reddish or pinkish-orange tympanic membrane may be noted because of increased vascularity of the middle ear. The Rinne test shows bone sound conduction to be equal to or greater than air conduction, an abnormal finding.

Patients with otosclerosis may choose conservative treatment, relying on a hearing aid to improve their ability to hear and interact with others. Sodium fluoride may be prescribed to slow bone resorption and overgrowth. Surgical treatment involves a stapedectomy and middle ear reconstruction or a stapedotomy. A *stapedectomy* is a microsurgical technique for removing the diseased stapes. A metallic prosthesis is then inserted, with one end connected to the incus and the other inserted into the oval window. *Stapedotomy* involves creation of a small hole in the footplate of the stapes and insertion of a wire or platinum ribbon prosthesis. An argon, KTP, or CO_2 laser may be used for surgery. Surgery usually restores hearing for the patient with otosclerosis.

Education and referral of the patient to appropriate community agencies are important nursing care priorities for the patient with otosclerosis. For the patient who chooses surgical treatment, nursing care is similar to that for other patients undergoing ear surgery (see Box 46.6).

The Patient with an Inner Ear Disorder

Disorders affecting the inner ear are much less common than disorders of the outer or middle ear. Inner ear disorders affect equilibrium and may also affect sensorineural hearing, the perception of sound. Labyrinthitis and Ménière disease are the most common diseases of the inner ear. Vertigo may be a disorder of the inner ear itself or a manifestation of other disorders.

Pathophysiology

The inner ear (also called the *labyrinth*) contains the cochlea and the semicircular canals. The hair cells and neurons that allow sound perception and transmission to the auditory center of the brain are in the cochlea. The semicircular canals filled with endolymph are the primary organs involved in maintaining equilibrium. Disruption of this portion of the ear by an inflammatory process or excess endolymph not only affects balance but may also result in permanent hearing loss (Sorenson et al., 2019).

Vertigo

Normally, the integration of input from the labyrinths, eyes, muscles, joints, and neural centers maintains balance and posture. This input and integration can be affected by disorders of the labyrinth, vestibular nerve or nuclei, eyes, cerebellum, brainstem, or cerebral cortex, causing vertigo. *Vertigo*, the sensation of movement when there is none, is a disorder of equilibrium. The sensation of whirling, rotation, or movement is described as either subjective or objective.

Labyrinthitis

Labyrinthitis, also called *otitis interna*, is inflammation of the inner ear. It is an uncommon disorder because the bony protection of the membranous labyrinth makes it difficult for organisms to enter the inner ear. However, bacteria, viruses, and other organisms may enter and infect the inner ear through the oval window during acute otitis media, through the cochlear aqueduct during meningitis, or through the blood. Viral labyrinthitis is suspected when the patient has a sudden onset of symptoms after an upper respiratory infection or when there is no evidence of concurrent otitis media. Labyrinthitis may also result from an autoimmune process of unknown etiology.

Ménière Disease

Ménière disease, also known as *endolymphatic hydrops*, is a chronic disorder characterized by recurrent attacks of vertigo with tinnitus and a progressive unilateral hearing loss. Ménière disease results from an excess of endolymph, the fluid in the membranous labyrinth of the inner ear. Although the precise pathophysiologic mechanism leading to accumulation of endolymph is unclear, it is thought to result from impaired filtration and excretion of the fluid by the endolymphatic sac (Sorenson et al., 2019). Excessive pressure resulting from the increased fluid volume causes neural organs of the cochlea to degenerate. The onset of Ménière disease may be gradual or sudden.

Risk Factors

Ménière disease affects men and women equally, with adults between the ages of 35 and 60 at highest risk (NIDCD, 2017c). The cause of Ménière disease is unclear, although the most common form of the disease is thought to result from viral injury to the fluid transport system of the inner ear. Other factors that may increase the risk for Ménière disease include trauma, bacterial infection, autoimmune processes, and selected drugs and toxins (Sorenson et al., 2019). A family history of the disease increases risk, suggesting a possible genetic link in some patients. There are no known environmental risk factors for labyrinthitis.

Manifestations

Patients with subjective vertigo report the sensation of being in motion in a stable environment. This is not always a sense of spinning; the patient may have a sense of tumbling or falling forward or backward. The sensation is reversed in objective vertigo; patients report a sensation of stability in a moving environment. This motion may be perceived as the room spinning around the patient or the ground rocking beneath the patient's feet. Dizziness, which may be mistaken for vertigo, is a sensation of unsteadiness, lack of balance, light headedness, or movement within the head. The person who is dizzy does not have the rotational sensation felt with vertigo.

Vertigo may be disabling, resulting in falls, injury, and difficulty walking. Attacks of vertigo are often accompanied by nausea and vomiting, nystagmus, and autonomic symptoms such as pallor, sweating, hypotension, and salivation. Vertigo is the hallmark manifestation of inner ear disorders. Labyrinthitis typically causes vertigo, sensorineural hearing deficit, and **nystagmus** (rapid involuntary eye movements). The vertigo of labyrinthitis is severe and often accompanied by nausea and vomiting. Any movement can aggravate the vertigo, and falling is a significant risk if the patient attempts to stand. Vertigo lasts days to weeks in labyrinthitis, making patient education a vital component of care. The involuntary rhythmic eye movements of nystagmus may not be present in all patients with labyrinthitis. When present, the eye movement is typically horizontal. Applying positive or negative pressure to the tympanic membrane of the affected ear may stimulate nystagmus, as will caloric testing (irrigating the ear canal with warm or cool water). Although nystagmus may also be a symptom of brainstem or cerebellar dysfunction, vertigo and hearing loss are not typically associated with those disorders. Hearing loss in the ear affected by labyrinthitis may be temporary or permanent. If inflammation destroys tissue of the membranous labyrinth, the hearing loss may be complete and permanent.

Ménière disease is characterized by recurrent attacks of vertigo, gradual loss of hearing, and tinnitus. Attacks may be preceded by a feeling of fullness in the ears and a roaring or ringing sensation. The sensorineural hearing loss and tinnitus are usually unilateral but can become bilateral.

Attacks of severe rotary vertigo occur abruptly and often unpredictably, lasting from minutes to hours. An attack may be linked to increased sodium intake, stress, allergies, vasoconstriction, or premenstrual fluid retention. As the disease continues, hearing loss progresses and the vertigo can be severe enough to cause immobility and nausea and vomiting. Attacks are often accompanied by hypotension, sweating, and nystagmus.

Interprofessional Care

The manifestations associated with inner ear disorders are similar, making testing necessary to establish a diagnosis. Once the diagnosis is determined, collaborative care is directed toward managing symptoms and preventing permanent hearing loss. Patients with labyrinthitis or an acute attack of Ménière disease may require hospitalization to manage the vertigo and its effects.

Diagnosis

The following diagnostic studies may be ordered:

- *Electronystagmography (caloric testing)* evaluates the vestibulo-ocular reflex by identifying eye movements (nystagmus) in response to changes in head position or instillation of warm or cool water into the ear canal. In patients with impaired vestibular function, the normal nystagmus response is blunted or absent. This portion of the test is contraindicated in patients who have a perforated tympanic membrane.
- *Rinne and Weber tests* of hearing show decreased air and bone conduction on the affected side if a sensorineural hearing loss is present. In Ménière disease, audiology shows sensorineural hearing loss involving the low tones.
- *X-rays and CT scans* of the petrous bones are used to evaluate the internal auditory canal. In patients with Ménière disease, the vestibular aqueducts may be shorter and straighter than normal.
- *A glycerol test* is conducted by giving the patient oral glycerol to decrease fluid pressure in the inner ear. An acute temporary hearing improvement is considered diagnostic for Ménière disease.

Medications

In Ménière disease, a diuretic such as acetazolamide (Diamox) or hydrochlorothiazide may be prescribed to reduce endolymphatic pressure. A central nervous system depressant such as diazepam (Valium) or lorazepam (Ativan) may halt an attack of vertigo. Parenteral droperidol (Inapsine) provides both a sedative and antiemetic effect, making it a useful drug for acute attacks. Antivertigo/antiemetic medications such as meclizine (Antivert), prochlorperazine (Compazine), or hydroxyzine hydrochloride (Vistaril) are prescribed to reduce the whirling sensation and nausea. Intratympanic gentamicin, injected through the tympanic membrane into the middle ear, has been shown to be effective in reducing the vertigo of Ménière disease. The gentamicin damages vestibular hair cells, effectively reducing attacks of vertigo while causing less hearing loss than traditional surgical approaches (Adams et al., 2017).

Treatment

Bedrest in a quiet, darkened room with minimal sensory stimuli and minimal movement provides the most comfort for the patient experiencing an acute attack of vertigo.

Between acute attacks, management of the patient with Ménière disease is directed at preventing future attacks and preserving hearing. A low-sodium diet (2 g/day) helps reduce labyrinthine pressure. A very low salt diet (1 g) may be prescribed if moderate sodium restriction is ineffective in controlling attacks. Patients should avoid tobacco, which causes vasoconstriction and can precipitate an attack, along with alcohol and caffeine.

Surgery

When episodes of vertigo cannot be controlled through medical interventions, surgery may be necessary. Surgical *endolymphatic decompression* relieves the excess pressure in the labyrinth; a shunt is then inserted between the membranous labyrinth and the subarachnoid space to drain excess fluid away from the labyrinths and maintain lower pressure. This procedure preserves hearing for most patients. Vertigo is relieved in approximately 70% of patients, but about half of patients undergoing this procedure continue to experience sensations of fullness and tinnitus.

Destruction of a portion of the acoustic nerve is an alternative to shunting procedures. In a *vestibular neurectomy*, the portion of cranial nerve VIII that controls balance and sensations of vertigo is severed. This procedure relieves vertigo for up to 90% of patients. Although there is a risk of damage to the cochlear portion of the nerve and resultant hearing loss, for most patients hearing loss stabilizes after neurectomy, even improving for some.

The surgery of last resort for Ménière disease is a *labyrinthectomy*. The labyrinth is completely removed, destroying cochlear function. This procedure is used only when hearing loss is nearly complete and vertigo is persistent. Although labyrinthectomy relieves vertigo in nearly all cases, the patient may remain unsteady and have continued problems with balance.

After surgery on the inner ear, the patient is positioned to minimize ear pressure and vertigo. Movement is restricted, and assistance is provided when the patient gets up. Antiemetics and antivertigo medications are used to manage symptoms resulting from disruption of the inner ear. Complications include infection and leakage of cerebrospinal fluid.

Nursing Care

The patient with an inner ear disorder has multiple nursing care needs related to the manifestations of the disorder.

Assessment

In addition to the following, assess the older patient for other medical causes of imbalance and dizziness, such as neurologic dysfunction, musculoskeletal and cardiovascular disorders, and endocrine problems.

- ***Health history:*** Medication use; presence of vertigo, tinnitus, nausea and vomiting, and hearing loss; balance problems; frequency and duration of symptoms, precipitating factors for an attack
- ***Physical assessment:*** Vital signs, general health; hearing, nystagmus, balance.

Priorities of Care

Maintaining safety is the priority of care for patients with inner ear disorders. Attacks of vertigo may occur without warning and can be so severe that the patient is unable to remain upright.

Diagnoses, Interventions, and Outcome

The risk for trauma due to attacks of vertigo in patients with inner ear disorders is great. If frequent attacks are accompanied by nausea, nutrition may be compromised. Constant or intermittent tinnitus can interfere with sleep and rest. Finally, because nearly all inner ear disorders are associated with some degree of hearing loss, which may be progressive, the patient has significant psychosocial needs.

Reduce Risk of Injury. Because of the unpredictable nature of attacks, the patient with vertigo due to an inner ear disorder needs to learn strategies for dealing with an acute episode. Because vertigo tends to be chronic except in acute labyrinthitis, the emphasis is on helping the patient develop strategies to reduce the frequency of attacks and the risk of injury.

Expected Outcome: Patient will remain free of injury.

The nurse will:

- Monitor for vertigo, nystagmus, nausea and vomiting, and hearing loss. *Monitoring is important to determine the severity of impairment, the duration of attacks, and the patient's ability to predict an impending attack.*
- Instruct to not get up without assistance during episodes of vertigo. *During attacks of vertigo, assistance reduces the risk of falling.*
- Teach to avoid sudden head movements or position changes. *Sudden movement may precipitate an attack of vertigo.*
- Administer prescribed medications as ordered, including antiemetics, diuretics, and sedatives. *These medications may reduce the frequency, severity, and duration of vertigo attacks.*
- Instruct to take the prescribed medication and lie down in a quiet, darkened room when an impending attack is sensed. *These measures help protect the patient from injury and may shorten the duration and reduce the severity of the attack.*
- Advise to pull to the side of the road and wait for the symptoms to subside if an attack occurs while driving. *Perception and judgment necessary for safe driving may be impaired during an acute attack; pulling off the road is vital to protect the safety of the patient and others.*
- Discuss the effect of unilateral hearing loss on the ability to identify the direction of sounds. To ensure safety, encourage the patient to use other senses (e.g., when crossing the street). *Just as depth perception changes when vision is lost in one eye, sound perception and differentiation of direction change when hearing is lost unilaterally.*

SAFETY ALERT: If a hospitalized patient has acute attack of vertigo, keep on bedrest with the side rails raised and the call light readily accessible. ■

Promote Adequate Sleep. The tinnitus often associated with inner ear disorders may be loud and continuous, interfering with the patient's ability to concentrate, relax, and sleep. It may be perceived as a continuous high-pitched whine or a buzzing, ringing, or humming sound. In some patients, it may have a pulsatile quality.

Expected Outcome: Patient will identify and use strategies to achieve restful sleep.

The nurse will:

- Refer for a complete hearing and ear examination if one has not been done. *Although most tinnitus is associated with hearing loss, often due to noise exposure, it may also be associated with treatable conditions such as impacted cerumen, hypertension, cerebrovascular disorders, and other conditions.*
- Discuss options for masking tinnitus to promote concentration and sleep:
  a. Ambient noise from a radio or sound system
  b. Masking device or white-noise machine
  c. Hearing aid that produces a tone to mask the tinnitus.
- Hearing aid that amplifies ambient sound. *These techniques or devices help mask the subjective perception of tinnitus, allowing the patient to focus on something other than the sound.*
- Discuss the possible risks and benefits of medications to treat tinnitus. *Many medications have been used to treat tinnitus; oral antidepressants such as nortriptyline (Aventyl, Pamelor) taken at bedtime have been shown to be most effective.*

Transitions of Care

Health promotion focuses on identifying patients with potential inner ear disorders. Persistent episodes of dizziness, ringing in the ears, balance problems, or loss of hearing should be reported to a healthcare provider. Patients diagnosed early may have a lower risk for injury and can be taught strategies for maintaining as near normal as possible their work and social lives.

Because disorders of the inner ear disrupt balance, safety is a primary focus of teaching. Assist the patient to identify possible hazards in the home environment. Discuss the following points during the teaching session:

- Change positions slowly, especially when ambulating
- Turn the whole body rather than just the head

- Sit down immediately with the onset of vertigo and lie down if possible
- Take prescribed antiemetic and antivertigo medications
- Wear medical alert identification
- If appropriate, discuss the surgical procedure, the immediate postoperative period, and the long-term effects of the surgery
- Discuss alternative communication techniques as needed
- Suggest the following resources: The Better Hearing Institute and Self-Help for Hard of Hearing People.

The Patient with a Vestibular Schwannoma

A *vestibular schwannoma* (or *acoustic neuroma*) is a benign tumor of the vestibular portion of cranial nerve VIII. It typically occurs in adults between the ages of 40 and 50. Vestibular schwannomas are common, accounting for about 9% of primary brain tumors. Although usually unilateral, people with neurofibromatosis type 2, a genetic disorder, frequently develop bilateral schwannomas (NIDCD, 2017e)

These tumors usually occur in the internal auditory meatus, compressing the auditory nerve where it exits the skull to the inner ear. If allowed to grow, the tumor eventually destroys the labyrinth, including the cochlea and vestibular apparatus. As the tumor expands, it erodes the wall of the internal auditory meatus. The tumor may eventually impinge on the brainstem and cerebellum, with development of obstructive hydrocephalus. Cranial nerves VII (facial) and V (trigeminal) are often affected by the expanding tumor; the tumor frequently wraps around the facial nerve.

Early manifestations of vestibular schwannoma are those associated with disorders of the inner ear: Tinnitus, unilateral hearing loss, and nystagmus. Dizziness or vertigo may occur. As the tumor expands and occupies increasing amounts of space in the closed cranium, the patient experiences neurologic signs related to the area of the brain affected.

The presence of the tumor can generally be identified on CT or MRI scans. X-ray films of the petrous pyramid of the temporal bone may show erosion caused by the tumor. The treatment of choice for vestibular schwannoma is surgical excision using microsurgery techniques or destruction of the tumor via stereotactic radiotherapy. Bevacizumab (Avastin), a drug that blocks blood vessel growth within tumors, may be beneficial in patients with neurofibromatosis type 2 (Adams et al., 2017).

Postoperative nursing care focuses on preserving cerebral function. Position the patient to minimize cerebral edema and monitor frequently for signs of increased intracranial pressure. Because the gag reflex may be affected, assess the patient carefully before food and fluids are allowed by mouth. Speech therapy is often prescribed for the patient after surgery. Because deficits may not resolve for a long time after surgery, education and support are vital components of nursing care for the patient. (See Chapter 42 for care of the patient undergoing craniotomy.)

The Patient with Hearing Loss

Hearing loss is a significant problem, affecting an estimated 15% of adults in the United States. The problem of hearing loss is particularly significant in older adults, affecting about 25% of people between the ages of 65 and 74 and 50% of those over age 75 (NIDCD, 2017d).

Hearing loss impairs the ability to communicate in a world filled with sound and hearing individuals. A hearing deficit can be partial or total, congenital or acquired. It may affect one or both ears. In some types of hearing loss, the ability to perceive sound at specific frequencies is lost. In others, hearing is diminished across all frequencies.

Patients with hearing loss often display signs that caregivers can recognize. The voice volume of the patient with impaired hearing frequently increases, and the patient positions the head with the better ear toward the speaker. The patient may frequently ask people to repeat what they have said or respond inappropriately to questions or statements. A question may elicit a blank look if the patient has not heard or understood its content.

Pathophysiology

Lesions in the outer ear, middle ear, inner ear, or central auditory pathways can result in hearing loss. The process of aging can also affect the structures of the ear and hearing. Hearing loss is classified as conductive, sensorineural, or mixed, depending on what portion of the auditory system is affected. Profound deafness is often a congenital condition.

Conductive Hearing Loss

Anything that disrupts the transmission of sound from the external auditory meatus to the inner ear results in a conductive hearing loss. The most common cause of conductive hearing loss is obstruction of the external ear canal. Impacted cerumen, edema of the canal lining, stenosis, and neoplasms may all lead to canal obstruction. Other causes of conductive loss include a perforated tympanic membrane, disruption or fixation of the ossicles of the middle ear, fluid, scarring, or tumors of the middle ear.

Sensorineural Hearing Loss

Disorders that affect the inner ear, the auditory nerve, or the auditory pathways of the brain may lead to a sensorineural hearing loss. In this type of hearing loss, sound waves are effectively transmitted to the inner ear. In the inner ear, however, lost or damaged receptor cells, changes in the cochlear apparatus, or auditory nerve abnormalities decrease or distort the ability to receive and interpret stimuli.

A significant cause of sensorineural hearing deficit is damage to the hair cells of the organ of Corti. In the United

States, noise exposure is the major cause, resulting in high-frequency hearing loss in 40 million Americans between age 20 and 69 (NIDCD, 2017d). Damage may result from either loud impulse noise (e.g., an explosion) or loud continuous noise (e.g., machinery). Exposure to a high level of noise (e.g., standing close to the stage or speakers at a concert) on an intermittent or continuing basis damages the hair and supporting cells of the organ of Corti. Ototoxic drugs also damage the hair cells; when combined with high noise levels, the damage is greater and resultant hearing loss more profound. Ototoxic drugs include aspirin, furosemide (Lasix), aminoglycosides, streptomycin, vancomycin (Vancocin), antimalarial drugs, and chemotherapy drugs such as cisplatin (Platinol). Other potential causes of sensorineural hearing loss include prenatal exposure to rubella, viral infections, meningitis, trauma, Ménière disease, and aging.

Tumors such as vestibular schwannomas (acoustic neuromas), vascular disorders, demyelinating or degenerative diseases, infections (bacterial meningitis in particular), or trauma may affect the central auditory pathways and produce a neural hearing loss.

Presbycusis

With aging, the hair cells of the cochlea degenerate, producing a progressive sensorineural hearing loss. In **presbycusis**, gradual hearing loss associated with aging, hearing acuity begins to decrease in early adulthood and progresses as long as the individual lives.

Tinnitus

Tinnitus is the perception of sound or noise in the ears without stimulus from the environment. The sound may be steady, intermittent, or pulsatile and is often described as a buzzing, roaring, or ringing.

Tinnitus is usually associated with hearing loss (conductive or sensorineural); however, the mechanism producing the sound is poorly understood. It is often an early symptom of noise-induced hearing damage and drug-related ototoxicity. Tinnitus is especially associated with salicylate, quinine, or quinidine toxicity. Other etiologies include obstruction of the auditory meatus, presbycusis, middle or inner ear inflammations and infections, otosclerosis, and Ménière disease. Most tinnitus, however, is chronic and has no pathologic importance.

Manifestations

With conductive hearing loss, there is an equal loss of hearing at all sound frequencies. If the level of sound is greater than the threshold for hearing, speech discrimination is good. Because of this, the patient with a conductive hearing loss benefits from amplification by a hearing aid.

Sensorineural hearing losses typically affect the ability to hear high-frequency tones more than low-frequency tones. This loss makes speech discrimination difficult, especially in a noisy environment. Hearing aids may not be useful because they amplify both speech and background noise. The increased sound intensity may actually cause discomfort for the patient.

With presbycusis, higher-pitched tones and conversational speech are lost initially. Hearing aids and other amplification devices are useful for most patients with presbycusis.

Because the hearing loss of presbycusis is gradual, the patient and family may not realize the extent of the deficit. The individual with impaired hearing may be described as unsociable or paranoid. The family may worry that the person is becoming increasingly forgetful, absentminded, or perhaps "senile." Depression, confusion, inattentiveness, tension, and negativism have been noted in older adults with hearing impairments. Functional problems such as poor general health, reduced mobility, and impaired interpersonal communication are also associated with hearing loss. Caregivers need to be alert for signs of impaired hearing such as cupping an ear, difficulty understanding verbal communication when the person cannot see the speaker's face, difficulty following conversation in a large group, and withdrawal from social activities.

Tinnitus that is intermittent or slight enough to be masked by environmental sounds is often well tolerated. When it is loud, continuous, and not responsive to treatment, tinnitus can be a significant stressor. It can interfere with ADLs, sleep, and rest.

Interprofessional Care

The best treatment for hearing loss is prevention. Patients need to know the risk for hearing damage and how to prevent it. Awareness of the effects of noise exposure, especially when combined with the ototoxic effects of aspirin or other drugs, is important to prevent sensorineural hearing loss.

Diagnosis

Hearing evaluation includes gross tests of hearing (such as the whisper test), the Rinne and Weber tests, and audiometry.

- ***Rinne and Weber tests*** compare air and bone sound conduction. When bone conduction of sound is better than air conduction, the hearing deficit is a conductive loss. The Rinne test can identify even mild conductive hearing losses. If both air and bone conduction are impaired, a sensorineural loss is indicated.
- ***Audiometry*** identifies the type and pattern of hearing loss. Specific sound frequencies are presented to each ear by either air or bone conduction.
- ***Speech audiometry*** identifies the intensity at which speech can be recognized and interpreted. ***Speech discrimination*** evaluates the ability to discriminate among various speech sounds.
- ***Tympanometry*** is an indirect measurement of the compliance and impedance of the middle ear to sound transmission. The external auditory meatus is subjected

to neutral, positive, and negative air pressure while the resultant sound energy flow is monitored.

- *Acoustic reflex testing* uses a tone presented at various intensities to evaluate movement of the structures of the middle ear.

Amplification

A hearing aid or other amplification device can help many patients with hearing deficits. These assistive devices do nothing to prevent, minimize, or treat the hearing loss itself. They amplify the sound presented to the hearing apparatus of the ear, which may bring the level of sound above the hearing threshold, allowing more accurate perception and interpretation of its meaning. When sound perception is distorted, a hearing aid may be less helpful because it simply amplifies the distorted sound.

Unfortunately, less than one-fifth of older patients with a hearing deficit have or use a hearing aid. Denial of the deficit, other health problems, poor visual acuity, decreased manual dexterity, and cost all contribute to this low usage. Hearing aids must be individually prescribed by an audiologist. Proper design, proper fit, and regular maintenance are necessary for their effectiveness.

All hearing aids include a microphone, amplifier, speaker, earpiece, and volume control. Most allow volume control, reduce background noise, and can be adjusted for the patient's pattern of hearing loss. Behind the ear and in-ear aids often include a telecoil, which amplifies sound from the telephone without feedback. These models may also allow direct audio input (e.g., from an MP3 player) or include Bluetooth capability for hands-free telephone use. Hearing aids are available in a variety of styles, each with advantages and disadvantages, as summarized in **Table 46.4**.

Table 46.4 Types of Hearing Aids

Type	Uses	Advantages	Disadvantages
Completely in canal	Mild to moderately severe hearing loss	■ Nearly invisible ■ Allows telephone use ■ Can be worn during exercise	■ Require good manual dexterity to insert, clean, and replace batteries
In the canal 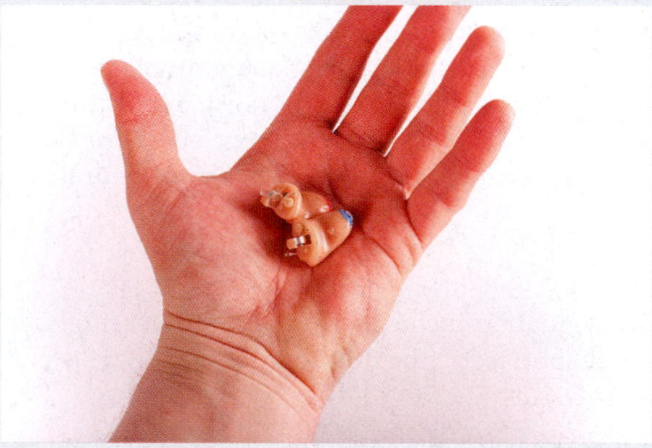	Mild to moderately severe hearing loss	■ Barely visible ■ Allows telephone use ■ May be worn during exercise ■ May include directional microphone depending on size of ear canal	■ Short battery life ■ Ear canal may feel plugged, causing discomfort ■ Too small for directional microphone ■ Vulnerable to wax and moisture
In the ear 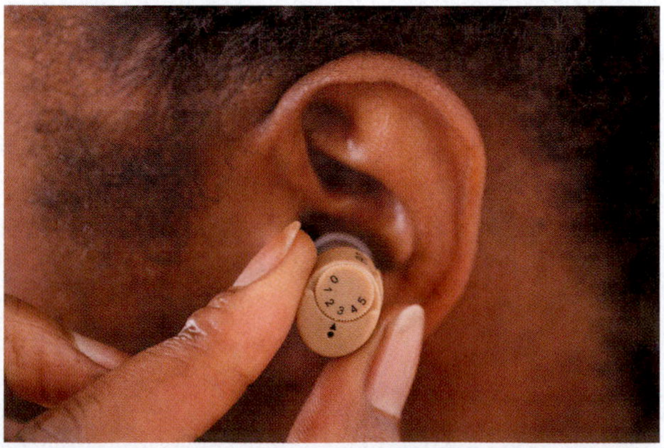	Mild to severe hearing loss	■ Allows greater amplification than canal hearing aids ■ Size allows features such as telecoil, directional microphone, and volume control ■ May be more comfortable than in-canal aids	■ More visible ■ May be difficult to manipulate for less dexterous individuals ■ Vulnerable to wax and moisture

Type	Uses	Advantages	Disadvantages
Behind the ear with earmold 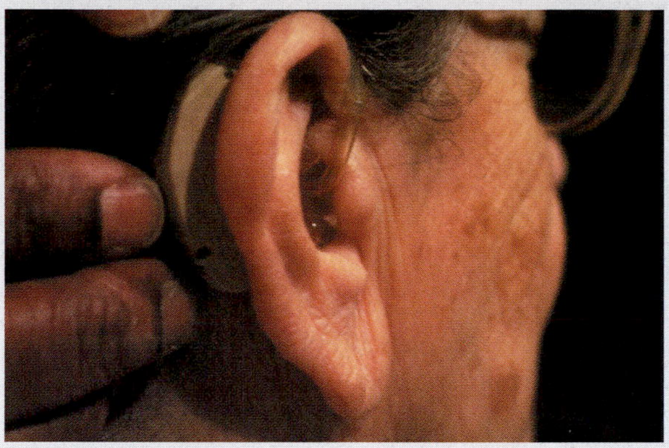	Mild to profound hearing loss	■ Most versatile and reliable ■ Allows finer amplification level adjustments ■ Easier to manipulate ■ Can be incorporated into temple of eyeglasses	■ Most visible ■ Earmold is vulnerable to wax and moisture ■ Earmold can cause canal to feel plugged and uncomfortable
Behind the ear open-fit	Mild to profound hearing loss	■ Comfortable, less visible ■ Works well in loud social settings ■ Less likely to be damaged by wax or cause ear canal to feel plugged	■ Manual controls are limited
Assistive listening device	Mild to profound hearing loss	■ May be used alone or with hearing aids or cochlear implants ■ Does not require a prescription ■ Helps separate speech from background noise or facilitate hearing when speaker is farther away ■ Can be used with telecoil, headphones, or earbuds	■ Requires separate amplifier unit

With both the in-canal and in-ear styles, cleaning is important. Small portals may become plugged with cerumen, interfering with sound transmission.

Patients with tinnitus may find a white-noise masking device helpful to promote concentration and rest. These devices conduct a pleasant sound to the affected ear, allowing the patient to block out the abnormal sound.

Surgery

Reconstructive surgeries of the middle ear, such as a stapedectomy or tympanoplasty, may help restore hearing with a conductive hearing loss. *Stapedectomy* is the removal and replacement of the stapes. This procedure is used to treat hearing loss related to otosclerosis.

In a *tympanoplasty*, the structures of the middle ear are reconstructed to improve conductive hearing deficits. Chronic otitis media with necrosis and scarring of the middle ear is a common indication for this type of surgery.

A device to strengthen sound vibrations is surgically attached to one of the ossicles in a middle ear implant. An external audio processor worn behind the ear transmits signals directly to the implant, bypassing the ear canal and tympanic membrane.

For the patient with a sensorineural hearing loss, a *cochlear implant* may be the only hope for restoring sound perception (NIDCD, 2017b). The cochlear implant consists of a microphone, speech processor, transmitter, receiver/stimulator, and electrodes (**Figure 46.19** ■). Its function is more similar to the way the ear normally receives and processes sounds than it is to a hearing aid. The microphone picks up sounds, sending them to the speech processor,

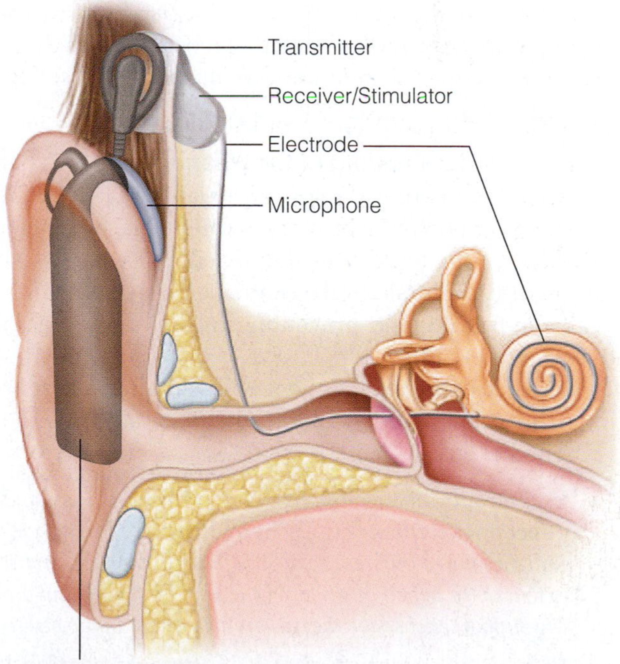
Transmitter
Receiver/Stimulator
Electrode
Microphone
Speech processor

Figure 46.19 ■ A cochlear implant for hearing loss.

which selects and processes useful sounds. The transmitter and receiver/stimulator receive signals from the speech processor, convert them to electrical impulses, and send these impulses to the electrodes for transmission to the brain.

Cochlear implants provide sound perception but not normal hearing. The patient is able to recognize warning sounds such as automobiles, sirens, telephones, and doors opening or closing. The implants also receive stimuli to alert them to incoming communication so they can focus on the person speaking. Many patients learn to interpret perceived sounds as words, especially when the hearing loss is acquired as an adult.

Nursing Care

In planning and implementing nursing care for the patient with a hearing deficit, the type and extent of hearing loss, the patient's adaptation to the loss, and the availability of assistive hearing devices are considered, as well as the patient's ability and willingness to use assistive devices.

Assessment

- ***Health history:*** Perceived ability to hear; effect of hearing loss on function and lifestyle; risk factors such as use of ototoxic medications, upper respiratory or ear infections, or noise exposure; presence of vertigo, tinnitus, unsteadiness, or imbalance
- ***Physical assessment:*** Apparent perception of normal speech; inspection of external ear, tympanic membrane; whisper, Rinne, and Weber tests; tests of balance and cranial nerve function.

Priorities of Care

In addition to health promotion activities to reduce the risk of hearing loss, the nurse's focus for the patient with a hearing impairment includes problems associated with the hearing deficit, impaired communication, and social isolation.

Diagnoses, Interventions, and Outcomes

Promote Understanding of the Hearing Loss. Whether the patient's hearing deficit is partial or total, impaired sound perception is the primary problem. The patient needs to understand what causes the deficit and what to expect for the future. Nursing interventions focus on maximizing available hearing and preventing further deterioration to the extent possible.

Expected Outcome: Patient will verbalize understanding of hearing loss, its evaluation, and management.

The nurse will:

- Encourage discussion about the hearing loss and its effect on activities of daily living. *Hearing loss affects each individual in a different way. The patient may be denying the extent of the deficit or grieving the loss. Listening and providing support encourage the patient to develop coping strategies.*
- Provide information about the type of hearing loss. Refer to an audiologist for evaluation of the hearing loss and possible exploration of amplification devices. *With improved understanding of the deficit, the patient can plan ways to compensate.*
- Replace batteries in hearing aids regularly and as needed. *Hearing aid batteries last approximately 1 week. If a battery is old or has been improperly stored, the life may be reduced further.*
- If the hearing aid has a toggle switch for microphone/telephone, be sure it is in the appropriate position. *This ensures proper amplification with the hearing aid.*

SAFETY ALERT: Check hearing aids for patency, cleaning out cerumen as necessary. ■

Promote Effective Verbal Communication. A hearing deficit impairs the patient's ability to receive and interpret verbal communication. A hearing loss affects the patient's ability to follow conversations, use the telephone, and enjoy television or other forms of entertainment.

Expected Outcome: Patient will interact appropriately and express understanding of caregiver instructions.

The nurse will:

- Use the techniques outlined in **Box 46.7** to improve communication.
- Be sure patient's hearing aid is properly placed, is turned on, and has fresh batteries. *The patient may not be aware that the hearing aid is not functioning well.*
- Do not place intravenous catheters in the dominant hand. *The patient may need to use that hand to write.*
- Rephrase sentences when there is difficulty understanding. *Hearing losses may affect different sound tones, making some words more difficult to comprehend. Using alternative words and phrases may increase the patient's ability to perceive the message.*
- Repeat important information. *The nurse makes sure that the patient understands the information.*
- Inform other staff about the patient's hearing deficit and effective strategies for communication. *Consistent use of effective strategies for communication decreases the patient's frustration.*

Promote Socialization. The patient with impaired hearing often becomes socially isolated. This isolation may be self-imposed because of difficulty communicating, especially in a group. Often, however, the isolation comes about gradually and without intention. The patient finds social settings such as family dinners or community gatherings increasingly difficult. Friends and family become frustrated trying to communicate with someone who has a hearing impairment, and invitations to participate in social activities dwindle.

Expected Outcome: Patient will engage appropriately in social activities.

The nurse will:

- Identify the extent and cause of the social isolation. Help to differentiate the reality of the isolation and its cause from the patient's perception of isolation. *Patients with impaired hearing may be unaware that they are isolated. Identifying factors that contribute to isolation may provide the needed impetus to remedy the hearing loss. Patients may also experience paranoid thinking as a result of impaired*

BOX 46.7

Techniques for Communicating with Patients with Hearing Loss

- Wave the hand or tap the shoulder before beginning to speak.
- If the patient wears hearing aids, ensure that they are clean and encourage the patient to wear them.
- When speaking, face your patient and keep your hands away from your face.
- Keep your face in full light.
- Reduce the noise in the environment before speaking.
- Use a low voice pitch with normal loudness.
- Use short sentences and pause at the end of each sentence.
- Speak at a normal rate, and do not overarticulate.
- Use facial expressions or gestures.
- Provide paper or electronic tablet for written communication.

Note that individuals with hearing impairments often lip-read, making good visibility of the speaker's face necessary. Excessive environmental noise interferes with the ability to perceive the message. Higher tones are typically lost with presbycusis and other types of hearing loss. Using short sentences and pausing give the patient time to interpret the message. Overarticulating makes it more difficult to follow the flow and to lip-read. Nonverbal cues and written messages enhance the patient's understanding.

communication and believe that friends and family have purposely begun to avoid interactions.

- Encourage to interact with friends and family on a one-to-one basis in quiet settings. *Patients with impaired hearing are more successful in understanding conversations that take place in small groups and quiet settings.*
- Treat with dignity and remind friends and family that a hearing deficit does not indicate loss of mental faculties. *Inappropriate responses due to a hearing deficit can cause others to perceive the patient as "stupid" or demented.*
- Involve in activities that do not require acute hearing, such as checkers and chess. *The patient has an opportunity to interact socially without the stress of straining to hear.*
- Refer the patient to an audiologist for evaluation and possible hearing aid fitting.
- Refer to resources such as support groups and senior citizen centers. *These groups provide new social outlets.*

Transitions of Care

Healthcare personnel can be instrumental in the early identification of hearing loss and in preventing hearing loss through education. It is important to promote environmental noise control and the use of ear protection. The Occupational Safety and Health Administration requires ear protection for work environments that consistently exceed 85 decibels. Teaching for primary prevention focuses on the following:

- Care of the ears and ear canals, including cleaning and treatment of infection
- Not placing objects into the ear canal
- Use of plugs to protect the ears during swimming or diving
- Avoiding intermittent or frequent exposure to loud noise
- Monitoring for side effects with ototoxic medications
- Hearing evaluation when hearing difficulty is present.

Teaching for home and community-based care for the patient with hearing loss focuses on managing the deficit and developing coping strategies. Referral to an audiologist for evaluation of the deficit and the usefulness of a hearing aid may be appropriate. In addition, discuss the following topics as appropriate for each patient:

- Use, care, and maintenance of a hearing aid
- Strategies for coping with the hearing deficit
- Voicing a preference for individual visits and small group interactions rather than large social functions
- Helpful resources include:
  a. American Academy of Audiology
  b. American Speech-Language-Hearing Association
  c. House Ear Institute
  d. National Institute on Deafness and Other Communication Disorders
  e. National Deaf Education Center
  f. Self-Help for Hard of Hearing People.

CHAPTER HIGHLIGHTS

46.1 Eye Disorders

Describe the pathophysiology and manifestations of eye disorders, and outline the interprofessional care and nursing care of patients with these disorders.

- Structures of the external eye are vulnerable to trauma and infection. Although usually minor, these problems can cause significant pain, scarring and clouding of the cornea, and loss or impairment of vision.
- Cataracts, glaucoma, age-related macular degeneration, and diabetic retinopathy are leading causes of visual impairment in the United States. Although these conditions cannot, in most cases, be prevented, they often can be treated or their progress slowed, preserving vision.

- Age, smoking, diabetes, radiation (sun exposure), and long-term use of certain drugs are risk factors for cataract development. Removal of the clouded lens with insertion of an intraocular lens is the treatment of choice for cataracts. Surgery is elective, performed only when the cataract significantly impairs the ability to maintain ADLs and recreational activities.
- Glaucoma is progressive loss of visual fields associated with increased intraocular pressure and impaired aqueous humor drainage. Open-angle or chronic glaucoma, the predominant form of the disorder, has few symptoms, making regular vision exams an important factor to preserve vision. It can be controlled using medications and, as needed, laser surgery to promote aqueous humor drainage.
- Angle-closure glaucoma is a medical emergency requiring immediate treatment to lower intraocular pressure to preserve vision. Angle-closure glaucoma usually affects only one eye; however, the patient is at risk for future attacks affecting the other eye.
- Age-related macular degeneration, a leading cause of blindness, cannot be effectively treated, although its progress may be slowed or halted through use of high-dose antioxidant vitamins and zinc if it is identified early. Macular degeneration affects the macula, the area of high-acuity central vision.
- Diabetic retinopathy eventually affects nearly all people with diabetes. It is a disease of the small blood vessels of the retina, leading to formation of aneurysms, retinal ischemia, and growth of fragile new vessels (neovascularization) that easily rupture, leading to hemorrhage. It is treated with laser surgery to seal fragile vessels.

46.2 Ear Disorders

Describe the pathophysiology and manifestations of ear disorders, and outline the interprofessional care and nursing care of patients with these disorders.

- Disruption of the integrity of any portion of the auditory pathway from the external ear through neural transmission to auditory centers of the brain can impact an individual's ability to hear and interpret sounds. Health promotion activities and prompt treatment of disorders are important measures to preserve hearing.
- Otitis media is related to auditory tube dysfunction, with impaired pressure equalization of the middle ear. Otitis media may be either serous (sterile) or infectious. Both cause acute discomfort with diminished hearing, snapping, popping, and possible vertigo and systemic symptoms. The risk of complications, including rupture of the tympanic membrane, damage to structures of the middle ear, and spread of infection to surrounding tissues, is greater with acute otitis media.
- Potential complications of acute otitis media include mastoiditis, chronic otitis media with tympanic membrane perforation, and cholesteatoma formation. Hearing loss in the affected ear is a possibility with these disorders. The primary treatment is prevention through adequate treatment of acute otitis media.
- Inner ear disorders can affect the perception of sound as well as equilibrium. When balance is affected, the patient is at significant risk for injury, making safety a nursing care priority.
- The primary manifestations of disorders of the inner ear are vertigo and possible hearing loss. Severe vertigo can interfere with safety, nutrition, and the patient's ability to maintain ADLs and life roles.
- Hearing loss affects people of all ages, although older adults are disproportionately affected. Impaired hearing significantly affects the ability to communicate, making it a major public health problem. Despite its prevalence, impaired hearing is often undiagnosed and untreated.
- The two major types of hearing loss are conductive and sensorineural. Presbycusis, hearing loss associated with aging, is a type of sensorineural hearing loss. Hearing loss may be accompanied by tinnitus, the perception of sound without an environmental stimulus. Amplification devices (hearing aids) are the primary treatment for hearing loss.

TEST YOURSELF NCLEX-RN® REVIEW

1. The nurse is caring for a group of residents in a long-term care facility, all of whom have moderate to severe hearing or vision impairment. What should the nurse identify as the highest priority of care for these residents?
   A. Maintaining resident safety
   B. Encouraging social interaction
   C. Promoting family relationships
   D. Preventing sensory deprivation
2. The nurse is teaching a patient with newly diagnosed glaucoma about the disease process. What should the nurse emphasize when teaching this patient?
   A. Contact the physician if further decline in vision is noticed.
   B. Use the prescribed eyedrops as directed on a continuing basis.
   C. Avoid coughing, sneezing, or straining to have a bowel movement.
   D. Turn the head side to side to compensate for impaired peripheral vision.

3. A patient with a history coronary artery disease and resultant of heart failure is prescribed medication for glaucoma. Which medication should the nurse question before providing to the patient? (Select all the apply.)
   A. timolol (Timoptic)
   B. latanoprost (Xalatan)
   C. dorzolamide (Trusopt)
   D. brimonidine (Alphagan)
   E. betaxolol (Betoptic)
4. The nurse is instructing a patient with Ménière disease on ways to prevent attacks of vertigo and tinnitus. What should the nurse include in this teaching? (Select all that apply.)
   A. Stop smoking.
   B. Follow a low-sodium diet.
   C. Avoid caffeine and alcohol.
   D. Sit down when an attack develops.
   E. Take prescribed antiemetic medications.
5. A patient is brought to the recovery room after having cataract surgery. Which action should the nurse immediately perform for this patient?
   A. Place the patient in a private room.
   B. Position the patient on the affected side.
   C. Place the patient in semi-Fowler position.
   D. Ensure the patient is in proximity to the nurses' station.
6. A patient is experiencing bright flashing lights throughout the field of vision. What is the most appropriate response by the nurse?
   A. Initiate immediate referral to an ophthalmologist.
   B. Advise to make an appointment to have blood pressure checked.
   C. Recommend the patient lie down until the sensation has passed.
   D. Reassure that this is not unusual and should resolve without treatment.
7. A patient is experiencing right ear pain. What should be included in the physical assessment of this patient? (Select all that apply.)
   A. Vital signs with temperature
   B. Manipulation of the ear pinna
   C. Inspection of the oral pharynx
   D. Palpation of cervical lymph nodes
   E. Inspection of the retina and cornea
8. An older patient is experiencing head stuffiness and ringing in the ears. What should the nurse do to help this patient?
   A. Notify the primary care physician.
   B. Inspect the ear canals for patency.
   C. Refer for evaluation by an audiologist.
   D. Provide nonprescription eardrops for daily use.
9. The nurse is caring for a patient with a severe hearing deficit. Which would be an appropriate goal to improve the patient's social interaction?
   A. Attend religious services of choice.
   B. Plan to have dinner with one or two friends weekly.
   C. Engage in activities such as card tournaments and dancing.
   D. Participate in senior center communal lunches at least twice per week.
10. During an assessment the nurse notes an absence of the red reflex in the patient's right eye. When questioned the patient responds that cataracts have been diagnosed and asks when they should be removed. How should the nurse respond? (Select all that apply.)
    A. "It appears that the right eye is due for surgery."
    B. "Cataracts can be removed any time that it is convenient for you."
    C. "Are you having difficulty reading or doing activities you enjoy?"
    D. "Are you starting to experience pain in your right eye or frequent headaches?"
    E. "Are you noticing a greater reduction in your vision?"

See Test Yourself answers in Appendix B.

REFERENCES

Adams, M. P., Holland, L. N., & Urban, C. (2017). *Pharmacology for nursing: A pathophysiologic approach* (5th ed.). Hoboken, NJ: Pearson Education.

American Academy of Ophthalmology. (2017). *Eye health statistics.* Retrieved from https://www.aao.org/newsroom/eye-health-statistics

Glaucoma Research Foundation. (2017). *Glaucoma facts and stats.* Retrieved from https://www.glaucoma.org/glaucoma/glaucoma-facts-and-stats.php.

Glaucoma Research Foundation. (2018). *The genetics of glaucoma.* Retrieved from https://www.glaucoma.org/glaucoma/the-genetics-of-glaucoma-what-is-new.php.

Kee, J. L. (2018). *Laboratory and diagnostic tests with nursing implications* (10th ed.). Hoboken, NJ: Pearson Education.

National Eye Institute (NEI). (2017a). *Age-related macular degeneration.* Retrieved from https://nei.nih.gov/health/maculardegen.

National Eye Institute (NEI). (2017b). *Cornea and corneal disease.* Retrieved from https://nei.nih.gov/health/cornea.

National Eye Institute (NEI). (2017c). *Data and statistics.* Retrieved from https://www.nei.nih.gov/eyedata.

National Eye Institute (NEI). (2017d). *Diabetic eye disease.* Retrieved from https://nei.nih.gov/health/diabetic.

National Eye Institute (NEI). (2017e). *Homepage.* Retrieved from https://www.nei.nih.gov.

National Federation of the Blind. (2017). *Blindness and low vision.* Retrieved from https://nfb.org/fact-sheet-blindness-and-low-vision.

National Institute on Deafness and Other Communication Disorders (NIDCD). (2017a). *Assistive devices for people with hearing, voice, speech, or language disorders.* Retrieved from http://www.nidcd.nih.gov/health/hearing/pages/Assistive-Devices.aspx.

National Institute on Deafness and Other Communication Disorders (NIDCD). (2017b). *Cochlear implants.* Retrieved from https://www.nidcd.nih.gov/health/cochlear-implants.

National Institute on Deafness and Other Communication Disorders (NIDCD). (2017c). *Ménière's disease.* Retrieved from https://www.nidcd.nih.gov/health/menieres-disease.

National Institute on Deafness and Other Communication Disorders (NIDCD). (2017d). *Statistics and epidemiology.* Retrieved from https://www.nidcd.nih.gov/health/statistics.

National Institute on Deafness and Other Communication Disorders (NIDCD). (2017e). *Vestibular Schwannoma.* Retrieved from https://www.nidcd.nih.gov/health/vestibular-schwannoma-acoustic-neuroma-and-neurofibromatosis.

Shearer, A. E., Hildebrand, M. S., & Smith, R. J. H. (2017). *Hereditary hearing loss and deafness overview.* Retrieved from https://www.ncbi.nlm.nih.gov/books/NBK1434/.

Sorenson, M., Quinn, L., & Klein, D. (2019). *Pathophysiology: Concepts of human disease.* Hoboken, NJ: Pearson Education.

ADDITIONAL RESOURCES

American Academy of Audiology
www.audiology.org

Genetics Home Reference
https://ghr.nlm.nih.gov

National Eye Institute
www.nei.nih.gov

National Institute on Deafness and Other Communication Disorders
https://www.nidcd.nih.gov

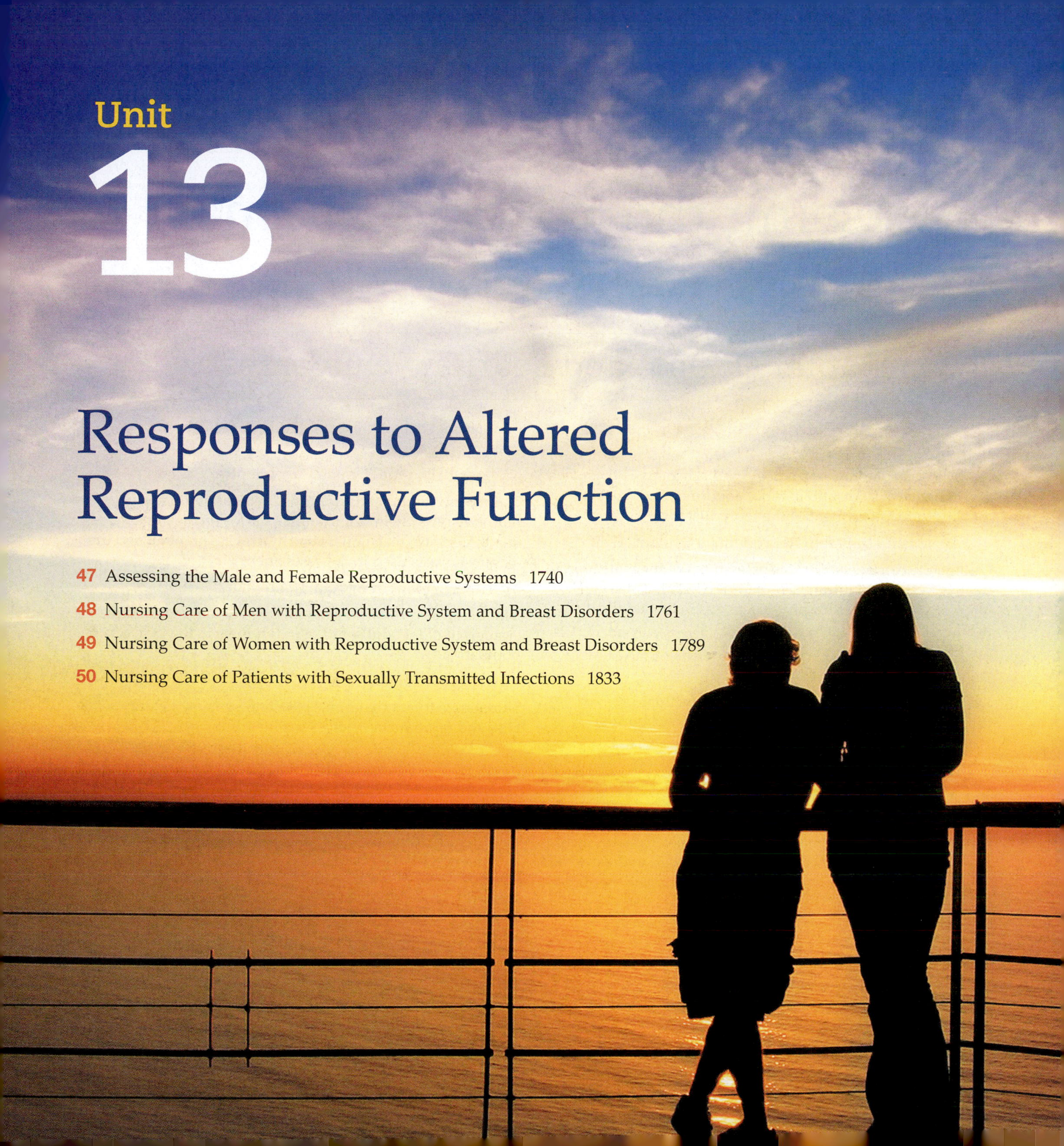

Unit 13

Responses to Altered Reproductive Function

Chapter 47

Assessing the Male and Female Reproductive Systems

Chapter Outline and Learning Outcomes

47.1 Anatomy, Physiology, and Functions of the Male Reproductive System 1741

Describe the anatomy, physiology, and functions of the male reproductive system, and identify abnormal findings that may indicate impairment of the reproductive system.

47.2 Assessing the Male Reproductive System 1742

Outline the components of the assessment of the male reproductive system, including topics for the health assessment interview, techniques for physical assessment, and the diagnostic tests used in the assessment.

47.3 Anatomy, Physiology, and Functions of the Female Reproductive System 1745

Describe the anatomy, physiology, and functions of the female eproductive system, and identify abnormal findings that may indicate impairment of the reproductive system.

47.4 Assessing the Female Reproductive System 1747

Outline the components of the assessment of the female reproductive system, including topics for the health assessment interview, techniques for physical assessment, and the diagnostic tests used in the assessment.

47.5 Assessment of Special Populations 1756

Differentiate considerations for assessing the reproductive systems of older adults and of individuals in the LGBTQI population.

47.6 Health Promotion 1757

Summarize topics that nurses teach to promote healthy sexuality and reproduction across the lifespan.

CLINICAL COMPETENCIES

- Assess male and female reproductive health status including physical comfort, values, preferences, and expressed needs.
- Identify, report, and document normal, abnormal, and unexpected assessments of the male and female reproductive systems.

KEY TERMS

androgens, 1742
anorgasmia, 1748
cis-gender, 1757
dyspareunia, 1748
estrogens, 1747
gender expression, 1757
gender identity, 1756
gynecomastia, 1743
impotence, 1742
menstrual cycle, 1747
menstruation, 1746
phimosis, 1743
progesterone, 1747
semen, 1741
testosterone, 1742
transgender, 1756

EQUIPMENT NEEDED

- Disposable gloves
- Water-soluble lubricant
- A good light source
- Sterile cotton swabs (for culture)
- Culture media (for culture)
- An endocervical brush and medium (for Pap test)
- Vaginal speculum of appropriate size

The reproductive organs in men and women share the functions of enabling sexual pleasure and reproduction. The reproductive organs, in conjunction with the neuroendocrine system, produce hormones important in biologic development and sexual behavior. Parts of the reproductive organs in men enclose and are integral to the function of the urinary system. The assessment of the reproductive system may be difficult for both the nurse and the patient and requires sensitivity on the part of the nurse when asking questions about topics that the patient may be hesitant to talk about. Skill in conducting physical examinations of an area of the body usually considered private is also required. The nurse must also respect the patient's sexual identity. Transgender patients may or may not have had gender reassignment surgery. Thus, while the patient identifies with one gender, there may be physiologic and anatomic concerns of the other gender that need to be addressed. When assessing the reproductive system, sensitivity and understanding of the patient's identity is important. Throughout the assessment, it is important to use the patient's chosen name and refer to them by their chosen pronoun. This is especially true for transgender patients (Eckstrand & Ehrenfeld, 2016).

47.1 Anatomy, Physiology, and Functions of the Male Reproductive System

The male reproductive system consists of the paired testes, the scrotum, ducts, glands, and penis (**Figure 47.1** ■). The breasts are also part of the male reproductive system.

The Breasts

The male breast is comprised primarily of an areola (circular pigmented area) and a small nipple. These lie over a thin disk of undeveloped breast tissue that may not be overtly different from surrounding tissue. Approximately one in three men have a firm area of breast tissue 2 cm or larger; the limits of normal size of this area have not been established. Some men have overdeveloped breasts, a condition called *gynecomastia*.

The Penis

The *penis* is the genital organ that encloses the urethra. It is homologous to the clitoris of the female. The penis is composed of a shaft and a tip called the *glans*, which is covered in the uncircumcised man by the *foreskin* (or *prepuce*). *Erection* of the penis occurs when erectile tissue is filled with blood in response to a reflex that triggers the parasympathetic nervous system to stimulate arteriolar vasodilation. The erection reflex may be initiated by touch, pressure, sights, sounds, smells, or thoughts of a sexual encounter. After ejaculation, the arterioles vasoconstrict, and the penis becomes flaccid.

The Scrotum

The *scrotum* hangs at the base of the penis, anterior to the anus, and regulates the temperature of the testes. The optimum temperature for sperm production is about 2 to 3 degrees below body temperature. When the testicular temperature is too low, the scrotum contracts to bring the testes up against the body. When the testicular temperature is too high, the scrotum relaxes to allow the testes to lie farther away from the body.

The Testes

The *testes* develop in the abdominal cavity of the fetus and then descend through the inguinal canal into the scrotum just before birth. They are homologous to the ovaries in females. These paired organs are each about 4 cm (1.5 in.) long and 2.5 cm (1 in.) in diameter. Each testis is divided into 250 to 300 lobules, with each lobule containing one to four seminiferous tubules. The testes produce sperm and testosterone. The *seminiferous tubules* are responsible for sperm production. *Leydig cells* (or *interstitial cells*) lie in the connective tissue surrounding the seminiferous tubules and produce testosterone. It is not unusual for one testes to be lower than the other.

The Ducts and Semen

The seminiferous tubules lead into the efferent ducts and become the rete testis. From the rete testis, 10,000 to 20,000 efferent ducts join the epididymis, a long coiled tube that lies over the outer surface of each testis. The *epididymis* is the final area for the storage and maturation of sperm. When a man is sexually excited, the epididymis contracts to propel the sperm through the vas deferens to the ampulla, where the sperm are stored until ejaculation.

The seminal vesicles produce most of the volume of seminal fluid. Seminal fluid is also made of secretions from the accessory sex organs, the epididymis, the prostate gland, and Cowper glands. Seminal fluid nourishes the sperm, provides bulk, and increases its alkalinity. An alkaline pH is essential to mobilize the sperm and ensure fertilization of the ova. Sperm mixed with this fluid is called **semen**. Each seminal vesicle joins its corresponding vas deferens to form an

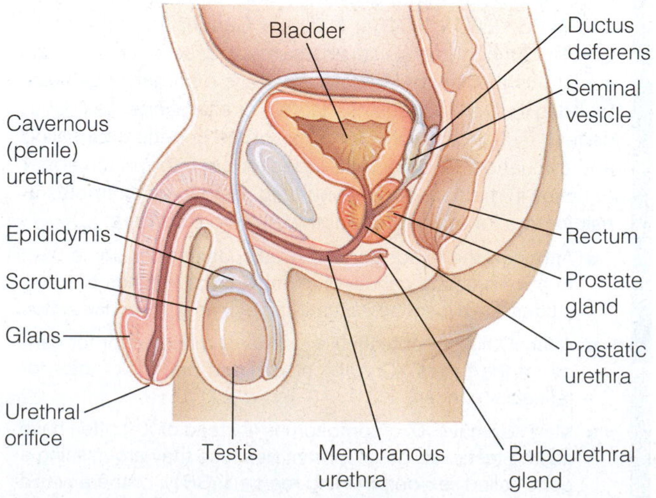

Bladder
Ductus deferens
Seminal vesicle
Cavernous (penile) urethra
Epididymis
Scrotum
Glans
Urethral orifice
Testis
Membranous urethra
Bulbourethral gland
Prostatic urethra
Prostate gland
Rectum

Figure 47.1 ■ The male reproductive system.

ejaculatory duct, which enters the prostatic urethra. During ejaculation, seminal fluid mixes with sperm at the ejaculatory duct and enters the urethra for expulsion. The total amount of semen ejaculated is 2 to 6 mL, although the amount varies. The total ejaculate of a healthy male contains from 20 million to 150 million sperm per milliliter.

The Prostate Gland

The *prostate gland* is about the size of a walnut. It encircles the urethra just below the urinary bladder and is surrounded by smooth muscle. Secretions of the prostate gland make up about one-third of the volume of the semen. These secretions enter the urethra through several ducts during ejaculation. Prostatic fluid helps activate sperm and has antibiotic properties thought to help prevent urinary tract infections in men.

Male Sex Hormones

The male sex hormones are called **androgens**. Most androgens are produced in the testes, although the adrenal cortex also produces a small amount. **Testosterone**, the primary androgen produced by the testes, is essential for the development and maintenance of sexual organs and secondary sex characteristics and for spermatogenesis. It also promotes metabolism, growth of muscles and bone, and libido (sexual desire) (Sorenson, Quinn, & Klein, 2019).

47.2 Assessing the Male Reproductive System

The structures and functions of the male reproductive system are assessed by a health assessment interview to collect subjective data, a physical assessment to collect objective data, and findings from diagnostic tests.

Health Assessment Interview

A health assessment interview to determine problems with the male reproductive system may be conducted during a health screening, may focus on a chief complaint (such as a discharge from the penis), or may be part of a total health assessment. Men may be embarrassed to discuss health problems or concerns involving their reproductive organs; it is important for the nurse to ask questions in a nonthreatening, matter-of-fact manner. Consider the psychologic, social, and cultural factors that affect sexuality and sexual activity. Use words that the man can understand, and do not be embarrassed or offended by the words he uses. The man may perceive the interview as less threatening if the discussion begins with more general questions and then progresses to specific questions, and if questions are asked in a way that gives him permission to describe behaviors and manifestations. For example, rather than asking a man if he has difficulty achieving or maintaining an erection, ask him to describe any changes he has noticed in his erections.

If the man has a reproductive health problem, analyze its onset, characteristics and course, severity, precipitating and relieving factors, and any associated symptoms, noting the timing and circumstances. For example, you may ask the man the following questions:

- "When did you first notice that you were having difficulty urinating?"
- "Did you use a different brand of condoms before you noticed the rash on your penis?"
- "Describe the changes that occurred in your ability to have an erection after you started taking medicine for high blood pressure."

In questioning the man about past medical history, ask about chronic illnesses such as diabetes, chronic kidney disease, cardiovascular disease, multiple sclerosis, spinal cord tumors or trauma, or thyroid disease. The effects of these illnesses as well as the treatment of the illnesses may cause **impotence** (inability to achieve or maintain an erection). The following drugs may cause erectile dysfunction: Antihypertensives, antidepressants, antispasmodics, beta-blockers, tranquilizers, sedatives, and histamine$_2$-receptor antagonists. Psychosocial stressors may also contribute to impotence.

If the man was born to a woman treated during pregnancy with diethylstilbestrol (DES), a drug used in the 1940s and 1950s to prevent miscarriage, he may have congenital deformities of the urinary tract as well as decreased semen levels. If the man had mumps as a child, sterility is possible. The risk for testicular cancer is greatest in men who have a history of an undescended testicle, an inguinal hernia, testicular swelling with mumps, a history of maternal use of DES or oral contraceptives, and a family history of testicular cancer (American Cancer Society [ACS], 2016b) (see the Genetic Considerations box).

Genetic Considerations

When conducting a health assessment interview and a physical assessment, it is important for the nurse to consider genetic influences on health of the adult. Several diseases of the male reproductive system have a genetic component. During the health assessment interview, it is especially important to ask about a family history of testicular or prostate cancer (ACS, 2016a; National Cancer Institute [NCI], 2018b). During the physical assessment, assess for any manifestations that might indicate a genetic disorder. If data are found to indicate genetic risk factors or alterations, ask about genetic testing and refer for appropriate genetic counseling and evaluation. Chapter 8 provides further information about genetics in medical-surgical nursing. Below are examples of risk factors for male reproductive system disorders.

- Although the exact genetic predisposition for some men to have prostate cancer is unknown, the findings of many studies have identified a family history as a major risk factor.
- A family history of testicular cancer is a risk factor for cancer of the testes. (Cryptorchidism can be a risk factor for testicular cancer.)
- Men who have XX chromosomes (instead of XY) often have altered testicular development because they are missing a gene called *sex-determining region Y (SRY)*, or there was a translocation during spermogenesis and the *SRY* is found on one of the X chromosomes

Male Reproductive System Assessments

Technique/Normal Findings	Abnormal Findings
Breast and Lymph Node Assessment	
Inspect and palpate both breasts, including areola and nipple. *Breast tissue should not be swollen, tender, or enlarged (although soft, fatty, and enlarged breast tissue does occur with obesity in men).*	■ A smooth, firm, mobile, tender disk of breast tissue behind the areola indicates **gynecomastia,** abnormal enlargement of the breast(s) in men. Gynecomastia requires additional investigation to determine the cause. ■ A hard, irregular, fixed nodule in the nipple area suggests carcinoma.
Palpate the axillary and supraclavicular lymph nodes. *Lymph nodes should not be palpable.*	■ Enlarged axillary nodes are common with infections of the hand or arm but may be caused by cancer. ■ Enlarged supraclavicular nodes may indicate metastasis.
External Genitalia Assessment	
Inspect and palpate the inguinal and femoral area for bulges. Ask the man to bear down or cough as you palpate (**Figure 47.2** ■). *There should be no bulging with coughing or bearing down.*	■ A bulge that increases with coughing or straining suggests a hernia.
Inspect the penis. If the man is uncircumcised, retract the foreskin or ask him to do so. *When nonerect, the penis is normally soft, flaccid, and nontender. The foreskin should be without lesions, of color equal with the penis, and should retract easily. The glans is normally free of lesions.*	■ **Phimosis** (tightness of prepuce that prevents retraction of foreskin) may be congenital or due to recurrent balanoposthitis (generalized infection of glans penis and prepuce). ■ Narrow or inflamed foreskin can cause paraphimosis, retraction of the foreskin that causes painful swelling of the glans. ■ Balanitis (inflammation of the glans) is associated with bacterial or fungal infections. ■ Ulcers, vesicles, or warts suggest an STI. ■ Nodules or sores seen in uncircumcised men may be cancer.
Inspect the external urinary meatus. Press the glans between the thumb and forefinger (**Figure 47.3** ■). Replace the foreskin, if appropriate. *The external urinary meatus is normally in the center of the glans, without redness or discharge.*	■ Erythema or discharge indicates inflammatory disease. Further assessment is required.
Inspect the skin on the shaft of the penis. *The skin on the shaft of the penis should be free of redness or lesions.*	■ Excoriation or inflammation suggests lice or scabies.
Palpate the shaft of the penis. *The shaft of the penis should not be tender.*	■ Induration with tenderness along the ventral surface suggests urethral stricture with inflammation.
Inspect the scrotum. Further assess any swelling in the scrotum using transillumination: Darken the room and place a lighted flashlight against the skin of the scrotum. *The normal scrotum and epididymis appear as dark masses with regular borders.*	■ A poorly developed unilateral or bilateral scrotum suggests cryptorchidism (failure of one or both testes to descend into the scrotum). ■ Swelling of the scrotum may indicate indirect inguinal hernia, hydrocele (accumulation of fluid in the scrotum), or scrotal edema. Swellings containing serous fluid will transilluminate. Swellings containing blood or tissue will not transilluminate.
Palpate each testis and epididymis. *The testes should not be tender or swollen.*	■ Tender, painful scrotal swelling occurs in acute epididymitis, acute orchitis, torsion of the spermatic cord, and strangulated hernia. ■ A painless nodule in the testis is associated with testicular cancer.
Prostate Assessment	
The prostate gland is assessed by digital rectal examination (DRE). Refer to Figure 21.19 in Chapter 21 for the technique used to palpate the prostrate through the rectal wall. This assessment is usually conducted by a physician or advanced practice nurse.	
With a gloved index finger, palpate the posterior surface of the prostate gland. *The prostate is normally nontender, with two lateral lobes that are divided, smooth, and about 2.5 cm (1 in.) long.*	■ Enlargement (1-cm protrusion into the rectum) with obliteration of the median sulcus suggests benign prostatic hypertrophy. ■ Enlargement with asymmetry and tenderness suggests prostatitis. ■ A hard irregular nodule is suspicious of carcinoma.

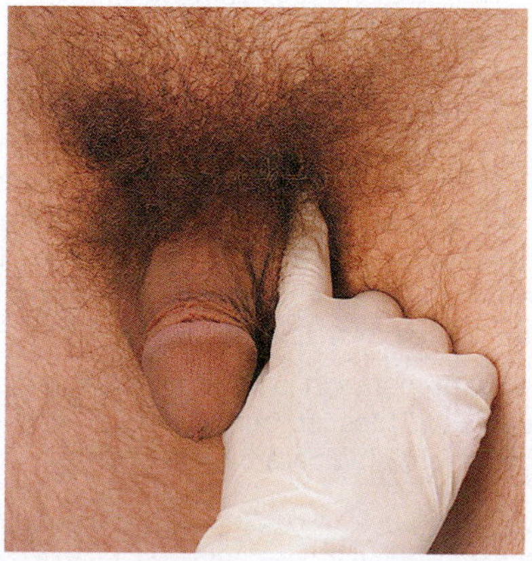

Figure 47.2 ■ Palpating the male inguinal area for bulges.

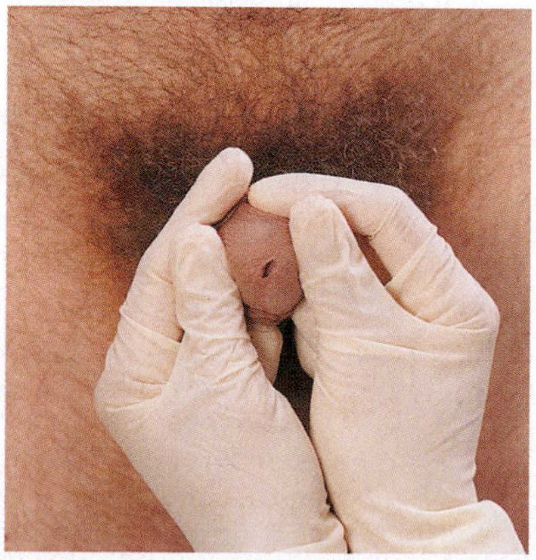

Figure 47.3 ■ Inspecting the external urinary meatus of the male.

Explore the lifestyle and social history of the man; the use of alcohol, cigarettes, or street drugs may affect sexual function. Unprotected sexual intercourse increases the potential for sexually transmitted infections (STIs) including HIV infection. Ask about sexual preference. Sexual intercourse with same-sex partners further increases the risk for HIV infection. Other questions about sexuality may include number of sexual partners; history of premature ejaculation, impotence, or other sexual problems; any history of sexual trauma; use of condoms or other contraceptives; and current level of sexual satisfaction.

Physical Assessment

Physical assessment of the male reproductive system may be performed as part of a total assessment or separately for men with known or suspected problems. If conducted as part of a total physical assessment, this is usually the final system to be assessed. Problems of the male reproductive system may involve the urinary system, making an assessment of both systems important (refer to Chapter 26 for assessment of the urinary system). The nurse must feel comfortable with the examination of patients of the opposite gender. If either the nurse or the patient is not comfortable, a nurse of the same gender should be asked to conduct this part of the assessment.

The male reproductive system is assessed by inspection and palpation. Explain the procedures for the examination thoroughly and in a matter-of-fact way to decrease anxiety and embarrassment. If the man is unfamiliar with his internal genitalia, charts may be used to demonstrate the parts that will be examined. Ask the man to empty his bladder, remove his clothing, and put on a gown or drape. The assessment may be done with the man sitting or standing. Expose only those body parts being examined to preserve modesty. Ensure that the examining room is warm and private. Put on gloves before beginning and wear them throughout the examination.

Diagnosis

The results of diagnostic tests of the structures and functions of the male reproductive system are used to support the diagnosis of a specific sexual problem, injury, or disease; to provide information to identify or modify the appropriate medications or treatments used to treat the disease; and to help nurses monitor the man's responses to treatment and nursing interventions. Diagnostic tests used to assess the male reproductive system are described in the Diagnostic Tests table. More information is included in the discussion of specific health problems or diseases in Chapter 48.

Regardless of the type of diagnostic test, the nurse is responsible for explaining the procedure and any special preparation needed, for assessing any medication use that might affect the outcome of the tests, for supporting the man during the examination as necessary, for ensuring the consent form is signed (if required), and for monitoring the results of the tests. The nurse is also responsible for postprocedure care and patient teaching for self-care at home (Kee, 2018).

Diagnostic Tests of the Male Reproductive System

NAME OF TEST	PURPOSE AND DESCRIPTION	RELATED NURSING INTERVENTIONS
Biopsy of the prostate	A biopsy of the prostate is conducted to help determine the cause of an elevated prostate-specific antigen (PSA) level and to diagnose cancer if a lump is found in the prostate. Various routes may be used to insert a biopsy needle into the prostate, through the rectum (transrectal), through the urethra (transurethral), or through the perineum. Transrectal ultrasound (TRUS) is often used to guide the placement of the needle during the procedure. The biopsy may be done in a physician's office, in an outpatient surgery unit or clinic, or in a hospital operating room.	Assess for a history of bleeding problems, allergies to medications, and if taking any anticoagulant medications (such as warfarin [Coumadin], heparin, enoxaparin [Lovenox], aspirin, or NSAIDs). If the biopsy is done with a local anesthetic, no other preparation is needed. If the biopsy is done transrectally, the patient may need an enema before the procedure. If the biopsy is done with general anesthesia, tell the patient he will be unable to eat or drink fluids for 8–12 h before the procedure, and that he may be given antibiotics. After the biopsy, advise the man to avoid strenuous activity for 4 hours. Explain that there may be some discomfort in the biopsy area for 1–2 days, there may be some blood in the urine or from the rectum, and semen may appear dark. Following a transurethral biopsy, a urinary catheter may remain in place for a few hours after the procedure. Excess bleeding, pain, inability to urinate, or signs of infection should be reported to the physician.
Gonorrhea culture	A culture is performed to evaluate for gonorrhea. A swab is used to collect a sample of discharge from the infected area (urethra, penis, anus, or throat), smeared on a slide, and a Gram stain is conducted to identify the organism (*Neisseria gonorrhoeae*). A urine sample is used in some tests.	No special preparation is needed. If test is positive, request referral to an STI testing center or clinic and emphasize need for treatment to eradicate the infection.

Diagnostic Tests
of the Male Reproductive System (*continued*)

NAME OF TEST	PURPOSE AND DESCRIPTION	RELATED NURSING INTERVENTIONS
Prostate-specific antigen (PSA)	A blood test used to screen for prostate cancer and to monitor treatment of prostate cancer. The American Cancer Society recommends that the decision to undergo routine prostate screening should be determined on an individual basis by the informed man and his physician. Normal value: 0–4.0 ng/mL	Inform the patient that transient increases in PSA occur following prostate palpation or rectal examinations; these procedures as well as prostate surgery should not be scheduled for 3 days before the PSA is done.
Prostate ultrasound (transrectal)	Transrectal ultrasound (TRUS) is conducted to evaluate prostate enlargement. Ultrasound is also used to identify testicular torsion or masses. Uses high-frequency sound waves, passed through tissues of various densities, to produce a visual graphic of tissue being examined.	Tell the patient to administer a Fleet enema about 1 h before the procedure (if ordered). Ask the patient to void and remove clothing from the waist down prior to the procedure. The patient may also be asked to avoid anticoagulants and antiplatelets, such as aspirin, before the procedure.
Semen analysis	Done to assess volume, motility and sperm count, and percent of abnormal sperm. *Normal values:* Volume: 1.5–5 mL Sperm count: 60–150 million/mL Motility: > 60% motile Normal forms: > 70%	Instruct the patient to refrain from use of alcohol for 24 hours and to abstain from intercourse for 3 days prior to the test. The patient is asked to bring in a fresh specimen (usually in a condom) within 2 h of ejaculation.
Syphilis screening tests ■ Venereal Disease Research Laboratory (VDRL) ■ Rapid plasma reagin (RPR) ■ Fluorescent treponemal antibody absorption (FTA-ABS)	These blood tests are conducted to screen for syphilis. Positive findings can be made within 1–2 weeks after primary lesion appears or 1–4 months after the initial infection. The FTA-ABS test is considered the most accurate and is often used if findings from the VDRL or RPR are questionable.	No special preparation is needed. If test is positive, request referral to an STI testing center or clinic and emphasize need for treatment to eradicate the infection.

47.3 Anatomy, Physiology, and Functions of the Female Reproductive System

The female reproductive system consists of the external genitalia (mons pubis, labia, clitoris, vaginal and urethral openings, and glands) and the internal organs (vagina, cervix, uterus, fallopian tubes, and ovaries). The breasts are a part of the women's reproductive organs. In women, the urethra and urinary meatus are separated from the reproductive organs; however, they are so close to each other that a health problem with one often affects the other.

The Breasts

The *breasts* (or *mammary glands*) are located between the third and seventh ribs on the anterior chest wall. They are supported by the pectoral muscles and are richly supplied with nerves, blood, and lymph (**Figure 47.4** ■). A pigmented area called the *areola* is located slightly below the center of each breast and contains sebaceous glands and a nipple. The nipple is usually protrusive and becomes erect in response to cold and stimulation. The breasts produce milk for the infant following delivery.

The breasts are made of adipose tissue, fibrous connective tissue, and glandular tissue. Cooper ligaments support the breast and extend from the outer breast tissue to the nipple, dividing the breast into 15 to 25 lobes. Each lobe is made of alveolar glands connected by ducts that open to the nipple.

The External Genitalia

The external genitalia are collectively called the *vulva*. They include the mons pubis, the labia, the clitoris, the vaginal and urethral openings, and glands (**Figure 47.5** ■).

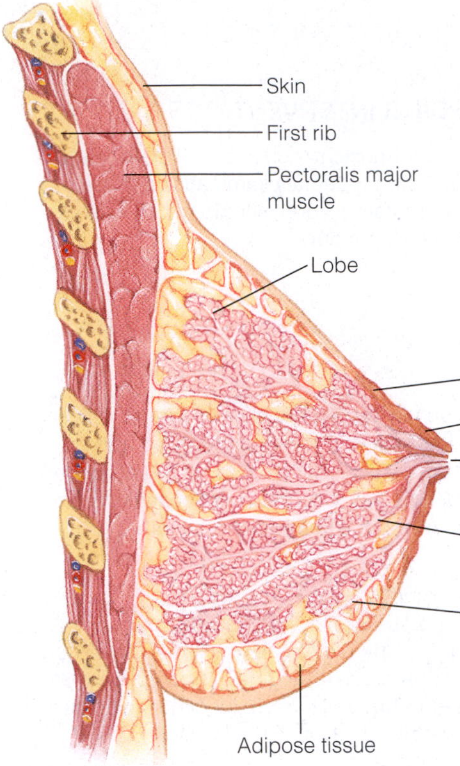
Skin
First rib
Pectoralis major muscle
Lobe
Areola
Nipple
Opening of lactiferous duct
Lactiferous duct
Suspensory ligament
Adipose tissue

Figure 47.4 ■ Structure of the female breast.

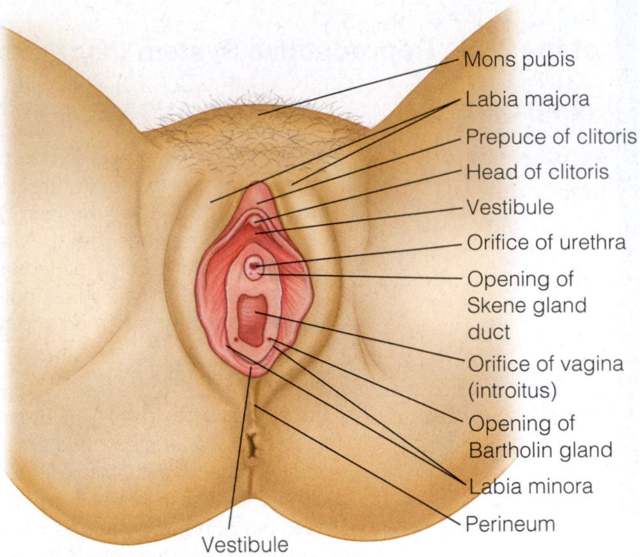
Mons pubis
Labia majora
Prepuce of clitoris
Head of clitoris
Vestibule
Orifice of urethra
Opening of Skene gland duct
Orifice of vagina (introitus)
Opening of Bartholin gland
Labia minora
Perineum
Vestibule

Figure 47.5 ■ The external organs of the female reproductive system.

The *mons pubis* is a pad of adipose (fat) tissue covered with skin and hair that lies anterior to the symphysis pubis. The labia are divided into two structures. The *labia majora*, outermost folds of skin and adipose tissue covered with hair, begin at the base of the mons pubis and end at the anus. The *labia minora*, usually light pink and hairless, are located between the clitoris and the base of the vagina and are enclosed by the labia majora.

The *vestibule* (the area between the labia) contains the openings for the vagina and the urethra as well as Bartholin and Skene glands. Prior to menopause, Bartholin and Skene glands secrete lubricating fluid during the sexual response cycle. The *clitoris* is an erectile organ analogous to the penis in the male. Like the penis, it is highly sensitive and distends during sexual arousal. The vaginal opening, called the *introitus*, is the opening between the internal and the external genitals. Prior to the first intercourse or trauma, the introitus is surrounded by a connective tissue membrane called the *hymen*. After menopause, Bartholin and Skene glands become dry because of the lack of estrogen.

The Internal Organs

The vagina, cervix, uterus, fallopian tubes, and ovaries are the internal organs of the female reproductive system (**Figure 47.6** ■). The ovaries are the primary reproductive organs in women and also produce female sex hormones. The vagina, uterus, and fallopian tubes serve as accessory ducts for the ovaries and a developing fetus.

The Vagina and Cervix

The *vagina* is a fibromuscular tube about 8 to 10 cm (3 to 4 in.) in length located posterior to the bladder and urethra and anterior to the rectum. The upper end contains the uterine cervix in an area called the *fornix*. The vagina serves as a route for the excretion of secretions (including menstrual fluid), as an organ of sexual response, and as a passageway for the birth of an infant. The walls of the vagina are usually moist and maintain a pH ranging from 3.8 to 4.2. This pH is bacteriostatic and is maintained by the action of the hormone estrogen and normal vaginal flora. Estrogen stimulates the growth of vaginal mucosal cells so that they thicken and have increased glycogen content. The glycogen is fermented to lactic acid by Döderlein bacilli (lactobacilli that normally inhabit the vagina), slightly acidifying the vaginal fluid. The cervix projects into the vagina and forms a pathway between the uterus and the vagina. The *cervix* is a firm structure, protected by mucus that changes consistency and quantity during the menstrual cycle and during pregnancy.

The Uterus

The *uterus* is a hollow, pear-shaped muscular organ with thick walls located between the bladder and the rectum. It has three parts: The fundus, the body, and the cervix. It is supported in the abdominal cavity by the broad ligaments, the round ligaments, the uterosacral ligaments, and the transverse cervical ligaments. The uterus receives the fertilized ovum and provides a site for growth and development of the fetus.

The uterine wall has three layers. The *perimetrium* is the outer serous layer that merges with the peritoneum. The *myometrium* is the middle layer and makes up most of the uterine wall. This layer has muscle fibers that run in various directions, allowing contractions during **menstruation** (the periodic shedding of the uterine lining in a woman of childbearing age who is not pregnant) or childbirth and

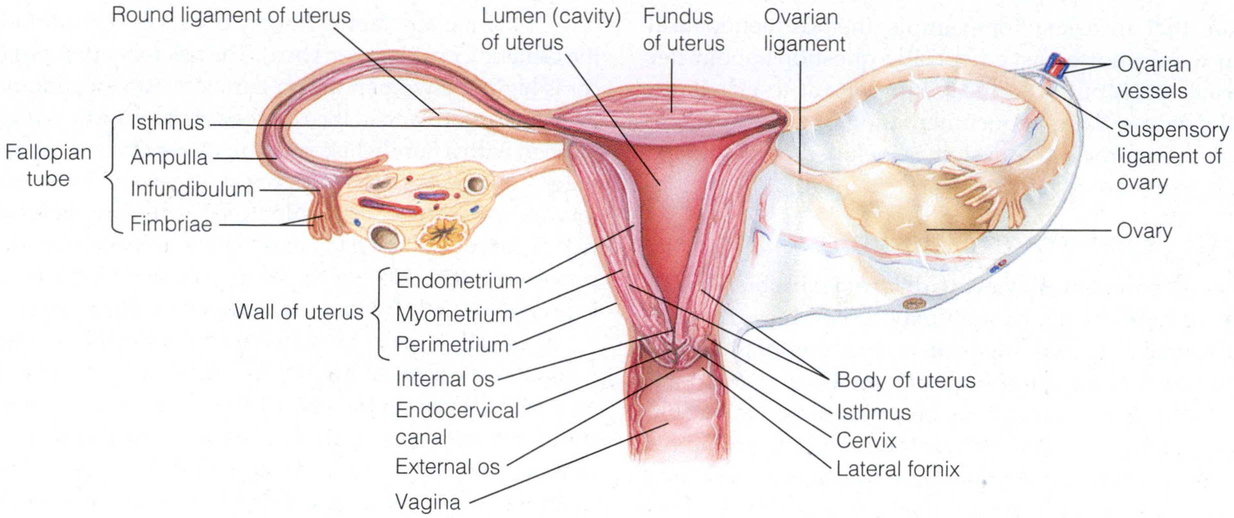
Round ligament of uterus
Lumen (cavity) of uterus
Fundus of uterus
Ovarian ligament
Ovarian vessels
Suspensory ligament of ovary
Ovary
Fallopian tube
Isthmus
Ampulla
Infundibulum
Fimbriae
Wall of uterus
Endometrium
Myometrium
Perimetrium
Internal os
Endocervical canal
External os
Vagina
Body of uterus
Isthmus
Cervix
Lateral fornix

Figure 47.6 ■ The internal organs of the female reproductive system.

expansion as the fetus grows. The *endometrium* lines the uterus; its outermost layer is shed during menstruation.

The Fallopian Tubes

The *fallopian tubes* are thin, cylindrical structures about 10 cm (4 in.) long and 2.5 cm (1 in.) in diameter. They are attached to the uterus on one end and are supported by the broad ligaments. The lateral ends of the fallopian tubes are open and made of projections called *fimbriae* that drape over the ovary. The fimbriae pick up the ovum after it is discharged from the ovary. The fallopian tubes are made of smooth muscle and are lined with ciliated, mucus-producing epithelial cells. The movement of the cilia and contractions of the smooth muscle move the ovum through the tubes toward the uterus. Fertilization of the ovum by the sperm usually occurs in the outer portion of a fallopian tube.

The Ovaries

The *ovaries* are flat, almond-shaped structures located on either side of the uterus below the ends of the fallopian tubes. They are homologous to the male's testes. The ovaries store the female germ cells (*ova*) and produce the female hormones estrogen and progesterone. A woman's total number of ova is present at her birth.

Female Sex Hormones

The ovaries produce estrogens, progesterone, and androgens in a cyclic pattern. **Estrogens** are steroid hormones that occur naturally in three forms: Estrone (E_1), estradiol (E_2), and estriol (E_3). Estradiol is the most potent and is the form secreted in greatest amount by the ovaries. Estrogens are essential for the development and maintenance of secondary sex characteristics. In conjunction with other hormones, they stimulate the female reproductive organs to prepare for growth of a fetus. Estrogens are responsible for the normal structure of skin and blood vessels. They also decrease the rate of bone resorption, promote increased high-density lipoproteins, reduce cholesterol levels, and enhance the clotting of blood. Estrogens also promote the retention of sodium and water.

Progesterone primarily affects the development of breast glandular tissue and the endometrium. During pregnancy, progesterone relaxes smooth muscle to decrease uterine contractions. It also increases body temperature. Androgens are responsible for normal hair growth patterns at puberty and may also have metabolic effects.

The Menstrual Cycle

The **menstrual cycle** begins with the menstrual phase, lasting from days 1 to 5. The inner endometrial (functionalis) layer detaches and is expelled as menstrual fluid (fluid and blood) for 3 to 5 days. As the maturing ovarian follicle begins to produce estrogen (days 6 to 14), the proliferative phase begins. In response, the functionalis layer is repaired and thickens, while spiral arteries increase in number and tubular glands form. Cervical mucus changes to a thin, crystalline substance, forming channels to help the sperm move up into the uterus.

The final phase, lasting from days 14 to 28, is the secretory phase. As the corpus luteum produces progesterone, the rising levels act on the endometrium, causing increased vascularity, changing the inner layer to secretory mucosa, stimulating the secretion of glycogen into the uterine cavity, and causing the cervical mucus again to become thick and block the internal os. If fertilization does not occur, hormone levels fall. Spasm of the spiral arteries causes hypoxia of the endometrial cells, which begin to degenerate and slough off as menstrual fluid.

47.4 Assessing the Female Reproductive System

The structures and functions of the female reproductive system are assessed by findings from diagnostic tests, a health assessment interview to collect subjective data, and a physical assessment to collect objective data. Information from the health assessment interview is used to individualize the questions that are asked; for example, the postmenopausal woman would not be asked specific questions about her menstrual cycle, but it would be important to ask about vaginal dryness. Sample documentation of an assessment of the female reproductive system is included following the physical assessment section.

Health Assessment Interview

A health assessment interview to determine problems with the female reproductive system may be conducted during a health screening, may focus on a chief complaint (such as severe menstrual cramping), or may be part of a total health assessment. Women may be embarrassed to discuss health problems or concerns involving their reproductive organs; it is important for the nurse to ask questions in a nonthreatening, matter-of-fact manner. Consider the psychologic, social, and cultural factors that affect sexuality and sexual activity. Use words that the woman can understand, and do not be embarrassed or offended by the words she uses. The woman may perceive the interview as less threatening if the discussion begins with more general questions and then progresses to specific questions, and if questions are asked in a way that gives the woman permission to describe behaviors and manifestations. For example, first ask a female patient about menstrual and childbirth histories before asking questions about STIs.

The focused interview for the female reproductive system is usually extensive. However, the questions may in many instances be tailored to the specific health problem of the woman. As with the assessment of other body systems, analyze and document the onset of the problem, its duration, frequency, precipitating and relieving factors, any associated symptoms, treatment, self-care, and outcome. For example, ask the woman the following questions:

- "Have you noticed vaginal bleeding after intercourse?"
- "Have you had vaginal bleeding when you did not expect to?"
- "Does over-the-counter medication relieve the vaginal itching and discharge?"
- "Have you had any fever or abdominal pain with this vaginal infection?"

Ask about menstrual history, sexual history, obstetric history, use of contraceptives, use of medications, and reproductive system examinations. Assess the use of condoms during intercourse; unprotected sexual intercourse increases the risk of STIs, including HIV infection. Ask about smoking; a history of smoking increases the risk of circulatory problems in the woman taking oral contraceptives and increases the risk for cancer of the cervix.

Chronic illnesses may affect the function of the female reproductive system. Diabetes mellitus increases the risk of vaginal infections and vaginal dryness, both of which interfere with sexual pleasure. Chronic heavy menstrual flow may result in anemia. Thyroid and adrenal disorders may affect secondary sex characteristics, the menstrual cycle, and the ability to become pregnant.

Obtaining any family history of cancer is important (see the Genetic Considerations box). The risk for endometrial cancer is higher in women with a family history of endometrial, breast, or colon cancer; the risk for ovarian cancer is higher in women with a family history of ovarian or breast cancer; and the risk for breast cancer is higher in women with a family history of breast cancer. Exposure to DES in utero increases the risk of cancer of the cervix and vagina. Exposure to asbestos poses a risk for cancer of the ovary. The risk for breast cancer is also greater if the woman has a history of fibrocystic disease.

Carefully explore any history of vaginal bleeding and vaginal discharge. Ask about the onset of vaginal bleeding, any related factors, the color (pink, red, dark red, brown), the character (thin, watery, presence of mucus, size and number of clots), the amount (spotting, how many pads or tampons in a specific amount of time), and relationship to menstrual cycle. Regarding vaginal discharge, ask about the onset, color (white, green, gray), character (thin, thick, curd-like), odor, itching, and rash.

Questions about sexuality may include sexual preference, number of sexual partners; history of **anorgasmia** (absence of orgasm), **dyspareunia** (painful intercourse), or other problems with intercourse; history of sexual trauma; use of condoms or other contraceptives; and current level of sexual satisfaction.

Physical Assessment

Physical assessment of the female reproductive system is usually conducted as part of a scheduled screening (e.g., an annual gynecologic examination) or for a specific reproductive health problem. If conducted as part of a total physical assessment, this is usually the final system to be assessed. The

Genetic Considerations

When conducting a health assessment interview and a physical assessment, it is important for the nurse to consider genetic influences on the health of the adult. Several diseases of the female reproductive system have a genetic component (NCI, 2018a). During the health assessment interview, it is especially important to ask about a family history of ovarian or breast cancer. During the physical assessment, assess for any manifestations that might indicate a genetic disorder. If data are found to indicate genetic risk factors or alterations, ask about genetic testing and refer for appropriate genetic counseling and evaluation. Chapter 8 provides further information about genetics in medical-surgical nursing. Below are examples of risk factors for female reproductive system disorders.

- There is a clear genetic link for some of the cases of both breast and ovarian cancer. Two breast cancer susceptibility genes have been identified: *BRCA1* and *BRCA2*. If a woman has either of these genes, she is at increased risk for having breast or ovarian cancer at some point in her life.
- A family history of endometrial, colon, or breast cancer increases a woman's risk for endometrial cancer.
- Turner syndrome is a disorder in a female caused by complete or partial absence of one of the two X chromosomes. The disorder is characterized by short stature, a webbed neck, and a lack of sexual development at puberty.

nurse must feel comfortable with the examination of patients of the opposite gender; if either the nurse or the patient is not comfortable, or if cultural beliefs prohibit examination by a nurse of the opposite gender, a nurse of the same gender should be asked to conduct this part of the assessment. Usually the internal portion of the examination is done by an advanced practice provider or physician, however, specially trained nurses may do the examination in certain circumstances. All nurses should be familiar with the procedure as the nurse is likely to be assisting with the examination.

The female reproductive system is assessed by inspection and palpation. Ask the woman to void before having the examination. Prior to the examination, collect all necessary equipment and explain the techniques to the woman to decrease anxiety. Put on disposable gloves before beginning the examination and wear them throughout. Ask the woman to remove her clothing and put on a gown. Ensure that the examining room is private and warm.

Explain the procedures for the examination thoroughly and in a matter-of-fact way to decrease anxiety and embarrassment. If the woman is unfamiliar with her reproductive organs, charts may be used to demonstrate the parts that will be examined. Carefully explain the procedure for the examination, and show the speculum to the woman. The assessment may be done with the woman in the sitting or supine position to examine the breasts and in the lithotomy position to assess the external genitalia and internal organs. Expose only those body parts being examined to preserve modesty.

The examination usually begins with inspection of the breasts with the woman in the sitting and supine positions. The nurse then helps the woman move to the lithotomy position on the examining table, with the feet in the stirrups and the buttocks even with the foot of the table. Older or frail women may not be able to tolerate this position. In this case, the woman is examined in the supine position or the left lateral position. Although the entire examination is described here, the internal examination is only conducted by a nurse with advanced practice in the procedure. However, nurses are often asked to assist with the examination and should be able to explain it to the woman.

Female Reproductive System Assessments

Technique/Normal Findings	Abnormal Findings
Breast Assessment	
Inspect both breasts simultaneously with the woman seated in the following positions: Arms at sides, arms overhead, hands pressed on hips, leaning forward. Inspect breast size, symmetry, contour, skin color, texture, venous patterns, and lesions. Lift the breasts, and inspect the lower and lateral aspects. *Breasts normally vary slightly in size and shape, and one breast may normally be larger than the other. Color should be consistent with the skin tone and texture smooth. There should be no redness, swelling, prominent veins, or lesions.*	■ Retractions, dimpling, and abnormal contours suggest lesions and should be further evaluated for malignancy. ■ Thickened, dimpled skin with enlarged pores (called *peau d'orange, orange peel*, or *pig skin*) and unilateral venous patterns are associated with malignancy. ■ Redness may be seen with infection or carcinoma.
Inspect the areolae and nipples. *The color of the areolae should be consistent with the woman's skin color (ranging from dark pink to dark brown), and Montgomery tubercles may be present. The nipples should be equal bilaterally in size, centrally located in each breast, and free of lesions or discharge. Nipples are usually everted, but may normally be inverted or flat.*	■ Peau d'orange may be noted first in the areola. ■ Recent unilateral inversion of the nipple or asymmetry in the directions in which the nipples point suggests cancer.
Palpate both breasts, axillae, and supraclavicular areas. **Figure 47.7** ■ illustrates a possible pattern for breast palpation. Various palpation patterns may be used as long as every part of each breast is palpated, including the *axillary tail* (also called *tail of Spence*), which is the breast tissue that extends from the upper outer quadrant toward and into the axillae. Ask the woman to assume a supine position with a small pillow under the shoulder and the arm over the head, and repeat the systematic palpation sequence. Describe identified masses by location, size, shape, consistency, tenderness, mobility, and delineation of borders. *Breasts should feel smooth, firm, and elastic, without palpable masses. Prior to the menstrual cycle, there may be increased nodularity and tenderness.*	■ Tenderness may be related to premenstrual fullness, fibrocystic disease, or inflammation. ■ Nodules in the tail of the breast may be enlarged lymph nodes. ■ Hard, irregular, fixed unilateral masses that are poorly delineated suggest carcinoma. ■ Bilateral, single or multiple, round, mobile, well-delineated masses are consistent with fibrocystic breast disease or fibroadenoma. ■ Swelling, tenderness, erythema, and heat may be seen with mastitis.
Palpate the nipple, then compress it between the thumb and index finger. Note the color of any discharge. *Nipples should be firm and elastic, normally without discharge (although some women normally have a clear discharge, and a milky substance may be expressed during pregnancy and lactation).*	■ Loss of nipple elasticity is seen in cancer. ■ Bloody or serous discharge is associated with intraductal papilloma. ■ Milky discharge not due to prior pregnancy and found on both sides suggests galactorrhea (lactation not associated with pregnancy or nursing), which is sometimes associated with a pituitary tumor. ■ Unilateral discharge from one or two ducts can be seen in fibrocystic breast disease, intraductal papilloma, or carcinoma.
Axillary Assessment	
Inspect and palpate the axillae. Palpate all sections of both axillae for palpable nodes (**Figure 47.8** ■). *There should be no redness, irritation, lesions, or enlarged lymph nodes on palpation.*	■ Rash may be due to allergy or other causes. ■ Signs of inflammation and infection may be due to infection of the sweat glands. ■ Enlarged axillary nodes are most often due to infection of the hand or arm but can be caused by malignancy. ■ Enlarged supraclavicular nodes are associated with lymphatic metastases from abdominal or thoracic carcinoma.

(continued)

Female Reproductive System Assessments (*continued*)

Technique/Normal Findings	Abnormal Findings
External Genitalia Assessment	
Help the woman to the lithotomy position with the knees flexed and separated.	
Inspect and palpate the labia majora. *The labia majora should be equal in size and free of lesions or bulging.*	■ Excoriation, rashes, or lesions suggest inflammatory or infective processes. ■ Bulging of the labia that increases with straining suggests a hernia. ■ Varicosities may be present on the labia.
Inspect the labia minora. Separate the labia majora for better visualization. *The labia minora should be symmetrical, dark pink and moist, without redness or lesions.*	■ Inflammation, irritation, excoriation, or caking of discharge in tissue folds suggests vaginal infection or poor hygiene. ■ Ulcers or vesicles may be manifestations of an STI.
Palpate the inside of the labia minora between thumb and forefinger. *There should be no nodules, ulcers, or lesions.*	■ Small, firm, round cystic nodules in labia suggest sebaceous cysts. ■ Wartlike lesions suggest condylomata acuminata (genital warts). ■ Firm, painless ulcers suggest chancre of primary syphilis. ■ Shallow, painful ulcers suggest herpes infection. ■ Ulcerated or red raised lesions in older women suggest vulvar carcinoma.
Inspect the clitoris. *The clitoris is normally not enlarged.*	■ Enlargement may be a symptom of a masculinizing condition.
Inspect the vaginal opening. *There should be no swelling, discoloration, lacerations, discharge, or lesions visible in the vaginal opening.*	■ Swelling, discoloration, or lacerations may be caused by trauma. ■ Discharge or lesions may be symptoms of infection. ■ Fissures or fistulas may be related to injury, infection, growth of a malignancy, or trauma.
Palpate Skene glands. Using the index finger, "milk" Skene glands on both sides and over the urethra and inspect for possible discharge (**Figure 47.9** ■). *There should be no discharge or tenderness present.*	■ Discharge from Skene glands and/or tenderness suggests infection.
Palpate Bartholin glands at the posterior labia majora (**Figure 47.10** ■). *There should be no masses, redness, swelling, or tenderness on palpation.*	■ A nontender mass in the posterolateral portion of the labia majora is indicative of a Bartholin cyst. ■ Swelling, redness, or tenderness, especially if unilateral, may indicate abscess of Bartholin glands.

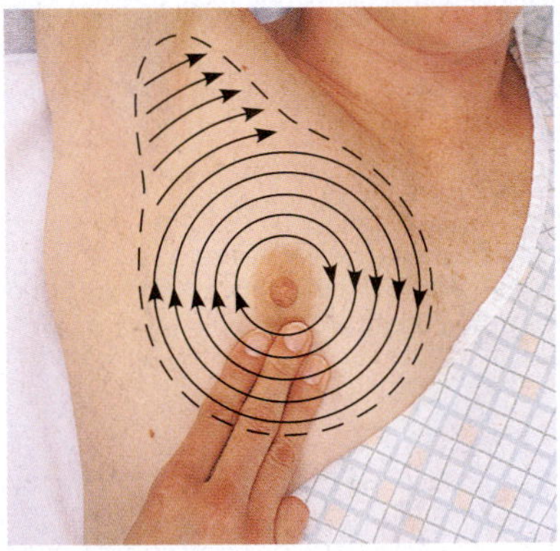

Figure 47.7 ■ Possible pattern for palpation of the breast.

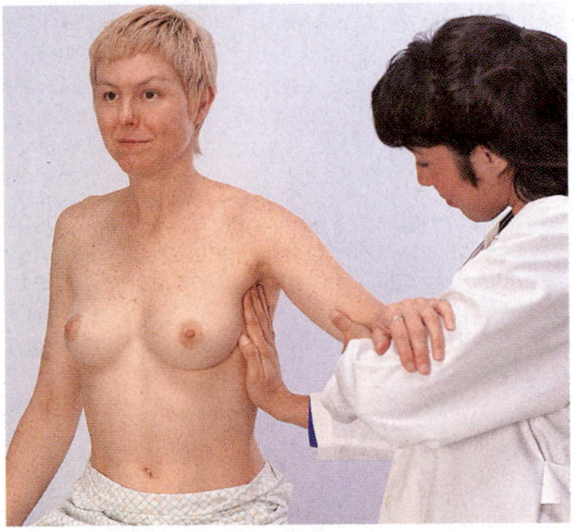

Figure 47.8 ■ Palpating the axillary lymph nodes.

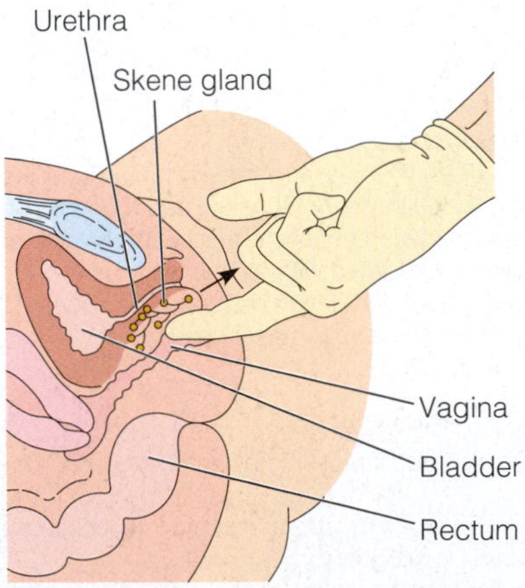
Urethra
Skene gland
Vagina
Bladder
Rectum

Figure 47.9 ■ Palpating Skene gland.

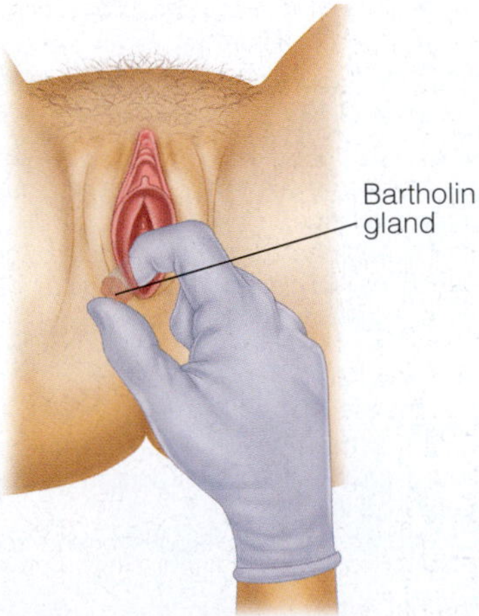
Bartholin gland

Figure 47.10 ■ Palpating Bartholin gland.

Technique/Normal Findings	Abnormal Findings
Inspect the vaginal orifice for bulging and urinary incontinence. Ask the woman to strain or "bear down." *No bulging should be visible with straining.*	■ Bulging of the anterior vaginal wall and urinary incontinence suggest a cystocele. ■ Bulging of the posterior wall suggests a rectocele. ■ Protrusion of the cervix or uterus into the vagina indicates uterine prolapse.
Inspect and palpate the perineum. *The perineum should be free of redness or lesions. Episiotomy scars are a normal finding.*	■ Inflammation, lesions, and growths may be seen in infections or cancer. ■ Fistulas may be the result of injury, trauma, infection, or growth of a malignancy.
Vaginal and Cervical Assessment	
This assessment is primarily conducted by a physician or an advanced practice nurse.	
Use a vaginal speculum to inspect the vaginal walls and cervix. See the guidelines in **Box 47.1**. *The vaginal opening varies, depending on age, sexual history, and vaginal births. Vaginal mucosa is normally pink and moist, without discharge or odor. There should be no bulging or loss of urine. The cervix is normally smooth and pink, without lesions, and has a consistency similar to the tip of the nose.*	■ Bluish color of the cervix and vaginal mucosa may be a sign of pregnancy. ■ A pale cervix is associated with anemia. ■ A cervix to the right or left of the midline may indicate a pelvic mass, uterine adhesions, or pregnancy. ■ Projection of the cervix more than 3 cm (about 1 in.) into the vaginal canal may indicate a pelvic or uterine mass. ■ Transverse or star-shaped cervical lacerations reflect trauma causing tearing of the cervix. ■ An enlarged cervix is associated with infection. ■ Nabothian cysts (small, white, or yellow raised, round areas on the cervix) are considered normal but may become infected. ■ Cervical polyps may be cervical or endometrial in origin.
Palpate the cervix, uterus, and ovaries. See the guidelines in **Box 47.2**. *The cervix can be moved slightly without discomfort. The uterus is normally at the level of the pubis, moves freely, and is nontender. The ovaries (about the size of a walnut) are firm, smooth, mobile, and slightly tender on palpation. The ovaries are not usually palpable 3–5 years after menopause. A small amount of clear drainage is normal.*	■ The uterus may be retroverted (tilted backward) or retroflexed (angled backward). ■ Pain on movement of the cervix during manual examination suggests pelvic inflammatory disease (PID). ■ Softening of the uterine isthmus (Hegar sign), softening of the cervix (Goodell sign), and uterine enlargement may be objective signs of pregnancy. ■ Firm, irregular nodules that vary greatly with size and are continuous with the uterine surface are likely to be myomas (fibroids). ■ Unilateral or bilateral smooth, compressible adnexal masses are found in ovarian tumors. ■ Profuse menstrual bleeding is seen with endometrial polyps, dysfunctional uterine bleeding (DUB), and use of an intrauterine device. ■ Irregular bleeding may be associated with endometrial polyps, DUB, uterine or cervical carcinoma, or oral contraceptives. ■ Postmenopausal bleeding is seen with endometrial hyperplasia, estrogen therapy, and endometrial cancer.

BOX 47.1

Guidelines for Intravaginal Assessment and Use of the Vaginal Speculum

The size of the speculum that is used for an internal examination of the female reproductive system depends on the age of the woman and the size of the vagina. Two types of specula are available. The Graves speculum is larger and is used most often for examinations of adult women. The Pederson speculum, which is narrower, may be used to examine adolescents or adult women who are virgins, have never had a baby, or who are postmenopausal with vaginal atrophy. The speculum should be warm. If cultures or smears are to be obtained, neither water nor gel should be used to warm or to lubricate the speculum.

If cells are to be taken for cytologic studies, the patient should not douche, use vaginal medications, or take a tub bath for 24 hours before the examination. Finally, the examination is usually deferred if the patient is menstruating or has a vaginal infection.

The general procedure is as follows:

1. Place the index and middle finger of one hand into the vagina, just inside the introitus, and press the fingers toward the rectum. Hold the speculum in the other hand.
2. Ask the patient to bear down, and insert the closed blades of the speculum into the vagina at an oblique angle until the ends of the blades reach the fingertips (see the accompanying figure). Withdraw the fingers and rotate the speculum to a transverse position.

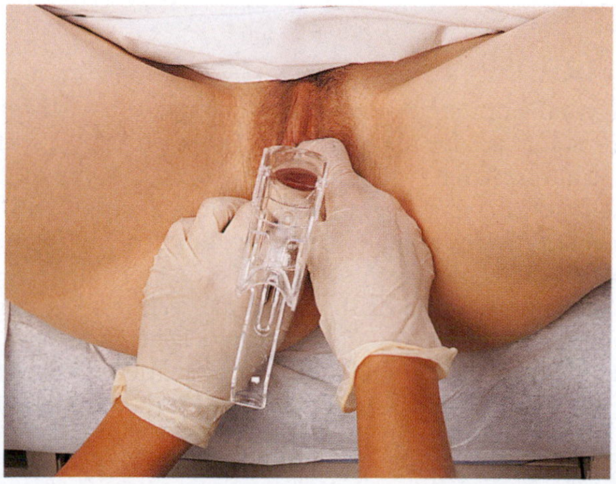

3. Continue to insert the speculum until it reaches the end of the vagina. Depress the lever of the speculum to open the blades. When the cervix is in full view, fix the depressed lever to an open position.
4. Inspect the cervix. The normal cervix is pink and midline. Assess color, position, size, projection into the vagina, surface and shape, and any discharge.

If a Pap test to collect cervical cells for cytologic studies is done, place the brush or spatula in the liquid vial and swirl at least 10 times to thoroughly mix specimen in medium.

If a yeast or bacterial culture is indicated, a specimen can be obtained by a trained provider. A cotton-tipped applicator is used and the inside walls of the vagina are gently wiped to obtain the specimen. The applicator is then placed into the culture medium according to agency protocol.

At the end of the examination, loosen the lever control and slowly withdraw the speculum, closing the blades slowly and rotating the speculum while observing all areas of the vaginal wall. Assess the color of the mucosa and the color and appearance of any discharge.

BOX 47.2
Guidelines for Bimanual Pelvic Examination

The bimanual pelvic examination is done to palpate the cervix, uterus, and ovaries. The examiner's hand that will be used intravaginally is held with the index and middle fingers extended, the thumb abducted, and the fourth and fifth fingers folded on the palm of the hand. The extended fingers are lubricated.

The general procedure is as follows:

1. Spread the labia with the thumb and finger of the opposite hand and insert the lubricated fingers into the vagina with the palm upward.
2. Place the opposite hand on the abdomen; it is used to press on the abdomen and gently move the internal genitals toward the intravaginal fingers (see the accompanying figure).
3. Ask the patient to take deep breaths to relax the abdominal wall.
4. Palpate the cervix, assessing size, contour, position, surface, consistency, tenderness, and mobility. The cervix should be freely movable and nontender.
5. Palpate the uterus by pressing downward on the abdomen while placing the intravaginal fingers in the anterior fornix and gently lifting against the abdominal hand. Assess the size, shape, surface, consistency, position, mobility, and tenderness of the uterus. The normal uterus is freely movable and nontender.
6. Palpate the adnexal areas, which surround the uterus and contain the fallopian tubes and ovaries. Because these structures are small, palpation may not be possible. If the ovaries are palpable, they should be smooth and firm. The normal ovary is sensitive to touch, firm, and highly movable.
7. Withdraw the fingers. Provide tissues for the patient's use in wiping the genital area.

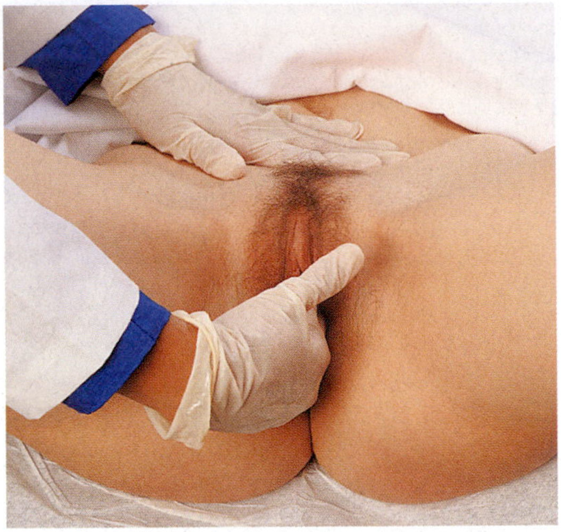

Diagnosis

The results of diagnostic tests of the structures and functions of the female reproductive system are used to monitor the health of female reproductive structures; to support the diagnosis of a specific sexual problem, injury, or disease; to provide information to identify or modify the appropriate medications or treatments used to treat the disease; and to help nurses monitor the woman's responses to treatment and nursing care interventions. Diagnostic tests to assess the female reproductive system are described in the accompanying Diagnostic Tests table. More information is included in the discussion of specific health problems or diseases in Chapter 49.

Regardless of the type of diagnostic test, the nurse is responsible for explaining the procedure and any special preparation needed, for assessing any medication use that might affect the outcome of the tests, for supporting the woman during the examination as necessary, for ensuring the consent form is signed (if appropriate), for documenting the procedures as appropriate, and for monitoring the results of the tests. The nurse is also responsible for post-procedure care and patient teaching for self-care at home (Kee, 2018).

Diagnostic Tests
of the Female Reproductive System

NAME OF TEST	PURPOSE AND DESCRIPTION	RELATED NURSING INTERVENTIONS
Breast biopsy ■ Fine-needle aspiration ■ Core needle biopsy ■ Vacuum-assisted mammotome ■ Open surgical biopsy	■ A fine-needle aspiration is conducted to withdraw fluid from cysts and may be used to sample cells from masses in the breast. A 22- to 25-gauge needle is used to collect five to six samples of fluid or cells. ■ A core needle biopsy is conducted to obtain a sample of tissue from a solid mass or calcium deposits in the breast. A 10-, 11-, or 12-gauge needle is used to collect five to six tissue samples. ■ A vacuum-assisted mammotome is primarily used to evaluate calcifications. An 11- or 14-gauge needle is inserted through a small (1/4-in.) incision and 8–10 samples are removed. ■ An open surgical biopsy is performed to evaluate breast masses, hard-to-reach lesions, multiple lesions, and masses with calcifications. A 4- to 5-cm (1.5- to 2-in.) incision is made and a golf ball–size (or larger) area of tissue is removed.	Explain that, depending on the physician, some procedures may be performed with or without a local anesthetic. Explain that a local anesthetic may be used, but no stitches are required for a fine-needle aspiration, a core needle biopsy, or mammotome. Explain that a local anesthetic will be administered and stitches will be used to close the incision for a large-core biopsy. For an open surgical biopsy, explain that a general anesthetic is usually used and that the incision will require stitches and leave a scar. For all types, wearing a bra, applying ice packs, and taking mild analgesics decrease discomfort postprocedure.
Breast cancer genetic testing (*BRCA1, BRCA2*)	This blood test is used to identify a predisposition to breast and ovarian cancers by mutations of the *BRCA1* and *BRCA2* genes. The genetic defect is passed to children by both the male and female parents.	Food and fluids are not restricted. Suggest the patient have genetic counseling, regardless of the test outcome. If a woman tests positive for this mutation, she may decide to have one or both breasts removed in an effort to prevent the development of cancer.
Breast ultrasound	This examination uses high-frequency sound waves passing through tissues to detect masses in the breast. It may be performed if lesions are identified by a mammogram.	Tell the woman not to apply ointment, body powder, or underarm deodorant prior to the test, or if present, to wash it off.
Chlamydia screening	This test is performed to screen for or diagnose chlamydial infections. A swab of cells from the infected area is taken and either smeared on a slide and analyzed or cultured. Although usually taken from the urethra, vagina, or cervix, cultures may also be taken from the throat and rectum. A urine sample can also be used in some settings (preferred method).	Assess if the woman is pregnant or has enlargement of inguinal lymph nodes. Withhold antibiotics (if prescribed) until after obtaining the specimen. Instruct not to douche before the examination. If the test is positive, emphasize need for treatment to eradicate the infection.
Colposcopy	A colposcopy may be done if a Pap test detects cell changes. The procedure, done in the health provider's office, uses a small binocular microscope to visualize the cervix. Acetic acid is applied to the cervix and abnormal cells turn white. A biopsy of the cervix and/or cryosurgery (freezing) of abnormal cells may be done during the procedure.	Instruct the woman to abstain from douching and intercourse for 48 hours prior to the examination. Assess for pregnancy, which may alter the procedure. Postprocedure: Tell the woman there may be slight vaginal bleeding for several days after the procedure, to abstain from vaginal intercourse for 1–2 days, and to take NSAIDs for discomfort or cramping.

(continued)

Diagnostic Tests
of the Female Reproductive System (*continued*)

NAME OF TEST	PURPOSE AND DESCRIPTION	RELATED NURSING INTERVENTIONS
Conization, cervical biopsy ■ LEEP (loop electrosurgical excision procedure) ■ LETZ (loop electrosurgical excision of transformation zone)	Conization, cervical biopsy, LEEP, or LETZ is done if a Pap test indicates abnormal cervical cells or cervical dysplasia. A cone-shaped portion of tissue surrounding the cervical os is removed for evaluation (most often for cervical cancer) or to treat cervical abnormalities. A thin wire electrode that transmits an electrical current is used to cut away the affected cervical tissue in LEEP and LETZ procedures; alternately, a cold knife or laser may be used. The procedure is usually done on an outpatient basis or at a surgery center.	Explain that an OTC analgesic may be recommended prior to the procedure or general, spinal, or epidural anesthesia may be required. If anesthesia is used, up to 4 h will be spent in recovery after the procedure before going home. Following the procedure, explain that the patient should not use tampons, douche, lift heavy objects, or have sexual intercourse for the recommended length of time, and that she should take showers (not tub baths). Explain that minor vaginal bleeding and discharge are expected for several days after the procedures and spotting may continue for about 3 weeks; perineal pads (not tampons) should be used. The physician should be called for bleeding heavier than a normal period, severe pain, fever, heavy vaginal discharge, or strong vaginal odor. OTC pain medication may be prescribed for pain and cramping.
Cultures for bacteria, *Candida* (yeast), or *Trichomonas*	A culture is performed to identify vaginal organisms or blood cells. A specimen of vaginal discharge is obtained with a swab, placed in solution, and examined under a microscope immediately after it is collected (referred to as a wet-mount).	Request the patient not douche before the examination.
Endometrial biopsy	An endometrial biopsy is performed to identify endometrial hyperplasia or endometrial cancer. The cervix is cleaned and tissue is obtained transcervically from the endometrium either by curettage or vacuum aspiration.	Explain that the procedure is briefly painful and causes vaginal bleeding for a few days. Advise to use perineal pads and avoid tampons and sexual intercourse while bleeding.
Gonorrhea culture	A culture is performed to evaluate for gonorrhea. A swab is used to collect a sample of discharge from the infected area (cervix, urethra, anus, or throat), smeared on a slide, and a Gram stain is conducted to identify the organism (*N. gonorrhoeae*). A urine sample is used in some tests (preferred method).	Instruct not to douche before the examination. If the test is positive, request referral to an STI testing center or clinic and emphasize need for treatment of the patient and her partner(s) to eradicate the infection.
HPV test (HPV DNA test, genital human papilloma test)	An HPV test is used as a screening tool for human papillomavirus (HPV) in women after the age of 30. It is usually conducted in conjunction with a pelvic examination and Pap smear. A finding of "low-grade changes" on the Pap test indicates the likely presence of HPV and the need for further testing. A positive test for HPV indicates an increased risk for cancer, but does not specify which type of HPV is present; HPV 16 and 18 are highly carcinogenic, other strains may carry a low risk for cancer.	Explain that the test should be done during a time when the woman is not menstruating and that she should not douche, use tampons, or use vaginal medications for at least 48 hours prior to the examination. Ask the woman to void prior to the examination. Explain that following the test there may be a small amount of vaginal bleeding or gray-green discharge; a panty liner may be used to avoid spotting clothing. Instruct her not to have intercourse until the healthcare provider says it is safe to do so.
Hysterosalpingogram	This test is conducted to diagnose causes of infertility and abnormalities of the uterus or fallopian tubes. A contrast medium is instilled through the cervix, through the uterus, and out the fallopian tubes while x-rays are taken. The test should be done on the seventh to the ninth day after the end of the menstrual period.	Assess for pregnancy, vaginal bleeding, or acute infection (all would contraindicate the test). Assess for allergy to seafood (iodine) or previous contrast media. A cleansing enema and douche may be ordered prior to the test. Inform the woman that there may be some bloody discharge for 3–4 days after the test; if it continues after that time, she should notify her healthcare provider.

Diagnostic Tests
of the Female Reproductive System (*continued*)

NAME OF TEST	PURPOSE AND DESCRIPTION	RELATED NURSING INTERVENTIONS
Laparoscopy	This examination is conducted to visualize the organs in the peritoneal cavity (uterus, fallopian tubes, ovaries) and to perform a tubal ligation. A fiberoptic scope is inserted through small abdominal incisions and carbon dioxide is inserted into the peritoneal cavity for better visualization. It is performed in an ambulatory surgery center. A microlaparoscopy uses much smaller instruments and is considered only minimally invasive, resulting in less postprocedure discomfort.	Instruct the woman not to smoke, eat, or drink fluids after midnight the day of the procedure. Depending on protocol, the woman may be asked to take laxatives and/or enemas to empty the bowel. Ask the woman to shower or bathe and remove nail polish and makeup the evening before the procedure. Ask the woman to void prior to the examination and explain that a general anesthetic will be used. Following the procedure, the woman remains in the recovery room for about 1 h and remains in the treatment center for 3–4 h. After voiding, the woman is discharged home. After the procedure, the woman will have medications for pain and may experience watery, pink-tinged drainage from the small abdominal incisions (the drainage usually lasts less than 48 hours). Explain that shoulder pain is common after the procedure (referred pain from the retained carbon dioxide gas); that some vaginal bleeding may occur and the woman should use a perineal pad; and to report excess bleeding, pain, or signs of infection to the physician.
Mammogram	Used to detect tumors in the breast. Breasts are flattened in the mammography machine and low-dose x-rays are taken. The American Cancer Society (2018) recommends annual mammography for women by age 45 and mammography every other year starting at 55.	Ask the woman if she is pregnant; if so, the test is contraindicated. Tell the woman not to apply ointment, body powder, or underarm deodorant prior to the test, or if present, to wash it off. Women should discuss the recommended frequency of mammography with their healthcare provider.
Papanicolaou test (Pap test)	This test is conducted to diagnose malignant and premalignant lesions of the cervix; to assess the effects of hormone replacement; identify viral, bacterial, fungal, and parasitic conditions; and to evaluate response to chemotherapy or radiation therapy to the cervix. Cells are obtained during a pelvic examination with a plastic spatula, a cotton swab, or an endocervical brush. The sample collected may be smeared on a glass slide or put into a special liquid preservative and then the cells in suspension are processed onto a slide. The cells are then stained and examined.	Explain that the test should be done during a time when the woman is not menstruating and that she should not have intercourse, douche, or use vaginal medications for at least 24 hours and preferably 48 hours prior to the examination. Ask about menstrual history, including any menstrual problems, last menstrual period, bleeding, and flow. Ask about vaginal discharge and vaginal itching. Assess medication use; vaginal antibiotics alter test results, so testing should be delayed if taking (Adams et al., 2017). Ask the woman to void prior to the examination.(*continued*)
Syphilis (dark-field examination)	See the Male Diagnostic Tests table.	
Syphilis screening tests ▪ Venereal Disease Research Laboratory (VDRL) ▪ Rapid plasma reagin (RPR) ▪ Fluorescent treponemal antibody absorption (FTA-ABS)	See the Male Diagnostic Tests table.	
Ultrasound (abdominal, vaginal)	An ultrasound is used to detect the presence of space-occupying lesions, such as fibroid tumors, cysts, abscesses, and neoplasms. The abdomen is coated with transducing gel, and a graphic visualization is made. For a vaginal ultrasound, a transducer is covered with a condom or vinyl glove coated with transducer gel and then introduced into the vagina.	Explain the need to increase intake of fluids and tell the woman not to void until the test is completed to ensure a full bladder (this lifts the pelvic organs higher in the abdomen and improves visualization).

47.5 Assessment of Special Populations

Assessing Older Adults

Myths, taboos, and stereotypes held by society may foster the belief that older adults are no longer interested in expressing their sexuality. But many older adults continue to enjoy their sexuality well into their 80s (Mayo Clinic, 2017; National Institute on Aging, 2017). As men age, changes in sexual function occur, mostly due to reduced levels of testosterone. Most older men require more stimulation to achieve an erection and orgasm, and they have shorter orgasms with less forceful ejaculation. A man's overall health, chronic health conditions, and prescription medications can all affect his sexuality. Nonetheless, it is possible for older men to enjoy sexual experiences, and nurses should promote expression of sexuality if their patients are interested.

Two commonly held myths are that menopause is the death of a woman's sexuality and that hysterectomy results in the inability to function sexually. Loss of sexual function is not an inevitable result of aging, although physical changes related to aging do affect the female sexual response. These physical changes, along with chronic conditions common in aging women, may alter a woman's sexual function. In addition, some medications used to treat the chronic conditions associated with aging can also alter the sexual response.

Changes in aging women's sexual function often begin in the perimenopausal period as estrogen levels decrease. Estrogen-sensitive cells are found throughout the central nervous system and the cardiovascular system. These cells are involved in the female sexual response. With menopause comes a decrease in the levels of estradiol, which affects nerve transmission and the response in the peripheral vascular system. As a result, the timing and degree of vasocongestion during the sexual response are affected. The capacity for vasocongestion decreases during the plateau phase, as does muscle tension. In the orgasmic phase, the contractions are fewer and less intense. During the resolution phase, vasocongestion subsides more quickly.

Age-related changes in the male and female reproductive systems are outlined in **Table 47.1**.

Assessing the LGBTQI Community

Health care disparities are numerous in the LGBTQI community. There are higher rates of HIV and other STIs along with lower rates for mammograms and Pap test screening (National LGBT Heath Education Center, 2016). The first step in decreasing healthcare disparities in this patient population is to understand terminology. **Gender identity** refers to a person's internal sense that they are a man or a woman or, in some cases, both or neither (Keuroghlian, Ard, & Makadon, 2017). For those patients who identify as **transgender**, this means the gender sex "assigned at birth" (male or female) does not

Table 47.1 **Age-Related Changes in the Male and Female Reproductive Systems**

Age-Related Change	Significance
Male Reproductive System	
Prostate Gland	
■ A significant number of older men have some degree of benign prostatic hyperplasia	Although aging does not cause prostate cancer, its incidence does increase with age.
Penis, Testes, and Scrotum	
■ Epithelial tissue and mucosa of seminal vesicles are thinner and have reduced capacity to hold fluid ■ Sclerosis of penile arteries and veins may occur	Although men may father children throughout life, the sperm count is reduced in some men. Changes in the vascular system of the penis may mean the aging man takes longer to achieve an erection and ejaculation or may be impotent.
Female Reproductive System	
Breasts	
■ Atrophy, with sagging of breast tissue ■ Linear strands may appear from shrinkage and fibrotic changes	Although aging does not cause breast cancer, the incidence rises in older women; age-related changes may make finding tumors more difficult.
External Genitalia	
■ Labia flatten, and vulvar adipose tissue and hair decrease ■ ↑ collagen and adipose tissues in the vaginal canal, resulting in loss of rugae and shortening and narrowing of vaginal canal ■ ↑ vaginal lubrication; epithelium becomes thinner and avascular ■ More alkaline pH of vagina ■ Cervix becomes smaller	Vagina is more easily irritated, increasing the risk of vaginal infections. Lubricants are necessary for comfortable intercourse.
Internal Organs	
■ Uterus shrinks ■ Fallopian tubes shrink and shorten ■ Ovaries are smaller and thicker ■ With menopause, production of estrogen decreases ■ Loss of estrogen may cause pelvic floor muscles to weaken ■ Loss of estrogen causes changes throughout the body, including loss of skin tone (wrinkling) and growth of facial hair	With the completion of menopause, the menstrual cycles end and the woman is infertile. Weakening of the pelvic floor muscles may contribute to involuntary incontinence with increased intra-abdominal pressure (as with coughing and sneezing). Skin is dry and thin.

correspond to their internal sense of gender identity, Those who identify as female (though "assigned" male at birth) may call themselves *transgender women, trans women*, or *male-to-female (MTF) persons*. The reverse is true for those who were "assigned" female sex at birth and identify as male. Those whose gender identity matches the sex assigned at birth are **cis-gender**. Gender identity does not indicate who someone has sexual relations with or which gender someone is attracted to. **Gender expression** describes a person's "outward manifestations of gender in relation to societal norms" (Keuroghlian et al., 2017). There is data that demonstrates that people who engage in same-sex intercourse do not necessarily identify themselves as gay, lesbian, or bisexual and may refer to themselves as men who have sex with men or women who have sex with women (National LGBT Heath Education Center, 2016).

The best way to be inclusive in the healthcare setting is for nurses and all healthcare providers to ask neutral-gender questions. Questions such as "Are you in a relationship?" and "What is the preferred pronoun you wish to go by?" are helpful in providing an inclusive environment. As always, nurses should ask all patients what name they would like to be addressed by during the healthcare interaction (Gelman, VanWagener, & Potter, 2015).

Routine health screenings for breast, ovarian, cervical, testicular, and prostate cancer should be offered for anyone who has an organ at risk. A transgender person may or may not have undergone sex reassignment surgery, so inclusive questions must be asked so that proper care is obtained. Nurses need to remember that historically the LGBTQI community was discriminated against and there are still a number of disparities that need to be overcome by the community. There are specific guidelines in relation to screening for sexually transmitted diseases. Men who have sex with men should be screened for HIV, gonorrhea (urine, rectal, and oral), and chlamydia at least annually. Other than Pap tests there are no clear guidelines for STI screening in women who have sex with women. Finally, for transgender patients, screening should be based on current organs and types of sexual encounters (Eckstrand & Ehrenfeld, 2016).

18.4 Health Promotion

Women and men need to be educated on healthcare promotion related to reproductive and sexual health. This is not only for younger women and men, but for adults throughout the lifespan. Besides nutrition, weight management, regular exercise, and not using any tobacco products, specific activities for health promotion related to reproductive and sexual health are important. Women should be familiar with the how their breasts look and feel and follow the current recommendations based on age and risk for breast cancer (ACS, 2018). Also, routine gynecologic examinations with/or without Pap screening should be completed based on current recommendations (American College of Obstetricians and Gynecologists, 2012). At all ages, men should perform routine testicular examinations (ACS, 2016b) and discuss with their healthcare provider when to start prostate cancer screening based on age and risk factors.

The nurse's role in assisting aging women to reach optimal sexual functioning centers on teaching them about the physiologic and psychologic changes associated with menopause. In addition, the nurse should instruct the woman in how the effects of chronic illness and the medications used to treat these illnesses affect sexual functioning. The woman should be taught the importance of maintaining a healthy lifestyle, which includes a balanced diet, weight-bearing and aerobic exercises, stress management, and routine health examinations.

For problems related to vaginal dryness and dyspareunia, the nurse can recommend water-soluble vaginal lubricants or vaginal gels before intercourse. Intercourse on a regular basis and estrogen replacement therapy can also be suggested for these problems. Estrogen replacement therapy, though, comes with risks, so women and their healthcare providers need to weigh the risks and benefits of hormone replacement therapy (usually vaginal cream for dryness) before use. Women who experience joint pain or other musculoskeletal pain due to conditions such as arthritis can benefit from instruction on how to adapt positions for intercourse. Finally, women (and men) with chronic lung disease can benefit from education on energy-sparing breathing-friendly positions and timing for sexual intercourse.

It is the role of the nurse to educate men about the changes in sexual functioning and to provide information about ways to achieve optimal sexual health. Beginning at the age of 15, all men should perform monthly testicular self-examination, as described in **Box 47.3**.

BOX 47.3
Testicular Self-Examination

- Examine your testicles when you are taking a warm shower or bath, or just after if you prefer to use a mirror to compare size.
- The scrotum, testicles, and hands should be soapy to allow easy manipulation of the tissue.
- Gently roll each testicle between the thumb and fingers of each hand. If one testicle is substantially larger than the other, or if you feel any hard lumps, consult your physician immediately.
- Normal scrotal contents may be confusing. Just above and behind the testicle is the epididymis. It feels soft and tender overall, although parts of it may be rather firm. This is normal. The spermatic cord, a small, round, movable tube, extends up from the epididymis. It feels firm and smooth. Of greatest concern is any hard lump felt directly on the testicle, even if it is painless.
- Choose a day of each month on which to examine yourself. Most men choose an easy day to remember, such as the first or last day of the month. Star this day on your calendar to help you remember.

CHAPTER HIGHLIGHTS

47.1 Anatomy, Physiology, and Functions of the Male Reproductive System

Describe the anatomy, physiology, and functions of the male reproductive system, and identify abnormal findings that may indicate impairment of the reproductive system.

- The male reproductive system contains both internal and external organs. There is an overlap between the reproductive system and the urinary system in male patients.
- Psychosocial factors including stress, anxiety, and grief influence sexual functioning. Sensitivity to cultural differences in discussions of reproductive function is important.

47.2 Assessing the Male Reproductive System

Outline the components of the assessment of the male reproductive system, including topics for the health assessment interview, techniques for physical assessment, and the diagnostic tests used in the assessment.

- Physical assessment of the male reproductive system includes inspection and palpation of external genitalia, palpation of internal reproductive organs, transillumination of the testes, assessment of inguinal areas, and assessment of the perianal area and rectum.
- Abnormal findings in the male reproductive system include lesions, disorders of the penis or scrotum, and inguinal hernias.

47.3 Anatomy, Physiology, and Functions of the Female Reproductive System

Describe the anatomy, physiology, and functions of the female reproductive system, and identify abnormal findings that may indicate impairment of the reproductive system.

- The female reproductive system undergoes cyclic changes in response to estrogen and progesterone levels. The female reproductive system manufactures ova for fertilization, transports fertilized ova for implantation, regulates production and secretion of hormones, and provides sexual stimulation and pleasure. Abnormal findings in the female reproductive system include inflammatory processes and problems with the external genitalia, the cervix, and the vagina.
- Psychosocial factors including stress, anxiety, and grief influence sexual functioning. Sensitivity to cultural differences in discussions of reproductive function is important.

47.4 Assessing the Female Reproductive System

Outline the components of the assessment of the female reproductive system, including topics for the health assessment interview, techniques for physical assessment, and the diagnostic tests used in the assessment.

- The external portion of the female reproductive system can be assessed by the registered nurse. The internal organs, however, are usually assessed by healthcare providers or specially trained nurses.
- The nurse should be familiar with the techniques of proper draping and assistance so the examination can be provided in comfort for the patient.

47.5 Assessment of Special Populations

Differentiate considerations for assessing the reproductive systems of individuals in the LGBTQI population.

- Most older men require more stimulation to achieve an erection and orgasm, and they have shorter orgasms with less forceful ejaculation. A man's overall health, chronic health conditions, and prescription medications can all affect his sexuality.
- Loss of sexual function in older women is not an inevitable result of aging, although physical changes related to aging do affect the female sexual response.
- The LGBTQI community presents unique concerns for care of the reproductive system. Sensitivity and acceptance are important in the care of these patients. The specific assessments and findings depend on the patients themselves.

47.6 Health Promotion

Summarize topics that nurses teach to promote healthy sexuality and reproduction across the lifespan.

- All patients should be educated to specific reproductive system health promotion. Nurses need to be current on the most up-to-date guidelines for screening based on gender, age, and risk factors for the patient.

TEST YOURSELF NCLEX-RN® REVIEW

1. While assessing a male patient who is obese, the nurse notes a normal change in the patient's breasts. What did the nurse most likely assess in this patient?
   A. Phimosis
   B. Absent areola
   C. Gynecomastia
   D. Enlarged axillary lymph nodes
2. The school nurse is preparing a lecture on the differences between the male and female reproductive anatomy. Which female structure should the nurse explain as being analogous to the penis in the male?
   A. Ovary
   B. Clitoris
   C. Labia majora
   D. Labia minora
3. An older male patient with prostate problems does not understand why this health problem causes a change in urination. What should the nurse say when responding to this patient's question?
   A. "The prostate gland presses on the bladder."
   B. "The prostate gland surrounds your urethra."
   C. "The prostate gland sits on top of the kidneys."
   D. "Your kidneys respond to prostate enlargement."
4. A nurse is working at a health fair. A patient asks about prostate health and what screening is suggested. How should the nurse respond? (Select all that apply.)
   A. "All men over age 50 should have a prostate exam and blood work done annually."
   B. "There is a test called a PSA that is used to help screen for prostate cancer."
   C. "All men who are sexually active should have a VDRL annually."
   D. "If you choose to be screened, blood work should be done at least 3 days after the physical exam."
   E. "Blood tests can be done, but they are expensive and not very accurate so I would not recommend you have it done."
5. The nurse is admitting a patient scheduled for a general anesthesia prostate biopsy today. The nurse would immediately notify the surgical team if the patient made which statement? (Select all that apply.)
   A. "I took a couple of ibuprofen for a headache yesterday."
   B. "We stopped for breakfast this morning, but I only got coffee."
   C. "I have a big conference call for work tomorrow."
   D. "I mowed the lawn yesterday so it won't have to been done for another week."
   E. "I have not taken any of my morning medications."
6. A female patient in menopause has a low estrogen level. Which should the nurse explain as potential changes that can occur with this low level of hormone? (Select all that apply.)
   A. Loss of skin tone
   B. Growth of facial hair
   C. Blood clots more easily
   D. Pelvic floor muscles weaken
   E. Increase in cholesterol
7. A young female patient is experiencing cessation of menstruation. Which biologic event should the nurse investigate first?
   A. Onset of puberty
   B. Onset of menopause
   C. Implantation of an embryo
   D. Beginning spermatogenesis
8. A patient is scheduled for a diagnostic test to detect cervical cancer. What information should the nurse provide? (Select all that apply.)
   A. "Schedule the test for when you will not be menstruating."
   B. "You will be scheduling a cervical culture examination."
   C. "Do not have intercourse for 2 days before the exam."
   D. "Use a cleansing douche the morning of the exam."
   E. "Schedule the exam sometime before lunch."
9. The nurse is preparing to assess a female patient's breasts. Which assessment techniques should the nurse use to determine abnormalities of the breast? (Select all that apply.)
   A. Palpation
   B. Aspiration
   C. Inspection
   D. Percussion
   E. Auscultation
10. A 72-year-old female patient reports suddenly having menstrual periods. What should the nurse respond to this patient?
    A. "Do you still have sexual activity?"
    B. "This is perfectly normal, even at your age."
    C. "Do you have menstrual cramps with the periods?"
    D. "Be certain to discuss that with the doctor."

See Test Yourself answers in Appendix B.

REFERENCES

American Cancer Society (ACS) (2016a). *American Cancer Society recommendations for prostate cancer early detection.* Retrieved from https://www.cancer.org/cancer/prostate-cancer/early-detection/acs-recommendations.html.

American Cancer Society (ACS). (2016b). *Testicular self-exam.* Retrieved from https://www.cancer.org/cancer/testicular-cancer/detection-diagnosis-staging/detection.html.

American Cancer Society (ACS). (2018). *American Cancer Society breast cancer screening guideline. Retrieved from* https://www.cancer.org/latest-news/special-coverage/american-cancer-society-breast-cancer-screening-guidelines.html.

American College of Obstetricians and Gynecologists. (2012). *Well-woman visit. Retrieved from* https://www.acog.org/Clinical-Guidance-and-Publications/Committee-Opinions/Committee-on-Gynecologic-Practice/Well-Woman-Visit.

Eckstrand, K. L., & Ehrenfeld, J. M. (Eds.). (2016). *Lesbian, gay, bisexual, and transgender health care: A clinical guide to preventive, primary and specialist care.* New York: Springer.

Gelman, M., VanWagenen, A., & Potter, J. (2015). *Principles for taking a LGBTQ-inclusive health history and conducting a culturally competent physical exam.* In H. J. Makadon, K. H. Mayer, J. Potter, & H. Goldhammer (Eds.), *The Fenway guide to lesbian, gay, bisexual and transgender health* (2nd ed.). Philadelphia, PA: American College of Physicians.

Kee, J. (2018). *Laboratory and diagnostic tests with nursing implications* (10th ed.). Upper Saddle River, NJ: Pearson.

Keuroghlian, A. S., Ard, K. L., & Makadon, H. J. (2017). Advancing health equity for lesbian, gay, bisexual and transgender (LGBT) people through sexual health education and LGBT-affirming health care environments. *Sexual Health, 14,* 119–122.

Mayo Clinic. (2017). *Sexual health.* Retrieved from https://www.mayoclinic.org/healthy-lifestyle/sexual-health/in-depth/senior-sex/art-20046465.

National Cancer Institute (NCI). (2018a). *Genetics of breast and gynecologic cancers (PDQ®)—Health Professional Version.* Retrieved from https://www.cancer.gov/types/breast/hp/breast-ovarian-genetics-pdq.

National Cancer Institute (NCI). (2018b). *Genetics of prostate cancer (PDQ®)—Health Professional Version.* Retrieved from https://www.cancer.gov/types/prostate/hp/prostate-genetics-pdq/.

National Institute on Aging. (2017). *Sexuality in later life.* Retrieved from https://www.nia.nih.gov/health/sexuality-later-life.

National LGBT Heath Education Center. (2016). *Understanding the health needs of LGBT people.* Retrieved from www.lgbthealtheducation.org/wp-content/uploads/LGBTHealthDisparitiesMar2016.pdf.

Sorenson, M., Quinn, L., & Klein, D. (2019). *Pathophysiology: Concepts of human disease.* Hoboken, NJ: Pearson Education.

ADDITIONAL RESOURCE

Services & Advocacy for Gay, Lesbian, Bisexual & Transgender Elders (SAGE)

www.sageusa.org

Chapter 48

Nursing Care of Men with Reproductive System and Breast Disorders

Chapter Outline and Learning Outcomes

CLINICAL COMPETENCIES

- Assess the functional health status of men with reproductive system and breast disorders and monitor, document, and report abnormal or unexpected manifestations and responses.
- Use current evidence and patient preferences to plan and implement optimal nursing care for men with reproductive and breast disorders.
- Prompt patient responses of values, preferences, and expressed needs as part of the clinical interview, implementation, and evaluation of care.
- Function competently within own scope of practice as a member of the healthcare team caring for men with reproductive and breast disorders.
- Apply quality measures, processes, and tools to improve outcomes for men with or at risk for reproductive and breast disorders.

KEY TERMS

benign prostatic hyperplasia (BPH), 1772
epididymitis, 1768
erectile dysfunction (ED), 1762
gynecomastia, 1785
hydrocele, 1767
impotence, 1762
libido, 1762
orchitis, 1768
phimosis, 1766
premature ejaculation, 1765
priapism, 1766
prostatitis, 1771
retrograde ejaculation, 1765
spermatocele, 1767
testicular torsion, 1768
varicocele, 1768

Men are subject to various disorders of the penis, scrotum and testes, prostate gland, and breast. These disorders may be inflammatory, structural, benign, or malignant. Young men are at increased risk for testicular cancer. Both benign and malignant conditions of the prostate gland become common as men age. Many of the disorders pose significant risk to the man's fertility and sexual and urinary function and some are life-threatening. This chapter discusses disorders of the male reproductive system, including disorders affecting sexual expression and the male breast. Because many of the treatments and disorders of the male reproductive system have the potential to affect erection and ejaculation, these problems are discussed first.

48.1 Disorders of Male Sexual Function

The Patient with Erectile Dysfunction

Erectile dysfunction (ED) is the inability of the male to attain and maintain an erection sufficient to permit satisfactory sexual intercourse. **Impotence**, a term often used synonymously with erectile dysfunction, may involve a total inability to achieve erection, an inconsistent ability to achieve erection, or the ability to sustain only brief erections. ED has many possible causes (**Table 48.1**) and may or may not be associated with a loss of **libido** (sexual desire).

The incidence of ED is difficult to estimate because many affected men may not report the disorder. It is estimated that as many as 30 million men in the United States have ED, and most are older than age 65 (National Institute of Diabetes and Digestive and Kidney Diseases [NIDDK], 2017). The incidence of the problem increases rapidly after age 50, although men of any age have reported at least one incident of ED. Most problems with erection are the result of a disease process, injury, or chemical substances (such as prescribed medications, alcohol, nicotine, cocaine, or marijuana) or other pathophysiologic process (Sorenson, Quinn, & Kline, 2019). Clinical studies have also found a correlation between obesity and ED; some studies report a probability increase of 70 to 90% for obese men to develop ED than normal-weight men (Maiorino, Bellastella, & Esposito, 2015). ED also occurs more often in men who smoke. Because impotence most often occurs in aging men, the discussion of pathophysiology focuses on this age group.

Pathophysiology

The underlying issue with ED is the disruption of the normal neurovascular events of the erectile process. These include age-related changes in sexual function that involve cellular and tissue changes in the penis, decreased sensory activity, hypogonadism, and the effects of chronic illness. In the penis, a change from elastic collagen to a more rigid collagen results in decreased distensibility (a less rigid erection). This, in turn, interferes with the veno-occlusive mechanism, which prevents blood from prematurely leaking out

Table 48.1 Common Causes of Erectile Dysfunction

Cause	Examples
Vascular	■ Atherosclerosis ■ Heart disease ■ Hyperlipidemia ■ Hypertension ■ Metabolic syndrome ■ Sickle cell disease ■ Stroke
Neurologic	■ Multiple sclerosis ■ Nerve disease ■ Parkinson disease ■ Spinal cord injury
Urologic	■ Direct injury to the penis that affects the nerves or vascular supply ■ Hypospadias and epispadias ■ Kidney failure ■ Peyronie disease
Endocrine	■ Abnormal prolactin levels ■ Diabetes mellitus ■ Hypogonadism ■ Low testosterone levels ■ Thyroid disease
Respiratory	■ Chronic obstructive pulmonary disease ■ Obstructive sleep apnea
Inflammatory	■ Prostatitis ■ Cystitis
Mechanical	■ Decreased penile distensibility ■ Congenital disorders ■ Morbid obesity ■ Hydrocele ■ Hip or pelvic fractures
Iatrogenic	*Medications including:* ■ Antidepressants ■ Antihistamines ■ Antihypertensives ■ Appetite suppressants ■ Cimetidine ■ Endocrinologic agents ■ Immunosuppressive agents ■ Tranquilizers *Procedures including:* ■ Bladder surgery ■ Colon surgery ■ Coronary artery bypass ■ Pelvic radiation or surgery ■ Radical cystectomy ■ Radical prostatectomy ■ Radiation therapy to pelvis ■ Spinal cord surgery
Lifestyle related	■ Alcohol use ■ Excessive caffeine use ■ Substance abuse ■ Lack of physical activity ■ Obesity/overweight ■ Tobacco use
Psychologic	■ Anxiety ■ Depression ■ Fatigue ■ Fear of sexual failure ■ Guilt ■ Compulsive food disorders ■ Low self-esteem ■ Relationship problems ■ Stress

Sources: Data from Adams, Holland, & Urban, 2017; American Psychiatric Association, 2013; Gerber, 2014; Mayo Clinic, 2018a.

of the penis into the general vasculature. Problems with this mechanism result in incomplete erections. Vibrotactile sensation over the skin of the penis declines with age: Some older men require longer stimulation to achieve an erection. Hypogonadism, common in aging men, results in decreased testosterone levels. There may be a relationship between lower androgen levels and erectile function.

Risk Factors

Many illnesses affect erectile function. Damage to arteries, smooth muscles, and fibrous tissues are the most common causes of impotence. Diseases such as diabetes, kidney disease, chronic alcoholism, atherosclerosis, and vascular disease are responsible for organic ED. Innervation and blood flow to the penis may be damaged from disease processes such as Parkinson disease and also during prostate surgery. Given the effects of aging on the vasculature of the penis, the increased incidence of chronic illness, and the multiple medications and treatments required to manage those illnesses, it is not surprising that many older men have problems with ED.

Manifestations

Manifestations of ED include the inability to achieve an erect penis to complete sexual intercourse. This can be either a completely flaccid penis or a partially erect penis that is not firm enough to achieve penetration.

Interprofessional Care

The management of men with ED is growing in importance and scale because the population as a whole is aging, with the incidence increasing proportionately. Another factor is the positive change in the willingness of men and their partners to discuss sexual concerns. Although sexuality is still a very sensitive and private area for most people, the knowledge that help is available is causing men to seek answers. Many older men are coming to know that loss of erectile function is not an inevitable part of aging.

Diagnosis

The diagnostic tests that may be ordered include laboratory studies, penile monitoring, and penile blood flow. Blood chemistry, complete blood count, lipid profile, urinalysis, testosterone, prolactin, thyroxin, and prostate-specific antigen (PSA) levels are measured to identify possible cardiovascular, metabolic, and endocrine problems that may be causing the dysfunction. Nocturnal penile tumescence and rigidity (NPTR) monitoring helps differentiate between psychogenic and organic causes. NPTR can be performed in a sleep laboratory, although home testing with portable devices is an alternative. The number and quality of erections occurring during REM sleep can be determined. Cavernosometry and cavernosography of the corpora are used to evaluate arterial inflow and venous outflow of blood in the penis.

Medications

ED can be treated with medications taken orally, injected directly into the penis, or inserted into the urethra at the tip of the penis.

Oral Medications. The oral medications used to treat ED include sildenafil citrate (Viagra), vardenafil hydrochloride (Levitra), or tadalafil (Cialis). Viagra and Levitra are taken an hour before sexual activity and enhance the effects of nitrous oxide to facilitate relaxation of the smooth muscle in the penis during sexual stimulation to increase blood flow. Both drugs should be taken no more than once a day. They should not be taken by men who are also taking nitrate-based medications because this may result in severe hypotension or serious cardiac side effects. It is recommended that men taking alpha-blockers to treat hypertension and prostate enlargement should only use these drugs if the baseline blood pressure is at least 90/60 mmHg, other treatments have been unsuccessful, and the patient is monitored closely by a physician (Lee, 2011). Tadalafil is a selective phosphodiesterase type 5 inhibitor that allows smooth muscle relaxation to facilitate inflow of blood into the penis. Different forms of tadalafil allow a single dose as a sustained-release medication that lasts for 36 hours or as a daily low-dose medication. In either case, an erection only occurs with sexual stimulation. Tadalafil should not be taken if the man is also taking nitrates, alpha-blockers, erythromycin or rifampicin (antibiotics), ketoconazole or itraconazole (antifungals), or protease inhibitors (for HIV). Men taking any of these medications should be told to call their healthcare provider for erections lasting more than 4 hours.

Injectable Medications. Hormone replacement therapy with testosterone injections or topical patches may be used for men with documented androgen deficiency and who do not have prostate cancer. Injectable medications, including papaverine and prostaglandin E injections, may be used. When injected directly into the penis, papaverine relaxes the arterioles and smooth muscles of the cavernosum, thus inducing tumescence (swelling). An erection usually develops that lasts from 30 minutes to 4 hours. Prostaglandin E functions much as papaverine does, but has fewer side effects. One problem with this treatment is its mode of delivery. There is a high attrition rate, and patients report dissatisfaction with lack of spontaneity, loss of interest in sex, physical limitations, cost, and, occasionally, pain. Alprostadil (Caverject) is another injectable medication that may be used to treat ED. It may be injected into the penis or placed in the urethra as a minisuppository.

Mechanical Devices

The vacuum constriction device (VCD) is a frequently prescribed mechanical device for ED. The VCD draws blood into the penis with a vacuum, trapping it there with a constricting band at the base of the penis. After the device is removed for intercourse, a single small band, often called an O-ring, is left at the base of the penis to maintain the erection. If the man can attain an erection but cannot maintain it, then an O-ring alone can be used.

Surgery

Surgical treatment for ED involves either revascularization procedures or implantation of prosthetic devices. Venous or arterial procedures are generally not successful. The result is often temporary because the underlying cause of the vascular insufficiency is usually not corrected. Implantation of penile prostheses is now common (**Figure 48.1** ■). Men are generally satisfied with their prostheses. Partners are also more likely to report satisfaction with the penile implant, although not to the same degree as patients. Some partners report that the implanted penis is harder than a normal erect penis and therefore causes pain. Also, the man can have intercourse for a prolonged period of time, and some partners do not find prolonged penetration enjoyable. Patient and partner teaching is necessary to ensure proper use of and satisfaction with the device. Counseling by a sex therapist may be needed to facilitate adaptation to the implant.

Lifestyle Changes

Depending on the cause of the ED, changes in lifestyle may improve the condition or decrease the progression of the problem. Smoking cessation, eating a healthy diet, and regular exercise may improve overall health and cardiovascular functioning. If the man is overweight, a weight loss program as well as avoidance of alcohol and practicing stress-reducing activities may be beneficial.

Nursing Care

Nurses in any healthcare setting may encounter men with ED, either through routine examinations or through assessment of patients' conditions and treatments that may incidentally cause ED. Nurses employed in clinics, operating rooms, and surgical units with urologic services commonly encounter men being treated for ED. Nurses in a variety of settings, including long-term care, encounter men who have had surgical interventions, such as penile implants.

Assessment

Assessment of ED includes a complete health history along with a detailed review of medications (both prescription and over the counter) and supplements. A detailed review of the complaint should be made, including asking such questions as:

- "How long has the issue been going on?"
- "Is the issue lack of erection, partial erection, or the inability to sustain an erection?"
- "Have there been any injuries or surgeries to the pelvic area?"

A complete physical should be performed along with the laboratory information described previously.

Priorities of Care

The priority of care is based on the man's wishes. Drug–drug interactions must be avoided and education on the therapy selected is important.

Diagnoses, Outcomes, and Interventions

Because nurses often complete a patient's health history, they are most likely to discover problems of ED. Once a problem is known, nurses are involved in providing information and emotional support and referring patients to healthcare providers or counselors. Although there are many possible nursing diagnoses, this section focuses on nursing care related to sexual dysfunction and self-esteem.

Promote Sexual Function. Many men who lose erectile function are not aware of the cause, which can induce anxiety and increase risk for depression. Often the man blames the loss on unrelated factors, such as age, a medication, a significant illness, or his sexual partner. Medications such as those used to treat hypertension (known to have ED as

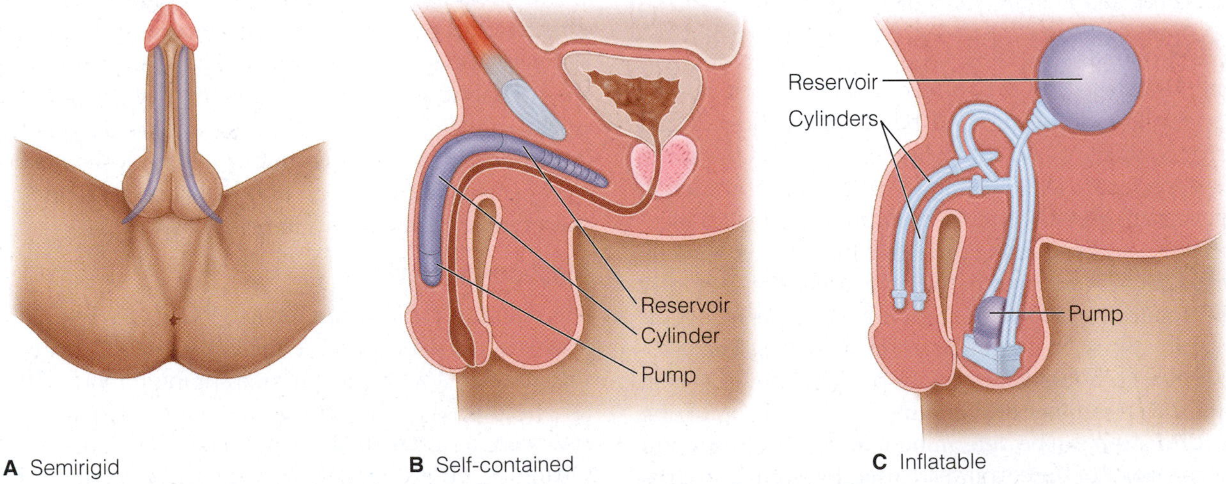
Reservoir
Cylinder
Pump
Reservoir
Cylinders
Pump
A Semirigid
B Self-contained
C Inflatable

Figure 48.1 ■ Types of penile implants. **A**, With semirigid rods implanted in the corpora cavernosa, the penis is always in a state of semi-erection, which may not be acceptable to the man. **B**, With a self-contained penile implant, the penis remains flaccid until the man compresses a pump at the head of the penis, which transfers fluid from a reservoir to a cylinder within the penis to achieve an erection. The man presses a release valve to return the fluid to the reservoir. **C**, With an inflatable penile implant, the penis remains flaccid until the man compresses a pump in the scrotum, which transfers fluid from an abdominal reservoir to cylinders in the corpora cavernosa to achieve an erection. Pressing a release valve returns the fluid to the reservoir.

a side effect) may not be taken as prescribed if the man believes this is the cause of the ED.

Expected Outcome: Patient will demonstrate willingness to discuss changes to sexual function and adapt modes of sexual expression to accommodate age-, medication-, or illness-related changes.

The nurse will:

- Assess for risk factors for ED. Be especially alert to men who have recently begun medications or had recent surgeries that could cause ED. *Awareness of risk factors helps the nurse prioritize care, although nurses must remember that almost all aging men have at least one risk factor for ED.*
- Assess for sexual dysfunction. Men have shown increasing willingness to discuss sexual concerns and expect nurses to be aware of the physiologic effects of their disease and side effects of treatment on all aspects of their health. *If a problem exists, information obtained in a sexual assessment guides the nurse in deciding if the next step should be patient teaching, referral, or both.*
- Conduct a detailed assessment of current sexual practices. *It is essential for healthcare providers to understand the patient and partner's sexual pattern in order to provide appropriate, individualized care.*
- Discuss previous methods of coping with ED. *Awareness of coping strategies can provide insight for the nurse and guide teaching.*
- Provide information about treatment options. *The man needs to know the details of the intervention, the chances for success, and the possible complications.*
- Encourage discussion of condition with partner. *It is not uncommon for men to withdraw from their partners, causing strain on the relationship and adding to the feelings of anxiety.*

Situational Low Self-Esteem. The man with ED often believes himself to be "less than a man." In addition, the insertion of a penile implant with a semirigid prosthesis may result in disturbances in body image related to changes in sexual activity as well as the appearance and embarrassment of a permanent semi-erection.

Expected Outcome: Patient will demonstrate self-esteem by use of effective coping strategies to deal with changes in body image.

The nurse will:

- Collect data during the health history, in a nonjudgmental manner, about physiologic function, other chronic illnesses, and feelings of sexual inadequacy. *This information is necessary to establish the database for individualized interventions.*
- If the man has had a penile implant, teach him and his partner how to use the pump, including how to inflate and deflate the device. Suggest he practice inflation and deflation during the postoperative period. Suggest wearing snug-fitting underwear with the penis placed in an upright position on the abdomen and loose trousers. Provide information about length of healing, and that sexual activity may resume within 6 to 8 weeks following surgery. *Practicing use of the pump will maintain the pump position and promote tissue growth around the implant. The type of clothing worn can improve the ability to conceal a semirigid prosthesis and decrease embarrassment. Recovery from surgery is necessary before resuming sexual activity.*

Many nurses find that men with ED and their partners have lived in isolation with the problem for many years. The partner may even be unaware of the problem, believing that the man is seeing someone else or that the man has lost his attraction to the partner. The man may have kept his problem a secret because an intense feeling of shame makes him unable to admit that he cannot perform sexually. Many men greet the information about the high incidence of ED with a sense of relief that they are not alone in having this problem. All men and their partners need to be aware of support services available to them (National Institute on Aging, 2017). Referral sources include the American Urological Association and the American Association of Sex Educators, Counselors, and Therapists.

The Patient with Ejaculatory Dysfunction

There are many types of ejaculatory dysfunction. **Retrograde ejaculation** (seminal fluid discharged into the bladder) may develop in older men, but it is usually related to surgery of the prostate or for testicular cancer. **Premature ejaculation** is the most common form of sexual dysfunction in men, and serotonin, dopamine, and oxytocin appear to play an important role in this condition (Allhof et al., 2014). Comorbidities such as diabetes can cause the problem as well. Delayed ejaculation can be related to aging changes, such as decreased vibrotactile sensation over the penis or decreased libido secondary to hypogonadism. Delayed ejaculation and inability to ejaculate at all may be caused by certain medications, such as antihypertensives, antidepressants, anxiolytics, and narcotics.

Among these problems, premature ejaculation has proved most responsive to medical management. Medications such as selective serotonin reuptake inhibitors (SSRIs), tricyclic antidepressants, and topical anesthetics are often prescribed. The man can also experiment with ways to decrease sensitivity (such as wearing condoms). Using relaxation and guided imagery can delay orgasm. Mechanical devices, such as constrictive rings around the base of the penis, can help the man delay ejaculation and sustain an erection.

Nursing care focuses on assessment of the problem and teaching for all types of ejaculatory dysfunction. The man's partner can be taught how to avoid excessive stimulation that would result in premature ejaculation. If the problem persists, the man should be referred to a specialist.

48.2 Disorders of the Penis

The Patient with Phimosis or Priapism

Although uncommon, phimosis and priapism can cause problems with urination and sexual activity. In some cases, they are considered a medical emergency because decreased blood flow to the penis may result in tissue ischemia and necrosis.

Pathophysiology

Phimosis is constriction of the foreskin in uncircumcised men so that it cannot be retracted over the glans penis. Phimosis may be congenital or it may be related to chronic infections under the foreskin, which lead to adhesions. The major problem with this condition is that it prevents adequate hygiene, which in turn may increase the risk of cancer of the penis. Phimosis may also interfere with urinary elimination and intercourse. In a related disorder, called *paraphimosis*, the foreskin is tight and constricted, and it is not able to cover the glans penis. The glans becomes engorged, edematous, and painful. Paraphimosis may result from long-term retraction of the foreskin, such as may occur in placement of an indwelling catheter in the uncircumcised male. The tight foreskin can result in ischemia of the glans.

Priapism is an involuntary, sustained, painful erection that is not associated with sexual arousal. The prolonged erection may result in ischemia and fibrosis of the erectile tissue with high risk of subsequent impotence. The disorder, classified as either primary or secondary, is caused by impaired blood flow in the corpora cavernosa. Primary priapism results from conditions such as tumors, infection, or trauma. Secondary priapism is caused by blood disorders (e.g., leukemia, sickle cell disease, and thrombocytopenia), neurologic disorders (e.g., spinal cord injury or stroke), renal failure, and some medications (e.g., papaverine, alcohol, marijuana, psychotropic drugs). Men who use intracavernous injection therapy or medications for ED are at risk for priapism.

Interprofessional Care

Severe phimosis or paraphimosis may require surgical circumcision. If infection is present, the appropriate antibiotic is administered.

Treatment of priapism varies, depending on the cause. Conservative measures include ice packs and analgesia. Under local or regional anesthesia, blood may be aspirated from the corpora cavernosa, followed by saline irrigation and intracavernous injection of phenylephrine, an Δ-receptor agonist. If necessary, surgery to create vascular shunts to maintain blood flow is performed. When priapism is prolonged, it increases the risk of subsequent ED.

Nursing Care

Assessment

Assessment for both conditions includes determining precipitating factors, medical history, and how noting how long the situation has been ongoing.

Priorities of Care

For both disease processes the priority is to prevent or minimize permanent damage to the penis.

Nursing care for the patient with phimosis focuses on prevention of further damage. Treating the cause of the phimosis is important. If an infection is the cause then completing the treatment plan along with meticulous skin hygiene to the penis is important. Untreated phimosis can lead to painful erections and frequent UTIs along with difficulty with urination. The best way to treat phimosis is to prevent it. Good hygiene of the penis with careful attention to gently pulling back the foreskin, cleaning the glans, then placing the foreskin back into position reduces risk of phimosis.

Nursing care for priapism focuses on assessing the penis, monitoring urinary output, and providing pain control. Assessment of the penis includes inspection for degree of erection and changes in color due to ischemia and palpation of the penis for firmness and degree of rigidity. Monitor urine output, assessing for oliguria or signs of acute urinary retention. Pain is treated with analgesics.

The man usually has moderate to severe anxiety related to pain, the treatment, and the threat to his sexual function. The treatment may sound bizarre and painful, especially because the area is already extremely sensitive. The man may be acutely embarrassed by the erection and needs reassurance that the nurse understands that the erection is not within his control. Risk factors for priapism should be discussed.

SAFETY ALERT: When inserting Foley catheters, nurses must be vigilant in preventing foreskin from staying retracted. After placement of the Foley catheter the foreskin should be back covering the glans. ■

The Patient with Cancer of the Penis

Cancer of the penis is a rare cancer in North America, occurring in less than 1% of all cancer patients with an estimated 2320 new cases and 380 deaths in 2018 (American Cancer Society [ACS], 2018b). Risk factors for penile cancer include having human papillomavirus infection, and men who are not circumcised are more likely not to be able to clear an HPV infection. It is not known if the immune system of the body actually rids the body of the infection or if there is suppression of the virus; however, there are no outward signs of the HPV virus (Sorenson et al., 2019). Age is a factor, and the greatest incidence is in men age 60 and above. It is lower in populations in which routine circumcision is practiced, although the correlation between circumcision and penile cancer is unclear. Phimosis and poor genital hygiene are risk factors, as are human papillomavirus (HPV) and HIV infections. Ultraviolet radiation exposure (such as that used to treat psoriasis) may also play a role (ACS, 2018f).

Pathophysiology

Squamous cell carcinoma accounts for 95% of all penile cancers (ACS, 2018e). The tumor usually develops as a nodular or wartlike growth or a red velvety lesion on the glans or foreskin. (Squamous cell carcinoma is illustrated in Chapter 16.) Penile cancer spreads to the superficial or deep inguinal nodes, and very late in the disease may spread to the bone, liver, or lungs. If the lesion is treated before inguinal node involvement, chances for a cure are good. Most of these lesions are painless but significant ulceration and bleeding may occur. Purulent, foul-smelling discharge may be evident under the foreskin. Occasionally, men with penile cancer may present with enlarged inguinal lymph nodes.

Interprofessional Care

Cancer of the penis is diagnosed by a biopsy of the lesion, including any suspicious inguinal lymph nodes. The cancer is staged according to the size of the tumor, extent of invasion, status of inguinal lymph nodes, and presence or absence of distant metastasis. Small, localized lesions may be treated with fluorouracil cream, external-beam radiation, laser therapy, or surgical excision. Larger lesions with superficial or deep infiltration of penile structures require partial or total amputation of the penis, although the goal is to preserve the penis as much as possible. Chemotherapy (discussed in Chapter 14) or radiation may also be used depending on the staging of the cancer.

Nursing Care

Education can help prevent this disease or provide early detection and cure. Advise parents and young men about recommendations for HPV vaccine (see Chapter 12 for more information about recommended immunizations). Teach men about genital hygiene (including retraction of the foreskin if uncircumcised and washing the glans penis while bathing or showering), the risks of unprotected sex, and the importance of using condoms. Instruct men to shield their genitals when having ultraviolet light therapy or using tanning salons. Discuss the importance of seeking prompt treatment for any lesion or abnormal drainage noted on the penis.

If the man has a penile amputation (penectomy), nurses can help in coping with the problems of a shortened or absent penis, including the potentially devastating effect on body image and self-concept. If a total penectomy is performed, the surgeon creates a perineal urethrostomy, preserving urinary continence. However, the man must void in the sitting position, reinforcing the feeling of loss. Dribbling of urine after voiding may be a problem for a few weeks. The man should be taught to perform careful perineal hygiene following surgery, using mild soap and water. Sitz baths may be helpful to relieve pain and to promote healing. If an inguinal lymph node dissection is performed, the man may experience persistent lymphedema of the lower extremities.

Radiation therapy may affect skin integrity and possibly cause irritation and stricture of the urethra. Radiation prior to surgery may impede incision healing. It is important to assess skin integrity and the man's ability to void. Leakage of urine from dribbling or catheters could also further irritate sensitive tissues.

48.3 Disorders of the Testis and Scrotum

The Patient with a Benign Scrotal Mass

Most scrotal masses are benign and can be managed in a manner that is satisfactory to the patient. The most common benign scrotal masses are hydroceles, spermatoceles, and varicoceles (**Figure 48.2** ■).

Pathophysiology

A **hydrocele**, the most common cause of scrotal swelling, is a collection of fluid within the tunica vaginalis. The swelling ranges from slightly larger than the testicle to larger than a grapefruit. Hydroceles may occur secondary to trauma, infection, or a tumor. The cause of chronic hydrocele in men over the age of 40 is an imbalance between production and reabsorption of fluid within the layers of the scrotum. A hydrocele may be differentiated from a solid mass by transillumination or ultrasound of the scrotum. If the hydrocele becomes large enough to cause embarrassment or significant pain, the fluid is aspirated and an agent is injected into the scrotal sac to sclerose the tunica vaginalis. Hydroceles are not associated with infertility.

A **spermatocele** is a mobile, usually painless mass that forms when efferent ducts in the epididymis dilate and form a cyst. It is thought to result from leakage of sperm due to trauma or infection. Treatment is usually not necessary. Spermatoceles are not associated with infertility.

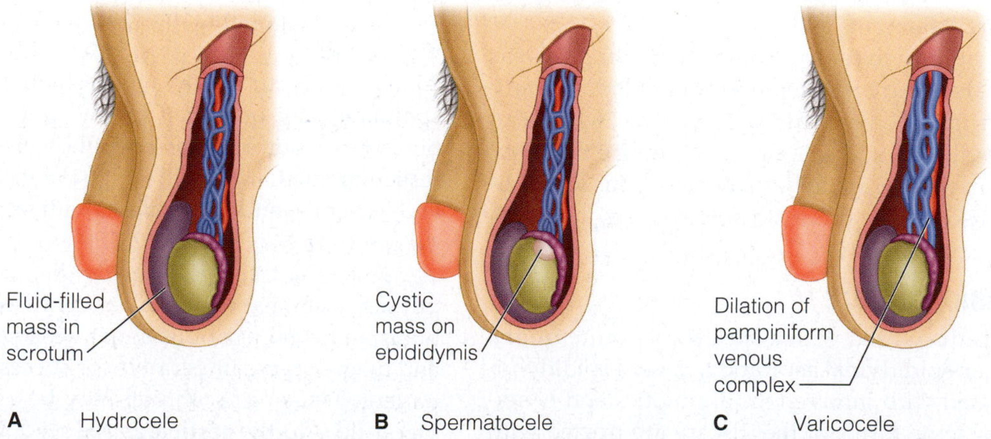
Fluid-filled mass in scrotum
Cystic mass on epididymis
Dilation of pampiniform venous complex
A Hydrocele
B Spermatocele
C Varicocele

Figure 48.2 ■ Common disorders of the scrotum. Hydroceles and spermatoceles do not usually require treatment unless they become large and cause pain. Varicoceles are usually treated to prevent infertility.

A **varicocele** is an abnormal dilation of a vein within the spermatic cord. Incompetent or congenitally missing valves allow blood to pool in the spermatic cord veins. The dilated vein forms a soft mass that may be painful. Most varicoceles occur on the left side. A major concern with this condition is that it can decrease blood flow through the testis, interfere with spermatogenesis, and cause infertility. Varicoceles can be felt by scrotal palpation and most often disappear when the man is in the supine position. Sonography is frequently used for diagnosis. If infertility is a concern, the spermatic vein may be ligated or occluded with a sclerosing agent or balloon catheter. If the varicocele is small and infertility is not a concern, a scrotal support is recommended.

Nursing Care

Nursing care focuses on reducing anxiety and teaching about comfort measures. Almost all men are aware of the possible pain associated with scrotal manipulation. They need information and reassurance about pain management if surgical treatment is necessary. External bleeding is minimal after surgery; however, some men do develop scrotal hematomas, manifested by scrotal edema and a purple discoloration.

The Patient with Epididymitis

Epididymitis is an infection or inflammation of the epididymis, the structure that lies along the posterior border of the testis. This disorder is more often seen in sexually active men who are less than 35 years of age.

Sexually transmitted urethritis caused by *Chlamydia trachomatis* or *Neisseria gonorrhoeae* is the usual precipitating factor for epididymitis in younger men. Men who practice unprotected anal intercourse may acquire sexually transmitted epididymitis from *Escherichia coli*, *Haemophilus influenzae*, *Cryptococcus*, or tuberculosis. In men older than age 35, epididymitis is often associated with a urinary tract infection or prostatitis. Chemical epididymitis is associated with an inflammatory response to the reflux of urine into the ejaculatory ducts from urethral strictures, congenital structural anomalies, or increased abdominal pressure from excessive heavy lifting. This type is usually self-limiting and does not require treatment.

Infectious epididymitis spreads by ascending the vas deferens from an already infected urethra or bladder. Early manifestations include pain and local edema, which can progress to erythema and edema of the entire scrotum, especially on the side of the involved epididymis. Complications of the disorder include abscess formation, infarction of the testis, and infertility.

Interprofessional Care

The infection is diagnosed with a specimen culture from a urethral swab or epididymal aspiration. Severe epididymitis may be treated with intravenous antibiotics and hospitalization. Less acute forms of the disease are treated with outpatient antibiotic therapy. The man's sexual partner should be treated with antibiotics if the causative organism is sexually transmitted.

Nursing Care

Nursing care involves symptomatic relief and teaching. Ice packs and a scrotal support may be applied to the scrotum to relieve pain. Ensure the man knows that complete resolution of the infection may take weeks to months and that treatment should continue until the infection is gone. Provide information about the possibility of infertility because the man may wish to seek evaluation for this problem at a later date. Instruction on sexually transmitted infection (STI) prevention may also be necessary if the epididymitis was caused by a sexually transmitted organism.

The Patient with Orchitis

Orchitis is an acute inflammation or infection of the testes. It most commonly occurs from an extension of a genitourinary infection or as a complication of a systemic illness. Infection may reach the testes through the vas deferens and the lymphatic and vascular channels. Trauma, including vasectomy and other scrotal surgeries, may cause inflammation of the testes.

The most common systemic infectious cause of orchitis in postpubertal men is mumps. Other causes include scarlet fever or pneumonia. The manifestations have a sudden onset, usually within 3 to 4 days after the swelling of the parotid glands. Manifestations include a high fever, increased WBCs, and unilateral or bilateral scrotal redness, swelling, and pain. If both testes are involved, permanent sterility may result (Sorenson et al., 2019).

Interprofessional Care

Treatment is supportive and symptomatic, including antibiotic therapy if urine cultures are positive. Bedrest, scrotal support and elevation, hot or cold compresses, and analgesics for pain are prescribed. If a hydrocele occurs, it is aspirated. Nursing care is similar to that of the patient with epididymitis and other scrotal disorders.

The Patient with Testicular Torsion

Testicular torsion, twisting of the spermatic cord resulting in sudden onset of scrotal swelling, pain, and nausea and vomiting, is a potential medical emergency (**Figure 48.3** ■). The condition occurs most often between birth and age 20, but can occur at any age. Testicular torsion may occur spontaneously, or it may follow trauma or physical exertion. The torsion of the arteries and veins decreases or stops testicular circulation with resultant vascular engorgement and ischemia, and it manifests with sudden severe pain in the scrotum (Mayo Clinic, 2018b).

Testicular torsion is usually diagnosed by history and physical examination. It may be confused with epididymitis but is much more serious in nature, so accurate assessment and diagnosis are imperative for successful outcome of the patient. Testicular scanning may be used to determine if blood flow to the testicle is reduced, or a prostate ultrasound may be done to identify masses or torsion. Surgical treatment, which involves detorsion of the testicle and fixation to the scrotum, must begin as quickly as possible. If

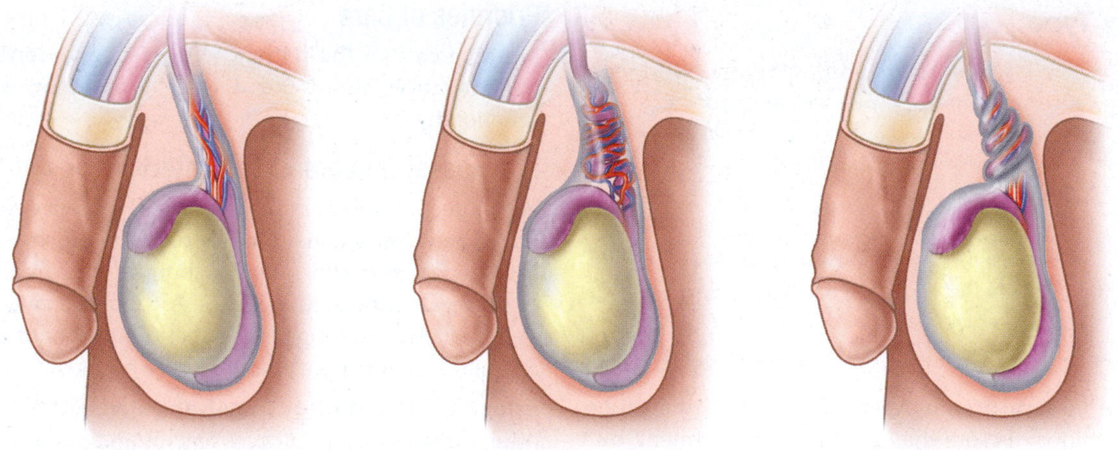
A Normal testicle
B Intravaginal torsion
C Extravaginal torsion

Figure 48.3 ■ The normal testicle **A**, compared with intravaginal torsion **B**, and extravaginal torsion **C**.

the testicle is necrotic or has sustained significant damage, an orchiectomy (surgical removal of a testes) is performed.

The Patient with Testicular Cancer

Testicular cancer accounts for only 1 in every 250 men; however, it is the most common cancer in men between the ages of 13 and 35 and can occur from infancy through old age. It is estimated that in 2018, over 9000 new cases of testicular cancer will be diagnosed (ACS, 2018d). Although the cause is unknown, Caucasian men are five times more likely to develop testicular cancer than are men of color. The incidence of testicular cancer has increased during the past several decades but survival from testicular cancer has improved dramatically as a result of treatment with effective combination chemotherapy. Testicular cancer is considered to be one of the most curable cancers, with a 95% 5-year survival rate for men living in the United States (ACS, 2018d).

The cause of testicular cancer is unknown, but both congenital and acquired factors have been associated with tumor development. About 5% develop in men with a history of undescended testicle (cryptorchidism).

Pathophysiology

Most testicular malignancies are germ cell tumors (Sorenson et al., 2019). Germ cell tumors are classified, depending on their origin and ability to differentiate, as seminomas and nonseminomas. Seminomas are the most common type and are believed to arise from the seminiferous epithelium of the testes. Nonseminomas contain more than one cell type; they include embryonal carcinoma, teratoma, choriocarcinoma, and yolk cell carcinoma. Testicular cancer may also arise from specialized cells of the gonadal stroma. These tumors are named for the cells from which they originate: Leydig cell, Sertoli cell, granulosa cell, and theca cell tumors.

Risk Factors

Risk factors for testicular cancer are:

- Age
- Cryptorchidism (undescended testicle)
- A family history of testicular cancer
- Cancer of the other testicle
- Other risk factors under investigation include occupational risks, presence of multiple atypical nevi, HIV infection, cancer in situ, and age (20% occur between the ages of 25 and 45) (ACS, 2018d).

Manifestations

The first sign of testicular cancer may be a slight, painless enlargement of one testicle. The man may also have an abdominal ache and a feeling of heaviness in the scrotum. Local spread of the cancer to the epididymis or spermatic cord is inhibited by the outer covering of the testicles, the tunica albuginea. Therefore, spread by lymphatic and vascular channels to other organs often causes distant disease before large masses develop in the scrotum. Lymphatic dissemination usually leads to disease in retroperitoneal lymph nodes, whereas vascular dissemination can lead to metastasis in the lungs, bone, or liver. Bilateral testicular cancer is unusual. Manifestations of metastasis include lower extremity edema, back pain, cough, hemoptysis, or dizziness. HCG-producing tumors may cause breast enlargement (gynecomastia). **Table 48.2** outlines the manifestations of testicular cancer by type.

Complications

Complications are rare with testicular cancer as most are discovered, diagnosed, and treated at an early stage. If the cancer has metastasized, then, depending on where the other sites are, complications can occur.

Interprofessional Care

Care focuses on diagnosis, elimination of the cancer, and prevention or treatment of metastasis. Once testicular cancer is suspected, the man undergoes a number of screening tests to help identify the disease and its stage. If the disease is confined to the testicle, it is classified as stage I. Stage II disease is limited to the testicle and regional lymph nodes. Stage III disease involves metastasis above the diaphragm

Table 48.2 Manifestations of Testicular Cancer by Type

Type	Manifestations
Common	■ Painless swelling on one testicle
Metastatic	■ Neck mass ■ Respiratory symptoms ■ Gastrointestinal disturbance ■ Lumbar back pain
Occasional	■ Dull ache in pelvis or scrotum ■ Painless nodule on one testicle
Uncommon	■ Acute pain in scrotum
Rare	■ Infertility ■ Gynecomastia

or extensive visceral involvement. Often, the man does not undergo biopsy before the beginning of treatment, but instead receives a definitive diagnosis after orchiectomy. Most men treated for testicular cancer will live a normal lifespan.

Diagnosis

Diagnosis may be made by various laboratory tests. Serum studies are done to identify tumor markers. Germ cell tumors produce biochemical markers such as human chorionic gonadotropin (hCG) and alpha-fetoprotein (AFP) that can be measured using radioimmunoassay techniques. Elevated levels provide strong evidence of testicular cancer. These markers are also measured after surgery to help determine the presence of residual disease that remains undetected by other means. Persistent elevation may indicate the need for further therapy. Serum lactate dehydrogenase (LDH) levels are elevated in testicular cancer and may be significantly elevated when metastatic disease is present. The LDH is a less specific indicator of testicular cancer than the hCG and AFP.

Medications

Progress in chemotherapy to treat testicular cancer is one of the chief reasons why curative rates are high. The patient with advanced disease receives platinum-based combination chemotherapy. Chemotherapy is discussed in Chapter 14.

Surgery

Radical orchiectomy, which removes the affected testicle and spermatic cord, is the treatment used in all forms and stages of testicular cancer. A modified retroperitoneal lymph node dissection that preserves the nerves necessary for ejaculation is often performed at the same time.

Radiation Therapy

Radiation therapy is used for stage I seminoma to treat cancer in the retroperitoneal lymph nodes, the most frequent site for distant metastasis. The man may experience temporary diarrhea, nausea, or a decline in bone marrow function, such as thrombocytopenia or leukopenia. These problems are usually mild and respond well to symptomatic treatment or time. Damage to the contralateral testicle is minimized by careful shielding. Pretreatment and post-treatment analyses of sperm number and function are necessary. The most common long-term complication is dyspepsia or ulcer disease. Radiation therapy is discussed in Chapter 14.

Nursing Care

Priorities of Care

Nursing care of the patient with testicular cancer focuses on education about the disease, treatment, and sexual functioning.

Diagnoses, Outcomes, and Interventions

Nursing care of the man with testicular cancer is complex. The nurse must consider the reactions to the diagnosis, the change in body image accompanying treatment, and sexual and reproductive issues. Although chances of a cure are excellent, the long-term effect on quality of life may be extensive, requiring a change in life goals.

Educate Patient About Postoperative Care. The nurse often initiates and reinforces teaching about what to expect after radical orchiectomy. The man's knowledge about surgery is assessed, and postoperative routines such as early ambulation are explained.

Expected Outcome: Patient will describe expected postoperative experience including pain management and surveillance for postoperative complications.

The nurse will:

- Explain pain control methods. In addition to the usual analgesics used to control postoperative incisional pain, ice bags may be applied to the scrotum. A scrotal support provides relief, especially when the patient ambulates. *Surgery results in incisional pain, and the scrotum is tender and slightly swollen.*
- Teach the manifestations of complications. The incision is closed with Steri-Strips or staples, and, although rare, wound dehiscence is possible. If the incision gapes open or if there is bleeding beyond slight oozing after 24 hours, contact the surgeon. Another rare complication is a hematoma in the scrotum caused by bleeding from the spermatic cord stump. Rapid onset of scrotal edema is a sign of this problem. *Because the man is usually discharged early, complications may not become apparent until he is at home.*

Promote Sexual Function. The effect of testicular cancer and its treatment on sexual and reproductive function is varied. If the man has a retroperitoneal lymph node dissection, severing of the sympathetic plexus may result in retrograde ejaculation or failure to ejaculate. Infertility may be caused by ejaculation disorders, surgery, chemotherapy, or radiation therapy.

Expected Outcomes: Patient will demonstrate willingness to discuss changes to sexual function. Patient adapts modes of sexual expression to accommodate testicular cancer treatment-related changes.

The nurse will:

- Assess the man's prediagnosis sexual function. To assess this area, the nurse must establish an atmosphere of openness and permission to discuss sexual concerns. After the initial shock of the diagnosis, men report intense concern about sexual and reproductive issues, which can be relieved only by information. *Knowledge of the man's usual sexual function is used to guide teaching.*

- Discuss the possibility of preserving sperm in a bank prior to treatment. *This option may help relieve the man's fears about his ability to father children in the future, but must be completed prior to initiating treatment with surgery, chemotherapy, or radiation therapy.*
- Help the patient cope with feelings about altered sexual function and appearance. Explain that testicular implants can be inserted to preserve appearance. *Many patients, regardless of whether they are in a significant relationship, deeply grieve the loss of the ability to father children. It is important to maintain body image despite disfiguring surgery.*

Delegating Nursing Care Activities

After surgery, activities such as routine vital sign monitoring, measuring urinary output, and assessing urine color can be delegated to unlicensed assistive personnel (UAPs).

Transitions of Care

Families need to be included in teaching for a variety of reasons. If the man is of reproductive age, he and his partner may have anxiety about the ability to have children and will require information. For a young single man, parents need information about the effect on sexual function and are often very involved in postoperative care. The man needs the support of the people he loves, and knowledgeable loved ones can give effective support.

Provide teaching and reinforcement of the need for follow-up, especially if the retroperitoneal lymph nodes were not surgically explored. For men with a risk for recurrence, surveillance with periodic physical examinations, chest x-ray films, tumor markers, and CT scans of the retroperitoneal nodes could continue for a minimum of 5 years and possibly 10 years after orchiectomy. Studies have found that men treated with chemotherapy are at an increased risk of developing cardiovascular disease and secondary malignancies. Men receiving both chemotherapy and radiation have an even higher rate of secondary malignancies. Educating men on the need to remain proactive in their healthcare throughout their lifetime is important (Thornton, 2016).

48.4 Disorders of the Prostate Gland

The Patient with Prostatitis

Prostatitis is a term used to refer to different types of inflammatory disorders of the prostate gland. *Chronic prostatitis/chronic pelvic pain syndrome (CP/CPPS)*, previously known as prostatodynia, is a condition in which the patient experiences the symptoms of prostatitis but shows no evidence of inflammation or infection.

Pathophysiology

The National Institute of Diabetes, Digestive and Kidney Diseases (NIDDK; 2014) has defined four types of prostatitis: Acute bacterial prostatitis, chronic bacterial prostatitis, CP/CPPS, and asymptomatic inflammatory prostatitis (**Table 48.3**).

Acute Bacterial Prostatitis

Acute bacterial prostatitis is usually caused by an ascending infection from the urethra or reflux of infected urine into the ducts of the prostate gland. The organism most often responsible for the infection is *E. coli*; other causative organisms include *Pseudomonas*, *Klebsiella*, and *Chlamydia*.

Chronic Bacterial Prostatitis

Men with chronic bacterial prostatitis often present with a history of recurrent urinary tract infections. The causative organisms are most often *E. coli*, *Proteus*, or *Klebsiella*. Calculi may form in the prostate and contribute to the chronicity of the problem.

Chronic Prostatitis/Chronic Pelvic Pain Syndrome

CP/CPPS is both the most common and the least understood of the syndromes (NIDDK, 2014). The actual etiology

Table 48.3 Categories and Manifestations of Prostatitis

Category	Manifestations
Acute bacterial prostatitis	■ Onset (may be abrupt): Obstruction, irritation, or pain upon voiding; frequency; and urgency ■ Slow or small urinary stream ■ Positive cultures of infectious organism ■ Nonurinary symptoms: Chills, fever, low back and pelvic floor pain
Chronic bacterial prostatitis	■ Urinary symptoms may be similar to those of the acute form, except less sudden, less dramatic, or even absent ■ Positive cultures of causative organism not always obtainable
Chronic prostatitis	■ Perineal, suprapubic, low back, or genital pain ■ Irritation upon voiding ■ Postejaculatory pain ■ Negative cultures of organisms
Chronic prostatitis/chronic pelvic pain syndrome	■ Pelvic, low back, or perineal pain ■ Irritation or obstruction upon voiding ■ Evidence of prostate inflammation may or may not be present ■ No urinary tract infection ■ Normal prostatic secretions ■ Pain when sitting
Asymptomatic inflammatory prostatitis	■ No symptoms ■ Elevated PSA

of CP/CPPS is not known, and there are many theories as to the cause, though no one theory has been proven (Franco et al., 2018). The two types (inflammatory and noninflammatory) are based on the presence or absence of white blood cells in the prostatic fluid. *Inflammatory prostatitis* is believed to be an autoimmune disorder, but the actual cause is unknown. The cause of noninflammatory prostatitis is not known, but is believed to be the result of a problem outside the prostate gland, such as obstruction of the bladder neck.

Asymptomatic Inflammatory Prostatitis

Asymptomatic inflammatory prostatitis is usually diagnosed when the man is undergoing assessment for another issue or during general healthcare screening (such as PSA testing). Treatment is usually not needed unless an underlying process is discovered.

Risk Factors

Risk factors for prostatitis include recent urinary tract infection or catheterization along with a transrectal biopsy. Other risk factors include sexually transmitted infection, HIV, dehydration, urethral stricture, and prostate calculi (Sorenson et al., 2019).

Manifestations

The onset of acute bacterial prostatitis may be abrupt, with manifestations of obstruction, irritation, or pain upon voiding, as well as frequency and urgency. The patient may have a slow or small urinary stream. Other manifestations include fever, chills, malaise, muscle and joint pain, low back and pelvic floor pain, painful ejaculation, and urethral discharge. The man often experiences dull, aching pain in the perineum and/or pain in the prostate gland, rectum, or lower back. On rectal examination, the prostate is enlarged and painful. Cultures will be positive for infectious organism.

The urinary symptoms of chronic bacterial prostatitis may be similar to those of the acute form, except less sudden, less dramatic, or even absent. The patient may experience urinary frequency and urgency, dysuria, low back pain, and perineal discomfort. Epididymitis may be associated with the prostatitis. Positive cultures of the causative organism are not always obtainable.

Men with inflammatory prostatitis have low back pain; urinary manifestations; pain in the penis, testicles, scrotum, lower back, and rectum; decreased libido; and painful ejaculations. They do not have bacteria in their urine, but do have abnormal inflammatory cells in prostatic secretions. Men with asymptomatic inflammatory prostatitis have no subjective manifestations, but are diagnosed when a biopsy or prostatic fluid examination is conducted.

Noninflammatory prostatitis has manifestations similar to those of inflammatory prostatitis, but no evidence of urinary or prostatic infection or inflammation can be found.

Complications

Complications include epididymitis, prostatic abscess, bacteremia, and potentially sepsis if not treated early.

Interprofessional Care

Diagnosis

It is often difficult to diagnose prostatitis. Urine and prostatic secretion examination and cultures are obtained to determine the presence and type of blood cells and bacteria. X-ray studies and ultrasound to visualize pelvic structures may also be useful.

Medications

Bacterial prostatitis is treated with appropriate antibiotics. Men with the chronic form must take antibiotics for up to 4 months and may still relapse as soon as the antibiotic is discontinued. Nonbacterial prostatitis and CP/CPPS do not usually respond satisfactorily to drug therapy, although relief from symptoms is possible. Nonsteroidal anti-inflammatory drugs are useful for pain, and anticholinergics may reduce voiding symptoms. Muscle relaxants and alpha-adrenergic blocking agents are also prescribed, depending on symptom severity. When pain is most severe, stress-reducing activities, warm baths, and avoidance of sitting have been reported to assist in pain reduction.

Nursing Care

Education is the focus of nursing care for the man with prostatitis. Teaching plans focus on symptom management. Men with acute and chronic bacterial prostatitis should be taught to increase fluid intake to around 3 L daily and to void often. These measures help decrease irritation when voiding. Increasing fiber intake to promote regular bowel movements helps ease the pain associated with defecation. Local heat, such as sitz baths, may be helpful to relieve pain and irritation. It is important to teach the man to finish the course of antibiotic therapy. Men with CP/CPPS need to know that the condition is not contagious. Referral sources for information include the National Kidney and Urologic Diseases Information Clearinghouse, the American Foundation for Urologic Disease, and the Prostatitis Foundation.

The Patient with Benign Prostatic Hyperplasia

Benign prostatic hyperplasia (BPH), an age-related, nonmalignant enlargement of the prostate gland, is a common disorder of the aging male (**Figure 48.4** ■). Benign hyperplasia (increased number of cells) begins at 40 to 45 years of age and continues slowly through the rest of life. It is estimated that more than one-half of all men over age 60 have BPH (Sorenson et al., 2019). Although the exact cause of BPH is unknown, risk factors include age, family history, race, and a diet high in meat and fats. The problem that brings men to a healthcare provider is the associated urinary dysfunction.

Pathophysiology

The two necessary preconditions for BPH are age of 48 or greater and the presence of testes. Men who are castrated before puberty do not develop BPH. The androgen that mediates prostatic growth at all ages is dihydrotestosterone (DHT), which is formed in the prostate from testosterone.

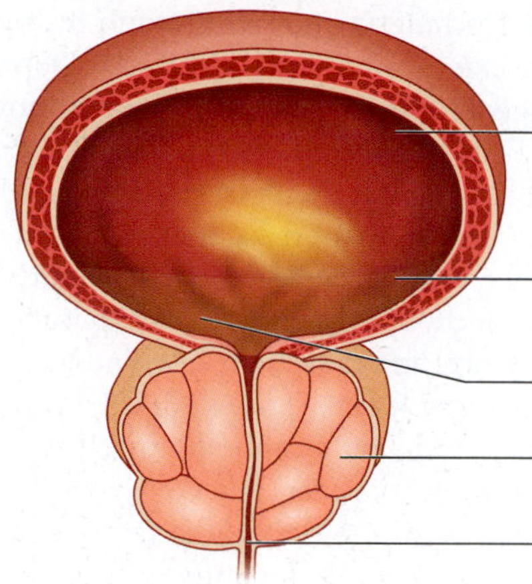
Bladder
Incomplete
emptying of bladder
Urine
Enlarged prostate
Compressed urethra

Figure 48.4 ■ In benign prostatic hyperplasia, the prostate enlarges, compressing the urethra. This can cause incomplete emptying of the bladder.

Although androgen levels decrease in aging men, the aging prostate appears to become more sensitive to available DHT. Estrogen, produced in small amounts in men, appears to sensitize the prostate gland to the effects of DHT. Increasing estrogen levels associated with aging or a relative increase in estrogen related to testosterone levels may contribute to prostatic hyperplasia.

BPH begins as small nodules in the periurethral glands, which are the inner layers of the prostate. The prostate enlarges through formation and growth of nodules (hyperplasia) and enlargement of glandular cells (hypertrophy). Enlargement occurs in an inward fashion, gradually compressing the urethra and resulting in the urologic symptoms associated with BPH. These changes occur over a long period of time. The pathophysiologic effects result from a combination of factors, including urethral resistance to the effects of BPH, intravesical pressure during voiding, detrusor muscle strength, neurologic functioning, and general physical health.

Risk Factors

Risk factors of BPH include being over 40 years of age and the presence of testosterone. Racial background may also play a role, as African American men and Hispanic men develop symptoms earlier than Caucasian American men (Sorenson et al., 2019).

Manifestations

The expanding prostatic tissue compresses the urethra and causes partial or complete obstruction of the outflow of urine from the urinary bladder (see Figure 48.4). The detrusor muscles hypertrophy to compensate for increased resistance to urinary flow; however, eventually decreased bladder compliance and bladder instability occur. As a result, the man with BPH has manifestations from urinary obstruction and a decrease in bladder contractibility and compliance. Urinary retention may become chronic, resulting in overflow incontinence with any increase in intra-abdominal pressure. There is little correlation between the size of the prostate gland and the urinary manifestations.

Complications

Unless the enlarging mass is reduced, multiple complications may occur. As urine is retained in the bladder, increasing bladder distention occurs. Diverticula (outpouchings) on the bladder wall result from the distention. The distention may also obstruct the ureters. Infection, more common in retained urine and in diverticula, may ascend from the bladder to the kidneys. Hydroureter, hydronephrosis, and renal insufficiency are additional possible complications.

Interprofessional Care

Care of men with BPH focuses on diagnosing the disorder, correcting or minimizing the urinary obstruction, and preventing or treating complications. Treatment is often determined by the severity of the manifestations and the presence of complications. Mild cases are often monitored over time and may remain stable or improve.

Diagnosis

It is important for clinicians to determine the actual cause of manifestations, differentiating them from those of infections, stones, urinary strictures, cancer of the prostate or bladder, and side effects of certain medications such as antihistamines and decongestants. A diagnosis of BPH involves both physical examination and laboratory tests. A digital rectal examination (DRE) is done to examine the external surface of the prostate; in BPH it is asymmetrical and enlarged. Examination of the creatinine levels of the blood is conducted to assess for kidney damage.

The urine is examined for WBCs, RBCs, and bacteria. Urinary function is assessed by measuring residual urine (amount of urine remaining in the bladder after voiding) with ultrasonography or postvoiding catheterization (more than 100 mL is considered high), and through uroflowmetry, which measures urine flow rate; normal is greater than 14 mL/sec. A finding of less than 10 mL/sec indicates obstruction.

Prostate-specific antigen (PSA) levels are obtained to rule out prostate cancer. PSA is a glycoprotein produced only in the cytoplasm of benign and malignant prostate cells; the serum level corresponds with the volume of both benign and malignant prostate tissue. Further information is provided in the next section under diagnosis of prostate cancer.

In addition, the man's own subjective experiences with BPH are included in the diagnosis and treatment. For example, the International Prostate Symptom Score and the American Urologic Association BPH Symptom Score questionnaires use scales of 0 (not at all) to 5 (almost always) to collect data about areas such as feeling as though the bladder did not empty with urinating, need to urinate within 2 hours after urinating, starting and stopping the stream several times while urinating, and straining to urinate. These questionnaires also ask how many times during the night the man gets up to urinate and how the man feels about having the disorder.

Medications

Treatment with medications is based on two considerations: The hyperplastic tissue is androgen dependent and smooth muscle contraction within the prostate can exacerbate urinary obstruction. The first consideration is usually addressed by treatment for mild prostate enlargement with finasteride (Proscar) or dutasteride (Avodart), antiandrogen agents that inhibit the conversion of testosterone to DHT and cause the enlarged prostate to shrink in size. These are usually only effective if the prostate is 40 mL or greater in size. They may cause impotence, decreased libido, and decreased volume of ejaculate. Patient and family education includes the information that crushed tablets should not be handled by pregnant women because the drug may be absorbed through the skin and be harmful to a male fetus.

Excessive smooth muscle contraction in BPH may be blocked with the alpha-adrenergic antagonists such as terazosin (Hytrin), doxazosin (Cardura), tamsulosin (Flomax), and alfuzosin (Uroxatral). These medications relieve obstruction and increase the flow of urine. They may cause orthostatic hypotension. If they are taken with phosphodiesterase inhibitors to treat ED, orthostatic hypotension effects are increased. Studies have found that using finasteride and doxazosin together is more effective than using each alone to relieve manifestations and prevent the progression of BPH, but medication side effects are increased as well as the costs of the medication. Patient and family teaching includes advice about making position changes slowly to avoid dizziness and accidental falls, how to take and record blood pressure, and to check with the healthcare provider before taking any OTC medication for coughs, colds, or allergies (because these medications may contain an adrenergic agent).

Surgery

Men who have urinary retention, recurrent urinary tract infection, hematuria, bladder stones, or renal insufficiency secondary to BPH are candidates for surgical intervention. Surgical treatment may be performed by minimally invasive surgery or through transurethral surgery, open surgery, or by laser surgery (**Figure 48.5** ■).

Minimally Invasive Surgery. Because medications are not effective for all men, a number of procedures have been developed to relieve the manifestations of BPH.

Microwaves are used to heat and destroy excess prostate tissue in a procedure called *transurethral microwave thermotherapy*. During the procedure, a cooling system protects the urinary tract. The procedure takes about an hour and can be performed on an outpatient basis. Although microwave procedures do not cure BPH, they do reduce urinary manifestations. The procedures do not cause impotence or incontinence.

The *transurethral needle ablation (TUNA)* system uses heat produced by radio-frequency waves to burn away a region of the enlarged prostate. Shields protect the urethra. TUNA improves the flow of urine through the urethra. It does not cause impotence or incontinence. This technique is performed for men with large prostates who are not good candidates for more invasive surgical procedures.

Transurethral Surgery. A *transurethral resection of the prostate (TURP)* is the surgical procedure used most often. Obstructing prostate tissue is removed using the wire loop of a resectoscope and electrocautery, inserted through the urethra (Figure 48.5A). No external incision is necessary. During the procedure the surgeon uses the resectoscope to remove obstructing tissue one piece at a time. The tissue is flushed into the bladder with fluid and then flushed out at the end of the operation. This surgery has potential risks, however, including postoperative hemorrhage or clot retention, inability to void, and urinary tract infection. Other possible complications are incontinence, impotence, and retrograde ejaculation.

In the *transurethral incision of the prostate (TUIP)* procedure, small incisions are made in the smooth muscle where the prostate is attached to the bladder. The gland is split to reduce pressure on the urethra. No tissue is removed, so this procedure is most appropriate for men with smaller prostate glands. TUIP can be done on an outpatient basis,

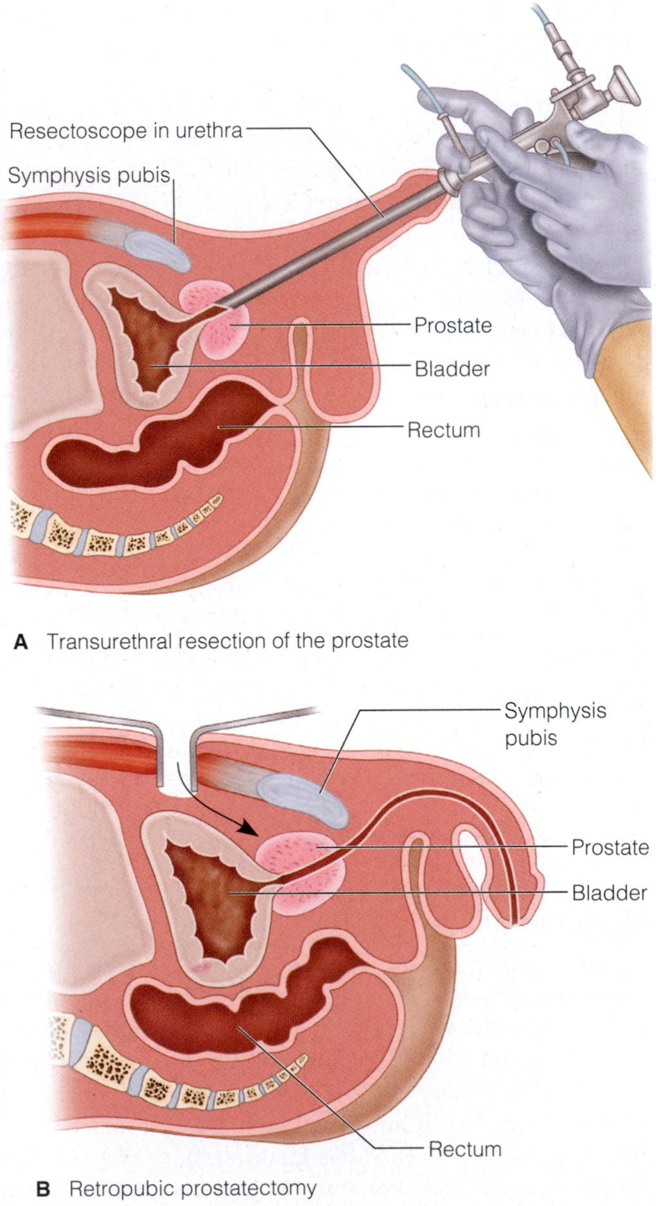
Resectoscope in urethra
Symphysis pubis
Prostate
Bladder
Rectum
A Transurethral resection of the prostate
Symphysis pubis
Prostate
Bladder
Rectum
B Retropubic prostatectomy

Figure 48.5 ■ **A**, In a transurethral resection of the prostate, a resectoscope inserted through the urethra is used to remove excess prostate tissue. **B**, In a retropubic prostatectomy, prostate tissue is removed through an abdominal incision.

and has the additional advantage of less risk of postoperative retrograde ejaculation than is associated with TURP or other prostatectomy procedures.

Open Surgery. When the prostate gland is very large, an open prostatectomy may be used. These procedures are discussed in the section on prostate cancer that follows. Nursing care for the patient having prostate surgery is outlined in **Box 48.1**.

Laser Surgery. In laser surgery, the surgeon uses a cystoscope to pass the YAG laser fiber through the urethra into

BOX 48.1
Nursing Care of the Patient Having a Prostatectomy

PREOPERATIVE CARE

- Assess the man's and family's knowledge about the surgery. *Some men are confused about the surgical approach because there are several quite different methods.*
- Inform the man that he will have a urinary catheter when he returns from surgery, and he may have a drain(s) in his incision. He also will be wearing antiembolic stockings or sequential pneumatic compression stockings. *This knowledge can reduce anxiety postoperatively and increase cooperation with postoperative care.*
- Ensure that a signed consent form is in the chart and that all other preoperative tasks, as outlined in Chapter 4, are done.
- Bowel preparation with a 2% neomycin enema may be ordered. *This cleanses the bowel if a perineal approach will be used.*
- Communicate willingness to address any concerns or anxiety. *Men may be anxious about the outcome of their surgery and potential long-term effects of the surgery on their sexuality. When a prostatectomy is performed for prostate cancer; additional fears include the extent of the cancer and surgery, chances for cure, and possible end-of-life issues.*

POSTOPERATIVE CARE

- Maintain the usual postoperative assessments and follow aseptic techniques in urinary drainage and irrigation care. Monitor vital signs closely for the first 24 hours and regularly thereafter. *The man who has had prostate surgery is at risk for hemorrhage and infection. Vital sign changes may be early manifestations of complications.*
- Maintain accurate intake and output records, including amounts of irrigating solution used. Frequently assess patency of any catheters and drains. Monitor color and character of urine. *Catheters may become occluded by blood clots or kinks, interfering with urinary drainage and increasing the risk of hemorrhage.*
- Assess and manage pain. *The man may have at least three types of pain: Incisional pain, bladder spasms, and abdominal cramps due to intestinal gas. Analgesics and nonsteroidal anti-inflammatory drugs (NSAIDs) are administered on a routine and prn basis to control incisional pain. Bladder spasms may be accompanied by strong urges to void and urine leakage around the catheter. Belladonna and opium (B&O) suppositories may be used to relieve bladder spasms.*
- Maintain antiembolic stockings or sequential compression stockings as prescribed, following agency protocol for assessments and times of removal. Assist with leg exercises and ambulation as ordered. *The man who has had prostate surgery is at risk for developing thromboemboli; these are important preventive measures.*
- Encourage the man to maintain a liberal fluid intake of 2 to 3 L a day. *Increased fluids reduce burning on urination after catheter removal and the risk of urinary tract infection.*

THE MAN WITH A TRANSURETHRAL RESECTION OF THE PROSTATE (TURP)

- For the first 24 to 48 hours, monitor for hemorrhage, evidenced by frankly bloody urinary output, presence of large blood clots, decreased urinary output, increasing bladder spasms, decreased hemoglobin and hematocrit, tachycardia, and hypotension. Notify the healthcare provider if any of these manifestations occur. *Postoperative hemorrhage may be either arterial or venous and may be precipitated by movement, bladder spasms, or an obstructed urinary drainage system.*
- Instruct the man with a three-way indwelling catheter with traction to keep the leg straight while the traction is applied. *A no. 18- to 22-Fr three-way catheter with a 30- to 45-mL balloon is usually inserted following a TURP. The inflated balloon is pulled down into the prostatic fossa and the catheter tubing is pulled down and secured to the man's leg with a urinary catheter attachment device to apply pressure against the operative site, preventing bleeding.*
- Explain that the presence of a urinary catheter will cause the sensation of needing to void, but it is important not to strain to try to void around the catheter or when having a bowel movement. Explain that bladder spasms, experienced as lower abdominal pressure or pain and a desire to urinate, may occur and medications may help with this issue. *Pressure on the urethra by the large catheter and on the internal sphincter by the catheter's balloon stimulate the micturition reflex. Straining to void or to have a bowel movement may stimulate bladder spasms and increase pain; it also may increase the risk for bleeding. Administer pain medications at regular intervals.*
- If the man has a continuous bladder irrigation (CBI), assess the catheter and the drainage tubing at regular intervals. Maintain the rate of flow of irrigating fluid to keep the output light pink or colorless. Assess the urinary output every 1 to 2 hours for color, consistency, amount, and presence of blood clots; assess for bladder spasms. *CBI is used to prevent the formation of blood clots, which could obstruct urinary output. Bladder distention resulting from output obstruction increases the risk of bleeding. Irrigating fluids are continuously infused and drained at a rate to keep urine light pink or colorless. Urine that is frankly bloody, contains many blood clots, or is decreased in amount, as well as bladder spasms, are indicators of obstruction and bleeding.*
- Assess for fluid volume excess and hyponatremia, called TURP syndrome, which is manifested by hyponatremia, decreased hematocrit, hypertension, bradycardia, nausea, and confusion. If these manifestations occur, notify the healthcare provider. *TURP syndrome results from the absorption of irrigating fluids during and after surgery. Untreated, it may result in dysrhythmias, seizures, or both.*
- If the man does not have CBI, follow agency procedure and healthcare provider orders for irrigating the indwelling catheter (usually when the urine is frankly bloody or has numerous larger blood clots or when bladder spasms increase). In most instances, using sterile technique, the catheter is gently irrigated with 50 mL of sterile irrigating solution at a time, until the obstruction is relieved or the urine is clear. Ensure equal input and output of irrigating fluid. *Intermittent irrigation may be used to prevent obstruction of urinary drainage.*
- Following catheter removal, assess the amount, color, and consistency of urine. Explain that the man may experience burning on urination, that dribbling after urination is a common experience, and that the urine may contain small blood clots after catheter removal. *The CBI and catheter are usually removed in the 24 to 48 hours following surgery. Urinary control may be*

(continued)

BOX 48.1
Nursing Care of the Patient Having a Prostatectomy (*continued*)

improved by teaching the man to start and stop the urine stream several times during each voiding and by practicing Kegel exercises. Regaining full control may take up to 1 year.

THE MAN WITH A RETROPUBIC PROSTATECTOMY

- Assess the abdominal incision (Figure 48.5B) for the presence of urine. *Because the bladder is not entered during a retropubic prostatectomy, no urine should be found on the dressing.*
- Assess the abdominal incision for increased or purulent drainage and the man for an increased temperature and pain. *These manifestations indicate the presence of infection.*

THE MAN WITH A SUPRAPUBIC PROSTATECTOMY

- Assess urinary output from both the suprapubic and the urethral catheters. *The man with a suprapubic prostatectomy often has two separate closed drainage systems: One from the suprapubic incision and one from a urethral catheter.*
- Assess the abdominal dressing for urinary drainage, and change saturated dressings frequently. Consult with a skin care specialist, if necessary. *Urine is highly irritating to the skin.*
- Following removal of the urethral catheter (usually 2 to 4 days after surgery) and based on healthcare provider orders, clamp the suprapubic catheter and encourage the man to void. Assess residual urine by unclamping the suprapubic catheter and measuring urinary output after voiding. *If residual urine is 75 mL or less with several voidings, the suprapubic catheter is removed.*

THE MAN WITH A PERINEAL PROSTATECTOMY

- Assess perineal incision for drainage and manifestations of infection. *Location of the incision in the perineum increases the risk of infection.*
- Do not take rectal temperatures or administer enemas. *Insertion of a thermometer or enema tubing into the rectum may precipitate bleeding.*
- Use a T-binder or padded scrotal support to hold the dressing in place. Following removal of the dressing and perineal sutures, heat lamps or sitz baths may be used. *The location of the dressing makes application difficult: Heat lamps or sitz baths provide heat and promote healing.*
- Teach the man to perform perineal irrigations with sterile normal saline as ordered and after each bowel movement. *Because of the proximity of the incision to the anus, special wound care is necessary to prevent infection.*

the prostate and then vaporizes obstructing prostate tissue with several short bursts of energy. An advantage of laser surgery is decreased blood loss and a more rapid recovery time. However, this method may not be as effective for larger prostates.

Other Treatments

Other treatments for BPH include minimally invasive procedures such as balloon urethroplasty and placement of intraurethral stents to maintain patency of the urethra. Balloon urethroplasty is a simple procedure in which a balloon-tipped catheter is inserted into the narrowed portion of the urethra and inflated. Inflation of the balloon widens the urethra, relieving obstruction. These procedures can be done as outpatient surgery.

Integrative Therapies

While previously the use of phytotherapy (the use of plants or plant extracts for medical treatment) was thought to be an option for men with BPH, a recent review of the literature demonstrates that phytotherapy is no more efficaciousness than placebo (Keehn, Taylor, & Lowe 2016), so healthcare providers should urge patients to use traditional therapies rather than complementary ones.

Nursing Care

There are many similarities between the nursing care of men with BPH and that of men with prostate cancer (see the section that follows).

Diagnoses, Outcomes, and Interventions

This section provides interventions related to education, urinary retention, reducing risk for infection, and risk for imbalanced fluid volume.

Educate Patients About BPH. Most men are unsure of the function of the prostate gland and even the prostate's exact location, though its relationship to sexual and urinary function is at least generally known. This lack of knowledge, coupled with the growing number of treatment options, is confusing to many men.

Expected Outcome: Patient will describe prostate anatomy and physiology and therapeutic options to treat BPH including medications and surgical options.

The nurse will:

- Explain the anatomy and physiology of the prostate gland, as well as normal changes that occur with aging. *Men must know about their bodies in order to make accurate decisions about treatment.*
- Discuss treatment options, including information about effects on erectile function, ejaculation, and fertility. Counsel the man to discuss specific concerns with his urologist. *Many different treatment options are available; the choice should be a mutual decision between the man, his partner, and the urologist.*
- Discuss effects of prostate surgery, including urinary retention and urinary incontinence. *These common transient postoperative effects are related to the surgical procedure and the postoperative indwelling catheter.*
- Explain to the man having a TURP that a catheter will be placed into the bladder, with the tubing taped to his inner thigh, and that irrigation fluid may be infusing into and out of the catheter for the first 36 to 72 hours following surgery. *The catheter and irrigation are necessary to remove blood clots from the bladder and allow drainage of urine. Gentle traction is applied to the catheter to apply pressure to the operative site (prostatic fossa) and prevent excessive bleeding.*

- Explain that, following removal of the catheter, he will most likely have urinary frequency and urgency. He may also experience dribbling of urine after voiding. Stress the importance of increasing oral fluid intake and regular Kegel exercises. *Urinary manifestations are related to the surgical procedure and the indwelling catheter. Increased fluid intake helps decrease dysuria. Kegel exercises strengthen periurethral muscles and decrease postvoiding urine leakage.*

Reduce Risk of Urinary Retention. Acute urinary retention is a potential complication of BPH, requiring immediate medical attention.

Expected Outcome: Patient will describe symptoms of urinary retention, medications, and actions to avoid development of urinary retention. Patient will demonstrate correct double-voiding technique to reduce urinary incontinence.

The nurse will:

- Teach the manifestations of acute urinary retention: Dysuria, overflow incontinence, bladder pain and distention, no urine output. *Acute urinary retention requires immediate medical attention.*
- Teach that the risk of developing urinary retention increases when the man with BPH takes OTC decongestant medications or prescription medications such as antidepressants, anticholinergics, calcium channel blockers, antipsychotics, and medications to treat Parkinson disease. *OTC decongestants may contain alpha-adrenergic agonists that increase smooth muscle tone of the prostate, bladder neck, and proximal urethra. The prescribed medications may relax detrusor muscle contractions. Both actions may increase the risk of urinary retention.*
- Suggest avoiding intake of large volumes of liquid at any one time. *A single intake of a large volume of liquid results in rapid bladder filling and increases the risk of urinary retention.*
- Teach how to use the double-voiding technique: Urinate, then sit on the toilet for 3 to 5 minutes, then urinate again. *This technique may relieve mild to moderate urinary retention.*

SAFETY ALERT: In addition to avoiding a large amount of fluids at one time, it is also important to teach the man to limit liquids that stimulate voiding, such as coffee and alcoholic beverages. ■

Reduce Risk for Infection. As with any invasive medical procedure, there is a risk of infection after prostate surgery.

Expected Outcome: Patient will describe symptoms of urinary tract infection and importance of early reporting of symptoms.

The nurse will:

- Monitor WBC and vital signs. *Infection is indicated by an increase in WBCs, body temperature, and pulse rate.*
- Maintain sterile procedures when changing irrigation fluids and emptying Foley catheter draining bag. *Sterile procedures are necessary to prevent infection.*

Promote Balanced Fluid Volume. A prostatectomy increases the risk for fluid volume imbalances as a result of excessive bleeding from the operative site (prostatic fossa) as well as absorption of irrigating fluid. Report manifestations indicating hypovolemic shock, excess bleeding, and/or TURP syndrome immediately.

Expected Outcome: Patient will describe symptoms that require immediate reporting: drop in blood pressure, increase in pulse, increase in postoperative bleeding.

The nurse will:

- Monitor pulse and blood pressure. *Manifestations of hypovolemic shock include an increasing pulse and a decreasing blood pressure.*
- Monitor color of drainage in urinary drainage bag (**Table 48.4**). *The appearance of urine and irrigation fluid in the urinary drainage bag is an excellent indicator of bleeding after a prostatectomy.*
- Monitor for manifestations of transurethral resection (TURP) syndrome: Nausea and vomiting, confusion, hypertension, bradycardia, and visual disturbances. *The absorption of isotonic bladder irrigating fluids during and after surgery may cause this hypervolemic, hyponatremic state. Treatment includes diuresis and, in severe cases, hypertonic saline administration.*

Delegating Nursing Care Activities

Routine vital signs along with measurements of intake and output can be delegated to appropriate personnel. The irrigation of any catheter should be done by the RN unless there is an instructional policy that differs. Ambulation is also important to prevent a number of complications and this can be delegated also.

Table 48.4 Urine Characteristics after Prostatectomy with Related Nursing Implications

Urine Color	Nursing Implications
Light red to red	Normal day of surgery and first postoperative day.
Very dark red	May indicate increased venous bleeding or inadequate dilution. Catheter at risk for occlusion. Increase flow rate of irrigant. If urine does not clear, notify healthcare provider.
Bright red	May indicate arterial bleeding. Increase flow rate of irrigant, monitor vital signs, and notify healthcare provider.
Contains blood clots	Occasional blood clot normal. If clots are frequent, catheter may become obstructed. Increase flow rate of irrigant.
Clear to light pink	Normal throughout hospitalization.

Transitions of Care

Depending on the man's choice of treatment, the procedure may be performed on an outpatient basis. The man having a TURP, although hospitalized for the surgery, may be discharged within 2 days after surgery if there are no complications. Discharge instructions after prostate surgery are outlined in **Box 48.2**. Home care often involves care of an indwelling urinary catheter. Teaching how to care for the catheter and drainage bag includes the following information:

- Change from the daytime leg drainage bag to a larger night drainage bag. A larger bag suspended from the bed frame at night permits gravity drainage of urine and prevents reflux of urine back into the bladder.
- Avoid strapping the leg bag on too tightly, which can decrease venous return and increase risk for thrombophlebitis and embolic complications such as pulmonary emboli.
- Place a soft cloth between the leg bag and thigh to decrease friction and absorb dampness under the bag, reducing the risk of skin irritation.
- Empty the leg bag every 3 to 4 hours during waking hours to prevent overfilling.
- Promptly report to the urologist any unexpected changes in urine color, consistency, or odor; hematuria; evidence of frank bleeding or large blood clots; or a lack of or significant decrease in urine output.

The Patient with Prostate Cancer

Cancer of the prostate is the most common type of cancer and the second leading cause of cancer deaths among men in North America (Sorenson et al., 2019). The greatest risk factor for prostate cancer is age; 85% of men with prostate cancer are diagnosed after the age of 65. The American Cancer Society states one in nine men will be diagnosed with prostate cancer in his lifetime (ACS, 2018c). Even though prostate cancer death rates are decreasing, this cancer still poses major health concerns and implications for healthcare for older men. Improved screening in the aging population has resulted in increasing numbers of men being diagnosed. Treating this cancer often proves to be more harmful than the cancer itself and does not improve mortality rates. Prostate cancer treatments can affect quality of life, with urinary and sexual dysfunction as well as complications from surgery itself. There is growing consensus that for many men, careful monitoring is more appropriate than treatment (Wilt et al., 2017). Still, for some men prostate cancer is more aggressive and ultimately contributes to their death. Because of these issues, debate exists concerning screening for prostate cancer. The American Cancer Society (2018c) recommends that screening be performed on an individual basis, dependent on risk factors and personal choice.

Prostate cancer is usually curable if detected early. However, all survival statistics need to be read cautiously. Definitions and other factors may influence the reported survival rate. Although, given this fact, prostate cancer has a good survival rate if the cancer has not spread too distant from the primary source. Many men are found to have prostate cancer on autopsy; usually the cancer has produced no manifestations or complications. If, however, the cancer has metastasized, outcomes are less positive and debilitation and death are a great possibility.

Pathophysiology

The prostate gland consists primarily of glandular epithelial cells. The exact etiology of prostate cancer is unknown, although androgens are believed to have a role in its development. Almost all primary prostate cancers are

BOX 48.2
Discharge Instructions after Prostate Surgery

- ***Activity:*** The healing period lasts from 4 to 8 weeks. Avoid strenuous activity and heavy lifting. Do not drive for 2 weeks, except for short rides. Do not take long walks; take stairs slowly and carefully. Continue exercises that you did in the hospital to prevent blood clots in the legs. You can take showers; avoid tub baths while the catheter is in place. If work is not strenuous, you may return in 4 weeks; otherwise, wait 6 to 8 weeks.
- ***Bleeding:*** Bleeding can occur any time after surgery. It is fairly common after a bowel movement, coughing, or increased exercise. If you notice blood in the urine, increase fluids and rest until the urine is clear. If heavy bleeding obstructs urine flow, call the healthcare provider immediately. Avoid aspirin and NSAIDs for at least 2 weeks.
- ***Bowel Movements:*** Keep bowel movements regular and soft to avoid pressure on the prostate area. Drink fruit juices, increase fiber in the diet, and take mild laxatives or stool softeners if needed.
- ***Diet:*** Resume your normal diet. Increase fluids to ten 8-oz glasses daily. Avoid alcohol unless otherwise approved by your healthcare provider.
- ***Sexual intercourse:*** Do not have sex for 6 weeks after surgery to avoid bleeding. You may still have erections even with the catheter in place. When you resume sex, ejaculate may flow back into the bladder; if so, you will expel little or no semen when having an orgasm.
- ***Urination:*** After your catheter is removed, you may experience some burning, stinging, or leakage for several weeks and you may pass small blood clots occasionally. These symptoms will disappear as the area heals. It is best to use pads to control leakage. Kegel exercises (see Box 27.3 in Chapter 27) can help gain urinary control.*Call your healthcare provider immediately if the following occurs:*

- You are unable to urinate.
- Bleeding is not controlled by fluids and rest or is excessive.
- You have chills and fever or severe abdominal pain.
- Your scrotum becomes swollen and tender.
- You have pain in one calf, chest pain, or difficulty breathing.

adenocarcinomas, and they develop in the peripheral zones of the prostate gland. This location increases the risk of local spread to the prostatic capsule. Despite its proximity to the rectum, spread to the bowel is uncommon because a tough sheet of fascia acts as an effective physical barrier.

As the tumor enlarges, it may compress the urethra, obstructing urinary flow. The tumor may metastasize and involve the seminal vesicles or bladder by direct extension. Metastasis by lymph and venous channels is common.

Risk Factors

In addition to age, race is a significant risk factor for prostate cancer, although the cause is unknown. Prostate cancer occurs more often and at an earlier age in Black men than in men of other races. Asians Americans and Native Americans have the lowest incidence of prostate cancer. Other risk factors being investigated are:

- Genetic and hereditary factors, with risk increased in men who have a family history of the disease. A father or brother having prostate cancer doubles a man's chances of developing it in his lifetime (ACS, 2018c).
- Having a vasectomy, believed to increase the levels of circulating free testosterone.
- Dietary factors, including a diet high in animal fat and excessive supplemental vitamin A.

Manifestations

Men with early-stage prostate cancer are often asymptomatic. Urinary manifestations depend on the size and location of the tumor and the stage of the malignancy. They are often much like manifestations of BPH: Urgency, frequency, hesitancy, dysuria, and nocturia. The man may also notice hematuria or blood in the ejaculate. Pain from metastasis to bones may occur with advanced disease. Manifestations of prostate cancer are outlined by body system in **Table 48.5**.

Complications

Death usually occurs secondary to debility caused by multiple sites of skeletal metastasis, especially to the vertebrae.

Table 48.5 Manifestations of Prostate Cancer by Body System

Body System	Manifestations
Genitourinary	■ Dysuria ■ Frequency of urination ■ Reduction in urinary stream ■ Nocturia ■ Hematuria ■ Abnormal prostate on digital rectal examination
Musculoskeletal	■ Bone or joint pain ■ Migratory bone pain ■ Back pain
Neurologic	■ Nerve pain ■ Bilateral lower extremity weakness ■ Bowel or bladder dysfunction ■ Muscle spasms
SYSTEMIC	■ Weight loss ■ Fatigue

The spinal cord may be compressed by tumors or by fractures of the spine, resulting in the possible loss of mobility and bowel and bladder function. Tumors may eventually involve bone marrow, resulting in severe anemias and impaired immune function.

Interprofessional Care

Care of the man with prostate cancer focuses on diagnosis, elimination or containment of the cancer, and prevention or treatment of complications. There are currently no clinical strategies to prevent the development of prostate cancer, although results of several large studies have demonstrated a reduced risk in men over age 55 that are treated with a 5α-reductase inhibitor such as finasteride (Propecia, Proscar) or dutasteride (Avodart). Education and early detection remain the major emphases for control of this disease.

The treatment of prostate cancer is complex and depends on the grade and stage of the cancer as well as the age, general health, and preference of the patient. In some cases, for example, when the patient with a slow-growing tumor is older or has a limited life expectancy, watchful waiting is the treatment of choice. Treatments for prostate cancer include surgery, radiation therapy, hormone manipulation, and chemotherapeutic agents.

Diagnosis

Although an increasing number of patients are now diagnosed with asymptomatic prostate cancer, many patients with prostate cancer have either locally advanced cancer or distant metastasis at the time of diagnosis. The definitive diagnosis can be made only by biopsy; however, other tests may suggest the presence of prostate cancer.

A digital rectal examination (DRE) will find the prostate gland nodular and fixed in prostate cancer. PSA levels are used to diagnose and stage prostate cancer and to monitor response to treatment. Levels depend on age, and there is no specific normal or abnormal level. An increase over time is more significant than one reading. The PSA test is used with a DRE to screen for prostate cancer in men age 48 to 76 years.

Transrectal ultrasonography (TRUS) may be used when the DRE is abnormal or if the PSA is elevated. In this test, a small probe is inserted in the rectum. The probe gives off sound waves that are reflected off tissues to provide a picture of the prostate on a video screen. Guided by this picture, the physician inserts a narrow needle through the rectal wall into the prostate gland to remove a tissue sample for examination (biopsy). Other tests that may be ordered include a urinalysis or cystoscopy. Bone scan, MRI, or CT scans may be performed to determine the presence of tumor metastasis.

Grade and stage help to determine prognosis and guide treatment decisions. Grade (cancer cell differentiation) is determined by the pathologist. Prostate cancer is staged with a variety of tests. **Table 48.6** outlines treatment options according to the stage of the cancer. The Moving Evidence into Action feature discusses how decision aids can help men with prostate cancer decide on the best course of treatment for them with their healthcare team.

Table 48.6 Prostate Cancer Staging and Treatment

Stage	Description	Treatment
I	Confined to prostate; nonpalpable, focal involvement; well differentiated	■ Observation and follow-up ■ Interstitial or external-beam radiation therapy ■ Prostatectomy
II	Confined to prostate, palpable, involves one or both lobes; poorly differentiated	■ Careful observation in selected patients ■ Prostatectomy ■ Interstitial or external-beam radiation therapy ■ Ultrasound-guided percutaneous cryosurgery
III	Extension of the tumor outside the prostate capsule, possible seminal vesicle involvement	■ External-beam radiation therapy ■ Interstitial radiation ■ Radical prostatectomy ■ Adjunctive hormone therapy ■ Palliative surgery (TURP)
IV	Extension of the tumor into surrounding tissues; lymph node involvement or distant metastasis	■ Hormone therapy ■ External-beam radiation therapy ■ Palliative treatment with radiation therapy and/or TURP ■ Radical prostatectomy with orchiectomy ■ Chemotherapy

Moving Evidence into Action

Clinical Issue

When faced with prostate cancer, men will face a number of decisions concerning treatment. This is a time of high stress and potential confusion. Decisional aids can help some men with this process.

External Evidence

A meta-analysis (Violette et al., 2015) examined studies that used decisional aids for men making treatment decisions concerning localized prostate treatment. The authors conclude that while the information provided with decisional aids is important, the data does not demonstrate the facilitation of shared decision making.

Internal Evidence

Most healthcare settings provide a number of different ways for knowledge to be transmitted to patients on treatment options. This can include written handouts, PowerPoint presentations, locally produced websites, and group presentations. Each institution and nurse must find the aid that is easiest for them and their patient to use. Comfort and familiarity with the decisional aid is important for the nurse.

Patient Considerations

Not all patients learn and acquire knowledge in the same fashion. The ability to go over the information at another time could be important for the patient. Patient education principles need to be included. Also use of technology needs to be determined. If the information is available on a website but the man does not have access to a computer in a private place, then this form of delivery of education materials is not helpful.

Putting the Pieces Together

When assisting with decisions on medical care, the nurse must work with the patient to determine the best way for the patient to receive the information. Decisional aids must be in a form that is acceptable to the patient, that the patient can readily use, and in a manner which the nurse can deliver the information.

References

Violette, P. D., Agoritsas, A., Alexander, P., Riikonen, J., Santti, H., Agarwal, A., . . . Tikkinenm, K. A. O. (2015). Decision aids for localized prostate cancer treatment choice: Systematic review and meta-analysis. *CA: A Cancer Journal for Clinicians*, *65*(3), 239–251.

Medications

Androgen deprivation therapy is used to treat but does not cure advanced prostate cancer. Many cells in the growing tumor are androgen dependent and either cease to grow or die if deprived of androgens. Response rates vary depending on the tumor sensitivity and other factors. Strategies to deplete androgen levels or block their effect vary from surgical orchiectomy (the most effective but least acceptable to the patient) to oral administration of hormonal agents (chemical castration). **Table 48.7** compares surgical and some hormone therapies to achieve androgen deprivation and the advantages and disadvantages of each. The treatment of prostate cancer is ever evolving.

Drugs such as degarelix (Firmagon), goserelin (Zoladex), and leuprolide (Lupron, others) are most commonly used to achieve androgen deprivation without orchiectomy. They may be administered orally or by depot injection. Hot flashes and ED are common adverse effects of these medications. Using these drugs in combination with an antiandrogen such as flutamide (Eulexin) or bicalutamide (Casodex) often reduces their adverse effects. Estrogens such as diethylstilbesterol (DES) may be used, but are associated with significant adverse effects (e.g., gynecomastia, hot flashes, ED) and a risk for thromboembolic disease.

Research is ongoing to demonstrate what mix of hormones is best and at what time in the perioperative period they are most effective. Hormonal therapy may also be used in conjunction with radiation therapy. Chemotherapy usually consists of cytotoxic agents. The biologic response modifier sipuleucel-T (Provenge) has been shown to improve

Table 48.7 Surgical and Selected Hormone* Therapies for Androgen Deprivation

Treatment	Advantages	Disadvantages
Orchiectomy	Inexpensive Immediate effect (i.e., men report diminished pain from metastasis in the recovery room)	Body image problems due to loss of testicles
Estrogen compounds (diethylstilbestrol)	Inexpensive Effects reversible	Increased risk of cardiovascular problems More likely to cause gynecomastia, hypertrophy of breast tissue
Luteinizing hormone-releasing hormone (LHRH) agonist (leuprolide)	Effects reversible No cardiovascular risk Monthly administration	Very expensive Subcutaneous injection route Slow onset: Up to 4 weeks
Steroidal antiandrogens (megestrol [Megace])	Effects reversible No cardiovascular risk Inexpensive	May not drop testosterone levels sufficiently Weight gain
Nonsteroidal antiandrogens (flutamide; often used in conjunction with LHRH)	Does not alter circulating androgens Blocks some side effects of LHRH May be effective if other methods fail	Very expensive

* All hormonal manipulations have the potential disadvantage of loss of libido, erectile dysfunction, hot flashes, and gynecomastia.

survival rates for prostate cancer patients and received FDA approval in 2010. This drug is mixed with the patient's immune cells and is administered by intravenous infusion to attack the tumor. Further studies of immunologic response drugs are currently in place to determine their effectiveness.

Surgery

Surgery for prostate cancer includes several types of prostatectomies. For very early disease in older men, cure may be achieved with a simple prostatectomy (such as TURP), discussed in the section on benign prostate hyperplasia. Following the surgery men usually experience erectile dysfunction for at least the first 3 months and return of sexual activity may take up to 2 years. Incontinence can also be a problem following prostatectomy surgery.

- ***Radical prostatectomy*** involves removal of the prostate, prostate capsule, seminal vesicles, and a portion of the bladder neck. In a laparoscopic radical prostatectomy (LRP), small incisions are made in the abdomen and a laparoscope is inserted and used to remove the prostate. Some surgeons use a robotic interface to perform this procedure.

  The most common radical prostatectomy techniques are:

  a. ***Retropubic prostatectomy*** is currently the favored method and is being combined with nerve-sparing techniques to improve erectile and bladder dysfunction problems. This form of surgery (see Figure 48.5B) allows visualization of the prostate bed and bladder neck and access to pelvic lymph nodes for biopsy.

  b. ***Perineal prostatectomy*** is often preferred for older men or those who are poor surgical risks. This approach requires less time, involves less bleeding and pain, and results in shorter hospital stays. A disadvantage to this approach is that lymph nodes cannot be accessed and require additional incisions to obtain.

  c. ***Suprapubic prostatectomy*** is rarely used, usually when problems with the bladder are expected. Control of bleeding is more difficult because the surgical approach is through the bladder.

For patients with stage III, locally advanced (beyond the prostatic capsule) cancer, surgery is controversial because of the likelihood of hidden lymph node metastasis and relapse. TURP is not performed as curative therapy but may be used to relieve urinary obstruction for men with advanced disease (stage III or IV).

Surgical intervention is now available for men with urinary sphincter insufficiency, which is the major cause of incontinence after prostatectomy. An artificial urinary sphincter is surgically implanted (**Figure 48.6** ■). To be eligible, the man must be able to manipulate the pump placed in the scrotum and have adequate cognitive function to know when a problem with the appliance occurs.

Potential complications of radical prostatectomy include erectile dysfunction, urethral stricture, fistula or other rectal injury, urinary incontinence, and risks from surgery and anesthesia.

Radiation Therapy

Radiation therapy may be used as a primary treatment for prostate cancer. Long-term problems of impotence and urinary incontinence occur less frequently, and survival rates are often comparable. Radiation may be delivered either by external beam or interstitial implants of radioactive seeds of iodine, gold, palladium, or iridium (brachytherapy). Interstitial radiation has a lower risk of impotence and rectal damage than external-beam radiation.

Immediate complications of radiation therapy include urethral stricture, cystitis, diarrhea, proctitis, rectal ulcer, and urinary incontinence. The following complications may appear months or years after radiation treatment: Erectile dysfunction, rectal/anal stricture, and bowel obstruction.

Radiation therapy has a palliative role for patients with metastatic prostate cancer, reducing the size of bone metastasis, controlling pain, and restoring function, such as continence or the ability to ambulate for patients with spinal

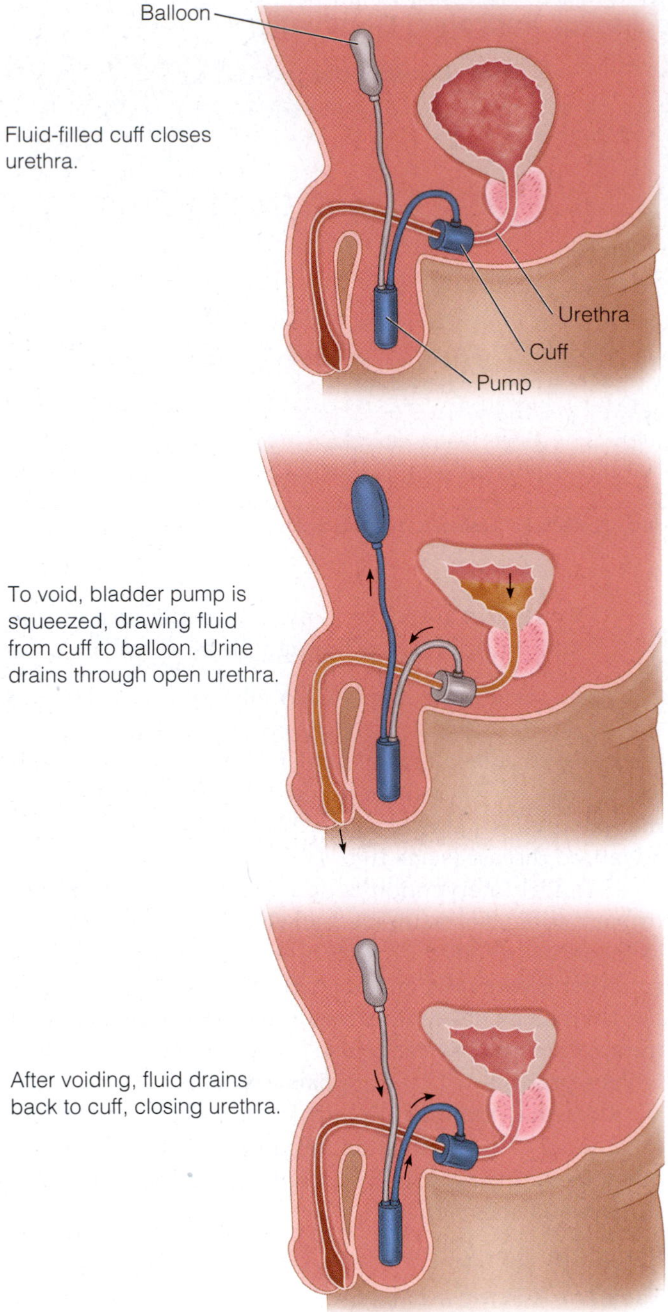
Balloon
Fluid-filled cuff closes urethra.
Urethra
Cuff
Pump
To void, bladder pump is squeezed, drawing fluid from cuff to balloon. Urine drains through open urethra.
After voiding, fluid drains back to cuff, closing urethra.

Figure 48.6 ■ Method of operation of an artificial urinary sphincter.

cord compression. Refer to Chapter 14 for nursing care of the patient receiving radiation therapy.

Nursing Care

Nurses plan and provide interventions to help prevent prostate cancer and to facilitate a return to functional health status. Interventions may range from teaching to using knowledge and skill in physical care following a radical prostatectomy. See the Case Study & Nursing Care Plan for a man having a radical prostatectomy on page 1784.

Assessment

Collect the following data through the health history and physical examination. Note that a digital rectal examination is an advanced nursing assessment.

- ***Health history:*** Risk factors, urinary elimination patterns and manifestations, hematuria, pain
- ***Physical assessment:*** DRE to assess prostate size, symmetry, firmness, and nodules.

Priorities of Care

Although the nursing care focus will differ depending on age of the man with prostate cancer, the stage of the disease, and the treatment plan, maintaining effective urinary elimination and helping the patient and family deal with the cancer diagnosis and treatment are priorities for nursing care.

Diagnoses, Outcomes, and Interventions

The nursing care of men with prostate cancer must be holistic, sensitive, and individualized. The nursing diagnoses discussed for the man with BPH may also be appropriate. This section focuses on problems with urinary incontinence, sexual function, and pain.

Promote Urinary Continence. Urinary incontinence is a disturbing complication following treatment for prostate cancer. Both radical prostatectomy and external-beam radiation therapy can cause incontinence, ranging from a drop or two when the patient lifts a heavy object (stress incontinence) to no control at all. Older men may experience urge incontinence, the involuntary passage of urine soon after a strong sense of urgency to void. Total and unpredictable loss of urine is classified as total incontinence. The man's reaction to incontinence may be significant even if the incontinence is not great. Many men have significant anxiety at the prospect of an incontinent episode in public because they feel shame and often guilt about the loss of control.

Expected Outcome: Patient will demonstrate urinary continence by recognizing the urge to void, managing independent toileting, and maintaining a predictable pattern of voiding.

The nurse will:

- Assess the degree of incontinence and its effects on lifestyle. *The nurse needs to determine previous urinary patterns and the type of incontinence currently being experienced to plan appropriate interventions.*
- Teach Kegel exercises to help restore continence. *Pelvic muscle or Kegel exercises can often either eliminate or improve stress incontinence.*
- Teach methods to control dampness and odor from stress incontinence as follows:
  a. Do not attempt to prevent accidental voiding by restricting fluids. *Not only will the man continue to have incontinent episodes, but also his urine will become concentrated, exacerbating the problem with odor.*
  b. Manage occasional episodes (one to three small-volume accidents per day) with absorbent pads

worn inside the underwear and changed as needed. Most pads are made with a polymer gel that controls odor. *Appropriate measures help promote good hygiene, decrease anxiety, and increase comfort.*

- Refer to physical therapy or a continence specialist for additional measures to promote continence. *Special exercises, restricting some types of fluid, and other measures such as bladder training can help the patient deal with incontinence.*
- Explore options such as an external collection device (external catheter or Texas catheter) for the man with total incontinence. *This device may improve the man's self-esteem and allow resumption of social activities.*
- Encourage verbalizing feelings about the impact of incontinence on quality of life. *The degree of incontinence does not necessarily correlate with the perceived level of suffering. Listening to these concerns with sensitivity can help the man work through these feelings and may allow him to move toward a healthy adaptation to his disability.*

Promote Sexual Function. Surgical treatment for prostate cancer may cause ED and changes in ejaculatory function. Hormone therapy for advanced prostate cancer lowers libido and may also cause ED. The diagnosis of cancer and body image changes caused by hormone therapy may lower self-esteem, which in turn can diminish sexual desire and willingness to interact sexually with a partner. Many older men are active sexually and fully capable of sustaining an erection. They are likely to fear the effect of treatment on their sexual health. They may allow this concern to guide their decision about the treatment course, or they may refuse all therapy because of this fear. Reactions vary greatly, and the nurse must maintain a nonjudgmental approach to education and support. It is also important to assess the spouse/partner's sexuality concerns because this will ultimately affect the man's decisions and well-being.

Expected Outcome: Patient will demonstrate willingness to discuss changes to sexual function and adapt modes of sexual expression to accommodate treatment-related changes.

The nurse will:

- Assess the man's pretreatment sexual function. *Knowledge of previous sexual function is necessary to plan appropriate interventions.*
- Teach the man about the actual or potential effects of therapy on sexual function. *The incidence of ED varies with different therapies for prostate cancer.*
- Provide an opportunity for the man and his partner to discuss implications of and concerns about the diagnosis and treatment of sexual function. A therapeutic approach to assessing how the man feels is to use an opening statement such as "Some men are very concerned about the effects of (type of treatment) on their ability to have an erection. Tell me how you feel about it." *The treatments for prostate cancer often affect the physiology of erection. The man and his partner need support and counseling during the period of adjustment.*
- Discuss medical and surgical treatments for ED (see the first section of this chapter). *Many men are as devastated by the loss of erectile function as they are by the diagnosis of cancer. Information about achieving erection and maintaining sexual intimacy is essential to quality of life.*
- Refer for sexual counseling as appropriate. *The man and his partner may require therapy beyond that provided by nurses.*

Manage Acute and Chronic Pain. There are many causes of pain in men with advanced prostate cancer. It is not unusual for a patient to have three or four types of pain simultaneously, all from different sources. The most common cause of pain is metastasis to the spinal column, usually the thoracic spine. Other sources of pain include fractures, lymphedema of the lower extremities, and muscle spasms. Because most men with prostate cancer are over the age of 65, many also have pain associated with preexisting conditions, such as osteoarthritis, unrelated to the cancer.

Expected Outcome: Patient will demonstrate adequate pain management through use of prescribed pharmacologic and nonpharmacologic interventions for pain relief.

The nurse will:

- Assess the intensity, location, and quality of the pain. *A cardinal rule of successful pain management is the importance of reducing or eliminating the cause of pain. Appropriate interventions are based on a careful assessment of the patient's pain.*
- Provide optimal pain relief with prescribed analgesics. *It is important for the man and his family to understand that pain medications should be used on a regular basis to maintain comfort and should not be delayed until pain is severe.*
- Teach the man and his family noninvasive methods of pain control. *Various modalities can be successful in alleviating pain or reducing its perception, thus enhancing the comfort of the patient* (refer to Chapter 9).

Transitions of Care

Nurses are in a unique position to increase public awareness about early detection of prostate cancer. Every encounter with men and their families—in clinics, hospital units, or in the home—is an opportunity to provide information about early detection and identify needs. Several studies have shown a positive correlation between increased awareness of and participation in prostate cancer screening procedures. The American Cancer Society provides free pamphlets about early detection of prostate cancer, which are useful in educating the public.

One risk factor that can be easily changed is diet. Men should know that they can lower their risk of prostate cancer by eating less red meat and fat. They should include fruits and vegetables as recommended in current USDA MyPlate guidelines; tomatoes, pink grapefruit, and watermelon are high in lycopenes that help prevent damage to DNA and may help lower prostate cancer risk.

All men should be given information about the limitations and benefits of testing for early detection and of treatment if diagnosed with prostate cancer, so they can make an informed decision. Men should be informed of the genetic predisposition in the development of prostate cancer. Men at high risk (men of African descent and those with a first-degree relative diagnosed at a younger age) should consider PSA testing.

Depending on the type of treatment, the following topics should be addressed in preparing the patient and his family for home care:

- For the man having a surgical procedure: Manifestations of infection and excessive bleeding, catheter care, wound care, pain management
- For the man receiving radiation therapy:
  a. Risk of radiation damage to others (none for external-beam radiation; if brachytherapy is used, sleep in a room alone for a week; avoid close contact with pregnant women, infants, and children)
  b. Condom use during sexual contact (ejaculate may be discolored, distressing sexual partner)
- The importance of keeping appointments with healthcare providers and having PSA testing if recommended and agreed on by the man, along with rectal examinations
- If appropriate, community services, such as support groups, home health nurses, and hospice
- Helpful resources:
  a. American Cancer Society
  b. American Urological Association
  c. National Cancer Institute.

Not all men with prostate cancer will have a cure or a control of the disease. The nurse must help the patient and his family cope with the fact the cancer is incurable and will lead to the death of the patient. General end-of-life care (pain control, symptom control) is important along with emotional support. Gerhart et al. (2016) reported an association between psychosocial distress and lower preference for palliative care services. The conclusion was patients with prostate cancer may benefit from additional emotional support as decisions are made concerning care and comfort.

Case Study & Nursing Care Plan

A Man with Prostate Cancer

William Turner, age 71, lives with his wife in a small retirement community in Florida. His wife had a stroke 2 years ago, and Mr. Turner does all the cooking and housework. He has been in good health for most of his life, having only "a small touch" of osteoarthritis in his knees and hands. He has noticed a gradual onset of urinary urgency and frequency during the past 2 years, but has never had incontinence. During a routine checkup, the nurse practitioner at the local health clinic performs a digital rectal examination and palpates a hard nodule on the surface of Mr. Turner's prostate. After his PSA is found to be elevated, he is referred to a urologist, who diagnoses prostate cancer. Mr. Turner chooses to have surgery, and a radical retropubic prostatectomy and lymph node dissection are performed. The lymph nodes are negative for metastasis. Following surgery, his recovery is uncomplicated. However, the nurse caring for Mr. Turner is concerned about his ability to care for his indwelling catheter because of his arthritis and his wife's physical disabilities from the stroke. The nurse makes a referral to a home health agency to ensure Mr. Turner can manage his care at home. An initial home health assessment is scheduled for the day after Mr. Turner is discharged from the hospital.

ASSESSMENT	DIAGNOSES	EXPECTED OUTCOMES
The home health nurse notes that the house is clean and neat. Mr. Turner is dressed, but still wearing his night urinary drainage bag, even though it is 1300. Mr. Turner tells the nurse that his main problem is going to get groceries because he is embarrassed to be seen with the drainage bag. He says he has not been able to remove the drainage bag and attach the leg bag because of his arthritis. Physical assessment findings reveal the pelvic incision to be healing without signs of infection. There is no tenderness in his calves, chest pain, or shortness of breath. The urine is yellow, without odor. Mr. Turner does state that he sees no need for the pelvic exercises because he is no longer in the hospital. He also expresses the belief that he is cured of cancer and questions the need for follow-up care.	■ Potential for urinary incontinence related to surgical procedure ■ Nonadherence to treatment plan related to inability to care for the urinary drainage system, not understanding need for postoperative exercises, and questions about follow-up care	■ Patient will regain urinary continence after catheter removal. ■ Patient will change the urinary drainage bag with the appropriate assistance. ■ Patient will verbalize the rationale for performing postoperative exercise. ■ Patient will verbalize the need for continued follow-up care.

PLANNING AND IMPLEMENTATION

- Discuss the possibility of stress incontinence after the catheter is removed.
- Reinforce the need for Kegel exercises while the catheter is still in place.
- Explore Mr. Turner's support system to identify people who could assist him with catheter care and arrange a teaching session with them.
- Teach Mr. Turner the importance of follow-up care, relating the care to the history of the disease.

EVALUATION

Good friends from Mr. Turner's church have assisted him with care of his drainage bag and have reminded him to do his Kegel exercises several times a day while the catheter is in place. When the catheter is removed, Mr. Turner has only a small amount of urine leakage after voiding. He understands that it may take several weeks for this to resolve. Efforts to help him understand the need for continued medical care are less successful. Mr. Turner continues to state that he is cured, his wife needs him, and he sees no need to go back to the doctor.

CLINICAL REASONING IN PATIENT CARE

1. Outline a teaching plan for Mr. Turner for potential skin irritation related to urinary incontinence.
2. As a result of Mr. Turner's refusal to have ongoing medical care, he might be labeled as noncompliant. Would you make this nursing diagnosis? Why or why not?
3. If you were the home health nurse making a home visit and found that Mr. Turner had no urinary drainage for 16 hours, what assessments would you make? How would you handle this problem?

See Evaluating Your Response in Appendix B.

48.5 Disorders of the Male Breast

The Patient with Gynecomastia

Gynecomastia, the abnormal enlargement of the male breast, is thought to result from a high ratio of estradiol to testosterone. It is common during puberty, when more than 30% of males experience gynecomastia, which usually resolves within a year after development (D'Amico & Barbarito, 2016). Any condition that increases estrogen activity or decreases testosterone production can contribute to gynecomastia. Conditions that increase estrogen activity include obesity, testicular tumors, liver disease, and adrenal carcinoma; conditions that decrease testosterone production include chronic illness such as tuberculosis or Hodgkin's lymphoma, injury, and orchitis. Drugs such as digitalis, opiates, and chemotherapeutic agents are also associated with gynecomastia. Gynecomastia after adolescence is usually bilateral. If it is unilateral, biopsy may be necessary to rule out breast cancer.

No treatment is necessary for the transient gynecomastia of puberty. If the condition becomes chronic, however, creating psychologic discomfort, surgery may be necessary to remove the subcutaneous breast tissue. When related to an underlying disorder, treatment of that disorder is required. In severe cases, tamoxifen is given to decrease estrogen activity.

Nursing care for the patient with gynecomastia includes education about the cause and treatment of the condition and emotional support for the psychosocial implications of this feminizing condition.

The Patient with Breast Cancer

Although male breast cancer is rare, accounting for about 1% of all breast cancer cases, it is as serious to the men who have it as it is to the women. In 2018 approximately 2500 men in the United States will be diagnosed with breast cancer and more than 450 men will die from breast cancer (ACS, 2018a). The etiology of male breast cancer is unclear; hormonal and perhaps environmental factors appear to be important. Genetics play a role as well: Men who inherit the *BRCA1* or *BRCA2* gene have an increased risk of developing breast cancer.

Male breast cancer is clinically and histologically similar to female breast cancer, although lobular cancer is rare in males. Most tumors are estrogen-receptor positive. Because many men believe that breast cancer is only a woman's disease, they often delay seeking medical attention for manifestations and thus may present with advanced disease.

Treatment of male breast cancer is much like the treatment of female breast cancer, beginning with lumpectomy or mastectomy, node dissection, and staging to determine the therapeutic options. Radiation, chemotherapy, and hormonal therapy (usually tamoxifen) are the conventional adjuncts to surgery. Castration (surgical removal of the testes) was previously used but current treatments consist of antiandrogen therapy resulting in tumor regression and prolonging life (ACS, 2018a).

Nursing care for the man with breast cancer is essentially the same as for the woman with breast cancer (see Chapter 49). The nurse has an opportunity to help the man and his family cope with the psychosocial effects of having breast cancer. He may feel embarrassment or shame about his condition as well as fear about the life-threatening nature of the disease. His family may share those feelings. By listening with understanding and empathy, the nurse can help the patient and family resolve their feelings and move toward healing.

CHAPTER HIGHLIGHTS

48.1 Disorders of Male Sexual Function

Describe the pathophysiology and manifestations of male sexual dysfunction, and outline the interprofessional care and nursing care of patents with erectile dysfunction.

- Many different illnesses, medications, and surgical procedures can affect male sexual function. It is important for nurses to initiate a conversation regarding sexual concerns with male patients.
- Psychologic issues can result from alterations in a man's sexual function at any age. Nurses must recognize patient values and preferences and demonstrate a sensitivity to the patient's concerns.
- Disorders of male sexual function include erectile dysfunction (ED) and ejaculatory dysfunction. Treatments include medications, mechanical devices, and surgical procedures. It is important for nurses to initiate a discussion of sexual concerns during assessments and to recognize that many male reproductive treatments and surgeries may result in sexual dysfunction.
- Disorders of the male reproductive system including scrotal masses, testicular infections and cancer, prostate enlargement and cancer, phimosis, and priapism may interfere with normal urination and sexual function.

48.2 Disorders of the Penis

Describe the pathophysiology and manifestations of disorders of the penis, and outline the interprofessional care and nursing care of patents with these disorders.

- Phimosis and priapism are disorders of the penis that can cause problems with urination and sexual activity and may in some cases be considered medical emergencies. The risk of cancer of the penis, although rare, is increased by phimosis, poor genital hygiene, and viral HPV and HIV infections.

48.3 Disorders of the Testis and Scrotum

Describe the pathophysiology and manifestations of disorders of the testis and scrotum, and outline the interprofessional care and nursing care of patents with these disorders.

- Benign scrotal masses include hydrocele, spermatocele, and varicocele. Epididymitis may be associated with a urinary tract infection, prostatitis, urethral strictures, or an STI.
- The testes may be infected (orchitis), twisted (testicular torsion), or develop cancer. Testicular cancer is the most common cancer in men between the ages of 15 and 40. Monthly testicular self-examination is critical to early detection and treatment of cancer.

48.4 Disorders of the Prostate Gland

Describe the pathophysiology and manifestations of disorders of the prostate gland, and outline the interprofessional care and nursing care of patents with these disorders.

- The prostate gland may be inflamed or infected (prostatitis), enlarged (benign prostatic hyperplasia), or may develop cancer. BPH is a common disorder of the aging male that causes problems with urination as the enlarging prostate gland constricts the urethra. Treatments include medications and various types of surgery, depending on the size of the prostate and the age and health status of the man.
- Cancer of the prostate is the most common type of cancer and the second leading cause of cancer deaths in American men. When diagnosed early, prostate cancer is curable. Diagnosis is often based on an increasing level of PSA and an abnormal DRE. The cancer is treated with surgery, radiation, or hormonal manipulation.

48.5 Disorders of the Male Breast

Describe the pathophysiology and manifestations of disorders of the breast, and outline the interprofessional care and nursing care of patents with these disorders.

- The male breast may become enlarged (gynecomastia) or develop cancer.

TEST YOURSELF NCLEX-RN® REVIEW

1. The nurse is conducting a health history with an older adult patient who had prostate surgery 18 months ago. Which statement should the nurse use to gather information about the patient's sexual concerns?
   A. "Do you miss having sex?"
   B. "Why do you think you should be sexually active at your age?"
   C. "Following your prostate surgery, when did you first notice you had problems with sexual intercourse?"
   D. "Tell me about your experience with sexual function since your prostate surgery."

2. The nurse is conducting a health teaching session for young men. Which information should the nurse include to reduce the risk of cancer of the penis? (Select all that apply.)
   A. Avoid tight pants and very hot showers.
   B. Wear a condom during sexual intercourse.
   C. Retract the foreskin of the penis when showering.
   D. Schedule diagnostic tests for HPV and HIV infections.
   E. Maintain a regular testicular self-examination schedule.
3. A male patient is diagnosed with gonorrhea. For which additional health problem should this patient be assessed?
   A. Hydrocele
   B. Epididymitis
   C. Gynecomastia
   D. Erectile dysfunction
4. The nurse is planning a teaching session on testicular cancer for high school students. Which information should the nurse include in this session? (Select all that apply.)
   A. It rarely occurs in brothers.
   B. The incidence increases with age.
   C. Severe pain and testicular swelling arethe initial manifestations.
   D. It occurs most between ages 13 and 35.
   E. It is more common in Caucasian men than men of color.
5. The nurse is teaching a male patient with chronic prostatitis about self-care measures at home. What should the nurse teach the patient to decrease discomfort? (Select all that apply.)
   A. Take warm baths
   B. Increase fiber intake
   C. Increase oral fluid intake to 3 L/day
   D. Take anti-inflammatory drugs.
   E. Avoid sexual activity
6. A male patient is being prepared for tests to diagnose prostate cancer. About which diagnostic tests should the nurse instruct the patient? (Select all that apply.)
   A. PSA level
   B. Sperm count
   C. Blood chemistry
   D. Pelvic ultrasound
   E. Digital rectal examination
7. The patient is being assessed for possible benign prostatic hyperplasia. Which assessment finding would the nurse attribute to this diagnosis?
   A. Rash on the lower abdomen
   B. Constipation
   C. Dribbling of urine
   D. Intermittent claudication
8. The nurse is caring for a male patient recovering from a TURP. The urinary drainage bag is filled with dark red fluid with obvious clots and the patient is experiencing painful bladder spasms. What should the nurse do first?
   A. Assess intake and output since surgery.
   B. Report the assessments to the urologist.
   C. Explain that bladder spasms are common following this surgery.
   D. Administer pain medication in the form of a B&O suppository.
9. The nurse is presenting an educational seminar for a group of male community members on prostate cancer. The nurse evaluates teaching to be effective if which statement is made following the presentation?
   A. "Prostate cancer is very aggressive and kills quickly."
   B. "My risk of prostate cancer will go up as I get older."
   C. "Since I am Native American, I have a higher risk of prostate cancer."
   D. "I have to get up to go to the bathroom in the middle of the night, so I guess I have it."
10. The nurse is participating on a community task force to reduce the risk of prostate cancer. What nutritional information should the nurse include to reduce the risk of this type of cancer?
    A. Increase fiber intake.
    B. Decrease lycopene intake.
    C. Avoid foods high in sodium.
    D. Decrease red meat and fat intake.

See Test Yourself answers in Appendix B.

REFERENCES

Adams, M. P., Holland, L. N., & Urban, C. (2017). *Pharmacology for nursing: A pathophysiologic approach* (5th ed.). Hoboken, NJ: Pearson Education.

Alhof, S. E., McMahon, C. G., Waldinger M. D., Serefpglu, E. C., Shindel A. W., Adlikan, P. G., . . . Toprres L. O. (2014). An update of the International Society of Sexual Medicine's guidelines for the diagnosis and treatment of premature ejaculation (PE). *Sexual Medicine*, 2(2), 60–90.

American Cancer Society (2018a). *Key statistics for breast cancer in men.* Retrieved from https://www.cancer.org/cancer/breast-cancer-in-men/about/key-statistics.html.

American Cancer Society (ACS). (2018b). *Key statistics for penile cancer.* Retrieved from https://www.cancer.org/cancer/penile-cancer/about/key-statistics.html.

American Cancer Society (ACS). (2018c). *Key statistics for prostate cancer.* Retrieved from https://www.cancer.org/cancer/prostate-cancer/about/key-statistics.html.

American Cancer Society (ACS). (2018d). *Key statistics for testicular cancer.* Retrieved from https://www.cancer.org/cancer/testicular-cancer/about/key-statistics.html.

American Cancer Society (ACS). (2018e). *Penile cancer stages.* Retrieved from https://www.cancer.org/cancer/penile-cancer/detection-diagnosis-staging/staging.html.

American Cancer Society (ACS). (2018f). *What are the risk factors for penile cancer?* Retrieved from https://www.cancer.org/cancer/penile-cancer/causes-risks-prevention/risk-factors.html.

American Psychiatric Association. (2013). *Diagnostic and statistical manual of mental disorders* (5th ed.). Arlington, VA: Author.

D'Amico, D., & Barbarito, C. (2016). *Health and physical assessment in nursing*. Hoboken, NJ: Pearson Education.

Franco, J. V. A., Turk, T., Jung, J. H., Xiao, Y. T., Iakhno, S., Garrote, V., & Vietto, V. (2018). Non-pharmacological interventions for treating chronic prostatitis/chronic pelvic pain syndrome. *Cochrane Database of Systematic Reviews*, Issue 1. Article No.: CD012551. DOI: 10.1002/14651858.CD012551.pub2.

Gerber, D. (2014). Sexual problems. In B. A. Magowan, P. Owen, & A. Thomson (Eds.), *Clinical obstetrics and gynaecology* (3rd ed., pp. 191–202). Philadelphia, PA: Elsevier Health.

Gerhart, J., Asvat, Y., Lattie, E., O'Mahony, S., Duderstein, P., & Hoerger M. (2016). Distress, delay of gratification and preference for palliative care in men with prostate cancer. *Psycho-oncology, 25*(1), 91–96.

Keehn, A., Taylor, J., & Lowe, F. C. (2016). Phytotherapy for benign prostatic hyperplasia. *Current Urology Report, 12*(7), 53.

Lee, M. (2011). Focus on phosphodiesterase inhibitors for the treatment of erectile dysfunction in older men. *Clinical Therapeutics, 33*(11), 1590–1608.

Maiorino, M. I., Bellastella, G., & Esposito, K. (2015). Lifestyle modifications and erectile dysfunction: What can be expected. *Asian Journal of Andrology, 17*(1), 5–10.

Mayo Clinic. (2018a). *Erectile dysfunction: Causes*. Retrieved from www.mayoclinic.org/diseases-conditions/erectile-dysfunction/basics/causes/con-20034244.

Mayo Clinic. (2018b). *Testicular torsion*. Retrieved from https://www.mayoclinic.org/diseases-conditions/testicular-torsion/symptoms-causes/syc-20378270.

National Institute on Aging. (2017). *Sexuality in later life.* Retrieved from https://www.nia.nih.gov/health/sexuality-later-life.

National Institute of Diabetes and Digestive and Kidney Diseases (NIDDK). (2014). *Prostatitis: Inflammation of the prostate.* Retrieved from https://www.niddk.nih.gov/health-information/urologic-diseases/prostate-problems/prostatitis-inflammation-prostate.

National Institute of Diabetes and Digestive and Kidney Diseases (NIDDK). (2017). *Erectile dysfunction (ED).* Retrieved from https://www.niddk.nih.gov/health-information/urologic-diseases/erectile-dysfunction.

Sorenson, M., Quinn, L., & Klein, D. (2019). *Pathophysiology: Concepts of human diseases*. Hoboken, NJ: Pearson Education.

Thornton, C. P. (2016). Best practice in teaching male adolescents and young men to perform testicular self-examinations: A review. *Journal of Pediatric Health Care, 30*(6), 518–527.

Violette, P. D., Agoritsas, A., Alexander, P., Riikonen, J., Santti, H., Agarwal, A., . . . Tikkinenm, K. A. O. (2015). Decision aids for localized prostate cancer treatment choice: Systematic review and meta-analysis. *CA: A Cancer Journal for Clinicians, 65*(3), 239–251.

Wilt, T. J., Jones, K. M., Barry, M. J., Andriole, G. L., Culkin, D., Wheeler, D., . . . Brawer, M. K. (2017). Follow-up of prostatectomy versus observation for early prostate cancer. *New England Journal of Medicine, 377*, 132–142.

ADDITIONAL RESOURCES

NIH Chronic Prostatitis Symptom Index
www.prostatitis.org/symptomindex.html

American Cancer Society
www.cancer.org

American Urological Society
www.urologyhealth.org

Lance Armstrong Foundation
www.laf.org

National Cancer Institute
www.cancer.gov

NIH Chronic Prostatitis Symptom Index
www.prostatitis.org/symptomindex.html

National Kidney and Urological Diseases Information Clearinghouse
www.niddk.nih.gov

Prostate Cancer Charity Specialist Nurse Helpline
www.prostate-cancer.org.uk/we-can-help/our-specialist-nurses

Prostatitis
www.prostatitis.org

The Testicular Cancer Resource Center
www.acor.org/TCRC/patient_links.html

Testicular Self-Examination
www.cancernetwork.com/PatientGuides/Testes_Examination.htm

Chapter 49

Nursing Care of Women with Reproductive System and Breast Disorders

Chapter Outline and Learning Outcomes

49.1 Disorders of Female Sexual Function 1790

Describe the pathophysiology and manifestations of disorders of female sexual function, and outline the interprofessional care and nursing care of patients with these disorders.

49.2 Menstrual Disorders 1791

Describe the pathophysiology and manifestations of menstrual disorders, and outline the interprofessional care and nursing care of patients with these disorders.

49.3 Perimenopause 1798

Describe the pathophysiology and manifestations of perimenopause, and outline the interprofessional care and nursing care of patients with this condition.

49.4 Structural Disorders 1801

Describe the pathophysiology and manifestations of structural disorders of the female reproductive system, and outline the interprofessional care and nursing care of patients with these disorders.

49.5 Disorders of Female Reproductive Tissue 1803

Describe the pathophysiology and manifestations of disorders of female reproductive tissue, and outline the interprofessional care and nursing care of patients with these disorders.

49.6 Disorders of the Female Breast 1816

Describe the pathophysiology and manifestations of disorders of the breast, and outline the interprofessional care and nursing care of patients with these disorders.

CLINICAL COMPETENCIES

- Assess the functional health status of women with reproductive system and breast disorders, and monitor, document, and report abnormal manifestations and responses.
- Use current evidence and patient preferences to plan and implement optimal nursing care for women with reproductive and breast disorders.
- Prompt patient responses of values, preferences, and expressed needs as part of the clinical interview, implementation, and evaluation of care.
- Function competently within own scope of practice as a member of the healthcare team caring for women with reproductive and breast disorders.
- Apply quality measures, processes, and tools to improve outcomes for women with or at risk for reproductive and breast disorders.

KEY TERMS

abnormal uterine bleeding (AUB), 1794
anorgasmia, 1790
dysmenorrhea, 1793
dyspareunia, 1790
endometriosis, 1806
fibrocystic changes (FCC), 1816
leiomyoma, 1805
lymphedema, 1820
menopause, 1798
premenstrual syndrome (PMS), 1791

Disorders of the female reproductive system range from menstrual cramps to life-threatening diseases such as cancer. Many of these disorders can occur at any point in a woman's adult life. They may affect her ability to bear children, her sexuality, and her sense of well-being as a woman. Women who experience reproductive system changes and disorders require a holistic approach to meet their physical, emotional, and educational needs. Because the ability to reproduce affects self-esteem, feelings of femininity, and general health, both sensitivity and understanding from caregivers are essential. Providing a medical and family history and undergoing diagnostic tests often require women to disclose personal, intimate information and have invasive procedures, which they may find embarrassing and uncomfortable. When providing care, nurses must consider the woman within the context of her culture, socioeconomic and educational level, sexual orientation, and lifestyle.

This chapter discusses female perimenopause, sexual function, menstrual disorders, structural disorders, disorders of reproductive tissues, and disorders of the breast. Sexually transmitted infections (STIs), including vaginal infections and pelvic inflammatory disease, are discussed in Chapter 50. Many of the disorders discussed in this chapter result in actual or potential health problems requiring nursing care based on similar nursing diagnoses. To avoid repeating those diagnoses and interventions for each disorder, they have been divided among the nursing care discussions as appropriate. Treatment of cancer with chemotherapy and radiation is discussed in Chapter 14. Disorders of female sexual function may result from the physical or emotional effects of the disorders discussed in this chapter and thus are discussed first.

49.1 Disorders of Female Sexual Function

A woman's body maintains the capacity for sexual activity for all of her life. In a typical sexual event, two physiologic sexual responses occur: Vasocongestion and myotonia. Sexual stimulation results in vasocongestion of the blood vessels surrounding the vagina, causing engorgement, increased lubrication, and genital swelling and enlargement. Arousal, or myotonia, increases muscular tension, resulting in voluntary and involuntary muscle contraction.

The Patient with Sexual Dysfunction

The sexual response cycle has four phases: Excitement, plateau, orgasm, and resolution. These phases always occur in the same sequence; however, the duration of each phase may vary. Sexual arousal typically ends in orgasm (climax), but sometimes fails to do so. A refractory period, or period in which the sexual organs are incapable of responding to stimulus, does not occur in the female. Multiple orgasms are physically possible in all women.

Although nurses may not conduct sexual counseling, they should be able to obtain a sexual history without embarrassment, discuss sexual concerns with women, and make appropriate referrals.

Pathophysiology

Disorders of sexual function include dyspareunia, inhibited sexual desire, and orgasmic dysfunction.

Dyspareunia

The woman with **dyspareunia** (pain during intercourse) may find it difficult to express her feelings to her partner. This condition may manifest itself as decreased desire or inhibited orgasm. Physical conditions, such as imperforate hymen, vaginal scarring, or vaginismus, may cause dyspareunia. *Vaginismus* is a rare condition in which the vaginal muscles at the introitus contract so tightly that an erect penis cannot be inserted. The muscle contraction without penetration may be painful for the woman. An early traumatic event, such as sexual abuse, fear of men, or rape, may contribute to this disorder. However, it is estimated that most dyspareunia is psychogenic in origin. The woman develops an anxiety–fear–guilt cycle in which negative thoughts become associated with the act of vaginal penetration, initiating a conditioned involuntary reflex. Other sexual activity may be pleasurable.

Inhibited Sexual Desire

Inhibited sexual desire may be a result of pathophysiologic processes or may be psychogenic in origin. Often, inhibited sexual desire is rooted deeply in childhood teaching or experiences that may be too painful to recall. Cultural and religious values can also affect the processing of sexual stimuli. Fear of pregnancy or STIs and depression also contribute to decreased libido.

Orgasmic Dysfunction

Inhibited female orgasm (**anorgasmia**) is a relatively common sexual problem among women. Primary anorgasmia, occurring in 10 to 15% of women, exists when a woman has never experienced an orgasm during the waking state, either through self-stimulation or intercourse. Secondary anorgasmia exists when a woman who previously experienced at least one orgasm in the past is no longer able to do so. Organic causes of anorgasmia include the presence of disease that results in general debilitation or that affects the sexual response cycle, and the use of drugs that depress the central nervous system (CNS).

Interprofessional Care

Although there is not currently a female version of Viagra, medications are being tested to treat female sexual-desire problems. These include tibolone, approved for use in Europe; yohimbine, a natural extract; and topical estrogens and testosterone creams. In 2015 the FDA approved flibanserin for hypoactive sexual desire disorder. However, there are many side effects with the medication and it has significant interactions with alcohol (Jaspers et al., 2016).

Nursing Care

Nursing care focuses on identifying the type of sexual dysfunction with a thorough history, including the onset, duration, frequency, and context or situation in which the problem occurs. Questioning the woman about medication use is important because many drugs can contribute to sexual dysfunction. Antidepressants—especially selective serotonin reuptake inhibitors (SSRIs) such as Celexa, Prozac, and Zoloft—contribute to lack of libido and delayed or absent orgasm (Adams, Holland, & Urban, 2017). The woman's partner should be included in discussions when possible.

Teach the woman and her partner about varied normal sexual responses. The goal is to increase self-awareness and understanding of communication and their relationship to sexual desire. Explain the differences in the behaviors that men and women consider sexually stimulating. Sex therapists may provide training in autostimulation techniques (masturbation) after inhibitions against this practice are discussed. Group therapy may be encouraged to help the woman discuss her problem and to decrease the sense of isolation it gives her.

49.2 Menstrual Disorders

Monthly menstruation normally involves some minor discomfort, including breast tenderness, a feeling of heaviness and congestion in the pelvic area, uterine cramping, and low back pain. Many women, however, experience more serious effects, both physiologic and psychologic. This section discusses premenstrual syndrome, dysmenorrhea, and abnormal uterine bleeding.

The Patient with Premenstrual Syndrome

Premenstrual syndrome (PMS) is a complex of manifestations (e.g., mood swings, breast tenderness, fatigue, irritability, food cravings, and depression) that are limited to 3 to 14 days before menstruation and relieved by the onset of menses. It is estimated that up to 30% of all adult women experience moderate to severe symptoms and up to 6.4% have such severe symptoms they can be diagnosed with *premenstrual dysphoric disorder (PMDD)* (Yonkers & Simoni, 2018).

The syndrome is seen less frequently during the teens and 20s, reaching a peak in women in their mid-30s. Major life stressors, age greater than 30, and depression are risk factors associated with PMS. Premenstrual syndrome can be a factor in absenteeism at school or work, decreased productivity, interpersonal relationship difficulties, and lifestyle disruption.

Pathophysiology

The pathophysiology of PMS is not clearly understood, and research has not supported a simple imbalance of hormones. Current thinking on the pathophysiology of PMS includes a progesterone metabolite influence of gamma aminobutyric acid (GABA) (Yonkers & Simoni, 2018). Also, there is evidence of estradiol and progesterone effects on serotonin and serotonin transporters and receptors (Chin & Mambiar, 2016; Yonkers & Simoni, 2018). There is also some evidence that altered calcium homeostasis and circadian rhythms have a role in PMDD (di Scalea & Pearlstein, 2017).

Risk Factors

The risk factors for PMS and PMDD include obesity, smoking, and early sexual abuse/trauma (Yonkers & Simoni, 2018). It is not clear whether anxiety and depression are risk factors for PMS and PMDD or if having PMS increases the risk of anxiety and depression. Finally, there is some evidence based on twin studies that there is a familial predisposition toward premenstrual disorders: Concordance rates are higher among monozygotic than dizygotic twins (Yonkers & Simoni, 2018).

Manifestations

Manifestations of PMS occur during the luteal phase of the menstrual cycle (7 to 10 days prior to the onset of the menstrual flow), abating when the menstrual flow begins. See the accompanying Multisystem Effects of PMS feature. Although PMS may produce a variety of physiologic and psychologic manifestations, the exact nature of these manifestations and their intensity are individualized for each woman with this disorder. The manifestations may even differ from month to month in the same woman.

Complications

Complications are more societal than physical. Women with PMS and PMDD may miss time from work and school or have impairment of quality of work. Quality of life can also be affected (Chin & Nambiar, 2016).

Interprofessional Care

If no organic cause can be identified for the premenstrual disorder, the goals of care are to relieve manifestations and to help develop self-care patterns that will help the woman anticipate and cope more effectively with future episodes of PMS. The treatment of PMS integrates this self-monitored record of manifestations, with regular exercise, avoiding caffeine, and a diet low in simple sugars and high in lean proteins (Chin & Nambiar, 2016; Yonkers & Simoni, 2018).

Diagnosis

There are no definitive diagnostic tests for PMS; instead, the regular recurrence of manifestations preceding the onset of menses for at least 3 months leads to a diagnosis.

Medications

There is a stepwise approach to the treatment of both PMS and PMDD. First-line therapies include nonpharmacologic approaches (discussed below in Integrative Therapies), then pharmacologic therapies. The first pharmacologic treatment is with SSRIs, which are prescribed for only the second half of the menstrual cycle. If there is no relief, the SSRIs are prescribed throughout the whole menstrual cycle. Interestingly, response to SSRIs for PMDD is rapid as compared to the time of response for depression (Yonkers & Simoni, 2018). If there is no or inadequate response to SSRIs, then use of the oral contraceptive Yaz for 24 out of 28 days should be prescribed, as this contraceptive has the best data demonstrating efficacy, although others can be prescribed (Yonkers & Simoni, 2018). Both SSRIs and oral contraceptives can be used together. If the above listed treatments do not work, then ovulation may be suppressed by the use of gonadotropin-releasing hormone (GnRH) agonists. Progesterone and antiprostaglandin agents such as nonsteroidal anti-inflammatory drugs (NSAIDs) may help relieve cramping. Diuretics may be prescribed to relieve bloating.

Multisystem Effects of PMS

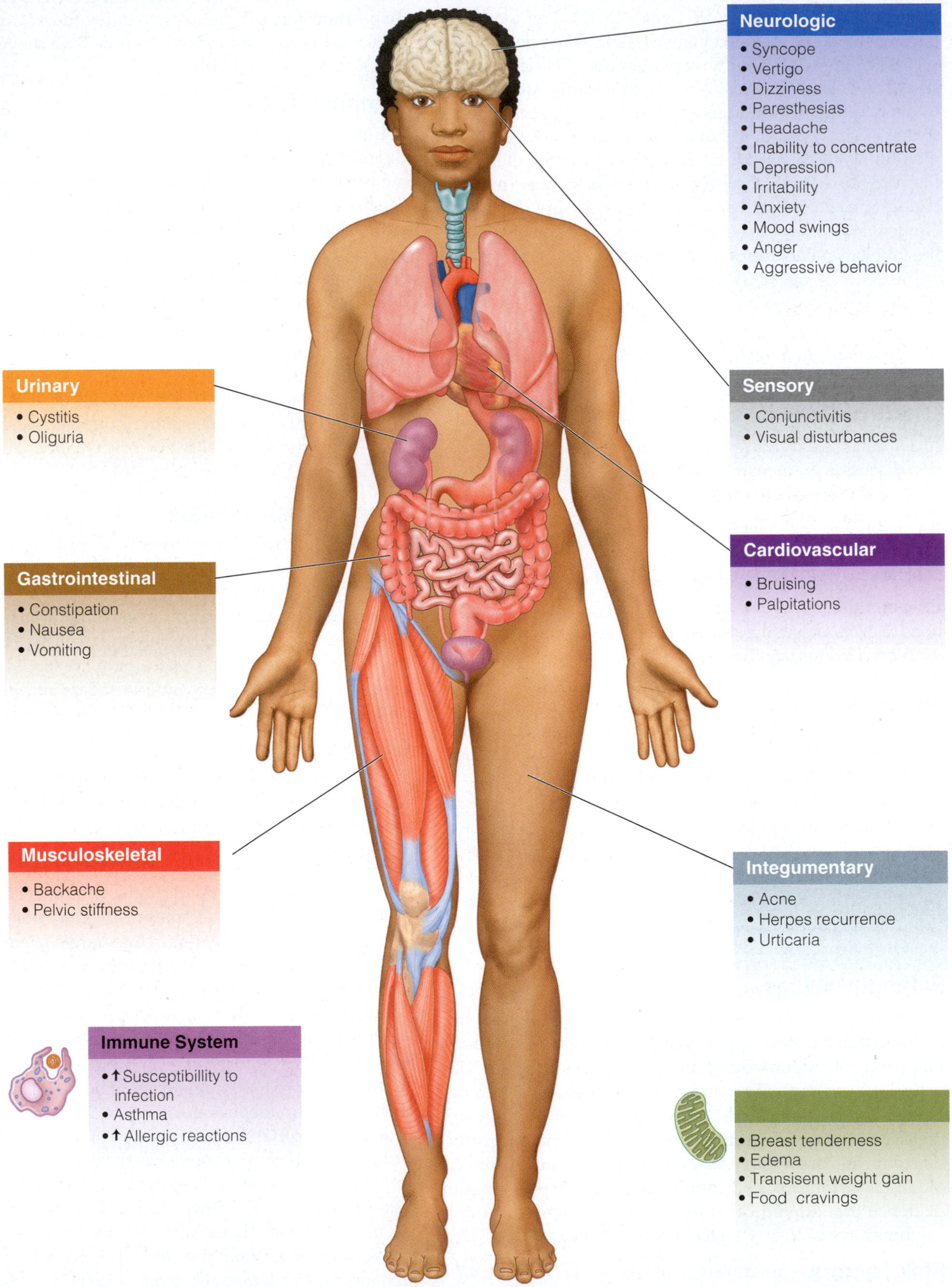
Neurologic
• Syncope
• Vertigo
• Dizziness
• Paresthesias
• Headache
• Inability to concentrate
• Depression
• Irritability
• Anxiety
• Mood swings
• Anger
• Aggressive behavior
Urinary
• Cystitis
• Oliguria
Sensory
• Conjunctivitis
• Visual disturbances
Gastrointestinal
• Constipation
• Nausea
• Vomiting
Cardiovascular
• Bruising
• Palpitations
Musculoskeletal
• Backache
• Pelvic stiffness
Integumentary
• Acne
• Herpes recurrence
• Urticaria
Immune System
• ↑ Susceptibillity to infection
• Asthma
• ↑ Allergic reactions
• Breast tenderness
• Edema
• Transient weight gain
• Food cravings

Nutrition

A diet high in complex carbohydrates during the late luteal phase may help some women. A healthy diet should be followed as excessive weight can lead to an increase in symptoms.

Integrative Therapies

The woman with PMS may find diet, exercise, relaxation, and stress management helpful.

- Increased intake of calcium (1000 mg per day) and vitamin B6 (50 to 100 mg per day) may be helpful (Yonkers & Simoni, 2018).
- Cognitive-behavioral therapy (CBT) may help some patients manage emotional symptoms.
- Herbal remedies that have demonstrated some efficacy are ginko biloba and St. John's wort (Yonkers & Simoni, 2018). However, before recommendation, a discussion about these complementary therapies with the health-care provider is recommended.
- Exercise is beneficial.
- Techniques for relaxation and stress management include deep abdominal breathing, meditation, muscle relaxation, and guided imagery.

Nursing Care

Assessment

Assessment for PMS and/or PMDD starts with the woman keeping track of her menstrual cycle and symptoms on a calendar for at least 2 months (Chin & Nambiar, 2016). There are a number of standardized calendars available.

Priorities of Care

The priority of care for a woman with either PMS or PMDD is relief (or at least decrease to a manageable level) of symptoms. Supporting the woman is important, as many treatments are tried to find the best one for the patient. This can be frustrating, so support from the nurse is needed during the process.

Diagnoses, Outcomes, and Interventions

Nursing care for the woman with PMS focuses on relieving manifestations. Most women experiencing PMS require interventions to manage pain and enhance coping.

Manage Acute Pain. The woman with PMS may have pain from headache (including migraine), menstrual cramps, excessive fluid retention, breast swelling, joint and muscle pain, and backache.

Expected Outcome: Patient will demonstrate adequate pain management through use of prescribed pharmacologic and nonpharmacologic interventions for pain and symptom relief.

The nurse will:

- Teach effective pharmacologic and nonpharmacologic self-care measures to relieve pain: Application of heat, relaxation techniques (such as breathing exercises, imagery techniques, or meditation), and exercise. *Heat relieves muscle spasms and dilates blood vessels, increasing blood supply to the pelvis and uterine muscles. Relaxation and exercise aid the release of naturally produced pain relievers called endorphins.*
- Review daily activities and suggest ways to balance rest periods and activity. *During rest periods, energy and oxygen requirements decrease, increasing the amount of energy and oxygen available to muscles.*
- Review manifestations and, if possible, correlate these with dietary patterns and activity levels. Encourage the woman to keep a diary of PMS manifestations. *Maintaining a diary of PMS manifestations, activity, and foods eaten can provide data to identify modifiable causes of discomfort.*
- If appropriate, suggest sexual activity as a way to lessen menstrual cramps. *Orgasm may help relieve dysmenorrhea.*

Promote Effective Coping. Many women experience mood swings during episodes of PMS, sometimes exhibiting self-destructive or aggressive behaviors toward others. These mood swings can interfere with a woman's ability to manage her responsibilities at home or at work.

Expected Outcome: Patient will demonstrate effective coping by use of strategies that reduce PMS symptoms.

The nurse will:

- Discuss CBT, if prescribed. *CBT can help with PMS symptoms and is the first-line therapy for treatment of PMS and/or PMDD.*
- Explore possible ways to rearrange or reschedule activities when experiencing PMS. *Planning ahead enables the woman to assume more control and promotes coping methods.*
- Explore what, if any, self-care measures have helped cope with mood alterations in the past. *Encourage healthful coping mechanisms, such as relaxation techniques and exercise. Some women may rely on alcohol or other drugs during PMS, which only exacerbate the manifestations.*

The Woman with Dysmenorrhea

Dysmenorrhea (pain or discomfort associated with menstruation) is estimated to occur in 40 to 95% of menstruating women (Iacovides, Avidon, & Baker, 2015). Primary dysmenorrhea is most often seen in girls who have just begun menstruating, becoming less severe after the mid-20s or giving birth. Secondary dysmenorrhea is most commonly seen when a woman is in her 20s and 30s, beginning after years of relatively painless menstrual periods.

Pathophysiology

In primary dysmenorrhea, prostaglandins are released from sloughing endometrial cells, causing myometrial contraction and vasoconstriction. As the muscles contract, uterine circulation is compromised, resulting in uterine ischemia and pain. These contractions can range from mild cramping to severe muscle spasms. Psychologic factors, such as anxiety and tension, may contribute to dysmenorrhea. Secondary dysmenorrhea is related to underlying pathologic conditions that involve scarring or injury to the reproductive tract. Endometriosis, fibroid tumors, chronic pelvic inflammatory disease, endometrial polyps, and use of an intrauterine device (IUD) may result in painful menses.

Manifestations

Manifestations of primary dysmenorrhea may be severe enough to disrupt activities of daily living, work, school attendance, and sexual function. They may include:

- Abdominal pain beginning with onset of menses and lasting 8 to 72 hours
- Pain radiating to lower back and thighs
- Headache
- Nausea and vomiting
- Diarrhea
- Fatigue
- Breast tenderness.

Interprofessional Care

Care of the woman with menstrual pain focuses on identifying the underlying cause, reestablishing functional capacity, and managing pain. A careful history and physical assessment are performed to rule out any underlying organic cause of dysmenorrhea. If no organic cause is found, the diagnosis is primary dysmenorrhea.

Diagnosis

Various diagnostic tests are performed to identify structural abnormalities, hormonal imbalances, and pathologic conditions that could cause menstrual pain.

Diagnosis is made based on findings from a pelvic examination and diagnostic procedures, including a Papanicolaou (Pap) test and cervical and vaginal cultures, ultrasound of the pelvis and vagina, and CT scan or MRI to detect structural abnormalities, malignancy, or infections. Laboratory tests used to assess possible causes of dysmenorrhea include FSH and LH levels to assess pituitary function, progesterone and estradiol levels to assess ovarian function, and thyroid function tests.

Laparoscopy is used to diagnose structural defects and blockages caused by scarring, endometriosis, tumors, and cysts (**Figure 49.1** ■). Care for the patient undergoing a laparoscopy is the same as for any patient undergoing general anesthesia and minimally invasive surgery. Patient teaching concerning pain afterward due to the insufflation of carbon dioxide during surgery should be noted as the woman may experience referred pain to the shoulders due to retained carbon dioxide. Educating the woman on what would be considered excessive bleeding after surgery and signs and symptoms of infection is also needed. An endometrial biopsy or a dilation and curettage (D&C) of the uterus may be performed to obtain tissue for evaluation or to relieve dysmenorrhea and heavy menstrual bleeding. (This procedure is discussed later in this chapter.)

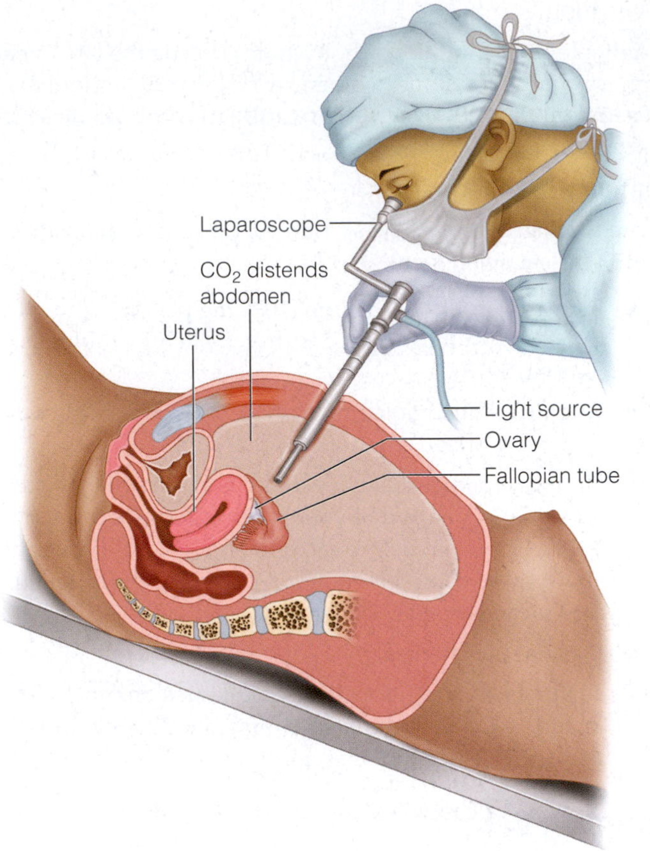
Laparoscope
CO_2 distends abdomen
Uterus
Light source
Ovary
Fallopian tube

Figure 49.1 ■ Laparoscopy. In this surgical procedure, a flexible, lighted instrument (laparoscope) is inserted through a periumbilical incision. Laparoscopy allows visualization of the pelvic cavity.

Medications

Dysmenorrhea may be treated with analgesics, prostaglandin inhibitors such as NSAIDs, or oral contraceptives (see **Medication Administration 49.A**).

Nursing Care

Nursing care for the woman with primary dysmenorrhea focuses on controlling manifestations and providing education about the normal physiology of the menstrual cycle and self-care measures. Care of the woman with secondary dysmenorrhea varies according to the underlying cause and is discussed in this chapter within sections on specific disorders. Nursing interventions previously described for the woman with PMS are also appropriate for the woman with dysmenorrhea.

The Woman with Abnormal Uterine Bleeding

Abnormal uterine bleeding (AUB), formerly known as *dysfunctional uterine bleeding (DUB)*, refers to vaginal bleeding that is usually painless but is abnormal in amount, duration, or time of occurrence (American College of Obstetricians and Gynecologists (ACOG), 2017a). A number of factors may predispose a woman to AUB. These factors include stress, extreme weight changes, use of oral contraceptive

Medication Administration 49.A

The Woman with Dysmenorrhea

EXAMPLES OF ORAL CONTRACEPTIVES

norethindrone and ethinyl estradiol (Brevicon, Norinyl)

norgestrel and ethinyl estradiol (Ovral)

Oral contraceptives inhibit ovulation and help reduce cramping and bleeding. Side effects of oral contraceptives include breast tenderness, weight gain, nausea, midcycle bleeding, mood swings, depression, chloasma (skin discoloration) on the face and chest, hypertension, vascular complications, vaginal candidiasis, migraines, and glucose intolerance. Oral contraceptives are contraindicated in women with personal or family history of breast cancer in first-degree relatives, hypertension, history of stroke or transient ischemic attack (TIA), smoking, history of estrogen-dependent cancer, pregnancy, liver disease, or thrombophlebitis.

Nursing Responsibilities

- Assess the patient for potential contraindications to drug therapy.

Health Education for the Patient and Family

- Take the drug as prescribed until the physician indicates otherwise or until side effects prevent you from continuing to take them.
- Be sure to take them at the same time every day.
- Report to the physician suspected pregnancy and any side effects such as nausea, rash, drowsiness, stomach pain, ringing in the ears, tenderness in the calf of the leg, and shortness of breath.
- Do not smoke while taking oral contraceptives because of the risk of developing a thrombus (blood clot).

Source: Data from Adams, et al., 2017.

agents or IUDs, and perimenopausal status. Abnormal uterine bleeding is usually related to hormonal imbalances or pelvic neoplasms, either benign or malignant. AUB, depending on cause, may occur in women from early to late adulthood. Abnormal uterine bleeding is a symptom and should be classified by the **PALM-COEIN** system for the underlying cause (ACOG, 2017b):

Polyp	**C**oagulopathy
Adenomyosis	**O**varian dysfunction
Leimyoma	**E**ndometrial
Malignancy and hyperplasia	**I**atrogenic
	Not otherwise classified.

Pathophysiology

The pathophysiology of AUB depends on the underlying cause. There may be a growth (either malignant or benign) in the uterus, abnormal hormonal levels, abnormal endometrial tissue, or other causes. Along with the classification system, there are more commonly used terms that patients may be more familiar with (ACOG, 2017b).

Current ACOG (2017b) classifications of AUB are:

- ***Heavy menstrual bleeding*** is characterized by excessive blood loss during menses.
- ***Intermenstrual bleeding*** is characterized by bleeding in between normal menses.
- ***Irregular uterine bleeding*** is characterized by unpredictable menses with more than 20 days between menses.

Women may be more familiar with previously used terminology (ACOG 2017b):

- ***Polymenorrhea:*** Frequent menstrual bleeding (frequency, 21 days or less)
- ***Menorrhagia*** (now called *heavy menstrual bleeding*): Prolonged or excessive uterine bleeding that occurs at regular intervals (the loss of 80 mL or more of blood that lasts for more than 7 days)
- ***Metrorrhagia:*** Irregular menstrual bleeding or bleeding between periods
- ***Menometrorrhagia*** (now called either *irregular* or *heavy uterine bleeding*): Frequent menstrual bleeding that is excessive and irregular in amount and duration.

Any bleeding after 1 year of absence of bleeding is called *postmenopausal bleeding*. The uterine bleeding may be caused by cervical polyps, endometrial polyps, endometrial hyperplasia, or uterine cancer. The possibility of cancer makes early evaluation and treatment essential.

One of the most common causes of abnormal uterine bleeding is hormonal imbalances, especially progesterone deficiency with relative estrogen excess, resulting in endometrial hyperplasia. Estrogen stimulates endometrial proliferation. However, without the support provided by progesterone, sloughing occurs, resulting in vaginal bleeding that may be irregular, prolonged, or profuse. Defects in the follicular phase shorten the proliferative phase of the menstrual cycle, resulting in spotting and breakthrough bleeding. Defects during the luteal phase result in excessive amount or duration of flow due to persistence of the corpus luteum. This leads to a deficiency of progesterone, resulting in vaginal bleeding. Anovulation (absence of ovulation) is associated with both estrogen and progesterone deficiencies. Emotional upsets or stress can cause hormonal imbalances and thus affect menstruation. Any of the causes of abnormal uterine bleeding described in the classification system should be addressed.

Interprofessional Care

The care of the woman with AUB focuses on identifying and treating the underlying disease. A careful history and physical examination are performed. Abdominal and pelvic examinations are performed to rule out abdominal masses. The woman may need to keep a menstrual history and basal body temperature chart for several months to determine whether ovulation is occurring.

Diagnosis

A variety of diagnostic tests are used to diagnose the cause of AUB. Diagnostic tests include a Pap test to rule out or identify cervical carcinoma; a pelvic or transvaginal ultrasound to identify luteal cysts, leiomyomas, or ovarian tumors; and an endometrial biopsy to obtain endometrial tissue for histologic examination. Depending on the suspected cause of the AUB, further testing may be needed.

Laboratory studies may include a complete blood count (CBC) to rule out a systemic disease, coagulant factors, PT and PTT to rule out clotting disorders, thyroid function studies, serum progesterone levels, and endocrine studies to evaluate pituitary and adrenal function (thyroid and pituitary dysfunction may be manifested by menstrual irregularities).

Medications

The use of pharmacologic agents is individualized depending on the underlying cause of the AUB. NSAIDs, which relieve cramping, may be the only treatment the woman desires once the underlying cause is known. Hormonal therapy or a hormonal releasing intrauterine device may be used. The key is to tailor the treatment to the underlying cause of the AUB and the woman's fertility desire and any comorbid conditions (Whitaker & Critchley, 2015). Oral iron supplements may be prescribed to replace iron lost through menstrual bleeding.

Surgery

Surgical intervention emphasizes the least invasive method that provides effective relief. These range from therapeutic D&C, to endometrial ablation, uterine artery embolization, myomectomy, and, lastly, hysterectomy.

Therapeutic D&C. In a therapeutic D&C, the cervical canal is dilated and the uterine wall is scraped. D&C is used to diagnose and treat AUB and other disorders of the female reproductive system. It may be performed to correct excessive or prolonged bleeding. D&C is contraindicated in any woman who has been taking anticoagulant drugs or whose condition precludes the use of regional or general anesthesia.

Discharge instructions for the patient who has a D&C include education about not inserting tampons or anything else into the vagina until all vaginal discharge has stopped and the woman has been seen for her postoperative visit. Also, the patient should be taught what the vaginal discharge will look like (bloody to brownish red with diminishing amounts) and signs/symptoms of infection.

Endometrial Ablation. In an endometrial ablation, the endometrial layer of the uterus is destroyed by using a laser, thermal balloon, or electrocautery. It is performed in women for whom childbearing has been completed and who do not respond to pharmacologic management or D&C. This procedure usually produces amenorrhea but there are cases where menstrual flow returns. A woman undergoing an endometrial ablation should understand that she should use contraception because her ovaries will function (i.e., produce hormones along with eggs) and fertilization can occur in the fallopian tubes.

Hysterectomy. Hysterectomy (surgical removal of the uterus) may be performed when medical management of bleeding disorders is unsuccessful or cancer is present, particularly if the woman no longer wishes to have children. Approximately 600,000 hysterectomies are performed each year in the United States, and one-third of all women have had a hysterectomy by age 60 (Centers for Disease Control and Prevention [CDC], 2015). In premenopausal women, the ovaries are usually left in place. In postmenopausal women, a total hysterectomy, or bilateral salpingo-oophorectomy with hysterectomy, may be performed; this procedure involves removal of the uterus, fallopian tubes, and ovaries.

Hysterectomy may be performed through an abdominal or a vaginal approach. The choice depends on the underlying disorder, the need to explore the abdominal cavity, and the preference of the surgeon and woman. When a hysterectomy is performed, the woman is hospitalized for 1 to 3 days and requires a recovery period of 4 to 6 weeks for an abdominal hysterectomy and 1 to 2 weeks for a vaginal and laparoscopic hysterectomy (see **Box 49.1**).

Abdominal hysterectomy is performed when a preexisting abdominal scar is present, when adhesions are thought to be present, or when a large operating field is necessary. For example, the woman with endometriosis is more likely to have an abdominal hysterectomy because endometrial tissue implants that may be present on other abdominal organs need to be removed. The surgical incision may be either longitudinal, made in the midline from umbilicus to pubis, or a Pfannenstiel incision, also known as the bikini cut. Vaginal hysterectomy, removal of the uterus through the vagina, is desirable when the uterus has descended into the vagina or if the urinary bladder or rectum has prolapsed into the vagina. Vaginal hysterectomy leaves no visible abdominal scar. A laparoscopy-assisted vaginal hysterectomy (LAVH) and a laparoscopic supracervical hysterectomy (LSH) are minimally invasive options to an open procedure. The recovery time following these procedures is often only 1 to 2 weeks.

Nursing Care

AUB usually causes anxiety. A woman's self-image, sexuality, or reproductive capacity may be threatened, and she may fear the possibility of cancer. She may be embarrassed to discuss her menstrual history, sexual history, and hygiene practices.

Assessment

Assessment for AUB includes the previously mentioned testing but one of the most important assessments that nurses can explain to a woman who is having AUB is maintaining a calendar of when and how much bleeding is occurring. This calendar will aid in the diagnosis of AUB.

Priorities of Care

Priorities of care for the patient with AUB include helping to relieve anxiety and promoting sexual function.

Diagnoses, Interventions, and Outcomes

Relieve Anxiety. The anxiety associated with abnormal uterine bleeding can be intense. Until the cause of the

BOX 49.1
Nursing Care of the Patient Having a Hysterectomy

PREOPERATIVE

- Encourage the woman to express feelings that may signal a negative self-concept. Correct any misconceptions. *Some women believe that hysterectomy means weight gain and the end of sexual activity.*
- Provide information about continuing to have regular gynecologic screenings. *If the cervix has not been removed, regular Pap tests should continue. Pelvic examination should continue regardless of removal of the cervix.*
- Teach the woman the Kegel exercise. *Hysterectomies can change the muscle tone of the pelvic floor. The exercise will help strengthen the pelvic floor.*

POSTOPERATIVE

- Monitor vital signs every 4 hours, auscultate lungs every shift, and measure intake and output. *These data are important indicators of hemodynamic status and complications.*
- Assess pain on a regular schedule, using a 1 (none) to 10 (severe) scale. Administer analgesics as prescribed. Splint incision, if present, to facilitate moving, coughing, and deep breathing. Assist with ambulation as prescribed. *Postoperative pain results from the surgery itself, as well as from gas pains prior to the return of peristalsis. Splinting the incision decreases pain from moving, turning, and deep breathing. Ambulation assists in the return of peristalsis.*
- Monitor for hemorrhage by keeping a perineal pad count and assessing abdominal dressing. Instruct the woman on how to conduct these assessments and to report abnormal findings to the surgeon. *As most women are discharged to home in 1 or 2 days, the woman's knowledge of possible hemorrhage is important.*
- Monitor voiding after surgery or after removal of a Foley catheter. *Voiding difficulty may occur after surgery or after the removal of a Foley catheter inserted prior to or during surgery. If the woman has not voided within 8 hours, notify the surgeon.*
- Instruct the woman about the manifestations of infection: Increased or a change in color or odor of drainage from the incision or perineal pads, general malaise, fever. If any of these occur, the woman should notify the surgeon. Discuss action of prescribed antibiotics and need to continue them until they are gone. *Early discharge mandates providing information about the risk for infection.*
- Explain the rationale for antiembolic or compression stockings and encourage leg exercises. Discuss manifestations of deep venous thrombosis (leg pain, redness, localized heat and swelling) and pulmonary embolism (cough, difficulty breathing, rapid heartbeat, chest pain) with importance of notifying the physician immediately if these occur. Instruct to avoid prolonged sitting in a chair that puts pressure behind the knees or sitting with legs crossed. *Positioning during surgery as well as postoperative edema and inactivity increase the risk for deep venous thrombosis, which in turn may break loose and travel to the lungs.*
- After an abdominal hysterectomy, instruct to restrict physical activity for 4 to 6 weeks. Heavy lifting, stair climbing, douching, tampons, and sexual intercourse should be avoided. The woman should shower, avoiding tub baths, until bleeding has ceased. *Infection and hemorrhage are the greatest postoperative risks; restricting activities and preventing the introduction of any foreign material into the vagina help reduce these risks.*
- Explain that appetite may be depressed and bowel elimination may be sluggish. *These are aftereffects of general anesthesia, handling of the bowel during surgery, and loss of muscle tone in the bowel while empty.*

bleeding is identified and has been addressed, the woman may fear cancer or other life-threatening conditions.

Expected Outcome: Patient will demonstrate anxiety relief related to abnormal uterine bleeding by focusing on knowledge about condition, treatment and surgical options, and interpersonal support systems.

The nurse will:

- Discuss the results of tests and examinations with the woman. *This allows for open exchange of information.*
- Provide information about the causes, treatments, risks, long-term effects of treatments, and prognosis. *This allows the woman to assume responsibility for her own health and become involved in her own treatment plan.*
- Evaluate coping strategies and psychosocial support systems. Teach coping strategies, if indicated. *The possibility of surgery or cancer represents a crisis for the woman and her support system. Support groups can provide assistance for the woman through crisis intervention.*

Promote Sexual Function. The woman with AUB may be unwilling to express herself sexually, particularly if bleeding is frequent or heavy. Additionally, fatigue may prevent her from participating in sexual activity.

Expected Outcome: Patient will demonstrate willingness to discuss changes to sexual function and will adapt modes of sexual expression to accommodate illness-related changes.

The nurse will:

- Offer information about engaging in sexual activity during menstruation. Explain that conception is possible during this time and that orgasm may help relieve symptoms. *Some women mistakenly believe that birth control measures are unnecessary during menstruation. Orgasm causes a release of tension and vascular congestion and frequently provides at least temporary relief of symptoms.*
- Provide an opportunity for the expression of concerns related to alterations in lifestyle and sexual functioning. *Some women have had a prolonged period of sexual abstinence related to DUB. Allowing women to verbalize concerns can assist them in working collaboratively with the healthcare provider to minimize the impact of illness and optimize function.*
- Encourage frequent rest periods. *This conserves energy and may allow sexual activities to resume.*
- Provide information about alternative methods of sexual expression. *Methods of sexual expression other than vaginal intercourse may satisfy the needs of both partners.*

Transitions of Care

Provide support, appropriate reassurance, and information to help the woman and her family better understand her disorder and the therapeutic interventions indicated. Teaching also includes self-care measures that help minimize the effects of AUB on the daily functioning of the woman. The following topics should be included:

- Administration and side effects of prescribed medications, including iron.
- The need to maintain a balanced diet, increasing iron-rich foods such as eggs, beans, liver, beef, and shrimp. Inform the woman that while orange juice may improve the absorption of iron, foods high in calcium and oxalic acid, such as spinach, may reduce its absorption.
- Importance of maintaining a fluid intake of 2000 to 3000 mL a day.
- The need to immediately report recurring episodes of AUB, particularly in postmenopausal women, to the healthcare provider.

49.3 Perimenopause

Menopause (referred to as *change of life*) is the permanent cessation of menses, a normal physiologic process as a woman ages. It is included here because it increases the risk of disorders of various aspects of women's health. In the United States, the average age of most women reaching menopause is age 52 (Shifren & Gass, 2014). Menopause occurs as a result of aging, surgical removal of the ovaries, or chemotherapy (this discussion focuses on natural menopause).

The Patient with Perimenopause

The climacteric, or perimenopausal, period denotes the time during which reproductive function gradually ceases. For most women, the perimenopausal period lasts several years. It begins with a decline in the production of the hormone estrogen, includes the permanent cessation of menstruation due to loss of ovarian function, and extends for 1 year after the final menstrual period, at which time a woman is said to be postmenopausal. The average woman will live one-third of her life after menopause.

Many women welcome the freedom from monthly menstrual periods and have relatively minor physical effects from the estrogen depletion. However, the hormonal changes that occur can be accompanied by side effects (discussed later in this section). Early menopause occurs between the ages of 40 and 45 and occurs in approximately 5% of women. Premature menopause refers to definitive cases of menopause in women who are younger than 40 (Shifren & Gass, 2014). Certain health risks increase after menopause, including heart disease, osteoporosis, macular degeneration, and breast cancer.

Physiology

The menopausal period marks the natural biologic end of reproductive ability. Surgical menopause occurs when the ovaries are removed in premenopausal women, dramatically reducing the production of estrogen and progestins. Chemical menopause often occurs during cancer chemotherapy, when cytotoxic drugs arrest ovarian function.

As ovarian function decreases, the production of estradiol (E_2), the most biologically active estrogen, decreases and is ultimately replaced by estrone as the major ovarian estrogen. Estrone is produced in small amounts and has only about one-tenth the biologic activity of estradiol. With decreased ovarian function, the second ovarian hormone, progesterone, which is produced during the luteal phase of the menstrual cycle, is also markedly reduced.

Manifestations

As estrogen decreases, various tissues are affected. There is a decrease in breast tissue, body hair, skin elasticity, and subcutaneous fat. The ovaries and uterus become smaller, and the cervix and vagina also decrease in size and become pale in color. These changes may result in problems with vaginal dryness, dyspareunia (painful intercourse), urinary stress incontinence, urinary tract infections (UTIs), and vaginitis. Vasomotor instability may cause hot flashes, palpitations, dizziness, and headaches. Other problems resulting from vasomotor instability include insomnia, frequent awakening, and perspiration (night sweats). The woman may experience mood and memory problems during the transition (Shifren & Gass, 2014).

Long-term estrogen deprivation results in an imbalance in bone remodeling and osteoporosis, leading to fractures and kyphosis. The risk for cardiovascular diseases increases in response to an increase in atherosclerosis (from an increase in the LDL-to-HDL cholesterol ratio). Manifestations of the perimenopausal period vary widely; some women experience severe symptoms, others experience moderate symptoms, and some women experience few or no symptoms. Manifestations may include:

- Menstrual cycles become erratic. Menstrual flow varies widely in amount and duration and eventually ceases.
- Vaginal, vulval, and urethral tissues begin to atrophy.
- Vaginal pH rises, predisposing the woman to vaginal infections.
- Vaginal lubrication decreases, and vaginal rugae decrease in number. This may result in dyspareunia, injury, and fungal infections.
- Vasomotor instability due to a decrease in estrogen may result in hot flashes and night sweats. A hot flash starts in the chest and moves upward toward the face and may last from seconds to several minutes.
- Psychologic symptoms may include moodiness, nervousness, insomnia, headaches, irritability, anxiety, inability to concentrate, and depression.

Interprofessional Care

Care of the woman experiencing menopausal symptoms focuses on relieving symptoms and minimizing postmenopausal health risks.

Diagnosis

As estrogen secretion diminishes, levels of follicle-stimulating hormone (FSH) and luteinizing hormone (LH) rise and remain elevated. A woman who has not menstruated for 1 full year or who has an increased FSH blood level is considered menopausal (Shifren & Gass, 2014).

Medications

Hormone replacement therapy (HRT) may be prescribed to alleviate severe manifestations of menopause, but only for a limited amount of time and only after a woman has been provided with known risks. A randomized trial of HRT by the Women's Health Initiative (2002) showed an increased risk for CHD in previously healthy women taking a commonly prescribed combination of estrogen and progestin. This well-controlled research study was terminated early when it showed a small but significant increased risk for coronary heart disease, stroke, pulmonary embolism, and invasive breast cancer in women taking HRT. HRT may include estrogen alone for women who have had a hysterectomy or a combination of estrogen and progestin. The addition of progestin stimulates monthly shedding of the interuterine lining, decreasing the risk of uterine cancer. HRT relieves hot flashes and night sweats and decreases problems of vaginal dryness and urogenital tissue atrophy, which can lead to painful intercourse and urinary incontinence. Long-term HRT may increase the risk for breast cancer, ovarian cancer, stroke, heart attack, and deep venous thrombosis. Recent trends in lowering dosages and eliminating the progesterone have been shown to decrease risks while limiting distressing menopausal manifestations; however, HRT should be used for the shortest period of time at the lowest dose possible (Shifren & Gass, 2014).

Selective estrogen receptor modulators (SERMs) such as raloxifene (Evista) and triphenylethylene (Tamoxifen) bind to estrogen receptors and exert site-specific effects in different target tissues. Tamoxifen and toremifene (a derivative of tamoxifen) have a beneficial effect on bone mineral density and serum lipids and decrease the risk of invasive breast cancer in women at high risk. They also provide an alternative to HRT for preventing osteoporosis.

Antidepressants may be prescribed as an off-label use for hot flashes and irritability. Both SSRIs and SRNIs have been used, but other than 7.5 mg of paroxetine (Paxil), all use is off label. Examples include fluoxetine (Prozac), venlafaxine (Effexor), and escitalopram (Lexapro) (Shifren & Gass, 2014). Possible side effects include headache, nausea, insomnia, anorexia, nightmares, diarrhea, and hypertension. Women over the age of 50 have an increased risk of bone fracture. Women should be told to discuss these medications with their physician prior to beginning or stopping use.

Nutrition

During menopause the rate of breast cancer increases. Multiple studies have demonstrated physical activity, maintaining a healthy weight, and decreasing alcohol consumption decreases the risk of breast cancer. The most recent of these studies followed a group of Mediterranean women (Masala et al., 2017). In this study, the authors conclude over 30% of breast cancer in postmenopausal women could be avoided by maintaining a healthy weight, exercising daily, and limiting alcohol consumption. The results of this study are in line with previous studies.

Integrative Therapies

As a result of the controversy surrounding the use of HRT, complementary and alternative therapies have become more popular. For example, phytoestrogens are estrogen-like substances found in some cereals, vegetables, legumes (including soy in tofu, tempeh, soymilk, and soy nuts), and herbs. Caution is recommended when using herbal therapies. The purity of the products is not assured, some have significant side effects (including irreversible liver damage, bleeding concerns), and they may interact with traditional medications. Healthcare professionals need to assess for the use of these therapies because some plant products may be harmful when combined with other drugs. The following complementary therapies are examples of those used by menopausal women to reduce associated discomforts (Taylor, 2015):

- Acupuncture
- Biofeedback
- Massage
- Soy supplements and food
- Herbs: *Cimicifuga racemosa* (black cohosh), *Vitex agnus castus* (chaste tree), *Rehmannia*, ginseng, Kava, dong quai, golden seal, flaxseed, valerian, and evening primrose
- Meditation and yoga.

Nursing Care

Nursing care during and after the menopausal period focuses on minimizing the symptoms associated with hormonal changes; reducing the risk of cardiovascular disease, cancer, and osteoporosis; and educating the woman about lifestyle changes important to health and well-being.

Assessment

Collect the following data through the health history and physical examination. When assessing the older woman, be aware of normal changes with aging.

- ***Health history:*** Problems with urinary frequency, urgency, or incontinence; menstrual history; sexual history; dyspareunia; use of alcohol, nicotine, and drugs; medications, sleep patterns, hot flashes, night sweats, changes in emotional responses
- ***Physical assessment:*** Height and weight, posture, vital signs, breast examination, pelvic examination, abdominal assessment.

Priorities of Care

Because menopause is a normal event, providing information to facilitate this life transition and promote health is the nursing care priority.

Diagnoses, Interventions, and Outcomes

Although each nursing care plan must be individualized, interventions often focus on problems with lack of information, sexuality, self-esteem, and a changing body image.

Provide Education. Because menopausal manifestations vary widely, it is difficult to predict their effect on an individual woman. However, the well-informed woman is better prepared to deal with whatever symptoms she experiences.

Expected Outcome: Patient will describe menopausal changes and therapeutic options to treat menopausal symptoms including diet, exercise, and pharmacologic options.

The nurse will:

- Discuss physiologic manifestations, such as hot flashes and night sweats. *The underlying cause of hot flashes is not known. Many physiologic effects of menopause are amenable to nonpharmacologic methods of relief, such as lifestyle changes.*
- Provide information about dietary recommendations. The recommended daily intake of calcium for women over age 50 is 1200 mg. *Some women need to use calcium supplements or calcium-containing antacid tablets to meet this requirement.*
- Emphasize the importance of weight-bearing exercise. *Weight-bearing exercise reduces the rate of bone loss, helps maintain optimum weight, and reduces cardiovascular risk.*
- Provide information about the benefits and risks of HRT. *Not every woman will need or want it. Every woman needs to understand both the risks and the benefits before deciding whether to use HRT.*
- Encourage the woman to obtain mammograms and Pap tests as recommended and also to be familiar with the tissues and consistency of her breasts. *The increased risk for cancer of the breast and pelvic reproductive organs makes healthcare provider screening during and after menopause even more important.*

Promote Sexual Function. Sexual dysfunction can occur during menopause. This can be due to vaginal dryness and atrophy from decrease in estrogen, which can interfere with sexual expression and satisfaction. Suggesting measures to help the woman and her partner cope with these changes can enable them to continue or resume a mutually satisfying sexual relationship.

Expected Outcome: Patient will demonstrate willingness to discuss changes to sexual function and treatment options and will adapt modes of sexual expression to accommodate menopausal-related changes.

The nurse will:

- Encourage expression of feelings and concerns about how menopause is changing her sex life, if appropriate. *Some women may not be comfortable discussing their intimate sexual behavior, however, this is an important topic for the nurse to discuss with the woman in a confidential, supportive, and empathic nature.*
- Explain that as women age, it may take longer for vaginal lubrication and orgasm to occur. This information is important to prevent the woman from believing something is wrong with her or her partner believing he or she is no longer interesting or sexually exciting. Suggest ways to increase vaginal lubrication, such as spending more time in foreplay and/or using water-soluble gels (e.g., Replens) or a vaginal HRT cream (if appropriate) for vaginal lubrication. *A more leisurely approach to sexual activity can be mutually gratifying for both the woman and her partner. Use of water-soluble gels and vaginal HRT cream can prevent vaginal pain and irritation and improve the quality of the sexual experience.*

Support Acceptance of the Aging Process. Each woman responds to the aging process in her own way, and most women have coping skills that adequately equip them to deal with the gradual changes associated with aging. Among the factors that may provoke a self-esteem disturbance are the loss of youth, a sense of emptiness as children leave home, and the need to redefine self-concept and roles as parenting becomes less important. Women who place a high value on their physical attractiveness may experience a painful psychologic response to the physical changes of menopause.

Expected Outcome: Patient will demonstrate acceptance by use of effective coping strategies to deal with changes in body image and function.

The nurse will:

- Discuss the importance of a healthy lifestyle in maintaining physical attractiveness. Identify risk factors and high-risk behaviors. *Lifestyle habits and behaviors affect many body systems and physical appearance. For example, cigarette smoking and overexposure to the sun make the skin age faster, contributing to wrinkles. Active women who exercise and eat a well-balanced diet look and feel better.*
- Encourage the woman to describe her perceptions of her own body. *How the woman views her body can lead to anxiety. Changes in body fat composition and hair growth patterns can all affect how a woman feels about her body. Information should be provided on how to minimize these changes.*
- Stress that certain physical characteristics of an individual cannot be changed; emphasize the importance of learning to recognize and appreciate one's own special strengths. *These help the woman gain acceptance and a realistic appraisal of self.*
- Refer, as appropriate, for dietary management, exercise, stress management, and cosmetic assistance (e.g., for aggravating facial hair). *These actions increase wellness and a positive sense of self.*

Transitions of Care

The American Cancer Society (ACS) recommends periodic cancer-related checkups (e.g., screening for cervical and breast cancer) beginning at age 20 or when the female becomes sexually active. Periodic mammography and colorectal cancer screening is initiated during perimenopause. Beginning at age 45, women should have periodic cholesterol and lipid profile tests. Women should undergo bone mineral density examination during perimenopause to establish a baseline. Refer to Table 3.5 in Chapter 3 for health screening recommendations. Health counseling should also include information about alcohol and tobacco use, sun exposure, diet and nutrition, exercise, and risk factors. Information regarding a woman's sexual practice should be discussed (although pregnancy is not possible after menopause, the sexually active woman may still be at risk for STIs). It is important to discuss the benefits of rest and exercise, as well as a diet that includes fruits, vegetables, and fiber.

49.4 Structural Disorders

Structural disorders of the female reproductive system include displacement disorders and fistulas. Structural disorders may occur in women of any age.

The Patient with Uterine Displacement

The uterus may be displaced within the pelvic cavity or may descend into the vaginal canal. Displacement of the uterus within the pelvic cavity is classified according to the direction of the displacement, as illustrated in **Figure 49.2 ■**.

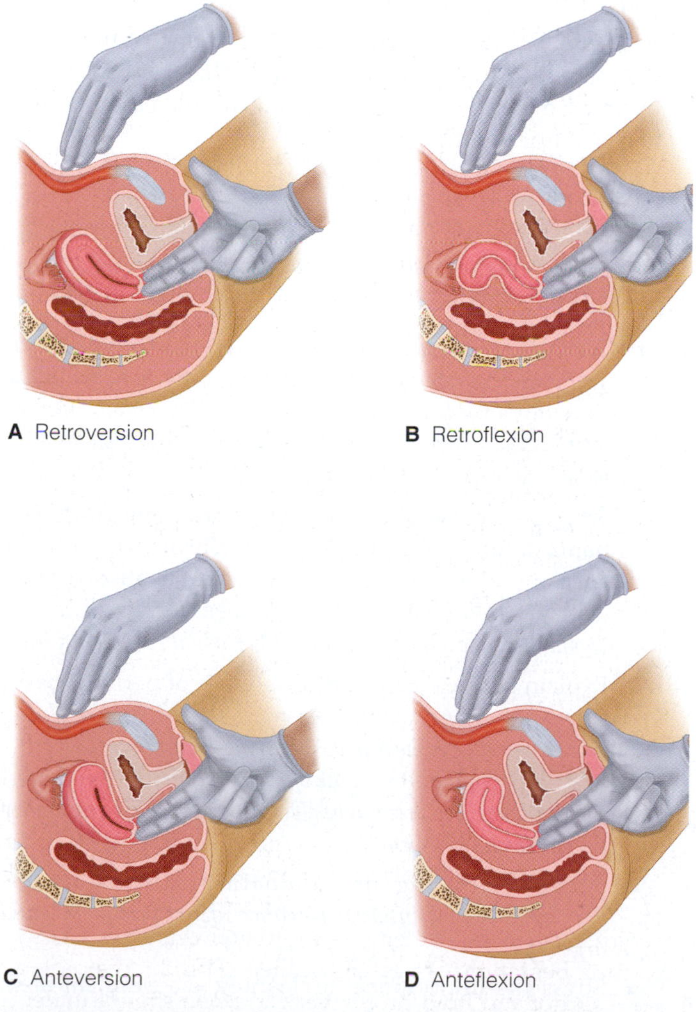
A Retroversion
B Retroflexion
C Anteversion
D Anteflexion

Figure 49.2 ■ Displacements of the uterus within the pelvic cavity. **A**, Retroversion is a backward tilting. **B**, Retroflexion is a backward bending. **C**, Anteversion is a forward tilting. **D**, Anteflexion is a forward bending.

Prolapse of the uterus into the vaginal canal can vary from mild to complete prolapse outside of the body. First-degree prolapse involves a descent of less than half the uterine corpus into the vagina. Second-degree prolapse involves the descent of the entire uterus into the vaginal canal so that the cervix is at the introitus to the vagina. Third-degree prolapse, or procidentia, is complete prolapse of the uterus outside the body, with inversion of the vaginal canal (**Figure 49.3 ■**). Prolapse of the uterus is often accompanied by cystocele (herniation of the bladder into the vagina) or rectocele (herniation of the rectum into the vagina).

Pathophysiology

Displacement or prolapse of the uterus, bladder, or rectum can be a congenital or an acquired condition. Congenital tilting or flexion of the uterus is rare. More commonly, tilting or flexion disorders in which the uterus remains within the pelvic cavity are related to the scarring and inflammation of pelvic inflammatory disease, endometriosis, pregnancy, and tumors.

Downward displacement of the pelvic organs into the vagina results from weakened pelvic musculature, usually attributable to stretching of the supporting ligaments and muscles during pregnancy and childbirth. Unrepaired lacerations from childbirth, rapid deliveries,

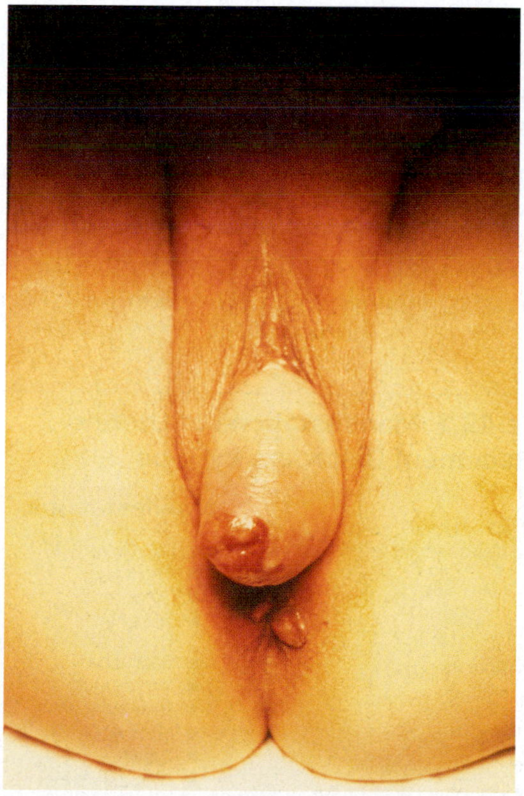

Figure 49.3 ■ Prolapse of the uterus can vary from mild to complete. In third-degree uterine prolapse, or procidentia, the uterus prolapses completely outside the body, with inversion of the vagina.

multiple pregnancies, congenital weakness, or loss of elasticity and muscle tone with aging may contribute to these disorders.

Manifestations

The manifestations of displacement disorders are outlined in **Table 49.1** by type. Complications can be recurrent urinary tract infections and chronic urinary retention.

Interprofessional Care

Interprofessional care focuses on identifying the cause of the structural disorder, correcting or minimizing the condition, relieving pain, preventing or treating infection, and supporting and educating the woman.

A careful history and physical examination are performed.

Diagnosis

Diagnosis of uterine displacement is made after physical examination. If herniation of the rectum or bladder is suspected, the woman is asked to bear down or cough during the examination so the prolapse can be palpated and any leakage of urine or feces visualized. A history of infections, multiple pregnancies in rapid succession, and rapid labors support this diagnosis.

Treatment may include Kegel exercises to strengthen weakened pelvic muscles. Kegel exercises can be useful in the early stages of downward displacement. These exercises are discussed in Chapter 27.

Nutrition

Obesity is a risk factor and can complicate successful treatment of a uterine prolapse. Maintaining a healthy weight or losing weight is important.

Surgery

Several surgical procedures are used to repair structural disorders. For women presenting with a cystocele, anterior colporrhaphy (repair of the cystocele) is the most common procedure. The anterior repair shortens the pelvic muscles, providing tighter support for the bladder. The Marshall-Marchetti-Krantz procedure involves resuspension of the urinary bladder in correct anatomic position. A rectocele is repaired with a posterior colporrhaphy, which shortens the pelvic muscles, providing a tighter support for the rectum. A prolapsed uterus may be surgically repositioned and the supporting muscles shortened to provide greater support. In postmenopausal women or women with procidentia, hysterectomy is the preferred treatment.

Pessary

When surgery is contraindicated, a pessary (a removable device) may be inserted into the vagina to provide temporary support for the uterus or bladder. At regular intervals, the pessary is removed, cleaned, and reinserted.

Table 49.1 Manifestations of Uterine Displacement Disorders by Type

Type	Manifestations
Uterine displacement within the pelvic cavity	■ Dysmenorrhea ■ Backache ■ Dyspareunia ■ Infertility
Uterine prolapse	■ Backache ■ Urinary incontinence ■ Bearing-down sensation ■ Hemorrhoids ■ Constipation ■ Dyspareunia
Cystocele/rectocele	■ Bearing-down sensation ■ Hemorrhoids ■ Constipation ■ Urinary incontinence ■ Fecal incontinence

Nursing Care

Nursing care focuses on education about the disorder, proposed treatments, and self-care measures for relief of symptoms.

Priorities of Care

Incontinence and anxiety are important topics for nurses to address the woman with a displacement.

Promote Urinary Continence. Relaxation of the pelvic floor can lead to stress incontinence. This can prove both troublesome and embarrassing and can increase the incidence of urinary tract infection.

Expected Outcome: Patient will demonstrate urinary continence, recognizing urge to void, performing perianal strengthening exercises, managing independent toileting, and maintaining a predictable pattern of voiding.

The nurse will:

- Teach Kegel exercises. *These exercises strengthen perineal muscle tone, minimize urinary leakage, and minimize descent of the bladder and rectum into the vagina. In postmenopausal women, estrogen supplements can also improve muscle tone in the perineal area.*
- Suggest the use of perineal pads (ranging from thin panty liners to full-thickness incontinence pads) or special underwear (such as Depends) to absorb urine leakage. *Using pads or undergarments often allows the woman to once again take part in her usual social activities.*
- Explain perineal care and proper use of perineal pads. *Cleansing the perineum from front to back and applying and removing perineal pads the same way minimizes cross infection from the anus to the vaginal and urethral openings. Incontinence pads need to be changed frequently to minimize surface bacterial counts.*
- Suggest reducing or eliminating caffeine intake. *Reducing caffeine intake can reduce urinary frequency and urgency.*
- Stress the importance of cleaning the perineal area. *Urine is very irritating to the skin.*

Relieve Anxiety. Anxiety is common among women with a displacement disorder. Many women have only a cursory understanding of their reproductive anatomy. This lack of knowledge often compounds the anxiety. The nurse can use drawings and models to explain structural disorders and the treatment options available.

Expected Outcome: Patient will demonstrate management of anxiety by use of effective coping strategies to deal with changes in body image related to the particular displacement disorder.

The nurse will:

- Encourage questions from the woman and her partner. *This helps assess the level of understanding so that teaching can be more effective.*
- Explain that the relief from discomfort and fatigue may positively influence sexual expression, and reassure the woman that the capacity for orgasm will not be affected. *Many women and their partners have major concerns about the effects of the disorder and its treatment on their sex life and capacity for sexual pleasure.*
- Explore coping mechanisms that have been previously successful. *This can help relieve anxiety and boost self-esteem.*

Transitions of Care

If medical treatment is used initially, teaching focuses on measures to relieve the manifestations, such as Kegel exercises, use of incontinence pads, or the use, care, and insertion of a pessary. Because obesity is a risk factor associated with relaxation of the pelvic and abdominal muscles, dietary counseling may be indicated. Preoperatively, a diet high in fiber may alleviate constipation, a particular concern during the postoperative period.

The Patient with a Vaginal Fistula

Pathophysiology

A *fistula* is an abnormal opening or passage between two organs or spaces that are normally separated or an abnormal passage to the outside of the body. Vaginal fistulas may be vesicovaginal or rectovaginal. A *vesicovaginal fistula* is an abnormal opening between the urinary bladder and the vagina, leading to incontinent leakage of urine through the vagina. A *rectovaginal fistula* (less common) is an abnormal opening between the rectum and vagina, causing incontinent leakage of stool or flatus through the vagina.

Fistulas may develop as a complication of childbirth, gynecologic or urologic surgery, or radiation therapy for gynecologic cancer. Cancer of the bladder is sometimes involved. The woman with a vaginal fistula often presents with a complaint of involuntary leakage of urine or flatus and symptoms of infection.

Interprofessional Care

Fistulas are usually diagnosed by pelvic examination. A vesicovaginal fistula can be diagnosed by instilling dye into the urinary bladder through a catheter and observing the vagina for leakage. If no leakage is detected, a tampon or vaginal pack is inserted into the vagina, and the woman is asked to ambulate. If an abnormal opening is present, the tampon will absorb the dye. Dye may also be injected intravenously because it is excreted by the kidneys. Urine and vaginal cultures may be performed to rule out infections. Antibiotics are administered if infection is present.

A small vaginal fistula may resolve spontaneously. Otherwise, surgery is performed after inflammation has subsided, often a period of several months. Rarely, in the presence of a large, highly inflamed rectovaginal fistula, a temporary colostomy is performed, allowing inflammation and irritation to subside (refer to Chapter 24).

Nursing Care

Nursing care for the woman with repair of a vaginal fistula is similar to that for the woman with a displacement disorder. Teaching is an important component of nursing care. Stress the importance of careful perineal cleansing to reduce irritation and prevent further tissue breakdown. Suggest perineal irrigation or sitz baths for cleansing. Perineal pads or special underwear may be used to absorb urine or fecal drainage. For the woman with a rectovaginal fistula, provide information about avoiding gas-forming foods to minimize embarrassment from odor.

49.5 Disorders of Female Reproductive Tissue

Both benign and malignant tissue disorders affect the female reproductive system. Benign tumors and cysts include Bartholin's gland cysts, cervical polyps, endometrial cysts and polyps, ovarian cysts, and uterine leiomyomas (fibroids). Endometriosis is a condition in which endometrial tissue implants outside the uterus in various locations in the pelvic cavity. Malignant tumors of reproductive tissue include cervical cancer, endometrial cancer, ovarian cancer, and vulvar cancer.

The Patient with Cysts or Polyps

A *cyst* is a fluid-filled sac. A *polyp* is a highly vascular solid tumor attached by a pedicle or stem. Cysts or polyps of the female reproductive system can occur in the vulva, cervix, endometrium, or ovaries; depending on the type, they may occur at any age.

Pathophysiology

Following are different types of female reproductive tissue cysts and polyps:

- ***Bartholin gland cysts*** are the most common cystic disorder of the vulva. These cysts are caused by the infection or obstruction of the Bartholin gland.
- ***Cervical polyps*** tend to occur in women over age 40 who have borne several children and have a history of using oral contraceptives. It is possible that cervical polyps develop from endocervical hyperplasia. The polyp develops at the vaginal end of the cervix, has a stem, and is highly vascular.

- ***Endometrial polyps*** are intrauterine overgrowths, similar to cervical polyps, and usually have a stalk. Although endometrial polyps are usually benign, some may be precancerous or malignant. Endometrial polyps usually affect women in perimenopause or menopause.
- ***Endometrial cysts*** (ovarian endometrioma) can develop on the ovary. They are caused by endometrial overgrowth and are often filled with old blood (the dark color leads to the label "chocolate cysts"). Endometrial cysts are the result of endometrial implants on the ovary and are associated with endometriosis.
- ***Ovarian cysts*** are classified as follicular cysts and corpus luteum cysts. *Follicular cysts* develop as a result of failure of the mature follicle to rupture or failure of an immature follicle to reabsorb fluid after ovulation. *Corpus luteum cysts* develop as a result of increased hormone secretion by the corpus luteum after ovulation. Most functional cysts regress spontaneously within two or three menstrual cycles.
- ***Polycystic ovarian syndrome (POS)*** is an endocrine disorder characterized by an excess of androgens and a long-term lack of ovulation. The exact cause is unknown. As a part of the disease, as many as 8 to 10 cysts form in the ovaries from a failure to release ova. Manifestations include amenorrhea or irregular menses, hirsutism, obesity, acne, hypertension, sleep apnea, and infertility. Women with POS often have insulin resistance and are at increased risk for type 2 diabetes, as well as heart disease, breast cancer, and endometrial cancer.

Manifestations and Complications

The causes and manifestations of benign cysts and polyps of the female reproductive system are presented in **Table 49.2**. Complications associated with cysts and polyps include infection, rupture, infertility, hemorrhage, and recurrence.

Interprofessional Care

Care focuses on identifying and correcting the disorder and preventing its recurrence. A health history and physical examination are performed. Examination of the reproductive tract reveals the presence of most cysts and polyps. The menstrual history may include menstrual irregularities.

Diagnosis

Diagnostic tests that may be used to diagnose cysts and polyps of the female reproductive system (and to eliminate the diagnosis of cancer) include a Pap test, an endometrial biopsy, a laparoscopy to visualize ovarian cysts, an ultrasound or x-ray to differentiate cysts from solid tumors, and/or a pregnancy test when luteal cysts are suspected. Laboratory analysis will demonstrate elevated LH and testosterone levels, as well as a reverse in FSH/LH in the woman with polycystic ovary syndrome (POS).

Medications

Antibiotics are used to treat infection or abscess, and oral contraceptives are used to promote regression of functional ovarian cysts. Clomiphene (Clomid, Serophene) may be prescribed to stimulate ovulation in the woman with POS who wishes to become pregnant. Metformin has been used off label as a method to combat the insulin resistance in some women with POS (Adams et al., 2017).

Surgery

Cervical polyps are visible through a vaginal speculum and are usually removed with a clamp. A transcervical approach is used to remove endometrial cysts or polyps. The specimen is sent to the laboratory for evaluation, and chemical or electrical cauterization may be applied after cyst removal. For Bartholin's gland cysts and any abscesses, the lesion is incised and drained, and a drainage device is left in place. Follicular cysts may be punctured through laser surgery, or a wedge resection of the ovary may be performed to restore ovulation. Rarely, oophorectomy (removal of the ovary) is performed if ovarian cysts are very large.

Table 49.2 Etiology and Manifestations of Benign Cysts and Polyps of the Female Reproductive System

Type	Etiologic Origin	Manifestations
Ovary		
Functional cysts	Ovulation—includes follicular cysts and corpus luteum cysts	May resolve spontaneously; can cause pain, menstrual irregularity, or amenorrhea
Polycystic ovarian syndrome	Unknown; possible hypothalamic–pituitary dysfunction	Hirsutism, obesity; amenorrhea or irregular menses; hyperinsulinemia; infertility
Chocolate cysts	Endometrial overgrowth; filled with old blood	Usually asymptomatic Abdominal or pelvic pain, peritonitis with rupture
Vulva		
Bartholin cysts	Obstruction or infection of Bartholin's gland	Pain, redness, perineal mass, dyspareunia
Endometrium		
Endometrial polyps	Unknown	Bleeding between periods
Cervix		
Cervical polyps	Unknown	Bleeding after intercourse or after activities involving heavy lifting

Nursing Care

Nursing care focuses on relieving pain and preventing recurrence and complications. Address the following topics for self-care at home:

- The condition, its treatment, and measures to relieve pain
- The importance of keeping follow-up appointments
- Manifestations of infection (for postsurgical care) and the need to notify the physician should they occur
- If cervical polypectomy is performed, advise use of external pads for 1 week; the woman should be able to recognize that saturating more than one pad in an hour indicates the need for immediate follow-up
- The importance of long-term follow-up care for the woman with POS.

The Patient with Leiomyoma

Leiomyomas (fibroids) are benign tumors that originate from smooth muscle of the uterus. They are the most common form of pelvic tumor and occurs in up to 80% of all women by age of 50 (Office on Women's Health, 2018).

Pathophysiology

The actual cause of fibroid tumors is not clearly understood, but there is a strong association with estrogen stimulation. Fibroid tumors usually develop in the uterine corpus and may be intramural, subserous, or submucous (**Figure 49.4 ■**).

Intramural fibroid tumors (the most common type) are embedded in the myometrium. They usually present as an enlargement of the uterus. Subserous fibroid tumors lie beneath the serous lining of the uterus and project into the peritoneal cavity. They may become pedunculated (on a stem) and displace or compress other tissues, such as the ureter or bladder. Submucous fibroid tumors lie beneath the endometrial lining of the uterus. They displace endometrial tissue and are more likely to cause bleeding, infection, and necrosis than the other types.

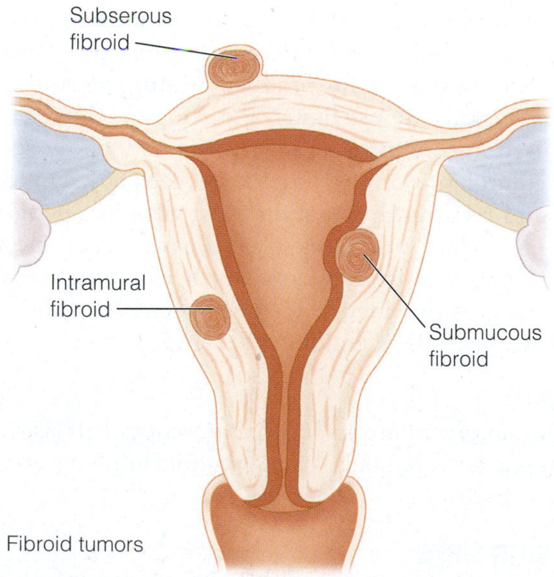
Subserous fibroid
Intramural fibroid
Submucous fibroid
Fibroid tumors

Figure 49.4 ■ Types of uterine fibroid tumors (leiomyomas). Intramural fibroid tumors lie within the uterine wall. Subserous fibroid tumors lie beneath the serous lining of the uterus and project into the peritoneum. Submucous fibroid tumors lie beneath the endometrial lining of the uterus.

Manifestations

Small tumors may be asymptomatic. The rate of growth varies, but they may increase in size during pregnancy or with use of oral contraceptives or HRT. Large fibroid tumors can crowd other organs, leading to pelvic pressure, pain, dysmenorrhea, menorrhagia, and fatigue. Depending on the location of the tumor, constipation and urinary urgency and frequency may occur.

Interprofessional Care

Treatment of the woman with uterine fibroids depends on the size and location of the tumors, the severity of the manifestations, and her age and childbearing status. Most fibroids grow as a woman ages, then shrink after menopause.

Diagnosis

Tests used to diagnose uterine fibroids may include an ultrasound to differentiate leiomyoma from endometriosis and a laparoscopy to visualize subserosal leiomyomas. In asymptomatic women who wish to bear children, the fibroid tumors are monitored for growth.

Medications

There are no medications to permanently shrink fibroids. Using birth control pills may decrease heavy vaginal bleeding. Medications that stop ovarian production of estrogen and progesterone (hormones necessary for fibroid growth) may provide a temporary decrease in manifestations. Injectable leuprolide acetate (Lupron) and nasal spray fluocinolone (Synalar) decrease bleeding and shrink the fibroids, but the tumors grow again when the medications are stopped. Long-term use of these medications is limited because of their side effects (hot flashes, vaginal dryness, and headaches).There is a significant risk of bone loss if treatment continues 6 months or more.

Surgery

Myomectomy, removal of the tumor without removing the entire uterus, is the surgical procedure of choice for young women who wish to retain reproductive capability. Laparoscopic laser technique is used for many women. A hysterectomy is performed if tumors are large and if bleeding or other problems continue in perimenopausal women. A nonsurgical method of treatment is a uterine fibroid embolization. In this procedure, a catheter is guided through the femoral artery to the uterus, where tiny particles are injected into the artery supplying the fibroid to cut off the fibroid's blood supply. This procedure requires only an overnight hospital stay with a return to normal activities in 1 week.

Nursing Care

If surgery is deferred, teaching emphasizes the importance of regular follow-up assessments to monitor tumor growth.

If a hysterectomy is performed, teaching emphasizes appropriate preoperative and postoperative care (refer to Box 49.1). Dietary modifications to increase iron intake, prevent constipation, and promote healing are important.

The Woman with Endometriosis

Endometriosis is a chronic inflammatory disease in which functional endometrial tissue is found outside the uterus (Sorenson, Quinn, & Klein, 2019). These implantations of endometrial tissue develop most commonly in the pelvic cavity, but also possibly in other areas of the body, such as the lungs. Endometriosis affects 10 to 15% of women of childbearing age and is more common in women who postpone childbearing. Risk factors for endometriosis include early menarche, regular periods with a cycle of less than 27 days, menses lasting more than 7 days, heavier flow, and increased menstrual pain. A history of the condition in first-degree female relatives places a woman at increased risk for endometriosis (Sorenson et al., 2019).

Pathophysiology

The cause of endometriosis is unclear, but several theories have been proposed. The metaplasia theory asserts that endometrial tissue develops from embryonic epithelial cells as a result of hormonal or inflammatory changes. The theory of retrograde menstruation suggests that menstrual tissue backs up through the fallopian tubes during menses, implants on various pelvic structures, and survives. The transplantation theory asserts that endometrial implants spread via lymphatic or vascular routes.

The abnormally located endometrial tissue responds to cyclic ovarian hormone stimulation, and bleeding at the time of menstruation occurs at the sites of implantation. Scarring, inflammation, and adhesions may develop. Endometrial implants on the ovary cause endometrial (chocolate) cysts, which are often filled with old blood and may rupture, causing peritonitis. Endometriosis is a slowly progressive disease, responsive to ovarian hormone stimulation. Thus, the implants regress during pregnancy and atrophy at menopause unless the woman is receiving HRT. Because progressive scarring may interfere with the ability to conceive, women with significant endometriosis are encouraged to have children early if they wish to do so.

Manifestations and Complications

Manifestations of endometriosis include:

- Heavy, throbbing pain of the lower abdomen and pelvis, radiating down the thighs and around the back (the degree of pain, however, is not indicative of the severity of the disease); pain can begin 2 to 3 days prior to menses and last for several days
- Feeling of rectal pressure and discomfort when having a bowel movement
- Dyspareunia
- Dysfunctional uterine bleeding
- Infertility.

The typical complication of endometriosis is infertility. With severe endometriosis that has spread to the abdominal cavity, bowel and urinary issues and obstructions can occur.

Interprofessional Care

Endometriosis may be difficult to diagnose, but a history of dysmenorrhea, dyspareunia, and infertility strongly suggests this diagnosis. Interventions depend on the severity of symptoms, the extent of the disease, and the woman's age and desire for childbearing. Treatment goals focus on pain management and restoring fertility.

Diagnosis

Diagnostic tests are ordered to rule out other medical conditions and identify the endometrial implants. The tests include a pelvic ultrasound and laparoscopy as well as a CBC with differential to rule out pelvic abscesses and infectious processes. A low hemoglobin and hematocrit may be noted if heavy menstrual bleeding accompanies endometriosis or tissue implants bleed significantly during menses.

Medications

A variety of medications may be used to decrease bleeding in and enlargement of the endometrial implants. Hormone therapy may include oral contraceptives. GnRH agonist therapy (e.g., goserelin [Zoladex], leuprolide [Eligard, Lupron], nafarelin [Synarel]) is used to lower estrogen, initiating a menopause-like state to shrink implants and reduce pain in most women. Oral or injectable progestin (such as Depo-Provera) increases progesterone levels similar to pregnancy, stopping ovulation and lowering estrogen to reduce the size of implants and relieve pain. Danazol, an anabolic steroid, suppresses release of FSH and LH by the pituitary to interrupt the cause of atrophy and involution of both normal and ectopic endometrial tissue. However, danazol may increase the risk of ovarian cancer and has masculinizing side effects. Aromatase inhibitors (*aromatase*, a protein responsible for producing estrogen, is found in the ovary, skin, adipose tissue, and ectopic endometrial tissue) used in combination with hormone therapy such as birth control pills or progestin have been shown to reduce pain and recurrence of endometrial growths. Long-term use of aromatase inhibitors (e.g., anastrozole, exemestane, letrozole) may cause bone loss. Further information about these drugs is provided in the later discussion of hormone therapy used to treat endometrial cancer.

Surgery

Surgical interventions include laparoscopy with laser ablation (excision or removal) of endometrial implants or a total hysterectomy.

Nursing Care

Nursing care includes providing pain relief, providing education about the condition and the treatment options, and helping the woman cope with treatment outcomes. The severity of the disease and its manifestations are not necessarily related. Advanced disease may exhibit few manifestations, whereas early disease may be quite painful. See the accompanying Case Study & Nursing Care Plan for a woman with endometriosis.

Priorities of Care

Anxiety related to the risk for loss of reproductive function is a priority diagnosis for the young woman with endometriosis.

Diagnoses, Interventions, and Outcomes

Interventions for pain, discussed previously, are also appropriate for the woman with endometriosis.

Reduce Anxiety. Anxiety about the unsure prognosis related to infertility is a particular problem for young women who plan to have a family in the future.

Expected Outcome: Patient will demonstrate management of anxiety by use of effective coping strategies to deal with uncertain prognosis and potential treatment options related to the particular cause of infertility.

The nurse will:

- Encourage expression of fears and anxiety about infertility, and answer questions honestly. *Knowledge helps relieve anxiety and fear.*
- Provide information on fertility awareness methods, including measurement of basal body temperature and other techniques for recognizing ovulation. *Understanding these techniques helps the woman and her partner optimize the conditions for conception.*

Transitions of Care

Explain the cause of the disorder and the various treatment options, including their side effects. Discuss fertility awareness methods and the risks and benefits of long-term use of oral contraceptives. Stress the importance of exercise, smoking cessation, and weight control. If surgical treatment is chosen, provide preoperative and postoperative teaching.

Case Study & Nursing Care Plan

A Woman with Endometriosis

Angela Hall is a 31-year-old married accountant. She relates a history of severe dysmenorrhea and menorrhagia, a feeling of pelvic heaviness, and pain that radiates down her thighs. Because of her discomfort, her husband has complained about the quality of their sex life and has expressed concerns about their plans for having children. Mrs. Hall reports being so tired she doesn't care whether she has sex or not, and, in fact, would really prefer not to: "Sex hurts so much, I just can't stand it." Endometriosis is suspected, and a diagnostic laparoscopy has been scheduled.

ASSESSMENT	DIAGNOSES	EXPECTED OUTCOMES
Christine Brigham, RN, NP, interviews Mrs. Hall and makes the following assessments: BP 110/70 mmHg, P 68 bpm, R 18/min, T 36.7°C (98.2°F). Mrs. Hall's weight is 59 kg (130 lb) and within normal limits for her height. Review of laboratory findings indicate a hemoglobin level of 9.8 g/dL (normal range: 12 to 16 g/dL) and a hematocrit of 33.1% (normal range: 35% to 45%). Physical examination reveals pelvic tenderness on manipulation of the cervix, and small masses that are palpable on abdominal/pelvic examination.	▪ Chronic pain related to endometrial pelvic implants ▪ Anxiety due to effect of endometriosis on fertility ▪ Need for education regarding diagnosis and treatment options ▪ Painful sex related to manifestations of endometriosis	▪ Patient will develop effective self-care measures to deal with the pain and discomfort. ▪ Patient will verbalize decreased anxiety. ▪ Patient will demonstrate understanding of the disease and treatment options. ▪ Patient will verbalize an improvement in sexual functioning and a decrease in interpersonal stress between herself and her husband.

PLANNING AND IMPLEMENTATION

- Identify the location, type, duration, and history of the pain.
- Recommend analgesics and heat therapy.
- Provide information on biofeedback, relaxation, and imagery to lessen pain.
- Discuss with Mr. and Mrs. Hall the causes of endometriosis and its manifestations.
- Encourage the Halls to discuss their feelings about the effect of the disease on their sex life, lifestyle, and fertility.
- Refer the couple to the local mental health center, if appropriate.

EVALUATION

Two years after the initiation of treatment, Mr. and Mrs. Hall have become parents of a baby girl. Mrs. Hall states that the discomfort and other manifestations of endometriosis have eased. Relaxation and imagery have effectively minimized her pain and brought about improvement in her function as wife, mother, and sexual partner. Counseling has improved the interpersonal and sexual relations between the Halls. Dietary management has improved her anemia, although the menorrhagia persists. The Halls are trying to have a second child, understanding the advantages of rapid succession of pregnancies. They will be followed in the nursing clinic and referred to a fertility clinic if conception does not occur within 1 year.

(continued)

CLINICAL REASONING IN PATIENT CARE

1. Explain the pathophysiologic basis for Mrs. Hall's anemia.
2. How would you handle the situation if Mr. and Mrs. Hall were extremely uncomfortable and embarrassed about discussing their sexual problems?
3. Develop a plan of care for Mrs. Hall's low self-esteem related to the manifestations of endometriosis.

See Evaluating Your Response in Appendix B.

The Patient with Cervical Cancer

Cancer of the cervix is the second most common cancer in women worldwide, and the 14th most common in women in the United States. The incidence is higher in Hispanic and Black women than in White women (ACS, 2018f). The American Cancer Society (2018f) estimates that in 2018 there will be approximately 13,000 new cases of invasive cervical cancer and 4000 women will die of cervical cancer. The death rate during the past 30 years has been reduced through effective screening for cervical cancer with the Pap test and the treatment of existing malignancies. Failure to have the recommended screenings and compliance with follow-up care after colposcopic procedures has been identified as a leading reason for development of the disease.

Pathophysiology

Most cervical cancers are squamous cell carcinomas that begin as neoplasia in the cervical epithelium. The strongest risk for cervical cancer is infection with the human papillomavirus (HPV). While most HPV infections are cleared by the body, sometimes the infection becomes chronic, which is strongly linked to cancer. There are other risk factors such as smoking and being overweight. There is also evidence that ether infection or co-infections with *Chlamydia trachomatis* can increase risk of cervical cancer. This could be due to the inflammatory effect of chlamydia either increasing the risk of a co-infection with HPV or the inflammatory effect preventing the body from clearing the HPV infection (Karin, Souho, Benlemlih, & Bennani, 2018). (*C. trachomatis* is discussed in Chapter 50.) Systems of grading of dysplastic changes in the cervix use the term *cervical intraepithelial neoplasia (CIN)* or the *Bethesda system* (which was updated in 2014) (Nayar & Wilbur, 2015). **Table 49.3** demonstrates the difference between the updated Bethesda system and the CIN classification. Once cancer has been diagnosed, the cancer is then classified by the International Federation of Gynecology and Obstetrics staging system, which uses clinical information, not what is found in surgery. If surgery is performed, then the American Joint Committee on Cancer staging can be used. The actual stages of both systems are the same (ACS, 2018c).

Cervical cancer spreads by direct invasion of accessory structures, including the vaginal wall, pelvic wall, bladder, and rectum. Although metastasis is most frequently confined to the pelvic area, distant metastasis may occur through the lymphatic system.

Risk Factors

Risk factors for cervical cancer include infection of the external genitalia and anus with HPV, first intercourse before 16 years of age, multiple sex partners or male partners with multiple sex partners, a history of STIs, and infection with HIV. Infection with HPV is the most important risk factor for cancer of the cervix. Other risk factors include smoking and poor nutritional status, obesity, multiple pregnancies, long-term use of birth control pills, family history of cervical cancer, and exposure to diethylstilbestrol (DES) in utero.

Manifestations

Preinvasive cancer is limited to the cervix and rarely causes manifestations. Invasive cancer causes vaginal bleeding after intercourse or between menstrual periods and a bloody or brown vaginal discharge that increases as the cancer progresses. These changes are subtle and may be more readily noticed by the postmenopausal woman. Manifestations of advanced disease include referred pain in the back or thighs, hematuria, bloody stools, anemia, and weight loss.

Interprofessional Care

The goals of treatment are to eradicate the cancer and minimize complications and metastasis. The type of treatment depends on the degree of malignant change, the size and location of the lesion, and the extent of metastasis.

Diagnosis

Tests used to diagnose cervical cancer include a Pap test, colposcopy, and cervical biopsy. A loop diathermy technique

Table 49.3 Classification Systems for Pap Tests

Dysplasia/Neoplasia	CIN (Cervical Intraepithelial Neoplasia)	Bethesda System
Benign	Benign inflammation	■ Normal ■ Atypical squamous cells of undetermined significance (ASCUS)
Mild dysplasia	CIN I	■ Low-grade squamous intraepithelial lesion (LSIL)
Moderate to severe dysplasia	CIN II/CIN III Carcinoma in situ Squamous cell carcinoma	■ High-grade SIL (HSIL) ■ Squamous cell carcinoma

(loop electrosurgical excision procedure [LEEP]) allows simultaneous diagnosis and treatment of dysplastic lesions found on colposcopy. This procedure is performed in the healthcare provider's office, using a wire for both cutting and coagulation during excision of the dysplastic region of the cervix. An MRI or CT of the pelvis, abdomen, or bones may be performed to evaluate the spread of the tumor. If the MRI or CT demonstrates metastases of the cancer, then an exploratory laparoscopy may be performed for staging.

Medications

Chemotherapy is used for tumors not responsive to other therapy, tumors that cannot be removed, or as adjunct therapy if metastasis has occurred (refer to Chapter 14).

Surgery

When combined with colposcopy, laser surgery is a viable treatment method if the cancer is limited to the cervical epithelium. Cryosurgery, which involves the use of a probe to freeze tissue, causing necrosis and sloughing, is also used for noninvasive lesions. Conization (**Figure 49.5** ■) is performed to treat microinvasive carcinoma when colposcopy cannot define the limits of the invasion. For invasive lesions, hysterectomy or radical hysterectomy (removal of the uterus, fallopian tubes, lymph nodes, and ovaries) is performed.

A *pelvic exenteration*—the removal of all pelvic contents, including the bowel, vagina, and bladder—may be performed if the cancer recurs without involvement of the lymphatic system. An *anterior exenteration* is the removal of the uterus, ovaries, fallopian tubes, vagina, bladder, urethra, and lymphatic vessels and nodes. An ileal conduit is created for excretion of urine (refer to Chapter 27). A *posterior exenteration* is the removal of the uterus, ovaries, fallopian tubes, bowel, and rectum. A colostomy is created for excretion of feces (refer to Chapter 24). This is an extensive procedure

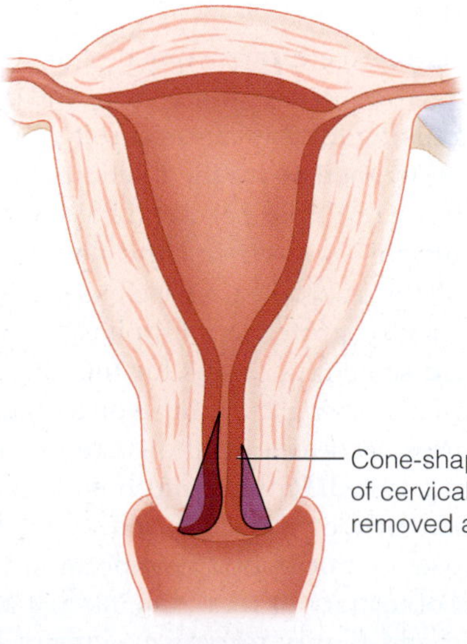
Cone-shaped area
of cervical tissue
removed and biopsied

Figure 49.5 ■ Conization, the surgical removal of a cone-shaped section of the cervix, is used to treat microinvasive carcinoma of the cervix.

with many possible complications, and it requires a lengthy recovering period.

Radiation and Chemoradiation Therapy

Radiation therapy is used to treat invasive cervical cancer. External radiation beam therapy and intracavitary cesium irradiation can be used. In some cases, chemotherapy medications that are known to be radiation sensitizing (such as cisplatin) can be used in conjunction with radiation. See Chapter 14 for more information about the types of radiation therapy and nursing care of the patient undergoing radiation therapy.

Targeted Therapies

A targeted therapy for cervical cancer is bevacizumab. Bevacizumab is used to prevent the tumor from creating blood vessels to keep nutrients from reaching the cancer cells. (NCI, 2018b).

Nursing Care

Nursing care involves helping the woman cope with the physical and psychologic effects of a potentially life-threatening illness, providing information needed to make informed decisions, and minimizing the adverse effects of therapy. Pain relief measures are important, as is grief work on the part of the woman and her family. The woman should be encouraged to perform self-care activities and resume normal everyday activities and sexual functioning to the extent possible. See the accompanying Case Study & Nursing Care Plan for a woman with cervical cancer on page 1811.

Assessment

Collect the following data through a health history and physical examination (refer to Chapter 47):

- ***Health history:*** History of STIs, sexual history, partner's sexual history, family history of cervical cancer, vaginal bleeding or discharge, smoking history, maternal treatment with DES
- ***Physical assessment:*** Pelvic examination, abdomen, lymph glands.

Priorities of Care

The priorities of nursing care for the woman with cervical cancer include helping the woman and her family cope with the physical and psychologic effects of this disease, providing information needed to make informed decisions, and minimizing the adverse effects of therapy.

Diagnoses, Interventions, and Outcomes

This section discusses nursing interventions for the woman who has been diagnosed with cervical cancer and requires surgical and/or radiation treatment. Other nursing diagnoses and interventions that may be appropriate for the woman with cervical cancer are discussed in the sections discussing other female reproductive system cancers.

Reduce Anxiety. Many people believe that cancer equals death; however, this is no longer true in many cases, especially with early diagnosis. For cervical cancer that is localized, the 5-year survival rate is 92% (ACS, 2018d).

Expected Outcome: Patient will discuss fears related to cervical cancer diagnosis and treatment by use of open communication and effective coping strategies.

The nurse will:

- Explain that many women with cervical cancer survive for 5 years or more and that the earlier the cancer is detected, the better the prognosis. *This gives the woman hope, an essential ingredient in recovery.*
- Allow adequate time for the woman and her partner to express their concerns and to ask questions. *Unexpressed feelings and fears and lack of understanding may cause the woman to view the situation as worse than it is.*
- Refer to a cancer counselor or support group for additional information. *Cancer survivors who visit patients in the hospital provide proof that people can survive the diagnosis and treatment of cancer and lead normal, productive lives.*

Promote Tissue Integrity. Surgery interrupts the integrity of the skin surface, providing a potential portal of invasion for bacteria. Radiation therapy causes an inflammatory response in the skin and mucous membranes within the field of radiation, creating further risk of tissue reaction and breakdown.

Expected Outcome: Patient will demonstrate skin integrity by supportive skin care to promote healing and reduce skin breakdown.

The nurse will:

- Teach wound and skin care, particularly if pelvic exenteration is performed. Irrigations with saline or solutions of saline and hydrogen peroxide are performed at intervals, with dry heat applied thereafter to dry the area. *Open and damaged tissue increases the risk for infection. Meticulous skin and wound care is necessary to prevent infection and further tissue destruction.*
- If appropriate, teach stoma care and care for the skin surrounding the stoma. (These procedures are discussed in Chapters 24 and 27.) *Urine and stool are irritating to the skin. Without proper care, the skin surrounding the stoma can become excoriated.*
- Apply non-oil-based lotions to skin surface. This may minimize itching and help maintain integrity. *Oil-based lotions are not recommended for tissue undergoing radiation.*
- Instruct the woman not to remove the markings used to localize the radiation beam to the target area. *Markings are used in future radiation treatments.*
- Monitor for evidence of fistula formation, and teach the woman to do the same. *Fistula formation is a potential complication of radiation to the pelvic or abdominal cavities. Vaginal fistulas may form between the vagina and the bladder or rectum. Fistulas may also develop between the bladder and rectum, resulting in the expulsion of stool in the urine or loss of urine through the anus.*

Transitions of Care

Encourage women to have their daughters (and sons for prevention of genital warts and spreading the virus to women) vaccinated with Gardasil to prevent cervical cancer, precancerous genital lesions, and genital warts due to HPV types 6, 11, 16, and 18 or a 9-valent HPV vaccine (Gardasil-9). Due to the evolving nature of immunization schedules based on new information, the CDC website should be consulted for the most up-to-date information. There has been controversy around the issue of vaccination for a sexually transmitted infection even though it prevents cancer. Many parents fear if they permit vaccination they are promoting premarital sex. Educating parents about the risks and the progression of HPV is important to ensure girls and boys are permitted to receive the vaccination. Legislation to mandate vaccination for HPV is pending in many states. Nurses should become familiar with and advocate for health-related legislation. While HPV vaccine has been recommended for cervical cancer, there is now a growing emphasis on males, not only for prevention of cervical cancer but also for oropharyngeal cancer as up to 70% of all oropharyngeal cancer can be attributed to HPV (CDC, 2017).

Recommendations for cervical cancer screening vary somewhat. The American Cancer Society (2018a) recommends that a woman should begin screening for cervical cancer at 21 years of age with the Pap test every 3 years. Cervical cancer screening with HPV DNA tests and Pap tests may be performed every 5 years for the woman over age 30 with previous normal results. Women 65 to 70 years of age and older who have had three or more normal Pap smears in the past 10 years may choose to stop cervical cancer screening. Screening for women who have had a total hysterectomy (including the cervix) is not recommended unless the surgery was done as a treatment for cancer. Women who have a hysterectomy without removal of the cervix should continue to follow ACS guidelines. If a woman is at high risk (e.g., due to DES exposure, HIV infection, or suppressed immune system for a number of reasons), then the ACS (2018a) recommends the woman follow the recommendation of her healthcare team. All women should discuss the schedule for examinations with their healthcare provider.

It is vital that nurses educate women of all ages about controlling risk factors for cervical cancer and about the importance of screening for this cancer throughout the lifespan. Teach young women about the relationship between early sexual activity, multiple partners, having a partner who has had multiple sex partners, and having sex with men who are not circumcised. Discuss safer sex alternatives and using condoms for protection. Emphasize the importance of continued screening exams for the older woman who may not see a gynecologic specialist on a regular basis.

Teaching varies according to the stage of the cancer and the treatment selected. Provide information concerning radiation, chemotherapy, or surgery, as indicated. Preoperative teaching focuses on postoperative expectations, including management of urinary or fecal diversion, if indicated. Help the woman and family recognize signs of infection and understand the importance of follow-up care. In addition, suggest the following resources: The American Cancer Society, the National Cancer Institute, and the Women's

Case Study & Nursing Care Plan

A Woman with Cervical Cancer

Anna Eliza Gillam is a 45-year-old divorced mother of four children ranging in age from 16 to 23. She was married at age 18 and had several sexual partners prior to her marriage. She has had three sexual partners since her marriage ended. A Pap smear taken 2 weeks ago showed atypical cells, and she has come in for a repeat test.

ASSESSMENT	DIAGNOSES	EXPECTED OUTCOMES
Judy Davis, RN, FNP, the admitting nurse, interviews Ms. Gillam and records the following assessment findings: BP 130/80 mmHg, P 72 bpm, R 18/min, T 37.3°C (99.2°F). Ms. Gillam weighs 142 lb (64.5 kg). Examination of the cervix reveals a large necrotic lesion at the 7 o'clock position. She has reduced her smoking to fewer than 10 cigarettes per day, and she does not drink alcohol. Ms. Gillam is extremely fearful and anxious and has told no one about her abnormal Pap smear. She reveals that she has had back pain radiating down her thighs for several months and a foul vaginal discharge that increases after intercourse. Until 2 weeks ago, she had not had a Pap smear for 5 years. Ms. Davis performs the repeat Pap smear, which is positive for squamous cell carcinoma of the cervix. A CT scan and lymphangiography are scheduled. Laparoscopy shows the disease to be widespread in the pelvic cavity.	■ Need for education related to treatment options ■ Acute pain due to metastasis and surgery ■ Potential for skin damage due to radiation therapy ■ Fear due to diagnosis of cervical cancer ■ Grief due to life-threatening illness and pain	■ Patient will gain knowledge to make informed decisions about treatment options. ■ Patient will develop strategies for pain control. ■ Patient will maintain skin and tissue integrity during radiation treatment. ■ Patient will express her feelings about the fear of cancer and death. ■ Patient will develop effective coping strategies for dealing with life-threatening illness and pain.

PLANNING AND IMPLEMENTATION

- Discuss treatment alternatives, including the prognosis with each option.
- Administer pain medications as prescribed.
- Inspect skin surfaces daily before and after radiation therapy.
- Provide information on biofeedback training and relaxation techniques for control of moderate pain.
- Assess for and assist with referrals for spiritual counseling because this has been shown to improve coping with life-altering cancer.
- Refer to a local cancer support group so that she can interact with cancer survivors.
- Refer Ms. Gillam to a social worker in preparation for her altered level of functioning.

EVALUATION

Ms. Gillam has begun radiation therapy following pelvic exenteration. She controls her pain with relaxation and imagery techniques, requiring only occasional analgesics. She uses a water-based lotion to soothe the skin surface and is careful not to remove the skin markings. She seems optimistic and has quit smoking. She and her family have continued to attend the cancer support group meetings. Ms. Gillam is planning for the future and has talked with her family about what it means to live with cancer.

CLINICAL REASONING IN PATIENT CARE

1. Compare and contrast your teaching plan for health promotion interventions to decrease the risks of cervical cancer for a young woman of 17 and an older woman of 70. Would they differ and, if so, how?
2. Develop a teaching plan to help Ms. Gillam cope with the effects of radiation.
3. During a home visit, Ms. Gillam tells the nurse that she has been so tired since beginning radiation treatments that all she can do is sit in her chair. Design a plan of care that addresses Ms. Gillam's fatigue.

See Evaluating Your Response in Appendix B.

Cancer Network. Cancer treatment can become a chronic, continuous treatment.

If the treatments are not curing or controlling the cancer, or if the woman chooses no treatment for advanced cervical cancer, a palliative care team consult should be requested. Discussions with the woman and her support systems as appropriate concerning pain management, fluids, and nutrition along with any other concerns are important.

The Patient with Endometrial Cancer

Endometrial cancer is the most frequently diagnosed cancer of the female reproductive organs in the United States. The ACS (2018g) estimates that in 2018 more than 63,000 women are diagnosed with endometrial cancer, and more than 11,350 women die annually from this disease. Most endometrial cancer is diagnosed in older women, with 60 as the average age of diagnosis. The incidence of endometrial cancer is higher in White women, but Black women are more likely to die from it. The overall 5-year survival rate is about 81%, but if found and treated early in the disease, that rate increases to over 95% (ACS, 2018i).

Pathophysiology

Most endometrial malignancies are adenocarcinomas that are slow to grow and metastasize. These cancers (classified as type 1 endometrial cancers) develop in the glandular cells or endometrial lining of the uterus (the same tissue that is shed each month during a normal menstrual period). Endometrial hyperplasia (excessive growth) is a precursor of endometrial cancer. A second and much less common type of tumor (classified as type 2 endometrial cancer) is not estrogen driven and occurs primarily in older menopausal women. These tumors are associated with endometrial atrophy and have a poorer prognosis (ACS, 2018j).

Tumor growth usually begins in the fundus, invades the vascular myometrium, and spreads throughout the female reproductive tract. Metastasis occurs by means of the lymphatic system, through the fallopian tubes to the peritoneal cavity, and to the rest of the body via the bloodstream. Target areas for metastasis include the lungs, liver, and bone. The International Federation of Gynecology and Obstetrics (FIGO) classification of endometrial cancer is outlined in **Table 49.4**.

Risk Factors

Significant risk factors for endometrial cancer are prolonged estrogen stimulation and obesity (ACS, 2018e). Other factors that increase risk are anovulatory menstrual cycles, increased number of menstrual cycles during one's lifetime, a high-fat diet, having cancer of the breast or ovary, prior radiation therapy of the pelvic region, atypical endometrial hyperplasia, decreasing ovarian function (as from menopause), estrogen-secreting tumors, and unopposed estrogen (e.g., estrogen therapy without progesterone) (ACS, 2018j). Medical conditions that may alter estrogen metabolism and increase the risk of endometrial cancer are diabetes mellitus, hypertension, and polycystic ovary disease. Tamoxifen, a drug that blocks estrogen receptor sites and is used to treat breast cancer, has a weak estrogenic effect on the endometrium and is also a risk factor. Endometrial cancer is the most commonly inherited gynecologic cancer. A family history of hereditary nonpolyposis colon cancer (HNPCC or Lynch syndrome) may mean that a woman has an inherited mutation that is a mismatch of repair genes and has a higher risk of developing endometrial cancer (ACS, 2018e). The risk for endometrial cancer is decreased by using birth control pills, use of an IUD without hormones to prevent pregnancy, and having multiple pregnancies.

Table 49.4 FIGO Staging Classification for Endometrial Cancer

Stage	Description
I	Tumor limited to endometrium or myometrium
II	Endocervical glandular involvement or invasion of cervical stroma
III	Metastasis or invasion of serosa, adnexa, vagina, and pelvic or para-aortic lymph nodes
IV	Tumor invasion of bladder or bowel mucosa; distant metastases

Manifestations

The major manifestation of endometrial hyperplasia or overt endometrial cancer is abnormal, painless vaginal bleeding. In menstruating women, this bleeding is manifested as heavy menstrual bleeding or metrorrhagia. In postmenopausal women, any bleeding is abnormal. Later manifestations include pelvic cramping, bleeding after intercourse, and lower abdominal pressure.

Complications

Complications of endometrial cancer are seen in the advanced stages. These complications include lymph node enlargement, pleural effusion, abdominal masses, and ascites. These complications may affect breathing and comfort and put pressure on different organs, limiting function.

Interprofessional Care

The goals of care for the woman with endometrial cancer are to eradicate the cancer and minimize complications and metastasis. Following diagnosis, there are four basic types of treatment for endometrial cancer: Surgery, radiation therapy, hormone therapy, and chemotherapy.

Diagnosis

Tests used to diagnose cancer of the endometrium include a transvaginal ultrasound to determine endometrial thickening (which may indicate hypertrophy or malignant changes) and an endometrial biopsy or a D&C to provide tissue for a definitive diagnosis (refer to Chapter 47 for further information). Other tests to determine the extent of the disease include chest x-ray; cystoscopy and intravenous pyelogram (IVP) to examine the urinary system; proctoscopy (to assess the rectum); CT scan, PET, or MRI to look for cancer cells and tissue changes; bone scans to identify metastasis; CBC (to identify anemia from bleeding); and a CA-125 blood test to identify the presence of markers for endometrial and ovarian cancers.

Surgery

After the diagnosis is confirmed, a total abdominal hysterectomy and bilateral salpingo-oophorectomy is performed for stage I cancer. A radical hysterectomy with node dissection is performed if the disease is stage II or beyond. Refer to Box 49.1 for nursing care of the patient undergoing a hysterectomy.

Radiation Therapy

Treatment with external-beam and internal (brachytherapy) radiation may be performed as a preoperative measure or as adjuvant treatment in advanced cases.

Hormone Therapy

Hormone therapy uses hormones or hormone-blocking drugs. They include:

- Progestins are progesterone-like drugs. Those used most commonly are medroxyprogesterone acetate (Provera, given by injection or orally) and megestrol acetate (Megace, given orally). These slow the growth of cancer cells. Side effects include hot flashes, night sweats, and weight gain. The drugs increase blood glucose levels in women with diabetes and may rarely cause serious blood clots.
- Tamoxifen is an antiestrogen drug also often used to treat breast cancer. It is useful against endometrial cancer because it prevents estrogens from stimulating growth of cancer cells. It does not cause bone loss, but can cause hot flashes and vaginal dryness; there is additionally an increased risk for serious blood clots in the legs.
- Gonadotropin-releasing hormone agonists (GnRH-a) lower estrogen levels. Examples are goserelin (Zoladex) and leuprolide (Lupron). These drugs are injected every 1 to 3 months. Side effects are menopausal manifestations and, with long-term use, osteoporosis.
- Aromatase inhibitors stop estrogen from being formed to lower estrogen levels. Examples include letrozole (Femara), anastrozole (Arimidex), and exemestane (Aromasin). Often used to treat breast cancer, these drugs are also believed to be helpful in treating endometrial cancer. They may be taken for years, may cause osteoporosis, and are still being studied.

Chemotherapy

A combination of drugs may be used to treat endometrial cancer, including doxorubicin (Adriamycin), cisplatin, carboplatin, and paclitaxel (Taxol). Two or more drugs are often combined for treatment. Chemotherapy is discussed in detail in Chapter 14.

Nursing Care

Assessment

Collect the following data through a health history and physical examination (refer to Chapter 47):

- ***Health history:*** Abnormal vaginal bleeding, menstrual history, use of estrogen (without progesterone) to treat menopausal symptoms, breast cancer treated with tamoxifen, childbearing status, presence of chronic illnesses, family history of hereditary nonpolyposis colon cancer
- ***Physical assessment:*** Height and weight, pelvic examination, abdomen, lymph glands.

Priorities of Care

For the woman who has undergone hysterectomy to treat endometrial cancer, acute pain and preventing surgical complications (infection, deep venous thrombosis, atelectasis) are the nursing care priorities.

Diagnoses, Interventions, and Outcomes

Nursing care involves helping the woman cope with the physical and psychologic effects of a potentially life-threatening illness, make informed decisions, and minimize the adverse effects of therapy. Pain relief is a key component of care, as is grief work on the part of the woman and family. Encourage the woman to perform self-care and resume normal activities of daily living.

Manage Pain. A total abdominal hysterectomy can result in severe and prolonged pain, not only from the surgical incision but also from the manipulation of internal organs during surgery. Abdominal viscera are highly vascular and easily bruised by handling.

Expected Outcome: Patient will demonstrate adequate pain management through use of prescribed pharmacologic and nonpharmacologic interventions for pain relief.

The nurse will:

- Administer analgesics as ordered. *Analgesics provide pain relief and promote early ambulation.*
- Encourage ambulation. *Ambulation facilitates the expulsion of flatus, which can cause distention as well as discomfort.*
- Apply heat to the abdomen, and recommend that the woman use a heating pad at home. *Heat dilates blood vessels, increasing blood supply to the pelvis, decreasing pain.*

Promote Healthy Body Image. For many women, the side effects of cancer treatment can be almost as difficult and painful as the disease itself. Although side effects of the different therapies vary among individuals, the woman's body image and quality of life are always affected. Such side effects as alopecia (hair loss), nausea and vomiting, fatigue, diarrhea, stomatitis, and surgical scarring disturb body image.

Expected Outcome: Patient will demonstrate appropriate self-esteem by use of effective coping strategies to deal with the temporary changes in body image and interventions to promote body image.

The nurse will:

- Review the side effects of the treatment regimen proposed and assist the woman to develop a plan to deal with these effects. *This promotes a sense of control.*
- Remind the woman and family that side effects are usually manageable and may be temporary. *Over-the-counter agents can be used to alleviate stomatitis. Frequent rest periods can relieve fatigue. Medications can be prescribed for nausea and vomiting and diarrhea.*

Promote Sexual Function. Altered sexuality may result from a feeling of unattractiveness, fatigue, or pain and discomfort. The woman's partner may fear that sexual activity will be harmful.

Expected Outcome: Patient will demonstrate willingness to discuss changes to sexual function and adapts modes of sexual expression to accommodate endometrial cancer treatment-related changes.

The nurse will:

- Encourage expression of feelings about the effect of cancer on their lives and sexual relationship. *Verbalizing feelings helps relieve stress and maximizes relaxation.*
- Suggest that the couple explore alternative sexual positions and coordinate sexual activity with rest periods and times that are relatively free from pain. *This creates a more favorable environment for satisfying sexual activity.*

Delegating Nursing Care Activities

Delegation of nursing care activities are the same for any patient undergoing surgery and or chemotherapy. Basic care and comfort activities, ambulation, and routine vital signs are all tasks that can be delegated as appropriate staffing allows.

Transitions of Care

All perimenopausal and postmenopausal women need annual pelvic examinations. The ACS recommends that at the time of menopause all women be informed of the risks and manifestations of endometrial cancer and strongly encouraged to report any unexpected bleeding or spotting to their healthcare provider. Those in high-risk groups are advised to have endometrial biopsies every 2 years, beginning at age 35. In addition, control of diseases such as diabetes mellitus and hypertension decreases the risk of endometrial hyperplasia.

The American Cancer Society recommends that, at the time of menopause, all women should be told about the risks and manifestations of endometrial cancer. They should be strongly encouraged to report any unexpected bleeding to their healthcare provider. Women with or at risk for hereditary nonpolyposis colon cancer should be offered annual screening for endometrial cancer with endometrial biopsy beginning at age 35.

Provide information about the specific treatment and prognosis. Explain the expected side effects of treatment used (refer to Chapter 14). Pain control measures are also an essential part of the teaching plan (refer to Chapter 9). The resources listed for the woman with cervical cancer are also appropriate for the woman with endometrial cancer.

If the treatments are not curing or controlling the cancer, or if the woman chooses no treatment for advanced endometrial cancer, a palliative care team consult should be requested. Discussions with the woman and support systems as appropriate concerning pain management, fluids, and nutrition along with any other concerns is important.

The Patient with Ovarian Cancer

Although ovarian cancer is the fourth most common gynecologic cancer in women in the United States, it is the fifth leading cause of cancer deaths among women (ACS, 2018h). In 2018, approximately 22,000 women were diagnosed with ovarian cancer and an estimated 14,000 died from the disease (ACS, 2018h). The cancer primarily develops in older women, with about two-thirds of the cases diagnosed in women ages 55 or older. Ovarian cancer is more common and has the highest mortality rate in White women (ACS, 2018h).

Pathophysiology

There are several types of ovarian cancers: Epithelial tumors, germ cell tumors, and gonadal stromal tumors. Most ovarian cancers are epithelial tumors, originating from the surface epithelium of the ovary. Ovarian cancer usually spreads by local shedding of cancer cells into the peritoneal cavity and by direct invasion of the bowel and bladder. Cancer cells in peritoneal fluid can implant in the intestines, bladder, and mesentery. Tumor cells also spread through the lymph and blood to such organs as the liver and across the diaphragm to involve the lungs. Both pelvic and para-aortic lymph nodes may be involved and tumor cells can block lymphatic drainage from the abdomen, resulting in ascites. FIGO staging for ovarian cancer is based on surgical and histologic evaluation (**Table 49.5**).

Risk Factors

There is about a four-fold increase in risk for ovarian cancer in women who have a first-degree relative with it. Twenty percent of all ovarian cancer cases are estimated to be due to an inherited mutation (mostly *BRCA1* and *BRCA2*) that increases risk (ACS, 2018h). There are other inherited mutations being studied for their relationship with ovarian cancer. Women with a Lynch syndrome mutation have an 8% higher risk of developing ovarian cancer (ACS, 2018h).

Risk factors also include increasing age, having no children or giving birth after age 35, early menarche and late menopause, infertility drugs, obesity, eating a high-fat diet, and a personal history of breast cancer. There is also a possibility that polycystic ovarian disease and hormone replacement therapy after menopause may place a woman at risk. Protective factors include long-term contraceptive use, a low-fat diet, having a child before the age of 25, tubal ligation, breastfeeding, and hysterectomy (ACS, 2018h).

Manifestations and Complications

In early stages, ovarian cancer generally causes no warning signs or manifestations. When manifestations do develop, they are often vague and mild, such as feeling full quickly, abdominal bloating, urinary urgency and/or frequency, and pelvic or abdominal pain. Other manifestations include fatigue, back pain, pain during intercourse, constipation,

Table 49.5 FIGO Staging Classification for Ovarian Cancer

Stage	Description
I	Growth limited to the ovaries
II	Growth involving one or both ovaries with pelvic extension
III	Tumor involving one or both ovaries, with peritoneal implants outside the pelvis or positive retroperitoneal or inguinal nodes
IV	Growth involving one or both ovaries with distant metastasis

and menstrual changes in women prior to menopause. Abnormal vaginal bleeding may occur if the endometrium is stimulated by a hormone-secreting tumor or if the tumor erodes the vaginal wall. An enlarged abdomen with ascites signals later-stage disease.

The complications of advanced ovarian cancer, with related assessments and treatment, are outlined in **Table 49.6**.

Interprofessional Care

As with other malignancies, care of the woman with ovarian cancer involves surgery to determine the stage of the tumor and to remove as much of the tumor as possible. Unfortunately, because there are no specific early manifestations, the disease may be well advanced prior to diagnosis. In younger women, an ovarian mass may be monitored for several menstrual cycles, but any ovarian mass must immediately be investigated in a postmenopausal woman. The treatment involves three modalities: Surgery, chemotherapy, and radiation therapy.

Diagnosis

Tests used in the diagnosis of ovarian cancer may include transvaginal or abdominal ultrasound, a CT scan of the abdomen and pelvis, an MRI of the abdomen, a PET scan, a laparoscopy, a colonoscopy, and/or an ovarian biopsy. The blood test most useful is a CA-125 antigen level. CA-125 is a tumor marker that is highly specific and elevated in epithelial ovarian cancer. Research is ongoing to develop a blood test to specifically identify ovarian cancer.

Surgery

In young women with stage I disease who wish to have children, treatment may be limited to removal of one ovary. Usually, however, total hysterectomy with bilateral salpingo-oophorectomy (removal of the ovaries and fallopian tubes) is performed. The omentum may be removed and biopsies of the peritoneum may be taken on initial surgery. If the tumor is extensive, then debulking is performed and other abdominal organs may be removed. If the cancer is advanced, chemotherapy prior to surgery may be provided. During surgery intraperitoneal chemotherapy can be administered. Treatment after surgery depends on the type, stage, and the woman's general state of health. Treatment after surgery can include chemotherapy (usually) and radiation therapy.

Chemotherapy

Combination chemotherapy, discussed in Chapter 14, is primarily used following surgery. The types of chemotherapy used in ovarian cancer are usually platinum (carboplatin IV and cisplatin intraperitoneal) and a taxane (paclitaxel or docetaxel). Other chemotherapies will be added depending on the type of ovarian cancer. Most if not all ovarian cancers will become resistant to the platinum-based chemotherapy (ASC, 2018h).

Radiation Therapy

Radiation therapy using external-beam or intracavitary implants is performed for palliative purposes only and is directed at shrinking the tumor at selected sites.

Nursing Care

Although individualized to each woman, nursing care is essentially the same as that provided for women with other gynecologic cancers and abdominal surgeries. However, research findings support the need for education because awareness of ovarian cancer manifestations and risk factors in the general population is low (ACS, 2018h). The side effects of treatment of cancer and generally poor prognosis diminish the woman's quality of life and involve major psychosocial implications (refer to Chapter 14).

Transitions of Care

Address the following topics in preparing the woman and her family for self-care:

- If a positive family history of breast, ovarian, or colon cancer exists, stress the importance of obtaining regular pelvic examinations. Inform women in this risk group that annual screening with transvaginal ultrasound and CA-125 measurements may be recommended.

Table 49.6 Complications of Advanced Ovarian Cancer and Related Assessments and Treatment

Complication	Assessments	Treatment
Ascites (accumulation of fluid in the abdominal cavity; a form of third spacing)	■ Abdominal distention ■ Shiny abdominal skin ■ Dullness on percussion of dependent areas ■ Dyspnea, constipation ■ Abdominal pain	Paracentesis (removing fluid from the abdomen)
Intestinal obstruction	■ Abdominal distention ■ Abdominal pain ■ Projectile vomiting ■ Constipation ■ Hyperactive bowel sounds	Nasogastric tube insertion, NPO
Deep venous thrombosis	■ Leg edema ■ Leg pain ■ Redness, warmth	Anticoagulants
Lymphedema (leg)	■ Edema of leg ■ Decreased range of motion ■ Tight, shiny skin on leg	Skin care, range-of-motion exercises, massage or physical therapy, compression bandaging

- It is crucial not to ignore manifestations such as indigestion, nausea, or urinary frequency because these seemingly unrelated manifestations may be early signs of ovarian tumors. Emphasize that ovarian cancer may be asymptomatic in the early stages.
- Discuss treatment options and their side effects and provide information on ways to minimize or manage side effects.
- Refer to hospice services when appropriate. The resources suggested for the woman with cervical cancer are also appropriate for the woman with ovarian cancer.

The Patient with Cancer of the Vulva

Cancer of the vulva is a relatively rare malignancy; it occurs most often in women over 60 years of age (Sorenson et al., 2019). The prognosis of vulvar carcinoma depends on the degree of invasion, general health status of the woman, presence of chronic diseases, and ability to withstand treatment.

The cause of vulvar cancer is unknown, but there is evidence to associate it with STIs, particularly HPV (Sorenson et al., 2019). Nearly 85% of malignant and premalignant cervical and vulvar lesions have been found to contain HPV DNA, HPV structural antigens, or both. Herpes simplex type 2 (HSV-2) infection and a history of leukoplakia (a precancerous lesion on the vulvar mucous membranes characterized by raised white patches) have also been associated with vulvar cancer. Other risk factors include smoking, HIV, precancerous lesions (vulvar intraepithelial neoplasia [VIN]), other genital cancers, and presence of melanoma or atypical moles.

Most vulvar cancers are epidermoid or squamous cell carcinomas. The primary site is usually the labia majora, but vulvar cancer is also found on the labia minora, clitoris, vestibule, and occasionally in multiple locations. Metastasis occurs by direct extension into the vagina, perineal skin, anus, and urethra. The cancer also spreads through the lymphatic system via the superficial and deep inguinal and femoral nodes and to the pelvic lymph nodes.

The manifestations of vulvar cancer include pruritus, wart-like growths, patchy changes in color or density of the vulva, vaginal bleeding, dysuria, or changes in a mole on the vulva. Inguinal lymph nodes may be enlarged. If lesions are present, they are biopsied. There are some topical treatments; however, surgical resection is the usual treatment. If lymph nodes are involved, radiation therapy is used postoperatively. Chemotherapy is reserved for distant metastases.

Nursing care is similar to that for the woman with endometrial cancer. The woman fears death as the ultimate outcome as well as the possible pain and suffering that surgery and other treatments may cause. Radical surgery represents a great loss to women of all ages.

49.6 Disorders of the Female Breast

Breast disorders are common conditions that primarily affect women (disorders of the male breast are discussed in Chapter 48). When a woman discovers a breast lump, her first response is often fear: Of breast cancer, of losing her breast, and perhaps of losing her life. Because American society views the breast as a significant component of feminine beauty, any problem that threatens the breast often strikes at the core of a woman's self-image.

Nurses play a critical role in the care of women experiencing breast disorders by providing education, support, and advocacy. Part of the nurse's role is educating women about normal breast tissue, common benign breast disorders, screening recommendations, and risk factors for breast cancer.

The Patient with a Benign Breast Disorder

Benign changes in a woman's breast tissue often correspond to hormonal changes of the menstrual cycle. Breast tissue also changes in response to nutritional, physical, and environmental stimuli. Benign breast disorders include fibrocystic breast changes, fibroadenomas, intraductal papillomas, duct ectasia, fat necrosis, and mastitis (**Table 49.7**).

Pathophysiology

Fibrocystic Changes

Fibrocystic changes (FCC) (fibrocystic breast disease) is the physiologic nodularity and breast tenderness that increases and decreases with the menstrual cycle. In the United States, an estimated 1 million women annually experience some of these changes, which include fibrosis, epithelial proliferation, and cyst formation. FCC is most common in women 30 to 50 years of age and is rare in postmenopausal women who are not taking hormone replacement (Santen, 2017).

FCC includes many different lesions and breast changes. The more common nonproliferative form does not increase the risk for breast cancer. The proliferative form, accompanied by giant cysts and proliferative epithelial lesions, does increase the risk for breast cancer.

Nonproliferative changes may be cystic or fibrous. Cystic change refers to the dilation of ducts in the subareolar, lobular, or lobe areas. Cysts often go unnoticed unless pain and tenderness is associated with menses. Fibrous changes are infrequent but can occur during the menstrual years. A firm, palpable mass, 2 to 3 cm in size, is typically located in the upper outer breast quadrant following an inflammatory response to ductal irritation.

Intraductal Disorders

An intraductal papilloma is a tiny, wartlike growth on the inside of the peripheral mammary duct that causes discharge from the nipple. The discharge may be clear and sticky or bloody. When more than one of these growths is present, the condition is called *intraductal papillomatosis*. This condition is most common in women in their 30s and 40s. The lesion must be investigated to rule out malignancy.

Mammary duct ectasia (plasma cell mastitis) is a palpable lumpiness found beneath the areola. Duct ectasia involves periductal inflammation, dilation of the ductal system, and

Table 49.7 Common Breast Disorders

Condition	Age	Pain	Nipple Discharge	Location	Consistency and Mobility	Diagnosis and Treatment
Duct ectasia	35–55 years; median age 40	Burning around nipple	Sticky, multicolored; usually bilateral	No specific location	Retroareolar mass with advanced disease	Open biopsy; local excision of diseased portion of breast
Fibroadenoma	15–39 years; median age 20	No	No	No specific location	Mobile, firm, smooth, well-delineated mass	Mammography, surgical or needle biopsy; excision of the tumor
Fibrocystic changes (FCC)	20–49 years; median age 30 (may subside with menopause)	Yes	May occur	Upper outer quadrant	Bilateral multiple lumps influenced by the menstrual cycle	Needle aspiration; observation; biopsy if there is an unresolved mass or mammographic changes
Intraductal papilloma	35–55 years; median age 40	Yes	Serous or sanguineous; usually unilateral from one duct	No specific location	Usually soft, poorly delineated mass	Pap smear of nipple discharge; biopsy; wedge resection
Mastitis, acute	Childbearing years	Tenderness, pain	No	No specific location	Generalized redness of overlying skin	Antibiotic therapy; incision and drainage if mastitis progresses to an abscess
Mastitis, chronic	Any age	Tenderness, pain; headache; high fever	No	No specific location	Generalized redness and swelling	Antibiotics, usually penicillin
Fat necrosis	Any age	Tenderness	No	No specific location	Firm, irregular, palpable	Surgical biopsy to rule out cancer

accumulation of fluid and dead cells that block the involved ducts. The condition usually occurs in perimenopausal women and is difficult to differentiate from cancer.

Manifestations

Women with fibrocystic changes experience bilateral or unilateral pain or tenderness in the upper, outer quadrants of their breasts and report that their breasts feel particularly thick and lumpy the week prior to menses. Nipple discharge may be present. Pain is due to edema of the connective tissue of the breast, dilation of the ducts, and some inflammatory response; some women report an increase in breast size. Multiple, mobile cysts may form, usually in both breasts (**Figure 49.6** ■). Fluid aspirated from these cysts ranges in color from milky white to yellow, brown, or green. If the fluid is tinged with blood, there is reason to suspect malignancy.

Manifestations of mammary duct ectasia include sticky, thick nipple discharge with burning and itching around the nipple and inflammation. The discharge may be green, greenish-brown, or bloody. Nipple retraction is often associated with duct ectasia in postmenopausal women.

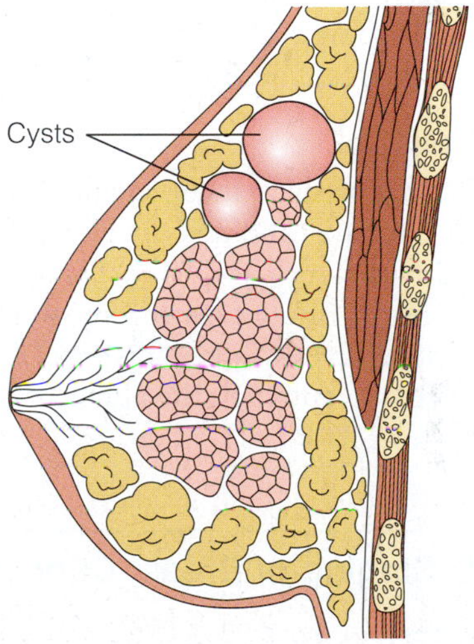
Cysts

Figure 49.6 ■ Fibrocystic breast changes.

Interprofessional Care

Diagnosis of FCC is based on complete history, physical examination, and imaging studies. A biopsy may be required for diagnosis. Analysis of nipple discharge, mammography, and possibly ductography may be used to diagnose ductal disorders. The affected duct is excised in an open biopsy procedure.

The treatment of FCC is usually symptomatic. Cyst aspiration may relieve pain and also allows examination of fluid to confirm the cystic nature of the disease. A well-fitting bra that provides good support worn day and night helps relieve discomfort. Some women report that eliminating xanthines (found in coffee, tea, cola, and chocolate) from the diet decreases symptoms. Aspirin, mild analgesics, local heat or cold, and vitamin E may help relieve breast pain. Hormone therapy is controversial because of the benign nature of the disease and potential adverse effects of therapy. Danazol, a synthetic androgen, may be prescribed for women with severe pain.

Nursing Care

When a woman presents with a breast mass, nursing responsibilities include taking a careful health history and facilitating follow-up care. If a palpable mass is present, it is important to ask how long the lesion has been present and whether the woman has noticed any pain associated with the mass, any change in its size, and any changes in association with the menstrual cycle.

In many cases, definitive diagnosis of the breast disorder requires surgical biopsy to rule out cancer. During the diagnostic process, the nurse can provide emotional support and education about diagnostic and therapeutic procedures, self-care and comfort measures, and resources to help the woman cope with the experience. Nursing care for the woman is similar to that for any patient with an open biopsy. It is also important to reassure the woman that these disorders are not breast cancer.

The Patient with Breast Cancer

Breast cancer is the unregulated growth of abnormal cells in breast tissue. Breast cancer is the most commonly occurring cancer in women and the second leading cause of cancer death in women in the United States. The ACS (2018b) estimates that more than 266,000 women were diagnosed with breast cancer in 2018, and approximately 40,900 women will die from breast cancer in 2018. The incidence rate of breast cancer has remained stable; however, the death rates have declined from a rate of approximately 25 deaths per 100,000 women in 2000 to 20 deaths per 100,000 women in 2015 (ACS, 2018b). There are racial differences in the incidence and mortality of breast cancer: Non-Hispanic White women have the highest incidence, but non-Hispanic Black women have the highest death rate based on most recent information (ACS, 2018b).

Pathophysiology

Possible causes of breast cancer include environmental, hormonal, reproductive, and hereditary factors. Two breast cancer susceptibility genes have been identified: *BRCA1* on chromosome 17 and *BRCA2* on chromosome 13. Current research has found that a family history of breast cancer is the greatest risk, even when the abnormal genes are not present. Changes in other genes that also might lead to inherited breast cancer are the *ATM* gene (normally helps repair damaged DNA), *CHEK2* gene (risk is greatly increased if mutated and there is a strong family history of breast cancer), *p53* gene (a tumor suppressor gene), and *PTEN* gene (normally helps regulate cell growth). There are now a number of models to predict breast cancer risk of an individual with or without genetic testing included (NCI, 2018b).

Cancer of the breast begins as a single transformed cell and is hormone dependent. Cancers of the breast are classified as noninvasive (in situ) or invasive, depending on the penetration of the tumor into surrounding tissue. Breast cancer may remain a noninvasive disease, or an invasive disease without metastasis, for long periods of time.

Breast cancer may be categorized as carcinoma of the mammary ducts, carcinoma of the mammary lobules, or sarcoma of the breast. Most breast cancers are adenocarcinomas and appear to arise in the terminal section of the breast ductal tissue. There are many histologic types of breast cancer, and only examples are described here. The most common type is infiltrating ductal carcinoma. Two atypical types of breast cancer are inflammatory carcinoma and Paget disease. *Inflammatory carcinoma of the breast*, a systemic disease, is the most malignant form of breast cancer. Edema with dimpling of the skin that results in the skin looking like the peel of an orange (peau d'orange) is usually present. *Paget disease* is a rare type of breast cancer involving infiltration of the nipple epithelium.

Breast cancer can metastasize to other sites through the bloodstream or lymphatic system. The common sites of metastasis of breast cancer are bone, brain, lung, liver, skin, and lymph nodes. The staging of the breast cancer (**Table 49.8**) provides important information for making decisions about treatment options and is also used as a basis for prognosis.

Table 49.8 Staging of Breast Cancer

Stage	Tumor	Node	Metastasis
0	T_{is}—Carcinoma in situ or Paget disease of the nipple	N_0—No regional lymph node metastasis	M_0—No evidence of distant metastasis
I	T_1—Tumor no larger than 2 cm	N_0	M_0
IIA	T_0—No evidence of primary tumor	N_1—Metastasis to movable ipsilateral	M_0
	T_1	axillary nodes	
	T_2—Tumor no larger than 5 cm	N_0	M_0
IIB	T_2	N_1	M_0
	T_3—Tumor larger than 5 cm	N_0	M_0
IIIA	T_0	N_2—Metastasis to ipsilateral fixed	M_0
	T_1	axillary nodes	
	T_2		
	T_3	N_1	M_0
		N_2	M_0
IIIB	T_4—Tumor of any size with direct extension to chest wall or skin	Any N	M_0
	Any T	N_3—Metastasis to ipsilateral internal mammary lymph nodes	M_0
IV	Any T	N_0 and N_1	M_1—Distant metastasis

Risk Factors

Of the various kinds of risk factors for breast cancer, some can be changed and some cannot. Those that cannot be changed are (NIC, 2018c):

- ***Age and gender.*** Women are 100 times more likely to have breast cancer than are men, with the risk increasing with age. Two out of three invasive breast cancers are found in women age 55 and older.
- ***Genetic risk factors.*** Approximately 5 to 10% of breast cancers are believed to result directly from genetic mutations inherited from a parent (see the discussion in the Pathophysiology section).
- ***Family history of breast cancer.*** Having a first-degree relative (mother, sister, or daughter) with breast cancer approximately doubles the risk and having two first-degree relatives increases it fivefold. Having a male family member with breast cancer also poses an increased risk.
- ***Dense breast tissue.*** Dense breast tissue (seen on a mammogram) has more glandular tissue and less fatty tissue, increasing the risk for the development of breast cancer.
- ***Personal history of breast cancer.*** A woman with cancer in one breast has a three- to fourfold increase in risk for developing a new cancer in the other breast or in a different part of the same breast.
- ***Previous chest irradiation.*** Radiation of the chest as a child or young woman for other cancer (such as Hodgkin lymphoma) significantly increases the risk. The risk is greatest in women who had irradiation during adolescent breast development.
- ***Menstrual history.*** Women who begin menstruating before the age of 12 or who have menopause after the age of 55 are at a slightly higher risk, probably the result of a higher lifetime exposure to estrogen and progesterone.

Lifestyle-related factors that increase breast cancer risk include recent use of oral contraceptives, not having children or having them after the age of 30, long-term use of HRT, not breast-feeding, drinking alcohol (especially two to five drinks daily), being overweight and obese (especially after menopause), and physical inactivity. In contrast, breastfeeding, moderate or vigorous physical activity, and maintaining a healthy body weight lower the risk for breast cancer.

Manifestations

The manifestations of breast cancer may include a nontender lump/mass or thickening in the breast (most often in the upper outer quadrant, the area with the most glandular tissue), abnormal nipple discharge, a persistent skin rash around the nipple area, nipple retraction, flaking or eruption near the nipple, dimpling of the skin, or a change in the position of the nipple. There may also be nipple pain, scaliness, ulceration, skin irritation, or discharge. Breast cancer is usually painless, but some women report a burning, stinging, or pricking sensation. Other manifestations include an unusual lump in the underarm or above the collarbone and dimpling, pulling, or retraction in an area of the breast. Many women with breast cancer have no manifestations and their tumors are detected by mammography. However, many breast cancers are found by the women themselves or by their partners.

Interprofessional Care

Diagnosis of breast cancer begins with detection, either detection of asymptomatic lesions discovered through screening or by a partner or symptomatic lesions discovered by the woman. Any palpable mass requires evaluation. Once the diagnosis is made, a number of treatment options are available. The choice of treatment depends on several factors, such as the stage of the cancer, the age of the woman, and the woman's preferences.

Diagnosis

Early detection of breast cancer is possible with clinical breast examination (CBE) and a mammogram (refer to Chapter 47 for further information). Mammography can detect breast tumors 2 years before they reach palpable size; most of these tumors have been present for 8 to 10 years. In addition, an ultrasound, MRI, or PET scan of the breast may be used to further identify breast tumors.

Other diagnostic tests include a percutaneous needle biopsy to define a cystic mass or fibrocystic changes and provide specimens for cytologic examination and a breast biopsy (**Figure 49.7** ■). In aspiration biopsy or fine-needle aspiration biopsy, a needle is used to remove cells or fluid from

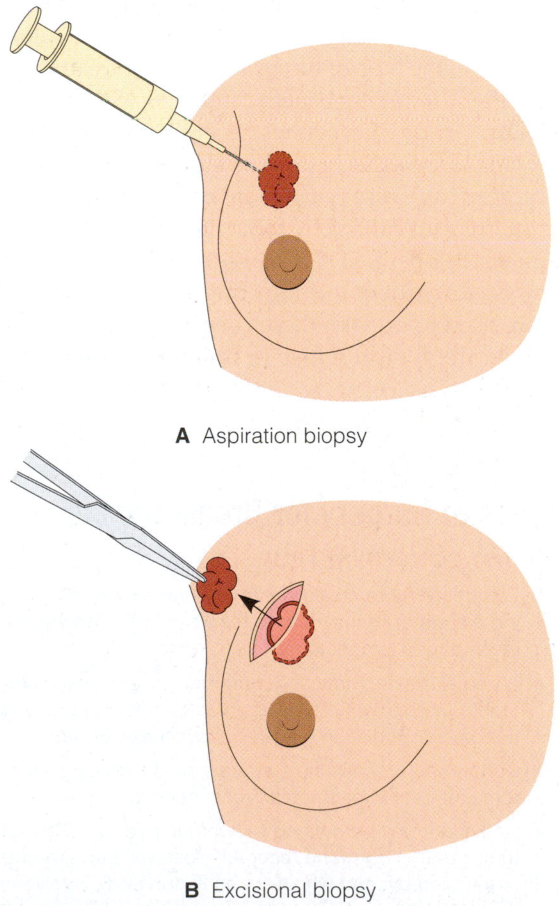
A Aspiration biopsy
B Excisional biopsy

Figure 49.7 ■ Types of breast biopsy. **A**, In an aspiration biopsy, a needle is used to aspirate fluid or tissue from the breast. **B**, In an excisional biopsy, tissue from the breast lesion is removed surgically.

the breast lesion. In many facilities, fine-needle aspiration biopsies are performed using a stereotactic biopsy device; mammography and a computer are used to guide the needle.

Molecular profiling of the tumor will guide treatment. Estrogen receptor (ER) and progesterone receptor (PR) along with human epidermal growth factor type 2 (HER2/neu) overexpression/amplification status are important in determining prognosis and treatment (NCI, 2018a). Other genetic testing can also be performed to assess prognosis.

Medications

In addition to the hormone therapy described later, bisphosphonates may be used to help strengthen and reduce the risk of fractures in bones weakened by metastatic breast cancer and may help prevent thinning of bone resulting from treatment with aromatase inhibitors or from early menopause as a side effect of chemotherapy. Examples include pamidronate (Aredia) and zoledronic acid (Zometa). Bisphosphonates have many side effects, including flulike manifestations and bone pain. A rare side effect is damage to the mandible, leading to loss of teeth or bone infection. All patients taking bisphosphonates should practice good oral hygiene and have regular dental checkups to help prevent this effect.

Surgery

The different types of surgeries used to treat breast cancer are outlined in **Box 49.2** and illustrated in **Figure 49.8** ■. The type of surgery used depends on the size of the tumor, the woman's age, the type of tumor, and the choice made by the woman after discussing benefits and risks with the surgeon.

Axillary node dissection is generally performed during surgery for all invasive breast carcinoma to stage the tumor. This surgery can cause **lymphedema** (accumulation of fluid in the soft tissues caused by removal of lymph channels) in the arm on the operated side, nerve damage, and adhesions. Nonsurgical methods of detecting lymph node involvement are used to prevent these complications and preserve the role of the lymph nodes in immune system function. Sentinel node biopsy prior to a node dissection is conducted by injecting a radioactive substance or dye into the region of the tumor. The dye is carried to the first (sentinel) lymph node to receive lymph from the tumor that would be the node most likely to contain cancer cells if metastasis has occurred. If the sentinel node is positive, more nodes are removed. If it is negative, further node evaluation is usually not indicated.

After a mastectomy, some women may choose to have their breast reconstructed. They report that surgical reconstruction of the breast simplifies their lives and restores a sense of body integrity. Other women choose to use a removable breast prosthesis, and some women are comfortable without reconstruction or a prosthesis. Breast reconstruction may be performed at the time of the mastectomy or at any time thereafter, depending on the woman's preference. A number of procedures may be used for the breast reconstruction (**Figure 49.9** ■). These include placement of a

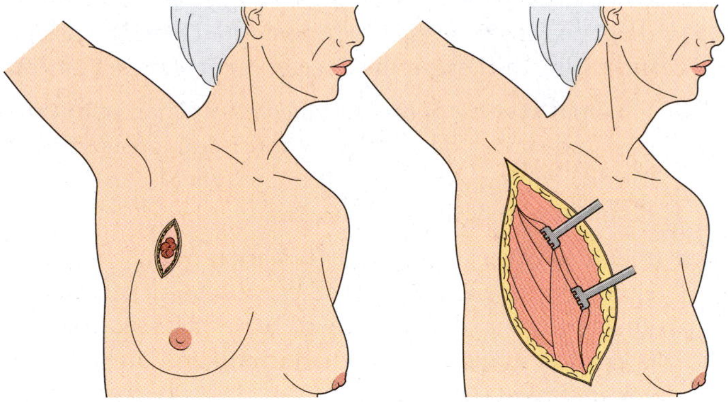
A Lumpectomy
B Modified radical mastectomy

Figure 49.8 ■ Types of breast surgeries. **A**, In a lumpectomy, only the tumor and a small margin of surrounding tissue are removed. **B**, In a modified radical mastectomy, all breast tissue and the underarm lymph nodes are removed, but the underlying muscles remain.

BOX 49.2
Types of Surgery for Breast Cancer

BREAST CONSERVING SURGERY

- Lumpectomy removes only the breast lump and a surrounding margin of tissue (refer to Figure 49.8A). Radiation is usually given after a lumpectomy.
- A partial mastectomy or quadrantectomy removes more tissue than a lumpectomy; a quadrantectomy removes one-fourth of the breast. Radiation usually follows these surgeries.
- Both breast-conserving surgeries are as effective as a mastectomy for stage I or stage II breast cancer.
- Radiation may be omitted for women over age 70 with a small tumor that is hormone receptor–positive, who are getting hormone therapy, and who have no lymph node involvement.
- Side effects of the surgeries can include pain, temporary swelling, risk for bleeding and wound infection, and hard scar formation.

MASTECTOMY

- A simple or total mastectomy removes the entire breast, but not axillary lymph nodes or muscles under the breast.
- A modified radical mastectomy removes the entire breast and some of the axillary lymph nodes (refer to Figure 49.8B).
- A skin-saving mastectomy, used for smaller tumors, leaves most of the skin over the breast (except the nipple and areola).
- A radical mastectomy (infrequently performed) removes the entire breast, axillary lymph nodes, and pectoral muscles under the breast.
- Side effects of these surgeries include postoperative pain, change in the shape of the breast, wound infection, hematoma formation, and seroma (buildup of clear fluid in the wound). If axillary lymph nodes are removed, the main long-term side effect in about one in four women is lymphedema of the arm.

submuscular implant, the use of a tissue expander followed by an implant, the transposition of muscle and blood supply from the abdomen or back, or using (most often) the transverse rectus abdominis myocutaneous (TRAM) free tissue flap. Information about breast reconstruction surgery is summarized in **Box 49.3**. Nursing care of the patient having a mastectomy is outlined in **Box 49.4**.

Radiation Therapy

Radiation therapy is typically used following breast cancer surgery to destroy any remaining cancer cells that could cause recurrence or metastasis. If a tumor is unusually large, radiation may be used to shrink the tumor prior to surgery. Radiation therapy is most commonly used in combination with lumpectomy for early stage (I or II) breast cancer. Palliative radiation therapy is also used to treat chest wall recurrences and some bone metastases to help control pain and prevent fractures. Radiation therapy is administered by external-beam or tissue implants.

External-beam radiation is most commonly used to treat breast cancer. It is performed on an outpatient basis, typically 5 days per week for 5 to 7 weeks. Treatment involves the entire breast; axillary lymph nodes may also be treated with radiation therapy. Intraoperative radiotherapy, available only at selected treatment centers, is provided by a single, concentrated dose of radiation. During surgery, a probe is inserted into the cavity created by the lumpectomy and radiation equivalent to 6 weeks of doses is emitted for about 25 minutes. Another method being researched is using higher doses of radiation over a shorter period of time following lumpectomy (called *accelerated breast irradiation*). This method has shown favorable results in cancer treatment while at the same time limiting the cost and time constraints placed on women compared with traditional radiation treatments.

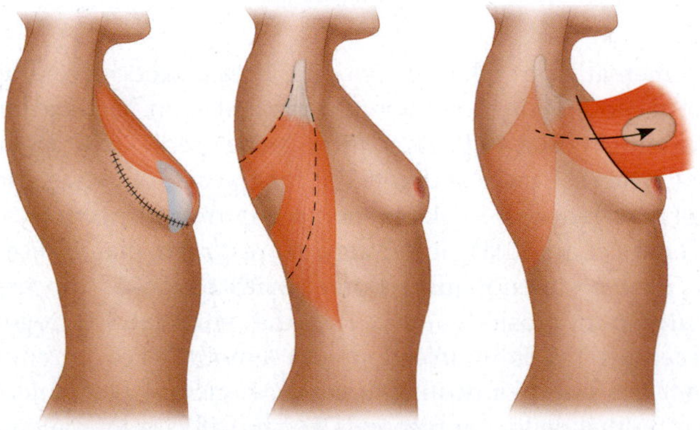
A Implant
B Latissimus dorsi musculocutaneous flap

Figure 49.9 ■ Types of breast reconstruction surgeries. **A**, A breast implant is inserted under the pectoris muscle. **B**, Autogenous procedures transfer a flap of skin, muscle, and fat from the donor site on the woman's body to the mastectomy site. The most frequently used donor muscle sites are the latissimus dorsi and the rectus abdominis (the TRAM flap).

In brachytherapy (internal radiation), radioactive seeds or pellets are placed directly into the breast tissue following lumpectomy. It may be used to provide a supplemental dose of radiation after external-beam radiation. Intracavity brachytherapy consists of inserting a small balloon attached to a small tube (that protrudes through the surgical site) into the cavity left by a lumpectomy. The balloon is filled with saline and a source of radioactivity is placed into the balloon and then removed. After 5 days of treatment, the balloon is removed. Interstitial brachytherapy is performed by inserting several small catheters into the breast around the lumpectomy. Radioactive pellets are inserted through the catheters for a short period of time each day and then removed. Clinical trials are being conducted to determine if these therapies might be used as the only source of radiation for women having a lumpectomy.

Chemotherapy

Chemotherapy has become the standard of care for the majority of breast cancer cases with axillary node

BOX 49.3
Breast Reconstruction Information

- Reconstruction can be done immediately after a mastectomy or at any time later on. Some surgeons believe that delayed reconstruction offers better cosmetic results.
- Reconstructive surgery can create a natural-looking breast that makes clothes fit better. Because it has no nerve endings, the reconstructed breast has no feeling or sensations.
- If a simple mastectomy is done, an implant approximately the same size as the other breast is placed under the pectoral muscle on the operative side. This creates a breast mound that closely resembles the natural breast in shape and softness. If the implant is placed over the pectoral muscle, a high degree of firmness may occur.
- With a simple mastectomy or modified radical mastectomy, a tissue expander may be used to replace the breast. The tissue expander is placed under the pectoral muscle and is gradually expanded with saline injections every 2 to 3 weeks to stretch the overlying skin and create a pocket. After a period of time, usually 1 to 2 months, the tissue expander is exchanged for a saline implant.
- Controversy exists about the health effects of silicone. While there is no conclusive evidence that silicone implants induce cancer or autoimmune disease, they are associated with hardening and pain due to contracture of the capsule around the implant. The implant may rupture, releasing silicone gel, or infection may occur. Saline-filled breast implants may be an alternative.
- With more extensive surgery such as radical mastectomy, a flap of skin, fat, or muscle is transferred from a donor site to the operative area. A new nipple may be created by using tissue from the opposite nipple or from the inner thigh.
- Reconstructive surgery may require multiple surgeries, including all the risks associated with anesthesia. As the complexity of the procedures increases, so does the risk of complications such as infection.
- To decrease the risk of a fibrous capsule forming around the implant, it is important to perform breast massage as instructed.

BOX 49.4
Nursing Care and Discharge Teaching of the Patient Having a Mastectomy

PREOPERATIVE

- Teach how to do deep-breathing exercises and use of incentive spirometry
- Education about plan for postoperative pain control, how long the dressing will be on, and any drains or other care the woman will need to perform upon discharge. By educating both pre- and postoperative, the teaching will be reinforced.

POSTOPERATIVE

- Encourage deep-breathing exercises and use of incentive spirometry every 4 hours.
- Monitor drainage from wound.
- Administer, as ordered, intravenous fluids and antibiotics.
- Instruct the woman how to control pain by using a patient-controlled analgesia device or requesting analgesics before pain becomes severe.
- Monitor the dressing for bleeding.
- Instruct the woman about the following to decrease anxiety, promote healing, and decrease postoperative risks:
    a. Numbness or feelings of "pins and needles" in the axillary area are common.
    b. Lying on one's back or on the side not operated on helps fluid drain from the site.
    c. Moving the arm on the operated side helps regain mobility; specific exercises will be prescribed for increasing mobility after the incisions have healed.
    d. Use caution when lifting heavy objects with the arm on the operated side.

DISCHARGE INSTRUCTIONS

- Discuss issues of lymphedema (LE) with the woman and ways to decrease it:
    a. Assess/monitor for manifestations of LE: Swelling in the affected area (usually the hand and arm), pain, fatigue, and changes in sensations (such as heaviness, numbness, or burning) in the affected area. Assess skin color, temperature, texture, scars, or lesions. Assess for tighter rings.
    b. Following surgery and while sleeping, elevate the affected arm higher than the shoulder on a pillow, but do not abduct it; the hand should be higher than the elbow.
    c. Explain about measures to control and/or reduce swelling and refer to a certified LE therapist: Compression bandaging, manual lymph drainage, exercises, wearing a LE sleeve.
- Teach the woman the following guidelines for preventing lymphedema:
    a. Avoid injury from very hot water, popping grease when cooking, and playing sports such as golf.
    b. Avoid tight clothing, jewelry, and elastic bands on the affected extremity.
    c. Avoid carrying a purse or briefcase on the affected side.
    d. Keep skin and nails clean and well cared for.
    e. Use cream or lotion to keep the skin moist.
    f. Treat small cuts with an antibiotic cream.
    g. Use a thimble when sewing or doing handwork.
    h. Wear gloves when gardening.
- Be careful about injury and infection on the affected side; wear rubber gloves when washing dishes and garden gloves when working outside. Request that caregivers do not perform blood pressures or venipunctures on the operative side to reduce the risk of injury and infection.
- Feelings of anxiety, sadness, and fear of looking at the incision are normal; mastectomy means abrupt change in body image. It is normal to mourn the loss of a breast and to fear the loss of one's life after a cancer diagnosis.
- Sexual intimacy can be affected by mastectomy; it often helps to be able to discuss potential sexual problems with one's partner, with a counselor, or with a breast cancer support group.

involvement. In late metastatic disease, chemotherapy becomes the primary treatment to prolong the woman's life. Neoadjuvant chemotherapy is chemotherapy given before surgery; it can shrink large tumors so they are small enough to be removed by a lumpectomy instead of a mastectomy. Adjuvant (additional) systemic therapy following primary treatment for early-stage breast cancer refers to the administration of chemotherapy and other pharmacologic agents after surgery. This type of therapy has been widely studied; its use reduces the rates of recurrence and death from breast cancer. For example, letrozole (Femara; an aromatase inhibitor) has reduced the risk of recurrence after surgery (in some cases more effectively than tamoxifen).

Hormone Therapy

Tamoxifen citrate (Nolvadex) and toremifene (Fareston) are oral medications that block estrogen activity. They are used to treat advanced breast cancer, as an adjuvant for early-stage breast cancer, and as a preventive treatment for women at high risk of developing breast cancer. Nursing implications for tamoxifen are presented in **Medication Administration 49.B**. Tamoxifen can be used to treat metastatic breast cancer and, if taken for 5 years following surgery, can reduce the risk of cancer reoccurrence by about half (Davies et al., 2011). Toremifene (Fareston) is mainly used to treat postmenopausal women with advanced cancers. Fulvestrant (Faslodex) is a drug that eliminates estrogen receptors. Given by injection once a month, it is currently only approved for postmenopausal women with advanced cancer that no longer responds to tamoxifen or toremifene.

Immunotherapy, using trastuzumab (Herceptin), is used to stop the growth of breast tumors that express the HER2/neu receptor (which binds an epidermal growth factor that contributes to cancer cell growth) on their cell surface. This drug is a recombinant DNA-derived monoclonal antibody that binds to the receptor, inhibiting tumor cell proliferation. It is given intravenously either once a week or as a larger dose every 3 weeks. Side effects include fever

Medication Administration 49.B

Tamoxifen

TAMOXIFEN (NOLVADEX)

Tamoxifen is the most widely prescribed breast cancer drug, commonly given to prevent recurrence of estrogen-positive breast cancer in postmenopausal women. It inhibits tumor growth by blocking the estrogen receptor sites of cancer cells. Tamoxifen increases a woman's risk of developing endometrial cancer, deep venous thrombosis (DVT), and pulmonary embolism.

Nursing Responsibilities

- Assess for potential contraindications to therapy.
- Assess liver function tests; tamoxifen may interfere with liver function.

Health Education for the Patient and Family

- If in childbearing years, use a nonhormonal, barrier form of contraception; tamoxifen has adverse effects on the developing fetus.
- Take the drug as prescribed until the physician indicates otherwise.
- Side effects commonly experienced by women taking tamoxifen are hot flashes, vaginal dryness, irregular periods, and weight gain.
- Do not smoke while taking tamoxifen; smoking further increases the risk of DVT.
- Promptly report any abnormal vaginal bleeding (nonmenstrual bleeding, bleeding after menopause) to your primary care provider.

Source: Adams, et al., 2017.

and chills, weakness, nausea and vomiting, cough, diarrhea, and headache. A more serious possible side effect is cardiac damage, leading to congestive heart failure. Other drugs that are used include lapatinib (Tykerb) and bevacizumab (Avastin), an oral drug that also targets the HER2 protein.

The aromatase inhibitors stop the production of estrogen in postmenopausal women by blocking the enzyme aromatase (which turns androgen into small amounts of estrogen in the body). The drugs, in oral form, are anastrozole (Arimidex), exemestane (Aromasin), and letrozole (Femara). In a comparison of aromatase inhibitors with tamoxifen in treating early-stage, hormone receptor–positive breast cancer in postmenopausal women, most physicians recommend an aromatase inhibitor as the best hormone therapy to start with because it has more benefits and fewer serious side effects (Breastcancer.org, 2018).

Integrative Therapies

There have been a number of studies of the use of integrative therapies in women undergoing breast cancer treatment. The therapies with the best supportive evidence are music therapy, stress management, and yoga. Herbal supplements are not to be used as many have adverse interactions with chemotherapy (Greenlee et al., 2014).

Nursing Care

Breast cancer is not one disease entity, but many, depending on the affected breast tissue, the tissue's estrogen dependency, and the age of the person at onset. The psychosocial effect of breast cancer extends beyond the fear and threat of death. The diagnosis may transform the woman's sense of self and lead to reintegration or negotiation of family relationships. See the accompanying Case Study & Nursing Care Plan for a woman with breast cancer on page 1828.

Assessment

Collect the following data through the health history and physical examination. Further focused assessments are described with nursing interventions.

- *Health history:* Family history of breast cancer, breast changes, nipple discharge, use of HRT, previous diagnostic tests and treatment for cancer, menstrual history, pregnancies, alcohol intake, physical activity, dietary history
- *Physical assessment:* Height and weight, breasts, axillary lymph glands.

Priorities of Care

Because lumpectomy and mastectomy are routinely performed in an ambulatory surgery basis and most continuing care (e.g., radiation therapy, chemotherapy) occurs in outpatient settings, education of the patient and her family is the nursing care priority.

Diagnoses, Outcomes, and Interventions

Although each woman has individual needs, nursing diagnoses prior to surgery are concerned with anxiety, decisional conflict, grief, risk for infection, risk for injury, and disturbed body image over the loss of a breast. Because the typical hospital stay is short, usually from 1 to 3 days, preoperative teaching is done on an outpatient basis.

Reduce Anxiety. A woman of any age with breast cancer is often anxious about the diagnosis, the surgery, the outcome of surgery if nodal involvement is found, and the possible changes in sexual and family relationships. Studies show that young women with breast cancer, a growing population, are particularly vulnerable to anxiety and other psychosocial effects, as are their spouses and their children. Young women with breast cancer often have a more aggressive disease and a lower survival rate when compared with older women with breast cancer (ACS, 2018b).

Expected Outcome: Patient will demonstrate anxiety relief related to breast cancer by focusing on knowledge about condition, treatment and surgical options, and utilization of interpersonal support systems.

The nurse will:

- Provide opportunities to express thoughts and feelings. In this process, the woman can name her fears. *Once the fears are named, the nurse may simply listen, educate, or dispel fears that stem from lack of understanding.*
- Discuss with the woman her knowledge of breast cancer. *Assessing the woman's knowledge of breast cancer helps the nurse plan more effective teaching.*

- Encourage discussion relating to immediate concerns about resuming her life at home and the changes she must make. *Anticipatory guidance can help her plan for and cope with changes in her life and relationships.*
- Explain the surgical procedure, including information about preoperative medications, anesthesia, and recovery. *Knowing what to expect helps to decrease anxiety.*
- Explain that it is normal to have decreased sensation in the surgical area. *Severed or damaged nerves reduce sensation.*

Support Thoughtful Decision Making. The woman with breast cancer must make life-changing decisions about treatment within a relatively brief and highly stressful time. Her age, menopausal status, and stage of cancer are only some of the factors that affect her decisions. Culture, values, lifestyle, socioeconomic status, and self-esteem are also considered.

Expected Outcome: Patient will demonstrate thoughtful decision making while deciding on healthcare choices.

The nurse will:

- Provide an opportunity for the woman to ask questions; answer questions as simply and directly as possible. Make eye contact and pay attention to body language. *During this time, the woman can process information and make informed decisions.*
- Focus on immediate concerns, and provide up-to-date written material for the woman to review. *Written material provides easy reference to information not processed immediately because of anxiety and stress.*
- Listen to the woman in a nonjudgmental manner during her decision-making process. *Nonjudgmental, empathic listening helps the woman process information and make informed decisions. Only she knows the context of her life.*
- If the woman wishes, provide opportunities for her to meet with other women who have had breast cancer surgery. *Not all women are ready to meet others in their situation, but opening the door to this resource is appropriate. The woman may choose to talk with these women after the surgery.*
- Facilitate a team approach with the surgeon, anesthesiologist, oncologist, plastic surgeon, and other health professionals. *Being the woman's advocate during this time of anxiety and decision making reduces the stress of coordinating multiple healthcare provider schedules.*

Facilitate the Grieving Process. Breast surgery, even a lumpectomy, alters the appearance of the breast. This loss of appearance, as well as the diagnosis of cancer, is expressed through grief.

Expected Outcome: Patient will demonstrate successful resolution of grief by adapting to changes in body image and role.

The nurse will:

- Listen attentively to expressions of grief and watch for nonverbal cues (failure to make eye contact, crying, silence). *Not all women will express grief clearly; sometimes unspoken grief is the most painful. Grief is relieved only when expressed in a nonthreatening environment.*

Moving Evidence into Action

Choosing When or Whether to Have Reconstruction Surgery

Clinical Issue

The decision to have breast reconstructive surgery after a mastectomy is an individualized decision. A woman and her healthcare team need to weigh a number of variables before a decision is made.

External Evidence

There are different rates of reconstructive surgery from 40% in White women to a low of 14% in low-acculturated Latina women. Lee et al. (2016) published research concerning how informed women are about breast reconstructive surgery after mastectomy. In a cross-sectional study using a standardized instrument, the mean knowledge score was only 58.8%. Women who were less educated, had lower income, and were single had lower scores. Knowledge of risks of reconstructive surgery were even lower. The authors conclude women in this study had only a modest knowledge base concerning breast reconstructive surgery.

Internal Evidence

Some breast cancer centers complete more reconstructive surgeries than others. Also differences in techniques depending on the type of mastectomy might not be available at all centers. Information concerning which reconstructive surgeries are available to the woman is important to provide for an informed decision. Also, information concerning surgeries that are possible but not available at the current center should also be discussed with the woman. Risks and benefits of each type of reconstructive surgery along with how surgery would fit into the treatment plan is important.

Patient Considerations

Exploring whether breast reconstructive surgery is important to the woman is essential. She may not want to undergo surgery or she may fear the costs associated with it. Some surgical techniques might not be available to the woman for a number of reasons. If there is a significant other, bringing that person into the discussion is important along with any family members the woman feels are supportive. Finally, giving the woman information about timelines (e.g., reconstructive surgery can be done immediately after the mastectomy or later) is important to help her make a decision.

Putting the Pieces Together

Decisions concerning breast reconstructive surgery are a personal choice. Complete information and exploration of feelings and meanings are an important part of the discussion.

Reference

Lee, C. N., Ubel, P. A., Deal, A. D., Blizard, L. B., Sepucha, K. R., Ollila, D. V., & Pignone, M. P. (2016). How informed is the decision about breast reconstruction after mastectomy?: A prospective, cross-sectional study. *Annals of Surgery, 264*, 1103–1109.

- Allow time to interact and do not rush interactions. *Taking time to be with the woman communicates caring.*
- Explain that it is normal to have periods of depression, anger, and denial after breast surgery. *All these feelings are appropriate expressions of grief.*
- If the woman wishes to do so, involve the partner in helping the woman cope with her grief. *Remember that the partner may also be grieving. Not all women want to share their grief, and not all partners are interested and supportive.*

Reduce Risk for Infection. Like any surgical patient, the woman who has breast surgery is at risk for infection. Removal of lymph nodes and the presence of a draining wound increase the risk.

Expected Outcome: Patient will describe symptoms of postoperative incisional infection and importance of early reporting of symptoms.

The nurse will:

- Assess the surgical dressings for bleeding, drainage, color, and odor every 4 hours for 24 hours and document your findings. Circle any visible bleeding and drainage on the dressing as a baseline for subsequent assessment. *Excessive bleeding or drainage signals postoperative complications that may require emergency attention.*
- Observe the incision and IV sites for pain, redness, swelling, and drainage. Assess the drainage system for patency and adequate suction; note the color and amount of drainage. *Careful observation for any signs of infection is essential because the woman's immune system is compromised. IV catheters should be placed on the uninvolved side only.*
- Change dressings and IV tubing using aseptic technique. *Moist dressings and intravenous tubing provide sites for bacterial growth. Routine dressing and IV tubing changes using aseptic technique reduce the risk for infection.*
- Encourage a protein-rich diet. Discuss the woman's nutritional status with the dietitian and request a consultation for the woman. *Adequate nutrition promotes healing and boosts the immune system.*
- Teach the woman how to care for the drainage system, if present (clean the site, empty the device, and record the amount, color, and type of drainage). *The woman is often discharged prior to removal of the drainage system and dressings and needs teaching to provide self-care.*
- At discharge, teach the woman to watch for and report to her healthcare provider the manifestations of infection: Fever, redness or hardness at the surgical site, or purulent drainage. *Any of these manifestations should be reported to the physician/surgeon. Knowing the signs and symptoms of infection prepares the woman to seek prompt treatment if infection occurs.*
- Explain that she may experience scaling, flaking, dryness, itching, rash, or dry desquamation of the skin, particularly after radiation therapy. *Impaired skin integrity increases the risk of infection.*
- Tell the woman to avoid deodorants and talcum powder on the affected side until the incision is completely healed. *These substances may irritate the skin and impede healing.*

Promote Good Tissue Integrity. Removal of the axillary lymph nodes puts the woman at risk for lymphedema (LE), a complication that involves an abnormal accumulation of lymph in the arm, shoulder, breast, or thoracic area. It is estimated that this complication affects as many as half of all breast cancer survivors. This complication may develop at any time following a mastectomy, but usually develops within the first 3 years after the surgery.

Expected Outcome: Patient will demonstrate skin integrity by supportive skin care to promote healing and reduce skin breakdown.

The nurse will:

- Assess/monitor for manifestations of LE: Swelling in the affected area (usually the hand and arm), pain, fatigue, and changes in sensations (such as heaviness, numbness, or burning) in the affected area. Assess skin color, temperature, texture, scars, or lesions. Ask about tighter rings. Measure the affected extremity 10 cm (4 in.) above and 5 cm (2 in.) below the olecranon process on a regular basis and record findings. *When an obstruction to the flow of lymphatic fluid develops, large proteins filter through the lymph vessels and accumulate in an area distal to the obstruction; fluid accumulates, causing tissue and skin changes. Accurate assessments are necessary to identify new-onset LE and to monitor already present LE for progression or improvement.*
- Use the nonsurgical side when obtaining blood pressure, blood draws, and starting IVs. *Compression of the arm on the surgical side may increase the risk of developing LE; if skin integrity is compromised, the risk for infection increases.*
- Elevate the affected arm higher than the shoulder on a pillow following surgery and while sleeping, but do not abduct it; the hand should be higher than the elbow. *Elevating the arm permits drainage, prevents swelling, and promotes circulation.*
- Instruct the woman to report any manifestations of infection, including increased swelling, pain, heat, and redness in the affected area, as well as fever and generalized malaise. *Infection may involve cellulitis or lymphangitis, requiring medical treatment with antibiotics. Infection may also precipitate or worsen existing LE.*
- Explain about measures to control and/or reduce swelling and refer to a certified LE therapist: Compression bandaging, manual lymph drainage, exercises, wearing a LE sleeve. *These lifelong measures can often control and even reduce the swelling of LE.*

Promote Healthy Body Image. Breast surgery can change the woman's body image. The surgical changes may be compounded by weight gain and other side effects of chemotherapy or hormone therapy. Self-esteem also affects adjustment to a changed body image.

Expected Outcome: Patient will demonstrate appropriate body image by use of effective coping strategies to develop acceptance of changes in her body.

The nurse will:

- Assess how the woman views her body. Discuss with the woman what image of herself she had prior to surgery. *Self-image is related to self-esteem. Discuss whether her self-image has changed.*
- Explain that redness and swelling in the scar will fade with time. *The knowledge that the scar will fade may give the woman a more realistic view of the changes.*
- Include the partner and family, if possible, when discussing the plan of care and activities of daily living (ADLs). Request consultation with a psychologist or other professional if the woman is interested. *Discussion with the partner and family can facilitate the woman's emotional healing process.*
- Offer pamphlets and suggest books and videos that might increase knowledge about what lies ahead. *Knowing what to expect can help the woman cope.*
- Encourage the woman to look at her incision when she feels ready; often the reality is not as frightening as the woman had imagined. Explain that it is normal to be afraid to look. *Reassurance that her behavior is normal decreases anxiety.*
- If the woman is interested in breast reconstruction, provide written material and encourage her to talk with a plastic surgeon and with women who have had reconstruction. *It is important for the woman to be fully informed about available options to make an informed decision.*

Transitions of Care

Although controversy exists about the ability of screening mammography to improve mortality rates for women under age 50, the ACS recommends an annual mammogram beginning at age 45. Women should talk to their healthcare provider around age 40 to assess when is the best time to start yearly mammograms. Once a woman reaches 55 years of age, the mammograms should be every other year, though women who wish to have mammograms every year should be allowed to do so. Regular mammograms should be continued for as long as the women is healthy and wants to continue. If a woman is at higher risk for breast cancer, then she and her healthcare provider should discuss routine screening options (ACS, 2015). A number of organizations recommend against breast self-examination or clinical breast examination based on the results of a 2008 meta-analysis (Kosters & Gotzche, 2008). All recommendations state that women should know how their breasts feel and should alert their healthcare provider of any changes.

Educational messages about breast cancer screening need to be culturally sensitive to the intended audience. Media campaigns promoting mammography often show young White women, an approach that has proved ineffective among women of color, although cancer screening is increasing in this population. By working with women of different races and cultures, nurses can help make breast cancer education more meaningful to women in these groups.

For surgery, most women will spend a day or two in the hospital. But all other treatments are done on an outpatient basis. Patients having radiation will be expected to travel to their radiation center daily for as long as 6 or 7 weeks. Care of the skin during radiation is important. Washing with a gentle soap and lukewarm water is important; however, any marks made by the radiologist should not be washed off. Use of hydrating lotions and creams to the area (but not right after treatment) is important as the skin can become dry and looked as if sunburned. The woman should check with her treating team first as they may have specific recommendations. Wearing soft clothing on the radiation site is important as the skin will be quite irritated. Some centers have nurses who specialize in the care of the skin in patients who are undergoing radiation treatment. Fatigue is also an issue for patients. These patients need to make sure they are getting plenty of sleep every night, taking time to relax, and nap as needed to conserve energy. Good nutrition will also help with healing and may decrease fatigue. If patients need help with shopping and/or transportation, there can be a number of resources available to the patient. Most cancer centers have at least a nurse or a social worker who can help the patient access community resources. There are resources for the significant other in the woman's life and family. Nurses should be familiar with the resources in their community or who to access for the resources.

If a patient is also getting chemotherapy, side effects will depend on the type of chemotherapy. In general, though, because chemotherapy targets rapidly dividing cells and is usually systemically given, any body system with rapidly dividing cells will be affected. Nausea and vomiting and diarrhea are the most common side effects of chemotherapy. Most treatment teams will prescribe some antiemetic medications to help decrease the nausea and vomiting. The patient should be encouraged to take these medications as ordered and not to wait until the symptoms are severe or try to "tough it out." Proper nutrition is important for healing during chemotherapy. Another issue is hair loss. When hair loss will occur depends on the chemotherapy. The woman should be aware of this and make plans ahead of time on how she will deal it. There are wigs especially designed for women undergoing chemotherapy along with head wraps and turbans; talking to other women who have gone through hair loss due to chemotherapy may help the person. Also depending on the length and type of chemotherapy, a woman may need to have an implantable intravenous access device inserted before starting treatment. Finally, if treatment is on an outpatient basis, arrangements for transportation may be needed. As with radiation, the treatment team nurse or social worker can assist in arranging transportation.

Long term, the woman that has had breast cancer is at risk for other cancers due to treatment and reoccurrences, depending on the genetics of the cancer. Types of cancer also depend on treatment for the initial occurrence. Cardiac problems and lung scarring can occur due to chest radiation. Secondary cancers due to chemotherapy can also occur. It is important for the woman to discuss any concerns related to long-term treatment issues before actual treatment starts.

Emotional support through all of this is extremely important. Patients with breast cancer can experience depression, anger, helplessness, and hopelessness. Talking to the treatment team is important. The nurse is usually on the front line for emotional support. Allowing the patient to voice concerns and helping them through the emotions can help the woman move forward with learning to live with cancer and/or as a cancer survivor. There are situations, however, when a referral to a mental health counselor is necessary. Comprehensive cancer centers usually have mental health counselors readily available to the patient along with experts in navigating long-term survivorship for a patient with cancer.

The woman with breast cancer and her family have much to learn to provide self-care at home. Address the following topics in preparation for home care:

- Manifestations of infection and the need to report any that occur to her healthcare provider.
- The importance of ADLs, such as eating, combing her hair, and washing her face.
- Postmastectomy exercises (see examples in **Figure 49.10** ■) and lymphedema care as approved by the healthcare provider and physical/occupational/LE therapist.

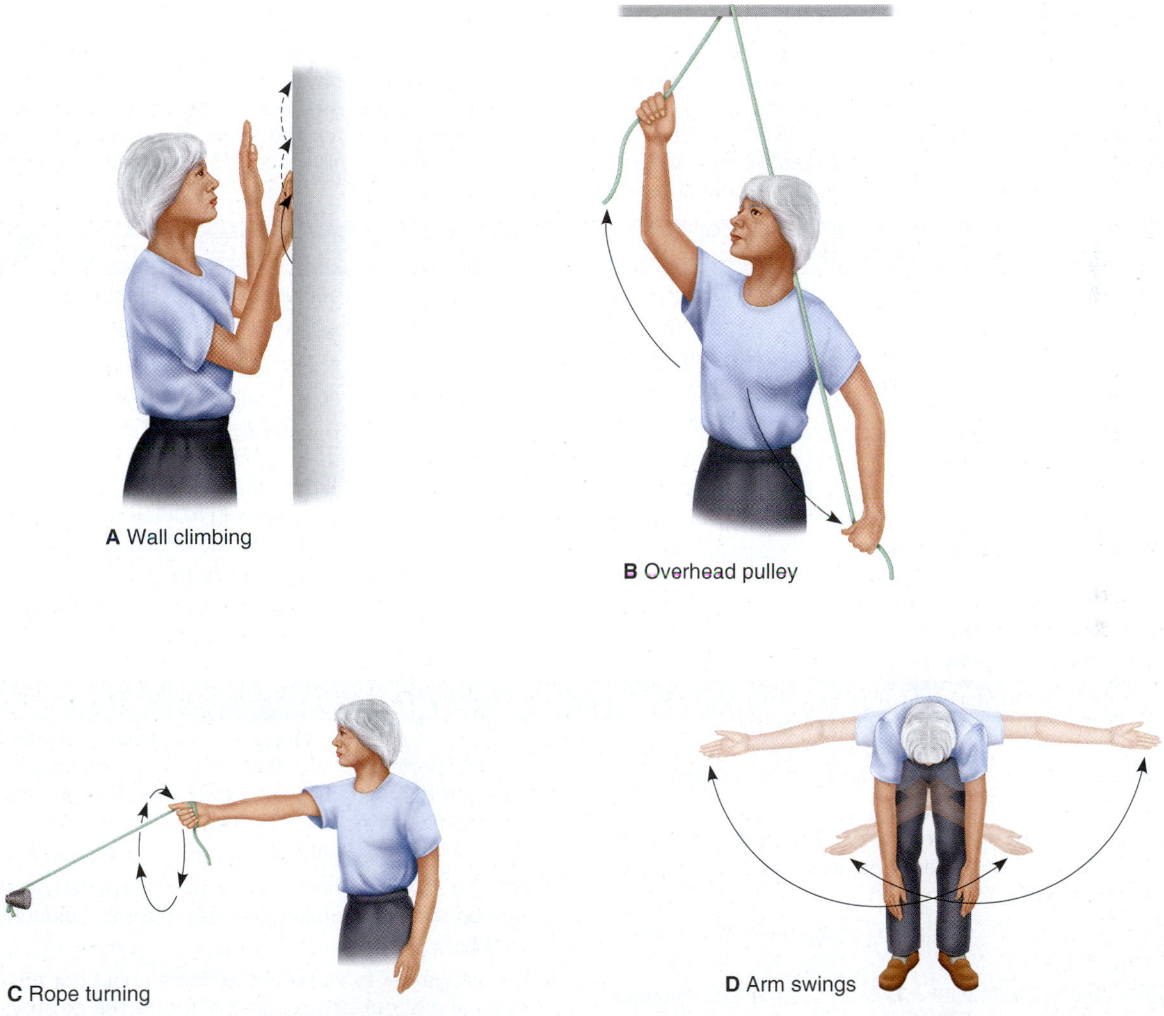
A Wall climbing
B Overhead pulley
C Rope turning
D Arm swings

Figure 49.10 ■ Examples of postmastectomy exercises. **A**, *Wall climbing:* Stand facing wall with toes 6 to 12 inches from wall. Bend elbows and place palms against wall at shoulder level. Gradually move both hands up the wall parallel to each other until incisional pulling or pain occurs. (Mark that spot on wall to measure progress.) Work hands down to shoulder level. Move closer to wall as height of reach improves. **B**, *Overhead pulley:* Toss 6-foot rope over shower curtain rod (or over top of a door that has a nail in the top to hold the rope in place for the exercise). Grasp one end of rope in each hand. Slowly raise operated arm as far as comfortable by pulling down on the rope on opposite side. Keep raised arm close to your head. Reverse to raise unoperated arm by lowering the operated arm. Repeat. **C**, *Rope turning:* Tie rope to door handle. Hold rope in hand of operated side. Back away from door until arm is extended away from body, parallel to floor. Swing rope in as wide a circle as possible. Increase size of circle as mobility returns. **D**, *Arm swings:* Stand with feet 8 inches apart. Bend forward from waist, allowing arms to hang toward floor. Swing both arms up to sides to reach shoulder level. Swing back to center, then cross arms at center. Do not bend elbows. If possible, do this and other exercises in front of mirror to ensure even posture and correct motion.

- The need for adequate rest and emotional support.
- Participation in a breast cancer support group and online information services and bulletin boards for sources of education and support.
- Prosthesis management, if this option is chosen. (A temporary lightweight prosthesis may be worn immediately after the drains and sutures have been removed from the surgical site. Because prostheses are expensive, a permanent one should not be purchased until the wound has completely healed. Prostheses are available at medical stores and many larger department stores. Most private and government insurance policies pay for the first prosthesis.)
- Helpful resources include Reach to Recovery, the American Cancer Society, the National Breast Cancer Coalition, and the National Lymphedema Network.

If the treatments are not curing or controlling the cancer or if the woman chooses no treatment for breast cancer, a palliative care team consult should be requested. Discussions with the woman and support systems, as appropriate, concerning pain management, fluids, and nutrition along with any other concerns is important. Refer to hospice when appropriate.

Case Study & Nursing Care Plan

A Woman with Breast Cancer

Rachel Clemments is a 42-year-old mother of two: Eva, age 12, and Lila, age 18. Because of a family history of breast cancer, she has been closely monitored (annual mammograms and a needle aspiration biopsy with negative findings) for 4 years prior to her diagnosis. Mrs. Clemments discovers a lump in her left breast while taking a shower. An incisional biopsy reveals invasive lobular carcinoma in the left breast. Mrs. Clemments is debating whether to have reconstructive breast surgery. One of her greatest concerns is how her illness will affect her ability to support and care for her daughters. The breast cancer diagnosis seems part of the family legacy. She wonders, "When will it happen to Lila? To Eva?"

ASSESSMENT	DIAGNOSES	EXPECTED OUTCOMES
During the history, Laura Nelson, RN, the nurse admitting Mrs. Clemments, learns that her mother, two of her aunts, and one sister had been diagnosed with breast cancer. Her mother and one of the aunts died before age 45. Physical assessment findings include T 37.0°C (98.5°F), BP 110/62 mmHg, P 65 bpm, R 14/min. Her weight is 54 kg (120 lb); she is 168 cm (66 in.) tall. Modified radical mastectomy is performed; histologic examination shows a 3-cm tumor; axillary node dissection shows that 4 of 16 lymph nodes are positive.	■ Potential for infection related to surgical incision ■ Acute pain related to surgery ■ Body image issues related to loss of breast ■ Need for education about the risks and benefits of treatment options ■ Fear related to disease process and prognosis	■ Patient will remain free of infection. ■ Patient will experience minimal pain or discomfort during her recovery. ■ Patient will maintain a positive body image, regardless of her decision about reconstruction. ■ Patient will evaluate the treatment options in relation to personal values and decide on a course of action. ■ Patient will identify the sources of her fear and demonstrate behaviors that may reduce fears.

PLANNING AND IMPLEMENTATION

- Teach her about hand hygiene and wound care.
- Assess her pain tolerance and administer analgesics as prescribed.
- Teach her to use caution when moving the arm on the operated side, to avoid lifting heavy objects, and to wear gloves when gardening.
- Encourage her to discuss her thoughts and feelings about her body changes.
- Suggest that she talk with a Reach to Recovery volunteer about her thoughts and feelings.
- Assess her interest in spiritual/religious support and refer, if appropriate.
- Discuss the use of a temporary prosthesis and later the fitting of a permanent prosthesis (6 to 8 weeks after surgery), the need to be fitted by an experienced person, and insurance reimbursement for the prosthesis.
- Discuss the possibility of attending a breast cancer support group where she can draw on the experiences of other women who have undergone mastectomy, chemotherapy, or radiation.
- Encourage her to verbalize her fears about her own prognosis and about her daughters' future risk of breast cancer; assess the need/interest for referral to psychologic counseling.

EVALUATION

At discharge, Mrs. Clemments has no signs of physical complications and is looking forward to being at home with her daughters as temporary caregivers. Mrs. Clemments met with a Reach to Recovery volunteer, who brought her a temporary prosthesis and booklets about postmastectomy exercises, chemotherapy, and breast reconstruction. The volunteer also referred her to a local cancer support group. Mrs. Clemments has talked about her concerns related to breast reconstruction. "I want to avoid anything that would increase the risk of complications. The possibility of recurrence and my fear for my daughters' future health are more than enough to worry about."

CLINICAL REASONING IN PATIENT CARE

1. What role could genetic counseling play in helping Mrs. Clemments and her daughters better understand the daughters' risk of breast cancer?
2. Describe the types of mastectomies and their implications for nursing care.
3. What medications might help minimize the side effects of chemotherapy?
4. Develop a plan of care for Mrs. Clemments who has stated that she is having trouble sleeping.

See Evaluating Your Response in Appendix B.

CHAPTER HIGHLIGHTS

49.1 Disorders of Female Sexual Function

Describe the pathophysiology and manifestations of disorders of female sexual function, and outline the interprofessional care and nursing care of patients with these disorders.

- Many different illnesses, medications, and surgical procedures may affect female sexual function. It is important for nurses to initiate a conversation regarding sexual concerns with female patients and respond in a caring, nonjudgmental manner.
- Disorders of sexual function include dyspareunia (pain during intercourse), inhibited sexual desire, and orgasmic dysfunction.

49.2 Menstrual Disorders

Describe the pathophysiology and manifestations of menstrual disorders, and outline the interprofessional care and nursing care of patients with these disorders.

- Premenstrual syndrome (PMS) is a complex of manifestations (e.g., mood swings, breast tenderness, fatigue, irritability, food cravings, and depression) that are limited to 3 to 14 days before menstruation and relieved by the onset of menses.
- Dysmenorrhea (pain or discomfort associated with menstruation), which is estimated to occur in 40 to 95% of menstruating women, may be primary or secondary.
- Abnormal uterine bleeding (AUB) refers to vaginal bleeding that is usually painless but is abnormal in amount, duration, or time of occurrence.

49.3 Perimenopause

Describe the pathophysiology and manifestations of perimenopause, and outline the interprofessional care and nursing care of patients with this condition.

- Menopause is the permanent cessation of menses, a normal physiologic process as a woman ages. Menopause is a normal physiologic life event but may result in many changes in the woman's body including osteoporosis, fractures, and cardiovascular disease.
- The perimenopausal period, which usually lasts for several years, denotes the time during which reproductive function gradually ceases. It begins with a decline in the production of the hormone estrogen, includes the permanent cessation of menstruation due to loss of ovarian function, and extends for 1 year after the final menstrual period, at which time a woman is said to be postmenopausal.

49.4 Structural Disorders

Describe the pathophysiology and manifestations of structural disorders of the female reproductive system, and outline the interprofessional care and nursing care of patients with these disorders.

- Disorders of the female reproductive system can include benign as well as malignant diagnoses. It is important to understand the emotional concerns of anxiety and fear of the diagnoses as well as the treatments.
- Uterine displacement occurs when the uterus prolapses into the pelvic cavity of the vagina. Treatments include Kegel exercises, use of a pessary, or surgical repair.
- A vaginal fistula is an abnormal opening between the vagina and bladder (vesicovaginal) or the vagina and rectum (rectovaginal). Minor fistulas may resolve on their own; most require surgical repair.

49.5 Disorders of Female Reproductive Tissue

Describe the pathophysiology and manifestations of disorders of female reproductive tissue, and outline the interprofessional care and nursing care of patients with these disorders.

- Cysts are fluid-filled sacs, while polyps are vascularized solid tumors that can develop on many of the structures of the female reproductive system. They can develop at any age. Treatment focuses on surgical removal and prevention of recurrence.
- Leiomyomas, commonly called fibroids, are benign tumors that arise from the smooth muscle wall of the uterus. Treatment depends on size, location, and impact on comfort or fertility.

- Endometriosis is a chronic inflammatory disease where functional endometrial tissue is found outside the uterus. Depending on the severity of the condition, fertility can be impacted. Treatment ranges from medical management to surgical intervention and is dependent on severity of the condition.
- Cancer of the cervix is common in women. Cervical cancer is linked to HPV infection and can be prevented or diagnosed early with cervical exams and Pap smears. Treatment includes surgery, chemotherapy, and radiation therapy.
- Endometrial cancer is the most common cancer of the female reproductive system. Treatment depends on stage of disease, ranging from chemotherapy to surgical intervention including hysterectomy.
- Ovarian cancer does not have clear-cut symptoms or early warning signs. Unfortunately, this results in late diagnosis, reducing curative treatment options. Treatment includes surgery, chemotherapy, and radiation therapy.
- Cancer of the vulva is rare. Treatment often requires surgical excision of the involved external genitalia, a loss for the patient.

49.6 Disorders of the Female Breast

Describe the pathophysiology and manifestations of disorders of the breast, and outline the interprofessional care and nursing care of patients with these disorders.

- Benign breast disorders often correspond to hormonal changes of the menstrual cycle.
- Breast cancer is one of the most common forms of cancer in women.
- Breast cancer treatment is based on stage and can range from nonsurgical treatment to radical mastectomy.
- Mammograms can detect breast cancer at an early stage. Education is necessary to encourage early diagnosis and prevention.

TEST YOURSELF NCLEX-RN® REVIEW

1. During a health assessment at a local clinic, a patient asks the nurse about the availability of sexual counseling. How should the nurse respond?
   A. "There may be a problem with insurance reimbursement."
   B. "Do you have a problem with sexual expression?"
   C. "Sexual problems often occur start occurring at about your age."
   D. "We can talk with your physician about getting a referral."
2. The nurse is reviewing the effects of long-term estrogen deprivation with a premenopausal patient. About which physical disorders should the nurse discuss that the patient might be at risk for developing in the future? (Select all that apply.)
   A. Fractures
   B. Osteoporosis
   C. Colon cancer
   D. Cervical cancer
   E. Cardiovascular disease
3. The nurse is conducting an educational seminar for postmenopausal women. A question is asked about alternatives to hormone replacement therapy. The nurse would include discussion about which substances?
   A. Tofu
   B. Almond milk
   C. Flaxseed
   D. Quinoa
   E. Ginseng
4. The nurse is teaching a female patient with a uterine displacement disorder about Kegel exercises. Which health problem should the nurse explain that these exercises help to reduce?
   A. Retroversion
   B. Menorrhagia
   C. Vaginal discharge
   D. Stress incontinence
5. The nurse is preparing a health promotion seminar for high school students. Which topic should the nurse include to reduce the risk of cervical cancer?
   A. Maintain a healthy weight
   B. Use birth control pills rather than condoms
   C. Eat a diet high in iron
   D. Avoid intercourse until after age 18
6. The nurse is discussing treatment options for a patient with PMS. The patient is unwilling to take medications. Which dietary changes should the nurse suggest? (Select all that apply.)
   A. Eat more lean proteins.
   B. Decrease simple carbohydrates.
   C. Decrease calcium intake.
   D. Take at least 50 mg of vitamin B6 daily.
   E. Decrease caffeine take.
7. A female patient with endometriosis is entering menopause. What should the nurse explain that occurs to endometrial implantations after menopause?
   A. Each implant enlarges.
   B. They tend to become malignant.
   C. The number of implants increases.
   D. They tend to atrophy and disappear.

8. The nurse is designing a home care teaching plan for a patient recovering from an abdominal hysterectomy. What interventions should be included in this plan? (Select all that apply.)
   A. For the first week spend much of the day sitting up in a chair
   B. Restrict heavy lifting for 4 to 6 weeks.
   C. Take tub baths until bleeding has stopped.
   D. Do not climb more than two flights of stairs a day.
   E. Report an increase in temperature or severe pain.
9. The nurse is preparing an educational session on women's health issues. Of the following female participants, which one would be most at risk for breast cancer?
   A. Age 45, dense breasts
   B. Age 23, two children
   C. Age 33, never pregnant
   D. Age 64, positive family history
10. A patient who had a mastectomy is being discharged. Which information should the nurse provide to help decrease development of lymphedema (LE)? (Select all that apply.)
   A. Do not play golf.
   B. Do not wear long sleeves.
   C. Wear gloves while gardening.
   D. Do not creams or lotions on the affected side.
   E. Carry your purse on the other side.

See Test Yourself answers in Appendix B.

REFERENCES

Adams, M. P., Holland, L.N., & Urban, C. (2017). *Pharmacology for nursing: A pathophysiologic approach* (5th ed.). Hoboken, NJ: Pearson Education.

American Cancer Society (2015). *Guidelines for breast cancer screening.* https://www.cancer.org/latest-news/american-cancer-society-releases-new-breast-cancer-guidelines.html.

American Cancer Society. (2018a). *The American Cancer Society guidelines for the prevention and early detection of cervical cancer.* Retrieved from https://www.cancer.org/cancer/cervical-cancer/prevention-and-early-detection/cervical-cancer-screening-guidelines.html.

American Cancer Society. (2018b). *Breast at a glance.* Retrieved from https://cancerstatisticscenter.cancer.org/#!/cancer-site/Breast.

American Cancer Society. (2018c). *Cervical cancer stages.* Retrieved from https://www.cancer.org/cancer/cervical-cancer/detection-diagnosis-staging/staged.html.

American Cancer Society. (2018d). *Cervical cancer statistics.* Retrieved from https://cancerstatisticscenter.cancer.org/?_ga=2.189567848.2130841238.1523217457-1252308240.1521986441#!/cancer-site/Cervix.

American Cancer Society. (2018e). *Endometrial cancer risk factors.* Retrieved from https://www.cancer.org/cancer/endometrial-cancer/causes-risks-prevention/risk-factors.html.

American Cancer Society. (2018f). *Key statistics for cervical cancer.* Retrieved from https://www.cancer.org/cancer/cervical-cancer/about/key-statistics.html.

American Cancer Society. (2018g). *Key statistics for endometrial cancer.* Retrieved from https://www.cancer.org/cancer/endometrial-cancer/about/key-statistics.html.

American Cancer Society. (2018h). *Special Section: Ovarian cancer.* Retrieved from https://www.cancer.org/content/dam/cancer-org/research/cancer-facts-and-statistics/annual-cancer-facts-and-figures/2018/cancer-facts-and-figures-special-section-ovarian-cancer-2018.pdf.

American Cancer Society. (2018i). *Uterine corpus statistics.* Retrieved from https://cancerstatisticscenter.cancer.org/?_ga=2.1572850.2130841238.1523217457-1252308240.1521986441#!/cancer-site/Uterine%20corpus.

American Cancer Society. (2018j). *What is endometrial cancer?* Retrieved from https://www.cancer.org/cancer/endometrial-cancer/about/what-is-endometrial-cancer.html.

American College of Obstetricians and Gynecologists. (2017a). *FAQ: Abnormal uterine bleeding*. Retrieved from https://www.acog.org/Patients/FAQs/Abnormal-Uterine-Bleeding.

American College of Obstetricians and Gynecologists. (2017b). *Gynecology data definitions (version 1).* Retrieved from https://www.acog.org/-/media/Departments/Patient-Safety-and-Quality-Improvement/reVITALize-Gynecology-Definitons-V1.pdf?dmc=1&ts=20180408T1621087595.

BreastCancer.Org. (2018). *Aromatase inhibitors.* Retrieved from www.breastcancer.org/treatment/hormonal/aromatase_inhibitors.

Centers for Disease Control and Prevention. (2015). *Key statistics from the National Survey of Family Growth.* Retrieved from www.cdc.gov/nchs/nsfg/key_statistics/h.htm#hysterectomy.

Centers for Disease Control and Prevention. (2017). *Sexually transmitted disease surveillance 2016.* Retrieved from https://www.cdc.gov/std/stats16/CDC_2016_STDS_Report-for508WebSep21_2017_1644.pdf.

Chin, L. N., & Nambiar, S. (2016). Management of premenstrual syndrome. *Obstetrics, Gynaecology and Reproductive Medicine, 27*, 1–6.

Davies, C., Godwin, J., Gret, R., Clarke, M., Cutter, D., Darby, S., . . . Peto, R. (2011). Relevance of breast cancer hormone receptors and other factors to the efficacy of adjuvant tamoxifen: Patient-level meta-analysis or randomized trails. *Lancet, 378*(9793), 771–784.

di Scalea, T. L., & Pearlstein, T. (2017). Premenstrual dysphoric disorder. *Psychiatric Clinics of North America, 40*, 201–216.

Greenlee, H., Balneaves, L. G., Carlson, L. E., Cohen, M., Deng, G., Hershman, D., . . . Tripathy, D. (2014). Clinical practice guidelines on the use of integrative therapies as supportive care in patients treated for breast cancer. *Journal of the National Cancer Institute Monographs, 50*, 346–358.

Iacovides, S., Avidon, I., & Baker, F. C. (2015). What do we know about primary dysmenorrhea today?: A critical review. *Human Reproduction Update, 21*(6), 762–778.

Jasper, L., Feys, F., Bramer, W. M., Franco, O. H., Leusink, P., & Lann, E. T. M. (2016). Efficacy and safety of flibanserin for the treatment of hypoactive sexual disorder in women: A systematic review and meta-analysis. *JAMA Internal Medicine, 176*(4), 432–462.

Karin, S., Souho, T., Benlemlih, B., & Bennani, B. (2018). Cervical cancer induction enhancement potential of *Chlamydia trachomatis*: A systematic review. *Current Microbiology*. [Epub ahead of print]

Kosters, J. P., & Gotzsche, P. C. (2008). Regular self-examination or clinical examination for early detection of breast cancer (review). *Cochrane Database of Systematic Reviews*, Issue 3, Article No. CD003373.

Lee, C. N., Ubel, P. A., Deal, A. D., Blizard, L. B., Sepucha, K. R., Ollila, D. V., & Pignone, M. P. (2016). How informed is the decision about breast reconstruction after mastectomy?: A prospective, cross-sectional study. *Annals of Surgery, 264*(6), 1103–1109.

Masala, G., Bendinelli, B., Assedi, M., Occhini, D., Zanna, I., Sieri, S., . . . Palli, D. (2017). Up to one-third of breast cancer cases in post-menopausal Mediterranean women might be avoided by modifying lifestyle habits: The EPIC Italy study. *Breast Cancer Research and Treatment*, 161(2), 311–320.

National Cancer Institute (NCI). (2018a). *Breast cancer treatment (PDQ®)—Health Professional Version*. Retrieved from https://www.cancer.gov/types/breast/hp/breast-treatment-pdq.

National Cancer Institute (NCI). (2018b). *FDA approved medications for cervical cancer*. Retrieved from https://www.cancer.gov/about-cancer/treatment/drugs/bevacizumab.

National Cancer Institute (NCI). (2018c). *Genetics of breast and gynecologic cancers (PDQ®)—Health Professional Version*. Retrieved from https://www.cancer.gov/types/breast/hp/breast-ovarian-genetics-pdq.

Nayar, R., & Wilbur, D. C. (2015). The Pap test and Bethesda 2014. *Acta Cytologica, 59*

Office on Women's Health. (2018). *Uterine fibroids*. Retrieved from https://www.womenshealth.gov/a-z-topics/uterine-fibroids.

Santen, R. J. (2017). Benign breast disease in women. *Endotext*. Retrieved from https://www.ncbi.nlm.nih.gov/books/NBK278994/.

Shifren, J. L., & Gass, M. L. S. (2014). The North American Menopause Society recommendations for clinical care of midlife women. *Menopause, 21*(1), 1038–1062.

Sorenson, M., Quinn, L., & Klein, D. (2019). *Pathophysiology: Concepts of human disease*. Hoboken, NJ: Pearson Education.

Taylor, M. (2015). Complementary and alternative approaches to menopause. *Endocrinology and Metabolism Clinics, 44*(3), 619–648.

Whitaker, L., & Critchley, H. O. D. (2015). Abnormal uterine bleeding: Best practice and research. *Clinical Obstetrics and Gynaecology, 34*, 54–65.

Women's Health Initiative. (2002). Risks and benefits of estrogen plus progestin in healthy postmenopausal women: Principal results from the Women's Health Initiative randomized controlled trial. *Journal of the American Medical Association, 288*, 321–333.

Yonkers, K. A., & Simoni, M. K. (2018). Premenstrual disorders. *American Journal of Obstetrics and Gynecology, 218*(1), 68–74.

ADDITIONAL RESOURCES

Centers for Disease Control and Prevention: Women's Reproductive Health

https://www.cdc.gov/reproductivehealth/womensrh/index.htm

Office on Women's Health, U.S. Department of Health and Human Services

https://www.womenshealth.gov

North American Menopause Society

www.menopause.org

Women's Health Initiative

https://www.whi.org/SitePages/WHI%20Home.aspx

Chapter 50

Nursing Care of Patients with Sexually Transmitted Infections

Chapter Outline and Learning Outcomes

50.1 Overview of Sexually Transmitted Infections 1833

Describe the characteristics of sexually transmitted infections, as well as key factors in their prevention and control.

50.2 Viral Sexually Transmitted Infections 1836

Describe the pathophysiology and manifestations of viral sexually transmitted diseases, including genital herpes and human papillomavirus, and outline the interprofessional care and nursing care of patients with these disorders.

50.3 Bacterial Sexually Transmitted Infections 1840

Describe the pathophysiology and manifestations of bacterial sexually transmitted diseases, including vaginal infection, chlamydia, gonorrhea, syphilis, and pelvic inflammatory disease, and outline the interprofessional care and nursing care of patients with these disorders.

CLINICAL COMPETENCIES

- With sensitivity and respect for diversity, assess the health status of patients with STIs and recognize, monitor, document, and report abnormal or unexpected manifestations.
- Determine priority nursing diagnoses and select and implement evidence-based and patient-centered nursing interventions for patients with STIs.
- Administer topical, oral, and injectable medications knowledgeably and safely.
- Integrate interprofessional care into care of patients with STIs.
- Provide teaching appropriate for prevention, control, and self-care of STIs.
- Revise plan of care as needed to provide effective interventions to promote, maintain, or restore functional health status of patients with STIs.

KEY TERMS

chancre, 1846
chlamydia, 1843
dyspareunia, 1842
genital herpes, 1836
gonorrhea, 1844
human papillomavirus (HPV), 1839
pelvic inflammatory disease (PID), 1849
sexually transmitted infections (STIs), 1833
syphilis, 1845

Infections transmitted by vaginal, oral, and anal intimate contact and intercourse are referred to as **sexually transmitted infections (STIs)**. Infections transmitted by sexual intercourse are also labeled as *sexually transmitted diseases (STDs)* or *venereal diseases*. STIs also include systemic diseases (such as tuberculosis, hepatitis, and HIV/AIDS) that can be transmitted from an infected person to a partner. This chapter discusses STIs that involve the urogenital system. Vaginal infections are included in this chapter because they are also included in the Centers for Disease Control and Prevention (CDC) treatment guidelines.

50.1 Overview of Sexually Transmitted Infections

Sexually transmitted infections include those caused by bacteria, *Chlamydiae*, viruses, fungi, protozoa, and parasites. Portals of entry for these agents of transmission include the mouth, genitalia, urinary meatus, anus, rectum, and skin. STIs have many consequences, and nurses have the responsibility of teaching sexually active patients how to prevent STIs, regardless of their gender, age, or sexual orientation.

Nurses have a critical role in the prevention of STIs by teaching patients about these diseases, their prevention, treatment, and potential complications.

Incidence and Prevalence

STIs have reached epidemic proportions in the United States and are on the increase worldwide. They are the most frequent infections encountered by professionals in the field of reproductive health and occur in more than half of all people at some point in their life. According to the CDC (2017b), in 2016 there were over 1.5 million cases of chlamydia, over 450,000 cases of gonorrhea, and over 27,500 cases of syphilis. All of these diseases are rising at a steady and alarming rate.

Women and infants are disproportionately affected by STIs. Many STIs are more easily transmitted from a man to a woman than from a woman to a man. Women often experience few early manifestations of the infection, delaying diagnosis and treatment. Furthermore, women are at greater risk for complications of STIs such as pelvic inflammatory disease (PID) and genital cancers.

Several factors help explain the escalating incidence of STIs. Earlier onset of intercourse, delay in finding marriage or monogamous co-habitating partners, and subsequent higher frequency in new partners or intercourse in general are related to higher incidences of STIs. In addition, since oral contraceptives were introduced to American women in 1961, they have replaced the condom as a birth control method for many couples. However, oral contraceptives do not protect against STIs, a fact of increasing importance.

STIs affect men and women of all ages, backgrounds, and socioeconomic levels. The incidence of STIs is highest in young adults ages 15 to 24 (CDC, 2017b). Multiple physiologic (i.e., route of transmission, depression), behavioral (i.e., lack of condom use, alcohol and drug use), and social (i.e., social networks, socioeconomic status) factors are associated with STIs. Healthcare disparities—access to quality healthcare and STI prevention services, healthcare-seeking behavior, poverty, lack of insurance or ability to pay—are additional factors contributing to the increased incidence of STIs in some populations (CDC, 2017c).

STIs have an epidemiologic synergy with each other. STIs such as syphilis, herpes simplex virus (HSV), and chancroid facilitate the transmission of HIV/AIDS, and the immune suppression caused by HIV potentiates the infectious process of other STIs. Individuals who are infected with STIs are at greater risk of acquiring HIV if they are exposed to the virus. This is the result of several factors: Genital ulcers create a portal of entry for HIV, nonulcerative STIs increase the concentration of cells in genital secretions that can be targets for HIV, and infection with both an STI and HIV results in an increased likelihood of having HIV in genital secretions and semen (CDC, 2017c).

Characteristics

Although various organisms cause STIs, they have several characteristics in common:

- Most can be prevented by consistent and correct use of latex condoms.
- They can be transmitted during oral, vaginal, and anal intercourse and, in the case of HSV and HPV, skin-to-skin contact through microfissures in skin and mucous membranes.
- For treatment to be effective, sexual partners of the infected person must also be treated.
- Two or more STIs frequently coexist in the same patient.

The complications of STIs in women include PID, ectopic pregnancy, infertility, chronic pelvic pain, neonatal illness and death, and genital cancer. Vaccination of preteens and teens before the onset of sexual activity can prevent HPV infection in men and women. Some bacterial STIs can be cured through appropriate early treatment with antibiotics. Others, such as genital herpes, are chronic conditions that can be managed but not cured because they are caused by viruses. The most serious STI is AIDS, which at this time is incurable. HIV and AIDS are discussed in Chapter 13. Treatment guidelines for STIs are updated regularly and are available from the CDC.

Prevention and Control

The prevention and control of STIs is based on the principles of education, prevention, detection, effective diagnosis, and treatment of infected persons and evaluation, treatment, and counseling of sexual partners of people who are infected.

Pre-exposure vaccination is an effective method of preventing the viral STIs HPV and hepatitis B. HPV-4 (Gardasil) is a quadrivalent HPV vaccine that prevents cervical cancer in women and genital warts in women and men. There is also a 9-valent HPV vaccine (Gardasil 9) that has come on the market and is becoming the standard of vaccination. The CDC recommends that it be given to girls and boys age 11 to 12 years and individuals age 13 to 26 years who have not previously been vaccinated; children as young as 9 years may be vaccinated (CDC, 2016). In 2018, the Food and Drug Administration approved Gardasil 9 for adults (both male and female) 27 through 45 years of age (FDA, 2018). For the most up-to-date vaccination schedule, check the CDC website. Hepatitis B vaccine is recommended for unvaccinated, uninfected individuals being evaluated for an STI and for men who have sex with men and for individuals who are injection-drug users (CDC, 2018c). Finally, there are recommendations for both preexposure to HIV medications in limited settings (e.g., where one partner is HIV positive and the other is not) and post–HIV exposure medications. Please refer to the CDC website as the recommendations are evolving as more research is done in the area. Please also refer to the CDC website for the most recent recommendations for screening for chlamydia, gonorrhea, syphilis, trichomonas, herpes, HIV, hepatitis B, and hepatitis C, as screening recommendations change on a regular basis.

The ability of the healthcare provider to obtain an accurate sexual history is essential to prevention and control efforts. Important information includes the number and gender of sexual partners, type of birth control used (if any), use of protection from STIs and HIV, sexual practices (e.g., vaginal, anal, oral), and any previous history of an STI or exposure to a partner known to have an STI. In the

Moving Evidence into Action

Preventing STIs in Minority Adolescents

Clinical Issue

Prevention of STIs is important, especially for adolescents at high risk. Minority adolescents are more likely to become infected with an STI. Reaching out to adolescents can be difficult. Use of technology may be the way to reach out.

External Evidence

In 2017 Chen et al. published the results of their pilot study in which they used a Web-based bilingual program for teaching the prevention of HIV/STIs, specifically targeting at-risk Mexican American adolescent girls. The participants were divided into two groups: One group received an HIV/STI prevention program and the other received nutritional counseling. The HIV/STI prevention program included how to respond to peer pressure, STI and pregnancy prevention, and the relationship between substance abuse and risky sexual behavior. Findings included that the participants found the culturally relevant case studies to be helpful, their sexual knowledge increased, and they were able to voice their concerns about STI prevention to their partners. Interestingly, though the participants identified as bilingual, they expressed difficulty with the Spanish-language content and used only the English-language content even though half spoke Spanish at home (Chen et al., 2017).

Internal Evidence

Nurses are the front line for HIV/STI prevention, independent of work setting. Nurses need to understand cultural differences and seek out resources when talking to patients concerning HIV/STI prevention. Local context is also important. Every community is different and nurses must understand the community they serve before implementing any educational programs. As evidenced in the small pilot study above, even those who identify as bilingual can have difficulties with one of the languages.

Patient Considerations

The patient's culture is important to take into account for HIV/STI education. Preferred language is important. Also, sensitivity to privacy and preferred method of education is important. Asking the patient how best he or she learns, what language is preferred, and other teaching/learning factors are important to assess.

Putting the Pieces Together

Nurses need to use what has been published that works for education on the patient population they serve in relation to HIV/STI prevention. However, assumptions need to be managed. As in the research presented above, while the education was designed as bilingual and the participants stated they were bilingual, all preferred the English version. Asking which language is the preferred language for learning is important.

Reference

Chen, A. C., Lightfoot, M., Szalacha, L. A., & Lindenberg, C. S. (2017). A pilot, Web-based HIV/STI prevention intervention targeting at-risk Mexican American adolescents: Feasibility, acceptability and lessons learned. *Journal of Nursing and Health Care, 4*(2).

United States approximately 45% of people with HIV/AIDS are age 50 and older, not only because the incidence of HIV in older people is increasing, but because treatments are helping people with the disease live longer (CDC, 2018a).

One approach to collecting accurate information about key areas of interest has been summarized by the CDC (2010) as the **Five Ps**. Nurses should ask patients about the following:

Partners
Prevention of pregnancy
Protection from STIs
Practice
Past history of STIs.

The full booklet to help all health care providers with taking a sexual history can be found at https://www.cdc.gov/std/treatment/sexualhistory.pdf.

The most effective way to prevent sexual transmission of HIV and most other STIs is to avoid sexual intercourse with an infected partner. It is recommended that both partners be tested for STIs, including HIV, before beginning to have sexual intercourse. If an individual chooses to have intercourse with an infected partner or one whose infection status is unknown, a new condom should be used for each act of intercourse. Some patients do not know how to properly use a condom or other barrier protections to prevent HIV/STIs or pregnancy. Even if the patient states he or she knows how to use a barrier method, this should be reviewed with the patient as there are misconceptions. See **Table 50.1** for a step-by-step guide to using a condom along with other information on barrier methods.

Prevention teaching for the person who is an injecting-drug user includes:

- Enroll or continue in a drug treatment program.
- Do not use injection equipment that has been used by another person. If equipment is shared, first clean the syringe and needle with bleach and water (to reduce the risk of HIV transmission).
- If needles can be legally obtained in the community, obtain and use clean needles.

Eliminating further transmission and reinfection of STIs is critical to control. For treatable STIs, this means that referral of sexual partners for diagnosis, treatment, and counseling is essential. Chlamydia, gonorrhea, syphilis, and chancroid are reportable diseases in every state; the CDC also collects HIV testing data from all states. When a health-care professional refers infected patients to a local or state department of health, every effort is made to identify and contact sexual partners. Reports of STI and HIV infections are maintained in strictest confidence and are protected by law from subpoena. Suggested resources for people with STIs are listed in **Box 50.1**.

Table 50.1 STI Barrier Guidelines

Barrier Protection	Teaching Topics
Male condoms	✔ Use a new condom with each act of sexual intercourse. ✔ Handle carefully to avoid damaging the condom. ✔ Be sure no air is trapped in the end of the condom. ✔ Put the condom on when the penis is erect and before genital contact with partner. ✔ Ensure adequate lubrication exists during intercourse, using only water-based lubricants (e.g., K-Y Jelly, Astroglide, AquaLube, and glycerine) with latex condoms. Oil-based lubricants, such as petroleum jelly, massage oil, mineral oil, or body lotions, can weaken latex. ✔ Nonlatex condoms made of polyurethane or other synthetic material protect against pregnancy and STIs; natural membrane condoms do not adequately protect against STIs and should not be used. ✔ Ensure adequate lubrication during vaginal and anal sex. ✔ Withdraw while the penis is erect and hold the condom firmly against the base of the penis during withdrawal.
Female condoms	✔ The female condom (Reality) is a lubricated polyurethane sheath with a ring on each end that is inserted into the vagina. It is an effective mechanical barrier to viruses.
Vaginal spermicides, sponges, diaphragms	✔ Spermicides used alone without condoms do not reduce the risk for cervical gonorrhea, chlamydia, or HIV infection. ✔ The diaphragm protects against cervical gonorrhea, chlamydia, and trichomoniasis, but not HIV.

BOX 50.1
Resources for Patients with STIs

- CDC National STD Hotline: https://www.usa.gov/federal-agencies/cdc-national-std-hotline
- CDC National Prevention Information Network: https://npin.cdc.gov
- National Center for HIV/AIDS, Viral Hepatitis, STD, and TB Prevention: https://www.cdc.gov/nchhstp/default.htm
- National HPV and Cervical Cancer Resource Center: http://vaccineresources.org/details.php?i=1339
- National Herpes Hotline: www.herpesonline.org/herpes-hotline/
- American Sexual Health Association: www.ashasexualhealth.org

Expedited partner therapy (EPT) is defined by the CDC (2010) as treatment of partners without an intervening personal assessment by a healthcare provider. EPT is one potential means of limiting the spread of STIs, and it may be implemented by any of several methods. The usual method for implementing EPT is *patient-delivered partner therapy (PDPT)*, wherein clinicians provide their patients with drugs intended for the partners or write prescriptions in the partners' names. Providing clear instructions for follow-up care is an important component of EPT. Although many public health agencies and personnel endorse it, EPT may fall outside legal guidelines for prescribing in many states and should not be used without clear direction.

50.2 Viral Sexually Transmitted Infections

The Patient with Genital Herpes

The herpes simplex viruses HSV-1 and HSV-2 both cause **genital herpes**, although most are caused by HSV-2. Like most STIs, genital herpes are most commonly found in young, sexually active adults and are associated with early onset of sexual activity and multiple sexual partners. Prevalence rates for HSV vary from 15 to 49% depending on age, gender, and race (CDC, 2017b). Exact incidence is unknown because HSV is not a reportable infection and some patients can have subclinical infections with no symptoms. While the overall percentage of young adults with genital herpes is decreasing, infection rates among non-Hispanic Blacks are significantly higher than among other populations (CDC, 2017b). There is no cure, and the treatments are primarily symptomatic.

Pathophysiology and Risk Factors

One hundred types of HSV viruses have been identified, with more than 30 affecting the urogenital area. HSV-2, the virus that causes genital herpes, is transmitted by sexual activity or during childbirth from an infected woman. HSV-1 is associated with cold sores, but may be transmitted to the genital area by oral intercourse or by self-inoculation through poor hand hygiene practices. HSV infections begin with an exposure to the virus by contact with infectious lesions or secretions. The virus then moves into the stratified squamous epithelium, stimulating the replication of the epithelium and infecting the neurons that innervate the area (Sorenson, Quinn, & Klein, 2019). HSV viruses are neurotropic viruses, meaning that they grow in neurons and can maintain their disease potential even when there are no manifestations. The virus ascends through the peripheral nerves to the dorsal root ganglia, where it can remain dormant. For unknown reasons, the virus may reactivate and return to the nerve root of the skin, causing lesions. During dormancy, the virus is impervious to treatment. Genital HSV-2 infection is more common in women (approximately one in four women) than it is in men (almost one in eight) (CDC, 2017b).

Risk factors for HSV are the same as for any STI. These include sexual intercourse without the use of a condom, oral sexual activities without the use of a barrier device, and multiple sexual partners.

Manifestations

Within 2 to 10 days after exposure to the herpes virus, painful red papules appear in the genital area. In men, the lesions generally occur on the glans or shaft of the penis. In women, the lesions commonly occur on the labia, vagina, and cervix. Anal intercourse or oral–anal sexual contact may result in lesions in and around the anus.

Soon after the papules appear, they form small, painful blisters filled with clear fluid containing virus particles (**Figure 50.1** ■). The blisters break, shedding the highly infectious virus and creating patches of painful ulcers that last 6 weeks (or longer if they become infected). Touching these blisters and then rubbing or scratching in another place can spread the infection to other areas of the body (*autoinoculation*).

The first outbreak of herpes lesions is called *first-episode infection*, with an average duration of 12 days. Subsequent occurrences, usually less severe, are termed *recurrent infections* (average duration of 4 to 5 days). The period between episodes is called *latency*, during which time the person remains infectious even though no symptoms are present. During latency, the virus withdraws into the nerve fibers that lead from the infected site to the lower spine, remaining dormant until recurrence, at which time it retraces its path to the genital area. There can be several recurrences within a year.

The manifestations of genital herpes include:

- Herpetic lesions
- Regional lymphadenopathy
- Headache
- Fever
- General malaise
- Dysuria
- Urinary retention
- Vaginal discharge
- Urethral discharge (men).

Prodromal symptoms of recurrent outbreaks of genital herpes can include burning, itching, tingling, or throbbing at the sites where lesions commonly appear. These sensations may be accompanied by pain in the legs, groin, or buttocks. Some authorities believe that prodromal symptoms signal increased levels of infectiousness, during which sexual contact should be avoided.

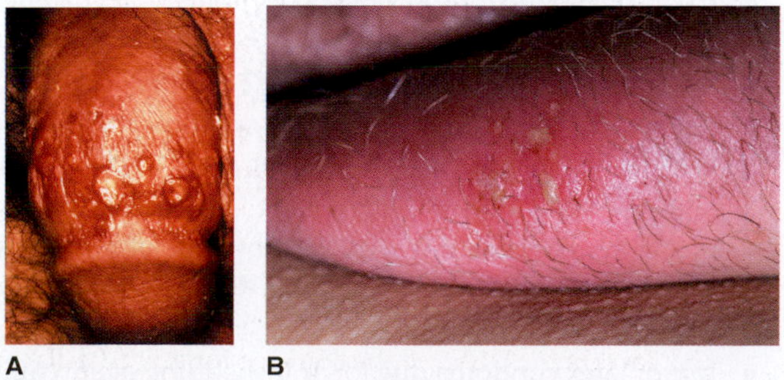

Figure 50.1 ■ Genital herpes on **A**, the penis, and **B**, the vulva.

A word of caution about clinical manifestations: Most people infected with HSV-2 are not aware they are infected. In fact, most people do not realize they have the infection until years after the infection is acquired.

Complications

Complications of HSV include increased risk for other STIs and HIV, the inability to void in severe cases, and rarely meningitis and proctitis. The most severe complications are found in babies born to mothers with active HSV infections (which might not be evident with lesions; the woman may be shedding the virus in her vagina). The baby exposed to the virus during the birthing process becomes infected, which can lead to brain damage, blindness, or even death. All women are screened early in pregnancy, and for those who are positive, screening right before birth is important. If the woman is shedding the virus in the vagina, then a cesarean section is scheduled to protect the newborn.

Interprofessional Care

Presumptive diagnosis of genital herpes is based on history and physical examination of the patient, including lesions and patterns of recurrence. Because there is no cure for genital herpes, treatment focuses on relieving symptoms and preventing spread of the infection. Patient education is essential to prevent further transmission of the disease and to help patients integrate management of a chronic disease into their lifestyles.

Diagnosis

Definitive diagnosis requires isolation of the virus in tissue culture. Ideally, tissue specimens should be obtained within 48 hours of the appearance of the blisters.

Medications

Acyclovir (Zovirax) helps reduce the length and severity of the first episode and is the treatment of choice for genital herpes. The oral form is considered most effective for a first episode as well as recurrences. It is given for 7 to 10 days or until lesions heal. Evidence shows that some strains of HSV are becoming resistant to acyclovir, particularly in people who are HIV positive. In those cases, foscarnet (Foscavir) is used. Other antivirals used for treatment and prevention are valacyclovir (Valtrex) and famciclovir (Famvir). Suppressive therapy using an antiviral (acyclovir, valacyclovir, or famciclovir) for recurrent genital herpes has been shown to reduce the frequency of outbreaks as well as the risk of transmission of the infection to an uninfected heterosexual partner (Adams, Holland, & Urban, 2017).

Nursing Care

In planning and implementing nursing care for the patient with genital herpes, the nurse needs to consider both short-term and long-term implications. Although the immediate priority is symptom relief and prevention of further transmission, the patient needs assistance to deal with the life-changing diagnosis of a chronic disease.

Assessment

See the Manifestations and Interprofessional Care sections for the assessment of the patient with genital herpes.

- Health history: Symptoms such as pain, burning, itching, tingling, or throbbing; presence of genital lesion(s); previous episodes; recent sexual activity with a new partner; use of safer sex practices and/or protection (e.g., condom)
- Physical assessment: Inspection for red, papular lesions on penis (men), labia or vagina (women), or around the anus (either).

Priorities of Care

Collaborating with the interprofessional team to ensure appropriate treatment of genital herpes while providing care that supports symptom relief, prevention of future transmission, and physical and psychologic responses to this diagnosis is a priority of nursing care. There can be acute pain with the infection.

Diagnoses, Outcomes, and Interventions

Nursing priorities discussed in this section focus on pain and sexual dysfunction.

Relieve Acute Pain. Herpetic lesions are very painful and can become infected. Because the virus resides in the nerve ganglia, pain may also occur in the legs, thighs, groin, or buttocks. Although acyclovir diminishes the pain of herpes and accelerates the healing process, additional measures can relieve the discomfort further.

Expected Outcome: Patient will demonstrate pain control as evidenced by use of prescribed and preventive measures.

The nurse will:

- Teach patient how to keep herpes blisters clean and dry. A gentle cleansing with soap and water is recommended, thoroughly drying the blisters afterward. It is important to wear loose cotton clothing that will not trap moisture and to avoid wearing tights, leggings, and jeans. *Keeping the lesions clean and dry reduces the possibility of secondary infection and speeds the healing process.*
- For dysuria, suggest pouring water over the genitals while urinating. Drinking additional fluids also helps dilute the acidity of the urine; however, fluids that increase acidity, such as cranberry juice, should be avoided. *These measures dilute the acid content of urine and thereby reduce the burning sensation.*
- Warm baths may be used to relieve pain. *The warm water is soothing and decreases pain from ulcers and an irritated urethral meatus. It also facilitates wound healing.*

Promote Healthy Self-Esteem. Patients who learn that they are infected with an incurable STI may believe they can no longer have a normal sex life. Fortunately, many people have learned to live with and manage genital herpes without infecting their partners or their children.

Expected Outcome: Patient will demonstrate self-esteem related to sexual patterns as evidenced by verbalization of self-acceptance.

The nurse will:

- Provide a supportive, nonjudgmental environment for the patient to discuss feelings and ask questions about what this diagnosis means to future sexual relationships. *Feelings of guilt, shame, and anger are natural responses to such a diagnosis and can lead to a total avoidance of sexual intimacy.*
- Provide information about suppressive therapy for the patient who is in a mutually monogamous heterosexual relationship. *Although suppressive therapy does not eliminate the need to avoid sexual contact during an outbreak, it has been shown to be safe and effective in reducing outbreak frequency and the risk of transmission to the sexual partner (CDC, 2017a).*
- Offer information about support groups and other resources for people with herpes such as the National Herpes Hotline (see Box 50.1). *Information about how others cope with this disease can offset feelings of shame and hopelessness.*

Delegating Nursing Care Activities

As appropriate and allowed by the designated duties and responsibilities of unlicensed assistive personnel, the nurse may delegate nursing care activities such as collecting vital signs and nonpharmacologic skin care.

Transitions of Care

As discussed previously, prevention is the key factor in relation to any STI transmission. Correct use of barrier protection for every sexual encounter is important. Monogamous relationships or limiting the number of sexual partners is important. For the patient with an acute infection, care involves symptom management, viral suppression with medications, and emotional support.

Health teaching for patients with chronic genital herpes involves helping them manage outbreaks of the disease with the least possible disruption in lifestyle and relationships. Understanding the disease process and factors that affect it helps the patient regain a sense of control and see the potential for future sexual intimacy without transmission of infection. The following topics should be addressed:

- How to recognize prodromal symptoms of recurrence and factors that seem to trigger recurrences (such as emotional stress, acidic food, sun exposure)
- The need for abstinence from sexual contact from the time prodromal symptoms appear until 10 days after all lesions have healed
- If lesions become infected, use of topical acyclovir (painful lesions can be protected with sterile petroleum jelly or aloe vera gel)
- Use of latex condoms due to viral shedding at any time and careful hygiene practices (such as not sharing towels or other personal items) even during latency periods.

The Patient with Human Papillomavirus

There are more than 100 **human papillomaviruses (HPV)**, 40 of which affect the genital area. The most concerning are types 16 and 18, which are oncogenic and are associated with cervical, penile, vulvar, vaginal, and certain oropharyngeal cancers. These two types of HPV account for approximately 66% of all cervical cancers in the United States (CDC, 2017b). Types 6 and 11 are not oncogenic, but cause approximately 90% of all reported genital warts. In most people, HPV infections are asymptomatic and resolve without treatment (CDC, 2018b). Currently, HPV is incurable.

Most HPV infections are asymptomatic or unrecognized. Approximately 42.5% of all sexually active people in the United States are infected with HPV (CDC, 2017b). Women are at greater risk for HPV genital infections because they have a larger mucosal surface area exposed in the genital area. Actual infections are not a reportable STI, so statistics quoted are based on estimates from other sources, though it is felt to be the most common sexually transmitted infection (CDC, 2017b).

Pathophysiology

Human papillomaviruses are most often transmitted through vaginal and anal sex. They can also be passed on during oral sex and genital-to-genital contact. The incubation period is 6 weeks to 8 months. HPV infects squamous epithelium, stimulating it to replicate and proliferate. Most HPV infections will have no clinical manifestations and resolve within 1 to 2 years. Some, however, do linger and may cause oncogenic complications or genital warts. The reasons why some resolve and others do not are unknown.

Risk Factors

Risk factors for HPV infection are the same as all other STIs: Having multiple partners and not using barrier protection for every sexual act. There are some known risk factors for HPV infection turning into cervical cancer, including long-term oral contraceptive use, having three or more pregnancies, cigarette smoking, and co-infections with HIV or other immune-compromising conditions (CDC, 2017d).

Manifestations

Most people with HPV do not have manifestations. When present, manifestations include single or multiple painless, soft, moist, pink, or flesh-colored swellings in the vulvovaginal area, perineum, penis, urethra, anus, groin, or thigh (**Figure 50.2** ■). In women, the growths may be in the vagina or on the cervix and be apparent only during a pelvic examination.

The four types of genital warts are:

- *Condyloma acuminata:* Cauliflower-shaped lesions that appear on moist skin surfaces such as the vagina or anus
- *Keratotic warts:* Thick, hard lesions that develop on keratinized skin such as the labia major, penis, or scrotum
- *Papular warts:* Smooth lesions that also develop on keratinized skin
- *Flat warts:* Slightly raised lesions, often invisible to the naked eye, that also develop on keratinized skin.

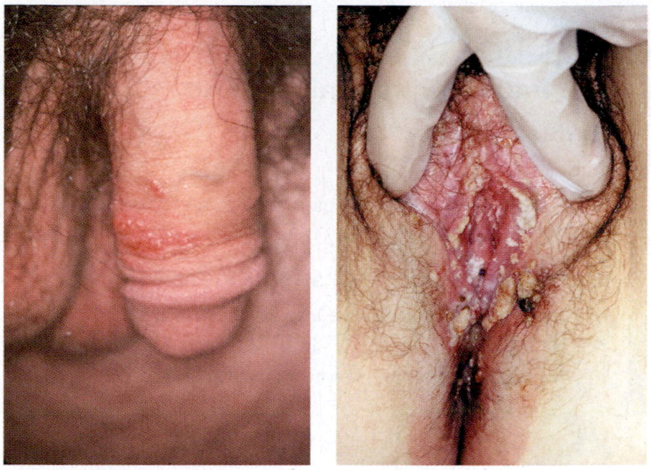
A B

Figure 50.2 ■ Genital warts (*condyloma acuminata*) on **A**, penis and **B**, the vulva.

Complications

The major complication from HPV infection is cancer. In females, the cancer is cervical, vaginal, and vulvar. In males, it is cancer of the penis. In both sexes, HPV infection can cause cancer of the anus, oropharynx, and tonsils. It is estimated that there are more than 37,000 new cases of cancer due to HPV infection every year (CDC, 2017b).

Interprofessional Care

Treatment is directed at removal of the warts, relief of symptoms, and health teaching to reduce the risk of recurrence and future transmission. Infection with HPV is considered chronic; however, research has shown that HPV becomes undetectable within 2 years in 90% of those infected (CDC, 2017b).

Diagnosis

Genital and anal warts are diagnosed primarily by clinical appearance. Cervical cell changes are identified by routine Papanicolaou (Pap) tests. An HPV DNA test can be used along with Pap testing to identify high-risk HPV subtypes.

Medications

Currently two vaccines can be used to prevent various types of HPV if given before the individual becomes sexually active. A quadrivalent vaccine, Gardasil, is available to protect against the four types of HPV that cause most cervical cancers and genital warts and a 9-valent HPV vaccine (Gardasil-9). Both vaccines are administered by intramuscular injections. Due to the evolving nature of immunization schedules based on new information, the CDC website should be consulted for the most up-to-date information. Special populations (e.g., men who have sex with men, HIV

Medication Administration 50.A

The Patient with Genital Warts

TOPICAL APPLICATION

imiquimod

Apply a thin layer to the affected area three times a week at bedtime then wash off the cream 6 to 10 hours after application.

Health Education for the Patient and Family

- Wash treated area before application and allow to dry for 10 to 15 minutes.
- Wash hands before applying to affected areas.
- Apply a thin layer of the cream and work in to the affected area until no longer visible.
- For penile warts in uncircumcised males, gently pull back the foreskin and wash area thoroughly before applying.
- Females should not apply directly into the vagina. Application to the labia may cause pain or swelling and difficulty urinating.
- Abstain from sexual activities until all lesions have healed.
- Use condoms to prevent future infections.

Source: Data from Shields, Fox, & Liebrecht, 2018.

positive, immunocompromised) should also receive the vaccination. The vaccine does not protect against an existing HPV infection.

Topical agents used to treat genital warts include podophyllotoxin, sinecatechins, and imiquimod, which can be applied by the patient (see **Medication Administration 50.A**).

Other Treatments

Genital warts may also be removed by cryotherapy, electrocautery, laser vaporization, or surgical excision. Carbon dioxide laser surgery is becoming increasingly common for removal of extensive warts.

Nursing Care

Health promotion activities for adults of all ages should include information about the causes, treatments, and prevention of HPV infections.

Assessment

See the Manifestations and Interprofessional Care sections for the assessment of the patient with HPV infection.

Priorities of Care

Collaborating with the interprofessional team to ensure appropriate treatment of HPV while providing care that supports treatment, prevention of future transmission, and physical and psychologic responses to this diagnosis is a priority of nursing care.

Diagnoses, Outcomes, and Interventions

Nursing interventions are primarily directed toward patient education.

Provide Patient Teaching. HPV is spread by contact with infectious lesions or secretions, with up to 70% of genital warts spread by people who do not know they have the infection. Although there is no known cure, it is essential to prevent secondary infections.

Expected Outcome: Patient will demonstrate knowledge about HPV by articulating vaccine efficacy, increased risk for cervical cancer, and transmission prevention activities.

The nurse will:

- Provide information to all women, particularly those who fall within the recommended age range and mothers of preteens and teens, about HPV vaccine and immunization recommendations. *A fully immunized population can have a significant impact on the incidence of and mortality related to cervical cancer.*
- Discuss the need for prompt treatment and the necessity for sexual abstinence until lesions have healed or consistent condom use while lesions are present. *This reduces the risk of reinfection and further transmission of the disease. Some studies have found that using condoms promotes the regression of HPV lesions in both men and women.*
- Discuss the increased risk of cervical cancer associated with HPV and the importance of an annual Pap smear for all sexually active females. *Understanding the risk, the patient will be more motivated to seek annual screening.*
- Stress the importance of thorough hand hygiene. *Hand hygiene is essential to prevent the spread of HPV.*

Delegating Nursing Care Activities

As appropriate and allowed by the designated duties and responsibilities of unlicensed assistive personnel, the nurse may delegate nursing care activities such as collecting vital signs and nonpharmacologic skin care.

Transitions of Care

Health teaching emphasizes the need for the patient and infected partners to return for regular treatment until lesions have resolved and to use condoms to prevent reinfection. Because of the increased risk of cervical cancer, annual Pap tests are essential for female patients.

50.3 Bacterial Sexually Transmitted Infections

The Patient with a Vaginal Infection

Yeasts, protozoa, or bacteria may infect the vagina. These infections can be sexually transmitted, but the male partner does not always have manifestations of the infection. Risk factors include the use of hormonal contraceptives or broad-spectrum antibiotics, obesity, diabetes, pregnancy, unprotected sexual activity, and multiple sexual partners. Manifestations of vaginal infections are outlined in **Table 50.2**.

Preventive measures include educating women about personal hygiene practices and safer sex. Women need to avoid frequent douching and wearing nylon underwear and/or tight pants. Unprotected sexual activity, particularly with multiple partners, increases the risk of vaginal infections.

Pathophysiology

Alterations in pH, changes in the normal flora, and low estrogen levels are conducive to the development of vaginal infections. When conditions are favorable, microorganisms invade the vulva and vagina.

Bacterial Vaginosis

Bacterial vaginosis (nonspecific vaginitis) is the most common cause of vaginal infection in women of reproductive age. *Gardnerella vaginalis* is one of the causative organisms, but others are also implicated. The relationship of sexual activity to this infection is not clear, though women who have never been sexually active are rarely affected. The infection is treated with oral or intravaginal antibacterial agents.

Candidiasis

Candidiasis (moniliasis or yeast infection) is caused by the organism *Candida albicans*, which has several strains of different virulence. *Candida* organisms are part of the normal vaginal environment in up to 50% of women, causing problems only when they multiply rapidly. When increased estrogen levels, antibiotics, diabetes mellitus, fecal contamination, or other factors alter the normal vaginal flora, the organism proliferates, resulting in a yeast infection. The infection is treated with oral or intravaginal antifungal agents.

Trichomoniasis

Trichomoniasis is caused by *Trichomonas vaginalis*, a protozoan parasite (**Figure 50.3** ■). It is the most common curable STI in young, sexually active women. In 2015, there were 139,000 initial visits for trichomoniasis (CDC, 2017b). Symptoms usually appear 5 to 28 days after exposure. It most commonly infects the vagina in women and the urethra in men. Trichomoniasis is treated with a single oral dose of metronidazole or tinidazole. As with all STIs, lack of using a barrier method during all sexual encounters is a risk factor.

Manifestations

The primary manifestation of bacterial vaginosis is a vaginal discharge that is thin and grayish-white and has a foul, fishy odor. The manifestations of candidiasis include an odorless, thick, cheesy vaginal discharge. This is often accompanied by itching and irritation of the vulva and vagina, with dysuria and dyspareunia (**Figure 50.4** ■).

With trichomoniasis, most men are asymptomatic; however, when symptomatic, they may complain of dysuria and urethral discomfort. Women have a frothy, green-yellow vaginal discharge with a strong fishy odor, often accompanied by itching and irritation of the genitalia.

Complications

Complications of bacterial vaginosis include PID, preterm labor, premature rupture of the membranes, and postpartum endometritis. With candidiasis, uncircumcised males may develop a yeast infection over the glans penis, manifested by itching and dysuria. Trichomoniasis increases a woman's risk of developing HIV if she is exposed and it may increase the risk of transmitting HIV to her sexual partner.

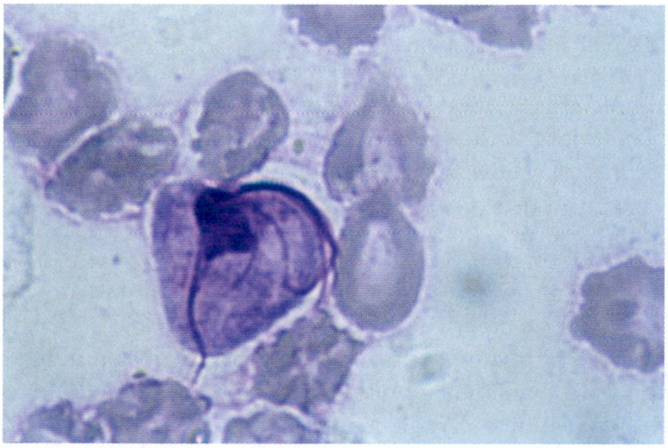

Figure 50.3 ■ Micrograph of *Trichomonas vaginalis* parasite.

Table 50.2 Manifestations and Nursing Care of Vaginal Infections

Infection	Type of Discharge	Typical Manifestations	Nursing Care
Candidiasis (*Monilia*, yeast)	Thick white patches adhering to cervix and vaginal wall, resembling cottage cheese; little odor	Itching of vulva and vaginal area, redness, painful intercourse	Teach perineal hygiene and proper use of vaginal applicators. Instruct the patient to complete the entire treatment.
Bacterial vaginosis	Thin, white, "milklike" or gray with fishy odor, especially when mixed with potassium hydroxide	None to mild itching or burning in vulvar area; clue cells on microscopic examination	Teach proper perineal hygiene. Instruct patient to complete treatment. Teach patient relationship of infection to PID.
Trichomoniasis	Frothy, yellow or white, foul odor	Burning and itching of vulva	Teach perineal hygiene. Instruct about need for both patient and her partner to complete treatment.
Atrophic vaginitis (senile vaginitis)	Thin, opaque discharge, occasionally blood tinged, odorless; pale, smooth, thin, dry vaginal walls	Painful intercourse, itching, vaginal dryness	Counsel patient on symptoms of menopause and sexual techniques to minimize trauma.

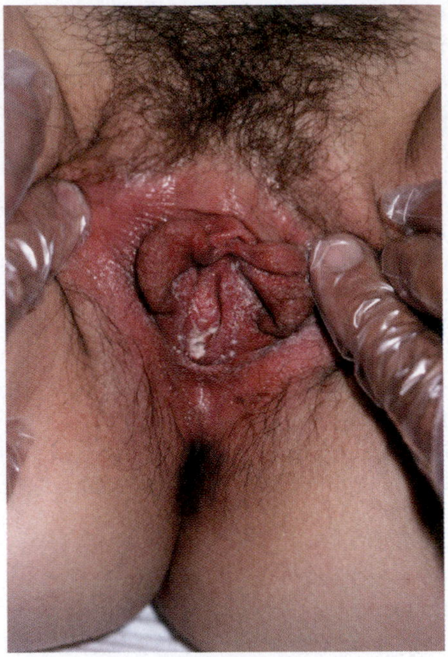

Figure 50.4 ■ Yeast infection on female genitalia.

Interprofessional Care

Interprofessional care focuses on identifying and eliminating the infection and preventing recurrence.

Diagnosis

Diagnostic tests vary with the suspected organism. Cervical cultures are examined to diagnose the causative organism. Trichomonas is identified by microscopically examining a specimen of vaginal discharge in saline. Ten percent potassium hydroxide is used to identify spores and filaments of *Candida*.

Medications

The pharmacologic treatment varies with the organism. The sexual partner of a woman with a *Trichomonas* infection must also be treated to prevent reinfection. Some antifungal agents are available without prescription, which can lead to self-medication with the incorrect agent or allow repeated infections to go unreported.

Nursing Care

Nursing care focuses on teaching the patient and, if necessary, the sexual partner, to comply with the treatment regimen, use safer sex practices, and prevent future transmission of the infection.

Assessment

Careful history taking may also reveal high-risk sexual practices that require intervention, particularly if the patient has had repeated infections. The initial presenting symptom for many HIV-positive women is vaginal candidiasis, which may not respond to over-the-counter treatments. Treatment with some antibiotics destroys normal vaginal flora, resulting in superinfection with yeast. Physical assessment will usually include a pelvic exam for women and cultures to diagnose the infection.

Priorities of Care

Collaborating with the interprofessional team to ensure appropriate treatment of vaginal infections while providing care that supports symptom relief, prevention of future transmission and recurrences, and physical and psychologic responses to the diagnosis is a nursing priority of care.

Diagnoses, Outcomes, and Interventions

Although each nursing care plan must be individualized, nursing priorities often include managing pain and educating patients.

Provide Patient Teaching. Many women are unaware of the causes of vaginal infections and the self-care measures to prevent and treat them. If possible, both the woman and her sexual partner should be taught the information.

Expected Outcome: Patient will demonstrate knowledge about vaginal infections by describing self-care measures and plans to adhere to plan of treatment.

The nurse will:

- Explain the transmission of the infection. Abstaining from sex or consistent condom use are the best ways to avoid transmission and reinfection. *A frank discussion of disease transmission and prevention with the woman and her partner can reduce the risk of reinfection.*
- The need to complete the course of treatment. *Many infections are asymptomatic in one partner. Incomplete treatment allows for recurrence of the infection and reinfection of the partner.*
- Advise women not to douche or use feminine hygiene sprays. *These interfere with the normal bacterial environment of the vagina, decreasing resistance to vaginal infection.*

Manage Acute Pain. The symptoms of vaginitis can include dysuria, painful excoriation or ulceration of tissue, and painful intercourse (**dyspareunia**). Often these symptoms can be relieved by relatively simple self-care measures.

Expected Outcome: Patient will demonstrate pain control as evidenced by use of prescribed and preventive self-care measures.

The nurse will:

- Suggest the use of cool compresses. *Cool compresses relieve itching.*
- Recommend sitz baths to alleviate discomfort. *Sitz baths cleanse the perineal area and the warmth is soothing to inflamed, irritated skin and mucous membranes.*
- Wear cotton underwear. *Cotton absorbs moisture and allows better air circulation than other types of material.*
- If infected with *Trichomonas*, avoid sexual contact until treatment is completed. *Treatment of the infected woman and her partner as well as sexual abstinence are necessary to facilitate healing and to prevent reinfection.*

See **Box 50.2** for additional comfort measures.

Delegating Nursing Care Activities

As appropriate and allowed by the designated duties and responsibilities of unlicensed assistive personnel, the nurse

BOX 50.2
Self-Care Comfort Measures

- Do not wear pantyhose, tights, or leggings; wear loose-fitting pants or skirts.
- Double-rinse underwear; do not use fabric softener on underwear.
- Do not use bubble bath, perfumed soaps, or feminine hygiene products.
- Use menstrual pads, not tampons.
- Use white, unscented toilet paper.
- Use a water-soluble lubricant for intercourse.
- Apply ice or a frozen blue gel pack wrapped in a towel to the vulva after intercourse to relieve burning.
- Rinse vulva with cool water after voiding and intercourse.

may delegate nursing care activities such as collecting vital signs and nonpharmacologic skin care.

Transitions of Care

Teaching focuses on eradicating the infection, preventing further disease transmission, and relieving discomfort associated with the condition. Educating the patient and her partner(s) about safer sex and improved genital hygiene practices can reduce the incidence of recurrence.

The Patient with Chlamydia

Chlamydia are a group of STIs caused by *Chlamydia trachomatis*, a bacterium that behaves like a virus, reproducing only within the host cell. The bacterium is spread by oral, vaginal, or anal intercourse and to the neonate by passage through the birth canal of an infected mother. The infections caused by *Chlamydia* include acute urethral syndrome, nongonococcal urethritis, mucopurulent cervicitis, and PID. Lymphogranuloma venereum (LGV) is an STI caused by several strains of *C. trachomatis*. LGV primarily affects men who have sex with men or women who have receptive anal intercourse (CDC, 2015b).

Chlamydia is the most commonly reported STI in the United States, affecting 475 to 497.3 cases per 100,000 people each year (CDC, 2017b). Of that number, more than half of reported cases occurred in women age 15 to 25 years.

Pathophysiology

C. trachomatis is an intracellular bacterial pathogen that resembles both a virus and bacteria. The organism enters the body as an elementary body, a form in which it is capable of entering uninfected cells. The infection begins when the organism enters a cell and changes into a reticulate body. The reticulate body divides within the cell, bursting the cell and infecting adjoining cells.

While the incubation period is from 1 to 3 weeks, chlamydia may be present for months or years without producing noticeable symptoms in women. Chlamydia typically invades cells of the cervix (in women) and urethra (in men and women). Because chlamydia is asymptomatic in most women until the uterus and fallopian tubes have been invaded, treatment may be delayed, resulting in devastating long-term complications. Nearly a third of men with urethral chlamydia are also asymptomatic. During delivery, pregnant women who have a chlamydial infection can pass the infection along to their infant, potentially resulting in ophthalmia neonatorum (which can lead to blindness) and/or pneumonia (Sorenson et al., 2019).

Risk Factors

Risk factors for chlamydial infection include intercourse during adolescence, unprotected sexual activity, and multiple sexual partners.

Manifestations

When present, manifestations include dysuria, urinary frequency, and vaginal discharge in women or urethral discharge in men. Patients may be asymptomatic; however, they are still potentially infectious.

Complications

If a chlamydial infection in women is not treated, it ascends into the upper reproductive tract, causing such complications as PID, which includes endometritis and salpingitis. Chronic pelvic pain may result. These infections are a major cause of infertility and ectopic pregnancy, a potentially life-threatening disorder in women. Complications of chlamydial infections in men include epididymitis, prostatitis, sterility, and Reiter syndrome. Routine screening for sexually active adolescents and young adults has been suggested by the CDC to minimize these serious complications in asymptomatic people (CDC, 2017b).

Interprofessional Care

Patients infected with *C. trachomatis* are treated with medications to eradicate the infection. Its prevalence, particularly in younger populations, makes widespread screening necessary if the disease is to be controlled. Because chlamydia is often asymptomatic, treatment is often begun on a presumptive basis.

Diagnosis

A urine specimen or swab of the vagina or endocervix, urethra, or rectum (as indicated) may be used to diagnose *C. trachomatis*. The specimen is cultured or subjected to tests for antibodies to chlamydia such as an enzyme-linked immunosorbent assay (ELISA), polymerase chain reaction (PCR), or nucleic acid amplification test (NAAT). NAATs performed on cervical and urethral swab specimens are highly sensitive and have become the diagnostic method of choice (CDC, 2015a).

Medications

The antibiotic recommended by the CDC for chlamydial infections in men and nonpregnant women is azithromycin (Zithromax) orally in a single dose or doxycycline (Adoxa, Apo-Doxy) orally for 7 days. Both sexual partners must be treated at the same time or prior to resuming sexual intercourse (CDC, 2015a).

Nursing Care

Assessment

Assessment of women for chlamydia is difficult as most women are asymptomatic. For women who are sexually active, yearly screening either through a cervical swab or a urine sample is recommended.

Nursing care of the patient with chlamydia focuses on eradication of the infection, prevention of future infections, and management of any chronic complications. Nursing priorities for the patient with chlamydia are the same as for patients with any STI. Interventions are similar to those discussed later in the section about gonorrhea and earlier for genital herpes.

Transitions of Care

Prevention for a chlamydial infection is the correct use of a barrier device (condom) during every sexual encounter.

Health teaching for the patient with chlamydia centers on the need to comply with the treatment regimen, refer partners for examination and necessary treatment, and the use of condoms to avoid reinfection. If the infection has progressed to PID (discussed later), the patient needs additional information on self-care and health promotion. The CDC (2017b) recommends annual screening for chlamydia for young, sexually active women and for young sexually active men in selected settings (adolescent and STD clinics, correctional facilities).

The Patient with Gonorrhea

Gonorrhea, also known as *GC* or *the clap*, is caused by *Neisseria gonorrhoeae*, a Gram-negative diplococcus. Gonorrhea is the second most common reportable communicable disease in the United States. In 2016 there were 468,514 new cases of gonorrhea, although not all cases are reported (CDC, 2017b).

Young adults (15 to 24 years old), and young women in particular, have the highest rate of gonorrhea infection. In men, the highest rate of infection is among those 20 to 29 years of age. Geographically, gonorrhea infection rates in the South are higher than in other parts of the United States (CDC, 2017b).

Pathophysiology and Risk Factors

The causative organism of gonorrhea is a pyogenic (pus-forming) bacteria that causes inflammation characterized by purulent exudate. Humans are the only host for the organism. Gonorrhea is transmitted by direct hetero- and homosexual intercourse and during delivery as the neonate passes through the birth canal. The portal of entry can be the genitourinary tract, eyes, oropharynx, anorectum, or skin. The incubation period is 2 to 7 days after exposure. The organism initially targets the female cervix and the male urethra. Without treatment, the disease ultimately disseminates (spreads widely) to other organs. In men, gonorrhea can cause acute, painful inflammation of the prostate, epididymis, and periurethral glands and can lead to sterility. In women, it can cause PID, endometritis, salpingitis, and pelvic peritonitis. Sexual behaviors and community prevalence are risk factors for gonorrhea (CDC, 2017b).

Manifestations

Manifestations of gonorrhea in men include dysuria and serous, milky, or purulent discharge from the penis (**Figure 50.5** ■). Some men also experience regional lymphadenopathy. About 20% of men and 80% of women remain asymptomatic until the disease is advanced. Women with symptoms experience dysuria, urinary frequency, abnormal menses (increased flow or dysmenorrhea), increased vaginal discharge, and dyspareunia.

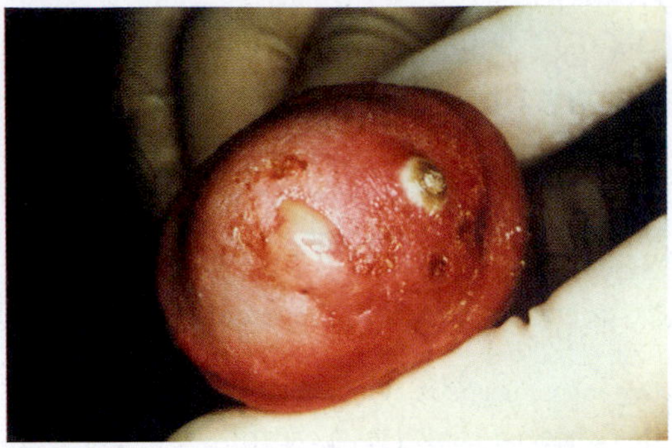

Figure 50.5 ■ Purulent penile discharge resulting from gonorrhea.

Anorectal gonorrhea is seen most often in homosexual men. The manifestations include pruritus, mucopurulent rectal discharge, rectal bleeding and pain, and constipation. Gonococcal pharyngitis occurs primarily in homosexual or bisexual men or heterosexual women after oral sexual contact with an infected partner. The manifestations include fever, sore throat, and enlarged lymph glands.

Complications

The complications of untreated gonorrhea in both men and women may be permanent and serious. They include:

- PID in women, leading to internal abscesses, chronic pain, ectopic pregnancy, and infertility
- Blindness, infection of joints, and potentially lethal infections of the blood in the newborn, contracted during delivery
- Epididymitis and prostatitis in men, resulting in infertility and dysuria
- Spread of the infection to the blood and joints
- Increased susceptibility to, and transmission of, HIV.

Interprofessional Care

The goals of treatment for the patient with gonorrhea include eradication of the organism and any coexisting disease and prevention of reinfection or transmission. It is important to emphasize the importance of taking all medications as prescribed and abstaining from sexual contact until the infection is cured in both patient and partners. Condom use to prevent future infections is essential, particularly for pregnant women whose partners may be infected.

Diagnosis

Diagnosis of gonorrhea is based on NAAT of specimens obtained from infected mucous membranes (cervix, urethra, rectum, or throat) or a urine specimen. Culture and sensitivity testing is performed for gonorrhea infection that is resistant to treatment. Testing for other STIs (especially chlamydia and syphilis) at the same time is recommended. Pregnant women are routinely screened during their first prenatal visit.

Medications

Per CDC recommendations, the treatment of *N. gonorrhoeae* has changed in recent years due to the emergence of antibiotic resistances. Now a dual therapy of ceftriaxone with azithromycin is the recommended treatment (CDC, 2017b). Because patients with gonorrhea are frequently also infected with *C. trachomatis*, concurrent treatment is recommended.

Nursing Care

In planning and implementing care for the patient with gonorrhea, the nurse considers the possible coexistence of other STIs such as syphilis and HIV, the impact of the disease and its treatment on the patient's lifestyle, and the likelihood of nonadherence to the treatment plan. See the Case Study & Nursing Care Plan for the patient with gonorrhea on page 1846.

Assessment

- Health history: Difficult or painful urination, frequency; discharge from penis or vagina; change in menses or painful intercourse (women); other symptoms such as sore throat, fever, swollen or tender lymph nodes; sexual activity including number of partners, use of safer sex practices including condom use; previous STIs and their treatment
- Physical assessment: Presence of penile, vaginal, or anal discharge, regional lymphadenopathy.

Signs and symptoms may be nonexistent as well, especially in women.

Priorities of Care

Collaborating with the interprofessional team to ensure adequate treatment of gonorrhea while providing care that supports the physical and psychologic responses to the infection is a priority of nursing care.

Diagnoses, Outcomes, and Interventions

Nursing diagnoses discussed in this section focus on nonadherence and impaired social interaction.

Promote Adherence with Therapeutic Regimen. Although one-time treatment with the recommended antibiotic is highly effective in curing gonorrhea, nonadherence to the doxycycline regimen may leave any coexisting chlamydial infection unresolved. Noncompliance with recommendations for abstinence, follow-up, or condom use fosters a high rate of reinfection. Failure to refer partners for examination and treatment also leads to reinfection.

Expected Outcome: Patient will demonstrate compliance with therapeutic regimen by reporting abstinence, utilization of safer sex interventions, and taking medications as prescribed related to the infection.

The nurse will:

- Reinforce the need to take all medications as directed and keep follow-up appointments to be sure no reinfection has occurred. Discuss the prevalence of gonorrhea and the potential complications if it is not cured. *The patient who understands the complications of incomplete or failed treatment is more likely to adhere to the medication regimen.*
- Discuss the importance of sexual abstinence until the infection is cured, referral of partners, and consistent and correct condom use to prevent reinfection. *Understanding that cure is possible and reinfection is avoidable helps the patient cope with the disease and its treatment and is likely to increase compliance.*

Promote Social Interaction. Diagnosis of any STI can make patients feel ashamed, guilty about their sexual behaviors, and unworthy to be with others.

Expected Outcome: Patient will demonstrate social interaction skills by communicating with friends and family members.

The nurse will:

- Provide privacy, confidentiality, and a safe, nonjudgmental environment for expression of concerns. Help the patient understand that gonorrhea is a consequence of sexual behavior, not a punishment, and that it can be avoided in the future. *Being treated with respect and privacy helps the patient realize that the disease does not change an individual's worth as a person. This knowledge enhances the patient's ability to relate to others.*

Transitions of Care

Health teaching focuses on helping patients understand the importance of (1) taking any and all prescribed medication, (2) referring sexual partners for evaluation and treatment, (3) abstaining from all sexual contact until the patient and partners are cured, and (4) using a condom to avoid transmitting or contracting infections in the future. Patients also need to understand the need for a follow-up visit 4 to 7 days after treatment is completed.

The Patient with Syphilis

Syphilis is a complex systemic STI caused by the spirochete *Treponema pallidum*, and it can infect almost any body tissue or organ. It is transmitted from open lesions during any sexual contact (genital, oral–genital, or anal–genital). The organism is highly susceptible to heat and drying, but can survive for days in fluids; thus, it may also be transmitted by infected blood or other body fluid such as saliva. The incubation period ranges from 10 to 90 days, averaging 21 days. If not treated appropriately, syphilis can lead to blindness, paralysis, mental illness, cardiovascular damage, and death. Syphilis often occurs with one or more other STIs, such as HIV/AIDS or chlamydial infection.

In 2000, the rate of syphilis infection reached its lowest level since reporting began in 1941. Unfortunately, since 2001, the rate of syphilis infection increased annually, with 27,814 cases of primary and secondary syphilis (8.7 cases per 100,000 people in the United States) reported in 2016 (CDC, 2017b).

Case Study & Nursing Care Plan

A Patient with Gonorrhea

Janet Cirit, a 33-year-old legal secretary, lives in a suburban Midwestern community. She is dating a man named Jim Adkins, who lives in an adjacent suburb. Ms. Cirit visits her gynecologist because her periods have become irregular and she is experiencing pelvic pain and an abnormal amount of vaginal discharge. Recently, she has developed a sore throat. The pelvic pain has begun to disrupt her sleeping pattern, and she is concerned that she might have cancer because her mother recently died of ovarian cancer.

ASSESSMENT

When Ms. Cirit arrives for her appointment at the gynecologist's office, Marsha Davidson, the nurse practitioner, interviews her. Ms. Davidson completes a thorough medical and sexual history, including questions about her menstrual periods, pain associated with urination or sexual intercourse, urinary frequency, most recent Pap test, birth control method, history of STI and drug use, and types of sexual activity. Ms. Cirit reports her symptoms and her concern about ovarian cancer. She also indicates that she is taking oral contraceptives and therefore sees no need for her boyfriend to use a condom because she believes their relationship is monogamous.

Physical examination reveals both pharyngeal and cervical inflammation and lower abdominal tenderness. Her temperature is 37.0°C (98.5°F). There are no signs or symptoms of pregnancy.

The gynecologist orders a Pap test and cultures of the cervix, urethra, and pharynx to evaluate for gonorrhea and chlamydial infection. Blood is drawn for WBC. Test results are positive for gonorrhea and negative for chlamydia. The WBC is slightly elevated, indicating possible salpingitis. Because Mr. Adkins has been Ms. Cirit's only sexual partner, it is clear that he is the source of infection and needs to be treated as well.

DIAGNOSES

- Acute pain related to the infectious process
- Anxiety due to shame and guilt because of having an STI
- Needs education related to possibility of reinfection

EXPECTED OUTCOMES

- Patient will experience relief of pain, indicating that the infection has been eradicated.
- Patient will verbalize that she has nothing to be ashamed of and that she has been wise to seek treatment as soon as symptoms occurred.
- Patient will verbalize that she will insist her partner use condoms during future sexual activity.

PLANNING AND IMPLEMENTATION

- Administer ceftriaxone IM and azithromycin PO as ordered.
- Emphasize the need for regular Pap smears and pelvic examinations because of the family history of ovarian cancer.
- Discuss feelings and concerns about the diagnosis of gonorrhea. Stress that such a diagnosis does not reflect on one's self-worth as a person.
- Teach how to talk with a future sexual partner about condom use.

EVALUATION

A week later during her follow-up visit, Ms. Cirit states that she is feeling much better and sleeping well at night since the pain has ended. She has terminated her relationship with Mr. Adkins and is considering joining a health club in the hope of increasing her level of fitness and perhaps meeting someone new.

CLINICAL REASONING IN PATIENT CARE

1. How are Ms. Cirit's manifestations related to the infectious process of gonorrhea?
2. Should the nurse have suggested that Ms. Cirit also be tested for HIV? Why or why not?
3. Develop a care plan for Ms. Cirit for helping her plan a discussion with Mr. Adkins about the diagnosis.

See Evaluating Your Response Appendix B.

Pathophysiology

Any break in the skin or mucous membrane is vulnerable to invasion by the spirochete. Once it has entered the system, the spirochete is spread through the blood and lymphatic system. Congenital syphilis is transferred to the fetus through the placental circulation. Syphilis is generally characterized by three clinical stages: Primary, secondary, and tertiary.

Primary Syphilis

The primary stage of syphilis is characterized by the appearance of a **chancre** (**Figure 50.6** ■) and by regional

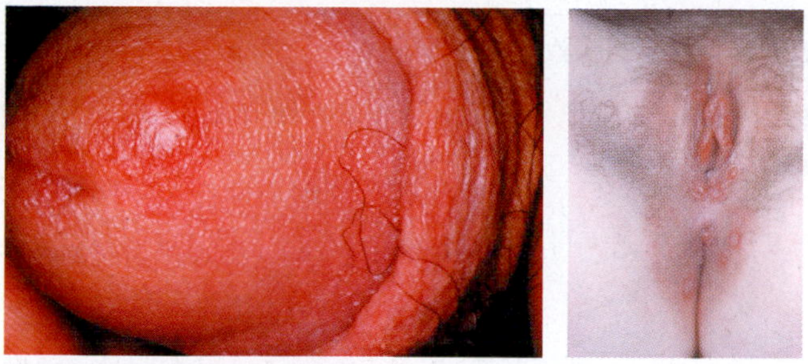

A B

Figure 50.6 ■ Chancre of primary syphilis on **A**, the penis, and **B**, the vulva.

enlargement of lymph nodes; little or no pain accompanies these early signs. The chancre appears at the site of inoculation (such as the genitals, anus, mouth, breast, fingers) 3 to 4 weeks after the infectious contact. In women, a genital chancre may go unnoticed, disappearing within 4 to 6 weeks. In both primary and secondary stages, syphilis remains highly infectious, even if no symptoms are evident.

Secondary Syphilis

Manifestations of secondary syphilis may appear any time from 2 weeks to 6 months after the initial chancre disappears. These symptoms can include a skin rash, especially on the palms of the hands or soles of the feet, mucous patches in the oral cavity; sore throat; generalized lymphadenopathy; condyloma lata (flat, broad-based papules, unlike the pedunculated structure of genital warts) on the labia, anus, or corner of the mouth; flulike symptoms; and alopecia. These manifestations generally disappear within 2 to 6 weeks, and an asymptomatic latency period begins.

Latent and Tertiary Syphilis

The latent stage of syphilis begins 2 or more years after the initial infection and can last up to 50 years. During this stage, no symptoms of syphilis are apparent, and the disease is not transmissible by sexual contact. It can be transmitted by infected blood, however. Thus, all prospective blood donors must be screened for syphilis. In two-thirds of all cases, the latent stage persists without further complications. Unless treated, the remaining one-third of infected people progress to late-stage or tertiary syphilis. In the presence of HIV infection, disease progression seems to be more rapid.

Two types of late-stage syphilis occur. Benign late syphilis, of rapid onset, is characterized by localized development of infiltrating tumors (*gummas*) in skin, bones, and liver, generally responding promptly to treatment. Of more insidious onset is a diffuse inflammatory response that involves the central nervous system and the cardiovascular system. Though the disease can still be treated at this stage, much of the cardiovascular and central nervous system damage is irreversible.

Risk Factors

The incidence of primary and secondary syphilis is highest in people 20 to 29 years of age and has increased in all age categories from 15 to 64 years. In 2016, men accounted for almost 90% of all cases of primary and secondary syphilis, and almost 60% of them were in men who have sex with men. Rates of primary and secondary syphilis increased in all ethnic groups in 2016 and were highest in Black populations (23.3 per 100,000). There is a high rate of co-infection with HIV (CDC, 2017b).

Manifestations

Each of the stages of syphilis has characteristic manifestations (see **Table 50.3**). The patient with syphilis may also experience a latency period when no signs of the disease are evident.

Interprofessional Care

The goals of treatment are to inactivate the spirochete and educate the patient about how to prevent reinfection or further transmission. Treatment includes antibiotic therapy and identification and referral of partners for testing and treatment if necessary, follow-up testing, and education about condom use to prevent reinfection of self and transmission of disease to partners. In addition, patients should be screened for chlamydial infection and advised to have an HIV test.

Diagnosis

Diagnosis of syphilis is complex because it mimics many other diseases. A careful history and physical examination are obtained, as well as laboratory evaluations of lesions and blood.

The VDRL (Venereal Disease Research Laboratory) and RPR (rapid plasma reagin) blood tests measure antibody production. People with syphilis become positive about 4 to 6 weeks after infection. However, these tests are not specific for syphilis and other diseases may also cause positive results. Additional tests are required for definitive diagnosis.

The FTA-ABS (fluorescent treponemal antibody absorption) test is specific for *T. pallidum* and can be used to confirm VDRL and RPR findings. It may be used for patients whose clinical picture indicates syphilis but who have negative VDRL results. In immunofluorescent staining a specimen is obtained from early lesions or aspiration of lymph nodes and is specially treated and examined microscopically for the presence of *T. pallidum*. Dark-field microscopy involves examining a specimen from the chancre for the presence of *T. pallidum* using a dark-field microscope.

Medications

The treatment of choice for all stages of syphilis in adults is penicillin G, given intramuscularly (IM) in a single dose. Patients allergic to penicillin are given oral doxycycline or tetracycline for 28 days. For those who have had syphilis more than a year, additional doses may be needed.

Treatment of syphilis may result in a severe reaction called the *Jarisch-Herxheimer reaction*, involving fever, musculoskeletal pain, tachycardia, and sometimes hypotension. This is not a reaction to the penicillin itself, but to the sudden and massive destruction of spirochetes by the penicillin

Table 50.3 Manifestations of Syphilis by Body System and Stage

System	Primary Syphilis	Secondary Syphilis	Tertiary Syphilis
Reproductive	■ Genital chancre (may be internal in female)	■ Condyloma lata	
Integumentary		■ Rash on palms of hands and soles of feet	■ Granulomatous lesions involving mucous membranes and skin
Gastrointestinal		■ Anorexia ■ Oral mucous patches	
Neurologic		■ Asymptomatic ■ Meningitis ■ Headache ■ Cranial neuropathies	■ Asymptomatic ■ Tabes dorsalis ■ Neurosyphilis ■ Seizures, hemiparesis, hemiplegia ■ Personality changes, hyperactive reflexes, Argyll Robertson pupil (pupils that do not constrict when exposed to light but will accommodate when looking at a near object), decreased memory, slurred speech, optic atrophy
Musculoskeletal		■ Arthralgias ■ Myalgia ■ Bone and joint arthritis ■ Periostitis	■ Gummas
Cardiovascular			■ Aortic insufficiency ■ Aortic aneurysm ■ Stenosis of openings to coronary arteries
Renal		■ Glomerulonephritis ■ Nephrotic syndrome	
Other	■ Regional lymphadenopathy	■ Generalized lymphadenopathy ■ Fever ■ Malaise ■ Hepatitis ■ Alopecia	

and the resulting release of toxins into the bloodstream. The Jarisch-Herxheimer reaction generally begins within 24 hours of treatment and subsides in another 24 hours. Treatment should not be discontinued unless symptoms become life-threatening.

Nursing Care

In planning and implementing nursing care for the patient with syphilis, the nurse needs to consider the patient's age, lifestyle, access to healthcare, and educational level. Although each patient has individualized needs, nursing diagnoses for the patient with syphilis would be the same as for any patient with an STI. See the Case Study & Nursing Care Plan for a patient with syphilis on page 1850.

Assessment

- Health history: Current or history of a painless genital lesion, rash on hands or feet, sore throat or flulike symptoms; recent and past sexual activity including number of partners, use of safer sex practices including condom use; previous STIs and their treatment
- Physical assessment: Inspection of genitalia for chancre or flat, broad-based papules; inspect palms and soles of feet for rash, mouth for mucous patches; palpate for lymphadenopathy.

Priorities of Care

Collaborating with the interprofessional team to ensure appropriate treatment of syphilis while providing care that supports symptom relief, prevention of future transmission, and physical and psychologic responses to this diagnosis is a priority of nursing care.

Diagnoses, Outcomes, and Interventions

Nursing priorities discussed in this section focus on reducing risk for injury and anxiety and promoting self-esteem.

Reduce Risk for Injury. If syphilis is not diagnosed and treated promptly and effectively, it can have devastating effects on all body systems, particularly the neurologic and cardiovascular systems, eventually leading to a painful death.

Expected Outcome: Patient will demonstrate adherence to the therapeutic regimen to reduce risk of infection progression.

The nurse will:

- Teach the importance of taking all prescribed medication. *Taking the prescribed antibiotic is important to ensure eradication of the infecting organism.*
- Encourage referral of sexual partners for evaluation and any necessary treatment. *Without treatment of both*

partners, reinfection can occur or the disease may be transmitted to other people through sexual activity.

- Teach abstinence from sexual contact until patient and partners are cured and to use condoms to prevent future infections. *Abstinence until the organism is eradicated prevents reinfection. Condoms provide barrier protection, reducing the risk of infection during sexual activity.*
- Emphasize the importance of returning for follow-up testing at 3- and 6-month intervals for early syphilis and 6- and 12-month intervals for late latent syphilis. *Follow-up testing is performed to ensure eradication of the disease.*
- Provide information about manifestations of reinfection. *Successful treatment of the disease does not prevent possible subsequent infections.*

Reduce Anxiety. The diagnosis of syphilis understandably causes the patient anxiety, not only about personal well-being but also about the well-being of partners and, in the expectant woman, her fetus.

Expected Outcome: Patient will demonstrate management of anxiety through information seeking and use of coping skills and relaxation techniques.

The nurse will:

- Emphasize that syphilis can be effectively treated, preventing the serious complications of late-stage disease. *This information provides a sense of control and helps decrease anxiety.*
- Teach the pregnant patient that taking medications as directed and returning each month for follow-up testing will help ensure the well-being of her baby. *Knowing that treatment can reduce the risk to her baby relieves anxiety and possibly increases compliance.*

Promote Healthy Self-Esteem. Living with any chronic disease can be damaging to an individual's self-esteem. However, the patient with syphilis needs additional support to cope with the stigma of this kind of infection. Unfortunately, the populations most affected by STIs often lack family and other social support networks.

Expected Outcome: Patient will demonstrate self-esteem related to sexual patterns as evidenced by verbalization of self-acceptance related to stigma of syphilis diagnosis.

The nurse will:

- Create an environment in which the patient feels respected and safe to discuss questions and concerns about the disease and its effect on his or her life. *Being treated with respect helps enhance self-esteem.*
- Provide privacy and confidentiality. *Patients are often embarrassed to discuss the intimate details of their sex lives.*
- Let patients know that the nurse and other healthcare providers care about them and the successful treatment of their disease. *Feeling valued enhances self-esteem.*

Transitions of Care

Education is an essential part of nursing care for the patient with any STI, and syphilis is no exception. The nurse emphasizes that untreated syphilis is a chronic disease that can be spread to others even though no symptoms are evident. Address the following topics:

- Taking all prescribed medication
- Referring sexual partners for evaluation and treatment
- Abstaining from all sexual contact as recommended by CDC guidelines
- Using condoms correctly and consistently to avoid transmitting or contracting infections in the future
- The need for follow-up testing (at 3 and 6 months for patients with primary or secondary syphilis and at 6 and 12 months for those with late-stage disease). If patients are HIV positive, follow-up visits are recommended 1, 2, 3, 6, 9, and 12 months after treatment.

The Patient with Pelvic Inflammatory Disease

Pelvic inflammatory disease (PID) is a term used to describe infection of the pelvic organs, including the fallopian tubes (*salpingitis*), ovaries (*oophoritis*), cervix (*cervicitis*), endometrium (*endometritis*), pelvic peritoneum, and the pelvic vascular system. PID can be caused by one or more infectious agents, including *Neisseria gonorrhoeae, Chlamydia trachomatis, Haemophilus influenzae*, and enteric Gram-negative rods. *N. gonorrhoeae* and *C. trachomatis* are responsible for most PID; dual infection with both agents is common.

PID is not a reportable disease in the United States; however, it is estimated that more than 4% of women in the United States have been treated for PID at some point during their lifetimes (Kreisel, Torrone, Bernstein, Hong, & Gorwitz, 2017). As a result of the infection, some women become infertile and the risk for ectopic pregnancies is increased by six times. The disease may also cause pelvic abscesses and chronic abdominal pain.

Sexually active women age 16 to 24 are most at risk. Risk factors include a history of sexually transmitted infection (especially gonorrhea and chlamydia), bacterial vaginosis, multiple sexual partners, douching, and previous PID. Barrier contraceptive devices such as condoms reduce the risk of PID.

The prognosis depends on the number of episodes, promptness of treatment, and modification of risk-taking behaviors. Prevention includes educating women, especially young women, regarding the causes and transmission of infection and methods of self-protection, such as avoiding unprotected sexual activity.

Pathophysiology

Pelvic inflammatory disease is usually polymicrobial (caused by more than one microbe) in origin, with gonorrhea and chlamydia being common causative organisms. Pathogenic organisms ascend from the vagina via the endocervical canal to the fallopian tubes and ovaries. The endocervical canal is slightly dilated during menstruation, allowing bacteria to enter the uterus. Once in the reproductive tract, the organisms rapidly multiply and ascend to the fallopian tubes and ovaries. The infection can extend beyond

Case Study & Nursing Care Plan

A Patient with Syphilis

Eddie Kratz, age 22, works as a bellman at a large hotel. For the past year, he has shared a small apartment with Maria Jones, who is 6 months pregnant with his child. Although he intends to marry Ms. Jones before the baby is born, he has continued a previous relationship with a woman named Justine Simpson. His sexual activities with Ms. Simpson have increased in frequency as Ms. Jones's pregnancy has advanced. Recently Mr. Kratz has noticed a swelling in his groin and a sore on his penis.

ASSESSMENT

When Mr. Kratz comes to the community clinic, he is interviewed by the NP, Sally Morovitz. She takes a thorough medical and sexual history, including questions about drug use, allergies, difficulty with urination, urinary frequency, itching or discharge from the penis, recent sexual activities, precautions taken against infection, history of STIs, and sexual function. She determines that Mr. Kratz has been having unprotected sex with both Ms. Jones and Ms. Simpson. He believes that Ms. Jones is not having sex with anyone except him, but he is not sure.

Physical assessment reveals a classic syphilitic chancre on the shaft of the penis and regional lymphadenopathy. A specimen of exudates from the chancre is sent for dark-field examination. Ms. Morovitz discusses with Mr. Kratz the likelihood that he has syphilis and the need to tell both Ms. Jones and Ms. Simpson so that they can be tested and, if necessary, treated. Ms. Morovitz also suggests that Mr. Kratz be tested for HIV because he has been having unprotected sex with two women, at least one of whom may be sexually active with other partners. He agrees, and blood is drawn for an ELISA test. Dark-field analysis of the chancre exudate confirms the diagnosis of syphilis; the ELISA results are negative for HIV.

DIAGNOSES

- Potential for injury to the patient, his partners, and the infant due to diagnosis of syphilis
- Needs education about the disease process, its transmission, and the need for treatment
- Stress and anxiety related to the diagnosis and its effect on his relationships

EXPECTED OUTCOMES

- Patient will acknowledge the importance of prompt treatment to cure syphilis.
- Patient will verbalize understanding for the need to abstain from sexual contact during treatment, complete all medications, return for follow-up visits, and use condoms to prevent reinfection.
- Patient will verbalize ability to cope with the effect of diagnosis and treatment on the relationship.
- Patient will verbalize decreased anxiety following education and treatment.

PLANNING AND IMPLEMENTATION

- Administer IM injection of penicillin G as ordered.
- Discuss the importance of abstaining from sexual activity until he and his partners are cured and of using condoms to prevent reinfection.
- Explain the need to return for follow-up testing in 3 months and again at 6 months. Provide a copy of the STI prevention checklist, and document that reminders need to be sent at 3- and 6-month intervals.
- Notify sexual partners that they need to come to the clinic for testing.
- Refer to a social worker for counseling about the effect of the disease on the couple's relationship.
- Teach the couple about the importance of treatment for the health of their infant.

EVALUATION

At the 3-month follow-up visit, the chancre on Mr. Kratz's penis has healed, and he reports that he is using a condom any time he has sex. Ms. Jones has also tested positive for syphilis and negative for HIV, so she, too, has been given penicillin G and verbal and written follow-up instructions, including follow-up until the infant is born. The couple is meeting every other week with the social worker and say that their relationship is improving. Ms. Simpson has received similar test results and has been given a prescription for doxycycline because she is allergic to penicillin.

CLINICAL REASONING IN PATIENT CARE

1. What manifestations might a patient with early syphilis experience?
2. List some appropriate questions for taking a sexual history when you suspect the presence of one or more STIs.
3. How might you counsel Mr. Kratz to help him break the news of the diagnosis to Ms. Jones?

See Evaluating Your Response in Appendix B.

the reproductive tract to involve the peritoneum (peritonitis or peritoneal abscess) or other abdominal organs.

Manifestations and Complications

Manifestations of PID include fever, purulent vaginal discharge, abnormal bleeding, lower abdominal or back pain, dyspareunia, and painful cervical movement. However, the manifestations may be so mild that the infection is not recognized. Complications include pelvic abscess, infertility, ectopic pregnancy, chronic pelvic pain, and pelvic adhesions. Abscess formation is common.

Interprofessional Care

The goals of treatment are to eliminate the infection and prevent complications and recurrence. The physical examination may reveal abdominal, adnexal, and cervical pain.

Diagnosis

Tests used in the diagnosis of PID may include a CBC with differential, which will show a markedly elevated WBC and an increased sedimentation rate. If a laparoscopy or laparotomy is done, it may reveal inflammation, edema, or hyperemia of the fallopian tubes or tubal discharge and, possibly, generalized pelvic involvement, abscesses, and scarring.

Medications

Combination antibiotic therapy with at least two broad-spectrum antibiotics administered IV or orally is the typical treatment for PID. If PID is not acute, outpatient antibiotic therapy is prescribed. In acute cases, however, the patient may be hospitalized. Analgesics are given, and antibiotics and fluids are administered intravenously. Commonly prescribed antibiotics include parental cefoxitin (Mefoxin) or clindamycin (Cleocin), plus gentamicin (Garamycin) or doxycycline (Vibramycin). Nursing implications for antibiotic use are discussed in Chapter 12.

Surgery

Surgery may be performed to drain an abscess or treat a life-threatening complication such as rupture of a fallopian tube or abscess.

Nursing Care

The goals of nursing care are to treat the infection and to prevent complications, such as scarring and infertility. The patient who is hospitalized maintains bedrest in the semi-Fowler position to promote drainage and to localize the infectious process in the pelvic cavity.

Assessment

See the Manifestations and Interprofessional Care sections for the assessment of the patient with pelvic inflammatory disease.

Priorities of Care

Collaborating with the interprofessional team to ensure adequate treatment of pelvic inflammatory disease while providing care that supports optimal function and physical and psychologic responses to the disorder is a priority of nursing care.

Diagnoses, Interventions, and Outcomes

Priorities of care for the patient with PID include reducing the risk for complications from the infection and patient education about complications.

Reduce Risk for Complications. PID can have severe, even life-threatening, complications. Scarring of fallopian tubes can lead to ectopic pregnancy or pelvic abscess. Infertility is a common complication, as are recurrent or chronic PID, chronic abdominal pain, pelvic adhesions, hysterectomy, and depression. The woman who has severe infection and manifestations may be hospitalized for treatment.

Expected Outcome: Patient will recover from PID without long-term sequelae.

The nurse will:

- Administer antibiotic therapy as ordered and monitor closely for adverse effects. *Antibiotics used in acute PID are potent agents; some can have serious side effects.*
- Practice thorough hand hygiene and strict adherence to standard precautions when handling perineal pads and linens. Appropriate disinfection of bedpans, toilet seats, linens, and utensils is also important. *These practices help avoid disseminating the infection to others.*

Provide Patient Teaching. PID is most common in young women, and many of them do not understand their own anatomy and physiology or STIs. Diagnosis and treatment of PID offer an opportunity to increase that understanding, thereby preventing complications and recurrent infection.

Expected Outcome: Patient will demonstrate knowledge about PID by verbalizing understanding of PID pathophysiology and consequences of untreated infection.

The nurse will:

- Explain how infection is spread and what measures to take to prevent future infection. *Understanding can improve compliance with treatment regimens and perhaps change high-risk behavior.*
- Explain the need to complete the treatment regimen and the importance of follow-up visits. If the patient or partner fails to take all of the medication as prescribed, the infection may not be completely cured. *Nonadherence and recurrence are common, particularly if follow-up appointments are not kept.*
- Teach proper perineal care, especially wiping from front to back. *This reduces transmission of fecal organisms to reproductive tissues and reduces the incidence of urinary tract infections.*
- Caution the patient about using tampons. Instruct the patient to change tampons or pads at least every 4 hours. *Menstrual flow and other discharges provide a favorable environment for microorganisms to multiply.*
- Provide information about safer sex practices and family planning. Instruct the patient to remove diaphragm within 6 hours after use. IUDs are contraindicated. Latex condoms offer the most effective protection against infection. *These measures help prevent recurrence of infection.*

- Teach the patient to report any unusual vaginal discharge or odor to the healthcare provider. *Treatment is most effective early in the disease process.*

Delegating Nursing Care Activities

As appropriate and allowed by the designated duties and responsibilities of unlicensed assistive personnel, the nurse may delegate nursing care activities such as collecting vital signs, measuring intake and output, and assisting with hygiene and activities as allowed.

Transitions of Care

Provide general information related to STIs. Teach measures to eradicate the infection and prevent recurrence and help the patient deal with the physical and psychosocial implications of treatment, including possible infertility. Inform the patient that the patency of the fallopian tubes can be evaluated after several menstrual cycles; this delay allows for complete resolution of the inflammatory process.

CHAPTER HIGHLIGHTS

50.1 Overview of Sexually Transmitted Infections

Describe the characteristics of sexually transmitted infections, as well as the key factors in their prevention and control.

- Sexually transmitted infections (STIs) are infections transmitted by sexual contact, including vaginal, oral, and anal intercourse. STIs affect women more than men and are more common in people who have multiple sexual partners, abuse drugs, and are of lower socioeconomic status.
- STIs can coexist in the same person and can be transmitted by either heterosexual or homosexual contact. Effective treatment mandates that both sexual partners be treated. Most STIs can be prevented by using latex condoms.

50.2 Viral Sexually Transmitted Infections

Describe the pathophysiology and manifestations of viral sexually transmitted diseases, including genital herpes and human papillomavirus, and outline the interprofessional care and nursing care of patients with these disorders.

- Genital herpes, caused by an infection with an HSV virus, is a commonly occurring STI in teens and young adults.
- There is no cure for genital herpes and treatment is primarily symptomatic. Nursing care is directed toward relieving the pain of the lesions, mitigating sexual dysfunction, and relieving anxiety.
- Human papillomavirus (HPV) is the most commonly occurring STI in the United States. Some strains cause genital warts, a chronic, incurable STI manifested by warts of various forms. Other strains cause no initial symptoms but are associated with cancers of the cervix, vulva, and penis, as well as oropharyngeal cancer.
- Infection with HPV poses a major risk for cervical cancer. A vaccine against the virus is recommended for adolescent boys and girls and young women.

50.3 Bacterial Sexually Transmitted Infections

Describe the pathophysiology and manifestations of bacterial sexually transmitted diseases, including vaginal infection, chlamydia, gonorrhea, syphilis, and pelvic inflammatory disease, and outline the interprofessional care and nursing care of patients with these disorders.

- Urogenital infections include vaginal infections (bacterial vaginosis, candidiasis, and trichomoniasis), chlamydia, gonorrhea, syphilis, and pelvic inflammatory disease (PID).
- Chlamydia, occurring most in young adults under age 25, is a bacterial infection that can spread to the uterus and fallopian tubes in women, causing PID, infertility, and ectopic pregnancy. Untreated chlamydia in men may result in epididymitis, prostatitis, sterility, and Reiter syndrome.
- Gonorrhea (caused by a bacteria) and syphilis (caused by a spirochete) affect both men and women and may infect the newborn as it moves through the birth canal in an untreated woman.
- Syphilis, if untreated, exists in the body in three stages, with the third stage lasting up to 50 years.
- Nursing care of gonorrhea and syphilis focus on education, preventing injury from complications, relieving anxiety, and supporting self-esteem.
- PID is an infection of the female pelvic organs and may be caused by one or more infectious agents.
- Sexually active young women between ages 16 and 24 are most at risk for PID. The prognosis depends on the number of episodes, promptness of treatment, and modification of risk-taking behaviors. The goals of nursing care are to treat the infection and prevent complications.

TEST YOURSELF NCLEX-RN® REVIEW

1. The nurse is preparing a community health session on sexually transmitted infections. Which population should the nurse emphasize as being most often affected by these infections?
   A. Men
   B. Women
   C. Older adults
   D. Adolescent males
2. The nurse is evaluating teaching provided to a patient with a sexually transmitted infection. Which patient statement indicates an understanding of the treatment for the infection?
   A. "I know I can never have sex again."
   B. "My sex partner and I must both take medication."
   C. "I will douche after every sexual encounter with my partner."
   D. "My sex partner does not have an infection, so won't need medication."
3. The nurse is teaching a male patient about using condoms to prevent sexually transmitted infections. What topics should the nurse include with this teaching? (Select all that apply.)
   A. Withdraw when the penis is erect.
   B. Use a new condom with each sex act.
   C. Handle carefully to ensure no damage.
   D. Ensure a small amount of air in the tip.
   E. Use oil-based lubricants, such as petroleum jelly.
4. While assessing a young male patient, the nurse notes blisters and ulcerations on the shaft of the penis. The patient reports he had "a similar rash a few months ago, but it went away." The nurse would assess for the presence of which additional symptoms of the most likely health problem? (Select all that apply,)
   A. Headache
   B. Nausea
   C. Fever
   D. Enlarged lymph nodes
   E. Regional edema
5. The nurse is preparing an educational session on genital warts for high school students. Which information about this sexually transmitted infection should the nurse include? (Select all that apply.)
   A. The infection cannot be cured.
   B. Cancer risk is higher in those affected.
   C. The infection is caused by a yeast organism.
   D. Many of those affected are unaware they are infected.
   E. The infection can be spread by any type of intercourse.
6. The nurse is counseling a young sexually active female patient diagnosed with a human papillomavirus genital infection. What screening test should the nurse recommend the patient have annually?
   A. Stool for occult blood
   B. Pelvic exam and Pap smear
   C. Breast exam and mammogram
   D. CBC to detect anemia and infection
7. A patient is concerned that she may have a vaginal yeast infection. The nurse would assess for the presence of which additional assessment findings to validate the patient's concern? (Select all that apply.)
   A. Report of painful intercourse
   B. Itching of vulvar area
   C. Drainage with a "fishy" odor
   D. Whitish drainage with curdled appearance
   E. Redness of vulvar area
8. The nurse is teaching a female patient with a sexually transmitted infection. What should the nurse recommend to relieve genital discomfort caused by the infection?
   A. Cut fingernails short.
   B. Douche frequently.
   C. Wear cotton underwear.
   D. Have sex more frequently.
9. The nurse is reviewing the mechanism of infection with the gonorrhea organism during health class with high school students. On which body parts should the nurse explain that the organism initially targets?
   A. Male prostate
   B. Female vulva and vagina
   C. Male urethra and female cervix
   D. Male and female external genitalia
10. A patient newly diagnosed with syphilis asks the nurse to explain the disease. What should the nurse include when teaching the patient about this sexually transmitted infection?
    A. Syphilis is caused by a virus.
    B. Syphilis is a systemic infection.
    C. Cases of syphilis are declining in the United States.
    D. Once the chancre is healed, the disease is cured.

See Test Yourself answers in Appendix B.

REFERENCES

Adams, M. P., Holland, L. N., & Urban, C. (2017). *Pharmacology for nursing: A pathophysiologic approach* (5th ed.). Hoboken, NJ: Pearson Education.

Centers for Disease Control and Prevention (CDC). (2010). Sexually transmitted diseases treatment guidelines. *Morbidity and Mortality Weekly Report, 59*(No. RR-12), 1–112.

Centers for Disease Control and Prevention (CDC). (2015a). *Chlamydia infections*. Retrieved from https://www.cdc.gov/std/tg2015/chlamydia.htm.

Centers for Disease Control and Prevention (CDC). (2015b). *Lymphogranuloma venereum (LGV)*. Retrieved from https://www.cdc.gov/std/tg2015/lgv.htm.

Centers for Disease Control and Prevention (CDC). (2016). *Parent and teen information on HPV*. Retrieved from https://www.cdc.gov/vaccines/parents/diseases/teen/hpv-indepth-color.pdf.

Centers for Disease Control and Prevention (CDC). (2017a). *Genital herpes treatment and care*. Retrieved from https://www.cdc.gov/std/herpes/treatment.htm.

Centers for Disease Control and Prevention (CDC). (2017b). *Sexually transmitted disease surveillance 2016*. Retrieved from https://www.cdc.gov/std/stats16/CDC_2016_STDS_Report-for508WebSep21_2017_1644.pdf.

Centers for Disease Control and Prevention (CDC). (2017c). *STIs and HIVE fact sheet*. Retrieved from https://www.cdc.gov/std/hiv/stdfact-std-hiv.htm.

Centers for Disease Control and Prevention (CDC). (2017d). *What are the risk factors for cervical cancer?* Retrieved from https://www.cdc.gov/cancer/cervical/basic_info/risk_factors.htm.

Centers for Disease Control and Prevention (CDC). (2018a). *HIV among people aged 50 and older*. Retrieved from https://www.cdc.gov/hiv/group/age/olderamericans/index.html.

Centers for Disease Control and Prevention (CDC). (2018b). *Human papillomavirus (HPV)*. Retrieved from https://www.cdc.gov/hpv/index.html.

Centers for Disease Control and Prevention (CDC). (2018c). *Prevention of hepatitis B virus infection in the United States: Recommendations of the advisory community on immunization practices*. Retrieved from https://www.cdc.gov/mmwr/volumes/67/rr/rr6701a1.htm.

Chen, A. C., Lightfoot, M., Szalacha, L. A., & Lindenberg, C. S. (2017). A pilot, Web-based HIV/STI prevention intervention targeting at-risk Mexican American adolescents: Feasibility, acceptability and lessons learned. *Journal of Nursing and Health Care, 4*(2).

Food and Drug Administration (FDA). (2018). *FDA approves expanded use of Gardasil 9 to include individuals 27 through 45 years old*. Retrieved from https://www.fda.gov/NewsEvents/Newsroom/PressAnnouncements/ucm622715.htm.

Kreisel, K., Torrone, E., Bernstein, K., Hong, J., & Gorwitz, R. (2017). Prevalence of pelvic inflammatory disease in sexually experienced women of reproductive age — United States, 2013–2014. *Morbidity and Mortality Weekly Report, 66*, 80–83.

Shields, K., Fox, K. L., & Liebrecht, C. M. (2018). *Pearson nurse's drug guide: 2018*. Hoboken, NJ: Pearson Education.

Sorenson, M., Quinn, L., & Klein, D. (2019). *Pathophysiology: Concepts of human disease*. Hoboken, NJ: Pearson Education.

ADDITIONAL RESOURCES

Centers for Disease Control and Prevention, Sexually Transmitted Diseases
www.cdc.gov/std/default.htm

The STI Foundation
www.stif.org.uk

World Health Organization, Sexual and Reproductive Health
www.who.int/reproductivehealth/topics/rtis/en/

Appendix A Standard Precautions

Standard precautions are designed to reduce the risk of transmission of microorganisms from both recognized and unrecognized sources of infection. They are the primary strategies for preventing nosocomial infections within institutions and are important to protect healthcare workers as well. Standard precautions apply to (1) blood; (2) all body fluids, secretions, and excretions except sweat, regardless of whether or not they contain visible blood; (3) nonintact skin; and (4) mucous membranes. Standard precautions are applied to all patients receiving care in any healthcare setting, regardless of their diagnosis or presumed infection status. Although these precautions are specifically designed for healthcare settings, they also may be implemented in providing home care or in other community-based care settings.

Hand Hygiene

- Avoid unnecessary touching of surfaces in the patient-care area.
- Perform hand hygiene (1) after touching blood, body fluids, secretions, excretions, and contaminated items, whether or not gloves are worn; (2) immediately after removing gloves, even if gloves appear to be intact; (3) between contacts with patients; and (4) when otherwise indicated to prevent transfer of organisms to other patients. You may need to wash your hands between tasks and procedures on the same patient to prevent cross-contaminating different body sites.
- Use soap and warm water for hand hygiene when hands are visibly dirty or contaminated with blood, other body fluids, or material containing body proteins.
- If hands are not visibly soiled, use an alcohol-based hand rub for routinely decontaminating hands in all other situations.

Personal Protective Equipment

Gloves

- Wear clean, nonsterile gloves when touching blood, body fluids, secretions, excretions, and contaminated items.
- Put on clean gloves just before touching mucous membranes and nonintact skin.
- Change your gloves between tasks and procedures on the same patient after contact with material that may contain a high concentration of microorganisms.
- Wear gloves for all invasive procedures such as performing venipuncture or other vascular or surgical procedures.
- Wear gloves if you have cuts, scratches, or other breaks in the skin.
- Remove gloves promptly after use, before touching noncontaminated items and surfaces, and before going to another patient; perform hand hygiene immediately after removing gloves.

Mask, Eye Protection, Face Shield

Wear a mask and eye protection or a face shield to protect mucous membranes of your eyes, nose, and mouth during procedures and patient-care activities that are likely to generate splashes or sprays of blood, body fluids, secretions, or excretions (including suctioning of the respiratory tract or endotracheal intubation). Wear a surgical mask when assisting with lumbar puncture or when material is injected into the spinal canal or subdural space.

Gown

Wear a gown (clean, disposable) to protect your skin and prevent soiling of clothing during procedures and patient-care activities that are likely to generate splashes or sprays of blood, body fluids, secretions, or excretions. Remove soiled gowns promptly, washing your hands immediately after gown removal.

Respiratory Hygiene/Cough Etiquette

Implement measures to control respiratory secretions of patients (and people accompanying them) with manifestations of a respiratory infection on entry into the healthcare setting:

- Post signs alerting patients to cover their mouths/noses when coughing or sneezing, to use and dispose of tissues, and to perform hand hygiene after contacting respiratory secretions.
- Provide tissues and no-touch receptacles (e.g., a waste container with a foot pedal) for tissue disposal.
- Provide instructions and resources (e.g., alcohol-based hand rub dispensers) for hand hygiene in or near patient waiting areas.
- As appropriate, offer masks to coughing patients, and encourage them to sit at least 3 feet away from other patients in the waiting area.

Environmental Control

Follow hospital procedures for routine care, cleaning, and disinfecting of environmental surfaces, beds, bed rails, bedside equipment, and other frequently touched surfaces.

Equipment

Handle used patient-care equipment that is soiled with blood, body fluids, secretions, and excretions in a way that prevents exposing your skin and mucous membranes, contaminating your clothing, and transferring microorganisms to other patients or environments. Ensure that reusable equipment is cleaned and appropriately reprocessed before using for the care of another patient.

Linens

Handle and transport linens soiled with blood, body fluids, secretions, and excretions in a manner that prevents exposing your skin and mucous membranes, contaminating your clothing, and transferring microorganisms to other patients and environments. Place soiled linens in leakage-resistant bags at the location where they are used.

Occupational Health and Bloodborne Pathogens

- Take care to prevent injuries when using needles, scalpels, and other sharps; when handling sharp instruments after procedures; when cleaning used instruments; and when disposing of used needles.
- Never recap used needles, manipulate them using both hands, or handle them in a manner that directs the point of a needle toward any part of your body. If it is necessary to protect the needle prior to disposal, use a one-handed "scoop" technique or mechanical device to hold the needle sheath.
- Do not remove used needles from disposable syringes by hand; do not bend, break, or otherwise manipulate used needles by hand.
- Place used disposable syringes and needles, scalpel blades, and other sharp items in appropriate puncture-resistant containers located as close as practical to the area in which the items were used.
- Place reusable syringes and needles in a puncture-resistant container for transport to the reprocessing area.
- Use mouthpieces, resuscitation bags, or other ventilation devices as an alternative to mouth-to-mouth resuscitation methods whenever possible.

Safe Injection Practices

When using needles, cannulas that replace needles, and intravenous delivery systems, do the following:

- Use aseptic technique to avoid contaminating sterile equipment.
- Needles, cannulas, and syringes are single-use items; never use the same syringe, needle, or cannula for more than one patient (even if used to enter or connect to a patient's IV fluid or administration set).
- Use intravenous fluid infusion and administration sets for one patient only and appropriately discard after using.
- Use single-dose vials of parenteral medications whenever possible; do not use the same single-dose vial for more than one patient or combine leftover contents with that from another vial.
- Use a sterile syringe and needle or cannula to access multiple-dose vials, if necessary to use; do not store the vial in the patient-care area and discard if sterility is compromised or questionable.

Patient Placement

Place patients who contaminate the environment or who do not (or are not expected to) assist in maintaining appropriate hygiene or environmental control (e.g., an ambulatory, confused patient with fecal incontinence) in a private room.

Source: Data from Centers for Disease Control and Prevention. (2017). *Standard precautions for all patient care.* Retrieved from https://www.cdc.gov/infectioncontrol/basics/standard-precautions.html.

Appendix B Answers, Rationales, and Cues

Chapter 1: Medical-Surgical Nursing in the 21st Century

Test Yourself NCLEX-RN Review Answers

1. **Correct answer**: D
   Rationale: Teamwork and collaboration foster open communication, mutual respect, and shared decision making to achieve quality patient care. Patient-centered care recognizes the patient or designee as the source of control and full partner in providing compassionate and coordinated care based on respect for patient's preferences, values, and needs. Quality improvement uses data to monitor the outcomes of care processes and improvement methods to design and test changes to continuously improve the quality and safety of healthcare systems. Evidence-based practice integrates best current evidence with clinical expertise and patient/family preferences and values for delivery of optimal healthcare. **Nursing Process**: Planning **Bloom's Taxonomy**: Understand
2. **Correct answer**: A, B, D, E
   Rationale: Foundational knowledge used in clinical reasoning includes knowing the profession, self, the case, the patient, and the person. Knowing the financial restraints is not an individual foundational source of knowledge. **Nursing Process**: Planning **Bloom's Taxonomy**: Understand
3. **Correct answer**: C
   Rationale: During the planning step, the nurse identifies the desired patient outcomes of care that are mutually established by the patient and nurse. The nurse will not focus on outcomes identified by the physician or family members since these may or may not be agreeable to the patient. The nurse will not plan patient care outcomes based on organizational policies and standards. **Nursing Process**: Planning **Bloom's Taxonomy**: Apply
4. **Correct answer**: D, B, A, E, C
   Rationale: The first step of the nursing process is assessment, during which patient needs are identified. From this step nursing diagnoses are established. The next step is planning, during which actions designed to meet the expected outcomes are identified. Implementation is placing the plan into action. The last step is evaluation, in which the plan is evaluated to determine the degree of goal and outcome achievement. It is during the evaluation step where the plan, goals, and outcomes may be changed to meet the patient's needs. **Nursing Process**: Implementation **Bloom's Taxonomy**: Apply
5. **Correct answer**: B
   Rationale: The knowledge base is considered the science of nursing. Holistic care is based on a philosophical view that interacting wholes are greater than the sum of their parts and emphasizes the uniqueness of the individual. Practice and clinical competency develop after the knowledge base is mastered. **Nursing Process**: Implementation **Bloom's Taxonomy**: Apply
6. **Correct answer**: A
   Rationale: A major component of the educator role is discharge planning, which is a systematic method of preparing the patient and family for exit from the healthcare agency and for maintaining continuity of care after the patient leaves the setting. As an advocate the nurse promotes the patient's rights to autonomy and free choice, speaks for the patient, mediates between the patient and other individuals, and/or protects the patient's right to self-determination. The caregiver role for the nurse today is both independent and collaborative. As a caregiver, nurses make assessments and plan and implement patient care based on nursing knowledge and skills. As a researcher, the nurse studies a broad variety of questions and issues in order to continually develop the knowledge of nursing. **Nursing Process**: Implementation **Bloom's Taxonomy**: Apply
7. **Correct answer**: C
   Rationale: As a patient advocate the nurse assists and supports patient decision making. These actions promote the patient's rights to autonomy and free choice. As a caregiver the nurse would perform range-of-motion exercises. As a researcher the nurse would analyze the effectiveness of exercise. As a manager, the nurse would delegate responsibilities for patient care to others. **Nursing Process**: Implementation **Bloom's Taxonomy**: Apply
8. **Correct answer**: D
   Rationale: As a leader/manager, the nurse assigns appropriate and effective work activities to other members of the healthcare team. As a caregiver, nurses make assessments and plan and implement patient care based on nursing knowledge and skills. As an advocate, the nurse promotes the patient's rights to autonomy and free choice, speaks for the patient, mediates between the patient and other persons, and/or protects the patient's right to self-determination. As a researcher, the nurse studies a broad variety of questions and issues in order to continually develop the knowledge of nursing. **Nursing Process**: Implementation **Bloom's Taxonomy**: Apply
9. **Correct answer**: A, D
   Rationale: Care bundles are interprofessional standards. Each bundle is used with a defined patient population in one location. Compliance with bundles is measured using all-or-nothing measurement, with a goal of 95% or greater. There are typically 3 to 5 interventions in a care bundle. The bundles are written by an interprofessional team. Bundle elements are descriptive, allowing for local customization and appropriate clinical judgment. **Nursing Process**: Planning **Bloom's Taxonomy**: Apply
10. **Correct answer**: B
    Rationale: When the nurse delegates nursing care activities to another person, that person is authorized to act in the place of the nurse, although the nurse retains the accountability for the activities performed. The nurse is ultimately responsible for the vital signs performed by UAP. The UAP cannot be responsible for delegated activities. The patient cannot be responsible for delegated responsibilities. The physician did not delegate the assessment of vital signs to UAP and cannot be responsible for this activity. **Nursing Process**: Implementation **Bloom's Taxonomy**: Understand

Chapter 2: Health and Illness in Adults

Test Yourself NCLEX-RN Review Answers

1. **Correct answer**: C
Rationale: Cognitive development affects whether people view themselves as healthy or ill and cognitive levels also may affect health practices. Although certain diseases have a higher rate of incidence in some cultural and ethnic groups than in others, the cultural background of an individual influences health values, behaviors, lifestyle, and illness behaviors. Genetic makeup affects personality, temperament, body structure, intellectual potential, and susceptibility to alterations in health. The components of an individual's lifestyle that affect health status include patterns of eating, use of chemical substances, exercise and rest patterns, and coping methods. Exposure to environmental hazards can lead to disease; however, the patient does not rate health according to lifestyle and environmental factors. **Nursing Process**: Assessment **Bloom's Taxonomy**: Apply

2. **Correct answer**: A
Rationale: Psychosocial stressors for the older adult include the illness of a spouse. Physical stressors for the older adult are those that could lead to a physical illness such as falling or having a 30-year smoking history. Pharmacologic effects on the older adult could develop from the use of over-the-counter pain medication. **Nursing Process**: Assessment **Bloom's Taxonomy**: Apply

3. **Correct answer**: B
Rationale: The nurse promotes health by teaching the activities that maintain wellness, by providing information about the characteristics and consequences of diseases when risk factors have been identified, and by supplying specific information about decreasing risk factors. The purpose of health teaching is not to diagnose diseases, explain the success of medication treatments for illnesses, or adhere to prescribed medication regimens. **Nursing Process**: Planning **Bloom's Taxonomy**: Apply

4. **Correct answer**: B, D, E
Rationale: Secondary prevention involves activities that emphasize early diagnosis and treatment of disease to effect an early cure or prevent disease progression such as obtaining regular physical examinations, obtaining specific treatment for illnesses, and screening for common diseases. Primary prevention focuses on activities and specific actions to prevent disease by eliminating risk factors for disease to the extent possible such as receiving recommended immunizations and eliminating the use of alcohol and cigarettes. **Nursing Process**: Planning **Bloom's Taxonomy**: Apply

5. **Correct answer**: D
Rationale: The stage of assuming a dependent role begins when an individual accepts the diagnosis and planned treatment for an illness. A physician or other healthcare provider usually provides validation of illness. People who believe that they are ill and are encouraged by others to contact a healthcare provider make an appointment for diagnosis, prognosis, and treatment of the illness. In the second stage of illness behavior, the person assumes the sick role, accepting the symptoms as indicative of an illness. In the first stage of an acute illness, an individual experiences symptoms such as pain, fever, bleeding, or swelling that signal a change in normal health. **Nursing Process**: Planning **Bloom's Taxonomy**: Apply

6. **Correct answer**: C
Rationale: The goal of transitional care is to improve the care and outcomes of chronically ill patients by improving the ability of patients and caregivers to manage care needs. Navigating through the healthcare system is a characteristic of care and disease management. Home healthcare is the delivery of services to restore or maintain the health of individuals and families in the home. Community care is an approach to manage acute or chronic health problems and to promote self-care. **Nursing Process**: Planning **Bloom's Taxonomy**: Analyze

7. **Correct answer**: B
Rationale: The patient-centered medical home is a primary care model that focuses on all levels of illness prevention. For people with chronic diseases, the goal of this approach is to provide comprehensive care with a focus on preventing acute disease crises. Reducing health disparities, increasing preventive services, and improving the patient–primary care relationship are additional goals of this delivery approach; however, they may or may not be appropriate for patients with chronic diseases. **Nursing Process**: Planning **Bloom's Taxonomy**: Apply

8. **Correct answer**: B
Rationale: Medicare will reimburse home care visits if specific criteria or needs are being met. One need is teaching about the care of a new health problem such as teaching a patient how to self-administer insulin for a new diagnosis of diabetes. Medicare does not reimburse visits made to support general health maintenance, health promotion, or patients' emotional or socioeconomic needs. Medicare will not reimburse for the emotional needs of a new widow, assistance with basic care such as bathing and dressing, or for socialization during mealtimes. **Nursing Process**: Planning **Bloom's Taxonomy**: Apply

9. **Correct answer**: A, B
Rationale: The disposal of toxic medications is a safety issue in the home. The nurse must address this issue with the patient, demonstrate safe disposal, and provide the necessary equipment for safe disposal. There is no indication that the patient should take medications that are not expired. Moving the expired medications to the back of the medication area is not effective. The nurse should not just take the medications and dispose of them. This could be interpreted as stealing from the patient. **Nursing Process**: Implementation **Bloom's Taxonomy**: Apply

10. **Correct answer**: A
Rationale: Infection control in the home centers on protecting patients, caregivers, and the community from the spread of disease. Health teaching is the single most important nursing intervention to control infection. Patients and caregivers need to know the importance of effective hand hygiene. The patient is recovering from bacterial pneumonia and may not need to be isolated from family members. The patient's disease process does not support the need to isolate bed linens and clothing from the rest of the family. The caregiver should be instructed to wash all of the family's eating utensils in hot soapy water and not just those of the patient who is recovering from an illness. **Nursing Process**: Implementation **Bloom's Taxonomy**: Apply

Chapter 3: Nursing Care of the Patient with Alterations in Sleep

Test Yourself NCLEX-RN Review Answers

1. **Correct answer**: B
Rationale: Rest is different than sleep, as during sleep hormones are released and short-term memories and learning are moved to long-term memories and learning. Rest and sleep do not have the same physiologic effects. People disengage from their environment while sleeping, not resting. In most cases sleeping is done in a recumbent position with eyes closed. **Nursing Process**: Planning **Bloom's Taxonomy**: Apply
2. **Correct answer**: B, D
Rationale: Exercising every day and avoiding use of electronic devices 1 to 2 hours before bedtime are both suggestions for improving sleep. Alcohol should be avoided before bedtime. Being exposed to bright light in the morning signals melatonin that sleep is over. The bed should be used only for sleep and sex. **Nursing Process**: Implementation **Bloom's Taxonomy**: Apply
3. **Correct answer**: C
Rationale: These devices often encourage the patient to seek treatment. Correlating the information from the device with the patient's experience of sleeping is the most valuable use of the data. The device should be worn on the nondominant arm. Accuracy in recording sleep is not related to how accurate the device measures heart rate. While it is true that the devices may not be very accurate, the nurse should not devalue the information being reported. **Nursing Process**: Implementation **Bloom's Taxonomy**: Apply
4. **Correct answer**: C
Rationale: Older adults tend to go to bed earlier and wake up earlier than do younger persons. Older adults often have multiple factors resulting in sleep disturbances, so there is no evidence that they sleep longer and better than young persons. Women in menopause have the same risk of obstructive sleep apnea, which causes snoring, as do older men. **Nursing Process**: Planning **Bloom's Taxonomy**: Understand
5. **Correct answer**: B, C, E
Rationale: Sleep deprivation can result in slowing of reflexes and can impair the immune system, resulting in higher risk for infection. Insulin resistance is increased, which results in increased fasting glucose and A1C levels. Heart rate tends to increase. **Nursing Process**: Implementation **Bloom's Taxonomy**: Apply
6. **Correct answer**: C
Rationale: Insomnia can become a self-reinforcing problem in which sleeplessness reduces the person's ability to cope with lack of sleep. Worrying about not sleeping can result in being unable to sleep. Even occasional insomnia should be addressed as each episode may lead to another, eventually becoming chronic in nature. Saying that people are genetically inclined to be poor sleepers is a hopeless statement for the person who cannot sleep. Chronic insomnia is not rare. **Nursing Process**: Implementation **Bloom's Taxonomy**: Apply
7. **Correct answer**: A
Rationale: Insomnia is diagnosed when the patient reports its presence. There is no definitive test such as serotonin level or brain wave measurements. Actigraphy may provide information about the degree of difficulty sleeping, but is not used to confirm the diagnosis of insomnia. **Nursing Process**: Implementation **Bloom's Taxonomy**: Apply
8. **Correct answer**: A, B
Rationale: Weight loss may be beneficial if the patient is obese. Most people experience OSA while back-sleeping, so devices to prevent this position may be helpful. An oral device may be used to bring the tongue forward away from the oropharynx. Daily exercise is not useful except if it helps with weight loss. Melatonin may induce sleep but will not prevent OSA. **Nursing Process**: Implementation **Bloom's Taxonomy**: Apply
9. **Correct answer**: D
Rationale: This feeling is associated with restless leg syndrome (RLS). The pathophysiology of RLS is related to dopamine levels in the brain. One of the limiting factors for producing dopamine is iron. Increasing iron stores may relieve symptoms. Sleeping in a cool room or with minimal covering on the legs is not shown to be helpful. Milk may interfere with iron absorption. **Nursing Process**: Implementation **Bloom's Taxonomy**: Analyze
10. **Correct answer**: C
Rationale: Sleep walking and sleep driving may occur when taking this medication, especially if any other central nervous system depressant is used concurrently. The patient should not drink alcohol while taking this medication. Sleep medications should be taken only for a limited time. The patient should go to bed immediately after taking this medication. **Nursing Process**: Evaluation **Bloom's Taxonomy**: Evaluate

Chapter 4: Nursing Care of the Patient Having Surgery

Evaluate Your Response to Clinical Reasoning in Patient Care

A Patient Having Surgery

1. Safety concerns include ambulating and not tripping over scatter rugs or clutter. See the information in Chapter 3 on safety in the home.
2. Medications used to prevent an occurrence such as infection are called prophylactic medications. Her risks for infection are from the surgical wound and microvascular circulation in bone. Teach her to take the complete course of antibiotics prescribed and about the possible side effects of the antibiotic. Encourage her to notify the physician if side effects or adverse events occur.
3. When blood stops flowing, it clots. Her immobility is a concern and puts her at risk for thrombosis and emboli. She has a risk for bleeding secondary to the anticoagulant and should inform healthcare providers such as dentists that she is taking the anticoagulant.
4. Consider Mrs. Overbeck's nutritional needs related to healing and age as well as her excess weight. She will need adequate protein, calcium, and vitamin D.

Test Yourself NCLEX-RN Review Answers

1. **Correct answer**: B
Rationale: The nurse's primary responsibility to informed consent is serving as a witness to the patient signature on the consent form. Defining the risks and benefits of the

surgery, explaining the right to refuse treatment or withdraw consent, and advising the patient and family about what is needed for the diagnosis are actions completed by the healthcare provider. **Nursing Process**: Implementation **Bloom's Taxonomy**: Understand

2. **Correct answer**: C
Rationale: The nurse has an extensive role in ensuring that education is provided at all phases of the perioperative process and that learning has occurred to reduce complications as patients have shorter lengths of stay and more patients have their surgical procedures performed on an outpatient basis. Although teaching about nutritional needs, pain control, and fluid and hydration status are important, the prevention of complications should take priority. **Nursing Process**: Implementation **Bloom's Taxonomy**: Apply

3. **Correct answer**: C
Rationale: Nonsteroidal anti-inflammatory drugs (NSAIDs) are used to treat mild to moderate postoperative pain. This category of drugs should be given soon after surgery unless contraindicated. Although NSAIDs may not be sufficient to control pain completely, they allow lower doses of opioid analgesics to be used. NSAIDs are not given during the postoperative period to increase amnesia, stimulate appetite, or improve renal function. **Nursing Process**: Implementation **Bloom's Taxonomy**: Apply

4. **Correct answer**: C
Rationale: Renal function is evaluated on the basis of glomerular filtration rate, which is estimated by using serum creatinine. When creatinine is increased renal impairment needs to be considered. Increased chloride, decreased hemoglobin, and decreased glucose may or may not influence the decision to continue with the surgical procedure and could be related to the patient's current treatment regimen or other health problems. **Nursing Process**: Implementation **Bloom's Taxonomy**: Apply

5. **Correct answer**: D, E
Rationale: The patient could have developed a deep venous thrombosis distal to the operative site. Common assessment findings include cramping in the involved calf and redness and edema of the area with a slightly elevated temperature. Bounding pedal pulse, poor muscle tone in the foot, and skin that is cool to the touch are not manifestations associated with a deep venous thrombosis. **Nursing Process**: Assessment **Bloom's Taxonomy**: Analyze

6. **Correct answer**: C
Rationale: In most organizations, orders written prior to surgery must be reordered following surgery because the patient's condition is presumed to have changed. The nurse should not resume the medications now because the healthcare provider has to determine the appropriate doses. Decreasing the doses by half for 36 hours is beyond the nurse's scope of practice. Withholding the medications until fully recovered from anesthesia is not an option because the healthcare provider needs to write new orders for the patient. **Nursing Process**: Implementation **Bloom's Taxonomy**: Apply

7. **Correct answer**: D
Rationale: Under anesthesia the manifestations of hypoglycemia are absent, so withholding insulin the morning of surgery when the patient is NPO is advisable. The patient is at risk for hyperglycemia during the surgery and will have blood glucose levels monitored throughout the procedure. The patient will not benefit from developing hypoglycemia during anesthesia since this can affect responses to anesthesia and recovery times. The patient most likely did not receive an extra dose of insulin the evening before the surgery, although the dosage may have been adjusted the previous evening. **Nursing Process**: Implementation **Bloom's Taxonomy**: Analyze

8. **Correct answer**: C
Rationale: After the first 36 to 48 hours for a patient recovering as expected, pain medications should be shifted to an as-needed basis. This helps to reduce medication adverse effects. Until that time the medication is given on a schedule. At this point NSAIDs should be the basis of pain therapy and opioid use should be diminishing and medications should be given orally. A strong sedative effect is not desired. **Nursing Process**: Implementation **Bloom's Taxonomy**: Apply

9. **Correct answer**: C, D, E
Rationale: Older adults are at more risk for hypothermia due to the cool environment in the operating room. They have decreased subcutaneous fat and reduced peripheral circulation that makes them at higher risk for pressure sores. Arthritic joints can cause postoperative pain due to intraoperative positioning and long anesthesia times. Immune function declines with aging, increasing risk of infection. Memory loss and hearing loss are not major concerns. **Nursing Process**: Planning **Bloom's Taxonomy**: Apply

10. **Correct answer**: A, B, C, D
Rationale: Normothermia reduces risk for infection, cardiac morbidity, myocardial ischemia, surgical bleeding, and patient discomfort. It is not implicated in the increase of respiratory drive. **Nursing Process**: Implementation **Bloom's Taxonomy**: Apply

Chapter 5: Palliative Care and End-of-Life Care

Evaluate Your Response to Clinical Reasoning in Patient Care

A Patient Experiencing Loss and Grief

1. Review the physical manifestations of grief described in the chapter and compare and contrast those with the ones verbalized by Mrs. Rogers.
2. Consider the benefits of including Mrs. Rogers's daughter in a meeting of the staff. What type of questions would be most useful in making the daughter feel a part of the plan of care? Why would a question such as "Why don't you do more for your mother?" be inappropriate?
3. Consider the losses Mrs. Rogers has experienced. Review the material in the chapter on responses to loss. Think about the reasons you would not say "Oh, you have a lot to live for." Think of two or three questions or statements that would help you assess the reason why Mrs. Rogers said this to you.

Test Yourself NCLEX-RN Review Answers

1. **Correct answer**: A, B, D, E
Rationale: Loss does result in change and culture exerts strong influence on grief and mourning. While mourning is visible, the feelings associated with loss can only be determined by the person who experiences it. Grief ranges from mildly discomforting to completely debilitating.

Successfully coping with loss is individual; some persons depend largely on their social network, some depend on family, and others are more private in their grief. **Nursing Process**: Planning **Bloom's Taxonomy**: Apply

2. **Correct answer**: A
   Rationale: In the anger stage, the person resists the loss, which in this case is directed toward the loss of health. The anger is often directed toward family and healthcare providers. A statement of denial would be "this cannot be happening to me." Bargaining is an attempt to postpone the reality of the loss by expressing a willingness to do anything to postpone the loss or change the prognosis. Depression is when the full impact of the actual or perceived loss is realized. The person prepares for the impending loss by working through the struggle of separation. **Nursing Process**: Assessment **Bloom's Taxonomy**: Understand
3. **Correct answer**: B, E
   Rationale: There are general ranges in the development of the concept of death. At age 12, the child begins to express interest in the afterlife and reflects the views of death learned from parents. This is also a time of recognizing death as irreversible and inevitable. Six- to 10-year-olds may believe their own death is avoidable and believe wishes can be responsible for death. Four- to 5-year-olds believe death is like sleeping and is reversible. **Nursing Process**: Evaluation **Bloom's Taxonomy**: Evaluate
4. **Correct answer**: B
   Rationale: Culture is the primary factor that dictates a family's rituals of mourning. While age, gender, and social support are also important, culture is the strongest factor. **Nursing Process**: Planning **Bloom's Taxonomy**: Remember
5. **Correct answer**: A
   Rationale: A living will is a legal document that formally expresses an individual's wishes regarding life-sustaining treatment in the event of terminal illness or permanent unconsciousness. It is not a type of durable power of attorney and usually does not designate a surrogate healthcare decision maker. It is the responsibility of the nurse as patient advocate to request and record the patient's preference for care and include it in the plan of care. The healthcare provider can write for a no-code order. The patient does not perform this task. **Nursing Process**: Implementation **Bloom's Taxonomy**: Apply
6. **Correct answer**: C
   Rationale: Hospice is a philosophy of care rather than a program of care. It is comprehensive and coordinated care for patients with limited life expectancy, provided at home, hospitals, and long-term care facilities, that reaffirms the right of every patient and family to fully participate in the final stages of life. It is based on a philosophy of death with comfort and dignity, encompassing biomedical, psychosocial, and spiritual aspects of the dying experience. Although most hospice care is provided in the home, it may also be provided in hospitals, long-term care facilities, or other community-based settings. **Nursing Process**: Implementation **Bloom's Taxonomy**: Apply
7. **Correct answer**: D
   Rationale: The nurse is ethically and morally responsible to uphold the wishes of the patient so the medication should not be provided. Giving the patient medication is not upholding the client's wishes. Changing the dose of pain medication is beyond the nurse's scope of practice. The nurse cannot discuss the patient's care decisions without the patient's permission. This would be a violation of the Health Insurance Portability and Accountability Act (HIPAA). **Nursing Process**: Implementation **Bloom's Taxonomy**: Apply
8. **Correct answer**: D
   Rationale: While all of these interventions are appropriate, the one that supports hearing is correct as this is thought to be the last sense lost in dying. **Nursing Process**: Implementation **Bloom's Taxonomy**: Apply
9. **Correct answer**: B
   Rationale: There is no maximum allowable dose for full agonist opioids such as morphine sulfate when caring for a patient who is dying. The dose should be increased to whatever is necessary to relieve pain. Only the patient can determine if pain is present. Pain medication should be provided as needed and necessary to control the dying patient's pain. Respiratory changes are not necessarily associated with the provision of pain medication and may occur as a part of the dying process. **Nursing Process**: Implementation **Bloom's Taxonomy**: Apply
10. **Correct answer**: B
    Rationale: An effective nurse–patient relationship begins with acceptance of the patient's feelings, attitudes, and values related to the loss. If the patient is ready to talk, listening and being present are the most appropriate interventions. The open-ended statement of acknowledging to the patient "This must be a difficult time for you" provides an opportunity for her to express her feelings as she recognizes the nurse's willingness to listen. The other responses do not support the nurse–patient relationship and will not help the patient resolve grief. **Nursing Process**: Implementation **Bloom's Taxonomy**: Apply

Chapter 6: Nursing Care of Patients with Problems of Substance Abuse

Evaluate Your Response to Clinical Reasoning in Patient Care

A Patient Having Withdrawal from Alcohol

1. Consider Mr. Russell's family history and the potential effect of his job loss on his self-esteem in developing your response to this question.
2. Think about Mr. Russell's BAL on admission to the ED and the circumstances of his accident. Also consider his safety while in the hospital, including the potential effects of anesthesia and alcohol withdrawal.
3. In developing a teaching plan, consider Mr. Russell's current nutritional status and elevated liver enzymes.
4. Consider the interactions of prescribed or over-the-counter medications with alcohol. What if the patient has not taken prescribed medications because of chronic alcoholism?
5. Review the effects of Antabuse. Make a list of possible interactions and side effects.
6. Impaired nutrition is an appropriate nursing diagnosis when a patient does not have sufficient nutritional intake to meet metabolic needs. What in Mr. Russell's history and physical assessment supports this diagnosis? What nutritional information should you provide?

Test Yourself NCLEX-RN Review Answers

1. **Correct answer**: B
   Rationale: The legal level of intoxication in many states is 0.08%. Toxic levels in excess of 0.5% can cause coma,

respiratory depression, peripheral collapse, and death. **Nursing Process**: Assessment **Bloom's Taxonomy**: Understand

2. **Correct answer**: C
Rationale: Questions should be asked in a nonthreatening, matter-of-fact manner, phrased as to not imply wrongdoing. For instance, a nonthreatening question such as "How much alcohol do you drink?" is preferable to the judgmental question "You don't drink too much alcohol, do you?" Open-ended questions that elicit more than a simple yes or no answer help to determine the direction of future counseling. Asking if the drinking has caused problems with the spouse is a judgmental question and should be avoided. **Nursing Process**: Assessment **Bloom's Taxonomy**: Analyze

3. **Correct answer**: D
Rationale: Thiamine depletion is thought to cause the Wernicke-Korsakoff syndrome observed in people with chronic alcoholism. This syndrome is characterized by nystagmus, ptosis, ataxia, confusion, coma, and possible death. This is why the nurse should plan to provide the patient with thiamine supplements. Thiamine is not provided to patients with chronic alcoholism to prevent acute pancreatitis, cirrhosis of the liver, or hepatic encephalopathy. **Nursing Process**: Planning **Bloom's Taxonomy**: Apply

4. **Correct answer**: B
Rationale: All CNS depressants, including alcohol, benzodiazepines, and barbiturates, have a potentially dangerous progression of withdrawal. Alcohol and the entire class of CNS depressants share the same withdrawal syndrome. Severe withdrawal or delirium tremens is a medical emergency that usually occurs 2 to 5 days following alcohol withdrawal and persists 2 to 3 days. Seizures may also occur, requiring the use of emergency equipment. Withdrawal from opiates, marijuana, amphetamines, hallucinogens, CNS stimulants, and amphetamines is not as severe as withdrawal from CNS depressants and alcohol. **Nursing Process**: Planning **Bloom's Taxonomy**: Apply

5. **Correct answer**: D, E
Rationale: Medications used to treat alcoholism include disulfiram (Antabuse). This medication is a form of aversion therapy that prevents the breakdown of alcohol, causing physical illness such as intense vomiting if taken while drinking alcohol. All forms of alcohol, including OTC cough and cold preparations, must be avoided. Disulfiram does not decrease the discomfort of withdrawal symptoms, decrease the pleasant effects of alcohol, nor does it block the manifestations of alcohol withdrawal. **Nursing Process**: Implementation **Bloom's Taxonomy**: Apply

6. **Correct answer**: B, C, E
Rationale: Haphazard personal appearance, if a new finding, can be a sign of substance abuse. People who abuse alcohol sometimes try to cover up the smell with perfume, mouthwash, or mints. When a patient denies receiving pain medication, the manager must consider the possibility of diversion. Working overtime to complete documentation is a common occurrence in nursing. Shift change admissions can be chaotic, leading to increased risk of medication error. **Nursing Process**: Assessment **Bloom's Taxonomy**: Analyze

7. **Correct answer**: A
Rationale: Far more women are dying of lung cancer than of breast cancer. Women who smoke do have an increased risk for stroke and heart disease. Women who smoke during pregnancy do have a higher risk for infertility. Smoking is the leading known cause of preventable death and disease among women. **Nursing Process**: Evaluation **Bloom's Taxonomy**: Evaluate

8. **Correct answer**: B
Rationale: It is recommended that patients wear a medical alert bracelet stating they are on naltrexone, in case of emergency medical treatment. Naltrexone can help reduce the craving for alcohol by blocking the pathways to the brain that trigger a feeling of pleasure when alcohol and other narcotics are used. Because naltrexone blocks opiate receptors, patients should avoid taking any narcotics, such as codeine, morphine, or heroin, while on naltrexone. There are other analgesics that the patient can still take with this medication. Products with alcohol do not necessarily have to be avoided while taking this medication. While on naltrexone, psychosocial treatments such as Alcoholics Anonymous meetings, individual counseling, or group therapy are important, as the desire to "take a break" from treatment can overcome the patient's motivation to continue taking the medication. **Nursing Process**: Evaluation **Bloom's Taxonomy**: Evaluate

9. **Correct answer**: C
Rationale: A realistic goal for patients who abuse substances is being able to identify healthy coping mechanisms, relaxation, and stress reduction techniques to decrease the risks of substance abuse. Many individuals with substance abuse problems are unable to use alcohol or drugs in moderation. Focusing on negative aspects of past behaviors and relationships could cause the person to seek substances to reduce the impact of the negative feelings. Many patients will not ever lose the craving for the substance so the goal of refraining from using substances until the cravings subside is not realistic. **Nursing Process**: Planning **Bloom's Taxonomy**: Apply

10. **Correct answer**: C
Rationale: Patients who abuse substances often have poor coping mechanisms, which lead them to make poor life choices. Cognitive decline can occur in patients with substance abuse, but it is typically a slow decline. Dehydration and weight loss are more common problems. If weight gain does occur, it is usually related to the patient's poor ability to cope with withdrawal symptoms. **Nursing Process**: Planning **Bloom's Taxonomy**: Analyze

Chapter 7: Nursing Care of Patients Experiencing Disasters

Evaluate Your Response to Clinical Reasoning in Patient Care

A Patient with Injuries from a Natural Disaster

1. Consider how Mr. Jones put himself at risk for infection (see Chapter 12). How could Mr. Jones have avoided exacerbating his skin lesions?

2. Because Mr. Jones has a history of elevated blood pressure that has not been consistently treated or monitored, cardiac status should be evaluated. Which tests are indicated? Also, could his decreased sensation and poor healing be related to cardiac impairment? Mr. Jones also has identifying data in his history and physical to suggest diabetes. Identify this data and tests that would be indicated.

3. Review risk factors for and causes and manifestations of infection in Chapter 12. Identify the factors that contributed to Mr. Jones's fever.
4. Consider Mr. Jones's environmental and personal situations. What information do you have about Mr. Jones that indicates a lack of interest in health maintenance? Are there signs of a change in outlook?

Test Yourself NCLEX-RN Review Answers

1. **Correct answer**: C
   Rationale: Although emergencies can typically be handled by available emergency services, disasters involve multiple services and agencies working together. Neither emergencies nor disasters can be controlled. Disasters can be natural or human generated. Disasters require the assistance of all available agencies in addition to local agencies. **Nursing Process**: Planning **Bloom's Taxonomy**: Understand
2. **Correct answer**: A, C, D, E
   Rationale: Communication and information sharing, developing policies and procedures, educating the community, and ensuring care for vulnerable populations are all disaster nursing competencies. Nurses seldom act as incident commanders at the scene of the disaster. **Nursing Process**: Assessment **Bloom's Taxonomy**: Analyze
3. **Correct answer**: D
   Rationale: Reverse triage is based on the principle of doing the greatest good for the greatest number of people. Reverse triage is not saving scarce resources for future use. It is also not saving victims who are in the most critical condition. Reverse triage is not done to test first responders on triage classification categories. **Nursing Process**: Implementation **Bloom's Taxonomy**: Apply
4. **Correct answer**: B
   Rationale: All of these assessments are important, but the patient's health literacy in the primary language is of greatest importance. The nurse must consider level of health literacy at all times and cannot assume the patient is health literate in the primary language. Whether the patient speaks any English, comfort with using an interpreter, and ability to read instructions written in English are all secondary to determining health literacy. **Nursing Process**: Assessment **Bloom's Taxonomy**: Analyze
5. **Correct answer**: C
   Rationale: Personal protective equipment is used to reduce the likelihood of occupational injury and/or illness. This equipment is not an absolute barrier against hazards. This equipment is to be used as needed but is not an expectation for all healthcare personnel to use. The use of personal protective equipment is in addition to adherence to universal precautions. **Nursing Process**: Implementation **Bloom's Taxonomy**: Apply
6. **Correct answer**: B
   Rationale: Decontamination cannot be completed in the hot zone because this is the area of greatest contamination. It is performed in the warm zone where initial emergency treatment may also begin. The patient should be decontaminated prior to entering the hospital. Decontamination may be necessary for biologic, chemical, or radiologic disasters **Nursing Process**: Evaluation **Bloom's Taxonomy**: Evaluate
7. **Correct answer**: D
   Rationale: A radiologic dispersion bomb or dirty bomb is a bomb that carries a radiologic signature and can cause contamination and radiation poisoning. A dirty bomb is not known to cause thermal injuries so burns will most likely not occur. Abdominal organ damage would be assessed for blunt trauma and not necessarily for a dirty bomb. Eye injuries are not associated with a dirty bomb but rather with a bright flash of light associated with nuclear detonation. **Nursing Process**: Implementation **Bloom's Taxonomy**: Apply
8. **Correct answer**: B
   Rationale: Reconstitution is an assessment of how well the community has achieved a new level of normal. Mitigation is reducing the harmful effects of the disaster. Evaluation is studying what did and did not work when responding to the disaster. Surge capacity is the local healthcare organizations' abilities to respond beyond normal services during a disaster. **Nursing Process**: Evaluation **Bloom's Taxonomy**: Apply
9. **Correct answer**: C
   Rationale: Older adults have individual needs. Some may be more independent than others regarding the degree of support needed in emergencies, whereas others may require multiple resources and support in an evacuation. Patients are not expected to take the lead in evacuation efforts in nursing homes. It is an expectation that all patients are removed from a facility in the event of evacuation. **Nursing Process**: Planning **Bloom's Taxonomy**: Apply
10. **Correct answer**: D, E
    Rationale: Nurses are often so involved in caring for others they tend to neglect themselves. In disaster situations, nurses may also suffer from loss while caring for others. As a result the nurse may feel overwhelmed and be as traumatized as the victims of the disaster. Simply giving nurses time off will not correct these problems. The mental health of the nurses is the focus of these meetings. All nurses do not always need the help of a mental health professional while working as a nurse. **Nursing Process**: Implementation **Bloom's Taxonomy**: Apply

Chapter 8: Genetic Implications of Adult Health Nursing

Test Yourself NCLEX-RN Review Answers

1. **Correct answer**: C
   Rationale: An individual with an autosomal recessive health problem inherited one altered gene from the mother and one from the father. Autosomal dominant disorders occur when only one altered gene is inherited from either the mother or the father. They tend to be more severe and are often lethal. In autosomal recessive health problems, the gene alteration occurred on a nonsex chromosome so both males and females have an equal chance of inheriting the altered gene from the parent. For an autosomal recessive health problem, the parents are carriers of the condition and will not usually exhibit manifestations of the health disorder. **Nursing Process**: Implementation **Bloom's Taxonomy**: Apply
2. **Correct answer**: D
   Rationale: With an X-linked recessive health problem, the altered gene appears on the X chromosome and the health problem will be expressed in all males. Since the female receives an X chromosome from both parents, the female will be a carrier. Because the female has two X chromosomes, the

health problem will not be expressed because the unaltered gene will compensate for the altered gene. The health problem is not transmitted through direct blood contact. **Nursing Process**: Implementation **Bloom's Taxonomy**: Apply

3. **Correct answer**: C
Rationale: It is a nurse's responsibility to explain what is involved in genetic testing. The nurse will use information on three generations to create a pedigree. The couple is seeking information on genetic testing prior to having children so the nurse should not suggest that testing be completed after the birth of a child. It is unknown if the couple will proceed with chromosome studies. It is unknown what genetic anomaly the couple is investigating and the impact of the anomaly on future children. **Nursing Process**: Implementation **Bloom's Taxonomy**: Apply

4. **Correct answer**: A
Rationale: Mitochondrial mutations are only passed from the mother. This is because mitochondria are primarily found in ova and not sperm. This is considered a matrilineal pattern of inheritance. An affected female will pass the condition on to her children; however, an affected male will not. The consequences of the altered gene on an X chromosome will be expressed in all males who inherit the altered chromosome. In autosomal dominant and recessive disorders, both males and females are affected equally. **Nursing Process**: Assessment **Bloom's Taxonomy**: Analyze

5. **Correct answer**: A
Rationale: Family history has been a part of nursing assessment, but the importance of obtaining a family history has increased knowledge of the interaction of genes and the environment. It is an inexpensive first "genetic screen," often underused by healthcare professionals. Obtaining a family history is not done to help the nurse focus the body system assessment. It also is not used to predict the health problems the patient will face in the future. This information is not used to validate Health and Human Services data on family health. **Nursing Process**: Implementation **Bloom's Taxonomy**: Apply

6. **Correct answer**: C
Rationale: When discussing the findings and recommendations with the patient newly diagnosed with a genetic disorder, much information will be provided. It is typical for the retention of information by a patient facing a new genetic diagnosis to be very low. The extra time is needed to ensure the patient understands as much as possible about the disorder at this time. While the information may be complex, it should be explained in simple terms, which should not take extra time. Extra time is not needed because the patient is resistant to learning or has difficulty learning. **Nursing Process**: Planning **Bloom's Taxonomy**: Apply

7. **Correct answer**: A, C, E
Rationale: Most genetic specialists will complete chromosomal studies and provide information for important decision making and about the natural history of the condition. Examining photographs of family members is not a part of a genetic referral. The genetics professional also will not prescribe medication to treat the disorder. **Nursing Process**: Implementation **Bloom's Taxonomy**: Apply

8. **Correct answer**: A, B, D, E
Rationale: Learning of this genetic predisposition commonly results in problems coping, realizing that a knowledge deficit exists, feeling powerless and that future health is predetermined, and having anxiety over what is to come. Some patients may consider suicide, but this is not a common response. **Nursing Process**: Planning **Bloom's Taxonomy**: Apply

9. **Correct answer**: C
Rationale: Coronary heart disease has a multifactorial inheritance pattern. Managing environmental and lifestyle factors is important to reduce the risk. A family history for mutation of the *MLH/MSH2* gene is not associated with CHD. Hematocrit levels are not indicated to evaluate risk. There is no information provided to support the need for statin or other drugs. **Nursing Process**: Implementation **Bloom's Taxonomy**: Apply

10. **Correct answer**: A, D
Rationale: GINA is a federal law designed to protect consumers from discrimination by employers and health insurance companies based on genetic information. This law has no provisions for long-term care or life insurance and does not mandate genetic testing for anyone. **Nursing Process**: Implementation **Bloom's Taxonomy**: Apply

Chapter 9: Nursing Care of Patients in Pain

Evaluate Your Response to Clinical Reasoning in Patient Care

A Patient Experiencing Chronic Pain

1. Review the factors that affect an individual's response to pain. What have you observed in your own family and friends, as well as patients for whom you have cared?
2. Reflect on the benefits and disadvantages of each alternative. Make your decision based on knowledge about pain and about medications for pain.
3. What factors in Ms. Akers's illness and treatment increase her risk for constipation? What would you include in the plan specific to fluid intake and diet?

Test Yourself NCLEX-RN Review Answers

1. **Correct answer**: A
Rationale: Chronic pain is defined as pain that has persisted long after the reason for the pain has healed or subsided. Low back pain is the most common cause of chronic pain. Somatic pain arises from nerve receptors originating in the skin, subcutaneous tissues, or deep body structures such as periosteum, muscles, tendons, joints, and blood vessels. Somatic pain may be either sharp and well localized or dull and diffuse. Visceral pain arises from body organs and is dull and poorly localized because of the low number of nociceptors. Visceral pain may be described as deep cramping, splitting or stabbing pain, intermittent pain, or colicky pain. Neuropathic pain is the result of hyperactive nociceptive stimulation. Neuropathic pain may be acute, is usually chronic, and is associated with conditions such as diabetic neuropathy or postherpetic neuralgia. This pain is described as gnawing, electric shock-like, burning, shooting, or tingling. **Nursing Process**: Planning **Bloom's Taxonomy**: Apply

2. **Correct answer**: B
Rationale: Initial or "fast" pain is sharp and well defined because the stimulus is transmitted along myelinated

A delta fibers to the thalamus and cerebral cortex. The smaller unmyelinated C fibers transmit the stimulus more slowly, producing a second or "slow" pain that is less well localized, dull, and throbbing. The gate-control theory of pain is a base for further research about pain-modulating systems. The change from acute sharp pain to dull throbbing pain does not indicate that the injury is less severe than initially perceived. **Nursing Process**: Assessment **Bloom's Taxonomy**: Analyze

3. **Correct answer**: A, B, D
Rationale: NSAIDs are more effective when taken on a scheduled basis for predictable pain rather than prn for occasional pain. These drugs can cause gastrointestinal bleeding and hypertension, necessitating regular follow-up. NSAIDs are not known to affect the respiratory tract and are not addictive. **Nursing Process**: Assessment **Bloom's Taxonomy**: Apply
4. **Correct answer**: B, C
Rationale: Transdermal patches are slowly absorbed, reaching a therapeutic level 12 to 72 hours after application. The drug can accumulate in the body tissues, leading to a toxic level accompanied by manifestations such as sleepiness or respiratory difficulty. A transdermal patch is applied to a clean, dry area on the upper torso. The patch is effective for about 72 hours. When transdermal therapy is initiated, the therapeutic level is not reached until approximately 12 to 24 hours have passed. Use of a heating pad may increase or enhance absorption. **Nursing Process**: Implementation **Bloom's Taxonomy**: Apply
5. **Correct answer**: C
Rationale: The quality of the pain is assessed through descriptive statements such as sharp, stabbing, aching, burning, stinging, deep, crushing, viselike, or gnawing. Asking where it hurts identifies the location or region of the pain. Rating the pain on a scale determines pain intensity. Asking if the pain affects sleep helps to determine how the pain impacts the patient's quality of life. **Nursing Process**: Assessment **Bloom's Taxonomy**: Apply
6. **Correct answer**: A
Rationale: Pain is a subjective response and the patient provides the most accurate information about its intensity. The nurse should provide the medication as prescribed. Behavioral responses to pain may or may not coincide with the patient's report of pain and are not always reliable cues to the pain experience. Pain assessment is considered the fifth vital sign and not taking action after learning of pain is a violation of regulatory agency expectations for accreditation. Additional information is needed before determining if the patient is developing a tolerance to the pain medication. **Nursing Process**: Implementation **Bloom's Taxonomy**: Apply
7. **Correct answer**: C, E
Rationale: Constipation is a common side effect of opioid narcotics, especially when used on a regular basis. The nurse should instruct the patient to increase intake of fluids and fiber in the diet to prevent constipation. If this does not relieve constipation, the nurse should suggest the patient contact the provider if additional measures such as laxatives are needed to manage constipation. Use of nonpharmacological methods of pain management may work with opioids to better control pain. It is outside of the nurse's scope of practice to prescribe medications so suggesting the use of diphenhydramine (Benadryl) should not be done. The nurse also cannot instruct a patient to stop taking a medication without discussing it with the physician. Opioid analgesics are not known to interfere with urination. **Nursing Process**: Implementation **Bloom's Taxonomy**: Apply
8. **Correct answer**: A
Rationale: The faces pain scale may be more accurate and effective for use with adults who have cognitive impairments. The family will not be able to accurately evaluate the patient's pain. Providing around-the-clock pain medication might result in overmedicating the patient. Physical responses and behavioral cues to pain are not always consistent. **Nursing Process**: Assessment **Bloom's Taxonomy**: Apply
9. **Correct answer**: A
Rationale: Respiratory depression is a symptom of excessive opioid dosage. Naloxone 0.4 to 2 mg is given intravenous push every 2 to 3 minutes to reverse respiratory depression. The patient is at risk for respiratory arrest, so just monitoring or just holding the next dose is not the primary action. Reversing the drug is more effective than rescue breathing alone. There is no indication that chest compressions are required. **Nursing Process**: Implementation **Bloom's Taxonomy**: Apply
10. **Correct answer**: A
Rationale: Meditation prompts the release of endorphins, which are natural opioid-like substances. Endorphins bind with opioid receptors in the CNS, which inhibits the transmission of pain signals. Meditation does not create a gate in the spinal cord to block pain signals. Meditation also does not change perception of pain in the brain. Meditation does not reduce the sensitivity of nociceptors in deep tissue. **Nursing Process**: Implementation **Bloom's Taxonomy**: Apply

Chapter 10: Nursing Care of Patients with Altered Fluid, Electrolyte, and Acid–Base Balance

Evaluate Your Response to Clinical Reasoning in Patient Care

A Patient with Hyperkalemia

1. Review the causes and manifestations of hyperkalemia.
2. What are the potential effects of hyperkalemia on cardiac conduction? At what level of hyperkalemia are these likely to be seen?
3. Review collaborative treatment measures to rapidly reduce potassium levels. Why would these be used with a K^+ of 8.5?
4. Think about the effects of anxiety on learning as you develop a plan to provide teaching to avoid future episodes of hyperkalemia. As you develop your plan, remember the potential long-term effects of chronic renal failure.

A Patient with Acute Respiratory Acidosis

1. Review normal gas exchange across the alveolar-capillary membrane and the processes that drive this exchange. Then review the role that carbon dioxide plays as a potential acid.
2. Describe the effect of acidosis on cerebral neurons. What manifestations of mental impairment may result?
3. Think about the ABCs as you prioritize implementation of these orders.
4. Consider risk factors for choking such as alcohol consumption, taking large bites of food, or inadequate chewing.

Test Yourself NCLEX-RN Review Answers

1. **Correct answer**: D
Rationale: Ringer solution is an isotonic, balanced electrolyte solution that can expand plasma volume and help restore electrolyte balance. Three percent saline solution is hypertonic and not used to expand body fluid volume. Solutions containing 0.45% sodium chloride are used as maintenance solutions. Solutions containing 10% dextrose are hypertonic and not used to expand body fluid volume. **Nursing Process**: Implementation **Bloom's Taxonomy**: Apply

2. **Correct answer**: C, D, E
Rationale: In fluid volume deficit, there is less volume in the vascular system, which decreases venous return and cardiac output, leading to manifestations of dizziness, orthostatic hypotension, and flat neck veins. The heart rate increases as compensation for lowered cardiac output. Dyspnea and respiratory crackles are associated with fluid volume excess. **Nursing Process**: Assessment **Bloom's Taxonomy**: Understand

3. **Correct answer**: A, D, E
Rationale: Frequent neurologic checks are necessary as hypernatremia draws water out of brain cells, causing them to shrink. As the brain shrinks, tension is placed on cerebral vessels, which may cause them to tear and bleed. Hypernatremia affects mental status and brain function including orientation to time, place, and person. Fluid replacement is the primary treatment for hypernatremia. Maintaining intravenous access is necessary for administration of fluids and possible emergency medications. There is no reason to limit the length of visits for the patient with hypernatremia. **Nursing Process**: Planning **Bloom's Taxonomy**: Apply

4. **Correct answer**: B
Rationale: Hypokalemia affects nerve impulse transmission, including the transmission of cardiac impulses. The patient may develop ECG changes and atrial or ventricular dysrhythmias. Oxygen therapy is not indicated for hypokalemia. There is no risk of seizures in the patient with hypokalemia. The patient with hypokalemia should be kept on bedrest; however, this is not the priority action for this patient. **Nursing Process**: Implementation **Bloom's Taxonomy**: Analyze

5. **Correct answer**: B, D, E
Rationale: Calcium should be taken with a full glass of water to allow maximum absorption. They should not be taken with food or milk. If possible, they should not be taken within 1 to 2 hours of other medications. Calcium does not need to be taken with meals. These supplements are not used as needed to treat tremulousness. **Nursing Process**: Evaluation **Bloom's Taxonomy**: Evaluate

6. **Correct answer**: B
Rationale: A positive Chvostek sign indicates increased neuromuscular excitability, commonly associated with both hypomagnesemia and hypocalcemia. Additional manifestations of hypomagnesemia include confusion, hallucinations, and possible psychoses. Administration of magnesium sulfate helps restore magnesium balance and neuromuscular function. Calcium chloride would be administered for manifestations of hypocalcemia. Insulin and glucose are used to treat hyperkalemia. Sodium bicarbonate is used in the treatment of hyperkalemia and metabolic acidosis. **Nursing Process**: Implementation **Bloom's Taxonomy**: Analyze

7. **Correct answer**: A
Rationale: pH of less than 7.35 indicates acidosis. The bicarbonate level is less than 22 mEq/L, which indicates a metabolic component. The $PaCO_2$ of 32 is less than 35 mmHg. This indicates respiratory compensation for the excess acid. None of these blood gas values supports respiratory acidosis or metabolic or respiratory alkalosis. **Nursing Process**: Assessment **Bloom's Taxonomy**: Analyze

8. **Correct answer**: A, B, E
Rationale: The slow respiratory rate leads to inadequate alveolar ventilation. As a result, carbon dioxide is not effectively eliminated from the blood, causing it to accumulate. This increases carbonic acid levels, leading to respiratory acidosis, as indicated by the low pH and high $PaCO_2$. Excess carbon dioxide causes vasodilation, leading to warm, flushed skin, particularly in acute respiratory acidosis. The bicarbonate level is initially unchanged in acute respiratory acidosis because the compensatory response of the kidneys occurs over hours to days. The increased carbon dioxide level will affect neurologic function and the patient will not be alert and oriented. **Nursing Process**: Assessment **Bloom's Taxonomy**: Apply

9. **Correct answer**: B
Rationale: Gastric suctioning removes highly acidic gastric secretions, increasing the risk of metabolic alkalosis. Gastric suctioning will not cause metabolic or respiratory acidosis. Respiratory alkalosis is caused by hyperventilation. **Nursing Process**: Assessment **Bloom's Taxonomy**: Understand

10. **Correct answer**: B
Rationale: The patient is demonstrating classic manifestations of respiratory alkalosis, a potential complication of mechanical ventilation when the rate or volume of ventilations is too high. Arterial blood gases (ABGs) provide the data necessary to confirm and treat this problem. The nurse should obtain recent ABG values before contacting the physician. An analgesic is not going to reduce the patient's symptoms because the respiratory rate on the ventilator is set too high. The nurse should obtain an ABG to validate the patient's manifestations before contacting the respiratory therapist to change or evaluate the ventilator settings. **Nursing Process**: Implementation **Bloom's Taxonomy**: Apply

Chapter 11: Nursing Care of Patients Experiencing Trauma and Shock

Evaluate Your Response to Clinical Reasoning in Patient Care

A Patient with Multiple Injuries

1. Decreased perfusion can result from hemorrhage. Which of Mrs. Souza's vital signs would support this diagnosis? What other assessments could you make that would further support this diagnosis?
2. Consider the physiology of cellular metabolism. How long do brain cells live without oxygen? What happens if circulation is improved but the airway is blocked?
3. What can cause restlessness? Consider comfort, elimination, oxygenation, emotional status, and immobility.
4. List the multiple possibilities for entry of pathogens into the human body. Would age and physical condition increase the risk? What about transmission from healthcare personnel?

A Patient with Septic Shock

1. Review the pharmacologic effects of vasopressors. Consider the pathologic basis for septic shock and how these medications may be effective.
2. Review the content on respiratory acidosis in Chapter 10. What do these findings tell you? What is present in Ms. Huang's physical status that would cause these manifestations?
3. Review the content about colloidal intravenous solutions in this chapter. What would you expect these solutions to do when they are administered? How does this correlate to cardiac output? How do you assess increased circulatory volume?

Test Yourself NCLEX-RN Review Answers

1. **Correct answer**: C
Rationale: The most common mechanical source of injury in all adult age groups is the motor vehicle. Guns are another common mechanical source of injury. Trauma from gunshot wounds has steadily increased during the past 20 years and remains a major reason for emergency department and trauma center admissions. An accidental fire is a thermal source of traumatic injuries. Swimming pools can lead to drowning, which is a physical source of traumatic injuries. **Nursing Process**: Planning **Bloom's Taxonomy**: Understand
2. **Correct answer**: C
Rationale: Maintenance of the airway is of the highest priority for the trauma patient. Other injuries or concerns such as fractures, a hemorrhage, or shallow respirations may distract the nurse away from assessing the airway; however, if the airway is not patent and the patient is unable to deliver oxygen to vital organs, all other interventions are futile. After an airway is established the nurse can assess for breathing, circulation, and then injuries. **Nursing Process**: Assessment **Bloom's Taxonomy**: Apply
3. **Correct answer**: A
Rationale: A pregnancy test is included for any woman of childbearing age in order to rule out the potential for pregnancy and fetal injury. Other tests that she is prescribed will depend on the type of injuries. Serum electrolytes are not specifically prescribed for trauma patients. A complete blood count evaluates the components of blood and will most likely be prescribed for all trauma patients regardless of the patient's gender. Blood type and crossmatch will also most likely be prescribed for all trauma patients regardless of the patient's gender. **Nursing Process**: Implementation **Bloom's Taxonomy**: Apply
4. **Correct answer**: A, C, E
Rationale: A hemolytic reaction is the most dangerous type of transfusion reaction and usually results from an ABO incompatibility. Manifestations of a hemolytic reaction include dyspnea, nausea and vomiting, and facial flushing. The patient is receiving blood for shock. An increase in blood pressure would be a desired outcome. An increase in body temperature of 0.3 degree is not significant when receiving a blood transfusion. **Nursing Process**: Assessment **Bloom's Taxonomy**: Analyze
5. **Correct answer**: A
Rationale: The endotoxins released from bacteria in septic shock stimulate the release of vasoactive proteins, causing peripheral vasodilation and decreased peripheral resistance. Obstructive shock is caused by an obstruction in the heart or great vessels that either impedes venous return or prevents effective cardiac pumping action. Cardiogenic shock occurs when the heart's pumping ability is compromised to the point that it cannot maintain cardiac output and adequate tissue perfusion. Hypovolemic shock is caused by at least a 15% decrease in intravascular volume. **Nursing Process**: Planning **Bloom's Taxonomy**: Analyze
6. **Correct answer**: D
Rationale: When the patient has suffered an injury that causes a hemorrhage, the bleeding must be controlled immediately. This may be done by applying direct pressure over the wound. Vessel clamps can only be used if a vessel is exposed. Limb elevation may slow the bleeding but will not stop it. Vasopressor application is not indicated. **Nursing Process**: Implementation **Bloom's Taxonomy**: Apply
7. **Correct answer**: B
Rationale: Trauma results from an abnormal exchange of energy between a host and a mechanism in a predisposing environment. The host is the person at risk of injury, and multiple factors influence the host's potential for injury, including preexisting illnesses. Recreational activities, psychosocial status, and previous history of traumatic injuries are not factors to determine the patient's ultimate extent of the current chest injury. **Nursing Process**: Assessment **Bloom's Taxonomy**: Apply
8. **Correct answer**: C
Rationale: The gastrointestinal organs normally receive 25% of the cardiac output through the splanchnic circulation. Shock constricts the splanchnic arterioles and redirects arterial blood flow to the heart and brain. This causes gastrointestinal organs to become ischemic and ulcerate. Stress ulcers can develop within hours of severe trauma and may hemorrhage within 2 to 10 days following the original cause of shock. Bleeding and translocation of bacteria can occur, resulting in anemia and septic shock. The patient would have other manifestations if liver lacerations, intracranial bleeding, or internal bleeding were occurring and increased temperature would not be likely in these conditions. **Nursing Process**: Assessment **Bloom's Taxonomy**: Analyze
9. **Correct answer**: A, C, E
Rationale: When administering nitroprusside (Nipride), the nurse should monitor the patient for signs of thiocyanate poisoning if the infusion lasts longer than 72 hours. Confusion is a potential adverse effect and should be reported. Other drugs should not be added to the solution. Urine output of more than 150 mL/hr is normal. Infiltrated intravenous sites should be assessed. Ice is not always the treatment of choice for infiltrated intravenous medications. **Nursing Process**: Implementation **Bloom's Taxonomy**: Apply
10. **Correct answer**: C
Rationale: Monitoring fluid status is essential in preventing shock and includes daily assessments of weight, fluid intake by all routes, measurable fluid loss, and fluid loss that must be estimated, such as profuse perspiration and wound drainage. The risk of neurogenic shock is increased in patients who have received spinal anesthesia. Preventive nursing care includes elevating the head of the bed 15 to 20 degrees following spinal anesthesia. Providing

immediate pain relief helps prevent the onset of cardiogenic shock. Nursing care to prevent septic shock includes careful and consistent hand hygiene. **Nursing Process**: Implementation **Bloom's Taxonomy**: Apply

Chapter 12: Nursing Care of Patients with Infections and Inflammation

Evaluate Your Response to Clinical Reasoning in Patient Care

A Patient with Acquired Immunity

1. Review the concept of acquired immunity and the discussion of immunization in this chapter. What effect could nonimmunized persons have on their family and community?
2. Consider current evidence regarding immunizations and immunization safety as you develop your response.
3. Identify possible systemic and local reactions associated with immunizations. List manifestations that the patient should report to the primary caregiver.

Test Yourself NCLEX-RN Review Answers

1. **Correct answer**: D
   Rationale: Acquired passive immunity is the result of a gamma globulin infusion following exposure to hepatitis A. This type of immunity is short lived and usually lasts only about 4 weeks. Natural passive immunity is acquired by the transfer of maternal antibodies to the fetus or neonate through the placenta or breast milk. Acquired active immunity occurs by immunization with an antigen, such as an attenuated live virus vaccine. Natural active immunity occurs after an infection with a pathogen, resulting in the production of antibodies. **Nursing Process**: Planning **Bloom's Taxonomy**: Understand
2. **Correct answer**: B
   Rationale: For the patient with an infection, the nurse should collect the specimen for culture and sensitivity (C&S) before the first dose of antibiotics is administered to ensure that the medication is effective against the microorganism. Assessing for a history of hypersensitivities and allergies would have been completed before the healthcare provider prescribed medication treatment. The medication should be provided after the C&S is obtained. The nurse would monitor for reactions to the prescribed anti-infective after providing the medication. **Nursing Process**: Implementation **Bloom's Taxonomy**: Apply
3. **Correct answer**: A
   Rationale: Prostaglandins are chemotactic substances that draw leukocytes to inflamed tissue. Aspirin inhibits prostaglandin synthesis and reduces fever, pain, and inflammation. Penicillin is an anti-infective that is used to kill bacteria. Morphine sulfate is an opioid analgesic that is used to control pain. Warfarin (Coumadin) is an anticoagulant and is not used to treat inflammation. **Nursing Process**: Implementation **Bloom's Taxonomy**: Apply
4. **Correct answer**: B
   Rationale: Banded neutrophils are immature white blood cells. An increase in the number of circulating bands indicates an infection. A low number of lymphocytes are seen in renal failure. A low number of basophils are seen in hyperthyroidism. An increased number of eosinophils may indicate an autoimmune disorder. **Nursing Process**: Assessment **Bloom's Taxonomy**: Analyze
5. **Correct answer**: B
   Rationale: Contact precautions reduce the risk of transmission by direct or indirect contact. Since the patient has a draining wound with methicillin-resistant *Staphylococcus aureus*, contact precautions are needed. Droplet precautions reduce the risk of droplet transmission of infectious agents that are generated during coughing, sneezing, talking, or suctioning. Airborne precautions reduce the risk of airborne transmission of infectious agent droplet nuclei or particles containing the infectious agent. Reverse precautions are a type of precaution used to protect a patient from being exposed to infectious microorganisms. This type of isolation is often used for the patient with neutropenia. **Nursing Process**: Implementation **Bloom's Taxonomy**: Apply
6. **Correct answer**: D
   Rationale: The inflammatory cytokines contribute to illness behaviors. Patients respond to increases in these chemicals with increased sleep, warmth-seeking behaviors, and reduced energy output. These are considered adaptive responses to illness. Interferons are a class of cytokine with broad antiviral and anticancer effects. Interferons also moderate the activity of NK cells and may be involved in preventing the spread of abnormal malignant cells. Neutrophils, monocytes, and macrophages, known as phagocytes, are the primary cells involved in phagocytosis. Once attracted to the inflammatory site, phagocytes select and engulf foreign material. The complement system consists of plasma proteins that are activated by a tissue injury or antigen–antibody reaction and are involved in both innate and adaptive immune responses. **Nursing Process**: Assessment **Bloom's Taxonomy**: Analyze
7. **Correct answer**: B, C, E
   Rationale: Neutrophilia is an increase in the numbers of circulating neutrophils and is a common response to infection, inflammation, or a stressful response. Neutrophilia occurs when the bone marrow responds to an increased need for phagocytes. Neutrophilia is not a result of bone marrow depression and does not mean that there is an expected average number of white blood cells. **Nursing Process**: Assessment **Bloom's Taxonomy**: Analyze
8. **Correct answer**: B, E
   Rationale: The patient should be instructed to apply heat for no longer than 20 minutes at a time to reduce the risk of tissue damage from burns. The patient should be instructed to increase fluid intake and to eat a well-balanced diet high in vitamins and minerals and with adequate protein and kilocalories for healing. Acutely inflamed tissue should be rested. This means that the patient should not engage in strenuous activity until the inflammation has subsided. All medication should be taken as prescribed. The course of antibiotics should be completed. **Nursing Process**: Implementation **Bloom's Taxonomy**: Apply
9. **Correct answer**: B, D, E
   Rationale: Nursing interventions to reduce the risk of healthcare-associated infections include encouraging patients to take deep breaths, washing hands with soap and water, and assessing intravenous sites by inspection and palpation. Adequate fluids should be provided and the use of invasive devices such as indwelling catheters should be avoided unless medically necessary. **Nursing Process**: Implementation **Bloom's Taxonomy**: Apply

10. **Correct answer**: C
Rationale: Wearing gloves, gowns, and goggles when there is a potential of body fluid splash or spray is considered a standard precaution. Needles should not be recapped. Preparing work surfaces by spraying with disinfectant is not part of standard precautions. The hands should be washed with antibacterial soap and water if visibly dirty or contaminated with blood. **Nursing Process**: Implementation **Bloom's Taxonomy**: Apply

Chapter 13: Nursing Care of Patients with Altered Immunity

Evaluate Your Response to Clinical Reasoning in Patient Care

A Patient with HIV Infection

1. Think about the effects of HIV and ART on body systems as well as Mr. Lu's current manifestations.
2. Review current data regarding ART and HIV prognosis. Review the section about ART and the ART medication administration box.
3. Consider using credible online resources to identify potential responses to this question by Mr. Lu.
4. Think not only about safer sex practices but also recommended prophylactic measures to prevent HIV infection in partners of infected patients.

Test Yourself NCLEX-RN Review Answers

1. **Correct answer**: A
Rationale: Anaphylaxis is the most severe form of type 1 immediate reactions. When an allergen is introduced for which there is circulating IgE specific to the allergen, a cascade leading to anaphylaxis is initiated. Hemolytic anemia can be associated with a type II cytotoxic hypersensitivity reaction. Graft rejection is a type of cell-mediated hypersensitivity response. Systemic lupus erythematosus is an autoimmune disorder. **Nursing Process**: Implementation **Bloom's Taxonomy**: Analyze
2. **Correct answer**: D
Rationale: Acute tissue rejection is the most common and treatable type of rejection episode that occurs between 4 days and 3 months after the transplant. Hyperacute tissue rejection occurs immediately to 2 to 3 days after the transplant of new tissue. Rejection episodes do not occur within 8 to 24 hours after the transplant. **Nursing Process**: Assessment **Bloom's Taxonomy**: Apply
3. **Correct answer**: C
Rationale: *Pneumocystis* pneumonia (PcP) is the most common pneumonia affecting patients with AIDS and is caused by *Pneumocystis jiroveci*, a common environmental organism that is not pathogenic in patients with intact immune systems. Cytomegalovirus causes disseminated viral infections in the patient with AIDS. *Toxoplasma gondii* and *Cryptococcus neoformans* are parasitic infections that commonly affect the central nervous system in patients with AIDS. **Nursing Process**: Assessment **Bloom's Taxonomy**: Analyze
4. **Correct answer**: C, E
Rationale: A positive HIV rapid antibody test likely indicates the presence of antibodies to HIV in the patient's blood. However, there are false positives to this test so additional testing is required. A positive HIV rapid antibody test is not a definitive test for AIDS. It does not say whether AIDS is or is not active in the patient's blood and does not predict development of AIDS in the future. **Nursing Process**: Implementation **Bloom's Taxonomy**: Apply
5. **Correct answer**: A, E
Rationale: Zidovudine (Retrovir, AZT) is the first antiretroviral agent approved for use with HIV infection. It is now generally reserved for second- or third-line regimens because it causes neutropenia. This medication causes anemia and not polycythemia. Zidovudine is not documented as causing cardio- or nephrotoxicity. **Nursing Process**: Assessment **Bloom's Taxonomy**: Apply
6. **Correct answer**: A
Rationale: When testing for allergies, epicutaneous or prick testing is generally done first to avoid a systemic reaction. This test may be followed by intradermal testing of allergens if a negative response to prick testing occurs. Inhalation is not a method for allergy testing. Sensitization to allergens is accomplished through subcutaneous injections. **Nursing Process**: Planning **Bloom's Taxonomy**: Apply
7. **Correct answer**: B
Rationale: When a hypersensitivity reaction is suspected, it is important to avoid any further exposure to the potential cause. The best way to do this is by replacing all tubing and attaching a new intravenous line primed with normal saline. Flushing the line and running normal saline attached at the Y connection does not reduce exposure to the blood product. It is more important to remove the agent causing the reaction than it is to give oxygen. The type and crossmatch is done prior to administering blood. **Nursing Process**: Implementation **Bloom's Taxonomy**: Analyze
8. **Correct answer**: A
Rationale: Protease inhibitors and nucleoside analogs are associated with serious metabolic problems such as diabetes mellitus. These medications do not cause lactose intolerance. Hashimoto's thyroiditis and systemic lupus erythematosus are autoimmune disorders and are not caused by specific medications. **Nursing Process**: Assessment **Bloom's Taxonomy**: Apply
9. **Correct answer**: D
Rationale: The priority when initiating or changing HIV drug therapy regimens is the patient's willingness to adhere to the drug regimen. Because the side effects can be difficult and challenging to overcome, many patients are not willing to continue with the therapy. Medication therapy for HIV and AIDS is expensive; however, adherence to the prescribed drug regimen is the priority. Accessing dental care and potential toxicities are important, but they are not considered priorities when initiating or changing the drug regimen in a patient who is HIV positive. **Nursing Process**: Planning **Bloom's Taxonomy**: Apply
10. **Correct answer**: D
Rationale: Lymphocyte immune globulin is used to prevent immediate transplant rejection and to treat steroid-resistant rejection episodes. Azathioprine is used to inhibit immune responses in autoimmune disorders. Large doses of corticosteroids used after a transplant are associated with significant adverse effects. MuromonabCD3 is a monoclonal antibody that binds with a surface antigen on T, B, and NK cells to prevent their activation and immune function. This medication is not used immediately after a transplant to prevent rejection. **Nursing Process**: Implementation **Bloom's Taxonomy**: Apply

Chapter 14: Nursing Care of Patients with Cancer

Evaluate Your Response to Clinical Reasoning in Patient Care

A Patient with Cancer

1. Review content on altered nutrition in Chapter 22 and the content in this chapter on nutritional status in patients with cancer. Make a list of diagnostic tests for malnutrition with normal values.
2. Consider the type of cancers Mr. Casey has been diagnosed as having. Where in the body do these malignancies commonly metastasize? What would cause the pain? Are there other causes of severe back pain that should be considered?
3. Review a pharmacology book for medications that increase appetite and make a list of those appropriate to Mr. Casey.
4. Review the content in Chapter 11 on septic shock and outline manifestations. Develop a plan of care for Mr. Casey that is structured by priority of nursing diagnoses.

Test Yourself NCLEX-RN Review Answers

1. **Correct answer**: C
   Rationale: Metastasis occurs when cells from a primary tumor site travel through the lymphatic system or bloodstream to find a secondary target. Mutation is an action that occurs within genetic material that can cause the development of neoplasms. Dysplasia develops when DNA loses control over cell differentiation. It occurs in response to adverse conditions and causes abnormal variations in cell size, shape, appearance, and usual arrangement. Carcinogenesis is a process in which normal cells are transformed into cancer cells. **Nursing Process**: Implementation **Bloom's Taxonomy**: Apply
2. **Correct answer**: C
   Rationale: Early in the disease process, threats to or changes in health status, physical discomfort, impaired role functioning, or even socioeconomic status can cause psychologic and emotional disturbance, such as fear, anxiety, or hopelessness. The patient may report insomnia and feelings of tension and apprehension. A patient with moderate or severe anxiety can be managed by counseling and teaching new coping skills. Encouraging the patient to express feelings about the cancer diagnosis is the most valuable and powerful intervention that could be offered. Antianxiety and sleep medication might be indicated if talking about the disease process does not help reduce anxiety and insomnia. The nurse will most likely document the patient's difficulty with sleep and anxiety in the medical record; however, this would not be the most appropriate initial intervention. **Nursing Process**: Implementation **Bloom's Taxonomy**: Apply
3. **Correct answer**: B, D
   Rationale: It is important not to rub or scratch the treated skin areas because this can cause skin breaks or irritation. Rubbing may also wipe off the ink markings, which are important landmarks to ensure that the radiation treatments are directed to the correct location. Mild soap may be used for daily cleaning. Lotions may be used, especially if the patient has lymphedema. Aluminum-containing products may interact with external-beam radiation and should be avoided. The patient should apply neither heat nor cold to the treated area. **Nursing Process**: Implementation **Bloom's Taxonomy**: Apply
4. **Correct answer**: D
   Rationale: Around-the-clock administration of antiemetic medications may be an effective measure to prevent nausea and vomiting associated with chemotherapy. Administering chemotherapy at bedtime will not prevent the development of nausea and vomiting resulting from the medication. It is not nutritionally sound to keep the patient on clear liquids or nothing by mouth status until daily chemotherapy treatments are completed. **Nursing Process**: Implementation **Bloom's Taxonomy**: Apply
5. **Correct answer**: D
   Rationale: Although all of these choices can be a result of chemotherapy, the one that is directly related to bone marrow suppression is a low platelet count of 50,000. The excessive numbers of immature leukocytes in the bone marrow diminish erythrocyte and thrombocyte or platelet production, resulting in secondary anemia, neutropenia, and thrombocytopenia. Cytotoxic drugs can affect hair cells, leading to alopecia. Anorexia and food aversion are common, but not related to bone marrow depression. Nausea and vomiting are caused by the chemotherapeutic medication, but are not an indication of bone marrow depression. **Nursing Process**: Assessment **Bloom's Taxonomy**: Analyze
6. **Correct answer**: A
   Rationale: Chemotherapy disrupts the cell cycle in various phases by interrupting cell metabolism and replication. It also works by interfering with the ability of the malignant cell to synthesize vital enzymes and chemicals. Different drugs work on some phases of the cell cycle and other drugs work through the entire cell cycle. Most chemotherapy involves combinations of drugs administered over varying periods of time according to different protocols. Chemotherapy does not promote the normal growth of cells. The side and toxic effects of chemotherapy vary with the drug used and the length of treatment. Tissues usually affected by cytotoxic drugs include mucous membranes, hair cells, bone marrow, and body organs such as the heart, lungs, bladder, kidney, and reproductive organs. **Nursing Process**: Evaluation **Bloom's Taxonomy**: Evaluate
7. **Correct answer**: C
   Rationale: External radiation therapy is when the radiation is initiated outside of the body, is directed toward the patient, and is set to deliver to a certain depth for a specified period of time. This exposure is meant to destroy the cancer cells with which the radiation comes into direct contact. Internal radiation is also called brachytherapy. With this approach radiation is given inside the body by implanting small amounts of radioactive material directly into a tumor or body cavity while avoiding scattering radiation to the surrounding tissues or organs. Biochemotherapy is the combining of biologic agents with chemotherapeutic drugs. Internal-beam radiation therapy is not a type of radiation therapy. **Nursing Process**: Implementation **Bloom's Taxonomy**: Apply
8. **Correct answer**: B
   Rationale: Tumor lysis syndrome, a life-threatening emergency for patients with cancer, is characterized by a combination of two or more metabolic abnormalities, including hyperuricemia, hyperphosphatemia, hyperkalemia, and/or hypocalcemia. White blood cell count would be monitored for septic shock. There is not a specific laboratory test to monitor spinal cord compression. Superior vena

cava syndrome is caused by the enlargement of a tumor adjacent to the superior vena cava, compressing the major blood vessel and leading to reduced blood flow to the heart. **Nursing Process**: Assessment **Bloom's Taxonomy**: Apply

9. **Correct answer**: A
   Rationale: The S phase is when DNA replication occurs. This is when the cell is beginning mitosis and the chromosomes multiply from 23 to 46. They then migrate toward each axis in preparation for division of the cell. In the M phase, the parent cell divides into two exact copy cells called daughter cells, each having identical genetic material. G1 is the beginning of the cell cycle. G2 occurs when the cell is preparing for mitosis. **Nursing Process**: Planning **Bloom's Taxonomy**: Apply
10. **Correct answer**: C, E
   Rationale: Oncogenes are abnormal genes that promote cell proliferation, are capable of triggering cancerous characteristics, and can be classified according to their overall function. A decrease in the body's immune surveillance may allow the expression of oncogenes, which can occur during times of stress or in response to certain carcinogens. Oncogenes do not promote cellular repair. They are not strictly regulated, nor do they stimulate a complex signaling process. **Nursing Process**: Planning **Bloom's Taxonomy**: Apply

Chapter 15: Assessing the Integumentary System

Test Yourself NCLEX-RN Review Answers

1. **Correct answer**: A
   Rationale: The dermis is the second, deeper layer of skin. Most of the hair follicles and sweat glands are located in the dermis. All layers of the skin through the dermis are burned. This includes the epidermis and its layers, two of which are the stratum basale and stratum spinosum. The stratum basale is the deepest layer of the epidermis and contains melanocytes, which produce the pigment melanin, and keratinocytes, which produce keratin. The next layer of the epidermis is the stratum spinosum, which contains abundant cells that arise from the bone marrow and migrate to the epidermis. Mitosis occurs at this layer. **Nursing Process**: Implementation **Bloom's Taxonomy**: Apply
2. **Correct answer**: B
   Rationale: Melanin is a pigment that forms a protective shield to protect the keratinocytes and the nerve endings in the dermis from the damaging effects of ultraviolet light. Melanocyte activity accounts for the difference in skin color in humans. Sebum is an oily substance that softens and lubricates the skin and hair and also decreases water loss from the skin. Carotene is a yellow-to-orange pigment found in areas of the body where the stratum corneum is thickest, such as the palms of the hands. This pigment is more abundant in the skins of persons of Asian ancestry and, together with melanin, accounts for the golden skin tone. Because the epidermis in White skin has very little melanin and is almost transparent, the color of the hemoglobin found in red blood cells circulating through the dermis shows through, causing the skin to appear pink. **Nursing Process**: Assessment **Bloom's Taxonomy**: Apply
3. **Correct answer**: B
   Rationale: Inspection is the first assessment technique to check the skin surface. After inspection the next assessment step is palpation of any skin areas that appear abnormal in order to get a better understanding of depth and size of any lesions. The assessment techniques of percussion and auscultation are not used to assess the integumentary status. **Nursing Process**: Assessment **Bloom's Taxonomy**: Apply
4. **Correct answer**: D
   Rationale: Erythema often occurs as a result of increased body temperature. This occurs when the capillaries in the skin dilate to release some of the heat caused from the increased body temperature. Pallor or paleness of the skin occurs with shock, anemia, or hypoxia from the reduction in number or oxygenation of red blood cells. Jaundice is a yellow-orange color caused by the breakdown of red blood cells or alteration in liver functioning. Cyanosis is a bluish color caused by poor oxygenation of hemoglobin. **Nursing Process**: Assessment **Bloom's Taxonomy**: Apply
5. **Correct answer**: B, D, E
   Rationale: During the health history the nurse should ask questions that focus on the precipitating cause of the itching such as the use of any new medications, soap, skin care agents, cosmetics, pets, travel, stress, or dietary changes. It is also important to identify when the symptom began and if the patient has ever had the symptom before this episode. It is redundant to ask a patient to explain how itching feels. Asking the patient why the itching is being scratched does not provide information about the possible cause. The patient's daily fluid intake will not provide sufficient information about the cause of the patient's itching. **Nursing Process**: Assessment **Bloom's Taxonomy**: Apply
6. **Correct answer**: A
   Rationale: When assessing skin turgor the skinfold should return rapidly to a normal position. Tenting (in which the skin remains in a pinched position for a few moments before returning to the normal position) commonly occurs in older patients who are thin. Decreased skin turgor is also a sign of dehydration. Pallor is skin paleness caused by anemia or hypoxia. Cyanosis is a bluish discoloration of the skin caused by reduced oxygenation of hemoglobin. Increased skin moisture may be associated with shock, fever, increased activity, or anxiety. Lesions can be ulcerated, scaly, asymmetric, linear, or grouped. **Nursing Process**: Assessment **Bloom's Taxonomy**: Apply
7. **Correct answer**: C
   Rationale: When documenting edema, 1+ is slight pitting without any obvious distortion; 2+ is a deeper pit without any obvious distortion; 3+ is an obvious pit and the extremity is swollen; and 4+ is a pit that remains with an obvious distortion. **Nursing Process**: Assessment **Bloom's Taxonomy**: Apply
8. **Correct answer**: D
   Rationale: Lichenification is rough, thickened, hardened areas of epidermis caused by chronic irritation from scratching or rubbing. Chronic dermatitis can cause lichenification. An ulcer is an area of skin erosion. A papule is an elevated, solid, palpable mass with a circumscribed border. Papules are smaller than 0.5 cm and include elevated moles, warts, and lichen planus. Atrophy is used to describe translucent, dry, paper-like or wrinkled skin surface resulting from thinning or wasting of the skin due to loss of collagen and elastin. **Nursing Process**: Assessment **Bloom's Taxonomy**: Apply
9. **Correct answer**: A, D
   Rationale: Pinpoint red dots with tiny radiating blood vessels that blanche with pressure are most likely spider

angiomas. These can be associated with liver disease or vitamin B deficiency. They are not related to poor hygiene, impairment of the immune system, or high sodium intake. **Nursing Process**: Assessment **Bloom's Taxonomy**: Apply

10. **Correct answer**: C
Rationale: Head lice may be seen as oval nits or eggs that adhere to the base of the hair shaft. Pustules may be related to an infection or tinea capitus. Greasy scaling is likely seborrhea and flakes in the hair can be dandruff or tinea capitus, requiring additional assessment. **Nursing Process**: Assessment **Bloom's Taxonomy**: Apply

Chapter 16: Nursing Care of Patients with Integumentary Disorders

Evaluate Your Response to Clinical Reasoning in Patient Care

A Patient with Herpes Zoster

1. Consider environmental, economic, and language barriers. What agencies in your own city or state exist to provide help? What can you do other than make referrals? If you do make a referral, to whom would it be?
2. Review skin assessment guidelines in Chapter 15. How would you determine that the lesions had not improved? What manifestations would indicate secondary infection of the lesions? What would you do next if the lesions are still very painful and have not improved?
3. Consider what issues the Rivera family may face if Mr. Rivera cannot work. Related factors include inadequate or inappropriate linkage with the healthcare system and poverty. Based on this information, what interventions would you use? How would you evaluate the effectiveness of your interventions?

A Patient with Malignant Melanoma

1. List reasons why people do not seek healthcare. Do you believe nurses can effect change? If so, what community activities would be most effective?
2. Consider attitudes toward the possibility of future illnesses. How would this affect your plan? What do you believe would be most effective in teaching this age group?
3. Think about what you know about taking prescribed antibiotics as well as the side effects of antibiotic therapy. What would you suggest that Mr. Sanders do?
4. Powerlessness is the perception that one's own actions will not significantly affect an outcome. Is this a common response to the diagnosis of cancer? Consider types of communications and interventions that would allow greater decision making for Mr. Sanders.

Test Yourself NCLEX-RN Review Answers

1. **Correct answer**: B, C
Rationale: The best way to help moisturize the skin is to apply a moisturizing agent after bathing. If used, bath oil should be added at the end of the bath since moist skin is more likely to retain the oil. Hot water can dry the skin, making the xerosis worse. A warm environment is not going to lubricate the patient's skin. Fabric softeners can cause skin irritations and should not be used. **Nursing Process**: Planning **Bloom's Taxonomy**: Apply
2. **Correct answer**: A
Rationale: Dysplastic nevi are larger than other nevi and may be flat, slightly raised, or appear as lesions with a darker, raised center and irregular border. Because dysplastic nevi can transform into malignant lesions, it is important to monitor them for changes in size, thickness, color, bleeding, or itching. If any of these changes occur, the person should seek immediate professional assessment. A keloid is a thickening of the skin caused by fibroblasts and type III collagen. A skin tag is a benign skin lesion that can become irritated and bleed. An angioma is a benign vascular tumor. **Nursing Process**: Assessment **Bloom's Taxonomy**: Analyze
3. **Correct answer**: C, E
Rationale: Psoriasis causes abnormal growth and division of epidermal cells, causing keratosis. The use of ultraviolet light therapy helps to slow down this cellular division, which decreases the lesions and keratosis associated with psoriasis. Eyes are shielded during the treatment. Ultraviolet light therapy does not need to be combined with hot baths to be effective. Ultraviolet-B light or narrowband UVB units may be purchased or constructed to be used in the patient's home. Ultraviolet light decreases the cellular division that causes keratosis and decreases itching. **Nursing Process**: Implementation **Bloom's Taxonomy**: Apply
4. **Correct answer**: D
Rationale: Actinic keratosis, also called senile or solar keratosis, is an epidermal skin lesion directly related to chronic sun exposure and photodamage. About 20% of actinic keratoses convert to squamous cell carcinoma. Folliculitis is a bacterial infection of the hair follicle, most commonly caused by *Staphylococcus aureus*. Pressure ulcers develop from external pressure that compresses blood vessels or from friction and shearing forces that tear and injure vessels. Pediculosis is an infestation with lice or parasites that live on the blood of an animal or human host. **Nursing Process**: Implementation **Bloom's Taxonomy**: Apply
5. **Correct answer**: D
Rationale: A linear pattern of painful vesicles indicates shingles, a varicella infection. The virus remains along a nerve from a previous infection with chickenpox. A rash of painful vesicles is not associated with acne, using tanning booths, or being sunburned as a child.
Nursing Process: Assessment **Bloom's Taxonomy**: Planning
6. **Correct answer**: D
Rationale: Anyone can have lice. They affect people of all social classes but are associated with crowded or unsanitary living conditions. Major infestations often occur in areas where many people are in close proximity, especially in the public school setting. Lice are a parasite and not a fungus. Pediculosis corporis is an infestation with body lice and pediculosis pubis is an infestation with pubic lice. **Nursing Process**: Implementation **Bloom's Taxonomy**: Remember
7. **Correct answer**: B
Rationale: Risk factors for the development of nonmelanoma skin cancer include fair skin, freckles, blue or green eyes, and blond or red hair. Alopecia, thin hair, and itching do not increase the risk of developing this skin disorder. Dark hair, dark or tanned skin, dry skin, and edema do not increase the risk of developing nonmelanoma skin cancer. **Nursing Process**: Planning **Bloom's Taxonomy**: Analyze
8. **Correct answer**: A
Rationale: A change in the color or size of a nevus is cause for concern when evaluating for the possibility of melanoma. Ichthyosis is an inherited dermatologic condition in which the skin is dry, fissured, and hyperkeratotic. The

surface of the skin has the appearance of fish scales. Psoriasis is a chronic immune skin disorder characterized by raised, reddened, round circumscribed plaques covered by silvery white scales. A carbuncle is a group of infected hair follicles. The lesion begins as a firm mass located in the subcutaneous tissue and the lower dermis. **Nursing Process**: Assessment **Bloom's Taxonomy**: Apply

9. **Correct answer**: B
   Rationale: Shearing forces result when one tissue layer slides over another. The stretching and bending of blood vessels cause injury and thrombosis. Patients in hospital beds are subject to shearing forces when the head of the bed is elevated and the torso slides down toward the foot of the bed. Pulling the patient up in bed also subjects the patient to shearing forces so, for this reason, always lift patients up in bed. In both cases, friction and moisture cause the skin and superficial fascia to remain fixed to the bed sheet, while the deep fascia and bony skeleton slide in the direction of body movement. The reason the patient is lifted is not related to stress on the patient's joints. Pulling a patient up in bed does not decrease tissue hypoxia. Lifting a patient up in bed is not done to provide a brief period of increased capillary circulation. **Nursing Process**: Implementation **Bloom's Taxonomy**: Apply

10. **Correct answer**: C
    Rationale: Dermabrasion is a skin treatment that helps to reduce the appearance of acne scarring and other skin imperfections. A skin flap is a piece of tissue whose free end is moved from a donor site to a recipient site while maintaining a continuous blood supply through its connection at the base or pedicle. Liposuction is a method of changing the contours of the body by aspirating fat from the subcutaneous layer of tissue. A blepharoplasty is a cosmetic surgery in which loose skin and protruding periorbital fat is removed from the upper and lower eyelids. **Nursing Process**: Implementation **Bloom's Taxonomy**: Apply

Chapter 17: Nursing Care of Patients with Burns

Evaluate Your Response to Clinical Reasoning in Patient Care

A Patient with a Major Burn

1. Review the effects of the major burn wound on the renal and gastrointestinal systems. What assessments would indicate effective fluid resuscitation?
2. What type of burns did Mr. Howard have on his arms? Consider the effect of compression on the peripheral vascular system. What assessments would you make to identify this complication?
3. Consider the type of pain the patient has. What do you think might happen if the narcotics were given by other routes, such as oral or intramuscular?
4. Review the effects of a major burn. Consider the damage to cell wall integrity and capillary beds. What effect does the shift of proteins and sodium have on intravascular volume?

Test Yourself NCLEX-RN Review Answers

1. **Correct answer**: A, C
   Rationale: During burn shock, potassium ions leave the intracellular compartment, predisposing the patient to developing cardiac dysrhythmias. Vast amounts of fluids are lost through the damaged skin, resulting in decreased intravascular fluid volume. This condition artificially increases hematocrit levels. Serum albumin is a measurement of nutritional status and is measured most often during the rehabilitative phase of burn management. During the early stages of the burn injury, renal blood flow and glomerular filtration rates are greatly reduced from the decreased intravascular blood volume and the release of antidiuretic hormone (ADH) by the posterior pituitary. The blood urea nitrogen level will increase. The shock of injury may result in a spike in blood glucose. **Nursing Process**: Assessment **Bloom's Taxonomy**: Analyze

2. **Correct answer**: B
   Rationale: A full-thickness burn involves all layers of the skin, including the epidermis, the dermis, and the epidermal appendages. The burn wound may appear pale, waxy, yellow, brown, mottled, charred, or nonblanching red. The wound surface is dry, leathery, and firm to the touch. There is no sensation of pain or light touch because pain and touch receptors have been destroyed. Superficial, superficial partial-thickness, and deep partial-thickness burns will still be very painful to the patient because the nerves remain intact or exposed. **Nursing Process**: Assessment **Bloom's Taxonomy**: Understand

3. **Correct answer**: D
   Rationale: The larger the surface area of the burn and the deeper the burn, the more at risk the patient is for burn shock. Although the pathophysiologic mechanisms of postburn vascular changes and fluid volume shifts are not clearly understood, burn shock is seen in patients with >40% of total body surface area burned. A high-voltage electrical accident will cause a deeper burn and because >50% of this patient's body is affected, this patient is at the highest risk. The patient with 10% TBSA and the patient with superficial burns are at less risk for developing burn shock. The patient with radiation burns from cancer treatment is also at a low risk for developing burn shock. **Nursing Process**: Assessment **Bloom's Taxonomy**: Analyze

4. **Correct answer**: A
   Rationale: Silver sulfadiazine (Silvadene) cream can cause neutropenia. It is important for the nurse to monitor the patient's WBC count daily to assess for any changes, which could indicate neutropenia. Signs of dehydration should be monitored if sulfa crystals develop in the patient's urine. Daily monitoring of serum electrolytes is not indicated for this medication. Pain medication is not necessary before applying this medication, although providing pain medication before a burn dressing change would be a part of routine nursing care. **Nursing Process**: Implementation **Bloom's Taxonomy**: Apply

5. **Correct answer**: B
   Rationale: The Consensus formula uses lactated Ringer or other balanced saline solution, administered at 2–4 mL × kg × % TBSA burn, with 50% of the total volume infused in the first 8 hours, and the remaining 50% over the next 16 hours. This would be 4 × 70 × 50% = 14,000 × 50% = 7000. The volume of 3000 mL is too low for either the 2 or the 4mL calculation. Both 10,500 mL and 14,000 mL are too high for either the 3 or the 4 mL calculation. **Nursing Process**: Implementation **Bloom's Taxonomy**: Apply

6. **Correct answer**: D
   Rationale: Hourly urine output is often used as an indicator of effective fluid resuscitation, with about

0.5 mL/kg/h for an adult considered adequate. Another indicator is heart rate; however, if fluid resuscitation is adequate, the rate should be fewer than 120 beats per minute or in the upper limits of normal for the patient's age. But the fear, anxiety, and pain that accompany burn injuries often increase heart rate. Blood pressure changes are less reliable because significant hypotension does not develop until volume losses exceed 30% due to the body's compensatory mechanisms. A steadily decreasing central venous pressure indicates inadequate fluid resuscitation. **Nursing Process**: Evaluation **Bloom's Taxonomy**: Analyze

7. **Correct answer**: B
   Rationale: A decreased left radial pulse is cause for alarm in this type and location of burn. This can be the first symptom seen in compartment syndrome and is a surgical emergency. The patient is going to have pain, fluid-filled vesicles, and blanching of the extremity, findings that are all consistent with deep partial-thickness burns. **Nursing Process**: Implementation **Bloom's Taxonomy**: Analyze

8. **Correct answer**: B
   Rationale: The "rule of nines" is a method of quickly estimating the percentage of TBSA affected by a burn injury. It is most useful in emergency situations but is not accurate for estimating TBSA in adults who are short, obese, or very thin. In this method, the body is divided into five surface areas—head, trunk, arms, legs, and perineum—and percentages that equal or total a sum of nines are assigned to each body area. Only partial- and full-thickness burns are included in the estimation. For this patient the calculation is as follows: anterior trunk = 18%, perineum = 1%, left arm = 9%. These are added together to equal 28%. The other percentage choices reflect an inaccurate use of the rule of nines. **Nursing Process**: Assessment **Bloom's Taxonomy**: Apply

9. **Correct answer**: B, C, D, E
   Rationale: Teaching injury prevention is a very important job in nursing. Burns are a common injury in the home. It is important to help older adults understand ways to help prevent burns. The water temperature of the water heater should not be set above 120°F. This can help prevent burns from water scalding. Wearing close-fitting clothing when cooking can help prevent shirt sleeves or scarves from catching on fire. Installing antiscald devices can also help prevent water burns. Because older adults often have decreased olfactory senses, having a neighbor routinely check for the odor of gas can help prevent fires. Smoke detector alarm batteries should be checked monthly. **Nursing Process**: Implementation **Bloom's Taxonomy**: Apply

10. **Correct answer**: A, E
    Rationale: A 15% carbon monoxide level would cause only mild manifestations of dizziness or nausea. Carbon monoxide levels of 21 to 40% will cause the manifestations of drowsiness and hypotension. Dark-red skin color occurs at levels over 60%. **Nursing Process**: Assessment **Bloom's Taxonomy**: Remember

Chapter 18: Assessing the Endocrine System

Test Yourself NCLEX-RN Review Answers

1. **Correct answer**: B
   Rationale: ADH (antidiuretic hormone) causes the distal tubules of the kidneys to reabsorb water, which would decrease the urine output. A decrease in the amount of ADH would cause an increase in urine output. ADH does not influence testosterone production or facial hair growth in women. **Nursing Process**: Assessment **Bloom's Taxonomy**: Analyze

2. **Correct answer**: C
   Rationale: A positive Trousseau sign occurs with low serum calcium levels. A positive test causes the fingers and hand to contract on the arm where a blood pressure cuff is inflated. The contraction is a carpal spasm. Palpating skin turgor assesses for hydration status. Skin color is assessed for oxygenation. The urine test for 17-ketosteroids is done to assess adrenal cortex, pituitary, and gonadal hormone function. **Nursing Process**: Assessment **Bloom's Taxonomy**: Apply

3. **Correct answer**: C
   Rationale: The glucocorticoids cortisol and cortisone affect carbohydrate metabolism by regulating glucose use in body tissues, mobilizing fatty acids from fatty tissue, and shifting the source of energy for muscle cells from glucose to fatty acids. Glucocorticoids are released in times of stress. Excessive amounts of glucocorticoids depress the inflammatory response and inhibit the effectiveness of the immune system. Excessive amounts of glucocorticoids do not affect maturation. The metabolic rate will be increased. The response to glucagon in the bloodstream is decreased. **Nursing Process**: Planning **Bloom's Taxonomy**: Apply

4. **Correct answer**: B, E
   Rationale: When assessing the endocrine system, it is important to look for manifestations of diabetes. One of the first manifestations is polydipsia, which is increased thirst. Tightness in rings may indicate increases in growth hormone. Questions about scar tissue, children's problems with urination, and abdominal pain do not focus on the patient's endocrine system assessment. **Nursing Process**: Assessment **Bloom's Taxonomy**: Apply

5. **Correct answer**: B
   Rationale: The thyroid gland is palpated to assess for size and consistency. This helps determine if the patient has an enlarged gland, which could indicate a goiter or the presence of nodules. The thyroid gland is not palpated to assess for pain, pulse rate, character, texture, edema, or movement. **Nursing Process**: Assessment **Bloom's Taxonomy**: Apply

6. **Correct answer**: C, E
   Rationale: Chvostek's sign, a test for hypocalcemia, is assessed by tapping a finger in front of the patient's ear at the angle of the jaw. A positive Chvostek sign causes facial grimacing due to repeated contractions of the facial muscle. A normal finding is no facial grimacing in response to tapping the patient's face in front of the ear. Depressing the skin over the shin would be assessing for edema. Pinching a fold of skin over the sternum is testing for skin turgor or hydration status. Inflating a blood pressure cuff above the antecubital space is assessing for Trousseau sign, which is another technique to assess for manifestations from a low calcium level. **Nursing Process**: Assessment **Bloom's Taxonomy**: Apply

7. **Correct answer**: B
   Rationale: Thyrotropic cells secrete thyroid-stimulating hormone (TSH), which in turn stimulates the synthesis and release of thyroid hormones from the thyroid gland.

Growth hormone (GH) is released by the anterior pituitary gland. Fasting blood sugar (FBS) is a laboratory test to measure blood glucose level after a period of fasting. Aldosterone is a mineralocorticoid released by the adrenal cortex. This hormone promotes kidney tubule reabsorption of sodium and water and excretion of potassium in response to elevated levels of potassium and low levels of sodium to increase blood pressure and blood volume. **Nursing Process**: Assessment **Bloom's Taxonomy**: Analyze

8. **Correct answer**: C
Rationale: Palpable thyroid nodules are considered an expected age-related change in the endocrine system. S1/S2l heart tones would be expected and not associated with the endocrine system. The older female patient might have an increase in facial hair because of the loss of estrogen. The pituitary gland is located within the cranium. The nurse will not be able to directly palpate this gland to determine size and consistency. **Nursing Process**: Assessment **Bloom's Taxonomy**: Analyze
9. **Correct answer**: A
Rationale: Rough, dry skin is often seen in patients with hypothyroidism. Smooth and flushed skin can be a sign of hyperthyroidism. Cold, clammy skin is not associated with any particular endocrine disorder. Hirsutism or excessive facial hair may indicate Cushing syndrome. **Nursing Process**: Assessment **Bloom's Taxonomy**: Apply
10. **Correct answer**: C
Rationale: Increased deep tendon reflexes are seen in hyperthyroidism. Tetany is assessed by using the Trousseau or Chvostek signs. Assessment for acromegaly will need to be done by measuring the patient's growth hormone level. Cushing syndrome is assessed by measuring adrenal cortex hormone levels. **Nursing Process**: Assessment **Bloom's Taxonomy**: Apply

Chapter 19: Nursing Care of Patients with Endocrine Disorders

Evaluate Your Response to Clinical Reasoning in Patient Care

A Patient with Graves Disease

1. What effect does increased TH have on metabolism and cardiac rate and stroke volume? How does this effect compare to that of sympathetic stimulation?
2. Consider the effect of elevating any body part, such as elevating your leg above heart level for a sprained ankle. How does this affect venous return?
3. You will need to consider Mrs. Manuel from both a medical and a surgical perspective. How would you teach her to care for her incision? With removal of most of the thyroid gland, what manifestations would you be sure she knew about? What should she do if these occur?

A Patient with Hypothyroidism

1. Make a list of changes in body systems that occur with aging and with decreased TH levels. How would you determine what assessment findings were abnormal?
2. Consider the effects of the following factors: weakness, fatigue, problems with memory. What would you recommend she do in her home to increase her safety?
3. Prepare a list of manifestations of hypothyroidism. Be sure they are in terms a patient would understand.

A Patient with Addison Disease

1. Review the functions of the hormones of the adrenal cortex in Chapter 18. Consider the effects of stress, and formulate your response with a rationale.
2. Review content on fluid imbalance in Chapter 10. Make a list of assessments you might make that would indicate severe dehydration. What is the pathophysiology of fluid loss in the patient with Addison disease?
3. Review content on sodium and potassium in Chapter 10 and make a list of foods you would suggest Addy eat.

Test Yourself NCLEX-RN Review Answers

1. **Correct answer**: D
Rationale: Graves' disease is the most common cause of hyperthyroidism and is considered an autoimmune disorder. It is sometimes associated with the presence of other autoimmune disorders such as myasthenia gravis, diabetes mellitus, celiac disease, and pernicious anemia. The serum of patients with Graves' disease has an antibody that binds to TSH receptors in the thyroid follicles and causes the thyroid cells to hyperfunction. When this antibody binds to the TSH receptors, it stimulates hormone synthesis and secretion, enlarging the gland. The cause is unknown, but there is a hereditary link. Graves' disease is seen eight times more often in women than in men and occurs most frequently between the ages of 20 and 40. Even though there is a genetic link with this disease, it is categorized as being an autoimmune disorder. Graves' disease does not develop in response to an allergy or an infection. **Nursing Process**: Implementation **Bloom's Taxonomy**: Apply
2. **Correct answer**: A
Rationale: Because the thyroid gland takes up iodine in any form, radioactive iodine (131^{I}) concentrates in the thyroid gland and damages or destroys thyroid cells so that they produce less thyroid hormone. Radioactive iodine is given orally and the patient will see results in 6 to 8 weeks. The patient is not hospitalized during treatment and does not require radiation precautions. This type of therapy is contraindicated in pregnant women because radioactive iodine crosses the placenta and can have negative effects on the developing fetal thyroid gland. Because the amount of gland destroyed is not readily controllable, the patient may develop hypothyroidism and require lifelong thyroid hormone replacement therapy. Adverse reactions include thyroiditis and cardiac instability due to liberation of stored thyroid hormone in the gland. Radioactive iodine does not impact the vascularity of the thyroid gland. **Nursing Process**: Implementation **Bloom's Taxonomy**: Apply
3. **Correct answer**: B
Rationale: When TH production decreases, the thyroid gland enlarges in a compensatory attempt to produce more hormones. The goiter that results is usually a simple or nontoxic form. People living in certain areas of the world where the soil is deficient in iodine, the substance necessary for TH synthesis and secretion, are more prone to become hypothyroid and develop simple goiter. In hypothyroidism the development of a goiter is associated with a lack of dietary iodine intake. A goiter does not develop because of excessive TH stimulating thyroid follicles. A goiter that develops in response to increased levels of TH is seen in hyperthyroidism. **Nursing Process**: Implementation **Bloom's Taxonomy**: Apply

4. **Correct answer**: D
Rationale: Cushing syndrome is a chronic disorder in which hyperfunction of the adrenal cortex produces excessive amounts of circulating cortisol or ACTH. The disorder also may occur as the result of pharmacologic therapy (iatrogenic Cushing). People who take steroids for long periods of time are at increased risk for developing the disorder. Acromegaly is caused by overproduction of growth hormone. Cortisone treatment for rheumatoid arthritis will not lead to the development of hypo- or hyperthyroidism. **Nursing Process**: Assessment **Bloom's Taxonomy**: Apply

5. **Correct answer**: C
Rationale: Addison disease is a disorder resulting from destruction or dysfunction of the adrenal cortex. The result is chronic deficiency of cortisol, aldosterone, and adrenal androgens, accompanied by skin pigmentation. Addisonian crisis is a life-threatening response to acute adrenal insufficiency. Triggers include surgery, acute systemic illness, trauma, or abrupt withdrawal of long-term corticosteroid therapy. Patients with Addison disease must learn to provide lifelong self-care that includes taking medications. The patient will need to learn how to self-administer steroids and the importance of carrying at all times an emergency kit containing parenteral cortisone and a syringe/needle. Medications for this disorder are to be taken continuously. Abruptly discontinuing the medication is dangerous. In the event of an illness or other stressor, the amount of medication the patient needs will be altered by the healthcare provider. **Nursing Process**: Evaluation **Bloom's Taxonomy**: Analyze

6. **Correct answer**: A, E
Rationale: Manifestations of SIADH occur as a result of water retention, hyponatremia, and serum hypo-osmolality. Blood volume expands, but the plasma is diluted. Aldosterone is suppressed and renal excretion of sodium increases. Water moves from the hypotonic plasma and the interstitial spaces into the cells. Urinary output decreases and the urine becomes very concentrated. Brain cells may swell, causing neurologic manifestations including both irritability and lethargy. Weight gain results from the retention of fluid. Constipation and hyperkalemia are not manifestations associated with SIADH. **Nursing Process**: Assessment **Bloom's Taxonomy**: Analyze

7. **Correct answer**: B
Rationale: Hyperparathyroidism results from an increase in the secretion of parathyroid hormone (PTH), which regulates normal serum levels of calcium. The increase in PTH affects the kidneys and bones, resulting in increased resorption of calcium and excretion of phosphate by the kidneys and increased release of calcium and phosphorus by bones. This leads to bone decalcification. Bone reabsorption results in pathologic fractures. Osteoporosis is a disease process of bone demineralization. The combination of the two health problems increases this patient's risk for injury from fractures. There is not enough information to determine if these disease processes will lead to fear, social isolation, or a risk for chronic low self-esteem. **Nursing Process**: Planning **Bloom's Taxonomy**: Analyze

8. **Correct answer**: C, E
Rationale: Increased serum calcium decreases neuromuscular excitability, which decreases bowel motility. Manifestations of the effect of hypercalcemia on the gastrointestinal tract include constipation. Hypercalcemia also affects the cardiovascular system, causing dysrhythmias. Hypercalcemia does not affect urine output. A positive Chvostek sign is a manifestation of hypocalcemia. Deep tendon reflexes are hyperactive in hypocalcemia, not hypercalcemia. **Nursing Process**: Assessment **Bloom's Taxonomy**: Apply

9. **Correct answer**: B
Rationale: Hypoparathyroidism results from abnormally low PTH levels. The most common cause is damage to or inadvertent removal of all of the parathyroid glands during thyroidectomy. The lack of circulating PTH causes hypocalcemia and an elevated blood phosphate level. The low calcium levels cause changes in neuromuscular activity, affecting peripheral motor and sensory nerves. The neuromuscular manifestations that result include numbness and tingling around the mouth and in the fingertips. Recovery from a thyroidectomy will not cause an Addisonian crisis, Cushing syndrome, or hyperparathyroidism. **Nursing Process**: Assessment **Bloom's Taxonomy**: Analyze

10. **Correct answer**: C
Rationale: In a patient with Cushing syndrome the skin becomes thinner, leading to the development of abdominal striae or stretch marks. This is due to the inhibition of fibroblasts by excessive glucocorticoids, leading to a loss of collagen and connective tissue. Excessive mineralocorticoids that reduce the absorption of calcium cause osteoporosis and compression fractures. Excessive cortisol changes protein metabolism and protein catabolism, which leads to muscle weakness and wasting. Excessive glucocorticoids affect normal carbohydrate metabolism and cause fat deposits in the abdomen, under the clavicles, over the upper back, and a round "moon" face. **Nursing Process**: Implementation **Bloom's Taxonomy**: Apply

Chapter 20: Nursing Care of Patients with Diabetes Mellitus

Evaluate Your Response to Clinical Reasoning in Patient Care

A Patient with T1D

1. How do the increased urinary output and increased osmolarity of the blood plasma affect the fluid status of the body? What is the response of the body to decreased intravascular volume?
2. Consider the effects of nicotine on blood vessels. How would these effects, when combined with the pathologic effects of long-standing hyperglycemia, affect blood vessel walls?
3. Review the information about chronic illness in Chapter 3. Powerlessness is a perceived lack of control over a situation and/or one's ability to significantly affect an outcome. What types of statements by a patient would help you make this nursing diagnosis?
4. Compare and contrast the developmental needs and tasks of the young adult and the older adult (see Chapter 2). Consider the teaching materials that might have to be adapted to physical changes in the older adult. Also consider similarities and differences in the management and complications of type 1 and type 2 diabetes.

Test Yourself NCLEX-RN Review Answers

1. **Correct answer**: D
Rationale: Immune-mediated type 1 diabetes mellitus leads to the destruction of beta cells and absolute insulin

deficiency. The rate of beta-cell destruction is variable, usually more rapid in infants and children and slower in adults. Idiopathic type 1 diabetes mellitus has no known cause. It is believed to be an inherited disorder and the needs for insulin may be intermittent. Type 2 diabetes mellitus is a disorder that ranges from insulin resistance to insulin deficiency. There is no immune destruction of beta cells. Maturity-onset diabetes mellitus is caused by a genetic defect within the beta cell that causes hyperglycemia to occur before the age of 25. **Nursing Process**: Assessment **Bloom's Taxonomy**: Analyze

2. **Correct answer**: B
   Rationale: Diabetic ketoacidosis (DKA) develops when there is a deficiency of insulin; this results in glucose deficiency at the cellular level. As the pathophysiology of untreated type 1 DM continues, the glucose deficit causes fat stores to break down to provide energy, resulting in mobilization of fatty acids with a subsequent ketosis. The lack of cellular glucose causes production of counterregulatory hormones. Glucose production by the liver increases, peripheral glucose use decreases, fat mobilization increases, and ketogenesis is stimulated. As a result of a loss of bicarbonate, which occurs when the ketone is formed, bicarbonate buffering does not occur, leading to metabolic acidosis. Diabetic ketoacidosis is not caused by decreased glucagon, low protein levels, excessive insulin, or a breakdown of glucose molecules. **Nursing Process**: Implementation **Bloom's Taxonomy**: Apply
3. **Correct answer**: B
   Rationale: The risks for developing type 2 diabetes mellitus include increasing age, obesity, and a sedentary lifestyle. Of the newly admitted patients, the one who is at the highest risk for developing type 2 diabetes mellitus is the 70-year-old patient who is overweight and sedentary. Normal weight, active lifestyle, and stress level do not contribute to the risk of developing this endocrine disorder. **Nursing Process**: Assessment **Bloom's Taxonomy**: Analyze
4. **Correct answer**: A, C, E
   Rationale: The person with diabetes mellitus is at risk for injury from multiple factors. Peripheral polyneuropathy manifests as numbness, tingling feeling in the feet; aching, burning, or shooting pain in the feet; feelings of cold feet; and impaired sensations of pain, light touch, two-point discrimination, and vibration. **Nursing Process**: Planning **Bloom's Taxonomy**: Analyze
5. **Correct answer**: C
   Rationale: Visual inspection of the feet each day is important in preventing more serious complications. Shoes should be purchased later in the day when feet are at their largest. Footwear should be worn at all times. The patient should be instructed to never walk barefoot. Foot wounds should be treated by a healthcare professional. **Nursing Process**: Evaluation **Bloom's Taxonomy**: Analyze
6. **Correct answer**: A, C, E
   Rationale: Insulin glargine (Lantus) and insulin detemir (Levemir) are clear, unlike other intermediate or long-acting insulins, and can accidentally be mistaken for regular insulin. These insulins should not be mixed with other insulins and are given subcutaneously. Regular insulin is short acting in 4 to 6 hours, whereas Lantus and Levemir are long acting in 24 to 28 hours. These insulins are not activated by vigorous agitation. These insulins are not inactivated by light. **Nursing Process**: Implementation **Bloom's Taxonomy**: Apply
7. **Correct answer**: B
   Rationale: Regular insulin is clear in appearance and is used for subcutaneous injection as well as IV insulin therapy. Other insulins such as NPH, glargine, and Humalog are suspensions and could be harmful if given by the IV route. Regular insulin is used in insulin infusions, as an IV bolus, or subcutaneously by itself or in combination with intermediate-acting insulins to provide better glucose control. **Nursing Process**: Implementation **Bloom's Taxonomy**: Understand
8. **Correct answer**: D
   Rationale: According to the American Diabetes Association diagnostic criteria, a hemoglobin A_1C greater than or equal to 6.5% indicates diabetes mellitus. The other laboratory values do not support the diagnosis of diabetes mellitus because they are below 6.5%. **Nursing Process**: Planning **Bloom's Taxonomy**: Apply
9. **Correct answer**: C
   Rationale: No intermediate- or long-acting insulin is given the day of surgery since dietary intake postoperatively is uncertain. Unless otherwise ordered, regular insulin is given at the usual dose to compensate for the anticipated stress-related increase in serum glucose until the patient is eating and drinking normally. If there is no food intake after surgery, intravenous dextrose is often prescribed with subcutaneous regular insulin. The insulin should not be chilled to slow absorption. The insulin does not need to be provided through the intravenous route. **Nursing Process**: Planning **Bloom's Taxonomy**: Apply
10. **Correct answer**: D
    Rationale: Although in theory any area of the body with subcutaneous tissue may be used for injections of insulin, certain sites are recommended. The rate of absorption and peak of action of insulin differ according to the site. The site that allows the most rapid absorption is the abdomen, followed by the subcutaneous tissue of the upper arm, thigh, and hip. Insulin sites are rotated within a given region with each injection. **Nursing Process**: Implementation **Bloom's Taxonomy**: Understand

Chapter 21: Assessing the Gastrointestinal System

Test Yourself NCLEX-RN Review Answers

1. **Correct answer**: A, B
   Rationale: Proteins are classified as either complete or incomplete. Complete proteins are found in animal products such as milk and eggs. Incomplete proteins are found in legumes and vegetables. Fruits are considered carbohydrates. Butter is considered a fat. **Nursing Process**: Implementation **Bloom's Taxonomy**: Apply
2. **Correct answer**: A
   Rationale: Vitamin K is synthesized by coliform bacteria in the large intestines. Evidence of a vitamin K deficiency includes bruising. A niacin deficiency could cause slow peristalsis. Poor wound healing could be a manifestation of a vitamin C deficiency. Keloid formation is not caused from a particular vitamin deficiency. **Nursing Process**: Assessment **Bloom's Taxonomy**: Understand
3. **Correct answer**: D
   Rationale: The serum amylase level is used to measure the secretion of amylase by the pancreas. It is used to diagnose acute pancreatitis, when amylase level peaks in 24 hours and then drops to normal in 48 to 72 hours. An elevated

amylase indicates that the pancreatic enzymes, released during acute pancreatic inflammation, are digesting their own tissues. Cheilosis or sores at the corners of the mouth are seen in vitamin B-complex deficiencies, especially riboflavin. The gallbladder stores bile, which is used to aid in the digestion of fats. An elevated serum amylase level is not associated with gastric reflux disease. **Nursing Process**: Planning **Bloom's Taxonomy**: Apply

4. **Correct answer**: C
   Rationale: While the patient might develop all of these health problems, the most likely is nutritional deficit. Difficulty swallowing and dry mouth may lead the patient to limit intake to soft, easily chewed and swallowed foods. This choice eliminates many vegetables and fruits, which support nutrition. **Nursing Process**: Assessment **Bloom's Taxonomy**: Analyze
5. **Correct answer**: C
   Rationale: In a patient with ascites, the level of dullness increases when the patient turns to the side. This finding is known as shifting dullness. Flatness is not an identified percussion tone. Resonance is a term used when assessing the lungs and thorax. Alternating amplitude is a term used when analyzing an electrocardiogram rhythm strip. **Nursing Process**: Assessment **Bloom's Taxonomy**: Apply
6. **Correct answer**: D, E
   Rationale: Internal hemorrhoids are clusters of dilated veins in swollen anal tissue and occur because of impaired venous return during evacuation of stool or increased abdominal pressure in pregnancy, causing distention of veins in the anus. These hemorrhoids may prolapse to the outside. Internal hemorrhoids are not a part of the lymphatic system, but are a part of the venous system. These structures are not bits of tissue that occur for no reason. **Nursing Process**: Implementation **Bloom's Taxonomy**: Apply
7. **Correct answer**: B, C, D
   Rationale: If the patient has an ostomy, the nurse should ask questions about the skin and associated care, consistency of stool, and foods that cause problems with flatus. Questions about appetite and hemorrhoids do not focus on the patient's ostomy. **Nursing Process**: Assessment **Bloom's Taxonomy**: Apply
8. **Correct answer**: C
   Rationale: A sample of stool is collected for gross and microscopic examination, as well as for form, consistency, and color. Gross examination includes volume and water content and the presence of any blood, pus, mucus, or excess fat. Microscopic examination identifies the presence of WBCs, unabsorbed fat, and parasites. Colonoscopy, barium enema, or CT of the abdomen is not needed to confirm the diagnosis of intestinal parasites. **Nursing Process**: Assessment **Bloom's Taxonomy**: Apply
9. **Correct answer**: B
   Rationale: A colonoscopy is the visual examination of the entire colon and is used to identify tumors, polyps, and inflammatory bowel disease and to dilate strictures. Because polyps have been documented as a risk factor for colon cancer, they are removed during the procedure to prevent future malignancies. Polyps are not removed to identify genetic disorders, facilitate further examination of the bowel, or decrease future problems with constipation. **Nursing Process**: Implementation **Bloom's Taxonomy**: Understand
10. **Correct answer**: A, B, D
    Rationale: Conditions that increase risk of colon cancer include age over 50; family member with colon cancer; history of endometrial, ovarian, or breast cancer; and previous diagnoses of colon inflammation, polyps, or cancer. Exposure to unpasteurized milk and having asthma are not known risks for colon cancer. **Nursing Process**: Assessment **Bloom's Taxonomy**: Analyze

Chapter 22: Nursing Care of Patients with Nutritional Disorders

Evaluate Your Response to Clinical Reasoning in Patient Care

A Patient with Obesity

1. Review the physiology of cholesterol formation in the body and the factors that affect this process.
2. Consider developmental stages and teaching strategies for adult learners.
3. Think about individual factors, family and support group influences, and cultural factors that may affect recommended weight loss and exercise strategies.

A Patient with Malnutrition

1. Review the physiology of albumin and cholesterol formation in the body.
2. Review Mrs. Morris's diet and compare it to the food pyramid or recommendations for food intake to formulate your response.
3. Consider cultural influences and the patient's preferred foods as you plan a diet that is high in calories and protein.

Test Yourself NCLEX-RN Review Answers

1. **Correct answer**: A, B, C
   Rationale: Overall, genetics, exercise, and intake are the biggest contributors to obesity. The patient's twin has a BMI in the obese range, the patient enjoys a sedentary hobby, and has a history of depression. Eating at home is typically healthier than eating out in restaurants or fast-food establishments. Increased time spent watching television is a major contributor to obesity. **Nursing Process**: Assessment **Bloom's Taxonomy**: Analyze
2. **Correct answer**: D
   Rationale: The nurse should assist the patient to create attainable goals that incorporate achievement of improved health outcomes. A pound of body fat is equivalent to 3500 kcal. To lose 1 pound an individual must reduce daily caloric intake by 500 kcal for 7 days or increase activity enough to burn the equivalent kilocalories. A weight loss goal of 1 to 2 pounds per week and a 10% reduction in body weight in 6 months of therapy is recommended. Research indicates most patients set unrealistic goals related to their "dream weight." Treatment focuses on reducing the health risks associated with obesity by changing both eating and exercise habits. There is no evidence to suggest that the patient is not able to adhere to the prescribed diet plan. The patient should not be encouraged to take time off from the diet and exercise plan. **Nursing Process**: Implementation **Bloom's Taxonomy**: Apply
3. **Correct answer**: A, B, D
   Rationale: Manifestations of protein-calorie malnutrition include thin hair, dry flaking skin, and a recent weight loss. The person with protein-calorie malnutrition will be

weak and listless. There is no specific bowel sound associated with protein-calorie malnutrition. **Nursing Process**: Assessment **Bloom's Taxonomy**: Analyze

4. **Correct answer**: A, C, E
Rationale: The patient should be positioned with the head of the bed elevated and should have a CPAP device in place. These interventions help to reduce pressure on the diaphragm and help to maintain upper airway patency. Surgery and anesthesia place an additional risk for cardiovascular complications on a patient who is already at significant risk for coronary heart disease. Adipose tissue does not heal well and is prone to infection. Strict aseptic technique must be used to prevent wound infections. Anesthesia agents can become sequestered in fatty tissues, resulting in slower clearance from the body. Monitoring for their effects is performed for a longer period of time than for those of normal weight. Adequate post-operative analgesia is essential to promote lung expansion and prevent respiratory complications. **Nursing Process**: Planning **Bloom's Taxonomy**: Analyze

5. **Correct answer**: B
Rationale: Patients with eating disorders require extended treatment of the disorder. Involvement of the family and social support persons is vital to success. Encourage family members to participate in teaching and nutritional counseling sessions. Discuss the value of family therapy to address issues that have contributed to the disorder. Emphasize the need to provide consistent messages of support for healthy eating habits. Refeeding is gradually introduced to avoid complications, so a weight gain of 2 lb per week would not be realistic. The patient should not be left alone after meals. Observing the patient during and after meals helps prevent disposal of food and purging behavior after eating. Consuming 2500 calories every day could lead to refeeding syndrome and would not be a realistic goal for this patient. **Nursing Process**: Planning **Bloom's Taxonomy**: Apply

6. **Correct answer**: D
Rationale: A BMI greater than 25 and central obesity as indicated by a waist–hip ratio of 1 or greater tend to have more intra-abdominal fat and higher levels of circulating free fatty acids. This places the patient at a higher risk for hypertension, elevated lipid levels, heart disease, stroke, and elevated insulin levels. These conditions have the greatest effect on health over time. The patient with obesity can be at risk for difficulty coping; however, this is not the priority. The patient with obesity may have diet education needs and may have had difficulty achieving weight loss goals; however, these problems are not the highest concern for the patient's health. **Nursing Process**: Planning **Bloom's Taxonomy**: Analyze

7. **Correct answer**: D, E
Rationale: Patients recovering from bariatric surgery should be instructed to avoid foods high in simple carbohydrates since this could precipitate dumping syndrome. Meals should be small and liquids and solids should not be taken together. Caffeinated carbonated liquids will not aid with weight loss. The patient should be encouraged to follow a specific eating plan to support behavior modification strategies. **Nursing Process**: Evaluation **Bloom's Taxonomy**: Evaluate

8. **Correct answer**: B, C, E
Rationale: Many contributing factors influence nutrition in the home-bound older adult, such as inability to shop for nutritional foods or the inability to afford and prepare nutritional food. There are also psychosocial issues of depression and loneliness since eating is a social affair; this could well influence the amount and proportion of caloric intake. Arranging the patient to be transported to a senior center for a meal may solve the weight loss issue and no further interventions may be necessary. Referral to the primary care provider is necessary. Diagnostic studies may be required after being examined by the primary care provider but are not the current priority. The patient does not need to be placed in a residential care facility because of unplanned weight loss. **Nursing Process**: Planning **Bloom's Taxonomy**: Applying

9. **Correct answer**: D
Rationale: The stress of surgery produces a state of hypermetabolism and catabolism, which increases energy expenditure and nutrient needs, resulting in protein-calorie malnutrition. Beginning oral intake of nutrients as soon as possible after surgery is the best way to prevent the development of this type of malnutrition. Measuring daily weights will provide information about fluid balance and not necessarily body weight. Aggressive pain management and intravenous fluids will not prevent the development of malnutrition. **Nursing Process**: Implementation **Bloom's Taxonomy**: Analyze

10. **Correct answer**: A
Rationale: The risk for postoperative complications after bariatric surgery is high. One of the postoperative complications with gastric bypass surgery is an anastomotic leak causing peritonitis. These manifestations could be related to this condition and the surgeon needs to be advised they are present. The patient is experiencing increasing abdominal pain and absent bowel sounds. These findings would not be consistent with effectiveness of analgesia. The patient should be maintained on bedrest until evaluated by the surgeon. The nurse needs to do more than chart the findings and monitor the patient. Peritonitis can be a life-threatening health problem. **Nursing Process**: Implementation **Bloom's Taxonomy**: Analyze

Chapter 23: Nursing Care of Patients with Upper Gastrointestinal Disorders

Evaluate Your Response to Clinical Reasoning in Patient Care

A Patient with Oral Cancer

1. Review the major risk factors for oral cancer and identify the populations most likely to have these risk factors.
2. Work with your classmates to plan (and implement) an education program, considering the developmental/teaching needs of this group of young people.
3. Think about the possible causes for Mr. Chavez's refusal to talk (remember that assessment is the first step of the nursing process). How will you identify factors contributing to his behavior?

A Patient with Peptic Ulcer Disease

1. Review the physiology of the gastric mucosal barrier and the pathogenesis of peptic ulcer disease and the effect of *H. pylori* infection on these processes.
2. Review physiologic responses to stress in your physiology or nursing fundamentals text; compare and apply this information with the physiology of the gastric mucosal barrier and the pathophysiology of ulcer development.

3. Consider Mr. Nassar's occupation and schedule, as well as the prescribed medications and when each should be taken.
4. Using journal and text resources as well as your classmates, identify as many stress reduction techniques as possible. Then sort your list into those that could be used while working and identify ways to effectively teach each technique.

A Patient with Gastric Cancer

1. Review the healing process and the normal physiology of the stomach as you formulate your answer to this question.
2. Consider the surgery, immediate postoperative care, and what the patient and family should expect in developing your teaching plan.
3. Review Chapter 14 and nursing care related to chemotherapy.
4. Again, review Chapter 14 for nursing care measures for patients with cancer; also review Chapter 22 for strategies to prevent and manage malnutrition.

Test Yourself NCLEX-RN Review Answers

1. **Correct answer**: A, B, E
   Rationale: The primary risk factors for oral cancer are smoking, drinking alcohol, and chewing tobacco. HPV may also contribute to the risk for oral cancer. Consumption of spicy foods and thumbsucking or pacifier use as a child are not risk factors for the development of oral cancer. **Nursing Process**: Assessment **Bloom's Taxonomy**: Apply
2. **Correct answer**: B, C
   Rationale: Placing the head of the bed on blocks and avoiding lying down for at least 2 hours after eating will help prevent backflow of gastric content into the esophagus by decreasing the pressure on the lower esophageal sphincter. Treatment for gastroesophageal reflux disease includes changing the diet and using proton-pump inhibitors, H_2 -receptor blockers, and in some cases, surgery. Peppermint and chocolate can aggravate gastroesophageal reflux and should be avoided. The patient should be instructed to take prescribed medication as ordered for the full course of therapy, even if symptoms are relieved. **Nursing Process**: Planning **Bloom's Taxonomy**: Apply
3. **Correct answer**: C, D
   Rationale: The ingestion of aspirin or other NSAIDs, corticosteroids, alcohol, and caffeine is commonly associated with the development of acute gastritis. Should vomiting occur, the patient should remain NPO for 2 to 4 hours after the last episode before gradually reintroducing clear liquids. Fully cooking all meat, poultry, and egg products is essential to prevent gastritis from contaminated food. The patient does not need to eat only bland food. The patient will not need yearly upper endoscopy exams. **Nursing Process**: Evaluation **Bloom's Taxonomy**: Evaluate
4. **Correct answer**: C
   Rationale: Erosion of a blood vessel with resultant hemorrhage is a significant risk for the patient with peptic ulcer disease. Acute bleeding can lead to hypovolemia and fluid volume deficit, which can lead to a decrease in cardiac output and impaired tissue perfusion. The problems of nausea, acute pain, and inability to care for self are important, but are not the priorities for the patient with a possible perforation from peptic ulcer disease. **Nursing Process**: Planning **Bloom's Taxonomy**: Analyze
5. **Correct answer**: A, B, C, E
   Rationale: Anemia may be a chronic problem after a major gastric resection. Iron is absorbed primarily in the duodenum and proximal jejunum; rapid gastric emptying or a gastrojejunostomy may interfere with adequate absorption. The cells of the stomach produce intrinsic factor, required for the absorption of vitamin B_{12}. Vitamin B_{12} deficiency leads to pernicious anemia. Vitamin B_{12} levels are routinely monitored following extensive gastric resections. Other nutritional problems seen following surgery include folic acid deficiency and decreased absorption of calcium and vitamin D and not vitamin C. **Nursing Process**: Planning **Bloom's Taxonomy**: Apply
6. **Correct answer**: B
   Rationale: Complications associated with radiation therapy to the esophagus include perforation and hemorrhage. Bright bleeding from the mouth could indicate perforation of the esophageal wall and vessel rupture. Weight loss and dysphagia are manifestations of esophageal cancer. Crackles in the base of the right lung could be due to atelectasis and not necessarily indicate a major respiratory problem. **Nursing Process**: Implementation **Bloom's Taxonomy**: Analyze
7. **Correct answer**: B
   Rationale: The medications used to treat PUD include agents to eradicate *H. pylori*, drugs to decrease gastric acid content, and agents that protect the mucosa. Eradication of *H. pylori* generally requires 14 days of therapy using a combination of two antibiotics with a proton-pump inhibitor or a bismuth compound. The patient needs to take the complete course of all medication as prescribed. The medications should be taken with sufficient water. Consuming yogurt or buttermilk might be appropriate if the patient is prone to developing a superinfection from antibiotic use. Omeprazole should be taken 30 minutes before breakfast on an empty stomach. **Nursing Process**: Implementation **Bloom's Taxonomy**: Apply
8. **Correct answer**: D
   Rationale: The discomfort of stomatitis is aggravated by eating. Using a topical anesthetic, such as a mouthwash of 2% viscous lidocaine diluted with water, can promote comfort and the ability to consume food and fluids orally. Smoking cessation will help prevent the development of stomatitis; however, this is not the reason that the patient has developed this health problem. Selecting appealing foods will not promote nutrition if the patient is experiencing mouth pain. A solution of saline, sodium bicarbonate, or a combination of saline/bicarbonate promotes comfort and healing when used after and between meals. Mouthwash would be too irritating to the oral tissue. **Nursing Process**: Implementation **Bloom's Taxonomy**: Apply
9. **Correct answer**: B
   Rationale: The surgeon should be notified. After surgery for esophageal cancer, do not move or manipulate the nasogastric tube. Low gastric suction should be maintained as prescribed. Manipulating or moving the nasogastric tube may disrupt suture lines, resulting in a leak into the mediastinum. Irrigating the tube with normal saline would be manipulating the tube and should not be done unless specifically ordered. The nurse needs to do more than chart the findings. **Nursing Process**: Implementation **Bloom's Taxonomy**: Apply

10. **Correct answer**: A, B, C
Rationale: When perforation occurs, gastric or duodenal contents enter the peritoneum, causing an inflammatory process and peritonitis. When an ulcer perforates, the patient has immediate, severe upper abdominal pain, radiating throughout the abdomen and possibly to the shoulder. The abdomen becomes rigid and boardlike, with absent bowel sounds. All food and fluids should be withheld and the physician notified. Placing the patient in Fowler or semi-Fowler position allows peritoneal contaminants to pool in the pelvis. The patient needs more help than pain medication or prescribed proton pump inhibitors. **Nursing Process**: Implementation **Bloom's Taxonomy**: Apply

Chapter 24: Nursing Care of Patients with Bowel Disorders

Evaluate Your Response to Clinical Reasoning in Patient Care

A Patient with Acute Appendicitis

1. Review the acute inflammatory response to an infectious process and the role WBCs play in the immune response.
2. Review Chapter 4. Consider factors such as incision size, abdominal muscle disruption, and manipulation of the bowel in developing your response.
3. Consider points such as pain management, resumption of activities, incision care, and potential complications in developing your teaching plan. Consider the patient's education and developmental stage as well.
4. Review the effects of anxiety on recovery and learning. Identify nursing measures to reduce situational anxiety.

A Patient with Ulcerative Colitis

1. Review normal functions of the small and large intestine. Review the usual location of an ileostomy. Review fluid volume deficit in Chapter 10 for manifestations and assessment data.
2. Think about the effect of chronic blood loss and review the effect of malnutrition on the hemoglobin and hematocrit.
3. Review the home care section of inflammatory bowel disease for teaching points to include.
4. Review nursing care for the patient with diarrhea, as well as the procedure for ileostomy care.

A Patient with Colorectal Cancer

1. Review peripheral innervation and impulse transmission in your anatomy and physiology textbook; think about how nerves in the rectal region are disrupted in an abdominoperineal resection. Also review the phantom pain phenomenon in Chapter 9.
2. Compare elimination through a colostomy with "normal" bowel elimination through the anus. How do they differ in terms of the passage of flatus?
3. Review the procedure for administering an enema in your fundamentals or skills textbook.
4. Consider what factors might contribute to a poor body image in a patient with a colostomy. Refer to Box 24.6.

Test Yourself NCLEX-RN Review Answers

1. **Correct answer**: A
Rationale: The nurse should first assess the duration and extent of diarrhea to include the number and character of the stools. Diarrhea is stool with a high water content, so refraining from all oral intake until the diarrhea subsides could exacerbate fluid and electrolyte imbalances caused by the diarrhea. The nurse should not prescribe or recommend the use of any medication. Once the nurse assesses the frequency and character of stools, the nurse can then assess if the patient has been exposed to spoiled food or contaminated water, which could be the source for the diarrhea. **Nursing Process**: Assessment **Bloom's Taxonomy**: Apply
2. **Correct answer**: A
Rationale: The acutely inflamed appendix can perforate within 24 hours, so rapid diagnosis and treatment are important. Because of this urgency and the low incidence of surgical complications, diagnostic testing and preoperative treatment may be limited. The patient is admitted to the hospital, and intravenous fluids and antibiotics are initiated. Oral food and fluids are withheld until a diagnosis is confirmed. Once the diagnosis is established, an appendectomy is performed. Preoperative skin preparation would be done once the decision is made for surgery. There may not be enough time to teach the patient about deep breathing and coughing and leg exercises. **Nursing Process**: Implementation **Bloom's Taxonomy**: Analyze
3. **Correct answer**: B, C
Rationale: Taking the medication after a meal reduces gastric distress. This drug increases sensitivity to the sun. Vitamin C and aspirin should be avoided while taking this drug. Fluid should be increased, not decreased. **Nursing Process**: Implementation **Bloom's Taxonomy**: Apply
4. **Correct answer**: B
Rationale: Steatorrhea is impairment in fat absorption leading to excess fat in feces. Steatorrhea and diarrhea typically occur with diseases of malabsorption because fat, water, and other nutrients are poorly absorbed, remaining in the bowel to be eliminated in the stool. Steatorrhea is not associated with colorectal cancer, alternating episodes of diarrhea and constipation, nor exposure to enterotoxins in food or water. **Nursing Process**: Assessment **Bloom's Taxonomy**: Apply
5. **Correct answer**: A, B, D, E
Rationale: Measures to prevent colon cancer that are considered to be effective and safe include consuming a diet high in fruits and vegetables and low in saturated fat and red meat, regular exercise, and maintaining a healthy weight. The patient should also follow the recommended testing schedule for the early detection of colorectal cancer beginning at age 50. Alcohol consumption should be limited. **Nursing Process**: Implementation **Bloom's Taxonomy**: Apply
6. **Correct answer**: A, C, D, E
Rationale: Accurate abdominal girth measurements allow for trending of decompression. Accurate intake and output monitors for fluid volume imbalances. Changes in amount or quality of NG tube drainage can indicate complications that should be addressed. Monitoring mental status helps to identify complications such as shock and electrolyte imbalance. **Nursing Process**: Assessment **Bloom's Taxonomy**: Apply
7. **Correct answer**: C
Rationale: It is most important to maintain the patency of the nasogastric tube to remove gastric secretions and air

that may apply pressure to the anastomosis site and cause failure of the suture line. Keeping the stomach decompressed is important to prevent vomiting that could also cause damage to the anastomosis site. Although important, monitoring bowel sounds is not the most important action for the nurse to take. The patient will be acutely ill and most likely not able to get out of bed. The patient should be placed on nothing by mouth status and should not be provided with a clear liquid diet. **Nursing Process**: Implementation **Bloom's Taxonomy**: Analyze

8. **Correct answer**: A, B, D
Rationale: A high-fiber diet is recommended. There is no need to avoid soup. Salad and whole-wheat bread is encouraged. Avoidance of foods with small seeds such as raspberries and popcorn is sometimes recommended. **Nursing Process**: Evaluation **Bloom's Taxonomy**: Evaluate
9. **Correct answer**: A, C, D, E
Rationale: Actions to prevent constipation include ingesting fresh fruits and vegetables, whole-wheat bread, and bran cereal since these food items supply roughage and fiber in the diet that can assist in the evacuation of fecal material. Adequate liquid is needed to prevent hard, formed stools that are difficult to pass. Taking daily laxatives can decrease the normal bowel reflex and lead to laxative dependency. **Nursing Process**: Implementation **Bloom's Taxonomy**: Apply
10. **Correct answer**: B, C
Rationale: The patient is prepared by taking a course of antibiotic prior to the transplant which is often done by enema. There is no indication that age over 45 is a restriction for donation. The patient does not need continued hospitalization based solely on the transplant. Donors are typically relatives and are closely screened for exposure to infectious diseases. This treatment is becoming more common. **Nursing Process**: Evaluation **Bloom's Taxonomy**: Evaluate

Chapter 25: Nursing Care of Patients with Gallbladder, Liver, and Pancreatic Disorders

Evaluate Your Response to Clinical Reasoning in Patient Care

A Patient with Cholelithiasis

1. Review the composition of gallstones, as well as the physiology of gallbladder function and bile. Research and discuss dietary practices of the Chickasaw tribe.
2. Review Chapter 4 for care related to a laparotomy (incision into the abdomen).
3. As you develop your plan, consider Mrs. Colbert's culture, job, and family obligations.

A Patient with Alcoholic Cirrhosis

1. Review the anatomy and physiology of the liver and its circulation, as well as the pathophysiology of cirrhosis and its complications.
2. Consult your nutrition textbook as needed for foods that are high in calories but low in protein and sodium. When planning for limited protein intake, be sure to include high-quality proteins and limit intake of lower-quality proteins such as legumes.
3. Review the pathophysiology of hepatic encephalopathy to develop your responses to this question.
4. Review therapeutic communication skills; consider what other members of the healthcare team and his family might be able to help Mr. Wright with these issues.

A Patient with Acute Pancreatitis

1. Review Chapter 6 for assessment data indicative of alcohol withdrawal.
2. Review both the pathophysiology of acute pancreatitis and the acute inflammatory process.
3. Consult your nutrition textbook or the American Dietetic Association website.
4. Consider what other members of the interprofessional team might be able to help with these issues.

Test Yourself NCLEX-RN Review Answers

1. **Correct answer**: A, E
Rationale: Cholelithiasis manifests as abrupt-onset RUQ pain that lasts 30 minutes to 5 hours. Nausea and vomiting are common. Pain that lasts 12 to 18 hours is related to cholecystitis as are chills and fever. Recurrent heartburn and acid reflux are findings associated with esophageal reflux disease. **Nursing Process**: Assessment **Bloom's Taxonomy**: Analyze
2. **Correct answer**: B, C, D
Rationale: Acute cholecystitis usually develops from a stone obstructing the cystic duct, preventing release of bile from the gallbladder. High-fat foods like gravies and peanut butter stimulate contraction of the obstructed gallbladder, causing pain. The patient should be instructed to call the physician if severe abdominal pain and a fever are experienced. A low-carbohydrate diet has a protective effect to reduce the incidence of gallstones and cholecystitis. An acutely inflamed gallbladder and ductal system increase surgical complexity and may necessitate open cholecystectomy. Infection is not an absolute contraindication to surgery. Foods and fluid should be withheld during episodes of acute pain. **Nursing Process**: Implementation **Bloom's Taxonomy**: Apply
3. **Correct answer**: C
Rationale: Hepatitis A is transmitted by the oral–fecal route from an infected person handling food, water, or fish or through direct contact without washing hands before handling food or after using the bathroom. Testing employees for the hepatitis A antigen will not prevent future outbreaks of the disease. Using gloves for handling food if cuts or scrapes are on the hands would be ineffective because this disease is not transmitted through the blood. If continued outbreaks occur, it might be necessary to have all employees immunized or consider another source of the infection. **Nursing Process**: Implementation **Bloom's Taxonomy**: Apply
4. **Correct answer**: A
Rationale: Hepatitis C is transmitted through contact with blood or body fluids. Alcohol and acetaminophen are irritating to the liver and should be avoided. The patient with hepatitis C is at risk for the development of liver cancer. A follow-up annual liver biopsy is not recommended for hepatitis C. **Nursing Process**: Evaluation **Bloom's Taxonomy**: Evaluate
5. **Correct answer**: C, D
Rationale: The hepatitis A virus is transmitted through the fecal–oral route and can be transmitted before manifestations of the disease including jaundice develop. It is

important to identify people who have had direct contact with the newly diagnosed patient because the incubation period is 2 to 6 weeks. The patient's immunization status will not help with exposure to the virus. Hepatitis A is not transmitted through body fluids. Hepatitis A does not manifest as blood in the feces. **Nursing Process**: Assessment **Bloom's Taxonomy**: Apply

6. **Correct answer**: D
Rationale: Bleeding esophageal varices are life-threatening and require intensive care management. Restoration of hemodynamic stability is the first priority. A central line is inserted and central venous and pulmonary artery pressures are monitored. The physician will determine if a nasogastric tube should be inserted. The head of the bed should be raised to prevent aspiration. Checking the stool for occult blood is not necessary to do at this time. **Nursing Process**: Implementation **Bloom's Taxonomy**: Apply
7. **Correct answer**: A
Rationale: The nurse should teach the patient to empty the bladder before the paracentesis to reduce the risk for bladder puncture. Excess flatus is not an adverse effect of a paracentesis. The nurse will cleanse the abdomen before the procedure. The patient does not need to do this at home. There are not restrictions on eating or drinking fluid after the procedure. **Nursing Process**: Implementation **Bloom's Taxonomy**: Apply
8. **Correct answer**: C
Rationale: Patients with cirrhosis and ascites may develop bacterial peritonitis. The inflammatory response to peritonitis worsens ascites by increasing the permeability of capillaries in the mesentery. The manifestations of spontaneous bacterial peritonitis may be subtle, with increased abdominal discomfort or pain, fever, increasing ascites, and worsening encephalopathy. The nurse should assess for enlargement of the abdomen, indicating increased ascities. A headache and nuchal rigidity are not applicable for the patient's manifestations. Neck vein distention and auscultating lung sounds do not focus on the patient's problem. Auscultating breath sounds is important, but does not match the patient's current symptoms. **Nursing Process**: Implementation **Bloom's Taxonomy**: Apply
9. **Correct answer**: C
Rationale: Gallstones are the leading cause of acute pancreatitis, with alcohol being the second leading cause. Since the patient reports no alcohol intake, the nurse does not need to ask if the patient formerly drank alcohol. Smoking and intravenous drug use are not risk factors for the development of acute pancreatitis. **Nursing Process**: Assessment **Bloom's Taxonomy**: Apply
10. **Correct answer**: A, B, D, E
Rationale: Nursing care for a patient recovering from a Whipple procedure includes using analgesics for pain control as prescribed, maintaining in the semi-Fowler position to facilitate lung expansion and reduce stress on the anastomosis and suture line, not repositioning the nasogastric tube to avoid disrupting the suture line, and frequently turning, deep breathing, and coughing to facilitate the drainage of pulmonary secretions. Ambulation will not occur until the patient's condition stabilizes. **Nursing Process**: Implementation **Bloom's Taxonomy**: Apply

Chapter 26: Assessing the Renal System

Test Yourself NCLEX-RN Review Answers

1. **Correct answer**: A
Rationale: Leakage of urine (urinary incontinence) is not a normal outcome of aging. Having to void during the night, urgency, and protein in the urine are all findings that are consistent with renal system changes in the older patient. **Nursing Process**: Assessment **Bloom's Taxonomy**: Analyze
2. **Correct answer**: A
Rationale: The dilution or concentration of urine is largely determined by antidiuretic hormone (ADH), secreted by the posterior pituitary gland in response to blood volume and serum osmolality. When serum osmolality increases or blood volume falls, ADH is secreted. Pores of the collecting tubules enlarge in response, and more water is reabsorbed. This is the mechanism that occurs with vomiting. Renin is released in response to a drop in blood pressure. Thyroxin and aldosterone are not released in response to decreases in blood volume. **Nursing Process**: Assessment **Bloom's Taxonomy**: Analyze
3. **Correct answer**: D
Rationale: The creatinine clearance test is a blood sample and 24-hour urine test is to evaluate glomerular filtration rate and renal function. This test determines the filtering ability of the glomeruli and the blood circulation to them. If the clearance is decreased, the glomeruli are damaged or the circulation is slowed. A renal scan evaluates kidney blood flow, location, size, and shape to assess kidney perfusion and urine production. A renal biopsy is performed to determine the cause of renal disease, to rule out cancer metastasis to the kidney, or if rejection is occurring with a kidney transplant. A routine urinalysis is an examination of the constituents of a urine sample to establish a baseline, provide data for diagnosis, or monitor treatment results. **Nursing Process**: Assessment **Bloom's Taxonomy**: Apply
4. **Correct answer**: B
Rationale: The prostate gland encircles the urethra at the base of the bladder in males. The spleen is located in the left upper abdominal quadrant and is not an organ of the renal system. The adrenal glands are located on the top of the kidneys. The pancreas is located in the mid to left region of the upper abdomen and is an organ of the renal system. **Nursing Process**: Assessment **Bloom's Taxonomy**: Understand
5. **Correct answer**: B, D
Rationale: Pain or burning with urination should be documented as dysuria. Nocturia is defined as two or more episodes of voiding during the night. This should be documented in the medical record. Pyuria is pus in the urine. Polyuria is frequent episodes of high-volume urination. Hematuria is blood in the urine. **Nursing Process**: Assessment **Bloom's Taxonomy**: Apply
6. **Correct answer**: A, B, E
Rationale: For an intravenous pyelogram, the nurse should assess for allergies to seafood or iodine since these could indicate an allergy to the contrast dye. Instruct the patient to complete ordered pretest bowel preparation, including a prescribed laxative or cathartic the evening before the test, and an enema or suppository the morning of the test. Oral hypoglycemic agents are contraindicated for use with

iodinated contrast. Food should not be eaten for 8 to 12 hours before the test, although clear liquids are permitted. There is no reason to withhold taking prescribed diuretics before the test. **Nursing Process**: Implementation **Bloom's Taxonomy**: Apply

7. **Correct answer**: A, B, E
Rationale: Before beginning the assessment, ask the patient to provide a clean-catch urine specimen if prescribed and give the patient a specimen cup. Assess the specimen for color, odor, and clarity before sending it to the laboratory. Examination will require that the patient change into a gown and a drape should be provided. The patient should be in the supine or sitting position for the beginning of the exam. Deep breaths are not necessary prior to assessing the renal system. Drinking water before the examination could cause the bladder to fill with urine, making the examination uncomfortable for the patient. **Nursing Process**: Assessment **Bloom's Taxonomy**: Apply

8. **Correct answer**: A, C, D
Rationale: The patient should avoid alcoholic drinks for at least 2 days after the procedure. Fluid intake should be increased. Urine may be slightly bloody for no more than three voidings. Slight burning is normal, but burning should not be significant. Decreased voiding is a reason to notify the surgeon. **Nursing Process**: Implementation **Bloom's Taxonomy**: Apply

9. **Correct answer**: C
Rationale: Bladder cancer is the fourth most common type of cancer in men. Genetic factors related to chromosome 9 are interrelated with risk factors such as smoking and exposure to industrial chemicals to cause bladder cancer. Hematuria may be a symptom of bladder cancer but is not genetic in nature. Incontinence is not usually associated with bladder cancer. A kidney infection is caused by bacteria or viruses. **Nursing Process**: Assessment **Bloom's Taxonomy**: Analyze

10. **Correct answer**: A
Rationale: Skin turgor is the best assessment technique to determine hydration of patients. Changes in skin turgor may indicate renal insufficiency with either excess fluid loss or retention. Kidney palpation is done to determine location and size of the organs. Auscultation of renal arteries is to determine changes in renal blood flow. Percussion for bladder dullness is performed to determine urinary retention. **Nursing Process**: Assessment **Bloom's Taxonomy**: Apply

Chapter 27: Nursing Care of Patients with Urinary Tract Disorders

Evaluate Your Response to Clinical Reasoning in Patient Care

A Patient with Cystitis

1. Consider the prescription provided for Mrs. Waisanen and its safe use.
2. See Chapter 12 for patient teaching about antibiotics and specific information about Mrs. Waisanen's prescription. Also refer to your pharmacology text and drug handbook or application.
3. Consider risk factors for UTI as well as factors affecting Mrs. Waisanen's immune function.
4. Consider the indications for short-course antibiotic therapy and the indications for conventional therapy. Think about factors such as cost, compliance, and the risk for adverse effects, as well as how antibiotics work to eradicate bacteria.
5. Identify why self-health management is a priority intervention for Mrs. Waisanen and the individual factors contributing to this diagnosis as you plan care.

A Patient with a Bladder Tumor

1. Consider Mr. Hussain's stated alcohol use and its potential effects on anesthesia and his postoperative recovery.
2. Review the risk factors for urinary tract tumors, looking for commonalities and considering the physiology of the bladder and urine formation and elimination.
3. Review Chapters 4 and 9 as you develop your response to Mr. Hussain's statement.
4. Remembering that patients rarely present with one isolated health problem, review Mr. Hussain's health history for possible contributing factors to these manifestations. Then review Chapter 6 for nursing care of the patient with substance abuse. Why might Mr. Hussain experience alcohol withdrawal after 2 to 3 days of hospitalization?
5. Considering the surgery performed and its potential effects on physical function and body image, use your nursing care planning book or guide to identify possible interventions and outcomes for this nursing priority.

Test Yourself NCLEX-RN Review Answers

1. **Correct answer**: B
Rationale: The use of a diaphragm and spermicidal compounds for birth control are risk factors for the development of urinary tract infections. The amount of milk consumed each day is not a factor in causing a urinary tract infection. Asking about a partner having similar symptoms is not the most pertinent question. Symptoms of a urinary tract infection are largely relieved within 24 to 48 hours of starting antibiotic therapy. The reoccurrence time factor of the UTI is too long to be a failure to complete antibiotic treatment the first time. **Nursing Process**: Assessment **Bloom's Taxonomy**: Apply

2. **Correct answer**: B, D, E
Rationale: The nurse needs to inform the patient that a urine culture in 10 days is done to ensure antibiotic therapy was effective. In a perimenopausal woman vaginal cream may maintain tissue integrity to prevent bacterial colonization of perineal tissues; instructions on cleansing may prevent further infections. In general, further diagnostic testing is not indicated for women experiencing three or fewer UTIs per year. Instrumentation of the urinary tract such as with a cystoscopy is a major risk factor for UTI. Imaging studies such as intravenous pyelography are used to evaluate for structural or functional abnormalities of the kidneys, ureters, and bladder. **Nursing Process**: Implementation **Bloom's Taxonomy**: Apply

3. **Correct answer**: D
Rationale: Increasing fluid intake to 2.5 to 3.0 L/day is recommended, regardless of stone composition. A higher fluid intake helps to ensure the production of approximately 2.0 to 2.5 L of urine a day and prevents the stone-forming salts from becoming concentrated enough to precipitate. The urine pH is helpful in identifying the type of stone. Calcium should not be provided until the type

of stone is identified because the majority of stones contain calcium. An indwelling urinary catheter is not routine treatment for urolithiasis. **Nursing Process**: Planning **Bloom's Taxonomy**: Apply

4. **Correct answer**: B
   Rationale: A stone that completely obstructs the ureter can lead to hydronephrosis and acute kidney injury on the affected side. The nurse should report symptoms such as dull flank pain or aching. Straining the urine can be done after the physician is notified of the change in the patient's condition. An analgesic can be provided after the physician is notified. There is no evidence to suggest the patient is retaining urine and would need a bladder scan. **Nursing Process**: Implementation **Bloom's Taxonomy**: Apply

5. **Correct answer**: B, C
   Rationale: Cigarette smoking is the primary risk factor for bladder cancer. The risk in smokers is twice that of nonsmokers. The chemicals and dyes used in the plastics, rubber, and cable industries; substances in the work environment of textile workers, leather finishers, spray painters, and petroleum workers; and high levels of arsenic in drinking water are also associated with a higher risk of bladder cancer. Additional risk factors for bladder cancer include residence in an urban area, chronic UTIs, and bladder calculi. The risk for bladder cancer appears to be reduced by increasing the intake of fluids and vegetables. Emptying the bladder every 2 hours and limiting the intake of coffee and other caffeinated beverages does not reduce the risk of developing bladder cancer. **Nursing Process**: Implementation **Bloom's Taxonomy**: Apply

6. **Correct answer**: A
   Rationale: Painless hematuria is the presenting sign in 75% of urinary tract tumors. Hematuria may be gross or microscopic and is often intermittent, causing delay in seeking treatment. The nurse should advise the participant to see a physician. Increasing fluids, tracking activities between urine color and activities, and waiting to notify the physician until pain or difficulty voiding occurs could delay potential diagnosis and treatment for bladder cancer. **Nursing Process**: Implementation **Bloom's Taxonomy**: Apply

7. **Correct answer**: B, E
   Rationale: The patient with a newly created continent ileal diversion with a continent reservoir will have to demonstrate self-catheterization since this is the only way to empty the reservoir. The patient should also be able to identify symptoms of electrolyte imbalance as the reservoir may reabsorb electrolytes. These behaviors indicate that teaching has been effective. There is no collection device for this diversion. This surgical procedure would have been performed for treatment of bladder cancer. Cloudy urine may occur as an effect of the urine on ileal mucosa. **Nursing Process**: Evaluation **Bloom's Taxonomy**: Evaluate

8. **Correct answer**: C
   Rationale: The priority for this patient is reducing the amount of incontinence. Stress incontinence should not be viewed as a normal result of aging, but as a treatable problem. Improved pelvic muscle strength helps retain urine and prevent stress incontinence by increasing urethral pressure. Exercises also decrease abnormal detrusor muscle contractions, decreasing pressure within the bladder. Being able to state the chronic and benign nature of the disorder and identifying products to protect clothing and furniture suggests this disorder is inevitable and untreatable. Fruit and vegetable intake should not be discouraged. **Nursing Process**: Planning **Bloom's Taxonomy**: Apply

9. **Correct answer**: A, B, C
   Rationale: Regular voiding schedules, wearing easily removed clothing, and reducing fluid intake after the evening meal all are techniques to help the patient manage incontinence. Feminine hygiene sprays are drying to the mucosal tissues and do not prevent incontinence. Acidic drinks like orange juice may irritate the bladder, increasing urge to void. **Nursing Process**: Implementation **Bloom's Taxonomy**: Apply

10. **Correct answer**: C
    Rationale: Intermittent catheterization carries a lower risk of infection than does an indwelling catheter and is preferred for patients who are unable to empty their bladder by voiding such as patients with spinal cord injury. Catheterizing the patient every 3 to 4 hours with a straight catheter prevents overdistension of the bladder. Increasing lower abdominal and bladder pressure with the Credé method can stimulate autonomic dysreflexia in some patients with spinal cord injuries. The patient with a spinal cord injury will have bladder retention and not be able to void spontaneously. Inserting an indwelling urinary catheter could lead to a urinary tract infection. **Nursing Process**: Implementation **Bloom's Taxonomy**: Apply

Chapter 28: Nursing Care of Patients with Kidney Disorders

Evaluate Your Response to Clinical Reasoning in Patient Care

A Patient with Acute Glomerulonephritis

1. Review Chapter 12 and the use of antibiotics to treat infection.
2. Research the potential complications and immune responses to group A beta hemolytic streptococcal infections.
3. Consider information about when to contact a healthcare provider and the appropriate use of antibiotics as you develop your teaching plan.
4. Review Mr. Chang's history and the risk factors for acute glomerulonephritis.
5. Review Chapter 26 for patient teaching and nursing responsibilities related to diagnostic studies.
6. Review the diagnostic tests used to differentiate different forms of glomerulonephritis.

A Patient with End-Stage Renal Disease

1. Consider the systemic effects of altered hematology, electrolyte, and renal function tests on functional health as you plan your nursing interventions.
2. Review Chapter 20 for nursing care of the patient experiencing complications of diabetes.
3. Review the usual onset, pathophysiology, and long-term effects of type 1 and type 2 diabetes (Chapter 20).
4. Consider the effects of urea and ammonia (both neurologic toxins) on brain function.

5. Consider the physiology of dialysis, the composition of dialysis solutions (dialysate), as well as potential planned and unplanned effects of peritoneal dialysis.

Test Yourself NCLEX-RN Review Answers

1. **Correct answer**: A, B
Rationale: The kidneys are instrumental in the regulation of blood pressure. Diabetes is the leading cause of end-stage renal disease. More adults over age 65 have kidney disease, but younger persons can also develop the disorder. Dialysis is a treatment, not a cure. In the United States, about 14% of adults have chronic kidney disease. **Nursing Process**: Evaluation **Bloom's Taxonomy**: Evaluate

2. **Correct answer**: B
Rationale: Polycystic kidney disease is a hereditary disease characterized by formation of fluid-filled cysts and massive kidney enlargement that affects both children and adults. This disease has two forms. The autosomal dominant form primarily affects adults and is common, affecting 1 in every 400 to 1000 people and accounting for approximately 4.5% of patients with end-stage renal disease in the United States. Genetic counseling and screening of family members for evidence of ADPD should be discussed. The autosomal recessive form is rare and is usually diagnosed prenatally or in infancy. Renal failure generally develops during childhood, necessitating kidney transplant or dialysis. **Nursing Process**: Implementation **Bloom's Taxonomy**: Apply

3. **Correct answer**: A, E
Rationale: Acute postinfectious glomerulonephritis or acute poststreptococcal glomerulonephritis is the most common form of glomerulonephritis. The usual initiating event for this disorder is an infection of the pharynx or skin with group A beta-hemolytic streptococcus. Staphylococcal or viral infections, such as hepatitis B, mumps, or varicella, can lead to a similar postinfectious acute glomerulonephritis. Acute postinfectious glomerulonephritis is not associated with gastrointestinal disorders, urinary tract infections, or musculoskeletal trauma. **Nursing Process**: Assessment **Bloom's Taxonomy**: Apply

4. **Correct answer**: C
Rationale: When recovering from acute glomerulonephritis, the patient is at risk for infection. A nutritionally sound diet with complete proteins is important to maintain nutritional status and support immune function. Complete proteins are preferred when total protein intake is restricted, as it may be in acute glomerulonephritis. Fluids may be restricted to reduce fluid overload, edema, and hypertension; however, the amount of the fluid restriction is individualized for each patient. Hemodialysis is indicated for acute or chronic kidney failure or injury. There is no need for the patient to remain on bedrest until the urine returns to clear yellow. **Nursing Process**: Evaluation **Bloom's Taxonomy**: Evaluate

5. **Correct answer**: B, D
Rationale: While providing postoperative care to a patient recovering from a partial nephrectomy, the nurse should note the placement, status, and drainage from ureteral catheters, stents, nephrostomy tubes, or drains and clearly label each drain. All catheters should not be connected to a single collection device. Catheters should only be irrigated as prescribed. Bright bleeding may indicate a surgical complication and should be reported to the surgeon. Cough suppressant medication is not a routine part of postoperative care of this patient. **Nursing Process**: Implementation **Bloom's Taxonomy**: Apply

6. **Correct answer**: C
Rationale: The most common causes of acute kidney injury are ischemia, sepsis, and exposure to nephrotoxins. The kidney is particularly vulnerable because of the amount of blood that passes through it. A fall in blood pressure or volume can cause ischemia of kidney tissues. Sepsis also produces hemodynamic effects with generalized vasodilation and a fall in GFR. Nephrotoxins in the blood damage renal tissue directly. Administering antihypertensive medications will not prevent the development of acute kidney injury. It is impossible to avoid all potentially nephrotoxic medications. When a nephrotoxic drug or substance must be used, the risk of AKI can be reduced by using the minimum effective dose, maintaining hydration, and eliminating other known nephrotoxins from the medication regimen. Although a history of diabetes or hypertension can increase a patient's risk of developing kidney disease, these health problems are not the most common cause of acute kidney injury in the intensive care unit. **Nursing Process**: Implementation **Bloom's Taxonomy**: Apply

7. **Correct answer**: B
Rationale: Prior to discharge the patient should have been instructed to avoid nephrotoxic drugs and chemicals for up to 1 year following an episode of acute kidney injury. During recovery, nephrons are vulnerable to damage by nephrotoxins such as NSAIDs, some antibiotics, radiologic contrast media, and heavy metals. Because alcohol can increase the nephrotoxicity of some materials, alcohol ingestion should also be discouraged. Fluid restriction may or may not be applicable for the patient. The patient recovering from acute kidney injury is not retaining urine and will not need to self-catheterize for residual urine. **Nursing Process**: Evaluation **Bloom's Taxonomy**: Evaluate

8. **Correct answer**: B, D
Rationale: Nursing care for the patient undergoing hemodialysis includes measuring weight and orthostatic blood pressure changes. These data provide baseline information to help evaluate the effects of hemodialysis. The patient who is hypotensive may not tolerate rapid fluid volume changes during dialysis. Monitoring laboratory values helps determine the effectiveness of the treatment and the timing of future dialysis sessions. Restricting fluid and protein intake would affect renal function but not necessarily the hemodialysis treatments. The patient may not have a urine output to assess specific gravity and pH. The extremity with the fistula should not be used for blood pressure assessment. **Nursing Process**: Planning **Bloom's Taxonomy**: Apply

9. **Correct answer**: C
Rationale: The patient's ability to state advantages and disadvantages of renal replacement therapies indicates understanding of treatment options and the ability to make informed decisions on treatment. Patients may be able to live independently or with the assistance of a part-time caregiver. Few patients perform hemodialysis in the home. Many people live for a number of years on dialysis, so hospice is not an immediate concern. **Nursing Process**: Planning **Bloom's Taxonomy**: Analyze

10. **Correct answer**: B
Rationale: Cloudy urine could be a manifestation of an infection. Prompt treatment is vital to preserve integrity of the transplanted organ in an immunosuppressed patient. The nurse needs to do more than record the finding. There is no evidence to support that the urinary catheter needs to be irrigated. Increasing the intravenous fluid rate would necessitate an order from a healthcare provider. **Nursing Process**: Implementation **Bloom's Taxonomy**: Apply

Chapter 29: Assessing the Cardiovascular and Lymphatic Systems

Test Yourself NCLEX-RN Review Answers

1. **Correct answer**: B
Rationale: Preload is the amount of cardiac muscle fiber tension, or stretch, that exists at the end of diastole, just before contraction of the ventricles. Preload is influenced by venous return and the compliance of the ventricles. It is related to the total volume of blood in the ventricles. Since hemorrhaging decreases the total volume of blood and venous return, the patient's cardiac output will decrease. Hemorrhaging will not increase afterload. Hemorrhaging will not affect cardiac muscle action potential. Hemorrhaging will decrease and not increase the ejection fraction. **Nursing Process**: Assessment **Bloom's Taxonomy**: Apply

2. **Correct answer**: D
Rationale: Pain intensity is assessed by using a pain rating scale that asks the patient to identify the amount of pain ranging from 0 to 10. Asking if the pain has moved into the left arm is assessing location. Asking if the pain is a pressure, burning, or tightness is assessing the quality and characteristics of the pain. Asking if the pain changes with activity assesses precipitating and aggravating factors. **Nursing Process**: Assessment **Bloom's Taxonomy**: Understand

3. **Correct answer**: C
Rationale: The apical impulse is a normal, visible pulsation in the area of the midclavicular line in the left fifth intercostal space. This location corresponds with the apex of the heart. The other anatomic locations would not be applicable when assessing the apical impulse. **Nursing Process**: Assessment **Bloom's Taxonomy**: Understand

4. **Correct answer**: A
Rationale: A heart rate of less than 60 beats/min is bradycardia. A heart rate that exceeds 100 beats per minute is tachycardia. Dysrhythmic refers to the rhythm of the heart, not specifically the rate. Apical is the location assessed, not the rate. **Nursing Process**: Implementation **Bloom's Taxonomy**: Understand

5. **Correct answer**: A, D, E
Rationale: Oxygen is carried by the hemoglobin molecule on the red blood cell. If this value is low, the patient will not be receiving sufficient oxygen to meet the body's demands. Manifestations of low oxygenation are fatigue, pallor, and dizziness. Low red blood cell counts do not cause nausea. Depending on the disease process, a low red blood cell count and subsequent low oxygenation levels could cause chest pain; however, fatigue and dizziness are the most prominent subjective effect of a low red blood cell count. **Nursing Process**: Assessment **Bloom's Taxonomy**: Apply

6. **Correct answer**: B, E
Rationale: Platelets release mediators required for clotting. If platelet counts are low, the clotting mechanism will be adversely affected. In the event a tissue injury occurs, the lack of platelets will cause bruising. Bleeding gums are also a possibility. Low platelet counts are not associated with varicose veins or enlarged lymph nodes. A low platelet count will not affect pulse pressure. **Nursing Process**: Assessment **Bloom's Taxonomy**: Apply

7. **Correct answer**:
Rationale: Peripheral vascular resistance is affected by blood viscosity and the length and diameter of arteries and arterioles. Sunken eyeballs indicate dehydration, which could cause the patient's blood to be more viscous. An elevated blood pressure indicates that the diameter and length of the arteries and arterioles are affecting the patient's blood pressure. Joint pain, bowel sounds, and fatigue do not indicate a problem with peripheral vascular resistance. **Nursing Process**: Assessment **Bloom's Taxonomy**: Analyze

8. **Correct answer**: A, B, C
Rationale: When assessing the carotid arteries, the nurse should inspect the arteries for pulsations, palpate the arteries for pulse rate, and auscultate the arteries for rhythm and other sounds. The techniques of percussion and deep palpation are not used when assessing the carotid arteries. **Nursing Process**: Assessment **Bloom's Taxonomy**: Apply

9. **Correct answer**: A
Rationale: A bruit is a murmur or blowing sound heard over stenosed vessels. A dysrhythmia is an abnormal heart rate or rhythm. A bigeminal pulse is a decrease in pulse amplitude every second beat. A hypokinetic or weak pulse is associated with decreased stroke volume. **Nursing Process**: Implementation **Bloom's Taxonomy**: Apply

10. **Correct answer**: C
Rationale: This patient is showing signs of arterial disruption including cyanosis, feeling cool to the touch, and the absence of pulses. The blood flow to this limb is insufficient, and the physician needs to be notified immediately. The lack of oxygen to the leg tissues is causing ischemia and limb pain. The nurse needs to do more than document the findings. Relaxation techniques will not be helpful to reduce the pain at this time. Asking how long the limb has been hurting does not address the urgency of the patient's problem. **Nursing Process**: Implementation **Bloom's Taxonomy**: Analyze

Chapter 30: Nursing Care of Patients with Coronary Heart Disease

Evaluate Your Response to Clinical Reasoning in Patient Care

A Patient with Coronary Artery Bypass Surgery

1. Identify Mr. Clements's modifiable risk factors as you develop your plan. What barriers might need to be overcome to implement strategies to reduce his risk factors?
2. What strategies can you use to overcome denial without creating hostility or impairing the patient–nurse relationship?
3. Consider traditional family roles as well as those roles that are unique to these individuals. Identify measures you can use to enlist the spouse's support.

4. Think about therapeutic communications as you formulate your response. Will your age or gender potentially affect your ability to respond effectively to these concerns? Would referral to another healthcare provider be appropriate?

A Patient with Acute Myocardial Infarction

1. Review immediate treatment measures for MI. Are other means available for reestablishing coronary artery perfusion? If you are in a rural area without immediate access to a cardiac catheterization lab, how will this affect your response?
2. Review the section of this chapter on dysrhythmias and their treatment. Research protocols for treating frequent PVCs in the post-MI patient at your clinical facility.
3. Review the goals of cardiac rehabilitation and Mrs. Williams's individual risk factors as you develop your teaching plan.
4. Consider the value of using a therapeutic response to Mrs. Williams's statement concerning smoking. Also consider the risks associated with cigarette smoke. How can you respond without supporting Mrs. Williams's desire to smoke and without precipitating anger or resistance? Review Chapter 6.

A Patient with Supraventricular Tachycardia

1. Review the effects of sympathetic and parasympathetic nervous system stimulation on cardiac function.
2. Review the section on supraventricular tachycardias, as well as the antidysrhythmic medications for other treatment options.
3. Use your pharmacology textbook as you develop your teaching plan.

Test Yourself NCLEX-RN Review Answers

1. **Correct answer**: A, E
   Rationale: Modifiable risk factors for the development of coronary artery disease include obesity, smoking, and physical inactivity. Physical activity should not be restricted. The patient can take active steps to modify any identified risk factors. People who do not drink alcohol should not be encouraged to start consuming it as a heart-protective measure. **Nursing Process**: Evaluation **Bloom's Taxonomy**: Evaluate
2. **Correct answer**: A, E
   Rationale: Lovastatin (Mevacor) is a first-line drug for treating hyperlipidemia and can cause myopathy. All patients should be instructed to report muscle pain and weakness or brown urine, which is an indication of muscle breakdown. Liver function tests are monitored during therapy because this drug may increase liver enzyme levels. No particular instruction is required regarding alcohol intake and this medication. This medication can be taken on an empty stomach. No specific dietary fat intake level is indicated for this medication. **Nursing Process**: Implementation **Bloom's Taxonomy**: Apply
3. **Correct answer**: C
   Rationale: Stable angina is the most common and predictable form of angina. It occurs with a predictable amount of activity or stress and usually occurs when the work of the heart is increased by physical exertion, exposure to cold, or by stress. Stable angina is relieved by rest and nitrates. Electrocardiogram changes are not seen with stable angina. Nocturnal pain is associated with Prinzmetal angina. Impaired cardiac output is associated with unstable angina. **Nursing Process**: Assessment **Bloom's Taxonomy**: Analyze
4. **Correct answer**: D
   Rationale: Acute coronary syndrome is a dynamic state in which coronary blood flow is acutely reduced, but not fully occluded. Myocardial cells are injured by the acute ischemia that results. The most important goal of care is to reestablish tissue perfusion through the use of medication or surgery. Poor peripheral circulation may occur, but this is not the priority. The patient's anxiety and need for information are also common problems, but can be addressed once the patient's primary problem has been addressed. **Nursing Process**: Planning **Bloom's Taxonomy**: Analyze
5. **Correct answer**: B
   Rationale: The cardiac catheter used to insert the stent is usually inserted via the femoral artery, a large, high-pressure vessel. The leg is maintained in extension for a prescribed period after the procedure to reduce the risk of bleeding, hematoma formation, or clot formation at the insertion site. The patient will not have chest tubes after this procedure. Intravenous lines should be continued until the healthcare provider determines they can be discontinued. Chest pain should be reported to the healthcare provider, not just treated, since this could indicate reocclusion of the coronary vessel. **Nursing Process**: Implementation **Bloom's Taxonomy**: Apply
6. **Correct answer**: A, B, D, E
   Rationale: Immediate treatment goals for the patient with an acute myocardial infarction are to reduce chest pain, reduce myocardial damage, decrease cardiac workload, and prevent complications. Increasing blood viscosity would increase potential for clotting and is not indicated. **Nursing Process**: Planning **Bloom's Taxonomy**: Apply
7. **Correct answer**: B, C
   Rationale: Fibrinolytic agents are drugs that dissolve clots and are given when access to cardiac catheterization for revascularization is not immediately available. These agents can also dissolve clots elsewhere in the body, so recent surgery is a potential contraindication. Depending on the mechanism and extent of the motor vehicle crash, fibrinolytic therapy may be contraindicated. Anxiety, obesity, and controlled hypertension are not contraindications. **Nursing Process**: Assessment **Bloom's Taxonomy**: Understand
8. **Correct answer**: B
   Rationale: Creatine kinase is an important enzyme for cellular function found principally in cardiac and skeletal muscle and the brain. CK levels rise rapidly with damage to these tissues, appearing in the serum 4 to 6 hours after an acute myocardial infarction, peaking within 12 to 24 hours, and then declining over the next 48 to 72 hours. The CK level correlates with the size of the infarction; the greater the amount of infarcted tissue, the higher the serum CK level. AST is a liver enzyme. The hematocrit level and APTT are within normal limits. **Nursing Process**: Assessment **Bloom's Taxonomy**: Analyze
9. **Correct answer**: C
   Rationale: Mobitz type II AV block is often associated with a large anterior myocardial infarction and has a high mortality rate. Pacemaker therapy may be necessary to maintain effective ventricular contractions and cardiac output. The nurse needs to do more than record the findings in

the patient's chart. The Fowler's position is not going to improve this potentially life-threatening dysrhythmia. Class IB drugs are used primarily to treat ventricular dysrhythmias, including PVCs and ventricular tachycardia. **Nursing Process**: Implementation **Bloom's Taxonomy**: Apply

10. **Correct answer**: A
Rationale: Sinus bradycardia may be well tolerated in some patients and assessment is needed before treating. If decreased mental status and hypotension are present, intravenous atropine may be indicated. Assessment of peripheral pulses and determination of an apical-radial pulse deficit can be done at a later time, if necessary. **Nursing Process**: Implementation **Bloom's Taxonomy**: Apply

Chapter 31: Nursing Care of Patients with Cardiac Disorders

Evaluate Your Response to Clinical Reasoning in Patient Care

A Patient with Heart Failure

1. Review the prescribed medications and their interactions. Do not forget to consider Mr. Jackson's age in assessing his risk for toxicity and interactions.
2. Review therapeutic communication skills and the use of open-ended statements to evaluate the underlying message of Mr. Jackson's statement.
3. Review exercise recommendations for the patient with heart failure as well as cardiac rehabilitation principles (Chapter 30).
4. Review the rationale for aspirin therapy in the patient with CHD and its effects on platelets and clotting as you formulate your response.
5. Review Chapter 42 for causes of stroke and the section of Chapter 30 on atrial fibrillation.

A Patient with Mitral Valve Prolapse

1. Review the pathophysiology and manifestations of MVP, as well as the general treatment measures for valve disorders.
2. Think about the effects of progressive conditioning on cardiac function.
3. Consider the anxiety associated with heart conditions and with a potentially progressive disorder that could affect childbearing and other life activities, as well as ultimately necessitate surgery.
4. Review the manifestations of MVP and of mitral regurgitation.

Test Yourself NCLEX-RN Review Answers

1. **Correct answer**: A
Rationale: Normal ejection fraction is 60%. An ejection fraction of 25% indicates severe impairment of ventricular function. With an ejection fraction of 25%, cardiac output is decreased. Ejection fraction does not measure the amount of blood remaining in the ventricles after systole. **Nursing Process**: Planning **Bloom's Taxonomy**: Analyze
2. **Correct answer**: C
Rationale: The main goals for care of heart failure are to slow its progression, reduce cardiac workload, improve cardiac function, and control fluid retention. A weight loss of 1 kg and crackles in the lung bases indicate control of fluid retention. A heart rate of 88 indicates reduced cardiac workload and improved cardiac function. The current treatment regimen is achieving the desired effect for this patient. There are no indications that more aggressive treatment is needed. The patient's condition has improved since admission. Because the patient continues to have crackles in the lungs, failure has not completely resolved. **Nursing Process**: Evaluation **Bloom's Taxonomy**: Evaluate
3. **Correct answer**: A, D, E
Rationale: In left-ventricular failure, the cardiac output falls and pressure in the pulmonary vascular system increases. Fatigue is a common early manifestation. Pulmonary congestion causes shortness of breath with minimal exertion. On auscultation of the lungs, inspiratory crackles may be heard in the lung bases. Jugular vein distention is a manifestation of right-ventricular failure. Chest pain with exercise can be due to angina pectoris or valvular disease. **Nursing Process**: Assessment **Bloom's Taxonomy**: Understand
4. **Correct answer**: B, D
Rationale: Calibrating and leveling the system during each shift ensures accuracy and consistency of measurements. To prevent infection, the tubing to the insertion site should be changed every 72 hours. There should be 300 mmHg of pressure on the flush solution at all times to prevent clot formation and catheter occlusion. The intravenous lines should not be secured to the bed linens. This could lead to accidental dislodging. Pressures should be measured between breaths so that intrathoracic pressure does not influence the reading. **Nursing Process**: Implementation **Bloom's Taxonomy**: Apply
5. **Correct answer**: A
Rationale: Morphine is administered intravenously to relieve anxiety and improve the efficacy of breathing. It is also a vasodilator that reduces venous return and lowers left atrial pressure. The nurse should provide the medication and monitor the patient's respiratory status. The medication should not be withheld to wait for the patient's respiratory status to improve. The medication order is correct as written and does not need to be questioned. The medication is not being used to treat chest pain. **Nursing Process**: Implementation **Bloom's Taxonomy**: Apply
6. **Correct answer**: D
Rationale: A pericardial friction rub, a grating sound, is a characteristic sign of pericarditis so it is expected, but should be documented in the patient's record. An electrocardiogram is not needed after auscultating this sound. The patient does not need to be resuscitated. The physician does not need to be notified with this auscultation sound. **Nursing Process**: Implementation **Bloom's Taxonomy**: Apply
7. **Correct answer**: D
Rationale: Antibiotic therapy effectively treats infective endocarditis in most cases. The goal of therapy is to eradicate the infecting organism from the blood and vegetative lesions in the heart. Since microorganisms may have a fibrin covering that protects them from antibiotic therapy, an extended course of multiple intravenous antibiotics is required. The patient will be fatigued and unlikely able to return to activities within 1 week of treatment. The condition is not benign and self-limiting. Cardiac transplantation is not a form of treatment for this health problem. **Nursing Process**: Planning **Bloom's Taxonomy**: Analyze

8. **Correct answer**: A, D, E
Rationale: The murmur of mitral valve stenosis would be heard during diastole when blood is flowing through the stenotic valve from the atrium to the ventricle at the apex of the heart. It is described as a low-pitched rumbling sound. There is a loud S_1 and a split S_2. S_3 and S_4 heart sounds are associated with aortic regurgitation. Muffled heart sounds are associated with cardiac tamponade. **Nursing Process**: Assessment **Bloom's Taxonomy**: Apply

9. **Correct answer**: C, E
Rationale: Lifetime anticoagulant therapy to prevent clot formation is necessary following insertion of a mechanical valve. Both types of valves can result in good hemodynamics. Biologic valves are prone to deterioration. Drugs to prevent tissue rejection are not needed after biologic valve replacement surgery. Infections are easier to treat after biologic valve replacement surgery **Nursing Process**: Implementation **Bloom's Taxonomy**: Apply

10. **Correct answer**: D
Rationale: In hypertrophic cardiomyopathy, manifestations may not develop until the demand for oxygen increases, such as with athletes during activity, causing sudden death due to a ventricular dysrhythmia. Hypertrophic cardiomyopathy is characterized by decreased compliance of the left ventricle and hypertrophy of the ventricular muscle mass. This impairs ventricular filling, leading to small end-diastolic volumes and low cardiac output. Hypertrophic cardiomyopathy may be asymptomatic for many years. Symptoms typically occur when increased oxygen demand causes increased ventricular contractility. They may develop suddenly during or after physical activity; in children and young adults, sudden cardiac death may be the first sign of the disorder. This type of cardiomyopathy does not lead to ventricle rupture during exercise. **Nursing Process**: Implementation **Bloom's Taxonomy**: Apply

Chapter 32: Nursing Care of Patients with Vascular and Lymphatic Disorders

Evaluate Your Response to Clinical Reasoning in Patient Care

A Patient with Hypertension

1. Review Mrs. Spezia's assessment data and the risk factors for primary hypertension.
2. Review the pathophysiology of primary hypertension and of obesity (Chapter 22), as well as the relationship between hypertension and coronary heart disease.
3. Think about resources that are available in your community for homeless people. Talk to community health and social service agencies to identify additional resources.
4. Correlate Mrs. Spezia's assessment data, the pathophysiology of hypertension, and the long-term effects of stress.

A Patient with Peripheral Vascular Disease

1. Review treatments for peripheral atherosclerosis, as well as lifestyle measures for preventing and treating atherosclerosis and coronary heart disease (Chapter 30).
2. Compare the pathophysiology of peripheral atherosclerosis, intermittent claudication, and coronary heart disease (Chapter 30) to identify similarities and differences.
3. Review the actions of beta-blockers and their role in angina prophylaxis.
4. Use your nursing care planning and nutrition textbooks to help develop your care plan.

A Patient with Deep Venous Thrombosis

1. Review the pathophysiologic processes of venous thrombosis and inflammation.
2. Think about questions you could ask for further information as well as potential resources for Mrs. Hipps.
3. Consider assessment data to evaluate Mrs. Hipps's limitations and resources, as well as community resources to help meet her needs.
4. Use your nursing diagnosis and care planning textbooks to develop your plan of care.

Test Yourself NCLEX-RN Review Answers

1. **Correct answer**: B
Rationale: The early stages of primary hypertension are typically asymptomatic, marked only by elevated blood pressure. Hypertension is defined as systolic blood pressure of 130 mmHg or higher or diastolic pressure of 80 mmHg or higher, based on the average of three or more readings taken on separate occasions. All elevated blood pressure readings should be investigated. Blood pressure elevations are initially transient but eventually become permanent. When symptoms do appear, they are usually vague. Headache, usually in the back of the head and neck, may be present on awakening, subsiding during the day. The patient needs to have the blood pressure rechecked before 3 months. **Nursing Process**: Implementation **Bloom's Taxonomy**: Apply

2. **Correct answer**: D
Rationale: Diet and exercise are both important factors in controlling hypertension. Following a diet is not sufficient. Salty foods such as pretzels and foods high in saturated fats should be avoided or reduced. Multiple daily servings of fruits and vegetables are encouraged. **Nursing Process**: Evaluation **Bloom's Taxonomy**: Evaluate

3. **Correct answer**: A, B
Rationale: Primary adverse effects of angiotensin II receptor blockers are persistent cough and first-dose hypotension. The medication should be taken before meals. Potassium supplements or potassium-based salt substitutes should not be taken with this medication. This medication should be taken as prescribed and not stopped without direction from the healthcare provider. **Nursing Process**: Implementation **Bloom's Taxonomy**: Apply

4. **Correct answer**: A
Rationale: Manifestations of acute arterial occlusion include cool or cold skin, pain, and pulselessness distal to the blockage. This is an emergency and the healthcare provider should be contacted immediately. Immediate embolectomy is the treatment of choice for acute arterial occlusion by an embolus to prevent tissue necrosis and gangrene. Heparin therapy is initiated to prevent further clot formation. Keeping the extremity lower than the heart promotes collateral blood flow. Even though ischemic tissue is easily damaged by minimal trauma such as shearing by bed linens, this can be done after the healthcare provider is notified of the patient's manifestations. **Nursing Process**: Implementation **Bloom's Taxonomy**: Apply

5. **Correct answer**: D
Rationale: Percutaneously inserted endovascular splints provide an alternative to surgery for abdominal aortic aneurysms. This reduces the surgical risk and faster recovery for an older patient. Type A aneurysms are treated surgically as soon as feasible. Type B aneurysms greater than 5 cm in diameter may be repaired, depending on the patient's operative risk factors. The risk of surgical repair is higher than the risk that the aneurysm will rupture for the older patient. Opening the abdomen for the surgical procedure increases the risk for postoperative infection. **Nursing Process**: Implementation **Bloom's Taxonomy**: Apply

6. **Correct answer**: B, E
Rationale: Manifestations of peripheral atherosclerosis include impaired sensation in the affected extremity. Toenails are thickened. The legs are pale when elevated, but often are dark red when dependent. The skin is often thin, shiny, and hairless, with discolored areas. Pulses may be decreased or absent, which means blood pressure in the affected extremity will be lower. **Nursing Process**: Assessment **Bloom's Taxonomy**: Analyze

7. **Correct answer**: B, E, A, D, C
Rationale: The nurse should first instruct in smoking cessation because nicotine causes vasoconstriction, further decreasing blood flow. Next, daily skin inspections are needed to look for breaks in integrity to prevent infections. Third, the patient should be instructed to provide foot care through regular cleansing, wearing cotton socks, and protecting the feet by wearing shoes. Fourth, the patient needs to engage in regular daily exercise to develop collateral circulation. And the last area is weight loss, if necessary, to keep the patient mobile. **Nursing Process**: Implementation **Bloom's Taxonomy**: Apply

8. **Correct answer**: C
Rationale: Anticoagulation is generally continued for at least 3 months. Regular follow-up is necessary to be sure prothrombin times remain within the desirable range for anticoagulation. The patient should use a recliner chair or footstool when sitting to prevent pooling of blood in the extremities. Patients should ambulate as soon as possible and maintain a schedule of regular ambulation and foot and ankle exercises throughout the day. The development of deep venous thrombosis is not because of an elevated cholesterol level. **Nursing Process**: Evaluating **Bloom's Taxonomy**: Evaluate

9. **Correct answer**: C
Rationale: Elevating the legs and wearing elastic stockings may relieve the discomfort associated with varicose veins. Surgical treatment of varicose veins is generally reserved for patients who are very symptomatic, experience recurrent superficial venous thrombosis, and/or develop stasis ulcers. Surgery will relieve the discomfort associated with varicose veins but may not be indicated for the patient. **Nursing Process**: Implementation **Bloom's Taxonomy**: Apply

10. **Correct answer**: A, B, C, D
Rationale: Careful skin and foot care is a high priority to prevent skin breakdown and potential infection in the patient with lymphedema. The foot of the bed is raised by 15 to 20 degrees at night to promote lymph flow. Diuretic therapy may be used intermittently when the condition is exacerbated by the menstrual cycle or seasonal variability. Elastic graduated compression stockings may be ordered for use during the day. Exercise is encouraged. **Nursing Process**: Implementation **Bloom's Taxonomy**: Apply

Chapter 33: Nursing Care of Patients with Hematologic Disorders

Evaluate Your Response to Clinical Reasoning in Patient Care

A Patient with Folic Acid Deficiency Anemia

1. Consider the effects of Mrs. Matthews's rapid weight loss on fluid balance, as well as the effects of tissue hypoxia on cardiac output.
2. Refer to this chapter and your nutrition text. Be sure to consider Mrs. Matthews's age in designing your menu.
3. Consider factors such as Mrs. Matthews's recent dietary history, the folic acid content of foods, and other pertinent factors in the history and physical assessment.
4. In addition to general factors to consider for the older adult (don't forget transportation among other factors), also consider the possible effect of Mrs. Matthews's recent loss and the grieving process.

A Patient with Acute Myelocytic Leukemia

1. Review the physiology of white blood cells and the immune and inflammatory responses.
2. Think about the risks created by hospitalization in terms of exposure to infection and invasive procedures.
3. Think about the effect of inability to perform self-care on self-esteem, self-confidence, and perception of power and control.
4. Use information provided in the nursing care and home care sections of this chapter as well as in Chapter 12.
5. Use your nursing care planning and fundamentals texts to develop your care plan.

A Patient with Hodgkin Disease

1. Review Chapter 14 and the effects of chemotherapy and radiation on cancer cells. Think about the advantages of combining these two therapies in terms of short- and long-term desired and adverse effects.
2. Consider the primary and potential risks for infection in community settings as you design your teaching plan. What teaching strategies will you use for a young adult with Mr. Quito's education and experience?
3. Review theories of development and the developmental tasks for the young adult.
4. Use your nursing fundamentals and nursing care planning texts for reference in developing your care plan.

A Patient with Hemophilia

1. Review the pathophysiology of hemophilia and its effect on the clotting process.
2. Consider both the ABCs and Maslow's hierarchy of needs as you respond to this question.
3. Think about the genetic transmission of hemophilia. How might Mr. Cruise's hemophilia affect any children that he has? Grandchildren?
4. Review your nursing fundamentals book, nursing skills book, and intravenous therapy text to develop your

teaching plan. Also consider previous learning and developmental levels.

5. What evidence supports this as an appropriate nursing diagnosis for Mr. Cruise?

Test Yourself NCLEX-RN Review Answers

1. **Correct answer**: D
Rationale: When anemia develops gradually and the RBC reduction is moderate, successful compensatory mechanisms may result in few symptoms except when the oxygen needs of the body increase due to exercise. There is a lack of hemoglobin to carry oxygen to the tissues. Tissue hypoxia may cause dyspnea on exertion. Tachycardia and elevated white blood cell counts might be associated with a specific type of anemia. Hematocrit levels can remain within normal limits with moderate anemia. **Nursing Process**: Assessment **Bloom's Taxonomy**: Apply

2. **Correct answer**: D, E
Rationale: During gastric resection, intrinsic factor production may decrease, leading to vitamin B_{12} deficiency anemia with associated neurologic deficits such as numbness and tingling of extremities and a sore, red, beefy tongue. Bone pain is associated with anemia caused by a reduction in red blood cell production. Steatorrhea is not a manifestation of anemia. Bronze skin color is a manifestation of thalassemia minor. **Nursing Process**: Assessment **Bloom's Taxonomy**: Analyze

3. **Correct answer**: B, C
Rationale: Prior to bone marrow transplant, chemotherapy or total body irradiation is used to destroy leukemic cells in the bone marrow. Normal blood cells are also destroyed, causing significant risk for infection and bleeding. The other problems are possible with this patient but would not be the highest priority when planning care for the patient receiving a bone marrow transplant. **Nursing Process**: Planning **Bloom's Taxonomy**: Analyze

4. **Correct answer**: A, B, D
Rationale: AML causes both neutropenia and thrombocytopenia, with resulting increased risk for infection and bleeding. A private room and oral hygiene help reduce infection risk, and a soft, bland diet reduces trauma to oral mucosal membranes. Invasive procedures such as rectal temperatures should not be performed because of the risk for bleeding. The patient does not need to be in airborne infection control precautions; however, individuals with respiratory illnesses should be restricted. **Nursing Process**: Implementation **Bloom's Taxonomy**: Understand

5. **Correct answer**: B
Rationale: The nurse should assess the patient's perception of body image through subjective information such as what the patient likes most and least about his body, preillness perception of people who are sick or have a disability, current understanding of health and limitations imposed by illness or treatment, and feelings about the illness and its effect on perception of self and others. The patient's comment may not be related to hair loss. The nurse should not instill false hope by telling the patient not to worry. The nurse has no way of knowing if the patient's comment is related to the inability to have children. **Nursing Process**: Implementation **Bloom's Taxonomy**: Apply

6. **Correct answer**: A, E
Rationale: Multiple-drug chemotherapy regimens are effective at different phases of the cell cycle, allowing lower doses of individual drugs to decrease adverse effects, reduce drug resistance, and produce more effective tumor destruction. This regimen is not used to target malignant cells in different organs. These medications will not prevent the development of adverse effects. The CHOP regimen is not used to support growth and development of normal cells. **Nursing Process**: Implementation **Bloom's Taxonomy**: Apply

7. **Correct answer**: B
Rationale: Pathologic fractures are a common and reoccurring problem with multiple myeloma. A new onset of severe pain may signal a pathologic fracture and needs to be reported. A back brace might be indicated; however, the new onset of pain needs to be reported and investigated first. Reassuring the patient that bone pain is an expectation of the disease process is not appropriate. The pain is new and should be reported. Knowing what medications the patient uses for pain control is important, but the onset of new pain should be reported. **Nursing Process**: Implementation **Bloom's Taxonomy**: Apply

8. **Correct answer**: D
Rationale: A platelet count of $60,000/mm^3$ is significantly low (normal 150,000 to $450,000/mm^3$), which increases the patient's risk of bleeding and bruising with minor trauma. More information is needed to determine if the INR of 4.0 is significant for this patient. A medication history and previous health history are required. A hematocrit of 28% would not cause bruising. A white blood cell count of $4,500/mm^3$ is below normal, which increases the patient's risk for infection and not bleeding. **Nursing Process**: Assessment **Bloom's Taxonomy**: Analyze

9. **Correct answer**: B
Rationale: Hemophilia A, the most common form, occurs in about 1 in 10,000 male births and is transmitted on the X chromosome: Each male offspring has a 50% risk of inheriting the defective gene. Each female offspring has a 50% risk of becoming a carrier. Von Willebrand disease affects about 1 in 100 to 500 people, usually inherited as an autosomal dominant trait. Offspring of an affected person has a 50% risk of inheriting the trait and the disorder. It is unknown if the husband has this type of hemophilia. **Nursing Process**: Implementation **Bloom's Taxonomy**: Apply

10. **Correct answer**: A
Rationale: When bleeding is the major manifestation of DIC, platelet concentrates are given to restore clotting factors and platelets. An infusion of platelets does not replace specific clotting factors. The infusion of platelets is not used to restore tissue oxygenation. The patient is experiencing intravascular clotting and medications will be used to prevent further clot formation. **Nursing Process**: Implementation **Bloom's Taxonomy**: Understand

Chapter 34: Assessing the Respiratory System

Test Yourself NCLEX-RN Review Answers

1. **Correct answer**: B
Rationale: The apex of each lung lies just below the clavicle. The base of each lung rests on the diaphragm. The

hilus, on the mediastinal surface of each lung, is where blood vessels of the pulmonary and circulatory systems and the primary bronchus enter and exit the lungs. The parietal pleura line the thoracic wall and mediastinum. **Nursing Process**: Assessment **Bloom's Taxonomy**: Apply

2. **Correct answer**: C
   Rationale: A familial history of lung cancer increases the risk of developing lung cancer, and small-cell lung cancer has a definite genetic component. Childhood obesity, family history of asthma, and frequent upper respiratory infections do not increase the risk of developing lung cancer. **Nursing Process**: Assessment **Bloom's Taxonomy**: Analyze
3. **Correct answer**: B
   Rationale: Bronchovesicular breath sounds are normal. The nurse should measure and record the vital signs as usual. The physician does not need to be notified of normal breath sounds. A respiratory treatment is not required. The nurse has not assessed breath sounds yet, so documenting the inability to hear the sounds would be incorrect data. **Nursing Process**: Assessment **Bloom's Taxonomy**: Apply
4. **Correct answer**: D, E
   Rationale: The organic chemical 2,3-DPG is formed in red blood cells and increases the release of oxygen from hemoglobin by binding to it during times of increased metabolism such as when body temperature increases. This binding alters the structure of hemoglobin to facilitate oxygen unloading. The increase in body temperature does not decrease respiratory rate or increase lung compliance. Oxygen unloading is enhanced and not inhibited. **Nursing Process**: Planning **Bloom's Taxonomy**: Analyze
5. **Correct answer**: A, B, C
   Rationale: A thoracentesis is done to obtain a specimen of pleural fluid for diagnosis, to remove excess pleural fluid, or instill medication. A large-bore needle is inserted through the chest wall and into the pleural space. Following the procedure, a chest x-ray is taken to check for a pneumothorax. A thoracotomy is not required. This is not an x-ray procedure. **Nursing Process**: Implementation **Bloom's Taxonomy**: Apply
6. **Correct answer**: A, B, C, E
   Rationale: In order to fully assess the patient's presenting problem the nurse should analyze its onset ("When did you first notice your cough?), characteristics, course, severity, precipitating and relieving factors ("Has anything you have tried made your cough go away"), and any associated symptoms ("Do you have pain in your chest when you cough?"), noting the time ("When do you have coughing episodes?") and circumstances. Everyone has coughed at some time in their life, so asking if the patient had ever coughed before does not provide useful information. **Nursing Process**: Assessment **Bloom's Taxonomy**: Apply
7. **Correct answer**: B
   Rationale: Wheezes are continuous musical sounds heard in the chest. Crackles are short, discrete, crackling, or bubbling sounds. A friction rub is a loud, dry, creaking sound. Murmurs are not typically heard during the assessment of breath sounds. **Nursing Process**: Implementation **Bloom's Taxonomy**: Apply
8. **Correct answer**: A
   Rationale: Breath sounds are absent over collapsed lung, surgical removal of lung, pleural effusion, and primary bronchus obstruction. The patient was admitted with pleural effusion, so breath sounds will be absent in that section of the lung. There are no other reasons in the patient's health history that would cause absent breath sounds. **Nursing Process**: Assessment **Bloom's Taxonomy**: Apply
9. **Correct answer**: B, D
   Rationale: When assessing breath sounds, the nurse should direct the patient to take slow, deep breaths through an open mouth. Holding the breath will not create any sounds. Breathing through the nose will not amplify the breath sounds. Repeating the number 99 assesses for lung consolidation, which may be done after the breath sounds assessment is complete. **Nursing Process**: Assessment **Bloom's Taxonomy**: Apply
10. **Correct answer**: A
    Rationale: Decreased diaphragmatic movement on the left side should be documented. This is an expected outcome with pneumothorax on the left since air movement and diaphragm movement would be decreased. The physician does not need to be notified with this finding. The assessment does not need to be repeated. Having the patient hold his or her breath is not going to change the finding. **Nursing Process**: Implementation **Bloom's Taxonomy**: Apply

Chapter 35: Nursing Care of Patients with Upper Respiratory Disorders

Evaluate Your Response to Clinical Reasoning in Patient Care

A Patient with Peritonsillar Abscess

1. Review the manifestations of upper respiratory infections.
2. Outline the management of these disorders.
3. Think about the primary uses of the nose, mouth, and pharynx as you consider nursing diagnoses related to upper respiratory disorders.

A Patient with Nasal Trauma

1. Consider other measures to restore the patient's sense of control over the situation. Consider the potentially traumatic effects of suction on the mucous membranes as well as possible infection control risks.
2. Review the implications and potential dangers of CSF leakage to help you develop your care plan.
3. Think about the benefits and drawbacks of immediate and delayed rhinoplasty.

A Patient with Total Laryngectomy

1. Review the options for speech rehabilitation. If available, practice using a speech generator. Practice esophageal speech.
2. Use your nursing care planning and nursing diagnoses handbook to develop your care plan. Consider Mr. Tom's age, occupation, and marital status in your plan of care.
3. Review Chapter 4 for surgical nursing care interventions, as well as your nursing fundamentals textbook for wound care strategies.
4. Consider measures to promote airway clearance and ventilation of all lung fields.

Test Yourself NCLEX-RN Review Answers

1. **Correct answer**: C
   Rationale: Over-the-counter topical nasal sprays are effective to relieve URI manifestations, but because the patient

has mild hypertension, the patient should discuss the use of this preparation with the healthcare provider before using. Antibiotics are not indicated for an acute URI. The use of vitamin C and zinc lozenges may not relieve the patient's symptoms. An over-the-counter decongestant may be contraindicated in the patient with hypertension and should not be recommended to this patient. **Nursing Process**: Implementation **Bloom's Taxonomy**: Apply

2. **Correct answer**: C
Rationale: Older adults have a high incidence of complications such as pneumonia when exposed to influenza. Preventing influenza by immunizing at-risk populations is an important aspect of care. Annual immunization for influenza is recommended for all at-risk patients, including older patients and residents of nursing homes. Avoiding crowds and using effective hand hygiene will help reduce the spread of microorganisms; however, an annual influenza vaccination is the best defense against contracting the health problem. Scheduling exercise programs indoors during the winter months will not reduce the risk of influenza and pneumonia in the older adult. **Nursing Process**: Planning **Bloom's Taxonomy**: Apply

3. **Correct answer**: A, B, C, D
Rationale: The nurse should focus on the importance of completing the entire course of prescribed antibiotics to achieve cure and prevent the development of antibiotic-resistant bacteria. A humidifier might be helpful to loosen secretions. Sleeping with the head of the bed elevated to a 45-degree angle and sleeping on the unaffected side is helpful. A liberal fluid intake will thin secretions. Warm, moist packs should be used on the area of tenderness and pain. **Nursing Process**: Implementation **Bloom's Taxonomy**: Apply

4. **Correct answer**: A
Rationale: Posterior nasal packing is very uncomfortable and can cause respiratory complications. Hypoxemia is common and supplementary oxygen is required. Although elevating the head of the bed facilitates ventilation, supplemental oxygen is the priority. Frequent oral hygiene would be required; however, supplemental oxygen is the priority. A cold compress decreases pain and promotes vasoconstriction, which will decrease bleeding and swelling but will not help with oxygenation. Supplemental oxygen is the priority for this patient. **Nursing Process**: Planning **Bloom's Taxonomy**: Analyze

5. **Correct answer**: C
Rationale: Fractures of other facial bones may accompany a broken nose, particularly when facial trauma is severe. Fractures in the nasoethmoidal or frontal region can disrupt the dura, causing CSF leakage or rhinorrhea. CSF rhinorrhea is suspected when watery nasal drainage tests positive for glucose. The nurse needs to do more than provide a box of tissues. Suctioning the nasopharynx would be contraindicated in the patient with facial trauma. Watery drainage is not expected after a nasal fracture. **Nursing Process**: Implementation **Bloom's Taxonomy**: Apply

6. **Correct answer**: A, B, C, D
Rationale: The manifestations of sleep apnea include loud, cyclic snoring, hypertension, morning headache, and daytime fatigue and sleepiness. Decreased oxygen saturation while awake is not a manifestation of obstructive sleep apnea. **Nursing Process**: Assessment **Bloom's Taxonomy**: Apply

7. **Correct answer**: C
Rationale: The most appropriate question would be for the nurse to ask how long the patient has been hoarse. Depending on the patient's response, asking about smoking or a sore throat might be appropriate. Hoarseness and a breathy voice quality are manifestations of benign vocal cord tumors. The usual symptom of glottic cancer is hoarseness or a change in the voice because the tumor prevents complete closure of the vocal cords during speech. The nurse needs to assess the patient before suggesting treatment with throat lozenges. **Nursing Process**: Assessment **Bloom's Taxonomy**: Apply

8. **Correct answer**: C
Rationale: Radiation therapy is often the treatment of choice for early laryngeal cancer and is extremely effective for treating glottic cancer, with cure rates equal to those achieved by surgery. Radiation therapy preserves the voice, although the tone or timber of the voice may be affected. This cancer does metastasize to other areas. Stage 1 laryngeal cancer does need to be treated. The patient will not lose the ability to speak. **Nursing Process**: Evaluation **Bloom's Taxonomy**: Evaluate

9. **Correct answer**: A, B, C, D, E
Rationale: Maintaining airway patency is of highest priority. The head may need additional support because of the removal of neck muscles. Regaining speech will require practice and assistance from a speech therapist. Loss of the voice will result in grieving; encouraging expression of feelings can facilitate gradual acceptance of the loss. **Nursing Process**: Implementation **Bloom's Taxonomy**: Apply

10. **Correct answer**: B, D, E
Rationale: Water sports are contraindicated due to the possibility of taking water in through the stoma. The area around the stoma should be kept clean and dry to prevent excoriation of the skin. Increased fluid intake helps to maintain mucosal moisture and loosen secretions. Clean technique is used for dressing changes in the home. Baths or showers may be used as long as the head is not submerged and water does not enter the stoma. **Nursing Process**: Implementation **Bloom's Taxonomy**: Apply

Chapter 36: Nursing Care of Patients with Ventilation Disorders

Evaluate Your Response to Clinical Reasoning in Patient Care

A Patient with Pneumonia

1. Review Mrs. O'Neal's assessment data and compare her history with identified risk factors for pneumonia.
2. Review normal immune and inflammatory responses and the role of white blood cells in these processes.
3. Review Chapter 11 and altered immune responses for the physiology and effects of anaphylactic shock.
4. Use your nursing care planning and nursing diagnosis textbooks to help develop your care plan.

A Patient with Tuberculosis

1. Consider available resources for patients with mental illness, as well as community and public health resources. Consider measures to ensure compliance with the prescribed treatment.

2. Contact your local public health department, the discharge planner for your unit, or the social services department in your clinical facility to help identify available resources.
3. Use the nursing care section under Pneumonia and your nursing diagnosis or care planning handbook as you develop your care plan.

A Patient with Lung Cancer

1. Review Chapter 14 and use your pharmacology text to research the effects of these drugs and the rationale for combination chemotherapy.
2. Use Chapter 14 and your pharmacology text to identify probable side effects of this treatment regimen. Then use your nursing care planning book to identify appropriate nursing diagnoses and interventions.
3. Review the pathophysiology and collaborative care sections for lung cancer to develop your response to this question.

Test Yourself NCLEX-RN Review Answers

1. **Correct answer**: C
Rationale: Adequate oxygenation is a priority for all patients. The nurse should apply the prescribed amount of oxygen to the patient first. The sputum specimen should be obtained before beginning the prescribed antibiotic. The meal tray would be of the least priority. **Nursing Process**: Implementation **Bloom's Taxonomy**: Apply
2. **Correct answer**: A, B, C, D, E
Rationale: Overall gray skin color and bluish tinge to lips indicate hypoxemia; supplemental oxygen is highest priority. Second, raise the head of the bed to promote chest expansion and alveolar ventilation. Assessment of oxygen saturation and breath sounds can be completed next. The physician should be contacted after the patient is receiving oxygen and assessments are completed. **Nursing Process**: Implementation **Bloom's Taxonomy**: Analyze
3. **Correct answer**: C
Rationale: The intradermal PPD is read by measuring the area of induration or hardness at the injection site. Redness or erythema at the site does not indicate a positive test. The test is read at 48 and 72 hours. Residing in a long-term care facility is not a relevant factor. **Nursing Process**: Evaluation **Bloom's Taxonomy**: Evaluate
4. **Correct answer**: C, E
Rationale: When teaching a patient who is taking INH, the nurse needs to include information on adverse effects such as numbness and tingling of extremities and how these effects need to be reported to the physician. The patient should also be made aware that periodic liver function studies are required. Rifampin may cause an orange-red coloration of saliva and urine. Ethambutol may affect red-green color discrimination and visual acuity. Periodic eye examinations are recommended. Aspirin may interfere with rifampin absorption and should not be taken concurrently. **Nursing Process**: Implementation **Bloom's Taxonomy**: Applying
5. **Correct answer**: B
Rationale: Smoking cessation is important with the diagnosis of lung cancer to prevent further damage from the chemicals in the cigarettes. Most people with lung cancer die within 1 year of the initial diagnosis. Successful treatment of lung cancer after the disease has spread is grim. The patient planning to do nothing but sit in an easy chair and wait to die indicates that teaching has not been effective. **Nursing Process**: Evaluation **Bloom's Taxonomy**: Evaluate
6. **Correct answer**: A, C
Rationale: Chest tube drainage that is red, free flowing, and exceeds 70 mL/h indicates hemorrhage and must be reported. Vital signs and level of consciousness are measured to evaluate cardiac output and hemodynamic stability. The drainage should not be emptied and pressure should not be applied to the chest tube insertion site. The nurse needs to notify the surgeon now and not wait for 30 minutes to reevaluate the patient's drainage. **Nursing Process**: Implementation **Bloom's Taxonomy**: Apply
7. **Correct answer**: C, E
Rationale: The patient having a thoracentesis needs to sit upright, leaning forward during the procedure to spread the rib cage for easier placement of the needle. Local anesthesia will prevent pain, but a feeling of pressure will occur during insertion. The patient should not cough as fluid is withdrawn. The patient does not need to breathe deeply when the needle is inserted. The patient only needs to remain positioned on the unaffected side for 1 hour after the procedure to allow the pleural puncture to heal. **Nursing Process**: Implementation **Bloom's Taxonomy**: Apply
8. **Correct answer**: A
Rationale: A patient with a fractured rib should be urged to use a small pillow to splint the area when coughing to reduce the movement of rib cage and pain. Providing adequate analgesia to promote breathing, coughing, and movement is the primary intervention. Bedrest is not required with a rib fracture. Rib belts, binders, and taping to stabilize the rib cage are not recommended because they may interfere with ventilation and lead to atelectasis. **Nursing Process**: Implementation **Bloom's Taxonomy**: Apply
9. **Correct answer**: A
Rationale: A respiratory rate of 36 indicates respiratory distress and is of greatest concern. Adventitious lung sounds like crackles can occur after an inhalation injury. Ashlike material in the sputum is expected after an inhalation injury. Pink mucous membranes and skin indicate adequate oxygenation. **Nursing Process**: Assessment **Bloom's Taxonomy**: Analyze
10. **Correct answer**: C
Rationale: Maintaining or restoring adequate alveolar ventilation and gas exchange is of highest priority for the patient with a pneumothorax. Loss of negative pressure in the pleural cavity and the resulting collapse of lung tissue can cause poor chest expansion and loss of alveolar ventilation. Pain, aspiration and other injury, and establishing effective breathing patterns are important concerns, but are not the highest priority for this patient. **Nursing Process**: Planning **Bloom's Taxonomy**: Analyze

Chapter 37: Nursing Care of Patients with Gas Exchange Disorders

Evaluate Your Response to Clinical Reasoning in Patient Care

A Patient with COPD

1. Review the processes by which cigarette smoke inflicts damage on lung tissue. Use your pediatric and pathophysiology texts for additional information.

2. Review the physiology of the respiratory drive, as well as the effects of chronic elevated carbon dioxide levels in the blood.
3. Review the manifestations of COPD and its complications as well as the section of this chapter on respiratory failure.
4. Use your nursing diagnosis handbook to help identify appropriate goals and interventions for this nursing diagnosis.

A Patient with ARDS

1. As you respond to this question, consider additional treatment measures for ARDS and respiratory failure. Also consider the potential long-term consequences and complications of intubation and mechanical ventilation. Discuss strategies for communicating with Ms. Adamson's family and supporting coping and decision making by Ms. Adamson and her family in an instance such as this.
2. Think about the precipitating factors for ARDS and the factors that may precipitate respiratory failure in a patient with COPD. Consider the probable overall respiratory and general health status of the individual affected by each of these conditions.
3. Review the precipitating factors for ARDS and discuss strategies to prevent them.
4. Use your nursing care planning book to identify appropriate goals and nursing interventions for this nursing diagnosis.

Test Yourself NCLEX-RN Review Answers

1. **Correct answer**: C
   Rationale: Bronchospasm and bronchoconstriction, increased mucous secretion, and airway edema narrow the airways and impair airflow during an acute attack of asthma. Both inspiratory and expiratory volumes are affected, decreasing the oxygen available at the alveolus for the process of respiration. Narrowed air passages increase the work of breathing, increasing the metabolic rate and tissue demand for oxygen. This is the priority patient problem. The problems related to anxiety, irregular respirations, and lack of knowledge are all important, but do not carry the highest priority for this patient. **Nursing Process**: Planning **Bloom's Taxonomy**: Analyze
2. **Correct answer**: C
   Rationale: Respiratory status can change rapidly during an acute asthma attack and its treatment. Slowed, shallow respirations with significantly diminished breath sounds and decreased wheezing may indicate exhaustion and impending respiratory failure. Immediate intervention is necessary so the healthcare provider needs to be notified. The healthcare provider might prescribe a chest x-ray. Asking the family members to leave is not a priority. Allowing the patient to rest undisturbed could eventually lead to respiratory arrest. **Nursing Process**: Implementation **Bloom's Taxonomy**: Apply
3. **Correct answer**: A, C
   Rationale: The patient should shake the canister vigorously to distribute the powder in the canister. The patient should rinse the mouth after using the inhaler to minimize systemic absorption. Press and hold the canister down while inhaling deeply and slowly for 3 to 5 seconds. Then hold the breath for 10 seconds, release pressure on the container, remove from the mouth, and exhale. Wait 20 to 30 seconds before repeating the procedure for a second puff. Administer anti-inflammatory inhaler doses after bronchodilators to facilitate transit of the medication to distal airways. **Nursing Process**: Implementation **Bloom's Taxonomy**: Apply
4. **Correct answer**: D, E
   Rationale: In the patient with chronic obstructive airway disease, air trapping and hyperinflation increase the anterior-posterior chest diameter, causing barrel chest. Accessory muscles of respiration are prominently used. Mental confusion, oxygen saturation levels below 85%, and 3+ pitting edema of the ankles and lower legs are not expected assessment findings and should be reported to the healthcare provider. **Nursing Process**: Assessment **Bloom's Taxonomy**: Analyze
5. **Correct answer**: A
   Rationale: During an acute exacerbation of COPD, keeping the SaO_2 above 90% is an appropriate goal. This goal must be individualized as some patients may no longer be able to obtain 90% saturation. However, this is the best of the goals listed. Lung function that has been lost from chronic obstructive pulmonary disease cannot be regained. Arterial blood gases will not be normal because the patient's oxygen and carbon dioxide levels are altered due to lung changes. The nurse should help the patient develop a smoking cessation plan to preserve remaining lung functioning. **Nursing Process**: Planning **Bloom's Taxonomy**: Analyze
6. **Correct answer**: C
   Rationale: Administering oxygen to patients with chronic elevated carbon dioxide levels in the blood can actually increase the $PaCO_2$, leading to increased somnolence and even respiratory failure. Close monitoring of level of consciousness and arterial blood gases during oxygen therapy is vital. Long-term oxygen therapy is used for severe and progressive hypoxemia. It also reduces the rate of hospitalization and increases length of survival. Oxygen may be used intermittently, at night, or continuously. For severely hypoxemic patients, the greatest benefit is seen with continuous oxygen. The patient with chronic obstructive pulmonary disease should be working on a smoking cessation plan. **Nursing Process**: Planning **Bloom's Taxonomy**: Analyze
7. **Correct answer**: A, C, D, E
   Rationale: Thick, tenacious, milky white sputum and fever indicate possible infection. Difficulty coughing up mucus and increased shortness of breath and fatigue indicate potential early manifestations of respiratory failure. Steatorrhea causing frequent, bulky, foul-smelling stools is a common manifestation as a result of associated pancreatic insufficiency. **Nursing Process**: Implementation **Bloom's Taxonomy**: Apply
8. **Correct answer**: B, C, E
   Rationale: These manifestations may indicate pulmonary embolism. Oxygen should be administered to support gas exchange and tissue oxygenation. The high-Fowler position facilitates oxygenation. Auscultating heart sounds can help detect cardiac compromise. Checking for Homans' sign would not be beneficial at this time. Pain medication should not be provided until a pain assessment is completed. **Nursing Process**: Implementation **Bloom's Taxonomy**: Apply
9. **Correct answer**: C
   Rationale: The manifestations of respiratory failure are caused by hypoxemia and hypercapnia, as well as the

underlying disease process. Dyspnea and headache are early signs. Hypoxemia causes dyspnea and neurologic symptoms such as restlessness, apprehension, impaired judgment, and motor impairment. Tachycardia and hypertension develop as the cardiac output increases in an effort to bring more oxygen to the tissues. As hypoxemia progresses, dysrhythmias, hypotension, and decreased cardiac output may develop. Increased carbon dioxide levels depress CNS function and cause vasodilation. **Nursing Process**: Assessment **Bloom's Taxonomy**: Apply

10. **Correct answer**: D
Rationale: A patent airway is necessary to maintain effective alveolar ventilation and gas exchange. Endotracheal suctioning as needed will ensure a patent airway for the patient. The supine position will not ensure effective alveolar ventilation. Providing oxygen as prescribed will not ensure effective alveolar ventilation. Increasing the tidal volume on the ventilator could cause lung tissue trauma. **Nursing Process**: Implementation **Bloom's Taxonomy**: Apply

Chapter 38: Assessing the Musculoskeletal System

Test Yourself NCLEX-RN Review Answers

1. **Correct answer**: B
Rationale: Long bones have a midportion, or shaft, called a diaphysis, and two broad ends, called epiphyses. Flat bones are thin and flat, and most are curved. Short bones, also called cuboid bones, include the bones of the wrist and ankle. Irregular bones are of various shapes and sizes. Irregular bones include the vertebrae, the scapulae, and the bones of the pelvic girdle. **Nursing Process**: Planning **Bloom's Taxonomy**: Apply
2. **Correct answer**: C
Rationale: Abduction is the term for moving an extremity away from the midline of the body. Flexion is bending a limb at the joint. Extension is straightening a limb at the joint. Adduction is moving a limb toward the midline of the body. **Nursing Process**: Assessment **Bloom's Taxonomy**: Apply
3. **Correct answer**: D
Rationale: Uric acid levels are used to diagnose and monitor the treatment of gout. Uric acid level has no relationship to bruising. A uric acid level is not used to diagnose rheumatoid arthritis. Uric acid level is not used to diagnose familial bone diseases. **Nursing Process**: Implementation **Bloom's Taxonomy**: Apply
4. **Correct answer**: A, B, D, E
Rationale: Age-related changes in the musculoskeletal system include decreased muscle mass and strength, reduced range of motion of joints because of a loss of elasticity of ligaments and tendons, and decreased height because of decreased bone mass, decreased calcium absorption, and thinning of intervertebral disks. Edema of the ankles, hips, and knees is not an age-related change of the musculoskeletal system. **Nursing Process**: Assessment **Bloom's Taxonomy**: Analyze
5. **Correct answer**: A, B, E
Rationale: In preparation for an electromyogram, the nurse should instruct the patient to avoid drinking fluids containing caffeine for 3 hours before the test, avoid smoking for 3 hours before the test, and to avoid taking medications such as muscle relaxants. Avoiding oral hypoglycemic agents before the test and alerting the healthcare provider with an allergy to shellfish would be appropriate if the patient were having a diagnostic test using contrast dye. **Nursing Process**: Implementation **Bloom's Taxonomy**: Apply
6. **Correct answer**: A, B
Rationale: Sticking out the tongue and clenching the teeth require strength in the jaw muscles. Closing the eyes tightly assesses ocular muscles and lids. Blowing out the cheeks tests facial muscle strength. Bending the head forward assesses neck muscles. **Nursing Process**: Assessment **Bloom's Taxonomy**: Apply
7. **Correct answer**: D
Rationale: Crepitation is a grating sound as the joint moves. Crackles are sounds created by fluid or mucus in the lungs. Arthritis is a health problem that can cause crepitation. Synovitis is inflammation of the synovial membrane lining the articular capsule of a joint. **Nursing Process**: Implementation **Bloom's Taxonomy**: Apply
8. **Correct answer**: A
Rationale: The ballottement test is used to assess for fluid in the knee joint. A positive ballottement test does not indicate an elbow deformity. This test is not used to assess for crepitus. Ballottement is not used to assess for a metatarsal infection. **Nursing Process**: Assessment **Bloom's Taxonomy**: Analyze
9. **Correct answer**: B
Rationale: Scoliosis is the term used to describe a lateral curve in the spine. Lordosis is an increased lumbar curve. Kyphosis is an exaggerated thoracic curvature of the spine. Musculosis is a fictitious health problem. **Nursing Process**: Assessment **Bloom's Taxonomy**: Apply
10. **Correct answer**: A, E
Rationale: The primary manifestations of altered musculoskeletal function are pain and limited mobility. Cyanosis and decreased pulses indicate a problem with blood flow. Exaggerated reflexes could indicate a neurologic problem and are not a common presenting problem with musculoskeletal disorders. **Nursing Process**: Assessment **Bloom's Taxonomy**: Apply

Chapter 39: Nursing Care of Patients with Musculoskeletal Trauma

Evaluate Your Response to Clinical Reasoning in Patient Care

A Patient with a Hip Fracture

1. Consider Mrs. Carbolito's age and the fact that she is postmenopausal. What effect does estrogen have on bone health? What might have increased her risk for falls?
2. Review the principles of traction application. What purpose does it serve prior to surgery? What words could you use that she would understand? Think about the effects of trauma, pain, and suddenly finding oneself in a strange environment on listening and understanding verbal communications.
3. List how each of these manifestations would affect skin integrity, food intake, and bone healing.

A Patient with a Below-the-Knee Amputation

1. Consider your role as a nurse and therapeutic communications techniques you could use in responding to Mr. Rocke.

You also may wish to review Chapter 5 in developing your response.

2. Review Mr. Rocke's subjective and objective assessment data, interprofessional care needs, and apparent stage of grieving to help prioritize nursing activities.
3. Review the roles of and resources available to various members of the interprofessional team.
4. Design a sequential plan for Mr. Rocke's self-care of the stump. Consider his readiness to learn and the complexity of the care. Is there a risk in letting him assume total responsibility from the beginning? Why or why not?
5. List the factors used to describe Mr. Rocke. How do these affect his ability or willingness to follow up with medical care? What community agencies are available where you live or go to school that would be good sources of assistance and support for Mr. Rocke?
6. Review the information about exercise. How would Mr. Rocke's choice not to do exercises affect his ability to use a prosthesis to walk?

Test Yourself NCLEX-RN Review Answers

1. **Correct answer**: D
   Rationale: Ice used on a sprained ankle immediately after injury will cause vasoconstriction of the blood vessels to decrease edema and pain. Ice is not used to increase white blood cells or lower the blood pressure or pulse. The use of ice does not promote venous return. **Nursing Process**: Implementation **Bloom's Taxonomy**: Understand
2. **Correct answer**: B
   Rationale: Since this is a compound fracture the skin is broken and tissue is damaged. There is a high risk of infection occurring in the bone, which is very difficult to treat. Instability and falling is the second highest priority. Transfers may require the assistance of more than one person, but this is not the highest priority. Depending on the cause of the fracture, the patient may be fearful, but the risk of infection is a higher priority. **Nursing Process**: Planning **Bloom's Taxonomy**: Apply
3. **Correct answer**: A
   Rationale: Pale, cold fingers in a patient with a cast could indicate decreased circulation to the hand. This finding needs to be investigated since the cast could be too tight or compartment syndrome could be developing. The fingers will be slightly edematous after an arm fracture occurs. Warm pink skin indicates adequate blood flow to the area. A pain rating of 2 on a scale from 0 to 10 indicates pain is being adequately controlled. **Nursing Process**: Assessment **Bloom's Taxonomy**: Analyze
4. **Correct answer**: B
   Rationale: After a fracture and during bone healing, osteoblasts continue to form collagen fibers and bone matrix, which are gradually mineralized with calcium and mineral salts. Sodium, potassium, and magnesium are not identified as minerals needed for bone healing. **Nursing Process**: Planning **Bloom's Taxonomy**: Apply
5. **Correct answer**: B, C, D, E
   Rationale: Pain and normal or decreased pulses are early signs of compartment syndrome. This is what was documented as occurring on the previous shift. Now the patient is experiencing later manifestations of compartment syndrome, which include weakness, cyanosis, tingling, and severe pain with passive flexion. Fever is not a manifestation of compartment syndrome. **Nursing Process**: Implementation **Bloom's Taxonomy**: Apply
6. **Correct answer**: C
   Rationale: The tail of the clot or the entire thrombus may dislodge and become an embolus, ultimately lodging in the pulmonary circulation (a pulmonary embolism). Patients with deep venous thrombosis of the lower extremity require careful monitoring of the respiratory system for manifestations of emboli. Deep venous thrombosis does not typically affect the renal, digestive, or hematologic systems. **Nursing Process**: Assessment **Bloom's Taxonomy**: Apply
7. **Correct answer**: A, C
   Rationale: Risk factors for CRPS include female gender and older age. This syndrome is not more frequent if the patient has a history of cardiac disease, if the injury is to an upper extremity rather than a lower extremity, or if the patient is fair-skinned with auburn hair. **Nursing Process**: Assessment **Bloom's Taxonomy**: Understand
8. **Correct answer**: A, B, D, E
   Rationale: The patient with a below-the-knee amputation should elevate the stump, keeping the knee extended. A knee immobilizer may be used to help maintain joint extension. All joints should receive either active or passive ROM exercises every 2 to 4 hours. The patient with an above-the-knee amputation should not sit for prolonged periods of time because this can lead to hip contracture. **Nursing Process**: Planning **Bloom's Taxonomy**: Apply
9. **Correct answer**: A, C
   Rationale: Phantom limb pain is distressing and difficult to manage. Some relief may be obtained with TENS or mirror therapy. There is no evidence that increasing vitamin D in the diet, decreasing fluid intake, or tightening the stump dressing is effective. **Nursing Process**: Implementation **Bloom's Taxonomy**: Apply
10. **Correct answer**: C
    Rationale: After a traumatic amputation of a digit, the nurse should instruct those present to wrap the amputated part in a clean cloth, place in a plastic bag, and put the bag on ice. Do not let the amputated part come into direct contact with the ice or water. This will preserve the amputated finger so that it can be surgically reattached. The person does need to be transported to the hospital but the amputated digit needs to be addressed. Warm water should not be used to preserve an amputated digit. The digit should not be taped to the patient. **Nursing Process**: Planning **Bloom's Taxonomy**: Apply

Chapter 40: Nursing Care of Patients with Musculoskeletal Disorders

Evaluate Your Response to Clinical Reasoning in Patient Care

A Patient with Osteoporosis

1. Use an Internet search engine to find the World Health Organization FRAX Fracture Risk Assessment Tool.
2. Identify data needed but not provided in the scenario to complete this assessment.
3. What is the purpose of this tool and how will you explain the results obtained to Mrs. Bauer? Explain the information in terms Mrs. Bauer can understand and relate to.

4. Review the effects of nicotine and caffeine on blood circulation to bones. What effect does alcohol play in bone loss?
5. Review foods that increase blood cholesterol levels. What is considered a normal cholesterol level? You may need to read content in Chapter 31. Knowing the patient needs calcium, what type of dairy products would you recommend?
6. List activities for the patient who is not able to be ambulatory. How many of the activities on your list would help prevent osteoporosis?

A Patient with Osteoarthritis

1. Review information about Parkinson disease, its treatment, and nursing care for the patient with Parkinson disease in Chapter 44.
2. Consider the manifestations of Parkinson disease and how those manifestations may affect Mr. Cerulli's ability to turn, cough, and deep breath as well as begin ambulating after surgery.
3. Using information in Chapter 44 and in your pharmacology text and drug handbook or application, identify potential interactions between medications used to manage Parkinson's disease, anesthetics, analgesics, and other medications likely to be prescribed for Mr. Cerulli. Also consider the effects of Parkinson disease and risks for common postoperative complications.
4. Review information about serum creatinine and BUN in a laboratory studies textbook or on the Web. What medications is Mr. Cerulli taking that may be affecting these findings? Consider what teaching is necessary related to these findings.
5. What assessments are significant for confusion? If necessary, review content related to confusion. Review Mr. Cerulli's history in the case study and determine factors that may have contributed to his risk for confusion before, during, and after surgery.
6. Acute confusion is defined as an abrupt onset of reversible disturbances in attention, cognition, psychomotor activity, level of consciousness, and/or sleep–wake cycle. What assessments could you make to support this diagnosis for Mr. Cerulli? What interventions might you design for this diagnosis?

A Patient with Rheumatoid Arthritis

1. Review the diagnostic criteria and tests used to establish the diagnosis of RA.
2. Use Chapter 38 and your laboratory and diagnostic tests handbook to identify other potential causes of abnormal test results.
3. Review Chapter 38 for the nursing implications and patient teaching related to diagnostic testing for RA.
4. Think about the role differences in a 40-year-old woman and a 72-year-old woman. On the other hand, consider the effects of a chronic illness that may have been present for 30 years. Would your plan differ? Why or why not?
5. Review information about chronic illness in Chapter 2. List the possible disabilities that may be caused by rheumatoid arthritis. How do you believe these would affect Mrs. James? What agencies in your community are available for support of people with this type of illness? Where would you go for literature to give Mrs. James?
6. Mrs. James is having trouble performing household tasks. Do you believe this is an appropriate nursing priority for Mrs. James? Why or why not? What interventions could be implemented for this problem?

Test Yourself NCLEX-RN Review Answers

1. **Correct answer**: A, B, C, D
   Rationale: The nurse should teach the patient taking alendronate (Fosamax) to take the medication with clear water only. The patient should avoid lying down for 30 to 60 minutes after taking the drug to prevent esophageal irritation. No food or fluids should be consumed for 30 minutes after taking the drug so as to not interfere with the drug's absorption. Calcium and vitamin D supplements are to be taken as prescribed. The tablet should not be crushed, broken, or chewed. **Nursing Process**: Implementation **Bloom's Taxonomy**: Apply
2. **Correct answer**: B, E
   Rationale: The pain of OA can often be managed through the use of mild analgesics such as acetaminophen or over-the-counter NSAIDs such as ibuprofen. Intra-articular hyaluronic acid (HA) is an option for patients with OA of the knee joint. An opioid analgesic may be necessary for patients with advanced OA whose pain is severe, but not for mild pain. Hormones and antibiotics are not used to treat osteoarthritis. **Nursing Process**: Implementation **Bloom's Taxonomy**: Apply
3. **Correct answer**: A, B, E
   Rationale: WBC count typically shows significant elevation as does the sed rate. The creatinine may be elevated if kidney function is affected. Hematocrit and alkaline phosphatase are not elevated. **Nursing Process**: Assessment **Bloom's Taxonomy**: Apply
4. **Correct answer**: B
   Rationale: In patients with osteoporosis and osteomalacia, fractures are a potential complication due to loss of bone mass or inadequate mineralization of bone matrix. Infection, blood clots, and contractures are not potential complications in osteoporosis or osteomalacia. **Nursing Process**: Planning **Bloom's Taxonomy**: Apply
5. **Correct answer**: D
   Rationale: Excessive weight contributes to the development of OA, especially in the hip and knee. Increasing body weight significantly increases the load placed on the knees during walking. A diet high in calcium has no effect on the development of osteoarthritis. Falls do not predispose an individual to developing osteoarthritis. Walking 30 minutes every day could help prevent the development of osteoarthritis. **Nursing Process**: Assessment **Bloom's Taxonomy**: Analyze
6. **Correct answer**: B, D, E
   Rationale: Deep vein thrombosis is a risk associated with orthopedic surgery. Sequential compression devices are used to lessen risk. Pain medications may result in constipation, so high-fiber diets are recommended. Initially the patient should not bear weight on the affected extremity. There is not a serious risk of joint dislocation in knee replacement. The patient should be mobile as soon as possible. **Nursing Process**: Planning **Bloom's Taxonomy**: Apply
7. **Correct answer**: B
   Rationale: Fever and weight loss are findings associated with rheumatoid arthritis. Stiffness relieved by activity is a manifestation of osteoarthritis. Abnormal joint findings are not limited to the hands in either RA or osteoarthritis.

Heberden nodes are characteristic of osteoarthritis. **Nursing Process**: Assessment **Bloom's Taxonomy**: Apply

8. **Correct answer**: C
Rationale: When a patient has ineffective protection the most important intervention is to practice careful hand hygiene because the patient is at risk for opportunistic and severe infections. Monitoring laboratory values, providing skin care, and administering prescribed medications are not interventions to address this patient problem. **Nursing Process**: Implementation **Bloom's Taxonomy**: Apply

9. **Correct answer**: C
Rationale: Lyme disease is an inflammatory disorder caused by the spirochete *Borrelia burgdorferi* that is transmitted primarily by ticks. Most cases of Lyme disease occur when an infected tick remains embedded for at least 24 hours. Lyme disease is not contracted through the bite of an infected mosquito. Brief contact with an infected tick will not cause the disorder. This disease is not transmitted through droplets from infected people. **Nursing Process**: Planning **Bloom's Taxonomy**: Apply

10. **Correct answer**: B
Rationale: Joint rest with no weight bearing is the typical activity prescription. Cultures of sputum, blood, and wounds are obtained. Arthroscopy or arthrotomy may be performed. A broad-spectrum antibiotic is ordered immediately, with changes after culture results are obtained. **Nursing Process**: Implementation **Bloom's Taxonomy**: Analyze

Chapter 41: Assessing the Nervous System

Test Yourself NCLEX-RN Review Answers

1. **Correct answer**: A
Rationale: The blood–brain barrier controls the environment within by allowing oxygen, carbon dioxide, lipids, glucose, and water into the capillaries but preventing entry of urea, creatinine, toxins, proteins, and antibiotics. The structure of neurons and cerebrospinal fluid circulation do not protect the brain from harmful substances. The brain has a large oxygen demand to prevent cerebral cell damage. **Nursing Process**: Assessment **Bloom's Taxonomy**: Understand

2. **Correct answer**: A, C, D, E
Rationale: Damage to lower motor neurons causes decreased muscle tone, muscle atrophy, fasciculations, and loss of reflexes. Damage to upper motor neurons results in increased muscle tone, decreased muscle strength, decreased coordination, and hyperactive reflexes. **Nursing Process**: Assessment **Bloom's Taxonomy**: Apply

3. **Correct answer**: A, B, D, E
Rationale: Cerebrospinal fluid (CSF) cushions the brain tissue and spinal cord, protects them from trauma, provides nourishment to the brain, and removes waste products. Glucose is needed in brain cells for normal cell and brain functioning. **Nursing Process**: Planning **Bloom's Taxonomy**: Apply

4. **Correct answer**: C, D
Rationale: Eyeball movement is controlled by the oculomotor and trochlear cranial nerves. The olfactory nerve controls sense of smell. The optic nerve is associated with vision. The trigeminal nerve controls sensation in several areas of the face and head and controls chewing. **Nursing Process**: Assessment **Bloom's Taxonomy**: Apply

5. **Correct answer**: C
Rationale: The sympathetic division of the ANS has the purpose of preparing the body to handle stressful events, such as almost being in an automobile crash, by increasing heart rate, force of contraction, vasodilation of coronary arteries, and increased mental alertness. The parasympathetic division of the ANS operates during nonstressful situations and causes pupil constriction, decreased heart rate, vasoconstriction of coronary arteries, constriction of the bronchioles, and increased peristalsis. Adrenergic is a term used to describe the effects of the neurotransmitter norepinephrine. Nerves that transmit impulses through the release of acetylcholine are called cholinergic. **Nursing Process**: Assessment **Bloom's Taxonomy**: Understand

6. **Correct answer**: A, B, C, E
Rationale: Assessment begins with history review. The skills of palpation, percussion, and inspection are used. Auscultation is not part of a typical neurologic system assessment. **Nursing Process**: Planning **Bloom's Taxonomy**: Apply

7. **Correct answer**: A
Rationale: A cotton ball and a safety pin would be used to assess sensations of light, dull, and sharp on the face. If the safety pin is used to assess sharp touch, the pin is to be discarded as a sharp after use. A measuring tape and pencil might be used to assess cranial diameter. Various scents would be used to assess CN I olfactory nerve function. A stethoscope is not used when assessing the neurologic system. **Nursing Process**: Assessment **Bloom's Taxonomy**: Apply

8. **Correct answer**: B
Rationale: There may be a normal decrease or absence of corneal reflex in those who wear contact lenses. Being over 50, taking a diuretic, and wearing dentures are not reasons this decrease will occur. **Nursing Process**: Assessment **Bloom's Taxonomy**: Apply

9. **Correct answer**: D
Rationale: The gag reflex is assessed by touching the back of the patient's throat with a tongue depressor. Safety pins, cotton balls, and stethoscopes are not used. **Nursing Process**: Assessment **Bloom's Taxonomy**: Apply

10. **Correct answer**: B, C, D
Rationale: In decorticate posturing the upper arms are close to the body; the elbows, wrists, and fingers are flexed; and the legs are extended with internal rotation. In decerebrate posturing the neck is extended, the arms are extended and pronated, and the feet are plantar flexed. **Nursing Process**: Assessment **Bloom's Taxonomy**: Apply

Chapter 42: Nursing Care of Patients with Intracranial Disorders

Evaluate Your Response to Clinical Reasoning in Patient Care

A Patient with a Seizure Disorder

1. List the teaching topics you would include for Ms. Carlson. Consider how her needs (e.g., for safety) would differ if she lived alone.
2. Describe statements you could use to help Ms. Carlson understand not only the dangers but also the legal issues involved. What if Ms. Carlson does not recognize these concerns?
3. What type of questions could you ask Ms. Carlson to determine why she feels this way? Would you personally find it embarrassing? How can you facilitate Ms. Carlson's understanding of this recommendation?

A Patient with a Stroke

1. What subjective manifestations does the patient with hypertension have? (Review content in Chapter 32.)
2. Consider referral to community resources as a volunteer tutor for adult literacy, gardening, and/or woodworking. Tutoring college students is another option.
3. Use statements that will encourage Mr. Boren to talk about his arm and how he feels about being unable to use it.

A Patient with a Subdural Hematoma

1. Review the manifestations of the types of intracranial hematomas. What assessments are specific to a subdural hematoma? Why is it important to know this?
2. What are some other interventions that might be used? How could family help? What if no family members are available?
3. Acute confusion is a sudden onset of changes in attention, cognition, psychomotor activity, level of consciousness, and/or sleep–wake cycle. What would you determine as priority nursing diagnoses and interventions for Mr. Lee?

A Patient with a Brain Tumor

1. Review content in the chapter on increased intracranial pressure and intracranial surgery. List collaborative and nursing interventions to decrease increased intracranial pressure.
2. What do these manifestations indicate? What would be your priority assessment? Who would you notify?
3. Practice the use of therapeutic communications and what response you would make.
4. Consider the reasons Ms. Lange feels powerless. What nursing interventions might decrease this feeling?

Test Yourself NCLEX-RN Review Answers

1. **Correct answer**: D
   Rationale: When there is damage to the reticular activating system or cerebral hemispheres, neural control of these centers is lost, and lower brainstem centers regulate breathing patterns by responding only to changes in $PaCO_2$, resulting in irregular respiratory patterns. Blood in the ventricles or subarachnoid space irritates the meninges and brain tissue, causing an inflammatory reaction and impairing absorption and circulation of cerebrospinal fluid. Reflexive motor responses may occur as brain function declines. Loss of oculocephalic reflexes indicates a deterioration in brainstem functioning. **Nursing Process**: Assessment **Bloom's Taxonomy**: Understand
2. **Correct answer**: A
   Rationale: The unconscious patient with a depressed or absent gag and swallowing reflex is at high risk for aspiration since saliva and any fluids taken by mouth could not be swallowed normally. There is no information to support that the patient has an ineffective breathing pattern. There is no information to support that the patient has increased intracranial pressure. There is also not enough information to support that the patient has imbalanced nutrition. In the absence of a gag reflex, nutrition can be provided through other, nonoral routes. **Nursing Process**: Planning **Bloom's Taxonomy**: Apply
3. **Correct answer**: D, E
   Rationale: Hyperosmotic agents (osmotic diuretics) draw fluid out of brain cells by increasing the osmolality of the blood. This helps to decrease intracranial pressure. The fluid is drawn into the circulating blood volume and is excreted as urine. These medications excrete water and leave behind solutes. Osmotic diuretics are not used to treat hyperthermia, prevent seizures, or prevent gastrointestinal hemorrhages. **Nursing Process**: Evaluation **Bloom's Taxonomy**: Evaluate
4. **Correct answer**: A
   Rationale: The level of brain dysfunction and the side of the brain affected may be assessed by motor responses. These responses are the most accurate identifier of changes in mental status. In altered LOC, asking the patient to "squeeze my hand" would be used to determine mental status changes. Other questions such as "Tell me your name," "Are you having trouble breathing?" and "Look at the light while it is shined in your eyes" will not accurately determine mental status changes in the patient. **Nursing Process**: Assessment **Bloom's Taxonomy**: Apply
5. **Correct answer**: A, C, D, E
   Rationale: A patient with an altered LOC would probably have blood glucose level checked for hypoglycemia, electrolytes checked for metabolic disturbances, liver function tests to evaluate hepatic function, and blood and urine toxicology studies to test for drug or alcohol toxicity. Urine white blood cell levels would not be indicated for the patient's health problem. **Nursing Process**: Planning **Bloom's Taxonomy**: Apply
6. **Correct answer**: D
   Rationale: Serum osmolality is an indicator of hydration status. The test measures the number of dissolved particles such as electrolytes, urea, and glucose in the serum. The complete blood count and urinalysis will not provide information about the patient's hydration status. Blood cultures are used to determine the presence of a bacterial infection in the blood. **Nursing Process**: Assessment **Bloom's Taxonomy:** Apply
7. **Correct answer**: B, E
   Rationale: Neurologic manifestations of a TIA vary according to the location and size of the cerebral vessel involved and have a sudden onset. Commonly occurring deficits include contralateral numbness or weakness of the leg, hand, forearm, and corner of the mouth; aphasia; and visual disturbances such as blurring. The patient may also experience a fleeting blindness of one eye. Eye pain is associated with a stroke of the vertebral artery. Loss of reflexes is associated with a contusion. Loss of sensation in the legs can be associated with a brain injury. Complete paralysis of the right arm and leg would indicate a stroke within the left cerebral hemisphere. **Nursing Process**: Assessment **Bloom's Taxonomy**: Analyze
8. **Correct answer**: A, C, D, E
   Rationale: The most important treatable conditions that increase the risk of stroke include hypertension, heart disease, hyperlipidemia, and diabetes. Having history of head trauma is not a major factor in contributing to a stroke. **Nursing Process**: Implementation **Bloom's Taxonomy**: Apply
9. **Correct answer**: D
   Rationale: The neurologic deficits that occur as a result of a stroke can often be used to identify its location. Because the motor pathways cross at the junction of the medulla and spinal cord, strokes lead to loss or impairment of sensorimotor functions on the side of the body opposite the side of the brain that is damaged. This effect, known as a contralateral

deficit, means that a stroke in the right hemisphere of the brain is manifested by deficits in the left side of the body and vice versa. Contralateral does not mean that the effects of the stroke are evident on both sides of the body, below the level of the stroke, or on the same side of the embolic event. **Nursing Process**: Planning **Bloom's Taxonomy**: Apply

10. **Correct answer**: B, D, E
Rationale: Supporting the head helps prevent stress on the operative site. Maintaining head and neck alignment prevents additional tension or pressure on the operative side. Respiratory distress may result from edema and hematoma formation, which may compress the trachea, making tracheostomy necessary. The patient should be positioned on the nonoperative side. The head of the bed should be flat or at 30 degrees. **Nursing Process**: Planning **Bloom's Taxonomy**: Apply

Chapter 43: Nursing Care of Patients with Spinal Cord Disorders and CNS Infections

Evaluate Your Response to Clinical Reasoning in Patient Care

A Patient with an SCI

1. What are the developmental tasks of a 19-year-old? How does the inability to meet these tasks affect emotional responses?
2. Think about questions that explore Mr. Valdez's fears in relation to sexuality. Practice questions and statements with friends until you are not embarrassed to ask them.
3. Consider how your own values and beliefs may differ from those of a patient.
4. What baseline assessments and information are necessary before developing a plan for urinary elimination needs? Why would self-catheterization be an option? What are the risks of long-term Foley catheterization?

A Patient with Bacterial Meningitis

1. List the environmental stimuli in the hospital setting. How could these be decreased? What effect do these stimuli have on cognition and behavior that is altered by an intracranial infection?
2. Think about how you would feel if Mr. Cook tried to hit you. How would you respond to him? To whom would you report this?
3. Why would Mr. Cook have pain? How would pain be manifested during the initial treatment period? Is it important to consider the respiratory effects of narcotics for him? Defend your answer.

Test Yourself NCLEX-RN Review Answers

1. **Correct answer**: B
Rationale: SCI at the C1–C4 level produces respiratory paralysis and the patient will be unable to breathe on his or her own, so a ventilator will be necessary to maintain respiratory function. The nerves controlling lung function have been injured. The patient does not have a lung injury. The use of a ventilator is not because the patient is unconscious. The use of a ventilator will not be temporary. **Nursing Process**: Implementation **Bloom's Taxonomy**: Apply
2. **Correct answer**: A, C
Rationale: Analgesics such as nonsteroidal anti-inflammatory drugs (NSAIDs) and narcotics are administered to reduce pain. Vasopressors are used in the immediate acute care phase to treat bradycardia or hypotension due to spinal and neurogenic shock. Antibiotics and antihistamines are not indicated in the acute care of a patient with a SCI. At this time, the use of corticosteroids is no longer part of the guidelines in initial treatment of SCI. **Nursing Process**: Implementation **Bloom's Taxonomy**: Apply
3. **Correct answer**: D, E
Rationale: Spinal shock is the response of the cord itself to injury. It involves temporary loss of reflex function below the level of injury at the cervical and upper thoracic spinal cord. There is loss of all sensations below the level of the injury. Spinal shock is not damage to the lower motor neurons. Spinal shock interrupts sympathetic nerve functioning. Spinal shock leads to a loss of sympathetic input to the blood vessels of the peripheral system and the heart, leading to unopposed vagal tone. Control of cardiovascular mechanisms is not lost but altered. **Nursing Process**: Implementation **Bloom's Taxonomy**: Apply
4. **Correct answer**: B
Rationale: Autonomic dysreflexia is triggered by stimuli that would normally cause abdominal discomfort, by stimulation of pain receptors, and by visceral contractions. The most common cause is from a full bladder resulting from a blocked urinary catheter. Diarrhea and respiratory problems do not cause autonomic dysreflexia. An elevated blood pressure is a manifestation of this disorder. **Nursing Process**: Assessment **Bloom's Taxonomy**: Apply
5. **Correct answer**: A, C
Rationale: In teaching prevention of back injuries, the nurse would incorporate principles of proper body mechanics, which include using large leg muscles to push when lifting and spreading the feet apart to widen the base of support. Bending from the waist to lift objects is dangerous; a squatting position should be used. Twisting should be avoided. **Nursing Process**: Implementation **Bloom's Taxonomy**: Apply
6. **Correct answer**: B, E
Rationale: To monitor for signs of nerve root compression after a cervical laminectomy, the nurse should assess hand grips, arm strength, the ability to move the fingers, and the ability to detect touch. Wiggling the toes would be used to assess for nerve compression after a lumbar laminectomy. Auscultation of heart sounds will not detect cervical root compression after a cervical laminectomy. A reflex hammer is not used to assess for a Babinski reflex. **Nursing Process**: Assessment **Bloom's Taxonomy**: Apply
7. **Correct answer**: C
Rationale: Sudden-onset numbness may indicate that spinal cord compression is occurring. Immediate action to relieve the compression may be necessary to prevent infarction and paralysis. Rating the numbness is not a primary intervention. Repositioning the patient may increase damage to the spinal cord. Waiting for 15 minutes to recheck the patient would delay definitive treatment. The numbness is not caused by a kinked indwelling catheter. **Nursing Process**: Implementation **Bloom's Taxonomy**: Analyze
8. **Correct answer**: D
Rationale: Pathogen entry into the CNS initiates the inflammatory response in the meninges, CSF, and ventricles. Meningeal vessels become engorged and permeability increases. Phagocytic white blood cells migrate into

the subarachnoid space, forming a purulent exudate that thickens and clouds the CSF and impairs its flow. Intracranial pressure can increase and not decrease with meningitis. Meningitis does not cause bleeding into the central nervous system. An elevated systemic white blood cell count does not affect the cognitive status. **Nursing Process**: Planning **Bloom's Taxonomy**: Apply

9. **Correct answer**: C
   Rationale: The best way to reduce the onset of West Nile disease is to control mosquitoes with repellants, insecticides, and protective clothing. Community programs such as spraying to destroy the insect larvae and eliminate breeding places, such as pools of stagnant water, should also be provided. Garbage pickup, sanitation services, and the washing of fruits and vegetables will not reduce the infestation of mosquitoes. **Nursing Process**: Planning **Bloom's Taxonomy**: Apply
10. **Correct answer**: A
    Rationale: A proton-pump inhibitor, such as pantoprazole (Protonix), is often prescribed to prevent stress-related gastric ulcers. This medication is not prescribed to encourage healing of gastric nerves, promote digestion of enteral feedings, or support healthy bacteria in the gastrointestinal tract. Cognitive Level: Analyzing; Nursing Process: Planning; Client Need: Physiological Integrity **Nursing Process**: Implementation **Bloom's Taxonomy**: Apply

Chapter 44: Nursing Care of Patients with Neurologic Disorders

Evaluate Your Response to Clinical Reasoning in Patient Care

A Patient with Alzheimer Disease

1. Think about what information you would need and how you would collect it. Consider such factors as the age and educational level of family members and stage of the patient's AD. What else would you need to know?
2. Review the suggested activities in this section of the chapter. What others can you think of or have you seen used successfully? Osteoarthritis often results in joint stiffness and pain as well as problems with mobility. Would this affect your interventions? If so, how could they be adapted?
3. Consider the type of foods that might be prepared, the timing of meals, and interventions that might be used to decrease agitation before or during meals.

A Patient with Multiple Sclerosis

1. Outline a typical day's activities for Mr. McMurphy that would provide a balance between activity and rest. What assessments would you make to evaluate the effectiveness of this plan?
2. Consider how respiratory infections are spread. Why is Mr. McMurphy at increased risk?
3. The potential for injury means that one is at risk as a result of environmental conditions interacting with the person's adaptive and defensive resources. What factors in this patient's history and physical status would support this diagnosis? What interventions would you include in the care plan and why?

A Patient with Parkinson Disease

1. Consider the adaptations that might be made to clothing and shoes. What adaptive devices might be useful?
2. What information would you need to know before you develop your interventions? Include information obtained from Mr. Ralph and what might be available in the community and the long-term care facility.
3. Chronic sorrow is a recurring pattern of sadness in response to continual loss. Consider the type of communications you would need to use with Mr. Ralph to identify his degree of sorrow. What other assessment might provide cues to support this diagnosis (think about eating and sleeping)? How might an activity such as reminiscence help?

Test Yourself NCLEX-RN Review Answers

1. **Correct answer**: A, D, E
   Rationale: Dementia is a general term used to describe the outcome of the death of neurons and the cognitive and behavioral manifestations of Alzheimer disease. The hallmark of dementia is impairment of both short- and long-term memory. Dementia is not an acute disorder and is not the primary manifestation of Guillain-Barre syndrome. **Nursing Process**: Assessment **Bloom's Taxonomy**: Analyze
2. **Correct answer**: B
   Rationale: Memory loss is usually the first sign of Alzheimer disease. Memory deficits are initially subtle and family members and friends may not suspect a problem until the disease progresses and manifestations become more noticeable. Inability to perform basic activities of daily living, loss of verbal communication, wandering, and changes in sleep patterns at night are later manifestations of the disease process. **Nursing Process**: Implementation **Bloom's Taxonomy**: Apply
3. **Correct answer**: A
   Rationale: Fatigue is a major problem for almost all patients diagnosed with multiple sclerosis. The patient with multiple sclerosis does not experience acute pain and is not necessarily at risk for aspiration or impaired gas exchange. **Nursing Process**: Planning **Bloom's Taxonomy**: Analyze
4. **Correct answer**: C, E
   Rationale: Immunomodulators are administered to patients with relapsing-remitting MS to prolong the time of onset to disability. Adrenocorticosteroids are used both to sustain a remission and to treat exacerbations of MS. Dopamine precursors are used in the treatment of Parkinson disease. Antibiotics and antihistamines are not used to treat multiple sclerosis. **Nursing Process**: Planning **Bloom's Taxonomy**: Apply
5. **Correct answer**: A, B, C, E
   Rationale: The onset of MS is usually between 20 and 40 years of age. There is no cure for the disease. The patient should be advised to avoid temperature extremes, such as hot showers or exposure to cold. Maintaining a relatively constant body temperature may prevent exacerbation of the disorder. Heat can delay impulse transmission across demyelinated nerves, which contributes to fatigue. Many people with MS experience a recurrent pattern of relapses and remissions. Many medications are available to aid in the treatment of this health problem. **Nursing Process**: Implementation **Bloom's Taxonomy**: Apply
6. **Correct answer**: D
   Rationale: The usual balance of dopamine (an inhibitory neurotransmitter) and acetylcholine (an excitatory neurotransmitter) in the brain is disrupted, and dopamine

no longer inhibits acetylcholine. The failure to inhibit acetylcholine is the underlying basis for the manifestations of Parkinson's disease. The cause of the disease is still unknown, but is believed to be the result of environmental and genetic factors, with genetic mutations especially implicated in early-onset Parkinson disease. This disease does not develop as an autoimmune response to a viral infection. **Nursing Process**: Implementation **Bloom's Taxonomy**: Apply

7. **Correct answer**: A, B, E
   Rationale: Parkinson disease is a common disorder in older adults, who are already at greater risk for falls resulting from orthostatic hypotension, osteoporosis, poor vision, and other problems causing disorientation and confusion. Tremors, altered gait, and impaired chewing and swallowing can cause nutritional problems and should be addressed. Constipation can also be an issue. There is no reason for the patient with Parkinson disease to avoid showers or baths. The skin is usually damp and oily, so bathing is needed. There is no reason to believe that the patient with Parkinson disease is at risk for medication overdose. **Nursing Process**: Implementation **Bloom's Taxonomy**: Apply
8. **Correct answer**: A
   Rationale: An antiglutamate was the first medication developed to treat ALS. It inhibits the presynaptic release of glutamic acid in the CNS and protects neurons against the excite-toxicity of glutamic acid. Anticholinergics and dopamine agonists are used to treat Parkinson disease. Anti-inflammatory medications may be used to treat Bell palsy. **Nursing Process**: Implementation **Bloom's Taxonomy**: Apply
9. **Correct answer**: A
   Rationale: When teaching patients about Bell palsy, the nurse needs to tell the patient that one side of the face will not move normally since the affected nerve supplies the muscles that produce expression on one side of the face. The disease does not affect lower extremity muscles. Pain from the ear along the jaw may precede the facial paralysis. There is no reason for the patient to boil home-canned foods since Bell palsy is not caused by botulism. **Nursing Process**: Implementation **Bloom's Taxonomy**: Apply
10. **Correct answer**: A, B, C
    Rationale: Manifestations of myasthenic crisis are severe muscle weakness, fast heartbeat, restlessness, difficulty breathing, and increasing difficulty swallowing or speaking. Incontinence of urine and depressed affect are not manifestations of this disorder. **Nursing Process**: Implementation **Bloom's Taxonomy**: Apply

Chapter 45: Assessing the Eye and Ear

Test Yourself NCLEX-RN Review Answers

1. **Correct answer**: C
   Rationale: When the cornea is touched, the patient will blink as a mechanism to protect it from foreign objects. Some tears are secreted when the cornea is touched; however, tearing is not excessive. The pupil should not dilate in response to the cornea being touched. Nystagmus is an involuntary rhythmic movement of the eyes and is associated with neurologic disorders and the use of some medications. **Nursing Process**: Assessment **Bloom's Taxonomy**: Analyze
2. **Correct answer**: B
   Rationale: Presbyopia develops in older adults as the lens of the eye loses its ability to adjust, requiring the patient to hold papers farther away in order to focus and read. Presbycusis is hearing loss associated with aging. Presbyopia is not associated with memory loss. **Nursing Process**: Assessment **Bloom's Taxonomy**: Analyze
3. **Correct answer**: C
   Rationale: A tuning fork is used to determine hearing and differentiate if hearing loss is conductive or sensorineural. A penlight is used to assess pupil dilation. An otoscope is used to assess the ear canal. An ophthalmoscope is used to assess the internal structures of the eye. **Nursing Process**: Assessment **Bloom's Taxonomy**: Apply
4. **Correct answer**: C, D
   Rationale: When testing for accommodation the pupils are assessed for dilation or constriction depending on the focus of an object. For a distant object the pupils should dilate. For a near object, the pupils should constrict. Rhythmical blinking is not a finding when testing for accommodation. The eyes move in six different directions when assessing for extraocular movements. The eyes moving in the direction that the head is turned are an abnormal finding when assessing for doll's-eyes. **Nursing Process**: Assessment **Bloom's Taxonomy**: Apply
5. **Correct answer**: C, E
   Rationale: Patients having a test of refraction will have the pupil dilated to examine the internal eye structures. The nurse should tell the patient that the pupils will be dilated with medication and may be enlarged for several hours. There is no special preparation by the patient prior to this exam. Dye is not used to complete refraction so an allergy to seafood is not an issue. The patient will not be blindfolded for a refraction test. This test does not cause discomfort. **Nursing Process**: Assessment **Bloom's Taxonomy**: Apply
6. **Correct answer**: A, B, D
   Rationale: Age-related changes to the inner ear include loss of ability to hear high-frequency sounds and possibly lost or decreased middle and low-frequency sounds. Vestibular structures degenerate, leading to balance and equilibrium problems. Sounds made from one's own body and speech being louder is an age-related change to the middle ear. Impacted cerumen and an itchy external ear canal are age-related changes to the external ear. **Nursing Process**: Assessment **Bloom's Taxonomy**: Analyze
7. **Correct answer**: D
   Rationale: The Snellen eye chart measures the patient's ability to read letters at a standard distance of 20 feet. The patient reads the smallest line possible, and the numbers on the side indicate visual acuity, for example, 20/20, 20/30. The Rosenbaum chart is used to assess for near vision. The confrontation test is used to assess for visual fields. Convergence is assessed by asking the patient to follow an object as it is moved toward the patient's eyes. **Nursing Process**: Assessment **Bloom's Taxonomy**: Apply
8. **Correct answer**: D
   Rationale: Hearing acuity is determined by using the whisper test. The examiner can whisper a word 1 or 2 feet behind the patient, asking the patient to repeat the word; this may provide a rough estimate of hearing acuity. The Rinne and Weber tests are performed with a tuning fork

and test conduction, not acuity. Audiometry is used to evaluate and diagnose conductive and sensorineural hearing loss. This test is performed with the patient sitting in a soundproof room and responding when sounds are heard. **Nursing Process**: Assessment **Bloom's Taxonomy**: Apply

9. **Correct answer**: A
Rationale: An age-related change in the lens of the eyes is a loss of elasticity and reduced ability to change shape and focus light. The lens becomes thicker and loses clarity. The patient may experience glare. A slow reaction to light is an age-related change to the pupils. Dry, itchy, burning eyes are age-related changes in the accessory eye structures. Age-related visual changes of the lens can result in difficulty accommodating for near vision. **Nursing Process**: Assessment **Bloom's Taxonomy**: Analyze

10. **Correct answer**: A, D
Rationale: The visual fields of the examiner, which must be normal for this assessment, are used as the standard. If the examiner does not have a normal visual field, then the results of this part of the exam will be inaccurate. The patient must be able to follow the examiner's instructions for this exam. The examiner can wear glasses. The patient does not need to wear corrective lenses nor have greater than 20/30 vision to assess visual fields. **Nursing Process**: Assessment **Bloom's Taxonomy**: Apply

Chapter 46: Nursing Care of Patients with Eye and Ear Disorders

Evaluate Your Response to Clinical Reasoning in Patient Care

A Patient with Glaucoma and Cataracts

1. What is the pathophysiology of glaucoma? How does a cataract affect glaucoma?
2. Consider the effects of corticosteroids on glaucoma. If Mrs. Rainey is to administer several medications at home, identify specific teaching guidelines for her.
3. Would you request a referral for home health visits? Why or why not? Think about the effect of transferring her for a brief admission to an assisted-living facility.

Test Yourself NCLEX-RN Review Answers

1. **Correct answer**: A
Rationale: Maintaining safety is the priority of care for patients with vision and hearing disorders. Preventing sensory deprivation would be the next priority for these residents. Encouraging social interaction and promoting family relationships would be of the lowest priority for these residents. **Nursing Process**: Planning **Bloom's Taxonomy**: Apply

2. **Correct answer**: B
Rationale: When teaching a patient with newly diagnosed glaucoma, the nurse should emphasize the importance of using eyedrops as prescribed on a continuing basis to control intraocular pressure and prevent vision loss. People with glaucoma often do not experience noticeable decline in vision. Avoiding coughing, sneezing, or straining with a bowel movement would be appropriate for the patient recovering from a corneal transplant or recovering from a detached retina. A loss of peripheral vision can occur in the patient with glaucoma; however, the patient is newly diagnosed and may not be experiencing this manifestation. **Nursing Process**: Implementation **Bloom's Taxonomy**: Apply

3. **Correct answer**: A, D, E
Rationale: Timolol and betaxolol are beta-adrenergic blockers that can decrease myocardial contractility and impair cardiac function in the patient with heart failure. These medications should not be prescribed to treat glaucoma if the patient has a history of heart failure. The adrenergic agonist brimonidine (Alphagan) is contraindicated in patients with coronary heart disease. Prostaglandin analogs such as latanoprost (Xalatan) are generally the drugs of choice for treating chronic glaucoma because they can be administered daily and have a low adverse effect rate. Dorzolamide (Trusopt) is a carbonic anhydrase inhibitor that decreases the production of aqueous humor and reduces intraocular pressure. It is used with other drugs to control pressures and may be used in patients for whom beta-blockers are contraindicated because of heart failure **Nursing Process**: Implementation **Bloom's Taxonomy**: Apply

4. **Correct answer**: A, B, C
Rationale: Between acute attacks, management of the patient with Ménière's disease is directed at preventing future attacks and preserving hearing. A low-sodium diet helps reduce labyrinthine pressure. Patients should avoid tobacco, which causes vasoconstriction and can precipitate an attack, along with alcohol and caffeine. Sitting down when an attack develops is a safety measure but will not prevent the onset of vertigo and tinnitus. Taking prescribed antiemetic medications will not prevent vertigo and tinnitus. **Nursing Process**: Implementation **Bloom's Taxonomy**: Apply

5. **Correct answer**: C
Rationale: Following eye surgery, the patient should be placed in the semi-Fowler or Fowler position on the unaffected side. Elevating the head of the bed and lying on the unaffected side reduce intraocular pressure in the affected eye. The patient should not be placed on the affected side. The patient does not need a private room nor does the patient need to be close to the nurses' station. **Nursing Process**: Implementation **Bloom's Taxonomy**: Apply

6. **Correct answer**: A
Rationale: Immediate referral to an ophthalmologist is necessary because the manifestations suggest a detached retina. Immediate treatment is necessary to preserve sight. Flashing lights are not associated with high blood pressure. Lying down might be indicated; however, the sensation is not going to pass. Flashing lights is not a usual occurrence and will not resolve without treatment. **Nursing Process**: Implementation **Bloom's Taxonomy**: Apply

7. **Correct answer**: A, B, C, D
Rationale: The patient could be experiencing otitis externa or otitis media and should have vital signs and body temperature assessed. The nurse should then manipulate the pinna to help differentiate between the pain associated with otitis externa and otitis media, inspect the oral pharynx for inflammation, and palpate cervical lymph nodes, which would indicate an infection. The retina and cornea do not need to be assessed in the patient experiencing ear pain. **Nursing Process**: Implementation **Bloom's Taxonomy**: Analyze

8. **Correct answer**: B
   Rationale: Aging is a risk factor for impaction because less cerumen is produced and it is harder and drier. When the ear canal becomes occluded with cerumen, the patient experiences a conductive hearing loss in the affected ear. Manifestations include a sensation of fullness, along with tinnitus and coughing due to stimulation of the vagal nerve. The nurse should inspect the ear canal for patency. The primary care physician does not need to be notified as of yet. The patient does not need to be evaluated by an audiologist. The nurse cannot determine interventions to treat the patient until an assessment is completed. **Nursing Process**: Assessment **Bloom's Taxonomy**: Apply
9. **Correct answer**: B
   Rationale: One-on-one social interactions in a quiet environment facilitate effective communication for the patient with a severe hearing deficit. Religious services may or may not help improve social interaction in the patient with a hearing deficit. Engaging in activities with a large number of people such as card tournaments, dancing, or community lunches will not help the patient be successful with hearing. **Nursing Process**: Planning **Bloom's Taxonomy**: Apply
10. **Correct answer**: C, E
   Rationale: Surgical removal of the cataract and lens is indicated when the cataract has developed to the point that vision and activities of daily living are affected. The nurse cannot diagnose when a cataract is ready to be removed. Cataracts may be removed prior to other health problems developing, which may or may not be convenient for the patient. Cataracts are not associated with eye pain or headaches. **Nursing Process**: Implementation **Bloom's Taxonomy**: Apply

Chapter 47: Assessing the Male and Female Reproductive Systems

Test Yourself NCLEX-RN Review Answers

1. **Correct answer**: C
   Rationale: Gynecomastia or abnormal enlargement of the breasts in men does occur with obesity. Phimosis is tightness of prepuce that prevents retraction of foreskin. Areolas are not typically absent in the male patient. Enlarged axillary lymph nodes are not a normal finding and would need to be further investigated. **Nursing Process**: Assessment **Bloom's Taxonomy**: Apply
2. **Correct answer**: B
   Rationale: In the female, the clitoris is an erectile organ analogous to the penis in the male. Ovaries produce eggs, which would be analogous to the male testicles. There are no male organs analogous to the labia majora and minora. **Nursing Process**: Implementation **Bloom's Taxonomy**: Apply
3. **Correct answer**: B
   Rationale: The explanation should explain that the prostate gland is about the size of a walnut. It encircles the urethra just below the urinary bladder and is surrounded by smooth muscle. The prostate gland does not press on the bladder. This gland does not sit on top of the kidneys. This gland does not have any effect on renal function. **Nursing Process**: Implementation **Bloom's Taxonomy**: Apply
4. **Correct answer**: B, D
   Rationale: The PSA blood test is available to screen for prostate cancer. It should be done at least 3 days after a rectal exam or prostate palpation. The American Cancer Society recommends that screening frequency be determined by the patient and physician on an individual basis. Annual screening is no longer recommended. VDRL does not screen for problems with the prostate. The nurse should never discourage the patient from being proactive about screening. **Nursing Process**: Implementation **Bloom's Taxonomy**: Analyze
5. **Correct answer**: A, B
   Rationale: Ibuprofen may increase bleeding risk and the patient should be NPO before this procedure. The patient should avoid strenuous activity after the procedure, so mowing the lawn yesterday was a good idea. A conference call for work should not be physically strenuous. **Nursing Process**: Implementation
   Bloom's Taxonomy: Analyze
6. **Correct answer**: A, B, D, E
   Rationale: With menopause, hormone production of estrogen decreases, which may cause pelvic floor muscles to weaken, loss of skin tone, and growth of facial hair. Estrogens are responsible for the normal structure of skin and blood vessels and reduce cholesterol levels. Estrogen enhances blood clotting. **Nursing Process**: Implementation
   Bloom's Taxonomy: Apply
7. **Correct answer**: C
   Rationale: When women of reproductive age become pregnant, menstruation normally stops until after delivery. Cessation of menstruation is not associated with the onset of puberty. The patient is young so menopause is not a consideration at this time. The patient is female so spermatogenesis is not a normal physiologic function of this patient. **Nursing Process**: Assessment **Bloom's Taxonomy**: Apply
8. **Correct answer**: A, C
   Rationale: The test used to detect cervical cancer is the PAP test and should be done when the patient is not menstruating. The patient should avoid intercourse for 24 to 48 hours prior to the test. The test is not a culture and a cleansing douche is contraindicated. There is no need to schedule the test for the morning. **Nursing Process**: Implementation **Bloom's Taxonomy**: Apply
9. **Correct answer**: A, C
   Rationale: The techniques of inspection and palpation are used to detect changes in breast tissue. The techniques of percussion and auscultation are not used when examining the breasts. Aspiration is not a physical examination technique. **Nursing Process**: Assessment **Bloom's Taxonomy**: Apply
10. **Correct answer**: D
   Rationale: Postmenopausal bleeding is seen with endometrial hyperplasia, estrogen therapy, and endometrial cancer. This is not normal and should be reported to the healthcare provider. Sexual activity does not cause vaginal bleeding. The presence or absence of cramps is not an issue. **Nursing Process**: Implementation **Bloom's Taxonomy**: Apply

Chapter 48: Nursing Care of Men with Reproductive System and Breast Disorders

Evaluate Your Response to Clinical Reasoning in Patient Care

A Man with Prostate Cancer

1. Why would Mr. Turner be at risk for altered skin integrity? Outline the interventions you would include on his teaching plan that would promote skin integrity as he cares for himself at home.
2. Noncompliance is defined as behaviors that do not coincide with the therapeutic plan agreed on by the person and the healthcare professional. Do you think Mr. Turner fully understood his treatment and agreed with his follow-up care? What could be done in the preoperative phase of Mr. Turner's care to better ensure his understanding and desire to have continued medical care?
3. What assessments indicate that Mr. Turner does or does not have bladder distention? Would you report this? If so, to whom?

Test Yourself NCLEX-RN Review Answers

1. **Correct answer**: D
   Rationale: The correct option opens the topic of sexual function and allows the patient to discuss concerns if they exist. The nurse should not assume the patient is not able to have sex, that there is a certain age that sex is no longer appropriate, or that the patient perceives problems with sex following the surgery. **Nursing Process**: Assessment **Bloom's Taxonomy**: Apply
2. **Correct answer**: B, C, D
   Rationale: In a health teaching session with young men, the nurse should tell them about the relationship between HPV infection and penile cancer, instructing young men who have not been vaccinated against HPV to wear a condom during sexual intercourse to reduce the risk of contracting this infection. Retracting the foreskin while showering and cleaning regularly to decrease the presence of secretions that can collect under the foreskin have also been shown to decrease the risk of penile cancer. Wearing tight pants and hot showers may influence sperm production. Testicular examination will not prevent penile cancer. **Nursing Process**: Implementation **Bloom's Taxonomy**: Apply
3. **Correct answer**: B
   Rationale: Sexually transmitted urethritis caused by *Neisseria gonorrhoeae* is the usual precipitating factor for epididymitis in younger men. Gonorrhea does not cause a hydrocele, gynecomastia, or erectile dysfunction. **Nursing Process**: Assessment **Bloom's Taxonomy**: Apply
4. **Correct answer**: D, E
   Rationale: Testicular cancer accounts for only a small percentage of all cancers in men; however, it is the most common cancer in men between the ages of 13 and 35 and can occur from infancy through old age. Caucasian men are five times more likely to develop testicular cancer than are men of color. Risk factors for testicular cancer include age and family history of the disorder. The first sign of testicular cancer may be a slight, painless enlargement of one testicle. **Nursing Process**: Planning **Bloom's Taxonomy**: Apply
5. **Correct answer**: A, B, C, D
   Rationale: Teaching plans for the man with prostatitis focus on symptom management. Men with chronic prostatitis should be taught to increase fluid intake to around 3 L daily. NSAIDs can help control discomfort. Increasing fiber intake to promote regular bowel movements helps ease the pain associated with defecation. Local heat, such as sitz baths, may be helpful to relieve pain and irritation. There is no need to avoid sexual activity. **Nursing Process**: Implementation **Bloom's Taxonomy**: Apply
6. **Correct answer**: A, E
   Rationale: The tests used to diagnose prostate cancer include a digital rectal examination (DRE) and prostate-specific antigen (PSA) level. A DRE will find the prostate gland nodular and fixed in prostate cancer. PSA levels are used to diagnose and stage prostate cancer, and to monitor response to treatment. Transrectal ultrasonography (TRUS) and not a pelvic ultrasound may be used when the DRE is abnormal or if the PSA is elevated. Blood chemistries and sperm counts are not used to diagnose prostate cancer. **Nursing Process**: Implementation **Bloom's Taxonomy**: Apply
7. **Correct answer**: C
   Rationale: The expanding prostatic tissue compresses the urethra and causes partial or complete obstruction of the outflow of urine from the urinary bladder. The detrusor muscles hypertrophy to compensate for increased resistance to urinary flow; however, eventually decreased bladder compliance and bladder instability occur. As a result, the man with BPH has manifestations from urinary obstruction and a decrease in bladder contractibility and compliance. Benign prostatic hyperplasia does not cause problems with skin integrity, bowel elimination, or peripheral vascular function. **Nursing Process**: Assessment **Bloom's Taxonomy**: Apply
8. **Correct answer**: B
   Rationale: The man who has had prostate surgery is at risk for hemorrhage. Catheters may become occluded by blood clots or kinks, interfering with urinary drainage and increasing the risk of hemorrhage. The nurse should speak with the urologist about this assessment. Bladder spasms are common and may be accompanied by strong urges to void and urine leakage around the catheter. Belladonna and opium (B&O) suppositories may be used to relieve bladder spasms; however, the nurse needs to report the assessment findings before medicating the patient. Assessing intake and output would not help the patient at this time. **Nursing Process**: Implementation **Bloom's Taxonomy**: Analyze
9. **Correct answer**: B
   Rationale: Aging is the primary risk for development of prostate cancer. Prostate cancer can be asymptomatic and slow growing. Risk is lower for men of Native American heritage. Nocturia is cause by many processes and is not a definitive symptom of prostate cancer. **Nursing Process**: Evaluation **Bloom's Taxonomy**: Evaluate
10. **Correct answer**: D
    Rationale: Diet high in animal fat increases risk of developing prostate cancer. Fiber is not identified as reducing the risk of prostate cancer. Lycopene and sodium are not

identified as increasing the risk of prostate cancer. **Nursing Process**: Implementation **Bloom's Taxonomy**: Apply

Chapter 49: Nursing Care of Women with Reproductive System and Breast Disorders

Evaluate Your Response to Clinical Reasoning in Patient Care

A Woman with Endometriosis

1. What is the relationship between Mrs. Hall's manifestations and a decreased RBC count? Review the information in Chapter 32 and list assessments you would make to identify anemia.
2. List nonthreatening questions you would use to begin the discussion. How might it help to ask these questions at the beginning of the interview? Then list questions that you might use to collect data about the couple's sexual history. Would you be embarrassed to ask them? If so, how might this in turn affect their responses?
3. Low self-esteem can be described as the state in which a person develops a negative perception of self-worth in response to a current situation. What information in Mrs. Hall's history might provide data to support this nursing diagnosis?

A Woman with Cervical Cancer

1. Consider developmental needs and how they differ by age. Also consider current options for preventing HPV infection and reducing the risk for cervical cancer.
2. Review the effects of radiation, discussed in Chapter 14.
3. Does fatigue differ from "feeling tired"? Can the fatigue from radiation be decreased? If so, how?

A Woman with Breast Cancer

1. Review the information in Chapter 8 and in this chapter on the genetic factors that pose a risk for developing breast cancer. How could you explain this in terms understandable by Mrs. Clemments and her daughters?
2. List the different types of mastectomies. Consider the implications of the differences, and how this would affect your nursing care.
3. Review the information on chemotherapy in Chapter 14. List the types of chemotherapy and its common side effects. Consider the classifications of medications that are used to treat these side effects.
4. What factors in Mrs. Clemments's treatment might disrupt the amount and quality of her sleep? What interventions might be used to improve her sleep pattern?

Test Yourself NCLEX-RN Review Answers

1. **Correct answer**: D
   Rationale: The best approach is to work with the patient and physician to establish referral to a sex counselor. The patient did not indicate that a problem existed, so the nurse's remarks should not be problem-oriented. Insurance reimbursement is not the first topic to consider. **Nursing Process**: Implementation **Bloom's Taxonomy**: Apply
2. **Correct answer**: A, B, E
   Rationale: Long-term estrogen deprivation results in an imbalance in bone remodeling and osteoporosis, leading to fractures and kyphosis. The risk for cardiovascular diseases increases in response to an increase in atherosclerosis. Colon and cervical cancer are not associated with long-term estrogen deprivation. **Nursing Process**: Implementation **Bloom's Taxonomy**: Apply
3. **Correct answer**: A, C, E
   Rationale: Tofu, flaxseed, and ginseng are alternatives to hormone replacement therapy. Soymilk, not almond milk, is also an alternative. Quinoa is not a known replacement. **Nursing Process**: Implementation **Bloom's Taxonomy**: Apply
4. **Correct answer**: D
   Rationale: Kegel exercises strengthen perineal muscle tone and minimize stress incontinence. They also minimize descent of the bladder and rectum into the vagina. Kegel exercises do not prevent retroversion of the uterus, menorrhagia, or vaginal discharge. **Nursing Process**: Implementation **Bloom's Taxonomy**: Apply
5. **Correct answer**: A
   Rationale: Obesity is a risk factor for developing cervical cancer. Condoms help to reduce infection with HPV and HIV, which increase risk. A diet high in iron is not a factor. First intercourse before age 16 is a risk factor. **Nursing Process**: Planning **Bloom's Taxonomy**: Apply
6. **Correct answer**: A, B, D, E
   Rationale: For a woman with PMS, the nurse would recommend an increase in lean proteins and a reduction of simple carbohydrates and caffeine. The patient should take 50 to 100 mg of vitamin B_6 daily and should increase calcium to 1000 mg per day. **Nursing Process**: Implementation **Bloom's Taxonomy**: Apply
7. **Correct answer**: D
   Rationale: Endometriosis is a slowly progressive disease, responsive to ovarian hormone stimulation. Endometrial implantations tend to atrophy and disappear after menopause since ovarian hormones no longer stimulate them. Endometrial implants do not enlarge, become malignant, or increase in number after menopause. **Nursing Process**: Implementation **Bloom's Taxonomy**: Apply
8. **Correct answer**: B, C, E
   Rationale: A teaching plan for home care of a woman following an abdominal hysterectomy should include no lifting to decrease chances of hemorrhage, showering rather than tub baths until bleeding has ceased, and reporting increase in temperature or pain. The patient should avoid sitting in a chair for long periods of time and should not climb stairs at all. **Nursing Process**: Planning **Bloom's Taxonomy**: Apply
9. **Correct answer**: D
   Rationale: The 64-year-old has two risks for breast cancer (age and positive family history). The other participants have none or only one risk (never pregnant, dense breasts). **Nursing Process**: Planning **Bloom's Taxonomy**: Analyze
10. **Correct answer**: A, C, E
    Rationale: Playing golf may cause injury, which would trigger LE. Gloves should be worn while washing dishes or gardening to help prevent injury. The patient should carry her purse, briefcase, or luggage with the unaffected arm. Long sleeves are not prohibited if they are not constrictive. Use of creams or lotions can help keep skin moist. **Nursing Process**: Implementation **Bloom's Taxonomy**: Apply

Chapter 50: Nursing Care of Patients with Sexually Transmitted Infections

Evaluate Your Response to Clinical Reasoning in Patient Care

A Patient with Gonorrhea

1. What manifestations does Ms. Cirit have that are typical of the disease? Would you make other assessments? If so, what are they?
2. Review the discussion of HIV in Chapter 13. Do you believe it is true that infection with gonorrhea may increase the risk of HIV? If so, how would you explain this to Ms. Cirit?
3. What communication techniques could you recommend to Ms. Cirit? What safety considerations should you recommend?

A Patient with Syphilis

1. Describe the assessments you would expect to find in a man or woman with early syphilis.
2. Consider topics such as number of sex partners, patterns of sexual activity, and use of safer sex practices. What other topics should be explored? How can you ask these questions without being embarrassed or embarrassing the patient?
3. List possible statements you might make. Do you believe this is a nursing responsibility? If you do not feel comfortable with this topic, what could you do?

Test Yourself NCLEX-RN Review Answers

1. **Correct answer**: B
   Rationale: Women and infants are disproportionately affected by STIs because women may not experience manifestations of the disease and pass the infection on to the infant through vaginal birth. Although the incidence of sexually transmitted infections is highest among young adults in general, women are affected more frequently than men. Men and older adults have lower incidence of sexually transmitted infections. **Nursing Process**: Implementation **Bloom's Taxonomy**: Apply
2. **Correct answer**: B
   Rationale: Both partners are treated for sexually transmitted infections to prevent reinfection from one to the other, since manifestations are not always demonstrated when the infection is present. Sex is not contraindicated after being treated for a sexually transmitted infection. Women should be advised not to douche because it interferes with the normal bacterial environment of the vagina, decreasing resistance to vaginal infection. Both partners need to be treated if one partner has a sexually transmitted infection. **Nursing Process**: Evaluation **Bloom's Taxonomy**: Evaluate
3. **Correct answer**: A, B, C
   Rationale: Topics of information when teaching a male to prevent an STI should include using a new condom with each sex act, careful handling to prevent damage to condom, and withdrawal from the vagina when the penis is erect, holding the condom against the base of the penis to prevent contamination of the penis. No air should be trapped in the end of the condom. Oil-based lubricants, such as petroleum jelly, massage oil, mineral oil, or body lotions, can weaken latex condoms and should not be used. **Nursing Process**: Implementation **Bloom's Taxonomy**: Apply
4. **Correct answer**: A, C, D
   Rationale: Within 2 to 10 days after exposure to the herpes virus, painful red papules appear in the genital area, but then disappear, only to return later. Additional manifestations of herpes incude lymphadenopathy, headache, and fever. Nausea and regional edema are not seen. **Nursing Process**: Assessment **Bloom's Taxonomy**: Analyze
5. **Correct answer**: A, B, E
   Rationale: Genital warts are caused by the human papillomavirus, which has no cure. Risk for cancer is increased. The infection can be spread by any form of intercourse and is often spread by those who do not know they are infected. Genital warts are caused by a virus and not a yeast infection. **Nursing Process**: Implementation **Bloom's Taxonomy**: Apply
6. **Correct answer**: B
   Rationale: Because of the increased risk of cervical cancer, annual Pap smears are essential for female patients with HPV. Checking the stool for occult blood is not done to determine the presence of cervical cancer caused by the human papillomavirus. A breast exam and mammogram are useful to detect the presence of breast cancer. The human papillomavirus does not cause anemia or an infection. **Nursing Process**: Implementation **Bloom's Taxonomy**: Apply
7. **Correct answer**: A, B, D, E
   Rationale: Vaginal yeast infection symptoms include painful intercourse, itching and redness of the vulvar area, and a thick whitish discharge that has a curdled appearance. "Fishy"-smelling drainage is common with bacterial vaginosis, not a yeast infection. **Nursing Process**: Assessment **Bloom's Taxonomy**: Apply
8. **Correct answer**: C
   Rationale: When teaching a woman with an STI experiencing severe genital discomfort, a simple recommendation is to wear cotton underwear because it absorbs moisture and provides for better airflow than other materials. The patient does not need to cut the fingernails short. Frequent douching should be avoided. Sex should be limited until the infection has been treated. **Nursing Process**: Implementation **Bloom's Taxonomy**: Apply
9. **Correct answer**: C
   Rationale: The organism that causes gonorrhea initially targets the female cervix and the male urethra. The organism does not initially target the prostate gland, the vulva, the vagina, or external genitalia. **Nursing Process**: Implementation **Bloom's Taxonomy**: Apply
10. **Correct answer**: B
    Rationale: Syphilis is a systemic infection caused by a spirochete that enters the blood and lymphatic systems. Cases of syphilis in the United States were declining until 2001, but are now escalating. The initial presentation of the disease is a chancre that will heal spontaneously. This does not mean the disease is cured. **Nursing Process**: Implementation **Bloom's Taxonomy**: Apply

Glossary

Abrasion Partial-thickness denudation of an area of integument, generally resulting from falls or scrapes.

Abscess Localized collection of pus.

Absence seizure (petit mal seizure) Type of generalized seizure characterized by a sudden brief cessation of all motor activity accompanied by a blank stare and unresponsiveness.

Accommodation Ability of the eye to adjust to variations in distance.

Accountable care organization (ACO) Organization aimed at providing accessible, comprehensive, and coordinated primary care focused on illness prevention for patients and families.

Achalasia Absence of peristalsis of the esophagus and high gastroesophageal sphincter pressure resulting in dilation and loss of tone in the esophagus.

Acidosis Condition in which the hydrogen ion concentration increases above normal (reflected in a pH below 7.35).

Acid Substance that releases hydrogen ions in solution.

Acne Disorder of the pilosebaceous (hair and sebaceous gland) structure, resulting in eruption of papules or pustules.

Acoustic neuroma or schwannoma Benign tumor of cranial nerve VIII.

Acquired immunity Immunity developed after exposure to a pathogen. See *Active immunity*.

Acquired immunodeficiency syndrome (AIDS) Final stage of HIV infection characterized by severe immune deficits and opportunistic infections.

Acromegaly Meaning literally "enlarged extremities," this is a condition resulting from excessive growth hormone secretion during adulthood.

Actigraphy Watchlike device that measures rest–activity levels continuously for up to 4 weeks.

Actinic keratosis Also called *senile* or *solar keratosis*, an epidermal skin lesion directly related to chronic sun exposure and photodamage.

Active immunity Production of antibodies or development of immune lymphocytes against specific antigens.

Active transport Movement of molecules across cell membranes and epithelial membranes against a concentration gradient; requires energy.

Acute coronary syndrome (ACS) Condition of unstable cardiac ischemia; includes unstable angina and acute myocardial ischemia with or without significant myocardial tissue injury.

Acute gastritis Benign, self-limiting disorder associated with ingestion of gastric irritants such as aspirin, alcohol, caffeine, or foods contaminated with certain bacteria.

Acute illness Illness that occurs rapidly, lasts for a relatively short time, and is self-limiting.

Acute kidney injury (AKI) Rapid decline in renal function with azotemia and fluid and electrolyte imbalances; also known as *acute renal failure*.

Acute lymphoblastic leukemia (ALL) Abnormal proliferation of lymphoblasts in the bone marrow, lymph nodes, and spleen; the most common type of leukemia in children and young adults.

Acute myeloblastic leukemia (AML) Uncontrolled proliferation of myeloblasts (granulocyte precursors) and hyperplasia of bone marrow and the spleen; the most common acute leukemia in adults.

Acute myocardial infarction (AMI) Necrosis (death) of myocardial cells.

Acute pain Pain of sudden onset that is usually self-limited and localized; it lasts for less than 6 months and has an identifiable cause, such as trauma, surgery, or inflammation.

Acute renal failure Abrupt onset of renal failure, also known as *acute kidney injury*.

Acute respiratory distress syndrome (ARDS) Noncardiac pulmonary edema and progressive refractory hypoxemia.

Acute tubular necrosis (ATN) Syndrome of abrupt and progressive decline in tubular and glomerular function.

Adaptive immune response Specific and systemic immune initiated by and directed against particular antigens.

Adaptive immunity Long-lasting and specific response of the lymphocytes to antigens.

Addiction Primary, chronic neurobiologic disease characterized by compulsive use of a substance despite negative consequences, such as health threats or legal problems.

Addison disease Primary adrenal insufficiency characterized by chronic deficiency of cortisol, aldosterone, and adrenal androgens and by skin pigmentation.

Addisonian crisis Life-threatening response to acute adrenal insufficiency. Triggers include surgery, acute systemic illness, trauma, or abrupt withdrawal of long-term corticosteroid therapy.

Advance directive Also called a *living will*, a document in which a patient formally states preferences for health care in the event that he or she later becomes mentally incapacitated and names a person who has durable power of attorney to serve as a substitute decision maker to implement the patient's stated preferences.

Adverse childhood experience (ACE) Exposure in childhood to psychological, physical, or sexual abuse; household dysfunction; substance abuse; and mental illness.

Aesthetic surgery See *Cosmetic surgery*.

Afterload Force the ventricles must overcome to eject their blood volume; the pressure in the arterial system ahead of the ventricles.

Agnosia Inability to recognize one or more subjects that were previously familiar; agnosia may be visual, tactile, or auditory.

Agranulocytosis Severe neutropenia, with less than 200 cells/μm.

Aid in dying End-of-life care option in which mentally competent, terminally ill adults can ask their physician to provide a prescription for medication that the patient can self-administer to end life peacefully.

Alcohol Alcohol and other CNS depressants act on other neurotransmitters in the brain such as gamma-aminobutyric acid (GABA). GABA is the most prevalent inhibitory neurotransmitter in the brain and has a major role in decreasing neuronal excitability. Alcohol creates an additive effect with GABA, further inhibiting arousal and depressing the autonomic nervous system.

Alcoholic cirrhosis (Laënnec's cirrhosis) End result of alcoholic liver disease.

Alkalis Bases that accept hydrogen ions in solution.

Alkalosis Condition where the hydrogen ion concentration decreases below normal (reflected in a pH above 7.45).

Alleles Different forms of a gene or DNA occupying the same place on a pair of chromosomes; an allele for each gene is inherited from each parent.

Allergy Hypersensitivity response to environmental or exogenous antigens.

Allograft Graft between members of the same species but who have different genotypes and HLA antigens. See also *Homograft*.

Alopecia Loss of hair; baldness.

Alzheimer disease (AD) Form of dementia characterized by progressive, irreversible deterioration of general intellectual functioning.

Amenorrhea Absence of menstruation.

Amphetamine Central nervous system stimulant that causes arousal and an elevation of mood with a sense of increased strength, mental capacity, self-confidence, and a decreased need for food and sleep.

Amputation Partial or total removal of a body part.

Amyotrophic lateral sclerosis (ALS) Progressive, degenerative neurologic disease characterized by weakness and wasting of the involved muscles, without any accompanying sensory or cognitive changes; also called *Lou Gehrig's disease*.

Analgesic A medication that reduces or eliminates the perception of pain.

Anaphylactic shock Shock resulting from a widespread hypersensitivity reaction (called *anaphylaxis*). The pathophysiology in this type of shock includes vasodilation, pooling of blood in the periphery, and hypovolemia with altered cellular metabolism.

Anaphylaxis Acute systemic type I hypersensitivity reaction that occurs in response to an injected antigen.

Anaplasia Regression of a cell to an immature or undifferentiated cell type.

Anasarca Severe, generalized edema.

Androgens Hormones synthesized in the testes, ovaries, and adrenal cortex that promote expression of male sex characteristics.

Anemia Abnormally low number of circulating RBCs, hemoglobin concentration, or both.

Anergy Inability to react to specific antigens.

Anesthesia Use of drugs to produce sedation, analgesia, reflex loss, and muscle relaxation during a procedure.

Aneurysm Abnormal dilation of a blood vessel, commonly at a site of a weakness or tear in the vessel wall.

Angina pectoris (angina) Chest pain resulting from reduced coronary blood flow that causes a temporary imbalance between myocardial blood supply and demand.

Angioma (hemangioma) Benign vascular tumor.

Anion gap Difference between the sum of two measured anions, chloride and bicarbonate, and the principal measured cation, sodium.

Ankylosing spondylitis Chronic inflammatory arthritis that primarily affects the axial skeleton, leading to pain and progressive stiffening and fusion of the spine.

Anorexia Loss of appetite.

Anorexia nervosa Eating disorder characterized by a body weight less than 85% of expected for age and height and an intense fear of gaining weight.

Anorgasmia Absence of orgasm.

Anosmia Inability to smell.

Anthropometric measurements Measurement of height, weight, triceps skinfolds, and midarm circumference.

Antibodies Immunoglobulin molecules that bind with an antigen to inactivate it.

Antibody-mediated (humoral) immune response Activation of B cells to produce antibodies to respond to antigens such as bacteria, bacterial toxins, and free viruses.

Anticipatory grieving Combination of intellectual and emotional responses and behaviors by which people adjust their self-concept in the face of a potential loss.

Antigen Substance capable of evoking a specific immune response; usually a protein that the body recognizes as foreign, causing an immune response to be stimulated.

Antigenic substances Agents such as microorganisms, cells and tissues from other humans or animals, and some inorganic substances that stimulate an immune response.

Aortic valve Semilunar valve between the left ventricle of the heart and the aorta. It prevents blood from flowing backward into the ventricle.

Aortitis Inflammation of the aorta, usually the aortic arch.

Aphasia Defective or absent language function.

Apical impulse Normal, palpable pulsation (thrust) in the area of the midclavicular line in the left fifth intercostal space. It can be seen on inspection in about half of the adult population.

Aplastic anemia Condition manifested by failure of the bone marrow to produce all three types of blood cells.

Apnea Cessation of breathing lasting from a few seconds to a few minutes.

Appendectomy Surgical removal of the appendix.

Appendicitis Inflammation of the vermiform appendix.

Applicability How well research findings can be applied to specific patient care.

Appraisal Judgment of the value of external evidence.

Apraxia Inability to carry out a motor pattern (such as drawing a figure) even when strength and coordination are adequate.

Areflexia Lack of normal reflexes.

Arterial blood gas (ABG) Laboratory test used to evaluate acid–base balance and gas exchange.

Arteriovenous (AV) malformation Congenital intracranial lesion, formed by a tangled collection of dilated arteries and veins, that allows blood to flow directly from the arterial into the venous system, bypassing the normal capillary network.

Arthoscopy Insertion of an arthroscope into a joint for diagnosis or treatment.

Arthralgia Joint pain.

Arthritis Joint inflammation.

Arthroplasty Reconstruction or replacement of a joint.

Ascites Excess fluid in the peritoneal cavity.

Asphyxiation Oxygen deprivation.

Assisted suicide Means to end a patient's life is provided to the patient with knowledge of the patient's intention.

Association Indicates only a relationship, not cause and effect in research.

Asthma Chronic inflammatory disorder of the airways that is characterized by recurrent episodes of wheezing, breathlessness, chest tightness, and coughing.

Astigmatism Condition that develops with abnormal curvature of the cornea or eyeball, causing the image to focus at multiple points on the retina.

Ataxia Uncoordinated, irregular gait and muscle movement; weakness.

Atelectasis Collapse of lung tissue following obstruction of the bronchus or bronchioles.

Atherosclerosis Form of arteriosclerosis in which deposits of fat and fibrin obstruct and harden the arteries.

Atopic dermatitis (eczema) Common inflammatory skin disorder of unknown cause.

Atrial kick Delivery of an additional bolus of blood to the ventricles resulting from atrial systole; occurs just prior to ventricular systole.

Atrial natriuretic peptide (ANP) Hormone released by atrial muscle cells in response to distention from fluid overload.

Aura Sensation preceding generalized seizure activity; may be a vague sense of uneasiness or an abnormal sensation.

Auscultatory gap Temporary disappearance of sound between the systolic and diastolic BP.

Autograft Transplant of the patient's own tissue (e.g., skin, bone marrow).

Autografting Transplanting of the patient's own tissue; the most successful type of tissue transplant.

Autoimmune disorder Failure of immune system to recognize itself, resulting in normal host tissue being targeted by immune defenses.

Autonomic dysreflexia Exaggerated sympathetic response that occurs in patients with spinal cord injuries at or above the T_6 level.

Autosomal dominant Genetic conditions that result from an altered gene on any of the 22 autosomes in spite of the fact that one unaltered or normal gene exists.

Autosomal recessive Genetic conditions that require two copies of an altered gene on any of the 22 autosomes to express the condition.

Autosome Single chromosome from any one of the 22 pairs of chromosomes not involved in sex determination (X or Y); humans have 22 pairs of autosomes.

Azotemia Increased blood levels of nitrogenous waste products.

B lymphocytes (B cells) Bursa-equivalent lymphocytes responsible for synthesizing antibodies in response to specific antigens.

Bacterial vaginosis Nonspecific vaginitis.

Bactericidal Capable of killing organisms without immune system intervention.

Bacteriostatic Inhibits growth of microorganisms, leaving the destruction to the host's immune system.

Bacteriuria Bacteria in the urine.

Balanced suspension traction Traction in which several forces of pull work in unison to raise and support the patient's injured extremity off the bed and maintain its alignment.

Balloon tamponade Application of pressure to stop esophageal bleeding using an inflatable balloon.

Bariatrics Healthcare science that focuses on patients who are extremely obese.

Basal cell cancer Epithelial tumor believed to originate either from the basal layer of the epidermis or from cells in the surrounding dermal structures.

Basal ganglia Deeply placed mass of gray matter in the brain.

Basal metabolic rate (BMR) Test to measure the energy used when the body is at rest; rarely used due to the availability of more accurate thyroid tests.

Base excess (BE) Calculated value also known as buffer base capacity. Base excess reflects the degree of acid–base imbalance by indicating the status of the body's total buffering capacity.

Base Substance that accepts hydrogen ions in solution.

Bell's palsy (facial paralysis) Disorder of the facial nerve (seventh cranial nerve), characterized by unilateral paralysis of the facial muscles.

Benign prostatic hyperplasia (BPH) Enlargement of the prostate gland.

Bereavement Time of mourning experienced after a loss.

Bile Greenish, watery solution containing bile salts, cholesterol, bilirubin, electrolytes, water, and phospholipids.

Biliary colic Severe, steady pain in the epigastric region or upper right quadrant of the abdomen caused by obstruction and increased pressure in the bile duct.

Binge-eating disorder Nutritional disorder characterized by recurrent episodes of binge eating—eating an excessive amount of food during a defined period of time and a sense of loss of control over eating during binge episodes.

Biofeedback Electronic method of measuring autonomic physiologic responses, such as brain waves, muscle contraction, and skin temperature, and then "feeding" this information back to the patient.

Biologic markers Stable segments of DNA important for the construction of chromosome maps.

Bioterrorism Use of an etiologic agent (disease) to cause harm or kill a population, food, and/or livestock.

Biotherapy Treatment that modifies the biologic processes that result in malignant cells, primarily through enhancing the person's own immune responses.

Bivalving Process of splitting a cast down both sides to alleviate pressure on the injured extremity.

Blood clot Venous thrombosis.

Blood flow Volume of blood transported in a vessel, in an organ, or throughout the entire circulation over a given period of time.

Blood pressure Tension or pressure exerted by blood against arterial walls.

Blunt trauma Type of trauma that occurs when there is no communication from the damaged tissues to the outside environment.

Body mass index (BMI) Used to identify excess adipose tissue, BMI is calculated by dividing the weight (in kilograms) by the height (in meters squared, m^2).

Bone marrow transplant (BMT) Infusion of bone marrow cells to restore bone marrow function after chemotherapy or radiation. Allogeneic BMT uses bone marrow cells from a donor; autologous BMT uses the patient's own bone marrow. See also *Stem cell transplant*.

Borborygmi Loud rushing bowel sounds.

Botulism Severe, life-threatening form of food poisoning caused by *Clostridium botulinum*.

Brachytherapy Type of radiation therapy in which the source of radiation is placed directly into or adjacent to the tumor, a technique that delivers a high dose to the tumor and a lower dose to normal tissue.

Bradycardia Heart rate of less than 60 beats per minute.

Bradykinesia Slowed movements due to muscle rigidity.

Bradypnea Abnormally low respiratory rate.

Brain abscess Infection with a collection of purulent material within the brain tissue.

Brain death Cessation of cerebral blood flow with global brain infarction and permanent loss of all brain function.

Brain death criteria Clinical signs used to determine whether a comatose patient is brain dead.

Breakthrough pain Pain that exceeds baseline chronic or persistent pain, with or without baseline analgesia.

Bronchiectasis Permanent abnormal dilation of one or more large bronchi and destruction of bronchial walls, usually accompanied by infection.

Bronchitis Inflammation of the bronchi (airways).

Bruit Adventitious sound heard during auscultation; of venous or arterial origin.

Buffer Substance that prevents major changes in pH by removing or releasing hydrogen ions.

Bulimia nervosa Eating disorder characterized by recurring episodes of binge eating followed by purge behaviors such as self-induced vomiting, use of laxatives or diuretics, fasting, or excessive exercise.

Burn Injury resulting from exposure to heat, chemicals, radiation, or electric current.

Burn shock Hypovolemic shock resulting from the shift of a massive amount of fluid from the intracellular and intravascular compartments into the interstitium following burn injury.

Bursitis Inflammation of the bursa.

Cachexia Wasted physical appearance characteristic of cancer and other chronic illnesses; characterized by rapid depletion of the body's protein, particularly in skeletal muscle, with less rapid loss of fat.

Caffeine Methylxanthine stimulant that increases the heart rate and acts as a diuretic.

Calculi Presence of abnormal concentration or stones in the body occur in the gallbladder, kidneys, ureters, bladder, or urethra.

Cancer Family of complex diseases with manifestations that vary according to body system and type of tumor cells involved; marked by uncontrolled growth and the spread of abnormal cells.

Candidiasis Infection of mucous membranes caused by *Candida albicans*, a yeastlike fungus.

Cannabis sativa Source of marijuana.

Carbuncle Group of infected hair follicles.

Carcinogen Cancer-causing agent.

Carcinogenesis Production or origin of cancer.

Carcinoma Tumor arising from epithelial tissue.

Cardiac arrest Sudden failure of the heart to pump.

Cardiac cycle Contraction and relaxation of the heart during one heartbeat.

Cardiac index (CI) Cardiac output adjusted for body size.

Cardiac output (CO) Amount of blood pumped by the ventricles into the pulmonary and systemic circulations in 1 minute.

Cardiac rehabilitation Long-term program of medical evaluation, exercise, risk factor modification, education, and counseling designed to limit the physical and psychologic effects of cardiac illness and improve the patient's quality of life.

Cardiac reserve Ability of the heart to respond to the body's changing need for cardiac output.

Cardiac tamponade Compression of the heart due to pericardial effusion, trauma, cardiac rupture, or hemorrhage.

Cardiogenic shock Shock that occurs when the heart's pumping ability is compromised to the point that it cannot maintain cardiac output and adequate tissue perfusion.

Cardiomegaly Enlargement of the heart.

Cardiomyopathy Primary abnormality of the heart muscle that affects its structural or functional characteristics.

Cardiovascular disease (CVD) Generic term for disorders of the heart and blood vessels.

Care bundle Small set of evidence-based interventions for a defined patient population and care setting aimed at improving patient outcomes.

Carpal spasm Decreased calcium levels cause the patient's hand and fingers to contract in response to occlusion of the blood supply by a blood pressure cuff (Trousseau sign).

Carpal tunnel syndrome Compression of the median nerve as a result of inflammation and swelling of the synovial lining of the tendon sheaths.

Carrier Any individual who carries a single copy of an altered gene or mutation for a recessive condition on one chromosome of a chromosome pair and an unaltered form of that gene on the other chromosome. A carrier is generally not affected by the gene alteration; on the average, each person in the general population is a carrier of five or six gene mutations for recessive disorders.

Carriers (related to infections) Harbor the pathogen without showing evidence of clinical disease.

Catabolism Biochemical process involving the breakdown of complex structures into simpler forms.

Cataract Opacification (clouding) of the lens of the eye.

Causation Indicates factor(s) that lead to an outcome.

Celiac disease (celiac sprue, nontropical sprue) Chronic hereditary disorder characterized by sensitivity to the gliadin fraction of gluten, a cereal protein.

Cell cycle Four phases that occur during growth and development of a cell.

Cell-mediated (cellular) immune response Direct or indirect inactivation of antigen by lymphocytes.

Cellulitis Localized infection of the dermis and subcutaneous tissue.

Central nervous system depressants Drugs, including barbiturates, benzodiazepines, paraldehyde, meprobamate, and chloral hydrate, that are subject to abuse.

Central obesity See *Upper body obesity*.

Central pain Related to a lesion in the brain that may spontaneously produce high-frequency bursts of impulses that are perceived as pain.

Central sleep apnea (CSA) Consolidation of a couple of different types of apnea including central sleep apnea with Cheyne-Stokes breathing (common with congestive heart failure), central apnea due to a medical disorder without Cheyne-Stokes breathing (due to failure of ventilatory control centers to initiate ventilator effort), and central sleep apnea due to a medication or substance.

Cerebral concussion Transient, temporary, neurogenic dysfunction caused by mechanical force to the brain.

Cerebral contusion Bruise on the surface of the brain.

Cerebral edema Increase in the volume of brain tissue due to abnormal accumulation of fluid in brain cells.

Cerumen Earwax.

Chalazion Granulomatous cyst or nodule of the lid.

Chancre Hard, syphilitic primary ulcer.

Cheilosis Cracks at corners of the mouth seen in vitamin B-complex deficiencies, especially riboflavin.

Chemotherapy Cancer treatment involving the use of cytotoxic medications to decrease tumor size, adjunctive to surgery or radiation therapy, or to prevent or treat suspected metastases.

Chlamydia Group of syndromes caused by *Chlamydia trachomatis*, a bacterium that behaves like a virus spreading within a host cell; spread by sexual contact and to the neonate by passage through the birth canal of an infected mother.

Cholecystectomy Removal of the gallbladder.

Cholecystitis Inflammation of the gallbladder, usually associated with stones in the cystic or common bile duct.

Cholelithiasis Formation of stones (calculi) within the gallbladder or biliary duct system.

Cholera Acute diarrheal illness caused by certain strains of *Vibrio cholerae*.

Chorea Jerky, rapid, involuntary movements.

Chromosome Genetic material carried by each cell; found in the cell nucleus.

Chronic bronchitis Excessive secretion of bronchial mucus characterized by a productive cough lasting 3 or more months in 2 consecutive years.

Chronic gastritis Disorders characterized by progressive and irreversible changes in the gastric mucosa.

Chronic hepatitis Chronic infection of the liver; the primary cause of liver damage leading to cirrhosis, liver cancer, and liver transplantation.

Chronic illness Condition that requires continuing management over a long period—years or even decades.

Chronic kidney disease (CKD) Presence of kidney damage for 3 or more months with loss of nephron units and decreased renal mass leading to progressive deterioration of glomerular filtration, tubular secretion, and reabsorption.

Chronic lymphocytic leukemia (CLL) Proliferation and accumulation of small, abnormal, mature lymphocytes in the bone marrow, peripheral blood, and body tissues; least common type of the major leukemias.

Chronic myelogenous leukemia (CML) Abnormal proliferation of all bone marrow elements, usually associated with a chromosome abnormality (the Philadelphia chromosome).

Chronic obstructive pulmonary disease (COPD) Chronic air flow obstruction due to chronic bronchitis and/or emphysema.

Chronic otitis media Condition involving permanent perforation of the tympanic membrane, with or without recurrent pus formation and often accompanied by changes in the mucosa and bony structures (ossicles) of the middle ear.

Chronic pain Prolonged pain, usually lasting longer than 6 months; pain that persists after the condition causing it has resolved; may be malignant or nonmalignant in origin.

Chronic sorrow Cyclical, recurring, and potentially progressive pattern of pervasive sadness experienced in response to continual loss, throughout the trajectory of an illness or disability.

Chronic stump pain Result of neuroma formation, causing severe burning pain.

Chronic venous insufficiency Chronic disorder of inadequate venous return.

Chvostek sign Contraction of the lateral facial muscles in response to tapping the face in front of the ear; caused by decreased blood calcium levels.

Chyme Thick, fluid mixture of food and gastric juices formed in the stomach during the digestive process.

Circulating nurse Registered nurse who coordinates and manages a wide range of activities before, during, and after surgical procedures.

Cirrhosis Progressive, irreversible disorder, eventually leading to liver failure; the end stage of chronic liver disease.

Clinical reasoning Complex process using cognition, metacognition, and discipline-specific knowledge to gather and analyze patient information, evaluate its significance, and weigh alternative actions.

Closed fracture (simple fracture) Break in continuity of bone with skin still intact.

Clubbing Enlargement and blunting of the terminal portion of the fingers; associated with chronic hypoxemia.

Cluster headache Severe, unilateral vascular headache that occurs in groups or clusters and is characterized by exacerbations and remissions; predominantly experienced by men age 20 to 40.

Coagulation Process of creating a fibrin meshwork that cements blood components together to form an insoluble clot.

Cocaine Highly addictive stimulant/euphoric drug extracted from the leaves of the coca plant.

Code of ethics Established and agreed-on group of principles of conduct that provides a frame of reference for nursing behaviors that are congruent with professional values.

Cold sore See *Herpes simplex*.

Cold zone Considered the safe zone during a disaster, it is adjacent to the warm zone and is the area where a more in-depth triage of victims would occur; survivors may find shelter in this area, and command-and-control vehicles would be found here as well as emergency transport vehicles.

Colectomy Surgical removal of the colon.

Collateral channels Connections between small arteries.

Collateral vessels Accessory pathways connected to the smaller arteries in the coronary system.

Colorectal cancer Malignant tumor arising from the epithelial tissues of the colon or rectum.

Colostomy Ostomy made in the colon.

Comedones Noninflammatory acne lesions.

Community-based care Centers on individual and family healthcare needs. The nurse practicing community-based care provides direct services to individuals to manage acute or chronic health problems and to promote self-care. The care is provided in the local community, is culturally competent, and is family centered.

Compartment Space enclosed by a fibrous membrane or fascia.

Compartment syndrome Condition in which excess pressure constricts the structures within a compartment and reduces circulation to muscles and nerves.

Complex regional pain syndrome Extremity pain that is severe, diffuse, and burning and accompanied by vasomotor changes that affect skin color and temperature.

Computer literacy Familiarity and skills to use a computer.

Conceptual variable Qualities of a variable of interest in research.

Concussion Brain injury resulting from a violent jar, shake, or impact with an object.

Conjunctivitis Inflammation of the conjunctiva.

Consanguinity Related by having a common ancestor; close blood relationship.

Conscious sedation Anesthesia that provides analgesia and amnesia, but in which the patient remains conscious. Patients are able to breathe independently and are cardiovascularly stable.

Consciousness Condition in which a person is aware of self and environment and is able to respond appropriately to stimuli; full consciousness requires both normal arousal and full cognition.

Constipation Infrequent (two or fewer bowel movements weekly) or difficult passage of stools.

Contact dermatitis Type of dermatitis caused by a hypersensitivity response or chemical irritation.

Continuous renal replacement therapy (CRRT) Form of hemodialysis in which blood is continuously circulated through a highly porous hemofilter from artery to vein or vein to vein.

Contractility Inherent capability of the cardiac muscle fibers to shorten.

Contracting Negotiation of a cooperative working agreement between the nurse and patient that is continuously renegotiated.

Contractures Permanent shortening of connective tissues.

Contralateral deficit Manifestations of a stroke on the side of the body opposite the side of the brain that is damaged.

Contusion Superficial tissue injury resulting from blunt trauma, such as a kick or blow from an object, that causes the breakage of small blood vessels and bleeding into the surrounding tissue.

Conventional weapons Weapons such as bombs and guns that are used more frequently than nonconventional terrorist weapons.

Convergence Moving the eyes inward toward the nose to see an object close to the face.

Co-occurring disorders Concurrent diagnosis of a substance-use disorder and a psychiatric disorder. One disorder can precede and cause the other, such as the relationship between alcoholism and depression.

Cor pulmonale Condition of right-ventricular hypertrophy and failure that results from long-standing pulmonary hypertension.

Core competencies Standards that a profession agrees are essential for a person to be deemed competent in his or her field.

Corneal reflex Closure of eyelids (blinking) due to corneal irritation.

Corneal ulcer Local necrosis of the cornea that may be caused by infection, exposure trauma, or the misuse of contact lenses.

Coronary heart disease (CHD) Heart disease caused by impaired blood flow to the myocardium.

Coryza (rhinorrhea) Profuse nasal discharge.

Cosmetic surgery (aesthetic surgery) One of two fields within plastic surgery. Cosmetic surgery enhances the attractiveness of normal features.

Crackles Discontinuous lung sounds heard by auscultation; can be fine or coarse. Produced by air passing over airway secretions or the opening of collapsed airways.

Crepitation Grating sound heard on movement of a joint.

Creutzfeldt-Jakob disease (CJD; spongiform encephalopathy) Rare, progressive neurologic disease that causes brain degeneration without inflammation.

Critical illness A subcategory of acute care where the patient typically requires life-sustaining treatment and intense monitoring involving specialized equipment.

Critical pathway Healthcare plan designed to provide care with a multidisciplinary, managed action focus; developed for specific diagnoses, usually those that are high volume, high risk, and high cost.

Critical thinking Self-directed thinking that is focused on what to believe or do in a specific situation.

CRNA Certified registered nurse anesthetist; a nurse certified in anesthesia administration.

Crohn's disease (regional enteritis) Chronic, relapsing inflammatory disorder affecting the gastrointestinal tract.

Crossing-over Process that occurs during meiosis in which homologous maternal and paternal chromosomes break and exchange corresponding sections of DNA and then rejoin; this process can cause an exchange of alleles between chromosomes and provides human diversity.

Cryosurgery Destruction of tissue by cold or freezing with agents such as fluorocarbon sprays, carbon dioxide snow, nitrous oxide, and liquid nitrogen.

Curettage Removal of lesions with a curette, a semisharp cutting instrument.

Curling ulcers Acute ulcerations of the stomach or duodenum that form following a burn injury.

Cushing disease Disorder caused by an adenoma, a tumor on the pituitary gland that causes overproduction of cortisol.

Cushing syndrome Chronic disorder caused by excessive amounts of circulating cortisol; also known as *hypercortisolism*.

Cushing ulcers Stress ulcers occurring as sequelae of head injury or central nervous system surgery.

Cutaneous melanoma See *Malignant melanoma*.

Cyanosis Bluish discoloration of the skin and mucous membranes due to oxygen deficiency.

Cystectomy Complete surgical removal of the urinary bladder and adjacent muscles and tissues.

Cystic fibrosis (CF) Inherited disorder of the exocrine glands that results in the secretion of abnormal amounts of mucus.

Cystitis Inflammation of the urinary bladder.

Cysts Benign closed sacs in or under the skin surface that are lined with epithelium and contain fluid or a semisolid material.

Cytokines Hormone-like polypeptides produced primarily by monocytes, macrophages, and T cells. Cytokines act as messengers of the immune system, facilitating communication between the cells to adjust or vary the inflammatory reaction or to initiate immune cell proliferation and differentiation.

Dawn phenomenon Rise in blood glucose between 4:00 AM and 8:00 AM that is not a response to hypoglycemia.

Death Irreversible cessation of circulatory and respiratory functions or irreversible cessation of all functions of the entire brain, including the brainstem.

Death anxiety Worry or fear related to death or dying.

Debridement Process of removing dead tissue from a wound.

Decerebrate posturing Abnormal posture with the neck extended; the jaw clenched; arms pronated, extended, and close to the sides; legs extended; and feet plantar flexed. Results from lesions of the midbrain, pons, or diencephalons.

Decorticate posturing Abnormal posture with the upper arms close to the sides; the elbows, wrists, and fingers flexed; the legs extended and internally rotated; and the feet plantar flexed. Results from lesions of the corticospinal tracts.

Deep venous thrombosis (DVT) Blood clot (thrombus) formation and inflammation within a deep vein, usually in the pelvis or lower extremities; a common complication of hospitalization, surgery, and immobilization.

Deformation Alteration of the spinal cord and soft tissues caused by abnormal movements from acceleration and deceleration forces.

Dehiscence Unintended separation of wound margins due to incomplete healing.

Dehydration Loss of water.

Delayed healing Healing that occurs at a slower rate than expected.

Delegation To effectively assign appropriate work activities to other members of the healthcare team. When the nurse delegates nursing care activities to another person, that person is authorized to act in the place of the nurse, while the nurse retains the accountability for the activities performed.

Delirium State of consciousness when the patient may be restless, confused, or agitated.

Delirium tremens (DT) Medical emergency usually occurring 3 to 5 days following alcohol withdrawal and lasting 2 to 3 days; characterized by paranoia, disorientation, delusions, visual hallucinations, elevated vital signs, vomiting, diarrhea, and diaphoresis.

Dementia Global impairment of cognitive function that is usually progressive and may be permanent; interferes with normal social and occupational activities.

Demyelination Destruction or removal of the myelin sheaths of nerves.

Dependent variable Variable that is impacted by a manipulated variable; commonly an outcome variable.

Depolarization Rapid inflow of sodium ions, causing an electrical change in which the inside of a cell becomes positive in relation to the outside.

Dermatitis Acute or chronic inflammation of the skin characterized by erythema and pain or pruritus.

Dermatome Area of skin innervated by cutaneous branches of a single spinal nerve.

Dermatophytes Fungi that cause superficial skin infections.

Dermatophytoses Superficial fungal infection of the skin; also called *ringworm*.

Descriptive statistics Statistics used to depict variations within a data set.

Detoxification Process of helping an addicted individual safely through withdrawal.

Diabetes insipidus Deficit of ADH causes excretion of large amounts of dilute urine, in some instances as much as 12 L/day. The patient has extreme thirst and drinks large volumes of water. If unable to replace the water loss, the patient becomes dehydrated and hypernatremic. Even though hyperosmolality is present, the urine is dilute and has a low specific gravity.

Diabetes mellitus (DM) Group of chronic disorders of the endocrine pancreas, all categorized under a broad diagnostic label. The condition is characterized by inappropriate hyperglycemia caused by a relative or absolute deficiency of insulin or by a cellular resistance to the action of insulin.

Diabetic ketoacidosis (DKA) Form of metabolic acidosis induced by stress in a person with type 1 diabetes.

Diabetic nephropathy Disease of the kidneys characterized by the presence of albumin in the urine, hypertension, edema, and progressive renal insufficiency.

Diabetic neuropathies Disorders of the peripheral nerves and the autonomic nervous system manifesting one or more of the following: sensory and motor impairment, muscle weakness and pain, cranial nerve disorders, impaired vasomotor function, impaired gastrointestinal function, and impaired genitourinary function.

Diabetic retinopathy Collective name for the changes in the retina that occur in the person with diabetes. The retinal capillary structure undergoes alterations in blood flow, leading to retinal ischemia and a breakdown in the blood retinal barrier.

Dialysate Dialysis solution.

Dialysis Diffusion of solute molecules across a semipermeable membrane from an area of higher concentration to one of lower concentration.

Diaphoresis Copious production of sweat.

Diarrhea Increase in the frequency, volume, and fluid content of the stool.

Diastolic blood pressure Minimum pressure maintained by elastic arterial walls during diastole (cardiac relaxation) to maintain blood flow through capillary beds; averages 80 mmHg in a healthy adult.

Dietary reference intakes (DRIs) Recommended intakes of nutrients (vitamins and elements).

Differentiation Process occurring over many cell cycles that allows cells to specialize in certain tasks.

Diffuse brain injury (DBI) Brain injury from a high-speed acceleration–deceleration accident with widespread disruption of axons in the white matter.

Diffuse esophageal spasm Nonperistaltic contraction of esophageal smooth muscle.

Diffusion Process by which solute molecules move from an area of high solute concentration to an area of low solute concentration to become evenly distributed.

Dilemma Choice between two unpleasant, ethically troubling alternatives.

Diplopia Unilateral or bilateral double vision.

Disability Degree of observable and measurable impairment.

Disaster Event that requires extraordinary efforts beyond those needed to respond to everyday emergencies.

Disease Literally meaning "without ease," this term describes alterations in structure and function of the body or mind. Diseases may have mechanical, biologic, or normative causes.

Diskectomy Removal of the nucleus pulposus of an intervertebral disk. Diskectomy may be performed alone or in conjunction with a laminectomy.

Dislocation Separation of contact between two bones of a joint.

Dissection (aortic) Life-threatening emergency caused by a tear in the intima of the aorta with hemorrhage into the media.

Disseminated intravascular coagulation (DIC) Disruption of hemostasis characterized by widespread intravascular clotting and bleeding; a syndrome that develops as a complication of many other disorders.

Distributive shock Also called *vasogenic shock*, this includes several types of shock that result from widespread vasodilation and decreased peripheral resistance.

Diverticula Saclike projections of mucosa through the muscular layer of the colon.

Diverticulitis Inflammation in and around the diverticular sac; typically affects only one diverticulum, usually in the sigmoid colon.

Diverticulosis Indicates the presence of diverticula.

Do-not-resuscitate (DNR or "no-code") order Usually written by the physician for the patient who has a terminal illness or is near death, this order is usually based on the wishes of the patient and family that no cardiopulmonary resuscitation be performed for respiratory or cardiac arrest.

Dominant Characteristic or gene that is apparent even when the relevant gene is present in only one copy; a person with a dominant gene usually expresses that gene trait.

Dopaminergic Activity that involves dopamine and its pathways in the brain.

Dual diagnosis Coexistence of substance abuse/dependence and a psychiatric disorder in one individual (used interchangeably with *dual disorder* and *co-occurring disorders*).

Dual disorder See *Dual diagnosis*.

Dumping syndrome Complication of partial gastrectomy characterized by nausea, weakness, sweating, palpitation, syncope, sensation of warmth, and occasionally diarrhea.

Duodenal ulcers Peptic ulcer disease affecting the duodenum.

Durable power of attorney Document that can delegate the authority to make health, financial, and/or legal decisions on a person's behalf. It must be in writing and must state that the designated person is authorized to make healthcare decisions.

Dwarfism Condition characterized by short stature; insufficient pituitary growth hormone is one cause.

Dysarthria Difficulty speaking.

Dysfunctional uterine bleeding (DUB) Vaginal bleeding that is usually painless but abnormal in amount, duration, or time of occurrence.

Dysmenorrhea Pain associated with menstruation.

Dyspareunia Painful intercourse.

Dysphagia Difficulty swallowing.

Dysphonia Change in the tone of voice.

Dysplasia Loss of DNA control over cell differentiation occurring in response to adverse conditions.

Dyspnea Difficult or labored breathing.

Dysrhythmia Abnormal heart rate or rhythm.

Dysuria Painful urination.

Ecchymosis Flat, irregularly shaped lesion (bruise) of varying size with no pulsation; caused by blood collecting under skin.

Ectopic beats Impulses originating outside normal conduction pathways of the heart.

Edema Accumulation of fluid in the body's tissues; an excess accumulation of fluid in the interstitial space.

Ejection fraction (EF) Percentage of total blood remaining in the ventricle at the end of diastole (relaxation); normal is 50 to 70%.

Electrical bone stimulation Application of electrical current at the fracture site to treat fractures that are not healing appropriately. The electrical stress increases the migration of osteoblasts and osteoclasts to the fracture site. Mineral deposition increases, promoting bone healing.

Electrocardiography Graphic recording of the heart's electrical activity detected and recorded through electrodes placed on the surface of the body.

Electrolytes Substances that dissociate in solution to form charged particles called *ions*.

Electronic medical records (EMRs) Electronic repository of all patient-related information. Commonly computer-based.

Electrosurgery Destruction or removal of tissue with high-frequency alternating current.

Embolic CVA Cerebrovascular accident occurring when a blood clot or clump of matter traveling through the cerebral blood vessels becomes lodged in a vessel too narrow to permit further movement.

Embolism Sudden obstruction of a blood vessel by a clot or debris.

Emergency Encompasses an unforeseen combination of circumstances calling for immediate action for a range of victims from one to many.

Emphysema Destruction of the walls of the alveoli, with resulting enlargement of abnormal air spaces.

Empyema Accumulation of purulent exudate in the pleural cavity.

Encephalitis Acute inflammation of the parenchyma of the brain or spinal cord.

End of life Final days or weeks of life when death is imminent.

End-stage renal disease Final stage of chronic renal failure in which the kidneys are unable to excrete metabolic wastes and regulate fluid and electrolyte balance adequately; characterized by a glomerular filtration rate of less than 5% of normal.

Endocarditis Inflammation of the endocardium.

Endometriosis Condition in which multiple, small implants of endometrial tissue develop throughout the pelvic cavity.

Endoscopy Inspection of organs or cavities of the body using an endoscope.

Endotoxins Found in the cell wall of Gram-negative bacteria, endotoxins are released only when the cell is disrupted. They act as activators of many human regulatory systems, producing fever, inflammation, and potentially clotting, bleeding, or hypotension when released in large quantities.

Enophthalmos Sunken appearance of the eyes.

Enteral nutrition Administration of liquid nutritional formulas to meet calorie and protein needs in patients unable to consume adequate food; also called *tube feeding*.

Enucleation Surgical removal of an eye.

Epicondylitis (tennis elbow, golfer's elbow) Inflammation of the tendon at its point of origin into the bone.

Epididymitis Infection or inflammation of the epididymis.

Epidural hematoma (extradural hematoma) Collection of blood between the dura and the skull.

Epilepsy Disorder characterized by chronic seizure activity.

Epistaxis Nosebleed.

Equianalgesia/equianalgesic Approximate equivalent doses of opioid analgesics as compared to morphine sulfate.

Erectile dysfunction Inability to attain and maintain an erection sufficient to permit satisfactory sexual intercourse.

Erosive gastritis See *Stress-induced (erosive gastritis)*.

Erysipelas Infection of the skin most often caused by group A *streptococci*.

Erythema Reddening of the skin.

Erythropoiesis Red blood cell production.

Eschar Hard, leathery crust that covers a burn wound and harbors necrotic tissue.

Escharotomy Surgical removal of eschar from the torso or extremity to prevent circumferential constriction.

Esophageal varices Enlarged, thin-walled veins that form in the submucosa of the esophagus.

Esophagojejunostomy Removal of the entire stomach with anastomosis of the distal esophagus to the jejunum.

Estrogen Hormone produced by the ovaries.

Ethics Principles of conduct. Ethical behavior is concerned with moral duty, values, obligations, and the distinction between right and wrong.

Euthanasia From the Greek for painless, easy, gentle, or good death, now commonly used to signify a killing prompted by a humanitarian motive.

Euthyroid Term describing normal thyroid hormone function.

Evaluation phase Final phase of disaster planning that involves a detailed review of a disaster relief program to determine if goals were met, to assess the program's impact on the community, and to identify lessons learned for the design of future plans.

Evidence-based practice (EBP) Practice of nursing in which the nurse makes clinical decisions on the basis of the best available current research evidence, his or her own clinical expertise including internal evidence of patient findings, and the needs and preferences of the patient.

Evisceration Protrusion of body contents through a surgical wound.

Exacerbation Period during chronic illness in which symptoms reappear.

Exfoliative dermatitis Inflammatory skin disorder characterized by excessive peeling or shedding of skin.

Exophthalmos Protrusion of the eyeballs.

Exotoxins Soluble proteins secreted into surrounding tissue by the microorganism; highly poisonous, causing cell death or dysfunction.

External evidence Relevant research findings related to a specified clinical question.

External otitis Inflammation of the ear canal.

Extracapsular fractures Fractures of the trochanteric region.

Extracorporeal shock-wave lithotripsy (ESWL; transcutaneous shock-wave lithotripsy) Noninvasive technique for fragmenting kidney stones using shock waves generated outside the body.

Faith community nursing Also known as *parish nursing*, a nontraditional, community-based way of providing health promotion and health restoration nursing interventions to specific groups of people.

Family Two or more persons joined by emotional closeness and shared bonds and who identify themselves as being part of a family.

Fascial excision Removing thin slices of a burn wound to the level of viable tissue; also known as fasciectomy.

Fasciculations Involuntary twitching.

Fasciectomy Removing thin slices of a burn wound to the level of viable tissue; also known as fascial excision.

Fat embolism syndrome (FES) Characterized by neurologic dysfunction, pulmonary insufficiency, and a petechial rash on the chest, axilla, and upper arms due to fat globules lodged in the pulmonary vascular bed or peripheral circulation.

Fecal impaction Rock-hard or putty-like mass of feces in the rectum.

Fecal incontinence Loss of voluntary control of defecation.

Fecalith Hard mass of feces.

Fibrocystic changes (FCC) Physiologic nodularity and breast tenderness that increases and decreases with the menstrual cycle.

Fibroid tumors (uterine leiomyoma) Solid benign tumors originating from smooth muscle of the uterus.

Fibromyalgia (fibrositis) Common rheumatic syndrome characterized by musculoskeletal pain, stiffness, and tenderness.

Filtration Process by which water and dissolved substances (solutes) move from an area of higher hydrostatic pressure to an area of lower hydrostatic pressure.

Fistula Abnormal opening or passage between two organs or spaces that are normally separated or an abnormal passage to the outside of the body.

Flaccidity Decreased muscle tone in disease or trauma of the lower motor neurons.

Flail chest Free-floating segment of the chest wall, resulting from two or more consecutive ribs fractured in multiple places.

Flap Piece of tissue whose free end is moved from a donor site to a recipient site while maintaining a continuous blood supply through its connection at the base or pedicle.

Flatus Gas in the digestive tract.

Fluid resuscitation Replacement of the extensive fluid and electrolyte losses associated with major burn injuries.

Fluid volume deficit (FVD) Decrease in intravascular, interstitial, and/or intracellular fluid in the body.

Fluid volume excess (FVE) Excess extracellular fluid resulting from retention of both water and sodium in the body.

Folic acid deficiency anemia Anemia resulting from folic acid deficiency, a necessary nutrient for DNA synthesis and RBC maturation.

Folliculitis Bacterial infection of the hair follicle, most commonly caused by *Staphylococcus aureus*.

Fracture Break in a bone usually due to trauma.

Freestanding outpatient surgical facilities Surgical units independent of a hospital with or without financial connections to a hospital or healthcare organization.

Friction rub Sound heard when two dry surfaces are rubbed together.

Frostbite Injury of the skin from freezing.

Full-thickness burn Burn that involves all layers of the skin, including the epidermis, dermis, and epidermal appendages.

Fulminant hepatitis Hepatitis with a rapid and severe onset and course.

Furuncle Often called a *boil*, but also an inflammation of the hair follicle.

Fusiform excision Removal of a full thickness of the epidermis and dermis, usually with a thin layer of subcutaneous tissue.

Fusion Insertion of a wedge-shaped piece of bone or bone chips (usually harvested from patient's iliac crest) between the vertebrae to stabilize them.

Galactorrhea Lactation not associated with pregnancy or nursing.

Gastric lavage Irrigation of the stomach with large quantities of normal saline.

Gastric mucosal barrier Protective barrier consisting of lipids, bicarbonate ions, and mucous gel that protects the stomach lining from the damaging effects of gastric juices.

Gastric outlet obstruction Obstruction of the pyloric region of the stomach and duodenum that impairs gastric outflow; a potential complication of peptic ulcer disease.

Gastric ulcers Ulcers of the stomach lining, usually in the lesser curvature and antrum; more common in older adults.

Gastritis Inflammation of the stomach lining.

Gastroduodenostomy (Billroth I) Excision of the pylorus of the stomach with the anastomosis of the upper stomach to the duodenum; commonly used partial gastrectomy procedure.

Gastroenteritis Inflammation of the gastrointestinal tract; not a specific disease, but a group of syndromes or a collection of related manifestations.

Gastroesophageal reflux Backward flow of gastric contents into the esophagus.

Gastroesophageal reflux disease (GERD) Reflux of acidic gastric contents into the lower esophagus.

Gastrojejunostomy (Billroth II) Subtotal excision of the stomach with closure of the duodenum and side-to-side anastomosis of the jejunum to the stomach; commonly used partial gastrectomy procedure.

Gastroparesis Slowed gastrointestinal motility resulting in dysphagia, anorexia, heartburn, nausea and vomiting, and slowed digestion with altered blood glucose control.

Gene Sequence of DNA on a chromosome that represents a fundamental unit of heredity; occupies a specific spot on a chromosome (gene locus).

Gene expression When the protein product of a gene is visible (e.g., through the presence of a body structure or identifiable through biochemical tests such as insulin or phenylalanine levels).

General anesthesia Deep sedation, which includes analgesia and muscle paralysis. This type of anesthesia requires respiratory maintenance without the aid of the patient's respiratory musculature.

Genital herpes (herpes simplex genitalis) Infection of the external genitalia caused by herpes simplex genitalis; transmitted by vaginal, anal, or oral–genital contact.

Genital warts (condyloma acuminatum, venereal warts) Sexually transmitted condition caused by the human papillomavirus.

Genotype Genes and the variations therein that a person inherits from his or her parents.

Germ cells Cells that give rise to a sperm or egg.

Gigantism Gigantism occurs when GH hypersecretion begins before puberty and the closure of the epiphyseal plates. The person becomes abnormally tall, often exceeding 7 ft (213 cm) in height, but body proportions are relatively normal.

Gingivitis Inflammation of the gums, characterized by redness and bleeding.

Gland Tissue that produces secretions or synthesizes hormones.

Glaucoma Condition characterized by increased intraocular pressure of the eye and a gradual loss of vision.

Glomerular filtration rate (GFR) Rate at which plasma is filtered through the glomeruli of the kidney.

Glomerulonephritis Inflammation of the capillary loops of the glomeruli.

Glossitis Inflammation of the tongue.

Glucocorticoid Group of hormones secreted by the adrenal cortex that regulate carbohydrate levels in the body.

Gluconeogenesis Formation of glucose from fats and proteins.

Glucose-6-phosphate dehydrogenase (G6PD) anemia Anemia due to a hereditary defect in RBC metabolism.

Glucosuria Excessive glucose in urine.

Glycogenolysis Breakdown of liver glycogen to glucose.

Goiter Enlarged thyroid gland resulting from both inadequate and excessive synthesis of thyroid hormones.

Gonorrhea (GC, clap) Infection caused by *Neisseria gonorrhoeae* that is transmitted by direct sexual contact or during delivery of a neonate by an infected mother.

Gout Metabolic disorder characterized by hyperuricemia and acute inflammatory arthritis triggered by urate crystallization within joints and deposits of insoluble urates in connective tissues of the body.

Grief Emotional response to loss and its accompanying changes.

Grieving Internal process the person uses to work through the response to loss.

Guillain-Barré syndrome (GBS) Acute demyelinating disorder of the peripheral nervous system characterized by progressive, usually rapid muscle weakness and paralysis.

Gynecomastia Breast enlargement in men.

Hallucinogens Drugs that produce hallucinations.

Hallux valgus (bunion) Enlargement and lateral displacement of the first metatarsal.

Hammertoe (claw toe) Dorsiflexion of the first phalanx with accompanying plantar flexion of the second and third phalanges.

Handicap Total adjustment to disability that limits functioning at a normal level.

Handoff When responsibility for care is transferred from one individual or care unit to another.

Hazardous materials Substances that pose a potential risk to life, health, or property if they are released because of their chemical, biologic, or physical nature.

Health The World Health Organization defines health as "A state of complete physical, mental, and social well-being, and not merely the absence of disease or infirmity."

Health–illness continuum Visual representation of health as a dynamic process, with high-level wellness at one extreme of the continuum and death at the opposite extreme.

Health information technology (HIT) System supported by the U.S. government designed to promote free exchange of health information while protecting patients' privacy and improving safety, efficacy, and quality of care.

Health literacy People's ability to obtain, process, communicate, and understand basic health information and services.

Healthcare-associated infections (HAIs) Infections acquired in a healthcare setting; also called *nosocomial infections*.

Healthcare surrogate Individual selected to make medical decisions when a person is no longer able to make them for him- or herself.

Heart block Block in the normal conduction pathways.

Heart failure Inability of the heart to pump adequate blood to meet the metabolic demands of the body.

Heave Excessive thrust.

Hemangioma See *Angioma*.

Hemarthrosis Collection of blood in a joint.

Hematemesis Blood in the vomit.

Hematochezia Blood in the stool.

Hematoma Contusion with a large amount of bleeding.

Hematopoiesis Blood cell formation.

Hematuria Blood in the urine.

Hemianopia Loss of half of the visual field of one or both eyes.

Hemiparesis Weakness of one side of the body.

Hemiplegia Paralysis in one-half of the body vertically.

Hemodialysis Procedure in which electrolytes, waste products, and excess water are removed from the body by diffusion and ultrafiltration as blood passes by an artificial semipermeable membrane outside the body.

Hemodynamics Study of the forces involved in blood circulation.

Hemoglobin Oxygen-carrying protein within RBCs; composed of the heme molecule and globin, a protein molecule.

Hemolysis Process of RBC destruction.

Hemolytic anemia Premature destruction (lysis) of RBCs.

Hemophilia Group of hereditary clotting factor disorders that lead to persistent and potentially severe bleeding.

Hemophilia A (classic hemophilia) Most common type of hemophilia, caused by clotting factor VIII deficiency.

Hemophilia B (Christmas disease) Hemophilia caused by factor IX deficiency.

Hemoptysis Bloody sputum.

Hemorrhage Rapid or excessive bleeding.

Hemorrhagic CVA (intracranial hemorrhage) Cerebrovascular accident occurring when a cerebral blood vessel ruptures.

Hemorrhoids (piles) Clusters of dilated veins in swollen anal tissue.

Hemostasis Control of bleeding.

Hemothorax Blood in the pleural space.

Hepatic encephalopathy Altered consciousness, mentation, and motor function affecting cirrhotic patients.

Hepatitis Inflammation of the liver, usually caused by a virus; may be acute or chronic.

Hepatorenal syndrome Renal failure accompanied by azotemia, sodium retention, oliguria, and hypotension in patients with cirrhosis and ascites.

Hernia Defect in the abdominal wall that allows abdominal contents to protrude out of the abdominal cavity.

Herniated intervertebral disk Rupture of the cartilage surrounding the intervertebral disk with protrusion of the nucleus pulposus.

Herniation Complication where the nucleus pulposus projects through the interrupted disk in a posterolateral direction, with compression of the associated nerve root. The resulting pressure on adjacent spinal nerves causes characteristic manifestations, which vary with the location and the amount of protruding disk material. Occasionally the herniation is central rather than posterolateral, with pressure on the spinal cord.

Herpes simplex (fever blister, cold sore) Acute viral infections of the skin and mucous membranes caused by two types of herpesvirus: HSV I and HSV II.

Herpes zoster (shingles) Viral infection of a nerve supplying a dermatome section of the skin caused by varicella zoster, the same herpesvirus that causes chickenpox.

Heterograft (xenograft) Skin obtained from an animal, usually a pig.

Heterozygous Nonidentical copies of a particular gene (different alleles) on the paired chromosomes.

Hiatal hernia Protrusion of part of the stomach through the esophageal hiatus of the diaphragm into the mediastinal cavity.

Hirsutism Increased growth of coarse hair, usually on the face and trunk.

Histocompatibility Ability of cells and tissues to survive transplantation without immunologic interference by the recipient.

Holistic healthcare Care in which all aspects of a person (physical, psychosocial, cultural, spiritual, and intellectual) are considered as essential components of individualized care.

Home care Services for patients who are in need of treatment or support to function effectively in the home environment.

Home healthcare Delivery of services to restore or maintain the health of individuals and families in the home.

Homeostasis Body's tendency to maintain a state of physiologic balance in the presence of constantly changing conditions.

Homograft (allograft) Human tissue (skin, cornea, organs) used in skin graft or tissue transplant.

Homologous Chromosomes that are members of the same pair and normally have the same number and arrangement of genes; usually one copy is from the mother and the other copy is from the father.

Homonymous hemianopia Impaired vision or blindness in one side of both eyes.

Homozygous Identical copies of a particular gene (same alleles) on both paired chromosomes.

Hordeolum (sty) Staphylococcal abscess that may occur on either the external or internal margin of the lid.

Hormone Chemical messengers secreted via body fluids that have specific targets where they increase or inhibit organ functions.

Hospice (hospice care) Special component of home care, designed to provide medical, nursing, social, psychologic, and spiritual care for terminally ill patients and their families. Hospice care relies on a philosophy of relieving pain and suffering and allowing the patient to die with dignity in a comfortable environment.

Hot zone Site of a disaster where a weapon was released or where contamination occurred.

Human genome Total amount of the DNA (genes) in an individual's cells.

Human-generated disasters Type of disasters the principle direct causes of which are identifiable human actions, deliberate or otherwise.

Human immunodeficiency virus (HIV) A retrovirus transmitted by direct contact with infected blood and body fluids that is responsible for AIDS.

Huntington disease Progressive, degenerative, inherited neurologic disease characterized by increasing dementia and chorea; also called *chorea*.

Hydrocele Fluid-filled mass within the scrotum.

Hydrocephalus Abnormal accumulation of cerebrospinal fluid within the cerebral ventricles.

Hydronephrosis Distention of the kidney pelvis and calyces with urine behind an obstruction.

Hydroureter Distention of the ureter with urine.

Hypercapnia Increased blood levels of carbon dioxide.

Hyperglycemia Elevated blood glucose levels, which causes osmotic diuresis and, if chronic, damages blood vessel epithelium and renal glomeruli.

Hyperopia (farsightedness) Condition in which the eyeball is short, causing the image to focus behind the retina.

Hyperosmolar hyperglycemic state (HHS) Condition of very high blood glucose with adequate insulin to prevent ketosis, a complication of type 2 DM.

Hyperparathyroidism Disorder that results from an increase in the secretion of parathyroid hormone (PTH), which regulates normal serum levels of calcium.

Hyperplasia Increase in the number or density of normal cells.

Hypersensitivity Exaggerated response of the immune system to an antigen.

Hypertension Excess pressure in the arterial portion of systemic circulation.

Hyperthyroidism Disorder caused by excessive production and delivery of thyroid hormone to the tissues.

Hypertrophic scar Overgrowth of dermal tissue that remains within the boundaries of the wound.

Hypervolemia Excess intravascular fluid.

Hyphema Bleeding into the anterior chamber of the eye, possibly as the result of blunt eye trauma.

Hypoglycemia Low blood glucose levels.

Hypoparathyroidism Disorder that results from abnormally low PTH levels. The most common cause is damage to or inadvertent removal of all of the parathyroid glands during thyroidectomy. The lack of circulating PTH causes hypocalcemia and an elevated blood phosphate level.

Hypothyroidism Disorder that results when the thyroid gland produces an insufficient amount of TH.

Hypovolemia Decreased circulating blood volume.

Hypovolemic shock Shock caused by a decrease in intravascular volume of 15% or more. This form of shock is caused by the loss of whole blood, blood plasma, or extracellular fluid.

Hypoxemia Decreased oxygen concentration in the blood, measured by PaO_2.

Hypoxia Insufficient supply of oxygen to the tissues.

Ichthyosis Inherited dermatologic condition in which the skin is dry, fissured, and hyperkeratotic; the surface of the skin has the appearance of fish scales.

Ileostomy Ostomy made in the ileum of the small intestine.

Illness Response a person has to a disease; integrates the patient's perception, as well as the pathophysiologic alterations and the psychologic effects of those alterations.

Immunity Protection of the body from disease.

Immunocompetent Possessing an immune system that can identify antigens and effectively destroy or remove them.

Immunocompromised Possessing an immune response that has been weakened by a disease or an immunosuppressive agent.

Immunoglobulin (Ig) Protein that functions as an antibody.

Immunosuppression Inability of the immune system to respond to an antigen. Occurs in response to disease or medications; may be intentional to prevent rejection of transplants or a side effect of some medications.

Impairment Disturbance in structure or function resulting from physiologic or psychologic abnormalities.

Impetigo Infection of the skin caused by either *Staphylococcus aureus* or beta-hemolytic streptococci.

Impotence Inability to achieve or maintain an erection.

Incidental pain Type of breakthrough pain that is predictable because it is associated with movement such as turning or coughing.

Increased intracranial pressure (IICP; intracranial hypertension) Sustained elevated pressure (10 mmHg or higher) within the cranial cavity.

Independent nursing care Care provided by nurses within the scope of their practice without the direction or supervision of a physician.

Independent variable Variable that is manipulated (commonly an intervention).

Infection Colonization by and multiplication of an organism within a host. The host can be any organism capable of supporting the nutritional and physical growth requirements of the microorganism, for example, humans.

Inferential statistics Statistics that are based on the laws of probability. These statistics allow generalizable conclusions.

Inflammation Complex, nonspecific, adaptive response to injury that brings fluid, dissolved substances, and blood cells into the interstitial tissues where the invasion or damage has occurred.

Inflammatory bowel disease (IBD) Chronic inflammation of the bowel common to a group of conditions that includes Crohn disease and ulcerative colitis.

Inflammatory phase First stage of wound healing that begins with the incision (either surgical or accidental) during which physiologic mechanisms are activated to maintain hemostasis and promote blood clotting.

Influenza Highly contagious viral respiratory disease characterized by coryza, fever, cough, and constitutional manifestations such as headache and malaise.

Information literacy Ability to locate, evaluate, and use appropriate facts effectively.

Information technology (IT) Mechanical infrastructure that supports the collection, recording, and utilization of patient information.

Informed consent Disclosure of risks associated with the intended procedure or operation to the patient. The language of the document varies according to statutory and common law of each state.

Inhalants Inhaled solvents categorized into three types: anesthetics, volatile nitrites, and organic solvents.

Innate immunity The body's natural barriers to infections and injury that provides a nonspecific, generic response to harmful events.

Insomnia Inability to fall asleep, stay asleep, or feel rested upon awakening.

Insulin Hormone that facilitates entry of glucose into fat and muscle cells for energy.

Insulin reaction Hypoglycemia in patients with type 1 diabetes mellitus.

Interdisciplinary care Care provided by members of the healthcare team in addition to medical professionals. Usually includes team members who address psychosocial and spiritual issues as well as physical care.

Intermittent claudication Cramping, aching ischemic pain in the calves, thighs, and buttocks that occurs with a predictable level of activity and is relieved by rest.

Internal evidence Type of evidence used in evidence-based practice that includes nursing expertise and results of quality improvement and outcome evaluation.

Interprofessional care Care delivered by intentionally created and usually relatively small work groups in health care as having a collective identity and shared responsibility for a patient or a group of patients.

Intimate partner violence (IPV) Physical violence, sexual violence, stalking, and psychologic aggression (including coercive acts) by a current or former intimate partner.

Intracerebral hematomas Collection of blood in the brain tissue, most often located in the frontal or temporal lobes.

Intracranial aneurysm Saccular outpouching of a cerebral artery that occurs at the site of a weakness in the vessel wall.

Intracranial hypertension See *Increased intracranial pressure.*

Intracranial pressure (ICP) Pressure within the cranial cavity, usually measured as the pressure within the lateral ventricles.

Intraductal papilloma Tiny wartlike growth on the inside of the peripheral mammary duct that causes discharge from the nipple.

Intraoperative phase Time during surgery, from beginning to end.

Iron deficiency anemia Most common type of anemia; results from inadequate iron for optimal RBC formation.

Irritable bowel syndrome (IBS) Motility disorder of the gastrointestinal tract characterized by alternating periods of constipation and diarrhea.

Ischemia Deficient blood flow to tissue resulting in reduced oxygen delivery.

Ischemic Deprived of oxygen.

Islets of Langerhans Hormone-producing cells (alpha cells, beta cells, and delta cells) scattered through the pancreas.

Isograft Tissue transplant where the donor and recipient are identical twins.

Jaundice Yellow-to-orange color visible in the skin and mucous membranes; most often the result of a hepatic disorder.

Joint arthroplasty Reconstruction or replacement of a joint.

Kaposi sarcoma (KS) Vascular malignancy (a tumor of the endothelial cells lining small blood vessels) that presents as vascular macules, papules, or violet lesions affecting the skin and viscera. It is often the presenting symptom of AIDS.

Keloid Elevated, irregularly shaped, progressively enlarging scar arising from excessive amounts of collagen in the stratum corneum during scar formation in connective tissue repair.

Keratin Keratin is a fibrous, water-repellent protein that gives the epidermis its tough, protective quality.

Keratitis Inflammation of the cornea.

Keratosis Any skin condition in which there is a benign overgrowth and thickening of the cornified epithelium.

Ketoacidosis Condition of very high blood glucose and insufficient insulin that results in accumulation of ketones and fatty acids in the blood; a form of metabolic acidosis.

Ketonuria Presence of ketones in the urine.

Ketosis Accumulation of ketone bodies produced during the oxidation of fatty acids.

Kidney failure Inability of the kidneys to effectively remove accumulated metabolites from the blood, leading to altered fluid, electrolyte, and acid–base balance.

Kindling Long-term changes in brain neurotransmission that occur after repeated detoxifications.

Kinesthesia Ability to perceive movement and sense of position.

Korotkoff sounds Sounds heard during auscultation of blood pressure.

Korsakoff psychosis Secondary dementia caused by thiamine (B_1) deficiency that may be associated with chronic alcoholism; characterized by progressive cognitive deterioration, confabulation, peripheral neuropathy, and myopathy.

Kussmaul respirations Deep, rapid respirations associated with compensatory mechanisms.

Kwashiorkor (protein energy malnutrition, PEM) Chronic protein deficiency with adequate calories to meet body needs.

Kyphosis Exaggerated thoracic curvature of the spine, common in older adults.

Labyrinthectomy Surgical removal of the labyrinth.

Labyrinthitis Inflammation of the inner ear.

Laceration Open wound that results from sharp cutting or tearing. Injuries to the integument are at risk for contamination from dirt, debris, or foreign objects.

Lacunar strokes Thrombotic stroke of smaller cerebral blood vessels in deeper parts of the brain or brainstem.

Laminectomy Removal of the lamina of the vertebrae.

Laparoscopic cholecystectomy Removal of the gallbladder using an endoscope.

Laryngectomy Removal of the larynx.

Laryngitis Inflammation of the larynx.

Late effects The health problems that occur months to years after the treatment for cancer has ended.

Leiomyoma See *Fibroid tumor*.

Leukemia Group of chronic malignant disorders of white blood cells and WBC precursors; characterized by replacement of bone marrow by malignant immature WBCs, abnormal immature circulating WBCs, and infiltration of malignant cells into other tissues.

Leukocytes Also called *white blood cells*, these are the primary cells involved in both nonspecific and specific immune system responses. These cells isolate the infecting organism or injury, destroy pathogens, and promote healing.

Leukocytosis Increase in the number of leukocytes in the blood (above 10,/mm^3), usually caused by infection.

Leukopenia Abnormal decrease of circulating leukocytes, usually below 5/mm^3; occurs when bone marrow activity is suppressed or when leukocyte destruction increases.

Leukoplakia Formation of white patches or spots on the mucous membranes or tongue; these lesions may become malignant.

Libido Sexual desire.

Lichen planus Benign inflammatory disorder of the mucous membranes and skin.

Lift More sustained cardiac thrust than normal.

Lipoatrophy Atrophy of subcutaneous tissue.

Liposuction Method of changing the contours of the body by aspirating fat from the subcutaneous layer of tissue.

Lithiasis Stone formation.

Lithotripsy Crushing of renal calculi.

Living will Document that provides written directions about life-prolonging proceures to provide instructions when a person can no longer communicate in a life-threatening situation.

Lobectomy Surgical removal of a single lobe of lung.

Locked-in syndrome Patient is alert and fully aware of the environment, but is unable to communicate through speech or movement as a result of blocked efferent pathways to the brain.

Lordosis Increased lumbar curve.

Loss Actual or potential situation in which a valued object, person, body part, or emotion that was formerly present is lost or changed and can no longer be seen, felt, heard, known, or experienced; may be temporary or permanent, complete or partial, objectively verifiable or perceived, physical or symbolic.

Lower body obesity (peripheral obesity) Waist-to-hip ratio of less than 0.8 in an obese individual.

Lung abscess Localized area of lung destruction or necrosis and pus formation.

Lung compliance Distensibility of the lungs.

Lyme disease Inflammatory disorder caused by a spirochete, *Borrelia burgdorferi*, which is transmitted primarily by ticks.

Lymphadenopathy Enlargement of lymph nodes (over 1 cm) with or without tenderness; may be caused by inflammation, infection, or malignancy of the nodes or the regions drained by the nodes.

Lymphangitis Inflammation of a lymphatic vessel.

Lymphedema Edema of an extremity due to accumulated lymph; may be primary or secondary, resulting from inflammation, obstruction, or removal of lymphatic vessels.

Lymphocytes Lymphocytes account for 20 to 40% of circulating leukocytes. Lymphocytes are the principal effector and regulator cells of specific immune responses.

Lymphoid tissues Connective tissues containing lymphocytes; include tissues of the bone marrow, thymus, lymph nodes, and spleen.

Lymphoma Malignancy of lymphoid tissue.

Macrophages Mature monocytes after settling into tissue; large phagocytes important in the body's defense against chronic infections.

Macular degeneration Destructive changes in the macula due to injury or gradual failure of the outer pigmented layer of the retina (the retinal layer adjacent to the choroid), which removes cellular waste products and keeps the retina attached to the choroid.

Malabsorption Condition in which nutrients are ineffectively absorbed by the intestinal mucosa, resulting in their excretion in the stool.

Malignant hypertension Hypertensive emergency, marked by a diastolic pressure greater than 120 mmHg.

Malignant hyperthermia Rare multifactorial genetic disorder that can be triggered by inhalational anesthetic gases and succinylcholine, a depolarizing neuromuscular blocker.

Malignant melanoma (cutaneous melanoma) Skin cancer that arises from melanocytes.

Malignant pain Pain associated with a life-threatening illness such as cancer but not limited to cancer pain.

Malnutrition Inadequate nutrient intake to meet body needs; may include deficiency of major nutrients (calories, carbohydrates, proteins, and fats) or micronutrients such as vitamins and minerals.

Man-made disasters Either accidental or intentional, they are complex emergencies, technological disasters, material shortages, and other disasters not caused by natural hazards.

Manifestations Signs and symptoms of a disease or condition caused by alterations in structure or function.

Marasmus (protein energy undernutrition) Insufficient protein and calorie intake to meet metabolic needs.

Mass casualty events Situations in which 100 or more casualties are involved, significantly overwhelming available emergency medical services, facilities, and resources.

Mastoidectomy Surgical removal of infected mastoid air cells.

Mastoiditis Bacterial infection of the mastoid process.

Maturity-onset diabetes of the young (MODY) Diabetes in young obese adults.

Mean arterial pressure (MAP) Average pressure in the arterial circulation throughout the cardiac cycle; product of cardiac output and systemic vascular resistance (SVR).

Medical-surgical nursing Health promotion, healthcare, and illness care of adults, based on knowledge derived from the arts and sciences and shaped by knowledge (the science) of nursing.

Meiosis Reduction of division of the cell occurring only in the sex cells of the testes and ovaries when the amount of genetic material is reduced in half (23 chromosomes).

Melanin Skin pigment that forms a protective shield to protect keratinocytes and nerve endings in the dermis from the damaging effects of ultraviolet light.

Melanoma Serious skin cancer that arises from the melanocytes; also known as *malignant melanoma*.

Melena Black, tarry stool that contains old, digested blood.

Ménière's disease Chronic disorder of unknown cause characterized by recurrent attacks of vertigo with tinnitus and a progressive unilateral hearing loss.

Meningitis Inflammation of the meninges of the brain and spinal cord.

Menopause Permanent cessation of menses.

Menorrhagia Excessive or prolonged menstruation.

Menstrual cycle Cyclic buildup of the uterine lining, ovulation, and sloughing of the lining occurring approximately every 28 days in nonpregnant females of childbearing age.

Menstruation Periodic shedding of the uterine lining in a woman of childbearing age who is not pregnant.

Metabolic syndrome Cluster of manifestations often associated with type 2 DM. Includes hypertension, visceral obesity, low HDL, high triglycerides, elevated C-reactive protein, and fasting glucose greater than 110mg/dL.

Metabolism Consisting of the breakdown of complex structures into simpler forms to produce energy (catabolism) and the combination of simpler molecules to produce and maintain more complex structures necessary to living organisms (anabolism).

Metaplasia Change in the normal pattern of differentiation such that dividing cells differentiate into cell types not normally found in that location in the body.

Metastasis Secondary tumor; the process by which spreading of malignant neoplasms occurs; the transfer of disease from one organ or part to another not directly connected with it.

Methicillin-resistant *Staphylococcus aureus* (MRSA) Strain of antibiotic-resistant *S. aureus* that colonizes the skin and nares.

Metrorrhagia Bleeding between menstrual periods; may be caused by hormonal imbalances, pelvic inflammatory disease, cervical or uterine polyps, uterine fibroids, or cervical or uterine cancer.

Microalbuminuria Protein in the urine.

Micturition Releasing urine from the urinary bladder (voiding).

Mild concussion Brain trauma resulting in a brief loss of consciousness that lasts from seconds to hours.

Minor trauma Injury to a single part or system of the body, usually treated in the hospital or emergency department.

Mitigation Action taken to prevent or reduce the harmful effects of a disaster on human health or property, it involves future-oriented activities to prevent subsequent disasters or to minimize their effects.

Mitosis Process of making new cells by cell division. Cell division through mitosis results in two cells called *daughter cells* that are genetically identical to the original cell, or *mother cell*, and to each other.

Mitral valve (bicuspid valve) Valve between the left atrium and ventricle in the heart; prevents blood from flowing backward into the atrium.

Monosomic (monosomy) When one member of the chromosome pair is missing, for example, Turner syndrome (45, XO).

Morbid obesity Weight greater than 100% over ideal body weight.

Morton's neuroma Tumor-like mass formed within the neurovascular bundle of the intermetatarsal spaces.

Mosaicism Chromosome variation or abnormality that occurs after fertilization during mitosis at an early cell stage so not all cells are affected with the variation; for example, a child who is mosaic for Down syndrome will have some cells with two copies of chromosome 21 and some that have an extra chromosome 21.

Mourning Actions or expressions of the bereaved, including the symbols, clothing, and ceremonies that make up the outward manifestations of grief.

Multifactorial Health conditions determined by multiple factors, including genetic and environmental factors, each having an additive effect.

Multiple-casualty incidents Incidents in which more than two but fewer than 100 persons are injured.

Multiple myeloma Malignancy in which plasma cells multiply uncontrollably and infiltrate the bone marrow, lymph nodes, spleen, and other tissues.

Multiple sclerosis (MS) Chronic demyelating autoimmune disease of the central nervous system.

Multiple trauma Most often the result of a motor vehicle crash, this type of trauma requires immediate intervention specifically focused on ensuring survival.

Murmur Sound made by turbulent blood flow through the heart.

Muscular dystrophy (MD) Group of inherited muscle diseases that cause progressive muscle degeneration and wasting.

Myasthenia gravis Chronic, progressive neuromuscular disorder characterized by fatigue and severe weakness of skeletal muscles.

Myelin sheaths Insulation of the neuron that facilitates conduction of impulses.

Myelodysplastic syndrome Group of blood disorders characterized by abnormal-appearing bone marrow and cytopenia (low numbers of circulating blood cells). Not a single disease; at least five variations of the disorder have been identified.

Myocarditis Inflammatory disorder of the heart muscle.

Myopia (nearsightedness) Condition in which the eyeball is elongated, causing the image to focus in front of the retina instead of on it.

Myringotomy Incision of the tympanic membrane.

Myxedema Systemic condition that develops from inadequate levels of thyroid hormone (hypothyroidism).

Myxedema coma Life-threatening complication of long-standing, untreated hypothyroidism, characterized by severe metabolic disorders (hyponatremia, hypoglycemia, lactic acidosis), hypothermia, cardiovascular collapse, impaired cognition, and coma.

Natural disasters Disasters caused by acts of nature or emerging diseases; some are unexpected and some are predictable through advanced meteorological technologies.

Natural killer cells (NK cells) Large, granular lymphocytes (found in the spleen, lymph nodes, bone marrow, and blood) that provide immune surveillance and resistance to infection and play an important role in the destruction of early malignant cells.

Nausea Unpleasant sensation of sickness or queasiness; may or may not be followed by vomiting.

Necrosis Tissue cell death.

Neglect syndrome (unilateral neglect) Disorder of attention. In this syndrome, the person cannot integrate and use perceptions from the affected side of the body or from the environment on the affected side and, hence, ignores that part.

Neoplasm Mass of new tissue (a collection of cells) that grows independently of its surrounding structures and has no physiologic purpose.

Nephrectomy Removal of the kidney.

Nephrotic syndrome Condition marked by massive proteinuria, hypoalbuminemia, hyperlipidemia, and edema.

Neuralgia Nerve pain.

Neurogenic bladder Dysfunctional urinary bladder due to lesion of central or peripheral nervous system.

Neurogenic shock Shock resulting from an imbalance between parasympathetic and sympathetic stimulation of vascular smooth muscle. If parasympathetic overstimulation or sympathetic understimulation persists, sustained vasodilation occurs and blood pools in the venous and capillary beds.

Neuropathic pain Pain resulting from abnormal impulse processing by the peripheral and central nervous systems following injury to the peripheral nerves.

Neuropathy Damage to peripheral nerves causing hyper- or hyposensation and leading to neuropathic pain and injury.

Neurotransmitters Substance (as norepinephrine or acetylcholine) that transmits nerve impulses across a synapse.

Neutropenia Decrease in circulating neutrophils.

Nevi (moles) Flat or raised macules or papules with rounded, well-defined borders.

Nicotine Stimulant found in tobacco that enters the system via the lungs (cigarettes and cigars) and oral mucous membranes (chewing tobacco as well as smoking).

Nociceptive pain Pain caused by stimulation of peripheral or visceral pain receptors.

Nociceptors Sensory nerve fibers that conduct pain impulses from the periphery to the central nervous system.

Nocturia Voiding two or more times at night.

Node Elements of the immune system connected by lymphatics. Upregulates immune function; does not synthesize hormones.

Non-Hodgkin lymphoma (NHL) Lymphoid tissue malignancies that do not contain Reed–Sternberg cells.

Nonconventional terrorist weapons Chemical, biological, and nuclear weapons of terrorism; used less frequently than conventional terrorist weapons.

Nonunion State that exists when the ends of a fracture fail to heal together.

Normal sinus rhythm (NSR) Normal heart rhythm, in which impulses originate in the sinus node and travel through normal conduction pathways without delay.

Nosocomial Pertaining to or occurring in a hospital.

Nosocomial infection Infection contracted during residence in a hospital or extended care facility.

Nuclear terrorism Use of a nuclear device to cause mass murder and devastation.

Nursing informatics Nursing specialty integrating nursing, computer science, and information science.

Nursing process Series of critical thinking activities nurses use as they provide care to patients; this logical approach to care ensures that patients receive comprehensive and effective care.

Nursing-sensitive quality indicators (NSQIs) Patient outcomes that are influenced significantly by quality nursing interventions.

Nutrients Substances found in food that are used by the body to promote growth, maintenance, and repair.

Nutrition Process by which the body ingests, absorbs, transports, uses, and eliminates food.

Nystagmus Rapid involuntary eye movements.

Obesity Excess of body fat (adipose tissue).

Obstructive shock Shock caused by an obstruction in the heart or great vessels that either impedes venous return or prevents effective cardiac pumping action.

Obstructive sleep apnea (OSA) Disorder of breathing during the night that is caused by the airway either partially or completely collapsing during the nighttime.

Occult blood/bleeding Blood or bleeding that is hidden or not readily apparent.

Office-based surgical suites Setting for many elective surgeries, although increasing malpractice insurance premiums have influenced their decline.

Oligomenorrhea Scant menses.

Oliguria Urine output of less than 400 mL in 24 hours.

Oncogene Gene capable of triggering cancerous characteristics.

Oncologic emergencies In caring for patients with cancer, nurses may encounter a number of emergency situations in which their role may be pivotal to the patient's survival. Most of these emergencies require astute observations, accurate judgments, and rapid action once the problem has been identified.

Oncology Study of cancer.

Onycholysis Separation of the distal nail plate from the nail bed.

Onychomycosis Fungal or dermatophyte infection of the nail plate.

Operational variable Description of how a research variable is measured (commonly a dependent variable).

Opiates Analgesics derived from the opium plant; produce analgesia by binding to opioid receptors within and outside the CNS; the most potent analgesics available, and the treatment of choice for acute moderate-to-severe pain. Examples include morphine, codeine, and fentanyl (Durgesic, Actiq). Also called *narcotic analgesics*.

Orchitis Infection or inflammation of the testicle.

Orthopnea Difficulty breathing when supine.

Orthostatic hypotension Decrease in systolic blood pressure of more than 10 to 15 mmHg and a drop in diastolic blood pressure on standing.

Osmosis Process by which water moves across a selectively permeable membrane from an area of lower solute concentration to an area of higher solute concentration.

Ossification Process of bone formation.

Osteitis deformans See *Paget disease of bone*.

Osteoarthritis (OA; degenerative joint disease) Most commonly occurring of all forms of arthritis; characterized by loss of articular cartilage in articulating joints and hypertrophy of the bones at the articular margins.

Osteoblast Cells that form bone.

Osteoclast Cells that resorb bone.

Osteomalacia (adult rickets) Metabolic bone disorder characterized by inadequate mineralization of bone matrix.

Osteomyelitis Infection within the bone that can lead to tissue death and necrosis.

Osteophytes Bony outgrowths often called *joint mice*.

Osteoporosis Literally defined as "porous bones," a metabolic bone disorder characterized by loss of bone mass, increased bone fragility, and an increased risk of fractures.

Osteotomy Incision into or transection of the bone.

Ostomy General term for an operation in which an artificial opening is created.

Otitis media Inflammation or infection of the middle ear.

Otorrhea Leakage of cerebrospinal fluid through the ear.

Otosclerosis Abnormal bone formation in the osseous labyrinth of the temporal bone causing the footplate of the stapes to become fixed or immobile in the oval window. The result is a conductive hearing loss.

Ovarian cycle Female cycle that occurs from puberty until menopause in which the production of ova occur.

Oxyhemoglobin Combined form of hemoglobin and oxygen; found in arterial blood, it carries oxygen to body tissues.

Pacemaker Pulse generator used to provide an electrical stimulus to the heart when the heart fails to generate or conduct its own at a rate that maintains the cardiac output.

$PaCO_2$ Partial pressure of carbon dioxide in arterial blood.

Paget disease of bone (osteitis deformans) Skeletal disorder that results from excessive osteoclastic activity; characterized by bone deformity, especially of the long bones of the lower limbs, the pelvis, the lumbar vertebrae, and the skull.

Pain Subjective response to both physical and psychologic stressors.

Pain threshold Point at which a stimulus elicits a pain response.

Pain tolerance Amount of pain a person can endure before responding to it.

Palliative care Area of care that has evolved out of the hospice experience, but exists outside of hospice programs and is not restricted to the end of life. Palliative care is focused on the relief of physical, mental, and spiritual distress for individuals who have an incurable illness and is used earlier in the disease experience than hospice care. The goal of palliative care is to prevent and relieve suffering by early assessment and treatment of pain and other physical, psychosocial, and spiritual needs to improve the patient's quality of life.

Pallor Lack of color; paleness of skin.

Pancreatitis Inflammation of the pancreas.

Pannus Granulation tissue that forms in joints affected by rheumatoid arthritis and leads to the formation of scar tissue that immobilizes the joint.

PaO_2 Partial pressure of oxygen in arterial blood.

Papilledema Swelling of the optic nerve.

Paracentesis Aspiration of fluid from the peritoneal cavity.

Paralytic ileus Impaired propulsion or forward movement of bowel contents.

Paraplegia Paralysis of the lower portion of the body, sometimes involving the lower trunk.

Parasites Organisms that live within, on, or at the expense of the patient.

Parenteral nutrition (PN or TPN) Intravenous administration of carbohydrates (high concentrations of dextrose), protein (amino acids), electrolytes, vitamins, minerals, and fat emulsions.

Paresthesia Abnormal sensation of the skin, such as numbness, burning, or pricking.

Parish nursing Nontraditional, community-based way of providing health promotion and health restoration nursing interventions to a spiritual community.

Parkinson disease (PD) Progressive, degenerative neurologic disease characterized by nonintentional tremor, bradykinesia, and muscle rigidity.

Paronychia Infection of the cuticle of the fingernails or toenails.

Paroxysmal Abrupt onset and termination.

Paroxysmal nocturnal dyspnea (PND) Attacks of acute shortness of breath that occur at night, waking up the patient.

Partial gastrectomy Removal of a portion of the stomach, usually the distal half to two-thirds.

Partial seizures Seizures that involve a restricted part of one cerebral hemisphere; may be simple partial (without loss of consciousness) or complex partial (with loss of consciousness).

Partial-thickness burn Burn that involves the entire dermis and the papillae of the dermis (superficial partial-thickness burn) or extends into the hair follicles (deep partial-thickness burn).

Passive immunity Temporary protection—provided by antibodies produced by other people or animals—against disease-producing antigens. Protection is gradually lost when these acquired antibodies are used up either by natural degradation or by combining with the antigen.

Pathogens Virulent organisms rarely found in the absence of disease.

Patient Person, family, or community with who and for who nursing care is designed and implemented.

Patient-centered medical home (PCMH) Accessible, comprehensive, and coordinated primary care focused on illness prevention for patients and families.

Patient-controlled analgesia (PCA) Pump with a control mechanism that allows the patient to self-manage pain.

Patient preferences Individualized patient experiences and values that are considered when determining evidence-based nursing care.

Patient Protection and Affordable Care Act (ACA) Landmark federal legislation enacted in 2010 and designed to provide access to healthcare services for more Americans and create new models of health care.

Pediculosis capitis Infestation with head lice.

Pediculosis corporis Infestation with body lice.

Pediculosis pubis Infestation with pubic lice (often called *crabs*).

Pelvic inflammatory disease (PID) Term used to describe infection of the pelvic organs.

Pemphigus vulgaris Chronic disorder of the skin and oral mucous membranes characterized by vesicle (blister) formation.

Penetrance Percentage or likelihood that an individual who has inherited a gene mutation will actually express the disease signs and symptoms in his or her lifetime.

Penicillin-resistant *Streptococcus pneumoniae* (PRSP) Infection transmitted by droplets from the respiratory tract; requires transmission-based droplet precautions.

Peptic ulcer/peptic ulcer disease (PUD) Break in the mucous lining of the gastrointestinal tract where it comes in contact with gastric juice; may affect any area of the gastrointestinal tract exposed to acid-pepsin secretions, including the esophagus, stomach, or duodenum.

Pericarditis Inflammation of the pericardium.

Perioperative nursing Specialized area of nursing practice that incorporates the three phases of the surgical experience: preoperative, intraoperative, and postoperative.

Peripheral vascular disease (PVD) Impaired blood supply to peripheral tissues, particularly the lower extremities.

Peripheral vascular resistance (PVR) Opposing forces or impedance to blood flow as the arterial channels become more and more distant from the heart.

Peristalsis Alternating waves of contraction and relaxation of involuntary muscles.

Peritoneal dialysis Procedure in which electrolytes, waste products, and excess water are removed from the body by diffusion using the peritoneum surrounding the abdominal cavity as the dialyzing membrane.

Peritonitis Inflammation of the peritoneum.

Pernicious anemia Anemia resulting from failure to absorb dietary vitamin B_{12} due to lack of intrinsic factor.

Persistent vegetative state (PVS) Condition of complete unawareness of self and the environment.

Personal protective equipment (PPE) Equipment used for the protection of personnel including gloves, masks, goggles, gowns, and biologic disposal bags (red bags); may also include hoods, helmets, head gear, and impermeable suits.

Pertussis (whooping cough) Highly contagious acute upper respiratory infection caused by the bacterium *Bordetella pertussis.*

Phagocytosis Process by which a foreign agent or target cell is engulfed, destroyed, and digested. Neutrophils and macrophages, known as phagocytes, are the primary cells involved in phagocytosis.

Phantom limb pain Confusing pain syndrome that occurs following surgical or traumatic amputation of a limb. The patient experiences pain in the missing body part even though there is complete mental awareness that the limb is gone.

Pharyngitis Acute inflammation of the pharynx.

Phenotype Expression of a person's entire physical, biochemical, and physiologic makeup, as determined by the individual's genotype and environmental factors.

Phimosis Constriction of the foreskin so that it cannot be retracted over the glans penis.

Physician orders for life-sustaining treatment (POLST) Form used for patients with serious, progressive, chronic illness that translates their wishes regarding life-sustaining treatment into actionable medical orders.

PICOT Format for evidence-based practice question. PICOT is a mnemonic for patient, intervention, comparison group, outcome, and time.

Plasmapheresis (plasma exchange) Removal of the plasma component from whole blood.

Plastic surgery Alteration, replacement, or restoration of visible portions of the body, performed to correct a structural or cosmetic defect.

Platelets (thrombocytes) Cell fragments that have no nucleus and cannot replicate.

Pleural effusion Collection of excess fluid in the pleural space.

Pleuritis Inflammation of the pleura.

Pneumonectomy Removal of an entire lung.

Pneumonia Inflammation of the lung parenchyma (the respiratory bronchioles and alveoli).

Pneumothorax Results when air enters the pleural space due to blunt and penetrating injuries to the chest.

Polycystic kidney disease Hereditary disease characterized by cyst formation and massive kidney enlargement.

Polycythemia (erythrocytosis) Excess RBCs characterized by a hematocrit higher than 55%.

Polydipsia Excessive thirst.

Polymorphisms DNA sequences that are natural variations in a gene usually having no adverse effects on the individual.

Polymyositis Systemic connective-tissue disorder characterized by inflammation of connective tissue and muscle fibers leading to muscle weakness and atrophy.

Polyp Mass of tissue that arises from the bowel wall and protrudes into the lumen.

Polyphagia Excessive eating.

Polysubstance abuse Simultaneous use of many substances.

Polyuria Excessive output of urine.

Portal hypertension Elevated pressure in the portal venous system that causes rerouting of blood to adjoining lower pressure vessels.

Portal systemic (hepatic) encephalopathy Impaired consciousness and mental status due to the accumulation of toxic waste products in the blood (ammonia in particular) as blood bypasses the congested liver.

Positive urine glucose Presence of glucose found in urine, however, not reliable as an indicator of hyperglycemia as glucose doesn't appear in the urine below the renal threshold of 180mg/dL.

Postanesthesia care unit (PACU) Hospital unit to which postsurgical patients are transferred for recovery.

Postconcussion syndrome Persistent headache, dizziness, irritability, insomnia, impaired memory and concentration, and learning problems following a concussion; may last for several weeks or up to 1 year.

Postoperative phase Period when a procedure or surgery has been completed and the patient is recovering from the stress associated with the surgery.

Postpoliomyelitis syndrome Complication of a previous infection by the poliomyelitis virus.

Prediabetes Impaired glucose tolerance.

Preload Amount of cardiac muscle fiber tension or stretch that exists at end diastole, just before ventricular contraction.

Premature ejaculation Common ejaculatory disorder in which semen is ejaculated before completion of sexual intercourse.

Premenstrual syndrome (PMS) Complex of symptoms characterized by irritability, depression, edema, and breast tenderness preceding the monthly menses.

Preoperative phase Time when preparation of the patient for surgery is conducted and completed.

Preparedness Actions that address preparations for and actions in dealing with the consequences of a disaster.

Presbycusis Age-related loss of the ability to hear high-frequency sounds; may occur because of cochlear hair cell degeneration or loss of auditory neurons in the organ of Corti.

Presbyopia Impaired near vision resulting from a loss of elasticity of the lens of the eye.

Pressure injury Ischemic lesion of the skin and underlying tissue caused by external pressure that impairs the flow of blood and lymph.

Priapism Sustained, painful erection that lasts at least 4 hours and is not associated with sexual arousal.

Primary care Comprehensive first-contact health and illness care across the lifespan.

Primary hypertension (idiopathic, essential) Persistently elevated systemic blood pressure.

Primary polycythemia (polycythemia vera) Neoplastic stem cell disorder characterized by overproduction of red blood cells and, to a lesser extent, white blood cells and platelets.

Professional boundaries Borders between the vulnerability of the patient and the power of the nurse.

Progesterone Hormone produced by the ovary; works with estrogen to control the menstrual cycle.

Proliferative phase Second stage of wound healing, which begins 2 to 3 days after the initial incision, where fibroblasts and vascular endothelial cells form granulation tissue.

Proptosis Forward displacement of the eye.

Prostatitis Inflammation of the prostate gland.

Protein-calorie malnutrition (PCM) Deficient protein and calories to meet metabolic needs.

Proteinuria Abnormal proteins in the urine.

Proto-oncogenes Normal genes that promote cell growth and repair.

Pruritus Subjective itching sensation producing an urge to scratch.

Psoriasis Chronic, noninfectious skin disorder that is characterized by raised, reddened, round circumscribed plaques covered by silvery white scales.

Psychogenic pain Pain that is experienced in the absence of any diagnosed physiologic cause or event.

Psychostimulants Drugs such as cocaine and amphetamines have a high potential for abuse. Euphoria is the main subjective effect associated with cocaine and amphetamines, leading to addiction.

Ptosis Drooping of the eyelid.

Pulmonary edema Abnormal accumulation of fluid in the interstitial tissue and alveoli of the lung.

Pulmonary embolism Sudden occlusion of blood flow in a portion of the pulmonary vascular system, causing a ventilation–perfusion imbalance and impaired gas exchange.

Pulmonary hypertension Condition in which the pulmonary arterial pressure is elevated to an abnormal level.

Pulmonic valve Semilunar valve between the right ventricle and the pulmonary artery.

Pulse Rhythmic pressure wave that can be felt over an artery.

Pulse deficit Condition in which the radial pulse is less than the apical pulse, indicating weak, inefficient left-ventricular contractions.

Pulse pressure Difference between the systolic and diastolic blood pressure.

Puncture wound Wound that occurs when a sharp or blunt object penetrates the integument.

Pupillary light reflex Reflex in which the pupil contracts in response to a bright light.

Pyelonephritis Upper urinary tract inflammation affecting the kidney and renal pelvis.

Pyoderma Purulent bacterial infection of skin.

Pyuria Pus in the urine.

Quadriplegia See *Tetraplegia*.

Qualitative research Research approach that focuses on a participant's experience and the perceived meaning of the situation of interest.

Quality assurance Process of ensuring quality control activities that evaluate, monitor, or regulate the standard of services provided to the consumer.

Quality improvement Systematic evidence-based methods used to evaluate and improve patient care.

Quantitative research Use of numerical computations and statistical analysis to answer empirical questions.

Rabies Viral (rhabdovirus) infection of the central nervous system transmitted by infected saliva that enters the human body through a bite or an open wound.

Radiation sickness One of the results of DNA mutation inside cells exposed to ionizing radiation.

Radiation therapy Therapy that uses radiation to kill a tumor, to reduce its size, to decrease pain, or to relieve obstruction.

Radiculopathy Condition in which one or more nerves, especially nerve roots, do not function normally.

Radiological dispersion bomb Also called a *dirty bomb*, consists of a conventional explosive such as trinitrotoluene (TNT) packed with radioactive waste by-products from nuclear reactors that discharges deadly radioactive particles into the environment.

Raynaud disease/phenomenon Disorders characterized by episodes of intense vasospasm in the small arteries and arterioles of the fingers and possibly the toes.

Reactive arthritis (ReA) (Reiter syndrome) Acute, nonpurulent inflammatory arthritis that complicates a bacterial infection of the genitourinary or gastrointestinal tracts.

Rebound tenderness Pain that occurs with withdrawal or release of pressure applied during abdominal palpation.

Recessive Characteristic that is apparent only when two copies of the gene encoding it are present, one from the mother and one from the father.

Reconstruction Recovery aspect of disaster response; during this period restoration, reconstitution, and mitigation take place.

Recovery Fifth of five stages of a disaster. Activities include rebuilding and returning to some semblance of "normalcy" but also includes mitigation activities or planning to prevent subsequent disasters or to minimize the effects of future disasters.

Red blood cells (RBCs, erythrocytes) Blood cells shaped like a biconcave disk that contain hemoglobin required for oxygen transport to body tissues; the most common type of blood cell.

Referral source Person recommending home care services and supplying the agency with details about the patient's needs. The source may be a physician, nurse, social worker, therapist, or discharge planner.

Referred pain Pain that is perceived in an area distant from the site of the stimuli.

Reflex sympathetic dystrophy Group of poorly understood posttraumatic conditions involving persistent pain, hyperesthesias, swelling, changes in skin color and texture, changes in temperature, and decreased motion.

Reflux, urinary Backflow of urine toward the kidneys.

Refraction Bending of light rays as they pass from one medium to another medium of different optical density.

Refractory period Period in which myocardial cells are resistant to stimulation.

Regional anesthesia Anesthesia that desensitizes the area to be operated but does not involve the full central nervous system or cause sedation.

Regurgitation (valvular) Backflow of blood through an incompletely closed valve into the area it just left.

Rehabilitation Process of learning to live to one's maximum potential with a chronic impairment and its resultant functional disability.

Reiter syndrome See *Reactive arthritis (ReA)*.

Reliability Describes the findings of a research study. Instrument reliability refers to the consistency of the measurement of the variable.

Remission Period in which symptoms are not experienced even though the disease is still clinically present.

Remodeling phase Final stage of wound healing where scar tissue is remodeled by a process of collagen synthesis and breakdown to increase strength.

Renal artery stenosis Narrowing of the renal artery.

Renal colic Acute, severe, intermittent pain in the flank and upper outer abdominal quadrant generally associated with acute obstruction of a ureter and resulting ureteral spasm.

Renal failure Condition in which the kidneys are unable to remove accumulated metabolites from the blood, resulting in altered fluid, electrolyte, and acid–base balance.

Renal impairment (decreased renal reserve) Glomerular filtration rate of approximately 50% of normal with normal BUN and serum creatinine levels.

Renal insufficiency Glomerular filtration rate of 20 to 50% of normal with azotemia and some manifestations of renal failure.

Renal transplant Surgical insertion of a functioning kidney.

Renin–angiotensin mechanism Intrinsic system that responds to renal perfusion; a fall in renal blood flow (e.g., due to low BP or cardiac output) stimulates renin release, ultimately leading to vasoconstriction and sodium and water retention and increased BP and cardiac output.

Repolarization Restoration of the resting cell membrane potential following generation of an action potential.

Research design Provides the structure for conducting a research study. The goal is maximum control of factors to reduce the potential that findings would be influenced by variables that were not part of the study.

Respiratory failure Inability of lungs to oxygenate the blood and remove carbon dioxide adequately to meet the body's needs, even at rest.

Respite care Short-term or intermittent home care, often using volunteers. These services exist to give the primary caregiver some relief from the burden of full-time care.

Response Occurs in the emergency stage of disaster response, after the impact of the disaster event has occurred, the community has been rapidly assessed for damage, and the types and extent of injuries suffered as well as the immediate needs of the community have been determined.

Rest Period of diminished activity, without disengagement from the environment, for mental and physical rejuvenation.

Restless legs syndrome A common sleep disorder where affected patients have a "creepy-crawly" or "pins-and-needles" feeling in their legs in the evening, which is relieved by movement, preventing the patient from falling asleep.

Reticular activating system (RAS) System of reticular neurons within the reticular formation that passes steady streams of impulses through thalamic relays in order to stimulate the cerebral cortex into wakefulness.

Retinal detachment Separation of the retina or sensory portion of the eye from the choroid.

Retinitis pigmentosa Hereditary degenerative disease characterized by retinal atrophy and loss of retinal function progressing from the periphery to the central region of the retina.

Retractions Pulling-in of the tissue of the precordium; a slight retraction just medial to the midclavicular line at the area of the apical impulse is normal and is more likely to be visible in thin patients.

Retrograde ejaculation Seminal fluid discharged into the bladder.

Reverse triage Working from the principle of the greatest good for the greatest number, reverse triage is an "upside-down triage" used in mass casualty events in which the victims who are most severely injured, requiring extensive resources with little chance of surviving, are treated last.

Rheumatic disorders Inflammatory diseases of connective tissues that affect joints, the muscles, and bones.

Rheumatic fever Systemic inflammatory disease caused by an abnormal immune response to pharyngeal infection by group A beta-hemolytic streptococci.

Rheumatic heart disease (RHD) Slowly progressive valvular deformity following acute or repeated attacks of rheumatic fever; characterized by rigid and deformed valve leaflets, fused valve commissures, and fibrosis of chordae tendineae.

Rheumatoid arthritis Chronic systemic autoimmune disease that causes inflammation of connective tissue, primarily in the joints.

Rhinitis Inflammation of the nasal cavities.

Rhinoplasty Surgical reconstruction of the nose.

Rhinorrhea Leakage of cerebrospinal fluid through the nose.

Rosacea Chronic facial condition that begins with erythema over the cheeks and nose and progresses to dark red skin color with enlarged pores.

Ruptured disk See *Herniated intervertebral disk.*

Salmonellosis Form of food poisoning caused by ingestion of foods contaminated with one or more varieties of *Salmonella* bacteria.

Sarcoidosis Systemic disease characterized by granulomas in the lungs, lymph nodes, liver, eyes, skin, and other organs.

Sarcoma Tumor arising from supportive tissues.

Sarcopenic obesity Process of muscle loss combined with increased body fat as people age, leading to a loss of function and reduced quality of life.

Scabies Parasitic infestation caused by the mite *Sarcoptes scabiei.*

Sciatica Pain over the sciatic nerve.

Scleroderma (systemic sclerosis) Hardening of the skin, a chronic condition characterized by the formation of excess fibrous connective tissue and diffuse fibrosis of the skin and internal organs.

Sclerotherapy Removal of benign skin lesions with a sclerosing agent that causes inflammation with fibrosis of tissue.

Scoliosis Lateral curvature of the spine.

Scrub person Prepares the sterile field, surgical supplies, and equipment for surgical procedures; also assists surgeon and physician assistant by passing instruments, suctioning blood, and maintaining the sterile field.

Seborrheic dermatitis Common and chronic inflammatory disorder of the skin that involves the scalp, eyebrows, eyelids, ear canals, nasolabial folds, axillae, and trunk. The cause is unknown.

Sebum Sebaceous glands are found all over the body except on the palms and soles. These glands secrete an oily substance called *sebum*, which softens and lubricates the skin and hair, decreases water loss from the skin in low humidity, and protects the body from infection by killing bacteria.

Secondary hypertension Elevated blood pressure resulting from an identifiable underlying process.

Second spacing Shift in fluid from the vascular space to the interstitial space.

Seizure Episode of excessive and abnormal discharge of electrical activity within the central nervous system.

Semen Fluid containing sperm secreted by the male reproductive system glands.

Seminoma Tumor from seminal or germ tissue.

Sepsis Life-threatening organ dysfunction caused by dysregulated host response to infection.

Septic arthritis Type of arthritis that develops when a joint space is invaded by a pathogen.

Septic shock One part of a progressive syndrome called *systemic inflammatory response syndrome (SIRS)*. Beginning with an infection, SIRS progresses to bacteremia, then sepsis, then septic shock, and finally multiple organ failure syndrome.

Septicemia Systemic disease associated with the presence of bacteria or their toxins in the blood.

Seroconversion Antibody response to a disease or vaccine.

Serum bicarbonate (HCO_3^-) Reflects the renal regulation of acid–base balance; often called the metabolic component of arterial blood gases. The normal HCO_3^- value is 22 to 26 mEq/L.

Severe acute respiratory syndrome (SARS) Lower respiratory illness of unknown etiology; spread by close person-to-person contact.

Sex chromosomes Chromosomes X or Y that indicate gender.

Sexually transmitted infection (STI; sexually transmitted disease, venereal disease) Any infection transmitted by sexual contact, including vaginal, oral, and anal intercourse.

Shigellosis (bacillary dysentery) Acute bowel infection caused by microorganisms of the *Shigella* genus.

Shingles See *Herpes zoster*.

Shock Clinical syndrome characterized by a systemic imbalance between oxygen supply and demand. This imbalance results in a state of inadequate blood flow to the peripheral tissues, causing life-threatening cellular dysfunction, hypotension, and oliguria.

Sickle cell anemia Hereditary, chronic hemolytic anemia characterized by episodes of sickling, during which RBCs become abnormally crescent shaped.

Sickle cell crisis Severe episodes of fever and intense pain that are the hallmark of sickle cell anemia.

Sickle cell disease Hereditary, chronic hemolytic anemia; characterized by episodes of *sickling*, during which RBCs become abnormally crescent shaped. The disorder is transmitted as an autosomal recessive genetic defect.

Sinusitis Inflammation of the mucous membranes of one or more of the sinuses.

Sjögren's syndrome Autoimmune disorder that causes inflammation and dysfunction of exocrine glands throughout the body.

Skeletal traction Application of a pulling force through placement of pins into the bone.

Skin graft Surgical method of detaching skin from a donor site and placing it in a recipient site, where it develops a new blood supply from the base of the wound.

Skin tags Soft papules on a pedicle.

Skin traction Traction in which the cradle-like sleeve placed around the extremity exerts its pulling force through the patient's skin.

Sleep Reversible disengagement from the environment; most humans sleep with their eyes closed, in a recumbent position, with regular breathing.

Sleep hygiene Series of practices and habits that help an individual achieve quality sleep.

Social determinants of health As defined by the World Health Organization, the conditions in which people are "born, grow, work, live, and age, and the wider set of forces and systems shaping the conditions of daily life."

Somatic cell Any cell in the body that is not a sex cell (ova and sperm).

Somatic pain Pain arising from nerve receptors originating in the skin or close to the surface of the body.

Somogyi phenomenon Morning rise in blood glucose to hyperglycemic levels following an episode of nocturnal hypoglycemia and a counterregulatory hormone response.

Spasticity Increased muscle tone in diseases involving the corticospinal motor tract.

Spermatocele Mobile, usually painless mass containing dead spermatozoa that forms in the epididymis.

Spinal cord injury (SCI) Injury to spinal cord, usually due to trauma.

Spinal cord tumors Benign or malignant, primary or metastatic tumor of the spinal cord.

Spinal shock Temporary loss of reflex function below the level of injury to the spinal cord.

Splenomegaly Enlargement of the spleen.

Sprain Tearing or stretching of a ligament that results from a twisting motion.

Sprue Chronic primary disorder of the small intestine in which the absorption of nutrients, particularly fats, is impaired.

Squamous cell carcinoma Malignant tumor of the squamous epithelium of the skin or mucous membranes.

Standard Statement or criterion that can be used by a profession and by the general public to measure quality of practice.

Starvation Inadequate dietary intake; the condition of being without food for long periods of time.

Statistical analysis Manipulation and testing of data in quantitative studies to determine if changes seen are due to the experiment or due to chance.

Status asthmaticus Severe, prolonged asthma that does not respond to routine treatment. Without aggressive therapy, status asthmaticus can lead to respiratory failure with hypoxemia, hypercapnia, and acidosis.

Status epilepticus Continuous seizure activity with only very short periods of calm occurring between intense and persistent seizures.

Steatorrhea Greasy, frothy, yellow stools resulting from excess fat in the feces.

Stem cell transplant (SCT) Alternative to bone marrow transplant. SCT results in complete and sustained replacement of the recipient's blood cell lines (WBCs, RBCs, and platelets) with cells derived from the donor stem cells. Donors must have tissue that is closely matched with that of the recipient.

Stem cells (hemocytoblasts) Bone marrow precursor cells for all blood cells.

Stenosis Condition where valve leaflets fuse together and are unable to open or close fully.

Stevens-Johnson syndrome A rare and serious condition of epidermal necrosis usually caused by an unpredictable reaction to medications or an infection.

Stoma Surface opening.

Stomatitis Inflammation of the oral mucosa.

Straight traction Pulling force applied in a straight line to the injured body part resting on the bed.

Strain Stretching or tearing of muscle fibers that results in bleeding into the tissues.

Stress incontinence Loss of usually less than 50 mL of urine occurring with increased abdominal pressure.

Stress-induced (erosive) gastritis Inflammation and superficial erosions of the gastric mucosa that may occur as a complication of other life-threatening conditions such as shock, severe trauma, major surgery, sepsis, burns, or head injury.

Striae Line above or below tissue that differs in color and texture from surrounding tissue.

Stridor High-pitched, harsh inspiratory sound indicative of upper airway obstruction.

Stroke (brain attack, cerebrovascular accident, CVA) Condition in which neurologic deficits occur as a result of decreased blood flow to a focal (localized) area of brain tissue from a blood clot, an embolus, or a cerebral vessel rupture.

Stroke volume (SV) Amount of blood pumped into the aorta with each contraction of the left ventricle.

Subdural hematoma Localized mass of blood that collects between the dura mater and the arachnoid mater.

Subluxation Partial separation (or dislocation) of the bones of a joint.

Substance abuse Use of any chemical in a fashion inconsistent with medical or culturally defined social norms despite physical, psychologic, or social adverse effects.

Substance dependence Severe condition occurring when the use of a chemical substance is no longer under an individual's control for at least 3 months. Continued use of the substance usually persists despite adverse effects on the person's physical condition, psychologic health, and interpersonal relationships (used interchangeably with addiction).

Substance use disorder (SUD) Disorder occurring when the recurrent use of alcohol and/or drugs causes clinically and functionally significant impairment, such as health problems, disability, and failure to meet major responsibilities at work, school, or home. According to DSM-5, the diagnosis of SUD is based on evidence of impaired control, social impairment, risky use, and pharmacological criteria.

Sudden cardiac death (SCD) Unexpected death occurring within 1 hour of the onset of cardiovascular symptoms.

Sundowning Behavioral change in Alzheimer disease characterized by increased agitation, time disorientation, and wandering during afternoon and evening hours.

Superficial burn Burn involving only the epidermal layer of the skin; most often results from damage from sunburn, ultraviolet light, minor flash injury (from a sudden ignition or explosion), or mild radiation burn associated with cancer treatment.

Surfactant Lipoprotein produced by the alveolar cells; interferes with adhesion of water molecules, reducing surface tension and helping to expand lungs.

Surge capacity Healthcare system's ability to rapidly expand beyond normal services to meet the increased demand for qualified personnel, medical care, and public health in the event of a large-scale disaster.

Surgery Invasive medical procedure performed to diagnose or treat illness, injury, or deformity. Although surgery is a medical treatment, the nurse assumes an active role in caring for the patient before, during, and after surgery.

Surgical debridement Process of excising a wound to the level of fascia (fascial excision) or sequentially removing thin slices of a burn wound to the level of viable tissue (sequential excision).

Surgical site infection (SSI) Infections that develop at surgical sites despite sterile precautions.

Surveillance Collecting and analyzing data to establish a baseline and determine a point at which there is a change or trend in the health of the population.

Syndrome of inappropriate ADH secretion (SIADH) Disorder characterized by high levels of ADH in the absence of serum hypo-osmolality. Manifestations of SIADH occur as a result of water retention, hyponatremia, and serum hypo-osmolality. Blood volume expands, but the plasma is diluted.

Synovitis Inflammation of the synovial membrane lining the articular capsule of a joint.

Syphilis Sexually transmitted infection caused by a spirochete that may invade almost any body tissue or organ. It enters the body through a break in the skin or mucous membranes, and can be transferred to the fetus through the placental circulation.

Systemic lupus erythematosus (SLE) Chronic, inflammatory immune complex connective tissue disease.

Systemic sclerosis (scleroderma) Hardening of the skin; a chronic disease characterized by the formation of excess fibrous connective tissue and diffuse fibrosis of the skin and internal organs.

Systole Phase during which the ventricles contract and eject blood into the pulmonary and systemic circuits.

Systolic blood pressure Arterial pressure wave produced by ventricular contraction (systole); averages 120 mmHg in healthy adults.

T lymphocytes (T cells) Type of lymphocyte that matures in the thymus gland.

Tachycardia Heart rate exceeding 100 beats per minute.

Tachypnea Abnormally rapid respiratory rate.

Tendonitis Inflammation of a tendon.

Tension headache Poorly localized headache characterized by ill-defined bilateral head aching, tightness, pressure, or a viselike feeling.

Tension pneumothorax Condition in which an injury to the chest allows air to enter but not escape the pleural cavity.

Terrorism Defined by the U.S. Department of Defense as the "calculated use of violence or the threat of violence to inculcate fear; intended to coerce or to intimidate governments or societies in the pursuit of goals that are generally political, religious or ideological."

Testicular torsion Twisting of the testes and spermatic cord.

Testosterone Male hormone produced in the testes.

Tetanus Disorder of the nervous system caused by a neurotoxin elaborated by *Clostridium tetani*.

Tetany Tonic muscular spasms.

Tetraplegia (formerly called quadriplegia) Injury to cervical segments of the cord, thus impairing function of the arms, trunk, legs, and pelvic organs.

Thalassemia Inherited disorder of hemoglobin synthesis in which either the alpha or beta chains of the hemoglobin molecule are missing or defective.

Third spacing Accumulation and sequestration of trapped extracellular fluid in an actual or potential body space as a result of disease or injury.

Thoracentesis Invasive procedure in which fluid (or occasionally air) is removed from the pleural space with a needle.

Thoracotomy Incision of the chest wall to gain access to the lung for surgery.

Thrill Palpable vibration over the precordium or an artery.

Thromboangiitis obliterans (Buerger disease) Occlusive vascular disease involving inflammation, spasm, and clot formation in small- and medium-sized peripheral arteries.

Thrombocytopenia Platelet count of less than 100 per milliliter of blood.

Thromboembolus Thrombus that breaks loose from the vessel wall.

Thrombophlebitis See *Venous thrombosis*.

Thrombotic cerebrovascular accident Cerebrovascular accident caused by occlusion of a vessel by a thrombus (a blood clot) on the interior wall of an artery.

Thrombus Blood clot that adheres to a vessel wall.

Thrust Visible pulsation.

Thyroid crisis or storm Extreme state of hyperthyroidism that is rare today because of improved diagnosis and treatment methods. Those affected are usually people with untreated hyperthyroidism (most often Graves' disease) and people with hyperthyroidism who have experienced a stressor, such as an infection, trauma, untreated diabetic ketoacidosis, or manipulation of the thyroid gland during surgery. Thyroid crisis is a life-threatening condition.

Thyroidectomy Surgical removal of the thyroid gland.

Thyroiditis Inflammation of the thyroid gland.

Thyrotoxicosis Another term for hyperthyroidism.

Tidal volume (TV) Amount of air (approximately 500 mL) moved in and out of the lungs with each normal, quiet breath.

Tinea capitis Fungal infection of the scalp.

Tinea corporis Fungal infection of the body.

Tinea pedis Fungal infection of the toenails and feet.

Tinnitus Perception of sound such as ringing, buzzing, or roaring in the ears.

Titrate To increase or decrease the dose in small increments.

Tolerable upper intake level (UL) Maximum level of daily nutrient intake that is likely to pose no risk of adverse effects.

Tolerance Cumulative state in which a particular dose of a chemical elicits a smaller response than before. With increased tolerance, the individual needs higher and higher doses to obtain the desired effect.

Tonic-clonic seizures Alternating contraction (tonic phase) and relaxation (clonic phase) of muscles during seizure activity.

Tonsillitis Acute inflammation of the palatine tonsils.

Tophi Small white nodules in subcutaneous tissue composed of urate deposits resulting from gout.

Total colectomy Surgical removal of the entire colon.

Total gastrectomy Removal of the entire stomach.

Total hip arthroplasty (THA) Replacement of both the femoral head and the acetabulum.

Total parenteral nutrition (TPN) Intravenous administration of carbohydrates (high concentrations of dextrose), protein (amino acids), electrolytes, vitamins, minerals, and fat emulsions.

Toxic epidermal necrolysis (TEN) Rare, life-threatening disease in which the epidermis peels off the dermis in sheets, leaving large areas of denuded skin.

Toxic megacolon Condition characterized by acute motor paralysis and dilation of the colon.

Traction Application of a straightening or pulling force to return or maintain the fractured bones in normal anatomic position.

Transcutaneous electrical nerve stimulation (TENS) Unit that consists of a low-voltage transmitter connected by wires to electrodes that are placed by the patient as directed by the physical therapist. The patient experiences a gentle tapping or vibrating sensation over the electrodes. The patient can adjust the voltage to achieve maximum pain relief.

Transdermal Medication absorbed through the skin without injection.

Transfusion Infusion of blood or blood components.

Transgender An umbrella term that covers a range of identities that transgress the social gender norms, including people whose gender identity differs from their anatomical sex or whose gender expression varies significantly from what is traditionally associated with that sex.

Transient ischemic attack (TIA) Brief period of localized cerebral ischemia that causes neurologic deficits lasting for less than 24 hours.

Transitional care Interventions designed to improve the ability of patients and caregivers to manage care needs in preparation for transitions from one healthcare setting to another or to home.

Transjugular intrahepatic portosystemic shunt (TIPS) Used to relieve portal hypertension and its complications of esophageal varices and ascites. A channel is created through the liver tissue using a needle inserted transcutaneously; an expandable metal stent is inserted into this channel to allow blood to flow directly from the portal vein into the hepatic vein, bypassing the cirrhotic liver. The shunt relieves pressure in esophageal varices and allows better control of fluid retention with diuretic therapy. Generally it is used as a short-term measure until liver transplant is performed.

Translocation Joining of a part of or a whole chromosome to another separate chromosome.

Trauma Injury to human tissues and organs resulting from the transfer of energy from the environment.

Traumatic brain injury (TBI) Traumatic insult to the brain capable of causing physical, intellectual, emotional, social, and vocational changes.

Tremors Rhythmic movement.

Triage Means "sorting"; continuous process in which patient priorities are reassigned as needed treatments, time, and the condition of the patients change.

Tricuspid valve Valve between the right atrium and right ventricle of the heart; prevents blood from flowing backward into the atrium.

Trigeminal neuralgia (tic douloureux) Chronic disease of the trigeminal cranial nerve (cranial nerve V) that causes severe facial pain.

Triglycerides Molecules of glycerol with fatty acids used to transport and store fats in body tissues.

Triple Aim Initiative launched by the Institute of Health Improvement aimed at simultaneously improving the patient care experience, improving the health of the population, and reducing the per capita costs of healthcare.

Trisomy 21 Possessing three chromosomes instead of the usual two as in trisomy 21 or Down syndrome where an additional copy of chromosome 21 is present.

Trousseau sign Contraction of the hand and fingers (carpal spasm) in response to occlusion of the blood supply by a blood pressure cuff; caused by decreased blood calcium levels.

Tuberculosis (TB) Chronic, recurrent infectious disease caused by *Mycobacterium tuberculosis*; usually affects the lungs, although any organ can be affected.

Tumor marker A protein molecule detectable in serum or other body fluids; used as a biochemical indicator of the presence of a malignancy.

Tympanoplasty Surgical reconstruction of the middle ear.

Type 1 diabetes One of two types of diabetes characterized by the destruction of beta cells, usually leading to absolute insulin deficiency.

Type 2 diabetes One of two types of diabetes, the characteristics of which may range from predominantly insulin resistance with relative insulin deficiency to a predominantly secretory defect with insulin resistance. There is no immune destruction of beta cells.

Ulcer Lesion of the skin or mucous membranes.

Ulcerative colitis Chronic inflammatory bowel disorder of the mucosa and submucosa of the colon and rectum.

Ultrafiltration Removal of excess body water using a hydrostatic pressure gradient.

Uniform Anatomical Gift Act Legislation that requires people to be informed about their options related to organ donation.

Unilateral neglect State in which a patient is unaware of and inattentive to one side of the body.

Upper body obesity (central obesity) Excess intra-abdominal fat characterized by a waist-to-hip ratio greater than 1 in men and 0.8 in women.

Urea End product of protein metabolism, eliminated in the urine.

Uremia Literally "urine in the blood"; the syndrome or group of symptoms associated with end-stage renal failure.

Ureteral stent Thin catheter inserted into the ureter to provide for urine flow and ureteral support.

Ureteroplasty Surgical repair of a ureter.

Urgency Sudden, compelling need to urinate.

Urinary calculi Calculi or stones in the urinary tract.

Urinary diversion Procedure to provide for urine collection and drainage following cystectomy. The most common urinary diversion is the ileal conduit.

Urinary drainage system Ureters, urinary bladder, and urethra.

Urinary incontinence (UI) Involuntary urination.

Urinary retention Incomplete emptying of the bladder.

Urine ketone tests Used to detect the presence of ketones in the urine.

Urolithiasis Development of stones within the urinary tract.

Urticaria Hives.

Vaccine Suspensions of whole or fractionated bacteria or viruses that have been treated to make them nonpathogenic.

Validity Soundness of the scientific methods used in a study including control to reduce bias. Instrument validity describes how well an instrument measures the concept or variable it is supposed to measure.

Valsalva maneuver Closing the glottis and contracting the diaphragm and abdominal muscles to increase intra-abdominal pressure.

Valvular heart disease Interference of blood flow to, within, and from the heart.

Vancomycin intermediate-resistant *Staphylococcus aureus* (VISA) Form of *S. aureus* with intermediate resistance to vancomycin.

Varicocele Dilation of the pampiniform venous complex of the spermatic cord.

Varicose veins Irregular, tortuous veins with incompetent valves.

Vasectomy Sterilization procedure in which a portion of the spermatic cord is removed.

Vasoconstriction Smooth muscle contraction that narrows the vessel lumen.

Vasodilation Smooth muscle relaxation that expands the vessel lumen.

Vasogenic shock See *Neurogenic shock*.

Venous thrombosis (thrombophlebitis) Blood clot (thrombus) formation on the wall of a vein, accompanied by inflammation of the vein wall and obstructed venous blood flow.

Ventilator-associated pneumonia Preventable secondary complication from intubation and mechanical support.

Vertigo Sensation of whirling or rotation.

Very-low-calorie diet (VLCD) Protein-sparing modified fast (400 to 800 kcal/day or less) under close medical supervision that may be used to treat significant obesity.

Vesicoureteral reflux Condition in which urine moves from the bladder back toward the kidney.

Visceral pain Pain arising from body organs. It is dull and poorly localized because of the low number of nociceptors.

Vital capacity Sum of TV (tidal volume) + IRV (inspiratory reserve volume) + ERV (expiratory reserve volume); approximately 4500 mL in healthy patients.

Vitamin B_{12} deficiency anemia Anemia due to inadequate vitamin B_{12} consumption or impaired absorption.

Vitiligo Abnormal patchy loss of melanin from the skin.

Volatile acids Acids eliminated from the body as a gas.

Volkmann contracture Common complication of elbow fractures; can result from unresolved compartment syndrome. Arterial blood flow decreases, leading to ischemia, degeneration, and contracture of the muscle.

Vomiting Forceful expulsion of the contents of the upper GI tract resulting from contraction of muscles in the gut and abdominal wall.

Von Willebrand disease Most common hereditary bleeding disorder, caused by a deficit of or defective von Willebrand factor.

Warm zone Adjacent to the hot zone of a disaster, the area where decontamination of victims or triage and emergency treatment takes place; also called the *control zone*.

Warts (verrucae) Lesions of the skin caused by the human papillomavirus.

Weaning Process of removing the patient from ventilator support and reestablishing spontaneous, independent respirations.

Weber test Test of hearing; a vibrating tuning fork is placed on the midline of the top of the head and the patient is asked to describe where the sound is heard. Normally, sound is heard equally in both ears.

Wellness Integrated method of functioning oriented toward maximizing an individual's potential within the environment.

Wernicke encephalopathy Caused by thiamine (B_1) deficiency and characterized by nystagmus, ptosis, ataxia, confusion, coma, and possible death. Thiamine deficiency is common in chronic alcoholism.

Wheezes Continuous, musical sounds caused by narrowing of the lumen in a respiratory passage.

White blood cells (WBCs, leukocytes) Blood cells that contribute to the body's defense against microorganisms.

Wild-type gene Most common type of gene; designated as normal.

Withdrawal Cessation of use of a substance to which an individual has become addicted.

Withdrawal symptoms Constellation of signs and symptoms that occurs in physically dependent individuals when they discontinue drug use.

X-linked Any gene found on the X chromosome or traits determined by such genes; also refers to the specific mode of inheritance of such genes. One altered gene on an X chromosome in a male can produce disease, such as hemophilia.

X-linked dominant Rare conditions with differential gender outcomes from an altered gene on the X chromosome. For example, if a male is affected, the condition is severe and often lethal. A family history of multiple male miscarriages may be a sign of an X-linked dominant condition.

X-linked recessive Result of an altered gene on the X chromosome. All males with this alteration will express the consequences due to only having one X chromosome. Females may not express the consequence if they have a second normal X chromosome.

Xenograft Transplant from an animal species to a human.

Xeroderma Chronic skin condition characterized by dry, rough skin.

Xerosis Dry skin.

Xerostomia Excessive dryness of the mucous membranes due to chemotherapy or radiation.

Zollinger–Ellison syndrome Peptic ulcer disease caused by a gastrinoma, or gastrin-secreting tumor of the pancreas, stomach, or intestines.

Credits

FM

ix: Gerene Bauldoff; Paula Gubrud; **x:** Margaret-Ann Carno

Unit Openers

cov, 0001: Natalia Gornyakova/Shutterstock; **0051**: Sean Lema/Shutterstock; **177**: NadyaEugene/Shutterstock; **451**: Maridav/Shutterstock; **cov, 547**: isarescheewin/Shutterstock; **633**: De Visu/Shutterstock; **853**: Diana Grytsku/Shutterstock; **951**: kovop58/Shutterstock; **1215**: rdonar/Shutterstock; **1393**: GaudiLab/Shutterstock; **cov, 1521**: Pavel1964/Shutterstock; **1671**: FreeBirdPhotos/Shutterstock; **1739**: Media Union/Shutterstock

Chapter 01

003: Tyler Olson/Shutterstock; Monkey Business Images/Shutterstock; **004:** Lighthunter/Shutterstock; GagliardiImages/Shutterstock; **007:** Pearson Education, Inc.; **013:** Photographee.eu/Shutterstock; **014:** Monkey Business Images/Shutterstock; **015:** Val lawless/Shutterstock

Chapter 02

024: PEARSON EDUCATION, . ., NURSING: A CONCEPT-BASED APPROACH TO LEARNING, VOLUME II, 3rd Ed., ©2019. Reprinted and Electronically reproduced by permission of Pearson Education, Inc., New York, NY.; **026:** Adriaticfoto/Shutterstock; **027:** Cecilie_Arcurs/E+/Getty Images; **029:** Steve Scold/Alamy Stock Photo; **030:** PEARSON EDUCATION, . ., NURSING: A CONCEPT-BASED APPROACH TO LEARNING, VOLUME I, 3rd Ed., ©2019. Reprinted and Electronically reproduced by permission of Pearson Education, Inc., New York, NY; **038:** Dmitry Lobanov/123RF; **039:** Corepics VOF/Shutterstock; **041:** Brian Eichhorn/Shutterstock; **042:** Alexander Raths/Shutterstock; Lisa F. Young/Shutterstock

Chapter 03

054: PEARSON EDUCATION, . ., NURSING: A CONCEPT-BASED APPROACH TO LEARNING, VOLUME II, 3rd Ed., ©2019. Reprinted and Electronically reproduced by permission of Pearson Education, Inc., New York, NY.; SORENSON, MATTHEW; QUINN, LAURETTA; KLEIN, DIANE, PATHOPHYSIOLOGY: CONCEPTS OF HUMANDISEASE, 1st Ed., ©2018. Reprinted and Electronically reproduced by permission of Pearson Education, Inc., NewYork, NY.; **058:** SORENSON, MATTHEW; QUINN, LAURETTA; KLEIN, DIANE, PATHOPHYSIOLOGY: CONCEPTS OF HUMANDISEASE, 1st Ed., ©2018. Reprinted and Electronically reproduced by permission of Pearson Education, Inc., NewYork, NY.; **060:** SORENSON, MATTHEW; QUINN, LAURETTA; KLEIN, DIANE, PATHOPHYSIOLOGY: CONCEPTS OF HUMANDISEASE, 1st Ed., ©2018. Reprinted and Electronically reproduced by permission of Pearson Education, Inc., NewYork, NY.; **062:** SORENSON, MATTHEW; QUINN, LAURETTA; KLEIN, DIANE, PATHOPHYSIOLOGY: CONCEPTS OF HUMANDISEASE, 1st Ed., ©2018. Reprinted and Electronically reproduced by permission of Pearson Education, Inc., NewYork, NY.

Chapter 04

070: Cathy Yeulet/123RF; **072:** PEARSON EDUCATION, . ., NURSING: A CONCEPT-BASED APPROACH TO LEARNING, VOLUME II, 3rd Ed., ©2019. Reprinted and Electronically reproduced by permission of Pearson Education, Inc., New York, NY.; PEARSON EDUCATION, . ., NURSING: A CONCEPT-BASED APPROACH TO LEARNING, VOLUME II, 3rd Ed., ©2019. Reprinted and Electronically reproduced by permission of Pearson Education, Inc., New York, NY.; **077:** CALLAHAN, BARBARA, CLINICAL NURSING SKILLS: A CONCEPT-BASED APPROACH, VOLUME III, 3rd Ed., ©2019. Reprinted and Electronically reproduced by permission of Pearson Education, Inc., New York, NY.; **078:** Image of Flowtron® Excel used with permission of Arjo Inc.; **079:** Rick Brady/Pearson Education, Inc.; Rick Brady/Pearson Education, Inc.; **085:** Tom Tracy Photography/Alamy Stock Photo; Tyler Olson/Fotolia; **094:** SORENSON, MATTHEW; QUINN, LAURETTA; KLEIN, DIANE, PATHOPHYSIOLOGY: CONCEPTS OF HUMANDISEASE, 1st Ed., ©2018. Reprinted and Electronically reproduced by permission of Pearson Education, Inc., NewYork, NY.; SORENSON, MATTHEW; QUINN, LAURETTA; KLEIN, DIANE, PATHOPHYSIOLOGY: CONCEPTS OF HUMANDISEASE, 1st Ed., ©2018. Reprinted and Electronically reproduced by permission of Pearson Education, Inc., NewYork, NY.; **095:** Rick Brady/Pearson Education, Inc.; Rick Brady/Pearson Education, Inc.; Chidkamol Nanta/Shutterstock

Chapters 04, 09

093, 206: Reprinted from WHO's cancer pain ladder for adults © 2018 WHO

Chapter 05

106: sturti/E+/Getty Images; David S. Holloway/Getty Images; **110:** Mark Gomez/Shutterstock; James.Pintar/Shutterstock; **112:** SORENSON, MATTHEW; QUINN, LAURETTA; KLEIN, DIANE, PATHOPHYSIOLOGY: CONCEPTS OF HUMANDISEASE, 1st Ed., ©2018. Reprinted and Electronically reproduced by permission of Pearson Education, Inc., NewYork, NY.; **117:** Pearson Education, Inc.

Chapter 06

127: mikedabell/GettyImages; **129:** PEARSON EDUCATION, . ., NURSING: A CONCEPT-BASED APPROACH TO LEARNING, VOLUME I, 3rd Ed., ©2019. Reprinted and Electronically reproduced by permission of Pearson Education, Inc., New York, NY; **134:** Aliaksandr Barouski/Shutterstock

Chapter 07

158: Sara Armas/Shutterstock; **159:** Brian L Stetson/Shutterstock; **160:** John Minchillo/AP Images; **161:** Elise Amendola/AP Images; **164:** Smallcreative/Shutterstock

Chapter 08

179: PEARSON EDUCATION, . ., NURSING: A CONCEPT-BASED APPROACH TO LEARNING, VOLUME I, 3rd Ed.,©2019. Reprinted and Electronically reproduced by permission of Pearson Education, Inc., New York, NY.; **180:** Mediscan/Alamy Stock Photo; **182:** BALL, JANE W.; BINDLER, RUTH C.; COWEN, KAY J., CHILD HEALTH NURSING, 3rd Ed., ©2014. Reprinted and Electronically reproduced by permission of Pearson Education, Inc., New York, NY.; **183:** Fortunata/Splash News/Alamy Stock Photo; BALL, JANE W.; BINDLER, RUTH C.; COWEN, KAY J., CHILD HEALTH NURSING, 3rd Ed., ©2014. Reprinted and Electronically reproduced by permission of Pearson Education, Inc., New York, NY.; **184:** BALL, JANE W.; BINDLER, RUTH C.; COWEN, KAY J., CHILD HEALTH NURSING, 3rd Ed., ©2014. Reprinted and Electronically reproduced by permission of Pearson Education, Inc., New York, NY.; **185:** Sacramento Bee/ZUMA Press Inc/Alamy Stock Photo; **189:** Ball, Jane W., Bindler, Ruth McGillis W., Cowen, Kay J., Child Health Nursing: Partnering with Children and Families, 3rd, © 2014. Reproduced by permission of Pearson Education, Inc., Upper Saddle River, New Jersey. ; KLUG, WILLIAMS.; CUMMINGS, MICHAEL R., CONCEPTS OF GENETICS, 7th, ©2003. Printed and Electronically reproduced by permission of Pearson Education, Inc., Upper Saddle River, New Jersey.

Chapter 09

199: SORENSON, MATTHEW; QUINN, LAURETTA; KLEIN, DIANE, PATHOPHYSIOLOGY: CONCEPTS OF HUMANDISEASE, 1st Ed., ©2018. Reprinted and Electronically reproduced by permission of Pearson Education, Inc., NewYork, NY.; **202:** SORENSON, MATTHEW; QUINN, LAURETTA; KLEIN, DIANE, PATHOPHYSIOLOGY: CONCEPTS OF HUMANDISEASE, 1st Ed., ©2018. Reprinted and Electronically reproduced by permission of Pearson Education, Inc., NewYork, NY.; **203:** SORENSON, MATTHEW; QUINN, LAURETTA; KLEIN, DIANE, PATHOPHYSIOLOGY: CONCEPTS OF HUMANDISEASE, 1st Ed., ©2018.

Reprinted and Electronically reproduced by permission of Pearson Education, Inc., NewYork, NY.; **212:** Roy Ramsey/Pearson Education; **213:** Praisaeng/Shutterstock; **217:** SORENSON, MATTHEW; QUINN, LAURETTA; KLEIN, DIANE, PATHOPHYSIOLOGY: CONCEPTS OF HUMANDISEASE, 1st Ed., ©2018. Reprinted and Electronically reproduced by permission of Pearson Education, Inc., NewYork, NY.

Chapter 10

228: SORENSON, MATTHEW; QUINN, LAURETTA; KLEIN, DIANE, PATHOPHYSIOLOGY: CONCEPTS OF HUMAN DISEASE, 1st Ed., ©2019. Reprinted and Electronically reproduced by permission of Pearson Education, Inc., New York, NY.; **229:** MARTINI, FREDERIC H.; NATH, JUDI L; RARTHOLOMEW, EDWIN F., FUNDAMENTALS OF ANATOMY & PHYSIOLOGY, 9th, Fig. 27.2, p. 1001 ©2012. Printed and Electronically reproduced by permission of Pearson Education, Inc., Upper Saddle River, New Jersey.; **233:** SORENSON, MATTHEW; QUINN, LAURETTA; KLEIN, DIANE, PATHOPHYSIOLOGY: CONCEPTS OF HUMAN DISEASE, 1st Ed., ©2019. Reprinted and Electronically reproduced by permission of Pearson Education, Inc., New York, NY.; **234:** SORENSON, MATTHEW; QUINN, LAURETTA; KLEIN, DIANE, PATHOPHYSIOLOGY: CONCEPTS OF HUMAN DISEASE, 1st Ed., ©2019. Reprinted and Electronically reproduced by permission of Pearson Education, Inc., New York, NY.; **236:** PEARSON EDUCATION, . ., NURSING: A CONCEPT-BASED APPROACH TO LEARNING, VOLUME I, 3rd Ed.,©2019. Reprinted and Electronically reproduced by permission of Pearson Education, Inc., New York, NY.; **256:** SORENSON, MATTHEW; QUINN, LAURETTA; KLEIN, DIANE, PATHOPHYSIOLOGY: CONCEPTS OF HUMAN DISEASE, 1st Ed., ©2019. Reprinted and Electronically reproduced by permission of Pearson Education, Inc., New York, NY.; **257:** SORENSON, MATTHEW; QUINN, LAURETTA; KLEIN, DIANE, PATHOPHYSIOLOGY: CONCEPTS OF HUMAN DISEASE, 1st Ed., ©2019. Reprinted and Electronically reproduced by permission of Pearson Education, Inc., New York, NY.; **266:** SORENSON, MATTHEW; QUINN, LAURETTA; KLEIN, DIANE, PATHOPHYSIOLOGY: CONCEPTS OF HUMAN DISEASE, 1st Ed., ©2019. Reprinted and Electronically reproduced by permission of Pearson Education, Inc., New York, NY.

Chapter 11

287: SORENSON, MATTHEW; QUINN, LAURETTA; KLEIN, DIANE, PATHOPHYSIOLOGY: CONCEPTS OF HUMANDISEASE, 1st Ed., ©2018. Reprinted and Electronically reproduced by permission of Pearson Education, Inc., NewYork, NY.; **288:** PEARSON EDUCATION, . ., NURSING: A CONCEPT-BASED APPROACH TO LEARNING, VOLUME II, 3rd Ed., ©2019. Reprinted and Electronically reproduced by permission of Pearson Education, Inc., New York, NY.; **291:** Kuttig - People/Alamy Stock Photo; paul cox/Alamy Stock Photo; Hercules Robinson/Alamy Stock Photo; Kathie Nichols/Alamy Stock Photo; **293:** SORENSON, MATTHEW; QUINN, LAURETTA; KLEIN, DIANE, PATHOPHYSIOLOGY: CONCEPTS OF HUMANDISEASE, 1st Ed., ©2018. Reprinted and Electronically reproduced by permission of Pearson Education, Inc., NewYork, NY.; **294:** Craig Stocks Arts/Shutterstock; ZUMA Press Inc/Alamy Stock Photo; **300:** Photo of the RotoRest® Critical Care Therapy System is copyrighted and used by permission of ArjoHuntLeigh Inc.; **305:** SORENSON, MATTHEW; QUINN, LAURETTA; KLEIN, DIANE, PATHOPHYSIOLOGY: CONCEPTS OF HUMANDISEASE, 1st Ed., ©2018. Reprinted and Electronically reproduced by permission of Pearson Education, Inc., NewYork, NY.; **307:** SORENSON, MATTHEW; QUINN, LAURETTA; KLEIN, DIANE, PATHOPHYSIOLOGY: CONCEPTS OF HUMANDISEASE, 1st Ed., ©2018. Reprinted and Electronically reproduced by permission of Pearson Education, Inc., NewYork, NY.; PEARSON EDUCATION, . ., NURSING: A CONCEPT-BASED APPROACH TO LEARNING, VOLUME II, 3rd Ed., ©2019. Reprinted and Electronically reproduced by permission of Pearson Education, Inc., New York, NY.; **315:** PEARSON EDUCATION, . ., NURSING: A CONCEPT-BASED APPROACH TO LEARNING, VOLUME II, 3rd Ed., ©2019. Reprinted and Electronically reproduced by permission of Pearson Education, Inc., New York, NY.

Chapter 12

323: PEARSON EDUCATION, . ., NURSING: A CONCEPT-BASED APPROACH TO LEARNING, VOLUME II, 3rd Ed., ©2019. Reprinted and Electronically reproduced by permission of Pearson Education, Inc., New York, NY.; **325:** PEARSON EDUCATION, . ., NURSING: A CONCEPT-BASED APPROACH TO LEARNING, VOLUME II, 3rd Ed., ©2019. Reprinted and Electronically reproduced by permission of Pearson Education, Inc., New York, NY.; PEARSON EDUCATION, . ., NURSING: A CONCEPT-BASED APPROACH TO LEARNING, VOLUME II, 3rd Ed., ©2019. Reprinted and Electronically reproduced by permission of Pearson Education, Inc., New York, NY.; **332:** SORENSON, MATTHEW; QUINN, LAURETTA; KLEIN, DIANE, PATHOPHYSIOLOGY: CONCEPTS OF HUMANDISEASE, 1st Ed., ©2018. Reprinted and Electronically reproduced by permission of Pearson Education, Inc., NewYork, NY.

Chapter 13

367: SORENSON, MATTHEW; QUINN, LAURETTA; KLEIN, DIANE, PATHOPHYSIOLOGY: CONCEPTS OF HUMANDISEASE, 1st Ed., ©2018. Reprinted and Electronically reproduced by permission of Pearson Education, Inc., NewYork, NY.; **368:** SORENSON, MATTHEW; QUINN, LAURETTA; KLEIN, DIANE, PATHOPHYSIOLOGY: CONCEPTS OF HUMANDISEASE, 1st Ed., ©2018. Reprinted and Electronically reproduced by permission of Pearson Education, Inc., NewYork, NY.; **369:** SORENSON, MATTHEW; QUINN, LAURETTA; KLEIN, DIANE, PATHOPHYSIOLOGY: CONCEPTS OF HUMANDISEASE, 1st Ed., ©2018. Reprinted and Electronically reproduced by permission of Pearson Education, Inc., NewYork, NY.; **370:** SORENSON, MATTHEW; QUINN, LAURETTA; KLEIN, DIANE, PATHOPHYSIOLOGY: CONCEPTS OF HUMANDISEASE, 1st Ed., ©2018. Reprinted and Electronically reproduced by permission of Pearson Education, Inc., NewYork, NY.; **372:** Hunna/Shutterstock; **376:** SORENSON, MATTHEW; QUINN, LAURETTA; KLEIN, DIANE, PATHOPHYSIOLOGY: CONCEPTS OF HUMANDISEASE, 1st Ed., ©2018. Reprinted and Electronically reproduced by permission of Pearson Education, Inc., NewYork, NY.; **388:** SORENSON, MATTHEW; QUINN, LAURETTA; KLEIN, DIANE, PATHOPHYSIOLOGY: CONCEPTS OF HUMANDISEASE, 1st Ed., ©2018. Reprinted and Electronically reproduced by permission of Pearson Education, Inc., NewYork, NY.; Nic Bothma/EPA/Newscom; **390:** Mediscan/Alamy Stock Photo; **394:** Mediscan/Alamy Stock Photo; **400:** Science Photo Library/Alamy Stock Photo

Chapter 14

416: SORENSON, MATTHEW; QUINN, LAURETTA; KLEIN, DIANE, PATHOPHYSIOLOGY: CONCEPTS OF HUMAN DISEASE, 1st Ed., ©2018. Reprinted and Electronically reproduced by permission of Pearson Education, Inc., New York, NY.; **418:** Simon Fraser/RVI, Newcastle upon Tyne/Science Source; **429:** © 2018 C. R. Bard, Inc. Used with permission.; © 2018 C. R. Bard, Inc. Used with permission.

Chapter 15

456: Blamb/Shutterstock; MANSEN, THOMAS, PATIENT-FOCUSED ASSESSMENT: THE ART AND SCIENCE OF CLINICAL DATAGATHERING, 1st Ed., ©2015. Reprinted and Electronically reproduced by permission of Pearson Education, Inc.,New York, NY.; **460:** Mediscan/Alamy Stock Photo; Southern Illinois University/Science Source; CLS Digital Arts/Shutterstock; Mediscan/Alamy Stock Photo; Scott Camazine/Science Source; **461:** Akkalak Aiempradit/Shutterstock; **462:** Dr. P. Marazzi/Science Source; SPL/Science Source; MANSEN, THOMAS, PATIENT-FOCUSED ASSESSMENT: THE ART AND SCIENCE OF CLINICAL DATAGATHERING, 1st Ed., ©2015. Reprinted and Electronically reproduced by permission of Pearson Education, Inc.,New York, NY.; **463:** MANSEN, THOMAS, PATIENT-FOCUSED ASSESSMENT: THE ART AND SCIENCE OF CLINICAL DATAGATHERING, 1st Ed., ©2015. Reprinted and Electronically reproduced by permission of Pearson Education, Inc.,New York, NY.

Chapter 16

473: Mediscan/Alamy Stock Photo; Pat Watson/Pearson Education, Inc.; **474:** Mediscan/Alamy Stock Photo; olavs/Shutterstock; **478:** Scott Camazine/Alamy Stock Photo; Dr. P. Marazzi/Science Source; Dr. P. Marazzi/Science Source; **479:** Mediscan/Alamy Stock Photo; **481:** SPL/Science Source; **484:** Dr. P. Marazzi/Science Source; National Archives and Records Administration; Center for Disease Control and Prevention (CDC); **488:** Clinical Photography, Central Manchester University Hospitals NHS Foundation Trust, UK/Science Source; **490:** Mediscan/Alamy Stock Photo; Milan Lipowski/Alamy Stock Photo;

493: Mediscan/Alamy Stock Photo; **495:** Dr. P. Marazzi/Science Source; Dr. P. Marazzi/Science Source; **498:** Dr. P. Marazzi/Science Source; **505:** Mediscan/Alamy Stock Photo; Mediscan/Alamy Stock Photo; Mediscan/Alamy Stock Photo; Scott Camazine/Alamy Stock Photo

Chapter 17

522: Anukool Manoton/Shutterstock; PEARSON EDUCATION, . ., NURSING: A CONCEPT-BASED APPROACH TO LEARNING, VOLUME I, 3rd Ed.,©2019. Reprinted and Electronically reproduced by permission of Pearson Education, Inc., New York, NY.; **523:** Biophoto Associates/Science Source; Dr M.A. Ansary/Science Source; **524:** PEARSON EDUCATION, . ., NURSING: A CONCEPT-BASED APPROACH TO LEARNING, VOLUME I, 3rd Ed.,©2019. Reprinted and Electronically reproduced by permission of Pearson Education, Inc., New York, NY.; PEARSON EDUCATION, . ., NURSING: A CONCEPT-BASED APPROACH TO LEARNING, VOLUME I, 3rd Ed.,©2019. Reprinted and Electronically reproduced by permission of Pearson Education, Inc., New York, NY.; **526:** PEARSON EDUCATION, . ., NURSING: A CONCEPT-BASED APPROACH TO LEARNING, VOLUME I, 3rd Ed.,©2019. Reprinted and Electronically reproduced by permission of Pearson Education, Inc., New York, NY.; **527:** PEARSON EDUCATION, . ., NURSING: A CONCEPT-BASED APPROACH TO LEARNING, VOLUME I, 3rd Ed.,©2019. Reprinted and Electronically reproduced by permission of Pearson Education, Inc., New York, NY.; **530:** PEARSON EDUCATION, . ., NURSING: A CONCEPT-BASED APPROACH TO LEARNING, VOLUME I, 3rd Ed.,©2019. Reprinted and Electronically reproduced by permission of Pearson Education, Inc., New York, NY.; **535:** James Stevenson/Science Source; **536:** Dr. P. Marazzi/Science Source; Leca/Science Source; **538:** Boucharlat/Science Source

Chapter 18

549: SORENSON, MATTHEW; QUINN, LAURETTA; KLEIN, DIANE, PATHOPHYSIOLOGY: CONCEPTS OF HUMAN DISEASE, 1st Ed., ©2019. Reprinted and Electronically reproduced by permission of Pearson Education, Inc., New York, NY.; Alfred Pasieka/Science Source; **550:** Pearson Education, Inc; **551:** annyart/123RF; **555:** Pearson Education, Inc.

Chapter 19

568: Medicshots/Alamy Stock Photo; Chris Pancewicz/Alamy Stock Photo; **581:** SORENSON, MATTHEW; QUINN, LAURETTA; KLEIN, DIANE, PATHOPHYSIOLOGY: CONCEPTS OF HUMAN DISEASE, 1st Ed., ©2019. Reprinted and Electronically reproduced by permission of Pearson Education, Inc., New York, NY.

Chapter 20

596: PEARSON EDUCATION, . ., NURSING: A CONCEPT-BASED APPROACH TO LEARNING, VOLUME I, 3rd Ed.,©2019. Reprinted and Electronically reproduced by permission of Pearson Education, Inc., New York, NY.; **600:** PEARSON EDUCATION, . ., NURSING: A CONCEPT-BASED APPROACH TO LEARNING, VOLUME I, 3rd Ed.,©2019. Reprinted and Electronically reproduced by permission of Pearson Education, Inc., New York, NY.; **608:** Medicshots/Alamy Stock Photo ; **610:** Lisa S./Shutterstock; Dexcom, Inc.; **615:** AJPhoto/Science Source; PEARSON EDUCATION, . ., NURSING: A CONCEPT-BASED APPROACH TO LEARNING, VOLUME I, 3rd Ed.,©2019. Reprinted and Electronically reproduced by permission of Pearson Education, Inc., New York, NY.; **620:** U.S. DEPARTMENT OF AGRICULTURE

Chapter 21

643: PEARSON EDUCATION, . ., NURSING: A CONCEPT-BASED APPROACH TO LEARNING, VOLUME II, 3rd Ed., ©2019. Reprinted and Electronically reproduced by permission of Pearson Education, Inc., New York, NY.; **643:** Pearson Education, Inc.; **645:** KTM_2016/iStock/Getty Images; Pearson Education, Inc.; Pearson Education, Inc.; **646:** Pearson Education, Inc.; Pearson Education, Inc.; **647:** Pearson Education, Inc.; Pearson Education, Inc.; **649:** Karan Bunjean/Shutterstock

Chapter 22

678: PEARSON EDUCATION, . ., NURSING: A CONCEPT-BASED APPROACH TO LEARNING, VOLUME II, 3rd Ed., ©2019. Reprinted and Electronically reproduced by permission of Pearson Education, Inc., New York, NY.; **684:** PEARSON EDUCATION, . ., NURSING: A CONCEPT-BASED APPROACH TO LEARNING, VOLUME I, 3rd Ed., ©2019. Reprinted and Electronically reproduced by permission of Pearson Education, Inc., New York, NY

Chapter 23

697: Cherries/Shutterstock; **701:** Mediscan/Alamy Stock Photo; **705:** PEARSON EDUCATION, . ., NURSING: A CONCEPT-BASED APPROACH TO LEARNING, VOLUME II, 3rd Ed., ©2019. Reprinted and Electronically reproduced by permission of Pearson Education, Inc., New York, NY.; **709:** SORENSON, MATTHEW; QUINN, LAURETTA; KLEIN, DIANE, PATHOPHYSIOLOGY: CONCEPTS OF HUMANDISEASE, 1st Ed., ©2018. Reprinted and Electronically reproduced by permission of Pearson Education, Inc., NewYork, NY.; **716:** PEARSON EDUCATION, . ., NURSING: A CONCEPT-BASED APPROACH TO LEARNING, VOLUME II, 3rd Ed., ©2019. Reprinted and Electronically reproduced by permission of Pearson Education, Inc., New York, NY.; Juan Gaertner/Shutterstock

Chapter 24

765: SORENSON, MATTHEW; QUINN, LAURETTA; KLEIN, DIANE, PATHOPHYSIOLOGY: CONCEPTS OF HUMANDISEASE, 1st Ed., ©2018. Reprinted and Electronically reproduced by permission of Pearson Education, Inc., NewYork, NY.; **766:** PEARSON EDUCATION, . ., NURSING: A CONCEPT-BASED APPROACH TO LEARNING, VOLUME II, 3rd Ed., ©2019. Reprinted and Electronically reproduced by permission of Pearson Education, Inc., New York, NY.; **767:** CNRI/Science Source; Dr. E. Walker/Science Source; Biophoto Associates/Science Source; **768:** PEARSON EDUCATION, . ., NURSING: A CONCEPT-BASED APPROACH TO LEARNING, VOLUME II, 3rd Ed., ©2019. Reprinted and Electronically reproduced by permission of Pearson Education, Inc., New York, NY.; **771:** PEARSON EDUCATION, . ., NURSING: A CONCEPT-BASED APPROACH TO LEARNING, VOLUME II, 3rd Ed., ©2019. Reprinted and Electronically reproduced by permission of Pearson Education, Inc., New York, NY.; **772:** Carol Williams/Pearson Education; **776:** SORENSON, MATTHEW; QUINN, LAURETTA; KLEIN, DIANE, PATHOPHYSIOLOGY: CONCEPTS OF HUMANDISEASE, 1st Ed., ©2018. Reprinted and Electronically reproduced by permission of Pearson Education, Inc., NewYork, NY.; **785:** David M. Martin, M.D./Science Source; David M. Martin, M.D./Science Source; **788:** SORENSON, MATTHEW; QUINN, LAURETTA; KLEIN, DIANE, PATHOPHYSIOLOGY: CONCEPTS OF HUMANDISEASE, 1st Ed., ©2018. Reprinted and Electronically reproduced by permission of Pearson Education, Inc., NewYork, NY.; **789:** PEARSON EDUCATION, . ., NURSING: A CONCEPT-BASED APPROACH TO LEARNING, VOLUME II, 3rd Ed., ©2019. Reprinted and Electronically reproduced by permission of Pearson Education, Inc., New York, NY.; **790:** PEARSON EDUCATION, . ., NURSING: A CONCEPT-BASED APPROACH TO LEARNING, VOLUME II, 3rd Ed., ©2019. Reprinted and Electronically reproduced by permission of Pearson Education, Inc., New York, NY.; **797:** SORENSON, MATTHEW; QUINN, LAURETTA; KLEIN, DIANE, PATHOPHYSIOLOGY: CONCEPTS OF HUMANDISEASE, 1st Ed., ©2018. Reprinted and Electronically reproduced by permission of Pearson Education, Inc., NewYork, NY.; **801:** SORENSON, MATTHEW; QUINN, LAURETTA; KLEIN, DIANE, PATHOPHYSIOLOGY: CONCEPTS OF HUMANDISEASE, 1st Ed., ©2018. Reprinted and Electronically reproduced by permission of Pearson Education, Inc., NewYork, NY.

Chapter 25

810: SORENSON, MATTHEW; QUINN, LAURETTA; KLEIN, DIANE, PATHOPHYSIOLOGY: CONCEPTS OF HUMANDISEASE, 1st Ed., ©2018. Reprinted and Electronically reproduced by permission of Pearson Education, Inc., NewYork, NY.; **811:** SORENSON, MATTHEW; QUINN, LAURETTA; KLEIN, DIANE, PATHOPHYSIOLOGY: CONCEPTS OF HUMANDISEASE, 1st Ed., ©2018. Reprinted and Electronically reproduced by permission of Pearson Education, Inc., NewYork, NY.; **816:** SORENSON, MATTHEW; QUINN, LAURETTA; KLEIN, DIANE, PATHOPHYSIOLOGY: CONCEPTS OF HUMANDISEASE, 1st Ed., ©2018. Reprinted and Electronically reproduced by permission of Pearson Education, Inc., NewYork, NY.; **817:** DONIYER YAKHSHIBAYEV/123RF; Garry Watson/Science Source; Dr. Thomas F. Sellers/Emory University/Centers for Disease Control and Prevention (CDC); **829:** SORENSON, MATTHEW; QUINN, LAURETTA; KLEIN, DIANE, PATHOPHYSIOLOGY: CONCEPTS OF HUMANDISEASE, 1st Ed., ©2018. Reprinted and Electronically reproduced by permission of Pearson Education, Inc., NewYork, NY.; **842:** CNRI/Science Source

Chapter 26

861-862: Pearson Education, Inc.

Chapter 27

874: SORENSON, MATTHEW; QUINN, LAURETTA; KLEIN, DIANE, PATHOPHYSIOLOGY: CONCEPTS OF HUMANDISEASE, 1st Ed., ©2018. Reprinted and Electronically reproduced by permission of Pearson Education, Inc., NewYork, NY.; **881:** PEARSON EDUCATION, . ., NURSING: A CONCEPT-BASED APPROACH TO LEARNING, VOLUME II, 3rd Ed., ©2019. Reprinted and Electronically reproduced by permission of Pearson Education, Inc., New York, NY.; **883:** GARO/PHANIE/Alamy Stock Photo; **898:** Adapted from Your Daily Bladder Diary, National Kidney and Urologic Diseases Information Center, National Institute of Diabetes and Digestive and Kidney Disease, National Institutes of Health.

Chapter 28

906: Arthur Glauberman/Science Source; **918:** Scott Camazine/Alamy Stock Photo; **922:** SORENSON, MATTHEW; QUINN, LAURETTA; KLEIN, DIANE, PATHOPHYSIOLOGY: CONCEPTS OF HUMANDISEASE, 1st Ed., ©2018. Reprinted and Electronically reproduced by permission of Pearson Education, Inc., NewYork, NY.; **928:** PEARSON EDUCATION, . ., NURSING: A CONCEPT-BASED APPROACH TO LEARNING, VOLUME II, 3rd Ed., ©2019. Reprinted and Electronically reproduced by permission of Pearson Education, Inc., New York, NY.; **930:** PEARSON EDUCATION, . ., NURSING: A CONCEPT-BASED APPROACH TO LEARNING, VOLUME II, 3rd Ed., ©2019. Reprinted and Electronically reproduced by permission of Pearson Education, Inc., New York, NY.; **931:** Doikanoi/Shutterstock; PEARSON EDUCATION, . ., NURSING: A CONCEPT-BASED APPROACH TO LEARNING, VOLUME II, 3rd Ed., ©2019. Reprinted and Electronically reproduced by permission of Pearson Education, Inc., New York, NY.; **936:** PEARSON EDUCATION, . ., NURSING: A CONCEPT-BASED APPROACH TO LEARNING, VOLUME II, 3rd Ed., ©2019. Reprinted and Electronically reproduced by permission of Pearson Education, Inc., New York, NY.

Chapter 29

953: PEARSON EDUCATION, . ., NURSING: A CONCEPT-BASED APPROACH TO LEARNING, VOLUME I, 3rd Ed.,©2019. Reprinted and Electronically reproduced by permission of Pearson Education, Inc., New York, NY.; **954:** PEARSON EDUCATION, . ., NURSING: A CONCEPT-BASED APPROACH TO LEARNING, VOLUME I, 3rd Ed.,©2019. Reprinted and Electronically reproduced by permission of Pearson Education, Inc., New York, NY.; **955:** PEARSON EDUCATION, . ., NURSING: A CONCEPT-BASED APPROACH TO LEARNING, VOLUME I, 3rd Ed.,©2019. Reprinted and Electronically reproduced by permission of Pearson Education, Inc., New York, NY.; PEARSON EDUCATION, . ., NURSING: A CONCEPT-BASED APPROACH TO LEARNING, VOLUME I, 3rd Ed.,©2019. Reprinted and Electronically reproduced by permission of Pearson Education, Inc., New York, NY.; **956:** PEARSON EDUCATION, . ., NURSING: A CONCEPT-BASED APPROACH TO LEARNING, VOLUME I, 3rd Ed.,©2019. Reprinted and Electronically reproduced by permission of Pearson Education, Inc., New York, NY.; **967:** PEARSON EDUCATION, . ., NURSING: A CONCEPT-BASED APPROACH TO LEARNING, VOLUME I, 3rd Ed.,©2019. Reprinted and Electronically reproduced by permission of Pearson Education, Inc., New York, NY.; **970:** PEARSON EDUCATION, . ., NURSING: A CONCEPT-BASED APPROACH TO LEARNING, VOLUME I, 3rd Ed.,©2019. Reprinted and Electronically reproduced by permission of Pearson Education, Inc., New York, NY.; PEARSON EDUCATION, . ., NURSING: A CONCEPT-BASED APPROACH TO LEARNING, VOLUME I, 3rd Ed.,©2019. Reprinted and Electronically reproduced by permission of Pearson Education, Inc., New York, NY.; **971:** Pearson Education, Inc.; **976:** Dr P. Marazzi/Science Source; PEARSON EDUCATION, . ., NURSING: A CONCEPT-BASED APPROACH TO LEARNING, VOLUME I, 3rd Ed.,©2019. Reprinted and Electronically reproduced by permission of Pearson Education, Inc., New York, NY.; **977:** Pearson Education, Inc.; Pearson Education, Inc.; **983:** PEARSON EDUCATION, . ., NURSING: A CONCEPT-BASED APPROACH TO LEARNING, VOLUME I, 3rd Ed.,©2019. Reprinted and Electronically reproduced by permission of Pearson Education, Inc., New York, NY.; PEARSON EDUCATION, . ., NURSING: A CONCEPT-BASED APPROACH TO LEARNING, VOLUME I, 3rd Ed.,©2019. Reprinted and Electronically reproduced by permission of Pearson Education, Inc., New York, NY.; **984:** PEARSON EDUCATION, . ., NURSING: A CONCEPT-BASED APPROACH TO LEARNING, VOLUME I, 3rd Ed.,©2019. Reprinted and Electronically reproduced by permission of Pearson Education, Inc., New York, NY.; PEARSON EDUCATION, . ., NURSING: A CONCEPT-BASED APPROACH TO LEARNING, VOLUME I, 3rd Ed.,©2019. Reprinted and Electronically reproduced by permission of Pearson Education, Inc., New York, NY.

Chapter 30

1013: PEARSON EDUCATION, . ., NURSING: A CONCEPT-BASED APPROACH TO LEARNING, VOLUME I, 3rd Ed.,©2019. Reprinted and Electronically reproduced by permission of Pearson Education, Inc., New York, NY.; **1014:** PEARSON EDUCATION, . ., NURSING: A CONCEPT-BASED APPROACH TO LEARNING, VOLUME I, 3rd Ed.,©2019. Reprinted and Electronically reproduced by permission of Pearson Education, Inc., New York, NY.; **1025:** PEARSON EDUCATION, . ., NURSING: A CONCEPT-BASED APPROACH TO LEARNING, VOLUME I, 3rd Ed.,©2019. Reprinted and Electronically reproduced by permission of Pearson Education, Inc., New York, NY.; **1040:** Floyd Jackson/Pearson Education, Inc.; **1041:** Richman Photo/Shutterstock; PEARSON EDUCATION, . ., NURSING: A CONCEPT-BASED APPROACH TO LEARNING, VOLUME I, 3rd Ed.,©2019. Reprinted and Electronically reproduced by permission of Pearson Education, Inc., New York, NY.; PEARSON EDUCATION, . ., NURSING: A CONCEPT-BASED APPROACH TO LEARNING, VOLUME I, 3rd Ed.,©2019. Reprinted and Electronically reproduced by permission of Pearson Education, Inc., New York, NY.; **1049:** PEARSON EDUCATION, . ., NURSING: A CONCEPT-BASED APPROACH TO LEARNING, VOLUME I, 3rd Ed.,©2019. Reprinted and Electronically reproduced by permission of Pearson Education, Inc., New York, NY.; Michal Heron/Pearson Education, Inc.; Michal Heron/Pearson Education, Inc.; Michal Heron/Pearson Education, Inc.

Chapter 31

1058: PEARSON EDUCATION, . ., NURSING: A CONCEPT-BASED APPROACH TO LEARNING, VOLUME I, 3rd Ed.,©2019. Reprinted and Electronically reproduced by permission of Pearson Education, Inc., New York, NY.; **1059:** PEARSON EDUCATION, . ., NURSING: A CONCEPT-BASED APPROACH TO LEARNING, VOLUME I, 3rd Ed.,©2019. Reprinted and Electronically reproduced by permission of Pearson Education, Inc., New York, NY.; **1060:** PEARSON EDUCATION, . ., NURSING: A CONCEPT-BASED APPROACH TO LEARNING, VOLUME I, 3rd Ed.,©2019. Reprinted and Electronically reproduced by permission of Pearson Education, Inc., New York, NY.; **1062:** PEARSON EDUCATION, . ., NURSING: A CONCEPT-BASED APPROACH TO LEARNING, VOLUME I, 3rd Ed.,©2019. Reprinted and Electronically reproduced by permission of Pearson Education, Inc., New York, NY.; **1063:** PEARSON EDUCATION, . ., NURSING: A CONCEPT-BASED APPROACH TO LEARNING, VOLUME I, 3rd Ed.,©2019. Reprinted and Electronically reproduced by permission of Pearson Education, Inc., New York, NY.; PEARSON EDUCATION, . ., NURSING: A CONCEPT-BASED APPROACH TO LEARNING, VOLUME I, 3rd Ed.,©2019. Reprinted and Electronically reproduced by permission of Pearson Education, Inc., New York, NY.; **1067:** PEARSON EDUCATION, . ., NURSING: A CONCEPT-BASED APPROACH TO LEARNING, VOLUME I, 3rd Ed.,©2019. Reprinted and Electronically reproduced by permission of Pearson Education, Inc., New York, NY.; **1078:** Dr. E. Walker/Science Source; **1085:** Biophoto Associates/Science Source; **1095:** JACOPIN/BSIP SA/Alamy Stock Photo

Chapter 32

1108: PEARSON EDUCATION, . ., NURSING: A CONCEPT-BASED APPROACH TO LEARNING, VOLUME I, 3rd Ed.,©2019. Reprinted and Electronically reproduced by permission of Pearson Education, Inc., New York, NY.; **1112:** PEARSON EDUCATION, . ., NURSING: A CONCEPT-BASED APPROACH TO LEARNING, VOLUME I, 3rd Ed.,©2019. Reprinted and Electronically reproduced by permission of Pearson Education, Inc., New York, NY.; **1122:** SORENSON, MATTHEW; QUINN, LAURETTA; KLEIN, DIANE, PATHOPHYSIOLOGY: CONCEPTS OF HUMAN DISEASE, 1st Ed., ©2019. Reprinted and Electronically reproduced by permission of Pearson Education, Inc., New York, NY.; **1125:** Chanawit Sitthisombat/123RF; **1128:** SORENSON, MATTHEW; QUINN, LAURETTA; KLEIN, DIANE, PATHOPHYSIOLOGY: CONCEPTS OF HUMAN DISEASE, 1st Ed., ©2019. Reprinted and Electronically reproduced by permission of Pearson Education, Inc., New York, NY.; **1135:** Richard Newton/Alamy Stock Photo; **1140:** PEARSON EDUCATION, . ., NURSING:

A CONCEPT-BASED APPROACH TO LEARNING, VOLUME I, 3rd Ed.,©2019. Reprinted and Electronically reproduced by permission of Pearson Education, Inc., New York, NY.; **1146:** SORENSON, MATTHEW; QUINN, LAURETTA; KLEIN, DIANE, PATHOPHYSIOLOGY: CONCEPTS OF HUMAN DISEASE, 1st Ed., ©2019. Reprinted and Electronically reproduced by permission of Pearson Education, Inc., New York, NY.; **1147:** Biophoto Associates/Science Source; **1149:** Mark Boulton/Alamy Stock Photo; **1152:** Sergio Azenha/Alamy Stock Photo

Chapter 33

1160: Casa nayafana/Shutterstock; Jarun Ontakrai/Shutterstock; **1161:** PEARSON EDUCATION, . ., NURSING: A CONCEPT-BASED APPROACH TO LEARNING, VOLUME I, 3rd Ed.,©2019. Reprinted and Electronically reproduced by permission of Pearson Education, Inc., New York, NY.; **1164:** SCIEPRO/Science Photo Library/Getty Images; SORENSON, MATTHEW; QUINN, LAURETTA; KLEIN, DIANE, PATHOPHYSIOLOGY: CONCEPTS OF HUMAN DISEASE, 1st Ed., ©2019. Reprinted and Electronically reproduced by permission of Pearson Education, Inc., New York, NY.; **1165:** SORENSON, MATTHEW; QUINN, LAURETTA; KLEIN, DIANE, PATHOPHYSIOLOGY: CONCEPTS OF HUMAN DISEASE, 1st Ed., ©2019. Reprinted and Electronically reproduced by permission of Pearson Education, Inc., New York, NY.; **1178:** PEARSON EDUCATION, . ., NURSING: A CONCEPT-BASED APPROACH TO LEARNING, VOLUME I, 3rd Ed.,©2019. Reprinted and Electronically reproduced by permission of Pearson Education, Inc., New York, NY.; **1179:** Jarun Ontakrai/123RF; Kateryna Kon/Shutterstock; **1180:** chirawan Somsanuk/123RF; **1182:** Tino Soriano/National Geographic Creative/Alamy Stock Photo; **1190:** Karan Bunjean/Shutterstock; **1196:** BSIP SA/Alamy Stock Photo; **1199:** Scott Camazine/Science Source; **1207:** PEARSON EDUCATION, . ., NURSING: A CONCEPT-BASED APPROACH TO LEARNING, VOLUME I, 3rd Ed.,©2019. Reprinted and Electronically reproduced by permission of Pearson Education, Inc., New York, NY.

Chapter 34

1218: Pearson Education; **1219:** PEARSON EDUCATION, . ., NURSING: A CONCEPT-BASED APPROACH TO LEARNING, VOLUME I, 3rd Ed.,©2019. Reprinted and Electronically reproduced by permission of Pearson Education, Inc., New York, NY.; **1221:** PEARSON EDUCATION, . ., NURSING: A CONCEPT-BASED APPROACH TO LEARNING, VOLUME I, 3rd Ed.,©2019. Reprinted and Electronically reproduced by permission of Pearson Education, Inc., New York, NY.; **1225:** Pearson Education; Pearson Education; Pearson Education; **1226:** Pearson Education

Chapter 35

1246: Scott Camazine / Alamy Stock Photo; **1261:** Pearson Education; Pearson Education; **1264:** Brian Chase/Shutterstock; **1267:** Clinical Photography, Central Manchester University Hospitals NHS Foundation Trust, UK/Science Source; **1268:** Dr M.A. Ansary/Science Source

Chapter 36

1282: PEARSON EDUCATION, . ., NURSING: A CONCEPT-BASED APPROACH TO LEARNING, VOLUME I, 3rd Ed.,©2019. Reprinted and Electronically reproduced by permission of Pearson Education, Inc., New York, NY.; PEARSON EDUCATION, . ., NURSING: A CONCEPT-BASED APPROACH TO LEARNING, VOLUME I, 3rd Ed.,©2019. Reprinted and Electronically reproduced by permission of Pearson Education, Inc., New York, NY.; **1286:** imagedb.com/Shutterstock; 72/Fotolia; Michal Heron/Pearson Education, Inc.; **1287:** Michal Heron/Pearson Education, Inc.; **1288:** PEARSON EDUCATION, . ., NURSING: A CONCEPT-BASED APPROACH TO LEARNING, VOLUME I, 3rd Ed.,©2019. Reprinted and Electronically reproduced by permission of Pearson Education, Inc., New York, NY.; **1297:** PEARSON EDUCATION, . ., NURSING: A CONCEPT-BASED APPROACH TO LEARNING, VOLUME I, 3rd Ed.,©2019. Reprinted and Electronically reproduced by permission of Pearson Education, Inc., New York, NY.; **1315:** SORENSON, MATTHEW; QUINN, LAURETTA; KLEIN, DIANE, PATHOPHYSIOLOGY: CONCEPTS OF HUMAN DISEASE, 1st Ed., ©2019. Reprinted and Electronically reproduced by permission of Pearson Education, Inc., New York, NY.; **1322:** PEARSON EDUCATION, . ., NURSING: A CONCEPT-BASED APPROACH TO LEARNING, VOLUME I, 3rd Ed.,©2019. Reprinted and Electronically reproduced by permission of Pearson Education, Inc., New York, NY.; PEARSON EDUCATION, . ., NURSING: A CONCEPT-BASED APPROACH TO LEARNING, VOLUME I, 3rd Ed.,©2019. Reprinted and Electronically reproduced by permission of Pearson Education, Inc., New York, NY.; PEARSON EDUCATION, . ., NURSING: A CONCEPT-BASED APPROACH TO LEARNING, VOLUME I, 3rd Ed.,©2019. Reprinted and Electronically reproduced by permission of Pearson Education, Inc., New York, NY.; PEARSON EDUCATION, . ., NURSING: A CONCEPT-BASED APPROACH TO LEARNING, VOLUME I, 3rd Ed.,©2019. Reprinted and Electronically reproduced by permission of Pearson Education, Inc., New York, NY.; **1324:** PEARSON EDUCATION, . ., NURSING: A CONCEPT-BASED APPROACH TO LEARNING, VOLUME I, 3rd Ed.,©2019. Reprinted and Electronically reproduced by permission of Pearson Education, Inc., New York, NY.

Chapter 37

1336: PEARSON EDUCATION, . ., NURSING: A CONCEPT-BASED APPROACH TO LEARNING, VOLUME I, 3rd Ed.,©2019. Reprinted and Electronically reproduced by permission of Pearson Education, Inc., New York, NY.; **1339:** vupulepe/Shutterstock; **1345:** PEARSON EDUCATION, . ., NURSING: A CONCEPT-BASED APPROACH TO LEARNING, VOLUME I, 3rd Ed.,©2019. Reprinted and Electronically reproduced by permission of Pearson Education, Inc., New York, NY.; **1347:** Michal Heron/Pearson Education, Inc.; **1348:** PEARSON EDUCATION, . ., NURSING: A CONCEPT-BASED APPROACH TO LEARNING, VOLUME I, 3rd Ed.,©2019. Reprinted and Electronically reproduced by permission of Pearson Education, Inc., New York, NY.; **1357:** Mediscan/Alamy Stock Photo; **1358:** PEARSON EDUCATION, . ., NURSING: A CONCEPT-BASED APPROACH TO LEARNING, VOLUME I, 3rd Ed.,©2019. Reprinted and Electronically reproduced by permission of Pearson Education, Inc., New York, NY.; **1374:** PEARSON EDUCATION, . ., NURSING: A CONCEPT-BASED APPROACH TO LEARNING, VOLUME I, 3rd Ed.,©2019. Reprinted and Electronically reproduced by permission of Pearson Education, Inc., New York, NY.; **1375:** Yon Marsh/Alamy Stock Photo; **1378:** PEARSON EDUCATION, . ., NURSING: A CONCEPT-BASED APPROACH TO LEARNING, VOLUME I, 3rd Ed.,©2019. Reprinted and Electronically reproduced by permission of Pearson Education, Inc., New York, NY.; **1382:** PEARSON EDUCATION, . ., NURSING: A CONCEPT-BASED APPROACH TO LEARNING, VOLUME I, 3rd Ed.,©2019. Reprinted and Electronically reproduced by permission of Pearson Education, Inc., New York, NY.

Chapter 38

1401: Pearson Education, Inc.; **1402:** Pearson Education, Inc.; Pearson Education, Inc.; Pearson Education, Inc.; **1403:** Pearson Education, Inc.; Pearson Education, Inc.; Pearson Education, Inc.; **1404:** Pearson Education, Inc.

Chapter 39

1419: PEARSON EDUCATION, . ., NURSING: A CONCEPT-BASED APPROACH TO LEARNING, VOLUME II, 3rd Ed., ©2019. Reprinted and Electronically reproduced by permission of Pearson Education, Inc., New York, NY.; **1424:** SORENSON, MATTHEW; QUINN, LAURETTA; KLEIN, DIANE, PATHOPHYSIOLOGY: CONCEPTS OF HUMANDISEASE, 1st Ed., ©2018. Reprinted and Electronically reproduced by permission of Pearson Education, Inc., NewYork, NY.; **1425:** Puwadol Jaturawutthichai/Alamy Stock Photo; **1427:** Pearson Education, Inc.; Rodolfo Arpia/Alamy Stock Photo; Pearson Education, Inc.; Pearson Education, Inc.; **1428:** Pearson Education, Inc.; Peter Alvey/Alamy Stock Photo; **1429:** SORENSON, MATTHEW; QUINN, LAURETTA; KLEIN, DIANE, PATHOPHYSIOLOGY: CONCEPTS OF HUMANDISEASE, 1st Ed., ©2018. Reprinted and Electronically reproduced by permission of Pearson Education, Inc., NewYork, NY.; SORENSON, MATTHEW; QUINN, LAURETTA; KLEIN, DIANE, PATHOPHYSIOLOGY: CONCEPTS OF HUMANDISEASE, 1st Ed., ©2018. Reprinted and Electronically reproduced by permission of Pearson Education, Inc., NewYork, NY.; Manny Crisostomo/MCT/Newscom; **1434:** Linda Gilliland/123RF

Chapter 40

1458: Mediscan/Alamy Stock Photo; **1461:** Mediscan/AlamyStockPhoto; **1466:** Scott Camazine/AlamyStockPhoto; **1469:** Edward Olive/123RF; **1477:** PEARSON EDUCATION, . ., NURSING: A CONCEPT-BASED APPROACH TO LEARNING, VOLUME II, 3rd Ed., ©2019. Reprinted and Electronically reproduced by permission of Pearson Education, Inc., New York, NY.; **1478:** Mediscan/Alamy Stock Photo; peterfactors/Shutterstock; **1488:** Mediscan/Alamy Stock Photo; **1489:** PEARSON EDUCATION, . ., NURSING: A CONCEPT-BASED

APPROACH TO LEARNING, VOLUME II, 3rd Ed., ©2019. Reprinted and Electronically reproduced by permission of Pearson Education, Inc., New York, NY.; **1493:** Mediscan/AlamyStockPhoto; **1496:** Centers for Disease Control and Prevention; **1497:** Jarva Jar/Shutterstock; **1507:** PEARSON EDUCATION, . ., NURSING: A CONCEPT-BASED APPROACH TO LEARNING, VOLUME II, 3rd Ed., ©2019. Reprinted and Electronically reproduced by permission of Pearson Education, Inc., New York, NY.; **1508:** SORENSON, MATTHEW; QUINN, LAURETTA; KLEIN, DIANE, PATHOPHYSIOLOGY: CONCEPTS OF HUMANDISEASE, 1st Ed., ©2018. Reprinted and Electronically reproduced by permission of Pearson Education, Inc., NewYork, NY.

Chapter 41

1524: PEARSON EDUCATION, . ., NURSING: A CONCEPT-BASED APPROACH TO LEARNING, VOLUME II, 3rd Ed., ©2019. Reprinted and Electronically reproduced by permission of Pearson Education, Inc., New York, NY.; **1527:** PEARSON EDUCATION, . ., NURSING: A CONCEPT-BASED APPROACH TO LEARNING, VOLUME II, 3rd Ed., ©2019. Reprinted and Electronically reproduced by permission of Pearson Education, Inc., New York, NY.; **1536:** Pearson Education, Inc.; Pearson Education, Inc.; **1537:** Pearson Education, Inc.; Pearson Education, Inc.; Pearson Education, Inc.; Pearson Education, Inc.; Pearson Education, Inc.; Pearson Education, Inc.; Pearson Education, Inc.; **1538:** Pearson Education, Inc.; Pearson Education, Inc.; Pearson Education, Inc.; PEARSON EDUCATION, . ., NURSING: A CONCEPT-BASED APPROACH TO LEARNING, VOLUME II, 3rd Ed., ©2019. Reprinted and Electronically reproduced by permission of Pearson Education, Inc., New York, NY.; PEARSON EDUCATION, . ., NURSING: A CONCEPT-BASED APPROACH TO LEARNING, VOLUME II, 3rd Ed., ©2019. Reprinted and Electronically reproduced by permission of Pearson Education, Inc., New York, NY.

Chapter 42

1547: PEARSON EDUCATION, . ., NURSING: A CONCEPT-BASED APPROACH TO LEARNING, VOLUME II, 3rd Ed., ©2019. Reprinted and Electronically reproduced by permission of Pearson Education, Inc., New York, NY.; **1559:** Michal Heron/Pearson Education.Inc; Michal Heron/Pearson Education.Inc; **1578:** PEARSON EDUCATION, . ., NURSING: A CONCEPT-BASED APPROACH TO LEARNING, VOLUME II, 3rd Ed., ©2019. Reprinted and Electronically reproduced by permission of Pearson Education, Inc., New York, NY.

Chapter 43

1603: Pearson Education, Inc.; Rodolfo Arpia/Alamy Stock Photo; **1610:** SORENSON, MATTHEW; QUINN, LAURETTA; KLEIN, DIANE, PATHOPHYSIOLOGY: CONCEPTS OF HUMANDISEASE, 1st Ed., ©2018. Reprinted and Electronically reproduced by permission of Pearson Education, Inc., NewYork, NY.; **1619:** Pearson Education, Inc.

Chapter 44

1631: ilusmedical/Shutterstock; **1642:** PEARSON EDUCATION, . ., NURSING: A CONCEPT-BASED APPROACH TO LEARNING, VOLUME II, 3rd Ed., ©2019. Reprinted and Electronically eproduced by permission of Pearson Education, Inc., New York, NY.; **1647:** John Birdsall/Alamy Stock Photo; **1648:** PEARSON EDUCATION, . ., NURSING: A CONCEPT-BASED APPROACH TO LEARNING, VOLUME II, 3rd Ed., ©2019. Reprinted and Electronically reproduced by permission of Pearson Education, Inc., New York, NY.; **1658:** Dr M.A. Ansary/Science Source; **1660:** Attapol Nowat/123RF; **1666:** Jo Ann Snover/Shutterstock

Chapter 45

1673: Pat Watson/Pearson Education, Inc.; **1677:** Pearson Education, Inc.; Pearson Education, Inc.; **1678:** Pearson Education, Inc.; Michal Heron/Pearson Education, Inc.; **1679:** Mediscan/Alamy Stock Photo; **1681:** Pearson Education, Inc.; Pearson Education, Inc.; memorisz/Shutterstock; **1683:** Todd Buck/Pearson Education, Inc.; **1685:** Pearson Education, Inc.; Pearson Education, Inc.; **1686:** Pearson Education, Inc.; Pearson Education, Inc.; Pearson Education, Inc.; **1687:** Prof. Tony Wright/Inst. of Laryngology & Otology/Science Source

Chapter 46

1694: Joe Miller, VD/Centers for Disease Control and Prevention (CDC); **1695:** PHUCHONG CHOKSAMAI/123RF; **1698:** Mediscan/Alamy Stock Photo; **1701:** Sorapop Udomsri/123RF; Gromovataya/Shutterstock; **1702:** Mediscan/Alamy Stock Photo; **1703:** PHUCHONG CHOKSAMAI/123RF; **1704:** Michal Heron/Pearson Education, Inc.; **1706:** Courtesy of National Eye Institute, National Institutes of Health; **1708:** Courtesy of National Eye Institute, National Institutes of Health; **1710:** Courtesy of National Eye Institute, National Institutes of Health; **1714:** Courtesy of National Eye Institute, National Institutes of Health; **1717:** Courtesy of National Eye Institute, National Institutes of Health; **1723:** Mediscan/Alamy Stock Photo; Mediscan/Alamy Stock Photo; **1732:** Andras Gyula Csontos/123RF; Andriy Popov/123RF; **1733:** Pearson Education, Inc.

Chapter 47

1743: Pearson Education, Inc.; Pearson Education, Inc.; **1750:** Pearson Education, Inc.; Pearson Education, Inc.; **1751:** Pearson Education, Inc.; **1752:** Pearson Education, Inc.

Chapter 48

1773: SORENSON, MATTHEW; QUINN, LAURETTA; KLEIN, DIANE, PATHOPHYSIOLOGY: CONCEPTS OF HUMANDISEASE, 1st Ed., ©2018. Reprinted and Electronically reproduced by permission of Pearson Education, Inc., NewYork, NY.

Chapter 49

1801: BSIP SA/Alamy Stock Photo

Chapter 50

1837: Centers for Disease Control and Prevention; SneSivan/Shutterstock; **1839:** Susan Lindsley/Centers for Disease Control and Prevention; Centers for Disease Control and Prevention; **1841:** BSIP SA/AlamyStockPhoto; **1842:** Biophoto Associates/Science Source; **1844:** Centers for Disease Control and Prevention; **1847:** BSIP SA/AlamyStockPhoto; Centers for Disease Control and Prevention

Index

Page numbers followed by *f* indicate figures and those followed by *t* indicate tables, boxes, or special features.

A

C

D

E

J

M

N

O

P

Q

R

V

W

X

Y

Z

Special Features

ASSESSMENT FEATURE

CASE STUDY & NURSING CARE PLAN

DIAGNOSTIC TESTS

GENETIC CONSIDERATIONS

MULTISYSTEM EFFECTS OF

PATHOPHYSIOLOGY ILLUSTRATED

MEDICATION ADMINISTRATION